AAOS
AMERICAN ACADEMY OF ORTHOPAEDIC SURGEONS

NAEMSP
National Association
of EMS Physicians®

Sanders' Paramedic Textbook

FIFTH EDITION

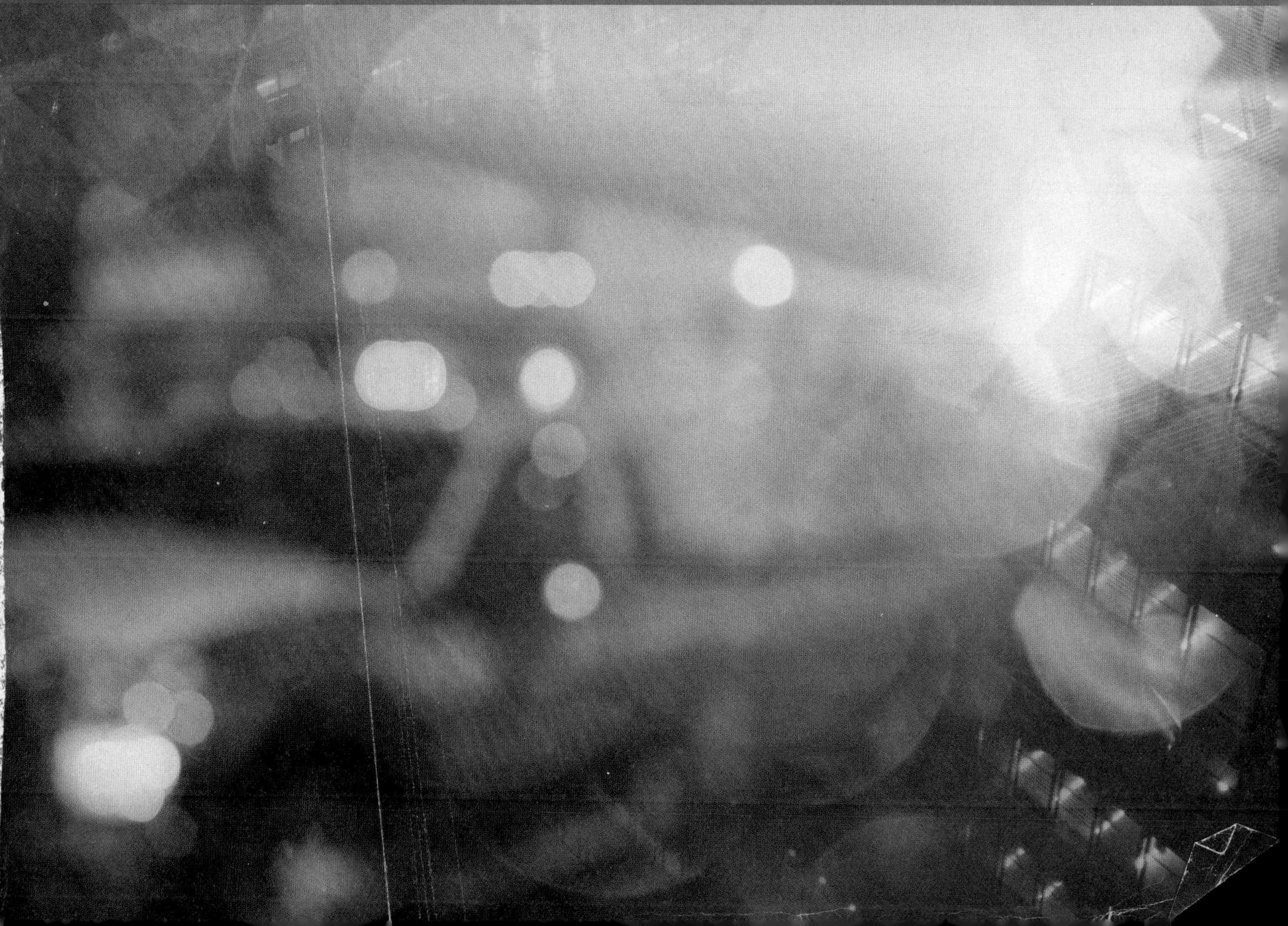

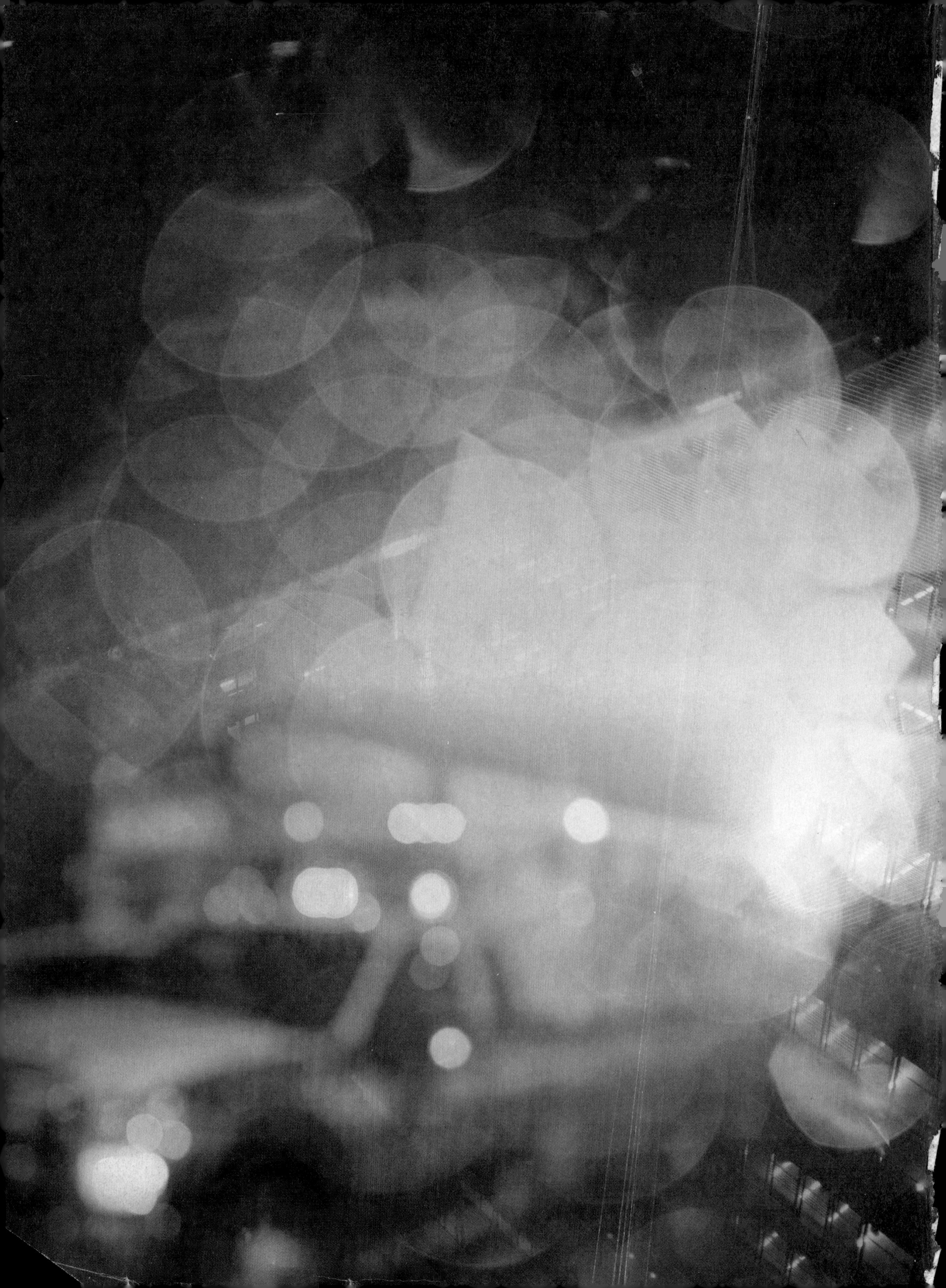

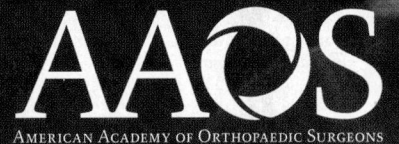

AAOS
AMERICAN ACADEMY OF ORTHOPAEDIC SURGEONS

NAEMSP
National Association of EMS Physicians®

Sanders' Paramedic Textbook

FIFTH EDITION

Mick J. Sanders, BS, MSA, EMT-P

Contributing Editor
Kim D. McKenna, PhD, MEd, RN, EMT-P

Medical Editors
David K. Tan, MD, FAAEM, FAEMS
Andrew N. Pollak, MD, FAAOS

Coeditor
Alfonso Mejia, MD, MPH, FAAOS, FAOA

JONES & BARTLETT
LEARNING

World Headquarters
Jones & Bartlett Learning
5 Wall Street
Burlington, MA 01803
978-443-5000
info@jblearning.com
www.jblearning.com
www.psglearning.com

Jones & Bartlett Learning books and products are available through most bookstores and online booksellers. To contact the Jones & Bartlett Learning Public Safety Group directly, call 800-832-0034, fax 978-443-8000, or visit our website, www.psglearning.com.

Substantial discounts on bulk quantities of Jones & Bartlett Learning publications are available to corporations, professional associations, and other qualified organizations. For details and specific discount information, contact the special sales department at Jones & Bartlett Learning via the above contact information or send an email to specialsales@jblearning.com.

AAOS
AMERICAN ACADEMY OF ORTHOPAEDIC SURGEONS

Editorial Credits
Chief Education Strategist:
Anna Salt Troise, MBA
Director, Publishing Partner Relationships:
Hans J. Koelsch, PhD
Senior Manager, Publishing Operations:
Joan Golembiewski
Senior Manager, Editorial: Lisa Claxton Moore
Senior Editor, Publications: Steven Kellert

NAEMSP
National Association of EMS Physicians®

Editorial Credits
Medical Editor: David K. Tan, MD
Executive Director: JerrieLynn Kind

56043-5

Production Credits

General Manager and Executive Publisher: Kimberly Brophy
VP, Product Development: Christine Emerton
Product Manager: Tiffany Sliter
Senior Editor: Barbara A. Scotese
Senior Editor: Carol B. Guerrero
Editorial Assistant: Jessica Sturtevant
Editorial Assistant: Ashley Procum
VP, Sales, Public Safety Group: Matthew Maniscalco
Production Editor: Kristen Rogers
Production Manager: Carolyn Rogers Pershouse
Director of Marketing Operations: Brian Rooney
Production Services Manager: Colleen Lamy
VP, Manufacturing and Inventory Control: Therese Connell
Composition: S4Carlisle Publishing Services
Cover Design: Kristin E. Parker
Text Design: Kristin E. Parker
Rights & Media Specialist: Robert Boder
Media Development Editor: Troy Liston
Cover & Title Page Images: © 400tmax/iStock/Getty Images, © Michael Mann/Getty Images
Printing and Binding: LSC Communications
Cover Printing: LSC Communications

Library of Congress Cataloging-in-Publication Data

Names: American Academy of Orthopaedic Surgeons, author. | Sanders, Mick J., author. | McKenna, Kim, author. | Tan, David K., editor. | Pollak, Andrew N., editor.
Title: Sanders' paramedic textbook / American Academy of Orthopaedic Surgeons, Mick Sanders, Kim McKenna, David K. Tan, Andrew N. Pollak.
Other titles: Mosby's paramedic textbook | Paramedic textbook
Description: Fifth edition. | Burlington, MA : Jones & Bartlett Learning, 2019. | Preceded by: Mosby's paramedic textbook / Mick J. Sanders ; physician advisers, Lawrence M. Lewis, Gary Quick ; contributing editor, Kim D. McKenna. 4th ed. c2012. | Includes bibliographical references and index.
Identifiers: LCCN 2018023771 | ISBN 9781284147827 (casebound)
Subjects: | MESH: Emergency Medical Services--methods | Emergencies | Emergency Medical Technicians
Classification: LCC RC86.7 | NLM WX 215 | DDC 616.02/5--dc23
LC record available at https://lccn.loc.gov/2018023771

6048

Printed in the United States of America
22 21 20 19 18   10 9 8 7 6 5 4 3 2 1

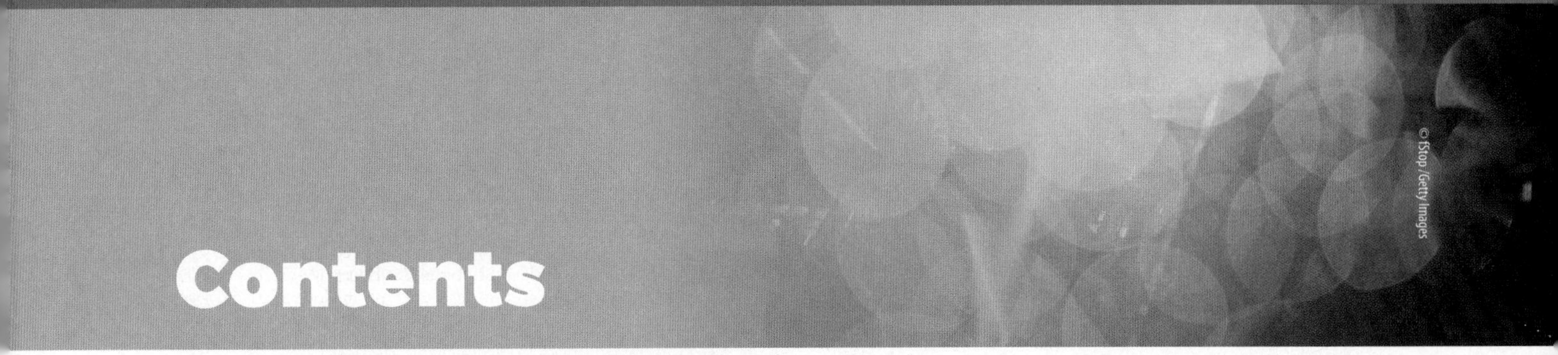

Contents

About the Author and Contributors

Mick J. Sanders, BS, MSA, EMT-P, received his paramedic training in 1978 from St. Louis University Hospitals. He earned a bachelor of science degree and a master of science degree from Lindenwood University in St. Charles, Missouri. He has worked in various health care systems as a field paramedic, emergency department paramedic, and EMS instructor. For 12 years, Mr. Sanders served as Training Specialist with the Bureau of Emergency Medical Services, Missouri Department of Health, where he oversaw EMT and paramedic training and licensure in St. Louis city and the surrounding metropolitan areas.

Kim D. McKenna, PhD, MEd, RN, EMT-P, is the Director of Education for the St. Charles County Ambulance District located in metropolitan St. Louis, Missouri. She is program director for the district's emergency medical technician and paramedic programs and leads a training staff that provides EMS education for district paramedics and for firefighters and emergency personnel within St. Charles County. Dr. McKenna has been teaching in EMS for more than 30 years. She formerly worked as an emergency and intensive care nurse and served as Chief Medical Officer for the Florissant Valley Fire Protection District. Dr. McKenna was the EMR Project Level Leader for the National EMS Education Standards project and was a member of the Board of Directors for the National Association of EMS Educators. She presently serves on the board of advisors for the Prehospital Care Research Forum.

David K. Tan, MD, FAAEM, FAEMS, is Associate Professor of Emergency Medicine and Chief of the Emergency Medical Services Section at Washington University School of Medicine and Barnes-Jewish Hospital in St. Louis, Missouri. Dr. Tan is an operational EMS physician and medical director for several police, fire, EMS, and US&R entities in greater St. Louis, Chairman of the Metropolitan St. Louis Emergency Transport Oversight Commission, Vice-Chair of the Missouri State Advisory Council on EMS, and President-Elect of the National Association of EMS Physicians.

Special Acknowledgment

In recognition of the contributions of the Physician Advisors for the first four editions of this textbook, the author and contributors thank:

Lawrence M. Lewis, MD, FACEP, Professor of Emergency Medicine at Washington University School of Medicine and Barnes-Jewish Hospital in St. Louis, Missouri.

Gary Quick, MD, FACEP (retired), Medical Director at Southwestern Medical Center, Lawton, Oklahoma, Associate Professor and Chair of the Department of Emergency Medicine at the University of Oklahoma Health Sciences Center in Oklahoma City, Oklahoma.

Acknowledgments

The American Academy of Orthopaedic Surgeons, the editors, and the authors wish to acknowledge and thank the many reviewers of this textbook, who devoted countless hours to intensive evaluation. The following organizations and individuals were involved in this extensive textbook revision.

Editorial Board

Mick J. Sanders, BS, MSA, EMT-P
St. Louis, Missouri

Kim D. McKenna, PhD, MEd, RN, EMT-P
Director of Education
St. Charles County Ambulance District
St. Peters, Missouri

David K. Tan, MD, FAAEM, FAEMS
Associate Professor of Emergency Medicine
Chief, Emergency Medical Services Section
Washington University School of Medicine and Barnes-Jewish Hospital
St. Louis, Missouri

Andrew N. Pollak, MD, FAAOS
The James Lawrence Kernan Professor and Chairman, Department of Orthopaedics, University of Maryland School of Medicine
Chief of Orthopaedics, University of Maryland Medical System
Medical Director, Baltimore County Fire Department
Director, Shock Trauma Go Team
Special Deputy US Marshal

Alfonso Mejia, MD, MPH, FAAOS, FAOA
Program Director, Orthopedic Surgery Residency Program
Vice Head, Department of Orthopedic Surgery
University of Illinois College of Medicine
Medical Director
Tactical Emergency Medical Support Physician
South Suburban Emergency Response Team
Chicago, Illinois

Authors of the Ancillaries

Kimberly Bailey, MA, NRP, CHSE, SCCEM
Emerging Infectious Disease Planner
SC DHEC Office of Public Health Preparedness
Columbia, South Carolina

Sharon F. Chiumento, BSN, EMT-P
Lead Instructor, Monroe Ambulance, University of Rochester
Guest Instructor, Monroe Community College
Rochester, New York

Stephen J. Rahm, NRP
Deputy Chief, Office of Clinical Direction
Co-chair, Centre for Emergency Health Sciences
Bulverde Spring Branch Emergency Services
Spring Branch, Texas

Brittany Ann Williams, DHSc, RRT-NPS, NREMT-P
Professor, Respiratory Care
Director, Clinical Education
Santa Fe College
Gainesville, Florida

Reviewers

Jonathan Adam Alford
Instructor/Clinical Coordinator of EMS Programs
Piedmont Virginia Community College
Charlottesville, Virginia

Andrew Bartkus, JD, RN, CEN, CCRN, CFRN, NREMT-P, FP-C
Sandoval Regional Medical Center
Rio Rancho, New Mexico

Dana Baumgartner, BS, NRP
Nicolet College
Rhinelander, Wisconsin

Jason Baumgartner, NRP, CCEMTP
Nicolet College
Rhinelander, Wisconsin

David S. Becker, MA, Paramedic, EFO
Columbia Southern University

Brandon B. Bleess, MD, FAAEM
Clinical Assistant Professor
University of Illinois College of Medicine
Peoria, Illinois

Robert Bowen
Arlington County Fire Department
Arlington, Virginia

Sabina A. Braithwaite, MD, MPH, FF/EMT-P, FACEP, FAEMS
Associate Professor and EMS Fellowship Director
Washington University School of Medicine
St. Louis, Missouri

Susan Smith Braithwaite, EdD, NRP
Western Carolina University
Cullowhee, North Carolina

Lawrence Brewer, MPH, NRP, FP-C
Rogers State University
Claremore, Oklahoma

Jason L. Brooks, MA, NRP
University of South Alabama

John T. Buttrick III, NRP, AAS
Thomas Nelson Community College
Hampton, Virginia

Aaron R. Byington, MA, NRP
Davis Technical College
Kaysville, Utah

Elliot Carhart, EdD, FAEMS
Jefferson College of Health Sciences
Roanoke, Virginia

Julie Chase, MSEd, FAWM, TP-C
Berryville, Virginia

Sharon F. Chiumento, BSN, EMT-P
University of Rochester, Monroe Ambulance
Rochester, New York

Cathy Cockrell, MHS, NRP
Western Virginia EMS Council
Roanoke, Virginia

Helen T. Compton, NRP
Mecklenburg County Lifesaving and Rescue Squad
Clarksville, Virginia

Scott Corcoran, MS, CIC, Paramedic
Erie Community College
Orchard Park, New York

Kent Courtney, NREMT, Paramedic
Emergency Specialist at Peabody Western Coal Company and owner of Essential Safety Training and Consulting
Rimrock, Arizona

Matthew A. Crawford, NREMT-P, UMBC-CCT
DCEMS and Emergency Training by Matt
Sutton, West Virginia

Mark A. Cromer, MS, MBA, NRP
Jefferson College of Health Sciences
Roanoke, Virginia

Mike Cronin, EMT-P/EMS-I
Director, Knox Technical Center
Chief, Utica EMS
Mount Vernon, Ohio

Sean Davis, MEd, CICNRP, EMS-I
Auburn Career Center
Concord, Ohio

Malcolm Edward Dean, Jr, MS, EMT-P
Jersey City Medical Center
Jersey City, New Jersey

Maia Dorsett, MD, PhD
Senior Instructor
University of Rochester Medical Center
Rochester, New York

Rommie L. Duckworth, LP
Founder and Director
New England Center for Rescue and Emergency Medicine
Sherman, Connecticut

Bob Elling, MPA, EMT-P
Educator, Author, and Advocate, High Quality Endeavors, Ltd
Lake Placid, New York
SMG Events Medic
Albany, New York
Olympic Regional Development Authority Medic
Lake Placid, New York

Wm. Travis Engel, DO, NRP, FP-C
Park Ridge, Illinois

Charles O. Erwin, EdD, NRP
University of South Alabama, Department of EMS Education
Mobile, Alabama

Reuben Farnsworth, CCP-C, NRP
President
RockStar Education and Consulting
Cedaredge, Colorado

Ronald Feller, Sr, MBA, NRP
Oklahoma City Community College

Adam C. Fritsch, NREMT-P, CCEMTP
Advanced Professional Healthcare Education, LLC
Wauwatosa, Wisconsin

Christopher B. Gage, BS, NRP, FP-C
Davidson County Community College
Thomasville, North Carolina

Fidel O. Garcia, Paramedic
President/Owner
Professional EMS Education
Grand Junction, Colorado

James W. Gardner
City of Santa Fe Fire Department (retired)
Santa Fe, New Mexico

John Gloede, BA, NRP, IC-II
Moraine Park Technical College
Fond du Lac, Wisconsin

Bill Grayson, NRP
Oklahoma City Community College
Oklahoma City, Oklahoma

Jeffrey R. Grunow, MSN, NRP, NCEE
Adjunct Instructor
Indian River State College
Fort Pierce, Florida

Kevin M. Gurney, MS, CCEMTP, I/C
Delta Ambulance
Waterville, Maine

Anthony S. Harbour, MEd, RN, NRP
Director
Southern Virginia EMS
Roanoke, Virginia

Phil Head III, BHS, NRP, FP-C, CP-C
Greenville Health System
Greenville, South Carolina

Donald H. Hiett, Jr, BS
Assistant Chief/Chief Medical Officer
Atlanta Fire Rescue Department (retired)
Atlanta, Georgia

Paul Hitchcock, NRP
Front Royal, Virginia

Mark A. Huckaby, NRP
OhioHealth EMS
Columbus, Ohio

Sandra Hultz, NRP, EMS
Faculty Instructor
Holmes Community College
Ridgeland, Mississippi

Joseph Hurlburt, BS, NRP, NREMT-P, EMT-P I/C
Instructor Coordinator/Training Officer
Rapid Response EMS
Romulus, Michigan

Darin Jackson, MDiv, Paramedic
Asheville-Buncombe Technical College
Asheville, North Carolina

Adam Johnson, NRP
Rhinelander Fire Department
Nicolet Area Technical College
NorthCentral Technical College
Rhinelander, Wisconsin

Melissa K. F. Johnson, NRP
Rappahannock Community College
Warsaw, Virginia

Jared Kimball, NREMT-P
Tulane Trauma Education
New Orleans, Louisiana

Timothy M. Kimble, AAS, NRP
Carilion Clinic Life Support Training Center
Roanoke, Virginia

Don Kimlicka, NRP, CCEMTP
Executive Director
Clintonville Area Ambulance Service
Clintonville, Wisconsin

Mark A. King, MA, EMT-P
Kennebec Valley Community College
Fairfield, Maine

Jason Kinlaw, BS, NRP
Navy Region Mid-Atlantic Fire and Emergency Services
Virginia Beach, Virginia

Ryan Kirk, Lieutenant, NRP, EC
Woodbridge, Virginia

Blake Klingle, MS, RN, CCEMTP
EMS Instructor/Coordinator
Waukesha County Technical College
Pewaukee, Wisconsin

Karen "Keri" Wydner Krause, RN, CCRN, EMT-P
Lakeshore Technical College
Cleveland, Wisconsin

Christopher Kroboth, MS, NRP, CCEMTP
Fairfax County Fire and Rescue
Fairfax, Virginia

Jim Ladle, BS, FP-C, CCP-C
South Jordan City Fire Department
South Jordan, Utah

Ricky Lyles, NRP
Southside Virginia Community College
Keysville, Virginia

Yogangi Malhotra, MD
Albert Einstein College of Medicine
New Rochelle, New York

Jeanette Mann, BSN, RN, NRP
Director of EMS Program
Dabney S. Lancaster Community College
Clifton Forge, Virginia

Brent Martin, JD, Attorney at Law
Farrell & Martin
St. Peters, Missouri

Michael A. Mattson
Spring Lake Park, Blaine, Mounds View (SBM) Fire Department
Blaine, Minnesota

Kevin McCarthy, MPA, NRP
Utah Valley University
Orem, Utah

Randy McCartney
Moraine Park Technical College
Fond du Lac, Wisconsin

Amanda McDonald, MA, NRP
University of South Alabama
Mobile, Alabama

Mike McEvoy, PhD, NRP, RN, CCRN
Albany Medical Center
Albany, New York

Steve McGraw
Prince William County (VA) Department of Fire and Rescue
Woodbridge, Virginia

Kristen McKenna, BS, NRP
University of South Alabama EMS Department
Mobile, Alabama

E. David Mejia, Paramedic
Director of Education
Delta Ambulance
Waterville, Maine

Nicholas Montelauro, BS, NRP, FP-C, NCEE
Terre Haute, Indiana

Gregory S. Neiman, MS, NRP, NCEE
VCU Medical Center
Richmond, Virginia

Jonathan R. Powell, BS, NRP
University of South Alabama Department of EMS Education
Mobile, Alabama

Lionel Powell, MEd, EMT-P
An Act of Caring
Salt Lake City, Utah

Steven T. Powell, AAS, NRP, EC
Rockingham County Department of Fire and Rescue
Harrisonburg, Virginia

Ernest K. Ralston, PG, CMAS, EMT-P
Center for Asymmetric Emergency Medicine and Training, Inc.
Centreville, Virginia

Jennifer Reese, BS, CCEMTP
Central Jackson County Fire Protection
Blue Springs, Missouri

Curtis A. Rhodes, AAS, NRP, CCEMTP
Gordon Cooper Technology Center
Shawnee, Oklahoma

Chris Rock, MSN, RN
Paramedic Program Director
City of Tacoma Fire Department
Tacoma, Washington

Hector Roman, RN, EMT-P
Tamarac Fire Rescue
Tamarac, Florida

Bryan Selvage, NRP, FP-C, CCEMTP
Cecil College
North East, Maryland

Jeb Sheidler, MPAS, NRP, PA-C, ATC
EMS Program Coordinator/Associate Professor, Rhodes State College
Training Officer, Bath Township Fire Department
Tactical Paramedic, Allen County Sheriff's Office
Lima, Ohio

Richard S. Shepard, BEd, EMT-P
South Florida State College
Avon Park, Florida

Warren W. Short, Jr, BS, NRP
Glen Allen, Virginia

Jeffrey E. Siegler, MD, FF/EMT-P
Instructor
Washington University School of Medicine
St. Louis, Missouri

Douglas P. Skinner, MPA, NRP, NCEE
Prince George's Community College
SCS Safety Health and Security Associates, LLC
Leesburg, Virginia

C. N. Jonathan Smith, FP-C, PNCCT, HCPC Paramedic, CCEMTP
Emergency Medical Training Group
Hampton, Middlesex, United Kingdom

Jamin Snarr, BSE, NREMTP
Northwest Arkansas Community College
Bentonville, Arkansas

Sandra Sokol, NREMT-Paramedic
Captain
Loudoun County Combined Fire Rescue System
Leesburg, Virginia

Mark Spangenberg, CCP, ECG-BC
Milwaukee Area Technical College
Milwaukee, Wisconsin

Tynell N. Stackhouse, MTh, NRP
Field Training Officer
Marion County EMS
Mullins, South Carolina

Bruce J. Stark, NRP
Lieutenant
Fairfax County Fire and Rescue Department
Fairfax, Virginia

Andrew W. Stern, MPA, MA, NRP, CCEMTP
Hudson Valley Community College
Troy, New York

Stephanie Stewart, MS, CRNA, APRN
Hartford EMS
Hartford, Connecticut

Richard Stump, NRP
Central Carolina Community College
Sanford, North Carolina

Bridgette B. Svancarek, MD, FAEMS
Assistant Professor
Washington University School of Medicine
St. Louis, Missouri

Benjamin D. Symonds, MPA, NRP
Kirkwood Community College
Cedar Rapids, Iowa

Amy E. Trujillo, BS, NREMT-P
Montana Medical Transport
Helena, Montana

Scott Vanderkooi, BS, NRP
Blue Ridge Community College
Weyers Cave, Virginia

Athanasios Viglis, NRP
Henrico County Division of Fire
Henrico, Virginia

Robert K. Waddell II, BS, EMT-P (retired)
SAM Medical, Inc.
Cedar Springs, Michigan

David M. Wade, MASc, Paramedic
Carrollton, Georgia

Jon Walker, NRP
Upper Valley Ambulance, Inc. (retired)
Fairlee, Vermont

Tom Watson, AS, AAS, Paramedic
Adjunct Instructor
Texas A&M University System, Texas Engineering Extension Service, Emergency Services Training Institute, EMS/Public Health Program
College Station, Texas

Christopher Weaver, NRP
Venture Crew 911
Lakewood, Colorado

William M. Wells, Sr, MEd, NRP
Technical College High School Brandywine Campus
Downingtown, Pennsylvania

Raymond C. Whatley, Jr, MBA, NRP
George Washington University
Emergency Health Services Program
Department of Clinical Research and Leadership School of Medicine and Health Sciences
Washington, DC

Kelly R. Whitacre, NRP, NCEE
Frederick County Fire and Rescue Department, Training Division
Winchester, Virginia

Michael H. Wilhelm, CRNA, APRN
IAA School of Nurse Anesthesia
East Hartford, Connecticut

Michael Wolczyz, EMT-P
Vista Health
Gurnee, Illinois

Thomas Worthington, MEd, EMT-P, EMSIC
Program Coordinator/Faculty
Schoolcraft College
Garden City, Michigan

Andy Yeoh
Pima Community College
Tucson, Arizona

First edition reviewers: National Association of EMTs Society of Paramedics Instructor/Coordinators Society; National Council of State EMS Training Coordinators; National Association of EMS Physicians; Thomas F. Anderson, PhD, RRT; Doug Austin, Jr; Vatche H. Ayvazian, MD; John Barrett, MD; David S. Becker; John E. Blue II, BS, EMT-P; Chip Boehm, RN, EMT-P; Kevin Brown, MD, MPH; Jeffrey A. Crill, RN, EMT-P; David DaBell, MD; Alice "Twink" Dalton; Theodore R. Delbridge, MD; Linda D. Dodge; Robert Elling, MPA, NREMT-P; Franklin E. Foster, JD; Bill Garcia, MICP; Mike Gray; Janet A. Head, MS, RN; Kenneth Hines; Steven Kidd; Mark A. Kirk, MD; Kevin Kraus, BS, EMT-P; Richard A. Lazar; Mark Lockhart, NREMT-P; Julie Long; Glenn H. Luedtke, NREMT-P; Mary Beth Michos, RN; Gary P. Morris; Keith Neely, EMT-P, MPA; Gregory Noll; Michael P. Peppers, PharmD; Dwight Polk, BA, NREMT-P; William Raynovich; Lou E. Romig, MD, FAAP; José V. Aalazar, BA, NREMT; Randy L. Sanders; Carol J. Shanaberger; JoAnn Shew, MSN, RN, CS; John Sinclair; Todd M. Stanford, BS, PA-C, MICP; Andrew W. Stern, MPA, NREMT-P; Mike Taigman; Vickie H. Taylor; Michael W. Turner; Patricia L. Westbrook, MS, CCC; Jason T. White; Sherrie C. Wilson, EMT-P, I/C; Monroe Yancie, NREMT-P; and Rodney C. Zerr.

Second edition reviewers: Joseph J. Acker, AHT, EMT-P; Richard Alcorta, MD, FACEP; Chandra Aubin, MD; Alan J. Azzara, JD, EMT-P; Catherine A. Parvensky Barwell, MEd, RN/EMT-P; James P. Boedeker, MD; William Brandes; David H. Brisson, RN, EMCA; Lawrence R. Brown, MD, PhD; Roy Edward Cox, Jr, MEd, EMT-P; Kevin Cunningham, BS, EMT-P; John Czajkowski; Heather Micholene Davis, MS, NREMT-P; Jeff G. DeGraffenreid, MEd, Paramedic; William H. Dribben, MD; William J. Dunne, MS, NREMT-P; Lisa Susan Etzwiler, MD, FAAP; Daryl Eustace; Edward Ferguson, MD; Janet Fitts, BSN, RN, CEN, EMT-P; Ken Fowke, BSc, EMA-II; Timothy Gridley; Larry Hatfield; Shirley A. Jones, MS Ed, MHA, EMT-P; Antoinette Kanne, MS, RN; Lisa Keenly, MD; Anthony C. Kessels; J. Steven Kidd; Jeffrey Levine, MD, FACS; James Linardos, MS, EMT-I; Michael Mullins, MD; Scott Mullins; Robert E. O'Connor, MD, MPH; Nathan Piemann, MD; Denise S. Pope, MSN, RN; John Eric Powell, MS, NREMT-P; Chris Richter, MD; Becky Ridenhour, PharmD; Cleeve Robertson, MD; S. Rutherford Rose, PharmD, FAACT; Stanley Sakabu, MD, FACS; Robert J. Schappert III; Roberta J. Secrest, PhD, PharmD; Sharon Smith, MD; Karen Snyder; Andrew W. Stern, MPA, MA, NREMT-P; Gail Stewart, BS, EMT-P, CHES; Robert Theriault, RCT (Adv), CCP (F); Eric Thompson, MD; Bryan Troop, MD, FACS, FCCM; Christina Wagner, MD; Bruce J. Walz, PhD; Roxanne Ward, RN; A. Keith Wesley, MD, FACEP; and Brian S. Zachariah, MD, MBA.

Third edition reviewers: Beth Lothrop Adams, MA, RN, NREMT-P; Patrick Black, BS, NREMT-P; Chip Boehm, RN, EMT-P/FF, EMS I/C; Kristen Borchelt,

NREMT-P; Angel Clark Burba, MS, NREMT-P; Heather Micholene Davis, MS, NREMT-P; Ken Davis, NREMT-P, CCEMTP, I/C; Bill Doss, EMT-P; Steven Dralle, BA, EMT-P; James W. Drake, MS, NREMT-P; Rudy Garrett, AS, NREMT-P, CCEMTP; Peter Glaeser, MD; Thomas James Gottschalk, NREMT-P, I/C, CCEMTP; Shawn Harthorn, EMT, MACS; Robert Hawkes, BA, BS, NREMT-P, CCEMTP; Seth Collings Hawkins, MD; Attila Hertelendy, MHSM, CCEMTP, NREMT-P, ACP; John C. Hopkins, EMT-P; Arthur Hsieh, MA, NREMT-P; I. Kevin Johnson, AS, BS, NREMT-P; Mark Lockhart, NREMT-P; Joanne McCall, RN, MA, CEN, SANE-A, CFN; Kirk E. Mittleman, AAS, BS, NREMT-P/Utah EMT-P; Taz Meyer, BS, EMT-P; Susan M. Caley Opsal, MS; David S. Pecora, MS, PA-C, NREMT-P; Eric Powell, EMT-P; Virginia K. Riedy, RN, NREMT-P; Becky Ridenhour, PharmD; Blaine Riggleman, EMT-P; Judith A. Ruple, PhD, RN, NREMT-P; Gordon M. Sachs, EFO, MPA; Gail Saxowsky, RNC, MPH; Janet L. Schulte, BS, NR-CCEMTP; Roberta J. Secrest, PhD, PharmD, RPh; Wayne Snyder, MPA, EMT-P; Robert Swor, DO, FACEP; Rob Theriault, EMCA, RCT(Adv), CCP(F); Mike Turner; Anne Walters; and Robert B. Wylie, BS, EFO, CFI.

Fourth edition reviewers: Mark "Sharky" Alexander, EMT-P, ACLS, PALS, DMT; David S. Becker, MA, EMT-P, EFO; Kristen D. Borchelt, RN, NREMTP; Robert P. Breese, EMT-P, MICP, CCEMTP, FP-C; Helen E. Burkhalter, BAS, NREMT-P/RN; Peter Connick, EMT-P, EMT I/C; Jon S. Cooper, Paramedic, NCEE; Thomas Czerniak, MS, EMT-Basic; Carolyn V. Daigneau, MSN ANCC Certification, RN, PNP-BC; Ken Davis, BA, EMT-P; John A. DeArmond, NREMT-P; Steven Dralle, MBA, LP; Dennis Edgerly, AAS, EMT-P; Harold C. Etheridge, Lic-P, NREMT-P; James M. Farmer, EMT-P, AOS, FF; Janet Fitts, BSN, RN, CEN, TNS, EMT-P; Jeffery S. Force, BA, NREMT-P; Scott Gilmore, MD, EMT-P; Mark Goldstein, MSN, RN, EMT-P I/C; Lynn Pierzchalski-Goldstein, Pharm D, RPH; Wes Hamilton, BSN, CCRN, CFRN, CTRN, NREMT-P, FP-C; Seth C. Hawkins, MD, FACEP, FAAEM, FAWM; Gary Hoertz, NREMT-P; Julie C. Leonard, MD, MPH; Reylon Meeks, PhD, RN; Laraine Moody, MSN, RN, CPNP-AC/PC; Ruth Novitt-Schumacher, MSN, RN; Joanne Onderko, MA, RN, CEN, CFN; Dennis Parker, MA, EMT-P, I/C; Deborah L. Petty, BS, CICP, EMT-P; Larry Richmond, AS, NREMT-P, CCEMTP; Randy L. Sanders; Kimberly Schmitzer, MA, NREMT-P; Michael E. Scott, BAS, Paramedic; Heather Seemann, BA, NREMT-P, FP-C, CCP-C, MLT (ASCP); Gale P. Sewell, MSN, RN, CNE; David M. Stamey, CCEMTP; Sara Stewart, RN, EMT-P; David L. Sullivan, PhD, NREMT-P; David K. Tan, MD, FAAEM, EMT-T; David M. Tauber, NREMT-P, CCEMTP, FP-C, NCEE; Mark A. Trueman, BS, NREMT-P; Keith Widmeier, NREMT-P, CCEMTP; and Brian J. Williams, BS, NREMT-P, CCEMTP.

Photoshoot Acknowledgments

We would like to thank the following people and institutions for their collaboration on the photoshoots for this project. Their assistance was greatly appreciated.

Technical Consultants and Institutions

UMass Memorial Paramedics, Worcester EMS
Worcester, Massachusetts

Richard A. Nydam, AS, NREMT-P
Training and Education Specialist, EMS
UMass Memorial Paramedics, Worcester EMS
Worcester, Massachusetts

Dudley Fire Department
Dudley, Massachusetts

Oxford Fire-EMS
Oxford, Massachusetts

Southbridge Fire Department
Southbridge, Massachusetts

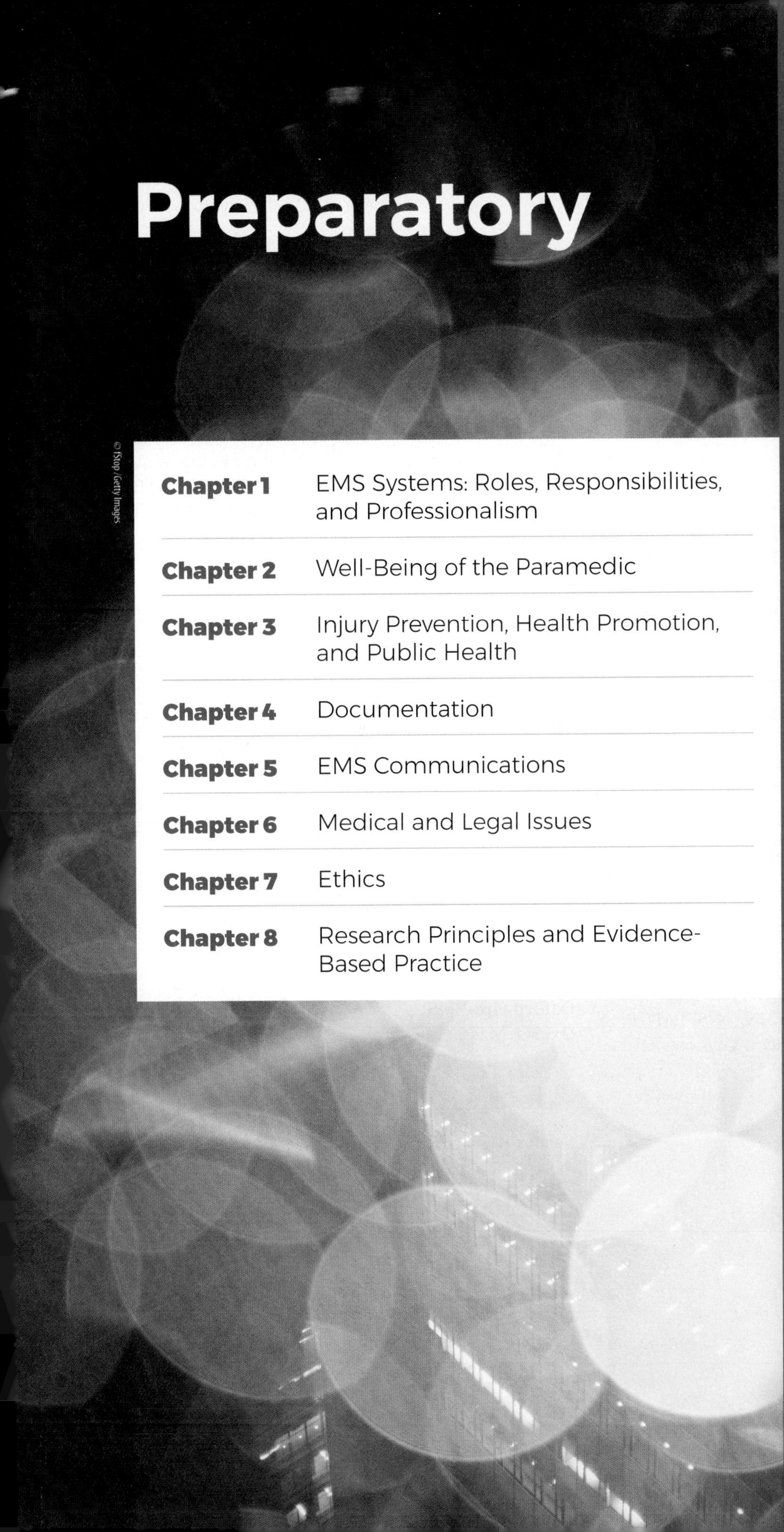

PART 1

Preparatory

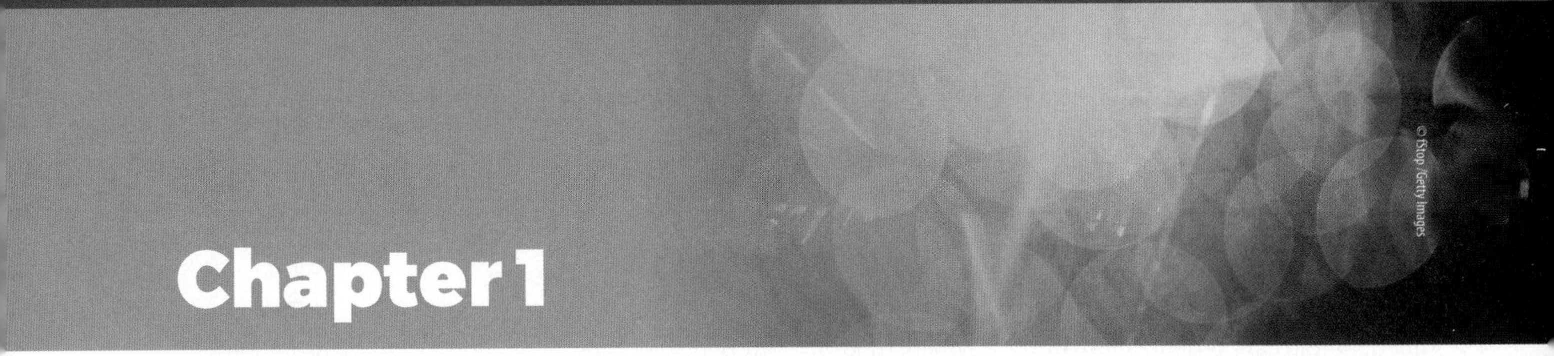

Chapter 1

EMS Systems: Roles, Responsibilities, and Professionalism

NATIONAL EMS EDUCATION STANDARD COMPETENCIES

Preparatory

Integrates comprehensive knowledge of the EMS system, safety/well-being of the paramedic, and medical/legal and ethical issues which is intended to improve the health of EMS personnel, patients, and the community.

Emergency Medical Services (EMS) Systems

- EMS systems (pp 5, 11–12)
- History of EMS (pp 5–10)
- Roles/responsibilities/professionalism of EMS personnel (pp 16–17, 18–22)
- Quality improvement (pp 23–27)
- Patient safety (pp 27–28)

OBJECTIVES

Upon completion of this chapter, the paramedic student will be able to:

1. Outline key historical events that influenced the development of EMS systems. (pp 5–10)
2. Identify the key elements necessary for effective EMS systems operations. (pp 11–12)
3. Outline the five components of the *EMS Education Agenda for the Future: A Systems Approach*. (pp 13–14)
4. Describe the benefits of continuing education. (p 14)
5. Differentiate among the training and roles and responsibilities of the four nationally recognized levels of EMS licensure/certification: Emergency Medical Responder, Emergency Medical Technician, Advanced Emergency Medical Technician, and Paramedic. (p 16)
6. List the benefits of membership in professional EMS organizations. (p 17)
7. Differentiate among professionalism, professional licensure, certification, registration, and credentialing. (p 18)
8. List attributes of the professional paramedic. (pp 19–20)
9. Describe the paramedic's role in patient care situations as defined by the US Department of Transportation. (pp 20–22)
10. Describe the benefits of each component of indirect and direct medical oversight. (pp 22–23)

11. Outline the role and components of an effective continuous quality improvement (CQI) program. (pp 23–27)
12. Recognize EMS activities that pose a high risk for patients. (p 28)
13. Describe actions paramedics may take to reduce the chance of errors related to patient care. (p 28)

KEY TERMS

accountable care organization (ACO) Payment models in which a health insurance entity, most commonly Medicare but private insurance as well, shares financial responsibility for all the health care received by a defined patient population with providers or health care organizations.

advanced life support (ALS) A level of care provided by paramedics or allied health professionals that includes advanced airway management, defibrillation, intravenous therapy, and medication administration.

basic life support (BLS) A level of care provided by people trained in first aid, cardiopulmonary resuscitation, and other noninvasive care.

certification A process by which a status or level of achievement is recognized by the granting of a document attesting to that level of status or achievement.

code of ethics A set of guidelines that are designed to set out acceptable behaviors for members of a particular group, association, or profession.

continuous quality improvement (CQI) A management approach to organizational performance that includes constant monitoring, evaluation, decisions, and actions.

credentialing A local process that allows a paramedic to practice in a specific EMS agency (or setting) in accordance with his or her level of certification and licensure.

direct medical oversight Physician-directed care provided in real time. The physician may be present on the scene or may provide direction through remote means; formerly known as online medical control.

emergency medical services A national network of services coordinated to provide aid and medical assistance from primary response to definitive care. The network involves personnel trained in rescue, stabilization, transport, and advanced management of traumatic and medical emergencies.

extended (expanded) scope of practice The expansion of health care services provided by EMS personnel in the prehospital setting.

indirect medical oversight The oversight of all medical components of an EMS system, including provider credentialing and education, protocol development, standing orders, quality assurance, and continuous quality improvement; formerly known as off-line medical control.

licensure A process by which a government entity regulates an occupation by granting authority (in the form of a license) to a person to take part in an activity.

managed care organization A network that provides patient care services to its members; includes health maintenance organizations and preferred provider organizations.

medical oversight The ultimate responsibility and authority for the medical actions of an EMS system; usually provided by one or more physicians.

mobile integrated health care (MIH) The provision of health care using patient-centered, mobile resources in the out-of-hospital environment that are integrated with the entire spectrum of health care and social service resources available in the local community.

paramedic A person who has completed training consistent with the *National EMS Education Standards*, including advanced training in clinical decision making, patient assessment, cardiac rhythm interpretation, defibrillation, drug therapy, and airway management.

patient care report (PCR) A document used in the prehospital setting to record all patient care activities and circumstances related to an emergency response.

reciprocity The practice of granting a person licensure or certification/registration based on licensure or certification/registration by another state, agency, or association.

registration The act of enrolling one's name in a register or book of record.

standing orders Specific interventions or actions that must be taken in specific situations by prehospital emergency care personnel without the need for direct medical oversight.

treatment protocols Guidelines that define the scope of prehospital intervention practiced by emergency services personnel.

The role of the paramedic is different than that of the "ambulance driver" of the past. Today's paramedics work in sophisticated EMS systems. They take part in an array of professional activities. These activities enhance the paramedic's ability to provide quality service and state-of-the-art patient care in the field and in less traditional health care settings.

EMS System Development

Assigning a time and place to the birth of organized prehospital emergency care is difficult. To understand the development of EMS, certain events from ancient times to the present must be considered.

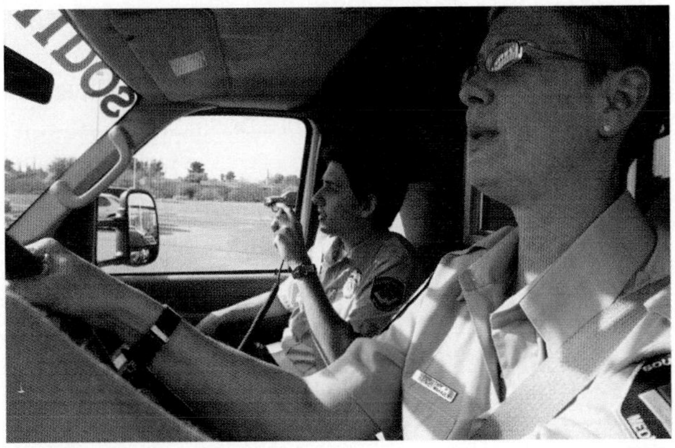

Organized prehospital emergency care has its roots in military medicine. Paintings of Roman battlefields suggest that some of the warriors cared for the injured. The first "ambulance" is thought to have been a covered cart used by one of Napoleon's surgeons, Dominique-Jean Larrey. He moved injured soldiers to treatment areas during the Napoleonic wars in the 1800s.[1] The first civilian ambulance services were established in Cincinnati and New York City in the 1860s. During the US Civil War, a scandal occurred when Walt Whitman and Matthew Brady reported that 3,000 wounded soldiers lay in the field for 3 days and 600 of these soldiers remained in the field for a week, during the 1862 Battle of Bull Run. In response, Surgeon General Jonathan Letterman created an ambulance service for each army corps. The service evacuated 10,000 wounded soldiers within 24 hours at the Battle of Antietam in 1862.[2]

CRITICAL THINKING

How would you feel about moving to an area with no advanced life support EMS?

Twentieth Century

Emergency medical services emerged as a nationwide system because of advances made by the military from World War I to the Vietnam War and the Iraq/Afghanistan conflicts. Death rates for battlefield casualties steadily decreased from 8% in World War I to 4.5% in World War II, to 2.5% during the Korean War, and less than 2% during the Vietnam War. From the invasion of Iraq in March 2003 through January 2007, 90.4% of all wounded troops survived.[3] Advances in field care for trauma patients, namely the initiation of medical care in the field and rapid evacuation, were the reason for the decreased death rates (BOX 1-1).[4,5] During World War I, wounded soldiers needed urgent care for injuries caused by machine guns and bombs. As a result, the military developed a battlefield ambulance corps. During World War II, the military moved wounded soldiers by airplane. Then during the Korean conflict, the military evacuated soldiers with helicopters. During the Vietnam conflict, the military improved urgent care and rapid evacuation with well-trained corpsmen. These efforts became the basis of prehospital care for the injured today.

Although the military made rapid progress in trauma care from the early 1900s through the mid-1960s, civilian prehospital care in the United States lagged behind. Care mostly was delivered by urban, hospital-based systems. These systems later developed into municipal services. Care also was provided by funeral directors and volunteers who had little or no training in emergency care. Most patients received minimal stabilization at the scene and were transported to the nearest hospital. The

BOX 1-1 Medical Care and Advances Made During Wartime

Civil War

- Railroads were used to evacuate casualties.
- Army still used ambulances much like Napoleon's.
- Death rate was very high because germs were unknown as the cause of infection; barns were used as hospitals.
- US Army set up the Medical Corps.
- Systemwide approach was instituted, which was used until the Vietnam War, with ambulances on the battlefield transporting the wounded to:
  - Aid stations
  - Field hospitals
  - Rear general hospitals

World War I

- Poor planning (no field hospitals) caused excessive evacuation times of 12 to 18 hours.
- High mortality rates (>20%).
- Most of those wounded died of hemorrhagic shock.
- No antibiotics were yet available; sepsis was common.
- Blood transfusions were just beginning to be used.
- Thomas half-ring femur splint was considered the greatest advancement in trauma care at this time.

World War II

- Evacuation time for wounded decreased to 4 to 6 hours.
- Antibiotics were developed.
- Plasma and blood transfusions became common.
- Hospitals were located closer to the front lines to decrease the time to surgery.
- Fixed-wing air transport began.

Korean War

- Evacuation time averaged 2 to 4 hours.
- Helicopter evacuation of wounded was introduced.
- Use of electrolyte solutions increased.
- Antibiotics became more effective.
- Surgical hospitals were located closer to the front lines.

Vietnam War

- Casualties were taken directly from the front lines to surgical hospitals by helicopter.
- Average evacuation time was 35 minutes.
- Average time to surgery was 1 to 2 hours.
- Civilian systems in that era never matched these time frames.

Iraq/Afghanistan conflicts

- Tourniquets were reintroduced.
- Hemostatic agents were developed.
- Concept of CAB (circulation-airway-breathing), a modification of the traditional ABC (airway-breathing-circulation) sequence, was developed for patients with exsanguinating hemorrhage.

realization that a person was more likely to survive a traumatic injury on a foreign battlefield than on a domestic city street made it clear that medical care should be initiated as soon as possible after the initial injury. This awareness led to the following two major landmarks in EMS development in 1966:

1. The National Academy of Sciences, National Research Council Committee on Trauma and Committee on Shock, published a white paper titled *Accidental Death and Disability: The Neglected Disease of Modern Society*. This document highlighted the significance of trauma as a public health threat and stressed the importance of emergency medical care. It listed recommendations to improve care for trauma victims. Eleven of these recommendations related directly to EMS (**BOX 1-2**).
2. The US Congress passed the Highway Safety Act of 1966. This act created the US Department of Transportation. Congress also created the National Highway Traffic Safety Administration (NHTSA), which provided legislative authority and funds to improve EMS and directed states to develop effective EMS programs. If the states did not develop effective EMS programs, they were subject to a loss of up to 10% of their federal highway construction funds. As a result of this act, states gave more than $142 million between 1968 and 1979 to develop EMS and early **advanced life support (ALS)** pilot programs.

CRITICAL THINKING

Which of the 11 elements identified in the white paper, *Accidental Death and Disability*, still need to be improved?

In 1973, Congress passed the Emergency Medical Service Systems (EMSS) Act.[6] This act paved the way for states to benefit from federal funds. The states could obtain the funds by forming regional EMS agencies. The act listed 15 vital components of the EMS system

BOX 1-2 Eleven Recommendations for EMS Identified in the White Paper

1. Extension of basic and advanced first aid training to greater numbers of the lay public
2. Preparation of nationally acceptable texts, training aids, and courses of instruction for rescue squad personnel, police officers, firefighters, and ambulance attendants
3. Implementation of recent traffic safety legislation to ensure completely adequate standards for ambulance design and construction, ambulance equipment and supplies, and the qualifications and supervision of ambulance personnel
4. Adoption at the state level of general policies and regulations pertaining to ambulance services
5. Adoption at district, county, and municipal levels of ways and means of providing ambulance services applicable to the conditions of the locality, control and surveillance of ambulance services, and coordination of ambulance services with health departments, hospitals, traffic authorities, and communication services
6. Initiation of pilot programs to determine the efficacy of providing physician-staffed ambulances for care at the site of injury and during transport
7. Initiation of pilot programs to evaluate automotive and helicopter ambulance services in sparsely populated areas and in regions where many communities lack hospital facilities adequate to care for seriously injured people
8. Delineation of radiofrequency channels and equipment suitable to provide voice communication between ambulances, emergency departments, and other health-related agencies at the community, regional, and national levels
9. Initiation of pilot studies across the nation for evaluation of models of radio and telephone installations to ensure effectiveness of communication facilities
10. Day-to-day use of voice communication facilities by the agencies serving emergency medical needs
11. Active exploration of the feasibility of designating a single nationwide telephone number to summon an ambulance

Reproduced from: Division of Medical Sciences, Committee on Trauma and Committee on Shock. *Accidental Death and Disability: the Neglected Disease of Modern Society*. Washington, DC: National Academy of Sciences, National Research Council; 1996, pp 35-36.

BOX 1-3 Fifteen Required Components of the EMS System

1. Manpower
2. Training
3. Communications
4. Transportation
5. Facilities
6. Critical care units
7. Public safety agencies
8. Consumers
9. Access to care
10. Transfer of patients
11. Medical record keeping
12. Consumer information and education
13. Review and evaluation
14. Disaster linkage
15. Mutual aid

(BOX 1-3). Also, the act required emergency care programs funded by the US Department of Health and Human Services to plan and put into practice a regional approach for emergency response and immediate care for trauma patients. This act played a major role in creating regional EMS systems from 1974 to 1981.

In 1981, funding for EMS development changed due to the Omnibus Budget Reconciliation Act.[7] This act consolidated EMS funding into state preventive health services block grants. As a result, funding under the EMSS Act was eliminated. These block grants were paid to state health departments instead of regional EMS organizations. Because these grants could be spent on projects other than EMS, the grants fell victim to politics and direct funding for EMS declined. Through cuts in funding and staff, the ability of NHTSA to support the US Department of Health and Human Services diminished. As a result, states had to develop and fund their own EMS systems, and the great growth that EMS experienced in the 1960s and 1970s declined. NHTSA continues to assist EMS development.[8] In 1988, NHTSA established

BOX 1-4 The 10 System Elements of the National Highway Traffic Safety Administration

1. Comprehensive EMS and trauma system legislation
2. Resource management and administration
3. Professional training
4. A communication system (9-1-1, communication centers, equipment, and the ability to communicate among ambulances, hospitals, fire departments, and police)
5. A transportation system (air, ground, and water)
6. Facilities (hospitals, trauma centers, specialty centers)
7. An inclusive trauma system fully integrated with emergency medical systems
8. Physician involvement (medical oversight)
9. Public information, education, and prevention
10. Data collection, quality improvement and evaluation, and research

Modified from: US Department of Transportation, National Highway Traffic Safety Administration. *EMS, Emergency Medical Services: NHTSA Leading the Way*. Washington, DC; 1996.

"10 System Elements" (the Statewide EMS Technical Assistance Program) as a recommended standard for EMS systems (**BOX 1-4**).

In 1996, NHTSA and the Health Resources and Services Administration (HRSA) published a consensus paper to help chart the course of EMS for the next 20 years. This document, the *EMS Agenda for the Future*,[8] was referred to as the *Agenda*. The *Agenda* was federally funded and completed by the National Association of EMS Physicians and the National Association of State EMS Directors. These organizations designed the *Agenda* to be used by government and private organizations at the national, state, and local levels. The intent of the document was to build a common vision for the future of EMS. The *Agenda* also was meant to help guide planning, decision making, and policy regarding EMS.

The *Agenda* made 14 suggestions for EMS focused on principles of public health and safety systems (**FIGURE 1-1**), including the EMS education system (described later in this chapter). The 14 attributes for EMS identified by the *Agenda* are the following:

1. Integration of health services
2. EMS research
3. Legislation and regulation
4. System finance
5. Human resources
6. Medical direction
7. Education systems
8. Public education
9. Prevention
10. Public access
11. Communication systems
12. Clinical care
13. Information systems
14. Evaluation

In 2017, NHTSA began to revise the *Agenda* based on the recommendation of key federal advisory committees. The new project, titled *EMS Agenda 2050: Envision the Future*, is slated to be complete in 2018.[9]

BOX 1-5 outlines other landmarks in EMS development.

DID YOU KNOW?

NEMSIS stands for the National Emergency Medical Services Information System. NEMSIS is the national repository used to store EMS data from every state in the nation. Since the 1970s, the need for EMS information systems and databases has been well established, and many statewide data systems have been created. However, these EMS systems vary in their ability to collect patient and systems data and allow analysis at a local, state, and national level. For this reason, the NEMSIS project was developed to help states collect more standardized elements and eventually submit the data to a national EMS database. This database is used in:

- Developing nationwide EMS training curricula
- Evaluating patient and EMS system outcomes
- Facilitating research efforts
- Determining national fee schedules and reimbursement rates
- Addressing resources for disaster and domestic preparedness
- Providing valuable information on other issues or areas of need related to EMS care

Reproduced from: What is NEMSIS? National EMS Information System website. https://nemsis.org/referenceMaterials/documents/NEMSIS%20Fact%20Sheet%206-2005.pdf. Accessed July 10, 2017.

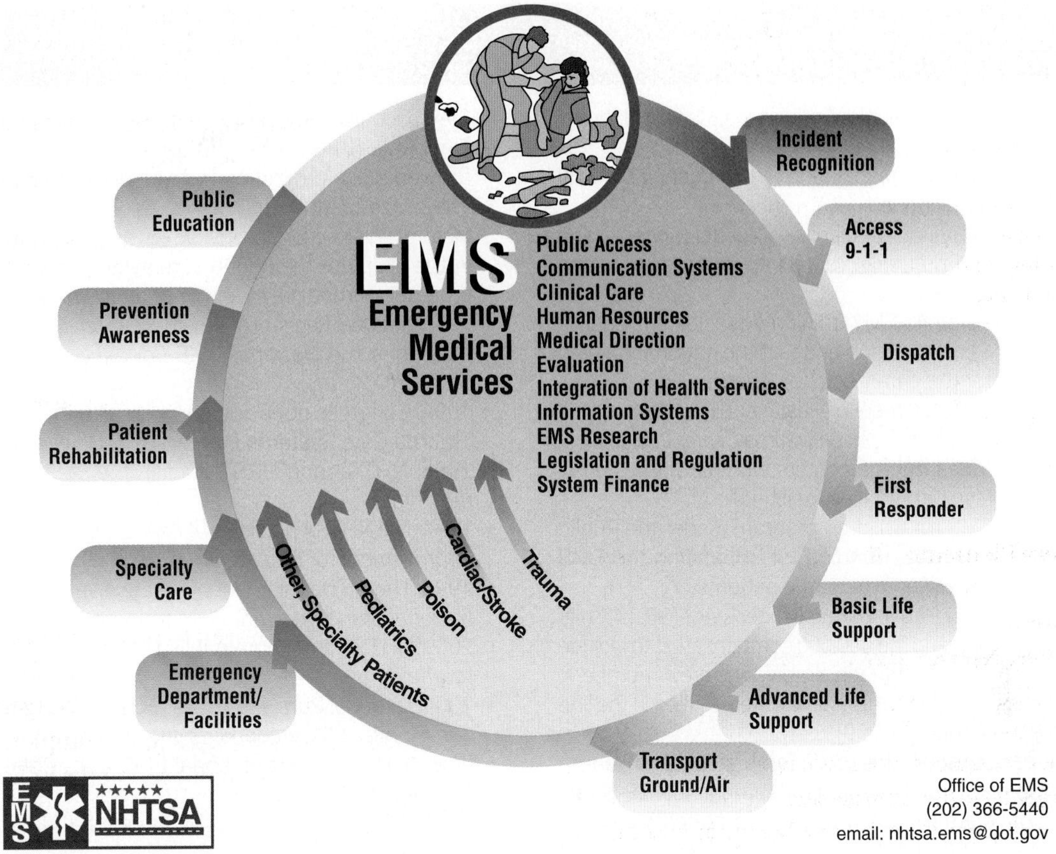

FIGURE 1-1 EMS: part of the health care system.

Modified from: the Emergency Medical Services for Children Innovation and Improvement Center, Houston, TX.

BOX 1-5 Other Landmarks in the Development of EMS

- Mid-1950s: The American College of Surgeons develops the first training programs for ambulance attendants.
- 1958: Dr. Peter Safar demonstrates the efficacy of mouth-to-mouth ventilation.
- 1960: Cardiopulmonary resuscitation is shown to be effective.
- 1967: Dr. Eugene Nagel trains Miami firefighters as paramedics at the University of Miami School of Medicine.
- 1968: The American Telephone and Telegraph Company (AT&T) designates 9-1-1 as the universal emergency telephone number.
- 1969: The US Department of Transportation and National Highway Traffic Safety Administration (NHTSA) develop the basic training course for emergency medical technicians (EMTs).
- 1969: The Committee on Ambulance Design develops *Ambulance Design Criteria*, a report to the US Department of Transportation and the NHTSA to complement the National Academy of Sciences–National Research Council's report titled *Medical Requirements for Ambulance Design and Equipment* (1968). This document recommends ambulance design standards and emergency equipment. The NHTSA agrees to issue matching federal funds to states that purchase vehicles meeting these standards.
- 1970: The National Registry of Emergency Medical Technicians is organized to standardize education, examinations, and certification of EMTs on a national level.
- 1972: President Richard Nixon directs the US Department of Health, Education, and Welfare to develop new ways to organize EMS, which results in $8.5 million in contracts being awarded to develop a model EMS system.
- 1972: The University of Cincinnati establishes the first residency program to train new physicians exclusively for the practice of emergency medicine.
- 1973: The star of life is adopted as the official symbol for EMS. The six blue bars of the star of life represent the six system functions of EMS: detection, reporting, response, on-scene care, care in transit, and transfer to definitive care.

(continued)

BOX 1-5 Other Landmarks in the Development of EMS *(continued)*

- 1974: President Gerald Ford proclaims the first National EMS Week.
- 1975: The National Association of Emergency Medical Technicians is founded.
- 1975: The American Medical Association accepts and approves the Paramedic role as an emergency health occupation.
- 1977: More than 40 EMT training agencies throughout the United States develop and test the national training standards for the paramedic for 2 years.
- 1980: The US Department of Health and Human Services releases the *Position Paper on Trauma Center Designation*, which describes trauma centers within EMS systems. The paper also categorizes facilities.
- 1984: The EMS for Children program, under the Public Health Act, provides funding for enhancing the EMS system to better serve pediatric patients.
- 1986: The 1979 Public Safety Officer's Act (SB 1479) is amended to expand the $50,000 compensation to include survivors of rescue squads, ambulance crew members, and public safety department volunteers killed in the line of duty (amended in 1990).
- 1990: President George H. W. Bush signs the Trauma Care Systems Planning and Development Act (HR 1602), which provides for annual grants to states based on geographic and population size to help establish and improve trauma systems. In 1995 Congress does not reauthorize funding for this act.
- 1991: Occupational Exposure to Bloodborne Pathogens; Final Rule (CFR 29 1910.1030) establishes standards for workplace protection from bloodborne diseases.
- 1993: The Institute of Medicine publishes *Emergency Medical Services for Children*, which points out deficiencies in the ability of the health care system to address the emergency medical needs of pediatric patients.
- 1993: National Registry of Emergency Medical Technicians publishes the *National EMS Education and Practice Blueprint*.
- 1995: Congress does not reauthorize funding under the Trauma Care Systems Planning and Development Act.
- 1996: NHTSA and HRSA publish the *EMS Agenda for the Future*.
- 1997: The NHTSA publishes *A Leadership Guide to Quality Improvement for Emergency Medical Services Systems*.
- 1998: The US Department of Transportation revises the *National Standard Curriculum* for paramedics.
- 2000: NHTSA and HRAA publish *EMS Education Agenda for the Future*.
- 2004: National Rural Health Association publishes *Rural and Frontier EMS Agenda for the Future*.
- 2005: NHTSA funds National EMS Core Content: The Domain of EMS Practice.
- 2007: NHTSA publishes the *National EMS Scope of Practice Model*.
- 2009: NHTSA publishes the *National EMS Education Standards*.

Health Care Reform and EMS

Because emergency medical services are part of the health care system, federal health care reform affects how prehospital emergency care is provided. **Managed care organizations** (eg, health maintenance organizations [HMOs], preferred provider organizations [PPOs], and other provider networks), because they control reimbursement for services provided by EMS, influence how EMS systems provide patient care choices for their clients (eg, emergency versus nonemergency response, resources, and personnel; transportation modes; and health care facility options). Currently, federal (Medicare) and state (Medicaid) insurance entities reimburse EMS agencies as suppliers of transportation rather than providers of health care. Most private insurance agencies, including managed care organizations, model their reimbursement after Medicare and Medicaid. In this system, insurers reimburse EMS agencies for care only if they transport a patient to the hospital.[10] In 2010, President Barack Obama signed into law the Patient Protection and Affordable Care Act (ACA). As part of an effort to better coordinate care for patients and stem the increasing cost of health care, the ACA included provisions for the development of **accountable care organizations (ACOs)**. ACOs are groups of physicians, hospital, and other health care providers who organize together to provide care for groups of patients, typically Medicare enrollees, while sharing the financial risk for that care with the insurer (typically Medicare).[11] In this model, if the health care cost of a patient is high, the groups of health care providers receives less money. ACOs are incentivized to develop innovative models to provide better care to patients and keep them out of the hospital. One of these models involves the employment of EMS personnel to reduce patient readmissions by helping coordinate care for patients, providing in-home follow-up care, and addressing social needs. This model, called community paramedicine or **mobile integrated health care (MIH)**, stresses that care is intended to be integrated with the entire health care system. Because of the link between reimbursement and transportation, sustainable funding and reimbursement for MIH will be important to the development of EMS.

NOTE

Medicare and Medicaid are the two insurance programs of the US government. Together, these insurance programs cover approximately 33% of the US population. These plans have rules that affect how patients qualify for EMS transportation. The rules also decide the conditions under which reimbursement for transportation will occur. In 2002, this reimbursement became standardized throughout the country through a consensus process involving national EMS agencies and the Centers for Medicare and Medicaid Services.

Modified from: Health insurance coverage of the total population. The Henry J. Kaiser Family Foundation website. http://kff.org/other/state-indicator/total-population/?currentTimeframe=0&sortModel=%7B%22colId%22:%22Location%22,%22sort%22:%22asc%22%7D.

Current Medical Services Systems

The current EMS system is a network of coordinated services that provides medical care to the community. The coordination was initiated by the NHTSA technical assessment program standards. These standards encouraged state EMS agencies not only to regulate their systems but to provide expertise to enhance their systems. Coordination of services ensures that patients are treated quickly and properly and that resources are used efficiently, potentially resulting in reduced health care costs (**FIGURE 1-2**) and improved patient outcomes.[8]

State EMS systems usually are made up of local and regional agencies that manage the delivery of prehospital care. Local agencies are responsible for providing day-to-day EMS to the community. Local agencies also work with regional and state agencies to create protocols and help set standards and guidelines. Local agencies provide data collection services and coordinate mutual aid and disaster planning. Most state EMS agencies have advisory councils to help organize EMS programs and activities. These councils are made up of medical professionals, paraprofessionals, consumers, and public and private agencies with an interest in EMS. The state agency is responsible for licensing and/or certification. In addition, the state enforces state EMS regulations and develops public education programs. Moreover, the state agency acts as a liaison with national agencies, some of which include NHTSA, the Federal Emergency Management Agency, Homeland Security, and the Maternal and Child Health Bureau of the Health Resources and Services Administration.

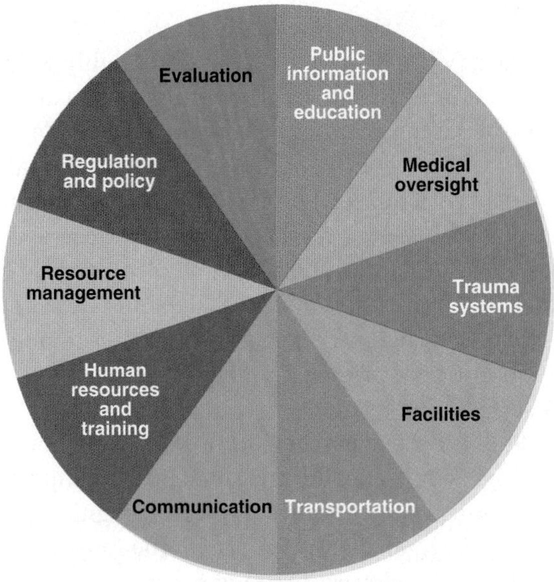

FIGURE 1-2 Ten components of the EMS system.

Modified from: National Highway Traffic Safety Administration, US Department of Transportation. *Emergency medical services: NHTSA leading the way*. Washington, DC: The Administration; 1995. www.nhtsa.dot.gov/people/injury/ems/agenda/emsman.html#Services.

DID YOU KNOW?

In December 1971, the television show *Emergency!* made its debut to millions of viewers. The series starred Randolph Mantooth as paramedic John Gage and Kevin Tighe as his partner, paramedic Roy DeSoto. This popular TV series contributed to a change in public attitudes about fire service and prehospital emergency care. It was also during this time that many fire departments expanded their services to include EMS response.

CRITICAL THINKING

How is the EMS system funded in your community?

EMS System Operations

The operations of an effective EMS system include public activation, emergency medical dispatch, prehospital care, hospital care, and rehabilitation.

Public Activation

Emergency public safety services are highly visible in the community. However, the public is not always aware of the complex nature of these services. People expect to have police and fire protection. They also expect to get a quick response with skilled personnel in a medical emergency. These expectations are due to years of available public safety service, public relations, press coverage, and national media. The public also expects such service because of their financial support in the form of taxes, donations, subscriptions for service, and user fees.

Public involvement in EMS, however, goes beyond funding. People are often at the scene of an injury or illness and play an important role in recognizing the need for emergency services. They sometimes administer first aid, help secure the scene, and gain access to the patient, and can be instrumental in managing a crisis. Educating the public is fundamental to the development of an effective EMS system. Paramedics build support for EMS by helping to develop and present public health care education and prevention programs (see Chapter 3, *Injury Prevention, Health Promotion, and Public Health*).

Once an emergency is recognized and a phone call for help is made, the response is coordinated. People usually contact communication centers and dispatch services by emergency phone numbers. Within most of the United States, the phone number 9-1-1 offers access to public safety services, including fire service, law enforcement, and EMS. The availability of emergency access through 9-1-1 continues to expand across the United States as areas adopt the system. In areas that do not have 9-1-1, other emergency phone numbers are typically available. These numbers can be promoted through public awareness programs and phone stickers. Other ways of engaging an emergency response include firebox pull stations, citizen band radios, voice over Internet protocol (VOIP), and cell phones. Chapter 5, *EMS Communications*, covers 9-1-1 in more detail.

Emergency Medical Dispatch

Emergency medical dispatch has been termed the "first, first responder."[12] Once a person activates the emergency response system, it is the responsibility of an emergency medical dispatcher to gather information from the caller and dispatch an appropriate and coordinated response. As the first point of contact with the emergency medical system, emergency medical dispatchers also provide callers with medical instructions before EMS arrives, which may include critical actions such as how to perform bystander cardiopulmonary resuscitation (CPR) or deliver a baby.

Prehospital Care

Ill or injured patients may need prehospital intervention and stabilization. Interventions may involve **basic life support (BLS)** and ALS skills. Initial prehospital care may be limited, providing only comfort and reassurance, depending on the situation (eg, entrapment, distance to the hospital, and availability of ALS). Care also may require electrocardiography performance and interpretation, motion restriction, noninvasive and invasive airway management, vascular access, medication administration, defibrillation, and external cardiac pacing.

Hospital Care

When a patient is transported to the emergency department, patient care resources expand and may include physicians, physician assistants, nurse practitioners, nurses, technicians, other support staff (eg, allied health counselors, social workers), and administrative staff. Patients often require resources and services beyond those offered in the emergency department, including diagnostic tests, surgery, cardiac catheterization, intensive care, physical therapy, pharmacy, nutrition services, and many others.

Rehabilitation

After patients have received definitive care in the hospital, many require some type of rehabilitation services. Rehabilitation often begins while the patient is still in the hospital and continues after hospital discharge. The services may be in the form of education and physical and occupational therapy, such as helping patients and families adjust to lifestyle changes after a stroke. Patients may also need retraining in activities of daily living (eg, bathing and preparing meals). Rehabilitation is designed to help patients regain any of the body functions lost due to illness or injury and to ensure the greatest possible independence is maintained.

EMS Education

In the past, EMS education was guided by the *National Standard Curriculum*. These guidelines for paramedics were last revised in 1998 and are no longer used. As previously discussed, the *EMS Agenda for the Future* was published by NHTSA in 1996 to provide a shared vision for the future of EMS. One of the goals of the *Agenda* was the development of robust educational systems for EMS professionals built on sound educational principles. These educational systems would prepare EMS providers to address the health care needs of the population and improve recognition of EMS as an allied health profession. The plan for this educational system was published in 2000 in the *EMS Education Agenda for the Future: A Systems Approach.* The *Education Agenda* described a five-component system to ensure quality in EMS education. The first three components have been further outlined in separate follow-up documents.

The five components include the following:

1. ***National EMS Core Content.*** The *National EMS Core Content* (*Core Content*) was published in 2005. The *Core Content* refers to the universal body of knowledge and skills for prehospital care. This project, led by the National Association of EMS Physicians and the American College of Emergency Physicians (ACEP), defined the entire domain of prehospital practice. It also identified the universal body of knowledge and skills for EMS personnel.
2. ***National EMS Scope of Practice Model.*** The *National EMS Scope of Practice Model* (*Scope of Practice*) was published in 2007. The *Scope of Practice* model divided the *Core Content* into levels of practice, defining the minimum knowledge and skills for each level—Emergency Medical Responder (EMR), Emergency Medical Technician (EMT), Advanced Emergency Medical Technician (AEMT), and Paramedic. Competencies required for the EMT, AEMT, and Paramedic levels assume mastery of the competencies for licensure at the previous level of training. Each person must demonstrate each skill within his or her scope of practice and for patients of all ages. In 2017, NHTSA hosted an expert panel to begin the revision process for this document.[13]
3. ***National EMS Education Standards.*** Development of the *National EMS Education Standards* (the *Standards*) was led by the National Association of EMS Educators (NAEMSE). The *Standards* replaced the *National Standard Curriculum*, which had been the cornerstone of EMS education since the 1960s. The *Standards* define the knowledge competencies and clinical behaviors and judgments that must be met at each licensure level, with the goal of meeting the practice guidelines as defined by the *National EMS Scope of Practice Model.* Content and concepts defined by the *National EMS Core Content* were also integrated within the *Standards.*[14] **BOX 1-6** outlines the timeline of these publications and standards.
4. **National EMS Certification.** National EMS Certification is a standard examination process for all provider levels that protects the public by ensuring the entry-level candidate has demonstrated entry-level competence. The education *Agenda* recommends that EMS students graduate from a nationally accredited EMS educational program to be eligible for National EMS Certification. This recommendation is to ensure consistency and quality in the performance of EMS personnel. National certification is critical to extending reciprocity to EMS personnel educated in other states (reciprocity is discussed later in the chapter).
5. **National EMS Education Program Accreditation.** Accreditation is a mechanism to ensure the quality of EMS education across institutions. The goal of accreditation is to ensure quality of education and to ensure that appropriate

BOX 1-6 Timeline of EMS Education Publications and Standards in the United States

- 1971: *AAOS: Emergency Care and Transportation of the Sick and Injured* (the "Orange Book," first edition)
- 1971: *EMT-Ambulance National Standard Curriculum*
- 1996: *EMS Agenda for the Future*
- 1998: National Standard Curriculum for EMT-Paramedic (revised)
- 2000: *Education Agenda for the Future: A Systems Approach*
- 2004: *National EMS Practice Analysis*
- 2006: *Emergency Medical Services at the Crossroads* (Institute of Medicine report)
- 2007: *National EMS Scope of Practice Model*
- 2009: *National EMS Education Standards*
- 2013: National Paramedic Program Accreditation
- 2017: National EMS reciprocity launched in 10 states
- 2017: Initiation of *EMS Agenda 2050* project
- 2017: Initiation of revision of *National EMS Scope of Practice Model*

educational infrastructures and resources are available for students in EMS programs. In 2013, the National Registry of Emergency Medical Technicians (NREMT) required EMS educational programs to be in the process of accreditation for their graduates to be eligible to take the registration examinations. Paramedic programs are accredited by the Commission on Accreditation of Allied Health Education Programs (www.caahep.org) on the advice of the Committee on Accreditation of Educational Programs for the Emergency Medical Services Professions. **FIGURE 1-3** is a diagram of the education model.[14]

NOTE

Each level in the EMS scope of practice represents a significant difference in skills, risk, knowledge, level of supervision and autonomy, judgment, and clinical decision making.

Continuing Education

Continuing education provides a way for all health care practitioners to retain their primary technical and professional skills. This ongoing effort is vital to professional competence because some skills learned during the initial course of study are not often used. Moreover, continuing education helps professionals stay current in the ever-changing field of health care, improving preparedness by teaching new and advanced skills and introducing fresh insights. New information, procedures, and resources that enhance patient care are continuously being developed to help maintain skill proficiency. Continuing education can take many forms, including the following:

- Conferences and seminars
- Lectures and workshops
- Quality improvement reviews
- Skill laboratories
- Simulations
- Certification and recertification programs
- Refresher training programs
- Journal studies
- Multimedia presentations
- Internet-based learning
- Case presentations
- Independent study

EMS Personnel Levels

Various levels of personnel and medical direction come together to make an effective prehospital EMS system. Personnel include dispatchers, EMRs, EMTs, AEMTs, and paramedics. Each level of EMS provider has satisfied training based on the *National EMS Education Standards.* The providers function as part of a comprehensive EMS response, under

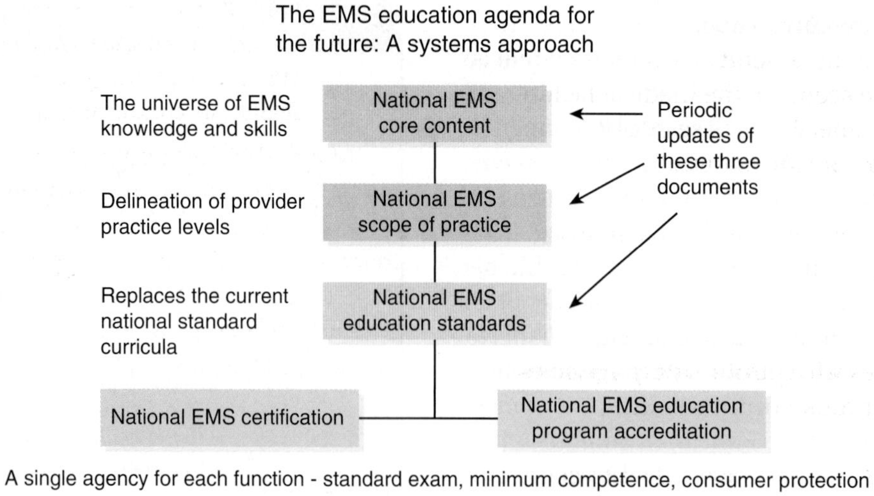

FIGURE 1-3 The EMS education system model.

Modified from: National Highway Traffic Safety Administration. *National EMS Education Standards.* Washington, DC: US Department of Transportation/National Highway Traffic Safety Administration; 2009.

medical oversight. The following descriptions of EMS practitioner levels are adapted from the *National EMS Education Standards.*[14]

Dispatcher

A dispatcher is a telecommunicator. The term *telecommunicator* applies to call takers, dispatchers, radio operators, data terminal operators, or any combination of such functions in a public service answering point located in a fire, police, or EMS communications center (see Chapter 5, *EMS Communications*). Although a dispatcher is not a recognized level of licensure in the *National EMS Scope of Practice Model*, the role is an integral part of the EMS system and serves as the primary contact with the public. The dispatcher directs the proper agencies to the scene. These agencies may include ground and air ambulances, fire departments, law enforcement, and utility services. An effective EMS dispatch communications system provides the following functions:

- **Receives and processes calls for EMS assistance.** The dispatcher receives and records calls for EMS assistance and selects an appropriate course of action for each call. To do this, the dispatcher must obtain as much information as possible about the emergency event, including the type of emergency, the caller's name, a call-back number, and the address. The dispatcher may also have to interact with distraught callers.
- **Dispatches and coordinates EMS resources.** The dispatcher directs the proper emergency vehicles to the correct address. This person also coordinates the emergency vehicles while en route to the scene, to the medical facility, and back to the operations base (**FIGURE 1-4**).
- **Relays medical information.** The dispatch center can provide a telecommunications channel among appropriate medical facilities and EMS personnel; fire, police, and rescue workers; and private citizens. This channel can consist of phone, radio, or biomedical telemetry.
- **Coordinates with public safety agencies.** The dispatcher aids communications between public safety resources (fire, law enforcement, rescue) and the EMS system, thereby coordinating services such as traffic control, escort, fire suppression, and extrication. The dispatcher must know the location and status of all EMS vehicles and whether support services are available. Larger systems use computer-aided dispatching, which provides for one or more of the following abilities:
  - Automatic entry of 9-1-1
  - Automatic interface to vehicle location with or without map display
  - Automatic interface to mobile data terminal
  - Computer messaging among multiple radio operators, call takers, or both
  - Dispatch note taking, reminder aid, or both
  - Ability to monitor response times, response delays, and on-scene times
  - Display of call information
  - Emergency medical dispatch review
  - Manual or automatic updates of unit status
  - Manual entry of call information
  - Radio control and display of channel status
  - Standard operating procedure review
  - Telephone control and display of circuit status

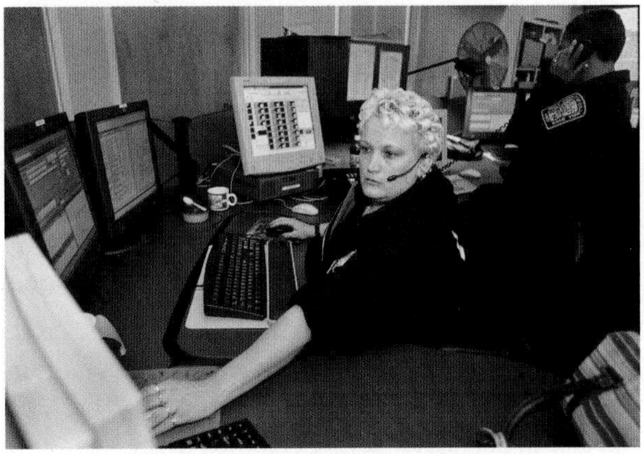

FIGURE 1-4 Computer dispatch console.

Many EMS and public service agencies require specialized training for their dispatch personnel. The dispatcher then can give prearrival instructions to the caller until EMS arrives. The training may include the US Department of Transportation training program for the emergency medical dispatcher, which is described further in Chapter 5, *EMS Communications*.

CRITICAL THINKING

What type of dispatching is provided in your community? Are dispatchers trained to the level of emergency medical dispatcher?

The EMR

The EMR may be the first medically trained person in an EMS system to arrive on a scene. These responders may include personnel from fire departments and law enforcement agencies. They also may include commercial medical response teams, athletic trainers, and others. The primary focus of the EMR is to initiate immediate lifesaving care to critical patients who access the EMS system. This person has the basic knowledge and skills necessary to provide basic lifesaving interventions while awaiting additional EMS response. The EMR can also assist higher-level personnel at the scene and during transport by providing basic interventions with minimal equipment. The EMR can do the following:

- Recognize the seriousness of the patient's condition or extent of injuries.
- Assess requirements for emergency medical care.
- Administer appropriate emergency medical care for life-threatening injuries related to airway, breathing, and circulation.

The EMT

The EMT is trained in all phases of basic life support. This training includes the use of automated external defibrillators and the administration of some emergency medications. The primary focus of the EMT is to provide basic emergency medical care and transport for critical and emergent patients who access the EMS system. EMTs perform interventions with the basic equipment typically found on an ambulance. They also assist paramedics in the care of patients during transport.

The AEMT

The AEMT was formerly known as EMT-Intermediate. The degree of training and skills that the AEMT practices varies between states and EMS systems. Training can include procedures such as insertion of airway adjuncts, administration of intravenous therapy, and administration of some emergency medications. The primary focus of the AEMT is to provide basic and limited advanced emergency medical care and transport for critical and emergent patients who access the EMS system.

The Paramedic

The **paramedic** is trained in all aspects of basic and advanced life support procedures that are relevant to prehospital emergency care. The paramedic has advanced training in patient assessment, clinical decision making, cardiac rhythm interpretation, defibrillation, drug therapy, and airway management (BOX 1-7). The paramedic provides emergency care based on advanced assessment skills and the formulation of a field diagnosis. The paramedic's specific roles and duties are discussed later in this chapter.

BOX 1-7 Description of the Paramedic Profession

The description of the paramedic profession provides the philosophy and rationale for the depth and breadth of coverage. The *EMT-Paramedic National Standard Curriculum* defines the position as follows:

- Paramedics have fulfilled requirements prescribed by an accrediting agency to practice the art and science of prehospital medicine under medical direction. Through performing assessments and providing medical care, their goal is to prevent and reduce mortality and morbidity caused by illness and injury. Paramedics primarily provide care to emergency patients in a prehospital setting.
- Paramedics possess knowledge, skills, and attitudes consistent with the expectations of the public and the profession. Paramedics recognize that they are an essential component of the continuum of care and serve as links to health resources.
- Paramedics strive to maintain high-quality, reasonable-cost health care by delivering patients directly to appropriate facilities. As advocates for patients, paramedics seek to be proactive in affecting long-term health care by working with other provider agencies, networks, and organizations. The emerging roles and responsibilities of the paramedic include public education, health promotion, and participation in injury- and illness-prevention programs. As the scope of service continues to expand, the paramedic will function as a facilitator of access to care and as an initial treatment provider.
- Paramedics are responsible and accountable to medical direction, the public, and their peers. Paramedics recognize the importance of research and actively participate in the design, development, evaluation, and publication of research. Paramedics seek to take part in lifelong professional development, perform peer evaluation, and assume an active role in professional and community organizations.

Modified from: National Highway Transportation Safety Administration. *EMT-Paramedic National Standard Curriculum*. Washington, DC: US Department of Transportation/National Highway Traffic Safety Administration; 1998.

Extended (Expanded) Scope of Practice

On a state or local level, health care services provided by EMS personnel in the prehospital setting have been expanded to address local health needs and gaps in the health care system, which is referred to as **extended (expanded) scope of practice.**[15] The role of these practitioners varies widely and includes community paramedics, critical care paramedics, tactical paramedics, and others. These specialists should be properly educated, credentialed by their system medical director, and operate within state EMS laws. In 2015, the National Association of EMS Officials (NASEMSO) proposed development of a national board to develop standards to guide models for each of these specialties.[16] Specialty certification helps ensure that EMS remains a vital part of the changing health care system.[17]

DID YOU KNOW?

Every 5 years, the NREMT conducts a *National EMS Practice Analysis.* The purpose of the study is to gather data on what EMS personnel actually do as part of their practice in providing emergency care. This analysis helps the NREMT to revise and tailor their certification examinations.

CRITICAL THINKING

What issues do you think your national EMS association should address to enhance patient care in your area?

National EMS Group Involvement

Many groups and organizations help to set the standards of EMS (BOX 1-8). These groups exist at the national, state, regional, and local levels. They take part in development, education, implementation, lobbying, and setting standards for EMS. Membership and participation in professional organizations help promote the professional status of the paramedic. These groups expose the paramedic to trends in emergency care, continuing education, and resource experts. The organizations also provide for national representation. They have a unified voice in other health care organizations and issues of national matters. Although the EMS standard-setting groups have many roles, their primary role is to set standards with input from members of the profession and the community. By doing so, they help ensure that the public is protected from people and agencies that do not meet professional standards for licensure and/or certification.

As the EMS system grew more complex, the need to coordinate initiatives and to meet the needs of all key stakeholder groups became evident. In response to this need, two federally appointed groups—the Federal Interagency Committee on Emergency Medical Services and the National EMS Advisory Council—were created and play an important role in shaping modern EMS.

The Federal Interagency Committee on Emergency Medical Services

Congress created the Federal Interagency Committee on Emergency Medical Services (FICEMS) in 2005. FICEMS helps coordinate federal agencies involved with state, local, tribal, or regional EMS and 9-1-1 systems. FICEMS recommends new or expanded programs and also identifies measures to improve federal agencies' efficiency with regard to EMS. Ten federal and one state agency serve on FICEMS.[18]

The National EMS Advisory Council

The National EMS Advisory Council (NEMSAC) was established in 2007. NEMSAC advises and consults with the Secretary of Transportation and FICEMS

BOX 1-8 National Organizations and Associations Involved in EMS

Air and Surface Transport Nurses Association
American Academy of Emergency Medicine
American Ambulance Association
American College of Emergency Physicians
American College of Surgeons
Association of Air Medical Services
Emergency Nurses Association
International Association of Fire Chiefs
International Association of Fire Fighters
International Association of Flight and Critical Care Paramedics
National Association of EMS Educators
National Association of EMS Physicians
National Association of Emergency Medical Technicians
National Association for Search and Rescue
National Association of State EMS Officials
National Registry of Emergency Medical Technicians
Special Operations Medical Association

regarding EMS issues. The council is composed of EMS industry and consumer representatives who serve 2-year terms. Although NEMSAC has no regulatory authority, it provides a knowledgeable independent voice to help guide federal EMS initiatives.[19]

> NOTE
> Some people believe that licensed professionals have greater status than those who are certified or registered. This belief is unfounded. A certification granted by a state and conferring a right to engage in a trade or profession is a form of licensure.

Licensure, Certification, Registration, and Credentialing

Paramedics are granted permission to practice their skills by three processes: licensure, certification, and registration. The exact wording of granting this permission varies by state.

Licensure

Licensure is a process of regulating occupations. In this process a license is granted by a government authority. The license allows a person to lawfully engage in a profession or activity. Most states and local authorities require that paramedics have a license.

Certification

Certification is a process by which a level of status or achievement is recognized by the granting of a document attesting to that level of status or achievement. In some states, a paramedic is certified to practice, which has the legal effect of a license.

Registration

Registration is the act of enrolling one's name in a register or book of record. For example, paramedics can be licensed or certified in their state and can be registered with the NREMT. The NREMT helps develop professional standards in the EMS industry. This organization verifies competencies for EMRs, EMTs, AEMTs, and paramedics by preparing and conducting certification examinations. Success on these examinations is the prerequisite for licensure in most states. Maintaining this national registration also simplifies the process of state-to-state mobility and **reciprocity** for its members (**BOX 1-9**).

BOX 1-9 Reciprocity for EMS Licensure

Recognition of EMS Personnel Licensure Interstate CompAct (REPLICA) is a multistate agreement allowing reciprocity for EMS licensure. This agreement permits EMS personnel licensed in a home state the legal right to practice in other states that have enacted REPLICA. In 2017, the compact was active in 10 states, with others considering legislation to join.

Modified from: Recognition of EMS Personnel Licensure Interstate Compact. National Registry of EMTs website. https://www.nremt.org/rwd/public/document/replica.

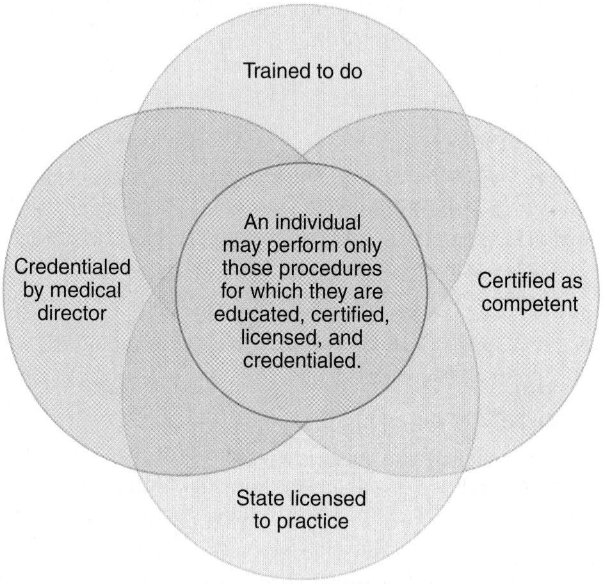

FIGURE 1-5 The relationship among education, certification, licensure, and credentialing.

Modified from: The National EMS Scope of Practice Model. National Highway Traffic Safety Administration website. https://one.nhtsa.gov/people/injury/ems/EMSScope.pdf.

Credentialing

Credentialing is a local process that allows a paramedic to practice in a specific EMS agency (or setting). Credentialing processes are typically guided by the local medical director (**FIGURE 1-5**).

Professionalism

Training and performance standards have helped to define EMTs and paramedics as health care professionals. The term *profession* refers to a body of knowledge or expertise. The members of such a field are often self-regulated through licensing or certification that confirms competence. In addition, most professions adhere to standards. These standards include initial and continuing education requirements. Professionalism refers to the way in which a person follows the standards of a profession. These standards may include conduct and performance standards. These standards also usually include adhering to a **code of ethics** approved by the profession (see Chapter 7, *Ethics*).

Health Care Professionals

Health care professionals conform to the standards of their profession. By providing quality patient care and striving for high standards, they instill pride in the profession and earn the respect of others. EMS professionals occupy positions of public trust and are highly visible role models. As such, the public has high expectations of EMTs and paramedics while they are both on and off duty. Therefore, professional conduct at all times and a commitment to excellence in daily activities complement the image of the EMS professional. Image and behavior are vital to establishing credibility and instilling confidence. The professional paramedic represents his or her employer; the EMS agency; the state, county, city, or district EMS office; and his or her peers.

Attributes of the Professional Paramedic

Many aspects of being professional can be applied to the role of the paramedic. Eleven of these attributes follow:[14]

1. **Integrity.** Integrity means being honest. Integrity may be the most important behavior for EMS professionals. The public assumes EMS professionals have integrity. Actions that show integrity include being truthful, being disciplined, and providing frequent communication and complete and correct documentation.
2. **Empathy.** Empathy is identifying with and understanding the feelings, situations, and motives of others. EMS professionals must always show empathy to patients, families, and other health care professionals. Traits of empathy include caring, compassion, and respect for others; understanding the feelings of the patient and family; being calm and helpful to those in need; and being supportive and reassuring of others.
3. **Self-motivation.** Self-motivation is the internal drive for merit and self-direction. Self-motivation can mean taking the lead to finish tasks, to improve behavior, and to follow through without supervision. Self-motivated people show enthusiasm for learning, are committed to **continuous quality improvement (CQI)** (described later in this chapter), and accept constructive feedback.
4. **Appearance and personal hygiene.** Paramedics are representatives of their profession. They must ensure that their clothing and uniforms are clean and in good repair. Personal hygiene is an important part of a paramedic's first impression.
5. **Self-confidence.** Paramedics must rely on themselves, often in difficult situations. One key task for paramedics is to assess their personal and professional strengths and weaknesses. Self-confidence shows that a paramedic is secure in his or her abilities.
6. **Communications.** An important part of the paramedic's profession is communicating. Paramedics must be able to convey key information to others verbally and in writing. They must speak clearly, write legibly, and listen actively. Finally, paramedics must be able to adjust communication strategies to various situations.
7. **Time management.** Time management involves organizing and prioritizing tasks to make the best use of time, such as being punctual, maintaining activity logs or to-do lists, and completing tasks and assignments on time.
8. **Teamwork and diplomacy.** The paramedic must be able to work well with others to achieve common goals. As a member of the EMS team, the paramedic must place the success of the team above personal success. To achieve common goals, paramedics support and respect other team members, are flexible and open to change, and communicate with coworkers to resolve problems (see Chapter 5, *EMS Communications*).
9. **Respect.** Respect means having regard for others and showing consideration and appreciation of their importance. Paramedics are polite and avoid the use of derogatory or demeaning terms. They know that being respectful brings credit to themselves, their associations, and their profession.
10. **Patient advocacy.** The paramedic is the patient's advocate. Paramedics should not attempt to impose their personal beliefs on patients or allow

personal biases (religious, ethical, political, social, or legal) to have an impact on the care they provide. Patient confidentiality must also be protected.

11. **Careful delivery of service.** Paramedics provide the highest quality patient care. With this care comes attention to detail and proper prioritization of care, which includes critical thinking skills. They also must evaluate their performance and attitude on every call. As part of the careful delivery of service, paramedics master and refresh their skills; perform full equipment checks; and ensure safe ambulance operations. Paramedics also follow policies, procedures, and protocols and comply with the orders of their supervisors and online medical direction.

CRITICAL THINKING

Which of these professional attributes represent your strengths? Which ones do you think you need to work on?

Roles and Responsibilities of the Paramedic

Paramedics provide patient care at an emergency scene, from an emergency scene to the hospital, between health care facilities, or in other health care settings as permitted by state and local laws. The paramedic's roles and duties can be divided into two groups: primary responsibilities and additional responsibilities[14] (BOX 1-10).

Primary Responsibilities

The paramedic must be prepared physically, mentally, and emotionally for the demands of the EMS profession. Preparation includes being committed to positive health practices (see Chapter 2, *Well-Being of the Paramedic*), maintaining adequate knowledge and skills of the profession, and having the proper equipment and supplies. The paramedic must respond to the scene in a safe and timely manner. Scene assessment considers personal safety; safety of the crew, patients, and bystanders; and the mechanism of injury or probable cause of illness.

On the scene, the paramedic quickly performs a patient assessment to determine the injury or illness. Integrating assessment findings with knowledge of disease or injury, the paramedic formulates a field impression, which also helps set priorities of care and transport. Paramedics who manage an emergency often follow protocols that include interacting with medical direction as needed. Paramedics provide care to minimize secondary injury.

After the patient's condition is stabilized in the field, the paramedic determines an appropriate transport destination. Transportation may be by ground or air ambulance. The type of transport needed for optimal patient care is based on the patient's condition, distance from the hospital, and travel time, among other factors. Knowledge of available resources, hospital designations, and categorization is required to choose the most appropriate facility (BOX 1-11). The hospital destination decision should be made jointly between the paramedic and the patient in cooperation with medical oversight. Knowledge of transfer agreements and local transport protocols is also helpful.

At the receiving facility, the paramedic gives staff members a handoff report that describes the patient's condition at the scene and during transport.

BOX 1-10 Roles and Responsibilities of the Paramedic

Primary Responsibilities

Preparation
Response
Scene assessment
Patient assessment
Recognition of injury or illness
Patient management
Appropriate patient disposition
Patient transfer
Documentation
Returning to service

Additional Responsibilities

Community involvement
Support of primary care efforts, such as in mobile integrated health care
Advocacy for public involvement in EMS
Participation in leadership activities
Personal and professional development

BOX 1-11 Specialized Care Facilities

Burn specialization center
Cardiac treatment center
Clinical laboratory service
Emergency department
Facility with acute hemodialysis capability
Facility with acute spinal cord or head injury management capability
Facility with reperfusion capability
Facility with special radiological capabilities
High-risk obstetric facility
Hyperbaric treatment center
Intensive care unit
Neurology center
Operating suite
Pediatric facility
Postanesthesia recovery room
Psychiatric facility
Rehabilitation facility
Stroke center
Substance abuse recovery center
Toxicology (including hazardous material or decontamination) service
Trauma center

The paramedic also needs to provide thorough and accurate written documentation in the **patient care report (PCR)**. The PCR should be completed as soon as possible, preferably at the hospital before the next call. The crew prepares the ambulance for return to service by replacing equipment and supplies (per agency protocol). Finally, the crew should review the call openly to identify ways to improve the care provided at the scene and during transport.

NOTE

Some EMS agencies organize community emergency response teams. These teams help prepare the public to respond to disaster-type emergencies. Members of the teams are trained to provide immediate help to victims, organize volunteers, and support first responder efforts.

Additional Responsibilities

Other duties of the paramedic include community involvement, support of primary care efforts, advocacy for public involvement in the EMS system, participation in leadership activities, and personal and professional development.

A paramedic can be a role model for the profession in many ways by participating as a leader in community activities. One way to improve the health of the community is by teaching CPR, first aid, and illness and injury prevention (see Chapter 3, *Injury Prevention, Health Promotion, and Public Health*). Such activities also create community awareness of the proper use of EMS resources. Programs that teach when, where, and how to use EMS and emergency departments promote the best use of health care resources. The integration of EMS with other health care and public safety agencies is strengthened through community outreach.

Communities and their health care organizations often enlist paramedics to support primary care efforts such as providing primary care patient follow-up in the patient's home. Paramedics can help to inform the public about alternatives to ambulance transportation, nonhospital emergency clinical providers, and freestanding emergency clinics.

Encouraging residents in the community to be involved in EMS improves the system and the community's health as a whole. They can help provide the information necessary to determine the needs and parameters for EMS use in the community. They can offer a personal view of quality improvement and possible solutions to problems. In addition, having involved residents from the community creates informed, independent advocates for the EMS system.

Paramedics can take part in leadership activities in their communities in many ways. One example is conducting primary injury prevention initiatives (activities and risk surveys). Another example is assisting media campaigns to promote EMS issues and other health programs (**FIGURE 1-6**) (see Chapter 3, *Injury Prevention, Health Promotion, and Public Health*).

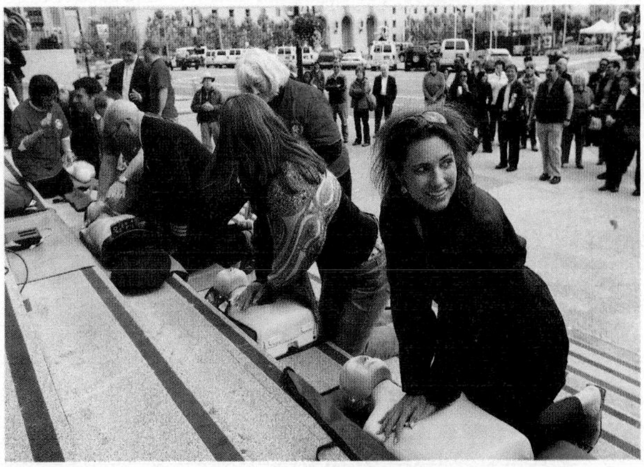

FIGURE 1-6 EMS outreach in the community.

Finally, a paramedic has a responsibility for personal and professional development. There are many ways to accomplish this, such as continuing education, student mentoring, membership in professional organizations, and participation in professional teams. Other methods include becoming involved in work-related issues that affect career growth, exploring alternative career paths in the EMS profession, conducting and supporting research initiatives, and being actively involved in legislative issues related to EMS.

Medical Oversight of EMS

Medical oversight refers to medical direction for the EMS system. The primary role of the physician medical director is to "ensure quality patient care."[20] The EMS medical director serves as a resource and as a patient advocate. One of the roles of the medical director is to credential EMS providers to work within an EMS system; in many areas, the medical director has the authority and responsibility to remove unsafe providers from practicing within the system.[21] The relationship between medical direction and the paramedic is critical to an effective EMS system. Medical directors and paramedics have the shared goal of excellent patient care. Close communication around patient care in real time allows for the provision of advanced and high-quality prehospital care.

The medical oversight physician should be educated as an EMS medical director and is ideally board certified in the subspecialty of EMS medicine.[22] A medical director must have knowledge of how the EMS system operates and full authority for medical direction. The medical director also is motivated to be involved in the following:[23]

- EMS system design and operations
- Education of EMS personnel
- Participation in personnel selection
- Participation in select training exercises or modules
- Participation in equipment selection
- Development of clinical protocols in cooperation with expert EMS personnel
- Participation in CQI and performance improvement
- Direct input on patient care
- Interface between EMS systems and other health care agencies
- Advocacy within the medical community
- Guidance as the "medical conscience" of the EMS system (advocating for quality and supervising patient care)
- Initial and ongoing credentialing to attest that the EMS providers have and maintain the knowledge, skills, and professional behaviors needed to safely practice in their system[24]
- Communication with external professional organizations

SHOW ME THE EVIDENCE

Researchers asked nationally registered EMS professionals how much contact they had with their medical director in the previous 6 months. For that period 62.5% of respondents indicated contact with the medical director during education, during a call review, or on the scene. Paramedics were more likely (78.5%) than were EMT-Intermediates (62.3%) or EMT-Basics (47.6%, $P < 0.001$) to have had contact with the medical director. Urban EMS professionals were more likely to have had medical director contact than were rural respondents (64.9% vs. 59.2%, $P < 0.001$).

Modified from: Studnek JR, Fernandez AF, Margolis GS, O'Connor RE. Describing the amount of medical director contact among nationally registered emergency medical services professionals, abstracted. *Prehosp Emerg Care.* 2008;12(1):115.

NOTE

An on-scene physician who is not the medical director may not be familiar with functions of EMS or medical oversight responsibilities. The lines of authority and responsibility for these physicians vary from state to state. Each EMS agency should have a policy that defines interaction with physicians on the scene.

Types of Medical Oversight

The two types of medical oversight are **indirect medical oversight** and **direct medical oversight.**[21,23] Both types ensure the quality of medical care in an EMS system.

Indirect medical oversight can be prospective or retrospective. Prospective oversight covers the authority to set treatment protocols (BOX 1-12). Such oversight also includes training for care and triage in the prehospital arena as well as the choice of equipment, supplies, and personnel. Retrospective oversight includes any actions that take place after the EMS

BOX 1-12 Protocols

Treatment protocols are written guidelines that define the scope of prehospital care for EMS personnel. The medical director of the EMS system or members of a regional EMS advisory group create them. The paramedic must follow the protocols unless advised otherwise by medical direction.

Standing orders are specific actions a paramedic must take in specific situations without the need for direct medical oversight. These orders are often a part of many protocols or treatment guidelines. Most protocols comply with national standards. They also comply with state EMS medical practice and regional guidelines. Examples of national standards include the American Heart Association guidelines for advanced cardiac life support and the American College of Surgeons guidelines for advanced trauma life support. Protocols define the standard of care for paramedic crews and online physicians. Often the paramedic acts strictly according to protocols, which eliminates delays in care during time-critical situations such as cardiac arrest, myocardial infarction, or stroke.

call. An example is reviewing a PCR and providing CQI. Direct medical oversight may be provided in person by the medical director or his or her designee if physically present on the scene. Online medical direction is a form of direct medical oversight.

Most prehospital care is provided following patient care protocols and standing orders, which vary by state. There are times, however, when a patient care issue falls outside the scope of established protocols or an unusual situation at the scene arises. In such cases, the paramedic may need to contact online medical direction by radio or phone to convey the patient's information and to receive orders through direct consultation with a physician or physician designee. This designee may be a registered nurse or physician assistant. The designee also may be a paramedic trained to give ALS orders in the medical direction system. Online medical direction allows for instant and specific care, telemetry, and CQI while paramedics are on the scene. As a rule, online medical direction supersedes established patient care protocols.[25]

Physician Bystanders

Some of the first ambulance personnel were physicians, a system still used in some countries. Currently, in the United States and Canada, there is seldom a medical director on the scene providing direct field supervision of EMS personnel. At times, however, a physician (physician intervener) may witness the injury or illness. Perhaps the patient's private physician is on the scene when EMS arrives. When this situation occurs, positive interaction between the on-scene physician and the EMS crew is essential.

If a physician who is not a medical director or the patient's physician is on the scene, EMS personnel must follow protocols. If no protocols are in place, the paramedic should immediately contact online medical direction. The policies of many EMS agencies require that the physician on the scene can assume responsibility for patient care and provide medical direction.[26] Together the physicians can make choices about the patient's care. With permission of medical direction, a bystander physician on the scene may take control of the patient's care. In some states, physician bystanders who want to assume care on the scene will be asked to show identification and sign an assumption of care form. By signing the form, the physician agrees to assume authority and responsibility of care and to ride with the patient to the hospital. If a physician on the scene advocates for care in opposition to medical direction, EMS personnel should attempt to remove the patient from the scene. In rare cases law enforcement may need to intervene to ensure that the scene is safe and the patient's care continues without interruption.[27]

Improving System Quality

A major goal of any EMS system is to continually evaluate and improve care. This goal requires both a retrospective evaluation of care that was provided (quality assurance) to identify areas that need improvement and the process of implementing and evaluating system-wide change (quality improvement). Together, these form the process of CQI, which is the ongoing study and improvement of a process, system, or organization (BOX 1-13). The Institute for Healthcare Improvement (IHI) developed the Triple Aim framework that describes an approach to optimizing health system performance (**FIGURE 1-7**).[28] New

BOX 1-13 Emergency Medical Services at the Crossroads

In the early 2000s the Institute of Medicine (now known as the National Academy of Medicine) established a committee to explore the strengths and limitations of the emergency care system in the United States and recommend strategies for improvement. The findings of this committee were published in 2007 in a report called *Emergency Medical Services at the Crossroads*. According to one of the central findings of this report, EMS was not well integrated within the health care system. In addition, many inconsistencies were found in the level of care provided from one region to the next. The report stressed that very little was actually known about the quality of care delivered by EMS, predominantly because there was no consensus regarding patient-centered measures of EMS quality. The panel recommended measures to improve integration of the EMS within the health care system and stressed the importance of developing evidence-based EMS performance indicators.

Modified from: Institute of Medicine. *Emergency Medical Services: At the Crossroads*. Washington, DC: The National Academies Press; 2007.

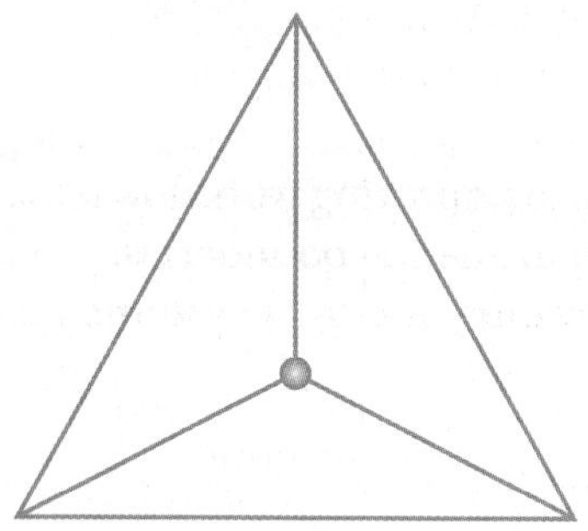

FIGURE 1-7 The Institute for Healthcare Improvement Triple Aim.

The IHI Triple Aim framework was developed by the Institute for Healthcare Improvement in Boston, Massachusetts (www.ihi.org).

system designs must be developed to simultaneously achieve the following:

- Improving the patient experience of care (including quality and satisfaction)
- Improving the health of populations
- Reducing the cost of health care

According to the National Academy of Medicine (formerly the Institute of Medicine), a quality health care organization is safe, effective, patient-centered, timely, efficient, and equitable.[29] In the past, quality assurance programs focused on evaluation of individual providers, often treating deviations in care with some type of punitive action. Health care has since evolved toward a focus on patient outcomes, such as survival or disability following a traumatic injury. As opposed to focusing on individual providers, CQI evaluates the entire EMS system. Key areas that are monitored in most EMS systems include:

- Medical direction
- Financing
- Training
- Communications
- Prehospital patient care and transport
- Interfacility transport
- Receiving facilities
- Specialty care units
- Dispatch
- Public information and education
- Disaster planning and mutual aid
- CQI activities include a review of the following:
  - Outcome measures of prehospital care (eg, scene times, procedure completion rates, and morbidity and mortality reviews)
  - Care while treatment is ongoing (concurrent reviews)
  - Written EMS PCRs (retrospective reviews)
  - Random or selected radio communication audio files
  - New procedures, equipment, or therapies

Input from CQI activities enables the EMS system to adapt treatment protocols and educational activities when needed. The most important feature of CQI is problem solving in a positive manner that includes all health care providers in the process (**FIGURE 1-8**). CQI stresses the value of enabling frontline personnel to perform their jobs well. With this group approach, all parties can be involved in elaborating on the cause of the problem. They can work together to develop remedies and can design a course of action to correct the problem. A plan is then enforced and the issue is reexamined to see whether the problem has been resolved (**BOX 1-14**).

CQI within an EMS system is an essential but often challenging process. EMS leaders should consider the following areas when seeking to improve quality within their organization:[8]

SHOW ME THE EVIDENCE

The 2007 US Metropolitan Municipalities' EMS Medical Directors' Consortium describes an evidence-based model to measure quality within suburban and urban EMS systems. The model includes specific key interventions and numbers-needed-to-treat that should be measured in the areas of ST-elevation myocardial infarction (STEMI), pulmonary edema, asthma, seizure, trauma, and cardiac arrest. The interventions to be evaluated in CQI are those that have been demonstrated by research to have a positive effect on patient outcome. For example, in a patient with trauma, prehospital records should be evaluated for scene time of less than 10 minutes and transport to a trauma center.

Modified from: Myers JB, Slovis CM, Eckstein M, et al. Evidence-based performance measures for emergency medical services systems: a model for expanded EMS benchmarking. *Prehosp Emerg Care*. 2008;12(2):141-151.

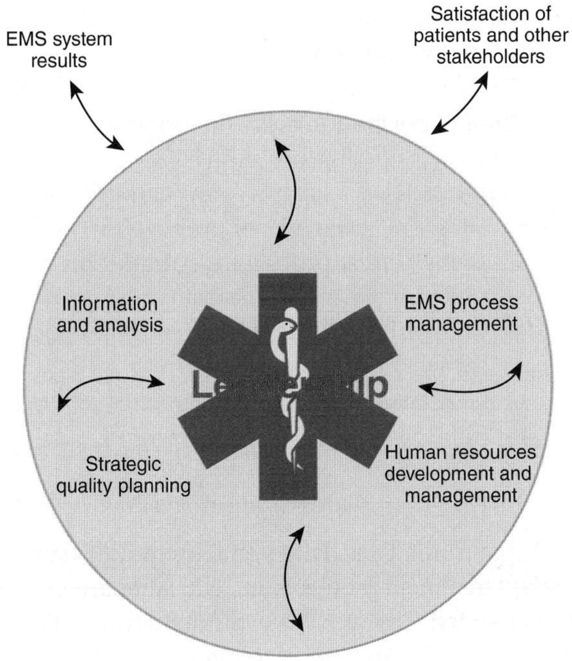

FIGURE 1-8 Leadership guide to quality improvement for EMS.

Modified from: A leadership guide to quality improvement for emergency medical services (EMS) systems. National Highway Traffic Safety Administration website. https://one.nhtsa.gov/people/injury/ems/Leaderguide/index.html.

1. **Leadership.** Leadership involves efforts by senior leadership and management. These people lead by example to integrate CQI into the strategic planning process and throughout the entire organization. Such integration promotes quality values and CQI techniques in work practices.
2. **Information and analysis.** Information and analysis involve managing and using the data needed for effective CQI. CQI is based on management by fact. Therefore, information and analyses are critical to CQI success.
3. **Strategic quality planning.** Strategic quality planning has three main parts. The first part is developing long- and short-term goals for structural, performance, and outcome quality standards. The second part is finding ways to achieve those goals. The third part is measuring the effectiveness of the system in meeting quality standards.
4. **Human resource development and management.** Human resource development and management focus on developing the full potential of the EMS workforce. This effort is guided by the principle that the entire EMS workforce is motivated to achieve new levels of service and value.
5. **EMS process management.** EMS process management concerns the creation and maintenance of high-quality services. Within the context of CQI, process management refers to the improvement of work activities. Process management also refers to improving work flow *across* functional or departmental boundaries.
6. **Emergency medical systems results.** Emergency medical systems must assess the results of quality-improvement initiatives and examine the success of the organization in achieving CQI.
7. **Satisfaction of patients and other stakeholders.** Emergency medical systems must ensure the ongoing satisfaction *of* patients and other stakeholders. Those internal and external to the EMS system must be satisfied with the services provided.

BOX 1-14 EMS Compass

EMS Compass is a project funded by NHTSA and led by the National Association of State EMS Officials. The project's goal is to develop a list of performance measures based on evidence and best practice. These measures can be used as key indicators of quality within an EMS system. Using standardized measures allows EMS agencies and the bodies that oversee them to have benchmarks against which to measure a program's outcomes over time.

Modified from: EMS Compass: improving systems of care through meaningful measures. National Association of State EMS Officials website. http://emscompass.org.

DID YOU KNOW?

In 2014, ACEP stated, "The most dangerous point in a patient's [emergency department] journey is the handoff and transition of care." Paramedics are involved in this high-risk process at least once during every call. Improvement in the process will reduce the chance of error.

Handoffs involve the transfer of rights, duties, and obligations from one person or team to another. A proper patient handoff ensures the appropriate continuity of care and safety. Verbal communication through a standardized process is the best way to transfer patient care. During a handoff, the health care team has an opportunity to provide information about the patient and to answer questions from the team at the receiving facility. The handoff information includes the patient's condition, the treatment provided, and any recent or anticipated changes in the patient's condition. A memory aid that can be used to provide structure in handoffs is called *I Pass the Baton* (**TABLE 1-1**).

Modified from: Welch S. 11—The Handoff. American College of Emergency Physicians website. www.acep.org/Membership/Sections/Quality-Improvement---Patient-Safety-Section/11---The-Handoff/.

TABLE 1-1 Transferring Patient Care Safely

I	Introduction	Formal introduction of the incoming/outgoing providers, including their roles and duties
P	Patient	Name, identifiers, age, sex, location
A	Assessment	Presenting chief complaint, vital signs, symptoms, and diagnosis
S	Situation	Current status and circumstances, including code status, level of certainty or uncertainty, recent changes, and response to treatment
S	Safety concerns	Critical laboratory values and reports, socioeconomic factors, allergies, and alerts, such as risk for falls
the		
B	Background	Comorbidities, previous episodes, current medication, and family history
A	Actions	Details regarding what actions were taken or are required and a brief rationale for those actions
T	Timing	Level of urgency and explicit timing, prioritization of actions
O	Ownership	Identification of who is responsible (nurse/doctor/team), including patient and family responsibilities
N	Next	Next steps in the patient's care plan and/or any anticipated changes

Modified from: Healthcare communications toolkit to improve transitions in care. Department of Defense Patient Safety Program website. https://www.oumedicine.com/docs/ad-obgyn-workfiles/handofftoolkit.pdf?sfvrsn=2.

SHOW ME THE EVIDENCE

Trained assistants observed and recorded 90 handoff reports given by EMS to the emergency department staff on high-acuity patients in a busy urban emergency department. Researchers evaluated the data and found that EMS personnel reported the chief concern for 78% of patients; description of the scene for 58%; and a complete set of vital signs 57% of the time. Pertinent physical examination, patient history, and overall assessment of the patient's condition were reported in less than 50% of cases. They concluded that increased training and a standardized approach to the handoff report is needed to reduce the risk to patients during this important transition of patient care.

Modified from: Goldberg SA, Porat A, Strother CG, et al. Quantitative analysis of the content of EMS handoff of critically ill and injured patients to the emergency department. *Prehosp Emerg Care*. 2017;*21*(1):14-17.

Benefits gained by applying these seven guidelines and recommendations include improvements in service and patient care delivery, economic efficiency, and profitability. They also help improve patient and community satisfaction and loyalty, and, most importantly, healthful outcomes.

Patient Safety

Patient safety is one of the most urgent health care challenges. In 1996, the Institute of Medicine launched an ongoing effort to assess and improve the nation's quality of care. The report brief of this initiative is titled *To Err Is Human: Building a Safer Health System.* This study found the following:[30]

- Health care in the United States is not as safe as it should—and can—be.
- At least 44,000 people, and perhaps as many as 98,000 people, die in hospitals each year as a result of medical errors that could have been prevented.
- Preventable medical errors in hospitals exceed attributable deaths to such causes as motor vehicle crashes, breast cancer, and AIDS.
- High error rates with serious consequences are most likely to occur in intensive care units, operating rooms, and emergency departments.
- Most errors are caused by faulty systems, processes, and conditions (BOX 1-15).

Although errors that directly lead to patient harm are most commonly recognized, an error does not need to have caused patient harm to be important in terms of patient safety. *Near misses* are events where an error occurred without causing patient harm. For example, the wrong drug is administered to a patient, but the mistake does not adversely affect the patient. Near misses represent opportunities to improve systems before patient harm occurs.

CRITICAL THINKING

The number of needlestick injuries in your agency has increased. How might the CQI process affect this situation?

SHOW ME THE EVIDENCE

A Survey of Paramedic Self-Reported Medication Errors

A survey about medication errors was given to paramedics in San Diego County, California. The survey tool was based on previous literature reviews and questions developed with previous CQI data. A total of 352 surveys were returned. Thirty-two (9.1%) responding paramedics reported committing a medication error in the preceding 12 months. Types of errors included dose-related errors (63%), protocol errors (33%), wrong route errors (21%), and wrong medication errors (4%). Issues identified as contributing to the errors included failure to triple check, infrequent use of the medication, dosage calculation error, and incorrect dosage given. Most of these errors were self-reported to the CQI representative (79.1%), with 8.3% being reported by the base hospital radio nurse, 8.3% found upon chart review, and 4.2% noted by the paramedic during the call but never reported.

Modified from: Vilke GM, Tornabene SV, Stepanski B, et al. Paramedic self-reported medication errors. *Prehosp Emerg Care*. 2007;11(1):80-84.

BOX 1-15 Types of Errors

Diagnostic

- Error or delay in diagnosis
- Failure to employ indicated tests
- Use of outmoded tests or therapy
- Failure to act on results of monitoring or testing

Treatment

- Error in the performance of an operation, procedure, or test
- Error in administering the treatment
- Error in the dose or method of using a drug
- Avoidable delay in treatment or in responding to an abnormal test
- Inappropriate (not indicated) care

Preventive

- Failure to provide prophylactic treatment
- Inadequate monitoring or follow-up of treatment

Other

- Failure of communication
- Equipment failure
- Other system failure

Reproduced from: Leape L, Lawthers AG, Brennan TA, Johnson WG. Preventing medical injury. *Qual Rev Bull*. 1993;19(5):144-149.

High-Risk Activities

Many activities in EMS can lead to medical errors, including poor clinical judgment, communication problems, dropping a patient (such as during a transfer), and patient refusal of care. In 2017, the Center for Patient Safety listed 10 additional priorities to improve patient and provider safety in EMS:[31]

1. Patient safety culture
2. Airway management
3. Bariatric care
4. Behavioral health encounters
5. Stretcher incidents
6. Medication mistakes
7. Pediatric care
8. Provider mental health
9. Crashes (ambulance and helicopter)
10. Transition of care

Many errors can be avoided by designing safe EMS systems that maintain skill proficiency, follow established rules and protocols, maintain team communications, and ensure an adequate knowledge base in patient care procedures and related EMS duties. Patient safety issues will be discussed throughout this text.

Strategies for EMS System Safety

EMS providers practice in a setting that poses a high risk of harm to EMS personnel, their patients, and the community. In 2013, a report sponsored by NHTSA, HRSA, and ACEP identified six strategies to promote a culture of safety in EMS:[32]

1. A just culture in EMS systems that balances fairness and accountability
2. Coordinated support and resources to promote safety in EMS
3. A data system to track responder injuries, adverse medical events, and adverse community events
4. EMS safety education initiatives
5. EMS safety standards
6. Requirement to report and investigate safety incident and near misses

Methods to Help Prevent Medical Errors in EMS

Methods to avoid medical errors in EMS can be grouped into environmental methods and individual methods.

Environmental methods that can help prevent medical errors include having clear and established protocols for procedures, ensuring that there is sufficient lighting for patient assessment and patient care procedures, and performing patient care duties with minimal interruptions. Examples include organizing and packaging drugs to avoid medication errors (eg, separating adult and pediatric drugs), securing equipment in the patient compartment of the ambulance, and safely securing adult and pediatric patients during transport.

Individual methods include the following personal actions to improve patient safety:

- **Practice reflection in action.** Think during an event (during action) while formulating a plan or performing a skill. Reflection in action allows the paramedic to make any necessary treatment changes to complete a task. Reflection in action promotes critical thinking and bridges the gap between knowing and doing.
- **Question assumptions.** Apply critical thinking to continuously seek out good ideas and new solutions. Doing so will help to set priorities and to problem solve.
- **Avoid reflection bias ("hindsight" bias).** Avoid the tendency to judge an event from a previous experience that had a bad outcome (eg, "I knew that was going to happen."). Reflection bias is the inclination to see events that have occurred in the past as more predictive than they really are of current events. Review the events after the fact and the outcome may be seen as more preventable. Replace hindsight with insight.
- **Use decision aids.** Use evidence-based decision aids and guidelines (eg, algorithms, pocket guides) to simplify decision making and improve patient safety. Decision aids can also facilitate the participation of patients in decisions about their care, when appropriate.
- **Ask for help.** A paramedic functions as part of a team. Don't hesitate to ask crew members or medical direction for help or advice, especially to verify a decision, drug dose, or procedure. Verbally check in with your partner before executing a task. Remember that patient safety comes first.

Summary

- Prehospital emergency care has its roots in the military.
- In the early 1900s through the mid-1960s, prehospital care in the United States was provided mostly by urban hospital-based systems. These systems later developed into municipal services. Care also was provided by funeral directors and volunteers who were not trained in these services.
- The operations of an effective EMS system include public activation, emergency medical dispatch, prehospital care, hospital care, and rehabilitation.
- EMS is composed of multiple levels of personnel, including dispatchers, emergency medical responders, EMTs, advanced EMTs, and paramedics. The levels are defined by distinct roles and duties, combining to make an effective prehospital EMS system.
- Professional groups and organizations help to set the standards of EMS. These groups exist at the national, state, regional, and local levels. The groups take part in development, education, and implementation. Being active in such a group helps to promote the status of the paramedic.
- Continuing education is crucial. It provides a way for all health care personnel to maintain technical and professional skills.
- Professionalism refers to the way in which a person conducts himself or herself. It also refers to how one follows the standards of conduct and performance established by the profession.
- The roles and duties of the paramedic can be divided into two categories: *primary* and *additional*.
- The two types of medical oversight are direct and indirect. Both are important. They help to ensure that the components of quality medical care are in place in an EMS system.
- A CQI program identifies and attempts to resolve problems in areas such as medical direction, financing, training, communication, prehospital management and transport, interfacility transfer, receiving facilities, specialty care units, dispatch, public information and education, audit and quality assurance, disaster planning, and mutual aid.
- Patient safety should be a high priority during every call. Errors that may cause injury or illness often involve handoffs, communication issues, medication issues, airway issues, lifting or moving of patients, ambulance crashes, and immobilization.

References

1. Lyons A, Petrucelli J. *Medicine: An Illustrated History*. New York, NY: Harry N Abrams; 1987.
2. McSwain NE. Prehospital care from Napoleon to Mars: the surgeon's role. *J Am Coll Surg*. 2005;201(4):651.
3. Goldberg MS. Death and injury rates of US military personnel in Iraq. *Mil Med*. 2010 Apr;175(4):220-226.
4. Division of Medical Sciences, Committee on Trauma and Committee on Shock. *Accidental Death and Disability: The Neglected Disease of Modern Society*. Washington, DC: National Academy of Sciences, National Research Council; 1966.
5. Manring MM, Hawk A, Calhoun J, Andersen RC. Treatment of war wounds: a historical review. *Clinical Orthop Relat Res*. 2002;467(8):2168-2191.
6. Emergency Medical Services Systems Act of 1973 (Public Law 93-154), 87 Stat. 594; 1973.
7. Omnibus Budget Reconciliation Act of 1981 (Public Law 97-35), 95 Stat 357; 1981.
8. *EMS Agenda for the Future*. National Highway Traffic Safety Administration website. https://one.nhtsa.gov/people/injury/ems/agenda/emsman.html. Accessed November 22, 2017.
9. *EMS Agenda 2050: Envision the Future*. National Highway Traffic Safety Administration website. http://emsagenda2050.org. Accessed November 10, 2017.
10. Munjal K, Carr B. Realigning reimbursement policy and financial incentives to support patient-centered out-of-hospital care. *JAMA*. 2013;309(7):667-668.
11. Barnes AJ, Unruh L, Chukmaitov A, van Ginneken E. Accountable care organizations in the USA: types, developments and challenges. *Health Policy*. 2014;118(1):1-7.
12. Clawson J, Dernocoeur K, Murray C. *Principles of Emergency Medical Dispatch*. 6th ed. Indianapolis, IN: Priority Press; 2015.
13. National EMS Scope of Practice Model Revision Project. National Association of State EMS Officials website. http://nasemso.org/Projects/EMSScopeOfPractice/. Accessed November 22, 2017.
14. National Highway Traffic Safety Administration. *National EMS Education Standards*. Washington, DC: US Department of Transportation/National Highway Traffic Safety Administration; 2009.
15. Expanded roles of EMS personnel. American College of Emergency Physicians website. https://www.acep.org/Physician-Resources/Policies/Policy-statements/EMS/Expanded-Roles-of-EMS-Personnel/. Updated April 2015. Accessed November 22, 2017.
16. A national strategy for EMS specialty certification. National Association of EMS Officials website. https://www.nasemso.org/Projects/EMSEducation/documents/National-Strategy-for-EMS-Specialty-Certification-020115.pdf. Published February 1, 2015. Accessed November 22, 2017.
17. National Highway Traffic Safety Administration. *The National EMS Scope of Practice Model*. Washington, DC: US Department of Transportation/National Highway Traffic Safety Administration; 2005.
18. FICEMS: Federal Interagency Committee on EMS. National Highway Traffic Safety Administration Office of EMS website. https://www.ems.gov/ficems.html. Accessed November 22, 2017.

19. NEMSAC: National EMS Advisory Council. National Highway Traffic Safety Administration Office of EMS website. https://www.ems.gov/nemsac.html. Accessed November 22, 2017.
20. Medical direction of emergency medical services. American College of Emergency Physicians website. https://www.acep.org/Clinical---Practice-Management/Medical-Direction-of-Emergency-Medical-Services/. Updated April 2005. Accessed November 22, 2017.
21. Pepe PE, Copass MK, Fowler RL, Racht EM. Medical direction of emergency medical services. In: Bass RR, Brice JJ, Delbridge TR, Gunderson MR, eds. *Emergency Medical Services: Clinical Practice and Systems Oversight*. Vol. Medical Oversight of EMS. Dubuque, IA: Kendall Hunt Publishing; 2009:24.
22. National Association of EMS Physicians. Physician oversight of emergency medical services. *Prehosp Emerg Care.* 2017;21(2):281-282.
23. Bass RR, Lawner B, Lee D, Nable JV. Medical oversight of EMS systems. In: Cone DC, Brice JH, Delbridge TR, Myers JB. eds. *Medical Oversight of EMS*. Vol. 2. 2nd ed. West Sussex, UK: Wiley; 2015.
24. Clinical credentialing of EMS providers. National Registry of Emergency Medical Technicians website. https://www.nremt.org/rwd/public/document/credentialing-ems. Published December 2016. Accessed November 22, 2017.
25. *A Leadership Guide to Quality Improvement for Emergency Medical Services (EMS) Systems*. National Highway Traffic Safety Administration website. https://one.nhtsa.gov/people/injury/ems/Leaderguide/index.html. Accessed November 22, 2017.
26. Out-of-hospital medical direction and the intervener physician. American College of Emergency Physicians website. https://www.acep.org/Clinical---Practice-Management/Out-of-Hospital-Medical-Direction-and-the-Intervener-Physician/. Updated January 2016. Accessed November 22, 2017.
27. Dees L. Family and bystanders. In: Cone DC, Brice JH, Delbridge TR, Myers JB, eds. *Emergency Medical Services: Clinical Practice and Systems Oversight*. Vol. 1. 2nd ed. West Sussex, UK: John Wiley & Sons; 2015:462-469.
28. Initiatives: The IHI Triple Aim. Institute for Healthcare Improvement website. http://www.ihi.org/Engage/Initiatives/TripleAim/Pages/default.aspx. Accessed November 22, 2017.
29. Richardson WC, Berwick DM, Bisgard JC, Bristow LR, Buck CR, Cassel CK. *Crossing the Quality Chasm: A New Health System for the 21st Century*. Washington, DC: Institute of Medicine; 2001.
30. Institute of Medicine: shaping the future for health. To err is human: building a safer health system. National Academy of Sciences website. http://www.nationalacademies.org/hmd/Reports/1999/To-Err-is-Human-Building-A-Safer-Health-System.aspx. Accessed July 18, 2017.
31. EMS forward: 10 topics that will move EMS forward in 2017. Center for Patient Safety website. http://www.centerforpatientsafety.org/emsforward/emsforward/. Accessed November 22, 2017.
32. Strategy for a national EMS culture of safety. National Highway Transportation and Safety Administration Office of EMS website. https://www.ems.gov/pdf/Strategy-for-a-National-EMS-Culture-of-Safety-10-03-13.pdf. Published October 2013. Accessed November 22, 2017.

Suggested Readings

Bigham BL, Buick JE, Brooks SC, Morrison M, Shojania KG, Morrison LJ. Patient safety in emergency medical services. *Prehosp Emerg Care*. 2012;16(1):20-35.

Brown WE, Dickinson PD, Misselbeck WJ, Levine R. Longitudinal emergency medical technician attribute and demographic study. *Prehosp Emerg Care*. 2002;6(4):433-439.

Institute of Medicine of the National Academies. *Future of Emergency Care Series: Emergency Medical Services at the Crossroads*. Washington, DC: National Academic Press; 2006.

Meisel ZF, Hargarte S, Vernick J. Addressing prehospital patient safety using the science of injury prevention and control. *Prehosp Emerg Care*. 2008;12(4):411-416.

National EMS Information System (NEMSIS) website. http://www.nemsis.org. Accessed November 22, 2017.

Page J. *The Magic of 3 A.M: Essays on the Art and Science of Emergency Medical Services*. Carlsbad, CA: JEMS Communications; 2002.

Page J. *The Modern History of EMS: Making a Difference 2.0* [DVD]. St. Louis, MO: Elsevier Mosby; 2004.

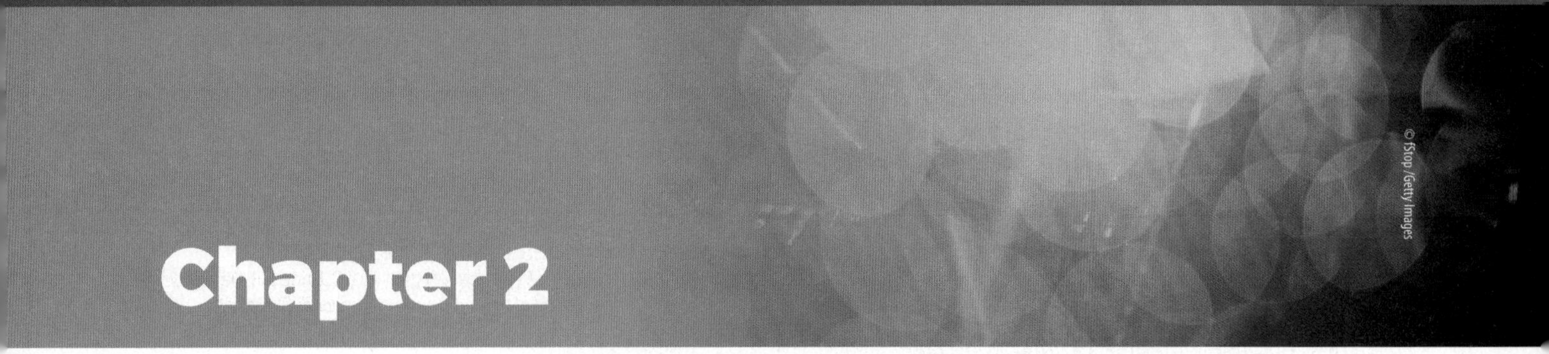
© fStop/Getty Images

Chapter 2

Well-Being of the Paramedic

NATIONAL EMS EDUCATION STANDARD COMPETENCIES

Preparatory

Integrates comprehensive knowledge of the EMS system, safety/well-being of the paramedic, and medical/legal and ethical issues which is intended to improve the health of EMS personnel, patients, and the community.

Workforce Safety and Wellness

- Provider safety and well-being (p 33)
- Standard safety precautions (pp 45–46)
- Personal protective equipment (p 47)
- Stress management (pp 56–58)
  - Understanding and dealing with death and dying (pp 60–62)
- Prevention of response-related injuries (pp 45–50)
- Prevention of work-related injuries (pp 45–50)
- Lifting and moving patients (p 48)
- Disease transmission (pp 45–48)
- Wellness principles (p 33)

Medicine

Integrates assessment findings with principles of epidemiology and pathophysiology to formulate a field impression and implement a comprehensive treatment/disposition plan for a patient with a medical complaint.

Infectious Diseases

Awareness of

- A patient who may have an infectious disease (pp 45–48)
- How to decontaminate equipment after treating a patient (Chapter 27, *Infectious and Communicable Diseases*)

Assessment and management of

- A patient who may have an infectious disease (Chapter 27, *Infectious and Communicable Diseases*)
- How to decontaminate the ambulance and equipment after treating a patient (Chapter 27, *Infectious and Communicable Diseases*)
- A patient who may be infected with a bloodborne pathogen (Chapter 27, *Infectious and Communicable Diseases*)
  - Human immunodeficiency virus (HIV) (Chapter 27, *Infectious and Communicable Diseases*)
  - Hepatitis B (Chapter 27, *Infectious and Communicable Diseases*)
- Antibiotic-resistant infections (Chapter 27, *Infectious and Communicable Diseases*)
- Current infectious diseases prevalent in the community (Chapter 27, *Infectious and Communicable Diseases*)

Anatomy, physiology, epidemiology, pathophysiology, psychosocial impact, presentations, prognosis, and management of

- HIV-related disease (Chapter 27, *Infectious and Communicable Diseases*)
- Hepatitis (Chapter 27, *Infectious and Communicable Diseases*)
- Pneumonia (Chapter 23, *Respiratory*)
- Meningococcal meningitis (Chapter 27, *Infectious and Communicable Diseases*)
- Tuberculosis (Chapter 27, *Infectious and Communicable Diseases*)
- Tetanus (Chapter 27, *Infectious and Communicable Diseases*)
- Viral diseases (see Chapter 23, *Respiratory*, Chapter 27, *Infectious and Communicable Diseases*, and Chapter 47, *Pediatrics*)
- Sexually transmitted disease (Chapter 27, *Infectious and Communicable Diseases*)

- Gastroenteritis (Chapter 28, *Abdominal and Gastrointestinal Disorders*, and Chapter 27, *Infectious and Communicable Diseases*)
- Fungal infections (Chapter 27, *Infectious and Communicable Diseases*)
- Rabies (Chapter 27, *Infectious and Communicable Diseases*)
- Scabies and lice (Chapter 27, *Infectious and Communicable Diseases*)
- Lyme disease (Chapter 27, *Infectious and Communicable Diseases*)
- Rocky Mountain spotted fever (Chapter 27, *Infectious and Communicable Diseases*)
- Antibiotic-resistant infections (Chapter 27, *Infectious and Communicable Diseases*)

OBJECTIVES

Upon completion of this chapter, the paramedic student will be able to:

1. Describe the components of wellness and associated benefits. (p 33)
2. Discuss the paramedic's role in promoting wellness. (pp 33, 44–49)
3. Outline the benefits of specific lifestyle choices that promote wellness, including proper nutrition, weight control, exercise, sleep, and smoking cessation. (pp 33–44, 51–52)
4. Identify risk factors for cardiovascular disease and cancer. (pp 44–45)
5. List measures to take to reduce the risk of infectious disease exposure. (pp 45–48)
6. Outline actions to take following a significant exposure to a patient's blood or other body fluids. (p 48)
7. Identify preventive measures to minimize the risk of work-related illness or injury associated with work-related stress, exposure to disease, lifting and moving patients, hostile environments, rescue situations, and vehicle operations. (pp 48–50, 56–58)
8. List signs and symptoms of addiction and addictive behavior. (p 51)
9. Distinguish between normal and abnormal anxiety and stress reactions. (pp 52–53)
10. Give examples of stress-reduction techniques. (pp 56–58)
11. Outline the components of critical incident stress management. (pp 58–59)
12. Given a scenario involving death or dying, identify therapeutic actions you may take based on your knowledge of the dynamics of this process. (pp 60–62)

KEY TERMS

adaptation A cellular response to stress of any kind that seeks to escape and protect from injury; a central part of the response to changes in the physiological condition.

addiction A compulsive, uncontrollable dependence on a substance, habit, or practice to such a degree that cessation causes severe emotional, mental, or physiological reactions.

adrenaline An endogenous adrenal hormone that helps prepare the body for energetic action.

anxiety A state or feeling of apprehension, uneasiness, agitation, uncertainty, or fear resulting from the anticipation of some threat or danger.

autonomic nervous system The part of the nervous system that regulates involuntary vital functions, including the activity of cardiac muscle, smooth muscle, and glands.

circadian rhythm A pattern based on a 24-hour cycle, especially repetition of certain physiological phenomena, such as sleeping and eating.

distress Negative, debilitating, or harmful stress.

eustress Positive, performance-enhancing stress.

posttraumatic stress disorder (PTSD) An anxiety disorder that can occur following a series of disturbing events or a single, emotionally traumatic incident.

standard precautions Measures used to reduce the risk of microorganisms in health care settings.

stress A nonspecific mental or physical strain caused by any emotional, physical, social, economic, or other factor that initiates a physiological response.

universal precautions Infection control practices in health care that are observed with every patient and procedure and that prevent exposure to bloodborne pathogens.

The paramedic has a demanding job that requires physical and mental well-being. By adopting a lifestyle that enhances personal wellness, paramedics can improve their health and prolong their careers. A healthful lifestyle also helps paramedics to serve as role models and coaches for others.

Wellness Components

Wellness has two main aspects: physical well-being and mental and emotional health. Both aspects are key to the paramedic's personal health and ability to safely deliver emergency care. They are also important to manage stressful events that are inherent in the profession.

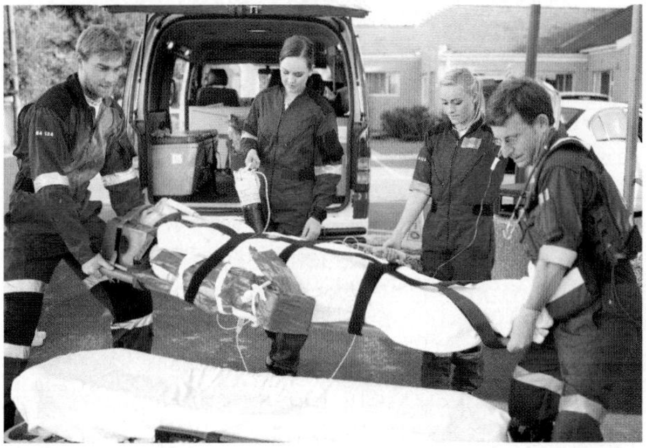

Physical Well-Being

Several factors play a major role in maintaining physical health, including good nutrition, physical fitness, ample sleep, and the prevention of illness and injury.

Nutrition

Nutrients are components of foods that provide the elements necessary for body function. The six categories of nutrients are carbohydrates, fats, proteins, vitamins, minerals, and water.

Carbohydrates are composed of carbon, hydrogen, and oxygen. Under normal circumstances, they serve as the body's source of fuel. Carbohydrates are obtained primarily from plant foods. Plants store carbohydrates as starch, which is made up of granules enclosed by cellulose walls that swell and burst when cooked. This feature makes cooked starchy foods easier to digest than raw, uncooked starchy foods. The only important source of animal carbohydrates is lactose (milk sugar).

All dietary fats contain a mixture of saturated and unsaturated fatty acids. Saturated fats raise the cholesterol levels in the blood by shutting down the process that normally removes excess cholesterol from the body. Unsaturated fats, which help rid the body of newly formed cholesterol, are further subdivided into polyunsaturated and monounsaturated fats. All polyunsaturated fats, including the omega-3 fats (fish oil), are considered important to human health. Monounsaturated fats are liquid vegetable oils. Like polyunsaturated fats, they may help decrease blood cholesterol levels (BOX 2-1). Trans fats are unsaturated fatty acids that are formed when vegetable oils are processed and made more solid or into a more stable liquid. Although trans fats are unsaturated, they appear similar to saturated fats in terms of their effect on blood cholesterol levels. A healthy diet should include good fats and limit saturated fats. Trans fat intake should be as low as possible.[1]

> NOTE
>
> Cholesterol is present in all foods of animal origin and is concentrated heavily in fat and in poultry skin. This white, waxy substance is found in every cell of an animal. Not all cholesterol is harmful; in fact, an adequate amount of cholesterol is needed for body functions. Cholesterol is manufactured in the liver and is carried through the bloodstream. Adding cholesterol to the diet is one of several dietary factors that can influence serum cholesterol levels and increase the risk of heart disease and stroke.
>
> *Modified from:* Grundy SM. Does dietary cholesterol matter? *Curr Atheroscler Rep*. 2016 Nov;18(11):68.

Proteins are made of hydrogen, oxygen, carbon, and nitrogen (and most contain sulfur and phosphorus). Proteins are vital to building body tissues during growth, maintaining those tissues, and repairing them. When proteins are digested, they break down into amino acids (classified as essential or nonessential). Essential amino acids are needed for body growth and cellular life. They must be obtained from food because they are *not* made in the body. Nonessential amino acids are not needed for body health and growth and can be made in the body. Proteins that contain all the essential amino acids are considered complete proteins; they are found in meats and dairy products. Proteins that are missing one or more essential amino acids are called incomplete proteins (eg, those in grains and vegetables). Proteins can be used as a source of energy but should be spared for their more important role in body health by the sufficient intake of carbohydrates.

Vitamins are organic substances that are present in minute amounts in foods. Because vitamins are crucial for metabolism and cannot be made in adequate amounts by the body, they must be obtained

BOX 2-1 A Primer on Fats and Oils

Not All Fats and Oils Are Created Equal

Fats and oils are made up of basic units called fatty acids. Each type of fat or oil is a mixture of different fatty acids.

- Saturated fatty acids can increase the risk of heart disease and stroke. They may raise both good and bad cholesterol levels. They are found chiefly in animal sources such as meat and poultry (fat), whole or reduced-fat milk, and butter. Some vegetable oils, such as coconut, palm kernel oil, and palm oil, also contain saturated fats. Saturated fats are usually solid at room temperature.
- Monounsaturated fatty acids and polyunsaturated fatty acids can lower bad cholesterol levels, provide essential fats the body cannot produce, and reduce the risk of cardiovascular disease. They are found in vegetable oils such as canola, olive, safflower, sesame, and peanut oils. Food such as avocados, nuts and seeds (eg, flaxseed, sunflower, walnuts), and fatty fish (eg, tuna, herring, lake trout, mackerel, salmon, sardines) also contain these types of fat.
- Trans–fatty acids are formed when vegetable oils are processed into margarine or shortening. Sources of trans fats in the diet include fried foods, snack foods, and baked goods made with "partially hydrogenated vegetable oil" or "vegetable shortening." Trans–fatty acids also occur naturally in some animal products such as dairy products. These fats can raise bad (low-density lipoprotein [LDL]) cholesterol levels and lower good (high-density lipoprotein [HDL]) cholesterol levels. They can increase the risk of cardiovascular disease and diabetes.

Cholesterol Is Different

Blood (serum) cholesterol and dietary cholesterol are two different types of cholesterol. Dietary cholesterol is found in foods of animal origin, such as egg yolks, organ meats, and full-fat dairy products. Blood cholesterol is a waxy substance that occurs naturally in the body. It is used to make the estrogen and testosterone sex hormones, as well as bile, which is needed for digestion. However, if the level of cholesterol in the blood is too high, cholesterol and other fats can stick to the artery walls.

Because blood cholesterol is waxy and cannot dissolve in water, it is carried through the blood in packages called lipoproteins. HDL is a "good" package for cholesterol, whereas LDL is a "bad" package for cholesterol. HDL cholesterol collects excess cholesterol in the blood and carries it to the liver, which then reprocesses or excretes the excess cholesterol. HDL may also help remove some of the cholesterol deposited on the artery walls. Excess LDL cholesterol can increase the risk of heart disease because it accumulates on the artery walls.

Modified from: American Heart Association. The facts on fats. November 2016. Available at: http://www.heart.org/HEARTORG/HealthyLiving/HealthyEating/Nutrition/FATS-The-Good-the-Bad-and-the-Ugly-Infographic_UCM_468968_SubHomePage.jsp.

BOX 2-2 Free Radicals and Antioxidants

Free radicals are natural by-products of chemical reactions in the body that can produce cellular injury. The buildup of these free radicals increases with age. Free-radical accumulation is thought to be the cause of many diseases, including cardiovascular disease, diabetes, and some cancers. Substances that can generate free radicals are found in fried foods, alcohol, tobacco smoke, pesticides, and air pollution, among other sources.

Antioxidants are free radical scavengers; that is, they reduce the formation of free radicals or react with and neutralize them, thereby making these substances nontoxic to cells. Antioxidants occur naturally in the body as well as in certain foods, such as fruits, vegetables, and whole grains. Beta carotene (a form of vitamin A) and vitamins C and E are popular antioxidant supplements that may have autoimmune and antiaging benefits.

through food or vitamin supplements. (An ample intake of vitamins through a balanced diet should make vitamin supplements unnecessary in healthy people.) Vitamins are classified as either water soluble or fat soluble. Water-soluble vitamins (vitamin C and the B-complex vitamins) cannot be stored in the body; they must be obtained from the daily diet. Fat-soluble vitamins (vitamins A, D, E, and K) can be stored in the body; therefore, while adequate intake of these vitamins over time is necessary, a daily dietary intake of these vitamins is often not required (**BOX 2-2**).

Minerals are inorganic elements that play a key role in biochemical reactions in the body. They include calcium, chromium, iron, magnesium, potassium, selenium, sodium, and zinc. Like vitamins, minerals come from the diet (**TABLE 2-1**).

TABLE 2-1 The ABCs of Nutrition

	Function	Source
Vitamins		
A	Essential to proper eye function; keeps skin, hair, and nails healthy; helps maintain healthy gums, glands, bones, and teeth; helps ward off infection; may protect against lung cancer	Liver,[a] dairy products,[a] fish, carrots, yellow squash, dark-green leafy vegetables, corn, tomatoes, papaya
B_1 (thiamine)	Helps convert carbohydrates into biological energy; promotes proper nerve function	Pork,[a] unrefined and enriched cereals, organ meats,[a] legumes, nuts[a]
B_2 (riboflavin)	Crucial in the production of energy in the body	Milk,[a] cheese,[a] yogurt,[a] green leafy vegetables, fruits, bread, cereals, meats[a]
B_3 (niacin)	Lowers cholesterol levels in blood only when taken in very high doses; may protect against cardiovascular disease	Yeast, meats[a] including liver,[a] cereals, legumes, seeds[a]
B_6	Essential for protein breakdown and absorption	Beef,[a] poultry,[a] fish, pork,[a] bananas, nuts,[a] whole grains, vegetables
B_{12}	Essential for the healthy function of nerve tissue	Meats,[a] meat products,[a] shellfish, fish, poultry,[a] eggs[a]
Biotin	Needed for breakdown of glucose (a type of sugar) and formation of certain fatty acids necessary for several important body functions, including metabolism and energy production	Meats,[a] poultry,[a] fish, eggs,[a] nuts,[a] seeds,[a] legumes, vegetables
C (ascorbic acid)	Strengthens the walls of blood vessels; keeps gums healthy; promotes healing of cuts and wounds	Strawberries, citrus fruits, tomatoes, cabbage, cauliflower, broccoli, greens
D	Helps build and maintain teeth and bones; needed so that the body can absorb calcium	Egg yolks,[a] fish and cod liver oil,[a] fortified milk and butter[a]
E	Helps form red blood cells, muscle tissue, and other tissues; may protect against cardiovascular disease	Poultry,[a] seafood, seeds,[a] nuts,[a] cooked greens, wheat germ, fortified cereals, eggs[a]
K[b]	Needed for normal clotting of blood	Spinach, broccoli, brussels sprouts, kale, turnip greens
Minerals		
Calcium	Helps build strong bones and teeth; promotes proper muscle and nerve function; helps blood to clot; helps activate enzymes needed to convert food to energy; may protect against the development of fragile, porous bones (osteoporosis)	Milk,[a] cheese,[a] yogurt,[a] buttermilk, other dairy products,[a] green leafy vegetables[b]
Chromium	Works with insulin to maintain normal blood glucose levels	Whole-grain cereals, condiments (black pepper, thyme), meat products,[a] cheeses[a]
Iron	Essential to make hemoglobin, the oxygen-carrying component of red blood cells	Red meat[a] and liver,[a] shellfish and fish, legumes, dried apricots, fortified breads and cereals
Magnesium	Activates enzymes needed to release energy in the body; promotes bone growth; needed to make cells and genetic material	Green leafy vegetables, beans, nuts,[a] fortified whole-grain cereals and breads, oysters, scallops

(continued)

TABLE 2-1 The ABCs of Nutrition *(continued)*

	Function	Source
Potassium	With sodium, helps to regulate the body's fluid balance; plays a major role in muscle contraction, nerve conduction, and beating of the heart	Bananas, citrus fruits, dried fruits, deep yellow vegetables, potatoes, legumes, milk,[a] bran cereal
Selenium	Interacts with vitamin E to prevent breakdown of cells in the body	Organ meats,[a] seafood, meats,[a] cereals and grains, egg yolks,[a] mushrooms, onions, garlic
Sodium	Helps maintain the body's fluid balance	Salt, processed foods, foods in brine, salted crackers and chips, cured meats, soy sauce (Note: Sodium is so prevalent that low intake is very rare; rather, the problem is avoiding excessive intake.)
Zinc	Boosts the immune system and helps fight disease; element in more than 100 enzymes—proteins that are essential to digestion and other functions	Red meats,[a] some seafoods, grains

[a] These foods are high in fat and/or cholesterol. Use sparingly or substitute low-fat versions, where possible.
[b] Green leafy vegetables and other foods rich in vitamin K can contribute to blood clotting. If you take a drug that prevents blood clotting, talk to your physician before changing your diet.
Modified from: US Department of Agriculture's Center for Nutrition Policy and Promotion, Washington, DC. Available at: www.cnpp.usda.gov.

Water is the most important nutrient because cellular function depends on a fluid environment. Water accounts for 50% to 60% of total body weight. Infants have the highest percentage of body water; older adults have the lowest. Water is obtained through consumption of liquids and fresh fruits and vegetables. It is also produced when food is oxidized during digestion.

NOTE

Diseases caused by vitamin deficiency (eg, scurvy, rickets, pellagra, beriberi) are common in less developed parts of the world but are rare in the United States and Western Europe. This decreased prevalence in more developed areas is largely due to the availability of many foods that have adequate amounts of vitamins. Making proper food choices can help to prevent diseases caused by vitamin deficiencies.

Dietary Recommendations

Numerous groups have provided, and continue to publish, recommendations for a healthful diet. Among these groups are the World Health Organization (WHO), the US Department of Agriculture (USDA), the US Department of Health and Human Services, and the US Food and Drug Administration (FDA). BOX 2-3 and BOX 2-4 detail dietary recommendations for the general population made by the American Heart Association and dietary recommendations for special populations made by the USDA, respectively.

CRITICAL THINKING

Does your average diet meet these guidelines? If not, in which areas do you need to make changes?

Food Guidance and Lifestyle Recommendations

In 2015, the USDA revised and simplified its original food guidance and lifestyle recommendations (which were made in 2010).[2] These recommendations are designed to educate the public and health professionals about diet and lifestyle for healthy Americans. The *2015–2020 Dietary Guidelines for Americans* provide recommendations that encourage healthy eating patterns, recognize that people will need to make shifts in their food and beverage choices to achieve a healthy pattern, and acknowledge that all segments of

BOX 2-3 Diet and Lifestyle Recommendations From the American Heart Association

Consume an overall healthy diet.
Aim for a healthy body weight:
- Body mass index (BMI): 18.5–24.9 kg/m^2

Aim for a desirable lipid profile:
- Low-density lipoprotein cholesterol (LDL-C):
  - Optimal: <100 mg/dL
  - Near or above optimal: 100–129 mg/dL
  - Borderline high: 130–159 mg/dL
  - High: 160–189 mg/dL
  - Very high: ≥190 mg/dL
- Triglycerides (TG): <150 mg/dL
- High-density lipoprotein cholesterol (HDL-C):
  - Men: >40 mg/dL
  - Women: >50 mg/dL

Aim for a normal blood pressure (BP):
- Systolic BP <120 mm Hg
- Diastolic BP <80 mm Hg

Be physically active.
Avoid use of and exposure to tobacco products.

Modified from: American Heart Association. Body mass index in adults (BMI calculator for adults). August 2014. Available at: http://www.heart.org/HEARTORG/HealthyLiving/WeightManagement/BodyMassIndex/Body-Mass-Index-BMI-Calculator_UCM_307849_Article.jsp#.Wc6P_bpFzIU.

BOX 2-4 *2015–2020 Dietary Guidelines for Americans*: Special Populations

Women Capable of Becoming Pregnant

- Choose foods that supply heme iron, which is more readily absorbed by the body; additional iron sources; and enhancers of iron absorption such as vitamin C–rich foods.
- Consume 400 mcg per day of synthetic folic acid (from fortified foods and/or supplements) in addition to food forms of folate from a varied diet.[a]

Women Who Are Pregnant or Breastfeeding

- Consume 8 to 12 ounces of seafood per week from a variety of seafood types.
- Due to their high methyl mercury content, limit white (albacore) tuna to 6 ounces per week and do not eat the following types of fish: tilefish, shark, swordfish, and king mackerel.
- If pregnant, take an iron supplement as recommended by an obstetrician or other health care provider.

People Age 50 Years and Older

- Consume foods fortified with vitamin B_{12}, such as fortified cereals or dietary supplements.

[a] Folic acid is the synthetic form of the nutrient, whereas folate is the form found naturally in foods.

Modified from: US Department of Agriculture. *Dietary guidelines for Americans*, 2015–2020. 8th ed. December 2015. Available at: https://health.gov/dietaryguidelines/2015/resources/2015-2020_Dietary_Guidelines.pdf.

our society have a role to play in supporting healthy choices. BOX 2-5 provides an overview of the new guidelines.

Healthy Body Weight

Ideal body weight is calculated by a formula that considers both height and weight to derive a body mass index (BMI). The BMI for most nonpregnant adults should be in the range of 18.5 to 24.9 kg/m^2. These fixed calculations are not appropriate for children because of the profound changes from birth to early adulthood (see Chapter 47, *Pediatrics*). People who maintain a normal BMI experience less joint or muscle pain and reduce the risk of development of cardiovascular disease, type 2 diabetes, hypertension, and some cancers. They often have a better quality of life because they are likely to have more energy and better sleep quality.

Maintaining a normal BMI is a challenge for some people because it requires balancing healthy eating

BOX 2-5 *2015–2020 Dietary Guidelines for Americans*: Key Recommendations

Have a healthy eating pattern that includes all foods within the calorie level appropriate for your age, sex, and activity level.

This diet should include:

- A variety of vegetables, including dark green, red, and orange vegetables; legumes (beans and peas); starchy vegetables; and other vegetables
- Grains (at least half should be whole grains)
- Fat-free or low-fat dairy, such as milk, yogurt, cheese, and fortified soy beverages
- A variety of proteins, including seafood, lean meats and poultry, eggs, legumes, nuts, seeds, and soy products

This diet should limit:

- Trans fats
- Saturated fats (less than 10% of calories per day)
- Added sugars (less than 10% of calories per day)
- Sodium (less than 2,300 mg per day)

Modified from: US Department of Agriculture. *Dietary guidelines for Americans, 2015–2020*. 8th ed. December 2015. Available at: https://health.gov/dietaryguidelines/2015/resources/2015-2020_Dietary_Guidelines.pdf.

(calories in) with physical activity (calories out). Key elements to losing or maintaining body weight include the following:

- Set realistic goals: make them short-term and measurable.
- Understand how much you eat by tracking your food intake.
- Manage portion sizes by reading food labels.
- Make smart dietary choices that fill you up and satisfy you.
- Aim for 150 minutes of moderate activity per week.[3]

The *2015–2020 Dietary Guidelines for Americans* stress that a person should engage in physical activity, show moderation in portion size, and choose the proper mix of food groups based on his or her sex, BMI, and level of physical activity. In 2011, the USDA introduced the MyPlate image as a dietary aid (**FIGURE 2-1**). This visual place setting is intended to simplify eating recommendations for the general public, using the following five food groups:

1. Grains, with half of all grains or more being eaten as whole grains
2. Vegetables (or 100% vegetable juice), emphasizing a mix of dark green vegetables, red and orange vegetables, starchy vegetables, dry beans and peas, and other vegetables
3. Fruits (fresh, canned, frozen, or dried) or 100% fruit juices
4. Dairy, including milk-based foods (fat-free or low-fat)
5. Protein, including meat, fish, eggs, and beans (proteins), processed soy products, and nuts and seeds, emphasizing low-fat and lean meats and at least 8 ounces of cooked seafood per week

MyPlate includes recommendations based on age, sex, and activity level. A person's specific daily nutrition recommendations can be obtained by visiting the ChooseMyPlate website (www.choosemyplate.gov/MyPlate-Daily-Checklist-input).

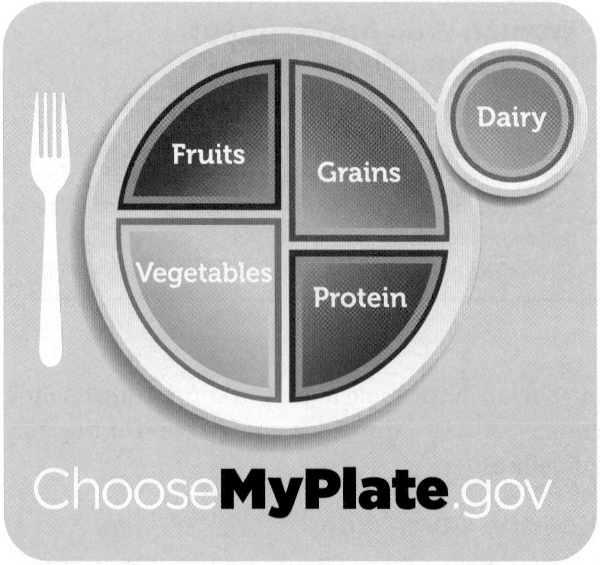

FIGURE 2-1 The MyPlate image is a visual place setting that is intended to simplify eating recommendations for the general public, using five food groups: grains, vegetables, fruits, dairy, and protein.

Courtesy of USDA

CRITICAL THINKING

Go to the ChooseMyPlate calculator (www.choosemyplate.gov/MyPlate-Daily-Checklist-input) and determine your recommended daily nutritional needs. How does the result compare with your current eating habits?

Principles of Weight Control. People who are overweight tend to be at higher risk for the development of certain illnesses—for example, high blood pressure, diabetes mellitus, heart disease, and some cancers. The tenets of weight control are to eat the right balance of foods in moderation, limit fat consumption, and exercise regularly (BOX 2-6).

Anyone committed to weight control for a healthier life should set realistic goals. For example, the general recommendation is a steady weight-loss goal of 0.5 to 1 pound per week. (Note that 3,500 calories is equal to 1 pound. An extra 500 calories per day results in a 1-pound gain per week; 500 fewer calories per day results in a 1-pound loss per week.) A healthful lifestyle effectively balances proper nutrition and exercise. A healthful diet includes a variety of foods that are low in fat, saturated fat, and cholesterol. It also includes plenty of whole-grain products, vegetables, and fruit (BOX 2-7) and modest amounts of simple sugars, salt, and sodium. Alcoholic beverages should be avoided or consumed only in moderation. Finally, a system for checking weight control progress is essential. Adjustments and professional advice sometimes may be needed to achieve weight control goals.

BOX 2-6 Getting a Handle on Fat

The *2015–2020 Dietary Guidelines for Americans* recommend that when possible, people should avoid trans fats, limit saturated fats to less than 10% of total calories per day, and replace saturated fat with healthier monosaturated and polyunsaturated fats. This eating pattern is important for the following reasons:

- Each gram of fat has more than double the calories of a gram of protein or carbohydrates.
- The body uses fewer calories to store the fat as excess weight.
- In complex carbohydrates, 23% of the calories are burned to make them into a usable form in the body; only 3% of fat calories are burned before they are "worn" on the hips or abdomen.
- Decreasing fat intake to less than 10% of daily calories is thought to help reduce cholesterol, decreases risk of heart disease, helps with weight loss, and reduces risk of diabetes.

Fat Content of Various Foods

- >90% fat: whipped cream, pork sausage, cooking oils, margarine, butter, gravy, mayonnaise
- >80% fat: spare ribs, bologna, cream cheese, salad dressing, high-fat steaks (T-bone, porterhouse, tenderloin, filet mignon)
- >70% fat: half-and-half dairy creamer, peanuts, hot dogs, pork chops, most cheeses and nuts, sirloin steak, bacon, lamb chops
- >60% fat: potato and corn chips, regular ground beef, ham, eggs
- >50% fat: round steak, pot roast, creamed soup, ice cream, sweet rolls
- >40% fat: whole milk, cake, doughnuts, french fries
- >30% fat: muffins, cookies, fruit pies, low-fat milk, cottage cheese, tuna, chicken, turkey
- >20% fat: lean fish, beef liver, ice milk
- >10% fat: bread, pretzels, whole grains, legumes
- <10% fat: sherbet, nonfat milk, most fruits and vegetables, baked potato

BOX 2-7 Fiber

The human body requires fiber to maintain good health and to fight disease. Fiber, which is found only in plant foods, may be either soluble or insoluble. Many authorities recommend a dietary intake of 20 to 35 g of fiber each day.

Soluble fiber helps control the blood glucose level. It also may lower the level of blood cholesterol. Examples of soluble fiber include fiber obtained from peas, beans, oats, barley, and some fruits and vegetables.

Insoluble fiber (found in whole grains and many vegetables) helps hold water in the colon and can reduce or prevent constipation. This type of fiber also may help prevent intestinal disease (eg, diverticulosis, hemorrhoids, and certain cancers).

DID YOU KNOW?

Food Labels 101

Understanding food labels and food content is important for a healthy diet. To make healthy eating choices, follow these steps when reading food labels (**FIGURE 2-2**):

1. **Start with the serving information at the top of the label.** This will tell you the size of a single serving and the total number of servings per container (package).
2. **Check the total calories per serving.** Pay attention to the calories per serving and how many servings you are really consuming if you eat the entire package. If you double the servings you eat, you double the calories and nutrients.
3. **Limit potentially harmful nutrients.** Limit the amounts of saturated fat and sodium you eat, and avoid trans fats. Choose foods with less of these nutrients when possible.

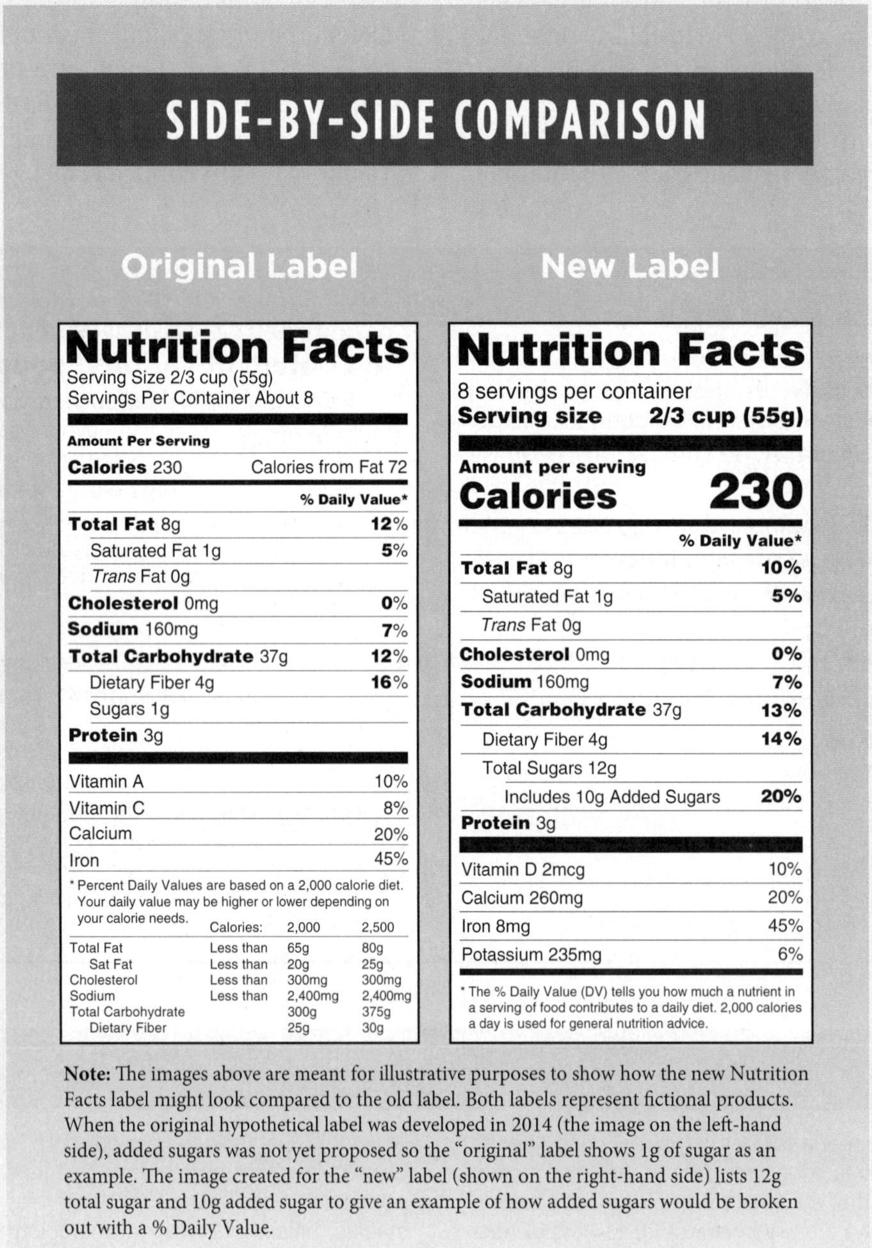
SIDE-BY-SIDE COMPARISON
Original Label
New Label
Nutrition Facts
Serving Size 2/3 cup (55g)
Servings Per Container About 8
Amount Per Serving
Calories 230 Calories from Fat 72
% Daily Value*
Total Fat 8g 12%
Saturated Fat 1g 5%
Trans Fat 0g
Cholesterol 0mg 0%
Sodium 160mg 7%
Total Carbohydrate 37g 12%
Dietary Fiber 4g 16%
Sugars 1g
Protein 3g
Vitamin A 10%
Vitamin C 8%
Calcium 20%
Iron 45%
* Percent Daily Values are based on a 2,000 calorie diet. Your daily value may be higher or lower depending on your calorie needs.
Calories: 2,000 2,500
Total Fat Less than 65g 80g
Sat Fat Less than 20g 25g
Cholesterol Less than 300mg 300mg
Sodium Less than 2,400mg 2,400mg
Total Carbohydrate 300g 375g
Dietary Fiber 25g 30g
Nutrition Facts
8 servings per container
Serving size 2/3 cup (55g)
Amount per serving
Calories 230
% Daily Value*
Total Fat 8g 10%
Saturated Fat 1g 5%
Trans Fat 0g
Cholesterol 0mg 0%
Sodium 160mg 7%
Total Carbohydrate 37g 13%
Dietary Fiber 4g 14%
Total Sugars 12g
Includes 10g Added Sugars 20%
Protein 3g
Vitamin D 2mcg 10%
Calcium 260mg 20%
Iron 8mg 45%
Potassium 235mg 6%
* The % Daily Value (DV) tells you how much a nutrient in a serving of food contributes to a daily diet. 2,000 calories a day is used for general nutrition advice.
Note: The images above are meant for illustrative purposes to show how the new Nutrition Facts label might look compared to the old label. Both labels represent fictional products. When the original hypothetical label was developed in 2014 (the image on the left-hand side), added sugars was not yet proposed so the "original" label shows 1g of sugar as an example. The image created for the "new" label (shown on the right-hand side) lists 12g total sugar and 10g added sugar to give an example of how added sugars would be broken out with a % Daily Value.

FIGURE 2-2 Components of a food label.

Courtesy of U.S. Food and Drug Administration

4. **Get enough beneficial nutrients.** Make sure you get enough of the beneficial nutrients such as dietary fiber, protein, calcium, iron, vitamins, and other nutrients you need every day.
5. **Consider the % Daily Value.** The % Daily Value (DV) tells you the percentage of each nutrient that is in a single serving, in terms of the daily recommended amount. As a guide, if you want to consume less of a nutrient (such as saturated fat or sodium), choose foods with a lower % DV—5% or less. If you want to consume more of a nutrient (such as fiber), seek foods with a higher % DV—20% or more.

Things to Remember

- The information shown in the Nutrition Facts panel is based on intake of 2,000 calories per day. You may need to consume less or more than 2,000 calories depending on your age, sex, activity level, and whether you are trying to lose, gain, or maintain your weight.
- When the Nutrition Facts label says a food contains "0 g" of trans fat, but includes "partially hydrogenated oil" in the ingredient list, it means the food contains trans fat, but less than 0.5 g per serving. So, if you eat more than one serving, you could quickly reach your daily trans fat limit.

Physical Fitness

Physical fitness can be described as a condition that helps people look, feel, and do their best (**FIGURE 2-3**). Physical fitness is highly individualized, so it varies from person to person. Physical fitness also is influenced by age, sex, heredity, personal habits, exercise, and eating habits.

There is solid evidence that regular physical activity reduces the risk of major illnesses and early death. According to the *2015–2020 Dietary Guidelines for Americans* and the Centers for Disease Control and Prevention (CDC), adults need at least 150 minutes of moderate-intensity physical activity, such as brisk walking, each week.[2,4] In addition, at least twice a week, they should perform exercises to strengthen all of the major upper and lower body muscle groups.[2,4]

Being physically fit offers many benefits, including the following:

- Decreased resting heart rate and blood pressure
- Increased oxygen-carrying capacity
- Enhanced quality of life
- Increased muscle mass and metabolism
- Increased resistance to injury
- Improved personal appearance and self-image
- Maintenance of motor skills throughout life

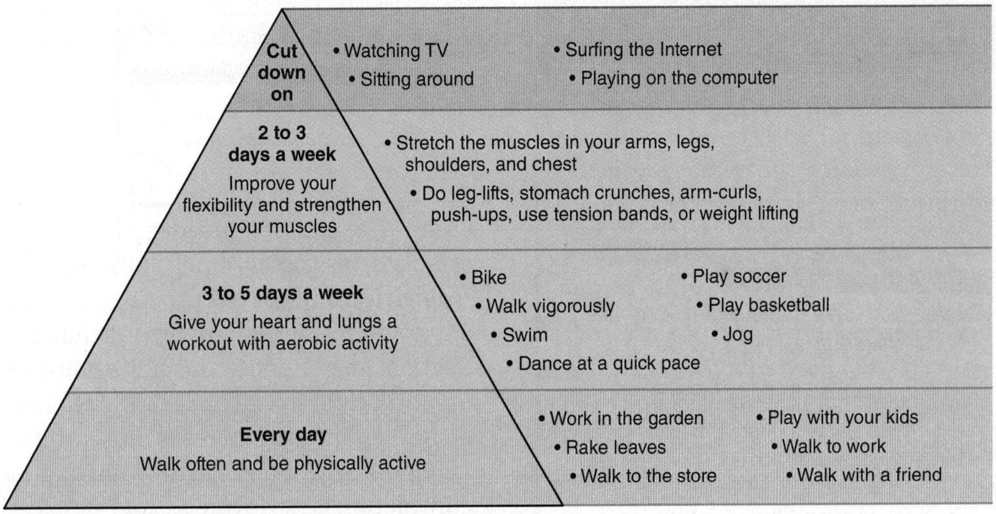

FIGURE 2-3 Exercise pyramid.

Cardiovascular Endurance. A physical examination is the first step before starting a fitness program. Another step is to have a fitness assessment performed by a certified physical trainer. The purpose of these assessments is to evaluate a person's current physical condition. These examinations establish the person's baseline weight, including BMI (**BOX 2-8**); measure blood pressure; and identify the presence of any potential health issues—for example, heart disease (including family history); arthritis or other bone problems; muscular, ligament, or tendon problems; and other known or suspected diseases. They also establish a heart rate target zone, which is a measure used to improve cardiovascular endurance through exercise. Ideally, the heart rate target zone should be maintained during exercise for 20 minutes to increase cardiovascular endurance.

NOTE

There is a simple way to determine the heart rate target zone. First, subtract the person's age in years from the established maximum heart rate of 220 beats/min. Then multiply this number by 70%.

Example for a 25-year-old:

$$220 - 25 = 195$$
$$195 \times 70 = 136 \text{ beats/min}$$

Muscle Strength. Another aspect of the fitness assessment tests muscular strength, power, mass, and endurance. Muscular strength is the ability of a muscle to exert force for a brief period. Muscular power is the ability to generate as much force as fast as possible. Muscular mass is the weight of muscles in a person's body, composed of skeletal muscles, smooth muscles, and the water contained in the muscles. Muscle endurance is the ability of a muscle or a group of muscles to sustain repeated contractions or to continue applying force against a fixed object. Many exercises improve muscle strength and endurance.

BOX 2-8 The Body Mass Index

Body mass index (BMI) is a widely used measurement of body fat that corrects for height. It is the only body fat index that conveys the risk of disease or death. A healthful BMI is defined as 19 to 25 kg/m^2; a BMI of 25 to 29 kg/m^2 indicates that the person is "moderately overweight," and a BMI of 30 kg/m^2 or more indicates that the person is "severely overweight."

To calculate your BMI, use the following formula:

1. Multiply your weight in pounds by 0.45.
   Example: 150 pounds × 0.45 = 67.5
2. Multiply your height in inches by 0.025.
   Example: 5 ft 9 in, or 69 inches × 0.025 = 1.725
3. Square the answer from step 2.
   Example: 1.725 × 1.725 = 2.976
4. Divide the answer in step 1 by the answer in step 3.
   Example: 67.5 ÷ 2.976 = BMI of 22.7

SHOW ME THE EVIDENCE

EMS personnel re-registering with the National Registry of Emergency Medical Technicians were surveyed to determine their existing medical conditions and key health indicators. The mean BMI for study participants was 27.69 kg/m^2, and 71.2% of participants were classified as having a high BMI (greater than or equal to 25). Three-fourths of respondents (75.3%) did not meet CDC recommendations for physical activity. EMS professionals with obesity were more likely to report existing health conditions. Conversely, those who met the CDC physical activity goals were less likely to report other medical conditions.

Modified from: Studnek JR, Bentley MA, Crawford M, Fernandez A. An assessment of key health indicators among emergency medical services professionals. *Prehosp Emerg Care*. 2010;14(1):14-20.

CRITICAL THINKING

Using Box 2-8, calculate your body mass index. Does it fall within the recommendations?

The tenets of training for muscle strength and endurance should consider isometric and isotonic exercises, resistance, repetitions, sets, and frequency. *Isometric* exercises refer to those in which the joint angle and muscle length do not change during contraction. An example is pushing against an immovable object such as a wall or door frame. These exercises do not significantly increase muscle bulk, but they do strengthen the muscle at the joint angle at which the contraction is performed. *Isotonic* exercises move a joint through a range of motion against resistance of a fixed weight. An example is lifting a barbell. These exercises add muscle bulk by creating tension within the muscle.

Resistance refers to the amount of weight moved or lifted during isotonic exercises. A repetition ("rep") refers to the full execution of an exercise from start to finish. A *set* is the number of times an exercise (rep) is done from start to finish, one after another, without any rest time. Frequency refers to the least number of workouts that will have a positive effect on muscle strength and endurance.

Muscular Flexibility. Flexibility refers to the ability to move joints and use muscles through their full range of motion. The fitness assessment tests flexibility in several ways. A lack of normal flexibility may lead to muscle strains and other injuries.

Muscular flexibility can be improved by stretching exercises. These exercises must be performed slowly, without a bouncing motion, and with mild intensity. A person should not strain or hold his or her breath and should feel no pain or discomfort. The type and frequency of stretching exercises performed should match the person's daily activities. For example, if daily work on an ambulance requires lifting patients, then regular stretching exercises specific to the paramedic's arms, back, thighs, calves, and hips would be helpful.

> CRITICAL THINKING
>
> How many minutes per week do you perform physical activities that raise your heart rate? What benefits does a paramedic gain by maintaining a high level of personal fitness?

The Importance of Sleep

Sleep plays an important role in being physically fit because it helps to rejuvenate a tired body. The average adult needs 7 to 8 hours of sleep each day. In emergency medical services (EMS), where rotating shifts and 24- and 48-hour work shifts are common, sleep deprivation may occur and interrupt the normal circadian rhythm.

Circadian is Latin for "about a day." The **circadian rhythm** is the physiological ebb and flow of the body as it relates to the rotation of the earth. This timing system is based roughly on the solar day, as the earth rotates in its course around the sun. For example, a person gets hungry or tired, or energetic or moody, at fairly set times each day as the body systems change. The levels of melatonin and cortisol affect the periods of sleepiness and wakefulness, respectively. The pineal gland secretes melatonin; the adrenal glands secrete cortisol. Release of these hormones is stimulated by the dark and is suppressed by light. Thus, when the line between night and day is disrupted on an ongoing basis (eg, by working rotating work shifts or responding to emergency calls in the early morning hours during a 24- or 48-hour shift), irritability, depression, loss of cognitive function/sharpness, and illness can result (BOX 2-9).

According to the Patient Safety Network of the Agency for Healthcare Research and Quality, fatigue is a "feeling of tiredness and decreased energy that results from inadequate sleep time or poor quality of sleep."[5] It is often associated with increased work duration or intensity. The effects of fatigue can impair cognitive function and the ability to make decisions. This impairment is of particular concern in situations

BOX 2-9 Getting Your Zs

Working nights, 24- and 48-hour shifts, and rotating shifts can prevent you from getting enough rest. Following are some helpful tips:

- Allow some time to unwind and relax before trying to go to sleep.
- Consider exercise before sleeping as a way to reduce stress.
- Avoid stimulants (eg, caffeine in coffee, soda, tea, and chocolate) during the last few hours of your work shift.
- Eat simple carbohydrates (eg, fresh fruit or yogurt) to release serotonin (a hormone that may help induce sleep).
- Keep your sleeping area cool and dark so that your body will think it is nighttime.
- Control your off-duty schedule to avoid reporting to work fatigued.
- Try to rest or nap if possible.
- Make sure your family and friends know about your work shifts and your sleeping schedule to minimize interruptions.
- Try to maintain your normal period of dedicated sleep time each day.
- Consult a physician about your sleep difficulties when needed.

where a health care worker needs to quickly assess, plan, and evaluate risks and execute interventions in a rapidly changing situation.

SHOW ME THE EVIDENCE

In 2012, Patterson et al. surveyed a convenience sample of EMS workers from around the United States to determine the association between poor sleep quality, fatigue, and self-reported safety outcomes in EMS. They received 547 responses from 30 EMS agencies. More than half of their respondents were classified as fatigued (55%, 95% confidence interval [CI], 50.7–59.3). The fatigued EMS respondents had 1.9 times greater odds of injury (95% CI, 1.1–3.3), 2.2 times greater odds of a medical error or adverse event (95% CI, 1.14–3.3), and 3.6 times greater odds of self-compromising behavior such as speeding (95% CI, 1.5–8.3) compared to their nonfatigued counterparts. The researchers concluded that fatigue was common in their sample of EMS workers and that fatigue may be associated with safety outcomes.

Modified from: Patterson PD, Weaver MD, Frank RC, et al. Association between poor sleep, fatigue, and safety outcomes in emergency medical services providers. *Prehosp Emerg Care.* 2012;16(1):86-97.

Shift-work studies have been done by numerous agencies, including the CDC and the National Institute for Occupational Safety and Health (NIOSH).[6] Findings in these studies suggest sleep loss has the following ramifications:

- Makes it easier to fall asleep at inappropriate times
- Affects performance both on and off the job
- Can lead to serious injuries
- Disrupts social and family life
- Increases health risks for digestive problems and heart disease

Other studies have shown that people who have disruptions in their circadian rhythms because of extended work shifts have increased risks of motor vehicle crashes, short-term decreases in cognition and neuropsychological performance, decreased job satisfaction, and an increased likelihood for making errors that result in patient care litigation.[5,7] Research and work shift studies are currently under way in EMS.[8] The goals of these studies are to help shift workers and their employers modify work schedules so that changes in normal biorhythms will have the fewest adverse effects on employee health and productivity.

CRITICAL THINKING

Do you get enough sleep? If not, which of the strategies listed in Box 2-9 should you try in an attempt to increase your hours of sleep?

Disease Prevention

There are many things a paramedic can do to help prevent serious personal illness. As health care professionals, paramedics must serve as role models in helping to prevent disease.

Cardiovascular Disease. Cardiovascular disease accounts for nearly 801,000 deaths each year in the United States.[9] For most people, cardiovascular disease can be altered through living a healthful life. Boosting cardiovascular endurance can help to prevent this disease. However, other steps can be taken:[9]

- Eliminating cigarette smoking and avoiding secondhand smoke
- Controlling high blood pressure
- Maintaining a normal BMI
- Getting at least 2.5 hours of moderate-intensity physical activity per week
- Assessing for and controlling diabetes
- Avoiding excessive alcohol intake
- Eating healthful foods
- Reducing stress
- Being aware of family health history
- Seeking evaluation of snoring
- Having regular health examinations
- Recognizing warning signs of heart attack and stroke

Cancer. The term *cancer* includes more than 100 diseases affecting nearly every part of the body. All of these diseases are potentially life threatening. The main cause of all cancer is a change or mutation to the DNA within a cell. Most common cancers are linked to one of three environmental risk factors: smoking, sunlight, or diet. Dietary factors are associated with some cancers of the gastrointestinal tract and may be linked to others, such as cancer of the breast, prostate, or uterus. Steps in preventing cancer include the following:

- Elimination of smoking
- A healthy diet and physical activity
- Limitation of sun exposure; use of sunscreen

- Regular physical examinations
- Attention to the warning signs (BOX 2-10)
- Periodic risk assessment

Infectious Disease Transmission

Guidelines. In 1987, the CDC developed recommendations for prevention of HIV transmission in health-care settings.[10] These recommendations, known as **universal precautions**, encouraged the use of blood and body fluid precautions for all patients, regardless of their infection status. Under these guidelines, it was assumed that body fluids of all patients were considered potentially infectious for HIV, HBV, and other bloodborne pathogens. The CDC also recommended that body substance isolation procedures (primarily the use of gloves) be taken for possible contact with all moist body substances. In 1991, the Occupational Safety and Health Administration (OSHA) mandated that universal precautions be the minimum standard of practice against occupational exposure to protect health care workers.[11]

> **BOX 2-10** The Seven Warning Signs of Cancer (CAUTION) as Designated by the American Cancer Society
>
> **C**hange in bowel or bladder habits
> **A** sore throat that does not heal
> **U**nusual bleeding or discharge
> **T**hickening or lump in the breast, testicle, or elsewhere
> **I**ndigestion or difficulty swallowing
> **O**bvious change in a wart, mole, or mouth sore
> **N**agging cough or hoarseness

> NOTE
>
> Universal precautions need to be followed with bloodborne diseases spread by pathogens such as hepatitis B and C viruses and HIV.

In 1996, the term **standard precautions** appeared in the revised CDC isolation guidelines.[12] These guidelines stated that standard precautions apply to all patients receiving health care, regardless of their diagnosis or presumed infection status. Standard precautions synthesize the major features of universal precautions and body substance isolation, which are the primary strategy to prevent the transmission of infectious agents to health care personnel, patients, and the general public at risk for exposure. Therefore, they apply to any healthcare delivery setting where patient care activities take place. The extent of precautions used is determined by the anticipated likelihood of exposure to blood, body fluids, or pathogens. Standard precautions include handwashing, gowning, wearing of mask, gloving, and the use of protective barriers (**TABLE 2-2**).

TABLE 2-2 Recommendations for Application of Standard Precautions for the Care of All Patients in All Healthcare Settings

Component	Recommendations
Hand hygiene	After touching blood, body fluids, secretions, excretions, contaminated items; immediately after removing gloves; between patient contacts
PPE Gloves	For touching blood, body fluids, secretions, excretions, contaminated items; for touching mucous membranes and nonintact skin
PPE Gown	During procedures and patient care activities when contact of clothing/exposed skin with blood/body fluids, secretions, and excretions is anticipated.
PPE Mask, eye protection (goggles), face shield	During procedures and patient care activities likely to generate splashes or sprays of blood, body fluids, secretions, especially suctioning, endotracheal intubation. During aerosol-generating procedures on patients with suspected or proven infections transmitted by respiratory aerosols, wear a fit-tested N95 or higher respirator in addition to gloves, gown and face/eye protection.
Soiled patient care equipment	Handle in a manner that prevents transfer of microorganisms to others and to the environment; wear gloves if visibly contaminated; perform hand hygiene.

(continued)

TABLE 2-2 Recommendations for Application of Standard Precautions for the Care of All Patients in All Healthcare Settings *(continued)*

Component	Recommendations
Environmental control	Develop procedures for routine care, cleaning, and disinfection of environmental surfaces, especially frequently touched surfaces in patient-care areas.
Textiles and laundry	Handle in a manner that prevents transfer of microorganisms to others and to the environment
Needles and other sharps	Do not recap, bend, break, or hand-manipulate used needles; if recapping is required, use a one-handed scoop technique only; use safety features when available; place used sharps in a puncture-resistant container
Patient resuscitation	Use a mouthpiece, resuscitation bag, or other ventilation devices to prevent contact with mouth and oral secretions
Patient placement	Prioritize for single-patient room if patient is at increased risk of transmission, is likely to contaminate the environment, does not maintain appropriate hygiene, or is at increased risk of acquiring infection or developing adverse outcome following infection.
Respiratory hygiene/cough etiquette (source containment of infectious respiratory secretions in symptomatic patients, beginning at initial point of encounter, eg, triage and reception areas in emergency departments and physician offices)	Instruct symptomatic persons to cover mouth/nose when sneezing/coughing; use tissues and dispose in no-touch receptacle; observe hand hygiene after soiling of hands with respiratory secretions; wear a surgical mask if tolerated or maintain spatial separation, >3 feet if possible.

Abbreviation: PPE, personal protective equipment

Modified from: Centers for Disease Control and Prevention. Guideline for Isolation Precautions: Preventing Transmission of Infectious Agents in Healthcare Settings (2007). https://www.cdc.gov/infectioncontrol/guidelines/isolation/appendix/standard-precautions.html. Accessed January 28, 2018.

In addition to standard precautions, transmission-based precautions have been developed for diseases that have multiple routes of transmission: airborne, droplet, and contact precautions.

- **Airborne precautions.** Infectious diseases that spread by tiny airborne droplet nuclei that can suspend in the air for long periods and travel far distances require the provider to follow airborne precautions. Airborne precautions require providers to wear an N-95 mask and patients to wear a surgical mask. Tuberculosis, measles, and chicken pox are examples of infectious diseases that spread by airborne means.
- **Droplet precautions.** Droplet precautions involve wearing mucous membrane protection, which includes a surgical mask and some form of eye protection. This level of protection is required when in the possible presence of an infectious disease that spreads by tiny droplets that travel short distances. Infectious diseases that require droplet precautions include influenza, respiratory syncytial virus, croup, meningococcal meningitis, whooping cough, and Ebola.
- **Contact precautions.** Contact precautions need to be used when caring for patients with certain known or suspected infectious disease. This level of precaution involves wearing a gown and gloves while caring for the patient. Examples of infectious diseases that require the use of contact precautions include methicillin-resistant *Staphylococcus aureus, Clostridium difficile* colitis, and vancomycin-resistant enterococcus.

Infectious Disease Prevention. Prevention of disease transmission—that is, infectious disease—must be a priority in daily EMS practice. Common sources of exposure to infectious agents in the prehospital setting include needlesticks and broken or scraped skin. Mucous membranes such as those that line the eyes, nose, and mouth also are a source for entry of infectious

TABLE 2-3 Personal Protective Equipment for Protection Against Transmission of HIV, Hepatitis B, and Hepatitis C

Activity	Disposable Gloves	Gown	Mask	Protective Eyewear
Bleeding control (spurting blood)	Yes	Yes	Yes	Yes
Bleeding control (minimal blood)	Yes	No	No	No
Emergency childbirth	Yes	Yes	Yes[a]	Yes[a]
Intravenous therapy	Yes	No	No	No
Endotracheal intubation	Yes	No	Yes	Yes
Oral or nasal suctioning	Yes	No	No	No
Administration of an injection	No	No	No	No

[a]If splashing is likely.

agents or microorganisms. Most infectious diseases can be avoided by practicing good personal hygiene and use of personal protective equipment (**TABLE 2-3**).

NOTE

A good rule of thumb for paramedics to follow in preventing exposure to infectious disease is this: *If it's wet and it isn't yours—don't touch it!*

To further defend against transmission of infectious diseases, OSHA requires that a periodic risk assessment be offered to staff, including regular testing for diseases such as tuberculosis and monitoring of vaccinations for infectious diseases (eg, hepatitis B). Other general guidelines to help prevent exposure to infectious diseases are summarized here:

1. Follow engineering and work practices. Maintain good personal health and hygiene habits. (Wash

DID YOU KNOW?

The Right Way to Wash Your Hands

The most important tool in your arsenal for preventing infection and protecting yourself from illness is washing your hands. Handwashing should be done whenever your hands are soiled. It should also be done between each patient contact, before eating, after using the restroom, and after coughing, sneezing, or blowing your nose. The CDC recommends vigorous scrubbing with warm soapy water for at least 15 seconds (or the time it takes to sing a short tune, such as "Happy Birthday").

There are five easy steps to proper handwashing:

1. **Wet** your hands under warm running water; apply soap.
2. **Rub** your hands with soap under warm running water.
3. **Scrub** your hands for a count of at least 15 seconds. Scrub all surfaces, including the back of your hands, and wrists. Clean between your fingers and under your fingernails.
4. **Rinse** your hands under clean warm water.
5. **Dry** your hands on a paper towel or with an air dryer, and use a towel to turn off the faucet.

When soap and water are not available, consider using alcohol-based disposable hand wipes or gel sanitizers. Gel sanitizers that contain at least 60% alcohol are more effective in killing bacteria and viruses than handwashing, and most contain ingredients that help prevent skin dryness. Alcohol sanitizers are not effective against *Clostridium difficile* spores, however.

Modified from: Mayo Clinic. Hand-washing: Do's and don'ts Available at: www.mayoclinic.org/healthy-lifestyle/adult-health/in-depth/hand-washing/art-20046253; and Cohen SH, Gerding DN, Johnson S, et al. Clinical practice guidelines for *Clostridium difficile* infection in adults: 2010 update by the Society for Healthcare Epidemiology of America (SHEA), and the Infectious Diseases Society of America (IDSA). *Infect Control Hosp Epidemiol.* 2010;31(5): 431-455. Available at: http://www.jstor.org/stable/10.1086/651706.

hands frequently and pay attention to general cleanliness.)
2. Maintain immunizations for tetanus, diphtheria, pertussis, polio, hepatitis B, MMR (measles, mumps, and rubella), and influenza.
3. Conduct a periodic screening for tuberculosis.
4. Practice standard precautions in all encounters with patients.
5. Properly clean, disinfect, and dispose of used materials and equipment immediately.
6. Use puncture-resistant containers to dispose of needles and other sharp objects.
7. Separate and label all soiled laundry (clothes, bed linens). Also separate and label all equipment. Do this until the items can be cleaned and disinfected properly.

In the event of a potential exposure to an infectious disease or a significant exposure to a patient's blood or body fluids, the paramedic should do the following:

1. Wash the area of contact with soap and water thoroughly and immediately.
2. Immediately document the situation in which the exposure occurred.
3. Describe actions taken to reduce chances of infection.
4. Comply with all required reporting responsibilities (eg, report the incident to the receiving hospital and to the proper designated officer in the local agency) and time frames.
5. Cooperate with incident investigation.
6. Be screened for antibody titers and potential infectious diseases.
7. Obtain proper immunization boosters.
8. Obtain a full medical follow-up.

Injury Prevention

The nature of EMS work exposes the paramedic to many risks. It has been estimated that the occupational fatality rate for EMS workers is similar to that of police and fire personnel and may be as much as three times the national average.[13]

For paramedics, injury may occur when lifting and moving patients, when a patient or bystander becomes violent, when participating in a hazardous rescue, or while driving to or from a call. The paramedic must be aware of these risks and be proactive to avoid a life- or career-ending injury.

Body Mechanics During Lifting and Moving. One in four EMS workers suffers a career-ending back injury within the first 4 years of employment, and back injury is the number one reason for leaving the EMS profession.[14,15] Almost one in two workers (47%) has sustained a back injury while performing EMS duties.[14] NIOSH estimates 6,000 body motion injuries occur each year to EMS workers, most of which are attributed to lifting, carrying, or transferring a patient and/or equipment.[16,17]

Using proper body mechanics during lifting and moving is crucial to avoid personal injury as well as injury to a partner or patient (BOX 2-11). Follow these guidelines when lifting and moving patients or equipment:

- Move a victim by yourself only if you can do so safely; get additional help if needed.
- Look where you are walking or crawling.
- Move forward rather than backward when possible.
- Take short steps, if walking.
- Bend at the hips and knees, while keeping the feet apart.
- Maintain the natural curvature of the spine when possible.
- Lift with the legs, not the back.
- Keep the load close to the body.
- Keep the patient's body in line when moving the patient.
- Use assistive devices to lift when possible.

NOTE

When preparing to lift, contract the abdominal muscles by pulling in the abdominal wall (sucking the belly button to the spine). The abdominal muscles are considered the core of the body. In addition, they help stabilize the back and help produce power and strength. Lift by extending through the hips and legs, not the back. ("Think with the hips" when lifting.) The body works from the center, outward. The hips are part of the "core" and more centralized than the legs, so extending through the hips first adds another muscle group to the lifting effort and also instantly provides greater strength and power for lifting. Incorporating the hips can also help prevent knee injuries.

Hostile Environments. Paramedics increasingly find themselves in hostile situations and are more likely than firefighters to experience patient-initiated violence and injuries.[18] There has been a steady increase

BOX 2-11 Prevention and Rehabilitation of Low Back Pain

The back is a complex system of ligaments, muscles, bones, nerves, and intervertebral disks—and all of these parts can be injured by improper lifting techniques. EMS workers are highly vulnerable to low back pain and injury. A common cause of these conditions is lordosis, an inward curvature in the lumbar spine that is normally present to some degree. Abnormal curvature in this area can result from poor posture and from being overweight with associated weak abdominal muscles.

Back injury can be prevented or lessened to a significant degree by being physically fit, performing regular stretching exercises, and following some general rules of lifting:

1. Know the weight (ask the patient's weight if you can, and add the weight of the equipment). Two people should work together to lift objects that weigh more than 60 pounds (27 kg).
2. Know your physical ability and limitations.
3. Keep your back positioned with a normal curvature.
4. Use your legs and abdominal muscles to support the weight; use your back muscles to maintain balance.
5. Keep the weight close to your body.
6. Communicate clearly and frequently with your partner.
7. When needed, call for additional help and use lift-assist devices.

If back pain or injury occurs when you are lifting, pushing, pulling, or stretching, tell a supervisor as soon as possible. Treatment for back pain usually begins with rest and ice or cold packs to lessen swelling. It also can include pain medicine and muscle relaxants. A rehabilitation program usually will follow the injury. Rehabilitation often includes exercises to improve abdominal muscle strength and to improve the control of the pelvis and the flexibility of the lower back.

Modified from: Ferno. Ferno: injury free. Available at: http://www.fernoems.com/injuryfree.

in the number of injuries related to violence on EMS calls. In 2017, NIOSH reported 2,000 such incidents, and these numbers will likely continue to rise.[16] A California study found that violence occurred on 8.5% of calls, with just over half of this violence directed toward EMS providers and the rest toward others.[19] Violence on an EMS call can include verbal threats and intimidation or physical assault, and is more likely to occur in responses with police or gang presence; when the patient has a psychiatric disorder; and in situations involving alcohol or illegal drugs.

An EMS scene is dynamic and should never be considered entirely safe. It is imperative that the paramedic maintain situational awareness throughout every response. It is also critical to recognize when a patient has become an attacker who intends to harm the EMS crew.[20] On all calls, paramedics should do the following:

- Carefully check the scene for safety concerns, and do not enter the scene if it is thought to be unsafe.
- Maintain situational awareness through all phases of the call.
- Coordinate all actions with law enforcement personnel.
- Maintain a safe distance when initially approaching patients and family members.
- Plan entrance and escape routes.
- Consider areas for concealment (a place to hide) or cover (something to shield from objects or gunfire).
- Above all, stay alert and be prepared for the unexpected.

Safely managing a violent scene requires special training. Several specialty courses are available that teach verbal and physical techniques to use in violent situations. The paramedic is encouraged to take one of these classes to learn strategies to defuse violent situations and, when verbal de-escalation does not work, physical maneuvers to escape a violent situation.

A situation involving violence also calls for unity among many emergency response agencies. As members of the response team, paramedics should take part in planning, training, and practice sessions. These sessions help to provide strategies for personal safety in hostile settings (see Chapter 55, *Crime Scene Awareness*).

Rescue Situations. Many personal safety issues arise in the case of rescue. Examples include exposure to hazardous materials, bad weather, extremes in temperature, fire, toxic gases, unstable structures, heavy equipment, road hazards, and sharp edges and fragments. In every rescue response, the priority is

SHOW ME THE EVIDENCE

The 2013 Longitudinal EMS Attributes and Demographics Study (LEADS) asked EMS personnel 14 questions related to violent encounters. The study found that more than two-thirds of the respondents (69%) experienced at least one form of violence in the preceding year, with verbal violence reported more frequently than physical violence. The odds of violent encounters were increased among EMS personnel working in urban settings and as the number of transports increased. Paramedics were almost three times more likely to experience violence than were emergency medical technicians. According to the researchers, this study highlights the need for education related to violence.

Modified from: Gormley MA, Crowe RP, Bentley MA, Levine R. A national description of violence toward emergency medical services personnel. *Prehosp Emerg Care*. 2016;20(4):439-447.

to assess the scene for hazards before entering that scene. All responders also must take personal protective measures. The paramedic should not enter a hazardous situation without proper personal protective equipment and training. In addition, the scene should be monitored constantly during the operation. A safe rescue requires proper use of protective gear, special training, and safe rescue practices (see Chapter 54, *Rescue Awareness and Operations*).

Safe Vehicle Operation. Safe operation of an emergency vehicle is important for personal safety and for the safety of the crew and patient and the public (see Chapter 52, *Ground and Air Ambulance Operations*). A 10-year review of 399 ambulance crashes found that most fatalities involved pedestrians, cyclists, or other vehicle operators not in the ambulance; most of these crashes occurred during emergency use and at intersections.[21] Many factors affect safe vehicle operations, including the following:

- Safe driving of the vehicle
- Selective use of lights-and-siren response
- Use of personal restraints for all occupants in the vehicle
- Safe and appropriate use of escorts to and from emergency scenes
- Attention to adverse environmental conditions (eg, inclement weather)
- Care when proceeding through intersections
- Safe ambulance design
- Safe parking at the emergency scene, including vehicle positioning strategies
- Due regard for the safety of all others

NOTE

Safe operations and personal safety on the roadways are of utmost importance. Emergency personnel should wear American National Standards Institute (ANSI) high-visibility safety vests over turnout gear. They should also minimize the time they spend on roadways.

CRITICAL THINKING

Is there any patient situation that would call for unsafe operation of a vehicle? Keep in mind that unsafe vehicle operation could risk the safety of those in the ambulance or in other vehicles.

Some EMS agencies require their employees to take a specialized driver's training class. One such program is the US Department of Transportation's Emergency Vehicle Operation Course. A program such as this allows EMS personnel to practice driving in a safe and controlled setting.

Safety Equipment and Supplies. Proper use of safety equipment and supplies is key to injury prevention for paramedics. Standards for protective clothing and equipment are established by OSHA. These and other standards (such as those set by the National Fire Protection Association) are used by many states, cities, and fire and EMS agencies to help ensure employee safety (see Chapter 53, *Medical Incident Command*). Safety equipment and supplies include the following:

- Body substance isolation equipment
- Head protection
- Eye protection
- Hearing protection
- Respiratory protection
- Gloves
- Boots
- Coveralls
- Turnout coat and pants
- Specialty equipment
- Reflective clothing

Mental and Emotional Health

EMS personnel encounter situations known to provoke strong emotions during work. In one study of EMS personnel, every person was exposed to a traumatic event such as the death of a child, abuse of a child or older adult, murder, suicide, or disaster.[22] These encounters take their toll on the emotional and mental health of the responder. One survey of more than 30,000 EMS personnel found that 6.8% were depressed, 6% were anxious, and 5.9% were stressed.[23] In this research, paramedics were found to have increased prevalence of depression and stress as compared to the general population. In addition, chronic and critical incident stressors have been shown to increase an EMS provider's risk of development of a posttraumatic stress reaction.[24]

Many factors play a role in mental and emotional health. For EMS personnel, it is important to be aware of "warning signs" that could indicate a potential problem (eg, signs of substance misuse and health disorders caused by anxiety and stress). Also key to maintaining good emotional health is realizing the value of having personal time; being connected with family, peers, and the community; and accepting the personal differences that make individuals unique.

Substance Misuse and Abuse Control

Health care workers and emergency responders are not immune to stressors that can lead to substance misuse and abuse. Studies have found that a substance abuse problem develops in approximately 10% of physicians and registered nurses in the United States[25,26] and approximately 25% of firefighters and law enforcement officers report problematic alcohol use.[27]

The misuse and abuse of drugs and other substances may lead to chemical dependency (**addiction**) (BOX 2-12). Such dependency may have a wide range of effects on physical and mental health, including damage to vital organs, cancer, increased risk for injuries, and mental impairment (see Chapter 33, *Toxicology*). Higher levels of alcohol abuse have been associated with the development of a posttraumatic stress reaction.[24] Warning signs of addiction and addictive behavior include the following:

- Using a substance to relieve tension
- Using an increasing amount of the substance
- Lying about using the substance
- Experiencing guilt about using the substance
- Avoiding discussion about using the substance
- Experiencing interference with daily activities as a result of substance abuse

CRITICAL THINKING

Do you know anyone who exhibits any of these warning signs?

Methods used to manage substance abuse depend on the type of substance being misused. Substance misuse or abuse control may call for professional counseling. Physician-controlled drug therapy and support programs also may be necessary.

Smoking Cessation

Cigarette smoking is a major health hazard. It is responsible for more than 480,000 deaths each year in the United States, including both deaths directly from smoking and from secondhand smoke.[28] Cigarette smoking has numerous negative health ramifications, including an increased risk of the following conditions, among others:

- Heart disease
- Stroke
- Chronic obstructive pulmonary disease
- Cancer
- Diabetes
- Erectile dysfunction
- Rheumatoid arthritis

BOX 2-12 Drugs and Substances That Are Often Misused or Abused

- Alcohol
- Central nervous system stimulants (eg, cocaine, amphetamines, methylphenidate)
- Cigarettes and other tobacco products
- Hallucinogens
- Inhalants
- Marijuana and its derivatives
- Opiates and opioids
- Depressants (barbiturates, benzodiazepines, sleep medications)
- Nonprescription substances
- Cough and cold preparations (dextromethorphan)
- Synthetic cannabinoids and cathinones (bath salts)

Some tobacco users prefer smokeless products. These products are also linked to serious health problems, including cancers and other diseases of the mouth, esophagus, and pancreas; early delivery and stillbirth (when used in pregnancy); and increased risk of death from heart disease and stroke.

Smokers often cite many reasons for continuing to smoke—for example, peer pressure, relief of stress, and weight control. Regardless of their reasons, most persons continue to smoke because of the addictive nature of nicotine, the stimulant found in tobacco. In addition, cigarettes contain other harmful chemicals such as hydrocarbons (tar) and carbon monoxide. Exposure to these chemicals is considered a health hazard for nonsmokers as well as smokers. Nonsmokers have an increased risk of the development of smoking-related illnesses through "passive smoking," or secondhand and thirdhand smoke.

Transitioning from cigarettes to e-cigarettes (vaping) is also unsafe. Because e-cigarettes are unregulated, it is difficult to know precisely what the solutions used in these devices contain. The nicotine present is known to be harmful to young users and persons who are pregnant.

Many resources and smoking cessation programs are available to people who want to quit smoking. Support groups and quit-smoking campaigns are sponsored by the American Heart Association, the American Cancer Society, government health agencies, and local health care organizations. Other smoking-cessation aids a person may use alone or with these programs include prescription and nonprescription drugs, such as varenicline (Chantix) and bupropion (Wellbutrin or Zyban). There are also many nicotine products that may be delivered by dermal patch, lozenge, nasal spray, or chewing gum. These products decrease the physical effects of smoking cessation. In a sense, they help to wean the smoker off nicotine (**BOX 2-13**).

> NOTE
>
> The frequency of exposures to e-cigarettes and nicotine liquid among young children is increasing rapidly and severe outcomes, including one death, have been reported. From January 2012 through April 2015, the National Poison Data System (NPDS) received 29,141 calls for nicotine and tobacco product exposures among children younger than 6 years, averaging 729 children per month. More than three-fourths of exposed children were younger than age 2 years.
>
> *Modified from*: Kamboj A, Spiller HA, Casavant MJ, et al. Pediatric exposure to e-cigarettes, nicotine, and tobacco products in the United States. *Pediatrics*. June 2016;137:6 e20160041.

Anxiety and Stress

Anxiety can be defined as worry or dread related to future uncertainties. **Stress** can result from the interaction of events that cause anxiety and affect the coping abilities of the person. Although stress can be positive

BOX 2-13 Body Changes When You Stop Smoking

Within 20 Minutes of Your Last Cigarette
Pulse and blood pressure drop.

Within 12 Hours of Your Last Cigarette
Carbon monoxide level in blood drops to normal.

Within 2 Weeks to 3 Months After Your Last Cigarette
Circulation improves.
Lung function increases.

Within 1 to 9 Months After Your Last Cigarette
Coughing and shortness of breath decrease.
Cilia regrow in lungs, increasing the ability to handle mucus, clean the lungs, and reduce infection.

Within 1 Year of Your Last Cigarette
The risk of heart disease is half that of someone who stills smokes.

Within 5 Years of Your Last Cigarette
The risk of cancers of the mouth, throat, esophagus, and bladder is cut in half.
Cervical cancer risk declines to that of a nonsmoker.
The stroke risk may fall to that of a nonsmoker after 2 to 5 years.

Within 10 Years of Your Last Cigarette
The lung cancer death rate is about half that of a smoker.
The risk of laryngeal and pancreatic cancer decreases.

Modified from: American Cancer Society. Benefits of quitting smoking over time. September 9, 2016. Available at: https://www.cancer.org/healthy/stay-away-from-tobacco/benefits-of-quitting-smoking-over-time.html.

(described later in this chapter), it is usually thought of as having a negative effect (eg, fear, depression, and guilt). Effective means of recognizing and coping with anxiety and stress are important for a lasting career in the EMS profession. Signs that you may need stress management assistance include the following:[29]

- Disorientation or confusion and difficulty communicating thoughts
- Difficulty remembering instructions
- Difficulty maintaining balance
- Decrease in patience, becoming easily frustrated and being uncharacteristically argumentative
- Inability to engage in problem solving and difficulty making decisions
- Unnecessary risk taking
- Tremors, headaches, or nausea
- Tunnel vision or muffled hearing
- Colds or flulike symptoms
- Limited attention span and difficulty concentrating
- Loss of objectivity
- Inability to relax when off duty
- Refusal to follow orders or to leave the scene
- Increased use of drugs/alcohol
- Unusual clumsiness

Personal Time for Meditation and Contemplation

Setting aside some personal time can boost mental and perhaps even physical health. This time can be spent meditating or contemplating. *Meditation* is a form of relaxation. To meditate, a person limits his or her awareness to a repeated or constant focus. The person may focus on something that holds some attraction (eg, controlled breathing, a pleasant site, a fragrance, or a mantra). This quiet time provides an uninterrupted period for thoughtful introspection (contemplation) of important things in a person's life. Most who practice meditation do so once or twice a day for 10 to 20 minutes.

> NOTE
>
> Spirituality is a unique quality of human existence. Spirituality should not be overlooked as a means for some to achieve mental and physical well-being.

Stress

As previously stated, stress can be either positive or negative. The responses to stress may be physical, emotional, or both. "Good" stress (**eustress**) is a positive response to stimuli; it is considered protective. "Bad" stress (**distress**) is a negative response to environmental stimuli; it is the source of anxiety and stress-related disorders.

Phases of the Stress Response

Hans Selye, an Austrian-born professor at the University of Montreal, coined the term *stress* in medical usage in 1950. Selye identified three stages in the stress response: alarm reaction, resistance, and exhaustion (**FIGURE 2-4**).[30] Selye called these phases the *general adaptation syndrome*, referring to the attempt of body and mind to deal with stressful events.

Alarm Reaction

The human body can prepare itself quickly to do battle or run from danger. This "fight-or-flight" reaction occurs when a situation threatens one's safety or comfort. This reaction is considered positive (eustress) in that it prepares people to be alert and to defend themselves. At first, the response of the body to stress is unaffected by the type of situation. The body reacts the same way to events that are pleasant or unpleasant, dangerous or exciting, happy or sad. The purpose of the response is to achieve top physical preparedness rapidly to cope with the event. Examples of situations that elicit the alarm reaction may include having an argument with a coworker, performing an unfamiliar patient care procedure, and taking part in the delivery of a healthy infant.

The alarm reaction is triggered by the **autonomic nervous system** (see Chapter 10, *Review of Human Systems*) and coordinated by the hypothalamus. The hypothalamus triggers the pituitary gland to release adrenocorticotropic hormone into the bloodstream, which in turn stimulates the production of glucose. Adrenocorticotropic hormone also increases the concentration of nutrients in the blood that provide energy and activates the adrenal glands to provide an intense sympathetic release of **adrenaline** and noradrenaline. These hormones cause the heart rate to increase, blood pressure to rise, and pupils of the eyes to dilate, which improves vision. Together these hormones relax the bronchial tree to permit deeper breathing, increase blood sugar (glucose) to increase the body's total energy, slow the digestive process, and shift blood supply to accommodate the clotting mechanism in case the body is wounded.

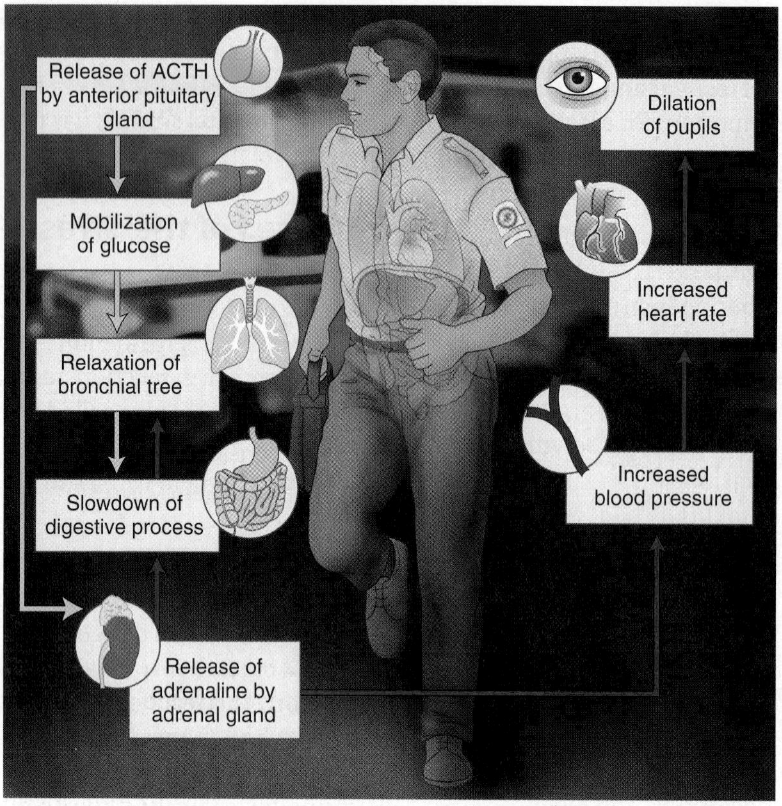

FIGURE 2-4 Physiological response to stress. During the alarm reaction, the release of adrenocorticotropic hormone (*yellow*) results in a sympathetic discharge of adrenaline (*red*). These stress hormones stimulate glucose production and cause the heart rate to increase, the blood pressure to rise, and the pupils to dilate. The bronchial tree relaxes for deep breathing, the digestive process slows, and the blood supply shifts to accommodate clotting mechanisms in case the body is wounded.

After these physiological events, the body is ready for an emergency (fight or flight) and can sometimes perform feats of strength and endurance far beyond its normal capacity.

The alarm reaction takes only seconds to become activated upon the first exposure of the body to a stressor. When the body realizes that an event is not dangerous or does not require the alarm reaction, the response stops. The person begins to adapt to the situation, and body functions subsequently return to normal.

Resistance

The stress response raises the affected person's level of resistance to the agent that provoked it and others like it. If a particular stress persists long enough, however, a person's reactions change. For example, a paramedic becomes accustomed to responding to emergency scenes in an ambulance using audible and visual warning devices, and eventually the alarm reaction that once occurred when lights and sirens were activated is no longer elicited.

Exhaustion

If negative stress continues over time, first coping mechanisms weaken and then resistance fails. For example, paramedics may appear to be unaffected by the stress of life-threatening emergencies, but all of their adaptive resources may have been used up to reach this stage of resistance. When their reservoir of adaptive resources no longer exists, resistance to other types of stress tends to decline as well. At that point, the body may be vulnerable to physical and psychological illness. Rest and recovery usually are needed before a person is ready for another emergency.

Factors That Trigger the Stress Response

Individual reactions to stress differ based on previous exposure to a specific type of stress, perception of the stressful event, and personal coping skills. Many factors can trigger the stress response:

- Loss of something that is of value
- Injury or threat of injury
- Poor health or nutrition
- Frustration
- Ineffective coping skills

A variety of factors specific to the EMS experience can produce stress. Environmental stressors include noise, bad weather, confined spaces, poor lighting, spectators, rapid response to the scene, threats to personal safety, and life-and-death decision making. Psychosocial stress may arise from family relationships and conflicts with coworkers, abusive patients, and similar sources. Personality stress relates to the way a person thinks and feels. For example, this kind of stress can include the need to be liked, a person's expectations, and feelings of guilt and anxiety. Given these many possible sources of stress, choosing a career in EMS requires developing an understanding of job-related stress and effective stress management.

Physiological and Psychological Effects of Stress

Anxiety is a common symptom of stress, and feeling anxious in certain situations or unusual circumstances is normal and healthy. This response provides a warning system that protects a person from being overwhelmed by a sudden stimulation. Anxiety also prepares a person to take action in critical situations; for example, it prepares the paramedic to make quick, correct decisions regarding the emergency. In addition, anxiety allows the paramedic to perform at maximal efficiency.

Sometimes stress is not reduced when the conflict or emergency is resolved, which may lead to an ongoing state of vigilance and alertness beyond the initial event. The paramedic then may begin to feel chronic anxiety. Chronic anxiety fails to stimulate effective coping. In such a case, anxiety interferes with thought processes and with relationships and work performance. This state may lead to a host of physical, emotional, cognitive, and behavioral effects (BOX 2-14). For example, a person may experience problems concentrating, lose the ability to trust others, or become isolated or withdrawn. Some warning signs may call for immediate evaluation and medical care, such as chest pain and difficulty breathing. The presence of one or more warning signs is an indicator

BOX 2-14 Warning Signs and Symptoms of Stress

Physical
- Cardiac rhythm disturbances
- Chest pain
- Difficulty breathing
- Nausea
- Profuse sweating
- Sleep disturbances
- Vomiting

Emotional
- Anger
- Denial
- Fear
- Feeling of being overwhelmed
- Inappropriate emotions
- Panic reactions

Cognitive
- Confusion
- Decreased level of awareness
- Difficulty making decisions
- Disorientation
- Distressing dreams
- Memory problems
- Poor concentration

Behavioral
- Changes in eating habits
- Crying spells
- Excessive silence
- Hyperactivity
- Increased alcohol consumption
- Increased smoking
- Withdrawal

of distress, but the absence of warning signs does not preclude the likelihood of a stress reaction.

Reactions to Stress

Certain types of people may be attracted to certain types of careers. For example, some believe that emergency services personnel have personality traits that attract them to action-oriented and risk-taking jobs.[31] However, no person is immune to potential conflicts in managing stress. Likewise, each person has unique means to deal with stressful situations.

Adaptation

Adaptation is a process that involves learning successful ways to deal with stressful situations. This process usually begins with the use of defense mechanisms, followed by development of coping skills, then problem solving, and finally mastery.

Defense mechanisms are adaptive functions of the personality that assist a person in adjusting to stressful situations and help a person to avoid dealing with problems (BOX 2-15). Denial, for example, is a defense mechanism. Denial might be used to separate a person from the event long enough to deal with a problem that normally would be overwhelming.

Coping is an active confronting process, which involves gathering information and using the information to change or adjust to a new situation. Some beneficial ways to cope include taking part in regular physical exercise and being involved in activities at work that result in financial rewards and increased productivity. Other positive ways to cope include finding humor in personal crises, and "talking through" stressful events with family, friends, and coworkers.

Paramedics may also use harmful or negative coping mechanisms. For example, some may become withdrawn or use alcohol or other drugs. Some may have angry outbursts toward family members and coworkers. Others may become silent. These negative coping mechanisms, which threaten interpersonal relationships with coworkers and loved ones, should be seen as signs that a person is having trouble dealing with stress.

Problem solving involves analyzing a problem and finding options to deal with the issue both now and in the future. This phase of the adaptation process allows a person to clearly identify the problem and determine a course of action. This is a healthy approach to everyday concerns.

Mastery refers to the ability to see multiple options and solutions for challenging situations. Mastery results from extensive experience and the use of effective coping mechanisms with situations that are very similar. Unfortunately, it may be difficult to achieve.

> **NOTE**
>
> Burnout can be the result of cumulative stress. This condition is characterized by physical and emotional exhaustion and negative attitudes. Burnout can develop when someone is exposed to chronic stress that cannot be managed with usual coping mechanisms.

Stress Management Techniques

To manage stress well, a person must recognize the early warning signs of anxiety. Some of the physical effects of anxiety a person may notice include the following:

- Heart palpitations
- Difficult or rapid breathing
- Dry mouth
- Chest tightness or pain
- Anorexia
- Lack of appetite, nausea, vomiting, diarrhea, abdominal cramps, flatulence, "butterflies"
- Flushing, diaphoresis (profuse sweating), body temperature fluctuation
- Urgency and frequency in urination
- Dysmenorrhea (painful menstruation), decreased sexual drive or performance
- Aching muscles, joints

Physical effects that may not be as noticeable include the following:

- Increased blood pressure and heart rate
- Increased blood glucose levels
- Increased adrenaline production by adrenal glands
- Reduced gastrointestinal peristalsis
- Pupillary dilation

> **CRITICAL THINKING**
>
> Compare your reactions while on a highly stressful call in the field to those you experience when stressed about school. How are those feelings similar to or different from each other?

BOX 2-15 Common Defense Mechanisms

Repression

Repression is thought to be the mechanism underlying all other defense mechanisms. Repression is the involuntary attempt to keep certain feelings or memories from reaching conscious awareness. Traumatic events, intolerable and dangerous impulses, and other unacceptable ideas are forced out of consciousness. This defense mechanism may be seen as a result of an approach–avoidance conflict, in which a person struggles between trying to recall or think about something and trying to avoid the topic because it creates fear. For example, if an EMS provider's coworker is killed while on duty, the person might have no recall of the event from the time they arrived at the scene until after the event. Once repressions form, they usually are difficult to abolish. The person must be reassured that no danger exists in recalling the event.

Regression

Regression is a return to earlier levels of emotional adjustment—perhaps a time when tension and conflict could be avoided. Of all the reactions to anxiety and danger, regression may be the most dramatic and debilitating. For example, an EMS worker might throw a temper tantrum because he was assigned driver status on a work shift when he thought he would have direct patient care duties.

Projection

Projection involves attributing one's own undesirable qualities, feelings, motives, or desires to someone else. It may appear as aggression toward others but is actually a form of self-anger. Often people wrongly label their own motives and the motives of others as part of projection. For example, if a paramedic crashes an emergency vehicle en route to a call, she may feel that others blame her for the crash; in reality, she is blaming herself.

Rationalization

Rationalizations occur when people feel the need to explain their behavior, perhaps as a result of social training. If the true explanation would cause anxiety or guilt, the person may try to prove that the behavior is "rational" and therefore worthy of the approval of self and others. For example, a paramedic performs a poor physical examination on a trauma patient and fails to discover a femur fracture. When questioned by medical direction, she might rationalize her actions by saying that the police were hurrying her to clear the scene.

Compensation

Compensation is trying to cover up for a real or imagined weakness by stressing a more positive trait or skill. This distraction conceals frustration and anxiety by focusing attention on some other behavior. For example, an EMS crew member who has weak clinical skills and feels inadequate at emergency scenes might compensate by becoming an instructor in water rescue.

Reaction Formation

Reaction formation is a defensive behavior that prevents unwanted desires from being expressed. The person exaggerates the opposite attitudes and behavior, thereby concealing the true motive. The original impulse is still present but is masked by actions or attitudes that do not cause anxiety or stress. For example, a paramedic might be outwardly friendly to a coworker whom she dislikes.

Sublimation

Sublimation—a form of substitution—entails changing undesirable urges so that they are socially acceptable. It requires that a person change focus or energy so that instinctual drives are substituted for ones that may result in a higher cultural achievement. For example, a paramedic may become angry upon seeing people die in drunk-driving crashes and start a public awareness program on the hazards of drinking and driving.

Denial

In denial, a person rejects elements of reality that would be intolerable if accepted. The person gains protection from the unpleasant reality by refusing to see it—either the event itself or the memory of it. For example, a person who has just lost a loved one may be unable to accept the reality of the loved one's death. Denial differs from repression, in that repression deliberately seeks to keep feelings or memories at a distance from the conscious mind, whereas denial does not require effort, in that the person remains unaware of the feelings or memories.

Substitution

Substitution is a defense mechanism that switches an activity or goal that is desired but unreachable with one that is reachable. It may involve the redirection of an emotion from the first object to a more acceptable one, often as the result of frustration. For example, a coworker is having marital problems but feels that it is unacceptable to argue with his spouse. He might displace, or substitute, a confrontation with his wife with irritable and hostile behavior toward other crew members.

Isolation

Isolation involves the separation of unacceptable impulses, acts, or ideas from their origin in memory. This defense mechanism removes the emotional charge from the event and prevents feelings from being linked to the memory. Isolation may be helpful to the paramedic who must turn off feelings until after a call. For example, a paramedic may also be a parent and may have to give care to a dying child without being overcome by emotions.

For paramedics, many warning signs of stress appear during the emergency response or within 24 hours after the event. Some aspects of the stress reaction, however, may be delayed for some time and may not appear for months or years after the event. If signs and symptoms of stress-related illness appear, the person should seek appropriate medical or psychological help.

Intervening to relieve stress is as important as recognizing the warning signs of stress. Methods one may use initially to manage stress include reframing, controlled breathing, progressive relaxation, and guided imagery. All of these methods require practice to perform them properly.

Reframing involves first looking at the situation from a different emotional viewpoint and then placing it in a different "frame" that fits the facts of another situation equally well. This technique acts to change the meaning of the situation.

Controlled breathing is a natural stress control technique in which a person concentrates on the depth and rate of breathing to achieve a calming effect. Controlled breathing may begin with deep breathing, followed by less deep breathing, and finally normal breathing. BOX 2-16 describes the controlled breathing technique known as tactical breathing.

Progressive relaxation is a stress reduction strategy in which the person systematically tightens and relaxes particular muscle groups (from head to toe or from toe to head). This sequence "fools" the brain into initiating muscle relaxation throughout the body.

Guided imagery is used in combination with meditation. Another person familiar with the technique acts as a guide during the stress response. The person experiencing stress then can focus on an image that helps relieve stress. (Once guided imagery is learned, a person can use the technique without prompting.)

Other ways to fight stress include being aware of personal limitations, taking part in peer counseling, and participating in group discussions. Proper diet, exercise, sleep, and rest can help to relieve stress as well. In addition, pursuing positive activities outside of EMS can promote a better balance between the demands of work and recreation.

The responsibility for personal health and well-being ultimately belongs to the individual. However, intervention programs may be available through EMS agencies, hospitals, and other groups.

BOX 2-16 Tactical Breathing

Tactical breathing (also known as square breathing) is a technique used by the military and some athletes to manage stress, to focus, and to stay calm when performing under pressure. The technique is thought to control the sympathetic (fight-or-flight) alarm reaction that is activated by stress, thereby allowing the person to perform better in high-risk situations. Simply described, tactical breathing involves counting to four for each step of the breathing process: Breathe in, count to four. Hold your breath, count to four. Exhale, count to four, and repeat (**FIGURE 2-5**).

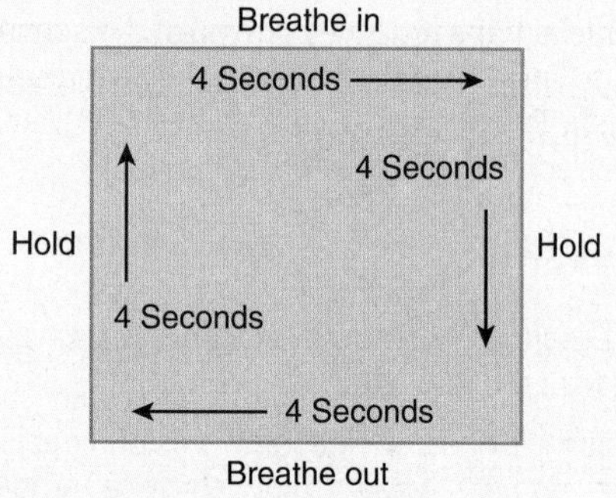

FIGURE 2-5 Tactical breathing.

Critical Incident Stress Management

Critical incident stress management (CISM), which evolved from the early 1970s concept of critical incident stress debriefing, is intended to help emergency workers who are exposed to a major incident cope with the stress created by that incident. CISM is based on a partnership between mental health professionals and peer group support. Although the benefits of CISM as a form of psychological first aid are debated,[32] CISM is designed to give emergency workers a chance to vent their feelings about a call or event that had a major effect. Because the evidence to date does not show that CISM has a clear benefit in reducing **posttraumatic stress disorder (PTSD)**, and may in fact worsen symptoms in some who attend, it is not recommended as a mandatory intervention (BOX 2-17).[33]

CISM aims to help emergency workers understand their reactions. It reassures them that what they are experiencing is normal and that others involved in the incident may be feeling the same way. The CISM process may be made available for one person or

BOX 2-17 Potential Situations for Critical Incident Stress Management

- Line-of-duty injury or death
- Disaster
- Emergency worker suicide
- Infant/child death
- Extreme threat to emergency worker
- Prolonged incident that ends in loss or success
- Victims known to operations personnel
- Death/injury of civilian caused by operations
- Other significant events

may include various members of the emergency team (eg, police, EMS crew members, firefighters, and emergency department staff).

NOTE

There are many programs available to EMS personnel and their families that can help manage stress. For example, the Code Green Campaign (Codegreencampaign.org) is a first responder–oriented mental health advocacy and education organization providing peer support, crisis referral, data collection, and education with the goal of improving the mental health of first responders everywhere. Other programs include agency-specific employee assistance programs, counseling, spouse support programs, family life programs, pastoral services, and periodic stress evaluations. These efforts and others can be good resources for the paramedic in dealing with stress on the job.

Posttraumatic Stress Disorder

PTSD is an anxiety disorder that can occur following a traumatic event:[34]

- Death of a child
- Caring for family members or a friend
- Caring for crime victims
- Caring for burn patients
- Combat or military exposure
- Child sexual or physical abuse
- Terrorist attacks
- Sexual or physical assault
- Serious incidents, such as a car crash
- Natural disasters, such as a fire, tornado, hurricane, flood, or earthquake

Recent studies have indicated that EMS personnel are more likely than the general public to develop PTSD.[35] The emotional difficulties that can result from dealing regularly with traumatic calls can lead to increased absenteeism from work, a troubled family life, and increased alcohol or other drug use. PTSD may also increase the risk of suicide.[36]

Four types of symptoms are associated with PTSD:[37]

- *Reexperiencing* is a mental "replay" of the event. It is often accompanied by strong, emotional reactions. This can occur during waking hours or during sleep (nightmares).
- *Avoidance* refers to efforts to evade activities, places, or people that remind those with the disorder of the traumatic event.
- *Numbing* is typically experienced as a loss of emotion, particularly positive feelings.
- *Arousal* reflects excessive psychological activation. Examples include a heightened sense of being "on guard" as well as difficulty with sleep and concentration that lasts more than 30 days.

The symptoms of PTSD are often managed with counseling, behavior therapy, and sometimes medication. Brief "time-out" periods from work (1 to 8 weeks) and support from coworkers and supervisors may also aid EMS personnel in their recovery (BOX 2-18).[38]

Coping strategies to reduce the incidence of PTSD vary by individual. Strategies shown to reduce traumatic stress include social support, purposeful problem-focused behaviors to address the situation, and positive reappraisal—that is, creating optimism to focus on personal and spiritual growth. Using "tough skin" coping mechanisms such as avoidance, escape, distancing, and anger have been found to worsen symptoms.[34]

CRITICAL THINKING

Imagine which type of call would be a critical incident for you personally.

BOX 2-18 Techniques for Reducing Crisis-Induced Stress

- Allow adequate rest for emergency workers.
- Provide food and fluid replacement.
- Limit exposure to the incident.
- Change assignments.
- Provide post-event defusing/debriefing.

Dealing With Death, Dying, Grief, and Loss

Death and dying will always be part of health care delivery. Medical science has given society the ability to postpone death in some instances and perhaps lessen its physical pain. However, the fight for self-preservation is still inevitably lost.

Patient and Family Needs

In the delivery of EMS, paramedics at times will give care to a dying person surrounded by loved ones. In such cases, the emotional needs of the dying patient, family, and loved ones should be of utmost importance (BOX 2-19). The patient and significant others will need to be comforted, given privacy, and treated with respect and dignity. Loved ones may need to express feelings of rage, anger, despair, and guilt. They may need the paramedic to provide control and direction for this solemn event. The paramedic's role in these cases is important and may be a determining factor in the way survivors adjust to their loss.

Stages of the Grieving Process

In 1968, Elisabeth Kübler-Ross began her work on the psychological aspects of death and dying. Kübler-Ross found that patients and loved ones dealing with the death process generally experience the following five stages:[39]

BOX 2-19 Palliative Care Versus Hospice Programs

Palliative care is specialized medical care for people with serious illness. Such care is focused on providing relief of symptoms and stress and on improving quality of life for both the patient and the family. Palliative care may include medication, counseling, and therapy. It may begin at the time of diagnosis and can be provided along with curative treatment.

Hospice programs began in England in 1967. Their goal is to help the terminally ill patient, family, and loved ones cope when death is expected. The hospice philosophy supports home care for the patient when possible. In addition, volunteers and health care professionals provide counseling and other psychological support to the patient and family during the death process. These programs play an important role in helping patients and their families accept death as a natural event in life.

1. *Denial* is characterized by disbelief: "No, not me." It is an expected response to news of a life-threatening illness or situation, which can be so overwhelming that it must be absorbed slowly. The patient seeks other opinions, verifies the accuracy of medical reports, or simply seems to ignore what he or she has been told. Denial is a valuable defense mechanism and is troubling only when no indication exists that the patient understands the seriousness of the situation. Most patients, families, and friends deny death to some degree so that they can continue with the daily business of living.
2. *Anger* can be viewed as the "Why me?" phase. This stage is probably the most difficult for persons who care about or are trying to help the dying person, because the person rejects all efforts to help or console him or her.
3. *Bargaining* is characterized by a "Yes, me, but . . ." frame of mind. The person admits the reality of being sick and of probably dying but tries to bargain for extension or quality of life. These bargains are often secret and rarely are kept. For example, a father might promise to be a "perfect patient" if only he can live to see his son's wedding.
4. *Depression* is the "Yes, me" reaction to anticipated death. It involves preparing to say, and actually saying, goodbye to everything and everyone a person has known and loved. The inherent sadness of this phase is appropriate and should be respected.
5. *Acceptance*, the simple and quiet "Yes," grows out of people's convictions that they have done what they could to be ready to die. Personal energy and interpersonal interests decrease significantly. During this phase, relatives and friends usually need more help than the dying person. The dying person's most important wish at this point is to not die alone.

NOTE

Dying patients and their loved ones may fluctuate between Kübler-Ross's stages and may or may not experience all five stages.

Paramedics rarely are involved in a patient's process of coming to terms with death. However, they often see the reactions of patients and families going through the death process. For example,

SHOW ME THE EVIDENCE

Researchers surveyed families of patients for whom EMS personnel terminated resuscitation of asystolic cardiac arrest in the field. They found that field resuscitation termination was accepted by the patients' families. The system had predefined termination criteria and a preplan that included a mechanism for family support (other than the EMS crew). Follow-up of these nontransported families in 3 to 6 months indicated that their grief adjustment trended more positively than that observed in families whose deceased family member was transported.

Modified from: Edwardsen EA, Chiumento S, Davis E. Family perspective of medical care and grief support after field termination by emergency medical services personnel. *Prehosp Emerg Care.* 2001;6(4):440-444.

denial may be obvious in some family members. These people may not appear to see or acknowledge the seriousness of a situation in which decisions about resuscitation must be made. Anger may be directed at the paramedic crew or other health care workers. Bargaining may occur as well: "Please save my child, and I promise that I'll always make her wear her seat belt!"

When it is necessary to give news of a sudden death to a family, the paramedic's initial contact can greatly influence the grief response. The paramedic should gather the family in a private area and advise them of the patient's death, with a brief account of the situation causing the death. The paramedic should use the words *death* or *dead* and should avoid euphemisms such as "he's passed on" or "she's no longer with us." It is important to be compassionate and allow time for the news to be absorbed and for questions to be asked. If they choose to do so, and the condition of the body makes it appropriate, the family members should be allowed to see the relative. They should be told in advance if resuscitation equipment is still connected to the patient. These efforts, along with empathic interaction with the family, help relatives deal with the loss of a loved one (BOX 2-20).

Needs of the Paramedic When Dealing With Death and Dying

Dealing with death is difficult for everyone, including the paramedic. When faced with death of a patient, the paramedic may experience some of the same stages of grief described earlier. These reactions are normal, and a great deal of effort to disguise or suppress these emotions may be required at the scene or while rendering care. However, the paramedic should discuss these feelings as soon as possible with friends, coworkers, and family in a constructive way that will lessen the emotional burden. Like others affected by the death, the paramedic will need a chance to process the incident and obtain closure. Accessing available resources, such as employee

BOX 2-20 Recommended Communication Strategies With Grieving Families: GRIEV_ING

- **G**ather: Gather the family; ensure that all members are present.
- **R**esources: Call for support resources available to assist the family with their grief (ie, chaplain services, ministers, family, friends).
- **I**dentify: Identify yourself, identify the deceased or injured patient by name, and identify the state of knowledge of the family relative to the events of the day.
- **E**ducate: Briefly educate the family as to the events that have occurred; educate them about the current state of their loved one.
- **V**erify: Verify that their family member has died. Be clear: Use the words "dead" or "died."
- **_** (Space): Give the family personal space and time for an emotional moment; allow the family time to absorb the information.
- **I**nquire: Ask if there are any questions, and answer them all.
- **N**uts and bolts: Inquire about organ donation, funeral services, and personal belongings. Offer the family the opportunity to view the body if appropriate.
- **G**ive: Give them your card and access information. Offer to answer any questions that may arise later. Always return their call.

Reproduced from: Hobgood C, Mathew D, Woodyard DJ, Shofer FS, Brice JH. Death in the field: teaching paramedics to deliver effective death notifications using the educational intervention "GRIEV_ING". Published June 27, 2013. Available at: http://www.tandfonline.com/doi/abs/10.3109/10903127.2013.804135?src=recsys&journalCode=ipec20.

assistance programs and counseling and pastoral services, can help the paramedic avoid the effects of cumulative stress.

> CRITICAL THINKING
> Have you experienced the death of a loved one? How did you or others who were close to the deceased react to the initial news of the death?

Developmental Considerations When Dealing With Death and Dying

The way people cope with their own death or the death of a loved one depends on their age, maturity, and understanding of death. The paramedic should be sensitive to the emotional needs of all age groups during this crisis. The following guidelines may be helpful when offering advice to family members who will be helping younger children or older adults cope with the death of a loved one.[40]

Children up to age 3 years probably will sense that something has happened in the family. They will realize that others are sad and crying. They also may be aware of increased activity in the household. The family should be urged to watch for changes in eating or sleeping patterns and for an increase in irritability. In addition, the family should be sensitive to the child's needs and try to maintain consistency in the child's routines and with significant persons in the child's life.

Children 3 to 6 years of age do not have a concept of the finality of death. They may believe that the person will return and may ask "when" continually. Members of this age group believe in "magical thinking" and may feel that they are responsible for the death. They also may believe that everyone else they love will die, too. The family should watch for changes in the child's behavior patterns with friends and at school, for difficulty sleeping, and for changes in eating habits. The family should emphasize that the child is not responsible for the death. They should also reinforce the fact that crying is normal when persons are sad and should encourage children to talk about their feelings.

Children 6 to 9 years of age are beginning to understand the finality of death. They want detailed explanations for the death and can differentiate fatal illness from just "being sick." Like 3- to 6-year-olds, these children may be afraid that other loved ones will die, too. Members of this age group may be uncomfortable with expressing their feelings and may act silly or embarrassed when talking about death. The paramedic should suggest to the family that they talk about the normal feelings of anger, sadness, and guilt and that they share their own feelings about death with the child. The family members should not hesitate to cry because crying will let the child know that expression of feelings is acceptable.

Children 9 to 12 years of age will typically show regression to an earlier stage of emotional response. However, some are aware of the finality of death and may want to know the details surrounding the event. They will be concerned with practical matters involving their lifestyle and may try to "act like an adult." The paramedic should suggest to the family that they set aside time to talk to the child about feelings and encourage the sharing of memories to aid in the grief response.

Older adults usually show concern for other family members. In addition, they may be worried about their further loss of independence and about financial matters at hand. Family members should be sensitive and understanding about these issues because they are real for this age group.

Summary

- Wellness has two main aspects: physical well-being and mental and emotional health.
- As health care professionals, paramedics have a responsibility to serve as role models in disease prevention.
- Persons who are overweight or have poor nutrition are at risk for the development of certain illnesses. A healthful diet includes a variety of foods that balance the number of calories appropriate for the person's age and sex with physical activity.
- Physical fitness can be described as a condition that helps people look, feel, and do their best. It includes cardiovascular endurance, muscle strength, and muscular flexibility.
- Adequate sleep is needed to prevent fatigue that can impair performance.
- Steps to reduce cardiovascular disease include improving cardiovascular endurance, eliminating cigarette smoking, controlling high blood pressure, maintaining a normal body fat composition, maintaining good total cholesterol/high-density lipoprotein ratio, monitoring triglyceride levels, controlling diabetes, avoiding excessive alcohol, eating healthy foods, reducing stress, and making a periodic risk assessment.
- Most common cancers are linked to one of three environmental risk factors: smoking, sunlight, and diet.
- The paramedic's duty is to be familiar with laws, regulations, and national standards that address issues of infectious disease. The paramedic also must take personal protective measures to guard against exposure.
- Actions to take after significant exposure include disinfection, documentation, incident investigation, screening, immunization, and medical follow-up.
- Injuries on the job can be minimized. Being aware of body mechanics during lifting and moving, securing help when necessary, and using lifting aids are good ways to avoid such injuries.
- Being alert for hostile settings is key to maintaining the paramedic's and others' safety at the scene.
- Prioritization of personal safety during rescue situations is wise, and paramedics must practice safe vehicle operation. They must use safety equipment and supplies as well.
- The misuse and abuse of drugs and other substances may lead to chemical dependency (addiction), which can have a wide range of effects on physical and mental health.
- Eustress ("good stress") is a positive response to stimuli and is considered protective. Distress ("bad stress") is a negative response to environmental stimuli and is the source of anxiety and stress-related disorders.
- Adaptation is a process in which a person learns effective ways to deal with stressful situations. This dynamic process usually begins with use of defense mechanisms, followed by development of coping skills, problem solving, and finally mastery.
- Critical incident stress management is designed to help emergency personnel understand their reactions to a call or event that had a major emotional impact. The process reassures them that what they are experiencing is normal and that others involved in the incident may be having the same feelings.
- Often news of a sudden death must be given to a family. The paramedic's initial contact can influence the grief process greatly.

References

1. The facts on fat. American Heart Association website. http://www.heart.org/HEARTORG/HealthyLiving/HealthyEating/Nutrition/FATS-The-Good-the-Bad-and-the-Ugly-Infographic_UCM_468968_SubHomePage.jsp. Updated November 2016. Accessed November 27, 2017.
2. *2015–2020 Dietary Guidelines for Americans*. 8th ed. US Department of Agriculture website. https://health.gov/dietaryguidelines/2015/resources/2015-2020_Dietary_Guidelines.pdf. Published December 2015. Accessed November 27, 2017.
3. Five steps to lose weight and keep it off. American Heart Association website. https://healthyforgood.heart.org/be-well/articles/5-steps-to-lose-weight-and-keep-it-off. Updated January 9, 2017. Accessed November 29, 2017.
4. How much physical activity do adults need? Centers for Disease Control and Prevention website. https://www.cdc.gov/physicalactivity/basics/adults/index.htm. June 4, 2015. Accessed November 29, 2017.
5. Fatigue, sleep deprivation, and patient safety. Agency for Healthcare Research and Quality, Patient Safety Network website. https://psnet.ahrq.gov/primers/primer/37/fatigue-sleep-deprivation-and-patient-safety. Updated November 2017. Accessed November 29, 2017.
6. Caruso C, Hitchcock EM, Dick RB, Russo JM, Schmit JM. *Overtime and Extended Work Shifts: Recent Findings on Illnesses, Injuries, and Health Behaviors.* Washington, DC: US Department of Health and Human Services, Centers for Disease Control and Prevention, National Institutes of Occupational Safety and Health; 2004.
7. Maltese F, Adda M, Bablon A, et al. Night shift decreases cognitive performance of ICU physicians. *Intens Care Med.* 2016;42(3):393-400.
8. Patterson PD, Higgins JS, Lang ES, et al. Evidence-based guidelines for fatigue risk management in EMS: formulating research questions and selecting outcomes. *Prehosp Emerg Care.* 2017;21(2):149-156.
9. How to help prevent heart disease—at any age. American Heart Association website. http://www.heart.org/HEARTORG/HealthyLiving/How-to-Help-Prevent-Heart-Disease---At-Any-Age_UCM_442925_Article.jsp#.WSndkzOZNp8. Updated April 3, 2017. Accessed November 29, 2017.
10. Centers for Disease Control and Prevention. Precautions to prevent transmission in health care settings, C virus (HCV) infection and HCV-related chronic disease. *MMWR.*1987; 36(suppl 2S):1S-18S.

11. Regulations (Standards - 29 CFR). Occupational Safety and Health Administration website. https://www.osha.gov/pls/oshaweb/owadisp.show_document?p_table=STANDARDS&p_id=10051#1910.1030(b). Accessed September 30, 2017.
12. Centers for Disease Control and Prevention. Hospital Infection Control Practices *Infect Control Hosp Epidemiol*.1996;17:53-80.
13. Maguire BJ, Hunting K, Smith G, Levick N. Occupational fatalities in emergency medical services. *Ann Emerg Med.* 2002;40(6):625-632.
14. Blau G, Chapman SA. Why do emergency medical services (EMS) professionals leave EMS? *Prehosp Disaster Med.* 2016;31(suppl 1):s105-s111.
15. EMS safety. NAEMT website. https://www.naemt.org/initiatives/ems-safety. Accessed December 19, 2017.
16. Reichard A, Marsh S, Olsavsky R, Morgantown WV. *Emergency Medical Services Workers: How Employers Can Prevent Injuries and Exposures.* Publication 2017–194. Washington, DC: US Department of Health and Human Services, Centers for Disease Control and Prevention, National Institute for Occupational Safety and Health; 2017.
17. Reichard AA, Marsh SM, Tonozzi TR, Konda S, Gormley MA. Occupational injuries and exposures among emergency medical services workers. *Prehosp Emerg Care.* 2017;21(4);420-431.
18. Taylor JA, Barnes B, Davis AL, Wright J, Widman S, LeVasseur M. Expecting the unexpected: a mixed methods study of violence to EMS responders in an urban fire department. *Am J Industrial Med.* 2016;59(2):150-163.
19. Grange JT, Corbett SW. Violence against emergency medical services personnel. *Prehosp Emerg Care.* 2009;6(2):186-190.
20. Defensive tactics 4 escaping mitigating surviving. DT4EMS website. http://dt4ems.com/. Accessed November 29, 2017.
21. Kahn CA, Pirralo RG, Kuhn EM. Characteristics of fatal ambulance crashes in the United States: an 11-year retrospective analysis. *Prehosp Emerg Care.* 2001;5(3):261-269.
22. Regehr C, Goldberg G, Hughes J. Exposure to human tragedy, empathy, and trauma in ambulance paramedics. *Am J Orthopsychiatry.* 2002;72(4):505-513.
23. Bentley MA, Crawford M, Wilkins JR, Fernandez AR, Studnek JR. An assessment of depression, anxiety, and stress among nationally certified EMS professionals. *Prehosp Emerg Care.* 2013;17(3):330-338.
24. Donnelly E. Work-related stress and posttraumatic stress in emergency medical services. *Prehosp Emerg Care.* 2012;16(1):76-85.
25. Oreskovich MR, Kaups KL, Balch CM, et al. Prevalence of alcohol use disorders among American surgeons. *Arch Surg.* 2012;147(2):168-174.
26. Star K. The sneaky prevalence of substance abuse in nursing. *Nursing.* 2015;45(3):16-17.
27. Firefighters, police and paramedics: hidden populations that need help. First Responders Recovery website. http://www.firstrespondersrecovery.com/firefighters-police-paramedics-hidden-populations-need-help/. Published July 27, 2015. Accessed November 29, 2017.
28. Smoking and tobacco use: fast facts. Centers for Disease Control and Prevention website. https://www.cdc.gov/tobacco/data_statistics/fact_sheets/fast_facts/index.htm. Updated November 16, 2017. Accessed November 29, 2017.
29. Tips for managing and preventing stress: a guide for emergency and disaster response workers. US Department of Health and Human Services, Substance Abuse and Mental Health Services Administration, Center for Mental Health Service website. https://store.samhsa.gov/shin/content/SMA11-DISASTER/SMA11-DISASTER-18.pdf. Accessed November 29, 2017.
30. Selye H. *The Stress of Life.* New York, NY: McGraw-Hill; 1956.
31. Salters-Pedneault K, Ruef AM, Orr SP. Personality and psychophysiological profiles of police officer and firefighter recruits. *Personality Individ Diff.* 2010;49(3):210-215.
32. Advisory Council on First Aid, Aquatics, Safety, and Preparedness. Scientific review: critical incident stress debriefing (CISD). American Red Cross website. https://www.yumpu.com/en/document/view/30398398/acfasp-scientific-review-critical-incident-stress-debriefing-cisd. Published June 2010. Accessed November 29, 2017.
33. PTSD: National Center for PTSD. Types of debriefing following disasters. US Department of Veterans Affairs website. https://www.ptsd.va.gov/professional/trauma/disaster-terrorism/debriefing-after-disasters.asp. Updated February 23, 2016. Accessed November 29, 2017.
34. Holland M. The dangers of detrimental coping in emergency medical services. *Prehosp Emerg Care.* 2011;15(3):331-337.
35. Walker A, McKune A, Ferguson S, Pyne DB, Rattray B. Chronic occupational exposures can influence the rate of PTSD and depressive disorders in first responders and military personnel. *Extreme Physiol Med.* 2016 Jul 15;5:8.
36. Martin C, Tran J. Correlates of suicidality in firefighter/EMS personnel. *J Affective Disorders.* 2017;208:177-183.
37. PTSD: National Center for PTSD. How is PTSD measured? US Department of Veterans Affairs website. https://www.ptsd.va.gov/public/assessment/ptsd-measured.asp. Updated August 10, 2015. Accessed September 30, 2017.
38. Coping in the aftermath of Hurricane Katrina: some brief guidance notes on stress, grief and loss for front line teams. International Medical Corp website. http://www.who.int/hac/techguidance/ems/IMC_Guidance_Stress_Grief_Loss.pdf. Accessed November 29, 2017.
39. Kübler-Ross E. *On Death and Dying.* New York, NY: Scribner; 1969.
40. Bassuk EL, Fox SS, Prendergast KJ. *Behavioral Emergencies.* Boston, MA: Little, Brown; 1983.

Suggested Readings

Bigham GL, Jensen JL, Tavares W, et al. Paramedic self-reported exposure to violence in the emergency medical services (EMS) workplace: a mixed-methods cross-sectional survey. *Prehosp Emerg Care*. 2014;18(4):489-494.

Grossman LCD, Christensen L. *On Combat: The Psychology and Physiology of Deadly Conflict in War and in Peace.* 3rd ed. Mascoutah, IL: Killology Research Group; 2012.

Martin-Gill, Barger C, Moore CG, et al. Effects of napping during shift work on sleepiness and performance in emergency medical services personnel and similar shift workers: a systematic review and meta-analysis. *Prehosp Emerg Care*. 2018;Jan 11:1-11.

Patterson PD, Weaver M, Hostler D, Guyette F, Callaway CW, Yealy D. The shift length, fatigue, and safety conundrum in EMS. *Prehosp Emerg Care.* 2012;16(4):572-576.

Temple JL, Hostler D, Martin-Gill C, et al. Systematic review and meta-analysis of the effects of caffeine in fatigued shift workers: implications for emergency medical services personnel. *Prehosp Emerg Care*. 2018;Jan 11:1-10.

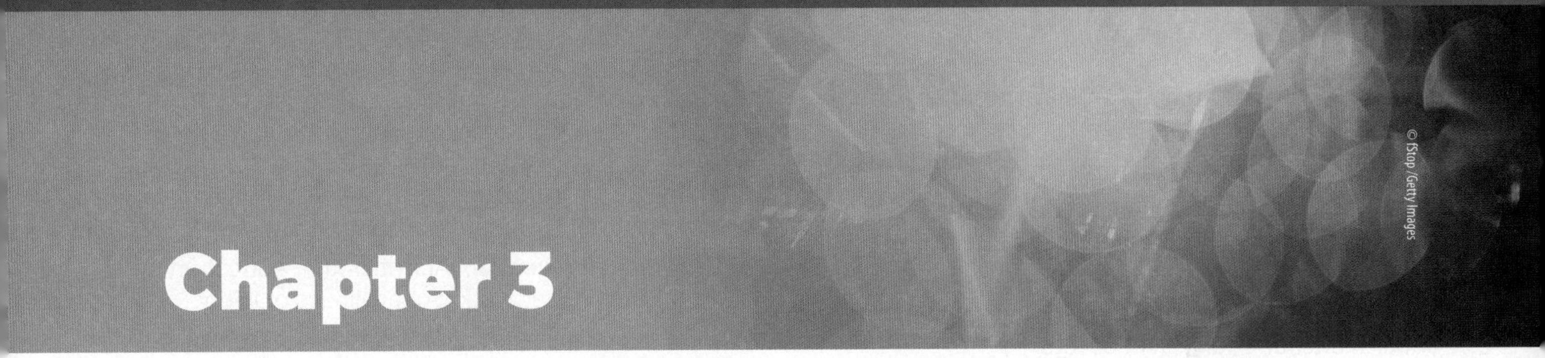

Chapter 3

Injury Prevention, Health Promotion, and Public Health

NATIONAL EMS EDUCATION STANDARD COMPETENCIES

Public Health

Applies fundamental knowledge of principles of public health and epidemiology including public health emergencies, health promotion, and illness and injury prevention.

OBJECTIVES

Upon completion of this chapter, the paramedic student will be able to:

1. Describe the epidemiology of trauma and disease in the United States. (p 66)
2. Define injury. (pp 67–68)
3. Describe the Haddon matrix and the injury triangle. (pp 68–70)
4. Relate how alterations in the epidemiologic triangle can influence injury and disease patterns. (pp 68–70)
5. Differentiate among primary, secondary, and tertiary health prevention activities. (p 70)
6. Describe public health goals and activities. (p 71)
7. Outline the aspects of the EMS system that make it a desirable resource for involvement in public health activities. (p 71)
8. Identify roles of the EMS community in health promotion and injury prevention. (pp 71–73, 75–77)
9. Describe essential activities for the active participation of EMS in community wellness activities. (pp 71–73)
10. List situations in which paramedics may participate in injury or disease prevention. (p 73)
11. Describe strategies to implement a successful injury or disease prevention program. (pp 74–75, 78–81)
12. Evaluate a situation to determine opportunities for injury or disease prevention. (p 75)
13. Identify resources necessary to conduct a community health assessment. (pp 77–78)

KEY TERMS

community health assessment An assessment of a target community to identify the needs and resources required to provide prevention and wellness promotion activities.

epidemiology The study of how disease is distributed within populations and the factors that influence that distribution.

injury Intentional or unintentional damage inflicted on a person. Examples include falls, assault, burns, and frostbite.

injury risks Any situations that increase a person's risk for sustaining an injury.

injury surveillance The ongoing systematic collection, analysis, and interpretation of injury data essential to the planning, implementation, and evaluation of public health practice.

primary injury prevention The practice of preventing an injury from occurring.

public health A field of medicine that deals with the physical and mental health of all people in a community.

secondary injury prevention Activities that minimize harm after an injury event occurs.

social determinants of health Factors that influence health, which include the conditions in which people are born, grow, work, live, and age and the conditions surrounding their daily life.

teachable moment The time after an injury has occurred when the patient and observers remain acutely aware of what has happened and may be more receptive to being taught ways that the event or illness could have been prevented.

tertiary injury prevention Activities that correct and prevent further deterioration of an illness or injury.

years of potential life lost The calculation obtained by subtracting the age of the victim's death from 65 (the average age of retirement); a measure of premature mortality.

A community has a duty to promote injury prevention. This prevention can occur in the form of leadership and educational activities. One goal of injury prevention is to decrease the incidence of preventable illness and injury. A final goal is to prevent people from needing costly medical care. As a member of the health care system, the paramedic can be a key resource in injury prevention programs.

Injury Epidemiology

According to the Centers for Disease Control and Prevention (CDC), **epidemiology** is the study of the distribution and determinants of health-related states or events, in specified populations, and the application of this study to the control of health problems. Unintentional **injury** is the leading cause of death among all people 1 to 44 years of age.[1] It is the fourth leading cause of death among all age groups, exceeded only by heart disease, cancer, and chronic lower respiratory disease.[2] In 2014, 199,756 injury-related deaths occurred in the United States.[3]

Unintentional injury results in more **years of potential life lost** before age 65 years than does any other cause of death. From a financial perspective,

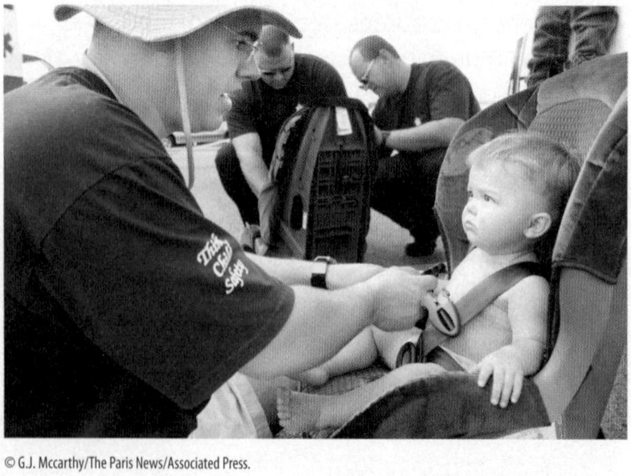

© G.J. Mccarthy/The Paris News/Associated Press.

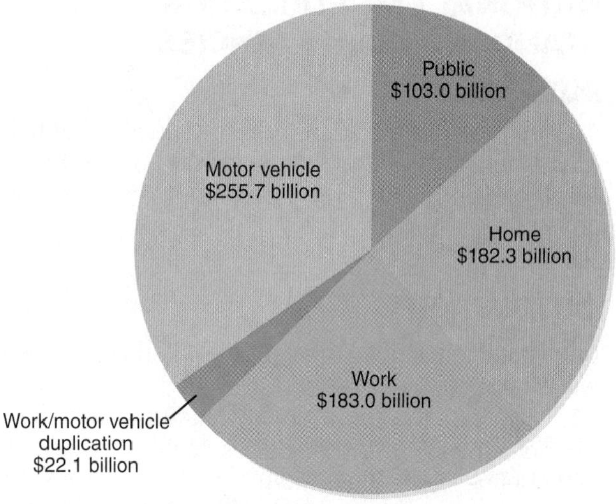

FIGURE 3-1 Cost of unintentional injuries by class in 2015.

Reproduced from: National Safety Council. *Injury Facts*. Itasca, IL: NSC; 2017.

fatal and nonfatal unintentional injury cost the United States $886.4 billion in 2015 (**FIGURE 3-1**). The quality of life lost from those injuries is valued at another $3,538.1 billion, for a total cost of $4,424.5 billion (**TABLE 3-1**).[4] In 2015 in the United States, more than 37 million visits to the emergency department (about 28%) were related to injury.[5]

Overview of Prevention

In the past, EMS was considered a form of reactive medical care, focused on treating illness and injury as opposed to their prevention. A complete system of

TABLE 3-1 Cost Equivalents of Fatal and Nonfatal Unintentional Injuries, 2015

The Cost of	Is Equivalent to
All injuries ($886.4 billion)	58 cents of every dollar paid in federal personal income taxes, *or*
	52 cents of every dollar spent on food in the United States
Motor vehicle crashes ($385.3 billion)	Purchasing 600 gallons of gasoline for each registered vehicle in the United States, or more than $1,800 per licensed driver
Work injuries ($142.5 billion)	15 cents of every dollar of corporate dividend to stockholders, *or*
	11 cents of every dollar of pretax corporate profits, *or*
	Exceeds the combined profits reported by the nine largest Fortune 500 companies
Home injuries ($254.7 billion)	A $365,000 rebate on each new single-family home built, *or*
	56 cents of every dollar of property taxes paid
Public injuries ($132.6 billion)	A $14.6 million grant to each public library in the United States, *or*
	A $103,000 bonus for each police officer and firefighter

Reproduced from: National Safety Council. *Injury Facts*. Itasca, IL: NSC; 2017.

NOTE

While you make a 10-minute speech about bicycle safety to a classroom of children, at least three people will be killed by unintentional injury. Another 772 suffer injuries requiring medical care. A death caused by unintentional injury occurs in the United States every 4 minutes.

National Safety Council. *Injury Facts*. Itasca, IL: NSC; 2017.

injury prevention is made up of several facets, with acute care being only one aspect (**FIGURE 3-2**). Currently, the focus of the public health arm of health care is prevention. Public health works to prevent illness and injury; it is proactive. EMS is able to work with public health agencies on both primary and secondary prevention strategies, discussed later.

Preventive strategies yield better outcomes than treatment strategies in terms of lives saved and money spent.[6] Identifying prevention strategies relies heavily on data collection. These data shed light on the nature of illness and injury within the EMS community as well as the effectiveness of prevention and management strategies. The success of prevention strategies also depends on teaching injury and illness prevention to patients and other members of the community. Paramedics have a unique opportunity to understand the illness and injury patterns that occur in the community and learn the characteristics and **injury risks** of the population they serve. Paramedics can then organize and participate in programs to reduce injuries and prevent illnesses.

DID YOU KNOW?

The National Health Interview Survey

The National Health Interview Survey is conducted annually by the National Center for Health Statistics. This survey samples US households to obtain data about the health status of household members, including any injuries that were sustained during the 5 weeks before the survey. The survey found that in 2014 most injuries occurred inside and outside the home (36% and 24%, respectively), followed by injuries at recreational or sports facilities (18%), and injuries on streets, highways, and parking lots (13%). The data collected by various government agencies and health organizations (discussed later in this chapter) help guide the focus of injury prevention initiatives in the United States.

Modified from: National Health Interview Survey, 2014. Centers for Disease Control and Prevention, National Center for Health Statistics website. https://ftp.cdc.gov/pub/health_Statistics/nchs/NHIS/SHS/2014_SHS_Table_P-8.pdf.

Definition of Injury

Injuries are commonly classified according to whether they are considered unintentional or intentional. A puzzling factor that hindered the study of injury

FIGURE 3-2 Conceptual diagram of working in health-promoting ways—a strategic framework.

Reproduced from: The Department of Health and Human Services. *Connecting care: chronic disease action framework for Tasmania 2009-2013*. Hobart: Tasmanian government; 2009. https://www.dhhs.tas.gov.au/__data/assets/pdf_file/0006/48390/Connecting_Care_Full_Version_web.pdf.

and therefore injury prevention was that injuries were considered accidents or random events that were not preventable. This belief is no longer held. According to the World Health Organization and the CDC,[7] injuries are caused by acute exposure to physical agents, such as mechanical energy, heat, electricity, chemicals, or ionizing radiation, interacting with the body in amounts or at rates that exceed the threshold of human tolerance. In some cases (eg, drowning and frostbite), injuries result from the sudden lack of essential agents such as oxygen or heat (see Chapter 36, *Trauma Overview and Mechanism of Injury*).

Poisoning is also included in the injury classification. In 2014, poisoning was the leading cause of unintentional death overall, followed by motor vehicle crashes, falls, and choking. This prevalence represents an 8% increase over the prior year. The top three drug categories associated with sudden and unexpected death were prescription opioids, heroin, and benzodiazepines.[4]

BOX 3-1 lists common terms related to illness and injury prevention.

The Injury Triangle and the Haddon Matrix

Injury is also a disease process. Three factors are necessary to cause an injury or illness: a host, an agent, and the environment. Together these three factors are known as the *injury triangle* (**FIGURE 3-3**). In the injury triangle, the victim is the host, energy expenditure is the agent, and the place external from the host where the agent and host interact over time is the environment. The injury event may take only a fraction of a

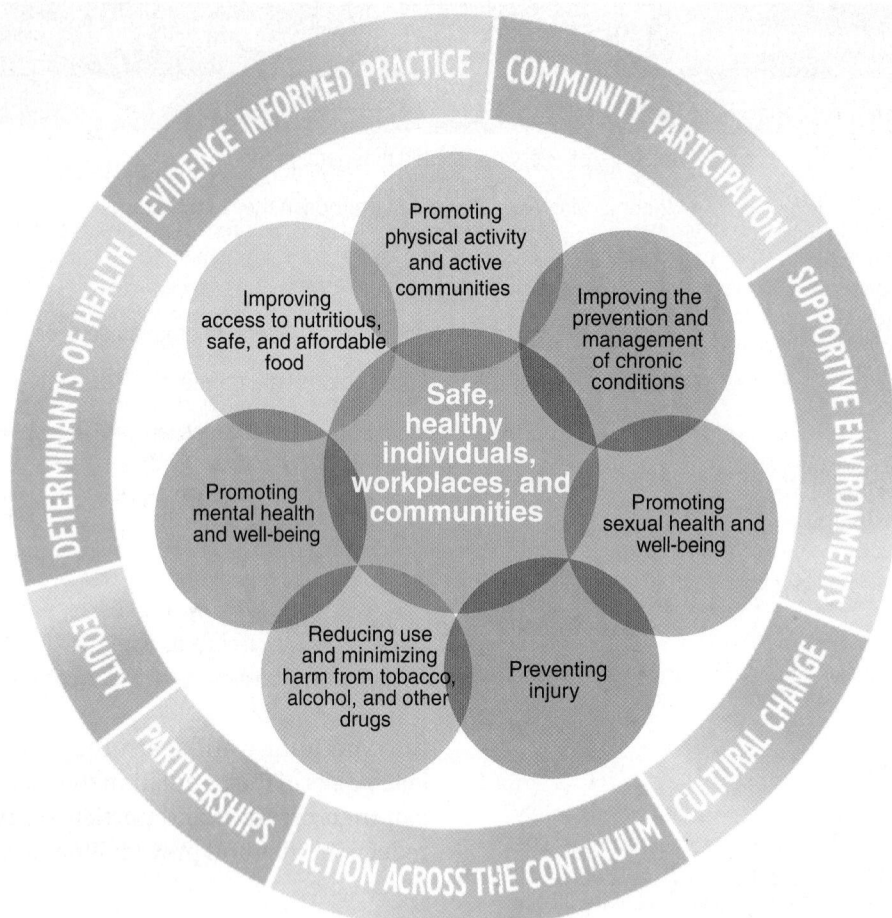

BOX 3-1 Injury and Illness Prevention Terminology

Health promotion. Process to help people understand causes of poor health and to improve their health.

Injury. Intentional or unintentional damage to a person resulting from acute exposure to thermal, mechanical, electrical, or chemical energy or from the absence of heat and oxygen.

Injury risk. Real or potentially hazardous situations that put people at increased risk for sustaining an injury.

Injury surveillance. The ongoing collection, analysis, and interpretation of injury data essential to the planning, implementation, and evaluation of public health practice; closely integrated with the timely dissemination of these data to those who need to know, with the final link in the chain being the application of these data to prevention and control.

Primary injury prevention. The practice of preventing an injury from occurring.

Secondary injury prevention. Activities that minimize harm after an injury event occurs.

Teachable moment. The time after an injury or acute illness when the patient and observers remain acutely aware of what has happened and may be more receptive to being taught ways that the event or illness could be prevented.

Tertiary injury prevention. Activities that correct and prevent further deterioration of an illness or injury.

Years of potential life lost. One measure of premature death calculated by subtracting the age of the victim's death from a predetermined end point (usually 65 years, the average age of retirement or average life expectancy).

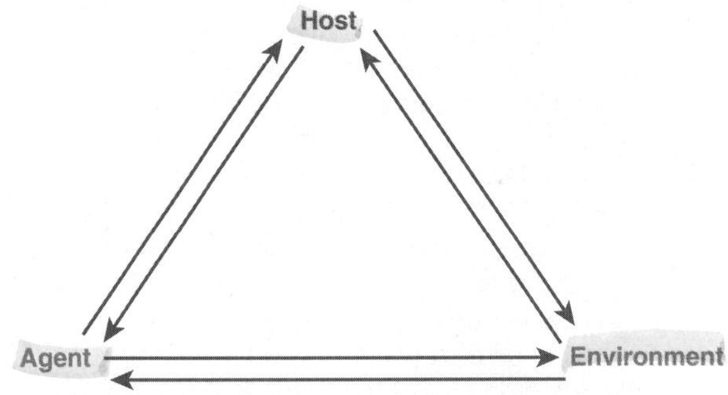

FIGURE 3-3 The injury triangle is a model developed by scientists for studying health problems. The triad constituted by the host (human), agent (cause), and environment (physical or social) is used to identify problems and determine the interventions necessary for prevention.

Modified from: The Centers for Disease Control and Prevention. Lesson 1: Understanding the epidemiologic triangle through infectious disease. Available at: https://www.cdc.gov/bam/teachers/documents/epi_1_triangle.pdf.

second, but the events that occur before an injury and the events that occur as a result of an injury may take place over seconds, months, or even years.

> NOTE
> Changing one or more of the factors in the injury triangle can alter disease or injury patterns.

In the mid-1960s, William Haddon (the "father" of injury prevention) developed an analytical tool, known as the Haddon matrix, to aid in understanding the entire injury sequence. Haddon added the factor of time in phases—preevent, event, and postevent (**TABLE 3-2**)—to the previous models used to address

TABLE 3-2 Haddon Matrix for Automobile Crashes

	Factor		
Phase	**Host**	**Agent**	**Environment**
Preevent	Impaired capabilities, age, fatigue, alcohol/drug use, driving experience, adherence to driving laws	Defective equipment, dirty windows, improper maintenance, equipment design	Road shoulder too narrow, poor lighting, weather conditions, highway not divided, inadequate notification signs, road design, and construction
Event	Injury threshold caused by aging, chronic disease, alcohol, use of restraints, ejection	Failure of doors, impact with sharp objects in the vehicle, vehicle size	Lack of guardrails, large trees near roadside, oncoming traffic
Postevent	Type or extent of injury, knowledge of first aid, alcohol	Bursting gas tanks, entrapment	Quality of rescue, EMS, hospitals, rehabilitation

the causes of injury. The Haddon matrix in Table 3-2 charts the events that may occur before, during, and after a car crash, which shows that injuries often result from a predictable and therefore preventable chain of events. The matrix also affirms that most injuries are linked with many causes.

The preevent phase of the matrix is the period before the release of injury-causing energy. During this time, the factors that affect the host are considered. Events in the preevent phase tend to influence the likelihood that an injury will occur. **Primary injury prevention** can take place at this time because the injury has yet to occur. The time frame can be seconds to years, depending on the events that come into play to cause the injury.

The event phase of the matrix is the period during which the injury occurs, usually within a fraction of a second to a few minutes. Events in this phase affect the transmission of energy. **Secondary injury prevention** is centered on reducing the severity of the injury as it is occurring.

The postevent phase of the matrix is the period after the injury has occurred, which can last from a few seconds to years. During this time, **tertiary injury prevention** takes place and traditional EMS exists to lessen the long-term adverse effects of the injury.

The Three Es of Injury Prevention

Three strategies typically have been used to establish injury prevention programs—education, enforcement, and engineering—known as the three Es. The combination of these strategies results in the most effective prevention efforts. Motivated paramedics can take key roles in these programs by participating in illness and injury prevention initiatives such as car seat safety checks or blood pressure monitoring programs.

Education

Education, the most often used approach in injury prevention, persuades people who are at high risk for injury or illness to change their behavior. Education informs people to adopt safety precautions and often requires them to make behavioral changes. Education is most effective when used with enforcement and engineering. Educational programs include the following:

- Alcohol and other drug prevention
- Burn prevention
- Drowning prevention
- Elder safety
- Fall prevention
- Pedestrian and bicycle safety
- Poison prevention
- School safety and school-based programs
- Sports safety
- Suicide prevention
- Violence prevention

SHOW ME THE EVIDENCE

A North Carolina EMS system developed a program called Welcome to the World. The program included 262 families, with children averaging 21 months of age. It found the following household characteristics:

- Ninety-eight percent of families (250/255) had a smoke detector, and 65% (140/215) had a fire extinguisher, with 77% (192/250) and 76% (107/140) of these respective devices functional.
- Twenty-seven percent (55/202) had a fire evacuation plan, and 33% (18/55) reported ever practicing their plan.
- For bathwater sites, 56% had temperatures measured lower than 120°F (48.9°C). Eighty-five percent (218/257) had medications and 53% (134/249) had household chemicals out of reach of children, but most reported storage in an unlocked location.
- Eighty-five percent (42/49) reported storing guns unloaded, and 45% (22/49) stored all guns in locked locations.

Paramedics distributed 63 smoke detectors, 46 fire extinguisher vouchers, 234 first-aid kits, and 225 educational packets.

Reproduced from: Hawkins ER, Brice JH, Overby BA. Welcome to the world: findings from an emergency medical services pediatric injury prevention program. *Pediatr Emerg Care*. 2007 Nov;23(11):790-795.

Enforcement

Enforcement can occur through the enforcement of laws. Laws require that people, manufacturers, and governments comply with certain safety practices that reduce risk; for example, most states have passed laws requiring use of seat belts in vehicles. Success also depends on the ability to enforce these laws, such as when lawsuits are brought against manufacturers of dangerous products. Enforcement strategies that have been proven to reduce vehicle-related injury include the following:

- Child restraint laws
- "Click It or Ticket" programs

- Motorcycle helmet laws
- Ignition interlock programs for repeat offenders
- Minimum legal drinking age laws
- Sobriety checkpoints to deter driving under the influence
- Speed limit enforcement
- Zero tolerance for young drivers

Engineering

Engineering refers to the design of products or spaces (eg, roads, car airbags, sprinkler systems in buildings). The design automatically provides protection from injury or decreases the likelihood that an incident will occur without the person ever having to make a change in behavior. Engineering is therefore considered a passive intervention. Although engineering has proved to be the most effective of the three Es, it is also the most expensive approach toward change. Engineering strategies used to prevent injury include the following:

- Disposable equipment
- Safe design of emergency vehicles
- Needleless syringes and injection ports
- Nonslip footwear and nonskid surfaces
- Retractable finger-stick lancets
- Vaccines
- Powered lifting devices

Basic Principles of Public Health

Most people know what is meant by the term *medical care*. And even though many people benefit from public health, they are less familiar with the term—specifically its missions and functions. Public health is different from medical care. Although there are many definitions of **public health**, the term can be defined as a field of medicine that deals with the physical and mental health of all people in a community. The focus of public health is more on prevention of disease than on treatment of disease. Important areas of public health include a community's water supply, waste disposal, air pollution, and food safety. Other examples of public health goals and accomplishments include the following:

- Widespread vaccination programs
- Clean drinking water and sewage systems
- Declines in infectious disease
- Fluoridated water supplies
- Reduction in use of tobacco products
- Prenatal care services

Public Health Laws, Regulations, and Guidelines

Laws, regulations, and guidelines for public health initiatives are provided by local, state, and governmental agencies. Others involved in public health include medical professionals such as physicians, nurses, and EMS personnel. Area hospitals, clinics, public service agencies, and other governmental and nongovernmental agencies also play important roles in providing public health services in a community.

EMS Involvement in Public Health

The United States has more than 826,000 EMS personnel.[8] As noted in *Emergency Medical Services: Agenda for the Future*, "People attracted to the EMS service are among society's best, and desire to contribute to their community's health. The composition of the EMS workforce reflects the diversity of the population it serves."[9] EMS personnel are a valuable resource for educating the public and promoting health because they are:

- Often the most medically educated people in rural settings
- Role models with high profiles
- Seen as the champions of patients and the community
- Welcome in homes, schools, and other settings
- Seen as authorities on injury and prevention
- Often the first to recognize situations that pose a risk for illness or injury (eg, unsanitary conditions and unsafe home environments)

> CRITICAL THINKING
>
> Did you ever have a class or program taught by a firefighter or paramedic when you were a child? How did you feel about him or her?

Essential Community Leadership Activities

For paramedics and other public service personnel to play active roles in community health and injury prevention programs, the community has the responsibility to assist and support paramedics in the following activities:

- Ensuring the safety of EMS personnel during a call.
- Providing community liaisons for injury prevention education to EMS personnel to establish successful injury and illness prevention programs.
- Supporting and promoting the collection and use of data on injury and illness.
- Obtaining financial support and resources for injury and illness prevention and management activities.
- Empowering paramedics to conduct injury and illness prevention and management activities.

EMS, through extended (expanded) scope of practice, perform some of these leadership activities for injury prevention and wellness.

EMS Personnel Safety

A basic first step for preventing injury and promoting wellness in a community is to protect the well-being of EMS personnel. Policies, such as traffic safety laws, and public education help to ensure EMS safety during an emergency response, while at the scene, and during patient transport. Protection of EMS personnel also can be enhanced with the help of law enforcement, fire service personnel, and other public service agencies.

All EMS personnel must have access to personal protective equipment according to Occupational Safety and Health Administration law. At a minimum, paramedics should have access to gloves, eyewear, gowns, and a facemask. This equipment reduces the risk of eye and skin injury. Other valuable safety equipment includes helmets to reduce head injury, reflective clothing to increase visibility, and steel-toed shoes to prevent foot injury. Tactical vests, used in some EMS systems, protect against penetrating chest trauma. Personal protective equipment also reduces disease transmission and exposure to hazardous chemicals. Community wellness programs for EMS personnel are an important component of preventing injury and illness and ensuring the safety of EMS providers during a call.

Community Liaisons

To help provide specific education and training, community leaders need to create a liaison between EMS programs and public and private specialty groups, including hospitals, other public health and safety agencies, safety councils, social services, religious organizations, and colleges and universities. Communication and cooperation among these groups can help EMS agencies determine the existing resources available in the community and target prevention activities and the establishment of programs to improve the health of the community.

Data Collection and Use

Data collection and management are important for tracking the effectiveness of programs within the community. After paramedics have connected with the community and programs are initiated or are up and running, policies that promote an effective process for collecting data need to be in place. The data collected contribute to local, state, and national **injury surveillance** programs—for example, the local hospital's trauma registry or the national Alzheimer's Prevention Registry, among others.

DID YOU KNOW?

Data Collection Registries

A registry (disease or trauma registry) is a file of uniform data that describes people who meet certain criteria. The registry collects medical and demographic data in an ongoing and systematic way to serve predetermined purposes, including (1) facilitating and coordinating rehabilitation and other needed services, (2) gathering data for injury prevention and control, (3) gathering data for health care planning, and (4) evaluating services provided to injured people.

The first computerized trauma registry was introduced in 1969 at Cook County Hospital in Chicago, Illinois. In 1985 the CDC began to promote the development of surveillance systems for clusters of injuries (sentinel injuries) at both the state and national levels. Since then, many states have developed statewide registries to track traumatic brain injuries, spinal cord injuries, and other classes of trauma. Federal agencies working with medical organizations and other groups help coordinate national-level standardizations of trauma registries. The Cardiac Arrest Registry to Enhance Survival provides a confidential method to collect national cardiac arrest data. EMS and health care professionals play a major role in gathering these data. Data collection helps in monitoring and evaluating the quality of trauma care and disease-specific care within health care systems.

Modified from: Pollock D. Trauma registries and public health surveillance of injuries. www.cdc.gov/nchs/data/ice/ice95v1/C11.pdf; Binder S, Corrigan JD, Langlois JA. The public health approach to traumatic brain injury: an overview of CDC's research and programs. *J Head Trauma Rehabil*. 2005;20(3):189-195; and Cardiac Arrest Registry to Enhance Survival website. https://mycares.net/sitepages/aboutcares.jsp.

Financial Support

The community needs to provide budgetary support for injury prevention programs. In addition, the community and EMS leaders need to initiate or attend meetings of local organizations that are involved or that are requesting involvement in injury prevention. EMS leaders may need to seek financial resources for fees and equipment, publicity, and networking with other injury prevention organizations. Grants can be obtained from state and national groups such as the CDC and Emergency Medical Services for Children to help fund injury and disease prevention initiatives. Grants may also be obtained from private donors, community block grants, and institutions. Although funding may not always be easy to obtain, EMS personnel have a duty to provide prevention education on any call where a preventable event has occurred.

EMS Personnel Involvement in Injury Prevention

The community, in addition to financially supporting injury prevention programs, must promote interest and involvement in injury prevention activities from EMS personnel. This support can influence individual participation in the following ways:

- Providing rotating assignments to prevention programs
- Providing salary for off-duty injury prevention activities
- Rewarding and/or remunerating participation for on-duty and off-duty prevention activities

Essential Paramedic Activities

It is essential for paramedics to practice personal injury prevention strategies, including the following:

- Personal wellness (eg, exercise and conditioning, fatigue-reduction strategies)
- Stress management (not just stress related to work, but also related to personal and family life)
- Use of personal protective equipment (eg, reflective clothing, helmets)
- Use of proper lifting and moving techniques and devices
- Appropriate use of audible and visual warning devices (eg, lights and sirens)
- Proper driving techniques (eg, safe approach to parking at, and exiting, the scene)
- Use of ambulance safety restraints for self, patient, and passenger
- Securing of equipment in patient care compartment
- Scene safety precautions, including on-scene survival techniques and resources
- Recognition of health hazards and high-crime areas
- Appropriate use of law enforcement
- Traffic control (eg, vehicles, bystanders)

Another essential activity in which paramedics must engage is review of illnesses and injuries common to the following populations and scenarios:

- Infancy (eg, low birth weight, mortality and morbidity)
- Childhood, including intentional, unintentional, or alleged intentional events
- Childhood violence to self and others
- Adults
- Geriatric patients
- Recreational activities
- Workplace hazards
- Day care centers (licensed and nonlicensed)
- Early release from the hospital
- Discharge from urgent care facilities or other outpatient facilities
- Signs of emotional stress that can signal other health problems
- Dangers of medication noncompliance
- Storage of medicine
- Self-medication, overmedication, and polypharmacy

SHOW ME THE EVIDENCE

For more than a decade, the National Highway Traffic Safety Administration's Special Crash Investigations teams have conducted investigations of serious ambulance crashes. Their findings revealed that 4 in 5 EMS providers in the back of the ambulance were not wearing seat belts at the time of a serious crash. Of the 45 providers in the patient compartment at the time of the crash, only 7 (16%) were wearing a seat belt at the time of the crash, meaning 38 (84%) were unrestrained. In addition, 11 of the providers (22%) driving the ambulance were not wearing seat belts.

Modified from: Smith N. A national perspective on ambulance crashes and safety. EMSWorld.com website. https://www.ems.gov/pdf/EMSWorldAmbulanceCrashArticlesSept2015.pdf. Accessed December 4, 2017.

Implementation and Prevention Strategies

In addition to the primary personal injury prevention strategies listed earlier, other key strategies exist. The paramedic needs to use these prevention strategies for patient care considerations and to recognize the signs and symptoms of exposure to danger and the need for outside assistance. EMS personnel must document primary care and injury data as well. Finally, on-scene education is essential.

Patient Care Considerations

The paramedic needs to identify signs and symptoms of suspected abuse and recognize potentially abusive situations. Such recognition helps to ensure the safety of the EMS crew and the patient (see Chapter 49, *Abuse and Neglect*). Preplanning for these events helps to identify outside resources that may play an important role in injury prevention. Examples include child protective services, abuse support groups, and rape/crisis intervention programs.

Recognition of Dangerous Situations

Personal safety is a priority for the paramedic. EMS personnel must stay alert for signs of dangerous situations, including recognizing general and specific environmental hazards that will help to assess a patient's need for preventive information and direction. Examples include the following:

- Safety hazards in the home
- Inadequate housing conditions
- Inadequate food and clothing
- Absence of protective devices (eg, smoke detectors)
- Hazardous materials (eg, lead-based paint and dangerous chemicals)
- Communicable disease (and potential for transmission)
- Signs of abuse or neglect
- Refusal to receive treatment after narcotic overdose

CRITICAL THINKING

Do you know a paramedic who was injured on the job? How did the injury occur? Can you identify any measures that could have prevented it?

Recognition of the Need for Outside Resources

Most communities have outside resources and services that are usually eager to assist with the development of injury prevention strategies. Such programs may be sponsored by municipal, community, and religious organizations. BOX 3-2 provides a list of outside resources and services that are available in most communities.

Documentation

Taking precise notes of patient care and primary injury data is crucial. This documentation offers a record of the events and assists others with the patient's care (see Chapter 4, *Documentation*). Gathering primary injury data is useful in designing injury prevention strategies. For example, a review of documentation may reveal that when horseback riders sustain serious

BOX 3-2 Outside Resources and Services

Municipal

Animal control services
Child protective services
Fire service personnel
Law enforcement personnel
Social services

Community

Abuse support groups for spouses, children, and older adults
Alternative health care services (eg, free clinics)
Alternative means of transportation
Alternative modes of education
Assistance with obtaining food, shelter, and clothing
Day care services
Disaster services (eg, American Red Cross)
Immunization programs
Managed care organizations
Mental health resources and counseling
Rape or crisis intervention
Rehabilitation programs
Services for the disabled
Substance abuse resources
Work-study programs

Religious

Family counseling
Grief support
Pastoral services
Support groups

head injuries (the primary injury), the rider is rarely wearing a helmet. Primary injury data include the following:

- Scene conditions
- Mechanism of injury
- Use of protective devices
- Absence of protective devices
- Risks at the scene
- Other factors as noted by the EMS agency

On-Scene Education

EMS response to an injury or near-injury may provide for a **teachable moment**, during which the patient and the family may be open to injury prevention tips and strategies. The paramedic can use this opportunity to assess environmental hazards and provide on-scene, one-on-one injury prevention education. The teachable moment involves a three-step process:[10]

1. **Observe the scene.** The first step is to look for contributing factors or hazards at the scene that may have caused the injury. Examples include floor rugs without a nonslip backing and inoperable smoke detectors.
2. **Gather information.** The next step is to gather information from observers. What did they see? Why do they think the injury occurred? Has this been a common occurrence? Patients, family members or bystanders, and first responders may have valuable insight about a situation that caused the injury.
3. **Make assessments.** The final step is to make treatment decisions from the information that has been gathered. The first assessment determines whether the situation is critical or noncritical. If the situation is critical, the focus must be on patient care. If the situation is noncritical, a teachable moment exists—one-on-one injury prevention counseling that may help to prevent another injury. Another assessment uses the information gathered through observation and history taking. These findings help the paramedic decide whether high-risk populations, behaviors, or settings exist and assist in creating the appropriate treatment.

Three common on-scene interventions are discussion, demonstration, and documentation. Discussion involves briefly talking about proper behavior or action with the person at risk in a patient-appropriate manner, which considers the patient's age and education. A paramedic's communication is always nonjudgmental, providing the facts to the patient in a positive, encouraging tone.

A paramedic can demonstrate proper behavior as an injury prevention strategy, for example, by replacing a safety cap on a pill bottle and explaining the importance of doing so to the patient, putting a new battery in a smoke detector, or removing a throw rug from a floor to avoid falls. These on-scene demonstrations can help prevent injuries.

The paramedic should document what was seen, heard, and done at the scene. A written history allows for timely, appropriate follow-up by the receiving personnel. Other injury prevention groups also can use written histories in their data-gathering efforts and for review within the EMS organization to improve established injury prevention programs.

NOTE

Paramedics at St. Charles County Ambulance District in Missouri are trying to capitalize on the teachable moment. In cases where patients are alert and oriented after resuscitation from opiate overdose, they are asked to consent to a follow-up visit. Those who grant permission are contacted by a mobile integrated health care (MIH) paramedic within 24 to 48 hours of their overdose. At that contact, they are assessed for referral and navigated to a substance abuse recovery program. The MIH team has negotiated a higher priority for admission for these patients (even those without insurance) to rehabilitation centers. Since the program's inception in 2017, more than half of those providing written consent have been connected with treatment.

Other Injury Prevention Roles in EMS

In addition to the injury prevention strategies previously discussed, EMS personnel can support legislative change through involvement in primary prevention programs. BOX 3-3 lists additional injury prevention roles.

CRITICAL THINKING

At some point, you probably will visit an older adult family member or friend. Can you identify any potential hazards that exist in that person's home?

BOX 3-3 Injury Prevention Strategies

Bicycle Safety
Bicycle helmet programs

Brain Injury
Brain injury prevention programs

Burns
Fire prevention programs
Smoke detector programs

Children
Babysitter training classes
Child abuse prevention programs
Child safety seat programs
Child safety programs
Drowning prevention programs
EMS for children (EMSC) programs
Parenting classes
Playground safety programs
Safe kids programs
Safe school programs
Swimming classes
Youth advocacy groups

Community Safety
Safe communities programs

Elderly
Programs to reduce falls in the elderly

Firearm Safety
Gun safety programs

Home Safety
Home assessment programs

Legal/Political
Being involved as an expert or advisor in the political process during the debate over laws dealing with the following:

- Child and adolescent safety laws
- Drunk driving laws
- Engineering regulations (building safety into a product)
- Gun legislation
- Helmet laws

The Internet can provide information on ways to prevent medical illness. Some of this material can be passed on to the paramedic's patients informally or through a program with handouts or public service activities. Possible topics include the following:

- Acquired immunodeficiency syndrome
- Cancer
- Cardiovascular health
- Childhood illnesses
- Influenza
- Healthful lifestyle
- Heat-related illness
- Medical conditions A to Z (CDC site)
- Parenting
- Premenstrual syndrome
- Senior citizen illnesses
- Stroke

Most local physician offices have brochures that EMS personnel can provide to patients.

Neurologic Injury
Head injury prevention programs

Nutrition
Proper nutrition programs

Occupational Safety
Occupational illness and injury prevention programs

Pedestrian Safety
Pedestrian safety programs

Poisoning
National Poisoning Prevention Week

Posttraumatic Stress Syndrome
Programs for EMS and other public safety personnel

Public Driving
Programs to prevent driving while intoxicated
Programs to prevent running of red lights
Programs to promote seat belt use

Rehabilitation
Rehabilitation support groups

Research
Universities throughout the United States research many illness and injury prevention strategies and often welcome input from EMS personnel in the form of volunteer work in data collection, ride-alongs with researchers, and assistance in the writing of the research documents. EMS personnel should search for injury prevention centers, illness prevention centers, EMS research centers, and schools of public health within colleges and universities in their local area, where they can find guidance for starting a program if one does not already exist.

Smoking
Smoking cessation programs

BOX 3-3 Injury Prevention Strategies *(continued)*

Substance Abuse

Addiction programs
Public Narcan distribution and education programs
Substance abuse prevention programs
Substance abuse prevention programs for youth

Suicide

Suicide prevention programs

Trauma

National Trauma Awareness Week

Violence

Violence prevention programs
Violence survivor programs

Note: This list is compiled from programs already in place. Some of these programs are national and some are local. Students should seek out programs that already exist in their area. If a program does not exist locally, chances are it exists somewhere in the United States. Students may search the Internet or other sources and find a comparable guide for starting a local program.

Participation in Prevention Programs

Development of effective prevention programs begins with a **community health assessment**. This assessment is needed before the intervention can take place. The assessment also is required before the education can begin.

Community Health Assessment

A systematic approach to a health assessment and prevention programs includes the following steps (**FIGURE 3-4**):

1. Gather information and identify the problem and population.
2. Identify prevention strategies.
3. Choose the best strategy.
4. Develop the plan.
5. Implement the plan.
6. Evaluate and revise the plan as needed.

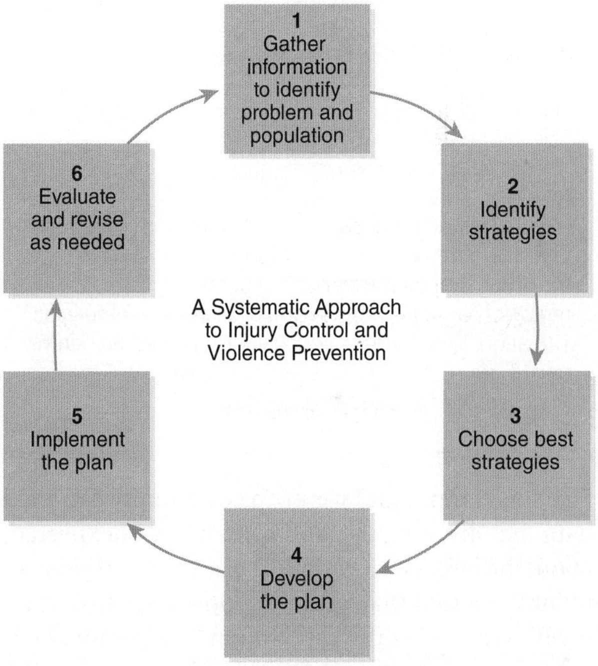

FIGURE 3-4 A systematic approach to health assessment and injury prevention programs.

Paramedics may have limited time and resources to allot to prevention and wellness promotion. To maximize their available time and resources, paramedics can perform a community health assessment to identify the target for community health education (**FIGURE 3-5**). This assessment often is a large undertaking and may be conducted more effectively through a group effort with other health agencies to evaluate the following:

- Population demographics
- Morbidity statistics
- Mortality statistics
- Crime and fire information
- Community resource allocation
- Hospital data (eg, emergency department visits and length of stay)
- Senior citizen needs
- Education standards
- Recreational facilities
- Environmental conditions
- Other factors

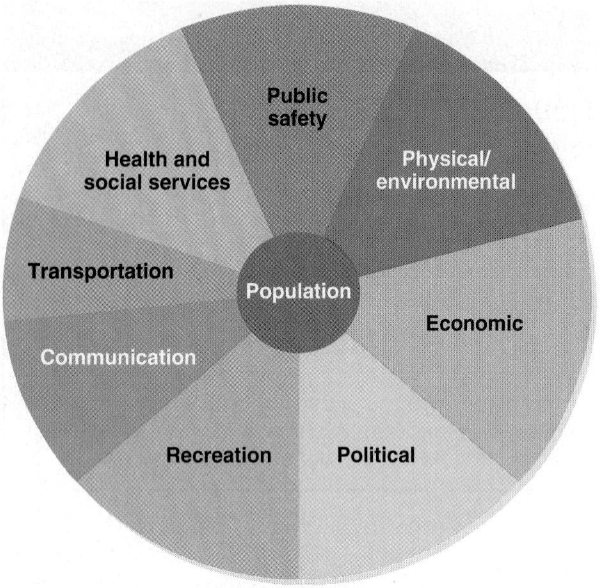

FIGURE 3-5 Community health assessment.

NOTE

Morbidity statistics refer to the disease rate of a population or geographic region. Mortality statistics refer to the number of deaths per unit of population in a specific region or for a specific age group, disease, or other classification. This number is usually expressed as deaths per 1,000, 10,000, or 100,000 (see Chapter 8, *Research Principles and Evidence-Based Practice*).

This "landscape" view of a community can yield data that are valuable, and sometimes unexpected, about the target population. The assessment also can identify factors that relate or contribute to certain health risks. After the assessment, the paramedic is able to target the areas in need of health education and then determine a fitting intervention. Ideally, the paramedic should compare the data from the assessment with those of another population with similar demographics, such as a city of similar size (BOX 3-4).

BOX 3-4 Community Health Information Sources

American Heart Association
American Red Cross
Births and deaths (including cause)
Call types and response times
Census data (public library, Internet)
Centers for Disease Control and Prevention
Chamber of Commerce
Clustering of illnesses and injuries
Communication
Crime rate statistics
Disaster planning
Distribution of age, sex, race, ethnicity
Distribution of grant monies
Education and literacy rates
Emergency coordinating council
EMS systems
Employment statistics
Environmental hazards (sanitation, air quality)
Federal Emergency Management Agency
Federal government
Fire service
Fire-related injuries and fatalities
Form of government
Geographic distribution
Health departments (city, county, state, Internet)
Health services and school lunch programs
Hospitals
Housing and tax information
Industry and economic figures
Infectious disease statistics
Law enforcement
Local government
Location and frequency of fires
National Safety Council
Newspapers, radio, and television stations
Parks and recreation
Population demographics
Religious organizations
Response times
School board
Socioeconomic status
State trauma registry statistics

Community Health Intervention

After identifying a health risk, the paramedic must implement a plan that attempts to reduce or eradicate the risk of illness or injury and improve the health of the community. Primary injury prevention activities prevent injury and disease from occurring; examples include seat belt education, laws requiring bicyclists to wear helmets, and vaccination programs. Secondary injury prevention activities minimize harm after the event happens to prevent complications from the injury or progression of disease; an example is health screenings to detect hypertension. Tertiary injury prevention activities correct and prevent further deterioration of an illness or injury; an example is

BOX 3-5 Prevention Activities

Primary Prevention Activities

Influenza/pneumococcal immunization
Smoking cessation
Preventive dental care
Car seat distribution and installation

Secondary Prevention Activities

General health screenings
Colonoscopy
Mammography
Blood pressure screenings

Tertiary Prevention Activities

Lowering cholesterol after myocardial infarction
Treating hypertension after stroke
Providing examinations for eye and foot problems in diabetic patients

providing EMS illness or injury prevention services in a community. The three types of prevention activities often overlap. BOX 3-5 provides examples of each activity.[11]

Community Health Education

An effective injury prevention program must serve the entire target population in a community. To do so, paramedics must understand the **social determinants of health** that affect a person's health, which include age, culture, religion, relationship status, and social and socioeconomic status, and the strategies needed to improve them.[12] Understanding the social determinants of health provides a foundation for health intervention programs.

Knowledge of the characteristics of the target group ensures proper training of paramedics to meet the needs of special groups before the prevention program is implemented. Examples include training emergency personnel to communicate effectively with the following people:

- Various ethnic, cultural, and religious groups
- Non–English-speaking populations
- Those with learning disabilities
- Those who are physically challenged

The paramedic must consider the reading level and age of the target population. Recognizing these considerations helps to prepare appropriate, effective educational materials. Before starting any type of large-scale educational program, the paramedic should test the program on a target audience to evaluate the appeal of the materials and ensure the message is understood. EMS personnel can provide community health education to promote illness and

DID YOU KNOW?

Immunization Programs

Paramedics are trained to administer medications and can play a vital role in immunization programs in a community. Numerous studies have demonstrated the feasibility of EMS agencies in administering vaccines. The programs followed CDC guidelines and were performed under strict medical oversight. Members of the community were recruited through public service campaigns to visit EMS stations, places of worship, retail establishments, and other public places to receive the vaccine. It was found that paramedics can safely provide immunizations and can sometimes reach populations who otherwise would not have received the medication.

In the event of a pandemic disease outbreak or other disease emergency requiring large-scale vaccination, it is likely that paramedics will provide vaccines and antiviral drugs at emergency dispensing sites in the community. (See Chapter 27, *Infectious and Communicable Disease*, and Chapter 57, *Bioterrorism and Weapons of Mass Destruction*, for more discussion.)

Modified from: Wiler JL, Pines, JM, Ward MJ, eds. *Value and Quality Innovations in Acute and Emergency Care*. Cambridge, UK: Cambridge University Press; 2017; Vaccine information statements (VISs). Centers for Disease Control and Prevention website. https://www.cdc.gov/vaccines/hcp/vis/index.html. Accessed December 4, 2017; Mosesso VN Jr, Packer CR, McMahon J, et al. Influenza immunizations provided by EMS agencies: the MEDICVAX project. *Prehosp Emerg Care*. 2003;7(1):74-78; Emergency dispensing site management. Massachusetts Department of Public Health website. http://sites.bu.edu/masslocalinstitute/2014/11/06/emergency-dispensing-site-management/. Accessed December 4, 2017; and Preparing for pandemic influenza: recommendations for protocol development for 9-1-1 personnel and public safety answering points, May 2007. US Department of Transportation website. https://www.ems.gov/pdf/preparedness/Resources/Pandemic_Influenza_Recommendations_For_911_And_PSAPS.pdf. Published May 3, 2007. Accessed December 4, 2017.

CRITICAL THINKING

What method of health education is most likely to change your personal behaviors? Would that same method be equally effective for a 5-year-old or a 70-year-old person?

injury prevention in numerous ways, including the following:

Verbal
- Lectures
- Informal discussions
- Informal teaching on an EMS call
- Podcasts
- Radio programs

Written/static visual
- Bulletin boards, exhibits
- Flyers, pamphlets, posters
- Models
- Slides, photographs

Dynamic visual
- Videotapes
- Television
- Internet resources (blogs, websites)

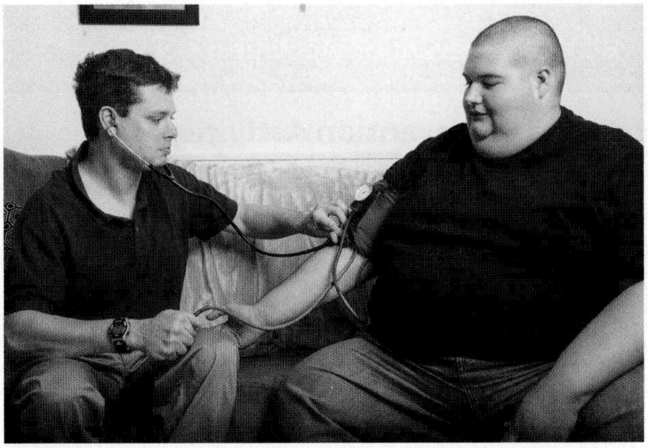

FIGURE 3-6 Mobile integrated health care professional.

Mobile Integrated Health Care and Community Paramedicine

Mobile integrated health care (MIH) is a role in EMS that combines public health and health care for paramedics. The MIH provider is often called a community paramedic (**FIGURE 3-6**). The role of the MIH paramedic varies widely based on community and local health system needs. Likewise, the specific services that MIH programs deliver vary widely based on community needs and the resources within the MIH program (**TABLE 3-3**). In a 2014 survey of 100 agencies with MIH programs, the National Association of Emergency Medical Technicians (NAEMT) found that each community reported different services based on the assessment of needs within their specific community. In many cases patients are referred from hospitals. Services can be provided by the MIH team quickly after discharge, eliminating the gap in patient care until traditional home health care providers can see the patient. Other sources of referral include other health care providers, EMS personnel, primary care physicians, and public health agencies.

Identifying gaps in health care in a community is required for the success of MIH programs. Although

TABLE 3-3 Mobile Integrated Health Care Programs

Program Types	Clinical Services
Readmission avoidance	Respiratory (oxygen saturation level, capnography, peak flow checks; continuous positive airway pressure; medication compliance checks)
Frequent EMS user management	Cardiovascular (blood pressure, 12-lead electrocardiogram, intravenous access)
Chronic disease management	Assessment (history and physical, weight, postinjury evaluation, stroke follow-up, ear examination)
Assessment and navigation to appropriate destinations	Laboratory services (point-of-care blood tests, urine and stool collection, throat swabs). Referral to substance abuse programs.
Primary care/physician extender	Medical services typically provided by a physician (monitoring, medication or fluid administration).

Note: Other services reported included discharge follow-up and wound care, prevention services for falls, social services, psychiatric needs, and patient education or health screening.

Modified from: Mobile integrated healthcare and community paramedicine (MIH-CP). National Association of Emergency Medical Technicians website. http://www.naemt.org/docs/default-source/community-paramedicine/naemt-mih-cp-report.pdf?sfvrsn=df32c792_4. Accessed January 29, 2018.

services and resources vary by state, most public state health departments have identified health needs by county or municipal levels of organization.[13] MIH programs should consult with these public health organizations, providers, hospital staff, clinics, health centers, home health agencies, and others engaged in meeting community needs.

Several challenges face MIH programs. Chief among them are financial sustainability and regulatory barriers. Only 36% of services surveyed by the NAEMT reported any revenue from these programs.[14] It will take meticulous data gathering and research to prove the safety, efficiency, and effectiveness of the MIH programs to ensure they can continue.

Summary

- EMS personnel are members of the community health care system. They can be an important resource in injury prevention.
- Unintentional injuries are the fifth leading cause of death. This cause is exceeded only by heart disease, cancer, stroke, and chronic obstructive pulmonary disease.
- The United States has more than 826,000 EMS personnel. This valuable human resource plays a major role in public education and community wellness activities.
- Paramedics play an active role in the health of a community. As such, the community has a responsibility to support paramedics by protecting EMS workers from injury, providing community liaisons to help establish injury and illness prevention programs, supplying support and promoting the collection and use of injury data, obtaining resources for primary injury prevention activities, and empowering paramedics to conduct primary injury prevention.
- Paramedics must have a basic knowledge of injury and illness prevention. They also should know about key strategies to monitor and manage chronic illness.
- The paramedic needs to note the signs and symptoms of abuse and abusive situations. In addition, the paramedic should notice exposure to danger.
- Paramedics should identify and use outside community resources. Also, they should document primary injury and illness data and contribute to appropriate databases.
- Paramedics should identify and properly employ the teachable moment.
- The paramedic must maximize time and resources by performing a community health assessment to identify target areas for community health education, keeping in mind the social determinants of health.
- To identify community education goals, the paramedic must understand several factors relating to illness or injury: (1) the extent or exposure to an agent, (2) the strength of the agent, (3) the susceptibility of the person (host), and (4) the biological, social, and physical environment.
- Primary injury prevention involves preventing an injury or illness from occurring. Secondary prevention, which includes screening to detect injury early, and tertiary prevention help to prevent further problems from an event that has already occurred.
- An effective injury prevention program must serve the whole target population in a community, taking into account the population's reading level and age. The paramedic can provide community health education in diverse ways, including written material and dynamic verbal and visual presentations.
- MIH programs help bridge the gap between prehospital and traditional health care. MIH programs provide a variety of nonemergency services based on the health needs of the community.

References

1. National Vital Statistics System, National Center for Health Statistics. Ten leading causes of death by age group, United States—2015. Injury Center. Centers for Disease Control and Prevention website. https://www.cdc.gov/injury/wisqars/pdf/leading_causes_of_death_by_age_group_2015-a.pdf. Accessed December 4, 2017.
2. National Vital Statistics System, National Center for Health Statistics. Number of deaths for leading causes of death. Centers for Disease Control and Prevention website. https://www.cdc.gov/nchs/fastats/leading-causes-of-death.htm. Accessed December 4, 2017.
3. National Center for Health Statistics. All injuries. Centers for Disease Control and Prevention website. https://www.cdc.gov/nchs/fastats/injury.htm. Updated May 3, 2017. Accessed December 4, 2017.
4. National Safety Council. *Injury Facts: 2017 Edition*. Itasca, NY: National Safety Council; 2017.
5. National Center for Health Statistics. National Health Interview Survey. Centers for Disease Control and Prevention website. https://www.cdc.gov/nchs/nhis/. Updated November 16, 2017. Accessed December 4, 2017.
6. The Healthcare Imperative: Lowering Costs and Improving Outcomes. Workshop Series Summary Institute of Medicine (US) Roundtable on Evidence-Based Medicine. Yong PL, Saunders RS, Olsen LA, eds. Washington, DC: National Academies Press; 2010.
7. Holder Y, Peden M, Krug E, Lund J, Gururaj G, Kobusingye O, eds. *Injury Surveillance Guidelines*. Geneva, Switzerland: World Health Organization; 2001.

8. The National Institute for Occupational Safety and Health, Division of Safety and Health. Workplace safety and health topics: emergency medical services workers. Centers for Disease Control and Prevention website. https://www.cdc.gov/niosh/topics/ems/. Updated September 8, 2017. Accessed December 4, 2017.
9. National Highway Traffic Safety Administration. *Emergency Medical Services: Agenda for the Future*. Washington, DC: National Highway Traffic Safety Administration; 1996.
10. Yancey AH II, Martinez R, Kellermann AL. Injury prevention and emergency medical services: *the "Accidents Aren't" program. Prehosp Emerg Care*. 2002(Apr-Jun);6(2):204-209.
11. Society, the individual and medicine: categories of prevention. University of Ottawa website. https://www.med.uottawa.ca/sim/data/Prevention_e.htm. Updated January 25, 2016. Accessed December 4, 2017.
12. Healthy people 2020: social determinants of health. Office of Disease Prevention and Health Promotion website. https://www.healthypeople.gov/2020/topics-objectives/topic/social-determinants-of-health. Accessed December 4, 2017.
13. NASEMSO CP-MIH Committee. Community health needs assessment for community paramedicine and mobile integrated healthcare. National Association of State EMS Officials website. https://www.nasemso.org/Projects/MobileIntegratedHealth/documents/CHNAs-Resources-for-CP-MIH-08May2017.pdf. Published May 2017. Accessed December 4, 2017.
14. Mobile integrated healthcare and community paramedicine (MIH-CP). National Association of Emergency Medical Technicians website. https://www.naemt.org/docs/default-source/MIH-CP/naemt-mih-cp-report.pdf. Published 2014. Accessed December 4, 2017.

Suggested Readings

Brownson RC, Baker EA, Deshpande AD, Gillespie KN. *Evidence-Based Public Health*. 3rd ed. New York, NY: Oxford University Press; 2018.

Brydges M, Denton M, Agarwal G. The CHAP-EMS health promotion program: a qualitative study on participants' view of the role of paramedics. *BMC Health Serv Res*. 2016;16:435.

Benney A, Hjermstad K, Wilcox M, eds. *Community Health Paramedicine*. Burlington, MA: Jones & Bartlett Learning; 2018.

Centers for Disease Control and Prevention, National Center for Injury Prevention and Control. *National Action Plan for Child Injury Prevention*. Atlanta, GA: Centers for Disease Control and Prevention; 2012.

Community paramedicine: mobile integrated health documents and resources. National Association of EMS Officials website. https://www.nasemso.org/Projects/MobileIntegratedHealth/Documents-Resources.asp. Accessed December 4, 2017.

Frieden TR. A framework for public health action: the health impact pyramid. *Am J Public Health*. 2010 April;100(4):590-595.

Krug EG, Sharma GK, Lozano R. The global burden of injuries. *Am J Pub Health*. 2000;90(4):523-526.

Schell SF, Luke DA, Schooley MW, et al. Public health program capacity for sustainability: a new framework. *Implementation Science*. February 2013;8:15.

Stanhope M, Lancaster J. *Public Health Nursing: Population-Centered Health Care in the Community*. 9th ed. Maryland Heights, MO: Elsevier; 2015.

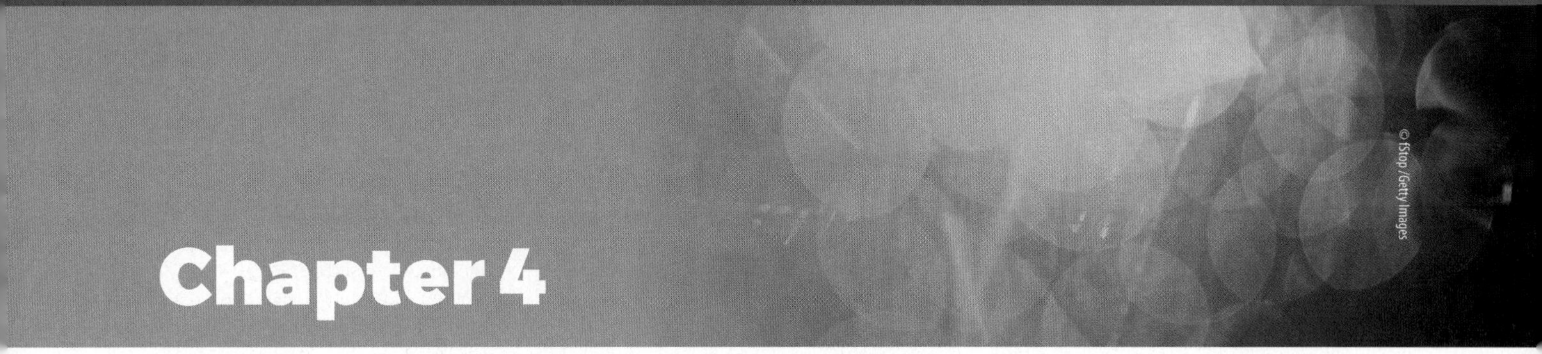

Chapter 4

Documentation

NATIONAL EMS EDUCATION STANDARD COMPETENCIES

Preparatory

Integrates comprehensive knowledge of EMS systems, the safety/well-being of the paramedic, and medical/legal and ethical issues which is intended to improve the health of EMS personnel, patients, and the community.

Documentation

- Recording patient findings (pp 84–85)
- Principles of medical documentation and report writing (pp 85–89)

OBJECTIVES

Upon completion of this chapter, the paramedic student will be able to:

1. Identify the purpose of the patient care report. (pp 84–85)
2. Describe the uses of the patient care report. (p 85)
3. Outline the components of an accurate, thorough patient care report. (pp 85–88)
4. Describe the elements of a properly written EMS document. (p 88)
5. Describe an effective system for documenting the narrative section of a prehospital patient care report. (pp 89–90)
6. Identify documentation considerations related to billing. (pp 90–91)
7. Identify important differences in the documentation of special situations. (pp 91–93)
8. Describe the appropriate method for revising or correcting the patient care report. (p 93)
9. Recognize consequences that may result from inappropriate documentation. (pp 93–94)

KEY TERMS

electronic patient care report (ePCR) An electronic program used in the prehospital setting to record all patient care activities and circumstances related to an emergency response.

military time A precise method of expressing time that is used by the armed forces and is based on a 24-hour clock.

narrative The portion of the patient care report that allows a provider to describe events during a call often not captured in prepopulated check boxes or drop-down menus.

objective information Information based on observable facts, such as clinical signs.

patient care report (PCR) A document used in the prehospital setting to record all patient care activities and circumstances related to a request for service.

pertinent negative findings Findings that warrant no medical care or intervention but that provide evidence of the thoroughness of the patient examination and the history of the event.

pertinent oral statements Statements made by the patient and other people at the scene.

pertinent positive findings Signs or symptoms that help substantiate the patient's condition.

subjective information Information based on opinions expressed by patients or others or information based on subjective feelings of the patient, such as clinical symptoms.

The patient care report is used to document the essential elements of patient assessment, care, and transport. It is a legal document, and in addition to contributing to good patient care, it can be good protection from liability action.

Importance of Documentation

Thorough written documentation by the EMS provider is important for many reasons (BOX 4-1). Documentation provides a tangible and legal record of an incident. This information is also used by physicians, nurses, and others involved in the patient's care after handoff from the EMS provider. Hospital staff members read the **patient care report (PCR)** to understand the patient's initial condition, identify the type of care given in the field, and determine whether time-critical treatment benchmarks were achieved. In addition, the EMS agency and medical director may use the PCR to bill for services provided, monitor care in the field, evaluate an individual paramedic's performance, and conduct review conferences and other educational forums. In summary, the four main reasons for charting patient care[1] are as follows:

- Demonstrate the continuity of the patient care provided.
- Create a legal record of the patient care provided.
- Assist in financial reimbursement and cost recovery for patient care services and equipment and supplies.
- Assist in quality improvement studies and EMS research.

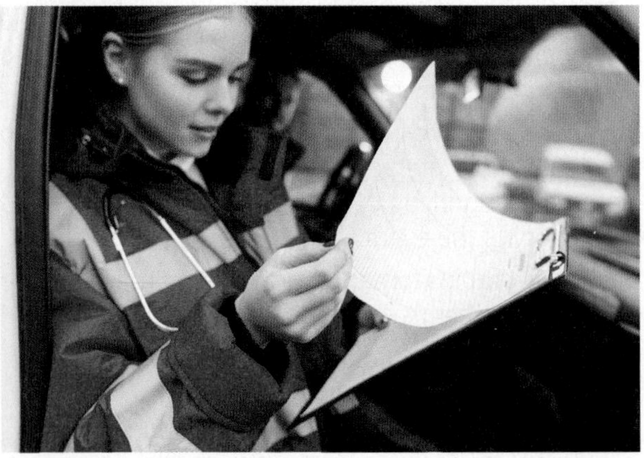

© LightField Studios/Shutterstock

BOX 4-1 Advantages of Written Documentation

Written documentation enables or provides:

- A tangible, legal record of the incident
- Validation of professionalism
- A medical audit
- Quality improvement
- Billing and administration information
- Data collection

NOTE

The requirements for retaining medical records vary throughout the United States and are dictated by each state. Most medical records (including PCRs) must be maintained for at least 10 years for adults. The requirements for minors vary widely, with most states requiring retention of these records until several years after the child reaches the age of majority. These records are kept as a safety measure in case legal action involving a claim of neglect arises. Thorough documentation is essential. It leads to good communication with other providers of care and accurate recall if litigation occurs.

Modified from: McWay D. *Legal Aspects of Health Information Management.* 4th ed. Clifton Park, NY: Cengage Learning; 2016; and Office of the National Coordinator for Health Information Technology. Records retention requirements by state. https://www.healthit.gov/sites/default/files/appa7-1.pdf. Accessed February 5, 2018.

Data collection and record keeping are important for identifying quality improvement issues (see Chapter 1, *EMS Systems: Roles, Responsibilities, and Professionalism*). Issues that may be identified through the PCR, and subsequently prompt policy changes to improve patient care, include the following:

- Minimizing the time spent at the scene with critical trauma patients
- Adding new medications to better manage some medical emergencies

- Changing the placement of emergency vehicles during peak response times in certain demographic areas

The PCR also documents any unique scene situations that may have affected patient care. For example, traffic may have caused a long response time. A trapped patient may have required prolonged extrication. The PCR and the data uploaded with it also help track certain patient care skills of the paramedic (eg, insertion of intravenous lines, intubation, electrocardiogram (ECG) interpretation, cardiopulmonary resuscitation performance, and defibrillation). The EMS agency's training division may require tracking of these skills as part of personnel records. In some states, documentation of advanced life support (ALS) skills may be required for relicensure or recertification.

General Considerations

The PCR is a legal document and part of the patient's medical record. The document should be legible and carefully detailed and should avoid slang terms and medical abbreviations that are not universally accepted. Chapter 9, *Medical Terminology*, identifies many of the medical abbreviations and symbols commonly used in EMS documentation.

The report should include all dates and response times, noted in **military time**. In addition, paramedics must describe any difficulties encountered en route or during patient treatment, extrication, or transport as well as observations at the scene, previous medical care provided (and by whom), and the time of patient extrication, if appropriate (BOX 4-2). Recording the times of all significant occurrences and interventions is useful to the receiving physician. In particular, the PCR provides a legal and accurate recording of the following incident times:

- Time of the call
- Time of dispatch
- Time of arrival at the scene
- Time at the patient's side
- Time(s) of vital signs assessments
- Time(s) of medication administration and certain medical procedures as defined by local protocol
- Time of departure from the scene
- Time of arrival at the medical facility (when a patient is transported)
- Time back in service

BOX 4-2 Data Included in the Patient Care Report

- Dates
- Response times
- Difficulties encountered en route
- Communication difficulties
- Scene observations
- Reasons for extended on-scene time
- Previous care provided
- Time of extrication
- Time of patient transport
- Reason for hospital selection (trauma center designation, patient choice, or other concerns)

NOTE

Most EMS agencies and patient care facilities use military time to chart patient care activities and to note other entries in the patient care record. Military time uses a 24-hour clock, which makes notation of AM or PM unnecessary. It is considered a precise method of expressing time. Military time begins at midnight (0000 hours).

NOTE

The National EMS Information System (NEMSIS) has developed a comprehensive list of all potential elements of information that would be collected about an emergency incident, known as the EMS Dataset. (Version 3 is the latest version available as of this text's publication.) These elements include all information that would be considered important from the perspectives of an EMS system, EMS personnel, and an EMS patient; thus, they provide documentation of both system performance and clinical care. The goal of NEMSIS is to create a national EMS database that contains information from local and state EMS agencies across the United States. Participants can use these data for both benchmarking and planning purposes. All states and territories have agreed to participate in and support the EMS data initiatives set by NEMSIS. As of this text's publication, only three states had not submitted data to the system, and all are working toward meeting that goal.

Modified from: National Highway Traffic Safety Administration, Office of EMS. NEMSIS: V3 national requisite elements. https://nemsis.org/technical-resources/version-3/version-3-national-requisite-elements/. Accessed February 5, 2018.

When testimony must be given years after an incident (see Chapter 6, *Medical and Legal Issues*), the PCR may be the only means by which a paramedic can recall accurately the events of an emergency response. A PCR that provides sufficient detail is critical.

SHOW ME THE EVIDENCE

A substantial amount of research has shown disparities in devices used to record time of EMS responses. When researchers from Pennsylvania and New York compared the accuracy of timing devices used on EMS calls to atomic time, they found the devices to be only 36.9% accurate. Although watches were used most often to record time on EMS calls, the time on cell phones (61.5%) was most accurate, followed by the time on watches (28.4%). None of the ambulance clocks was within 1 minute of accuracy.

Modified from: Frisch AN, Dailey MW, Heeren D, Stern M. Precision of time devices used by prehospital providers. *Prehosp Emerg Care*. 2009;13(2):247-250.

CRITICAL THINKING

Documentation of specific times on the PCR is important. How can this information be useful?

The Narrative

The **narrative** section of the PCR provides a chronological account of the call. The creation of a narrative is essential to ensure an effective and complete patient care record. It summarizes the incident history and care in a manner that is easily shared between caregivers. The narrative facilitates continuity of care and provides a place for EMS to document facts that do not fit into fixed data fields.

Paramedics should write the narrative concisely and clearly, using simple words. They should not use uncommon abbreviations or unnecessary terms or include duplicate information. Paramedics should use the standard report format established by their EMS system's medical direction. Adherence to a standardized format can aid quality improvement efforts, which are often based on reviews of PCR data.

Components of the PCR's narrative include the following:

- Dispatch complaint and information
- Initial contact
- All patient care activities (including medications and treatments administered, in addition to care provided by others at the scene prior to EMS arrival)
- Pertinent oral statements
- Initial assessment and vital signs
- Chief complaint or concern
- Pertinent significant medical history
- Time of hospital contact
- Time of physician's orders and advice (name of physician)
- Detailed information related to physical examination findings
- Pertinent positive and negative examination findings
- Treatments and the reason they were performed
- Patient's response to treatment
- Changes in the patient's status
- Vital signs reassessment
- ECG interpretation
- Diagnostic readings (eg, capnography, pulse oximetry, serum glucose)
- Use of support services
- Measures used to move the patient
- Destination and reason for selecting that destination
- Time of delivery and patient's condition on arrival at destination
- Name of receiving health care worker
- Signature of paramedic

Pertinent findings may be classified as positive or negative. Both types should be documented in the PCR, because both can help determine the course of treatment. **Pertinent positive findings** are signs or symptoms that help substantiate the patient's condition. Examples of positive findings include difficulty breathing, numbness or paralysis, and altered mental status. **Pertinent negative findings** are findings that warrant no medical care or intervention but show

NOTE

Paramedics should never use documentation to creatively reconstruct patient care. If the paramedic did not document the care, it is rational to presume that it was not done. Conversely, if the care was not done, the paramedic should not document it. Falsifying a patient care record, in addition to being unethical, may constitute Medicare fraud and abuse, a violation of the False Claims Act, or both.

SHOW ME THE EVIDENCE

Researchers reviewed the records of 4,744 trauma patients in King County, Washington, and studied whether either basic life support (BLS) requests for advanced life support (ALS) response to the scene or physiologic findings on the scene were associated with in-hospital mortality. Using multivariate analyses, they found that patients for whom one or more measures of patient physiology (ie, systolic blood pressure, pulse, respiratory rate, or Glasgow Coma Scale score) were missing on the record had double the risk of death. No difference of risk of death was identified in situations where BLS providers called for ALS assistance to the scene.

Although the researchers initially suspected that this relationship could be explained by higher patient acuity requiring more care on the scene, the conclusions did not change even after they adjusted the data for injury severity. The researchers also considered whether EMS training, proficiency, scene leadership, staffing, and resources might explain their findings. Although the exact cause of this variation in death rates was not determined, the authors suggested the presence versus absence of data on the PCR could serve as a quality measure to trigger further analysis and performance improvement in a trauma system.

Modified from: Laudermilch DJ, Schiff MA, Nathens AB, Rosengart MR. Lack of emergency medical services documentation is associated with poor patient outcomes: a validation of audit filters for prehospital trauma care. *J Am Coll Surg*. 2010;2:220-227.

the thoroughness of the paramedic's examination of the patient and the history of the event and can help rule out some clinical conditions. Examples of negative findings include the absence of diminished breath sounds, the absence of skin rashes, and the absence of abdominal tenderness. BOX 4-3 describes the documentation of pertinent negative findings related to medications.

BOX 4-3 Medications Given: Showing Positive Action Using Pertinent Negatives

When a medication is required by protocol but is not given, pertinent negatives can be used to explain why. This scenario might occur when a patient with chest pain has taken a proper dose of aspirin in accordance with the dispatcher's prearrival instructions. Appropriate documentation shows this information as a medication given, prior to arrival, with the best estimated time of its administration, and qualifies the medication as "medication already taken" using the pertinent negative.

Pertinent oral statements are statements made by the patient and others on the scene and should be documented. Statements that may have an effect on patient care or resolution of the situation can relate to the following:

- Mechanism of injury
- Patient's behavior
- Aid given before arrival of EMS
- Safety-related information (including disposition of weapons)
- Information of interest to crime scene investigators
- Disposition of valuable personal property (eg, jewelry and wallets)

Paramedics can use quotation marks to indicate any direct statements made by patients or others that suggest suicidal intention or possible criminal activity.

Additionally, paramedics need to document details in the PCR narrative such as unsuccessful attempts at endotracheal intubation or the patient's response to treatment and the use of support services and mutual aid assistance (eg, helicopter, coroner, or rescue or extrication team).

A paper-based report requires a paramedic's signature. For most types of **electronic patient care reports (ePCRs)**, the unique password used to sign in constitutes an electronic signature when the report is submitted.

CRITICAL THINKING

Why should you note the previous care given by bystanders in your report?

The PCR should list everyone who took part in the patient's care before delivery to the emergency department (ED). Because a copy of the report is placed in the patient's hospital medical record, paramedics may need to leave a completed copy at the receiving hospital. This means that the report must be completed in a timely fashion so it is available to the hospital quickly.

NOTE

Even electronic reports that allow automatic selections require a narrative. The narrative tells the story of the call in a coherent sequence. Details such as the patient's appearance, the appearance of the patient's home or vehicle, the mechanism of injury, and specific statements made by the patient often are not included in an electronic report if a narrative is not written.

If possible, the report should be left with the patient at the hospital or transmitted to this facility immediately.

NOTE

The National Association of State EMS Officials has developed guidelines for universal documentation that emphasize important aspects of narrative writing for EMS responders. These guidelines include recommended formats for the narrative section of the PCR.

Modified from: National Association of EMS Officials. *National Model EMS Clinical Guidelines, Version 2.0*. NASEMSO website. https://nasemso.org/Projects/ModelEMSClinicalGuidelines/index.asp. Published September 2017. Accessed November 30, 2017.

Elements of a Properly Written EMS Document

A properly written EMS document is accurate and complete, legible, timely, unaltered, and free of nonprofessional or extraneous information.

- **Accurate and complete.** All relevant information must be provided in the narrative and check-box sections of the report; this ensures accuracy. Completion of all areas of the report (even a section that was unused) is the sign of a precise, thorough document. The paramedic should make sure medical terms, abbreviations, and acronyms are used properly and spelled correctly.
- **Legible.** Handwritten reports must be easy for others to read. Check-box markings should be clear and consistent throughout all pages of the report.
- **Timely.** Ideally, the documentation is completed immediately after the paramedic completes the patient care. Delays in recording can result in serious omissions, which may be interpreted as negligence in patient care.
- **Unaltered.** If an error is made during documentation of a handwritten PCR, the paramedic should draw a single line through the error and then date and initial the error (**FIGURE 4-1**). Any changes to a completed ePCR should be done following proper "revision/correction" protocols with the date and time of revision.
- **Free of nonprofessional and extraneous information.** The PCR must be free of jargon, slang, personal bias, libelous or slanderous remarks, and irrelevant opinions or impressions.

FIGURE 4-1 Correction of a patient care report.

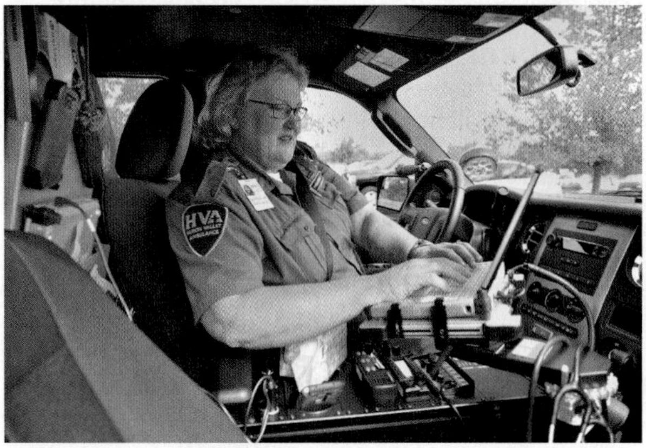

FIGURE 4-2 Paramedic completing an electronic patient care report.

These same five principles of documentation apply to ePCRs (**FIGURE 4-2**) and other computer-generated forms. Related documentation (eg, ECG or capnography tracings, photographs, insurance information) should be properly labeled and attached, scanned, or uploaded with the report.

NOTE

An EMS report is confidential. Paramedics must comply with all patient privacy provisions as outlined by the policies of their agency and by the Health Insurance Portability and Accountability Act (see Chapter 6, *Medical and Legal Issues*).

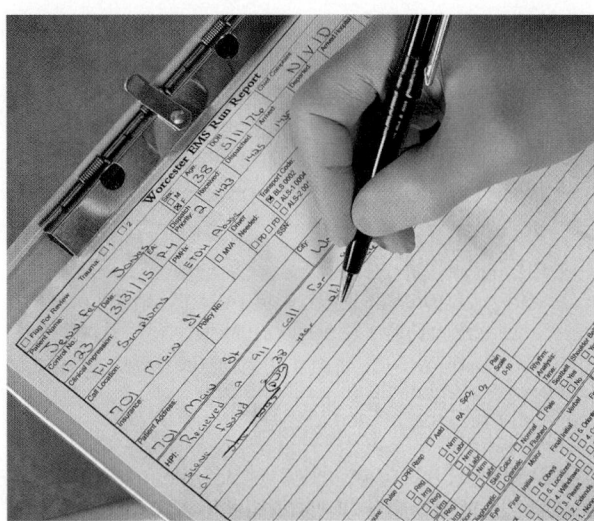

Systems of Narrative Writing

As with all other aspects of emergency care, paramedics should develop a systematic approach to writing the PCR narrative. Although many approaches can be used for this purpose, the best practice is to adopt only *one* approach and to use it consistently, which helps prevent omissions in report writing. Additionally, maintaining consistency in formatting makes it easy for others who use the report (eg, hospital physicians, quality improvement officers, billing personnel) to find information quickly.

In the past, EMS providers were poorly trained in documentation. It is important for training programs to emphasize proper documentation strategies and to allow for sufficient practice.

Regardless of the system used, the paramedic must make sure **objective information** (facts), rather than **subjective information** (opinion), is the focus of the report.

> NOTE
>
> Objective information is supported by facts and direct observation (eg, obvious deformity). Subjective information cannot be supported by facts (eg, the patient says he or she is depressed). In the narrative, subjective information should be entered in the patient's own words when possible, enclosed within quotation marks. Some subjective information, such as observations in a patient's home suggestive of child abuse, needs to be reported to medical direction.

Narrative Formats

Formats that have been established to organize the narrative include the SAMPLE history (presented in detail in Chapter 17, *History Taking*), the SOAP format, the CHART format, and the CHEATED charting method. Other approaches also may be used to write the narrative, including the head-to-toe physical approach; a review of primary body systems approach; a chronological, call-incident approach; and a patient management approach.

SAMPLE History

The elements of the *SAMPLE history* include the following:

- **S**igns and symptoms
- **A**llergies
- **M**edications
- **P**ast medical history
- **L**ast meal or oral intake
- **E**vents before the emergency

SOAP Format

The SOAP format can be used to organize a patient report for most patient care encounters. It includes the following elements:

- **Subjective data.** All of the patient's symptoms, including the chief complaint, associated symptoms, history, current medications, and allergies, in addition to information provided by the patient, bystanders, and family.
- **Objective data.** Pertinent physical examination information, including vital signs, level of consciousness, physical examination findings, ECG data, pulse oximetry readings, and blood glucose determinations.
- **Assessment data.** The paramedic's clinical impression of the patient based on subjective and objective data.
- **Plan of patient management.** Treatment that has been provided and any requests for additional treatment.

CHART Format

The CHART format is an alternative to the SAMPLE and SOAP methods. It includes the following elements:

- **Chief complaint or concern.** The patient's primary complaint (chest pain) or the chief concern (unresponsive).
- **History.** The history of the current illness or injury, including where and how the patient was found, any significant medical history, the patient's current health status, and a review of systems.
- **Assessment.** The paramedic's general impression, vital signs, physical examination findings, diagnostic tests, and field diagnosis.
- **Rx (treatment).** Treatment provided based on protocols or direct orders from online medical direction and the patient's response to that treatment.
- **Transport.** Transport mode, destination, and the rationale for choosing that location; patient changes in condition en route to other destination; where the patient was delivered and to whom patient handoff was given; and any patient changes in condition during transport.

CHEATED Charting Method

The CHEATED charting method begins with the initial patient contact and ends when the patient is delivered to the ED. It includes the following elements:

- **Chief complaint or chief concern.** The reason the patient or others requested EMS assistance.
- **History.** Past and present medical history, nature of incident, and mechanism of injury.
- **Examination.** The physical assessment.
- **Assessment.** General impression and diagnosis.
- **Treatment.** Any care rendered.
- **Evaluation.** The patient's response to the care provided (improvement or deterioration).
- **Disposition.** The transfer of patient care to another health care professional.

Head-to-Toe Physical Approach

Paramedics often use the head-to-toe physical approach to record their findings after performing a full head-to-toe physical examination. Findings are noted in the narrative in the same order as they occurred in the examination. For example, findings from the examination of the patient's head are noted first (eg, pupillary response). The paramedic ends by noting circulatory findings (eg, the character of a pedal pulse or capillary refill) from the examination of the patient's extremities.

When findings are documented using this approach, it is important to be specific about the locations of significant wounds, devices, or injuries. Documenting "wound found on the right upper chest" is too vague. Instead, write "2.5 cm linear wound with no subcutaneous fat visible and minimal bleeding found on the right anterior chest approximately 5 cm inferior to the clavicle at the midclavicular line."

Primary Body Systems Approach

A review of primary body systems approach may be used when the examination is performed for a chief complaint that focuses on one body system. For example, for a patient who reports chest pain and for whom myocardial infarction is suspected, the paramedic would limit the findings to the cardiorespiratory system. Findings may include a description of the patient's pain, vital signs, ECG findings, associated breathing difficulties, significant medical history, allergies, and medication use.

Chronological, Call-Incident Approach

The chronological, call-incident approach begins by noting the time of arrival at the patient's side and the initial examination findings, the times of vital signs assessment and reassessment, and a chronological listing of all patient care interventions performed at the scene and en route to the ED. This format is considered less desirable, as other parties (eg, hospital care providers) may have difficulty retrieving key information efficiently when reading the report. This type of report may be used to document the events surrounding a patient with major trauma who requires extended on-scene time, such as during a cardiac arrest event, when numerous medications are administered and procedures are performed.

Patient Management Approach

The patient management approach, also called the medical narrative approach, is used to organize and record the complete patient management plan. A report created using this format covers the emergency response from start to finish. The paramedic might describe in detail how the patient was found, which interventions were performed and why, and any important assessment findings. The patient management approach differs slightly from the other narrative formatting options described here in that it provides a more complete picture of the events at the scene, during care, and during transport of the patient.

Billing Considerations

Although a paramedic's primary focus is on patient care, reimbursement for service is critical to maintain the operating budget of most EMS systems. Paramedics need to ensure that their patient care documentation meets the requirements necessary to collect payment for their services. Without supporting documents, appropriate wages, supplies, and equipment maintenance are not possible.

By taking a few extra minutes to document carefully and to obtain necessary supporting documents, paramedics can increase the chances that their system will be paid for the call. In almost all cases, signatures from the patient or the guardian giving permission to release information and bill the call should be obtained. This information can be gathered later, but waiting greatly reduces the chance of collection and timely payment.

For most nonemergency scheduled transports, the burden of documentation for reimbursement is even greater. The following elements are important to ensure billing documentation requirements are met for non–9-1-1 patient transports:

- A physician certification statement about why ambulance transport is needed. This statement does not guarantee reimbursement, but it is an important supporting document.
- Documentation (if available) about why the patient needs transport by ambulance as opposed to other means. For example, merely documenting that oxygen is needed is not sufficient; many patients have home oxygen supplies and travel without using an ambulance. Documenting that the patient needs oxygen because the home oxygen delivery system is not adequately maintaining the normal oxygen saturation is preferred. If the patient is confined to bed, document the reason for this status; then note how the patient was moved to the stretcher to more fully justify the need for ambulance transport.

CRITICAL THINKING

How many meanings can you think of for the word *lethargic*? Look up the definition. Should you use this word to document a patient's mental status? Why?

Special Considerations in Documentation

Several considerations in the documentation of patient care deserve special mention, some of which include a patient's refusal of care or transport, situations and events in which transportation is not needed, interagency and interfacility transfers, mass-casualty situations, and exposure or injury reporting. Other special situations (eg, legal reporting, caring for intoxicated patients, and cases of abuse and neglect) are discussed in Chapter 6, *Medical and Legal Issues* **TABLE 4-1**.

Patient's Refusal of Care or Transport

A patient's refusal of care or transport is a major area of potential liability for paramedics and EMS agencies (see Chapter 6, *Medical and Legal Issues*). Thorough documentation of these situations is crucial and should include the following elements:[1]

- Clinical information that suggests the patient possesses decision-making capacity. This information is far more than simply noting "A and O × 3" (alert and oriented to person, place, and time), but rather should illustrate capacity indicators such as, but not limited to, intact immediate and delayed recall, simple math ability, abstract and concrete thinking ability, and the ability to follow simple directions.
- The physical assessment findings.
- The paramedic's advice to the patient about the benefits of treatment and the risks associated with refusing care.
- The advice provided by online medical direction.
- The signatures of any witnesses to the event, according to local protocol.
- Any care provided.
- Aftercare instructions given to the patient or others.
- A statement that the patient was told to call again if he or she changes his or her mind or if the condition worsens.
- A complete narrative, including quotations or statements made by others.

If the patient refuses care or transport, the paramedic should document the incident in exacting detail (Table 4-1). When possible, friends or family members should be encouraged to stay with the patient.

Cases in Which Care and Transport Are Not Needed

At times, care and transport of a patient are not required, perhaps because of the patient's condition or because a request for help is canceled. After evaluating the patient or the scene, the paramedic may determine that circumstances do not warrant EMS transport (eg, for a car crash without injuries, a lift assist, or a patient who has left the scene). At this point, the paramedic should advise the dispatch center and document the event. If the EMS unit is canceled en route to the scene, the paramedic should make note of the canceling authority and the time of the cancellation. The canceling authority, for example, may be the dispatch center or the EMS supervisor. As with refusal of care, thorough documentation of

TABLE 4-1 Documenting Refusal of Care

Component to Document	Details to Document
Patient level of consciousness and orientation	• Alert and oriented to person, place, time, and location
Evidence that patient has decision-making capacity	• Patient can repeat back recent events, follow directions, understand instructions
Physical assessment	• List pertinent positive and negative history and physical examination findings relevant to the situation • Record vital signs appropriate to complaint • Include documentation that patient does not display evidence of intoxication with drugs or alcohol (if relevant)
Risks of refusal	• Explain possible benefits of treatment and consequences of refusing care from minor to very serious • Document specific information provided to patient related to abnormal findings and why they are of concern
Medical direction	• Note whether medical direction was contacted; who was contacted; advice medical direction provided
Care provided	• Detail the interventions performed
Aftercare instructions	• Provide instructions to patient about how to care for the illness or injury (verbal and sometimes written) • Tell patient-related signs or symptoms that would indicate worsening of his or her condition • Instruct patient to call again if condition worsens or if patient changes their mind
Narrative	• Detail the sequence of events, including quotes or statements made by others • Note names and relationship of others on the scene who encouraged patient to be treated
Signatures	• Patient (based on protocol) signs a statement indicating their wish to refuse treatment and/or transport • Witness other than the partner if possible (preferably law enforcement officer) to attest the patient signed the refusal

these events can protect the paramedic from potential liability (see Chapter 6, *Medical and Legal Issues*), depending on your local protocols.

Interagency and Interfacility Transfers

Interagency transfers are those in which patient care duties are assigned (or "turned over") to another EMS unit. For example, a BLS unit may intercept an ALS unit that is better able to manage the patient's needs, or a fire rescue squad that provided initial emergency care but that does not have transport duties or capabilities may turn over transport duties for a patient in critical condition to air ambulance personnel for speedier transport to a hospital. Documentation, tracking, and reporting systems should be established for these situations and followed consistently.

Interfacility (hospital to hospital) transfers occur between hospitals and other facilities as approved by medical direction. They are arranged by the sending hospital to maximize the patient's safety and care. Some interfacility transfers are done for critical care patients, such as pediatric trauma patients, patients with severe burns, transplant candidates, patients with ST-segment elevation myocardial infarction, and patients with indwelling medical devices that support life (see the Appendix B, *Advanced Practice Procedures for Critical Care Paramedics*). In some cases, medical personnel from the sending hospital may accompany the patient during the interfacility transfer. Such personnel include physicians, critical care nurses, respiratory therapists, or other specialty care professionals. Most sending hospitals have special interfacility transfer forms that document care en route, identify any standing orders, and document the transfer of patient care at the new destination. For the EMS personnel providing the transport, it is important to document the hospital personnel's names, titles, and reasons for accompanying the patient in the ambulance.

Some patients are transferred because of insurance requirements or to receive specialized care not available at the sending hospital. A standard PCR is used to document these transfers, with the reason for the transfer (eg, a burn unit is available at the receiving hospital) clearly stated in the report.

Mass-Casualty Events

A major incident may result in a large number of patients, and comprehensive documentation may have to be postponed at such an incident until patients have been triaged and transported for definitive care (see Chapter 53, *Medical Incident Command*). These are difficult and unusual situations; in these circumstances, the paramedic should follow local documentation procedures.

Exposure and Injury Reporting

EMS agencies have special forms for documenting and reporting a possible unprotected exposure to infectious disease, hazardous chemicals, or a job-related injury. These reports are developed by the local EMS agency and their legal advisers. They must follow state and federal guidelines, as well as those established by the Occupational Safety and Health Administration and the Centers for Disease Control and Prevention, if applicable. (Reporting of a possible exposure to infectious disease or hazardous chemicals is discussed in detail in Chapter 27, *Infectious and Communicable Diseases*, and Chapter 56, *Hazardous Materials Awareness*.)

Paramedics who have been injured on the job or who believe that they may have been exposed to an infectious disease should follow agency protocol and do the following:

1. Immediately contact the EMS supervisor or designated officer.
2. Seek medical care.
3. Thoroughly document the event.

Document Revision and Correction

As noted previously, a PCR sometimes must be revised or corrected. Most EMS agencies provide separate report forms for this purpose. If a separate report is needed, the paramedic should do the following:

- Make the revision or correction as soon as the need for it is realized.
- Note the purpose of the revision or correction and the reason the information did not appear on the original document.
- Note the date and time the revision or correction was made.
- Make sure the revision or correction was made by the original author of the document.

Acceptable methods of making revisions or adding information to a document vary by agency. Some include making the change to the original form; on a paper form, such changes must be initialed, and the date and time must be noted. Electronic patient reports typically have a built-in mechanism to track the changes. All changes must be truthful and accurately represent the facts from the call. The paramedic should follow the policies set by the EMS agency and medical direction for revising or correcting reports.

CRITICAL THINKING

Consider this situation: Your supervisor asks you to change your documentation so that the insurance company will pay for the transport. What would you do?

Consequences of Inappropriate Documentation

Incorrect or incomplete documentation can have serious consequences that have medical and legal implications. With an inaccurate, incomplete, or illegible PCR, subsequent caregivers may provide improper care to a patient. In an example scenario, a paramedic fails to mention that a patient with a possible myocardial infarction is allergic to amiodarone. The patient later becomes unconscious in the ED as a result of a ventricular rhythm disturbance. Amiodarone, an antidysrhythmic agent, might be administered, but in this case it could prove lethal for the patient. A thorough PCR completed in a professional manner may influence the decision of an attorney considering the merits of an impending lawsuit for negligence or malpractice. (The attorney's decision may also be influenced if the documentation is not thorough and professional.)

Documentation should never become routine or superficial (**BOX 4-4**). Good documentation should be completed in a timely manner and with careful attention to detail. This helps ensure that the PCR is medically and legally sound.

BOX 4-4 Documentation Responsibilities of the Paramedic

The paramedic's professional responsibilities with regard to documentation include the following:

- View the task of documentation as one of utmost importance.
- Assume responsibility for self-assessment of all documentation.
- Appreciate the importance of good documentation to all health care personnel.
- Strive to set a good example in the completion of the documentation task.
- Respect the confidential nature of an EMS report.

NOTE

Recently there has been a trend toward sharing patient information across health care systems in an effort to improve quality, efficiency, and timeliness of patient care. Health information exchanges (HIEs) are secure systems that permit real-time sharing of patient health information accessible to EMS, the health system, and the patient. A paramedic with full access to an HIE could use this system to perform the following tasks:

- Search a patient's records on the scene to determine health history, allergies, and do-not-resuscitate orders.
- Alert the hospital about the patient's status prior to arrival.
- File the patient report directly within the health system's electronic health record (EHR) system.
- Reconcile the EHR information to find the patient's outcome.
- Secure billing information.
- Perform quality improvement.

Modified from: Office of the Coordinator for Health Information Technology. Health information exchange and emergency medical services. 2016. https://www.healthit.gov/sites/default/files/HIE_Value_Prop_EMS_Memo_6_21_16_FINAL_generic.pdf. Accessed February 5, 2018.

Summary

- The PCR is used to document the key elements of patient assessment, care, and transport.
- Four important reasons for written documentation are that the medical community involved in the patient's care uses it; it is a legal record; it is important for reimbursement; and it is essential to data collection.
- The PCR should include dates and response times, difficulties encountered, observations at the scene, previous medical care provided, a chronological description of the call, and significant times.
- A properly written EMS document is accurate and complete, legible, timely, unaltered, and free of nonprofessional or extraneous information.
- Many approaches can be used to write the narrative. The paramedic should adopt only one approach and use it consistently to prevent omissions in report writing.
- Documentation should provide details necessary for billing purposes; reimbursement is critical to ensure the EMS agency's long-term success.
- Special documentation is necessary when a patient refuses care or transport, when care or transport is not needed, and for mass-casualty events.
- Most EMS agencies have separate forms for revising or correcting the patient care report.
- Incorrect or incomplete documentation may have medical and legal implications.

Reference

1. National Association of State EMS Officials. *National Model EMS Clinical Guidelines. V.11-14.* NASEMSO website. https://nasemso.org/Projects/ModelEMSClinicalGuidelines/documents/National-Model-EMS-Clinical-Guidelines-23Oct2014.pdf. Accessed November 30, 2017.

Suggested Readings

Helferich G. The dos and don'ts of documentation. *JEMS/EMS Insider* website. http://www.jems.com/ems-insider/articles/2016/06/the-dos-don-ts-of-documentation.html. Published June 3, 2016. Accessed November 30, 2017.

Helferich G. How to write good patient care reports, part 1: collecting patient information. *JEMS* website. http://www.jems.com/ems-insider/articles/2016/09/how-to-write-good-patient-care-reports-part-1-collecting-patient-information.html. Published September 14, 2016. Accessed November 30, 2017.

Lippincott Williams & Wilkins. *Chart Smart: The A-to-Z Guide to Better Nursing Documentation.* 3rd ed. Philadelphia, PA: Lippincott Williams & Wilkins; 2009.

McWay D. *Legal Aspects of Health Information Management.* 4th ed. Clifton Park, NY: Cengage Learning; 2016.

Milewski R, Lang R. *EMS Documentation: Field Guide.* 3rd ed. Burlington, MA: Jones & Bartlett Learning; 2013.

National Association of State EMS Officials. *National Model EMS Clinical Guidelines, Version 2.0.* NASEMSO website. https://www.nasemso.org/documents/National-Model-EMS-Clinical-Guidelines-Version2-Sept2017.pdf. Published September 2017. Accessed November 30, 2017.

National Highway Traffic Safety Administration. *The National EMS Education Standards.* Washington, DC: US Department of Transportation/National Highway Traffic Safety Administration; 2009.

Page WW. Why documentation is part of good patient care. EMS1 website. https://www.ems1.com/ems-products/ePCR-Electronic-Patient-Care-Reporting/articles/2124085-Why-documentation-is-part-of-good-patient-care/. Published March 10, 2015. Accessed November 30, 2017.

Regulations (standards—29 CFR). Table of contents: bloodborne pathogens, 29 CFR 1910.1030. US Department of Labor, Occupational Safety and Health Administration website. https://www.osha.gov/pls/oshaweb/owadisp.show_document?p_id=10051&p_table=STANDARDS. Accessed November 30, 2017.

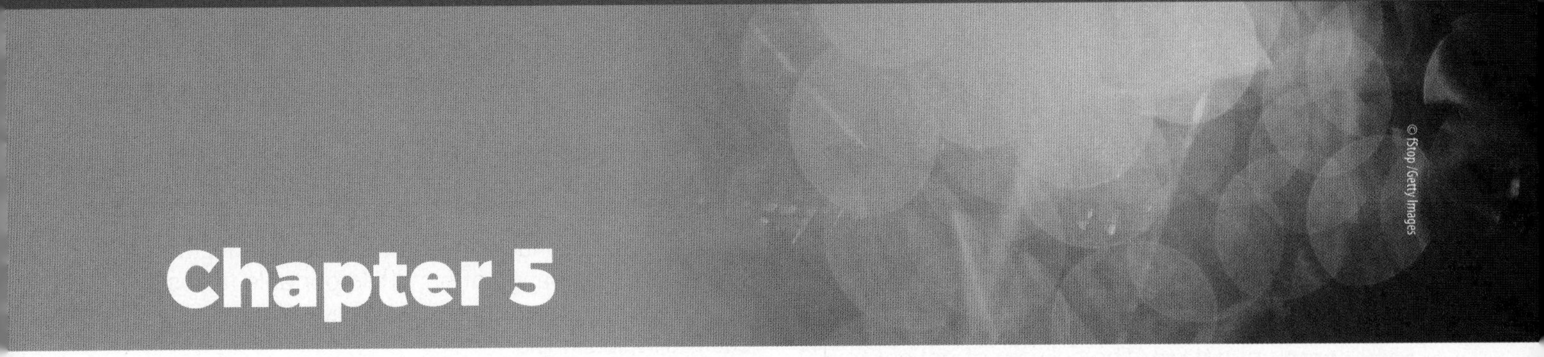

Chapter 5

EMS Communications

NATIONAL EMS EDUCATION STANDARD COMPETENCIES

Preparatory

Integrates comprehensive knowledge of the EMS system, safety/well-being of the paramedic, and medical/legal and ethical issues which is intended to improve the health of EMS personnel, patients, and the community.

EMS System Communication

Communication needed to

- Call for resources (p 109)
- Transfer care of the patient (p 113)
- Interact within the team structure (p 107, and Chapter 20, *Assessment-Based Management and Clinical Decision Making*)
- EMS communication system (pp 98, 107, 109–110)
- Communication with other health care professionals (pp 107–109, 112–114)
- Team communication and dynamics (p 107, and Chapter 20, *Assessment-Based Management and Clinical Decision Making*)

OBJECTIVES

Upon completion of this chapter, the paramedic student will be able to:

1. Describe the role of communications in EMS. (pp 98, 107)
2. Define common EMS communications terms. (pp 98–100)
3. Describe the regulation of EMS communications. (p 100)
4. Distinguish between EMS frequency ranges. (pp 100–102)
5. Outline the elements of an EMS communications system. (pp 103–106)
6. Describe the characteristics of EMS communications operation modes. (pp 104–105)
7. Outline the phases of the communications that occur during a typical EMS event. (p 106)
8. Outline the basic model of communications. (pp 107–108)
9. Outline techniques for relaying EMS communications clearly and effectively. (pp 108–109, 112–114)
10. Describe ways to communicate effectively using the primary modes of EMS communications. (pp 108–109, 112–114)
11. Describe the role of dispatching as it applies to prehospital emergency medical care. (pp 109–112)
12. Outline procedures for EMS communications. (pp 112–114)

KEY TERMS

communication The process by which one person or group transmits information to others.

communications systems The science and technology of communicating, especially by electronic means.

decoding The process by which the intended meaning of information is interpreted.

EMS communications The delivery of patient and scene information (either in person, in writing, or through communications technology) to other members of the emergency response team.

encoding The process by which information is organized through a medium or channel.

Federal Communications Commission (FCC) A federal agency that regulates interstate and international communications by radio, television, wire, satellite, and cable in all 50 states, the District of Columbia, and US territories.

half-duplex mode A communications mode in two frequencies that allows data to flow in one direction or the other, but not both at the same time.

multiplex mode A communications mode that allows multiple data streams to be aggregated onto a single carrier signal, which may then be transmitted via a single transmission medium, such as radio or telephone.

repeater A device that is used to increase the effective communications range of handheld portable radios, mobile radios, and base station radios by retransmitting received radio signals.

simplex mode A communications mode in which information can be transmitted or received in only one direction at a time on a single frequency. Simultaneous transmission cannot occur.

team dynamics The unseen forces that operate in a team between different groups of people; will enable a group of people to act as one.

telemedicine Technologic communications that allow the transmission of photographs, video, and other information directly from the scene to a hospital for physician evaluation and consultation.

trunked radio system A sophisticated computer-controlled radio system that uses multiple frequencies and repeaters.

EMS communications *refers to the delivery of information about the patient and the scene. The information may be delivered in person, in writing, or through various electronic devices to other members of the emergency response team. These members include telecommunicators, EMS personnel, emergency response workers, EMS system control and administration staff, and medical direction. This chapter addresses the complexities of communications that are vital aspects of the EMS system.*

Communications Systems

Communications systems allow public service agencies to exchange information. These systems are crucial in an emergency event to ensure scene safety and to communicate with telecommunicators and other emergency personnel who are involved in the incident. Communications systems also provide a means to convey patient information to medical direction and others involved in the patient's care. Communications systems are composed of various technologies, including radio frequencies and specialized equipment. The terms used to describe emergency communications systems and technologies are specific to the industry (BOX 5-1).

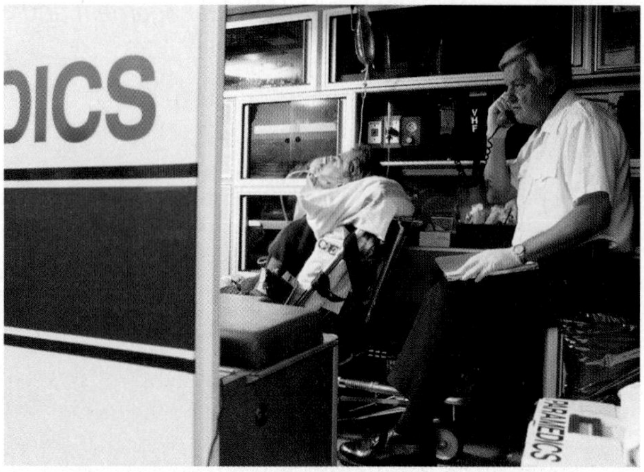

BOX 5-1 Communications Terminology

9-1-1. A three-digit telephone number used to facilitate reporting of an emergency that requires a response by a public safety agency.

9-1-1 service area. The geographic area that has been granted authority by a state or local government body to provide 9-1-1 service.

Abandoned call. A call placed to 9-1-1 in which the caller disconnects before the call can be answered by the public safety answering point (PSAP) telecommunicator.

Advanced mobile phone service. The analog or digital radio interface used in wireless telephone systems.

All relay. Forwarding of pertinent information by a PSAP telecommunicator to the appropriate response agency; not to be confused with telephone relay service.

Alternate PSAP. A PSAP designated to receive calls when the primary PSAP is unable to do so.

Alternate routing. A system for routing 9-1-1 calls to one or more designated alternate locations if all 9-1-1 trunks to a primary PSAP are busy or out of service. Alternate routing may be activated on request or automatically, if detectable, when 9-1-1 equipment fails or the PSAP itself is disabled.

Amplitude modulated. The encoding of a carrier wave by variation of its amplitude (wave height) in accordance with an input signal.

Attendant position. The call-taking location in which the telecommunicator answers and responds to calls.

Automatic alarm and automatic alerting device. Any automated device that can access the 9-1-1 system for emergency services upon activation but that does not provide for two-way communication. Many states prohibit dialing of 9-1-1 by an automated device.

Automatic call distributor. Equipment that automatically distributes incoming calls to available PSAP call takers in the order the calls are received or queues calls until a call taker becomes available.

Automatic location identification. The automatic display at the PSAP of the caller's telephone number, the address or location of the telephone, and supplementary emergency services information.

Automatic number identification (ANI). The telephone number associated with the access line from which a call originates.

Automatic vehicle location (AVL). A means for determining the geographic location of a vehicle and transmitting this information to a point where it can be used.

Backup PSAP. Typically, a disaster recovery answering point that serves as a backup to the primary PSAP and that is not located in the same place as the primary PSAP.

Basic 9-1-1. An emergency telephone system that automatically connects 9-1-1 callers to a designated answering point. Call routing is determined only by the originating central office. Basic 9-1-1 typically does not support ANI or automatic location identification.

Caller hold. The capability of the PSAP to maintain control of a 9-1-1 caller's access line, even if the caller hangs up.

Calling party's number. The callback number associated with a wireless telephone; similar to ANI for wireline telephones.

Cell. The wireless telecommunications (cellular or PCS) antenna serving a specific geographic area.

Circuit route. The physical path between two terminal locations.

Computer-aided dispatch. A computer-based system that aids PSAP telecommunicators by automating selected dispatching and recordkeeping activities.

Consolidated PSAP. An arrangement in which one or more public safety agencies choose to operate as a single 9-1-1 entity.

Dedicated trunk. A telephone circuit used for a single purpose, such as transmission of 9-1-1 calls.

Direct dispatch. The performance of 9-1-1 call answering and dispatching by personnel at the primary PSAP.

Diverse routing. The practice of routing circuits along different physical paths to prevent total loss of 9-1-1 service in the event of a facility failure.

Emergency call. A telephone request for public safety agency emergency services that requires immediate action to save a life, report a fire, or stop a crime. It may include other situations as determined locally.

Emergency ring back. The ability of a PSAP telecommunicator to ring the telephone on a held circuit (a basic 9-1-1 feature); requires calling party hold; also known as *re-ring*.

Emergency service trunks. Message trunks capable of providing ANI, connecting the serving central office of the 9-1-1 calling party and the designated enhanced 9-1-1 control office.

Enhanced 9-1-1 (E9-1-1). An emergency telephone system that includes network switching, database, and customer premises equipment elements capable of providing selective routing, selective transfer, fixed transfer, ANI, and automatic location identification.

Forced disconnect. The capability of a PSAP attendant to disconnect a 9-1-1 call even if the calling party remains off the hook; used to prevent overloading of 9-1-1 trunks.

Global positioning system (GPS). A satellite-based technology for determining location.

Highway call box. A telephone enclosed in a box and placed along a highway that allows a motorist to summon emergency and nonemergency assistance; rapidly becoming obsolete.

Management information system. A program that collects, stores, and collates data into reports to allow interpretation and evaluation of information such as performance, trends, and traffic capacities.

Master street address guide. A database of street names and house number ranges within their associated communities defining emergency service zones and

(continued)

BOX 5-1 Communications Terminology *(continued)*

their associated emergency service numbers to enable proper routing of 9-1-1 calls.

National Emergency Number Association. A not-for-profit corporation established in 1982 to further the goal of "one nation, one number." The association is a networking source that promotes research, planning, and training. It strives to educate, set standards, and provide certification programs, legislative representation, and technical assistance for implementing and managing 9-1-1 systems.

Primary PSAP. A PSAP to which 9-1-1 calls are routed directly from the 9-1-1 control office.

Public safety answering point (PSAP). A facility equipped and staffed to receive 9-1-1 calls. A primary PSAP receives the calls directly. If the call is relayed or transferred, the next receiving PSAP is designated a secondary PSAP.

Selective routing. The routing of a 9-1-1 call to the proper PSAP based on the location of the caller. Selective routing is controlled by the emergency service number, which is derived from the customer's location.

Telecommunicator. As used in 9-1-1, a person trained and employed in public safety telecommunications. The term applies to call takers, dispatchers, radio operators, data terminal operators, or any combination of such functions in a PSAP.

Trunk. Typically, a communication path between central office switches or between the 9-1-1 control office and the PSAP.

Trunking. A method for a computerized radio system to provide network access to many users by sharing a set of frequencies instead of providing them individually.

Reproduced from: National Emergency Number Association Technical Committee and PSAP Operational Standards Committee: *NENA master glossary of 911 terminology*, Arlington, VA, Version 15, March 29, 2011, The National Emergency Number Association.

Radio communications in the United States are regulated by the **Federal Communications Commission (FCC)**. The FCC develops rules and regulations for the use of all radio equipment and frequencies. In addition to the FCC, state and local governments may have rules and regulations for radio operations. Paramedics must be knowledgeable about these agencies and must follow their guidelines. The primary functions of the FCC include the following rules and regulations for Title 47 of the Code of Federal Regulations:

- Licensing and allocating broadcast frequencies
- Establishing technical standards for radio equipment
- Establishing and enforcing rules and regulations for equipment operation, including monitoring frequencies for appropriate use and spot-checking for appropriate licenses and records

CRITICAL THINKING

Why are these rules and regulations needed for good EMS communications?

Public Service Radio Frequencies

Land mobile radio (LMR) systems include most of the radio transmission technologies currently used by public service agencies. The radio frequencies are assigned for use by the FCC.[1] According to FCC rules, LMR systems are allowed to operate in portions of the radio spectrum called *bands.* They include very high frequency (VHF), ultra high frequency (UHF), 700-megahertz (MHz), and 800-MHz (BOX 5-2) bands. Many EMS agencies use encrypted frequencies to protect the privacy of medical communications.

BOX 5-2 Land Mobile Radio System Radio Frequency Bands

Very high frequency (VHF)
Low band: 30 MHz to 50 MHz (usually used for long-range or large-area coverage)[a]
High band: 152 MHz to 174 MHz (usually used for medium-range, medium-area coverage)[a]
Ultra high frequency (UHF) (usually used for short-range, smaller-area coverage)
700 MHz[a]
800 MHz[a]

[a]Megahertz (MHz) is a unit of alternating current or electromagnetic wave frequency equal to one million hertz (1,000,000 Hz). The gigahertz (GHz) is equal to one billion hertz (1,000,000,000 Hz), or 1,000 MHz.

For public safety radio, VHF may be defined as low band and high band. A number of VHF low-band

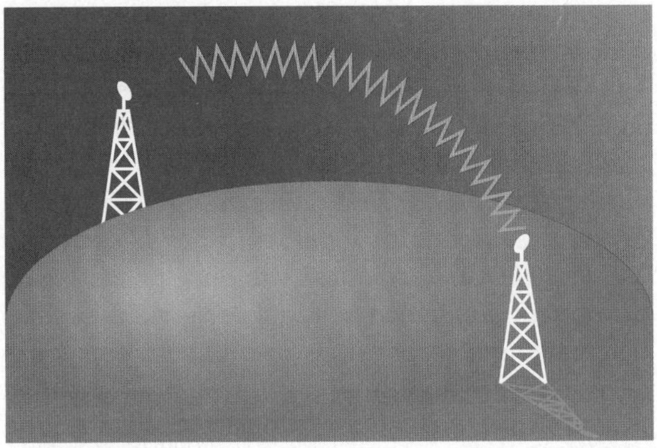

FIGURE 5-1 VHF low band.

and VHF high-band frequencies are assigned strictly to two-way use or one-way paging. VHF low-band signals (**FIGURE 5-1**) generally have the greatest range and usually cover a greater distance than VHF high band or UHF band. However, these low-band signals follow the curvature of the earth's surface; therefore, they are subject to noise interference and physical or structural interference. Consequently, although these signals have the best range, they may not provide the best coverage.

VHF high-band signals (**FIGURE 5-2**) generally have medium range. They travel in straight lines rather than following the curvature of the earth. This virtual "straight line" characteristic means that high-band signals more easily reflect around buildings and other structures. These signals may provide better radio coverage in some areas, although they are now primarily used in rural areas.

UHF-band signals (**FIGURE 5-3**) generally have a limited range. They are more "straight line sensitive" than VHF high-band signals. However, the ability of the UHF band to reflect or bounce around buildings exceeds that of the VHF high band. In metropolitan areas, the UHF band may be the most effective frequency. Of the three bands, UHF is the least susceptible to noise interference and can reach into and out of structures more easily.

The 700- and 800-MHz signals generally have a limited range because they travel in a straighter line than do VHF high-band signals. As such, the 700- and 800-MHz spectra are best suited for use in urban areas. Cell phone companies also use the 800-MHz band. This can cause congestion and can interfere with public service communications, especially

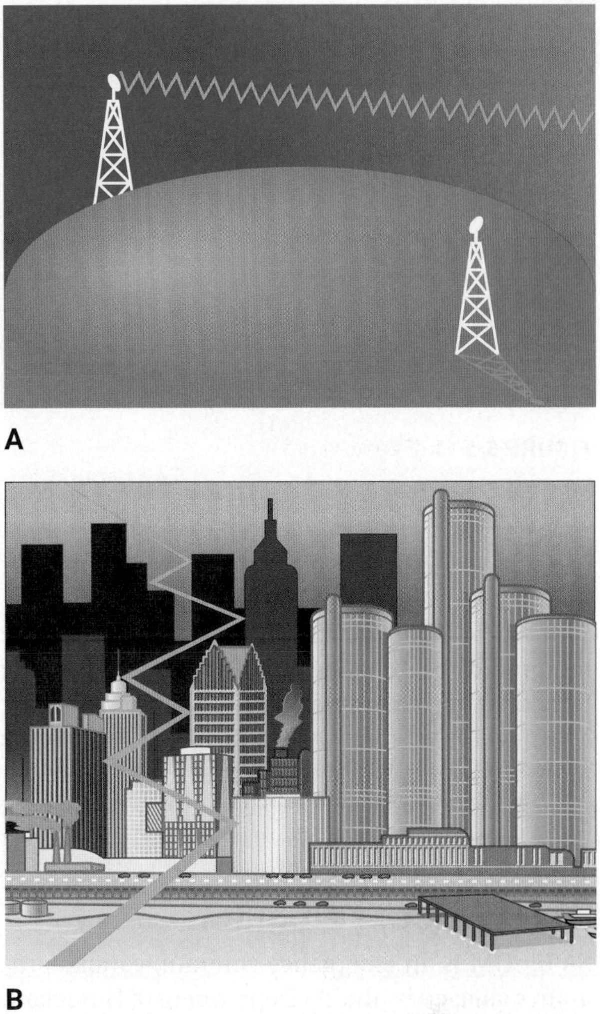

FIGURE 5-2 VHF high band. **A.** VHF high band travels in straight lines. **B.** Straight line travel allows high-band signals to more easily reflect around buildings and other structures.

during a large-scale incident or major disaster. This type of communications gridlock occurred during the 9/11 attacks on the World Trade Center in New York City in 2001. Work is underway to "reband" the 800-MHz system, thus increasing the space of the frequencies to accommodate the communications needs of commercial carriers and public service agencies.[2]

Narrow-Band Technology

Older technology used frequency assignments that were spaced 25 kHz (0.025 MHz) apart. With the growth of public service use, the 150- to 174-MHz and 421- to 512-MHz bands have become congested, and limited frequency is available for implementation

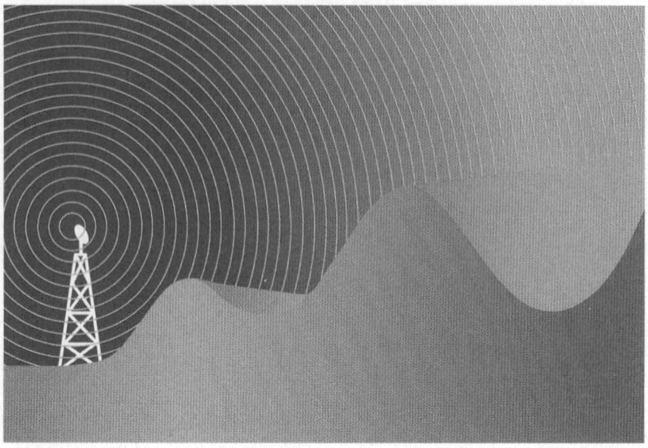

FIGURE 5-3 UHF band.

© Jones & Bartlett Learning.

of new systems or existing systems. As of January 1, 2013, all public safety LMR systems operating in the 150- to 174-MHz and 421- to 470-MHz bands were required to begin using at least 12.5-kHz spacing technology (commonly referred to as *narrowbanding*). The new technology enables licensees to operate more efficiently with narrower channel bandwidth or an increased number of voice paths or higher data rate per channel.[3]

The SAFECOM Program

SAFECOM is an emergency communications program managed by the US Department of Homeland Security (DHS). SAFECOM provides research, development, testing and evaluation, guidance, tools, and templates on interoperable communications-related issues to state, local, tribal, and federal emergency

> **NOTE**
>
> In 2004, the 4.9-GHz Public Safety frequency band was opened for transmission of broadband wireless data, voice, and video communications in public service applications. All state, local, and federal governmental agencies working with state and local public safety systems are eligible for 4.9-GHz licensing. The 4.9 GHz supports a wide variety of broadband applications, including wireless networks for incident scene management, mesh networks, Wi-Fi hotspots, and voice over IP (VoIP).
>
> *Modified from:* 4.9 GHz in Public Safety. Strix Systems website. http://www.strixsystems.com/4.9Ghzinpublicsafety.aspx. Accessed December 19, 2017.

response agencies.[4] SAFECOM and its partners work to improve the interoperability of multijurisdictional and intergovernmental communications through collaboration with emergency responders and policy makers across all levels of government.[5]

As part of SAFECOM's mission, the DHS developed the *National Interoperability Field Operations Guide* (*NIFOG*), a technical reference pocket guide of spectrum reference material designed for use by field personnel responsible for emergency response and spectrum coordination during both planned events and emergency situations (**FIGURE 5-4**). The *NIFOG* contains tables of nationwide interoperability channels, communications references, and tables of commonly used frequencies. The guide also includes an organized listing of the national mutual aid channels and other reference materials.[6]

The P25 Standard

The P25 standard, also known as Project 25, was initiated by the Association of Public Safety Communications

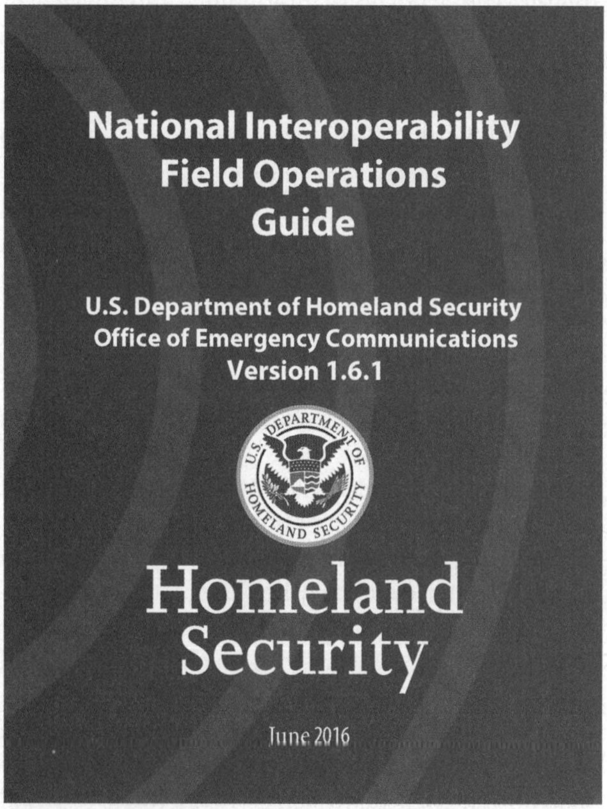

FIGURE 5-4 *National Interoperability Field Operations Guide.*

Courtesy of US Department of Homeland Security.

Officials to accomplish the primary goal of having interoperable LMR equipment.[7] P25 is a suite of standards developed to provide secure digital voice and data communications systems suited to public safety and first responders. P25 development is open and user-driven to allow competing products from multiple vendors to be interoperable. The standards are constantly being enhanced and refined in several phases of development.

Radio equipment that is compatible with P25 standards allows users from different agencies (federal, state, provincial, or local level, or any other agency) or areas to communicate directly with each other via two-way radios. A key element of the P25 standard is that P25 digital equipment must be compatible with older analog mobile and portable radios. This compatibility allows adopters of the P25 standard to purchase new system equipment without replacing all of their older radios.

Land Mobile Radio Systems Technologies

Radio systems used by public service agencies are wireless, usually composed of base stations, mobile and portable transceivers, and repeaters.

Base Station Radios

Base station radios are located in fixed positions, such as public safety answering points, dispatch centers, and hospitals. They tend to have the most powerful transmitters, with output powers of up to 275 watts. Base station radios use antennas that are usually located on a high spot, such as a hill, mountain, or tall building, to ensure optimum transmission and reception. Base station radios often have multiple channels and frequency bands, and may serve as central hubs for radio systems. A network is required to connect the different base stations to the same communications system.

Mobile Transceivers

Vehicle- or aircraft-mounted transmitters usually operate at lower outputs than do base stations. They provide a range of 10 to 15 miles over average terrain. Transmission over flat land or water increases this range. However, range is reduced when transmission occurs over mountainous terrain, dense foliage, or urban areas with tall buildings. Transmitters with higher outputs are available and may offer greater ranges for transmission. Multichannel units are preferred over single-channel radios because an EMS system uses many channels.

Portable Transceivers

Portable transceivers are handheld or hand-carried devices (often called *portables*). They are used when the paramedic is working away from the emergency vehicle. Because portable transceivers operate at much lower power than do mobile or base station radios, they usually have a limited range. Many systems boost the signal through a mobile or vehicular repeater. Portable transceivers may be single-channel or multichannel units.

Repeaters

A **repeater** is used to increase the effective communications range of a handheld portable radio, mobile radio, or base station radio by retransmitting received radio signals. Repeaters act as a special type of long-range transceiver located on a high spot, covering a large geographic area. They receive transmissions from a low-power portable or mobile radio on one frequency. At the same time, they retransmit it at a higher power on another frequency. Repeaters may be fixed or vehicle-mounted; EMS systems often use both. Repeaters are needed for large geographic areas.

Encoded Radio Signals

Most radio systems have multiple repeaters and use Continuous Tone-Coded Squelch System (CTCSS) private line tones to identify which repeater is being accessed. CTCSS is an inaudible tone that accompanies a voice during radio transmission. The transmit tone is referred to as the *encode* tone and the receiver tone is referred to as the *decode* tone. CTCSS is part of a repeater's receiver that allows only signals with the "proper tone" to access or open the receiver. Encoded radio signals cut down on interference and permit the use of multiple receivers on the same frequency. This technology is especially important for rural EMS units operating in different parts of their service area because they may need to use different repeaters that share the same frequency pair.[8]

Selective call encoders look like the buttons of a push-button phone. When activated, the encoder transmits tone pulses or pairs of tones over the air. Receivers with decoders recognize the specific codes, and the audio circuits of the receivers open. Two-tone sequential paging alerts personnel using two pairs of specific frequency tones to address pagers and alert monitors selectively. A selective-address system usually has a code for calling all units within radio range (all call).

Modes of Radio Transmission

Any type of data transmission can be characterized by the direction of the signal. The three modes of transmission commonly used in emergency communications are classified as simplex, half-duplex, and multiplex.

Simplex Mode

The **simplex mode** (**FIGURE 5-5**) requires a transmitter and receiver at each end of the communications path. Both elements operate on the same frequency and the data are transmitted in only one direction. That is, only one end may operate at a time. Examples of data transmission using simplex mode are television or radio broadcast stations. As a rule, simplex mode is generally used in public safety communications for only short-range communication, such as tactical on-scene communications, and the communications path can easily become overcrowded at a busy scene.

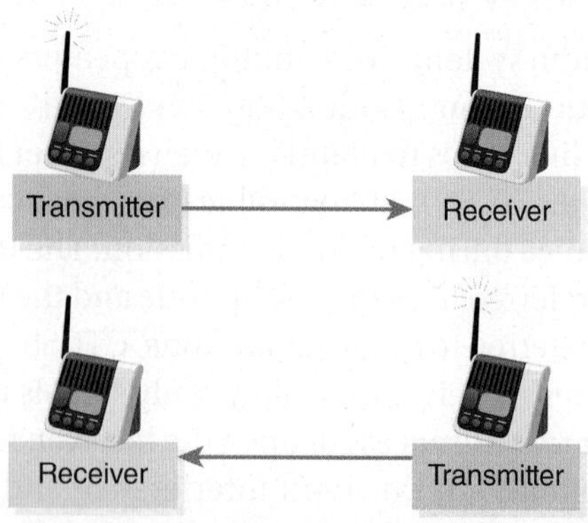

FIGURE 5-5 Simplex mode requires a transmitter and a receiver at each end of the communications path, both operating on the same frequency. In this mode, only one end may operate at a time.

Half-Duplex Mode

The **half-duplex mode** (**FIGURE 5-6**) uses two frequencies that allow data to flow in one direction or the other, but not both at the same time. With this type of transmission, each end of the connection transmits in turn. An example of half-duplex mode is a handheld portable radio. Full-duplex mode allows transmission in both directions simultaneously. An example is a telephone.

Multiplex Mode

The **multiplex mode** (**FIGURE 5-7**) allows multiple data streams to be aggregated onto a single carrier

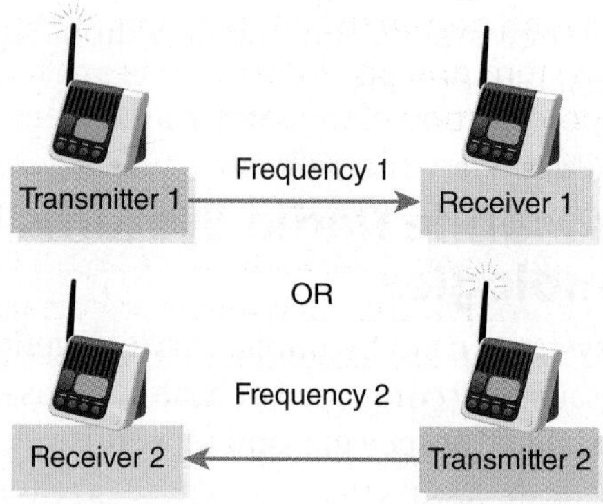

FIGURE 5-6 Half-duplex mode uses two frequencies that allow data to flow in one direction or the other, but not both at the same time.

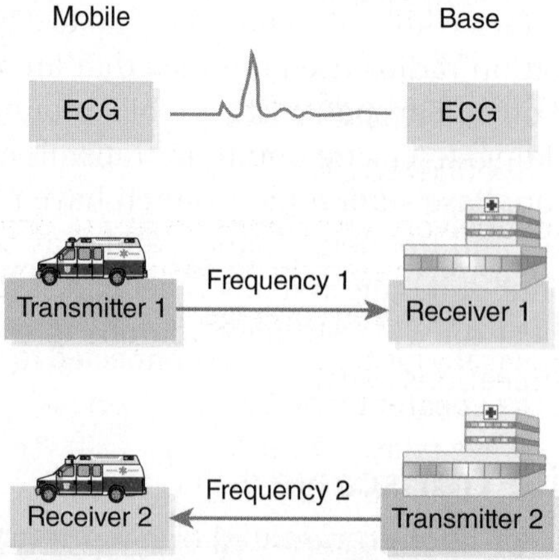

FIGURE 5-7 Multiplex mode is most commonly used in EMS communications to transmit both voice and electrocardiogram tracings.

signal, which may then be transmitted via a single transmission medium, such as a radio or telephone. Multiplex EMS communications systems use a single radio carrier signal to send this information. This is a one-way process. It does not allow simultaneous two-way voice communications unless it is a part of a full-duplex system. Stereo signals in commercial FM (frequency modulated) radio and voice and electrocardiogram data in EMS communications are examples of multiplex technology.

Trunked Radio Systems

A **trunked radio system** is a sophisticated computer-controlled radio system. The system uses multiple frequencies and repeaters. Each repeater is not typically assigned to a particular frequency. Individual repeaters operate on the entire frequency spectrum of the system and are located to cover a specific geographic portion of the service area. They are frequently located so that their coverage areas overlap, which prevents "dead spots" if an individual repeater goes off line. Each radio in the system can be set to a range of individual channels, sometimes called "modes," which are assigned for specific purposes (dispatch, tactical, hospital). When a user initiates a transmission, or "call," the system assigns a frequency pair from its pool of frequencies. The call is then routed through the appropriate repeaters so that the two parties have a clear two-way communications path. Once the call is completed, the frequencies are returned to the pool, allowing more efficient use of available frequencies.[9]

Satellite Receivers and Terminals

Satellite receivers sometimes are used, depending on the area and the terrain, to ensure that low-power units are always within coverage. The satellite receivers are strategically located and are connected to the base station or repeater by dedicated phone lines, radio, or microwave relay. "Voting systems" automatically select the best audio signal. These systems pick up the signal from among multiple satellite receivers and the main base station receiver. (This technology is also used in other types of communications systems, such as global positioning systems [GPS] and geographic information systems [GIS].)

Commonly available satellite terminals incorporate ground stations and transportable stations. They provide voice, data, and video communications. Portable satellite terminals are useful when other systems are not available. For example, they may be used during major disasters.

Cell Phones

Many EMS systems use cell phones as an alternative to their other radio equipment. One benefit of cell phones is that they have more channels. In addition, a cell phone offers a reasonably secure link between EMS workers and area hospitals. A cell phone also allows the online physician to speak directly with the patient. However, the use of cell phones for emergency services also has some disadvantages. For example, network usage might limit channel access. In addition, high network usage may create problems in maintaining continuous communications in some areas, which would be especially problematic in a community disaster. Other concerns are a lack of priority access and the issue that calls cannot be monitored by other members of an emergency response team. Another issue of concern is that cell phones can lead to potential breaches in patient

DID YOU KNOW?

The Integrated Public Alert and Warning System (IPAWS) is a group of alert and warning tools designed to protect life and property. Government authorities warn the public of serious emergencies using various elements of IPAWS from a central system controller. The IPAWS tools include the Emergency Alert System (EAS), Wireless Emergency Alerts (WEA), the National Oceanic and Atmospheric Administration (NOAA) Weather Radio, and other public systems. The EAS broadcasts emergency messages to the public via cable and wireless television systems, radio, and satellite information portals. The WEA allows public safety entities to transmit cell phone alerts to any cell phone that can display text messages. This system sends urgent messages such as Amber alerts (for abducted children) and extreme weather or major emergency declarations. These warnings are initiated by authorized government entities.

Modified from: Integrated public alert and warning system. Federal Emergency Management Agency website. https://www.fema.gov/integrated-public-alert-warning-system. Updated October 31, 2017. Accessed December 19, 2017.

privacy by way of camera-equipped smart devices. For these reasons, many EMS agencies that use cell phones have a backup option, such as backup radio communications capabilities.

Digital Modes

Digital communication modes include digital phones, telemetry, facsimile ("fax") transmissions, and digital signals used in some wireless phone, paging, and alerting systems. Telemetric communications and facsimiles are transmitted using electronic signals that are converted into audio tones. These tones are converted back into electronic signals by the receiver decoder. The signals then can be displayed or printed. Transmission of a patient's electrocardiogram is an example of telemetry.

Computer Technologies

Computer technology (eg, that used with automated external defibrillators [AEDs] and other devices) is capable of "saving" (preserving a record of) every step of data entry. Computers allow for (1) documentation in near real time, (2) sorting of information in many categories, (3) creation of multiple reporting formats, and (4) quick online and retrieval system data access. Computer terminals also are used by some communications centers to dispatch units automatically to a scene. As with most technologies, computer devices are subject to human error and machine limitations. Therefore, they require regular upgrades and user education.

Advances in EMS communications technology and **telemedicine** continue to proceed at a rapid pace. Video cameras, fax machines, cellular networks, and the Internet now allow photographs, videos (including movie-type imaging), and other information to be sent directly from the scene to a hospital for physician evaluation and consultation.

Phases of Communications During a Typical EMS Event

A typical EMS event involves five phases of communications.[8] The first phase is the occurrence of the event. The second phase is the detection of the need for emergency services. The third phase is the notification and emergency response. The fourth phase is the arrival of the EMS responders, treatment of the patient, and preparation for transport. (Treatment may require consultation with medical direction.) Following transport of the patient, the fifth phase is preparation of the EMS crew for the next response.

In most areas, the public requests help by a phone call. This call goes to a communications center or public safety answering point (PSAP). Most PSAPs are law enforcement based, and in larger communities and cities, a secondary PSAP is used to handle calls for fire suppression and medical services. Communications specialists receive the call. In the most modern systems, details about the origin of the call and any history of a response to that locale are displayed automatically on a console (**FIGURE 5-8**). The call taker uses digital technology to send these details to the telecommunicator, who sends a response unit to the scene. In many PSAP systems, the caller is given prearrival instructions by emergency medical dispatchers or other qualified personnel. The communication with the caller ideally continues until the first EMS unit arrives at the scene.

The EMS unit is dispatched to the scene. The paramedic crew advises the communications center of its response and arrival status by radio or electronically using a computer data terminal. The paramedics provide care at the scene of the emergency. They prepare ("package") the patient for transport and then deliver the patient to the receiving facility. After reporting has been completed, the paramedics make the EMS vehicle ready for the next emergency call.

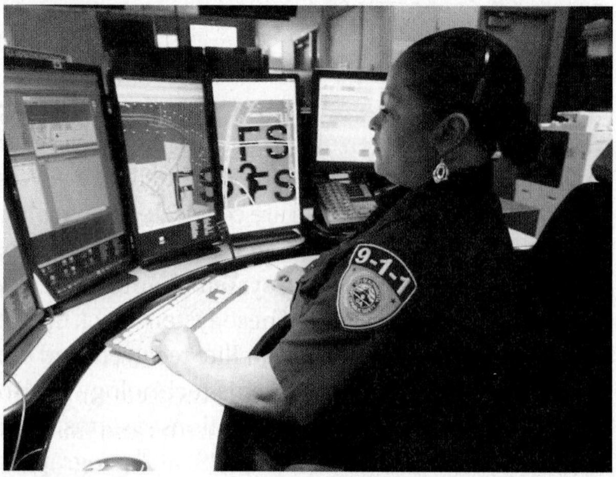

FIGURE 5-8 Communications console (dispatch).

Courtesy of Brendan Keefe, WXIA-TV.

DID YOU KNOW?

Vehicle Telemetry

Vehicle telemetry systems (eg, OnStar, Tele-Aid, eCall, Uconnect, and others) are installed on some newer automobiles. These systems provide advanced automatic crash notification. This feature uses a collection of sensors that send crash data to an adviser if the vehicle is involved in a moderate or severe front, rear, or side-impact crash. The data may include information on the severity of the crash, the direction of impact, airbag deployment, multiple impacts, and a rollover. Advisers relay this information to emergency dispatchers, helping them to determine the appropriate emergency response needed. Telemetry systems can pinpoint the location of the vehicle if it is equipped with a GPS. Since OnStar launched its program in 1996, the company responds to more than 100,000 emergency calls every month.

Modified from: Mello MJ, Kerr HD, Cheng D, Sochor MR, McAteer KE. Motor vehicle safety: an update for emergency medicine practitioners. American College of Emergency Physicians website.https://www.acep.org/search.aspx?searchtext=Clinical-%20intelligent%20transport%20systems&pgsize=10&filter=acep,news,ecfy,media. Accessed December 19, 2017; and OnStar reaches 1 billion customer interactions. Pressroom Europe website. http://media.gm.com/media/intl/en/opel/news.detail.html/content/Pages/news/intl/en/2015/opel/07-29-onstar-reaches-1-billion-customer.html. Published July 29, 2015. Accessed December 19, 2017.

NOTE

As described in Chapter 1, *EMS Systems: Roles, Responsibilities, and Professionalism*, a telecommunicator is a person trained in public safety telecommunications. The term applies to call takers, dispatchers, radio operators, data terminal operators, or any combination of such functions in a public safety answering point located in a fire, police, or EMS communications center.

Role of Communications in EMS

Verbal, written, and electronic communications allow the delivery of information between the person requesting help and the telecommunicator and between the telecommunicator and the paramedic. Communications occur among the paramedic, patient, hospital, and direct/online medical direction (if needed) and between the paramedic and hospital personnel who receive the patient on arrival at the emergency department (**FIGURE 5-9**). Good communication occurs only when key elements are in place. These elements make up the basic model of communications.

Basic Model of Communications

Communications can be verbal, nonverbal, or written. They serve a vital information function in the course of decision making. **Communication** is the process by which one person or group transmits meaning to others. The basic model of communications describes the relationships between an idea, encoding, a sender, a medium or channel, a receiver, decoding, and feedback (**FIGURE 5-10**).

NOTE

The elements of successful communication apply to *all* types of communication between people. This includes communications with friends, family, coworkers, other emergency personnel, and other health care professionals. Successful communication is an important part of **team dynamics**.

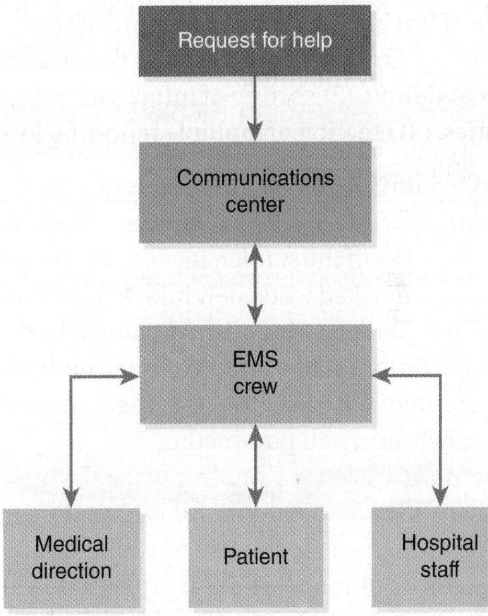

FIGURE 5-9 EMS communications.

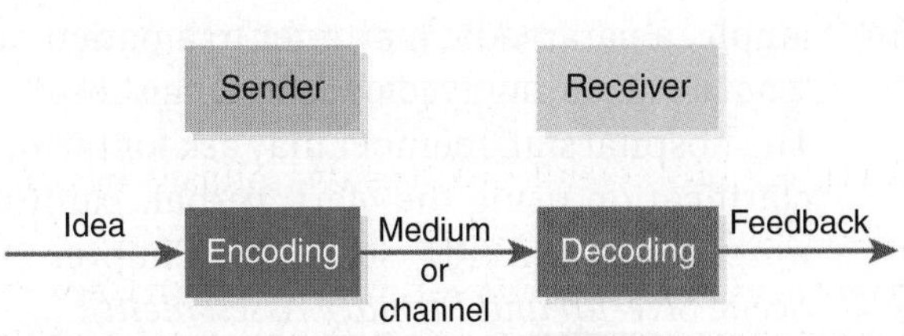

FIGURE 5-10 Basic model of communication.

The idea is the meaning that is intended in the communication. Conveying the idea requires two steps. First, the sender must organize the intended meaning through a medium or channel; this is called **encoding**. For example, the medium or channel may be written or verbal, facial or body expression, or voice modulation. Second, the communication must be interpreted by the receiver; this is called **decoding**. The receiver provides feedback that indicates the idea was received. If the communication is fully successful, the idea intended by the sender will overlap with the feedback provided by the receiver (ie, the receiver interprets, or decodes, the idea exactly as intended by the sender.) Four common barriers can prevent successful communication.[10]

1. **Attributes of the receiver.** Different people react in different ways to the same message or idea. A variety of personal reasons may affect the interpretation of the message. These reasons may include cultural differences, language barriers, or sensory deficits. For example, a patient from one culture may find personal touch comforting, whereas a patient from another culture may be offended by touching.
2. **Selective perception.** People tend to listen to only part of an idea or message and block out other information. This tendency may stem from a variety of reasons, such as values, mood, or motives of the sender. Ideas or messages also may be blocked when new information conflicts with a person's established values, beliefs, or expectations. For example, a paramedic supervisor may not welcome or respect the input of a newly licensed paramedic.
3. **Semantic issues.** Commonly used words may have different meanings for different people. A common issue is the use of vague or abstract words or phrases. These words invite varying interpretation. Another problem is the use of medical terms and technical language (jargon) that the receiver may not understand. For example, a paramedic may refer to a patient as "comatose" during a radio report to the hospital. The hospital staff member may ask for further clarification using the *a*lert, *v*erbal, *p*ainful, *u*nresponsive (AVPU) scale (see Chapter 18, *Scene Size-up and Primary Assessment*).
4. **Time pressures.** Time pressures can lead to distortions in communications. When people are pressed for time, there can be a tendency to bypass or "short circuit" normal channels. In these cases, the immediate demands of the situation are met. However, several unintended consequences can result. For example, a paramedic may not document the medications administered at the scene to a patient in cardiac arrest, resulting in confusion about the next appropriate drug to be used.

CRITICAL THINKING

What tends to happen to you when you are talking with someone who continually interrupts you?

Paramedics should reflect on this basic model of communications and the common barriers that block good communication. It is essential for paramedics to recall these key elements when conveying information to or receiving information from telecommunicators, coworkers, patients, bystanders, medical direction, and hospital personnel.

Proper Verbal Communications During an EMS Event

During an EMS event, the role of proper verbal communications is to exchange system and patient information with other members of the response team. Communications must be done according to local protocol and patient privacy standards and regulations (see Chapter 4, *Documentation*, and Chapter 6, *Medical and Legal Issues*).

The terms used in EMS communications should be clear and conveyed in a short narrative form. Avoid using technical or semantic jargon that cannot be understood clearly by all parties. Some EMS systems use a code (eg, a *10 code*) to shorten radio transmissions; however, the meanings of these codes vary by jurisdiction. The English language, however, usually is preferred for written and verbal messages, especially for mutual-aid and large-scale, multijurisdiction events.[11] Paramedics should keep in mind that many radio and phone communications are recorded. These recordings may be replayed for patient care audits, media broadcasts, and disciplinary hearings, and also during legal proceedings. Professional conduct is important in all communications. In many communities, members of the public use scanners to monitor emergency services. Paramedics, therefore, must take steps to preserve a patient's confidentiality. They should not speak the patient's name or use descriptive phrases over unsecured airwaves. They should also be mindful of patient privacy issues and of regulations relating to the Health Insurance Portability and Accountability Act (HIPAA) (Chapter 6, *Medical and Legal Issues*).

Technologic Advances in the Collection and Exchange of Information

As technology evolves, it alters the way EMS personnel gather and exchange information. Technology reduces the reliance on more traditional means of verbal and written communications. Examples of such advances include portable wireless voice and data devices, satellite terminals, GPS for tracking emergency vehicles, diagnostic devices, and laptop or tablet computers (**FIGURE 5-11**). These and other devices can allow for real-time capture of EMS events and data. In addition, they can allow advanced notification and reduce the time to in-hospital diagnosis and therapy. Again, the paramedic should be aware of patient privacy issues and HIPAA regulations and follow agency protocol (see Chapter 6, *Medical and Legal Issues*).

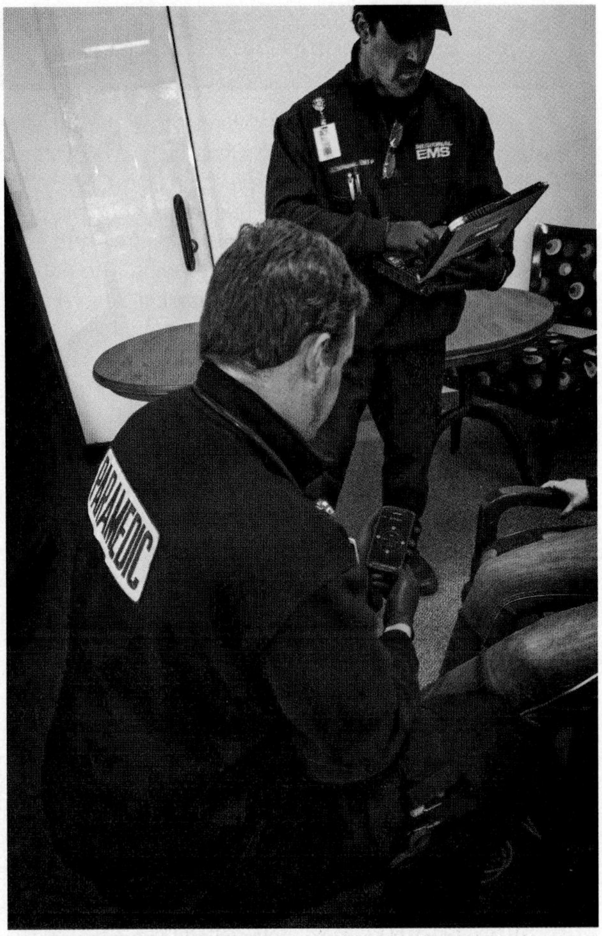

FIGURE 5-11 Computer used for EMS documentation.

Reproduced with permission from Pulsara.

> NOTE
>
> Smartphones and tablet devices can send patient information from a scene to a receiving hospital or a host computer. The data can then be transferred electronically into a final report and patient record. This electronic information has the same legal status as a written document. The data take the place of the paper record of the incident.

Components and Functions of Dispatch Communications Systems

The dispatch communications system is the public safety answering point (BOX 5-3). The following are some of the functions of an effective EMS dispatch communications system:[12]

- **Receive and process calls for EMS assistance.** Calls for EMS assistance are received and recorded by the dispatcher, who selects an appropriate course of action for each call. This function involves obtaining as much information as possible about the emergency event, including the caller's name, callback number, and address; it also may involve conversing with distraught callers. In addition, emergency care instructions may be provided while the EMS crew is dispatched.
- **Dispatch and coordinate EMS resources.** The dispatcher directs the proper emergency vehicles to the correct address. In addition, the dispatcher coordinates the movements of emergency vehicles while en route to the scene, to the medical facility, and back to the operations base.
- **Relay medical information.** The dispatcher may provide a telecommunications channel between appropriate medical facilities and EMS

BOX 5-3 9-1-1, Enhanced 9-1-1, and Computer-Aided Dispatch Systems

In 1988, the number 9-1-1 was designated as the universal emergency telephone number (Chapter 1, *EMS Systems: Roles, Responsibilities, and Professionalism*). The number, chosen by the American Telephone and Telegraph Company (AT&T), offers the public a toll-free means of reaching a public safety answering point. The nation's 9-1-1 centers receive about 240 million calls each year. It is estimated that as many of 80% of them originate from wireless devices. Although the 9-1-1 service has become a fixture in most parts of the United States, currently it is not available in all areas.

More recent developments, enhanced 9-1-1 (E9-1-1) and wireless E9-1-1 are used in many areas of the country to allow for automatic caller location and identification. E9-1-1 shows the number and address of the caller on a terminal at the communications center.

The most advanced centers use a computer-aided dispatch system that monitors the available resources. The system makes an assignment based on access and routes for the ambulance closest to the map grid shown on the terminal. GPS allows the telecommunicator or system status controller to determine which unit is closest to the origin of the call by air miles or by road miles if an intelligent map (also known as a "smart map") is used automatically to route the unit closest to the scene. That unit is then sent to the scene. The telecommunicator monitors the call from beginning to end and records status changes using digital media (eg, tapes, CDs, or DVDs).

Modified from: 9-1-1 statistics. National Emergency Number Association (NENA) website. http://www.nena.org/page/aboutfaq2017. Accessed December 19, 2017.

personnel; firefighters, the police, and rescue workers; and private citizens. The channel may consist of telephone, radio, or biomedical telemetry.

- **Coordinate with public safety agencies.** The dispatcher provides for communications between public safety units (fire department, law enforcement, rescue workers) and elements of the EMS system. This communication enables services such as traffic control, escort, fire suppression, and extrication. The dispatcher ensures an integrated, well-coordinated system. To accomplish this, the dispatcher must know the location and status of all EMS vehicles. The dispatcher also must know the availability of support services (eg, utility companies, coroner). In larger systems, computer-aided dispatching may be used. This advanced technology allows one or more of the following capabilities or functions:
  - Automatic emergency medical dispatch
  - Automatic entry of 9-1-1
  - Automatic call notification/request for assistance
  - Automatic interface to automatic vehicle location (AVL), with or without map display (**FIGURE 5-12**)
  - Automatic interface to mobile data terminal
  - Computer messaging among multiple radio operators, call takers, or both
  - Dispatch note taking, reminder aid, or both
  - Emergency medical dispatch review
  - Manual or automatic updates of unit status
  - Manual entry of call information
  - Radio control and display of channel status
  - Standard operating procedure review
  - Telephone control and display of circuit status

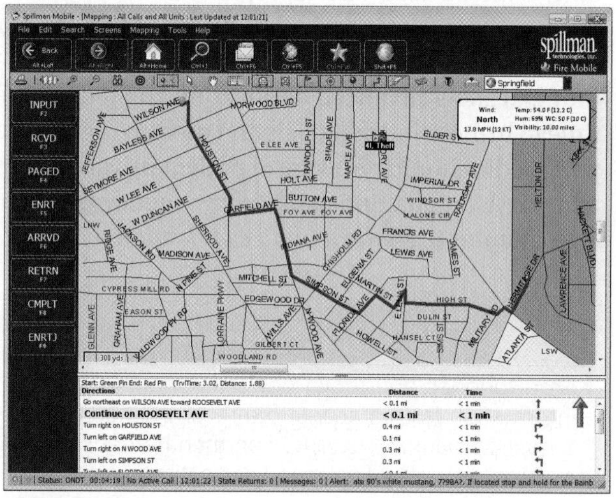

FIGURE 5-12 Automatic vehicle location mapping system in an ambulance cab.

Reproduced with permission from Spillman Technologies, a Motorola Solution Company.

SHOW ME THE EVIDENCE

EMS calls from a 2-year period in an emergency medical dispatch system in a California suburb that totaled 500 or more calls in one dispatch category were compared with the prehospital patient care report for those same calls. The researchers wanted to see whether the dispatch code predicted prehospital use of medications and other interventions. They found that the emergency medical dispatch system had "only a modest ability" to predict which patients would need advanced life support interventions. More medicines were given to patients with shortness of breath, chest pain, diabetic problems, and altered mental status.

Modified from: Sporer KA, Johnson NJ, Clement CY, Youngblood GM. Can emergency medical dispatch codes predict prehospital interventions for common 9-1-1 call types? *Prehosp Emerg Care*. 2008;12:470-478.

DID YOU KNOW?

Wireless Enhanced 9-1-1

The rules established by the FCC for wireless enhanced 9-1-1 (E9-1-1) are intended to improve the effectiveness and reliability of wireless 9-1-1 services by providing 9-1-1 dispatchers with additional information on wireless 9-1-1 calls. The wireless E9-1-1 rules apply to all wireless licensees, broadband Personal Communications Services (PCS) licensees, and certain Specialized Mobile Radio (SMR) licensees.

The FCC has divided its wireless E9-1-1 program into two parts, phase I and phase II. Under phase I, within 6 months of a valid request by a local PSAP, wireless carriers must provide the PSAP with the telephone number of the originator of a wireless 9-1-1 call and the location of the cell site or base station transmitting the call.

Under phase II, within 6 months of a valid request by a PSAP, wireless carriers must begin providing more precise information to PSAPs—specifically, the caller's latitude and longitude. This information must meet FCC accuracy standards, generally to within 164 to 984 feet (50 to 300 m), depending on the type of technology used. The deployment of E9-1-1 requires the development of new technologies and upgrades to local 9-1-1 PSAPs, in addition to coordination among public safety agencies, wireless carriers, technology vendors, equipment manufacturers, and local wireline carriers.

Modified from: Enhanced 9-1-1: wireless services. Federal Communications Commission website. https://www.fcc.gov/general/enhanced-9-1-1-wireless-services. Accessed December 19, 2017.

Dispatcher Training

Many EMS and public safety agencies require specialized medical training for their dispatch personnel. This training may include the Association of Public Communications Officials and Emergency Medical Dispatch Program (which is based on the National Standard Curriculum for Emergency Medical Dispatch, established by the National Highway Traffic Safety Administration). Emergency medical dispatchers are trained to do the following:[13]

- Use locally approved emergency medical dispatch guide cards (customized to local protocols and EMS response priorities).
- Quickly and properly determine the nature of the call.
- Determine the priority of the call.
- Dispatch the appropriate response.
- Provide the caller with instructions to help treat the patient until the responding EMS unit arrives.

A background of training in EMS helps the telecommunicator understand functions of the EMS

SHOW ME THE EVIDENCE

A prospective, experimental, before-and-after trial was conducted in a small Connecticut city with a population of 125,000 in which a first responder fire department engine company was routinely dispatched on most EMS calls. The purpose of the study was to see whether changing the emergency medical dispatch protocol would reduce the call volume of first responder engine companies without affecting patient safety. Before the protocol was implemented, engine companies responded to 84.3% of calls. In the after phase, they were dispatched to 39.1% of EMS calls. The researchers estimated that only 0.55% of patients were undertriaged, but they cautioned that these results may not be applicable to all EMS systems because of the diversity of response modes and dispatch protocols. They concluded that in their system, emergency medical dispatch protocols can safely limit the number of first responder runs.

Modified from: Cone D, Galante N, MacMillan DS. Can emergency medical dispatch systems safely reduce first-responder call volume? *Prehosp Emerg Care*. 2008;12:479-485.

system, personnel capabilities, and equipment limitations. The training also arms the dispatcher with the protocols for giving prearrival instructions, such as performing cardiopulmonary resuscitation or administering aspirin to a patient with a coronary event. These protocols may mitigate the event before the EMS unit arrives.

A variety of dispatching systems and procedures are in place across the United States. Some are the simple call received–ambulance dispatched types; others are the more advanced call prioritization–prearrival instructions systems.

Call Prioritization–Prearrival Instructions Systems

In a call screening–prearrival instructions system, an emergency medical dispatcher, paramedic, or nurse determines the type of assistance needed for an emergency call. This role may involve referring the caller to other services, choosing a basic life support or an advanced life support response, selecting a private or public EMS agency, and determining the appropriate use of audible and visual warning devices.

CRITICAL THINKING

What are some possible consequences of a dispatching error?

NOTE

First Responder Network Authority (FirstNet) was created as part of the Middle Class Tax Relief and Job Creation Act of 2012. The mission of FirstNet is to coordinate the creation and operation of a public safety high-speed nationwide wireless broadband network. This system provides one interoperable platform for public safety data communications. When complete, the system is designed to fill gaps in communication in rural areas; carry high-speed data, location information, images, and video reliably and securely; and ensure that first responder communication has priority during emergencies and large-scale events.

Modified from: First Responder Network Authority (FirstNet) website. https://www.firstnet.gov. Accessed December 19, 2017.

While dispatching the proper unit, the dispatcher can give the caller prearrival instructions. These instructions are crucial for several reasons:

- They provide the caller with instant help.
- They complement the call prioritization process.
- They allow the dispatcher to give updated information to responding units.
- They may be lifesaving in critical incidents.
- They provide emotional support for the caller, bystander, or victim.

Procedures for EMS Communications

Most EMS systems use a standard radio communications protocol. This protocol includes the desired format for message transmission and key words and phrases. This format aids professional and efficient radio communication within the system. General guidelines for radio communications include the following:

- Think before you speak (ie, formulate the message) to ensure that the communication will be effective.
- Key the microphone for 2 to 3 seconds before speaking.
- Speak at close range (2 to 3 inches) when talking into a microphone.
- Speak slowly and clearly. Enunciate each word distinctly and avoid words that are difficult to hear.
- Speak in a normal pitch without emotion.
- Be brief and concise. Break up long messages into shorter ones.
- Avoid codes unless they are systems-approved. Avoid dialect or slang.
- Advise the receiving party when the transmission has been completed.
- Confirm that the receiving party has received the message.
- Always be professional, polite, and calm.

CRITICAL THINKING

Can you think of three reasons why a concise EMS radio report is essential?

A
O
B
A
R

A
A
A
A
A

DID YOU KNOW?

NATO Alphabet Chart

The NATO alphabet assigns code words to the letters of the English alphabet acrophonically (ie, the code word, through its unambiguous pronunciation, represents the letter intended). This system ensures uniform pronunciation of critical combinations of letters and numbers, making them more easily understood by those who transmit and receive voice messages. It also ensures the intelligibility of voice signals over radio links.

A–Alpha	**B**–Bravo	**C**–Charlie	**D**–Delta	**E**–Echo	**F**–Foxtrot
G–Golf	**H**–Hotel	**I**–India	**J**–Juliet	**K**–Kilo	**L**–Lima (*Lee-ma*)
M–Mike	**N**–November	**O**–Oscar	**P**–Papa	**Q**–Quebec	**R**–Romeo
S–Sierra	**T**–Tango	**U**–Uniform	**V**–Victor	**W**–Whiskey	**X**–Xray
Y–Yankee	**Z**–Zulu				

Relaying Patient Information

A standard format of transmission may be developed as a protocol for some EMS agencies. This format allows the best use of communications systems because (1) it limits radio air time, (2) physicians can receive details quickly about the patient's condition, and (3) it reduces the chance that any critical details will be omitted. (Patient assessment findings are presented in Section 5 of the text.)

Patient information can be reported to the hospital or dispatcher by radio or phone. Although the order of information delivery may vary by EMS system and scenario, the radio report should be brief and concise and should contain the following information:

- Unit and personnel identification
- Description of the scene or incident
- Patient's age, sex, and approximate weight (if drug orders are needed)
- Patient's chief complaint or chief concern
- Associated symptoms
- Brief pertinent history of the present illness or injury
- Pertinent medical history, medications, and allergies
- Pertinent physical examination findings, such as:
 - Level of consciousness
 - Vital signs
 - Neurologic examination
 - General appearance and degree of distress
 - Electrocardiogram results (if applicable)
 - Diagnostic findings (eg, serum glucose level)
- Trauma index or Glasgow Coma Scale score (if applicable)
- Other pertinent observations and significant findings
- Any treatment given
- Estimated time of arrival
- Request for orders from or further questions for the medical direction physician

General Procedures for the Exchange of Information

When communicating with medical direction, the paramedic should repeat all orders received from the physician. Any order that is unclear should be confirmed. The paramedic should also repeat all drug orders for confirmation. The receiving hospital should be informed of any significant changes in the patient's status before and during transport. General procedures for the exchange of information include the following:

- Protect the patient's privacy.
- Use proper unit numbers, hospital numbers, names, and titles.
- Avoid slang and profanity.
- Use the echo procedure (repeat what was heard) when receiving directions from the dispatcher or physician.
- Obtain confirmation that the message was received.

When performing the handoff of patient care to the receiving facility (see Chapter 6, *Medical and Legal Issues*), the paramedic should make the final verbal report to the person who will be assuming responsibility for the patient. This report may be only a short update if the person receiving the patient has been following the care given in the field and en route to the emergency department. If this person is not familiar with the patient, the report should be complete. In either case, all pertinent information about the patient should be conveyed during the handoff.

Summary

- Communication is the process by which one person or group transmits information to others. The sender encodes a message that the receiver decodes. Four barriers to communication include the attributes of the receiver, selective perception, semantic issues, and time pressures.
- EMS communications refer to the delivery of information. Information relating to the patient and the scene is delivered to other key members of the emergency response team.
- Proper verbal and written communications allow the delivery of information between the members of the emergency team, the patient, and the community. Communications should be brief, clear, and confidential.
- In the United States, the Federal Communications Commission (FCC) regulates communications over the radio. Paramedics must be familiar with and follow the rules and guidelines of the FCC and those of state and local regulatory agencies.
- EMS frequency ranges include VHF bands and UHF bands.
- EMS communications involve both simple and complex systems. A simple system includes a desktop transceiver and two-way radio. Complex systems include high-power communications capabilities.
- Operation modes used in EMS communications include the simplex mode, which permits only one person to talk at a time; the half-duplex mode, which allows data to flow in one direction, but not at the same time; and the multiplex mode, which allows multiple data streams to be aggregated onto a single carrier that can then be retransmitted.
- The functions of an effective dispatch communications system include receiving and processing calls for EMS assistance, dispatching and coordinating EMS resources, relaying medical information, and coordinating with public safety agencies. Some emergency dispatchers provide prearrival instructions for patient care.
- Typical EMS events have five phases: (1) the occurrence of the event; (2) detection of the need for emergency services; (3) notification and emergency response; (4) EMS arrival, treatment of the patient, and preparation of the patient for transport; and (5) EMS preparation for the next response.
- Establishing a standard format for transmission of patient information is important. It allows the best use of communications systems by reducing the use of radio air time, allowing physicians to receive details about the patient quickly, and reducing the chance that any critical details will be omitted.

References

1. Radio spectrum allocation. Federal Communications Commission website. https://www.fcc.gov/engineering-technology/policy-and-rules-division/general/radio-spectrum-allocation. Accessed December 19, 2017.
2. 800 MHz spectrum: land mobile radio for public safety. Federal Communications Commission website. https://www.fcc.gov/general/800-mhz-spectrum. Accessed January 3, 2018.
3. Narrowbanding overview. Federal Communications Commission website. https://www.fcc.gov/general/narrowbanding-overview. Accessed December 19, 2017.
4. The SAFECOM Program. Federal Communications Commission website. https://www.fcc.gov/safecom-program. Accessed December 19, 2017.
5. SAFECOM, FirstNet and EMS: Interoperability and Communication in the Future. National Highway Traffic Safety Administration website. https://www.ems.gov/newsletter/july2013/safecom_ems.htm. Accessed December 19, 2017.
6. US Department of Homeland Security, Office of Emergency Communications. *National Interoperability Field Operations Guide*. Version 1.6.1. US Department of Homeland Security website. https://www.dhs.gov/sites/default/files/publications/National%20Interoperability%20Field%20Operations%20Guide%20v1%206%201.pdf. Published June 2016. Accessed December 19, 2017.
7. Spectrum management: Project 25. APCO International website. https://www.apcointl.org/spectrum-management/resources/interoperability/p25.html. Accessed December 19, 2017.
8. US Fire Administration, US Department of Homeland Security, Federal Emergency Management Agency. *Voice Radio Communications Guide for the Fire Service*. US Fire Administration website. https://www.usfa.fema.gov/downloads/pdf/publications/voice_radio_communications_guide_for_the_fire_service.pdf. Published June 2016. Accessed December 19, 2017.
9. National Highway Traffic Safety Administration. *Paramedic National Standard Curriculum*, Washington, DC: National Highway Traffic Safety Administration; 1998.
10. Szilagyi A, Wallace M. *Organizational Behavior and Performance*. 5th ed. Glenview, IL: Addison-Wesley; 1990.
11. US Department of Homeland Security. Plain language guide: making the transition from ten codes to plain language. Federal Emergency Management Agency website. https://www.fema.gov/media-library-data/20130726-1824-25045-1506/plain_language_guide.pdf. Accessed December 19, 2017.
12. National Highway Traffic Safety Administration. *Emergency Medical Dispatch: National Standard Curriculum*. Washington, DC: US Government Printing Office; 1996.
13. APCO Institute. *Emergency Medical Dispatch Services*. South Daytona, FL: APCO Institute; 2009.

Suggested Readings

APCO Project 25: Statement of Requirements. APCO International website. https://www.apcointl.org/images/pdf/SOR-2010.pdf. Published March 3, 2010. Accessed December 19, 2017.

Carhart E. Applying crew resource management in EMS: an interview with Captain Sully. *EMSWorld* website. http://www.emsworld.com/article/12268152/applying-crew-resource-management-in-ems-an-interview-with-capt-sully. Published October 11, 2016. Accessed December 19, 2017.

Federal Standard 1037C: Glossary of Telecommuncation Terms. Institute for Telecommunications Sciences website. https://www.its.bldrdoc.gov/fs-1037/fs-1037c.htm. Accessed December 19, 2017.

Greenwood MJ, Heninger J. Structured communication for patient safety in emergency medical services: a legal case report. *Prehosp Emerg Care.* 2010:14(3):345-348.

Institute of Medicine, Committee on the Future of Emergency Care in the United States Health System. *Emergency Medical Services—At the Crossroads: Future of Emergency Care*. Washington, DC: Institute of Medicine; 2007.

McGinnis K. Communications. In: Cone DC, Brice JH, Delbridge TR, Meyer JB, eds. *Medical Oversight of EMS Systems.* Vol. 2. West Sussex, UK: Wiley; 2015.

National Highway Traffic Safety Administration. *Emergency Medical Services: Education Agenda for the Future*. Washington, DC: National Highway Traffic Safety Administration; 1996.

NENA standards and other documents. NENA website. http://www.nena.org/?page=Standards. Accessed December 19, 2017.

Spectrum management: Project 25. APCO International website. https://www.apcointl.org/spectrum-management/resources/interoperability/p25.html. Accessed December 19, 2017.

US Department of Commerce, National Telecommunications and Information Administration. Land mobile spectrum planning options appendix: sharing trunked public safety radio systems among federal, state, and local organizations. National Telecommunications and Information Administration website. https://www.ntia.doc.gov/page/land-mobile-spectrum-planning-options-appendix. Accessed December 19, 2017.

US Department of Transportation, Office of the Assistant Secretary for Research and Technology, and Intelligent Transportation Systems Joint Program Office. Next-generation 9-1-1: research overview. Intelligent Transportation Systems Joint Program Office website. https://www.its.dot.gov/research_archives/ng911/index.htm. 2017. Accessed December 19, 2017.

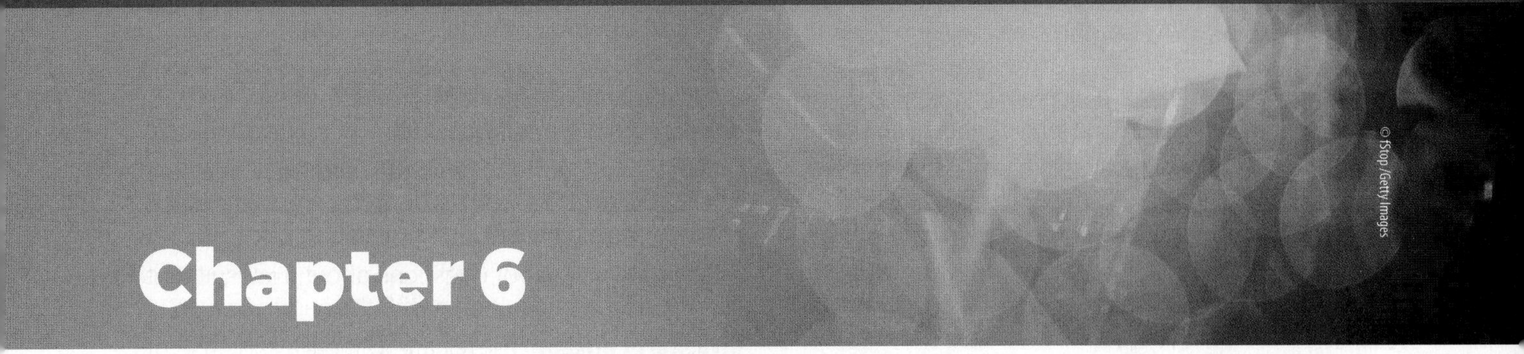

Chapter 6

Medical and Legal Issues

NATIONAL EMS EDUCATION STANDARD COMPETENCIES

Preparatory

Integrates comprehensive knowledge of the EMS system, safety/well-being of the paramedic, and medical/legal and ethical issues which is intended to improve the health of EMS personnel, patients, and the community.

Medical/Legal and Ethics

- Consent/refusal of care (pp 131–135)
- Confidentiality (pp 129–130)
- Advance directives (pp 138–141)
- Tort and criminal actions (p 120)
- Evidence preservation (p 143)
- Statutory responsibilities (p 119)
- Mandatory reporting (pp 121–122)
- Health care regulation (pp 119–120)
- Patient rights/advocacy (p 129)
- End-of-life issues (pp 138–141)
- Ethical principles/moral obligations (see Chapter 7, *Ethics*)
- Ethical tests and decision making (see Chapter 7, *Ethics*)

OBJECTIVES

Upon completion of this chapter, the paramedic student will be able to:

1. Describe the basic structure of the legal system in the United States. (p 120)
2. Explain how laws affect the paramedic's practice. (pp 120–123)
3. List situations the paramedic is legally required to report in most states. (pp 121–122)
4. Describe the four elements of a claim of negligence. (pp 125–126)
5. Describe measures paramedics may take to protect themselves from claims of negligence. (pp 126–129)
6. Describe the paramedic's responsibilities regarding patient confidentiality. (pp 129–130)
7. Outline the process for obtaining expressed, informed, and implied consent. (p 132)
8. Describe actions to be taken in a refusal of care situation. (pp 133–134)
9. Describe legal complications relating to consent. (pp 134–135)
10. Describe legal considerations in situations that require the use of force. (p 135)
11. Describe legal considerations related to patient transport. (pp 135–136)
12. Outline legal implications related to resuscitation and death of a patient. (pp 136–138)
13. Describe advance directives and other end-of-life planning considerations. (pp 138, 140–142)
14. List the paramedic's responsibilities at a crime scene. (pp 142–143)
15. Outline the characteristics of an effective written or electronic patient care report. (pp 143–144)

KEY TERMS

abandonment The act of terminating medical care without legal excuse or of turning care over to personnel who do not have the training and expertise appropriate for the patient's medical needs.

administrative law Regulations developed by a government agency to provide details about the function and process of the law.

advance directive A legal document in which a person specifies what should be done for his or her health if the person is unable to make medical decisions because of injury, illness, or lack of decision-making capacity.

assault The act of creating apprehension or fear; also, unauthorized handling and treatment of a patient.

battery Physical contact with a person without consent and without legal justification.

borrowed servant A legal doctrine that refers to a servant who serves two "masters" (eg, an emergency medical technician [EMT] who is employed by a municipality but who is supervised by a paramedic).

breach of duty A breach of a professional duty to act.

civil law An area of law that deals with "private" complaints brought by one person (the plaintiff) against another person (the defendant); also known as *tort law*.

common law Law that comes from societal acceptance of customs or norms of behavior over time; also known as *case law* or *judge-made law*.

compensable damages Damages awarded in a lawsuit that may include medical expenses, lost earnings, conscious pain and suffering, and wrongful death.

criminal law A type of law in which the federal, state, or local government prosecutes people for violating a law.

decision-making capacity Patients' ability to make their own health care decisions.

defamation Saying something untrue about a person's character or reputation without legal privilege or the person's consent.

dependent practice A type of medical practice in which the provider offers a certain type of care that falls under the same scope of practice as a physician but that requires medical oversight.

deposition A testimony taken under oath in a location other than a courtroom.

discovery The judicial process in which documents are exchanged and depositions and interrogatives are taken.

duty to act The duty of a party to take necessary action to prevent harm to another party. This duty may be formal or contractual.

emancipation The state of being legally released from parental control and supervision.

expressed consent Verbal or written consent to treatment.

false imprisonment Intentional and unjustifiable detention of a person.

Good Samaritan laws State laws that are passed to encourage people to help others in an emergency without fear of litigation (being sued), if not expressly abrogated by statute.

implied consent The presumption that an unconscious or incompetent person would consent to lifesaving care.

informed consent Consent obtained from a patient after all facts necessary for the person to make a reasonable decision have been explained.

interrogative A set of questions about a lawsuit that is answered in consultation with the party's lawyer.

invasion of privacy The release, without legal cause, of details about a patient's private life that might expose the person to ridicule, notoriety, or embarrassment.

involuntary consent Consent to treatment granted by authority of law.

legislation Laws made by legislative branches of government.

libel False statements about a person with malicious intent or reckless disregard for the falsity of the statements; includes statements made in writing or through the mass media.

malfeasance A wrongful or unlawful act.

mandatory reporting The requirement by law that health care professionals report certain types of cases, such as abuse and neglect.

medical malpractice Professional negligence by act or omission by health care personnel in which the care provided deviates from accepted standards of practice in the medical community and causes injury to the patient.

medical malpractice insurance A type of professional liability insurance that protects health care professionals from medical acts and omissions that cause harm or injury.

medical practice act A law that governs the practice of medicine.

misfeasance A legal act that is performed in a manner that is harmful or injurious.

negligence Failure to use such care as reasonably prudent EMS personnel would use in similar circumstances.

nonfeasance Failure to perform a required act or duty.

physician orders for life-sustaining treatment (POLST) An approach to end-of-life planning that emphasizes patients' wishes regarding the medical treatment they receive.

protected health information (PHI) Any information about health status, provision of health care, or payment for health care that can be linked to a specific person.

proximate cause Proof that a negligent act or lack of action caused an injury or worsened an existing injury.

punitive damages Damages awarded in a lawsuit that may be in excess of compensable damages; damages meant to punish the person at fault and to deter others from causing such harm in the future.

regulations Standards promulgated by a government authority pursuant to a legislative grant that have the force and effect of law.

scope of practice Regarding EMS personnel, the range of duties and skills that paramedics are allowed and expected to perform when necessary.

settlement An agreement to accept an amount of money in exchange for a promise not to pursue a legal claim.

slander False statements about a person.

standard of care The action and prudence that a reasonable person in the same or similar circumstances would exercise in providing care to a patient.

statutes Formal written enactments of a legislative authority that governs a state, city, or county.

tort A personal harm or injury caused by civil versus criminal wrongs.

transcript A formal record of questions and answers that may be used during a trial.

vicarious liability A form of liability in which an employer or supervisor is liable for the negligent actions of another person, even though the employer or supervisor was not directly responsible for the wrongdoing.

Historically, only hospitals and physicians were affected by **medical malpractice** *because EMS personnel were not expected to meet professional standards of patient care. However, with state and national certification, licensure, and the paramedic's role as a health care professional, medical liability for EMS personnel and their employers has become a real concern.*

Legal Duties and Ethical Responsibilities

The paramedic's legal duties are to the patient, the employer, the medical director, and the public. These duties are defined by **statutes** and **regulations** that are based on commonly accepted standards of medical care. As do other health care professionals, paramedics have ethical responsibilities in addition to their legally mandated duties. These ethical responsibilities include the following:

- Responding with respect to the physical and emotional needs of every patient
- Maintaining mastery of skills
- Participating in continuing education and refresher training
- Critically reviewing one's own performance and taking steps to improve it
- Reporting honestly
- Respecting confidentiality
- Working cooperatively and with respect with other emergency personnel and health care professionals
- Staying current on new concepts and modalities

Failure to perform EMS duties properly can result in civil or criminal liability. As described in this chapter, the best legal protection is providing appropriate assessment and care to the patient. This care should be coupled with correct and full written documentation.

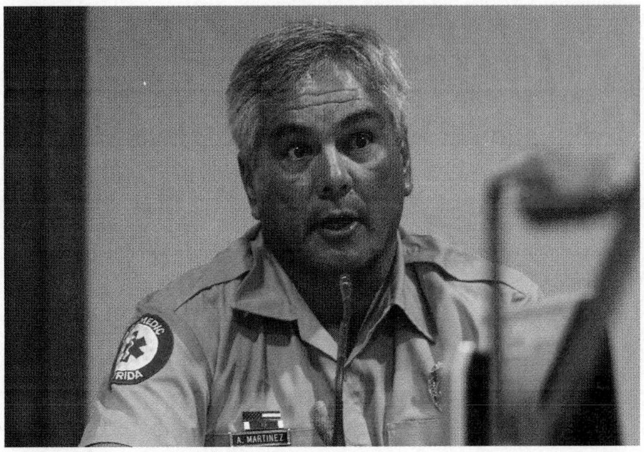

© Elaine Litherland/AP Images

NOTE

Laws pertaining to patient care delivery vary by state. Every paramedic should be thoroughly familiar with, and comply with, his or her responsibilities defined by the applicable regulatory statutes. State EMS laws and regulations can often be found on state government websites. If necessary, the paramedic should consult with a private attorney experienced in EMS law. The information in this chapter is general information and is not intended to be a complete guide to the legislative system, EMS laws, or regulations of any state.

The United States Legal System

The structure of the legal system in the United States is composed of five types of law:[1]

- **Legislation** is law made by legislative branches of government. Examples of these branches include city councils, district boards, general assemblies, and Congress. The power of these bodies to make law is defined by statutes, state constitutions, and, in the case of Congress, the US Constitution.
- **Administrative law** refers to regulations developed by a government authority that have the force and effect of law. An example is the general requirement for paramedic licensure. These regulations may address areas such as examinations, licenses, and maintenance of records. Regulatory agencies may hold disciplinary hearings on the revocation or suspension of licenses. An example of a regulatory agency is a state EMS bureau.
- **Common law** is also known as case law or judge-made law. This law is derived from society's acceptance of customs or norms of behavior over time and is based on the decisions of judges within the state and federal judicial systems. These court decisions may help define acceptable conduct, negligence, and the interpretation of state statutes and regulations that apply to EMS patient care.
- **Criminal law** is designed to protect society. Under this type of law, the federal, state, or local government prosecutes people for violating a law—that is, for a "public" complaint. Such violations may be punishable by fine or imprisonment or both.
- **Civil law** (tort law) deals with "private" complaints brought by one person (the plaintiff) against another person (the defendant). These complaints allege that an illegal act or wrongdoing (**tort**) occurred for which the plaintiff asks the court to award damages. Most EMS activities that result in litigation are civil suits.

How Laws Affect the Paramedic

To avoid litigation, paramedics must be knowledgeable about issues related to medical malpractice and ensure that they follow the laws and regulations that apply to their profession. They also must know how these issues can affect patient care activities.

Scope of Practice

Scope of practice for paramedics refers to the range of duties and skills they are allowed and expected to perform when necessary. These duties, which are set by state law or regulation, are typically based on the National EMS Scope of Practice Model recommendations developed by the National Highway Traffic Safety Administration.[2] The scope of practice defines the boundaries between the paramedic and the layperson, as well as the boundaries between professionals (eg, EMTs, paramedics, and physicians).[2] For example, the scope of practice for most paramedics in most states includes endotracheal intubation, administration of medications, and other basic and advanced life support (ALS) procedures. A scope of practice violation may result in disciplinary action by a state agency and may sometimes be considered a criminal offense.

> CRITICAL THINKING
>
> Why is it necessary to define the scope of practice for a profession?

Medical Direction

As is explained in Chapter 1, *EMS Systems: Roles, Responsibilities, and Professionalism,* medical direction is a required component of paramedic practice. In most states, the paramedic does not work "under the license" or as an agent of the physician who serves as medical director. Paramedics are agents of the EMS agency that employs them, not agents of the medical director. The legal relationship between a paramedic and the medical director is one of supervision, meaning that the physician is responsible for overseeing the medical practice of the paramedic. This supervision may take the form of direct (online) or indirect (off-line) medical oversight. The medical director credentials paramedics to verify their competence, writes protocols, participates in continuing medical education, and performs quality improvement as part of this supervisory relationship. Thus, the medical director has the authority to withdraw the credentials to practice medicine for those paramedics under his

WHEN DRIVING MUST CLEAR EACH LANE OF TRAVEL

or her supervision, but would not be responsible for making a decision to terminate a paramedic's employment with the EMS agency.

Medical Practice Act

A **medical practice act** is a law that governs the practice of medicine. Medical practice acts are put in place to protect the public and the health care profession. This legislation varies by state but may include the following elements:

- Designates restricted acts and prohibits certain tasks from being performed by nonphysicians
- Authorizes physicians to oversee and supervise certain tasks performed by nonlicensed personnel
- Provides for the authorization and the withdrawal of **dependent practice**—for example, how and to what extent paramedics may perform medical acts as a function of their licensure or certification

> NOTE
>
> Dependent providers include paramedics, physician assistants, advanced practice registered nurses, surgical assistants, physical therapists, and other health care professionals who provide care that may overlap with that of physicians. Dependent providers must receive medical oversight and supervision from physicians who authorize them to apply their skills within a limited scope of practice. The laws and regulations governing this relationship vary by state.
>
> ---
>
> *Modified from*: Hafter J, Fedor V. *EMS and the Law*. Sudbury, MA: Jones & Bartlett Publishers; 2003.

Licensure and Certification

Paramedic licensure or certification (or both) may be required by state or local authorities. Licensure is a legal process of occupational regulation. In this process a government agency (eg, a state medical board) grants permission for a person who meets established qualifications to engage in a profession. Certification may be granted by a training entity, a governmental body (eg, a city, county, or state), or a nongovernmental certifying agency or professional association, if permitted by state statutes or regulations. An example of a group that provides certification is the National Registry of Emergency Medical Technicians, which certifies that paramedics meet the minimal standard of practice. Certification is often a prerequisite for licensure. The terms *certification* and *licensure* often are used to refer to the same process. When certification is granted by the state and confers a right to engage in a trade or profession, it is actually a license.

> CRITICAL THINKING
>
> How do licensure and certification help ensure the safety of your community?

Motor Vehicle Laws

Motor vehicle laws usually define the standards for equipping and operating emergency vehicles. Like most laws, they vary by state. Emergency vehicle operations and motor vehicle codes are addressed further in Chapter 52, *Ground and Air Ambulance Operations*.

> NOTE
>
> Criminal statutes do not always require proof of intent or intentional conduct for an action to be seen as criminal in nature. For example, an emergency vehicle crash caused by reckless driving may result in a civil suit and criminal prosecution against EMS personnel. Excessive speed, failure to consider road and weather conditions, and improper use or nonuse of audible and visual warning devices are key areas of liability for all emergency drivers. The paramedic should be well aware of state motor vehicle codes and laws that apply to emergency vehicle operations.

Mandatory Reporting Requirements

Paramedics and health care workers may be required by law to report certain cases—a practice called **mandatory reporting**. Mandatory reporting usually applies to cases involving abuse or neglect of children (all states) or older adults (most states). It may also apply to include cases involving gunshot wounds, stab wounds, animal bites, and some communicable diseases (BOX 6-1). The content of the report and to whom it must be made are set by law, regulation, or policy. Local protocols established by medical direction and the EMS agency may give guidance in these areas. Some states apply penalties if mandatory reporting is not satisfied.

BOX 6-1 Cases Requiring Mandatory Reporting in Most States

- Neglect or abuse of children
- Neglect or abuse of older adults
- Gunshot wounds
- Stab wounds
- Animal bites
- Certain communicable diseases

Some state laws related to child abuse and neglect specifically include human trafficking in the mandatory reporting requirements.

Modified from: Atkinson HG, Curnin KJ, Hanson NC. US state laws addressing human trafficking: education of and mandatory reporting by health care providers and other professionals. *J Hum Trafficking*. 2016;2(2):111-138.

Many reporting statutes provide immunity for the person who reports the situation. These statutes prohibit lawsuits against people who file reports or offer a defense in court in the event of a lawsuit. This type of protection lessens the fear of legal consequences for the person who makes the report if it turns out to be false or unfounded.

CRITICAL THINKING

Imagine that your state requires all cases involving gunshot wounds to be reported. A patient has a flesh wound caused by a small-caliber gunshot. The patient refuses care and begs you not to tell anyone so that her privacy will be protected. What would you do?

Protection for the Paramedic

Some state and federal regulations provide legal protection for the paramedic. Examples include notification of exposure to infectious disease, protection provided by immunity statutes, and laws that describe special crimes against EMS personnel. These regulations vary by state and local jurisdictions.

Notification of Infectious Disease Exposure. Part G of the Ryan White Comprehensive AIDS Resources Emergency Act of 1990 (PL 101-381) requires that emergency responders be advised if they have been exposed to certain infectious diseases. These diseases include hepatitis, tuberculosis, bacterial (meningococcal) meningitis, rubella (German measles), and human immunodeficiency virus (see Chapter 27, *Infectious and Communicable Diseases*). The 1990 act also requires that EMS employers name a designated officer to coordinate communications between the hospital and the emergency response organization in the event of an exposure. The responder is to be notified within 48 hours of determination of the exposure so that postexposure management procedures can be taken.

In December 2006, the Ryan White Treatment Modernization Act of 2006 (PL 109-415) was signed into law. The part of the law in the original act that covered notification of disease exposure to first responders was stricken from the legislation. In 2009, the language that was dropped from the bill in 2006 was reinstated.[3]

In addition to the Ryan White Act, many states have laws that require emergency responders to be notified if they have been exposed to an infectious disease.

CRITICAL THINKING

Reflect on the time before the Ryan White Act of 1990. At that time, why would some health care facilities not report significant infectious disease exposures to EMS personnel?

Immunity Statutes. Protection of state and other government entities from litigation derives from an ancient English common law. This immunity (often referred to as sovereign immunity) was originally based on the concept that "the king can do no wrong." In modern law, it means that the actions for which government agencies can be held liable because of negligent acts of their employees are limited.[4] Since the 1950s, however, the trend in many states has been to discard this doctrine or limit its application. In some states, for example, immunity, if exercised, may apply only to the government agency and not to the individual employee or operator of an emergency vehicle. Governmental immunity statutes vary throughout the United States; therefore, EMS personnel may or may not be protected by them.

All 50 states have some form of **Good Samaritan laws**. The intent of these laws is to encourage people to help others in an emergency without fear of a lawsuit. As a rule, a person who gives emergency first aid in good faith, without expecting to be paid, and in a manner that another person with similar training would, is covered by these laws. However, these laws generally do not protect health care workers from acts of gross negligence, reckless disregard, or willful or wanton misconduct. They also generally do not apply to paid, on-duty EMS personnel.

Some states have enacted other forms of Good Samaritan laws that protect EMS personnel and other health care professionals from liability from injuries caused by a Good Samaritan act when there is no legal duty to act. To trigger this protection, the actions must be voluntary, and they must be a good-faith effort to help without gross negligence or willful misconduct.[5]

CRITICAL THINKING

Imagine that your state has no Good Samaritan laws or similar protections. Would this affect your decision about whether to stop and aid an ill or injured person while off duty?

Special Crimes Against a Paramedic. During the course of performing their duties, paramedics may become victims of assault or battery. To deter crimes against paramedics, some localities have enacted ordinances that provide the same level of protection for EMS personnel as for law enforcement personnel. These ordinances make it illegal to harm or threaten to harm EMS crews or to obstruct patient care. Every paramedic should maintain situational awareness and work closely with the dispatch center and police to avoid dangerous situations when possible. *If the scene is not reasonably safe, the EMS crew should immediately retreat from the scene and not enter the area until law enforcement has arrived and secured the scene.*

The Legal Process

A malpractice lawsuit against a paramedic proceeds through a series of specific steps (**FIGURE 6-1**). It begins with an incident in which a person (the plaintiff) perceives that he or she has been injured as a result of negligent patient care. The plaintiff hires an attorney who conducts a case investigation to determine the merit of the complaint. This investigation may include examining patient care reports (PCRs), textbooks, journal articles, and local protocols. If the attorney believes the plaintiff's case has merit based on expert testimony that deviation from the standard of care caused harm (required in many states), a complaint is prepared and filed in court. The complaint outlines the negligent conduct that resulted in the alleged injury. After the complaint has been filed in court, the complaint and a summons are served on the defendant, and the litigation process is initiated. The summons, which is usually served by a sheriff or other authorized person, requires that the defendant answer the complaint or risk automatically losing the case. At this point, the defendant and all parties involved (eg, the paramedic, ambulance service, and hospital) usually retain attorneys to defend against the lawsuit.

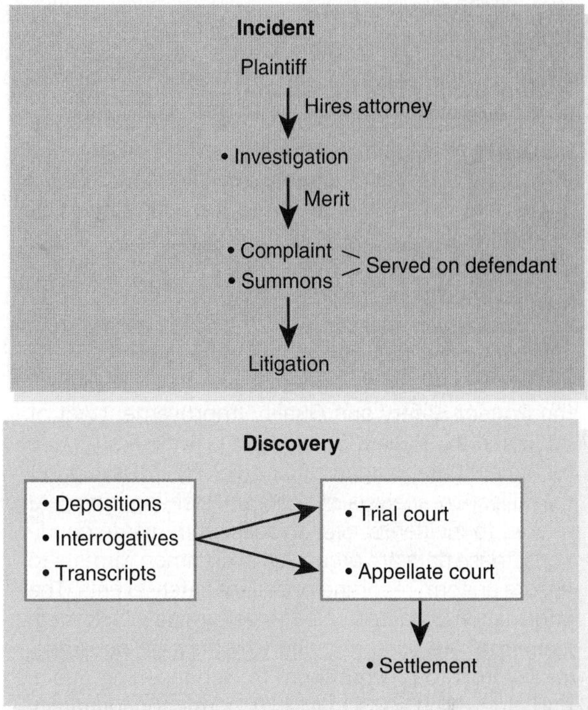

FIGURE 6-1 Anatomy of a lawsuit.

The next step in the legal process, known as **discovery**, usually involves the exchange of documents and the taking of depositions and interrogatives. **Deposition** is a testimony taken under oath

NOTE

Patient Safety Organizations

In July 2005, Congress passed the Patient Safety and Quality Improvement Act of 2005 in response to the Institute of Medicine's groundbreaking report, *To Err Is Human*, which characterized the many types of medical errors that were occurring in the US health care system. Three years later, the Patient Safety Rule was established to help identify problems related to patient safety by collecting data from a variety of health care providers; its implementation is overseen by the Agency for Healthcare Research and Quality. Together, the Patient Safety and Quality Improvement Act of 2005 and the Patient Safety Rule provide a structure for Patient Safety Organizations (PSOs). PSOs support the collection, analysis, sharing, and learning from data related to incidents, near misses, and unsafe conditions; these data are organized in common formats to ensure uniform reporting of patient safety events. The information collected helps to determine which medical errors are occurring and why they are occurring, in an effort to prevent them from happening again. Participation in a PSO provides some confidentiality and privilege protections (so that organizations do not have to introduce the protected information in a legal proceeding) when certain requirements are met. PSOs are intentionally differentiated from most regulatory and mandatory reporting programs that also collect health care–related data.

An EMS agency that participates in a PSO can obtain the following protections:

- Call review documentation
- Documentation and conversations related to investigations of incident reports
- Internal studies of medication and other types of errors
- Case reviews by the agency's medical director
- Regional quality committee meetings (certain conditions must be present)
- Most any electronic or paper documentation, notes, and data related to the agency's safety and quality improvement processes

Reproduced from: Patient safety organization (PSO) for EMS. Center for Patient Safety website. www.centerforpatientsafety.org/emsforward/pso/. Accessed December 21, 2017.

at a location other than in a courtroom. The person giving the deposition answers questions from the attorney for the other side. A court reporter types the questions and answers stated during the deposition and prepares a **transcript** that may be used during the trial. When a person gives a deposition, his or her attorney should always be present. An **interrogative** is a set of questions about the lawsuit that is answered in consultation with the party's lawyer; this information is then given to the lawyer for the other side. During discovery, each side is entitled to receive all key information having to do with the lawsuit. Other documents that may be gathered during discovery are PCRs, computer dispatch records, and recordings of radio messages related to the incident. Quality improvement materials (described in Chapter 1, *EMS Systems: Roles, Responsibilities, and Professionalism*) are "discoverable" in some states.

CRITICAL THINKING

Consider a scenario in which you need to describe a case that occurred 5 years ago. How important would your written documentation of that case be?

After discovery, the case is settled out of court, dismissed or adjudicated, or goes to trial. In a trial, each party presents its side of the case. Based on the evidence, expert opinions, and testimonies, a judge or jury determines liability and any damages to be awarded to the plaintiff, if any. Either side may appeal the decision of the trial court, but the appeal usually can be based only on errors in law made by the trial court.

Settlement may occur at any stage during the litigation. As part of the settlement, the plaintiff sometimes agrees to accept an amount of money in exchange for a promise not to pursue the claim. After the settlement, and as a condition of the settlement, the case is dismissed.

NOTE

The legal process may involve both trial and appellate courts. A trial court determines the outcome of individual cases; this outcome may be determined by a judge or by a jury. The appellate court hears appeals of decisions by trial courts or other appeals courts. Decisions reached in the appellate court may set a precedent for later cases of a similar nature.

Legal Accountability of the Paramedic

Paramedics are responsible for acting in a way that is reasonable and prudent. They should provide a level of care and transport consistent with their education, training, and local protocol. If paramedics fail to meet these responsibilities, the result may be legal liability.

> NOTE
> Almost anyone can be sued, regardless of the validity of the complaint, as long as an expert is willing to attest to a deviation from the standard of care that led to some injury. A lawsuit itself is not an indication of guilt or wrongdoing unless the allegations are proved and they establish a basis for liability.

Components of Negligence

Lawsuits involving patient care usually result from civil claims of **negligence**—that is, the failure to act as a reasonable, prudent paramedic would act in similar circumstances. In most states, four elements must be present to prove negligence: (1) A duty to act existed, (2) the actions performed were at a level that deviated from the standard of care (**breach of duty**), (3) damage to the patient or other person (plaintiff) occurred, and (4) the breach was the proximate cause of the damage.

> CRITICAL THINKING
> Certain ALS interventions pose a greater risk of causing harm to the patient compared with basic life support (BLS) skills. As a paramedic, which ALS interventions do you think you will perform that have this increased risk?

Duty to Act

Paramedics assume a "duty" to provide emergency care when requested while working for an EMS system. This duty may be formal (contractual) or informal (volunteer). Once a paramedic assumes the **duty to act**, the paramedic must continue to act. That is, the duty must not be interrupted until (1) patient care has been transferred to another health care worker whose training and experience meet the patient's needs, (2) it is abundantly clear that the patient no longer needs assistance, or (3) the patient–caregiver relationship is terminated by the patient. Among the paramedic's duties are the following:

- Respond and render care.
- Obey laws and regulations.
- Operate emergency vehicles reasonably and prudently.
- Provide care and transport to the expected standard.
- Provide care and transport consistent with the scope of practice, applicable medical protocols, and any medical direction provided by a physician legally authorized to do so.
- Continue care and transport through to its appropriate conclusion.

> NOTE
> The authorization of dependent practice between a physician and a paramedic may be effective only when the paramedic is on duty, unless other protections are provided by some form of a Good Samaritan law. Therefore, an off-duty paramedic who provides emergency care usually must act in a BLS capacity unless the paramedic has specific authorization from medical direction and state law to perform ALS procedures while off duty.

Breach of Duty

As mentioned earlier, for negligence to exist, the plaintiff first must prove two of the required elements: that the paramedic had a duty to act and that the actions performed were at a level that deviated from the **standard of care** (breach of duty). The paramedic must exercise the degree of care, skill, and judgment that any other similarly trained paramedic would provide under similar circumstances. This standard of

> NOTE
> The standard of care refers to the action and prudence that a reasonable person in the same or similar circumstances, with the same resources, would exercise in providing care to a patient. The standard of care may vary, depending on the situation; however, the scope of practice should not. The scope of practice describes a paramedic's authority (vested by the state through licensing) to engage in or perform an activity but does not specify whether a paramedic should engage in an activity or perform a procedure. It is a description of what a licensed person legally can and cannot do.
>
> *Modified from*: Moffett P, Moore G. The standard of care: legal history and definitions; the bad and good news. *West J Emerg Med*. 2011 Feb;12(1):109-112; and National Highway Traffic Safety Administration. National EMS scope of practice model. EMS.gov website. https://www.ems.gov/pdf/education/EMS-Education-for-the-Future-A-Systems-Approach/National_EMS_Scope_Practice_Model.pdf. Published February 2007. Accessed December 21, 2017.

care is established by court testimony and referenced to public codes, standards, criteria, and guidelines related to the situation. Many states consider national standards when defining acceptable care. If the paramedic violated written national or state standards, the plaintiff may more easily prove breach of duty.

Breach of duty may occur by **malfeasance** (performing a wrongful or unlawful act), **misfeasance** (performing a legal act in a manner that is harmful or injurious), or **nonfeasance** (failure to perform a required act or duty). In some cases, negligence may be so obvious that it does not require extensive proof. The Latin phrase *res ipsa loquitur* means "the thing speaks for itself." This phrase implies that the facts are so clear that without a doubt the injury could have been caused only by negligence. Negligence per se means that negligence is shown by the fact that a statute or ordinance was violated and injury resulted.

Damage to the Patient or Another Person

The third element of negligence is proof of damage—in other words, proof that the plaintiff suffered **compensable damages**. These damages may include medical expenses, lost earnings, conscious pain and suffering, permanent disability, and wrongful death. **Punitive damages** may be awarded in excess of compensable damages and reflect the reckless disregard for human life or outrageous conduct that the defendant engaged in. These damages are meant to punish the person at fault and to deter others from causing such harm in the future. Punitive damages usually are not covered by malpractice insurance (discussed later in the chapter).

Proximate Cause

Finally, the plaintiff must prove that the negligent act or lack of action caused the injury or made an existing injury worse—a condition known as **proximate cause**. The plaintiff also must prove that the injury or further harm was foreseeable by the paramedic. The element of proximate cause sometimes is difficult to establish. Expert witnesses may be called upon to provide proof of proximate cause by addressing issues of duty, standard of care, and conflicting views of causation. For example, was a cervical spine injury caused by the car crash or was it the result of rescue efforts by the EMS crew? Negligent conduct is possible in areas other than direct patient care, such as when a patient is transported to a medical facility contrary to medical direction advice, trauma center designation, or other known special patient care needs and facility capabilities. Another example, failure to maintain equipment, supplies, or vehicles, may be identified as the proximate cause in a case. Negligent or reckless driving also is a source of potential liability.

> CRITICAL THINKING
>
> Do you think an effective quality management program can reduce an EMS agency's risk of negligence lawsuits? Explain your reasoning.

Defenses to Negligence Claims

Training, competent patient care skills, and full documentation of all patient care activities all are excellent ways for health care professionals to protect themselves against claims of negligence. Other defenses to negligence are described here, along with their pros and cons.

1. Good Samaritan laws
   - Generally do not protect EMS personnel from acts of gross negligence, reckless disregard, or willful or wanton misconduct
   - Generally do not prohibit the filing of a lawsuit
   - May provide coverage for paid or volunteer EMS personnel
   - Vary from state to state
2. Government immunity
   - Trend is toward limiting protection
   - May protect only the government agency, not EMS personnel
   - Varies from state to state
3. Statute of limitations
   - Limits the number of years after an incident during which a lawsuit can be filed
   - Is set by law and may differ for cases involving adults and children
   - Varies from state to state
4. Contributory negligence
   - Plaintiff may be found to have contributed to his or her own injury
   - Damages awarded may be reduced or eliminated based on the plaintiff's contribution to the injury

SHOW ME THE EVIDENCE

A descriptive study was performed as a retrospective review of litigation against ambulance services in England over the previous 10 years. In the 272 cases found by the authors, the most common reason given for the lawsuit was "lack of assistance or care," followed by failure or delay in treatment or diagnosis. The authors concluded that ambulance services should focus on areas including obstetric care, recognition of spinal injury, and decisions not to transport.

Modified from: Dobbie A, Cooke M. A descriptive review and discussion of litigation claims against ambulance services. *Emerg Med J*. 2008;25:455-458.

Liability Insurance

All practicing active health care professionals should have adequate liability insurance. An especially important type of liability insurance to carry is **medical malpractice insurance**. These policies offer coverage for legal defense and potential judgments against the policyholder. Malpractice insurance falls into two groups: primary policies and umbrella policies.

Primary policies, which are personal policies, offer limited coverage for the types of risks against which the professional is insured. For example, a policy with a $100,000 limit pays up to that amount for covered damages caused by the insured.

CRITICAL THINKING

Which type of liability insurance protects you now as an emergency medical technician? Which type of liability insurance protects you as a student paramedic in a clinical experience?

Umbrella policies are liability insurance policies carried by employers of paramedics, such as an ambulance service or a hospital. These policies often have additional limited coverage that applies to on-duty employees who perform activities within the scope of practice authorized by the employer, policy, or protocol. A $1 million umbrella policy, for example, covers damages caused by the insured in excess of those limits in the underlying primary policy. The amount of coverage provided by such umbrella policies varies by hospital and EMS agency, and it may not cover the employee's liability. In such a case, a separate individual policy may be desirable.

A variety of companies offer the individual insurance coverage. Group plans often are less expensive, though, and may offer better coverage than the more costly individual policies.

Special Liability Concerns

Several liability concerns are unique to prehospital care. One issue is the liability of the medical director. Another issue is the liability for "borrowed servants." Concerns also may arise relating to civil rights.

Liability of the Paramedic Medical Director. As stated earlier, paramedics function as dependent providers who are supervised by the EMS agency's medical director. As a result, the medical director oversees the practice of the paramedic. Although the functions and responsibilities of a medical director vary by state, generally the medical director is not responsible for the actions of paramedics under his or her supervision, especially for acts of omission, gross negligence, or willful misconduct. Instead, the medical director generally is responsible for providing appropriate supervision and oversight, and for setting standards and protocols that are consistent with current standards of care.[6] Other responsibilities of the medical director include training and remedial education for paramedics under the medical director's supervision. Some states provide liability protection for medical directors and their designees, including emergency department (ED) hospital physicians and nurses who are authorized to provide on-line medical direction for an EMS agency.

Vicarious liability arises from an employer–employee relationship in which an employer is liable for the negligent actions of an employee, even though the employer was not directly responsible for the injury caused by the employee. Because the paramedic is not an employee of the medical director physician, vicarious liability generally does not apply. The employer of the paramedic (government or EMS agency), however, may have some vicarious liability for the actions of its employees.[7]

Liability for Borrowed Servants. **Borrowed servant** is a legal doctrine that refers to a servant who serves two "masters." An example is an EMT who is employed by a municipality but supervised by a paramedic. This doctrine can create liability for the supervising paramedic as well as for the employer (through vicarious liability). The amount of liability for the supervising paramedic depends on the degree of supervision and control given to the paramedic by the employer.

The borrowed servant doctrine is based on the theory that when a person has control over someone else's employee, he or she should be responsible for that person's acts, even though no employer–employee relationship exists. Paramedics who normally have full supervisory control over EMTs must protect the patient's interests by making sure the EMTs perform patient care properly.

Civil Rights. The first civil rights measure, which prohibited discrimination based on race, was enacted in 1866.[8] Since then, civil rights laws have been modified several times to make it illegal to discriminate by reason of race, color, sex, religion, national origin, and, in the case of health care, ability to pay (BOX 6-2). In the case of a municipal ambulance service, a patient could bring a claim under the civil rights act for several possible violations in addition to discrimination, including treatment and transport without proper consent.

Another civil rights law, the Rehabilitation Act of 1973 (revised in 2015), prohibits discrimination against handicapped people solely based on the person's handicap.[9] This act applies to any program or activity that receives federal funding, which may include EMS agencies that receive Medicare or Medicaid reimbursement. Title II of the Americans with Disabilities Act also allows for equal accessibility for public services by people with disabilities. This includes receiving appropriate patient care regardless of disease condition, including communicable diseases such as acquired immune deficiency syndrome, infection with human immunodeficiency virus, and tuberculosis.

Section 1557 of the Patient Protection and Affordable Care Act builds on other nondiscrimination laws by extending protection against discrimination to people covered under any health program that receives funding from or is administered by the US Department of Health and Human Services.[10] Thus, this provision applies to services that accept Medicare and Medicaid payments. One element of this section ensures that people with limited English proficiency have meaningful access to covered health services.

BOX 6-2 COBRA and OBRA

The Consolidated Omnibus Budget Reconciliation Act (COBRA) took effect in 1986. It has since been revised several times and is now known as the Emergency Medical Treatment and Active Labor Act (EMTALA). EMTALA addresses the medical screening, stabilization, and transfer of patients who have emergency medical conditions or who are in active labor for Medicare-participating hospitals. These services must be provided without discriminating against patients based on their ability to pay, insurance status, national origin, race, creed, or color. The act also addresses the issue of "patient dumping," which is the transfer, diversion, or premature discharge of patients from a hospital because they are unable to pay.

COBRA set penalties of up to $20,000 for each violation, but subsequent amendments via the Omnibus Budget Reconciliation Act (OBRA 1989, 1990, and 1993; revised 2000 and 2003) clarified and strengthened enforcement of the COBRA rules. It also raised the maximum possible fine to $104,826 per infraction for hospitals with 100 or more beds. (Fines are periodically adjusted, based on inflation.) In addition, patients may sue for injury in civil court if a hospital violates EMTALA. Hospitals that incur costs related to another hospital's violation of EMTALA can bring suit to recover damages.

The major provisions of COBRA include the following:

- Medical screening within the capabilities of the hospital's emergency department, including ancillary services available to it to determine whether an emergency medical condition exists
- Treatment until the condition resolves or stabilization of the patient at a referring hospital (legal and financial responsibility), unless the patient refuses to consent to treatment
- Provision of appropriate transfer methods after making sure the patient's condition is stable and the person has consented to the transfer
- Requirement that specialty hospitals must accept transfers from nonspecialty medical centers that are unable to treat specific medical conditions
- Requirement to report to the Centers for Medicare and Medicaid Services (CMS) or appropriate state agency if a hospital receives a transfer of an unstable patient from another hospital
- Whistle blower protection for physician and hospital staff

Modified from: Emergency Medical Treatment and Active Labor Act. Centers for Medicare and Medicaid Services website. https://www.cms.gov/Regulations-and-Guidance/Legislation/EMTALA/index.html. Updated March 26, 2012. Accessed December 20, 2017; and American College of Emergency Physicians. EMTALA. American College of Emergency Physicians website. https://www.acep.org/news-media-top-banner/emtala/. Accessed December 20, 2017.

Covered entities must take reasonable steps to meet these requirements, which may include ensuring access to language assistance services (oral or written), and posting information about patient rights in the top 15 languages spoken by people with limited English proficiency within the state.

Protection Against Negligence Claims

Paramedics must be aware of the various ways that patient care activities can pose a threat of litigation for negligence. The best protections against such claims are those associated with excellence in the paramedic role:

- Education, training, continuing education, and skills retention
- Appropriate quality improvement
- Appropriate medical direction (online and offline)
- Accurate, thorough documentation (see Chapter 4, *Documentation*)
- Professional attitude and demeanor

> CRITICAL THINKING
>
> Think back to a call you ran as an emergency medical technician that did not go well and in which the patient did not do well. Did that call include any of the elements of negligence? Which measures could you take to prevent the recurrence of that type of situation?

Paramedic–Patient Relationships

The relationship formed between the paramedic and the patient during a patient care encounter is a legal one. Consequently, legal issues may arise from the provision of patient care. These issues include confidentiality, consent (including the occasional use of force to restrain a patient), and transport.

Confidentiality

Paramedics have a legal and ethical duty to protect a patient's privacy. Information from a patient usually can be conveyed without the patient's consent to other health care workers involved in the patient's care. For example, such information may include a history of communicable disease. Similarly, paramedics may report to law enforcement personnel and testify in court about information obtained from a patient about an incident or crime. However, potential liability for invasion of privacy and defamation (libel or slander, discussed later) exists in other cases. Liability claims may arise when information is released with malicious intent or reckless disregard. Potential liability also exists in cases in which **protected health information (PHI)** is released to people who are not legally entitled to the information. BOX 6-3 summarizes the key elements of the Health Insurance Portability and Accountability Act of 1996 (HIPAA), the federal law that governs the use of PHI.

Definition of Confidentiality

Information related to a patient's history, assessment findings, and any treatment rendered generally is considered confidential information. This information can be in an electronic, written, or verbal format, and it includes information transmitted by social media such as tweets, social media posts, or photos of the patient, his or her vehicle, or anything individually identifiable.[11] As a rule, the release of this information for purposes other than treatment, payment (eg, filing insurance claims), or ambulance service operations requires written permission from the patient or legal guardian. Exceptions to this general rule include the following:[12]

- Federal, state, or local law that requires release of information
- Health care fraud and abuse detection
- Certain public health activities, such as reporting a birth, death, or disease, as required by law, as part of a public health investigation; to report child or adult abuse or neglect or domestic violence; to report adverse events, such as product defects; or to notify a person about exposure to a possible communicable disease, as may be required by law
- Health oversight activities, including audits or government investigations, inspection, disciplinary proceedings, and other administrative or judicial actions undertaken by the government by law to oversee the health care system
- Judicial and administrative proceedings as required by a court or an administrative order or in some cases in response to a subpoena or other legal process
- Law enforcement activities in limited situations, such as when a warrant has been issued for the

BOX 6-3 Health Insurance Portability and Accountability Act

The privacy provisions of the Health Insurance Portability and Accountability Act of 1996 (HIPAA) were published in 2003 by the US Department of Health and Human Services. Further revisions were made in 2013. Compliance with the privacy rule is mandatory.

HIPAA requires all health care providers to do the following:

- Protect the privacy of patients' protected health information, disclosing the minimum amount needed for treatment (unless requested by a health care provider for treatment), payment, and operations.
- Safeguard that information physically, electronically, and administratively.
- Grant certain rights to patients regarding that information.

Compliance with HIPAA is required for health plans (payers of health care), health care clearinghouses (facilitators of electronic data exchange between standard and nonstandard formats for payers and providers), and health care providers who conduct certain financial and administrative transactions electronically. These groups, which are known as *covered entities*, must comply with certain standards regarding the release of PHI. They also must comply with the coding of electronic transactions. In addition, they must maintain proper security measures for electronic information.

EMS agencies are direct providers of health care to patients. They generate protected health records that have information that identifies a person (eg, name, Social Security number, and address). These records also contain medical information about the person, such as an injury or illness and the treatments provided. If an EMS agency transmits or has ever transmitted this protected health information electronically in connection with any of the transactions designated under HIPAA (eg, billing or fund transfers), it is a covered entity and is subject to HIPAA regulations.

Modified from: HIPAA for professionals. US Department of Health and Human Services, Office of Civil Rights website. https://www.hhs.gov/hipaa/for-professionals/index.html. Updated June 16, 2017. Accessed December 20, 2017; and Recent HIPAA changes. *HIPAA Journal* website. https://www.hipaajournal.com/recent-hipaa-changes/. Accessed December 20, 2017.

request or when the information is needed to locate a suspect or stop a crime
- Military, national defense and security, and other special government functions
- Efforts to avert a serious threat to the health and safety of a person or the public at large
- Workers' compensation purposes and in compliance with workers' compensation laws
- Use by coroners, medical examiners, and funeral directors to identify a deceased person, determine the cause of death, or carry out their duties as authorized by law
- Use by organizations that handle organ procurement or organ, eye, or tissue transplantation (if the patient is an organ donor), or by an organ donation bank, as necessary to facilitate organ donation and transplantation
- Research purposes (subject to strict oversight)
- Use when caring for patients who are inmates or in the custody of a law enforcement official, as needed (1) for the correctional institution to render health care, (2) to protect the patient's health or the health and safety of others, or (3) for the safety and security of the correctional institution or law enforcement

In some cases, confidential patient information may need to be released without the patient's consent. The paramedic must adhere to all reporting requirements and procedures established by HIPAA, state and local laws, the EMS agency, and medical direction. Even then, only the minimum necessary details should be released.

Violation of HIPAA provisions can be costly—and increases based on the number of violations committed by an agency and the level of negligence. The maximum penalty is $1.5 million per infraction.[13]

CRITICAL THINKING

If your local police department has a naloxone program for victims of opiate overdose, are the police officers who administer this medication bound by the privacy protections of HIPAA?

Improper Release of Information

In addition to federal government penalties for HIPAA violation, improper release of confidential information or the release of inaccurate information can result in liability. Civil liability may come into play in two areas: invasion of privacy and defamation (libel and/or slander).

Invasion of Privacy. **Invasion of privacy** is the release, without legal justification, of details about a patient's private life that might expose the person to ridicule, notoriety, or embarrassment. For example, a paramedic is caring for a public official who was in a car crash. After the call, the paramedic tells everyone at the ambulance base that the official had a Nazi tattoo on his left shoulder. A custodian at the base hears the discussion and tells his wife, who works at the official's office building. The next day, a flyer is distributed with a caricature of the official in the back of an ambulance with this tattoo. Within a few days, the EMS agency is contacted by the official's attorney, who claims an invasion of privacy. (The fact that the information released is true is not a defense for invasion of privacy.)

NOTE

Posting anything on social media related to a patient can put the paramedic at risk for claims of invasion of privacy or libel. This includes printed words, recorded sounds, or images related to the call. The result can be civil liability, federal fines, and termination of employment.

Modified from: West G. *Legal Aspects of Emergency Services.* Burlington, MA: Jones & Bartlett Learning; 2016.

CRITICAL THINKING

Have you ever been in a situation in which you or a colleague said something about a patient that you think may have violated confidentiality? What did you do about it?

Defamation. **Defamation** refers to a statement made about a person's character or behavior that is either untrue or made without legal privilege or the person's consent. **Libel** refers to false statements about a person made in writing or through the mass media with malicious intent or reckless disregard for the falsity of the statements. **Slander** refers to false verbal statements about a person made with malicious intent or reckless disregard for the falsity of the statements. If the paramedic in the previous example had lied about the official's tattoo, he or she could be sued for slander, and the office worker who made and distributed the flyer could be sued for libel.

Consent

The rights of patients have been defined and clarified both by legislation and by the judicial system through malpractice litigation. A basic concept of law and medical practice is that the patient has rights, though these rights are subject to the patient's **decision-making capacity**. In particular, patients have the right to choose which medical care and transport they will receive.

NOTE

In defining a defamatory statement, the courts have looked to whether the statement exposed the plaintiff to public hatred, contempt, ridicule, or degradation. Proof must exist of actual harm to the person's reputation.

Modified from: Pozgar G. *Legal and Ethical Essentials of Health Care Administration.* 2nd ed. Burlington, MA: Jones & Bartlett Learning; 2014.

CRITICAL THINKING

Imagine being called to care for a patient who clearly is having signs and symptoms of a heart attack but is alert and refusing care. How would you feel? Which strategies would you use to try to persuade the patient to allow you to provide care and transport?

To give consent, the patient must be of legal age and must be able to make a reasoned decision about the following:

- Nature of the illness or injury
- Treatment recommended
- Risks and dangers of treatment
- Alternative treatments and associated risks
- Dangers of refusing treatment (including transport)

SHOW ME THE EVIDENCE

Fraess-Phillips conducted a literature review to determine whether paramedics can safely decide which nonurgent patients require ambulance transport. In the 11 studies included in the review, the triage agreement between the paramedics and receiving emergency department physicians in the study group was generally poor. Fraess-Phillips concluded that there is insufficient evidence to support the contention that paramedics can safely determine which nonurgent patients should be refused transport.

Modified from: Fraess-Phillips AJ. Can paramedics safely refuse transport of non-urgent patients? *Prehosp Disaster Med.* 2016;313(6):667-674.

Types of Consent

Informed consent is patient consent that signifies the person knows, understands, and agrees to the care rendered. This consent is given based on full disclosure of the information. Verbal or written consent to the treatment is called **expressed consent**. Consent also can be expressed nonverbally by actions (such as the patient nodding his or her head) or simply by the patient allowing care to be provided.

> NOTE
>
> Consent generally must be obtained before treatment is initiated. However, paramedics do not have to obtain the same degree of informed consent as do other health care personnel. For example, in-hospital staff members must obtain a higher degree of consent. Because the paramedic is working in an emergency situation, the patient must only agree to, or at least must not object to, the general nature of the treatment.

Implied consent presumes that an unconscious person without decision-making capacity who needs emergency care would consent to lifesaving care if able to do so. Unconscious patients and victims of shock, head injury, and alcohol or other drug intoxication are examples of patients to whom emergency care should be provided in the absence of informed consent. Be aware, however, that a patient with decision-making capacity who regains normal mental status can revoke consent at any time during care and transport. This pattern is commonly seen in situations involving patients with diabetes who are treated for unconsciousness due to hypoglycemia and then refuse transport after regaining consciousness.

Involuntary consent refers to treatment that is granted by the authority of law. An example is caring for patients who are held involuntarily for mental health evaluation. Another example is patients who may be held under arrest or who are in protective custody. The paramedic must follow established policies and procedures when providing care to these patients. Note that law enforcement personnel may not order a paramedic to treat a patient who has decision-making capacity and who objects to the treatment.

Special Consent Situations

Situations may arise in which obtaining consent for treatment is difficult. Such cases may involve minors, adults who lack competence (ie, have been legally deemed unable to make their own decisions), patients in an institution, or prisoners. In such cases, consent for medical care may need to be obtained from a parent, legal guardian, representative of a state agency, or other legal authority. If a delay in obtaining consent would pose a threat to the patient's life, however, the person should be treated. EMS personnel should be familiar with state laws governing these unique circumstances and should follow agency protocols. When a situation arises with consent issues, paramedics should *always* make sure medical direction is sought and involved in the decision-making process, and they should carefully document all events.

> DID YOU KNOW?
>
> *Competence* is a legal term. Competence is presumed unless a court has determined that a person is incompetent. A judicial declaration of incompetence may be global or limited (eg, financial matters, medical decisions). *Decision-making capacity* is a clinical term that is task specific (eg, specific medical decisions). EMS providers and other medical professionals determine capacity; they do not determine competence.
>
> *Reproduced from*: Orr RD. Competence, capacity, and surrogate decision-making. Published March 9, 2004. The Center for Bioethics & Human Dignity, Accessed at, https://cbhd.org/content/competence-capacity-and-surrogate-decision-making.

Minors. In most states, a person is a minor until age 18 years. Consent of the minor's parent or legal guardian is needed to provide medical treatment and transport unless the child meets specific legal exceptions to consent. All minors may be treated and transported using implied consent in specific situations:

- The child's life or health is in danger due to the emergency condition.
- The legal guardian is not available or not able to give consent.
- Treatment and transport cannot be safely delayed until consent can be obtained.
- The treatment addresses only the immediately life-threatening condition.[14]

Threats in this situation include both life-threatening conditions and other urgent conditions such as fractures, infections, and pain. It is important to document the nature of the threat. In addition, all attempts to contact the parents or guardians should be noted in the patient report.

Minors and Exceptions to Legal Consent. There are three situations in which minors are permitted to seek medical care without parental consent: emancipation, the mature minor exception, and exceptions based on specific medical conditions. All states specify the conditions under which each exception is permitted.

Emancipation is the legal release of a minor from parental control and supervision. Emancipation may include minors who are married, who have active-duty status in the armed forces, or who are living independently and are self-supporting. An example of the latter is college students who do not live at home or do not receive financial aid. In addition, some states consider minors who are parents or pregnant to be emancipated. An emancipated minor has the right to either consent to or refuse medical treatment and transport.

Many states also have a mature minor exception to parental consent, which usually applies to children 14 years of age and older who display sufficient maturity and intelligence to understand treatment choices and to weigh the risks and benefits of medical care. Typically, a physician or in some cases a court makes the decision about whether this exception applies based on the state laws.

The final exception for parental consent relates to specific medical conditions. In particular, minors may be allowed to access mental health services, treatment for addiction to drugs or alcohol, and treatment related to pregnancy, contraception, or sexually transmitted diseases without their parents' permission.

Adults Without Decision-Making Capacity. Regarding obtaining consent, providing emergency care for adults without decision-making capacity is similar to caring for minors. These patients may not be able legally to give or refuse consent. Decision-making capacity may be impaired by a number of factors, such as disease, injury, anxiety, mental illness, intellectual disability, and alcohol or other drug use. The patient may not be mentally able to make sound decisions about his or her care. Therefore, the emergency doctrine of treating and transporting without consent should be applied. Emergency care should be provided without consent only when a life-threatening illness or injury exists and only when a legal guardian is not present to grant or refuse consent. The paramedic should involve medical direction in these decisions.

NOTE

Not all emergency treatment and transport situations involve a life-threatening illness or injury. Some states provide civil liability protection for failure to secure consent when no person qualified to give consent is reasonably available and the EMS provider acts in good faith and without knowledge of facts negating consent.

Modified from: Shickich B, Joye S. Consent to healthcare: general rules. In: Fox H, ed. *Washington Health Law Manual.* 4th ed. Washington State Society of Healthcare Attorneys and Washington State Hospital Association. http://www.wsha.org/wp-content/uploads/HLM_Chapter2A.pdf. Published 2016. Accessed December 21, 2017.

Prisoners or Arrestees. Incarceration or detention generally does not eliminate a person's right to make choices about medical treatment. However, a prisoner or arrestee may have a limb- or life-threatening injury or illness and may refuse to give consent. In these cases, the court or law enforcement agency that has the patient in custody sometimes may authorize treatment. The authority of law provides consent through the emergency doctrine. Paramedics who often provide care in prison settings should be aware of local and state laws regarding consent for this population.

Refusal of Care or Transport. An adult with decision-making capacity has the right to refuse medical care, even if the choice could result in death or permanent disability. Refusal of care may be based on religious beliefs, inability to pay, fear, or lack of understanding of medical procedures. Paramedics should be sensitive to these concerns; they should explain each procedure carefully and answer any questions the patient has. Documentation of this effort on the PCR is prudent.

Involving medical direction, law officers, family members, and friends at the scene may help persuade the patient to accept care and transport. Despite these efforts, however, some patients may still refuse care. If this occurs, the paramedic should make sure before leaving that the patient understands that he or she can call again for help despite the initial refusal. In addition,

NOTE

When a patient refuses care or transport, the paramedic should try to ensure that the patient has decision-making capacity. The following steps may be helpful:

1. Make a visual assessment that includes responsiveness, level of consciousness, orientation, obvious injuries, respiratory distress, and gait.
2. Make an initial assessment to evaluate airway, breathing, circulation, and disability.
3. Measure vital signs, including pulse, blood pressure, and respiratory rate and effort. Use pulse oximetry or blood glucose testing (or both) when clinically indicated.
4. Perform a focused examination as dictated by the patient's complaint (if any).
5. Make sure the patient understands the nature of his or her condition and the medical consequences of the patient's medical care decision.
6. Consult with medical direction and thoroughly document the event.

family members or friends should be encouraged to stay with the patient, if possible. Cases involving refusal of care are a major cause of lawsuits against EMS agencies. The paramedic should always consult with medical direction about these cases.

When attempting to provide care to any patient who refuses care, the paramedic should thoroughly document the event. The names and addresses of others who witnessed the event should be recorded, as should all attempts to obtain consent. In addition, the paramedic should advise the patient of the medical risks of refusing care and record this advice on the PCR. Law enforcement officers and other allied health professionals at the scene should be asked to make similar records of the event. Many EMS systems require the paramedic to obtain a "release of liability" signed by the patient and a disinterested witness. The release should note the refusal of care or of transport, or both (**FIGURE 6-2**), and an acknowledgment that risks of refusal have been explained and understood.

Some EMS systems require EMS crews to contact medical direction while at the scene. At that time, the paramedics review the case with the physician or physician designee. Medical direction personnel may discuss the situation with the patient while the call is recorded. This policy may be useful in suppressing legal action. Nevertheless, the most critical legal document of refusal is the written PCR prepared by the paramedic.

NOTE

Parents and legal guardians who are authorized to give consent have the right to refuse treatment for a child, provided they have decision-making capacity. If the parent or guardian refuses to consent to care and transport in a situation that poses a risk of death, disability, or serious harm to the child, contact medical direction. If despite the physician's advice and after careful communication with the parent or guardian consent for treatment and transport is still being withheld, the physician online may direct the paramedic to contact law enforcement for additional assistance.

Modified from: Committee on Pediatric Emergency Medicine and Committee on Bioethics, American Academy of Pediatrics. Policy statement: consent for emergency medical services for children and adolescents. *Pediatrics*. 2011;128(2):427-433.

Legal Complications Related to Consent

Four other key legal issues are related to consent: abandonment, false imprisonment, assault, and battery. These events may result in a civil or criminal violation.

- **Abandonment** is the improper termination of care or the turning over of care to personnel without the training and expertise appropriate for the patient's medical needs. Abandonment may occur at the scene or when the patient is delivered to the ED. Examples include allowing an emergency medical responder to provide care for a patient who requires ALS care and placing a patient in critical condition in the care of an unlicensed ED "tech" at the receiving hospital without first advising a nurse or physician.

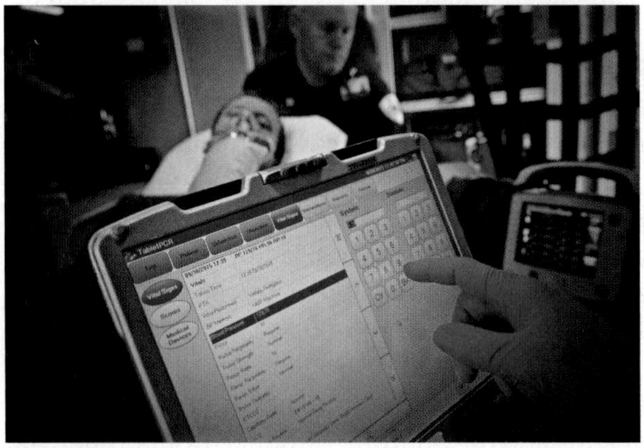

FIGURE 6-2 Electronic refusal form.

Provided with permission by ZOLL Medical.

- **False imprisonment** is the intentional and unjustifiable detention of a person. Examples include a patient who was transported without consent or who was restrained without proper cause or authority.
- **Assault** is the creation of apprehension or fear, or the unauthorized handling and treatment of patients. An example is threatening to restrain a patient unless the patient "quiets down."
- **Battery** refers to physical contact with a person without the person's consent and without legal cause. An example is drawing a patient's blood without permission or authorization.

The paramedic can prevent problems in these other areas of liability by using good judgment. In addition, the paramedic must be sensitive to any special needs of the patient in crisis. Unusual situations or actions should be recorded on the PCR. Medical direction and law enforcement should be involved when needed.

Use of Force

Occasionally, reasonable force or restraints may be needed to deal with unruly or violent patients. These patients may be unable to make sound decisions about their care because of a behavioral emergency, for example, or because of an altered level of consciousness caused by injury, substance abuse, or illness.

Most law enforcement agencies have the authority to place a patient in protective custody, thereby permitting some patients to be treated. EMS personnel should become involved in restraining patients only when this measure can be done safely and there is reason to suspect that patients are a threat to themselves or others. Agency protocols should be followed when restraint of patients is necessary. Some protocols require that violent patients be put in protective custody by law enforcement personnel before paramedics become involved in patient care. The use of reasonable force to restrain a patient must always be humane and should never be punitive. (Physical restraint and the use of sedative drugs [chemical restraint] to help subdue a patient are described in Chapter 34, *Behavioral and Psychiatric Disorders*.)

Transport

As previously stated, once the paramedic has assumed the duty to act and has begun patient care, the paramedic must continue care until (1) the patient is transferred to another health care worker with training and expertise appropriate for the patient's medical needs, (2) the patient clearly no longer needs care, or (3) the patient ends the patient-caregiver relationship. A key aspect of this continuum of care is patient transport.

Use of Emergency Vehicle Operating Privileges

In operating the emergency vehicle, the driver must conform to laws, regulations, and policies. The driver also must operate the vehicle in a manner that safeguards the patient, crew, and public. In most states, operators of emergency vehicles usually are given right-of-way privileges, allowing the driver to do the following:[15]

- Travel slightly faster than the posted speed limit.
- Drive the wrong way in opposing traffic or on one-way streets against other traffic.
- Safely enter and pass through intersections on a red light.
- Use audible and visual warning devices appropriately.
- Park in unauthorized areas.

CRITICAL THINKING

Your supervisor decides that exceeding the posted speed limit (even with audible and visual warning devices) is too dangerous to the community, so the supervisor disallows this practice on all calls. What will you do?

Paramedics should be aware of the laws in their state regarding the operation of ambulances and should not violate those laws. Driving at a speed exceeding the speed limit and the use of audible and visual warning devices, when permitted, are examples of privileges that sometimes are abused. Most states recommend that ambulances not exceed the posted limits by more than 10 miles per hour during response or patient transport. At least one state does not permit ambulances to exceed the speed limit, whereas another permits EMS units to travel up to 15 miles per hour higher than the speed limit[15] (see Chapter 52, *Ground and Air Ambulance Operations*).

New recommendations suggest that states permit lights and sirens use at the posted speed limit, and only when the patient outcome may be affected by the potential time saved—a condition that typically is present in fewer than 5% of responses. Further, it has been recommended that all states require ambulances to come to a full stop before entering an intersection against traffic.[15]

Choice of Patient Destination

The choice of hospital to which the patient is taken should be based on the patient's needs and the hospital's capabilities. If possible, the paramedic should honor the patient's choice, with disclosure to the patient, if it is the case, that the patient will be required to pay for the difference in mileage for transport to a more distant hospital than the closest hospital capable of attending to the patient's needs. Examples of conditions that may limit hospital selection include hospitals on diversion status because of patient load and the need for specialty care that can be provided only at designated facilities (BOX 6-4). Protocols for hospital selection must be established. In addition, medical direction should be involved when a patient's choice of hospital cannot be honored. For example, some EMS agencies use a "nearest hospital" rule, even if the nearest hospital is not the facility requested by the patient.

Payer Protocols

In some cases, health care plan restrictions may affect when and where a patient can be taken for medical care that is covered by those plans. For example, Medicare, which is the largest single payer for ambulance services in the United States,[16] has complex rules about the types of services and patient transports that are eligible for reimbursement. Paramedics must have a basic understanding of these programs so that the EMS agency can be paid for its services. In addition, such knowledge helps paramedics during discussions with patients about which services are likely to be covered by their insurance policies.

In emergencies involving a threat to life or limb, payer protocols should not be a factor in providing patient care or transport to the closest appropriate facility. Even so, the paramedic must provide a full description of patient care activities on the PCR. Thorough reporting is crucial, because some claims are rejected for reimbursement simply because of poor documentation.

Resuscitation Issues

Issues involving resuscitation are complex, often posing legal and ethical considerations for the patient, family, EMS crew, and medical direction. Resuscitation issues that relate directly to EMS include withholding or stopping resuscitation (termination of resuscitation), advance directives, and potential organ donation.

BOX 6-4 Categorization of Hospital Resource Capabilities

In the early 1970s, the American Medical Association recommended categorization of hospital emergency services as a means to clarify hospital capabilities. In 1990, a task force of the American College of Surgeons' Committee on Trauma published *Resources for Optimal Care of the Injured Patient* (most recently revised in 2014), which describes four levels of trauma centers based on resources, admissions, staff, research, and education involvement.

- Level I institutions can provide total care for every aspect of injury. The trauma center is qualified to care for the most severely injured patient, especially in the surgical critical care setting.
- Level II institutions provide care similar to that provided in Level I facilities but without the same level of focus on research and trauma prevention; they often also serve as the primary care institutions in less populated areas.
- Level III institutions provide services such as assessment, resuscitation, emergency surgery, and stabilization. Patients may be transferred to higher-level institutions as needed.
- Level IV institutions are usually located in rural areas. They assess injured patients and arrange transfer to a higher-level trauma center. These facilities must have 24-hour emergency coverage by a physician or midlevel provider. Resuscitation teams and transfer plans must be in place at Level IV centers.

Categorization of hospital resources identifies hospitals capable of handling trauma patients. It also enables EMS personnel to transport patients rapidly to the most appropriate medical facility. Based on the guidelines established by the American College of Surgeons, some state government agencies have designated certain institutions as trauma centers. Other specialized care facilities, such as pediatric trauma centers, burn centers, hyperbaric centers, and poison treatment centers, provide care for critically ill or injured patients with special needs.

Modified from: Committee on Trauma, American College of Surgeons. *Resources for Optimal Care of the Trauma Patient: 2014.* Chicago, IL: American College of Surgeons; 2014.

Consent for Resuscitation

As stated previously, informed adult patients with decision-making capacity have the right to refuse medical care, including cardiopulmonary resuscitation (CPR). This right does not depend on the presence or absence of terminal illness, the agreement of family members, or approval of physicians. As a rule, patients who are pulseless should be resuscitated (unless directed otherwise by a physician), until one of the following occurs:[17]

- Restoration of effective, spontaneous circulation and ventilation
- Transfer of care to a senior emergency medical professional
- The presence of reliable criteria indicating irreversible death
- Inability of the health care provider to continue because of exhaustion or dangerous environmental hazards or because continued resuscitation places the lives of others in jeopardy
- Presentation of a valid do not resuscitate (DNR) order (BOX 6-5)
- Online authorization from medical direction or by prior medical protocol for termination or resuscitation

Withholding Resuscitation

There are cases where no DNR order is present in which it is appropriate to withhold resuscitation. As a rule, CPR should generally be withheld in the following circumstances:

- Performing CPR would cause risk of harm or death to the rescuer.
- There are obvious signs of clinical death, such as rigor mortis or dependent lividity (BOX 6-6).
- A valid advance directive (described later) or a valid DNR order is present.[17]

According to the American Heart Association, unwitnessed deaths in the presence of known serious, chronic, debilitating disease or in the terminal state of fatal illness may be a reliable criterion in some settings for deciding whether to withhold CPR.[17] When in doubt, however, the paramedic should begin resuscitation and consult medical direction.

The National Association of EMS Physicians and the American College of Surgeons Committee on Trauma have developed a position statement to provide guidance on when it is appropriate to withhold resuscitation in patients with traumatic cardiac arrest. Resuscitative efforts may be withheld in the following circumstances:[18]

BOX 6-5 Do Not Resuscitate Orders

Orders that specify no CPR attempts (ie, do not resuscitate [DNR], do not attempt resuscitation [DNAR], and no CPR) are the result of a decision made between the patient and the physician that CPR should be withheld in the event of cardiac arrest. However, such orders do not limit other forms of treatment, such as oxygen, fluid replacement, and drug administration. Some nursing home orders specify the levels of care and support to be provided; for example, the orders may specify no intubation.

BOX 6-6 Physiologic Changes That Occur After Death

Within minutes after death, postmortem changes begin to occur in the body. The surface of the skin becomes pale and yellowish; body temperature falls and reaches that of the environment within 24 hours; blood pressure and muscle tension decrease; and the pupils become dilated. Blood and fluids begin to drain away from the face, nose, and chin as gravity causes blood to settle in the most dependent (ie, lowest) tissues. This drainage results in a blue-purple discoloration in the tissues known as postmortem lividity.

Within 6 hours after death, muscle stiffening occurs as a result of chemical changes in the body, a phenomenon known as rigor mortis. Smaller muscles in the face usually are affected first. Rigor mortis is followed by a stiffening of the entire body within 12 to 14 hours.

Signs of tissue decay usually are obvious within 24 to 48 hours after death, depending on environmental temperatures. Rigor mortis diminishes and the body becomes flaccid within 12 to 14 hours. As the body decays, the skin loosens from the underlying tissues, and swelling and bloating become evident.

- In trauma patients with injuries that are obviously incompatible with life. Examples include hemicorporectomy (translumbar amputation) and decapitation.
- In patients with blunt or penetrating trauma when signs of death such as rigor mortis or dependent lividity are present.
- In patients with blunt trauma who, on EMS arrival, are found to be apneic, pulseless, and without organized electrocardiographic (ECG) activity.
- In patients with penetrating trauma who, on arrival of EMS, are found to be pulseless and apneic and there are no other signs of life, including spontaneous movement, ECG activity, and pupillary response.

Resuscitation would not be attempted in pulseless apneic adults during a multiple-casualty incident. This decision, which is made during triage, allows resources to be used more effectively for care of living patients.

Policies for determining death in the field should be established by medical direction in accordance with state and local protocols. In addition to the factors mentioned earlier, determination of death usually is confirmed by the following signs:

- No spontaneous electrical activity in the heart, as confirmed by an electrocardiogram in several leads
- No spontaneous respirations
- Absent cough and gag reflex
- No spontaneous movement
- No response to painful stimuli
- Fixed and midpoint pupils

In some cases, the paramedic may have difficulty determining whether resuscitation should be initiated. For example, a family member may request CPR for a patient despite the existence of a DNR order. In this situation (or if the paramedic suspects that the DNR order is invalid), the paramedic should initiate resuscitation and contact medical direction.

When paramedics encounter an apparent death in the field, they should take the following steps:

- Contact medical direction and follow established state and local protocols.
- Document any observations or unusual findings at the scene.
- Notify appropriate authorities per protocol (eg, the police and the coroner).
- Disturb the scene as little as possible.
- Provide emotional support to surviving family members and loved ones at the scene.

CRITICAL THINKING

You are called to care for a debilitated older adult in full cardiac arrest. The family members tell you that they want nothing done and are sobbing and begging you not to resuscitate the patient. They do not have the written documentation needed by your agency to verify the DNR order. What do you do? How would you feel about your decision?

Termination of Resuscitation

The American Heart Association's 2015 guidelines also list criteria for termination of resuscitation.[19] Specifically, they suggest that resuscitative efforts stop when the arrest is unwitnessed by EMS personnel and there is no return of spontaneous circulation before transport if no defibrillation was performed. An end-tidal carbon dioxide reading of less than 10 mm Hg after 20 minutes of CPR is another factor to consider when deciding to terminate resuscitation.

The determination to stop resuscitation in the prehospital setting should be made by EMS authorities and medical directors, who generally should ensure the following:

- Airway management has been successfully performed.
- Vascular access has been achieved, and appropriate medications and defibrillation for ventricular fibrillation or pulseless ventricular tachycardia have been administered according to advanced cardiac life support protocols.
- Persistent asystole or agonal ECG patterns ("dying heart rhythms") are present, and no reversible causes have been identified (see Chapter 21, *Cardiology*).

Advance Directives

In 1991, Congress passed the Patient Self-Determination Act of 1990.[20] Among other things, this law required all facilities that accept Medicare- or Medicaid-covered patients to recognize any kind of **advance directive**. Advance directives require interpretation by a physician and must be formulated into a treatment plan. These legal documents inform health care personnel of a patient's wishes in the event the person becomes incapacitated and unable to convey these wishes directly. The person's wishes may include treatment or the withholding of treatment. Examples of such directives are a *durable power of attorney for health care* and a DNR order (**FIGURE 6-3**). Many states

OUTSIDE THE HOSPITAL DO-NOT-RESUSCITATE (OHDNR) ORDER

I, ______________________________, authorize emergency medical services personnel to
(name)
withhold or withdraw cardiopulmonary resuscitation from me in the event I suffer cardiac or respiratory arrest. Cardiac arrest means my heart stops beating and respiratory arrest means I stop breathing.

I understand that in the event that I suffer cardiac or respiratory arrest, this OHDNR order will take effect and no medical procedure to restart breathing or heart functioning will be instituted.

I understand this decision will **not** prevent me from obtaining other emergency medical care and medical interventions, such as intravenous fluids, oxygen or therapies other than cardiopulmonary resuscitation such as those deemed necessary to provide comfort care or to alleviate pain by any health care provider (e.g. paramedics) and/or medical care directed by a physician prior to my death.

I understand I may revoke this order at any time.

I give permission for this OHDNR order to be given to outside the hospital care providers (e.g. paramedics), doctors, nurses, or other health care personnel as necessary to implement this order.

I hereby agree to the "Outside The Hospital Do-Not-Resuscitate" (OHDNR) Order.

Patient – Printed or Typed Name	Date
Patient's Signature or Patient Representative's Signature	Date

REVOCATION PROVISION

I hereby revoke the above declaration.

Patient's Signature or Patient Representative's Signature	Date

I AUTHORIZE EMERGENCY MEDICAL SERVICES PERSONNEL TO WITHHOLD OR WITHDRAW CARDIOPULMONARY RESUSCITATION FROM THE PATIENT IN THE EVENT OF CARDIAC OR RESPIRATORY ARREST.
I affirm this order is the expressed wish of the patient/patient's representative, medically appropriate and documented in the patient's permanent medical record.

Attending Physician's Signature **(Mandatory)**		Date
Attending Physician – Printed or Typed Name	Attending Physician's License No.	Attending Physician's Telephone No.
Address – Printed or Typed		Facility or Agency Name

THIS OHDNR ORDER SHALL REMAIN WITH THE PATIENT WHEN TRANSFERRED OUTSIDE THE HEALTH CARE FACILITY.

Emergency Medical Services personnel shall not comply with an outside the hospital do-not-resuscitate order when the patient or the patient's representative expresses to such personnel in any manner, before or after the onset of a cardiac or respiratory arrest, the desire to be resuscitated or if the patient is or is believed to be pregnant.

Statutory citation 190.600-190.621 RSMo
9/07

FIGURE 6-3 Advance directive.

also have passed legislation regarding *living wills* and the *right to die with dignity,* which provide for advance directives for patients with a terminal illness. Another type of end-of-life planning, **physician orders for life-sustaining treatment (POLST)**, has been adopted in many states (BOX 6-7). Medical direction must establish and implement policies for dealing with all types of advance directives.

The EMS crew may be dispatched to a dying patient who has asked not to be resuscitated. In such a case,

NOTE

EMS and medical direction should work closely with the families and physicians of terminally ill patients in private homes and hospice programs to ensure that these people make appropriate use of the EMS system and know when to call 9-1-1. Even though resuscitation may not be indicated, EMS personnel may be needed to manage pain and to treat an acute medical illness or a traumatic injury and to provide transport to a hospital. Policies must be set and adopted by local or state EMS authorities (or addressed in state statutes) to allow people to decline resuscitation attempts but still have access to other emergency medical care and ambulance transport.

BOX 6-7 Physician Orders for Life-Sustaining Treatment

Although not an advance directive, the National POLST Paradigm is an approach to end-of-life planning that emphasizes patients' wishes regarding the medical treatment they receive. The program (which may go under various names in different states) is recommended for patients with serious illness or frailty who will likely die within the year. A POLST form consists of a set of signed medical orders based on shared decision making between patients and their family and their physician. The POLST form is legally binding, which means EMS providers may follow its instructions without concern of legal repercussions, and the form should be incorporated into the EMS agency's protocols. The patient should have the original POLST form, and copies are placed in the medical record and, in some cases, in a state registry. **TABLE 6-1** lists the primary differences between a POLST form and an advance directive form. A POLST form and an advance directive are designed to work together; a patient can have both forms.

Modified from: National POLST Paradigm website. http://polst.org/wp-content/uploads/2017/03/2017.03.27-POLST-vs.-ADs.pdf. Accessed December 21, 2017.

TABLE 6-1 Differences in POLST and Advance Directive Forms

	POLST Paradigm Form	Advance Directive
Type of document	Medical order	Legal document
Who completes the document?	Health care professional (which health care professional can sign varies by state)	Individual
Who should have one?	Any seriously ill or frail individual (regardless of age) whose health care professional wouldn't be surprised if he/she died in the year	All competent adults
What document communicates	Specific medical orders	General treatment wishes
Can this document appoint a surrogate decision-maker?	No	Yes
Surrogate decision-maker role	Can engage in discussion and update or void form if patient lacks capacity	Cannot complete
Can emergency personnel follow this document?	Yes	No
Ease in locating/portability	Patient has original; a copy is in patient's medical record. A copy may be in a state registry (if the state has a registry)	No set location. Individuals must make sure surrogates have most recent version.
Periodic review	Health care professional responsible for reviewing with patient or surrogate.	Patient is responsible for periodically reviewing.

Reproduced with permission from National POLST Paradigm.

the crew should contact medical direction immediately so that decisions can be made about the patient's care. If medical direction determines that the patient is not to receive medical intervention to prolong life, paramedics should provide reasonable measures of comfort. Emotional support to family members and loved ones also is important during this time.

Potential Organ Donation

Each day in the United States, about 84 people receive organ transplants, but another 20 people on the waiting list die because not enough organs are available to meet the demand for donated organs[21] (BOX 6-8). The donation of organs and tissues and the transplantation process are complex, and they require the coordinated efforts of many health care professionals. Paramedics can play a key role in the evaluation of potential donors by identifying appropriate patients, establishing communication with medical direction, and providing emergency care to help maintain viable organs.

Identifying likely donors who are dead or near dead is a vital role for EMS agencies in organ procurement. Paramedics can identify a donor by searching for a donor card (FIGURE 6-4) or looking for a notation on a driver's license that indicates the person's intent to be a donor or not to be a donor. Another strategy is to talk with the patient's next of kin about the patient's intent to donate tissue or organs at death (BOX 6-9). Even if the patient has no donor card or other document, the family still has the right to make the decision to donate. Tissue procurement organizations provide special training for EMS personnel that can teach them how to approach the family about organ donation.

Once the patient has been identified as a potential donor, paramedics should contact medical direction. The proper organ procurement agencies should then be notified. These agencies are staffed 24 hours a day to assist in all aspects of the donation, including gathering the proper documentation. The paramedic should carefully and thoroughly record

BOX 6-8 The Wait for Organ Transplantation

Every 10 minutes, a new name is added to the national transplant waiting list. **TABLE 6-2** gives the statistics that reflect the national patient waiting list for organ transplant on December 15, 2017, as reported by the United Network for Organ Sharing (UNOS). UNOS is a private, nonprofit organization that has a contract with the federal government to manage the nation's organ transplant system.

Modified from: Waiting list candidates by organ type—all patient states based on OPTN data as of December 15, 2017. United Network for Organ Sharing website. https://www.unos.org/data/transplant-trends/waiting-list-candidates-by-organ-type/. Accessed December 21, 2017.

TABLE 6-2 Transplant Statistics

Transplant Type	Patients Waiting
Heart	3,941
Heart/lung	42
Intestine	255
Kidney	96,120
Kidney/pancreas	1,609
Liver	14,051
Lung	1,379
Pancreas	908
Total	**118,305**[a]

[a]UNOS policies allow patients to be listed with more than one transplant center (multiple listing); therefore, the number of registrations is greater than the actual number of patients. Also, some patients are waiting for more than one organ; therefore, the total number of patients is less than the sum of patients waiting for each organ.

Modified from: Waiting list candidates by organ type—all patient states based on OPTN data as of December 15, 2017. United Network for Organ Sharing website. https://www.unos.org/data/transplant-trends/waiting-list-candidates-by-organ-type/. Accessed December 21, 2017.

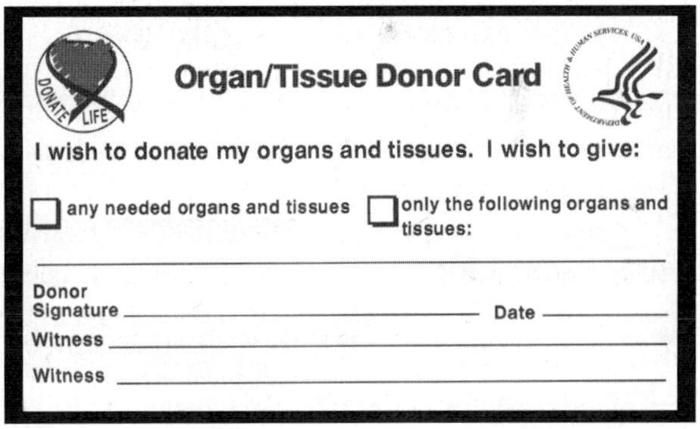
Organ/Tissue Donor Card
I wish to donate my organs and tissues. I wish to give:
any needed organs and tissues
only the following organs and tissues:
Donor Signature ______ Date ______
Witness ______
Witness ______

FIGURE 6-4 Organ donor card.

Courtesy of the US Department of Health and Human Services

BOX 6-9 Legal Next of Kin

When a patient dies in the prehospital setting, organ and tissue donation should be offered as an option to the surviving family members, regardless of the decision to transport the patient to the hospital. Obtaining consent for organ or tissue donation is a delicate subject, and the paramedic should approach the issue with compassion and in a positive manner. As part of this process, the paramedic must obtain consent from the next of kin. This relationship is defined by law and may vary by state. The accepted legal order is generally defined as follows:

1. Spouse (even if separated but not divorced)
2. Adult son or daughter (older than 18 years)
3. Parents (for any unmarried child)
4. Siblings (in the event both parents are deceased and the donor is unmarried or divorced with no adult children)
5. Legal guardian

Modified from: Scoles EF, Halbach EC, Roberts PG, Begleiter MD. *Problems and Materials on Decedents Estates and Trusts.* 7th ed. New York, NY: Aspen; 2006.

BOX 6-10 Criteria for Brain Death

Brain death has been defined as the state of a person who has sustained either (1) irreversible cessation of circulatory and respiratory functions or (2) irreversible cessation of all functions of the entire brain, including the brainstem. These clinical findings usually are confirmed in the hospital by electroencephalogram or a brain flow scan. Only after brain death has been confirmed and the time of death noted does organ donation become a possibility. In most states, brain death must be declared by two separate physicians, and neither physician can be involved in the removal or transplantation of the organs.

Modified from: Schmie S, Horby L. International guideline development for the determination of death. *Intens Care Med.* 2014;40(6):788-797.

all patient care activities, vital signs assessments, and scene observations/events (eg, presence of drug paraphernalia) that may affect the agency's evaluation of the potential donor.

Two general groups of donors are distinguished: living and cadaver (deceased organ donors). Living donors may donate a kidney or a single lobe of the liver or lung. Deceased donors may donate the heart, liver, kidneys, lungs, pancreas, and intestines. In 2014, hands and faces were added to this organ transplant list. Deceased donors may also donate the corneas, various tissues (skin, heart valves, bone, tendons, stem cells, bone marrow, blood, and platelets). These donors must meet the criteria for brain death (BOX 6-10). In addition, the donor's heartbeat and circulation must be maintained until the vital organs have been harvested. More than 125 million people have registered as organ donors, but only about 3 in 1,000 actually die in such a way that allows for organ donation.[22]

Donors after cardiac death represent a subset of potential donors who do not meet the brain death criteria but have suffered some catastrophic event from which they will not recover. If life support is withdrawn and consent to organ donation is obtained, then organ recovery will proceed after cardiac death ensues.

The paramedic plays a key role in helping to maintain viable organs in the prehospital setting by preserving organ function. This is accomplished by airway management and by proper fluid resuscitation to maintain blood pressure and organ perfusion (see Chapter 35, *Shock*). For all nontransported people who die at the scene, eye care should be provided using lubrication and saline solution or a commercial product (eg, Lacri-Lube). In addition, the eyes should be taped closed so that donation of the corneas can continue to be an option for the family.

Crime Scene Responsibilities

Paramedics play two important roles in the management of crime and other incident scenes. First, they provide patient care (the primary focus).

BOX 6-11 Crime Scene Preservation

Lifesaving procedures always take precedence over forensic considerations. However, the paramedic should disturb a crime scene as little as possible so as to help preserve evidence. Some forensic considerations include the following:

- Park the ambulance away from skid marks, tire prints, or other evidence.
- Follow the same path to and from the ambulance and patient.
- Avoid stepping on blood stains.
- Do not touch or move weapons or other environmental clues unless absolutely necessary for patient care.
- Document the exact condition of the patient and the wound's appearance on arrival at the scene, including the environment of the patient and the body's position in relation to objects and doorways.
- If possible, cut or tear clothing along a seam to avoid altering tears made by a penetrating object. Do not cut through a hole made in the clothing by a wounding object.
- Do not shake clothing. Keep all clothing in a paper bag rather than a plastic bag that may alter evidence. Do not give clothing to the victim's family members.
- Save any avulsed tissue for forensic pathologic examination.
- If a bullet is retrieved, place it in a padded container to prevent marring and secure the evidence until it is delivered to the authorities; obtain a receipt.
- Document any dying declarations made by patients.
- Report all actions and alterations made to the crime scene to the police.

Modified from: US Department of Transportation, National Highway Traffic Safety Administration. EMT-paramedic national standard curriculum. EMS.gov website. https://www.ems.gov/pdf/education/Emergency-Medical-Technician-Paramedic/Paramedic_1998.pdf. Published 1998. Accessed December 21, 2017.

Second, they help preserve evidence at the scene when possible.

Personal safety always is the first priority in any emergency response, but especially in crime scenes. If the scene is not safe and cannot be made safe, the EMS crew should not enter the area until it has been made as reasonably safe as practical by law enforcement personnel.

CRITICAL THINKING

Consider this scenario: At the scene of a shooting, you see a patient with slow, gasping respirations, but the police will not let you enter the crime scene. How do you think you would feel? What would you do?

When responding to a crime scene, paramedics should be in direct radio communication with law enforcement officers at the scene. They can provide the paramedics with information on scene safety, the number of patients, and the need for additional resources, which may include more EMS vehicles or personnel, air medical transport, fire service or specialized rescue units, and hazardous materials teams. If the police are not on the scene or if the EMS crew is the first to respond, paramedics should maintain contact with the dispatch center so that appropriate information can be relayed to law enforcement officials. Paramedics must always keep in mind that law enforcement officers are in charge of the crime scene; paramedics are in charge of patient care. EMS crews should work closely with law enforcement officers, who also provide protection for the EMS crew.

In addition to providing patient care, the paramedic should observe and document the overall scene and make an effort to protect potential evidence (BOX 6-11). Steps for ensuring scene safety include the following:

- Approach the scene only after it has been made reasonably safe by law enforcement.
- Approach the scene from a direction that appears safe and allows for easy exit.
- Maintain constant radio contact with the police or dispatch.
- Survey and assess the scene before approaching the patient.
- Keep all unnecessary people away from the patient.
- Initiate conversations with bystanders only when necessary.

Documentation

As described in Chapter 4, *Documentation*, the PCR serves several functions. A particularly important function is providing a legal record of the patient care delivered in the field. This report also becomes a permanent part of the patient's hospital record. Documentation of the legal record of care can be either written or recorded electronically.

The paramedic's record of an emergency call is one of the first items reviewed in the case of a lawsuit for negligence or malpractice. Memory is not infallible, and claims may not be filed until years after an event occurred. In this scenario, EMS personnel may be expected to testify to events that took place years earlier. To refresh their memory about details while testifying, paramedics are allowed to refer to written reports.

Not surprisingly, then, accuracy and attention to detail are crucial in documentation for legal purposes. The characteristics of an effective written or electronic PCR include the following:

- **It is completed promptly.** The PCR is a record made "in the course of business," not long after the event. Timely completion is essential to the PCR becoming part of the hospital record.
- **It is completed thoroughly.** The PCR should cover assessment, treatment, and other relevant facts. The report should paint a complete, clear picture of the patient's condition and the care provided.
- **It is completed objectively.** The paramedic should make observations, rather than stating assumptions or conclusions. The use of emotional and value-laden words or phrases should be avoided.
- **It is completed accurately.** Descriptions should be as precise as possible; the paramedic should not use abbreviations or jargon that is not commonly understood.
- **It is protected to maintain confidentiality.** The paramedic should follow the EMS agency's policy for the release of patient information. When possible, the paramedic should obtain the patient's consent before such release. All records, whether paper or electronic, should be stored in a secure location, with access limited by department policy.

All patient care records must be maintained in a secure location at least for the duration of the statute of limitations. This statute varies by state but generally ranges from 2 to 6 years for personal injury or professional liability (malpractice) lawsuits. Patient records involving minors may have to be kept for a longer time, because the statute of limitations may not begin until the minor reaches 18 years of age. (This requirement also varies from state to state.)

CRITICAL THINKING

Think back to your first call in which a patient refused medical care. Can you remember the exact details of the patient's level of consciousness, what you told the patient about the risks of refusing care, and what you told the patient to do if the problem got worse? Do you think all those facts are in the written documentation of that call in the event of litigation?

Summary

- The structure of the US legal system includes five types of law: legislation, administrative law, common law, criminal law, and civil law. The law requires that paramedics perform within their scope of practice and follow all legal guidelines applicable to their practice.
- To safeguard against litigation, paramedics must be knowledgeable about legal issues and recognize how these issues affect their practice as health care providers.
- Under mandatory reporting requirements, paramedics and health care workers may be required by law to report some cases, such as those involving abuse or neglect of children and older adults, gunshot wounds, stab wounds, animal bites, and some communicable diseases.
- Some states and federal agencies require notification of EMS personnel of exposure to infectious disease. Also, some states have passed immunity statutes that protect EMS personnel from lawsuits in some circumstances, as well as laws that describe special crimes against EMS personnel.
- Lawsuits related to patient care usually stem from civil claims of negligence—that is, the failure to act as a reasonable, prudent paramedic would act in such circumstances.
- Paramedics can protect themselves against claims of negligence by ensuring they have sufficient training, by demonstrating competent patient care skills, and by fully documenting all patient care activities.
- Details about a patient that are related to the patient's history must be kept confidential. Any assessment findings are considered protected health information, as is any treatment given. As a rule, the release of these details requires written permission from the patient or legal guardian.

- Adults with decision-making capacity, who are capable of understanding the risks and benefits of their decision, have the right to refuse care—even if that decision could result in death or permanent disability.
- Four legal complications related to consent are abandonment, false imprisonment, assault, and battery.
- An adult patient with decision-making capacity has certain rights, including the right to decide which medical care to receive and where and whether he or she will be transported.
- Once the paramedic begins to care for a patient, the paramedic's legal responsibility for that patient does not end until patient care is transferred to another member of the health care system or the patient clearly no longer requires care.
- Legal issues related to patient transport include the level of care provided during transport, use of the emergency vehicle operating privileges, choice of patient destination, and payer protocols.
- Resuscitation issues that relate directly to EMS personnel include withholding or stopping resuscitation, advance directives, potential organ donation, and death in the field.
- EMS personnel play two important roles when responding to a crime scene: providing patient care and preserving evidence at the scene when possible.

References

1. Burnham W. *Introduction to the Law and Legal System of the United States.* 6th ed. St. Paul, MN: West Academic Publishing; 2017.
2. National Highway Traffic Safety Administration. National EMS scope of practice model. EMS.gov website. https://www.ems.gov/pdf/education/EMS-Education-for-the-Future-A-Systems-Approach/National_EMS_Scope_Practice_Model.pdf. Published February 2007. Accessed December 21, 2017.
3. Ryan White Care Act extension success, October 2009. *EMS Insider.* 2009;36:10.
4. Maggiore WAW. Legal issues. In: Cone DC, Brice JH, Delbridge TR, eds. *Emergency Medical Services: Clinical Practice and Systems Oversight.* Vol. 2. 2nd ed. West Sussex, UK: John Wiley and Sons; 2015:160-181.
5. Good Samaritans law and legal definition. USLegal website. https://definitions.uslegal.com/g/good-samaritans/. Accessed December 21, 2017.
6. Cone D. *Emergency Medical Services: Clinical Practice and Systems Oversight.* 2nd ed. Hoboken, NJ: John Wiley and Sons; 2015.
7. Maggiore WA. Liability for EMS licensing: whose license is it anyway? *J Emerg Med Serv* website. http://www.jems.com/articles/2011/02/liability-ems-licensing.html. Published February 2, 2011. Accessed December 21, 2017.
8. Jefferies J, Karlan PS, Low PW, et al. *Civil Rights Actions: Enforcing the Constitution.* 3rd ed. New York, NY: Foundation Press; 2013.
9. Rehabilitation Act of 1973 [As amended through P.L. 114-95, Enacted December 10, 2015], 29 USC 701 CFR. Office of the Legislative Counsel website. https://legcounsel.house.gov/Comps/Rehabilitation%20Act%20Of%201973.pdf. Accessed December 21, 2017.
10. Office of Civil Rights, US Department of Health and Human Services. Section 1557: ensuring meaningful access for individuals with limited English proficiency. US Department of Health and Human Services website. https://www.hhs.gov/civil-rights/for-individuals/section-1557/fs-limited-English-proficiency/index.html. Updated August 25, 2016. Accessed December 21, 2017.
11. West G. *Legal Aspects of Emergency Services.* Burlington, MA: Jones & Bartlett Learning; 2016.
12. Office of Civil Rights, US Department of Health and Human Services. HIPAA for professionals. US Department of Health and Human Services website. https://www.hhs.gov/hipaa/for-professionals/index.html. Updated June 6, 2017. Accessed December 21, 2017.
13. McCallion T. Feds make sweeping changes to HIPAA privacy and security rules. *J Emerg Med Serv* website. http://www.jems.com/articles/2013/02/feds-make-sweeping-changes-hipaa-privacy.html. Published February 28, 2013. Accessed December 21, 2017.
14. Committee on Pediatric Emergency Medicine and Committee on Bioethics, American Academy of Pediatrics. Policy statement: consent for emergency medical services for children and adolescents. *Pediatrics.* 2011;128(2):427-433.
15. Kupas DF. *Lights and Siren Use by Emergency Medical Services (EMS): Above All Do No Harm.* Washington, DC: National Highway Traffic Safety Administration; 2017.
16. NAEMT position statement: Medicare reimbursement. National Association of Emergency Medical Technicians website. https://www.naemt.org/docs/default-source/advocacy-documents/positions/6-11-10_Medicare_Reimbursement.pdf?sfvrsn=0. Adopted June 11, 2010. Accessed December 21, 2017.
17. Mancini ME, Diekema DS, Hoadley TA, et al. 2015 American Heart Association guidelines update for cardiopulmonary resuscitation and emergency cardiovascular care, Part 3: ethical issues. *Circulation.* 2015;132(suppl):S383-S396.
18. Case A, Zive D, Cook J, Schmidt TA. End-of-life issues. In: Cone DC, Brice JH, Delbridge TR, eds. *Emergency Medical Services: Clinical Practice and Systems Oversight.* Vol. 1. 2nd ed. West Sussex, UK: John Wiley and Sons; 2015:444-452.
19. American Heart Association. Highlights of the 2015 American Heart Association guidelines update for CPR and ECC. CPR and First Aid: Emergency Cardiovascular Care website. https://eccguidelines.heart.org/wp-content/uploads/2015/10/2015-AHA-Guidelines-Highlights-English.pdf. Published 2015. Accessed December 21, 2017.
20. HR 4449—Patient Self-Determination Act of 1990. 101st Congress (1989–1990). Congress.gov website. https://www.congress.gov/bill/101st-congress/house-bill/4449. Accessed December 21, 2017.
21. US Department of Health and Human Services. Organ donation statistics. OrganDonor.gov website. https://organdonor.gov/statistics-stories/statistics.html#glance. Accessed December 21, 2017.
22. Strickland A. Organ donation 101. Harriet F. Ginsburg Health Sciences Library website. https://ucfmedlibrary.wordpress.com/2017/02/09/organ-donation-101/. Published February 9, 2017. Accessed December 21, 2017.

Suggested Readings

Hafter J, Fedor V. *EMS and the Law*. Rosemont, IL: American Academy of Orthopaedic Surgeons; 2004.

Hill P, Bishop E, Hamilton S, Morrell J, Ellington S. *Emergency Services Law and Liability*. Bristol, UK: Jordans Ltd; 2006.

Isaacs SM, Cash C, Antar O, Fowler RL. The case against EMS red lights and siren responses. *J Emerg Med Serv* website. http://www.jems.com/articles/print/volume-42/issue-2/features/the-case-against-ems-red-lights-and-siren-responses.html. Published February 1, 2017. Accessed December 21, 2017.

West G. *Legal Aspects of Emergency Services*. Burlington, MA: Jones and Bartlett Learning; 2016.

[a]UNOS policies allow patients to be listed with more than one transplant center (multiple listing); therefore, the number of registrations is greater than the actual number of patients. Also, some patients are waiting for more than one organ; therefore, the total number of patients is less than the sum of patients waiting for each organ.

Modified from: Waiting list candidates by organ type—all patient states based on OPTN data as of December 15, 2017. United Network for Organ Sharing website. https://www.unos.org/data/transplant-trends/waiting-list-candidates-by-organ-type/. Accessed December 21, 2017.

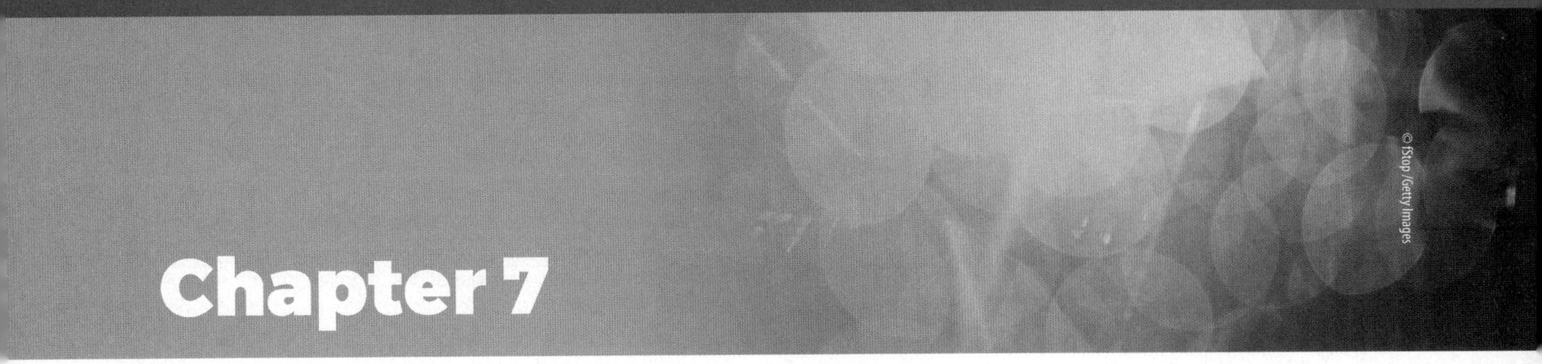

Chapter 7

Ethics

NATIONAL EMS EDUCATION STANDARD COMPETENCIES

Preparatory

Integrates comprehensive knowledge of the EMS system, safety/well-being of the paramedic, and medical/legal and ethical issues, which is intended to improve the health of EMS personnel, patients, and the community.

Medical/Legal and Ethics

- Consent/refusal of care (see Chapter 6, *Medical and Legal Issues*)
- Confidentiality (see Chapter 6, *Medical and Legal Issues*)
- Advance directives (see Chapter 6, *Medical and Legal Issues*)
- Patient rights/advocacy (see Chapter 6, *Medical and Legal Issues*)
- End-of-life issues (see Chapter 6, *Medical and Legal Issues*)
- Ethical principles/moral obligations (pp 148–152)
- Ethical tests and decision making (pp 152–153)

OBJECTIVES

Upon completion of this chapter, the paramedic student will be able to:

1. Define ethics and bioethics. (p 148)
2. Distinguish between professional, legal, and moral accountability. (pp 151–152)
3. Describe the role of ethical tests in resolving ethical dilemmas in health care. (p 152)
4. Outline strategies for resolving ethical conflicts. (pp 153–154)
5. Discuss specific prehospital ethical issues, including the allocation of resources, decisions surrounding resuscitation, confidentiality, and consent. (pp 154–155)
6. Identify ethical dilemmas that may arise with regard to care in futile situations, the obligation to provide care, patient advocacy, and the paramedic's role as physician extender. (pp 155–156)

KEY TERMS

autonomy The principle of self-determination; that is, a person's ability to make moral decisions, including those affecting personal medical care.

beneficence A duty to confer benefits; the practice of good deeds; an obligation to benefit others or to seek their good.

bioethics The systematic study of moral dimensions, including the moral vision, decisions, conduct, and policies of the life sciences and health care.

ethics The discipline relating to right and wrong, moral duty and obligation, moral principles and values, and moral character; a standard for honorable behavior designed by a group with expected conformity.

moral injury The psychological impact of witnessing events that conflict with one's personal morals, or acting in a way that contradicts one's morals.

morals The personal standards that a person uses to distinguish right from wrong.

unethical Conduct that fails to conform to moral principles, values, or standards.

Ethical dilemmas will always be a part of prehospital care. At times paramedics must perform duties that may involve conflicts in moral judgment. Examples include issues of patient confidentiality, patient's rights, and honoring a do not resuscitate order. Such ethical issues are dynamic. The ethical dilemmas of today may be decided by law tomorrow.

Ethics Overview

Paramedics make ethical choices on almost every shift. Issues such as consent, refusal, confidentiality, and end-of-life choices often involve ethical dilemmas. Ethical dilemmas may occur in every phase of an emergency medical services (EMS) call.[1] Having a framework for making ethical decisions is essential. This framework is especially important on calls when there is incomplete information and little time to delay.

Ethics is the field relating to right and wrong, duty and obligation, principles and values, and character.[2] Ethics is a basis for honorable actions designed by a group with expected conformity. **Morals** are the standards that a person uses to distinguish right from wrong. The term **unethical** refers to conduct that fails to conform to these moral principles, values, or standards.[3] Ethical decisions are based on an appraisal of moral judgments—a concept that places the responsibility on individuals.

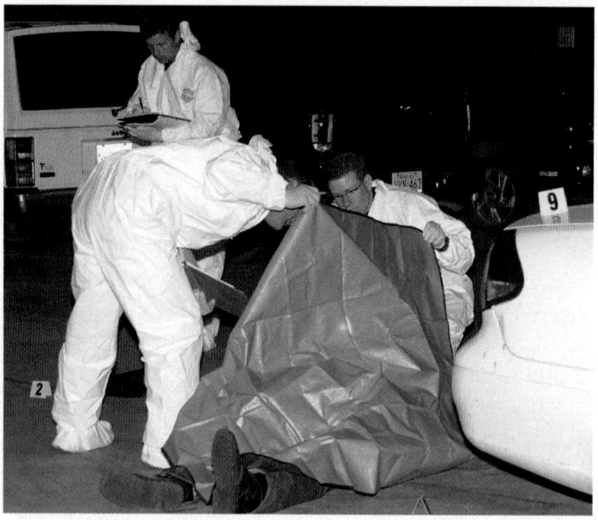

© Jack Dagley Photography/Shutterstock.

The concept of ethics dates back to the ancient Greek philosophers such as Hippocrates, Socrates, Plato, and Aristotle. They turned the focus of philosophy toward questions of ethics and virtue (how one should live) and away from ideas of choice and fate, which traditionally had been guided by astrology.

DID YOU KNOW?

The Difference Between Morals and Ethics

The difference between morals and ethics can seem confusing. The two concepts have similarities, but a basic, subtle difference exists. Morals define personal character. Ethics stresses a social system in which those morals are applied. In other words, ethics points to standards or codes of behavior expected by the group to which a person belongs. This group could be a social group, a religion, a company, a profession, or even a family. Therefore, although a person's moral code usually is unchanging, the ethics that the person practices can depend on the groups to which he or she belongs.

To help clarify the difference between morals and ethics, consider the following examples:

- **Example 1.** A defense attorney must defend a man she believes is guilty of murder. The attorney believes that murder is wrong and immoral and that this person would be a danger to society if found not guilty and released. However, the legal system and the ethics of the profession to which she belongs require that her client be defended as vigorously as possible. Her client also must receive a fair trial. In this case, the attorney's ethics must override her personal morals.
- **Example 2.** In most parts of the world, a doctor may not euthanize a patient, even at the patient's request, because it is against the ethical standards for health care professionals. However, the same doctor may personally believe in a patient's right to die; this belief represents his or her own morality.

These philosophers laid the basis for a science of medical ethics (bioethics), the analysis of choice in medicine (BOX 7-1).[4]

Bioethics is the systematic study of moral dimensions, including the moral vision, decisions, conduct, and policies of the life sciences and health care. Bioethics uses a variety of ethical methodologies in an interdisciplinary setting.

All paramedics face ethical issues during the course of their careers. Most issues deal with the patient's right to self-determination and the paramedic's duty to provide patient care (BOX 7-2). The concept of the patient's right to self-determination is known as

BOX 7-1 The Earliest Hippocratic Oath

The Oath of Hippocrates is a brief statement of principles. It is thought to have been conceived during the 4th century BCE. The oath protected the rights of the patient. It also addressed the moral character of the physician as a healer. The Hippocratic oath was modified in the 10th or 11th century to eliminate references to pagan gods. The oath remains an expression of ideal conduct for the physician.

I swear by Apollo the physician and Asclepius and Hygieia and Panaceia and all the gods and goddesses, making them my witnesses, that I will fulfill according to my ability and judgment this oath and this covenant:

To hold him who has taught me this art as equal to my parents and to live my life in partnership with him, and if he is in need of money to give him a share of mine, and to regard his offspring as equal to my brothers in male lineage and to teach them this art—if they desire to learn it—without fee and covenant; to give a share of precepts and oral instruction and all the other learning to my sons and to the sons of him who has instructed me and to pupils who have signed the covenant and have taken an oath according to the medical law, but to no one else.

I will apply dietetic measures for the benefit of the sick according to my ability and judgment; I will keep them from harm and injustice.

I will neither give a deadly drug to anybody if asked for it, nor will I make a suggestion to this effect. Similarly I will not give to a woman an abortive remedy. In purity and holiness I will guard my life and my art.

I will not use the knife, not even on sufferers from stone, but will withdraw in favor of such men as are engaged in this work.

Whatever houses I may visit, I will come for the benefit of the sick, remaining free of all intentional injustice, of all mischief and in particular of sexual relations with both female and male persons, be they free or slaves.

What I may see or hear in the course of treatment or even outside of the treatment in regard to the life of men, which on no account one must spread abroad, I will keep to myself, holding such things shameful to be spoken about.

If I fulfill this oath and do not violate it, may it be granted to me to enjoy life and art, being honored with fame among all men for all time to come; if I transgress it and swear falsely, may the opposite of all this be my lot.

BOX 7-2 Commonly Accepted Bioethical Values

Allocation of resources. Consistent access to quality medical services; the distribution of health-related services among various people and uses.

Autonomy. Self-determination; a person's ability to make moral decisions, including those affecting personal medical care. The three components of autonomy are agency (awareness of oneself as having desires and intentions and acting on them); independence (absence of influences that so control what a person does that it cannot be said the person wants to do it); and rationality (rational decision making).

Beneficence. A duty to act in the interest of the patient's welfare; the practice of good deeds; an obligation to benefit others or seek their good.

Confidentiality. The presumption that certain information will not be revealed to others without the patient's permission. Confidentiality, like privacy, is valued because it protects individual preferences and rights.

Nonmaleficence. The prevention of harm, from the Hippocratic tradition that established *primum non nocere* ("Above all, do no harm"); a prohibition against actions with foreseeable harmful effects.

Personal integrity. Adherence to a personal set of values and moral standards.

autonomy, and the concept of the paramedic's duty to provide patient care that is of benefit to the patient is known as **beneficence**.

Many ethical and other value choices can be made instinctively, by drawing on longstanding personal beliefs, commitments, and habits. For example, most people believe it is wrong to steal, to be deceitful, or to commit murder. In health care, however, paramedics are faced with life issues that involve a patient. The patient may have beliefs, commitments, and habits that are different from the paramedic's personal experience. Throughout history, guidance in these situations has been provided through a variety of professional codes. These codes represent the collective wisdom of a group. The Code of Ethics for EMS Practitioners by the National Association of Emergency Medical Technicians (BOX 7-3) and the Code of Ethics for Emergency Physicians by the American College of Emergency Physicians (BOX 7-4) are examples of professional codes.

As with professional codes, an individual's personal code of ethics consists of principles of proper conduct. It is a vital reflection on one's life and incorporates values that can help one make moral choices. For the paramedic, a personal code of ethics must take into account professional, legal, and moral responsibilities (BOX 7-5).

BOX 7-3 Code of Ethics for EMS Practitioners

Professional status as an EMS Practitioner is maintained and enriched by the willingness of the individual practitioner to accept and fulfill obligations to society, other medical professionals, and the EMS profession. As an EMS practitioner, I solemnly pledge myself to the following code of professional ethics:

- To conserve life, alleviate suffering, promote health, do no harm, and encourage the quality and equal availability of emergency medical care.
- To provide services based on human need, with compassion and respect for human dignity, unrestricted by consideration of nationality, race, creed, color, or status; to not judge the merits of the patient's request for service, nor allow the patient's socioeconomic status to influence our demeanor or the care that we provide.
- To not use professional knowledge and skills in any enterprise detrimental to the public well-being.
- To respect and hold in confidence all information of a confidential nature obtained in the course of professional service unless required by law to divulge such information.
- To use social media in a responsible and professional manner that does not discredit, dishonor, or embarrass an EMS organization, co-workers, other health care practitioners, patients, individuals or the community at large.
- To maintain professional competence, striving always for clinical excellence in the delivery of patient care.
- To assume responsibility in upholding standards of professional practice and education.
- To assume responsibility for individual professional actions and judgment, both in dependent and independent emergency functions, and to know and uphold the laws which affect the practice of EMS.
- To be aware of and participate in matters of legislation and regulation affecting EMS.
- To work cooperatively with EMS associates and other allied healthcare professionals in the best interest of our patients.
- To refuse participation in unethical procedures, and assume the responsibility to expose incompetence or unethical conduct of others to the appropriate authority in a proper and professional manner.

Modified from: Gillespie CB., Code of Ethics and EMT Oath. National Association of Emergency Medical Technicians website. https://www.naemt.org/about-ems/emt-oath. Updated June 14, 2013. Accessed January 16, 2018.

BOX 7-4 Code of Ethics for Emergency Physicians

Emergency physicians shall:

1. Embrace patient welfare as their primary professional responsibility.
2. Respond promptly and expertly, without prejudice or partiality, to the need for emergency medical care.
3. Respect the rights and strive to protect the best interests of their patients, particularly the most vulnerable and those with impaired decision making capacity.
4. Communicate truthfully with patients and secure their informed consent for treatment, unless the urgency of the patient's condition demands an immediate response or another established exception to obtaining informed consent applies.
5. Respect patient's privacy and disclose confidential information only with consent of the patient or when required by an overriding duty such as the duty to protect others or to obey the law.
6. Deal fairly and honestly with colleagues and take appropriate action to protect patients from health care providers who are impaired or incompetent, or who engage in fraud or deception.
7. Work cooperatively with others who care for, and about, emergency patients.
8. Engage in ongoing study to maintain the knowledge and skills necessary to provide high quality care for emergency patients.
9. Act as responsible stewards of the health care resources entrusted to them.
10. Support societal efforts to improve public health and safety, reduce the effects of injury and illness, and secure access to emergency and other basic health care for all.

These principles were adapted by the American College of Emergency Physicians' Board of Directors in June 2016.

BOX 7-5 Perspectives on Ethical Living

Socrates. The unexamined life is not worth living. Know thyself. Morality is the necessity of the heart. The soul is that which is.
Plato. Justice is the harmony of all virtues. Truth belongs to the mind.
Aristotle. Sense reveals only individual existence. The universal is immanent in the individual. Man finds his ethics only in his natural self-realization.
Zoroastrianism and Parsis. Good thoughts, good words, good deeds. The Reality is one, the wise by many men call it.
Buddhism. Let a man lift himself up by his own self; let him not depress himself; for he himself is his friend and he himself is his enemy.
Confucianism. Seek to be in harmony with all your neighbors.
Taoism. Being in one's inmost heart in kindly sympathy with all things.
Christianity. Love thy neighbor as thyself.
Judaism. Perform righteousness on earth that ye may find treasures in heaven.
Islam. Do what God likes, and avoid what He dislikes.

CRITICAL THINKING

Which of the perspectives on ethical living presented in Box 7-5 best speaks to your personal philosophy?

SHOW ME THE EVIDENCE

Adams and colleagues conducted a study to identify the ethical conflicts experienced by prehospital personnel. A single observer interviewed a convenience sample of 607 paramedics. (These researchers cautioned against applying their results to the broad EMS population, because their sample was not random.)

The authors found ethical conflicts in 14.4% of the paramedics' responses. Ethical dilemmas were related to informed consent (27%), the duty of paramedics in threatening situations (19%), requests to limit resuscitation (14%), patients' decision-making capacity (17%), resource allocation (10%), confidentiality (8%), truth telling (3%), and training (1%).

Another study, which appeared in the *Turkish Journal of Emergency Medicine*, identified four categories in which prehospital ethical issues can arise: the process before medical interventions, dangerous situations and safe driving, the treatment process, and end-of-life care. These categories show that ethical issues can arise at any point throughout the spectrum of prehospital care.

Modified from: Adams J, Siminoff L, Wolfson A. Ethical conflicts in the prehospital setting. *Ann Emerg Med*. 1992;21:1259-1265; Erbay H. Some ethical issues in prehospital emergency medicine. *Turk J Emerg Med*. 2014;14(4):193-198.

Professional Accountability

As professionals, paramedics conform to a standard set by their level of training and regional practice. Paramedics are accountable to the patient, the medical director, and the EMS system for meeting this standard of care, and they can face legal accountability if the standard is not met. Duties include commitment to high-quality patient care, continuing education, skill proficiency, and licensure and/or certification. A paramedic who is accountable to the profession is more likely to provide good patient care and make ethical decisions.

Legal Accountability

Through patient care activities, the paramedic also assumes a role in the health care legal system (see Chapter 6, *Medical and Legal Issues*). Legal issues often are intertwined with ethical issues. However, ethics is not synonymous with law. Many ethical decisions occur outside the boundaries of the law, and many legal decisions may not be ethical. An example is a patient who has a living will in a state in which the legality of advance directives has not been resolved. Another example is a terminally ill patient who requests assisted suicide in a state where the practice is illegal. The paramedic should consider the importance of legal accountability as it relates to medical ethics and abide by the law when ethical conflicts occur.

Moral Accountability

Moral accountability refers to personal ethics—that is, personal values and beliefs. Combining moral, legal, and professional accountability may be difficult in an emergency. At times, the paramedic must draw on personal ethics to resolve conflicts among these roles and duties. Moreover, the paramedic must decide on a course of action. When dealing with ethical questions, paramedics should remember the following key points:[5,6]

1. **Emotion is not a reliable determinant for ethical decision making.** Rational decision making relies on research and prudence to determine what is right. Remember, however, that in the prehospital setting it may not be possible to make a fully informed decision. All available information should be considered and acted upon according to one's experience and ethical framework.
2. **Global protocols are meant to guide, not dictate.** If paramedics encounter an unfamiliar situation, they are likely to make a poor or even an unethical decision. In these circumstances, paramedics should consult with medical direction, coworkers, a supervisor, or a set of guidelines or other resources. Consultation is better than limiting oneself to one's own knowledge base or principles. At times, input from patients and their loved ones can be a key source of information and can lead to a better decision.
3. **Once the ethical question has been answered, the answer becomes a "rule" to guide behavior, at least in that particular setting.** Paramedics should follow that rule, and use it as an established guideline moving forward. Experience addressing ethical dilemmas in the field will build a foundation for future ethical issues that may be encountered.

Ethical Tests in Health Care

The most basic question of ethical tests in health care is, "What is in the patient's best interest?" However, doing what is best, or what one thinks is best, is not enough to justify actions. One must determine what the patient wants. The paramedic can do this using statements by the patient (if the patient has decisional capacity) and written statements. Family input is helpful if the patient shows altered mental status or a lack of decisional capacity.

The role of "good faith" in making ethical decisions should be balanced with the wishes of the patient and the family. Whether an act is done in good faith can be determined by answering the question, "Am I doing my best to help and not harm my patient?"

DID YOU KNOW?

The Heinz Dilemma

Lawrence Kohlberg was a well-known theorist in the field of moral development. During his research, he posed a moral dilemma (called the Heinz dilemma) to young children and asked for a specific course of action to three scenarios. A brief description of each scenario follows.

1. A woman was near death from a unique cancer. A physician had developed a drug that could cure her. The cost of the drug was $4,000 per dose, but it cost the physician only $2,000 to produce it. The woman's husband (Heinz) could raise only $2,000. He asked the physician who developed the drug to accept the $2,000 and said that he would pay the remaining $2,000 at a later date. The physician refused. *Should Heinz break into the laboratory to steal the drug for his wife? Why or why not?*
2. Heinz broke into the laboratory and stole the drug. The break-in and theft were reported in newspapers the next day. A police officer (Officer Brown), a friend of Heinz, remembered seeing him the previous evening running away from the laboratory. *Should Brown report what he saw? Why or why not?*
3. Officer Brown reported what he saw. Heinz was arrested and brought to court. If convicted, he would face up to 2 years in prison. Heinz was found guilty. *Should the judge sentence Heinz to prison? Why or why not?*

Kohlberg was not interested so much in the answers to the questions in each scenario being wrong or right. He was more interested in the reasoning behind the participants' decisions. The responses were then classified into various stages of reasoning in his theory of moral development.

Modified from: Kohlberg L. *Essays on Moral Development: The Philosophy of Moral Development.* Vol 1. San Francisco, CA: Harper & Row; 1981.

NOTE

With regard to answering ethical questions, no one knows all the answers. None of the tools or techniques works in every case to arrive at the "right" decision. Nonetheless, paramedics are accountable for personal and professional actions and decisions. Seeking counsel and guidance in such decisions is always prudent.

The global concept of health care is providing patient benefit and avoiding harm. It recognizes and respects the patient's autonomy. The concept also recognizes the various legal issues that affect the delivery of health care (BOX 7-6).

BOX 7-6 Global Concepts of Ethical Health Care

For an ancient Greek physician (as described by Hippocrates in Epidemics), therapeutic activity was subject to the following rules:

- Help the patient, or at least to do no harm.
- Refrain from interfering if the illness is incurable and inevitably mortal.
- Insofar as possible, attack the cause of the disease therapeutically.

Today, these global concepts of ethical health care can be stated as follows:

- Provide patient benefit.
- Do no harm.

Modified from: Doctor interview. Researchomatic website. http://www.researchomatic.com/doctor-interview-163692.html. Published 2013. Accessed February 8, 2018.

Rapid Approach to Ethical Problems in an Emergency

A method of ethical case analysis, or "rules of thumb" process, has been designed as a way to deal rapidly with ethical problems in an emergency.[7] The steps of this process are as follows:

1. Ask yourself whether you have experienced a similar ethical problem in the past. If so, use that experience as a precedent for this problem and follow the previously established rule. (The paramedic must evaluate these rules periodically.)
2. If you have not already experienced a similar ethical problem, buy time for deliberation and for consulting with coworkers and medical direction.
3. If buying time for deliberation is not an option, use a set of three tests to help you make a decision (**FIGURE 7-1**):[7]
   - **Test 1 (impartiality test).** Would you accept the action if you were in the patient's place? The impartiality test helps correct partiality or personal bias.
   - **Test 2 (universalizability test).** Would you feel comfortable having this action performed in all relevantly similar circumstances? The universalizability test helps do away with moral decision difficulty.
   - **Test 3 (interpersonal justifiability test).** Are you able to provide good reasons to justify and defend your actions to others? The interpersonal justifiability test requires that the paramedic define reasons for proceeding that others would approve.

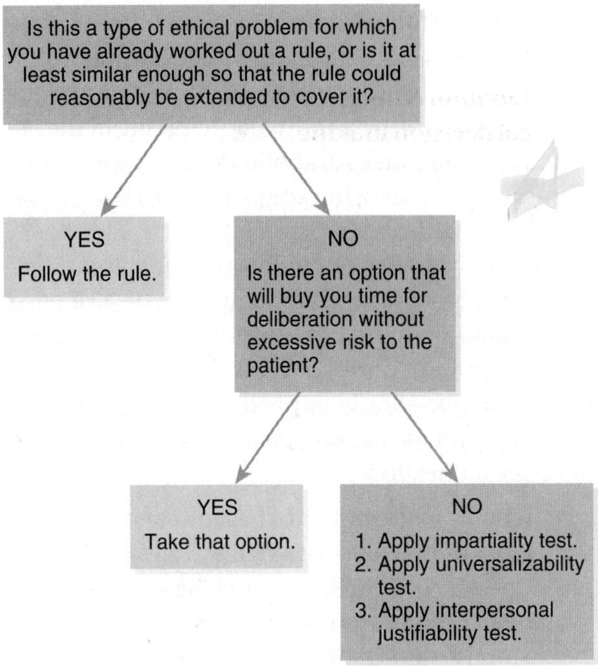

FIGURE 7-1 Rapid approach to resolving ethical problems in an emergency.

If all three tests can be answered in the affirmative, there is a fair probability that the action falls within the scope of being ethically acceptable. Even though disagreement may occur about a specific set of values, general agreement often exists about what constitutes wrong actions.

Resolving Ethical Dilemmas

At times, ethical dilemmas can be difficult to resolve. This may be the case when global concepts of health care are in conflict. Resolution of these conflicts can be guided by the health care community and the public. The role of the health care community in resolving these conflicts is to set standards of care, provide research and treatment protocols, and to prospectively and retrospectively review decisions and policies. The intent of these reviews is to educate the paramedic and improve the quality of patient care.

The role of the public in managing ethical conflicts in medicine includes creating laws, setting public policy, and allocating resources to protect the patient's rights. It also includes participating in the use of advance directives and other self-determination documents to make the patient's wishes known (see Chapter 6, *Medical and Legal Issues*).

Some of the more common ethical issues encountered in paramedic practice are described in this section. Sample case studies are provided to help illustrate some of these concepts. For each case study, the paramedic should apply the rapid approach to emergency medical problems and answer the following ethical questions:

1. What is in the patient's best interest?
2. What are the patient's rights?
3. Does the patient understand the issues at hand?
4. What is the paramedic's professional, legal, and moral accountability?

Allocation of Resources

Fairness in the allocation of resources and obligations is a commonly accepted bioethical value and is incorporated into society-wide health care policies. This perceived right to universal access to an adequate level of health care is a complex economic issue that is affected by the need to contain health care costs. Two factors affect true parity in the allocation of resources. The first is a person's access to health insurance. Even if a person has health insurance, the plan may define which medical services are covered or excluded. The second is treatment decisions made when resources are inadequate to meet patient care needs. This may occur, for example, during a disaster involving multiple casualties. When rationing of care is required, it should be based on ethically oriented criteria.[7]

The allocation of resources (medical rationing) is more of a policy issue than it is a clinical concept. However, allocation can pose ethical dilemmas in prehospital care, as illustrated in the following case study.

Case Study 1

A paramedic crew has been dispatched to the home of a 74-year-old man. The man complains of chest pain and shortness of breath. The patient is in obvious distress and provides a significant cardiac history. He asks to be taken to the Veterans Administration hospital (30 miles away), where he had heart surgery several years ago. Based on the patient's history, the physical examination findings, and the electrocardiogram (ECG), the paramedic crew (in consultation with medical direction) elects to take the patient to a closer hospital so that his condition can be stabilized. The patient becomes anxious and complains of increasing chest pain. He tells the paramedic crew that he has no medical insurance and demands to be taken to the Veterans Administration hospital.

Confidentiality

Most people are considered to have a basic right to privacy. The principle of confidentiality refers to a person's private and personal information. This information should not be disclosed by a health care professional without the patient's consent. Doing so is illegal and may violate state and federal laws and the regulations established by the Health Insurance Portability and Accountability Act (HIPAA), described in Chapter 6, *Medical and Legal Issues.*

In some cases, however, the release of such information may be required by law. An example of such a case is the disclosure to others involved in the patient's care that a patient has tested positive for infection with the human immunodeficiency virus (HIV). However, conflict between ethics and confidentiality may arise, particularly if the public health would benefit from the disclosure of confidential information, as described in the following case study.

Case Study 2

A paramedic crew has been dispatched to a motor vehicle collision. A young man's car struck another car head-on, killing the driver of that car. The young man, who is the patient, is shaken but has only minor injuries. As the patient is prepared for transport, he confides to the paramedic that he had used cocaine shortly before the crash. He asks the paramedic to keep the information confidential and not to tell the police officers at the scene.

> CRITICAL THINKING
>
> Your partner uses the phone number from a patient care report to contact the patient and ask for a date. Do you think that action violates any ethical principles? If so, which ones?

Consent

As explained in Chapter 6, *Medical and Legal Issues*, patients with decisional capacity have a legal right to decide on the medical care they will receive. This right is a basic element of the relationship between the patient and physician and is described in the American Medical Association's Principles of Medical Ethics. This right also can be inferred from the Code of Ethics for EMS Practitioners. Cases in which patients refuse lifesaving care can produce legal and ethical conflicts, as shown in the following case studies.

Case Study 3

A paramedic crew has been dispatched to a restaurant where an older adult woman has collapsed. She has suffered cardiac arrest, and a waiter is performing cardiopulmonary resuscitation (CPR). The ECG monitor reveals ventricular fibrillation. Defibrillation is delivered, but the rhythm remains unchanged. As resuscitation measures are continued, the woman's husband says to the paramedics, "She said she didn't want this. Her living will is at home. Please stop what you're doing and let her go."

Case Study 4

A paramedic crew has been dispatched to an office building where a 55-year-old woman collapsed at a business meeting. She is alert and oriented, complains of chest pain, and is pale and diaphoretic. The paramedics advise the patient of the possibility of a heart attack and the need for immediate care and transport. The patient insists on waiting until after the meeting has concluded to seek medical care on her own and asks the EMS crew to leave.

Error Disclosure

A recent trend in health care is the practice of truth telling and error disclosure after an adverse patient event. Although most people would agree that telling the patient or family that an error was made is the ethical thing to do, the fear of legal consequences has typically prevented doing so. Recent evidence has found that agencies who implement this practice have not seen unfavorable legal outcomes. Patients not only have a right to know an error was made, but research has shown that they want to know. A full explanation and apology should be provided, along with assurance that measures are in place to prevent a subsequent similar incident. While this practice is recommended, it should be implemented using very carefully crafted department policies.[8]

Care in Futile Situations

An action is seen as futile if it serves no purpose or is totally ineffective. A paramedic providing care in a case that may be futile should consult with medical direction. Consultation can help the paramedic decide on a course of action. An example of a futile situation in health care is continuing resuscitation initiated by bystanders when the patient clearly has expired. Another example is providing life support measures for a patient who has fatal injuries. The definition of futility may pose an ethical dilemma, especially when a dispute or lack of agreement exists about the goals of treatment. Providing CPR to a patient when rescuers believe the patient has irreversible brain damage can cause ethical conflict. Not all futility judgments are controversial. For example, CPR is futile in patients with obvious signs of death, such as decapitation, rigor mortis, tissue decomposition or extreme dependent lividity.[9]

CRITICAL THINKING

You arrive at a home where you find a 3-month-old baby who obviously has been dead for several hours. The mother is screaming, "Help her! Help her!" Your partner decides to proceed with advanced life support care even though it is clearly futile. Is this decision ethical?

Obligation to Provide Care

In the prehospital setting, the paramedic's duty to provide care is seldom an issue; the patient's request for emergency services presents a legal duty to act. In other areas of health care, though, an obligation to provide care other than emergency care may be affected by several factors. Examples include a patient's ability to pay for service, the patient's insurance, or other economic factors. As described in Chapter 6, *Medical and Legal Issues*, some laws protect well-meaning caregivers from liability (eg, Good Samaritan legislation). Other laws protect patients from unethical health care practices (eg, the Emergency Medical Treatment and Active Labor Act [EMTALA]). An example of such practices is "economic triage," in which evaluation of the impact of the patient's care is based on fiscal aspects important to the hospital. Another example is "patient dumping," in which a patient who is not in stable condition is transferred or discharged from a hospital for financial reasons.

Patient Advocacy and Paramedic Accountability

While providing care, the paramedic serves as the patient's advocate. This advocacy may conflict at times with the paramedic's accountability to the patient, the physician medical director, and the health care system (eg, health maintenance organization [HMO] protocols). In such a case, the paramedic should discuss all options with medical direction. As a rule, it is prudent and ethical to err on the side of providing for the needs of the patient when conflict arises. Examples of ways in which a paramedic can serve as the patient's advocate include the following:

- Educating patients about the delivery of health care and the role they can play to help change the nation's health care system
- Intervening when it is in the patient's best interest, particularly when the patient cannot communicate[10]
- Making sure health care decisions are made by patients and their physicians and are based on the patient's medical needs, not financial considerations
- Informing patients of health care reform initiatives in the federal, state, and private sectors
- Promoting patient access to reliable information about state-of-the-art medical technologies and treatments
- Promoting fairness and equality in America's health care system

Paramedic's Role as Physician Extender

As a physician extender, the paramedic generally is responsible for following the orders of the medical director or the director's designee. However, sometimes these orders may not seem appropriate. For example, the paramedic may believe that a medication order is contraindicated for the patient (such as giving narcotics when the patient is hypotensive). Or a medication may be medically acceptable but may not be in the patient's best interest (eg, an order for an intravenous drug to treat asthma before the patient's inhaler has been tried).

The converse also can occur. For example, a paramedic might request treatment in a situation in which the field diagnosis is not certain, or the physician may lack information needed to approve the request. When a conflict occurs between medical direction and the paramedic, communication is the key to resolving short-term and long-term concerns.

CRITICAL THINKING

How are ethical issues involved in each of the following aspects of an EMS call?

1. Problems associated with finding an address
2. Stigmatization of patients
3. Interventions in dangerous situations
4. Safe driving
5. Dealing with difficult patients
6. Difference of opinion with other health care providers
7. Telling the truth to patients

Modified from: Erbay H. Some ethical issues in prehospital emergency medicine. *Turkish J Emerg Med*. 2014;14(4):193-198.

NOTE

Moral Injury

In their careers, paramedics witness cruelty, loss, and suffering that can take its toll on their own lives and emotional well-being. **Moral injury**, or moral suffering, is the "emotional and spiritual impact of participating in, witnessing, and/or being victimized by actions and behaviors which violate one's core moral values and behavioral expectations of self or others." The term was coined by the military, and in recent years the concept has been applied to the health care setting. Moral injury can be caused by merely seeing events that conflict with one's own morals, or it may occur when paramedics feel as though they acted in a way that contradicts their personal morals. Unresolved feelings of anguish from moral injury can lead to depression and suicidal thoughts or actions. It is important that paramedics recognize moral injury and seek counseling to help work through the distress it causes.

Modified from: Moral Injury Project. What is moral injury? Syracuse University website. http://moralinjuryproject.syr.edu/about-moral-injury/. Accessed January 16, 2018; and Butts JB, Rich KL. *Nursing Ethics: Across the Curriculum and Into Practice*. 4th ed. Burlington, MA: Jones & Bartlett Learning; 2016.

Ethical Leadership in Paramedicine

Leadership is a key aspect of the paramedic role. Effective leaders are committed to ethical conduct. Ethical conduct applies to interactions with patients, the community, and other members of the EMS team. The community expects ethical behaviors from public safety professionals, and as leaders within that system, it is imperative that paramedics model those practices.

Reflection on one's own ethical life can begin by asking five questions:

1. Did I practice any virtues today?
2. Did I do more good than harm today?
3. Did I treat people with dignity and respect today?
4. Was I fair and just today?
5. Was my community better because I was in it? Was I better because I was in my community?[11]

On the surface, these seem like simple questions, and most people would readily respond in the affirmative to each. Faced with the complexities of the stressful EMS work environment, however, paramedics may find these questions more complicated. It requires work every day of a paramedic's career to continue to confidently say, "Yes, I am leading an ethical life as a paramedic leader."

Summary

- Ethics is the discipline relating to right and wrong, duty and obligation, moral principles and values, and moral character. Morals refers to standards that a person uses to distinguish right from wrong. Bioethics is the science of medical ethics.
- Most ethical issues paramedics face in their careers deal with a patient's right to self-determination and the paramedic's duty to provide patient care.
- Paramedics must meet a standard established by their level of training and regional practice. They must abide by the law when ethical conflicts occur.
- Two concepts of ethical health care are to provide patient benefit and to do no harm.
- The rapid approach to resolving ethical issues is a process that involves reviewing past experiences; deliberation (if possible); and/or performing the impartiality test, universalizability test, and interpersonal justifiability test to reach an acceptable decision.
- All resources must be allocated fairly. This is an accepted bioethical value.
- A health care professional is not allowed to reveal details supplied by the patient to others without the patient's consent. This is the principle of confidentiality.
- Patients with decisional capacity have a legal right to decide on the medical care they will receive. In some cases, patients refuse lifesaving care. These cases can produce legal and ethical conflicts.
- Advance directives, living wills, and other self-determination documents can help the paramedic make decisions about the appropriateness of resuscitation in the prehospital setting.
- Other areas likely to raise ethical questions in the prehospital setting include error disclosure, providing care in futile situations, and the paramedic's obligation to provide care.
- While providing care, the paramedic serves as the patient's advocate. The paramedic also serves the role of physician extender.
- Ethical leadership is a key aspect of the paramedic role.

References

1. Erbay H. Some ethical issues in prehospital emergency medicine. *Turk J Emerg Med.* 2014;14(4):193-198.
2. Sanderson B. *History of Ethics to 30 BC: Ancient Wisdom and Folly.* Santa Barbara, CA: World Peace Communications; 2002.
3. American Medical Association, Council on Ethical and Judicial Affairs. *Code of Medical Ethics: Current Opinions With Annotations.* Chicago, IL: American Medical Association; 2009.
4. Veatch R. *Medical Ethics.* 2nd ed. Sudbury, MA: Jones & Bartlett Publishers; 1997.
5. National Highway Traffic Safety Administration. *EMT-Paramedic National Standard Curriculum.* Washington, DC: US Department of Transportation; 1998.
6. Bourn S. Through traffic keep right. *J Emerg Med Serv.* 1996;21(5):26.
7. Iserson KV, Sanders AB. *Ethics in Emergency Medicine.* 2nd ed. Tucson, AZ: Galen Press; 1995.
8. Lu DW, Adams JG. Ethical challenges. In: Cone DC, Brice JH, Delbridge TR, Myers JB, eds. *Emergency Medical Services: Clinical Practice and Systems Oversight.* Vol 2. 2nd ed. West Sussex, England: Wiley and Sons; 2015.
9. Mancini ME, Diekema DS, Hoadley TA, et al. 2015 American Heart Association guidelines update for cardiopulmonary resuscitation and emergency cardiovascular care, part 3: ethical issues. *Circulation.* 2015;132(suppl):S383-S396.

10. Robertson B. A brief on patient rights. EMS Reference website. https://www.emsreference.com/articles/article/brief-patient-rights. Published November 2, 2016. Updated January 5, 2017. Accessed February 9, 2018.

11. National Association of Emergency Medical Technicians. *Ethics and Personal Leadership*. Burlington, MA: Jones & Bartlett Learning; 2015: 36.

Suggested Readings

Awdish RLA. A view from the edge—creating a culture of caring. *New Engl J Med.* 2017;376(1):7-9.

Breaux P. Leadership ethics in EMS. EMSWorld website. https://www.emsworld.com/article/10712788/leadership-ethics-ems. Published May 10, 2012. Accessed February 9, 2018.

Ethical challenges in emergency medical service. *Prehosp Disaster Med.* 1993 April-June;8(2):179-182.

Malina D. Liberty versus need—our struggle to care for people with serious mental illness. *New Engl J Med.* 2016;375(15):1490-1495.

Shapiro MF. Considering the common good—the view from seven miles up. *New Engl J Med.* 2016;374:2006-2007.

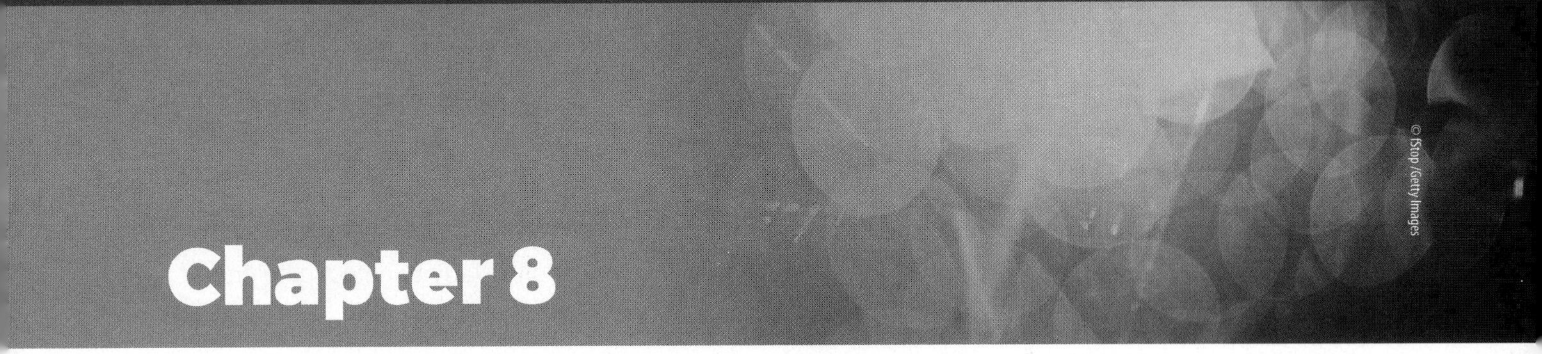

Chapter 8

Research Principles and Evidence-Based Practice

NATIONAL EMS EDUCATION STANDARD COMPETENCIES

Preparatory

Integrates comprehensive knowledge of the EMS system, safety/well-being of the paramedic, and medical/legal and ethical issues which is intended to improve the health of EMS personnel, patients, and the community.

Research

- Impact of research on emergency medical responder (EMR) care (p 161)
- Data collection (pp 167–168, 170)
- Evidence-based decision making (pp 169–171)
- Research principles to interpret literature and advocate evidence-based practice (pp 161–169)

OBJECTIVES

Upon completion of this chapter, the paramedic student will be able to:

1. Explain the importance of EMS research. (p 161)
2. Outline the 10 steps in performing research. (pp 161–169)
3. Describe the differences between types of EMS research. (pp 163–165)
4. Define evidence-based practice. (pp 169–170)
5. Describe the criteria for evaluating a research paper. (pp 170–171)

KEY TERMS

alternative time sampling Sampling to prevent bias by assigning a treatment group based on the day, week, or month in which patients are encountered in a study.

bias A systematic error introduced into sampling or testing that results in the deviation of the results of a study from the actual "truth."

blinding A research specification that dictates that parties are not made aware of the study, treatment, or outcome to be measured.

confidence interval An estimate of the range of likely values in the source population (the true value) based on the given study sample value, where a narrow range indicates more certainty about the value than does a wide range.

confounding variables Unmeasured variables that may affect the results of an experiment.

convenience sampling The process of choosing the people who are easiest to reach, or sampling that is easily done. The sample does not represent the entire population.

descriptive statistics A form of statistics that does not try to conclude (infer) anything about a subject that goes beyond the data; can be qualitative or quantitative.

evidence-based medicine Medical practice that is based on current scientific evidence.

exclusion criteria Criteria that exclude a patient from eligibility for a particular research study; defined on a study-by-study basis.

hypothesis A statement of the relationship between two or more variables.

inclusion criteria Criteria that a patient must meet to be eligible for a particular research study; defined on a study-by-study basis.

inferential statistics A form of statistics that enables the researcher to conclude (infer) whether the relationships seen in a sample are likely to occur in the larger population.

institutional review board (IRB) A committee that performs critical oversight functions (scientific, ethical, and regulatory) for research conducted on human subjects.

level of significance The likelihood that a finding in research data is due to chance; the probability of rejecting the null hypothesis if it is true.

mean The arithmetic average of a group being studied.

median A descriptive statistic that is found by first arranging the measurements according to size from smallest to largest, then choosing the measurement in the middle; the midpoint of a distribution score.

mode The number that occurs more often than any other number in a set of data.

nuisance variables Variables that can make drawing accurate conclusions from a study difficult.

null hypothesis An exact statement that the results occur by chance (the opposite of the hypothesis).

number needed to harm (NNH) The number of patients, on average, who need to be exposed to a treatment or risk factor for one person to have an adverse effect.

number needed to treat (NNT) The number of patients, on average, who need to be treated to prevent one additional bad outcome.

parameter An aspect of a population that is difficult or impossible to measure and so is estimated using a sample population.

population A large group of people, places, or objects that are the main focus of a scientific query.

power The ability of a study to detect difference if a difference really exists. It is based on the sample size (number of subjects) and effect size (difference in outcomes between the groups).

qualitative analysis The non-numerical organization and interpretation of observations.

quantitative analysis Research data that are measured and analyzed numerically.

random sample A subset from the larger population of a study chosen randomly and entirely by chance.

sampling error Error that results from observation of a sample rather than the whole population.

selection bias A distortion of evidence or data that arises from the way the data are collected.

standard deviation An estimate of the average deviation from the mean, measured in the same units as the original data.

statistically significant A descriptive term used when the observed phenomenon represents a significant departure from what might be expected by chance alone.

statistics A summary of characteristics of numerical facts or data.

systematic sampling A statistical method that involves the selection of a population from an ordered sampling so as to ensure equal probability.

unblinding A research specification by which all parties are made aware of the study, treatment, and outcome to be measured.

EMS systems are committed to providing effective and efficient health care to acutely ill and injured patients. As the National Highway Traffic Safety Administration has said, EMS agencies face a challenge today. Practices have been based on tradition and expert opinion. They need to be transformed into practices based on guidelines and protocols that have been developed through thoughtful, systematic examination of scientific evidence and data.[1] Paramedics must have a basic knowledge of research principles. This knowledge is necessary for conducting research and interpreting published studies. Paramedics also must be willing to help collect research data, which provide important information for the continued development of EMS care.

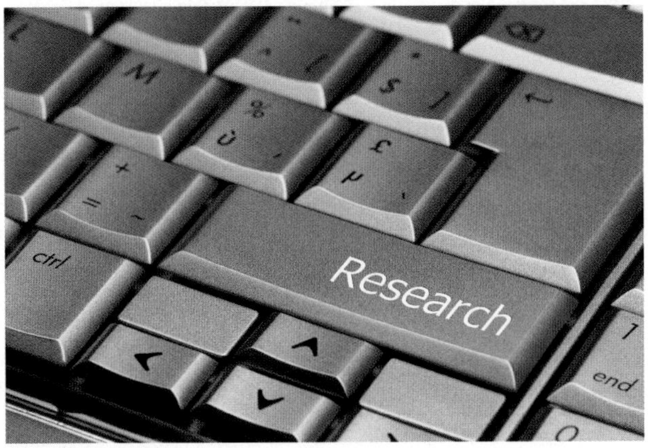

EMS Research

Research is a desirable activity for an EMS system and is vital to improving patient care. This process involves gathering data to answer clinically valuable questions, such as which procedures, techniques, and equipment are clinically beneficial versus those that do not improve outcomes or cause patient harm. Thus, research is essential to the evolution of EMS. The National EMS Research Agenda, published in 2001, states, "Research is essential to ensure that the best possible care is provided in the prehospital setting."[1] The aims of this agenda[2] were further advanced in a consensus research project in 2005 that developed target areas for clinical research in EMS. In 2014, the Federal Interagency Committee for Emergency Medical Services reaffirmed this focus in its strategic plan, which incorporated an objective to support data collection and research that leads to the development of evidence-based prehospital guidelines.[3]

Research is based on data and can improve patient care by leading to changes in professional standards, training, equipment, and procedures. In addition, EMS research increases respect for EMS professionals (BOX 8-1).

BOX 8-1 Importance of Research in Emergency Medical Services

- Production of outcome-based research
- New procedures, medications, and treatment
- Quality assurance
- Improved patient outcomes
- Professionalism

CRITICAL THINKING

What are your thoughts about research?

NOTE

The Longitudinal Emergency Medical Technician Attributes and Demographics Study (LEADS) project is hosted by the National Registry of Emergency Medical Technicians (NREMT) and is conducted each year. This study is designed to describe the EMS population in the United States, including their work activities, working conditions, and job satisfaction. LEADS, which began in August 1998, is led by a team of researchers made up of state EMS directors, state EMS training coordinators, EMS system managers, emergency physicians, EMS educators, survey researchers, and staff of the NREMT. The NREMT is a leader in the areas of research in EMS education and practice. For more information about the LEADS project, see www.nremt.org/rwd/public.

Basic Principles of Research

This chapter describes 10 basic steps for conducting research[4] (**FIGURE 8-1**):

1. Prepare a question.
2. Write a hypothesis.
3. Decide what to measure and the best way to measure it.
4. Define the population.
5. Determine the study design.
6. Seek institutional review board (IRB) approval of the study.
7. Obtain informed consent if needed.
8. Gather data after conducting pilot trials.
9. Analyze the data with an awareness of the pitfalls in interpreting the data.
10. Determine what to do with the research product (publish, present, perform follow-up studies).

NOTE

Paramedics should search the medical literature for related research when seeking evidence or before undertaking their own studies. This research should be evaluated for validity and reliability (described later in this text). Reference sources for literature review include peer-reviewed studies, government publications, and literature searches on the Internet using reliable sources such as MEDLINE on PubMed (www.ncbi.nlm.nih.gov/pubmed/).

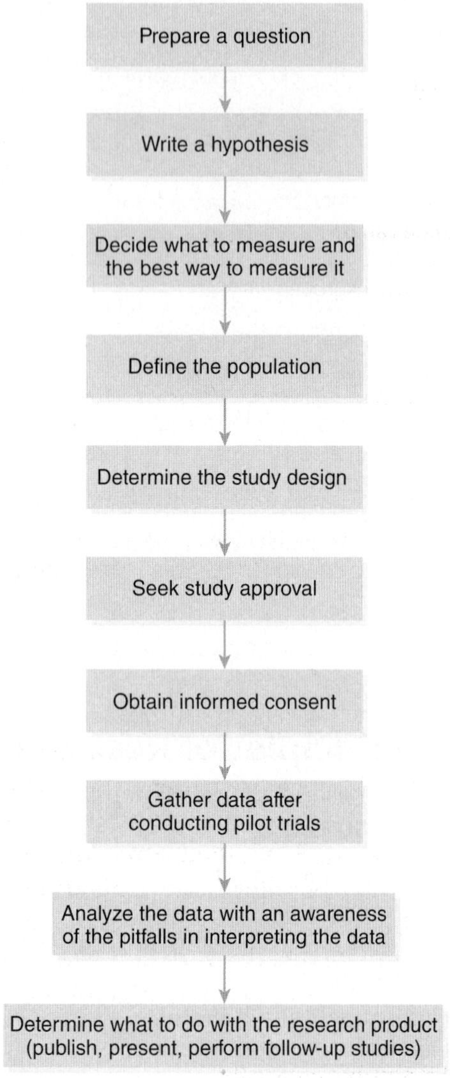

FIGURE 8-1 Ten steps for conducting research.

Prepare a Question

EMS research begins with the identification of a specific problem or question. The research then is carried out using standard research methods. Examples of problems or questions specifically related to EMS might include the following:

- Which factors predict success for paramedic students on the National Registry of Emergency Medical Technicians written examination?
- Is the incidence of complications greater with prehospital peripheral vascular access than with hospital peripheral vascular access?
- Does the paramedic uniform influence a patient's satisfaction?
- What is the incidence of violence in an EMS system?
- Does the paramedic's shift length influence the number of medical errors?
- Does performance of prehospital electrocardiography change survival rates for patients with acute myocardial infarction?
- Does prehospital intubation improve outcomes for patients with traumatic brain injury?
- Does the use of mechanical cardiopulmonary resuscitation improve outcomes in prehospital cardiac arrest?

When an area of clinical interest has been identified, it is of utmost importance to review the current literature to determine what is already known and optimize the objectives of the study.

> CRITICAL THINKING
> Can you think of any EMS-related questions that you would be interested in studying?

Write a Hypothesis

After a problem or question to be studied has been identified, the researcher must define a statement to be tested by the study. This statement, which is called the **hypothesis**, proposes the relationship between two or more variables. A variable is any factor or entity that can vary in amount or type. For example, the problem might be the ability of one drug to lower a patient's blood pressure more effectively than another drug. A hypothesis for the drug study might be that drug A lowers blood pressure better and with fewer side effects than drug B. The variables would include each drug being studied and the blood pressure. Other variables such as age and sex might also be considered.

Decide What and How to Measure

When the hypothesis has been defined, the next step is to decide what to measure and the best way to measure it. Using the previously described drug study, for example, the research may be focused on patients of a certain age, sex, or weight. It may also be limited to the effects of only a small number of antihypertensive drugs (eg, a specific angiotensin-converting enzyme inhibitor and a specific beta blocker.)

Define the Population

The next step in the research process is to define the **population** for the study. For a study to be clinically relevant, the population should be carefully chosen based on the research question. The population is formally defined using **inclusion criteria** and **exclusion criteria**, which specify which people are and are not eligible to participate in the study. For example, a study to evaluate an intervention for cardiac arrest could include all patients who receive prehospital cardiopulmonary resuscitation in a specific region over a specific period. Exclusion criteria could include age younger than 18 years, nonshockable rhythm, return of spontaneous circulation prior to EMS arrival, and existence of a do not resuscitate order. Inclusion and exclusion criteria help minimize the influence of specific **confounding variables**.

As it is typically impossible to research an entire population, research studies use a sample of the population to draw conclusions about the entire population. Ideally, to minimize **bias**, the sample is selected in such a way that every member of the population has an equal chance of being included in the sample. For example, drawing a **random sample** prevents **selection bias** (placing the best or worst patients in a study group). The researcher can ensure random sampling with the use of computer software programs, random digits, and even flipping a coin. Another way to limit bias is with **systematic sampling**. With this method, patients are put into groups in the order in which they are encountered in the prehospital setting. For example, the first patient seen is put into group A, the second into group B, the third into group A, and so on. The researcher also can use **alternative time sampling** to prevent bias by assigning a treatment group based on the day, week, or month in which patients are encountered in the study. **Convenience sampling**, which is based on choosing a readily available group, is the least preferred method. For example, patients might be assigned to groups when a particular person or crew is working.

Even when researchers use carefully designed methods, however, **sampling error** may occur. Such errors result from the fact that even the best sample will not work perfectly to represent the population, because of the chance inclusion of one person in the study group rather than the chance inclusion of someone else.

> NOTE
>
> A **parameter** is a numerical quantity or attribute of a population that is estimated using data collected from that population. For example, determining the exact age (hour of birth) of all patients in a group is nearly impossible; therefore, age is estimated using a sample population. **Nuisance variables** are issues that complicate the process of drawing accurate conclusions from a study by increasing background variability. An example is the use of audible and visual warning devices that can contribute to a rise in a patient's blood pressure. Parameters and nuisance variables are difficult to identify, control, prevent, or eliminate.

Determine the Study Design

A study design is a plan for conducting a study. Not all research study designs are equally effective. Study designs vary in terms of their size, degree of bias, and ability to control for confounding variables. In turn, these designs lead to differences in how confidently the results of the research can be used in clinical practice. The goal is to select the experimental design that balances feasibility, cost, and usefulness (**FIGURE 8-2**).

The first step in selecting a study design is to determine the study method. Study methods vary in terms of whether they follow patients over time, whether they study events as they occur or instead look backward in time, and whether they intervene with study subjects or instead simply observe them. The following study methods are widely used:

- **Descriptive method.** A research design in which events are monitored and analyzed without any attempt to manipulate or alter the outcome.
- **Cross-sectional method.** A research design in which a group of subjects is studied during a specified (usually short) period.

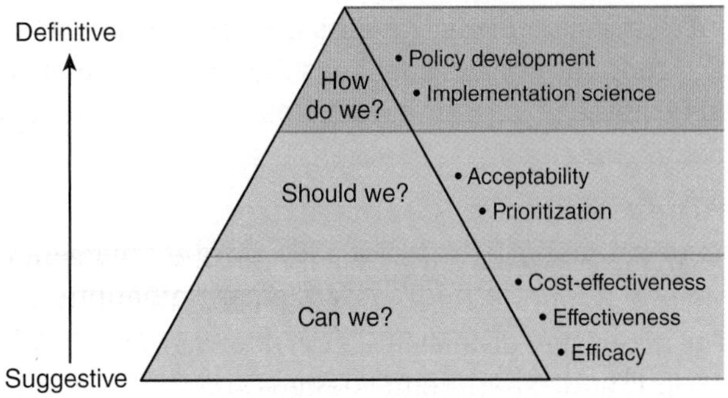

FIGURE 8-2 Key considerations when selecting a study design.

- **Longitudinal method.** A research design in which members of a sample population are followed forward over time.
- **Retrospective method.** A research design in which the specific question, hypothesis, and data collection are defined after the data already exist.
- **Prospective method.** A research design in which the specific question, hypothesis, and data collection are defined before the study begins.
- **Experimental method.** A research design in which an intervention is introduced and the effects are monitored for an outcome.

The research method is intimately connected to the overall design because it determines whether the overall design is descriptive or analytical.[5]

Descriptive Designs

Descriptive designs are the simplest of the study designs and are used primarily to generate hypotheses for future work. Because they do not control for confounding variables, descriptive studies are unable to draw a causal relationship between variables. For example, a descriptive study might identify that paramedics regularly experience fatigue while at work but not determine why they do.

Although descriptive studies may use simple designs, they can have powerful results. The main types of descriptive studies include case reports/series and cross-sectional designs.

- Case reports and case series analyze individual cases or events. They can give insight into new diseases or presentations. Because they review the experience of only one person or a few people, they do not represent a true sample of the population and their results cannot be extrapolated to the general population.
- Cross-sectional designs analyze data from a population at a specific point in time. Surveys are a typical example of a cross-sectional design.

Analytical Designs

Analytical designs collect data that are then evaluated for a cause-and-effect relationship between variables. The main types of analytical designs are observational designs and experimental designs.

- Observational designs include case-control, cohort, and before–after studies. Case-control studies compare participants by their outcomes, whereas cohort studies compare participants by exposure to a risk factor or intervention. For example, if a researcher designed an observational study to address the relationship between smoking and cancer, a case-control study might compare patients with lung cancer to patients without lung cancer on the basis of how much they had smoked, whereas a cohort study might compare patients who smoked with patients who did not smoke on the basis of how often lung cancer developed. A before–after study compares the same population before and after an intervention. This design is very common in EMS quality improvement research, where outcomes are compared before and after a protocol or equipment change.
- Experimental designs are studies in which the researcher assigns an intervention (exposure) to a participant and then follows the participants to measure specific outcomes. Ideally, patients are randomly assigned to their intervention arm to minimize selection bias.

NOTE

Correlation and Causation: What Do They Mean?

When a researcher finds a connection or association between two or more variables, it is called a correlation. The correlation can be in a positive direction where all variables go up (eg, as texting while driving increases, crashes increase), or it can be in a negative direction where some variables go up and some go down (eg, as seat belt use increases, fatal crashes decrease). However, in order to prove causation (ie, that one variable directly causes the other), the variables must be properly controlled and measured using methods that are statistically valid. An example would be studying seat belt use and distracted driving data obtained from patient interviews following a vehicle crash. It is much more difficult to prove causation than it is to prove correlation. When reading media reports or scientific papers, the paramedic should critically question whether the correlation between two variables can be treated as having a causal relationship.

As mentioned earlier, each study is likely to contain some form of bias, and the goal of good study design is to minimize this influence on the results. One technique for minimizing bias is **blinding**, which is used to limit the effects of the researchers' or participants' beliefs on the results of the study (assessment bias).

In a single-blind method, one party (the patient, the paramedic, or the person gathering the data) is unaware of (blinded to) the treatment at the time it is given. For example, in a study to evaluate the effectiveness of a drug to treat nausea, some patients may be given the study drug, and others a placebo (ie, an inactive substance that is physically indistinguishable from the study drug). The paramedic, but not the patient, would know if the patient received a placebo or study drug, which would eliminate some bias.

In a double-blind study, both the parties administering the intervention and the research subject (in the previous example the patient and the paramedic) are unaware of which intervention is being administered. Note that in the double-blind scenario, there is still a party, the researcher, who knows which intervention is being administered.

In a triple-blind study, the study participant, the care provider, and the researcher are all unaware of which intervention the participant received. The outcomes of the study cannot be evaluated until the researcher is unblinded. **Unblinding** refers to making all parties aware of the study, treatment, and outcome to be measured.

When a research report is evaluated, the study design should be considered before drawing conclusions based on the results. The strength of evidence that research provides can range from very weak (expert opinion) to very strong (meta-analysis) (**FIGURE 8-3**).

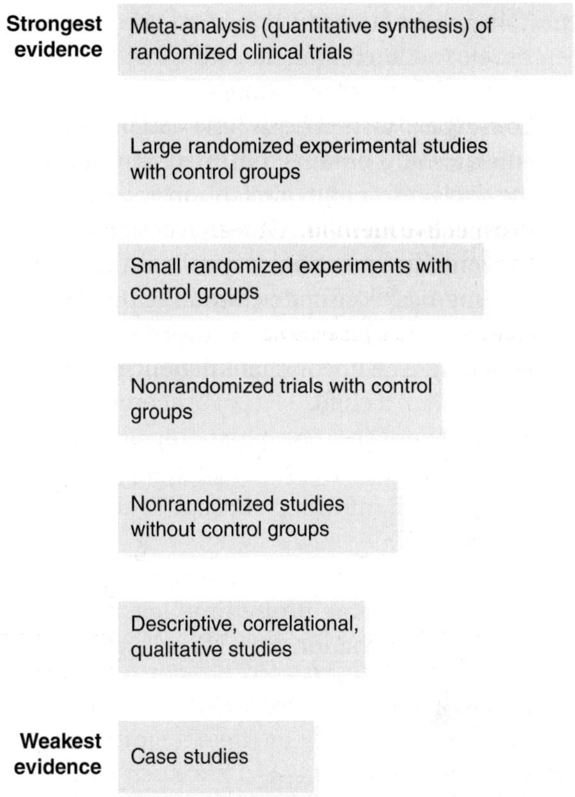

FIGURE 8-3 Quality of evidence ranges from very weak (expert opinion) to very strong (meta-analysis).

> CRITICAL THINKING
> Why might experimental trials be difficult to perform in EMS? Why is it important to conduct such trials?

Seek Institutional Review Board Approval of the Study

When planning for research involving human subjects, researchers use an **institutional review board (IRB)** as a touchstone for advice and a source of approval for the study. IRBs (also known as independent ethics committees or ethical review boards) came into widespread use as a result of a mandate from the US Public Health Services in 1966.[6] This mandate required a review by a "committee of institutional associates" for any federally funded research that used human subjects. In the United States, regulations have empowered IRBs to approve research, require modifications in planned research before approval, or disapprove research. These regulations were developed by the US Food and Drug Administration and the Department of Health and Human Services (specifically the Office for Human Research Protections). An IRB performs critical oversight functions for research conducted on human subjects to protect their safety. To receive IRB approval, the research is required to be scientific, ethical, and regulatory.

> CRITICAL THINKING
> Why do you think the development of IRBs was needed for research?

Obtain Informed Consent

A subject who voluntarily agrees to take part in the research project gives informed consent. Informed consent recognizes that the subject has decisional capacity and understands what is being presented. With respect to EMS research and the problems associated with obtaining informed consent in emergency situations, alternatives to informed consent have been developed, including the following:[4]

- **Consent at a distance.** The base station physician educates and obtains informed consent from the subject by radio or telephone.
- **Consent by proxy.** The paramedic obtains informed consent from a surrogate who is authorized to give medical consent on behalf of the patient, such as a medical power of attorney, a relative on behalf of an unconscious patient, or a parent on behalf of a child.
- **Stepped consent.** The paramedic provides the subject with a brief overview of the experimental therapy. Full informed consent is obtained at the hospital.
- **Cohort consent.** Permission is obtained to enter the study at some future time (eg, during an asthma exacerbation or sickle cell crisis).
- **Deferred consent.** This type of consent is used during resuscitation; the subject's condition is stabilized and the person receives experimental therapy without permission, after which the family is approached for traditional informed consent.
- **Surrogate consent.** Surrogate consent is consent from someone other than the patient. It varies by state, but if the patient has no designated medical power of attorney, most states use a hierarchy starting with a spouse, proceeding to an adult child, and ending with a close friend. The surrogate consents to whether the patient will participate in the treatment based on the surrogate's desires and wishes and not by evaluating the treatment as to its appropriateness.
- **Consent jury.** A lay panel determines certain aspects of the experimental protocol, particularly potential risks and complications that must be presented during a request for consent.

DID YOU KNOW?

Institutional Review Boards

Currently most IRBs involved in EMS research consist of physicians, attorneys, psychologists, ethicists, allied health professionals, and lay members of the community. In fact, most peer-reviewed EMS journals ask for a record that the research was approved by an IRB. IRBs seek to reduce the risk of patients unknowingly entering into research that could harm them in any way. In 2016, the US Department of Health and Human Services updated the regulations for research practice (CFR title 21, part 56; revised, 2016). These regulations are observed by most IRBs.

1. Risks to subjects are minimized by using procedures consistent with sound research design that do not unnecessarily expose subjects to risk and, whenever appropriate, by using procedures already being performed on the subjects for diagnostic or treatment purposes.
2. Risks to subjects are reasonable in relation to anticipated benefits, if any, to subjects, and the importance of the knowledge that may reasonably be expected to result. In evaluating risks and benefits, the IRB should consider only risks and benefits that may result from the research (as distinguished from risks and benefits of therapies that subjects would receive even if not participating in the research). The IRB should not consider possible long-range effects of applying knowledge gained in the research (eg, the possible effects of the research on public policy) as among the research risks that fall within the purview of its responsibility.
3. Selection of subjects is equitable. In making this assessment, the IRB should take into account the purposes of the research and the setting in which the research will be conducted. The IRB should be particularly cognizant of the special problems of research involving vulnerable populations such as children, prisoners, pregnant women, people with mental disability, and economically or educationally disadvantaged people.
4. Informed consent will be sought from each prospective subject or the subject's legally authorized representative in accordance with and to the extent required by federal regulations related to protection of human subjects.
5. Informed consent will be appropriately documented in accordance with and to the extent required by federal regulations related to protection of human subjects.
6. When appropriate, the research plan makes adequate provision for monitoring the data collected to ensure the safety of subjects.
7. When appropriate, adequate provisions are made to protect the privacy of subjects and to maintain the confidentiality of data.
8. When some or all of the subjects are likely to be vulnerable to coercion or undue influence (eg, children, prisoners, pregnant women, people with mentally disability, or economically or educationally disadvantaged people), additional safeguards are included in the study to protect the rights and welfare of these subjects.

Modified from: Code of Federal Regulations title 21, part 56. https://www.accessdata.fda.gov/scripts/cdrh/cfdocs/cfcfr/CFRSearch.cfm?CFRPart=56&showFR=1. US Food and Drug Administration website. Updated August 14, 2017. Accessed December 1, 2017.

NOTE

Exceptions to obtaining informed consent may be permitted in some emergency research. To be granted this waiver, the researchers must prove that they have informed the community about the research and must solicit feedback from the community about the proposed research. This process is known as community consultation and public disclosure. It can be accomplished in a number of ways, depending on the community and the specific group targeted for the research.

In 2010, the National Registry of Emergency Medical Technicians surveyed more than 65,000 EMS providers to seek their opinions on this type of consent. Almost all of the 36% of survey respondents agreed that EMS research is important; however, only one-third thought that it was acceptable to enroll patients without their consent to learn about a new treatment, and less than half were willing to enroll in a similar study. The researchers suggested that the opinions of this group meant that it would be important to meet with EMS providers and address these concerns before conducting prehospital research involving exceptions from informed consent.

Modified from: Jasti J, Fernandez AR, Schmidt TA, Lerner EB. EMS provider attitudes and perceptions of enrolling patients without consent in prehospital emergency research. *Prehosp Emerg Care*. 2015;20(1):22-27.

SHOW ME THE EVIDENCE

The following study demonstrates an example of community consultation to perform research. Nelson and colleagues collected a cross-sectional, standardized survey conducted by two sets of random-digit telephone surveys, paper surveys at community meetings, and web-based surveys. Their goal was to comply with federal law that allows research to be conducted using very strict criteria without having prior consent of the patient. The surveys were done to fulfill the law's requirement for community consultation and public disclosure. The authors found that community meetings were poorly attended and that phone surveys were effective for gauging public opinion. However, they recommended targeted surveys to reach special populations.

Modified from: Nelson M, Schmidt TA, Delorio NM, McConnell KJ, Griffiths DE, McClure KB. Community consultation methods in a study using exception to informed consent. *Prehosp Emerg Care*. 2009;12:417-425.

Gather and Analyze Data

Data from the research study should be gathered after conducting pilot trials and analyzed using statistical methods. The term **statistics** refers to numerical facts or data. These facts or data are classified into groups and are often organized into charts to present key details about a subject. Statistics can be descriptive or inferential.

Descriptive Statistics

Descriptive statistics does not try to conclude (infer) anything about a subject that goes beyond the data. This type of statistics describes the sample of objects or people being studied. It does not infer anything from the data, but simply reports the data. Descriptive statistics can be qualitative or quantitative.

Qualitative analysis is the organization and interpretation of observations; it is non-numerical, using text and few numbers to describe the research findings. The sample size in qualitative research usually is very small. Interviews, analysis of written text, and focus groups are often used to gather data in this type of research. The conclusions reveal key underlying dimensions and patterns in a group, allowing the researcher to propose themes, trends, or theories related to the group. Findings from qualitative studies can provide rich detail not obtainable through pure numerical data analysis. For example, in 2012 Leonard et al. tried to understand factors that influenced EMS partnerships in prehospital research.[7] To answer their research question, the team conducted focus group interviews using a structured interview process. During their data analysis of the transcripts of these interviews, they identified 17 barriers and 12 motivators for EMS personnel participation in research. Their findings provided the foundation for a model to plan and facilitate prehospital research.

Quantitative analysis in descriptive statistics uses the mean, median, and mode to describe numeric data such as the most commonly occurring values in a sample. The **mean** is the arithmetic average of the group (eg, the average age of the people in the sample). The **median** (also called the 50th percentile) is found by first arranging the measurement according to size from smallest to largest and then choosing the one in the middle (or the mean of the two measurements that are nearest to the middle). The median frequently is used to divide a sample into two halves. The **mode** is the number that occurs more often than any other number in a set of data.

The following is an example of quantitative analysis:

> Your sample has 13 participants. Their ages are 53, 53, 53, 54, 55, 55, 56, 57, 59, 60, 64, 71, and 79. The mean (average) age of the group is 59.15 years; the median (middle) age is 56; and the mode age is 53.

To further explore how the mean describes the sample, the researcher calculates the **standard deviation**. The standard deviation measures how much variability there is from the mean in the research data.

Inferential Statistics

Inferential statistics is a type of quantitative analysis used to infer whether the relationships seen in a sample are likely to occur in the larger population. The researcher can use these statistics to decide whether the results of the study support or contradict the initial hypothesis. To do this, the researcher states a **null hypothesis**. A null hypothesis is a default position, such as that a specific treatment has no effect or that the results are a chance of variation (the opposite of what the researcher expects to prove). In US courts, the null hypothesis is that the accused person is assumed to be innocent until proved guilty beyond a reasonable doubt. If this assumption cannot be rejected, the accused goes free—which does not always mean that the accused is actually innocent, just that guilt has not been definitively proven. A research hypothesis is the opposite of the null hypothesis—the finding that the research expects to prove. In the court system, the research hypothesis would be that the accused person is guilty until proved innocent.

> **NOTE**
>
> The level of sureness with which a null hypothesis can be rejected is called the **confidence interval**, which measures the probability that the true value of a measurement lies within the range of two values. The confidence increases as the confidence interval narrows.
>
> Confidence intervals are often stated at the 95% level, which means that 95% of the time the confidence interval will contain the true value of a measurement for the population of interest. For example, if large random samples are repeatedly taken from the same population and used to create 95% confidence intervals for the population average, approximately 95% of the intervals should contain the true population average.

When a statistical test reveals that the probability is rare that a set of results is attributable to chance alone, this result is called **statistically significant**. Statistically significant means that the observed phenomenon represents a significant departure from what might be expected by chance alone.

Generally, the **level of significance** refers to the probability of the event occurring as a result of chance. The level of significance is the acceptable risk of sampling errors and is established through mathematical equations. The level of significance (*P* value) is usually designated as 0.05 (1 chance in 200) or 0.01 (1 chance in 100) that the difference between two groups is larger than expected as a result of chance alone (too large to be reasonably attributed to chance). Researchers must set their level of significance before they begin their research.

The **power** of a study reflects its ability to detect a difference between groups when such a difference exists. In EMS research, the power of a study is determined by the incidence of a disease or outcome and by the number of participants (sample size). For example, if a particular outcome is rare, a very large sample size would be needed to determine whether an intervention changes outcomes.

> **NOTE**
>
> Increasingly, EMS research in which an intervention is evaluated includes the **number needed to treat (NNT)** and the **number needed to harm (NNH)** in the results. The NNT is the number of patients who need to be treated to prevent one additional bad outcome. It is the estimated number of patients who need to be treated with the proposed intervention rather than the standard treatment before one additional patient will benefit when there are two possible outcomes. The NNH is the number of patients, on average, who need to be exposed to a treatment or risk factor before one person will have an adverse effect.
>
> *Modified from*: Altman DG. Confidence intervals for the number needed to treat. *BMJ*. 1998;317(7168):1309-1312. https://www.ncbi.nlm.nih.gov/pmc/articles/PMC1114210/. Accessed September 15, 2017; and Centre for Evidence-Based Medicine. Number needed to treat (NNT). August 14, 2012. http://www.cebm.net/number-needed-to-treat-nnt/.

Determine What to Do With the Results

The final step in EMS research is to determine what to do with the results of the study. Several options are available, including publishing the results, presenting the results, and performing follow-up studies.

Publishing the Results

The findings from research may be published in a professional journal for peer evaluation. Publication in a peer-reviewed journal means that several experts in the field being studied have reviewed the research to assess its quality. The peer reviewers may recommend the article be accepted as written, accepted with minor or major revisions, or rejected. Most medical peer-reviewed journals require evidence that an IRB has approved any research involving human subjects. Examples of EMS-related peer-reviewed journals are *Prehospital Emergency Care, Annals of Emergency Medicine,* and *Prehospital and Disaster Medicine.* (Sometimes just an abstract, or summary, of the research is published. Published abstracts have not always gone through the same rigorous peer-review process as a full article.) The format for writing a manuscript for scientific literature typically has five basic sections:

1. The introduction provides a brief historical background of the research and describes any previously published research. The introduction provides both a rationale for the study and the research hypothesis (or hypotheses).
2. The methods section describes how the experiment was done so that it can be replicated by other researchers and so that readers can assess the validity of the methodology. This section should identify the inclusion or exclusion criteria for the study (how patients were chosen) as well as the statistical methods used to analyze the data. It is important to read this section carefully to determine how to interpret the results and to decide whether they are transferrable to another system.
3. The results section contains the research findings. It provides answers to the study questions and summarizes the data obtained by the researcher (eg, tables and figures).
4. The discussion section includes the author's interpretation of the research findings and implications of the findings. Limitations of the project are also given here. This section frequently offers suggestions for improving the study through follow-up research.
5. The conclusion provides a succinct summary of the four preceding sections (BOX 8-2).

Presenting the Results and Performing Follow-Up Studies

Clinical studies can lead to improvements in patient outcomes. Presenting the results of a study—to peers, professional organizations, and higher education institutions—can help put research into practice.

Follow-up studies may be done through, and funded by, collaborative efforts with public agencies, corporations, and foundations. They may also be funded and supported by state and federal government programs that support research consortia. (A consortium is a group of people and/or organizations that pool resources and information to achieve a common goal.) Examples of such consortia in the EMS field include the Pediatric Emergency Care Applied Research Network (PECARN), which focuses on pediatric emergency care, and the Resuscitation Outcomes Consortium (ROC), which focuses on research related to prehospital cardiopulmonary arrest and severe traumatic injury.

Evidence-Based Practice

For too long, prehospital care has been driven more by intuitive thinking about what is right rather than by evidence.[8] A system-wide process is needed to

BOX 8-2 Fifteen Steps for Evaluating and Interpreting Research

1. Was the research peer reviewed?
2. What was the research hypothesis?
3. Was the study approved by an IRB and conducted ethically?
4. What was the population studied?
5. What were the inclusion and exclusion criteria for the study?
6. Which method was used to draw a sample of patients?
7. How many patient groups participated?
8. How were patients assigned to groups?
9. Which type of data was gathered?
10. Does the study appear to have enrolled a sufficient number of patients?
11. Does the study fail to account for any potential confounding variables?
12. Were the data properly analyzed?
13. Is the author's conclusion logical and based on the data?
14. Could the results apply in local EMS systems?
15. Are the patients in the study similar to those seen in the local EMS system?

ensure that prehospital care is based on current and scientific evidence—that is, to facilitate evidence-based practice, also known as **evidence-based medicine**. Evidence-based medicine involves translating the best science into EMS clinical policies and individual paramedic decision making. Already, many medical specialties have developed evidence-based guidelines (EBGs) for specific conditions, such as traumatic brain injury, spinal injury, and ST-segment elevation myocardial infarction. (These conditions are addressed in other chapters in the text.)

In 2016, the National Association of EMS Physicians developed a consensus document to establish a process to create EBGs for EMS.[9] Its framework includes the establishment of a guidelines consortium that connects researchers to various EMS groups; promotion of research to support EBGs; development of EBGs for EMS; education of EMS providers about the EBGs; implementation of EMS EBGs; evaluation of prehospital EBGs; and identification of funding sources for the process.

NOTE

The National Guideline Clearinghouse (NGC) is a public resource for evidence-based, clinical practice guidelines and expert commentaries, which can be found using the NGC's research tools. The mission of the NGC is to provide physicians and other health professionals with an accessible means of obtaining objective, detailed information on clinical practice guidelines. Another goal of the NGC is to disseminate practice guidelines for implementation and use.

Modified from: National Guideline Clearinghouse, Agency for Healthcare Research and Quality, US Department of Health and Human Services. https://www.guideline.gov. Accessed December 1, 2017.

High-quality patient care requires use of procedures that have been proven useful in improving patient outcomes.[10] To obtain this evidence, paramedics should participate in EMS research, data collection, and sharing of information obtained through research. These efforts aid in the design of a system-wide process for prehospital care that reflects the current state of scientific evidence (**FIGURE 8-4**).

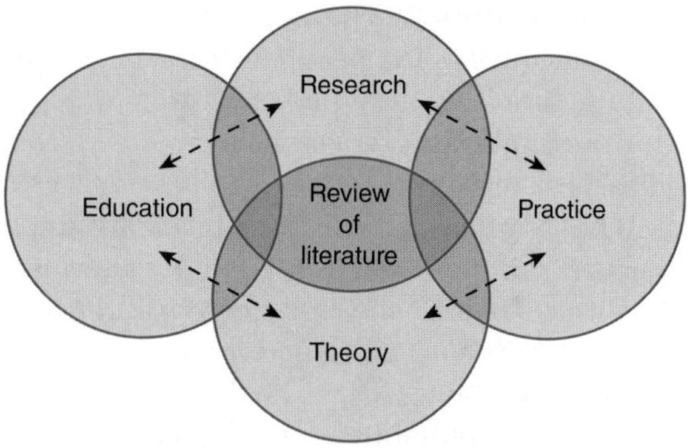

FIGURE 8-4 Relationship of the review of the literature to theory, research, education, and practice.

Modified from: LoBiondo-Wood G, Haber J. *Nursing Research: Methods and Critical Appraisal for Evidence-Based Practice*. 8th ed. St. Louis, MO: Elsevier/Mosby; 2010.

Reviewing Research

Paramedics should read research articles critically to determine whether the findings are relevant to their practice. When reviewing research articles, the following components should be carefully studied:[11]

- **Population.** Is the sample adequate and is it similar to your practice? For example, a study that evaluates response times without lights and sirens conducted in a rural setting may not be relevant to an urban EMS system. Similarly, if a study is conducted in an area that has a significantly different ethnic makeup than your practice area, this setting could influence the results if the study subject involves disease processes that are more prevalent in certain ethnic communities.
- **Inclusion and exclusion criteria.** A study of patients with chest pain that did not include patients older than age 65 years, for example, would eliminate a key group at risk for heart disease and death.
- **Data collection.** Is there anything that could have influenced the data collection? If the study used the experimental method, how were the groups randomized? Was the method clearly described? Could the method have varied based on the person delivering care? Were the conditions in the control group and the experimental group the same?
- **Results.** Are the numbers presented clearly? When percentages are presented, are the underlying numbers reported? If a statistically significant difference was seen in the outcome, is it also clinically significant?
- **Discussion and conclusion.** Is the conclusion consistent with the results reported? Did the

authors properly report correlations and relationships, rather than predictions? Did they link the research to relevant literature? Were the limitations of the study pointed out clearly? Did the researchers make specific suggestions for future research? Did you identify any major flaws in the conclusion?

- **Relation of the research to your practice.** Does the research suggest an area of improvement for your system? Does it suggest an area that should be monitored in your quality improvement program? Is there a reason to seek out more literature on the same subject to propose a change in your system?

NOTE

It is important that researchers not overstate their findings. The journal peer review process evaluates the study findings and may suggest that the authors revise their discussion and conclusion if the findings are beyond what their results actually show. The study may be designed only to demonstrate that there is a relationship between variables (correlation) and not that one variable predicts a particular outcome (causation). The power of a study to predict rather than suggest a relationship is based on the research methods and design.

Summary

- The paramedic must be familiar with research principles. This knowledge is needed to conduct research, collect research data, and interpret published studies.
- Research is essential to improving patient care.
- The 10 steps for conducting EMS research are (1) prepare a question, (2) write a hypothesis, (3) decide what to measure and how to measure it, (4) define the population, (5) determine the study design, (6) seek IRB approval, (7) obtain informed consent, (8) gather data after conducting pilot trials, (9) analyze the data, and (10) present the data.
- The two main types of research designs are descriptive designs and analytical designs.
- Descriptive statistics does not try to infer anything about a subject that goes beyond the data. It includes both qualitative analysis, which provides a non-numerical description of the population, and quantitative analysis, which evaluates the data using numbers.
- Inferential statistics infers whether the relationships seen in a sample are likely to occur in the larger population. In this type of study, researchers develop a null hypothesis.
- EMS care should be evidence based; that is, interventions and procedures should be proven to benefit the patient.
- Paramedics should read research articles critically to determine whether the article is relevant to their practice.

References

1. National Highway Traffic Safety Administration, Maternal and Child Health Bureau. *National EMS Research Agenda.* Washington, DC: Health Resources Administration; 2001.
2. Sayre MR, White LJ, Brown LH, McHenry S. National EMS research agenda. *Prehosp Emerg Care.* 2001;6(suppl 3):S1-S43.
3. Federal Interagency Committee on Emergency Medical Services. *FICEMS Strategic Plan* (DOT HS 811 990). Washington, DC: Federal Interagency Committee on Emergency Medical Services; 2014.
4. Menegazzi J. *Research: The Who, What, Why, When and How.* Wilmington, OH: Ferno-Washington; 1994.
5. Lerner EB, Cone DC, Yealy DM. EMS research basics. In: Cone D, Brice JH, Delbridge TR, Myers JB, eds. *Emergency Medical Services: Clinical Practice and Systems Oversight.* 2nd ed. Hoboken, NJ: John Wiley & Sons; 2015:401-409.
6. Hicks S. *How the Past Influenced Human Research Protection Legislation.* Washington, DC: US Department of Health and Human Services; 2007.
7. Leonard JC, Scharff DP, Koors V, et al. A qualitative assessment of factors that influence emergency medical services partnerships in prehospital research. *Acad Emerg Med.* 2012;19(2):161-173.
8. National Highway Traffic Safety Administration, Office of EMS. *EMS Update.* Washington, DC: National Highway Traffic Safety Administration; Fall 2008–Winter 2009.
9. Martin-Gill C, Gaither JB, Bigham BL, Myers JB, Kupas DF, Spaite D. National prehospital evidence-based guidelines strategy: a summary for EMS stakeholders. *Prehosp Emerg Care.* 2016;20(2):175-183.
10. National Highway Traffic Safety Administration. *The National EMS Education Standards.* Washington, DC: US Department of Transportation/National Highway Traffic Safety Administration; 2009.
11. Pyrczak F. *Evaluating Research in Academic Journals: A Practical Guide to Realistic Evaluation.* 5th ed. Glendale, CA: Pyrczak Publishing; 2013.

Suggested Readings

American College of Emergency Physicians. Online evidence-based emergency medicine (EBEM). *Annals of Emergency Medicine* website. http://www.annemergmed.com/content/sectII. Accessed December 1, 2017.

Brown LH, Criss EA, Prasad NH, Larmon B. *An Introduction to EMS Research*. Upper Saddle River, NJ: Pearson Education; 2002.

Jacobsen KH. *Introduction to Health Research Methods: A Practical Guide*. Burlington, MA: Jones & Bartlett Learning; 2017.

Office of EMS, National Highway Traffic Safety Administration. Progress on evidence-based guidelines for prehospital emergency care (DOT HS 811 643). National Highway Traffic Safety Administration website. http://www.nhtsa.gov/staticfiles/nti/pdf/811643.pdf. Published January 2013. Accessed December 1, 2017.

Prehospital Care Research Forum. Articles. UCLA Center for Prehospital Care website. https://www.cpc.mednet.ucla.edu/pcrf/articles. Accessed December 1, 2017.

Prehospital evidence-based practice program (PEP). Dalhousie University, Division of Emergency Medical Services. https://emspep.cdha.nshealth.ca. Accessed January 29, 2018.

Salkind NJ. *Statistics for People Who (Think They) Hate Statistics*. 6th ed. Thousand Oaks, CA: Sage; 2017.

PART 2

Anatomy and Physiology

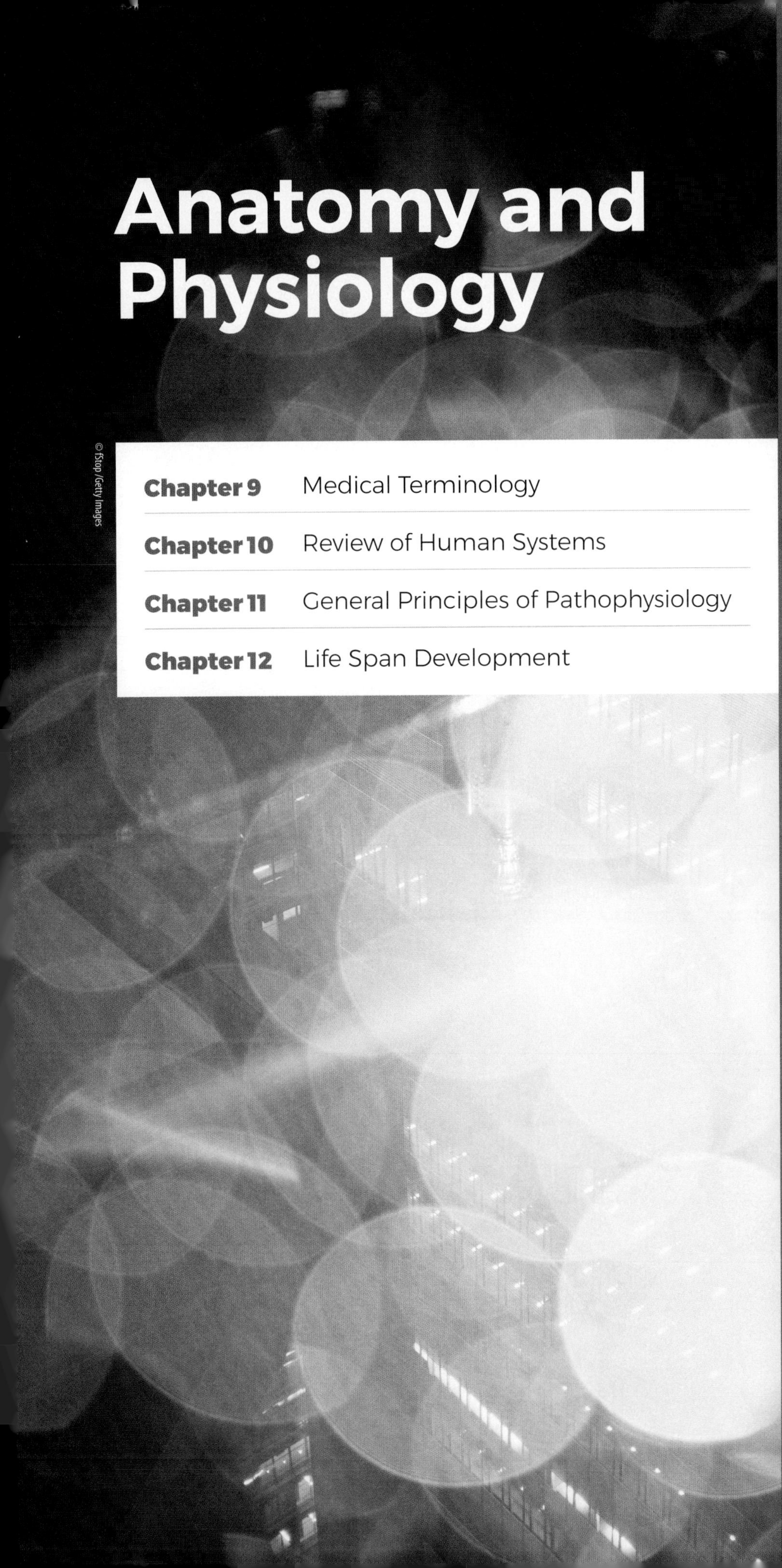

© fStop/Getty Images

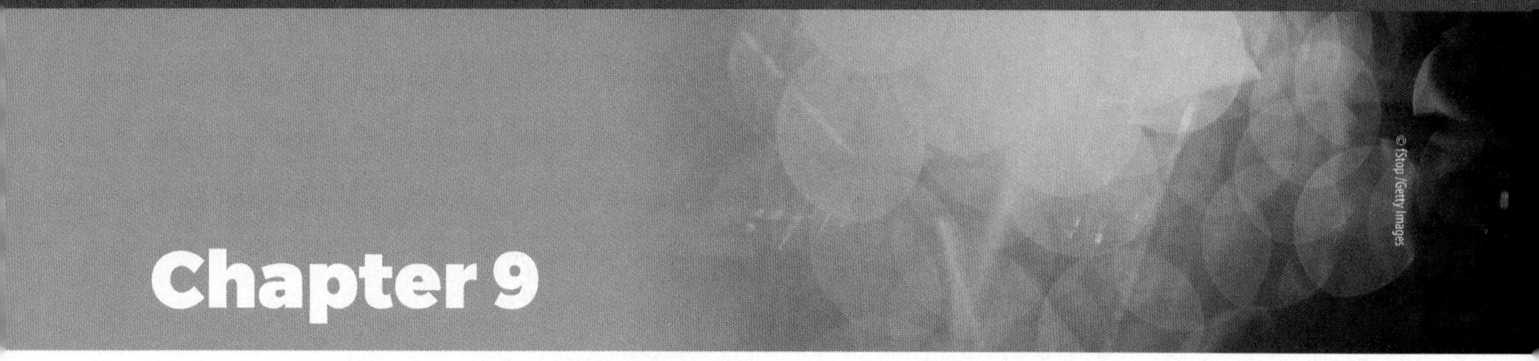

Chapter 9

Medical Terminology

NATIONAL EMS EDUCATION STANDARD COMPETENCIES

Medical Terminology

Uses foundational anatomic and medical terms and abbreviations in written and oral communication with colleagues and other health care professionals.

OBJECTIVES

Upon completion of this chapter, the paramedic student will be able to:

1. Explain the use of medical terms to describe organs and processes. (pp 176–177)
2. Explain the role of a root word, prefix, suffix, and combining vowels in a medical term. (pp 177–181)
3. Interpret selected examples of medical root words, prefixes, suffixes, and combining vowels. (pp 178–181)
4. Distinguish between singular and plural forms of medical terms. (p 181)
5. Use accepted medical abbreviations appropriately. (pp 181–187)
6. Differentiate between similar medical terms and abbreviations. (pp 182–188)
7. Pronounce medical terms correctly. (pp 188–189)

KEY TERMS

combining vowel A vowel often used between root words and suffixes or between two or more root words.

eponym A term that is derived from a person's name.

homonym A word that has the same pronunciation as another word but a different meaning, and often a different spelling (in which case it can more specifically be referred to as a *homophone*).

prefix A word part that appears at the beginning of a word. In the medical context, a prefix often describes location or intensity.

root word The foundation of a term. In the medical context, a root word may be combined with other word parts to describe a particular structure or condition.

suffix A word part that appears at the end of a word. In the medical context, a suffix often describes a patient's condition or diagnosis.

A necessary skill and expectation for working in the health care profession is the ability to speak and understand the language of medicine. This skill is required for conveying patient information to other members of the heath care team. In addition, medical terminology is accurate and universally understood. It provides a clear and concise way to document patient care activities.

The Language of Medicine

The language of medicine offers intriguing challenges both to medical historians and to linguists. The oldest written sources of Western medicine are Hippocrates' writings from the fourth and fifth centuries BC. Hippocrates's work marked the beginning of the Greek era in regard to the language of medicine—an era that continued even after the Roman conquest. During the Renaissance (14th to 17th centuries), however, the Greek language was not widely understood, and many Greek words were translated into Latin. As a result of this history, most medical terms currently are derived from Greek, and many have Latin roots. Medical terms that describe a disease are usually of Greek origin, whereas medical terms used to describe anatomy are usually of Latin origin.[1]

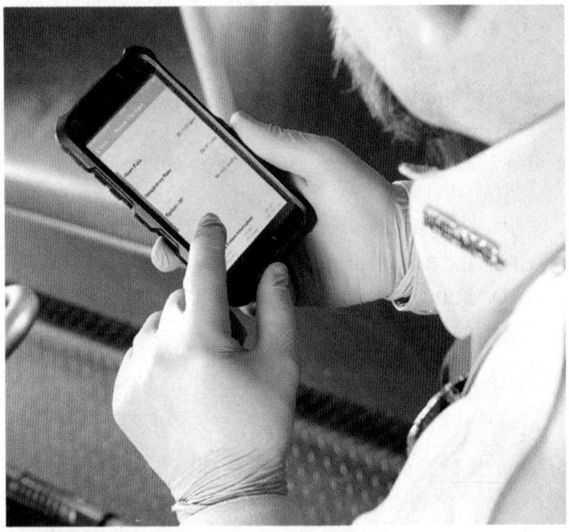

NOTE

Most major medical journals are written in English. In addition, English has become the language of choice at international medical conferences. Newer medical terms are being coined from ordinary English words. Examples include *bypass*, *shunt*, *pacemaker*, and *screening*. Non-English-speaking countries often translate these terms into their own language. These countries also accept and use English abbreviations, such as AIDS (acquired immunodeficiency syndrome) and CPR (cardiopulmonary resuscitation).

TABLE 9-1 Examples of Medical Terms

Body Structures and Systems
Aden/o: Gland
Cardi/o: Heart
Cyt/o: Cell
Hist/o: Tissue
Neur/o: Nerve
Viscer/o: Internal organs
Anatomic Regions and Locations
Anteroposterior: Pertaining to both the front and the back
Bilateral: Pertaining to two sides
Caudal: Pertaining to the tail
Cephalic: Pertaining to the head
Dorsal: Pertaining to the back
Diseases and Other Health Problems
Aphagia: Without swallowing (inability to swallow)
Carcinoma: Cancerous tumor (malignant)
Dyspnea: Difficulty breathing
Neoplasm: New growth (of abnormal tissue or tumor)
Sepsis: Systemic infection
Medical and Surgical Procedures
Appendectomy: Surgical removal of the appendix
Endoscopy: Visual examination of a hollow organ or body cavity
Hemodialysis: Removal of impurities from the blood
Laryngoscopy: Visual examination of the larynx
Nephrectomy: Surgical removal of a kidney
Medical Instruments
Capnometer: Used to measure carbon dioxide
Ophthalmoscope: Used to evaluate the eye
Otoscope: Used to evaluate the inner ear
Oximeter: Used to measure oxygen
Sphygmomanometer: Used to measure blood pressure
Diagnostic Tests
ABGs: A test performed on arterial blood to determine levels of oxygen, carbon dioxide, and other gases
CT scan: Computerized imaging of body organs in sectional slices
MRI: An imaging technique in which magnetic and radio waves are used to produce images of organs and tissues in all three planes of the body
PPD skin test: A test performed on people who have been recently exposed to tuberculosis
Ultrasonography: An imaging technique in which scans are obtained through the use of high-frequency sound waves

Abbreviations: ABGs, arterial blood gases; CT, computed tomography; MRI, magnetic resonance imaging; PPD, purified protein derivative

Word Parts: The Building Blocks of Medical Terminology

Medical terms are used to describe the following (**TABLE 9-1**):

- Body structures and systems
- Anatomic regions and locations

- Diseases and other health problems
- Medical and surgical procedures
- Diagnostic tests
- Medical instruments

Most medical terms can be broken down into word parts. Commonly used word parts include *prefixes, suffixes, root words,* and *linking* or *combining vowels.* Knowledge of the basic word parts can help paramedics understand medical terminology and use it correctly (**FIGURES 9-1** and **9-2**).

- **Root word**. Forms the foundation of the medical term
- **Prefix**. Occurs before the root word
- **Suffix**. Occurs after the root word
- **Combining vowel**. Links one or more root words to other parts of the medical term

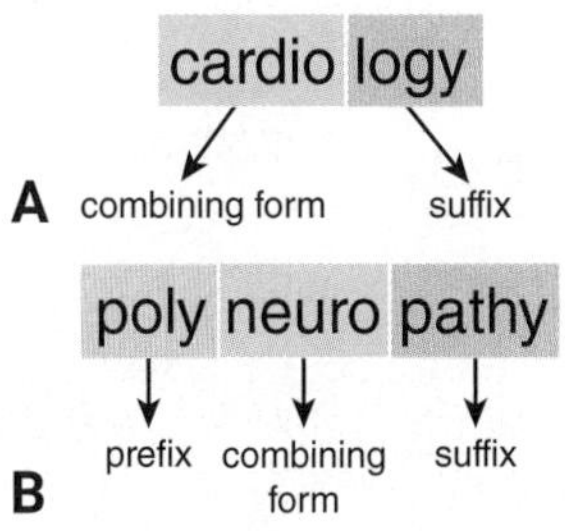

FIGURE 9-1 The relationship of prefixes, suffixes, and combining words. **A.** *Cardiology* means "study of the heart"; *cardi/o* is the combining form (*cardi* + *o*), and *-logy* is the suffix. **B.** *Polyneuropathy* means "disease of many nerves"; *poly-* is the prefix, *neur/o* is the combining form (*neur* + *o*), and *-pathy* is the suffix.

Modified from: How to understand medical terminology. https://www.wikihow.com/Understand-Medical-Terminology. Accessed October 31, 2017.

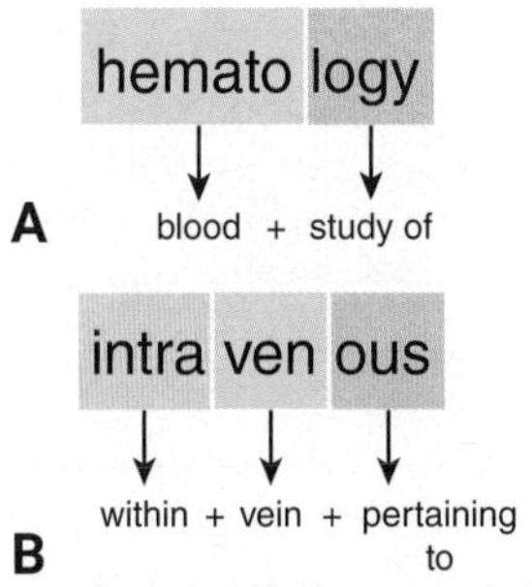

FIGURE 9-2 Root words form the foundation of a medical term. **A.** *Hematology* is broken down as follows: *-logy* (study of) + *hemat/o* (blood) = study of the blood. **B.** Intravenous is broken down as follows: *-ous* (pertaining to) + *intra-* (within) + *ven/o* (vein) = pertaining to within a vein.

Modified from: WikiHow. How to Understand Medical Terminology. Accessed at, https://www.wikihow.com/Understand-Medical-Terminology.

Root Words

The root word is the foundation or building block of the medical term (Figure 9-2); it is the part of the word to which prefixes, suffixes, and combining vowels may (or may not) be attached. A medical term may include one or more root words that are usually derived from Latin or Greek nouns, verbs, or adjectives. For example, *cardiopulmonary* begins with the root word *cardio*, which means "heart"; the next root word is *pulmonary*, which means "lungs." Therefore, *cardiopulmonary* refers to the cardiac and respiratory systems. Other common root words are listed in **TABLE 9-2**.

> NOTE
>
> Most medical terms have at least one root word, but do not have to have either a prefix or a suffix. For example, the term *sternocleidomastoid* can be divided into three root words: *stern, cleid,* and *mastoid.* The sternocleidomastoid is a muscle that has attachments at the sternum, the clavicle, and the mastoid. Some medical terms are not composed of word parts. These nondecodable terms must be memorized. Examples include *cataracts, asthma, diagnosis,* and *suture*.

Prefixes

A prefix is one or more syllables found at the beginning of a word, before the root word. In medical terminology, a prefix often describes location, a unit of measure, or intensity. For example, the word *abnormal* begins with the prefix *ab*, which means "away from." This prefix is followed by the root *normal*, which means "within a balance." Therefore, *abnormal* describes something that is not within balance. Other common prefixes are listed in **TABLE 9-3**.

Suffixes

A suffix appears at the end of a word. In medical terminology, a suffix often describes a patient's condition or diagnosis. For example, *bronchitis* begins with the root word *bronchi* (a respiratory structure). The root word, *bronchi*, is followed by the suffix *itis*, which means "inflammation." Therefore, *bronchitis* describes inflammation of the bronchi. Other common suffixes are listed in **TABLE 9-4**.

Combining Vowels

Combining vowels are also known as *linking vowels.* Combining vowels make medical terms easier to pronounce. The vowel most often used is *o*. An

TABLE 9-2 Common Root Words

Root Word	Meaning	Root Word	Meaning
adeno-	gland	*mal-*	bad
arter-	artery	*meningo-*	meninges
arthro-	joint	*myo-*	muscle
asthenia-	weakness	*nephro-*	kidney
bio-	life	*neuro-*	nerve
bucc-	cheek	*noct-*	night
burs-	pouch or sac	*oculo-*	eye
carc-	cancer	*orchi-*	testicle
cardio-	heart	*osteo-*	bone
caut-	to burn	*oto-*	ear
cephalo-	head	*ov-*	egg
cerv-	neck	*pariet-*	wall
chole-	bile	*phago-*	to eat
chondro-	cartilage	*pharyngo-*	throat
cysto-	bladder	*phlebo-*	vein
cyto-	cell	*photo-*	light
dermo-	skin	*pneumo-*	air
edem-	swelling	*procto-*	rectum
entero-	intestine	*pseud-*	false
eryth-	red	*psych-*	mind
eti-	cause	*pyo-*	pus
febr-	fever	*rhino-*	nose
flex-	to bend	*sclero-*	hardness
gastro-	stomach	*sept-*	wall
glyco-	sugar	*somat-*	body
gyn-	female	*stern-*	chest
hemo-	blood	*tact-*	to touch
hepato-	liver	*thoraco-*	chest
hydra-	water	*uro-*	urinary
iod-	distinct	*varic-*	dilated vein
leuko-	white	*vaso-*	vessel

TABLE 9-3 Common Prefixes

Prefix	Meaning	Example
a-, an-	without, lack of	apnea (without breath) anemia (lack of blood)
ad-	to, toward	adhesion (something stuck to or remaining close to)
angio-	vessel	angiogram (the study of vessels)
ante-	before, forward	antenatal (occurring or formed before birth)
anti-	against, opposed to	antipyretic (against fever)
arter-	artery	arteriogram (study of arteries)
arthro-	pertaining to a joint	arthroscopy (inspection of a joint)
bi-	two	bilateral (both sides)
bio-	life	biology (the study of life)
brady-	slow	bradycardia (slow heart rate)
cardi-	pertaining to the heart	cardiography (recording the movements of the heart)
cerebr-	brain	cerebral (pertaining to the brain)
cerv-	neck	cervical (pertaining to the neck)
chole-	pertaining to bile	cholelithiasis (stones in the gallbladder)
contra-	against, opposite	contrastimulant (against stimulating)
cost-	pertaining to a rib	costal margin (margin of the lower limit of the ribs)
cyst-	pertaining to the bladder or any fluid-containing sac	cystitis (inflammation of the urinary bladder)
cyt-	cell	cytology (the study of cells)
di-	twice, double	diplopia (double vision)
dys-	with difficulty	dyspnea (difficulty breathing)
ecto-	out from	ectopic (out of place)
hyper-	above, excessive, beyond	hypertension (high blood pressure)
inter-	between	intercostal (between the ribs)
micro-	tiny, small	microcirculation (movement of blood in the smallest blood vessels)
post-	after, following, behind	postpartum (following childbirth)
retro-	behind, backward	retroperitoneum (abdominal cavity behind the peritoneum)

TABLE 9-4 Common Suffixes

Suffix	Meaning	Example
-algia	pertaining to pain	neuralgia (pain along a nerve)
-centesis	puncturing	thoracentesis (puncturing into a pleural space)
-cyte	cell	leukocyte (white cell)
-ectomy	a cutting out	tonsillectomy (surgical removal of the tonsils)
-emia	blood	anemia (a decrease in blood hemoglobin)
-esthesia	sensation	anesthesia (without sensation)
-genic	causing	carcinogenic (cancer causing)
-ology	science of	psychology (the science or study of behavior)
-osis	condition	psychosis (condition of the mind)
-ostomy	creation of an opening	gastrostomy (artificial opening into the stomach)
-paresis	weakness	hemiparesis (one-sided weakness)
-pathy	disease	neuropathy (disease of the peripheral nerves)
-phagia	eating	polyphagia (excessive eating)
-phasia	speech	aphasia (loss of the power of speech)
-plasty	repair of, tying of	angioplasty (repair of damaged vessels)
-pnea	breathing	dyspnea (difficulty breathing)
-rhythmia	rhythm	dysrhythmia (variation from a normal rhythm)
-rrhagia	bursting forth	hemorrhage (flowing of blood)
-rrhea	flowing	pyorrhea (discharge of pus)
-scopy	examination by inspection	laparoscopy (examination of the abdominal cavity with a laparoscope)
-uria	pertaining to urine	polyuria (excessive secretion of urine)

NOTE

Antonyms are pairs of root words, prefixes, or suffixes that have opposite meanings. Examples of medical antonyms include *anterior* (front) and *posterior* (back), *bio* (life) and *necro* (death), *brady* (slow) and *tachy* (fast), and *superior* (above) and *inferior* (below).

NOTE

An easy way to learn medical terminology is to use an organized approach to examine the word parts of a medical term. One way to analyze a medical term is to begin with the suffix. Then look at the prefix. The remaining part is the root word. Put the three parts of the term together into a definition of the word.

Example: Pericardial
The suffix is *-al* (pertaining to), the prefix is *peri-* (around), and the root word is *cardio* (heart). The definition, then, is "pertaining to around the heart."

example of the use of a combining vowel is shown in the earlier Note box for the term *sternocleidomastoid: stern-***o***-cleid-***o***-mastoid.* Other vowels, namely *i* and *a,* are also used. Combining vowels often are used between root words and suffixes, as well as between two or more root words. They are not used between prefixes and root words. **TABLE 9-5** presents guidelines for the use of combining vowels.

Plural Forms of Medical Terms

As do words in any language, medical terms need both a singular form and a plural form. Because most medical terms are Greek or Latin in origin, some unusual rules must be followed to change a singular word into its plural form. These rules are presented in **TABLE 9-6**.

Medical Abbreviations, Acronyms, and Symbols

Communication and documentation of medical information require thoroughness, precision, and

TABLE 9-5 Guidelines for Using Combining Vowels

1. When a word root and a suffix are connected, a **combining vowel** *is used* **if the suffix** *does not begin* **with a vowel**.

   arthr-**o**-pathy

2. When a word root and a suffix are connected, a **combining vowel** *usually is not used* **if the suffix** *begins* **with a vowel**.

   hepat-ic

3. When two word roots are connected, a **combining vowel** *usually is used* **even if vowels are present at the junctions**.

   oste-**o**-arthr-it-is

4. When a prefix and a word root are connected, a **combining vowel** *is not used*.

   sub-hepat-ic

Reproduced from: LaFleur Brooks M, *Exploring Medical Language*. 7th ed. St. Louis, MO: Mosby; 2009.

TABLE 9-6 Guidelines for Pluralizing Medical Terms

Guideline	Singular Form	Plural Form
1. If the term ends in *a*, the plural is formed by adding an *e*.	bursa vertebra	bursae vertebrae
2. If the term ends in *ex* or *ix*, the plural is formed by changing *ex*/*ix* to *ices*.	appendix cervix	appendices cervices
3. If the term ends in *is*, the plural is formed by changing the *is* to *es*.	diagnosis metastasis neurosis	diagnoses metastases neuroses
4. If the term ends in *itis*, the plural is formed by dropping the *s* and adding *des*.	arthritis meningitis	arthritides meningitides
5. If the term ends in *nx*, the plural is formed by changing the *x* to *g* and adding *es*.	larynx phalanx	larynges phalanges
6. If the term ends in *on*, the plural is formed by dropping the *on* and adding *a*.	criterion ganglion	criteria ganglia
7. If the term ends in *um*, the plural is formed by changing *um* to *a*.	diverticulum ovum	diverticula ova
8. If the term ends in *us*, the plural is formed by changing *us* to *i*.	alveolus bronchus malleolus	alveoli bronchi malleoli

Reproduced from: Russell WJ. *Medical Terminology by the Mnemonic Story System*. Bloomington, IN: Xlibris Corp; 2006.

accuracy. Medical abbreviations, acronyms, and symbols are a form of medical shorthand, intended to promote efficient communication and documentation. They will achieve those aims only if they are used correctly and are universally understood by other members of the heath care team. Many EMS systems develop lists of agency-approved medical abbreviations; paramedics should not use abbreviations other than the approved versions. **BOX 9-1** lists some of the more common medical abbreviations, acronyms, and symbols used in EMS systems.

BOX 9-1 Common Medical Abbreviations Used by EMS Systems

°C	degrees Centigrade
°F	degrees Fahrenheit
ABG	arterial blood gas
ac	before meals
ACS	acute coronary syndrome
ad lib	freely as desired
ADHD	attention-deficit/hyperactivity disorder
ADL	activity of daily living
AED	automated external defibrillator
AF	atrial fibrillation
AICD	automatic implanted cardioverter-defibrillator
AIDS	acquired immunodeficiency syndrome
ALS	amyotrophic lateral sclerosis
AM	morning
AMA	against medical advice
AMI	acute myocardial infarction
amp	ampule
ARC	AIDS-related complex
ARDS	acute respiratory distress syndrome
AS	aortic stenosis
ASD	atrial septal defect
BE	barium enema
bid	two times a day
BLS	basic life support
BM, bm	bowel movement
BMR	basal metabolic rate
BNP	brain natriuretic peptide
BP	blood pressure
BPAP	bilevel positive airway pressure
BPH	benign prostatic hypertrophy
BPM	beats per minute
BSA	body surface area
BUN	blood urea nitrogen
BVM	bag-valve mask
c/o	complains of
Ca	calcium, cancer, carcinoma
CAD	coronary artery disease
cap	capsule
CAT	computed axial tomography
cath	catheter, catheterize, catheterization
CBC	complete blood count
CBR	complete bed rest
CC	chief complaint
CCU	coronary care unit, critical care unit
CDC	Centers for Disease Control and Prevention
CHF	congestive heart failure
CHO	carbohydrate

BOX 9-1 Common Medical Abbreviations Used by EMS Systems *(continued)*

Cl	chlorine	**ECF**	extracellular fluid
cm	centimeter	**ECG**	electrocardiogram
cm^3	cubic centimeter	**ECT**	electroconvulsive therapy
CNS	central nervous system	**ED**	emergency department
CO	carbon monoxide	**EDC**	estimated date of confinement
CO_2	carbon dioxide	**EDD**	estimated date of delivery
COPD	chronic obstructive pulmonary disease	**EEG**	electroencephalogram
CPAP	continuous positive airway pressure	**EKG**	electrocardiogram
CPK	creatine phosphokinase	**elix**	elixir
CPR	cardiopulmonary resuscitation	**EMG**	electromyogram
CRP	C-reactive protein	**EPAP**	expiratory positive airway pressure
CSF	cerebrospinal fluid	**ER**	emergency room
CT	computed tomography	**ESR**	erythrocyte sedimentation rate
CVA	cerebrovascular accident, costovertebral angle	**ESRD**	end-stage renal disease
CVP	central venous pressure	**$ETCO_2$**	end-tidal carbon dioxide
D&C	dilation and curettage	**ETOH**	ethyl alcohol
D_5W	5% dextrose in water	**FAST**	focused assessment with sonography for trauma
dc	discontinue	**Fe**	iron
DIC	disseminated intravascular coagulation	**FEV**	forced expiratory volume
diff	differential blood count	**FHR**	fetal heart rate
dil	dilute	**FRC**	functional residual capacity
DJD	degenerative joint disease	**FUO**	fever of unknown origin
dL	deciliter	**Fx, fx**	fracture, fractional urine test
DM	diabetes mellitus	**g, gm, Gm**	gram
DNR/ DNAR	do not resuscitate/do not attempt resuscitation	**GCS**	Glasgow Coma Scale
DOE	dyspnea on exertion	**GERD**	gastroesophageal reflux disease
DVT	deep vein thrombosis	**GI**	gastrointestinal
dx	diagnosis	**grava I, II, III, etc.**	pregnancy 1, 2, 3, etc.
EBV	Epstein-Barr virus	**gt, gtt**	drop, drops
		GTT	glucose tolerance test

(continued)

BOX 9-1 Common Medical Abbreviations Used by EMS Systems *(continued)*

GU	genitourinary
GYN, Gyn	gynecologic
H_2O	water
H^+	hydrogen ion
h/o	history of
H&P	history and physical examination
HAV	hepatitis A virus
Hb	hemoglobin
HBV	hepatitis B virus
Hct	hematocrit
HCV	hepatitis C virus
Hg	mercury
Hgb	hemoglobin
HIV	human immunodeficiency (AIDS) virus
HSV	herpes simplex virus
HTN	hypertension
I&O	intake and output
IBD	irritable bowel disease
IC	inspiratory capacity
ICP	intracranial pressure
ICU	intensive care unit
Ig	immunoglobulin
IgA, IgD, etc.	immunoglobulin A, immunoglobulin D, etc.
IM	intramuscular
IN	intranasal
INR	international normalized ratio
IO	intraosseous
IPAP	inspiratory positive airway pressure
IPPB	intermittent positive pressure breathing
ITD	impedance threshold device
IV	intravenous
IVP	intravenous push; intravenous pyelogram
IVPB	intravenous piggyback
J	joules
K	potassium
kg	kilogram
KUB	kidney, ureters, and bladder (radiograph)
KVO	keep vein open
L	liter
L&A	light and accommodation
LBBB	left bundle branch block
LLE	left lower extremity
LLL	left lower lobe
LLQ	left lower quadrant
LMP	last menstrual period
LNMP	last normal menstrual period
LP	lumbar puncture
LR	lactated Ringer solution
LUE	left upper extremity
LUL	left upper lobe
LUQ	left upper quadrant
LV	left ventricle
LVAD	left ventricular assist device
LVH	left ventricular hypertrophy
m	meter
MAP	mean arterial pressure
max	maximum
mcg	microgram
MCH	mean corpuscular hemoglobin
MCHC	mean corpuscular hemoglobin concentration

BOX 9-1 Common Medical Abbreviations Used by EMS Systems *(continued)*

mg	milligram
Mg	magnesium
MG	myasthenia gravis
MI	myocardial infarction
MICU	medical intensive care unit
min	minute(s), minimum
mL	milliliter
mm	millimeter
mm^3	cubic millimeter
mm Hg	millimeters of mercury
MOI	mechanism of injury
MRI	magnetic resonance imaging
MS	multiple sclerosis
mV	millivolt
N	nitrogen
Na	sodium
NG	nasogastric
NICU	neonatal intensive care unit
NIPPV (NPPV)	noninvasive positive pressure ventilation
NOI	nature of illness
NPA	nasopharyngeal airway
NPO	nothing by mouth
NS	normal saline or not significant
O_2	oxygen
OCD	obsessive compulsive disorder
OD	overdose
OG	orogastric
OPA	oropharyngeal airway
ORIF	open reduction and internal fixation
OT	occupational therapy
OTC	over-the-counter
oz	ounce
$Paco_2$	partial pressure of carbon dioxide (arterial blood)
Pao_2	partial pressure of oxygen (arterial blood)
para I, . . . II, etc.	unipara, bipara, etc.
PAT	paroxysmal atrial tachycardia
pc	after meals
PCI	percutaneous coronary intervention
Pco_2	partial pressure of carbon dioxide
PCP	pulmonary capillary pressure, phencyclidine
PCV	packed cell volume
PCWP	pulmonary capillary wedge pressure
PE	pulmonary embolism, physical examination
PEEP	positive end-expiratory pressure
PEF	peak expiratory flow
per	through, by way of
PERRLA	pupils equal, round, and reactive to light and accommodation
PET	positron emission tomography
PG	prostaglandin
pH	hydrogen ion concentration (acidity and alkalinity)
PID	pelvic inflammatory disease
PIH	pregnancy-induced hypertension
PKU	phenylketonuria
PM	postmortem
PM	evening
PMS	premenstrual syndrome

(continued)

BOX 9-1 Common Medical Abbreviations Used by EMS Systems *(continued)*

PND	paroxysmal nocturnal dyspnea, postnasal drip
PO, po	orally
Po_2	partial pressure of oxygen
PPD	purified protein derivative
ppm	parts per million
prn	when required, as often as necessary
PRVC	pressure-regulated volume control
PSVT	paroxysmal supraventricular tachycardia
PT	physical therapy; prothrombin time
PTSD	posttraumatic stress disorder
PTT	partial thromboplastin time
PVC	premature ventricular complex
q	every
q2h	every 2 hours
q3h	every 3 hours
q4h	every 4 hours
qh	every hour
qid	four times a day
qn	every night
qns	quantity not sufficient
R/O	rule out
RA	rheumatoid arthritis
RBBB	right bundle branch block
RDS	respiratory distress syndrome
Rh^+	positive Rh factor
Rh^-	negative Rh factor
RHD	rheumatic heart disease
RLE	right lower extremity
RLL	right lower lobe
RLQ	right lower quadrant
RML	right middle lobe
ROM	range of motion
ROS	review of systems
ROSC	return of spontaneous circulation
RSI	rapid-sequence intubation
RSV	respiratory syncytial virus
RUE	right upper extremity
RUL	right upper lobe
RUQ	right upper quadrant
Rx	take; treatment
SB	sternal border
sec	second(s)
sib	sibling
SICU	surgical intensive care unit
SIDS	sudden infant death syndrome
Sig	write on label
SIMV	synchronized intermittent ventilation
SL	sublingual
SLE	systemic lupus erythematosus
sol	solution, dissolved
sos	if necessary
sp gr, SG, sg	specific gravity
Spco	saturated pressure of carbon monoxide
SpMet	saturated pressure of methemoglobin
Spo_2	saturated pressure of oxygen
SSS	sick sinus syndrome, short-stay surgery
stat	immediately
STD	sexually transmitted disease
STEMI	ST-elevation myocardial infarction

BOX 9-1 Common Medical Abbreviations Used by EMS Systems *(continued)*

STI	sexually transmitted infection
Sub-Q, subQ	subcutaneous
susp	suspension
T_3	triiodothyronine
T_4	tetraiodothyronine
T&A	tonsillectomy and adenoidectomy
TAH	total abdominal hysterectomy
TB, TBC	tuberculosis
TCP	transcutaneous pacing
Tdap	tetanus, diphtheria, acellular pertussis
TdP	torsades de pointes
TIA	transient ischemic attack
tid	three times a day
TKO	to keep open
TPN	total parenteral nutrition
TPR	temperature, pulse, and respirations
UA	unstable angina; urinalysis
URI	upper respiratory infection
UTI	urinary tract infection
VC	vital capacity
VD	venereal disease
VDH	valvular disease of the heart
VDRL	Venereal Disease Research Laboratory (test for syphilis)
VF	ventricular fibrillation
VS	vital signs
VSD	ventricular septal defect
V_T	tidal volume
VT	ventricular tachycardia
WBC	white blood cell, white blood count
WNL	within normal limits
WPW	Wolff-Parkinson-White syndrome

NOTE

Many medical abbreviations and acronyms may have common, multiple meanings. For example, the abbreviation *PE* may be used for *physical examination, pulmonary edema*, or *pulmonary embolism*. Therefore, it is important for every EMS agency or medical direction system to have an approved list of medical abbreviations and acronyms. This list helps ensure precision in documentation. It also facilitates patient assessments and patient histories. In addition, approved lists may provide for medical legal protection if cases are reviewed for litigation.

Eponyms and Homonyms

An **eponym** is a term that is derived from a person's name. For example, a disease, surgical procedure, or test is often named after someone involved in its creation or discovery. Common medical eponyms include the following terms:

- Alzheimer disease, named after the German neurologist Alois Alzheimer
- Apgar score, named after the American anesthesiologist Virginia Apgar
- Down syndrome, named after the English physician John Hayden Down
- Heimlich maneuver, named after the German physician Henry J. Heimlich
- Lou Gehrig disease, named after the famous New York Yankees baseball player
- Macintosh laryngoscope, named after the New Zealand physician Sir Robert Reynolds Macintosh
- Parkinson disease, named after the English physician James Parkinson

It is considered acceptable to drop the possessive apostrophe and letter *s* from most eponyms. The trend in possessive usage varies among countries, journals, and diseases.

A **homonym** is a word that has the same pronunciation as another word but a different meaning, and often a different spelling (in which case it can more specifically be referred to as a *homophone*). Although homonyms are common in everyday English (eg, feet/feat, meet/meat, peal/peel), they are rare in medical terminology. Examples include humerus and humerous, lyse and lice, plane and plain, pleural and plural, venous and Venus.

Do Not Use List

The Joint Commission (formerly known as the Joint Commission on Accreditation of Healthcare Organizations) created a "Do Not Use" list of abbreviations in 2004.[2] This list, which is updated annually, is intended to eliminate the use of abbreviations, acronyms, symbols, and drug dose designations that could be confusing or dangerous and that might result in errors. Many EMS agencies and health care facilities use this list as part of their documentation protocol (**TABLE 9-7**).

SHOW ME THE EVIDENCE

Brunetti and colleagues found that nearly 5% of the errors reported to Medmarx, a national database for medication errors, were related to abbreviation use. Many of the abbreviations involved in the errors were on the official "Do Not Use" list of abbreviations established by The Joint Commission.

Modified from: Brunetti L, Santell JP, Hicks RW. The impact of abbreviations on patient safety. *Joint Comm J Qual Patient Saf.* 2007;33:576-583.

Pronunciation of Medical Terms

Correct spelling and pronunciation of medical terms are necessary for good communication and are skills that health care professionals are expected to have. A good way to learn (and remember) the spelling and pronunciation of medical terms is to first consider the way the terms are built. This is done by analyzing the root words, prefixes, and suffixes described earlier in the chapter. Understanding root words and memorizing these terms and their correct spelling can help paramedics build a medical vocabulary.

The pronunciation of medical terms often varies, because no "rigid rules" exist. In addition, medical terms often are pronounced somewhat differently even among medical professionals. For some medical terms, more than one pronunciation is considered

TABLE 9-7 The Joint Commission's "Do Not Use" Abbreviations List[a]

Do Not Use	Potential Problem	Use Instead
> (greater than)	Misinterpreted as the number 7 (seven) or the letter *L*	Write *greater than.*
U, u (unit)	Mistaken for the number 0 (zero), the number 4 (four), or *cc*	Write *unit.*
IU (International Unit)	Mistaken for IV (intravenous) or the number 10 (ten)	Write *international unit.*
Q.D., QD, q.d., qd (daily) Q.O.D., QOD, q.o.d., qod (every other day)	Mistaken for every other Period after the *Q* mistaken for *I* and the *O* mistaken for *I*	Write *daily*; write *every other day.*
Trailing zero (X.0 mg)[b] Lack of leading zero (.X mg)	Decimal point is missed	Write *X mg.* Write *0.X mg.*
MS MSO_4 and $MgSO_4$	Can mean morphine sulfate or magnesium sulfate Confused for one another	Write *morphine sulfate.* Write *magnesium sulfate.*

[a]Applies to all orders and all medication-related documentation that is handwritten (including free-text computer entry) or on preprinted forms.

[b]Exception: A "trailing zero" may be used only where required to demonstrate the level of precision of the value being reported, such as for laboratory results, imaging studies that report size of lesions, or catheter/tube sizes. It may not be used in medication orders or other medication-related documentation.

acceptable (**TABLE 9-8**). A common example is *angina*: It can be pronounced with the emphasis on the first syllable and a short *i* (AN-ji-na) or with the emphasis on the second syllable and a long *i* (an-JĪ-na). Some medical terms look alike and sound alike but have very different meanings.

TABLE 9-8 Guide to Pronunciation of Medical Terms

The following is a simple guide for practicing the pronunciation of medical terms. The pronunciations are only approximate; however, they are adequate to meet the needs of the beginning student.

In respelling for pronunciation, words are minimally distorted to indicate phonetic sound.

Examples:
- doctor (dok-tor)
- gastric (gas-trik)

A special mark, called the *macron* (¯), is used to indicate long vowel sounds.

Examples:
- donate (dō-nāt)
- hepatoma (hep-a-tō-ma)
- ā as in *ate*, *say*
- ē as in *eat*, *beet*, *see*
- ī as in *I*, *mine*, *sky*
- ō as in *oats*, *so*
- ū as in *unit*, *mute*

Vowels with no markings have the short sound.

Examples:
- discuss (dis-kus)
- medical (med-i-kal)
- a as in *at*, *lad*
- e as in *edge*, *bet*
- i as in *itch*, *wish*
- o as in *ox*, *top*
- u as in *sun*, *come*

The primary accent is indicated by capital letters, and the secondary accent (which is stressed but not as strongly as the primary accent) is indicated by italics.

Examples:
- altogether (*all*-tū-GETH-er)
- pancreatitis (*pan*-krē-a-TĪ-tis)

Modified from: LaFleur Brooks M, LaFleur Brooks *D. Exploring Medical Language*. 7th ed. St Louis: Elsevier; 2009.

NOTE

Paramedics who can spell a medical term accurately usually can also pronounce it correctly.

The pronunciation of medical terms is best perfected by using the word frequently and by saying the word aloud. If the paramedic is unsure of any word, he or she should check the correct spelling and pronunciation in a medical dictionary.

DID YOU KNOW?

Confusing Medical Terms

Some medical terms look alike and sound alike, but have very different meanings. Some common terms that are easily confused include the following:

- *Arterio* means "artery." *Athero* means "plaque or fatty substance." *Arthro* means "joint."
- The *ileum* is a part of the small intestine. *Ilium* means "part of the hip bone."
- *Mucous* means "resembles mucus." *Mucus* is the substance secreted from the membranes.
- *Myco* means "fungus." *Myelo* means both "bone marrow" and "spinal cord." *Myo* means "muscle."
- *Palpation* is an examination technique. *Palpitation* means "a pounding racing heart."
- *Pyelo* refers to the renal pelvis. *Pyo* means "pus."
- *Viral* means "related to a virus." *Virile* means "having masculine traits."

Summary

- Medical terminology is the language of medicine. It is important to know the language to interpret patient information and communicate it to other health care personnel.
- Medical terms are used to describe body structures, systems, and functions; anatomic regions and locations; diseases and other health problems; medical and surgical procedures; diagnostic tests; and medical instruments.
- Medical terms are broken down into several parts. These parts include root words, prefixes, suffixes, and combining vowels.
- Root words describe a structure or condition. They may be combined with other root words, a prefix, and/or a suffix.
- A prefix is a root syllable at the beginning of a root word that often describes location or intensity.
- A suffix comes at the end of a root word and often describes a condition or diagnosis.
- Combining vowels join syllables in medical terms to make them easier to pronounce.
- Medical terms are interpreted by analyzing each word part and then combining them to determine the meaning.
- Specific rules govern the conversion of medical terms from the singular form to the plural form. For example, *vertebra* becomes *vertebrae*; *diagnosis* becomes *diagnoses*; *phalanx* becomes *phalanges*; and *alveolus* becomes *alveoli*.
- Medical abbreviations, acronyms, and symbols are a form of medical shorthand that can make communication among medical professionals more efficient. It is important for paramedics to use only the abbreviations approved within their EMS system.
- Paramedics must be able to pronounce medical terms correctly so that their intended meaning is communicated clearly.

References

1. Wulff H. The language of medicine. *R Soc Med.* 2004;97:187-188.
2. Facts about the official "do not use" list of abbreviations. The Joint Commission website. https://www.jointcommission.org/facts_about_do_not_use_list/. Accessed December 7, 2017.

Suggested Readings

Chabner DE. *Medical Terminology: A Short Course.* 7th ed. St. Louis, MO: Elsevier; 2009.

Fremgen BF, Frucht SG. *Medical Terminology: A Living Language.* 6th ed. Boston, MA: Pearson; 2016.

Stanfield PS, Hui YH, Cross N. *Essential Medical Terminology.* 4th ed. Burlington, MA: Jones & Bartlett Learning; 2014.

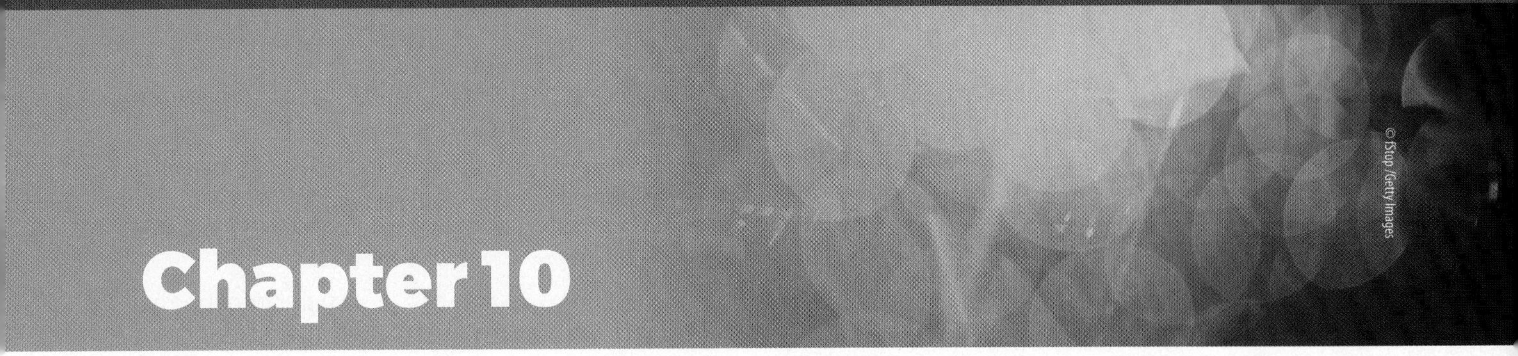
© fStop /Getty Images

Chapter 10

Review of Human Systems

NATIONAL EMS EDUCATION STANDARD COMPETENCIES

Anatomy and Physiology

Integrates a complex depth and comprehensive breadth of knowledge of the anatomy and physiology of all human systems.

OBJECTIVES

Upon completion of this chapter, the paramedic student will be able to:

1. Discuss the importance of human anatomy as it relates to the paramedic profession. (pp 199, 200)
2. Describe the anatomic position. (pp 199–200)
3. Properly interpret anatomic directional terms and body planes. (pp 200, 201)
4. List the structures that compose the axial and appendicular regions of the body. (p 200)
5. Define the divisions of the abdominal region. (pp 200–201)
6. List the three major body cavities. (pp 200, 202)
7. Describe the contents of the three major body cavities. (p 202)
8. Discuss the functions of the following cellular structures: the cytoplasmic membrane, the cytoplasm (and organelles), and the nucleus. (pp 202–206)
9. Describe the process by which human cells reproduce. (pp 206–207)
10. Differentiate and describe the following tissue types: epithelial tissue, connective tissue, muscle tissue, and nervous tissue. (pp 207–209)
11. For each of the 11 major organ systems in the human body, label a diagram of anatomic structures, list the functions of the major anatomic structures, and explain how the organs of the system interrelate to perform the specific functions of that system. (pp 209–261)
12. For the special senses, label a diagram of the anatomic structures of the special senses, list the functions of the anatomic structures of each sense, and explain how the structures of the senses interrelate to perform their specialized functions. (pp 261–265)

KEY TERMS

abdominal aorta The portion of the descending aorta that passes from the aortic hiatus of the diaphragm into the abdomen, where it divides into the two common iliac arteries.

acetabulum The large, cup-shaped articular cavity at the juncture of the ilium, the ischium, and the pubis that contains the ball-shaped head of the femur.

action potential A change in membrane potential in an excitable tissue that acts as an electrical signal and is propagated in an all-or-none fashion.

adenosine triphosphate (ATP) A nucleotide composed of adenosine, an organic base, with three phosphate groups attached to it. It stores energy in muscles.

adipose tissue A specialized connective tissue that stores lipids; also known as fat tissue.

aerobic oxidation A biochemical reaction that increases the positive charges on an atom or the loss of negative charges in the presence of oxygen.

afferent division The division of the peripheral nervous system that transmits impulses from the periphery to the central nervous system.

afferent neurons Neurons that carry action potentials from the periphery to the central nervous system.

aldosterone A steroid hormone produced by the adrenal cortex to regulate the sodium and potassium balance in the blood.

alveoli Minute air sacs in the lungs through which gas exchange takes place between alveolar air and pulmonary capillary blood.

amino acids Organic chemical compounds composed of one or more basic amino groups and one or more acidic carboxyl groups.

anatomic position The position of standing erect with the feet and palms facing the examiner.

anterior The front, or ventral, surface.

antidiuretic hormone (ADH) A hormone produced in the posterior pituitary gland that regulates the balance of water in the body by accelerating the resorption of water.

anus The distal end or outlet of the rectum.

aorta The main and largest artery in the body.

appendicular region The region consisting of the limbs, or extremities.

appendicular skeleton The bones of the upper and lower extremities.

aqueous humor The clear, watery fluid that circulates in the anterior and posterior chambers of the eye.

arachnoid layer The delicate, weblike, middle membrane that covers the brain.

areola The circular, pigmented area surrounding the nipple.

areolar connective tissue A loose tissue that consists of delicate webs of fibers and a variety of cells embedded in a matrix of soft, sticky gel.

arterioles Small branches of arteries.

arteriovenous anastomoses Vessels that allow blood to flow from arteries to veins without passing through capillaries; also known as arteriovenous shunts.

atria The two upper chambers of the heart (singular, atrium).

atrial natriuretic factor (ANF) A peptide released from the atria when atrial blood pressure is increased. It lowers blood pressure by increasing urine production, thereby reducing blood volume.

atrioventricular node An area of specialized cardiac muscle that receives the cardiac impulse from the sinoatrial node and conducts it to the bundle of His.

atrioventricular valve A valve in the heart through which blood flows from the atria to the ventricles.

auricle The part of the external ear that protrudes from the head; also known as the pinna.

autonomic nervous system The division of the peripheral nervous system that acts as a control system for visceral processes. It functions largely below the level of consciousness.

autonomic reflexes Any of a large number of normal reflexes governing and regulating the functions of the viscera

autophagia A condition in which the body obtains nutrition through consumption of its own tissues.

axial region The region consisting of the head, neck, thorax, and abdomen.

axial skeleton The bones of the head, neck, and torso.

bacteria Single-celled microorganisms that cause an infection characteristic of that species.

basophils White blood cells that promote inflammation.

bicuspid valve One of the two atrioventricular valves located between the left atrium and the ventricle; also known as the mitral valve.

bile A bitter, yellow-green secretion of the liver that is stored in the gallbladder.

blood The fluid and its suspended, formed elements that circulate through the heart, arteries, capillaries, and veins.

bone A highly specialized form of hard, connective tissue. It consists of living cells and a mineralized matrix.

bony labyrinth Part of the inner ear. It contains the membranous labyrinth.

Bowman capsule The expanded beginning of a renal tubule.

bronchioles Small branches of the bronchi.

bulbourethral glands Small glands located just below the prostate gland that lubricate the terminal portion of the urethra and contribute to seminal fluid; also known as the Cowper glands.

bundle of His A band of fibers in the myocardium through which the cardiac impulse is transmitted from the atrioventricular node to the ventricles.

calcaneus The heel bone, the largest of the tarsal bones.

cancellous bone Lattice-like tissue normally present in the interior of many bones, where spaces usually are filled with marrow; also known as spongy bone.

capillaries Tiny vessels that connect arterioles to venules.

cardiac muscle A special striated muscle of the myocardium that contains dark, intercalated disks at the junctions of the abutting fibers. It is characterized by special contractile abilities.

cardiac output The volume of blood pumped each minute by the heart.

cardiac sphincter A ring of muscle fibers at the juncture of the esophagus and the stomach.

carina A downward and backward projection of the lowest tracheal cartilage, forming a ridge between the openings of the right and the left primary bronchi.

carpal bones The bones of the carpus, or wrist.

cartilage Firm, smooth, nonvascular connective tissue.

cartilaginous joints Joints that are slightly movable.

cecum A cul-de-sac constituting the first part of the large intestine.

cell The functional basic unit of life.

central nervous system (CNS) The system composed of the brain and spinal cord.

centrioles Usually paired organelles that lie in the centrosome.

centrosome A specialized zone of cytoplasm close to the nucleus that contains two centrioles.

cerebellum The second largest part of the brain. It plays an essential role in coordinating normal movements.

cerebral cortex A thin layer of gray matter, made up of neuron dendrites and cell bodies, that comprises the surface of the cerebrum.

cerebrospinal fluid (CSF) The fluid that fills the subarachnoid space in the brain and spinal cord and is found in the cerebral ventricles.

cerebrum The largest and uppermost part of the brain. It controls consciousness, memory, sensations, emotions, and voluntary movements.

cervix The lower part of the uterus.

chromatin granules The material within the cell nucleus from which chromosomes are formed.

chromosomes Organized structures of deoxyribonucleic acid (DNA) and protein that are found in cells.

chyme The semifluid mass of partly digested food passed from the stomach into the duodenum.

cilia Small, hairlike processes on the outer surfaces of some cells.

clitoris Erectile tissue in the vestibule of the vagina.

compact bone Hard, dense bone that usually is found at the surface of skeletal structures, as distinguished from cancellous bone.

conjunctiva A mucous membrane that covers the anterior surface of the eyeball and the lining of the eyelids.

connective tissue Tissue that supports and binds other body tissues and parts.

cornea The convex, transparent, anterior part of the eye.

coronary arteries The two arteries that arise from the base of the aorta and carry blood to the muscle of the heart.

costal cartilages Cartilages that connect the sternum and the ends of the ribs. They allow the chest to move in respiration.

coxae The hip joints; the head of the femur and the acetabulum of the innominate bone.

cranial vault The eight skull bones that surround and protect the brain; the brain case.

cricoid cartilage The most inferior laryngeal cartilage.

cricothyroid membrane The membrane joining the thyroid and cricoid cartilages.

cytoplasm All of the substance of a cell other than the nucleus.

cytoplasmic membrane The plasma membrane.

deoxyribonucleic acid (DNA) A type of nucleic acid that makes up the genetic material of cells.

dermatomes Areas of skin surface supplied by a single spinal nerve.

dermis Dense, irregular connective tissue that forms the deep layer of the skin.

diaphragm The dome-shaped, musculofibrous partition that separates the thoracic and abdominal cavities.

diaphysis The shaft of a long bone, consisting of a tube of compact bone that encloses the medullary cavity.

diencephalon The parts of the brain between the cerebral hemispheres and the mesencephalon.

differentiation A process in which cells become specialized in one type of function or act in concert with other cells to perform a more complex task.

dorsal root A sensory component that conveys afferent nerve processes to the spinal cord.

ductus deferens A thick, smooth muscular tube that allows sperm to exit from the epididymis through the ejaculatory duct; also known as the vas deferens.

duodenum The first subdivision of the small intestine.

dura mater The outermost layer of the meninges.

efferent division The division of the peripheral nervous system that transmits action potentials from the central nervous system to effector organs such as muscles and glands.

efferent neurons Neurons that carry impulses away from the central nervous system to the periphery.

electrolytes Cations or anions in solution that conduct an electrical current.

endocrine glands Glands that secrete hormones into the blood rather than through a duct.

endocrine system A collection of glands that produce and secrete hormones.

endoplasmic reticulum A network of connecting sacs or canals that wind through the cytoplasm of a cell, serving as a miniature circulatory system for the cell.

enzymes A protein produced by living cells that catalyzes chemical reactions in organic matter.

eosinophils White blood cells that inhibit inflammation. These readily stain with acidic dyes.

epicardium The portion of the serous pericardium that covers the heart's surface; also known as the visceral pericardium.

epidermis The outer portion of the skin. It is formed of epithelial tissue that rests on or covers the dermis.

epididymis A tightly coiled tube, lying along the top of and behind the testes, where sperm matures.

epidural space The space above or on the dura.

epiglottis A lidlike cartilage that overhangs the entrance to the larynx.

epiphyseal plate The site of bone elongation; also known as the growth plate.

epithelial tissue The cellular covering of internal and external surfaces of the body, including the lining of vessels and other small cavities.

erection The condition of hardness, swelling, and elevation observed in the penis and to a lesser degree in the clitoris, usually caused by sexual arousal.

erythrocytes Red blood cells.

esophagus The muscular canal extending from the pharynx to the stomach.

eukaryotes Cells with a true nucleus. They are found in all higher organisms and in some microorganisms.

eustachian tube The auditory canal, which extends from the middle ear to the nasopharynx; also known as the auditory tube.

exocrine gland A gland that secretes chemicals and hormones into a duct.

external ear The portion of the ear that includes the auricle and external auditory meatus. It terminates at the eardrum.

extracellular Occurring outside a cell or cell tissues or in cavities or spaces between cell layers or groups of cells.

extracellular matrix Nonliving chemical substances located between connective tissue cells.

femur The thigh bone, which extends from the pelvis to the knee; the largest and strongest bone in the body.

fibrous connective tissue A connective tissue that consists mainly of bundles of strong, white collagenous fibers arranged in parallel rows.

fibrous joints Joints that are immovable.

fibula A bone of the lower leg, lateral to and smaller than the tibia.

flat bones Bones that have a thin, flattened shape, such as certain skull bones, the ribs, the sternum, and the scapulae.

gallbladder A pear-shaped excretory sac on the visceral surface of the right lobe of the liver. It serves as a reservoir for bile.

ganglia A group of nerve cell bodies in the peripheral nervous system.

glomerulus The mass of capillary loops at the beginning of each nephron.

glottic opening The vocal cords and the space between them.

glycoproteins A large group of conjugated proteins in which the nonprotein substance is a carbohydrate.

Golgi apparatus Specialized endoplasmic reticulum that concentrates and packages materials for secretion from the cell.

gray matter The gray tissue that makes up the inner core of the spinal column.

hematopoietic tissue Tissue related to the process of formation and development of various types of blood cells.

hemoglobin A complex protein–iron compound in the blood that carries oxygen to the cells from the lungs and carbon dioxide away from the cells to the lungs.

hepatic artery The branch of the aorta that delivers blood to the liver.

histamine An amine released by mast cells and basophils that promotes inflammation.

homeostasis A state of equilibrium in the body with respect to functions and composition of fluids and tissues.

humerus The largest bone of the upper arm, comprising a body, head, and condyle.

hymen A mucous membrane that may partly or entirely occlude the vaginal outlet.

hyoid bone The U-shaped bone between the mandible and the larynx.

hypothalamus A portion of the diencephalon of the brain that activates, controls, and integrates the peripheral autonomic nervous system, endocrine processes, and many somatic functions, such as body temperature, sleep, and appetite.

ileum The distal portion of the small intestine.

iliac crest The upper free margin of the ilium.

ilium One of the three bones that make up the innominate bone.

inferior Toward the feet; below a point of reference in the anatomic position.

inferior vena cava The vein that returns blood from the lower limbs and the greater part of the pelvic and abdominal organs to the right atrium.

inflammatory response A tissue reaction to injury or an antigen. It may include pain, swelling, itching, redness, heat, and loss of function.

inguinal canal The passage through the lower abdominal wall that transmits the spermatic cord in the male and the round ligament in the female.

inner ear The part of the ear that contains the sensory organs for hearing and balance.

integumentary system The largest organ system in the body, consisting of the skin and accessory structures.

intercellular Occurring between or among cells.

interstitial fluid Fluid that occupies the space outside the blood vessels and/or outside the cells of an organ or tissue.

intracellular Occurring within cell membranes.

intraocular pressure Pressure within the eye that keeps the eye inflated.

ions Atoms or groups of atoms that carry a charge of electricity by virtue of having gained or lost one or more electrons.

iris The colored contractile membrane of the eye that can be seen through the cornea.

irregular bones Bones that are not representative of the other three categories (long, short, or flat bones).

ischium One of the three parts of the hipbone. It joins the ilium and the pubis to form the acetabulum.

jejunum One of the three portions of the small intestine.

joint capsule A well-defined structure that encloses a joint.

jugular notch The superior margin of the manubrium, which is palpated easily at the anterior base of the neck; also known as the suprasternal notch.

kidney One of the pair of organs that cleanse the body of the waste products continually produced by metabolism.

Krebs cycle A sequence of enzymatic reactions, involving the metabolism of carbon chains of sugar, fatty acids, and amino acids, that yield carbon dioxide, water, and high-energy phosphate bonds.

lacrimal gland The tear gland located in the superolateral corner of the orbit.

large intestine The portion of the digestive tract comprising the cecum; the appendix; the ascending, transverse, and descending colons; and the rectum.

laryngopharynx The lowest part of the pharynx.

larynx The voice box, located just below the pharynx.

lateral recumbent A position in which the patient lies on the right or left side.

left atrium One of the four chambers of the human heart. It receives oxygenated blood from the lungs and pumps it into the left ventricle.

lens The crystalline portion of the eye.

leukocytes White blood cells.

limbic system The part of the brain involved with emotions and olfaction.

lipid bilayer The central layer of the cytoplasmic membrane. It is composed of a double layer of lipid molecules.

lipoproteins Conjugated proteins in which lipids form an integral part of the molecule. They are synthesized primarily in the liver.

liver An organ in the upper abdomen that aids in digestion and removes waste products and cellular debris from the blood; the largest solid organ in the human body.

long bones Bones that are longer than they are wide, such as the humerus, ulna, radius, femur, tibia, fibula, and phalanges.

loop of Henle The U-shaped portion of the renal tubule.

lymph nodes Encapsulated masses of lymphoid tissue found among lymph vessels.

lymph nodules Small, densely packed spherical nodes or aggregations of lymph cells embedded in the reticular meshwork of the lymphatic system. They are found mainly in the tonsils, spleen, and thymus.

lymphatic system The network of vessels, ducts, nodes, valves, and organs involved in protecting and maintaining the internal fluid environment of the body.

lymphocytes A type of white blood cell formed in lymphoid tissue.

lysosomes Membranous-walled organelles that contain enzymes, which enable the lysosome to function as an intracellular digestive system.

macrophages Phagocytic cells in the immune system.

mammary glands External accessory sex organs in females; the breasts.

medial malleolus The rounded process on the medial side of the ankle joint.

mediastinum The area of the body that includes the trachea, esophagus, thymus, heart, and great vessels.

medulla The lowest part of the brainstem, which controls vital functions; an enlarged extension of the spinal cord; also known as the medulla oblongata.

meninges Fluid-containing membranes surrounding the brain and spinal cord.

mesencephalon One of the three parts of the brainstem; also known as the midbrain.

mesentery A continuous abdominal organ composed of a double fold of peritoneum that holds other abdominal organs to the body wall.

metabolism The culmination of all chemical processes that take place in living organisms.

metacarpals The five bones that extend from the carpus to the phalanges.

metatarsals The five bones that compose the metatarsus.

middle ear An air-filled space in the temporal bone that contains the auditory ossicles.

mitochondria Small, spherical, rod-shaped or thin filamentous structures in the cytoplasm of cells; a site of adenosine triphosphate production.

mitosis Cell division that results in two daughter cells with exactly the same number and type of chromosomes as the mother cell.

monocytes A type of white blood cell found in the lymph nodes, spleen, bone marrow, and loose connective tissue.

mons pubis The prominence caused by a pad of fatty tissue over the symphysis pubis in the female.

motor neuron A neuron that innervates muscle fibers.

mucus The viscous, slippery secretion of mucous membranes and glands.

mycoplasmas A genus of microscopic organisms that lack rigid cell walls; considered the smallest free-living organisms.

myofilaments Extremely fine, molecular, threadlike structures that help form the myofibril of muscle. Thick myofibrils are formed of myosin, and thin myofilaments are formed of actin.

nephron The functional unit of the kidney.

neuroglia The supporting or nonneuronal tissue cells of the central and peripheral nervous system.

neurons The functional units of the nervous system, consisting of the nerve cell body, the dendrites, and the axon.

neutrophils Small, phagocytic white blood cells with a lobed nucleus and small granules in the cytoplasm.

nucleoplasm The protoplasm of the nucleus, as contrasted with that of the cell.

nucleus The central controlling body within a living cell.

obturator foramen A large opening on each side of the lower portion of the hipbone, formed posteriorly by the ischium, superiorly by the ilium, and anteriorly by the pubis.

oculomotor nerve The third cranial nerve, which contains sensory and motor fibers. It provides for movement of most of the muscles of the eye, for constriction of the pupil, and for accommodation of the eye to light.

olfactory Of or pertaining to the sense of smell.

oocytes Incompletely developed ova.

optic nerve The nerve that carries visual signals from the eye to the crossing of the optic tracts.

organ A structure made up of two or more kinds of tissues organized to perform a more complex function than any one tissue alone.

organelles Various particles of living substance that are bound within most cells, such as the mitochondria, the Golgi apparatus, the endoplasmic reticulum, the lysosomes, and the centrioles.

ovarian follicles Spherical cell aggregations in the ovary that contain an oocyte.

ovaries The pair of female gonads found on each side of the lower abdomen beside the uterus.

pancreas A fish-shaped, nodular gland located across the posterior abdominal wall in the epigastric region of the body. It secretes various substances, including digestive enzymes, insulin, and glucagon.

parasympathetic nervous system The subdivision of the autonomic nervous system, usually involved in activating vegetative functions such as digestion, defecation, and urination.

parietal peritoneum The serous membrane that covers the body cavity wall.

patella A flat, triangular bone at the front of the knee joint; the kneecap.

penis The external reproductive organ of the male.

pericardial sac The sac that surrounds the heart.

perineum The pelvic floor and associated structures occupying the pelvic outlet, bounded anteriorly by the pubic symphysis, laterally by the ischial tuberosities, and posteriorly by the coccyx.

periosteum Tough connective tissue that covers the bone.

peripheral nervous system (PNS) A subdivision of the nervous system consisting of nerves and ganglia.

phagocytosis The process by which cells ingest solid substances, such as other cells, bacteria, bits of necrosed tissue, and foreign particles.

phalanges The bones of the fingers and toes.

phospholipids A class of compounds, widely distributed in living cells, that contain phosphoric acid, fatty acids, and a nitrogenous base.

pia mater The innermost layer of the meninges. It directly covers the brain.

pituitary gland A small gland attached to the hypothalamus. It supplies numerous hormones that govern many vital processes.

plasma membrane The outer covering of a cell that contains the cellular cytoplasm; also known as the cell membrane.

platelets Fragments of a cell. These initiate the clotting process.

pleural cavity The area of the body that surrounds the lungs.

pleural space The potential space between the visceral layer and the parietal layer of the pleura.

polysaccharides Carbohydrates that contain three or more molecules of simple carbohydrate.

pons The part of the brainstem between the medulla and the midbrain.

portal vein A vein in the liver that conveys the blood to the inferior vena cava through the hepatic veins.

posterior The back, or dorsal, surface.

precapillary sphincters Smooth muscle sphincters that regulate blood flow through a capillary.

prokaryotes Cells without a true nucleus; instead, nuclear material is scattered throughout the cytoplasm.

prone A position in which the patient lies on the stomach (facedown).

prostate gland The gland that lies just below the male bladder. Its secretion is one of the components of semen.

puberty The period of life when the ability to reproduce begins.

pubis One of a pair of pubic bones that, with the ischium and the ilium, form the hipbone and join the pubic bone from the opposite side at the pubic symphysis.

pulmonary surfactant Certain lipoproteins that reduce the surface tension of pulmonary fluids, allowing the exchange of gases in the alveoli of the lungs and contributing to the elasticity of pulmonary tissue.

pulmonary trunk The large elastic artery that carries blood from the right ventricle of the heart to the right and left pulmonary arteries.

pulmonary veins The veins that carry oxygenated blood from the lung to the left atrium.

pupil The opening in the center of the iris that regulates the amount of light entering the eye.

Purkinje fibers Myocardial fibers that are a continuation of the bundle of His and that extend into the muscle walls of the ventricles.

radius One of the bones of the forearm. It lies parallel to the ulna.

rectum The segment of the large intestine continuous with the descending sigmoid colon just proximal to the anal canal.

red marrow Specialized soft tissue found in many bones of infants and children; in the spongy bone of the proximal epiphyses of the humerus and femur; and in the sternum, ribs, and vertebral bodies of adults. It is essential in the manufacture of red blood cells.

renal pyramids Pyramidal masses seen on longitudinal section of the kidney. They contain part of the loop of Henle and the collecting tubules.

respiration The process of the molecular exchange of oxygen and carbon dioxide in the body's tissues.

reticular activating system A functional system in the brain that is essential for wakefulness, attention, concentration, and introspection.

reticular formation A small, thick cluster of neurons nestled in the brainstem that controls breathing, the heartbeat, blood pressure, level of consciousness, and other vital functions.

retina The nervous tunic of the eye. It is continuous with the optic nerve.

retroperitoneal Behind the peritoneum.

ribonucleic acid (RNA) A nucleic acid found in the nucleus and the cytoplasm of cells that transmits genetic instructions from the nucleus to the cytoplasm. In the cytoplasm, RNA functions in the assembly of proteins.

ribosomes The "factories" in cells, in which protein is synthesized.

right atrium One of the four chambers of the human heart. It receives deoxygenated blood from the body through the venae cavae and pumps it into the right ventricle.

sarcomere The contractile unit of skeletal muscle. It contains thick and thin myofilaments.

sclera The opaque membrane covering the eyeball.

scrotum The sac of skin that contains the testes.

sebaceous glands Glands of the skin, usually associated with a hair follicle, that produce sebum.

sebum The secretion of sebaceous glands. It prevents drying of the skin and protects against invasion by some bacteria.

semen The male reproductive fluid.

seminal vesicle One of two glandular structures that empty into the ejaculatory ducts. Its secretion is one of the components of semen.

septum A thin wall dividing two cavities or masses of soft tissue.

serum Blood plasma without its clotting factors.

short bones Bones that are approximately as broad as they are long, such as the carpal bones of the wrist and the tarsal bones of the ankle.

sinoatrial node An area of specialized heart tissue that generates the cardiac electrical impulse.

sinuses The cavities in the bones of the skull that connect to the nasal cavities by small channels.

skeletal muscle Muscle tissue that appears microscopically to consist of striped myofibrils; also known as striated muscle and voluntary muscle.

small intestine The longest portion of the digestive tract. It is divided into the duodenum, jejunum, and ileum.

smooth muscle One of two kinds of muscle. It is composed of elongated, spindle-shaped cells in muscles not under voluntary control, such as smooth muscle of the intestines, stomach, and other visceral organs. Also known as visceral muscle, involuntary muscle, and nonstriated muscle.

somatic nervous system The part of the nervous system composed of nerve fibers that send impulses from the central nervous system to skeletal muscle.

somatomotor neurons Neurons that innervate skeletal muscles.

spermatogenesis The process of development of spermatozoa.

spermatozoa The male sex cells, which are composed of a head and a tail. Sperm contains genetic information transmitted by the male.

spinal nerves Thirty-one pairs of nerves formed by the joining of the dorsal and ventral routes that arise from the spinal cord.

spleen A large, highly vascular lymphatic organ situated in the upper part of the abdominal cavity between the stomach and the diaphragm. It responds to foreign substances in the blood, destroys worn-out erythrocytes, and is a storage site for red blood cells.

sternal angle The point at which the manubrium joins the body of the sternum; also known as the angle of Louis.

sternoclavicular joint The double gliding joint between the sternum and the clavicle.

sternomanubrial joint The articulation between the upper two parts of the sternum, the manubrium and the sternal body.

sternum The elongated, flattened bone that forms the middle portion of the thorax.

subarachnoid space The area below the arachnoid membrane but above the pia mater that contains cerebrospinal fluid.

subclavian vein The continuation of the axillary vein in the upper body. It extends from the lateral border of the first rib to the sternal end of the clavicle, where it joins the internal jugular to form the brachiocephalic vein.

subcutaneous tissue The adherent layer of adipose tissue just below the dermal layer; also known as the hypodermis.

subdural space The space between the dura mater and the arachnoid.

superior Situated above or higher than a point of reference in the anatomic position.

superior vena cava The vein that returns blood from the head and neck, upper limbs, and thorax to the right atrium.

supine A position in which the patient lies on the back (faceup).

sweat glands Glands that produce sweat or viscous organic secretions; also known as sudoriferous glands.

sympathetic nervous system A subdivision of the autonomic nervous system that usually is involved in preparing the body for physical activity.

symphysis pubis The joint that connects the coxal bones of the pelvis.

synapse Any junction between nerve cells and other nerve cells, muscle cells, gland cells, or sensory receptors. It serves to transmit action potentials from one cell to another.

synovial joints Joints that are freely movable.

system Interconnected functions or organs in which a stimulus or an action in one area affects all other areas.

tarsal bones The bones of the ankle.

taste buds The peripheral taste organs that are distributed over the tongue and the roof of the mouth.

testes The male gonads, which produce the male sex cells, or sperm.

thalamus Tissue located just above the hypothalamus. It helps to produce sensations, associates sensations with emotions, and plays a part in arousal.

thymus A single, unpaired gland located in the mediastinum. The primary central gland of the lymphatic system.

thyroid membrane The fibrous membrane that joins the hyoid and the thyroid cartilages.

tibia The second longest bone of the skeleton. It is located at the medial side of the leg.

tonsils Large collections of lymphatic tissue beneath the mucous membrane of the oral cavity and pharynx.

trachea A cylindrical tube in the neck composed of cartilage and membrane. It conveys air to the lungs.

tricuspid valve The valve located between the right atrium and the right ventricle.

tunic One of the enveloping layers of a part; one of the coats of a blood vessel; one of the coats of the eye; one of the coats of the digestive tract.

tympanic membrane The cellular membrane that separates the external ear from the middle ear; also known as the eardrum.

ulna One of the bones of the forearm.

ureters A pair of tubes that carry the urine from the kidneys into the bladder.

urethra A small tubular structure that drains urine from the bladder. In men, it also serves as a passageway for semen during ejaculation.

urinary bladder The muscular, membranous sac in the pelvis that stores urine for discharge through the urethra.

uterine tubes A pair of ducts that open at one end into the uterus and at the other end into the peritoneal cavity, over the ovary; also known as the fallopian tubes.

uterus The hollow, pear-shaped internal female organ of reproduction.

uvula The cone-shaped process hanging down from the soft palate that helps prevent food and liquid from entering the nasal cavities.

vagina The part of the female genitalia that forms a canal from the orifice through the vestibule to the uterine cervix.

vascular tunic The choroid, ciliary body, and iris.

ventral root The nerve that conveys efferent nerve processes away from the spinal cord.

ventricles Small cavities; in the human systems context, this term usually refers to the right and left ventricles of the heart.

viruses Minute, parasitic microorganisms without independent metabolic activity that can replicate only within a cell of a living plant or animal host.

visceral peritoneum The serous membrane that covers the abdominal organs.

visceral reflexes Reflexes mediated by autonomic nerves and initiated in the viscera.

vitreous humor The transparent, jellylike material that fills the space between the lens and the retina of the eye.

vocal cords The two folds of elastic ligaments covered by mucous membrane that stretch from the thyroid cartilage to the arytenoid cartilage. Vibration of the vocal cords is responsible for voice production; also known as the true vocal cords.

vulva The external genitalia of the female.

xiphoid process The smallest of three parts of the sternum. It articulates caudally with the body of the sternum and laterally with the seventh rib.

yellow marrow Specialized soft tissue (mainly adipose) found in the compact bone of most adult epiphyses.

Human anatomy is the study of how the human body is organized. The paramedic must know anatomy to assess a patient by body region. This knowledge also helps the paramedic communicate well with other members of the health care team.

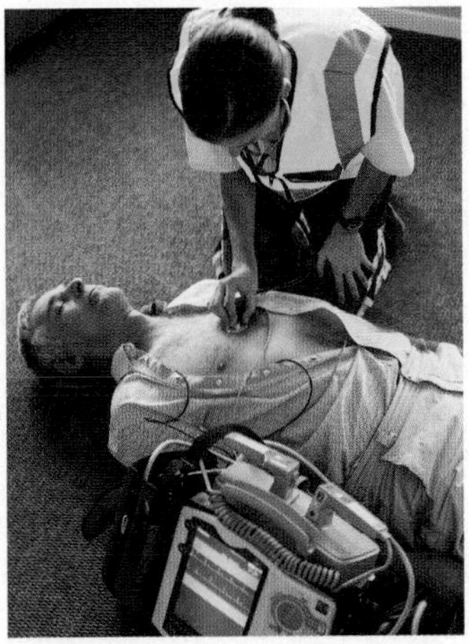

Anatomy Overview

Understanding the relationship between human anatomy and normal body function is the center of all patient care. As professionals, paramedics must have knowledge of anatomy to educate their patients, to advocate for their patients' health, and to ensure the most appropriate care is provided.

Terminology

To ensure that all health care providers have a common understanding of terminology, directional terms used by medical professionals refer to the human body in the **anatomic position**. This position describes a person standing erect with the feet and palms facing the examiner. A patient in the **supine** position is lying on the back (faceup). A patient in the **prone** position is lying on the stomach (facedown). A patient in the **lateral recumbent** position is lying on the right or left side. Regardless of the patient's specific position, the paramedic should always report patient information with reference to the anatomic position[1] (**FIGURE 10-1**).

> SHOW ME THE EVIDENCE
>
> In 2012, Lim and colleagues piloted a 3-hour human cadaver training workshop for second-year undergraduate paramedic students. The workshop aimed to provide the students with an opportunity to refine a range of procedural skills and to experience first-hand the differences in human anatomy compared to manikin-based simulation alone. A total of 114 students attended the workshop, and 96 evaluations were included in the analysis, representing a return rate of 84%. The researchers found statistically significant improvement in anatomic knowledge and improved confidence in performing procedural skills after the workshop. The researchers concluded that cadaver training provides an effective adjunct to simulated learning and clinical placements.
>
> *Modified from:* Lim D, Bartlett S, Horrocks P, Grant-Wakefield C, Kelly J, Tippett V. Enhancing paramedics procedural skills using a cadaveric model. *BMC Med Educ.* 2014;14:138.

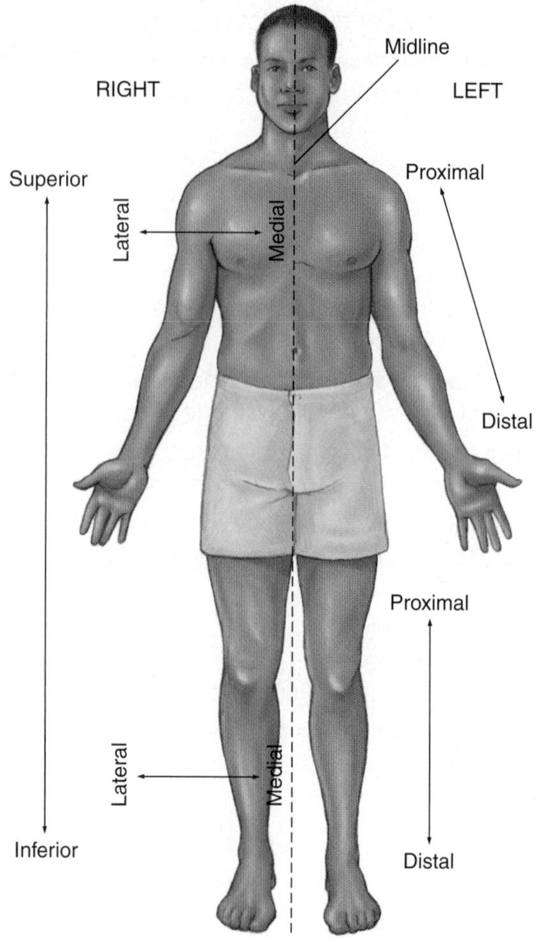

FIGURE 10-1 Anatomic position. A person in the anatomic position stands with the feet and the palms of the hands facing forward, with the thumbs to the outside.

Directional terms, such as *up* or *down, front* or *back*, and *right* or *left*, also are expressed in anatomic terminology (**TABLE 10-1**). These terms always refer to the patient, not the examiner (eg, the patient's left arm).

Anatomic Planes

The relationships of internal body structures are organized into anatomic planes. These planes may be viewed as imaginary straight-line divisions of the human body (**FIGURE 10-2**). The sagittal plane runs vertically through the middle of the body, creating right and left sections. A plane that is to one side of the midline is said to be parasagittal. The transverse (or horizontal) plane divides the body into top and bottom sections, known as **superior** and **inferior** sections. The frontal (or coronal) plane divides the body into front and back sections, known as **anterior** and **posterior** sections.

Body Regions

The human body is divided into a number of regions,[2] a division that helps to organize anatomic structures. The **appendicular region** consists of the limbs, or extremities. The **axial region** includes the head, neck, thorax, and abdomen. The abdomen usually is divided into four quadrants: right upper, right lower, left upper, and left lower (**FIGURE 10-3**). The dividing lines between the abdominal quadrants consist of two imaginary divisions, which run horizontally through the umbilicus and vertically from the **xiphoid process** through the **symphysis pubis**.

Body Cavities

The three major cavities of the human body are the thoracic cavity, the abdominal cavity, and the pelvic

TABLE 10-1 Directional Terms

Term	Definition
Left	Toward the left side
Right	Toward the right side
Superior	Situated above another structure (usually synonymous with "cephalic")
Inferior	Situated below another structure (usually synonymous with "caudal")
Cephalic	Toward the head of the body
Caudal	Toward the distal end of the spine
Proximal	Closer than another structure to the point of attachment to the trunk
Distal	Farther than another structure from the point of attachment to the trunk
Medial	Toward the midline of the body
Lateral	Away from the midline of the body
Anterior	The front of the body (synonymous with "ventral")
Posterior	The back of the body (synonymous with "dorsal")
Ventral	Pertaining to the front
Dorsal	Pertaining to the back

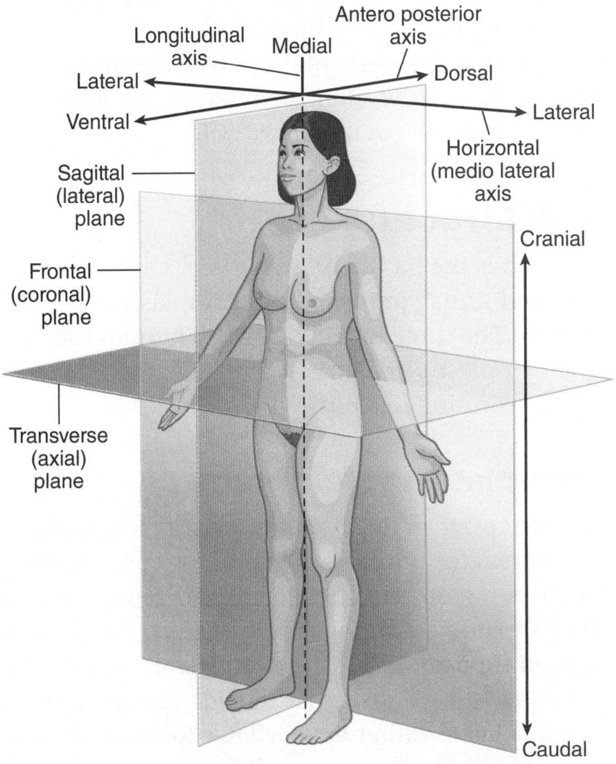

FIGURE 10-2 Body planes.

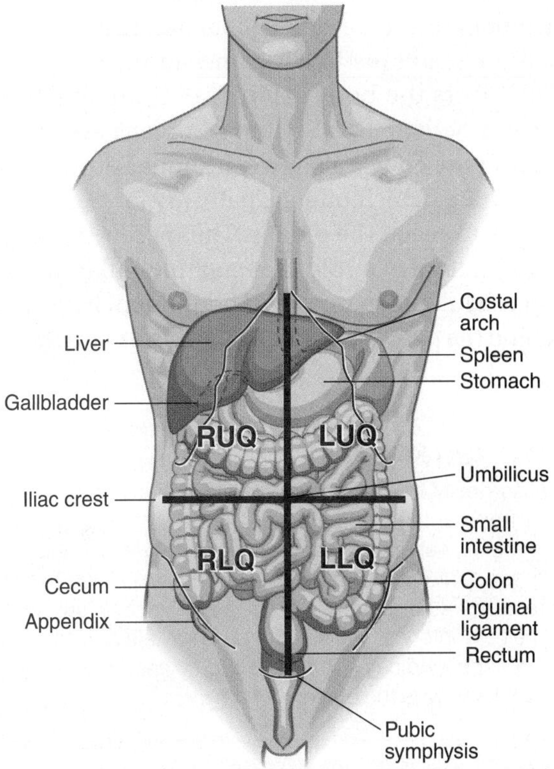

FIGURE 10-3 Abdominal quadrants.

cavity (**FIGURE 10-4**). The thoracic cavity is divided into two portions by a midline structure known as the **mediastinum**. The mediastinum includes the trachea, esophagus, thymus, heart, and great vessels. The lungs are located on either side of this midline structure. The thoracic cavity is surrounded by the rib cage and separated from the abdominal cavity by the diaphragm.

The thorax contains two pleural cavities (which contain the lungs) and a pericardial cavity (which contains the heart). Each of these cavities is lined with a serous membrane. The visceral serous membrane comes in contact with the organ, whereas the parietal serous membrane comes in contact with the cavity wall. These membranes produce a thin, lubricating film of fluid; this fluid reduces the friction that occurs during movement of organs against other organs or body cavities.

An imaginary plane divides the abdominal cavity from the pelvic cavity. In this plane, the division is drawn between the symphysis pubis and the sacral promontory—that is, the projecting portion of the pelvis at the base of the sacrum. The abdominal and pelvic cavities are lined with a thin sheet of membranous tissue that secretes serous fluid. The serous membrane that covers the abdominal organs is known as the **visceral peritoneum**; the serous membrane that covers the body cavity wall is known as the **parietal peritoneum**. Peritoneal organs are held in place at the body wall by a continuous organ called **mesentery**, which offers a pathway for nerves and vessels to reach the organs. The mesentery is also thought to play a role in regulating inflammation and coagulation pathways. Abdominopelvic organs behind the peritoneum are said to be **retroperitoneal**, meaning behind the peritoneum. These organs include the kidneys, adrenal glands, pancreas, portions of the colon, and the urinary bladder. The pelvic cavity is enclosed by the bones of the pelvis. The abdominal and pelvic cavities often are referred to collectively as the *peritoneal* or *abdominopelvic cavity.*

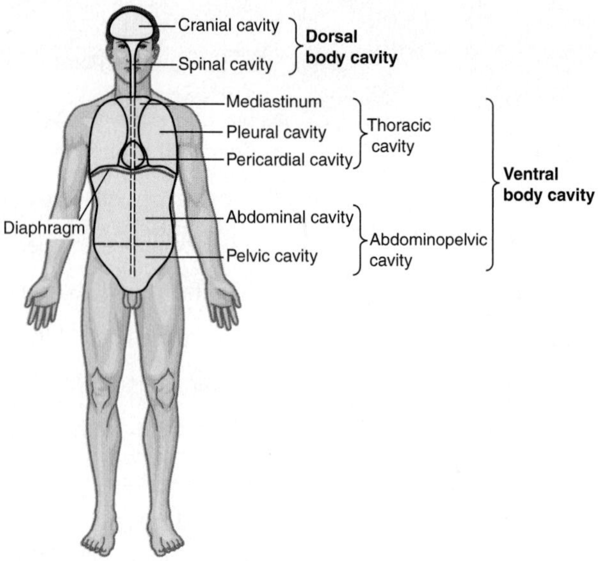

FIGURE 10-4 Body cavities. The thoracic cavity includes the two pleural cavities and the pericardial cavity. The abdominopelvic cavity contains the abdominal cavity and the pelvic cavity.

DID YOU KNOW

Historically, the mesentery was thought to be made up of fragmented, separate structures. Recent research, however, has shown that it is actually one continuous organ that reaches from the duodenum down to the rectum. Although its function is still unclear, studying the mesentery as a distinct organ may aid researchers in understanding dysfunction and diseases caused by problems with the mesentery.

Modified from: Coffey JC, O'Leary DP. The mesentery: structure, function, and role in disease. *Lancet Gastroenterol Hepatol.* 2016;1(3):238-247.

Cell Structure

The **cell** is the basic unit of life. Cells are highly organized units composed of protoplasm, or living matter. The three main parts of all human cells are the cytoplasmic membrane (**plasma membrane**), cytoplasm, and nucleus.

Cytoplasmic Membrane

The **cytoplasmic membrane** encloses the **cytoplasm** and forms the outer boundary of the cell. The cytoplasmic membrane has two layers of **phospholipids** (phosphate-containing fat molecules), which form a fluid framework for the cytoplasmic membrane (**FIGURE 10-5**). Substances outside this membrane are labeled as either **extracellular** (outside of cells) or **intercellular** (between cells); substances inside the cytoplasmic membrane are termed **intracellular**. The functions of the cytoplasmic membrane are to

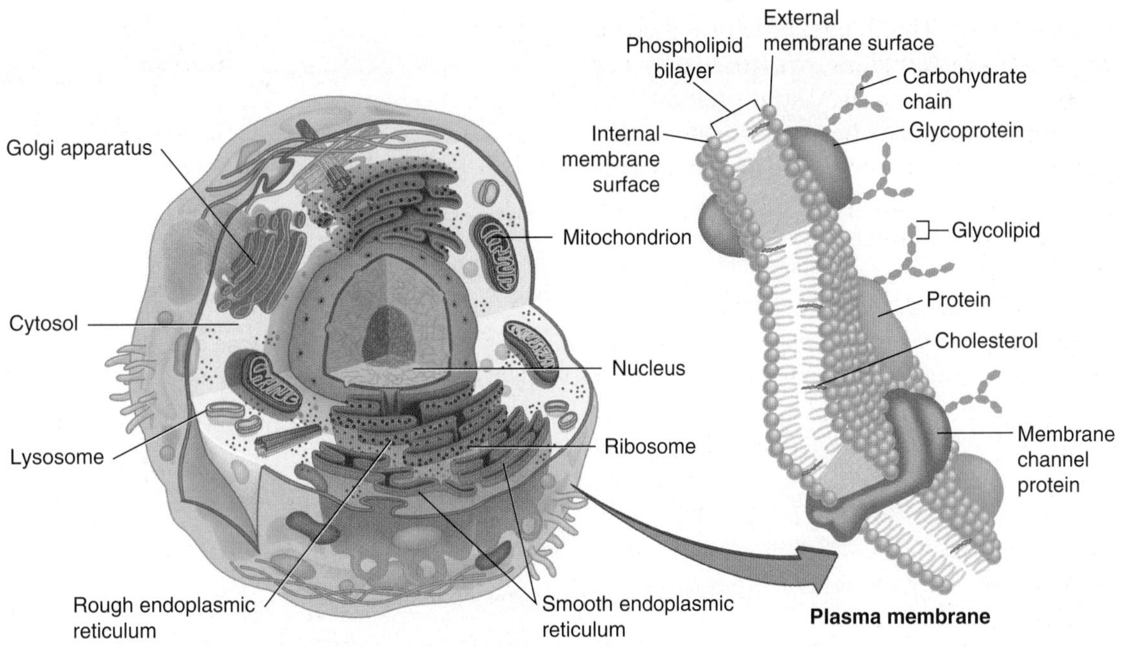

FIGURE 10-5 Fluid mosaic model of the plasma membrane.

enclose and support the cell contents and regulate what moves into and out of the cell.

The central layer of the cytoplasmic membrane is a **lipid bilayer**—in other words, a layer composed of a double layer of lipid molecules. The lipid bilayer has a liquid quality, such that protein molecules "float" on the inner and outer surfaces. Some of these proteins have carbohydrate molecules bound to them. The protein molecules are thought to function as membrane channels, carrier molecules, receptor molecules, **enzymes**, or structural supports in the membrane (see Chapter 11, *General Principles of Pathophysiology*).

Cytoplasm

The cytoplasm lies between the cytoplasmic membrane and the nucleus. The nucleus is visible as a round or spherical structure in the center of the cell. Specialized structures in the cytoplasm, known as **organelles**, perform functions important to the cell's survival (**TABLE 10-2** and **FIGURE 10-6**).

The **endoplasmic reticulum** is a chain of connecting sacs or canals that winds through the cytoplasm of the cell. In essence, the endoplasmic reticulum serves as a tiny circulatory system for the cell. The tubular passages or canals in the endoplasmic reticulum carry proteins and other substances through the cytoplasm of the cell from one area to another. The two types of endoplasmic reticulum are smooth endoplasmic reticulum and rough endoplasmic reticulum. Smooth endoplasmic reticulum is found in cells that handle or produce fatty substances, and it also plays a part in detoxification processes through the chemical action of enzymes. Rough endoplasmic reticulum is found in cells that produce proteins to be secreted for use outside the cell.

Ribosomes are the "factories" in the cells where protein is synthesized. These macromolecules consist of protein and **ribonucleic acid (RNA)** and are composed of thousands of atoms. Ribosomes usually are bound to the endoplasmic reticulum but also are found free in cytoplasm. They form complexes with strands of RNA, which provides the blueprint for the new protein through its contents, the body's genetic code. To form the new proteins, individual **amino acids** are attached in long chains via peptide bonds.

The **Golgi apparatus** concentrates and packages materials (including proteins) for secretion from the cell. This organelle consists of tiny sacs composed of smooth endoplasmic reticulum, which are stacked one on top of the other near the nucleus. The Golgi apparatus sometimes chemically modifies proteins by synthesizing and attaching carbohydrate molecules to the proteins to form **glycoproteins** or by attaching lipids to the proteins to form **lipoproteins**.

TABLE 10-2 Major Cell Structures and Their Functions

Structure	Function
Centrioles	Play a role in cell reproduction.
Cilia	Short, hairlike extensions on the free surfaces of some cells capable of movement.
Endoplasmic reticulum	Ribosomes attached to rough endoplasmic reticulum synthesize proteins; smooth endoplasmic reticulum synthesizes lipids and certain carbohydrates.
Flagella	Single projections of cell surfaces that are much larger than cilia; the only example in human beings is the "tail" of a sperm cell.
Golgi apparatus	Synthesizes carbohydrates, combines them with proteins, and packages the product as globules of glycoproteins.
Lysosomes	The "digestive system" of the cell.
Mitochondria	Synthesize adenosine triphosphate; the "powerhouses" of the cell.
Nucleoli	Play an essential role in the formation of ribosomes.
Nucleus	Dictates protein synthesis, thereby playing an essential role in other cell activities—namely, active transport, metabolism, growth, and heredity.
Plasma membrane	Serves as the boundary of the cell. Protein and carbohydrate molecules on the outer surface of the plasma membrane perform various functions; for example, they serve as markers that identify the cells of each individual or as receptor molecules for certain hormones.
Ribosomes	Synthesize proteins; the "protein factories" of the cell.

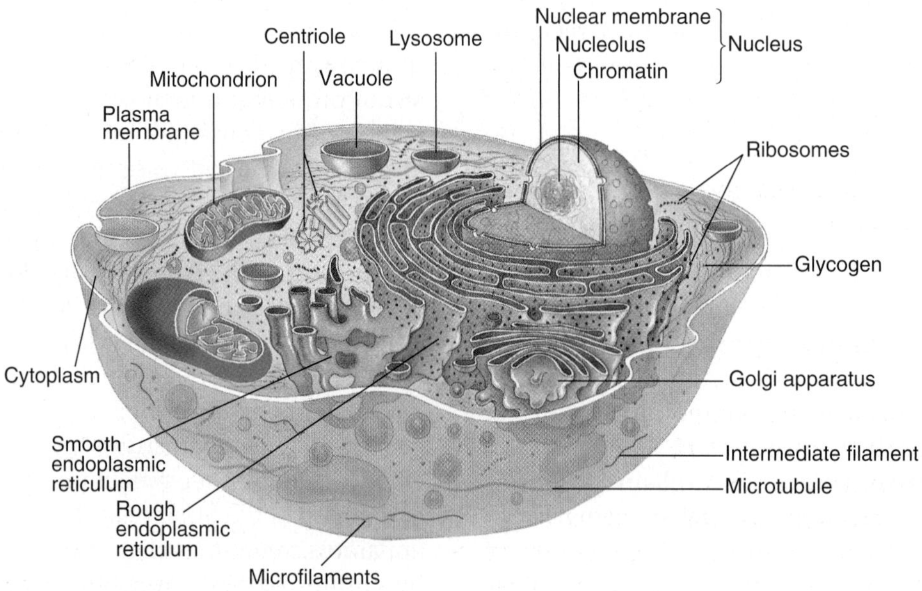

FIGURE 10-6 Structure of a cell.

These concentrated globules move slowly outward to and through the cell membrane. At this point, the globules break open and spill their contents. **Mucus** is an example of a product of the Golgi apparatus.

Lysosomes are membranous-walled organelles that contain enzymes, which enable them to function as intracellular digestive systems. For example, some enzymes digest nucleic acids, proteins, **polysaccharides**, and lipids. Certain white blood cells (leukocytes) have large numbers of lysosomes that contain enzymes to digest engulfed bacteria. If tissues are damaged, these powerful enzymes may escape from ruptured lysosome sacs into the cytoplasm, where they digest both damaged and healthy cells. Lysosomes also digest organelles of cells that are no longer functional, a process called **autophagia**.

The **mitochondria** are the "power plants" of the cell. These organelles, which are found throughout the cell, serve as the site of **aerobic oxidation**. In the mitochondria, energy derived from the efficient **metabolism** of nutrients and oxygen via the **Krebs cycle** (further described in Chapter 11, *General Principles of Pathophysiology*) is used to synthesize high-energy triphosphate bonds, such as **adenosine triphosphate (ATP)**. These triphosphate bonds are the energy source for the muscles, nerves, and overall function of the body.

CRITICAL THINKING

A patient has severe lung disease and poor oxygenation. What effect will this have on cellular energy production?

Centrioles are paired, rod-shaped organelles that lie at right angles to each other in a specialized zone of the cytoplasm known as the **centrosome**. Each centriole is composed of microtubules, which play an important role in the process of cell division.

Nucleus

At some point in their existence, all human cells contain a **nucleus**, in which the genetic material of the cell is located. The nucleus is a large, membrane-bound organelle that ultimately controls all other organelles in the cytoplasm. The nucleus may be spherical, elongated, or lobed, depending on the type of cell in which it is found. The nucleus usually is located near the center of the cell; however, some cells, such as red blood cells (erythrocytes), lose their nucleus as they develop. Other cells, such as certain bone cells, have more than one nucleus. The most significant feature for categorizing cells is the presence or absence of a nucleus.

The cell nucleus is surrounded by a nuclear membrane, which encloses the **nucleoplasm**. The nucleoplasm contains a number of specialized structures, including the nucleolus and the chromatin granules. The nucleolus consists of **deoxyribonucleic acid (DNA)**, which contains the genetic blueprint for the body's RNA, and protein, which makes ribosomes. These ribosomes ultimately migrate through the nuclear membrane into the cytoplasm of the cell and produce proteins. **Chromatin granules** are threadlike structures

DID YOU KNOW?

Human Genome Project

October 1, 2015, marked the 25th anniversary of the launch of the Human Genome Project (HGP), which was completed in 2003. The HGP has led to the discovery of more than 1,800 disease-related genes and more than 2,000 genetic tests for human conditions. The original goals of the project were the following:

- Identify all of the approximately 20,000 to 25,000 genes found in human DNA.
- Determine the sequences of the three billion chemical base pairs that make up human DNA.
- Store this information in databases.
- Improve tools for data analysis.
- Transfer related technologies to the private sector.
- Address the ethical, legal, and social issues (ELSI) that might arise from the project.

A genome is all the DNA in an organism, including its genes. Genes carry information for making all the proteins required by all organisms. These proteins determine, among other things, how the organism looks, how well its body metabolizes food or fights infection, and sometimes even how it behaves.

Knowledge of the effects of DNA variations among people may lead to revolutionary new ways to diagnose, treat, and perhaps prevent some of the thousands of disorders that affect human beings. Besides providing clues to understanding human biology, learning about nonhuman DNA sequences or organisms can lead to an understanding of their natural capabilities. This knowledge can then be applied to solving challenges in health care, agriculture, energy production, environmental remediation, and carbon sequestration.

Modified from: Human Genome Project. US Department of Health and Human Services, National Institutes of Health, website. https://report.nih.gov/NIHfactsheets/ViewFactSheet.aspx?csid=45&key=H#H. Updated March 29, 2013. Accessed December 26, 2017.

made up of proteins and DNA. During cell division, the chromatin condenses to form the 23 pairs of **chromosomes** characteristic of human cells. The information in nuclear DNA determines most of the chemical events that occur within the cell.

The basic functions of the nucleus are cell division and control of genetic information. Not all cells are capable of continuous division, and some cells (eg, nerve cells) cannot reproduce.

Major Classes of Cells

Free-living cells of multicellular "social" organisms are divided into two major classes based on the organization of their genetic material. The two main types of cells are **eukaryotes** ("true nucleus") and **prokaryotes** ("before nucleus").

Eukaryotes are larger than prokaryotes, have a more extensive intracellular anatomy, and have a separate membrane-bound nucleus that holds the genetic material (chromosomes, DNA). The fluid filling eukaryotic cells is divided into the nucleoplasm (inside the nuclear membrane) and the cytoplasm (outside the nuclear membrane). Nearly all human body cells are eukaryotes, as are those of most living organisms. Exceptions are **bacteria**, cyanobacteria (blue-green algae), and **mycoplasmas**, which are prokaryotes; bacteria and mycoplasmas cause many diseases in human beings and other animals. **Viruses** have a close association with cells but are not classified as cells.

In prokaryotic cells, the genetic material and enzymes required for energy production, cell growth, and cell division are contained in the jellylike cytoplasm, which in turn is surrounded by the plasma membrane. Unlike eukaryotes, these cells have a simple internal organization. Prokaryotes do not have a nucleus that is bound by a plasma membrane, and their DNA is attached to the plasma membrane.

Chief Cellular Functions

Cells have evolved in myriad ways to fulfill specific tasks in the human body. Through **differentiation** (maturation), cells become specialized in one type of function or act in concert with other cells to perform a more complex task. (Stem cells—a class of undifferentiated cells that are able to differentiate into any kind of specialized cell types—are discussed in **BOX 10-1**.) For example, red blood cells carry out only one function: They transport respiratory gases around the body. In contrast, the cells in the pancreas synthesize and secrete large amounts of the digestive enzymes required to break down foods. The seven chief cellular functions are as follows:

1. Movement (muscle cells)
2. Conductivity (nerve cells)
3. Metabolic absorption (kidney and intestinal cells)
4. Secretion (mucous gland cells)
5. Excretion (all cells)
6. Respiration (all cells)
7. Reproduction (most cells)

Cell Reproduction

All human cells, with the exception of reproductive (sex) cells, reproduce by **mitosis**. In this process, cells divide to multiply; one cell divides to form two cells. Many cell types in the body (eg, epithelial, liver, and

BOX 10-1 Stem Cells: A Brief Overview

Stem cells come from two main sources: embryonic stem cells and adult stem cells. Research involving the use of embryonic stem cells is controversial, as it involves the destruction of human embryos. Less controversial sources of acquiring stem cells include using cells from adults, amniotic fluid and membrane, the umbilical cord, breast milk, and bone marrow. These methods do not raise the same kinds of legal, religious, moral, and ethical concerns that arise with embryonic stem cell research—but stem cells from those sources also do not have the same potential as embryonic stem cells to develop into specialized cell types.

At present, the most widely used stem cell–based therapy is bone marrow transplantation, which is used to treat blood cancers such as leukemia and lymphoma.

Modified from: Stem cells: what they are and what they do. Mayo Clinic website. http://www.mayoclinic.org/tests-procedures/stem-cell-transplant/in-depth/stem-cells/ART-20048117. Published March 23, 2013. Accessed December 26, 2017;
Stem cell information: stem cell basics. US Department of Health and Human Services, National Institutes of Health website. https://stemcells.nih.gov/info/basics.htm. Accessed June 27, 2017.

bone marrow cells) undergo cell division throughout a person's life. Other cell types (eg, nerve and skeletal muscle cells) divide until near the time of birth, but no longer divide in the extrauterine human.

Body Tissues

The characteristics of cell structure and composition are used to classify tissue types. Four main types of tissue make up the many organs of the body: epithelial tissue, connective tissue, muscle tissue, and nervous tissue.

> CRITICAL THINKING
> Think about the role of each of the tissue types. Compare these roles with the types of materials used to construct a building. How does each tissue type serve as a component for building a body?

Epithelial Tissue

Epithelial tissue covers surfaces or forms structures derived from body surfaces (eg, glands). This tissue consists almost entirely of cells that have little or no intercellular material between them. It forms continuous sheets that contain no blood vessels. Epithelium covers the outside of the body and also lines the digestive tract, the blood vessels, and many body cavities.

Epithelial tissues can be subdivided by the shape and arrangement of the cells found in each type. When classified according to shape, epithelial cells are described as squamous (flat and scalelike), cuboidal (cube-shaped), or columnar (taller than they are wide). When classified according to arrangement, epithelial cells are described as simple (a single layer of cells of the same shape), stratified (multiple layers of cells of the same shape), or transitional (several layers of cells of differing shapes).

Connective Tissue

Connective tissue is the most abundant and widely distributed type of tissue in the body. It consists of cells separated from each other by intercellular material, known as the **extracellular matrix**. This nonliving matrix gives most connective tissue its fundamental characteristics and is the basis for separating connective tissue into seven subgroups.

Areolar Connective Tissue

Areolar connective tissue is a loose tissue that consists of delicate webs of fibers and a variety of cells embedded in a matrix of soft, sticky gel. It serves as the "loose packing" material of most organs and other tissues, and attaches the skin to the underlying tissues. The areolar connective tissue contains three major types of protein fibers: collagen, reticulum, and elastin.

Adipose Tissue

Adipose tissue (fat tissue) is a specialized connective tissue that stores lipids. Because lipids take up less space per calorie than carbohydrates or proteins, adipose tissue acts not only as an insulator and protector, but also as a site of energy storage.

Fibrous Connective Tissue

Fibrous connective tissue is made up mainly of bundles of strong, white collagenous fibers in parallel rows; tendons are an example. Fibrous connective tissue is characterized by its high strength and inelasticity.

Cartilage

Cartilage is made up of cartilage cells (chondrocytes). These cells are located in tiny spaces and are distributed throughout a somewhat rigid matrix. The makeup of cartilage varies by its location and ultimate role. For example, hyaline cartilage is found at articulating surfaces and is firm and smooth. Fibrocartilage is more flexible and supple. Cartilage makes up part of the human skeleton and covers the articulating surfaces of bones. In addition, it forms the major skeletal tissue of the embryo before it is replaced by bony tissue.

The type of cartilage depends on the relative amounts of collagen, elastin, and ground substance. Ground substance is composed of nonfibrous protein and other organic molecules and fluid. Increased amounts of collagen or elastin allow cartilage to spring back after being compressed. Because blood vessels do not penetrate the substance of cartilage, cartilage heals slowly after injury.

Bone

Bone is a highly specialized form of hard, connective tissue that consists of living cells and a mineralized

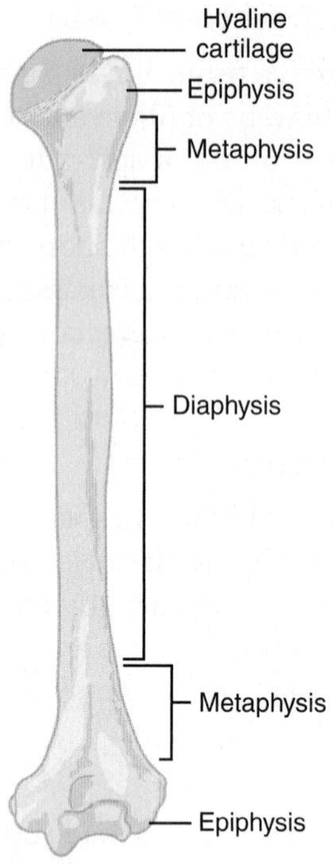

FIGURE 10-7 Long bone.

matrix. The strength and rigidity of this matrix allow bone to support and protect other tissues and organs.

Bones are classified according to their shape. **Long bones** are longer than they are wide (**FIGURE 10-7**). The humerus, ulna, radius, femur, tibia, fibula, and phalanges are examples. **Short bones** are about as broad as they are long. Examples include the carpal bones of the wrist and the tarsal bones of the ankle. **Flat bones** have a thin, flattened shape; examples include certain skull bones, the ribs, the sternum, and scapulae. **Irregular bones** do not fit any of the other three categories; they include the vertebrae and facial bones.

Each growing long bone consists of a **diaphysis** (shaft), an *epiphysis* at the end of each bone, and an **epiphyseal plate** (growth plate). The epiphyseal plate is the site of bone elongation. When bone growth stops, this plate becomes ossified, at which point it is called the epiphyseal line. An injury to this area can impair bone growth if it is not recognized and treated properly (see Chapter 43, *Orthopaedic Trauma*).

Bones contain both large and small cavities. An example of a large cavity is the medullary cavity in the diaphysis. Smaller cavities include the epiphyses of long bones and cavities found throughout the interior of other bones. These spaces are filled with **yellow marrow** (mainly adipose tissue) or **red marrow** (the site of blood cell formation). Blood supply to most bones is excellent. Therefore, some bones, such as the tibia and sternum, are suitable choices for venous access by means of intraosseous infusion (described in Chapter 14, *Medication Administration*). This rich blood supply also means that bone can repair itself much more readily than cartilage can.

Bones can also be classified as cancellous or spongy bone and compact bone. **Cancellous bone** has spaces between the plates of the bone and resembles a sponge. **Compact bone** is essentially solid.

> CRITICAL THINKING
>
> Intraosseous infusion is a critical intervention that can save a life when it is used to administer fluids and drugs. This infusion requires the insertion of a needle into the marrow of long bones. Why could failure to identify anatomic landmarks or to place the needle correctly in a child's epiphysis be harmful?

Blood

Blood is a unique connective tissue in that the matrix between the cells is liquid. The liquid matrix of blood allows it to flow rapidly through the body. Blood carries nutrients, oxygen, waste products, and other materials.

Hematopoietic Tissue

Hematopoietic tissue is the connective tissue in the marrow cavities of bones. This tissue is also found in organs such as the spleen, tonsils, and lymph nodes. It is responsible for the formation of blood cells and cells of the lymphatic system that are important in the defense against disease.

Muscle Tissue

Muscle tissue is a contractile tissue and is the force behind all body movement. It is highly specialized to contract or shorten forcefully. Muscle tissue is classified as skeletal, cardiac, and smooth (visceral) muscle, according to the anatomic location and function. When classified by appearance, muscle is striated or nonstriated. When classified by function, muscle is voluntary (consciously controlled) or involuntary (not normally consciously controlled). The three types of muscles are striated voluntary (skeletal) muscle, striated involuntary (cardiac) muscle, and nonstriated involuntary (smooth) muscle.

Skeletal muscle, which attaches to bones, represents a large portion of the total weight of the human body. Contraction of these muscles is responsible for body movement. **Cardiac muscle**—the muscle of the heart—contracts to pump blood throughout the body. **Smooth muscle** is widespread throughout the body and is responsible for a variety of functions, including movement in the digestive, urinary, and reproductive systems.

Nervous Tissue

Nervous tissue is characterized by its ability to conduct an electrical signal, also known as **action potential**. Nervous tissue consists of two basic kinds of cells: neurons and neuroglia.

Neurons, or nerve cells, are the actual conducting cells of nervous tissue. Each neuron has three major parts: cell body, dendrite, and axon. The cell body contains the nucleus and is the site of general cell functions. Dendrites and axons are nerve cell processes (projections of cytoplasm surrounded by membrane). Dendrites receive electrical impulses and conduct them toward the cell body, whereas axons usually conduct impulses away from the cell body. Neurons have many sizes and shapes, especially in the brain and spinal cord.

Neuroglia are the support cells of the brain, spinal cord, and peripheral nerves. These cells are divided into several subgroups that nourish, protect, and insulate neurons.

Organ Systems

An **organ** is a structure made up of two or more kinds of tissues that are organized to perform a more complex job than any one tissue can perform. A **system** is a group of organs arranged to perform a more complex job than any one organ can perform (**FIGURE 10-8**). The human body has 11 major organ systems:[3]

1. Integumentary system
2. Skeletal system
3. Muscular system
4. Nervous system
5. Endocrine system
6. Circulatory system
7. Lymphatic system
8. Respiratory system
9. Digestive system
10. Urinary system
11. Reproductive system

Integumentary System

The **integumentary system** is the largest organ system of the body. It consists of the skin and accessory structures, such as hair, nails, and a variety of glands. The functions of this system include protecting the body against injury and dehydration. The integumentary system also defends against invading microorganisms and regulates temperature.

> CRITICAL THINKING
>
> Consider your knowledge of the functions of the skin. Which signs, symptoms, or complications would you expect in a patient with burns covering half the body?

Skin

The skin is a sheet-like organ composed of two distinct layers of tissue, the epidermis and the dermis (**FIGURE 10-9**). The **epidermis**, or outermost layer of the skin, consists of tightly packed epithelial cells. Cells of the innermost layer of the epidermis can undergo mitosis and can repair themselves if injured. Because of this characteristic, the body can maintain an effective barrier against infection, even when subjected to injury and normal wear and tear.

The **dermis**, which is the deeper of the two layers of the skin, is largely made up of connective tissue. It is much thicker than the epidermis and contains collagenous and elastic fibers. The dermis also contains a specialized network of nerves and nerve endings, which provide sensory information about pain, pressure, touch, and temperature. At various levels of the dermis are muscle fibers, hair follicles, sweat and sebaceous glands, and many blood vessels.

The layers of the skin are supported by a thick layer of loose connective tissue and fat called **subcutaneous tissue**. Subcutaneous tissue insulates the body from temperature extremes, serves as a source of stored energy, and acts as a shock absorber to protect underlying tissue from injury.

Hair

Hair formation begins when cells of the epidermal layer of the skin grow into the dermis, forming a small

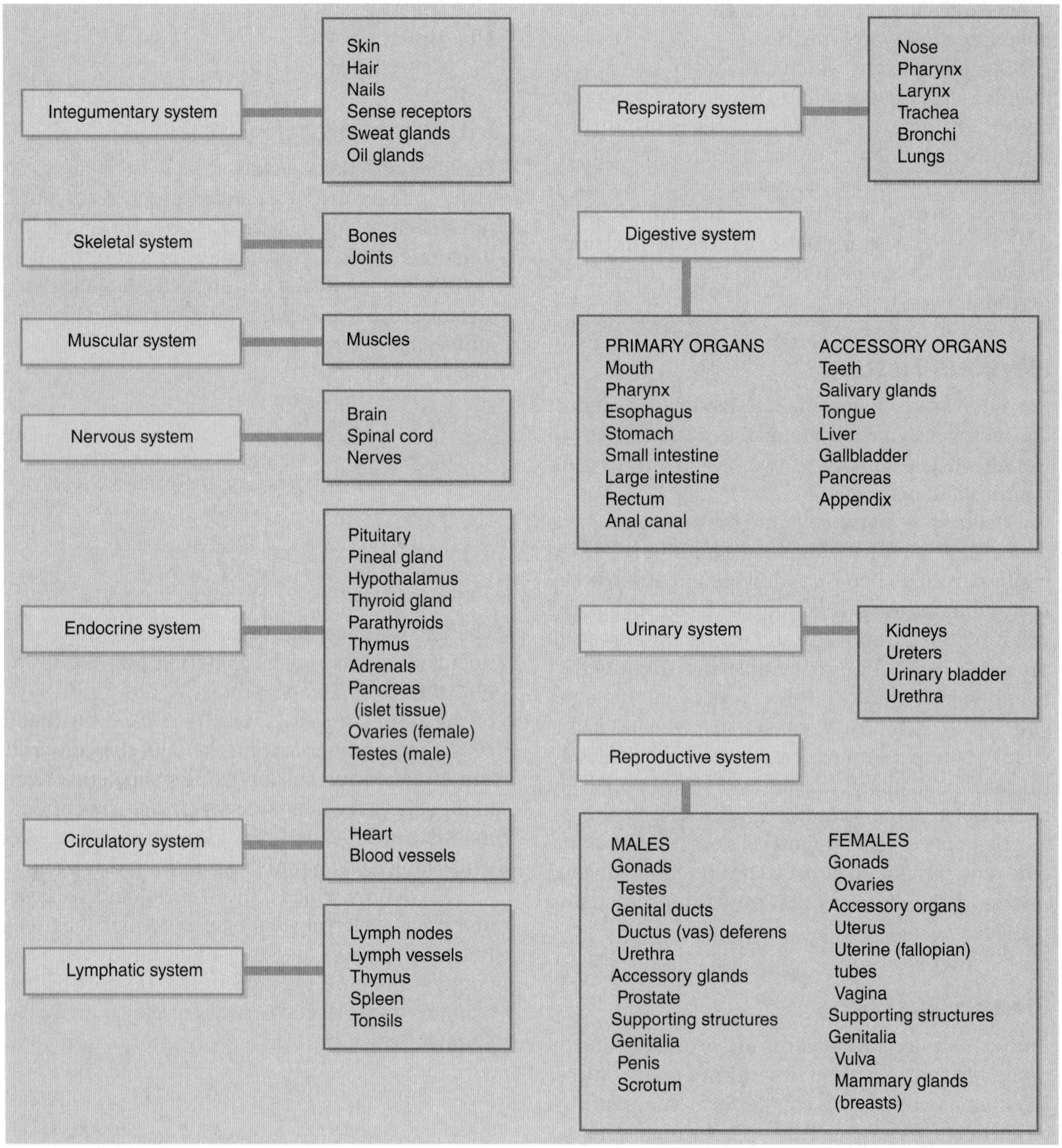

FIGURE 10-8 Body systems and their organs.

tube, the hair follicle. Hair growth begins from a small cluster of cells known as the hair papilla. The part of the hair that lies hidden in the follicle is known as the root, and the visible part is the shaft. The arrector pili are smooth muscles associated with each hair follicle. Movement of the hair follicle by the arrector pili produces pressure on the skin (resulting in "goose bumps") and pulls the hairs upward.

Nails

Nails are produced by cells in the epidermis. The visible part of the nail is the nail body. The root of the nail lies in a groove and is hidden by a fold of skin known as the cuticle. The crescent-shaped white area of the nail, the lunula, is most visible on the thumbnail. This is where the majority of nail

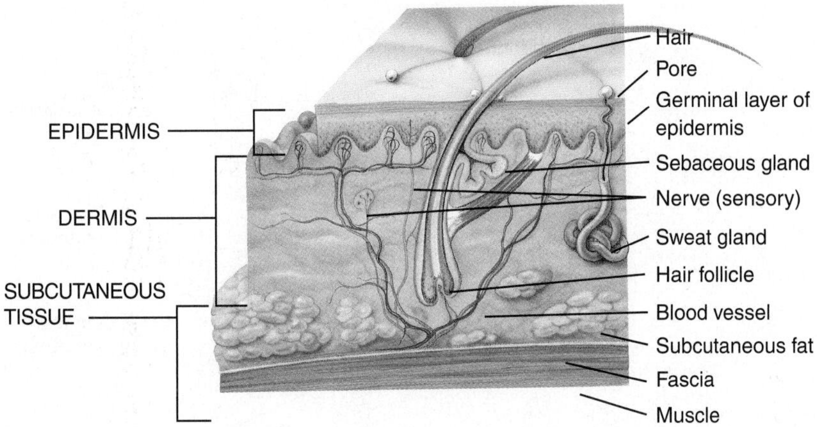

FIGURE 10-9 Microscopic view of the skin.

growth comes from. The nail bed that lies under the nail contains many blood vessels. Thus, in healthy people, this layer of epithelium appears pink through the translucent nail body.

Glands

The major glands of the skin are the sebaceous and sweat glands. Most **sebaceous glands** are found in the dermis and secrete oil (**sebum**) that prevents drying of the hair and skin and protects against some bacteria. Sebum secretion increases during adolescence, stimulated by increased blood levels of the sex hormones. Other skin glands include the ceruminous glands of the external auditory meatus, which produce cerumen (earwax), and the mammary glands.

Sweat glands (sudoriferous glands) are the most numerous skin glands. They usually are classified as merocrine or apocrine, according to their mode of secretion. Merocrine sweat glands (the most common) open directly onto the surface of the skin through sweat pores. The coiled portion of the gland produces sweat—a fluid that is mostly water but also contains some salts (mainly sodium chloride) and small amounts of ammonia, urea, uric acid, and lactic acid. As the body temperature rises, the sweat glands produce sweat; evaporation of the sweat cools the body. Apocrine glands usually open into hair follicles. These glands, which are found in the axillae and genitalia and around the anus, become active at puberty through the influence of sex hormones. Apocrine glands secrete an organic substance that is odorless when released but is quickly metabolized by bacteria to cause body odor.

> CRITICAL THINKING
> The ability to sweat is impaired in the older adult population. What implications for health does this have?

Skeletal System

The skeletal system consists of bones and associated connective tissues, including cartilage, tendons, and ligaments. The skeletal system offers a rigid framework for support and protection of the body, including the internal organs. It also provides a system of levers on which muscles act to produce body movements.

The skeletal system contains 206 bones. Bones are divided into two groups, the axial skeleton and the appendicular skeleton (**FIGURE 10-10**).

Axial Skeleton

The **axial skeleton** is made up of the skull, hyoid bone, vertebral column, and thoracic cage. The skull is composed of 28 bones, which are divided into three groups: the auditory ossicles, the cranial vault, and the facial bones (**FIGURE 10-11**). The six auditory ossicles (three on each side of the head) are located inside the cavity of the temporal bone and play a role in hearing. The **cranial vault** consists of eight bones that surround and protect the brain: the *occiptal* bone, two *temporal* bones, two *parietal* bones, and the *sphenoid, ethmoid,* and *frontal* bones.

The 14 facial bones form the structure of the face in the anterior skull but do not contribute to the cranial vault. They include the *maxilla, mandible,* and *zygomatic, palatine, nasal, lacrimal, vomer,* and

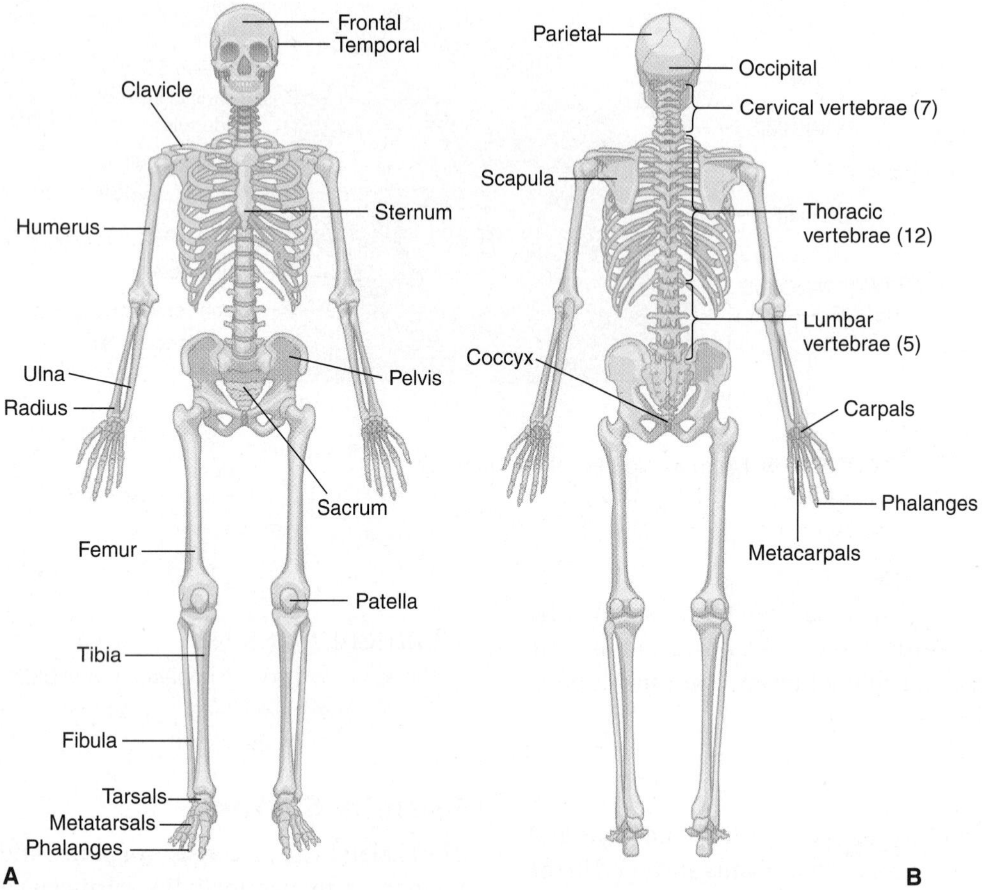

FIGURE 10-10 Anterior view **(A)** and posterior view **(B)** of the skeleton.

inferior nasal concha bones. The frontal and ethmoid bones contribute to the cranial vault and the face.

The **hyoid bone** is attached to the skull by muscles and ligaments and "floats" in the superior aspect of the neck, just below the mandible. This bone serves as the attachment point for several important neck and tongue muscles.

The vertebral column consists of 33 bones, which can be divided into five regions: 7 cervical vertebrae, 12 thoracic vertebrae, 5 lumbar vertebrae, 5 sacral vertebrae (fused), and 4 (the number of bones can range from 3 to 5) coccygeal vertebrae (fused) (**FIGURE 10-12**). The weight-bearing portion of each vertebra is a bony disk called the body. Intervertebral disks are located between the bodies of adjacent vertebrae. These disks serve as shock absorbers for the vertebral column, provide additional support for the body, and prevent the vertebral bodies from rubbing against each other. The spinal cord is protected by the vertebral arch and the dorsal portion of the body. A transverse process extends laterally from each side of the arch, and a single spinous process is present at the point of junction. Much vertebral movement is accomplished by the contraction of skeletal muscles attached to the transverse and spinous processes.

The thoracic cage protects vital organs in the thorax and prevents the thorax from collapsing during respiration. The thoracic cage consists of the thoracic vertebrae, 12 pairs of ribs with their associated **costal cartilages**, and the **sternum** (**FIGURE 10-13**).

The superior seven ribs (the true ribs) articulate with the thoracic vertebrae and attach directly through their costal cartilages to the sternum. The inferior five ribs (the false ribs) articulate with the thoracic vertebrae but do not attach directly to the sternum. The 8th, 9th, and 10th ribs are joined to a common cartilage, which is attached to the sternum. The 11th and 12th ribs are "floating" ribs that have no attachment to the sternum.

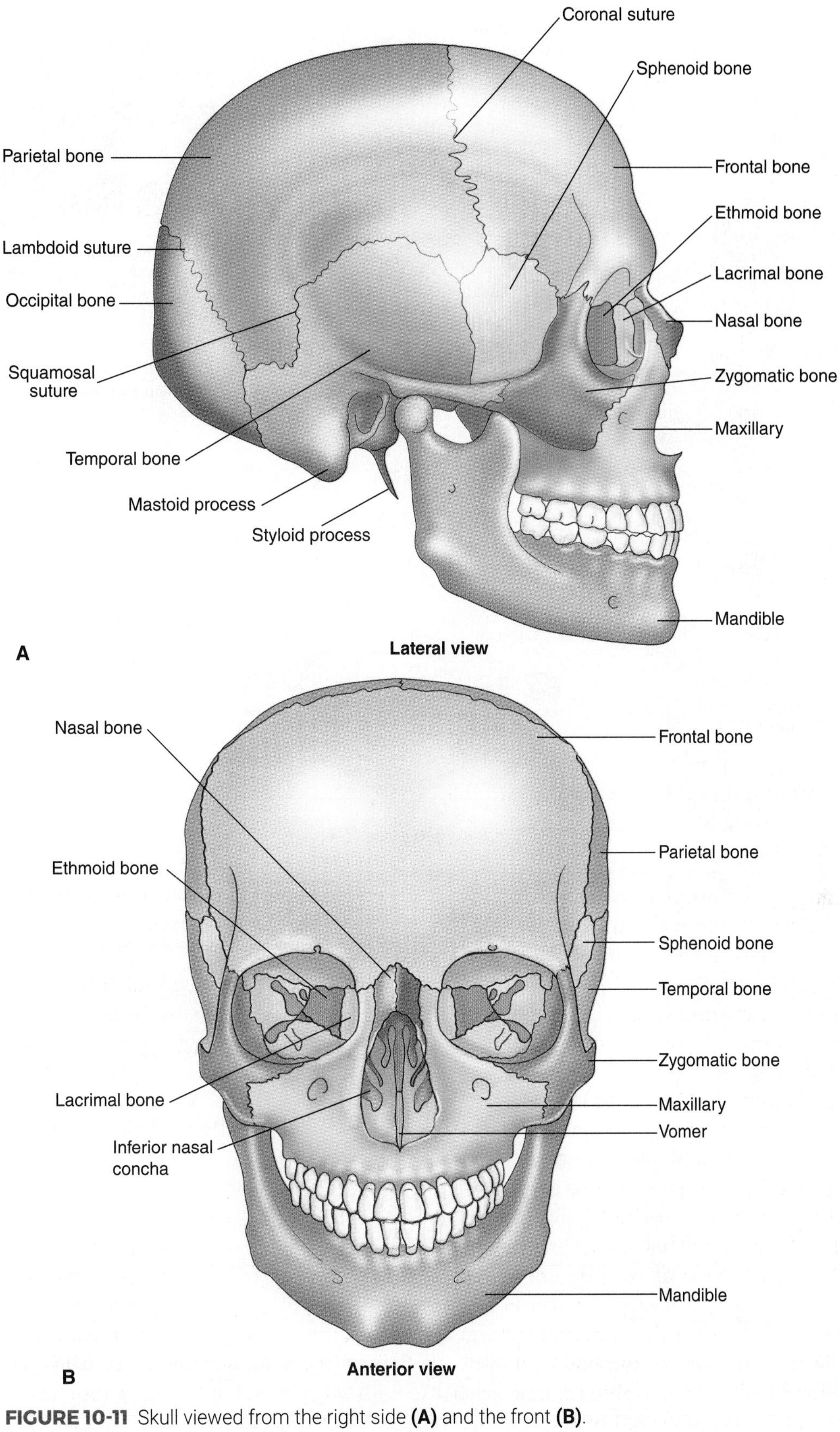

FIGURE 10-11 Skull viewed from the right side **(A)** and the front **(B)**.

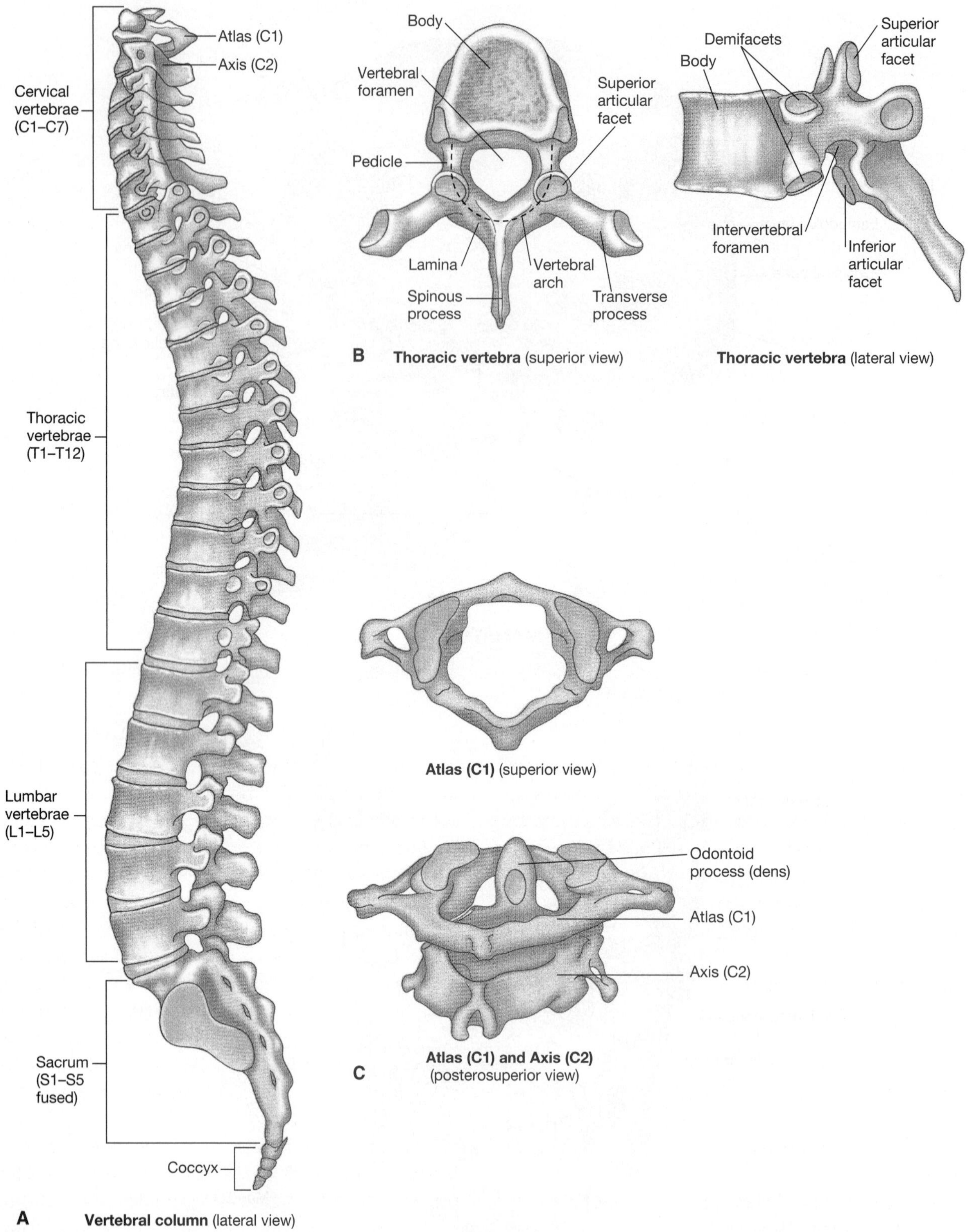

FIGURE 10-12 A. Vertebral column viewed from the left side. **B.** Superior and lateral views of the thoracic vertebra. **C.** Views of the atlas (C1) and axis (C2).

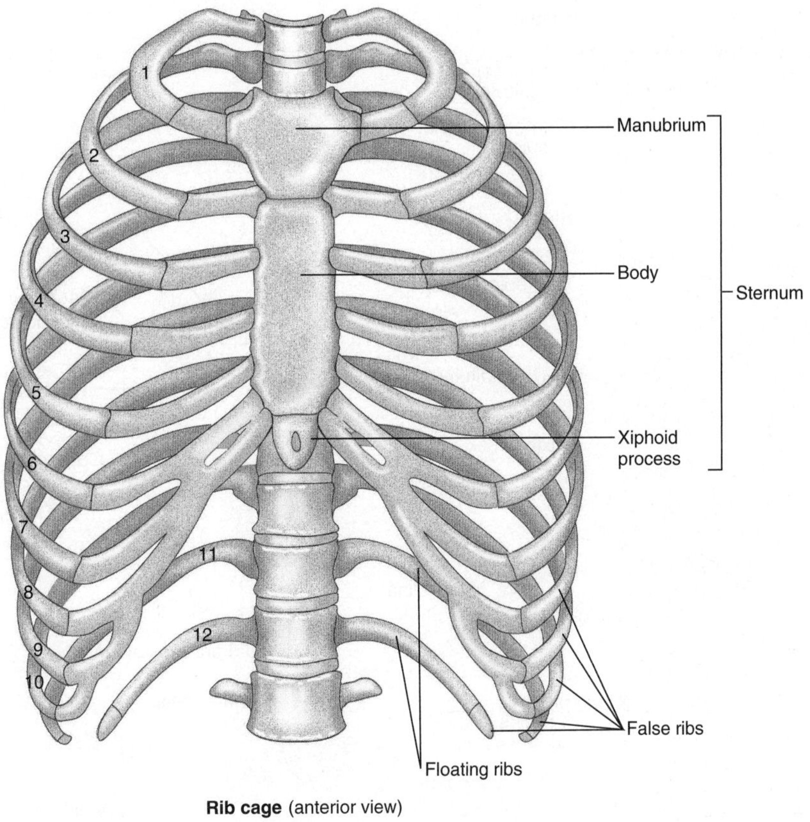

FIGURE 10-13 Thoracic cage. Note the costal cartilages and their articulations with the body of the sternum.

The sternum is divided into three parts: the manubrium, the body, and the xiphoid process. The superior margin of the manubrium, known as the **jugular notch** (also known as the suprasternal notch), can be easily palpated at the anterior base of the neck. The point where the manubrium joins the body of the sternum is the **sternal angle** (also known as the angle of Louis). The second rib is found lateral to the sternal angle and is used clinically as a starting point for counting the other ribs.

Appendicular Skeleton

The **appendicular skeleton** consists of the bones of the upper and lower extremities. It also includes their girdles, by which those extremities are attached to the body.

The scapula and clavicle form the pectoral girdle, which attaches the upper limbs to the axial skeleton. The direct point of attachment between the bones of the appendicular and axial skeletons occurs at the **sternoclavicular joint** between the clavicle and the sternum.

The **humerus** is the second longest bone in the body. The head of the humerus articulates with the scapula. The greater and lesser tubercles are located on the lateral and anterior surfaces of the proximal end of the humerus; they act as sites of muscle attachments. The humerus articulates with the **radius** and **ulna** at its distal end. The capitulum (lateral aspect of the humerus) articulates with the head of the radius; the trochlea (medial aspect of the humerus) articulates with the ulna. Proximal to the trochlea and capitulum are the medial and lateral epicondyles, respectively. These sites act as muscle attachments for the muscles of the forearm. **FIGURE 10-14** illustrates the bones of the upper extremity.

The large bony process of the ulna (the olecranon process) can be felt at the point of the elbow. This process fits into a large depression on the posterior surface of the humerus known as the olecranon fossa. The structural relationship between these two processes makes movement of the joint possible. The distal end of the ulna has a small head that articulates with the radius and wrist bones. The posterior-medial

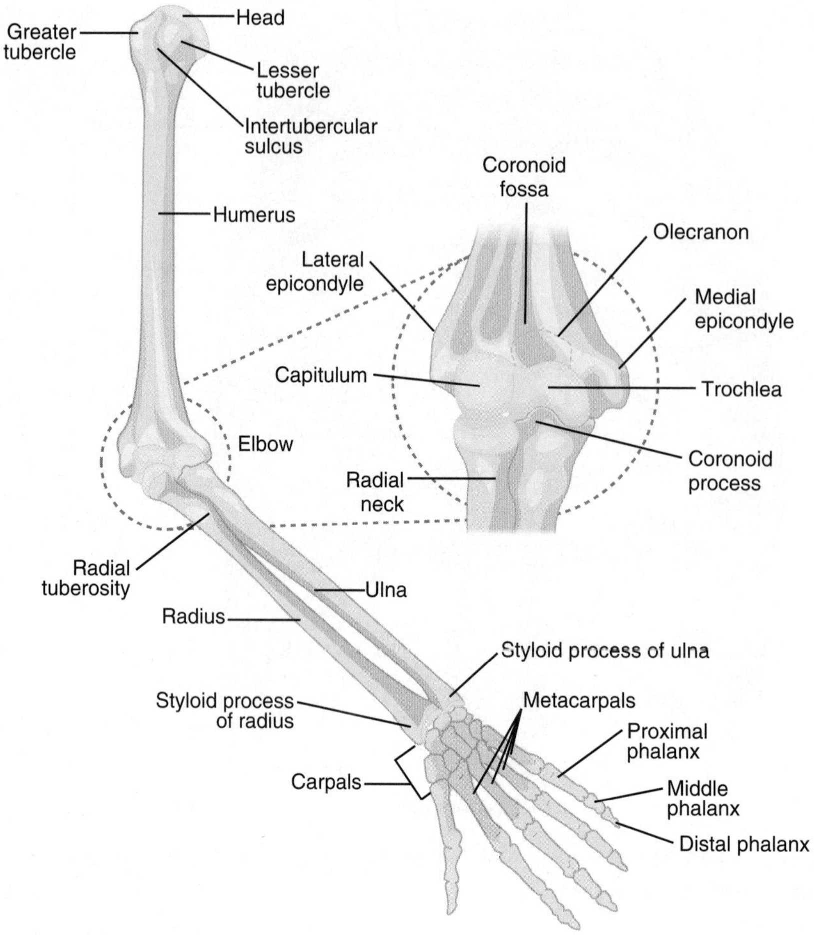

FIGURE 10-14 Bones of the upper extremity.

side of this head has a small styloid process to which the ligaments of the wrist are attached. The proximal end of the radius articulates with the humerus. The medial surface of the head constitutes a smooth cylinder where the radius rotates against the radial notch of the ulna. Major anterior arm muscles (biceps brachii) are attached to the radial tuberosity.

The wrist is composed of eight carpal bones, which are arranged in two rows of four each. Five **metacarpals** are attached to the **carpal bones** and constitute the bony framework of the hand. Fourteen **phalanges** make up the five digits of the hand. Each thumb has two phalanges, and each finger has three.

The pelvic girdle, which attaches the legs to the trunk (**FIGURE 10-15**), consists of two **coxae** (hip bones), located on each side of the pelvis. Each coxa surrounds a large **obturator foramen**, through which muscles, nerves, and blood vessels pass to the leg. A fossa called the **acetabulum** is located on the lateral surface of each coxa; it serves as the point of articulation of the lower limb with the girdle. During development, each coxa is formed by the fusion of three separate bones: the **ilium**, the **ischium**, and the **pubis**. The superior portion of the ilium—the **iliac crest**—ends anteriorly as the anterior-superior iliac spine and posteriorly as the posterior-superior iliac spine.

The **femur** is the longest bone in the body. It has a well-defined neck as well as a prominent rounded head that articulates with the acetabulum. The proximal shaft has two tuberosities: a greater trochanter, which is lateral to the neck, and a smaller or lesser trochanter, which is inferior and posterior to the neck. Both trochanters serve as attachment sites for muscles that attach the hip to the thigh. The distal end of the femur has medial and lateral condyles that articulate with the tibia. Located laterally and

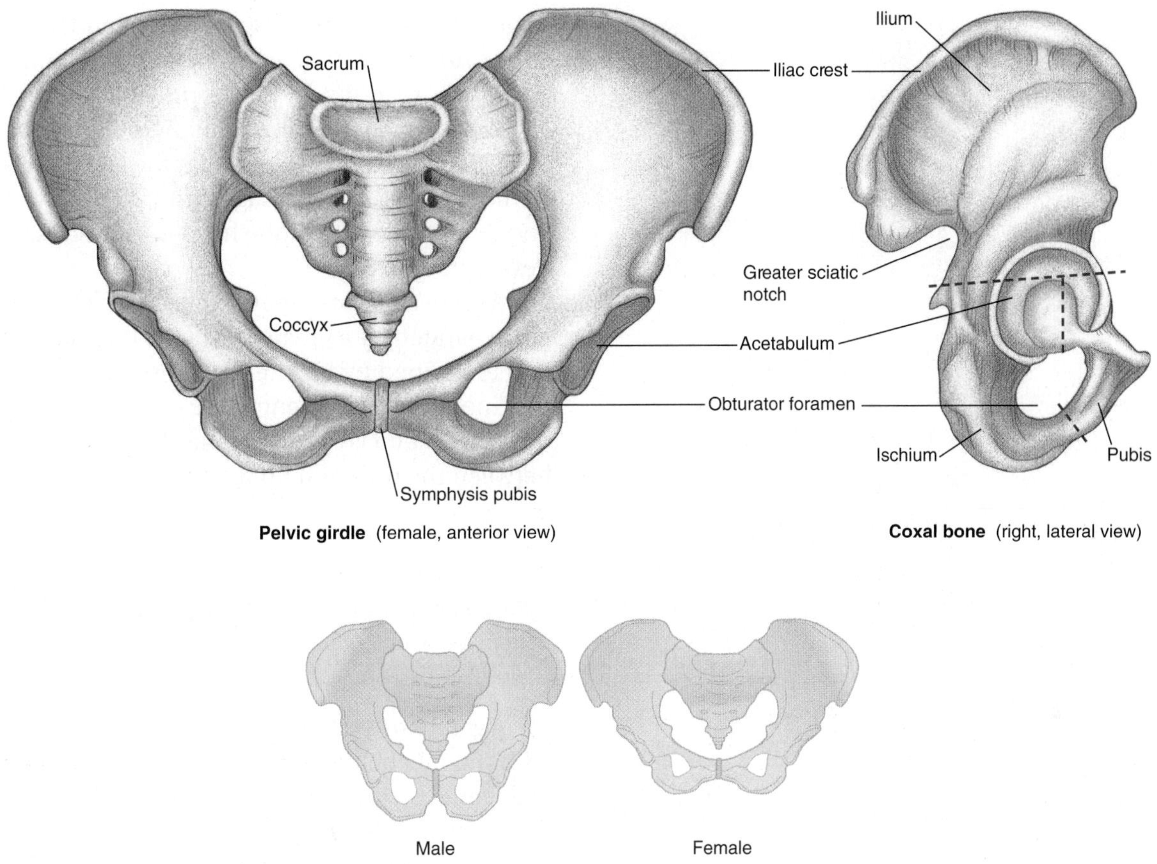

FIGURE 10-15 Complete pelvic girdle (anterior view).

proximally to the condyles are the medial and lateral epicondyles, which are sites of muscle and ligament attachment. **FIGURE 10-16** illustrates the bones of the lower extremity.

> **CRITICAL THINKING**
> Why should you anticipate blood loss when large bones are fractured?

Distally, the femur also articulates with the **patella**, which is located in a major tendon of the thigh muscle. The patella provides mechanical advantage to the quadriceps muscle in its function of straightening the knee.

The two bones of the lower leg are the tibia and the fibula. The **tibia**, which is the larger of the two, supports most of the weight of the leg. A tibial tuberosity can be seen and palpated just inferior to the patella. The proximal end of the tibia has flat medial and lateral condyles that articulate with the condyles of the femur. The distal end of the tibia forms the **medial malleolus**, which helps to form the medial side of the ankle joint.

The **fibula** does not articulate with the femur, but it does have a small proximal head that articulates with the tibia. The distal end of the fibula forms the lateral malleolus to create the lateral aspect of the ankle joint.

The foot consists of seven **tarsal bones** (**FIGURE 10-17**). The talus articulates with the tibia and the fibula to form the ankle joint. The **calcaneus** is located inferior and slightly lateral to the talus, supporting the bone. The calcaneus protrudes posteriorly where the calf muscles attach to it. The calcaneus is identified easily as the heel. The foot consists of tarsals, **metatarsals**, and phalanges. These bones are arranged in a manner similar to the metacarpals and phalanges of the hand, with the great toe being analogous to the thumb. The ball of the foot is the junction between the metatarsals

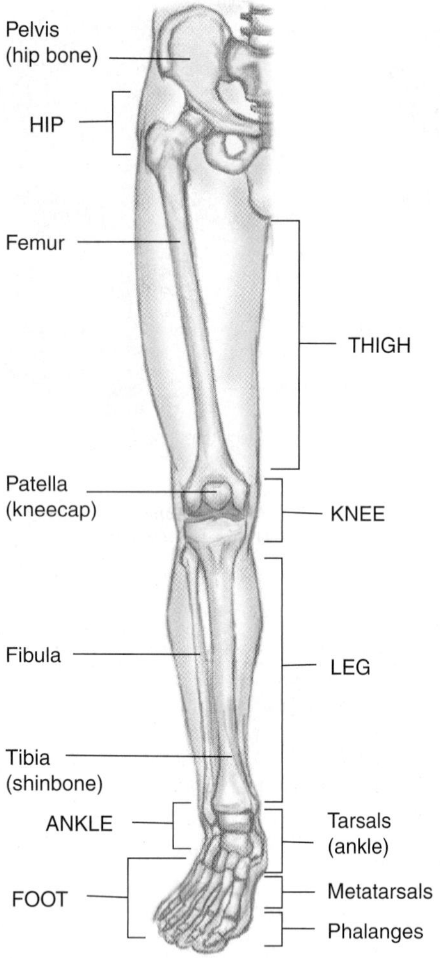

FIGURE 10-16 Bones of the lower extremity.

and the phalanges. Strong ligaments and leg muscle tendons normally hold the foot bones firmly in their arched position.

Biomechanics of Body Movement

With the exception of the hyoid bone, every bone in the body connects to at least one other bone.

The connections, or joints, commonly are named according to the bones or portions of bones that are united at the joint. The three major classifications of joints are fibrous joints, cartilaginous joints, and synovial joints.

Fibrous Joints. **Fibrous joints** consist of two bones united by fibrous tissue; these joints have little or no movement. Fibrous joints are further classified, based on their structure, as sutures, syndesmoses, or gomphoses. Sutures (seams between flat bones) are located in the skull bones and may be completely immobile in adults. In newborns, the sutures have gaps between them, called fontanels (**FIGURE 10-18**); these gaps are fairly wide so that the skull can "give" during birth to allow passage through the birth canal and to allow growth of the head during subsequent development.

A syndesmosis is a fibrous joint in which the bones are separated by a greater distance than in a suture and are joined by ligaments. These ligaments may provide some movement of the joint. An example of this type of joint is the distal tibia fibular syndesmosis, between the tibia and fibula (**FIGURE 10-19**).

> CRITICAL THINKING
> Why might the structure of the skull sutures be a disadvantage in the case of head trauma in an adult?

A gomphosis consists of a peg that fits into a socket, with the peg being held in place by fine bundles of collagenous connective tissue. The joints between the teeth and the sockets along the processes of the mandible and maxilla are examples of gomphoses.

Cartilaginous Joints. **Cartilaginous joints** unite two bones by means of hyaline cartilage (synchondroses) or fibrocartilage (symphyses). A synchondrosis allows only slight movement at the joint. A common example of this type of joint is the epiphyseal plate of a growing bone. Another example is the cartilage rod found between most of the ribs and the sternum. Symphyseal joints are slightly movable because of the flexible nature of the fibrocartilage. Symphyses include the junction between the manubrium and the body of the sternum in adults, the symphysis pubis of the pelvis, and the intervertebral disks.

Synovial Joints. **Synovial joints** contain synovial fluid, which is a thin lubricating film that allows considerable movement between articulating bones. Most joints that unite the bones of the appendicular skeleton are synovial. The articular surfaces of bones in synovial joints are covered with a thin layer of hyaline cartilage, which provides a smooth surface where the bones meet. The joint is enclosed by a **joint capsule** that consists of an outer fibrous capsule and an inner synovial membrane. The synovial membrane lines the joint and produces synovial fluid. Synovial joints

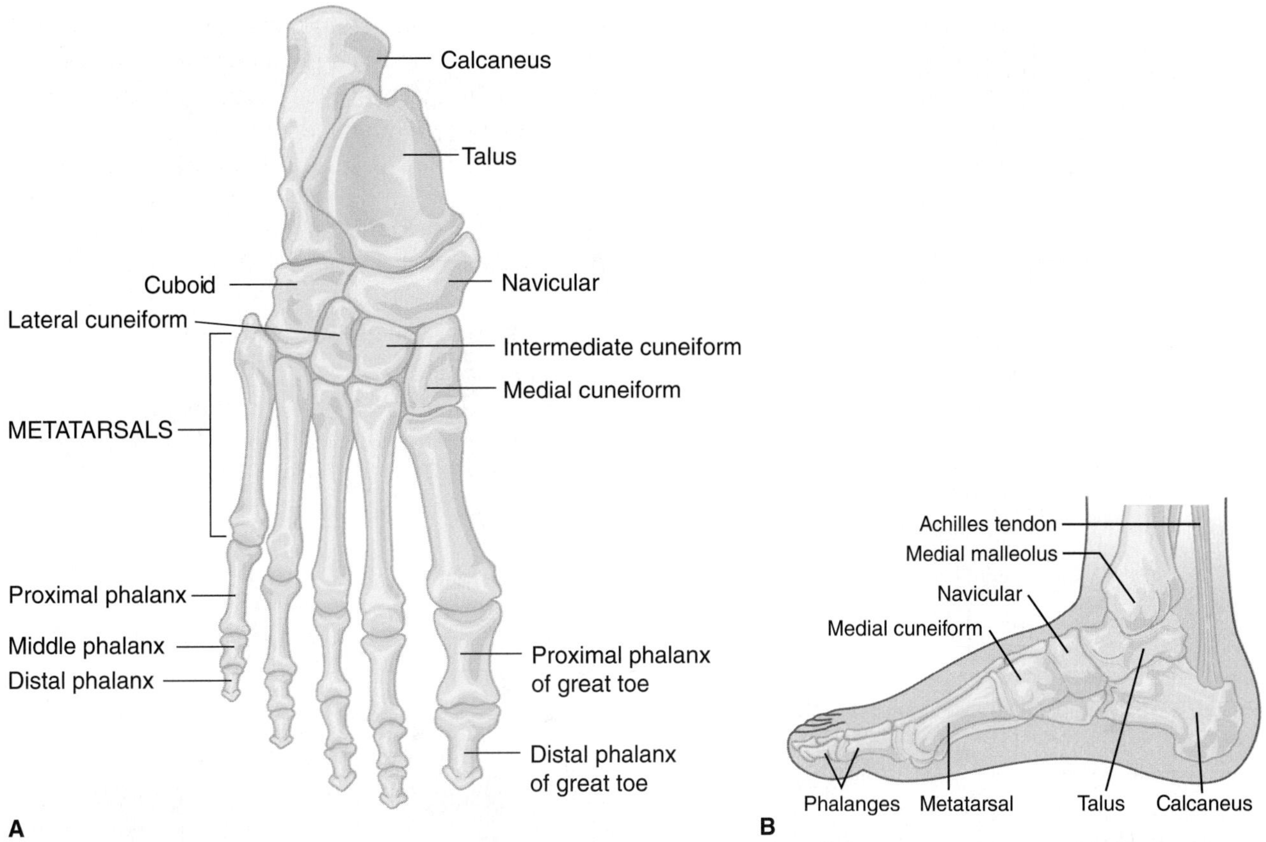

FIGURE 10-17 Bones of the right ankle and foot. **A.** Dorsal view. **B.** Medial view.

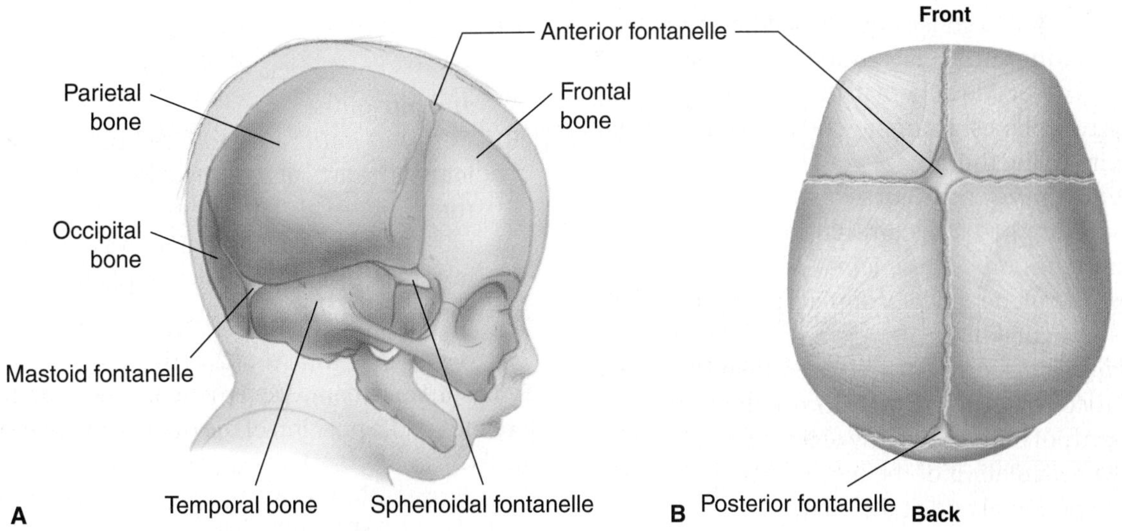

FIGURE 10-18 Infant skull showing the fontanels. **A.** Lateral view. **B.** Superior view.

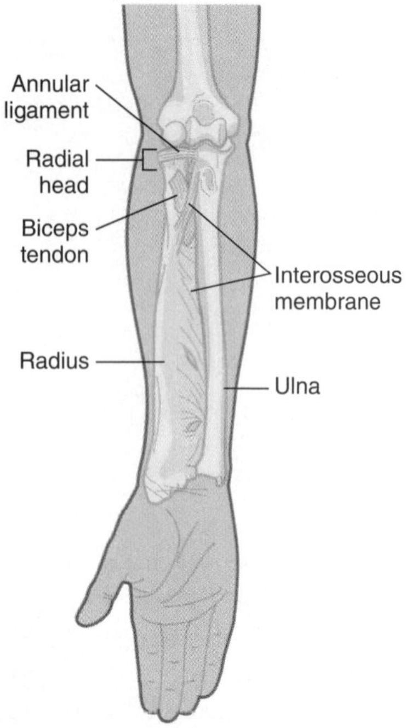

FIGURE 10-19 Radioulnar syndesmosis of the right forearm.

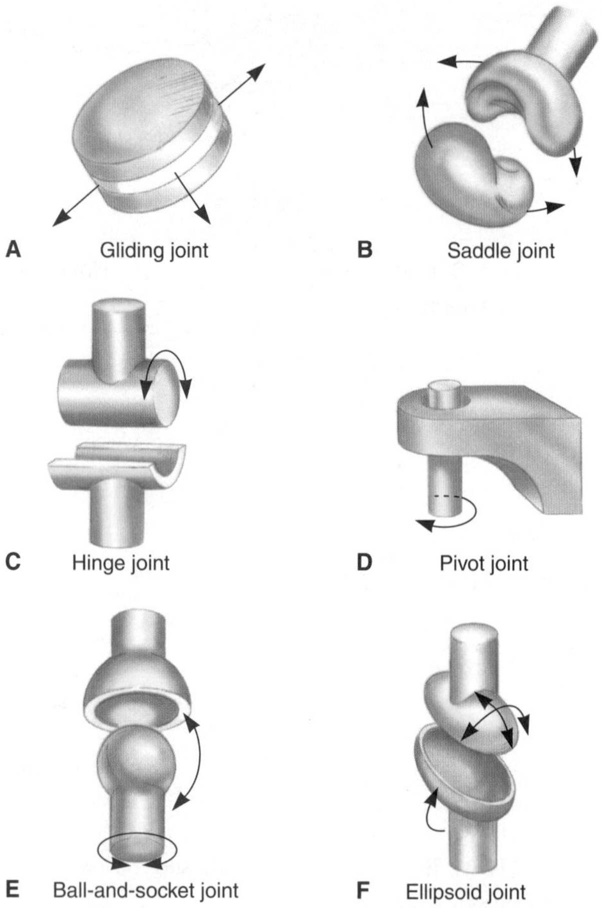

FIGURE 10-20 Types of synovial joints and selected examples. **A.** Plane or gliding. **B.** Saddle. **C.** Hinge. **D.** Pivot. **E.** Ball-and-socket. **F.** Ellipsoid.

are classified into six divisions according to the shape of the adjoining articular surfaces (**FIGURE 10-20**):

1. *Plane* or *gliding joints* consist of two opposed flat surfaces that are approximately equal in size. Examples: the articular processes between the vertebrae.
2. *Saddle joints* consist of two saddle-shaped articulating surfaces oriented at right angles to each other. Movement in these joints can occur in two planes. Example: the carpometacarpal joint of the thumb.
3. *Hinge joints* consist of a convex cylinder in one bone applied to a corresponding concavity in another bone. These joints permit movement in one plane only. Examples: the joints of the elbow and knee.
4. *Pivot joints* consist of a relatively cylindrical bony process, which rotates within a ring composed partly of bone and partly of ligament. Example: the articulation of the head of the radius with the proximal end of the ulna.
5. *Ball-and-socket joints* consist of a ball (head) at the end of one bone and a socket in an adjacent bone into which a portion of the ball fits. These joints allow wide ranges of movement in almost any direction. Examples: the shoulder and hip joints.
6. *Ellipsoid joints* are modified ball-and-socket joints. The articular surfaces are ellipsoid, rather than spherical. The shape of the joint limits movement, making it similar to a hinge motion, but the motion occurs in two planes. Example: the atlantooccipital joint.

Types of Movement. Movement may be described as it relates to the position of the body[3]—in other words,

CRITICAL THINKING

Why would it be helpful to other providers to use movement terms in your radio report or written patient care report?

TABLE 10-3 Body Movement Terminology

Term	Definition
Flexion	Bending
Extension	Straightening out
Protraction	Movement in the anterior direction
Retraction	Movement in the posterior direction
Abduction	Movement away from the midline
Adduction	Movement toward the midline
Inversion	Turning inward
Eversion	Turning outward
Excursion	Movement from side to side
Rotation	Movement of a structure around its axis
Circumduction	Movement in a circular motion
Pronation	Rotation of the forearm so that the anterior surface is down
Supination	Rotation of the forearm so that the anterior surface is up
Elevation	Movement of a structure in a superior direction
Depression	Movement of a structure in an inferior direction
Opposition	Movement of the thumb and little finger toward each other
Reposition	Movement of a structure to its original position

as motion away from the anatomic position or motion toward it. **TABLE 10-3** lists examples of each type of movement; also see **FIGURES 10-21** through **10-25**.

Muscular System

The three primary functions of the muscular system are movement, postural maintenance, and heat production. As previously discussed, the major types of muscles are skeletal, cardiac, and smooth muscle

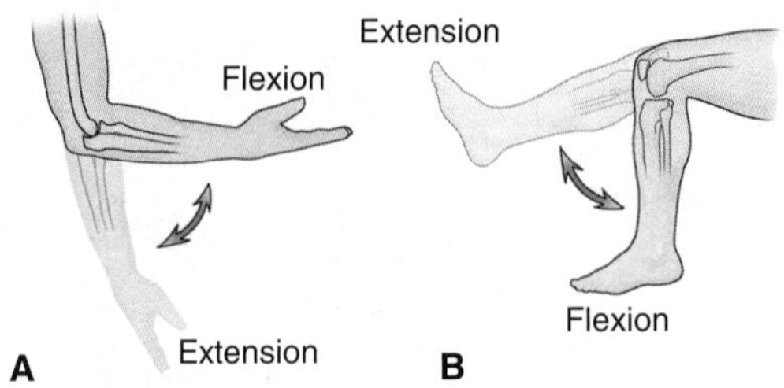

FIGURE 10-21 Flexion and extension of the elbow **(A)** and the knee **(B)**.

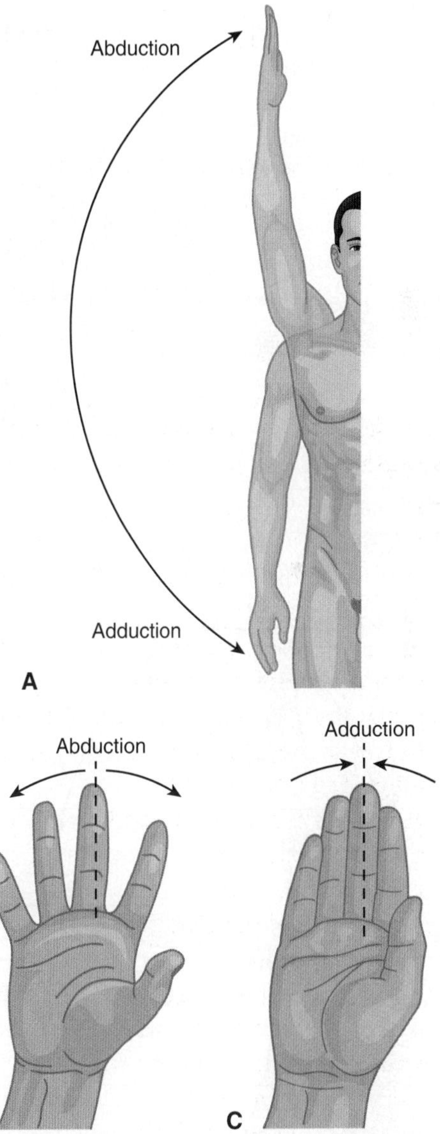

FIGURE 10-22 Abduction and adduction of the upper extremity **(A)**, and abduction **(B)** and adduction **(C)** of the fingers.

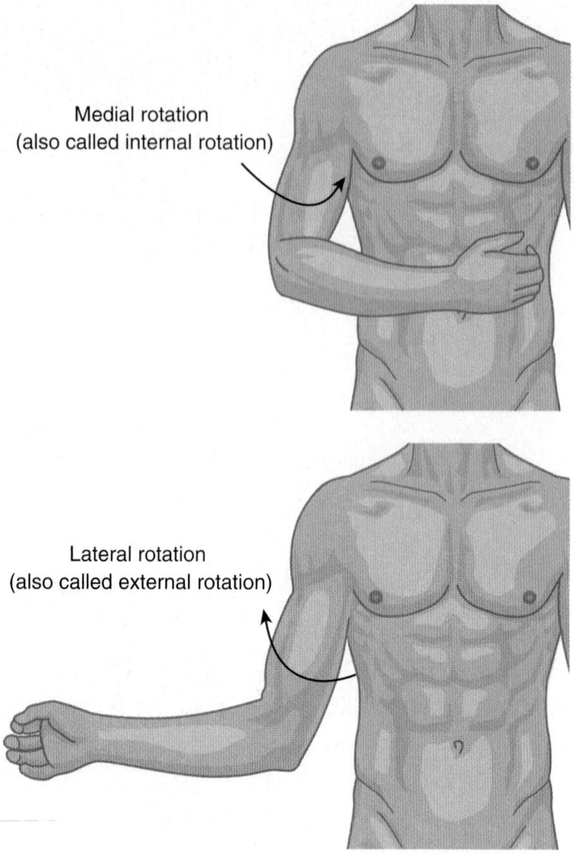

FIGURE 10-23 Medial and lateral rotation of the humerus.

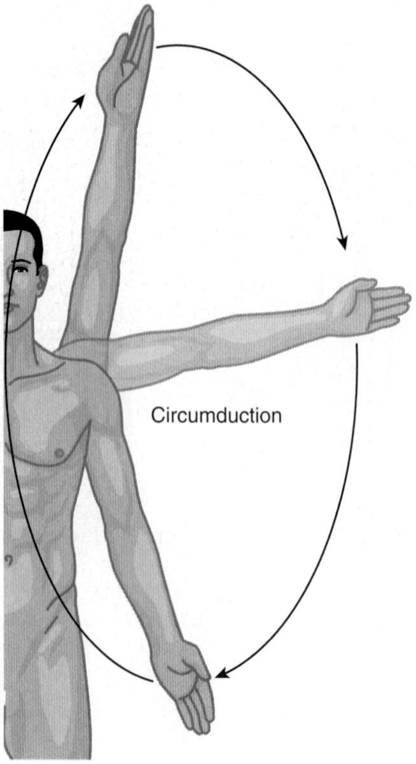

FIGURE 10-24 Circumduction of the shoulder.

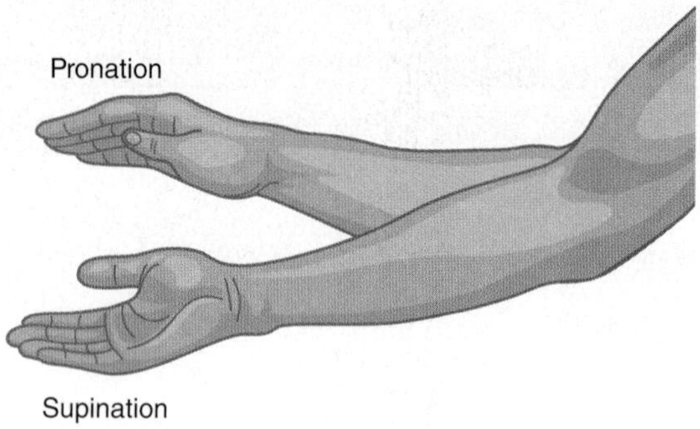

FIGURE 10-25 Pronation and supination.

(**TABLE 10-4**). Skeletal muscle is far more common than other types of muscle in the body and is the focus of this section. Cardiac and smooth muscle are presented later in this text. **FIGURE 10-26** illustrates the body's musculature.

Physiology of Skeletal Muscle

Muscle tissue is made up of specialized contractile cells or muscle fibers. Skeletal muscle contracts in response to electrochemical stimuli. Nerve cells regulate the function of skeletal muscle fibers by controlling the series of events that result in muscle contraction.

Each skeletal muscle fiber is filled with thick and thin threadlike structures called **myofilaments**. The thick myofilaments are formed from the protein myosin; the thin myofilaments are composed of the protein actin. The **sarcomere**, or contractile unit of skeletal muscle, contains both thick and thin myofilaments. During the contraction process, energy obtained from ATP molecules enables the two types of myofilaments to slide toward each other, shortening the sarcomere and eventually the entire muscle.

A nervous impulse enters the muscle fiber through a specialized nerve known as a **motor neuron**. The point of contact between the nerve ending and the muscle fiber is the neuromuscular junction, or **synapse** (**FIGURE 10-27**). Each muscle fiber receives a branch of an axon, and each axon innervates more than a single muscle fiber. When a nerve impulse passes through this junction, specialized chemicals are released, causing the muscle to contract.

CRITICAL THINKING

Suppose exposure to a chemical nerve weapon caused too much chemical stimulation at the synapse for the muscles of the eye. What might you find in your examination of the eye?

TABLE 10-4 Comparison of Muscle Types

Features	Skeletal Muscle	Cardiac Muscle	Smooth Muscle
Location	Attached to bones	Heart	Walls of hollow organs, blood vessels, eyes, glands, and skin
Cell shape	Long and cylindrical (1–40 mm in length; may extend the entire length of a muscle; 10–100 μm in diameter)	Cylindrical and branched (100–500 μm in length; 100–200 μm in diameter)	Spindle-shaped (15–200 μm in length, 5–10 mcg in diameter)
Nucleus special features	Multiple, peripherally located	Single, centrally located Intercalated disks join the cells to each other	Single, centrally located
Striations	Yes	Yes	No
Control	Voluntary	Involuntary	Involuntary
Capable of spontaneous contraction	No	Yes	Yes
Function	Moves body	Pumps blood	Moves food through the digestive tract, empties the urinary bladder, regulates blood vessel diameter, changes pupil size, contracts many gland ducts, moves hair, and other functions

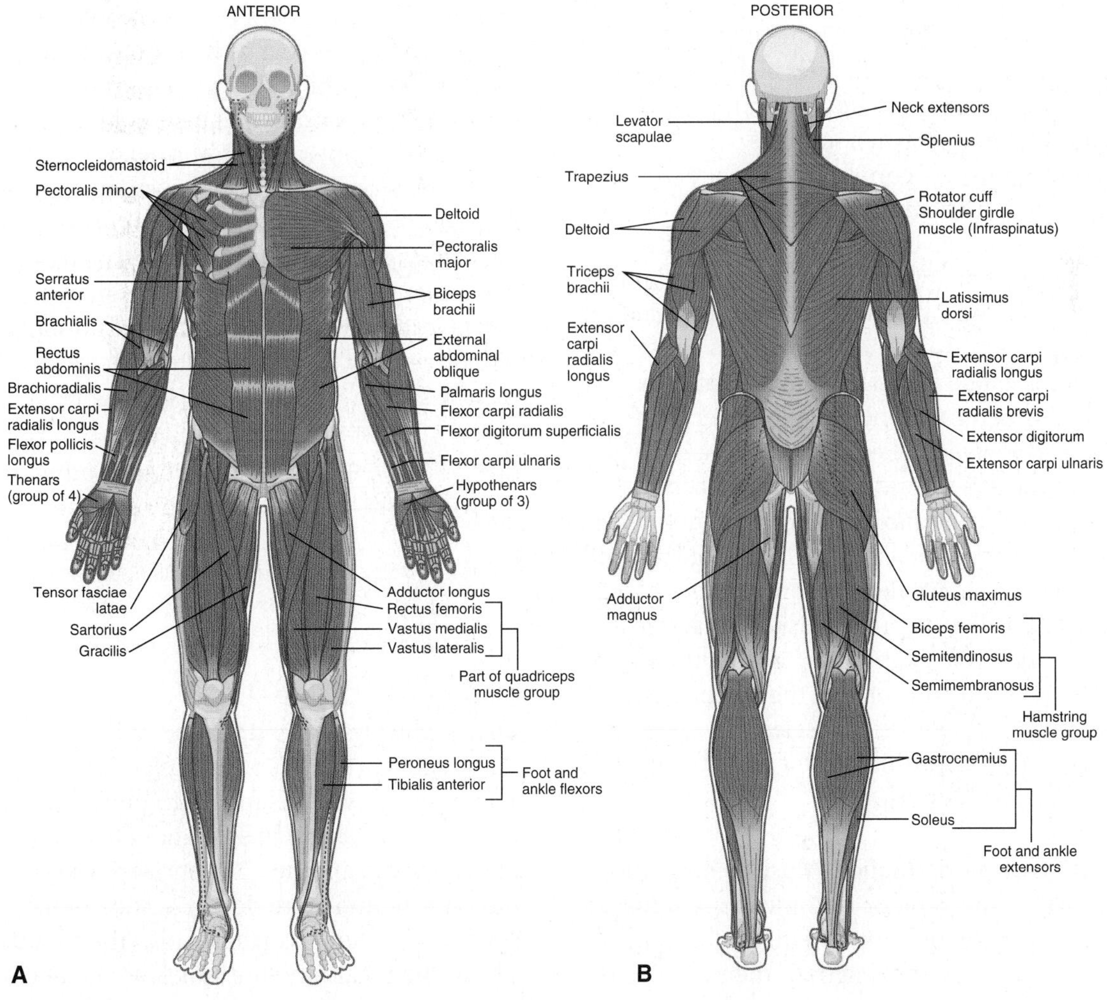

FIGURE 10-26 **A.** Anterior view of the body's musculature. **B.** Posterior view of the body's musculature.

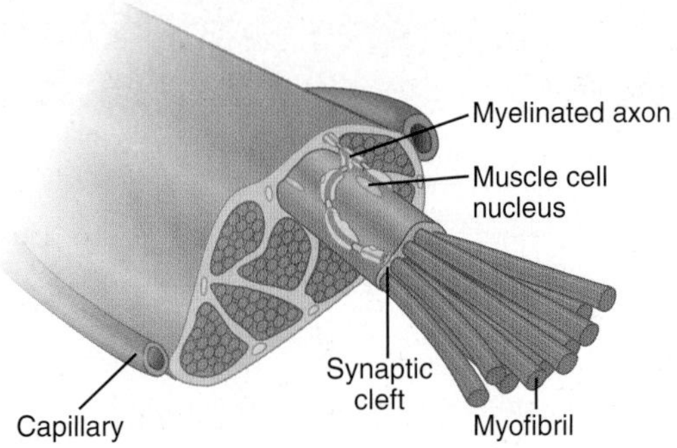

FIGURE 10-27 Neuromuscular junction.

Skeletal Muscle Movement

Most muscles extend from one bone to another and cross at least one joint. Muscle contraction causes most body movements by pulling one of the bones toward the other across the movable joint. The origin is the end of the muscle attached to the more stationary of the two bones; the insertion is the end of the muscle attached to the bone undergoing the greatest movement. Some muscles of the face are not attached to bone at both ends, but rather attach to the skin, which moves when muscles contract.

As some muscles contract and others relax at the same time, movement is created. Muscles that work together to cause movement are called *synergists.* A muscle that opposes another muscle (moves the structure in an opposite direction) is called an antagonist. The muscle that is the main cause of a movement is called the prime mover. For example, the biceps brachii, brachialis, and triceps brachii muscles are involved in flexion and extension of the forearm at the elbow joint. The biceps brachii is the prime mover during flexion, and the brachialis is the synergistic muscle. When the biceps brachii and the brachialis muscles flex the forearm, the triceps brachii relaxes; thus, the triceps is the antagonist. In contrast, during extension of the forearm, the triceps brachii is the prime mover, and the biceps and brachialis are the antagonistic muscles. The synergists and antagonists coordinate their activity, making movement occur smoothly.

Types of Muscle Contraction. Muscle contractions can be either isometric or isotonic, depending on the type of contraction that predominates. In isometric contractions, the length of the muscle does not change, but the amount of tension increases during the contraction. Isometric contractions are responsible for the constant length of the postural muscles of the body. During isotonic contractions, the amount of tension created by the muscle is constant, but the length of the muscle changes. An example of isotonic contraction is the movement of the arms or fingers. Most muscle contractions are a mix of the two types of contractions.

Postural Maintenance. Postural maintenance is a result of muscle tone, meaning the constant tension produced by muscles of the body for long periods. This tone keeps the back and legs straight, the head in an upright position, and the abdomen from bulging. These positions balance the distribution of weight. Therefore, they put less strain on muscles, tendons, ligaments, and bones.

Heat Production. The energy needed to create muscle contraction is derived from ATP. Most of the energy released in the breakdown of ATP during a muscular contraction is used to shorten the muscle fibers. Some energy, though, is lost as heat during the chemical reaction. The normal body temperature is, in large part, attributable to this metabolism in skeletal muscle. If the body temperature drops below a certain level, the nervous system induces shivering—that is, rapid contractions of skeletal muscle that produce shaking rather than coordinated movements. This kind of muscle movement increases heat production up to 18 times that of resting levels. The heat created during shivering can exceed that from moderate exercise, and it helps to raise the body temperature to its normal range.

CRITICAL THINKING

Children younger than 3 months cannot shiver. How will this affect prehospital care for patients in this age group?

Nervous System

The nervous system and the endocrine system are the main regulatory and coordinating systems of the body. The nervous system sends out information rapidly, via nerve impulses that are conducted from one area of the body to another. The endocrine system sends out information more slowly, by means of chemicals secreted by ductless glands into the bloodstream. These chemicals and hormones then are circulated

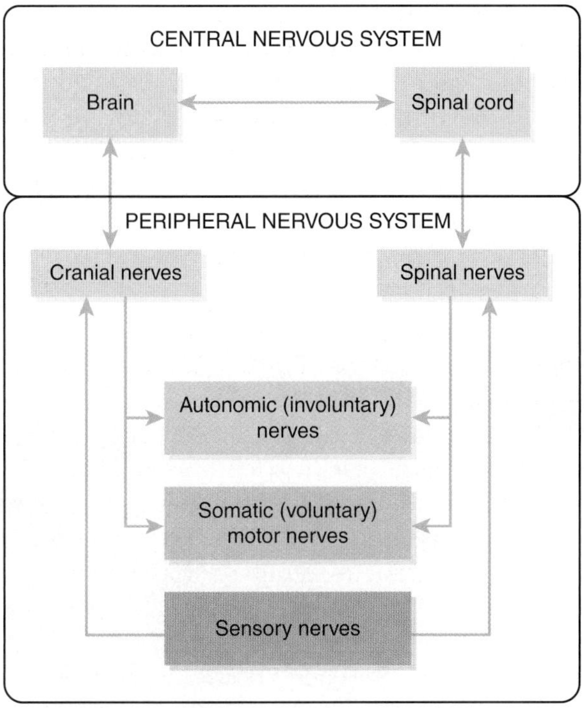

FIGURE 10-28 Divisions of the nervous system.

© Jones & Bartlett Learning.

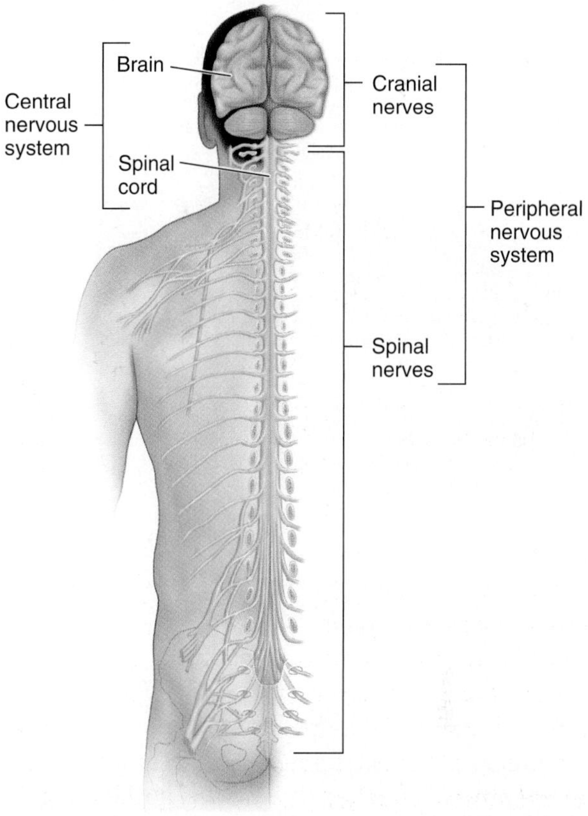

FIGURE 10-29 The central nervous system consists of the brain and spinal cord. The peripheral nervous system consists of the cranial nerves, which arise from the brain, and the spinal nerves, which arise from the spinal cord.

© Jones & Bartlett Learning.

to other parts of the body. The constancy of the internal environment of the body, called **homeostasis**, is a steady state that is sustained to a large degree by these regulatory and coordinating actions.

Divisions of the Nervous System

The human body has a single nervous system, although some of its subdivisions are referred to as separate systems. Each subdivision has structural and functional aspects that distinguish it from the others (**FIGURE 10-28**).

The **central nervous system (CNS)** is made up of the brain and spinal cord. These organs are encased in and protected by bone, and the brain and spinal cord are continuous with each other. The **peripheral nervous system (PNS)** consists of the nerves and ganglia. The **ganglia** are collections of nerve cell bodies located outside the CNS. A total of 43 pairs of nerves originate from the CNS to form the PNS: The cranial nerves (12 pairs) originate from the brain, and the spinal nerves (31 pairs) originate from the spinal cord. The **afferent division** transmits action potentials from the sensory organs to the CNS. The **efferent division** transmits action potentials from the CNS to effector organs such as muscles and glands (**FIGURE 10-29**). The efferent division is further divided into the **somatic nervous system**, which transmits

impulses from the CNS to skeletal muscle, and the **autonomic nervous system**, which transmits action potentials from the CNS to smooth muscle, cardiac muscle, and certain glands.

> **CRITICAL THINKING**
> How are the cranial nerves like the Supreme Court?

Central Nervous System

As stated earlier, the CNS consists of the brain and spinal cord. The adult brain has four major regions: the brainstem (consisting of the medulla, pons, and midbrain), the diencephalon (which includes the thalamus and hypothalamus), the cerebrum, and the cerebellum (**FIGURE 10-30**). **TABLE 10-5** describes the functions of these divisions.

Brainstem. The brainstem connects the spinal cord to the remainder of the brain and is responsible for

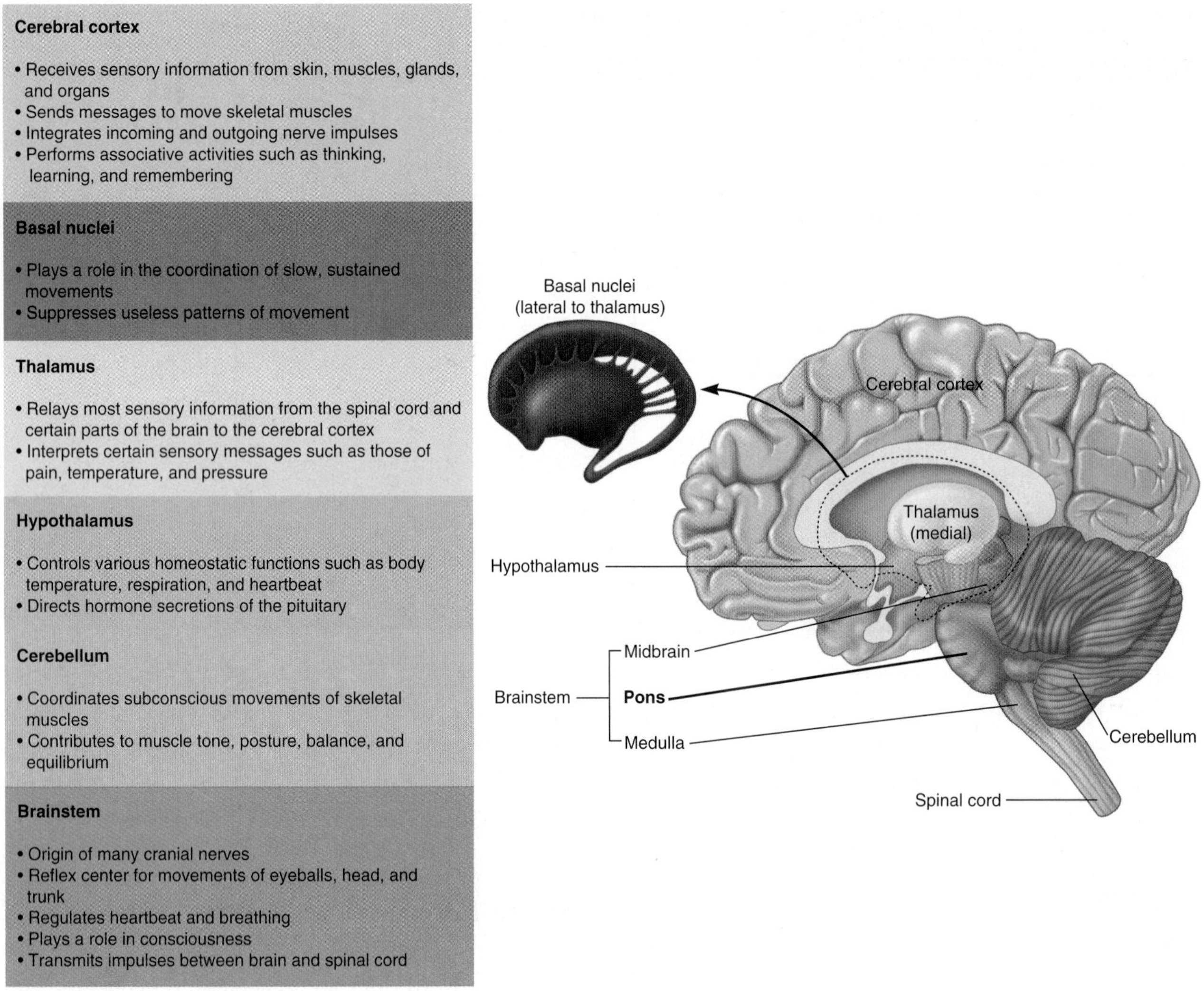

Cerebral cortex
• Receives sensory information from skin, muscles, glands, and organs
• Sends messages to move skeletal muscles
• Integrates incoming and outgoing nerve impulses
• Performs associative activities such as thinking, learning, and remembering
Basal nuclei
• Plays a role in the coordination of slow, sustained movements
• Suppresses useless patterns of movement
Thalamus
• Relays most sensory information from the spinal cord and certain parts of the brain to the cerebral cortex
• Interprets certain sensory messages such as those of pain, temperature, and pressure
Hypothalamus
• Controls various homeostatic functions such as body temperature, respiration, and heartbeat
• Directs hormone secretions of the pituitary
Cerebellum
• Coordinates subconscious movements of skeletal muscles
• Contributes to muscle tone, posture, balance, and equilibrium
Brainstem
• Origin of many cranial nerves
• Reflex center for movements of eyeballs, head, and trunk
• Regulates heartbeat and breathing
• Plays a role in consciousness
• Transmits impulses between brain and spinal cord
Basal nuclei (lateral to thalamus)
Cerebral cortex
Thalamus (medial)
Hypothalamus
Brainstem
Midbrain
Pons
Medulla
Cerebellum
Spinal cord

FIGURE 10-30 Regions of the brain.

many essential functions. All but 2 of the 12 cranial nerves enter or exit the brain through the brainstem.

The **medulla**, also known as the medulla oblongata, is the most inferior portion of the brainstem. It acts as a conduction pathway for ascending and descending nerve tracts. It controls several body functions, such as regulation of the heart rate, blood vessel diameter, breathing, swallowing, vomiting, coughing, and sneezing.

The section of the brainstem known as the **pons** contains ascending and descending nerve tracts.

> CRITICAL THINKING
>
> A patient has an injury that affects the medulla. What is the initial prehospital management priority? Why?

This structure relays information from the cerebrum to the cerebellum. In addition, the pons houses the sleep center and respiratory center that, along with the medulla, help control breathing.

The midbrain, or **mesencephalon**, is the smallest region of the brainstem. The midbrain is involved in hearing through audio pathways in the CNS. It is also involved in visual reflexes such as visual tracking of moving objects and turning of the eyes. Other parts of the midbrain help regulate the automatic functions that require no conscious thought—for example, coordination of motor activities and muscle tone.

The **reticular formation** comprises a group of nuclei scattered throughout the brainstem. It receives axons from a large number of sources, especially from the nerves that innervate the face. The reticular formation and its connections are collectively known as the

TABLE 10-5 Functions of Major Divisions of the Brain

Brain Area	Function
Brainstem	
Medulla	Two-way conduction pathway between the spinal cord and higher brain centers; cardiac, respiratory, and vasomotor control centers
Pons	Two-way conduction pathway between areas of the brain and other regions of the body; influences respiration
Midbrain	Two-way conduction pathway; relay point for visual and auditory impulses
Diencephalon	
Hypothalamus	Regulation of body temperature, water balance, sleep-cycle control, appetite, and sexual arousal
Thalamus	Sensory relay station from various body areas to cerebral cortex; emotions and alerting or arousal mechanisms
Cerebellum	Muscle coordination; maintenance of equilibrium and posture
Cerebrum	Sensory perception, emotions, willed movements, consciousness, and memory

reticular activating system. This system is involved in the sleep–wake cycle and plays an important role in arousing and maintaining consciousness. Coma after head injury results from damage to the reticular activating system.

Diencephalon. The **diencephalon** is the part of the brain between the brainstem and the cerebrum. Major components of this organ include the thalamus and hypothalamus. The **thalamus**—the largest portion of the diencephalon—receives sensory input from various sense organs of the body and relays these impulses to the **cerebral cortex**. The thalamus also has other functions, such as influencing mood and general body movements linked with strong emotions such as fear or rage.

The **hypothalamus** is a major controller in the brain; it acts as a gatekeeper in determining which information is passed along to the cerebrum. The hypothalamus is an active participant in emotions, hormonal cycles, and sexuality. **TABLE 10-6** summarizes the various functions of the hypothalamus.

Cerebrum. The **cerebrum** is the largest portion of the brain. It is divided into left and right hemispheres, and each hemisphere is divided into lobes named for the bones that lie over them (**FIGURE 10-31**).

The frontal lobe is important in voluntary motor function, motivation, aggression, and mood. The parietal lobe is the major center for the reception and evaluation of most sensory information, except for smell, hearing, and vision. The occipital lobe functions in the reception and integration of visual input; this lobe is not distinctly separate from other lobes. The temporal lobe receives and evaluates olfactory and auditory input; it plays a key role in memory. A thin layer of **gray matter**, made up of neuron dendrites and cell bodies, composes the surface of the cerebrum (cerebral cortex).

The **limbic system** is made up of portions of the cerebrum and diencephalon. This system influences emotions, visceral responses to those emotions, motivation, mood, and sensations of pain and pleasure.

Cerebellum. The **cerebellum**—the second largest part of the human brain—is involved in gross motor coordination and helps produce smooth movements. A major job of the cerebellum is to compare impulses from the motor cortex with those from moving structures (eg, the position of the body or of body parts that innervate the joints and tendons of the structure being moved). If the cerebellum detects a difference between the intended movement and the actual one, it sends impulses to the motor cortex and the spinal cord to correct the discrepancy. Loss of cerebellar functioning results in inability to make exact movements.

Spinal Cord. The spinal cord lies within the spinal column and extends from the occipital bone to the

TABLE 10-6 Hypothalamic Functions

Function	Description
Autonomic	Helps control heart rate, urine release from the bladder, movement of food through the digestive tract, and blood vessel diameter.
Endocrine	Helps regulate pituitary gland secretions and influences metabolism, ion balance, sexual development, and sexual functions.
Muscle control	Controls muscles involved in swallowing and stimulates shivering in several muscles.
Temperature regulation	Promotes heat loss when the hypothalamic temperature increases by increasing sweat production (anterior hypothalamus); promotes heat production when the hypothalamic temperature decreases by triggering shivering (posterior hypothalamus).
Regulation of food and water intake	Hunger center promotes eating, and satiety center inhibits eating; thirst center promotes water intake.
Emotions	Large range of emotional influences over body functions; directly involved in stress-related and psychosomatic illnesses and with feelings of fear and rage.
Regulation of the sleep–wake cycle	Coordinates responses to the sleep–wake cycle with other areas of the brain (eg, the reticular activating system).

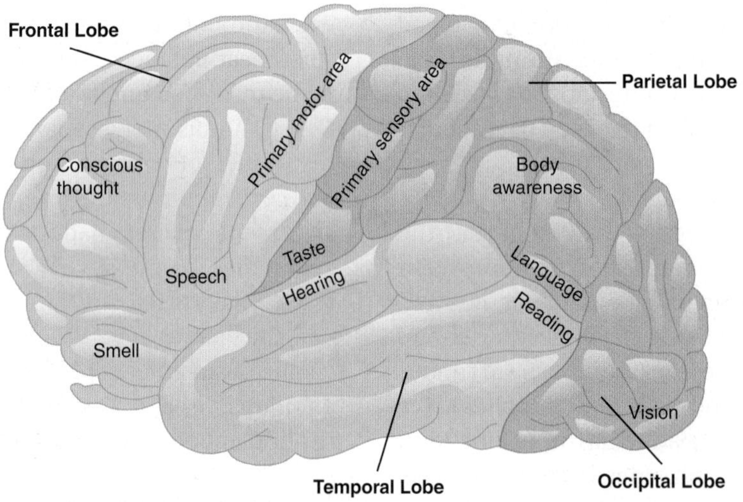

FIGURE 10-31 Lobes of the cerebrum.

level of the second lumbar vertebra. The spinal cord has a central gray portion and a peripheral white portion. The white matter consists of nerve tracts, and the gray matter consists of nerve cell bodies and dendrites. The **dorsal root** conveys afferent nerve processes to the cord, and the **ventral root** conveys efferent nerve processes away from the cord. Spinal ganglia, or dorsal root ganglia, contain the cell bodies of sensory neurons (**FIGURE 10-32**).

CRITICAL THINKING

An older adult patient has a new onset of staggering gait. Which area of the brain do you suspect has altered function?

The spinal cord is the main reflex center of the body. It produces **autonomic reflexes** and **visceral reflexes**, among others. Examples include increased heart rate in response to decreased blood pressure and the stretch reflex (knee-jerk reflex). The body also demonstrates withdrawal reflexes, such as removing a

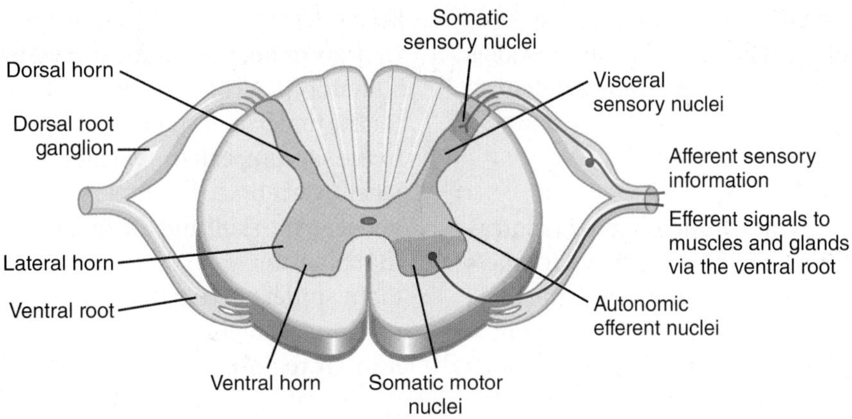

FIGURE 10-32 Dissection of a cervical segment of the spinal cord.

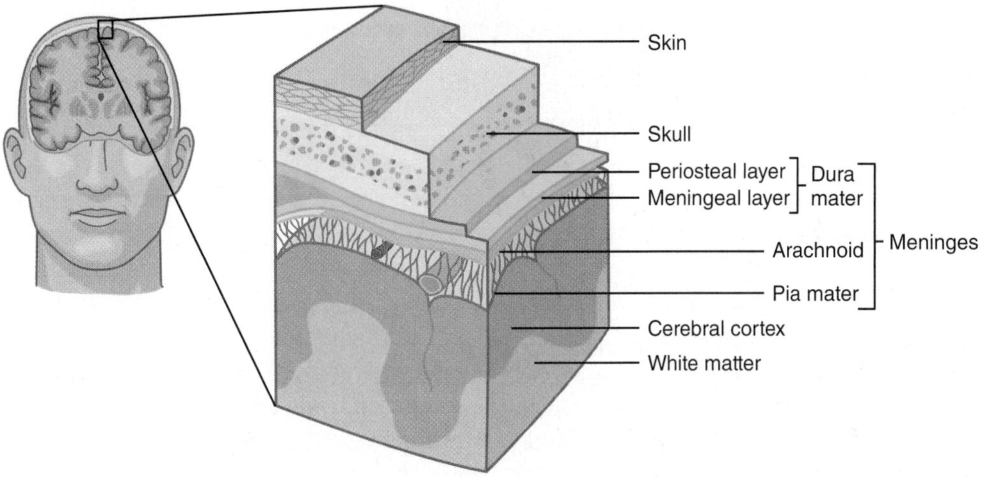

FIGURE 10-33 Meningeal coverings of the brain and spinal cord.

limb or other body part from a painful stimulus. The spinal cord tracts carry impulses to the brain in afferent, ascending tracts, as well as motor impulses from the brain in efferent, descending tracts. (Ascending and descending pathways are addressed further in Chapter 24, *Neurology.*)

The organs of the nervous system are surrounded by a tough, fluid-containing membrane known as the **meninges**, which is itself surrounded by bone. The meninges contain three connective tissue layers. The most superficial and thickest layer is the **dura mater**, which consists of two layers around the brain and one layer around the spinal cord. The two layers of the dura mater are fused around most of the brain but are separate in several places. The dura mater of the brain is attached tightly and is continuous with the **periosteum** of the cranial vault, whereas the dura mater of the spinal cord is separated from the periosteum of the vertebral canal by the **epidural space.**

The **arachnoid layer** is the second meningeal layer. The space between this layer and the dura mater, known as the **subdural space**, contains a small amount of serous fluid. The third meningeal layer, called the **pia mater**, lies external to a basement membrane formed by special cells called the glia limitans, which completely envelops the CNS. The space between the pia mater and the arachnoid layer, known as the **subarachnoid space**, is filled with blood vessels and cerebrospinal fluid (**FIGURE 10-33**).

The **cerebrospinal fluid (CSF)** is similar to plasma and **interstitial fluid** (the fluid that occupies the space outside the blood vessels). CSF bathes the brain and spinal cord and acts as a cushion around the CNS. It is formed continually from fluid filtering out of the blood in a network of brain capillaries and cells known as the choroid plexus. CSF fills the ventricles of the brain, the subarachnoid space, and the central canal of the spinal cord.

Peripheral Nervous System

The PNS collects information from numerous sources inside the body and on the body surface. It relays this information by way of afferent fibers to the CNS, which then evaluates the information. Efferent fibers in the PNS relay information from the CNS to various parts of the body, primarily to muscles and glands.

Spinal Nerves. The **spinal nerves** arise from many rootlets along the dorsal and ventral surfaces of the spinal cord. All of the 31 pairs of spinal nerves, except for the first pair of spinal nerves and the spinal nerves in the sacrum, exit the vertebral column through adjacent vertebrae. The first pair of spinal nerves exits between the skull and the first cervical vertebra, while the spinal nerves in the sacrum exit through the bone. Eight spinal nerve pairs exit the vertebral column in the cervical region, 12 in the thoracic region, 5 in the lumbar region, 5 in the sacral region, and 1 in the coccygeal region (**FIGURE 10-34**).

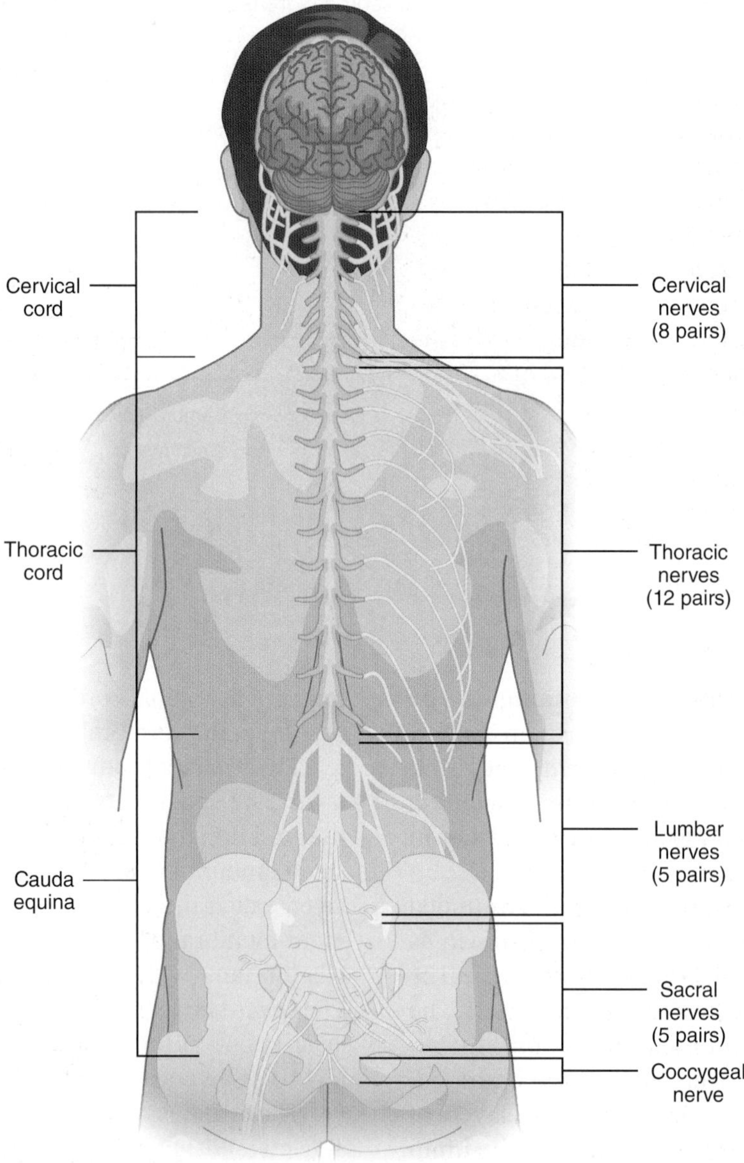

FIGURE 10-34 Spinal cord and spinal nerves.

Each spinal nerve except the first has a specific cutaneous sensory distribution. Detailed mapping of the skin surface reveals a close relationship between the source on the cord of each spinal nerve and the level of the body it innervates. The paramedic should understand this relationship when examining a patient with a spinal cord injury. The skin surface areas supplied by a single spinal nerve are known as **dermatomes** (**FIGURE 10-35**).

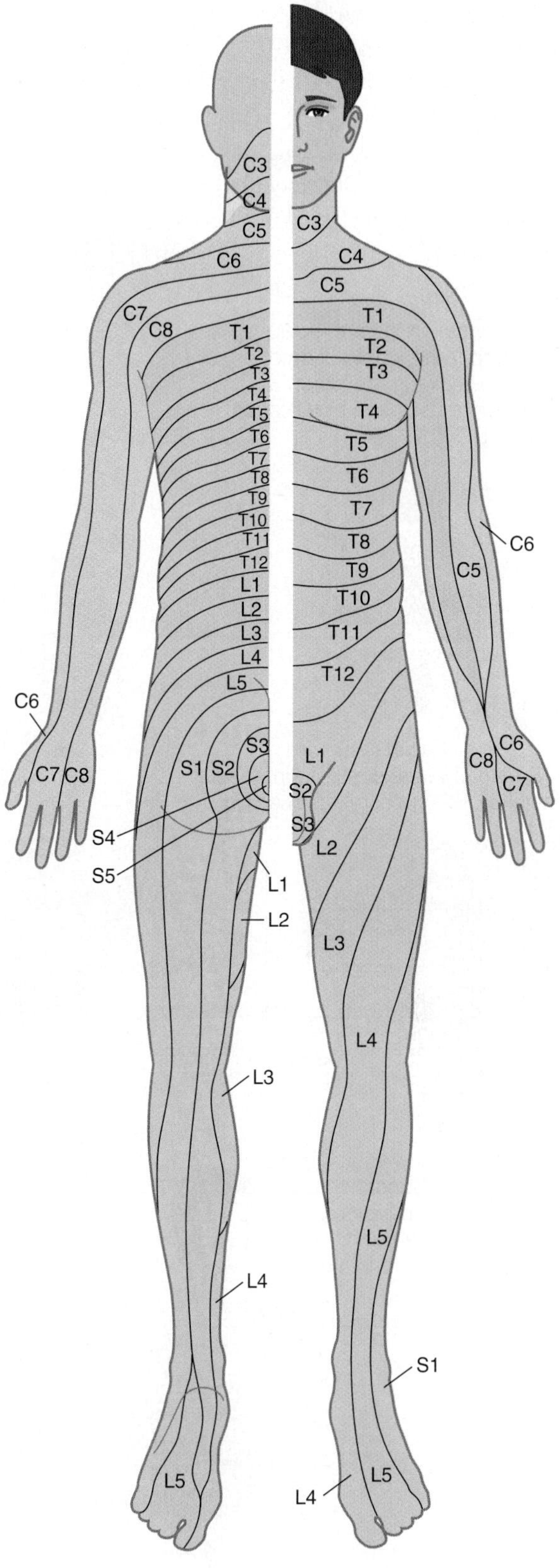

FIGURE 10-35 Dermatome map. Letters and numbers indicate the spinal nerves innervating a given region of the skin.

> CRITICAL THINKING
>
> Does a person with a spinal cord injury at the C5 level have movement in the hands?

Cranial Nerves. The 12 cranial nerves are divided into three general groups based on their function: sensory, somatomotor and proprioception, and parasympathetic (**FIGURE 10-36**). Sensory functions include the special senses, such as vision, as well as the more general senses, such as touch and pain. Somatomotor functions control the skeletal muscles through motor neurons. Proprioception provides the brain with information about the position of the body and its various parts, including joints and muscles. Parasympathetic function involves the regulation of glands, smooth muscle, and cardiac muscle (functions of the autonomic nervous system). Some cranial nerves have only one of the three functions; others have multiple functions (**TABLE 10-7**).

Autonomic Nervous System

As stated earlier, the PNS is made up of afferent and efferent neurons. **Afferent neurons** carry action potentials from the periphery to the CNS; **efferent neurons** carry action potentials from the CNS to the periphery. Afferent neurons provide data to the CNS that may trigger somatomotor and autonomic reflexes. Thus, these neurons cannot be easily categorized based on their function. In contrast, efferent neurons clearly differ structurally and functionally and can be classified into the somatomotor nervous system or the autonomic nervous system on that basis.

Somatomotor neurons innervate skeletal muscles, so they play a key role in locomotion, posture, and equilibrium. The movements controlled by the somatomotor nervous system usually are conscious movements. The effect of these neurons on skeletal

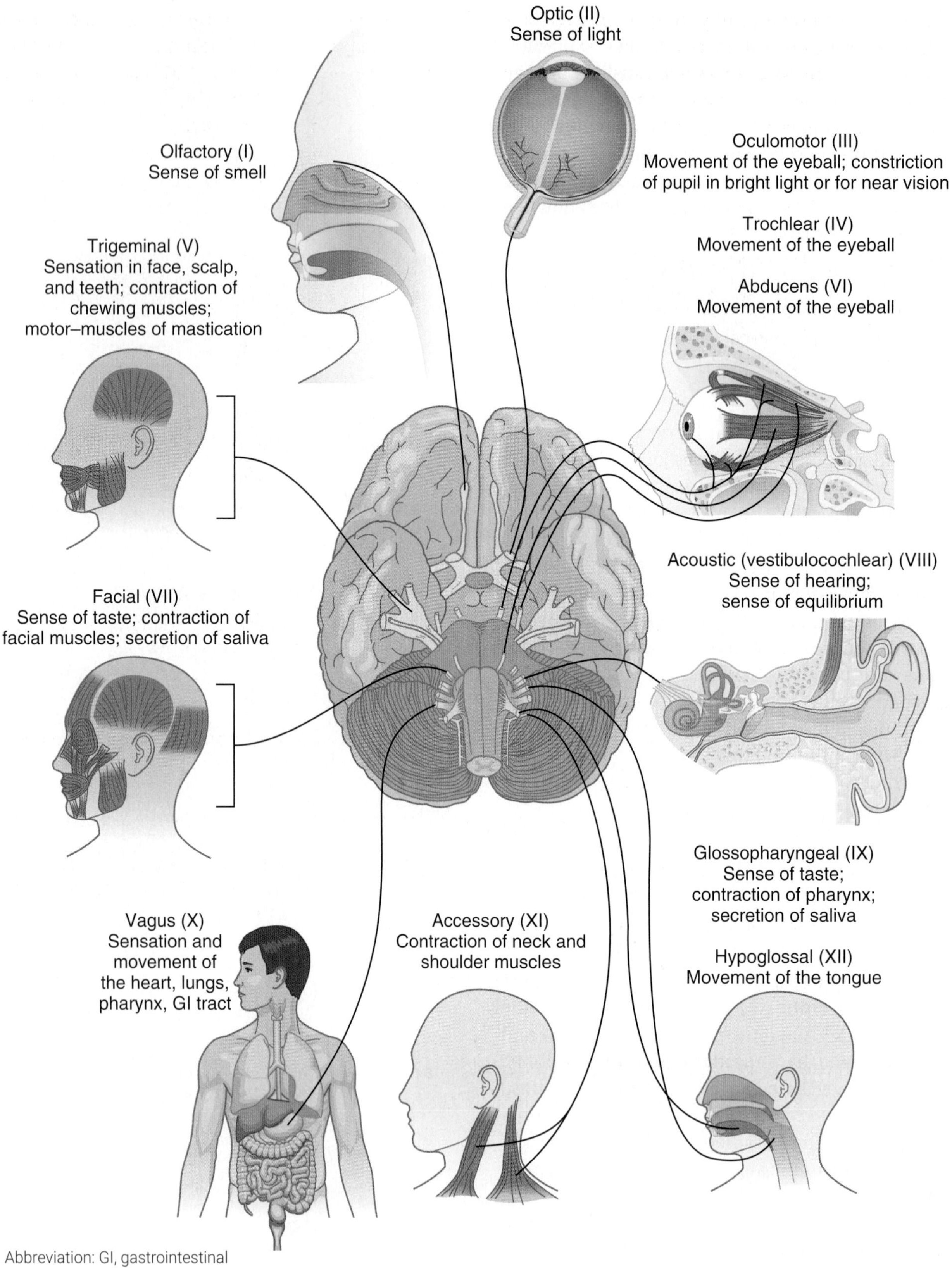
Optic (II)
Sense of light
Olfactory (I)
Sense of smell
Oculomotor (III)
Movement of the eyeball; constriction of pupil in bright light or for near vision
Trochlear (IV)
Movement of the eyeball
Abducens (VI)
Movement of the eyeball
Trigeminal (V)
Sensation in face, scalp, and teeth; contraction of chewing muscles; motor–muscles of mastication
Acoustic (vestibulocochlear) (VIII)
Sense of hearing; sense of equilibrium
Facial (VII)
Sense of taste; contraction of facial muscles; secretion of saliva
Glossopharyngeal (IX)
Sense of taste; contraction of pharynx; secretion of saliva
Vagus (X)
Sensation and movement of the heart, lungs, pharynx, GI tract
Accessory (XI)
Contraction of neck and shoulder muscles
Hypoglossal (XII)
Movement of the tongue

Abbreviation: GI, gastrointestinal

FIGURE 10-36 Origins of the cranial nerves.

muscle is always excitatory. By comparison, neurons of the autonomic nervous system innervate smooth muscle, cardiac muscle, and glands and are usually controlled unconsciously. The effect of autonomic neurons on their target tissue is inhibitory or excitatory.

The autonomic nervous system is made up of two divisions, the **sympathetic nervous system** and the **parasympathetic nervous system**. Both of these divisions consist of autonomic ganglia and nerves. The action potentials in sympathetic neurons generally prepare a person for physical activity. Parasympathetic stimulation, however, activates vegetative functions such as digestion, defecation, and urination.

The functions of the autonomic nervous system help to maintain or quickly restore homeostasis (**TABLE 10-8**). Many internal organs receive fibers

TABLE 10-7 Functions of the Cranial Nerves

Nerve	Name	Impulse Conduction	Functions
I	Olfactory	From nose to brain	Sense of smell
II	Optic	From eye to brain	Vision
III	Oculomotor	From brain to eye muscles	Eye movements, pupillary constriction
IV	Trochlear	From brain to external eye muscles	Eye movements
V	Trigeminal	From skin and mucous membranes of head and from teeth to brain; also from brain to chewing muscles	Sensations of face, scalp, and teeth; chewing movements
VI	Abducens	From brain to external eye muscles	Turning eyes outward
VII	Facial	From taste buds of tongue to brain; from brain to facial muscles	Sense of taste; contraction of muscles of facial expressions
VIII	Vestibulochochlear (acoustic)	From ear to brain	Hearing; sense of balance
IX	Glossopharyngeal	From throat and taste buds of tongue to brain; also from brain to throat muscles and salivary glands	Sensation of throat, taste, swallowing movements; secretion of saliva
X	Vagus	From throat, larynx, and organs in thoracic and abdominal cavities to brain; also from brain to muscles of throat and to organs in thoracic and abdominal cavities	Sensations of throat and larynx and of thoracic and abdominal organs; swallowing, voice production, slowing of heartbeat, acceleration of peristalsis
XI	Spinal accessory	From brain to certain shoulder and neck muscles	Shoulder movements, turning movements of head
XII	Hypoglossal	From brain to muscles of tongue	Tongue movements

TABLE 10-8 Functions of the Autonomic Nervous System

Visceral Effectors	Sympathetic Control	Parasympathetic Control
Heart muscle	Accelerates heartbeat	Slows heartbeat
Smooth Muscle		
Of most blood vessels	Constricts blood vessels	None
Of blood vessels in skeletal muscles	Dilates blood vessels	None

(continued)

TABLE 10-8 Functions of the Autonomic Nervous System *(continued)*

Visceral Effectors	Sympathetic Control	Parasympathetic Control
Smooth Muscle		
Of the digestive tract	Decreases peristalsis; inhibits defecation	Increases peristalsis
Of the anal sphincter	Stimulates—closes sphincter	Inhibits—opens sphincter for defecation
Of the urinary bladder	Inhibits—relaxes bladder	Stimulates-contracts bladder
Of the urinary sphincters	Stimulates—closes sphincter	Inhibits—opens sphincter for urination
Of the eye:		
Iris	Stimulates radial fibers—dilation of pupil	Stimulates circular fibers—constriction of pupil
Ciliary	Inhibits—accommodation for far vision (flattening of lens)	Stimulates—accommodation for near vision (bulging of lens)
Of hairs (pilomotor muscles)	Stimulates—goose bumps	No parasympathetic fibers
Glands		
Adrenal medulla	Increases epinephrine secretion	None
Sweat glands	Increase sweat secretion	None
Digestive glands	Decrease secretion of digestive juices	Increase secretion of digestive juices

from parasympathetic and sympathetic divisions (**FIGURE 10-37**) and are therefore continually bombarded by impulses from these systems. These impulses influence the function of these organs in opposite or antagonistic ways. For example, the heart receives sympathetic impulses that increase the heart rate as well as parasympathetic impulses that decrease the heart rate. The ratio between these two forces determines the actual heart rate.

CRITICAL THINKING

You administer a drug that blocks the action of the parasympathetic nervous system. What happens to the patient's heart rate?

Endocrine System

The **endocrine system** is made up of glands, which secrete hormones into the circulatory system (**FIGURE 10-38**). The endocrine and nervous systems have considerable functional and anatomic overlap. Some neurons secrete regulatory chemicals that function as hormones (neurohormones), such as antidiuretic hormone, into the circulatory system. Other neurons innervate **endocrine glands** and influence their secretory activity. Some hormones secreted by these glands, however, affect the nervous system.

Hormones, including neurohormones, are classified as proteins, polypeptides, derivatives of amino acids, or lipids (ie, steroids or derivatives of fatty acids). Hormones are dissolved in blood plasma and quickly become distributed throughout the body. In general, the amount of hormone that reaches the target tissue directly correlates with the concentration of the hormone in the blood. **TABLE 10-9** lists endocrine glands, hormones, and their functions.

Some hormones are present in fairly constant levels in the circulatory system. For example, concentrations of thyroid hormones in the blood vary within only a small range. Amounts of other hormones change suddenly in response to certain stimuli. For example, epinephrine is released in large amounts in response to stress or exercise; its concentration therefore can change quite dramatically. Still other hormone levels change in fairly constant cycles. Reproductive hormones, for example, increase and decrease cyclically in women during their reproductive years.

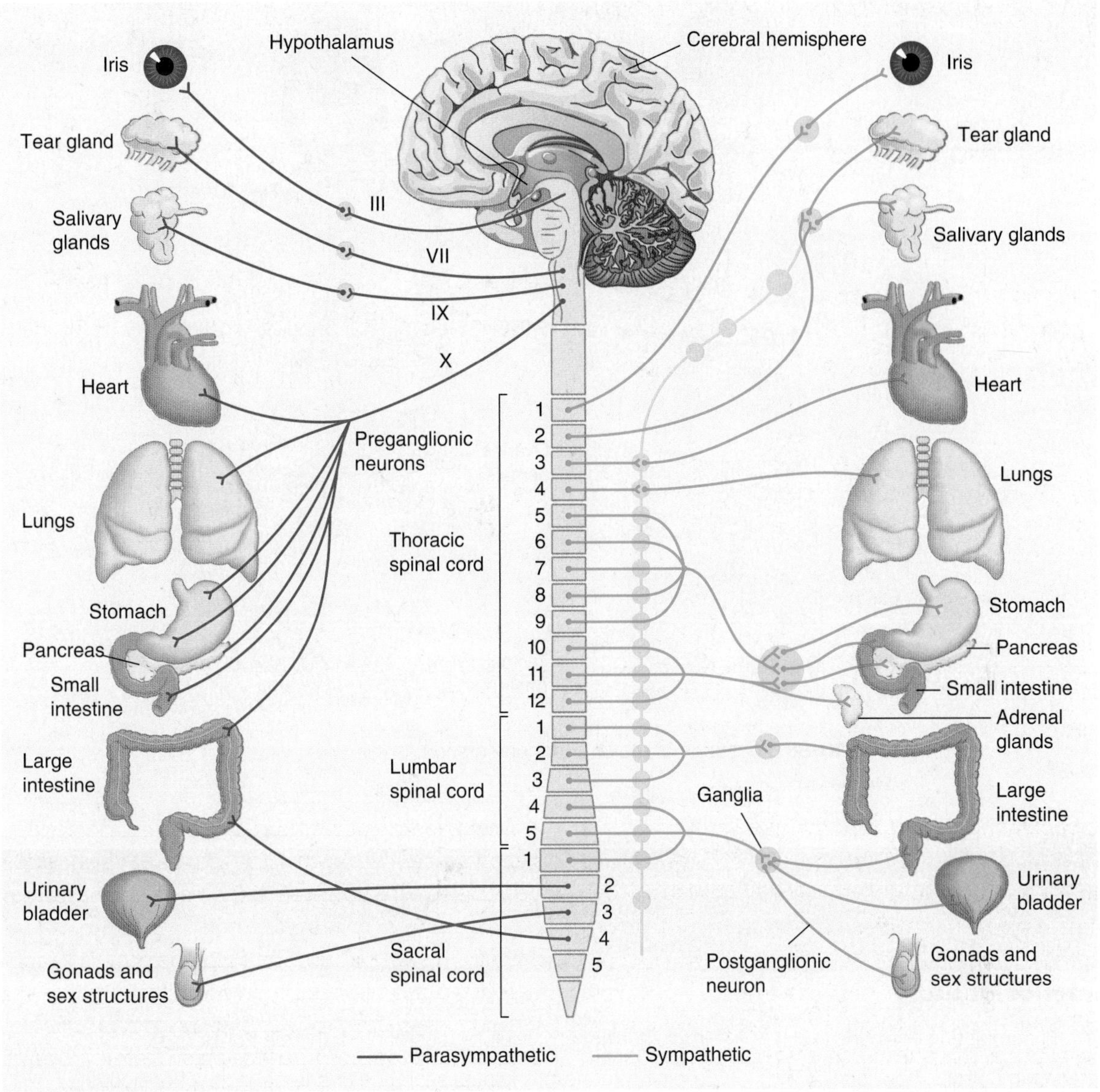

FIGURE 10-37 Innervation of major target organs by the autonomic nervous system. The parasympathetic fibers are highlighted in red, and the sympathetic fibers are highlighted in blue.

Circulatory System

The blood vessels found throughout the body carry blood to and from all tissues. Blood performs a number of important functions: (1) It transports nutrients and oxygen to tissues, (2) it carries carbon dioxide and waste products away from tissues, (3) it carries hormones produced in the endocrine glands to their target tissues, (4) it plays a key role in temperature regulation and fluid balance, and (5) it protects the body from bacteria and foreign substances. These and other functions of blood help to maintain homeostasis.

Blood Components

Blood is a special form of connective tissue that consists of cells and cell fragments (*formed elements*) surrounded by a liquid intercellular matrix (plasma). Approximately 95% of the volume of formed elements consists of red blood cells (erythrocytes). The remaining 5% consists of white blood cells (leukocytes) and cell fragments called *platelets*.

Plasma. Plasma is a pale yellow fluid composed of approximately 92% water and 8% dissolved or

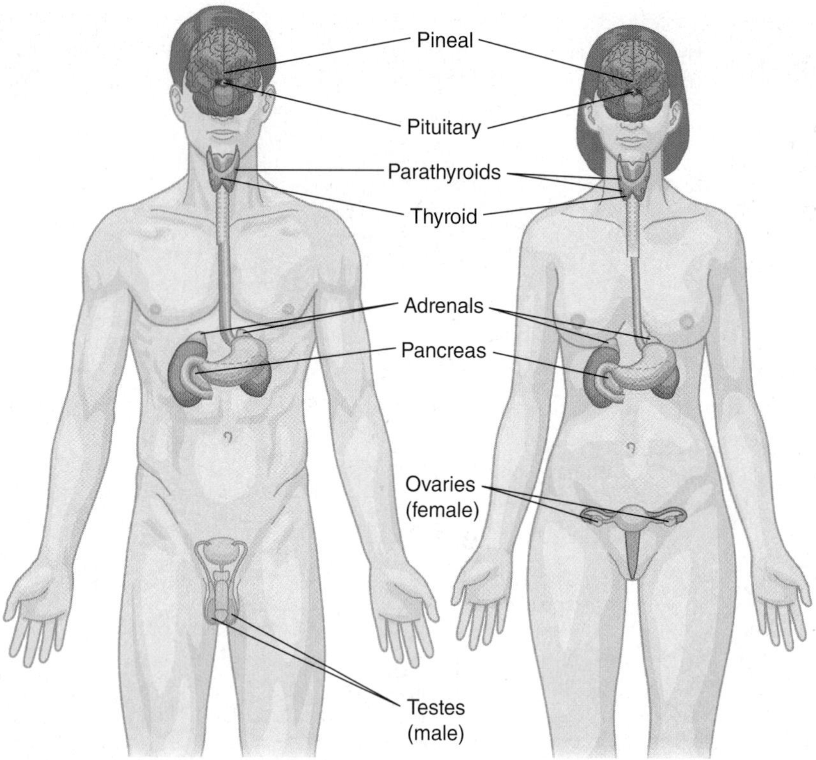

FIGURE 10-38 Locations of major endocrine glands.

TABLE 10-9 Endocrine Glands, Hormones, and Their Functions

Gland/Hormone	Function
Anterior Pituitary	
Thyroid-stimulating hormone (TSH)	Tropic hormone; stimulates secretion of thyroid hormones
Adrenocorticotropic hormone (ACTH)	Tropic hormone; stimulates secretion of adrenal cortex hormones
Follicle-stimulating hormone (FSH)	Tropic hormone *Female:* Stimulates development of ovarian follicles and secretion of estrogens *Male:* Stimulates seminiferous tubules of testes to grow and produce sperm
Luteinizing hormone (LH)	Tropic hormone *Female:* Stimulates maturation of ovarian follicle and ovum; stimulates secretion of estrogen; triggers ovulation; stimulates development of corpus luteum (luteinization) *Male:* Stimulates interstitial cells of the testes to secrete testosterone
Melanocyte-stimulating hormone	Stimulates synthesis and dispersion of melanin pigment in the skin
Growth hormone	Stimulates growth in all organs; mobilizes food molecules, causing an increase in blood glucose concentration
Prolactin (lactogenic hormone)	Stimulates breast development during pregnancy and milk secretion after pregnancy
Posterior Pituitary[a]	
Antidiuretic hormone (ADH)	Stimulates retention of water by the kidneys and helps to maintain water metabolism by conserving body water and reducing the loss of water in urine
Oxytocin	Stimulates uterine contractions at the end of pregnancy; stimulates the release of milk into the breast ducts

TABLE 10-9 Endocrine Glands, Hormones, and Their Functions *(continued)*

Gland/Hormone	Function
Hypothalamus	
Releasing hormones (several)	Stimulate the anterior pituitary to release hormones
Inhibiting hormones (several)	Inhibit secretion of hormones by the anterior pituitary
Thyroid	
Thyroxine (T_4), triiodothyronine (T_3)	Stimulate the energy metabolism of all cells
Calcitonin	Inhibits the breakdown of bone; decreases blood calcium concentration
Parathyroid	
Parathyroid hormone (PTH)	Stimulates the breakdown of bone; causes an increase in blood calcium concentration
Adrenal Cortex	
Mineralocorticoids: aldosterone	Regulate electrolyte and fluid homeostasis
Glucocorticoids: cortisol (hydrocortisone)	Stimulate gluconeogenesis, causing an increase in blood glucose concentration; also have anti-inflammatory, anti-immunity, and antiallergy effects
Sex hormones (androgens)	Stimulate sexual drive in the female but have negligible effects in the male
Adrenal Medulla	
Epinephrine (adrenaline), norepinephrine	Prolong and intensify the sympathetic nervous response during stress
Pancreatic Islets	
Glucagon	Stimulates liver glycogenolysis, increasing the blood glucose concentration
Insulin	Promotes glucose entry into all cells, decreasing the blood glucose concentration
Ovary	
Estrogens	Promote development and maintenance of female sexual characteristics
Progesterone	Promotes conditions required for pregnancy
Testis	
Testosterone	Promotes development and maintenance of male sexual characteristics
Thymus	
Thymosin	Promotes development of immune system cells
Placenta	
Chorionic gonadotropin, estrogens, progesterone	Promote conditions required during early pregnancy
Pineal	
Melatonin	Inhibits tropic hormones that affect the ovaries; may be involved with the internal clock of the body
Heart (Atria)	
Atrial natriuretic hormone (ANF)	Regulates fluid and electrolyte homeostasis

[a]Posterior pituitary hormones are synthesized in the hypothalamus but are released from axon terminals in the posterior pituitary.

TABLE 10-10 Classes of Blood Cells

Cell Type	Function
Erythrocyte	Oxygen and carbon dioxide transport
Neutrophil	Immune defenses (phagocytosis)
Eosinophil	Defense against parasites
Basophil	Inflammatory response
B lymphocyte	Antibody production (precursor of plasma cells)
T lymphocyte	Cellular immune response
Monocyte	Immune defenses (phagocytosis)
Platelet	Blood clotting

suspended molecules. Plasma contains proteins such as *albumin, globulins,* and *fibrinogen.* When the proteins that produce clots are removed from the plasma, the remaining fluid is called **serum**.

Formed Elements. Three formed elements of blood are erythrocytes, leukocytes, and platelets or thrombocytes (cell fragments) (**TABLE 10-10**). Formed elements are produced in the embryo and fetus. After birth, they are also produced in tissues such as the liver, thymus, spleen, lymph nodes, and red bone marrow.

Erythrocytes are the most numerous of the formed elements. One drop of male blood contains approximately 5.2 million erythrocytes; one drop of female blood contains approximately 4.5 million erythrocytes. The major erythrocyte contents include lipids, ATP, and the enzyme carbonic anhydrase. The main component of erythrocytes is **hemoglobin**, the protein that gives blood its red color. The primary functions of erythrocytes are to transport oxygen from the lungs to the various tissues of the body and to transport carbon dioxide from the tissues to the lungs. Under normal conditions, approximately 2.5 million erythrocytes are destroyed and replaced by the body each second. The average erythrocyte circulates for 120 days.

CRITICAL THINKING

If the number of erythrocytes drops, a person may become short of breath during mild exertion. Why does this happen?

Leukocytes are white blood cells that do not contain hemoglobin; thus, they have a clear appearance when viewed under a microscope. The several types of leukocytes play a role in guarding the body against invading microorganisms and removing dead cells and debris. Some leukocytes are grouped by their appearance—that is, based on the presence or absence of cytoplasmic granules. The granular leukocytes include neutrophils, eosinophils, and basophils. The nongranular leukocytes are named according to nuclear morphology and major site of proliferation; they include lymphocytes and monocytes.

- **Neutrophils** are the most common type of leukocyte in the blood. These cells normally remain in the circulation for 10 to 12 hours, then move into tissues to seek out and destroy bacteria and other foreign matter—a process called **phagocytosis**. Neutrophils also secrete lysosomes that can destroy certain bacteria. Neutrophils usually survive for 1 to 2 days after leaving the circulation.
- **Eosinophils** leave the circulation and enter the tissues during an inflammatory reaction. Their numbers usually are elevated in the blood of people with allergies and certain parasitic infections. These cells have phagocytic properties but play a less important role in this regard compared to neutrophils.
- **Basophils** are the least common of all leukocytes. Like eosinophils, basophils leave the circulation and migrate through tissues (where they are called mast cells) to play a role in allergic and inflammatory reactions. In addition, they release *heparin,* which inhibits blood clotting. Basophils also release **histamine**, which is important to the **inflammatory response** (see Chapter 2, *Well-Being of the Paramedic*).
- **Lymphocytes** are the smallest of all leukocytes. They are capable of migrating through the cytoplasm of other cells. The many different types of lymphocytes play a major role in immunity, including antibody production. Lymphocytes originate in bone marrow and are most abundant in lymphoid tissues—that is, the **lymph nodes**, **spleen**, **tonsils**, **lymph nodules**, and **thymus**.
- **Monocytes** are the largest of the leukocytes. They remain in the circulation for about 3 days before changing into **macrophages**. These large "eating" cells migrate through various tissues. An increase in the number of monocytes is common in patients with chronic infections.

Platelets are cell fragments that are produced in bone marrow. They are 40 times as common in blood as leukocytes. Platelets play a key role in preventing blood loss by forming plugs that seal holes in small vessels and by forming clots that seal off larger wounds in the vessels.

Cardiovascular System

The heart and cardiovascular system are responsible for circulating blood throughout the body. The cardiovascular system is discussed in detail in Chapter 21, *Cardiology*.

The heart is a muscular pump consisting of four chambers—two **atria** and two **ventricles**. The adult heart is shaped like a blunt cone and is about the size of a closed fist. The blunt, rounded point of the heart is the *apex*, and the larger, flat portion at the opposite end is the *base*.

The heart lies obliquely in the mediastinum of the thoracic cavity in the pericardial cavity. The base is directed posteriorly and slightly superiorly. The apex is directed anteriorly and slightly inferiorly. Two-thirds of the mass of the heart lies to the left of the midline of the sternum (**FIGURE 10-39**).

Pericardium. The pericardium, or **pericardial sac**, surrounds the heart. It has a fibrous outer layer (fibrous pericardium) and a thin inner layer (serous pericardium). The portion of the serous pericardium that lines the fibrous pericardium is the parietal pericardium; the portion that covers the heart surface is the visceral pericardium (**epicardium**). The cavity between the parietal pericardium and the visceral pericardium normally contains a small amount of pericardial fluid, which reduces friction as the heart moves within the pericardial sac.

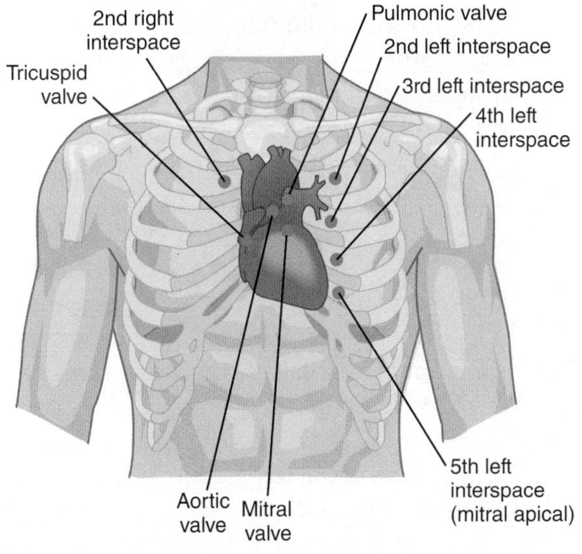

FIGURE 10-39 Location of the heart in the thorax.

> CRITICAL THINKING
> Why would a sudden increase in the amount of pericardial fluid be harmful?

Coronary Vessels. Seven large veins normally carry blood to the heart: Four **pulmonary veins** carry blood from the lungs to the left atrium, the **superior vena cava** and **inferior vena cava** carry blood from the body to the right atrium, and the coronary sinus carries blood from the walls of the heart to the right atrium. Two arteries, the aorta and the pulmonary trunk, exit the heart. The **aorta** carries blood from the left ventricle to the body; the **pulmonary trunk** carries blood from the right ventricle to the lungs. The right and left **coronary arteries**, which exit the aorta near the point where the aorta leaves the heart, supply the heart muscle with oxygen and nutrients (**FIGURE 10-40**).

Heart Chambers and Valves. The right and left chambers of the heart are separated by a **septum**. The interatrial septum separates the **right atrium** and the **left atrium**. The interventricular septum separates the two ventricles. The atria open into the ventricles through the atrioventricular canals. An **atrioventricular valve** on each atrioventricular canal is composed of cusps or flaps. These valves allow blood to flow from the atria into the ventricles, while preventing blood from flowing back into the atria. The atrioventricular valve between the right atrium and right ventricle has three cusps; it is called the **tricuspid valve**. The atrioventricular valve between the left atrium and left ventricle has two cusps; it is called the **bicuspid valve** (or mitral valve). Heart chambers and valves are shown in **FIGURE 10-41**.

The aorta and pulmonary trunk possess both aortic and pulmonary semilunar valves. These valves meet in the center of the artery to block blood flow. Blood flowing out of the ventricles pushes against each valve, forcing it open. However, when blood flows back from the aorta or pulmonary trunk toward the ventricles, the valves close.

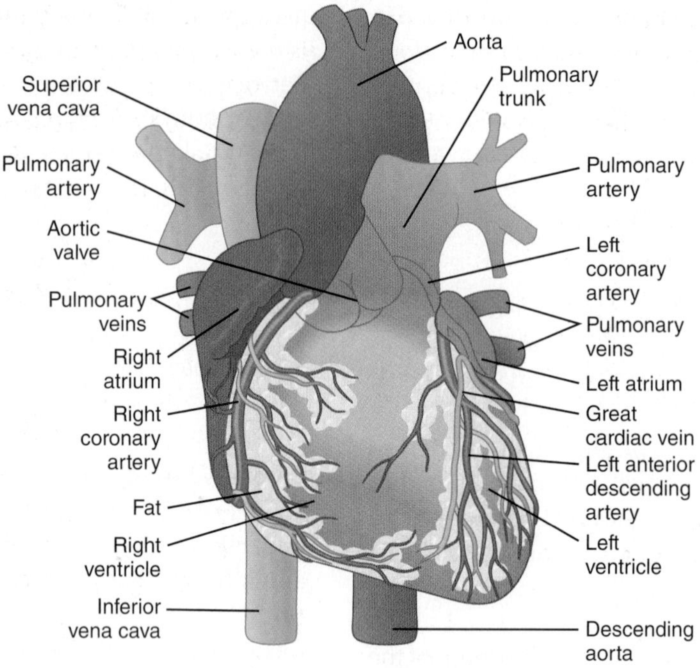

FIGURE 10-40 Anterior surface of the heart.

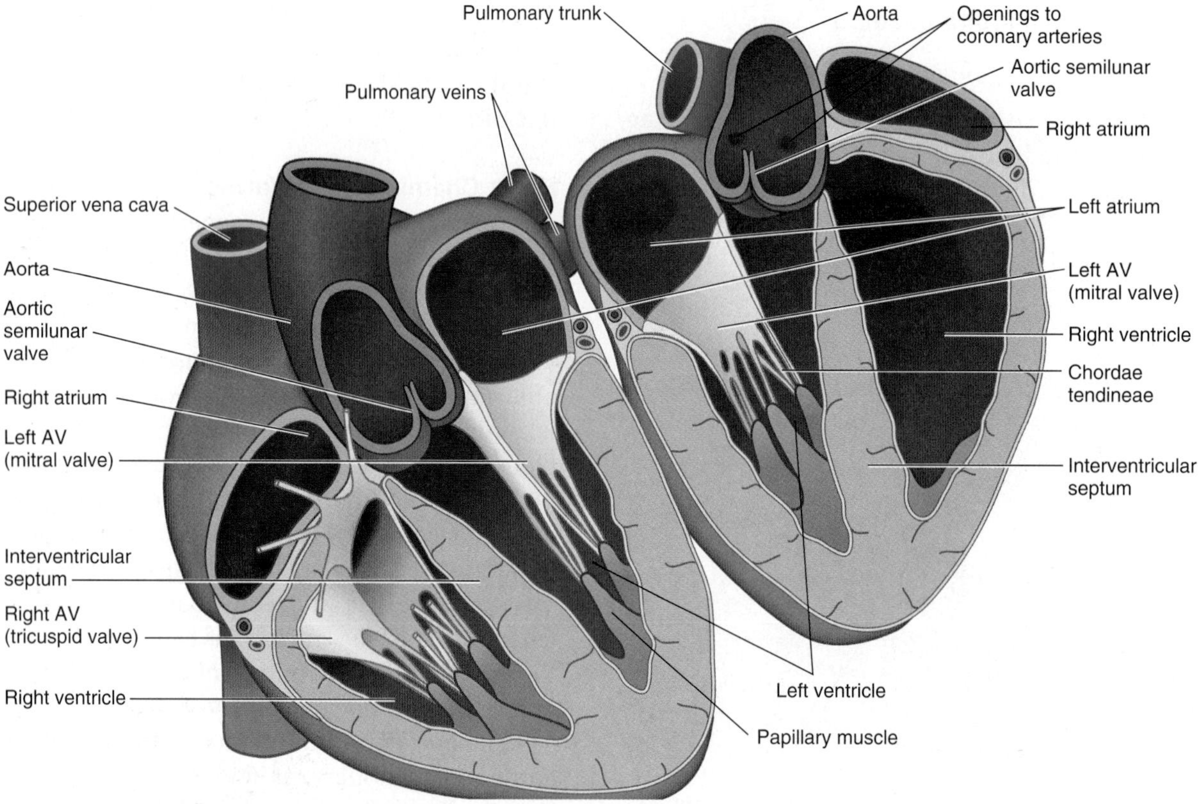

Abbreviation: AV, atrioventricular

FIGURE 10-41 Internal view of the heart.

Conduction System of the Heart. The muscle tissue of the heart has the unique ability to engage in spontaneous, rhythmic self-excitation. This excitation occurs by way of four structures embedded in the wall of the heart: the **sinoatrial node**, the **atrioventricular node**, the **bundle of His**, and the **Purkinje fibers** (**FIGURE 10-42**).

Impulse conduction normally begins in the sinoatrial node. From there, the impulse spreads in all directions through both of the atria, causing an atrial contraction. As the electrical impulses reach the atrioventricular node, they are relayed to the ventricles through the bundle of His and the Purkinje fibers. This impulse conduction causes both of the ventricles to contract shortly after the atrial contraction.

Route of Blood Flow Through the Heart. This text presents blood flow through the heart by discussing right and left heart circulation (**FIGURE 10-43**). It is important to remember that both atria contract at the same time, with the contraction being followed shortly thereafter by essentially simultaneous contraction of both ventricles. This knowledge is key to understanding clearly the electrical impulses of the heart, pressure changes, and heart sounds that are discussed in other chapters.

Blood enters the right atrium from the systemic circulation via the inferior and superior venae cavae; it enters from the heart muscle via the coronary sinus. Most of this blood passes into the right ventricle as the ventricle relaxes after the previous contraction. When the right atrium contracts, the blood remaining in the atrium is pushed into the ventricle. The contraction of the right ventricle pushes blood against the tricuspid valve, forcing it to close. The contraction also pushes blood against the pulmonary semilunar valve, forcing this valve to open. This flow allows blood to enter the pulmonary trunk. The pulmonary trunk divides into left and right pulmonary arteries that carry blood to the lungs. In the lungs, the blood releases carbon dioxide and picks up oxygen.

> CRITICAL THINKING
>
> A clot forms in the right atrium of the heart. Will it be circulated to the extremities? Why?

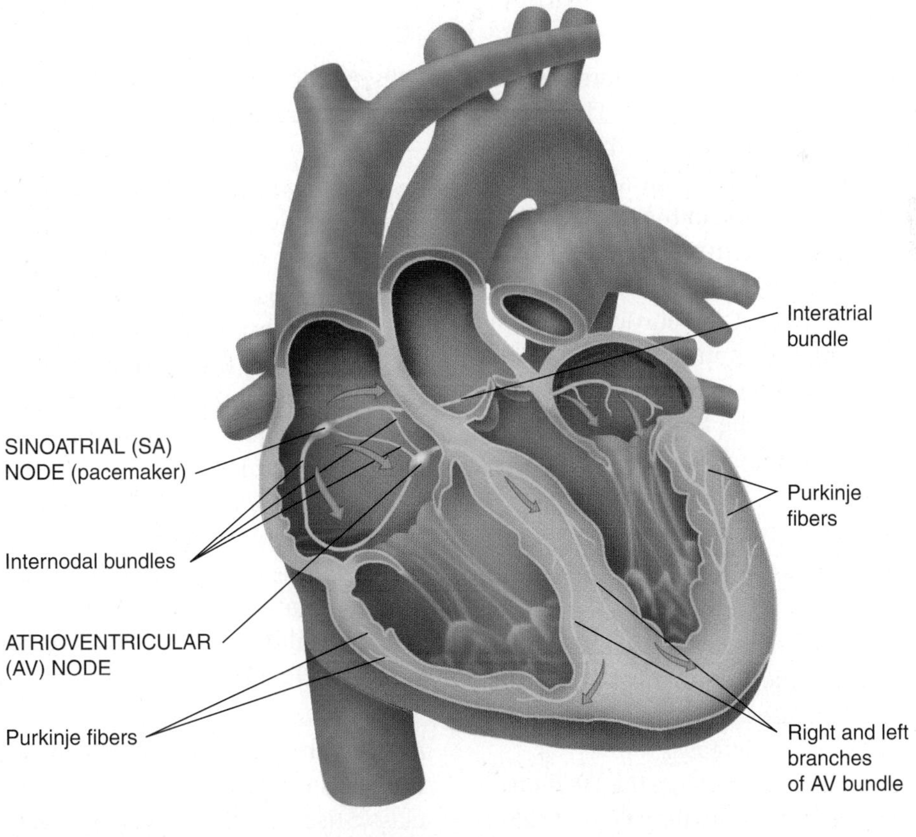

FIGURE 10-42 Conduction system of the heart.

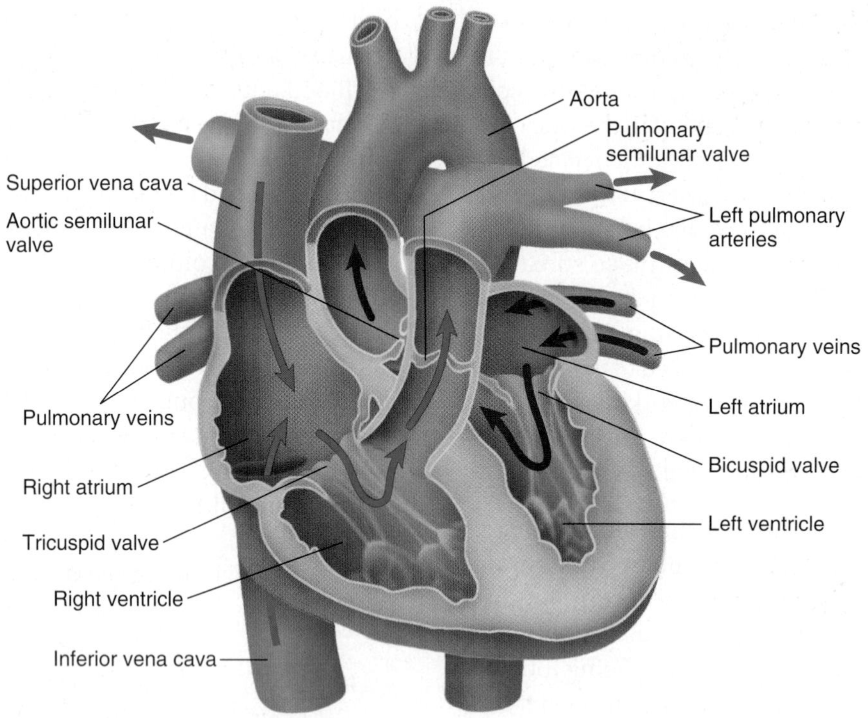

FIGURE 10-43 Frontal section of the heart showing the four chambers and the direction of blood flow through the heart.

Blood returning from the lungs enters the left atrium through four pulmonary veins. The blood passing from the left atrium to the relaxed left ventricle opens the bicuspid valve. The contraction of the left atrium completes the filling of the left ventricle.

Contraction of the left ventricle pushes blood against the bicuspid valve, closing this valve. The pressure of the blood against the aortic semilunar valve causes it to open, which in turn allows blood to enter the aorta. Blood flowing through the aorta is distributed to all parts of the body except for the pulmonary vessels in the lungs.

Peripheral Circulation

Blood is pumped from the ventricles of the heart into large elastic arteries. These arteries branch repeatedly to form many gradually smaller arteries. As these vessels become smaller, the amount of elastic tissue in the arterial wall decreases. At the same time, the amount of smooth muscle increases.

Blood flows from the **arterioles** into the **capillaries**, and then from these capillaries into the venous system. Compared with artery walls, vein walls are thinner and contain less elastic tissue and fewer smooth muscle cells. As veins approach the heart, the walls increase in diameter and thickness.

Capillary Network. Arterioles supply blood to each capillary network (**FIGURE 10-44**). Blood flows through this network and into the venules. The ends of the capillaries closest to arterioles are arterial capillaries; the ends closest to venules are venous capillaries.

Blood flow through arterioles may continue through metarterioles (which are short vessels that connect arterioles to capillaries; also referred to as arterial capillaries) and into a thoroughfare channel to a venule in a relatively constant way; alternatively, blood may enter the capillary circulation. Flow in the capillaries is regulated by smooth muscle cells known as **precapillary sphincters**. The major role of the capillaries is the exchange of nutrients and waste products.

Arteries and Veins. Except in capillaries and venules, the walls of blood vessels consist of three layers of elastic tissue and smooth muscle; each is known as a **tunic**. The three layers are the tunica intima (inner layer), the tunica media (middle layer), and the tunica

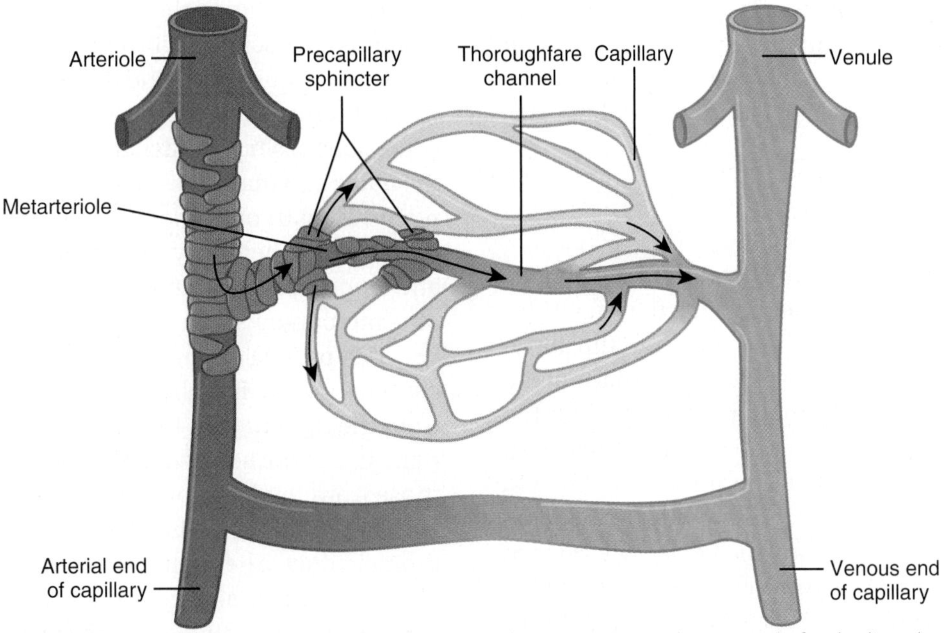

FIGURE 10-44 Capillary network. The metarteriole, giving rise to the network, feeds directly from the arteriole into the thoroughfare channel, which feeds into the venule. The network forms numerous branches that transport blood from the thoroughfare channel and may return to the thoroughfare channel.

adventitia (outer layer). The thickness and composition of each layer vary with the type and diameter of the blood vessel.

Large elastic arteries often are called conducting arteries, because they have the largest diameter. These vessels have more elastic tissue and less smooth muscle than do any other arteries. Medium and small arteries have fairly thick muscular walls and well-developed elastic membranes. These vessels are called distributing arteries because the smooth muscle allows these vessels partially to regulate blood supply to various body regions, through the processes of constriction and dilation. Arterioles are the smallest arteries in which the three tunics can be detected. Like small arteries, arterioles can vasodilate and vasoconstrict.

Venules have only a few isolated smooth muscle cells and are similar in structure to the capillaries. These vessels collect blood from the capillaries and transport it to small veins, which in turn transport the blood to the medium-size veins. Nutrient exchange occurs across the walls of the venules, but as the small veins increase in thickness, the degree of nutrient exchange decreases.

As venules increase in diameter, the vessels become veins whose walls consist of a continuous layer of smooth muscle cells. Medium-size and large veins collect blood from small veins and deliver it to the large venous trunks. Large veins transport blood from the medium-size veins to the heart.

Large-diameter veins have valves that allow blood to flow to, but not from, the heart. Medium-size veins have many valves, and the veins of the lower extremities have more valves than do those of the upper extremities. These valves help prevent the backflow of blood, especially in dependent tissues.

Arteriovenous anastomoses allow blood to flow from arteries to veins without passing through capillaries. Natural arteriovenous shunts occur in large numbers in the soles of the feet, the palms, and the nail beds, where they regulate body temperature. Pathologic shunts can result from injury or tumors. These shunts can cause a direct flow of blood from arteries to veins. Severe shunts may lead to "high-output" heart failure from increased venous return to the heart and its resultant demand on **cardiac output** (see Chapter 21, *Cardiology*).

Pulmonary Circulation

Blood from the right ventricle is pumped into the pulmonary trunk. This trunk splits into the right and left pulmonary arteries, which move blood to the respective lungs, where oxygen and carbon dioxide are exchanged. Two pulmonary veins exit each lung and enter the left atrium; they are the only veins in the body that carry oxygenated blood. Pulmonary arteries are the only arteries in the body that carry deoxygenated blood.

Systemic Circulation

Oxygenated blood enters the heart from the pulmonary veins. The blood passes through the left atrium first into the left ventricle, and then into the aorta. From the aorta, blood is distributed to all parts of the body. The arteries of systemic circulation include the aorta, coronary arteries, arteries of the head and neck, arteries of the upper and lower limbs, the thoracic aorta and its branches, the **abdominal aorta** and its branches, and the arteries of the pelvis. The veins of systemic circulation include coronary veins, veins of the head and neck, veins of the upper and lower limbs, veins of the thorax, veins of the abdomen and pelvis, and the hepatic portal system, which transports blood from the digestive tract to the liver (**FIGURE 10-45**).

Lymphatic System

The **lymphatic system** includes lymph, lymphocytes, lymph nodes, tonsils, the spleen, and the thymus gland. It is considered part of the circulatory system because it consists of a moving fluid that comes from the body and returns to the blood. Unlike the circulatory system, the lymphatic system carries fluid only away from the tissues. It has three basic functions: (1) to help maintain fluid balance in tissues, (2) to absorb fats and other substances from the digestive tract, and (3) to act as part of the body's immune defense system.

The lymphatic system begins in the tissues as lymph capillaries. Unlike blood capillaries, lymph capillaries contain a series of one-way valves, which allow fluid to enter the capillary but prevent fluid from passing back into the interstitial spaces. Almost all body tissues have lymph capillaries; the exceptions are the CNS, bone marrow, and tissues without blood vessels (eg, cartilage, epidermis, and cornea). Lymph capillaries join to form larger lymph capillaries that resemble small veins.

Lymph nodes are distributed along various lymph vessels. Most lymph passes through at least one such node before entering the blood. The node filters the lymph as it passes through, removing microorganisms and foreign substances, and thereby preventing them from entering the general circulation. Three major collections of lymph nodes are located on each side of the body: inguinal nodes, axillary nodes, and cervical nodes. If a part of the body is inflamed or otherwise diseased, the nearby lymph nodes become swollen and tender as they accumulate—and limit the spread of—microorganisms and foreign substances.

After passing through lymph nodes, lymph vessels converge toward the right or left **subclavian vein**. Vessels from the right thorax, the upper right limb, and the right side of the head enter the right lymphatic duct; those from the left thorax, the left upper extremity, and the left side of the head and neck enter the larger thoracic duct. The right lymphatic duct opens into the right subclavian vein, whereas the thoracic duct ends by entering the left subclavian vein. All fluid drained from the tissue spaces eventually returns to the venous circulation.

Lymph serves a unique transport role, in that it returns tissue fluid, proteins, fats, and other substances to the general circulation. The lymphatic system does not form a closed ring or circuit, as does the true circulatory system. Once lymph has formed, it flows only once through its system of lymphatic vessels before draining into the right and left subclavian veins.

> CRITICAL THINKING
> Why might a chronic cocaine abuser have a higher risk of sinus infection?

Respiratory System

Oxygen is a basic element needed for normal cell metabolism, while carbon dioxide is a major waste product of this process. The organs of the respiratory system and the cardiovascular system transport oxygen to individual cells and transport carbon dioxide from the cells to the lungs. In the lungs, the carbon dioxide is released into the air.

The respiratory system is a complex part of the human body. The aim of this section is to familiarize the paramedic student with the respiratory anatomy. (Further discussion of the respiratory system

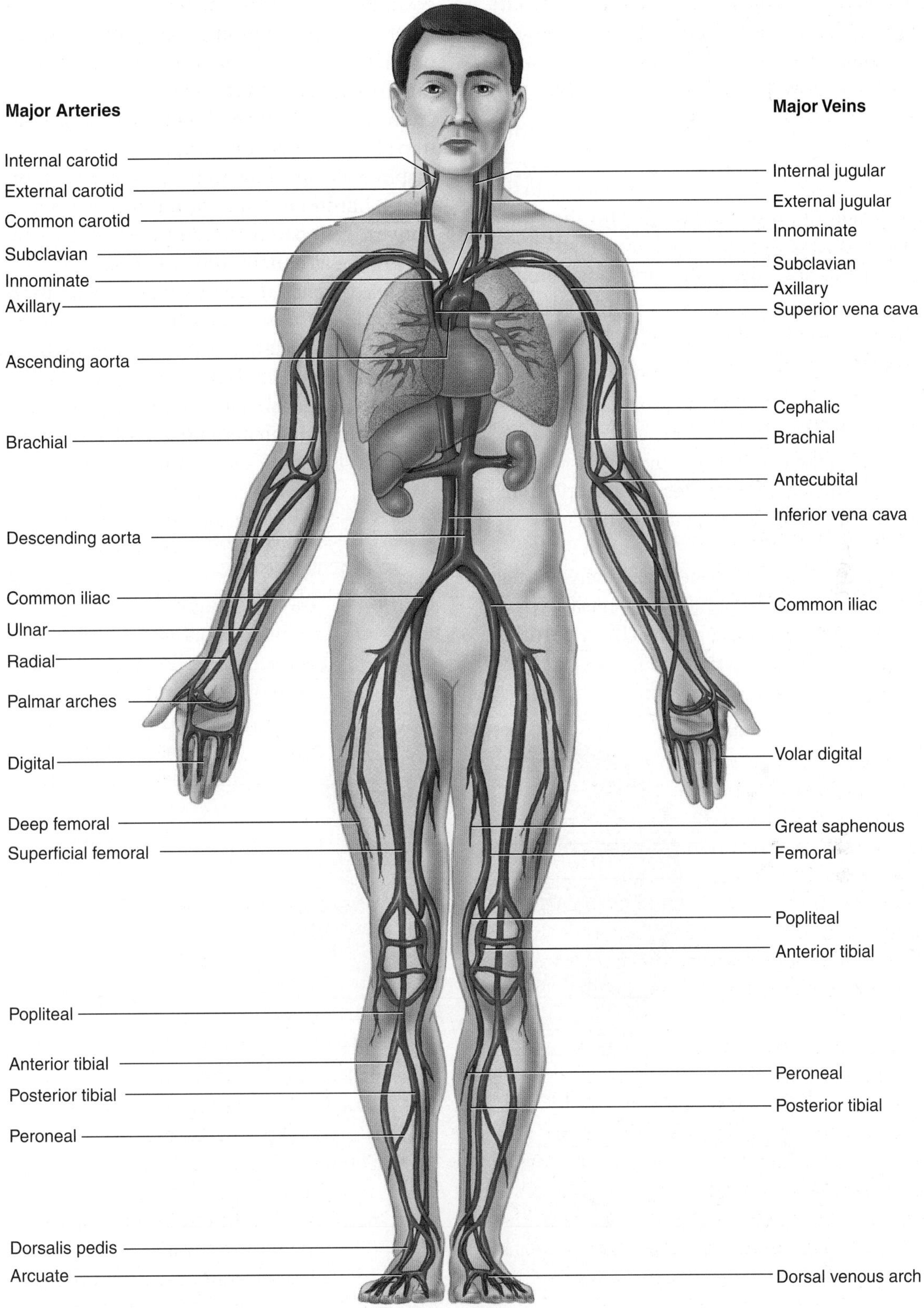

Major Arteries
Internal carotid
External carotid
Common carotid
Subclavian
Innominate
Axillary
Ascending aorta
Brachial
Descending aorta
Common iliac
Ulnar
Radial
Palmar arches
Digital
Deep femoral
Superficial femoral
Popliteal
Anterior tibial
Posterior tibial
Peroneal
Dorsalis pedis
Arcuate
Major Veins
Internal jugular
External jugular
Innominate
Subclavian
Axillary
Superior vena cava
Cephalic
Brachial
Antecubital
Inferior vena cava
Common iliac
Volar digital
Great saphenous
Femoral
Popliteal
Anterior tibial
Peroneal
Posterior tibial
Dorsal venous arch

FIGURE 10-45 Principal arteries and veins of the body.

is presented in Chapter 15, *Airway Management, Respiration, and Artificial Ventilation.*)

Airway Anatomy

The structures of the respiratory system are divided into the upper airway and the lower airway—a classification based on their locations relative to the **glottic opening** (ie, the vocal cords and the space between them). For the purpose of this text, all airway structures above the glottis are considered to be part of the upper airway. All structures below the glottis are considered to be part of the lower airway (**FIGURE 10-46**).

Upper Airway Structures

The entrance to the respiratory tract begins with the nasal cavity. This cavity includes the nasopharynx, oropharynx, laryngopharynx, and larynx.

Nasopharynx. Air passes into the nasal cavity through the nostrils, or nares. The right and left nasal cavities are separated by the nasal septum, a bony partition covered with a mucous membrane. This membrane has a rich blood supply that warms and humidifies the nasal lining and the inspired air as it passes through the nose. Inside each nostril, a slight enlargement, known as the vestibule, is lined with coarse hairs that trap foreign substances carried into the nasal cavity by inspired air. The floor of the nasal cavity is composed of the hard palate; the lateral walls are formed by bony ridges coated with respiratory mucosa, which are known as conchae or turbinates.

Two patches of yellow-gray tissue lie just beneath the bridge of the nose and make up the olfactory membranes. Located in the roof of the nasal cavity, these membranes contain the receptors for the sense of smell. The nasal cavities also connect to the middle ear cavities through the auditory (or eustachian) tubes.

CRITICAL THINKING

A woman has undergone a radical mastectomy (removal of breast and lymph tissue). Why might she have a chronically swollen arm?

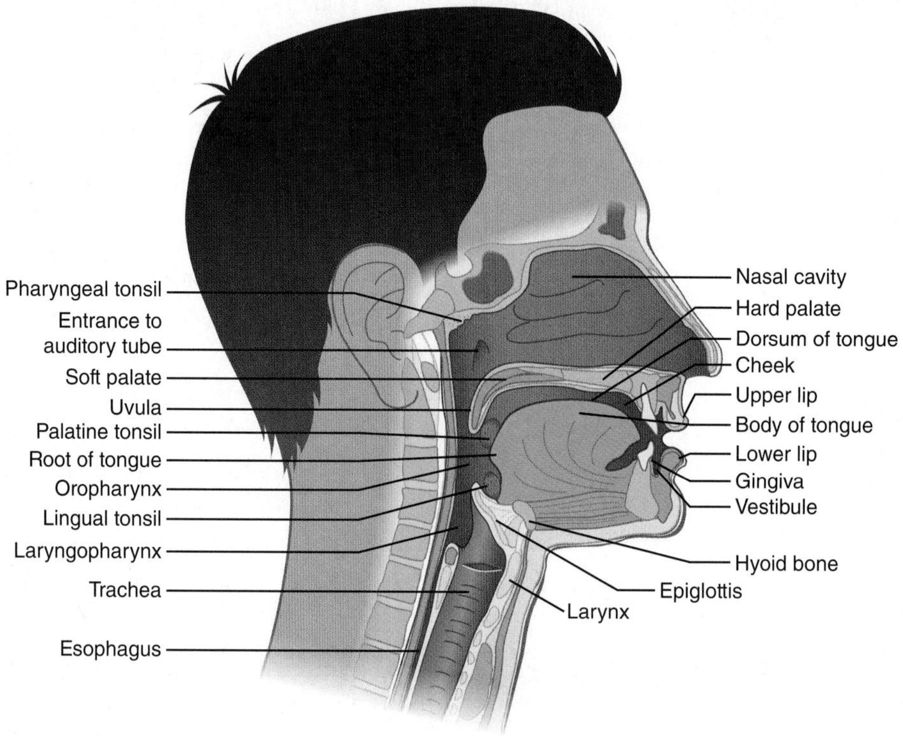

FIGURE 10-46 Airway structures.

Sinuses are cavities in the bones of the skull that connect to the nasal cavities by small channels (**FIGURE 10-47**). The four groups of sinuses, each of which is named for the skull bone in which it lies, are the frontal sinuses, above the eyebrows; the maxillary sinuses (the largest sinuses), in the cheekbones; the ethmoid sinuses, just behind the bridge of the nose; and the sphenoid sinuses, in a bone that cradles the brain, slightly anterior to the **pituitary gland**. These hollow chambers are lined with mucous membranes that secrete mucus into the nasal cavities. They are thought to help add resonance to the voice and to reduce the weight of the skull.

The back of each nasal cavity opens into the nasopharynx—the superior part of the pharynx. The nasopharynx extends from the internal nares to the level of the **uvula**. Like the nasal cavity, the nasopharynx is lined with mucous membrane.

Oropharynx. At the level of the uvula, the nasopharynx ends and the oropharynx begins. The oropharynx extends down to the level of the **epiglottis**. Anteriorly, the oropharynx opens into the oral cavity, which consists of the lips, cheeks, teeth, tongue (which is attached to the mandible), hard and soft palates, and palatine tonsils. The palatine tonsils and the pharyngeal tonsils (located in the roof and posterior wall of the nasopharynx) form a partial ring of lymphoid tissue that surrounds the respiratory tract. This ring is completed by the lingual tonsils, which lie on the floor of the oropharyngeal passageway at the base of the tongue.

Laryngopharynx. The **laryngopharynx** extends from the tip of the epiglottis to the glottis and the **esophagus**. It is lined with mucous membrane, which protects the internal surfaces from abrasion.

Larynx. The laryngopharynx opens into the **larynx**, which lies in the anterior neck (**FIGURE 10-48**). The larynx serves three main functions: (1) It is the air passageway between the pharynx and the trachea, (2) it is a protective sphincter that prevents solids and liquids from passing into the respiratory tree, and (3) it is involved in the production of speech.

The larynx consists of an outer casing of nine cartilages connected to each other by muscles and ligaments. Six of the nine cartilages are paired; three are unpaired. The largest, most superior of the cartilages is the unpaired thyroid cartilage, or Adam's apple. This prominence is hardly visible in children or adult females but is readily visible in males after

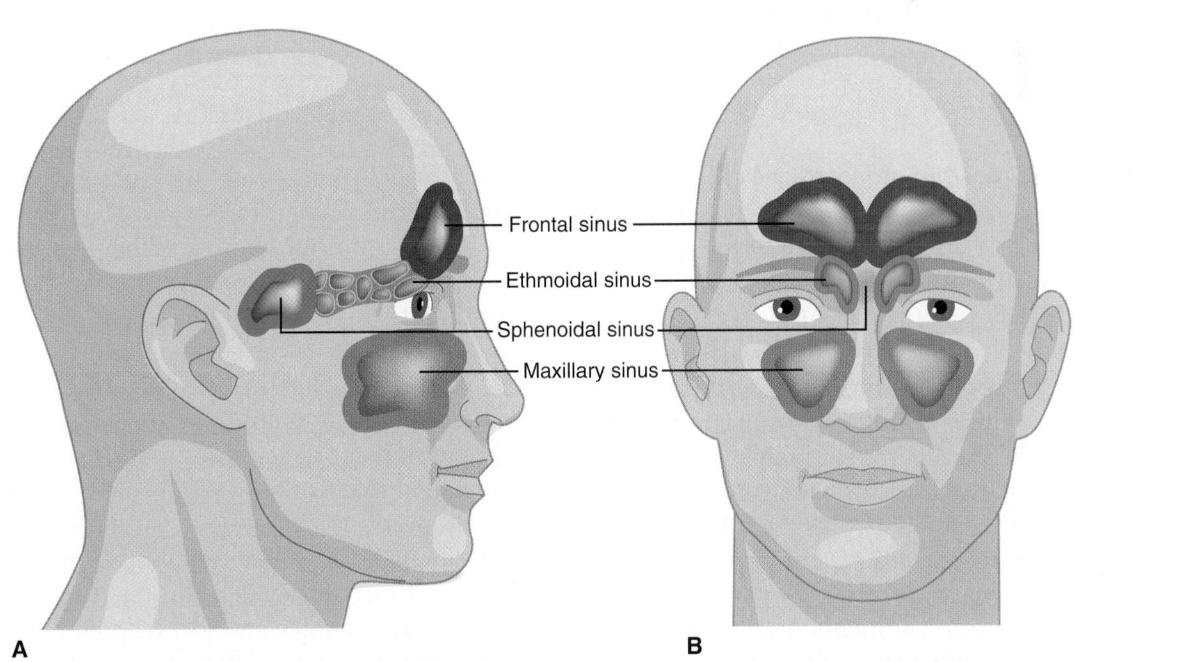

FIGURE 10-47 Paranasal sinuses. **A.** Side view. **B.** Front view.

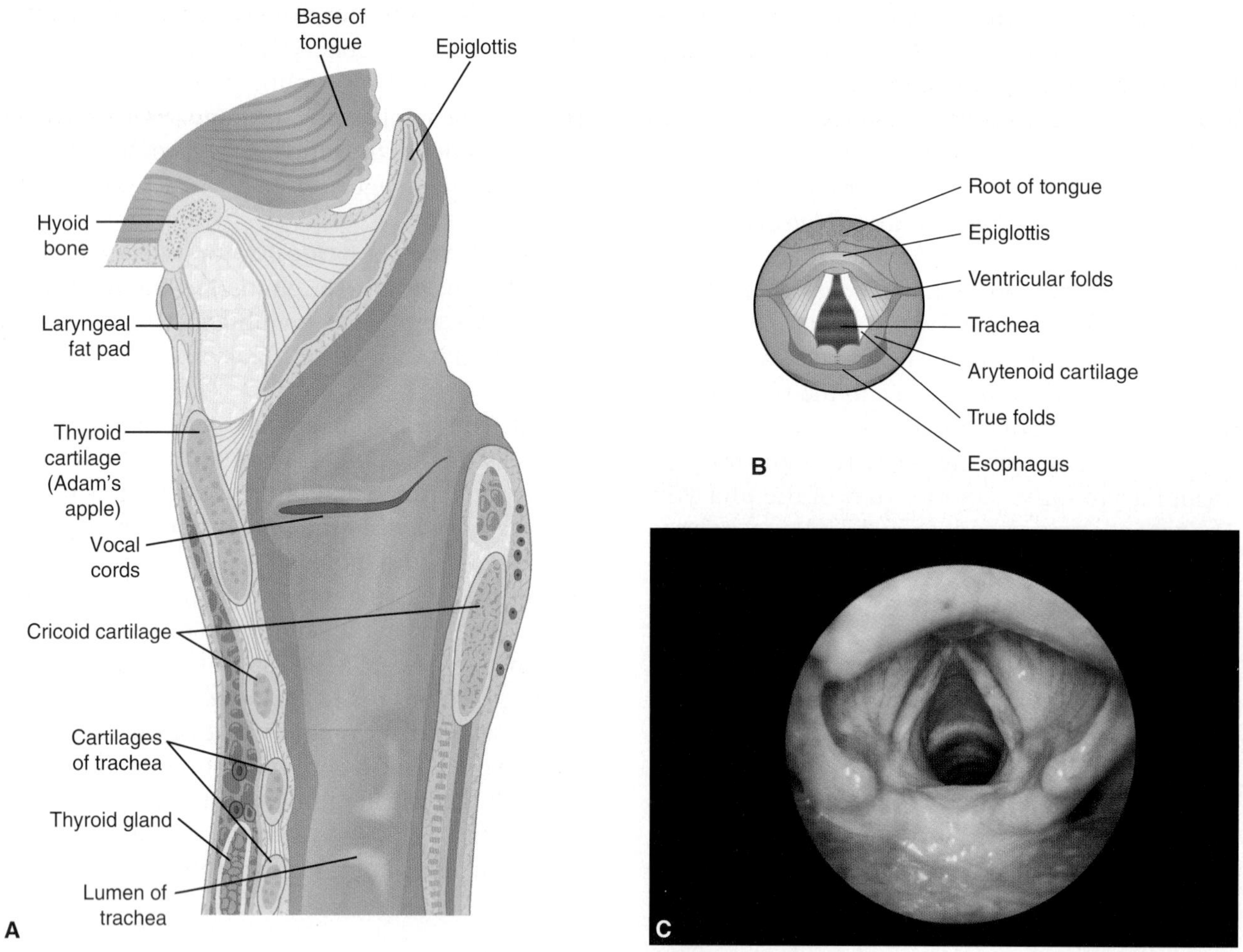

FIGURE 10-48 Larynx. **A.** Sagittal section. **B.** Superior view. **C.** View obtained with an endoscope.

puberty. The most inferior cartilage of the larynx is the unpaired **cricoid cartilage**. The only complete cartilaginous ring in the larynx, it forms the base of the larynx on which all other cartilages rest. The third unpaired cartilage is the epiglottis.

The six paired cartilages are stacked in two pillars between the cricoid cartilage and the thyroid cartilage. The largest, ladle-shaped, inferior cartilages are known as the arytenoid cartilages. The middle, horn-shaped pair are known as the corniculate cartilages. The smallest, wedge-shaped, most superior cartilages are known as the cuneiform cartilages.

The U-shaped hyoid bone is tucked beneath the mandible. As previously mentioned, the hyoid is the only bone of the human body that does not articulate with another bone. The hyoid bone helps to suspend the airway by anchoring the muscles (particularly those of the tongue) to the jaw. The fibrous membrane that joins the hyoid and the thyroid cartilage is called the **thyroid membrane**. The membrane joining the thyroid and cricoid cartilages is called the **cricothyroid membrane**.

Two pairs of ligaments extend from the anterior surface of the arytenoid to the posterior surface of the thyroid cartilage. The superior pair forms the vestibular folds, or false vocal cords, which are not involved directly in the production of voice sounds. The inferior pair of ligaments composes the **vocal cords**, or true vocal cords, which participate directly in the production of voice sounds. When a person talks, air expelled from the lungs rushes up the throat to the larynx. In the larynx, the air creates sound by vibrating the vocal cords. Muscles tighten the folds of the cords to produce the high-pitched tones and relax the cords to produce the deeper tones. The lips, tongue, and jaw further modify the sounds into intelligible words.

CRITICAL THINKING

Why can't a person talk when an endotracheal tube is correctly positioned in the trachea?

Lower Airway Structures

Below the glottis are the structures of the lower airway and lungs. These structures include the trachea, the bronchial tree (primary bronchi, secondary bronchi, and bronchioles), the alveoli, and the lungs (**FIGURE 10-49**).

Trachea. The trachea is the air passageway from the larynx to the lungs. It is composed of dense connective tissue and smooth muscle reinforced with 15 to 20 C-shaped pieces of cartilage that form an incomplete ring. This ring protects the trachea and maintains an open passage for air. The adult trachea is approximately 0.6 inch (1.5 cm) in diameter and 3.5 to 5.9 inches (9 to 15 cm) long.

NOTE

A centimeter is equal to 0.4 inch. One inch is equal to 2.54 cm.

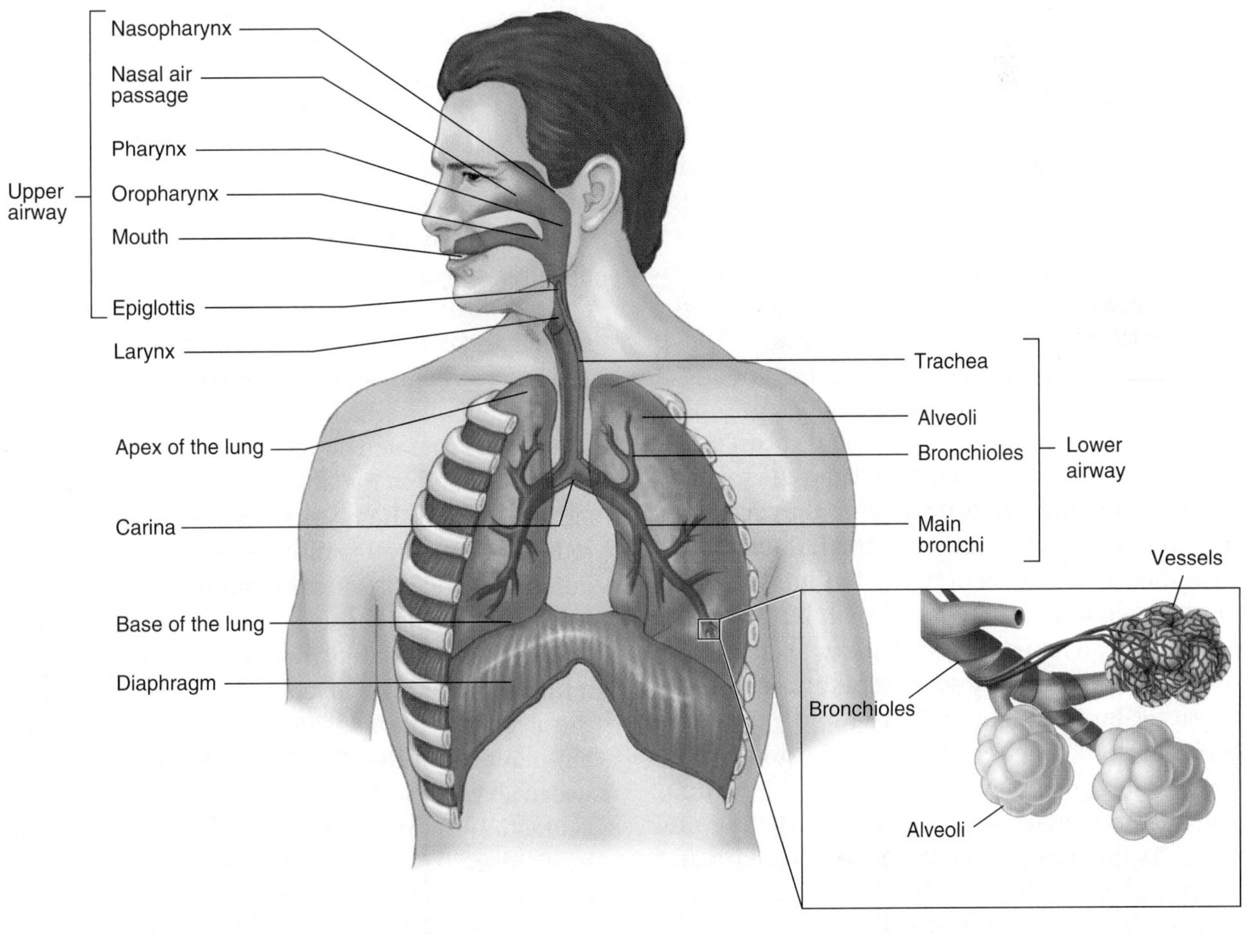

FIGURE 10-49 Structural plan of the respiratory system. The inset shows alveolar sacs; the exchange of oxygen and carbon dioxide takes place through the walls of the grapelike alveoli.

The trachea is located anterior to the esophagus and extends from the larynx to the fifth thoracic vertebra. It is lined with ciliated epithelium that contains many goblet cells. These cilia protect the lower airway by sweeping mucus, bacteria, and other small particles toward the larynx. At the larynx, the mucus and its contents may be expelled through coughing, or they may enter the esophagus, where they are swallowed and digested. Constant exposure to some irritants (eg, cigarette smoke) may produce a tracheal epithelium that lacks cilia and goblet cells. When this protective mechanism is disrupted, mucus and bacteria may contribute to disease.

Bronchial Tree. The lower airway may be thought of as resembling an inverted tree; the many subdivisions become narrower and shorter until they terminate at the alveoli. The large branches are primary bronchi, which divide into smaller secondary bronchi and bronchioles.

The trachea divides into the right and left primary bronchi at the level of the angle of Louis (the **sternomanubrial joint**). The point of bifurcation of the trachea into the right and left main stem bronchi is called the **carina**. The right primary bronchus is shorter, wider, and more vertical than its left counterpart. Like the trachea, the primary bronchi are lined with ciliated epithelium. They are supported by C-shaped cartilage rings. As the bronchi sequentially branch into smaller subdivisions, however, the amount of cartilage decreases. The bronchi also become more and more muscular until no cartilage is present.

The primary bronchi extend from the mediastinum to the lungs. They divide into the secondary bronchi as they enter the right and left lungs. Two secondary lobar bronchi in the left lung conduct air to its two lobes; three in the right lung conduct air to its three lobes. The secondary bronchi then divide into the tertiary segmental bronchi; there are 10 tertiary bronchi in the right lung and nine in the left lung. The tertiary bronchi extend to the individual segments of each lobe of the lung (lobule). The bronchial tree continues to branch several times. As the cartilage continues to decrease and the diameter is reduced to about 0.04 inch (1 mm), the bronchi become **bronchioles**.

CRITICAL THINKING

What is the benefit of having many bronchiole branches?

NOTE

One millimeter is equal to 0.04 inch. One inch is equal to 25.4 mm.

The walls of the bronchioles are devoid of cartilage. Their muscles are sensitive to certain circulating hormones, such as epinephrine. Contraction and relaxation of these muscles alter resistance to airflow. The bronchioles can constrict if the smooth muscle contracts forcefully—for example, during an asthma exacerbation.

Bronchioles continue to divide into ever-smaller passageways—first into terminal bronchioles and ultimately into respiratory bronchioles. Each respiratory bronchiole comprises a series of alveolar ducts, which end as grapelike clusters of tiny, hollow air sacs called alveoli. The exchange of oxygen and carbon dioxide in the lungs takes place in the alveoli (see Chapter 15, *Airway Management, Respiration, and Artificial Ventilation*).

Alveoli. The **alveoli**, which are the functional units of the respiratory system, are the main constituent of lung tissue. Collectively, the two lungs contain approximately 300 million alveoli. The wall of an alveolus consists of a single layer of epithelial cells and elastic fibers. These fibers permit the alveolus to stretch and contract during breathing.

Each alveolus is surrounded by a fine network of blood capillaries, which are arranged so that air in the alveolus is separated by a thin respiratory membrane from the blood in the alveolar capillaries. The large surface area of the respiratory membrane may be reduced by respiratory diseases, such as emphysema and lung cancer. As a consequence, such diseases restrict the exchange of oxygen and carbon dioxide.

Alveoli are coated with **pulmonary surfactant**, a thin film made by alveolar cells. This fluid keeps the alveoli from collapsing. In addition, pores in the alveolar membrane allow for a limited flow of air between alveoli. This collateral ventilation offers some protection for an alveolus that has been occluded by disease.

CRITICAL THINKING

One effect of toxic smoke inhalation is destruction of pulmonary surfactant. Why won't oxygen therapy alone always help? Which intervention might help?

Lungs. The lungs are large, paired, spongy organs; their main function is **respiration**. Although smooth muscle is present in the bronchioles of the lungs, the lungs actually expand and contract during the respiratory cycle as a result of the expansion of the thoracic cavity during inspiration and its elastic recoil during expiration. The lungs are attached to the heart by the pulmonary artery and veins. The two lungs are separated by the mediastinum and its contents (ie, the heart, blood vessels, trachea, esophagus, lymphatic tissues, and vessels). The point of entry for the bronchi, vessels, and nerves of each lung is known as the hilum, or root, of each lung.

At birth, the lungs are rose pink. By adulthood, however, they are slate gray with dark patches because of the particulate matter that is inhaled and deposited in the tissues. An adult lung weighs less than 2 pounds (0.9 kg).

Each lung is conical, with the base resting on the **diaphragm** and the apex extending to a point approximately 1 inch (2.5 cm) superior to each clavicle. The right lung is divided into three lobes. The left lung is slightly smaller than the right and is divided into two lobes. Each lobe is divided into lobules separated by connective tissue. Major blood vessels and bronchi do not cross this connective tissue, which can allow a diseased lobule to be removed surgically, leaving the remaining lung relatively intact. The left lung has 9 lobules, and the right lung has 10 lobules.

Each lung lies within a separate **pleural cavity**. The lungs are attached to each other only at the point of entry of the bronchi, vessels, and nerves of each lung (**FIGURE 10-50**). The two layers of the pleura (the visceral layer and the parietal layer) are so close that they are almost in contact with each other. The pleurae are separated by a thin fluid that acts as a lubricant, allowing the pleural membranes to slide past each other during respiration.

Between the two pleurae is a potential space known as the **pleural space**. When significant chest wall injury or a pathologic pulmonary condition occurs, the pleural space may become filled with air (pneumothorax) or blood (hemothorax). Another fluid that may accumulate in the pleural space—most commonly because of congestive heart failure—is transudates. By comparison, exudates can accumulate in this space as a result of infectious or malignant conditions.

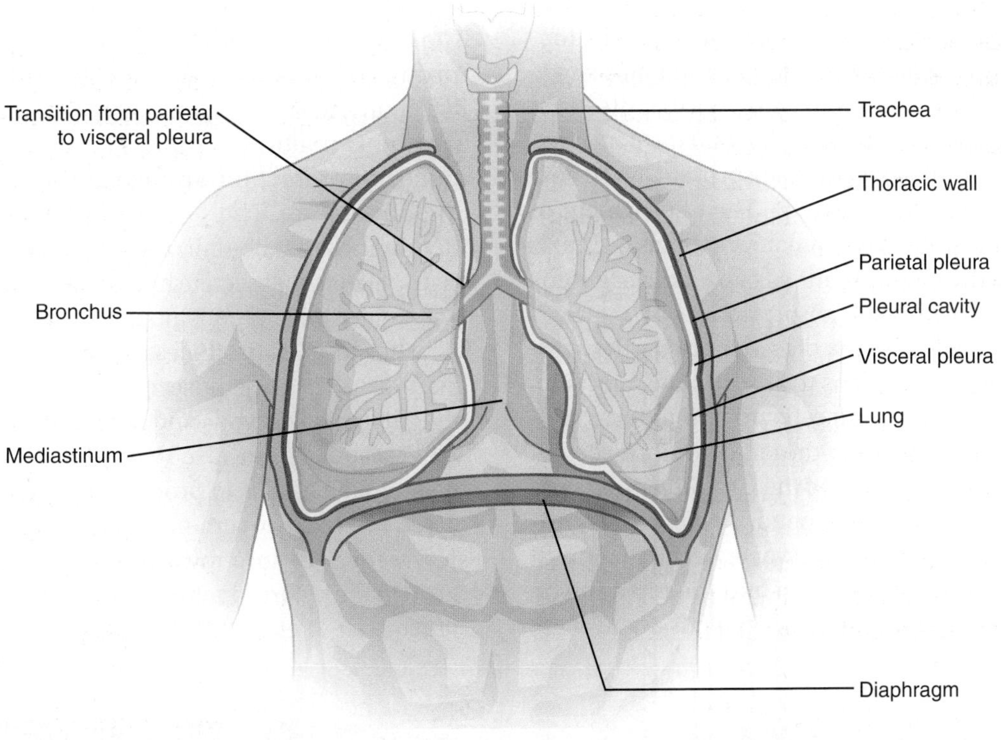

FIGURE 10-50 Lungs within the pleural cavities.

Digestive System

The digestive system provides the body with water, **electrolytes**, and other nutrients used by cells. To accomplish this task, the digestive system is specialized to ingest food. It propels this food through the gastrointestinal tract (digestive tract), with the nutrients from that food being absorbed across the wall of the lumen of the gastrointestinal tract. As food moves through the digestive system, secretions are added to liquefy and digest it. These secretions also provide lubrication for the food during its passage. The processes of secretion, movement, and absorption are regulated by nervous and hormonal mechanisms.

The gastrointestinal tract is an irregularly shaped tube, into which associated accessory organs (mainly glands) secrete fluid. The first part of the digestive tract comprises the oral cavity. The salivary glands and tonsils are accessory organs of the oral cavity. The oral cavity opens posteriorly into the pharynx, the pharynx opens inferiorly into the esophagus, and the esophagus opens inferiorly into the stomach (through the muscular **cardiac sphincter**). In the stomach, small glands secrete acids and enzymes that help with digestion. The cardiac sphincter stops food from reentering the esophagus when the stomach contracts.

The stomach opens into the **duodenum**, the first section of the small intestine. Important accessory structures in this segment of the gastrointestinal tract are the **liver**, the **gallbladder**, and the **pancreas**. The **jejunum**, the major site of absorption, is the next segment of the **small intestine**. The last segment of the small intestine is the **ileum**, which has a similar function to the jejunum but has fewer digestive enzymes and provides less absorption.

The last section of the digestive tract is the **large intestine**, which functions to absorb water and salts and to concentrate undigested food into feces. The major accessory glands of the large intestine secrete mucus. The first segment of the large intestine is the **cecum** with its attached appendix. The cecum is followed by the ascending, transverse, descending, and sigmoid portions of the colon and the rectum. The **rectum** joins the anal canal, which ends at the **anus**.

Oral Cavity

Saliva contains salivary amylase, an enzyme that begins the chemical digestion of carbohydrates. In addition, saliva prevents bacterial infection in the mouth by washing the oral cavity with substances that have a weak antibacterial action. Salivary gland secretion is stimulated by the parasympathetic and sympathetic nervous systems; the parasympathetic nervous system controls salivation in the relaxed state.

The teeth chew food in the mouth to break it up, which aids swallowing and processing. Food then is swallowed by voluntary and involuntary actions. The pharynx elevates to receive the food from the mouth. As the pharyngeal muscles contract, the upper esophageal sphincter relaxes, the esophagus opens, and the food is pushed into the esophagus. During this phase of swallowing, the vocal folds are moved medially. The epiglottis is tipped posteriorly to close the entrance of the airway and prevent aspiration.

Muscular contractions in the esophagus occur in peristaltic waves, which push the food through the esophagus toward the stomach. The contractions cause the cardiac sphincter (also known as the lower esophageal sphincter) to relax, and they then push the food into the stomach.

Stomach

The stomach acts primarily as a storage area and mixing chamber for ingested food. Although some digestion and absorption occur in the stomach, these are not its major functions. The stomach secretes mucus to protect the surface of the stomach wall and duodenum. The stomach is lined by mucous membranes that contain thousands of microscopic gastric glands that secrete hydrochloric acid, intrinsic factor, gastrin, and pepsinogen.

The stomach produces approximately 2.1 to 3.2 quarts (2 to 3 L) of gastric secretions each day. Secretion is regulated by nervous and hormonal mechanisms. The ingested food is mixed well with the secretions of the stomach glands to produce a semisolid mixture called **chyme**. Movements resembling peristalsis slowly force chyme toward the pyloric sphincter, through the pyloric opening, and into the duodenum (**FIGURE 10-51** and **FIGURE 10-52**).

> NOTE
>
> One liter is equal to 1.06 quarts. One gallon is equal to 3.79 L.

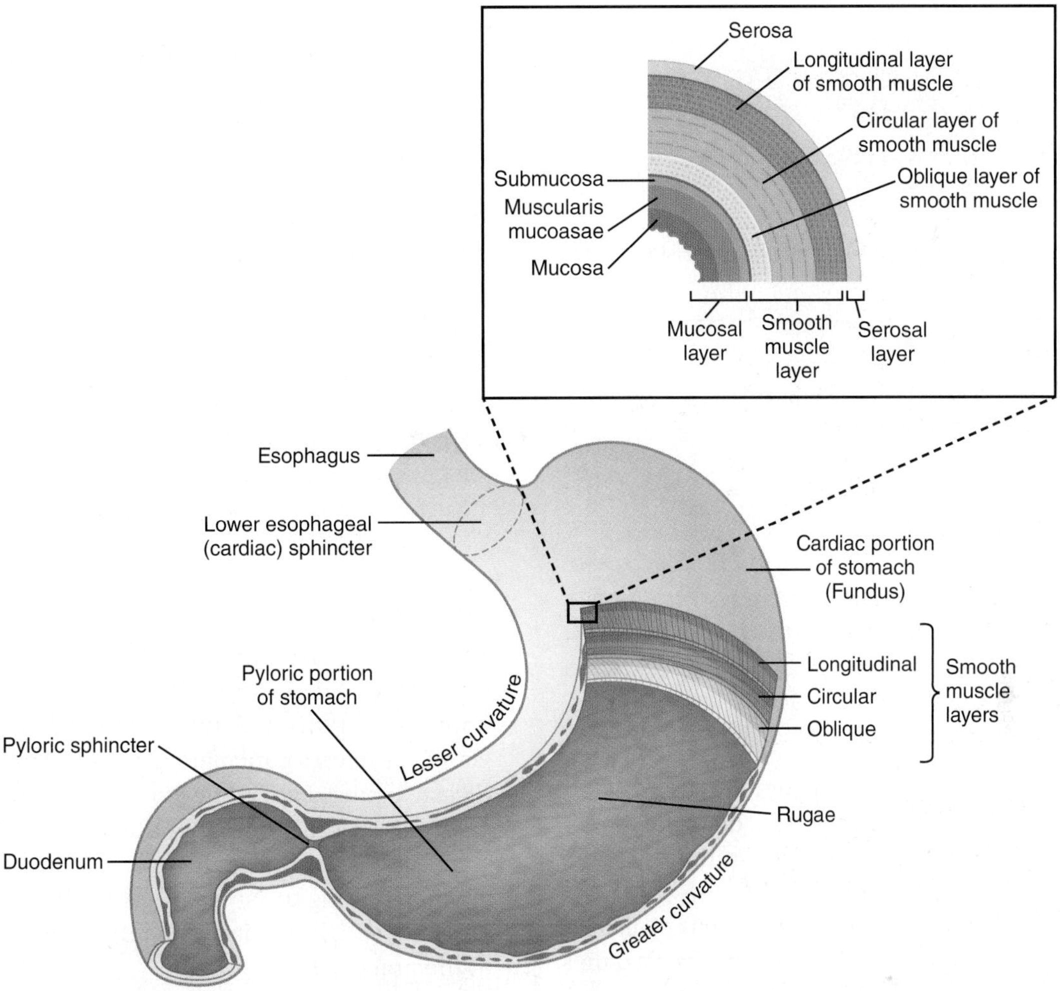

FIGURE 10-51 Muscle layers of the stomach wall.

Small Intestine

The mucosa of the small intestine produces secretions that contain mucus, electrolytes, and water. These substances lubricate the intestinal wall and protect the intestine from the acidic chyme and digestive enzymes. In addition, secretions of the liver and pancreas enter the small intestine to aid the digestive process.

The main functions of the small intestine are the mixing and propulsion of chyme and the absorption of fluid and nutrients. Peristaltic contractions move the chyme through the small intestine toward the ileocecal sphincter. At this point, the chyme enters the cecum. When the chyme causes the cecum to distend, the sphincter closes. This closure slows the rate of movement of chyme from the small intestine into the large intestine. Closure also prevents material from returning to the ileum from the cecum.

CRITICAL THINKING

What might happen if the excretion of protective mucus in the small bowel is impaired?

Liver

The liver—the largest internal organ—lies just under the diaphragm in the upper regions of the abdominal cavity. This highly vascular organ gets its blood supply from two sources, the **hepatic artery** and the

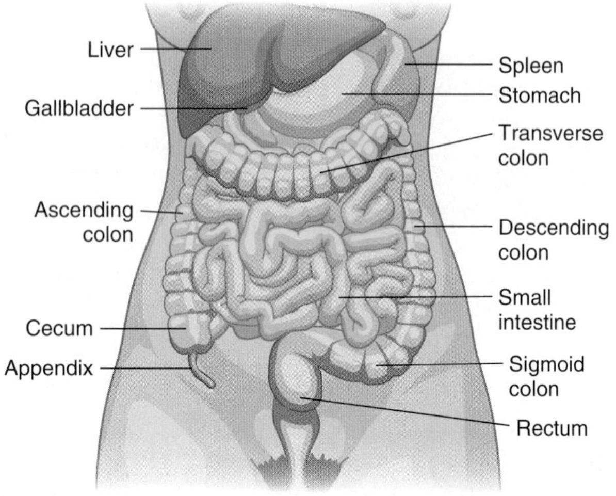

FIGURE 10-52 Organs of the digestive system. Chyme passes from the stomach into the duodenum (the first portion of the small intestine) and then to the large intestine.

portal vein. The liver plays a major role in iron metabolism, plasma protein production, detoxification of drugs and other substances circulating in plasma, and many other biochemical pathways.

The liver secretes approximately 600 to 1,000 mL of **bile** each day. Bile contains no digestive enzymes, but it dilutes stomach acid and emulsifies fats. Most bile salts are reabsorbed in the ileum and are carried back to the liver in the blood; the remaining bile salts are lost through feces.

> NOTE
> One teaspoon is equal to approximately 5 mL. One tablespoon volume is equal to approximately 15 mL.

In addition to secreting bile, the liver has other functions that are needed for healthy survival. The liver plays a major role in the metabolism of certain foods and helps maintain a normal blood glucose concentration. This organ serves as a line of defense against many by-products of metabolism that are toxic if they collect in the body. Blood proteins (eg, albumin, fibrinogen, globulins, and clotting factors) also are made and released into the circulation by the liver.

Gallbladder

Bile is secreted regularly by the liver and is stored in the gallbladder. When chyme containing lipid or fat enters the duodenum, the gallbladder is stimulated by the hormones cholecystokinin and secretin (secreted by the intestinal mucosa). As a result of this stimulation, the gallbladder contracts, forcing concentrated bile into the small intestine. The only role of the gallbladder is to concentrate and store the bile made by the liver.

> CRITICAL THINKING
> When is the person who suffers from gallstones (cholelithiasis) most likely to have pain? Why?

Pancreas

The pancreas is both an endocrine gland and an **exocrine gland**. As an endocrine gland, it secretes hormones (eg, insulin) into the blood. As an exocrine gland, it secretes pancreatic juice—the most critical digestive juice. Pancreatic juice consists of digestive enzymes, sodium bicarbonate, and alkaline substances that neutralize the hydrochloric acid in the chyme entering the small intestine. It also contains amylase, which continues the digestion that began in the oral cavity.

Large Intestine

Chyme moves through the small intestine in 3 to 5 hours. Its passage through the large intestine, however, takes 18 to 24 hours. Processes involving the absorption of water and salts, the secretion of mucus, the action of microorganisms, and the conversion of chyme produce feces. Feces remain in the colon until eliminated through defecation.

The contents of the large intestine are forced toward the anus by peristaltic contractions, which occur three or four times per day. During the movement of chyme through the large intestine, bacteria act on material that escaped digestion in the small intestine. As a result of this action, more nutrients may be released and absorbed. Some of the bacteria also synthesize vitamin K, a vitamin needed for normal blood clotting, and produce the vitamin B complex. Once formed, these vitamins are absorbed from the large intestine and enter the blood.

Distention of the rectal wall by feces starts the defecation reflex, which causes weak contractions and relaxations of the internal anal sphincter. The external anal sphincter (under conscious cerebral control) stops the passage of feces out of the rectum until it is relaxed. During defecation, pressure in the abdominal cavity increases; this pressure forces the contents of the colon through the anal canal and out the anus.

Urinary System

The urinary system is made up of two kidneys, two ureters, the urinary bladder, and the urethra. This system works with other body systems to maintain homeostasis by removing waste products from the blood and by helping to maintain a constant body fluid volume and composition. In addition, the kidneys play a role in the control of red blood cell production and metabolism of vitamin D.

> CRITICAL THINKING
> Think about patients with renal failure. Why should you anticipate anemia and decreased calcium levels?

Kidneys

Each **kidney** is shaped much like a bean. The two kidneys lie on the posterior abdominal wall behind the peritoneum, on either side of the vertebral column near the lateral border of the psoas muscles. The superior pole of each kidney is protected by the rib cage. The right kidney is slightly lower than the left kidney because of the superior position of the liver. A fibrous renal capsule surrounds each kidney, along with a dense deposit of adipose tissue that protects the kidney from injury.

The kidney is divided into an outer cortex and an inner medulla. The medulla consists of a number of triangular divisions called the **renal pyramids**, which extend into the cortex (**FIGURE 10-53**). The papilla is the innermost end of a pyramid. Several large urinary tubes (calyces) extend to the renal pelvis from the kidney tissue.

The basic functional unit of the kidney is the **nephron**. Each nephron is made up of a large terminal

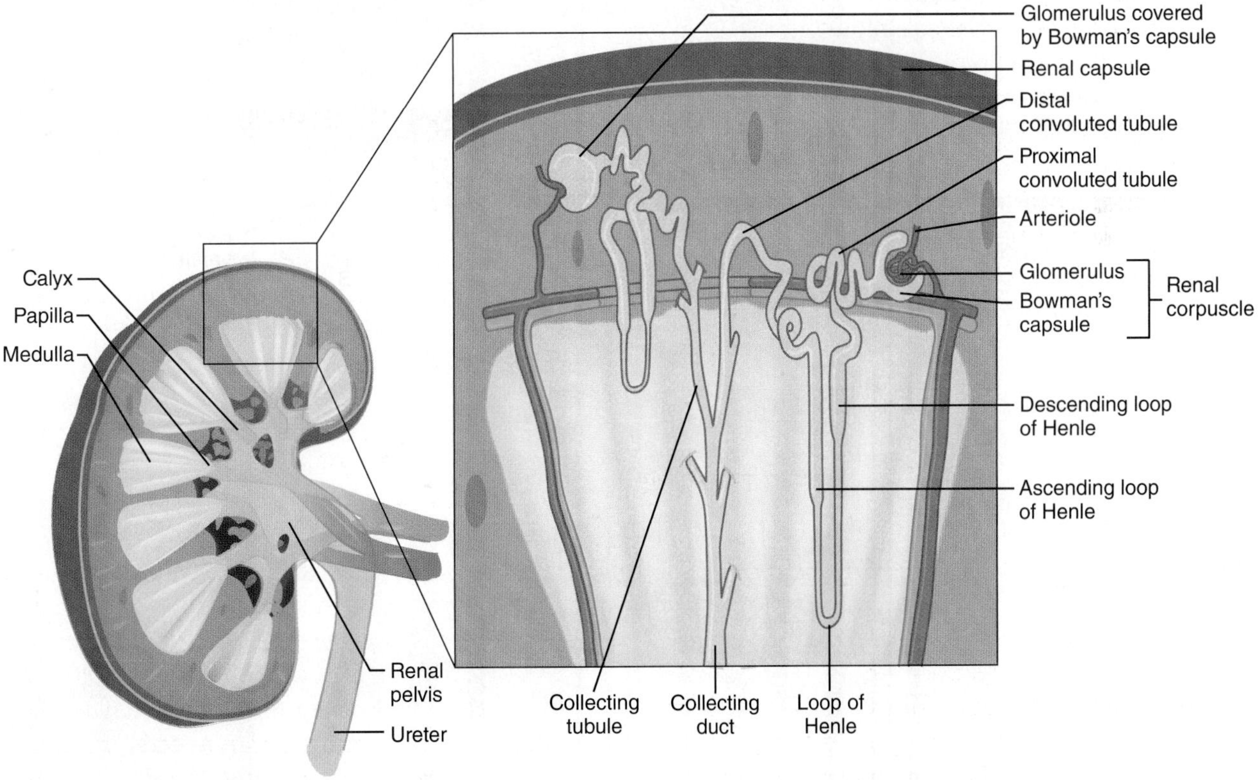

FIGURE 10-53 Magnified section of a renal pyramid.

end (called a renal corpuscle), a proximal convoluted tubule, the **loop of Henle**, and a distal convoluted tubule. The distal convoluted tubule empties into a collecting duct, which carries the urine from the cortex of the kidney to the calyces. The terminal end of the nephron is enlarged to form the **Bowman capsule**. The wall of the Bowman capsule is indented to form a double-walled chamber occupied by a network of blood capillaries known as the **glomerulus**. Together, the glomerulus and the Bowman capsule form the renal corpuscle.

Ureters, Urinary Bladder, and Urethra

The **ureters** extend from the renal pelvis to the urinary bladder. The triangular area of the bladder wall between the two ureters and the urethra is called the trigone. This region differs from the rest of the bladder wall in that it does not expand during bladder filling.

The **urinary bladder** is a hollow, muscular organ that lies in the pelvic cavity just posterior to the pubic symphysis. The size of the bladder depends on the volume of urine. **FIGURE 10-54** depicts the male and female urinary bladders.

> CRITICAL THINKING
> Why is the bladder more susceptible to injury when full than when empty?

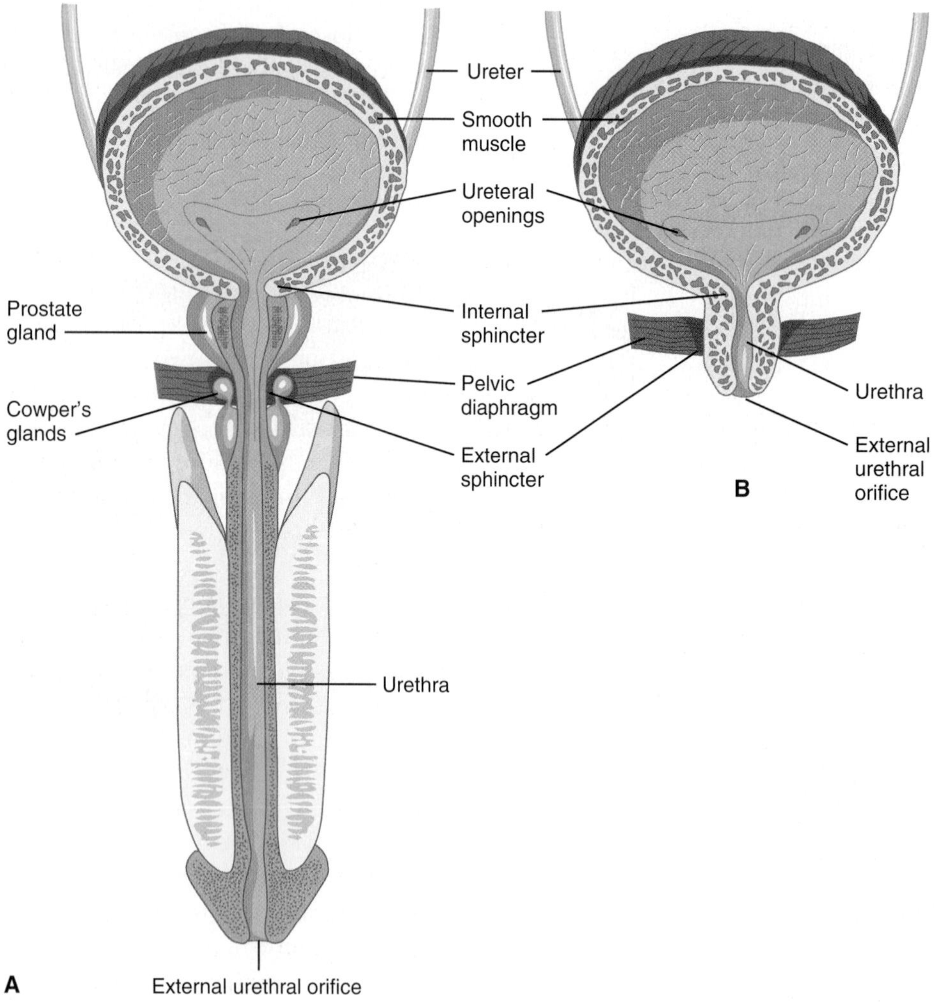

FIGURE 10-54 Longitudinal sections of **(A)** the male urinary bladder and related structures, and **(B)** the female urinary bladder and related structures.

At the junction of the urethra and the urinary bladder, smooth muscle of the bladder forms the internal urinary sphincter. The external urinary sphincter surrounds the urethra as the urethra extends through the pelvic floor. These sphincters control the flow of urine through the urethra. In the male, the urethra extends to the end of the penis, where it opens to the outside. The female urethra, which is much shorter than the male urethra, opens into the vestibule anterior to the vaginal opening.

Urine Production

Nephrons are the structural parts of the kidney where urine is produced. The more than 2 million nephrons form urine in a three-step process of filtration, reabsorption, and secretion (**FIGURE 10-55**):

1. Blood flowing through the glomeruli of the kidney exerts pressure that pushes water and small dissolved molecular substances out of the glomeruli and into the Bowman capsule. Simply stated, glomerular blood pressure causes filtration through the glomerular capillaries. Glomerular filtration normally occurs at the rate of 125 mL/min or 180 L/day (glomerular filtration rate). Approximately 90% of this filtrate is reabsorbed; the remainder is excreted as urine. Healthy people produce 1 to 2 L of urine per day.
2. Upon leaving the renal capsule, the filtrate flows through the proximal convoluted tubule, the loop of Henle, and the distal convoluted tubule, and finally into the collecting duct. During this process, many substances in the filtrate are reabsorbed by the blood capillaries around the tubules and reenter the general circulation. Substances that are reabsorbed include water, glucose and other nutrients, and most of the sodium and other **ions** in the filtrate.
3. In the process of secretion, substances move into urine in the distal convoluted tubules and collecting ducts from blood in the capillaries around these structures. Reabsorption moves substances out of the urine and into the blood; secretion, however, moves substances out of the blood and into the urine. Secreted substances include hydrogen and potassium ions, ammonia, and certain drugs.

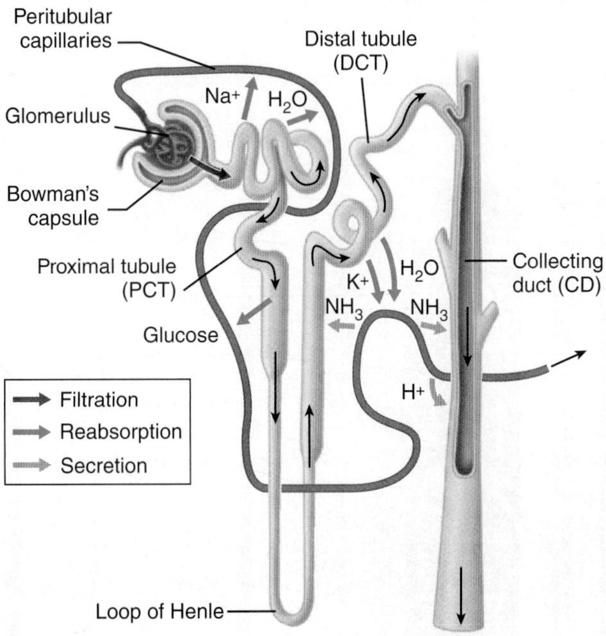

FIGURE 10-55 Formation of urine. The steps in urine formation in successive parts of a nephron are filtration, reabsorption, and secretion.

Urine Regulation

The body usually can control the amount and makeup of the urine it secretes via hormonal mechanisms, autoregulation, and sympathetic nervous system stimulation.

Aldosterone is a steroid hormone secreted by the adrenal gland. It passes through the circulatory system from the adrenal gland to the kidney. Aldosterone stimulates the tubules to reabsorb sodium salts and water.

Antidiuretic hormone (ADH), which is secreted by the posterior pituitary gland, tends to reduce the amount of urine produced by making distal and collecting tubules permeable to water, thereby increasing water reabsorption. As a result, water is retained by the body in the presence of ADH.

Atrial natriuretic factor (ANF) is a hormone secreted from the cells in the right atrium of the heart when the pressure in the right atrium increases. ANF inhibits ADH secretion and reduces the kidneys' ability to concentrate urine. As a result, the body produces a large volume of dilute urine.

Prostaglandins and kinins are substances formed in the kidneys that affect kidney function. These substances are believed to influence the rate of filtrate formation and sodium ion reabsorption.

Autoregulation is the ability of the kidneys to maintain a stable glomerular filtration rate over a wide range of systemic blood pressures. When small increases in glomerular capillary pressure occur, the rate of filtrate formation increases substantially. Therefore, large increases in the arterial blood pressure increase the rate of urine production. Conversely, when the arterial blood pressure decreases, urine production decreases. Through autoregulation, the kidneys change the degree of constriction or dilation of the arterioles in the renal capsule to maintain glomerular capillary pressure and urine production within normal limits over a wide range of arterial blood pressures.

Sympathetic neurons innervate the blood vessels of the kidney. The sympathetic stimulation that occurs in response to severe stress, intense exercise, or circulatory shock constricts the small arteries and the afferent arterioles, which in turn reduces renal blood flow.

Reproductive System

Most organs and systems of the human body are the same in the male and the female, with a notable exception—the reproductive systems. The male reproductive system produces **spermatozoa** and transfers the spermatozoa to the female. The female reproductive system produces **oocytes** and receives the spermatozoa, thereby enabling fertilization, conception, gestation, and birth.

Male Reproductive System

The male reproductive system consists of the testes, epididymis, ductus deferens, urethra, seminal vesicles, prostate gland, bulbourethral glands, scrotum, and penis (**FIGURE 10-56**).

The **testes** are ovoid organs in the scrotum that develop as retroperitoneal organs in the abdominopelvic cavity. The testes move from the abdominal cavity to the scrotum by way of the **inguinal canal**—a structure found in both men and women. Normally the inguinal canal is closed, but it persists as a weak spot in the abdominal wall where the testes pass through it. If the inguinal canal weakens or ruptures, an inguinal hernia may result.

Interstitial cells of the testes secrete the male hormone testosterone. Before **puberty** (12 to 14 years of age), the testes are relatively simple. At the time of puberty, however, the interstitial cells increase in number and size, and the production of spermatozoa begins. The testes contribute approximately 5% of the seminal fluid (**semen**).

The final maturation of spermatozoa occurs in the **epididymis**, a convoluted, comma-shaped structure located on the posterior side of the testis. Infection

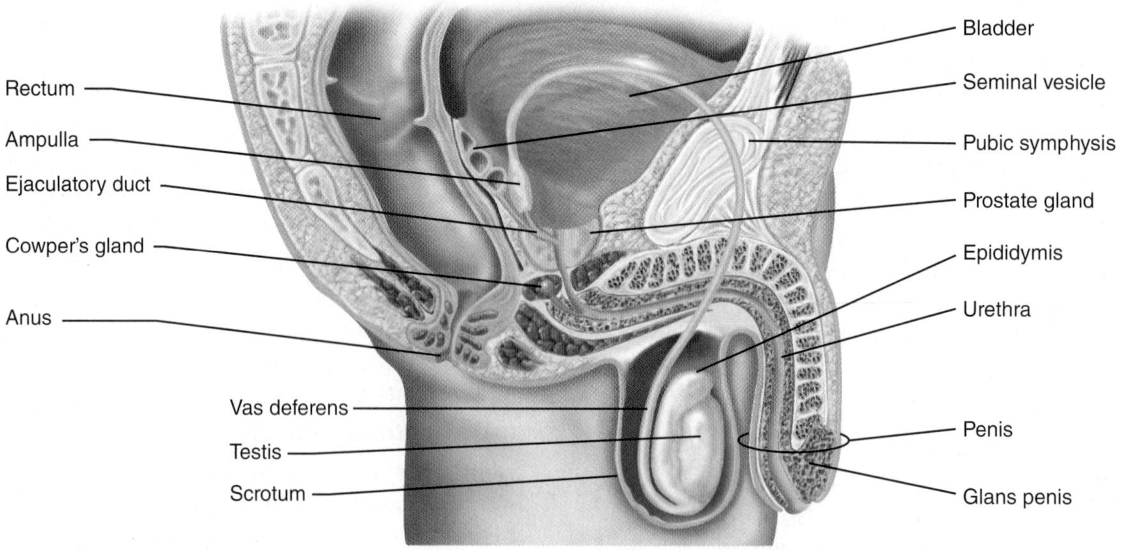

FIGURE 10-56 Sagittal section of the male pelvis.

or injury can block a single epididymis or both of them, leading to infertility.

The **ductus deferens** (also called the vas deferens) emerges from the tail of the epididymis. This duct ascends to the seminal vesicle, finally associating with the blood vessels and nerves that supply the testis. These structures and their coverings constitute the spermatic cord. The ductus deferens and the spermatic cord structures ascend and pass through the inguinal canal to enter the abdominal cavity. The ductus deferens crosses the lateral wall of the cavity, travels over the ureter, and loops over the posterior surface of the urinary bladder to approach the prostate gland. It is surrounded by smooth muscle, which helps propel sperm through the duct.

The **urethra** is a passageway for urine and male reproductive fluids. It can be divided into three parts: the prostatic portion (which passes through the prostate gland), the membranous portion (which extends from the prostatic urethra through the muscular floor of the pelvis), and the spongy portion (which extends the length of the penis).

The **seminal vesicle** is a sac-shaped gland that lies adjacent to each ductus deferens. A short duct from the seminal vesicle joins the ductus deferens to form the ejaculatory duct. These ducts project into the prostate gland and end by opening into the urethra. Seminal vesicles produce approximately 60% of the seminal fluid.

The **prostate gland** consists of glandular and muscular tissue. Approximately the size and shape of a walnut, it is located dorsal to the symphysis pubis at the base of the bladder and surrounds the prostatic urethra and the two ejaculatory ducts. Some 20 to 30 small prostatic ducts secrete prostatic fluid into the prostatic urethra. The prostate gland contributes about 30% of the seminal fluid.

The **bulbourethral glands** are a pair of small glands located near the membranous portion of the urethra. In young adults, each of these glands is approximately the size of a pea, but they decrease in size with age. In these compound mucous glands, a series of small ducts unite to form a single duct that exits from each gland. The two bulbourethral glands enter the spongy urethra at the base of the penis. They add secretions to semen, contributing approximately 5% of the seminal fluid.

The **scrotum** is divided into two internal compartments by a connective tissue septum. Beneath the skin of the scrotum is a layer of superficial fascia (loose connective tissue) and a layer of cutaneous muscle (dartos muscle). The dartos and cremaster muscles of the abdomen are crucial for regulating temperature in the testes—a function that is required for **spermatogenesis**. These muscles pull the testes near the body in cold temperatures and allow the testes to descend away from the body in warm temperatures and during exercise.

CRITICAL THINKING

If a patient's prostate gland is greatly enlarged by benign or malignant disease, which symptoms would you expect?

The **penis** consists of three columns of erectile tissue. Engorgement of this tissue with blood causes the penis to enlarge and become firm, producing an **erection**. The penis is the male organ of copulation and functions in the transfer of spermatozoa from the male to the female.

Female Reproductive System

The female reproductive organs consist of the ovaries, uterine (or fallopian) tubes, uterus, vagina, external genital organs, and mammary glands. The internal reproductive organs lie within the pelvis between the urinary bladder and the rectum. These organs are held in place by a group of ligaments (**FIGURE 10-57**).

The small **ovaries** are attached to the posterior of the broad ligament called the mesovarium. Two other ligaments associated with the ovary are the suspensory ligament and the ovarian ligament. The ovarian arteries, veins, and nerves traverse the suspensory ligament and enter the ovary through the mesovarium. Each ovary has a dense outer portion—the cortex—as well as a looser inner portion called the medulla. Many small vesicles, called **ovarian follicles** (each of which contains an oocyte), are distributed throughout the cortex.

The **uterine tubes** are ducts for the ovaries. Each tube is located along the superior margin of the broad ligament and opens right into the peritoneal cavity to receive the oocyte. Once inside the uterine tube, the oocyte is transported by cilia and peristaltic contractions of the smooth muscle in the uterine tube.

The **uterus** is approximately the size and shape of a medium-size pear. It is oriented in the pelvic cavity with the larger rounded portion (the fundus)

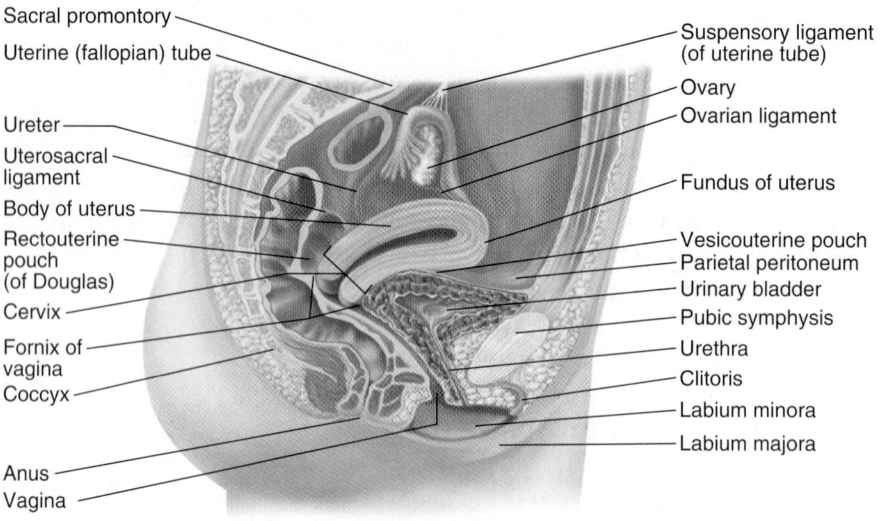

FIGURE 10-57 Sagittal section of the female pelvis.

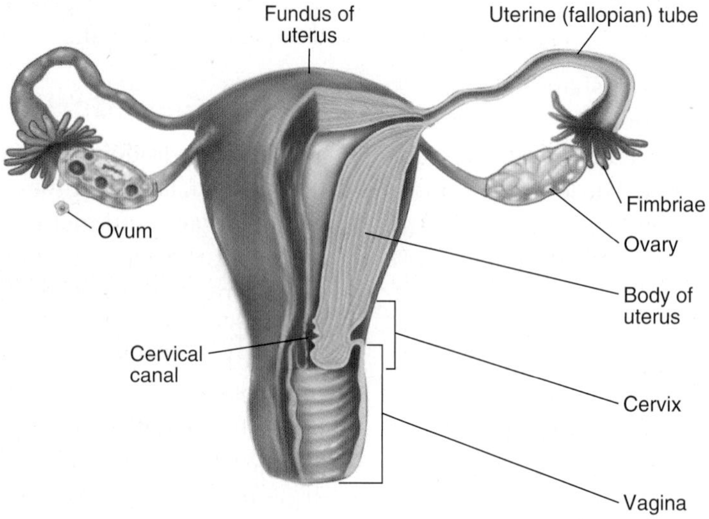

FIGURE 10-58 Internal anatomy of the female pelvis.

directed superiorly and the narrower portion (the **cervix**) directed inferiorly. The main portion of the uterus (the body) is positioned between the fundus and the cervix. The major ligaments that hold the uterus in place are the broad ligament, round ligaments, and uterosacral ligaments (**FIGURE 10-58**).

The **vagina** is the female organ of copulation; it functions to receive the penis during intercourse. Extending from the uterus to the outside of the body, the vagina provides a passageway both for menstrual flow and for childbirth. The smooth muscle layer of the vagina allows the organ to increase in size to accommodate the penis during intercourse and to stretch greatly during delivery. The vaginal orifice is covered by a thin mucous membrane called the **hymen**. The openings in the hymen usually are enlarged during the first sexual intercourse but also may be perforated or torn during strenuous exercise.

The external genitalia, referred to as the **vulva**, consist of the vestibule and its surrounding structures (**FIGURE 10-59**). The vestibule is the space into which the vagina and urethra open. It is bordered

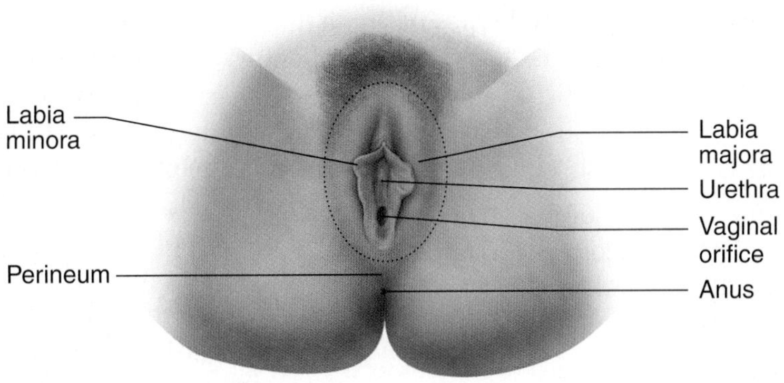

FIGURE 10-59 Female external genitalia.

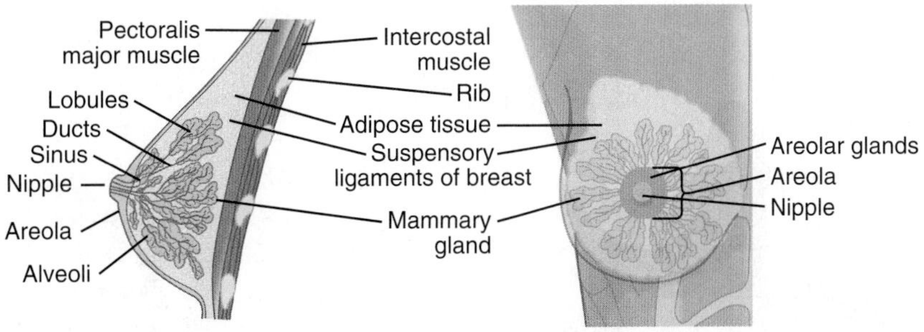

FIGURE 10-60 Mammary glands and duct system of the right breast.

by a pair of thin, longitudinal skin folds called the labia minora. A small erectile structure, called the **clitoris**, is located in the anterior margin of the vestibule. The two labia minora unite over the clitoris to form a fold of skin known as the prepuce. Lateral to the labia minora are two prominent folds of skin called the labia majora. These folds unite anteriorly in an elevation over the pubic symphysis to form the **mons pubis**. Most of the time, the labia majora are in contact with each other. They conceal the deeper structures within the vestibule.

The **perineum** is divided into triangles by perineal muscles. The urogenital triangle contains the external genitalia. The posterior anal triangle contains the anal opening. The region between the vagina and the anus, the clinical perineum, sometimes tears during childbirth.

The **mammary glands** are the organs of milk production. They are located in the breasts, or mammae. Externally, the breasts of males and females have a raised nipple surrounded by a circular pigmented **areola**. Nipples are sensitive to tactile stimulation and may become erect in response to sexual arousal. The areolae normally have a slightly bumpy surface due to the presence of areolar glands just below their surface. Secretions from these glands protect the nipple and areola from chafing during nursing.

Female breasts begin to enlarge during puberty (usually between ages 12 and 13 years) under the effects of two sex hormones, estrogen and progesterone. Each adult female mammary gland consists of 15 to 20 glandular lobes covered by adipose tissue. Each lobe has a single lactiferous duct that subdivides to form smaller ducts, each of which supplies a lobule. These ducts expand at their ends to form secretory sacs, or alveoli, which secrete milk during nursing (**FIGURE 10-60**).

Special Senses

Senses provide the brain with information about the outside world. Four senses are recognized as special senses: (1) smell, (2) taste, (3) sight, and (4) hearing and balance. The sense of touch now is considered a general sense, which consists of several types of nerve endings scattered throughout the body and not localized to a specific area.

Olfactory Sense Organs

The smell receptors for the fibers of the **olfactory** (first cranial) nerve lie in the mucosa of the upper part of the nasal cavity (**FIGURE 10-61**). Most of the nasal cavity is involved with respiration; only a small part is devoted to smell.

The dendrites of olfactory neurons extend to the epithelial surface of the nasal cavity, where they form vesicles. These vesicles have long **cilia**, which lie in a thin, mucous film on the epithelial surface. When olfactory cells are stimulated by molecules in the air, the resulting nerve impulses travel through the olfactory nerves in the olfactory bulb and olfactory tract. In the olfactory tract, the impulses enter the thalamic and olfactory centers of the brain. There, the nervous impulses are interpreted as specific odors.

The exact mechanism of olfactory stimulation is not understood clearly. The range of smells is thought to be just a combination of seven main odors: (1) camphoraceous, (2) musk, (3) floral, (4) peppermint, (5) ethereal, (6) pungent, and (7) putrid. Olfactory receptors are sensitive to even slight odors but are

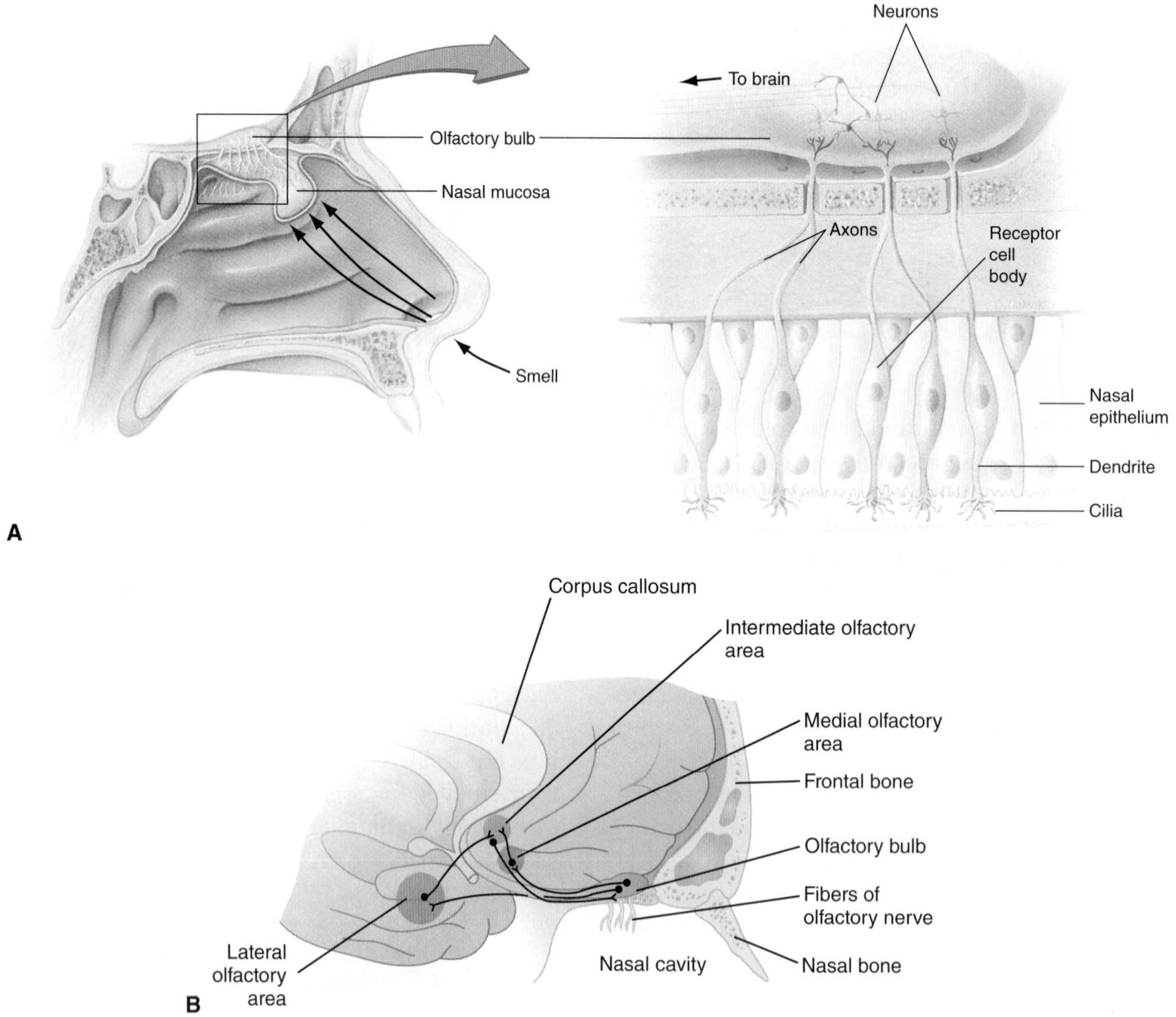

FIGURE 10-61 Olfactory structures. **A.** Midsagittal section of the nasal area showing the locations of major olfactory sensory structures. **B.** Major olfactory integration centers of the brain. Gas molecules stimulate olfactory cells in the nasal epithelium. Sensory information is conducted along nerves in the olfactory bulb and olfactory tract to sensory processing centers in the brain.

A: © Jones & Bartlett Learning; **B:** *Modified from:* McCance KL, Huether SE. *Pathophysiology: The Biologic Basis for Disease in Adults and Children*. 5th ed. St. Louis, MO: Mosby; 2005.

fatigued easily. Thus, the olfactory system quickly adapts to ongoing stimulation, such that a certain odor may cease to be noticed in a short time. This is a key factor to consider when dealing with hazardous materials incidents (see Chapter 56, *Hazardous Materials Awareness*).

Taste

Taste is a function of multiple nerves in the tongue, soft palate, uvula, and upper esophagus, including cranial nerves VII and IX. The primary sensations of taste are sour, salty, sweet, bitter, and savory. These tastes can be sensed by all parts of the tongue, with the sides of the tongue being more sensitive than the middle overall.[4]

The **taste buds** are sensitive to each of the primary sensations. The average adult has between 2,000 and 4,000 taste buds that are renewed weekly. Most taste buds are located in specific areas on the tongue, although some are located on the palate, lips, throat, smooth muscles of the airway, and gastrointestinal tract. The sensory cells of taste buds and associated nerve fibers are responsible for passing information for a particular perception of flavor on to the brain. Alterations in taste can be caused by injury, medication, oral infections, and aging.

Visual System

The visual system includes the eyes, the accessory structures (eyelids, eyebrows, eyelashes, and tear glands), and the optic nerve, tracts, and pathways. The second cranial nerve (**optic nerve**) conducts impulses from the eye to the brain, where these impulses create the sensation of vision. The third cranial nerve (**oculomotor nerve**) conducts impulses from the brain to the muscles of the eye, where they cause contractions that constrict the pupil and move the eye.

> CRITICAL THINKING
>
> Why is an examination of the eyes a key part of the neurologic evaluation?

Anatomy of the Eye

The eye is composed of three layers: the fibrous tunic, consisting of the sclera and cornea; the vascular tunic, consisting of the choroid, ciliary body, and iris; and the nervous tunic, consisting of the retina (**FIGURE 10-62**).

The **sclera** is the firm, opaque, white outer layer of the eye. It helps to maintain the shape of the eye, protects the internal structures of the eye, and provides

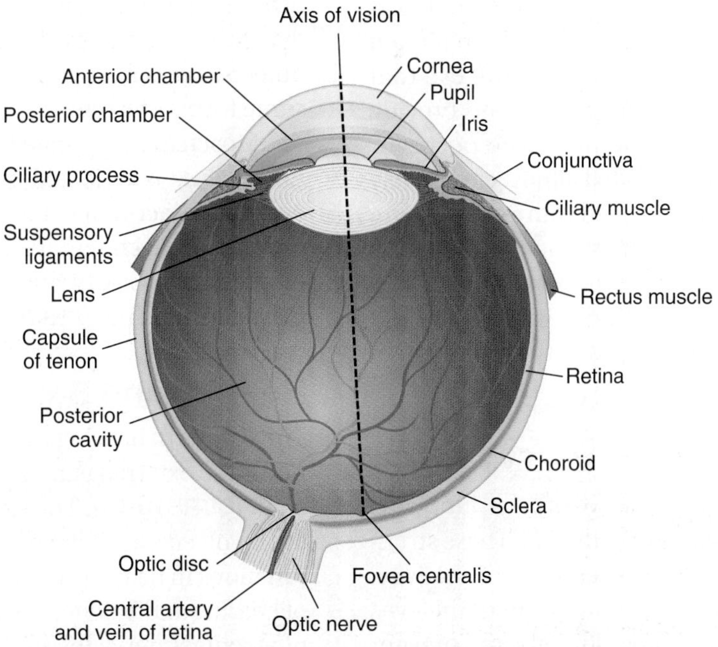

FIGURE 10-62 Horizontal section through the left eyeball. The eye is viewed from above.

an attachment point for the muscles that move the eye. The sclera is continuous with the meningeal layers of the brain that extend along the optic nerve. The **cornea** is continuous with the sclera. The cornea is an avascular, transparent structure that permits light to enter the eye. It also bends and refracts entering light.

The **vascular tunic** contains most of the blood vessels of the eyeball. The part of this layer associated with the sclera is the choroid. Anteriorly, the vascular tunic consists of the ciliary body and the iris. The ciliary body includes both ciliary muscles (which can change the shape of the lens) and complex capillaries involved in producing **aqueous humor**. The **iris**—the colored part of the eye—consists mainly of smooth muscle that surrounds the **pupil**. Light enters through the pupil, and the iris regulates the amount of light by controlling the size of the pupil.

The **retina** consists of an outer pigmented retina and an inner sensory layer, which responds to light. The sensory layer contains photoreceptor cells, called rods and cones, and numerous relay neurons. Rods are the receptors for night vision; cones are the receptors for daytime and color vision.

Compartments of the Eye

The two compartments of the eye are separated by a **lens**. The lens is suspended between the two eye compartments—that is, the anterior and posterior chambers—by ligaments. The anterior chamber is filled with aqueous humor, a fluid that helps maintain **intraocular pressure** (pressure within the eye that keeps the eye expanded), refract light, and provide nutrition for the anterior chamber. The posterior chamber of the eye is surrounded almost completely by the retina. This chamber is filled with a transparent, jellylike substance called **vitreous humor**. Like the aqueous humor, the vitreous humor helps maintain intraocular pressure. In addition, it helps to hold the retina in place and functions in the refraction of light in the eye.

Accessory Structures of the Eye

The accessory structures of the eye protect, lubricate, move, and aid in the function of the eye. These structures include the eyebrows, eyelids, conjunctivae, and lacrimal gland. The eyebrows protect the eyes by providing shade from direct sunlight and prevent perspiration from running into the eyes. The eyelids help regulate the amount of light entering the eyes and protect the eyes from foreign objects. Blinking, which normally occurs about 25 times per minute, helps lubricate the eyes by spreading tears over their surfaces. The **conjunctiva** is a thin, transparent mucous membrane that covers the inner surface of the eyelids and the outer surface of the sclera.

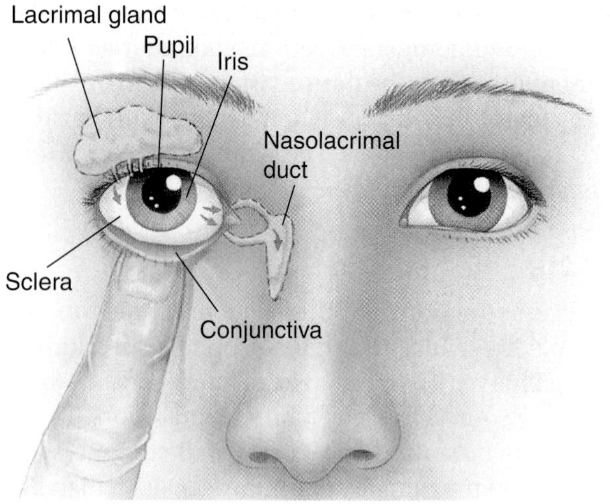

FIGURE 10-63 Lacrimal structures of the eye.

The **lacrimal gland** makes lacrimal fluid (tears) that leaves the gland through several ducts, passing over the anterior surface of the eyeball. This gland, which is located in the superolateral corner of the orbit, makes tears that moisten the surface of the eye, lubricate the eyelids, and wash away foreign objects. Tears also contain lysosomes that destroy some forms of bacteria.

Most tears evaporate from the surface of the eye. Excess fluid is collected in the medial corner of the eye by the lacrimal canals through a punctum (the opening of each canal). The lacrimal canals open into a lacrimal sac, which in turn continues into the nasolacrimal duct (**FIGURE 10-63**).

Hearing and Balance

The organs of hearing can be divided into three portions: the external ear, the middle ear, and the inner ear (**FIGURE 10-64**). The external ear and middle ear are involved only in hearing. The inner ear, however, functions in hearing and balance. The special senses of hearing and balance are transmitted by the vestibulocochlear nerve (eighth cranial nerve).

The **external ear** includes the **auricle** (also called the pinna) and the external auditory meatus, which opens into the external auditory canal. The auricle,

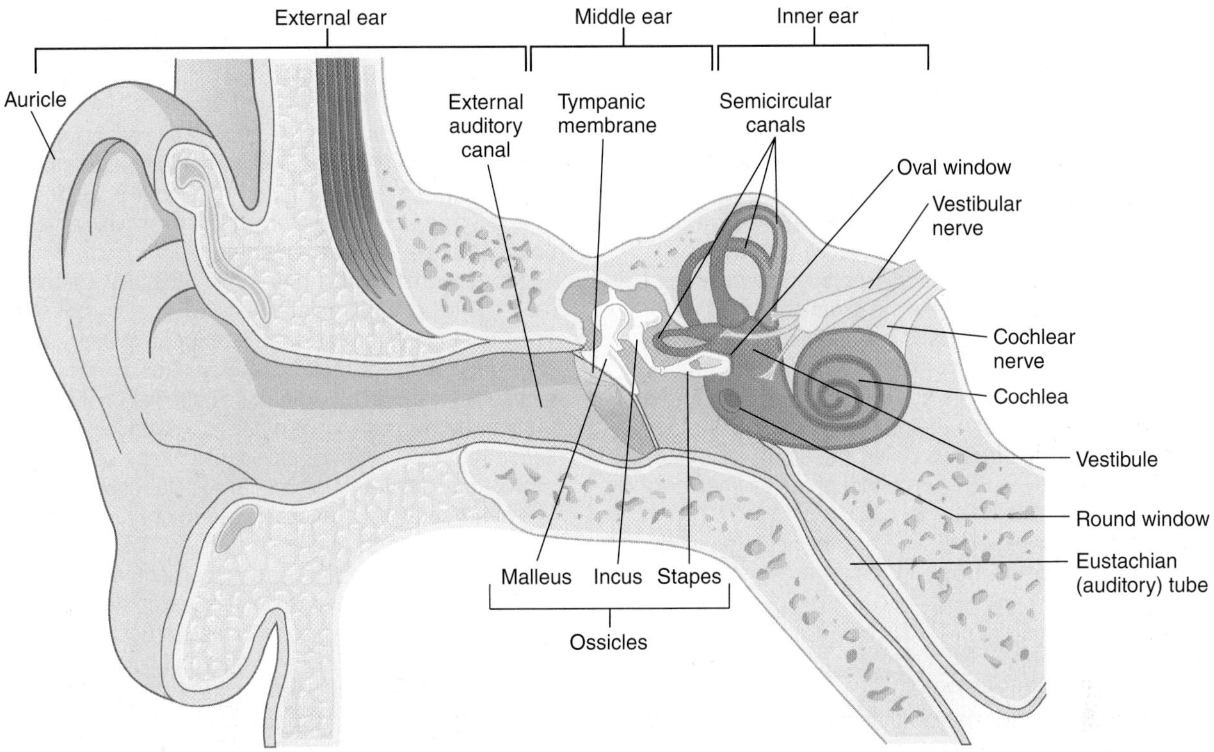

FIGURE 10-64 External, middle, and inner ear.

which is shaped to collect sound waves, directs sound waves toward the external auditory meatus. From the meatus, sound waves travel through the auditory canal to the eardrum (**tympanic membrane**), causing this membrane to vibrate. The external auditory canal is lined with hairs and ceruminous glands (ie, glands that make cerumen).

The **middle ear** is an air-filled space in the temporal bone that contains the auditory ossicles. The auditory ossicles of the middle ear (called the malleus, incus, and stapes) transmit vibrations from the tympanic membrane to the oval window. The middle ear is connected to the inner ear by two membrane-covered openings—the round window and the oval window. Two other openings that are not covered by membranes offer a passageway for air from the middle ear. One opens into the mastoid air cells; the other, known as the auditory (or eustachian) tube, opens into the pharynx.

The **eustachian tube** allows for the equalization of air pressure between the outside air and the middle ear cavity. Children have shorter eustachian tubes. Consequently, bacteria can travel more easily from infected areas in the throat to the middle ear. This difference between children and adults is responsible for the increased frequency of earaches and ear infections in children.

The **inner ear** holds the sensory organs for hearing and balance. It consists of interconnecting tunnels and chambers in the **bony labyrinth**. The bony labyrinth is divided into three regions: the vestibule, the cochlea, and the semicircular canals. The vestibule and semicircular canals are involved primarily in balance; the cochlea is involved in hearing. The hearing sense organ, which lies inside the cochlea, is called the organ of Corti. In young, healthy people, the frequencies that can be detected by the ear range (over octaves) from 20 to 20,000 cycles per second.

Inside the bony labyrinth is another set of membranous tunnels and chambers called the membranous labyrinth, which is filled with a clear fluid called endolymph. The space between the membranous and bony labyrinths is filled with a fluid called perilymph. Both endolymph and perilymph are similar to CSF.

CRITICAL THINKING

Besides pain and impaired hearing, which other symptoms would you look for in a patient with an inner ear problem?

Summary

- The paramedic must understand human anatomy fully. This understanding helps the paramedic organize a patient assessment by body region. Knowledge of anatomy also helps the paramedic communicate well with medical direction and other members of the health care team.
- The anatomic position refers to a person standing erect with the feet and palms facing the examiner.
- Directional terms are expressed in anatomic terminology—for example, *up* or *down* (superior or inferior), *front* or *back* (anterior or posterior), and *right* or *left*. These terms are always respective to the patient, not the examiner. Internal body structure is classified into anatomic planes of the human body, which can be thought of as imaginary straight-line divisions.
- The appendicular region of the body includes the limbs, or extremities. The axial region consists of the head, neck, thorax, and abdomen.
- The abdomen usually is divided into four quadrants: upper right, lower right, upper left, and lower left.
- The three major cavities of the human body are the thoracic cavity, the abdominal cavity, and the pelvic cavity.
- The thoracic cavity contains the trachea, esophagus, thymus, heart, great vessels, lungs, and the cavities and membranes that surround them. The abdominopelvic cavity is surrounded by membranes and contains organs and blood vessels.
- At the cellular level, the cytoplasmic membrane encloses the cell's cytoplasm and forms the outer boundary of the cell. Organelles found in the cytoplasm perform functions that are vital to the cell's survival. The cell's nucleus is a large, membrane-bound organelle that ultimately controls all of the other organelles in the cytoplasm.
- All human cells, except for the reproductive (sex) cells, reproduce by a process known as mitosis. In this process, cells divide to multiply.
- Four main types of tissue make up the many organs of the body: epithelial tissue, connective tissue, muscle tissue, and nervous tissue. Epithelial tissue covers surfaces and forms structures. Connective tissue is made of cells separated from each other by intercellular material, known as the extracellular matrix. Muscle tissue is contractile tissue and is responsible for movement. Nervous tissue has the ability to conduct electrical signals, known as action potentials.
- A system is a group of organs arranged to perform a more complex function than any one organ can perform alone. The 11 major organ systems in the body are the integumentary, skeletal, muscular, nervous, endocrine, circulatory, lymphatic, respiratory, digestive, urinary, and reproductive systems.
- The integumentary system consists of the skin and accessory structures such as the hair, nails, and a variety of glands. The functions of the integumentary system include protecting the body against injury and dehydration, defending against infection, and regulating temperature.
- The skeletal system consists of bone and associated connective tissues, including cartilage, tendons, and ligaments. This system provides a rigid framework for support and protection as well as a system of levers on which muscles act to produce body movements.
- The three primary functions of the muscular system are movement, postural maintenance, and heat production.
- The nervous system and the endocrine system are the major regulatory and coordinating systems of the body. The nervous system rapidly transmits information throughout the body by means of nerve impulses. The endocrine system sends information more slowly by means of chemicals secreted by ductless glands into the bloodstream.
- The heart and cardiovascular system are responsible for circulating blood throughout the body. Blood transports nutrients and oxygen to tissues, carries carbon dioxide and waste products away from tissues, carries hormones produced in endocrine glands to their target tissues, plays a key role in temperature regulation and fluid balance, and protects the body from bacteria and foreign substances.
- The lymphatic system is made up of lymph, lymphocytes, lymph nodes, tonsils, the spleen, and the thymus gland. It has three basic functions: to help maintain fluid balance in tissues; to absorb fats and other substances from the digestive tract; and to play a role in the body's immune defense system.
- The organs of the respiratory system and the cardiovascular system bring oxygen to cells and carry carbon dioxide away from cells to the locations where this waste product is released into the air. The entrance to the respiratory tract begins at the nasal cavity and includes the nasopharynx, oropharynx, laryngopharynx, and larynx. Below the glottis are the structures of the lower airway and lungs, including the trachea, bronchial tree, alveoli, and lungs.
- The digestive system provides the body with water, electrolytes, and other nutrients used by cells. The gastrointestinal tract is an irregularly shaped tube into which associated accessory organs (mainly glands) secrete fluid.
- The urinary system works with other body systems to maintain homeostasis by removing waste products from the blood and helping maintain a constant body fluid volume and composition. The urinary system comprises two kidneys, two ureters, the urinary bladder, and the urethra.
- The male reproductive system makes and transfers spermatozoa to the female; the female reproductive system makes oocytes and receives the spermatozoa for fertilization, conception, gestation, and birth. The male reproductive system consists of the testes, epididymis, ductus deferens, urethra, seminal vesicles, prostate gland, bulbourethral glands, scrotum, and penis. The female reproductive organs consist of the ovaries, uterine (or fallopian) tubes, uterus, vagina, external genital organs, and mammary glands.
- Senses provide the brain with information about the outside world. Four senses are recognized as special senses: smell, taste, sight, and hearing and balance.

References

1. Ball JW, Dain JE, Flynn JA, Solomon BS, Stewart RW. *Seidel's Guide to Physical Examination*. 8th ed. St. Louis, MO: Elsevier; 2014.
2. Patton KT, Thibodeau GA. *Anatomy and Physiology*. 9th ed. St. Louis, MO: Saunders/Elsevier; 2013.
3. VanPutte C, Regan J, Russo AF, Seeley RR. *Seeley's Anatomy and Physiology*. 11th ed. New York, NY: McGraw-Hill; 2017.
4. How does our sense of taste work? US National Library of Medicine PubMed Health website. https://www.ncbi.nlm.nih.gov/pubmedhealth/PMH0072592/. Accessed February 12, 2018.

Suggested Readings

An online examination of human anatomy and physiology. Get Body Smart website. https://www.getbodysmart.com/. Accessed December 28, 2017.

Gould B, Dyer R. *Pathophysiology for the Health Professions*. 5th ed. St. Louis, MO: Elsevier/Saunders; 2014.

InnerBody website. http://www.innerbody.com. Accessed December 28, 2017.

McCance K, Huether S. *Pathophysiology: The Biologic Basis for Disease in Adults and Children*. 7th ed. St. Louis, MO: Mosby; 2015.

SEER training modules: cancer registration and surveillance modules. US Department of Health and Human Services, National Institutes of Health, National Cancer Institute website. https://training.seer.cancer.gov/modules_reg_surv.html. Accessed December 28, 2017.

Web anatomy. University of Minnesota website. http://msjensen.cbs.umn.edu/webanatomy/. December 28, 2017.

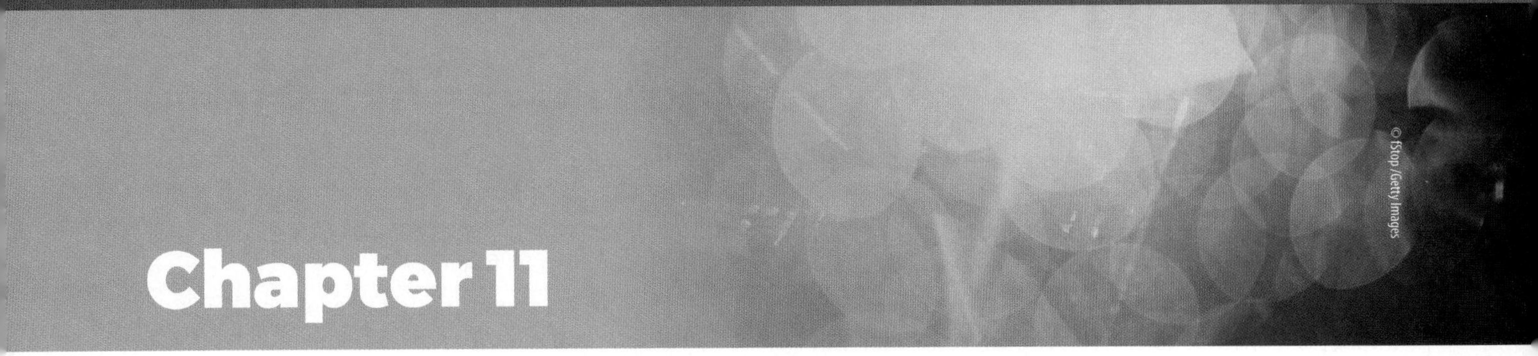

Chapter 11

General Principles of Pathophysiology

NATIONAL EMS EDUCATION STANDARD COMPETENCIES

Pathophysiology

Integrates comprehensive knowledge of pathophysiology of major human systems.

OBJECTIVES

Upon completion of this chapter, the paramedic student will be able to:

1. Describe the normal characteristics of the cellular environment and the key homeostatic mechanisms that strive to maintain an optimal fluid and electrolyte balance. (pp 273–280)
2. Outline pathophysiologic alterations in water and electrolyte balance and list their effects on body functions. (pp 280–287)
3. Describe the treatment of patients with particular fluid or electrolyte imbalances. (pp 282–287)
4. Describe the mechanisms in the body that maintain normal acid–base balance. (pp 287–289)
5. Outline pathophysiologic alterations in acid–base balance. (pp 289–296)
6. Describe the management of a patient with an acid–base imbalance. (pp 291–296)
7. Describe the changes in cells and tissues that occur with cellular adaptation, injury, neoplasia, aging, or death. (pp 296–302)
8. Outline the effects of cellular injury on local and systemic body functions. (pp 301–302)
9. Outline the causes, adverse systemic effects, and compensatory mechanisms associated with hypoperfusion. (pp 302–306)
10. Describe the ways in which the inflammatory and immune mechanisms respond to cellular injury or antigenic stimulation. (pp 309–312)
11. Explain how changes in immune status and the presence of inflammation can adversely affect body functions. (pp 310–312)
12. Describe the impact of stress on the body's response to illness or injury. (pp 316–319)
13. Describe factors that influence disease. (pp 320–321)
14. Describe changes in body functions that can occur as a result of genetic and familial disease factors. (pp 322–325)

KEY TERMS

acid–base balance The body's balance between acidity and alkalinity.

acidosis A condition marked by a high concentration of hydrogen ions (ie, a pH below 7.35).

acids Compounds that yield hydrogen ions when dissociated in solution.

active transport A carrier-mediated process that can move substances against a concentration gradient; assisted by enzymes and requires energy.

aerobic Of or pertaining to the presence of air or oxygen.

afterload The total resistance against which blood must be pumped; also known as peripheral vascular resistance.

aldosterone A steroid hormone produced by the adrenal cortex to regulate the sodium and potassium balance in the blood.

alkalosis A condition marked by a low concentration of hydrogen ions (ie, a pH above 7.45).

allergens Antigens that can produce hypersensitivity reactions in the body.

allergy A hypersensitivity reaction to intrinsically harmless antigens, most of which are environmental.

alpha-adrenergic receptors Any of the postulated adrenergic components of receptor tissues that respond to norepinephrine and to various blocking agents.

ammonium ions The monovalent cations symbolized by NH_4^+.

anaerobic Of or pertaining to the absence of oxygen.

anaphylaxis An exaggerated, life-threatening hypersensitivity reaction to an antigen.

angiotensin I The inactive form of angiotensin, formulated by the stimulation of renin, which is converted to angiotensin II.

angiotensin II A potent vasoconstrictor that also acts to stimulate the secretion of antidiuretic hormone.

angiotensin-converting enzyme (ACE) A circulating enzyme that participates in the body's renin-angiotensin system, which mediates extracellular volume and arterial vasoconstriction by converting angiotensin I to angiotensin II.

anion An ion with a negative charge.

antibodies Proteins produced by the body that destroy or inactivate specific substances (antigens) that have entered the body.

antigens Substances (usually proteins) that are capable of generating an immune response causing the formation of an antibody that reacts specifically with that antigen.

anuria The inability to urinate; the cessation of urine production; a diminished urinary output of less than 100 to 250 mL per day.

areflexia A neurologic condition characterized by the absence of reflexes.

arterioles Small branches of arteries that lead into capillaries.

arteriovenous anastomoses Vessels that allow blood to flow from arteries to veins without passing through capillaries; also known as an arteriovenous shunts.

ascites An abnormal intraperitoneal accumulation of fluid containing large amounts of protein and electrolytes.

atherosclerosis A common arterial disorder characterized by yellow plaques of cholesterol, lipids, and cellular debris in the inner layers of the walls of large and medium-size arteries.

atrial natriuretic factor A peptide released from the atria when atrial blood pressure is increased. It lowers blood pressure by increasing urine production, thus reducing blood volume.

atrophy Decrease in size (shrinkage) of a cell, which adversely affects cell function.

autoimmunity An abnormal characteristic or condition in which the body reacts against constituents of its own tissues.

autolysis The spontaneous disintegration of tissues or cells by the action of their own autogenous enzymes.

B lymphocytes The lymphocytes responsible for antibody-mediated immunity.

bacteremia The presence of bacteria in the blood.

bases Chemical compounds that combine with acids to form salts; also known as alkalis.

beta-adrenergic receptors Any of the postulated adrenergic components of receptor tissues that respond to epinephrine and various blocking agents.

bicarbonate An alkaline substance in the blood that participates in the transport of carbon dioxide and in the regulation of pH.

bivalent cation An ion with two positive charges.

botulism An often fatal form of food poisoning caused by the bacillus *Clostridium botulinum*.

capillaries Tiny branching vessels that connect arterioles to venules; the site where most gas exchange occurs between the blood and tissues.

capillary network A complex, interconnected structure where a single blood cell traveling from an arteriole to a venule via a capillary bed passes through capillary segments.

capsid A protein coat that encloses a virus.

carbonic acid An aqueous solution of carbon dioxide.

carbonic anhydrase The enzyme that converts carbon dioxide into carbonic acid.

cardiac output The volume of blood pumped each minute by the ventricles.

carrier-mediated transport Movement that occurs across membranes to move substances against a concentration gradient, from areas of lower concentration to areas of higher concentration.

carrier molecule A protein that combines with solutes on one side of a membrane, transporting the solute to the other side. It is used in mediated transport mechanisms.

cathartics Substances that accelerate defecation.

cation An ion with a positive charge.

central nervous system ischemic response An increase in blood pressure caused by vasoconstriction that occurs when oxygen levels are too low, carbon dioxide levels are too high, or pH is too low in the medulla.

chemotactic factors Biochemical mediators that are important in activating the inflammatory response.

complement system A group of proteins that coat bacteria. The proteins then either help kill the bacteria directly or assist neutrophils (in the blood) and macrophages (in the tissues) to engulf and destroy the bacteria.

concentration gradient The concentration difference between two points in a solution divided by the distance between the points.

congenital Present at birth.

cortisol A steroid hormone that occurs naturally in the body.

cytochromes Proteins in the liver that play a role in drug detoxification.

dehydration An excessive loss of water from the body tissues. It may follow prolonged fever, diarrhea, vomiting, acidosis, and other conditions.

diabetes mellitus A complex disorder of carbohydrate, fat, and protein metabolism that primarily results from partial or complete lack of insulin secretion by the beta cells of the pancreas or occurs because of defects in the insulin receptors.

diffusion The process by which solid, particulate matter in a fluid moves from an area of higher concentration to an area of lower concentration, resulting in an even distribution of the particles in the fluid.

diuretics Medicines that help increase excretion of water from the body.

dysplasia Abnormal cellular growth.

dysrhythmias Variations from a normal rhythm.

edema The accumulation of fluid in the interstitial spaces.

endotoxins Toxins contained in the cell walls of some microorganisms, especially gram-negative bacteria.

exotoxins Toxins secreted or excreted by a living organism.

extracellular fluid The fluid found outside the cells, including that in the intravascular and interstitial compartments.

facilitated diffusion A carrier-mediated process that moves substances into or out of cells from a high to a low concentration.

glycolysis An anaerobic process during which glucose is converted to pyruvic acid.

hemodialysis A procedure in which impurities or wastes are removed from the blood. It is used in treating renal insufficiency and various toxic conditions.

hemoglobin A complex protein–iron compound in the blood that carries oxygen to the cells from the lungs and carbon dioxide away from the cells to the lungs.

hydrogen ion The acidic element in a solution.

hypercalcemia A higher-than-normal concentration of calcium in the blood.

hyperemia An increase in organ blood flow.

hyperkalemia A higher-than-normal concentration of potassium in the blood.

hypermagnesemia A higher-than-normal concentration of magnesium in the blood.

hypernatremic dehydration The loss of more water than sodium.

hyperphosphatemia High levels of phosphate in the blood.

hyperplasia An excessive increase in the number of cells.

hypersensitivity An altered immunologic reactivity to an antigen.

hypersensitivity reactions A pathologic immune response to an antigen.

hypertonic A term used to describe a solution that has a greater concentration of solutes than does another solution, giving it a higher osmotic pressure than the pressure of body cells. Cells may shrink as water is pulled out of the cell into the area of higher solute concentration.

hypertrophy An increase in the size of a cell.

hypocalcemia An abnormally low level of calcium in the blood.

hypokalemia A lower-than-normal concentration of potassium in the blood.

hypomagnesemia A lower-than-normal concentration of magnesium in the blood plasma.

hyponatremic dehydration The loss of more sodium than water.

hypoperfusion Severely inadequate circulation that results in insufficient delivery of oxygen and nutrients necessary for normal tissue and cellular function; may cause shock.

hypophosphatemia Low levels of phosphate in the blood.

hypotonic A term used to describe a solution that has a lower concentration of solutes than does another solution.

hypoxemia A lower-than-normal oxygen content of the blood as measured in an arterial blood sample.

immune response A defense function of the body that produces antibodies to destroy invading antigens and malignancies.

infarction Tissue death from lack of oxygen.

inflammatory response A tissue reaction to injury or to an antigen. It may include pain, swelling, itching, redness, heat, and loss of function.

interstitial fluid Fluid that occupies the space outside the blood vessels and/or outside the cells of an organ or tissue.

intracellular fluid The fluid found in all body cells.

ischemia A state of insufficient perfusion of oxygenated blood to a body organ or part.

isoimmunity Production by an individual of antibodies from members of the same species, such as anti-Rh antibodies in an Rh-negative person; also called alloimmunity.

isotonic A term used to describe a solution in which its solute concentration is the same as the solute concentration of another solution with which it is compared.

isotonic dehydration Excessive loss of sodium and water in equal amounts.

ketone bodies The normal metabolic products of lipid and pyruvate within the liver. Excessive production leads to their excretion in urine.

Krebs cycle A sequence of enzymatic reactions involving the metabolism of carbon chains of sugar, fatty acids, and amino acids to yield carbon dioxide, water, and high-energy phosphate bonds.

lactate A salt of lactic acid.

lactic acidosis A disorder characterized by an accumulation of lactic acid in the blood, resulting in a lowered pH in muscle and serum.

leukocytosis An abnormal increase in the number of circulating white blood cells.

malaise A vague feeling of weakness or discomfort.

mast cells Specialized cells of the inflammatory response.

mediated transport mechanisms Mechanisms that use carrier molecules to move large, water-soluble molecules or electrically charged molecules across cell membranes.

membrane permeability A quality of cell membranes that permits the passage of solvents and solutes into and out of cells.

metaplasia A change from one cell type to another that is better able to tolerate adverse conditions; a conversion into a form that is not normal for that cell.

metarterioles Small peripheral blood vessels that contain scattered groups of smooth muscle fibers in their walls. They are located between the arterioles and the true capillaries.

multiple organ dysfunction syndrome (MODS) The progressive failure of two or more organ systems after a severe illness or injury.

necrosis Death of a cell or group of cells as the result of disease or injury.

negative feedback mechanisms Mechanisms that tend to produce a response that balances a change in a system.

neoplasia New and abnormal development of cells, which may be benign or malignant.

nonelectrolytes Substances with no electrical charge.

oliguria A diminished capacity to form or pass urine.

osmolality The osmotic pressure of a solution.

osmosis The diffusion of solvent (water) through a membrane from a less concentrated solution to a more concentrated solution.

osmotic pressure The minimum pressure required to prevent the movement of a solution across a semipermeable membrane.

overhydration Water excess or water intoxication.

paresthesia A sensation of numbness, tingling, or "pins and needles."

partial pressure The pressure exerted by a single gas.

pathophysiology The abnormal functions and diseases of the human body.

pH An inverse logarithm of the hydrogen ion concentration.

phagocytosis The process by which cells ingest solid substances such as other cells, bacteria, bits of necrosed tissue, and foreign particles.

pitting edema Observable indentation of body tissues that persists after applying pressure to an area swollen from fluid accumulation.

polyuria Excessive excretion of urine.

postcapillary sphincter The smooth muscle sphincter at the venous end of a capillary that regulates blood flow out of the capillary.

precapillary sphincter The smooth muscle sphincter at the arterial end of a capillary that regulates blood flow into the capillary.

preload The amount of blood returning to the ventricle.

renin A proteolytic enzyme secreted by the kidneys that is involved in the release of angiotensin; plays an important role in the maintenance of blood pressure.

renin-angiotensin-aldosterone mechanism The mechanism for regulating levels of sodium and water.

respiratory acidosis An abnormal condition characterized by an increased arterial partial pressure of carbon dioxide, excess carbonic acid, and an increased plasma hydrogen ion concentration (pH).

respiratory alkalosis An abnormal condition characterized by decreased arterial partial pressure of carbon dioxide, decreased hydrogen ion concentration, and increased blood pH.

Rh factor An antigenic substance present in the erythrocytes of most people. A person lacking the Rh factor is Rh negative.

semipermeable membranes Membranes that allow some fluids and substances to pass through them but not others, usually dependent on size, shape, electrical charge, or other chemical properties of the substance or fluid.

shock Hypoxia at the cellular level.

solutes Substances dissolved in solution.

Starling hypothesis The concept that describes the movement of fluid across the capillary wall (net filtration).

stroke volume The volume of blood ejected from one ventricle in a single heartbeat.

systemic vascular resistance The total resistance against which blood must be pumped; also known as afterload.

T lymphocytes The lymphocytes responsible for cell-mediated immunity.

tetany The involuntary contraction of skeletal muscles.

total pressure The combination of the pressures exerted by all the gases in any mixture of gases.

toxoids Toxins that have been treated with chemicals or with heat to reduce their toxic effects but still retain their antigenic power.

virulence The relative harmfulness or severity of a pathogen.

Chapter 10, Review of Human Systems, *describes anatomy and physiology—the structure and function of the human body. This chapter discusses* ***pathophysiology****—the abnormal functions and diseases of the human body. Paramedics need to understand the physical and biologic principles of disease. This knowledge will help them to anticipate, direct, and provide appropriate care to their patients.*

NOTE

This chapter is intended to provide an introduction and overview of pathophysiology. Additional discussions of disease processes are presented throughout this textbook as indicated by subject matter.

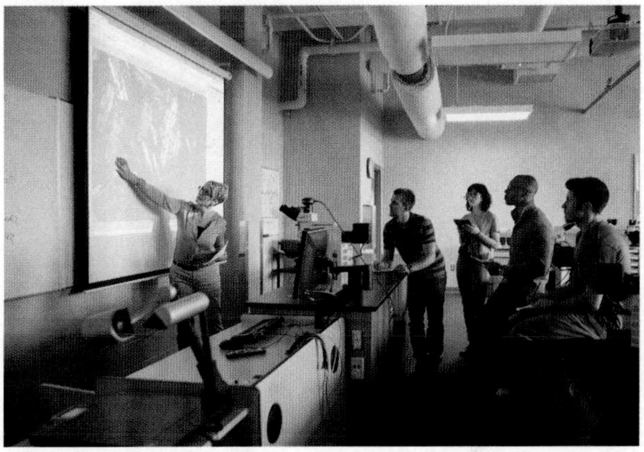

© Hero Images / Getty images

Cellular Physiology: Basic Cellular Review

As discussed in Chapter 10, *Review of Human Systems,* the cell is the basic unit of higher life forms. All cells have various key components and structures. These include cell membranes, membranes that isolate individual cells and separate each cell's internal (cellular) environment from its external environment, and enzymes, proteins that mediate biochemical processes. Other key components and structures are the internal membranes that encapsulate chemicals, and the genetic material for replication. Cells form the four basic types of tissue:

- Epithelial tissue
- Connective tissue (including hematologic tissue)
- Muscle tissue
- Nervous tissue

The cells of the human body live in a fluid environment that consists mainly of water. Body water is essential because it is the medium in which all metabolic reactions occur and the body's health depends on precise regulation of the volume and composition of this fluid. The body has two fluid compartments: the intracellular fluid and the extracellular fluid (**FIGURE 11-1**).

Intracellular and Extracellular Fluid

Total body water in humans makes up between 45% to 75% of total body weight. About two thirds of this is intracellular fluid, and one third is extracellular fluid. **Intracellular fluid** is the fluid found inside all body cells. **Extracellular fluid** is the fluid found outside the cells. This includes the intravascular and interstitial compartments. The extracellular fluid between the cells and outside the vascular bed (ie, connective tissue, cartilage, and bone) is known as **interstitial fluid**. This category also includes special fluids, such as cerebrospinal fluid and intraocular fluid.

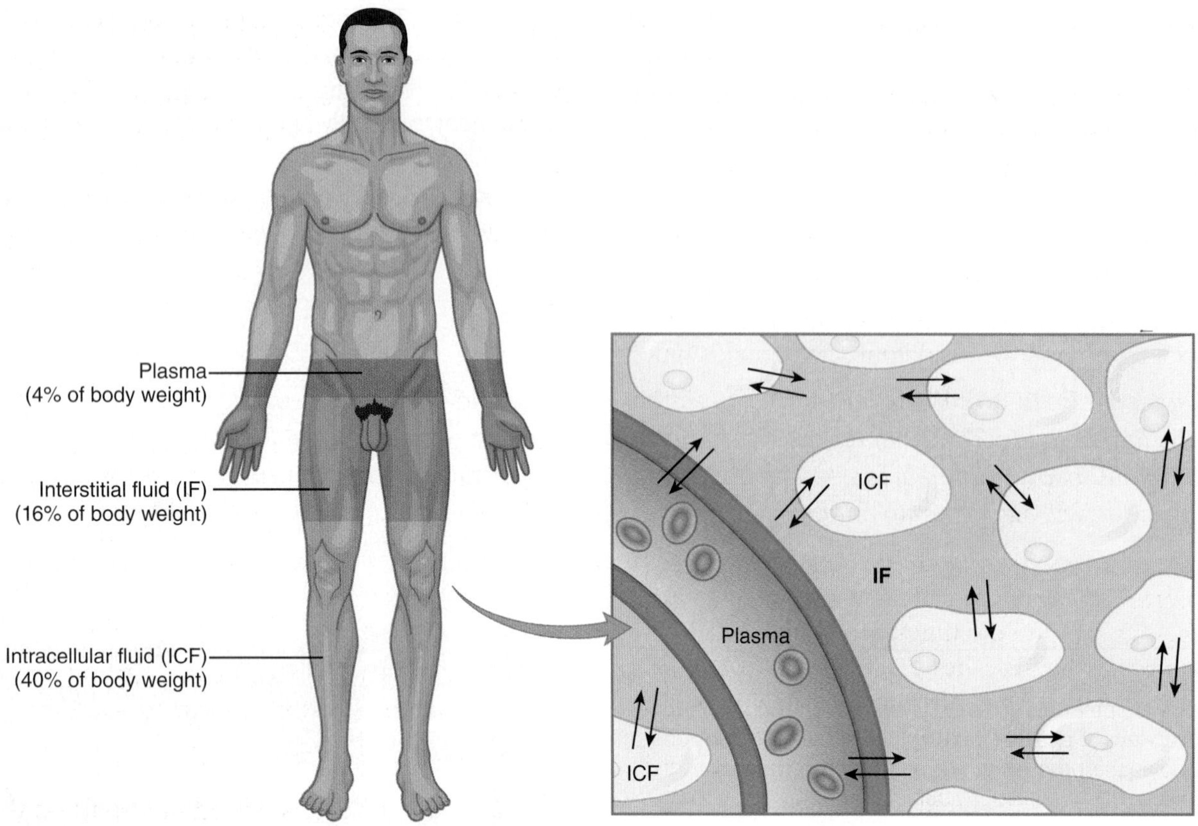

FIGURE 11-1 Fluid compartments of the body.

Aging and the Distribution of Body Fluids

Body mass consists mainly of water. In fact, water accounts for 50% to 60% of total body weight in adults. The distribution and amount of total body water (TBW) vary according to age. For example, about 80% of a newborn's body weight is TBW. During childhood, TBW decreases to 60% to 65% of body weight, and it declines further with age (**TABLE 11-1**). TBW in the older adult population decreases to 45% to 55%, increasing the risk of dehydration and electrolyte abnormalities (see Chapter 48, *Geriatrics*).

NOTE

In older adults, the normal reduction in TBW becomes a significant factor if fever or dehydration is present. With illness or injury, loss of body fluids can be severe or life threatening.

TABLE 11-1 Total Body Water Relative to Body Type

Body Build	Adult Male (% TBW)	Adult Female (% TBW)	Infant (% TBW)
Normal	60	50	70
Lean	70	60	80
Obese	50	42	60

Abbreviation: TBW, total body water

Water Movement Between Intracellular Fluid and Extracellular Fluid

Body fluids constantly move from one compartment to another. In healthy people, the volume in each compartment remains about the same. To keep the volume stable, the body uses **osmosis**, **diffusion**, and **mediated transport mechanisms**. To understand illness and disease, the paramedic first must understand how fluids in the body move and how changes in these fluids can occur.

Osmosis

For the body to function well, molecules must be able to move within a cell or across cell membranes. Membranes separate fluid compartments. Most of these membranes allow water to pass freely. They also regulate the flow of **solutes** (substances dissolved in solution) on the basis of size, shape, electrical charge, or other chemical properties. These membranes are referred to as **semipermeable membranes**. Channels in these membranes permit the passage of solutes. The channels may be open at all times to specific solutes, or they may be closed at times, depending on the cell's composition. Because the cell membrane can regulate the flow of solutes, the cell can maintain homeostasis (stability in the body's internal environment).

Osmosis is the spontaneous net movement of solvent molecules through a semipermeable membrane into a region of higher solute concentration, in the direction that tends to equalize the solute concentrations on the two sides (**FIGURE 11-2**). The semipermeable membrane blocks the transport of salts or other solutes between the two solutions of different concentrations. The pressure that prevents the flow of fluid across a semipermeable membrane is **osmotic pressure**; it is the pressure required to maintain cellular equilibrium. Osmotic pressure depends on two factors: (1) the number and molecular weight of particles on each side of the cell membrane and (2) the **membrane permeability** to these particles.

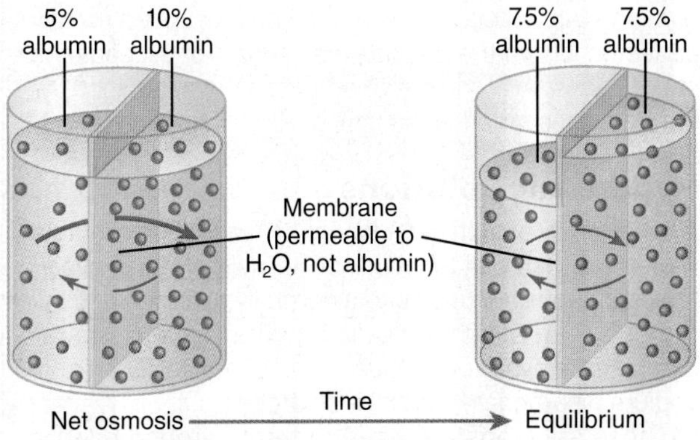

FIGURE 11-2 Osmosis is the net movement of solvent molecules through a semipermeable membrane. The membrane shown in this diagram is permeable to water but not to albumin. Because there are relatively more water molecules in 5% albumin than in 10% albumin, more water molecules osmose from the more dilute solution into the more concentrated solution (as indicated by the larger arrow in the diagram on the left) than osmose in the opposite direction. Therefore, the overall direction of osmosis is toward the more concentrated solution. Movement across the membrane continues until the concentrations of the solution equalize.

NOTE

With gases, the driving force of osmosis is produced by the partial pressures of the dissolved gases (eg, oxygen, nitrogen, carbon dioxide) and water. In any mixture of gases, the combination of the pressures exerted by all the gases is the **total pressure**. The pressure exerted by a single gas is the **partial pressure**. The partial pressure of a gas in a mixture is denoted by the letter *P* preceding the gas (eg, the partial pressure of oxygen [Po_2] or the partial pressure of carbon dioxide [Pco_2]) (see Chapter 15, *Airway Management, Respiration, and Artificial Ventilation*).

When a living cell is placed in a solution that has a higher solute concentration (and a lower water concentration) than that inside the cell, the solution is called a **hypertonic** solution. When the cell is placed in this solution, the osmotic pressure exerted on it produces a net movement of water out of the cell. This causes the cell to dehydrate, shrink, and possibly die.

Likewise, when a living cell is placed in a solution that has a lower solute concentration (and a higher water concentration) than that inside the cell, the solution is called a **hypotonic** solution. Osmotic pressure draws water from the solution into the cell. The net movement of water into the cell causes it to swell and possibly burst (lyse).

NOTE

Electrolytes are salt substances whose molecules dissociate into charged components in water, producing positively and negatively charged ions. An ion with a positive charge is called a cation. An ion with a negative charge is called an anion. Sodium is the most abundant cation in the extracellular fluid. It is responsible for the osmotic balance of the extracellular fluid space. Potassium is the most abundant cation in the intracellular fluid. It maintains the osmotic balance of the intracellular fluid space. The body also has **nonelectrolytes** (substances with no electrical charge), such as glucose and urea.

A cell may be placed in a solution that has the same solute and water concentrations as the solution inside the cell. This solution is called **isotonic**. Isotonic solutions have no net movement of water molecules (**FIGURE 11-3** and BOX 11-1).

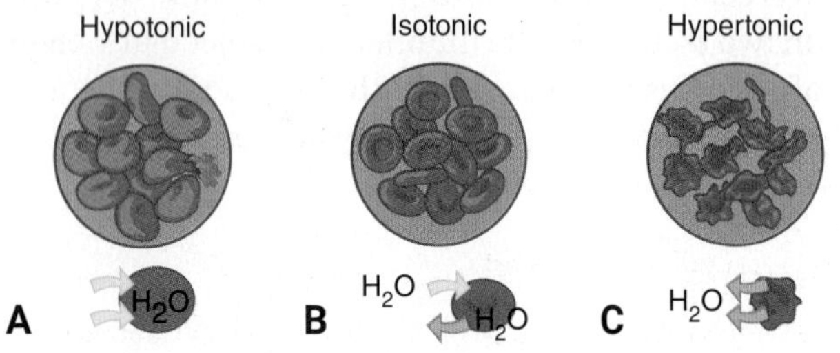

FIGURE 11-3 Effects of hypotonic, isotonic, and hypertonic solutions on red blood cells. **A.** The hypotonic solution, which has a low ion concentration, causes swelling and lysis of the cells. **B.** In the isotonic solution, which has a normal ion concentration, the cells keep their normal shape. **C.** The hypertonic solution, which has a high ion concentration, causes shrinkage (crenation) of the cells.

Diffusion

Diffusion is a result of the constant motion of all the atoms, molecules, or ions in a solution. It is a passive process in which molecules or ions move from an area of higher concentration to an area of lower concentration (**FIGURE 11-4**). An area of high concentration has more solute particles than does an area of low concentration. More solute particles move from the higher concentration to the lower one. Once at equilibrium, the movement of solutes in one direction is balanced by equal movement in the opposite direction.

The concentration of a solute may be greater at one point in the solvent than it is at another point. This means that a **concentration gradient** exists. Solutes diffuse down their concentration gradients from high to low concentration until equilibrium is achieved. Some nutrients enter and some waste products leave the cell by diffusion. Maintenance of the proper intracellular concentrations of certain substances depends on this process.

BOX 11-1 Fluid Replacement Therapy

Intravenous therapy is based on hypertonic, hypotonic, and isotonic properties.

Hypotonic Solutions

A hypotonic solution has a lower solute concentration than that of normal cells. When a hypotonic solution is infused into a normally hydrated patient, water is drawn from the solution into the cells. Hypotonic solutions containing dextrose supply the patient with calories. Those containing sodium replenish salt and water. They are used to hydrate patients. They are used to prevent dehydration as well. An example of a hypotonic solution is 2.5% dextrose in water. Another is 0.45% normal saline (½NS). Although 5% dextrose in water (D_5W) is technically isotonic, it acts physiologically as a hypotonic solution. This is because the solute (glucose) is quickly metabolized to carbon dioxide and water.

Isotonic Solutions

In an isotonic solution, the concentration of solute molecules is the same as that found in most normal cells. When an isotonic solution is infused into a normally hydrated patient, water is neither drawn out of the cells nor moved into them. Rather, water stays in the vascular space. Isotonic solutions are usually given to replace extracellular fluid. This fluid may have been depleted as a result of blood loss or severe vomiting. An isotonic solution may be prescribed for any patient in whom the chloride loss equals or exceeds the sodium loss. An example of an isotonic solution is 0.9% normal saline. Another is lactated Ringer solution.

Hypertonic Solutions

A hypertonic solution has a higher concentration of solute molecules than that found in normal cells. When a hypertonic solution is infused into a normally hydrated patient, it draws water from the cells into the vascular space. Examples of hypertonic solutions are mannitol (Osmitrol), sodium bicarbonate, and 50% dextrose (D_{50}).

These solutions are used to treat cerebral edema (mannitol), metabolic acidosis (bicarbonate), and profound hypoglycemia (D_{50}). Past studies suggested that some hypertonic solutions (eg, Dextran and sodium chloride [3% and 7.5%, respectively]) should be used for volume restoration after trauma. More recent evidence finds no benefit to the use of hypertonic saline, with or without dextran, in general trauma patients.

Modified from: Metheny NM. *Fluid and Electrolyte Balance*. 5th ed. Burlington, MA: Jones & Bartlett Learning; 2012; Udeani J. Hemorrhagic shock treatment and management. Medscape website. http://emedicine.medscape.com/article/432650-treatment. Updated May 27, 2015. Accessed February 1, 2018; and de Crescenzo CD, Gorouhi F, Salcedo ES, Galante JM. Prehospital hypertonic fluid resuscitation for trauma patients: a systematic review and meta-analysis. *J Trauma Acute Care Surg*. 2017;82(5):956-962.

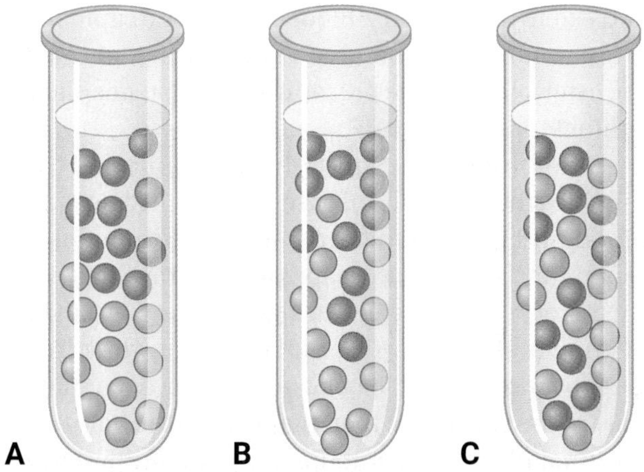

FIGURE 11-4 Diffusion. **A.** A solution (red, representing one type of molecule) is layered onto another solution (blue, representing a second type of molecule). A concentration gradient exists that favors the passage of red molecules into the blue solution because the blue solution has no red molecules. Likewise, a concentration gradient exists that favors the passage of blue molecules into the red solution because the red solution has no blue molecules. **B.** Red molecules move with their concentration gradient into the blue solution, and the blue molecules move with their concentration gradient into the red solution. **C.** Red and blue molecules are distributed evenly throughout the solution. Even though the red and blue molecules continue to move randomly, equilibrium exists. This means that no net movement occurs because no concentration gradient exists.

CRITICAL THINKING

What happens to a raisin that is put into a cup of water and left there for an hour? Why does this change occur? Is the water hypotonic, hypertonic, or isotonic relative to the inside of the raisin? Does a concentration gradient exist?

Mediated Transport Mechanisms

A number of vital molecules (eg, glucose) cannot enter most cells by diffusion. Also, several products (eg, some proteins) cannot exit most cells by diffusion. Mediated transport mechanisms are required to move large, water-soluble molecules or electrically charged molecules across the cell membranes. These mechanisms use carrier molecules. A **carrier molecule** is a protein that combines with a solute molecule on one side of a membrane. It then changes shape, passes through the membrane, and releases the solute molecule on the other side (**FIGURE 11-5**).

Carrier-mediated transport can be divided into two types: active transport and facilitated diffusion.

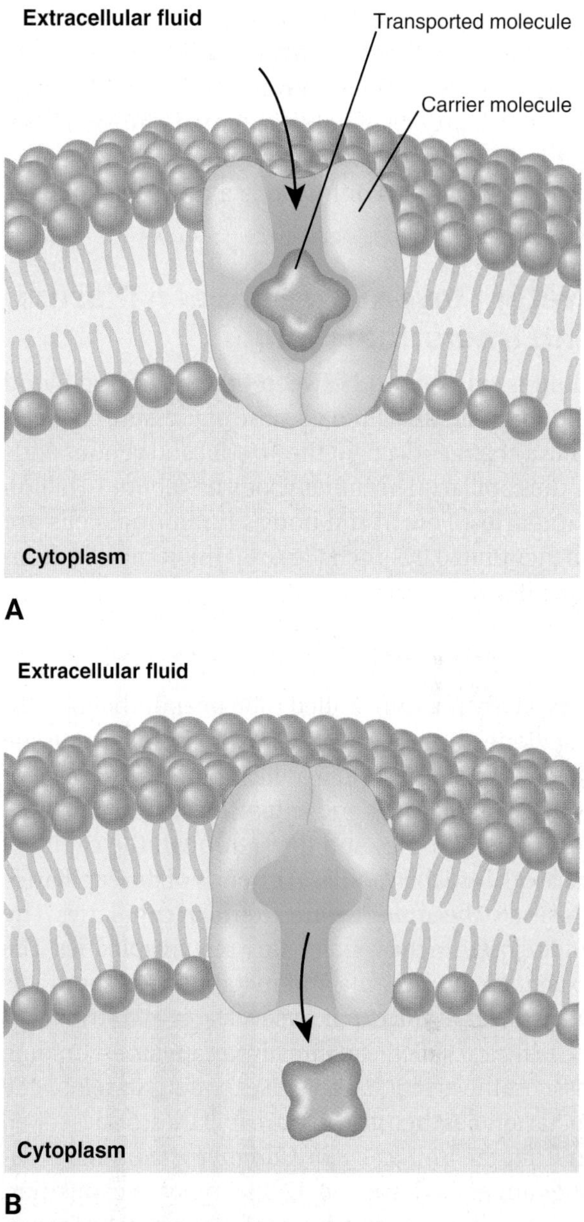

FIGURE 11-5 Mediated transport by a carrier molecule. **A.** The carrier molecule binds with a molecule on one side of the plasma membrane and changes shape. **B.** The molecule is released on the other side of the plasma membrane.

Active transport moves substances against a concentration gradient, from areas of lower concentration to areas of higher concentration. The cell must expend energy to work against this concentration gradient. Active transport occurs at a faster rate than does diffusion.

Facilitated diffusion moves substances into and out of cells from an area of higher concentration to an area of lower concentration. For these materials, the direction of movement is with the concentration gradient. As with active transport, this movement occurs more quickly than in normal diffusion. However, unlike in active transport, facilitated diffusion does not require the cell to expend energy. The moving force in facilitated diffusion is a downhill concentration gradient.

Water Movement Between Plasma and Interstitial Fluid

Fluid is transferred between the circulating blood and the interstitial fluid because of pressure changes. These changes occur at the arterial and venous ends of the capillary. The human body has about 10 billion capillaries. Few of the body's functional cells are farther than 0.001 inch (20 to 30 micrometers) from a capillary.

Anatomy of the Capillary Network

A capillary is a thin-walled tube of endothelial cells. **Capillaries** do not have elastic or connective tissue or smooth muscle that would impede the transfer of water and solutes. Blood enters the **capillary network** from the arterioles and flows through the capillary network into the venules. The ends of the capillaries closest to the arterioles are arteriolar capillaries. The ends closest to the venules are venous capillaries. The exchange of nutrients and metabolic end products takes place at the capillary level.

The arterioles lead directly to capillaries. In some tissues, the **arterioles** give rise to **metarterioles**. The metarterioles then give rise to capillaries. As described in Chapter 10, *Review of Human Systems*, most tissues appear to have two distinct types of capillaries: true capillaries and thoroughfare channels. From a metarteriole, blood may flow into a thoroughfare channel that connects arterioles and venules directly, bypassing the true capillaries. Blood flow through thoroughfare channels is relatively constant. From the thoroughfare channels, fluid commonly exits and reenters the network of true capillaries.

The capillaries of some tissues have small cuffs of smooth muscle. These cuffs, which encircle the proximal and distal portions of the capillary, are known as capillary sphincters. The sphincter at the arterial end is known as the **precapillary sphincter**. The sphincter at the venous end is known as the **postcapillary sphincter**. These sphincters control capillary blood flow by opening and closing the entrance and exit to the capillary. Blood flow in true capillaries is not uniform. It depends on the contractile state of the arterioles and the precapillary and postcapillary sphincters (if present).

The blood flow through the capillaries that provides the exchange of gases and solutes between blood and tissue is referred to as nutritional flow. Blood that bypasses the capillaries in traveling from the arterial to the venous side of the circulation is known as nonnutritional, or shunt, flow. True **arteriovenous anastomoses** (AV shunts) occur naturally in the sole of the foot, the palm of the hand, the terminal phalanges, and the nail bed. These shunts are important for the regulation of body temperature. Some evidence suggests the presence of AV shunts upstream from the capillary sphincters.[1]

Sympathetic fibers innervate all blood vessels of the body, except for the capillaries, the capillary sphincters, and most metarterioles. Sympathetic innervation of blood vessels includes both vasoconstrictor and vasodilator (vasomotor) fibers. However, the vasoconstrictor fibers are the most important in regulating blood flow. During normal circulation in the healthy body, when arterial blood pressure is adequate, arterioles are open (although with some vasomotor tone), AV shunts are closed, and about 20% of the capillaries are open at any given time (**FIGURE 11-6**).

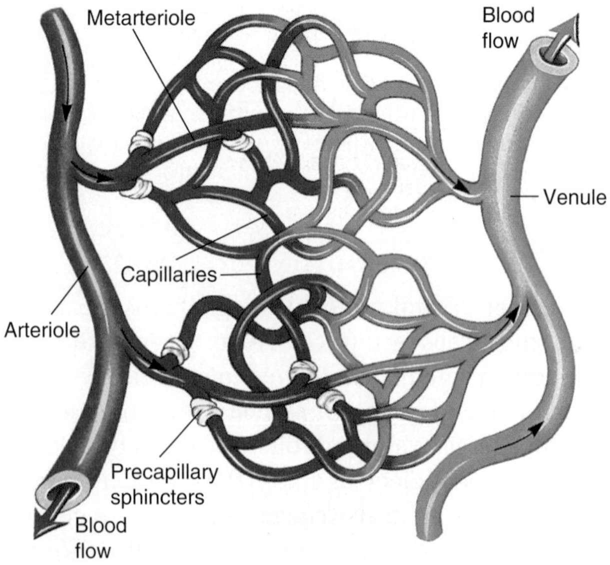

FIGURE 11-6 Microcirculation. The precapillary sphincters (circular structures) regulate blood flow from arterioles into the capillaries. The arrows indicate the direction of blood flow.

Diffusion Across the Capillary Wall. Tissue cells do not exchange material directly with blood. The interstitial fluid always acts as a "middleman." Nutrients must diffuse across the capillary wall into the interstitial fluid to enter cells. Metabolic end products, such as carbon dioxide and lactic acid, first must move across cell membranes into interstitial fluid to diffuse into the plasma.

At the arteriole end of the capillary, the forces moving fluid out of the capillary are greater than the forces attracting fluid into it. At the venous end, these forces are reversed. Therefore, more fluid is attracted into the capillary at the venous end. Hydrostatic and osmotic pressures are the two forces responsible for this movement of fluid. The hydrostatic pressure (created with each heartbeat) forces water out of the arterial end of the capillary. The osmotic pressure results from the presence of plasma proteins (mostly albumin), which are too large to pass through the wall of the capillary; this pressure is referred to as blood colloid osmotic pressure or oncotic pressure.

At the venous end of the capillary, the hydrostatic pressure is lower. The concentration of proteins in the capillary increases slightly because of the movement of fluid out of the arteriolar end. The result is a greater plasma protein concentration and a greater colloid osmotic pressure. Consequently, nearly all the fluid that leaves the capillary at its arteriolar end reenters the capillary at its venous end. The remaining fluid enters the lymphatic capillaries and eventually returns to the general circulation. The movement of fluid across the capillary wall is called net filtration. It is best described by the **Starling hypothesis**:[2]

Net filtration = Forces favoring filtration –
Forces opposing filtration

The forces favoring filtration include capillary hydrostatic pressure and the interstitial oncotic pressure. The forces opposing filtration are the plasma oncotic pressure and the interstitial hydrostatic pressure.

Fluid also may be exchanged across the capillary wall as a result of the cyclic dilation and constriction of the precapillary sphincter. When this sphincter dilates, the pressure rises in the capillary and forces fluid to move into the interstitial spaces. When the precapillary sphincter constricts, the pressure in the capillary drops and the fluid moves into the capillary (**FIGURE 11-7**).

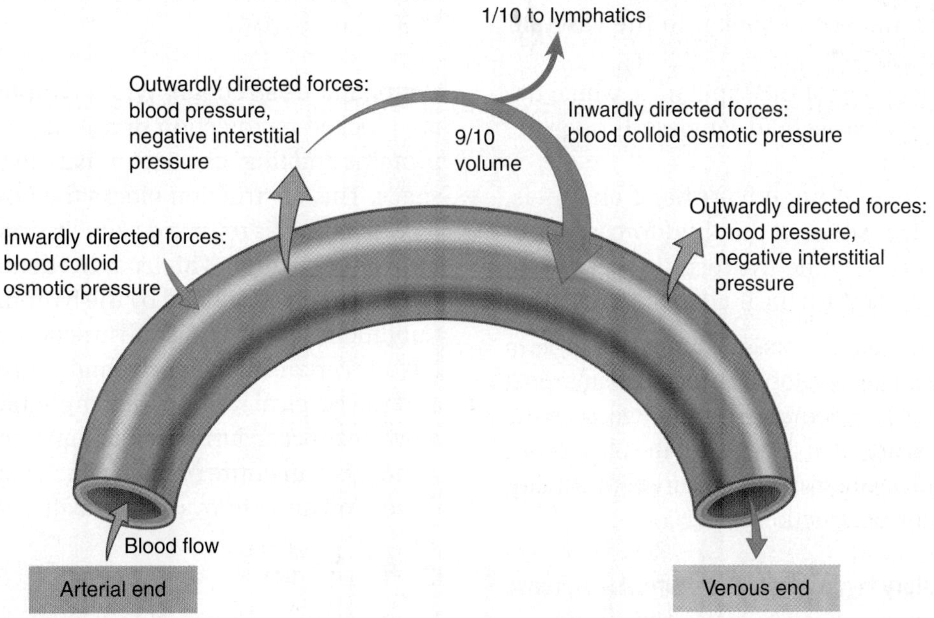

FIGURE 11-7 Total pressure differences between the inside and the outside of the capillary at its arteriolar and venous ends. At the arteriolar end, the sum of the forces causes fluid to move from the capillaries into the tissues. At the venous end, the sum of the forces attracts fluid into the capillary. About 9⁄10 of the fluid leaving the capillary at the arteriolar end reenters it at the venous end while the remainig 1⁄10 goes into lymphatic capillaries.

Capillary and Membrane Permeability

A key factor in the movement of fluid across the capillary wall is the integrity of the capillary membrane. Changes in membrane permeability may allow plasma proteins to escape into the interstitial space. The resultant increase in interstitial oncotic pressure changes the relationship defined by the Starling hypothesis. It leads to osmotic movement of water into the interstitial space, resulting in tissue edema.

Alterations in Water Movement

Edema is a problem of fluid distribution that results in the accumulation of fluid in the interstitial spaces. It can be caused by any condition that leads to a net movement of fluid out of capillaries and into the interstitial tissues. It does not always indicate a fluid excess.

Pathophysiology of Edema

The normal flow of fluid through the interstitial spaces depends on the following four factors:

1. The capillary hydrostatic pressure that filters fluid from the blood through the capillary wall
2. The oncotic pressure exerted by the proteins in the blood plasma, which attracts fluid from the interstitial space back into the vascular compartment
3. The permeability of the capillaries, which determines how easily fluid can pass through the capillary wall
4. The presence of open lymphatic channels, which collect some of the fluid forced out of the capillaries by the hydrostatic pressure of the blood and return the fluid to the circulation

When any of these four factors is disturbed, changes in water movement can develop. The mechanisms most often responsible for edema are (1) an increase in the hydrostatic pressure, (2) a decrease in the plasma oncotic pressure, (3) an increase in capillary permeability, and (4) lymphatic obstruction.

Increased Capillary Hydrostatic Pressure. An increase in hydrostatic pressure can be caused by venous obstruction or sodium and water retention. With venous obstruction, the hydrostatic pressure of fluid in the capillaries can become great enough to cause fluid to escape into the interstitial spaces. Conditions that can lead to venous obstruction and edema include thrombophlebitis (the formation of a blood clot and inflammation in a vein), chronic venous disease, hepatic obstruction (blockage of hepatic veins or common bile duct), tight clothing around an extremity, and prolonged standing.

Sodium and water retention can cause an increase in circulating fluid volume (volume overload) and edema. Congestive heart failure and renal failure are two conditions associated with sodium and water retention.

Decreased Plasma Oncotic Pressure. Decreases in plasma albumin concentration lead to a decrease in the plasma oncotic pressure. As a result, fluid moves into the interstitial space. This condition most often results from liver disease or protein malnutrition.

Increased Capillary Permeability. Increases in capillary permeability result in greater than normal filtration of fluid into the interstitial space. This condition usually is associated with allergic reactions. It also is linked to inflammation and the immune response triggered by trauma. (The immune response is described later in this chapter.) Examples of such trauma are burns or crushing injuries. In such cases, proteins escape from the vascular bed, causing decreased capillary oncotic pressure and increased fluid oncotic pressure. The result is edema.

Lymphatic Obstruction. When lymphatic channels are blocked by infection or are surgically removed, proteins and fluid can accumulate in the interstitial space. This obstruction blocks the normal pathway by which fluid is returned from the interstitial space into the circulation. This leads to edema in the region that normally is drained by the lymphatic channels. Conditions that can cause obstruction in the channels include certain malignancies and parasitic infections, and the surgical removal of lymphatics. Surgical removal may occur during a radical mastectomy (surgical removal of an entire breast), which usually includes dissection and removal of the axillary lymph nodes.

Clinical Manifestations of Edema

Edema may be localized or generalized. Localized edema usually is limited to an injury site, such as a sprained ankle, or an organ system. An affected organ system may be the brain (cerebral edema) or the lungs (pulmonary edema). Edema of specific organs such as the brain, lungs, or larynx can be life threatening.

Generalized edema is more widespread. It is most obvious in dependent parts of the body. It usually is noted first in the legs and ankles after prolonged standing or sitting. It is noted in the sacrum and buttocks when the person is lying down. Generalized edema usually causes weight gain, swelling, and puffiness. It is often linked to other symptoms caused by an underlying illness. In industrialized countries, the diseases that most often cause generalized edema are heart disease, kidney disease, and liver disease. In developing countries, the most common causes are malnutrition and parasitic disease.[3] When edematous tissue is compressed with a finger (eg, over the ankle or tibia), the fluid is pushed aside, leaving a "pit" or indentation that gradually refills with fluid. This condition is called **pitting edema** (BOX 11-2). The accumulation of fluid in the peritoneal cavity is a condition called **ascites**.

BOX 11-2 Pitting Edema Scale

- +1 Minor pitting of the skin without visible deformation; depression disappears quickly.
- +2 No obvious distortion of the skin; depression typically normalizes within 10 to 15 seconds.
- +3 Noted deformity of the skin; depression produces a definite pit that persists longer than 1 minute.
- +4 Obvious gross deformity of the skin (see photo); depression produces a very deep pit that persists longer than 2 minutes.

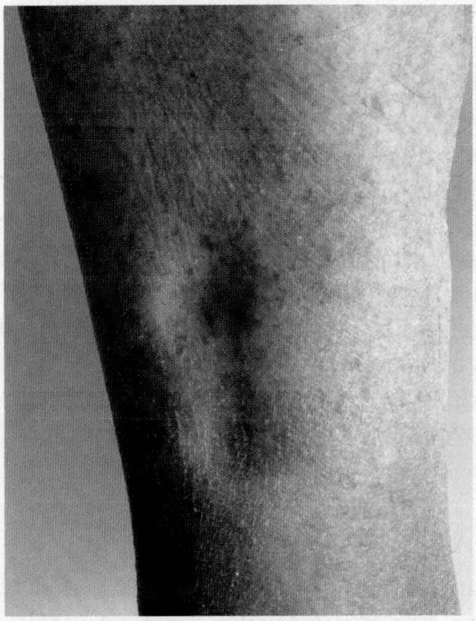

CRITICAL THINKING

The rest, ice, compression, and elevation (RICE) treatment is used for swelling from a sprained ankle. Why does this treatment reduce tissue edema?

Water Balance, Sodium, and Chloride

Water follows the osmotic gradient established by changes in the sodium concentration. Therefore, sodium and water balance are closely related.

Water Balance

Water balance is mainly regulated by antidiuretic hormone (ADH) (see Chapter 10, *Review of Human Systems*). The secretion of ADH and the perception of thirst help regulate water balance. Release of ADH is triggered by an increase in the plasma **osmolality** (the osmotic pressure of a solution). It also may be triggered by a decrease in the circulating blood volume and a decline in venous and arterial pressures. An increase in plasma osmolality stimulates hypothalamic neurons (called osmoreceptors), causing the person to feel thirsty. It also increases the release of ADH from the posterior pituitary gland (neurohypophysis).

In response to the release of ADH, water is reabsorbed into the plasma from the distal renal tubules and collecting ducts of the kidneys. This action reduces the amount of water lost in the urine. Also, as the water is reabsorbed, the plasma osmolality decreases, returning to normal. Volume-sensitive receptors, as well as pressure-sensitive receptors (baroreceptors, which are found in the heart and great vessels), also can stimulate the release of ADH when body fluids are depleted. These fluids may be lost from conditions such as vomiting, diarrhea, or excess sweating.

NOTE

Volume-sensitive receptors and baroreceptors are nerve endings that are sensitive to changes in volume and pressure, respectively. Volume-sensitive receptors are located in the right and left atria and the thoracic vessels. Baroreceptors are found in the aorta, pulmonary arteries, and carotid sinus.

Sodium and Chloride Balance

Sodium is the major extracellular fluid **cation**. Chloride is the major extracellular fluid **anion** and provides electroneutrality in relation to sodium. Increases or decreases in chloride concentration occur in proportion to changes in sodium concentration. Along with chloride and bicarbonate, sodium regulates osmotic forces and therefore water balance.

Sodium balance is regulated by **aldosterone** (a hormone secreted by the adrenal cortex). Secretion of aldosterone is triggered by a decrease in sodium levels. It also is triggered by an increase in potassium levels. Aldosterone causes the distal tubules of the kidneys to increase both the reabsorption of sodium and the secretion of potassium.

The enzyme **renin** also is secreted by the kidneys. This secretion occurs when the circulating blood volume is reduced or the sodium–water balance is disrupted. Renin catalyzes the conversion of a plasma protein (angiotensinogen) and stimulates the formation of **angiotensin I**. Angiotensin I is converted to **angiotensin II** by **angiotensin-converting enzyme (ACE)**, an enzyme found in the lungs. Angiotensin II is a potent vasoconstrictor. It acts to stimulate the secretion of ADH, which results in the reabsorption of sodium and water. It also results in an increase in the systemic blood pressure (described later in the chapter). This mechanism for regulating levels of sodium and water is known as the **renin-angiotensin-aldosterone mechanism** (**FIGURE 11-8**).

Atrial natriuretic hormone also helps to regulate sodium concentration by promoting the secretion of sodium in the urine. One result is a decrease in tubular reabsorption of sodium. Another result is a subsequent loss of sodium and water. **Atrial natriuretic factor** is a hormone released from the atrial cells of the heart. (It is described in Chapter 10, *Review of Human Systems*, and later in this chapter.) This peptide hormone also helps control the balance of sodium and water by promoting renal elimination of sodium.

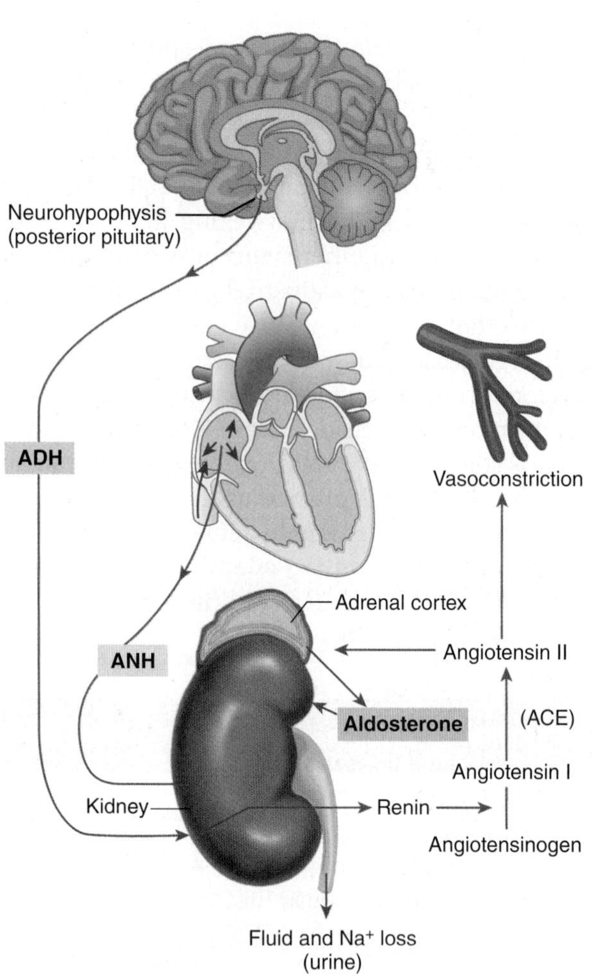

Abbreviations: ACE, angiotensin-converting enzyme; ADH, antidiuretic hormone; ANH, atrial natriuretic hormone

FIGURE 11-8 Three mechanisms that influence total plasma volume. The antidiuretic hormone mechanism and renin-angiotensin-aldosterone mechanism tend to increase water retention and thus increase total plasma volume. The atrial natriuretic hormone mechanism antagonizes these mechanisms by promoting water loss and thus promoting a decrease in total plasma volume.

Alterations in Sodium, Chloride, and Water Balance

In the healthy body, homeostatic mechanisms maintain a constant balance between the intake and the excretion of water. The water gained each day basically equals the water lost. The body gains water mainly in two ways: (1) when a person drinks fluids and eats moist foods and (2) when water is formed through the oxidation of hydrogen in food during the metabolic process. The body loses water through the kidneys as urine, through the bowel as feces, through the skin as perspiration, through exhaled air as vapor, and by the excretion of tears and saliva. Two abnormal states of body fluid balance can occur. If the water lost exceeds the water gained, a water deficit occurs. This is **dehydration**. If the water gained exceeds the water lost, a water excess occurs. This is **overhydration**.

Dehydration

Dehydration may occur in three ways. **Isotonic dehydration** is excessive loss of sodium and water in equal amounts. **Hypernatremic dehydration** is the loss of

CRITICAL THINKING

Consider the causes of dehydration and your knowledge of anatomy and physiology. What two age groups do you think are at highest risk for dehydration? Why?

more water than sodium. **Hyponatremic dehydration** is the loss of more sodium than water.

Isotonic Dehydration. Possible causes of isotonic dehydration include the following:

- Loss of water and electrolytes
  - Vomiting or diarrhea
  - Excess laxative use
  - Fistulas
  - Gastrointestinal suction
  - Polyuria
  - Fever
  - Excessive sweating
  - Third-space fluid shifts[4]
- Decreased fluid intake
  - Anorexia
  - Nausea
  - Inability to acquire fluids
  - Depression

Signs and symptoms may include the following:

- Dry skin and mucous membranes
- Poor skin turgor
- Longitudinal wrinkles or furrows of the tongue
- **Oliguria** (decreased urinary output of <30 mL/h in adults)
- **Anuria** (essentially no urinary output [≤100 mL in 24 hours])
- Acute weight loss (except when third-space fluid loss is present)
- Postural (orthostatic) hypotension (systolic blood pressure drop >20 mm Hg when patient stands)
- Rapid pulse
- Delayed capillary refill
- Elevated blood urea nitrogen (BUN)
- Decreased level of consciousness (late)
- Depressed or sunken fontanels in infants

Treatment for isotonic dehydration, if the patient has signs of shock, requires administering an intravenous infusion of an isotonic solution. The solution has a solute concentration equal to that of blood (0.9% sodium chloride [normal saline] or lactated Ringer solution typically is used). If signs of shock resolve or are not present, ½NS is indicated.[4] If no signs of shock are present and the patient can drink, fluids can be given orally.

NOTE

Third spacing occurs when injury, inflammation, or ischemia causes a change in capillary permeability. Conditions such as hip fracture, major surgery, burns, intestinal obstruction, inflamed abdominal organs, sepsis, pancreatitis, or ascites can cause large amounts of fluid shifts from the blood vessels to areas where the fluid cannot be used for normal body tasks, such as a body cavity, the bowel, or inflamed tissue. This shift does not lower the net amount of fluid in the body. The problem is that the leaked fluid is nonfunctional.

Hypernatremic Dehydration. Possible causes of hypernatremic dehydration include the following:

- Excessive use or misuse of diuretics
- Continued intake of sodium in the absence of water consumption
- Excessive loss of water with little loss of sodium
- Profuse, watery diarrhea

Signs and symptoms may include the following:

- Dry, sticky mucous membranes
- Flushed, doughy skin
- Intense thirst
- Oliguria or anuria
- Increased body temperature
- Altered mental status

Treatment for hypernatremic dehydration is volume replacement, which usually begins with isotonic fluids because the patient often has both salt and water depletion, with the water supply being more depleted. Isotonic fluids are relatively hypotonic in these patients. Rehydration for hypernatremic dehydration should be done slowly (often over 2 days) to avoid cerebral edema.[5]

Hyponatremic Dehydration. Possible causes of hyponatremic dehydration include the following:

- Use of diuretics
- Excessive perspiration (heat-related illness)
- Salt-losing renal disorders
- Increased water intake (eg, excessive use of water enemas)

Signs and symptoms may include the following:

- Abdominal or muscle cramps
- Seizures

- Rapid, thready pulse
- Diaphoresis (profuse sweating)
- Cyanosis

Treatment for hyponatremic dehydration is intravenous fluid replacement (ie, normal saline or lactated Ringer solution). Occasionally, hypertonic saline is given (eg, in seizures caused by hyponatremia).

SHOW ME THE EVIDENCE

Dehydration

Researchers at the Illinois Fire Institute measured firefighter hydration before and after a 3-hour firefighting training exercise. They assessed the usefulness of salivary measures to assess hydration status in the firefighters. They compared nude body weight changes to the urine color, specific gravity, osmolality, and salivary osmolality for 35 firefighters who participated. They found their subjects lost an average of 1.1 ± 0.8 kg (1.4%) of body mass. Of the nine who lost greater than 2% of body weight, seven were dehydrated when they started the training. They calculated that 2,200 mL of fluid would need to be consumed to balance fluid loss in firefighters hydrated at the outset of training. Portable serum osmolality tests showed a stronger correlation with hydration status than did urine measures. The researchers concluded that firefighters should hydrate prior to training. They suggest that using tests, such as salivary measurement, should be investigated further.

Modified from: Horn GP, DeBlois J, Shalmyeva I, Smith DL. Quantifying dehydration in the fire service using field methods and novel devices. *Prehosp Emerg Care.* 2012;16(3):347-355.

Overhydration

Because overhydration is an increase in body water, it results in a decrease in the solute concentration. This water excess may result from administration of excessive intravenous fluids, heart failure, renal failure, Cushing syndrome (from prolonged steroid use), or cirrhosis of the liver. Signs and symptoms of overhydration may include the following:

- Shortness of breath
- Puffy eyelids
- Ascites
- Peripheral edema
- **Polyuria** (voiding of a large volume of urine within a given time)
- Distended veins
- Moist crackles in the lungs
- Bounding pulse
- Acute weight gain
- Pulmonary edema (if severe)

Treatment for overhydration depends on the cause. It usually includes administration of **diuretics** and water and sodium restriction. In some cases, only one method is indicated. When profound hyponatremia is associated with overhydration (a low serum sodium level and associated seizures or altered consciousness), administration of hypertonic saline may be indicated.

Electrolyte Imbalances

In addition to water and sodium imbalances, disturbances may occur in the balance of electrolytes other than sodium. These electrolytes include potassium, calcium, and magnesium (**TABLE 11-2**).

Potassium. Potassium is the major positively charged ion in intracellular fluid. The body must keep potassium levels within a narrow range. This allows normal nerve impulse conduction, cardiac electrical function, skeletal muscle contraction, and intracellular acid–base balance. Normal potassium losses cannot be avoided;

TABLE 11-2 Electrolyte Concentrations of Intracellular and Extracellular Fluid

Predominant Cations	Normal Adult Range
Intracellular	
Potassium (K^+)	3.5–5.0 mEq/L
Magnesium (Mg^+)	1.5–2.0 mEq/L
Extracellular	
Sodium (Na^+)	135–145 mEq/L
Predominant Anions	**Normal Adult Range**
Intracellular	
Phosphate (PO_4^{3-})	50–60 units/L
Extracellular	
Chloride (Cl^-)	90–108 mEq/L
Bicarbonate (HCO_3^-)	22–30 mEq/L

however, these losses usually are minimal. In addition, they usually can be replaced through the diet. About 80% of excess potassium is excreted by the kidneys.[4] Potassium imbalances interfere with neuromuscular function and may cause cardiac rhythm disturbances (**dysrhythmias**). These disturbances may even include sudden cardiac death.

Hypokalemia is an abnormally low level of potassium in the blood. It can be caused by reduced dietary intake (rare), gastrointestinal losses from vomiting or diarrhea, alkalosis, hypomagnesemia, or medications—most commonly diuretics, but steroids, beta agonists (albuterol, terbutaline), insulin, and others have also been implicated. The most common cause of hypokalemia in the United States is the use of diuretics. About 80% of patients who are receiving diuretics become hypokalemic.[6] Mild hypokalemia is often well tolerated in patients who are not taking digoxin. Signs and symptoms of moderate to severe hypokalemia may include the following:

- **Malaise**
- Skeletal muscle weakness
- Cardiac dysrhythmias
- Hyperglycemia
- Decreased reflexes
- Weak pulse
- Rhabdomyolysis
- Hypertension
- Anorexia
- Vomiting
- Constipation
- Excessive thirst (rare)

In-hospital treatment of hypokalemia involves intravenous or oral administration of potassium. Administration of intravenous potassium should be given using established safety protocols.

> CRITICAL THINKING
> What common illness mimics many of the signs and symptoms of fluid and electrolyte imbalance?

Hyperkalemia is an abnormally high level of potassium in the blood. This condition may be caused by acute or chronic renal failure, burns, crush injuries, severe infection, excessive use of potassium salts, and a shift of potassium from the cells into the extracellular fluid (such as occurs in acidosis, described later in this chapter). Medications that may cause hyperkalemia include ACE inhibitors (eg, lisinopril), potassium-sparing diuretics (eg, spironolactone), beta blockers (eg, atenolol), nonsteroidal anti-inflammatory drugs (eg, ibuprofen), and others. A falsely elevated serum potassium level may occur in a specimen if it is drawn when the patient's fist is clenched and unclenched repeatedly or if prolonged tight tourniquet application occurs during the blood draw. Signs and symptoms of hyperkalemia may include the following:

- Cardiac conduction disturbances (peaked T waves, bradycardia, ventricular dysrhythmias)
- Irritability
- Abdominal distention
- Nausea
- Diarrhea
- Oliguria
- Weakness (an early sign) and paralysis (a late sign of severe hyperkalemia)

Treatment for hyperkalemia involves measures to either move potassium from the extracellular fluid to the intracellular fluid, protect the heart from its effects, or eliminate it from the body. Measures that cause potassium to move intracellularly include intravenous administration of glucose and insulin. Nebulized albuterol acts additively with insulin to promote intracellular movement of potassium through stimulation of beta-2 adrenergic receptors. By decreasing the acidity of the extracellular environment, sodium bicarbonate also causes potassium to move back into the cells. Calcium protects the heart from the potentially lethal effects of elevated potassium, and it should be administered when there are electrocardiographic changes or dysrhythmias. These measures temporize the effects of hyperkalemia but do not reduce the amount of potassium in the body. Potassium may be eliminated through the urine by the administration of intravenous fluids or diuretics. In patients with severe hyperkalemia or renal failure, **hemodialysis** is indicated.

Calcium. Calcium is a **bivalent cation** (an ion with two positive charges). It is essential for a variety of body functions, including neuromuscular transmission, cardiac action potential, cell membrane permeability, hormone secretion, growth and ossification of bones, and muscle contraction (including smooth, cardiac, and skeletal muscle). Calcium intake in a balanced diet usually is sufficient for normal body needs. Calcium is excreted through urine, feces, and perspiration. Parathyroid hormone increases serum calcium, whereas calcitonin and calcitriol decrease the amount of calcium in the blood.

Hypocalcemia is an abnormally low level of calcium in the blood. It may result from endocrine dysfunction (mostly underactivity of the parathyroid gland). It may also result from renal insufficiency, pancreatitis, magnesium imbalance, alkalosis, alcoholism, some drugs, a decreased intake or malabsorption of calcium, or sepsis. Another cause of hypocalcemia is a deficiency of, malabsorption of, or inability to activate vitamin D (which is responsible for calcium absorption). Signs and symptoms of hypocalcemia may include the following:

- **Paresthesia** (numbness or tingling sensation)
- **Tetany** (muscle twitching)
- Abdominal cramps
- Muscle cramps
- Neural excitability
- Personality changes
- Abnormal behavior
- Convulsions
- Heart failure
- Electrocardiographic abnormalities (prolonged QT interval, dysrhythmias)
- Laryngeal spasm
- Depression, psychosis

In-hospital treatment for hypocalcemia involves intravenous administration of calcium. Calcium salt and vitamin D may be given orally for maintenance.

Hypercalcemia is an abnormally high level of calcium in the blood. The primary causes are cancerous tumors and parathyroid overactivity. A small number of cases are related to diuretic therapy, immobilization, and excessive administration of vitamin D (as in the treatment of osteoporosis). Calcium can be deposited in various body tissues, including many organ systems, such as the skeletal, gastrointestinal, central nervous, renal, neuromuscular, and cardiovascular systems. Signs and symptoms of hypercalcemia include the following:

- Decreased muscle tone
- Decreased deep tendon reflexes
- Renal stones
- Increased urination
- Anorexia, nausea, vomiting
- Altered mental status, seizures, coma
- Deep bone pain
- Cardiac dysrhythmias
- Hypertension

The treatment of hypercalcemia is aimed at controlling the underlying disease. It may include hydration and/or drug therapy to decrease the calcium level. In-hospital therapy for severe hypercalcemia most commonly includes aggressive hydration with normal saline. Hemodialysis may be needed in patients with heart failure or renal insufficiency.

NOTE

Changes in the level of phosphate in the blood also can occur, possibly resulting in hypophosphatemia or hyperphosphatemia. **Hypophosphatemia**, an abnormally low serum phosphate level, may be caused by malnutrition, uncontrolled diabetes mellitus, sepsis, and chronic alcoholism. **Hyperphosphatemia**, an abnormally high serum phosphate level, is associated with renal failure, high intake of phosphate, or movement of phosphorus from the intracellular to the extracellular space.

Modified from: Metheny NM. *Fluid and Electrolyte Balance*. 5th ed. Burlington, MA: Jones & Bartlett Learning; 2012.

Magnesium. Like calcium, magnesium is a bivalent cation. It activates many enzymes. Magnesium is distributed throughout the body approximately as follows: 40% to 60% in an insoluble state in muscle and bone, 30% in the cells, and 1% in the serum.[7] Magnesium is excreted by the kidneys. Its physiologic effects on the nervous system resemble those of calcium.

Hypomagnesemia is an abnormally low level of magnesium in the blood. It may be encountered in alcoholism, diabetic ketoacidosis, malabsorption disorders, starvation, diarrhea, diuresis, diuretic use, and diseases that cause hypocalcemia and hypokalemia. The condition is characterized by increased irritability of the central nervous and cardiovascular systems. Signs and symptoms of hypomagnesemia include the following:

- Tremors
- Ataxia
- Vertigo
- Depression
- Psychosis
- Seizures or myoclonus (muscle spasms)
- Nausea or vomiting
- Diarrhea

- Hyperactive deep reflexes
- Confusion (including hallucinations)
- Cardiac dysrhythmias (prolonged QT interval may lead to cardiac arrest)

Treatment for significant, symptomatic hypomagnesemia involves intravenous administration of a solution that contains magnesium. Magnesium sulfate should be given to treat torsades de pointes associated with hypomagnesemia. (Torsades de pointes is a type of ventricular dysrhythmia, described in Chapter 21, *Cardiology*.)

Hypermagnesemia is an abnormally high level of magnesium in the blood. It is quite rare and occurs mainly in patients with chronic renal insufficiency. It also can occur in patients who take large amounts of magnesium-containing compounds. Examples of such compounds are **cathartics** (eg, magnesium citrate, magnesium sulfate) and antacids (eg, magnesium hydroxide). Hypermagnesemia causes central nervous system depression, profound muscular weakness, and **areflexia** (absence of reflexes). It also causes cardiac rhythm disturbances that may lead to sudden death. Signs and symptoms of hypermagnesemia include the following:

- Sedation
- Confusion
- Muscle weakness
- Respiratory paralysis

The most effective treatment for hypermagnesemia is hemodialysis. It can return blood levels to normal in about 4 hours. Calcium salts may be given parenterally as well. These act as an antagonist to magnesium. Administration of intravenous glucose and insulin also drives magnesium back into the cells. This treatment can be used in emergencies when respiratory depression or cardiac conduction defects are present.

Acid–Base Balance

Acids are produced by the body through normal metabolism. Two types of acids are produced: respiratory acids (culminating in carbon dioxide) and nonrespiratory (metabolic) acids. **Bases** are used in metabolic disturbances to return the body's plasma to normal pH. For physiologic functioning, the balance between acids and bases must be kept in a narrow range. The body's main regulators of **acid–base balance** are the lungs and the kidneys. The lungs secrete respiratory acids and the kidneys secrete metabolic acids.

pH

A **hydrogen ion** is a proton with a positive charge. In chemistry, a hydrogen ion is created when a hydrogen atom loses or gains an electron. A hydrogen ion that loses its charge is marked with a positive sign (H+). A hydrogen ion that gains a charge is marked with a negative sign (H–). Acids are materials that release or donate hydrogen ions. Bases (alkaline substances) receive, or absorb, hydrogen ions. Thus, they neutralize positively charged ions. The concentration of hydrogen ions is expressed as the **pH** (the potential for hydrogen), which is the negative logarithm of the hydrogen ion concentration. Consequently, the higher the concentration of H+, the lower the pH and the more acidic the solution. A small change in pH is very important: The strength of an acid or a base changes by 10 times with each unit change of pH. For example, a pH that changes by 0.3 unit (eg, from 7.4 to 7.1) doubles the concentration of hydrogen ions (BOX 11-3). The pH is neutral (7.0) when equal numbers of positive and negative ions are present. A solution increases in acidity as the pH decreases. It increases in alkalinity (basicity) as the pH rises (**FIGURE 11-9**).

Buffer Systems

Because a healthy body is sensitive to changes in the concentration of hydrogen ions, it attempts to maintain the pH of extracellular fluid within a range of 7.35 to 7.45. This pH level is maintained through several compensatory mechanisms: carbonic acid–bicarbonate buffering, renal buffering, and protein buffering. Lung function is also essential to acid–base homeostasis. These mechanisms are stimulated by changes in the pH. They require normal organ function to effectively maintain acid–base balance.

BOX 11-3 pH Values

A solution of pH 1 is 1 million times as acidic as a solution of pH 7.
pH 2 is 100,000 times as acidic as pH 7.
pH 3 is 10,000 times as acidic as pH 7.
pH 4 is 1,000 times as acidic as pH 7.
pH 5 is 100 times as acidic as pH 7.
pH 6 is 10 times as acidic as pH 7.
pH 7 is neutral (distilled water).
pH 8 is $\frac{1}{10}$ as acidic as pH 7, or 10 times as alkaline.
pH 9 is $\frac{1}{100}$ as acidic as pH 7, or 100 times as alkaline.

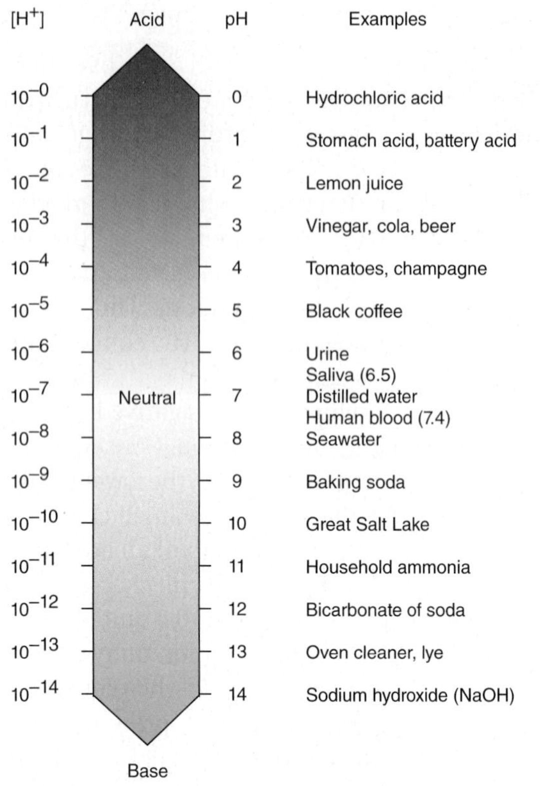

FIGURE 11-9 The pH scale. A pH of 7 is considered neutral. Values less than 7 are acidic (the lower the number, the more acidic the substance). Values greater than 7 are basic (the higher the number, the more basic the substance). Representative fluids and their approximate pH values are listed.

Carbonic Acid–Bicarbonate Buffering. Bicarbonate, carbon dioxide, and carbonic acid are always present in a dynamic balance in the blood. **Bicarbonate** (HCO_3^-) arises from the transport of carbon dioxide in the blood. Carbon dioxide (CO_2), a by-product of cellular respiration, is dissolved in the blood, where it is converted to **carbonic acid** (H_2CO_3) by **carbonic anhydrase** (an enzyme found mainly in red blood cells). Most of the carbonic acid then dissociates into hydrogen and bicarbonate ions. Because of the effects of carbonic acid or sodium bicarbonate, the buffering must occur through the lungs or kidneys. As such, the pH can be increased or decreased in one of three ways: (1) by the renal system that excretes or retains sodium bicarbonate; (2) by the respiratory system that excretes or retains carbonic acid, or its component carbon dioxide; or (3) by both systems acting together. At a physiologic pH of 7.4, the normal ratio of carbonic acid to bicarbonate is 1:20 (1 part of carbonic acid to every 20 parts of sodium bicarbonate), as summarized by the following chemical equation:

$$CO_2 + H_2O \leftrightarrow H_2CO_3 \leftrightarrow H^+ + HCO_3^-$$

Bicarbonate may bind with a cation to form base bicarbonate (eg, $NaHCO_3$). The ratio of carbonic acid to base bicarbonate determines the pH. When there is 1 milliequivalent (mEq) of carbonic acid for each 20 mEq of base bicarbonate in the extracellular fluid, the pH stays within normal limits.

> **NOTE**
> An mEq is a unit of measure, applied to electrolytes, that expresses the combining power of a substance:
>
> mEq= (mg × valence)/molecular weight
>
> (An mEq is 1⁄1,000 of an equivalent.)

The carbonic acid–bicarbonate compensatory mechanism is triggered immediately by changes in pH. The respiratory rate helps maintain this balance (**FIGURE 11-10**). This is the most important buffering system in extracellular fluid. It can buffer up to 90% of the hydrogen ions in extracellular fluid and has little effect on the cells.[8]

Renal Buffering. The kidneys help maintain an acid–base balance through three mechanisms: (1) the recovery of bicarbonate, which is filtered into the tubules; (2) the excretion of hydrogen ions against

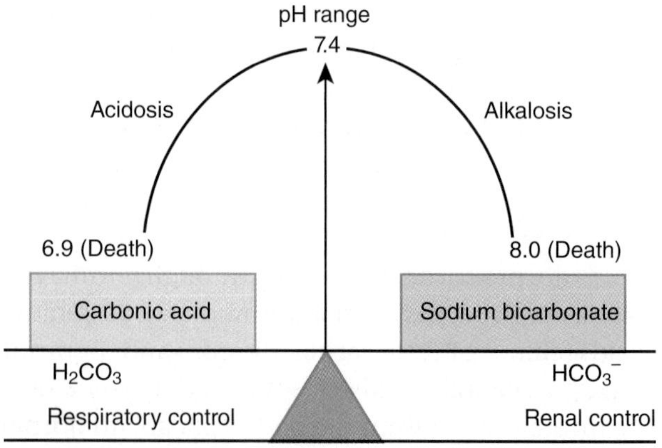

FIGURE 11-10 Bicarbonate buffer system. When body fluids are in acid–base balance, the ratio of bicarbonate (HCO_3^-) to carbonic acid (H_2CO_3) normally is 20:1, and the pH is between 7.35 and 7.45.

a gradient to acidify the urine; and (3) the excretion of **ammonium ions** (NH_4^+), each of which carries a hydrogen ion with it. The renal system compensates for acid–base imbalances slowly. The kidneys can take several hours to days to restore the pH to the normal physiologic range.

Protein Buffering. Both intracellular and extracellular proteins have negative charges. Both also can serve as buffers for changes in the pH. However, most proteins are inside cells. Protein buffering, therefore, is mainly an intracellular buffer system. **Hemoglobin** is an excellent intracellular buffer because it can bind with hydrogen ions (forming a weak acid) and carbon dioxide.

After oxygen is released in the peripheral tissues, hemoglobin binds with carbon dioxide and hydrogen ions. As the blood reaches the lungs, these actions are reversed. Hemoglobin binds with oxygen, releasing carbon dioxide and hydrogen ions. The released hydrogen ions combine with bicarbonate ions, forming carbonic acid. The carbonic acid dissociates into carbon dioxide and water. Then the lungs exhale the carbon dioxide. Therefore, in normal circumstances, respirations help maintain pH. The respiratory centers are more responsive to pH changes than to changes in the oxygen level of the tissues. For this reason, the amount of carbon dioxide in the blood (and hence the pH), rather than the need for oxygen in the tissues, controls the rate of breathing in healthy people. Within minutes of a decrease in the pH, alveolar ventilation increases in an effort to lower the carbon dioxide concentration.

NOTE

The concentration of carbonic acid is controlled by the lungs. (Carbonic acid is dissolved carbon dioxide.) The concentration of bicarbonate is controlled by the kidneys.

Lungs. Any disruption in ventilation impacts acid–base balance. The ability of the lungs to adapt to changes in pH is an essential part of the compensatory mechanism.[4] Ventilation helps maintain normal pH by regulating the amount of carbon dioxide in the blood. When the pH declines because of lack of bicarbonate, the patient hyperventilates to blow off carbon dioxide (an acid) and raises the pH. When the bicarbonate rises in metabolic alkalosis, the minute volume declines to help raise the pH back toward normal. This homeostatic mechanism of the lungs depends on healthy lung and neurologic function to work properly. Abnormal pulmonary function can actually cause, rather than compensate for, acid–base imbalances.

Acid–Base Imbalance

Acid–base balance is maintained mainly through two factors: a respiratory element and a metabolic element. Any condition that increases the concentration of carbonic acid or decreases the concentration of base bicarbonate causes **acidosis**. Any condition that increases the concentration of base bicarbonate or decreases the concentration of carbonic acid causes **alkalosis**. When discussing acid–base imbalance, it is important to remember that acidosis means that the pH is more acidic than normal, and alkalosis means that the pH is less acidic than normal (BOX 11-4). Also, a patient can have more than one contributing disorder at the same time (eg, respiratory acidosis and metabolic alkalosis, described later). When two disturbances are present, one is usually the primary disturbance while the other represents the body's attempt to compensate.

Acidosis

The accumulation of acid and the resulting acidosis (pH below 7.35) cause the pH to be more acidic compared with the normal pH of 7.4. (A decrease in pH means an increase in acidity.) A discussion of respiratory and metabolic acidosis follows.

BOX 11-4 Typical Acid–Base Measurements

Normal arterial pH range: 7.35–7.45 (7.40)
Normal arterial P_{CO_2} range: 35–46 mm Hg (40 mm Hg)
Normal serum bicarbonate (HCO_3^-) concentration range: 22–26 mEq/L (24 mEq/L)

pH	P_{CO_2}	HCO_3^-
7.35 to 7.45	35–46 mm Hg	22–26 mEq/L
↑ Acidosis	↓ CO_2 = pH ↑	↓ HCO_3^- = pH ↓
↓ Alkalosis	↑ CO_2 = pH ↓	↑ HCO_3^- = pH ↑

Respiratory Acidosis. Primary **respiratory acidosis** is caused by the retention of carbon dioxide, which leads to an increase in the Pco_2. This state usually is caused by an imbalance in the production of carbon dioxide and its elimination through alveolar ventilation (**FIGURE 11-11**). Respiratory acidosis can be summarized by the following chemical equation:

$$\downarrow \text{Respiration} = \uparrow CO_2 + H_2O \rightarrow \uparrow H_2CO_3 \rightarrow \uparrow H^+ + HCO_3^-$$

Reductions in alveolar ventilation are the result of respiratory failure, which may be caused by the following:

- Neuromuscular impairment causing diaphragmatic weakness (eg, opiate overdose, airway obstruction, traumatic brain injury)
- Obstructive lung disease (eg, asthma, chronic obstructive pulmonary disease, obstructive sleep apnea)
- Medications (eg, opiates, sedatives, hypnotics)
- Chest wall injury (eg, flail chest, pneumothorax)

Some patients are at increased risk for hypoventilation and can decompensate quickly. These patients include people who are morbidly obese, have tight abdominal binders or dressings, have significant pain after surgery, or are experiencing abdominal distention from cirrhosis or bowel obstruction.[4]

> NOTE
> In primary respiratory acidosis, the abnormality is failure of the lungs to excrete carbon dioxide efficiently.

When the respiratory system is unable to adequately excrete carbon dioxide, the body's renal system must

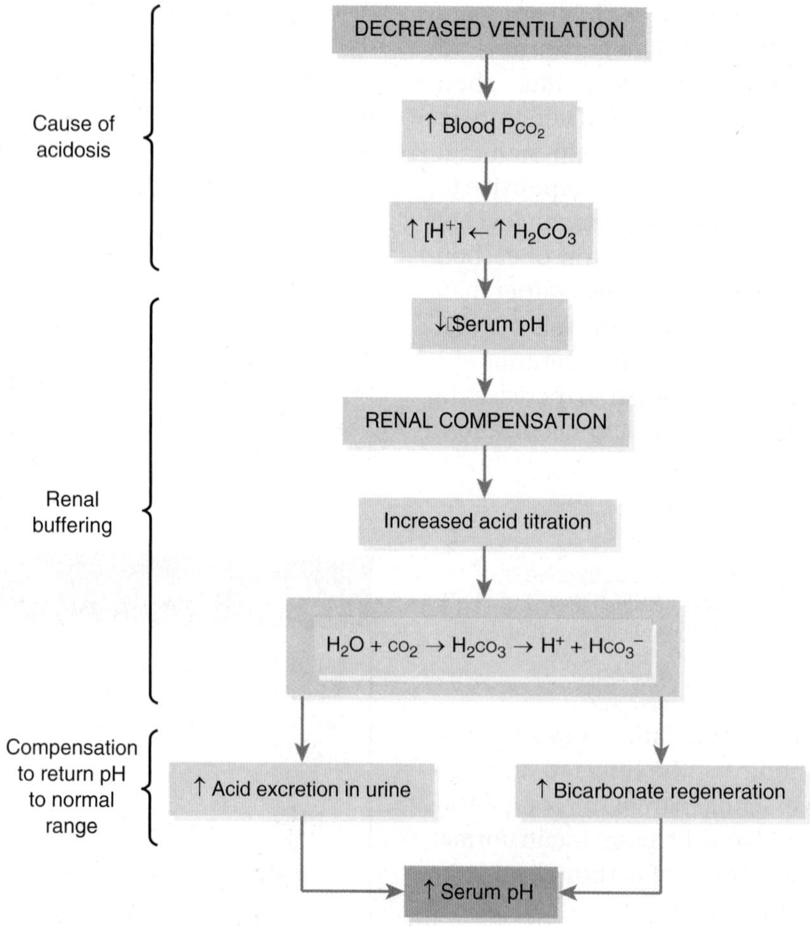

Abbreviations: co_2, carbon dioxide; H^+, hydrogen ion; Hco_3^-, bicarbonate; H_2co_3, carbonic acid; H_2O, water; Pco_2, partial pressure of carbon dioxide

FIGURE 11-11 Respiratory acidosis. An excess of carbon dioxide in the body results in acidosis.

> NOTE
>
> End-tidal capnography can help determine the severity of respiratory distress by providing a breath-by-breath measurement of a patient's ventilation. It can also provide real-time feedback on the patient's response to treatment. Capnography is further discussed in Chapter 15, *Airway Management, Respiration, and Artificial Ventilation*, and in Chapter 23, *Respiratory*.

compensate by conserving bicarbonate and excreting more hydrogen ions to help bring the pH into normal limits. Compensation by the kidneys is slow. Thus, respiratory acidosis is treated by improving ventilation to improve carbon dioxide elimination. This may be done by assisting ventilations to decrease the Pco_2. Supplemental oxygen also should be given to help correct any accompanying **hypoxemia** (which itself can lead to acidosis). After ventilation is established, any reversible causes, such as opiate overdose, should be corrected.

> CRITICAL THINKING
>
> What kind of acid–base imbalance exists in a patient you have just defibrillated and resuscitated from cardiac arrest? How will you treat that imbalance?

Metabolic Acidosis. Metabolic acidosis results from a buildup of acid or a loss of base. When excessive acid is produced by the body, the acid spills into the extracellular fluid and consumes some bicarbonate buffers. The result is an increase in acid and a decrease in available base (**FIGURE 11-12**). Metabolic acidosis can be summarized by the following equation:

$$\uparrow H^+ + HCO_3^- \rightarrow \uparrow H_2CO_3 \rightarrow H_2O + \uparrow CO_2$$

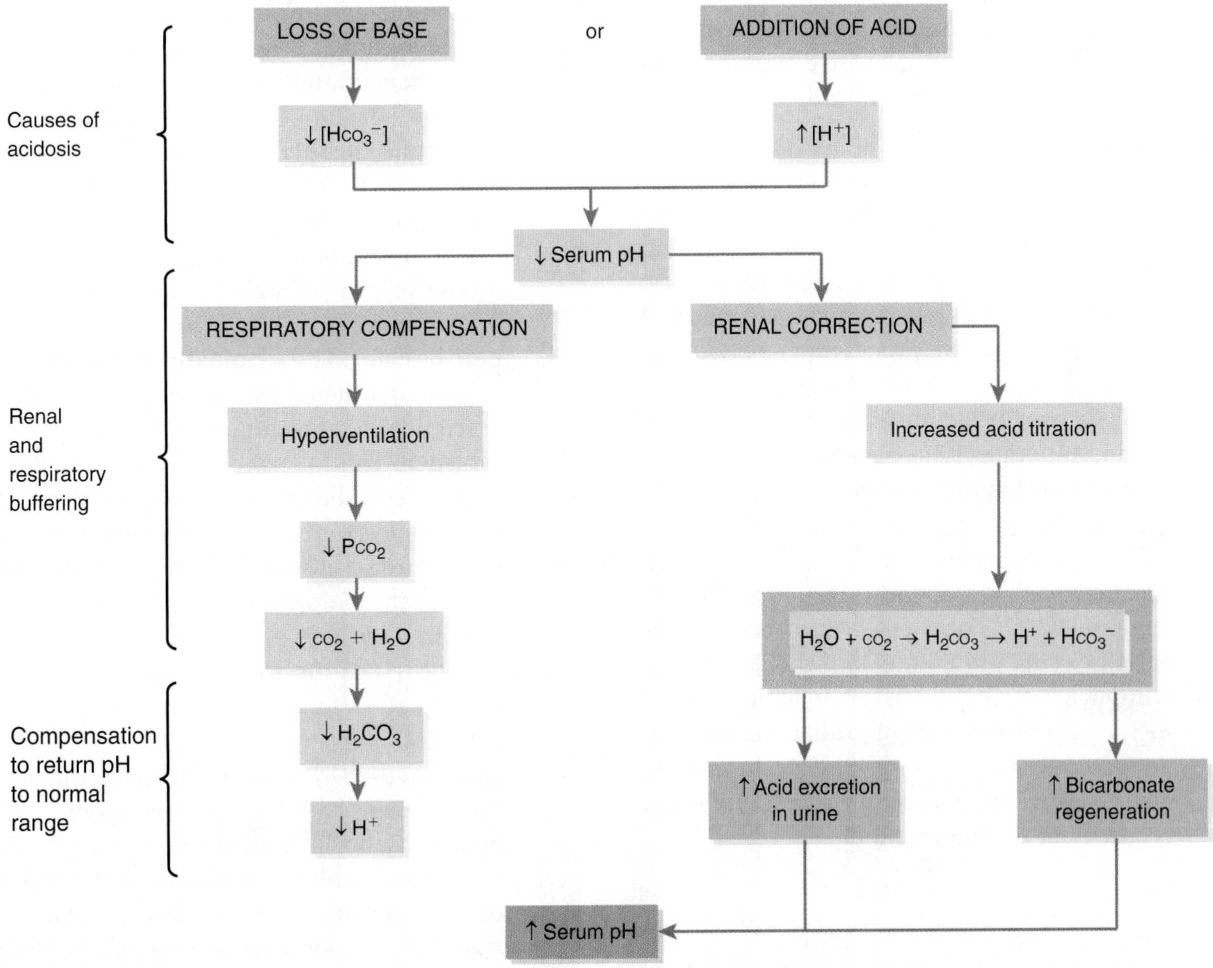

Abbreviations: CO_2, carbon dioxide; H^+, hydrogen ion; HCO_3^-, bicarbonate; H_2CO_3, carbonic acid; H_2O, water; Pco_2, partial pressure of carbon dioxide

FIGURE 11-12 Metabolic acidosis. With an excess of metabolic acids, bicarbonate is consumed and hydrogen ions are liberated, resulting in a primary metabolic acidosis.

Modified from: McCance KL, Huether SE. *Pathophysiology: The Biologic Basis for Disease in Adults and Children*. 6th ed. St. Louis, MO: Mosby; 2010.

The increase in available hydrogen ions forces the reaction to the right, decreasing the amount of base bicarbonate.

NOTE

Metabolic acidosis occurs when the amount of acid generated by the body exceeds the body's buffering capacity.

The healthy respiratory system instantly tries to compensate for the acidosis by increasing the rate and depth of breathing to reduce carbon dioxide levels; this causes a compensatory respiratory alkalosis. As the carbon dioxide concentration falls, so does the concentration of carbonic acid, moving the pH toward normal. In addition, the kidneys excrete more hydrogen ion to equilibrate the excess acid in the extracellular fluid.

The most common forms of metabolic acidosis encountered in the prehospital setting are lactic acidosis, diabetic ketoacidosis, acidosis caused by renal failure, acidosis caused by ingestion of toxins (poisons), and diarrheal dehydration.

- **Lactic acidosis.** Lactic acid is created when a large number of cells are inadequately oxygenated. This results in a shift from **aerobic** (with oxygen) to **anaerobic** (without oxygen) metabolism. The end product of anaerobic metabolism is lactic acid. The lactic acid releases hydrogen ions and becomes **lactate**. This process creates systemic acidosis. Normally, the liver changes lactate back into glucose, or lactate is oxidized to carbon dioxide and water. When lactic acid is produced faster than it is metabolized, **lactic acidosis** occurs. The most common causes of systemic lactic acidosis are extreme exertional states (eg, seizures), **ischemia** (reduced blood supply) in large muscles or organs (eg, mesenteric ischemia), circulatory failure, and shock. Specific complications associated with lactic acidosis include decreased force of cardiac contraction, decreased peripheral response to catecholamines, hypotension and shock, and cardiac muscle that is refractory to defibrillation.

CRITICAL THINKING

Think about the last time you ran so fast you had a muscle cramp. What acid–base changes were occurring inside your body? How did your body compensate for those changes?

Treatment of lactic acidosis involves reestablishing tissue perfusion and cardiac output. This allows the liver to regenerate bicarbonate by metabolizing lactate to carbon dioxide and water. Vigorous rehydration to support circulation and optimization of oxygenation may also be indicated. Correction of lactic acidosis often depends on identification and rectification of the underlying cause.

- **Diabetic ketoacidosis.** Ketoacidosis usually is a complication of **diabetes mellitus**. It also may be seen in people who are alcoholics (alcoholic ketoacidosis). Diabetic ketoacidosis usually results when a patient fails to take adequate insulin. It also may develop when the need for insulin increases. The body may need more insulin, for example, in cases of infection or trauma. Insulin is required for many cells to absorb glucose. With impaired glucose utilization, fatty acids are metabolized, producing **ketone bodies** and releasing hydrogen ions. When large amounts of ketone bodies exceed the ability of the body's buffering system to compensate, the result is acidosis and a decrease in blood pH. Prehospital care for patients with diabetic ketoacidosis involves administration of normal saline for volume repletion. (The pathophysiology of diabetes mellitus is further addressed in Chapter 25, *Endocrinology*.)
- **Acidosis caused by renal failure.** The kidneys help maintain acid–base balance by reabsorbing or secreting either bicarbonate or hydrogen ions as needed. This keeps the pH constant. Renal failure affects the compensatory mechanisms of the kidneys to varying degrees. Patients with moderate to severe renal failure often have mild to moderate acidosis. Acidosis results because the failing kidneys are unable to excrete the acid waste products efficiently. These waste products are the result of normal metabolic processes.
- **Acidosis caused by ingestion of toxins.** Ingestion of some toxins, such as ethylene glycol, methanol, and salicylate, a component of aspirin, can cause metabolic acidosis. (It should be noted that aspirin toxicity actually begins as a respiratory alkalosis via central effects [early] that is then followed by a metabolic acidosis because of metabolic effects.) These and other toxins lead to the production of toxic metabolites that may result in acid–base disorders. These

disorders are characterized by metabolic acidosis and compensatory respiratory alkalosis. Treatment for various toxic ingestions frequently includes gastrointestinal evacuation but also may require hemodialysis, diuresis, hydration to promote excretion, and specific antagonistic or antidotal therapy.

- **Acidosis caused by diarrhea.** Prolonged and frequent diarrhea causes loss of bicarbonate and fluid. Chloride ions become concentrated and cause metabolic acidosis. This condition is compounded by dehydration that can lead to shock.

> NOTE
> In a patient with oliguric renal failure, administration of intravenous fluids may rapidly lead to overhydration.

Alkalosis

Alkalosis (pH above 7.45) causes the blood and body fluids to be less acidic compared with the normal pH of 7.4. (An increase in pH means a decrease in acidity.)

Respiratory Alkalosis. Hyperventilation produces primary respiratory alkalosis by decreasing the Pco_2 (**FIGURE 11-13**). **Respiratory alkalosis** can be summarized by the following chemical equation:

$$\uparrow \text{Respiration} = \downarrow CO_2 + H_2O \rightarrow \downarrow H_2CO_3 \rightarrow \downarrow H^+ + HCO_3^-$$

When carbonic acid is lacking because of excessive elimination of carbon dioxide, the blood pH rises. The kidneys must then excrete bicarbonate ions and retain hydrogen ions to return the pH to normal. Treatment

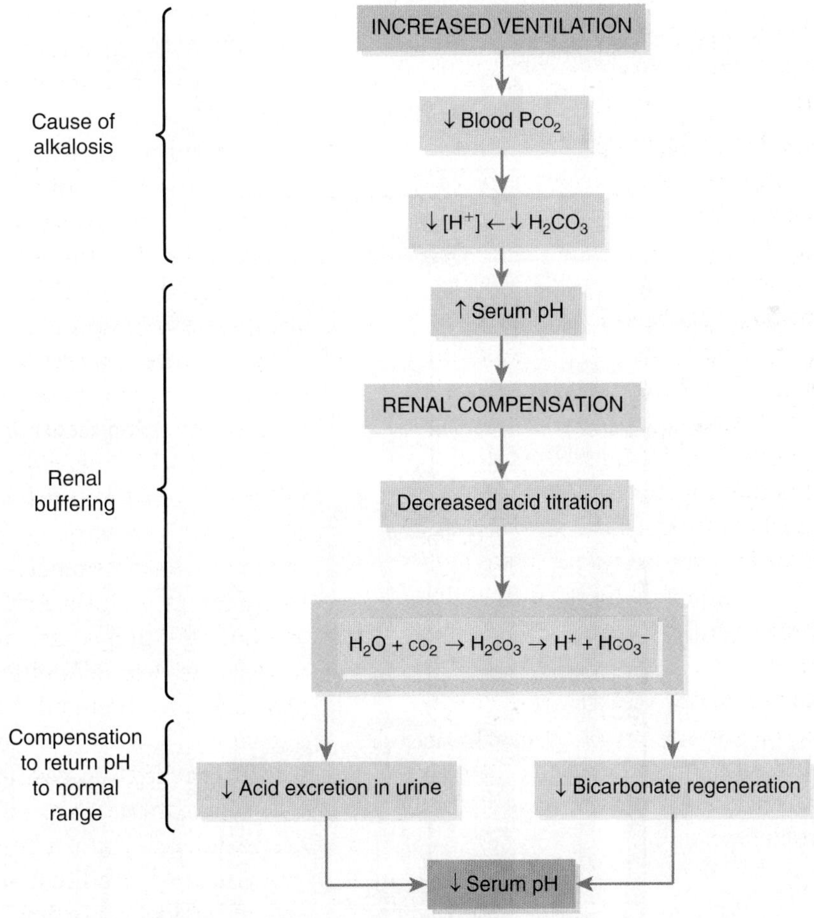

Abbreviations: CO_2, carbon dioxide; H^+, hydrogen ion; HCO_3^-, bicarbonate; H_2CO_3, carbonic acid; H_2O, water; Pco_2, partial pressure of carbon dioxide

FIGURE 11-13 Respiratory alkalosis. A deficit of carbon dioxide results in respiratory alkalosis.

> NOTE
> Respiratory alkalosis is caused by hyperventilation. Hyperventilation lowers the Pco_2 in the alveoli (the air cells in the lungs) and subsequently the Pco_2 in the blood.

of respiratory alkalosis is directed at correcting the underlying cause of the hyperventilation. If the patient is on a ventilator, the setting can be adjusted to reduce minute volume. Although anxiety can lead to hyperventilation, many patients become anxious when they are experiencing a serious underlying condition. When anxiety appears to be the cause, provide calming measures to assist the patient with slow, controlled breathing.

Metabolic Alkalosis. Primary metabolic alkalosis (rare) most often results from loss of hydrogen ions (from vomiting or gastric suction), ingestion of large amounts of absorbable base sodium bicarbonate (baking soda) or calcium carbonate (antacids), or excessive intravenous administration of alkali (eg, intravenous injection of sodium bicarbonate). Endocrine problems, such as hyperaldosteronism or Cushing syndrome, and the use of diuretics also may be a factor (**FIGURE 11-14**). Metabolic alkalosis can be summarized by the following chemical equation:

$$\downarrow H^+ + HCO_3^- \rightarrow \uparrow H_2CO_3^- \rightarrow H_2O + CO_2$$

The loss of hydrogen ions is the initial cause of a primary metabolic alkalosis. This loss may result from vomiting (loss of hydrochloric acid), suctioning of gastric contents, or increased renal excretion of hydrogen ions in the urine. When vomiting occurs, gastric acid (ie, hydrochloric acid) is lost, but volume also is depleted.

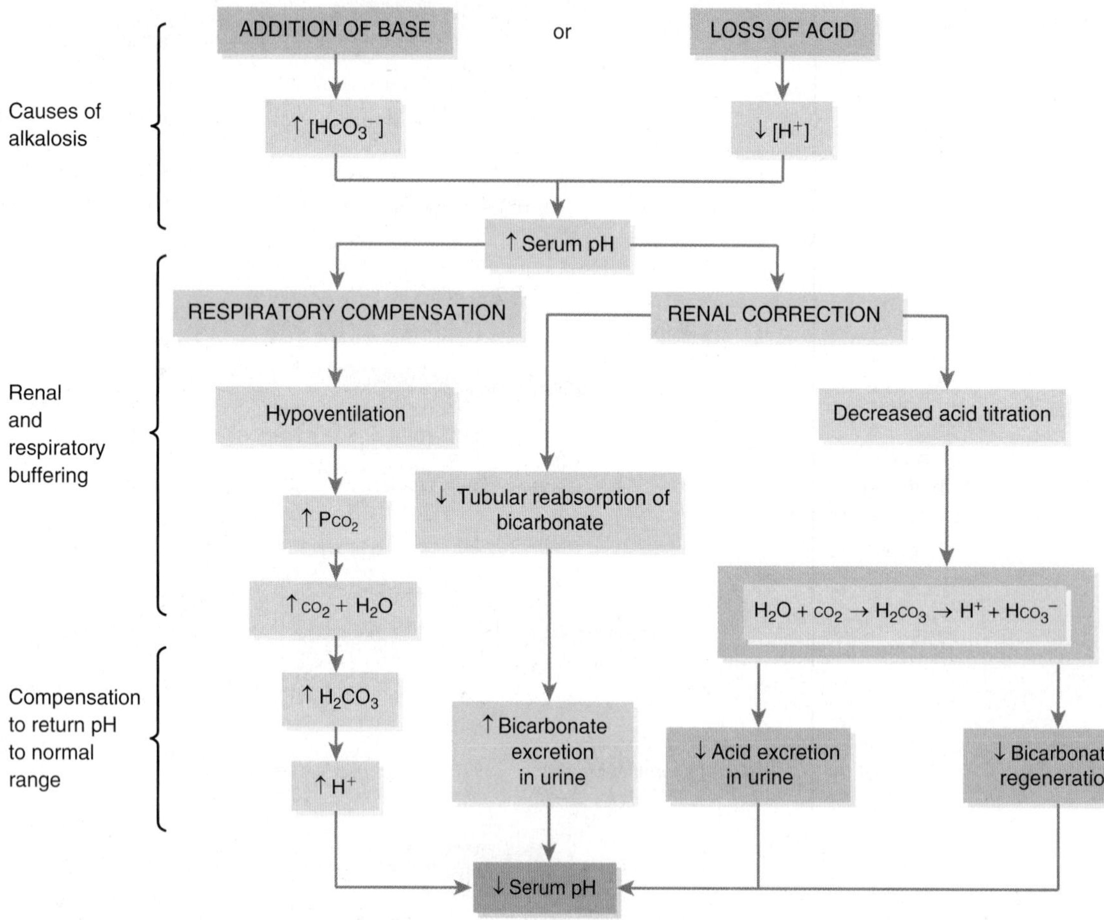

Abbreviations: CO_2, carbon dioxide; H^+, hydrogen ion; Hco_3^-, bicarbonate; H_2co_3, carbonic acid; H_2O, water; Pco_2, partial pressure of carbon dioxide

FIGURE 11-14 Metabolic alkalosis. An excess of bicarbonate results in metabolic alkalosis.

Modified from: McCance KL, Huether SE. *Pathophysiology: The Biologic Basis for Disease in Adults and Children.* 6th ed. St. Louis, MO: Mosby; 2010.

The loss of potassium from the chronic use of diuretics or an excess of adrenal corticotropic hormones causes the kidneys to reabsorb potassium and increase hydrogen ion excretion. This action, coupled with a shift of potassium from the cells into the blood in exchange for hydrogen ions, can result in a net increase in bicarbonate level and lead to metabolic alkalosis.[4]

Initially, the respiratory system tries to compensate by retaining carbon dioxide, and compensatory respiratory acidosis develops in the patient. However, this mechanism is limited by the development of hypoxemia. (Hypoventilation causes a rise in the Pco_2 and a decrease in the Po_2; these actions stimulate respiration.)

Treatment of metabolic alkalosis is aimed at correcting the underlying condition. Volume depletion, if present, should be corrected using isotonic solutions. Hypokalemia may require correction with potassium replacement.

Mixed Acid–Base Disturbances

Many conditions, such as various forms of shock, may cause mixed abnormalities of acid–base regulation. Simultaneous respiratory and metabolic alterations are commonly seen in patients who are in shock. These alterations develop because pathophysiologic changes occur in both the respiratory and the metabolic components of the acid–base system (BOX 11-5; also see **TABLE 11-3**). Examples of mixed acid–base disturbances include the following:

- Combined respiratory and metabolic acidosis
- Metabolic acidosis and respiratory alkalosis

BOX 11-5 Acid-Base Determination and Other Laboratory Studies

Blood Gas Analysis

Blood gas values are measured for two reasons: one reason is to determine whether the patient is well oxygenated. The second reason is to determine the patient's acid–base status. Most often, blood gas values are measured in a sample of arterial blood obtained in a heparinized syringe (see Appendix, *Advanced Practice Procedures for Critical Care Paramedics*). Arterial samples are used for this test more often than venous samples because arterial samples provide more direct information about the ability of the lungs to oxygenate blood and remove carbon dioxide.

Acid-Base Determination

The patient's acid–base status is assessed by measuring the Pco_2 and the pH of the arterial blood. The pH level indicates whether an acid or a base state is present. The Pco_2 value indicates whether a respiratory component is a factor in the acidosis or alkalosis. (For example, it may show whether alveolar hypoventilation or hyperventilation is present.) Table 11-3 summarizes the abnormalities that occur in acid–base disturbances.

Currently, paramedics are not expected to determine the pH by blood gas analysis in the prehospital setting. Pulse oximetry allows continual assessment of the arterial oxygen saturation. End-tidal capnography, which measures exhaled carbon dioxide, can indirectly quantify carbon dioxide levels in the blood and help determine whether the patient is likely to have a primary respiratory acid–base problem or is compensating for a metabolic acid–base disturbance.

TABLE 11-3 Acid-Base Disturbances

pH	Initial Chemical Change	Primary Acid-Base Disturbance	Compensatory Response	
<7.4	↑ Pco_2	Respiratory acidosis	Metabolic alkalosis	↑ HCO_3^-
>7.4	↓ Pco_2	Respiratory alkalosis	Metabolic acidosis	↓ HCO_3^-
<7.4	↓ HCO_3^-	Metabolic acidosis	Respiratory alkalosis	↓ Pco_2
>7.4	↑ HCO_3^-	Metabolic alkalosis	Respiratory acidosis	↑ Pco_2

Abbreviations: HCO_3^-, bicarbonate; Pco_2, partial pressure of carbon dioxide

- Respiratory acidosis and metabolic alkalosis
- Combined respiratory and metabolic alkalosis

Acid–base balance can be a difficult concept to master. When providing emergency care, the paramedic should remember the following primary points:

1. The normal pH of blood is 7.4. A decrease in pH indicates an increase in acidity (more acid than normal); an increase in pH indicates a decrease in acidity (less acid than normal).
2. Acid–base balance has two components: a respiratory (carbon dioxide) factor and a nonrespiratory (metabolic) factor.
3. Respiratory acidosis is caused by an increase in the carbon dioxide level of the blood and body fluids as a result of inadequate breathing. The treatment of respiratory acidosis involves improving ventilation to lower the carbon dioxide level. Respiratory alkalosis results from hyperventilation.
4. Metabolic acidosis is caused by hypoperfusion. The treatment of metabolic acidosis involves reestablishing tissue perfusion and cardiac output. Metabolic alkalosis is rare.
5. The body always seeks to maintain a normal blood pH. When an acid–base disturbance develops, the body will attempt to compensate via the lungs (faster) and/or the kidneys (slower).

Alterations in Cells and Tissues: Injury and Disease

Certain concepts are crucial to an understanding of the disease process. One of these concepts is the way that cells and tissues react to injury, both structurally and functionally. Changes in the structure and function of cells and tissues can result from cellular adaptation, injury, **neoplasia** (actual formation of a tumor), aging, and death.

Cellular Adaptation

Cells adapt to their environment (**FIGURE 11-15**). They do so to escape and to protect themselves from injury.

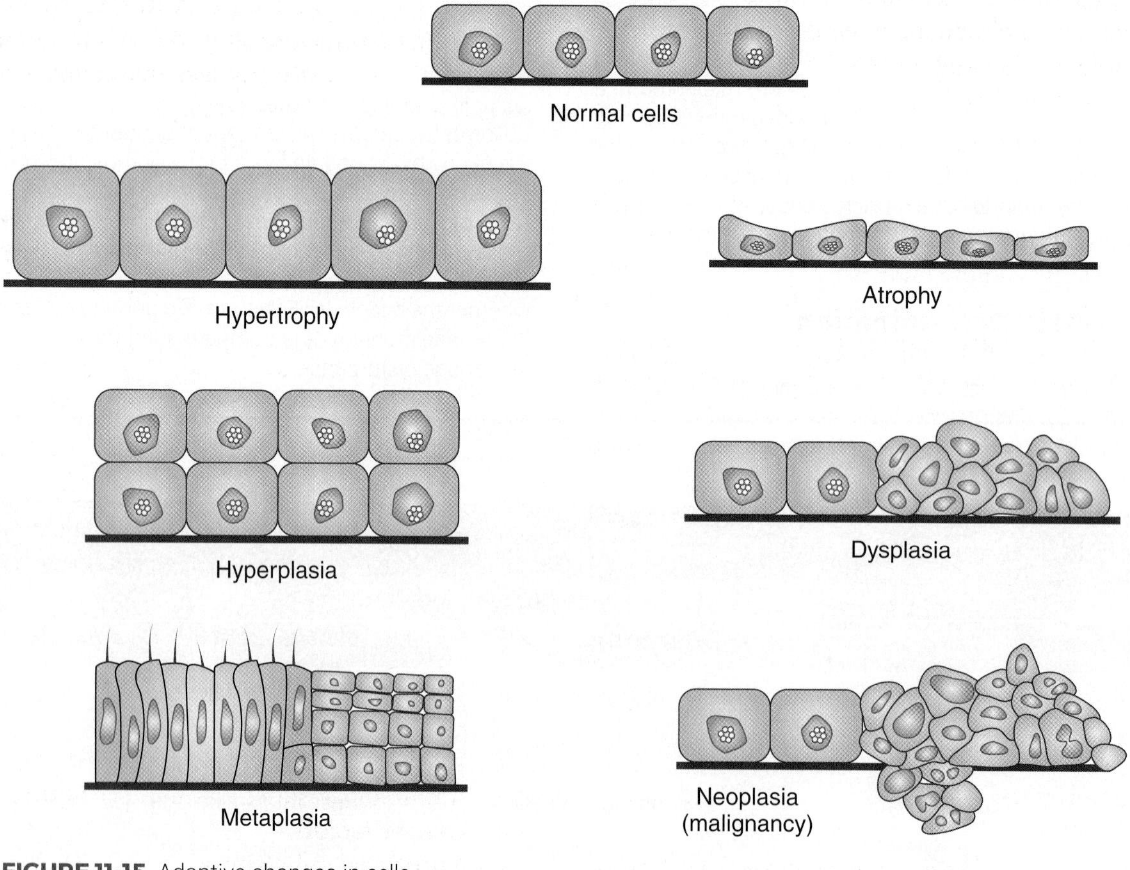

FIGURE 11-15 Adaptive changes in cells.

Adaptations are common and are a central part of the response to changes in the physiologic condition. In many instances, the adaptation allows the cell to function more efficiently. For this reason, it can be difficult to distinguish between a pathologic response and an extreme adaptation to changing conditions. The following is a list of the five most significant adaptive changes in cells:

1. Atrophy (a decrease in cell size)
2. Hypertrophy (an increase in cell size)
3. Hyperplasia (an excessive increase in the number of cells)
4. Metaplasia (a change from one cell type to another that is better able to tolerate adverse conditions; a conversion into a form that is not normal for that cell)
5. Dysplasia (abnormal changes in mature cells)

Atrophy is a decrease in cellular size that adversely affects cell function. It can affect any organ; however, it is seen most often in skeletal muscle, the heart, the secondary sex organs, and the brain. Causes include decreased use, chronic inflammation, poor nutrition or starvation, inadequate hormonal or nervous stimulation, and reduced blood supply. An example of atrophy is a skeletal muscle that is reduced in size because of prolonged wearing of a cast. Atrophy may be reversed (in some cases) when normal function is restored.

Hypertrophy is an increase in the size of cells. It occurs without an increase in the number of that type of cell. Along with the increase in the size of the cells comes an increase in the size of the affected organ. Hypertrophy results when cells must do more work to achieve a task. Examples of "normal" or physiologic hypertrophy are the development of large muscles in a weight lifter, increased growth of the uterus during pregnancy, and the development of sexual organs in adolescence (initiated by sex hormones). Examples of pathologic hypertrophy are enlargement of the heart (myocardial hypertrophy) and of the kidneys (which also can be physiologic).

> CRITICAL THINKING
>
> What happens to muscle strength when the muscle cells are affected by each of these conditions: atrophy, hypertrophy, and hyperplasia?

Hyperplasia is an excessive increase in the number of cells that results in an increase in the size of a tissue or an organ. Hyperplasia occurs in response to increased demand. It may be a pathologic event or it may be a normal adaptive mechanism that allows certain organs to regenerate (compensatory hyperplasia). The formation of a callus is an example of compensatory hyperplasia. Another example is benign prostatic hyperplasia. An example of pathologic hyperplasia is endometrial hyperplasia. This condition can cause excessive menstrual bleeding. Hyperplasia and hypertrophy often occur together.

Metaplasia is a change into a form that is not normal for that cell. It also can be seen as the reversible replacement of normal tissue cells by other cells that may be better able to tolerate poor environmental conditions. An example of metaplasia is the change that occurs in the bronchial lining as a result of smoking. The normal ciliated epithelial cells are replaced by nonciliated squamous epithelial cells. The latter cells are more resistant to irritation. (Bronchial metaplasia can be reversed if the person quits smoking.) Chronic inflammation of the cervix also can result in metaplasia.

Dysplasia is the development of abnormal changes in mature cells. The cells vary in size, shape, and color, and their relationship to one another also is abnormal. Dysplastic changes frequently are seen as precancerous. These changes occur most often in epithelial tissue, are often the result of chronic irritation or inflammation, and frequently are found in cells near cancerous cells. Dysplasia is not considered a true cellular adaptation. Rather, it is seen as an atypical hyperplasia.

Cellular Injury

Many processes can injure a cell. The mechanisms involved in cellular injury are complex. The specific site of injury often is characteristic of a certain pathologic process. As a rule, cellular injury occurs if the cell is unable to maintain homeostasis as a result of the following factors:

1. Hypoxic injury
2. Free radical-induced injury
3. Chemical injury
4. Infectious injury (eg, bacteria, viruses)
5. Immunologic and inflammatory injury
6. Genetic factors
7. Nutritional imbalances
8. Physical agents

Hypoxic Injury

Hypoxic injury is the most common cause of damage to a cell. It may result from a decrease in the amount of oxygen in the air, the loss of hemoglobin or altered hemoglobin function, a decrease in the number of red blood cells, diseases of the respiratory or cardiovascular system, external compression (eg, in trauma), or poisoning and loss of **cytochromes** (proteins in the liver that play a role in drug detoxification). Hypoxic injury commonly is a result of **atherosclerosis** (narrowing of the arteries) and thrombosis (complete blockage of an artery or a vein by a blood clot). Prolonged ischemia leads to **infarction**, or cell death (see Chapter 21, *Cardiology*). Atherosclerosis and thrombosis can lead to gangrene, myocardial infarction, and stroke.[9]

> NOTE
>
> Cells need an adequate supply of oxygen. Without oxygen they cannot generate enough energy to maintain the mechanisms (ion pumps) that move some substances across the cell membrane. Lack of oxygen also causes cellular swelling.

Free Radical Injury

The chemical process that reduces oxygen to water requires several steps. That conversion produces intermediate chemicals (superoxide, hydrogen peroxide, and hydroxyl radical) that are toxic to cells. These free radicals can form bonds with carbohydrates, lipids, and proteins within cell membranes and damage them. Harmful effects of free radicals include membrane, organelle, and cellular destruction. The body has some mechanisms to rid itself of small amounts of free radicals. The best defense is to minimize their production.[7,10]

Chemical Injury

Many chemical agents can damage a cell. Examples include heavy metals (eg, lead), carbon monoxide, ethanol, drugs, and complex toxins. Some of these chemicals injure cells directly (eg, curare and cyanide). Others, when metabolized, produce a toxin that affects the cells (eg, carbon tetrachloride [CCl_4]).

The injury begins with a biochemical interaction. The interaction occurs between a toxic substance and an integral part of the cell's structure. Some drugs and toxins (eg, salicylate, certain venoms) affect the cellular membrane. This interaction can damage the plasma membrane, leading to increased permeability, cellular swelling, and irreversible cellular injury (see Chapter 31, *Hematology*). Other toxins, such as carbon monoxide, mainly affect the cytochrome system found in the mitochondria. This leads to a halt in oxidative metabolism. Other toxins affect the genetic material (a primary target for chemotherapeutic drugs).

Infectious Injury

The **virulence** of microorganisms, such as bacteria and viruses, depends on their ability to survive and reproduce in the human body. The disease-producing potential of microorganisms depends on their ability to do the following:

- Invade and destroy cells
- Overcome the organism's defense system
- Produce toxins
- Produce **hypersensitivity reactions**

Bacteria. The survival and growth of bacteria are determined by the success of the body's defenses and also depend on the bacteria's ability to resist these mechanisms (see Chapter 27, *Infectious and Communicable Diseases*). Many bacteria that survive and multiply in the body produce toxins that can injure or destroy cells and tissues. The toxins take two forms: **exotoxins** (toxins secreted or excreted by a living organism) and **endotoxins** (toxins contained in the cell walls of some living organisms).

Bacteria secrete exotoxins when they have been produced by viruslike particles called bacteriophages. These particles carry the genetic material needed to make the toxin. Exotoxins are produced by a microorganism and are then excreted into the medium surrounding the microorganism. Exotoxins have highly specific effects that are produced by the release of exotoxins as metabolic products during bacterial growth. Several of the streptococci (bacteria that cause sore throats and rheumatic fever) produce an exotoxin. The bacterium *Clostridium botulinum,*

> NOTE
>
> **Toxoids** are modified (harmless) toxins. They are used as vaccines so that the body can develop specific **antibodies** to them. The best-known toxoid is tetanus toxoid, which is made from tetanus toxin.

which causes the severe food poisoning known as **botulism**, also produces an exotoxin.

Endotoxins are complex molecules. They are contained in the cell walls of some bacteria. Endotoxins are released during treatment with antibiotics or when the cell walls disintegrate. Examples of bacteria that produce endotoxins are gonococci and meningococci (the bacteria that cause gonorrhea and meningitis, respectively). Endotoxins do not stimulate the production of strong antibodies. For this reason, it has not been possible to develop vaccines against endotoxin-bearing bacteria. Instead, to fight these bacteria, the body uses a group of proteins collectively called the **complement system**. These proteins coat the bacteria and then either help kill the microorganisms directly or aid neutrophils (in the blood) or macrophages (in the tissues) in the process of microorganism destruction. The reticuloendothelial system (composed of cells in the spleen, lymph nodes, liver, bone marrow, lungs, and intestines) works with the lymphatic system to dispose of the debris produced by the immune system's attack on invading organisms.

Bacteria that make endotoxins are also called pyrogenic bacteria because they activate the inflammatory process. They also produce fever directly through the release of cell membrane toxins. As part of the inflammatory process, white blood cells are released from the bone marrow. This process is the cause of the increased white blood cell count that is commonly found with infection. Inflammation also increases capillary permeability, allowing substances that destroy bacteria to migrate from the capillaries to the site of infection (see Chapter 27, *Infectious and Communicable Diseases*). Fever is caused by the release of endogenous pyrogens (proteins that act on the thermoregulatory centers of the hypothalamus). These proteins are released by macrophages or by circulating white blood cells that are attracted to the injury site.

CRITICAL THINKING

Will treating a fever with antipyretic drugs cause the body to rid itself of the toxin that caused the fever?

Uncommonly, a bacterial toxin may induce an immunologic response upon first exposure. Hypersensitivity develops the next time the person is exposed to the toxin, and the result is an inflammatory response. At times, the response is so extreme that it results in the person, rather than the bacteria, dying. For example, the complement system can activate blood clotting and can cause platelets to aggregate and form "clumps" that block blood vessels.

The net effect of overactivation of the complement system by endotoxins is the blockage of small blood vessels in the lungs (with the clumps) and the formation of tiny blood clots in small arteries elsewhere in the body. However, this type of life-threatening reaction is rare. Moreover, the complement system normally acts as an efficient defense against most bacterial toxins without causing any damage. (Hypersensitivity reactions are further described later in this chapter and in Chapter 26, *Immune System Disorders*).

NOTE

When the body's defenses fail and microorganisms multiply in the blood, **bacteremia** develops. Bacteremia may lead to septicemia, a severe systemic infection in which pathogens are present in the bloodstream. The endotoxins (along with a number of proteins involved in the inflammatory response) cause vasodilation. Vasodilation reduces blood pressure and oxygen delivery, resulting in shock. Other signs of an inflammatory response to bacteremia may include chills, fever, and an altered level of consciousness. Rashes or red streaks also may be associated with bacteremia. (The red streaks are indicative of lymphatic channel inflammation or lymphangitis.)

CRITICAL THINKING

In septic shock, cell membrane permeability increases. This allows fluids to leak out of the blood vessels more freely. How could this condition affect cardiac output?

Viruses. Viruses cause many human diseases, including the common cold, influenza, chickenpox, smallpox, hepatitis, herpes, and acquired immunodeficiency syndrome (AIDS), the result of infection with the human immunodeficiency virus (HIV). Viruses are intracellular parasites that work very differently from bacteria (**FIGURE 11-16**). Viruses lack much of the machinery that allows bacterial cells and other types of cells to grow rapidly and multiply. They can reproduce only by infecting the living cells of host tissue. (They often destroy the host cell.) Viruses usually consist of a protein coat (**capsid**) that encloses a core of nucleic acid. They have no organelles and therefore have no metabolism. They do not produce endotoxins or exotoxins.

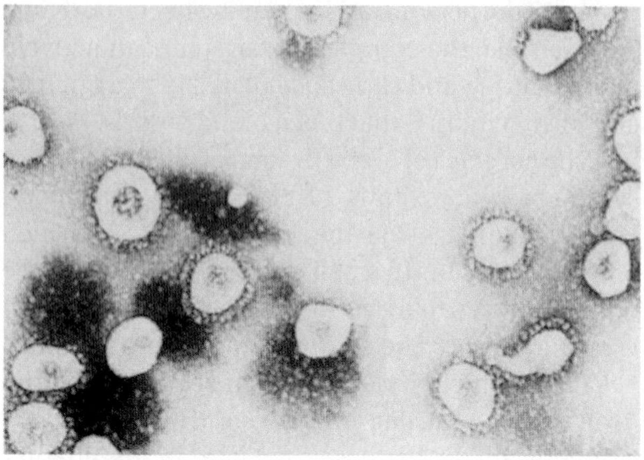

FIGURE 11-16 Coronavirus particles.

Courtesy of U.S. Department of Health Education and Welfare, Public Health Service, Centers for Disease Control and Prevention, Atlanta, GA.

Viruses need host cell proteins to replicate. Cells are thought to engulf the virus particles by surrounding them with part of the cell membrane. Once inside the cell, the virus loses the capsid and begins to replicate the viral nucleic acids. Some viruses cause the cell to burst. Others replicate without destroying the cell.

The capsid enables the virus particle to resist **phagocytosis**, even though viruses often trigger a very strong immune response. Viruses can rapidly cause permanent and lethal injury in hosts, regardless of the host's state of immunosuppression. Rabies, smallpox, and influenza are examples of viral diseases that are highly infectious and have high rates of illness (morbidity) and death (mortality).

NOTE

Phagocytosis is the process of ingestion of solid substances by cells. Substances ingested may include other cells, bacteria, pieces of necrosed (dead) tissue, and foreign particles.

Viral infections are easier to prevent than to treat. Vaccines have proven to be the best guard against viral disease (BOX 11-6). The signs and symptoms of viral illness are based on the type and location of the cells infected. For this reason, certain viruses tend to cause respiratory illness (eg, influenza), whereas others cause gastroenteritis (enteroviruses), central nervous system disease (eg, St. Louis B encephalitis, rabies), or liver disease (hepatitis).

BOX 11-6 Influenza Vaccines

Human influenza viruses are categorized into three major types: A, B, and C. Influenza A and B cause most of the outbreaks in the United States. These viruses mutate every few years. The mutations allow the virus to escape containment by the immune system. This is true even if a person had a previous influenza infection. Each year, virologists and epidemiologists analyze cultures from the southern hemisphere (where the flu season occurs during the northern hemisphere's summer). They try to determine which strains are likely to appear in the upcoming flu season and use this information to prepare effective vaccines. If the expected strain strikes, the vaccine reduces the risk of influenza by about 50% to 60% in those who have been vaccinated. It is estimated that the influenza vaccine prevented 71,000 hospitalizations in 2015–2016. It takes about 2 weeks after the vaccination to build antibodies (see Chapter 27, *Infectious and Communicable Diseases*).

Modified from: Centers for Disease Control and Prevention, National Center for Immunization and Respiratory Diseases. Influenza (Flu). Centers for Disease Control and Prevention website. https://www.cdc.gov/flu/index.htm. Updated 2017. Accessed December 4, 2017.

Immunologic and Inflammatory Injury

Cellular membranes are damaged by direct contact with cellular and chemical components of the immune and inflammatory responses. These components include phagocytic cells (monocytes, neutrophils, and macrophages) and substances such as antibodies, lymphokines, complements, and proteases (see Chapter 27, *Infectious and Communicable Diseases*, and Chapter 33, *Toxicology*). If the cell membrane is injured or if the transport mechanism (which moves potassium into the cell and sodium out of it) begins to fail, the intracellular water level increases and causes the cell to swell. If the swelling continues, the cell eventually may rupture.

Injurious Genetic Factors

Genetic disease results from a chromosomal abnormality or a defective gene. These genetic defects are usually inherited (eg, sickle cell anemia) or may result from spontaneous mutations (eg, most mutations that cause cancer). Some genetic disorders can alter the cell's structure and function and can cause changes in the structural or metabolic component of the specific target cells. Huntington disease and muscular dystrophy are examples of conditions caused by such disorders (see Chapter 32, *Nontraumatic Musculoskeletal Disorders*).

> NOTE
> The term **congenital** refers to any abnormality that is present at birth. Despite its presence from the time of birth, the abnormality may not be detected until much later.

Injurious Nutritional Imbalances

Cells need adequate amounts of essential nutrients to function normally. If the needed nutrients are not obtained through the diet and transported to the cells, pathophysiologic effects are possible. Damage can also occur if excessive amounts of nutrients are consumed and transported to the cells. Examples of conditions caused by injurious nutritional imbalances include protein–calorie malnutrition, obesity, hyperglycemia, scurvy, and rickets.

Injurious Physical Agents

Many physical agents can damage cells and tissues. Examples of physical agents (including environmental agents) that can cause cellular or tissue injury include the following:

- Temperature extremes (eg, hypothermic and hyperthermic injury)
- Changes in atmospheric pressure (eg, blast injury, decompression sickness)
- Ionizing radiation (eg, radiation injury)
- Nonionizing radiation (eg, radio waves, microwaves)
- Illumination (light injury [eg, vision injury, skin cancer])
- Mechanical stresses (eg, noise-induced hearing loss, overuse syndromes)

Manifestations of Cellular Injury

An injured cell may show various types of abnormalities in its form and structure. These are known as morphologic abnormalities. The two most common abnormalities of this type are cellular swelling and fatty change. Cellular injury is indicated by both local and systemic signs.[7]

Cellular Manifestations

In injured cells (and in some healthy cells), several substances accumulate. They include fluids and electrolytes, triglycerides (lipids), glucose, calcium, uric acid, protein, melanin, and bilirubin. These substances normally are present in certain cells of the body. However, abnormal intracellular accumulation may lead to cellular damage. In addition, injured cells may be unable to rid themselves of excessive amounts of water, sodium, or calcium, leading to increased injury. If water, sodium, or calcium continues to accumulate, the cells become permanently damaged.

Macrophages ingest debris from injured cells. Some macrophages circulate throughout the body. Others remain fixed in tissues (eg, the liver and the spleen). Phagocytes migrate to injured tissue where they engulf dying cells and abnormal extracellular substances. As more phagocytes migrate to injured tissue to engulf the metabolites, the affected tissue begins to swell. Phagocytosis by the fixed macrophages of the reticuloendothelial system causes enlargement of the liver (hepatomegaly) or the spleen (splenomegaly). This condition is seen with many diseases that are associated with abnormal accumulation of various metabolic products (amyloidosis) or abnormal cells (hemolytic disease).

Cellular Swelling. The swelling in injured cells results from membrane changes that allow potassium to leak rapidly out of the cell and sodium and water to enter the cell. Because the increase in intracellular sodium concentration increases the osmotic pressure, more water is drawn into the cell. If the swelling affects all cells in an organ, the organ increases in weight and becomes distended. Cellular swelling usually is reversible.

> NOTE
> Inflammation is associated with cellular swelling. This is true whether the cause is infection, trauma, or an autoimmune reaction. Inflammation is often accompanied by fever.

Fatty Change. Fatty change occurs when the enzyme systems that metabolize fat are impaired or overwhelmed. When this happens, lipids accumulate inside the cell. This condition is common in liver cells (fatty liver) because these cells are actively involved in the metabolism of fat. Hepatic metabolism and secretion of lipids are crucial to proper body function. For this reason, deficiencies in these processes lead to major pathologic changes. Alcohol abuse is a common cause of fatty liver. It usually is a precursor to cirrhosis.

Systemic Manifestations. Cellular injury produces many systemic manifestations, including fever, malaise, loss of well-being, change in appetite, altered heart rate, an abnormal rise in white blood cells (**leukocytosis**), and pain. Testing of extracellular fluid may reveal the presence of cellular enzymes released by injured cells or tissue.

Cellular Death and Necrosis

A cell dies if it has been irreparably damaged. Shortly after cell death, structural changes begin to occur in the nucleus and cytoplasm. The lysosome (a membranous sac of digestive enzymes found in many cells) begins to undergo membrane breakdown. This releases the lysosomal enzymes, which begin to digest the cell. The nucleus shrinks and dissolves or breaks into fragments (BOX 11-7).

Necrosis is the death of cells or tissues caused by injury or disease. It also can occur by cellular self-destruction (**autolysis**). Different types of necrosis tend to occur in different organs or tissues. The type may indicate the cause of cellular injury. Necrotic changes take several hours to develop. They are easy to recognize on histologic examination by their structure and staining characteristics.

BOX 11-7 Normal Cellular Aging and Death

Cellular aging and death are common processes. They are natural functions of the cell cycle. As the cell ages, it becomes less efficient in executing its functions. It also is more at risk of damage from harmful environmental agents. With progressive damage, cells lose their ability to repair themselves. In time, they begin to malfunction. Changes in immunologic cells slowly lead to decreased immunity and an increased risk of infectious disease. Malignancies increase with age because of decreased immunity and an increased incidence of malignant transformation in various cells. Other examples of the manifestations of aging in cells include gray hair, reduced muscle mass, menopause, arteriosclerosis, memory and vision impairment, and arthritis.

Hypoperfusion and Shock

The term **hypoperfusion** is used to describe decreased circulation of blood and nutrients to tissues and organs. If hypoperfusion is prolonged or becomes systemic, **shock** develops, which can lead to permanent cellular dysfunction and death. Hypoperfusion can be caused by a number of medical and traumatic conditions.

Pathogenesis

Hypoperfusion often is the result of a decrease in cardiac output. Decreased cardiac output, if prolonged, leads to shock (hypoxia at the cellular level), multiple organ dysfunction syndrome, and other disease states associated with impaired cellular metabolism.

Decreased Cardiac Output

Cardiac output (also known as the cardiac minute volume) is the total amount of blood pumped by the ventricles each minute. It is usually expressed in liters per minute (L/min). Cardiac output is a crucial determinant of organ perfusion. It depends on several factors, including the strength of contraction, the rate of contraction, and the amount of available blood returning through the veins (venous return) to the ventricles (**preload**).

NOTE

Cardiac output is determined by multiplying the heart rate by the stroke volume (ie, the volume of blood ejected by the ventricles during each heartbeat). For example, if the ventricles contract 64 times per minute and eject 70 mL of blood with each contraction, the cardiac output would be 64 beats per minute multiplied by 70 mL per beat, or 4.48 L/min.

Compensatory Mechanisms

Under both normal and pathologic circumstances, the body prevents tissue hypoperfusion by using compensatory mechanisms to manage blood pressure and cardiac output. These include a number of **negative feedback mechanisms**. A negative feedback mechanism is any mechanism that tends to balance a change in a system. A number of negative feedback mechanisms are crucial to the process of maintaining cardiac output and tissue perfusion. These mechanisms include baroreceptor reflexes, chemoreceptor reflexes, the central nervous system ischemic response, hormonal mechanisms, reabsorption of tissue fluids, and splenic discharge of stored blood (seen in animals but minimal in humans).

Baroreceptor Reflexes. Baroreceptors (**FIGURE 11-17A**) are pressure-sensitive nerve endings found in the heart and great vessels. They keep blood pressure and cardiac output within a normal range. Normal blood pressure produces a constant, low-level stimulation of the baroreceptors. When the blood pressure moves out of the normal range, either up or down, stimulation of the baroreceptors increases (**BOX 11-8**). The baroreceptor reflexes then act to correct the condition. If the arterial blood pressure increases, the baroreceptor reflexes act to lower blood pressure. Likewise, if the arterial blood pressure decreases, the baroreceptor reflexes act to increase blood pressure[11] (see Figure 11-17A).

When baroreceptor stimulation ceases because of a fall in arterial pressure, the negative feedback mechanism evokes several cardiovascular responses (see Box 11-8). Vagal (parasympathetic) stimulation is reduced, and sympathetic response is increased. The increase in sympathetic impulses results in increased **systemic vascular resistance**. It also results in an increase in the heart rate and **stroke volume**. Sympathetic responses also cause generalized arteriolar vasoconstriction that reduces the size of the vascular

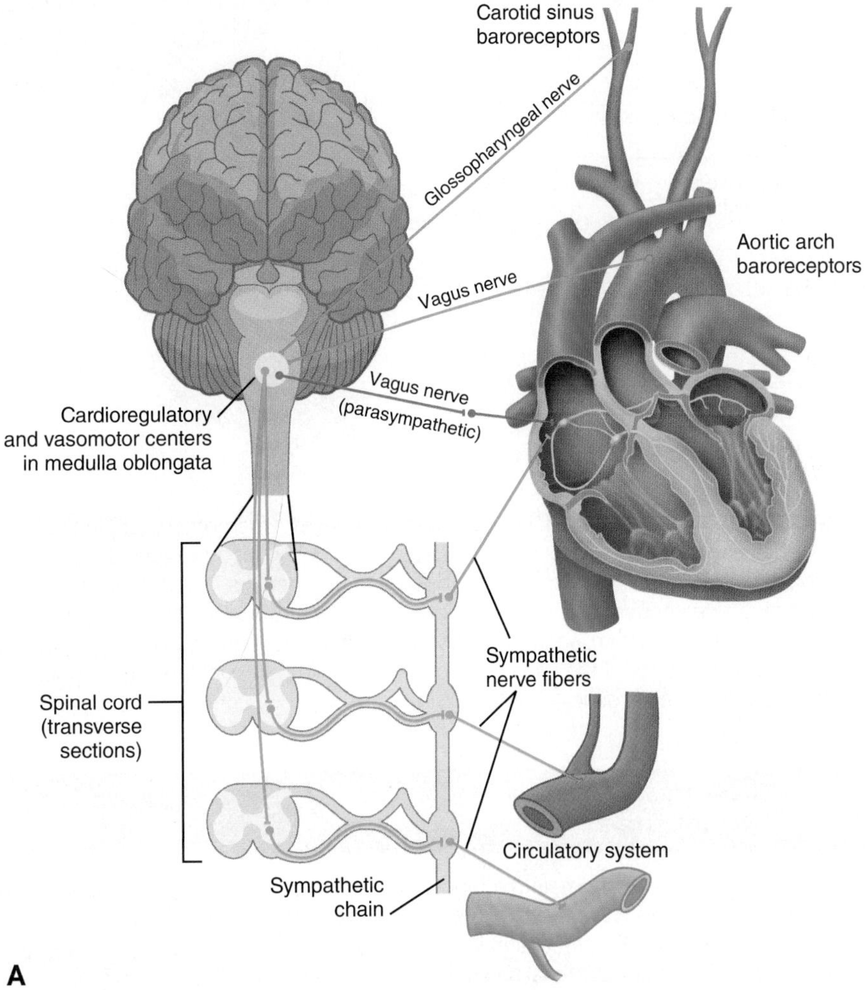

FIGURE 11-17 A. Baroreceptor reflexes. Baroreceptors in the carotid sinuses and the aortic arch detect changes in blood pressure. Impulses are conducted to the cardioregulatory and vasomotor centers. The heart rate can be decreased by the parasympathetic system; the heart rate and stroke volume can be increased by the sympathetic system. The sympathetic system can also constrict or dilate blood vessels.

(continued)

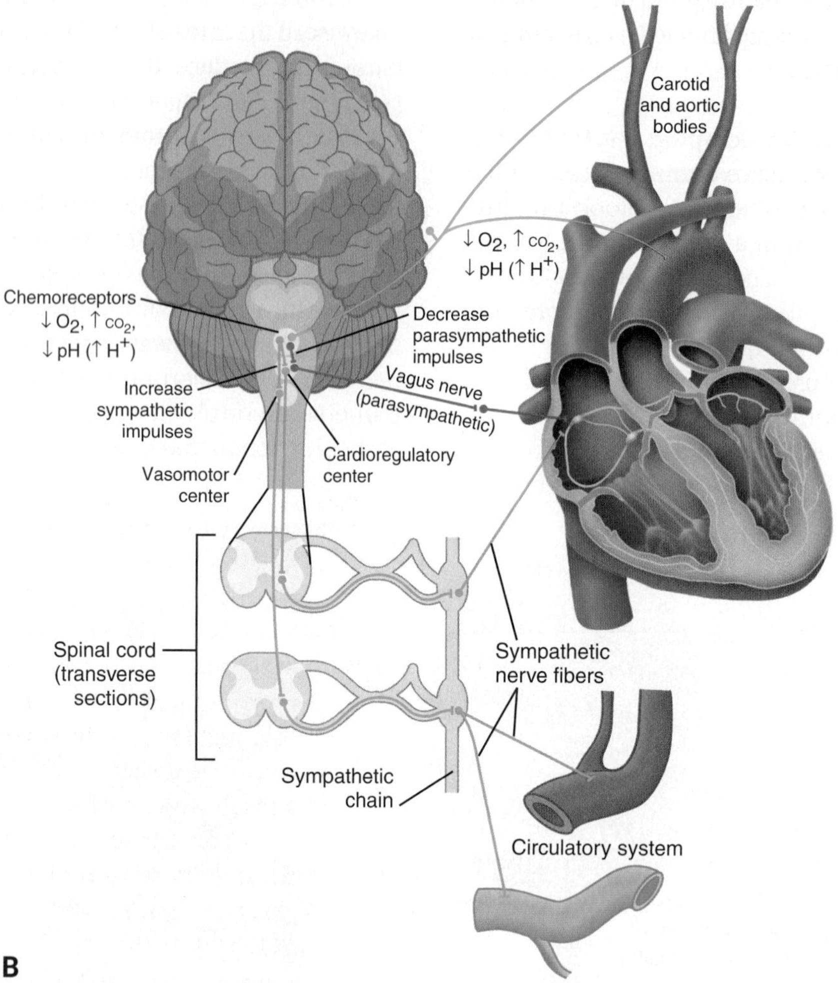

FIGURE 11-17 *(continued)* **B.** Chemoreceptor reflexes. Chemoreceptors in the medulla and carotid and aortic bodies detect changes in blood oxygen, carbon dioxide, or pH levels. Impulses are conducted to the medulla. In response, the vasomotor center can cause constriction or dilation of blood vessels through the sympathetic system, and the cardioregulatory center can cause changes in the pumping activity of the heart through the parasympathetic and sympathetic systems during emergency situations.

BOX 11-8 Baroreceptor Responses to Changes in Blood Pressure: Sympathetic Nervous System

Baroreceptors (see Figure 11-17A) help maintain blood pressure and cardiac output in two ways. Both of these are negative feedback mechanisms. Baroreceptors lower blood pressure in response to increased arterial pressure. They also increase blood pressure in response to decreased arterial pressure. Normal blood pressure partially stretches the arterial walls so that the baroreceptors produce a constant, low-level frequency stimulation. This stimulation increases progressively from a lower pressure limit of 60 mm Hg to a maximum at 180 to 200 mm Hg. Impulses from the baroreceptors travel through the vagus and the Hering nerve to the glossopharyngeal nerve. There, they inhibit the vasoconstrictor center of the medulla and excite the vagal center. These impulses result in vasodilation in the peripheral circulatory system. They also cause a decrease in the heart rate and strength of contraction. The combined effect is a decrease in arterial pressure.

When low blood pressure stimulates a response in the baroreceptors, the effects on the heart include increases in the strength and rate of contraction. Peripheral effects include arteriolar constriction, decreased blood vessel size, and increased peripheral vascular resistance.

compartment. As the veins constrict, blood is shifted into the central circulation. This shift, coupled with the constriction of blood vessels in the skin, muscles, and viscera, helps maintain perfusion of the central organs. The vasoconstriction in these peripheral vascular beds results in the characteristic pale, cool skin seen in patients experiencing hypovolemic shock.

NOTE

Systemic vascular resistance is the resistance to blood flow in the systemic circulation (small arteries, arterioles, venules, veins). **Afterload** is the systemic vascular resistance on the left side of the heart. It is the pressure against which the left ventricle must contract to eject its contents.

NOTE

Baroreceptors adapt within 1 to 3 days to the ambient pressure in the immediate locale. They therefore do not regulate the average blood pressure on a long-term basis.

Chemoreceptor Reflexes. When low arterial pressure leads to hypoxemia, acidosis, or both, peripheral chemoreceptor cells are stimulated. These cells are found in the carotid and aortic bodies. Because of the location of these bodies, the chemoreceptor cells have a vast blood supply. When the Po_2 or pH decreases, chemoreceptor cells stimulate the vasomotor center of the medulla. At the same time, the rate and depth of ventilation are increased to help eliminate excess carbon dioxide. It also helps to maintain acid–base balance. Chemoreceptors (**FIGURE 11-17B**) are more involved in the regulation of respiration than in the regulation of the cardiovascular rate and rhythm or blood pressure. However, during profound hypotension or acidosis, chemoreceptors will produce vasoconstriction. This vasomotor stimulation results in enhanced peripheral vasoconstriction, which is initiated by the baroreceptors.

Central Nervous System Ischemic Response. Blood flow to the vasomotor center of the medulla can be reduced enough to cause ischemia. When this condition occurs, the neurons in the vasomotor center become excited, raising the arterial blood pressure. This effect is known as the **central nervous system ischemic response**. The degree of sympathetic vasoconstriction can be intense. It can be so intense that it elevates the arterial pressure for as long as 10 minutes, sometimes to more than 200 mm Hg. If the ischemia lasts longer than a few minutes, the vagal centers are activated. Activation of the vagal centers results in vasodilation in the periphery and bradycardia (a slowed heart rate). Like the chemoreceptor reflex, the central nervous system ischemic response functions only in emergency situations. It is not activated until the arterial blood pressure falls below 50 mm Hg.

Hormonal Mechanisms. Several hormonal mechanisms also help to control arterial pressure through negative feedback. These include the adrenal medullary mechanism, the renin-angiotensin-aldosterone mechanism, and the vasopressin mechanism.

- **Adrenal medullary mechanism.** When sympathetic stimulation of the heart and blood vessels increases, stimulation of the adrenal medulla also increases. The hormones secreted by the adrenal medulla are epinephrine and norepinephrine. The effect of these hormones on the cardiovascular system is very similar to that produced by the sympathetic nervous system. As a result, the heart rate, the stroke volume, and vasoconstriction increase.
- **Renin-angiotensin-aldosterone mechanism.** As described earlier, renin is an enzyme that changes the structure of the plasma protein angiotensinogen, thereby producing angiotensin I. Angiotensin I, in turn, is converted by ACE (mostly in the lungs), creating angiotensin II (active angiotensin).

NOTE

ACE inhibitors are drugs that block the conversion of the precursor angiotensin I to the active molecule angiotensin II. As a result, blood pressure is lowered and less stress is placed on the heart. Examples of ACE inhibitors include captopril (Capoten), enalapril (Vasotec), and lisinopril (Prinivil).

Angiotensin II causes vasoconstriction in the arterioles and to a lesser degree in the veins. This vasoconstriction results in increased peripheral vascular resistance, increased venous return to the heart, and a resultant increase in blood pressure. Angiotensin II also stimulates the release of aldosterone. Aldosterone acts on the kidneys to conserve sodium and water.

The renin-angiotensin-aldosterone mechanism is an important regulatory loop for increasing the blood pressure in circulatory shock. It takes about 20 minutes to become effective in hypovolemia caused by hemorrhagic shock. It remains active for about 1 hour.

CRITICAL THINKING

You are assessing your patient's radial pulse. What compensatory changes can you evaluate while doing this?

- **Vasopressin mechanism.** When the blood pressure drops or the concentration of solutes in the plasma increases (increased serum osmolality), the hypothalamic neurons are stimulated. This causes the anterior pituitary to increase secretion of vasopressin, or ADH. ADH acts directly on the blood vessels. It causes vasoconstriction within minutes after a rapid fall in the blood pressure. ADH also reduces the rate of urine production by enhancing reabsorption of water. This helps to maintain blood volume and blood pressure.

NOTE

Atrial natriuretic factor also helps to control arterial pressure through a negative feedback mechanism. Its release is triggered by a rise in atrial pressure. (This rise is usually a sign of volume overload.) Atrial natriuretic factor increases the rate of urine production. Loss of water through the urine decreases blood volume, which results in a decrease in the atrial pressure. Atrial natriuretic factor is the only hormone that decreases blood volume and blood pressure.

Reabsorption of Tissue Fluids. Arterial hypotension, arteriolar constriction, and reduced venous pressure during hypovolemia lower the blood pressure in the capillaries (hydrostatic pressure). This decrease promotes reabsorption of interstitial fluid into the vascular compartment. Large amounts of fluid may be drawn into the circulation during hemorrhage. It has been estimated that about 0.25 mL/min per kilogram of body weight, or 1 L/h in an adult male, can be autoinfused from the interstitial spaces after acute blood loss.

Splenic Discharge of Blood. Some of the blood that circulates through the spleen continues through the microcirculation. It is stored in an area called the venous sinuses. The venous sinuses can store more than 300 mL of blood. Sudden reductions in blood pressure cause the sympathetic nervous system to stimulate constriction of these sinuses. Constriction can expel as much as 200 mL of this blood into the venous circulation to help restore blood volume or pressure in the circulation.

SHOW ME THE EVIDENCE

Researchers at Fort Sam Houston in Texas evaluated the ability of end-tidal carbon dioxide ($ETCO_2$) to track reductions in blood volume. They recruited 50 healthy volunteers and placed them in a device that generated lower body negative pressure (LBNP) to redistribute blood volume to the lower extremities and simulate central blood loss. Vital signs, including mean arterial pressure, stroke volume, and $ETCO_2$, were measured at each increment of simulated volume loss. The researchers found that all variables except respiratory rate declined as LBNP increased. Stroke volume and $ETCO_2$ most closely correlated with increments of simulated blood loss. Their findings were limited by the large individual subject baseline $ETCO_2$ variability. They suggest that monitoring trends rather than absolute values of $ETCO_2$ during blood volume loss may be useful to detect changes in patients.

Modified from: McManus JG, Ryan KL, Morton MJ, Rickards CA, Cooke WH, Convertino VA. Limitations of end-tidal CO_2 as an early indicator of central hypovolemia in humans. *Prehosp Emerg Care*. 2008;12(2):199-205.

NOTE

An increase in preload or afterload or a decrease in stroke volume can lead to volume overload and pulmonary edema. This, in turn, can reduce tissue perfusion and impair cellular metabolism (see Chapter 21, *Cardiology*).

Types of Shock

Shock is defined as hypoxia at the cellular level and is classified according to the primary cause (BOX 11-9). Although these classifications are separate and distinct, two or more types may be combined. Brief descriptions of the five types of shock are given here. A more detailed discussion of shock is presented in Chapter 35, *Shock*.

- Hypovolemic shock is most often caused by hemorrhage. It also may be caused by severe dehydration. In either case, circulating volume is lost.
- Cardiogenic shock results when the heart's pumping action cannot deliver adequate circulation

BOX 11-9 Common Etiologic Classifications of Shock

Hypovolemic shock
Cardiogenic shock
Obstructive shock
Distributive shock
- Neurogenic shock
- Anaphylactic shock
- Septic shock

for tissue perfusion despite an adequate amount of circulating blood volume.
- Neurogenic shock results most often from spinal cord injury that is accompanied by loss of sympathetic vasomotor tone.
- Obstructive shock occurs when there is an obstruction of blood flow into or out of the heart (eg, cardiac tamponade, tension pneumothorax).
- Distributive shock occurs when systemic vascular resistance drops, leading to leakage of the intravascular volume. This most commonly occurs as a response to severe inflammation, such as in anaphylaxis or sepsis.

Regardless of the classification, the underlying defect in shock is lack of oxygen delivery or utilization at the cellular level.

Multiple Organ Dysfunction Syndrome

Multiple organ dysfunction syndrome (MODS) (also known as multi-organ failure) is the progressive failure of two or more organ systems following an acute threat.[12,13] This occurs after a severe illness or injury. Septic shock is a common cause of MODS. However, it may follow any period of prolonged shock, regardless of the cause (see Chapter 35, *Shock*) and carries a high degree of mortality.

Pathophysiology

Any process that triggers the body's inflammatory response (eg, trauma, sepsis, burn injury) may initiate MODS. The syndrome begins with vascular endothelial damage that is caused by the release of endotoxins and inflammatory mediators into the circulation. When the vascular endothelium is damaged, it becomes permeable and allows fluid and cells to leak into the interstitial spaces. This, in turn, contributes to hypotension and hypoperfusion. The release of mediators activates three major plasma enzyme cascades, or processes: complement, coagulation, and kallikrein/kinin.

The plasma protein cascade systems are responsible for mediating the inflammatory response. Each system consists of a series of inactive enzymes (proenzymes). These inactive enzymes are converted to active enzymes. This action initiates a cascade in which the substrate (a substance changed by an enzyme in a chemical reaction) of the activated enzyme is the next component of the system.

The complement cascade activates phagocytes and induces further inflammation and damage to the endothelium. As a result of the endothelial damage, coagulation becomes uncontrolled and results in the formation of microvascular thrombi and tissue ischemia. Activation of the kallikrein/kinin system releases bradykinin (a potent vasodilator), which contributes to low systemic vascular resistance. The overall effect of these three systems is a hyperinflammatory and hypercoagulable state that leads to edema formation, cardiovascular instability (hypotension), and clotting abnormalities. These inflammatory processes alter the normal pathways both of systemic blood flow and of blood flow in the individual organs. The result is a hyperdynamic circulation where the cardiovascular system responds to a decrease in systemic vascular resistance by an elevation in cardiac output that is above normal. It is also marked by an increase in the amount of blood returning to the heart through the veins. Blood is shunted past some regional capillary beds. Changes in capillary permeability allow the formation of interstitial edema. As a result, the delivery of oxygen to the tissues is decreased. In addition, the capillaries become blocked by tiny blood clots and by clumps of inflammatory cells. The resultant ischemia contributes to MODS.

The same hormonal responses that help conserve volume in shock cause the body to enter into a hypermetabolic (catabolic) state, altering carbohydrate, fat, and lipid metabolism to meet the increased demand for energy. In time, the sympathetic drive and the hyperdynamic circulation place great demands on the heart. The net result is depletion of oxygen and fuel supplies. The decrease in oxygen delivery to the cells, the hypermetabolism, and the associated myocardial depression create an imbalance in oxygen supply and demand. This imbalance is soon followed by tissue hypoxia with cellular acidosis and

BOX 11-10 Scores to Quantify Severity of MODS

Organ failure or dysfunction is a process rather than an acute event. Organ dysfunction occurs on a continuum from minor to severe, and severity may vary over time. Organ failure usually develops over a period of days to weeks following an initial episode of shock. Multiple scoring tools have been developed to quantify the severity of organ dysfunction. One of the most commonly used tools is the Sequential Organ Failure Assessment (SOFA) score. The purpose of the SOFA score is to facilitate assessment of organ failure in patients with sepsis by quantifying its severity over time. The score includes six organ systems—respiration, coagulation, liver, cardiovascular, central nervous system, and renal—which are each scored daily using clinical and diagnostic criteria from 0 (normal) to 4 (most abnormal). As may be expected, a higher SOFA score is associated with higher mortality.

A recent study demonstrated that in patients with infection, a SOFA score of 12 had a 50% mortality rate, with this number climbing at higher SOFA scores. The association with disease severity in patients with underlying infection led the Society of Critical Care Medicine to advocate for incorporation of the SOFA score into the clinical definition of sepsis syndromes in 2016. The SOFA score has also been used to assess degree of organ dysfunction following cardiac arrest and severe trauma.

Modified from: Vincent JL, Moreno R, Takala J, et al. The SOFA (Sepsis-related Organ Failure Assessment) score to describe organ dysfunction/failure. On behalf of the Working Group on Sepsis-Related Problems of the European Society of Intensive Care Medicine. *Intensive Care Med.* 1996;22:707-710; Singer M, Deutschman CS, Seymour CW, et al. The Third International Consensus Definitions for Sepsis and Septic Shock (Sepsis-3). *JAMA.* 2016; 315(8):801-810; Seymour CW, Liu VX, Iwashyna TJ, et al. Assessment of Clinical Criteria for Sepsis for the Third International Consensus Definitions for Sepsis and Septic Shock (Sepsis-3). *JAMA.* 2016;315(8):762-774; Cour M, Bresson D, Hernu R, Argaud L. SOFA score to assess the severity of the post-cardiac arrest syndrome. *Resuscitation.* 2016;102:110-115; and Ulvik A, Kvåle R, Wentzel-Larsen T, Flaatten H. Multiple organ failure after trauma affects even long-term survival and functional status. *Crit Care.* 2007;11(5):R95.

impaired cellular function. Finally, multiple organ failure begins (BOX 11-10 and **FIGURE 11-18**). No specific therapy exists for MODS. However, early detection is crucial because it allows supportive measures to be started immediately.

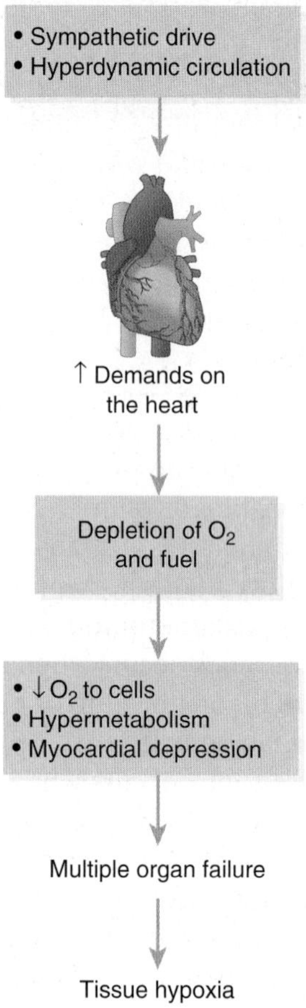

FIGURE 11-18 Multiple organ dysfunction syndrome.

Impairment of Cellular Metabolism

Energy is required for nearly all cellular activities that support life. The active transport pumps in the cell membrane consume a large portion of the cell's energy and use it to maintain a normal fluid and electrolyte composition inside the cell. Adenosine triphosphate (ATP) and other high-energy phosphate molecules provide the fuel for all the energy-related functions of the cell. In the healthy body, most cellular metabolism is aerobic metabolism. Anaerobic metabolism occurs when the metabolic need for energy exceeds the oxygen supply. However, anaerobic metabolism can supply only a small fraction of the energy produced by aerobic metabolism; anaerobic metabolism generates 2 ATP molecules for every molecule of glucose, and aerobic metabolism generates 36 ATP molecules for every molecule of glucose. By itself, anaerobic metabolism cannot meet the body's energy needs.

Glucose is a key fuel for the production of energy. It is the only fuel that can be used anaerobically under conditions of cellular hypoxia (as occurs in a state of shock). Under these conditions, glucose is metabolized to lactate and pyruvate. This produces a net sum of two ATP molecules. If oxygen is present (aerobic metabolism), pyruvate enters the **Krebs cycle**. The Krebs cycle is a sequence of reactions that breaks down a molecule of pyruvic acid into molecules of carbon dioxide and water (**FIGURE 11-19**). It is 18 times more efficient at producing ATP than is glycolysis (glycolysis is the breakdown of glucose to lactate). The Krebs cycle cannot occur in the absence of oxygen. Anaerobic production of ATP is inefficient. Thus, with anaerobic metabolism, the rate of **glycolysis** must be greatly increased to meet the body's energy demands. This leads to an increase in the production of lactic acid and resultant metabolic acidosis.

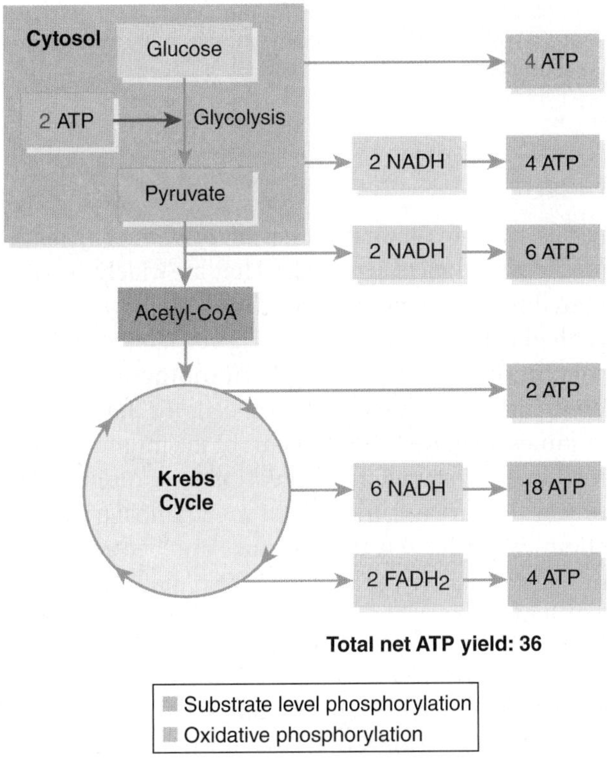

Abbreviations: Acetyl CoA, acetyl coenzyme A; ATP, adenosine triphosphate; $FADH_2$, flavin adenine dinucleotide hydroquinone form; NADH, nicotinamide adenine dinucleotide (reduced)

FIGURE 11-19 Krebs cycle.

As tissue metabolites (and hydrogen ions) continue to accumulate, they stimulate vasodilation. This vasodilation opposes the hormonally regulated constriction of the precapillary sphincters, thereby reducing the body's ability to continue vital tissue perfusion by maintaining the proper size of the vascular compartment. The postcapillary sphincters are more resistant to the vasodilating effects of tissue metabolites, and they stay constricted long after the precapillary sphincters dilate. This action increases the capillary hydrostatic pressure. The result is fluid loss from the vascular space into the interstitial space. In addition, the insufficient energy production of anaerobic metabolism affects the cell's ability to maintain a normal sodium–potassium differential across the cell membrane. Intracellular potassium leaks out of the cell; sodium leaks into the cell. This abnormal sodium–potassium differential creates cellular swelling and a decreased transmembrane potential. Energy production is further impaired. Finally, the cells are irreversibly damaged.

Self-Defense Mechanisms

The body's first lines of defense against illness and injury are the external barriers. These include the skin and the mucous membranes of the digestive, respiratory, and genitourinary tracts. These structures form a barrier between the internal organs and the environment (see Chapter 27, *Infectious and Communicable Diseases*). When they are breached, chemicals, foreign bodies, or microorganisms are allowed to enter cells and tissues. The second and third lines of defense then are activated. These are the **inflammatory response** and the **immune response**, respectively.

Inflammatory Response

Inflammation is a local reaction to cellular injury. The response may be triggered by physical, thermal, or chemical damage. It also may be caused by microbial infection. When a microbial invasion occurs, this line of defense is activated. It prevents further invasion of the pathogen by isolating, destroying, or neutralizing the microorganism. As a rule, the response is protective and is considered beneficial. However, if the response is sustained or directed toward the host's own **antigens**, healthy tissue may be destroyed.

NOTE

An antigen is a substance (usually a protein) that may stimulate the formation of an antibody. The antigen reacts specifically with that antibody. Specific antibodies bind to specific antigens when the two fit together. The attachment of antibodies aids in the neutralization of antigens. It also aids in their removal from the body.

Stages of the Inflammatory Response

The inflammatory response may be divided into three separate stages: the cellular response to injury, the vascular response to injury, and phagocytosis.

Cellular Response to Injury. Metabolic changes occur with any type of cellular injury. The most common primary effect of cellular injury is damage to the cell's aerobic metabolism and ATP-generating process (oxidative phosphorylation). This leads to a decrease in energy reserves. When the energy sources are depleted, the sodium–potassium pump can no longer work effectively. The cell begins to swell as sodium ions accumulate. The organelles in the cell also swell. This swelling, along with increasing acidosis, leads to further impairment of enzyme function and further deterioration of the cell's membranes. In time, the membranes of the cellular organelles begin to leak. The release of hydrolytic enzymes by the lysosomes contributes further to cellular destruction and autolysis. As the cellular contents are dissolved by enzymes, the inflammatory response is stimulated in surrounding tissues.

Vascular Response to Injury. After cellular injury, localized **hyperemia** (an increase in organ blood flow) develops as the surrounding arterioles, venules, and capillaries dilate. The associated increase in filtration pressure and capillary permeability causes fluid to leak from the vessels into the interstitial space and creates edema. Leukocytes (particularly neutrophils and monocytes) begin to collect along the vascular endothelium. As a result of the release of **chemotactic factors** (chemicals that attract white blood cells to the site of inflammation), they soon migrate to the injured tissue.

Phagocytosis. Phagocytosis is the process by which leukocytes engulf, digest, and destroy pathogens. The circulating macrophages are also responsible for clearing the injured area of dead cells and other debris. Intracellular phagocytosis is the ingestion of bacteria and dead cell fragments. It occurs at the site of tissue invasion. It may extend into the general circulation if the infection becomes systemic. Intracellular phagocytosis stimulates the release of chemicals that induce lysis of the leukocytes. These leukocytes combine with dead organisms, proteins, and fluid to form an inflammatory exudate (commonly known as pus). This exudate is a by-product of the inflammatory process associated with bacterial infection. Exudate may be watery (serous exudate), as is seen with blisters; thick and clotted (fibrinous exudate), as is seen with lobar pneumonia; or pus filled (purulent exudate), as is seen with cysts or abscesses. If bleeding occurs, the exudate is described as hemorrhagic exudate.

CRITICAL THINKING

Consider these signs or symptoms: heat, redness, pain, and swelling. What pathophysiologic inflammatory response causes each of these?

Mast Cells

As described in Chapter 10, *Review of Human Systems*, **mast cells** are specialized cells. They are widely distributed throughout connective tissues. Their cytoplasm is filled with granules containing vasoactive amines (histamine, serotonin) and chemotactic factors. When tissue is injured, the mast cells discharge their granules (degranulation) as part of the inflammatory response. Mast cell degranulation is stimulated by physical injury (eg, thermal or mechanical trauma), chemical agents (eg, toxins, snake and bee venoms), or hypersensitivity reactions. It also may be a direct result of the activity of complement components.

Local and Systemic Response to Acute Inflammation

Acute inflammation may be characterized by both local and systemic effects (**FIGURE 11-20**). Local responses include vascular changes (vasodilation and increased vascular permeability) and the formation of exudate. Systemic responses include fever, leukocytosis, and an increase in the level of circulating plasma proteins.

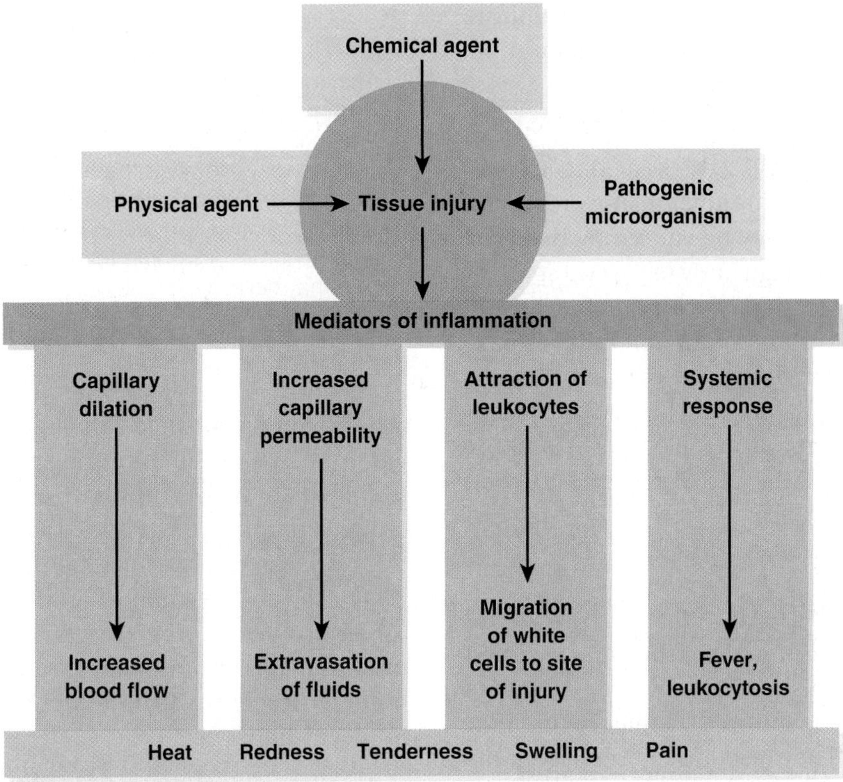

FIGURE 11-20 Inflammation.

Modified from: Crowley L. *Introduction to Human Disease*. 3rd ed. Boston, MA: Jones and Bartlett Publishers; 1992:67.

NOTE

Systemic Inflammatory Response Syndrome Criteria

In 1992 (revised in 2016), a definition for systemic inflammatory response syndrome (SIRS) was introduced to characterize a clinical response to a nonspecific insult of either infectious or noninfectious origin. The SIRS criteria along with other screening tools (ie, SOFA, quick SOFA [qSOFA], and Logistic Organ Dysfunction System [LODS]) attempt to identify patients with an increased risk for sepsis, septic shock, or a severe outcome. SIRS is defined by two or more of the following variables in a patient:

- Fever or hypothermia above 38°C (100.4°F) or below 36°C (96.8°F)
- Heart rate of more than 90 beats per minute
- Respiratory rate of more than 20 breaths per minute or $Paco_2$ of less than 32 mm Hg
- Abnormal white blood cell count (leukocytosis, leukopenia, or bandemia).

Note: SIRS variables are useful for emergency medical services (EMS) providers because three of the four criteria need no special equipment for determination.

There is still no clinical tool to help prehospital providers identify infected patients at greater risk of poor outcome prior to laboratory results. However, some EMS systems provide a SIRS alert notification to the receiving facility so appropriate resources are mobilized prior to the patient's arrival. In some cases, the prehospital SIRS protocol includes drawing blood for culture and antibiotic administration prior to arrival at the emergency department.

Modified from: Kaplan L. Systemic inflammatory response syndrome. Medscape website. https://emedicine.medscape.com/article/168943-overview. Updated September 13, 2017. Accessed February 2, 2018; Bone RC, Balk RA, Cerra FB, et al. Definitions for sepsis and organ failure and guidelines for the use of innovative therapies in sepsis. The ACCP/SCCM Consensus Conference Committee. American College of Chest Physicians/Society of Critical Care Medicine. *Chest*. 1992;101(6):1644-1655; Willoughby J, Damodaran A, Belvitch P. Diagnostic differences between SOFA scores and SIRS criteria in an ICU cohort. *Am J Resp Crit Care Med*. 2017;195:A1918. http://www.atsjournals.org/doi/abs/10.1164/ajrccm-conference.2017.195.1_MeetingAbstracts.A1918. Accessed February 2, 2018; and Tusgul S, Carron P-N, Yersin B, Calandra T, Dami F. Low sensitivity of qSOFA, SIRS criteria and sepsis definition to identify infected patients at risk of complication in the prehospital setting and at the emergency department triage. *Scand J Trauma Resusc Emerg Med*. 2017;25:108.

The characteristic signs of localized inflammation are heat, redness, tenderness, swelling, and pain.

Responses to Chronic Inflammation

Chronic inflammation lasts 2 weeks or longer. It can result from a persistent acute inflammatory response. This type of response may be caused by bacterial contamination by a foreign body (eg, wood splinter, glass), persistent infection, or continued exposure to an antigen. If the inflammatory process is severe or prolonged, the body attempts to repair or replace tissue that has been damaged. The body produces connective tissue fibers and new blood vessels for use in the repair process. If the area of tissue destruction is large, scar tissue forms.

Immune Response

The skin and the inflammatory response are the first two defense mechanisms the body uses to protect itself from injurious agents (see Chapter 26, *Immune System Disorders*). They respond to every agent using the identical nonspecific mechanism. However, the immune response is specific to each individual pathogen. Immunity may be natural, present at birth, or acquired. Acquired immunity develops through exposure to a specific antigenic agent or pathogen. It can be induced through vaccination (immunization) against certain infectious diseases. An example of such a disease is measles.

Acquired immunity is further classified as humoral immunity and cell-mediated immunity. Humoral immunity is associated with the production of antibodies that combine with and eliminate foreign material. Cell-mediated immunity is characterized by the formation of a group of lymphocytes that attack and destroy foreign material (see Chapter 27, *Infectious and Communicable Diseases*). Cell-mediated immunity is the body's best defense against viruses, fungi, parasites, and some bacteria. It also is the mechanism the body uses to reject transplanted organs.

CRITICAL THINKING

Consider hepatitis B, feline leukemia, and chickenpox. What kind of immunity protects you from each of these infections?

NOTE

The immune response is affected by age. Infants are born with immature immune systems and rely on antibodies passed from their mother to protect them from disease. However, the cells of the immune system become less efficient with age. Older people become more susceptible to disease. The aging immune system also becomes less able to eliminate abnormal cells that may develop.

Induction of the Immune Response

An antigen is a substance that reacts with preformed components of the immune system. For example, it may react with lymphocytes and antibodies. An antigen may be a molecule or a molecular complex. An immunogen is a specific type of antigen, one that also can bring about, or induce, the formation of antibodies. (Some antigens, therefore, are not immunogens because they are unable to induce the immune response.) To be immunogenic, the antigenic molecule must be:

- Sufficiently foreign to the host
- Sufficiently large
- Sufficiently complex
- Present in sufficient amounts

The immune response is triggered after foreign materials have been cleared from the area of inflammation. After phagocytes digest the pathogens, antigenic material appears on their surface. The antigen is recognized by receptors on lymphocytes as foreign, or "non-self." Then, a chain of events is set in motion to destroy or neutralize the antigen. This chain of events involves two primary changes that occur among the lymphocytes. Some mature into plasma cells (derived from **B lymphocytes**), which produce antibodies. Others mature into sensitized lymphocytes (**T lymphocytes**) that are capable of interacting directly with the foreign antigen to neutralize or destroy it. (The immune response is presented in more detail in Chapter 26, *Immune System Disorders*, and Chapter 27, *Infectious and Communicable Diseases*.)

Blood Group Antigens

In the early 1900s, researchers discovered that human blood had individual variations. A donor's blood was separated into plasma and red blood cell components

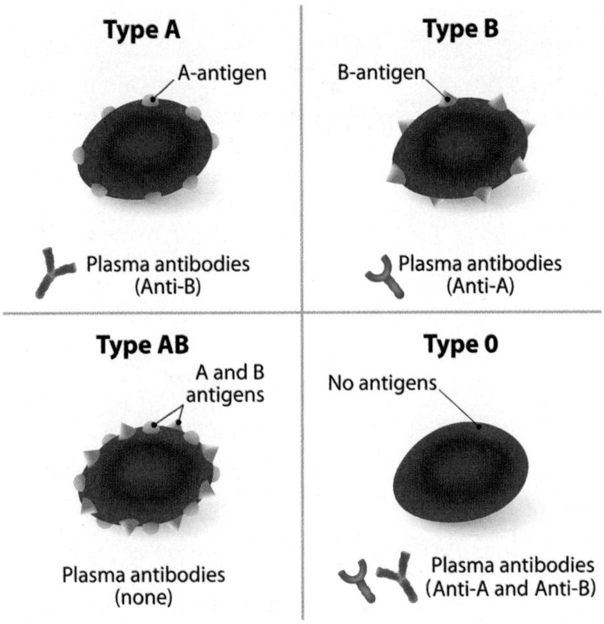

FIGURE 11-21 ABO blood groups. In type A blood, the red blood cells have type A surface antigens and the plasma has type B antibodies. In type B blood, the red cells have type B surface antigens and the plasma has type A antibodies. In type AB blood, the red cells have both type A and type B surface antigens but no plasma antibodies. In type O blood, the red cells have no ABO surface antigens but the plasma has A and B antibodies.

and mixed with separated blood samples from another donor. Two reactions were noted. When combined with foreign plasma, the red cells either clumped together (agglutinated) or showed no change. Scientists also found that two distinct agglutinins (substances on red blood cells that act as antigens) were responsible for the clumping. Based on possible combinations of these antigens, four types of human blood were identified: A, B, AB, and O (**FIGURE 11-21**).

Type A blood has anti-B antibodies in the plasma; therefore, it clumps type B blood. Type B blood has anti-A antibodies; therefore, it clumps type A blood.

> NOTE
>
> Immune tolerance refers to the ability of the immune system to allow self-antigens (versus non–self-antigens) to exist by preventing their recognition by lymphocytes and antibodies.

Type AB blood has neither antibody. People with this blood type can be given any of the four types of blood (universal recipient). Type O blood has both anti-A and anti-B antibodies but no antigens. It can be given to patients with any blood type. Type O blood has become known as the universal donor.

> SHOW ME THE EVIDENCE
>
> This research evaluated patients who received prehospital blood product transfusion during critical care transport. The authors conducted a retrospective review of records of patients who were transported from the scene or another facility by a single air medical agency from 2004 to 2012. The air medical service, based in Pennsylvania, Ohio, and Maryland, was primarily staffed by a nurse/paramedic team trained in critical care. They found that 1,440 patients received blood products during transport. Of these, 75% were medical cases (most common issue was gastrointestinal bleeding), and only 25% were trauma. The most common products transfused were packed red blood cells (62%), followed by fresh-frozen plasma (17.5%). Of the group transfused, the 30-day mortality was 22.5% and the need for emergent surgery was 27%. Additional transfusions were administered after hospital arrival in 47% of patients. The researchers found that the volume of packed red blood cells transfused was associated with higher morbidity and mortality.
>
> *Modified from*: Mena-Munoz J, Srivastava U, Martin-Gill C, Suffoletto B, Callaway CW, Guyette FX. Characteristics and outcomes of blood product transfusion during critical care transport. *Prehosp Emerg Care.* 2016;20(5):586-593.

Rh Factor

In the late 1940s, another determinant in human blood was discovered: the **Rh factor**. The acronym Rh was taken from the word rhesus, the species of monkey used in the research. Researchers found that when the blood of a rhesus monkey was injected into a rabbit, the rabbit's immune system developed antibodies. When a sample of the rabbit's plasma was mixed with a sample of human red blood cells, the human cells usually agglutinated (Rh positive). About 85% of Americans have Rh-positive blood. Incompatibility between Rh-positive and Rh-negative blood can cause a harmful immune response (eg, through transfusion or during childbirth). The percentages of ABO and Rh blood groups in the population are shown in **TABLE 11-4**.

TABLE 11-4 ABO and Rh Blood Groups

	Caucasian	African American	Latin American	Asian
O positive	37%	47%	53%	39%
O negative	8%	4%	4%	1%
A positive	33%	24%	29%	27%
A negative	7%	2%	2%	0.5%
B positive	9%	18%	9%	25%
B negative	2%	1%	1%	0.4%
AB positive	3%	4%	2%	7%
AB negative	1%	0.3%	0.2%	0.1%

Modified from: Learn about blood types. American Red Cross website. http://www.redcrossblood.org/learn-about-blood/blood-types.html. Accessed February 2, 2018.

Variances in Immunity and Inflammation

The immune responses usually are protective. They help to protect the body from harmful microorganisms and other injurious agents. At times, however, these responses may be inappropriate and may have undesirable effects.

Hypersensitivity: Allergy, Autoimmunity, and Isoimmunity

Hypersensitivity is an altered immunologic reactivity to an antigen. It results in a pathologic immune response upon reexposure. These abnormal responses include allergy, autoimmunity, and isoimmunity. **Allergy** refers to an exaggerated immune response that is provoked by environmental **allergens**. **Isoimmunity** is production by an individual of antibodies from members of the same species, such as anti-Rh antibodies in an Rh-negative person (also blood transfusions, transplanted organs). **Autoimmunity** is an immune response against the host's own cells (self-antigens). Of these three responses, allergy is the most common. It also is usually the least life threatening (see Chapter 26, *Immune System Disorders*).

Autoimmunity is responsible for some diseases, including the following:

- Graves disease
- Rheumatoid arthritis
- Myasthenia gravis
- Immune thrombocytopenic purpura
- Systemic lupus erythematosus
- Multiple sclerosis

Mechanisms of Hypersensitivity

Hypersensitivity reactions may be immediate or delayed. With immediate hypersensitivity, antibodies present in the serum trigger an antigen–antibody reaction upon reexposure. Mild reactions of this type include itching and hives. Severe reactions may include life-threatening respiratory distress and **anaphylaxis** (see Chapter 26, *Immune System Disorders*).

Delayed hypersensitivity reactions are a product of cell-mediated immunity. In these reactions, the body develops hypersensitivity after exposure to a foreign antigen from bacteria, parasites, or other microorganisms. The reaction may take from several hours to 2 days to appear and may reach maximal severity several days later. An example of a delayed hypersensitivity reaction is the response against grafted tissue. The results of contact with poison ivy are a more common example.

IgE Reactions. Antibodies, or immunoglobulins, are produced by plasma cells in response to antigenic stimulation. Five distinct classes of immunoglobulins are produced in humans (BOX 11-11). Immunoglobulin E (IgE) accounts for less than 1% of the antibodies in normal serum. It is responsible for immediate (type I) hypersensitivity reactions. With type I reactions, the

BOX 11-11 Classes of Immunoglobulins

IgG Immunoglobulins

IgG immunoglobulins account for 70% to 75% of the antibodies in normal serum. IgG is most abundant in blood. However, it also is found in lymph, cerebrospinal, synovial, and peritoneal fluid and in breast milk. It is the main antibody involved in secondary immune responses. IgG is the only immunoglobulin that crosses the placenta, and it provides temporary immunity in neonates.

IgM Immunoglobulins

IgM immunoglobulins account for about 5% to 10% of the antibodies in normal serum. Most anti-A or anti-B antibodies are of the IgM class. IgM is produced early in the immune response and triggers the increased production of IgG in acute infections and the complement fixation required for an effective antibody response.

IgA Immunoglobulins

IgA immunoglobulins account for about 15% of the antibodies in normal serum. This immunoglobulin is found in blood, secretions such as tears and saliva, and the respiratory tract, stomach, and accessory organs. IgA combines with a protein in the mucosa and defends body surfaces against invading microorganisms.

IgE Immunoglobulins

IgE immunoglobulins account for less than 1% of the antibodies in normal serum. IgE is found in some tissues and on the surface membranes of basophils and mast cells. IgE is responsible for immediate hypersensitivity reactions.

IgD Immunoglobulins

IgD immunoglobulins account for less than 1% of the antibodies in normal serum. The precise biologic function of IgD is unknown.

response is mediated through IgE, which is bound to mast cells or basophils. When an antigen reacts with an IgE molecule bound to a mast cell or circulating basophil, these cells promptly release a host of chemical mediators into the extracellular space. The target organs and the manifestations of the reaction vary, ranging from hives to hay fever to asthma to life-threatening anaphylaxis (see Chapter 26, *Immune System Disorders*).

NOTE

Hypersensitivity reactions are divided into four distinct types: type I (IgE-mediated allergic reactions), type II (tissue-specific reactions), type III (immune complex–mediated reactions), and type IV (cell-mediated reactions). These types are further described in Chapter 26, *Immune System Disorders*.

Immunity and Inflammation Deficiencies

Immunity and inflammation deficiencies describe the failure of these mechanisms of self-defense to function at normal capacity. The source of the deficiency may be primary or secondary. Primary immune deficiencies are hereditary. Secondary immune deficiencies are acquired and are much more common. Acquired immune deficiencies may be caused by infection. Examples include HIV, cancer (in particular, the leukemias), immunosuppressive drugs, and aging. Whether the source is present at birth or acquired, the deficiency usually is caused by a disruption in the function of the lymphocytes, although neutrophil dysfunction also has been described. Research is underway to find replacement therapies for immune deficiencies (BOX 11-12).

Primary Immune Deficiencies

Primary immune deficiencies are genetically determined. They typically manifest during infancy and childhood as recurrent or unusual infections. These deficiencies are classified by the part of the immune system that is deficient, absent, or defective.[14]

Secondary Immune Deficiencies

Acquired immune deficiencies (BOX 11-13) may be classified into the following groups:

- Nutritional deficiencies (eg, severe deficits in calorie or protein intake)

BOX 11-12 Replacement Therapies for Immune Deficiencies

Intravenous replacement of infection-fighting antibodies (immunoglobulins)
Transplantation of cells and tissue
Blood component transfusions
Biologic therapy (eg, monoclonal antibodies)
Gene therapy

BOX 11-13 Acquired Immune Deficiency Disorders[a]

The following are associated with acquired immune deficiency disorders:

- Aging
- Alcoholic cirrhosis
- Anesthesia
- Diabetes
- Down syndrome
- Immunosuppressive treatment
- Infants born with immature immune systems
- Infection (eg, maternal rubella during pregnancy [congenital], maternal cytomegalovirus infection [during pregnancy], measles, leprosy, tuberculosis)
- Malignancies (eg, Hodgkin disease, leukemia, myeloma)
- Malnutrition
- Pregnancy
- Sickle cell anemia
- Stress caused by surgery or emotional trauma

[a]Note: Immunity tends to decrease with age. This is due in part to age-related changes and conditions that impair immunity. Examples include diabetes, chronic kidney disease, and the use of certain drugs that are more common among older adults.

- Iatrogenic deficiencies (deficiencies caused by some form of medical treatment)
- Deficiencies caused by trauma (eg, bacterial infection, burns)
- Deficiencies caused by stress (depressed immune function)
- AIDS

NOTE

AIDS currently is the best-known example of acquired dysfunction of the immune system. HIV causes AIDS. Without access to antiretroviral medications, patients die from opportunistic infections and malignancies. The disease was first identified in 1981. Since then it has become a global health problem. In 2015, an estimated 36.7 million people were living with HIV/AIDS worldwide (see Chapter 27, *Infectious and Communicable Diseases*).

Modified from: HIV/AIDS. *Global Health Observatory (GHO) Data*. World Health Organization website. http://www.who.int/gho/hiv/en/. Accessed February 2, 2018.

CRITICAL THINKING

Think about a time when you or someone close to you became ill because of an acquired immune deficiency. What kind of deficiency caused it? Was it preventable?

Stress and Disease

Prolonged emotional or psychological stress can result in physical illness. This type of illness can produce disturbances in three important areas: cognition, emotion, and behavior. The growing evidence of the link between stress and disease has created a field of science called psychoneuroimmunology. Psychoneuroimmunology is the study of the three-way interaction of the emotional state, the central nervous system, and the body's defense against external infection and abnormal cell division (**FIGURE 11-22**).

Neuroendocrine Regulation of Stress

As described in Chapter 2, *Well-Being of the Paramedic*, the sympathetic nervous system is activated during the stress response. Stress causes the adrenal glands to release catecholamines (epinephrine, norepinephrine, and dopamine) into the bloodstream (**TABLE 11-5**). At the same time, the hypothalamus

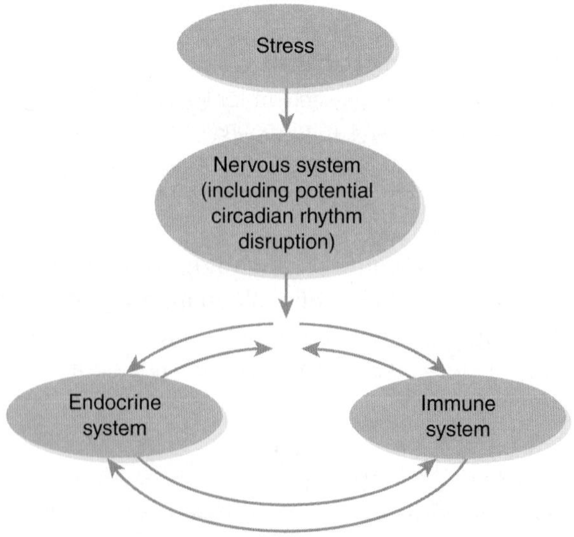

FIGURE 11-22 Interaction of the emotional state, the central nervous system, and the body's defense against infection and abnormal cell division.

TABLE 11-5 Physiologic Effects of Catecholamines

Organ	Process or Result[a]
Brain	Increased blood flow Increased glucose metabolism
Cardiovascular system	Increased rate and force of contraction Peripheral vasoconstriction
Pulmonary system	Increased oxygen supply Bronchodilation Increased ventilation
Muscle	Increased glycogenolysis (breakdown of glycogen) Increased contraction Increased dilation of skeletal muscle vasculature
Liver	Increased glucose production Increased gluconeogenesis (synthesis of glucose from noncarbohydrate sources) Increased glycogenolysis Decreased glycogen synthesis
Adipose tissue	Increased lipolysis (breakdown of fats) Increased fatty acids and glycerol
Skin	Decreased blood flow
Skeleton	Decreased glucose uptake and utilization (decreases insulin release)
Gastrointestinal and genitourinary tracts	Decreased protein synthesis
Lymphoid tissue	Increased protein breakdown (lymphoid tissue shrinks)

[a]Some of these responses require the presence of glucocorticoids (eg, cortisol) for maximal activity.

Reproduced from: McCance K, Huether S. *Pathophysiology: The Biologic Basis for Disease in Adults and Children*. 7th ed. St. Louis, MO: Elsevier; 2014.

stimulates the pituitary gland to release the hormones ADH, prolactin, growth hormone, and adrenocorticotropic hormone (ACTH). ACTH, in turn, stimulates the cortex of the adrenal gland to release cortisol (**TABLE 11-6**).[15]

Catecholamines

Catecholamines act by stimulating two major classes of receptors: **alpha-adrenergic receptors** and **beta-adrenergic receptors**. These two classes are further subcategorized into alpha-1 receptors, alpha-2 receptors, beta-1 receptors, and beta-2 receptors.

- Alpha-1 receptors are postsynaptic. They are located on the effector organs (eg, blood vessels, skeletal muscle). The main role of the alpha-1 receptors is to stimulate the contraction of smooth muscle. The alpha-2 receptors are found on the presynaptic nerve endings. Stimulation of the alpha-2 receptors serves as a negative feedback mechanism by inhibiting further release of norepinephrine.
- The beta-1 receptors are located mainly in the heart. Beta-2 receptors are located primarily in the bronchiolar and arterial smooth muscle. The beta receptors perform several functions: stimulate the heart; dilate bronchioles and blood vessels in skeletal muscle, brain, and heart; and aid in glycogenolysis. Epinephrine activates both the alpha and the beta receptors (**TABLE 11-7**); norepinephrine mainly excites the alpha receptors. (Alpha and beta receptors are discussed in more detail in Chapter 13, *Principles of Pharmacology and Emergency Medications*.)

TABLE 11-6 Physiologic Effects of Cortisol

Function	Effects
Carbohydrate and lipid metabolism	Diminishes peripheral uptake and utilization of glucose, promotes gluconeogenesis in liver cells, enhances gluconeogenic response to other hormones, promotes lipolysis in adipose tissue
Protein metabolism	Increases protein synthesis in liver and depresses protein synthesis (including immunoglobulin synthesis) in muscle, lymphoid tissue, adipose tissue, skin, and bone; increases plasma level of amino acids; stimulates deamination (an oxidative reaction related to protein breakdown) in liver
Inflammatory function	Decreases circulating eosinophils, lymphocytes, and monocytes; increases release of polymorphonuclear leukocytes from bone marrow; decreases accumulation of leukocytes at site of inflammation; delays healing; permissive for vasoconstrictive action of norepinephrine
Lipid metabolism	Promotes lipolysis in extremities and lipogenesis (fat formation) in face and trunk
Immune reserve	Decreases tissue mass of all lymphoid tissues (eg, decreases protein synthesis); promotes rapid decrease in circulating lymphocytes, eosinophils, basophils, and macrophages; inhibits production of interleukin-1 and interleukin-2 and consequently blocks cell-mediated immunity and generation of fever
Digestive function	Promotes gastric secretion
Urinary function	Enhances urinary excretion
Connective tissue	Decreases proliferation of fibroblasts in connective tissue (thereby delaying healing)
Muscle	Maintains normal contractility and maximal work output for skeletal and cardiac muscle
Bone	Decreases bone formation
Vascular system and myocardial function	Maintains normal blood pressure, increases responsiveness of arterioles to constrictive action of adrenergic stimulation, optimizes myocardial performance
Central nervous system	Modulates perceptual and emotional functioning (although mechanism for this is unknown), which are essential for normal arousal and initiation of daytime activity

Reproduced from: McCance K, Huether S. *Pathophysiology: The Biologic Basis for Disease in Adults and Children*. 7th ed. St. Louis, MO: Elsevier; 2014.

TABLE 11-7 Physiologic Actions of Alpha and Beta Receptors

Receptor	Physiologic Actions
Alpha-1 receptor	Increased glycogenolysis; smooth muscle contraction (blood vessels, genitourinary tract)
Alpha-2 receptor	Smooth muscle relaxation (gastrointestinal tract); smooth muscle contraction (some vascular beds); inhibition of lipolysis, renin release, platelet aggregation, and insulin secretion
Beta-1 receptor	Stimulation of lipolysis, myocardial contraction (increased rate, increased force of contraction)
Beta-2 receptor	Increased hepatic gluconeogenesis; increased hepatic glycogenolysis; increased muscle glycogenolysis; increased release of insulin, glucagon, and renin; smooth muscle relaxation (bronchi, blood vessels, genitourinary tract, gastrointestinal tract)

Reproduced from: McCance K, Huether S. *Pathophysiology: The Biologic Basis for Disease in Adults and Children*. 7th ed. St. Louis, MO: Elsevier; 2014.

Cortisol

Cortisol (hydrocortisone) circulates in the plasma and mobilizes substances that are needed for cellular metabolism. The main metabolic effect of cortisol is the stimulation of gluconeogenesis. It also enhances the elevation of blood glucose level by reducing glucose utilization. Cortisol also acts as an immunosuppressant; it reduces the reproduction of lymphocytes, particularly among the T lymphocytes. This, in turn, leads to a decrease in cellular immunity.

Cortisol also reduces the migration of macrophages into an inflamed area. It reduces phagocytosis, partly by stabilizing the lysosomal membranes. This decrease in immune cell activity may be beneficial because it prevents immune-mediated tissue damage. Two factors—the type of stress event and the length of exposure to the stressor—determine whether the effects of cortisol are adaptive or destructive.

Role of the Immune System

Many immunologic conditions and diseases seem to be triggered by stress (**TABLE 11-8**). However, the exact mechanisms that link stress to these diseases and conditions have not yet been clearly defined. It is believed that the immune, nervous, and endocrine systems communicate through complex pathways. Also, they may be affected by factors involved in the stress reaction.

TABLE 11-8 Examples of Stress-Related Diseases and Conditions

Target Organ or System	Disease or Condition
Cardiovascular system	Coronary artery disease Hypertension Stroke Disturbances of heart rhythm
Muscles	Tension headaches Muscle contraction backache
Connective tissues	Rheumatoid arthritis (autoimmune disease) Related inflammatory diseases of connective tissue
Pulmonary system	Asthma (hypersensitivity reaction) Hay fever (hypersensitivity reaction)
Immune system	Immunosuppression or deficiency Autoimmune diseases
Gastrointestinal system	Ulcer Irritable bowel syndrome Diarrhea Nausea and vomiting Ulcerative colitis
Genitourinary system	Diuresis Impotence Frigidity
Skin	Eczema Neurodermatitis Acne
Endocrine system	Diabetes mellitus Amenorrhea
Central nervous system	Fatigue and lethargy Aggression Overeating Depression Insomnia Impaired learning and memory

Reproduced from: McCance K, Huether S. *Pathophysiology: The Biologic Basis for Disease in Adults and Children*. 7th ed. St. Louis, MO: Elsevier; 2014.

Interrelationship of Stress, Coping, and Illness

As noted earlier in this chapter and in Chapter 2, *Well-Being of the Paramedic*, the damage caused by stress is determined by the nature, intensity, and duration of the stressors. It also is affected by the way in which a person perceives the stressors and how well the person is able to cope with them. The ability to notice the signs and symptoms of stress and to use stress management tactics is crucial to good health. Stress-reduction techniques include meditation, exercise, and guided imagery. In healthy people, such methods can help prevent harmful physiologic and psychological illness arising from stress.

Genetics and Familial Diseases

People are born with a genetic predisposition to the development of certain diseases. The genetics of some diseases, like hemophilia or sickle cell anemia, are well understood (see Chapter 31, *Hematology*). Patients either have no genetic predisposition, are carriers of the disease, or have the disease. Other disease processes (like arthritis, diabetes mellitus, and hypertension) certainly are linked to genetics but are strongly associated with environmental factors as well. Medical researchers attempt to reduce the incidence or severity of these inherited medical conditions through environmental manipulation.

Factors Causing Disease

Factors that cause disease may be simplistically classified as genetic or social and environmental. However, there is a strong interaction between the two classifications (BOX 11-14). For example, genes cannot exert their effects without an environment in which to operate, and environmental factors act differently on different people. Conversely, the environment may be the same, but people have unique genetic makeups. Therefore, the interaction between genetics and environment is complex.

Genetic Factors

Heredity is governed by the laws of chance and probability. This situation exists because each pair of chromosomes is sorted at random when packaged into eggs and sperm. More than 19,000 genes are involved in a person's genetic makeup. Thus, the range of variation is huge. Different types of genetic diseases can arise and occur because of individual genetic changes or because of abnormalities involving an entire chromosome.

Sometimes mistakes occur when chromosomes are packaged. These mistakes result in rearrangement of the chromosomes. Widespread chromosomal abnormalities lead to diseases such as Down syndrome or Turner syndrome. More commonly, an individual abnormal gene on the chromosome is passed on, resulting in the production of a dysfunctional protein. This type of genetic defect is responsible for sickle cell anemia and hemophilia. Some conditions may involve more than one gene (ie, they are polygenic) and a number of factors, but they still may have a strong inherited component. These diseases include coronary artery disease, hypertension, and cancer.

BOX 11-14 Environmental Influence in Genetic Selection

The gene that causes sickle cell anemia was recognized to be much more common in environments in which malaria was prevalent. People with sickle cell disease have sickle-shaped red blood corpuscles that clog the capillaries. This condition often proves fatal. However, in people who are carriers of the sickle cell trait, fewer than 1% of the red corpuscles are abnormal. These people do not die of sickle cell anemia, and they are more resistant to malaria than are people who do not carry the sickle cell trait. Thus, the trait provided protection, and its prevalence increased as a result of natural selection.

NOTE

Genes are unchangeable units of inheritance. However, the way genes work (gene expression or epigenetics) can be affected by environmental factors, such as food, drugs, or exposure to toxins (see Box 11-14).

Social and Environmental Factors

Many common chronic diseases may occur because of the influence of social and environmental factors, some of which may cause a predisposition to the development of disease (**TABLE 11-9**; also see Table 11-10). Important social and environmental factors include the following:

- Microorganisms and immunologic exposure
- Personal habits and lifestyle
- Chemical substances
- Physical environment
- Psychosocial environment

The goal in preventing disease is to find the genetic, social, and environmental influences that lead to major diseases. This knowledge will help people who have specific susceptibilities to make changes to certain social and environmental factors to lessen their risk for the development of an illness. Scientists generally recognize five determinants of health of a population (**FIGURE 11-23**):

1. Genes and biology (eg, sex, age)
2. Health behaviors (eg, alcohol use, injection drug use [needles], unprotected sex, smoking)
3. Social environment or social characteristics (eg, discrimination, income, gender)
4. Physical environment or total ecology (eg, where a person lives, crowding conditions)
5. Health services or medical care (eg, access to quality health care, having or not having insurance)

Age and Sex

Age and sex also seem to play a role in the incidence of familial (hereditary) diseases. This is especially true for diseases that are not caused by a single genetic

TABLE 11-9 Social and Environmental Factors That Affect the Occurrence of Disease

Factors	Examples
Microorganisms and immunologic exposure	Bacteria Viruses Fungi Protozoa Vectors (eg, insects and animals) Allergens
Personal habits and lifestyle	Smoking Physical exercise Dietary intake Unprotected sex
Chemical substances	Toxins Pollutants Medications and substance abuse Solvents, fumes Contaminants
Physical environment	Climate Radiation Physical trauma Geographic location (eg, sun exposure, altitude) Community (eg, water and food supplies)
Psychosocial milieu	Family status (eg, bereavement, loss, status change) Stress Coping skills Social isolation Social customs

defect. In the polygenic disorders, the combined effects of genes and environment over time play a role. These combined influences may result in diseases linked to age-related changes in metabolism. This relationship may explain why heart disease, hypertension, and cancer are seen more often in people older than 40 years.

A person's sex is associated with specific diseases that arise from hormonal and anatomic differences. Two examples are breast cancer in women and testicular cancer in men. Lifestyle and environmental differences in gender-related activities also may play a role. These differences may be responsible for the predisposition

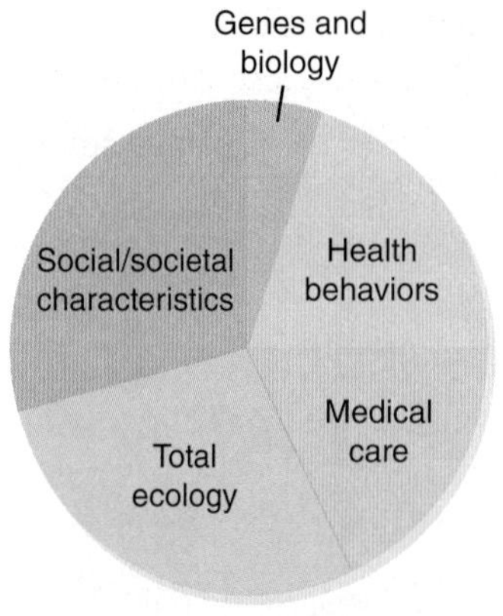

FIGURE 11-23 Social determinants of health.

Modified from: National Center for HIV/AIDS, Viral Hepatitis, STD, and TB Prevention. NCHHSTP social determinants of health: frequently asked questions. Centers for Disease Control and Prevention website. https://www.cdc.gov/nchhstp/socialdeterminants/faq.html. Updated March 21, 2014. Accessed February 2, 2018.

to some diseases. An example of the combined effects of sex/gender, lifestyle, and environmental combinations is the higher rate of lung cancer and coronary artery disease in men who smoke cigarettes.

Analyzing the Risk of Disease

Epidemiologists are researchers who study disease "rates" and analyze risk factors. Disease rates help to describe the occurrence of disease. Risk factors are indicators of a person's predisposition to the development of a disease.

Disease Rates

Three statistics are commonly used to assess the impact of a disease on a society: incidence rate, prevalence rate, and mortality rate. The incidence rate refers to the number of new cases detected during a given period per the number of people in the population surveyed. The prevalence rate refers to the number of people living with the disease per the number of people in the population surveyed.[16] The mortality rate refers to the number of people who died from the disease during a given period per the number of people in the population surveyed.[17]

Risk Factor Analysis

The presence of certain risk factors in any group of people is linked to an increased disease rate in that group. Diseases may have causal and noncausal risk factors. With causal risk factors, removal or elimination of the risk factors delays or prevents the disease. Noncausal risk factors can help predict a person's chances

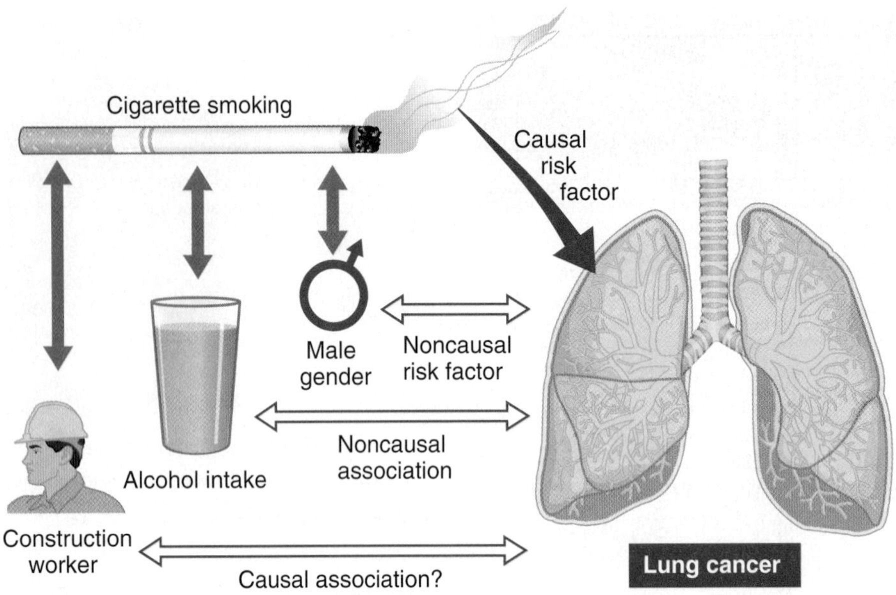

FIGURE 11-24 Causal and noncausal risk factors and associations.

for the development of the disease, but they have no direct effect on the underlying cause (**FIGURE 11-24**). Risk factors, as the term suggests, indicate a person's risk of developing a disease; however, they cannot precisely predict whether a person will develop a disease.

Combined Effects and Interaction of Risk Factors

When one or more risk factors interact, the individual effects of risk factors may be greatly magnified. For example, some risk factors alone may pose little or no danger of disease. However, if another risk factor is added, the danger increases substantially.

Familial Disease Tendency

In some families, members of the family (brothers and sisters, parents and children, spouse pairs, twins) are more prone to some diseases than are the people of the general population. Often the familial risk factors are genetic or shared factors in the environment. For example, illnesses such as heart disease and pulmonary disease may run in a family because of a shared genetic trait or because the family members decided to smoke or consume a diet high in fat, or both.

> CRITICAL THINKING
>
> Think about how many risk factors you have for heart disease. Which of these factors are genetic and which ones could you eliminate by modifying your habits or environment?

Aging and Age-Related Disorders

Advanced age is a risk factor for many diseases, such as heart attack, stroke, and cancer. This risk factor likely represents the cumulative effects of genetics and social and environmental factors. Disorders related to age occur throughout life. Some disorders, such as dental cavities and "strep throat," are more common in younger age groups. The degenerative disorders (eg, arthritis) are more common in older age groups. A correlation between aging and age-related disorders can be drawn by examining the leading causes of death by age group (**FIGURE 11-25**).

Common Familial Diseases and Associated Risk Factors

People who are at high risk can take steps to avoid many familial diseases (**TABLE 11-10**). Some risk factors have overlap between genes, a person's lifestyle, and the environment. While the genetic component may not be modifiable, the person's lifestyle or environment may be. For example, obesity contributes to many disease processes, and the factors leading to obesity are often a combination of genetic and environmental.

10 Leading Causes of Death by Age Group, United States – 2015

Rank	<1	1-4	5-9	10-14	15-24	25-34	35-44	45-54	55-64	65+	Total
1	Congenital Anomalies 4,825	Unintentional Injury 1,235	Unintentional Injury 755	Unintentional Injury 763	Unintentional Injury 12,514	Unintentional Injury 19,795	Unintentional Injury 17,818	Malignant Neoplasms 43,054	Malignant Neoplasms 116,122	Heart Disease 507,138	Heart Disease 633,842
2	Short Gestation 4,084	Congenital Anomalies 435	Malignant Neoplasms 437	Malignant Neoplasms 428	Suicide 5,491	Suicide 6,947	Malignant Neoplasms 10,909	Heart Disease 34,248	Heart Disease 76,872	Malignant Neoplasms 419,389	Malignant Neoplasms 595,930
3	SIDS 1,568	Homicide 369	Congenital Anomalies 181	Suicide 409	Homicide 4,733	Homicide 4,863	Heart Disease 10,387	Unintentional Injury 21,499	Unintentional Injury 19,488	Chronic Low. Respiratory Disease 131,804	Chronic Low. Respiratory Disease 155,041
4	Maternal Pregnancy Comp. 1,522	Malignant Neoplasms 354	Homicide 140	Homicide 158	Malignant Neoplasms 1,469	Malignant Neoplasms 3,704	Suicide 6,936	Liver Disease 8,874	Chronic Low. Respiratory Disease 17,457	Cerebro-vascular 120,156	Unintentional Injury 146,571
5	Unintentional Injury 1,291	Heart Disease 147	Heart Disease 85	Congenital Anomalies 156	Heart Disease 997	Heart Disease 3,522	Homicide 2,895	Suicide 8,751	Diabetes Mellitus 14,166	Alzheimer's Disease 109,495	Cerebro-vascular 140,323
6	Placenta Cord. Membranes 910	Influenza & Pneumonia 88	Chronic Low. Respiratory Disease 80	Heart Disease 125	Congenital Anomalies 386	Liver Disease 844	Liver Disease 2,861	Diabetes Mellitus 6,212	Liver Disease 13,278	Diabetes Mellitus 56,142	Alzheimer's Disease 110,561
7	Bacterial Sepsis 599	Septicemia 54	Influenza & Pneumonia 44	Chronic Low Respiratory Disease 93	Chronic Low Respiratory Disease 202	Diabetes Mellitus 798	Diabetes Mellitus 1,986	Cerebro-vascular 5,307	Cerebro-vascular 12,116	Unintentional Injury 51,395	Diabetes Mellitus 79,535
8	Respiratory Distress 462	Perinatal Period 50	Cerebro-vascular 42	Cerebro-vascular 42	Diabetes Mellitus 196	Cerebro-vascular 567	Cerebro-vascular 1,788	Chronic Low. Respiratory Disease 4,345	Suicide 7,739	Influenza & Pneumonia 48,774	Influenza & Pneumonia 57,062
9	Circulatory System Disease 428	Cerebro-vascular 42	Benign Neoplasms 39	Influenza & Pneumonia 39	Influenza & Pneumonia 184	HIV 529	HIV 1,055	Septicemia 2,542	Septicemia 5,774	Nephritis 41,258	Nephritis 49,959
10	Neonatal Hemorrhage 406	Chronic Low Respiratory Disease 40	Septicemia 31	Two Tied: Benign Neo./Septicemia 33	Cerebro-vascular 166	Congenital Anomalies 443	Septicemia 829	Nephritis 2,124	Nephritis 5,452	Septicemia 30,817	Suicide 44,193

Data Source: National Vital Statistics System, National Center for Health Statistics, CDC.
Produced by: National Center for Injury Prevention and Control, CDC using WISQARS™.

Centers for Disease Control and Prevention
National Center for Injury Prevention and Control

FIGURE 11-25 Ten leading causes of death by age group.

Reproduced from: Centers for Disease Control and Prevention. Data Source: National Vital Statistics System, National Center for Health Statistics, CDC. Produced by: National Center for Injury Prevention and Control, CDC using WISQARS™.www.cdc.gov/injury/images/lc-charts/leading_causes_of_death_age_group_2015_1050w740h.gif. Accessed December 4, 2017.

TABLE 11-10 Common Familial Diseases and Associated Social and Environmental Risk Factors

Disease	Social and Environmental Risk Factors
Immunologic Disorders	
Asthma and other allergies	Dog and cat dander, cockroaches, dust, pollen, mold, or other allergens; tobacco smoke exposure; infections (some pneumonias, respiratory syncytial virus)
Cancer	
Breast cancer	Obesity, sedentary lifestyle, high dietary fat intake, alcohol ingestion, hormone changes, having no children or first child after age 30 years, hormone therapies
Colorectal cancer	Inadequate fiber intake, high dietary fat intake
Lung cancer	Tobacco smoke, environmental pollutants (radon, asbestos, workplace agents, including diesel exhaust), air pollution, prior lung radiation, beta carotene
Endocrine Disorders	
Diabetes mellitus type 1 (insulin-dependent)	Viral infection, cold weather, early dieting (less common in those who were breastfed)
Diabetes mellitus type 2 (non–insulin-dependent)	Obesity, diet high in sugar and low in fiber, sedentary lifestyle, chronic pesticide or air pollution exposure
Cardiovascular Disorders	
Coronary artery disease	Sedentary lifestyle, alcohol ingestion, smoking, obesity, stress, increased blood pressure, elevated blood lipids and cholesterol.
Cardiomyopathies	Infection, obesity, alcohol ingestion
Mitral valve prolapse	Infection
Hypertension and stroke	Diet high in fat and salt and low in potassium, sedentary lifestyle, obesity, tobacco use, excessive alcohol ingestion
Renal Disorders	
Gout	Obesity, diet high in purines (liver, dried beans), lead exposure, medications (diuretics, salicylates, niacin, levodopa [used to treat Parkinson disease], cyclosporine [immune suppressant])
Kidney stones	Obesity, diet high in salt or protein or low in calcium, excessive alcohol ingestion, low fluid intake, endocrine disorders, medications (thiazide diuretics, ACE inhibitor, antihypertensives)
Gastrointestinal Disorders	
Malabsorption Disorders	
Ulcerative colitis	Negative association with appendectomy before 10 years of age, NSAID (ibuprofen, aspirin) use
Crohn disease	Smoking, diet, antibiotic use, NSAID use
Peptic ulcers	NSAID use, infection (*Helicobacter pylori*), tumors
Gallstones	High dietary fat intake, obesity, dieting, rapid weight loss, sedentary lifestyle, medication use (some antibiotics, thiazide diuretics, female hormones)
Obesity	Diet high in fat, sugar, and total calories, sedentary lifestyle, illnesses (Cushing disease, polycystic ovary syndrome), medication use (steroids, some antidepressants)

TABLE 11-10 Common Familial Diseases and Associated Social and Environmental Risk Factors *(continued)*

Disease	Social and Environmental Risk Factors
Neuromuscular Disorders	
Multiple sclerosis	Virus, possible links to lack of natural vitamin D, smoking
Alzheimer disease	Decreased mental stimulation later in life, head injury, heart disease, stroke
Psychiatric Disorders	
Schizophrenia	Possible links to developmental trauma, growing up in urban environment, minority group (first and second generation immigrant), and cannabis use
Depression	Chronic illness, chronic pain, some drug treatments (some antihypertensives, hormone, antiulcer, antituberculosis, Parkinson disease, immunomodulatory, and psychotropic drugs)

Abbreviations: ACE, angiotensin-converting enzyme; NSAID, nonsteroidal anti-inflammatory drug

Summary

- Two facts highlight the importance of body water. First, body water is the medium in which all metabolic reactions occur. Second, the precise regulation of the volume and composition of body fluids is essential to health. Water follows osmotic gradients established by changes in sodium concentrations; therefore, sodium balance and water balance are closely related.
- Two abnormal states of body fluid balance can occur. If the water gained exceeds the water lost, a state of water excess, or overhydration, exists. If the water lost exceeds the water gained, a state of water deficit, or dehydration, exists.
- In addition to fluid imbalances, disturbances in the balance of electrolytes (other than sodium) may occur. These electrolytes include potassium, calcium, and magnesium. Imbalances of these electrolytes can interfere with neuromuscular function. They may even cause cardiac rhythm disturbances.
- The treatment of isotonic dehydration may include volume replacement with isotonic or occasionally hypotonic solutions. The treatment of hypotonic dehydration may involve intravenous replacement with normal saline or lactated Ringer solution. Occasionally hypertonic saline (eg, in seizures caused by hyponatremia) is used. Interventions for overhydration depend on the cause. These interventions may include water restriction, administration of a diuretic, or, if hyponatremia is present, administration of saline.
- In-hospital treatment of hypokalemia involves intravenous or oral potassium replacement. Management of hyperkalemia may involve potassium restriction, intravenous administration of glucose and insulin, nebulized albuterol, sodium bicarbonate, or calcium.
- Treatment of hypocalcemia involves intravenous administration of calcium ions. The management of hypercalcemia may include controlling the underlying disease and aggressive hydration.
- Hypomagnesemia typically is corrected by the administration of intravenous magnesium sulfate. The most effective treatment for hypermagnesemia is hemodialysis. Calcium salts that antagonize magnesium may also be given.
- The healthy body is sensitive to changes in the concentration of hydrogen ions (pH). It tries to maintain the pH of extracellular fluid at 7.4. This is accomplished through three interrelated compensatory mechanisms: carbonic acid–bicarbonate buffering, protein buffering, and renal buffering.
- Metabolic acidosis occurs when the amount of acid generated exceeds the body's buffering capacity. The four most common forms of metabolic acidosis encountered in the prehospital setting are lactic acidosis, diabetic ketoacidosis, acidosis resulting from renal failure, and acidosis caused by ingestion of toxins. Treatment for metabolic acidosis is aimed at correcting the underlying cause.
- Loss of hydrogen ions is the initial cause of metabolic alkalosis. This may be caused by vomiting (hydrochloric acid loss), suctioning of gastric contents, or increased renal excretion of hydrogen ion in the urine. Treatment is directed at correcting the underlying condition. Volume depletion, if present, should be corrected with isotonic solutions.
- Respiratory acidosis is caused by the retention of carbon dioxide, which leads to an increase in the partial pressure of carbon dioxide (Pco_2). This condition usually is caused by ventilator insufficiency that results in an imbalance in the production of carbon dioxide and its elimination from the alveoli. Treatment for respiratory acidosis involves improving ventilation quickly to eliminate carbon dioxide.
- Hyperventilation may produce respiratory alkalosis by decreasing the Pco_2. Treatment of respiratory alkalosis is directed at correcting the underlying cause of the hyperventilation.
- Paramedics must understand the processes of disease. This requires knowledge of the structural and functional

reactions of cells and tissues to injurious agents. Changes in cells and tissues can be caused by adaptation, injury, neoplasia, aging, or death.

- An injured cell may have an abnormal physical shape or size. Cell injury has both cellular and systemic effects.
- Certain factors cause disease. For the most part, these factors may be classified as genetic or environmental. However, a strong interaction occurs between the two.
- The terms *hypoperfusion* and *shock* are used to describe inadequate tissue circulation. Negative feedback mechanisms important in maintaining tissue perfusion are baroreceptor reflexes, chemoreceptor reflexes, the central nervous system ischemia response, hormonal mechanisms, reabsorption of tissue fluids, and splenic discharge of stored blood.
- The external barriers are the body's first line of defense against illness and injury. These barriers include the skin and the mucous membranes of the digestive, respiratory, and genitourinary tracts. When these barriers are breached, chemicals, foreign bodies, or microorganisms are allowed to penetrate cells and tissues. Then the second and third lines of defense are activated. These are the inflammatory response (second) and the immune response (third). Both the external barriers and the inflammatory response respond to all organisms using the identical nonspecific mechanism. The immune response is specific to individual pathogens.
- Immune responses usually are protective. They help to protect the body from harmful microorganisms and other injurious agents. At times, these responses may be inappropriate. They may even have undesirable effects. Examples of inappropriate responses include hypersensitivity and immunity or inflammation deficiencies.
- Many immune-related conditions and diseases are associated with stress. However, the exact mechanisms causing these illnesses have not yet been clearly defined. It is believed that the immune, nervous, and endocrine systems communicate through complex pathways and that they may be affected by factors involved in the stress reaction.
- Factors that cause disease are complex. They may involve genetic or environmental factors or a combination of both. Age and sex/gender also influence illness.

References

1. Jacob M, Chappell D, Becker BF. Regulation of blood flow and volume exchange across the microcirculation. *Crit Care.* 2016;20(1):319.
2. Sherwood L. *Human Physiology.* 9th ed. Boston, MA: Cengage Learning; 2016.
3. How the other half dies: the major causes of death and disease in developing countries. International Medical Volunteers Association website. http://www.imva.org/pages/deadtxt.htm. Accessed February 2, 2018.
4. Metheny NM. *Fluid and Electrolyte Balance.* 5th ed. Sudbury, MA: Jones and Bartlett Learning; 2012.
5. Kim SW. Hypernatemia: successful treatment. *Electrolyte Blood Press.* 2006;4(2):66–71.
6. Garth D. Hypokalemia in emergency care. Medscape website. http://emedicine.medscape.com/article/767448-overview. Updated April 5, 2017. Accessed February 2, 2018.
7. McCance KL, Huether SE. *The Biologic Basis for Disease in Adults and Children.* 7th ed. St. Louis, MO: Elsevier; 2014.
8. Infusion Nurses Society. *Journal of Infusion Nursing: Infusion Therapy Standards of Practice.* Norwood, MA: INS; 2016.
9. American Heart Association. *Atherosclerosis.* Dallas, TX: American Heart Association; 2017.
10. Fridovich I. Oxygen toxicity: a radical explanation. *J Exp Biol.* 1998;201(Pt8):1203-1209.
11. VanPutte C, Rean J, Russo AF, Seeley RR. *Seeley's Anatomy and Physiology.* 11th ed. New York, NY: McGraw Hill; 2017.
12. Tilney NL, Bailey GL, Morgan AP. Sequential system failure after rupture of abdominal aortic aneurysms: an unsolved problem in postoperative care. *Ann Surg.* 1973;178(2):117-122.
13. Bone RC, Balk RA, Cerra FB, et al. Definitions for sepsis and organ failure and guidelines for the use of innovative therapies in sepsis. The ACCP/SCCM Consensus Conference Committee. American College of Chest Physicians/Society of Critical Care Medicine. *Chest.* 1992;101(6):1644-1655.
14. Fernandez J. Overview of Immunodeficiency Disorders. MSD Manual website. http://www.msdmanuals.com/professional/immunology-allergic-disorders/immunodeficiency-disorders/overview-of-immunodeficiency-disorders. Updated August 2016. Accessed February 3, 2018.
15. McVicar A, Ravalier JM, Greenwood C. Biology of stress revisited: intracellular mechanisms and the conceptualization of stress. *Stress Health.* 2014;30(4):272-279.
16. Bonis PAL. Glossary of common biostatistical and epidemiological terms. UpToDate website. https://www.uptodate.com/contents/glossary-of-common-biostatistical-and-epidemiological-terms?source=search_result&search=prevalence&selectedTitle=1~150. Updated February 22, 2016. Accessed February 3, 2018.
17. Dicker RC, Coronado F, Koo D, Parrish RG. Frequency measures. In: CDC, ed. *Principles of Epidemiology in Public Health Practice.* 2nd ed. Atlanta, GA: Centers for Disease Control and Prevention; 2011.

Suggested Readings

Hsieh A. A delicate balance: understanding acid-base issues in EMS patients. EMS1.com website. https://www.ems1.com/ems-products/Capnography/articles/276334048-A-delicate-balance-Understanding-acid-base-issues-in-EMS-patients/. Published June 15, 2017. Accessed February 3, 2018.

Lazenby R. *Handbook of Pathophysiology.* 4th ed. Lippincott Williams & Wilkins; 2011.

Long B, Koyfman A. Clinical mimics: an emergency medicine-focused review of sepsis mimics. *J Emerg Med.* 2017;52(1):34-42.

Shane B, Hales M. *Principles of Pathophysiology.* New South Wales, Australia: Pearson; 2012.

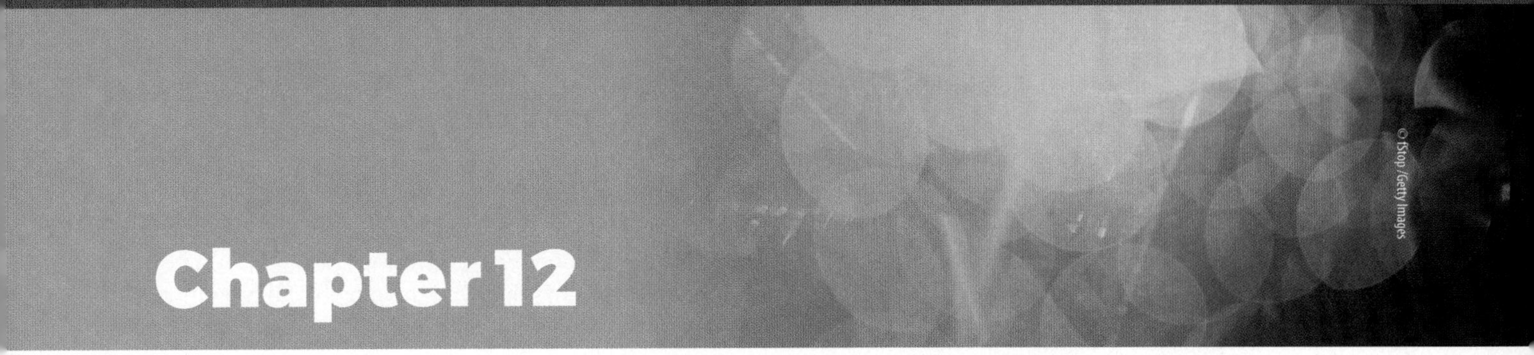

© fStop/Getty Images

Chapter 12

Life Span Development

NATIONAL EMS EDUCATION STANDARD COMPETENCIES

Life Span Development

Integrates comprehensive knowledge of life span development.

OBJECTIVES

Upon completion of this chapter, the paramedic student will be able to:

1. Describe the normal vital signs and body system characteristics of the newborn, neonate, infant, toddler, preschooler, school-aged child, adolescent, young adult, middle-aged adult, older adult, and advanced-old-age adult. (pp 328–336, 338–343)
2. Identify key psychosocial features of the infant, toddler, preschooler, school-aged child, adolescent, young adult, middle-aged adult, older adult, and advanced-old-age adult. (pp 332–337, 339–342)
3. Explain the effect of peer relationships and other factors on a child's psychosocial development. (pp 335–336, 339)
4. Discuss the physical and emotional challenges faced by the older adult. (pp 341–345)

KEY TERMS

adolescent A person 13 to 18 years of age.

advanced old age A new age category that includes people older than 75 years.

attachments Physical and emotional bonds that develop between infants and their family members or caregivers.

Babinski reflex A reflex movement in which the great toe bends upward when the outer edge of the sole is stroked.

cognitive development The construction of thought processes, including remembering, problem solving, and decision making, from childhood through adolescence to adulthood.

early adulthood An age category that includes people 19 to 40 years of age.

frailty A geriatric syndrome characterized by exhaustion, slowed performance, weakness, weight loss, and low physical activity.

infant A child 1 month to 1 year of age.

late adulthood An age category that includes people 61 to 75 years of age.

menarche The first menstruation and the commencement of the cyclic menstrual function.

menopause The cessation of menses.

middle adulthood An age category that includes people 41 to 60 years of age.

Moro (startle) reflex A normal infant response elicited by a sudden loud noise. The infant flexes the legs, makes an embracing gesture with the arms, and usually gives a brief cry.

neonate An infant from birth to 1 month of age.

newborn An infant within the first few hours of life.

palmar grasp A normal infant response in which the infant curls the fingers in response to a touch on the palm of the hand.

passive immunity Immunity acquired by transmission of antibodies from the mother, through placental transfer, to the fetus; a form of acquired immunity in which antibodies against disease are acquired naturally.

periodontal disease Disease that affects tissues that surround or support the teeth.

preschooler A child 3 to 5 years of age.

puberty The period of life when the ability to reproduce begins.

reciprocal socialization A term that refers to a child's temperament and the responses it elicits from adults and family members. This interaction forms the basis for early social interactions with others and with the child's environment.

reproductive maturity The time at which a person has attained the ability to reproduce.

rooting reflex A normal infant response elicited by touching or stroking the side of the cheek or mouth, causing the infant to turn the head toward that side and to begin to suck.

school age An age category that includes children 6 to 12 years of age.

self-concept The accumulation of knowledge about one's self, including beliefs regarding personality traits, physical characteristics, abilities, values, goals, and roles.

self-esteem A person's overall evaluation or appraisal of his or her own worth.

separation anxiety The anxiety that a child experiences when separated from the primary caregiver. It is a normal reaction during infancy.

sucking reflex A normal infant response in which touching the infant's lips with the nipple of a breast or bottle causes involuntary sucking movements.

temperament The characterization of a person's behavior, as defined by how the person interacts with the environment. It is the basis on which children develop relationships.

terminal decline A theory that older adults experience an overall slowdown or gradual decline of cognitive abilities in the absence of dementia.

terminal drop A theory that a decline in intelligence in older adulthood may be caused by the person's conscious or unconscious perception of coming death.

toddler A child 1 to 2 years of age.

Paramedics provide care to patients from all age groups. Often a patient's complaints are directly related to the growth and developmental characteristics common for that person's age group. Therefore, it is important that paramedics study and understand the physiologic and psychosocial development of human beings at different stages in life.

NOTE

The *National EMS Education Standards* provide general descriptions of development across the life span. Age ranges for groups may differ slightly from other references in this and other textbooks. The age groups presented in this chapter are infants (birth to 1 year of age), toddlers (1 to 2 years of age), preschoolers (3 to 5 years of age), school-age children (6 to 12 years of age), adolescents (13 to 18 years of age), early adulthood (19 to 40 years of age), middle adulthood (41 to 60 years of age), late adulthood (61 to 75 years of age), and advanced old age (older than 75 years).

Pediatric data adapted from: American Heart Association. *Pediatric Advanced Life Support*. Dallas, TX: American Heart Association; 2015.

Newborn

The term **newborn** is used for infants in the first few hours of life (**FIGURE 12-1**). A child younger than 1 month is known as a **neonate**. The term **infant** is used for a child 1 month to 1 year of age.

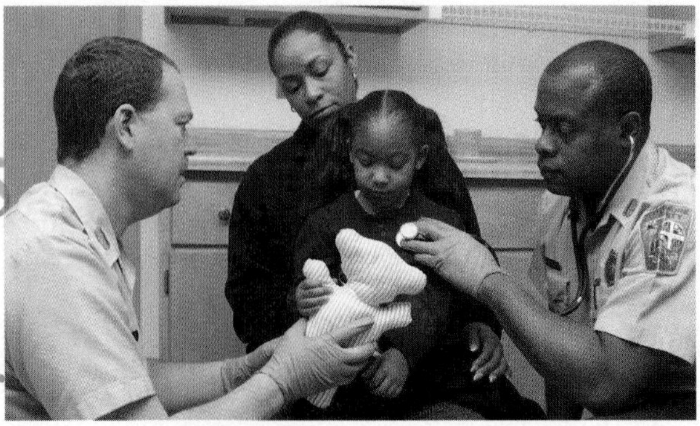

Vital Signs

During the first 30 minutes of life, the newborn's heart rate is 100 to 200 beats/min. By 1 year of age, the heart rate averages 120 beats/min. At birth, the

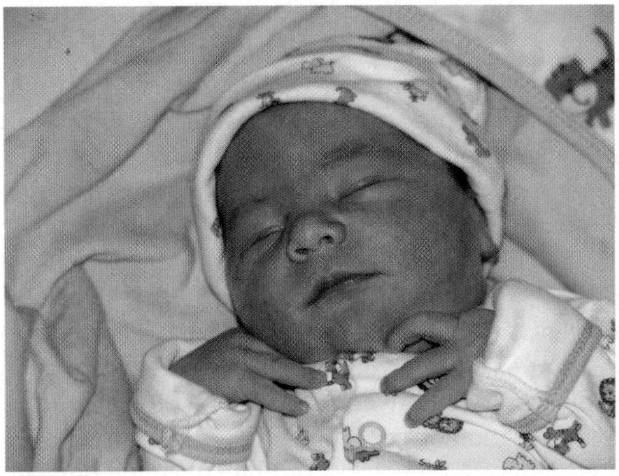

FIGURE 12-1 Newborn.

Courtesy of Mick Sanders.

CRITICAL THINKING

Why are newborn, neonate, and infant considered distinct stages?

respiratory rate usually is 40 to 60 breaths/min. This rate drops to 30 to 40 breaths/min within a few minutes after delivery. By 1 year of age, a rate of 25 breaths/min is considered normal. The average systolic blood pressure increases from 70 mm Hg at birth to 90 mm Hg at 1 year. Body temperature during infancy ranges from 98°F to 100°F (36.7°C to 37.8°C).

Weight

A full-term newborn normally weighs 7 to 8 pounds (3 to 3.5 kg). The newborn's head accounts for about 25% of the total body weight; its circumference is equal to that of the newborn's chest. For the first few days of life, the total body weight may decrease 5% to 10% as a result of excretion of extracellular fluid (fluid outside the cells). By the second week of life, the birth weight has been regained, and the neonate's weight exceeds the newborn weight. Although some infants gain weight faster than others, most gain an average of 5 to 6 ounces (140 to 168 g) per week. The increase in an infant's body weight should follow a

NOTE

One kilogram (kg) is equal to 2.2 pounds (lb). One gram (g) is equal to 0.035274 ounce (oz). These and other equivalents are described in Chapter 14, *Medication Administration*.

CRITICAL THINKING

What considerations for patient care are necessary based on the size of the infant's head?

steady upward curve at about 1 ounce (30 g) per day during the first month of life. At this rate, the birth weight will be doubled within 4 to 6 months and tripled within 9 to 12 months. Monitoring the infant's weight every few weeks is a good way to keep track of development.

Cardiovascular System

A newborn's body must make some physiologic changes to survive outside the womb. For example, the cardiovascular system must begin to work apart from the maternal circulation. Shortly after birth, the ductus venosus, ductus arteriosus, and foramen ovale constrict; these structures are unique to the fetal circulation. They close permanently within the first year of life. This results in an increase in systemic vascular resistance and increases in aortic, left ventricular, and left atrial pressures. In addition, pulmonary vascular resistance decreases. This change occurs because the lungs expand as the newborn begins to breathe, which reduces the pulmonary arterial, right ventricular, and right atrial pressures (see Chapter 45, *Obstetrics*, and Chapter 46, *Neonatal Care*). The left ventricle of the newborn's heart becomes stronger during the first year of life.

Respiratory System

Fetal lungs are filled with fluid. During delivery, the thorax is compressed and the lung fluid is drained as the newborn gasps for air. Once the newborn gasps, the remaining lung fluid is absorbed through the lymphatic and pulmonary circulations. These strong first breaths open the alveoli and allow subsequent respirations to occur more easily. The principal support for the chest wall comes from the accessory muscles rather than the bones; however, these muscles are

NOTE

Infants and small children are "belly breathers." They require full diaphragmatic excursion to produce normal respirations. Children continue to use the abdominal muscles to breathe until approximately 7 years of age, when they typically become "chest breathers."

immature and tire easily. The normal practice of using the accessory muscles for breathing increases the infant's susceptibility to the accumulation of lactic acid in the blood (lactic acidosis). In addition, collateral ventilation between the alveoli and bronchioles is decreased because newborns have fewer alveoli.

A baby's short, narrow airway is less stable than that of an adult. Breathing occurs primarily through the nose during the first month of life. When infection or stress occurs, the baby breathes more rapidly and may quickly lose body heat and fluids.

Nervous System

A healthy newborn can respond to a wide variety of stimuli and has a range of reflexes (**TABLE 12-1**). Many of these reflexes, such as the reflexes associated with breathing and eating, are essential for life outside the womb. Other important reflexes are those that result from stress or discomfort. For example, obstruction of the airway may trigger a sneeze or cough. Facial stimulation causes the baby to make sucking movements with the lips (**sucking reflex**) and to turn the head and move the lips toward the touch (**rooting reflex**). Crying may indicate hunger, pain, or discomfort from heat or cold. Some reflexes appear to have no useful purpose and gradually disappear during the first few months of life. These include the **Babinski reflex**, the **Moro (startle) reflex**, and the **palmar grasp**.

> NOTE
>
> The Babinski reflex is a normal response in infants and young children. However, in an older child or adult, it may indicate damage to the brain or spinal cord (see Chapter 40, *Spine and Nervous System Trauma*).

Sleep is thought to be important to normal functioning of the brain. Newborns sleep an average of 16 to 18 hours a day. Sleep and wakefulness are evenly distributed over 24 hours. This sleep pattern gradually decreases to 14 to 16 hours a day with a 9- to 10-hour concentration of sleep at night. By 4 months of age, an infant generally sleeps through the night but can be easily roused.

During the first year of life, an infant makes major advances in physical and mental skills. The brain and nervous system gradually mature during this period. To make room for brain growth, the posterior fontanel (unclosed joint between the bones of the skull) remains open until about 3 months of age. The anterior fontanel remains open for 9 to 18 months after birth. The anterior fontanel usually is level with or slightly below the surface of the skull. It is a good indicator of adequate hydration. With dehydration, the anterior fontanel may fall below the level of the skull and appear sunken (**FIGURE 12-2**). By the end of the first year, the development of mature nerves is virtually complete. The muscles have matured to

TABLE 12-1 Reflexes Associated With Infancy

Reflex	Test	Normal Finding
Babinski	The examiner gently strokes the sole of the infant's foot.	The toes spread outward and upward.
Moro	A loud or startling noise is made near the infant.	The infant stretches the arms and legs, spreads the fingers, and then hugs self.
Palmar grasp	The examiner puts an object or a finger in the infant's palm.	The fingers curl around the object or finger.
Rooting	The examiner gently touches the infant's cheek or an area near the lips.	The infant's head turns toward the stimulation, and the mouth puckers.
Stepping	The examiner holds the infant upright with the feet touching a solid surface.	The infant makes stepping movements that resemble walking.
Sucking	The infant's mouth comes in contact with the nipple of a breast or bottle.	The infant's lips begin to pucker and suck.
Tonic neck	The infant is placed in the supine position.	The infant turns the head and then extends the arm and leg on the side of the body toward which the head is turned.

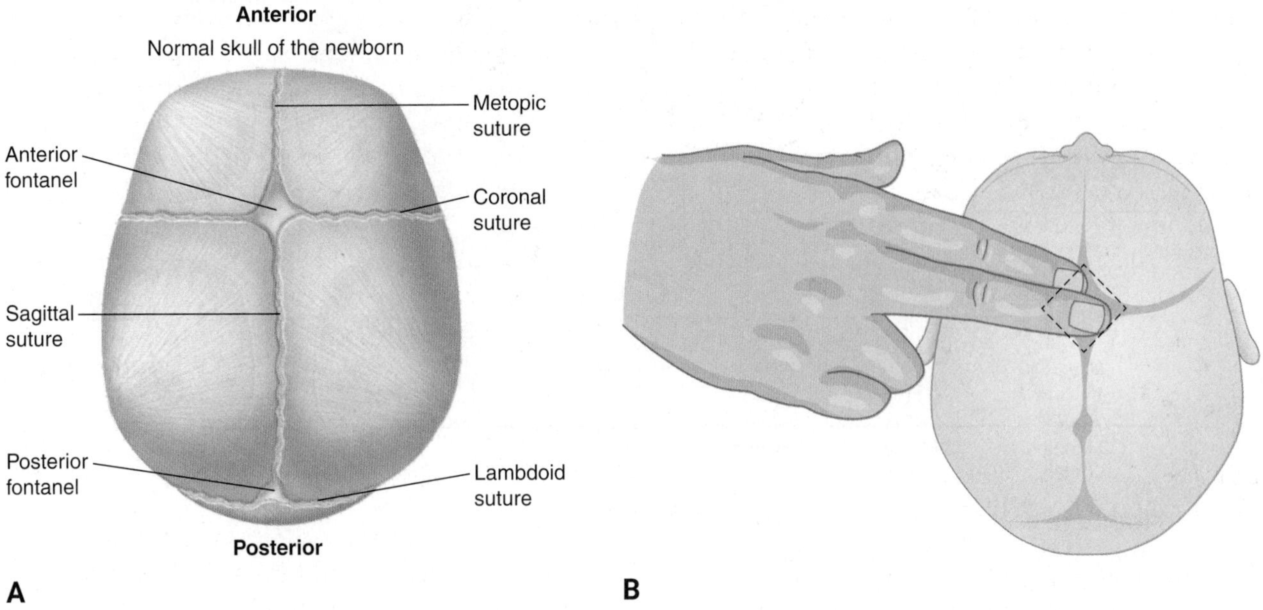

FIGURE 12-2 **A.** Location of the sutures and fontanels. **B.** Palpation of the anterior fontanel.

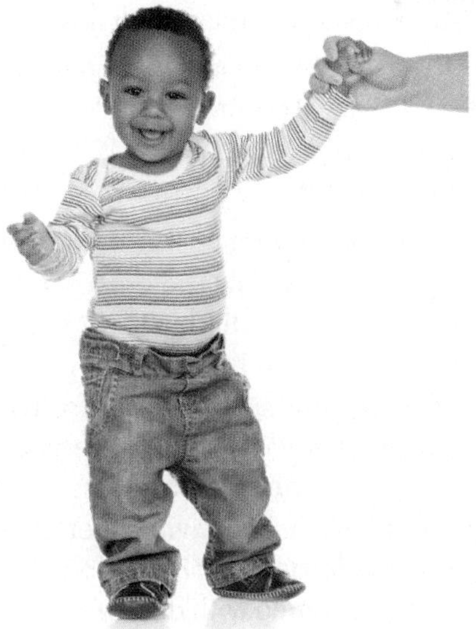

FIGURE 12-3 Infant.

the point that many infants can stand and walk with little or no assistance (**FIGURE 12-3**).

Musculoskeletal System

At birth, the only hard bones are in the fingers. As long bones mature, hormones acting on the cartilage in the epiphyses of growing bones result in the deposition of calcium salts and the replacement of soft cartilage with hard bone. The epiphyseal plate lengthens, and bones thicken as new layers of bone are deposited on existing bone. Factors that influence bone growth include genetics, the production of growth hormone and thyroid hormone, nutrition, and the child's general health status. In infants, muscle weight accounts for about 25% of the entire musculoskeletal system. Motor control in the infant moves from head to toe and from the core to the periphery of the body. Therefore, infants should be able to lift the head before they are able to sit; also, they can crawl before they can walk.[1] The arms and legs are proportionately smaller in the infant. These proportions change throughout the life span (**FIGURE 12-4**).

Immune System

Infants are born with enough **passive immunity** from disease to protect them until they can make their own antibodies. Passive immunity arises from the mother's antibodies, which are passed through the blood to the fetus. If the infant is breastfed, the antibodies also are passed through the mother's milk. Passive immunity lasts only about 6 months after birth. After that interval, childhood immunizations against disease (eg, pertussis, diphtheria, tetanus) usually are recommended (see Chapter 47, *Pediatrics*).

Metabolism

An infant's metabolic rate is much higher than that of older children or adults. Infants consume more

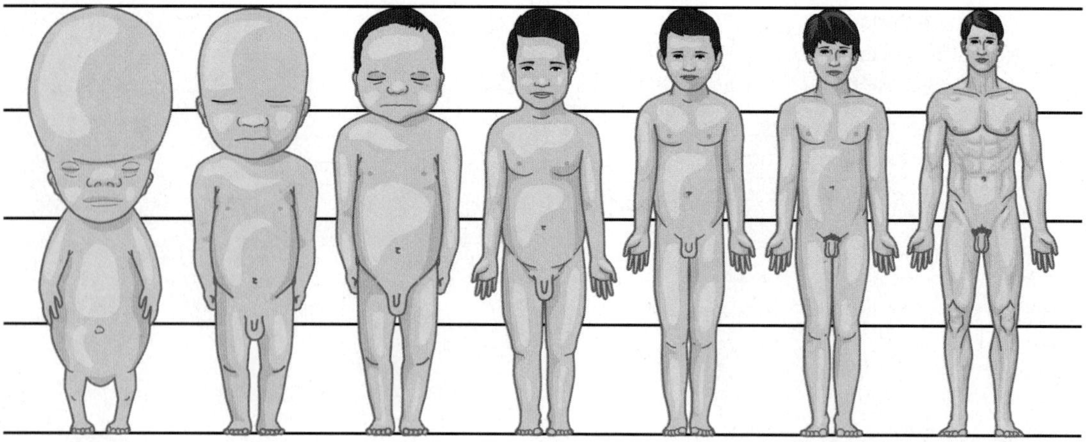

FIGURE 12-4 Changes in body proportions with growth.
Modified from: McKinney ES et al: *Maternal child nursing*, ed 3, St Louis, 2009, Saunders.

fluids, calories, minerals, and vitamins per pound. They also lose more fluid from the respiratory and integumentary systems than do older children. Because of these increased fluid losses, infants are predisposed to dehydration, thus increasing their risk for the development of heat- and cold-related illnesses.

Other Developmental Milestones

Development during infancy depends on the interaction of heredity and the environment. Growth and development should be compared with standard growth charts showing norms. BOX 12-1 lists some developmental milestones from birth to 12 months of age.

Psychosocial Development

An infant's relationship with the caregiver (usually the mother) is a major factor in psychosocial development. This person is the baby's main source of comfort. The caregiver also represents the baby's main means of coping with stresses in the environment, such as fear, pain, and anxiety. Erik Erikson, a proponent of the psychosocial theory, saw human development as the interaction between a person's genes and the environment.[2] He theorized that life moves through a series of overlapping stages. Each stage is marked by a crisis that must be resolved. According to Erikson, the most critical stage, which occurs in infancy (up to 18 months of age), is the trust versus mistrust stage.[2] This stage is based on the infant's knowledge of two things: (1) that the surroundings are safe and predictable and (2) that causes and effects can be anticipated. For example, parental care is warm and loving, but punishment may result from not following rules. Consistency, or lack of it, in this type of care is the basis for trust versus mistrust issues.

Temperament

Temperament is a characterization of a person's behavior, as defined by how the person interacts with the environment. It is the basis on which children form relationships. A child's temperament and the responses this temperament elicits from adults form the foundation for early social interactions. (Early social interactions are the child's interactions with others and with his or her environment.) This process is known as **reciprocal socialization**. A baby's first interactions, combined with developmental changes, lead to specific relationships, as follows:

- During the first few weeks of life, infants are not much affected by an adult's appearance. The only exception is when the infant is fed.
- From about the start of the fourth week, infants begin to direct actions at the adults. Emotional reactions also appear at this time. The baby shows obvious signs of pleasure at the sight and sound of adults, especially the primary caregiver.
- During the second month, more complex and sensitive reactions emerge. These include smiling and vocal sounds aimed at the mother. Animated behavior is shown during interactions.

BOX 12-1 Developmental Milestones (Birth Through 12 Months)

Growth and development should be compared with standard growth charts showing established norms. It is important to remember that infants move through these stages at different rates.

1 Month
- Brings hands within range of eyes and mouth
- Keeps hands in tight fists
- Recognizes some sounds

2 Months
- Tracks objects with eyes
- Recognizes familiar faces

3 Months
- Moves objects to mouth with hands

4 Months
- Salivation increases with impaired swallowing
- Reaches out to people

5 Months
- Sleeps through the night without food
- Gains weight to twice birth weight
- Eruption of teeth may begin

6 Months
- Sits upright in high chair
- Makes one-syllable sounds (*ma, mu, da, di*)

7 Months
- Fears strangers
- Quickly changes from crying to laughing

8 Months
- Responds to "No"
- Sits without assistance

9 Months
- Responds to adult anger
- Pulls self to standing position
- Explores objects by sucking, chewing, and biting

10 Months
- Recognizes own name
- Crawls well

11 Months
- Attempts to walk unaided
- Shows frustration at restrictions

12 Months
- Walks with assistance
- Gains weight to three times birth weight

- By 3 months of age, the infant has formed a need for social interactions. That need continues to grow and is nourished by adults until the end of the second or the beginning of the third year. At that time, a need for peer interaction develops.

As the infant grows, his or her interactions become more complex. Bonding develops between the infant and family members. These bonds are considered **attachments**. For example, at 4 months of age, an infant shows perceptual discrimination by visually tracking the caregiver. At 9 months of age, an infant cries when the mother leaves, which is a demonstration of **separation anxiety**.

Separation from true attachments (eg, separation from a parent) may result in a series of behaviors. The first is protest (loud crying, extreme restlessness, and rejection of all adults). Second is despair (nonstop crying, inactivity, and withdrawal). Third is detachment (a renewed but distant interest in surroundings, even if the caregiver comes back). Some psychologists believe that attachments continue through a person's life span.

When possible, the parent should be allowed to hold the child during the assessment. This accomplishes two goals: first, the child and parent will be less anxious; second, the assessment will be easier to perform if the child is calm and not crying.

Toddler and Preschool Years

A child 1 to 2 years of age generally is considered a **toddler**. A child 3 to 5 years of age is considered a **preschooler** (**FIGURE 12-5**).

Vital Signs

A toddler's heart rate usually is 98 to 140 beats/min. In preschoolers the heart rate is 80 to 120 beats/min. Respirations for toddlers and preschoolers average 20 to 37 breaths/min. A normal systolic blood pressure for toddlers is 86 to 106 mm Hg, and for preschoolers it is

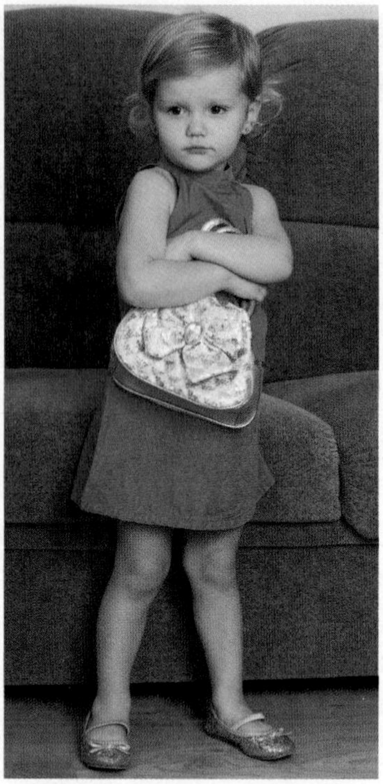

FIGURE 12-5 Preschooler.

89 to 112 mm Hg. The normal body temperature for both age groups is 96.8°F to 99.6°F (36°C to 37.6°C).

Review of Body Systems

As children enter the toddler and preschool age groups, changes occur in some body systems:

- **Cardiovascular system.** As the capillary beds become better developed, they are better able to assist in the body's thermoregulation. Hemoglobin levels approach those of adults.
- **Respiratory system.** The ear, nose, and throat structures in toddlers and preschoolers are similar to those in infants. Although infants are at greatest risk for serious respiratory illness, toddlers and preschoolers may acquire such infections in nursery school or preschool. Repeated upper respiratory tract infections may occur, but they are rarely an indication of underlying disease in toddlers and preschoolers. The use of respiratory muscles changes from primarily abdominal to chest muscles as the child nears school age.
- **Nervous system.** Myelination (the maturation of nerve cells) begins in the third trimester of pregnancy and continues for about 10 to 12 years. This process eventually provides for a smooth flow of neural impulses throughout the brain, increasing cognitive development. Even so, by 2 years of age much of the nervous system is completely developed. The brain weight is about 90% that of the adult brain. Visual acuity averages 20/30. Hearing essentially is mature by 3 to 4 years of age.
- **Musculoskeletal system.** Muscle mass and bone density increase. Most children walk well with a normal gait by 2 years of age. Fine motor skills (eg, scribbling with a pencil, stacking building blocks) become evident in toddlers and preschoolers.
- **Immune system.** Passive immunity no longer protects toddlers and preschoolers. They become more susceptible to minor respiratory and gastrointestinal infections.
- **Endocrine system.** The endocrine organs mature and increase production of growth hormone, insulin, and corticosteroid. Children in the toddler and preschool age groups gain an average of 6 pounds (2.9 kg) per year.
- **Renal system.** The kidneys are well developed by 2 years of age. At this time, many children begin to gain control of bladder and bowel functions. Specific gravity is a measure of the concentrating ability of the kidneys. This value and other measurements of urinary function are similar to those in adults (see Chapter 29, *Genitourinary and Renal Disorders*).

Psychosocial Development

By 2 years of age, children have developed unique personality traits and moods, as well as specific likes and dislikes. Basic language skills are mastered by 3 years of age. Refinement of these skills continues through childhood. Toddlers and preschoolers also begin to recognize the difference between men and women. They begin to model themselves after people of their own sex. BOX 12-2 lists other social milestones in the development of toddlers and preschoolers.

> **NOTE**
>
> Toddlers are active and have a brief attention span. At this age, they are at risk for falls, choking, pedestrian–motor vehicle crashes, and burn injuries. Just as with infants, many toddlers do not verbalize feelings of pain or fear directly. Toddlers often have a comfort item, such as a blanket or special toy. When possible, allow the child to hold this item during assessment and transport.

BOX 12-2 Social Milestones in Children 1 to 5 Years of Age

1 to 3 Years

- Can combine two different words
- Can complete some word phrases
- Follows directions
- Can point to a named part of the body
- Shows symbolic play when playing with toys
- Can remove some clothing

3 to 5 Years

- Can give first and last name
- Recognizes colors
- Speech is understandable to strangers
- Completes short sentences and questions
- Can state name of a friend
- Begins to accept temporary absence of primary caregiver
- Plays independently in the presence of other children
- Shows increased level of confidence
- Shows sympathy at appropriate times (eg, when another child is injured)
- Likes to hear and tell stories

CRITICAL THINKING

Reassuring and nonthreatening language should be used when treating toddlers and preschoolers. Consider how a 3-year-old child might interpret statements such as, "I'm going to give you a shot" or "You'll feel a stick in your arm."

Peer Relationships

Peer relationships offer a source of information about the child's world outside the family and expose the child to other types of families. In the toddler and preschool age groups, peer bonds are formed with others near the same age and maturity. These relationships often begin during play. Play may involve exploring a new toy, acting out fantasies, or using the imagination for new situations. Play also allows children to develop the ability to play simple games and competitive games with rules. These experiences can lead to problem-solving skills and cognitive development. Play that involves others fosters interpersonal relationships. Toward the end of the preschool period, children begin to form lasting friendships. The importance of peer bonds and peer-group functions increases throughout childhood.

Other Factors That Can Affect Psychosocial Development

Other key factors can have a significant effect on psychosocial development in the toddler and preschool age groups. Two of these factors are divorce and exposure to aggression or violence.

About half of marriages in the United States end in divorce.[3] Several factors determine the effect divorce has on toddlers and preschoolers. These factors include the child's age, cognition, social competencies, and sense of dependence on or independence from the parents. Common reactions to divorce in young children include depression, withdrawal, fear of abandonment, and fear that their parents no longer love them. The parents' ability to recognize and respond to the child's needs is important for helping the child deal with the effects of divorce.

Exposure to violence may increase a child's acceptance of this type of behavior. For example, some children may regularly watch television shows or video games with aggressive overtones. These children may model their behavior on these activities. It is particularly important that parents screen shows and play activities for children in the toddler and preschool age groups.

NOTE

Exposure to alcohol or other drugs can be a negative factor in a child's behavior. Drug or alcohol abuse in the home environment increases the risk for child abuse. Child abuse is not limited to abuse by parents, but parents account for 80% of offenders. Abuse can be inflicted by babysitters, relatives, domestic partners, or casual acquaintances. Abuse occurs at every socioeconomic level and often is precipitated by a stressful situation in the family (eg, unemployment, marital problems, chronic illness, poverty).

Modified from: Children's Bureau, Administration for Children and Families, US Department of Health and Human Services. Child maltreatment: 2015. Administration for Children and Families website. http://www.acf.hhs.gov/programs/cb/research-data-technology/statistics-research/child-maltreatment. Updated October 12, 2017. Accessed January 6, 2018.

School-Age Years

Children are considered **school age** from 6 to 12 years of age (**FIGURE 12-6**). The heart rate in this age group is 70 to 120 beats/min, the respiratory rate is 15 to 20 breaths/min, the systolic blood pressure is 80 to 110 mm Hg, and the body temperature averages 98.6°F (37°C).

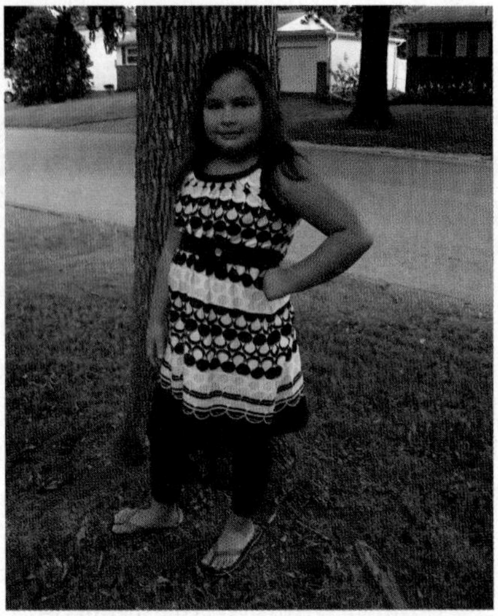

FIGURE 12-6 School-age child.

Courtesy of Mick Sanders.

> **NOTE**
> School-age children are more independent. Children of this age often begin to play sports. Injuries in school-age children may be related to bicycle or other wheeled activities and to other sports. Failure to wear proper protective equipment often accounts for some of these injuries.

Review of Body Systems

The growth of children in the school-age years is slower and steadier than it is during infancy and the toddler and preschool years. School-age children gain an average 6.6 cm (2.5 inches) in height per year. (Note: 2.54 centimeters [cm] is equal to 1 inch.) Most body functions reach adult levels in this age group. BOX 12-3 presents several important developmental milestones for school-age children.

- **Nervous system.** About 95% of the skull's growth is complete by 10 years of age. In addition, children's skills and abilities become more varied as their nervous and musculoskeletal systems develop. Brain function increases in both hemispheres. The child's ability to concentrate and learn develops rapidly in this age group.
- **Reproductive system.** The reproductive system becomes active when a child reaches puberty. Puberty is brought about by increasing levels of sex hormones in the body. For both sexes, these hormone levels begin increasing before any external signs appear. The timing of puberty varies greatly. On average, it starts 2 years earlier in girls (between ages 8 and 13 years) than in boys (between ages 13 and 15 years).

BOX 12-3 Developmental Milestones in School-Age Children (6 to 12 Years)

Physical Development

- Weight gain begins to consist more of muscle than fat; physical strength increases.
- Psychomotor skills (eg, throwing, jumping, running) improve.
- Girls experience a "growth spurt" between ages 8 and 13 years; boys' growth spurt comes between ages 13 and 15 years.
- Body changes indicate approaching puberty.
- Proportions of face and body become closer to those of adults.
- Eyes reach maturity in size and function.
- Permanent teeth begin to develop.
- Right- or left-handedness becomes well established.

Cognitive, Social, and Emotional Development

- Child is permitted more self-regulation with less supervision in the family setting.
- Parents usually spend less time with the child.
- Child's moral reasoning capabilities develop.
- Child gradually gains an understanding of the concept of death.
- Sexual interest grows rapidly with the onset of puberty.
- Friendships become based on loyalty and mutual support.
- Social skills of giving, receiving, and sharing are learned.

- **Lymphatic system.** The lymphatic system plays a key role in fighting disease and infection. This system undergoes many changes throughout a child's growth until puberty, when growth slows. Until that time, the lymphatic tissues in school-age children are proportionally larger than those in adults.

Psychosocial Development

Between the ages of 6 and 12 years, the child's world expands outward from the family. At this time, relationships are formed with friends, teachers, coaches, caregivers, and others. As interactions with others increase, the school-age child begins to compare himself or herself with others, thus developing a self-concept. Some situations can create stress and affect self-esteem. Self-esteem is often based on external factors (eg, popularity with peers, experience of rejection, emotional support from family and friends) and appears to be higher in the early years of school age. Low self-esteem can have damaging effects in later development.

Psychosocial development varies with each person. Some children seem mature, whereas others seem immature. During this stage, behavior may depend on the child's mood and experience with various types of people. It may even be determined simply by what happened on a certain day. In addition, school-age children begin to face the normal challenges of daily life. Fear of new situations (eg, attending school) and peer pressure are predictable stressors for this age group.

Moral development occurs over time through experience. For school-age children, control of behavior begins to shift from external sources (eg, what parents believe is right or wrong) to more internal self-control. With this internal control, these children justify the morality of their choices.

Many theories attempt to explain moral development. Kohlberg's theory proposes six stages, extending from about 4 years of age through adulthood. The stages occur at three age-related levels of development: preconventional reasoning, conventional reasoning, and postconventional reasoning (BOX 12-4).[4] Most experts agree that loving, caring, and positive bonds play key roles in moral education.

SHOW ME THE EVIDENCE

Researchers in New York performed a retrospective chart review to determine the accuracy of weight estimates by prehospital personnel on children from birth to age 17 years. They compared estimated weights from prehospital patient care reports to measured weight at the hospital. After exclusions, 199 records were analyzed. The mean age of patients included was 9.8 years (± 5.9). EMS personnel accurately estimated weights in 164 of 199 patients (82.4%); estimated weights were within 10.8% (standard deviation ± 10.5) of the actual weights. Of the 35 inaccurate weight recordings (17.6%), 16 were underestimated. The study was underpowered to make conclusive statements; however, it appears that weight estimation was less accurate in patients aged 9 years or younger and in those presenting with seizure or cardiac arrest.

Modified from: Lim CA, Kaufman BJ, O'Connor J, Cunningham SJ. Accuracy of weight estimates in pediatric patients by prehospital emergency medical services personnel. *Am J Emerg Med.* 2013;31(7):1108-1112.

BOX 12-4 Kohlberg's Stages of Moral Development

Preconventional Reasoning (About 4 to 10 Years)

From 4 to 10 years of age, children respond to cultural control mainly to avoid punishment and attain satisfaction. The first two stages of moral development occur at this level:

- **Stage 1—Punishment and obedience.** Children obey rules and orders to avoid punishment; the child has no concern about moral rectitude.
- **Stage 2—Naïve instrumental behaviorism.** Children obey rules but only out of pure self-interest. They are vaguely aware of fairness to others but only for their own satisfaction. The concept of reciprocity comes into play (ie, "You scratch my back, I'll scratch yours.").

Conventional Reasoning (About 10 to 13 Years)

From 10 to 13 years of age, children desire approval both from individual people and from society. They not only conform, they actively seek to support society's standards. The next two stages occur at this level:

- **Stage 3—Good boy/good girl mentality.** Children seek the approval of others. They begin to judge behavior by intention (eg, "She meant to do well.").
- **Stage 4—Law and order mentality.** Children are concerned with authority and with maintaining the social order. Correct behavior is "doing one's duty."

Postconventional Reasoning (13 Years and Older)

If true morality (an internal moral code) is to develop, it appears during these years. The person does not appeal to other people for moral decisions. Such decisions are made by an "enlightened conscience." The final two stages of moral development occur at this level:

- **Stage 5—The person makes moral decisions legalistically or contractually.** This means that the best values are those supported by law, because they have been accepted by society as a whole. If a conflict arises between human need and the law, people work to change the law.
- **Stage 6—An informed conscience defines what is right.** A person's actions are not based on fear, a need for approval, or legal demands, but on the person's own internalized standards of right and wrong.

Modified from: Kohlberg L. A cognitive-developmental analysis of children's sex-role concepts and attitudes. In: MacCoby E, ed. *The Development of Sex Differences.* Stanford, CA: Stanford University Press; 1966.

Adolescence

A person 13 to 18 years of age is an **adolescent** (**FIGURE 12-7**). Normal vital signs for this age group are a heart rate of 60 to 100 beats/min, respirations of 12 to 20 breaths/min, a systolic blood pressure of 110 to 131 mm Hg, and a body temperature of 98.6°F (37°C). Adolescence is the final phase of change in growth and development. Organs, including the heart, kidneys, spleen, and liver, rapidly increase in size. Blood chemistry values are nearly the same as those in adults (see Chapter 31, *Hematology*). Activity of the sebaceous glands causes the skin to toughen. Growth of bone and muscle mass is nearly completed during the 2- to 3-year adolescent growth spurt.

During adolescence, a person reaches **reproductive maturity**. In girls, the first external sign of puberty is a change in one or both nipples. The nipples change into what is known as a breast bud. A few months later, pubic hair and underarm hair begin to grow, and the breasts enlarge. Within about 2 years after the appearance of the breast bud and after body fat reaches 18% to 20% of body weight, **menarche** (first menstruation) usually occurs. Changes in the endocrine system cause the release of gonadotropin, luteinizing hormone, and follicle-stimulating hormone. These hormonal substances promote estrogen and progesterone production. Progesterone affects breast development and the menstrual cycle. Estrogen causes the development of the female secondary sex characteristics, such as disposition of subcutaneous fat in the breast, thighs, and buttocks and the development of axial and pubic hair. Estrogen also promotes the buildup of endometrium in the uterus.

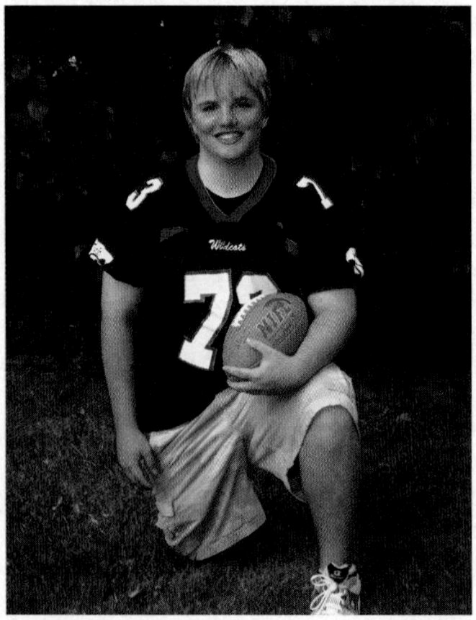

FIGURE 12-7 Adolescent.

Courtesy of Mick Sanders.

NOTE

In 2015, almost 230,000 babies were born to women aged 15 to 19 years. This represented an 8% decline from the prior year. Teen pregnancies carry extra health risks for the mother and the baby. Teenagers often do not receive timely prenatal care, and they have a higher risk for pregnancy-related high blood pressure and its complications. These babies have a higher incidence of premature birth and low birth weight.

Modified from: Division of Reproductive Health, National Center for Chronic Disease Prevention and Health Promotion. Reproductive health: teen pregnancy. Centers for Disease Control and Prevention website. https://www.cdc.gov/teenpregnancy/about/index.htm. Updated May 9, 2017. Accessed January 7, 2018; National Institutes of Health, US Department of Health and Human Services. Teenage pregnancy. MedlinePlus website. https://medlineplus.gov/teenagepregnancy.html. Updated December 6, 2017. Accessed January 7, 2018.

In boys, gonadotropin promotes testosterone production. Testosterone is a hormone produced by the testes. It causes the development of the male secondary sex characteristics. These include color and texture changes in the scrotum and an increase in the size of the testes. With these changes, the penis begins to enlarge and assume an adult shape, and pubic hair grows. At about 14 years of age, a boy's first ejaculation of semen occurs during masturbation or sleep. Other male secondary sex characteristics that occur during late adolescence and early adulthood include deepening of the voice and growth of facial hair, underarm hair, and sometimes chest hair.

The development of secondary sex characteristics in both sexes coincides with the last period of rapid growth in adolescence. Rapid growth usually is preceded by an increase in body fat. This body fat decreases during the period of growth and increases again in later years. Girls retain more fat than boys do in the subcutaneous tissue in the areas of the breasts, thighs, and buttocks. Boys gain an average of 8 inches (20 cm) in height before age 21 years, when growth usually stops. Growth in girls is less dramatic and is usually complete by age 18 years. During the period of rapid growth in adolescence, the hands and feet grow first. The arms and legs then begin to lengthen, and the shoulders become broader. Finally, the trunk of the body grows. The bones of the upper and lower jaw also grow. As a result, the face can change dramatically in appearance within a short time, especially in boys.

Psychosocial Development

In addition to physical changes, adolescence usually involves some emotional turmoil (BOX 12-5). Adolescents may "try on" identities. These young people also begin to develop their adult personality. Conflicts with parents over school, manners, dress, hygiene, curfews, and other topics are common because the adolescent has begun to express independence. Because of these conflicts, most adolescents draw away from their parents. At the same time, they may emotionally move more toward their peers. Friendships with others who are also trying on various identities may result in the use of alcohol and other drugs, sexual experimentation, and extreme forms of behavior or dress. Antisocial behavior tends to peak at about the eighth- or ninth-grade level.

In the teenage years, both boys and girls are very concerned about their appearance. Comparisons continually are made among peers. Concerns about body image are common in this age group, including weight issues, body odor, acne, and dandruff. All these

CRITICAL THINKING

It may be best to interview the adolescent and the parents separately. Why might this approach be important?

NOTE

Learning to drive an automobile occurs during adolescence. Motor vehicle crashes represent the top cause of death in children of this age. Suicide and homicide are other leading causes of death in adolescents in the United States. According to the Centers for Disease Control and Prevention, most of these homicides and about 40% of the suicides involve a firearm. Adolescent deaths from drug overdoses, particularly involving opioids, more than doubled from 1999 (1.6 per 100,000) to 2015 (3.7 per 100,000).

Modified from: Heron M. Deaths: leading causes for 2014. *Natl Vital Stat Rep.* 2016;65(5):1-96; Hedegaard H, Warner M, Miniño AM. Drug overdose deaths in the United States, 1999–2015. NCHS data brief, no 273. Hyattsville, MD: National Center for Health Statistics; 2017.

BOX 12-5 Psychosocial Development of Adolescents (13 to 18 Years)

Some variations from the following descriptions are to be expected. Also, some characteristics and traits may be affected by other developmental issues.

13 to 14 Years

- Struggles with identity issues
- Displays moodiness
- Develops close friendships
- Pays less attention to parents
- Interests and clothing styles are influenced by peer groups
- Shows ability to work
- Has same-sex friends
- Develops need for privacy
- Experiments with body (masturbation)
- May experiment with cigarettes, alcohol, and marijuana
- Has capacity for abstract thought

14 to 17 Years

- Becomes self-involved
- Shows extreme concern with body image and sexual attractiveness
- Examines personal and inner experiences
- Channels sexual and aggressive energies into creative activities (eg, poetry, writing, music)
- Develops feelings of sexual love and passion
- Selects role models
- Shows greater capacity for setting goals

17 to 18 Years

- Develops secure personal identity
- Shows greater emotional stability
- Has heightened sense of humor
- Shows pride in work
- Shows stable interests and concern for others
- Has higher level of concern for the future
- Develops clear sexual identity and ability for sensual love
- Shows gradual interest in adult behavior
- Accepts social norms and cultural traditions
- Can set goals and follow through with plans

conditions can arise from the hormonal changes associated with adolescence. During adolescence, many teenagers, especially girls, become obsessed with weight loss. They may try fad diets to control their figures. Eating disorders are common in this age group. Obsession with weight loss may lead to bulimia, anorexia nervosa, and severe depression. Depression and suicide are common among adolescents.

Early Adulthood

Early adulthood spans the period from 19 to 40 years of age (**FIGURE 12-8**). Average vital signs for this age group are a heart rate of 60 to 100 beats/min, respirations of 12 to 20 breaths/min, a systolic blood pressure of 90 to 140 mm Hg, and a body temperature of 98.6°F (37°C). At the onset of early adulthood, between 18 and 26 years of age, men and women are reaching their physical peak. Lifelong habits and routines develop. Body systems are at their optimum performance. This also is the age group in which pregnancy is most likely to occur. However, the aging process has begun. Some of the effects of aging (eg, slowed reaction times, hearing loss, vision deficiencies) gradually become evident during this stage of life.

Good health in early adulthood tends to be centered on lifestyle and physical fitness. Unintentional injury is the leading cause of death in this age group.[5] Poisoning (with opioids causing more than one-half of the poisonings) is now the leading cause of death in this group, followed by suicide, motor vehicle crashes, and homicide.

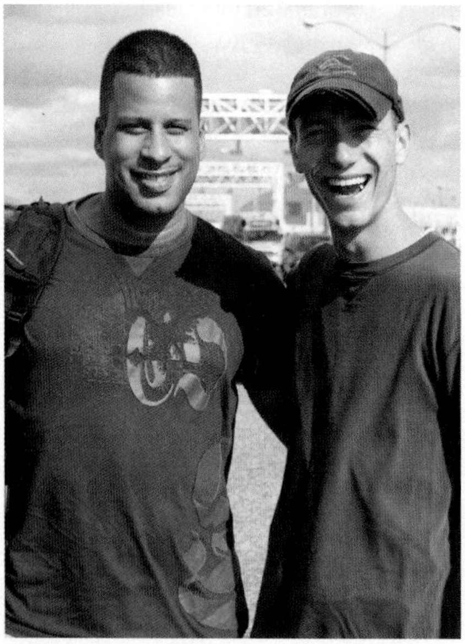

FIGURE 12-8 Early adulthood.

Courtesy of Mick Sanders.

Psychosocial Development

The ability to love usually is well developed by early adulthood. This includes both romantic and affectionate love. Also, newly formed families bring on new challenges and stresses during this period. The highest levels of job stress are felt in this age group. Even so, fewer psychological issues related to well-being arise during early adulthood than during any other phase of life. Most people in this age group focus their attention on career and family as part of their psychosocial development. Their pursuits include the following:

- Selecting a mate
- Learning to live with a marriage partner
- Raising children
- Managing a home
- Finding a congenial social group
- Developing adult leisure activities
- Selecting a secure and stable occupation
- Establishing and maintaining an economic standard of living

Middle Adulthood

Middle adulthood extends from 41 to 60 years of age (**FIGURE 12-9**). The average vital signs are the same as for early adulthood. Also, body systems continue

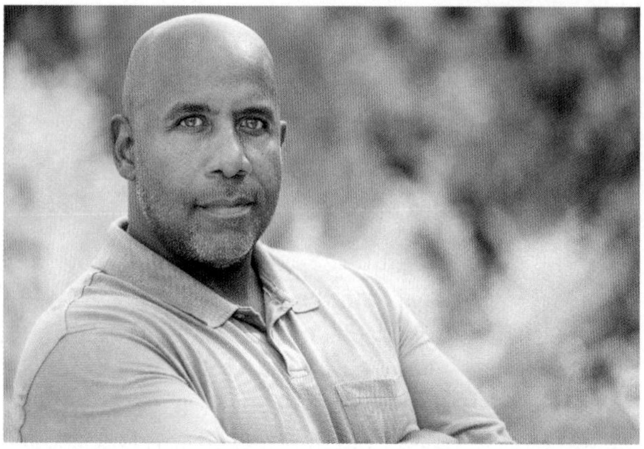

FIGURE 12-9 Middle adulthood.

© pixelheadphoto digitalskillet/Shutterstock.

to work at a high level. However, the physiologic aspects of aging may become more obvious during this stage. For example, cardiovascular health becomes a concern. Hearing and vision changes occur. **Periodontal disease** may develop. Weight control becomes more difficult. Cancer tends to strike often; it is the top cause of death in this age group, followed by heart disease.[5] For women, **menopause**, which ends a woman's ability to reproduce, normally occurs between ages 45 and 55 years.

Psychosocial Development

Middle adulthood generally is a productive time for social and professional recognition. It often is a period of financial security. However, because of the physical changes that occur in this phase of life, a person in middle adulthood often becomes concerned with the "social clock." The person may feel a sense of time pressure to meet lifelong goals. Common causes of stress in this age group include financial commitments and responsibility for the care of elderly parents. Another stressor is concern for young adult children who have moved out and are on their own. As the last child leaves home, many parents experience a feeling of depression or a sense of loss (empty nest syndrome), whereas others feel a sense of freedom and enjoy a greater chance for self-fulfillment.

DID YOU KNOW?

In about 3% of US households, grandparents and their grandchildren live together. Most of these households (67%) are maintained by the grandparents, who are often the primary caregivers for children in their home.

Modified from: Ellis RR, Simmons T. Coresident grandparents and their grandchildren: 2012. Population characteristics. US Census Bureau website. https://www.census.gov/content/dam/Census/library/publications/2014/demo/p20-576.pdf. Published October 2014. Accessed January 7, 2018.

Some adults in middle age experience a "midlife crisis." They may make sudden and sometimes irrational changes in their life (similar to the identity issues seen in the teenage years). This sudden desire to make life changes may be the result of many factors, such as health worries, a change in physical appearance as a result of aging, or a change in the level of sexual activity with a spouse. However, most middle-aged adults tend to approach problems in their lives more as challenges than as threats. Important goals, for example, often are (1) to help their children to be responsible and happy adults, (2) to accept and adjust to aging parents, and (3) to accept the physiologic changes of middle age.

Late Adulthood

People 61 to 75 years of age are in **late adulthood** (**FIGURE 12-10**). Vital signs in this age group depend on the person's health status. Moreover, vital signs are affected by the physiologic changes in body systems that normally occur during this stage of life. A person's life span is determined by health, genetics, and other factors. Cancer, heart disease, and chronic obstructive pulmonary disease are the leading causes of death during this period.[5] In addition, older adults take more prescribed and over-the-counter medications than do younger adults, increasing the risk for harmful drug interactions, misuse, and abuse.

DID YOU KNOW?

According to *The State of Aging and Health in America 2013*, 72 million Americans—1 in 5—will be 65 years or older by 2030. By 2050, this group will consist of nearly 89 million people.

Modified from: Centers for Disease Control and Prevention. *The State of Aging and Health in America 2013*. Atlanta, GA: Centers for Disease Control and Prevention, US Department of Health and Human Services; 2013.

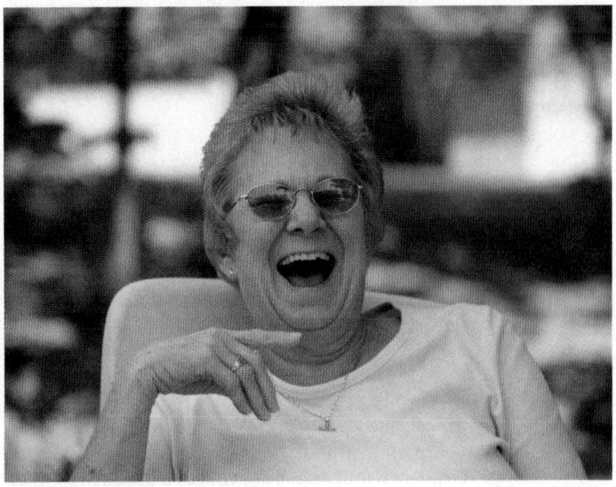

FIGURE 12-10 Late adulthood.

Courtesy of Mick Sanders.

Review of Body Systems

Body system changes associated with late adulthood vary from person to person (**FIGURE 12-11** and BOX 12-6). They also vary from organ to organ and from function to function (see Chapter 48, *Geriatrics*). Some body changes occur dramatically, whereas others occur gradually. Some functions even remain constant well into old age. This variation can be seen in several systems. For example, a decrease in cardiac output and the ability to metabolize carbohydrates becomes evident early on. Changes in skin texture and hair color occur throughout late adulthood. The speed of nerve conduction and the manufacture of red blood cells do not decline until late old age.

Psychosocial Development

The attitude of society toward age can either enhance or detract from an older person's sense of self-worth. Some cultures credit wisdom to age; others consider older adults to be more of a burden. For people who enjoy good health and retirement, late adulthood is a time of happiness and personal fulfillment. For others, this period is marked by financial burdens and physical and emotional challenges.

Financial Burdens

Most people in late age begin to accept and adjust to retirement. They also adjust to having a reduced income. However, they face new issues. For example, some must pay for health care, and they may need to establish new living arrangements. About 95% of older adults live in their own homes, choosing not to reside in home care facilities such as nursing homes and assisted care communities. The financial requirements for either type of living arrangement can be a burden for older adults and their family. For example, an older person living at home may require in-home

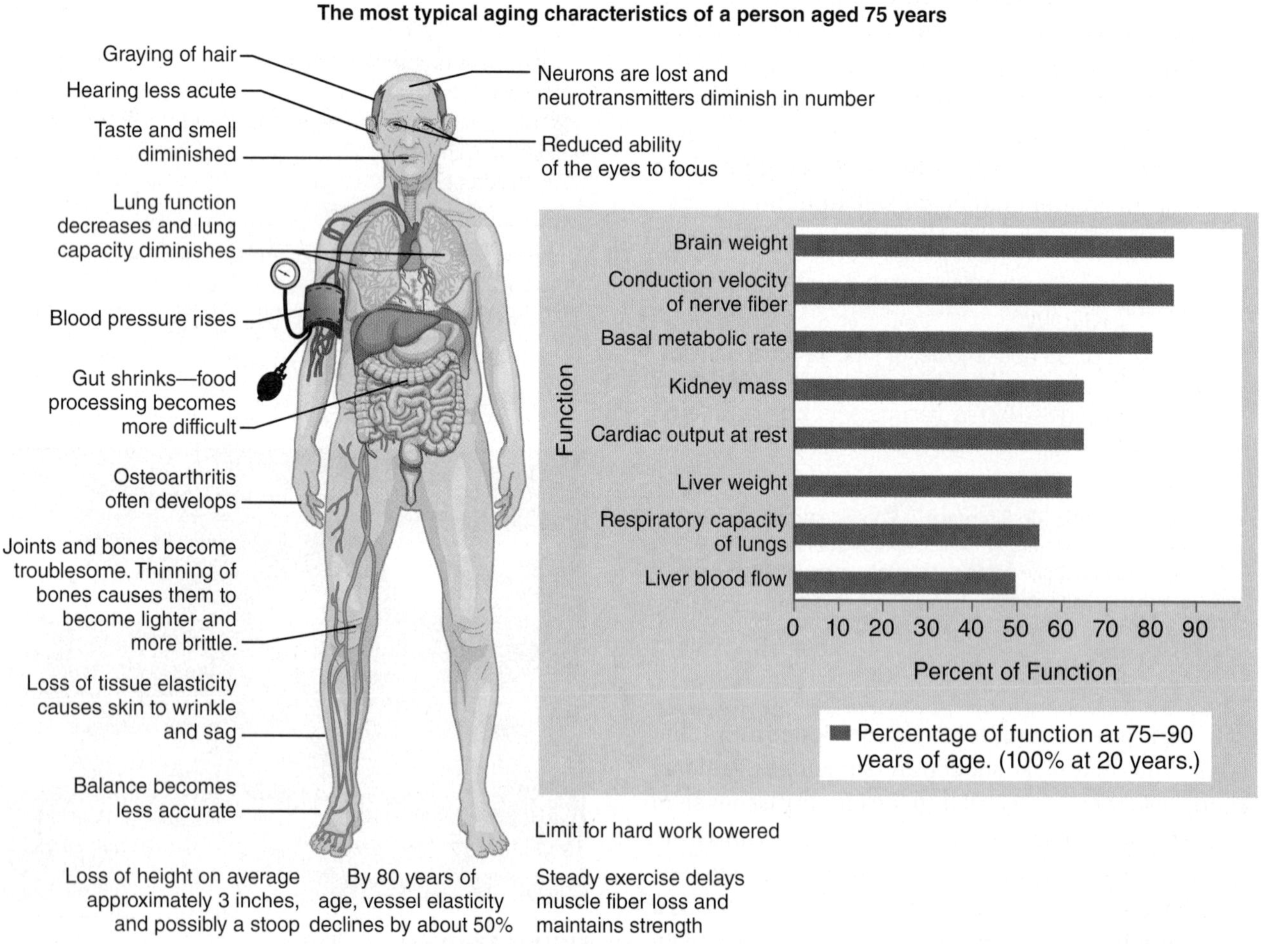

FIGURE 12-11 Body changes that occur in late adulthood.

BOX 12-6 Physiologic Changes Associated With Late Adulthood

Cardiovascular System

- Functional changes occur as blood vessels thicken and peripheral resistance increases.
- By 80 years of age, vessel elasticity declines by about 50%.
- Blood flow to organs decreases.
- Baroreceptor sensitivity is reduced, and blood pressure tends to rise.
- Increased workload of the heart causes cardiomegaly (enlarged heart), changes in the mitral and aortic valves, and decreased myocardial elasticity.
- The heart becomes less able to respond to exercise.
- The number of pacemaker cells in the heart diminishes, resulting in dysrhythmias (tachycardias are not well tolerated).
- The functional blood volume and platelet count decrease.
- The number of red blood cells decreases in late old age.
- Iron levels are poor.

Respiratory System

- Functional changes occur in the mouth, nose, and lungs.
- Lung function decreases, and lung capacity diminishes.
- The elasticity of the diaphragm declines, and the chest wall weakens.
- Diffusion through the alveoli diminishes from lifelong exposure to pollutants.
- Less oxygen becomes available for uptake by the blood.
- Coughing becomes ineffective because of weakened chest wall function and bone structure.

Nervous System

- Neurons are lost, and neurotransmitters diminish in number.
- Some taste buds are lost, and the olfactory sense diminishes.
- Pain perception decreases.
- The kinesthetic sense (sense of body movement) is lessened.
- Visual acuity diminishes.
- Reaction time declines.
- Hearing changes occur.
- The sleep–wake cycle is disrupted.

Musculoskeletal System

- Muscle mass is replaced by fibrous tissue.
- Progressive bone loss occurs, and changes in bones and joints become troublesome.
- Balance becomes less accurate.
- Osteoarthritis often develops.
- Shrinking of vertebral disks leads to loss of height and stooping posture.

Gastrointestinal System

- Secretion of saliva and gastric juices is reduced.
- Peristalsis and gastrointestinal secretions decrease.
- The esophageal sphincter becomes less effective, and internal intestinal sphincters lose tone.
- Vitamin and mineral deficiencies occur.
- Changes in the liver affect the metabolism of some drugs and foods.

Endocrine System

- Glucose metabolism and the production of insulin decrease.
- Production of triiodothyronine (T_3) by the thyroid gland declines.
- Production of cortisol decreases by about 25%.
- The pituitary gland becomes about 20% less effective.
- Women's reproductive glands begin to atrophy.

Renal System

- About 50% of the nephrons in the kidneys are lost.
- The filtration surface in the kidneys is reduced.
- Salt and water balance is compromised.
- Abnormal glomeruli become more common.
- The frequency of urination and the amount of urine eliminated decrease.

SHOW ME THE EVIDENCE

In 2010, researchers in Nova Scotia, Canada, performed a retrospective review of all prehospital patient records in their province. They found 63,076 adult emergency responses, 48.6% of which were for people age 65 years or older. The most commonly reported incident for transported and nontransported patients was a fall. Of those older adults transported, the most common conditions were cardiovascular (13.7%), respiratory (13.5%), trauma (15.9%), and gastrointestinal (13.4%). Nontransports represented 12% of the calls for this population. Notably, on-scene time was 30% greater for the nontransport calls. Because these results were comparable to results found in the United States, the researchers thought their findings will help inform the health system about the need for alternative services for this growing age group.

Modified from: Goldstein J, Jensen JL, Carter AJ, Travers AH, Rockwood K. The epidemiology of prehospital emergency responses for older adults in a provincial EMS system. *Can J Emerg Med.* 2015; 17(5):491-496.

health and home care services to assist with tasks of daily living. An older person who lives in a home care facility may need constant nursing care and other types of supervision. These situations, plus the cost of health insurance, prescription medicines, and other health care needs, can create financial burdens, even for those who plan well for their retirement. In 2015, about 4.2 million older adults in the United States were living below the poverty level, and 2.9 million households with a resident 65 years or older had food insecurity.[6]

CRITICAL THINKING

In an older patient's home, what clues may indicate that the person is under a financial strain or burden?

Cognitive and Emotional Challenges

In addition to the physical challenges linked to aging and the related health consequences, older adults face cognitive challenges, such as a decline in cognition, and emotional challenges, such as facing the dying or death of a companion.

Aging does not always produce a decline in brain function. However, some conditions can cause a loss of mental faculties. Such conditions include circulatory disorders and some diseases common in older adults (eg, Parkinson disease). Problems with short-term memory, learning, attention, and judgment may develop. This decline in mental capability is an important concern and a cause of depression in older adults.

Cognitive Aging. Research on cognitive aging has demonstrated a strong association between age and several aspects of cognition. This research has led to theories of **terminal decline** and **terminal drop**.[7]

Terminal decline is an overall slowdown or gradual decline of cognitive abilities in the absence of dementia. Examples of this decline include a drop in key mental skills, such as verbal ability, spatial reasoning, and perceptual speed, which are not a routine part of the aging process. This phase can occur as much as 15 years before death and may be associated with early heart disease, insufficient physical and mental exercise, and perhaps undetectable dementia.[8]

Terminal drop refers to a period of decline that is interrupted by an acceleration of cognitive impairment that may be caused by a person's conscious or unconscious perception of coming death.[9] Such a perception may cause the person to begin withdrawing from his or her daily life anywhere from a few weeks up to 5 years before death. Terminal drop may become evident by changes in mood or mental functioning or by the way the body responds. It also may be linked to the presence of a disease (eg, cancer).

Death and Dying of a Companion. The dying or death of a partner can be one of the most stressful events in life. The ways in which a person deals with the death or imminent death of a partner are based on several factors, including the person's cultural or religious views, the cause and timing of death, the length and type of relationship, the person's quality of life before death, and the support of friends, family, and organizations. Most people experience a variety of emotions in dealing with death and dying. These range from initial denial to final acceptance (see Chapter 2, *Well-Being of the Paramedic*).

Advanced Old Age

As the life span has increased, a new category representing people older than 75 years has been added.[1] This category is known as **advanced old age**. Heart disease is the leading cause of death in this age group, followed by Alzheimer disease and other dementias, and then stroke.[10]

The process of aging described in late adulthood continues in this group. Social and physical changes can cause people in this age group to withdraw and lose independence. For many, the need to move into assisted care or other care facilities may increase their feelings of loneliness and their dependence on others. The incidence of dementia also increases with advanced old age. It is during this time that people often begin to accept their mortality and may make arrangements for end-of-life care, which may include preparing a final will and making loved ones aware of the medical care they wish to receive or deny (eg, do- not- resuscitate orders, physician orders for scope of treatment [see Chapter 6, *Medical and Legal Issues*]).

Frailty

Frailty is a syndrome found in about 25% of adults 85 years of age and older. It is characterized by exhaustion (low energy level), slowed performance (walking speed), weakness (grip strength), unintentional weight loss (> 10 pounds [4.5 kg] in a year), and low physical activity. These signs and symptoms develop over time. Older adults in whom frailty has been diagnosed have worse health. They often suffer from an increased incidence of falls, disability after incidents, hospitalization, and mortality.[11,12]

Summary

- A newborn is a baby in the first hours of life. A neonate is a baby from birth to 1 month. An infant is a child 1 month to 1 year of age.
- The newborn normally weighs 7 to 8 pounds (3 to 3.5 kg). This weight typically triples in 9 to 12 months. The infant's head accounts for about 25% of the total body weight.
- At birth, structures unique to fetal circulation constrict and normally close within the first year of life. Fluid is expelled from the lungs during the first few breaths. Respiratory muscles and alveoli are not fully developed.
- Infants are born with protective reflexes related to breathing, eating, and stress or discomfort.
- At birth, the anterior and posterior fontanels are open. Bone growth occurs at the epiphysis of the bones.
- Some passive immunity is conferred at birth and through the mother's breast milk.
- The caregiver is the major factor in the infant's psychosocial development.
- Temperament is a characterization of a person's behavior, as defined by how the person interacts with the environment.
- Toddlers are children 1 to 2 years of age. Preschoolers are children 3 to 5 years of age.
- The hemoglobin level in toddlers and preschoolers approaches that of adults. The brain in this age group is about 90% of the adult brain weight. Muscle mass and bone density increase. Walking occurs by 2 years of age, and fine motor skills develop. Control of the bowel and bladder is achieved.
- Peer relationships, divorce, and exposure to aggression and violence affect a child's development.
- School-age children range from 6 to 12 years of age. Physical growth slows, but brain function and the ability to learn quickly develop in this age group. Many children reach puberty during this time. Self-esteem and moral development are critical at this age.
- Adolescents are 13 to 18 years of age. The growth of bone and muscle mass is nearly complete in this age group. Reproductive maturity has been reached. Adolescence often involves some emotional turmoil, and antisocial behavior may be seen.
- Early adulthood spans the period from 19 to 40 years of age. Lifelong habits and routines develop. Body systems are at their optimal performance.
- Middle adulthood extends from 41 to 60 years of age. The physiologic aspects of aging become more apparent in this age group. Menopause in women occurs during this stage.
- Late adulthood occurs between 61 and 75 years of age. Body system changes vary widely from person to person, but the systemic changes of aging become apparent. Some adults in this age group face financial, physical, and emotional challenges.
- Advanced old age, a new age category, begins at 75 years of age.

References

1. Leifer G, Fleck E. *Growth and Development Across the Lifespan*. 2nd ed. St. Louis, MO: Elsevier; 2013.
2. Erikson E. *Childhood and Society*. 2nd ed. New York, NY: WW Norton; 1963.
3. Marriage and divorce. American Psychological Association website. http://www.apa.org/topics/divorce/. Accessed January 8, 2018.
4. Kohlberg L. A cognitive-developmental analysis of children's sex-role concepts and attitudes. In: MacCoby E, ed. *The Development of Sex Differences*. Stanford, CA: Stanford University Press; 1996.
5. National Vital Statistics System, National Center for Health Statistics, Centers for Disease Control and Prevention. Ten leading causes of death by age group, United States—2015. Centers for Disease Control and Prevention website. https://www.cdc.gov/injury/wisqars/pdf/leading_causes_of_death_by_age_group_2015-a.pdf. Accessed January 8, 2018.
6. Economic security for seniors facts. National Council on Aging website. https://www.ncoa.org/news/resources-for-reporters/get-the-facts/economic-security-facts/. Accessed January 8, 2018.
7. Palmore E, Cleveland W. Aging, terminal decline, and terminal drop. *J Gerontol*. 1976;31(1):76-81.
8. Mozes A. Mental skills can decline years before dying. *Washington Post* website. http://www.washingtonpost.com/wp-dyn/content/article/2008/08/27/AR2008082702464.html. Published August 27, 2008. Accessed January 8, 2018.

9. MacDonald SW, Hultsch DF, Dixon RA. Aging and the shape of cognitive change before death: terminal decline or terminal drop? *J Gerontol B Psychol Sci Soc Sci.* 2011;66(3): 292-301.
10. World Health Organization, Global Health Observatory Data. Top 10 causes of death: situation and trends; 2015. World Health Organization website. http://www.who.int/gho/mortality_burden_disease/causes_death/top_10/en/. Accessed January 8, 2018.
11. Xue QL. The frailty syndrome: definition and natural history. *Clin Geriatr Med.* 2011;27(1):1-15.
12. Fedarko NS. The biology of aging and frailty. *Clin Geriatr Med.* 2011;27(1):27-37.

Suggested Readings

Feldman RS. *Development Across the Life Span*. 8th ed. London, UK: Pearson; 2018.

Kahn JH, Magauran BG, Olshaker J. *Geriatric Emergency Medicine*. New York, NY: Cambridge University Press; 2016.

Kail RV, Cavanaugh JC. *Human Development: A Life-Span View*. 3rd ed. Boston, MA: Cengage Learning; 2016.

Kuther T. *Lifespan Development: Lives in Context*. Thousand Oaks, CA: Sage Publications; 2017.

Torpy JM, Lynm C, Glass RM. Frailty in older adults. *JAMA.* 2006;296(18):2280.

Pharmacology

PART 3

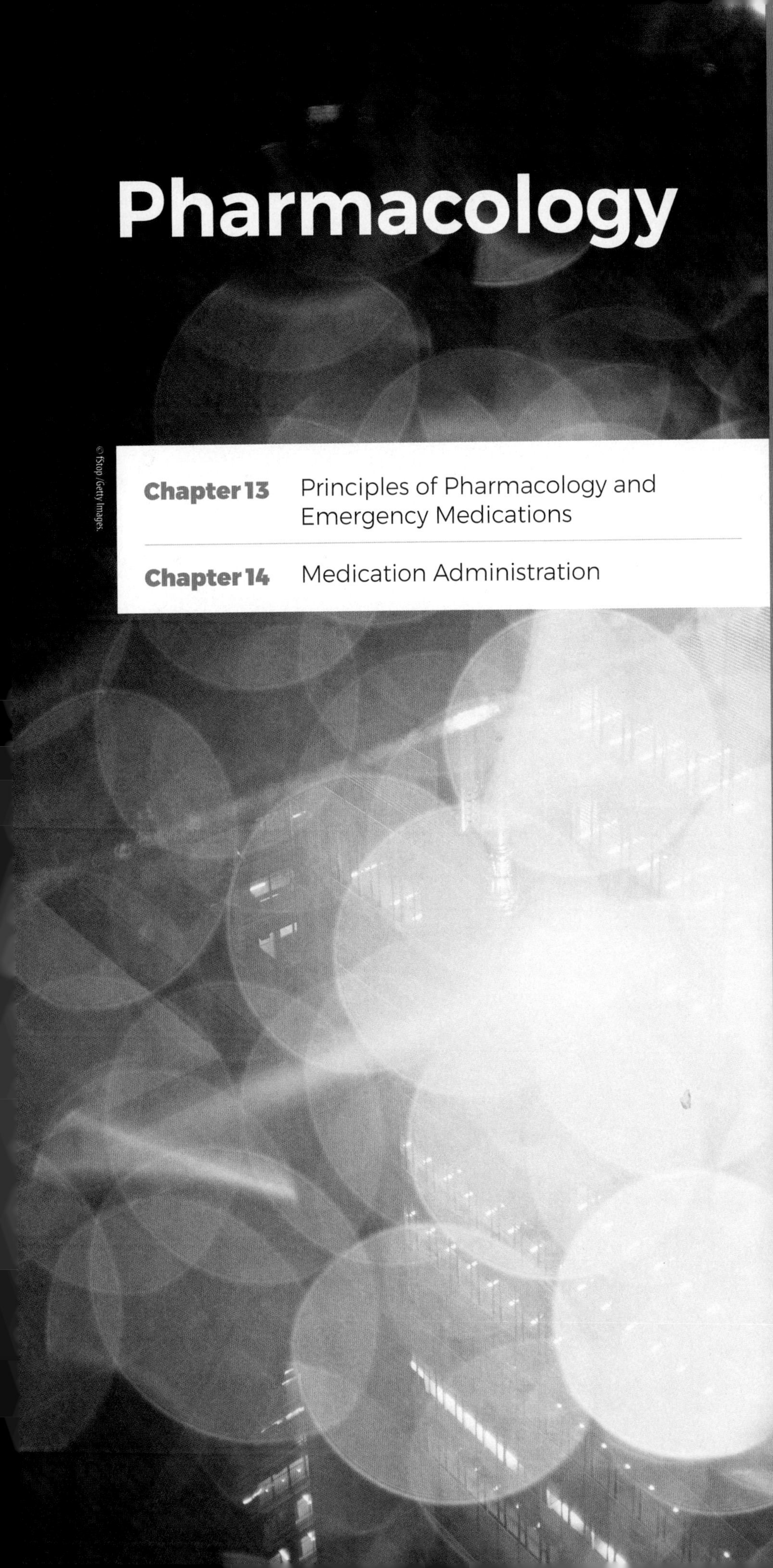

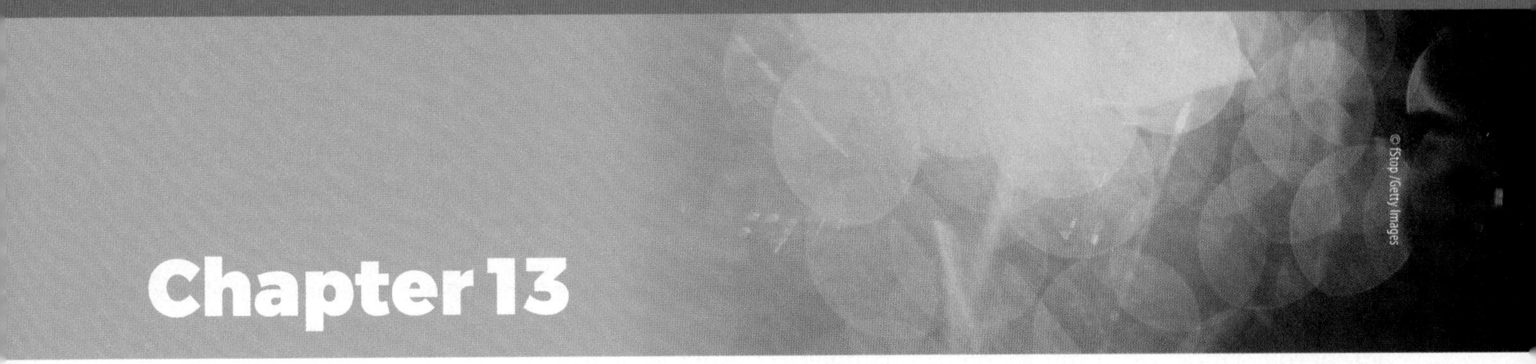

Chapter 13

Principles of Pharmacology and Emergency Medications

NATIONAL EMS EDUCATION STANDARD COMPETENCIES

Pharmacology

Integrates comprehensive knowledge of pharmacology to formulate a treatment plan intended to mitigate emergencies and improve the overall health of the patient.

Principles of Pharmacology

- Medication safety (p 354, and Chapter 14, *Medication Administration*)
- Medication legislation (pp 354–356)
- Naming (p 353)
- Classifications (pp 355–356, 370, 379, 384, 386, 388, 390, 391, 392, 394–396, 401, 408, 414)
- Schedules (p 355)
- Pharmacokinetics (p 358)
- Storage and security (p 370)
- Autonomic pharmacology (pp 375–384)
- Metabolism and excretion (pp 363–365)
- Mechanism of action (pp 366–370)
- Phases of medication activity (pp 357–366)
- Medication response relationships (pp 367–368)
- Medication interactions (pp 369–370)
- Toxicity (p 368)

OBJECTIVES

Upon completion of this chapter, the paramedic student will be able to:

1. Define the term *drug*. (p 353)
2. Identify the four types of drug names. (p 353)
3. Explain the meaning of drug terms that are necessary to interpret information in drug references safely. (pp 353, 357)
4. Outline drug standards and legislation and the enforcement agencies pertinent to the paramedic profession. (pp 354–357)
5. Discuss factors that influence drug absorption, distribution, and elimination. (pp 358, 361–365)
6. Distinguish between characteristics of routes of drug administration. (pp 359–361)
7. Describe how drugs react with receptors to produce their desired effects. (pp 366–367)
8. List variables that can influence drug interactions. (pp 369–370)
9. Describe the paramedic's responsibilities to understand drug profiles. (p 370)
10. Distinguish among drug forms. (pp 370–371)
11. Identify special considerations for administering pharmacologic agents to pregnant patients, pediatric patients, and older patients. (pp 371–375)
12. Outline drug actions and care considerations for a patient who is given drugs that affect the nervous, cardiovascular, respiratory, endocrine, and gastrointestinal systems. (pp 375, 381–406)

KEY TERMS

absorption The process by which drug molecules are moved from the site of entry into the body into the general circulation.

acetylcholine A neurotransmitter, widely distributed in body tissues, with the primary function of mediating the synaptic activity of the nervous system.

adrenergic Of or pertaining to the sympathetic nerve fibers of the autonomic nervous system, which use epinephrine or epinephrinelike substances as neurotransmitters.

agonist A drug that combines with receptors and initiates the expected response.

alpha-adrenergic receptor Any one of the postulated adrenergic components of receptor tissues that responds to norepinephrine and to various blocking agents.

antagonist An agent designed to inhibit or counteract the effects of other drugs or undesired effects caused by normal or hyperactive physiologic mechanisms.

anticholinergic Of or pertaining to the blocking of acetylcholine receptors, resulting in inhibition of transmission of parasympathetic nerve impulses.

beta-adrenergic receptor Any of the postulated adrenergic components of receptor tissues that respond to epinephrine and various blocking agents.

biologic half-life The time required to metabolize or eliminate half the total amount of a drug in the body.

biotransformation The process by which a drug is converted chemically to a metabolite.

blood–brain barrier An anatomic-physiologic feature of the brain thought to consist of walls of capillaries in the central nervous system and surrounding glial membranes. Its function is to prevent or slow the passage of chemical compounds from the blood into the central nervous system.

blood coagulation A process that results in the formation of a stable fibrin clot that entraps platelets, blood cells, and plasma.

chemical name The exact designation of a chemical structure as determined by the rules of chemical nomenclature.

cholinergic Of or pertaining to the effects produced by the parasympathetic nervous system or drugs that stimulate or antagonize the parasympathetic nervous system.

contraindications Medical or physiologic factors that make it harmful to administer a medication that would otherwise have a therapeutic effect.

controlled substance Any drug defined in the categories of the Comprehensive Drug Abuse Prevention and Control Act (also known as the Controlled Substances Act) of 1970.

cumulative action The effect that occurs when several doses of a drug are administered or when absorption occurs more quickly than removal by excretion or metabolism, or both.

distribution The transport of a drug through the bloodstream to various tissues of the body and ultimately to its site of action.

drug Any substance taken by mouth; injected into a muscle, blood vessel, or cavity of the body; or applied topically to treat or prevent a disease or condition.

drug interaction Modification of the effects of one drug by the previous or concurrent administration of another drug, thereby increasing or diminishing the pharmacologic or physiologic action of one or both drugs.

drug–protein complex A complex formed by the attachment of a drug to proteins, mainly albumin.

drug receptors Parts of a cell (usually an enzyme or large protein molecule) with which a drug molecule interacts to trigger its desired response or effect.

dystonia A condition characterized by local or diffuse changes in muscle tone, resulting in painful muscle spasms, unusually fixed postures, and strange movement patterns.

effective dose 50 (ED_{50}) The amount of drug that produces a therapeutic response in 50% of those who take it.

effector organs Muscles or glands that respond to nerve impulses from the central nervous system.

endorphins Peptides secreted in the brain that have pain-relieving effects similar to morphine.

excretion The elimination of toxic or inactive metabolites, primarily by the kidneys. The intestines, lungs, and mammary, sweat, and salivary glands also may be involved.

first-pass metabolism The initial biotransformation of a drug during passage through the liver from the portal vein that occurs before the drug reaches the general circulation.

generic name The official, established name assigned to a drug.

idiopathic Arising from an obscure or unknown cause.

idiosyncrasy An abnormal or peculiar response to a drug.

loading dose A large quantity of drug that temporarily exceeds the capacity of the body to excrete the drug.

maintenance dose The amount of a drug required to keep a desired steady state of drug concentration in tissues.

neurotransmitters Chemicals that are released from neurons at the presynaptic nerve fiber.

nonselective beta-blocking agents Agents that block $beta_1$- and $beta_2$-receptor sites.

official name The name of a drug that is followed by the initials USP (*United States Pharmacopeia*) or NF (*National Formulary*), denoting its listing in one of the official publications; usually the same as the generic name.

orphan drugs Medications that have been developed specifically to treat rare medical conditions.

parenteral Of or pertaining to any medication route other than the alimentary canal.

partial reabsorption Reabsorption from the renal tubule by passive diffusion.

pharmaceutics The science of dispensing drugs.

pharmacology The science of drugs used to prevent, diagnose, and treat disease.

pharmacodynamics The study of how a drug acts on a living organism.

pharmacokinetics The study of how the body handles a drug over a period of time, including the processes of absorption, distribution, biotransformation, and excretion.

placebo An inactive substance or a less-than-effective dose of a harmless substance. It is used in experimental drug studies to compare the effects of the inactive substance with those of the experimental drug.

placental barrier A protective biologic membrane that separates the blood vessels of the mother and the fetus.

potentiation Enhancement of the effect of a drug, caused by concurrent administration of two drugs in which one drug increases the effect of the other.

selective beta-blocking agents Agents that block $beta_1$ or $beta_2$ receptors.

summation The combined effects of two drugs that equal the sum of the individual effects of each agent.

synergism The combined action of two drugs that is greater than the sum of each agent acting independently.

tardive dyskinesia A potentially irreversible neurologic disorder characterized by involuntary repetitious movements of the muscles of the face, limbs, and trunk.

therapeutic action The desired, intended action of a drug.

therapeutic index A measurement of the relative safety of a drug.

therapeutic range The range of plasma concentrations that is most likely to produce the desired drug effect with the least likelihood of toxicity; the range between minimal effective concentration and toxic level.

tolerance A physiologic response that requires that a drug dosage be increased to produce the same effect formerly produced by a smaller dose.

trade name The trademark name of a drug, designated by the drug company that sells the medication.

untoward effects Side effects that prove harmful to the patient.

Pharmacology *can be defined as the science of drugs used to prevent, diagnose, and treat disease. Pharmacology deals with the interactions between living systems and chemical molecules. The paramedic must have a thorough understanding of a drug and its actions before it is administered. This understanding will help to ensure maximum effectiveness and will reduce the potential for harm.*

NOTE

The drug information presented in this section conforms to current medical literature, to manufacturers' monographs, and to the clinical practice of the general medical community at the time of publication. Although every effort has been made to ensure accuracy and completeness, the authors, editors, medical advisers, and publisher disclaim liability for any discrepancies, incongruities, undetected errors, omissions in content, or reader misunderstanding. Local protocol for drug administration may vary from the information presented in this chapter. The paramedic should follow the guidelines established by medical direction.

Historical Trends in Pharmacology

The science of pharmacology may date back as early as 10,000 to 7,000 BC.[1] Medicinal herbs are thought to have been among the plants grown by humans in the Neolithic period. Yet whether the herbs were thought to have healing properties is not known. A number of medicines are mentioned in the Bible. Some of these include gums, spices, oils, and maybe even narcotics. Drugs derived from plants were used heavily throughout the Middle Ages. They were used as digestives, laxatives, and diuretics (**FIGURE 13-1**).

Courtesy of Kim McKenna.

The concept of "chemical medicine" was born in the 17th century. Some preparations introduced during the 17th and 18th centuries are still in use today. Opium (morphine) is a good example of one drug still in use. Accurate studies of drug dosage in the 19th century led to the development of manufacturing facilities to produce drugs. In addition, knowledge of the expected actions of these drugs became more exact. Important drug discoveries in the 20th and 21st centuries (eg, insulin, antibiotics, fibrinolytics) have had major effects on common illnesses such as diabetes, bacterial infections, and cardiovascular disease.

Modern health care and pharmaceutics are undergoing many changes due in large part to consumer awareness of disease prevention. Changes also come from the consumers' drive to take responsibility for their health and wellness. The health care and pharmaceutical industries actively seek to develop new drugs, treatments, cures, or other methods to prevent diseases that affect aging, everyday living, or life span. The federal government also provides incentives to pharmaceutical companies to research and develop less profitable drugs, called **orphan drugs**. These drugs treat rare, chronic diseases such as hemophilia, leprosy, Cushing syndrome, and Tourette syndrome.

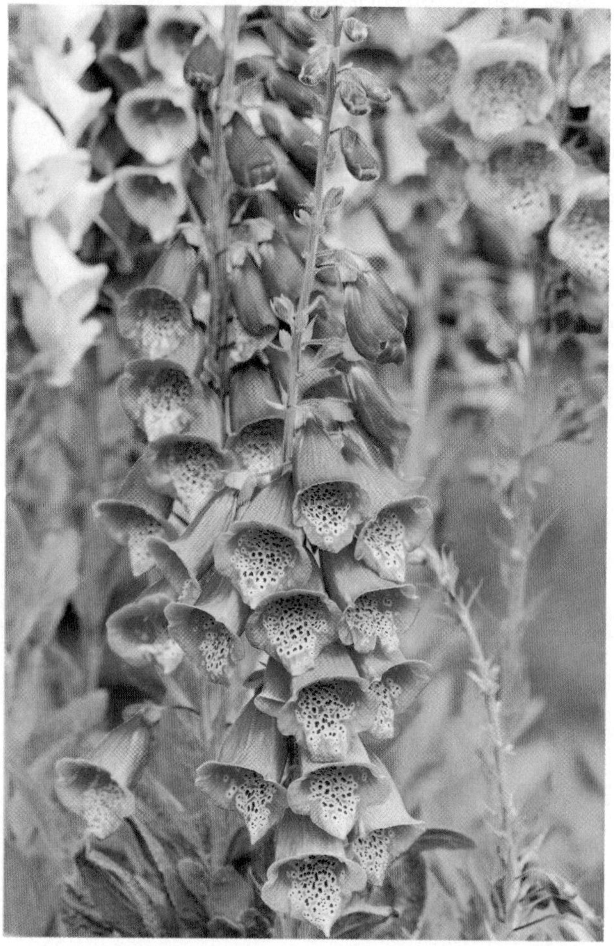

A

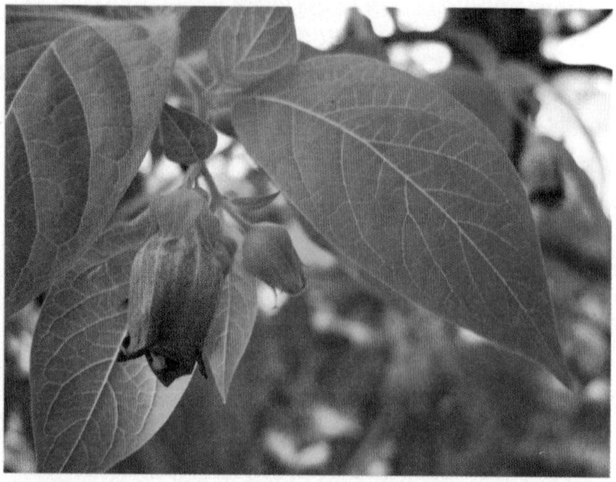

B

FIGURE 13-1 A. Foxglove. **B.** Deadly nightshade. These are the plant sources of digoxin and atropine, respectively.

A: © Mariola Anna S/Shutterstock; **B:** © Heike Brauer/Shutterstock.

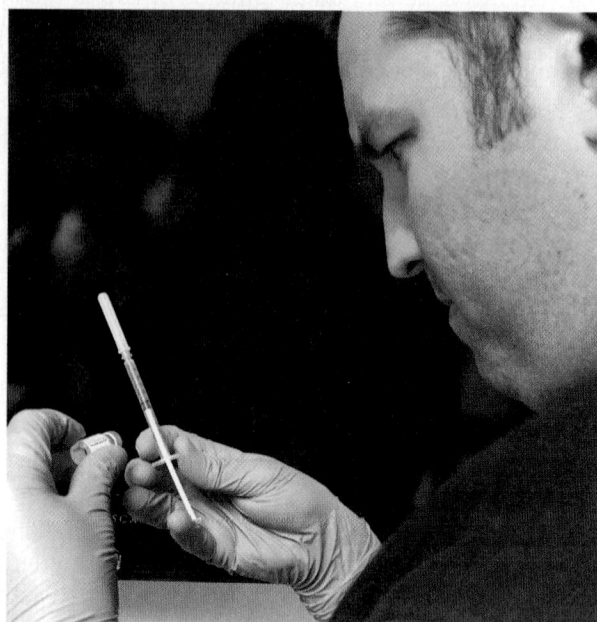

NOTE

The term *orphan drug* refers to a medication that has been developed specifically to treat a rare medical condition (an orphan disease). The assignment of orphan status to a disease and to any drugs developed to treat it is a matter of public policy in many countries. Medical breakthroughs have resulted from these assignments. Some of these medical advancements would not have otherwise been achieved because of the expense of drug research and development.

Investigational drugs are drugs that are under study and not yet approved by the US Food and Drug Administration (FDA) for sale in the United States. The most common way patients receive these drugs is by taking part in clinical trials. Specific criteria must be met to receive an investigational drug outside of a clinical trial. In general, these drugs are provided free of charge.

Drug Names

A **drug** may be defined as "any substance taken by mouth, injected into a muscle, blood vessel, or cavity of the body, or applied topically to treat or prevent a disease or condition."[2] Drugs have been identified or derived from five major sources: plants (alkaloids, glycosides, gums, and oils), animals and humans, minerals or mineral products, microorganisms, and chemical substances made in the laboratory (BOX 13-1).

Drugs can be identified by the following four types of names:

1. **Chemical name.** The chemical name is an exact description. It describes the chemical composition of the drug. It also describes its molecular structure.
2. **Generic name (nonproprietary name).** This name often is an abbreviated form of the chemical name. The generic name is used more commonly than the chemical name. Generic drugs usually have the same therapeutic efficacy as nongeneric drugs. However, they generally are less expensive. The generic name is the official name approved by the US FDA.
3. **Trade name (brand or proprietary name).** The trade name is a trademark name designated by the drug company that sells the medication. Trade names are proper nouns, and the first letter is capitalized. This text shows the trade name in parentheses after the generic name of the drug. The trade name usually is suggested by the first manufacturer of the drug.

BOX 13-1 Examples of Drugs and Their Sources

Plant Sources
Digoxin
Morphine sulfate
Atropine sulfate

Animal and Human Sources
Epinephrine
Insulin
Adrenocorticotropic hormone

Mineral or Mineral Product
Calcium chloride
Iodine
Iron
Sodium bicarbonate

Microorganism Sources
Penicillin
Streptomycin

Laboratory-Produced Chemicals
Diazepam (Valium)
Lidocaine (Xylocaine)
Midazolam (Versed)

4. **Official name.** The official name of a drug is followed by the initials USP (*United States Pharmacopeia*) or NF (*National Formulary*). These initials denote the listing of the drug in one of the official publications. In most cases, the official name is the same as the generic name.

An example of the four names for a drug would be as follows:

Chemical name: 17-allyl-4,5α-epoxy-3,14-dihydroxy-morphinan-6-one-hydrochloride
Generic name: naloxone hydrochloride
Trade name: Narcan
Official name: naloxone hydrochloride USP

Sources of Drug Information

Several publications offer information on various drugs, their preparation, and recommended administration. These references include the *American Medical Association Drug Evaluations*, the *American Hospital Formulary Service Drug Information*, medication package inserts, the *Physicians' Desk Reference*, and

> DID YOU KNOW?
>
> Approval from the US FDA is the final step in the process of drug development. The first step is for the new drug to be tested in the laboratory. If the results are promising, the drug company or sponsor must apply for FDA approval to test the drug in people. This application is called an Investigational New Drug (IND) Application. Once the IND is approved, clinical trials can begin. Clinical trials are research studies to determine the safety and to measure the effectiveness of the drug in people. Once clinical trials are completed, the sponsor submits the study results in a New Drug Application (NDA) or Biologics License Application (BLA) to the FDA. This application is carefully reviewed; if the drug is found to be reasonably safe and effective, it is approved.
>
> *Modified from*: Access to investigational drugs. National Cancer Institute website. https://www.cancer.gov/cancertopics/factsheet/therapy/investigational-drug-access. Reviewed August 4, 2009. Accessed December 13, 2017.

the *Nursing Drug Reference* (BOX 13-2). Paramedics should be familiar with these and other emergency pharmacology manuals. It is particularly important for paramedics to be familiar with drugs that often are administered in the prehospital setting. Reliable Internet sources and computer application software (eg, Lexicomp, Micromedex, UpToDate) for handheld devices (eg, personal digital assistants [PDAs], smartphones) also can be a good source of information about pharmacotherapeutics. In addition, the findings of current research can be found on the Internet. This research provides details about certain drug studies and treatments.

Drug Standards and Legislation

Before 1906, little control was exercised over the use of medications. Drugs often were sold or distributed by traveling medicine men, drugstores, mail order companies, and both legitimate and self-proclaimed physicians. The ingredients of drugs were not required to be listed. In fact, many drug products contained opium, heroin, and alcohol, which could be potentially harmful to the user.

In 1906, Congress passed the Pure Food and Drug Act, which was meant to protect the public from mislabeled or adulterated drugs. The act prohibited the use of false and misleading claims for drugs. The act also restricted the sale of drugs with a potential for abuse (**TABLE 13-1**). The act designated the *United States Pharmacopeia* and the *National Formulary* as official standards and empowered the federal government to enforce these standards. In 1980, the United States Pharmacopeial Convention purchased the *National Formulary*. This purchase made the *United States Pharmacopeia* the only official book of drug standards in the United States. In addition to the

BOX 13-2 Drug References

American Medical Association Drug Evaluations. *Drug Evaluations* provides information on drug groups, dosages, prescribing information, and usage. It also covers valid clinical applications of drug use that differ from those approved by the FDA thus far.

Hospital Formulary. The *Hospital Formulary*, a manual published by the American Society of Hospital Pharmacists, provides an overview in monograph form of nearly every available (approved and unapproved) drug in the United States. The formulary is updated regularly and is available in all hospital pharmacies and in many emergency departments. The *Hospital Formulary* is considered by many to be the most reliable source of information on medications and drugs.

Medication package inserts. Most medications are packaged with written literature describing product use. These inserts provide valuable information as new drugs are introduced, and the health care professional should consult them to become familiar with the product.

Physicians' Desk Reference. The *Physicians' Desk Reference*, published yearly by the Medical Economics Company, is a concise compilation of drug information, including FDA-approved indications, contraindications, and adverse effects. In addition to providing product information through several cross-referenced indexes, the textbook serves as an identification guide by showing actual-size, color pictures of commonly prescribed medications. The *Physicians' Desk Reference* also lists emergency telephone numbers for poison control centers throughout the United States.

Nursing Drug Reference. The *Nursing Drug Reference* is published yearly and includes nursing considerations, side effects, adverse reactions, precautions, interactions, and contraindications for drug and intravenous therapy. The textbook contains an alphabetical listing of commonly prescribed drugs and detailed monographs for drugs recently approved by the FDA.

TABLE 13-1 Controlled Substances

Characteristics	Dispensing Restrictions	Examples
Schedule I		
Has high abuse potential Has no accepted medical use; for research, analysis, or instruction only May lead to severe dependence	Approved protocol is required.	Heroin, lysergic acid diethylamide (LSD), marijuana (cannabis), methaqualone, 3,4-methylenedioxymethamphetamine (MDMA; ecstasy), peyote
Schedule II		
Has high abuse potential Has accepted medical uses May lead to severe physical or psychological dependence, or both	Electronic or written prescription is necessary (signed by the practitioner); only emergency dispensing is permitted without written prescription (only required amount may be prescribed for emergency period). No prescription refills are allowed. Container must have warning label.[a]	Amphetamine, cocaine, dextroamphetamine, fentanyl, hydrocodone (combination products with less than 15 milligrams per dose), hydromorphone, meperidine, methadone, methamphetamine, methylphenidate, oxycodone
Schedule III		
Has less abuse potential than drugs in schedules I and II Has accepted medical uses May lead to moderate to low physical dependence or high psychological dependence	Electronic, written, or oral prescription is required. Prescription expires in 6 months. No more than five refills are allowed in a 6-month period. Container must have warning label.[a]	Anabolic steroids, ketamine, testosterone, and products containing less than 90 milligrams of codeine per dose
Schedule IV		
Has lower abuse potential compared with schedule III drugs Has accepted medical uses May lead to limited physical or psychological dependence	Electronic, written, or oral prescription is required. Prescription expires in 6 months, with no more than five refills allowed. Container must have warning label.[a]	Alprazolam, carisoprodol, diazepam, lorazepam, pentazocine with naloxone, propoxyphene, propoxyphene with acetaminophen, ultram, zolpidem
Schedule V		
Has low abuse potential compared with schedule IV drugs Has accepted medical uses May lead to limited physical or psychological dependence	Drug may require written prescription or may be sold without prescription (check state law).	Attapulgite, difenoxin with atropine, diphenoxylate, pregabalin, and products with less than 200 milligrams of codeine or per 100 milliliters

[a]The warning must read "Caution: Federal law prohibits the transfer of this drug to any person other than the patient for whom it was prescribed."

Modified from: Drug Scheduling. United States Drug Enforcement Administration website. https://www.dea.gov/druginfo/ds.shtml. Accessed March 23, 2018.

United States Pharmacopeia, other drug standards and legislation are listed in BOX 13-3.

Standardization of drugs is necessary because drugs made by different manufacturers (brand name versus generic) may vary significantly in strength and activity. The strength, purity, or effectiveness of a drug can be measured through chemical analysis in a lab. This process is known as assay. A concentration of a drug can be determined by comparing its effect on an organism, animal, or isolated tissue to that of a drug that produces a known effect. This process is known as bioassay (biologic assay). Bioassay is used to measure the bioequivalence, or relative therapeutic effectiveness, of two chemically equivalent drugs.

BOX 13-3 History of Drug Standards and Legislation

1912: Congress passed the Sherley Amendment prohibiting fraudulent therapeutic claims.
1914: The Harrison Narcotic Act was passed to control the sale of narcotics and to help curb drug addiction or dependence. This was the first narcotic act to be passed by any nation, and it established the word *narcotic* as a legal term.
1938: Prompted by more than 100 deaths in 1937 from ingestion of a diethylene glycol solution of sulfanilamide, the federal Food, Drug, and Cosmetic Act was passed. This act contained a provision to prevent marketing of a new drug before it was tested properly. In addition, the act required that the label list all ingredients used in preparing the drug and the directions for drug use.
1952: The Durham-Humphrey Amendment changed the 1938 drug act, restricting the dispensing of legend (prescription) drugs. Legend drugs must bear the legend "Caution: Federal law prohibits dispensing without prescription."
1962: The Kefauver-Harris Amendment required that the safety and efficacy of a new drug be proved before the drug could be approved for use.
1970: The Comprehensive Drug Abuse Prevention and Control Act (also known as the Controlled Substances Act) superseded the Harrison Narcotic Act of 1914. The Controlled Substances Act classifies a controlled substance by its use and abuse potential. Drugs are classified into numbered schedules from schedule I (drugs with highest abuse potential) to schedule V (drugs with lowest abuse potential) (see Table 13-1).

NOTE

The Controlled Substances Act was passed in 1970. A **controlled substance** is any drug that is defined in the categories of the act. These categories include opium and its derivatives, hallucinogens, depressants, and stimulants. It is illegal for any person to possess a controlled substance, unless the substance was obtained by a valid prescription or physician's order. A person may also possess a controlled substance if the possession of the drug is pursuant to actions in the course of professional practice. The authority for use of controlled substances and other prescription drugs is a function of state agencies. These agencies operate under restrictions of the federal government. The restrictions are provided by the federal Drug Enforcement Agency. Paramedics and other allied health workers who administer drugs should be familiar with state laws governing the administration and storage of drugs. They also should be familiar with the record-keeping requirements. Violations of the act are punishable by fine or imprisonment, or both.

Drug Regulatory Agencies

In July 1973 the Drug Enforcement Agency, an agency of the Department of Justice, became the sole legal drug enforcement body in the United States. Other regulatory bodies or services include the following:

CRITICAL THINKING

News stories often feature miracle drugs. These drugs are used in other countries but are not yet available in the United States. They are not available because they lack FDA approval. Why would the FDA not automatically approve drugs already known to be helpful in the international market?

- **Food and Drug Administration.** The FDA is responsible for enforcing the federal Food, Drug, and Cosmetic Act of 1938. The FDA may seize offending goods and criminally prosecute people involved.
- **Public Health Service.** The Public Health Service is an agency of the US Department of Health and Human Services. One of the duties of the Public Health Service is to regulate biologic products, which include viruses, therapeutic serums, antitoxins, or analogous products applicable in the prevention or cure of human diseases or injuries. The agency examines and licenses these products and inspects and licenses the establishments that produce them.
- **Federal Trade Commission.** The Federal Trade Commission is an agency of the federal government directly responsible to the President of the United States. Its principal action with respect to drugs lies in its power to suppress false or misleading advertising aimed at the public.
- **Canadian drug control.** In Canada the Health Protection Branch of the Department of National Health and Welfare is responsible for administering and enforcing the Food and Drugs Act, the Proprietary or Patent Medicine Act, and the Narcotics Control Act.
- **International drug control.** International control of drugs began in 1912 when the first "Opium Conference" was held at The Hague. Various international treaties were adopted, obligating governments to control narcotic substances. These treaties were consolidated in 1961 into one document, known as the *Single Convention on*

Narcotic Drugs, which became effective in 1964. Later the International Narcotics Control Board was established to enforce this law.

CRITICAL THINKING

Your patient is acutely ill. She reports taking only an herbal medicine, which is not found in standard drug reference materials. Where can you or the medical staff find information about these alternative therapies?

NOTE

It is crucial for the paramedic to perform a thorough patient assessment. The paramedic also must obtain a pertinent medical (and drug) history from the patient. Being able to recognize and understand the reasons why certain drugs are prescribed for certain conditions or diseases is important. This knowledge can help establish a field diagnosis for the patient based on the assessment and physical findings. By having a thorough understanding of drug actions/interactions, the paramedic should be able to use the right drug to manage the illness, disease, or condition.

General Properties of Drugs

Drugs may act in the body in many ways. Some of these actions are desirable (a therapeutic effect). Others are considered undesirable or even harmful (a side effect). Drugs also may interact with other drugs, which may produce uncommon and frequently unpredictable effects. (Allergic reactions to drugs are discussed in Chapter 26, *Immune System Disorders*.) In addition, drugs generally exert several effects rather than a single effect.

Drugs do not confer any new functions on a tissue or organ; they only modify existing functions. As is described later in this chapter, the actions of a drug are achieved by a biochemical interaction between the drug and certain tissue components in the body (usually receptors). A drug that interacts with a receptor to stimulate a response is known as an **agonist**. A drug that attaches to a receptor but does not stimulate a response is called an **antagonist**. BOX 13-4 contains other pharmacologic terms and their definitions.

To produce the desired effect, a drug first must enter the body. Then the drug must reach appropriate concentrations at its site of action. This process is influenced by three phases of drug activity: the pharmaceutical phase, the pharmacokinetic phase, and the pharmacodynamic phase.

BOX 13-4 Pharmacologic Terminology

Antagonism. The opposition of effects between two or more medications that occurs when the combined (conjoint) effect of two drugs is less than the sum of the drugs acting separately.

Contraindications. Medical or physiologic factors that make it harmful to administer a medication that would otherwise have therapeutic value.

Cumulative action. The tendency for repeated doses of a drug to accumulate in the blood and organs, causing increased and sometimes toxic effects. It occurs when several doses are administered or when absorption occurs more quickly than removal by excretion or metabolism.

Depressant. A substance that decreases a body function or activity.

Drug allergy. A systemic reaction to a drug resulting from previous sensitizing exposure and the development of an immunologic mechanism.

Drug dependence. A state in which withdrawal of a drug produces intense physical or emotional disturbance; previously known as habituation.

Drug interaction. Beneficial or detrimental modification of the effects of one drug by the prior or concurrent administration of another drug that increases or decreases the pharmacologic or physiologic action of one or both drugs.

Idiosyncrasy. Abnormal or peculiar responses to a drug (accounting for 25% to 30% of all drug reactions) thought to result from genetic enzymatic deficiencies or other unique physiologic variables and leading to abnormal mechanisms of drug metabolism or altered physiologic effects of the drug.

Potentiation. The enhancement of effect caused by the concurrent administration of two drugs in which one drug increases the effect of the other drug.

Side effect. An undesirable and often unavoidable effect of using therapeutic doses of a drug; an action or effect other than those for which the drug was originally given.

Stimulant. A drug that enhances or increases body function or activity.

Summation. The combined effect of two drugs such that the total effect equals the sum of the individual effects of each agent (1 + 1 = 2).

Synergism. The combined action of two drugs such that the total effect exceeds the sum of the individual effects of each agent (1 + 1 = more than 2).

Therapeutic action. The desired, intended action of a drug.

Tolerance. Decreased physiologic response to the repeated administration of a drug or chemically related substance, possibly necessitating an increase in dosage to maintain a therapeutic effect (tachyphylaxis).

Untoward effect. A side effect that proves harmful to the patient.

Pharmaceutical Phase

Pharmaceutics is the science of dispensing drugs. One aspect of this field is the study of the ways in which the forms of drugs (solid or liquid) influence pharmacokinetic and pharmacodynamic activities (described in the following sections). All drugs must be in solution to cross the cell membranes to achieve absorption. The term *dissolution* refers to the rate at which a solid drug goes into solution after ingestion. The faster the rate of dissolution, the more quickly the drug can be absorbed.

Pharmacokinetic Phase

Pharmacokinetics is the study of how the body handles a drug over time, including the processes of absorption, distribution, biotransformation, and excretion. These factors affect a patient's response to drug therapy.

Drug Absorption

Absorption involves the movement of drug molecules from the entry site to the general circulation. The degree to which drugs attain pharmacologic activity depends partly on the rate and extent to which they are absorbed. The rate and extent in turn depend on the ability of the drug to cross the cell membrane. The drug crosses the membrane through the processes of passive diffusion and active transport (described in Chapter 11, *General Principles of Pathophysiology*). Most drugs enter the cell by passive diffusion. Yet some drugs require a carrier-mediated mechanism to assist them across the membrane.

Absorption begins at the site of administration. The rate and extent of absorption depend on the following factors:[3]

- **The nature of the absorbing surface (cell membrane) the drug must traverse.** If a drug must pass through a single layer of cells such as the intestinal epithelium, transport is faster than if the drug must pass through several layers of cells (eg, the skin). In addition, the greater the surface area of the absorbing site, the greater the absorption and the quicker the drug takes effect. For example, the small intestine offers a large absorption area, whereas the stomach has a relatively small absorption surface area.
- **Blood flow to the site of administration.** A rich blood supply enhances absorption, and a poor blood supply delays it. For example, a patient with diminished blood flow may not respond to intramuscular administration of a drug because diminished circulation reduces absorption. In contrast, intravenous administration of a drug immediately places the drug in the circulatory system, where it is absorbed completely and delivered to its target tissue.
- **The solubility of the drug.** The more soluble the drug, the more rapidly it is absorbed. For example, drugs that are prepared in oily solutions are absorbed more slowly than are drugs dissolved in water or in isotonic sodium chloride.
- **The pH of the drug environment.** In solution, many drugs exist in an ionized (electrically charged) and nonionized (uncharged) form. A nonionized drug is lipid (fat) soluble and readily diffuses across the cell membrane. An ionized drug is lipid insoluble and generally does not cross the cell membrane. Most drugs do not ionize fully following administration. Rather, they reach an equilibrium between their ionized and nonionized forms, allowing for the nonionized form to be absorbed. Both the mechanism and the extent of ionization depend on whether the drug is an acid or a base. An acidic drug such as aspirin is relatively nonionized and does not dissociate well in an acidic environment such as the stomach; therefore it is absorbed easily in the stomach. A drug that is basic in the same acidic environment tends to ionize and is not absorbed easily through the gastric membrane. The reverse occurs when the drug is in an alkaline medium.
- **The drug concentration.** Drugs administered in high concentrations tend to be absorbed more rapidly than those administered in low concentrations. In some situations, administration of a **loading dose** (large dose) first that temporarily exceeds the capacity for excretion of the drug is necessary. This large dose rapidly establishes a therapeutic drug level at the receptor site. A **maintenance dose** (smaller dose) then can be administered to replace the amount of drug excreted. Thus loading doses are based more on the volume of distribution (of which body size is an important component) and less on capacity for excretion (eg, renal failure). Maintenance doses are exactly the opposite.
- **The form of the drug dosage.** Drug absorption can be manipulated by pharmaceutical processing. An example is a combination of an active drug with another substance that is slowly released or a drug that resists digestive action (eg, those with enteric coatings).

CRITICAL THINKING

Consider a common condition seen in the prehospital setting. This condition requires that drugs be given at higher than usual doses to achieve therapeutic levels. What is the condition?

Routes of Drug Administration

The mode of drug administration affects the rate at which onset of action occurs. Route of administration also may affect the therapeutic response that results. The routes of drug administration are categorized as follows:

- Enteral (administration along any portion of the gastrointestinal tract)
- Parenteral (administration by any route other than the gastrointestinal tract)
- Pulmonary (administration by inhalation or through an endotracheal tube)
- Topical (administration by application to the skin and mucous membranes)

The route of administration greatly influences drug absorption (**TABLE 13-2**). Chapter 14, *Medication Administration*, describes the methods used to administer drugs by various routes.

TABLE 13-2 Comparison of Drug Absorption Rates by Common Routes of Administration

Route	Rate of Absorption
Enteral	Slow
Sublingual	Rapid
Subcutaneous	Slow
Intramuscular	Moderate
Intravenous	Immediate (no absorption required)
Endotracheal	Rapid
Intraosseous	Immediate
Pulmonary	Rapid
Topical	Moderate
Intranasal	Rapid

BOX 13-5 Emergency Drugs Administered via the Enteral Route

Activated charcoal
Aspirin

Enteral Route. Drugs administered along any portion of the gastrointestinal tract are said to use the enteral route (**BOX 13-5**). Administration may be orally, rectally, or through a gastric tube. The enteral method of giving drugs is the safest, most convenient route. This route also is the most economical route of administration. Yet the enteral route is the least reliable and slowest of the common routes because of the frequent changes in the gastrointestinal environment (eg, changes in food contents, emotional state, and physical activity). This route allows four types of absorption: oral absorption, gastric absorption, absorption from the small intestine, and rectal absorption.

- **Oral absorption.** The oral cavity has a rich blood supply. However, little absorption normally occurs in the mouth. Certain drugs, such as nitroglycerin (Nitrostat) tablets and some hormones, are prepared to be absorbed orally. When administered by sublingual or buccal routes, these drugs rapidly dissolve in the salivary secretions and are absorbed by the oral mucosa. Drugs that are absorbed in the upper gastrointestinal tract enter the systemic circulation. They initially bypass gastrointestinal fluids and the liver. Drugs absorbed in the stomach and intestines pass through the portal vein system of the liver. They are subject to **first-pass metabolism** in the liver. (First-pass metabolism refers to the concentration of a drug being reduced before it reaches the systemic circulation. It will be further described later in this chapter.) In the sublingual route, the drug is placed under the tongue. The tablet or spray dissolves in the salivary secretions. The effects of sublingual medication usually are clear within a few minutes. With buccal administration the drug is placed between the teeth and mucous membrane of the cheek. As in the sublingual route, absorption by buccal administration usually is rapid. Orally dissolving (disintegrating) tablets are placed on the tongue and disintegrate in less than 30 seconds after contact with saliva.[4]

CRITICAL THINKING

Nitroglycerin spray may be more effective in geriatric patients than is the tablet form. Why do you think this is the case?

- **Gastric absorption.** The stomach also has a rich blood supply but is not considered an important site of drug absorption. The length of time a medication remains in the stomach varies, depending on the pH of the environment and gastric motility. As previously described, weakly acidic drugs tend to remain nonionized. These drugs are absorbed readily into the circulation. In comparison, basic drugs ionize in the stomach and are absorbed poorly. Altering the gastric emptying rate may alter the rate and extent of drug absorption. Many drugs are administered on an empty stomach with sufficient water (8 ounces [237 mL]) to ensure rapid passage into the small intestine. Other drugs cause gastric irritation and usually are given with food.
- **Absorption from the small intestine.** The small intestine has a rich blood supply. Thus it has a larger absorption area than the stomach has. Most drug absorption occurs in the upper part of the small intestine. The pH of intestinal fluid is alkaline, which increases the rate of absorption of basic drugs. Prolonged exposure allows more time for drug absorption. An increase in intestinal motility (eg, diarrhea) decreases exposure to the intestinal membrane and diminishes absorption.
- **Rectal absorption.** The surface area of the rectum is not large. However, the rectum is vascular and capable of drug absorption. Drugs administered rectally are subject to erratic absorption because of rectal contents, local drug irritation, and the uncertainty of drug retention. Fifty percent of a drug that has been administered rectally is estimated to bypass the liver after absorption. This makes first-pass metabolism by the liver following rectal administration less than that of an orally given dose.

CRITICAL THINKING

The drugs given rectally in emergencies usually are anticonvulsants. Why do you think this route would be chosen over the oral or intravenous route?

BOX 13-6 Emergency Drugs Administered via the Parenteral Route

Adenosine (Adenocard)
Amiodarone (Cordarone)
Atropine
Dextrose 50%
Diazepam (Valium)
Diphenhydramine (Benadryl)
Dopamine (Intropin)
Epinephrine (Adrenalin)
Fentanyl (Sublimaze)
Lorazepam (Ativan)
Midazolam (Versed)
Morphine
Naloxone (Narcan)
Ondansetron (Zofran)
Oxytocin (Pitocin)
Sodium bicarbonate
Verapamil (Isoptin)

Parenteral Route. Drugs administered by injection are said to use the **parenteral** route (BOX 13-6). The commonly used parenteral routes for administering medications include the following:

- **Subcutaneous route.** A subcutaneous injection is given beneath the skin into the connective tissue or fat immediately beneath the dermis. This route is used only for small volumes of drugs (0.5 mL or less) that do not irritate tissue. The rate of absorption usually is slow and can provide a sustained effect.
- **Intramuscular route.** An intramuscular injection is given into the skeletal muscle. Absorption generally occurs more rapidly than with a subcutaneous injection because of greater tissue blood flow.
- **Intravenous route.** An intravenous injection is given directly into the bloodstream, bypassing the absorption process. This route produces an almost immediate pharmacologic effect. Most intravenous drugs should be administered slowly to help limit adverse reactions.
- **Intradermal route.** An intradermal injection is made just below the epidermis. This route primarily is used for allergy testing and to administer local anesthetics. Drugs given by this route are not absorbed into the general circulation.
- **Intraosseous route.** An intraosseous injection is given directly into the bone marrow cavity

of pediatric and adult patients through an established intraosseous infusion system. Agents infused by this method are thought to circulate via the medullary cavity of the bone. Through the numerous venous channels of long bones, fluids or drugs rapidly enter the central circulation. The length of time from injection to entry into the systemic circulation is thought to equal that of the intravenous route.[5] All emergency medications can be administered intraosseously.[6]

- **Endotracheal route.** Access to the endotracheal route generally is through an endotracheal tube, which allows drug delivery into the alveoli and systemic absorption via the capillaries of the lungs. Administration of drugs via an endotracheal tube usually is reserved for situations in which an intravenous or intraosseous line cannot be established. Medications that can be administered by the endotracheal tube include naloxone (Narcan), atropine, vasopressin (Pitressin), epinephrine (Adrenalin), and lidocaine (Xylocaine). Administration of 2 to 2.5 times the recommended intravenous dose (diluted in 10 mL of normal saline) is recommended when medication is given by this route.[7]

NOTE

A mnemonic for the five medications that may be administered via the pulmonary route through an endotracheal tube is *NAVEL*, which stands for *n*aloxone, *a*tropine, *v*asopressin, *e*pinephrine, and *l*idocaine.

Pulmonary Route. Medication can be administered by inhalation in the form of gas or fine mist (aerosol). The most commonly used inhalation medications are bronchodilators (BOX 13-7). However, the pulmonary circulation can absorb a number of other medications if necessary, such as nitrous oxide/oxygen for pain relief.

Because of the large surface area and the rich capillary network of the alveoli, drug absorption into the bloodstream is rapid. Bronchodilators and steroids can be given by inhalation devices, such as a nebulizer (described in Chapter 14, *Medication Administration*). A nebulizer propels the drug into alveolar sacs. Drugs that are given by a nebulizer device produce mainly local effects. Occasionally, nebulized drugs can produce unwanted systemic effects. An example of these effects is an elevated heart rate (tachycardia).

BOX 13-7 Emergency Drugs Administered via the Pulmonary Route

Albuterol (Proventil, Ventolin)
Amyl nitrite
Racemic epinephrine (Micronefrin)
Levalbuterol (Xopenex)
Metaproterenol (Alupent)
Nitrous oxide/oxygen (Nitronox)
Oxygen

BOX 13-8 Emergency Drugs Administered via the Topical Route

Lidocaine (lidocaine gel)
Nitropaste (Nitro-Bid ointment)

Topical Route—Skin. In most cases, drugs applied topically to the skin and mucous membranes are absorbed rapidly (BOX 13-8). Only lipid-soluble compounds are absorbed through the skin. The skin acts as a barrier to most water-soluble compounds. To prevent adverse systemic effects, intact skin surfaces should be used as an administration site. Massaging the skin helps to promote drug absorption because it dilates capillaries and increases local blood flow.

Topical Route—Nasal. As described in Chapter 10, *Review of Human Systems*, the nasal mucosa is highly vascular. The delivery of medication via the intranasal route results in rapid absorption of the medication into the bloodstream and cerebrospinal fluid, which results in therapeutic drug levels that are effective in the management of seizures, pain, hypoglycemia, opiate overdose, and other medical conditions (BOX 13-9). Using the intranasal route greatly reduces the risk of needlestick injury. Some vaccines are also administered by the intranasal route in select patient groups, including live attenuated influenza vaccine (LAIV) and influenza virus vaccine live (Intranasal FluMist) (see Chapter 14, *Medication Administration*).

Drug Distribution

Distribution is the transport of a drug through the bloodstream. The drug is transported to various tissues of the body and ultimately to its site of action.

BOX 13-9 Emergency Drugs Administered via the Nasal Route

Diazepam (Valium)
Dexmedetomidine (Precedex)
Fentanyl (Sublimaze)
Glucagon
Haloperidol (Haldol)
Ketamine (Ketalar)
Ketorolac (Toradol)
Lidocaine (Xylocaine)
Lorazepam (Ativan)
Midazolam (Versed)
Naloxone (Narcan)

After a drug has entered the circulatory system, it is distributed rapidly throughout the body. The rate at which distribution occurs depends on the permeability of capillaries to the drug molecules.

To review, lipid-soluble drugs readily cross capillary membranes to enter most tissues and fluid compartments. Lipid-insoluble drugs require more time to arrive at their point of action. Cardiac output and regional blood flow also affect the rate and extent of distribution into body tissues. Generally, a drug is distributed first to organs that have a rich blood supply. These organs include the heart, liver, kidneys, and brain. Then, depending on its composition, the drug enters tissue with a lesser blood supply, such as muscle and fat.

Drug Reservoirs. Drugs may accumulate at certain locations that act as storage sites. At these sites, the drugs form reservoirs by binding to specific tissues. As serum levels decline, tissue-bound drug is released from its storage site into the bloodstream. The released drug maintains the serum drug levels and may permit sustained release of the drug over time, which allows continued pharmacologic effect at the receptor site. Plasma protein binding and tissue binding are the two general processes that create drug reservoirs.

As drugs enter the circulatory system, they may attach to plasma proteins (mainly albumin), forming a **drug–protein complex**. The extent to which this binding occurs affects the intensity and duration of the effect of the drug. Because the albumin molecule is too large to diffuse through the membrane of the blood vessel, it traps the bound drug in the bloodstream. A drug bound to plasma protein is pharmacologically inactive, and the protein becomes a circulating drug reservoir. The free drug (non–protein-bound drug) exists in proportion to the protein-bound fraction and is the only portion of the drug that is biologically active. As the free drug is eliminated from the body, the drug–protein complex dissociates, and more drug is released to replace the free drug that was metabolized or excreted. This process is summarized in the following equation:

$$\text{Free drug} + \text{Protein} \rightleftharpoons \text{Drug–protein complex}$$

Albumin and other plasma proteins provide a number of binding sites. Two drugs, however, can compete for the same site and displace each other. Certain combinations of drugs may be given at the same time. As a result, this competition can have serious consequences. For example, a patient taking the anticoagulant drug warfarin (Coumadin) may be given quinidine (eg, Quinaglute Dura-Tabs). The quinidine may displace some of the protein-bound warfarin, causing warfarin toxicity that can lead to severe hemorrhage.

Other factors that influence the binding ability of a drug include the concentration of plasma proteins (especially albumin), the number of binding sites on the protein, the affinity (attraction) of the drug for the protein, and the acid–base balance of the patient. Various disease states, such as liver disease, alter the ability of the body to metabolize many medications. These alterations result from a decrease in serum albumin levels (albumin is manufactured by the liver) and a decrease in hepatic metabolism. These factors and others may result in more free drug being available for distribution to tissue sites (increased free drug fraction and enhanced pharmacologic response).

A second type of "drug pooling" occurs in fat tissue and bone. Lipid-soluble drugs have a high affinity for adipose tissue, where these drugs are stored. Because fat tissue has low blood flow, it serves as a stable reservoir for drugs. Some lipid-soluble drugs can remain in body fat for as long as 3 hours after administration. Other drugs (eg, tetracycline) have an unusual affinity for bone. These drugs accumulate in bone after being absorbed onto the bone crystal surface.

CRITICAL THINKING

Tetracycline typically is not given to pregnant women because of the harmful effects it has on the development of the baby's teeth. Why would it affect the teeth?

Barriers to Drug Distribution. The blood–brain barrier and the placental barrier are protective membranes. These membranes prevent the passage of certain drugs into these body sites. The **blood–brain barrier** consists of a single layer of capillary endothelial cells. These cells line the blood vessels entering the central nervous system and are tightly joined at common borders by continuous intercellular junctions. This special arrangement permits only lipid-soluble drugs, such as general anesthetics and barbiturates, to be distributed into the brain and cerebrospinal fluid. Drugs that are poorly soluble in fat (eg, many antibiotics) have trouble passing this barrier and therefore cannot enter the brain.

The **placental barrier** is made up of membrane layers. These layers separate the blood vessels of the mother and the fetus. Like the blood–brain barrier, the placental barrier is not permeable to many lipid-insoluble drugs. Thus the placenta offers some protection to the fetus. However, the placenta does allow the passage of certain non–lipid-soluble drugs. Examples of these are steroids, narcotics, anesthetics, and some antibiotics. If these drugs are given to the pregnant mother, they may affect the developing embryo or fetus or the neonate. (Pregnancy category ratings for drugs are described later in this chapter.)

Biotransformation

After absorption and distribution, the body eliminates most drugs, first by biotransformation and then by excretion. **Biotransformation** (metabolism) is a process in which drugs are chemically converted to metabolites (smaller components). The purpose of biotransformation usually is to "detoxify" a drug and render it less active. The liver is the primary site of drug metabolism. However, other tissues also can be involved. Some of these include the plasma, kidneys, lungs, and the intestinal mucosa.

Orally administered drugs that are absorbed through the gastrointestinal tract normally travel to the liver before entering the general circulation. When this occurs, a large amount of the drug may be metabolized before reaching the systemic circulation. This is known as first-pass metabolism. This process reduces the amount of drug that is available for distribution in the body. Medications affected by this initial biotransformation in the liver may be given in higher dosages or administered parenterally (intravenously or intramuscularly) to bypass the liver.

People metabolize drugs at variable rates. For example, patients with liver, renal, or cardiovascular disease are expected to have prolonged drug metabolism. Infants with immature metabolic capacity and older adults with degenerative metabolic function experience depressed biotransformation. If drug metabolism is delayed, drug accumulation and cumulative drug effects may occur. Therefore the paramedic may need to consider dosage reductions (particularly maintenance doses) for patients in these categories (**FIGURE 13-2**).

Excretion

Excretion is the elimination of toxic or inactive metabolites. The kidney is the primary organ for excretion. However, the intestine, the lungs, and the mammary, sweat, and salivary glands also may be involved.

Excretion by the Kidneys. A drug can be excreted in the urine unchanged. Or, a drug can be excreted as a chemical metabolite of its previous form. Renal excretion consists of three mechanisms: passive glomerular filtration, active tubular secretion, and partial reabsorption (**FIGURE 13-3**).

Passive glomerular filtration is a simple filtration process. Filtration can be measured as the glomerular filtration rate (described in Chapter 10, *Review of Human Systems*). The glomerular filtration rate is the total quantity of glomerular filtrate formed each minute in all nephrons of both kidneys. (This measure is usually expressed in milliliters.) The availability of a drug for glomerular filtration depends on its free concentration in plasma. Unbound drugs and water-soluble metabolites are filtered by the glomeruli. Drugs highly bound to protein do not pass through this structure.

After filtration, lipid-soluble compounds are reabsorbed by the renal tubules. Thus they reenter the systemic circulation. Water-soluble compounds are not reabsorbed. Therefore they are eliminated from the body. Because of the proportional relationship between free and bound drug, as free drug is filtered from the blood, bound drug is released from its binding sites into the plasma. The rate of excretion and the **biologic half-life** of the drug (described later in this chapter) depend on how quickly bound drug is released.

CRITICAL THINKING

You pick up a patient at the renal dialysis center for chest pain and a decreasing level of consciousness. Which medications can be administered safely; which ones should be avoided; and which medicines would need to be given at a reduced dose?

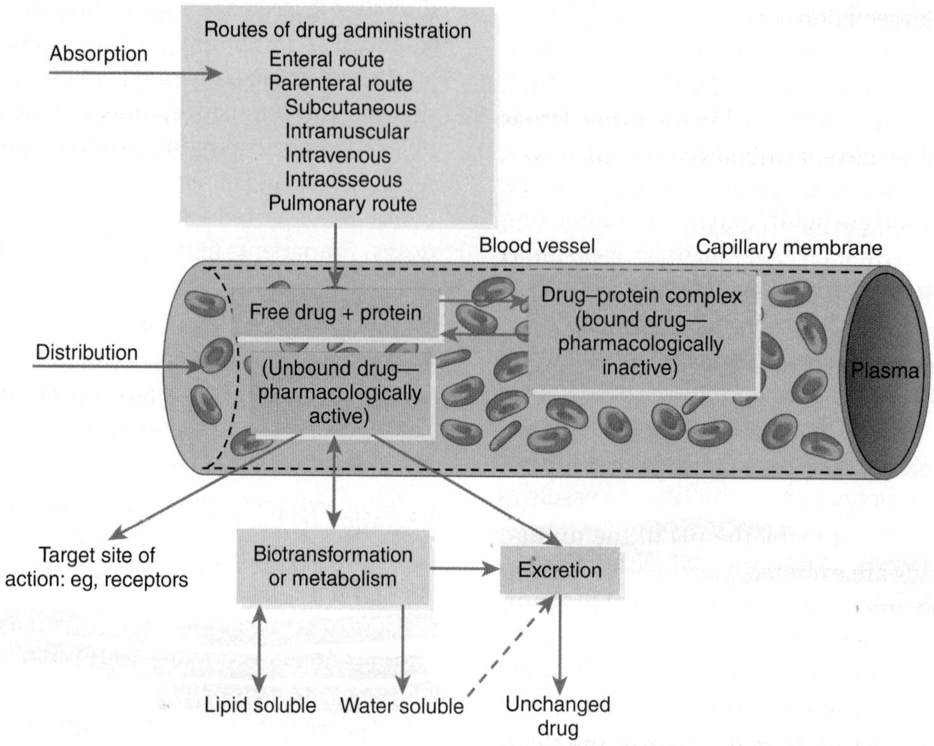

FIGURE 13-2 Pharmacokinetic phase of drug action, showing absorption, distribution, biotransformation, and excretion of drugs. Only free drug is capable of movement for absorption, distribution to the target site of action, biotransformation, and excretion. The drug–protein complex represents bound drugs; because the molecule is large, it is trapped in the blood vessel and serves as a storage site for the drug.

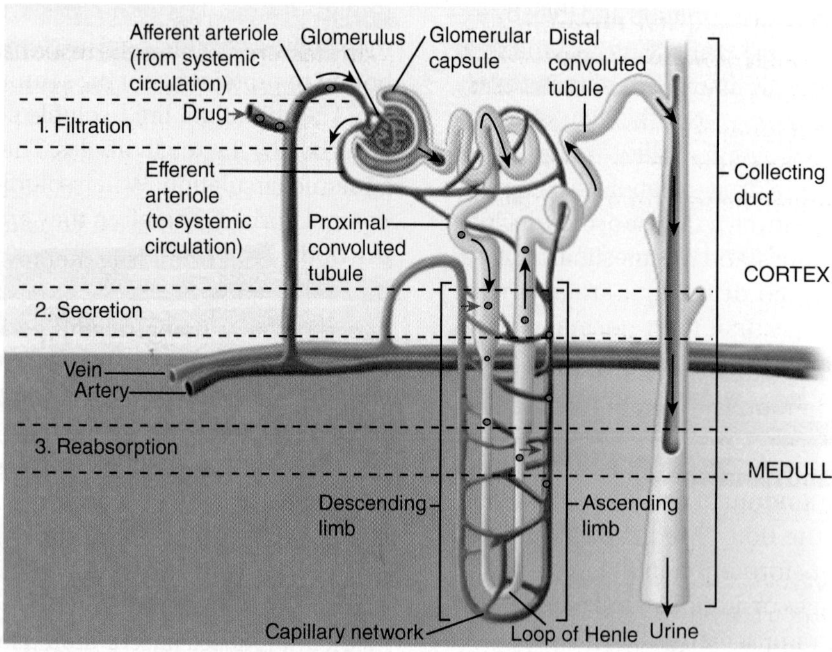

FIGURE 13-3 Renal drug excretion process.

Active tubular secretion occurs in the renal tubules, where free drug can be transported or secreted from the blood across the structure called the proximal tubule and from there deposited in the urine. Drugs actively secreted by the renal tubules can compete with other drugs for the same active transport process. The interaction of amiodarone (Cordarone) and digoxin (Lanoxin) is an example of a competitive drug interaction, in which the first drug reduces the removal or clearance of the second drug. (The term *clearance* refers to the complete removal of a drug by the kidneys.) The result of this competition for removal is an increase in the plasma concentration of the second drug.

Partial reabsorption is the reabsorption from the renal tubule by passive diffusion. Such reabsorption can be influenced greatly by the pH of the tubular urine. Weak acids are excreted more readily in alkaline urine. They are secreted more slowly in acidic urine because they are ionized in alkaline urine but nonionized in acidic urine. The reverse is true for weak bases. For example, an increase in urinary pH decreases the reabsorption and increases the clearance of weak acids such as furosemide (Lasix) and aspirin. However, a decrease in urinary pH increases the clearance of weak bases such as amphetamine and tricyclic antidepressants.

As a rule, substances that are completely or almost completely excreted by the normal kidney can be removed by an artificial process, hemodialysis, that resembles glomerular filtration (see Chapter 28, *Abdominal and Gastrointestinal Disorders*). Hemodialysis can be used to remove a wide variety of substances, although it is not very effective for drugs that are highly tissue- or protein-bound. Moreover, hemodialysis is of limited benefit for the removal of rapidly acting toxins.

Excretion by the Intestine. Drugs are eliminated through the intestine by biliary excretion. After liver metabolism, the metabolites are carried in bile and passed into the duodenum. The metabolites then are eliminated with the feces. Some drugs are reabsorbed by the bloodstream and returned to the liver and then later excreted by the kidneys.

Excretion by the Lungs. Some drugs can be eliminated by the lungs, such as general anesthetics, volatile alcohols, and inhaled bronchodilators. Certain factors can alter drug elimination via the lungs, including the rate and depth of respiration and cardiac output. Deep breathing and an increase in cardiac output (which increases pulmonary blood flow) promote excretion. However, respiratory compromise and decreased cardiac output may occur during illness or injury and can prolong the period required to eliminate drugs through the lungs.

Excretion by the Sweat and Salivary Glands. Sweat is an unimportant means of drug excretion. However, this process can cause various skin reactions and can discolor the sweat. Drugs excreted in saliva usually are swallowed and are eliminated in the same manner as other orally administered medicines. Certain substances given intravenously, such as adenosine (Adenocard) and calcium chloride, can be excreted into saliva, which may cause the person to complain about the "taste of the drug" even though it was given intravenously.[8]

Excretion by the Mammary Glands. Many drugs or their metabolites are excreted through the mammary glands in breast milk. Nursing mothers are advised not to take any medicine except under the supervision of a physician. Mothers usually are advised to take prescribed medicines immediately after breastfeeding, which diminishes any risk to the infant.

Factors That Influence the Action of Drugs

Many factors can alter the response to drug therapy, including age, body mass, sex, pathologic state, genetic factors, psychological factors, environment, and time of administration. The paramedic should recognize these factors and should consider individual responses. The paramedic also must consider complications that may result from drug therapy.

Age. Generally, pediatric and geriatric patients are known to be highly sensitive to drugs. In a child, this sensitivity results in part from the immature hepatic and renal systems. In an older adult, sensitivity results from the natural decline of these systems. These aspects of body function can reduce the efficiency of excretory and metabolic mechanisms. The older patient also may have underlying disease processes that can create unexpected responses to drug therapy. Medication doses for children usually are modified based on body weight or surface area (see Chapter 47, *Pediatrics*).

Q17

Body Mass. Many drugs are given according to body mass (kilograms). An indirect relationship exists between body mass and the final concentration of drug in a patient for any given dosage (ie, the larger the patient, the lower the concentration for any given dose of drug). The average adult drug dose is calculated on the basis of drug quantity needed to produce a particular effect when administered to 50% of the population. This population includes only people between the ages of 18 and 65 years who weigh about 150 pounds (68 kg). Therefore the appropriate drug doses for children who weigh less than 150 pounds and are younger than 18 years are always based on body mass.

Sex. Drug effects differ in men and women. These differences result partly from size differences. Women usually are smaller in body mass than men are. Thus they may have higher concentrations of a drug when the standard dose is administered without consideration of size. Differences in the relative proportions of fat and water in the bodies of men and women also can cause variations in drug distribution.

Environment. Drugs that affect mood and behavior may be susceptible to the person's environment and the personality of the user. For example, sensory deprivation and sensory overload may affect a person's response to a drug. The physical environment also can affect the actions of some drugs for some people. For example, temperature extremes and changes in altitude may increase sensitivity to some drugs.

CRITICAL THINKING

You can alter the environment in the ambulance. How might you do this to promote the action of pain-relieving drugs that have been administered to a patient?

Time of Administration. As previously described, the presence or absence of food in the gastrointestinal tract affects the manner in which drugs are tolerated and absorbed. Other factors that may influence drug activity and reactions to drug therapy include a person's biologic rhythms (eg, sleep–wake cycles and circadian rhythms, described in Chapter 2, *Well-Being of the Paramedic*).

Pathologic State. Illness or injury and the severity of symptoms also can play a role in a person's sensitivity to drugs. Illness or injury can affect the type and amount of drug needed to achieve a desired effect. In addition, underlying disease processes such as circulatory, hepatic, or renal dysfunction can interfere with the physiologic actions of the drug and drug elimination.

Genetic Factors. Genetics can alter the response of some people to a number of drugs. Examples of genetic factors include inherited diseases or enzyme deficiencies and altered receptor site sensitivities. The results of genetic abnormalities may manifest as idiosyncrasies (peculiar responses to a drug) or may be mistaken for drug allergies.

Psychological Factors. A patient's belief in the effects of a drug may strongly influence and potentiate drug effects. For example, a **placebo** (eg, a sugar pill) can have the same result as a pharmacologic agent if the patient thinks it will have the desired effect. In contrast, patient hostility and mistrust can lessen the perceived effects of a drug. The paramedic can enhance the action of a drug by telling the patient that the drug is going to work and when it will take effect.

Pharmacodynamic Phase

Pharmacodynamics is the study of how a drug acts on a living organism, which includes the pharmacologic response observed relative to the concentration of the drug at an active site in the organism. As stated earlier, drugs do not confer any new function on a tissue or organ of the body; rather, they modify existing functions. Most drug actions are thought to result from a chemical interaction between the drug and various receptors throughout the body. The most common form of drug action is the drug–receptor interaction (**BOX 13-10**).

Drug–Receptor Interaction

It is generally believed that most drugs bind to **drug receptors** to produce their desired effect. According to this theory, a specific portion of the drug molecule (the active site) selectively combines or interacts with some molecular structure (the reactive site on the cell surface or within the cell). This interaction produces a biologic effect. These reactive cellular sites are known as receptors.

The relationship of a drug to its receptor may be thought of as a key fitting into a lock (**FIGURE 13-4**). The

BOX 13-10 Drug–Receptor Interaction Terms

Affinity. The propensity of a drug to bind or attach itself to a given receptor site.

Agonist. A drug that combines with receptors and initiates the expected response.

Antagonist. An agent that inhibits or counteracts effects produced by other drugs or undesired effects caused by normal or hyperactive physiologic mechanisms.

Efficacy (intrinsic activity). The ability of a drug to initiate a desired biologic activity as a result of binding to a receptor site.

Noncompetitive antagonist. An agent that combines with different parts of the receptor mechanism and inactivates the receptor so that the agonist cannot be effective regardless of its concentration. Noncompetitive antagonist effects are considered to be irreversible or nearly so.

Partial antagonist. An agent that binds to a receptor and stimulates some of its effects but may antagonize the action of other drugs with greater efficacy. Antagonists frequently share some structural similarities with their agonists.

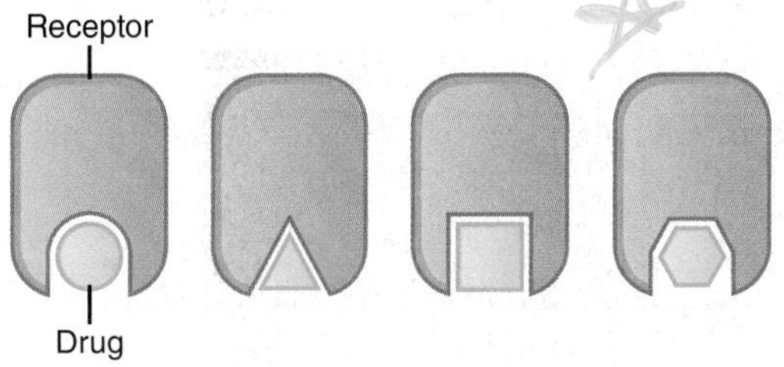

FIGURE 13-4 Lock and key fit between a drug and the receptors through which it acts. The site on the receptor that interacts with a drug has a definite shape (four examples are shown here). A drug that conforms to that shape can bind and produce a biologic response.

drug represents the key; the receptor represents the lock. The drug molecule with the best fit to a receptor produces the best response. Following absorption, a drug is believed to gain access to a receptor after it leaves the bloodstream and is distributed to tissues that contain receptor sites. To review, drugs that bind to a receptor and cause an expected physiologic response are referred to as agonists. Conversely, drugs that bind to a receptor and prevent a physiologic response or other drugs from binding are referred to as antagonists.

Drug-Response Assessment

In the prehospital setting the response to drug therapy often can be assessed by observing the effect of the drug on specific physical findings. Examples include monitoring blood pressure after administration of an antihypertensive medication and assessing pain relief after administration of an analgesic.

Each drug has its own characteristic rate of absorption, distribution, biotransformation, and excretion. Thus the effectiveness of some drugs cannot be monitored solely by the patient's response. For example, medications such as theophylline, digoxin, and phenytoin (Dilantin) must reach a certain concentration at the target site to achieve the desired effect. Tissue concentrations often are proportional to and can be estimated from drug levels in the blood determined by laboratory analysis. Therapeutic drug levels in the blood, or serum, generally indicate ranges in tissue drug concentration that produce the desired therapeutic response.

Plasma-level profiles (BOX 13-11) demonstrate the relationship between the concentration of drug in the plasma and the effectiveness of the drug over time (**FIGURE 13-5**). These profiles depend on the rate of absorption, distribution, biotransformation, and excretion after drug administration.

BOX 13-11 Plasma-Level Profile Terms

Duration of action. The period from onset of drug action to the time when a drug effect is no longer seen.

Loading dose. A bolus of a drug given initially to attain a therapeutic plasma concentration rapidly.

Maintenance dose. The amount of drug necessary to maintain a steady therapeutic plasma concentration.

Minimum effective concentration. The lowest plasma concentration that produces the desired drug effect.

Onset of action or latent period. The interval between the time a drug is administered and the first sign of its effect.

Peak plasma level. The highest plasma concentration attained from a dose.

Termination of action. The point at which the effect of a drug is no longer seen.

Therapeutic range. The range of plasma concentrations most likely to produce the desired drug effect with the least likelihood of toxicity (the range between minimum effective concentration and toxic level).

Toxic level. The plasma concentration at which a drug is likely to produce serious adverse effects.

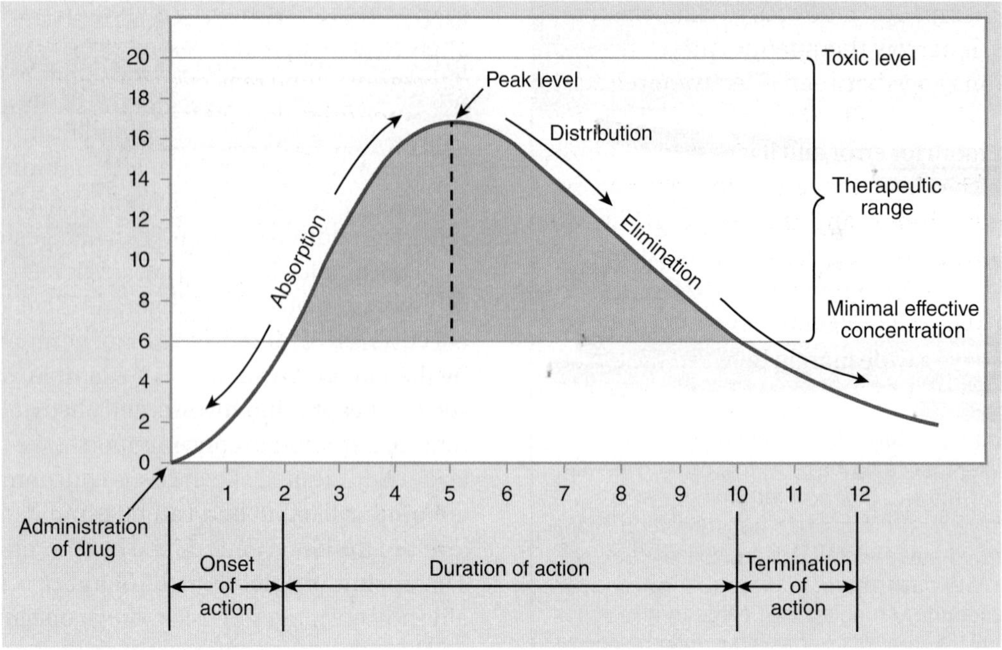

FIGURE 13-5 Plasma-level profile of a drug.

The **therapeutic range** for most drugs is based on the concentration that provides the highest probability of response with the least risk of toxicity. The dosage (loading and maintenance) required to achieve a therapeutic concentration varies because of the previously described factors that influence the actions of drugs: age, body mass, sex, pathologic state, and genetic and psychological factors. In most patients, doses in the therapeutic range have a high probability of producing the desired effect and a low probability of toxicity. However, some patients fail to respond to doses in the therapeutic range. Still others may develop drug toxicity.

Biologic Half-Life

The rate of biotransformation and excretion of a drug determines its biologic half-life. The biologic half-life is defined as the time it takes to metabolize or eliminate 50% of a drug in the body. For example, a 100-mg injection of a drug is given. Its half-life is 4 hours. Thus 50 mg will be eliminated in the first 4 hours, 25 mg (half of the remaining 50 mg) will be eliminated in the second 4 hours, and so on. A drug is considered to be eliminated from the body after five half-lives have passed.

The half-life of a drug is crucial when determining the frequency of administration. A drug that has a short half-life (eg, 2 to 3 hours) must be administered more often to maintain a therapeutic range than a drug with a long half-life, such as 12 hours. The half-life of a drug may be lengthened considerably in people with liver dysfunction or renal disorders. These and other disease processes may require a reduction in drug dosage, or the interval between doses may have to be lengthened.

> CRITICAL THINKING
>
> Adenosine is an intravenous antidysrhythmic medicine. Adenosine has a half-life of only 1 to 3 seconds. How will this brief half-life influence the speed and frequency of administration of this drug?

Therapeutic Index

The **therapeutic index** is a measurement of the relative safety of a drug. The index represents the ratio between two factors. The first factor is lethal dose 50 (LD_{50}). This is the dose of a drug that is lethal in 50% of laboratory animals tested. The second factor is **effective dose 50 (ED_{50})**. This is the dose that produces a therapeutic effect in 50% of a similar population. The therapeutic index (TI) is calculated as follows:

$$TI = \frac{LD_{50}}{ED_{50}}$$

Q30

A wide therapeutic index range indicates a drug is fairly safe. A narrow therapeutic index means the concentration range between effective levels of the drug and lethal levels of the drug is small. Therefore, there is little room for error and it is easy to administer a toxic dose. The closer the ratio is to 1, the narrower the therapeutic index, and the greater the danger in administering the drug. In certain drugs, such as digoxin, the difference between the effective dose and the lethal dose is small. In contrast, drugs such as naloxone have a wide margin between the effective dose and the lethal dose (**FIGURE 13-6**).

Drug Interactions

Many variables can influence drug interactions, including intestinal absorption, competition for plasma protein binding, biotransformation, action at the receptor site, renal excretion, and alteration of electrolyte balance. Not all drug interactions are dangerous; some may even be beneficial.

Some drug–drug interactions are clinically significant and can be dangerous. The paramedic should be aware of common drug–drug interactions. In addition, the paramedic should seek medical direction before giving drugs concurrently. (See the Appendix, *Emergency Drug Index*.) The following drugs are associated with clinically significant drug–drug interactions:

- Anticoagulants
- Tricyclic antidepressants
- Monoamine oxidase inhibitors
- Amphetamines
- Digitalis glycosides
- Diuretics
- Antihypertensives

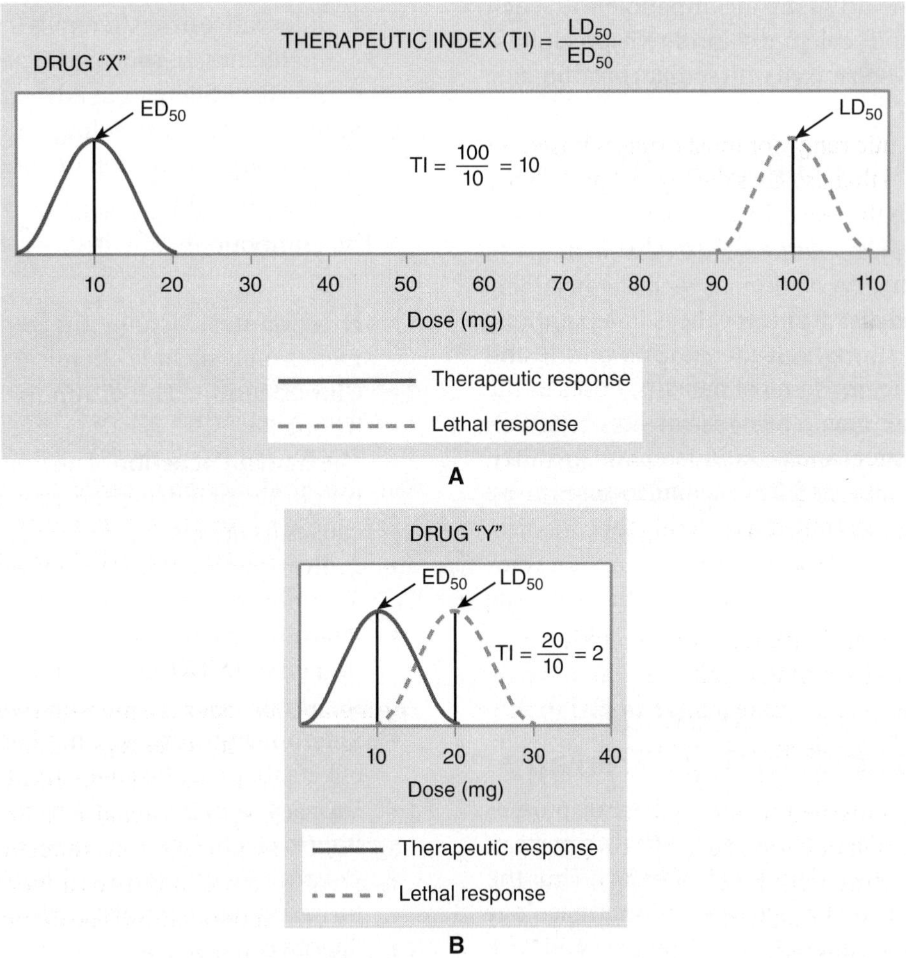

FIGURE 13-6 Plasma-level profile of a drug. **A.** High therapeutic index. **B.** Low therapeutic index.

Other factors that can influence drug interactions include the following:

- Drug-induced malabsorption of food and nutrients
- Food-induced malabsorption of drugs
- Enzyme alterations that affect the metabolism of food or drugs
- Alcohol consumption
- Cigarette smoking that affects drug metabolism or excretion
- Food-initiated alteration of drug excretion

NOTE

Grapefruit and its juice can boost blood levels of some drugs as much as 1,000%. This effect occurs through liver enzyme inhibition. Emergency drugs that can be affected include verapamil (Isoptin) and midazolam (Versed).

Finally, some drugs are incompatible with each other. For example, calcium chloride will precipitate (or crystallize) when mixed with sodium bicarbonate.

Drug Forms, Preparations, and Storage

Drugs and drug preparations are available in many forms (BOX 13-12). Each one has specific indications, advantages, and disadvantages. These preparations are explained throughout the chapter and in the Appendix, *Emergency Drug Index*.

Certain rules should guide the manner in which drugs are secured, stored, distributed, and justified. The paramedic should follow agency protocol and also local and state regulations. Emergency medical services (EMS) personnel must be aware that temperature, light, moisture, and shelf life can affect drug potency and effectiveness.

Drug Profiles and Special Considerations in Drug Therapy

A paramedic should be familiar with the drug profiles of any drug he or she administers. Not all aspects of drug profiles can be committed to memory. Thus the paramedic should make regular use of pharmacology references (eg, handbooks, pocket guides) and seek medical direction as needed. Paramedics are legally, morally, and ethically responsible for safe and effective drug administration (see Chapter 14, *Medication Administration*). As part of the professional practice of patient management, paramedics must do the following:

- Use correct precautions and techniques when administering medications
- Observe and document the effects of drugs
- Be current in their knowledge base regarding changes in trends in pharmacology
- Establish and maintain professional relationships with other members of the health care team
- Understand pharmacodynamics of the drugs they administer
- Carefully evaluate patients to identify drug indications and contraindications
- Take a drug history from patients that includes the following information:
  - Prescribed medications (name, strength, daily dosage)
  - Over-the-counter medications
  - Vitamins
  - Alternative drug therapies (eg, homeopathic medicines, herbal medicines)
  - Any drug allergies or adverse drug reactions
- Strictly adhere to standing orders or protocols for drug administration or consult with online medical direction

The components of a drug profile include the following:

- **Drug names.** Usually the generic and trade names; may include chemical names
- **Classification.** The group to which the drug belongs
- **Mechanism of action.** The pharmacodynamic properties of a drug; the way in which a drug causes its effects
- **Indications.** Conditions for which the drug is administered, as approved by the FDA
- **Pharmacokinetics.** How the body handles the drug over time; includes absorption, distribution, biotransformation, excretion, and onset and duration
- **Side/adverse effects.** Untoward or undesired effects that may be caused by the drug
- **Dosages.** The amount of drug to be administered
- **Routes of administration.** How the drug is given
- **Contraindications.** Conditions in which it may be harmful to administer the drug
- **Special considerations.** How the drug may affect pediatric patients, geriatric patients, pregnant patients, and other special groups (described next)
- **Storage requirements.** How the drug should be stored

BOX 13-12 Various Forms of Drug Preparations

Preparations for Oral Use

Liquids

Aqueous solution: substance dissolved in water and syrups
Aqueous suspension: solid particles suspended in liquid
Emulsion: fat or oil suspended in liquid with an emulsifier
Spirits: alcohol solution
Elixir: aromatic, sweetened alcohol and water solution
Tincture: alcohol extract of plant or vegetable substance
Fluid extract: concentrated alcoholic liquid extract of plant or vegetables
Extract: syrup or dried form of pharmacologically active drug, usually prepared by evaporating a solution

Solids

Capsule: soluble case (usually gelatin) that contains liquid, dry, or beaded drug particles
Tablet: compressed, powdered drugs in the form of a small disk
Troche or lozenge: medicated tablets that dissolve slowly in the mouth
Powder or granules: loose or molded drug substance for administration with or without liquids

Preparations for Parenteral Use

Ampule: sealed glass container for liquid injectable medication
Vial: glass container with rubber stopper for liquid or powdered medication
Cartridge or Tubex: single-dose unit of parenteral medication to be used with a specific injecting device

Intravenous Infusions (Suspended on Hanger at Bedside)

Flexible collapsible plastic bags (25 to 250 mL): used for continuous infusion of fluid replacement with or without medications
Intermittent intravenous infusions: usually secondary intravenous setup of a small plastic bag (25 to 250 mL) to which medication is added. The infusion runs as a "piggyback," hung separately from the primary intravenous infusion via a secondary administration tubing set usually for 20 to 120 minutes. The primary intravenous solution is run between medication doses or may be co-infused if the solutions are compatible
Heparin or saline lock: a port site for direct administration of intermittent intravenous medications without the need for primary intravenous solution

Preparations for Topical Use

Liniment: liquid suspension for lubrication that is applied by rubbing
Lotion: liquid suspension that can be protective, emollient, cooling, astringent, antipruritic, or cleansing
Ointment: semisolid medicine in a base for local protective, soothing, astringent, or transdermal application for systemic effects (nitroglycerin, scopolamine, estrogen)
Paste: thick ointment primarily used for skin protection
Plasters: solid preparations that are adhesive, protective, or soothing
Cream: emulsion that contains aqueous and oily bases
Aerosol: fine powder or solution in a volatile liquid that contains a propellant

Preparations for Use on Mucous Membranes

Drops for eyes, ears, or nose: aqueous solutions with or without gelling agent to increase retention time in the eye
Topical instillation of aqueous solution of medications: usually for topical action but occasionally for systemic effects (enema, douche, mouthwash, throat spray, gargle)
Aerosol sprays, nebulizers, and inhalers: aqueous solutions of medication delivered in droplet form to the target membrane, such as the bronchial tree (bronchodilators)
Nasal drugs: an alternative route for drugs with poor bioavailability and high–molecular-weight compounds such as peptides, steroids, and vaccines
Foam: powder or solution of medication in volatile liquid with propellant (vaginal foams for contraception)
Suppositories: usually medicinal substances mixed in a firm but malleable base (cocoa butter to facilitate insertion into a body cavity [rectum or vagina])

Miscellaneous Drug Delivery Systems

Intradermal implants: pellets that contain a small deposit of medication and are inserted into a dermal pocket; they are designed to allow medication to leach slowly into tissue and usually are used to administer hormones such as testosterone or estradiol
Micropump system: small, external pump attached by belt or implanted that delivers medication via a needle in a continuous steady dose (insulin, anticancer chemotherapy, opioids, treatment of spasticity)
Membrane delivery systems: drug-laden membranes are instilled into the eye to deliver a steady flow of medication (pilocarpine or corticosteroids)

Special Considerations in Drug Therapy

Special considerations in drug therapy must be taken into account when a paramedic is caring for pregnant patients, pediatric patients, and older adult patients.

Pregnant Patients

Before administering any drug to a pregnant patient, the paramedic should consider the expected benefits and the possible risks to the fetus. Drugs given to a pregnant patient may cross the placental barrier and

PEDS DRUGS ARE MORE OFTEN WEIGHT BASED

harm the fetus or may be communicated to a newborn during breastfeeding. The FDA established a scale to indicate drugs that may be harmful to a fetus during pregnancy; these letter categories, however, will be phased out (BOX 13-13).

In 2014, the FDA published a final rule titled Content and Format of Labeling for Human Prescription Drug and Biological Products: Requirements for Pregnancy and Lactation Labeling, which is also known simply as the Pregnancy and Lactation Labeling Rule (PLLR). The PLLR will phase out the use of pregnancy letter categories and will change and combine sections pertaining to pregnancy and lactation.

Pediatric Patients

Special considerations for administration of drugs to pediatric patients are presented here and throughout the text. Following is a summary of the pharmacokinetics that influence dosing principles in the neonate, infant, and pediatric populations.

Age. The effects of drugs are unpredictable among infants because of the variation in the development and maturation of the different organ systems.

CRITICAL THINKING

Drug doses vary for pediatric and neonatal patients. They are almost always related to weight. How can you ensure accuracy of dosing for these patients in critical situations when seconds count, even though you know the wrong dose calculation could be lethal?

Absorption. Drug absorption in infants and children follows the same basic principles as it does in adults. A factor that influences drug absorption is blood flow at the site of intramuscular or subcutaneous administration. Blood flow usually is determined by the patient's cardiovascular function. Certain physiologic conditions might reduce blood flow to the muscle and subcutaneous tissue, including shock, vasoconstriction, and heart failure. The smaller muscle mass of the infant further complicates drug absorption because of diminished peripheral perfusion to these areas. For orally administered drugs, underlying gastrointestinal function may influence drug absorption.

Liquids and suspensions disperse quickly in gastrointestinal fluids and therefore are more readily absorbed than tablet or capsule forms. Increases in peristalsis (eg, diarrheal conditions) and lowered gastrointestinal enzyme activities tend to decrease overall absorption of orally or rectally administered medications.

Distribution. Most drugs are distributed in body water. Increases in total body water and extracellular volume therefore can increase the volume of the distribution. Compared with adults, infants have proportionately higher volumes of total body water (70% to 75% compared with 50% to 60%). Infants also have a higher ratio of extracellular to intracellular fluid (40% compared with 30%); higher dosages of water-soluble drugs may be needed to have effective blood levels in the newborn.

Another key factor that affects drug distribution is drug binding to plasma proteins. In general, protein binding of drugs is reduced in the infant; therefore the concentration of free drug in plasma is increased, which can result in a greater drug effect or toxicity. The blood–brain barrier in the infant is much less effective than in adults, which allows drugs greater access to this area.

Biotransformation. Various liver enzyme systems for metabolism generally mature unevenly. The infant therefore has a decreased ability to metabolize drugs. This condition predisposes the infant to developing toxicity from drugs metabolized by the liver. In addition, many drugs given to infants have slower renal clearance times and longer half-lives in the body. The paramedic must adjust dosages based on age and weight.

Elimination. The glomerular filtration rate is much lower in newborns than in older infants, children, and adults. Therefore drugs eliminated through renal function are cleared from the body slowly in the first few weeks of life. Renal excretory mechanisms progress to maturity after 1 year of age. Before that age, excretion of some substances through the renal system may be delayed because of immaturity, which may result in higher serum levels and a longer duration of action than intended.

Older Adult Patients

Key changes in drug responses occur with age in most people. Factors associated with aging that significantly affect pharmacokinetics include the likelihood of

BOX 13-13 Current and New Pregnancy Category Ratings for Drugs

Drugs have been categorized by the FDA according to the level of risk to the fetus. These categories are listed for each drug under Pregnancy Safety and are interpreted as follows:

Category A. Controlled studies in women fail to demonstrate a risk to the fetus in the first trimester, and there is no evidence of risk in later trimesters; the possibility of fetal harm appears to be remote. Examples include levothyroxine and folic acid.

Category B. Either (1) animal reproductive studies have not demonstrated a fetal risk but there are no controlled studies in pregnant women or (2) animal reproductive studies have shown an adverse effect (other than decreased fertility) that was not confirmed in controlled studies on women in the first trimester, and there is no evidence of risk in later trimesters. Examples include metformin, hydrochlorothiazide, and amoxicillin.

Category C. Either (1) studies in animals have revealed adverse effects on the fetus and there are no controlled studies in women or (2) studies in women and animals are not available. Drugs in this category should be given only if the potential benefit justifies the risk to the fetus. Examples include tramadol, gabapentin, amlodipine.

Category D. There is positive evidence of human fetal risk, but the benefits for pregnant women may be acceptable despite the risk, as in life-threatening diseases for which safer drugs cannot be used or are ineffective. An appropriate statement must appear in the "Warnings" section of the labeling of drugs in this category. Examples include lisinopril, lorazepam, and losartan.

Category X. Studies in animals or humans have demonstrated fetal abnormalities, there is evidence of fetal risk based on human experience, or both; the risk of using the drug in pregnant women clearly outweighs any possible benefit. The drug is contraindicated in women who are or may become pregnant. An appropriate statement must appear in the "Contraindications" section of the labeling of drugs in this category. Examples include atorvastatin, simvastatin, and warfarin.

The PLLR became effective June 30th, 2015. The PLLR requires changes to the content and format for information presented in prescription drug labeling to assist health care providers in assessing benefit versus risk and in subsequent counseling of pregnant women and nursing mothers who need to take medication, thus allowing them to make informed and educated decisions for themselves and their children. The PLLR removes pregnancy letter categories—A, B, C, D and X. The PLLR also requires the label to be updated when information becomes outdated. **FIGURE 13-7** compares current prescription drug labeling with the new PLLR labeling requirements.

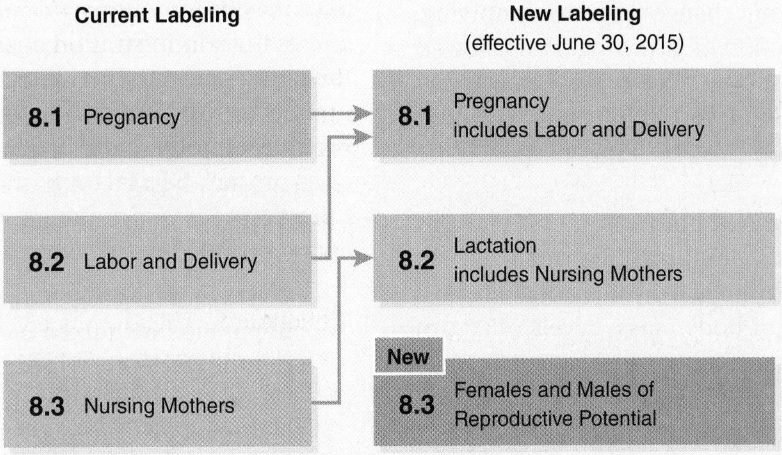

FIGURE 13-7 Comparison of Pregnancy and Lactation Labeling Rules: 1979 versus 2015.

Courtesy of U.S Food & Drug Administration.

[a]Only included when there are recommendations or requirements for pregnancy testing and/or contraception before, during, or after drug therapy, and/or there are human and/or animal data suggesting drug-associated effects on fertility and/or preimplantation loss effects.

Modified from: Lyons A, Petrucelli R. *Medicine: An Illustrated History*. New York, NY: Abradale Press; 1987.

multiple diseases requiring the use of several drugs (also referred to as polydrug usage). In addition, nutritional problems, decreased ability to metabolize drugs, and the possibility of decreased drug dosing compliance for a variety of reasons can influence the effects of drugs. This summary is meant to serve as a review of the pharmacokinetics that influence dosing principles in the older adult.

Age. Declines in the functional capacity of most major organ systems begin in young adulthood. These changes continue throughout life. Older adults do not lose specific function at a quicker rate as compared to young and middle-aged adults; rather, they have less physiologic reserves. Decreases in physiologic function (glomerular filtration rate, cardiac function, maximal breathing capacity) generally are accepted as beginning by age 45 years. Decreased renal function has the greatest impact on medication administration and drug clearance.

Absorption. Little evidence exists of major changes in drug absorption with age. Conditions associated with age, however, may alter the rate at which some drugs are absorbed, including altered nutritional habits, greater consumption of nonprescription drugs (eg, antacids, laxatives), and changes in gastric emptying. The reduced production of gastric acid and slowed gastric motility may have an impact and may result in unpredictable rates of dissolution and absorption of weakly acidic drugs.

Distribution. Changes in body composition have been noted in the older adult, including reduced lean body mass, reduced total body water, and increased fat as a percentage of body mass. Levels of serum albumin—which binds many drugs, especially weak acids—also usually decline. This decline affects drug distribution; it decreases protein binding of drugs, resulting in an increase in the amount of free drug in the circulation. Thus the ratio of bound to free drug in these patients may be significantly altered.

Biotransformation. The ability of the liver to metabolize drugs does not appear to decline consistently with age for all drugs. But disorders common with aging can impair liver function, such as congestive heart failure. Hepatic recovery from injury, such as that caused by alcohol or viral hepatitis, declines as well.

Certain drugs generally are believed to be metabolized more slowly in older adults because of decreased liver blood flow, which may lead to drug accumulation and toxicity. The paramedic must use caution when administering repeated doses of a medication that is metabolized primarily in the liver (eg, lidocaine) to a patient with a history of liver disease. Older patients with severe nutritional deficiencies also may have impaired hepatic function.

Elimination. Renal function is the most important factor for clearance of most drugs from the body. A natural reduction in renal function occurs with aging and usually is caused by loss of functioning nephrons and a decrease in blood flow. Both of these conditions result in a decreased glomerular filtration rate. A decrease in renal function caused by decreases in renal blood flow also may occur because of congestive heart failure. Renal impairment may result in a prolongation of the half-life of many drugs and the possibility of accumulation to toxic levels. Other reversible conditions (eg, dehydration) can cause further reduction in the renal clearance of drugs.

Drug Administration Problems. Older adults commonly do not comply with their drug therapy. Noncompliance may be intentional or unintentional and rarely affects the administration of emergency drugs. Still, the paramedic must be familiar with the most common factors that contribute to drug administration problems in older adults, because noncompliance or errors may be a factor in the patient's condition. Common causes of noncompliance and medication errors include the following:

- The expense of drugs may lead to noncompliance in patients with fixed incomes. Older patients may not take prescribed medications routinely or may be unwilling to receive medications in emergency situations.
- Noncompliance in taking prescribed medications may result from forgetfulness or confusion, especially if the patient has several prescriptions and different dosing intervals.
- Older patients may forget instructions on the need to complete medication because symptoms have disappeared. Disappearance of symptoms often is regarded by the patient as the best reason to stop the therapy.
- Errors in self-administered medications may result from physical disabilities such as arthritis or visual impairment.

- Noncompliance may be deliberate. A patient may be opposed to taking a drug because of past experiences or side effects of the drug. Drug effects such as fatigue related to beta blockers or frequent urination when taking a diuretic may influence a patient to stop taking drugs as prescribed. A careful drug history is especially important when caring for older adults. The paramedic should remember that a patient has the right to refuse medication.

Drugs That Affect the Nervous System

The actions of many drugs depend on which branch of the autonomic nervous system they affect and whether the branch is stimulated or inhibited by drug therapy. The paramedic must understand how pharmacology relates to the anatomy and physiology of the nervous system, which is the focus of this section. BOX 13-14 provides a list of drugs that affect the nervous system.

As described in Chapter 10, *Review of Human Systems*, the central nervous system (CNS) consists of the brain and spinal cord. The CNS serves as the collection point for nerve impulses (**FIGURE 13-8**). The peripheral nervous system consists of cranial and spinal nerves and all their branches (those nerves outside the CNS). The peripheral nervous system connects all parts of the body to the CNS. The somatic nervous system controls functions that are under conscious, voluntary control such as skeletal muscles and sensory neurons of the skin. The autonomic nervous system, comprised mostly of motor nerves, controls functions of involuntary smooth muscles, cardiac muscles, and glands.

BOX 13-14 Emergency Drugs: Nervous System

Atropine
Diazepam (Valium)
Dopamine (Intropin)
Epinephrine (Adrenalin)
Etomidate (Amidate)
Fentanyl (Sublimaze)
Hydromorphone (Dilaudid)
Ketamine (Ketalar)
Lorazepam (Ativan)
Magnesium sulfate
Midazolam (Versed)
Morphine (Astramorph PF)
Naloxone (Narcan)
Succinylcholine (Anectine)

The peripheral (sensory) nervous system receives stimuli from the body. The CNS interprets these stimuli. The peripheral (motor) nervous system initiates responses to the stimuli. Together, the visceral afferent and visceral efferent nerve fibers form the autonomic nervous system. In contrast, the somatic afferent and somatic efferent nerve fibers form the somatic nervous system. Thus, the autonomic nervous system and the somatic nervous system can be regarded as subdivisions of the peripheral nervous system.

Autonomic Division of the Peripheral Nervous System

The autonomic division of the peripheral nervous system provides almost every organ with a double set of nerve fibers: sympathetic (also known as **adrenergic**) and parasympathetic (also known as **cholinergic**). The cell bodies of the neurons in these two divisions are located in different areas of the CNS. They also exit the spinal cord at different levels. The sympathetic fibers exit from the thoracic and lumbar regions of the spinal cord. The parasympathetic fibers exit from the cranial and sacral portions of the spinal cord.

The sympathetic and parasympathetic systems generally work as physiologic antagonists on **effector organs**. That is, one division carries impulses that inhibit a certain function, and the other division usually carries impulses that augment that function. As a rule, the sympathetic system prepares the body for vigorous muscular activity, stress, and emergencies (fight or flight). The sympathetic nervous system tends to affect widespread areas of the body for sustained periods. In contrast, the parasympathetic system lowers muscular activity, operates during nonemergency situations, conserves energy, and produces selective and localized responses of short duration. The sympathetic and parasympathetic systems operate at the same time, yet one usually has more dominant effects at any given time.

Autonomic innervation by the sympathetic and parasympathetic nervous systems involves a two-neuron chain. This chain exists in a series between the CNS and the effector organs. This two-neuron chain is composed of a preganglionic neuron, located in the CNS, and a postganglionic neuron, located in the periphery. The functional

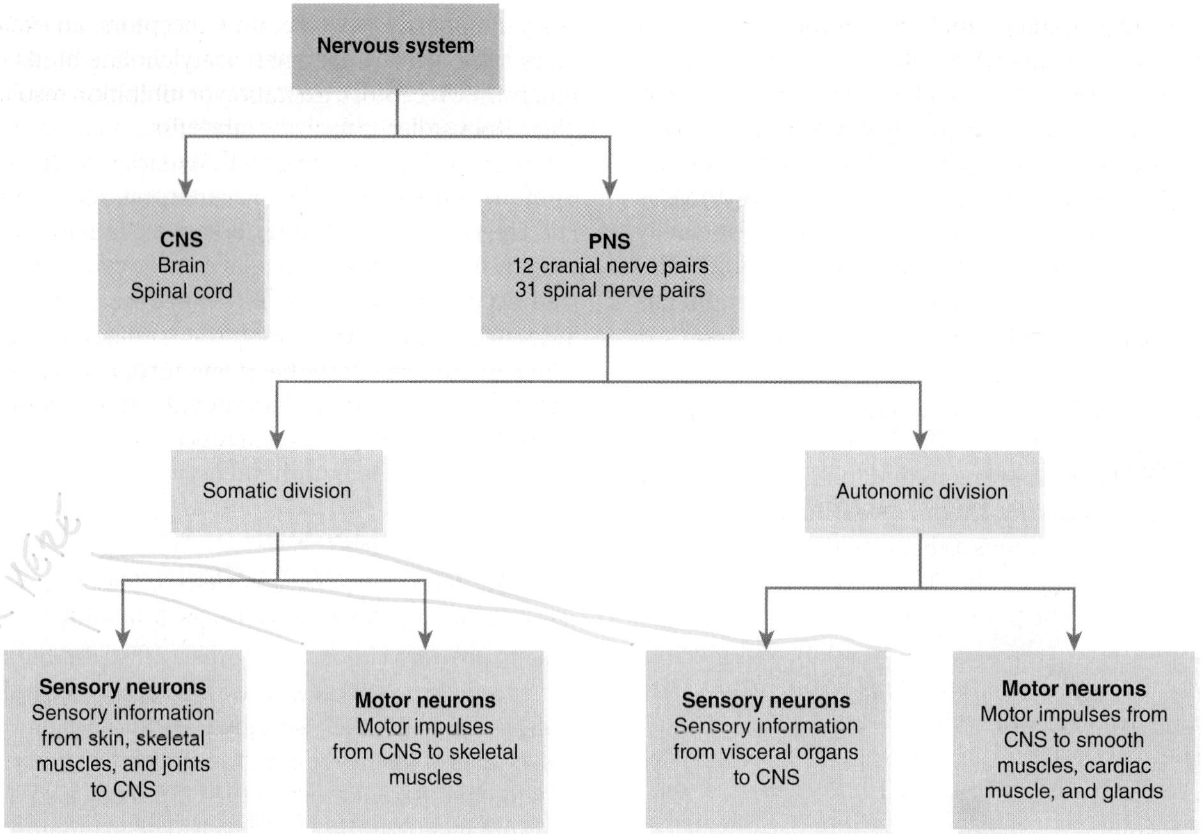

Abbreviations: CNS, central nervous system; PNS, peripheral nervous system

FIGURE 13-8 Overview of the nervous system.

junction between these two neurons is known as a synapse. The preganglionic fibers pass between the CNS and the nerve cell bodies in the peripheral nervous system (ganglia). The postganglionic fibers pass between the ganglia and the effector organ. Many of the sympathetic ganglia lie close to the spinal cord. Others lie about midway between the spinal cord and the effector organ. The parasympathetic ganglia lie close or within the walls of the effector organ. The difference in location of the ganglia in these two divisions is the anatomic reason for the widespread responses caused by the sympathetic division versus the localized responses caused by the parasympathetic division.

Neurochemical Transmission

Most neurons are separated electrically from each other. Because of this separation, the fibers communicate by way of **neurotransmitters**, which are chemicals that are released from one neuron at the presynaptic nerve fiber. These neurotransmitters then cross the synapse where they may be accepted by the next neuron at a specialized site called a receptor. (Neurotransmitters bind only to specific receptors on the postsynaptic membranes that recognize them.) The neurotransmitter then is deactivated or taken up into the presynaptic neuron.

In the sympathetic and parasympathetic divisions, the neurotransmitter for the preganglionic fiber at the junction between the preganglionic fiber and the synapse is **acetylcholine**. The neurotransmitter at the junction between the parasympathetic postganglionic fiber and the effector cell is also acetylcholine. Fibers that release acetylcholine are known as cholinergic fibers. All preganglionic neurons of the autonomic division and all postganglionic neurons of the parasympathetic division are cholinergic.

NOTE

All preganglionic nerves use the same neurotransmitter: acetylcholine.

The neurotransmitter between the sympathetic postganglionic fiber and the effector cell is norepinephrine. This chemical is a member of the catecholamine family. Fibers that release norepinephrine are known as adrenergic fibers. (This term is derived from noradrenaline, the British name for norepinephrine.) Most postganglionic neurons of the sympathetic division are adrenergic; that is, they release norepinephrine. However, a few are cholinergic. The actions of the autonomic nervous system depend on the interaction between the neurotransmitter released by the ganglionic cells and the receptor effector cells. For example, stimulation of the sympathetic nerves causes excitatory effects in some organs and inhibitory effects in others. Likewise, parasympathetic stimulation causes excitation in some organs but inhibition in others.

> NOTE
> Two different neurotransmitters exist for postganglionic neurons. All parasympathetic postganglionic neurons release acetylcholine onto their target tissue. Most sympathetic postganglionic neurons release norepinephrine onto their target tissue.

The parasympathetic and sympathetic systems function continuously. Most organs, however, are controlled predominantly by one or the other of the two systems.

Transmission of Nerve Impulses in the Autonomic Nervous System

Both branches of the autonomic nervous system have multiple receptors. The variety among neurotransmitters and receptors accounts for the differences in response to stimulation of sympathetic and parasympathetic nerves (excitatory or inhibitory).

The parasympathetic nervous system has nicotinic and muscarinic receptors (**FIGURE 13-9**). Nicotinic receptors (stimulated by nicotine) are found at the neuromuscular junctions of skeletal muscles. They also are found on the postganglionic neurons of the parasympathetic nervous system. Muscarinic receptors (stimulated by the mushroom poison muscarine) are found at the neuromuscular junction of cardiac and smooth muscle. They also are found on glands and on the postganglionic neurons of the sympathetic nervous system. Drugs that can activate nicotinic receptors typically do not activate muscarinic receptors. The difference between nicotinic and muscarinic receptors is crucial in drug therapy. For example, when acetylcholine binds to nicotinic receptors, an excitatory response occurs. When acetylcholine binds to muscarinic receptors, excitation or inhibition results. This response depends on the target tissue in which the receptors are found (**TABLE 13-3**). When acetylcholine binds to muscarinic receptors in cardiac muscle, the heart rate slows. When it binds to muscarinic receptors in smooth muscle cells of the gastrointestinal tract, the rate and amplitude of contraction increase. Atropine blocks muscarinic but not nicotinic receptor sites. (Thus atropine affects the heart rate but does not cause paralysis.) A drug such as curare (a nicotinic receptor blocker), however, causes paralysis.

> NOTE
> The two types of cholinergic receptors are nicotinic receptors and muscarinic receptors. Nicotinic responses are of fast onset and short duration and are excitatory. Nicotinic receptors are associated with preganglionic neurons of both branches of the autonomic nervous system. Muscarinic receptors are of slow onset and long duration and may be excitatory or inhibitory. These receptors are associated with the neuromuscular junction. The two major types of adrenergic receptors are alpha and beta. Both receptors can be excitatory or inhibitory.

> CRITICAL THINKING
> Imagine that your patient has eaten some poisonous mushrooms containing muscarine. What signs or symptoms related to pulse rate would you expect? What signs or symptoms related to gastrointestinal tract activity should be evident? Lastly, what signs or symptoms related to pupil diameter should be present?

For the sympathetic (adrenergic) nervous system, the major receptor types belong to two structural categories: the **alpha-adrenergic receptors** and the **beta-adrenergic receptors** (and their subgroups). Norepinephrine binds to and activates both types of receptor molecules. Yet norepinephrine has more affinity for alpha (α) receptors. The hormone epinephrine is produced by the adrenal medulla and is classified as an adrenergic substance. Epinephrine has nearly equal affinity for both receptors. In tissues containing alpha- and beta (β)-receptor cells, one type is more abundant. As a result, that type has a predominant effect. Both receptors can be excitatory or inhibitory. For example, beta receptors are stimulatory in cardiac

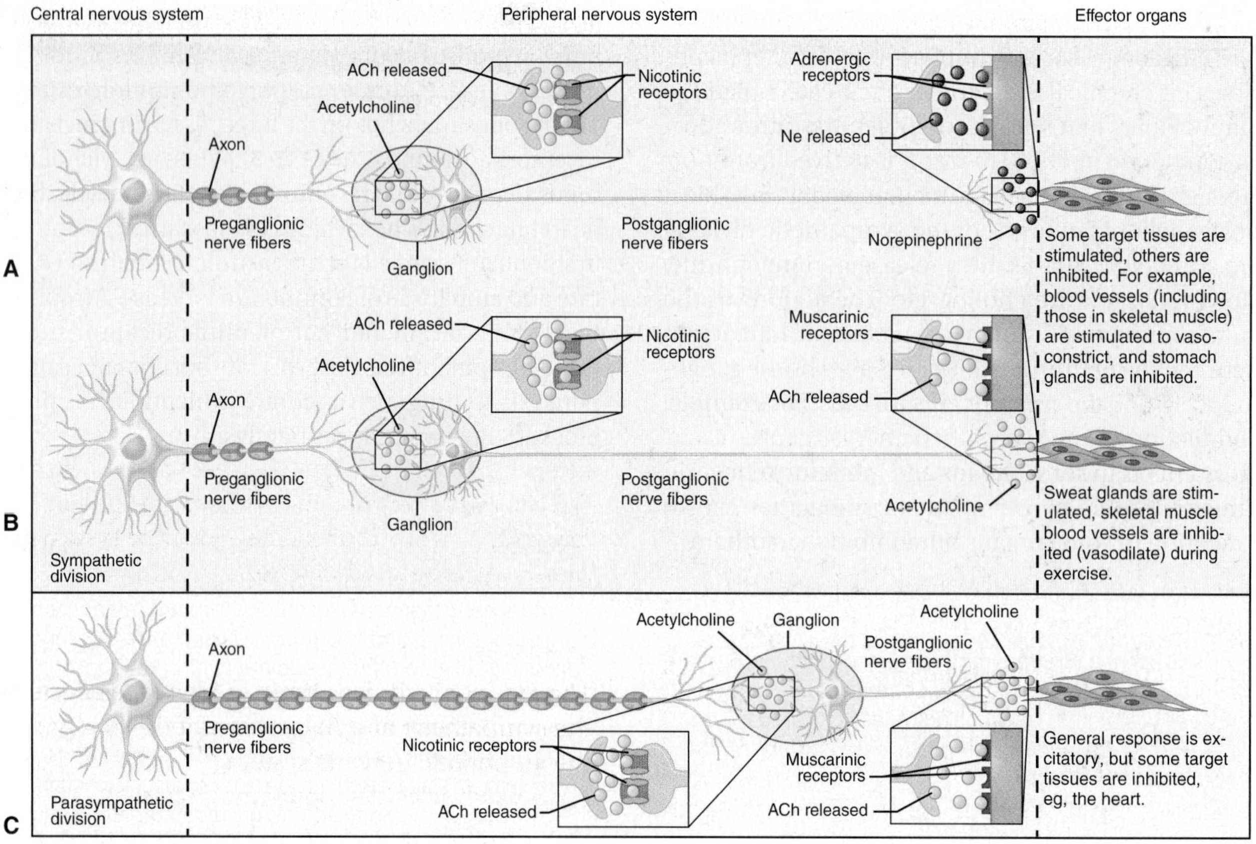

Abbreviations: ACh, acetylcholine; NE, norepinephrine

FIGURE 13-9 Nicotinic, muscarinic, and adrenergic receptors in the autonomic nervous system and their target tissues. Nicotinic receptors are found on the cell bodies of sympathetic and parasympathetic postganglionic cells in the autonomic ganglia. **A.** Adrenergic receptors are found in most target tissues innervated by the sympathetic division. **B.** Some sympathetic target tissues have muscarinic receptors. **C.** The parasympathetic nervous system uses acetylcholine as its primary neurotransmitter.

TABLE 13-3 Sites for Muscarinic and Nicotinic Actions of Acetylcholine

Site	Muscarinic Actions[a]	Nicotinic Actions
Cardiovascular		
Blood vessels	Dilation	Constriction
Heart rate	Slowed	Increased
Blood pressure	Decreased	Increased
Gastrointestinal		
Tone	Increased	Increased
Motility	Increased	Increased
Sphincters	Relaxed	None
Glandular secretions	Increased salivary, lacrimal, intestinal, and sweat secretion	Initial stimulation and then inhibition of salivary and bronchial secretions
Other		
Skeletal muscle	None	Stimulation

TABLE 13-3 Sites for Muscarinic and Nicotinic Actions of Acetylcholine *(continued)*

Autonomic ganglia	None	Stimulation
Eye	Pupil constriction	None
	Decreased accommodation	None
Blocking agent	Atropine	Tubocurarine
Remarks	Above effects increase as dosage increases	Increased dosage inhibits effects and causes receptor blockade

[a] Usual sites for therapeutic effects.

muscle. Yet they are inhibitory in intestinal smooth muscle (**TABLE 13-4**).

Drugs That Affect the Autonomic Nervous System

The nervous and endocrine systems are responsible for controlling and coordinating body functions. These two systems share three characteristics: a high level of integration in the brain, the ability to influence functions in distant regions of the body, and the extensive use of negative feedback mechanisms (described in Chapter 11, *General Principles of Pathophysiology*). One main difference between the two systems is the mode of transmission of information.

The endocrine system transmission is chiefly chemical. The information moves via bloodborne hormones. The hormones are not targeted for a specific organ. Instead, they diffusely affect many cells and organs at the same time. In contrast, the nervous system mainly relies on rapid electrical transmission of information over nerve fibers. Chemical impulses carry signals only between nerve cells and their effector cells in a localized manner, perhaps affecting only a few cells. (Drugs that affect the endocrine system are presented later in this chapter.)

Classifications

The autonomic drugs mimic or block the effects of the sympathetic and parasympathetic divisions of the autonomic nervous system (BOX 13-15). These drugs can be classified into four groups:

1. Cholinergic (parasympathomimetic) drugs, which mimic the actions of the parasympathetic nervous system
2. Cholinergic-blocking (parasympatholytic) drugs, which block the actions of the parasympathetic nervous system
3. Adrenergic (sympathomimetic) drugs, which mimic the actions of the sympathetic nervous system or the adrenal medulla
4. Adrenergic-blocking (sympatholytic) drugs, which block the actions of the sympathetic nervous system or adrenal medulla

BOX 13-15 Anatomic and Functional Terms for the Autonomic Nervous System

The anatomic names and functional terms for the autonomic nervous system often are used interchangeably: sympathetic or adrenergic, and parasympathetic or cholinergic. The terms *parasympathomimetic* and *sympathomimetic* mean to mimic or to produce an effect similar to activation of either system. The words *parasympatholytic* and *sympatholytic* mean to block the normal effects seen with activation of either system. The term *anticholinergic* is synonymous with *parasympatholytic*.

Anatomic Name	Functional Term	Primary Neurotransmitter
Sympathetic	Adrenergic	Norepinephrine
Parasympathetic	Cholinergic	Acetylcholine

TABLE 13-4 Autonomic Innervation of Target Tissues

Organ	Effect of Sympathetic Stimulation[a]	Effect of Parasympathetic Stimulation[a]
Heart		
Muscle	Increased rate and force (b)	Slowed rate (c)
Coronary arteries	Dilation (b),[b] constriction (a)[b]	Dilation (c)
Systemic blood vessels		
Abdomen	Constriction (a)	None
Skin	Constriction (a)	None
Muscle	Dilation (b, c), constriction (a)	None
Lungs, bronchi	Dilation (b)	Constriction (c)
Liver	Release of glucose into blood (b)	None
Skeletal muscles	Breakdown of glycogen to glucose (b)	None
Metabolism	Increase of up to 100% (a, b)	None
Glands		
Adrenal glands	Release of epinephrine and norepinephrine (c)	None
Salivary glands	Constriction of blood vessels and slight production of thick, viscous secretion (a)	Dilation of blood vessels and thin, copious secretion (c)
Gastric glands	Inhibition (a)	Stimulation (c)
Pancreas	Inhibition (a)	Stimulation (c)
Lacrimal glands	None	Secretion (c)
Sweat glands		
Merocrine glands	Copious, watery secretion (c)	None
Apocrine glands	Thick, organic secretion (c)	None
Gut		
Wall	Decreased tone (b)	Increased motility (c)
Sphincter	Increased tone (a)	Decreased tone (c)
Gallbladder and bile ducts	Relaxation (b)	Contraction (c)
Urinary bladder		
Wall	Relaxation (b)	Contraction (c)
Sphincter	Contraction (a)	Relaxation (c)
Eye		
Ciliary muscle	Relaxation for far vision (b)	Contraction for near vision (c)
Pupil	Dilation	Constriction (c)
Erector pili muscles	Contraction (a)	None
Blood	Increased coagulation (a)	None
Sex organs	Ejaculation (a)	Erection (c)

[a](a) Mediated by alpha receptors; (b) mediated by beta receptors; (c) mediated by cholinergic receptors.

[b]Normally blood flow through coronary arteries increases as a result of sympathetic stimulation of the heart because of increased demand by cardiac tissue for oxygen. In experiments that isolate the coronary arteries, however, sympathetic nerve stimulation, acting through alpha receptors, causes vasoconstriction. The beta receptors are relatively insensitive to sympathetic nerve stimulation but can be activated by drugs.

Cholinergic Drugs. As described earlier, acetylcholine plays a key role in the parasympathetic and sympathetic divisions of the nervous system. Acetylcholine has two major effects in the nervous system: (1) a stimulant effect on the ganglia, adrenal medulla, and skeletal muscle (the nicotinic effect) and (2) stimulant effects at postganglionic nerve endings in cardiac muscle, smooth muscle, and glands (the muscarinic effect). Drugs that affect nicotinic or cholinergic receptor sites on autonomic ganglia are ganglionic-stimulating drugs (eg, nicotine and nicotine gum) and ganglionic-blocking drugs (eg, mecamylamine).

Cholinergic drugs (choline esters) act directly with cholinergic receptors on postsynaptic membranes, or they act indirectly by inhibiting the enzyme that normally destroys acetylcholine. This inhibition results in an accumulation of acetylcholine. This in turn causes a longer and more intense response at various effector sites. Cholinergic drugs have little therapeutic value. For the most part, they are not thought of as emergency drugs. The main exception to this is physostigmine (Antilirium), which is an indirect-acting cholinergic drug. Physostigmine may be used to manage extreme cases of poisoning resulting from atropine-type drugs (see Chapter 33, *Toxicology*). Indirect-acting cholinergic drugs are used to treat myasthenia gravis, a condition characterized by weakness of the skeletal muscles (described in Chapter 32, *Nontraumatic Musculoskeletal Disorders*). These drugs work to elevate the concentration of acetylcholine at myoneural junctions. This in turn increases muscle strength and function.

Cholinergic-blocking (**anticholinergic**) agents have many uses in emergency medicine. These drugs work by blocking the muscarinic effects of acetylcholine. Thus they decrease the action of acetylcholine on its effector organ.

The best known cholinergic-blocking drug used in emergency care is atropine. Atropine is a belladonna alkaloid that acts as a competitive antagonist. Atropine works by occupying muscarinic receptor sites. This action prevents or reduces the muscarinic response to acetylcholine. Large doses dilate the pupils, inhibit accommodation of the eyes, and increase the heart rate by blocking the cholinergic effects of the heart. Synthetic substitutes for atropine have been created to obtain only the antispasmodic effects of the drug. (For example, they may be used to treat gastric and duodenal ulcers.) These synthetic drugs include dicyclomine (Bentyl) and glycopyrrolate (Robinul).

Adrenergic Drugs. Adrenergic drugs are designed to produce activities like those of neurotransmitters. The three types of adrenergic agents are direct acting, indirect acting, and dual acting (direct and indirect).

Three naturally occurring catecholamines are present in the body: epinephrine, norepinephrine, and dopamine. Epinephrine acts mainly as an emergency hormone. Epinephrine is released by the adrenal medulla. Norepinephrine acts as a vital neurotransmitter of nerve impulses. Dopamine is a precursor of epinephrine and norepinephrine. Dopamine has a neurotransmitter role of its own in certain parts of the CNS. Examples of synthetic catecholamine drugs and the three endogenous catecholamines are epinephrine, norepinephrine (Levophed), dopamine (Intropin), and dobutamine (Dobutrex).

Catecholamines depend on their ability to act directly with alpha and beta receptors. Two subgroups of alpha receptors have been identified. These are alpha$_1$ and alpha$_2$. Alpha$_1$ receptors are postsynaptic receptors. They are located on the effector organs. The chief role of the alpha$_1$ receptor is to stimulate contraction of smooth muscle. In the vasculature, this results in an increase in blood pressure. Alpha$_2$ receptors are found on presynaptic and postsynaptic nerve endings. When stimulated, presynaptic receptors inhibit the further release of norepinephrine. Like alpha$_1$ receptors, alpha$_2$ postsynaptic receptors produce vasoconstriction to increase resistance in blood vessels and thus increase blood pressure.

Beta receptors are subdivided into beta$_1$ and beta$_2$ receptors based on their response to drugs. However, the division also follows anatomic distinctions. Beta$_1$ receptors are located mainly in the heart. Beta$_2$ receptors are located mainly in the bronchiolar and arterial smooth muscle. Beta receptors stimulate the heart; dilate bronchioles; dilate blood vessels in the skeletal muscle, brain, and heart; and aid in glycogenolysis (the breakdown of glycogen to glucose) (**TABLE 13-5**).

> NOTE
>
> Use of a memory aid to differentiate the physiologic effects of beta receptors may be helpful: A person has one heart (beta$_1$ effects) and two lungs (beta$_2$ effects).

Norepinephrine acts mainly on alpha receptors. It causes almost pure vasoconstriction of the blood vessels. Epinephrine acts on alpha and beta receptors. It produces a mixture of vasodilation and vasoconstriction. This effect depends on the number of alpha and beta receptors present in the target tissue. The

TABLE 13-5 Actions of Autonomic Nervous System Neuroreceptors

Effector Organ or Tissue	Receptor	Adrenergic Effect	Cholinergic Effect
Eye, iris			
Radial muscle	α_1	Contraction (mydriasis)	None
Sphincter muscle		None	Contraction (miosis)
Eye, ciliary muscle	β_2	Relaxation for far vision	Contraction for near vision
Lacrimal glands	None		Secretion
Nasopharyngeal glands	None	None	Secretion
Salivary glands	α_1	Secretion of potassium and water	Secretion of potassium and water
	β	Secretion of amylase	None
Heart			
SA node	β_1	Increased heart rate	Decreased heart rate; vagus arrest
Atrial	β_1	Increased contractility and conduction velocity	Decreased contractility; shortened action potential duration
AV junction	β_1	Increased automaticity and propagation velocity	Decreased automaticity and propagation velocity
Purkinje system	β_1	Increased automaticity and propagation velocity	None
Ventricles	β_1	Increased contractility	None
Arterioles			
Coronary	α_1, β_2	Constriction, dilation	Dilation
Skin and mucosa	α_1, α_2	Constriction	Dilation
Skeletal muscle	α, β_2	Constriction, dilation	Dilation
Cerebral	α_1	Constriction (slight)	None
Pulmonary	α_1, β_2	Constriction, dilation	None
Mesenteric	α_1	Constriction	None
Renal	α_1, β_1, β_2,	Constriction, dilation	None
Salivary glands	α_1, α_2	Constriction	Dilation
Veins, systemic	α_1, β_2	Constriction, dilation	None
Lung			
Bronchial muscle	β_2	Relaxation	Contraction
Bronchial glands	α_1, β_2	Decreased secretion; increased secretion	Stimulation
Stomach			
Motility	α_1, β_2	Decreased (usually)	Increased
Sphincters	α_1	Contraction (usually)	Relaxation (usually)

Effector Organ or Tissue	Receptor	Adrenergic Effect	Cholinergic Effect
Secretion	None	Inhibition	Stimulation
Liver	α, β_2	Glycogenolysis and gluconeogenesis	Glycogen synthesis
Gallbladder and ducts	None	Relaxation	Contraction
Pancreas			
Acini	α	Decreased secretion	Secretion
Islet cells	α_2, β_2	Decreased secretion; increased secretion	None
Intestine			
Motility and tone	α_1, β_1, β_2	Decreased	Increased
Sphincters	α_1	Contraction (usually)	Relaxation (usually)
Secretion	α_2	Inhibition	Stimulation
Adrenal medulla	None	None	Secretion of epinephrine and norepinephrine (nicotinic effect)
Kidney			
Renin secretion	α_1, β_1	Decreased; increased	None
Ureter			
Motility and tone	α_1	Increased	Increased
Urinary bladder			
Detrusor muscle	β_2	Relaxation (usually)	Contraction
Trigone and sphincter	α_1	Contraction	Relaxation
Sex organs, male	α_1	Ejaculation	Erection
Skin			
Pilomotor muscles	α_1	Contraction	None
Sweat glands	α_1	Localized secretion	Generalized secretion
Fat cells	α_2; $\beta_1(\beta_3)$	Inhibition of lipolysis; stimulation of lipolysis	None
Pineal gland	β	Melatonin synthesis	None

Abbreviations: α, alpha; β, beta; AV, atrioventricular; SA, sinoatrial.

following are the most important alpha and beta activities in humans:

1. Alpha activities
   - Vasoconstriction of arterioles in the skin and splanchnic area, resulting in a rise in blood pressure and peripheral shunting of blood to the heart and brain from the shifting of blood volume
   - Pupil dilation
   - Relaxation of the gut
2. Beta activities
   - Cardiac acceleration and increased contractility
   - Vasodilation of arterioles supplying the skeletal muscle
   - Bronchial relaxation
   - Uterine relaxation

Indirect-acting adrenergic drugs act indirectly on receptors by triggering the release of the catecholamines norepinephrine and epinephrine. These chemicals then activate the alpha and beta receptors.

Dual-acting adrenergic drugs have indirect and direct effects. Ephedrine (ephedrine sulfate) is an example of a drug in this group.

Adrenergic-blocking agents may be classified into alpha- and beta-blocking drugs. Alpha-blocking drugs block the vasoconstricting effect of catecholamines and are used in certain cases of hypertension. They also are used to help prevent necrosis when norepinephrine or dopamine has leaked, or extravasated, into the tissues. They have limited clinical application in the prehospital setting.

NOTE

All drugs with alpha effects should be administered through a secure intravenous line. This line should be well positioned in a large vein because of the possibility of extravasation and tissue necrosis.

Beta-blocking agents have greater clinical application. They often are used in emergency care. These drugs block beta receptors. They inhibit the action of beta receptors at the effector site. Beta-blocking agents are grouped into **selective beta-blocking agents** and **nonselective beta-blocking agents.** The selective blocking agents block $beta_1$ or $beta_2$ receptors. The nonselective beta-blocking agents block $beta_1$- and $beta_2$-receptor sites. Selective $beta_1$-blocking agents also are known as cardioselective blockers because they block the $beta_1$ receptors in the heart with minimal $beta_2$ activities in the lungs. Examples of important selective $beta_1$-blocking agents are metoprolol (Lopressor, Toprol-XL) and atenolol (Tenormin). These drugs are antihypertensives and antidysrhythmics. They are used in managing hypertension. They also are used in select patients with suspected myocardial infarction and high-risk unstable angina.

Nonselective beta-blocking agents inhibit beta receptors in the smooth muscle both of the bronchioles and of the blood vessels. Examples include the antianginal antihypertensives nadolol (Corgard) and propranolol (Inderal), and the antihypertensive labetalol (Normodyne, Trandate). (Labetalol also has some alpha-blocking activity.)

CRITICAL THINKING

Physicians usually will not prescribe a nonselective beta blocker such as propranolol for patients with a history of asthma. Explain why this is true.

Narcotic Analgesics and Antagonists

Narcotic analgesics relieve pain. Narcotic antagonists reverse the effects of some narcotic analgesics. Pain has two components: First is the sensation of pain, which involves the nerve pathways and the brain, and second is the emotional response to pain, which may be a result of the patient's anxiety level, previous pain experience, age, sex, and culture. BOX 13-16 lists and defines classifications of pain.

Opiates are drugs that contain or are extracted from opium. The term *opioid* refers to synthetic drugs. These drugs have pharmacologic properties that are similar to those of opium or morphine. Morphine is the chief alkaloid of opium. Opioids work by binding with opioid receptors in the brain and other body organs, thus altering the patient's perception of pain and the emotional response to a pain-causing stimulus. Opioid analgesics include morphine, codeine,

NOTE

Endorphins serve as the body's own supply of "opiates." Endorphins are produced by the pituitary gland and the hypothalamus during strenuous exercise, excitement, pain, and orgasm. They resemble the opiates in their abilities to produce analgesia by binding to opiate receptors, thereby blocking pain. They also produce a sense of well-being. Endorphins work as "natural pain relievers," whose effects may be enhanced by other medications.

BOX 13-16 Classifications of Pain

Acute pain. Pain sudden in onset that usually subsides with treatment (eg, pain associated with acute myocardial infarction, acute appendicitis, renal colic, or traumatic injuries)

Chronic pain. Persistent or recurrent pain that is difficult to treat (eg, pain that accompanies cancer and rheumatoid arthritis)

Referred pain. Visceral pain felt at a site distant from its origin (eg, pain from a myocardial infarction felt in the arm)

Somatic pain. Pain arising from skeletal muscles, ligaments, vessels, or joints

Superficial pain. Pain arising from the skin or mucous membrane

Visceral pain. "Deep" pain arising from smooth musculature or organ systems that may be difficult to localize and is often described as dull or aching

COX

hydromorphone (Dilaudid), meperidine (Demerol), fentanyl (Duragesic, Sublimaze), methadone (Dolophine, Methadose), oxycodone (OxyContin, Percodan, Tylox, Percocet), hydrocodone (Lortab, Vicodin), and propoxyphene (Darvon, Dolene).

Opioid analgesics may produce undesirable effects such as nausea and vomiting, constipation, urinary retention, orthostatic hypotension, respiratory depression, and CNS depression. Most of these effects can be avoided by careful administration and close patient monitoring.

Opioid antagonists block the effects of opioid analgesics by displacing the analgesics from their receptor sites. (Examples of such effects are opioid-induced respiratory depression and sedation.) Naloxone, naltrexone (Trexan), and nalmefene (Revex) are opioid antagonists.

Opioid agonist–antagonist agents have analgesic and antagonist effects. They are thought to have pharmacokinetic and adverse effects similar to those of morphine. These agents, such as pentazocine (Talwin), nalbuphine (Nubain), and buprenorphine (Suboxone), may antagonize some opioid receptors competitively, although they may have varying degrees of agonist effect at other opioid receptor sites. These drugs generally have a lower potential for creating dependency than do opioid analgesics. In addition, withdrawal symptoms may be initiated in addicts but are not as severe as those of the opioid agonist drugs.

NOTE

Carfentanil is a synthetic opioid that was made to tranquilize elephants and other large mammals. Because it is 10,000 times more potent than morphine and 100 times more potent than fentanyl and is sold as heroin, it has caused a significant number of overdose deaths. It is of particular concern to EMS and other first responders because it can be absorbed through the skin or inhaled by first responders, causing serious illness. (See Chapter 33, *Toxicology*.)

Modified from: DEA issues carfentanil warning to police and public. US Drug Enforcement Administration website. https://www.dea.gov/divisions/hq/2016/hq092216.shtml. Published December 22, 2016. Accessed December 13, 2017.

Non-narcotic Analgesics

Non-narcotic analgesics act by a peripheral mechanism that interferes with local mediators released when tissue is damaged. These mediators stimulate nerve endings, causing pain. When non-narcotic analgesics are used, the nerve endings in damaged tissues are stimulated less often. This mechanism differs from that of narcotic analgesics, which act at the level of the CNS. An example of a non-narcotic analgesic is ketorolac (Toradol), a nonsteroidal anti-inflammatory drug (NSAID) that exhibits analgesic activity. Other non-narcotic analgesics include cyclooxygenase (COX) inhibitors and oral NSAIDs such as ibuprofen (eg, Advil), naproxen (eg, Aleve), and acetaminophen (described later in this chapter).

Q21

CRITICAL THINKING

A non-narcotic analgesic may be selected instead of a narcotic for a paramedic returning to work on the ambulance. Why?

Anesthetics

Anesthetic drugs are CNS depressants. They have a reversible action on nervous tissue. The three major types of anesthesia are general, regional, and local. General anesthesia is achieved by intravenous or inhalation routes and is the most common type of anesthesia used during surgery to induce unconsciousness. Regional anesthesia is obtained by injecting a local anesthetic drug. The drug is injected near a nerve trunk or at specific sites in a large region of the body (eg, spinal block). Local anesthesia is achieved topically to produce a loss of sensation. Local anesthesia also can be achieved by injection to block an area surrounding an operative field, making it insensitive to pain (BOX 13-17).

Antianxiety and Sedative-Hypnotic Agents and Alcohol

Antianxiety agents, sedative-hypnotic agents, and alcohol are presented together because of their similarities in pharmacologic action. Antianxiety agents are used to reduce feelings of apprehension, nervousness, worry, or fearfulness.

Sedatives and hypnotics are drugs that depress the CNS, produce a calming effect, and help induce sleep (BOX 13-18). The major difference between a sedative and a hypnotic is the degree of CNS depression induced by the agent. For example, a small dose of an agent administered to calm a patient is called a sedative; a

BOX 13-17 Anesthetics

Inhalation Anesthetics

Gases
Cyclopropane
Nitrous oxide/oxygen (Nitronox)

Volatile Liquids
Halothane (Fluothane)
Methoxyflurane (Penthrane)
Enflurane (Ethrane)
Isoflurane (Forane)
Sevoflurane (Ultane)
Desflurane (Suprane)

Intravenous Anesthetics

Ultrashort-Acting Barbiturates
Thiopental sodium (Pentothal)
Thiamylal sodium (Surital)
Methohexital sodium (Brevital Sodium)

Nonbarbiturates
Etomidate (Amidate)
Fentanyl (Sublimaze)
Sufentanil (Sufenta)
Alfentanil (Alfenta)
Propofol (Diprivan)

Dissociative Anesthetics
Ketamine (Ketalar)

Neuroleptic Anesthetics
Droperidol-fentanyl (Innovar injection)

Local Anesthetics

Topical
Benzocaine (Anbesol)
Ethyl chloride cocaine
Lidocaine (Xylocaine)
Tetracaine (Pontocaine)

Injectable
Lidocaine (Xylocaine)
Procaine (Novocain)

larger dose of the same agent sufficient to induce sleep is called a hypnotic. Thus an agent may be a sedative or a hypnotic, depending on the dose used.

As stated before, alcohol has actions that are characteristic of sedative-hypnotic or antianxiety drugs. Alcohol is a major source of drug abuse and dependency.

Scattered throughout the brainstem is a group of nuclei, collectively called the reticular formation. The reticular formation and its neural pathways compose a system known as the reticular activating system (described in Chapter 10, *Review of Human Systems*). This system is involved with the sleep–wake cycle. Through these pathways, the reticular activating system collects incoming signals from the senses and viscera. The system then processes and passes these signals to the higher brain centers. The reticular activating system determines the level of awareness to the environment. Thus the reticular activating system also governs actions and responses to the environment. Antianxiety and sedative-hypnotic agents and alcohol act by depressing this system.

BOX 13-18 The Physiology of Sleep

Sleep can be viewed as a series of rhythms. Each has its own brain wave patterns. These rhythms can be divided into two major categories: rapid eye movement (REM) and non–rapid eye movement (non-REM). During sleep, a person moves through REM sleep. Then the person moves through four stages of non-REM sleep. REM, or active, sleep is the time of irregular body activity, vivid dreaming, and REM. During REM sleep, the eyes move back and forth under the closed lids as they follow the action of a dream. The heart rate, blood pressure, and respirations may become irregular. During non-REM sleep, the person drifts out of wakeful awareness. The muscles relax, and the blood pressure, heartbeat, and breathing begin to decline. The brain sends signals to the arms, legs, and other large muscles to stop moving. At that point, "sleep paralysis" occurs. The first REM period lasts nearly 10 minutes. The whole cycle repeats itself usually four to five times each night. Each cycle lasts an average of 90 minutes. As the night continues, REM periods lengthen and non-REM periods shorten. The final REM period of the night may last as long as 1 hour.

Classifications

Two prototypical groups of drugs are used to treat anxiety and to induce sleep. These are the benzodiazepines and barbiturates, respectively. Benzodiazepines make up the drug class most often used today to treat anxiety and insomnia. Barbiturates compose an older drug class with many uses. These uses range from sedation to anesthesia.

Benzodiazepines. Benzodiazepines were introduced in the 1960s as antianxiety drugs. Currently they are among the most widely prescribed drugs in clinical medicine, partly because of their wide therapeutic index. Mortality and morbidity from an oral overdose is rare, unless taken with other CNS depressants, such as alcohol.[9] Benzodiazepines are thought to work by binding to specific receptors in the cerebral cortex and limbic system. (These systems together govern emotional behavior.) These drugs are highly lipid soluble and are distributed widely in the body tissues. They also are highly bound (more than 80%) to plasma protein. Benzodiazepines reduce anxiety and are a sedative-hypnotic, muscle relaxant, and anticonvulsant. All benzodiazepines are schedule IV drugs because of their potential for abuse. Commonly prescribed benzodiazepines are alprazolam (Xanax), clonazepam (Klonopin), diazepam (Valium), flurazepam (Dalmane), midazolam (Versed), lorazepam (Ativan), and temazepam (Restoril).

CRITICAL THINKING

Consider that you are preparing to reduce a dislocated shoulder. Why would a benzodiazepine be preferred over a narcotic?

NOTE

Flumazenil (Romazicon) is a specific benzodiazepine receptor antagonist. Flumazenil has been shown to be effective in reversing benzodiazepine-induced sedation and coma (see Chapter 33, *Toxicology*, and the Appendix, *Emergency Drug Index*).

Modified from: Rosen P, Barkin R. *Emergency Medicine: Concepts and Clinical Practice*. 8th ed. St Louis, MO: Mosby; 2014.

Barbiturates. Barbiturates were once the most commonly prescribed class of medications for sedative-hypnotic effects. However, they virtually have been replaced by the benzodiazepines. Barbiturates are divided into four classes according to their duration of action: ultrashort acting, short acting, intermediate acting, and long acting. The differences in onset and duration of action depend on their lipid solubility and protein-binding properties. Ultrashort-acting barbiturates commonly are used as intravenous anesthetics, such as thiopental sodium (Pentothal). These drugs act rapidly and can produce a state of anesthesia in a few seconds.

Short-acting barbiturates produce an effect in a short time (10 to 15 minutes). They also peak over a short period (3 to 4 hours) and are rarely used to treat insomnia. These barbiturates, such as pentobarbital (Nembutal) and secobarbital (Seconal), more often are used for preanesthesia sedation and in combination with other drugs for psychosomatic disorders.

Intermediate-acting barbiturates have an onset of 45 to 60 minutes. They peak in 6 to 8 hours. Short-acting and intermediate-acting barbiturates, such as amobarbital (Amytal) and butabarbital (Butisol), produce similar patient responses.

Long-acting barbiturates require more than 60 minutes for onset. They peak over 10 to 12 hours. These agents, such as mephobarbital (Mebaral) and phenobarbital (Luminal), are used to treat epilepsy and other chronic neurologic disorders (see Chapter 24, *Neurology*) and also are used to sedate patients with severe anxiety.

Miscellaneous Sedative-Hypnotic Drugs. The previously discussed drug classes do not include all of the antianxiety and sedative-hypnotic drugs. In fact, a number of other antianxiety and sedative-hypnotic drugs do not fall into these classes. These agents are more similar to barbiturates than to benzodiazepines because they are generally shorter acting. Examples of miscellaneous drugs with antianxiety and sedative-hypnotic effects are chloral hydrate (Noctec), eszopiclone (Lunesta), and zolpidem (Ambien). In addition to these drugs, antihistamines such as hydroxyzine (Vistaril, Atarax) have pronounced sedative effects. Etomidate (Amidate) is another nonbarbiturate, hypnotic anesthetic used for premedication for tracheal intubation and cardioversion.

Alcohol Intake and Behavioral Effects

Alcohol is a general CNS depressant that can produce sedation, sleep, and anesthesia. In addition, alcohol enhances the sedative-hypnotic effects of other drug classes, including all general CNS depressants, antihistamines, phenothiazines, narcotic analgesics, and tricyclic antidepressants. If alcohol is taken with other drugs, this enhancement could result in coma or death. Blood alcohol levels are measured in milligrams per deciliter (mg/dL). Characteristic behavioral effects can be predicted based on the amount of alcohol consumed and blood alcohol levels. Behavioral effects associated with alcohol intake are described further in Chapter 33, *Toxicology*.

Anticonvulsants

Anticonvulsant drugs are used to treat seizure disorders. The most notable of these disorders is epilepsy. Epilepsy is a neurologic disorder characterized by a recurrent pattern of abnormal neuronal discharges within the brain. These discharges result in a sudden loss or disturbance of consciousness, sometimes associated with motor activity, sensory phenomena, or inappropriate behavior. Epilepsy is estimated to occur in 0.5% to 1% of the population. In 50% of these cases, the cause is unknown (primary or idiopathic epilepsy). Secondary epilepsy is epilepsy that can be traced to trauma, infection, a cerebrovascular disorder, or some other illness. (Epilepsy is discussed further in Chapter 24, *Neurology*.)

Anticonvulsant drugs work by depressing the excitability of neurons that fire to initiate the seizure. These drugs also suppress the neurons responsible for the spread of the seizure discharge. Anticonvulsants are presumed to modify the ionic movements of sodium, potassium, or calcium across the nerve membrane. Thus they reduce the response to incoming electrical or chemical stimulation. Benzodiazepines also stimulate major inhibitory neurotransmitters in the CNS. Many patients need drug therapy throughout their lives to control seizure disorders.

Several drugs are available for the control of seizure disorders. The choice of drug depends on the type of seizure disorder (generalized, partial, or status; described in Chapter 24, *Neurology*). The choice of drug also depends on the patient's tolerance and response to the prescribed medication. **BOX 13-19** presents classes of anticonvulsant drugs.

BOX 13-19 Classes of Anticonvulsant Drugs

Barbiturates

Phenobarbital (Luminal)

Benzodiazepines

Clonazepam (Klonopin)
Diazepam (Valium)
Lorazepam (Ativan)

Hydantoins

Fosphenytoin (Cerebyx)
Phenytoin (Dilantin)

Succinimides

Ethosuximide (Zarontin)
Zonisamide (Zonegran)

Other

Carbamazepine (Tegretol)
Divalproex (Depakote)
Gabapentin (Neurontin)
Lamotrigine (Lamictal)
Magnesium sulfate
Topiramate (Topamax)
Valproic acid (Depakene)
Levetiracetam (Keppra)

CNS Stimulants

Drugs that stimulate the CNS are classified by where they exert their major effects in the nervous system: on the cerebrum, on the medulla and brainstem, or in the hypothalamic limbic regions. All CNS stimulants work to increase excitability by blocking activity of inhibitory neurons or their respective neurotransmitters or by enhancing the production of the excitatory neurotransmitters. Some of the more common CNS stimulant drugs are anorexiants and amphetamines.

Anorexiants

Anorexiants are appetite suppressants that are used to treat obesity. They work by producing a direct stimulant effect on the hypothalamic and limbic regions and may have this effect on other areas of the nervous system as well. Examples of anorexiants include phendimetrazine (Plegine) and mazindol (Mazanor, Sanorex).

A new class of drugs, gastrointestinal lipase inhibitors (or fat blockers), such as orlistat (Xenical), block the absorption of about 30% of dietary fat. These drugs sometimes are used to manage obesity along with a reduced-calorie diet.

DID YOU KNOW?

At one time, a two-drug combination of fenfluramine and phentermine (Fen-Phen) was used to manage obesity. The combination was withdrawn from the market in 1997. It was found to have serious complications, including potentially fatal primary pulmonary hypertension and valvular heart disease.

Amphetamines

Amphetamines stimulate the cerebral cortex and reticular activating system, which increases alertness and responsiveness to environmental surroundings.

Amphetamines mainly are used to treat attention-deficit/hyperactivity disorder (ADHD), attention-deficit disorder (ADD), and narcolepsy. ADHD is seen mostly in children and adolescents and is characterized by a short attention span and impulsive behavior. (ADHD and ADD are described further in Chapter 34, *Behavioral and Psychiatric Disorders.*)

People with narcolepsy experience excessive drowsiness, sudden sleep attacks during daytime hours, and sometimes sleep paralysis. Medications used to treat these disorders include methamphetamine (Desoxyn), amphetamine-mixed salts (Adderall), and dextroamphetamine tablets and elixir. Nonamphetamine CNS stimulants used to treat ADHD and ADD include methylphenidate (Ritalin, Concerta), atomoxetine (Strattera), and pemoline (Cylert). Paradoxically, amphetamines and other stimulants have a calming effect on people with ADHD. Likely, the drugs achieve this effect by increasing neurotransmitter levels of dopamine.

Psychotherapeutic Drugs

Psychotherapeutic drugs include antipsychotic agents, antidepressants, and lithium. These drugs are used to treat psychoses and affective disorders, especially schizophrenia, depression, and mania (see Chapter 34, *Behavioral and Psychiatric Disorders*).

CNS and Emotions

The neurotransmitters acetylcholine, norepinephrine, dopamine, serotonin, and monoamine oxidase have a major effect on emotion (**FIGURE 13-10**). Alterations in the levels of these chemicals are linked to changes in mood and behavior. Drug therapy alleviates symptoms by temporarily modifying unwanted behavior.

> NOTE
>
> Acetylcholine is released from central neural tissue into the cerebrospinal fluid during activity. Norepinephrine and dopamine have widespread inhibitory effects. They influence functions such as sleep and arousal, affect, and memory. Serotonin levels affect mood and behavior. Monoamine oxidase is an enzyme that inactivates dopamine and serotonin, both of which are produced during intense emotional states.

Antipsychotic Agents

The main use of antipsychotic drugs is to treat schizophrenia. This class of drugs is the only clearly effective treatment for this condition. There are other psychiatric indications for the use of antipsychotic drugs. These drugs are used to treat Tourette syndrome. They also are used to control disturbing behavior in patients with senile dementia associated

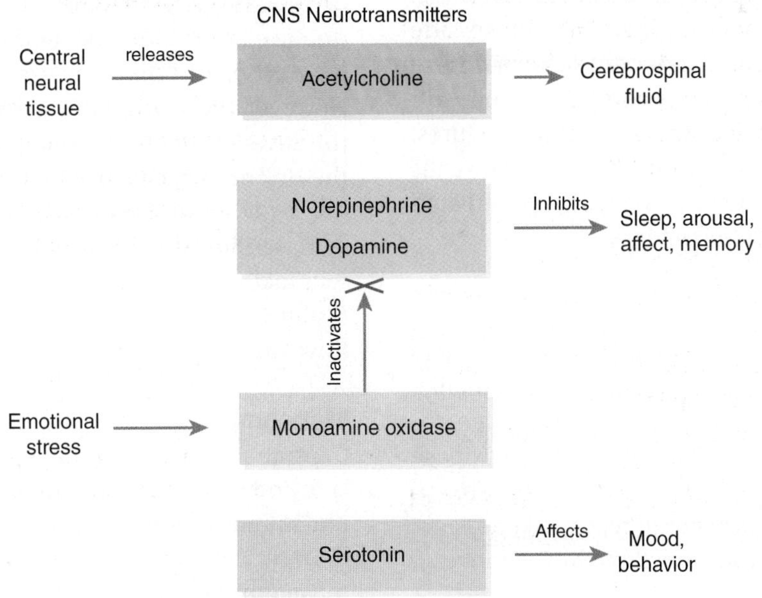

Abbreviation: CNS, central nervous system

FIGURE 13-10 Neurotransmitters in the brain and their effects on emotion.

with Alzheimer disease, but only after nonpharmacologic interventions have been attempted. Effective antipsychotic (neuroleptic) drugs block dopamine receptors in specific areas of the CNS. These drugs can be classified into the following groups:

- Phenothiazine derivatives
  - Chlorpromazine (Thorazine)
  - Thioridazine (Mellaril)
  - Fluphenazine (Prolixin)
- Butyrophenone derivatives
  - Haloperidol (Haldol)
- Dihydroindolone derivatives
  - Molindone (Moban)
- Dibenzoxazepine derivatives
  - Loxapine (Loxitane)
- Thienbenzodiazepine derivatives
  - Olanzapine (Zyprexa)
- Atypical agents
  - Clozapine (Clozaril)
  - Risperidone (Risperdal)

With continued use of certain antipsychotics, some patients develop supersensitivity of dopamine receptors. This supersensitivity can lead to tardive dyskinesia or dystonia. **Tardive dyskinesia** is a potentially irreversible neurologic disorder characterized by involuntary repetitious movements of the muscles of the face, limbs, and trunk. Other identifying features include excessive blinking of the eyelids, lip smacking, tongue protrusion, foot tapping, and side-to-side rocking. **Dystonia** is characterized by local or diffuse changes in muscle tone. This condition can result in painful muscle spasms, unusually fixed postures, and strange movement patterns. A patient who calls 9-1-1 reporting an acute onset of dystonia is treated with diphenhydramine (Benadryl).

Antidepressants

Antidepressants are used to treat affective disorders (mood disturbances), including depression, mania, and elation. Tricyclic antidepressants, selective serotonin reuptake inhibitors, and monoamine oxidase inhibitors are prescribed for depression; lithium (an antimanic drug) is the preferred treatment for mania (see Chapter 34, *Behavioral and Psychiatric Disorders*).

Tricyclic Antidepressants. Tricyclic antidepressants, such as nortriptyline (Pamelor) and amitriptyline (Elavil), are thought to treat depression by increasing levels (blocking the reuptake) of the neurotransmitters norepinephrine and serotonin. Excessive doses of these drugs (eg, tricyclic antidepressant overdose) have the potential for cardiac dysrhythmias and cardiovascular collapse (see Chapter 33, *Toxicology*).

> **NOTE**
>
> Depression may be exogenous or endogenous. Exogenous depression results from a person's response to a loss or disappointment (eg, "the blues"). This type of depression is considered a normal reaction to the precipitating event. It is usually temporary and remits without the use of drug therapy. Endogenous depression, however, lasts 6 months or longer. This type of depression is characterized by the absence of external causes; it may be the result of genetic or biochemical alterations. Antidepressants often are needed to treat endogenous depression. Depression is discussed further in Chapter 34, *Behavioral and Psychiatric Disorders*.

> **CRITICAL THINKING**
>
> You know that tricyclic antidepressants increase the levels of norepinephrine. Thus what side effects might you expect in an overdose?

Selective Serotonin Reuptake Inhibitors. Selective serotonin reuptake inhibitors work to block the reabsorption or reuptake of serotonin, thus making more of the chemical available to the brain. These drugs do have some side effects; for example, insomnia, headache, and diarrhea are common complaints. However, these drugs often treat depression without the adverse effects of other antidepressants, such as the dry mouth caused by tricyclic antidepressants or the dietary restrictions mandated by monoamine oxidase inhibitors. Examples of selective serotonin reuptake inhibitors are fluoxetine (Prozac), sertraline (Zoloft), paroxetine (Paxil), escitalopram (Lexapro), fluvoxamine (Luvox), and citalopram (Celexa).

Monoamine Oxidase Inhibitor Antidepressants. Central-acting monoamines, especially norepinephrine and serotonin, are thought to cause depression and mania. Monoamine oxidase is an enzyme found in nerve cells and is thought to be produced during tense emotional states. The enzyme is responsible for metabolizing norepinephrine within the nerve. Monoamine oxidase inhibitors block this enzyme, which leads to increased levels of norepinephrine. Examples of monoamine oxidase inhibitors used to treat depression include isocarboxazid (Marplan), phenelzine (Nardil), and tranylcypromine (Parnate). Monoamine oxidase inhibitors also are used as antihypertensive agents (described later in this chapter).

NOTE

The monoamine oxidase inhibitors used in psychiatric practice are irreversible inhibitors of both forms (A and B) of brain monoamine oxidase. These drugs are rarely used today because of their potentially dangerous interactions with dietary tyramine and other agents that have sympathomimetic or serotoninergic properties.

Modified from: Goldman L, Schafer AI. *Goldman-Cecil Medicine*. 25th ed. Philadelphia, PA: Elsevier Saunders; 2016.

Lithium. Lithium is a cation that is closely related to sodium. Both cations are transported actively across cell membranes. However, lithium cannot be pumped as effectively out of the cell as sodium and therefore accumulates in the cells, resulting in a decrease in intracellular sodium concentration and possibly improvement in manic symptoms. In addition, lithium appears to enhance some of the actions of serotonin, may decrease levels of norepinephrine and dopamine, and appears to block the development of dopamine receptor supersensitivity that may accompany long-term therapy with antipsychotic agents. Lithium carbonate is used to treat manic disorders, such as bipolar disorder. Toxicity is common because lithium has a narrow therapeutic range

Drugs for Specific CNS–Neuromuscular Dysfunction

Several movement disorders result from an imbalance of dopamine and acetylcholine. Two of the most common are Parkinson disease (including parkinsonism syndromes) and Huntington disease.

Parkinson Disease

Parkinson disease is a chronic disabling disease characterized by rigidity of voluntary muscles. Parkinson disease also is characterized by tremor of the fingers and extremities. The most common risk factors are increasing age, male sex, and pesticide exposure.[10] Parkinson disease has also been reported after acute encephalitis or cases of carbon monoxide or metallic poisoning or from the use of some illicit drugs. The disease is thought to result from an abnormally low concentration of dopamine. Parkinsonism syndromes mimic the symptoms of Parkinson disease and are usually of an unknown cause (**idiopathic**) but may result from treatment with antipsychotic drugs (drug-induced parkinsonism) that block dopaminergic receptors (eg, haloperidol, metoclopramide [Clopra, Emex], and phenothiazines). Symptoms of Parkinson disease include the following:

- Immobile facial expression (parkinsonism facies)
- Bobbing of the head
- Resting tremor
- Pill-rolling of the fingers
- Shuffling gait
- Forward flexion of the trunk
- Loss of postural reflexes

Huntington Disease

Huntington disease is an inherited disorder characterized by progressive dementia and involuntary muscle twitching (chorea). Like Parkinson disease, Huntington disease is thought to be related to an imbalance of dopamine, acetylcholine, and perhaps other neurotransmitters.

Drugs With Central Anticholinergic Activity

Drugs that inhibit or block acetylcholine are referred to as anticholinergic. They work by restoring the normal dopamine–acetylcholine balance in the brain. Common anticholinergic agents include benztropine (tablets and injections), ethopropazine hydrochloride, and ipratropium (Atrovent). Another commonly prescribed anticholinergic is donepezil (Aricept) that is used to treat dementia in patients with mild-to-moderate Alzheimer disease.

Drugs That Affect Dopamine in the Brain

Three classifications of drugs affect dopamine in the brain: those that release dopamine, those that increase brain levels of dopamine, and dopaminergic agonists (BOX 13-20). Levodopa (l-dopa) is a drug that increases brain levels of dopamine. Levodopa is the current drug of choice in the treatment of movement disorders associated with dopamine–acetylcholine imbalance.

Monoamine Oxidase Inhibitors

Two types of monoamine oxidase inhibitors have been identified: monoamine oxidase A, which metabolizes

BOX 13-20 Drugs That Affect Dopamine in the Brain

Amantadine (Symmetrel)
Bromocriptine (Parlodel)
Carbidopa-levodopa (Sinemet)
Levodopa (Larodopa)
Pergolide (Permax)

norepinephrine and serotonin, and monoamine oxidase B, which metabolizes dopamine. Selegiline (Deprenyl) is a selective inhibitor of monoamine oxidase B that delays the breakdown of dopamine. Selegiline often is used along with levodopa because it enhances and prolongs the antiparkinsonism effects of levodopa. (Selegiline allows the dose of levodopa to be reduced.)

Skeletal Muscle Relaxants

Skeletal muscle contraction is evoked by a nicotinic cholinergic transmission process. Just as the autonomic ganglionic transmission can be modified by drugs, so too can skeletal muscle contractions. Skeletal muscle relaxants can be classified as central-acting relaxants, direct-acting relaxants, and neuromuscular blockers.

Central-Acting Muscle Relaxants

Central-acting drugs are used to treat muscle spasms. They are thought to work by producing CNS depression in the brain and spinal cord. Antispastic agents include carisoprodol (Soma), cyclobenzaprine (Flexeril), and diazepam.

Direct-Acting Muscle Relaxants

Direct-acting muscle relaxants directly affect skeletal muscles to produce muscle relaxation. This results in a decrease in muscle contraction. Dantrolene (Dantrium) is an example of a direct-acting muscle relaxant.

Neuromuscular Blockers

Neuromuscular-blocking drugs produce complete muscle relaxation and paralysis by binding to the nicotinic receptor for acetylcholine at the neuromuscular junction. Neuromuscular nerve transmission is thus blocked and remains blocked for a variable period depending on the type and amount of neuromuscular blocker used.

EASIEST TO USE

Neuromuscular blockers sometimes are used to achieve total paralysis before endotracheal intubation (described in Chapter 15, *Airway Management, Respiration, and Artificial Ventilation*), to relieve muscle spasms of the larynx, to suppress tetany, to treat depression resulting from electroconvulsive therapy, and to allow for breathing control by a respirator. Because these blocking agents can produce complete paralysis, a patient's breathing must be supported and the effectiveness of ventilation and oxygenation must be monitored closely. (These muscle relaxants do not inhibit pain or seizure activity.) Examples of neuromuscular blockers include rocuronium (Zemuron), vecuronium (Norcuron), cisatracurium (Nimbex), and succinylcholine (Anectine).

NOTE

The two types of neuromuscular-blocking drugs are depolarizing agents and nondepolarizing agents. Depolarizing agents (eg, succinylcholine) substitute themselves into the neuromuscular junction. They bind to receptors for acetylcholine and have a rapid onset and brief duration of action. This makes them the drug of choice for endotracheal intubation. Nondepolarizing agents bind to the receptors for acetylcholine at the neuromuscular junction. They do this without initiating depolarization of the muscle membrane. Nondepolarizing agents (eg, rocuronium) have a longer onset and duration than depolarizing agents.

Drugs That Affect the Cardiovascular System

The heart consists of many interconnected branching fibers or cells that form the walls of the two atria and two ventricles (see Chapter 10, *Review of Human Systems*). Some of these cells are specialized to conduct electrical impulses, others contraction. All of these cells are nourished through a profuse network of blood vessels (coronary vasculature). Cardiac drugs are classified by their effects on these tissues. BOXES 13-21 and 13-22 list cardiac drugs and the pharmacologic terms that describe their actions.

Cardiac Glycosides

Cardiac glycosides are naturally occurring plant substances that have characteristic effects on the heart. These compounds contain a carbohydrate molecule (sugar). When combined with water, the molecule is converted into a sugar plus one or more active substances. Glycosides may work by blocking certain

BOX 13-21 Emergency Drugs: Cardiovascular System

Drugs Used to Treat Dysrhythmias

Adenosine (Adenocard)
Amiodarone (Cordarone)
Atropine

Beta-Adrenergic Blockers
Atenolol (Tenormin)
Metoprolol (Lopressor, Toprol-XL)

Calcium Channel Blockers
Diltiazem (Cardizem)
Verapamil (Isoptin)

Other
Dopamine (Intropin)
Lidocaine (Xylocaine)
Magnesium
Procainamide (Pronestyl)

Drugs Used to Impact Cardiac Output and Blood Pressure

Calcium chloride
Digoxin (Lanoxin)
Dobutamine (Dobutrex)
Dopamine (Intropin)
Epinephrine (Adrenalin)
Nitroglycerin (Nitrostat, Tridil)
Norepinephrine (Levophed)
Vasopressin (Pitressin)

BOX 13-22 Pharmacologic Terms to Describe Actions of Cardiovascular Drugs

Chronotropic. Chronotropic drugs affect heart rate. If the drug accelerates the heart rate (eg, epinephrine), it is said to have a positive chronotropic effect. A drug that decreases the heart rate (eg, diltiazem) is said to have a negative chronotropic effect.

Dromotropic. Dromotropic drugs affect conduction velocity through the conducting tissues of the heart. If a drug accelerates conduction, it is said to have a positive dromotropic effect. Examples of drugs with positive dromotropic effects include isoproterenol and phenytoin. Drugs with negative dromotropic effects (eg, verapamil and adenosine) delay conduction.

Inotropic. Inotropic drugs strengthen or increase the force of cardiac contraction (a positive inotropic effect). Some examples include digoxin, dobutamine, and epinephrine. A drug that weakens or decreases the force of cardiac contraction has a negative inotropic effect. An example of such a drug is metoprolol.

ionic pumps in the cellular membrane, which indirectly increases the calcium concentration to the contractile proteins. A key cardiac glycoside, digoxin, is used to treat heart failure and to manage certain tachycardias (see Chapter 21, *Cardiology*).

Digitalis glycosides affect the heart in two distinct ways. First, they increase the strength of contraction. This is a positive inotropic effect. Second, they have a dual effect on the electrophysiologic properties of the heart. They have a modest negative chronotropic effect, causing slight slowing of the heart rate. Digitalis glycosides also have a profound negative dromotropic effect, decreasing conduction velocity of impulses in the heart.

Many patients who take cardiac glycosides experience side effects at one time or another because of the narrow therapeutic index of the drugs. The symptoms may be neurologic, visual, gastrointestinal, cardiac, or psychiatric and are often vague and can easily be attributed to a viral illness. A high index of suspicion in patients taking cardiac glycosides who report experiencing flulike symptoms is important. The most common side effects of cardiac glycosides are anorexia, nausea or vomiting, visual disturbances (flashing lights, altered color vision), and dysrhythmias (cardiac rhythm disturbances), usually slowing of the heart rate with varying degrees of blocked conduction (see Chapter 21, *Cardiology*).

NOTE

Proarrhythmias are serious dysrhythmias that are generated by antidysrhythmic agents. All antidysrhythmic drugs have some degree of proarrhythmic effects. The sequential use of two or more antidysrhythmic drugs compounds these effects. As a rule, it is best not to use more than one agent to manage dysrhythmias (unless absolutely necessary).

The toxic effects of cardiac glycosides are dose related. These effects may be increased by the presence of other drugs, such as diuretics. These other drugs may predispose the patient to cardiac rhythm disturbances. Dysrhythmias may include bradycardias, tachycardias, and even ventricular fibrillation. For these reasons, patients taking these drugs require close monitoring. Treatment for digitalis toxicity may include correction of electrolyte imbalances, neutralization of the free drug, and use of antidysrhythmics. A patient with a low potassium level is much more likely to develop digoxin toxicity.

Antidysrhythmics

Antidysrhythmic drugs are used to treat and prevent disorders of cardiac rhythm. The pharmacologic agents that suppress dysrhythmias may do so by direct action on the cardiac cell membrane (vasopressin), by indirect action that affects the cells (metoprolol), or both.

Cardiac rhythm disturbances may be caused by a number of factors. Factors include ischemia, hypoxia, acidosis or alkalosis, electrolyte abnormalities, excessive catecholamine exposure, autonomic influences, drug toxicity, or scarred and diseased tissue. Dysrhythmias result from disturbances in impulse formation, disturbances in impulse conduction, or both.

Classifications

Antidysrhythmic drugs have been classified into categories based on their fundamental mode of action on cardiac muscle. Drugs that belong to the same class do not always produce identical actions. However, all antidysrhythmic drugs have some ability to suppress automaticity.

> NOTE
>
> Local protocols and standing orders assist and guide EMS personnel. These orders often are established to allow paramedics to use certain drugs in certain cases. With these orders in place, paramedics can act without seeking medical direction. One such example is antidysrhythmic drugs for a patient with specific cardiac conduction disturbances. Another is first-line cardiac life support drugs for a patient in cardiac arrest.

Class I. Class I drugs are sodium channel blockers. These drugs work to slow conduction. They are divided further into subclasses (Ia, Ib, and Ic) based on the extent of sodium channel blockade. Examples of Class Ia drugs include quinidine, disopyramide (Norpace), and procainamide (Pronestyl). Class Ib drugs decrease or have no effect on conduction velocity. Examples include lidocaine. Class Ic drugs profoundly slow conduction and are indicated only for control of life-threatening ventricular dysrhythmias. An example of a Class Ic drug is flecainide (Tambocor).

> CRITICAL THINKING
>
> How might the signs of shock in a patient taking digoxin or propranolol vary from what might be expected normally?

Class II. Class II drugs are beta-blocking agents. These drugs reduce adrenergic stimulation of the heart. An example is metoprolol.

Class III. Class III drugs produce potassium channel blockade, which increases the contractility. Unlike other antidysrhythmic agents, drugs in this class do not suppress automaticity. They also have no effect on conduction velocity. These drugs are thought to cease dysrhythmias that result from the reentry of blocked impulses. An example of such a drug is amiodarone.

Class IV. Class IV drugs are also known as *calcium channel blockers*. These drugs are thought to work by blocking the inflow of calcium through the cell membranes of the cardiac and smooth muscle cells. This action depresses the myocardial and smooth muscle contraction, decreases automaticity, and in some cases decreases conduction velocity. Examples of calcium channel blockers include verapamil (Isoptin) and diltiazem (Cardizem, Tiazac).

Other: Variable Mechanism. Some antidysrhythmic drugs work by other or unknown mechanisms (direct nodal inhibition). These drugs are sometimes referred to as Class V and include adenosine, digoxin, and magnesium sulfate.

Antihypertensives

High blood pressure affects as many as 75 million adults in the United States[11] and has been related directly to an increased incidence of stroke, cerebral hemorrhage, heart and renal failure, and coronary heart disease. The exact mechanism of action of many antihypertensive drugs is unknown. The ideal antihypertensive drug should accomplish the following:

- Maintain blood pressure within normal limits for various body positions
- Maintain or improve blood flow without compromising tissue perfusion or blood supply to the brain
- Reduce the workload of the heart
- Have no undesirable side effects
- Permit long-term administration without intolerance

Classifications

Certain drugs are used to reduce blood pressure in patients with chronic hypertension. These drugs usually are given in low-dose combinations and are titrated (gradually adjusted) to effect. These drugs include diuretics, sympathetic-blocking agents (sympatholytic drugs), vasodilators, angiotensin-converting enzyme inhibitors, calcium channel blockers, and the newer class, angiotensin II receptor antagonists.

Diuretics. Diuretics, which cause a loss of excess salt and water from the body by the kidneys, are the drugs of choice in managing hypertension. They often are used with other antihypertensive agents. The decrease in plasma and extracellular fluid volume decreases preload and stroke volume. The decrease in fluid volume has a direct effect on the size of the arterioles, resulting in lowered blood pressure and an initial decline of cardiac output that is followed by a decrease in peripheral vascular resistance. These responses result in a lowering of the blood pressure.

Thiazides are diuretics that work well to lower blood pressure. Many antihypertensive agents cause retention of sodium and water; thiazides, such as hydrochlorothiazide, may be given concomitantly (along with other drugs) to help prevent this side effect.

Loop diuretics, such as furosemide, are strong, short-acting agents that inhibit sodium and chloride reabsorption in the loop of Henle and cause excessive loss of potassium. They also cause an increase in the excretion of sodium and water. Loop diuretics have fewer side effects than do most other antihypertensives. However, hypokalemia and profound dehydration can be a result of their use. These agents are prescribed to patients who have renal insufficiency and also may be given to patients who cannot take other diuretics.

> NOTE
>
> Many drugs are excreted by the kidneys. Thus patients with renal system dysfunction (acute or chronic renal failure) may accumulate drugs in their systems. These patients often require modifications in drug doses and dosing intervals. These changes are in addition to diet modification and fluid restriction.

Potassium-sparing agents, such as spironolactone (Aldactone), can be effective as an antihypertensive when they are used in combination with other diuretics because they promote sodium and water loss without a loss of potassium. These agents are used to treat hypertensive patients who become hypokalemic from other diuretics. They also can be used by patients who are apparently resistant to the antihypertensive effects of other diuretics. Potassium-sparing agents are also used to treat some edematous states, such as cirrhosis of the liver with ascites.

Sympathetic-Blocking Agents. Sympathetic-blocking agents may be classified as beta-blocking agents and adrenergic-inhibiting agents. Beta-blocking agents are used to treat cardiovascular disorders, including patients with suspected myocardial infarction, high-risk unstable angina, and hypertension. These drugs work by decreasing cardiac output and inhibiting renin secretion from the kidneys. Both actions result in lower blood pressure. Beta-blocking drugs compete with epinephrine for available beta-receptor sites as well. This inhibits tissue and organ response to beta stimulation. Examples of beta-blocking agents include the following:

- Beta$_1$-blocking agents (cardioselective)
  - Acebutolol (Sectral)
  - Atenolol
  - Metoprolol
- Beta$_1$- and beta$_2$-blocking agents (nonselective)
  - Labetalol (also has alpha$_1$-blocking properties)
  - Nadolol
  - Propranolol

Adrenergic-inhibiting agents work by modifying the actions of the sympathetic nervous system. They are effective antihypertensive drugs. Arterial pressure is influenced through various mechanisms of the heart, blood vessels, and kidneys. Sympathetic stimulation increases the heart rate and force of myocardial contraction, constricts arterioles and venules, and causes the release of renin from the kidneys. Blocking this sympathetic stimulation can reduce blood pressure.

Adrenergic-inhibiting agents are classified as centrally acting adrenergic inhibitors or peripheral adrenergic inhibitors. The mechanism by which many of these agents work is unknown. Generally, most of these agents are believed to have multiple sites of action. Examples include the following drugs:

- Centrally acting adrenergic inhibitors
  - Clonidine hydrochloride (Catapres)
  - Methyldopa (Aldomet)
  - Prazosin hydrochloride (Minipress)
- Peripheral adrenergic inhibitors
  - Doxazosin (Cardura)
  - Guanethidine sulfate (Ismelin)

- Reserpine (Sandril, Serpasil)
- Phentolamine (Regitine)
- Phenoxybenzamine (Dibenzyline)
- Terazosin (Hytrin)

Vasodilator Drugs. Vasodilator drugs act directly on the smooth muscle walls of the arterioles, veins, or both. They lower peripheral resistance, thus lowering blood pressure. This effect stimulates the sympathetic nervous system and also activates the baroreceptor reflexes. In turn, heart rate, cardiac output, and renin release increase. Medications that inhibit the sympathetic response usually are given with vasodilator drugs.

In addition to their use as antihypertensives, some vasodilator drugs work to treat angina pectoris (ischemic chest pain). For example, nitrates dilate veins and arteries. Their dilating effects on veins lead to venous pooling of blood. They also reduce the amount of blood return to the heart. Thus these effects reduce left ventricular end-diastolic pressure and volume (the volume of blood in the left ventricle at the end of filling) (see Chapter 21, *Cardiology*). The subsequent decrease in wall tension helps to reduce myocardial oxygen demand and also relieves the chest pain of myocardial ischemia. Vasodilator drugs are classified as arteriolar dilators and arteriolar and venous dilators. Examples of each include the following:

- Arteriolar dilator drugs
  - Hydralazine (Apresoline)
  - Minoxidil (Loniten)
- Arteriolar and venous dilator drugs
  - Sodium nitroprusside (Nipride, Nitropress)
  - Nitrates and nitrites
  - Amyl nitrite inhalant
  - Isosorbide dinitrate (Isordil, Sorbitrate)
  - Nitroglycerin sublingual tablet
  - Nitropaste (Nitro-Bid ointment, Nitrol)
  - Intravenous nitroglycerin (Tridil)

Angiotensin-Converting Enzyme (ACE) Inhibitor Drugs. As described in Chapter 11, *General Principles of Pathophysiology*, the renin-angiotensin-aldosterone system plays a key role in maintaining blood pressure. This system also plays a key role in sodium and fluid balance. A disturbance in this system can result in hypertension, edema, and congestive heart failure. In addition, kidney damage can result in an inability to regulate the release of renin through normal feedback mechanisms. This causes elevated blood pressure in some patients.

Angiotensin II is a strong vasoconstrictor that raises blood pressure and also causes the release of aldosterone. Aldosterone contributes to sodium and water retention. By inhibiting conversion of the precursor angiotensin I to the active molecule angiotensin II (a process triggered by ACE), the renin-angiotensin-aldosterone system is suppressed and blood pressure is lowered. Examples of ACE inhibitors include captopril (Capoten), enalapril (Vasotec), benazepril (Lotensin), fosinopril (Monopril), lisinopril (Prinivil, Zestril), and quinapril (Accupril).

Calcium Channel Blockers. Calcium channel–blocking agents such as verapamil, amlodipine (Norvasc), felodipine (Plendil), and diltiazem reduce peripheral vascular resistance by inhibiting the contractility of vascular smooth muscle. They dilate coronary vessels through the same mechanism. The effects of these drugs are important in treating hypertension, decreasing the oxygen requirements of the heart (through decreased afterload), and increasing oxygen supply (by abolishing coronary artery spasm), thus relieving the causes of angina pectoris. The various drugs in this class differ in degree of selectivity for coronary (and peripheral) vasodilation or decreased cardiac contractility.

Angiotensin II Receptor Antagonists. Angiotensin II receptor antagonists are a newer class of antihypertensive agent. They block the renin-angiotensin-aldosterone system more completely than do ACE inhibitors. They lower blood pressure by selectively inhibiting the actions of angiotensin II receptors, which include vasoconstriction, renal tubular sodium reabsorption, aldosterone release, and stimulation of central and peripheral sympathetic activity. These drugs are used to manage hypertension in patients with adverse effects from ACE inhibitors (eg, dry cough). The drugs appear to be equally effective in lowering systolic and diastolic pressure. They also are being studied for their effectiveness in treating congestive heart failure, diabetic nephropathy, and vascular diseases such as atherosclerosis. Drugs in this classification include candesartan (Atacand), irbesartan (Avapro), losartan (Cozaar, Hyzaar), olmesartan (Benicar), telmisartan (Micardis), and valsartan (Diovan) (**FIGURE 13-11**).

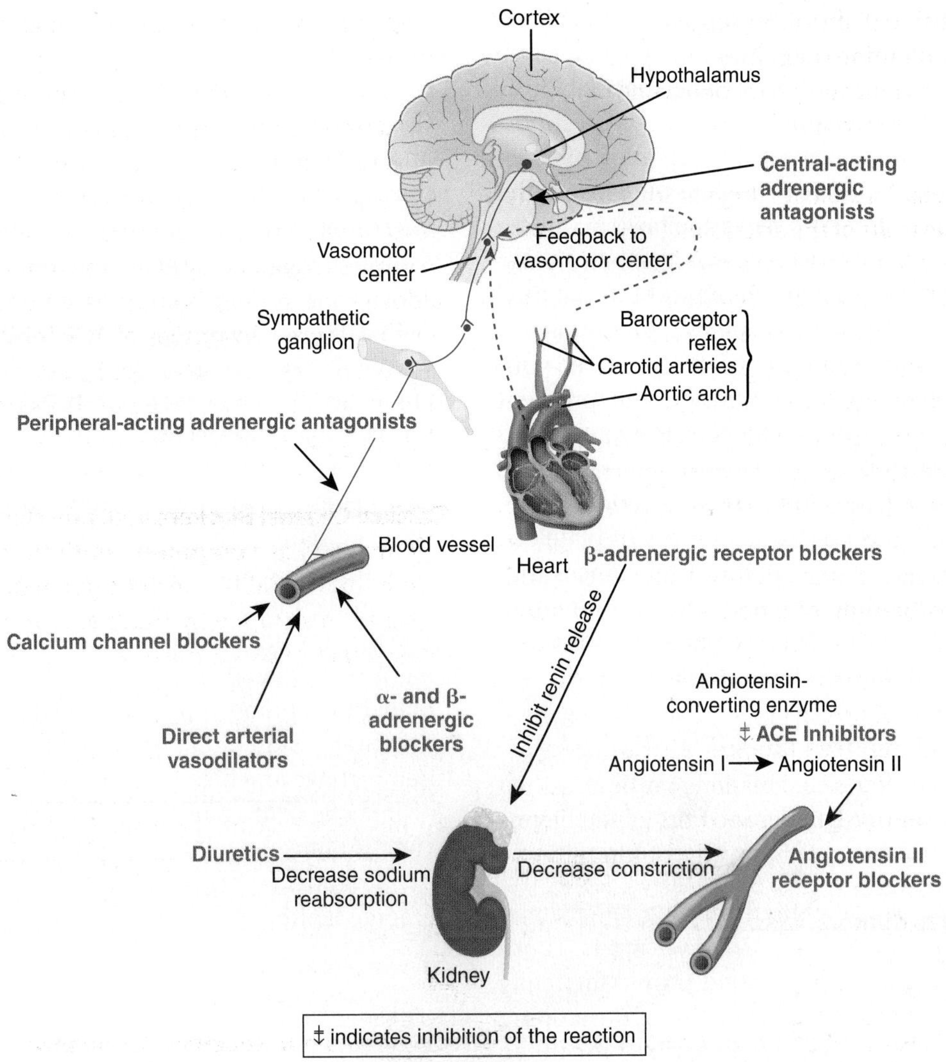

FIGURE 13-11 Sites of action of antihypertensive agents.

Drugs That Affect the Blood

Bleeding and thrombosis are altered states of hemostasis. An understanding of the drugs that affect blood coagulation and the use of fibrinolytic agents and blood components is crucial. In the prehospital arena, these concepts will assist in the management of patients. Drugs discussed in this section include anticoagulants, antihemophilic agents, hemostatic agents, antifibrinolytic agents, blood and blood components, and antihyperlipidemic drugs.

Anticoagulants

As described in Chapter 10, *Review of Human Systems*, platelets are small cell fragments in the blood. They provide the initial step in normal repair of blood vessels. **Blood coagulation** is a process that results in the formation of a stable fibrin clot that entraps platelets, blood cells, and plasma. The end result of this process is called a blood clot or thrombus. Abnormal thrombus formation is the major cause of myocardial infarction (from coronary thrombosis) and stroke (from cerebral vascular thrombosis) (see Chapter 21, *Cardiology*).

Thrombus formation can occur in both the venous and arterial systems. An example of thrombosis in the venous system is pulmonary embolus and deep vein thrombosis. The three major risk factors for various thromboses are stasis, localized trauma, and hypercoagulable states. Stasis (reduced blood flow) results from immobilization or venous insufficiency and is responsible for the increased incidence of deep vein thrombosis in many bedridden patients. Localized trauma may initiate the clotting cascade and may cause arterial and venous thrombosis. Hypercoagulability is the increased likelihood of blood to become abnormally thick and thus increase the formation of fibrin complexes in the blood vessels and is the cause of the increased incidence of deep vein thrombosis in women who take birth control pills. Hypercoagulability is also a factor in clotting problems for many of the familial thrombotic disorders (see Chapter 21, *Cardiology*).

Arterial thrombi commonly are associated with atherosclerotic plaques, hypertension, and turbulent blood flow that damages the endothelial lining of blood vessels. Damage to the endothelium causes platelets to stick and aggregate (clump) in the arterial system. Arterial thrombi are composed mostly of platelets, but they also involve the chemical substances that contribute to the coagulation process (in particular, fibrinogen and fibrin). Myocardial infarctions and strokes are often the result of arterial thrombi.

Agents That Affect Blood Coagulation

Drugs that affect blood coagulation may be classified as antiplatelet, anticoagulant, and fibrinolytic agents. They each act at a different phase in the clotting process.

Antiplatelet Agents. Drugs that interfere with platelet aggregation are known as antiplatelet drugs. These drugs sometimes are prescribed prophylactically (as a precaution) for patients at risk of developing arterial clots. They also are prescribed for those who have suffered myocardial infarction or stroke. Antiplatelet agents also are given to patients with certain valvular heart diseases, valvular prostheses (replacement valves), and various intracardiac shunts (a passage that allows blood to flow from one part of the heart to another). Among the most common oral antiplatelet drugs are aspirin, dipyridamole (Persantine), clopidogrel (Plavix), ticagrelor (Brilinta), and ticlopidine (Ticlid), and newer drugs such as prasugrel (Effient) and cangrelor (Kengreal). These are sometimes prescribed in combinations such as aspirin and dipyridamole (Aggrenox).

> **NOTE**
>
> Platelet adhesion, activation, and aggregation that result in the formation of an arterial thrombus are pivotal in the pathogenesis of acute coronary syndromes (acute myocardial infarctions). Studies indicate that the administration of a glycoprotein IIb/IIIa receptor antagonist may reduce ischemic complications after plaque fissure or rupture. (These drugs inhibit glycoprotein receptors in the membrane of platelets and help prevent platelet aggregation.) These drugs may be included along with aspirin, heparin, and beta blockers during in-hospital reperfusion therapy for select patients. Examples of glycoprotein IIb/IIIa inhibitors include abciximab (ReoPro), eptifibatide (Integrilin), and tirofiban (Aggrastat).

Anticoagulant Agents. Anticoagulant drug therapy is used to prevent intravascular thrombosis. The therapy works by decreasing blood coagulability. Such therapy commonly is used to prevent postoperative thromboembolism. Anticoagulant agents also are used during hemodialysis and in reperfusion therapy for some patients with acute coronary syndromes (see Chapter 21, *Cardiology*). Anticoagulant therapy is a preventive measure against future clot formation. The therapy has no direct effect on a blood clot that has formed already or on ischemic tissue injured by inadequate blood supply as a result of a thrombus. The major side effect of anticoagulant therapy is hemorrhage and bleeding complications. Examples of anticoagulant agents include warfarin and heparin. Heparin must be administered by injection.

Several newer classes of oral anticoagulants have emerged. Although they are very expensive, patients

> **NOTE**
>
> Natural (unfractionated) heparin and its derivative, low-molecular-weight heparin (LMWH), are effective and indicated for the prevention of venous thromboembolism. Heparin also is indicated for the treatment of venous thrombosis, pulmonary embolism, and acute myocardial infarction. In addition, heparin is administered to patients who undergo cardiac surgery using cardiac bypass, vascular surgery, and coronary angioplasty; in patients with coronary stents; and in selected patients with coagulation disorders.
>
> Natural heparin is usually administered in the hospital. It is given intravenously and requires laboratory monitoring. LMWH (eg, enoxaparin [Lovenox, Clexane]) may be given intravenously or subcutaneously in weight-adjusted doses. LMWH may be given in the out-of-hospital or home setting. LMWH is given in the prehospital setting to some patients with ischemic chest pain and myocardial infarction (see Chapter 21, *Cardiology*).
>
> *Modified from:* Hirsh J, Warkentin TE, Shaughnessy SG, et al. Heparin and low-molecular-weight heparin mechanisms of action, pharmacokinetics, dosing, monitoring, efficacy, and safety. *Chest*. 2001;119:64S-94S.

find them more convenient than warfarin. Unlike with warfarin, food does not interfere with their effects and patients do not require frequent blood tests to assure their effectiveness.

The factor Xa inhibitor medications block clotting factor Xa to prevent clot formation. They are used to prevent deep vein thrombosis and pulmonary embolism and to reduce the risk of stroke in patients who have atrial fibrillation. Factor Xa inhibitors include apixaban (Eliquis), edoxaban (Savaysa), fondaparinux (Arixtra), and rivaroxaban (Xarelto).[12] Presently, there is no FDA-approved reversal agent for these anticoagulants, although several are in development.

Dabigatran (Pradaxa) is a direct thrombin inhibitor used to prevent stroke in patients with atrial fibrillation and to prevent deep vein thrombosis and pulmonary embolism following hip replacement. The drug idarucizumab (Praxbind) is available to reverse the effects of dabigatran when needed.[13]

SHOW ME THE EVIDENCE

A retrospective chart review evaluated whether EMS providers ascertained anticoagulant and antiplatelet use in older adults with head trauma. The researchers included 2,110 patients from 5 EMS agencies and 11 hospitals in Sacramento County, California. The researchers found there was acceptable agreement between prehospital and hospital records with regard to documentation of warfarin use, but not with direct oral anticoagulants (dabigatran, rivaroxaban, and apixaban) or with other platelet use. They concluded that the use of these drugs is common in older adults with head trauma; however, some of these drugs were not documented in the patient report. Given the increased risk of traumatic intracranial hemorrhage in patients taking these agents, there is a need to improve in this area.

Modified from: Nishijima DK, Gaona S, Waechter T, et al. Do EMS providers accurately ascertain anticoagulant and antiplatelet use in older adults with head trauma? *Prehosp Emerg Care*. 2017;21(2):209-215.

Fibrinolytic Agents. Fibrinolytic drugs dissolve clots after their formation by promoting the digestion of fibrin. Fibrinolytic therapy is used to treat acute myocardial infarction in patients when the onset of symptoms is less than 12 hours and percutaneous coronary intervention is not available within 90 minutes of the first medical contact.[14] Fibrinolytic therapy also has become the treatment of choice in managing some stroke patients and is used in treatment of frostbite when vascularity is compromised. The goal is to reestablish blood flow and prevent ischemia and tissue death. Fibrinolytic therapy also has been used in acute pulmonary embolism, deep vein thrombosis, and peripheral arterial occlusion. Fibrinolytics are used in the prehospital setting in some areas of the United States. These drugs include anistreplase (also known as anisoylated plasminogen streptokinase activator complex [APSAC]; Eminase), alteplase (t-PA), reteplase (Retavase), streptokinase (Streptase), and tenecteplase (TNKase) (see Chapter 21, *Cardiology*, and the Appendix, *Emergency Drug Index*).

CRITICAL THINKING

Fibrinolytics have the potential to dissolve clots. This in turn may reverse the serious effects of myocardial infarction and stroke. So why are fibrinolytics not given to everyone who is suspected of having these conditions?

Antihemophilic Agents

Hemophilia (further described in Chapter 31, *Hematology*) is a group of hereditary bleeding disorders in which the affected person lacks one of the factors needed for the coagulation of blood. These disorders are characterized by persistent and uncontrollable bleeding that can occur after even a minor injury. Bleeding may occur into joints, the urinary tract, and at times the CNS. Hemophilia *A* is the classic form of hemophilia and is caused by a deficiency of factor VIII. Hemophilia *B* results from a deficiency in factor IX complex. Replacement therapy of the missing clotting factor can be effective in managing hemophilia. These include factor VIII (Factorate), factor IX (Konyne), and antiinhibitor coagulant complex (Autoplex).

NOTE

Coagulation factors refer to the 13 proteins contained in blood plasma. These proteins interact to produce a blood clot.

Hemostatic Agents

Hemostatic agents hasten clot formation, which in turn reduces bleeding. Systemic hemostatic agents (eg, Amicar, Cyklokapron) generally are used to control rapid blood loss after surgery by inhibiting fibrinolysis. Topical hemostatic agents (eg, Gelfoam, Nova-Cell) are used to control capillary bleeding during surgical and dental procedures.

Hemostatic agents are now being used in the prehospital setting and in combat medical care. Celox, Combat Gauze (cotton gauze with Kaolin), and QuickClot ACS work by absorbing plasma from blood, thereby reducing clotting times. The Tactical Combat Casualty Care Committee of the US military recommended cotton gauze with Kaolin as its only hemostatic agent in 2009 because it was the most effective and safest (see Chapter 37, *Bleeding and Soft-Tissue Trauma*).[15]

Hemorrhagic Agents

Hemorrheologic agents are used to treat peripheral vascular disorders caused by pathologic or physiologic obstruction (eg, arteriosclerosis). These drugs improve blood flow by increasing viscosity and increasing red blood cell (RBC) flexibility and tissue oxygenation. An example of a hemorrheologic agent is pentoxifylline (Trental).

Antifibrinolytic Agents

Tranexamic acid (TXA; Cyklokapron, Lysteda) is an antifibrinolytic drug that prevents the breakdown of clots. The agent was initially used for dental procedures to reduce bleeding in patients who had clotting disorders. The US military studied the use of TXA to reduce bleeding after battlefield injuries.[15] Civilian research is currently underway. Early results suggest the need for blood products is reduced in patients who receive this drug.[16] A guidance document from the National Association of EMS Physicians suggests that it be administered carefully within specific situations.[17]

Blood and Blood Components

The healthy body maintains a normal balance of blood and its components. However, illness and injury such as hemorrhage, burns, and dehydration may impair this balance and require replacement therapy (see the Appendix, *Advanced Practice Procedures for Critical Care Paramedics*).

Knowledge of how to manage an imbalance of blood or blood components is crucial. The usual treatment of choice is to replace the sole blood component that is deficient. Replacement therapy may include transfusing the following:

- Whole blood (red blood cells and plasma; rarely used)
- Packed red blood cells (red blood cells without plasma)
- Fresh-frozen plasma (plasma without red blood cells or platelets)
- Plasma expanders (dextran)
- Platelets
- Cryoprecipitate (multiple clotting factors)
- Fibrinogen (found in fresh frozen plasma and cryoprecipitate)
- Albumin
- Gamma globulins (antibodies)

Antihyperlipidemic Drugs

Hyperlipidemia refers to an excess of lipids in the plasma. Several types of hyperlipidemia occur; all are associated with elevated levels of cholesterol and triglycerides (described in Chapter 2, *Well-Being of the Paramedic*). This condition is thought to play a role in the development of atherosclerosis. Thus antihyperlipidemic drugs sometimes are used along with diet and exercise to control serum lipid levels (BOX 13-23).

Drugs That Affect the Respiratory System

Disorders of the respiratory system that may require dug therapy are those associated with infection and obstructive airway disease. Drugs discussed in this section include bronchodilators, mucokinetic drugs, and oxygen and other respiratory agents (BOX 13-24).

BOX 13-23 Antihyperlipidemic Drugs

Statins

Atorvastatin (Lipitor)
Fenofibrate (Tricor)
Fluvastatin (Lescol)
Gemfibrozil (Lopid)
Lovastatin (Mevacor)
Pravastatin (Pravachol)
Simvastatin (Zocor)
Rosuvastatin (Crestor)

Others

Colesevelam (Welchol)
Ezetimibe (Zetia)
Fenofibrate (Lipofen, TriCor, Antara)
Fenofibric acid (Fibricor, Trilipix)
Nicotinic acid (Niacin)

BOX 13-24 Emergency Drugs: Respiratory System

Albuterol (Proventil, Ventolin)
Levalbuterol (Xopenex)
Epinephrine (Adrenalin) 1:1,000
Ipratropium (Atrovent)
Magnesium sulfate
Racemic epinephrine (Micronefrin)

The respiratory system includes all structures that are involved in the exchange of oxygen and carbon dioxide. Serious narrowing of any portion of the respiratory tract may be an indication for drug therapy. Emergencies involving the respiratory system usually are caused by reversible conditions such as asthma, emphysema with infection, and foreign body airway obstruction (see Chapter 15, *Airway Management, Respiration, and Artificial Ventilation*).

Smooth muscle fibers line the tracheobronchial tree. They directly influence the diameter of the airways. The bronchial smooth muscle tone is maintained by impulses from the autonomic nervous system. Parasympathetic fibers from the vagus nerve stimulate bronchial smooth muscle through the release of acetylcholine. This neurotransmitter interacts with the muscarinic receptors on the membranes of the cell, producing bronchoconstriction.

Sympathetic fibers mainly affect beta$_2$ receptors in the lungs through the release of epinephrine from the adrenal medulla and the release of norepinephrine from the peripheral sympathetic nerves. The epinephrine reaches the lungs via the circulatory system. Epinephrine interacts with beta$_2$ receptors to produce smooth muscle relaxation and bronchodilation. Thus the beta$_2$ receptor plays the dominant role in bronchial muscle tone. (Although beta$_1$ receptors also are found on bronchial smooth muscle, their ratio to beta$_2$ receptors is 1:3.)

Bronchodilators

Bronchodilator drugs are the primary treatment for obstructive pulmonary disease such as asthma, chronic bronchitis, and emphysema. These drugs are classified as sympathomimetic drugs, anticholinergic drugs, or xanthine derivatives. Many of these drugs are administered by inhalation via a nebulizer or pressure cartridge (see Chapter 23, *Respiratory*).

Sympathomimetic Drugs

Sympathomimetic drugs are grouped according to their effects on receptors. Nonselective adrenergic drugs have alpha, beta$_1$ (cardiac), and beta$_2$ (respiratory) activity. Nonselective beta-adrenergic drugs have beta$_1$ and beta$_2$ effects. Selective beta$_2$-receptor drugs act primarily on beta$_2$ receptors in the lungs (bronchial smooth muscle). BOX 13-25 summarizes the alpha, beta$_1$, and beta$_2$ activities of the adrenergic drugs used as bronchodilators.

Nonselective adrenergic drugs stimulate alpha and beta receptors. The alpha activity lessens vasoconstriction to reduce mucosal edema. Beta$_2$ activity produces bronchodilation and vasodilation. Undesirable beta$_1$ effects include an increase in heart rate and force of contraction, and undesirable beta$_2$ effects include

BOX 13-25 Alpha, Beta$_1$, and Beta$_2$ Activities of Inhaled Adrenergic Drugs Used as Bronchodilators

Alpha Effects (Vasoconstriction)
Vasoconstriction
Increased blood pressure
Decreased bronchial congestion
Increased duration of action for coadministered beta$_2$ drugs

Beta$_1$ Effects
Cardiac stimulation
Increased heart rate
Increased force of contraction
Possible palpitations and dysrhythmias
Relaxation of gastrointestinal tract
Some bronchodilation and increased heart rate
Fewer effects than with subcutaneous administration

Beta$_2$ Effects
Bronchiole dilation
Stimulation of skeletal muscles (tremors)
Vasodilation (mainly in blood vessels supplying muscle)
Glycogenolysis

CNS Effects
Anxiety
Dizziness
Insomnia
Irritability
Nervousness
Sweating
Lower incidence of systemic effects than with subcutaneous administration

muscle tremors and CNS stimulation. Examples of nonselective adrenergic drugs include nonprescription epinephrine inhalation aerosol (Bronkaid Mist, Primatene Mist) and epinephrine inhalation solution. Racemic epinephrine inhalation solution (Micronefrin) is another nonselective adrenergic drug that is used mainly to manage upper airway swelling associated with croup (see Chapter 23, *Respiratory*).

Nonselective beta-adrenergic drugs are not selective for $beta_2$ receptors and therefore have a wide range of effects (described earlier in this chapter). This class of drug is no longer recommended for the management of asthma.[18] Examples of nonselective beta-adrenergic drugs include epinephrine (eg, Adrenalin, Asmolin), ephedrine (Ephed II), and ethylnorepinephrine (Bronkephrine), each of which has some alpha activity; isoproterenol inhalation solution (Aerolone, Vapo-Iso, Isuprel); and isoproterenol inhalation aerosol (Isuprel Mistometer, Norisodrine Aerotrol).

The action of $beta_2$-selective drugs lessens the incidence of unwanted cardiac effects caused by $beta_1$ adrenergic agents. Patients with hypertension, cardiac disease, or diabetes can better tolerate this group of bronchodilators. Examples of selective $beta_2$-receptor drugs include albuterol (Proventil, Ventolin), levalbuterol (Xopenex), pirbuterol (Maxair), bitolterol (Tornalate), salmeterol (Serevent), formoterol (Foradil aerolizer), and isoetarine (Bronkosol).

NOTE
Some bronchodilators act rapidly ("rescue inhalers"), whereas others provide slow relief. If a patient claims to have used his or her inhaler, it is important to ask the patient which inhaler was used.

Anticholinergic Bronchodilator

Ipratropium is an inhaled bronchodilator. Because it is an anticholinergic, ipratropium prevents acetylcholine from attaching to the muscarinic receptors on smooth muscle cells. This allows bronchiolar smooth muscle to relax and causes bronchodilation.[18]

Xanthine Derivatives

The xanthine group of drugs includes caffeine, theophylline, and theobromine. These drugs relax smooth muscle (particularly bronchial smooth muscle), stimulate cardiac muscle and the CNS, increase diaphragmatic contractility, and promote diuresis through increased renal perfusion. The action of various theophylline compounds depends on the concentration of theophylline, which is the active ingredient. Theophylline products vary in their rate of absorption and therapeutic effects. Aminophylline (Somophyllin, Aminophyllin), dyphylline (Dilor, Droxine, Lufyllin), and theophylline (Bronkodyl, Theo-Dur, Elixophyllin, Somophyllin-T) are some of the many theophylline-containing preparations. Theophylline preparations are not a first-line drug in the treatment of acute reactive airway disease such as asthma. This is because of their high side effect profile and slow onset of action.

Other Respiratory Drugs

A number of other drugs can be used to treat asthma and other obstructive pulmonary diseases. These drugs include prophylactic asthmatic agents such as cromolyn sodium (Intal, sodium cromoglycate), aerosol corticosteroid agents such as beclomethasone dipropionate (Vanceril inhaler, Beclovent), dexamethasone (Decadron), antileukotrienes such as montelukast (Singulair) and zafirlukast (Accolate), and glycopyrrolate. These drugs reduce the allergic or inflammatory response to a variety of stimuli. They also have an effect on bronchial smooth muscle. In the acute care setting, intravenously administered steroids (eg, methylprednisolone [Solu-Medrol]) may be given in an attempt to decrease the inflammatory response and improve airflow.

Mucokinetic Drugs

Mucokinetic drugs are used to move respiratory secretions along the tracheobronchial tree. These agents work by altering the consistency of these secretions, enabling them to be removed from the body more easily. People with chronic pulmonary disease often use mucokinetic drugs. These drugs help to clear their respiratory passages and also improve ciliary activity in the airways. Mucokinetic drugs include diluents (water, saline solution), aerosols, and mucolytic drugs or expectorants (Mucomyst).

NOTE
Mucus is a normal secretion produced by the surface cells in the mucous membranes. Sputum is an abnormal viscous secretion. Sputum consists mainly of mucus. Sputum originates in the lower respiratory tract.

Oxygen and Other Respiratory Agents

Oxygen is mainly used to treat hypoxia and hypoxemia. Oxygen is a colorless, odorless, and tasteless gas. It is essential for sustaining life. (Oxygen and oxygen delivery are described in detail in Chapter 15, *Airway Management, Respiration, and Artificial Ventilation.*)

Direct Respiratory Stimulants

Direct respiratory stimulants are known as analeptics. These act directly on the medullary center of the brain to increase the rate and depth of respirations. These drugs are considered inferior to mechanical ventilatory measures to treat respiratory depression and to counteract drug-induced respiratory depression caused by anesthetics. An example of a direct respiratory stimulant is doxapram (Dopram).

Reflex Respiratory Stimulants

Spirits of ammonia is given by inhalation and acts as a reflex respiratory stimulant. The noxious vapor is used sometimes in cases of fainting. The vapor works by irritating sensory nerve receptors in the throat and stomach. These nerve receptors send afferent messages to the control centers of the brain to stimulate respiration. Because ammonia has the potential to cause pulmonary irritation and worsen respiratory conditions, it is no longer routinely used in emergency care.

Respiratory Depressants

Respiratory depressants include opiates and barbiturate drugs previously described. Respiratory depression is a common side effect of these drugs. However, they seldom are given to intentionally inhibit rate and depth of respiration.

Cough Suppressants

The cough is a protective reflex to expel harmful irritants. It may be productive when removing irritants or secretions from the airway, or nonproductive (dry and irritating). When the cough is prolonged or secondary to an underlying disorder, treatment with antitussive drugs may be indicated. BOX 13-26 presents a few narcotic and non-narcotic antitussive agents.

BOX 13-26 Narcotic and Non-narcotic Antitussive Agents

Narcotic Agent

Codeine

Non-narcotic Agents

Benzonatate (Tessalon)
Dextromethorphan (Sucrets, Robitussin DM)

Antihistamines

Histamine is a chemical mediator found in almost all body tissues. The concentration is highest in the skin, lungs, and gastrointestinal tract. The body releases histamine when exposed to an antigen, such as pollen or insect stings. This antigen exposure results in increased localized blood flow, increased capillary permeability, and swelling of the tissues. In addition, histamine produces contractile action on bronchial smooth muscle.

Allergic responses involving histamines and other chemical mediators include local effects such as angioedema, eczema, rhinitis (runny nose), urticaria (hives), and asthma. Systemic effects from the release of histamine and certain other mediators may result in anaphylaxis (see Chapter 26, *Immune System Disorders*).

Antihistamines compete with histamine for receptor sites. Thus they prevent the physiologic action of histamine. Two types of histamine receptors are H_1 receptors (these act mainly on the blood vessels and the bronchioles) and H_2 receptors (these act mainly on the gastrointestinal tract). In addition to blocking some actions of histamine, antihistamines have anticholinergic or atropinelike action. This may result in tachycardia, constipation, drowsiness, sedation, and inhibition of secretions. Most antihistamines have a local anesthetic effect as well. This effect may soothe the skin irritation caused by an allergic reaction. The chief clinical use of antihistamines is for allergic reactions. However, they also sometimes are prescribed to control motion sickness or as a sedative or antiemetic. Examples of antihistamines are dimenhydrinate (Dramamine), diphenhydramine, hydroxyzine, promethazine (Phenergan), and the newer H_1-receptor antagonists—for example, loratadine (Claritin), cetirizine (Zyrtec), and fexofenadine (Allegra).

Serotonin

Serotonin is a naturally occurring vasoconstrictor material found in platelets and in the cells of the brain and intestine. It has several pharmacologic actions, which are exerted on various smooth muscles and nerves. Serotonin is not administered as a drug but has a major influence on other drugs and some disease states. It is helpful in repairing damaged blood vessels, stimulates smooth muscle contraction, and acts as a neurotransmitter in the CNS, where it has an effect on sleep, pain perception, and some mental illnesses.

Selective Serotonin Reuptake Inhibitors

Selective serotonin reuptake inhibitors are drugs that block the absorption (reuptake) of serotonin in the brain, making more serotonin available. They mainly affect the levels of serotonin and not the levels of other neurotransmitters. These drugs, also known as serotonin antidepressants, are used to ease symptoms of moderate to severe depression and anxiety disorders. Selective serotonin reuptake inhibitors include citalopram, escitalopram, fluoxetine, and sertraline.

Antiserotonins

Antiserotonins are serotonin antagonists that inhibit responses to serotonin and its influence on other drugs and disease states. Specific antiserotonins block smooth muscle contraction and vasoconstriction and inhibit the action of serotonin in the brain. Some antiserotonins are used to treat vascular headaches and allergic disorders. Examples of these drugs include cyproheptadine (Periactin). Lysergic acid diethylamide (LSD) is a type of antiserotonin drug.

Drugs That Affect the Gastrointestinal System

As described in Chapter 10, *Review of Human Systems*, the gastrointestinal system is composed of the digestive tract, the biliary system, and the pancreas. The primary function of the gastrointestinal system is to provide the body with water, electrolytes, and other nutrients used by cells. Drug therapy for the gastrointestinal system can be divided into two groups: drugs that affect the stomach and drugs that affect the lower gastrointestinal tract. In emergency care, conditions of the stomach or gastrointestinal tract that may require drug therapy usually are limited to nausea and vomiting (BOX 13-27).

BOX 13-27 Emergency Drugs: Gastrointestinal System

Activated charcoal
Diphenhydramine (Benadryl)
Hydroxyzine (Vistaril)
Metoclopramide (Reglan)
Ondansetron (Zofran)
Prochlorperazine (Compazine)
Promethazine (Phenergan)

Drugs That Affect the Stomach

Conditions of the stomach that may require drug therapy include hyperacidity, hypoacidity, ulcer disease, nausea, vomiting, and hypermotility.

Antacids

Antacids buffer or neutralize hydrochloric acid in the stomach. They are prescribed for the relief of symptoms associated with hyperacidity, including peptic ulcer, gastritis, esophagitis, heartburn, and hiatal hernia. Common over-the-counter antacids include Alka-Seltzer, Gaviscon, and Rolaids.

Antiflatulents

Antiflatulents prevent the formation of gas in the gastrointestinal tract. Gas retention is a common condition with diverticulitis, ulcer disease, and spastic or irritable colon (see Chapter 28, *Abdominal and Gastrointestinal Disorders*). These drugs sometimes are used along with antacids. Simethicone (Mylicon) is an example of an antiflatulent.

Digestants

Digestant drugs promote digestion in the gastrointestinal tract by releasing small amounts of digestive enzymes in the small intestine. Examples of digestants include pancreatin (Hi-Vegi-Lip) and pancrelipase (Pancreaze, Creon).

Emetics and Antiemetics

Vomiting is usually an involuntary action that is coordinated by the emetic center of the medulla. Vomiting may be initiated through the CNS as a secondary reaction to emotion, pain, or disequilibrium (motion sickness); through irritation of the mucosa of the gastrointestinal tract or bowel; or through stimulation from the chemoreceptor trigger zone of the medulla by circulating drugs and toxins (eg, opiates, digitalis).

Emetics. Emetics induce vomiting. They rarely are administered today as part of the treatment for drug overdoses and poisonings. These drugs include apomorphine and syrup of ipecac. The treatment of drug overdoses and poisoning is addressed further in Chapter 33, *Toxicology*.

Antiemetics. Drugs used to treat nausea and vomiting include antagonists of histamine, acetylcholine, and dopamine as well as other drugs. These drugs work best when they are given before nausea and vomiting have begun rather than afterwards. For example, drugs used to treat motion sickness or vertigo should be taken 30 minutes before traveling. Common antiemetics include scopolamine (Transderm Scop), dimenhydrinate, diphenhydramine, hydroxyzine, meclizine (Antivert), promethazine, prochlorperazine (Compazine), and ondansetron (Zofran).

NOTE

Cannabinoids are drugs that are derived from hemp plants. They have been used experimentally to prevent vomiting in patients who receive cancer chemotherapy. Examples of these drugs include dronabinol (Marinol) and nabilone (Cesamet). These drugs use a synthetic derivative of the active ingredient in marijuana.

SHOW ME THE EVIDENCE

Researchers in California prospectively investigated the effect of ondansetron administered by intravascular (IV), intramuscular (IM), or orally dissolving tablet (ODT) routes. In the 6 months of data collection, they evaluated the effect of administration of this drug to 2,071 EMS patients who had nausea and vomiting (64% IV; 4% IM; 33% ODT). Eight patients had adverse effects. The largest decrease in nausea score was in the IV group, followed by IM and ODT. They concluded that ondansetron is safe and effective to treat nausea in out-of-hospital patients.

Modified from: Salvucci AA, Squire B, Burdick M, Luoto M, Brazzel D, Vaezazizi R. Ondansetron is safe and effective for prehospital treatment of nausea and vomiting by paramedics. *Prehosp Emerg Care*. 2011:15(1);34-38.

Cytoprotective Agents

Cytoprotective agents are drugs that protect cells from damage. They are used along with other drugs to treat peptic ulcer disease by protecting the gastric mucosa. Examples of these drugs include sucralfate (Carafate) and misoprostol (Cytotec).

H_2-Receptor Antagonists

As described previously, the action of histamine is mediated through H_2 receptors. Histamine has been associated with gastric acid secretion. H_2-receptor antagonists block the H_2 receptors. They reduce the volume of gastric acid secretion and its acid content. Examples of H_2-receptor antagonists include cimetidine (Tagamet), ranitidine (Zantac), and famotidine (Pepcid).

Proton Pump Inhibitors

Proton pump inhibitors are used for treatment of symptomatic gastroesophageal reflux disease, short-term treatment of erosive esophagitis, and maintenance of erosive esophagitis healing. Some agents also are approved for use with antibiotics to treat *Helicobacter pylori* infection (associated with duodenal ulcers). The proton pump (potassium adenosine triphosphate enzyme system) is the final pathway for secretion of hydrochloric acid by the parietal cells of the stomach. Proton pump inhibitors decrease hydrochloric acid secretion by inhibiting the actions of the parietal cells. In addition, the gastric pH of the stomach is altered. Examples of proton pump inhibitors include esomeprazole (Nexium), lansoprazole (Prevacid), omeprazole (Prilosec), pantoprazole (Protonix), dexlansoprazole (Dexilant), and rabeprazole (Aciphex).

Drugs That Affect the Lower Gastrointestinal Tract

Constipation and diarrhea are two common conditions of the lower gastrointestinal tract. Both conditions may require drug therapy. Drugs used to manage these conditions include laxatives and antidiarrheals.

Laxatives

Laxatives produce defecation. They are used to evacuate the bowel and to soften hardened stool for easier passage. Situations that may indicate the need for laxative use include the following:

- Constipation
- Neurologic diseases (eg, multiple sclerosis, Parkinson disease)
- Pregnancy
- Rectal disorders
- Drug poisoning
- Surgery and endoscopic examination

Numerous types of laxatives are available. Many can be purchased without a prescription. Examples include saline laxatives (Epsom salt, Milk of Magnesia), stimulant laxatives (Dulcolax, castor oil, Ex-Lax), bulk-forming laxatives (Mitrolan, Metamucil), lubricant laxatives (mineral oil), fecal moistening agents (Colace, glycerin suppositories), and those used for bowel evacuation (GoLYTELY, Chronulac). Regular or excessive use of laxatives is common in older adults and in people with eating disorders. Laxative abuse may result in permanent bowel damage and electrolyte imbalance.

Antidiarrheal Drugs

Antidiarrheal drugs are used to reduce an abnormally high frequency of bowel evacuation. Common causes of acute and chronic diarrhea include bacterial or viral invasion, drugs, diet, and numerous disease states (eg, diabetes insipidus, inflammatory bowel syndromes). Drugs used to treat diarrhea include the following:

- Adsorbents
    - Bismuth subsalicylate (Pepto-Bismol)
- Anticholinergics
    - Donnatal
- Opiates
    - Paregoric
    - Codeine
- Other agents
    - Diphenoxylate (Lomotil)
    - Loperamide (Imodium)

Drugs That Affect the Eye and Ear

Drug therapy is sometimes indicated in the assessment and management of acute, subacute, and chronic conditions of the eye and ear that may threaten the senses of vision and hearing.

Drugs That Affect the Eye

Drugs used to treat eye disorders include antiglaucoma agents, mydriatics and cycloplegics, anti-infective/anti-inflammatory agents, and topical anesthetics.

Antiglaucoma Agents

Glaucoma is an eye disease in which the pressure of the fluid in the eye is abnormally high (see Chapter 22, *Diseases of the Eyes, Ears, Nose, and Throat*). The pressure causes compression or obstruction of the small internal blood vessels of the eye, the fibers of the optic nerve, or both, which results in nerve fiber destruction and partial or complete loss of vision. Glaucoma is a common eye disorder in people older than 60 years and is responsible for 15% of blindness in adults in the United States.[19] Agents used to reduce the pressure in chronic glaucoma include cholinergic and anticholinesterase drugs. Some of these drugs (eg, pilocarpine) dilate the pupil of the eye, and some constrict the pupil; others (eg, acetazolamide) slow the secretion of aqueous fluid. If these drug therapies fail, surgery may be indicated. If glaucoma is diagnosed early, drugs can control it for a lifetime. Most physicians recommend testing for glaucoma every 2 years after age 35 years.

Mydriatic and Cycloplegic Agents

Mydriatic and cycloplegic agents are applied topically and cause dilation of the pupils and paralysis of accommodation to light. They are used to treat inflammation and to relieve ocular pain by helping the eye to rest. These drugs are used during routine eye examinations and in ocular surgery as well. Examples of these drugs include atropine ophthalmic solution, cyclopentolate hydrochloride ophthalmic solution (Cyclogyl), homatropine ophthalmic solution (Isopto Homatropine), epinephrine, and oxymetazoline (OcuClear).

> **CRITICAL THINKING**
>
> You are caring for an older adult patient. This patient had mydriatic eye drops instilled by an ophthalmologist. If you did not know this history, what might you consider after your physical examination of this patient?

Anti-infective/Anti-inflammatory Agents

Anti-infective and anti-inflammatory agents are used to treat eye conditions such as conjunctivitis, stye, and keratitis (corneal inflammation caused by bacterial infection). Examples of these drugs include bacitracin (Baciguent), chloramphenicol (Chloroptic), erythromycin (Ilotycin), and natamycin (Natacyn).

Topical Anesthetic Agents

Local anesthetics are used to prevent pain in surgical procedures and eye examinations. They also are used in the treatment of some eye injuries (eg, a corneal abrasion). These drugs usually have a rapid onset (within 20 seconds) and last 15 to 20 minutes. Examples of these drugs include proparacaine (Ophthaine, Alcaine) and tetracaine (Ak-T-Caine, Pontocaine). Other eye medications include artificial tear solutions and lubricants to provide additional moisture, irrigation solutions, and antiallergic agents to relieve symptoms of itching, tearing, and redness. Many of these drugs and solutions are available without a prescription.

Drugs That Affect the Ear

Drugs used to treat disorders of the external ear canal include antibiotics, steroid/antibiotic combinations, and miscellaneous preparations. These drugs include the following:

- Antibiotics used to treat infections
  - Chloramphenicol (Chloromycetin Otic)
  - Gentamicin sulfate (Garamycin)
- Steroid/antibiotic combinations used to treat superficial bacterial infections
  - Neomycin sulfate/polymyxin B sulfate/hydrocortisone (Cortisporin Otic)
  - Neomycin/colistin/hydrocortisone (Coly-Mycin S Otic)
- Miscellaneous preparations used to treat earwax accumulation, inflammation, pain, fungal infections, and other minor conditions
  - Boric acid in isopropyl alcohol (Aurocaine 2)
  - Triethanolamine with chlorobutanol in propylene glycol (Cerumenex)

People with inner ear infections or serious illness associated with hearing impairment may require antibiotics with systemic effects, following physician evaluation. These actions will help to prevent complications (see Chapter 22, *Diseases of the Eyes, Ears, Nose, and Throat*).

Drugs That Affect the Endocrine System

The endocrine system works to control and integrate body functions. BOX 13-28 presents emergency drugs that affect the endocrine system. Information from various parts of the body is carried via bloodborne hormones to distant sites. Hormones are natural chemical substances. They act after they have been secreted into the bloodstream from endocrine glands (ductless glands that secrete internally). These glands include the anterior and posterior pituitary, thyroid, parathyroid, and adrenal glands and the thymus, pancreas, testes, and ovaries. Hormones from the various endocrine glands work together to regulate vital processes, including the following:

- Secretory and motor activities of the digestive tract
- Energy production
- Composition and volume of extracellular fluid
- Adaptation (eg, acclimatization and immunity)
- Growth and development
- Reproduction and lactation

BOX 13-28 Emergency Drugs: Endocrine System

Dexamethasone (Decadron)
Dextrose 50%, 25%, 10%
Glucagon
Insulin
Methylprednisolone (Solu-Medrol)
Oxytocin (Pitocin, Syntocinon)

BOX 13-29 Drugs That Affect the Anterior and Posterior Pituitary Gland

Anterior Pituitary Gland Drugs

Used to treat growth failure in children caused by growth hormone deficiency:
Somatrem (Protropin)
Somatropin (Humatrope)

Posterior Pituitary Gland Drugs

Used to treat the symptoms of diabetes insipidus resulting from antidiuretic hormone deficiency:
Vasopressin (Pitressin)

Drugs That Affect the Pituitary Gland

As described in Chapter 10, *Review of Human Systems*, the hormones of the anterior and posterior pituitary gland are important for regulating the secretion of other hormones in the body. BOX 13-29 lists drugs that affect the anterior and posterior pituitary. (Disorders of the endocrine glands are described further in Chapter 25, *Endocrinology*.)

Drugs That Affect the Thyroid and Parathyroid Glands

The thyroid hormone controls the rate of metabolic processes and is required for normal growth and development. Parathyroid hormone regulates the level of ionized calcium in the blood. Parathyroid hormone

BOX 13-30 Drugs That Affect the Thyroid and Parathyroid Glands

Thyroid Drugs

Used to treat hypothyroidism and to prevent goiters:
Thyroxine
Iodine products
Levothyroxine (Synthroid, Levoxyl)

Parathyroid Drugs

Used to treat hyperparathyroidism:
Vitamin D
Calcium supplements

does this through the release of calcium from bone, the absorption of calcium from the intestine, and the regulation of calcium excretion by the kidneys.

Disorders of the thyroid gland include goiter (enlargement of the thyroid gland), hypothyroidism (thyroid hormone deficiency), and hyperthyroidism (thyroid hormone excess). Disorders of the parathyroid include hypoparathyroidism and hyperparathyroidism. BOX 13-30 lists the drugs used to treat these disorders (see Chapter 25, *Endocrinology*).

Drugs That Affect the Adrenal Cortex

The adrenal cortex secretes three major classes of steroid hormones: glucocorticoids (cortisol), mineralocorticoids (primarily aldosterone), and sex hormones. Glucocorticoids raise blood glucose level, deplete tissue proteins, and suppress the inflammatory reaction. Mineralocorticoids regulate electrolyte and water balance. Sex hormones are estrogen, progesterone, and testosterone and are produced in small amounts by men and women. The sex hormones have little physiologic effect under normal circumstances. BOX 13-31 lists drugs that affect the adrenal cortex. Two disorders of the adrenal cortex are Addison disease (adrenal cortical hypofunction) and Cushing disease (adrenal cortical hyperfunction) (see Chapter 25, *Endocrinology*).

BOX 13-31 Drugs That Affect the Adrenal Cortex

Glucocorticoids

Betamethasone (Celestone)
Dexamethasone (Decadron)
Methylprednisolone (Solu-Medrol)
Triamcinolone (Aristocort)

Mineralocorticoids

Desoxycorticosterone acetate (DOCA)
Fludrocortisone (Florinef)

Adrenal Steroid Inhibitors

Aminoglutethimide (Cytadren)
Metyrapone (Metopirone)

Drugs That Affect the Pancreas

As described in Chapter 10, *Review of Human Systems*, the pancreas is an exocrine gland and an endocrine gland. The exocrine portion secretes hormones into ducts, providing digestive juices to the small intestine. The endocrine portion of the pancreas consists of pancreatic islets (islets of Langerhans). These cells produce the hormones that directly enter the circulatory system.

Hormones of the Pancreas

The pancreatic hormones play a key role in regulating the concentration of certain nutrients in the circulatory system. The pancreas secretes two major hormones: insulin and glucagon.

Insulin is the primary hormone that regulates glucose metabolism. In general, insulin increases the ability of the liver, adipose tissue, and muscle to take up and use glucose. Glucose not immediately needed for energy is stored in the skeletal muscle, liver, and other tissues. This stored form of glucose is called glycogen.

Glucagon mainly influences the liver, although it has some effect on skeletal muscle and adipose tissue. In general, glucagon stimulates the liver to break down glycogen so that glucose is released into the blood. Glucagon also inhibits the uptake of glucose by muscle and fat cells. The balancing action of these two hormones protects the body from hyperglycemia (high blood sugar) and hypoglycemia (low blood sugar).

This balance of hormonal actions is important when one considers the metabolic problems that can occur in diabetes mellitus. The relationship of glucagon and insulin to other hormones and substances such as dextrose 50% and thiamine (vitamin B_1) is addressed in Chapter 25, *Endocrinology*. BOX 13-32 lists drugs that affect the pancreas.

Drugs That Affect the Reproductive System

Drugs that affect the reproductive system are primarily used to restore homeostasis of the female and male hormones, which are produced by the endocrine glands. Drugs are also used to prevent pregnancy, to improve fertility, and to enhance sexual function.

The Female Reproductive System

Drugs that affect the female reproductive system include synthetic and natural substances such as hormones, oral contraceptives, ovulatory stimulants, and drugs used to treat infertility.

Female Sex Hormones

Two main types of hormones are secreted by the ovary: estrogen and progesterone. Supplemental estrogen is indicated for estrogen deficiency or replacement, for treatment of breast cancer, and as prophylaxis for osteoporosis in postmenopausal women (controversial). Progesterone (and synthetic progestins) may be used to treat hormonal imbalance, endometriosis, and specific cancers and to prevent pregnancy when used properly.

BOX 13-32 Drugs That Affect the Pancreas

Insulin Preparations

Rapid Acting
Insulin lispro (Humalog)
Insulin aspart (NovoLog)

Short Acting
Regular (Humulin R, Novolin R)

Intermediate Acting
NPH (Humulin N, Novolin N)
Lente (Humulin L, Novolin N)

Long Acting
Insulin Detemir (Levemir)
Insulin Glargine (Lantus)

Oral Hypoglycemic Agents
Glimepiride (Amaryl)
Glipizide (Glucotrol)
Glyburide (Micronase, Diabeta)
Metformin (Glucophage)
Pioglitazone (Actos)

Combination Drugs
Glyburide/metformin (Glucovance)
Glipizide/metformin (Metaglip)

Hyperglycemic Agents
Dextrose
Diazoxide (Proglycem)
Glucagon
Oral glucose (Glutose, Insta-Glucose)

Oral Contraceptives

Oral contraception is the most effective form of birth control and is known as "the pill." Oral contraception is a combination of estrogen and progesterone. This combination results in the suppression of ovulation (see Chapter 30, *Gynecology*). Several types of oral contraceptives and drug combinations are available. All are nearly 100% effective in preventing pregnancy when taken properly.

DID YOU KNOW?

Emergency contraception is a method of preventing pregnancy to be used after a contraceptive fails or after unprotected sex. It is not for routine use. Emergency contraceptives (Previn and Plan B) are also known as postcoital pills, or morning-after pills. They contain the hormones estrogen and progestin (levonorgestrel), either separately or in combination. Emergency contraceptives can reduce the chance of pregnancy when taken as directed up to 72 hours (3 days) after unprotected sex. These drugs are approved by the FDA for women 17 years of age and older. They are available without prescription and do not require parental consent.

Modified from: FDA's decision regarding plan B: questions and answers. US Food and Drug Administration website. https://www.fda.gov/Drugs/EmergencyPreparedness/BioterrorismandDrugPreparedness/ucm109795.htm. Updated December 7, 2015. Accessed January 26, 2018.

Ovulatory Stimulants and Infertility Drugs

The absence of ovulation in women is anovulation. The condition, which may be pathologic in women with abnormal bleeding or infertility, sometimes is treated with gonadotropins, thyroid preparations, estrogen, and synthetic agents. One example of a drug used to induce ovulation and increase fertility is clomiphene citrate (Clomid).

NOTE

Certain drugs are used during labor and delivery. These drugs help to increase (oxytocin [Pitocin]) or decrease (ritodrine [Yutopar]) uterine contractility. In prehospital care, oxytocin is used to control hemorrhages that occur after the delivery of the infant and placenta (see Chapter 45, *Obstetrics*).

The Male Reproductive System

The male sex hormone is testosterone. Adequate amounts of this hormone are needed for normal development and for the maintenance of male sex characteristics.

Testosterone therapy is indicated for the treatment of hormone deficiency (eg, testicular failure), impotence, delayed puberty, female breast cancer, and anemia. The choice of dosage and length of therapy depend on the diagnosis, age of the patient, and intensity of side effects or adverse reactions. An example of an oral testosterone drug is methyltestosterone (Metandren).

Drugs That Affect Sexual Behavior

Sexual drive (libido) can be affected by psychological, social, and physiologic factors or by a combination of these. Negative effects of these factors can result in a lack of interest in sexual activity in men and women and impotence in men.

Drugs That Impair Libido and Sexual Gratification

Some drugs interfere with sympathetic nervous stimulation. At times they may cause sexual dysfunction. Drugs may interfere with the nervous system mechanisms (directly and indirectly) that are responsible for sexual arousal. Examples of such drugs include antihypertensives, antihistamines, antispasmodics, sedatives and tranquilizers, antidepressants, alcohol, and barbiturates.

Drugs That Enhance Libido and Sexual Gratification

A patient may change medicines (under physician supervision) to avoid drug-induced sexual dysfunction. In addition, a patient may be prescribed drugs to enhance libido and sexual gratification. Drugs that enhance sexual function include levodopa (L-DOPA), tadalafil (Cialis), vardenafil (Levitra), and sildenafil citrate (Viagra).

NOTE

The administration of nitroglycerin or nitrate/nitrite medications is contraindicated in patients who have taken Cialis, Levitra, or Viagra within the previous 24 to 48 hours because the combination can cause a lethal drop in blood pressure. Other drugs that may produce untoward effects in patients taking drugs to enhance sexual gratification include some antibiotics, antivirals, and some antihypertensive medications. The paramedic should question the patient about the use of sexual enhancement drugs before administering any of these medications.

Modified from: Jones & Bartlett Learning. *2017 Nurse's Drug Handbook*. 16th ed. Burlington, MA: Jones & Bartlett Learning; 2017.

Drugs Used in Neoplastic Diseases

Neoplastic disease refers to any abnormal growth, whether malignant or benign. All types of cancer fall into the category of malignant neoplastic disease. Although cancer may occur in any part of the body, it is observed primarily in the lungs, breast, colorectum, and prostate.[20]

Antineoplastic Agents

Antineoplastic agents are used in cancer chemotherapy. They are used to prevent the increase of malignant cells (BOX 13-33). These drugs do not directly kill tumor cells. Rather they interfere with cell reproduction or replication through various mechanisms.

NOTE

Any person who handles antineoplastic agents should be trained properly in safety procedures. These drugs are considered cytotoxic (toxic to human cells).

BOX 13-33 Antineoplastic Agents[a]

Doxorubicin (Adriamycin)
5-Fluorouracil (Adrucil)
Mechlorethamine (Mustargen)
Methotrexate (Amethopterin, MTX)
Streptozocin (Zanosar)
Cistiplatin (Platinol-AQ)
Carmustine (BCNU)
Chlorambucil (Leukeran)
Cyclophosphamide (Cytoxan)
Melphalan (Alkera)
Tamoxifen (Nolvadex)
Interferon

[a]Varies greatly, depending on the type of cancer.

Antineoplastic agents are nonselective. They are injurious to all cells in the body. Side effects from these drugs may include infection, hemorrhage, nausea and vomiting, and changes in bowel function. Short-term toxicity from these agents may affect the pulmonary, cardiovascular, renal, and integumentary systems. Prehospital care for these patients mainly is supportive and is aimed at providing comfort measures and emotional support.

Drugs Used in Infectious Disease and Inflammation

Infection and inflammation are two of the body's primary defenses against trauma or foreign invasion. Infection and inflammation are managed with antibiotics, antifungals, and antiviral medications.

Antibiotics

Antibiotics, which kill or suppress the growth of organisms, are used to treat local or systemic infection. Antibiotics disrupt the bacterial cell wall by disturbing the functions of the cell membrane or by interfering with the metabolic functions of the cell. This group of drugs includes penicillins, cephalosporins, and related products; macrolide antibiotics; tetracyclines; fluoroquinolones; and miscellaneous antibiotic agents (eg, metronidazole [Flagyl], spectinomycin [Trobicin]). Antibiotics are much more toxic to bacteria than they are to patients. Some antibiotics, though, may produce hypersensitivity, which can lead to a fatal reaction if the drug is given to a sensitized patient (see Chapter 26, *Immune System Disorders*).

> NOTE
> In time, some bacteria that are at first sensitive to antibiotics may become resistant to them. The bacteria develop ways to evade the effect of a drug. Widespread use and misuse of antibiotics lead to the development of resistant strains of bacteria. Bacterial resistance may even complicate treatment when a person is infected with an antibiotic-resistant organism.

Penicillins

Penicillins are active against gram-positive and some gram-negative bacteria (BOX 13-34). Penicillins are used to treat many infections, including tonsillitis, pharyngitis, bronchitis, and pneumonia. Examples of penicillins include amoxicillin (Amoxil), ampicillin (Amcill), dicloxacillin (Dynapen), and penicillin V potassium (Pen Vee K). Penicillin can produce severe anaphylactic reactions.

> **BOX 13-34** Gram Stain
>
> Gram stain is an iodine-based stain used to differentiate various types of bacteria. Examples of gram-positive bacteria are staphylococci, streptococci, and pneumococci. Examples of gram-negative bacteria are gonococci and meningococci.

Cephalosporins

Cephalosporins (and related products) resemble penicillins; yet they are active against gram-positive and gram-negative bacteria. Cephalosporins are used widely to treat ear, throat, and respiratory tract infections. They also are useful for treating urinary tract infections. Urinary tract infections often are caused by bacteria that are resistant to penicillin-type antibiotics. Examples of cephalosporins and related products include cefazolin (Ancef), cephalothin (Keflin), cephalexin (Keflex), and cefotaxime (Claforan). A small number of patients who are allergic to penicillins are also allergic to cephalosporins; however, recent studies suggest that the chance of cross-reactivity with cephalosporins and penicillin allergy is less than 2%.[21] With newer-generation cephalosporins, it is virtually 0%.

Macrolide Antibiotics

Macrolides (erythromycins) are used to treat infections of the skin, chest, throat, and ears. Macrolides are useful for treating pertussis (whooping cough), Legionnaires' disease, and pneumonia (see Chapter 27, *Infectious and Communicable Diseases*). Examples of erythromycin drugs include Eryc, EMycin, E.E.S, and Erythrocin. Other antibacterial agents include azithromycin (Zithromax) and clarithromycin (Biaxin).

Tetracyclines

Tetracyclines are active against many gram-negative and gram-positive organisms (broad-spectrum). Tetracyclines commonly are used to treat conditions such as acne, bronchitis, syphilis, gonorrhea, and certain types of pneumonia. Examples of tetracyclines include demeclocycline (Declomycin), doxycycline (Vibramycin), and tetracycline (Achromycin). Tetracyclines may discolor developing teeth. Thus they usually are not prescribed for children younger than 12 years or for pregnant women.

> CRITICAL THINKING
> Explain how antibiotics and infectious organisms work like a lock and key.

Fluoroquinolones

Fluoroquinolone antibiotics are the treatment of choice for some human gastrointestinal infections, particularly severe foodborne illness caused by *Campylobacter* or *Salmonella* bacteria. They are also used to treat urinary tract infections, bone and joint infections, some types of pneumonia, and other human illness. Examples of fluoroquinolones include ciprofloxacin (Cipro), gatifloxacin (Tequin), and levofloxacin (Levaquin).

Antifungal and Antiviral Drugs

As discussed, people can be infected by bacterial organisms; in addition, they can be infected by fungi and viral diseases.

Antifungal Drugs

Some fungi are harmlessly present at all times in areas of the body such as the mouth, skin, intestines, and vagina. These fungi are prevented from multiplying through competition from bacteria. The actions of the immune system also prevent them from multiplying. Fungal infections are more common and serious in people taking antibiotics long term (antibiotics destroy the bacterial competition), in those who are immunosuppressed as a complication of illness (eg, infection with the human immunodeficiency virus [HIV]), and in those who are taking corticosteroids or immunosuppressant drugs (described later in this chapter). Fungal infections can be classified broadly into superficial infections, subcutaneous infections, and deep infections (BOX 13-35). Examples of antifungal drugs include tolnaftate (Tinactin), fluconazole (Diflucan), and nystatin (Mycostatin). About 50 species of fungi can cause illness and sometimes fatal disease in humans.

BOX 13-35 Categories of Fungal Infections

Examples of Superficial Infections

Candidiasis (thrush): Affects the genitals or inside of the mouth and vaginal and intertriginous areas
Tinea (including ringworm, athlete's foot, jock itch): Affects external areas of the body

Examples of Subcutaneous Infections (Rare)

Mycetoma (Madura foot): Occurs in tropical countries
Sporotrichosis: May follow inoculation of spores through a puncture or scratch

Examples of Deep Infections

Aspergillosis
Blastomycosis
Candidiasis (that spreads from its usual site to the esophagus, urinary tract, or other internal sites)
Cryptococcosis
Histoplasmosis

Antiviral Drugs

To date, few effective drugs exist to treat minor viral infections such as colds. In fact, few drugs exist for use in any viral infections. Because symptom onset is relatively delayed with viral diseases, patients may delay seeking medical treatment. Drug therapy, thus, is difficult because the disease is established. Some viral infections are trivial and harmless (eg, warts). Yet others are serious diseases such as influenza, rabies, acquired immunodeficiency syndrome (AIDS), and probably some types of cancers (**TABLE 13-6**).

Many agents have been tested as antiviral drugs. However, few have been proved to work against specific virus-infected cells without toxic effects to uninfected cells. Examples of specific antiviral drugs include acyclovir (Zovirax) and valacyclovir (Valtrex),

> NOTE
> Some antiviral drugs may shorten the duration of symptoms from the influenza viruses, if taken early in the illness. These drugs include oseltamivir (Tamiflu) and zanamivir (Relenza). These drugs are effective against some A and B influenza viruses. Others include amantadine (Symmetrel) and rimantadine (Flumadine). These drugs are effective against influenza virus A (see Chapter 27, *Infectious and Communicable Diseases*).

TABLE 13-6 Common Viruses and Viral Diseases or Conditions

Viral Family	Diseases or Conditions
Papovavirus	Warts
Adenovirus	Cold sores, genital herpes, chickenpox, herpes zoster (shingles), congenital abnormalities (cytomegalovirus)
Picornavirus	Poliomyelitis, viral hepatitis A and B, respiratory tract infections, myocarditis, rhinovirus (common cold)
Togavirus	Yellow fever, encephalitis
Orthomyxovirus	Influenza
Paramyxovirus	Mumps, measles, rubella
Coronavirus	Common cold
Rhabdovirus	Rabies
Retrovirus	Acquired immunodeficiency syndrome, degenerative brain disease, possibly cancer

which is effective against herpes infection. Others are zidovudine (Retrovir, AZT, ZDV), lamivudine (Epivir), and the combination drug lamivudine/zidovudine (Combivir). At present, these drugs are used to treat HIV infection. Oseltamivir, peramivir (Rapivab), and zanamivir are antiviral drugs recommended to treat seasonal influenza.[22]

Protease Inhibitors

The complete mechanism of action of protease inhibitors is not understood clearly. Yet they appear to inhibit the replication of retroviruses (eg, HIV) in acute and chronically infected cells. (A retrovirus is a virus that travels and tries to enter host cells with a ribonucleic acid (RNA) genome.) Side effects and adverse reactions of these drugs include nausea and vomiting, headache, malaise, fever, and flulike symptoms. Examples of protease inhibitors include indinavir (Crixivan), ritonavir (Norvir), and saquinavir (Invirase).

> NOTE
> The administration of protease inhibitors to a health care worker who has been exposed to body fluids that may contain HIV is no longer a postexposure prophylaxis recommendation by the Centers for Disease Control and Prevention. These drugs were removed because their side effects prevented many patients from completing their full treatment. Presently a combination of antiviral drugs is used.
>
> *Modified from*: Kuhar DT, Henderson DK, Struble KA, et al. Updated US Public Health Service guidelines for the management of occupational exposures to human immunodeficiency virus and recommendations for postexposure prophylaxis. *Infect Control Hosp Epidemiol*. 2013;34:875–92.

Other Antimicrobial Drugs and Antiparasitic Drugs

Various drugs are used to treat atypical microbial infection (eg, *Mycobacterium tuberculosis, M leprae*) and infection and disease caused by parasite and insect vectors (eg, trichomoniasis, malaria). BOX 13-36 lists examples of these drugs and their classifications.

> NOTE
> Malaria is still a prevalent disease in tropical areas and may be carried into the United States by refugees, immigrants, and travelers. Tuberculosis is on the rise in people with AIDS. Tuberculosis also is increasing in people who are homeless, people who abuse drugs, and people taking immunosuppressant drugs.

Anti-inflammatory and Nonsteroidal Anti-inflammatory Drugs

Anti-inflammatory drugs and NSAIDs are used to reduce pain, decrease fever, and decrease inflammation. NSAIDs have been prescribed extensively throughout the world. More than 70 million prescriptions for NSAIDs are written each year in the United States. With over-the-counter use included, more than 30 billion doses of NSAIDs are consumed annually in the United States alone.

Inflammation

Inflammation is a defense mechanism of body tissues in response to physical trauma, foreign biologic and chemical substances, surgery, radiation, and electricity. Regardless of the event producing inflammation, the response is similar. For example, if bacterial infection or an injury to the tissues occurs, chemical mediators

BOX 13-36 Antimicrobial and Antiparasitic Drugs

Antimalarial Agents
Chloroquine phosphate (Aralen)
Hydroxychloroquine (Plaquenil)
Atovaquone plus proguanil (Malarone)
Quinine (Quinamm) (plus doxycycline, tetracycline, or clindamycin)
Mefloquine (Lariam)

Antitubercular Agents
Isoniazid (Isozid, INH)
Rifampin (Rifadin)
Rifabutin
Rifapentine
Ethambutol
Pyrazinamide

Antiamebic Agents
Emetine
Iodoquinol (Yodoxin)
Paromomycin (Humatin)

Antihelminthic Agents
Diethylcarbamazine (Hetrazan)
Mebendazole (Vermox)

Antiprotozoal Agents
Metronidazole (Flagyl)

Leprostatic Agents
Clofazimine (Lamprene)
Dapsone (DDS)

Cephalosporins
Cephalexin (Keflex)
Cefazolin (Ancef)
Cefaclor (Ceclor)
Cefprozil (Cefzil)
Cefuroxime (Ceftin)
Ceftriaxone (Rocephin)
Cefdinir (Omnicef)
Cefepime (Maxipime)

Fluoroquinolones
Ciprofloxacin (Cipro)
Levofloxacin (Levaquin)
Moxifloxacin (Avelox)

Penicillins
Amoxicillin (Amoxil)
Ampicillin (Polycillin)
Dicloxacillin (Dynapen)
Penicillin G
Penicillin V

are released or activated. These mediators cause vasodilation and increased blood flow (localized warmth and redness at the site). This process brings phagocytes and other leukocytes to the area. The process prevents the spread of infection by limiting the infected site. Finally, phagocytes clean the area. The damaged tissues are repaired.

Inflammation can be localized or systemic. Local inflammation is confined to a specific area of the body. Symptoms include redness, heat, swelling, pain, and loss of function. Systemic inflammation occurs in many parts of the body. In addition to local symptoms at the inflammation site, red bone marrow produces and releases large numbers of neutrophils that promote phagocytosis, pyrogens stimulate fever production, and increased vascular permeability in severe cases may result in decreased blood volume. Drugs used to treat inflammation or its symptoms may be classified as analgesic-antipyretic drugs and NSAIDs. A number of medications have both properties.

Analgesic-Antipyretic Drugs

An antipyretic drug is one that reduces fever. The temperature-regulating mechanism of the body is located in the anterior hypothalamus. (This is known as the thermostat of the body.) Normally, the set point of this hypothalamic center is about 98.6°F (37°C). When an inflammatory response occurs in the body, endogenous pyrogens are released by the phagocytic leukocytes. This response produces fever. Analgesic-antipyretic drugs work by reversing the effect of the pyrogen on the hypothalamus. Thus the set point of the hypothalamus is returned to normal. The analgesic effects of these drugs act on peripheral pain receptors to block activation. Examples of these drugs include the following:

- Acetaminophen (eg, Datril, Tylenol, Panadol)
- Aspirin/acetylsalicylic acid (ASA) (eg, Aspergum, Bayer Aspirin)
- Aspirin (buffered) (eg, Aluprin, Bufferin, Alka-Seltzer)

Nonsteroidal Anti-inflammatory Drugs

Aspirin is the prototype of the NSAID. New drugs also have been developed, and like aspirin they are analgesic, antipyretic, and anti-inflammatory. These drugs often are prescribed for patients with various inflammatory conditions. One such condition is rheumatoid arthritis. The new drugs also often are prescribed for those who cannot tolerate aspirin. In addition, these drugs may be used to treat painful joint disorders (with or without inflammation) such as osteoarthritis, low back pain, and gout. One should note that like aspirin, the other NSAIDs may decrease platelet activity. This could result in gastrointestinal bleeding. Long-term use of some NSAIDs has been linked to an increased risk for heart attack and stroke (see Chapter 32, *Nontraumatic Musculoskeletal Disorders*).[23]

> NOTE
>
> Gout is a metabolic disease associated with high levels of uric acid in the blood (hyperuricemia). Gout is characterized by attacks of acute pain, swelling, and tenderness of joints. The condition is treated with uricosuric drugs, colchicine, steroids, and NSAIDs.

NSAIDs are thought to act by inhibiting specific enzymes so that prostaglandins (substances that promote inflammation and pain) are not formed. Examples of these drugs include the following:

- Aspirin (eg, Bayer Timed-Release, Bufferin)
- Diflunisal (Dolobid)
- Ibuprofen (eg, Advil, Motrin, Nuprin)
- Indomethacin (Indocin)
- Naproxen (Anaprox, Aleve, Naprosyn)
- Sulindac (Clinoril)
- Ketorolac (Toradol)
- COX-2 inhibitors
  - Celecoxib (Celebrex)
  - Valdecoxib (Bextra)

Drugs That Affect the Immunologic System

As described earlier in this chapter and in Chapter 11, *General Principles of Pathophysiology*, the immunologic system is composed of cells and organs. These cells and organs defend the body against invasion by foreign substances. Organs and tissues of the immune system include the spleen, tonsils, lymph nodes, and thymus (**FIGURE 13-12**).

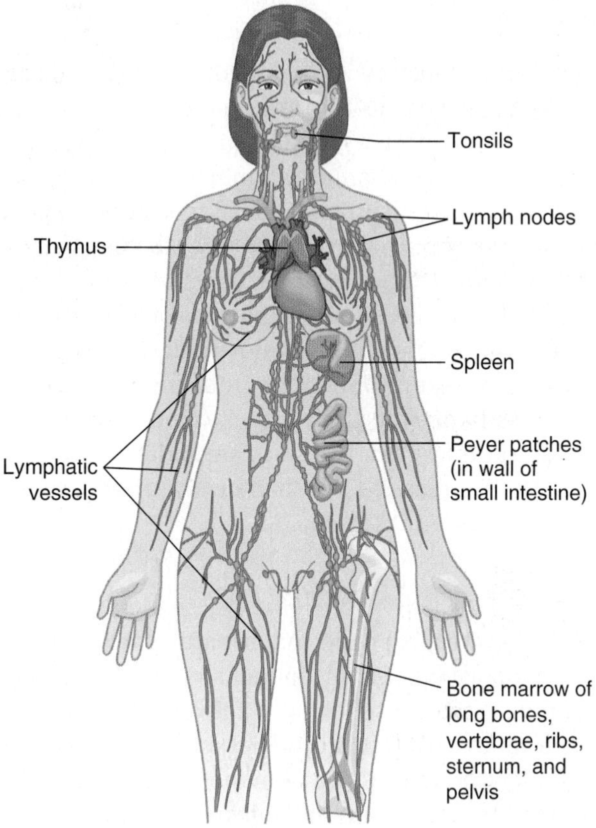

FIGURE 13-12 Organs and tissues of the immune system.

Drugs Used to Treat the Immune System

97

Immunosuppressants

Immunosuppressant drugs reduce the activity of the immune system. They do this by suppressing the production and activity of lymphocytes. These drugs are given after transplant surgery to help prevent the rejection of foreign tissues. They also are administered to halt the progress of autoimmune disorders when other treatments are ineffective. Examples of immunosuppressant drugs include antirejection drugs (used in organ transplantation), anticancer drugs, and corticosteroids.

> CRITICAL THINKING
>
> It would be important to know that a patient with an altered level of consciousness is taking an immunosuppressant drug. Why is this?

Immunomodulating Agents

Immunomodulating agents are drugs that increase the efficiency of the immune system. These agents activate the immune defenses or modify a biologic response to an unwanted stimulus. These drugs include vaccines that protect against specific infectious agents. One group of drugs belonging to this group is the interferons. (They are used to treat viral infections such as hepatitis C and certain types of cancer.) Another drug in this group is zidovudine. (Zidovudine is used to treat AIDS.) Some immunomodulating agents enhance the ability of a vaccine to stimulate the immune system. Thus they are added to the vaccine for this reason (see Chapter 27, *Infectious and Communicable Diseases*).

Serums and Vaccines

Serum is the clear fluid that separates from blood when blood clots. Serum contains salts, glucose, and proteins. Serum also includes antibodies formed by the immune system. Antibodies are formed to fight against infection. Serum from the blood of a person (or in rare cases an animal) infected with a microorganism usually contains antibodies. Therefore that serum may protect against that microorganism if the serum is injected into someone else. This relationship forms the basis for passive immunization (see Chapter 27, *Infectious and Communicable Diseases*).

> **NOTE**
>
> The two main types of immunization are passive and active. In passive immunization, antibodies are injected into a person. The antibodies provide instant but short-lived protection against specific disease-causing bacteria, viruses, or toxins. Active immunization stimulates the body to make its own antibodies. These antibodies fight against such microorganisms and confer longer-lasting immunity.

Vaccines contain killed or modified microorganisms (live attenuated organisms) that usually do not cause the disease. The vaccines are given to a person to produce specific immunity. This immunity may be for a disease-causing bacterial toxin, virus, or bacterium (active immunization). The infectious agent may invade the body at a later time, during which the sensitized immune system quickly produces antibodies to destroy the agent or the toxin it produces. Examples of live attenuated vaccines are those given to protect against measles, mumps, rubella, yellow fever, and polio. Diphtheria and tetanus vaccines contain inactivated bacterial toxins. Cholera, typhoid fever, pertussis, rabies, viral hepatitis B, influenza, and Salk injected polio vaccines contain killed organisms. (In the case of hepatitis B, the vaccine contains only part of the hepatitis B virus. See Chapter 27, *Infectious and Communicable Diseases.*)

> DID YOU KNOW?
>
> **Immunoglobulin**
>
> Immunoglobulin (IG) is a sterilized solution obtained from pooled human blood plasma that contains the immunoglobulins (or antibodies) required for protection against infectious agents that cause various diseases. Antibodies are substances in the blood plasma that fight infections. Our bodies create antibodies (or immunity) against disease-causing agents when infections occur. These antibodies can protect us from becoming ill if we are exposed to the same infectious agents sometime in the future. When someone is given IG, that person is using other people's antibodies to help fight or prevent an illness from occurring. This protection is temporary and should not be confused with getting an immunization, which provides longer-term protection.
>
> Special IG formulations are produced from donors with high levels of antibodies against cytomegalovirus immune globulin (CMVIg), hepatitis B (hepatitis B immune globulin, HBIG), rabies (rabies immune globulin, RIG), respiratory syncytial virus (RSV) monoclonal antibody (RSVAb), tetanus (tetanus immune globulin, TIG), and varicella (chickenpox) (varicella-zoster immune globulin, VZIG). Immune globulins are sometimes called gamma globulins or immune serum globulins. IG administered by injection persists in the body for several months. The protective effect of the injection disappears after approximately 3 months. If risk of exposure to disease continues, the person may require additional IG.
>
> *Modified from: Canadian Immunization Guide: Part 5—Passive Immunization.* Government of Canada website. https://www.canada.ca/en/public-health/services/publications/healthy-living/canadian-immunization-guide-part-5-passive-immunization.html?wbdisable=true. Updated November 2013. Accessed January 26, 2018.

Summary

- A drug is any substance taken by mouth; injected into a muscle, blood vessel, or cavity of the body; or applied topically to treat or prevent a disease or condition.
- Drugs can be identified by four types of names. These include the chemical name; generic or nonproprietary name; trade, brand, or proprietary name; and official name.
- The Drug Enforcement Agency is the sole legal drug enforcement body in the United States. Other regulatory bodies or services include the US Food and Drug Administration; the Public Health Service; the Federal Trade Commission; in Canada, the Health Protection Branch of the Department of National Health and Welfare; and for international drug control, the International Narcotics Control Board.
- Drugs do not confer any new functions to a tissue or organ; they only modify existing functions. A drug that interacts with a receptor to stimulate a response is known as an agonist. A drug that attaches to a receptor but does not stimulate a response is called an antagonist.
- Pharmacokinetics is the study of how the body handles a drug over a period of time.
- The degree to which drugs attain pharmacologic activity depends partly on the rate and extent to which they are absorbed. Absorption in turn depends on the ability of the drug to cross the cell membrane. The rate and extent of absorption depend on the nature of the cell membrane the drug must cross, blood flow to the site of administration, solubility of the drug, pH of the drug environment, drug concentration, and drug dosage form.
- The route of drug administration influences drug absorption. These routes can be classified as enteral, parenteral, pulmonary, and topical.
- Distribution is the transport of a drug through the bloodstream to various tissues of the body and ultimately to its site of action. After absorption and distribution, the body eliminates most drugs. The body first biotransforms the drug and then excretes the drug. The kidney is the primary organ for excretion; however, the intestine, lungs, and mammary, sweat, and salivary glands also may be involved.
- The blood–brain barrier and the placenta are barriers to distribution of some drugs.
- Many factors can alter the response to drug therapy, including age, body mass, sex, pathologic state, time of administration, genetic factors, and psychological factors.
- Most drug actions are thought to result from a chemical interaction. This interaction is between the drug and various receptors throughout the body. The most common form of drug action is the drug–receptor interaction.
- Many variables can influence drug interactions, including intestinal absorption, competition for plasma protein binding, biotransformation, action at the receptor site, renal excretion, and alteration of electrolyte balance.
- Paramedics are legally, morally, and ethically responsible for the safe and effective administration of each drug they provide to a patient.
- Elements of the drug profile the paramedic should know include the following: drug names, classification, mechanism of action, indications, pharmacokinetics, side/adverse effects, dose, route of administration, contraindications, special considerations, and storage requirements.
- Alterations in drug administration may be needed when caring for children, pregnant patients, or older adults.
- Autonomic drugs mimic or block the effects of the sympathetic and parasympathetic divisions of the autonomic nervous system. These drugs are classified into four groups: cholinergic (parasympathomimetic) drugs, cholinergic-blocking (parasympatholytic) drugs, adrenergic (sympathomimetic) drugs, and adrenergic-blocking (sympatholytic) drugs.
- Narcotic analgesics relieve pain. Narcotic antagonists reverse the narcotic effects of some analgesics. Non-narcotic analgesics interfere with local mediators released when tissue is damaged in the periphery of the body. These mediators stimulate nerve endings and cause pain.
- Anesthetic drugs are central nervous system (CNS) depressants that have a reversible effect on nervous tissue. Antianxiety agents are used to reduce feelings of apprehension, nervousness, worry, or fearfulness. Sedatives and hypnotics are drugs that depress the CNS. They produce a calming effect. They also help induce sleep. Alcohol is a general CNS depressant that can produce sedation, sleep, and anesthesia.
- Antianxiety agents are used to reduce feelings of apprehension, nervousness, worry, or fearfulness. Sedatives and hypnotics are drugs that depress the CNS, produce a calming effect, and help induce sleep. Alcohol has characteristics of both of these drug groups.
- Anticonvulsant drugs are used to treat seizure disorders. Most notably they treat epilepsy.
- All CNS stimulants work to increase excitability. They do this by blocking the activity of inhibitory neurons or their respective neurotransmitters or by enhancing the production of the excitatory neurotransmitters.
- Psychotherapeutic drugs include antipsychotic agents, antidepressants, and lithium. These drugs are used to treat psychoses and affective disorders, especially schizophrenia, depression, and mania.
- Movement disorders such as Parkinson disease can result from an imbalance of dopamine and acetylcholine. Drugs that inhibit or block acetylcholine are referred to as anticholinergic. Three classes of drugs affect brain dopamine levels: those that release dopamine, those that increase brain levels of dopamine, and dopaminergic agonists.

- Skeletal muscle relaxants can be classified as central acting, direct acting, and neuromuscular blockers.
- Cardiac drugs are classified by their effects on specialized cardiac tissues. Cardiac glycosides are used to treat congestive heart failure and certain tachycardias. Antidysrhythmic drugs are used to treat and prevent disorders of cardiac rhythm. The pharmacologic agents that suppress dysrhythmias may do so by direct action on the cardiac cell membrane (lidocaine), by indirect action that affects the cell (metoprolol), or both. The four classes of antidysrhythmic drugs are sodium channel blockers, beta blockers, potassium channel blockers, and calcium channel blockers.
- Antihypertensive drugs used to reduce blood pressure are classified into six major categories: diuretics, sympathetic-blocking agents (sympatholytic drugs), vasodilators, calcium channel blockers, angiotensin-converting enzyme (ACE) inhibitors, and angiotensin II receptor antagonists.
- Antihemorrheologic agents are used to treat peripheral vascular disorders. These disorders are caused by pathologic or physiologic obstruction (eg, arteriosclerosis). These agents improve blood flow to ischemic tissues.
- Drugs that affect blood coagulation may be classified as antiplatelet, anticoagulant, or fibrinolytic agents. Drugs that interfere with platelet aggregation are known as antiplatelet or antithrombic drugs. Anticoagulant drug therapy is designed to prevent intravascular thrombosis. The therapy decreases blood coagulability. Fibrinolytic drugs dissolve clots after their formation. These drugs work by promoting the breakdown of fibrin.
- Hemophilia is a group of hereditary bleeding disorders. These disorders involve a deficiency of one of the factors needed for the coagulation of blood. Replacing the missing clotting factor can help manage hemophilia.
- Hemostatic agents accelerate clot formation, thus reducing bleeding. Systemic hemostatic agents are used to control blood loss after surgery. They work by inhibiting the breakdown of fibrin. Topical hemostatic agents are used to control capillary bleeding. They are used during surgical and dental procedures. Antifibrinolytic drugs prevent destruction of existing clots.
- The treatment of choice in managing a loss of blood or blood components is to replace the blood component that is deficient. Replacement therapy may include transfusing whole blood (rare), packed red blood cells, fresh-frozen plasma, plasma expanders, platelets, cryoprecipitate, fibrinogen, albumin, or gamma globulins.
- Antihyperlipidemic drugs sometimes are used along with diet and exercise to control serum lipid levels, which may include high levels of cholesterol and triglycerides.
- Bronchodilator drugs are the primary form of treatment for obstructive pulmonary disease such as asthma, chronic bronchitis, and emphysema. These drugs may be classified as sympathomimetic drugs, anticholinergic agents, and xanthine derivatives.
- Mucokinetic drugs are used to move respiratory secretions, excessive mucus, and sputum along the tracheobronchial tree.
- Oxygen is used chiefly to treat hypoxia and hypoxemia.
- Direct respiratory stimulant drugs act directly on the medullary center of the brain. These drugs are analeptics. They increase the rate and depth of respiration.
- A cough may be prolonged or result from an underlying disorder. In such a case, treatment with antitussive drugs may be indicated.
- The main clinical use of antihistamines is for allergic reactions. They also are used to control motion sickness or as a sedative or antiemetic.
- Drug therapy for the gastrointestinal system can be divided into drugs that affect the stomach and drugs that affect the lower gastrointestinal tract. Antacids buffer or neutralize hydrochloric acid in the stomach. Antiflatulents prevent the formation of gas in the gastrointestinal tract. Digestant drugs promote digestion in the gastrointestinal tract. They do this by releasing small amounts of hydrochloric acid in the stomach. Drugs used to treat nausea and vomiting include antagonists of histamine, acetylcholine, and dopamine as well as other drugs, the actions of which are not understood clearly.
- Cytoprotective agents and other drugs are used to treat peptic ulcer disease by protecting the gastric mucosa. H_2-receptor antagonists block the H_2 receptors. They also reduce the volume of gastric acid secretion and its acid content. Proton pump inhibitors decrease hydrochloric acid secretion by inhibiting the actions of the parietal cells.
- Two common conditions of the lower gastrointestinal tract may require drug therapy: constipation and diarrhea. Drugs used to manage these conditions include laxatives and antidiarrheals.
- Drugs used to treat eye disorders include antiglaucoma agents, mydriatics, cycloplegics, anti-infective/anti-inflammatory agents, and topical anesthetics.
- Drugs used to treat disorders of the ear include antibiotics, steroid/antibiotic combinations, and miscellaneous preparations.
- The endocrine system works to control and integrate body functions. A number of drugs are used to treat disorders of the anterior and posterior pituitary, the thyroid and parathyroid glands, and the adrenal cortex.
- The pancreatic hormones play a key role in regulating the amount of certain nutrients in the circulatory system. The two main hormones secreted by the pancreas are insulin and glucagon. Imbalances in either of these may necessitate drug therapy. This therapy is meant to correct metabolic derangements. Oral hypoglycemic agents help lower blood glucose level by a variety of mechanisms.
- Drugs that affect the female reproductive system include synthetic and natural substances such as hormones (estrogen and progesterone), oral contraceptives, ovulation stimulants, and drugs used to treat infertility.

- The male sex hormone is testosterone. Adequate amounts of this hormone are needed for normal development and maintenance of male sex characteristics.
- Erectile dysfunction drugs are used to enhance sexual function.
- Antineoplastic agents are used in cancer chemotherapy to prevent the increase of malignant cells.
- People can be infected by bacterial organisms, fungi, and viruses.
  - Antibiotics are used to treat local or systemic infection. This group includes penicillins, cephalosporins, and related products; macrolide antibiotics; tetracyclines; fluoroquinolones; and miscellaneous antibiotic agents.
  - Examples of antifungal drugs include tolnaftate (Tinactin), fluconazole (Diflucan), and nystatin (Mycostatin).
  - Few drugs exist to treat viral infections. One antiviral drug is acyclovir (Zovirax). This drug is effective against herpes infection. Another drug is zidovudine (Retrovir, AZT), which currently is used to treat human immunodeficiency virus infection.
- Drugs used to treat inflammation or its symptoms may be classified as analgesic-antipyretic drugs and nonsteroidal anti-inflammatory drugs. A number of medications have both properties.
- Immunosuppressant drugs reduce the activity of the immune system. They do this by suppressing the production and activity of lymphocytes. These drugs are prescribed after transplant surgery. They can help to prevent the rejection of foreign tissues. They also are sometimes given to halt the progress of autoimmune disorders.
- Immunomodulating agents are drugs that help the immune system to be more efficient. They do this by activating the immune defenses and by modifying a biologic response to an unwanted stimulus.
- Serum contains antibodies, which are agents of immunity. The antibodies can protect against an organism if the serum is injected into someone else. This process forms the basis for passive immunization. Vaccines are composed of killed or altered microorganisms. They are administered to a person to produce specific immunity to a disease-causing bacterial toxin, virus, or bacterium (active immunization).

References

1. Lyons A, Petrucelli R. *Medicine: An Illustrated History*. New York, NY: Abradale Press; 1987.
2. O'Toole M, ed. *Mosby's Medical, Nursing, and Allied Health Dictionary*. 10th ed. St Louis, MO: Elsevier; 2017.
3. McKenry L, Salerno E. *Mosby's Pharmacology in Nursing*. 22nd ed. St Louis, MO: Mosby; 2005.
4. US Department of Health and Human Services, Food and Drug Administration, and Center for Drug Evaluation and Research. Guidance for industry: orally disintegrating tablets. Food and Drug Administration website. https://www.fda.gov/downloads/Drugs/.../Guidances/ucm070578.pdf. Published December 2008. Accessed January 26, 2018.
5. Buck M. Intraosseous administration of drugs in infants and children. *Pediatr Pharm*. 2006;12(12).
6. Tay ET. Intravenous access. Medscape website. http://reference.medscape.com/article/80431-overview. Updated April 12, 2017. Accessed January 26, 2018.
7. *Guidelines 2000 for Cardiopulmonary Resuscitation and Emergency Cardiovascular Care*. International Consensus on Science. Dallas, TX: American Heart Association; 2000.
8. Gahart B, Nazareno AR. *2018 Intravenous Medications: A Handbook for Nurses and Health Professionals*. 34th ed. St Louis, MO: Mosby; 2018.
9. Mowry B, Spyker D, Brooks DE, Zimmerman A, Schauben JL. 2015 Annual Report of the American Association of Poison Control Centers' National Poison Data System (NPDS): 33rd Annual Report. *Clin Toxicol (Philadelphia)*. 2016;54(10):924-1109.
10. Beard JD, Steege AS, Ju J, Lu J, Luckhaput SE, Schubauer-Bergan MK. Mortality from amyotrophic lateral sclerosis and Parkinson's disease among different occupational groups—United States, 1985–2011. *Morb Mortal Wkly Rep*. 2017;66(27):718-722.
11. National Center for Chronic Disease Prevention and Health Promotion, Division for Heart Disease and Stroke Prevention. High blood pressure facts. Centers for Disease Control and Prevention website. https://www.cdc.gov/bloodpressure/facts.htm. Updated November 30, 2016. Accessed January 26, 2018.
12. Connors JM. Antidote for factor Xa anticoagulants. *N Engl J Med*. 2015;373:2471-2472.
13. Jones & Bartlett Learning. *2017 Nurse's Drug Handbook*. 16th ed. Burlington, MA: Jones & Bartlett Learning; 2017.
14. American Heart Association. *Advanced Cardiac Life Support*. Dallas, TX: American Heart Association; 2016.
15. Davids NB, Mabry RL. Hemorrhage control. In: Cone DC, Brice JH, Delbridge TR, eds. *Emergency Medical Services: Clinical Practice and Systems Oversight*. Vol 1. 2nd ed. West Sussex, UK: John Wiley & Sons Ltd; 2015.
16. Neeki MM, Dong F, Toy J, et al. Efficacy and safety of tranexamic acid in prehospital traumatic hemorrhagic shock: outcomes of the Cal-PAT Study. *West J Emerg Med*. 2017;18(4):673-683.
17. Fischer PE, Bulger EM, Perina DG, et al. Guidance document for the prehospital use of tranexamic acid in injured patients. *Prehosp Emerg Care*. 2016;20(5):557-559.
18. US Department Health and Human Services, National Institutes of Health, National Heart Lung and Blood Institute. *Guidelines for the Diagnosis and Management of Asthma (EPR-3)*. National Heart Lung and Blood Institute website. https://www.nhlbi.nih.gov/files/docs/guidelines/asthsumm.pdf. Published October 2017. Accessed January 26, 2018.
19. Goldman L, Schafer AL. *Goldman-Cecil Medicine*. 25th ed. Philadelphia, PA: Elsevier Saunders; 2016.
20. Worldwide data. World Cancer Research Fund International website. http://www.wcrf.org/int/cancer-facts-figures/worldwide-data. Accessed January 26, 2018.

21. Bhattacharya S. The facts about penicillin allergy: a review. *J Adv Pharmaceutical Technol Res.* 2010;1(1):11-17.
22. Centers for Disease Control and Prevention, National Center for Immunization and Respiratory Diseases (NCIRD). Influenza antiviral medications. Centers for Disease Control and Prevention website. https://www.cdc.gov/flu/professionals/antivirals/summary-clinicians.htm. Updated October 26, 2017. Accessed January 26, 2018.
23. American Heart Association News. Non-steroidal anti-inflammatory drugs Q&A. American Heart Association website. http://news.heart.org/nsaids-qa/. Accessed January 26, 2018.

Suggested Readings

Brunton L, Chabner B, Knollmann B. *Goodman and Gilman's Pharmacological Basis of Therapeutics*. 12th ed. New York, NY: McGraw-Hill; 2016.

Bledsoe B, Claydon D. *Prehospital Emergency Pharmacology*. 7th ed. New York, NY: Pearson; 2011.

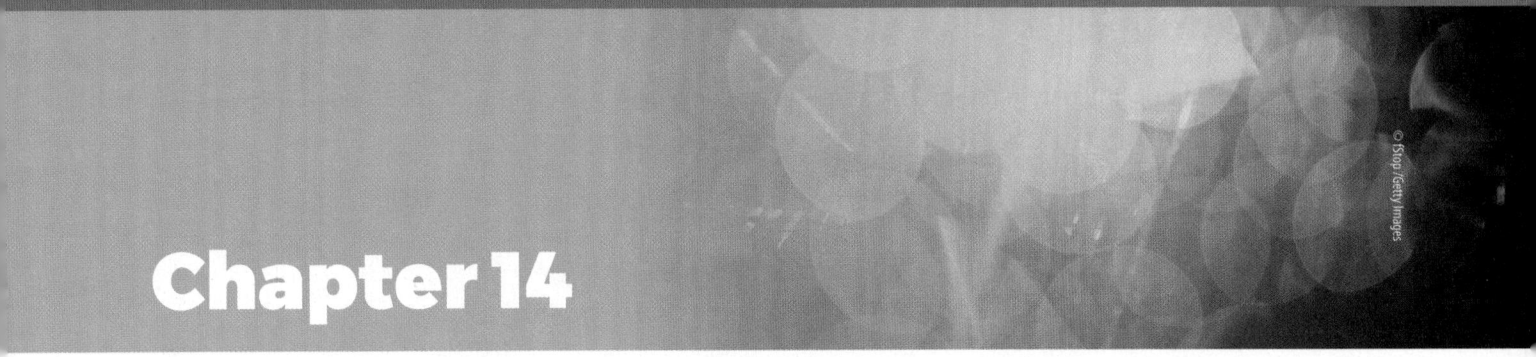

Chapter 14

Medication Administration

NATIONAL EMS EDUCATION STANDARD COMPETENCIES

Pharmacology

Integrates comprehensive knowledge of pharmacology to formulate a treatment plan intended to mitigate emergencies and improve the overall health of the patient.

Medication Administration

- Routes of administration (pp 434–435, 439–444, 457, 459, 461, 462, 464, 466)
- Self-administer medication (pp 434, 459, 461–466)
- Peer-administer medication (pp 434–466)
- Assist/administer medications to a patient (pp 434–466)
- Within the scope of practice of the paramedic, administer medications to a patient (pp 434–466)

OBJECTIVES

Upon completion of this chapter, the paramedic student will be able to:

1. Convert selected units of measurement into the metric and household systems. (pp 422–424)
2. Identify the steps in the calculation of drug dosages. (pp 425–428)
3. Calculate the correct volume of drug to be administered in a given situation. (pp 425–428)
4. List measures for ensuring the safe administration of medications. (pp 428, 430–431)
5. Describe actions paramedics should take if a medication error occurs. (pp 431–432)
6. List measures for preserving asepsis during parenteral administration of a drug. (pp 432–434)
7. Explain drug administration techniques for the enteral and parenteral routes. (pp 434–450, 453–459)
8. Compute the correct rate for an infusion of drugs or intravenous fluids. (pp 444–445)
9. Describe the steps for safely initiating an intravenous infusion. (pp 445–450)
10. Identify complications and adverse effects associated with intravenous access. (pp 450–453)
11. List the steps for safely initiating intravenous access. (pp 453–457)
12. Describe the steps for safely initiating an intraosseous infusion. (pp 459–460)
13. Explain drug administration techniques for the transmucosal, transdermal, inhalation, and endotracheal routes. (pp 459–466)
14. Identify special considerations in the administration of pharmacologic agents to pediatric patients. (pp 466–467)
15. Explain the technique for obtaining a venous blood sample. (pp 467–469)
16. Describe the safe disposal of contaminated items and sharps. (p 469)

KEY TERMS

air embolism The presence of air bubbles in the bloodstream.

catheter fragment embolism The shearing or detachment of an intravenous catheter, allowing the embolus to travel in the bloodstream.

cellulitis An infectious condition of the skin resulting in inflammation that is characterized most commonly by local heat, redness, pain, and swelling, and occasionally by fever, malaise, chills, and headache.

centimeter A metric unit of length equal to 1/100 (ie, 0.01) of a meter, or 0.3937 inch.

deciliter A metric unit of volume equal to 1/10 (ie, 0.1) of a liter.

embolus A blockage or free-moving thrombus in a blood vessel.

extravasation The passage or escape of blood, serum, or lymph into the tissues.

gram A metric unit of mass equal to $^1/_{1,000}$ (ie, 0.001) of a kilogram.

hematoma formation The infiltration of blood into the tissues at the site of venipuncture.

household system A common system of measurement that includes the glass, cup, tablespoon, teaspoon, drop, quart, and pint.

Infiltration The process by which a fluid passes into tissues.

kilogram A metric unit of mass equal to 1,000 grams, or 2.2046 pounds.

liter A metric unit of capacity equal to 1 cubic decimeter, 61.025 cubic inches, or 1.0567 liquid quarts.

medical asepsis The removal or destruction of disease-causing organisms or infected material.

meter A metric unit of length equal to 1,000 millimeters.

metric system A system of measurement that includes the meter, liter, and gram.

microgram A metric unit of mass equal to $^1/_{1,000,000}$ (ie, 0.000001) of a gram.

milligram A metric unit of mass equal to $^1/_{1,000}$ (ie, 0.001) of a gram.

milliliter A metric unit of capacity equal to $^1/_{1,000}$ (ie, 0.001) of a liter.

millimeter A metric unit of length equal to $^1/_{1,000}$ (ie, 0.001) of a meter

necrosis The death of tissue.

phlebitis Inflammation of a vein, often accompanied by the formation of a clot; also known as thrombophlebitis.

pulmonary embolism The blockage of a pulmonary artery by foreign matter, such as fat, air, tumor tissue, or a thrombus that usually arises from a peripheral vein.

sepsis Infection.

sloughing The separation of tissue.

thromboembolism A condition in which a blood vessel is blocked by an embolus carried in the bloodstream from the site of formation of the clot.

thrombosis The formation of a blood clot (thrombus) in a blood vessel.

transdermal drug administration Administration of drugs that are absorbed through the skin.

The ability to gain venous access safely and to administer prescribed medications are key elements of professional paramedic practice. This chapter addresses techniques for drug administration. It also emphasizes the paramedic's patient care responsibilities with regard to medication therapy.

NOTE

Math skills are important in the administration of drugs. These skills include multiplication and division, figuring percentages, and working with Roman numerals, fractions, decimal fractions, and proportions. Paramedics must have a good working knowledge of these principles and must be adept at calculations.

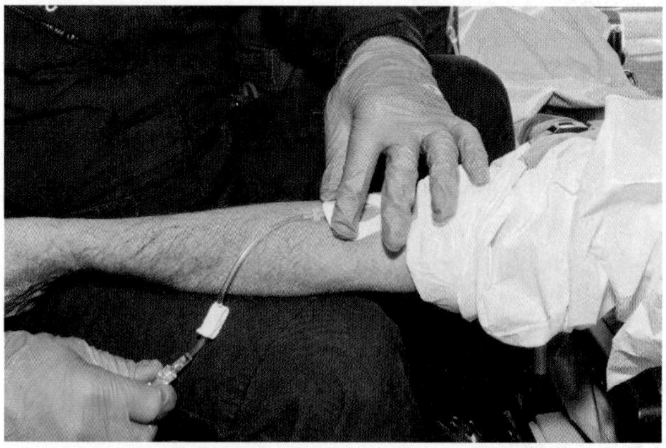

Mathematical Equivalents Used in Pharmacology

Two systems for measuring drug dosages are in common use today: the **metric system** and the common **household system** (BOX 14-1). Each system deals with units of mass and volume. A physician may use either of these systems in ordering drugs.

Metric System

The French developed the metric system of weights and measures in the late 1700s. Although the US Congress declared it to be the official measurement

BOX 14-1 Systems of Equivalents

Metric System

1 g = 0.001 kg
1 g = 1,000 mg
1 L = 1,000 mL

Household System

1 lb = 16 oz
1 pt = 1/2 qt = 1/8 gal
1 pt = 16 fl oz = 32 T
1 T = 3 t
1 t = 5 mL
1 T = 15 mL
1 pt = 480 mL
1 qt = 960 mL
1.0 gal = 3.84 L

Abbreviations: fl oz, fluid ounce; g, gram; gal, gallon; L, liter; lb, pound; mg, milligram; mL, milliliter; pt, pint; qt, quart; t, teaspoon; T, tablespoon

system in the United States in 1866,[1] use of the metric system is not required in the United States. The metric system, however, has been adopted by US medical sciences and pharmacies, and most countries around the world use this system. The International System of Units is the modern form of the metric system; its name is often abbreviated as SI, from the French *Le Système International d'Unités.*

The basic SI units of measurement are the **meter**, the unit for linear measurement; the **liter**, the unit for capacity or volume; and the **gram**, the unit for weight. A meter is slightly longer than a yard, a liter is slightly more than a quart, and a gram is slightly more than the weight of a metal paper clip.

The basic units of the metric system can be divided or multiplied by 10, 100, or 1,000 to form secondary units; these secondary units therefore differ from each other by 10 or some multiple of 10. Subdivisions of these basic units are made when the decimal within a number is moved to the left. Multiples of the basic units are made when the decimal is moved to the right. The names of the secondary units are formed by putting a Greek or Latin prefix on the primary unit (**TABLE 14-1**).

The meter (m) is the unit of length from which the other metric units of length are derived (**FIGURE 14-1**). The **centimeter** (cm) and the **millimeter** (mm) are the primary linear measurements used in medicine. For example, they are used to measure the size of body organs and to measure blood pressure.

TABLE 14-1 Common Metric Prefixes

Prefix	Meaning
kilo-	1,000 times greater
deci-	10 times less
centi-	100 times less
milli-	1,000 times less
micro-	1,000,000 times less

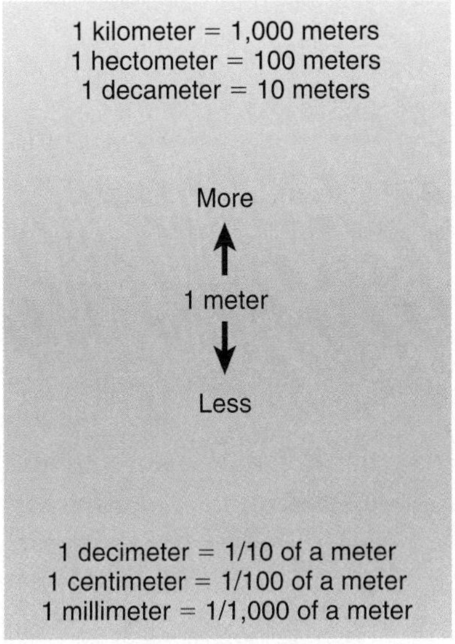

FIGURE 14-1 The meter measures length.

The liter (L) is the unit of capacity or volume (**FIGURE 14-2**). A fractional part of a liter is expressed in milliliters (mL) or cubic centimeters (cc). The liter is equal to 1,000 mL (1,000 cc). A **milliliter**, therefore, is 1/1,000 (ie, 0.001) of a liter. A **deciliter** is 1/10 (ie, 0.1) of a liter. The National Institute of Standards and Technology recommends that the units of measure *ml*, or *mL*, and *dl*, or *dL*, be used to express fractional parts of a liter.

The gram (g) is the metric unit used to weigh drugs and various pharmaceutical preparations (**FIGURE 14-3**). The gram equals the weight of 1 mL of distilled water at 39.2°F (4°C). A **kilogram** (kg) is equal to 1,000 grams, or 2.2 pounds. A **milligram** (mg) is equal to 1/1,000 (ie, 0.001) of a gram. A **microgram** (mcg) is equal to 1/1,000,000 (ie, 0.000001) of a gram.

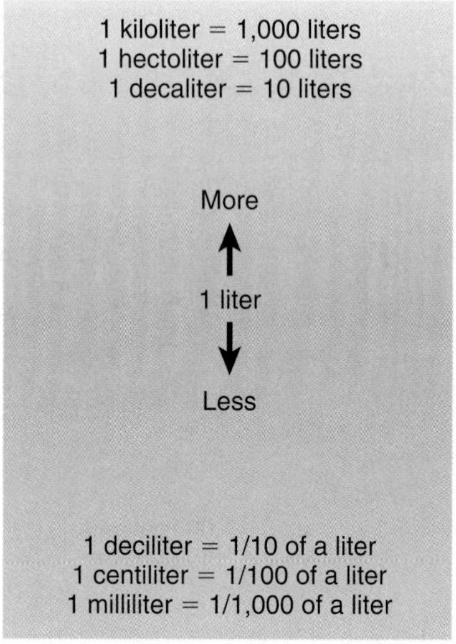

FIGURE 14-2 The liter measures capacity.

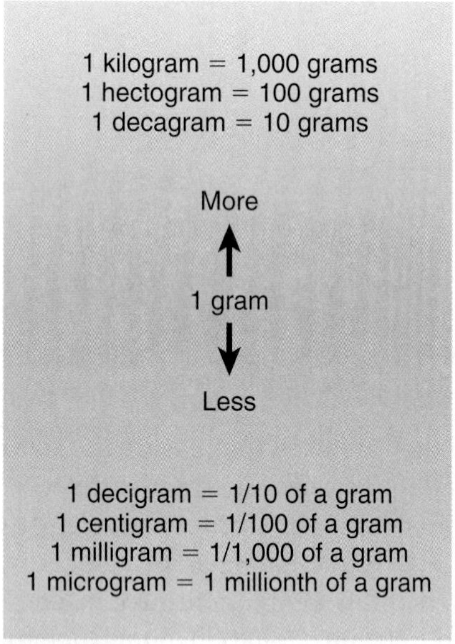

FIGURE 14-3 The gram measures weight.

Metric Style of Notation

The National Institute of Standards and Technology recommends the following style of metric notation except when it conflicts with the proper use of English:[2]

- Units are not capitalized (gram, not Gram).
- Unit abbreviations are not followed by a period (mL, not m.L. or mL.).
- A single space is left between the quantity and the symbol (24 kg, not 24kg).
- Unit abbreviations are not pluralized (kg, not kgs).
- As a rule, fractions are not used, only decimal notation (0.25 kg, not ¼ kg).
- For numeric quantities less than 1, a 0 (zero) is placed to the left of the decimal point (0.75 mg, not .75 mg).
- Trailing zeros should not be used after a decimal point (2 mg, not 2.0 mg).

CRITICAL THINKING

Placing a zero to the left of the decimal point reduces the likelihood of a drug dosing error. Why?

Household System

Standard (ie, exact) measures of the household system are not available in most homes, so household measurements are only approximations. For example, the average coffee cup may hold 5 to 9 ounces or more, and the average household teaspoon may hold 4 to 6 mL of liquid.

The household units for weight are pounds and ounces. The household conversion needed most often in emergency drug therapy is pounds to kilograms: 1 kg = 2.2 pounds. When the weight of an adult patient is converted from pounds to kilograms, the whole number can be rounded up when the number to the right of the decimal point is 5 or greater. For example, 70.9 kg could be rounded up to 71 kg.

Temperature Conversions

The *Fahrenheit* and *Celsius* (centigrade) temperature scales are used to measure temperature (**FIGURE 14-4**). On the Fahrenheit scale, water freezes at 32° and boils at 212°. On the Celsius scale, water freezes at 0° and boils at 100°. Throughout most of the world, the Celsius scale is the preferred temperature scale used in scientific and engineering fields. Most of the general population in the United States is more accustomed to the Fahrenheit scale, however, because the Fahrenheit scale is widely used by the US media in weather forecasts.

Normal body temperature is 98.6°F, or 37°C. A simple formula can be used to convert temperatures. To convert a Celsius reading to Fahrenheit, multiply

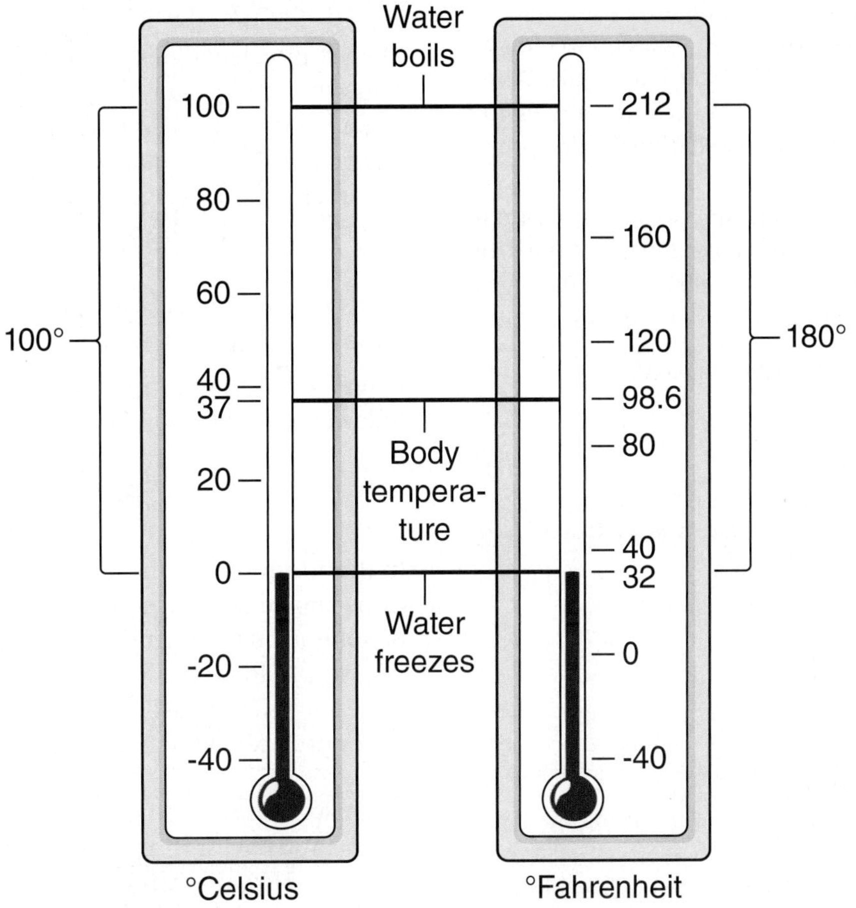

FIGURE 14-4 Comparison of the Celsius and Fahrenheit temperature scales.

the Celsius reading by 9⁄5, or 1.8; then add 32. To convert a Fahrenheit reading to Celsius, subtract 32 from the Fahrenheit reading; then multiply by 5⁄9, or 0.555.

> NOTE
> Remember these temperature conversion formulas:
> Celsius to Fahrenheit: (°C × 9⁄5) + 32, or (°C × 1.8) + 32
> Fahrenheit to Celsius: (°F − 32) × 5⁄9, or (°F − 32) × 0.555

Drug Calculations

While providing emergency care, the paramedic must calculate adult and pediatric drug dosages and infusion rates, as well as the strength of drug solutions and diluted solutions. These tasks involve using basic math skills in a logical order, which requires a working knowledge of decimals, fractions, ratios, and proportions. This section presents commonly used equations used for drug calculations that are accepted in the medical community. Other drug calculation methods may work as well.

Calculation Methods

Calculation methods must be precise and reliable. To perform drug calculations, paramedics should do the following:

- Convert all units of measure to the same unit and system.
- Check the computed dosage to determine whether it is reasonable.
- Use one dosage calculation method consistently.

Conversion of Units of Measure

Most emergency drug preparations do not require conversion, because most drugs are packaged in milligrams and administered in milligrams. However, some drugs, such as dopamine, are packaged in milligrams but administered in micrograms (mcg). These drugs must be converted to like units. When conversion to like units is required, the conversion must be completed before calculating the drug dose.

Example. You are to administer dopamine at a rate of 800 mcg per minute. You have 200 mg of the drug in 250 mL of solution. Convert 800 mcg to 0.8 mg so that both measures of weight are in the same units:

$$800 \text{ mcg} \div 1{,}000 = 0.8 \text{ mg}$$

CRITICAL THINKING

Imagine that you failed to convert the 800 mcg of dopamine to 0.8 mg in this example. Would you overdose or underdose the patient?

NOTE

Math tip: Move the decimal point to the right when multiplying (converting the measurement to smaller units). Move it to the left when dividing (converting the measurement to larger units).

When the dose is given per unit of weight (kg), the patient's weight must be converted from pounds to kilograms. This conversion should be done before calculating the total dose to be given.

Example. You are to give 1 mg/kg of lidocaine to a patient who weighs 132 pounds. Divide 132 by 2.2 to convert pounds to kilograms (132 pounds = 60 kg). The total dose is 1 mg/kg multiplied by 60 kg, which equals 60 mg.

$$132 \text{ lb} \div 2.2 = 60 \text{ kg}$$

$$1 \text{mg/kg} \times 60 \text{ kg} = 60 \text{ mg}$$

Assessment of Computed Doses

Many emergency drugs are packaged in units that contain enough drug for a normal adult dose. After computations are performed, the paramedic should decide whether the answer is reasonable.

Example. You are to administer 8 mg of diazepam. It is supplied in a 2-mL ampule that contains 10 mg of the drug. Therefore, a reasonable calculation of volume would be less than 2 mL.

Methods of Calculation

Many drug calculations can be performed almost intuitively, because many drugs are packaged to supply one adult dose. However, a paramedic should never rely on intuitive calculations, no matter how simple the drug dose may seem. The three methods of calculation discussed in this section are most widely used.

Method 1: Basic Formula ("Desire Over Have")

In method 1, information must be substituted in the following formula:

$$\frac{D}{H} \times Q = X$$

In this formula, *D* is the desired dose to be given, *H* is the known dose on hand, *Q* is the unit of measure or volume on hand, and *X* is the unit of measure to be given. Many consider "desire over have" to be the easiest formula to use. It works for nearly all emergency drug calculations.

Example. You are to administer 25 mg of diphenhydramine. You have a 10-mL vial that contains 50 mg of the drug. How many milliliters will you give? Using the "desire over have" formula, calculate the dose.

$$\frac{25 \text{ mg}}{50 \text{ mg}} \times 10 \text{ mL} = X$$

$$\frac{25}{5} \times 1 \text{ mL} = X$$

$$5 \times 1 \text{ mL} = X$$

$$X = 5 \text{ mL}$$

NOTE

Math tip: When using the basic formula, always divide the bottom number into the top number.

Method 2: Ratios and Proportions

Method 2 uses ratios and proportions to calculate the drug dosage. A ratio compares two numbers and is the same as a fraction. When used to calculate drug doses, a ratio refers to the weight or quantity of a drug in solution. For example, the ratio of 10 mg of morphine in 1 mL of solution is 10 mg to 1 mL. A proportion is an equation made up of two ratios; it states that the two ratios are equal. For example, ⅔ is equal to ⁴⁄₆

(2:3 :: 4:6); therefore the ratios are equivalent and the proportions are true.

To use method 2, the equation must be set up to ensure that the same units of measure are stated in the same sequence (eg, mg: mL = mg: x mL). x is the quantity (eg, mL) to be solved. The formula can be expressed as

Dose on Hand : Volume on Hand :: Desired Dose : Desired Volume

Example. You are to administer 40 mg of furosemide. You have 100 mg of the drug in 10 mL of solution. How many milliliters will you give? Calculate the dose using ratios and proportions:

$$100 \text{ mg} : 10 \text{ mL} :: 40 \text{ mg} : x \text{ mL}$$

Multiply inside numbers (means) and outside numbers (extremes). Drop the unit of measurement terms.

Means

$$100 \text{ mg} : 10 \text{ mL} :: 40 \text{ mg} : x \text{ mL}$$

Extremes

Solve the proportion by dividing both sides of the equation by the number before the multiplication symbol, × (100, in this example).

$$\frac{100x}{100} \times \frac{400}{100} = 4 \text{ mL}$$

> NOTE
>
> Math tip: Remember the phrases *middle for means* and *end for extremes*. In a proportion, the product of the means is always equal to the product of the extremes.

To check your answer, multiply the means and then multiply the extremes. The sum product will be equal if the proportion is true.

$$\left.\begin{array}{l} 100 \times 4 = 400 \\ 10 \times 40 = 400 \end{array}\right\} \text{Sum parts are equal}$$

Method 3: Dimensional Analysis

Dimensional analysis works well for complex drug calculations—for example, those that call for several conversions of a similar basic dimensional unit so that all units of measure are changed to like units (eg, milligrams). Dimensional analysis is based on the same tenet as the basic formula, but it does not require memorization of the "desire over have" equation. All conversion factors are set up in one equation and are separated by multiplication signs.

> NOTE
>
> Math tip: When using dimensional analysis, convert all units to the easiest math operation. This reduces the chance of error.

Example. You are to administer 0.8 mg of naloxone. The drug is packaged in 1 mL of solution containing 0.4 mg of the drug.

Step 1. Set up the equation, placing the desired unit of measure in the answer to the left of the equal sign. Place the first factor to the right of the equal sign. Make sure it is the same unit as the answer.

$$\text{mL} = \frac{1 \text{ mL}}{0.4 \text{ mg}} \times \frac{0.8 \text{ mg}}{1}$$

Step 2. Cancel like units of measure in the numerator and denominator, and reduce the fraction, if needed:

$$\text{mL} = \frac{1 \text{ mL}}{0.4 \cancel{\text{mg}}} \times \frac{0.8 \cancel{\text{mg}}}{1}$$

> NOTE
>
> Math tip: The only unit remaining after canceling the like units should be the unit of the answer. If this is not the case, the equation is set up incorrectly.

Step 3. Multiply the numerators and then the denominators.

$$\text{mL} = \frac{1 \text{ mL}}{0.4} \times \frac{0.8}{1}$$

Step 4. Divide the numerator by the denominator to solve the equation.

$$\text{mL} = \frac{0.8 \text{ mL}}{0.4} = 2 \text{ mL}$$

Calculating Drug Dosages for Infants and Children

The doses of some medications for infants and children are administered in the same proportion to body weight as the doses for adults. Others are given in very reduced doses, due to differences in children's ability to metabolize the drug. In general, the total dose administered to a child rarely exceeds a normal adult dose (see Chapter 13, *Principles of Pharmacology and Emergency Medications*).

Paramedics often calculate pediatric drug doses in the prehospital setting by using memory aids—such as charts, tapes, pocket guides, and dosage wheels (**FIGURE 14-5**)—or after consulting with medical direction. Some of the memory aids, such as personal electronic devices and cell phone apps, include drug calculation software (**FIGURE 14-6**). The most precise way to calculate a pediatric drug dose is based on the child's body surface area. (Body surface area as a function of weight is discussed in Chapter 47, *Pediatrics.*) The wisest course is to have someone double-check the dose before a medication is administered to a child.

NOTE

Paramedics who administer a medication do so by the authority provided by medical direction. The paramedic has both a professional and a legal responsibility to follow all patient management protocols, policies, and procedures. These policies specify the regulations of drug administration, including policies on the stocking and supply of drugs.

Drug Administration

During the administration of any drug, safety should always be a high priority.

Safety Considerations and Procedures

In the prehospital setting, paramedics should carefully follow all standing orders and protocols for drug therapy. Specifically, they should take the following precautions:

- Make sure any medication orders received from medical direction are fully understood. Repeat all orders back to medical direction for confirmation, stating the name of the drug, the dose, and the route by which it is to be given. If the order is unclear or if there is reason to question the order, ask medical direction to repeat it.
- In the emergency department or other patient care areas, make sure there is a written or electronic order for every medication administered.
- Verify the patient's name on the person's armband or identification tag and scan the tag (per protocol for electronic recordkeeping).
- Verify that the patient is not allergic to the medication.
- Strictly follow these five patient rights of drug administration: Make sure the right patient receives the right dose of the right drug via the right route at the right time.
- Some sources add documentation as the sixth right of medication administration. It is essential to document the drug administration accurately and thoroughly.

In addition, paramedics should follow these guidelines during drug administration:

- Focus on the procedure and avoid distractions (including when preparing the medicines).
- Make a habit of reading the drug label and comparing it to the medication order at least three times before administration:
  1. When removing the drug from the drug kit or supply area
  2. When preparing the medication for administration
  3. Just before administering the drug to the patient (before the container is discarded)
- Check for the correct route of administration. Some medications can be prepared for administration by several routes—for instance, either intramuscular or intravenous.
- Make sure the information on the label matches the prescriber's order.
- Never give a medicine from an unlabeled container. Also, never give a medicine from a container on which the label is not legible.
- If unsure about the drug calculation, have a coworker check it. Alternatively, contact medical direction for verification.
- Handle multidose vials carefully and with aseptic technique, so as to prevent drugs from being wasted or contaminated.
- When preparing more than one injection, always label the syringe immediately. Keep the medication container with the syringe. Do not

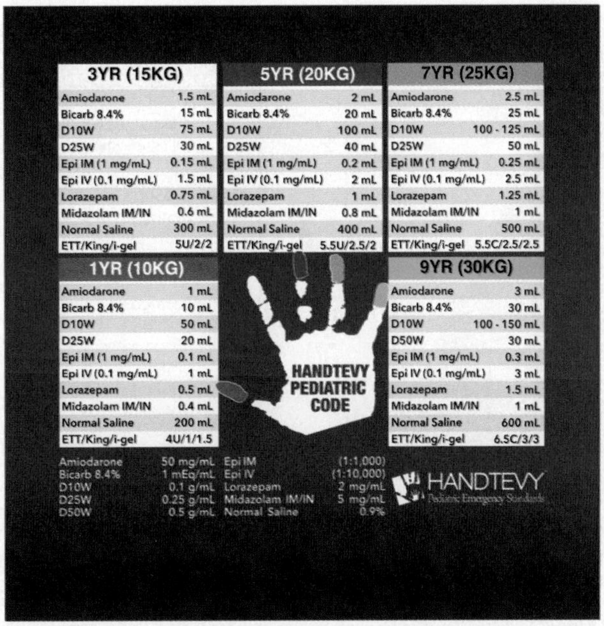

A

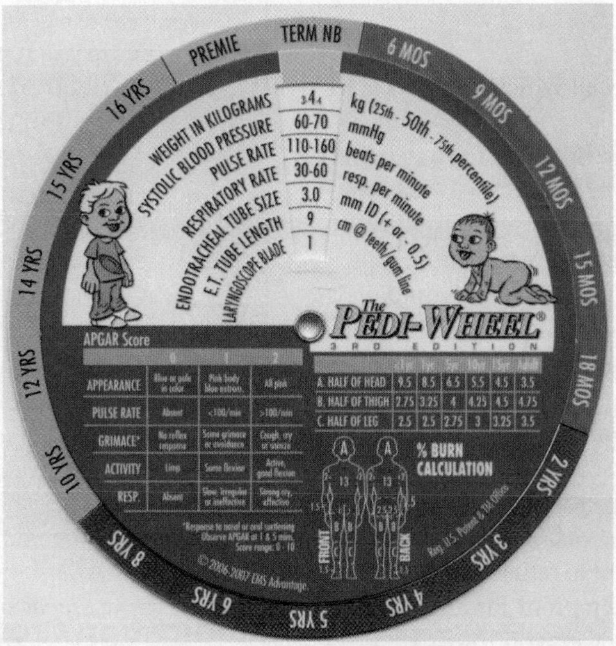

B

FIGURE 14-5 A. The Handtevy badge buddy is a quick-reference card that allows providers to determine medication volumes prior to the patient encounter. The badge buddy is a piece of a comprehensive system of care which utilizes customized dosing guides and an integrated mobile application. To use the Handtevy Method: 1. On your hand, count the age in years; 2. Then count the weight in kilograms; 3. Once the weight is known, the volume dosages are easily obtainable. For complete information on the Handtevy Method, refer to www.Handtevy.com. **B.** Pedi Wheel. Select the patient's age to find average weight in kilograms, systolic blood pressure, pulse rate, respiratory rate, endotracheal tube (ET) size, ET tube length, and laryngoscope blade.

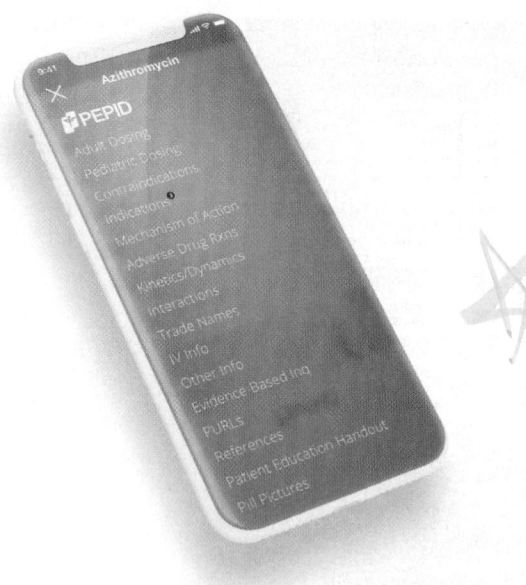

FIGURE 14-6 Drug references are available on wireless devices.

Image used with permission from PEPID LLC Medical Information Services.

rely on memory to recall which solution is in which syringe.

- Never administer a medicine that is unlabeled and that was prepared by someone else. In doing so, the paramedic accepts the responsibility for accuracy, dose, and correct medication.
- Never administer a medication that is outdated. Likewise, never give one that looks discolored, cloudy, or in any other way unusual, or as if someone has tampered with it.
- If the patient or a coworker expresses doubt or concern about a medication or dose, recheck it. Do not administer it until everyone is certain that no error has been made. Remember that the patient has the right to refuse a medication.
- Carefully monitor the patient for any adverse effects. Monitor for at least 5 minutes after giving the medication. (Intramuscular and oral medicines may require longer monitoring.)
- Document all medications given, including the name of the drug, the dosage, and the time and route of administration. When documenting administration of parenteral medications, note the site of injection. Record the patient's response, including both adverse and intended effects.
- Follow government guidelines and local emergency medical services (EMS) policies regarding the return and disposal of any unused medication.

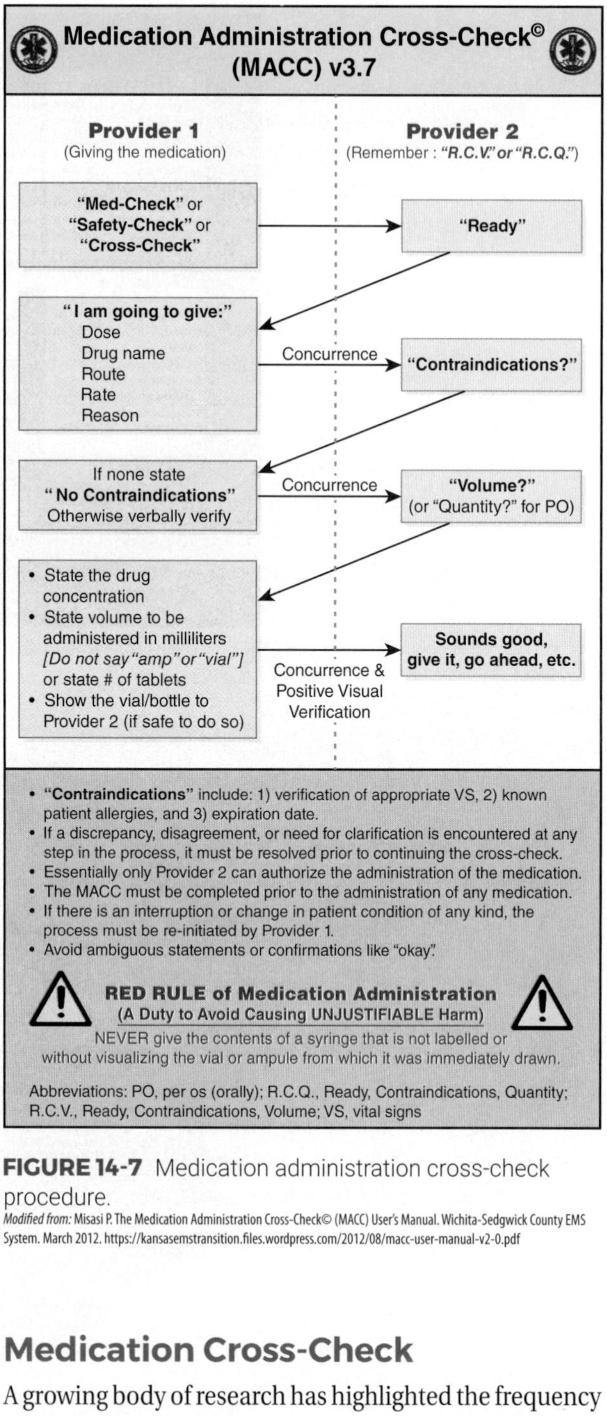

FIGURE 14-7 Medication administration cross-check procedure.

Modified from: Misasi P. The Medication Administration Cross-Check© (MACC) User's Manual. Wichita-Sedgwick County EMS System. March 2012. https://kansasemstransition.files.wordpress.com/2012/08/macc-user-manual-v2-0.pdf

Medication Cross-Check

A growing body of research has highlighted the frequency of prehospital medication errors. Alarmingly, many of these errors occur when drugs are administered to children.[3] The prehospital setting—with its rapid pace, chaotic environment, and poor light—makes it even more challenging to calculate, measure, and administer the correct and intended medication.

In an attempt to reduce the incidence of medication errors, many departments have implemented a safety cross-check procedure (**FIGURE 14-7**). This procedure should be followed when administering every medication, every time. This process was pioneered by Sedgwick County EMS in Kansas.

To complete this procedure, the paramedic administering the medication alerts a team member by stating, "Med-check." Providing closed loop communication, the team member responds by stating, "Ready." Then the person administering the medication states, "I am going to give <medication name> <dose> for <indication>." If the teammate has no objection, he or she replies with the query, "Contraindications?" If there are none, the first team member says, "None." The partner then asks, "Volume?" In response, the person giving the medication states the volume, while at the same time showing the syringe with the medication that has been measured as well as the container with the label containing the name of the drug clearly visible. If all appears correct, the final response is, "Give it."

With practice, this sequence can be performed quickly, even in life-threatening and time-sensitive situations. It is during these very situations that paramedics are especially vulnerable to making errors. Using this system on a routine basis increases paramedics' confidence that they will not make an error.[4]

If there is no paramedic partner available, the cross-check procedure can be performed with an emergency medical technician (EMT) partner. While the EMT is not expected to know proper medication indications and doses, he or she can verify that the name of the medication stated by the paramedic is the name on the label. Likewise, this procedure can be performed when the paramedic is alone in the patient compartment during transport. The mere act of pausing and saying the planned action aloud can permit reflection that can reduce the incidence of errors.

NOTE

A multidose vial should be discarded after a single patient use. Proper aseptic technique should always be followed.

CRITICAL THINKING

Your clinical preceptor hands you an unlabeled syringe of medication and tells you to give it by intramuscular injection. What do you do?

Medication Errors

Medication errors (adverse drug events) occur with some frequency. An estimated 1.5 million people (hospital patients and nursing home residents) receive the wrong medicine or the incorrect dose of medicine in the United States each year. Of these, about 7,000 people die annually.[5] Common causes of medication errors include the following:

- The prescriber ordered the wrong dose of medication.
- Drug calculations were incorrect.
- Drugs were administered by the wrong route.
- The drug was given to the wrong patient.
- The wrong drug was given to the patient.

If a medication error occurs, paramedics should do the following:

- Accept responsibility for the error.
- Immediately advise medical direction or the prescriber.

NOTE

Most injectable medications are given as their mass concentration (mg/mL or mcg/mL). For only a few drugs (eg, *epinephrine*) is the concentration expressed as a ratio or percentage. Calculations involving these expressions are error prone because (1) practitioners may not recognize or understand the difference between dose concentrations (eg, 1:1,000 or 1 mg/mL and 1:10,000 or 0.1 mg/mL) and (2) numbers in the thousands are easily confused, because they have so many zeros (eg, at a quick glance, 1,000 may be mistaken for 10,000). Paramedics should be especially careful when administering *epinephrine*. They should always have a coworker double-check the dose and route of administration, which can help prevent a life-threatening drug error.

SHOW ME THE EVIDENCE

A survey of nationally registered paramedics sought to describe training and practice related to pediatric drug administration, exposure to pediatric drug dose errors, and safety culture among paramedics. In the 1,014 surveys that met the researchers' inclusion criteria, almost half (43%) of respondents knew of a case where an EMS provider administered the incorrect pediatric drug dose. More than one-half believed that their initial paramedic program did not provide enough pediatric training. Almost 20% said their agency had an anonymous error-reporting system, and approximately one-half felt they could report an error without fear of discipline. The authors concluded that pediatric drug-dosing safety can be improved.

Modified from: Hoyle JD Jr, Crowe RP, Bentley MA, Beltran G, Fales W. Pediatric prehospital medication dosing errors: a national survey of paramedics. *Prehosp Emerg Care*. 2017;21(2):185-191.

- Assess and monitor the patient for effects of the drug.
- Document the error as required by local and state drug administration policies and those of the medical direction institution.
- Modify personal practice to avoid a similar error in the future.
- Follow EMS agency procedures for documentation and quality improvement activities.

Medical Asepsis

Medical asepsis is the removal or destruction of disease-causing organisms or infected material. Medical asepsis is performed by using "clean" technique (rather than sterile technique). Clean technique includes hygienic measures, cleaning agents, antiseptics, disinfectants, and barrier fields.

NOTE

Sterile technique—also known as surgical asepsis—means using sterile equipment and sterile fields that are free of all forms and types of life. Clean technique focuses on destroying or inhibiting only pathogens (not all forms and types of life).

Antiseptics and Disinfectants

Antiseptics and disinfectants are chemical agents that are used to kill specific groups of microorganisms (BOX 14-2 and **TABLE 14-2**). They generally are not very effective against spores of bacteria and fungi, many viruses, and some resistant bacterial strains. Disinfectants are used only on nonliving objects and are toxic to living tissue. Antiseptics are applied only to living tissue and are more dilute, to prevent cell damage. Some chemical agents, such as alcohol and some chlorine compounds, have both antiseptic and disinfectant properties.

Currently, chlorhexidine is the preferred antiseptic for vascular access in most settings because it is fast acting and kills gram-positive bacteria, gram-negative bacteria, and fungi without these organisms developing resistance. Chlorhexidine is often supplied in a solution that also contains alcohol to provide more rapid and sustained reductions in bacteria.

NOTE

Several new disinfection methods are under consideration by the Environmental Protection Agency (EPA) and the Food and Drug Administration (FDA):

- Surfacine: A persistent antimicrobial drug coating that can be applied to inanimate and animate objects
- Orthophthalaldehyde: A high-level disinfectant with reduced exposure time
- Superoxidized water: An antimicrobial drug that can be applied to animate and inanimate objects

Modified from: Rutala WA, Weber DJ. New disinfection and sterilization methods. Centers for Disease Control and Prevention website. https://wwwnc.cdc.gov/eid/article/7/2/70-0348_article. Updated April 17, 2012. Accessed January 10, 2018.

BOX 14-2 Examples of Antiseptics and Disinfectants

Antiseptics

Chlorhexidine
Povidone-iodine
Alcohol (isopropyl, ethyl, or propanol)

Disinfectants

Cidex (orthophthalaldehyde)
Glutaraldehyde
Hydrogen peroxide (7.5% solution)
Peracetic acid

Modified from: Accini S. Top ten disinfectants to control HAIs. Hospital Management website. http://www.hospitalmanagement.net/features/featureppc-disinfectants-hai-globaldata/. Published May 14, 2012. Accessed January 10, 2018.

Standard Precautions in Medication Administration

As described in Chapter 2, *Well-Being of the Paramedic*, standard precautions include a group of infection prevention strategies to prevent the transmission of infectious agents to health care personnel, patients, and the general public who risk exposure. It applies to all patients, regardless of suspected or confirmed infection status. It can be best accomplished by following infection control practices with every patient and patient care procedure. (Standard precautions and personal protective measures are also described in Chapter 27, *Infectious and Communicable Diseases.*)

TABLE 14-2 Sterilization and Disinfection Methods for Equipment Used by Paramedics[a]

Organisms Destroyed	Methods	Uses
Sterilization		
All forms of microbial life, including high numbers of bacterial spores	Steam under pressure (autoclave), gas (ethylene oxide), dry heat, or immersion in an EPA-approved chemical sterilant for a prolonged period (eg, 6–10 hours or according to the manufacturer's instructions). *Note*: Liquid chemical sterilants should be used only on instruments that cannot be sterilized or disinfected with heat.	Instruments or devices that penetrate the skin or come into contact with normally sterile areas of the body (eg, scalpels, needles). Use of disposable invasive equipment eliminates the need to reprocess these items. When indicated, however, arrangements should be made with a health care facility for reprocessing of reusable invasive instruments.
High-Level Disinfection		
All forms of microbial life except high numbers of bacterial spores	Hot water pasteurization (176°F to 212°F [80°C to 100°C] for 30 minutes), or exposure to an EPA-registered chemical sterilant, except for a short exposure time (10–45 minutes or as directed by the manufacturer).	Reusable instruments or devices that come into contact with mucous membranes (eg, laryngoscope blades, endotracheal tubes).
Intermediate-Level Disinfection		
Mycobacterium tuberculosis, vegetative bacteria, most viruses, and most fungi but not bacterial spores	EPA-registered hospital disinfectant chemical germicides with a label claim of tuberculocidal activity; commercially available hard-surface germicides; or solutions with at least 500 parts per million (ppm) free available chlorine (a 1:100 dilution of common household bleach—approximately 1 cup of bleach per 1 gallon of tap water).	Instruments and equipment that come into contact only with intact skin (eg, stethoscopes, blood pressure cuffs, splints) and that have been visibly contaminated with blood or bloody body fluids. Surfaces must be cleaned of visible material before the germicide is applied.
Low-Level Disinfection		
Most bacteria, some viruses, some fungi, but not *Mycobacterium tuberculosis* or bacterial spores	EPA-registered hospital disinfectants (no label claim for tuberculocidal activity).	Routine housekeeping or removal of soiling in the absence of visible blood contamination.
Environmental Disinfection		
	Any cleaner or disinfectant agent intended for environmental use.	Environmental surfaces that have become soiled and that should be cleaned and disinfected (eg, floors, woodwork, ambulance seats, countertops).

Abbreviation: EPA, Environmental Protection Agency

[a]To ensure the effectiveness of any sterilization or disinfection process, equipment and instruments first must be thoroughly cleaned of all visible soiling.

Before administering drugs, paramedics should follow handwashing procedures.[6] They also should follow gloving procedures when indicated. Face shields should be used during administration of endotracheal (ET) drugs and whenever splashing of blood or body fluids is likely.

NOTE

Handwashing is the most crucial step in reducing the risk of transmission of organisms from one person to another or from one site to another on the same patient. Handwashing protects both the paramedic and the patient. If soap and water are not available, a sanitizing gel, foam, or wipe should be used.

Enteral Administration of Medications

Enteral medications are drugs that are administered and absorbed through the gastrointestinal tract. Enteral drugs are administered by the oral, gastric, or rectal route.

Oral Route

The oral route is the most frequently used method of drug administration. Before taking an oral medication, the patient should be in an upright or sitting position. The pill, tablet, or capsule should be placed in the patient's mouth and swallowed with enough fluid (4 to 8 ounces [118 to 237 mL]) to make sure the drug reaches the stomach. Some oral drugs, such as ondansetron, are placed on the tongue and allowed to dissolve without water. Medication should not be administered orally if the patient cannot swallow or does not have an effective gag reflex.

Many oral drugs are manufactured in both solid and liquid forms (BOX 14-3). If the medication is in a liquid suspension, the stock bottle or unit dose should be shaken thoroughly before the drug is poured for administration. A drug not packaged as a unit dose should be measured in a medicine cup or a medicine dropper or by syringe.

CRITICAL THINKING

Think of some clinical situations in which oral administration of a drug would not be the best technique. Why is this so?

BOX 14-3 Forms of Solid and Liquid Oral Medications

- Caplets
- Capsules
- Time-released capsules
- Lozenges
- Pills
- Tablets
- Elixirs
- Emulsions
- Suspensions
- Syrups

NOTE

Orally dissolving (or disintegrating) drugs are gaining in popularity. These medicines are supplied in a tablet or wafer form. They dissolve within seconds when placed on the tongue. This property speeds their time of onset, eliminates the need for water, and decreases the risk of choking. Absorption begins in the oral cavity and continues through the gastrointestinal tract. The antiemetic ondansetron is often administered by this route.

Administration of Medications by Gastric Tube

Most drugs that can be given orally can also be given via a gastric tube. Orogastric tubes are placed through the mouth and into the esophagus and stomach. Nasogastric tubes are placed through the nose and esophagus and into the stomach. Before giving a drug by this route, the paramedic must make sure the tube has been inserted correctly (see Chapter 28, *Abdominal and Gastrointestinal Disorders*). Correct insertion can be confirmed by aspirating the patient's stomach contents and checking that the pH is acidic

NOTE

The traditional method of auscultating the epigastric area to confirm correct tube placement is not considered reliable. The two approved methods for gastric tube confirmation are radiography and measuring the pH of the aspirate.

Modified from: Lemyze M. The placement of nasogastric tubes. *CMAJ*. 2010;182(8):802.

(between 0 and 4). Once correct insertion has been verified, the drug is administered through the tube, followed by a small amount of water (about 30 mL). The water flushes the drug and helps to maintain the patency of the tube. One drug that is given by gastric tube in emergency care is activated charcoal.

Rectal Administration of Medications

Some drugs, such as suppositories, are routinely administered by the rectal route (BOX 14-4). Other drugs can be given by the rectal route when vascular access cannot be established. Emergency drugs that can be given rectally include diazepam and lorazepam (**FIGURE 14-8**).

BOX 14-4 Procedure for Administering Drugs Rectally[a]

1. Carefully restrain the patient. If the patient is a child and it is possible to do so, place the child in a knee–chest or lateral recumbent position with the legs flexed at the hips and the knees.
2. Draw the drug dose into a syringe and remove the needle. (A slightly higher dose may be required because absorption is incomplete. Consult medical direction.)
3. Insert the lubricated syringe just beyond the external sphincter, aiming just above the junction of the skin and mucous membranes and toward the rectal wall.
4. Inject the solution into the rectum.
5. Aid drug retention by squeezing the buttocks together with manual pressure.

[a]Although the procedure is described for a child, it also is appropriate for adults.

Parenteral Administration of Medications

Parenteral drugs are administered outside the gastrointestinal tract, usually as injections. Drugs may be administered parenterally by the intradermal, subcutaneous, intramuscular, intravenous, and intraosseous routes. (Transdermal medications also are discussed in this chapter.) Blood collection procedures (ie, phlebotomy procedures) are discussed later in this chapter.

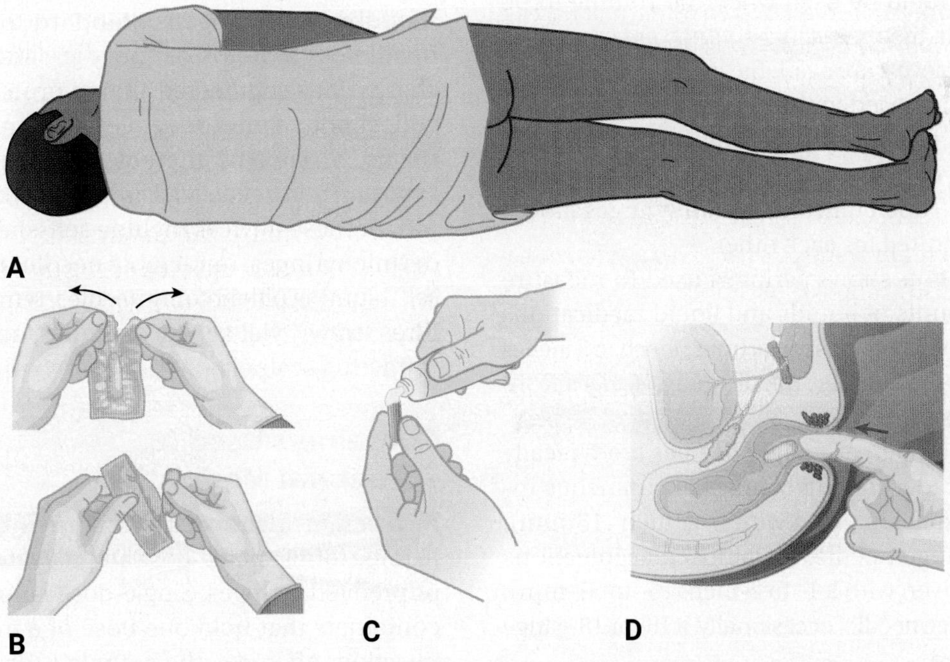

FIGURE 14-8 Rectal drug administration. **A.** Position the patient in the lateral recumbent position and drape. **B.** Unwrap the suppository and remove it from the package. **C.** Apply a water-soluble lubricant. **D.** Gently insert the suppository about 1 inch (3 cm) past the internal sphincter.

> NOTE
>
> Parenteral administration of drugs can be very hazardous, because drugs given by injection are usually considered irretrievable; that is, the injection cannot be undone. Also, a slight risk of infection exists, because the skin is broken. Other possible hazards associated with parenteral administration include pain with drug administration, cellulitis or abscess formation, necrosis, skin sloughing, nerve injury, prolonged pain, and periostitis (inflammation of connective tissue covering bones). The use of aseptic technique, ensuring an accurate drug dosage, finding the proper site for the injection, and administering the injection at the proper rate are essential to minimize the risk of harm.

Equipment Used for Injections

Syringes and Needles

The choice of syringe and needle depends on three factors: (1) the route of administration, (2) the characteristics of the fluid (eg, aqueous or oil based), and (3) the volume of medication. Syringes in common use today are made of disposable plastic. Sizes range from 1-mL tuberculin and insulin syringes to 60-mL irrigation syringes.

Tuberculin syringes, which are marked in 0.01-mL gradients, should be used when the volume to be given is small. Insulin syringes, which are marked in 1-unit increments, are available in 0.5-mL and 1-mL volumes. When used with the specified strength of insulin, this type of syringe allows the patient to draw up the correct dose easily without doing any calculations. Tuberculin and insulin syringes should not be substituted for each other.

FIGURE 14-9 shows syringes used to measure varying amounts of liquids and liquid medications accurately. Needle lengths range from ⅜ inch to 3 inches (10 to 76 mm) or longer; needle gauge ranges from 12 gauge (large lumen) to 30 gauge (small lumen). Smaller-lumen (larger-gauge) needles are typically used for intradermal injections. Subcutaneous injections usually are given with a ⅝-inch (16-mm), 23- or 25-gauge needle. Intramuscular injections usually are given with a 1- to 2-inch (25- to 51-mm), 19- or 21-gauge needle; occasionally, a 16- or 18-gauge needle is used.

In 2000, Congress passed the Healthcare Worker Needlestick Prevention Act to revise the bloodborne pathogens standard to include safer medical devices. The following year, the Occupational Safety and Health Administration (OSHA) amended its Bloodborne Pathogens Standard to recommend needleless systems or "needle-safe" devices (ie, sharps with engineered sharps protection), which collect body fluids or deliver medications without the use of a needle, thereby helping prevent blood exposure and needlestick injuries (BOX 14-5). Examples of these devices include self-sheathing hypodermic syringes, retractable needles for injections, self-blunting phlebotomy needles, retracting lancets, filter straws, vial access cannulas, and disposable retracting scalpels.

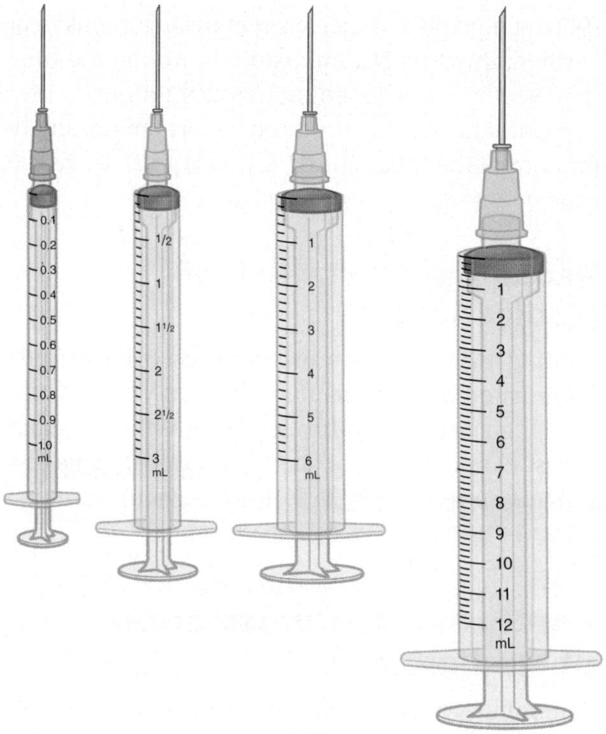

FIGURE 14-9 Types of syringes.

Containers Used for Parenteral Medications

Medications given by injection usually are supplied in three forms: single-dose ampules, multidose vials, or prefilled syringes. Single-dose ampules are glass containers that hold one dose of a medication for injection. After use, the ampule is discarded into a sharps container. Multidose vials are glass containers that come with rubber stoppers; they permit several medication doses to be withdrawn for injection. In most

BOX 14-5 Prevention of Needle and Sharps Injuries

Each year, health care workers experience 385,000 sharps-related injuries, 40% of which involve a safety-designed needle. Health care workers are at highest risk for infection with the hepatitis B virus (HBV), hepatitis C virus (HCV), and human immunodeficiency virus (HIV) caused by needlestick and sharps injury. However, transmission of other diseases also is possible, including syphilis, herpes simplex, herpes zoster, Rocky Mountain spotted fever, and tuberculosis. The following precautions can help prevent exposure to these pathogens:

- Paramedics should get help when administering infusion therapy or injections to uncooperative patients.
- Needles should not be recapped, purposely bent or broken by hand, removed from disposable syringes, or otherwise manipulated by hand. If a needle must be recapped or removed because there is no alternative or because a specific medical procedure requires it, the paramedic should use a mechanical device or a one-handed technique. Needleless products should be used when available.
- Disposable syringes and needles, scalpel blades, and other sharp items should be placed in puncture-resistant containers for disposal immediately after use.

Modified from: National Institute for Occupational Safety and Health. Sharps injuries. Stop Sticks Campaign. Centers for Disease Control and Prevention website. https://www.cdc.gov/niosh/stopsticks/sharpsinjuries.html. Reviewed June 26, 2013. Accessed January 10, 2018; National Institute for Occupational Safety and Health. Sharps injuries: bloodborne pathogens. Stop Sticks Campaign. Centers for Disease Control and Prevention website. https://www.cdc.gov/niosh/stopsticks/bloodborne.html. Updated September 28, 2010. Accessed January 10, 2018.

cases, multidose vials are intended for single-patient use. Using a vial more than once without using proper aseptic technique has been associated with contamination and outbreaks of hepatitis B and C.[7]

To prepare a prescribed medication for injection, the paramedic should choose the appropriate needle and syringe. The size of the syringe must be in proportion to the volume of solution to be given. To withdraw medication from an ampule or vial, the paramedic should follow these steps:

1. Assemble the equipment (antiseptic swab or gauze, syringe, 18-gauge filter needle or filter straw to withdraw medication if using an ampule, and appropriate-gauge needle for injection).
2. Compute the volume of medication to be given. Confirm the five rights of medication administration aloud.
3. If using a vial (**FIGURE 14-10**):
   - Clean the rubber stopper with antiseptic.
   - Inject a volume of air into the vial equivalent to the amount of solution to be withdrawn. (This prevents the formation of a vacuum in the vial. A vacuum can make the solution difficult to withdraw.) Withdraw the volume required, and remove the syringe from the vial.

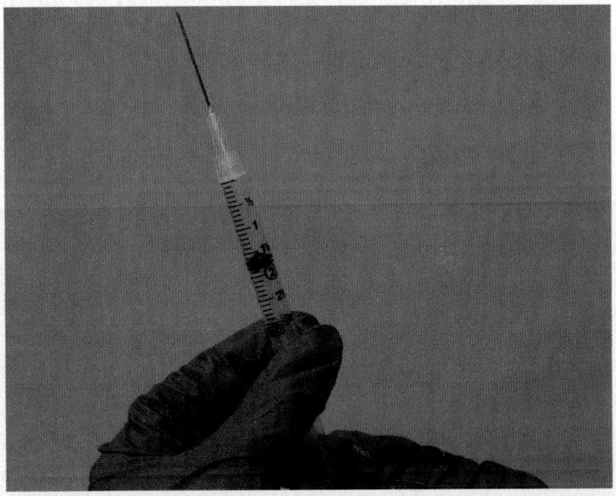

A

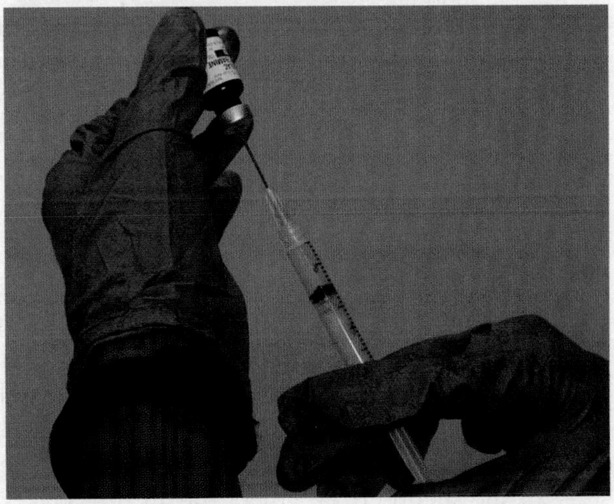

B

FIGURE 14-10 Withdrawing medication from a vial. **A.** Determine the amount of medication that is needed and draw that amount of air into the syringe. **B.** Inject the air into the drug vial and draw the drug into the syringe.

   - Gently push in the plunger of the syringe to expel air from the solution.
4. If using an ampule (**FIGURE 14-11**):
   - Lightly tap or shake the ampule to dislodge any solution from the neck of the container.
   - Wrap the neck of the glass ampule with an antiseptic swab or gauze dressing to protect the fingers.
   - Grasp the ampule, snap off the top, and discard the top in an appropriate medication disposal container. (The ampule is designed to break easily when pressure is exerted at the neck.)
   - Carefully insert an 18-gauge filter needle or filter straw into the solution, without allowing it to touch the edges of the ampule, and draw the solution into the syringe.
   - Carefully remove the 18-gauge needle or filter screw and discard it in the appropriate container. Attach the needle to be used for injection.
   - Gently push in the plunger of the syringe to expel air.

Mixing Medications. Two compatible drugs can be mixed into one injection if the total volume of the dosage is within accepted limits. For example, this technique can be used with butorphanol and hydroxyzine. When mixing medications, it is crucial not to contaminate one with the other and to maintain aseptic technique. Any doubt about compatibility should be discussed with medical direction. It also can be verified by consulting a proper reference, such as a drug compatibility chart. To mix medications, the paramedic should follow these steps:

1. Use only one syringe to mix the drugs.
2. Aspirate a volume of air equivalent to the dose of the first drug. Inject the air into vial A, making sure the needle or vial access cannula does not touch the solution. Withdraw the needle or vial access cannula.
3. Aspirate a volume of air equivalent to the dose of the second drug. Inject the air into vial B. Withdraw the required medication from vial B.
4. Put a new sterile needle or vial access cannula on the syringe and insert it into vial A. Be careful not to push in the plunger or expel the drug from the syringe into the vial. Doing so would pose a risk of infection and result in mixing of the drugs.

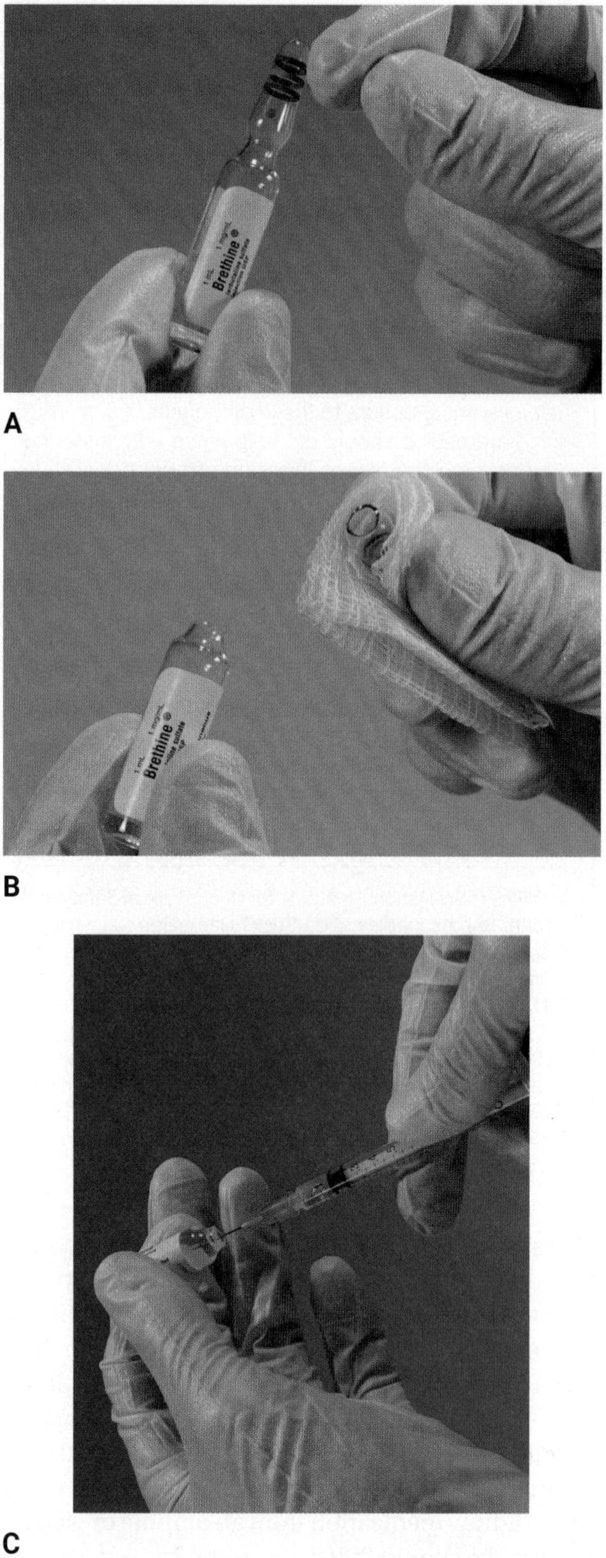

FIGURE 14-11 Withdrawing medication from an ampule. **A.** Tap the ampule to remove drug from the neck. **B.** Break off the top of the ampule with a gauze pad. **C.** Use a filter straw or filter needle to withdraw the medication from the ampule.

5. Withdraw the desired amount of the drug from vial A into the syringe.
6. Put a new sterile needle on the syringe and administer the injection.

> NOTE
>
> Some medications are dry powders that must be reconstituted before administration. An example is glucagon.
>
> Carefully read the manufacturer's information. Use the correct amount of the diluent prescribed for this purpose. Always mix the diluent and powder in the closed vial before withdrawing the dose. Some drugs are packaged in a vial that contains the diluent and powder in two compartments (eg, Mix-o-Vial, Act-o-Vial).

Prefilled Syringes. Several manufacturers make prefilled syringes (**FIGURE 14-12**). The techniques for activating and using these products vary. Paramedics should be familiar with the devices used by their particular EMS system. The technique for activating a common type of prefilled syringe is as follows:

1. Calculate the volume of medication to be administered. Confirm the five rights of medication administration aloud.
2. Remove the protective caps from the syringe barrel and medication cartridge.
3. Screw the cartridge into the syringe barrel.
4. Gently push in the plunger of the syringe to expel air.

Preparing the Injection Site

The injection site is prepared by cleansing the area using aseptic technique. The steps in preparing the injection site are as follows:

1. Thoroughly scrub the site with the appropriate antiseptic cleanser to remove dirt, dead skin, and other surface contaminants.
2. If using a chlorhexidine-based preparation, scrub the area up and down and then side to side. If using other products, clean the site with overlapping, concentric circles and moving outward from the site.
3. Allow the site to dry.

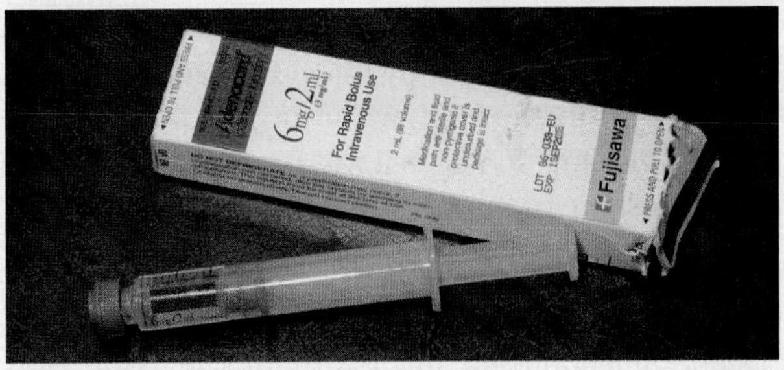

FIGURE 14-12 Prefilled medication syringe.

Intradermal Injections

An intradermal injection is administered just below the epidermis, or outer layer of skin (**FIGURE 14-13** and **FIGURE 14-14**). This site is commonly used for allergy testing and for administration of local anesthetics. A tuberculin syringe typically is used for intradermal injections, and the volume injected usually is less than 0.5 mL. Common sites for intradermal injections are the medial surface of the forearm and the back.

The steps for administering an intradermal injection are as follows:

1. Choose the injection site and cleanse the skin surface. Confirm the five rights of medication administration aloud.

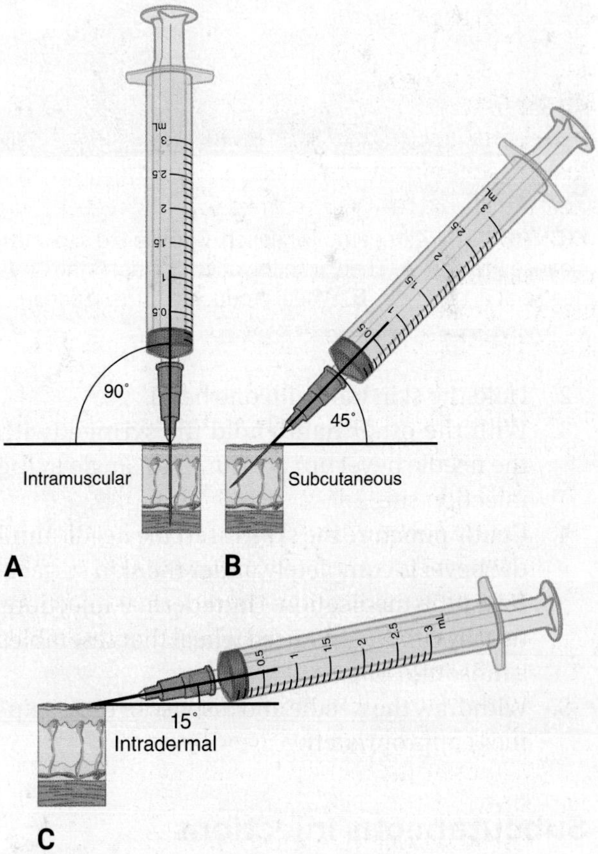

FIGURE 14-13 Comparison of angle of injection and deposition of medication for intramuscular **(A)**, subcutaneous **(B)**, and intradermal injections **(C)**.

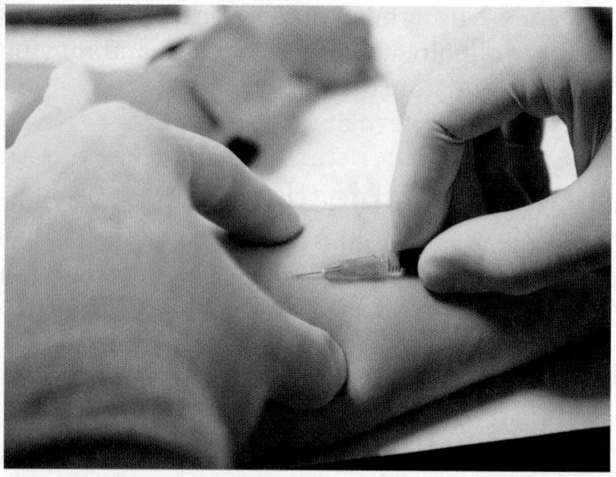

A

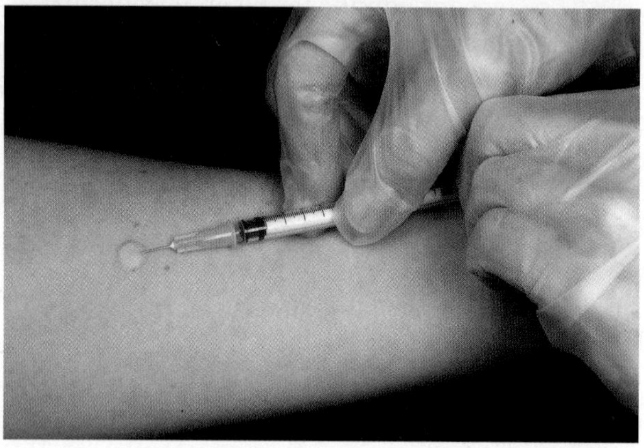

B

FIGURE 14-14 Intradermal injection. Choose the site and cleanse the skin. **A.** Then, with the bevel up, insert the needle at a 15° angle. **B.** Wheal produced by the injection.

2. Hold the skin taut with one hand.
3. With the other hand, hold the syringe (with the needle bevel up) at a 10° to 15° angle to the injection site.
4. Gently puncture the skin. Insert the needle until the bevel is completely under the skin surface. Inject the medication. (Intradermal injections usually produce a raised wheal that resembles a mosquito bite.)
5. Withdraw the needle and dispose of the equipment appropriately.

Subcutaneous Injections

Subcutaneous injections are given to place medication below the skin into the subcutaneous layer (**FIGURE 14-15**). The volume of such an injection usually is less than 0.5 mL. It is administered through a ½- or ⅝-inch (13- or 16-mm), 23- or 25-gauge needle. In the prehospital setting, the drug most often given by this route is epinephrine.

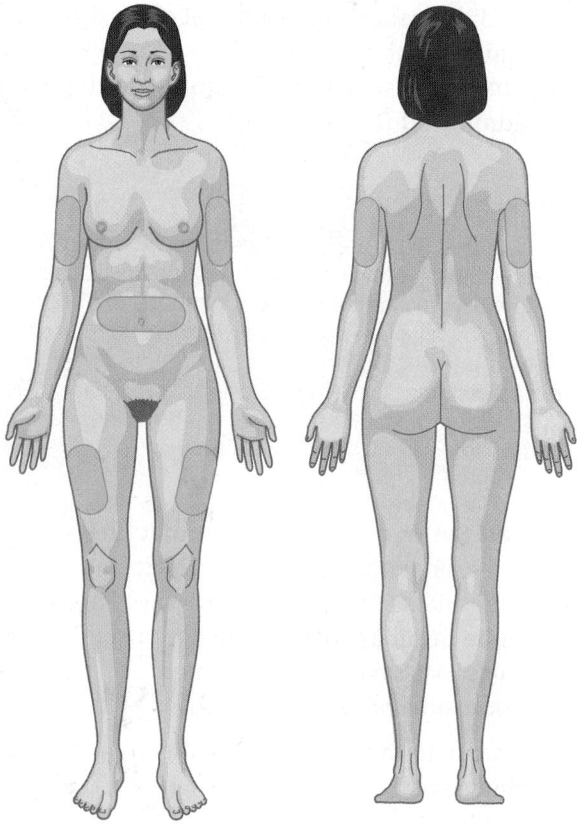

FIGURE 14-15 Sites commonly used for subcutaneous injections.

The steps for subcutaneous injections are as follows (**FIGURE 14-16**):

1. Choose the injection site and cleanse the area with an antiseptic. Confirm the five rights of medication administration aloud.
2. Elevate the subcutaneous tissue by gently pinching the injection site.
3. With the needle bevel up, insert the needle at a 45° angle in one quick motion.
4. Gently but smoothly inject the medication.
5. After the injection, withdraw the needle at the same angle at which it was inserted. Apply direct pressure to the site.

Intramuscular Injections

Deeper injections are made into muscle tissue; thus, they pass through the skin and subcutaneous tissue.

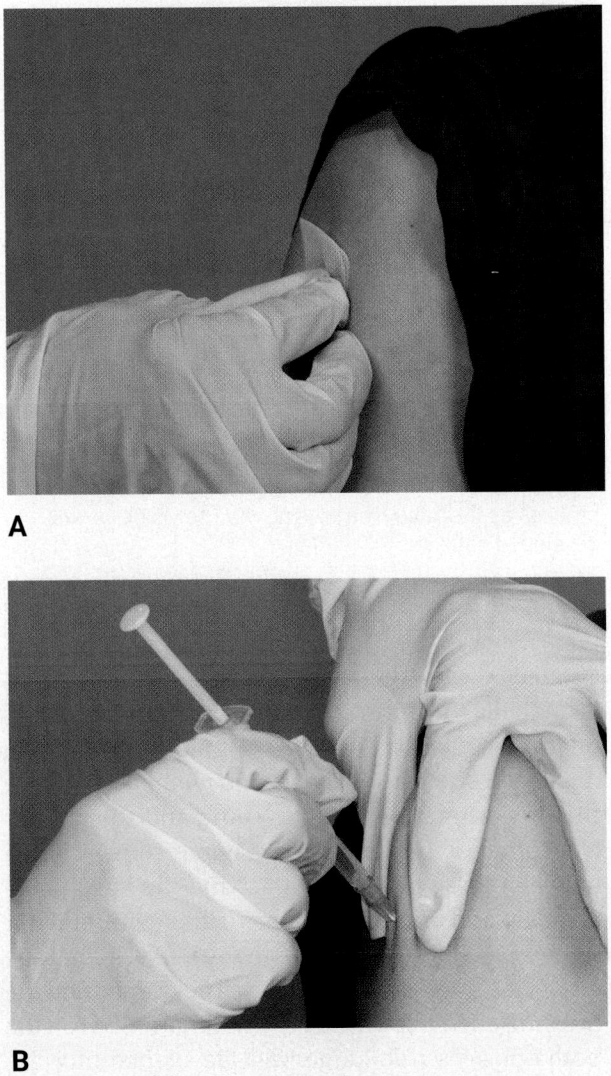

FIGURE 14-16 Subcutaneous injection. **A.** Cleanse the skin. **B.** Grasp the skin to maximize the amount of subcutaneous tissue available and insert the needle. Aspirate unless contraindicated and slowly inject the medication. Discard the needle and syringe in an appropriate sharps container.

Intramuscular injections are given when a drug is too irritating to be injected subcutaneously or when a greater volume or faster absorption is desired. (Irritation still may occur with administration by this route.) A maximum volume of 5 mL may be given by intramuscular injection in a large muscle mass (eg, gluteal muscle).

The type of needle used depends on four factors: (1) the site of the injection, (2) the condition of the tissue, (3) the size of the patient, and (4) the type of drug to be injected (ie, small-lumen needles are used for thin solutions, and larger-lumen needles are used for suspensions and oils). Because the muscle layer is below the subcutaneous layer, a longer needle generally is used (usually 1½ inches [38 mm] and 19 or 21 gauge). The procedure for administering an intramuscular injection is similar to that described for intradermal and subcutaneous injections (**FIGURE 14-17**), except that the needle is inserted at a 90° angle. Also, the skin is held taut, not pinched. In addition, after inserting the needle, the paramedic pulls back slightly on the plunger (ie, aspirates) to ensure needle placement. If no blood is aspirated, the medication is injected.

NOTE

The Centers for Disease Control and Prevention (CDC) recommends that aspiration not be performed when administering immunizations intramuscularly in the recommended sites. The CDC advises using the vastus lateralis when administering vaccines intramuscularly for children less than 2 years of age. If there is adequate muscle in those older than 2 years, the deltoid may be used.

Modified from: National Center for Immunization and Respiratory Diseases. Vaccine administration. Centers for Disease Control and Prevention website. https://www.cdc.gov/vaccines/pubs/pinkbook/vac-admin.html. Updated September 8, 2015. Accessed January 10, 2018.

Several muscles are commonly used for intramuscular injections—the deltoid muscle, the gluteal muscles (dorsogluteal site), the vastus lateralis muscle, the rectus femoris muscle, and the ventrogluteal muscle. The deltoid muscle is located in the upper arm and forms a triangular shape, with the base of the triangle along the acromion process and the peak of the triangle ending approximately one-third of the way down the lateral aspect of the upper arm (**FIGURE 14-18**). This muscle is used primarily for vaccinations involving only a small volume of drug, because it is small and can accommodate only small doses of injection (1 mL or less). This site is not used in children younger than 1 year. When injections are made in the deltoid muscle, care must be taken to avoid hitting the radial nerve. The patient should be sitting upright or lying flat and should be told to relax the arm muscles.

The dorsogluteal site consists of several gluteal muscles, though the gluteus medius muscle is most often used for injections. The dorsogluteal site can be

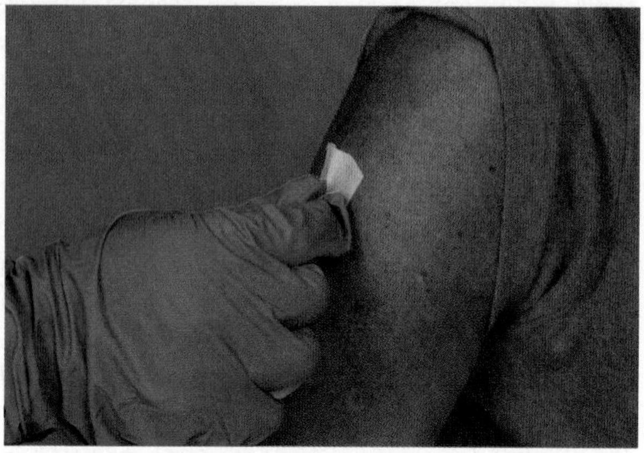

A

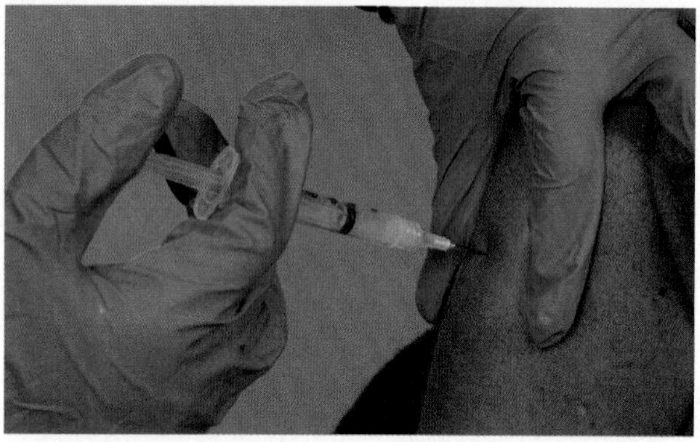

B

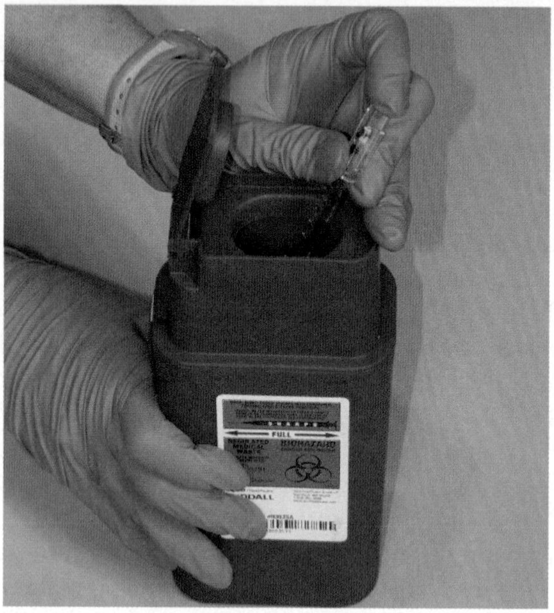

C

FIGURE 14-17 Intramuscular injection. **A.** Choose the site and cleanse the skin. **B.** Pull the skin tight, insert the needle, aspirate, and then slowly inject the medication. **C.** Discard the needle and syringe in an appropriate sharps container.

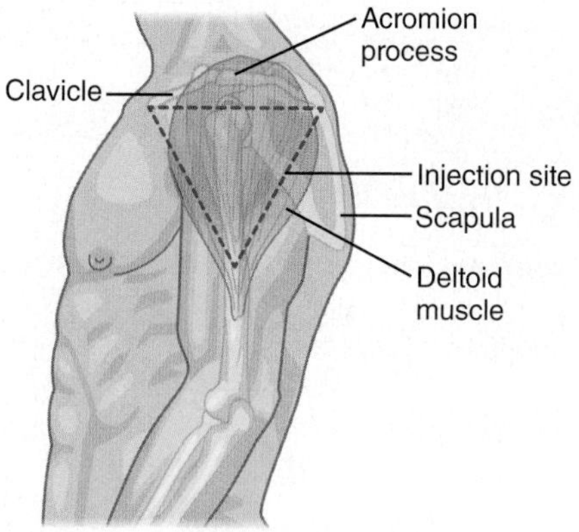

FIGURE 14-18 The injection site for the deltoid muscle roughly forms an inverted triangle, with the acromion process as the base. The muscle may be visible in well-developed patients.

defined in two ways (**FIGURE 14-19**). The first method is to divide the buttocks on one side into imaginary quadrants; the medication is administered into the upper outer quadrant. The second method is to locate the posterior superior iliac spine and the greater trochanter of the femur. An imaginary line is drawn between these two landmarks, and the injection is given up and out from this line. This site should not be used for children younger than 3 years. In that age group, the muscles are not yet well developed and the proximity of the sciatic nerve (the largest nerve in the body) poses a risk. Large, well-developed muscles can accommodate an injection of up to 5 mL, but volumes exceeding 3 mL may be uncomfortable for the patient. When an injection is administered at the dorsogluteal site, the patient should lie prone, pointing inward to promote muscle relaxation.

The vastus lateralis and the rectus femoris muscles lie side by side in the thigh. To identify the necessary landmarks, the paramedic should place one hand on the patient's upper thigh and one hand on the lower thigh. The area between the hands is the middle third of the thigh and the middle third of the underlying muscle (**FIGURE 14-20**). The vastus lateralis lies lateral to the midline and is the preferred injection site for children. It is well developed in virtually all patients and has few major blood vessels and nerves that can be injured. The rectus femoris is located in the midline of the middle third of the thigh. This site is most often used for self-injection because of its accessibility. Acceptable volumes for injection in the

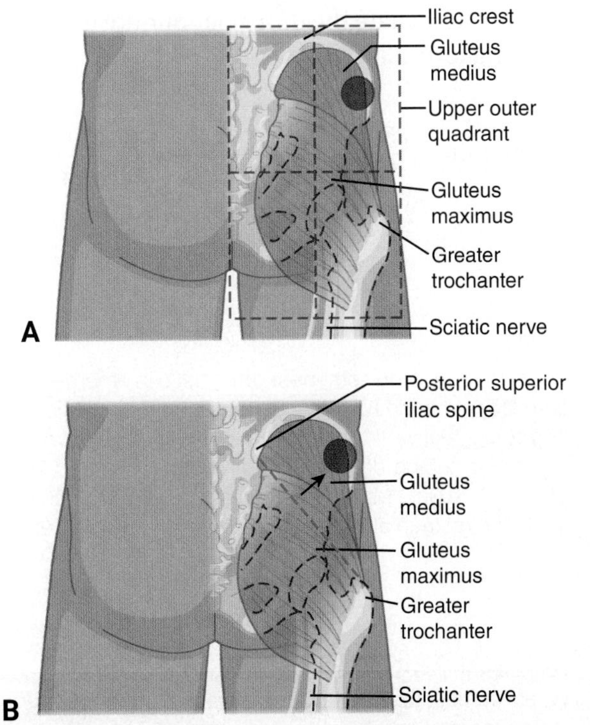

FIGURE 14-19 The injection area for the dorsogluteal site can be defined in two ways. **A.** Divide the buttocks on one side into imaginary quadrants. Use the center of the upper outer quadrant as the injection site. **B.** Locate the posterior superior iliac spine and the greater trochanter by palpation, and draw an imaginary line between the two. The injection site should be above and out from that line.

© Jones & Bartlett Learning.

vastus lateralis and rectus femoris muscles vary with the age of the patient and the size of the muscle. Up to 5 mL may be injected into a well-developed adult. The patient should be sitting upright or lying supine and should be advised to relax the muscles.

The ventrogluteal muscle is accessible when the patient lies in a supine or lateral recumbent position. The paramedic should palpate the greater trochanter using the palm, with the index finger pointing to the anterior superior iliac spine. The paramedic's remaining three fingers should extend toward the iliac crest. The injection is made into the center of the V formed by the fingers (**FIGURE 14-21**). This injection site, which may be used for all patients, is a desirable site because it has no large nerves or fat tissue. In the adult, this muscle may accommodate up to 5 mL of drug.

Intravenous Therapy

Intravenous (IV) cannulation is used to gain access to the body's circulation. It is indicated for three reasons: (1) to administer fluids, (2) to administer drugs, and (3) to obtain specimens for laboratory testing. The IV route puts the drug directly into the bloodstream, which bypasses all barriers to drug absorption.

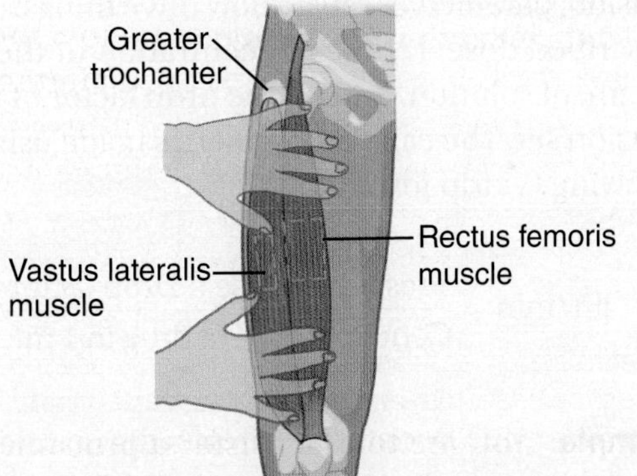

FIGURE 14-20 The injection sites for the vastus lateralis muscle and the rectus femoris muscle can be defined through landmarks. Place one hand below the greater trochanter; place the other hand above the knee. The space between the two hands defines the middle third of the underlying muscle. The rectus femoris is on the anterior thigh; the vastus lateralis is on the lateral side.

© Jones & Bartlett Learning.

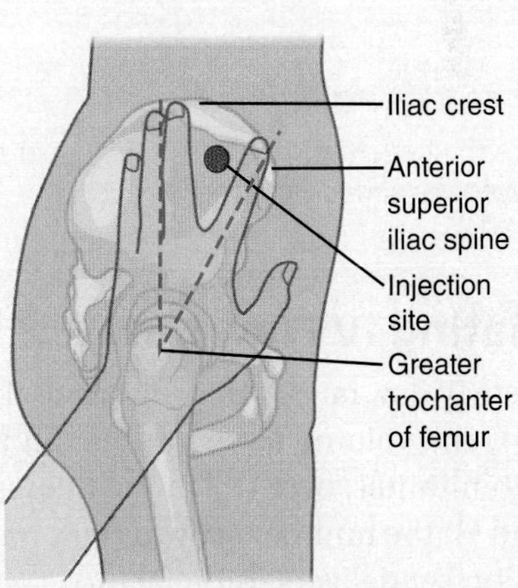

FIGURE 14-21 The injection site for the ventrogluteal muscle is defined by placing the palm of one hand on the trochanter of the femur. A "V" is then made with the fingers of that hand. One side runs from the greater trochanter to the anterior superior iliac spine; the other side runs from the greater trochanter to the iliac crest. The injection is made into the center of the V.

© Jones & Bartlett Learning.

NOTE

Many children fear pain from injections and efforts to obtain vascular access. Several strategies are known to reduce pain during injection (if not contraindicated by the patient's medical condition):

- Breastfeeding infants younger than 12 months who are receiving injections
- Administering a few drops to one-half a teaspoon of a sugar solution to an infant prior to the injection
- Rapidly administering the injection
- Rubbing or stroking the skin near the injection site before and during the injection with moderate intensity—may decrease pain in children 4 years of age and older (also appropriate for adults)
- Distracting the child by having the parent/caregiver joke with the child or by playing music (ie, not talking about the injection)

Modified from: National Center for Immunization and Respiratory Diseases. Vaccine administration. Centers for Disease Control and Prevention website. https://www.cdc.gov/vaccines/pubs/pinkbook/vac-admin.html. Updated September 8, 2015. Accessed January 10, 2018.

NOTE

Some intramuscular medications (eg, promethazine) should be administered into a large muscle. In such cases, the paramedic should use one of the leg or hip injection sites.

CRITICAL THINKING

What are the benefits of choosing the upper extremity for intravenous access in an adult?

Calculating IV Flow Rates

To calculate IV flow rates, paramedics must know three factors: (1) the volume to be infused; (2) the period of time, in minutes, over which the fluid is to be infused; and (3) the number of drops (gtt) per milliliter the infusion set delivers (drop factor). The flow rate can then be calculated using the following equation:

$$\text{gtt/min} = \frac{\text{Volume to be infused} \times \text{Drop factor}}{\text{Duration of infusion (minutes)}}$$

Example. You are to give a patient 250 mL of normal saline over 90 minutes. Your infusion set delivers 10 gtt/mL. Calculate the drops per minute using the preceding formula.

$$\text{gtt/min} = \frac{250\ \cancel{\text{mL}} \times 10\ \text{gtt}/\cancel{\text{mL}}}{90\ \text{minutes}} = \frac{2500\ \text{gtt}}{90\ \text{min}}$$
$$= 27.7 \text{ or } 28\ \text{gtt/min}$$

NOTE

The two IV infusion sets most often used in emergency care are microdrip tubing and macrodrip tubing. Microdrip tubing delivers the infusion at a rate of 60 gtt/mL; macrodrip tubing delivers the infusion at a rate of 10, 15, or 20 gtt/mL. Math tip: When a drop factor of 60 is used, the gtt/min always equals the mL/hour infusion.

CRITICAL THINKING

When is it best to use microdrip tubing? When is it better to use macrodrip tubing?

Calculating Infusion Rates

Paramedics may need to administer medications by continuous IV infusion. Calculating the correct drip rate is crucial to avoid overdosing or underdosing of the patient (BOX 14-6 and BOX 14-7). To properly calculate and give a prescribed drug by continuous infusion, paramedics must know three things: (1) the prescribed dose, (2) the concentration of the drug in 1 mL of solution, and (3) the drop factor of the IV infusion set. The calculation then is made using the following IV drip formula:

$$\text{gtt/min} = \frac{\text{Prescribed dose} \times \text{Drop factor}}{\text{Concentration of drug in 1 mL}}$$

Example. You are to administer a procainamide infusion at 3 mg/min. You have 1 g of the drug in 250 mL of 5% dextrose in water (D_5W). The infusion set delivers the infusion at a rate of 60 gtt/mL. How many drops per minute will you deliver?

Convert all units to like measurements and calculate the concentration of the drug in 1 mL:

$$1\ \text{g} \times 1{,}000 = 1{,}000\ \text{mg}$$

$$1{,}000\ \text{mg} \div 250\ \text{mL} = 4\ \text{mg/mL}$$

BOX 14-6 "Clock" Method of Calculating Flow Rates

Visualizing a clock can help paramedics calculate the flow rate for an IV medication. For example, if the concentration of a drug in solution is 4 mg/mL, microdrip tubing is used that delivers 1 mL in 60 drops, and 60 drops are delivered in 1 minute, then 4 mg will be delivered with every 60 drops of solution. Picturing a clock where 4 mg and 60 drops are at the 12 position, you can calculate that 15 drops/min will deliver 1 mg/min, 30 drops will deliver 2 mg/min, and 45 drops will deliver 3 mg/min. You can use this same method with any drug in solution when microdrip tubing is used.

Lidocaine Infusion Clock

- Mix 2 g of lidocaine in 500 mL of 5% dextrose in water or normal saline (or 1 g in 250 mL) = 4 mg/mL.
- Infusion dose range = 2–4 mg/min.
- When administered with a microdrip (60 gtt/mL) IV administration set, lidocaine drip rates resemble a seconds "clock":

60 gtt/min = 4 mg/min

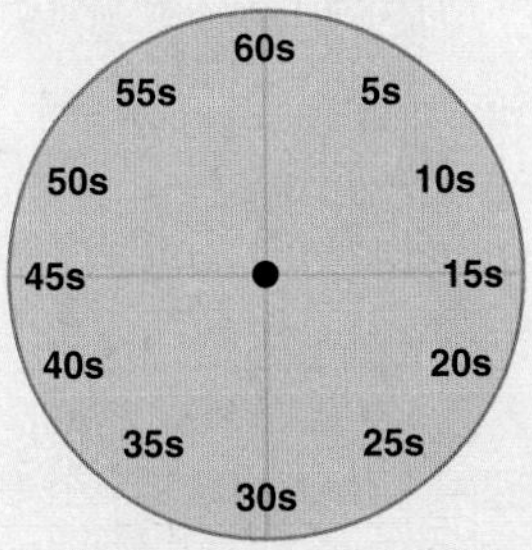

30 gtt/min = 2 mg/min

BOX 14-7 Shortcut for Calculating Dopamine Drips

Dopamine is a very strong drug, and calculating the correct dose of this medication can daunt even the best mathematician. The following is a shortcut for calculating dopamine infusions using 60 drops/min IV tubing and a standard mixture of drug in solution (eg, 400 mg in 250 mL or 800 mg in 500 mL—both yield a 1,600 mcg/mL concentration).

Formula

$$\frac{\text{Dose} \times \text{Weight (kg)} \times 60 \text{ gtt/mL}}{1{,}600} = \text{Drops per minute}$$

Example

You are to administer 5 mcg/kg of dopamine per minute to a patient who weighs 75 kg.

$$\frac{5 \text{ mcg} \times 75 \text{ kg} \times 60 \text{ gtt/mL}}{1{,}600} = 14 \text{ drops per minute}$$

Calculate the drops per minute using the IV drip formula:

$$\text{gtt/min} = \frac{3 \text{ mg/min} \times 60 \text{ gtt/mL}}{4 \text{ mg in } 1 \text{ mL}} = \frac{180}{4} = 45 \text{ gtt/min}$$

IV Fluid Administration

In the prehospital setting, the route of choice for fluid therapy is through a peripheral vein in an extremity. If the arms have no major injury, upper extremity veins should be used. (Some EMS agencies advise against using upper extremity sites if a major injury to the neck or upper thorax has occurred on that side.) If upper extremity sites are not available, lower extremity sites may be used. IV fluids often used in the prehospital setting include normal saline, lactated Ringer solution, and mixtures of glucose and water. For the most part, normal saline and lactated Ringer solution are used for fluid replacement. They also are used as a means of administering a drug.

Types of IV Catheters

The three main types of IV catheters are (1) the hollow needle (butterfly) type, (2) the indwelling plastic catheter over a hollow needle (eg, Protective Cath, Autoguard, Acuvance Safety) (**FIGURE 14-22**), and (3) the indwelling plastic catheter inserted through a hollow needle (eg, Intracath), though this type is seldom used in the prehospital setting.

Hollow needles are not advised for IV fluid replacement in the prehospital setting, because stabilizing

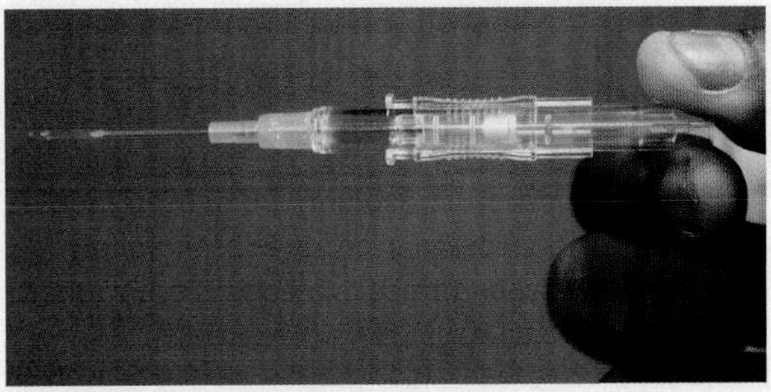

FIGURE 14-22 An intravenous catheter.

the needle is very difficult. In some cases, a butterfly catheter may be used for a pediatric patient if it can be stabilized adequately. Stabilization sometimes can be achieved by using armboards or other immobilization devices. In the prehospital setting, use of the over-the-needle catheter is preferred. This type of catheter is easily secured. Also, it is more comfortable for the patient.

Peripheral IV Insertion

Areas commonly used for peripheral IV therapy are the hands and the arms, including the antecubital fossae (AC space). Other sites are the long saphenous veins in the leg and the external jugular veins in the neck, although the incidences of embolism (described later) and infection are higher at these two sites. **FIGURE 14-23**, **FIGURE 14-24**, and **FIGURE 14-25** show sites and techniques for peripheral cannulation.

Another factor in the selection of a puncture site for IV therapy is the patient's clinical status. Injuries or diseases involving an extremity interfere with the use of veins in that extremity for venipuncture or venous cannulation. Examples of such conditions include trauma, infection at the site, dialysis fistula, and a history of mastectomy.

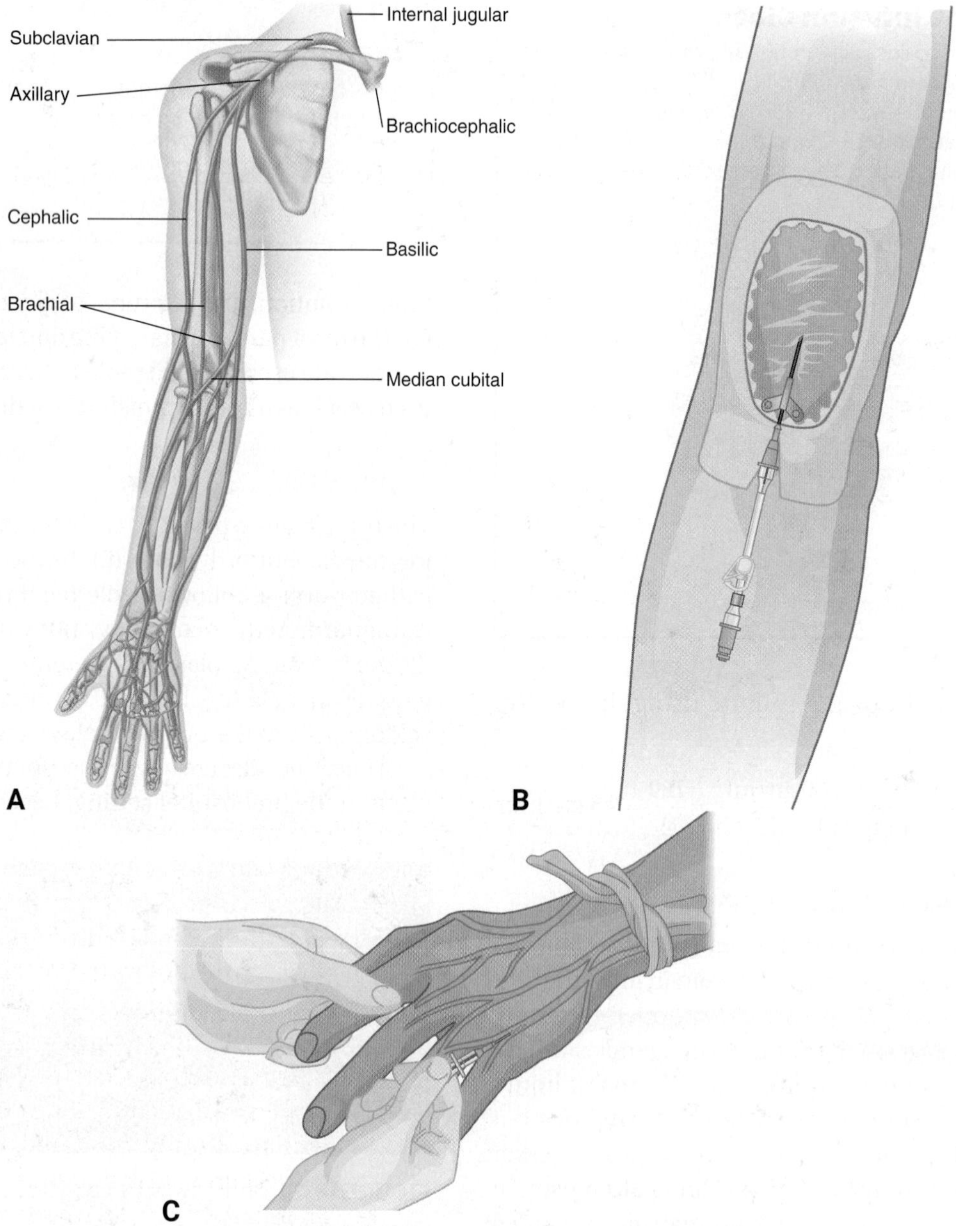

FIGURE 14-23 **A.** Veins of the upper extremity. **B.** Antecubital venipuncture. **C.** Dorsal hand venipuncture.

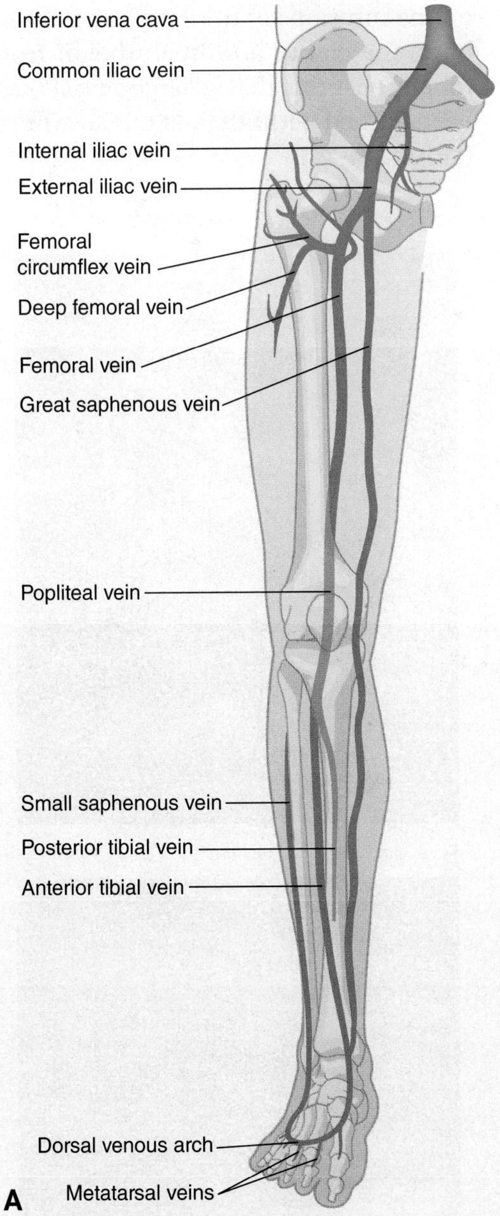

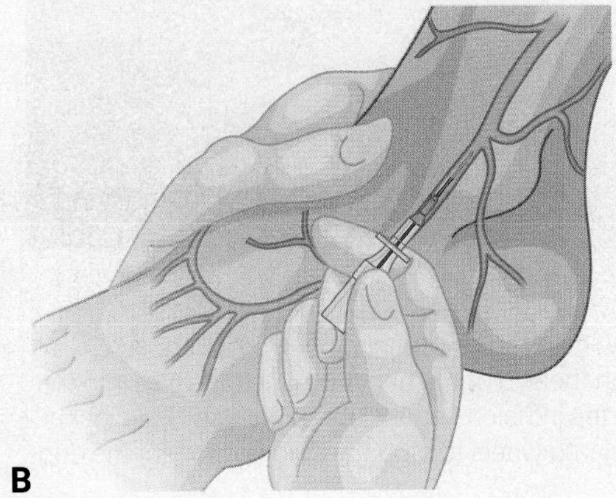

FIGURE 14-24 **A.** Long (great) saphenous vein. **B.** Venipuncture of the long saphenous vein.

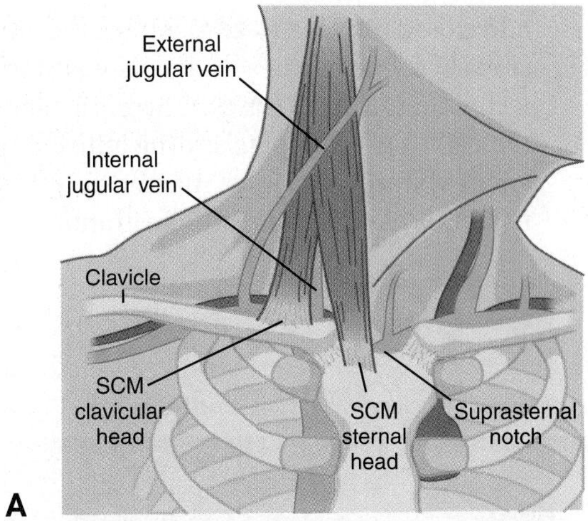

Abbreviation: SCM, sternocleidomastoid

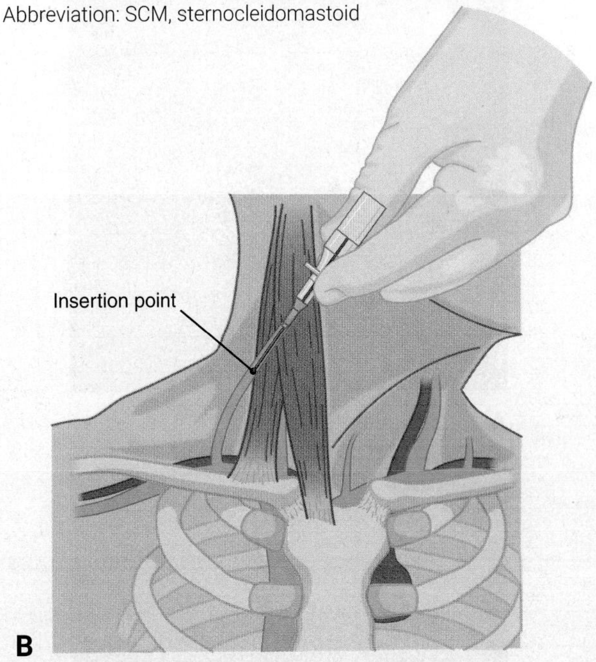

FIGURE 14-25 **A.** Anatomy of the external jugular vein. **B.** External jugular venipuncture.

To perform peripheral venous insertion of a cannula, follow these steps:

1. If the patient is conscious, explain the procedure. Give the reason IV therapy is necessary and describe the procedure. Confirm the five rights of medication administration aloud.
2. Assemble the equipment.
   - Inspect the fluid for proper solution, clarity, particulate matter, protective covers on tail ports, and expiration date. Never use fluids that are cloudy, outdated, or in any way suspect for contamination.
   - Prepare the microdrip or macrodrip infusion set. Check that tubing is not tangled, protective covers are present on both ends, and the flow clamp is positioned close to the drip chamber

and closed (**FIGURE 14-26A**). Attach the infusion set to the bag of solution using aseptic technique (**FIGURE 14-26B**). (Microdrip tubing typically is used for precise drug infusions or small-volume infusions; macrodrip tubing usually is used for fluid administration.)

3. Clamp the tubing and squeeze the reservoir on the infusion set until it fills halfway. Then open the clamp and flush the air from the tubing, ensuring that all large air bubbles have been flushed (**FIGURE 14-26C**). Close the clamp (**FIGURE 14-26D**).

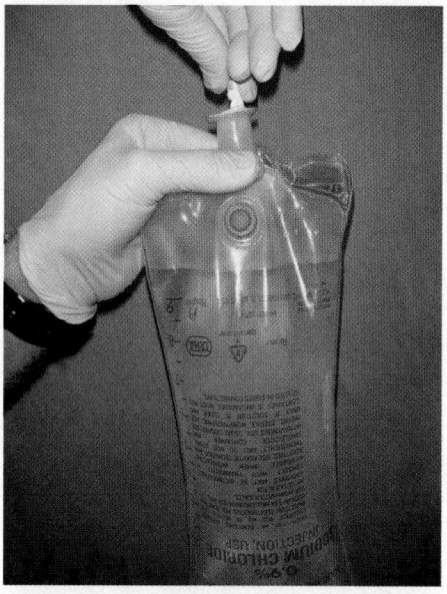

A

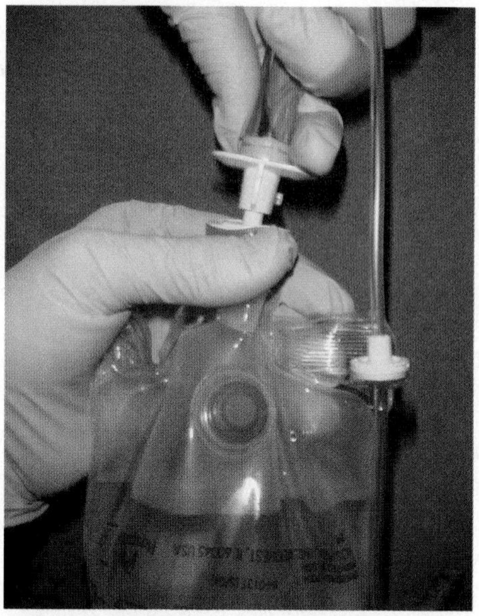

B

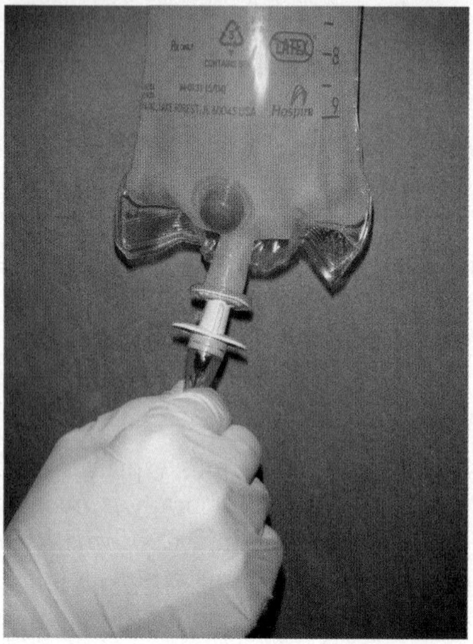

C

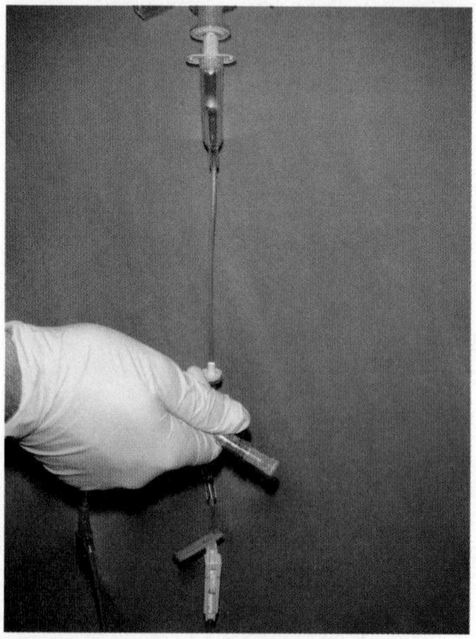

D

FIGURE 14-26 Intravenous (IV) infusion set up. **A.** Ensure that the correct administration set is chosen (microdrip or macrodrip). **B.** Remove the protective covering on the end of the bag and slide the spike into the IV bag port. **C.** Clamp the tubing and squeeze the reservoir on the infusion set until it fills halfway. Then open the clamp and flush the air from the tubing. **D.** Turn the roller clamp wheel to stop the fluid flow or set the drip rate per the required dose.

4. Select the catheter. Use a large-bore catheter (14 to 16 gauge) for fluid replacement; use a smaller-bore catheter (18 to 20 gauge) for to keep open (TKO) lines and saline locks. TKO lines are used to maintain hydration and to establish a channel for IV medication if needed.
5. Prepare other equipment:
   - Antiseptic to cleanse the skin
   - Sterile dressings or 4 × 4 gauze pads
   - Adhesive tape, torn or cut into several strips
   - Syringes and Vacutainers for blood samples
   - Tourniquet (blood pressure cuff may be used)
6. Put on gloves for personal and patient protection.
7. Select the puncture site (**FIGURE 14-27A**). If using an upper extremity, allow the patient's arm to hang dependent and apply the tourniquet

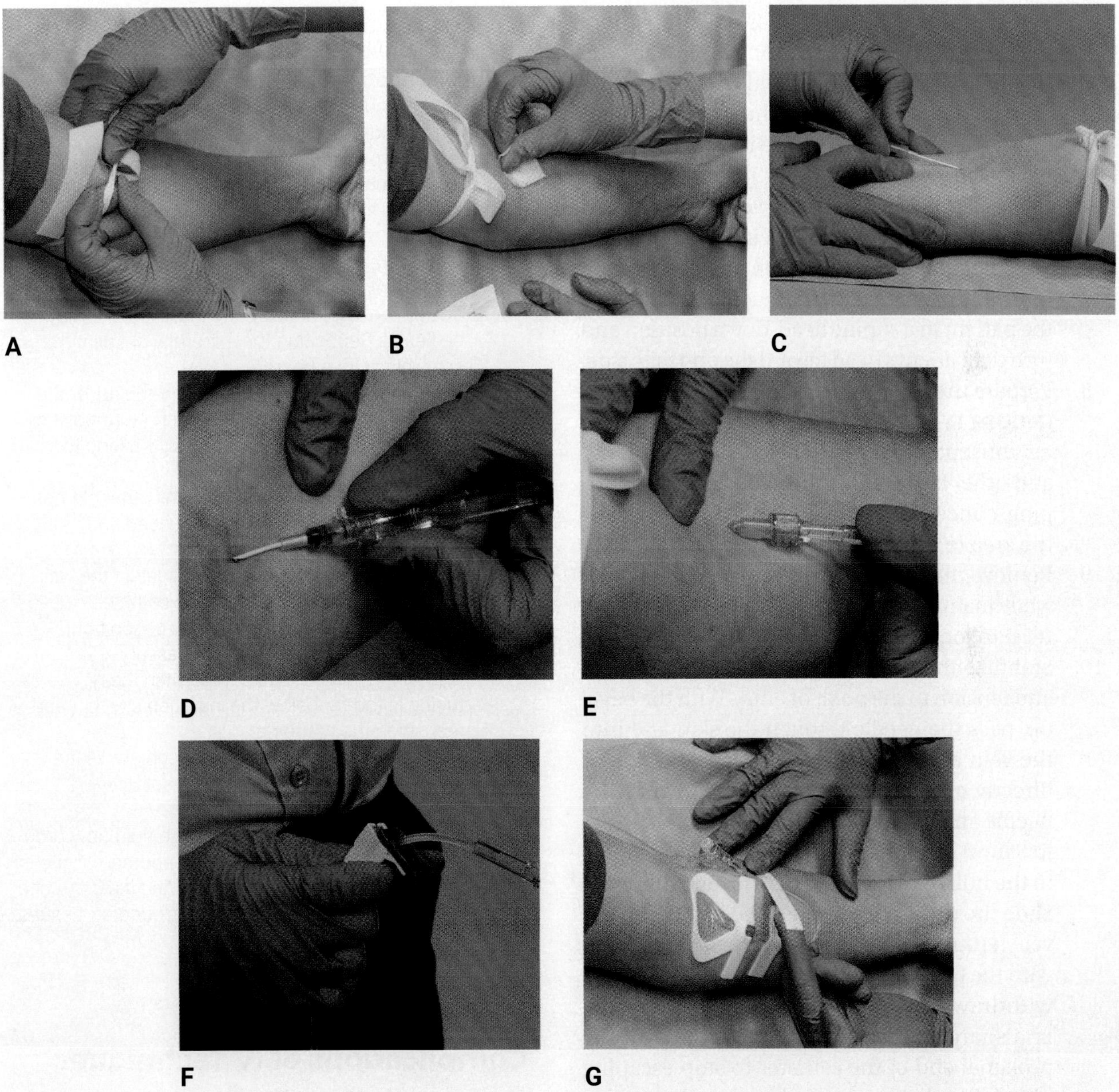

FIGURE 14-27 Intravenous (IV) catheterization technique. **A.** Apply a tourniquet above the desired site, and identify the vein. **B.** Cleanse the site. **C.** Stabilize the vein and pass the needle into the vein from the side or directly on top. **D.** Feel for a "pop" as the catheter slides over the needle and into the vein. While stabilizing the catheter, withdraw the needle into the protective sheath. **E.** While stabilizing the catheter, withdraw the needle into the protective sheath. Release the tourniquet and attach the IV line. **F.** Open the tubing clamp. Adjust the infusion to begin at the prescribed flow rate. **G.** Apply a dressing and secure it. Make sure the needle has been discarded in an appropriate container.

several inches above the antecubital space. (The tourniquet should be just tight enough to tamponade venous vessels but not so tight as to occlude arterial flow.) When selecting a suitable vein, begin by looking at the dorsum of the hand and forearm (unless another site is indicated). Choose a vein that is fairly straight and easily accessible. The forearm is a better choice than the hand because it allows hand movement and is more easily secured after cannulation. If a second puncture attempt is necessary, the second puncture should always be proximal to the first puncture. Therefore the vein selected for initial cannulation should be the most suitable distal vein. Avoid veins near joints, where immobilization is difficult, and veins near injured areas. If the long saphenous vein is chosen, begin site selection near the medial malleolus of the foot. To locate the external jugular vein, place the patient in a supine head-down position and turn the patient's head toward the opposite side.

8. Prepare the puncture site and cleanse the area (**FIGURE 14-27B**). Thoroughly clean the site with an antiseptic to remove dirt, dead skin, blood, and other surface contaminants. Use overlapping, concentric circles moving outward. Allow the area to dry.
9. Remove the IV catheter from the package and, while maintaining sterility, inspect for burrs and twist to loosen the hub.
10. Stabilize the vein by applying distal pressure and tension to the point of entry. With the bevel up, pass the needle through the skin and into the vein at a 35° to 45° angle from the side or directly on top (**FIGURE 14-27C**). Advance the needle and catheter about 0.125 to 0.25 inch (3 to 6 mm) beyond the point where blood return in the hub of the needle was first encountered. Slide the catheter over the needle and into the vein (**FIGURE 14-27D**). (Do not touch the catheter with the fingers.) While stabilizing the catheter, withdraw the needle. Dispose of the needle in a sharps container. Apply pressure on the proximal end of the catheter to stop escaping blood. Obtain blood samples, if needed, with a syringe or Vacutainer.
11. Release the tourniquet and attach the IV tubing (**FIGURE 14-27E**). Open the tubing clamp and allow the fluid infusion to begin at the prescribed flow rate (**FIGURE 14-27F**). Assess for infiltration.
12. Cover the puncture site with an occlusive dressing to ensure asepsis and to secure the line (**FIGURE 14-27G**). Anchor the tubing and secure the catheter. Catheter movement can increase the risk of phlebitis and cause migration of pathogens along the cannula into the vein.
13. Document the infusion procedure.

DID YOU KNOW?

Troubleshooting an Intravenous Infusion

If IV fluids are not flowing well or have completely stopped flowing, the paramedic should attempt to correct the problem before abandoning the IV site. Troubleshooting of an IV infusion should begin at the patient and proceed to the IV bag. The following are some common problems and solutions to consider for IV flow problems:

1. Make sure the tourniquet has been removed. If it is still in place, remove it.
2. The patient's joint above the insertion site may be flexed. Reposition the extremity or splint the extremity with a board.
3. The patient may be lying on the IV tubing, or the tubing may be kinked, restricting flow. Reposition the patient. Secure the tubing using a loop to prevent kinking.
4. Make sure the flow clamp and any other clamps are open. Adjust the clamp as needed and recalculate the drop rate.
5. The catheter tip may be lodged against the wall of the vein. Gently reposition the catheter.
6. The securing tape or device may be too tight, restricting flow. Reapply it if necessary.
7. Gravity may prevent fluid flow when the IV tubing is too far below the insertion site. Lift and reposition the IV tubing.
8. The IV bag may not be high enough above the insertion site. Raise the bag at least 3 feet (0.9 m) above the insertion site.

If these attempts do not resolve the fluid flow problem, remove the IV line and choose another IV site in the opposite extremity, if possible. If the insertion site is swollen or is leaking fluid into surrounding tissues (infiltration), remove the catheter.

Complications of IV Techniques

Approximately 330 million IV catheters are sold in the United States each year.[8] Although IV therapy is a crucial aspect of medical treatment for acute illnesses, cancer, surgery, anesthesia, and trauma, it can have complications—notably, local complications, systemic complications, infiltration, and air embolism.

NOTE

More than 85% of hospitalized patients receive some type of IV therapy, and many of these IV lines are established in the prehospital setting. To help hospital personnel understand when it may be time to change these IV access points, it is important for paramedics to document the following information when inserting an IV line:

- Type, length, and gauge of the catheter inserted
- Date and time of insertion
- Number and location of attempts
- Any complications with placement of the IV line
- Name of the vein
- Type of dressing applied to the site
- How the patient tolerated the procedure
- Any comments the patient made about the insertion procedure
- Name of the person inserting the device

Modified from: Iyer PW, Levin BJ, eds. *Nursing Malpractice*. 3rd ed. Tucson, AZ: Lawyer & Judges Publishing; 2007.

Local Complications

Local complications may involve hematoma formation, thrombosis, cellulitis, phlebitis, and sloughing and necrosis of tissue.

- **Hematoma formation** is the collection of blood or fluids at the site of injection or cannulation. The hematoma usually is small enough that it resolves spontaneously. Thus, this local complication rarely requires surgical treatment, drainage, or other interventions.
- **Thrombosis** is the formation of a blood clot (thrombus) inside a blood vessel when the vessel is injured. A clot that remains in place can become a **thromboembolism** and enter the circulatory system.
- **Cellulitis** is a potentially serious bacterial infection of connective tissue, which is associated with severe inflammation of dermal and subcutaneous skin. This condition can be caused by the introduction of normal skin flora after an injection or cannulation. Cellulitis appears as a swollen, red area of skin that feels hot and tender and can spread to any part of the body. Cellulitis usually is treated with antibiotics.
- **Phlebitis** is inflammation of a vein. This local complication is common after insertion of an IV catheter, especially if the catheter is too large for the vein or is left in place longer than 48 hours. Phlebitis causes localized redness and warmth at the IV site. It may extend a short distance along the course of the cannulized vein. This condition, which increases the risk of clot formation in a vein, is treated with anti-inflammatory medicines.
- **Sloughing** and **necrosis** of tissue can occur from infiltration of some IV medications (eg, dextrose 50%, sodium bicarbonate, epinephrine, potassium, digoxin, calcium, dopamine, and promethazine). Sloughing (the separation of tissue) and necrosis (tissue death) can be prevented by taking care to choose a stable vein of adequate size for drug administration. Frequent monitoring of the IV site for position and patency before, during, and after drug administration is important as well.

Systemic Complications

Systemic complications include sepsis, pulmonary embolism, catheter fragment embolism, and arterial puncture.

- **Sepsis** is a bacterial infection in the bloodstream. It can be caused by the use of contaminated equipment, poor aseptic technique, and prolonged IV therapy. Signs and symptoms of sepsis include a body temperature greater than 100.4°F (38°C) or less than 96.8°F (36°C), profuse sweating, nausea and vomiting, diarrhea, abdominal pain, tachycardia, hypotension, an increased white blood cell count, and altered mental status. Treatment includes the use of broad-spectrum antibiotics (see Chapter 31, *Hematology*).
- **Pulmonary embolism** is the sudden blocking of an artery in the lung, caused by a collection of solid material (**embolus**) brought through the bloodstream. It also may occur as a result of air bubbles introduced through an IV catheter (air embolism, described later). Signs and symptoms include a sudden onset of chest pain, shortness of breath, tachycardia, and hypotension. The patient should be placed on high-concentration oxygen and a cardiac monitor and should be transported for evaluation and treatment by a physician. (Pulmonary embolism is further described in Chapter 23, *Respiratory*.)
- **Catheter fragment embolism** can occur during the insertion of an IV catheter. It can result if part of the catheter becomes sheared off (detached), allowing the embolus to travel in the bloodstream, and when there is motion at the cannula and

the hub. An example is a catheter that is poorly secured or placed at areas of flexion. Reinsertion of a needle through the catheter during IV insertion can also produce a fragment embolism. Signs and symptoms include sharp pain at the insertion site, chest pain, and tachycardia. If a catheter fragment embolism is suspected, the IV infusion should be stopped, the vein should be palpated for the catheter tip, and a venous tourniquet should be applied above the tip to prevent further movement of the fragment.

NOTE

A needle should never be reinserted through a catheter. If IV insertion fails, the catheter should be removed, and a new IV catheter should be placed. When IV therapy is discontinued, the catheter should be examined to verify that it is intact and has not been sheared.

- Most arteries lie deep within the tissues, but some may lie close to the surface. Inadvertent arterial puncture during IV therapy is noted by the presence of pulsating and bright red blood in the catheter hub. Arteries are not suited for drug administration. In addition, arterial puncture can cause diminished blood supply to areas nourished by the affected artery. If arterial puncture occurs, the catheter should be removed and direct pressure applied to the site for at least 5 minutes. (Apply direct pressure for at least 10 minutes if the patient is on anticoagulant therapy.) A new IV line should be placed, and the incident should be well documented on the patient care report.

NOTE

Nerves, tendons, and ligaments can all be injured during IV therapy as a result of improper technique or lack of knowledge of anatomy. The patient may complain of intense pain, numbness, and an electric shock–type pain if a nerve is damaged. Injuries to nerves, tendons, and ligaments may be temporary or permanent. Patient management includes removing the IV catheter, inserting a new IV line, and providing careful documentation.

Infiltration

Infiltration may occur when the needle or catheter has been displaced or when blood or fluid leaks from around the catheter and escapes into the tissues (**extravasation**). It also can occur if a vein is punctured more than once during initiation of IV access. Signs and symptoms include the following:

- Coolness of the skin at the puncture site
- Swelling at the puncture site, with or without pain
- Sluggish or absent flow rate

If infiltration is suspected, the paramedic should lower the fluid reservoir to a dependent position to check for the backflow of blood into the tubing. (The absence of backflow suggests infiltration.) If any of the signs and symptoms are present, the IV flow should be discontinued (BOX 14-8), and the needle or catheter should be removed immediately. Moreover, a pressure dressing should be applied to the site. An alternative puncture site should be chosen and the infusion restarted with new equipment. In addition, the incident should be documented. Medication should not be injected into an IV line if there is a possibility it has infiltrated.

Air Embolism

Air embolism is uncommon but can be fatal when it occurs. The volume of air the venous bloodstream can tolerate is thought to be between 200 and 300 mL. However, arterial air embolism can cause ischemia or infarction in organs even when only small volumes are present.[9]

The embolism is caused by air entering the bloodstream via the catheter tubing. The risk of air embolism is greatest when a catheter is passed into the central circulation, where negative pressure may actually pull in air. Air can enter the circulation either upon insertion of the catheter or when the tubing is disconnected to replace solutions or add new extension

BOX 14-8 Discontinuation of an Intravenous Infusion

To discontinue an IV infusion and remove the IV catheter, follow these steps:

1. Put on gloves.
2. Carefully remove any securing tape and dressings.
3. Close the drip chamber to stop the flow of fluid.
4. Place sterile gauze over the insertion site and apply gentle pressure with one hand. With the other hand, quickly withdraw the catheter, pulling straight back from the angle of insertion. Check that the catheter is intact.
5. Apply firm pressure to the insertion site for 2 to 5 minutes to prevent bleeding or bruising.
6. Cover the insertion site with a bandage.
7. Appropriately dispose of all equipment.

BOX 14-9 Replacement of Intravenous Solutions

When a bag of IV fluids must be replaced during an infusion, the paramedic should prepare all equipment in advance and follow these steps:

1. Close the roller clamp. Hold the infusing bag upside down in one hand and remove the spike from the old container. Discard the old bag.
2. Quickly insert the spike chamber into the new bag. Assure the chamber is 1/3 to 1/2 full.
3. Tap or flick the IV tubing to allow air bubbles (if present) to rise to be expelled from the tubing into the drip chamber.
4. After the air has been expelled, adjust the flow rate of the infusion.
5. Document the time the IV fluids were replaced.

tubing (BOX 14-9). With subsequent pumping, blood foaming occurs in the heart. If enough air enters the heart chamber, it can impede the flow of blood, which in turn can lead to shock. Signs and symptoms of air embolism include hypotension; cyanosis; weak, rapid pulse; and loss of consciousness.

If air embolism is suspected, take the following steps:

1. Close the tubing.
2. Turn the patient on the left side with the head down. If air has entered the heart chambers, this position may keep the air in the right side of the heart and away from the right ventricular outflow tract.
3. Check the tubing for leaks.
4. Administer 100% oxygen.
5. Notify medical direction.

Accidental disconnection of the IV tubing—for example, during patient movement—can cause an air embolism. The chance of an air embolism can be minimized by making sure all tubing connections are secure. Also, fluid containers should be changed before they are empty.

IV Medications

Medications can be given directly into the vascular system via the venous route by injection or infusion. An IV injection can be administered through a previously established IV infusion line, heparin or saline lock, or implantable port (eg, Port-A-Cath, Hickman catheter). It also can be administered directly into the vein with a sterile needle or butterfly device. An IV infusion is given by adding a drug to an infusing IV solution (eg, normal saline). Another method is to dilute the drug in a larger volume of fluid and administer the medication as an IV push, or through a volume control, in-line device (eg, burette, Volutrol, infusion pump) (FIGURE 14-28). Sometimes the medication is given by intermittent infusion through an existing infusion site (IV piggyback or secondary set).

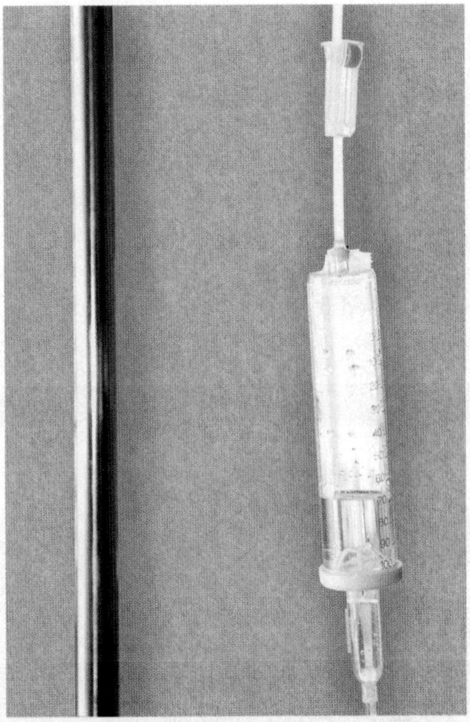

FIGURE 14-28 Buretrol, a volume control device.

IV injections normally involve a small amount of medication, called an IV push or IV bolus medication. To give such an injection (FIGURE 14-29), after verifying the correct dose and volume, the paramedic should clean the most proximal needleless port of the IV line with antiseptic. The medication is then injected slowly (usually over 1 to 3 minutes). The rate of injection depends on the type of medication, its indication, and the patient's response. Most types of IV tubing have a one-way valve to prevent the backflow of medication. If such a valve is not present or cannot be identified, the tubing above the injection site should be clamped or the infusion stopped during drug administration. After the injection, the infusion of fluids is continued.

IV infusions for drug administration can take several forms. To add a medication to the IV fluid (eg, normal saline) that is infusing in an established

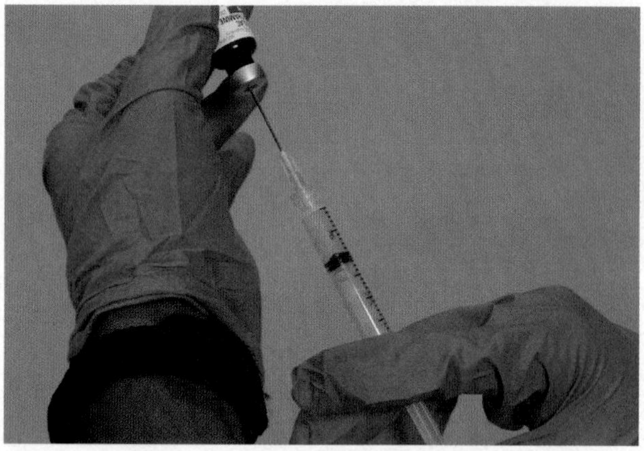

A

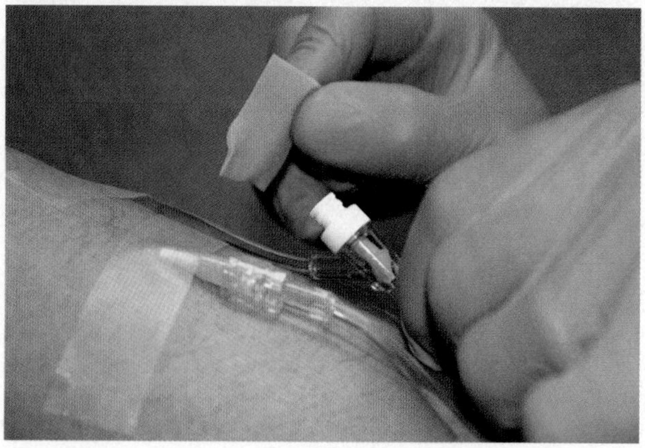

B

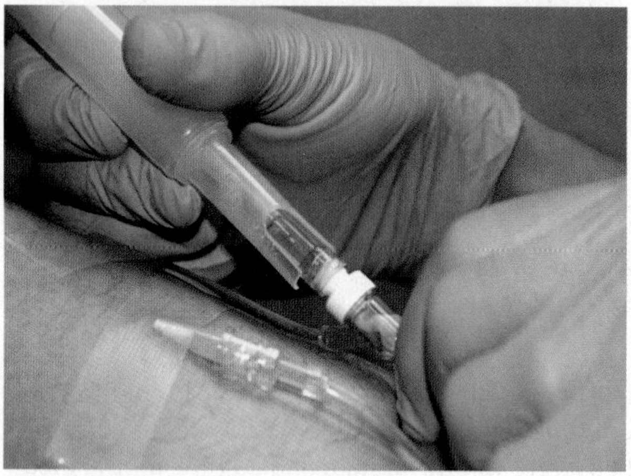

C

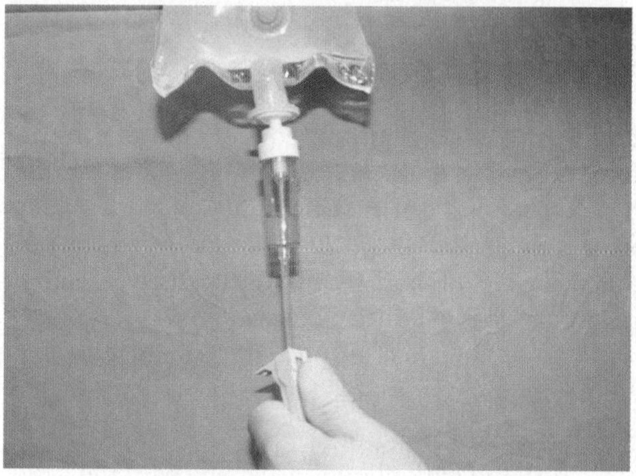

D

FIGURE 14-29 Administration of a drug by the intravenous (IV) route. **A.** Prepare the correct volume of the drug. **B.** Clean the injection port. **C.** Insert the tip of the syringe into the luer port, pinch the line, and inject the drug. **D.** Dispose the syringe and then briefly flush the IV line.

IV line, the paramedic should follow these steps (**FIGURE 14-30**):

1. Compute the volume of the drug to be added to the IV bag.
2. Draw up the prescribed dose into a syringe. If prefilled syringes are used, note the volume of medication in the syringe and the dose to be used. Confirm the five rights of medication administration aloud.
3. Clean the rubber sleeve of the IV bag with an antiseptic.
4. Puncture the rubber sleeve (if a needle is used) and inject the prescribed medication into the fluid reservoir.
5. Withdraw the needle (if not using a needleless system) and discard the needle and syringe.

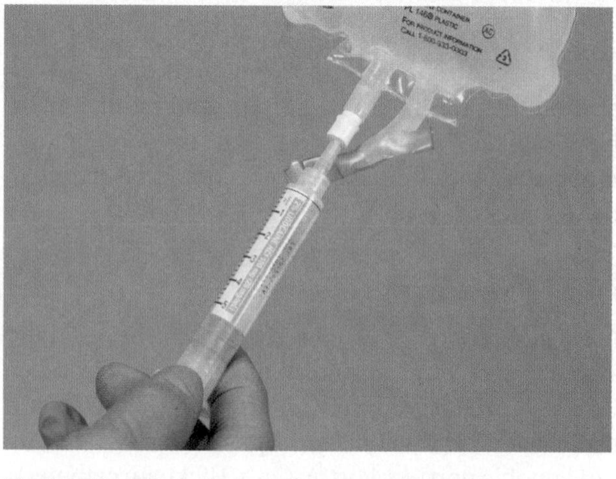

FIGURE 14-30 Adding medication to an intravenous bag.

Gently mix the medication with the fluid by agitating the IV bag.

6. Label the IV bag with (1) the name of the medication added, (2) the amount of the medication added, (3) the resultant concentration of the medication in the reservoir, (4) the date and time the infusion was prepared, and (5) the name of the paramedic who prepared the infusion.
7. Calculate the rate of administration in drops per minute as prescribed.

A number of in-line volume control devices allow more accurate delivery of medication diluted in precise amounts of fluids than can be achieved by simply setting the drip rate manually. These devices often are used to give IV medications to children and adults who need precise doses. Medications that can readily cause toxicity when given too rapidly (eg, antidysrhythmics, vasopressors) are well suited to this delivery method. In-line devices include electronic flow rate regulators that regulate the amount of fluid administered by means of a magnetically activated metal ball valve. They also include infusion pumps that exert pressure on tubing or fluid by pumping against pressure gradients (**FIGURE 14-31**). When using such an in-line volume control device, paramedics should be familiar with the device before using it and follow the instructions of the equipment's manufacturer. Other mechanical (nonelectric) devices are available (eg, Dial-A-Flow) and are used by some EMS agencies to closely regulate the flow rate.

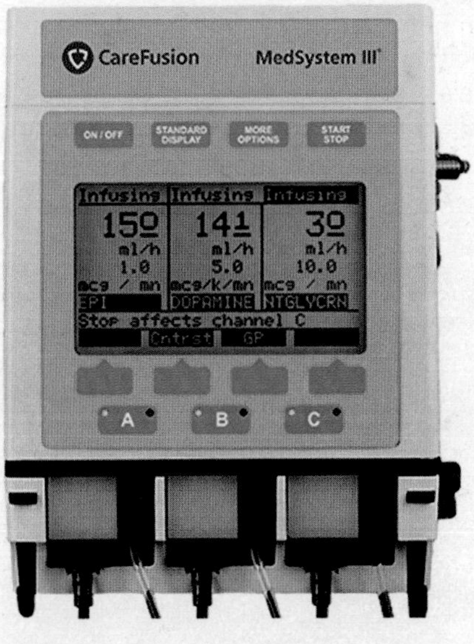

FIGURE 14-31 Intravenous infusion pump.

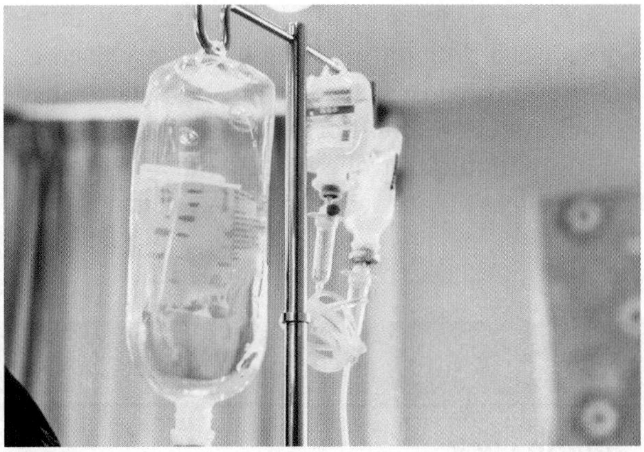

FIGURE 14-32 Intravenous piggyback setup.

Intermittent infusions are given via a setup that is "piggybacked" secondary to the primary IV infusion. The piggyback medication is hung in tandem and connected to the primary setup (**FIGURE 14-32**). Most intermittent diluted drug infusions (except lidocaine and dopamine) are meant to have a total infusion time of 20 or 30 minutes to 1 hour, though the precise time depends on the drug and the patient's response. To prepare an intermittent infusion, the paramedic should follow these steps:

1. Prepare the prescribed medication using the medication cross-check. Confirm the five rights of medication administration aloud. Add the medication to the secondary IV solution.
2. Flush the air out of the secondary administration set. Attach a 1-inch (25-mm), 18-gauge needle if a needleless system is not available.
3. Clean the medication port of the primary infusion tubing. Insert the tubing from the piggyback medication while maintaining sterility.
4. Tape the needle (if present) or carefully secure the tubing to the medication port.
5. Calculate the flow rate of the secondary infusion in drops per minute.
6. Clamp the tubing of the primary infusion to allow the piggyback medication to infuse. Open the piggyback line flow clamp. Adjust the flow rate to the desired dose. After administration of the piggyback medication, restart the primary infusion. Discard the piggyback equipment.
7. Always label the bag with the medication.
8. Monitor the patient and document the medication's effects.

Another device used to administer a drug intravenously is a drug pump. Drug pumps are used by patients who need a slow injection of medication in the home or elsewhere—for example, cancer chemotherapy, patient-controlled analgesia, and insulin. These devices may consist of a syringe with a battery attachment, a pager device, or a large pump that regulates the injection of medication. Drug pumps are used to give medication subcutaneously, intravenously, or, in some cases, into the epidural space. They also can be attached to indwelling vascular devices such as a Port-A-Cath or Hickman catheter (BOX 14-10).

BOX 14-10 Indwelling Vascular Devices

Saline Lock

A saline lock is a peripheral IV cannula that has no attached IV tubing (**FIGURE 14-33**). These devices, which allow ready access to peripheral veins, are used for brief administration of medications. They also are used for IV therapy that is administered frequently on an outpatient basis (eg, chemotherapy). The cannula is filled with saline solution, which prevents clotting when the device is not in use. In some inpatient settings, heparin is used instead of normal saline for the flush.

To gain access to the peripheral vein, draw 4 mL of normal saline into a syringe. Use aseptic technique. Flush 2 mL of the normal saline through the lock reservoir before and after infusion of the prescribed medication or IV fluid. After IV therapy, inject 3 mL of 0.9% normal saline into the reservoir (to keep the lock patent). It is preferred to use normal saline in a prefilled syringe to reduce the risk of medication error.

Central Venous Access Devices

Four types of central venous access devices (CVADs) are available: nontunneled catheters, tunneled catheters, peripherally inserted central catheters (PICCs), and implanted ports (**FIGURE 14-34**). The tip of the CVAD rests in the superior vena cava. (The tip of a femoral CVAD is placed in the inferior vena cava.) If the tip moves into the atria, complications can occur. Nontunneled CVADs are inserted through the skin into the subclavian vein; they can be inserted in an emergency. Tunneled CVADs are silicone catheters inserted into the subclavian vein in the operating room or radiographic procedure room. These devices, which are designed to stay in place for years, include Hickman, Broviac, Groshong, Hohn, and Leonard catheters. Peripherally inserted central catheters usually are introduced through a vein in the antecubital fossa. They are designed for short-term treatment (up to 6 months). Because PICCs are longer than the other CVADs, drawing blood or infusing fluids quickly through these lines sometimes is more difficult.

Paramedics may or may not be trained to access CVADs. It is important to verify that this skill is authorized by protocol before attempting to perform it in the field.

Most CVADs have a volume of 1 to 3 mL. Be careful not to introduce air when drawing blood, administering drugs, or initiating IV fluids, because an air embolus could result. Follow these steps to access a tunneled, nontunneled, or peripherally inserted CVAD:

1. Prepare the equipment (use only 10-mL or larger syringes; smaller syringes can create high pressure and damage the catheter).
2. Draw up 3 to 5 mL of normal saline (at least twice the volume of the catheter).
3. Put on gloves. Use aseptic technique.
4. Explain the procedure to the patient. Confirm the five rights of medication administration aloud.
5. Clamp the catheter with the attached clamp or padded smooth shunt clamp. (Groshong catheters have a built-in valve and should not be clamped.)

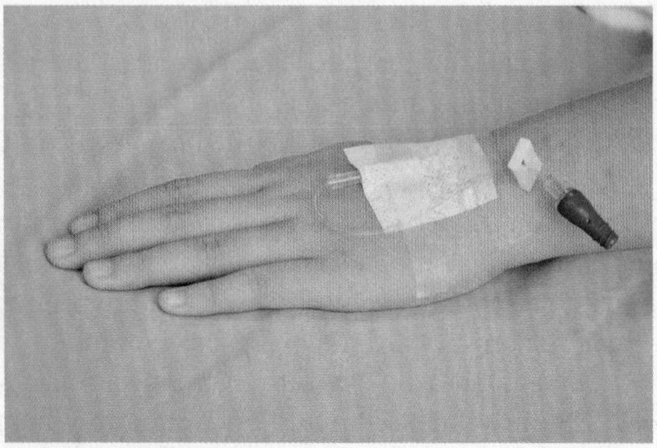

FIGURE 14-33 Saline lock.

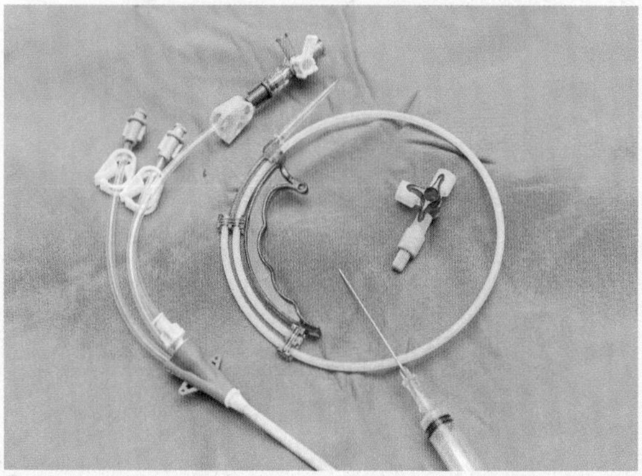

FIGURE 14-34 Example of a triple lumen device.

6. Wipe the site with povidone-iodine and allow it to dry.
7. Connect the syringe and unclamp the catheter. Withdraw 5 mL blood. *If blood cannot be withdrawn, do not use the catheter.*
8. Replace the clamp.
9. Attach the syringe of normal saline to the catheter. Remove the clamp and flush (do not use excessive pressure).
10. Replace the clamp and remove the syringe.
11. Connect the IV tubing to the catheter. Make sure the tubing is free of air.
12. Remove the clamp and begin the infusion.
13. Tape the connection site between the tubing and catheter. Administer fluids and drugs.

Implantable Ports

An implantable port is a CVAD that is surgically inserted in a pocket under the skin (**FIGURE 14-35**). It has a self-sealing septum over a small chamber or reservoir.

Each time the port is used, the skin must be punctured by a needle. A special, noncoring Huber needle should be used, as a regular needle could damage the port, requiring immediate surgery.

Implantable ports should not be accessed in the ambulance if the patient is stable. If the septum is punctured or the port becomes infected, a surgical technique is needed to replace it. The steps for accessing the port are as follows:

1. Palpate the skin and locate the port.
2. Use sterile technique to clean the area first with alcohol and then with povidone-iodine.
3. Feel for the edge of the port housing and stabilize the port with one hand.
4. Insert the Huber needle through the skin and port septum until contact is made with the back of the port.
5. Confirm correct placement by aspirating blood.
6. Flush with saline and connect the IV tubing (make sure it is free of air).
7. Cover the Huber needle with a transparent dressing. Start the infusion.

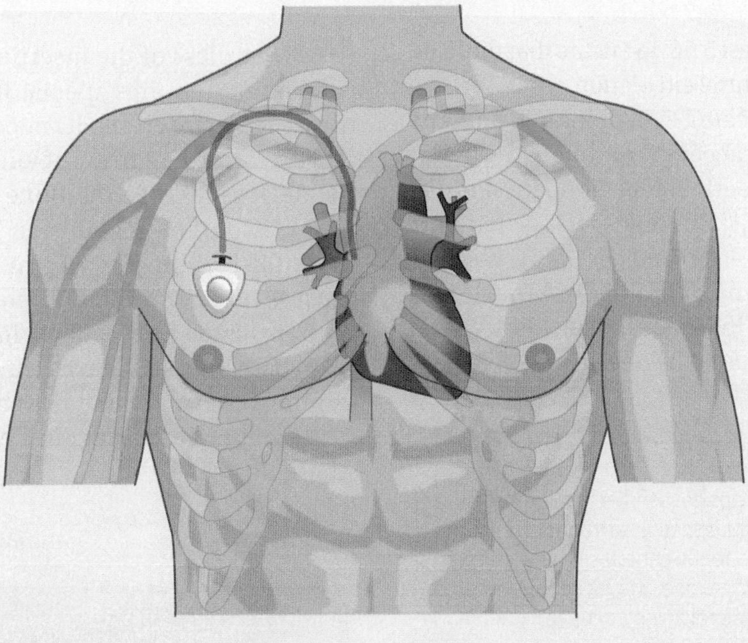

FIGURE 14-35 Port-A-Cath.

NOTE

To prevent damage to central venous catheters, paramedics should:

- Use a clamp on the clamping sleeve provided on silicone catheters.
- Avoid using scissors or other sharp objects around the device.
- Use only small-gauge needles (22 to 25 gauge) with a needle length of 1 inch (25 mm) or less when accessing the injection port.
- Administer fluids or medications gently (never force them).

Intraosseous Medications

Studies have shown that intraosseous (IO) infusion is relatively safe and effective in both children and adults.[10] Fluids and drugs infused through IO access pass quickly from the marrow cavities of long bones into the sinusoids, then move into large venous channels and emissary veins, and finally enter the systemic circulation. Normal saline, lactated Ringer solution, D_5W, plasma, blood, and most advanced life support medications may be infused quickly by this route (**FIGURE 14-36**). Drugs administered by the IO route should be followed

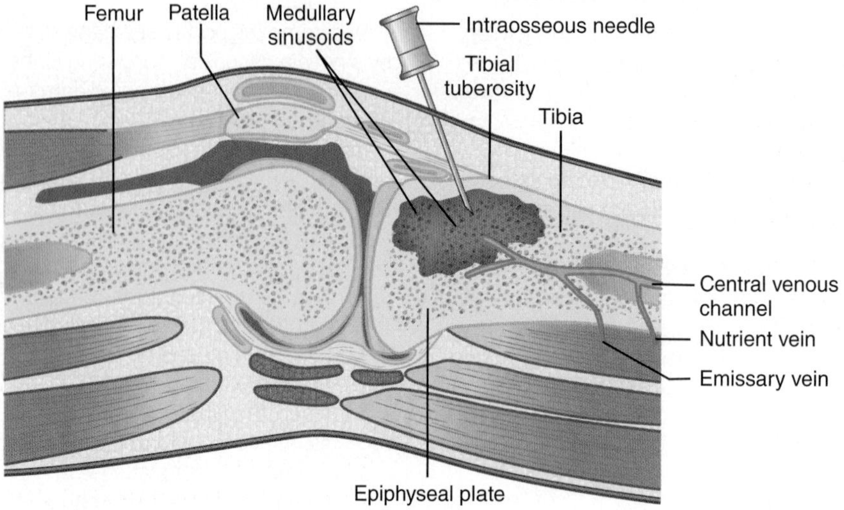

FIGURE 14-36 Obtaining intraosseous access.

by a saline flush of at least 5 mL to ensure that the drug is delivered into the central circulation.

IO infusion is indicated in ill or injured patients who require vascular access for administration of drugs or fluids when peripheral cannulation is difficult or unobtainable.[10] Examples include patients with cardiopulmonary arrest and peripheral vascular collapse (as in shock, major trauma, or burns). This procedure also may be indicated in patients in whom vascular access is impaired by obesity or edema.

> **NOTE**
> The intraosseous (IO) space can be thought of as a "noncollapsible vein." This space is surrounded by bone and is directly connected to the central circulation. In the absence of trauma to the bone, the IO space remains patent, even when peripheral veins collapse.

The site of choice for initiation of this procedure varies based on the patient and the condition. In many EMS systems, it is the tibia, just below the tubercle on the anteromedial surface. Alternative sites in children are the femur, just above the lateral condyles in the midline, and the head of the humerus (preferred location in many systems). In adults, alternative sites are the sternum, just below the sternal notch; the tibia; the medial malleolus; and the head of the humerus. The bones of adults are slightly more difficult to penetrate than the bones of children.

Regardless of the insertion site chosen, the IO procedure requires special IO devices, which are designed to insert the IO needle safely through the cortex into the marrow of long bones. Commercial IO devices include the Bone Injection Gun (BIG), Cook Disposable IO Infusion Needle (Sur-Fast Needle), EZ-IO infusion system (**FIGURE 14-37**), First Access for Shock and Trauma (FAST1) IO infusion system, FAST1 Sternal IO infusion system, New Intraosseous (NIO) device, and Jamshidi IO needle, among others. Paramedics should carefully follow the manufacturer's recommendations when using these devices.

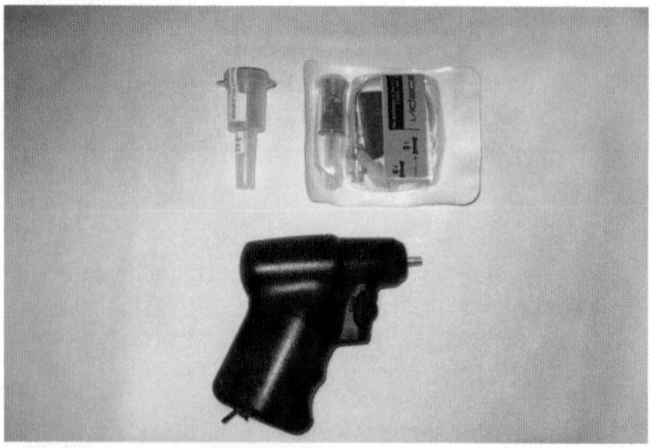

FIGURE 14-37 EZ-IO device.

Necessary Equipment for IO Infusion

- Antiseptic
- Tape
- Bone marrow needle or commercial IO needle with insertion gun
- IV extension tubing
- IV tubing (based on patient need)
- IV fluids (specified by medical direction): normal saline, lactated Ringer solution
- Pressure infusion bag or pump

Insertion Technique

The procedure for initiating an IO infusion in the tibia is described as follows:

1. Put on gloves for personal and patient protection.
2. Identify the appropriate site (**FIGURE 14-38A**).
3. Clean the site as previously described for peripheral cannulation (**FIGURE 14-38B**).
4. Prepare the needle for insertion and stabilize the site (**FIGURE 14-38C**). Insert the needle at the proper angle pointing away from the epiphyseal plate. Advance it to the periosteum.
5. Using a boring or screwing motion (or the device-specific technique), advance the needle until it penetrates the bone marrow (usually noted by decreased resistance and a slight popping [trapdoor] sensation) (**FIGURE 14-38D**).
6. Remove the stylet and dispose of it in the proper sharps container (**FIGURE 14-38E**).
7. Infuse saline by syringe or aspirate it (if recommended by manufacturer) to ensure placement of the needle while assessing for infiltration. Confirmation is completed if it flows without infiltration.
8. Secure the needle with tape or a securing device, if so equipped (although the needle usually is well stabilized by the bone). Attach an extension tubing to lessen the chance of rocking the IO needle and causing leakage.
9. Attach standard IV tubing and regulate fluids to infuse under pressure as prescribed by medical direction (**FIGURE 14-38F**).
10. Apply a dressing to the site.
11. Monitor the patient and document the procedure.

Contraindications

- Fracture of the site or proximal to the site
- Traumatized extremity
- Cellulitis
- Burns that may be infected by the technique
- Congenital bone disease

Potential Complications

Technical Complications

- Subperiosteal infusion from improper placement
- Penetration of the posterior wall of the medullary cavity, resulting in soft-tissue infusion
- Slow infusion from clotting of marrow

Systemic Complications. IO devices are short-term emergency devices. They usually are removed within 24 hours of insertion to prevent systemic complications, such as the following:

- Osteomyelitis (occurs in fewer than 0.6% of cases, usually with prolonged infusion)
- Fat embolism (rare)
- Slight periostitis at the injection site (usually clears within 2 to 3 weeks)
- Infection (acceptably low rate, comparable to that with other infusion techniques)
- Fracture

Transmucosal Medication Administration

Body cavities are lined by membranes coated with thick mucus. The mucus linings of the sublingual, buccal, and nasal tissues provide good sites for emergency medication administration. They offer some advantages over the oral route, including fast, noninvasive absorption into the systemic circulation. In addition, drugs given through the transmucosal surface do not undergo first-pass metabolism in the liver. Drugs that readily attach to or penetrate the submucosal surface are suitable for this route of delivery.[11] In EMS care, the sublingual, buccal, and intranasal sites are used to administer medication.

Sublingual Drugs

The most frequently prescribed sublingual drugs are nitrates (eg, nitroglycerin), which are used to treat angina pectoris. Other sublingual drugs used in emergency care include lorazepam, which is used to treat anxiety, and captopril, which is used to manage congestive heart failure.

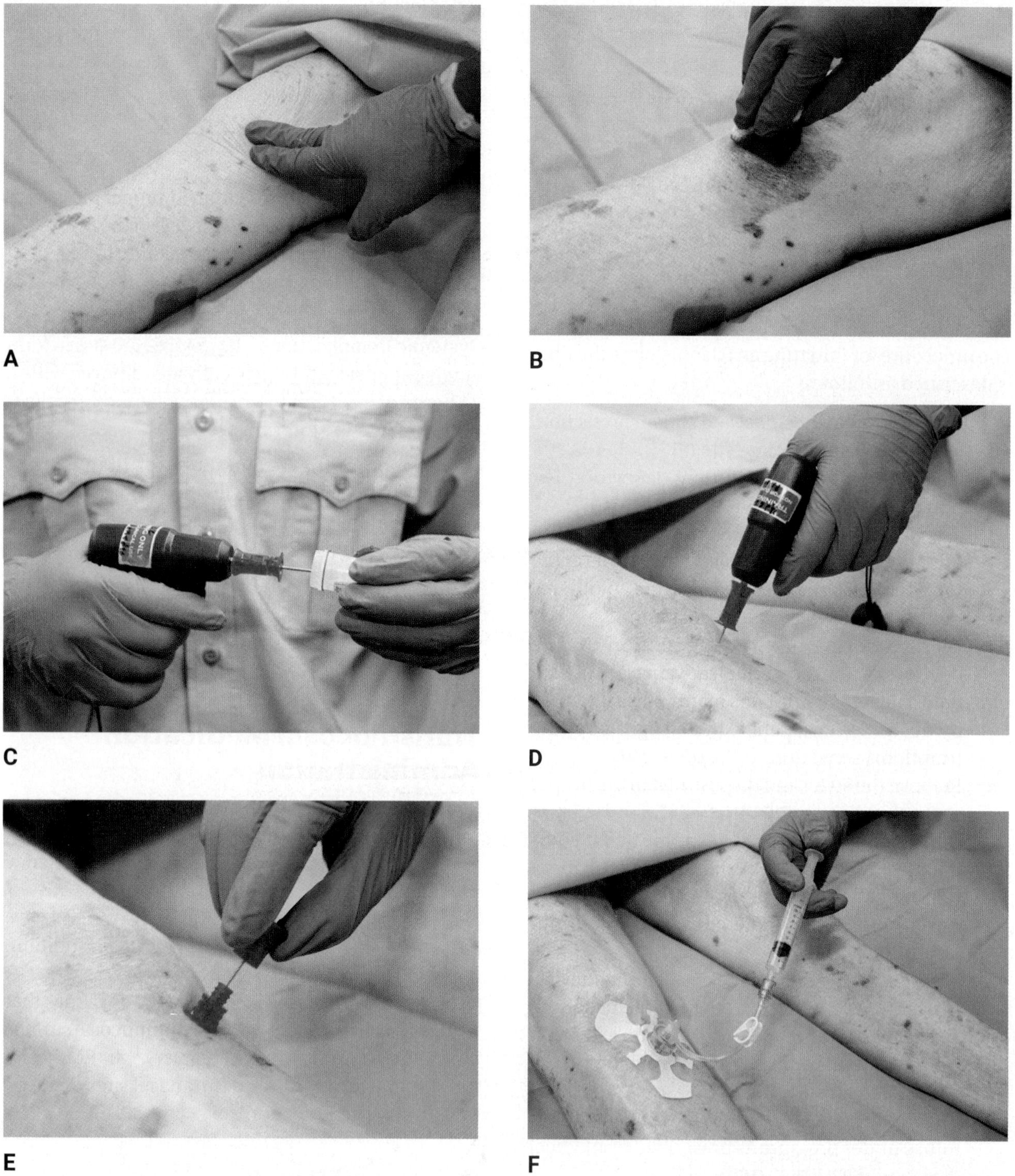

FIGURE 14-38 Intraosseous infusion. **A.** Assess the site. **B.** Clean the site. **C.** Attach the needle to the EZ-IO gun and remove the protective cover. **D.** Stabilize the site, insert the needle at a 90-degree angle, advance the needle until a "pop" is felt, then remove the stylet. **E**. Remove the stylet from the catheter. **F.** Attach the syringe and extension set to the intraosseous needle. Flush with normal saline to ensure proper placement. Assure flow and secure the site.

Sublingual tablets should be placed under the tongue, where they dissolve. The patient should not drink fluids while the drug is being absorbed. If the patient inadvertently swallows the tablet, the effects are diminished and delayed. Older adults have decreased saliva, so absorption of sublingual drugs can be slow and unpredictable in these patients.

Buccal Drugs

Buccal drugs are held between the patient's cheek and gum, where they dissolve to achieve their desired effects. As with sublingual drugs, the patient should not drink fluids while the drug is being absorbed. Glucose gel preparations are an example of an emergency medication administered via the buccal route. This route should not be used for patients with altered level of consciousness, for patients who cannot swallow, or for patients who have an ineffective gag reflex.

Intranasal Drugs

Over the past 10 years, the use of atomized intranasal drugs in EMS care has increased. Giving drugs by this route of administration has some advantages. For example, because the nasal route is needleless, giving intranasal drugs eliminates the risk of needlestick injury. Also, nasal drugs can be administered safely in a moving ambulance or rescue vehicle. The nasal route may be preferred with combative patients and small children and when IV access is difficult to obtain. Drugs given by this route act quickly on the brain because they are absorbed close to the brain—their desired site of action. They also do not undergo first-pass metabolism through the liver (like oral medicines), so their serum concentration remains high.

Only drugs that have molecules that are easily absorbed and cross a lipid membrane (those with high lipophilicity) can be administered by this route. Many emergency medications are approved for nasal administration, including diazepam (Valium), fentanyl (Sublimaze), glucagon, haloperidol (Haldol), lidocaine (Xylocaine), lorazepam (Ativan), midazolam (Versed), ketamine (Ketalar), and naloxone (Narcan). Any drug that can cause hypotension should not be administered intranasally unless an IV line has been established.

Several limitations apply to administration of drugs by the intranasal route. Most importantly, not all medications can be given by this route. Also, drug effectiveness is limited if the patient has nasal congestion or damaged nasal mucosa. Only small volumes can be given intranasally: The ideal drug volume is 0.3 mL, although up to 1 mL can be administered in each nostril. The drug volume should be split and half of the total volume given in each nare.

Equipment Needed to Administer Intranasal Medications

The device used to administer an intranasal medication must be able to atomize the drug into a fine spray so it can be appropriately dispersed into the nasal cavity for absorption. Several commercial devices are available for this purpose.

Most paramedics administer intranasal medication using a syringe that contains the medicine and a nasal atomizer that separates the medicine into a fine mist (**FIGURE 14-39**). When intranasal medicines are given by nonparamedic personnel or by the patient's family members, a commercial device is often used. This drug delivery device is prefilled with the medication and is attached to an atomizer for ease of use (**FIGURE 14-40**). The cost of these prefilled devices is much higher than the cost of the medication by itself.

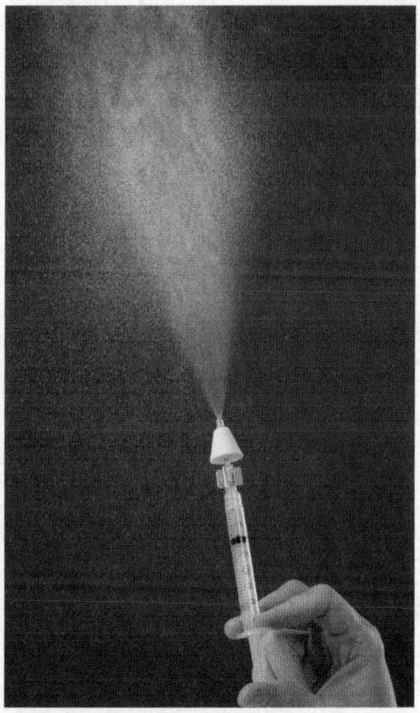

FIGURE 14-39 A nasal atomizer.

Courtesy of LMA North America

Intranasal Drug Administration Technique

Intranasal drug administration places the medication on the mucosal layer of the nasal cavity (**FIGURE 14-41**). The steps for administering a drug via this route are as follows:

1. Measure the appropriate dose and an additional amount to account for the dead space in the device (dead space varies from 0.06 mL to 0.15 mL depending on device—consult your protocol).[12] Confirm the five rights of medication administration aloud.
2. Place the atomizer on the syringe and secure it firmly.
3. Place the atomizer firmly into one nostril, aiming toward the top of the ear on the same side.
4. Hold the top of the patient's head with your free hand to stabilize it.
5. Squeeze briskly on the syringe to deliver half the dose.
6. Place the atomizer in the other nostril and squeeze the syringe forcefully to administer the second half of the medicine. If the syringe is not squeezed forcefully, the medicine may drip or run down the nasopharynx and will not be atomized into a mist to distribute onto the nasal membranes.

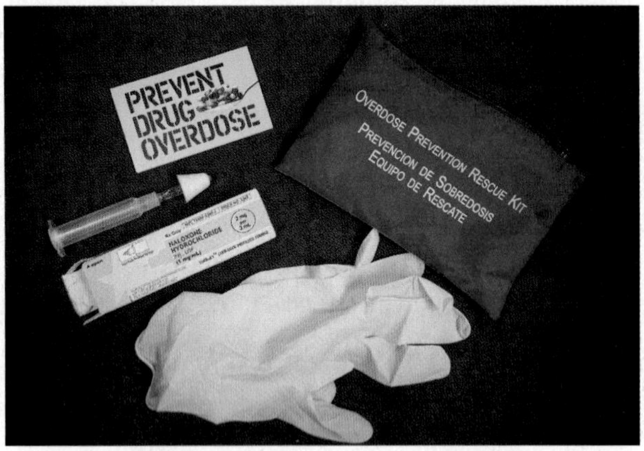

FIGURE 14-40 Prefilled naloxone drug delivery devices—used to counteract the effects of opioid overdose—rely on use of a nasal atomizer.

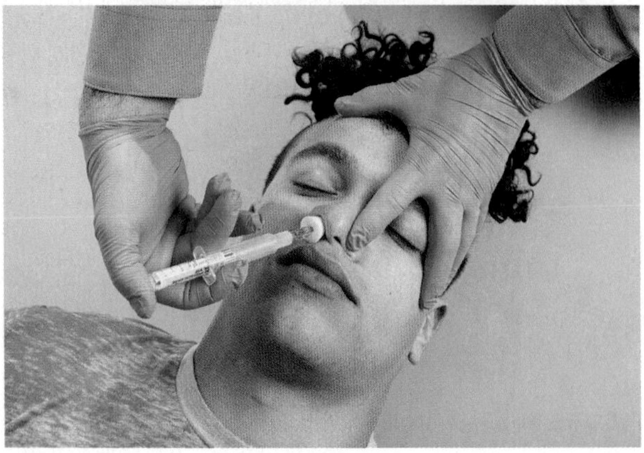

FIGURE 14-41 Nasal administration of naloxone.

SHOW ME THE EVIDENCE

An emergency pharmacist and an emergency physician inspected the medication-carrying and storage practices of nine advanced life support ambulance agencies within five counties. Their findings were then rated by two EMS medical directors to determine the level of risk with each. In total, they found 38 medication safety issues: 16 were considered high risk, 14 were moderate risk, and 8 posed low risk for harm. Issues found included expired medicines, container-labeling problems, medications stored in look-alike containers in the same compartment, and crystalloid IV fluids stored next to infusion bags with premixed medication. The researchers concluded that understanding the nature of these issues may lead to changes that can reduce the likelihood of medication-related errors and the risk of patient harm.

Modified from: Kupas DF, Shayhorn M, Green P, Payton TF. Structured inspection of medications carried and stored by emergency medical services agencies identified practices that may lead to medication errors. *Prehosp Emerg Care*. 2012;16(1):67-75.

Administration of Transdermal Medications

Transdermal drug administration (or *percutaneous* drug administration) is the administration of drugs that are absorbed through the skin. Medications delivered via this route include topical drugs and drugs for the eye and ear.

Topical Drugs

In addition to the various emollients and antibiotic ointments, the most commonly used transdermal emergency medication is nitroglycerin. Two types of topical nitroglycerin preparations are available: nitropaste and transdermal nitroglycerin delivery patches. These can be applied to any clean, dry area of the upper arm or hair-free portion of the chest. Nitropaste, which has a lanolin-petrolatum base, is applied in 0.5-inch (1-cm) increments with special papers to measure the dose. Transdermal nitroglycerin patches have an adhesive back (**FIGURE 14-42**). They are available in a solid or semisolid form, depending on the manufacturer. Paramedics should always wear gloves when applying or removing these medications to prevent inadvertent self-absorption of the drug. (More information is available in the Appendix, *Emergency Drug Index*.) The onset of drug action for transdermal medications is slower and the duration is longer than those given by parenteral routes.

Drugs such as fentanyl, scopolamine, clonidine, and estrogen are also used in patch form. These drug patches can affect the patient unfavorably during illness. Paramedics should be able to recognize the different types of patches and should remove them if indicated. Usual sites for the patches are behind the ear and on the chest, back, hip, and upper arms. If these medications are ingested orally by children, they can cause lethal overdose.

Drugs for the Eye, Nose, and Ear

Eye medications usually are supplied in the form of drops or ointments. To administer these drugs, the paramedic should have the patient lie down or sit with the head tilted back. Stabilizing the patient's head with one hand, the paramedic uses the thumb or fingers of the other hand to pull down the lower lid gently. The medication should be applied into the conjunctival sac of the lower lid—never onto the eyeball (**FIGURE 14-43**).

Nose drops administered to act on nasal tissue (as opposed to systemically) are best administered with the patient lying down with the head over the edge of a bed in a midline position. The drops are instilled into each nostril. The patient should be instructed not to blow the nose for several minutes to allow absorption of the drug. To administer a drug via the nasal route, the paramedic should instruct the patient to hold the head upright or tilted back and to block one nostril. The patient then inhales through the open nostril while squeezing the spray applicator to release the atomized drug. Allergy and decongestant medications are two examples of medications administered by this route.

Ear medications usually are provided in the form of drops. The patient should lie down with the affected ear up. With adults or children older than 3 years, the paramedic should gently pull the top of the ear up and back and up to straighten the ear canal. The prescribed number of drops is then instilled. In children younger than 3 years, the ear is pulled down and straight back. The patient should remain in the ear-up position for about 10 minutes to allow the medicine to disperse. To prevent contamination of the drops, the paramedic should not allow the tip of the dropper to come into contact with the ear canal. Placing a cotton ball in the ear canal after administration of the drug may reduce seepage of the drops onto the face.

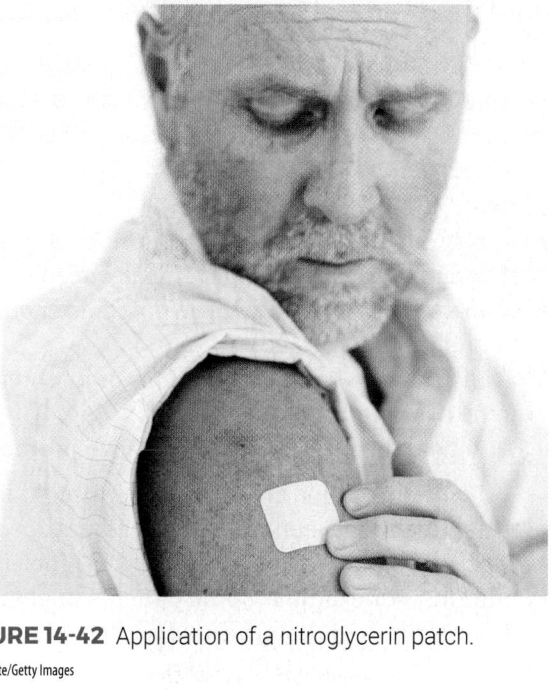

FIGURE 14-42 Application of a nitroglycerin patch.

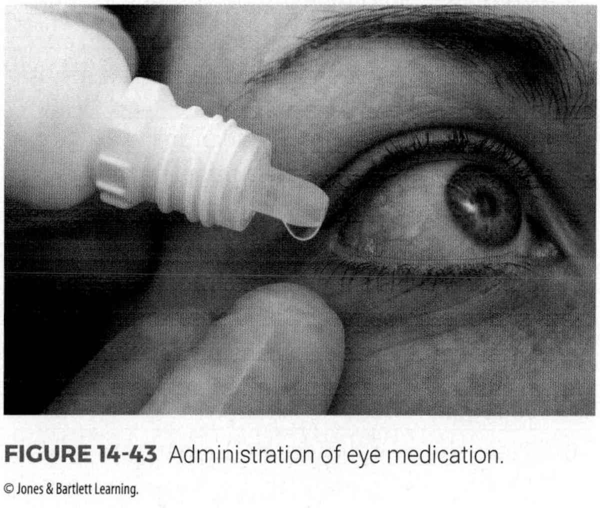

FIGURE 14-43 Administration of eye medication.

Administration of Inhaled Drugs

In addition to oxygen and nitrous oxide, several other drugs are administered by means of inhalation. These include bronchodilators, corticosteroids, antibiotics, and mucokinetic agents delivered through aerosolization.

Aerosols are liquid or solid particles of a substance dispersed in gas or solution. The effectiveness of aerosolization therapy depends on the number of droplets that can be suspended in the gas or solution, the rate of oxygen or gas flow, the particle size (diameter in microns), output (cubic centimeters per minute [cc/min]), and the rate and depth of the patient's breathing. Rapid, shallow breathing reduces the number and retention of droplets that reach the deep bronchioles of the lungs. The delivery of drugs by this method has certain advantages over other routes—specifically, rapid onset of the drug's effect and fewer or less-intense systemic side effects.

Aerosols are made by devices called *nebulizers.* Intermittent positive pressure breathing (IPPB) devices are designed for in-hospital use. Out-of-hospital devices include metered-dose inhalers (pressure cartridges) and handheld nebulizers. Handheld nebulizers operate by means of a compressed air or oxygen source regulated by a flowmeter.

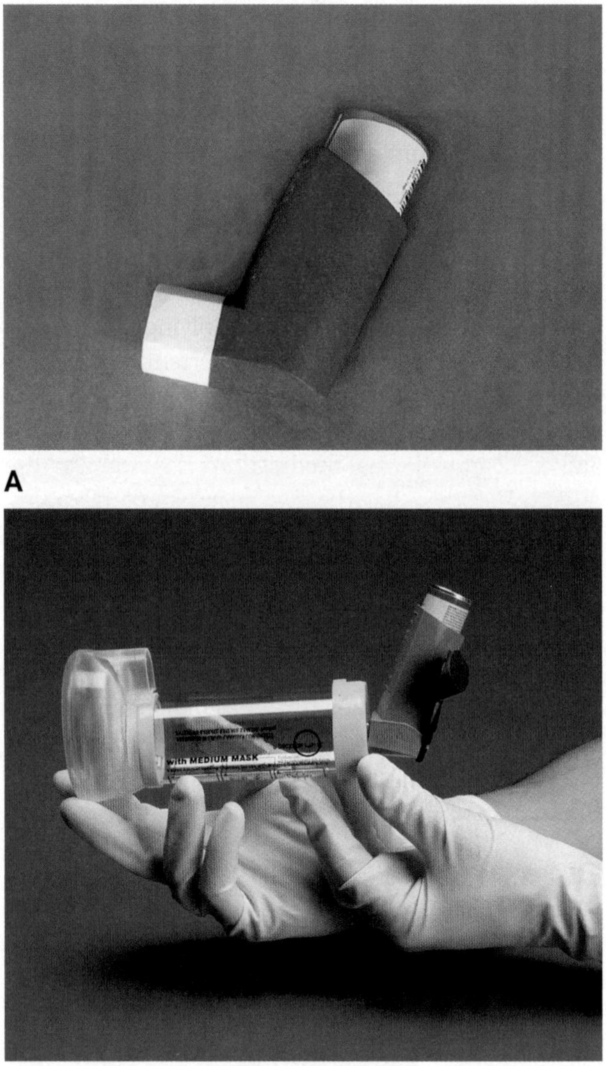

A

B

FIGURE 14-44 **A.** Metered-dose inhaler (MDI). **B.** MDI with an extender or spacer.

Metered-Dose Inhaler

The metered-dose inhaler (MDI) is a commonly used device in aerosol therapy (**FIGURE 14-44**). It is convenient and delivers a measured dose with each push of the cartridge. MDIs usually are prescribed for self-treatment of asthma. Other medications prepared in MDIs are ipratropium and albuterol.

Paramedics should follow these steps to administer a drug by MDI:

1. Confirm the five rights of medication administration aloud.
2. Remove the mouthpiece and protective cap from the canister (the drug container) of the MDI.
3. Insert the canister stem into the hole inside the mouthpiece.
4. Shake the canister and mouthpiece well.
5. Hold the MDI close to the patient's mouth, with the MDI's nozzle down. Instruct the patient to exhale, pushing as much air from the lungs as possible.
6. Place the mouthpiece in the patient's mouth. Instruct the patient to close the lips loosely around it, with the tongue underneath the mouthpiece. As the patient inhales deeply over 2 to 3 seconds, press down on the canister quickly and then release it.
7. Instruct the patient to hold his or her breath 5 to 10 seconds before exhaling.
8. Repeat the procedure according to protocol.

MDI medications are often administered using aerochambers (spacers). These devices are especially beneficial for children and for patients with problematic conditions. For example, some patients might need additional time to inhale the medication, others may lack coordination, and still others may be hampered by a high level of anxiety or by a diminished ability to inhale slowly and deeply in coordination with dispensing the medication. Aerochambers allow the patient to receive the maximum benefit of the drug and do not require exact synchronization of breathing with operation of the MDI. If a spacer is used with the MDI, follow the manufacturer's instructions to prime it if it is new or has not been used for a week or more. Instruct the patient to inhale deeply but not enough to make the spacer whistle.

CRITICAL THINKING

What happens to the medication if the patient does not use the MDI properly?

Handheld Nebulizers

Handheld nebulizers are another means of administering some medications via inhalation in the prehospital setting. Various manufacturers make disposable nebulizer kits. The kits usually include a mouthpiece or aerosol mask, oxygen tubing, and reservoir tubing (**FIGURE 14-45**). These devices are attached to a nonhumidified portable or on-board oxygen source and use the Bernoulli principle to create an aerosol mist (sometimes referred to as a *jet* or *pneumatic nebulizer*). Medications appropriate for nebulization therapy include albuterol, racemic epinephrine, ipratropium, levalbuterol, and metaproterenol.

Specific procedures for administering a drug via nebulizer may vary slightly, depending on the patient's ability to tolerate the treatment by mouthpiece or mask. A tight seal around the mouthpiece is required, so the patient must be able to cooperate during treatment.

Both the mouthpiece and the mask methods have advantages. With treatment by mouthpiece, less of the drug is wasted. However, patients with severe dyspnea who are mouth breathers tolerate mask administration much better.

To administer a medication with a handheld nebulizer, paramedics should follow these steps:

1. Using aseptic technique, mix the prescribed drug with a specified amount of normal saline and then instill it into the nebulizer. Some medications come in a packaged unit dose and have a fixed amount of diluent (usually 0.9% normal saline). Confirm the five rights of medication administration aloud.
2. Attach the nebulizer to a T-piece and mouthpiece, and connect it with tubing to the unit delivering nonhumidified oxygen (for the hypoxic patient) or compressed air. (If the patient cannot use the mouthpiece, a nebulizer face mask may be used in its place.)
3. Adjust the oxygen flowmeter according to the manufacturer's recommendations (usually a rate of 4 to 6 L/min) to create a steady, visible mist. (This rate usually offers a steady mist without too much wastage of medication. The higher the flow rate, the greater the medication use.) If an aerosol mask is used, the oxygen flow rate should be regulated according to the manufacturer's recommendations (usually 6 to 8 L/min). This prevents the buildup of exhaled carbon dioxide in the mask.
4. When the mist is visible, begin treatment. Instruct the patient to inhale slowly and deeply by mouth. Have the patient hold a breath for 3 to 5 seconds before exhaling, so as to ensure topical deposition of the aerosol particles deep within the tracheobronchial tree. Inhalation and exhalation should continue until the aerosol canister is depleted of the medication. Repeat treatments usually are not given more often than every 15 to 20 minutes (usually to a maximum of three treatments). Treatment of severe asthma, however, may include continuous administration of nebulized beta agonists, tailored to the patient's response.

The patient must be cooperative to undergo nebulization therapy. He or she must be able to follow

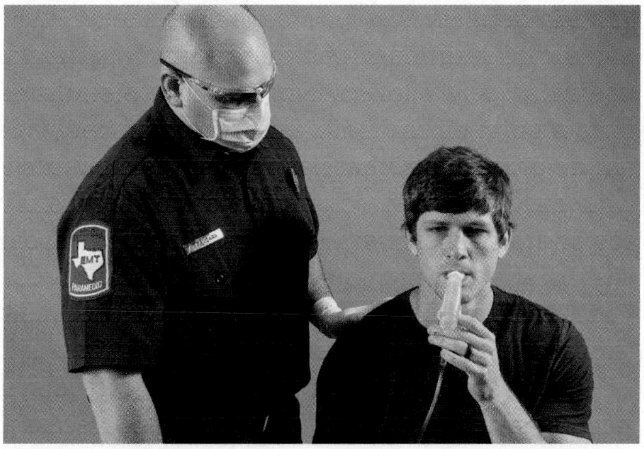

FIGURE 14-45 Administration of medication with a handheld nebulizer.

instructions to breathe deeply so that the drug can be absorbed. If the patient is unable to inhale the drug sufficiently or if bronchospasm is too severe, administration of the medication via another route should be considered. Nebulizer treatments may be administered to a patient who is artificially ventilated by placing the drug into the ventilation circuit of the bag-mask device or ventilator. It is important to regulate the flow of oxygen to the correct rate. If too little or too much flow is given for the device, the medicine will not aerosolize to the particle size needed to penetrate to the desired site of action.

Notable changes in the patient's heart rate or dysrhythmias may occur during nebulization therapy. If these occur, treatment should be stopped and medical direction should be contacted for further orders. Paramedics and ambulance crews should avoid the medication vapor stream during nebulization therapy.

Administration of Endotracheal Drugs

The ET route is an alternative route of drug administration. It may be used when IV or IO access cannot be established and other routes are not appropriate for the situation. Absorption through the ET route is unpredictable and less effective than the IV or IO routes, so the ET drug dose must be increased. Emergency drugs that may be administered by this route are naloxone, atropine, vasopressin, epinephrine, and lidocaine (memory aid: *NAVEL*).

When giving medication by this route, paramedics should follow these steps (**FIGURE 14-46**):

1. Make sure the ET tube is in the correct position. Placement can be checked by direct visualization and by auscultation (see Chapter 15, *Airway Management, Respiration, and Artificial Ventilation*).
2. Make sure oxygenation and ventilation of the patient's lungs are adequate.
3. Prepare the medication so that it is 2 to 2.5 times the IV dose. Dilute the adult dose to 10 mL with normal saline (or prepare a 10-mL normal saline flush, per protocol). Confirm the five rights of medication administration aloud.
4. Remove the air source from the ET tube. Inject the medication through a catheter deep into the tube, or inject it directly into the tube, and follow it with a normal saline flush (per protocol). (Some ET tubes have a drug port; with these tubes, the air source need not be removed for drug administration.)
5. Resume ventilations with one to two full ventilations. This step helps ensure that the medication penetrates as deeply as possible into the pulmonary tree, which enhances absorption.
6. Monitor the patient for the desired therapeutic effect and for any side effects.

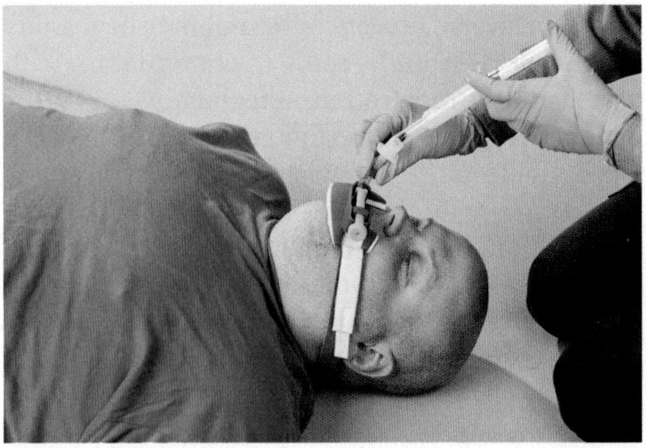

FIGURE 14-46 Administration of a drug through an endotracheal tube.

Special Considerations for Pediatric Patients

Administering drugs to infants and children can be quite difficult, especially in emergency situations. The following guidelines may be helpful for this process:

- Try to establish a positive relationship with the child. Accept fearful or anxious behavior as a natural response.
- Be honest with the child when explaining a medication or procedure that will be unpleasant or painful.
- If appropriate, allow the child to help administer the medication (eg, by holding the medicine cup or by placing a pill in the mouth).
- When administering oral liquid drugs to infants or small children, hold the child (or have the parent hold the child) in a semireclined position. Place the oral medication syringe or administration device alongside the tongue. Slowly inject the medication, allowing the child to swallow small amounts at a time.
- Use mild physical restraint only if it is required. Explain to the child why it is needed.

- Enlist the assistance of parents or other caregivers when possible.
- When parenteral medications are required, stabilize the injection site well and give the injection quickly. Two or more people should be available to hold a child older than 4 years, even if the child promises to "be still."
- Remember when administering medications that the younger and smaller the child, the smaller the margin for error.

SHOW ME THE EVIDENCE

Michigan researchers performed a mixed-methods study using both quantitative (cross-sectional, observational) and qualitative research designs. In the study, they evaluated prehospital provider performance during simulated care of a child with altered mental status, seizures, and respiratory arrest. The researchers found errors in airway management, oxygen delivery, glucose measurement, cardiopulmonary resuscitation, and drug administration. The error rate was 47% for diazepam administration and 60% for midazolam administration. These medication errors were traced to causes including incorrect weight estimate, incorrect use of the Broselow length-based emergency tape, incorrect recollection of doses, problems calculating doses under stress, errors converting doses, inaccurate measurement of volumes, improper use of prefilled syringes, and failure to cross-check doses with partners. The researchers concluded that this exercise was helpful in finding causes of errors in pediatric care. On the basis of the conclusions, they identified 14 recommendations to reduce errors in the care of pediatric patients in their system.

Modified from: Lammers R, Bryrwa M, Fales W. Root causes of errors in a simulated prehospital pediatric emergency. *Acad Emerg Med*. 2015;19(1):37-47.

Obtaining a Blood Sample

Venous blood samples often are obtained in the prehospital setting for glucose testing and for laboratory determinations performed in the hospital. If possible, these samples should be obtained when an IV line is established and always before any fluids are infused. If blood for serum potassium is being drawn, avoid having the patient pump the fist to make the veins more prominent or to increase the blood flow, as this practice can cause potassium levels to be falsely high.

When obtaining a blood sample from an IV site, the paramedic should follow these steps:

1. Prepare all equipment in advance.
2. After removing the needle from the IV catheter, exert manual pressure above the IV site to prevent the free flow of blood from the catheter.
3. While stabilizing the site, insert the Vacutainer into the hub of the IV catheter.
4. Push blood collection vacuum tubes (**TABLE 14-3**) into the barrel of the Vacutainer to draw blood from the IV catheter.
5. After obtaining the required specimens, attach the IV tubing and begin infusion.
6. Gently invert sample tubes that are intended to prevent clotting three to four times.
7. Label the sample with the patient's name and the time and date it was obtained.

CRITICAL THINKING

Why should a venous blood sample never be drawn above an IV infusion site?

TABLE 14-3 Types of Blood Sample Tubes and Order of Blood Draws

To prevent contamination of tubes with additives from other tubes, it is important to draw the tubes in a *specific* order, called the *order of the draw.* The following is the collection sequence for evacuated tubes when multiple tubes must be drawn:[a]

1. Yellow top or bottles: Sterile/blood cultures
2. Royal blue: Red label for trace metal analysis
3. Light blue coagulation tube. If only coagulation tests are ordered *and* a butterfly catheter is used, draw a discard tube to collect the air in the tubing. If this is not done, a short draw (insufficient amount of blood for the sample) results, which will be rejected by the laboratory.
4. Red: Nonadditive
5. Red Gel separator tube (speckled or "tiger" top)
6. Green (heparin)
7. Green/gray mottled PST with heparin
8. Lavender/purple top and/or pink EDTA
9. Gray top (oxalate/fluoride tube)

(continued)

TABLE 14-3 Types of Blood Sample Tubes and Order of Blood Draws *(continued)*

Stopper Color	Additive/ Preservative	Tests Done on Blood Sample	Comments
Green	Heparin	Electrolytes, glucose; cardiac enzymes	Invert tube several times. Heparin prevents blood from clotting without killing cells.
Gray	Oxalate/fluoride	Blood alcohol Lactate levels Fasting glucose assays	
Lavender	EDTA anticoagulant	Blood cell count, hemoglobin, hematocrit, erythrocyte sedimentation rate Glycohemoglobin A1c T8 for human immunodeficiency virus	Invert tube several times to prevent clotting (do not shake). EDTA tubes are used to collect samples for whole-blood hematology testing.
Light blue	Sodium citrate	Prothrombin time, activated partial thrombin time, fibrinogen levels d-Dimer	Tube must be filled completely. Invert tube several times to prevent clotting. Sodium citrate tubes are used to collect samples primarily for coagulation studies. Such tests often are needed for patients with bleeding problems (eg, in the abdomen, brain, or elsewhere)
Red	None	Serum electrolytes, liver and other enzymes, therapeutic drug levels, blood bank procedures	The tube need not be inverted, because the objective is to produce a clot. Some companies make tubes with clot activators, which hasten clotting to speed testing.
Yellow	Glass particles to speed up clotting process	All immunology tests	Tubes with clot activators

Abbreviations: EDTA, ethylenediaminetetraacetic acid; PST, plasma separator tube

[a]University of Michigan Health System, Department of Pathology. Blood bank: FAQs. University of Michigan website. https://www.pathology.med.umich.edu/blood-bank/faq. Accessed January 12, 2018.

Modified from: Specimen collection. Becton, Dickinson and Company website. http://www.bd.com/en-us/offerings/capabilities/specimen-collection. Accessed January 12, 2018.

If no IV line is to be used, the paramedic may obtain the blood sample using a Vacutainer (**FIGURE 14-47**) or a needle and syringe and then transfer the sample to an evacuation tube. The steps for obtaining a blood sample using a needle and syringe are as follows:

1. Apply a tourniquet above the selected site.
2. Cleanse the site as previously described for venipuncture.
3. Using an 18- or 20-gauge needle attached to a 10- or 12-mL syringe, enter the vein.
4. With an even, steady motion, draw back on the plunger to obtain the sample.
5. After the sample has been obtained, release the tourniquet, withdraw the needle, and apply manual pressure to the site.

FIGURE 14-47 Obtaining a blood sample with a Vacutainer.

6. Immediately transfer the sample to the appropriate evacuation tube. Do not force additional blood into the tube; each tube has the correct amount

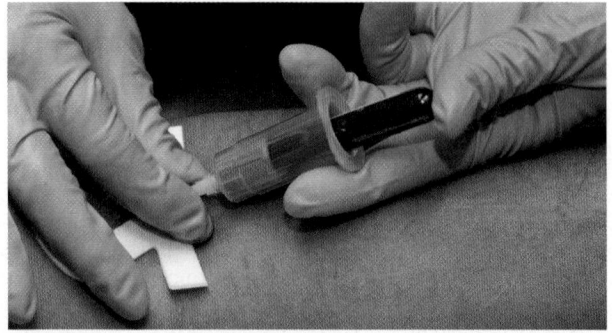

of vacuum for the amount of blood required in the vial. Forcing blood into a vacuum tube can cause expulsion of contents and can lead to unnecessary injury or exposure to contents.

7. Gently invert sample tubes that are not intended to clot three to four times.
8. Label the sample with the patient's name and the time and date it was obtained.

Disposal of Contaminated Items and Sharps

Needles and other sharp objects can injure the patient, the paramedic, coworkers, and others. They also can be a source of infection with hepatitis or the human immunodeficiency virus (HIV). The Centers for Disease Control and Prevention recommends that needles not be capped, bent, or broken before disposal. Rather, they should be discarded with the syringe intact in a special container (ie, sharps container) that is clearly marked (**FIGURE 14-48**). These containers should be puncture- and leakproof. When full (as indicated by the "Full" line, which usually is no more than three-fourths of the space), the container should be discarded according to established policies for disposition of contaminated items and sharps.

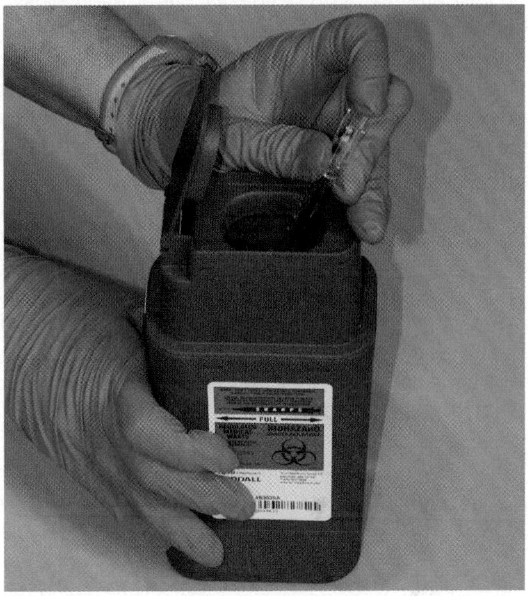

FIGURE 14-48 Disposal of a needle in a sharps container.

Summary

- Systems for measuring drug dosage include the metric system and the common household system. Each system deals with units of mass and volume, and each may be used by a physician when ordering drugs.
- Paramedics should choose a drug calculation method that is precise and reliable. When performing such calculations, paramedics should:
  1. Convert all units of measure to the same size and system.
  2. Assess the computed dosage to determine whether it is reasonable.
  3. Use one method of dose calculation consistently.
- Many drug calculations can be performed almost intuitively. Nevertheless, paramedics should never rely on intuitive calculations. Methods of calculation include the basic formula ("desire over have"), ratios and proportions, and dimensional analysis.
- Intravenous flow rates can be calculated using the following formula:

$$\text{Drops/min} = \frac{\text{Volume to be infused} \times \text{Drops/mL of infusion set}}{\text{Total time of infustion (min)}}$$

- Safety procedures should be a high priority during the administration of any medication. The paramedic must ensure the five rights of medication administration: The *right* patient must receive the *right* dose of the *right* drug via the *right* route at the *right* time and should always confirm these points out loud.
- If a medication error occurs, paramedics should take responsibility for their actions. They should quickly advise medical direction of the error and should assess and monitor the patient for effects of the drug. They must also document the error as required by local, state, and medical direction policies. Finally, they must change their personal practice to prevent similar errors from happening in the future.
- Medical asepsis is accomplished by using clean technique, which involves hygienic measures, cleaning agents, antiseptics, disinfectants, and barrier fields.
- Enteral drugs are administered and absorbed through the gastrointestinal tract. They are given by the oral, gastric, and rectal routes.
- Parenteral drugs are administered outside the intestine and are usually injected. They are given by the intradermal, subcutaneous, intramuscular, intravenous, and intraosseous routes.
- In the prehospital setting, the route of choice for fluid replacement is through a peripheral vein in an extremity. The over-the-needle catheter generally is preferred in this setting.
- Possible complications associated with intravenous (IV) drug administration techniques include local complications, systemic complications, infiltration, and air embolism.

- Fluids and drugs that are infused by the intraosseous (IO) route pass from the marrow cavities into the sinusoids, then into large venous channels and emissary veins, and finally into the systemic circulation.
- A commonly employed site of choice for IO infusions in children and adults is the tibia, one to two fingerbreadths below the tubercle on the anteromedial surface. Other sites for IO infusions include the distal tibia, humerus, and sternum (adults).
- Some drugs are readily absorbed through the mucous membranes (transmucosal administration) or skin (transdermal administration). Medications administered by the transmucosal route include sublingual drugs, buccal drugs, and nasal drugs; those administered by the intradermal route include topical drugs and drugs for the eye and ear.
- In addition to oxygen and nitrous oxide, several other drugs are administered by means of inhalation, including bronchodilators, corticosteroids, antibiotics, and mucokinetic agents delivered through aerosolization. These medications may be provided by means of a metered-dose inhaler or a handheld nebulizer.
- The endotracheal route may be used when IV or IO access cannot be established and other routes are not appropriate for the situation, although this route is the least reliable in terms of systemic absorption and efficacy. Medications sometimes administered by this route include naloxone, atropine, vasopressin, epinephrine, and lidocaine
- Administering drugs to infants and children can be quite difficult, especially in emergency situations. The younger and smaller the child, the smaller the margin for error when giving medications.
- If possible, venous blood samples should be obtained when IV access is established and before any fluids are infused. If no IV line is to be used and a blood sample is still needed, it must be obtained with a needle and syringe (or a special vacuum needle and sleeve).
- The Centers for Disease Control and Prevention recommends that needles not be capped, bent, or broken before disposal. Rather, they should be left on the syringe and discarded in an appropriate, clearly marked container that is puncture- and leakproof.

References

1. Moseley R. *Everything You Always Wanted to Know About Metrics But Didn't Know Who to Ask*. Valdese, NC: R&R Enterprises; 1978.
2. Thomson A, Taylor B. *Guide for the Use of the International System of Units (SI)*. NIST Special Publication 811. Gaithersburg, MD: National Institute of Standards and Technology, US Department of Commerce; 2008.
3. Hoyle JD Jr, Crowe RP, Bentley MA, Beltran G, Fales W. Pediatric prehospital medication dosing errors: a national survey of paramedics. *Prehosp Emerg Care*. 2017;21(2):185-191.
4. Misasi P, Keebler J, Braithwaite S. Paramedics believe verbal verification with a team mate reduces medication errors more than mental verification alone. *Ann Emerg Med*. 2013;62(4):S47-S48.
5. Institute of Medicine. *Preventing Medication Errors*. Washington, DC: National Academies Press; 2007.
6. Centers for Disease Control and Prevention. Handwashing: clean hands save lives. Centers for Disease Control and Prevention website. https://www.cdc.gov/handwashing/index.html. Updated December 8, 2017. Accessed January 12, 2018.
7. Institute for Safe Medication Practices. ISMP safe practice guidelines for adult IV push medications. Institute for Safe Medication Practices website. http://www.ismp.org/Tools/guidelines/ivsummitpush/ivpushmedguidelines.pdf. Published 2015. Accessed January 12, 2018.
8. Hadaway L. Short peripheral intravenous catheters and infections. *J Infusion Nurs*. 2012;35(4):230-240.
9. McCarthy CJ, Behravesh S, Naidu S, Oklu R. Air embolism: practical tips for prevention and treatment. *J Clin Med*. 2016;5(93).
10. Weiser G, Hoffmann Y, Galbraith R, Shavit I. Current advances in intraosseous infusion: a systematic review. *Resuscitation*. 2012;83:20-26.
11. Mitra AK, Kwatra D, Vadlapudi AD. *Drug Delivery*. Burlington, MA: Jones & Bartlett Learning; 2015.
12. Teleflex. MAD Nasal: intranasal mucosal atomization device. Teleflex website. http://www.lmaco.com/sites/default/files/940699-000001_MADNasal_UsageGuide_Sheet_1605_V2.pdf. Published 2016. Accessed January 12, 2018.

Suggested Readings

Brown M, Mulholland J. *Drug Calculations: Ratio and Proportion Problems for Clinical Practice*. 10th ed. St. Louis, MO: Mosby/Elsevier; 2016.

McKenna KD. The top 10 things you need to know to reduce medication errors. EMS Reference website. https://www.emsreference.com/articles/article/top-10-things-you-need-know-reduce-medication-errors. Updated November 27, 2015. Accessed January 12, 2018.

Plumlee R. EMS develops process to reduce medication errors. *Wichita Eagle* website. http://www.kansas.com/news/article1114743.html. Updated May 5, 2013. Accessed January 12, 2018.

Airway

PART

4

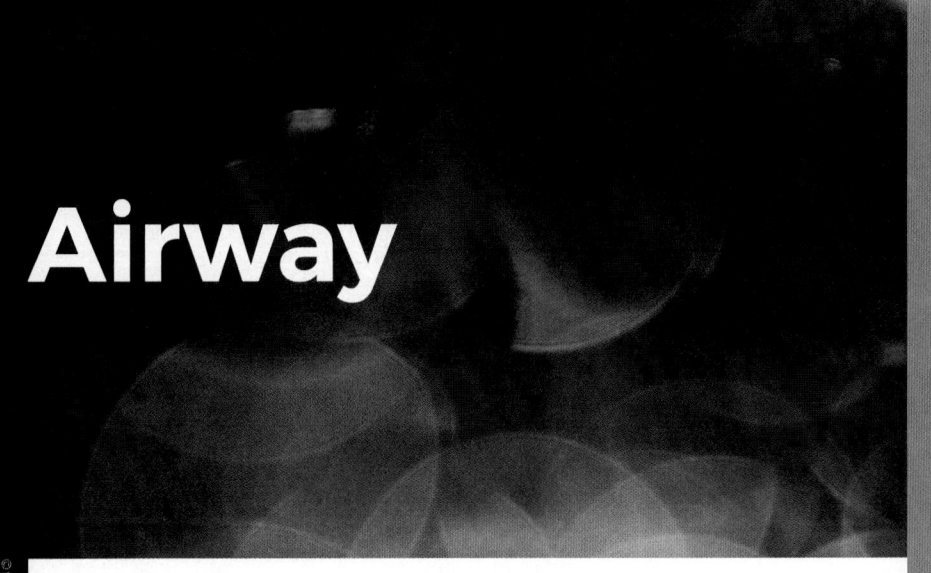

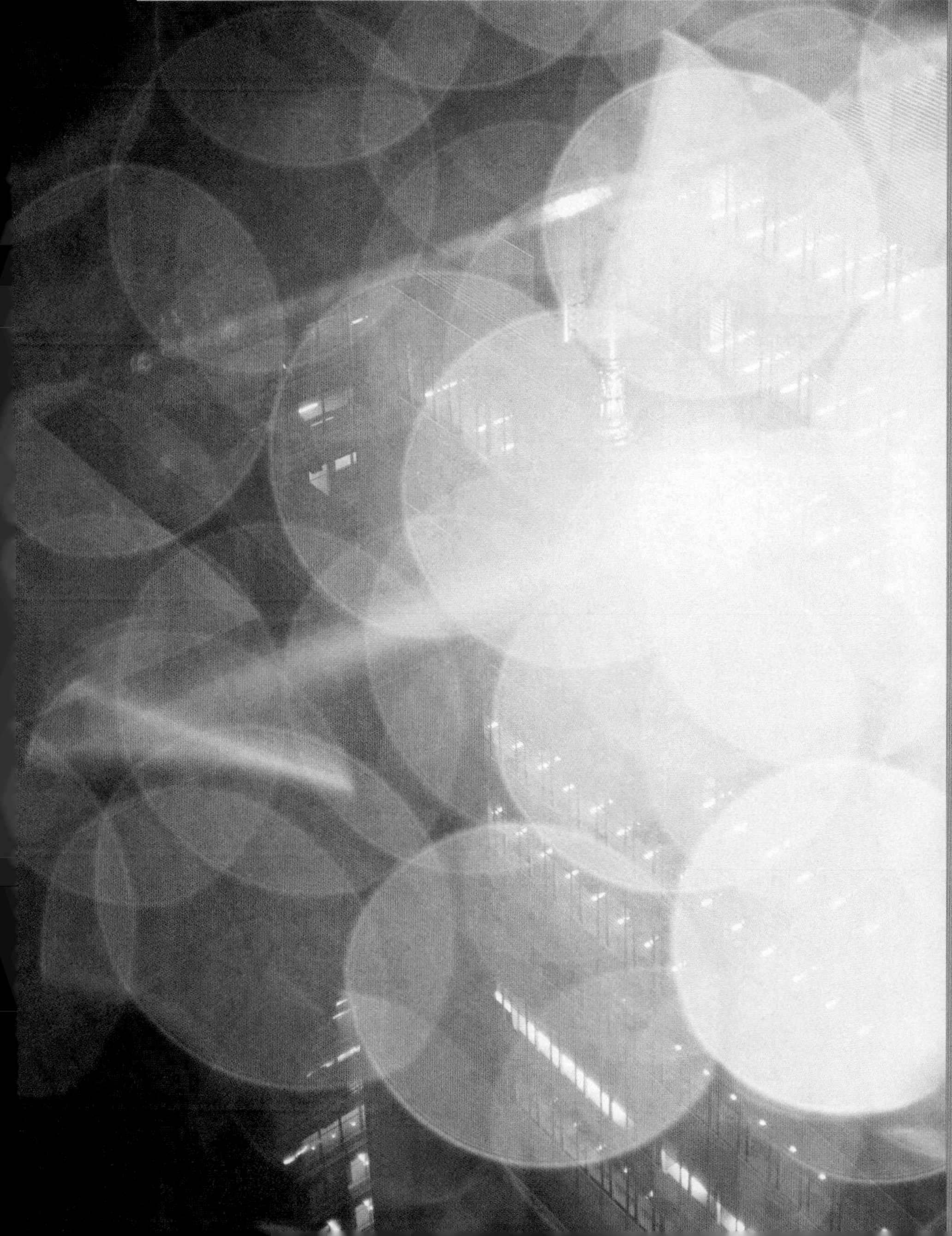

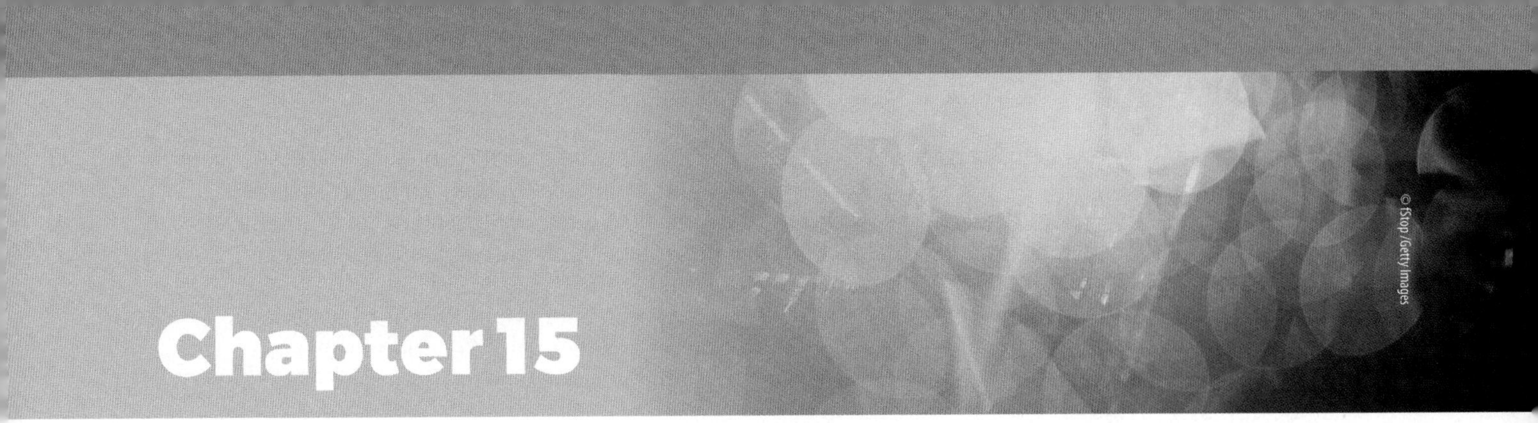

Chapter 15

Airway Management, Respiration, and Artificial Ventilation

NATIONAL EMS EDUCATION STANDARD COMPETENCIES

Airway Management, Respiration, and Artificial Ventilation

Integrates complex knowledge of anatomy, physiology, and pathophysiology into the assessment to develop and implement a treatment plan with the goal of ensuring a patent airway, adequate mechanical ventilation, and respiration for patients of all ages.

Airway Management

- Airway anatomy (pp 476–481)
- Airway assessment (pp 481–488, 508–511)
- Techniques of ensuring a patent airway (pp 526–527, 532–537)

Respiration

- Anatomy of the respiratory system (pp 476–481)
- Physiology and pathophysiology of respiration (pp 481–488)
  - Pulmonary ventilation (pp 481–483)
  - Oxygenation (pp 492–495, 497)
  - Respiration (pp 497–502)
    - External (p 481)
    - Internal (p 481)
    - Cellular (p 481)
- Assessment and management of adequate and inadequate respiration (pp 510–511, 516–573)
- Supplemental oxygen therapy (pp 510–516)

Artificial Ventilation

Assessment and management of adequate and inadequate ventilation

- Artificial ventilation (pp 519–526)
- Minute ventilation (p 488)
- Alveolar ventilation (pp 488, 496)
- Effect of artificial ventilation on cardiac output (pp 494–495, 519, 526)

OBJECTIVES

Upon completion of this chapter, the paramedic student will be able to:

1. Describe the anatomy of the airway and respiratory structures. (pp 476–481)
2. Distinguish between respiration, pulmonary ventilation, and external and internal respiration. (p 481)
3. Explain the mechanics of ventilation and respiration. (pp 481–488)
4. Explain how partial pressures of gases in the blood and lungs relate to atmospheric gas pressures. (pp 488–489)
5. Describe pulmonary circulation. (pp 489–497)
6. Explain the process of exchange and transport of gases in the body. (pp 489–495)
7. Describe voluntary, nervous, and chemical regulation of respiration. (pp 498–502)
8. Discuss the assessment and management of airway obstruction. (pp 503, 505–507)
9. Explain variations in the assessment and management of airway and ventilation problems in pediatric patients. (pp 505–506, 521, 524–525, 534, 538–539, 553–554, 561–562, 567, 568, 572)
10. Describe risk factors and preventive measures for pulmonary aspiration. (pp 507–508)

11. Outline the assessment of airway and breathing. (pp 508–511)
12. Describe the indications, contraindications, and techniques for delivering supplemental oxygen. (pp 510–516)
13. Discuss the methods of patient ventilation based on the indications, contraindications, potential complications, and use of each method. (pp 516–525)
14. Describe the use of manual airway maneuvers and mechanical airway adjuncts based on the indications, contraindications, potential complications, and techniques for each. (pp 526–527, 532–537)
15. Describe effective techniques for verifying proper placement of endotracheal and peritracheal airway devices. (pp 547, 555–560)

KEY TERMS

accessory muscles Muscles that sometimes assist in breathing. They include the scalene muscles and the sternocleidomastoid, deep muscles of the neck and thorax, posterior neck and back muscles, pectoralis major, pectoralis minor, and abdominal muscles.

alveoli Minute air sacs in the lungs through which gas exchange takes place between alveolar air and pulmonary capillary blood.

anatomic dead space The volume of the conducting airways from the external environment down to the terminal bronchioles.

apneustic center A group of neurons in the pons that has a stimulatory effect on the inspiratory center.

atelectasis An abnormal condition characterized by the collapse of lung tissue. It prevents respiratory exchange of oxygen and carbon dioxide.

atmospheric pressure The pressure of the gas around us, which varies with differences in altitude. At sea level, it is 760 mm Hg.

bilevel positive airway pressure (BPAP) Airway support that combines partial ventilatory support and continuous positive airway pressure. It allows the pressure to vary during each breath cycle.

Bohr effect The property of hemoglobin by which an increasing concentration of protons and/or carbon dioxide reduces the oxygen affinity for hemoglobin.

Boyle's law A gas law that states pressure and volume are inversely related, assuming a constant temperature.

capnography The combination of a capnometric reading (numeric value) and a capnogram (graph/drawing).

carina A downward and backward projection of the lowest tracheal cartilage. It forms a ridge between the openings of the right and left primary bronchi.

compliance The ease with which the lungs and thorax expand during pressure changes. The greater the compliance, the easier the expansion.

continuous positive airway pressure (CPAP) Airway support that transmits positive pressure into the airways of a spontaneously breathing patient throughout the respiratory cycle at a constant pressure.

Dalton's law A law stating that the total pressure exerted by a mixture of gases is equal to the sum of the partial pressure of gases.

diaphragm The dome-shaped, musculofibrous partition that separates the thoracic and abdominal cavities.

diffusion The process by which solid, particulate matter in a fluid moves from an area of higher concentration to an area of lower concentration, resulting in an even distribution of the particles in the fluid.

expiration Breathing out (exhalation); normally a passive process.

expiratory reserve volume The amount of gas that can be forcefully exhaled after expiration of the normal tidal volume.

external respiration The transfer (diffusion) of oxygen and carbon dioxide between the inspired air and pulmonary capillaries.

extubation Removal of an endotracheal tube.

Fick principle The assumption that the amount of oxygen delivered to an organ is equal to the amount of oxygen consumed by that organ plus the amount of oxygen carried away from that organ. This principle is used to determine cardiac output.

gag reflex A normal neural response triggered by touching the soft palate or posterior pharynx.

Henry's law A law stating that at a constant temperature, the amount of gas that dissolves in a liquid is directly proportional to the partial pressure of that gas in equilibrium with that liquid.

Hering-Breuer reflex A reflex in which afferent impulses from stretch receptors in the lungs arrest inspiration. Expiration then occurs. Inflation and deflation reflexes are triggered to prevent overinflation of the lungs.

hypocapnia A state of diminished carbon dioxide in the blood; also called hypocarbia.

hypoxemia A lower than normal oxygen content of the blood as measured in an arterial blood sample.

hypoxia A state of decreased oxygen content at the tissue level.

hypoxic drive The low arterial oxygen pressure stimulus to respiration that is mediated through the carotid bodies.

inadvertent hyperventilation Excessive ventilation that is thought to result in increased intrathoracic pressure and decreased coronary perfusion pressure; also known as rescuer hyperventilation.

inspiration The act of drawing air into the lungs.

inspiratory reserve volume The maximum volume of air that can be inspired after inspiration of tidal volume.

intercostal muscles Internal and external muscles between the ribs that contract to raise the ribs, thereby increasing the front-to-back (anterior–posterior) and side-to-side dimensions of the chest cavity.

internal respiration The transfer (diffusion) of oxygen and carbon dioxide between the capillary red blood cells and the tissue cells.

intrapulmonic pressure The pressure of the gas in the alveoli.

intrathoracic pressure The pressure in the pleural space; also known as the intrapleural pressure.

left main stem bronchus One of two main bronchi that branch from the trachea at the level of the carina.

lobules Small lobes or subdivisions of a lobe.

lower airway Airway structures below the glottis.

mediastinum The area of the body that includes the trachea, esophagus, thymus, heart, and great vessels.

minute volume The amount of gas inhaled or exhaled in 1 minute. It is found by multiplying the tidal volume by the respiratory rate.

oxyhemoglobin Oxygenated hemoglobin.

partial pressure The pressure exerted by a single gas.

phrenic nerve A nerve composed mostly of motor nerve fibers that produce contractions of the diaphragm; also provides sensory innervation for many components of the mediastinum and pleura.

physiologic dead space The sum of the anatomic dead space plus the volume of any nonfunctional alveoli.

pneumotaxic center A group of neurons in the pons that have an inhibitory effect on the inspiratory center.

positive end-expiratory pressure (PEEP) Airway support that maintains a degree of positive pressure at the end of exhalation.

pressure gradient The force produced by differences between atmospheric pressure, intrapulmonic pressure, and intrathoracic pressure.

pressure support A spontaneous mode of ventilation in which a ventilator delivers support with the preset pressure value for the patient's own respiratory rate.

pulmonary surfactant Certain lipoproteins that reduce the surface tension of pulmonary fluids, allowing the exchange of gases in the alveoli of the lungs and contributing to the elasticity of pulmonary tissue.

pulmonary ventilation The movement of air into and out of the lungs. This process brings oxygen into the lungs and removes carbon dioxide.

pulsus paradoxus An abnormal decrease in systolic blood pressure in which it drops more than 10 to 15 mm Hg during inspiration compared with expiration.

rapid sequence induction (RSI) The administration of a potent sedative or induction agent and a neuromuscular blocking agent at the same time to achieve optimal intubation conditions in less than 1 minute.

residual volume The volume of air remaining in the lungs after a maximum expiratory effort.

respiration The process of molecular exchange of oxygen and carbon dioxide in the body's tissues.

respiratory membrane The membrane in the lungs, formed by the wall of an alveolus and the wall of a capillary, across which gas exchange with the blood occurs.

right main stem bronchus One of two main bronchi that branch from the trachea at the level of the carina.

secondary bronchi Branches from a primary bronchus that conduct air to each lobe of the lungs.

sternal angle The point at which the manubrium joins the body of the sternum; also known as the angle of Louis.

surfactant Lipoproteins that reduce the surface tension of pulmonary fluids.

terminal bronchioles The ends of the conducting airways.

tidal volume The volume of air inspired or expired in a single, resting breath.

torr A non–Système International unit of pressure defined as 1 standard atmosphere divided by 760, or about 1 mm Hg.

total pressure The combination of pressures exerted by all the gases in any mixture of gas.

upper airway Airway structures above the glottis.

vallecula A furrow between the glossoepiglottic folds on each side of the posterior oropharynx.

ventilation The mechanical movement of air into and out of the lungs that makes respiration possible.

ventilation/perfusion mismatch Any condition leading to interference of airflow at the alveolar level or blood flow at the pulmonary capillary level.

vocal cords The two folds of elastic ligaments covered by mucous membrane that stretch from the thyroid cartilage to the arytenoid cartilage. Vibration of the vocal cords is responsible for voice production. Also known as the true vocal cords.

An inadequate airway coupled with ineffective ventilation is a major cause of preventable death and cardiopulmonary complications in both medical and trauma patients. A thorough understanding of the respiratory system and mastery of airway management and ventilation are essential aspects of prehospital emergency care.

The Airway: Anatomy

Successful management of the airway requires an understanding of the upper and lower airway structures and functions. For the purpose of this text, all airway structures above the glottis are considered the **upper airway**. All structures below the glottis are considered the **lower airway** (**BOX 15-1** and **FIGURE 15-1**). Airway anatomy is presented in Chapter 10, *Review of Human Systems*; the following discussion serves as a review.

Upper Airway

The human airway has two openings, the nose and the mouth. Air passes through the nose into the nasopharynx. This is the superior part of the pharynx. Air passes through the mouth into the oropharynx. The nasopharynx ends and the oropharynx begins at the level of the uvula. The oropharynx extends to the level of the epiglottis. The laryngopharynx (also known as the hypopharynx) extends from the tip of the epiglottis to the glottis and esophagus. The laryngopharynx opens into the larynx, which lies in the anterior neck (**FIGURE 15-2**).

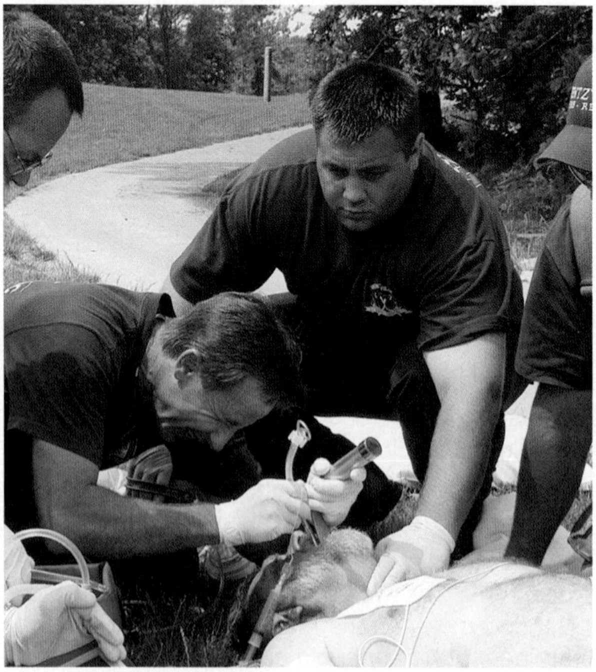

Courtesy of Ray Kemp, St. Charles, MO.

BOX 15-1 Structures of the Upper and Lower Airways

Upper Airway Structures

Nasopharynx
Frontal, maxillary, ethmoid, sphenoid sinuses
Oropharynx
Laryngopharynx
Larynx

Lower Airway Structures

Trachea
Bronchial tree
Alveoli
Lungs

NOTE

An important anatomic landmark in the laryngopharynx is the vallecula. The **vallecula** is a depression just behind the root of the tongue and between the folds of the throat and epiglottis. This area identifies where the curved blade of the laryngoscope is placed during endotracheal (ET) intubation to facilitate direct visualization of the glottis. (ET intubation is described later in this section.)

When visualizing a patient's airway, remember that the floor of the nose is the roof of the mouth.

The larynx consists of an outer casing of nine cartilages. These cartilages are connected to each other by muscles and ligaments. Six of the nine cartilages

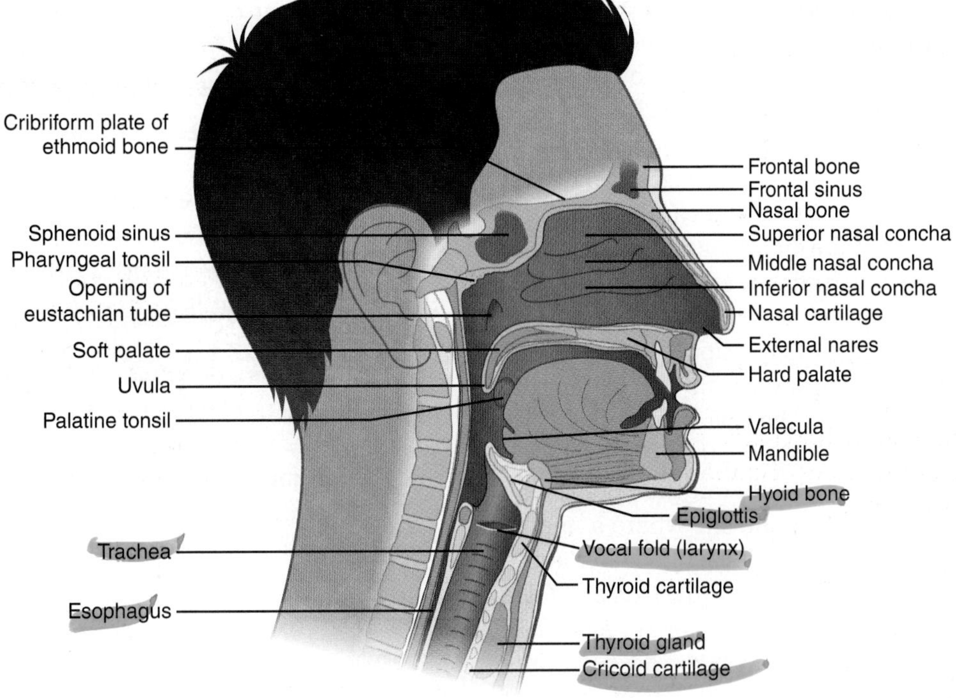

FIGURE 15-1 Midsagittal section through the upper airway.

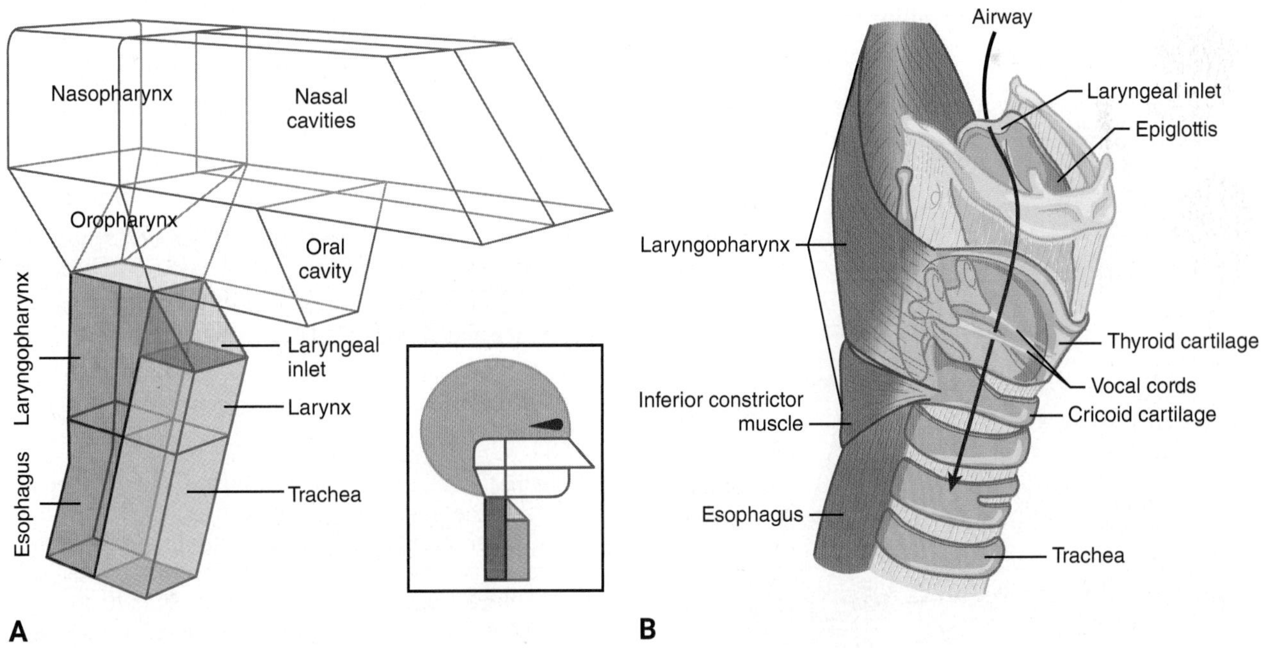

FIGURE 15-2 Specialized structures of the neck. **A.** Conceptual view. **B.** Anatomic view.

are paired; three are unpaired. The unpaired thyroid cartilage is the largest, most superior of the cartilages. This structure is also known as the Adam's apple. The most inferior cartilage of the larynx is the unpaired cricoid cartilage. This cartilage is the only complete cartilage ring in the larynx. The third unpaired cartilage is the epiglottis. The six paired cartilages are stacked in two pillars between the cricoid cartilage and the thyroid cartilage. They are the arytenoid cartilages, the corniculate cartilages, and the cuneiform cartilages. The U-shaped hyoid bone is located beneath the mandible. The hyoid bone helps support the airway by anchoring muscles to the jaw. The thyroid membrane joins the hyoid bone and the thyroid cartilage. The fibrinous membrane between the thyroid and cricoid cartilage is known as the cricothyroid membrane. The cricothyroid membrane is the site where a needle cricothyrotomy is performed (described later in the chapter). The larynx also contains the true and false vocal cords. As described in Chapter 10, *Review of Human Systems*, the **vocal cords** regulate the flow of air to and from the lungs for the production of voice sounds (**FIGURE 15-3**). The ET tube is passed through the open vocal cords of the larynx during ET intubation. The larynx extends from the lower part of the pharynx to the trachea. On either side of the larynx is a recess called the piriform sinus. Foreign materials that are swallowed may become lodged in these areas.

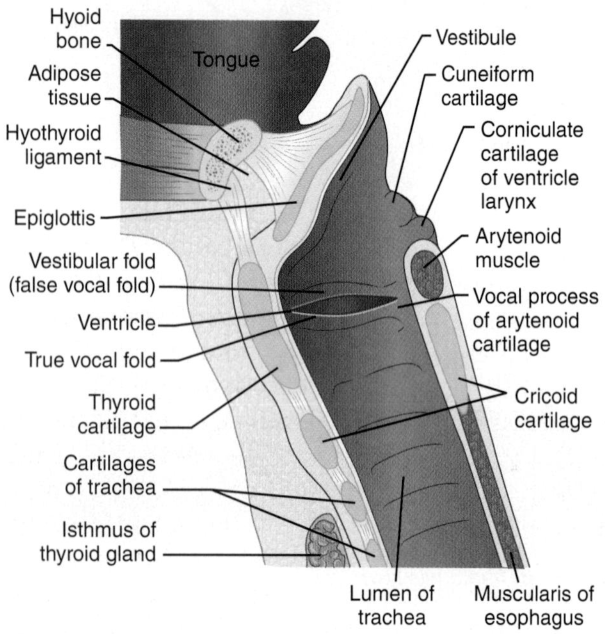

FIGURE 15-3 Vocal cords.

Lower Airway

The trachea lies anterior to the esophagus. It is the air passage from the larynx to the lungs. The trachea begins at the border of the cricoid cartilage and ends where it bifurcates into the right and left main bronchi; this bifurcation is at the level of the **sternal angle**. The trachea is composed of 16 to 20 incomplete cartilaginous rings. These rings open posteriorly to allow slight collapse so food can pass easily through the esophagus that is located just posterior to the trachea.

The **carina** is a downward and backward projection of the last tracheal cartilage. It forms a ridge that separates the opening of the **right main stem bronchus** and the **left main stem bronchus**. The carina occurs between the division of the two main stem bronchi at the sternal angle (also known as the angle of Louis).

> NOTE
> The right main bronchus is wider, shorter, and more vertical than the left one is. As such, the right main bronchus is the more common site of foreign body obstruction. It is also the more common site of main stem bronchus intubation when the ET tube is inadvertently inserted too far.

The right and left main bronchi pass from the bifurcation of the trachea to the lungs to form the bronchial tree. The right and left main bronchi further branch into **secondary bronchi**. They divide again into tertiary segmental bronchi and finally **terminal bronchioles**. The terminal bronchioles are the smallest airways without alveoli. The terminal bronchioles divide into respiratory bronchioles and then alveolar ducts (**FIGURE 15-4**).

> NOTE
> Like the trachea, the bronchi are supported by cartilaginous rings. As the bronchi branch into smaller subdivisions, the amount of cartilage decreases and the bronchi become increasingly muscular. This decrease in cartilage continues until no cartilage is present. Bronchial smooth muscle has $beta_2$ adrenergic receptors. Therefore, the muscles are sensitive to certain hormones (eg, epinephrine). The muscles also are sensitive to $beta_2$ receptor drugs such as albuterol. Stimulation of the $beta_2$ adrenergic receptors causes the bronchial smooth muscles to relax, resulting in bronchodilation.

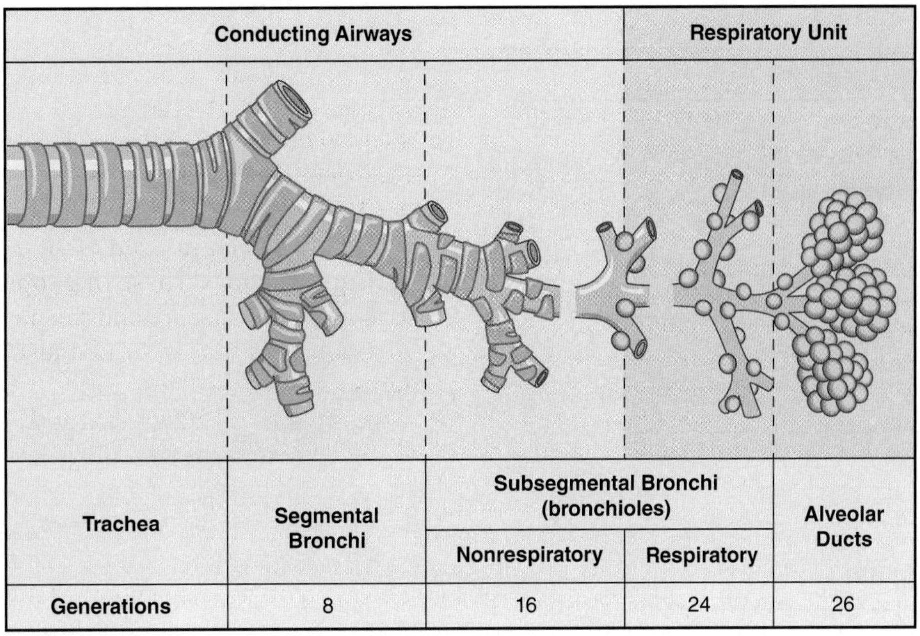

FIGURE 15-4 Structures of the lower airway.

The **alveoli** are the functional units of the respiratory system. They make up most of the lung tissue. The alveoli also are where most of the respiratory gas exchange takes place. Together the two lungs have about 300 million alveoli.[1] Each alveolus is surrounded by a fine network of blood capillaries. The capillaries are arranged so that air in the alveolus is separated from the blood by a thin **respiratory membrane**. The alveoli are coated with **pulmonary surfactant**. The surfactant is a thin film produced by the alveolar cells that prevents the alveoli from collapsing.

The lungs are large, paired, spongy organs that are attached to the heart by pulmonary arteries and veins. The two lungs are separated by the **mediastinum**. The contents of the mediastinum include the heart, blood vessels, trachea, esophagus, lymphatic tissue, and lymphatic vessels. Each lung is shaped like a cone, with its base resting on the diaphragm. The left lung is smaller than the right and is divided into two lobes. The right lung has three lobes. Each lobe is divided into **lobules**. The left lung has 9 lobules, and the right lung has 10 lobules. Both lungs are surrounded by a separate pleural cavity. The two layers of pleura are visceral (inner layer) and parietal (outer layer). They are separated by serous fluid that acts as a lubricant to allow the pleural membranes to slide past each other during breathing. The primary function of the lungs is **respiration** (the exchange of oxygen and carbon dioxide between an organism and the environment) (**FIGURE 15-5**).

NOTE

Respiration should not be confused with ventilation. **Ventilation** is the mechanical movement of air into and out of the lungs. Ventilation makes respiration possible.

Support Structures of the Airway

The support structures of the airway include the thoracic cage, the phrenic nerve, and the mediastinum.

As described in Chapter 10, *Review of Human Systems*, the thoracic cage protects vital organs. It also prevents collapse of the thorax during ventilation. The thoracic cage consists of the thoracic vertebrae, ribs and their associated costal cartilages, and the sternum (**FIGURE 15-6**). Muscles involved in ventilation include the **intercostal muscles** and the **diaphragm**. The intercostal muscles and **accessory muscles** (described later in this chapter) are used only during exercise, exertion, or distress. They are not used during quiet breathing. The diaphragm is the most important muscle for ventilation. When the diaphragm contracts, the abdominal contents are pushed downward and

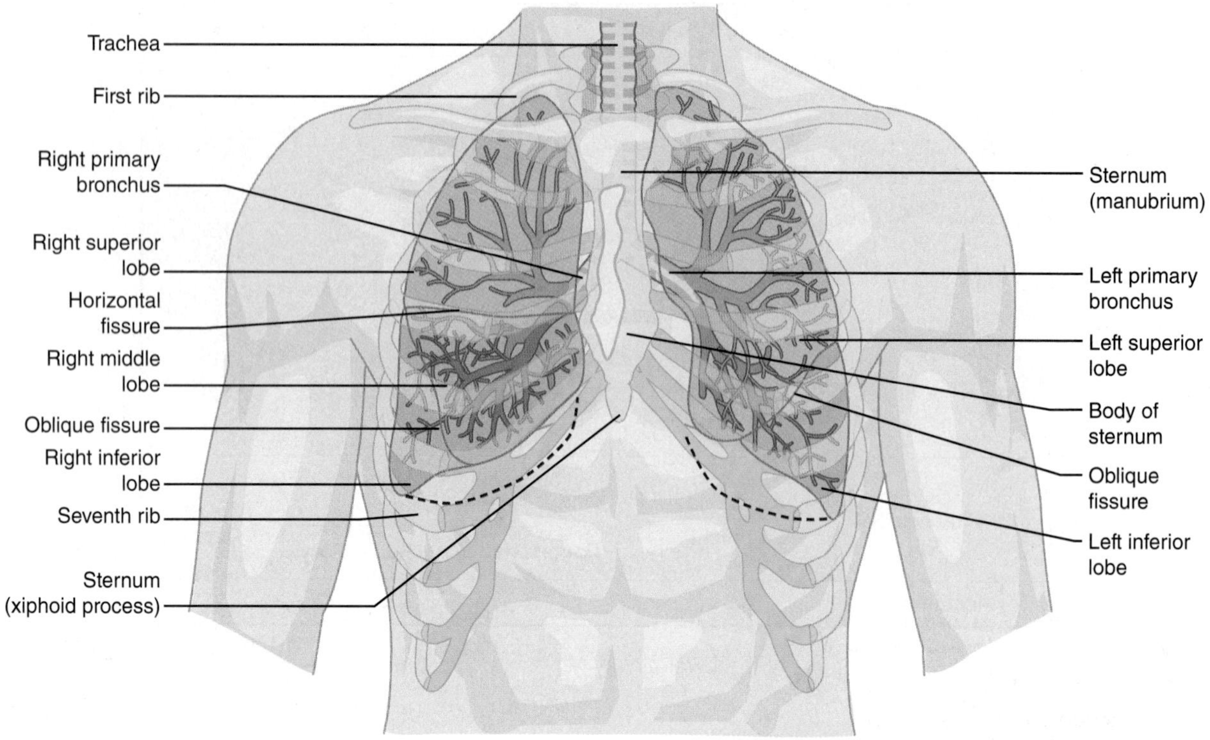

FIGURE 15-5 Lungs. The trachea is an airway that branches to form an inverted tree of bronchi and bronchioles. Note that the right lung has three lobes and the left lung has two lobes. Fissures are boundaries between the lobes.

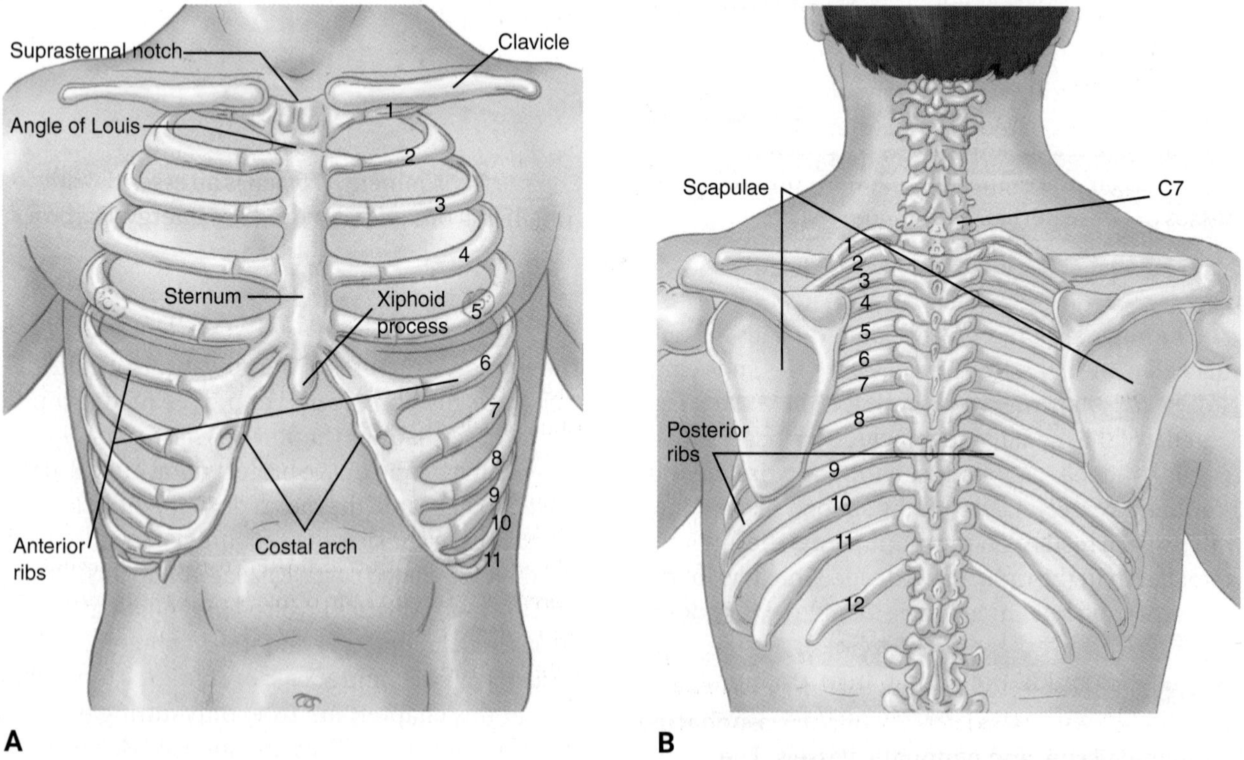

FIGURE 15-6 Thorax and underlying structures. **A.** Anterior view. **B.** Posterior view.

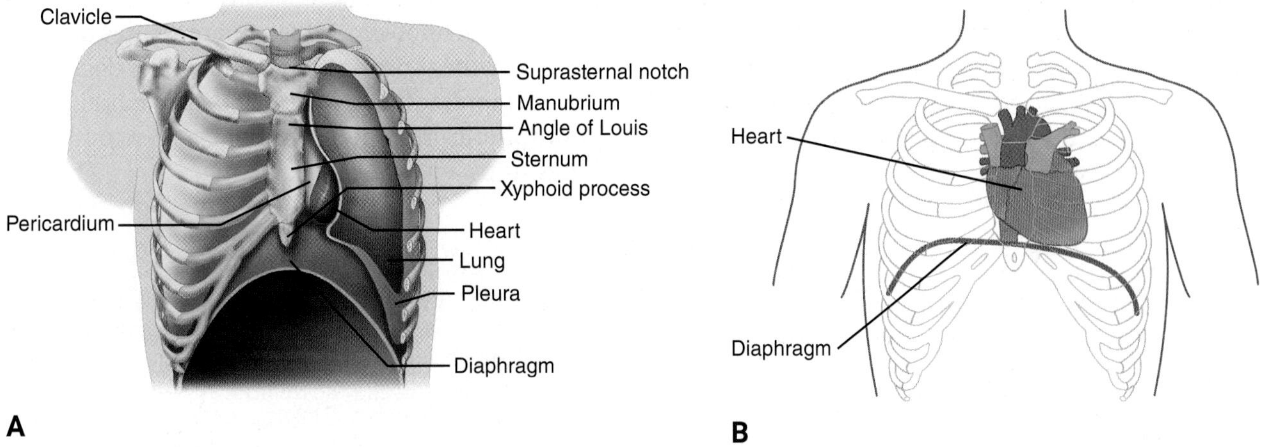

FIGURE 15-7 **A.** Anterior (frontal) view of the mediastinum. **B.** The position of the heart.

the intercostal muscles move the ribs upward and outward. This movement increases the volume and decreases the pressure in the thoracic cavity.

The **phrenic nerve** is composed mostly of motor nerve fibers. These motor nerve fibers produce contractions of the diaphragm. The phrenic nerve also provides sensory innervation for many components of the mediastinum and pleura; further, it provides sensory innervation for the upper abdomen, especially the liver, and the gallbladder. The right phrenic nerve passes over the brachiocephalic artery and right atrium, and then crosses the root of the right lung anteriorly. It leaves the thorax by passing through an opening in the diaphragm. The left phrenic nerve passes over the pericardium of the left ventricle and enters the diaphragm separately.

> NOTE
>
> The phrenic nerve originates from the spinal cord between C3 and C5. Injury to the spinal cord at the C3 level or above eliminates phrenic nerve function of all of the intercostal muscles in the chest wall, which makes it impossible for the patient to initiate contraction of the diaphragm or the chest wall. Because these two functions are essential in allowing inspiration and therefore ventilation to occur, a patient with this injury will not able to breathe on his or her own (see Chapter 41, *Chest Trauma*).

As stated earlier, the contents of the mediastinum include the heart, blood vessels, trachea, esophagus, lymphatic tissue, and lymphatic vessels. The mediastinum is the central compartment of the thoracic cavity and therefore is a supporting structure of the respiratory system. It lies between the right and left pleura in and near the median sagittal plane of the chest. It extends from the sternum in front to the vertebral column behind. It is continuous with the loose connective tissue of the neck and extends inferiorly onto the diaphragm. The mediastinum contains all the thoracic viscera except the lungs (**FIGURE 15-7**).

Respiratory Physiology: Mechanics of Respiration

As described previously, respiration is the exchange of oxygen and carbon dioxide between an organism and the environment. Oxygen is an essential nutrient for a living organism to produce energy. Carbon dioxide is a by-product of energy production that must be removed from the body. For this gas exchange to occur, air must move freely into and out of the lungs. The mechanical process of bringing oxygen into the lungs and removing carbon dioxide is known as **pulmonary ventilation**.

The two phases of respiration are external respiration and internal respiration. **External respiration** is the transfer (diffusion) of oxygen and carbon dioxide between the inspired air and pulmonary capillaries. **Internal respiration** is the transfer (diffusion) of oxygen and carbon dioxide between the capillary red blood cells and the tissue cells.

Pressure Changes and Ventilation

Gas flows from an area of higher pressure or concentration to an area of lower pressure or concentration in a process known as **diffusion**. This means for gas to flow into the lungs, a **pressure gradient** is required. This pressure gradient is produced by differences between atmospheric pressure, intrapulmonic pressure, and intrathoracic pressure (also known as intrapleural pressure).

> CRITICAL THINKING
>
> Think of two medical conditions that could impair (1) external respiration and (2) internal respiration.

Atmospheric pressure is the pressure of the gas around us. It varies with differences in altitude. At sea level, it is 760 mm Hg. **Intrapulmonic pressure** is the pressure of the gas in the alveoli. Depending on the size of the thorax, this pressure varies a little above and below 760 mm Hg. The intrapulmonic pressure also depends on whether it is measured during inspiration or expiration. **Intrathoracic pressure** is the pressure in the pleural space. It normally is less than the atmospheric pressure (usually 751 to 754 mm Hg). However, it may exceed the atmospheric pressure during coughing or straining during bowel movements.

During **inspiration** the chest wall expands to increase the size of the thoracic cavity and expand the lungs. Increasing the size of the thoracic cavity decreases the pressure in the pleural space. This relationship is explained by **Boyle's law**, which states the pressure of a gas is inversely proportional to its volume. Therefore, the expansion of the thoracic cavity (resulting from muscle movement) decreases the pressure in the pleural space. As the thorax expands, the lung space increases because of the negative pressure created in the pleural space. This increases the size of the intrapulmonic space and causes a drop in the intrapulmonic pressure of about 1 mm Hg below the atmospheric pressure. The pressure gradient between the intrapulmonic space and atmosphere results in gas flowing into the lungs. At end inspiration, the thorax and alveoli stop expanding. The intrapulmonic pressure becomes equal to the atmospheric pressure, and gas no longer moves into the lungs (**FIGURE 15-8**).

As the chest wall relaxes during **expiration**, the muscles of ventilation are at rest. The process of inspiration reverses. Elastic recoil causes the thorax and lung space to decrease in size, which increases the intrapulmonic pressure about 1 mm Hg above the pressure in the atmosphere. The pressure gradient results in gas flow out of the lungs. At the end of expiration, the opposing forces and pressures become equal and the thoracic volume no longer decreases. The intrapulmonic pressure becomes equal to the atmospheric pressure, and gas movement out of the lungs stops (**FIGURE 15-9**).

> NOTE
>
> Boyle's law states that as the pressure of a gas decreases, its volume expands. Conversely, as the pressure of a gas increases, its volume decreases. (Pressure is inversely proportional to volume.) Simply put, during inspiration, when the diaphragm and intercostal muscles contract, the volume in the chest increases, negative pressure occurs, and air enters the lungs. This process is reversed during expiration.

Muscles of Ventilation

Expansion of the lungs and thorax is caused by the movement of the diaphragm and the internal and external intercostal muscles (**FIGURE 15-10**). On inspiration, the diaphragm contracts and the dome of the diaphragm flattens. This increases the superior–inferior dimension of the chest cavity. The internal and external intercostal muscles also contract, which raises the ribs and increases the front-to-back (anterior–posterior) and side-to-side dimensions of the chest cavity.

> CRITICAL THINKING
>
> How does interruption of the chest wall from a stab wound change the mechanics of breathing?

Expiration is usually a passive motion. During expiration, relaxation of the diaphragm and internal intercostal muscles allows the elastic recoil properties of the lungs to reduce the size (or volume) of the thoracic cavity (**FIGURE 15-11**). The ease with which the lungs and thorax expand during inspiration is known as **compliance**. The greater the compliance, the easier the expansion. Diseases that reduce compliance increase the energy required for breathing. Examples of such diseases are asthma, bronchitis, and pulmonary edema. Other diseases, such as emphysema, increase lung compliance by breaking down the elastic fibers that surround lung tissue. This breakdown may be the result of overstretching of the fibers from chronic coughing. These patients have no problem inflating

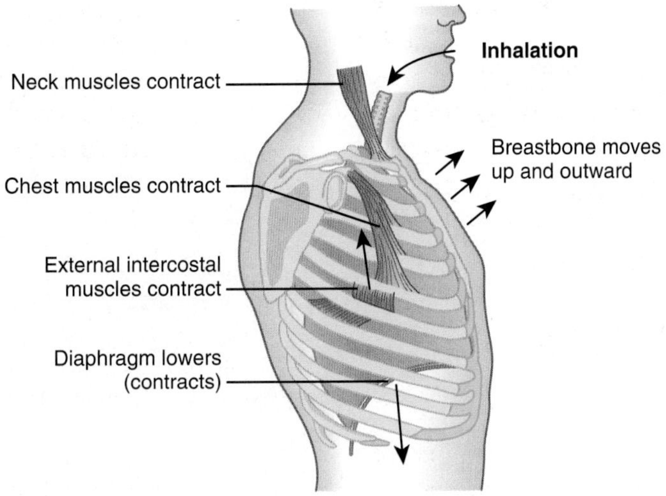

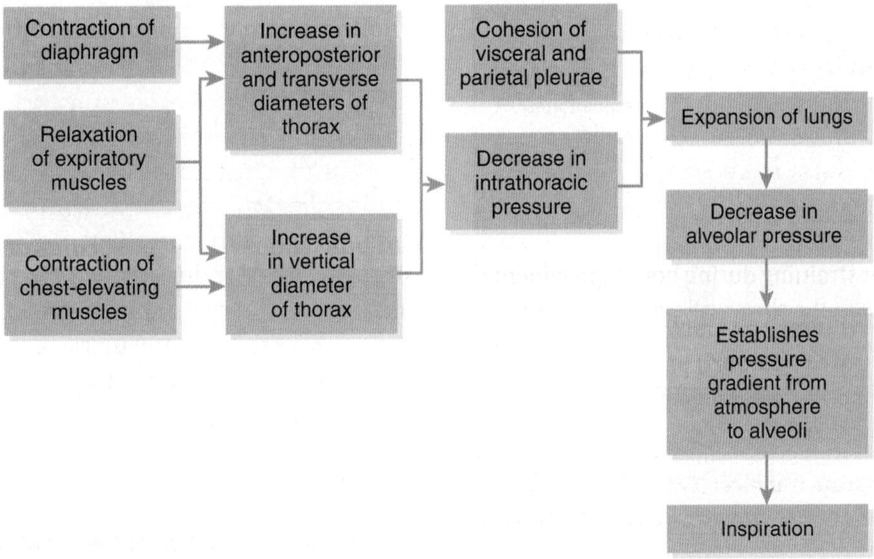

FIGURE 15-8 Mechanics of inspiration.

the lungs but have extreme difficulty exhaling air (see Chapter 23, *Respiratory*).

Work of Breathing

In people who are healthy, the energy needed for normal, quiet breathing is less than 5% of the total body expenditure.[2] Factors that increase the amount of energy needed for ventilation include loss of pulmonary surfactant (eg, from smoke inhalation), an increase in airway resistance (eg, from asthma), or a decrease in pulmonary compliance (eg, from cystic fibrosis). These factors can increase the energy requirement to as much as 30% of the total body expenditure.[3]

The pulmonary alveoli have a tendency to collapse. This is the result of recoil caused by the elastic fibers and the surface tension of the alveolar walls. The surface tension is created because water molecules are attracted to each other in the alveolar membrane. Pulmonary surfactant lowers the surface tension by intermingling with the water molecules to reduce the cohesive force. This action helps prevent collapse of the alveolus at the end of expiration.

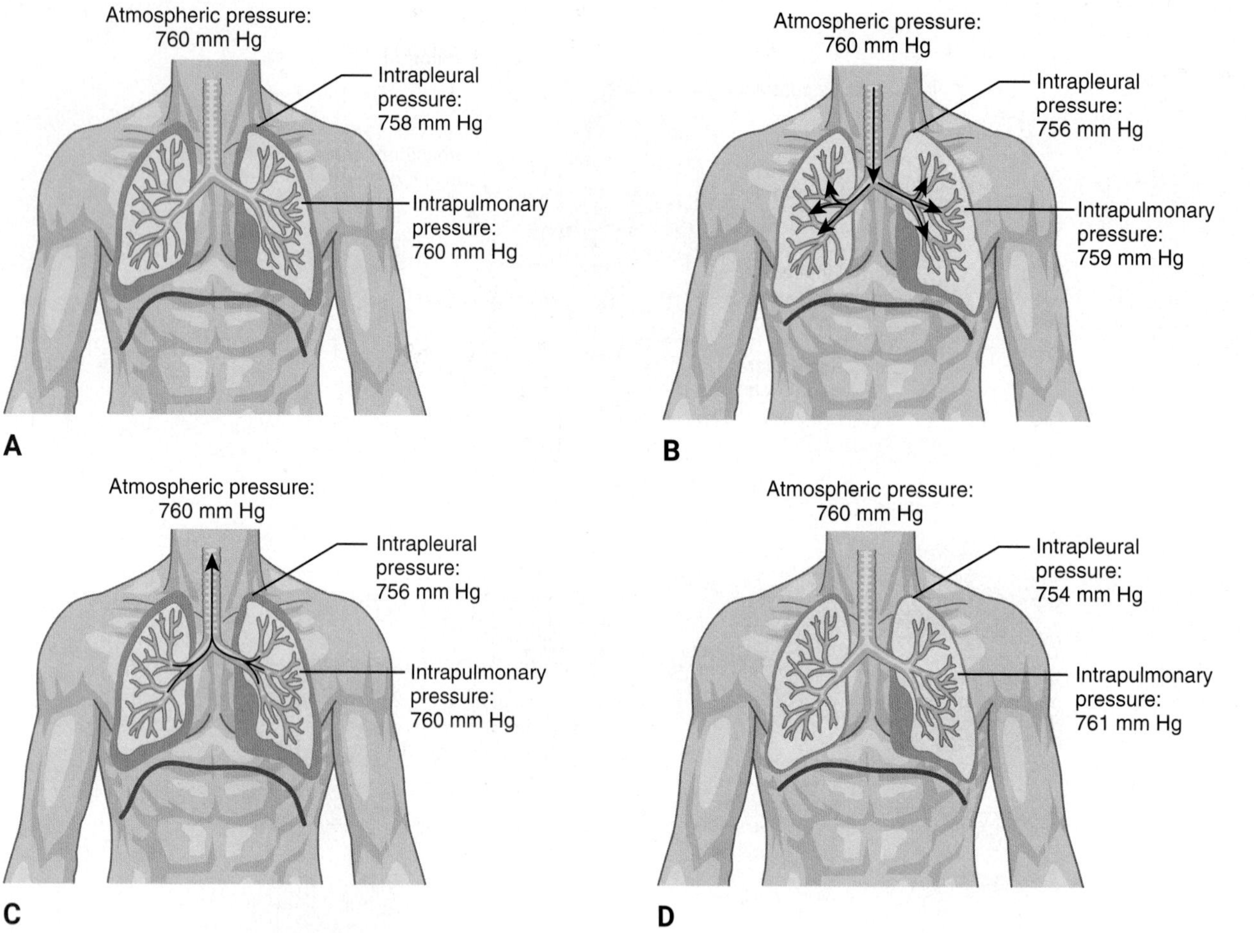

FIGURE 15-9 Pressure changes during inspiration and expiration. **A.** At the end of expiration, intrapulmonary pressure equals atmospheric pressure, and no movement of air occurs. **B.** During inspiration, the volume of the pleural space increases, causing the pressure in the intrapulmonary spaces (alveoli) to decrease. Air then flows from the outside of the body, where the pressure is greater (760 mm Hg), into the alveoli, where it is lower (759 mm Hg). **C.** At the end of inspiration, intrapulmonary pressure again equals atmospheric pressure, and no movement of air occurs. **D.** During expiration, the volume of the pleural spaces decreases, causing the intrapulmonary pressure to increase. Because the intrapulmonary pressure exceeds the atmospheric pressure, air flows out of the lungs.

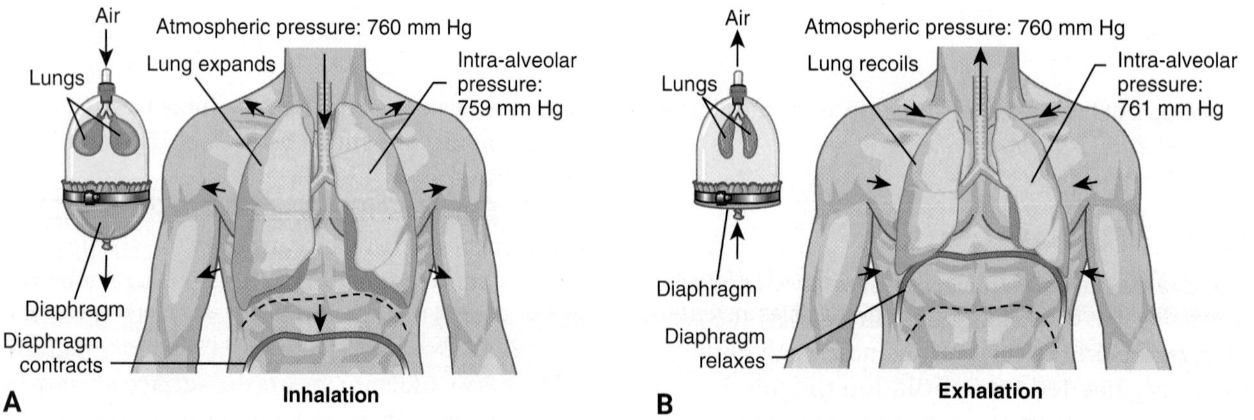

FIGURE 15-10 During inhalation, the diaphragm contracts, increasing the volume of the thoracic cavity. The increase in volume results in a decrease in pressure, which causes air to rush into the lungs. During expiration, the diaphragm returns to an upward position, reducing the volume of the thoracic cavity. Air pressure increases and forces air out of the lungs.

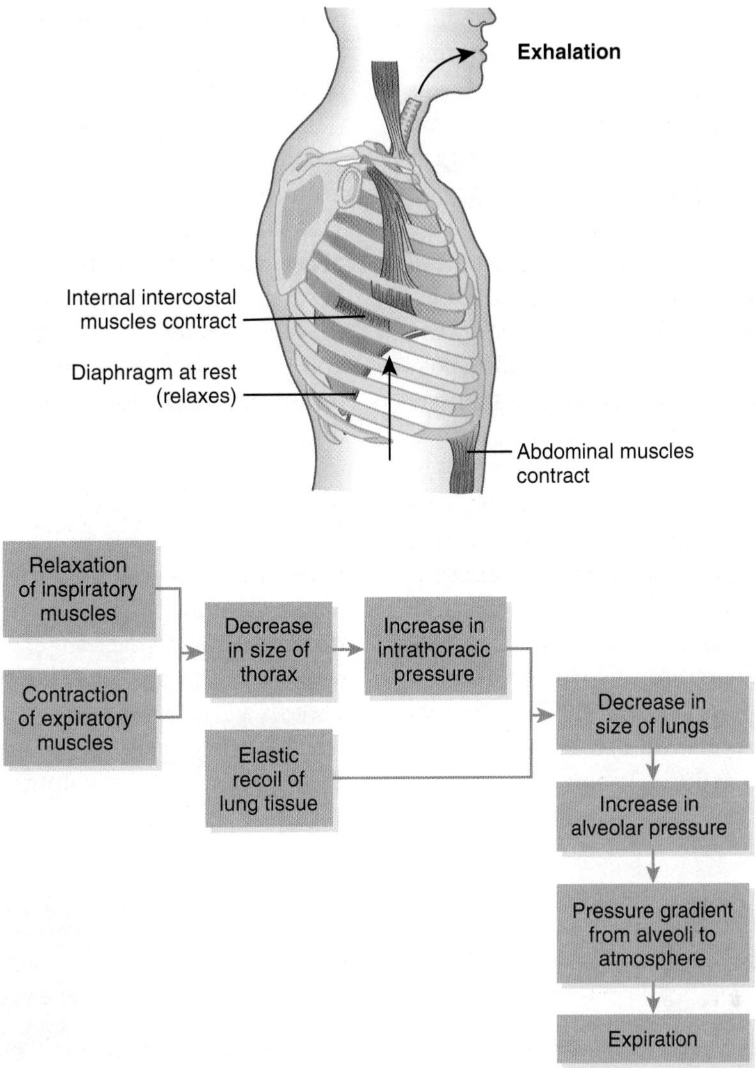

FIGURE 15-11 Relaxation of the diaphragm and contraction of the chest-depressing muscles (the internal intercostal muscles) reduce the thoracic volume. This reduced volume increases pressure in the lungs, pushing air out.

NOTE

Atelectasis is the collapse (diminished volume) of all or part of the lung. This condition can be caused by obstruction, such as from a foreign body, tumor, or mucus plugging. It also may be caused by compression (eg, pneumothorax). A deficiency in surfactant (eg, decreased production or inactivation of surfactant) is another cause. Continuous positive airway pressure (CPAP), bilevel positive airway pressure (BPAP), and positive end-expiratory pressure (PEEP) can prevent the collapse of alveoli. These airway therapies increase the amount of gas that remains in the lungs at the end of expiration, thus preventing the collapse of alveoli and decreases the work of breathing in patients who have respiratory distress. (CPAP and PEEP are described later in this chapter and in Chapter 23, *Respiratory*.)

Surfactant is composed of lipoproteins that reduce the surface tension of pulmonary fluids. Surfactant is constantly being replenished by certain alveolar cells. Its production is thought to be stimulated by normal ventilation. If this production decreases, as occurs in pneumonia, very high ventilation pressures may be needed to produce lung expansion.

Viscous and frictional forces often play the central role in impeding airflow into and out of the lungs. Much of the resistance to airflow is provided by the upper airways of the respiratory tract. The nasal passages cause about 50% of the total airway resistance during nose breathing. The mouth, pharynx, larynx, and trachea account for approximately 20% to 30% of airway resistance during quiet mouth breathing. This resistance may increase to about 50% during times of increased ventilation (eg, during vigorous exercise).[4]

Airway resistance falls greatly as the bronchial tree continues to branch toward the alveoli. Still, the presence of airway secretions or bronchiolar constriction can lead to increased airway resistance. These factors may occur separately. More often, they occur at the same time, such as in asthma. When resistance to airflow increases, the usual pressure gradient needed for ventilation is inadequate. Therefore, muscular effort is needed to create a larger pressure gradient.

Structural changes in the lungs or thorax as a result of trauma or disease also may increase the amount of work needed for effective ventilation. This increased work usually is obvious from the use of accessory muscles during labored breathing. The accessory muscles include the scalene muscles and the sternocleidomastoid, deep muscles of the neck and thorax, posterior neck and back muscles, pectoralis major, pectoralis minor, and the abdominal muscles (**FIGURE 15-12**).

Lung Volumes and Capacities

At rest, the average adult breathes about 12 to 24 times a minute. One-fifth of this inspired air never reaches the alveoli for gas exchange. Instead, it fills the upper respiratory tract and lower nonrespiratory bronchioles.[5] This area is referred to as **anatomic dead space**. The term **physiologic dead space** refers to the anatomic dead space plus the volume of any nonfunctional

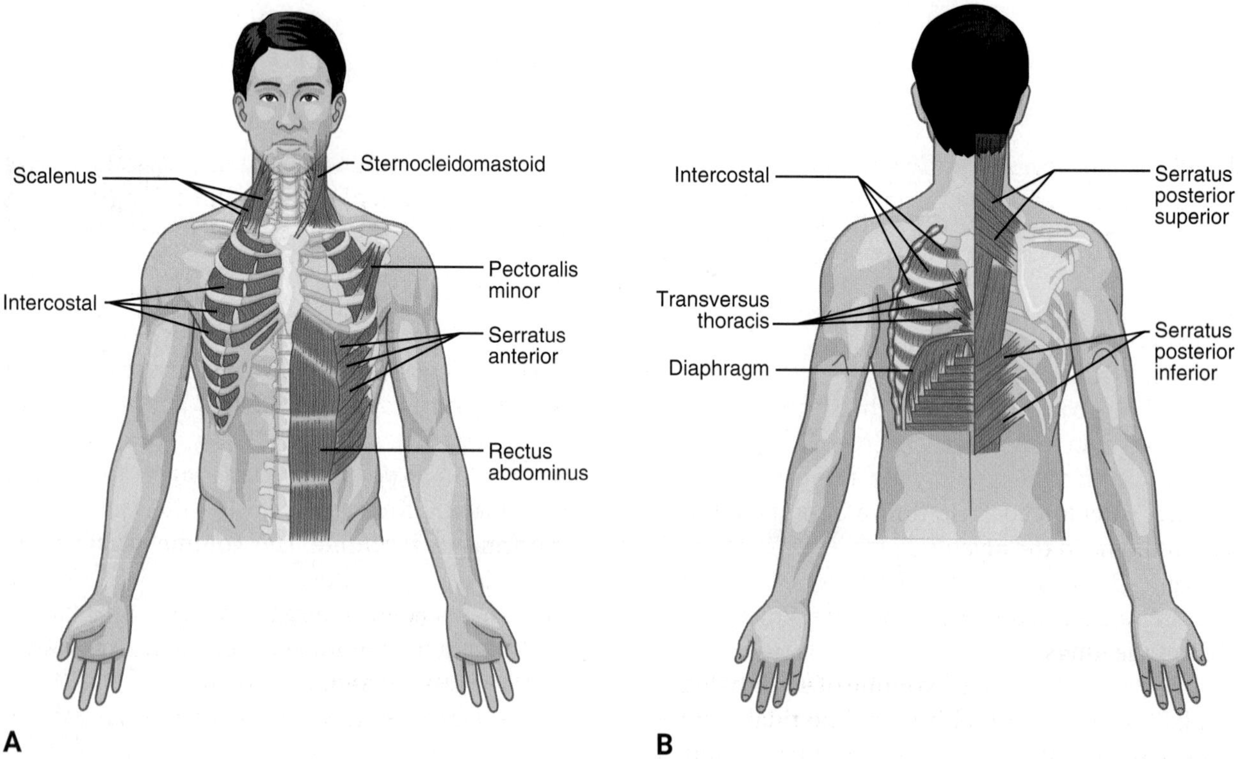

FIGURE 15-12 Muscles of ventilation. **A.** Anterior view. **B.** Posterior view.

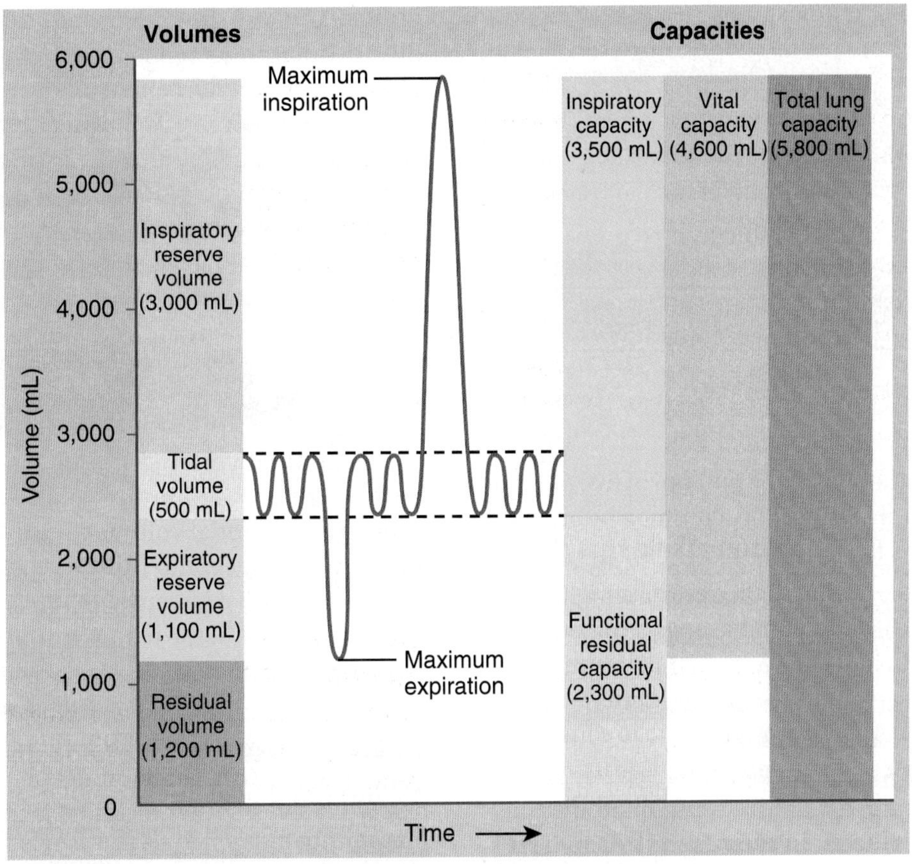

FIGURE 15-13 Lung volumes and capacities. Tidal volume during resting conditions.

alveoli. Usually the anatomic and physiologic dead spaces are nearly identical. However, this is not always the case. In patients with respiratory diseases, such as emphysema, the alveolar walls begin to degenerate. The destruction of these walls can increase the size of the physiologic dead space up to 10 times that of the anatomic dead space (**FIGURE 15-13**).

The lungs can hold about eight times the amount of air brought in by a normal resting inhalation. From the first breath of life, the lungs are never fully emptied. Even after forced expiration, a "residual volume" of air remains in the alveoli. This residual volume is replenished slowly. At least 16 breaths, and at certain times more, are needed to renew the residual volume of air in the lungs.[6]

The **tidal volume** is the volume of gas inhaled or exhaled during a normal breath. The tidal volume of the average adult is about 500 to 600 mL. Of this, 150 mL remains in the anatomic dead space (the bronchi, bronchioles, and other prealveolar structures) until it is exhaled during the next respiratory cycle. Therefore, 150 mL of the atmospheric gas inhaled during each inspiration never reaches the alveoli. It is merely moved into and out of the airways. A paramedic observing the rise and fall of a patient's chest is indirectly observing tidal volume.

The **inspiratory reserve volume** is the amount of gas that can be forcefully inhaled after inspiration of the normal tidal volume. This amount is usually 3,000 mL. The **expiratory reserve volume** is the amount of gas that can be forcefully exhaled after expiration of the normal tidal volume. This volume usually is less than the inspiratory reserve volume (about 1,100 mL). The **residual volume** is the gas that remains in the respiratory system after forced expiration. The normal residual volume is about 1,200 mL.[4]

The combined measurements of tidal volume, inspiratory reserve volume, expiratory reserve volume, and residual volume constitute the maximum volume to which the lungs can be expanded.

Pulmonary Capacities	
Tidal volume + Inspiratory reserve volume **Inspiratory capacity (3,500 mL)**	Expiratory reserve volume + Residual volume **Functional residual capacity (2,300 mL)**
Inspiratory reserve volume + Tidal volume + Expiratory reserve volume **Vital capacity (4,600 mL)**	Vital capacity + Residual volume **Total lung capacity (5,800 mL)**

FIGURE 15-14 Pulmonary capacities.

Pulmonary capacities are the sum of two or more pulmonary volumes. The more common pulmonary capacities are as follows (**FIGURE 15-14**):

- **Inspiratory capacity.** Inspiratory capacity is the tidal volume plus the inspiratory reserve volume. This capacity reflects the amount of gas a person can inspire maximally after a normal expiration (about 3,500 mL).
- **Functional residual capacity.** Functional residual capacity is the expiratory reserve volume plus the residual volume. This capacity reflects the amount of gas remaining in the lungs at the end of a normal expiration (about 2,300 mL).
- **Vital capacity.** Vital capacity is the volume of gas that can move on deepest inspiration and expiration or the sum of the inspiratory reserve volume, the tidal volume, and the expiratory reserve volume. This capacity is about 4,600 mL.
- **Total lung capacity.** Total lung capacity is the sum of the vital capacity and the residual volume (about 5,800 mL).

CRITICAL THINKING

Consider a severe burn that encircles the chest. Which respiratory volumes are affected?

Minute Volume and Minute Alveolar Ventilation

The **minute volume** is the amount of gas inhaled or exhaled in 1 minute. It is found by multiplying the tidal volume by the respiratory rate. For example, a patient's respiratory rate may be 10 breaths/min, and the resting tidal volume may be 500 mL. Thus, the average minute volume is 5 L/min.

Much of the gas that is inspired during breathing fills the anatomic dead space before reaching the alveoli. That air therefore is unavailable for gas exchange. The amount of inspired gas available for gas exchange during 1 minute is referred to as the minute alveolar ventilation. The minute alveolar ventilation is calculated by subtracting the amount of dead space from the tidal volume and then multiplying the result by the respiratory rate:

$$\text{Minute alveolar ventilation} = (\text{Tidal volume} - \text{Dead space}) \times \text{Respiratory rate}$$

If the tidal volume or the respiratory rate, or both, increase, the minute volume also increases. Likewise, if the tidal volume or the respiratory rate, or both, decrease, the minute volume decreases. The paramedic must note the depth of breathing (tidal volume) and the respiratory rate to determine whether the patient's respiratory status is adequate.

Measurement of Gases

As described in Chapter 11, *General Principles of Pathophysiology*, the mixture of gases that make up the atmosphere exerts a combined partial pressure (**Dalton's law**). This pressure is measured in millimeters of mercury (mm Hg), or **torr** (1 torr = 1/760 of a standard atmosphere, or about 1 mm Hg), based on the percentage of a particular gas (**TABLE 15-1**). The atmospheric pressure at sea level (760 mm Hg) represents 100%. Nitrogen makes up about 78.62% of the volume of dry atmospheric gas at sea level. The partial pressure that results from nitrogen is calculated by multiplying 78.62% by 760 mm Hg. This equals 597 mm Hg, or a partial pressure of nitrogen (PN_2) of 597 torr. Oxygen accounts for 20.84% of the volume of atmospheric gas. The partial pressure of oxygen (PO_2), therefore, is found by multiplying 20.84% by 760 mm Hg. This equals 159 mm Hg, or a PO_2 of 159 torr (**FIGURE 15-15**).

NOTE

To review: According to Dalton's law, in any mixture of gases, the combination of the pressure exerted by all the gases is the **total pressure**. The pressure exerted by a single gas is the **partial pressure**. The partial pressure of a gas in a mixture is denoted by a *P* preceding the gas. For example, the partial pressure of oxygen is PO_2. The partial pressure of carbon dioxide is PCO_2.

TABLE 15-1 Concentration of Gases

Gas	Concentration
Atmospheric Gases	
Nitrogen	597 torr (78.62%)
Oxygen	159 torr (20.84%)
Carbon dioxide	0.3 torr (0.50%)
Water (vapor)	3.7 torr (6.2%)
Alveolar Gases	
Nitrogen	569 torr (74.9%)
Oxygen	104 torr (13.7%)
Carbon dioxide	40 torr (5.2%)
Water (vapor)	47 torr (6.2%)

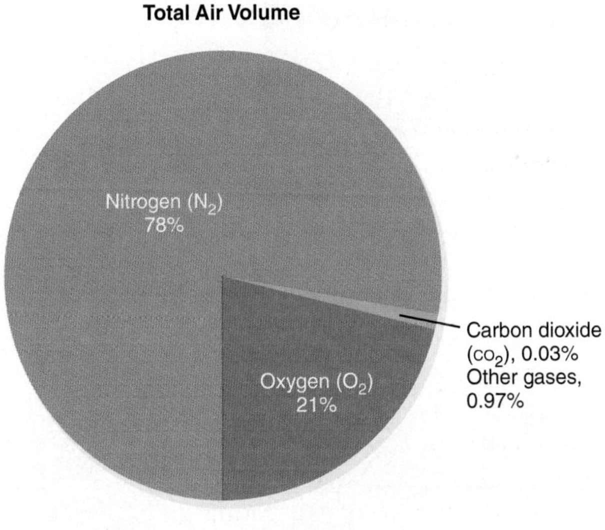

FIGURE 15-15 Partial pressure of gases in atmospheric air.

Another partial pressure can be measured when gas comes into contact with water. The water molecules convert into a gas, evaporate, and exert a partial pressure. This partial pressure is known as water vapor pressure (PH_2O).

The compositions of alveolar gas and dry atmospheric gas are not the same. This difference is a result of several factors: humidification of the air entering the respiratory system by the body, the exchange of oxygen and carbon dioxide between the alveoli and the blood, and incomplete emptying of the alveoli with expiration.

Pulmonary Circulation

The process of gas exchange in the lungs is the opposite of that which occurs in the tissues throughout the rest of the body. As inspired gas enters the lungs, the respiratory system brings oxygen to the blood and removes carbon dioxide. Blood that is low in oxygen returns to the heart from all parts of the body. Passing through the right side of the heart, the blood flows into either lung through the pulmonary artery where it then flows into the smaller pulmonary arterioles. From here the flow is directed into capillaries that surround each of the hundreds of millions of alveoli inside the lungs (**FIGURE 15-16**).

The alveoli are now filled with a high concentration of oxygen molecules and a low concentration of carbon dioxide molecules as a result of the inhaled air. They have the pressure gradient required for gas exchange. Oxygen molecules move into the surrounding capillaries at the same time that carbon dioxide molecules move into the alveoli to be exhaled. The blood is now rich in oxygen as it flows through the pulmonary venules into the pulmonary veins. From there it flows into the left atrium and then into the left ventricle. Next, it flows back out through the aorta to the body's tissues. To supply enough oxygen to the body tissues, an alveolus fills and empties more than 15,000 times in a day of normal breathing.[7]

Exchange and Transport of Gases in the Body

The volume of oxygen taken up in the lungs can be measured. It can be calculated from the difference in the amount of oxygen in inspired and expired air. The volume of carbon dioxide that is eliminated can be determined in a similar way.

As noted in Chapter 10, *Review of Human Systems*, metabolism is defined as all the chemical changes that occur in the body. In a healthy body with a constant metabolism, the relationship between tissue carbon dioxide production and oxygen consumption is fixed.

At rest, the combined consumption of all the body cells is about 200 mL of oxygen per minute. About the same amount of carbon dioxide is produced by the cells. Because about 20% of atmospheric gas is oxygen, the total oxygen inspired is 20% multiplied

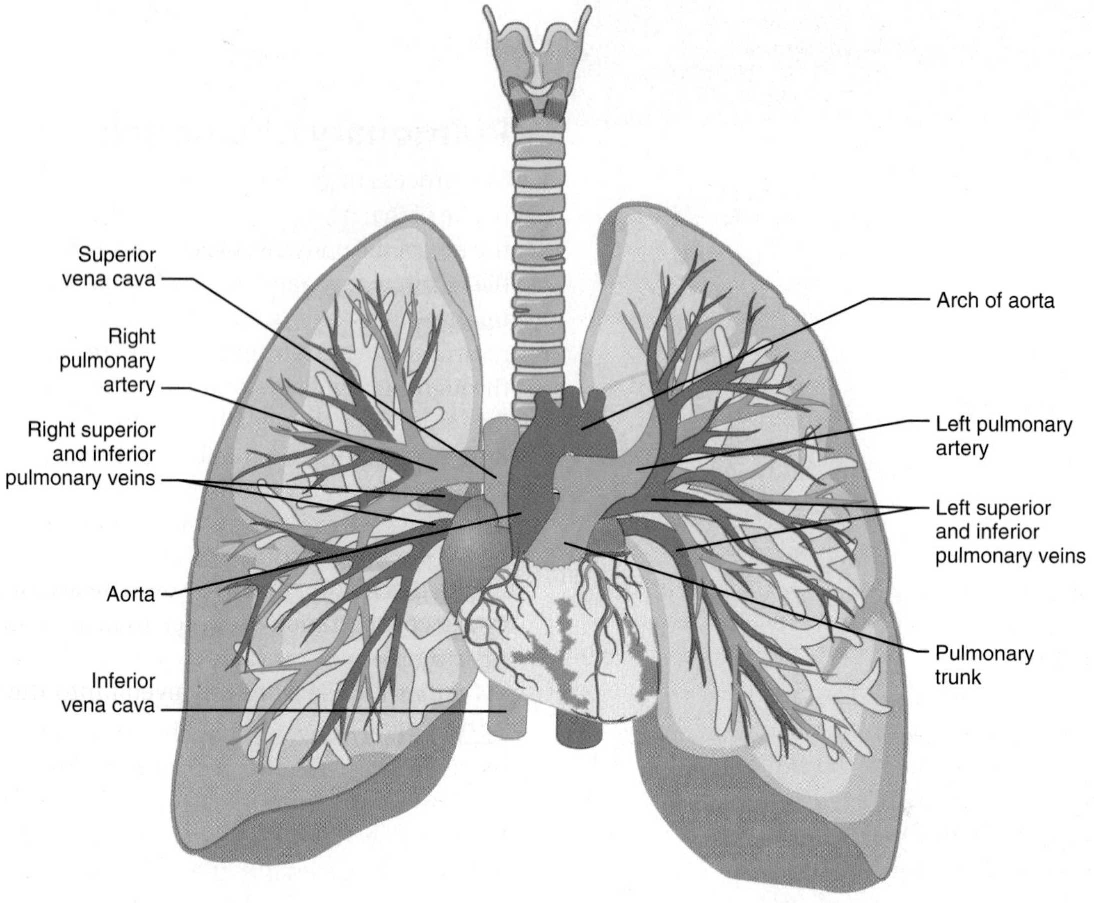

FIGURE 15-16 Pulmonary circulation.

by 5 L total gas inhaled per minute, or about 1 L of oxygen per minute. Of this, 200 mL crosses the alveoli into the pulmonary capillaries. The remaining 800 mL is exhaled. The 200 mL of oxygen is added to the quantity of oxygen already in the pulmonary capillaries. It is then transported to body tissues by the circulatory system. After the body cells use the necessary oxygen, the oxygen remaining in the blood returns to the heart and lungs. This exchange of oxygen and carbon dioxide is carried out by the passive process of diffusion. As described in Chapter 11, *General Principles of Pathophysiology*, diffusion is the tendency for molecules in solution to move from an area of higher concentration to an area of lower concentration.

Diffusion

Molecules of gases are in constant, random motion. This motion is fueled by collisions with other molecules. If the blood is divided by a permeable barrier, such as a capillary wall or cell membrane, many gas molecules come in contact with and cross the barrier. The likelihood is much greater that highly concentrated molecules will strike and cross the membrane than will less concentrated molecules. Thus, the concentration of molecules on either side of a permeable membrane tends to equilibrate (**FIGURE 15-17**).

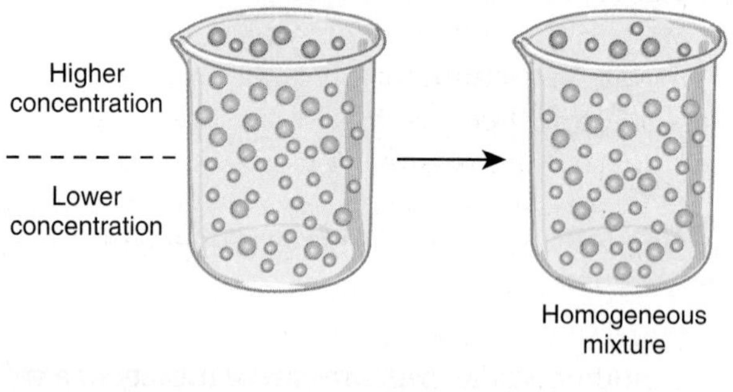

FIGURE 15-17 Random movement of gas proceeds from a higher concentration to a lower concentration until a homogeneous mixture of gases is achieved.

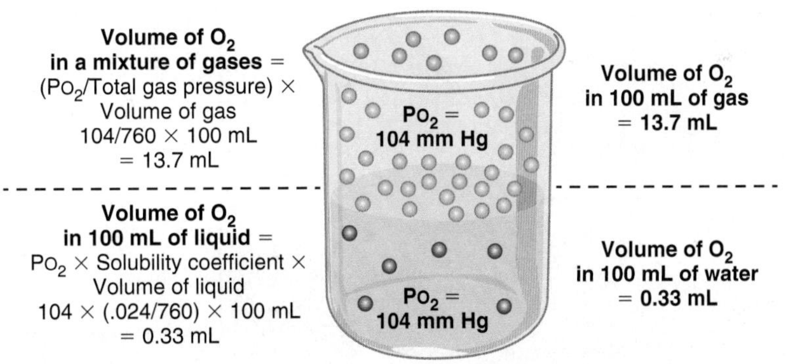

Abbreviations: mL, milliliters; O_2, oxygen; Po_2, partial pressure of oxygen

FIGURE 15-18 At equilibrium, the concentration of a gas in a liquid is determined by the partial pressure of the gas and by the solubility of the gas in the liquid at atmospheric pressure (760 mm Hg) and 98.6°F (37°C). In this illustration, the values relate to pressure within the alveoli.

The diffusion of gases through liquid is determined by the pressure of the gases. It also is determined by the solubility of the gases in liquid (**FIGURE 15-18**). When a free gas comes into contact with liquid, the number of gas molecules that dissolve in the liquid is directly proportional to the pressure of the gas (**Henry's law**). When the free gas pressure is higher than the pressure of the gas in the liquid, enough molecules dissolve in the liquid to allow the free gas pressure to equal the dissolved gas pressure.

Conversely, if a liquid containing a dissolved gas at a high pressure is exposed to a free gas at a lower pressure, gas molecules leave the liquid and enter the free gas until the pressures become equal (the general gas law). This is the underlying theme of the exchange of gases between the cells and the capillary blood throughout the body. Because the partial pressure of the free gas (Po_2) in the lungs is greater than the partial pressure of the dissolved oxygen in the bloodstream, oxygen diffuses from the lungs to the blood. The Po_2 in the blood is higher than that in the peripheral tissues. Thus oxygen diffuses from the blood into the tissues.

In addition to its pressure, the solubility of a gas is a factor. The solubility of gases in a liquid affects the behavior of the gases. The ease with which gases dissolve determines the absolute number of gas molecules that diffuse through the liquid at a given pressure. For example, a liquid may be exposed to two different gases at the same pressure. The number of molecules of each gas that diffuse may not be the same because of the differing solubilities of the two gases.

Blood entering the pulmonary capillaries is systemic venous blood that has been circulated to the lungs via the pulmonary arteries. The Pco_2 is relatively high in this blood; the Po_2 is low. The alveoli have a greater concentration of oxygen than does the blood entering the pulmonary capillaries. Thus, oxygen molecules diffuse from the alveoli into the blood. Carbon dioxide moves from the blood, where it is more concentrated, into the alveoli, where it is less concentrated (**FIGURE 15-19**).

NOTE

Oxygen and carbon dioxide do not readily dissolve in blood plasma. Transport molecules are required. Transport molecules include hemoglobin for oxygen and bicarbonate and hemoglobin for carbon dioxide.

The blood flowing through the pulmonary capillaries is separated from the alveolar air by a thin layer of tissue known as the respiratory membrane. The membrane is composed of the alveolar wall (surfactant, epithelial cells, and basement membrane), interstitial fluid, and the wall of the pulmonary capillary (basement membrane and endothelial cells). The differences in the partial pressures of oxygen and carbon dioxide on the two sides of the membrane result in diffusion. Oxygen moves into the blood and carbon dioxide into the alveoli. With this diffusion, the capillary blood Po_2 level rises. The capillary blood Pco_2 level falls. Diffusion of these gases stops when alveolar and capillary partial pressures equalize. In healthy people, this gas exchange occurs so quickly that the blood leaving the lungs to be pumped through the arteries has nearly the same Po_2 (80 to 100 mm Hg) and Pco_2 (35 to 40 mm Hg) as alveolar air.

The diffusion of gases at the alveolar–capillary level can be affected in several ways. Some respiratory

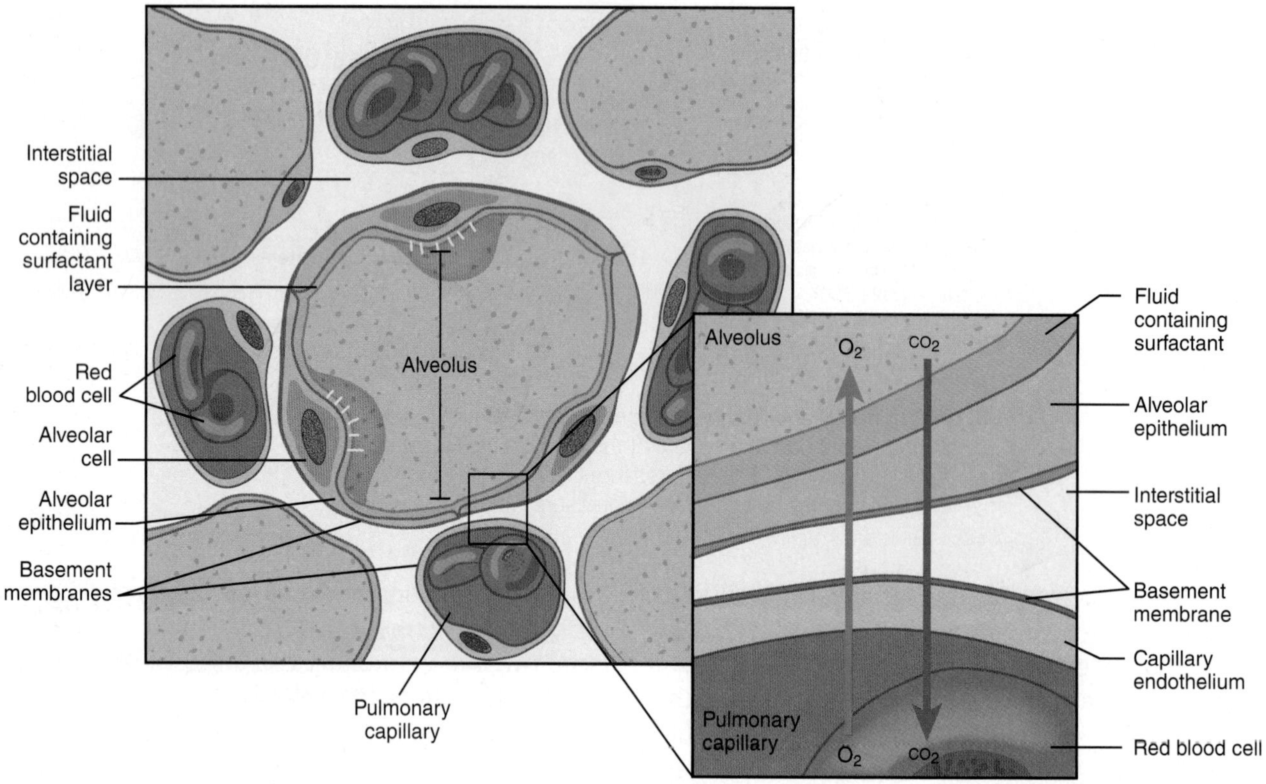

FIGURE 15-19 Gas exchange structure of the lung. Each alveolus is continually ventilated with fresh air. The inset shows a magnified view of the respiratory membrane composed of the alveolar wall (fluid coating, epithelial cells, and basement membrane), interstitial fluid, and the wall of a pulmonary capillary (basement membrane and endothelial cells). The gases, carbon dioxide (CO_2) and oxygen (O_2), diffuse across the respiratory membrane.

diseases (eg, emphysema) destroy and collapse the alveolar walls. This damage results in the formation of fewer but larger alveoli. The degenerative process reduces the total area available for diffusion. In other diseases, the alveolar–capillary membrane becomes thick or less permeable, forcing the gas molecules to travel farther, and the rate of diffusion is reduced. An example of such a disease is pulmonary edema. With this condition, fluid collects in the alveoli and pulmonary interstitial space. Consequently, gases must diffuse through a thicker than normal layer of fluid and tissue.

Oxygen Content of Blood

Oxygen is present in the blood in two forms: (1) physically dissolved in the blood and (2) chemically bound to hemoglobin (Hb) molecules. Compared with carbon dioxide and nitrogen, oxygen is relatively insoluble in water. Only 0.3 mL of oxygen can be dissolved in 100 mL of blood at the normal alveolar and arterial Po_2 of 100 mm Hg. In contrast, 197 mL of oxygen (about 98%) is carried in red blood cells. In red blood cells, it is chemically bound to hemoglobin (**oxyhemoglobin**) (**FIGURE 15-20**).

> NOTE
>
> Hematocrit is a blood test that measures the percentage of blood volume occupied by red blood cells. Normal values are about 46% for men and about 38% for women.

Hemoglobin can unload carbon dioxide and absorb oxygen 60 times faster than blood plasma can. When fully converted to oxyhemoglobin (Hbo_2), each hemoglobin molecule can carry four molecules of oxygen. At this point, the hemoglobin molecule is said to be fully saturated. Hemoglobin nears full saturation at a Po_2 of 80 to 100 mm Hg.

The degree to which hemoglobin combines with oxygen increases rapidly when the Po_2 is 10 to 60 mm Hg. This is because about 90% of total hemoglobin is combined with oxygen when the Po_2 is 60 mm Hg. Further increases in Po_2 produce only small increases

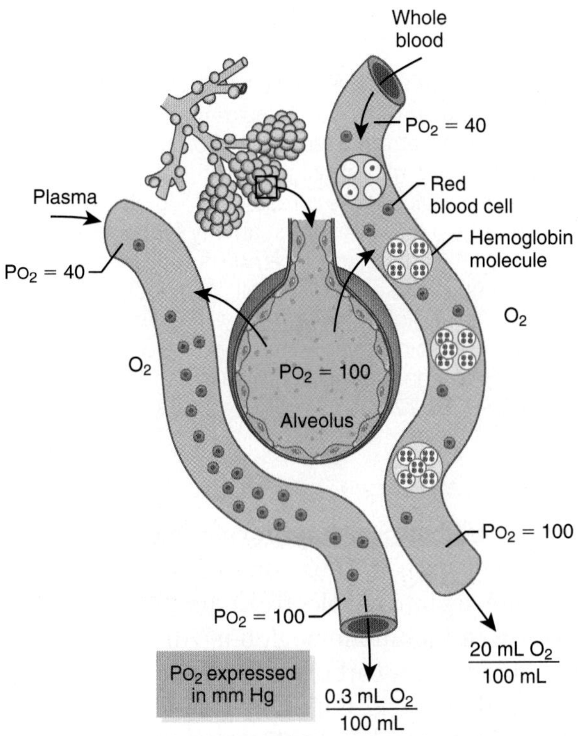

Abbreviations: O_2, oxygen; Po_2, partial pressure of oxygen

FIGURE 15-20 Oxygen-carrying capacity of the blood. If blood consisted only of plasma, the maximum amount of oxygen that could be transported would be only about 0.3 mL per 100 mL of blood. However, because the red blood cells contain hemoglobin molecules, which act as "oxygen sponges," the blood can actually carry up to 20 mL of dissolved oxygen (O_2) per 100 mL of blood.

in the amount of oxygen bound to hemoglobin. If the Po_2 falls slightly, the amount of oxyhemoglobin decreases only slightly. It still provides adequate oxygenation to tissues (**FIGURE 15-21**).

NOTE

The concept of the body adapting to higher Po_2 values is important when dealing with patient situations involving excessive exercise or cardiac and pulmonary disease. The Po_2 in the blood plasma is the most important factor in determining the extent to which oxygen combines with hemoglobin. However, oxyhemoglobin does not contribute to the Po_2 of the blood. Only the physically dissolved oxygen molecules can create gas pressure. This oxygen uptake by hemoglobin molecules removes dissolved oxygen from blood plasma. It also maintains a low Po_2, allowing diffusion to continue (see Figure 15-21). (Laws that affect gas pressures [eg, Boyle's law, Dalton's law, and Henry's law] are further described in Chapter 44, *Environmental Conditions*.)

NOTE

If the oxygen saturation as measured by arterial blood sampling (Sao_2) is 100%, the partial pressure of arterial oxygen (Pao_2) can range from 80 to 500 mm Hg. This explains the rationale to maintain Sao_2 at less than 100% after return of spontaneous circulation (ROSC). Although too much oxygen can be toxic, too little oxygen is far more dangerous than too much oxygen.

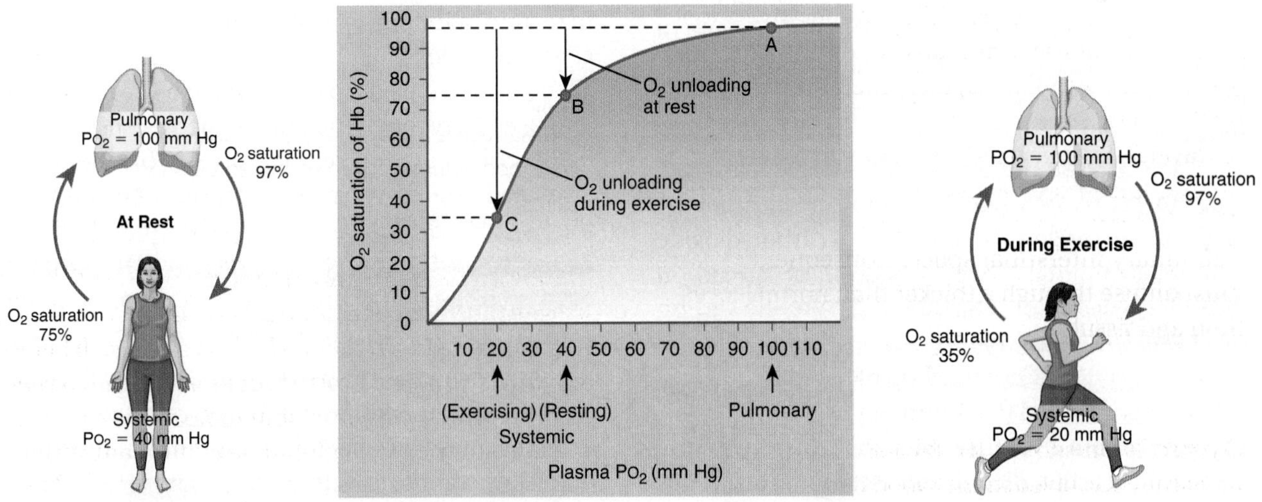

FIGURE 15-21 Oxygen (O_2) unloading at rest and during exercise. At rest, fully saturated hemoglobin (Hb) unloads almost 25% of its O_2 when it reaches the low partial pressure of oxygen (Po_2) environment (40 mm Hg) in systemic tissues (left inset). During exercise, the tissue Po_2 is even lower (20 mm Hg). Consequently, fully saturated Hb unloads about 70% of its O_2 (right inset). As the graph shows, a slight drop in the tissue Po_2 (from B to C) greatly increases O_2 unloading.

Venous blood entering the lungs has a Po_2 of 40 mm Hg and a hemoglobin saturation of 75%. Oxygen diffuses from the alveoli (because of its higher Po_2 of 100 mm Hg) into the plasma. This diffusion raises the plasma Po_2, producing an increase in the uptake of oxygen by the hemoglobin molecules. In the tissue capillaries, this process is reversed. As the blood enters the capillaries, the plasma Po_2 is greater than the Po_2 in the fluid surrounding the capillaries. This state causes diffusion across the capillary membranes to the cells of the tissues.

NOTE

Diagnostic tests that can be used in the field to monitor the oxygen content of blood and the effectiveness of ventilation include pulse oximetry monitoring, peak expiratory flow testing, and end-tidal carbon dioxide ($ETCO_2$) monitoring. (These techniques are described later in this chapter and in Chapter 23, *Respiratory*.)

NOTE

The way in which a patient's lungs are ventilated can change the pH of blood. It also may enhance or hinder oxygenation at the tissue level. For example, carbon dioxide levels may be high (resulting in a drop in pH in capillary blood). As a result, hemoglobin does not bind oxygen as well (oxygen affinity for hemoglobin is low). On the other hand, if carbon dioxide levels are low (resulting in a rise in pH in capillary blood), the oxygen binds hemoglobin more tightly (the oxygen affinity for hemoglobin is high). The response of hemoglobin affinity to changes in pH is called the **Bohr effect** (**FIGURE 15-22**; also see Figure 15-23).

Carbon Dioxide Content of Blood

As described in Chapter 11, *General Principles of Pathophysiology*, the amount of carbon dioxide produced by the body is relatively constant. It is determined by the body's rate and type of metabolism. If the metabolic rate increases, such as during exercise, more carbon dioxide is produced. In contrast, as the metabolic rate decreases, such as during sleep, less carbon dioxide is produced. Certain types of metabolic processes also result in increased carbon dioxide production. An example is anaerobic metabolism that occurs in the absence of oxygen. Another example is the body's production of ketoacids when metabolism occurs in the absence of insulin.

Carbon dioxide is transported in the blood in three major forms: plasma, blood proteins, and bicarbonate ions. As with oxygen, the solubility of carbon dioxide in water is minimal. It accounts for 8% of the carbon dioxide carried in plasma. About 20% of the carbon dioxide is present in blood proteins (including hemoglobin). About 72% is in the form of bicarbonate ions. When arterial blood flows through tissue capillaries, oxyhemoglobin gives up oxygen to the tissues. At the same time, carbon dioxide diffuses from the tissues into the blood. As a result, a small amount of the carbon dioxide dissolves in the plasma.

As described in Chapter 11, *General Principles of Pathophysiology*, oxygen-free hemoglobin binds more readily to carbon dioxide than hemoglobin binds with oxygen. Thus, some of the carbon dioxide that diffuses into red blood cells binds to hemoglobin to form carbaminohemoglobin (HbNHCOOH). The remainder of the carbon dioxide reacts with water to form carbonic acid. Carbonic acid then dissociates to form a hydrogen ion and bicarbonate. Bicarbonate, in contrast to carbon dioxide, is very soluble in water. Venous blood rich in carbon dioxide is returned to the lungs. Because the blood Pco_2 is greater than that in the alveoli, carbon dioxide from the blood diffuses into the alveoli. From there it is exhaled and eliminated from the body (**FIGURE 15-23**).

Factors That Influence Blood Oxygenation

In healthy people, the process of breathing fully oxygenates the blood at the alveolar–capillary level. It also allows carbon dioxide to be eliminated. The movement and use of oxygen in the body to perfuse tissues can be described by the Fick principle. (This method is also used to measure cardiac output.) According to the **Fick principle**, the amount of oxygen the lungs deliver to the blood is directly related to the amount of oxygen the body consumes. The movement and use of oxygen are based on the following conditions:

1. An adequate amount of oxygen must be available to saturate the hemoglobin on red blood cells as they pass by alveolar membranes in the lungs. This condition requires adequate ventilation of the lungs through the patient's airway, a high fraction of inspired oxygen (FIO_2), and minimal obstruction to the diffusion of oxygen across the alveolar–capillary membrane.

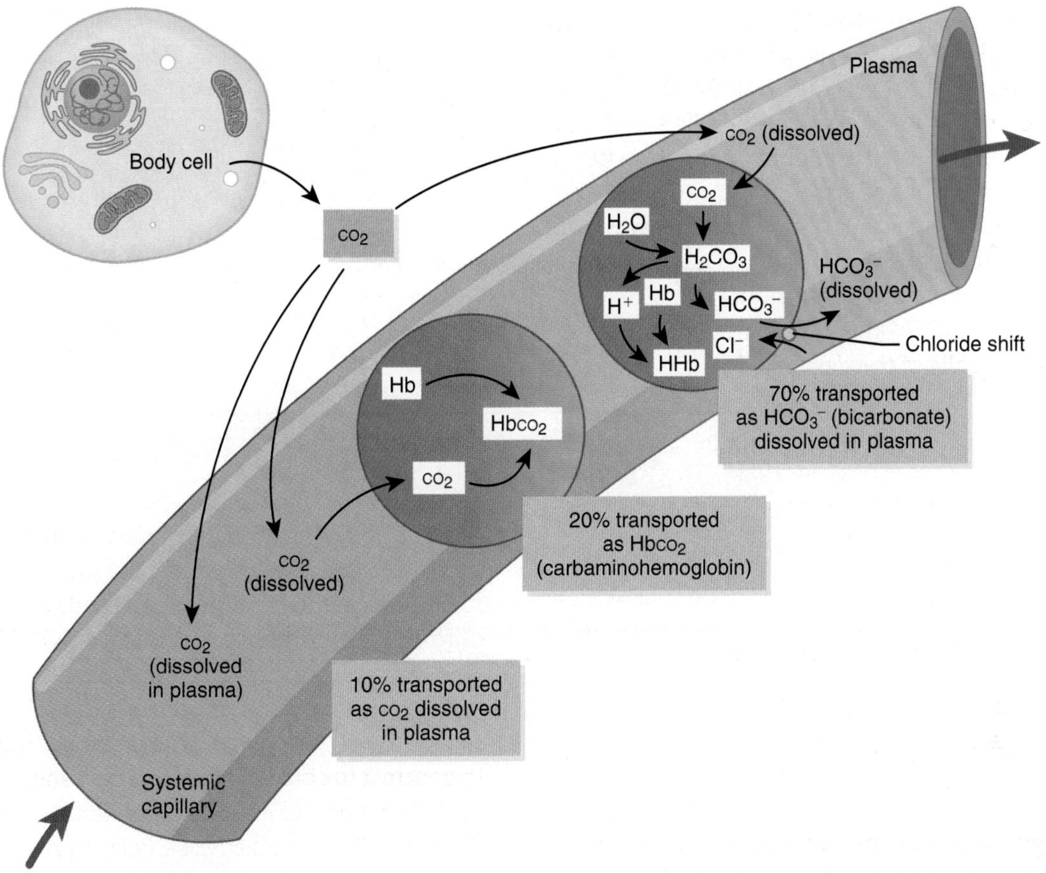

Abbreviations: Cl-, chloride; CO_2, carbon dioxide; H^+, hydrogen ion; HCO_3^-, bicarbonate; H_2CO_3, carbonic acid; H_2O, water; Hb, hemoglobin; $HbCO_2$, carbaminohemoglobin; HHb, un-ionized hemoglobin; O_2, oxygen; PO_2, partial pressure of oxygen

FIGURE 15-22 Interaction of the partial pressure of oxygen and the partial pressure of carbon dioxide (PCO_2) on gas transport by the blood. An increase in the PCO_2 in systemic tissues decreases the affinity between hemoglobin and oxygen. This appears as a right shift of the oxygen–hemoglobin dissociation curve. A right shift can also be caused by a decrease in the plasma pH.

2. The red blood cells must be circulated to the tissue cells. This condition requires adequate cardiac function, an adequate volume of blood flow, and proper routing of blood through the vascular channels.
3. The red blood cells must be able to load oxygen in the pulmonary capillaries. They also must be able to unload the oxygen at the site of peripheral tissue cells. This condition requires normal hemoglobin levels, circulation of the oxygenated red blood cells to the tissues in need, close approximation of the cells to the capillaries to allow for diffusion of oxygen, and ideal conditions of pH, temperature, and other factors.

> **NOTE**
> In medical care, the FIO_2 in a gas mixture is expressed as a number from 0 (0%) to 1 (100%). For example, the FIO_2 of normal room air is 0.21 (21%). The FIO_2 can be manipulated with airway devices that provide supplemental oxygen.

Hypoxemia is a state of decreased oxygen content of the arterial blood. It may lead to **hypoxia** (decreased oxygen content at the tissue level). Some abnormal conditions can result in inadequate blood oxygenation (BOX 15-2). These conditions are described later in this chapter and throughout this text by subject matter.

Blood Volume Circulation Disturbances

Disturbances in the effective circulation of blood can affect the body's ability to nourish the tissues

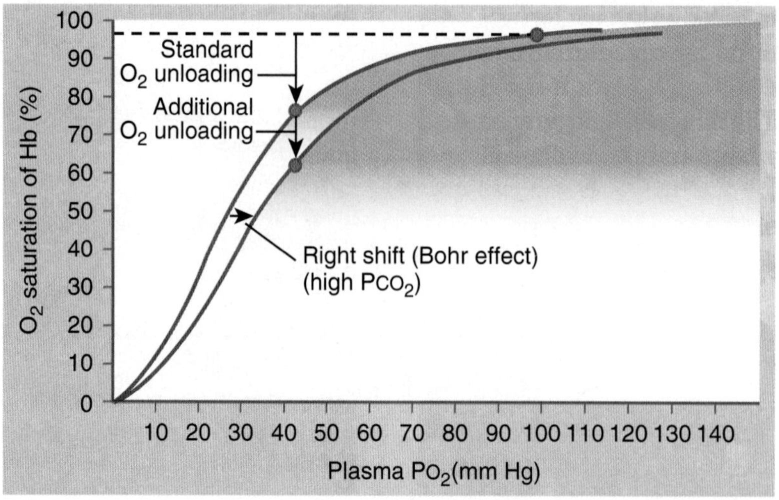

Abbreviations: Hb, hemoglobin; mm Hg, millimeters of mercury; O_2, oxygen; PCO_2, partial pressure of carbon dioxide; PO_2, partial pressure of oxygen

FIGURE 15-23 Carbon dioxide transport in the blood. Carbon dioxide (CO_2) dissolves in the plasma. Some of the dissolved CO_2 enters red blood cells (RBCs) and combines with hemoglobin (Hb) to form carbaminohemoglobin. Some of the CO_2 enters RBCs and combines with water to form carbonic acid (H_2CO_3); this process is facilitated by an enzyme (carbonic anhydrase) present inside each cell. H_2CO_3 then dissociates to form a hydrogen ion (H^+) and bicarbonate (HCO_3^-). The H^+ combines with the Hb. The HCO_3^- diffuses down its concentration gradient into the plasma. As HCO_3^- leaves each RBC, chloride enters. This phenomenon is known as the chloride shift. It prevents an imbalance in charge.

Modified from: Patton KT, Thibodeau GA. *Anatomy and Physiology*. 7th ed. St. Louis, MO: Mosby; 2007.

DID YOU KNOW?

Ventilation/Perfusion Ratio

In respiratory physiology, the ventilation/perfusion ratio ($\dot{V}/\dot{Q}$ ratio) is a measurement used to assess the efficiency and adequacy of the matching of two variables: alveolar ventilation and pulmonary perfusion:

$\dot{V}$ (ventilation)—the air that reaches the lungs

$\dot{Q}$ (perfusion)—the blood that reaches the lungs

These two variables constitute the main determinants of the blood oxygen concentration. The matching of these two variables is vital to life. The $\dot{V}/\dot{Q}$ ratio can be affected by circulation disturbances in blood volume that may result from cardiorespiratory disease, trauma, and systemic illness.

The $\dot{V}/\dot{Q}$ ratio can be measured by using a $\dot{V}/\dot{Q}$ scan. This imaging test gauges the circulation of air and blood in a patient's lungs. The ventilation part of the test evaluates the ability of air to reach all parts of the lungs. The perfusion part of the test evaluates how well the blood circulates within the lungs. Normally, alveolar ventilation is about 4 liters per minute (L/min), and pulmonary capillary blood flow (perfusion) is about 5 L/min. Therefore, the normal $\dot{V}/\dot{Q}$ ratio is 4:5, or 0.8. An area with no ventilation ($\dot{V}/\dot{Q} = 0$) is called a shunt. An area with no perfusion ($\dot{V}/\dot{Q}$ of infinity) is called dead space. An increased $\dot{V}/\dot{Q}$ ratio is seen with disorders in which ventilation is greater than perfusion (increased PaO_2, decreased partial pressure of arterial carbon dioxide [$PaCO_2$]). Examples of such disorders include pulmonary embolism and pneumothorax. A decreased $\dot{V}/\dot{Q}$ ratio is seen with disorders in which perfusion is greater than ventilation and there is an increased shunting of blood. Examples of these disorders include obstructive lung diseases that cause alveolar hypoventilation.

Although the $\dot{V}/\dot{Q}$ ratio is not a prehospital evaluation tool, it is important that paramedics understand the relationship between alveolar ventilation and pulmonary perfusion. It also is important that they understand the way **ventilation/perfusion mismatch** (ventilated alveoli that are not perfused or perfused alveoli that are not ventilated) can affect patients with respiratory compromise.

Modified from: Kumar BU. *Handbook of Mechanical Ventilation*. 2nd ed. Philadelphia, PA: Jaypee Brothers Medical Publishers; 2016.

BOX 15-2 Abnormal Conditions That Can Affect Blood Oxygenation

Depressed Respiratory Drive
Head injury
Central nervous system depressants (anesthetics, narcotics, sedatives)

Paralysis of Respiratory Muscles
Spinal injury
Toxic exposure
Neuromuscular disease

Increased Resistance in the Respiratory Airways
Asthma
Bronchitis
Emphysema
Congestion

Decreased Compliance of the Lungs and Thoracic Wall
Interstitial lung disease
Infection (pneumonia, tuberculosis)
Lung cancer
Connective tissue diseases
Chronic pulmonary hypertension

Chest Wall Abnormalities
Chest wall injury (flail chest)
Scoliosis
Eschar (full-thickness burn contractions)

Decreased Surface Area for Gas Exchange
Emphysema
Tuberculosis
Pneumonia
Atelectasis

Increased Thickness of the Respiratory Membrane
Pulmonary edema (caused by heart failure, pneumonia, infections)
Interstitial fibrosis

Ventilation/Perfusion Mismatch[a]
Asthma
Pneumonia
Pulmonary embolus
Pulmonary edema
Myocardial infarction
Respiratory distress syndrome
Shock

Reduced Capacity of the Blood to Transport Oxygen
Anemias
Hemoglobin alterations
Carbon monoxide poisoning
Methemoglobinemia

[a]Ventilated alveoli that are not perfused or perfused alveoli that are not ventilated.

and maintain adequate cellular oxygenation. These circulation disturbances can result from cardiac disease, hypovolemia, and problems with systemic vascular resistance.[8] The heart rate must be capable of circulating blood through the vascular system for adequate tissue perfusion (BOX 15-3). Conditions that can negatively affect blood circulation include conduction disturbances, tachycardia, bradycardia, and inadequate preload that diminishes stroke volume. The role of the autonomic nervous system and medications that affect alpha and beta stimulation of the heart also are important for adequate cardiac function.

Hypovolemia (from hemorrhage or dehydration) decreases the amount of blood circulating to the tissues. Finally, vascular resistance in the systemic circulation (total peripheral resistance) must be adequate to maintain blood pressure and cardiac output. One factor that affects total peripheral resistance is the capacitance of blood vessels (functioning precapillary arterioles). Another is the smooth muscle effects initiated by alpha and beta cholinergic receptors. As described in Chapter 11, *General Principles of Pathophysiology*, total peripheral resistance can be affected by hypoxia, acidosis, and the effectiveness of the buffer systems, temperature changes, neural factors, and catecholamines.

Regulation of Respiration

Respiration is controlled by a number of factors. The rate, depth, and pattern of breathing are crucial elements the paramedic needs to evaluate. When any of

BOX 15-3 Blood Volume Circulation Disturbances

Blood circulation disturbances can occur as a result of conditions that affect vascular resistance, cardiac disease that affects cardiac output, injury, and systemic illness.

Changes in Vascular Resistance

Orthostatic hypotension
Oncotic fluid pressure
Hydrostatic fluid pressure
Capacitance of the venules and veins

Cardiac Disease Affecting Cardiac Output

Heart rate (tachycardia, bradycardia)
Stroke volume (preload, afterload)
Alpha and beta stimulation of the heart
Conduction disturbances
Congestive heart failure

Injury

Head, chest, and spinal trauma
Blood loss
Shock

Systemic Illness

Acid–base disturbances
Anemia
Infection
Renal disease
Respiratory disease
Dehydration

Modified from: National Highway Traffic Safety Administration. *The National EMS Education Standards*. Washington, DC: US Department of Transportation/National Highway Traffic Safety Administration; 2009.

these elements are abnormal, the paramedic needs to consider the various mechanisms responsible for controlling them.

Voluntary Control of Respiration

Breathing is mainly an involuntary process. Within limits, however, the pattern of respiration can be consciously altered. For example, voluntary hyperventilation can lead to a decrease in the blood P_{CO_2}, vasodilation of the peripheral blood vessels, a decrease in blood pressure, or a combination of these effects. Hyperventilation causes excessive loss of exhaled carbon dioxide, which produces **hypocapnia**, resulting in cerebral vascular constriction, reduced cerebral perfusion, paresthesia (tingling sensation), dizziness, or even feelings of euphoria.

Breathing also can be affected by voluntary apnea. An example of this is when children hold their breath. In such cases, the arterial blood P_{CO_2} increases, whereas the P_{O_2} decreases. As the apneic period continues, the abnormal levels of P_{CO_2} and P_{O_2} trigger the respiratory centers. These changes in the levels override the child's conscious control of breathing. If loss of consciousness occurs, the respiratory center resumes normal function.

CRITICAL THINKING

If a prolonged, deep breath is held, what vagal effects might the patient experience?

Nervous Control of Respiration

The inspiratory muscles are the diaphragm and intercostal muscles. These are composed of skeletal muscle. They cannot contract unless they are stimulated by nerve impulses. The two phrenic nerves responsible for moving the diaphragm originate from the third, fourth, and fifth cervical spinal nerves. The 11 pairs of intercostal nerves originate from the 1st through the 11th thoracic spinal nerves. The nerve impulses that control these respiratory muscles originate in neurons of the medulla and form several groups that control breathing. Collectively, these neural groups

NOTE

The respiratory center in the medulla is bilateral. Each lateral area is made up of two groups of neurons: the dorsal respiratory group (DRG) and the ventral respiratory group (VRG). The DRG is involved in the generation of respiratory rhythm. This group is primarily responsible for inspiration. The VRG has both inspiratory and expiratory neurons. This group plays a secondary role in inspiratory activity, after the DRG. The neurons in the VRG remain almost inactive during normal quiet respiration. When the respiratory drive for increased pulmonary ventilation becomes greater than normal, respiratory signals spill over into the VRG from the DRG area. The VRG then contributes to the respiratory drive. The VRG is responsible for motor control of inspiratory and expiratory muscles during exercise. Together, these two groups of neurons are responsible for the basic rhythm of ventilation.

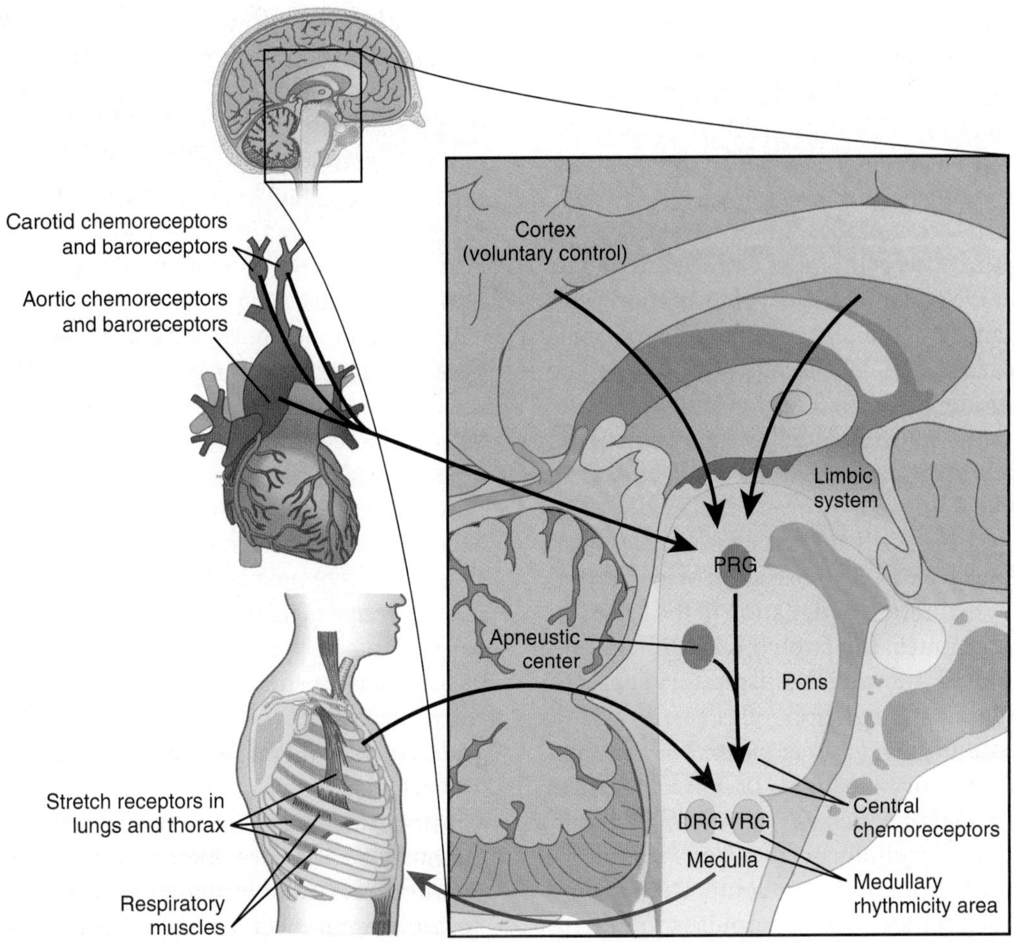

Abbreviations: DRG, dorsal respiratory group; PRG, pontine respiratory group; VRG, ventral respiratory group

FIGURE 15-24 Regulation of breathing. The dorsal respiratory group and ventral respiratory group of the medulla represent the medullary rhythmicity area. The pontine respiratory group (pneumotaxic center) and apneustic center of the pons influence the basic respiratory rhythm by means of neural input to the medullary rhythmicity area. The brainstem also receives input from other parts of the body; information from chemoreceptors, baroreceptors, and stretch receptors can alter the basic breathing pattern, as can emotional (limbic) and sensory input. Despite these subconscious reflexes, the cerebral cortex can override the "automatic" control of breathing to some extent to allow such activities as singing or blowing up a balloon. Black arrows show flow of information to the respiratory control centers. The red arrow shows the flow of information from the control centers to the respiratory muscles that drive breathing.

form the medullary respiratory center. This inspiratory and expiratory center is influenced by the pons, the hypothalamus, the reticular activating system, and the cerebral cortex. The center is innervated by afferent activity in the vagus, glossopharyngeal, and somatic nerves (**FIGURE 15-24**). It also contains chemoreceptors that will alter breathing based on changes in pH.

The inspiratory center neurons are spontaneously active. They exhibit a pattern of activity followed by fatigue and then activity again. When active, they send impulses along the spinal cord to the phrenic and intercostal nerves. These impulses stimulate the muscles of inspiration. (Head and spinal trauma, stroke, and some diseases can interrupt nervous control.)

The expiratory center is inactive during quiet respiration. The exact nervous system mechanisms that control the activity of this center are unknown. However, the expiratory center appears to be stimulated when the activity of the inspiratory center increases. (For example, this may occur during heavy or labored breathing.) When activated, the expiratory center counters the inspiratory center, responding to a forceful inspiration with a forceful expiration.

Two distinct neural mechanisms are responsible for the basic respiratory rhythm established by the inspiratory and expiratory centers: the **Hering-Breuer reflex** and the **pneumotaxic center**.

The Hering-Breuer reflex limits inspiration and prevents overinflation of the lungs via the vagus nerve. The vagus nerve conveys sensory information from the thoracic and abdominal organs. Some of the vagus nerve fibers end in stretch or inflation receptors in the walls of the bronchi, bronchioles, and lungs. When the stretch receptors are stimulated by expansion of the lungs, information is communicated by the vagus nerve to the medulla. The medulla produces discharges of inhibitory impulses. This, in turn, causes inspiration to stop (inflation reflex). The cessation of inspiration is followed by expiration or deflation of the lungs. As expiration continues, the stretch receptors are no longer stimulated, allowing the inspiratory center to become active again (deflation reflex).

The pneumotaxic center is located in the pons above the respiratory center in the medulla. It has an inhibitory effect on the inspiratory center. When the activity of the inspiratory center stops, inhibitory impulses from the pneumotaxic center stop, freeing the inspiratory center to send impulses to initiate inspiration again. The pneumotaxic center appears to be active only in labored breathing. Its activity prevents overexpansion of the lungs during rapid breathing. In quiet breathing, the stretch receptors (Hering-Breuer reflex) are the main control mechanisms for rhythmic breathing.

The **apneustic center** is located in the lower portion of the pons. Nerve impulses from this area stimulate the inspiratory center. The apneustic center neurons are constantly active during normal respiratory rates. However, they are overridden by the pneumotaxic center when the demand for increased ventilation arises.

CRITICAL THINKING

What change in breathing would you expect in a patient who has an injury affecting the pons?

Chemical Control of Respiration

The activities of the respiratory centers are determined by changes in oxygen and carbon dioxide concentrations. They also are determined by the hydrogen ion concentration (pH) of body fluids, such as cerebrospinal fluid. The partial pressure of carbon dioxide is the major factor that controls respiration.[9]

The chemoreceptive area in the medulla has neurons that are sensitive to changes in carbon dioxide and pH levels. An increase or decrease in the plasma P_{CO_2} is accompanied by changes in pH. An increase in the P_{CO_2} and the resulting decrease in pH adversely affect cellular metabolism. Excess carbon dioxide must be eliminated to return the pH to normal. For example, the body responds to an increase in P_{CO_2} of 5 mm Hg with an increase in ventilation of 100%. In contrast, a decrease in P_{CO_2} inhibits ventilation. The carbon dioxide created by normal metabolism is allowed to accumulate and return the P_{CO_2} to normal. Through these adaptive measures, the P_{CO_2} is kept within a normal range of 35 to 45 mm Hg (**FIGURE 15-25**).

Compared with pH and carbon dioxide levels, oxygen plays a small part in regulating respiration. However, if the P_{O_2} levels in the arterial blood fall and the pH and P_{CO_2} are held constant, ventilation increases.

Chemoreceptors monitor the arterial P_{O_2}. They are located in the medulla and peripherally at the bifurcation of the common carotid arteries and in the arch of the aorta. These peripheral receptors are known as the carotid and aortic bodies. The carotid and aortic bodies are in intimate contact with the arterial blood of the great vessels; therefore, their blood supply is greater than their use of oxygen. Moreover, the P_{O_2} of their tissues is very close to that of arterial blood. The nerve fibers from these bodies enter the brainstem and synapse with the neurons of the medulla, initiating a respiratory response.

Carbon dioxide and hydrogen ion concentrations are the major regulators of respiration. However, a reduced P_{O_2} in the arterial blood can play a part in regulating respiration. When a patient is hypotensive (eg, in shock), the P_{O_2} in the arterial blood may fall to low levels. This reaction stimulates the sensory receptors in the carotid and aortic bodies. Their stimulation, in turn, leads to an increased rate and depth of ventilation. This process can occur without a significant change in the blood P_{CO_2}. However, it usually is accompanied by metabolic acidosis, which occurs secondary to anaerobic metabolism (as described in Chapter 11, *General Principles of Pathophysiology*).[9]

P_{O_2} plays a role in respiratory regulation at high altitudes. At these altitudes, the barometric pressure

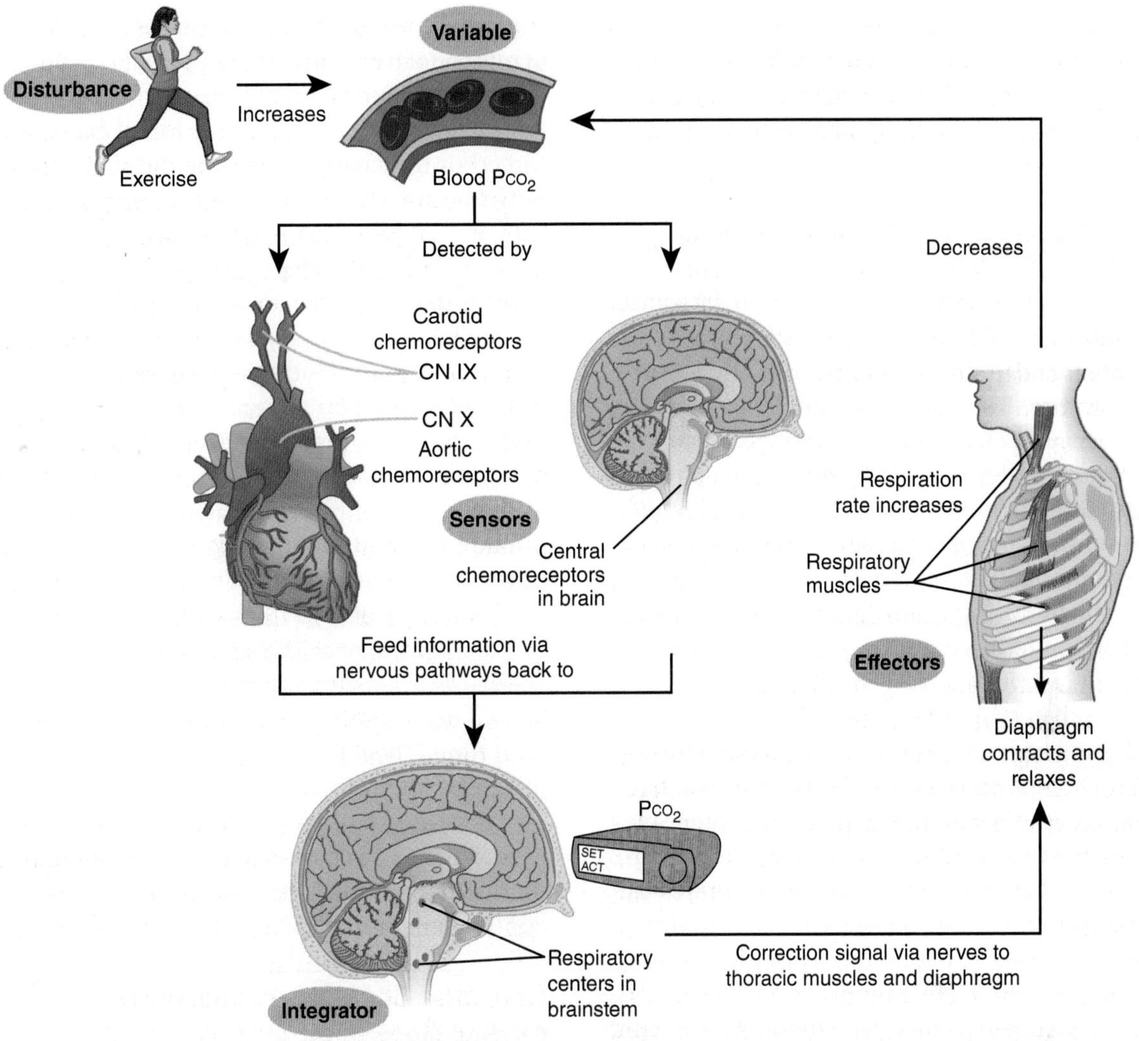

Abbreviations: CN, cranial nerve; Pco_2, partial pressure of carbon dioxide

FIGURE 15-25 Negative feedback control of respiration. The diagram summarizes the feedback loop by which the respiratory rate is increased in response to a high plasma partial pressure of carbon dioxide (Pco_2). Increased cellular respiration during exercise causes a rise in the plasma Pco_2. This rise is detected by central chemoreceptors in the brain and perhaps by peripheral chemoreceptors in the carotid sinus and aorta. Feedback information is relayed to integrators in the brainstem. The integrators respond to the increase in Pco_2 above the set point by sending nervous correction signals to the respiratory muscles, which act as effectors. The effector muscles increase their alternating contraction and relaxation, thereby increasing the rate of respiration. As the respiration rate increases, the rate of carbon dioxide loss from the body increases and the Pco_2 drops accordingly. This process brings the plasma Pco_2 back to its set point value.

is low, which means the Po_2 is lower. This causes the Po_2 in the arterial blood to also drop. The low Po_2 levels stimulate the carotid and aortic bodies. Lowered barometric pressure does not affect the body's ability to eliminate carbon dioxide. The increase in ventilation (triggered by the lowered arterial Po_2) results in a drop in the carbon dioxide levels in the blood.

Patients with severe emphysema or chronic bronchitis have chronically elevated Pco_2 levels. These patients may rely on the low Po_2 as the stimulus for ventilation (**hypoxic drive**). In diseases with chronic elevation of Pco_2, the chemoreceptors become less sensitive to a high carbon dioxide level. For many years, it was thought that the rise in $Paco_2$ with increased oxygen in these patients was the result of a blunting of the hypoxic drive, but it is more likely due to the Haldane effect. It is for this reason that chronic obstructive pulmonary disease (COPD) patients should be maintained on the lowest level of oxygen required to keep oxygen saturation (Spo_2) between 88% and 92%, but oxygen should not be withheld for fear of causing respiratory depression.[10]

Control of Respiration by Other Factors

A number of other factors may play a role in the control of respiration. These factors include body temperature, drugs and medications, pain, emotion, and sleep.

An increase in body temperature can affect the respiratory center neurons. Such an increase may be caused by a febrile illness or an increase in physical activity. The increase can cause an increase in ventilation. In contrast, major decreases in body temperature can lower the ventilation rate. An extreme example of this can occur during severe hypothermia. With this condition, patients can appear almost apneic (see Chapter 44, *Environmental Conditions*).

Some drugs, such as epinephrine, stimulate ventilation. They do so by promoting cellular metabolism during stressful events and vigorous exercise. However, drugs such as diazepam and morphine may reduce ventilations. A person who takes an overdose of narcotics, benzodiazepines, or barbiturates can become apneic.

Pain anywhere in the body may produce a reflex stimulation of ventilation. Examples include performing a sternal rub on a patient or stepping into a cold shower. Also, certain emotions, such as laughing or crying, require an increase in the movement of air into and out of the lungs. Situations involving fear and anger cause rapid breathing.

As the body's activity and metabolism slow, so does the formation of impulses to stimulate the respiratory centers. During times of decreased activity, ventilation also decreases.

Modified Forms of Respiration

The cough reflex and the sneeze reflex are protective mechanisms. The function of each is to dislodge foreign matter or irritants from the respiratory passages. Coughing generally is preceded by an inspiration of greater than normal force (about 2.5 L of gas). The glottis then closes, and the muscles of the thorax contract forcibly. This causes an increase in intrapulmonic pressure. The pressure change in the lungs increases to about 100 mm Hg.[11] When this pressure is reached, the vocal cords part, and air escapes from the lungs at high velocity. This air carries foreign materials and particles of mucus out of the lungs.

Sneezing is a violent expulsion of gas. The gas is forced or directed through the nasal cavity. It may occur because of nasal irritants, stimulation of the fifth cranial nerve (trigeminal nerve) in the nose, or exposure to bright lights. During the sneeze reflex, the uvula and the soft palate are depressed to direct air through both the nasal passages and the oral cavity.

Other forms of modified respiration include the sigh and the hiccup (in rare cases, these are chronic disorders). Sighing is a slow, deep inspiration followed by a prolonged expiration. This modified respiratory effort is thought to be a protective reflex to hyperinflate the lungs and to reexpand alveoli that might have been collapsed (atelectasis).

The hiccup results from a spasmodic contraction of the diaphragm with the sudden inspiration cut short by the closure of the glottis. Hiccups serve no known useful physiologic purpose and usually stop with time. They almost always represent a benign, insignificant event; however, in rare situations, they may indicate a pathologic condition, such as a tumor in the lung or an abscess in the abdomen impinging on the diaphragm. Typically, these episodes of hiccupping are more prolonged and frequent.

Special Considerations in Older Patients

Respiratory disorders create distinctive problems for the older patient. As a result of aging, the respiratory function of older patients may be compromised. Pulmonary changes that occur as a result of aging reduce vital capacity (**FIGURE 15-26**). They also increase the physiologic dead space. Ventilation/perfusion mismatch also tends to increase, leading to a gradually lowered Po_2. The changes in pulmonary physiology include the following:[4]

1. Mechanics of ventilation
   - Decreased chest wall compliance
   - Decreased respiratory muscle mass and strength
   - Decreased elastic recoil
2. Perfusion, ventilation, and gas exchange
   - Decreased uniformity of breathing, especially when supine
   - Increased physiologic dead space
   - Decreased alveolar surface for gas exchange

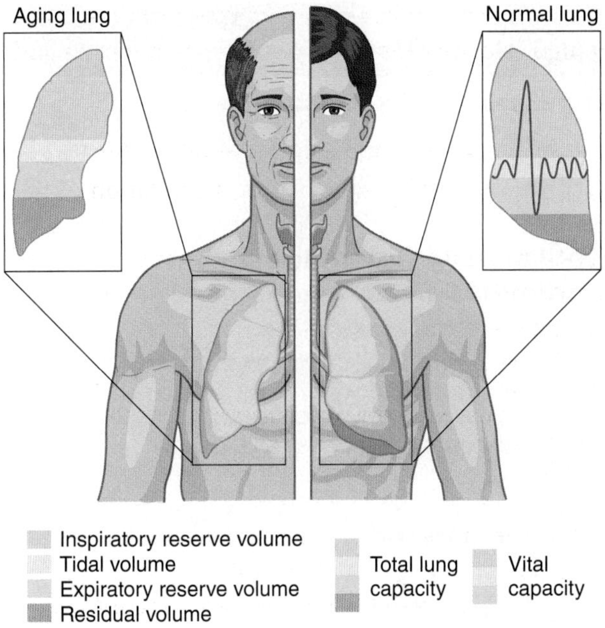

FIGURE 15-26 Changes in lung volumes with aging. Note particularly the decrease in vital capacity and the increase in residual volume that occur with aging.

3. Exercise capacity
   - Decreased work capacity of respiratory muscles
   - Decreased efficiency of ventilation
4. Regulation of ventilation
   - Decreased responsiveness of chemoreceptors
5. Sleep and breathing
   - Decreased ventilatory drive
   - Decreased upper airway muscle tone
   - Decreased arousal and cough reflexes
6. Lung defenses
   - Decreased upper airway function
   - Decreased mucociliary function
   - Decreased immune functions

As a person ages, the body's arterial Po_2 falls. Yet no significant change in arterial Pco_2 occurs. Several methods have been developed to calculate the expected Po_2 in older people. One method is to keep in mind that a person who is 70 years old is expected to have a Po_2 of 70 mm Hg. Using this value as a baseline, the expected change is a decrease in Po_2 of 1 mm Hg for every year older than 70 years, or an increase in Po_2 of 1 mm Hg for every year younger than 70 years. For example, a person who is 75 years old would be expected to have a Po_2 of 65 mm Hg. A person who is 65 years old would be expected to have a Po_2 of 75 mm Hg.[12]

These changes predispose the older person to respiratory failure. It is important that older patients with respiratory compromise from any cause receive immediate intervention, oxygenation, and ventilatory support.

Respiratory Pathophysiology

Many conditions can cause respiratory compromise and hypoxia (**TABLE 15-2**). Some of these conditions are described in this chapter and throughout the text by subject matter.

Upper Airway Obstruction

A common cause of poor ventilation is upper airway obstruction. In patients who are conscious, this type of obstruction typically is caused by inhalation of food, a foreign body, or fluid (vomitus, saliva, blood, neutral liquids). In any patient who has poor ventilation from any cause, the most important lifesaving maneuvers a paramedic can perform are establishing and maintaining a clear airway. This should always be a first-order priority of patient care. Early detection, early intervention, and education of the general public in basic life support (BLS) measures are major factors in preventing unnecessary deaths from airway compromise.

> NOTE
>
> Brain damage may occur 4 to 6 minutes after interruption of breathing and circulation. After 6 minutes of circulatory arrest, brain damage almost always occurs. In as few as 10 minutes of circulatory arrest, the most vulnerable cells in the brain are fatally injured.
>
> *Modified from*: Kirino T. Delayed neuronal death. *Neuropathology*. 2000;20:S95-S97.

Foreign Body Airway Obstruction

About 4,500 deaths each year result from foreign body obstruction of the airway.[13] Immediate removal of the obstruction might have prevented the resulting hypoxemia, unconsciousness, and cardiopulmonary arrest. The management of foreign body airway obstruction by health care professionals, as recommended by the American Heart Association, is summarized in **TABLE 15-3**.

TABLE 15-2 Conditions That Can Cause Respiratory Compromise

Interruption of Nervous Control
Drugs
Trauma
Muscular dystrophy
Poliomyelitis
Neuromuscular junction blocking agent

Structural Damage to the Thorax
Chest trauma

Bronchoconstriction
Respiratory diseases
Inhaled toxins
Anaphylaxis

Disruption of Airway Patency
Infection
Trauma/burns
Foreign body obstruction
Allergic reaction
Unconsciousness (loss of airway tone)

Oxygen Deprivation
Suffocation
Strangulation
Oxygen-deficient atmosphere

External Respiration (Environmental Factors)
Altitude
Closed environment
Toxic or poisonous environment

Internal Respiration (Pathology Related to Changes in Alveolar–Capillary Gas Exchange)
Emphysema
Pulmonary edema
Pneumonia
Environmental/occupational exposure
Drowning

Ventilation Deficiencies
Tachypnea
Mechanical ventilation with noncompliant lungs
Breathing against an elevated diaphragm

Decreases in Lung Compliance
Pneumonia
Cystic fibrosis
Trauma

Ventilation/Perfusion Mismatch
Ventilation Defects
Pulmonary edema
Pneumonia
Atelectasis
Obstruction caused by mucus plugs
Increased dead space ventilation as a result of emphysema

Perfusion Defects
Pulmonary emboli
Disruption of normal chest architecture

Disruption in Oxygen Transport With Diminished Oxygen-Carrying Capacity
Anemia
Blood loss
Hemotoxins

Disruption in Effective Circulation
Shock
Blood loss
Diminished peripheral resistance
Cardiac failure
Emboli
Increased capillary permeability

Disruptions at the Cellular Level
Acid–base disturbances
Poisons/toxins
Blood glucose changes
Hormone effects
Drugs
Hypoxia

TABLE 15-3 EMS Management of Foreign Body Airway Obstruction

Condition	Objectives	Adult (and children ≥1 year old)	Infant (<1 year old)
Conscious patient	1. Assessment: Check for signs of cyanosis, silent cough, inability to speak or breathe.	Ask, "Are you choking?" Determine whether patient can cough or speak.	Observe for breathing difficulty.
	2. Act to relieve obstruction.	Perform subdiaphragmatic abdominal thrusts until object is expelled or patient loses consciousness. Consider chest thrusts if patient is obese or pregnant or if initial actions are ineffective.	Give five back blows. Give five chest thrusts until the object is expelled or the baby becomes unresponsive.
Patient who loses consciousness		Lower to the ground and initiate chest compressions.	
	3. Start CPR.	Begin chest compressions. No pulse check needed.	
	4. Give rescue breaths after 2 minutes.	Open airway with head tilt–chin lift maneuver. Check for foreign body and remove with fingers if easily accessible. Attempt rescue breathing.	
		Repeat steps 3 and 4 until obstruction is relieved or until advanced procedures become possible (ie, use of Magill forceps or cricothyrotomy).	
Unconscious patient suspected to have foreign body airway obstruction	1. Assessment: Determine unresponsiveness.	Tap or gently shake shoulder. Shout, "Are you okay?"	Tap or gently shake shoulder.
	2. Position patient.	Turn on back as unit, supporting head and neck; position faceup, arms by sides.	
	3. Open airway, check for breathing and pulse.	Open airway with head tilt–chin lift maneuver. Look for breathing or gasping. Palpate carotid pulse.	Open airway with head tilt–chin lift maneuver without hyperextension. Look for breathing; palpate brachial pulse.
	4. Begin CPR.	Perform 30 chest compressions.	Perform 30 chest compressions (15 if there are two rescuers).
	5. Attempt to ventilate.	Check for foreign object each time you open the airway. Attempt to ventilate.	
	6. Prepare to perform advanced procedures.	Check for foreign object each time you open the airway until advanced procedures become possible (ie, use of Magill forceps or cricothyrotomy).	

Abbreviation: CPR, cardiopulmonary resuscitation

Modified from: American Heart Association. *Basic Life Support*. Dallas, TX: American Heart Association; 2015.

Airway Obstruction in a Conscious Patient

About 80% of the approximately 3,000 deaths each year from foreign body aspiration occur in children.[14] Peanuts are a commonly aspirated food. However, hot dogs caused the most deaths. There are also many nonfood items that cause foreign body obstruction in children. These objects include coins, balloons, small toy parts, pen caps, dice, safety pins, medicine syringes, and marbles.[15] Meat is the most common cause of foreign body airway obstruction in conscious adults. Factors associated with choking include large, poorly chewed pieces of food, an elevated blood alcohol level, and poorly fitting dentures. The patient often is middle-aged or older.

Large food particles and other foreign bodies can block the airway, potentially causing hypoventilation of lower lung segments. The size of the particle determines which airway is obstructed and to what extent.

Most aspirated foreign bodies are found in the right main stem bronchus and the lower lobe.[16] The left main stem bronchus branches from the trachea at a 45° to 60° angle. Thus, foreign body occlusion of this bronchus is less likely than of the right main stem bronchus, which is shorter, wider, and more vertical. When the larynx or trachea is completely obstructed, the victim can die of asphyxiation within minutes.

> CRITICAL THINKING
> How can you relieve a foreign body airway obstruction using only your hands?

Foreign bodies may cause partial or complete airway obstruction. A patient with a partially obstructed airway usually can speak and cough forcefully in an effort to expel the object. If air exchange is adequate, the rescuer should not intervene.[17] A patient with a partial obstruction should be monitored closely. The person should be encouraged to persist with spontaneous coughing and breathing efforts. If the obstruction persists or air exchange becomes severely compromised (evidenced by a silent cough, wheezing, increased respiratory difficulty, decreased air movement, and cyanosis), the patient should be managed as though a complete airway obstruction exists.

Patients with complete airway obstruction cannot speak (aphonia), exchange air, or cough. They often clutch their throat with both hands (universal choking sign). These patients need immediate rescuer intervention. Complete airway obstruction causes hypoxemia. It can lead to an acute myocardial infarction in patients with atherosclerotic cardiovascular disease. Airway obstruction leads to cardiac arrest in all patients if not corrected within minutes.

Airway Obstruction in an Unconscious Patient

Although upper airway obstruction may lead to loss of consciousness and cardiopulmonary arrest, a state of unconsciousness itself may cause an airway obstruction, usually from the tongue falling back against the oropharynx.[17]

The tongue is attached to the mandible by the muscles that form the floor of the mouth. The normal tone of these muscles allows for air exchange by keeping the posterior pharynx open. If a patient is unconscious or has neuromuscular dysfunction, relaxation of these muscles may cause the airway to be blocked by the tongue. Airway obstruction by the tongue is common in the following situations:

- Cardiac arrest
- Trauma
- Stroke
- Intoxication with alcohol, barbiturates, or psychotropic drugs
- Paralysis caused by muscle relaxants
- Myasthenia gravis
- Fractured facial and nasal bones

Laryngeal Spasm and Edema

Spasmodic closure of the vocal cords often is caused by an aggressive intubation technique. (ET intubation is discussed later in this chapter.) It also may occur during **extubation** (removal of the ET tube), especially if the patient is semiconscious. Laryngeal spasm is best managed with aggressive ventilation and a forceful upward pull on the jaw. At times it may require the use of muscle relaxants. Maintaining steady pressure against the cords with the ET tube sometimes overcomes the spasmodic closure.

Swelling of the glottic and subglottic tissues of the airway can close off the larynx. The formation of edema may result from inflammatory or mechanical causes such as epiglottitis, croup, allergic reaction, thermal injuries, strangulation, or blunt trauma. Associated swelling may partially or completely obstruct the airway. Aggressive airway management (including the consideration for cricothyrotomy if unable to intubate or ventilate) is required for the patient's survival when such swelling occurs.

Fractured Larynx

The most common cause of external trauma to the larynx is a motor vehicle crash. If a trauma patient has localized laryngeal pain on palpation or swallowing, stridor, hoarseness, difficulty with speech (dysphonia), or hemoptysis (coughing up blood), a fracture of the larynx should be suspected. Laryngeal injury can result in a lack of support for the vocal cords. This may cause them to collapse into the tracheal-laryngeal opening, obstructing the airway. Subcutaneous emphysema, dysphagia (difficult swallowing), and throat discomfort that increases with coughing or swallowing indicate the possibility of an impending airway obstruction as a result of a fracture. The paramedic should remain alert to the possibility of laryngeal fracture because laryngeal edema can rapidly close off the airway.

Certain types of injury may cause laryngeal fracture. Examples include a clothesline injury and blunt trauma to the neck. A laryngeal fracture requires rapid intervention. Cricothyrotomy may be required. The paramedic must carefully evaluate the status of the airway to determine whether there is an immediate need to secure an open airway before laryngeal edema and hemorrhage cause complete closure.

Tracheal Trauma

Trauma to the trachea is rare but serious. The most common site of tracheal injury is the area bordered by the cricoid cartilage and the third tracheal ring. This injury seldom occurs as an isolated event. More often it is associated with injuries to the surrounding esophagus and cervical spine. Central nervous system injuries and abdominal and thoracic trauma also usually accompany tracheal injury. (Tracheal trauma is described in more detail in Chapter 39, *Head, Face, and Neck Trauma.*)

Aspiration Below the Glottis

Aspiration is the active inhalation of any nongaseous foreign substance into the lung. It often occurs when fluids, such as vomitus, saliva, blood, or neutral liquids, enter the airway. Depending on the type and degree of aspiration, the syndrome may cause spasm, mucus production, atelectasis, a change in pH (if the substance is acidic), or coughing. Prevention of aspiration is far superior to any known treatment. Aspiration is prevented mainly by controlling and maintaining the airway. Paramedics should always be prepared for the chance of aspiration in patients with a diminished level of consciousness.

The average adult stomach has a capacity of 1.4 L and manufactures an additional 1.4 L of gastric juices in each 24-hour period. Hydrochloric acid is manufactured by special cells in the gastric mucosa. With the assistance of a protein-dissolving enzyme (pepsin), this acid helps break down large pieces of food into smaller ones. Vomitus contains not only partially digested food particles but also acidic gastric fluid.

Saliva is a watery, slightly acidic fluid. It is secreted in the mouth by the major salivary glands and the smaller salivary glands in the mucous membranes that line the mouth. Saliva contains the digestive enzyme amylase. This enzyme helps break down carbohydrates. Saliva also contains a number of other substances, including minerals (eg, sodium, calcium, and chloride), proteins, mucin (the principal constituent of mucus), urea, white blood cells, debris from the lining of the mouth, and bacteria.

The consequences of aspiration of neutral liquids (liquids that are neither acidic nor basic) are easier to reverse with supportive therapy than are the consequences of aspiration of acids or bases. Nonetheless, aspiration of a large volume of neutral liquids also is associated with a high mortality rate.

Pathophysiology of Aspiration

Three conditions are associated with a high risk of aspiration: (1) a diminished level of consciousness or other neurologic dysfunction, (2) iatrogenic obstructions, and (3) mechanical disturbances of the airway and gastrointestinal (GI) tract.

A diminished level of consciousness may be caused by trauma, alcohol or other drug intoxication, a seizure disorder, cardiopulmonary arrest, a stroke, or central nervous system dysfunction. The common element of these conditions is depression or loss of the gag reflex, with or without a full stomach. The **gag reflex** is a normal neural reflex triggered by touching the soft palate or posterior pharynx.

Iatrogenic obstructions (ie, those caused by medical procedures) are a common type of mechanical obstruction. This type of obstruction results from the use of various devices to control upper airway problems. Examples include removal of certain airway devices (risk of vomiting on removal), placement of a nasogastric (NG) tube (the artificial opening through the esophageal sphincter increases the risk of regurgitation and aspiration), and intubation, which requires an adequate seal at the tracheal orifice to prevent aspiration. These mechanical airway devices are discussed later in this chapter.

Other mechanical or structural problems that may lead to a high risk of aspiration include tracheostomy and esophageal motility disorders, such as hiatal hernia and esophageal reflux. Radiation treatment for head or neck cancers can increase the likelihood of aspiration. Other patients at risk include those with intestinal obstructions and those fed by gastric tube.

The chance of aspiration increases whenever vomiting occurs. Vomiting follows stimulation of the vomiting center of the medulla. This stimulation can result from irritation anywhere along the GI tract, from information passed to the medulla from the frontal lobes of the brain, or from disturbances in the balance mechanism (vestibular system) of the inner ear. Once this center is stimulated, the following seven events occur:[18]

1. A deep breath is taken.
2. The hyoid bone and larynx are elevated. This opens the pre-esophageal sphincter.
3. The opening of the larynx closes.
4. The soft palate is elevated, closing the posterior nares.
5. The diaphragm and the abdominal muscles contract forcefully. This compresses the stomach and increases the intragastric pressure.
6. The lower esophageal sphincter relaxes. The stomach contents are propelled into the lower esophagus.
7. If the patient is unconscious or unable to protect the airway, pulmonary aspiration may occur.

Effects of Pulmonary Aspiration

The severity of pulmonary aspiration depends on the pH of the aspirated material, the volume of the aspirate, and whether particulate matter (eg, food) and bacterial contamination are present in the aspirate. It generally is accepted that severe pulmonary damage occurs when the pH of an aspirated material is 2.5 or lower. When the pH is below 1.5, the patient usually dies. The mortality rate among patients who aspirate grossly contaminated material (as occurs in bowel obstruction) approaches 100%.

The toxic effects on the lungs of gastric acid (which has a pH below 2.5) can be equated with those of chemical burns.[19] These severe injuries produce pulmonary changes such as destruction of surfactant-producing alveolar cells, alveolar collapse and destruction, and destruction of pulmonary capillaries. The permeability of the capillaries increases with massive flooding of the alveoli and bronchi with fluid. The resulting pulmonary edema creates areas of hypoventilation, shunting, and severe hypoxemia. The massive fluid shift from the intravascular area to the lungs also may produce hypovolemia severe enough to require volume replacement.

> **NOTE**
>
> The risk of pulmonary aspiration can be minimized by continuously monitoring the patient's mental status, properly positioning the patient to allow for drainage of secretions, administering prophylactic antiemetics, limiting ventilatory pressures to prevent gastric distention, and using suction devices and esophageal or ET intubation. Airway protection should be provided if the risk of aspiration exists. It also should be provided promptly after an occurrence of aspiration.

Essential Parameters of Airway Evaluation: Ventilation

Evaluation of the respiratory system is presented in depth in Chapter 19, *Secondary Assessment and Reassessment*. This discussion is limited to essentials of airway evaluation that are used to identify immediate signs of life-threatening airway compromise. The essential parameters of airway evaluation are rate, regularity, and effort, in addition to recognition of airway problems that might indicate respiratory distress.

> NOTE
>
> This section serves as a review of techniques of airway assessment and airway management used by emergency medical responders (EMRs), emergency medical technicians (EMTs), and advanced emergency medical technicians (AEMTs). It also addresses advanced procedures used by paramedics.

Rate, Regularity, and Effort

The normal respiratory rate in a resting adult is 12 to 20 breaths/minute. Regularity is defined as a steady inspiratory and expiratory pattern. Breathing at rest should be effortless. It also should be marked by only subtle changes in rate or regularity.

Patients in respiratory distress often compensate for their inability to breathe easily by sitting upright with the head tilted back (upright sniffing position), leaning forward on the arms (tripod position), or lying with the head and thorax slightly elevated (semi-Fowler position). These patients frequently avoid lying flat, or supine.

> CRITICAL THINKING
>
> Why would lying flat on the back (ie, in the supine position) most likely worsen respiratory distress?

Recognition of Airway Problems

Respiratory distress may be caused by upper or lower airway obstruction, inadequate ventilation, impairment of the respiratory muscles, ventilation/perfusion mismatch, diffusion abnormalities, or impairment of the nervous system. Dyspnea often is associated with hypoxia.

> NOTE
>
> Recognition and management of respiratory failure are crucial to the patient's survival. The brain can survive only a few minutes of anoxia. All therapies will fail if the airway is not adequate.

Observation Techniques

Visual clues can aid the recognition of airway problems. Paramedics should note the patient's preferred position to facilitate breathing. They also should assess the rise and fall of the patient's chest. Other visual clues to respiratory distress include the following:

- Gasping for air
- Cyanosis
- Nasal flaring
- Pursed-lip breathing
- Retraction of the accessory muscles (intercostal or subcostal muscles, suprasternal notch, and supraclavicular fossa during respirations) (**FIGURE 15-27**)

Auscultation, Palpation, and Percussion Techniques

Air movement can be evaluated by listening to respirations without using a stethoscope (**FIGURE 15-28**) or by using a stethoscope to assess bilateral lung fields. Palpation of the chest wall helps determine the presence or absence of paradoxical (contrary) motion of the chest wall, inspiration, expiration, and any retraction of accessory muscles. Percussion may be helpful in some circumstances. This technique can be used to help determine the presence of air or fluid, such as blood in the chest cavity when diminished breath sounds or unequal chest wall movement is present (see Chapter 19, *Secondary Assessment and Reassessment*).

Other Signs of Respiratory Distress

Other signs that indicate possible causes of respiratory distress include resistance or decreased compliance

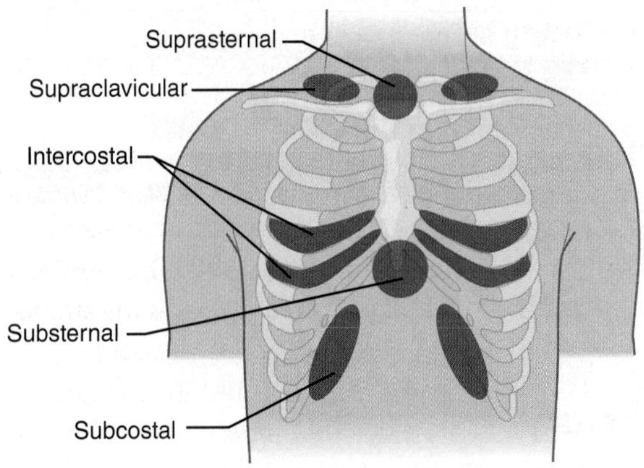

FIGURE 15-27 Areas of chest muscle retraction.

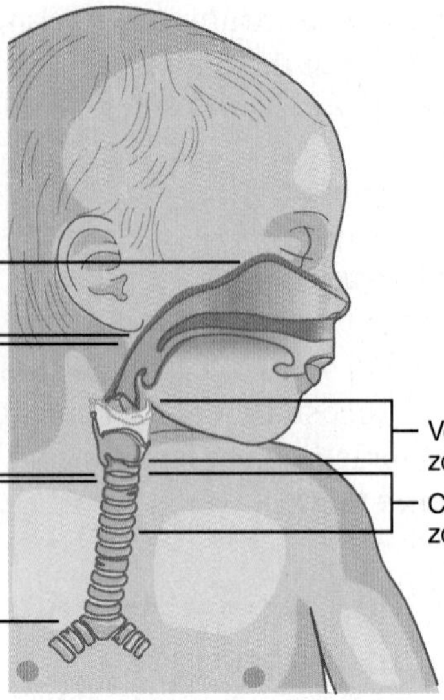

FIGURE 15-28 A loud, gasping snore suggests enlarged tonsils or adenoids. With inspiratory stridor, the airway is compromised at the level of the supraglottic larynx, vocal cords, subglottic region, or upper trachea. Expiratory stridor, or central wheeze, results from narrowing or collapse of the lower trachea or bronchi. Airway noise during both inspiration and expiration often represents a fixed obstruction of the vocal cords or subglottic space. Hoarseness or a weak cry is a by-product of obstruction of the vocal cords. If a cough is croupy or low pitched, a tracheal disorder should be suspected.

when assisting or delivering respirations with a bag-mask device (seen in asthma, COPD, and tension pneumothorax) and the presence of pulsus paradoxus.

> NOTE
>
> **Pulsus paradoxus** is an exaggeration of the normal blood pressure variation that occurs with breathing. It is defined as a fall in systolic pressure of 10 mm Hg or more on spontaneous inspiration. At times it is associated with a change in the quality of the pulse. The condition occasionally is observed in patients with asthma or COPD and in cardiac tamponade (see Chapter 41, *Chest Trauma*). Pulsus paradoxus is difficult to measure. The paramedic should rely on more obvious signs and symptoms of respiratory distress.

History

Obtaining a history to determine the progression and duration of the dyspneic event also helps guide the direction of patient care. For example, the paramedic should ask whether the event was sudden in onset or occurred over time. If it occurred over time, the length of that period should be determined. The paramedic also should ask whether any known causes or triggers initiated the difficulty breathing and whether the respiratory distress is continuous or recurring. Other questions that should be asked in obtaining a patient's history include the following:

- What makes it better?
- What makes it worse?
- Do any other symptoms occur at the same time (eg, cough, chest pain, fever)?
- Has any treatment with drugs been attempted?
- Has the patient taken all medications and treatments as prescribed?

It also is crucial to determine whether the patient has been previously evaluated or hospitalized for this condition and whether the person has ever been intubated because of respiratory problems.

Changes in the Respiratory Pattern

As previously stated, the breathing process should be comfortable, regular, and performed without distress. Abnormal respiratory patterns are commonly seen in ill or injured patients (**FIGURE 15-29** and **BOX 15-4**). Recognizing these patterns may help paramedics determine the proper patient care.

Inadequate Respiration

Inadequate respiration can occur when the body cannot compensate for increased oxygen demand or cannot maintain a normal range of oxygen–carbon dioxide balance. Numerous factors can cause inadequate ventilation and respiration, including infection, trauma, brainstem injury, and a noxious or hypoxic atmosphere. A patient with respiratory compromise may have a number of symptoms and various respiratory rates and breathing patterns. Some medical experts distinguish between inadequate ventilation (usually defined by the P_{CO_2}) and inadequate oxygenation but normal ventilation, as seen in pulmonary embolus and often pneumonia.

Supplemental Oxygen Therapy

Oxygen therapy is the administration of oxygen at concentrations greater than that in ambient air (21%). The administration of supplemental oxygen is an

HAVE YOU EVER BEEN
ITUBATED BEFORE ?
L YES= PUCKER

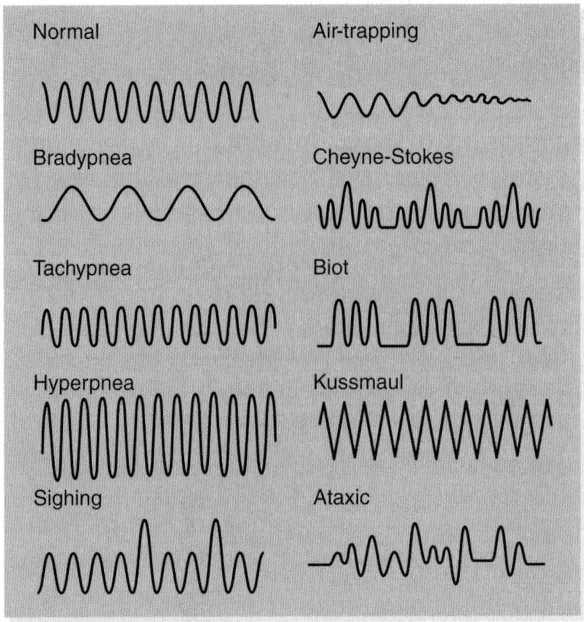

Some Influences on the Rate and Depth of Breathing

The rate and depth of breathing will increase with	The rate and depth of breathing will decrease with
Acidosis (metabolic)	Alkalosis (metabolic)
Anxiety	Central nervous system lesions (cerebrum)
Aspirin poisoning	Myasthenia gravis
Oxygen need (hypoxemia)	Narcotic overdoses
Pain	Obesity (extreme)
Central nervous system lesions (pons)	

FIGURE 15-29 Patterns of respiration. In the patterns shown in the blue box above, the horizontal axis indicates time; the vertical swings indicate the relative depth.

essential element of appropriate management for a wide range of clinical conditions with symptoms and manifestations of hypoxia. The safe implementation of oxygen therapy with appropriate monitoring is an integral component of emergency care. The clinical goals of oxygen therapy are to (1) treat hypoxia, (2) decrease the work of breathing, and (3) decrease myocardial work.

Oxygen Sources

The most common form of oxygen used in the prehospital setting is pure oxygen gas, delivered in liters per minute (L/min). This gas is stored under pressure in stainless steel or lightweight alloy cylinders (**FIGURE 15-30**). These cylinders have been color coded

BOX 15-4 Abnormal Respiratory Patterns

Agonal respiration. A type of breathing that usually follows a pattern of gasping succeeded by apnea. It generally indicates the onset of respiratory arrest or the breathing pattern of a dying person.

Ataxic pattern. A type of cluster or irregular breathing pattern characterized by a series of inspirations and expirations. Ataxic respiration usually is associated with a structural or compressive lesion in the medullary respiratory centers.

Biot pattern. A respiratory pattern involving irregular respirations varying in depth and interrupted by intervals of apnea (absence of breathing). Although similar to Cheyne-Stokes respiration, this pattern lacks the repetitiveness of that type and often is irregular. Biot respiration usually is seen in patients with head injuries who have increased intracranial pressure. Unlike Cheyne-Stokes respiration, the Biot ataxic pattern frequently produces ventilatory failure and may lead to apnea.

Bradypnea. A persistent respiratory rate slower than 12 breaths/minute. This abnormal rate may be a result of the patient guarding against respiratory discomfort caused by chest wall injury, respiratory failure, stroke, pulmonary infection, or narcotic poisoning. However, bradypnea is more commonly caused by respiratory drive depression that occurs secondary to neurologic disturbances.

Central neurogenic hyperventilation. A pattern of breathing marked by rapid and regular ventilations at a rate of about 25 breaths/minute. Increasing regularity, rather than rate, is an important diagnostic sign, because it indicates an increasing depth of coma.

Cheyne-Stokes respiration. A regular, periodic pattern of breathing with equal intervals of apnea followed by a crescendo–decrescendo sequence of respirations. Cheyne-Stokes respirations are thought to represent a level of cortical dysfunction of the brain. Although some children and older adults breathe in this pattern during sleep, it is usually seen in patients who are seriously ill or injured.

Eupnea. Normal breathing.

Hyperventilation. A persistent, rapid, deep respiration that often results in hyperpnea. Compared with tachypnea, hyperpnea usually is slower and much deeper. Its causes include exercise, anxiety, metabolic disturbances (eg, diabetic ketoacidosis), and central nervous system illness.

Kussmaul respiration. An abnormally deep, very rapid sighing respiratory pattern characteristic of diabetic ketoacidosis or other metabolic acidosis.

Tachypnea. A persistent respiratory rate that exceeds 20 breaths/minute. It may be common in patients who are in pain, frightened, or anxious. The many other causes of tachypnea include fractured ribs, pneumonia, pneumothorax, pulmonary embolus, and pleurisy.

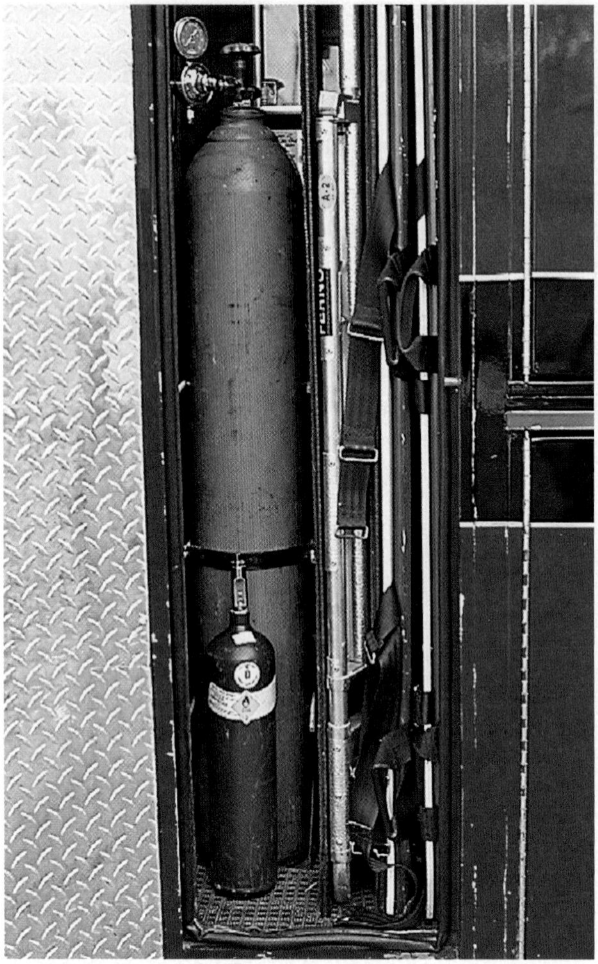

FIGURE 15-30 Oxygen tanks in outer ambulance compartment.

by the US Pharmacopeia to distinguish various compressed gases. Steel green and white cylinders have been assigned to all grades of oxygen. Stainless steel and aluminum cylinders are not painted. Common sizes of oxygen cylinders (and their factors) used in emergency care include the following (**BOX 15-5**):

Oxygen cylinders are filled under a pressure of 2,000 to 2,200 pounds per square inch (psi). Therefore, safety is critical when this equipment is handled. The paramedic should make sure the correct regulator is firmly attached before moving an oxygen cylinder. Also, a cylinder should never be handled by the neck assembly alone. Most oxygen cylinders are considered "empty" at 200 psi (the safe residual pressure). As a rule, tanks with less than 500 psi are too low to keep in service.

BOX 15-5 Calculating Oxygen Tank Life

This method can be used to estimate the amount of oxygen available in an oxygen cylinder. First, subtract the safe residual pressure (200 psi) from the tank pressure. Second, multiply the result by the tank's factor (cylinder constant). This equals the volume of gas. Third, divide the volume of gas by the liters per minute (L/min) delivery. This equals the tank life in minutes.

Example

The tank pressure in an E cylinder is 650 psi. You are delivering 6 L/min of oxygen to the patient.

Step 1. Subtract the safe residual pressure from the tank's psi:

$$650 - 200 = 450$$

Step 2. Multiply the result by the E cylinder factor to obtain the volume of gas:

$$450 \times 0.28 = 126$$

Step 3. Divide the volume of gas by the L/min delivery to determine the tank life in minutes:

$$126 \div 6 = 21 \text{ minutes}$$

Liquid Oxygen

Liquid oxygen (LOX) has been cooled to its aqueous state. However, it converts to a gaseous state when warmed. The liquid form is used by some air medical services and by other emergency medical services (EMS) agencies when the weight and space that a standard oxygen system occupies must be considered. The main advantage of liquid oxygen is that a much larger volume of gaseous oxygen can be stored in an aqueous state. One disadvantage of liquid oxygen is that it is more expensive than pressurized oxygen. Another is the fact that the units generally require upright storage. Finally, special requirements are necessary for large-volume storage and cylinder transfer.

Regulators

High-pressure regulators are used to transfer cylinder gas from tank to tank. They are attached to cylinder stems and allow cylinder gas to be delivered under high pressure. Therapy regulators are used to deliver a safe pressure of oxygen to patients (**FIGURE 15-31**). They are attached to the cylinder stem. Therapy regulators work through a regulator mechanism whereby

FIGURE 15-31 Therapy regulator.

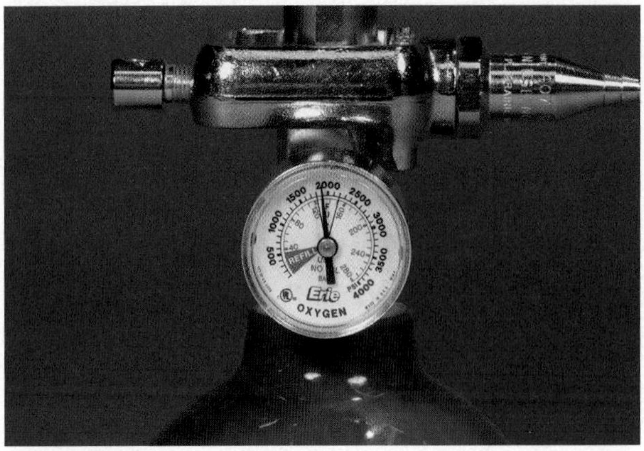

FIGURE 15-32 Flowmeter.

50 psi escape pressure is reduced ("stepped down") to 30 psi for safe delivery to the patient.

NOTE

Therapy regulators (used for delivery of oxygen to patients) are attached to smaller oxygen cylinders by a yoke assembly with a pin index safety system. This system prevents the paramedic from using a regulator with the wrong type of gas. It requires that the yoke pins match the corresponding holes in the valve assembly for oxygen to be delivered. Larger oxygen cylinders have valve assemblies with a threaded outlet specific to medical oxygen.

Flowmeters

Flowmeters control the amount of oxygen delivered to the patient (**FIGURE 15-32**). These devices are connected to the pressure regulator. They are adjusted to deliver oxygen at a set number of liters per minute. Some EMS agencies attach disposable humidifiers to the flowmeter. The humidifier provides moisture to the dry oxygen coming from the supply cylinder. Humidified oxygen is desirable for long-term oxygen administration and for patients with croup, epiglottitis, or bronchiolitis (see Chapter 23, *Respiratory*).

Oxygen Delivery Devices

Patients who have spontaneous respirations can receive supplemental oxygen through several different oxygen delivery devices. These include a nasal cannula, simple face mask, partial rebreather mask, nonrebreather mask, and Venturi mask (**TABLE 15-4**). Each of these devices has advantages and disadvantages.

TABLE 15-4 Oxygen Delivery Devices

Device	Flow Rate (L/min)	Oxygen Delivered
Nasal cannula	1–6	24%–44%
Simple face mask	6–10	35%–60%
Partial rebreather mask	6–10	35%–60%
Nonrebreather mask	10–15	80%–95%
Venturi mask	4–8	24%–50%

Abbreviation: L/min, liters per minute

Nasal Cannula

The nasal cannula (**FIGURE 15-33**) delivers low-concentration oxygen through two small plastic prongs placed into the nostrils. Nasal cannulas should not be used in patients with poor respiratory effort, severe hypoxia, or apnea. They also should not be used in patients who breathe primarily through the mouth. As a rule, the nasal cannula is well tolerated. However, a standard nasal cannula does not deliver high-volume/high-concentration oxygen. The relationship of approximate oxygen concentrations to liter per minute flow is listed in **TABLE 15-5**. Recall that room air has an oxygen concentration of approximately 21%.

Obtaining oxygen concentrations of greater than 30% to 35% is difficult with a standard nasal cannula because the patient continues to breathe through the

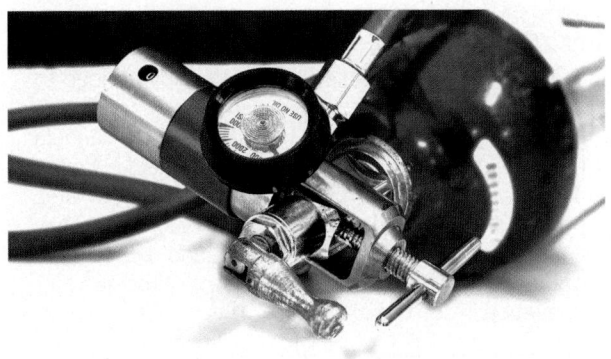

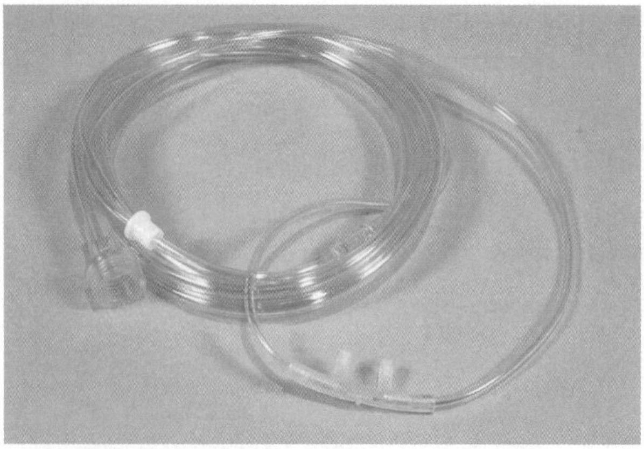

FIGURE 15-33 Nasal cannula.

TABLE 15-5 Approximate Oxygen Concentration for Liters per Minute Flow

Liters per Minute	Oxygen Concentration
1	24%
2	28%
3	32%
4	36%
5	40%
6	44%

mouth during oxygen administration. The mouth breathing reduces the concentration of oxygen inspired through the nose. The device also is ineffective if the patient's nose is blocked by blood or mucus. For these reasons, use of the nasal cannula is limited to patients who would benefit from low-concentration oxygen delivery. This may include some patients with chest pain and patients with chronic pulmonary disease. The maximum oxygen flow rate for a standard nasal cannula is 6 L/min.

Simple Face Mask

The simple face mask (**FIGURE 15-34**) is a soft, clear plastic mask that conforms to the patient's face. Small perforations in the mask allow atmospheric gas to be mixed with oxygen during inhalation and permit the patient's exhaled air to escape. Oxygen concentrations of 35% to 60% can be delivered through this device with a flow rate of 6 to 10 L/min. A flow rate of less than 6 L/min can produce an accumulation of carbon dioxide in the mask; therefore, oxygen delivery through any face mask should always exceed this minimum. Flow rates above 10 L/min do not enhance oxygen concentration. All masks must be well fitted to the patient's face for optimal benefit because leaks reduce the oxygen concentration.

> NOTE
>
> High-flow nasal cannula (HFNC) therapy is used to treat acute respiratory distress syndrome and respiratory failure in critical care settings. The HFNC cannula has wide prongs that are designed to deliver flow rates as high of 50 to 60 L/min in adults. These flow rates provide an oxygen concentration of 90% to 100%. They can also provide a mild CPAP effect and reduce work of breathing. These benefits may prevent the need for intubation in some patients.
>
> *Modified from*: Beachey W. *Respiratory Care Anatomy and Physiology*. 4th ed. St. Louis, MO: Elsevier; 2018; Nishimura M. High-flow nasal cannula oxygen therapy in adults: physiological benefits, indication, clinical benefits, and adverse effects. *Respir Care*. 2016;61(4):529-541.

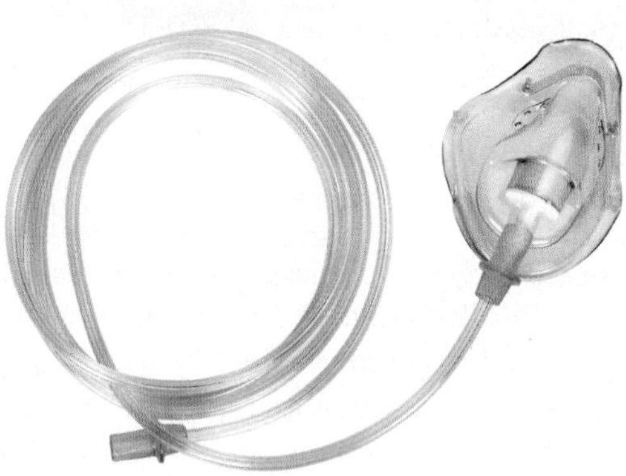

FIGURE 15-34 Simple face mask.

Partial Rebreather Mask

The partial rebreather mask (**FIGURE 15-35**) has an attached oxygen reservoir bag. The bag should be filled before the patient uses the mask. This device has vent ports covered by one-way disks that allow a portion of the patient's exhaled gas to enter the reservoir bag and be reused. The remainder of the carbon dioxide–loaded gas escapes into the atmosphere. Oxygen concentrations of 35% to 60% can be delivered with a flow rate that prevents the reservoir

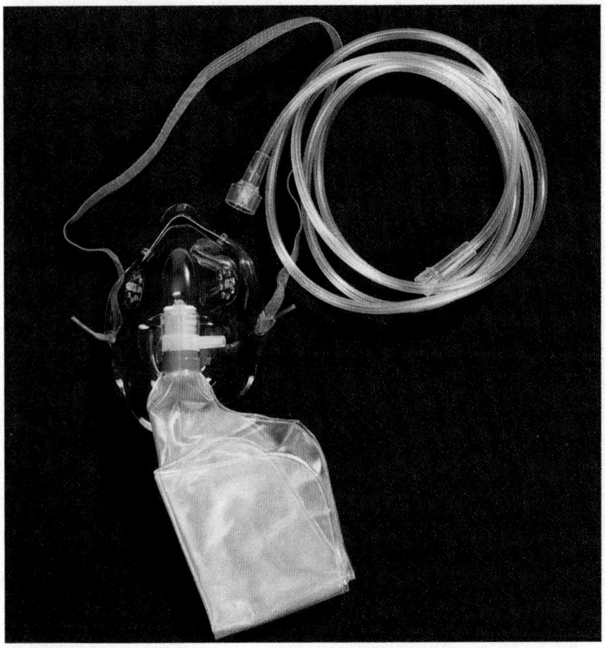

FIGURE 15-35 Partial rebreather mask.

© Jones & Bartlett Learning.

bag from collapsing completely on inspiration. Partial rebreather masks should not be used in patients with apnea or poor respiratory effort. As with the simple face mask, delivery of volumes above 10 L/min with this device does not enhance oxygen concentration.

Nonrebreathing Mask

The nonrebreathing mask (**FIGURE 15-36**) is similar in design to the partial nonrebreather mask. However, a flutter valve assembly in the mask piece stops the patient's exhaled air from returning to the reservoir bag. This device delivers oxygen concentrations up to 95%. The flow rate must be adequate to keep the reservoir bag partially inflated during inspiration. (Patients with severe respiratory distress may need up to 20 L/min to maintain inflation of the reservoir bag.) Paramedics should make sure the mask is seated firmly over the patient's mouth and nose. They also should make sure the reservoir bag is never less than two-thirds full. This device most often is used in patients who need high-concentration oxygen delivery (10 to 15 L/min). As with other masks, it should not be used in patients with apnea or poor respiratory effort.

CRITICAL THINKING

What could happen if the oxygen source is disconnected from a nonrebreathing mask?

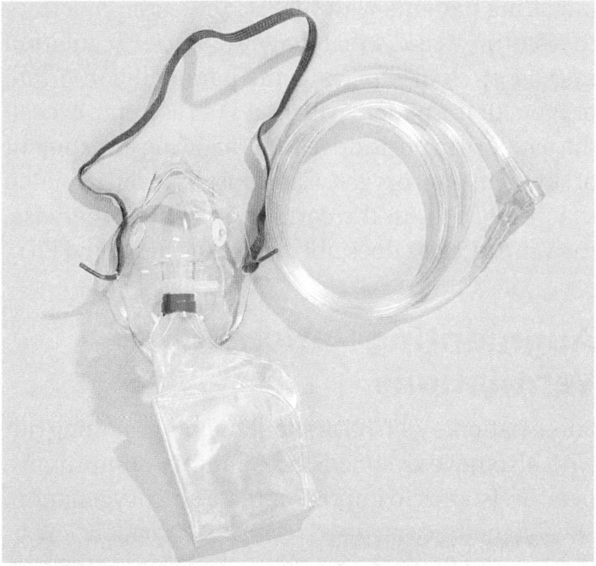

FIGURE 15-36 Nonrebreathing mask.

© Jones & Bartlett Learning

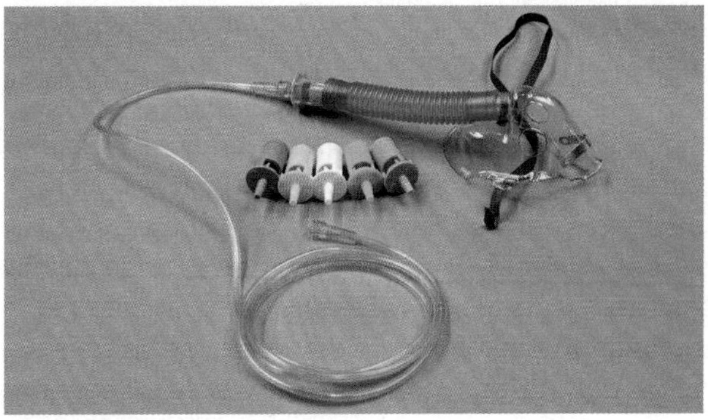

FIGURE 15-37 Venturi mask.

© Jones & Bartlett Learning.

Venturi Mask

The Venturi mask (**FIGURE 15-37**) is a high-airflow oxygen entrainment delivery device. It delivers a precise F_{IO_2} at typically low concentrations. The device originally was designed to deliver 30% to 40% concentrations. However, it since has been adapted to deliver higher oxygen percentages. The Venturi mask uses "jet mixing" of atmospheric gas and oxygen to achieve the desired mixture.

Color-coded adapters in various sizes are attached to the mask to control the oxygen flow rate. (Standard-sized adapters are 3, 4, and 6 L/min.) The color codes and adapters state the exact liter flow to use to obtain the precise F_{IO_2}. Choosing a different liter flow greatly alters the F_{IO_2} delivered. The various Venturi masks deliver 24% to 50% oxygen. They are advised for patients who rely on a hypoxic respiratory drive, including patients with COPD. The main benefit of the Venturi mask is that it allows precise regulation of the FIO_2. It also permits the paramedic to titrate oxygen for the patient with COPD so as not to exceed the patient's hypoxic drive while allowing enrichment of supplemental oxygen. Care must be taken to match the proper FIO_2 to the correct flow rate. Otherwise, the Venturi mask does not deliver the indicated FIO_2.

Augmenting Patient Ventilations

Some patients who have spontaneous breathing but who also have dyspnea or respiratory compromise need assistance to improve airflow and oxygenation. Several methods are used to improve a patient's arterial oxygenation using noninvasive positive pressure ventilation (NIPPV). These methods include CPAP and BPAP. CPAP and BPAP can improve oxygenation by ensuring positive pressure during spontaneous breathing, reducing the work of breathing, preventing atelectasis, and allowing for nebulized drug administration. In addition, it can have beneficial hemodynamic effects on heart failure patients by reducing the preload, afterload, and left ventricle compliance (in part secondary to increasing the intrathoracic pressure).[20] These methods also may prevent the need for intubation and the associated risks and complications of this invasive airway procedure. The general indication for NIPPV is dyspnea with early respiratory failure in patients who can protect their airway and are awake.[21] Specific indications and contraindications for CPAP and BPAP are presented in BOX 15-6.

Continuous Positive Airway Pressure

Continuous positive airway pressure (CPAP) transmits positive pressure into the airways of a spontaneously breathing patient throughout the respiratory cycle. The increase in airway pressure allows for better diffusion of gases and reexpansion of collapsed alveoli. These effects improve gas exchange and reduce work of breathing. CPAP can be applied invasively in a patient with spontaneous breathing (through an ET tube). It also can be applied noninvasively (noninvasive ventilation [NIV]) through a face or nose mask. Mask CPAP is provided through a tight-fitting face mask that is connected to a ventilator or battery-operated or oxygen-driven breathing circuit. This breathing circuit may have a fixed or an adjustable FIO_2 and a fixed or an adjustable pressure valve that delivers pressures of 4 to 20 centimeters of water (cm H_2O) or more (**FIGURE 15-38**).[21] A normal adult CPAP protocol for most EMS agencies ranges from 5 to 10 cm H_2O.[21] CPAP is not a leak-tolerant system.

BOX 15-6 Indications and Contraindications for CPAP and BPAP

Indications

Acute respiratory distress syndrome
Asthma
Bronchiolitis
COPD
Congestive heart failure with pulmonary edema
Cystic fibrosis
Pneumonia
Some neuromuscular conditions
Submersion (drowning) incidents

Contraindications

Respiratory arrest
Patients who are unconscious or sedated
Upper airway trauma
Hypotension or shock
Facial/chest trauma
Pneumothorax
Barotrauma
Inability to maintain mask seal
Stoma or tracheotomy
Serious dysrhythmias
Nausea or vomiting
GI bleeding or recent GI surgery

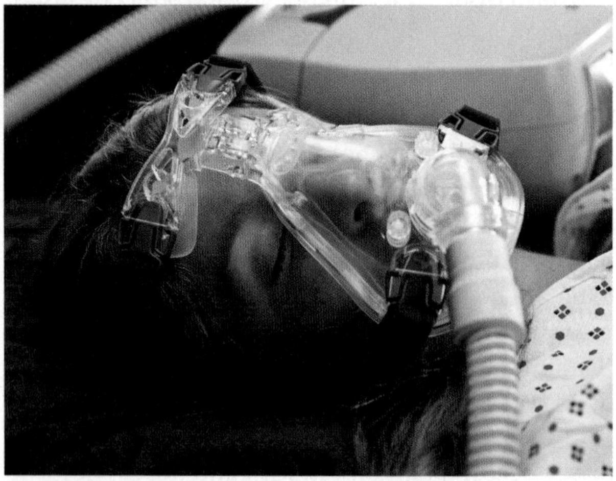

FIGURE 15-38 A patient on continuous positive airway pressure.

NOTE

Noninvasive ventilation (NIV; NIVPP) refers to positive pressure ventilation delivered through a noninvasive interface (ie, nasal mask, face mask, or nasal plugs), rather than an invasive interface (eg, ET tube). The procedure is sometimes indicated for patients with acute respiratory failure who do not require intubation. It is contraindicated in patients with impaired consciousness or severe hypoxemia and in patients with copious respiratory secretions. NIV is administered through the application of positive pressure via a sealed face mask, nasal mask, or mouthpiece using CPAP and BPAP modes of ventilatory support. Possible indications for NIV include the following:

- COPD, with emphysema and/or bronchitis
- Pneumonia
- Heart failure/pulmonary edema
  - Acute lung injury
  - Acute respiratory distress syndrome
  - Asthma
- Drowning
- Obesity hypoventilation syndrome
- Neuromuscular disease
- Chest wall disorders
- Breathing impairment due to a spinal cord injury

Modified from: British Thoracic Society Standards of Care Committee. BTS guideline. Non-invasive ventilation in acute respiratory failure. BMJ Journals website. http://thorax.bmj.com/content/57/3/192. Accessed February 6, 2018.

NOTE

CPAP is generally well tolerated by patients. However, CPAP may have adverse effects on the circulation or pulmonary system, especially at higher pressures. Such effects include decreased venous return, decreased cardiac output, and pulmonary barotrauma. All patients should be closely monitored for signs and symptoms of adverse effects. If CPAP is used, start with low pressures (5 to 10 cm H_2O) and increase in increments of 2 cm H_2O as tolerated by the patient to a maximum of 20 cm H_2O. Respiratory goals may include an exhaled tidal volume greater than 7 mL/kg, decreased respiratory distress, oxygen saturation greater than 94%, and perhaps most important, patient comfort.

Modified from: Mosesso VN, Jameson AM. Oxygenaton and ventilation. In: Cone D, Brice JH, Delbridge TR, Myers JB, eds. *Emergency Medical Services: Clinical Practice and Systems Oversight*. 2nd ed. West Sussex, England: Wiley and Sons; 2015:159-173.

CPAP, in addition to its use in patients with pulmonary edema, may benefit patients with obstructive airway disease. (Nasal CPAP is used in the home for patients with a history of sleep apnea.) Patients who receive CPAP usually are quite anxious. About 5 minutes after the mask is applied, the patient should be observed for signs and symptoms of improvement, including reduced effort of breathing, increased ease in speaking, slowing respiratory and heart rate, and increased Pao_2. The patient is likely to require extensive coaching and reassurance from the paramedic. Use of CPAP with standard drug therapy to treat pulmonary edema has been shown to reduce mortality and the need for intubation.[22] (Early hospital notification allows for CPAP to be available on arrival at the emergency department [ED].)

SHOW ME THE EVIDENCE

A team of researchers from North America and Europe conducted a meta-analysis to evaluate the effectiveness of prehospital CPAP and BPAP in treating respiratory failure. After identifying 2,284 citations on the topic, they found 8 meeting their inclusion criteria (randomized or quasirandomized). Seven included individual patient data that could be analyzed in the meta-analysis. They found that prehospital CPAP appears to reduce mortality (odds ratio [OR], 0.41; 95% credible interval [CrI], 0.20 to 0.77) and intubation rates (OR, 0.32; 95% CrI, 0.17 to 0.62) in acute respiratory failure. The analysis of BPAP data was inconclusive.

Modified from: Goodacre S, Stevens JW, Pandor A, et al. Prehospital noninvasive ventilation for acute respiratory failure: systematic review, network meta-analysis, and individual patient data meta-analysis. *Acad Emerg Med*. 2014;21(9):960-970.

CRITICAL THINKING

What benefits are there for the patient when ET intubation can be avoided by using CPAP or BPAP to treat respiratory distress?

Bilevel Positive Airway Pressure

Bilevel positive airway pressure (BPAP), also known as biphasic positive airway pressure, combines partial ventilatory support and CPAP. This combination allows the pressure to vary during each breath cycle. When the patient inhales, the pressure is similar to CPAP. When the patient exhales, the pressure drops, making it easier to breathe. BPAP is applied by face

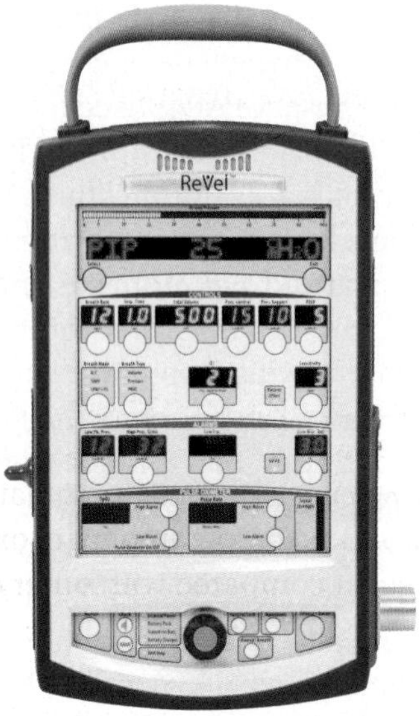

FIGURE 15-39 Bilevel positive airway pressure machine.

mask or nose mask through a NIV device with two settings (**FIGURE 15-39**). The device provides a pressure difference between inspiratory positive airway pressure (IPAP) and expiratory positive airway pressure (EPAP). This difference represents the **pressure support** being delivered to the patient. Typical initial BPAP settings are IPAP of 10 cm H_2O and EPAP of 5 cm H_2O.[21] These settings are adjusted as needed based on the patient's response. BPAP is a leak-tolerant system; that is, the unit can respond and adjust to leaks. It allows IPAP and EPAP settings to be titrated (adjusted) to reach a desired range of pressure support (described later). In some patients with respiratory distress caused by COPD, pulmonary edema, pneumonia, or asthma, BPAP may eliminate the need for ET intubation. It has been shown to improve COPD exacerbation more quickly than does CPAP.

> **NOTE**
>
> With BPAP, the IPAP setting may range from 4 to 24 cm H_2O, and the EPAP setting may range from 2 to 20 cm H_2O. Typical initial settings for BPAP are 10 cm H_2O IPAP and 5 cm H_2O EPAP. These settings presume that the pressure differences allow patient tolerance and training. When using BPAP, the paramedic should remember that the inspiratory pressure must be maintained higher than the expiratory pressure at all times to ensure biphasic flow.
>
> *Modified from*: Noninvasive airway management techniques: how and when to use them. EB Medicine website. https://www.ebmedicine.net/topics.php?paction=showTopicSeg&topic_id=58&seg_id=1094. Accessed February 6, 2018.

Procedure for Administering CPAP

Methods for delivering CPAP vary by device and by the manufacturer's guidelines. The following are general guidelines.

1. Treat the patient's underlying conditions as needed.
2. Assess for indications and contraindications.
3. Place the patient in a sitting position or similar position of comfort.
4. Assess vital signs and lung sounds before and during therapy. (The systolic pressure should be above 100 mm Hg.) Vital signs should be assessed every 5 minutes.
5. Monitor the electrocardiograph (ECG), oxygen saturation, and $ETCO_2$ levels.
6. Explain the procedure to the patient.
7. Anticipate and control anxiety.
8. Provide coaching as needed.
9. Connect CPAP to oxygen source; begin CPAP pressure at 5 to 7.5 cm H_2O.
10. Apply the mask and check for air leaks. Use head straps if needed and if tolerated by the patient.
11. Administer nebulized medications as indicated.
12. Treatment should be given continuously throughout transport to the ED. CPAP therapy should be continued until arrival in the ED; however, CPAP may be stopped if the patient cannot tolerate the mask, if the airway requires suctioning or intervention, if respiratory distress worsens, if hypotension develops, or if a pneumothorax is suspected.

Note: Intermittent positive pressure ventilation and/or intubation should be considered if the patient is removed from CPAP therapy in the prehospital setting. Some patients require intubation in the prehospital setting even with CPAP therapy. Intubation should be considered in the following situations:

- Deterioration of mental status
- Increase in $ETCO_2$ level
- Decrease in SpO_2 level
- Progressive fatigue
- Ineffective tidal volume
- Respiratory or cardiac arrest

FIGURE 15-40 Positive end-expiratory pressure valve.

Reproduced with permission from Ambu.

Positive End-Expiratory Pressure

As do CPAP and BPAP, **positive end-expiratory pressure (PEEP)** maintains a degree of positive pressure at the end of exhalation. PEEP is given to patients who have been intubated and who are receiving mechanical ventilation. Positive pressure at the end of exhalation keeps the alveoli open and helps reinflate previously collapsed alveoli.

In the prehospital setting, ventilatory support with PEEP can be provided by a transport ventilator or through a PEEP valve. These valves are hollow cylinders that have a weight in the lumen (eg, a Boehringer valve or other special PEEP delivery device) (**FIGURE 15-40**). The PEEP device is connected to the expiratory port of a bag-mask device. The valve is available in pressures of 5, 10, and 15 cm H_2O. It creates PEEP by forcing the patient to exhale against the weight of the metal ball. Most transport ventilators have built-in PEEP controls.

Rescue Breathing and Mechanical Ventilation

Ventilation of a patient can be provided by several methods in the prehospital setting. These methods include rescue breathing (mouth-to-mask, mask-to-nose, mask-to-stoma), bag-mask devices, and automatic transport ventilators (ATVs). The following discussion of ventilation methods follows the recommendations of the American Heart Association.[23]

NOTE

Providing ventilations with barrier protection should always be a priority when performing rescue breathing. Mouth-to-mask, mask-to-nose, and mask-to-stoma ventilations are presented here for a complete discussion.

Rescue Breathing

As discussed previously, inspired air has an oxygen concentration of about 21%. Of this 21%, about 4% is used by the body, and the remaining 17% is exhaled. Ventilation by rescue breathing can provide adequate oxygenation to a patient with respiratory insufficiency.

Rescue breathing has some advantages: No equipment is needed, and it is immediately available. However, it also has disadvantages. One disadvantage is the limitation of the vital capacity of the rescuer. (About 500 to 600 mL is needed to ventilate an adult.) Another drawback is the low amount of oxygen delivered in expired air compared with other methods of ventilation with supplemental oxygen. Also, a rescuer may have difficulty forcing air past any obstructions in the airway. Transmission of a communicable disease through direct body fluid contact is a risk. Complications common to all rescue breathing techniques include the following:

- Hyperinflation of the patient's lungs
- Gastric distention

NOTE

Rescuer hyperventilation is also known as **inadvertent hyperventilation**. This condition commonly occurs during the delivery of cardiopulmonary resuscitation (CPR) when a patient in cardiac arrest is ventilated excessively. Excessive ventilation is thought to result in increased intrathoracic pressure that causes decreased venous return and decreased coronary perfusion pressure. Rescuer hyperventilation is believed to have a negative effect on survival rates for patients who have suffered cardiac arrest (see Chapter 21, *Cardiology*). Impedance threshold devices (ITDs) with pressure-sensitive valves are available to limit the influx of air during chest wall compressions. The ITD also lowers intracranial pressure during the decompression phase of CPR. This reduced intracranial pressure, combined with increased cardiac output, may result in greater cerebral perfusion. Studies, however, have yet to determine the relative contribution of the ITD to improved outcome.

Modified from: American Heart Association. 2015 American Heart Association guidelines for cardiopulmonary resuscitation and emergency cardiovascular care. *Circulation.* 2015;132(18)(suppl 2):S313-S314; Graham R, McCoy MA, Schultz AM, eds. *Strategies to Improve Cardiac Arrest Survival: A Time to Act.* Board on Health Sciences Policy. *Treatment of Cardiac Arrest: Current Status and Future Directions.* Washington, DC: National Academies Press; 2015; Wigginton JG. The inspiratory impedance threshold device for treatment of patients in cardiac arrest. Business Briefing: Long-term Healthcare, 2005. *Emerg Med Rev.* 2005:58-61.

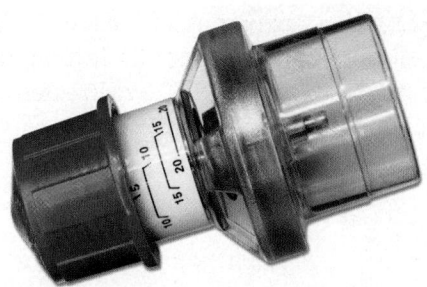

- Blood or body fluid contact concerns
- Rescuer hyperventilation

CRITICAL THINKING
What are two harmful effects of gastric distention during artificial ventilation?

Mouth-to-Mask Method

Mouth-to-mask devices are used to protect the rescuer during manual ventilation. These masks are constructed of a clear, flexible material. They are available with one-way valves, bacterial filters, and ports for supplemental oxygen delivery (**FIGURE 15-41**). They are made by several manufacturers and are available in a variety of sizes. The mouth-to-mask technique offers several advantages:

- It eliminates direct contact with the patient's mouth and nose.
- It provides more effective ventilation than does the mouth-to-mouth method or a bag-mask device.
- It reduces the risk of disease transmission.
- It allows delivery of supplemental oxygen.
- The one-way valve eliminates exposure to exhaled gases and sputum.
- The mask is easy to apply.

Technique. The mask device can be used in patients with or without spontaneous respirations (**FIGURE 15-42**).

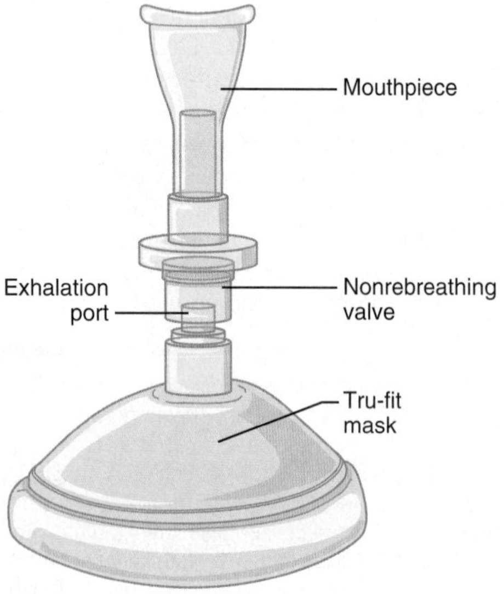

FIGURE 15-41 Mouth-to-mask device.

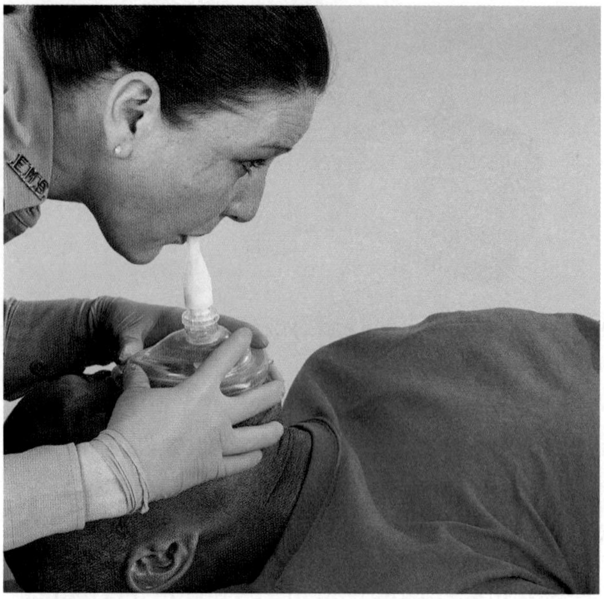

FIGURE 15-42 Mouth-to-mask ventilation technique (cephalic technique).

To apply the mask, the paramedic should follow these steps:[23]

1. If no spinal injury is suspected, position the patient with optimum head tilt and chin lift. Use an oropharyngeal or a nasopharyngeal airway if the patient is unconscious. (If a spinal injury is suspected, spinal precautions should be followed.)
2. Connect the one-way valve to the mask. Oxygen tubing should be connected to the inlet port with an oxygen flow rate of 10 to 12 L/min. Using supplemental oxygen provides a higher concentration of oxygen in the inspired air. An oxygen flow rate of 10 L/min, combined with rescuer ventilations, can supply an oxygen concentration of 50%.
3. Position yourself at the patient's head (cephalic technique) or side (lateral technique). Clear the airway of secretions, vomitus, and foreign objects. Place the mask on the patient's face and create an airtight seal. Using the thumb side of the palm with both hands, apply pressure to the sides of the mask. If using the cephalic technique, apply upward pressure to the mandible just in front of the earlobes, using the index, middle, and ring fingers of both hands while maintaining head tilt. If using the lateral technique, seal the mask

by placing the index finger and thumb of the hand closer to the top of the patient's head along the border of the mask, and place the thumb of the other hand along the lower margin of the mask. Place the remaining fingers of the hand closer to the patient's feet and lift the jaw while performing a head tilt–chin lift.

4. Blow into the opening of the mask, observing chest rise and fall.
5. Remove the mask from the patient's face to allow for passive exhalation.
6. Deliver another breath (as described in step 4).
7. Continue rescue breathing at a rate of 10 to 12 breaths/min (1 breath every 5 to 6 seconds), as needed. If an advanced airway is placed, reduce the rate to 8 to 10 breaths/minute (1 breath every 6 to 8 seconds).

Mouth-to-mask breathing can ventilate patients effectively. If supplemental oxygen is used with the face mask, provide a minimum flow rate of 10 to 12 L/min.

Mask-to-Nose Method

Mask-to-nose ventilation is very similar to the technique described for mouth-to-mask rescue breathing. The differences in the mask-to-nose method are as follows:[23]

- If no spinal injury is suspected, the rescuer must keep one hand on the patient's forehead to maintain an open airway while using the other hand to close the patient's mouth. (If a spinal injury is suspected, the jaw-thrust without head-tilt technique should be used. The rescuer's cheek is used to seal the patient's mouth.)
- The patient's nose is left open.
- The mask is placed over the patient's nose with as tight a seal as possible. A smaller size may be needed when ventilating over the nose only.
- During passive exhalation by the patient, the rescuer's mouth is removed from the mask and the patient's mouth is opened for exhalation. The head-tilt or jaw-thrust position must be maintained.

Mask-to-nose ventilation may be appropriate for patients who have injuries to the mouth and lower jaw and for patients with missing teeth or dentures (which makes a tight seal around the mouth difficult).

Ventilation of Infants and Children

To provide ventilations to infants and children, the paramedic should use the mouth-to-mask-and-nose technique:[23]

1. Position the patient with a slight head tilt and chin lift sufficient to open the airway. Hyperextension of a pediatric patient's neck may block the airway. (Use spinal precautions as needed [see Chapter 40, *Spine and Nervous System Trauma*].)
2. During ventilation, the mask should cover both the mouth and the nose of the infant or small child up to 1 year of age.
3. Exhale into the mask until the chest rises.
4. When allowing for passive exhalation, break contact with the mask.
5. Provide ventilations at a rate of 12 to 20 breaths/min (1 breath every 3 to 5 seconds). When an advanced airway has been placed, reduce the rate to 8 to 10 breaths/minute (1 breath every 6 to 8 seconds).
6. Deliver each breath over 1 second.
7. Make sure the chest rises.

Mask-to-Stoma Method

A stoma is a temporary or permanent surgical opening in the neck of a patient who has had a laryngectomy or tracheostomy (**FIGURE 15-43**). The airway of such a patient has been surgically interrupted. The larynx is no longer connected to the trachea (**BOX 15-7**).

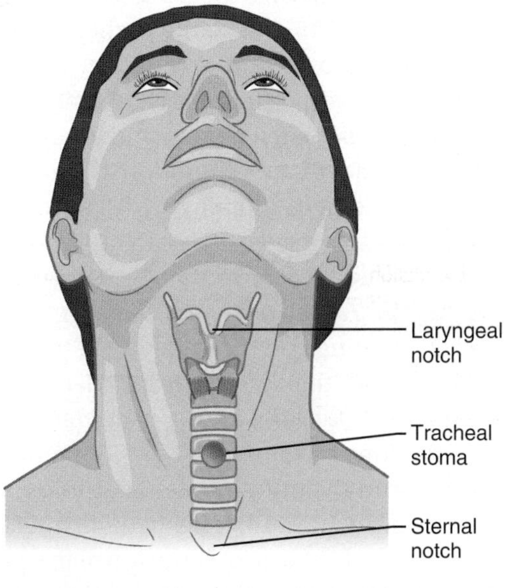

FIGURE 15-43 Stoma.

BOX 15-7 Special Considerations for Patients Who Have Had a Laryngectomy

When providing care for a patient who has had a laryngectomy, paramedics sometimes may need to suction the tracheostomy tube or remove, clean, and replace a tube that has become obstructed by mucus. (Patients who have had a laryngectomy have a less effective cough. As a result, mucus plugs often obstruct breathing tubes.)

The steps for suctioning and replacing an obstructed tracheostomy tube are as follows:

1. Attempt to ventilate the patient.
2. Inject 3 mL of sterile saline down the trachea.
3. Step 2 usually results in coughing. If it does not, instruct the patient to exhale.
4. Insert the suction catheter into the trachea to the depth recommended by the caregiver or until resistance is met (without negative pressure).
5. Step 4 usually results in coughing. If it does not, instruct the patient to cough or exhale.
6. Suction while withdrawing the catheter.

If the breathing tube cannot be cleared and requires replacement, follow these steps:

1. Lubricate a same-sized tracheostomy tube or ET tube (5 mm or larger for an adult). Most patients have a "go bag" with a spare tracheostomy tube.
2. Loosen the tracheostomy ties or securing device.
3. Deflate the tracheal tube cuff (if present) by aspirating the sterile water out of the cuff.
4. Instruct the patient to exhale.
5. Remove the tracheostomy tube.
6. Quickly and gently insert the new tracheostomy tube until the flange rests against the skin.
7. Remove the obturator.
8. Inflate the cuff.
9. Verify the patency and proper placement of the tube.

Stenosis (spontaneous narrowing of a stoma) is rare and may be life threatening. It also makes replacing a tracheostomy tube difficult or impossible. When stenosis is a factor, a replacement tracheostomy or smaller-size ET tube must be placed before total obstruction occurs.

Modified from: American Heart Association. 2015 American Heart Association guidelines for cardiopulmonary resuscitation and emergency cardiovascular care. *Circulation*. 2015;132(18)(suppl 2):S313-S314.

The stoma created by a laryngectomy is large and round; the edge of the tracheal lining can be seen attached to the skin. The stoma in tracheostomy patients usually is no more than several millimeters in diameter. Some tracheostomy tubes have external devices attached to permit speaking or to humidify secretions (**FIGURE 15-44**). Remove these devices before attempting to suction or ventilate.

Stomas and breathing tubes may become clogged with secretions, encrusted mucus, and foreign matter, leading to inadequate ventilation. If cleaning is needed, wipe the neck opening with gauze. If the breathing tubes are clogged, they can be removed or suctioned. The tracheostomy tube or stoma is suctioned by passing a sterile suction catheter through the external opening into the trachea. Do not insert the catheter more than 3 to 5 inches (7 to 12 cm) into the trachea. Once the airway is partially open, begin ventilations by the mouth-to-stoma method (mouth-to-stoma ventilation is bacteriologically cleaner than the mouth-to-mouth method) by using a pediatric-size pocket mask over the top of the stoma or by securing the airway with an ET tube placed through the stoma.

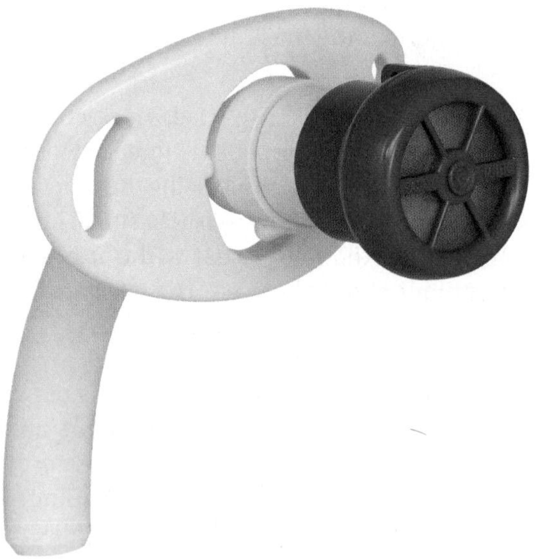

FIGURE 15-44 Passy Muir valve.

Image courtesy of Passy Muir, Inc. Irvine, CA.

The technique for stoma ventilation is basically the same as that for other methods of artificial ventilation. However, the patient's head should be kept straight (rather than tilted back), with the shoulders slightly elevated. This position allows more effective ventilation. If the patient's chest does not rise or if air is heard to escape through the patient's upper airway, the patient may be a "partial neck breather." These patients are able to inhale and exhale some air through their nose and mouth. If this occurs, the patient's nostrils must be pinched closed and the mouth sealed with the palm of one hand during ventilation. Alternately, ventilation over the nose and mouth can be attempted while occluding the stoma. Note that some patients who have a tracheostomy (such as those who had a laryngectomy) do not have an intact airway path between their upper airway and the stoma. Attempting to ventilate these patients in this manner will be unsuccessful.

Bag-Mask Devices

Bag-mask devices consist of a disposable self-inflating bag with a nonrebreathing valve (**FIGURE 15-45**). They can be used with a mask, an ET tube, or another invasive airway device. A bag-valve unit may have the following components:[24]

1. Suction ports to clear the airway
2. A medication administration port
3. A non–pop-off valve
4. Ports to sample ETCO$_2$
5. An oxygen inlet port at the back of the bag or by an oxygen reservoir
6. A nonrebreathing valve

The device should perform in all common environmental conditions and under extremes of temperature. It should be available in both adult and pediatric sizes. The mask should be clear to detect vomiting early.

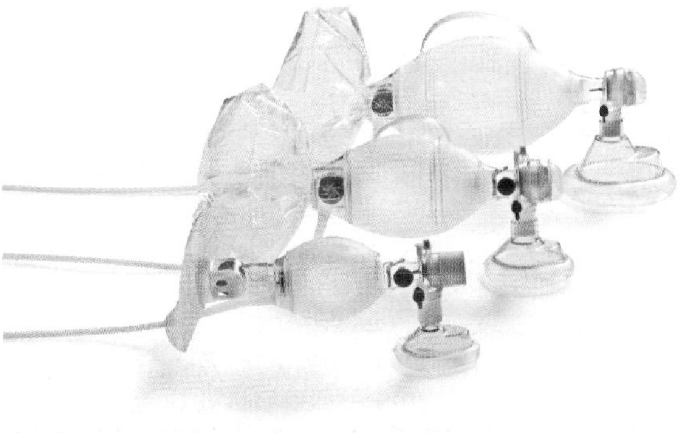

FIGURE 15-45 Disposable and reusable adult and pediatric bag-mask devices.

Reproduced with permission from Ambu.

> **NOTE**
>
> All paramedics should be proficient in delivering effective oxygenation and ventilation with a bag-mask device to adults, children, and infants.
>
> *Modified from*: American Heart Association. 2015 American Heart Association guidelines for cardiopulmonary resuscitation and emergency cardiovascular care. *Circulation.* 2015;132(18 suppl 2):S313-S314.

When the bag-mask device is compressed, air is delivered to the patient through a one-way valve. The air inlet to the bag is closed during delivery. When the bag is released, the patient's expired gas passes through an exhalation valve into the atmosphere. This design prevents the patient's exhaled air from reentering the bag-mask device. As the patient exhales, atmospheric air and supplemental oxygen from the reservoir refill the bag.

Use of the bag-mask device is difficult because of the problem of creating an effective seal between the mask and the patient's face while maintaining an open airway. It is easier when two rescuers use the device. One should hold the mask and maintain the airway while the other compresses the bag with two hands.[25]

When properly used, the bag-mask device has many benefits. The rescuer can provide a wide range of inspiratory pressures and volumes to adequately ventilate patients of varying sizes and underlying pathologic conditions. It can be used to assist patients with shallow respirations. It performs adequately in extremes of environmental temperatures. Oxygen concentrations ranging from 21% (room air concentration) to nearly 100% (using supplemental oxygen and a reservoir) can be achieved. In addition, manual compression of the bag can give the rescuer a sense of the patient's lung compliance, which is an advantage over mechanical methods of ventilation.

Technique

Ventilation with the bag-mask device is best accomplished when the patient has been intubated with an ET tube or a supraglottic device (eg, the King LT-D airway, laryngeal mask airway [LMA], or i-gel, which are described later in this chapter). If the patient has not been intubated, the bag-mask device may be used as follows:

1. The rescuer is positioned at the top of the patient's head.
2. If no spinal injury is suspected, place the patient in the optimum head tilt–chin lift position, with the patient's head elevated in extension. (If a spinal injury is suspected, spinal precautions should be used.) If the jaw-thrust maneuver does not produce an open airway, use the head tilt–chin lift maneuver.
3. Clear the airway of secretions, vomitus, and foreign objects. If the patient is unconscious, insert an oropharyngeal or a nasopharyngeal airway. The patient's mouth should remain open under the mask.
4. Connect an oxygen source. Then flush the reservoir with high-concentration oxygen.
5. Place the mask on the patient's face, making a tight seal. This can be accomplished by placing the thumb on the nose area and an index finger on the chin and then spreading the remaining fingers along the mandible (EC-clamp). The anterior displacement of the mandible must be maintained. To compress the bag, the rescuer's other hand presses the bag against his or her body (eg, the thigh), or another rescuer (if available) compresses the bag with two hands. The bag should be compressed smoothly, delivering approximately 500 to 600 mL over 1 second (for the average adult) to produce visible chest rise.

Pediatric Considerations

Smaller bag-mask devices are needed for infants and children. These specially sized devices help reduce the risk of overinflation and barotrauma. Bag-mask devices are used mainly for pediatric patients who are in respiratory arrest. Bag-mask devices equipped with a fish mouth– or leaf flap–operated outlet valve should not be used to provide supplemental oxygen to an infant or a child breathing spontaneously. If the valve fails to open during inspiration, the child receives only the exhaled gases from within the mask itself. For this reason, bag devices for ventilation of full-term neonates, infants, and children should have a minimum volume of 450 to 500 mL.[26] At least 10 to 15 L/min of oxygen flow is needed to maintain an adequate oxygen volume in the reservoir of a pediatric bag (**FIGURE 15-46**). Overventilation should be avoided because it can cause barotrauma and impair venous return. Recent evidence suggests that pediatric bag-mask devices may deliver sufficient volumes to ventilate adults.[27]

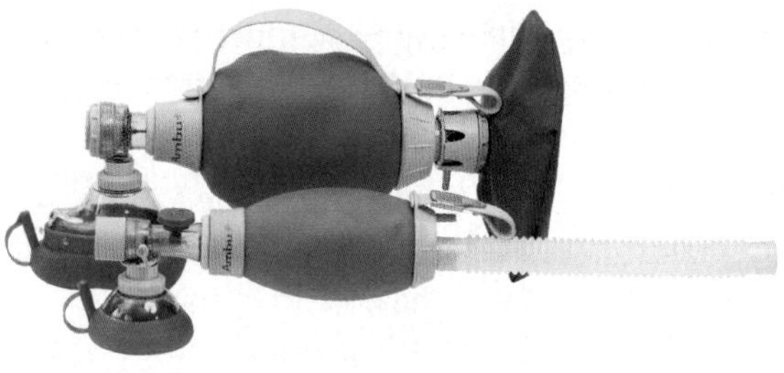

FIGURE 15-46 Pediatric bag-mask device.

SHOW ME THE EVIDENCE

A recent study enrolled 50 EMS providers from an urban fire-based EMS agency with 14.96 mean years of experience to determine if they could provide ventilations with a pediatric-sized bag-mask device that would be sufficient to ventilate adult patients. Only 1.5% of all breaths delivered with the pediatric bag-mask device during the ventilation scenarios were below the recommended tidal volume. A greater percentage of breaths delivered in the recommended range occurred when the pediatric bag-mask device was used (17.5% versus 5.1%, $P < 0.001$). Median volumes for each scenario were 570.5, 664.0, and 663.0 mL for the pediatric bag-mask device and 796.0, 994.5, and 981.5 mL for the adult bag-mask device. In all three categories of airway devices, the pediatric bag-mask device provided lower median tidal volumes ($P < 0.001$). The results suggest that ventilating an adult patient is possible with a smaller, pediatric-sized bag-mask device. The tidal volumes recorded with the pediatric bag-mask device were more consistent with lung-protective ventilation volumes.

Modified from: Siegler J, Kroll M, Wojcik S, Moy HP. Can EMS providers provide appropriate tidal volumes in a simulated adult-sized patient with a pediatric-sized bag-valve-mask? *Prehosp Emerg Care*. 2017;21(1):74-78.

NOTE

A child's flat nasal bridge makes achieving a mask seal difficult. In addition, compressing the mask against the face may result in obstruction. The mask seal is best achieved with jaw displacement using two rescuers to provide bag-mask ventilation.

Technique. The following procedure is used to artificially ventilate a pediatric patient with a bag-mask device:

1. Make sure the mask fits properly by using a length-based resuscitation tape or by measuring from the bridge of the nose to the cleft of the chin.
2. Make sure the mask is properly positioned and sealed. Place the mask over the mouth and nose (do not compress the eyes). With one hand, place a thumb on the mask at the apex and place the index finger on the mouth at the chin (like a C-clamp). With gentle pressure, push down on the mask to establish an adequate seal. Maintain the airway by lifting the bony prominence on the chin, with the remaining fingers placed on the mandible, forming an *E*. Avoid putting pressure on the soft area under the chin.
3. Provide ventilations at a rate of 12 to 20 breaths/min.
4. Deliver each breath over 1 second; both rescuers should make sure it produces visible chest rise.
5. Assess bag-mask ventilation by observing adequate rise and fall of the chest, by listening for lung sounds at the third intercostal space and midaxillary line, and by checking for improvement in skin color or heart rate, or both (see Chapter 19, *Secondary Assessment and Reassessment*).

CRITICAL THINKING

What should you do if you find that ventilating a nonintubated patient suddenly has become more difficult?

Automatic Transport Ventilators

Several types of time-cycled, gas-powered, ATVs are available. One commonly used in prehospital emergency care is the Autovent. The use of other more sophisticated transport ventilators is increasing. Presently, most are used for interhospital transport of patients who require ventilatory support (see the Appendix, *Advanced Practice Procedures for Critical Care Paramedics*). Most ATVs consist of a plastic control module. This module is connected by tubing to any 50-psi gas source (eg, air or different concentrations of oxygen, including 100% oxygen). Depending on the model, the exit valve of the control module is connected by one or two tubes to the patient valve assembly to deliver selected tidal volumes for adults and for children). Another control selects respiratory rates based on age. New models include other features such as inspiratory time. (Most ATVs are not to be used in children younger than 5 years.) Most units provide an oxygen flow rate of 40 L/min. This flow remains constant despite changes in the patient's airway or lung compliance.

NOTE

ATVs should have a default rate of 10 breaths/minute for adults and 20 breaths/minute for children. The paramedic should be able to adjust the rate once the patient has been intubated with a tracheal tube or alternative airway.

Modified from: American Heart Association. 2015 American Heart Association guidelines for cardiopulmonary resuscitation and emergency cardiovascular care. *Circulation*. 2015;132(18)(suppl 2):S313-S314.

The volume of gas delivered by the automatic ventilator is determined by the length of time the manual trigger is depressed or by the inspiratory effort of the spontaneously breathing patient. Most units are designed to limit the inspiratory pressure to 60 to 80 cm H_2O. When this pressure is reached, an alarm sounds and excess gas flow is vented off, preventing possible lung damage. On an intubated patient, or on a patient with an inserted supraglottic airway (SGA) device, ATVs allow the paramedic to perform other tasks. Most ATVs should not be used in patients who are awake, who have an obstructed airway, or who have increased airway resistance (eg, pneumothorax, asthma, pulmonary edema).

> **NOTE**
>
> Spontaneous breathing produces negative intrathoracic pressure during inspiration. It also plays an important role in maintaining cardiac output. It does this by enhancing venous return to the heart. Ventilations that are assisted with positive pressure ventilation using ATVs or bag-mask devices produce positive intrathoracic pressure during inspiration. This reduces venous return and, secondarily, cardiac output. That is, cardiac output decreases as air pressure increases. The paramedic should remember that assisted ventilations can impair cardiac output, even in patients with healthy hearts. This effect is exaggerated when the patient is ventilated at an excessive rate or tidal volume. This can be particularly harmful in cardiac arrest patients. The paramedic should consider use of an ITD to limit the influx of air in the lungs.
>
> *Modified from*: Demestiha TD, Pantazopoulos IN, Xanthos TT. Use of the impedance threshold device in cardiopulmonary resuscitation. *World J Cardiol*. 2010;2(2):19-26.

Airway Management

Science and technology have produced many devices for providing airway management. However, the paramedic must not neglect basic airway management procedures. A basic procedure that secures a safe and functional airway may be better than a more technically difficult procedure. Airway management should progress rapidly from the least to the most invasive procedures and devices (**FIGURE 15-47**). Paramedics

> **NOTE**
>
> Unconscious patients lack the muscular tone and control to maintain a patent airway. For this reason, an airway must be established and maintained in the initial assessment of all unconscious patients. Most injuries severe enough to cause loss of consciousness are severe enough to cause spinal injury. Spinal precautions should be considered in trauma patients who need airway management or ventilatory support.

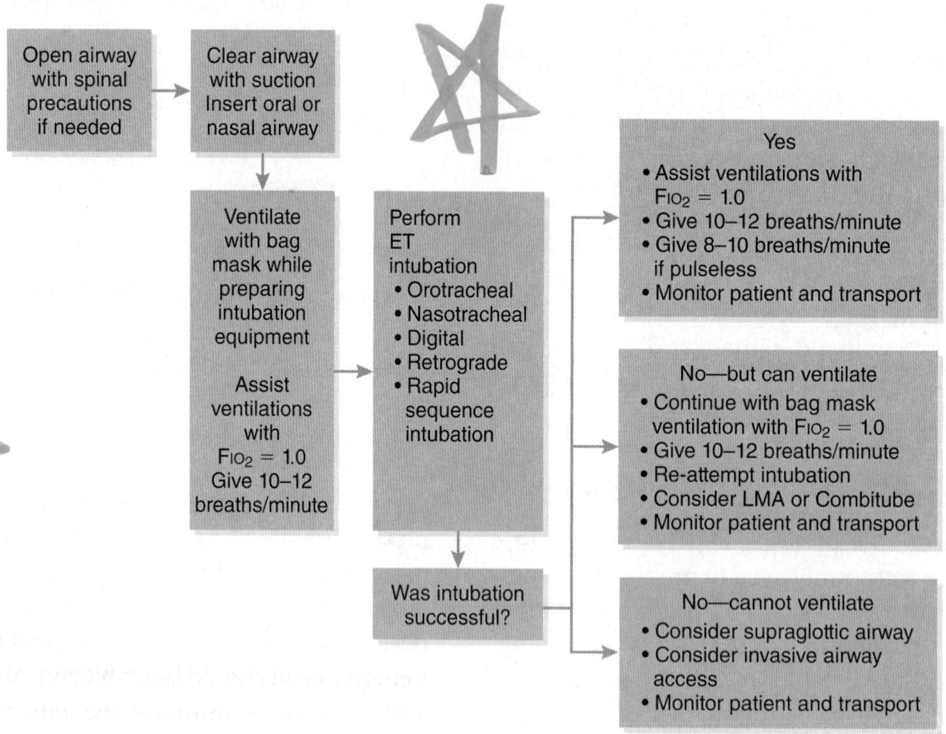

Notes:

Indications for emergency ET intubation are (1) the inability of the rescuer to adequately ventilate the unconscious patient with a bag and mask, and (2) the absence of protective reflexes (coma or cardiac arrest).

If more than one intubation attempt is required, there should be a period of adequate ventilations between attempts. Correct tube placement should be verified with primary and secondary confirmation methods.

Abbreviations: ET, endotracheal; FIO_2, fraction of inspired oxygen

FIGURE 15-47 Advanced airway management.

BOX 15-8 Personal Protective Equipment

The Centers for Disease Control and Prevention recommends that health care workers, in addition to taking the normal precautions for personal protection from communicable diseases, use masks, eyewear (eg, safety glasses, face shields), and gowns when splashing of blood or other body fluids is likely. During airway management, patients often vomit and cough. Exposure to blood and other body fluids is possible. Because of these possibilities, the paramedic should observe barrier precautions.

also should make sure they are always equipped with the appropriate personal protective equipment for these procedures (BOX 15-8).

Manual Techniques for Airway Management

Manual techniques for airway management include the head tilt–chin lift method, the jaw-thrust method, and the jaw-thrust without head-tilt method. The paramedic should not use manual maneuvers to open the airway in patients who are responsive or when attempts to open the patient's mouth are met with resistance. All such maneuvers are hazardous if spinal injury is a factor. In addition, none of these maneuvers protects against aspiration.

The head tilt–chin lift maneuver (**FIGURE 15-48**) is preferred for opening the airway when a spinal injury is not suspected. The head tilt is performed by placing one hand on the victim's forehead and applying firm backward pressure with the palm to tilt the head back. The fingers of the other hand then are placed under the bony part of the lower jaw (near the chin) and lifted to bring the chin forward. These fingers support the jaw and help maintain the head-tilt position.

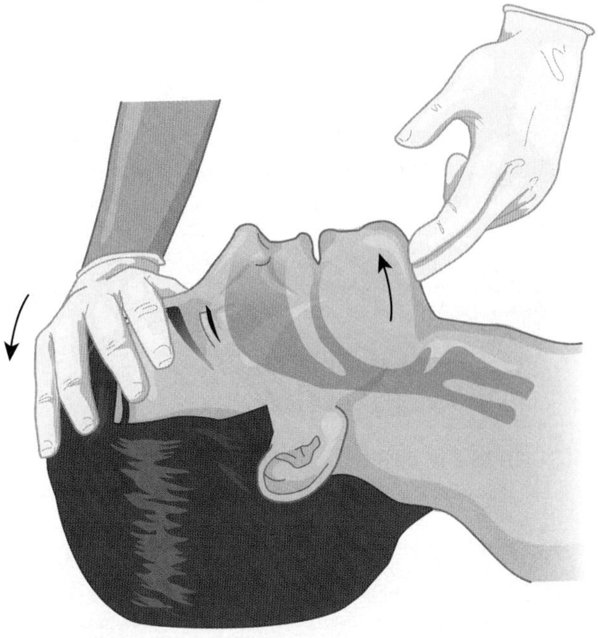

FIGURE 15-48 Head tilt–chin lift maneuver.

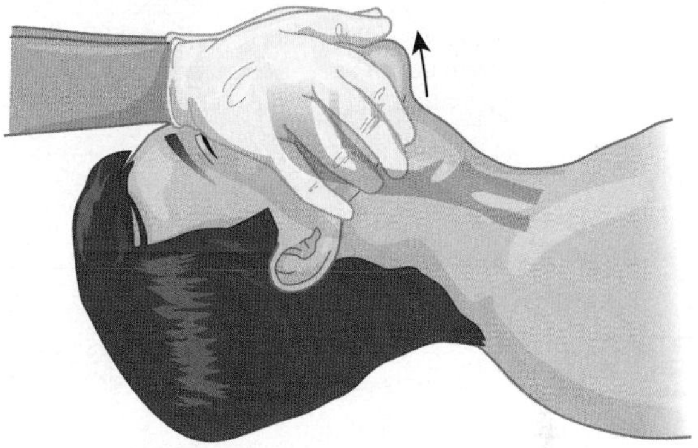

FIGURE 15-49 Jaw-thrust maneuver.

The jaw-thrust maneuver (**FIGURE 15-49**) may be used to gain additional forward displacement of the mandible if no spinal injury is suspected. This positioning is achieved by grasping the angles of the patient's lower jaw and lifting with both hands, one on each side. This technique displaces the mandible forward while tilting the head back. However, if the paramedic is unable to open the airway with the jaw-thrust maneuver, the head tilt–chin lift maneuver should be performed. An open airway remains the highest priority, even for an unresponsive trauma victim.

If a spinal injury is suspected, the jaw-thrust without head-tilt maneuver (**FIGURE 15-50**) should be used to open the airway. During this maneuver, the patient's head should be stabilized. Also, the cervical spine should be immobilized with neutral, in-line stabilization. The jaw-thrust maneuver should then proceed without extension of the neck.

Suction

Suction can be used to remove vomitus, saliva, blood, food, and other foreign objects that might block the airway or increase the likelihood of pulmonary

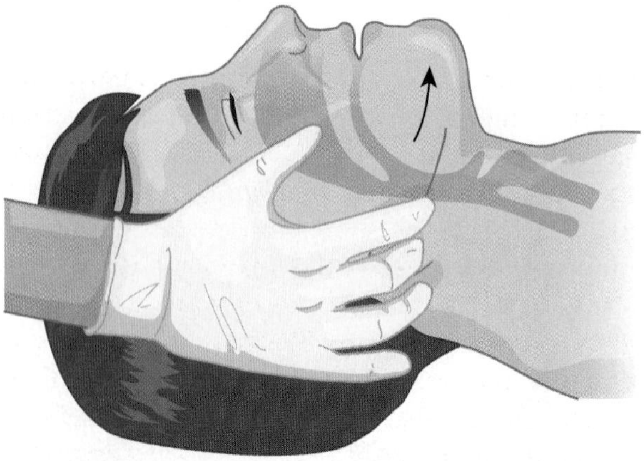

FIGURE 15-50 Jaw-thrust without head-tilt maneuver.

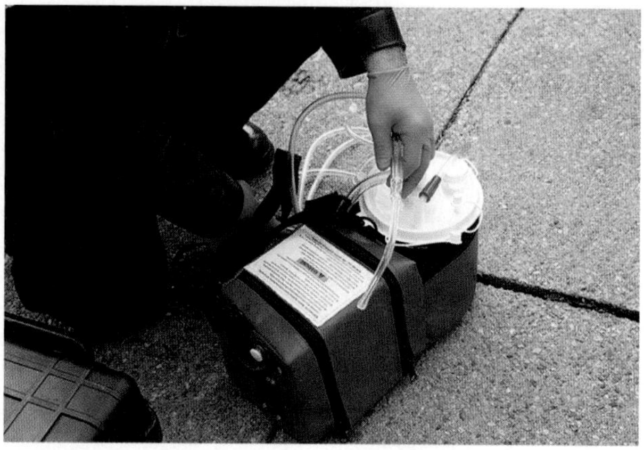

FIGURE 15-52 Portable suction unit.

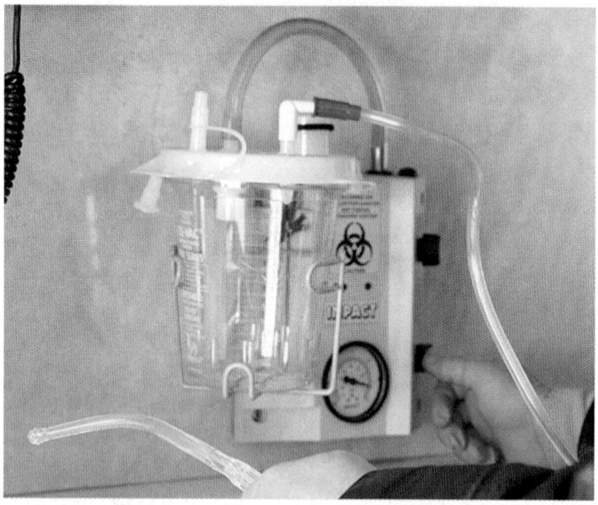

FIGURE 15-51 Fixed suction unit.

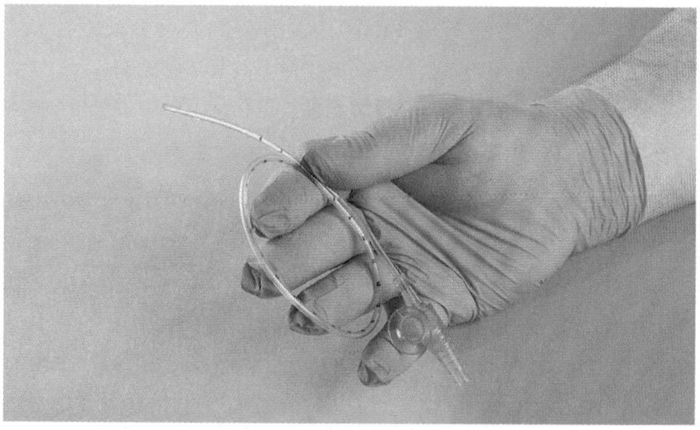

FIGURE 15-53 Soft (whistle-tip) suction catheter.

aspiration by inhalation. Many factors can predispose a person to aspiration. For this reason, every patient should be considered a possible aspiration victim.

Suction Devices

Fixed and portable mechanical suction devices are available through a number of manufacturers. Fixed suction devices (**FIGURE 15-51**) are mounted in patient care areas of hospitals and nursing homes. They also are used in many emergency vehicles. These systems are electrically operated by vacuum pumps or powered by the vacuum produced by a vehicle engine manifold. Fixed suction devices furnish an air intake of at least 40 L/min. They provide a vacuum of more than 300 mm Hg when the tube is clamped.

Portable suction devices may be oxygen or air powered, electrically powered, or manually powered (**FIGURE 15-52**). To operate effectively, these devices should furnish an air intake of no less than 20 L/min.

Suction Catheters

Suction catheters are used to clear secretions and debris from the oral cavity and airway passages. The two broad classifications of catheters are whistle-tip suction catheters and tonsil-tip suction catheters.

The whistle-tip catheter is a narrow, flexible tube. It is used primarily for tracheobronchial suctioning to clear secretions through either an ET tube or the nasopharynx (**FIGURE 15-53**). Some are supplied in a protective sheath that maintains sterility when the intubated trachea is suctioned. The flexible catheter is designed with molded ends and side holes to cause minimal trauma to the mucosa. It should be lubricated

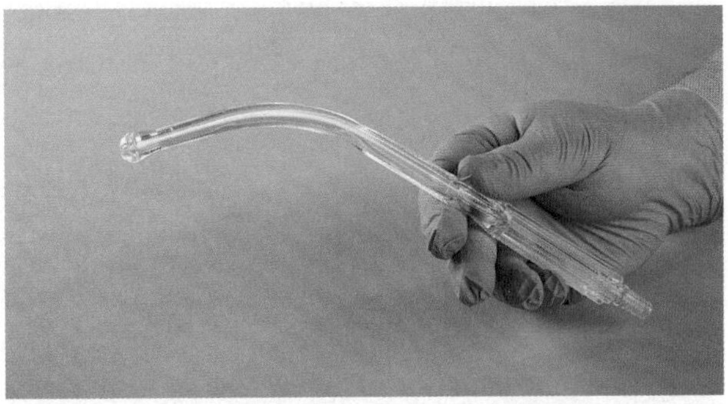

FIGURE 15-54 Rigid (tonsil-tip, or Yankauer) suction catheter.

before insertion. A side opening in the proximal end is covered with the thumb to produce suction. Using sterile technique, the paramedic advances the catheter to the desired location. Suction is applied intermittently as the catheter is withdrawn.

The tonsil-tip (Yankauer) suction catheter is a rigid pharyngeal catheter. It is used to clear secretions, blood clots, and other foreign material from the mouth and pharynx (**FIGURE 15-54**). The device is carefully inserted into the oral cavity under direct visualization. It is then slowly withdrawn while suction is activated.

Before any suctioning is begun, all equipment should be checked. For adults, the suction should be set between minus 80 and minus 120 mm Hg. If possible, the patient's lungs should be oxygenated with 100% oxygen for at least 2 minutes before suction is initiated. Suction should not be applied for longer than 10 seconds in adult patients.[28] It should not be applied for longer than 5 seconds in pediatric patients. If more suctioning is needed, the patient's lungs should be reoxygenated first. Possible complications from suctioning include the following:

- Sudden hypoxemia that occurs secondary to decreased lung volume during the application of suction
- Severe hypoxemia that may lead to cardiac rhythm disturbances and cardiac arrest
- Airway stimulation that may increase arterial pressure and cardiac rhythm disturbances
- Coughing that may result in increased intracranial pressure with reduced blood flow to the brain and increased risk of herniation in patients with head injury
- Bradycardia related to vagal stimulation
- Soft-tissue damage to the respiratory tract

Tracheobronchial Suctioning

Before tracheobronchial suctioning is performed through an ET tube (**FIGURE 15-55**), the patient should be oxygenated with 100% oxygen for 30 to 60 seconds.[29] For tracheal suctioning, a Y- or T-piece or a lateral opening should lie between the suction tube and the source of the on–off suction control. Using sterile technique, the paramedic advances the catheter to the desired location (about the level of the carina). Suction is applied intermittently by closing the side opening as the catheter is withdrawn in a rotating motion. The patient's cardiac rhythm should be monitored throughout the procedure. If dysrhythmias or bradycardia develops, suctioning should stop. The patient then should be manually ventilated and oxygenated. Before suctioning is resumed, the patient should again be ventilated with 100% oxygen for 30 to 60 seconds.

> **NOTE**
> It may be necessary to instill 3 to 5 mL of sterile saline down the ET tube to loosen secretions before suctioning.

Gastric Distention

Gastric distention results from the trapping of air in the stomach. As the stomach enlarges, it pushes against the diaphragm and interferes with lung expansion. The abdomen becomes more and more distended (especially in small children). Resistance may be felt to bag-mask ventilation.

Management of gastric distention begins by slightly increasing the bag-mask ventilation inspiratory time. Large-volume suction should be readily available. If possible, the patient should be placed in a left lateral recumbent position. Gastric distention that cannot be managed with these techniques may require insertion of a gastric tube (**FIGURE 15-56**).

Gastric Tubes

Gastric distention is very common in patients who are ventilated but have not been intubated. Gastric decompression for gastric distention or vomiting control can be achieved through nasogastric (NG) or orogastric (OG) emptying or decompression of the stomach. Gastric decompression is done with extreme caution in patients who have esophageal trauma or esophageal disease. Gastric decompression should

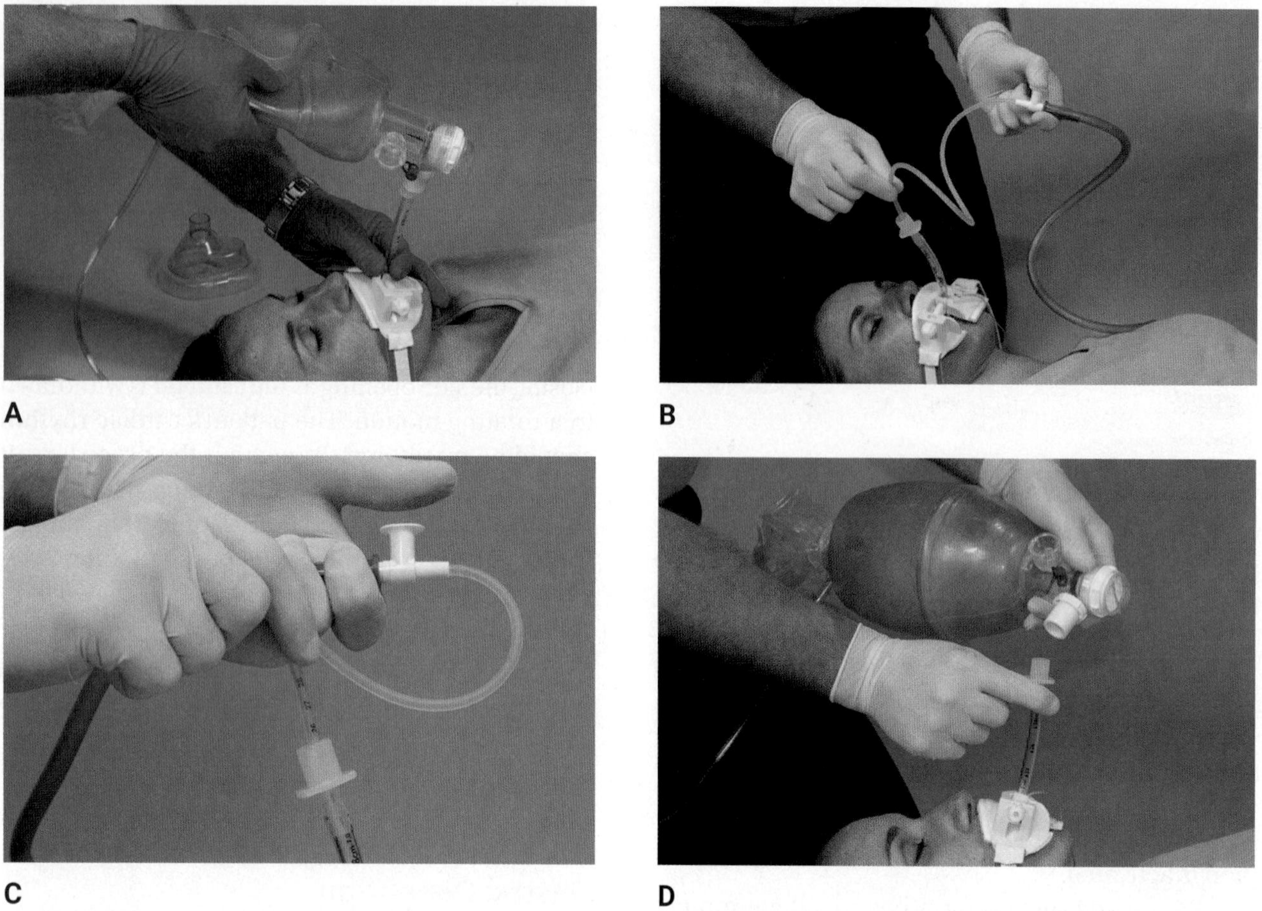

FIGURE 15-55 Tracheobronchial suctioning. **A.** Preoxygenate the patient. **B.** Introduce the suction catheter through the endotracheal tube without suction. **C.** Withdraw the catheter with suction intermittently applied while observing the electrocardiographic rhythm. **D.** Ventilate the patient and reevaluate the respiratory status. In-line capnography should always be used to confirm tube placement. Monitor tube position before and after suctioning.

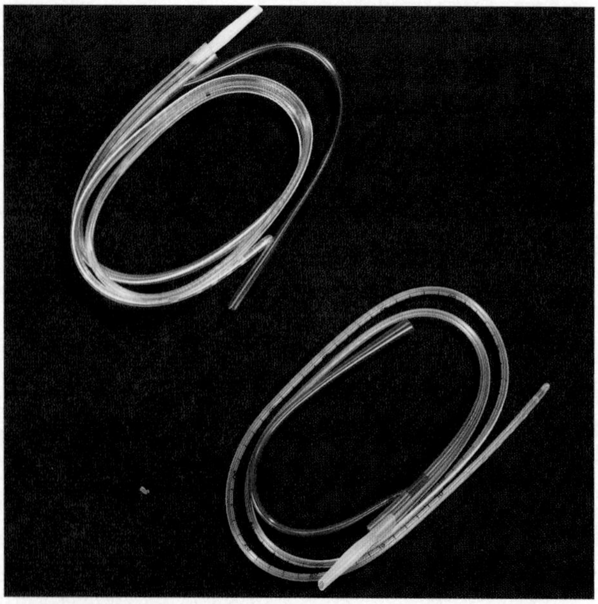

FIGURE 15-56 Nasogastric/orogastric tubes.

not be performed if an esophageal obstruction is present. NG decompression should not be attempted in a patient with facial trauma.

NG Decompression

1. Prepare the patient. Position the patient in a high Fowler position (if condition permits).
   - Place the head in a neutral position.
   - Preoxygenate and monitor oxygen saturation as measured by arterial blood sampling (Sao_2).
   - Instill a topical anesthetic per protocol (check for allergies).
   - Select the larger nostril.
2. Measure the NG tube from the patient's nose to the ear and from the ear to the xiphoid process to determine the correct insertion length. Lubricate the tube with viscous lidocaine or water-soluble lubricant per protocol (**FIGURE 15-57**).
3. Advance the tube gently along the nasal floor and into the stomach. (Having the patient swallow

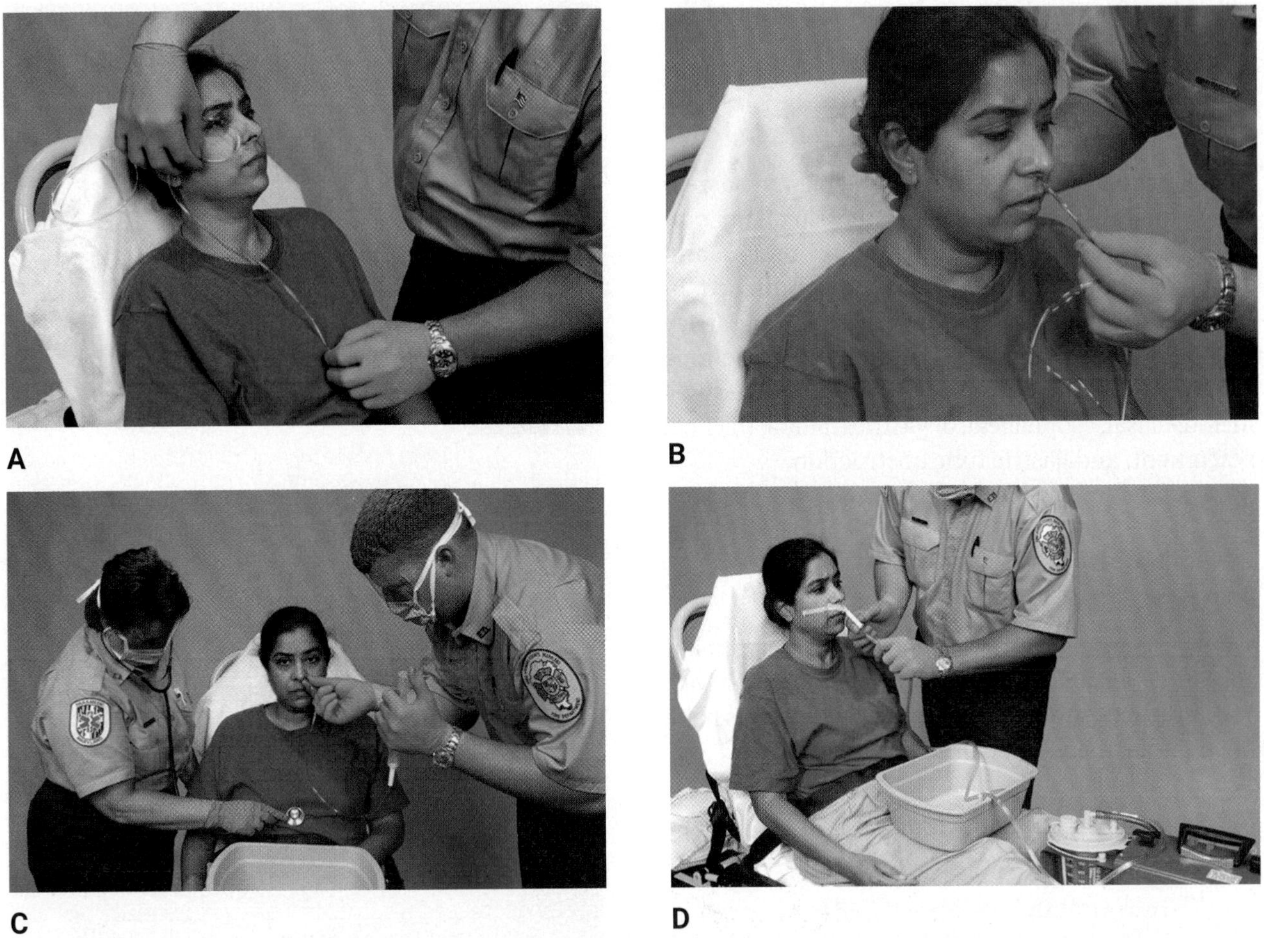

FIGURE 15-57 Insertion of a nasogastric tube. **A.** Position the patient. Measure the tube from the nose to the ear and from the ear to the xiphoid process. **B.** Lubricate the tube and insert it into the larger nostril. Advance the tube to the proper length. **C.** Verify correct placement of the tube by aspirating gastric contents. **D.** Secure the tube and attach the suction unit.

during insertion may help advance the tube into the esophagus and prevent tracheal insertion.) If the patient is conscious and starts to cough vigorously, do not advance the tube during inspiration.

4. Using a penlight, visualize the posterior pharynx to be sure the tube is not coiled in the back of the throat.
5. Confirm placement per agency protocol.
   - Aspirate gastric contents in the NG tube.
   - Check aspirate with color-coded pH paper. A pH of 1.0 to 4.0 indicates gastric placement.[30]
   - Tube placement is confirmed by radiograph in the hospital.
6. Secure the NG tube in place and attach to suction if indicated.

OG Decompression

1. Prepare the patient and tube as described for NG insertion.

DID YOU KNOW?

Some clinical sites no longer use auscultation as a method to verify NG tube placement. pH testing and radiographic verification are used instead. Aspiration of gastric contents provides a means of measuring fluid pH and of verifying placement of the tube tip in the GI tract. The aspirate is obtained by attaching a catheter-tipped syringe to the end of the tube and pulling back gently on the syringe. (The aspirate usually is cloudy and green, off-white, tan, bloody, or brown.) The pH of the aspirate is measured with color-coded pH paper that is graded in whole numbers from 1 to 11. Gastric secretions usually are highly acidic (preferably 4 or lower), compared with intestinal aspirates (usually greater than 4) or respiratory secretions (usually greater than 5.5).

Modified from: Perry AG, Potter P, Ostendorf WR, Laplante N. *Clinical Nursing Skills and Techniques*. 9th ed. St. Louis, MO: Elsevier; 2018.

2. Introduce the OG tube down the midline of the oropharynx and into the stomach.
3. Confirm placement. Secure the OG tube as described for NG insertion.

Complications of Gastric Decompression. Whatever the method chosen, gastric decompression is uncomfortable for the patient. It may induce nausea and vomiting even when the gag reflex is suppressed. In addition, gastric tubes interfere with mask seals. They also interfere with visualization of airway structures during intubation. Complications of the procedures include nasal, esophageal, or gastric trauma; tracheal placement; and gastric tube obstruction.

Mechanical Adjuncts in Airway Management

The use of mechanical devices for airway management should never delay manual opening of the airway. These devices should be used only after efforts have been made to open the airway manually.

Nasopharyngeal Airway (Nasal Airway)

Nasal airways (**FIGURE 15-58**) are used to maintain an open airway passage in unconscious patients or in patients who are responsive but not alert enough to control their own airway. Insertion of a nasal airway may be useful as a temporary airway maintenance maneuver. It may be used to control the airway in patients with seizures or possible cervical spine injury. It also may be used before nasotracheal intubation (described later in this chapter). In addition, it can serve as a guide for insertion of an NG tube.

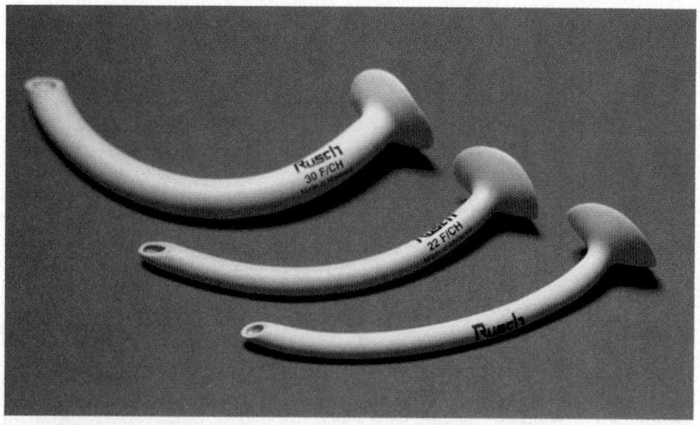

FIGURE 15-58 Nasal airways.

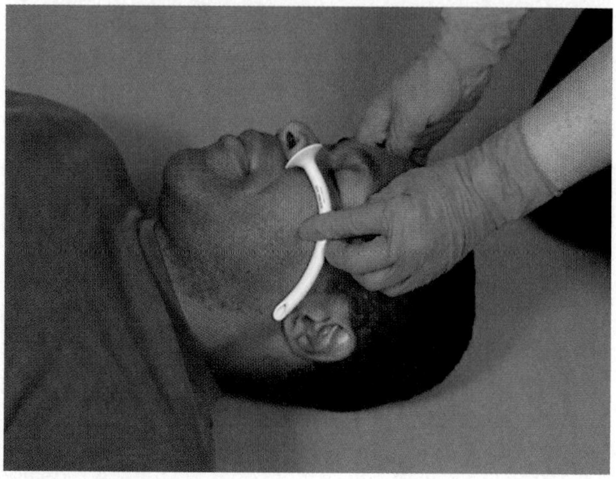

FIGURE 15-59 Measuring a nasal airway.

> CRITICAL THINKING
>
> Think about two or three specific patient conditions that would warrant the use of a nasal airway.

Description

Nasal airways are soft and pliable, have a gentle curve, and have a flared outer end. They are available in a variety of sizes to accommodate infants and adults. They range in length from 17 to 20 cm (about 7 to 8 inches) and in diameter from 12 to 36 French. As with most other catheters, the French scale system is used to indicate internal diameter. Each unit of the scale equals about one-third of 1 millimeter. A 21 French catheter, for example, is 7 mm (about 0.3 inch) in diameter. The following are recommended sizes of nasopharyngeal airways:

- Large adult: internal diameter of 8 to 9 mm (0.3 to 0.35 inch), or 24 to 27 French
- Medium adult: internal diameter of 7 to 8 mm (about 0.3 inch), or 21 to 24 French
- Small adult: internal diameter of 6 to 7 mm (about 0.25 inch), or 18 to 21 French

To determine the correct size for a patient, the paramedic should choose an airway with a tube length equal to the distance from the tip of the patient's nose to the earlobe (**FIGURE 15-59**). The paramedic should use the guide on a length-based resuscitation tape to select the proper size for pediatric airway devices.

Insertion

The nasal airway should be lubricated with a water-soluble lubricant to help ease the airway through the nasal cavity. The device is placed in the nostril with the beveled tip (designed to protect nasal structures) directed toward the nasal septum. The airway is gently passed close to the midline, along the floor of the nostril, following the natural curve of the nasal passage. The airway should not be forced. If resistance is encountered, rotating the tube slightly may help, or insertion can be attempted through the other nostril (**FIGURE 15-60**).

After insertion, the nasal airway rests in the posterior pharynx behind the tongue. If the patient begins to gag, the tube may be stimulating the posterior pharynx. It may be necessary to remove the airway or withdraw it 0.5 to 1 cm (0.25 to 0.5 inch) and reinsert it. The paramedic should maintain displacement of the mandible with either the head tilt–chin lift or the jaw-thrust without head-tilt maneuver when using this airway.

Advantages

- A nasal airway is well tolerated by conscious and semiconscious patients with an intact gag reflex.
- Insertion is a quick procedure.
- A nasal airway may be used when insertion of an oropharyngeal airway is contraindicated or difficult because of oral trauma or soft-tissue injury.

Possible Complications

- Long nasal airways may enter the esophagus.
- The airway may precipitate laryngospasm and vomiting in patients with a gag reflex.
- The airway may injure the nasal mucosa, causing bleeding and possibly airway obstruction.
- Small-diameter airways may become obstructed by mucus, blood, vomitus, and the soft tissues of the pharynx.
- A nasal airway does not protect the lower airway from aspiration.
- Suctioning through a nasal airway is difficult.

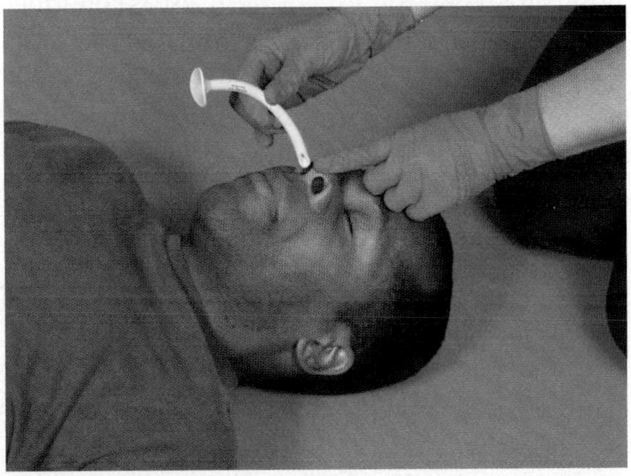

FIGURE 15-60 Insertion of a nasal airway.

Oropharyngeal Airway (Oral Airway)

Oral airways are designed to prevent the tongue from obstructing the glottis. They are indicated in unconscious or semiconscious patients who have no gag reflex and in intubated patients who are trying to bite the ET tube.

Description

The oral airway is a semicircular device designed to hold the tongue away from the posterior wall of the pharynx. Most oropharyngeal airways are made of disposable plastic. The two types of airways most often used are the Guedel airway and the Berman airway. The Guedel airway is distinguished by its tubular design. The Berman airway is distinguished by the airway channels along each side of the device (**FIGURE 15-61**).

Like nasopharyngeal airways, oral airways are available in a variety of sizes ranging from infant to adult. The size is based on the distance in millimeters from the flange to the distal tip. The proper size for the patient may be determined by placing the airway next to the patient's face so that the flange is at the level of the central incisors and the bite block segment is

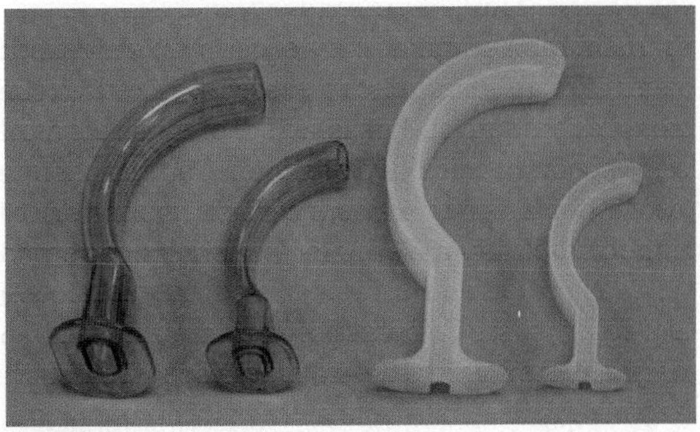

FIGURE 15-61 Oral airways.

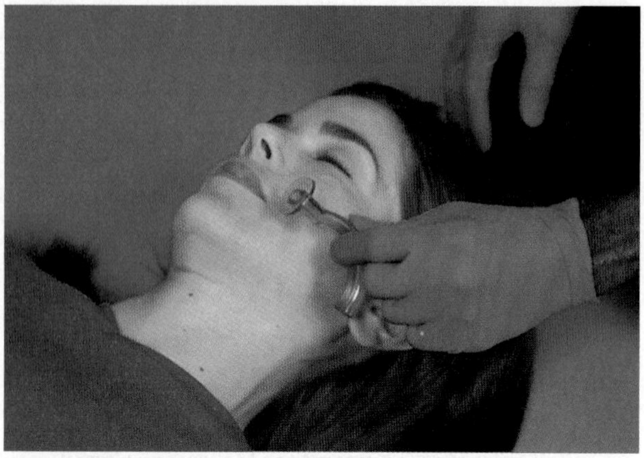

FIGURE 15-62 Measuring an oral airway.

parallel to the hard palate. The airway should extend from the corner of the mouth to the tip of the earlobe or the angle of the jaw (**FIGURE 15-62**). The following sizes are recommended[26]:

- Large adult: 100 mm (about 4 inches), which is Guedel size 5
- Medium adult: 90 mm (about 3.5 inches), which is Guedel size 4
- Small adult: 80 mm (about 3.1 inches), which is Guedel size 3

Insertion

Before an oral airway is inserted, the mouth and pharynx should be cleared of all secretions, blood, or vomitus. In an adult or older child, the oral airway may be inserted upside down or at a 90° angle (**FIGURE 15-63A**). This approach helps the paramedic avoid catching the tongue during insertion. As the oral airway passes the crest of the tongue, it is rotated into the proper position. It should be situated against the posterior wall of the oropharynx.

A different method of insertion is recommended for pediatric patients (**FIGURE 15-63B**). (It also can be used in adults.) A tongue blade or bite stick is used to displace the tongue inferiorly and anteriorly. The airway then is inserted and moved posteriorly toward the back of the oropharynx, following the normal curve of the oral cavity. Regardless of the method of insertion, care must be taken to prevent trauma to the face and oral cavity. In addition, the paramedic should make sure the patient's lips and tongue are not caught between the teeth and the airway.

Proper placement of the airway is confirmed by observable chest wall expansion. It also is confirmed by good breath sounds on auscultation of the lungs during ventilation. It is important to remember that even with an oral airway in place, the patient's head must be kept in proper position. This helps ensure a patent airway.

> CRITICAL THINKING
> Why is the alternative method of oral airway insertion used for infants and young children?

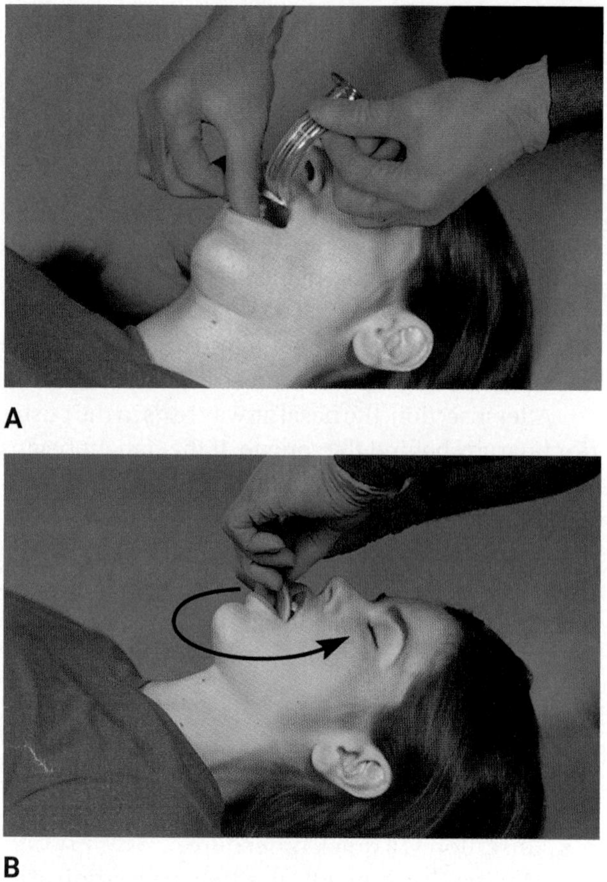

FIGURE 15-63 A. Inserting an oral airway upside down. **B.** Rotate oral airway 180 degrees after partial insertion to conform to contour of tongue.

Advantages

- An oral airway secures the tongue forward and down, away from the posterior pharynx.
- It provides easy access for airway suction.
- It serves as a bite block to protect an ET tube and the airway in the event of seizures.

Possible Complications

Even experienced paramedics may have difficulty managing the patient's airway in some situations (**BOX 15-9**), highlighting the importance of ongoing

BOX 15-9 Difficult Airway

A "difficult airway" can be defined as a clinical situation in which an experienced practitioner has difficulty with mask ventilation, tracheal intubation, or both. The airway should be examined before airway management in all patients. Examination is done to identify physical characteristics that may indicate the presence of or potential for a difficult airway. Paramedics should assess the following airway features.

Feature	Sign of Difficult Airway
Length of upper incisors	Relatively long
Relation of maxillary and mandibular incisors with normal jaw closure	Prominent overbite
Visibility of uvula	Not visible when tongue is protruded (eg, larger than Mallampati class II)
Shape of palate	Highly arched or very narrow
Length of neck	Short
Thickness of neck	Thick
Range of motion of head and neck	Inability to touch tip of chin to chest or extend neck

Mallampati Signs as Indicators of Difficult Intubation

Class I (soft palate, uvula, fauces, pillars visible)—No difficulty
Class II (soft palate, uvula, fauces visible)—No difficulty
Class III (soft palate, base of uvula visible)—Moderate difficulty
Class IV (hard palate only visible)—Severe difficulty

The following also may be indicators of a potentially difficult airway:

- Immobilized trauma patient
- Morbidly obese patient
- Child
- Limited jaw opening
- Upper airway conditions (eg, angioedema, burns, neck injury, epiglottitis)
- Facial trauma
- Laryngeal trauma

If a difficult airway is evident, advanced airway management is required, as presented in the algorithm in **FIGURE 15-64**.

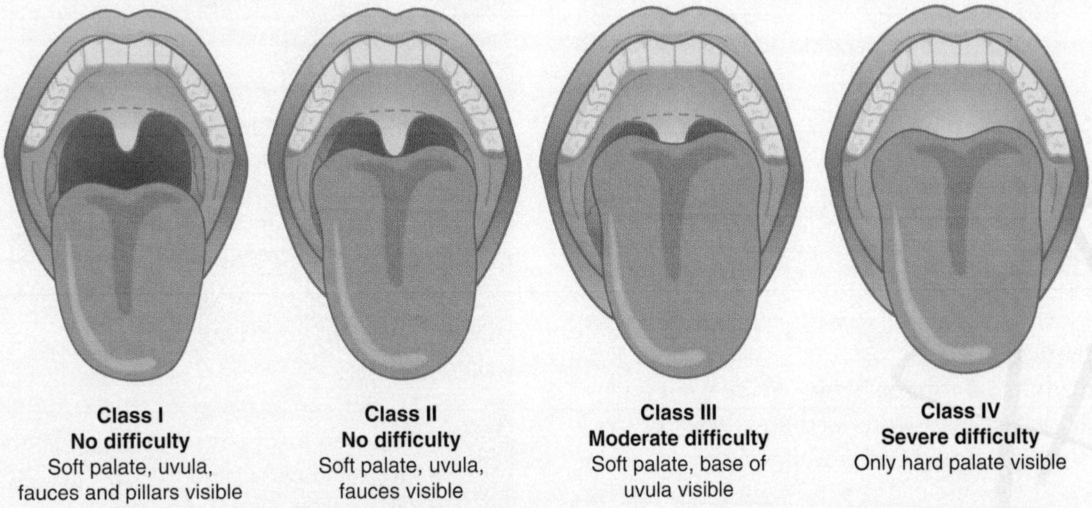

Reproduced from: Tariq S, Deshpande J. Preoperative assessment. In: McInerny TK, Adam HM, Campbell DE, DeWitt TG, Foy JM, Kamat DM, eds. *American Academy of Pediatrics Textbook of Pediatric Care*. Itasca, IL: American Academy of Pediatrics; 2017.

Modified from: Apfelbaum JL, Hagberg CA, Caplan RA, Blitt CD, Connis RT. Practice guidelines for management of the difficult airway: an updated report by the American Society of Anesthesiologists Task Force on Management of the Difficult Airway. *Anesthesiology*. 2013;118(2):251-270.

Airway Management

Airway Management Indicated

↓

Manual cervical spine stabilization

↓

Essential Skills
Manual clearing of airway
Manual maneuvers
• Trauma jaw thrust
• Trauma chin lift
Suctioning
Basic adjuncts
• Oropharyngeal airway
• Nasopharyngeal airway

↓

Advanced skills?

No / Yes

No:
Assist ventilations F_{IO_2} >0.85
↓
Complete primary survey
↓
Rapid transport

Yes:
Intubation skills?

No / Yes

No:
Supraglottic airway
↓
Assist ventilations F_{IO_2} >0.85
↓
Complete primary survey
↓
Rapid transport

Yes:
ET intubation
• Orotracheal[a]
• Nasotracheal[b]
↓
Successful[c]

Yes / No

Yes:
Assist ventilations F_{IO_2} >0.85
↓
Complete primary survey
↓
Rapid transport

Notes:
[a]Face-to-face intubation may be used if patient position is an issue for performing traditional orotracheal intubation; pharmacologically assisted intubation may be used to facilitate orotracheal intubation if properly trained and authorized.

[b]Blind nasotracheal intubation should only be used in spontaneously breathing patients.

[c]Intubation should be limited to three attempts, and proper placement should be confirmed.

[d]Ventilation attempted using essential skills in combination with bag-mask device.

[e]Retrograde intubation may be performed if properly trained and authorized.

[f]Digital intubation should only be attempted in unconscious, apneic patients.

[g]Percutaneous transtracheal catheter ventilation; surgical cricothyrotomy may be performed if properly trained and authorized.

Difficult Airway

No:
Able to ventilate?[d]

Yes / No

Yes:
Options
• Essential skills
• Supraglottic airway
• Retrograde intubation[e]
• Digital intubation[f]
↓
Assist ventilations F_{IO_2} >0.85
↓
Complete primary survey
↓
Rapid transport

No:
Options
Supraglottic airway
↓
Able to ventilate?

Yes / No

No: Invasive airway access[g]

↓

Assist ventilations F_{IO_2} >0.85
↓
Complete primary survey
↓
Rapid transport

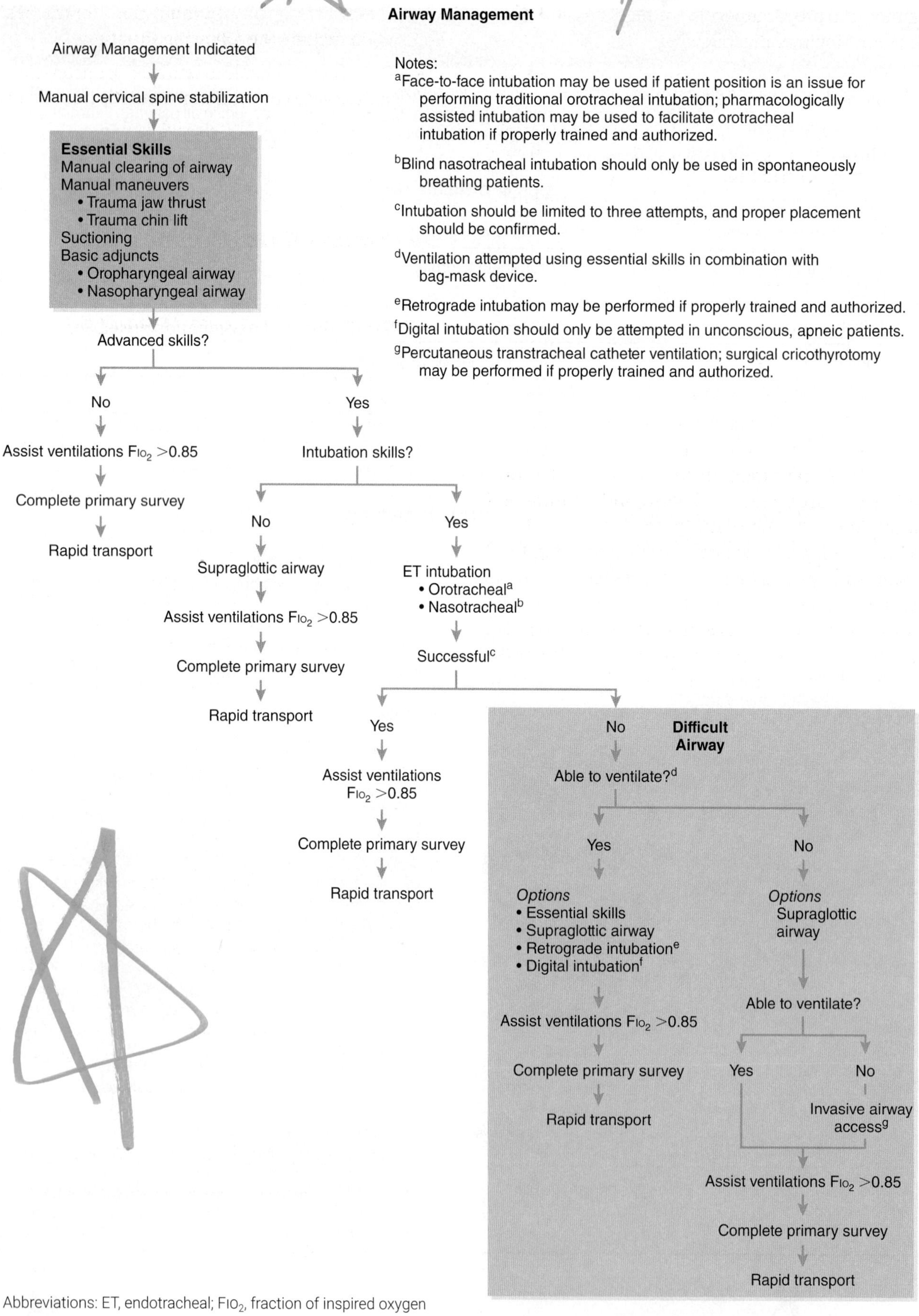

Abbreviations: ET, endotracheal; F_{IO_2}, fraction of inspired oxygen

FIGURE 15-64 Difficult airway algorithm.

training and preparedness in the field. Possible complications include the following:

- Oral airways that are too small may fall back into the oral cavity, resulting in blockage of the airway.
- Long airways may press the epiglottis against the entrance of the trachea, producing a complete airway obstruction.
- The airway may stimulate vomiting and laryngospasm in a patient with a gag reflex.
- The airway does not protect the lower airway from aspiration.
- Improper insertion may push the tongue back, causing it to obstruct the airway.

Advanced Airway Procedures

Advanced airway procedures described in this text include subglottic and supraglottic procedures (BOX 15-10). The subglottic procedures are ET intubation, digital or blind intubation, and nasotracheal intubation. The supraglottic procedures include the LMA, esophageal-tracheal Combitube, King LT-D airway, and i-gel. All these procedures require special training. Before performing advanced airway procedures, the paramedic must either receive authorization from medical direction or be operating under written protocols. The paramedic also should be aware that long-term complications may result from these procedures. This risk exists even when the procedures are performed properly. Such complications include aspiration, tracheal stenosis, transient dysphagia, and voice changes.

Endotracheal Intubation

Tracheal intubation is the most definitive technique for controlling the airway in patients who are unable to maintain an open airway. Indications for tracheal intubation include the following situations:

- The rescuer is unable to ventilate an unconscious patient with conventional methods (mouth-to-mask method, bag-mask device).
- The patient cannot protect his or her own airway (coma, respiratory, and cardiac arrest).
- Prolonged artificial ventilation is needed.

The advantages of tracheal intubation are:

- The airway is isolated, which prevents aspiration of material into the lower airway.
- Ventilation and oxygenation are easier.

BOX 15-10 Advanced Airway Procedures

Subglottic Procedures

ET intubation
Digital or blind intubation
Nasotracheal intubation

Supraglottic Procedures

LMA
i-gel
King LT-D airway
Esophageal-tracheal Combitube

SHOW ME THE EVIDENCE

Researchers in Cincinnati, Ohio, performed a meta-analysis to determine if patient outcomes from prehospital cardiac arrest were different in those who received ET intubation compared with those who had a SGA placed. The exclusion criteria included trauma, pediatrics, physician or nurse intubators, rapid sequence intubation, video intubation, and older airway devices. Ten observational studies evaluated included over 34,000 ET intubation and 41,000 SGA patients. ROSC, survival to hospital admission, and neurologically intact survival were significantly higher in the ET intubation group than in the SGA group. Survival to hospital discharge was not statistically different.

That same year, some of the same researchers reached a slightly different conclusion.

Researchers examined data from 10,691 adult prehospital cardiac arrests from the Cardiac Arrest Registry to Enhance Survival (CARES) database. In these cases, they compared neurologically intact survival rates (survival) after cardiac arrest based on whether the airway was managed with ET intubation, SGA, or no advanced airway. They found that patient survival was higher in the ET intubation group (5.4%) compared with the SGA group (5.2%). Compared with SGA, the odds of survival in the ET intubation group was higher (OR, 1.44; 95% CI, 1.10–1.88). However, the group with no advanced airway had the highest rate of survival (18.6%). When compared with ET intubation or SGA, the odds of survival were significantly greater (OR, 4.24; 95% CI, 3.46–5.20). The authors caution that their findings must be viewed in light of the methods and that a prospective study is needed to confirm their results.

Modified from: Benoit JL, Gerecht RB, Steuerwald MT, McMullan JT. Endotracheal intubation versus supraglottic airway placement in out-of-hospital cardiac arrest: a meta-analysis. *Resuscitation*. 2015;93:20-26; McMullan J, Gerecht R, Bonomo J, et al; CARES Surveillance Group. Airway management and out-of-hospital cardiac arrest outcome in the CARES registry. *Resuscitation*. 2014;85(5):617-622.

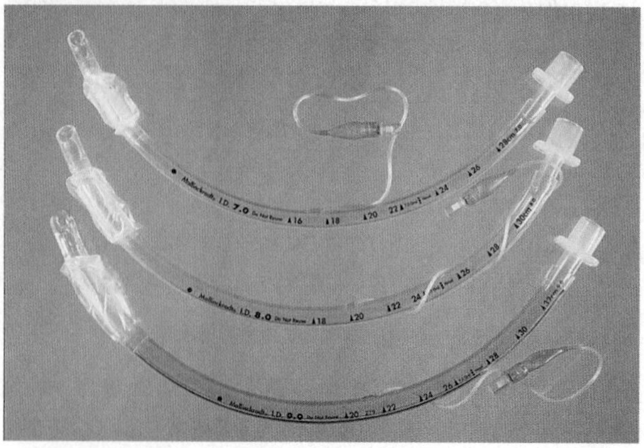

FIGURE 15-65 Endotracheal tubes.

- Suctioning of the trachea and bronchi is easier.
- Wasted ventilation and gastric insufflation are prevented during positive pressure ventilation.
- A route is provided for administration of some medications (eg, naloxone, atropine, vasopressin, epinephrine, and lidocaine [NAVEL]).

Description

The common ET tube is a flexible tube open at both ends (**FIGURE 15-65**). The proximal end has a standard 15-mm (about 0.6-inch) adapter. This adapter connects to various oxygen delivery devices for positive pressure ventilation. The end of the tube that is inserted into the trachea is beveled to aid placement between the vocal cords. The adult tube size (5 or larger) has a balloon cuff that closes off the remainder of the tracheal opening. This cuff prevents aspiration of fluids around the tube. It also minimizes air leakage during ventilation. The cuff is attached to a small tube. This tube has a one-way inflating valve with a port designed to fit a standard syringe. A properly positioned ET tube with the cuff inflated allows administration of high concentrations of oxygen at controlled pressures.

> NOTE
>
> Some EMS medical directors prefer the use of supraglottic procedures over subglottic procedures to initially secure a patient's airway. Paramedics should follow protocols and standing orders when providing advanced airway care.

In addition to the common ET tube, specialized variations are available. An example is a tube with medication ports for ET drug administration.

ET Tube Sizes

The markings on the ET tube indicate the internal diameter of the tube in millimeters. (The tubes are available in graduated sizes from 2.5 to 10 mm.) The length of the tube from the distal end is indicated in centimeters at several levels. Recommended ET tube sizes are 7- to 8-mm (about 0.3-inch) internal diameter for men and 7-mm (about 0.25-inch) internal diameter for women.[23] Tube sizes are expressed simply as "size 6" or "size 7," without the millimeter designation.

Infant and pediatric ET tubes are available with and without balloon cuffs. Children younger than 8 to 10 years have a circular narrowing at the level of the cricoid cartilages. This narrowing serves as a functional cuff. It minimizes air leakage at the cricoid ring. Accordingly, uncuffed ET tubes are sometimes used for this age group (see Chapter 23, *Respiratory*).

Various methods can be used to determine the correct ET tube size for infants and children. Tracheal tube size for children older than 1 year may be estimated using one of the following equations:[26]

Uncuffed tube:

$$\text{Tracheal tube size (mm)} = \frac{\text{Age (yr)}}{4} + 4$$

Cuffed tube:

$$\text{Tracheal tube size (mm)} = \frac{\text{Age (yr)}}{4} + 3.5$$

A more reliable method for selecting the correct ET tube size is to use length-based resuscitation tapes (for children up to 77 pounds [35 kg]) (see Chapter 47, *Pediatrics*). Suggested sizes for ET tubes and suction catheters for adult and pediatric patients are listed in **TABLE 15-6**.

Necessary Equipment

A laryngoscope is required for visualization of the glottis during tracheal intubation. Although various makes are available, all have a number of features in common. The standard laryngoscope includes a handle made of plastic or stainless steel. The handle contains the batteries for the light source and attaches to a plastic

TABLE 15-6 Tracheal Tube and Suction Catheter Sizes[a]

Approximate Age/Size (Weight)	Internal Diameter of Tracheal Tube (mm)	Suction Catheter Size (French)
Premature infant (<1 kg [2 pounds])	2.5	5
Premature infant (1–2 kg [2–4 pounds])	3.0	5 or 6
Premature infant (2–3 kg [4–7 pounds])	3–3.5	6 or 8
Infant (6–9 kg [13–20 pounds])	3.0 cuffed 3.5 uncuffed	8
Toddler (10–11 kg [22–24 pounds])	3.5 cuffed 4.0 uncuffed	10
Small child (12–14 kg [26–31 pounds])	4.0 cuffed 4.5 uncuffed	10
Child (15–18 kg [33–40 pounds])	4.5 cuffed 5.0 uncuffed	10
Child (19–23 kg [42–51 pounds])	5.0 cuffed 5.5 uncuffed	10
Large child (24–29 kg [44–64 pounds])	6 cuffed	10
Adolescent/Small adult (30–36 kg [66–80 pounds])	6.5 cuffed	12
Adult female	7 cuffed	12 or 14
Adult male	7 or 8 cuffed	14

[a]These sizes are approximations and should be adjusted on the basis of clinical experience.

Tracheal tube selection for a child should be based on the child's size or age. One size larger and one size smaller should be allowed for individual variation. Color coding based on length or on the size of the child may facilitate approximation of correct tracheal tube size.

Modified from: American Heart Association. 2010 American Heart Association guidelines for cardiopulmonary resuscitation and emergency cardiovascular care. *Circulation*. 2010;122(18)(suppl 3):S639-S946.

or stainless steel blade with a bulb placed in the distal third. The electrical contact between the blade and the handle is made at a connection point called the fitting. The indentation of the blade is attached to the bar of the handle. When the blade is elevated to a right angle with the laryngoscope handle, the blade snaps into place and the bulb lights (**FIGURE 15-66**). (Failure of the bulb to light may be the result of a loose connection between the bulb and the bulb socket, a damaged bulb, or faulty batteries.) Other necessary equipment includes a 10-mL syringe for cuff inflation, water-soluble lubricant, and suction equipment.

Fiberoptic intubation handles and blades improve visualization during intubation by eliminating shadows, which sharpens the focus. The fiberoptic set has the bulb in the handle. The light is transmitted through the blades along fiberoptic strands compressed within it. This improved visualization is less pronounced in disposable kits.

Two types of blades (available in various sizes) are used with the laryngoscope: a straight blade, such as the Miller, Wisconsin, or Flagg blade (**FIGURE 15-67**), and a curved blade, such as a MacIntosh blade (**FIGURE 15-68**). The tip of a straight blade is applied directly to the epiglottis to expose the vocal cords. Advocates of the straight blade claim it provides more exposure of the glottis and less need for a stylet. It may also provide better visualization of anterior airways

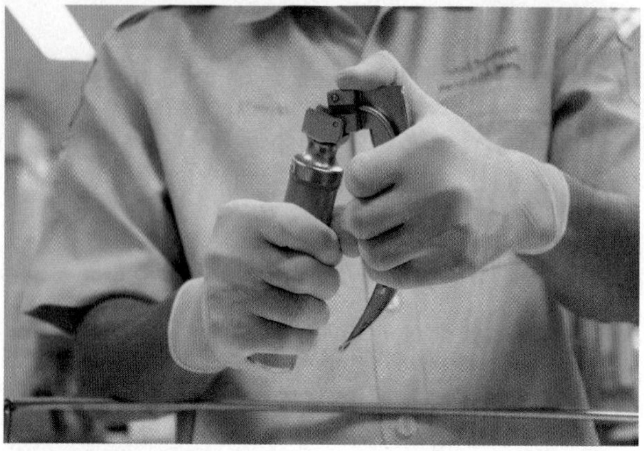

FIGURE 15-66 Attaching a blade to the handle of a laryngoscope.

© Kamon_Wongnon/Shutterstock

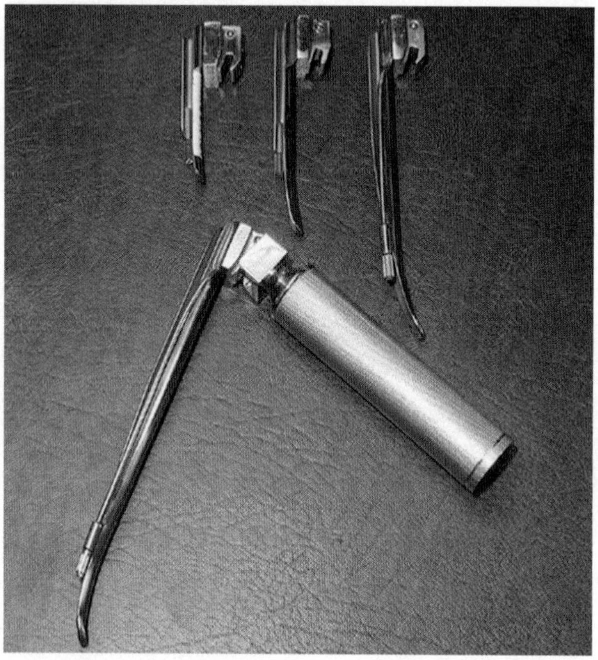

FIGURE 15-67 Types of straight laryngoscopic blades.

© Jones & Bartlett Learning.

and airways with a large epiglottis. A straight blade usually is recommended for infant intubation. This is because it provides greater displacement of the tongue into the floor of the mouth and better visualization of the glottic structures.

CRITICAL THINKING

Ask several paramedics and anesthesiologists which laryngoscope blade they prefer and why.

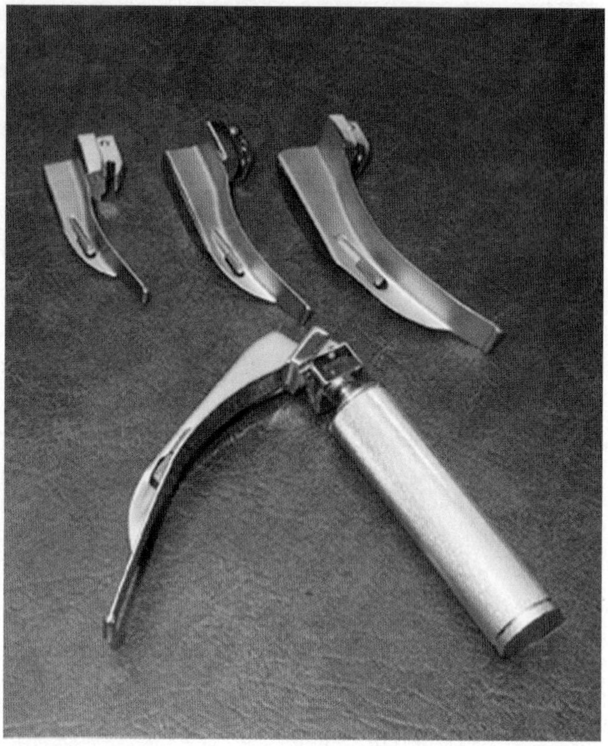

FIGURE 15-68 Types of curved laryngoscopic blades.

© Jones & Bartlett Learning.

The curved blade design is intended to be inserted into the vallecula. Placement of the blade displaces the tongue to the left to elevate the epiglottis without touching it. Advocates of the curved blade claim it reduces the chance of dental trauma. They also claim it provides more room for passage of the ET tube. The choice of blade is a matter of personal preference and the patient's anatomy. Paramedics should acquire expertise in using both curved and straight blades; some patients can be intubated more easily with one type than the other. Occasions also may arise when only one type of blade is available. Versatility with both curved and straight blades may improve the patient's chances of survival.

A malleable stylet (preferably plastic coated) may be inserted through the ET tube before intubation (**FIGURE 15-69**). The stylet conforms to any desired configuration and may facilitate proper placement of the ET tube. If used, the stylet must be recessed 1 to 2 inches (2.5 to 5 cm) from the distal end of the ET tube to prevent injury to the patient. Recession of the stylet tip is maintained by bending the proximal end of the stylet over the proximal rim of the adapter so that it does not advance through the lumen with

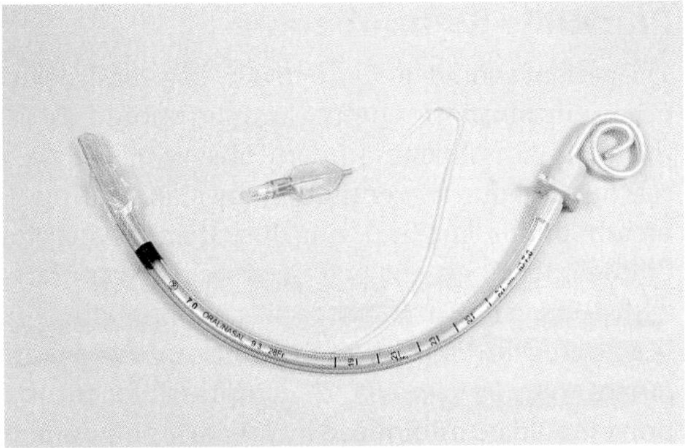

FIGURE 15-69 Endotracheal tube with malleable stylet.

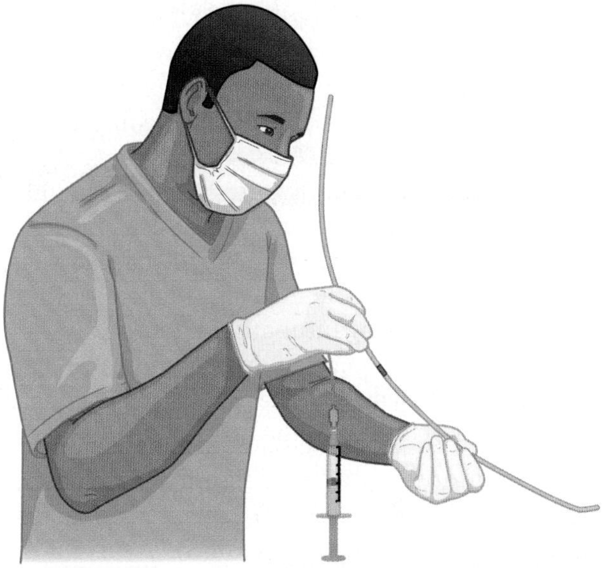

FIGURE 15-70 Gum elastic bougie (tube introducer).

manipulation of the ET tube. If the stylet is allowed to extend beyond the distal end of the tube, the mucosal surface of the larynx or trachea or the vocal cords may be damaged. A gum elastic bougie (**FIGURE 15-70**) or tube introducer can be used to assist with ET tube placement. It is a type of semirigid stylet. This flexible device is placed in the trachea under direct visualization using a laryngoscope. Because it is smaller and more rigid than the ET tube, it can pass through the vocal cords more easily. The "hockey stick" bend on the end of the bougie allows the operator to feel it pass over the tracheal rings as it bumps against each of them. The tracheal tube then is passed over the bougie and into position in the trachea.[31]

NOTE

Lighted stylets, or "light wands," are available to assist in intubation. (They are useful only in low-light environments and are intended only for adult patients.) These devices have a high-intensity light at the distal end. The light is powered by a small battery housing at the operator end (**FIGURE 15-71**). This device aids placement of the ET tube, because the paramedic can see the light from the end of the ET tube passing through the soft tissues of the neck. Lighted stylets also can be used to help verify placement after intubation by other methods. Once the cuff has been inflated and lung sounds auscultated, the stylet is advanced through the ET tube. A bright light below the thyroid cartilage indicates proper placement. If the illumination creates a dim, indistinct light, the esophagus probably has been intubated.

An optical stylet is a malleable light wand, similar to other light wands that allow airway visualization. It consists of a stainless steel sheath with illumination fibers and a fiberoptic bundle to provide a clear view of the airway. The stylet can be used with a separate camera and monitor system on its own or with an optical eyepiece (**FIGURE 15-72**). Lighted stylets and the optical stylet are used infrequently in EMS.

Magill forceps (**FIGURE 15-73**), a scissors-style clamp with circular tips, are also used for airway management. This instrument may be used to help direct the tip of the ET tube into the larynx during intubation and to remove some foreign bodies (BOX 15-11).

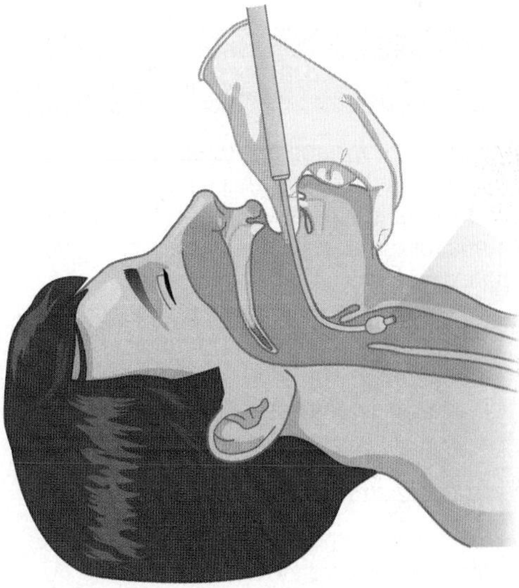

FIGURE 15-71 Fiberoptic intubation. The endotracheal tube is inserted with the aid of a lighted stylet.

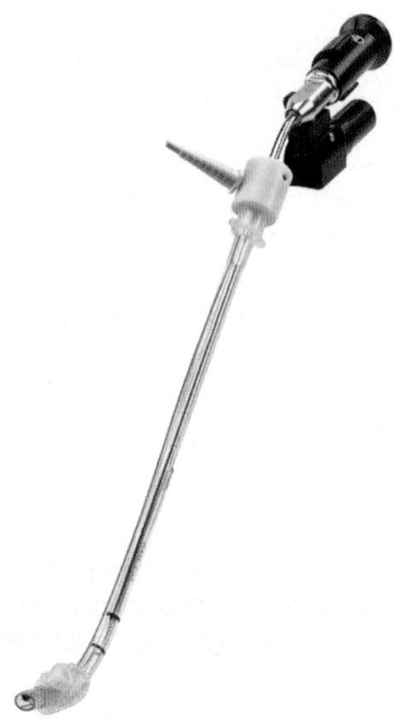

FIGURE 15-72 Shikani Seeing Optical Stylet.

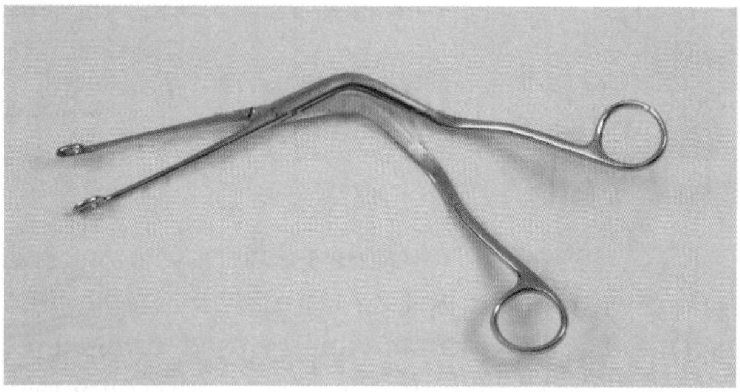

FIGURE 15-73 Magill forceps.

Preparing for Intubation

The patient should be ventilated by bag-mask device before intubation. The paramedic should assess the adequacy of ventilation by observing the chest rise and fall during ventilation, by auscultating for breath sounds, and by noting the patient's skin color. Before intubation, the patient should be ventilated with 100% oxygen. In a pulseless patient, the goal is to avoid interrupting chest compressions for longer than 10 seconds. Interruptions for intubations should be minimized by preparing equipment beforehand. Ideally, chest compressions should not be interrupted for the placement of the tube. If that is not possible, CPR should be paused only long enough to pass the tube. Chest compressions should resume immediately after the tube is distal to the vocal cords. When more than two attempts are required, the patient should receive adequate ventilation, oxygenation, and chest compressions before each attempt. The patient's lungs should then be ventilated and hyperoxygenated for 15 to 30 seconds by other means before intubation is attempted again if the patient is not in cardiac arrest. Pulse oximetry and the ECG should be monitored continuously during intubation attempts.

Before intubation, all equipment should be examined and tested for defects. The paramedic should check the integrity of the cuff of the ET tube by inflating the balloon with 5 to 8 mL of air and checking for leaks in the cuff or inlet port. The blade of the laryngoscope

BOX 15-11 Removal of Foreign Bodies by Direct Laryngoscopy

Direct laryngoscopy and use of Magill forceps to remove foreign bodies should be attempted only after manual techniques for clearing the airway have proved unsuccessful. The steps for removing a foreign body from the airway by direct laryngoscopy are as follows:

1. Assemble the necessary laryngoscopic equipment. (Have suction ready for immediate use in case of vomiting.)
2. Place the supine patient in the sniffing position (see Figure 15-75) with the head extended.
3. Ventilate the patient with supplemental oxygen if possible.
4. Insert the laryngoscope, visualizing the glottic opening and surrounding structures.
5. If foreign matter is seen, grasp it with Magill forceps and remove it from the airway.
   Note: Forceps removal of foreign matter should be attempted only with direct visualization of the obstruction. Even then, caution must be exercised to avoid soft-tissue damage caused by the teeth of the forceps.
6. If spontaneous respirations resume within 5 seconds, remove the blade of the laryngoscope and monitor the patient.
7. If spontaneous respirations do not resume, insert an ET tube, administer 100% oxygen, and assess the patient's circulatory status.

If complete foreign body obstruction of the upper airway cannot be relieved, needle cricothyrotomy or transtracheal jet insufflation may be warranted. These advanced airway procedures provide oxygenation if they are inserted below the obstruction until tracheal intubation or tracheostomy can be performed in a controlled setting.

NOTE

Multiple and prolonged airway insertion efforts during cardiac arrest may result in impaired systematic circulation and delivery of oxygen. Apneic oxygenation is the passive flow of oxygen into the alveoli during apnea. This passive movement occurs to the differential rate between alveolar oxygen absorption and carbon dioxide excretion, producing a mass flow of gas from the upper respiratory tract into the lungs. Passive oxygenation in apneic patients prior to intubation can be provided through the nares using a standard nasal cannula or a HFNC. These methods have been studied in critical care settings and have been found to reduce the degree of hypoxia in apneic patients. The paramedic should follow intubation policies and procedures established by medical direction.

Modified from: Benoit JL, Prince DK, Wang HE. Mechanisms linking advanced airway management and cardiac arrest outcomes. *Resuscitation*. 2015;93:124-127; Russotto V, Cortegiani A, Raineri SM, Gregoretti C, Giarratano A. Respiratory support techniques to avoid desaturation in critically ill patients requiring endotracheal intubation: a systematic review and meta-analysis. *J Crit Care*. 2017;41:98-106.

should be snapped into place to examine the light bulb. The bulb should be secured in its socket and checked for brightness ("light, bright, and tight").

Anatomic Considerations

The ET tube may be passed into the trachea through the mouth (orotracheal method) or through the nose (nasotracheal method). The orotracheal method is used most often. It is performed under direct visualization of the glottic opening. The nasotracheal route basically is a "blind" (nonvisualized) technique. The following anatomic structures are key landmarks during intubation:

- The trachea is in the midline of the neck with the superior entry at the level of the glottic opening. With orotracheal intubation, the vocal cords should be visualized while the tube is passed to ensure entry into the trachea.
- The uvula is suspended from the midline of the soft palate. It is used as a guide for correct placement of the laryngoscope.
- The epiglottis is attached to the base of the tongue. It should be visualized and elevated to expose the glottis and vocal cords. Cricoid pressure may help the paramedic better visualize the entrance of the trachea by pushing it slightly posterior (**BOX 15-12**).

BOX 15-12 Application of Cricoid Pressure

Applying pressure to the solid ring of the cricoid cartilage (Sellick maneuver) can occlude the esophagus and may improve visualization of the vocal cords during intubation. Studies suggest that cricoid pressure can interfere with effective ventilation. It is no longer recommended for routine use during ventilation during adult cardiac arrest. Complications include laryngeal trauma with excessive force and esophageal rupture from unrelieved high gastric pressures.

Modified from: American Heart Association. 2015 American Heart Association guidelines for cardiopulmonary resuscitation and emergency cardiovascular care. *Circulation*. 2015;132(18)(suppl 2):S313-S314.

The trachea extends to the level of the second intercostal space anteriorly, at which point it divides into the left and right main stem bronchi. The right main bronchus branches off at a very slight angle to the trachea, whereas the left branches at a 45° to 60° angle.

NOTE

An ET tube that has been advanced too far most often enters the right main bronchus, bypassing and occluding the origin of the left main bronchus. If this occurs, atelectasis and pulmonary insufficiency of the left lung may result. Therefore, evaluation of ET tube placement by auscultation of both lungs is crucial. With proper ET tube placement, breath sounds should be of almost equal intensity over the two lung fields. Certain pathologic conditions (eg, pneumothorax, hemothorax, surgical removal of a lung) may result in unequal breath sounds even when an ET tube is in the proper position.

Orotracheal Intubation

In preparation for orotracheal intubation, a patient who is not a trauma victim should be placed in the sniffing position (**FIGURE 15-74**). In this position, the neck is flexed at the fifth and sixth cervical vertebrae. The head is extended at the first and second cervical vertebrae. This position aligns the three axes of the mouth, pharynx, and trachea (the oropharyngolaryngeal axis), allowing direct visualization of the larynx (**FIGURE 15-75**). When trauma is not a factor, placing a few layers of towels under the patient's head to elevate it may be helpful.

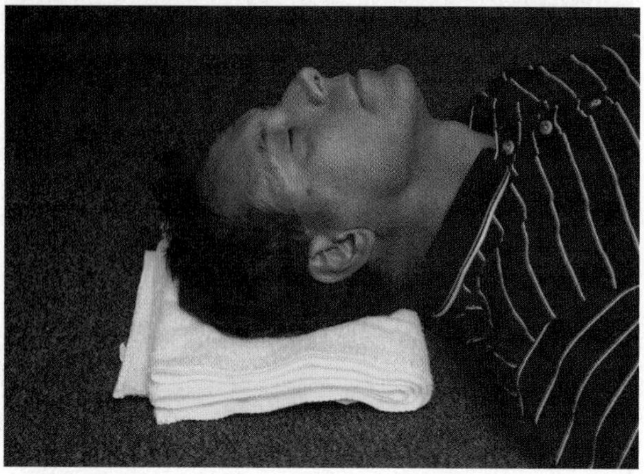

FIGURE 15-74 Sniffing position.

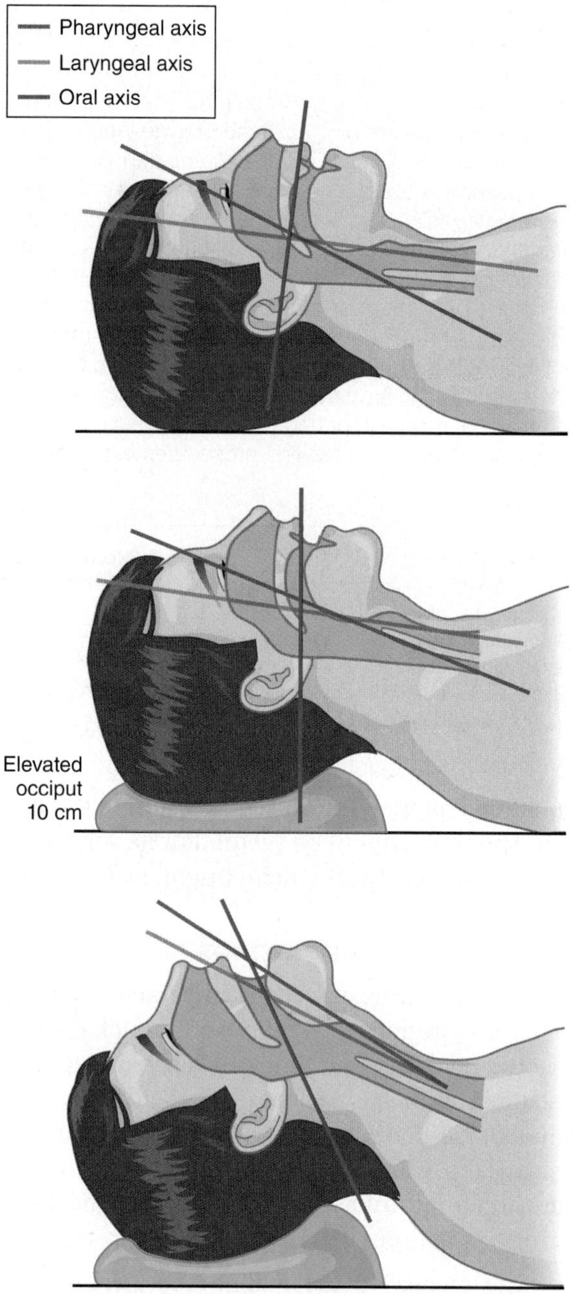

FIGURE 15-75 Oropharyngolaryngeal axis.

A stethoscope, stylet, and suction equipment (with large-bore catheters) should be readily available. As for all advanced airway procedures, the patient's lungs should be ventilated with 100% oxygen before intubation. In addition, the patient should be monitored using Spo_2, and capnography monitoring should be prepared. The orotracheal intubation procedure is as follows (**FIGURE 15-76**):

1. Position yourself at the patient's head.
2. Inspect the oral cavity for secretions and foreign material. Suction the mouth and pharynx if needed.
3. Open the patient's mouth with the fingers of the right hand. Retract the patient's lips on the teeth or gums to avoid pinching them in the blade. The "crossed-finger technique" also may be useful in opening the patient's mouth. To perform this procedure, cross the right thumb and index finger to form an X. Place the thumb on the patient's lower incisors and the index finger on the patient's upper incisors; apply crossed-finger pressure to open the patient's mouth.
4. Grasp the lower jaw with the right hand and draw it forward and upward. Remove any dentures.
5. Holding the laryngoscope in the left hand, insert the blade into the right side of the mouth, displacing the tongue to the left. Move the blade toward the midline and the base of the tongue and identify the uvula. It is essential to work gently and avoid pressure on the lips and teeth.
6. When using a curved blade, advance the tip of the blade into the vallecula, the space between the base of the tongue and the pharyngeal surface of the epiglottis (**FIGURE 15-77**). When using a straight blade, insert the tip over the epiglottis (**FIGURE 15-78**). The glottic opening is exposed by exerting upward traction on the handle. Never use a prying motion with the handle, and do not use the teeth as a fulcrum.
7. Advance the ET tube through the right corner of the mouth and, under direct vision, through the vocal cords (**FIGURE 15-79**). If a stylet has

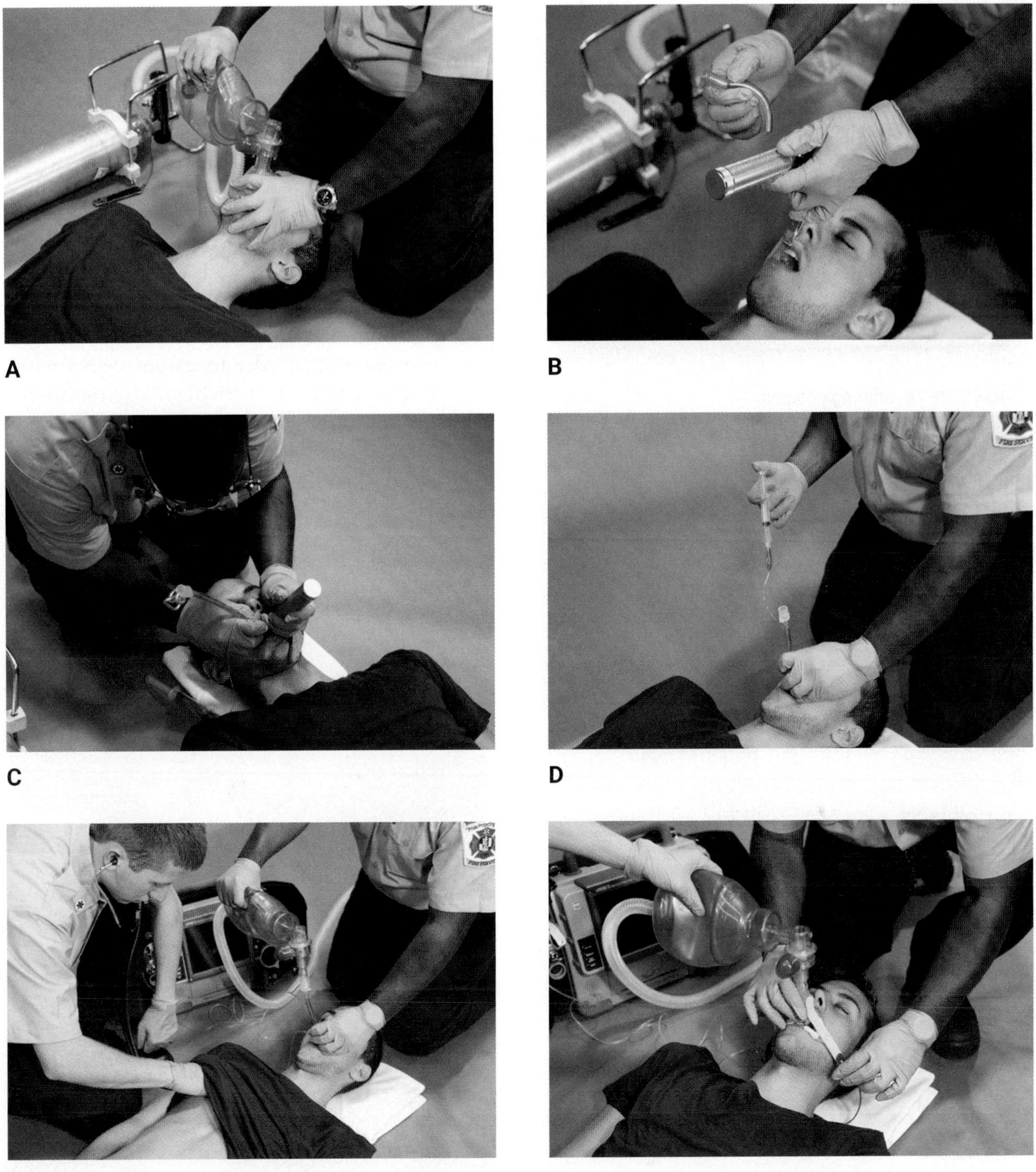

FIGURE 15-76 Orotracheal intubation. **A.** Before intubation, ventilate the patient's lungs with 100% oxygen. **B.** Hold the laryngoscope in the left hand and insert the blade into the right side of the patient's mouth, displacing the tongue to the left. **C.** Advance the endotracheal (ET) tube through the right corner of the mouth and, under direct vision, through the vocal cords. **D.** Inflate the cuff with about 6 to 7 mL of air. Ventilate the patient's lungs with a mechanical airway device. **E.** Confirm correct placement of the ET tube by primary and secondary confirmation methods. In-line capnography should always be used to confirm tube placement. Monitor tube position. **F.** Secure the ET tube in place and provide ventilatory support with supplemental oxygen.

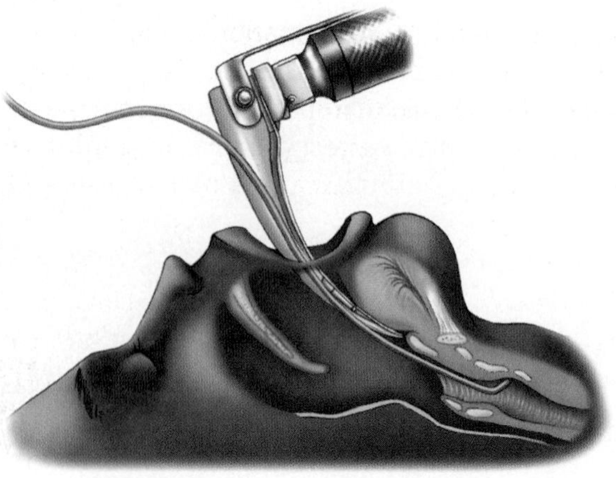

A

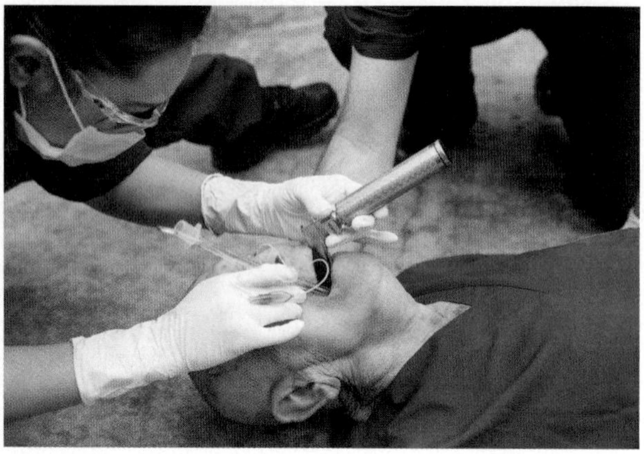

B

FIGURE 15-77 **A.** The curved blade tip goes into the vallecula as shown in this figure of a gum elastic bougie. **B.** Relax your arms and gently advance the blade until the anatomy can be visualized.

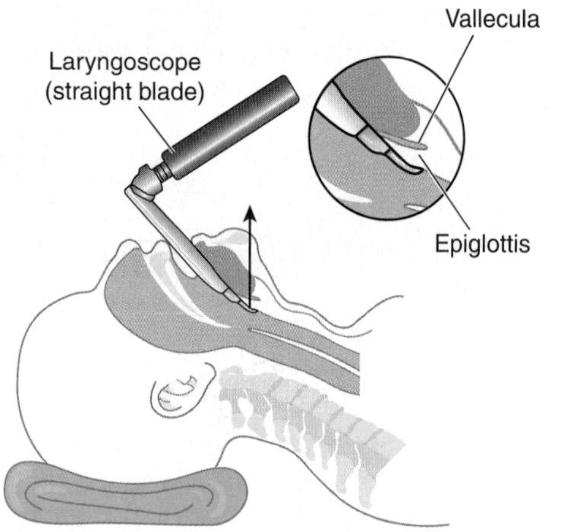

FIGURE 15-78 A straight laryngoscopic blade is used to lift the epiglottis, directly exposing the vocal cords.

been used, it should be removed from the tube after the tube passes through the cords into the trachea.

8. After viewing the vocal cords, make sure the proximal end of the cuffed tube has advanced past the cords about 1 to 2.5 cm (0.5 to 1 inch). The tip of the tube should then be halfway between the vocal cords and the carina (**FIGURE 15-80**). This position allows some displacement of the tube tip during flexion or extension of the patient's neck without extubation or movement of the tip into the main stem bronchus. In the average adult, the distance from teeth to carina is 27 cm (about 11 inches). The paramedic should check the depth markings on the ET

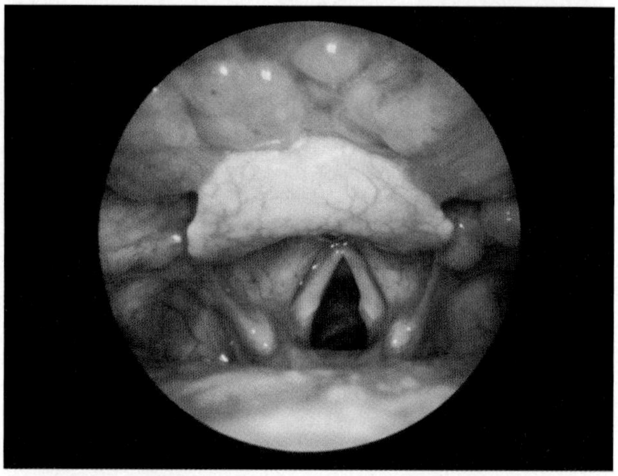

FIGURE 15-79 View of the vocal cords.

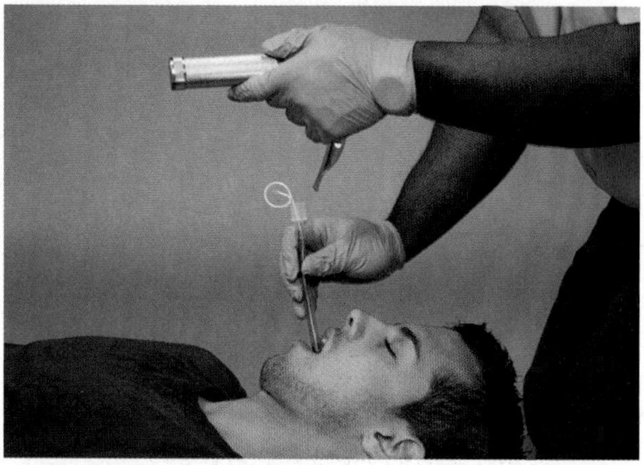

FIGURE 15-80 When inserted to the correct depth, the tip of the tube will be halfway between the vocal cords and the carina.

tube during intubation. In the average adult, the tube is properly positioned when the patient's teeth are between the 19 and 23 cm marks on the tube. This depth places the tip of the tube 2 to 3 cm (0.75 to 1.5 inches) above the carina. The average tube depth in men is 22 cm (about 9 inches) ("teeth and tube at 22"). The average tube depth in women is 21 cm (about 8.5 inches).

9. Inflate the cuff with about 6 to 7 mL of air to prevent any air leaks around the tracheal cuff seal.[32]
10. Attach the tube to a mechanical airway device and ventilate the patient's lungs.
11. During ventilation, confirm accurate tube placement using primary and secondary confirmation methods.[23]

Primary Confirmation Methods

Initially confirm proper tube placement by auscultating over the epigastrium, the midaxillary region, and the anterior chest line on the right and left sides of the chest. If stomach gurgling is present or chest expansion is absent, immediately deflate the cuff and remove the tracheal tube. Reattempt intubation after oxygenating the patient's lungs with 100% oxygen for 15 to 30 seconds. When appropriate tube placement has been confirmed, reconfirm and note the tube mark at the front of the patient's teeth. Secure the tube to the patient's head and face with tape or a commercially available device. Then reevaluate lung sounds to ensure that the tube was not inadvertently repositioned. Finally, insert an oral airway or bite block to prevent the patient from biting down and blocking the airway.

> NOTE
>
> If breath sounds are decreased or absent in the left lung, the orotracheal tube may have passed into the right main stem bronchus, effectively bypassing the origin of the left main bronchus. If this is the case, the cuff should be deflated and the tube withdrawn 1 to 2 cm (about 0.5 to 0.75 inch). The cuff then should be reinflated, and tube placement should be verified as explained previously.

Secondary Confirmation Methods

A second method of determining correct tube placement requires the use of mechanical devices. These devices include $ETCO_2$ detectors, esophageal detectors, and pulse oximetry for patients who have a perfusing rhythm. These devices are described later in this chapter. Tube confirmation should be include clinical and mechanical methods. Do not rely on a single method. Capnography is considered the gold standard. Confirm correct placement immediately after intubation and each time a patient is moved.

Video Laryngoscopy

Video laryngoscopy devices are available and increasingly used in EMS systems. They are appropriate for both oral and nasal intubation procedures. Video laryngoscopes improve the glottis view, increase intubation success, and decrease time to intubation when appropriately used. Visualization of the glottis is improved in these laryngoscopes by optical or video magnification. These devices include the C-MAC, GlideScope, McGrath, Storz, Airway Scope, and others. Using an enhanced optical laryngoscope, the glottis can be visualized and intubation performed while viewing a video monitor. Like other advanced airway techniques, intubation using these devices requires special training that is manufacturer specific, as well as authorization from medical direction. Any patient who meets the criteria for intubation (described earlier) can be intubated with a video laryngoscope (**FIGURE 15-81**).[33]

Video-assisted intubation involves inserting a video laryngoscope into the patient's mouth and then into the pharynx. Upon visual confirmation of the glottic opening, the ET tube is advanced through a specially designed channel or alongside the laryngoscope. The tube is placed in the trachea under direct vision, using the video monitor.

Digital (Blind) Intubation

Before the advent of laryngoscopes, intubation was performed by the intubator inserting his or her fingers

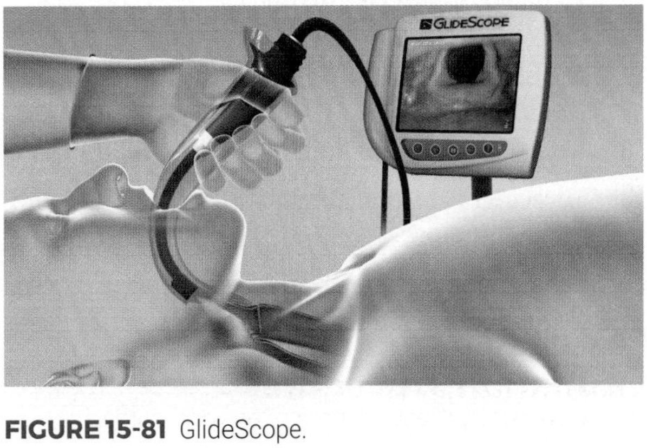

FIGURE 15-81 GlideScope.

into the patient's mouth. The fingers were used to guide the ET tube into the trachea. Digital intubation is not a common prehospital procedure. However, it may be necessary in cases of patient entrapment, in patients whose airway is blocked from view by large amounts of blood or other secretions, or if equipment fails. Digital intubation also may be used in certain disaster or tactical situations in which victims are widespread and equipment is in short supply. The procedure for digital (blind) intubation is as follows (**FIGURE 15-82**):

1. Position yourself at the patient's left side. If a spinal injury is suspected, have a second rescuer maintain in-line spinal immobilization.
2. Ventilate the patient with 100% oxygen before intubation.
3. Use a bite stick or other device to hold the patient's mouth open. This helps protect the inserted fingers.
4. Bend the tube and stylet combination into a J or hockey stick configuration or use the gum elastic bougie.[31]
5. Insert your gloved left middle and index fingers into the patient's mouth. Alternating fingers, "walk" down the patient's tongue, pulling the tongue and epiglottis away from the glottic opening.
6. When you feel a flap of cartilage covered by the mucous membrane with your middle finger, you have reached the epiglottis. Maintain contact and advance the ET tube with your right hand. Use the index finger of your left hand as a guide. The index finger maintains the tube position against the middle finger, leading the tip of the tube into the glottic opening. It may be helpful for a second rescuer to perform the Sellick maneuver (cricoid pressure) for better visualization of the airway.
7. Once the cuff of the ET tube passes the tips of the inserted fingers, inflate the cuff, remove the stylet, and verify placement in the usual manner.
8. Secure the tube as previously described.

Correct ET tube placement should be confirmed often. At a minimum, reconfirm placement each time a patient is moved or has a sudden change in condition.

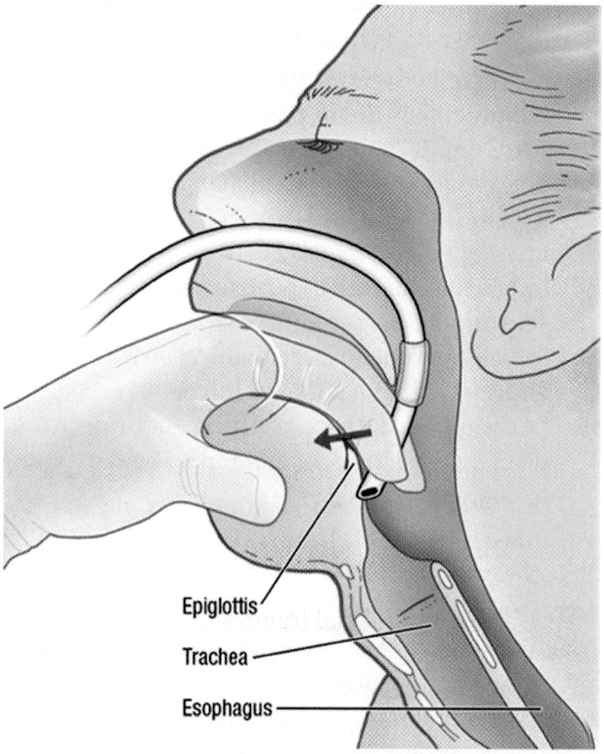

A

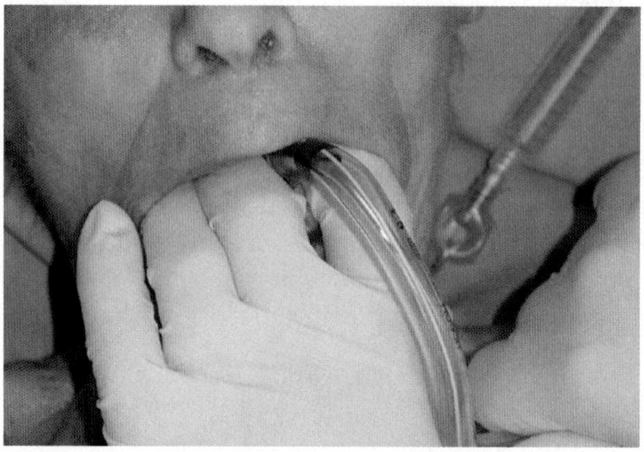

B

FIGURE 15-82 **(A)** demonstrates manually-assisted nasotracheal intubation; **(B)** illustrates manually-assisted orotracheal intubation. Both are valid techniques.

A: Reproduced from Emergency Medicine Procedures, Second Edition. Eric F. Reichman, PhD, MD.McGraw-Hill Education. © 2013; **B:** © American Academy of Orthopaedic Surgeons.

Potential Complications From Intubation Procedures

- Intubation of the esophagus
- Intubation of a bronchus
- Lacerated lips or tongue (oral)
- Dental trauma from the laryngoscope (oral)
- Lacerated pharyngeal or tracheal mucosa
- Tracheal rupture
- Avulsion of an arytenoid cartilage
- Vocal cord injury
- Vomiting and aspiration of stomach contents
- Significant release of epinephrine and norepinephrine, leading to hypertension, tachycardia, or cardiac rhythm disturbances

- Vagal stimulation (particularly in infants and children), resulting in bradycardia and hypotension
- Increased intracranial pressure in patients with a head injury
- Hypoxia related to prolonged intubation attempts
- Displacement when the patient moves or is moved

In addition, rupture of the cuff, inflation port malfunction, or severance or kinking of the inflation tube may cause cuff malfunction and air leakage.

Nasotracheal Intubation

At times nasotracheal intubation may be the airway procedure of choice. This may be the case in patients who have spontaneous respirations, when laryngoscopy is difficult, or when the motion of the cervical spine must be limited. Examples of such conditions include the following:

- Major maxillofacial trauma
- Angioedema (as may be seen in anaphylaxis or allergic reactions)
- Trismus (as seen in status epilepticus)

These and other situations may make aligning the oropharyngolaryngeal axis difficult, thus ruling out successful orotracheal intubation. It should be noted that nasotracheal intubation is a blind procedure. It carries a high risk of improper tube placement, because the paramedic cannot visualize the vocal cords.

In general, conscious patients tolerate a nasotracheal tube better than an orotracheal tube. Also, a nasotracheal tube often causes less trauma to the tracheal mucosa, because the tube moves less inside the trachea with head motion than does an orotracheal tube. If time allows, the paramedic should prepare the patient using a vasoconstrictor spray and topical anesthetic. Examples of these products are phenylephrine spray and lidocaine jelly. These measures may make the patient more comfortable. They also reduce the risk of nasal hemorrhage, which may occur secondary to the procedure. If time allows, placement of a soft nasopharyngeal airway before the procedure may show which nostril is more passable. Doing so also may compress the mucosa, allowing less traumatic placement of the ET tube.

> NOTE
>
> Nasotracheal intubation is contraindicated in patients who are apneic, who have midfacial fractures or nasal fractures, or who are suspected of having a basilar skull fracture.

Insertion

The procedure for inserting a nasotracheal tube is as follows (**FIGURE 15-83**):[23]

1. Choose a cuffed ET tube that is 1 mm smaller than optimal for oral intubation. (Most ET tubes are designed for both orotracheal and nasotracheal intubation. Some longer ET tubes are designed specifically for this procedure. A ringed ET tube [Endotrol] also is available that controls the tip of the ET tube, aiding entry into the trachea.) Prepare and check all needed equipment (balloon cuff, syringe, suction, stethoscope). Stylets are not used in nasotracheal intubation, because the stylet reduces flexibility and increases the risk of injury during blind insertion.
2. Ventilate the patient with 100% oxygen before intubation.
3. Lubricate the ET tube with a water-soluble or lidocaine jelly.
4. Insert the tube with the flange facing the nasal septum. Advance the tube along the nasal floor of the nostril that is clearer and more direct. If both nostrils appear open, advance through the larger nostril first. If the chosen nostril is impassable, try the other nostril before selecting an ET tube that is 0.5 mm smaller in diameter.
5. Stand beside the patient with one hand on the tube and the thumb and index finger of the other hand palpating the larynx. The curve of the tube should follow the natural curve of the airway. Gently advance the tube while rotating it medially 15° to 30° until maximal airflow is heard through the tube. (Airflow sounds can be amplified by placing a simple device called the Beck airway airflow monitor [BAAM] whistle on the end of the ET tube.) Gently and swiftly advance the tube during early inspiration. Voluntary tongue extrusion in cooperative patients is helpful. Otherwise, the tongue can be wrapped with gauze and pulled forward. Flexion of the neck (if no spinal instability is suspected) and posterior pressure on the thyroid cartilage may help position the larynx.
6. Externally observe the advancement of the tube toward the carina. Misting or condensation on the tube should be evident as the tube approaches tracheal placement. This condensation occurs because the patient's exhaled breath has a high concentration of water vapor. The water vapor promptly condenses on exposure to cooler room

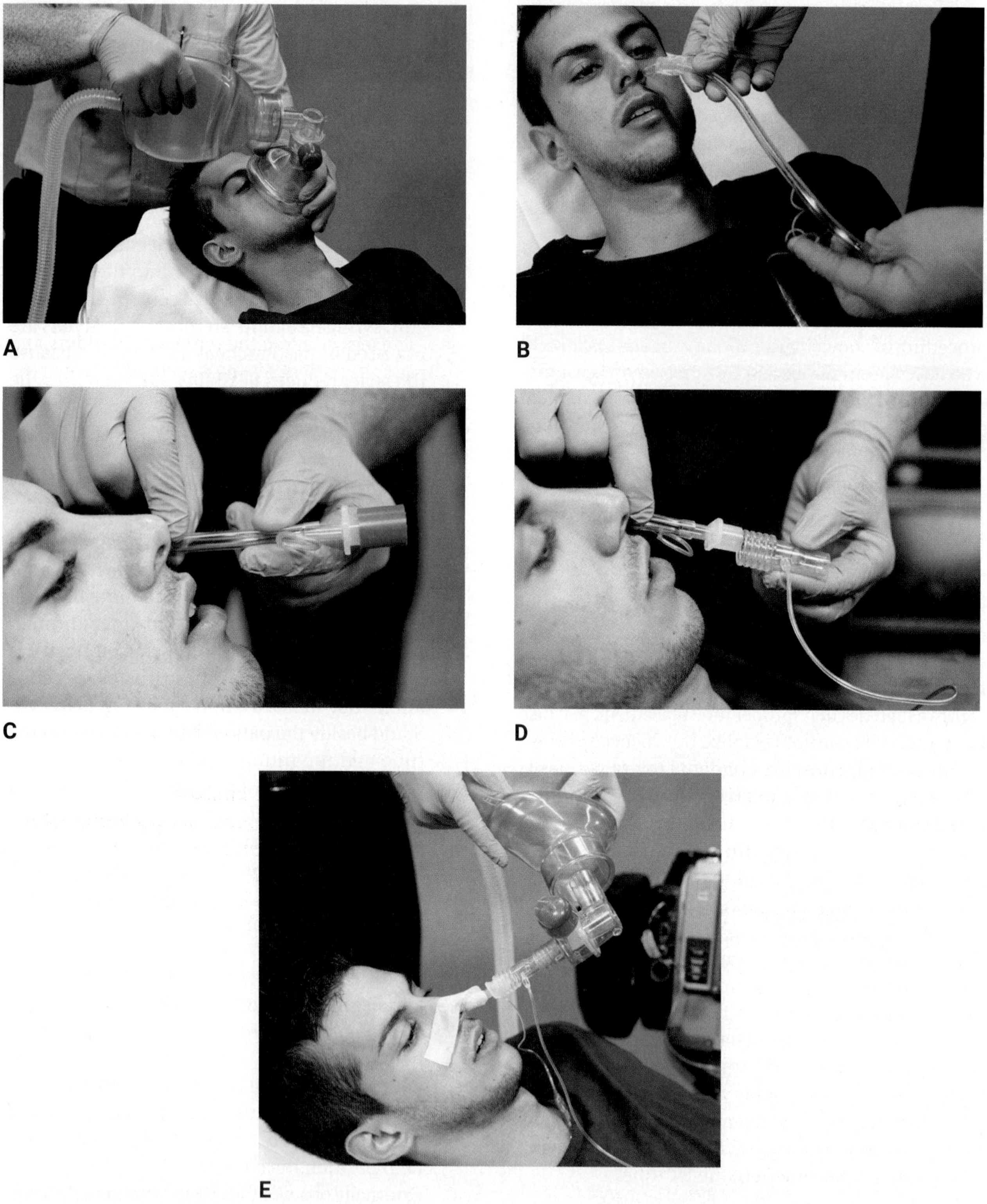

FIGURE 15-83 Nasotracheal intubation. **A.** Oxygenate the patient while the nasotracheal tube is prepared and lubricated. **B.** Insert the tube into the larger nostril. **C.** Listen for airflow over the tube as it is advanced. Ensure the patient is unable to speak. **D.** Attach the $ETCO_2$ detector (waveform capnography preferred) to the nasotracheal tube. **E.** Secure the tube and monitor the patient.

air. However, tube misting is not always a reliable indicator of proper tube position.

7. On completion of intubation, verify proper tube placement as described earlier. Inflate the cuff with about 6 to 7 mL of air and secure the tube in place. Ventilations may then be assisted with supplemental oxygen, or the patient's lungs can be ventilated by mechanical means.
8. If intubation fails, withdraw the tube and redirect it after ventilating and oxygenating the patient. It may be possible to recognize tube misplacement by inspecting and palpating the neck for bulges.

Possible Complications

- Epistaxis
- Sinusitis
- Vagal stimulation
- Injury to the nasal septum or turbinates
- Retropharyngeal laceration
- Vocal cord injury
- Avulsion of an arytenoid cartilage
- Esophageal intubation
- Intracranial tube placement if the patient has a basilar skull fracture

Intubation With Spinal Precautions

Nasal or oral intubation may be performed in patients suspected of having a spinal injury. The procedure is as follows:

1. Auscultate for bilateral breath sounds while manual or mechanical ventilations are in progress. This provides a baseline.
2. One rescuer should apply manual in-line stabilization from the patient's side. The rescuer places the hands over the patient's ears. The little fingers should be under the occipital skull. The thumbs should be on the face over the maxillary sinuses. Stabilization (without distraction) should be maintained in a neutral position throughout the procedure. Thin padding under the patient's head may be necessary to maintain neutral, in-line positioning.

NOTE

Intubation of patients suspected of having a spinal injury is risky and should be performed in a manner approved by medical direction. If the paramedic elects to intubate the trachea of a patient suspected of having a spinal injury, in-line stabilization must be maintained. Two trained rescuers are required. Video-assisted devices may be helpful in these situations.

Modified from: American College of Surgeons. *Upper Airway Management: Advanced Trauma Life Support*. 9th ed. Chicago, IL: American College of Surgeons; 2012.

Several alternative positions for intubation may be used to accommodate unusual space and environmental conditions. In one method of intubation, the primary paramedic is positioned at the patient's head. The legs straddle the patient's shoulders and arms, and the patient's head is secured between the paramedic's thighs. The grip of the primary rescuer in this position and of the other rescuer (from the side) prevents the head from moving during the intubation. In this position, the primary paramedic may need to lean back to visualize the vocal cords. With another method, the primary paramedic lies prone at the patient's head, and the other rescuer (at the patient's side) maintains the in-line position alone (**FIGURE 15-84**). The left lateral decubitus, kneeling, sitting, or straddle positions may be used in some situations (**FIGURE 15-85**).

Face-to-Face Orotracheal Intubation

Face-to-face orotracheal intubation (**FIGURE 15-86**) may be used when the paramedic cannot take a position above the patient's head (eg, the patient is in a sitting position). In this method of intubation, a second rescuer maintains in-line immobilization

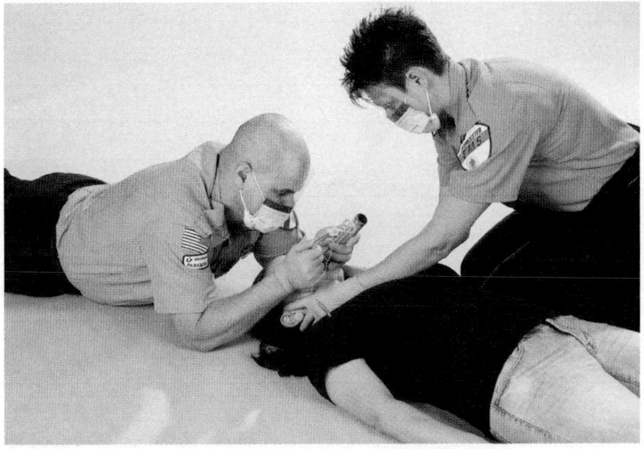

FIGURE 15-84 Intubation in a prone position.

of the patient's neck and head from behind the patient. The primary rescuer takes a position facing the patient. The patient's mouth is opened with the left hand. The laryngoscope is held in the right hand, and the blade is inserted into the patient's mouth, following the normal curve of the tongue. After visualizing the vocal cords from a position above the patient's mouth, the primary rescuer passes an ET tube between the cords with the left hand. The cuff is inflated and the syringe removed. The patient then is ventilated with a bag-mask device. After proper placement has been confirmed as previously described, the ET tube is secured in place. Video laryngoscopy devices can be helpful when spinal motion needs to be restricted and in face-to-face situations.

Extubation

The ET tube is not usually removed in the prehospital setting. However, the patient may develop intolerance to the tube. Also, sedating the patient to improve tolerance may not be possible. In such cases, medical direction may advise extubation. If time allows, the patient's lungs first should be ventilated with 100% oxygen. To remove the ET tube, the paramedic should tilt the patient or backboard to one side and proceed as follows:

1. Have suction available. (The oral cavity and the area above the cuff should be suctioned before the ET tube is removed.)
2. Deflate the cuff completely.

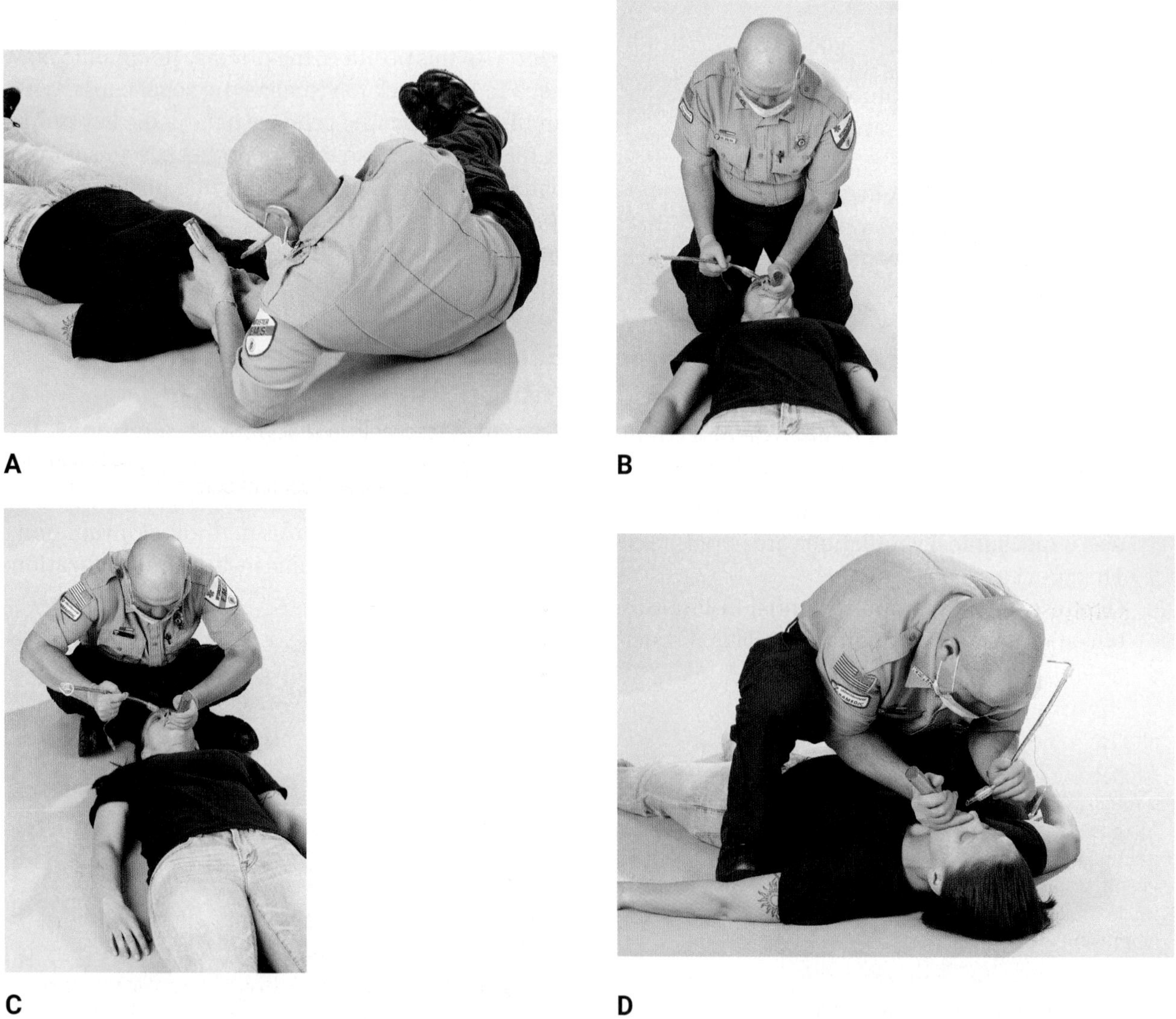

FIGURE 15-85 Intubation positions. **A.** Left lateral decubitus. **B.** Kneeling. **C.** Sitting. **D.** Straddle.

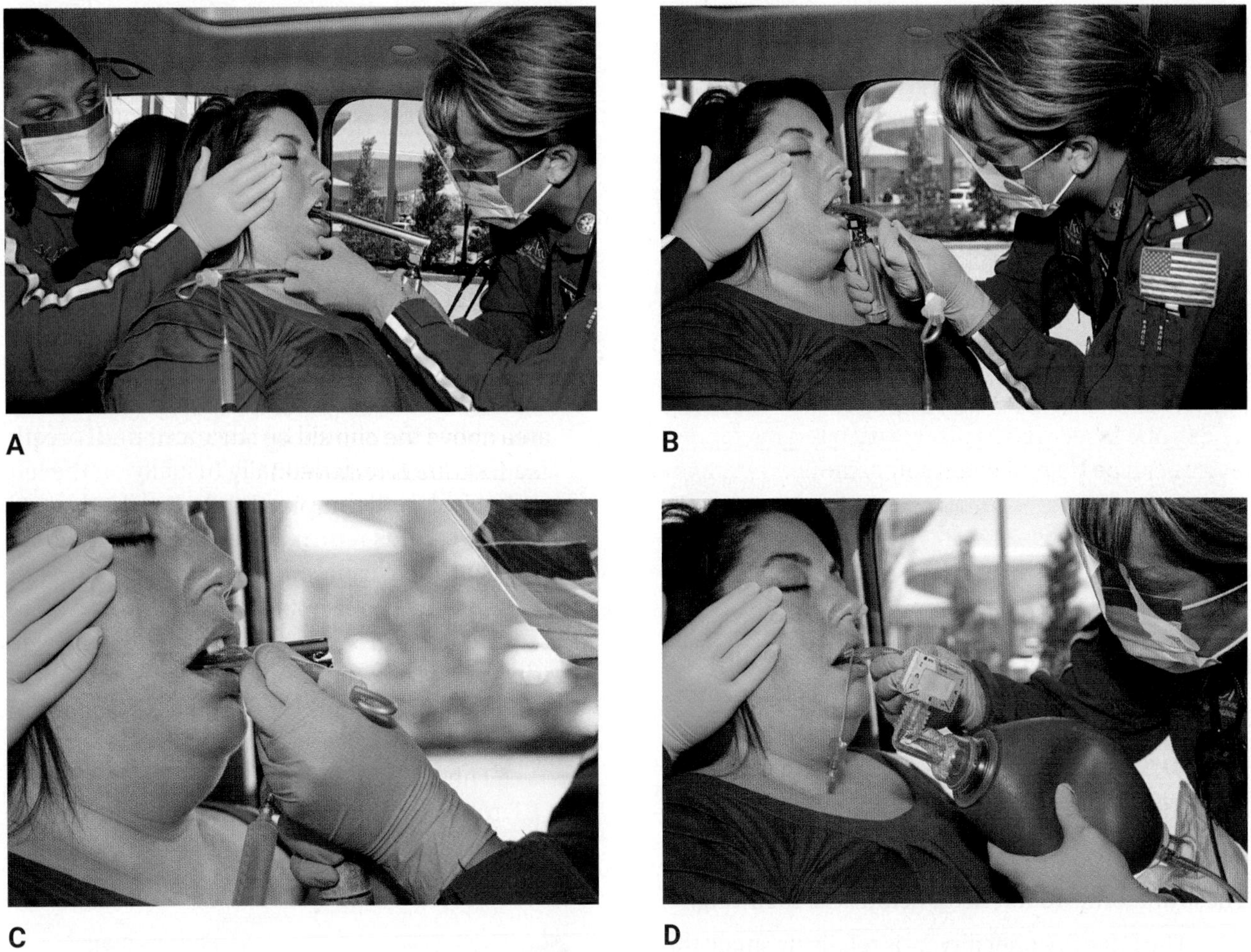

FIGURE 15-86 Face-to-face orotracheal intubation. **A.** One rescuer maintains in-line immobilization. The primary rescuer takes a position facing the patient and opens the person's mouth. The primary rescuer then should follow these steps: **B.** Hold the laryngoscope in the right hand and insert it into the patient's mouth. **C.** With the left hand, pass the endotracheal tube into the mouth and through the vocal cords. **D.** Inflate the cuff. Ventilate the patient and confirm correct placement of the tube. Secure the tube in place.

3. Swiftly withdraw the tube on cough or expiration.
4. Assess the patient's respiratory status.
5. Provide high-concentration oxygen; assist ventilations as needed.

> NOTE
> Patients who are awake are at high risk of laryngospasm immediately after extubation. Also, they may be difficult to reintubate should respiratory distress or failure recur.

Advantages of ET Intubation

- It provides complete airway control.
- It helps prevent aspiration.
- It prevents gastric distention.
- Positive pressure ventilation can be delivered.
- It allows tracheal suctioning.
- High concentrations of oxygen and large volumes of ventilation can be delivered.
- It may provide a route for administration of some drugs.

Special Considerations for Pediatric Intubations

Pediatric intubation remains a controversial topic. Evidence reviewing pediatric prehospital airway management shows an 81% to 83% success rate for ET intubation. However, in one large analysis, that rate dropped to 76% for nonphysicians.[34] In another, $ETCO_2$ was used during only 37% of pediatric intubations.[35]

SHOW ME THE EVIDENCE

Hansen and colleagues reviewed the 2012 National EMS Information System (NEMSIS) data for children younger than 18 years to describe airway interventions and their success. Airway interventions were performed in about 4.5% of 950,000 pediatric patients from 40 states. Of those patients, 1.5% had undergone an advanced airway procedure (eg, ET intubation, cricothyrotomy, alternate airway, CPAP, BPAP, bag-mask ventilation, or other ventilation). ET intubation was performed in 3,124 patients, with an overall success rate of 81.1% (95% confidence interval [95% CI], 79.7–82.6). A lower rate of success was achieved during cardiac arrest and in children aged 1 to 12 months.

Modified from: Hansen M, Lambert W, Guise JM, Warden CR, Mann NC, Wang H. Out-of-hospital pediatric airway management in the United States. *Resuscitation.* 2015;90:104-110.

Most paramedics intubate infants and children infrequently. Because of this, research has shown no improvement in either survival or neurologic outcomes as compared to bag-mask ventilation. Others have shown worse outcomes or extended scene times.[36,37]

In addition to the differences in airway and ventilation procedures for pediatric patients, the anatomic differences of the pediatric airway must be considered.[23] These anatomic differences include the following:

1. The infant's upper airway is relatively small; the tongue is disproportionately large. Therefore, posterior displacement of the tongue easily obstructs the airway. In addition, the larger tongue of the pediatric patient tends to make laryngoscopy more difficult. Have another rescuer pull on a corner of the mouth to increase visualization.
2. The epiglottis is shaped like the Greek letter omega (Ω). It is narrower and longer in children than in adults. Because of this, the epiglottis is more difficult to control with a laryngoscopic blade. The larynx lies more anteriorly in relation to the base of the tongue than in the adult. It also is elevated under the base of the tongue, making visualization more difficult. The glottic opening is at the third cervical vertebra in premature neonates, the third to fourth cervical vertebrae in term neonates, and the fourth to fifth cervical vertebrae in adults.
3. During the first few months of life, the infant's vocal cords slope from back to front. As a result, the ET tube frequently gets hung up in the angle formed by the cords. This problem can be minimized by rotating the ET tube or by having a second rescuer perform the Sellick maneuver during intubation.
4. The cricoid cartilage is the narrowest part of the airway in the infant and young child. As the child reaches 8 to 10 years of age, the vocal cords become the narrowest part. This remains the case into adulthood.
5. The distance from the vocal cords to the carina varies and can be correlated with the patient's height. This distance is about 2 to 2.5 inches (4 to 5 cm) at birth and 3 to 3.5 inches (6 to 7 cm) by 6 years of age. During placement of the ET tube, the tube should be advanced until breath sounds are lost unilaterally (usually on the left side). It should then be withdrawn slowly until breath sounds return, indicating that the tube tip is at the carina. After the return of breath sounds, the tube should be withdrawn 0.75 to 1.5 inches (2 to 3 cm) farther, placing it at a safe distance above the carina and below the cords. The tube then should be secured with tape or a commercial device.

   The correct depth of the insertion for an ET tube in children older than 2 years can be approximated by adding one-half of the patient's age to 12:

$$\text{Depth of insertion (cm)} = \frac{\text{Patient's age}}{2} + 12$$

   Alternatively, the depth of insertion can be estimated by multiplying the internal diameter of the tube by 3:[26]

$$\text{Depth of insertion (cm)} = \text{ET tube internal diameter} \times 3$$

6. Children use the diaphragm as the major muscle for ventilation. They require full diaphragmatic excursion to breathe. Gastric distention caused by swallowing air or artificial ventilation can inhibit the child's respiratory efforts. Infants are nose breathers until 3 to 5 months of age.
7. Deciduous teeth begin to develop at about 6 months. These are lost between 6 and 8 years of age. They may become dislodged during airway procedures such as intubation and oral airway insertion and by the child biting on the airway.

During any airway procedure, the paramedic should remember that the airway structures of children are very fragile and easily damaged. Therefore, great care must be taken not to injure these patients.

Adjuncts to Aid Confirmation of Endotracheal Tube Placement

Several adjuncts often can help the paramedic determine correct ET tube placement. These include $ETCO_2$ detectors, bulb- or syringe-type esophageal detection devices, and pulse oximeters. As stated previously, confirmation of tube placement requires more than one method of assessment.

End-Tidal Carbon Dioxide Detectors

Capnography is the measurement of carbon dioxide concentrations in exhaled air. This measurement is made possible by $ETCO_2$ detectors. $ETCO_2$ detectors help verify placement of the ET tube. They also are designed to reveal inadvertent esophageal intubation. These devices provide a noninvasive estimate of alveolar ventilation, carbon dioxide production, and arterial carbon dioxide content. Their use as an adjunct to assessment of ET tube placement is essential.[23,26] Some capnometers can be used in patients who have not been intubated (ie, using a device that resembles a nasal cannula). They may be helpful in determining the effectiveness of ventilation and EMS treatments.

Three types of carbon dioxide detectors are available: disposable colorimetric devices, electronic capnometry devices, and capnography devices. Colorimetric devices contain a chemical indicator that is sensitive to carbon dioxide (**FIGURE 15-87**). When the detector is attached to the ET tube, the color of the indicator changes with elevated carbon dioxide. These elevations would be expected in the trachea but not in the esophagus. A memory aid for colorimetric devices is as follows: yellow (yes) indicates that the ET tube is correctly placed in the trachea; tan indicates that the ET tube may not be in the trachea; (think about it) and purple (problem) indicates a problem (the ET tube is not in the trachea). Colorimetric devices provide limited information and can be used only for short periods. Exposure to secretions may render them ineffective (**FIGURE 15-88**).

A capnometer is an electronic device for measuring the $ETCO_2$. The monitor probe or sampling tubing is connected between the advanced airway device and the ventilation device. Because capnometers display

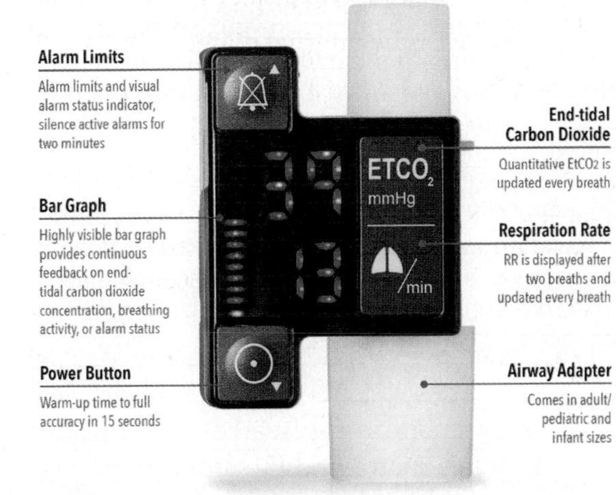
Alarm Limits
Alarm limits and visual alarm status indicator, silence active alarms for two minutes
Bar Graph
Highly visible bar graph provides continuous feedback on end-tidal carbon dioxide concentration, breathing activity, or alarm status
Power Button
Warm-up time to full accuracy in 15 seconds
ETCO2
mmHg
/min
End-tidal Carbon Dioxide
Quantitative EtCO2 is updated every breath
Respiration Rate
RR is displayed after two breaths and updated every breath
Airway Adapter
Comes in adult/pediatric and infant sizes

FIGURE 15-87 Digital (or electronic) end-tidal carbon dioxide detector.

Image used with permission from Masimo Corporation.

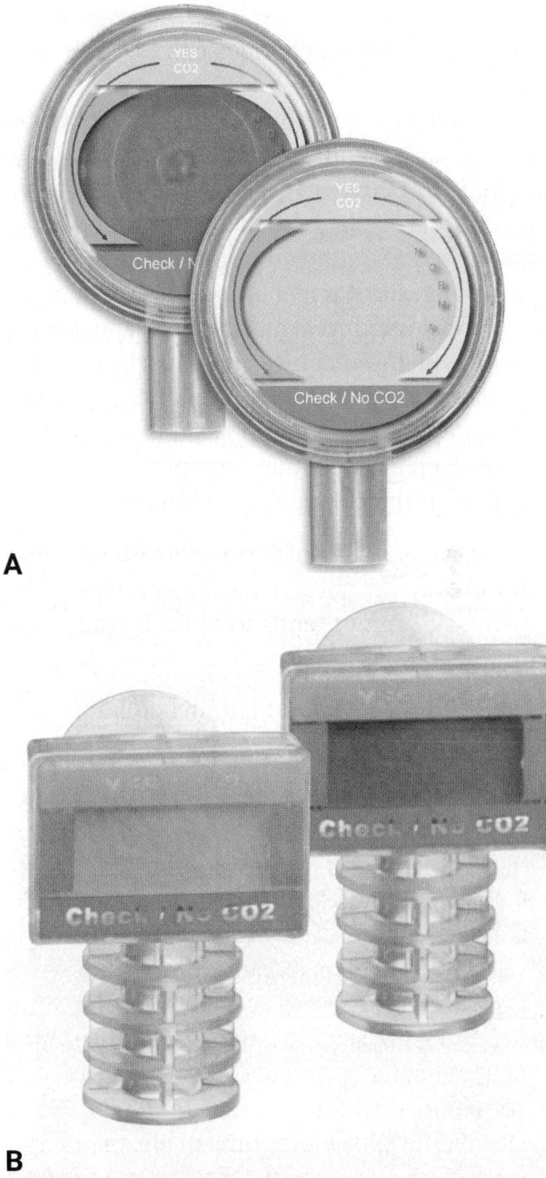
YES
CO2
Check / No CO2
A
B

FIGURE 15-88 Colorimetric end-tidal carbon dioxide detector. **A.** Adult. **B.** Pediatric.

Reproduced with permission from Westmed, Inc.

NOTE

The color indicators of colorimetric carbon dioxide detectors can be affected by vomitus. They also can be affected if the patient recently drank a carbonated beverage (if the ET tube is placed in the esophagus).

NOTE

Cardiac output is low during CPR. Consequently, colorimetric devices may show no color change even when the ET tube is in the trachea. In such cases, a second method of confirming tube placement should be used, such as an esophageal detector device.

a numeric $ETCO_2$ value, changes can be measured over time.

Capnography is a method of measuring carbon dioxide that displays and records both a numeric value for the $ETCO_2$ and a dynamic waveform. This method provides a visual display of the rate, depth, and effectiveness of the patient's ventilation (**FIGURE 15-89**). It does not measure oxygenation. Because carbon dioxide is a waste product of metabolism, capnography also provides an indirect measure of perfusion. This is important during CPR. A decline in $ETCO_2$ values may indicate that chest compressions are not fast enough or deep enough. Capnographic waveforms also can provide information about bronchoconstriction (BOX 15-13). When the terminal bronchioles are constricted, the upslope of the capnographic waveform resembles a shark's fin. This finding is related to uneven emptying of air from the narrowed airways. Paramedics can monitor the capnographic waveform to evaluate the effectiveness of bronchodilator treatment (see Chapter 23, *Respiratory*).

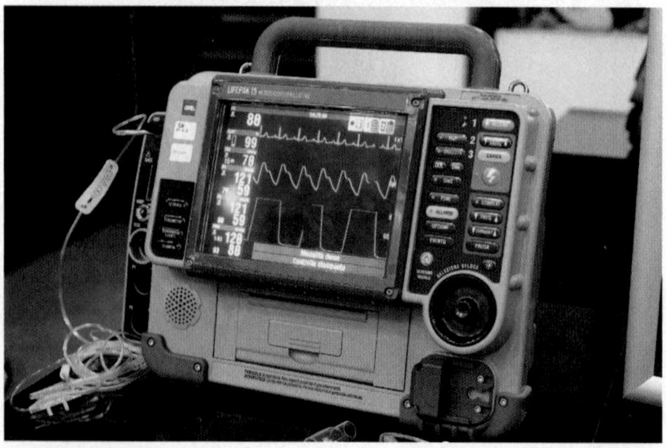

FIGURE 15-89 Monitor displaying continuous capnographic waveform.

Continuous capnography readings can be obtained in intubated and nonintubated patients. Using the $ETCO_2$ values to help assess the patient and the

SHOW ME THE EVIDENCE

Wirtz and colleagues sought prospectively to find the incidence of unrecognized prehospital ET tube misplacement in patients arriving at two EDs in New York City from 17 EMS agencies from February 2003 to June 2004. Only one agency used $ETCO_2$ detectors. Paramedics intubated 132 patients during the study period. Eleven ET tubes were placed in the esophagus, and one was placed in the hypopharynx. In addition, 15% of patients had right main stem intubation on arrival at the ED. Eleven of 12 patients with unrecognized esophageal intubation died.

Modified from: Wirtz D, Ortiz C, Newman D, Zhitomirsky I. Unrecognized placement of endotracheal tubes by ground prehospital providers, *Prehosp Emerg Care*. 2007;11:213-218.

NOTE

Capnography provides a breath-by-breath measurement of a patient's ventilation. It therefore can quickly reveal a trend in a patient's condition and provide early warning of a decline in a patient's respiratory status. Capnography is useful for monitoring patients with asthma, congestive heart failure, diabetes, shock, pulmonary embolus, acidosis, and other conditions. A high $ETCO_2$ reading in a patient with altered mental status or severe dyspnea may indicate hypoventilation and the need for tracheal intubation.

SHOW ME THE EVIDENCE

Silvestri and coworkers performed a prospective observational study for 10 months in 2002 on all adult and pediatric patients who had prehospital ET intubation and were taken to a level I trauma center. Use of continuous $ETCO_2$ monitoring was available but not required by all the participating EMS systems. During this period, 153 patients who arrived at the trauma center had been intubated and met the study criteria. Continuous $ETCO_2$ monitoring was used for 93 patients (61%); none of these patients had unrecognized misplaced intubation. In the group in which continuous $ETCO_2$ monitoring was not used, 13 patients had esophageal intubation and 1 patient had hypopharyngeal placement. This constituted a 23% misplacement rate.

Modified from: Silvestri S, Ralls G, Krauss B, et al. The effectiveness of out-of-hospital use of continuous end-tidal carbon dioxide monitoring on the rate of unrecognized misplaced intubation within a regional emergency medical services system. *Ann Emerg Med*. 2005;45:497-502.

NOTE

Capnography also can be used as an early indication of ROSC. Studies have shown that when a patient experiences ROSC, the first indication often is a sudden rise in the $ETCO_2$ level. This rise occurs as the rush of circulation washes untransported carbon dioxide from the tissues. Likewise, a sudden drop in the $ETCO_2$ may indicate the patient has lost pulses, and CPR may need to be initiated.

Modified from: Kodali BS, Urman RD. Capnography during cardiopulmonary resuscitation: current evidence and future directions. *J Emerg Trauma Shock*. 2014;7(4):332-340.

effectiveness of interventions is crucial. $ETCO_2$ values can help detect hypoventilation, hyperventilation, and ET tube misplacement. Paramedics must monitor it continuously en route to detect with preventable abnormalities that could contribute to a poor outcome.[38]

CRITICAL THINKING

Your patient is in full arrest. The measurements from your $ETCO_2$ detector are inconclusive. Also, you cannot get the oxygen saturation monitor to work. You are not sure whether you hear breath sounds clearly. What should you do?

BOX 15-13 Capnographic Waveforms

Capnographic waveforms on the monitor screen are condensed to provide assessment information in a 4-second view. Printouts of waveforms provide the same information in "real time" and may differ in duration from that of the monitor screen. The following are example waveforms for both intubated and nonintubated patients.[a]

Normal Ranges

Arterial $Paco_2$: 35–45 mm Hg
Capnographic $ETCO_2$: 35–45 mm Hg (4–6 vol%)

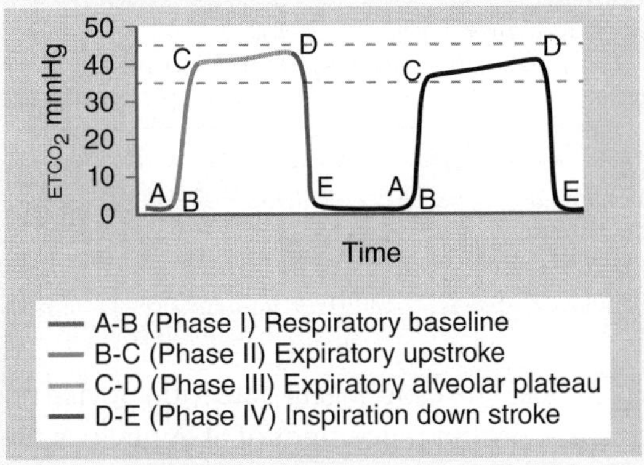

Normal capnography tracing:

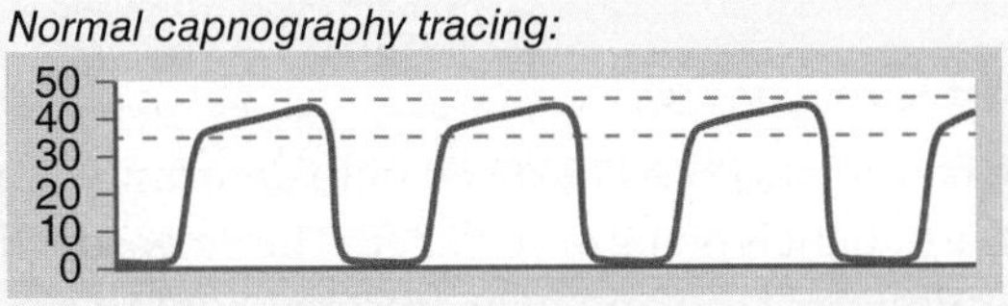

Intubated Patients

In an intubated patient, capnography may be used to:

- Verify ET tube placement
- Monitor or detect ET tube dislodgement
- Monitor loss of circulatory function
- Assess the adequacy of CPR compressions
- Confirm ROSC

Examples

Tube dislodged:

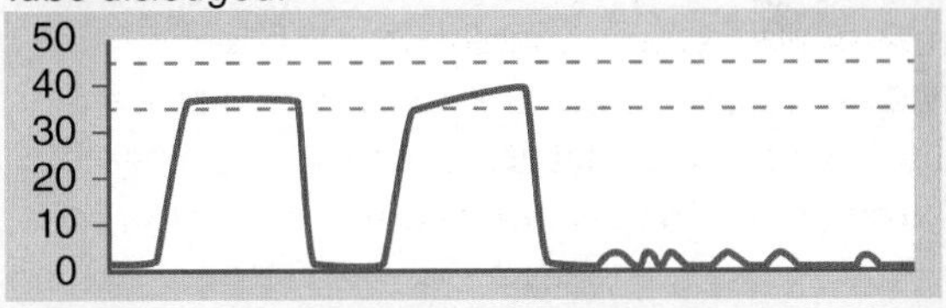

ET tube cuff problem or partial obstruction:

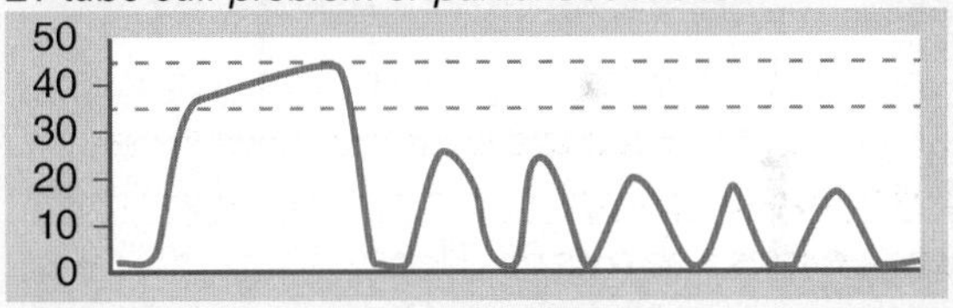

Return of spontaneous circulation:

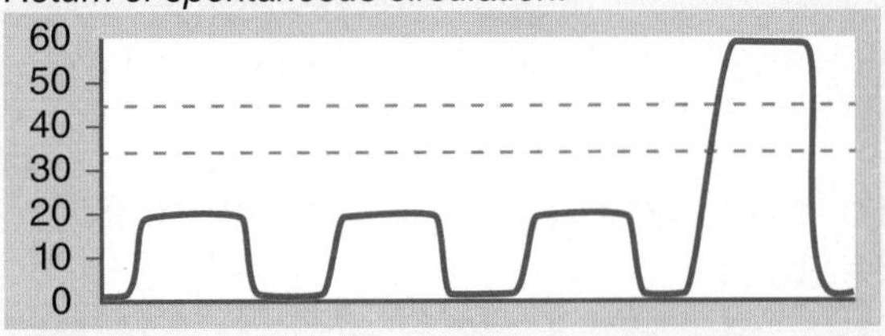

Nonintubated Patients

In a nonintubated patient, capnography may be used to:

- Assess asthma and COPD
- Document and monitor procedural sedation
- Detect apnea or inadequate breathing
- Measure hypoventilation
- Evaluate hyperventilation

BOX 15-13 Capnographic Waveforms *(continued)*

Examples

"Shark-fin" appearance during bronchospasm:

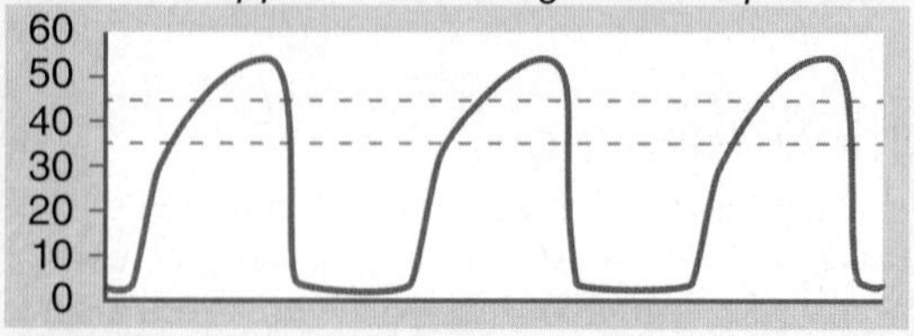

Hypoventilation:

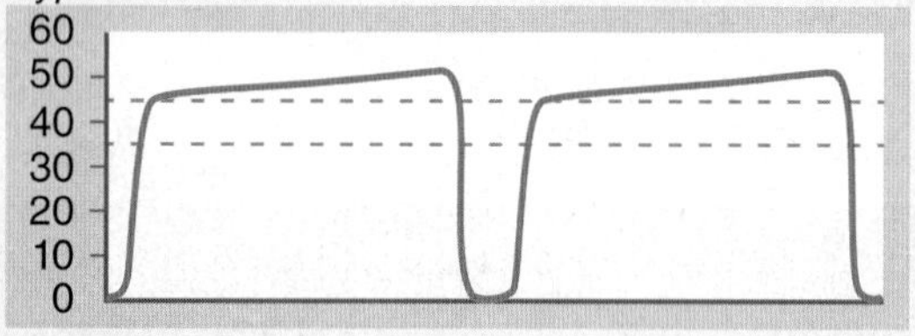

Hyperventilation:

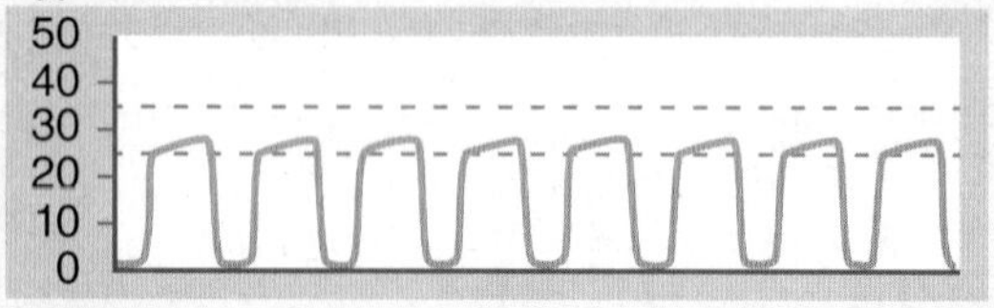

Irregular breathing:

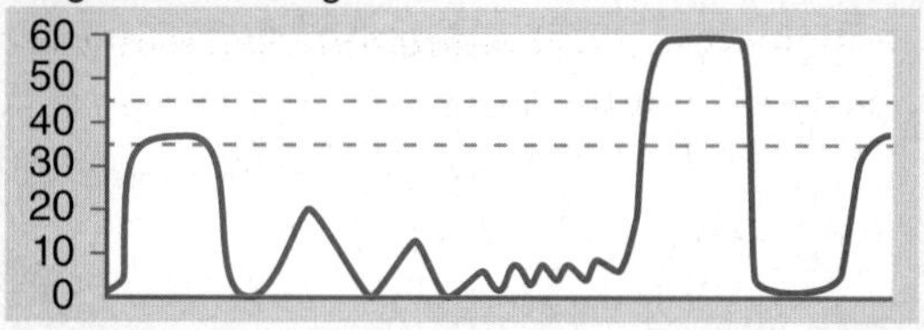

Causes of Elevated $ETCO_2$

- Decreased ventilation secondary to:
  - Head trauma
  - Overdose
  - Respiratory failure (severe asthma, COPD)
  - Sedation
  - Stroke
  - Increased carbon dioxide production
  - Fever
  - Shivering
- Return of circulation after cardiac arrest
- Tourniquet release
- Sodium bicarbonate administration
- Thyroid storm

Causes of Low $ETCO_2$

- Ventilation problem
  - Esophageal intubation
  - Airway obstruction
- Inadequate blood flow
  - Cardiac arrest (lower if poor compressions; lower values predict poor outcome)
  - Tension pneumothorax
  - Pericardial tamponade
- Ventilation/perfusion mismatch
  - Pulmonary embolism
- Decreased production of carbon dioxide
  - Hypothermia
- Sampling error
  - Inadequate tidal volume delivery
  - Carbon dioxide sampling tubing blocked

[a]The level of sedation and severity of conditions may affect the respiratory rate and $ETCO_2$ level.
Modified from: Ornato JP, Peberdy, MA. Prehospital end-tidal carbon dioxide monitoring – it's not all hot air. *JEMS*. 1993.

Bulb- and Syringe-Type Esophageal Detectors

Esophageal detection devices (eg, the Toomey syringe) are attached to the end of the ET tube immediately after intubation (**FIGURE 15-90**). They operate on the principle that the esophagus is a collapsible tube. As such, a vacuum is created when air is removed from the esophagus. Air is removed from the esophagus when the bulb device is compressed or when air is withdrawn by the syringe device if the ET tube is in the esophagus. If the ET tube has been correctly placed in the trachea, the bulb device easily refills with air or the syringe device is easily aspirated when the plunger is pulled back. The esophageal detection device does not confirm proper placement of SGA devices.

Pulse Oximetry

Pulse oximeters (**FIGURE 15-91**) help determine how well the patient is being oxygenated. They measure the transmission of red and near-infrared light through arterial beds. Hemoglobin absorbs red and infrared light waves differently when it is bound with oxygen (oxyhemoglobin) than when it is not (reduced hemoglobin). Oxyhemoglobin absorbs more infrared than red light. Reduced hemoglobin absorbs more red than infrared light. Pulse oximetry (Spo_2) indirectly

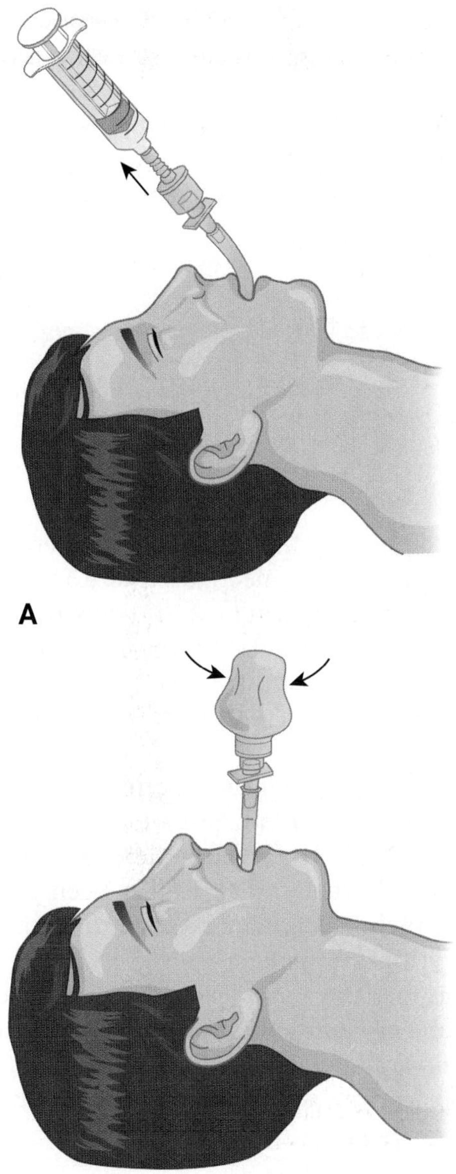

FIGURE 15-90 Esophageal intubation detector. **A.** Syringe. **B.** Bulb.

reveals the arterial saturation (Spo_2) by measuring this difference in absorption.

The oximeter probe is placed on an area of thin tissue, such as a finger, toe, or earlobe. One side of the probe sends wavelengths of light through the arterial bed. The other side detects the presence of red or infrared light. Using this balance of red and infrared colors, the oximeter calculates the oxygen saturation of the blood and displays it on the monitor screen.

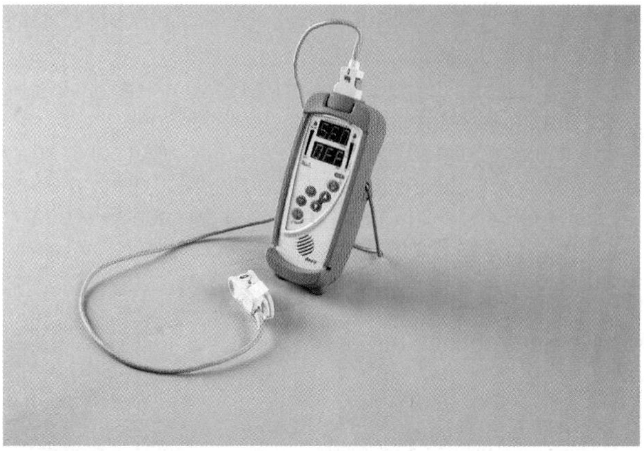

FIGURE 15-91 Pulse oximeter.

BOX 15-14 Oxygen Saturation and Partial Pressure

With 90% saturation: Po_2 drops to 60 mm Hg
With 75% saturation: Po_2 drops to 40 mm Hg
With 50% saturation: Po_2 drops to 27 mm Hg

The percentage of hemoglobin saturated with oxygen is denoted as the Spo_2. It depends on a number of factors, including the Pco_2, pH, temperature, and whether the hemoglobin is normal or altered. The lower range of normal for the Spo_2 is 93% to 95%. The upper range is 99% to 100%. Once the Spo_2 falls below 90% (corresponding to a Po_2 of 60 mm Hg), further decreases are associated with a marked decline in oxygen content (BOX 15-14).

NOTE

Comprehensive assessment of a patent's ventilation and perfusion status requires blood gas analysis (an in-hospital procedure). As described in Chapter 11, *General Principles of Pathophysiology*, blood gas analysis is used to assess pH, the partial pressure of arterial carbon dioxide, bicarbonate, and base deficit. (Methods used to obtain arterial blood gas samples are presented in the Appendix, *Advanced Practice Procedures for Critical Care Paramedics*.)

Difficulties and inaccuracies may result from the use of pulse oximeters. Therefore, paramedics should consider them only as another tool to assist the monitoring of a patient's oxygenation levels.

NOTE

Recent research has suggested that in some conditions, such as general respiratory distress, oxygen therapy should be regulated to maintain the Spo_2 level between 93% and 96%. Likewise, beginning in 2010, the American Heart Association began to recommend oxygen therapy for treatment of stroke, or myocardial infarction when the Spo_2 is less than 94%. Oxygen continues to be recommended for all patients who are dyspneic or who have signs of heart failure or shock.

Modified from: Oost J, Daya M. Respiratory distress. In: Cone D, Brice JH, Delbridge TR, Myers JB, eds. *Emergency Medical Services: Clinical Practice and Systems Oversight*. 2nd ed. West Sussex, England: Wiley and Sons; 2015:143-158; American Heart Association. 2010 American Heart Association guidelines for cardiopulmonary resuscitation and emergency cardiovascular care. *Circulation*. 2010;122(18)(suppl 3):S639-S946.

Circumstances that may produce false readings include the following:[39]

- Dyshemoglobinemia, which is hemoglobin saturation with compounds other than oxygen (eg, carbon monoxide, methemoglobin, anemia)
- Excessive ambient light (sunlight, fluorescent lights) on the oximeter's sensor probe
- Patient movement
- Hypotension
- Hypothermia/vasoconstriction
- Patient use of vasoconstrictive drugs
- Jaundice

Supraglottic Airway Devices

SGAs, also referred to as extraglottic airways, have been used in operating rooms for decades. They have become very popular and widely adopted in the prehospital realm because of their simplicity, ease of use, ease of training, speed of deployment, and classification as a BLS airway device. There are several different SGA devices available on the market, and the selection of one over another is largely based on training, experience, and local preferences. More common SGA tools used by EMS personnel include the LMA, i-gel, King LT-D, and esophageal-tracheal Combitube.

Laryngeal Mask Airway

The LMA is an advanced airway control device. It may be used in the prehospital setting when conventional ET intubation is unsuccessful, when access to the patient is limited, when an unstable neck injury may be present, or when appropriate positioning of the patient for tracheal intubation is impossible.[23] Some LMAs also allow ET intubation through the device. This option allows for easier placement of the tube.

AFTER 3 INTUBATION ATTEMPTS

NOTE

The LMA does not offer full protection against aspiration. However, aspiration is uncommon with this device. A small number of patients cannot be ventilated adequately with the LMA. Also, it is contraindicated in conscious patients and in those with an intact gag reflex.

Description. The LMA is available in several sizes, ranging from size 1 for neonates to size 5 for adults. It consists of a proximal tube with standard adapters for connecting ventilatory devices. The tube is connected to a distal mask that is inflated by means of a pilot tube and balloon (**FIGURE 15-92**).

Insertion. The LMA is inserted through the mouth into the pharynx. It is advanced until resistance is felt as the distal portion of the tube locates in the hypopharynx. When the device has been properly inserted, the black line marked on the LMA rests midline against the patient's upper lip. Inflating the cuff seals the larynx and leaves the distal opening of the tube just above the glottis, providing a clear, secure airway. After the pilot cuff has been inflated, proper placement is confirmed by observing equal

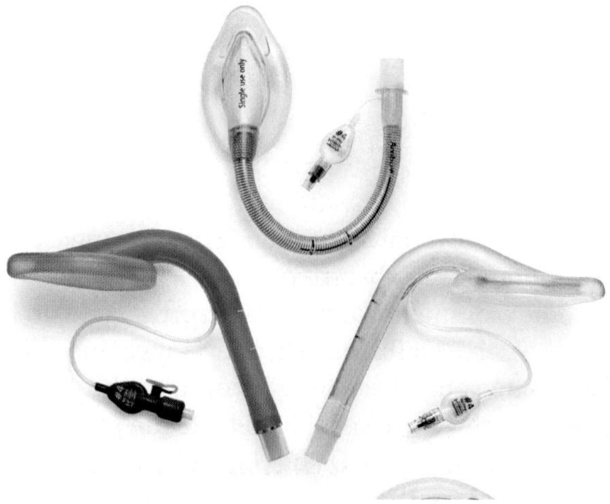

FIGURE 15-92 Laryngeal mask airways.

Courtesy of Ambu, Inc.

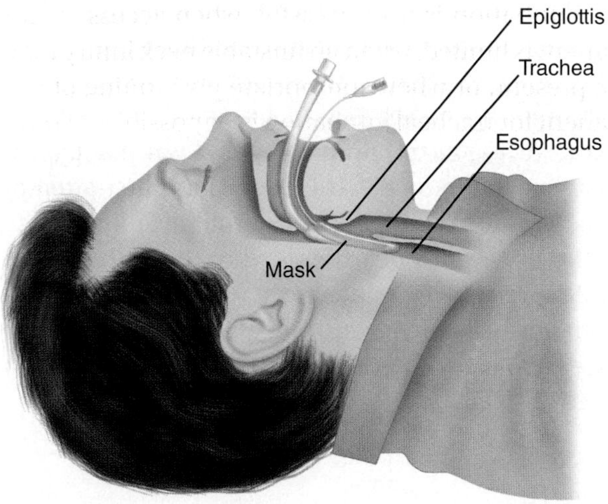

FIGURE 15-93 A patient with a laryngeal mask airway.

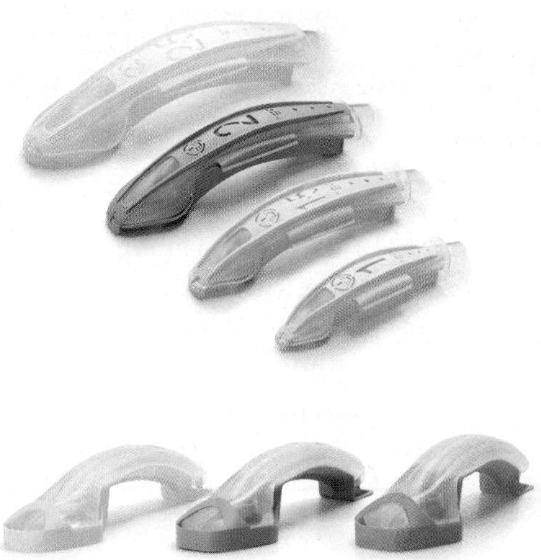

FIGURE 15-94 The i-gel airway.

rise and fall of the chest, by ensuring bilateral breath sounds, and with $ETCO_2$ detectors and pulse oximetry monitoring (in a patient who has a perfusing rhythm) (**FIGURE 15-93**). Use of the LMA requires special training and authorization from medical direction. The LMA may be difficult to maintain during patient movement, which can make it difficult to use during patient transport.

Necessary Additional Equipment

- Water-soluble lubricant
- Syringes
- Bag-mask device
- Oxygen source and connecting tubing
- Suction equipment
- Stethoscope
- One or more confirmation devices

Common Advantages

- Less skilled training or maintenance is required than for ET intubation.
- Laryngoscopy and visualization of the vocal cords are not required.
- Minimal spinal movement is required for insertion.
- ET intubation can be achieved through some LMAs.

Common Disadvantages

- The patient must be unresponsive and have no gag reflex.
- Not all patients can be adequately ventilated with the LMA.
- The airway must be removed when the patient becomes responsive or agitated.
- The airway does not provide as much protection from aspiration as the ET tube provides.
- It is appropriate for short-term use only.

Common Contraindications

- Presence of a gag reflex
- Caustic ingestion
- Esophageal trauma or disease

i-gel

The i-gel is a type of LMA that has a soft gellike noninflatable cuff (**FIGURE 15-94**). It is designed to rest over the larynx. The insertion is the same as that for the LMA, except that no inflation is needed. The indications and contraindications are also the same. Evidence suggests the i-gel airway is easier to place than the standard LMA is, taking less than 5 seconds to insert.[40] The airways are color coded and are available in four pediatric sizes and three adult sizes (**BOX 15-15**). The straps that come with the i-gel must be firmly secured to ensure it remains in place during transport.

King LT-D Airway

The King LT-D airway (laryngeal tube) is a disposable supraglottic device designed for positive pressure ventilation as well as for patients who are breathing

BOX 15-15 i-gel Airway Sizes

Pediatric

1.0 (pink): 2–5 kg (4–11 pounds)
1.5 (light blue): 5–12 kg (11–26 pounds)
2.0 (gray): 10–25 kg (22–55 pounds)
2.5 (white): 25–35 kg (55–77 pounds)

Adult

3.0 (yellow): 30–60 kg (66–132 pounds)
4.0 (green): 50–90 kg (110–198 pounds)
5.0 (orange): >90 kg (>198 pounds)

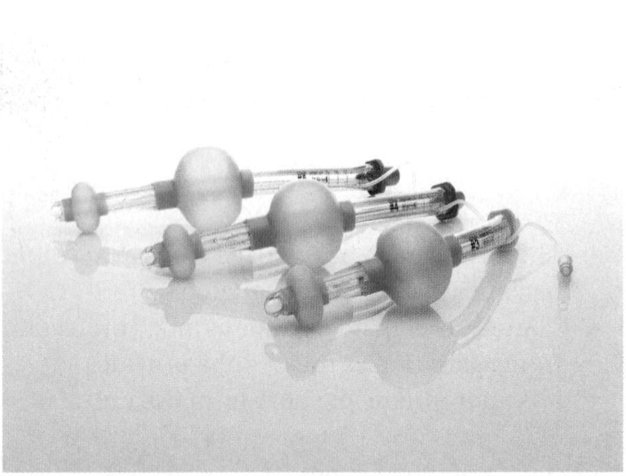

FIGURE 15-95 King LT-D airways.

spontaneously. It is an alternative to mask ventilation and tracheal intubation.

The King LT-D airway has a single tube that is placed only into the esophagus. (The tube's large size and short length virtually eliminate the possibility of placement into the trachea.) The tube is curved and has a proximal and distal cuff. As with the esophageal-tracheal Combitube, a large balloon is inflated in the oropharynx. At the same time, a smaller cuff is inflated in the esophagus by the same port that inflates the large cuff. Ventilations are delivered by attaching a bag-mask device to the proximal end of the tube. With each ventilation, the air escapes through holes in the tube between the cuffs. Some King LT-D airways also provide for passage of tubes for gastric decompression. The King LT-D is available in multiple sizes, based on a patient's height, although the smallest size is designed for a 26-pound (12-kg) patient (**FIGURE 15-95**).

Use of the King LT-D airway is indicated when tracheal intubation cannot be established in two attempts and when a patient is unable to adequately maintain his or her airway, has an altered mental status (Glasgow Coma Score of 8 or lower), or has respiratory compromise. This device has a first-attempt success rate of about 85%.[41] Contraindications to use of the airway include patients who are less than 4 feet (1.2 m) tall, have an intact gag reflex, have ingested caustic substances, and have known esophageal disease. **FIGURE 15-96** describes the insertion of a King LT-D airway.

NOTE

The King LT-D airway may be considered before tracheal intubation if significant access issues exist (eg, prolonged entrapment) or if a difficult intubation is anticipated.

Before the airway is inserted, the cuff should be tested for integrity and then deflated. Lubricant is applied to the back side of the airway, with care taken not to clog the holes in the tube. The patient's head should be placed in a neutral position, observing spinal precautions if indicated. Before insertion, the patient's lungs are preoxygenated with 100% oxygen. The patient's mouth should be opened using a head-tilt or chin-lift maneuver. The tube is advanced gently behind the base of the patient's tongue while the tube is rotated back to the midline. The tube's blue orientation line should face the patient's chin. The tube then is gently advanced until the base of the connector is aligned with the patient's teeth or gums. The airway is inflated with the appropriate volume of air.

The bag-mask device is connected to the adaptor on the tube, and ventilations are provided. While providing ventilations, the paramedic gently withdraws the tube until ventilation compliance becomes easy and free flowing. Cuff inflation may be adjusted if necessary to maintain a seal of the airway at the peak ventilatory pressure used. Correct placement is confirmed by listening for equal and bilateral breath sounds, observing chest rise and fall, verifying the presence of $ETCO_2$, and monitoring for a stable or rising SpO_2. The device is secured, and placement of a bite block should be considered.

The position of the King LT-D airway should be rechecked after each patient movement, on transfer of care to another provider, and after an ascent or a descent of more than 1,000 feet (305 m).

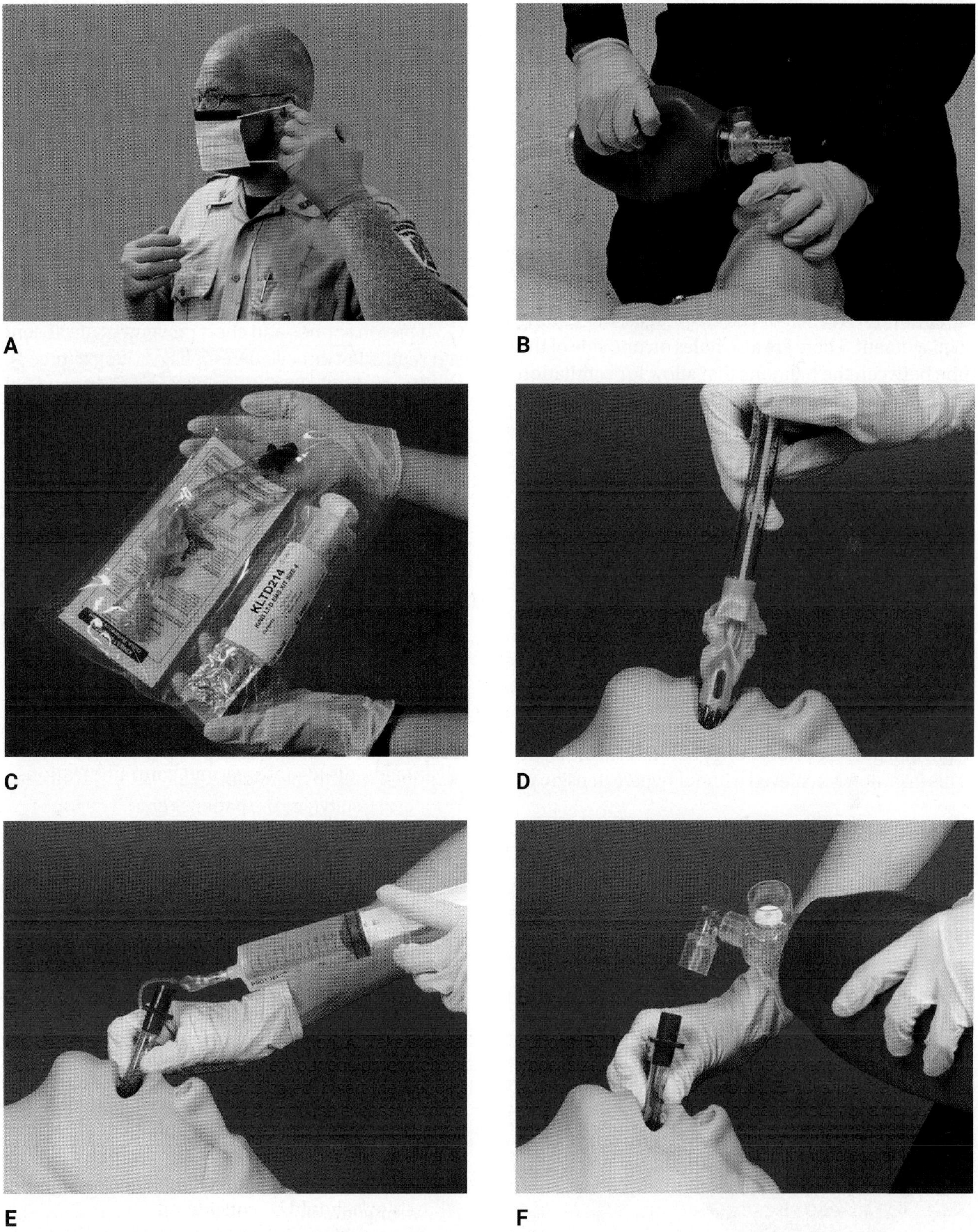

FIGURE 15-96 King LT-D airway insertion. **A.** Take standard precautions. **B.** Preoxygenate the patient with a bag-mask device with 100% oxygen. **C.** Gather your equipment; choose the proper size of airway. **D.** Place the patient's head in a neutral position, unless contraindicated. Insert the lubricated airway into the midline of the mouth. **E.** Advance the tip beyond the base of the tongue. Do not use excessive force. Inflate the cuffs with the recommended amount of air or just enough to seal the device. **F.** Attach the tube to the ventilation device and verify proper placement by primary and secondary confirmation methods. In-line capnography should always be used to confirm tube placement. Monitor tube position.

Esophageal-Tracheal Combitube

The esophageal-tracheal Combitube (ETC, Combitube) allows for either esophageal or tracheal insertion. With the advent of newer, smaller devices that are easier to insert, use of the ETC has declined. The ETC takes almost twice the time to insert as the King airway.[42] It is a plastic tube with twin lumens that are separated by a partition wall. One tube resembles an ET tube and has an open distal end. The other tube is blocked by an obturator at the distal end. Both tubes use low-pressure balloons that provide a seal for either the trachea or the esophagus, depending on placement. There are also holes on one side of the tube between the balloons that allow for ventilation through tube 1. When inflated, the large pharyngeal balloon fills the space between the base of the tongue and the soft palate, anchoring the tube in position. The Combitube usually finds its way into the esophagus because of the stiffness and curve of the tube and the shape and the structure of the pharynx. The Combitube is another option for airway control when ET intubation is indicated, but is unsuccessful or unavailable.

Insertion. The Combitube is inserted by gently guiding the device into the esophagus or trachea (**FIGURE 15-97**). The tube should be inserted into the midline and to a depth that puts the printed ring at the level of the teeth. (This insertion is achieved without hyperextension or flexion of the patient's head. It also is done without visualization of the glottic opening.) The pharyngeal and distal balloons then are inflated. This design isolates the oropharynx above the upper balloon and the esophagus (or trachea) below the lower balloon. Ventilation is at first provided through the esophageal lumen. (This is due to the significant chance of esophageal placement with blind insertion.) In this position, air passes into the pharynx and beyond the glottis into the trachea. The placement is confirmed by the primary and secondary confirmation methods described previously.

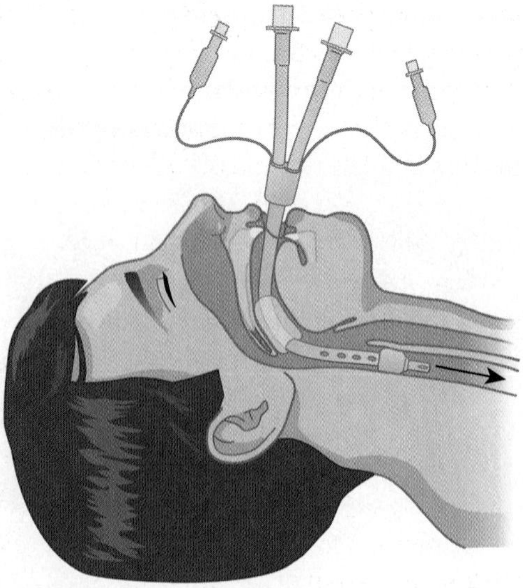

FIGURE 15-97 Placement of the esophageal-tracheal Combitube airway.

If breath sounds and chest movement are absent with ventilation through the esophageal lumen (tube 1), ventilation should be performed through the tracheal lumen (tube 2) without changing the position of the airway. Air passes through this lumen directly into the trachea. Placement is confirmed in the usual manner.

Necessary Equipment

- Water-soluble lubricant
- Syringes
- Bag-mask device
- Oxygen source and connecting tubing
- Suction equipment
- Stethoscope
- $ETCO_2$ device

The various kinds of balloon-system devices share advantages, disadvantages, and contraindications.

Advantages

- Airways cannot be placed improperly.
- Less skill training or skill maintenance is needed than for ET intubation.
- Minimal spinal movement is required for insertion.
- Suctioning is easy.

Disadvantages

- The patient must be unresponsive and without a gag reflex.
- The airway must be removed when the patient becomes responsive or agitated.
- Proper identification of the tube's location may be difficult, leading to ventilation through the wrong lumen.
- The trachea cannot be suctioned when the tube is in the esophagus.
- The airway should be replaced with an ET tube as soon as possible.

- Complications may include upper airway bleeding, esophageal laceration, esophageal perforation, and mediastinitis.[42]

Contraindications

- Patient height less than 5 feet (1.5 m) or age younger than 14 years
- Caustic ingestion
- Esophageal trauma or disease
- Presence of a gag reflex

Pharmacologic Adjuncts to Airway Management and Ventilation

Sedation sometimes is used in airway management and ventilation to reduce anxiety, induce amnesia, and decrease the gag reflex. Possible indications for sedation include combative patients, patients who require aggressive airway management but who are too alert to tolerate intubation, and agitated trauma patients. Three medications commonly used for drug-assisted intubation (DAI) are etomidate (a nonbarbiturate hypnotic), ketamine (a dissociative anesthetic), and midazolam (a short-acting benzodiazepine) often combined with fentanyl (a synthetic opioid analgesic) or other pain medication. Pain medication should be considered with the sedative because intubation is a painful procedure.

Paralytic Agents in Emergency Intubation

Although controversial in the prehospital setting, paralysis after appropriate sedation may be used for emergency intubation. Paralysis involves the use of neuromuscular blocking drugs. These drugs are indicated for combative patients who need to be intubated. For instance, a patient suffering a head injury may be agitated and combative. These drugs should not be used in the following situations:

- Patients who will be difficult to ventilate (eg, patients with facial hair)
- Patients who will be difficult to intubate (eg, patients with short necks, obstructions)

> NOTE
>
> Paralyzing a patient for intubation is associated with significant risk and is not an authorized procedure in many EMS systems. If permitted by state EMS law, the procedure requires advanced training and authorization from medical direction.

Pharmacology

The use of medication to facilitate intubation is increasing. Most ground EMS agencies do not credential paramedics to administer paralytic drugs. It is not a generally expected competency of entry-level paramedics. Other types of medication-assisted intubation (MAI) or DAI are widely accepted. The protocols to intubate using MAI or DAI typically include etomidate, fentanyl, or morphine and midazolam or ketamine. These medications sedate but do not paralyze patients. A joint policy on DAI created by the American College of Emergency Physicians, American College of Surgeons Committee on Trauma, and National Association of EMS Physicians acknowledged the benefits and potential harm associated with this procedure. These organizations recommended that a prehospital DAI program include strict medical oversight. This oversight should include training on the medications, intubation, and backup airway maneuvers; quality assurance; standardized protocols to include drug storage; resources for continuous patient monitoring to confirm patient status and proper airway placement; and research to identify appropriate use of DAI.[43]

As described in Chapter 13, *Principles of Pharmacology and Emergency Medications*, neuromuscular blockers produce skeletal muscle paralysis. They do this by binding to the nicotinic receptor for acetylcholine (ACh) at the neuromuscular junction. To review, this junction is the point of contact between the nerve ending and the muscle fiber (see Chapter 10, *Review of Human Systems*). When nerve impulses pass through this junction, ACh and other chemicals are released. This release causes the muscle to contract. The two types of neuromuscular blocking drugs are depolarizing agents and nondepolarizing agents. Neuromuscular blockers should not be administered to patients until sufficient sedation has been achieved.

Depolarizing agents invade the neuromuscular junction and bind to the receptors for ACh. These drugs produce depolarization of the muscular membrane. Thus, they often lead to fasciculations (uncontrollable muscle twitching). These drugs also may lead to some muscular contractions. An example of a depolarizing agent is succinylcholine. Succinylcholine has a rapid onset of action. Yet it has the briefest duration of action of all the neuromuscular blocking drugs. This makes it the drug of choice for emergency ET intubation.

Nondepolarizing agents also bind to the receptors for ACh. However, they block the uptake of ACh at the neuromuscular junction without initiating depolarization of the muscle membrane. Examples of nondepolarizing drugs include vecuronium and rocuronium. These drugs have a longer onset and duration than depolarizing agents have.

Neuromuscular blocking agents produce complete paralysis. Consequently, ventilatory support must be provided. Ventilation and oxygenation must be closely monitored to ensure that they are adequate. If the patient is conscious, the paramedic should explain the effects of the medication before administering it. Lidocaine given before administration of a neuromuscular blocking agent may blunt any increase in intracranial pressure associated with intubation (though this is a controversial topic, with studies showing mixed results).[44] Finally, diazepam, etomidate, midazolam, ketamine, or a different sedative approved by medical direction should be used in any conscious patient before a blocking agent is administered; neuromuscular blocking agents do not inhibit pain or seizure activity (**TABLE 15-7**).

Rapid Sequence Intubation

Rapid sequence induction (RSI) involves the administration of a potent sedative or induction agent and a neuromuscular blocking agent at the same time to achieve optimal intubation conditions in less than 1 minute.[45] The blocking agent most often used is succinylcholine (see the Appendix, *Emergency Drug Index*). In addition to providing optimal intubation conditions, RSI also minimizes the risk of aspiration of gastric contents. RSI is indicated in the following situations:[46]

- Emergency intubation is warranted.
- The patient has a higher risk of aspiration because of food or liquid in the stomach.
- Intubation is predicted to be successful (ie, the patient does not have a difficult airway).
- If intubation fails, ventilation is predicted to be successful.

RSI is not indicated for patients in cardiac arrest or for deeply comatose patients when immediate intubation is required. Relative contraindications include concern that intubation or mask ventilation would be unsuccessful; significant facial or laryngeal edema, trauma, or distortion; or a spontaneously breathing patient who requires upper airway muscle tone and positioning (eg, upper airway obstruction, epiglottitis).[23]

NOTE

Rapid sequence induction is not within the national scope of practice of the paramedic. Special training, credentialing, and authorization from medical direction are required in most states.

RSI is an organized approach to ET intubation. It involves specific steps and actions that lead to rapid sedation and paralysis without positive pressure ventilation once the procedure begins. The purpose of RSI is to achieve optimum and rapid tracheal intubation in patients at risk for aspiration. The procedure is intended to take the patient from a conscious, breathing state to a state of unconsciousness. This intervention is accomplished with complete neuromuscular paralysis. Intubation is performed without interposed mechanical ventilation. The six steps of RSI (ie, the six Ps) are preparation, preoxygenation, pretreatment, paralysis (with sedation), placement of the tube, and postintubation management (BOX 15-16 and BOX 15-17).

CRITICAL THINKING

How would you decide whether a patient needs more sedation after a paralytic has been given?

Technique

1. **Preparation**
   - Assess the patient for difficulty of intubation (eg, using the Mallampati score [see Box 15-9]).
   - Prepare all drugs and equipment.
   - Make sure the patient has one or more patent IV lines.
   - Explain the procedure to the patient.
2. **Preoxygenation (done simultaneously with preparation)**
   - Preoxygenate the patient with 100% oxygen for 5 minutes (an essential step of the "no bagging" approach of RSI).
   - Consider using a pulse oximeter.

TABLE 15-7 Drugs Commonly Used for Pharmacologically Assisted Intubation

Drug	Dose (Adult) IV/IO	Dose (Pediatric) IV/IO	Indications	Complications/ Side Effects
Pretreatment				
Oxygen	High concentration Assist ventilation as needed to achieve oxygen saturation of 100% if possible	High concentration Assist ventilation as needed to achieve oxygen saturation of 100% if possible	All patients undergoing pharmacologically assisted intubation	—
Lidocaine	1–2 mg/kg	1–2 mg/kg	Brain injury	Seizure
Induction of Sedation				
Midazolam (Versed)	0.1–0.3 mg/kg (maximum single dose, 10 mg)	0.1–0.3 mg/kg (maximum single dose, 10 mg)	Sedation	Respiratory depression/ apnea, hypotension
Fentanyl (Sublimaze)	2–5 mcg/kg	2–5 mcg/kg	Sedation	Respiratory depression/apnea, hypotension, bradycardia
Etomidate	0.2–0.4 mg/kg (limit 1 dose)	0.2–0.4 mg/kg	Sedation, induced anesthesia	Apnea, hypotension, vomiting
Ketamine	1–2 mg/kg	1–2 mg/kg	Dissociative anesthetic	Hypertension, tachycardia, increased secretions, laryngospasm, emergence reactions
Chemical Paralysis				
Succinylcholine	1–1.5 mg/kg	1–1.5 mg/kg (children); 2 mg/kg (infants)	Muscle relaxation and paralysis (short duration)	Hyperkalemia, muscle fasciculations
Rocuronium	0.6–1.2 mg/kg	0.6–1.2 mg/kg	Paralysis after sedation (nondepolarizing)	Hypotension or hypertension
Vecuronium	0.1–0.2 mg/kg	0.1–0.3 mg/kg	Paralysis after sedation (nondepolarizing)	Hypotension

Abbreviations: IV, intravenous; IO, intraosseous

Modified from: American Heart Association. *2015 Handbook of Emergency Cardiovascular Care for Healthcare Providers*. Dallas, TX: American Heart Association; 2015.

BOX 15-16 Six Ps of Rapid Sequence Induction

1. Preparation
2. Preoxygenation
3. Pretreatment
4. Paralysis (after sedation)
5. Placement of the tube and confirmation of placement
6. Postintubation management

Modified from: American Heart Association. *2015 Handbook of Emergency Cardiovascular Care for Healthcare Providers*. Dallas, TX: American Heart Association; 2015.

3. **Pretreatment (done 3 minutes before intubation)**
   - Consider giving lidocaine to protect against a rise in intracranial pressure and to prevent laryngospasm.
   - Consider giving beta-blockers or opioids to reduce a sympathoadrenal response (eg, a rise in blood pressure) to intubation.
4. **Paralysis (with sedation)**
   - Administer a sedative and analgesic (per protocol) to produce unconsciousness and pain control. This should be immediately followed by a rapid push of the neuromuscular blocker (see the Appendix, *Emergency Drug Index*).

BOX 15-17 Protocol for Rapid Sequence Induction (RSI)

1. Make sure the required equipment is available.
   - Oxygen supply
   - Bag-mask of appropriate size and type
   - Nonrebreathing mask
   - Laryngoscope with blades
   - ET tubes
   - Gum elastic bougie
   - Surgical and alternative airway equipment
   - RSI medications
   - Materials or devices to secure ET tube after placement
   - Suction equipment
   - Monitors ($ETCO_2$, SaO_2, ECG)
2. Make sure at least one patent IV line is present (two are preferable).
3. Preoxygenate the patient using a nonrebreathing mask or bag-mask with 100% oxygen. Preoxygenation for 3 to 4 minutes is preferred.
4. Apply cardiac and pulse oximetry monitors.
5. If the patient is conscious, use sedative agents.
6. Consider administration of sedative agents and lidocaine if potential or confirmed traumatic brain injury is a factor.
7. Use analgesic medications also, because none of the medications routinely used for induction or paralysis provide pain relief.
8. After administration of paralytic agents, manipulate the thyroid cartilage with pressure directed posteriorly and cephalad to optimize view of the glottic opening (external laryngeal manipulation).
9. Confirm tube placement immediately after intubation with $ETCO_2$. Continuous cardiac and pulse oximeter monitoring is also required during and after RSI. Reconfirm tube placement continuously throughout transport and with specific attention paid each time the patient is moved.
10. Use repeat doses of sedative and paralytic agents as needed, but never administer paralytic without sedatives.

Procedure

1. Assemble the required equipment.
2. Make sure the intravenous (IV) lines are patent.
3. Preoxygenate the patient with 100% oxygen for approximately 3 to 4 minutes if possible.
4. Place the patient on cardiac and pulse oximeter monitors.
5. Administer a sedative (eg, midazolam) if appropriate.
6. Administer an analgesic, such as fentanyl, if appropriate.
7. If traumatic brain injury is possible or has been confirmed, medical direction may recommend the administration of lidocaine 2 to 3 minutes before administration of a paralytic agent.
8. For pediatric patients, administer atropine 1 to 3 minutes before paralytic administration to minimize the vagal response to intubation. The use and effectiveness of atropine for this purpose is controversial. The paramedic should follow guidelines established by medical direction.
9. Administer a short-acting paralytic agent (eg, succinylcholine) intravenously. Paralysis and relaxation should occur within 30 seconds. Using the Sellick maneuver may also be helpful.
10. Insert an ET tube. If initial attempts are unsuccessful, precede repeat attempts with preoxygenation.
11. Confirm ET tube placement using primary and secondary methods to include $ETCO_2$.
12. If repeated attempts to achieve ET intubation fail, consider placement of an alternative or surgical airway.
13. Use a long-acting paralytic agent (eg, vecuronium) to continue paralysis.
14. Repeat doses of sedative medications also may be needed.

Note: Requirements vary with individual patients.

Modified from: American College of Surgeons Committee on Trauma. *Prehospital Trauma Life Support*. 8th ed. St. Louis, MO: Elsevier; 2016; Ali MS, Bakri MH, Mohamed HA, Shebab H, Taher AI. External laryngeal manipulation done by the laryngoscopist makes the best laryngeal view for intubation. *Saudi J Anaesth*. 2014;8(3):351-354.

- Monitor the airway for vomiting as the patient loses consciousness. (Once neuromuscular blockade has been established, active vomiting cannot occur.)
- Do not initiate ventilations unless the patient's oxygen saturation falls below 90%.
- Within 45 seconds of administration of succinylcholine, the patient will be relaxed enough for intubation.

5. **Placement**
   - Perform orotracheal intubation and confirm proper placement of the tube.

6. **Postintubation management**
   - Secure the tube in place.
   - Begin mechanical ventilation.
   - Monitor the patient continuously.

If RSI is unsuccessful and the patient cannot be intubated, the airway should be managed by other means (eg, ETC, bag-mask device, cricothyrotomy).

Note: Succinylcholine directly depolarizes all motor end plates, simultaneously causing fasciculations and a rise in these pressures. Premedication with vecuronium, administered in a dosage of 0.01 mg/kg, can prevent these pressure rises (see the Appendix, *Emergency Drug Index*).[45]

Needle Cricothyrotomy

Needle cricothyrotomy is also known as percutaneous transtracheal ventilation and translaryngeal cannula ventilation. It may be valuable in the initial stabilization of a patient whose airway cannot be managed by the usual manual measures. It also may be valuable in patients who cannot be intubated by oral or nasal means or who have complete airway obstruction. It is a temporary procedure. It provides oxygenation when the airway is obstructed as a result of edema of the glottis, fracture of the larynx, or severe oropharyngeal hemorrhage. Needle cricothyrotomy requires special training and authorization from medical direction. Needle cricothyrotomy is rarely performed in the prehospital setting.

Description

Needle cricothyrotomy uses cannulation of the trachea below the glottis to oxygenate and ventilate a patient's lungs.

Necessary Equipment

- A 12- or 14-gauge over-the-needle catheter with a 10-mL or 20-mL syringe
- Antiseptic swabs
- Adhesive tape or appropriate ties
- Pressure-regulating valve and pressure gauge attached to a high-pressure (30 to 60 psi) oxygen supply (Most oxygen tanks and regulators can provide 50 psi at 15 L/min or when opened toflush.)
- High-pressure tubing connecting the high-pressure regulating valve to a hand-operated release valve (5-foot [1.5-m] tubing is recommended.)
- 3.0-mm ET adapter (or 3-mL syringe) and bag-mask device if jet ventilation is not available; alternatively, a 3-mL syringe without the plunger can serve as an adapter to the cricothyrotomy catheter
- A release valve connected by tubing to the catheter (This release valve may be provided by using a Y- or T-connector, a push-button device, or a three-way stopcock directly attached to the high-pressure tubing, or by cutting a hole in the oxygen line to provide a "whistle stop" effect.)

Technique

The steps in needle cricothyrotomy are as follows (**FIGURE 15-98**):

1. Make sure the patient is supine. Also make sure the cricothyroid membrane has been identified. (If a spinal injury is suspected, in-line stabilization may be provided as for nasal and tracheal intubation.)
2. Stabilize the larynx using the thumb and middle finger of one hand. With the other hand, palpate the small depression below the thyroid cartilage (the Adam's apple). Slide the index finger down to locate the cricothyroid membrane.
3. Insert the needle of the syringe downward through the midline of the membrane at a 45° angle toward the patient's carina. Apply negative pressure to the syringe during insertion. The entrance of air into the syringe indicates that the needle is in the trachea.
4. Advance the catheter over the needle toward the carina and remove the needle and syringe. Take care not to kink the catheter when removing the needle and syringe. Dispose of the needle in a sharps container.
5. Hold the hub of the catheter or secure it to prevent accidental dislodgement while providing ventilation. Remove the end of the oxygen tubing from the hub of the cannula and connect it to the oxygen regulator. Provide for a release valve as described previously.
6. Observe for chest rise and auscultate breath sounds.
7. Ventilate at a rate of 1 second for inflation and at least 2 seconds for exhalation.

When the release valve is closed, oxygen under pressure is introduced into the trachea. The pressure is adjusted to a level that allows adequate lung expansion. The patient's chest must be observed

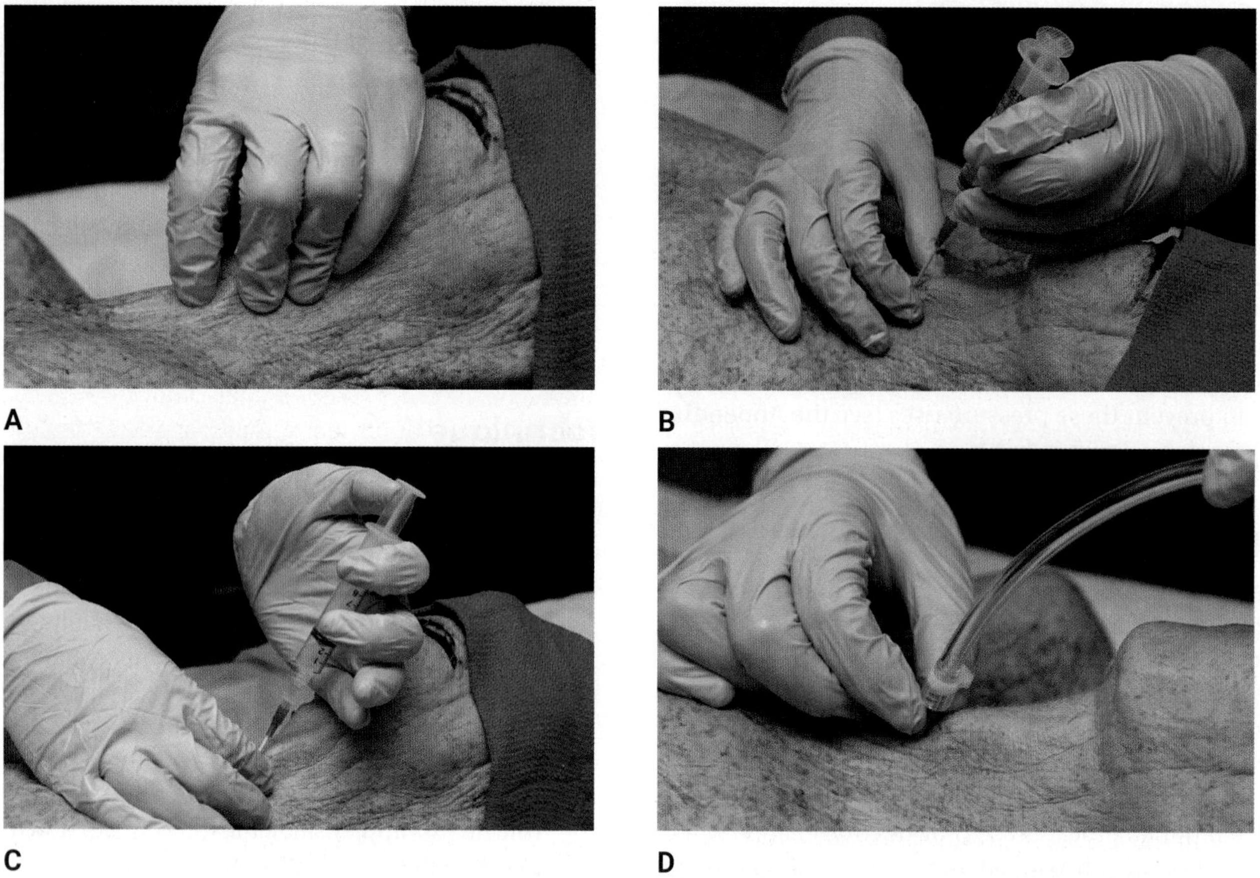

FIGURE 15-98 Needle cricothyrotomy. **A.** Stabilize the larynx and identify the cricothyroid membrane. **B.** Insert the needle of the syringe downward through the midline of the membrane at a 45° angle toward the carina. **C.** While inserting the needle, draw back on the plunger of the syringe. If air enters the syringe, the needle is in the trachea. **D.** After advancing the catheter and removing the needle and syringe, stabilize the catheter and connect the end of the oxygen tubing from the hub of the cannula to the oxygen regulator. Provide for a release valve. (If jet ventilation is not available, attach a 3-mL endotracheal (ET) tube adapter or 3-mL syringe without the plunger to the catheter. Then attach the bag-mask device to the ET tube adapter or syringe and provide ventilations.)

CRITICAL THINKING

What conditions could make it difficult to locate the anatomic landmarks for needle or surgical cricothyrotomy?

closely. The release valve must be opened to allow for exhalation. The correct ratio of inflation to deflation varies, depending on whether upper airway obstruction is present. For an open upper airway, an inspiratory-to-expiratory ratio of 1 to 2 seconds is recommended.[47] A longer inflation-to-deflation ratio may be needed to prevent barotrauma (injuries caused by excessive pressures [eg, pneumothorax]) when the upper airway is obstructed.[48]

NOTE

If the chest remains inflated during exhalation, a complete upper airway obstruction may be present. In such cases, a longer expiratory time should be allowed. If this does not produce adequate deflation, a second large-bore catheter may be inserted through the cricothyroid membrane next to the first one. If the chest remains distended, a cricothyrotomy should be performed.

Advantages

- Needle cricothyrotomy is a minimally invasive surgical procedure.
- It can be initiated quickly.
- When performed by a trained paramedic, it is simple, inexpensive, and potentially effective.
- Minimal spinal movement is needed for insertion.

Disadvantages

- The technique is an invasive procedure.
- Constant monitoring is required.
- The airway is not protected.
- The procedure does not allow for efficient elimination of carbon dioxide.
- The patient's lungs can be ventilated adequately only for 30 to 40 minutes.[49]

Possible Complications

- High pressure during ventilation and air entrapment may cause pneumothorax.
- Hemorrhage may occur at the insertion site. The thyroid and esophagus also may be perforated if the needle is advanced too far.
- Hypoventilation may occur from inadequate volume.
- False placement may occur.
- Direct suctioning of secretions is impossible.
- Subcutaneous emphysema may occur.

Removal

Needle cricothyrotomy is a temporary emergency procedure. It provides time for the use of other airway management techniques. The catheter should be removed only after successful orotracheal or nasotracheal intubation or after a cricothyrotomy or a tracheostomy has been performed. Removal involves withdrawing the catheter and dressing the wound.

Surgical Cricothyrotomy

Surgical cricothyrotomy is a procedure that paramedics may be authorized to perform in some EMS systems. It allows rapid entrance to the airway through the cricothyroid membrane. The procedure can be performed quickly. It is much faster and easier than a tracheostomy and much more reliable than a needle cricothyrotomy. In addition, it does not require manipulation of the cervical spine.

Description

Cricothyrotomy can provide ventilation and oxygenation when airway control is not possible by other means. It should not be performed on patients who can be orally or nasally intubated. Few situations require this surgical procedure. Relative indications for cricothyrotomy include severe facial or nasal injuries that preclude oral or nasal intubation, massive midfacial trauma, possible spinal trauma preventing adequate ventilation, anaphylaxis, angioedema, and chemical inhalation injuries. Like needle cricothyrotomy, surgical cricothyrotomy requires special training and authorization from medical direction.

> NOTE
>
> Remember: Cricothyrotomy should be considered only when you cannot intubate *and* cannot ventilate. If you cannot intubate but you can ventilate, then do not cut the neck.

Necessary Equipment

Commercially prepared cricothyrotomy kits are available through several manufacturers (**FIGURE 15-99**). If such a kit is not available, the following equipment is required:

- Scalpel blade
- Size 6 (preferred) or size 7 ET tube or tracheostomy tube
- Tracheal hook (if available)
- Antiseptic solution
- Oxygen source
- Suction device
- Bag-valve device

Technique

In patients suspected of having a spinal injury, in-line stabilization should be maintained throughout the procedure. If possible, the neck should be cleaned with alcohol or another antiseptic solution. The steps in the surgical procedure are as follows (**FIGURE 15-100**):

1. Locate the anatomic landmarks of the neck. Identify the cricothyroid membrane.

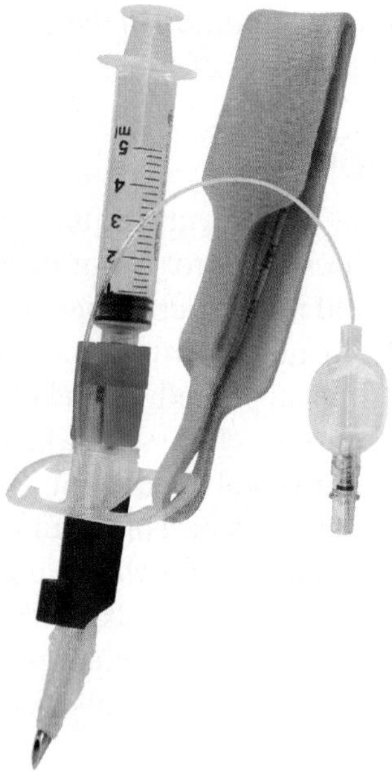

FIGURE 15-99 Quicktrach II kit.

2. Make a 0.75-inch (2-cm) vertical incision with the scalpel through the skin at the level of the cricothyroid membrane. Increase the size of the opening by inserting the scalpel handle and rotating it 90°. Be careful not to lose your opening by using a tracheal hook, if available.
3. Place a size 6 or 7 ET tube or tracheostomy tube through the opening. Inflate the cuff and secure the tube to prevent dislodgement.
4. Provide ventilation by a bag-mask device with the highest available oxygen concentration.
5. Determine the adequacy of ventilation. This can be done through bilateral auscultation and observation of chest rise and fall.
6. Use a secondary confirmation method, such as $ETCO_2$.

Possible Complications

- Prolonged procedure time
- Hemorrhage
- Aspiration
- Possible misplacement
- False passage
- Perforation of the esophagus
- Injury to the vocal cords and carotid and jugular vessels lateral to the incision (the patient must be immobilized)
- Subcutaneous emphysema

Contraindications

- Inability to identify anatomic landmarks
- Underlying anatomic abnormality (eg, tumor, subglottic stenosis)
- Tracheal transection
- Acute laryngeal disease caused by trauma or infection
- Small child younger than 10 years (In these patients, insertion of a 12- to 14-gauge catheter over the needle may be safer than a surgical cricothyrotomy).

NOTE

Use of a smaller-diameter ET tube may aid successful placement and will not damage the larynx. Once the tube is in the airway, the paramedic should be careful not to advance it more than a few centimeters. This helps prevent main stem intubation.

Removal

In the prehospital setting, no attempt should be made to remove ET tubes used during an emergency cricothyrotomy.

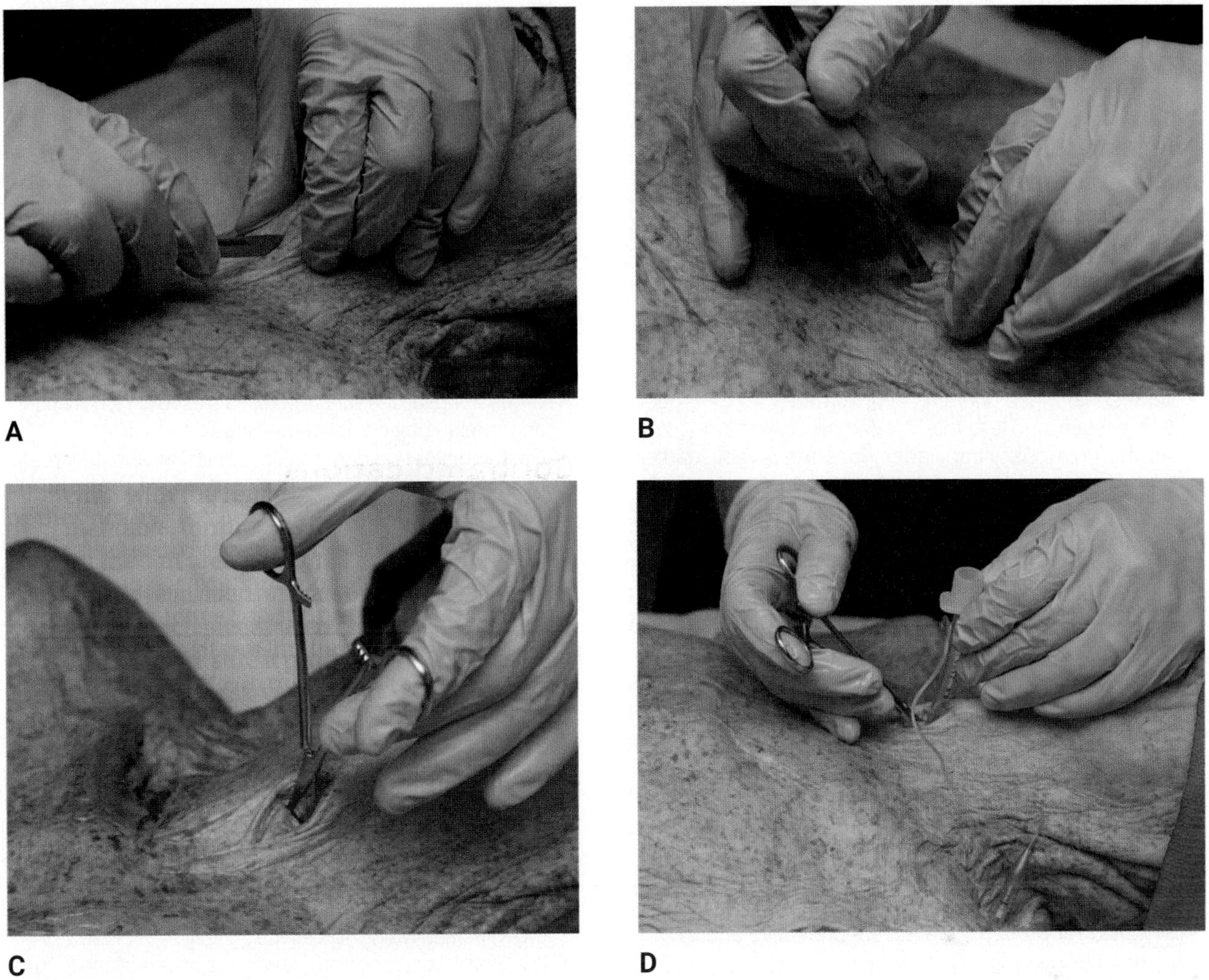

FIGURE 15-100 Surgical cricothyrotomy. **A.** Make a vertical incision through the cricothyroid membrane. **B.** Open the hole by twisting the handle of a scalpel in it. **C.** Or, open the hole with a clamp. **D.** Insert the endotracheal tube. Here, the tube has been shortened.

Summary

- The upper airway opens at the nose and mouth and extends to the glottic opening.
- Structures of the lower airway include the trachea, the right and left main stem bronchi, the secondary and tertiary bronchi, the bronchioles, and the functional units of the lungs, the alveoli.
- The base of each lung rests on the diaphragm. The right lung has three lobes, and the left has two.
- The primary muscles of ventilation are the diaphragm and the intercostal muscles.
- The phrenic nerve innervates the diaphragm.
- Respiration is the exchange of oxygen and carbon dioxide between an organism and the environment. Pulmonary ventilation involves the movement of gas into and out of the lungs.
- External respiration is the transfer of gases between the inspired air and pulmonary capillaries. Internal respiration is the transfer of gases between the blood and tissue cells.
- During inspiration, the size of the thoracic cavity increases. This increased size creates negative pressure inside the chest relative to atmospheric pressure, allowing air to rush into the lungs.

- During exhalation, the chest muscles relax passively, and air is forced out of the lungs.
- The work of breathing increases if surfactant is lost, airway resistance increases, or pulmonary compliance decreases.
- The normal adult respiratory rate is 12 to 20 breaths/min.
- No gas exchange occurs in the anatomic dead space. The physiologic dead space includes the anatomic dead space plus any nonfunctional alveoli.
- Tidal volume is the amount of gas inhaled or exhaled with each normal breath.
- The respiratory rate multiplied by the tidal volume equals the minute volume.
- Atmospheric gas contains approximately 79% nitrogen, 21% oxygen, and less than 1% carbon dioxide.
- As the pulmonary capillaries pass the alveoli, carbon dioxide diffuses into the alveoli and oxygen diffuses into the pulmonary capillaries.
- Oxygen is carried in the blood on hemoglobin. A small amount is also dissolved in the plasma. The amount of oxygen dissolved in the blood influences the extent to which oxygen binds with hemoglobin. The normal partial pressure of arterial blood oxygen is 80 to 100 mm Hg. Venous partial pressure of oxygen (Po_2) in the lungs is only 40 mm Hg; as a result, oxygen diffuses easily from the alveoli into the pulmonary capillaries.
- The respiratory centers normally are controlled by the pH of body fluids, which is influenced by carbon dioxide levels. Oxygen plays a role in the regulation of breathing in abnormal situations.
- Body temperature, medications, pain, emotion, and sleep also influence breathing.
- Modified forms of respiration are protective and include coughing, sneezing, and sighing.
- Older adults experience changes in ventilation and respiration that lead to a gradual decline in Po_2.
- Respiratory compromise and hypoxia can be caused by interruption of nervous control, structural damage to the thorax, bronchoconstriction, disruption of airway patency, oxygen deprivation, environmental factors, changes in alveolar–capillary gas exchange, ventilation deficiencies, decreases in lung compliance, ventilation/perfusion mismatch, disrupted oxygen transport, disrupted circulation, or cellular disruptions.
- Upper airway obstruction can rapidly cause death if not corrected.
- Aspiration is the inhalation of food, fluid, or foreign bodies into the lungs. It can cause airway obstruction and chemical damage with collapse of alveoli.
- The paramedic must assess the rate, regularity, and rhythm of breathing and must note the patient's position, skin color, and heart rate. A thorough patient history should be obtained.
- Respiratory distress may be caused by upper or lower airway obstruction, inadequate ventilation, impairment of the respiratory muscles, ventilation/perfusion mismatch, diffusion abnormalities, or impairment of the nervous system.
- Supplemental oxygen is administered to increase the oxygen content in pulmonary capillaries and to help the patient compensate.
- Oxygen gas is administered by a variety of devices that regulate the concentration of oxygen delivered to the patient.
- Patient ventilation is provided by several methods, including rescue breathing (mouth to mask, mask to nose, mouth to stoma), mouth-to-mask breathing, bag-mask devices, and automatic transport ventilators.
- Airway management should progress from the least to the most invasive methods. Airway management begins with manual maneuvers.
- Oropharyngeal or tracheal suction is used to remove liquids and foreign objects from the airway.
- Gastric distention can impair ventilation, and it increases the risk of aspiration. Orogastric or nasogastric tubes are inserted to reduce gastric distention.
- After manual airway maneuvers have been performed, mechanical adjuncts can be used to maintain the airway. Nasopharyngeal airways are used to maintain the airway in patients with a gag reflex. An oropharyngeal airway is inserted in patients with no gag reflex.
- Advanced airways include those that intubate the trachea as well as blind insertion devices such as the laryngeal mask airway, i-gel, King LT-D airway, and esophageal-tracheal Combitube airway.
- Endotracheal (ET) intubation permits direct ventilation of the trachea, protection against aspiration, and a route for administering some medications. The ET tube may be inserted orally or nasally (in breathing patients). Adjuncts to assist with intubation include the stylet, tube introducer (bougie), and Magill forceps.
- It is essential to confirm proper placement of the ET tube. Methods of confirmation include auscultating the breath sounds, checking for gastric sounds, using an esophageal detector device, and measuring the end-tidal carbon dioxide and oxygen saturation.
- The laryngeal mask airway and i-gel are inserted blindly into the hypopharynx in unresponsive patients with no gag reflex.
- An esophageal-tracheal Combitube is a twin-lumen airway placed blindly in unconscious patients with no gag reflex. In most cases the distal lumen is positioned in the esophagus, and inflation of balloons in the hypopharynx permits ventilation through tube 1. In rare cases, when the distal lumen is positioned in the trachea, the patient is ventilated through tube 2.
- Sedation and pain management are often used in airway management and ventilation to reduce pain and anxiety, induce amnesia, and decrease the gag reflex.
- In some EMS systems, neuromuscular blocking agents are used with sedation to permit ET intubation.
- When an airway cannot be introduced through the nose or mouth and the patient cannot be ventilated, needle or surgical cricothyrotomy may be performed to access the airway by creating an opening in the cricothyroid membrane in the neck.

References

1. Thibodeau GA, Patton KT. *Anatomy and Physiology*. 9th ed, St. Louis, MO: Elsevier; 2013.
2. Sherwood L. *Human Physiology: From Cells to Systems*. 9th ed. Boston, MA: Cengage Learning; 2016.
3. Peate I, Wild K, Muralitharan N, eds. *Nursing Practice: Knowledge and Care*. Hoboken, NJ: Wiley-Blackwell; 2014.
4. Beachey W. *Respiratory Care Anatomy and Physiology*. 4th ed. St. Louis, MO: Elsevier; 2018.
5. Quinn M, Bhimji SS. Anatomy, airway, anatomic dead space. In: StatPearls (Internet). Treasure Island, FL: StatPearls Publishing; October 6, 2017. https://www.ncbi.nlm.nih.gov/books/NBK442016/. Accessed February 7, 2018.
6. Beamis J, Mathur P, Mehta AC, eds. *Interventional Pulmonary Medicine*. 2nd ed. Bethesda, MD: Informa Health Care; 2010.
7. Bogdanov K. *Biology in Physics: Is Life Matter?* Orlando, FL: Academic Press; 2002.
8. Scanlon V, Sanders T. *Essentials of Anatomy and Physiology*. 6th ed. Philadelphia, PA: FA Davis Company; 2015.
9. McCance KL, Huether SE. *Pathophysiology: The Biologic Basis for Disease in Adults and Children*. 7th ed. St. Louis, MO: Mosby; 2015.
10. Abdo WF, Heunks LM. Oxygen-induced hypercapnia in COPD: myths and facts. *Crit Care*. 2012;16(5):323.
11. Khurana I. *Essentials of Medical Physiology*. India: Elsevier; 2009.
12. Kahn HK, Magauran BG Jr. *Geriatric Emergency Medicine: Principles and Practice*. New York, NY: Cambridge University Press; 2014.
13. National Safety Council. *Injury Facts*. 2017 ed. Itasca, NY: National Safety Council; 2017.
14. Altkorn R, Chen X, Milkovich S, et al. Fatal and non-fatal food injuries among children (aged 0–14 years). *Int J Pediatr Otorhinolaryngol*. 2008;72(7):1041-1046.
15. Nichols BG, Visotcky A, Aberger M, et al. Pediatric exposure to choking hazards is associated with parental knowledge of choking hazards. *Int J Pediatr Otorhinolaryngol*. 2012;76(2):169-173.
16. Munter DW. Trachea foreign bodies. Medscape website. http://emedicine.medscape.com/article/764615-overview. Updated December 12, 2016. Accessed February 7, 2018.
17. American Heart Association. *Basic Life Support*. Dallas, TX: American Heart Association; 2015.
18. US Department of Transportation, National Highway Traffic Safety Administration. *EMT-Paramedic: National Standard Curriculum*. EMS.gov website. https://www.ems.gov/pdf/education/Emergency-Medical-Technician-Paramedic/Paramedic_1998.pdf. Accessed February 7, 2018.
19. Goldman L, Schafer AI, eds. *Goldman's Cecil Medicine*. 24th ed. Philadelphia, PA: Elsevier Sanders; 2012.
20. Luecke T, Pelosi P. Clinical review: positive end-expiratory pressure and cardiac output. *Crit Care*. 2005;9(6):607-621.
21. Daily JC, Wang HE. Noninvasive positive pressure ventilation: resource document for the National Association of EMS Physicians Position Statement. *Prehosp Emerg Care*. 2011;15(3):432-438.
22. Goodacre S, Stevens JW, Pandor A, et al. Prehospital noninvasive ventilation for acute respiratory failure: systematic review, network meta-analysis, and individual patient data meta-analysis. *Acad Emerg Med*. 2014;21(9):960-970.
23. American Heart Association. 2015 American Heart Association guidelines for cardiopulmonary resuscitation and emergency cardiovascular care. *Circulation*. 2015;132(18)(suppl 2):S313-S314.
24. American Heart Association. *ACLS Provider Manual*. Dallas, TX: American Heart Association; 2016.
25. Joffe AM, Hetzel S, Liew EC. A two-handed jaw-thrust technique is superior to the one-handed "EC-clamp" technique for mask ventilation in the apneic unconscious person. *Anesthesiology*. 2010;113(4):873-879.
26. American Heart Association. *Pediatric Advanced Life Support*. Dallas, TX: American Heart Association; 2015.
27. Siegler J, Kroll M, Wojcik S, Moy HP. Can EMS providers provide appropriate tidal volumes in a simulated adult-sized patient with a pediatric-sized bag-valve-mask? *Prehosp Emerg Care*. 2017;21(1):74-78.
28. American Heart Association. *Advanced Cardiac Life Support*. Dallas, TX: American Heart Association; 2016.
29. American Association for Respiratory Care. AARC Clinical Practice Guidelines. Endotracheal suctioning of mechanically ventilated patients with artificial airways 2010. *Respir Care*. 2010;55(6):758-764.
30. Perry AG, Potter P, Ostendorf WR, Laplante N. *Clinical Nursing Skills and Techniques*. 9th ed. St. Louis, MO: Elsevier; 2018.
31. Carlson JN, Wang HE. Airway procedures. In: Cone D, Brice JH, Delbridge TR, Myers JB, eds. *Emergency Medical Services: Clinical Practice and Systems Oversight*. 2nd ed. West Sussex, England: Wiley and Sons; 2015:110-130.
32. Carhart E, Stuck LH, Salzman JG. Achieving a safe endotracheal tube cuff pressure in the prehospital setting: is it time to revise the standard cuff inflation practice? *Prehosp Emerg Care*. 2016;20(2):273-277.
33. Guyette FX, Wang HE. EMS airway management. In: Cone D, Brice JH, Delbridge TR, Myers JB, eds. *Emergency Medical Services: Clinical Practice and Systems Oversight*. 2nd ed. West Sussex, England: Wiley and Sons; 2015:89-109.
34. Hubble MW, Brown L, Wilfong DA, Hertelendy A, Benner RW, Richards ME. A meta-analysis of prehospital airway control techniques part I: orotracheal and nasotracheal intubation success rates. *Prehosp Emerg Care*. 2010;14(3):377-401.
35. Hansen M, Lambert W, Guise JM, Warden CR, Mann NC, Wang H. Out-of-hospital pediatric airway management in the United States. *Resuscitation*. 2015;90:104-110.
36. DiRusso S, Sullivan T, Risucci D, Nealon P, Slim M. Intubation of pediatric trauma patients in the field: predictor of negative outcome despite risk stratification. *J Trauma*. 2005;59(1):84-91.
37. Gausche M, Lewis RJ, Stratton SJ, et al. Effect of out-of-hospital pediatric endotracheal intubation on survival and neurological outcome. *JAMA*. 2000;283(6):783-790.
38. Holmes J, Peng J, Bair A. Abnormal end-tidal carbon dioxide levels on emergency department arrival in adult and pediatric intubated patients. *Prehosp Emerg Care*. 2012;16(2):210-216.
39. World Health Organization. *Pulse Oximetry Training Manual*. Geneva, Switzerland: WHO Press; 2011.
40. Middleton PM, Simpson PM, Thomas RE, Bendall JC. Higher insertion success with the i-gel supraglottic airway in out-of-hospital cardiac arrest: a randomised controlled trial. *Resuscitation*. 2014;85(7):893-897.
41. Martin-Gill C, Prunty HA, Ritter SC, Carlson JN, Guyette FX. Risk factors for unsuccessful prehospital laryngeal tube placement. *Resuscitation*. 2015;86:25-30.

42. Ostermayer DG, Gausche-Hill M. Supraglottic airways: the history and current state of prehospital airway adjuncts. *Prehosp Emerg Care*. 2014;18(1):106-115.
43. ACEP Board of Directors. Drug-assisted intubation in the prehospital setting. *Clinical and Practice Management*. American College of Emergency Physicians website. https://www.acep.org/Physician-Resources/Policies/Policy-statements/EMS/Drug-Assisted-Intubation-in-the-Prehospital-Setting/. Published April 2011. Accessed February 7, 2018.
44. Lafferty KA, Windle ML, Dillinger R, Talavera F, Schraga ED. Medications used in tracheal intubation. Medscape website. https://emedicine.medscape.com/article/109739-overview#a2. Updated June 20, 2017. Accessed February 7, 2018.
45. Lafferty K, Dillinger R. Rapid sequence induction. Medscape website. http://emedicine.medscape.com/article/80222-overview. Updated March 23, 2017. Accessed February 7, 2018.
46. Marx JA, Hockberger R, Walls R. *Rosen's Emergency Medicine: Concepts and Clinical Practice*. 5th ed. St. Louis, MO: Mosby; 2002.
47. National Registry of Emergency Medical Technicians. *2015 Paramedic Psychomotor Competency Portfolio (PPCP)*. Columbus, OH: National Registry of Emergency Medical Technicians; 2015.
48. Hsu CW, Sun SF. Iatrogenic pneumothorax related to mechanical ventilation. *World J Crit Care Med*. 2014;3(1):8-14.
49. Roberts JR, Hedges JR. Surgical cricothyrotomy. *Clinical Procedures in Emergency Medicine*, ed 5. Philadelphia, PA: Elsevier; 2010.

Suggested Readings

American College of Emergency Physicians. Verification of endotracheal tube placement: policy statement. *Ann Emerg Med*. 2009;54:141-142.

Benger J, Coates S, Davies R, et al. Randomised comparison of the effectiveness of the laryngeal mask airway supreme, i-gel and current practice in the initial airway management of out of hospital cardiac arrest: a feasibility study. *Br J Anaesth*. 2016;116(2):262-268.

Brown CA, Sakles JC, Mick NW. *The Walls Manual of Emergency Airway Management*. Philadelphia: PA: Wolters Kluwer; 2017.

Crewdson K, Lockey DJ, Røislien J, Lossius HM, Rehn M. The success of pre-hospital tracheal intubation by different pre-hospital providers: a systematic literature review and meta-analysis. *Crit Care*. 2017;21(1):31.

Gilpin R. Gas exchange for EMS providers. *EMS Reference* website. https://www.emsreference.com/articles/article/gas-exchange-ems-providers-0. Published January 6, 2017. Accessed February 7, 2018.

Guyette F, Greenwood M, Neubecker D, Roth R, Wang HE. Alternate airways in the prehospital setting (resource document to NAEMSP position statement). *Prehosp Emerg Care*. 2007;11(1):56-61.

Hagberg CA. *Benumof and Hagberg's Airway Management*. 3rd ed. Elsevier Saunders; 2013.

Moy HP. Evidence-based EMS: out-of-hospital BiPAP vs. CPAP. Is one any better than the other? *EMS World*. 2016:45(1):36-38.

National Association of EMS Physicians. Alternate airways in the out-of-hospital setting: position statement of the National Association of EMS Physicians. *Prehosp Emerg Care*. 2007;11:248-250.

Patient Assessment

PART

5

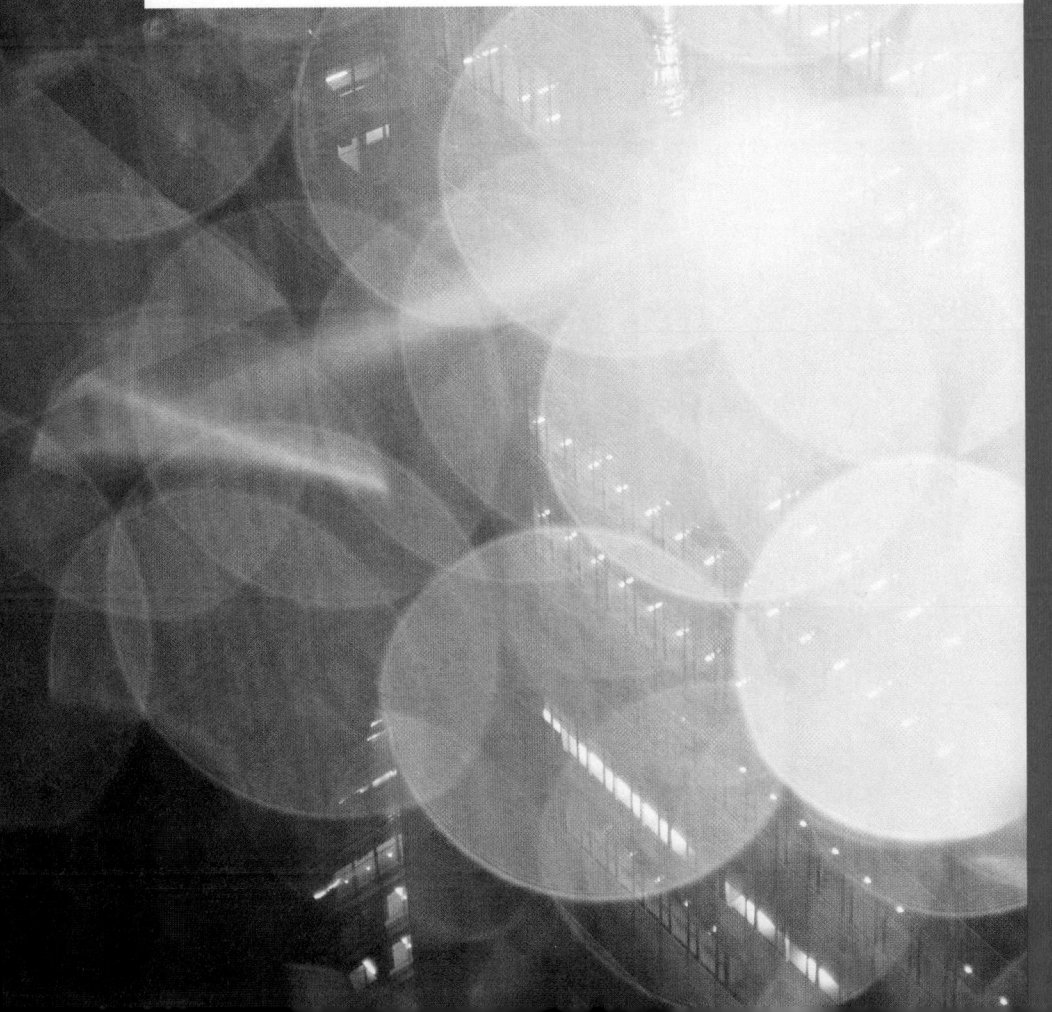

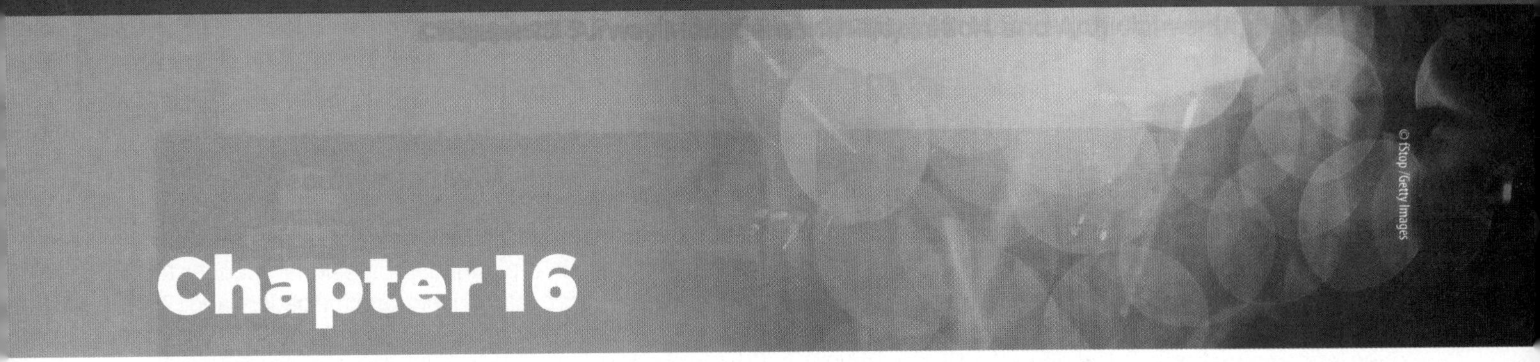

© fStop /Getty Images

Chapter 16

Therapeutic Communications

NATIONAL EMS EDUCATION STANDARD COMPETENCIES

Preparatory

Integrates comprehensive knowledge of the EMS system, safety/well-being of the paramedic, and medical/legal and ethical issues which is intended to improve the health of EMS personnel, patients, and the community.

Therapeutic Communication

Principles of communicating with patients in a manner that achieves a positive relationship

- Interviewing techniques (pp 584–587)
- Adjusting communication strategies for age, stage of development, patients with special needs, and differing cultures (pp 589–591, 593–594)
- Verbal defusing strategies (pp 587–588)
- Family presence issues (p 580)
- Dealing with difficult patients (pp 589–592)
- Factors that affect communication (pp 582–584)

OBJECTIVES

Upon completion of this chapter, the paramedic student will be able to:

1. Define therapeutic communications. (p 580)
2. List the elements of the communication process. (pp 580–582)
3. Identify internal factors that influence effective communications. (pp 582–583)
4. Identify external factors that influence effective communications. (p 584)
5. Explain the elements of an effective patient interview. (pp 584–587)
6. Summarize strategies for gathering appropriate patient information. (pp 587–588)
7. Discuss methods of assessing the patient's mental status during the patient interview. (pp 588–589)
8. Describe ways the paramedic can improve communication with a variety of patients: (1) those who are unmotivated to talk; (2) hostile patients; (3) children; (4) older adults; (5) patients who are hard of hearing; (6) patients who are visually impaired; (7) disabled patients with service animals; (8) patients under the influence of drugs or alcohol; (9) sexually aggressive patients; (10) lesbian, gay, bisexual, and transgender patients; and (11) patients whose cultural traditions are different from those of the paramedic. (pp 589–594)
9. Describe methods to communicate in a culturally sensitive manner. (p 593)

KEY TERMS

closed-ended questions Questions asked in a narrative form that can be answered with a "yes" or "no."

cultural imposition The forcing of one's beliefs, values, and patterns of behavior on people from another culture.

decoding The act of interpreting symbols and format (either written or verbal).

empathy The ability to see a situation from the viewpoint of the person experiencing it.

encoding The act of placing a message in an understandable format (either written or verbal).

ethnocentrism The belief that one's own life is the most acceptable or best; acting in a superior manner toward another culture's way of life.

leading questions Questions that persuade the patient to respond in a particular way, usually in a way that confirms the paramedic's assumptions.

open-ended questions Questions asked in a narrative form that cannot be answered with a "yes" or "no."

private space The region surrounding a person that the person regards as his or hers; also known as personal space.

sympathy The expression of one's feelings about another person's problem.

therapeutic communications The use of communication techniques in a planned, professional manner to (1) foster a positive relationship with the patient and (2) facilitate a shared understanding of information between the patient and the paramedic. These two outcomes aid in the attainment of the desired patient care goals.

Therapeutic communications can have several important effects; namely, it can improve the paramedic's interaction with the patient, ensure better patient care, defuse potentially violent situations or prevent them from escalating, and reduce the risk of lawsuits.

Communication

Communication is the basic element of human interaction. It involves both verbal and nonverbal behavior, as well as all the symbols and clues people use to convey and receive meaning.[1] **Therapeutic communications** refers to the use of communication techniques in a planned, professional manner to (1) foster a positive relationship with the patient and (2) facilitate a shared understanding of information between the patient and the paramedic. These two outcomes aid in the attainment of the desired patient care goals.

The process of communication has several elements. The paramedic must be aware of each element to interact effectively with a patient. Each element is crucial, and information and meaning can be gained or lost if any one element is changed (**FIGURE 16-1**). To achieve good communication, all participants must take equal responsibility for their part in the process. Communication is successful only when each person clearly understands the message.

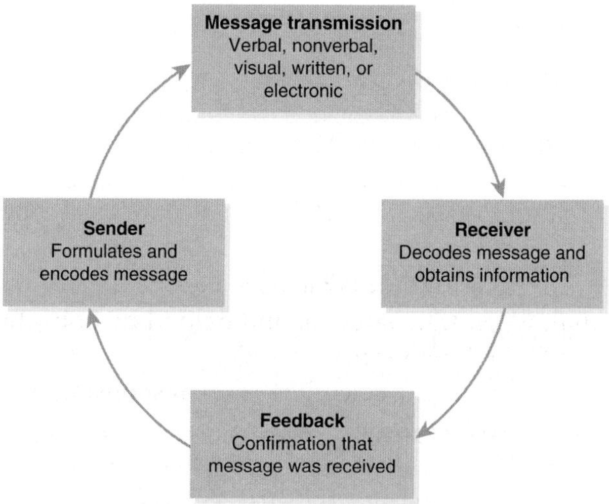

FIGURE 16-1 The process of communication.

NOTE

This chapter deals with communication between paramedics and their patients. However, these suggestions and techniques also can be used to improve communication between bystanders, the patient's family members, crew members, nurses, physicians, dispatchers, and other emergency personnel.

Elements of the Communication Process

Communication is a dynamic process that includes six elements: the source, encoding, the message, decoding, the receiver, and feedback.

Source

Verbal communication uses spoken or written words (common symbols) to express ideas or feelings. This expression is the source of the communication. The common symbols used in therapeutic communications should be simple, short, and direct to avoid confusion. **BOX 16-1** lists methods that can be used to achieve clarity in verbal communications.

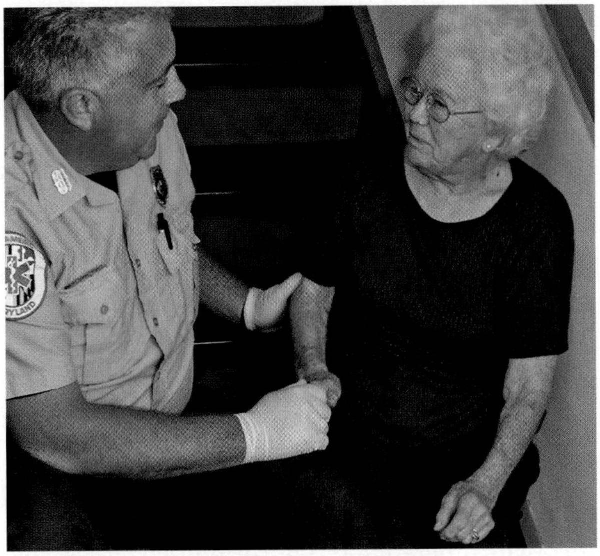

CRITICAL THINKING

Think about the last time you had a misunderstanding with someone. Would any of the techniques listed in Box 16-1 have improved the situation?

Encoding

Encoding is the act of placing a message in a format that, when translated, is understood by both the sender and the receiver. The format may be either written or verbal. Encoding is the responsibility of the sender (encoder), because the sender defines the content and emotional tone of the message. In the process of communication, the sender role may pass from one person to another as information is exchanged. For example, the paramedic may initially be the sender of the message by asking a patient for information. When the patient responds, he or she assumes the role of the sender.

BOX 16-1 Techniques for Verbal Communication

- Use fewer words to avoid confusion.
- Use words that express an idea simply.
- Do not use vague phrases.
- Use examples (including demonstrations) if they will make the message easier to understand.
- Repeat the important parts of a message.
- Do not use technical jargon.
- Speak at an appropriate speed or pace.
- Do not pause for long periods or quickly change the subject.

Message

The message is the information that is sent or expressed by the sender. It should be clear, organized, and communicated in a manner familiar to the person receiving it. The message may include verbal and nonverbal symbols (eg, spoken words, facial expressions, gestures). As a rule, the more ways (or formats) in which a message is communicated, the more likely the receiver is to understand it. For example, combining soothing words and a reassuring touch for a patient in pain communicates the message of compassion better than does using spoken words alone.

Not all symbols have universal meaning. For example, a reassuring touch might be welcome to people of certain cultures, whereas members of other cultures may find it offensive. Thus, when interacting with community members, paramedics must take into account the cultural differences of people in their service area. They should also consider how they will deal with a language barrier before attempting to send a message.

NOTE

It is estimated that one in five US residents (almost 62 million people) speaks a language other than English at home. Slightly less than one-half (44%) of these foreign-language speakers were born in the United States. In 2013, the languages spoken by at least 1 million people living in the United States were Spanish, Chinese, Tagalog, Vietnamese, French, Korean, and Arabic.

Modified from: Camarota SA, Zeigler K. One in five US residents speaks foreign language at home, record 61.8 million. Center for Immigration Studies website. https://cis.org/One-Five-US-Residents-Speaks-Foreign-Language-Home-Record-618-million. Published October 3, 2014. Accessed January 21, 2018.

Decoding

Decoding is the interpretation of symbols and formats, which prompts the receiver to respond to the sender's message. The decoding process can fail if symbols or words sent in the message are unfamiliar to either party. It also can fail if interpretation of the message is based on different understandings of symbols or format. For example, the word *pain* may mean horrific discomfort to one person but may mean a mild annoyance to another. When communicating with patients, the paramedic must carefully select words that cannot easily be misinterpreted.

NOTE
Some medical conditions, such as a stroke, can make it more difficult for a person to encode or decode a message.

Receiver

The receiver is essentially the decoder—that is, the person intended to understand the message. As with the role of sender, the role of receiver switches back and forth between participants during the communication process.

CRITICAL THINKING
Have you ever attended a class in which nothing made sense? Contemplate the reason you did not understand the content. Was it an encoding problem or a decoding problem?

Feedback

Feedback is the receiver's response to the sender's message. The quality of the feedback reveals whether the intended meaning of the message was received. If the intended meaning was not received, the sender must clarify the message by modifying its content, resending it, and then reassessing the new feedback. Like the message itself, feedback may be verbal or nonverbal.

Internal Factors in Effective Communication

To communicate well with patients, paramedics must genuinely like people. They must be able to empathize with others and recognize internal biases. They also must have the ability to listen (BOX 16-2). Each of these internal factors plays an important role in therapeutic communications.

Liking Others

As a "helping profession," health care depends on the relationships forged between patients and health

BOX 16-2 Active Listening Attitudes and Guidelines

1. Listen to understand, not to ready yourself to reply, contradict, or argue. This attitude is extremely important.
2. Remember that understanding involves more than simply knowing the dictionary meaning of the words used. It requires paying attention to the patient's tone of voice, facial expressions, and overall behavior.
3. Look for clues to what the patient is trying to say. Try to put yourself in the patient's shoes; that is, try to see the world as the patient sees it. Accept the patient's feelings as facts that must be taken into account, whether you share them or not.
4. Put aside your own views and opinions while communicating with the patient. Realize that you cannot listen to yourself inwardly and at the same time truly listen to the patient.
5. Control your impatience. Listening is faster than talking. The average person speaks about 120 words per minute, whereas people can listen to about 400 words per minute. Do not jump ahead of the patient: Give him or her enough time to tell the story. A patient does not always say what the paramedic expects to hear.
6. Do not prepare an answer while you listen. Get the whole message before deciding what to say. The patient's last sentence may put a whole new slant on what was said before.
7. Show the patient that you are alert and interested. This encourages the patient and improves communication.
8. Do not interrupt. Ask questions only to obtain more information. Do not try to trap the patient or force him or her into a corner.
9. Expect the patient's use of words to differ from yours. Do not quibble about terms; try to determine what was meant.
10. Your purpose is the opposite of a debater's goal. Look for areas of agreement, not for weak spots to attack with a barrage of counterpoints.
11. Before giving an answer in a particularly difficult discussion, summarize what you understand the patient to have said. If the patient disagrees with this version, clear up the contested points before giving your own views.
12. Let patients describe themselves and their interests, position, and opinions.

Modified from: Legal Advocates for Abused Women. Crime Victim Advocacy Center website. https://www.supportvictims.org/legal-advocates-for-abused-women. Accessed January 21, 2018.

care personnel. These relationships are based on trust and caring. In fact, they cannot be achieved unless health care personnel feel genuine concern for others and understand human strengths and weaknesses. Patients must trust paramedics and believe that they want to care for their needs. Paramedics can foster this trust by accepting patients as individuals.

Empathy

Empathy is the ability to see a situation from the viewpoint of the person experiencing it. It is widely accepted as a clinical aspect of a helping profession. **Sympathy**, by comparison, is the expression of one's feelings about another person's problem. Unlike sympathy, empathy uses sensitive and objective communication, which helps patients explain and explore their feelings so that problem solving can occur (BOX 16-3).

BOX 16-3 Empathy Versus Sympathy

The following case shows the difference between empathy and sympathy, and illustrates how empathy can help the paramedic soothe the patient and gain his trust.

Your emergency medical services (EMS) crew is sent to the home of a 60-year-old man with substernal chest pain. When you arrive, you find the patient sitting on the living room sofa with his wife. The couple are upset and afraid that he might die. Your crew begins standard procedures for a possible heart attack and prepares to transport the patient to the emergency department.

On the way to the hospital, the paramedic and the patient, who is accompanied by his wife, have the following conversation:

Paramedic: Even though you're feeling better, I can tell you're worried and afraid.

Patient: Yes, I am. I'm afraid I'm going to die.

Paramedic: Would you like me to explain to you and your wife what will happen after we arrive in the emergency department? I can also explain what the doctors and nurses will do to make sure you get the best possible care.

Patient: Yes, we would like that very much.

The use of empathy, shown in this conversation, allows the paramedic to accomplish three things: (1) calm the patient and his wife, (2) provide the couple with useful information, and (3) partly address their concerns. If the paramedic had used sympathy alone (eg, "I understand how you feel, but don't worry, everything will be okay."), the patient's fears would have been ignored. Also, the problem of the couple's agitation would not have been improved.

Ability to Listen

Listening is an active process that requires complete attention and practice. To be an effective listener, the paramedic should follow these guidelines:[2]

1. Face patients while speaking.
2. Maintain natural eye contact to show a willingness to listen.
3. Assume an attentive posture (avoid crossing the legs and arms, because this stance may convey a defensive attitude).
4. Avoid distracting body movements (eg, wringing the hands, tapping the feet, or fidgeting with an object).
5. Nod in acknowledgment when patients talk about important points or look for feedback.
6. Lean toward the speaker to communicate involvement.

One device for remembering ways to improve communication is the listening ladder (BOX 16-4). This device includes six steps of listening, which can easily be remembered with the mnemonic LADDER (Look at the speaker, Ask questions, Do not interrupt, Do not change the subject, Empathize, and Respond).[3]

BOX 16-4 The Ladder of Listening

Look at the speaker (for example, your patient or colleague). Eye contact shows that you are willing to listen.

Ask questions when you wish to clarify something the patient (or other speaker) said. However, wait to ask these questions until after the patient has finished.

Do not interrupt. You may be tempted to interrupt to seek clarification; instead, save your questions for when the patient is finished.

Do not change the subject. Changing the subject before your patient (or other speaker) is ready could indicate to him or her that you do not wish to listen.

Empathize. You may show concern through verbal and nonverbal body language. For example, nod in response to important points, or when the patient (or other speaker) seeks feedback.

Respond. For example, lean slightly toward the patient (or other speaker) to show that you are engaged and listening. When the patient pauses, use phrases such as "I see" or "I understand", but do not be insincere; if you do not understand, wait for your patient to finish, then ask for clarification.

Modified from: Mahal, A. (2015). Facilitator's and Trainer's Toolkit: Engage and Energize Participants for Success in Meetings, Classes, and Workshops. Technics Publications.

External Factors in Effective Communication

Effective communication requires a suitable setting. The paramedic has control over a number of the external factors that affect the setting, including privacy, interruptions, eye contact, and personal dress. Control of these factors results in a better interaction between the paramedic and the patient.

Privacy, Interruptions, and the Physical Environment

When possible, the paramedic should ensure privacy during the encounter. This helps to eliminate distractions and to reduce any inhibitions the patient may feel. Interruptions should be kept to a minimum. Noise and interference should be minimized, and the patient interview should be initiated away from distracting equipment. When possible, the lighting should be adequate.

The paramedic should be aware of the patient's **private space**—that is, the region surrounding a person that the person regards as his or hers. Private space (also known as personal space) is a form of subconscious personal protection that varies by person and by culture. Some patients may become defensive if this space is invaded, and entering this space usually causes the patient to back away.

Eye Contact

The paramedic should maintain eye contact with the patient as much as possible, even when taking notes. Eye contact is a type of nonverbal communication that can help express gentleness, sincerity, and authority and can help make the patient feel safe and secure. If possible, the paramedic should be positioned at eye level (equal seating) with the patient.

> NOTE
>
> Most patients are comfortable with note taking. They understand it may be difficult for the paramedic to remember all details. If concerns arise, the paramedic should explain the purpose of taking notes as part of a thorough assessment.

Personal Dress

Communication with a patient begins with first impressions—the patient's impression of the paramedic, as well as the paramedic's impression of the patient. Paramedics' appearance should be professional. Their clothing should be clean and should meet professional standards (eg, uniforms provided by the EMS agency). These standards help the patient instantly identify the paramedic as a professional and help to set the tone of the paramedic–patient encounter.

Patient Interview

In the paramedic–patient encounter, the ability to conduct a successful patient interview may be as important as physical assessment skills. The information gathered during this interview often helps to decide the direction of the physical examination. The patient interview should be initiated early and should continue throughout the patient encounter.

Because of the emergency nature of their work, paramedics often think in terms of specific illnesses and injuries. They often must categorize patients into general groups, such as trauma or medical cases. However, good emergency care requires the paramedic to view each patient as an individual. Moreover, it requires the paramedic to attend to each patient's needs in a caring, concerned, and receptive manner.

Communication Techniques

The paramedic should approach the conscious patient and make a personal introduction by name and title: "Hello. My name is [name], and I am a paramedic with [name of EMS agency]. What's your name?" This kind of verbal exchange with the patient will provide information about the person's level of consciousness and sensorium, and may also provide information on any hearing or speech impediments and language barriers. During the introduction, the paramedic should maintain eye contact with the patient.

Nonverbal cues should be used to gain the patient's trust and cooperation, which can in turn help the paramedic provide the best care for the patient. Nonverbal communication is not always positive, however. It can send a message of negative feelings and can convey the insecurities of both the patient and the paramedic. Voice inflection, facial expression, and body position are examples of nonverbal cues that may reflect anger, fear, or impatience. Similarly, performing patient care procedures with trembling, sweaty hands may make the patient question the paramedic's skills.

Touch is a form of communication that can show compassion and reassurance. Small gestures can help comfort a person in distress—for example, holding a patient's hand or squeezing a shoulder. Experience and familiarity with patient care activities will help the paramedic determine the appropriateness of these gestures.

In talking with patients, the paramedic must listen to what is said and interpret what is said. Patients may say they feel fine, yet their appearance and tone of voice may indicate that they are ill and afraid. If paramedics are unsure of the real message in a patient's response, they should ask additional questions that will help them better understand what the patient is trying to communicate.

Most patients do not understand medical terminology, and many have only a vague understanding of the way their bodies work. For these reasons, common words and phrases that are easy to understand should be used during the patient interview. The paramedic should guide and direct this interview without manipulating the patient's response. Specifically, the paramedic should avoid asking **leading questions** or, if possible, **closed-ended questions**, in favor of asking **open-ended questions**, which encourage a free-form response. For example, the paramedic should ask, "When did this pain begin?" rather than "Did the pain begin this morning?"

DID YOU KNOW?

Open-Ended Versus Closed-Ended Questions

Open-ended questions are asked in a narrative form. They cannot be answered with a "yes" or "no," so they encourage the patient to talk.

Closed-ended questions can be answered with a "yes" or "no." They are restrictive and may not provide much information.

Open-Ended Questions	Closed-Ended Questions
How can I help you?	Can I help you?
Can you tell me about the pain in your chest?	Do you have chest pain?
How are you feeling today?	Do you feel better today than yesterday?
When was your last meal?	Did you eat today?
What medicines do you take?	Do you take any medicines?
What examples can you give me?	Can you give me an example?
Where else do you hurt?	Is this the only place that hurts you?
Can you tell me how this happened?	Has this happened before?
Can you describe your pain?	Does your pain feel sharp?
What else would you like to ask me?	Does this answer your question?

NOTE

Open-ended questions:

- Are asked in a narrative form.
- Encourage the patient to talk.
- Do not restrict the areas of response.

The paramedic should ask only one question at a time, and the patient should be given ample time to answer this question before another question is asked. If the patient's response does not seem relevant to the question, the response should be clarified. Paramedics should be flexible. They should not discount the patient's experiences or information.

If possible, the paramedic should answer all questions asked by the patient. However, this does not mean that paramedics must provide a full explanation for each inquiry. Rather, a sensitive response that addresses the question is adequate. Paramedics should choose an answer carefully and should try to ensure the answer does not increase the patient's anxiety.

Responses

Many different tactics and responses can be used to conduct a successful patient interview (BOX 16-5). For example, the paramedic may use silence, which gives the patient more time to gather his or her thoughts. The paramedic also may echo (paraphrase) a patient's words. Echoing allows the paramedic to clarify or expand on the information provided. It also lets the patient know that the paramedic is listening. Empathy can be used to encourage a patient to talk more openly. Other tactics include asking a patient to clarify confusing statements and forcing the patient to focus on one factor of the interview (confrontation). At times the paramedic may need to interpret

BOX 16-5 Helpful Techniques for the Patient Interview

- **Silence.** Gives patients more time to gather their thoughts.
- **Reflection.** Allows patients to clarify or expand on the information provided; the technique used is generally echoing (ie, paraphrasing) of the patients' words.
- **Empathy.** Encourages patients to talk more openly.
- **Clarification.** Allows patients to rephrase a word or thought that is confusing to the paramedic.
- **Confrontation.** Focuses patients' attention on one specific factor of the interview.
- **Interpretation.** Links events; makes associations or implies a cause; is based on observation or conclusion.
- **Explanation.** Provides information to patients; encourages sharing of facts or objective information.
- **Summary.** Provides a review of the interview; asking open-ended questions can encourage patients to clarify details.

information by linking events, making associations, or inferring a cause based on what can be seen or concluded. Additional information (explanation) also can be given to a patient in an effort to persuade the person to share facts or objective information. Finally, the paramedic can summarize information by asking open-ended questions that can be used to review and to clarify important details.

Traps in Interviewing

Paramedics must be aware of some traps that can be damaging to the patient interview. These include the following:

- Providing false reassurance
- Offering poor or unwanted advice
- Showing approval or disapproval
- Giving an opinion that takes away the patient's part in decision making
- Changing the subject inappropriately
- Stereotyping the patient or complaint
- Using professional jargon
- Talking too much
- Asking leading or biased questions
- Interrupting the patient
- Asking the patient "Why" questions (these can be viewed as accusations)
- Being defensive in response to criticism

Developing a Good Rapport With the Patient

Skill in developing good rapport with a patient requires experience and practice. In most patient encounters, paramedics can follow some general guidelines to help establish good rapport:

1. Put patients at ease by letting them know you (the paramedic) are "on their side"—that is, you respect the patient's comments and are there to help.
2. Be alert for and respond to visual clues that a patient needs help.
3. Show compassion.
4. Assess the patient's level of understanding and insight. Use words and explanations at the person's level.
5. Show expertise.

CRITICAL THINKING

A suicidal patient keeps telling you that you do not care about him. Which communication techniques could you use to persuade this patient that you are truly concerned about him?

Overcoming Language Barriers

Language barriers may potentially hinder effective communication during the patient interview. These barriers may take the form of linguistic barriers (people speaking different languages) as well as use of dialects (people who technically speak the same language but have a different way of speaking). Language disabilities—such as stuttering, dysphonia, articulation disorders, and hearing loss—can also prevent effective communication. To overcome potential barriers to effective communication, the paramedic should follow these guidelines:

1. Speak slowly and clearly. Focus on enunciation and slow your speech.
2. Ask for clarification if you are not absolutely sure your message was understood. Enlist the help of friends or family members at the scene.
3. Use plain language. Avoid jargon and the use of technical terms.
4. Consider using visual aids, such as pictures or diagrams.
5. Be respectful and patient.

SHOW ME THE EVIDENCE

Dispatchers and EMS providers from New Mexico and South Africa were surveyed and interviewed to identify methods they used to communicate when faced with language barriers on the job. Telecommunicators indicated that third-party telephonic interpreter services were most effective if available. Altering the dispatcher's or provider's normal speech pattern—for example, speaking more slowly or loudly, and using repetition or rephrasing—were also identified as helpful ways to clarify understanding during patient interviews.

EMS participants noted that delays in accessing interpreters over the telephone often forced them to resort to other strategies for communicating with patients with language barriers. Field providers indicated they rely on bystanders, coworkers, or nonverbal communications, even though these methods had a number of disadvantages. One-third used digital applications on their mobile devices in situations involving language barriers, but noted that these methods permitted only yes/no answers to questions, thereby limiting communication.

Modified from: Tate RC, Hodkinson PW, Meehan-Coussee K, Cooperstein N. Strategies used by prehospital providers to overcome language barriers. *Prehosp Emerg Care.* 2016;20(3):404-414. doi: 10.3109/10903127.2015.1102994.

Strategies for Obtaining Information

Patients generally communicate with health care personnel in one of three ways. First, they may pour out information in the form of complaints. Second, they may reveal some problems while hiding others they think are embarrassing. Third, they may hide the most embarrassing parts of their problem from the paramedic (and personally deny the issue). The best way to obtain information from the patient is to use techniques based on use of open-ended and closed-ended (direct) questions. These techniques include resistance, shifting focus, recognizing defense mechanisms, and distraction.

NOTE

Closed-ended questions allow the paramedic to obtain specific information that focuses on a certain aspect of the patient's condition. "What part of your back hurts?" and "When was your last meal?" are two examples of closed-ended questions. This type of questioning is also helpful when a patient has difficulty speaking.

Resistance

Often a patient is reluctant to give information for one of two reasons. First, the patient may prefer to maintain a certain personal image and be afraid of losing that image. Second, the patient may fear that the paramedic will respond with rejection and ridicule. Being nonjudgmental will help paramedics obtain information from both types of patients (BOX 16-6). To develop a trusting relationship, the paramedic must be willing to talk to the patient about any condition in a professional manner.

Shifting Focus

Sometimes a patient may be hesitant to discuss an obvious problem. In this situation, the paramedic may have to shift the focus of the questions away from that problem. For example, a man with groin pain at first may describe the pain (especially to a female paramedic) as being in his "lower back." By shifting the focus of questioning to low back pain, the paramedic can use another group of questions that focus on the presence or absence of radiating pain. This new angle of questioning can make patients feel more comfortable when describing their condition.

Defense Mechanisms

As described in Chapter 2, *Well-Being of the Paramedic*, paramedics should recognize common defense mechanisms and, if possible, try to anticipate their use. For example, a distraught parent with a seriously

BOX 16-6 Approaching Sensitive Issues

Discussing sensitive issues can be awkward for both the patient and the paramedic. Such issues might include alcohol use, sexual subjects, and suicide risk. Even so, these issues must not be avoided when the information is needed to ensure good patient care. The paramedic should use the following guidelines when sensitive issues are discussed with patients:

- Make sure privacy is maintained.
- Be confident, direct, and firm with questions.
- Do not apologize for asking a sensitive question.
- Do not be judgmental.
- Use words that are understandable, but do not be patronizing.
- Be patient and proceed slowly.

ill child may show regression or denial. The parent may be unable to provide needed information at the emergency scene. Confrontation may be required in these and similar situations to force the parent to deal with key issues. Confrontation can clarify roles and can help others identify problems and goals. This technique should be used carefully, however—that is, only to obtain information critical for medical care. Confrontation must be performed in a professional way, thereby allowing the patient to become aware of inconsistencies in interfering behavior or thoughts.

Distraction

Paramedics may use distraction to help patients recognize irrational thoughts or behavior. This type of behavior may be seen in hostile situations in which patients "act out." In such cases, paramedics need to point out the unacceptable behavior and educate patients about its self-defeating nature. Often, this distraction prompts patients to let the paramedic control the situation until they can gain self-control. When dealing with an angry or hostile patient, paramedics should use the following approach:

- Avoid raising their voices to match the angry person's tone.
- Have the person identify and describe the cause of anger.
- Restate the cause of the anger.
- Offer a solution (if possible) or empathize and acknowledge the person's feelings.

Methods of Assessing Mental Status During the Interview

Three methods can be used to assess a patient's mental status: observation, conversation, and exploration. (Assessment of the level of consciousness is discussed in more detail in other chapters.)

Observation

The first step in assessing mental status is to observe the patient. Paramedics should note the patient's appearance, level of consciousness, and normal or abnormal body movements. Physical characteristics, dress, and grooming can provide clues to the patient's well-being, social status, religion, culture, and self-concept. Conscious patients generally are alert and able to speak intelligently. Body movements (eg, gestures, facial expressions) should be appropriate for the situation. Abnormal body movements—for example, unusual posture or gait, or clenched fists—may indicate an unstable situation.

Conversation

Conversation with patients should reveal whether they know who they are, where they are, and the day or date (ie, whether they are oriented to person, place, and time). If the patient knows these things, the remote, recent, and intermediate facets of memory probably are intact. The patient should be able to speak at a normal pace and with even flow. Responses should not have long pauses or rapid shifts (although such nuances vary regionally according to minor cultural differences). During normal conversation, the patient should be able to demonstrate clear thinking, a normal attention span, and the ability to concentrate on and understand the discussion.

> NOTE
>
> Evaluating a patient's orientation to person, place, and date (oriented × 3) also can include other parameters. Some health care professionals use time or event (eg, most recent holiday) as a fourth component in the assessment (oriented × 4).

A patient's responses to the environment (affect) also should be appropriate for the situation. Normal reactions to stress may include autonomic responses, such as sweating, trembling, and odd facial movements (eg, muscle twitching around the mouth, nose, and eyes). Reactive movements, such as not holding eye contact during conversation, should be noted. Other actions may indicate that a patient is uncomfortable or anxious—for example, grooming movements, such as fixing the hair and straightening the clothes.

Exploration

Exploration offers a way to assess the patient's emotions. For example, by observing that the patient's mood is anxious, excited, or depressed and by noting the patient's energy level, the paramedic can gauge the patient's mental status. Exploration can be done simply by interacting with the patient, with the paramedic taking care to observe the appropriateness of behaviors and ideas. An objective assessment must consider the patient's culture and educational background, as well as his or her values, beliefs, and previous experiences.

Because time is often a consideration when providing emergency care, the following "basic" questions can be used during exploration with patients of various cultures:[4]

1. What do you think caused your problem?
2. Why do you think it started when it did?
3. What does your sickness do to you? How does it work?
4. How severe is your sickness? How long do you expect it to last?
5. What problems has your sickness caused you?
6. What do you fear about your sickness?
7. What kind of treatment do you think you should receive?
8. What are the most important results you hope to receive from this treatment?

CRITICAL THINKING

The mental status examination is crucial, both for medical reasons and for legal reasons. Why do you think this is so?

Special Interview Situations

At times paramedics may have to use special skills to interact successfully with a patient who is uncooperative or frightened or who has a disability (also see Chapter 17, *History Taking*).

Patients Who Do Not Talk

Although most patients are more than willing to talk, some need more time and encouragement through various techniques to participate in a successful interview. Difficult interviews generally stem from four sources:[5]

1. The patient's condition may affect the ability to speak.
2. The patient may fear talking because of psychological disorders, cultural differences, safety, or age.
3. The patient may have a cognitive impairment.
4. The patient may want to deceive the paramedic.

The following techniques may be useful for communicating with a patient who is unmotivated to talk:

- Start the interview in the normal way. If the patient does not talk, review the nature of the call as received from the dispatch center. Take time to develop a rapport with the patient.
- Use open-ended questions to get a response. If this approach is unsuccessful, try direct questions.
- Provide positive feedback when the patient provides appropriate responses.
- Make sure the patient understands the question. Consider whether a language barrier or a hearing difficulty is a factor.
- Continue asking questions to obtain the information needed to provide treatment. (Nonessential information may be difficult to obtain.)
- Question family members or others at the scene. If the patient has been uncommunicative for a long period, try to rule out a disease or disorder as the reason.
- Use summary and interpretation of events or conditions. Also, ask the patient if the summary and interpretation are correct.
- Ask the patient questions about the care provided, equipment used, or the paramedic profession in an attempt to create conversation. If the patient responds, answer all questions fully (not with one-word answers).
- Realize that all of the information needed may not be obtained.
- Observe the patient's affect, and record these observations. This information sets a mental status baseline for later evaluations.
- Consider asking questions for which answers are known. Comparing the answers received to the known answers helps to gauge the patient's credibility.

NOTE

Patients who are unconscious or unresponsive may be able to receive stimuli. Hearing is thought to be the last sensation lost with unconsciousness and the first regained with consciousness. The paramedic must not say anything near an unconscious patient that would not be said if the patient were fully conscious.

Modified from: Sisson R. Effects of auditory stimuli on comatose patients with head injury. *Heart Lung.* 1990;19(4):373-378.

Hostile Patients

As part of ensuring their personal safety, paramedics should be alert for signs that a situation could potentially turn violent. Signs expressed by the patient, or by others on the scene, that may indicate the potential for violence include clenched fists, a rising voice level, or a threatening facial expression. Further, paramedics, through dispatch information or past experience, may know that the patient or others on scene have a history of violence toward others. If such a situation exists or is expected, the EMS crew should retreat from the scene and request the help of law enforcement officers. If safe retreat is not an option, the paramedics should stay far enough away from the patient to ensure their personal safety (see Chapter 34, *Behavioral and Psychiatric Disorders*).

The following guidelines can be used when interviewing a hostile patient:

- Try to use normal interviewing techniques.
- Never leave the patient alone without adequate assistance.
- Set limits and establish boundaries with the patient.
- Explain the advantages of cooperation to the patient.
- Follow local protocol for dealing with hostile patients, including the use of physical and chemical restraints.

Patients With Age-Related Factors

Communicating with children and older adults should not be difficult or a challenge. Therapeutic communication works best when the paramedic takes into account the common developmental characteristics of a particular age group (see Chapter 12, *Life Span Development*).

Communicating With Children

When communicating with children, the paramedic often must establish rapport with two people—the child and the parent. With children 1 to 6 years old, most conversation should be directed first to the parent. (Offering a toy may distract the child while the parent is interviewed.) The paramedic should be aware that information from the parent is that person's point of view, and the parent might be feeling defensive. Paramedics should not be judgmental if the parents had not provided proper care or safety for the child before EMS arrival. (Be observant but not confrontational.)

The paramedic should gradually begin to make contact with the child during the parent interview. This can be done by moving to eye level to speak with the child and by using a quiet, calm voice. It should be remembered that children are especially responsive to nonverbal cues. BOX 16-7 lists special considerations for communicating with children of various ages. (Assessing pediatric patients is discussed in detail in Chapter 47, *Pediatrics.*)

BOX 16-7 Tips for Communicating With Children of Various Ages

- Infants respond best to firm, gentle handling and a quiet, calm voice. Older infants may have stranger anxiety. If possible, the parent should remain in view of the child.
- Preschoolers see the world only from their perspective and base everything on past experience. Use short sentences and give concrete explanations (eg, "You will need to hold still so that I can splint your arm and make you feel better.").
- Adolescents want to be adults. Treat them with respect and use age-appropriate words. Do not talk to or treat them as if they were small children.

Communicating With Older Adults

Many older adults are dealing with age-related diseases and the inevitability of death. Interviewing older adults may take longer than interviewing younger people. Older patients may tire easily, and some may have physical disabilities that distort speech. Touch is generally important to most older adults. When interviewing an older person, the paramedic should always use the patient's last name and a title (eg, Mr., Mrs., or Ms.) unless the patient requests otherwise. In addition, the patient should be able to see the paramedic's face easily. Eye contact should be maintained, and speech should be clear and slow. Using short, open-ended questions and talking with family members usually are the best approaches for the patient interview with an older adult. (Assessing the older adult is addressed in detail in Chapter 48, *Geriatrics.*)

Patients Who Are Hard of Hearing

When dealing with a patient with a hearing impairment, the paramedic should determine the patient's preferred method of communicating—for example, lipreading (speechreading), signing, or writing. Writing often is the best prehospital method for communicating with a deaf patient. If the patient prefers lipreading, the paramedic should (1) face the patient squarely, (2) ensure lighting is adequate, (3) speak slowly using short words and phrases, and (4) enunciate clearly. Because many deaf patients lip-read, paramedics must speak clearly in full view of these patients. It is important to note that some deaf patients may nod "yes" even if they do not understand the question.

If a patient is thought to be hard of hearing or deaf, the paramedic should try to gain the person's attention. This can be done by a gentle touch or by slowly waving the hands in front of the patient. The paramedic also may try speaking a little more loudly or speaking into the patient's ear if the person is not wearing a hearing aid. If a hearing-impaired patient needs to be transported to a medical facility, the paramedic should inform the emergency department staff as soon as possible about the impairment. This prearrival information allows arrangements to be made for personnel to aid in communications with the patient. (Offering advance information to the receiving facility is also a good practice with patients who do not speak English.)

Finger-spelling and simple sign language are easy to learn. Developing skills with these techniques can assist the paramedic in communicating with deaf patients in the prehospital setting.

Patients Who Are Visually Impaired

When communicating with a patient who cannot see, paramedics should ascertain whether the patient also has a hearing impairment (although it is unusual for sightless people to be deaf as well). Paramedics should identify themselves in a normal voice. All questions about the emergency scene and the surroundings should be answered. In addition, all examination and treatment procedures should be explained in detail before touching the patient.

Disabled Patients With Service Animals

If a person who is visually impaired or otherwise disabled has a service dog and the situation permits, the two should not be separated. If the dog was injured during the emergency event or the owner cannot safely control its behavior, the dispatch center should be quickly advised so that special arrangements can be made to care for the dog.

Several important points relate to service animals. The Americans With Disabilities Act applies only to service dogs. The requirement to permit ambulance transport of the service animal does not apply to other species, although the paramedic may use discretion based on the needs of the patient and on departmental policies.

1. If unsure that the animal companion is a service animal, the paramedic may legally ask only whether it is a service dog required for a disability and which work or task the dog has been trained to perform.[6] The paramedic may not ask for documentation of the disability related to the dog's status. Likewise, the service animal is not required to wear a vest, identification tag, or harness.[7]
2. A paramedic may not deny access to the ambulance to a service dog because of a crew member's allergies or fear of the dog if a reasonable accommodation can be made.
3. The service animal should be permitted to ride in the ambulance unless the dog's presence would interfere with the ability to treat the patient.
4. The service dog must be harnessed, leashed, or tethered unless the patient's disability prevents that type of restraint. In those cases, the patient must maintain control of the animal. If the paramedic feels the dog is out of control, it may be removed from the ambulance.

Patients Under the Influence of Street Drugs or Alcohol

If street drugs or alcohol plays a part in an emergency, paramedics should ensure their personal safety. They should also be prepared for unpredictable patient behavior. (The assistance of law enforcement officers may be needed to ensure scene safety.) During the patient interview, paramedics should ask simple and direct questions. Paramedics should avoid any action that the patient may view as a threat or confrontation (see Chapter 33, *Toxicology*, and Chapter 34, *Behavioral and Psychiatric Disorders*).

Sexually Aggressive Patients

Paramedics should confront male or female patients who make improper sexual advances, so as to ensure that the patient is aware of the professional role of the paramedic. Paramedics should document unusual incidents and record the names and statements of witnesses who observed inappropriate conduct. If possible, sexually aggressive patients should receive care from paramedics of the same gender. It also is best to have a chaperone or witness present during the care and transport of the patient. Some EMS agencies use audio devices during transport to record all interactions with sexually aggressive patients; the use of these devices may require the patient's legal consent.

LGBTQ Patients

Lesbian, gay, bisexual, transgender, queer (or questioning their sexual identity) (LGBTQ) patients may present with some health issues and life obstacles that are more frequent in this population than in heterosexual patients. For example, physical and sexual assault (including intimate-partner violence), depression and other anxiety disorders, substance abuse, and suicidal ideations are common in LGBTQ populations (BOX 16-8).

When communicating with LGBTQ patients, paramedics should employ techniques to lower barriers to effective treatment and to support disclosure and dialogue. They should use sensitive and inclusive language when discussing relationships with LGBTQ patients, and should not make assumptions about a patient's sexual identity or sexual behavior. The transgender patient may be undergoing transition from one gender to another. If the gender identity of the patient is not clear, ask whether the patient identifies as male or female to appropriately refer to the patient as he or she prefers. Maintain good eye contact and avoid any awkward body language that may be interpreted as discrimination.

LGBTQ patients' partners and spouses should be afforded the same consideration and care as the family members of any other patient group. Laws relating to next-of-kin and medical decision making for spouses of LGBTQ patients vary, so paramedics should be familiar with the laws relating to this issue within their state. Regardless of the law, it is important to provide appropriate communication and comfort to the patient's loved ones.

BOX 16-8 LGBTQ Health/Life Facts

Compared to non-LGBTQ people:

- LGBTQ youth are two to three times more likely to attempt suicide.
- LGBTQ youth are more likely to be homeless.
- Lesbians are less likely to get preventive services for cancer.
- Gay men are at higher risk of human immunodeficiency virus (HIV) and other sexually transmitted diseases (STDs), especially those in communities of color.
- Lesbians and bisexual females are more likely to be overweight or obese.
- People who are transgender have a high prevalence of HIV/STDs, victimization, mental health issues, and suicide.
- Older adults who are LGBTQ face additional barriers to health because of isolation and a lack of social services and culturally competent providers.
- LGBTQ populations have the highest rates of tobacco, alcohol, and other drug use.

Modified from: Healthypeople.gov Lesbian, gay, bisexual, and transgender health. Updated December 8, 2017. https://www.healthypeople.gov/2020/topics-objectives/topic/lesbian-gay-bisexual-and-transgender-health.

NOTE

To effectively and compassionately care for LGBTQ patients, paramedics should be familiar with the following terms:

Bisexual. A sexual orientation in which a person is sexually attracted to both males and females.

Cis-gender. A gender identity that is the same as the person's sex at birth.

FTM (Female-to-Male). A person who is born female and whose gender identity is male.

Gay. A sexual orientation in which a person is primarily sexually attracted to people of the same gender or sex. Both males and females can be gay.

Gender affirming. Behaviors and/or treatments that affirm a transgender person's identity (eg, hormone therapy).

Gender discordance. A mismatch between a person's sex at birth and his or her perceived gender identity.

Gender expression. Behavior, clothing, or personal traits that communicate a person's gender identity.

Lesbian. A female whose primary sexual attraction is toward the same gender or sex.

MTF (Male-to-Female). A person who is born male and whose gender identity is female.

Queer. A gender identity that is neither strictly male nor female.

Sexual orientation. Sexual attraction to a particular gender.

Transgender. A gender identity that does not align with the person's sex at birth.

Transitioning. The process of adopting a different gender identity.

Transcultural Considerations

Culture can influence how patients and family interpret and respond to an injury or illness. Therefore, it is important to consider the patient's cultural perspective to provide optimal care. Culture affects a variety of social factors that influence health (ie, social determinants of health), shaping how a person interprets his or her illness and how a patient and family respond to illness.

Both historically and in the present day, some cultural groups have faced disparities in health care that can cause them to view even well-meaning paramedics with suspicion and that affect their interactions with health care professionals in general. Several studies have found disparities persist even when controlling for insurance type and socioeconomic class.[8,9] It is likely that factors such as bias and inadequate communication contribute to these disparities in care. For example, a 2011 report found that African Americans, American Indians, and Alaska Natives received inferior care compared to Caucasians on 40% of evidence-based core health measures; Asians' care was worse than Caucasians' care on 20% of these core measures; and Hispanics' care was worse than Caucasians' care on 60% of those same indicators.[10]

Paramedics must also be aware that they may be viewed as a cultural stereotype to the patient and family. For this reason, the roles of everyone involved in providing care (paramedics, patient, and family members) must be clearly understood. BOX 16-9 outlines ways to improve patient–provider interactions when caring for patients of other cultures.

Two pitfalls that paramedics must avoid when speaking with patients of a different culture are ethnocentrism and cultural imposition. **Ethnocentrism** is the belief that one's own culture is the most acceptable or best. It may prompt someone to act in a superior manner toward another culture's way of life. **Cultural imposition** is the forcing of one's beliefs, values, and patterns of behavior on people from another culture. Paramedics do not fall into these pitfalls on purpose, but they must be sensitive to how their actions and words may be seen by members of another culture.

The following factors should also be considered when communicating with patients of another culture:

- Some cultures expect health care workers to have all the answers to their illness.
- Different cultures accept illness or injury in different ways.
- Nonverbal cues (eg, handshaking, touching) are perceived differently in different cultures.

BOX 16-9 Seven Lessons to Learn About Cross-Cultural Communication

1. Don't assume sameness.
2. What you think of as normal behavior may only be cultural.
3. Familiar behaviors may have different meanings.
4. Don't assume that what you meant is what was understood.
5. Don't assume that what you understood is what was meant.
6. You don't have to like or accept different behaviors, but you should try to understand where they come from.
7. Most people do behave rationally, you just have to discover the rationale.

Modified from: Storti, C. (1999). *Figuring Foreigners Out: A Practical Guide*. Reproduced by permission of Nicholas Brealey Publishing.

- Some cultures consider direct eye contact to be impolite or aggressive; patients may avert their eyes during an interview.
- Paramedics should not use touch as a means of reassurance with members of different cultural groups, because touch may be easily misunderstood.
- Language barriers may present communication difficulties, even when an interpreter is used (BOX 16-10).
- Personal space is often defined by culture, but it also varies by each person (BOX 16-11).

When trying to interview a patient from a different culture to understand the illness and then negotiate care, the LEARN mnemonic can be helpful:[11]

- **L**isten to the patient's perception of the problem.
- **E**xplain how the paramedic views the patient's problem.
- **A**cknowledge cultural differences and the similarities and differences between the patient's and paramedic's perceptions.
- **R**ecommend the appropriate care.
- **N**egotiate the care, incorporating some of the patient's cultural views and wishes when possible.

CRITICAL THINKING

Have you ever tried to communicate with someone who spoke a different language? Which strategies did you use?

BOX 16-10 General Guidelines for Working With an Interpreter

Paramedics are sometimes asked to assist a patient who does not speak English. Often someone in the home or at the scene can help the paramedic communicate with the patient. When working with an interpreter, follow these guidelines:

1. Explain to the interpreter the key information you are trying to get before you begin the interview.
2. Ask a child to interpret only if no adult interpreter is available.
3. Speak directly to the patient or to a family member when asking questions. Doing so establishes the primary relationship with that person (not the interpreter). It also allows you to observe nonverbal clues.
4. Ask questions that require one response at a time. For example, ask, "Do you have pain?" rather than "Do you have any pain, trouble breathing, or nausea?"
5. Try not to interrupt the patient, family member, or interpreter when that person is speaking.
6. Do not make comments about the patient or family to the interpreter; the patient or family may know some English.
7. Use simple language. Do not use medical terms for which other languages may have no similar words.
8. Be sensitive to cultural differences related to issues such as pregnancy or death and dying.
9. After the interview, if time permits, ask for the interpreter's impressions and observations of the interview.

Modified from: Hockenberry MJ, Wilson D. *Wong's Nursing Care of Infants and Children.* 10th ed. St. Louis, MO: Elsevier Mosby; 2015.

BOX 16-11 General Guidelines on Personal Space[a]

Intimate Zone

- 0 to 1.5 feet (0 to 0.5 m).
- Visual distortion occurs.
- Best for assessing breath and other body odors.

Personal Distance

- 1.5 to 4 feet (0.5 to 1.2 m).
- Perceived as an extension of the self.
- Speaker's voice is moderate.
- Body odors are not apparent.
- Much of the physical assessment occurs at this distance.

Social Distance

- 4 to 12 feet (1.2 to 3.7 m).
- Used for impersonal business transactions.
- Perceptual information is much less detailed.
- Much of the patient interview occurs at this distance.

Public Distance

- 12 feet (3.7 m) or farther.
- Interaction with others is impersonal.
- Speaker's voice must be projected.
- Subtle facial expressions are imperceptible.

[a]These are only general guidelines. Many factors—such as age, gender, and geographic location—affect a person's definition of personal space. Some cultures are more comfortable at a variety of distances when communicating.

Modified from: Potter PA, Perry AG, Stockert PA, Hall A. *Essentials for Nursing Practice.* 8th ed. St. Louis, MO: Elsevier Mosby; 2015.

Summary

- Therapeutic communications is both a planned act and a professional act. Through this type of communication, the paramedic, working with the patient, obtains information that is used to meet patient care goals.
- Communication is a dynamic process that includes six elements: the source, encoding, the message, decoding, the receiver, and feedback.
- To effectively communicate with patients, paramedics must genuinely like people, be able to empathize with others, and have the ability to listen.
- Good communication requires a favorable physical environment. Factors such as privacy, interruption, eye contact, and personal dress are external influences that can be controlled, thereby enabling the paramedic to better communicate with the patient.
- The information gained through the patient interview often determines the direction of the physical examination. During the interview, the paramedic should take care to see each patient as an individual and meet that patient's needs in a caring, concerned, and receptive way.

- Open-ended and closed-ended (direct) questions can be used to obtain information from the patient. Helpful interview techniques may include resistance, shifting focus, recognizing defense mechanisms, and distraction.
- The first step in therapeutic communications is to assess the patient's mental status. This can be done by observing the patient's appearance and level of consciousness and by looking for normal versus abnormal body movements. During normal conversation, the patient should be able to show clear thinking, a normal attention span, and the ability to concentrate on and understand the discussion. The patient's responses to the environment (ie, affect) should be appropriate to the situation.
- Difficult interviews generally arise from four types of situations: (1) The patient's condition may affect the ability to speak; (2) the patient may fear talking because of psychological disorders, cultural differences, or age; (3) a cognitive impairment may be present; or (4) the patient may want to deceive the paramedic.
- Paramedics should avoid ethnocentrism and cultural imposition when caring for patients from other cultures.

References

1. Satir V. *The New Peoplemaking.* Palo Alto, CA: Science & Behavior Books; 1988.
2. Potter PA, Perry AG, Stockert PA, Hall A. *Essentials for Nursing Practice.* 8th ed. St. Louis, MO: Elsevier Mosby; 2015.
3. Moore M. *Embracing the Mystery.* Madison, WI: MJM Publishing; 1999.
4. Kleinman A. *Patients and Healers in the Context of Culture.* Berkeley, CA: University of California Press; 1980.
5. Rathus SA. *Psychology: Concepts and Connections.* 10th ed. New York, NY: Wadsworth Publishing; 2012.
6. US Department of Justice, Civil Rights Division, Disability Rights Section. Service animals. ADA.gov website. https://www.ada.gov/service_animals_2010.htm. Published July 12, 2011. Accessed January 22, 2018.
7. US Department of Justice, Civil Rights Division, Disability Rights Section. Frequently asked questions about service animals and the ADA. ADA.gov website. https://www.ada.gov/regs2010/service_animal_qa.html. Published July 20, 2015. Accessed January 22, 2018.
8. Blendon RJ, Buhr T, Cassidy EF, et al. Disparities in physician care: experiences and perceptions of a multi-ethnic America. *Health Affairs.* 2008;27(2):507–517.
9. Harris DR, Andrews R, Elixhauser A. Racial and gender differences in use of procedures for black and white hospitalized adults. *Ethn Dis.* 1997;7(2):91-105.
10. Agency for Healthcare Research and Quality. Disparities in health care quality among racial and ethnic minority groups: selected findings from the 2010 national healthcare quality and disparities reports. Agency for Healthcare Research and Quality website. https://www.ahrq.gov/sites/default/files/wysiwyg/research/findings/nhqrdr/nhqrdr10/minority.pdf. Published 2010. Accessed January 22, 2018.
11. Campinha-Bacote J. Delivering patient-centered care in the midst of a cultural conflict: the role of cultural competence. *Online J Issues Nurs.* 2011;16(2). http://www.nursingworld.org/MainMenuCategories/ANAMarketplace/ANAPeriodicals/OJIN/TableofContents/Vol-16-2011/No2-May-2011/Delivering-Patient-Centered-Care-in-the-Midst-of-a-Cultural-Conflict.html. Accessed January 22, 2018.

Suggested Readings

Agency for Healthcare Research and Quality. Health literacy universal precautions toolkit, 2nd ed. Consider culture, customs, and beliefs: Tool #10. Agency for Healthcare Research and Quality website. https://www.ahrq.gov/professionals/quality-patient-safety/quality-resources/tools/literacy-toolkit/healthlittoolkit2-tool10.html. Published February 2015. Accessed January 22, 2018.

Brainard C. EMS transport of service dogs and support animals. *J Emerg Med Serv.* July 1, 2017. http://www.jems.com/articles/print/volume-42/issue-7/features/ems-transport-of-service-dogs-support-animals.html. Accessed January 22, 2018.

Culture, language and health literacy. Health Resources and Services Administration website. http://www.hrsa.gov/culturalcompetence/index.html. Reviewed May 2017. Accessed January 22, 2018.

Heron S, Kazzi A, Martin ML, eds. Monograph on cultural competency. University of Virginia School of Medicine website. https://www.med-ed.virginia.edu/courses/culture/. Published 2009. Accessed January 22, 2018.

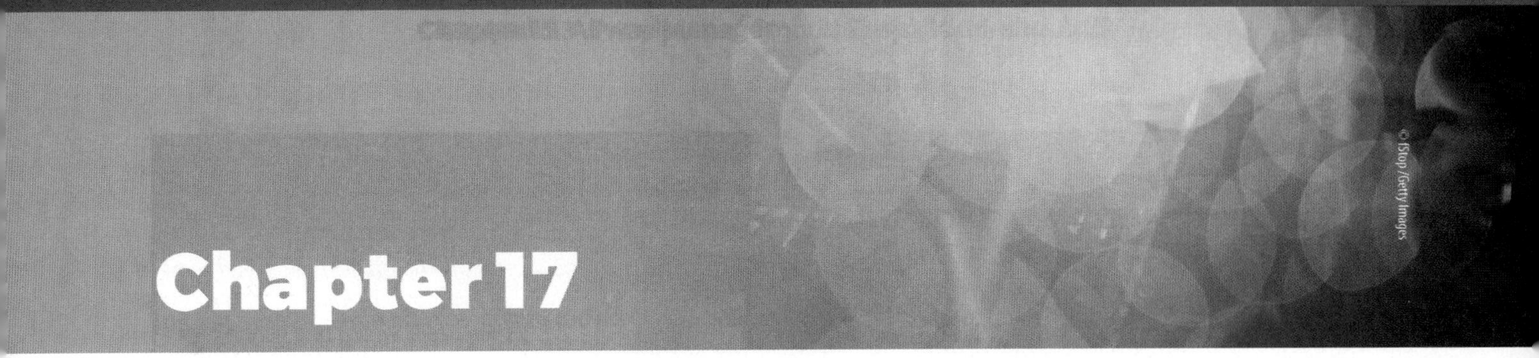
© iStop/Getty Images

Chapter 17

History Taking

NATIONAL EMS EDUCATION STANDARD COMPETENCIES

Assessment

Integrate scene and patient assessment findings with your knowledge of epidemiology and pathophysiology to form a field impression. Use clinical reasoning to develop a list of differential diagnoses, modify the assessment, and formulate a treatment plan.

History Taking

- Determining the chief complaint (p 600)
- Investigation of the chief complaint (pp 599–603)
- Mechanism of injury/nature of illness (p 600)
- Past medical history (pp 602–603)
- Associated signs and symptoms (p 601)
- Pertinent negatives (p 603)
- Components of the patient history (p 598)
- Interviewing techniques (pp 599–600, 605)
- How to integrate therapeutic communication techniques and adapt the line of inquiry based on findings and presentation (pp 599–602)

OBJECTIVES

Upon completion of this chapter, the paramedic student will be able to:

1. Describe the purpose of effective history taking in prehospital patient care. (p 598)
2. List the content of the patient history. (p 598–599)
3. Outline effective patient interviewing techniques to facilitate history taking. (pp 599–603)
4. Describe how the paramedic uses clinical reasoning. (pp 606–607)
5. Outline the process to determine differential diagnoses. (pp 606–608)
6. Identify strategies to manage special challenges in obtaining a patient history. (pp 606, 608–610)

KEY TERMS

chief complaint A patient's primary complaint; usually the reason for the EMS response.

chief concern The paramedic's primary concern related to the patient condition.

clinical decision making A contextual, continuous, and evolving process, in which data are gathered, interpreted, and evaluated so as to select an evidence-based choice of action.

clinical reasoning Use of the results of questions to think about associated problems and body system changes related to the patient's complaint.

current health status A focus on the patient's current state of health, environmental conditions, and personal habits.

differential diagnosis The process of weighing the probability of one disease versus that of other diseases possibly accounting for a patient's illness.

family history Illness or disease in a patient's family or family's background that may be relevant to the patient complaint.

history taking The process of gathering information during the patient interview.

opening questions Questions that determine why the patient is seeking medical care or advice.

past medical history A patient's medical background, which may offer insight into the patient's current problem.

present illness The chief complaint. Identification of the present illness is supported by a full, clear, chronologic account of the symptoms.

History taking *refers to the process of gathering details during an interview with a patient. History taking provides an account of medical and social events in a patient's life. It also indicates environmental factors that may affect the patient's condition. Obtaining a patient history gives structure to patient assessment and often is crucial to establish priorities in patient care.*

Components of the Patient History

The patient history that is obtained in the prehospital setting is focused on the patient's problem or the reason EMS was summoned (a problem-based history). It has several purposes.[1] First, the patient history identifies life-threatening conditions that require immediate intervention. That is, it gives full attention to the "needs of the moment." The patient history provides information that leads to appropriate care for the patient, whose condition is determined to be either emergent (life threatening), urgent (not life threatening), or nonemergent (stable). In addition, the patient history identifies the potential for life threats to arise as well as the existence of a current life threat.

Finally, the patient history can be expanded, when appropriate, to allow opportunities for patient education. It can also allow opportunities to provide service referrals to agencies and organizations that can help the patient and/or family with specific health care needs.

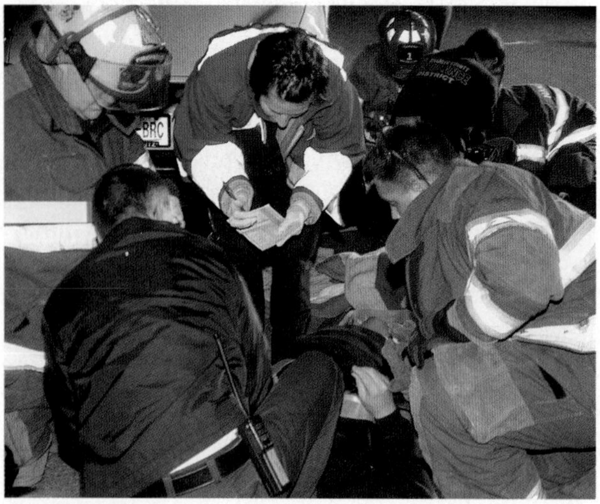
Courtesy Ray Kemp, St. Charles, MO.

Content of the Patient History

The patient history is made up of several parts. Each of these parts has a specific purpose, which offers a "snapshot" of the patient and his or her condition. BOX 17-1 lists the parts of a patient history, as described in this chapter.

The patient history should include the date and time when the history was obtained. It should also

BOX 17-1 Content of the Patient History

Date and Time

Identifying Data
- Age
- Sex
- Race/ethnicity
- Occupation
- Weight

Source of Referral
- Patient referral
- Referral by others

Source of History
- Patient
- Family
- Friends
- Police
- Others

Reliability
- Variable (memory, trust, motivation)
- Determined at the end of the evaluation

Chief Complaint or Chief Concern
- Main part of history
- One or more symptoms for which the patient is seeking medical care

Present Illness
- Identifies the chief complaint
- Provides a chronologic account of the patient's symptoms

Medical History

Current Health Status

Review of Body Systems

include any appropriate identifying information for the patient (eg, age, sex, weight, race and ethnicity, occupation). Identifying information can be key, as illustrated in the following scenario:

> Your crew has been dispatched to a "sick case." On arrival, you find a woman who is ill with flu-like symptoms. Her symptoms include nausea, vomiting, and diarrhea. During your interview, she tells you that she is a 49-year-old businesswoman. She has just returned to the United States from an extended visit to her birthplace in Southeast Asia. In addition to the chance of gastrointestinal illness or food poisoning, you now suspect that she could be ill from an endemic disease (ie, a disease prevalent in a population or geographic region).

Documentation should include the source of the referral and patient history. For example, did the patient request EMS assistance, or did a family member, friend, law enforcement officer, or bystander initiate the EMS response?

The paramedic also must decide whether the source of the referral and patient history is reliable, as illustrated in the following scenario:

> Your crew has been dispatched to a car crash. The driver of the car is a 17-year-old boy who has minor injuries. His speech is slurred, and his breath smells of an odor resembling alcohol. He denies alcohol or other drug use to you and the law enforcement officers at the scene. Is this patient history reliable?

The chief complaint (explained later in this chapter) is the main part of the patient history; it is the reason why EMS was summoned. After identifying the chief complaint, the paramedic obtains a history and description of the present illness or injury. This history provides a chronologic account of the patient's symptoms. The paramedic then questions the patient about any past medical history and current health status. Finally, the paramedic performs a review of body systems appropriate to the patient's symptoms or complaint (see Chapter 19, *Secondary Assessment and Reassessment*).

Techniques of History Taking

As described in Chapter 16, *Therapeutic Communications*, it is important to "set the stage" for a good paramedic–patient encounter. This is done by establishing a good first impression and by ensuring that the environment is conducive to free-flowing communication. The paramedic should do the following to encourage the patient to share information honestly and openly:

- Establish a professional demeanor with the patient.
- Ensure patient comfort and provide a safe environment.
- Greet the patient by name or surname and avoid use of demeaning terms (eg, "Granny," "Pop," "Hon").
- Avoid entering the patient's personal space.
- Inquire about the patient's feelings.
- Be sensitive to the patient's feelings and experiences.
- Watch for signs of uneasiness.
- Use language that is appropriate and easily understood.
- Ask open-ended questions and direct questions (if needed).

> NOTE
> The paramedic's demeanor and appearance are very important in "setting the stage." Just as the paramedic is watching the patient, so the patient will be watching the paramedic.

Opening questions are questions that determine why the patient is seeking medical care or advice. Such questions may incorporate facilitation, reflection, clarification, empathetic responses, confrontation, and interpretation, and may involve asking patients about their feelings.

- **Facilitation.** Use posture and positive actions or words to encourage the patient to say more. Maintain eye contact and use phrases such as "Go on" and "I'm listening." These phrases encourage the patient to continue talking.
- **Reflection.** Repeat or "echo" what the patient tells you. This response encourages additional responses. Reflection usually will not bias the patient's story or interrupt the patient's train of thought.
- **Clarification.** Ask questions to better grasp vague statements or words.
- **Empathy.** Demonstrate that you understand the patient's feelings by identifying with his or her condition. This will help to gain the patient's trust.

- **Confrontation.** Some issues may necessitate confronting patients about their feelings. For example, a paramedic might ask a patient who is severely depressed, "Have you ever thought about killing yourself?"
- **Interpretation.** When appropriate, go beyond confrontation and make an inference from the patient's response. For example, the paramedic might draw an inference from the patient who says, "I think I'm going to die"—namely, that the patient may be gravely ill.
- **Asking patients about their feelings.** Use the therapeutic techniques described in Chapter 16, *Therapeutic Communications*, to encourage patients to explain how they feel.

Chief Complaint

The **chief complaint** is the patient's primary complaint and is usually the reason for the EMS response. The complaint may be verbal (eg, complaint of chest pain) or nonverbal (eg, a facial grimace that indicates pain or distress). Most chief complaints are characterized by pain, abnormal function, a change in the patient's normal state, or an unusual observation made by the patient (eg, heart palpitations).

> NOTE
>
> When exploring the chief complaint, it is important to ask every patient:
> - "What do you think is wrong with you?"
> - "What are your specific concerns about your condition?"
> - "What do you think caused your problem?"
>
> The patient's answers to these questions may be very relevant.

The paramedic's primary concern related to the patient's condition is termed the **chief concern** and may not be synonymous with the patient's chief complaint. A chief complaint may be misleading or a problem may be more serious than the complaint indicates. For example, the patient who has fallen down a flight of steps may complain of an injured ankle, but the physical examination may reveal possible internal injuries. Or, the patient may have fallen because of sudden paralysis on one side of the body related to a stroke. In addition, patients often modify or substitute their chief complaint, perhaps to hide a problem they find embarrassing or difficult to discuss. For example, a chief complaint of vaginal bleeding might be described by the patient as "a heavy period," when the bleeding was actually an abrupt hemorrhage that occurred during intercourse. Likewise, a chief complaint of "frequent headaches" may be substituted for feelings of depression with suicidal thoughts. Determining the *true* reason for the patient's concern is one of the skills of history taking.

After identifying the patient's chief complaint (and managing any life-threatening situations), the paramedic should obtain a history of the present illness and any relevant medical history.

> NOTE
>
> The true needs of the patient may not be the stated chief complaint.

> CRITICAL THINKING
>
> Which illnesses or injuries could cause a chief complaint of confusion?

History of Present Illness

The **present illness** refers to the chief complaint and is supported through a full, clear, and chronologic account of the patient's symptoms. Obtaining a full history of the present illness takes skill—that is, skill in asking proper questions related to the chief complaint and in interpreting the patient's response. For example, a patient's complaint of low back pain suggests a muscle strain. During direct questioning in the interview, however, the patient might reveal a history of a burning sensation with urination and a low-grade fever for the past several days, which suggests a urinary tract infection. Thus the history of the present illness may be more crucial than the obvious chief complaint.

The mnemonic OPQRST helps define the patient's complaint by focusing on essential elements of assessment (BOX 17-2); its elements are explored further in the following subsections. Use of this or another memory device (eg, the SOCRATES survey; BOX 17-3) will help lead the paramedic through a thorough series of questions to better understand the chief complaint.

The paramedic should take notes while obtaining the health history. Most patients realize that it is difficult to remember all details and accept note taking.

BOX 17-2 OPQRST Mnemonic

Onset. What were you doing when the pain started? Do you have a history of this problem? Was it sudden or gradual in onset?
Provocation/palliation. What brought on the symptoms? What makes the symptoms better? What makes them worse?
Quality. What does the pain feel like? Is it sharp, dull, burning, or tearing?
Region/radiation. Where is the symptom? Where does it go? Is it in one or more areas?
Severity. On a scale of 0 to 10, with 0 being no pain and 10 being the worst, what number would you give your pain or discomfort?
Timing. How long have you had this symptom? When did it start? When did it end? How long did it last?

BOX 17-3 SOCRATES Survey

Site
Onset (eg, sudden, gradual)
Character (eg, dull, sharp, stabbing)
Radiation
Associated symptoms (eg, what else did you notice?)
Time, course, duration
Exacerbating and relieving factors
Severity (using a scale of 0 to 10)

Onset

Onset identifies what the patient was doing when the pain began and whether there is any history of a similar episode. Attention should also be paid to the setting at the time when the signs or symptoms began. Questions to ask to obtain this information may include the following:

- "Did the pain or discomfort begin suddenly, or did it occur gradually over time?"
- "When did you last feel well?"
- "What were you doing when the pain started?"
- "Did the pain begin during a period of activity or while you were at rest?"
- "Have you ever had this type of pain or discomfort before? If so, is it the same or is it different than what you're experiencing now?"
- "Does anyone else at the scene have similar signs or symptoms?"

Provocation/Palliation

Provocation and palliation refer to precipitating factors associated with the patient's complaints. Questions to ask to identify precipitating factors may include the following:

- "What makes your pain or discomfort better?"
- "What makes your pain or discomfort worse?"
- "Does the pain increase or decrease when you take a breath?"
- "Does lying down or sitting up affect your level of discomfort?"
- "Have you taken any medications for your symptoms? If so, did the medications make you feel better?"

Quality

Quality refers to how the patient perceives the pain or discomfort. Questions to ask to determine quality of the pain include the following:

- "What does the pain feel like?"
- "Can you describe the pain to me?"
- "Is the pain sharp or dull?"
- "Is the pain constant, or does it come and go?"

Region/Radiation

Region and radiation refer to the location of the pain and whether it is localized or associated with pain elsewhere in the body. Questions to ask to identify region and radiation include the following:

- "Where is the pain?"
- "Can you point with one finger to the exact location of the pain?"
- "Does the pain stay in the same place or does it move?"
- "If the pain moves, where does it go? Does the pain go to more than one area?"

Severity

Severity refers to how the patient rates the level of the pain or discomfort. This rating also provides a baseline for future evaluation of the patient's pain. Questions to ask the patient include the following:

- "On a scale of 0 to 10, with 0 being the least and 10 being the worst pain you can imagine, how would you rate your pain or discomfort?"
- "How bad is the pain?"

> SHOW ME THE EVIDENCE
>
> Australian paramedic researchers conducted a survey to identify how ambulance personnel access health information and to determine the barriers preventing them from doing so. In addition, the researchers wondered whether a lack of information could lead to a less than optimal care plan, which could be improved if that information were available. Of the 302 respondents, 94.4% felt they were not able to access health information about a patient for whom they provided care. Of those, 90.7% felt this unavailability of health information resulted in a less than optimal care path for their patients. Many (81.5%) said that information was easier to access during weekday business hours. Notably, 77.2% of respondents said they could not gain timely access to a patient's resuscitation status or end-of-life wishes. The researchers concluded that timely access to patient health information is vital to make appropriate patient care and transport decisions.
>
> *Modified from*: Zorab O, Robinson M, Endacott R. Are prehospital treatment or conveyance decisions affected by an ambulance crew's ability to access a patient's health information [published online October 7, 2015]? *BMC Emerg Med*. 2015;15(26).

- "Does the intensity of the pain vary, or does it stay the same?"
- "Have you had this type of pain before? If so, how is this pain different, or is it exactly the same?" (**FIGURE 17-1**)

Timing

Timing refers to the duration of the pain or discomfort. Questions to ask to clarify the duration of the patient's pain or discomfort include the following:

- "How long have you been feeling this way?"
- "Have you had this same type of pain before, and if so, how long did it last?"
- "When did the pain or discomfort start?"
- "How long did the pain or discomfort last?"
- "When did the pain or discomfort end?"

Past Medical History

An important element of history taking is obtaining the patient's **past medical history**. This step can occur after the paramedic gains a good grasp of the

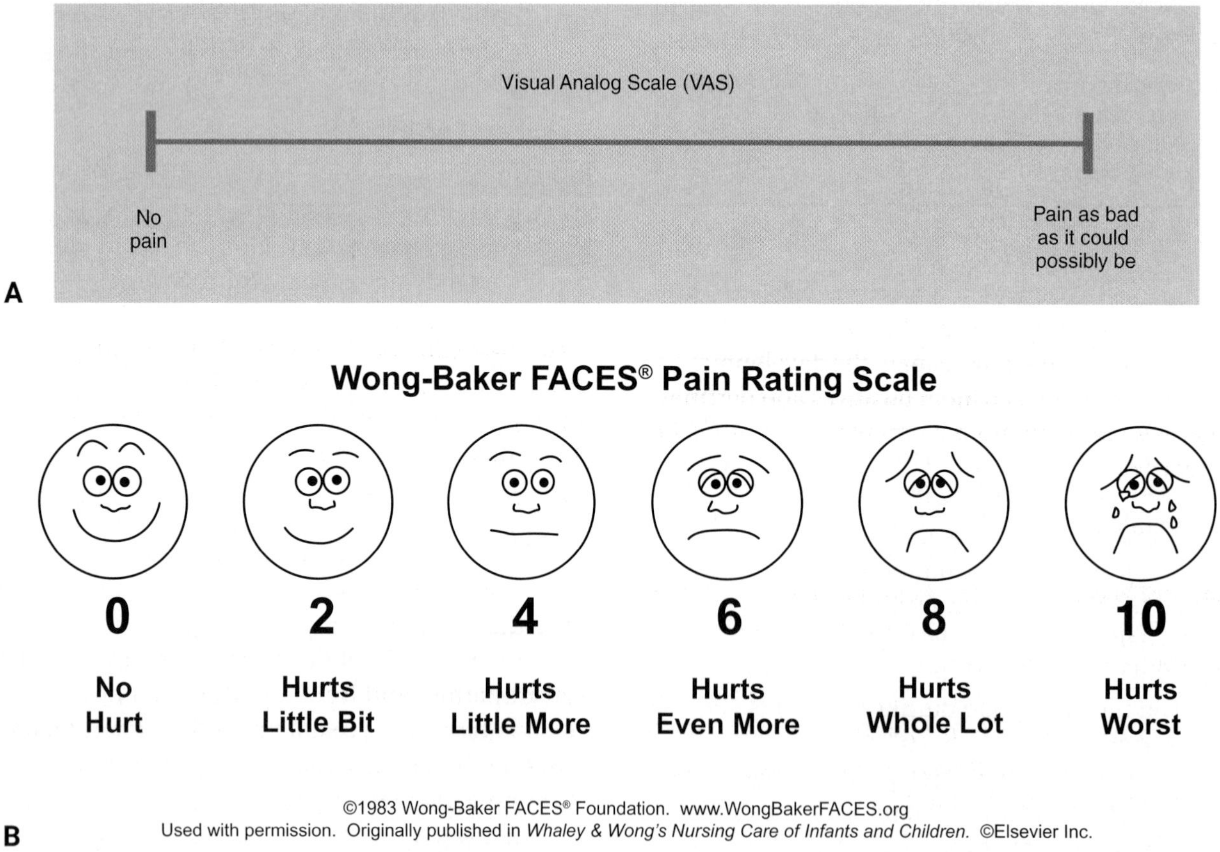

FIGURE 17-1 A. Visual analog pain scale. **B.** Wong-Baker FACES pain rating scale, originally developed for children and patients with language barriers.

A: © Jones & Bartlett Learning; **B:** Wong-Baker FACES Foundation (2018). Wong-Baker FACES® Pain Rating Scale. with permission from http://www.WongBakerFACES.org.

BOX 17-4 Elements of the SAMPLE Survey

Signs and symptoms
Allergies
Medications
Pertinent past medical history
Last oral intake
Events leading up to the illness or injury

patient's chief complaint. The past medical history may include, for example, diabetes, cardiac disorders, or respiratory disorders. This history may add insight into the patient's current state. Important past medical history information may include the following:

- General state of health
- Medications
- Allergies and nature of allergic reactions
- Childhood illnesses
- Adult illnesses
- Psychiatric illnesses
- Previous injuries
- Physical disability attributable to previous illness or injury
- Surgeries
- Hospitalizations

A variety of memory devices are used to recall key questions for gathering medical history. One example is the SAMPLE survey (BOX 17-4). Regardless of the patient's past medical history, these important, direct questions should be asked of every patient, as the answers can be significant in the development of a field impression. Pertinent positives and pertinent negatives can help build a complete picture of the patient's medical history.

Current Health Status

A **current health status** focuses on a patient's current state of health. It also considers personal habits and environmental conditions (BOX 17-5). Details regarding allergies, medications, last oral intake, and family history can be crucial to the patient's current health status. Female patients with abdominal pain should be questioned about their last menstrual period (if of childbearing age). All patients with abdominal pain should be asked about their last bowel movement. Finally, the paramedic should identify events that occurred before the emergency.

BOX 17-5 Personal Habits and Environmental Conditions

Personal Habits

Tobacco use
Use of alcohol, other drugs, and related substances
Diet
Screening tests
Immunizations
Sleep patterns
Exercise and leisure activities
Use of safety measures
Home situation, spouse, or significant other
Physical abuse or violence
Sexual history
Daily life
Important experiences
Religious beliefs
Patient outlook

Environmental Conditions

Home conditions: housing, cleanliness, temperature, economic circumstances, pets and their health
Occupation: description of past and current work; exposure to heat, cold, and industrial toxins; similar complaints of illness among coworkers
Travel: exposure to contagious diseases, residence in tropics, water and milk supply, other possible sources of infection
Military record: geographic areas, exposure to chemicals

Medications

The paramedic should ask whether the patient takes any medications on a regular basis and, if so, for what reasons. Often patients do not know why they are taking some medicines. Paramedics must be familiar with common medications to help narrow the differential diagnosis. Many print and online references can be used for this purpose. In addition to information about prescribed medicines, information about the use of over-the-counter medicines is important. Likewise, the paramedic should ask about the use of herbs, naturopathic, and homeopathic medicines. This line of questioning should include the reason and frequency of use. If possible, the paramedic should determine whether the patient takes the medications as prescribed and when the last dose was taken.

The medication history may offer clues to the chief complaint. For example, a patient with diabetes may have taken insulin but may have eaten at odd

DID YOU KNOW?

Family and Social History

A family history can give clues to possible predisposition to medical illness. Certain diseases and health conditions tend to run in families, including heart disease, cancer, hypertension, and stroke. Family history can also provide insight into why a patient or family member may be anxious about the possibility of contracting a particular disease. For example, a man with a sister and aunt in whom schizophrenia developed in their late 20s might be overly concerned that his son's irrational behavior is a sign of the same disease. When obtaining a medical history of family members or blood relatives, the paramedic should ask about family members' health and ages and the causes of death for parents, siblings, spouse, and children.

A patient's social history can also shed light on aspects of a patient's life that may be affected by or connected to illness risk factors. The following topics may be appropriate to explore as part of history taking:

- Family (marriage, children)
- Dynamics in the home
- Dynamics in the workplace
- Financial circumstances
- Activities (work and leisure)

Other elements of a social history that may affect risk factors for illness include smoking, drinking, and drug use (past or current); sexual habits; current and previous occupation(s); and any recent travel abroad. Family pets and exposure to animals or birds can be important as well and should be part of the patient's social history.

NOTE

Many people have a life-threatening allergy to latex. Latex is a common substance found in EMS care equipment.

intervals. Other examples in which the medication history may inform the differential diagnosis include a patient with chest pain who takes various cardiac drugs, an irrational patient who takes prescribed sedatives, and a trauma patient who takes blood-thinning drugs.

In some cases it is helpful to examine the prescription fill date to determine whether the patient has been taking the medications as prescribed. Older adults with dementia may neglect to take medications or take them more often than prescribed.

The patient's medications, or a list of medications, should be transported to the hospital with the patient. This permits the emergency department staff to more fully evaluate the medications and compliance with medication instructions. The medication handoff to hospital staff should be documented thoroughly.

CRITICAL THINKING

What would you do if you could not recognize the names or indications for the patient's home medicines?

The patient's medication history may not always be relevant to the problem at hand. At other times, the history can point to potential problems that may be seen during the patient care episode. In addition, it is wise to directly ask a patient if he or she has taken specific drugs if they may potentially interact with the proposed care. For example, before giving nitroglycerin, the paramedic should ask a male patient if he has taken any drugs for erectile dysfunction such as tadalafil (Cialis), vardenafil (Levitra), or sildenafil (Viagra). Administration of nitroglycerin to patients who have recently taken these drugs can cause life-threatening hypotension.

NOTE

Paramedics should also question patients about alcohol use and illicit drug use. A direct line of questions is best. For example, the paramedic might say, "Mr. Jones, it is policy to ask all patients these questions, so please don't be offended. Have you used alcohol today? Have you taken any tablets or inhaled any drugs today that were not prescribed for you? Have you injected any drugs?"

Last Oral Intake

The time of the last meal or fluid intake is important when considering potential airway problems in a patient who loses consciousness or whose condition begins to deteriorate. Determining the patient's last oral intake also may help rule out some problems such as food poisoning and food allergies. For example, symptoms of certain types of food poisoning do not usually appear for several hours. In contrast, in patients who are sensitive to certain foods, for example, peanut oil and shellfish, an allergic reaction would develop immediately after eating or otherwise coming in contact with these foods. Oral intake can also point to some illnesses. For example, a patient with undiagnosed or uncontrolled diabetes may report excessive hunger or thirst. Some older adults may have inadequate food intake related to inability to procure or prepare food, leading to a state of malnutrition that leaves them more vulnerable to multiple health conditions.

> NOTE
>
> The time of the patient's last oral intake may be important and may help to determine the appropriateness of surgery or ED procedures that require sedation. Generally, if a patient has consumed any food or drink within the previous 6 to 8 hours, surgery is delayed if possible. Clear liquids, however, can be consumed closer to the time of surgery, so ask the patient when and what he or she ate. The delay is intended to prevent the patient from aspirating the stomach contents, especially during the induction of anesthesia. If immediate surgery is indicated after recent oral intake, a nasogastric tube is generally inserted to evacuate the patient's stomach before the surgical procedure begins.

Family History

A **family history** of illness or disease may be relevant to the chief complaint. The paramedic should establish whether the patient has a family history of heart disease, high blood pressure, cancer, tuberculosis, stroke, diabetes, kidney disease, current contagious illness, or other ailments. The paramedic also should note the presence or absence of hereditary diseases—for example, hemophilia or sickle cell anemia—during the interview. Through experience, the paramedic will develop a "personal" line of questioning to further analyze a patient's particular symptoms.

Last Menstrual Period

The paramedic should obtain a menstrual history when interviewing female patients between the ages of 12 and 55 years who have abdominal pain. The paramedic should ask the patient when her last period was and if it was normal for her. This questioning may prompt the patient to discuss other significant symptoms, such as vaginal discharge, bleeding, and pregnancy history. The patient's response determines the need to pursue additional questions regarding contraceptive use, venereal disease, urinary tract infections, and ectopic pregnancy (see Chapter 30, *Gynecology*).

Last Bowel Movement

The paramedic should ask a patient about his or her bowel habits to determine whether they have been normal or abnormal. A patient with abdominal pain may describe a recent history of diarrhea, constipation, or bloody bowel movements. This information will be helpful to the receiving physician when assessing the patient for bowel obstruction, dehydration, or lower gastrointestinal bleeding. As part of this line of questioning, the paramedic also should ask the patient about any symptoms of abnormal urinary function. These symptoms may include blood in the urine, urethral discharge, pain or burning with urination, frequent urination, or the inability to void (see Chapter 29, *Genitourinary and Renal Disorders*).

Events Before the Emergency

The paramedic should ask the patient and bystanders about events or actions that occurred before the emergency. For example, was a fainting episode preceded by exertion or straining? Did a loss of consciousness occur before or after a fall? The paramedic should attempt to correlate any event with the progression of an illness or injury.

Getting More Information

With experience, paramedics learn to communicate with more skill and to obtain a more complete picture of a patient's illness or injury. By honing their interview skills, they become able to obtain more information about a symptom or complaint. In addition, they become more adept at using clinical reasoning to evaluate associated problems and possible effects on body systems. Defining the attributes of a symptom may require the paramedic to ask direct questions and to address sensitive topics, such as alcohol or other drug use, physical abuse or violence, and sexual issues. When questioning a patient about sensitive issues, the paramedic should follow these guidelines:

1. Remember that privacy is essential with all patients, regardless of age or sex.
2. Be direct and firm, and do not apologize for asking a question.
3. Avoid confrontation.
4. Be nonjudgmental.
5. Use language that is easily understood but not patronizing.
6. Encourage the patient to ask any relevant questions.
7. Document carefully and use the patient's words (noted by quotation marks) when possible.

Clinical Reasoning

The depth and focus of the patient interview depend on the specifics of the case at hand. In every situation, however, the paramedic should gather as much information as possible at the scene and during transport to the hospital. Questions to the patient should be selected based on the patient's chief complaint and current problem. The paramedic then uses the answers to think about possible associated problems and body system changes related to the patient's complaint—a process known as **clinical reasoning**. By comparison, **clinical decision making** is a contextual, continuous, and evolving process, in which data are gathered, interpreted, and evaluated so as to select an evidence-based choice of action—that is, to make a decision about care.[2]

Clinical reasoning requires integrating the patient's history with the physical assessment findings. It also requires knowledge of anatomy, physiology, and pathophysiology to direct appropriate questions to the patient. The answers to the questions are analyzed by the paramedic as they are received. As such, the paramedic must be prepared to change the direction of questioning based on careful evaluation of the answers.

The Process of Clinical Reasoning

Clinical reasoning should begin with the broad range of systems that could contribute to the patient's complaint. The paramedic then identifies the patient's current symptoms, past medical history, and abnormal symptoms and physical findings, which are subsequently analyzed by anatomic location. During the process of clinical reasoning, the paramedic must consider all systems found in that location that may cause or contribute to the patient's problem and must interpret the patient-specific findings in terms of a pathologic process (**TABLE 17-1**).

Forming a Differential Diagnosis

During clinical reasoning, the possible body systems involved must be narrowed down or ruled out (**FIGURE 17-2**). Doing so allows the paramedic to develop a working hypothesis of the nature of the problem—that is, the **differential diagnosis**. In this process, the paramedic weighs the probability of one disease versus that of other diseases that might potentially account for the patient's illness. The differential diagnosis is then tested with questions and assessments relating to systems with similar types of signs and symptoms. Finally, the competing possibilities are considered and the paramedic selects the most likely problem to treat (**FIGURE 17-3**). Careful attention must be paid to the signs and symptoms that do not fit with the working diagnosis.

NOTE

Before completing the patient history, the paramedic should ask every patient these three questions:

- Is there anything else you would like to tell me that I haven't asked you about?
- Is there anything you are worried about that we have not discussed?
- Do you have any questions for me?

Special Challenges

History taking often presents special challenges. Each patient is unique, so each patient encounter is slightly different from all others. The paramedic must be able to adapt quickly to the special requirements of each encounter and obtain the needed information quickly. Some challenges that commonly affect history taking are discussed in this section.

Silence

Silence is often uncomfortable and has many meanings and uses. For example, patients may use silence to collect thoughts, recall details, or decide whether they trust the paramedic. Silence also can defuse an emotionally tense event effectively. The paramedic should stay alert for nonverbal clues of distress or anxiety such as a worried expression or loss of eye contact, which often precede a silent period during the patient encounter. As a rule, when patients are ready to talk again, they will express feelings more clearly.

A patient's silence also may result from a paramedic's lack of sensitivity, understanding, or compassion. To avoid this type of patient withdrawal during the encounter, the paramedic should incorporate an appropriate, caring "bedside manner" as part of good patient care.

Overly Talkative Patients

Interviewing talkative patients can be frustrating when the paramedic has only limited time to obtain a health history. Although there are no perfect solutions in these situations, the following techniques may be helpful:

TABLE 17-1 Assessment by Body Systems

General symptoms	Fever, chills, malaise, fatigue, night sweats, weight changes
Skin, hair, and nails	Rashes, itching, swelling
Musculoskeletal	Joint pain, loss of motion, swelling, redness, warmth, deformity
Head and neck	
General	Headache, loss of consciousness
Eyes	Visual acuity, blurred vision, diplopia, photophobia, pain, vision changes, flashes of light (photopsia)
Ears	Hearing loss, pain, discharge, tinnitus, vertigo
Nose	Sense of smell, rhinorrhea, obstruction, epistaxis, postnasal discharge, sinus pain
Throat and mouth	Sore throat, bleeding, pain, dental issues, ulcers, changes in taste
Endocrine system	Thyroid enlargement, temperature intolerance, skin changes, swelling of hands and feet, weight changes, polyuria, polydipsia, polyphagia, changes in body and facial hair
Reproductive system	
Male	Erectile dysfunction, penile discharge, testicular pain
Female	Menstrual regularity, last menstrual period, dysmenorrhea, vaginal discharge, bleeding, pregnancy, contraception use
Chest and lungs	Dyspnea, cough (productivity/description), wheezing, hemoptysis, tuberculosis status
Heart and blood vessels	Chest pain (onset, duration, quality, provocation, palliation), palpations, orthopnea, edema, past cardiac evaluation and tests
Hematologic system	Anemia, bruising, fatigue
Lymphatic system	Enlarged or tender lymph nodes
Gastrointestinal system	Appetite, digestion, food allergies or intolerance, heartburn, nausea, vomiting (frequency, color, texture, contents), diarrhea, hematemesis, bowel regularity, stool changes (frequency, color, texture, odor), flatulence, jaundice, past gastrointestinal evaluation and tests
Genitourinary system	Dysuria, pain (flank, suprapubic), frequency, urgency, nocturia, hematuria, polyuria, sexually transmitted infections
Neurologic system	Seizures, syncope, loss of sensation, weakness, paralysis, loss of coordination or memory, twitches, tremors
Behavioral or psychiatric disorders	Depression, mood changes, difficulty concentrating, anxiety, suicidal or homicidal ideation, irritability, sleep disturbances, fatigue on waking

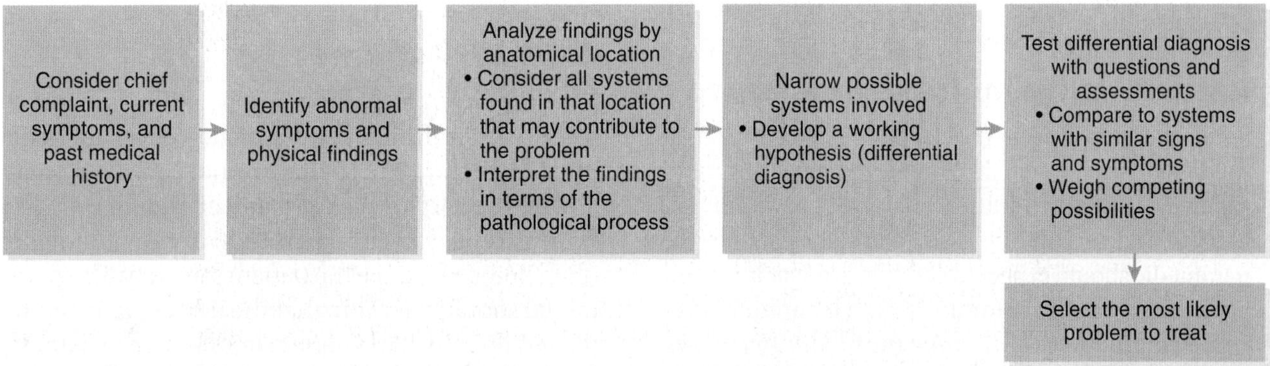

FIGURE 17-2 Review of body systems.

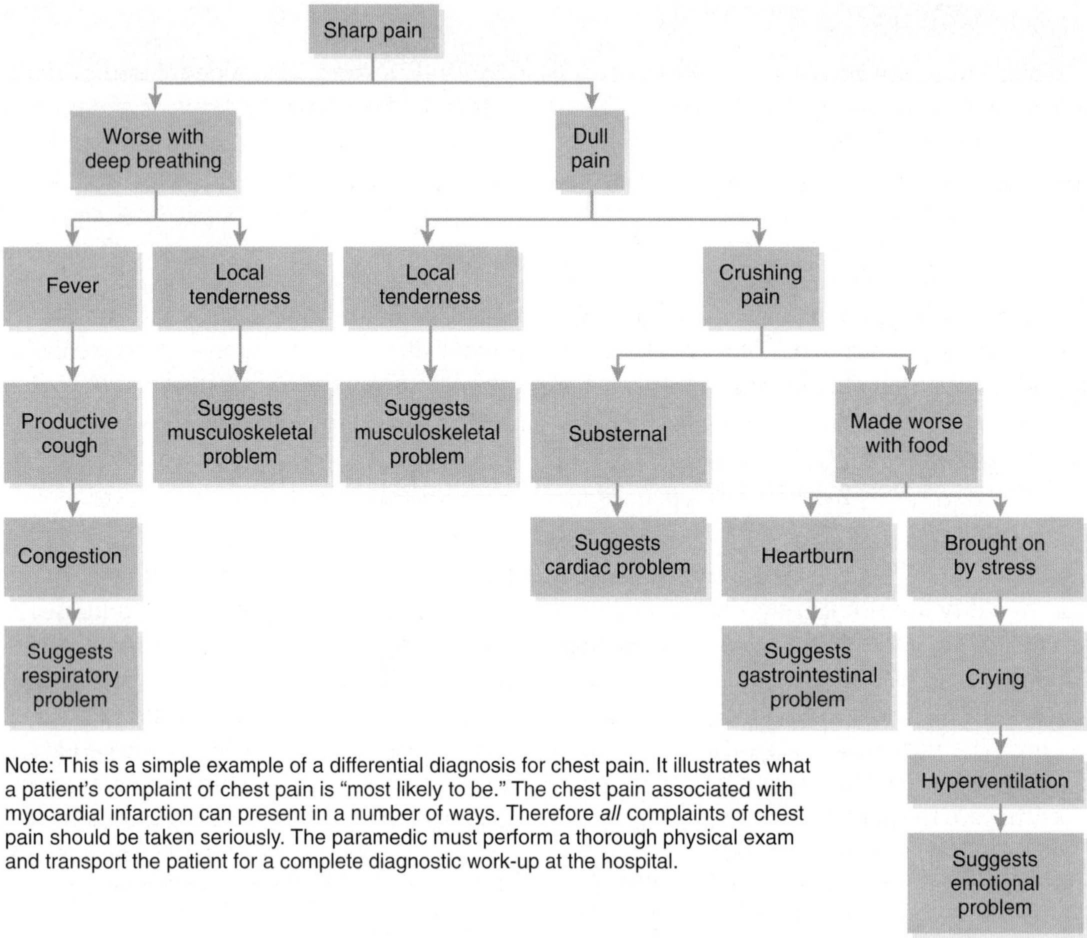

FIGURE 17-3 Differential diagnosis sample—chest pain.

- Accept a less comprehensive history.
- Let the patient speak freely for the first several minutes.
- Ask questions that invite brief "yes" or "no" answers when appropriate.
- Summarize the patient's comments frequently.
- Refocus the discussion as needed.

Patients With Multiple Symptoms

Some patients (especially older patients) have a longer medical history because of age, chronic illness, and medication use. In addition, many older patients are likely to have multiple illnesses. With such patients, the paramedic should expect to conduct a longer interview and should use the communication techniques presented in Chapter 16, *Therapeutic Communications*. These techniques will help patients with multiple symptoms focus on the most relevant aspects of the chief complaint.

CRITICAL THINKING

Often patients identify multiple problems during history taking. As a paramedic, you have to identify the chief complaint. Which single question would you ask?

Anxious Patients

It is normal for the patient, family, and bystanders to be anxious in an emergency situation. The paramedic must be sensitive to the nonverbal clues of anxiety and be supportive in a calm and confident way. The professional and caring attitude of the paramedic often helps to reduce the patient's anxiety. The paramedic should be aware that the anxiety may not be related directly to the illness or injury. For example, an older patient on a fixed income may worry about the cost of a hospital stay, and a victim of a car crash may worry about liability and losing car insurance.

False Reassurance

The paramedic may be tempted to provide false reassurance in certain cases—to say "It's all right" or "Everything's going to be okay." Although these statements may comfort an ill or injured patient, they should be avoided. False reassurance or over-reassurance may block open dialogue between the paramedic and the patient. The paramedic should reassure the patient that the patient's medical condition is understood and that good patient care is available. Patients also will be comforted to know that the outcome is hopeful (if appropriate) and that they will be treated with dignity and respect during their care. These verbal reassurances generally work well in most patient care situations.

Anger and Hostility

Anger and hostility are not too far removed from anxious behavior, in that they are natural responses in some emergency situations. The paramedic should expect these reactions at times to be displaced toward the EMS crew. The paramedic must always ensure personal and scene safety. However, displaying anger and hostility toward the patient is never appropriate. A much more effective approach includes maintaining a calm, confident manner and setting limits on acceptable behavior. Acknowledge the patient's emotion and reassure the patient you are there to help resolve the problem. Maintain a normal vocal tone and volume to avoid escalating the situation.

Intoxication

Patients who are intoxicated with alcohol or other drugs should be managed with caution. Their behavior may be difficult to predict. Intoxicated patients should not be challenged or aggravated. Similar to managing patients who are angry or hostile, the paramedic must ensure scene safety and set limits on acceptable behavior. If the scene is not secure, the paramedic should call for assistance from law enforcement personnel.

Crying

Crying can reduce tension and may help reestablish the patient's emotional stability during an emergency. If the patient's crying is excessive or uncontrollable, the paramedic should wait for the patient to calm down. Direct eye contact with the patient will demonstrate compassion and help control the patient's crying. Reducing exhaustive crying conserves energy and promotes comfort.

Depression

Communicating with a depressed patient can be difficult. Many types and causes of depression exist (see Chapter 34, *Behavioral and Psychiatric Disorders*), but the depression seen in an emergency often is due to moderate to high anxiety. Depression also may be enhanced by alcohol or substance use. The paramedic should use the communication techniques described previously when taking the history for anxious patients. If possible, the paramedic should identify the seriousness of the patient's depression and encourage evaluation by a physician.

Sexually Attractive or Seductive Patients

Sometimes paramedics and patients may be sexually attracted to each other. The paramedic should accept these feelings as normal but ensure that they do not affect his or her behavior. If a patient becomes seductive or makes sexual advances, the paramedic should firmly set limits of what is acceptable, making it clear that the relationship is a professional one. As discussed in Chapter 16, *Therapeutic Communications*, providing same-sex care often is the best practice. If this is not possible, an extra caregiver (or a chaperone) should stay with the patient.

Confusing Behavior or Histories

Emergency situations are often intense, and emotions can run high. In this setting, the paramedic should expect to encounter confusing histories and inappropriate or abnormal behavior. Factors that may contribute to these sometimes chaotic situations include mental illness, delirium, dementia, drug use, illness, and injury. Though it may be challenging, the paramedic should try to identify a pattern of patient behavior (eg, signs and symptoms consistent with a certain disorder). In addition, the paramedic should attempt to lead the patient in an appropriate line of questioning.

It is also important to avoid bias in these situations: It is all too easy to attribute a patient's behavior to intoxication or mental illness without considering other treatable and emergent conditions. Rule out life threats such as hypoxia, hypoglycemia, or head injury.

Developmental Disabilities

The paramedic should not overlook the ability of patients with intellectual disabilities to provide adequate information. Patients with developmental disabilities should be interviewed just like other patients, using easily understood words and phrases. An obvious omission in such a patient's answers reveals the need for more questioning, and perhaps questions that need to be stated more clearly. If the patient has severe intellectual impairment, the paramedic should try to obtain information from family or friends (see Chapter 50, *Patients With Special Challenges*).

Communication Barriers

As discussed in Chapter 16, *Therapeutic Communications*, barriers to communication may result from social or cultural differences. These barriers also may arise because of sight, speech, or hearing impairments. The paramedic should seek assistance in ensuring adequacy of communication during history taking with such patients if possible. Family members, translators, and people with special training in communicating with the blind or the deaf may be helpful in these situations.

Talking With Family and Friends

Friends and family are often present at the scene of an emergency. The paramedic should consider them a good source of information, especially when the patient cannot provide all of the necessary information because of illness or injury. Sometimes family or friends are unavailable and more patient information is needed. In these cases, the paramedic should try to locate a third party (eg, a neighbor) who can help supply the missing details.

Summary

- Obtaining a patient history offers structure to the patient assessment. The history often identifies life threats and sets priorities in patient care.
- Content of the patient history includes the onset and duration of signs and symptoms, identifying data, source of referral, history, reliability, chief complaint, present illness, past medical history, current health status, and review of body systems.
- The paramedic should ensure patient comfort by not entering the patient's personal space unless necessary, being sensitive to the patient's feelings, and watching for signs of uneasiness.
- During the history taking, the paramedic should use appropriate language and ask open-ended and direct questions. The paramedic should use therapeutic communication techniques as well.
- Clinical reasoning requires integrating the patient's history with the physical assessment findings. It also requires knowledge of anatomy, physiology, and pathophysiology to direct appropriate questions to the patient.
- Differential diagnosis is the process of weighing the probability of one condition versus others as accounting for a patient's illness.
- Many challenges can affect history taking, including silent or talkative patients, patients with multiple symptoms, and anxious, angry, or hostile patients. The paramedic also may encounter intoxication, crying, depression, and sexually attractive or seductive patients.
- Paramedics should avoid providing false reassurance and should recognize that confusing behaviors and histories are not unusual in emergency situations.
- Two other issues that can affect history taking are developmental disabilities and communication barriers. In such cases, talking with family and friends can help clarify the patient's chief complaint and history.

References

1. National Highway Traffic Safety Administration. *The National EMS Education Standards*. Washington, DC: US Department of Transportation/National Highway Traffic Safety Administration; 2009.
2. Faucher C. Differentiating the elements of clinical thinking. *Optometric Educ.* 2011;36(3):140-145. http://journal.opted.org/articles/Volume_36_Number_3_CriticalThinking.pdf. Accessed January 29, 2018.

Suggested Readings

Ball JW, Dains JE, Flynn JA, Solomon BS, Stewart RW. *Seidel's Guide to Physical Examination*. 8th ed. St. Louis, MO: Mosby; 2015.

Lord B. The assessment of pain in paramedic practice. *EMS Reference*. https://www.emsreference.com/articles/article/assessment-pain-paramedic-practice-0. Published November 2015. Accessed January 29, 2018.

Page D, Rosenberger P. On-scene EMS access to past medical history may improve care. *J Emerg Med Serv*. http://www.jems.com/articles/print/volume-41/issue-5/departments-columns/research-review/on-scene-ems-access-to-past-medical-history.html. Published March 30, 2016. Accessed December 20, 2017.

Potter PA, Perry AG, Hall A. *Fundamentals of Nursing*. 8th ed. St. Louis, MO: Elsevier Mosby; 2015.

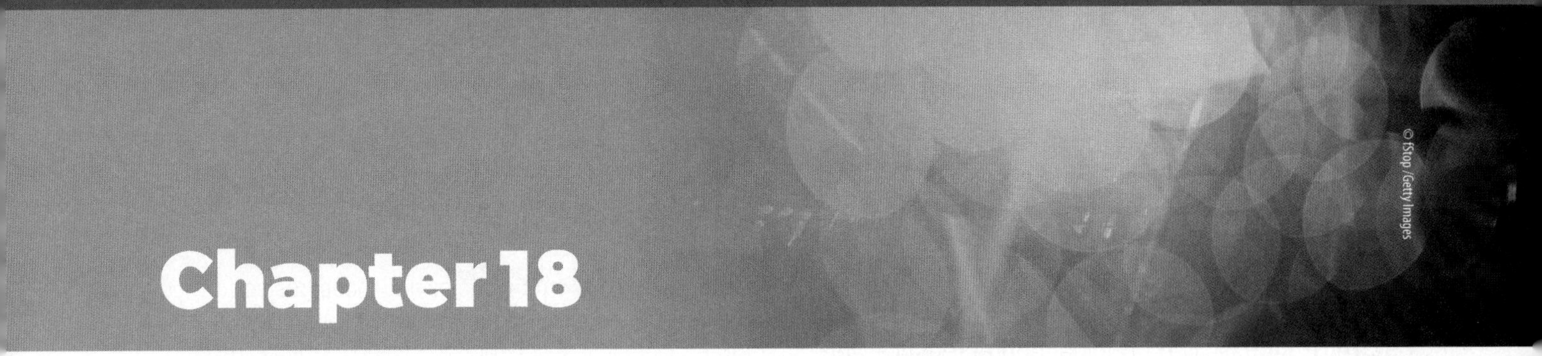

Chapter 18

Scene Size-up and Primary Assessment

NATIONAL EMS EDUCATION STANDARD COMPETENCIES

Assessment

Integrate scene and patient assessment findings with your knowledge of epidemiology and pathophysiology to form a field impression. Use clinical reasoning to develop a list of differential diagnoses, modify the assessment, and formulate a treatment plan.

Scene Size-up

Scene safety (pp 613–616)
Scene management (p 616)

- Impact of the environment on patient care (p 617)
- Addressing hazards (pp 617–618)
- Violence (pp 614–615)
- Need for additional or specialized resources (p 613)
- Standard precautions (pp 618–619)
- Multiple patient situations (p 619)

Primary Assessment

Primary assessment for all patient situations (pp 621–626)

- Initial general impression (pp 621–622)
- Level of consciousness (pp 622–623)
- ABCs (pp 623–625)
- Identifying life threats (p 626)
- Assessment of vital functions (p 626)

Begin interventions needed to preserve life (pp 623–624, 626)
Integration of treatment/procedures needed to preserve life (p 626)

OBJECTIVES

Upon completion of this chapter, the paramedic student will be able to:

1. Describe the purpose of scene size-up. (pp 612–613)
2. Outline the components of scene size-up. (pp 612–613)
3. Recognize factors that may contribute to an unsafe scene. (pp 613–616)
4. Describe scene evaluation techniques. (p 616)
5. Identify steps in scene management. (p 616)
6. Outline measures to lower the risks associated with illness or injury at an unsafe scene. (pp 617–619)
7. Identify additional resources that may be needed to manage multiple-patient incidents. (p 619)
8. Identify the priorities in each component of the patient assessment. (pp 619–626)
9. Outline the critical components of the primary assessment. (pp 619–620)
10. Describe findings in the primary survey that may indicate a life-threatening condition. (pp 622–625)
11. Discuss interventions for life-threatening conditions that are identified in the primary survey. (pp 622–626)
12. Distinguish priorities in the care of the medical versus trauma patient. (p 626)

Note: The terms *primary assessment* and *primary survey* are sometimes used interchangeably. This text uses primary assessment to refer to the combination of scene size-up and the initial patient evaluation, with the primary survey of the patient being a critical component. Both terms refer to the initial evaluation of a patient encounter to establish scene safety and to recognize and manage life-threatening conditions.

KEY TERMS

general impression An immediate assessment of the environment and the patient's chief complaint used to determine whether the patient is ill or injured and the nature of illness or the mechanism of injury.

mechanism of injury The nature of the force exerted on the body that produced physical injury.

nature of illness The principal characteristics and causes of an illness.

personal protective equipment (PPE) Clothing or specialized equipment that provides some protection to the wearer from environmental or infectious hazards.

primary assessment The combination of scene size-up and the initial patient evaluation used to establish scene safety and to recognize and manage life-threatening conditions.

primary survey A critical component of the primary assessment that focuses on the initial evaluation of a patient to recognize and manage life-threatening conditions.

priority patients Patients who need immediate care and transport.

resuscitative measures Life-saving measures performed immediately, such as airway control, ventilatory assistance, control of severe bleeding, and cardiopulmonary resuscitation.

safe staging area An area away from the emergency scene that provides for safety.

scene size-up An assessment of the scene to promote scene safety for the paramedic crew, patient(s), and bystanders; includes determination of additional resources that may be needed to manage the scene adequately.

situational awareness A state of constant vigilance for changes in the scene or in the patient.

The prehospital environment is a place of uncertainty and is subject to many potential hazards. Therefore, the assessment of both the scene and the patient, and all of the information the assessment conveys, is critical to personal safety and appropriate patient care.

Scene Size-up

Scene size-up refers to a quick assessment of an emergency scene. Scene size-up and personal safety must be the initial priority for every emergency medical services (EMS) response. These steps begin with information about the patient and scene provided by dispatch. This information helps to ensure scene safety for the paramedic crew and other response agencies, patients, and bystanders. It also allows the paramedic to mentally prepare for the patient's potential medical needs and decide on the required resources needed to best manage the patient and the scene. The goals of scene size-up are to quickly gather facts about the situation, analyze problems and potential problems, and determine the appropriate response. Scene size-up is a continuous evaluation of the scene with a focus on maintaining **situational awareness** for changing conditions.

> NOTE
> Scene size-up continues until the incident has been successfully managed and completed.

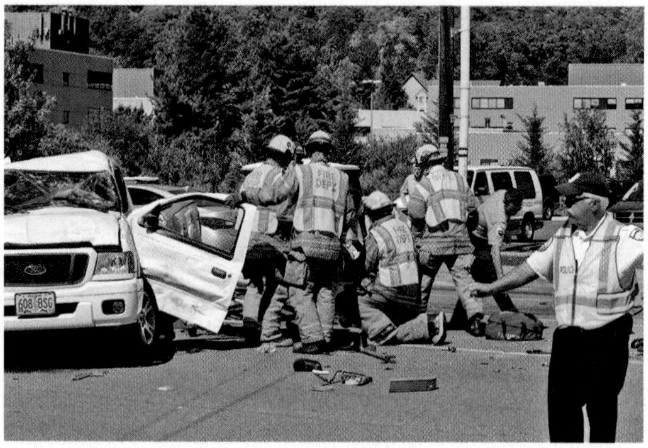

When a call is received for an emergency response, the dispatcher should provide as much pertinent information as possible. Information from the dispatch center that helps in scene size-up includes the following:[1]

- Exact location
- Type of location (eg, industrial, highway, residence)
- Number of patients

- Type of situation (eg, difficulty breathing, vehicle crash, domestic violence, assault)
- Known or potential hazards on the scene (eg, scene not secure, possible toxic exposure)
- Prearrival instructions given (hemorrhage control, cardiopulmonary resuscitation [CPR], exiting building)
- Unique issues (eg, key boxes, known medical or access problems)

Obtaining this information and regular updates from the dispatch center will help the paramedic determine the need for additional resources, either before arrival or after assessing the scene and the patient. These resources may include a supervisor, additional ambulances, fire-rescue services, mutual aid, utility services (eg, electrical power lines and gas lines), law enforcement, air medical services, and hazardous materials teams (BOX 18-1). These resources may be required to render the scene safe for entry, to stabilize a potential hazard on scene, or to ensure that patients receive the needed level of care for their injury or illness.

BOX 18-1 Resources That May Be Needed to Manage a Scene

Special equipment for extrication and fire suppression
Additional medical supplies and equipment
Aeromedical transport
EMS physician scene response
Specialized rescue teams
Hazardous materials decontamination
Traffic and crowd control
Utility services
Animal control
Additional lighting
Hospital and/or emergency department (ED) bed availability
Coroner
Public health resources

CRITICAL THINKING

What type of information might you obtain from dispatch that would make you concerned that a hazardous materials incident exists?

Scene Safety

Many factors can affect scene safety in an emergency response. Examples include environmental hazards, the presence of hazardous substances, violence, and rescue-related hazards (BOX 18-2) (see section on EMS Operations).

BOX 18-2 Possible Hazards at an Emergency Scene

Environmental hazards
- Inclement weather
- Extremes in temperatures
- Slick or icy conditions
- Poor or inadequate lighting

Hazardous substances
- Chemical
- Biologic
- Nuclear
- Explosive

Violence
- Patient
- Bystanders
- Animals
- Crime scenes

Rescue-related hazards
- Extrication
- Road operation dangers
- Specialized rescue situations

Environmental Hazards

Dealing with the environment is a unique aspect of prehospital care (see Chapter 44, *Environmental Conditions*). Hot weather conditions can expose the patient to thermal injury. For example, a patient could sustain thermal burns from being placed on a spine board that is left uncovered on hot asphalt. Likewise, heat-related illness (hyperthermia) can quickly escalate if the EMS crew does not take immediate measures to remove the patient from the hot environment. All patients who are at risk for hyperthermia should be moved to a cooler environment to begin care.

Cold weather poses many challenges as well. An ill or injured patient is less able to regulate body temperature, allowing hypothermia to develop quickly. Infants and young children are particularly susceptible to this risk. Patients who are at risk for hypothermia should be immediately sheltered from the wind and moved to a warm environment. Wet clothing should be quickly removed, and the patient should be covered with warm, dry blankets. Warming measures may need to be initiated. Mortality is significantly increased in critical trauma patients who become hypothermic, which can occur even in temperate weather.[2] Paramedics need to initiate aggressive measures to prevent hypothermia, including administering warm intravenous fluids and limiting heat loss by covering the patient and warming the ambulance compartment.

Caring for patients in a thunderstorm can be dangerous to everyone on the scene. Patients should be quickly moved to a location that is protected from lightning and other storm hazards. The paramedic should assume that wires downed from high winds are charged and dangerous until trained personnel verify their safety.

Some environmental hazards warrant specialized rescue teams and additional resources. An example is water rescue of a patient who is in the water or has fallen through ice. Low light conditions can make patient assessment difficult and can easily contribute to personal injury. Portable light should be available to properly assess for hazards. Large rescue scenes should be properly lit by requesting additional resources.

Hazardous Substances

Chemical, biologic, radiologic, and explosive hazards may be encountered from industrial accidents or terrorist incidents. Paramedics should be alert to dispatch information that indicates the potential for any of these hazards. Reports of large numbers of patients with similar signs or symptoms should signal the potential for one of these incidents.

Assessment of a scene with a possible hazardous materials spill should be carefully planned. Scene assessment should begin at a distance using binoculars to look for indicators of hazardous materials. Indicators include identifying hazardous materials placards, container shape, and smoke or vapor clouds. In industrial settings, the material safety data sheet (MSDS) should be provided to responders. These data sheets supply pertinent information regarding toxicity, exposure risks, and decontamination. Hazardous materials scenes should not be entered until they have been secured and made safe by specialized teams, which may include law enforcement personnel, hazardous materials teams, or public health specialists. Specific information related to this type of response is presented in Chapter 56, *Hazardous Materials Awareness*, and Chapter 57, *Bioterrorism and Weapons of Mass Destruction*.

Violence

Many factors can contribute to a violent scene. An example is a domestic violence situation, which may not be immediately obvious, even after arrival on scene. Another example is verbal aggression toward the EMS crew out of concern for the safety and well-being of a loved one. Drugs or behavioral illness can also alter a patient's behavior and create a dangerous situation. When patients or others on the scene display aggressive or violent behavior, the EMS crew should safely retreat from the scene until it has been secured by law enforcement personnel. In addition, agencies should have a mechanism that allows crews to advise officials that they are in a potentially dangerous situation without using plain language (eg, a panic button on the radio or a specific code that is transmitted over the air).

Paramedics should be alert for the potential presence of weapons at any scene. Traditional weapons include knives and guns. Other objects within reach of the patient also can be used as a weapon. Examples include tools, kitchen appliances, and household chemicals. In some states, concealed weapons are legal. All patients should be asked if they are carrying anything that could injure the provider. This may be a knife, gun, other weapon, or hypodermic needles if drug use is suspected. Dangerous items should be safely removed and secured as dictated by department policy (**FIGURE 18-1**).

Dogs or other pets can be a hazard to rescuers, particularly if they perceive their owner may be harmed. If dangerous animals are unsecured, the patient or a family member should be asked to contain them. If that is not possible, local animal control specialists should be summoned (**FIGURE 18-2**).

When responding to a known violent crime scene, the EMS crew should remain at a safe distance. This staging position should be maintained until law enforcement personnel have secured the area. Many crime scenes are not completely safe, even when law enforcement personnel are present. The paramedic should stay alert for clues that a dangerous situation may ensue or escalate. They should also maintain

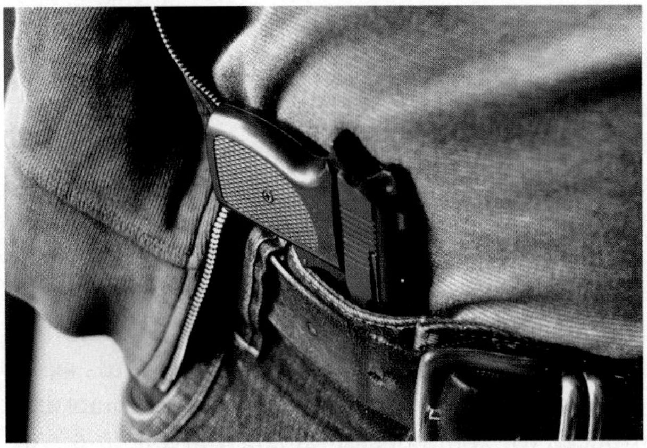

FIGURE 18-1 During your assessment, simply moving the jacket may reveal a concealed weapon.

NOTE

Paramedics should always keep in mind that a scene that appears safe can quickly become unsafe. All public service agencies play an important role in ensuring the safety of emergency response personnel. Each responder should maintain situational awareness throughout the call and share information as appropriate, either concurrently or following the incident. EMS and other responders are in a unique position to "see something, say something" about observations at the scene that may present as an immediate or potential future hazard to people at the scene or a larger population.

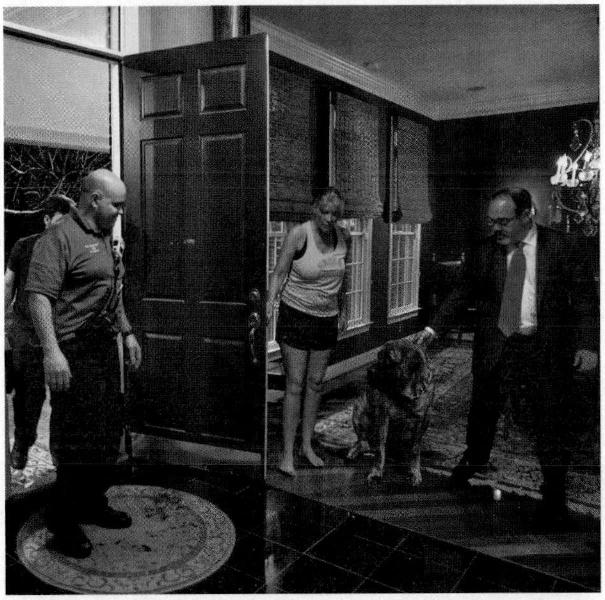

FIGURE 18-2 Paramedics preparing to enter a home with a large dog.

awareness of issues related to crime scenes and preserve evidence whenever possible (see Chapter 55, *Crime Scene Awareness*).

Rescue-Related Hazards

Scenes involving rescue can be dangerous. Common motor vehicle crash safety issues include close proximity of moving traffic, patient extrication activities, sharp metal, broken glass, unstable vehicles, and leaking fluids that increase the risk of fire. If it is safe to approach a patient in a vehicle involved in a crash, the paramedic should put the patient's vehicle in park, turn off the ignition, and secure the keys before beginning patient care. The extrication itself may create additional hazards related to the use of rescue cutting and spreading tools, a shifting vehicle, electric vehicle batteries, or the possibility that an air bag may suddenly deploy (see Chapter 54, *Rescue Awareness and Operations*). Paramedics should not remain in the vehicle during extrication unless properly trained and wearing appropriate protective equipment (**FIGURE 18-3**).

Each time a paramedic enters a roadway to provide care, there is a risk of being struck by moving traffic. Measures to reduce this risk should be taken on all roadway calls, regardless of the roadway speed limit. If the incident is on a busy roadway, emergency vehicles can be quickly positioned to provide protection for emergency personnel. The ambulance should be positioned in a safe location. Other emergency vehicles and response personnel should park their units in a manner that shields the ambulance and the involved vehicles from oncoming traffic. Providers should follow

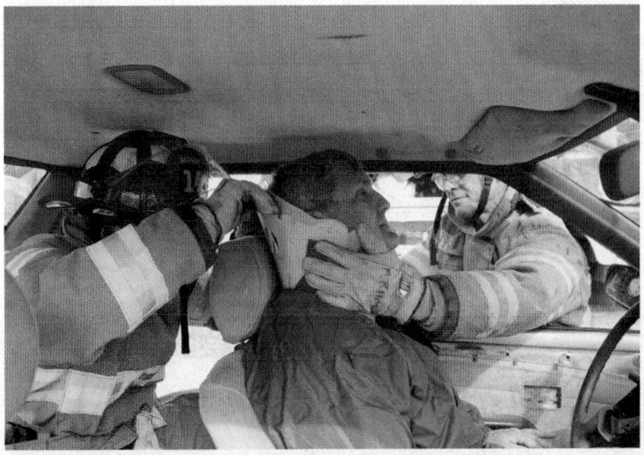

FIGURE 18-3 Paramedics should wear appropriate protective equipment during an extrication procedure.

departmental policies and wear appropriate American National Standards Institute (ANSI) Class 2 reflective vests (traffic vests) and other appropriate protective gear to improve rescuer visibility (**FIGURE 18-4**). When possible, a safety officer should be assigned to monitor the scene. Egress from the roadway should be made as quickly as possible. Safe roadway operations will be further addressed in Chapter 52, *Ground and Air Ambulance Operations*.

Specialized rescue requires advanced training and equipment. Examples include high- and low-angle rescue, trench rescue, confined space rescue, water rescue, and unstable structure rescue. Each specialized rescue event can pose a variety of unusual hazards. Paramedics who are not trained in these special rescue situations should not assist with the rescue or enter the scene until it has been made safe (**FIGURE 18-5**) (see Chapter 54, *Rescue Awareness and Operations*).

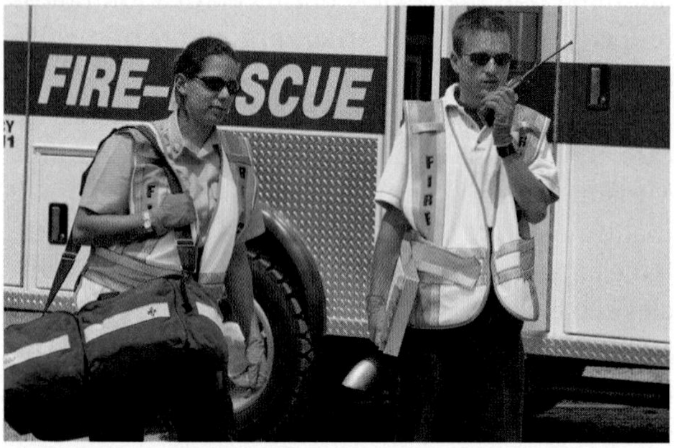

FIGURE 18-4 Reflective ANSI Class 2 vests.

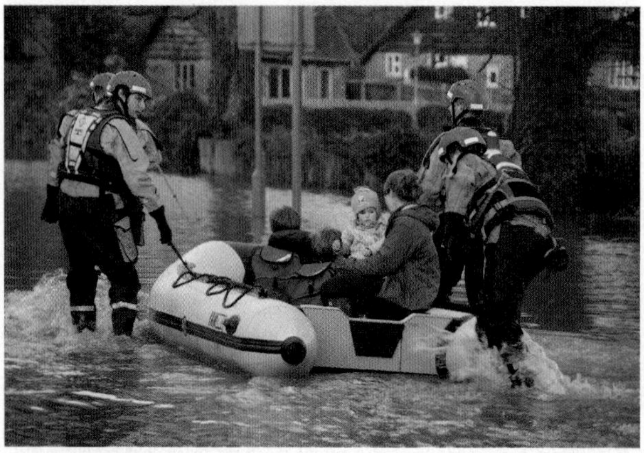

FIGURE 18-5 Water rescue.

Evaluation of the Scene

When evaluating the scene, the paramedic must always ask, "Is the scene safe?" If the scene is not safe and cannot be made reasonably safe, the scene should not be entered. Rather, the EMS crew should remain in a **safe staging area** and request additional resources to secure the scene. Only when the scene is secured should EMS personnel enter the area. When possible, it is best to enter the scene with another first responder.[3] If no obvious safety hazards exist, the paramedic should establish patient contact and proceed with patient assessment (**FIGURE 18-6**). Although there are situations where it may be possible to quickly improve scene safety, it must be stressed that making a scene safe to enter should be considered only when it can be done without accepting significant risk to the paramedic or the patient.

Scene Management

Successful and safe management of an emergency scene requires many considerations. Specific considerations to be discussed in this chapter relate to the following:

- Impact of the environment on patient care
- Scene hazards
- Violent scenes and crime scene preservation
- Need for additional/specialized resources
- Standard precautions
- Multiple patient situations

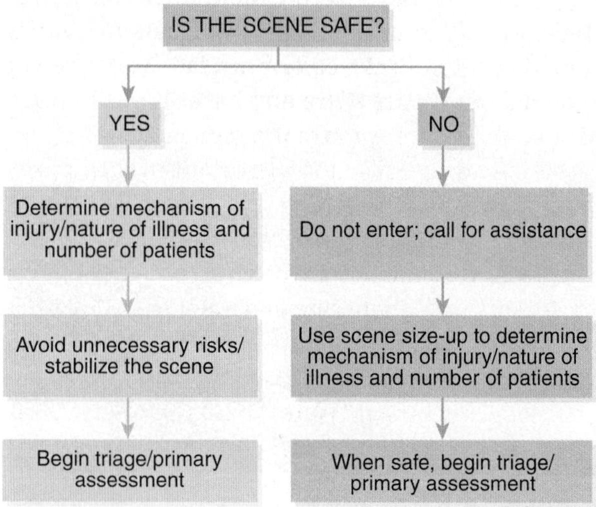

FIGURE 18-6 Scene safety algorithm.

SHOW ME THE EVIDENCE

From July 2010 to July 2014, The National Institute for Occupational Safety and Health, in collaboration with the National Highway Traffic Safety Administration, conducted a follow-up survey on EMS workers seen in EDs to compile a list of occupational injuries and exposures sustained among this population. The survey consisted of interviewing a sample of the 89,100 EMS workers treated in EDs over that period. Of those contacted, 572 workers (74%) completed the telephone interview. Sprains and strains accounted for more than 40% of the injuries. Body motion injuries were the most common event, with 90% related to lifting, carrying, or transferring a patient or equipment. This type of event was followed by exposure to harmful substances (with 21% related to needlestick injury). Most injuries (83%) occurred while on a call. Researchers estimate that motor vehicle incidents account for 8% of injuries and assaults or violence for 7% of other injuries reported.

Modified from: Reichard AA, Marsh SM, Tonozzi TR, Konda S, Gormley MA. Occupational injuries and exposures among emergency medical services workers. *Prehosp Emerg Care.* 2017;21(4):420-431.

Impact of the Environment on Patient Care

A quick visual survey of the scene should be made on every emergency call. For medical calls, the paramedic should first determine the **nature of illness**. This determination involves observing the patient's surroundings for possible clues to the nature of the emergency. For example, are there empty pill bottles or drug paraphernalia nearby? Is the patient wearing a medical alert necklace or bracelet? Are there any unusual odors? Are there any hazards at the scene that could suddenly make the scene unsafe?

For trauma calls, it is important to quickly determine the **mechanism of injury** (see Chapter 36, *Trauma Overview and Mechanism of Injury*). Visual clues can be significant in directing patient care and in anticipating patient care that may be needed while at the scene and during transport. For example, was a steering wheel, dashboard, or window damaged in a motor vehicle crash? Were the occupants in the car wearing personal restraints? Did the airbag deploy? Was the patient wearing a helmet in a motorcycle crash? What is the length of the knife that was used to stab the victim? Are there any hazards at the scene that could suddenly make the scene unsafe?

CRITICAL THINKING

Case Study

You respond to a residence for an "accidental injury." When you arrive, you find a tearful pregnant woman and her boyfriend. Her boyfriend says she fell down the stairs. The patient is quiet and appears fearful. You note bruising on her upper arms, face, and abdomen, and other injuries not consistent with a fall down the stairs.

How can you make this scene safer for both you and your patient?

Scene Hazards

As stated previously, all emergency scenes should be assessed for any pertinent environmental conditions or hazards. To ensure scene safety, any controllable hazard must be addressed. Environmental conditions and hazards that could affect patient care or the safety of patients, bystanders, or emergency personnel include the following:

- Weather or extreme temperatures
- Toxins and gases
- Secondary collapses and falls
- Unstable conditions
- Weapons

After making the scene safe for the paramedic, the safety of the patient becomes the next priority. The paramedic should attempt to correct any hazards that might threaten the health or safety of the patient. If a hazard cannot be alleviated, the patient should be moved to a safer environment. Likewise, any condition that poses a threat to bystanders should be minimized by moving the bystanders to a safer area.

Additional and specialized resources may be needed to address hazards at the scene. These resources should be requested as soon as the need for them is

CRITICAL THINKING

Case Study

You are dispatched to a residence for multiple patients with a headache and vomiting. The power is out because of severe storms. When you arrive on the scene, you hear the sound of a generator running in the house.

What actions can you take as you arrive on the scene to treat these patients in a manner that is safe for both you and your patients?

recognized. The need for additional resources should be anticipated quickly when the scene is initially scanned for mechanism of injury or nature of illness. For example, if there are multiple patients, additional ambulances will be needed. The fire service will be needed if there are fire or electrical hazards, chemical spills, biologic threats, unsafe structures, and rescue or extrication requirements. Utility services may be required to manage downed power lines or to secure natural gas lines. Law enforcement personnel may be needed to control traffic, to manage bystanders, and to contain any violence at the scene (see Chapter 54, *Rescue Awareness and Operations*).

If a patient is armed and there is any question of safety, the paramedic should retreat until law enforcement indicates the weapon has been secured. In many parts of the country, it is legal to carry a concealed firearm. These weapons may be visible in the patient's home or found while performing the physical examination. It is advised not to move firearms unless there is an immediate threat. When possible, ask the patient or appropriate family member to secure the weapon in his or her home prior to transport. If law enforcement is present, officers should assist in securing the weapon. If a weapon is discovered with a patient who appears to present no immediate danger, and law enforcement is not available, the firearm should be moved and placed in a locked container if available. When moving the firearm, keep the finger off the trigger and hammer and point the barrel in a direction away from others. Do not attempt to unload or otherwise manipulate the gun.[3]

NOTE

In general, paramedics should never enter a scene or approach a patient if the threat of violence exists. The EMS crew should retreat from the scene and remain in a safe area until the scene has been secured by law enforcement personnel. If the scene is not safe and cannot be made safe, do not enter.

Standard Precautions

As discussed in Chapter 2, *Well-Being of the Paramedic*, the use of standard precautions should be part of any EMS response. Standard precautions apply to all patients, regardless of suspected or confirmed infection status, and are the primary strategy to prevent the transmission of infectious agents. Standard precautions include washing the hands; wearing a gown, mask, and gloves; and using protective barriers, when indicated.[4]

CRITICAL THINKING

Case Study

You are dispatched for a woman with abdominal pain. As you enter the patient's bedroom, you note that she is screaming, "The baby is coming! The baby is coming!"

How can you minimize your risk of exposure to blood or bloody body fluids on this call?

Personal Protective Equipment

Personal protective equipment (PPE) includes any clothing or specialized equipment that provides some protection to the wearer from environmental or infectious hazards (**FIGURE 18-7**). PPE protects the paramedic and other emergency personnel from substances that may pose a health or safety risk. PPE should be appropriate for the potential hazard. (PPE is further addressed in the section on EMS Operations.) Examples of PPE include the following:

- Boots with steel insoles and steel toe protection
- Impact-resistant helmet with ear protection and chinstrap

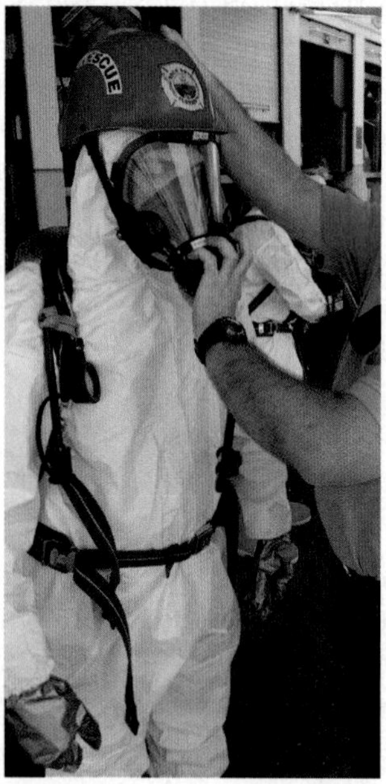

FIGURE 18-7 Example of personal protective equipment.

- Turnout gear
- Heat-resistant outerwear
- Reflective clothing
- Ballistic vests in high crime areas
- Safety glasses
- Hearing protection
- Self-contained breathing apparatus (SCBA)
- Latex, nitrile, or leather gloves or slip-resistant waterproof gloves
- Equipment for standard precautions

Multiple-Patient Situations

When responding to an incident where there are multiple patients, the paramedic should anticipate the need for additional support. Sometimes, the dispatch center has made this determination and requested assistance before EMS arrives at the scene. If there are multiple patients, the first unit establishes command and initiates the incident command system (ICS). Additional and specialized resources that may be needed are based on the nature of the incident. These resources may include additional ambulances and/or air medical service, additional manpower to sort and care for the injured, additional medical supplies, special equipment for extrication and fire suppression, specialized rescue teams, utility services, hazardous materials decontamination, and traffic and crowd control.

The goals of managing an event with multiple patients are to ensure scene safety, protect the patients, and protect the bystanders. Bystanders will need to be removed from the patient care area and isolated from the scene. Barricades may need to be erected and manned by law enforcement personnel to ensure the goals of managing the event. Large-scale scenes or major incidents will likely require a command structure to safely manage the scene. These command structures are known as an ICS or an incident management system (IMS). These systems organize interagency functions and responsibilities of emergency personnel and public service agencies at the scene. Command structures play a vital role in scene management whenever available resources are insufficient to manage the number of casualties or the type of emergency. (Command systems are described in detail in Chapter 53, *Medical Incident Command.*) Examples of major incidents include the following:

- Highway crashes
- Air crashes
- Major fires
- Train derailments
- Building collapse
- Acts of violence or terrorism
- Search and rescue operations
- Hazardous materials releases
- Natural disasters

CRITICAL THINKING

Case Study

Your unit is the first to arrive at the scene of the call dispatched as a "motor vehicle crash." You find a school bus that left the roadway and rolled. You see multiple injured children. The bus has major damage, and smoke is rising from the engine compartment. As you begin triage, your partner calls dispatch to establish command, to provide a brief size-up of the situation, and to request fire, rescue, and additional ambulances. Several parents in their cars have already arrived at the scene.

What challenges will you face in managing this scene?

Patient Assessment Priorities

After ensuring that the scene is safe and that needed resources are available or have been requested (**FIGURE 18-8**), paramedics can initiate patient assessment (**FIGURE 18-9**). Patient assessment involves the following priorities:[1]

1. Primary survey
2. Integration of immediate life-saving interventions
3. Evaluation of the priority of patient care and transport

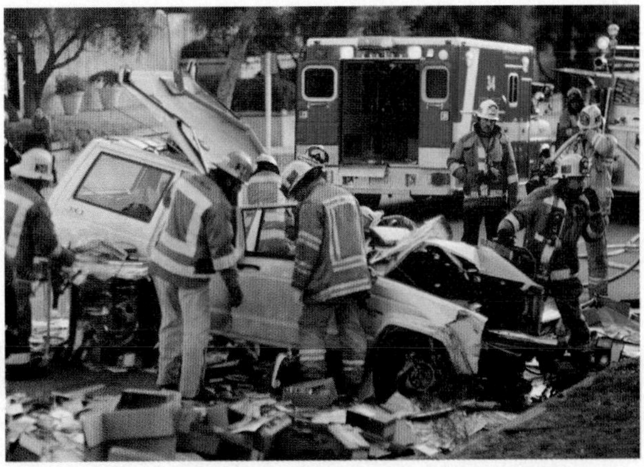

FIGURE 18-8 Many resources may be needed at an emergency scene.

Patient Assessment

Scene Size-up

Ensure scene safety
Determine mechanism of injury/nature of illness
Take standard precautions
Determine number of patients
Consider additional/specialized resources

Primary Assessment

Form a general impression
Assess level of consciousness
Assess for and control exsanguinating hemorrhage (life-threatening bleeding)
Assess the airway: identify and treat life threats
Assess breathing: identify and treat life threats
Assess circulation: identify and treat life threats
Perform primary assessment
Determine priority of patient care and transport

History Taking

Investigate the chief complaint (history of present illness)
Obtain SAMPLE history

Secondary Assessment: Medical or Trauma

Systematically assess the patient
- Secondary assessment and/or focused assessment
  Assess vital signs using the appropriate monitoring device

Reassessment

Repeat the primary assessment
Reassess vital signs
Reassess the chief complaint
Recheck interventions
Identify and treat changes in the patient's condition
Reassess the patient
- Unstable patients: every 5 minutes
- Stable patients: every 15 minutes

FIGURE 18-9 Components of patient assessment.

Primary Survey

The **primary survey** is a critical component of the **primary assessment** that focuses on the initial evaluation of a patient to recognize and manage life-threatening conditions. It is performed on all patients to establish priorities of care, which may include immediate **resuscitative measures** (BOX 18-3). The primary survey consists of the paramedic's **general impression** of the patient. This general impression is initially based on the patient's age and appearance. Components of the primary survey include assessment of the patient's level of consciousness, airway, breathing, and circulation (ABCs). The order of assessment and intervention priority varies between trauma and medical patients.

General Impression of the Patient

The general impression is the paramedic's initial assessment of the setting and the patient's chief complaint. It is formed based on information from the scene size-up and the primary and possibly secondary survey. The paramedic uses the general impression to determine whether the patient appears stable, as described in the following examples:

- **Appears stable.** A 35-year-old man with stable vital signs, no significant past medical history, and a complaint of abdominal pain and vomiting
- **Appears stable, but could become unstable.** A 61-year-old man with stable vital signs, history of anticoagulation for atrial fibrillation and one episode of melena
- **Appears unstable.** A 35-year-old woman with hypotension and tachycardia, complaining of abdominal pain and reporting a recent positive pregnancy test

Forming a general impression of the patient involves a visual assessment as he or she is approached, followed by a rapid primary survey to identify and immediately manage life threats. If no life threat is identified in the primary survey, a quick, structured secondary survey may uncover findings that could reveal the patient to be unstable.

As the scene is entered, the general setting should be observed for any clues of illness, injury, or mechanism of injury. The following factors help the paramedic form a general impression:

- **Position.** Is the patient upright? Prone? Contorted in an unusual position? In the tripod position?
- **Work of breathing.** Is the patient breathing quietly or struggling to breathe?
- **Apparent attentiveness.** Are the patient's eyes closed or open? As you approach the patient or speak to the patient, does he or she turn to look at you? Is he or she staring blankly?

BOX 18-3 Immediate Resuscitation

Some immediate resuscitation measures should be initiated while conducting the primary survey. These interventions should be limited to life-saving measures, such as control of exsanguinating hemorrhage, airway control, ventilatory assistance, and CPR, immediately after recognizing the need for them.

For medical patients in cardiac arrest, immediate resuscitation begins at the scene and includes CPR and advanced cardiac life support (ACLS) interventions. For significantly injured trauma patients, most resuscitative measures should be performed en route to the receiving hospital. Immediate resuscitative measures and priorities for medical and trauma patients are as follows:

Immediate Resuscitative Measures for Medical Patients

Airway-Breathing-Circulation

- Airway and breathing: Open airway, clear airway if needed, bag-mask ventilation assistance as needed
- Circulation:
  - Chest compressions or CPR
  - ACLS interventions for unstable patients
    - Electrical therapy if unstable or in arrest (eg, defibrillation, cardioversion, external pacing)
  - Medication or fluid resuscitation therapy
  - Intravenous or intraosseous access

Immediate Resuscitative Measures for Trauma Patients

eXsanguinating hemorrhage-Airway-Breathing-Circulation (XABC)

- eXsanguinating hemorrhage: Control of life-threatening bleeding (direct pressure, tourniquet)
- Airway and breathing: Open airway, clear airway if needed, bag-mask ventilation assistance as needed, needle chest decompression if indicated
- Circulation: Evaluate pulse, skin color, moisture, and temperature.
- Cervical spine immobilization if indicated
- Venous access for fluid administration to be provided en route

AVPU

- **Skin color.** Is the patient pale, diaphoretic, pink, or cyanotic?
- **Any obvious wounds noted.** Is there any bleeding or gross deformity evident?
- **Any body fluids noted.** Is there any visible blood, vomit, urine, or feces?
- **Any odor noted.** Is there a sweet or fruity odor to the patient's breath (diabetes mellitus), or smell of decomposition (necrotic tissue) or melena (gastrointestinal bleeding)?

Stability of the Patient

- **Patients who appear stable.** These patients usually require only minimal care at the scene and are unlikely to have immediately life-threatening illness or injury. They are conscious and alert, and their vital signs are within normal limits. Stable patients may not require immediate transport for physician evaluation.
- **Patients who appear stable, but who may become unstable, are injured, or have underlying illness or disease.** These patients may be conscious and alert, and their vital signs may or may not be within normal limits. Findings on the primary and secondary survey, together with the patient history, will lead the paramedic to potential causes of their complaint. These findings may also help identify those patients who could become unstable or require specialized care or specific interventions. History of an injury or an underlying illness or disease can alert the paramedic that a possible decline in the patient's status may occur. Patients who are potentially unstable should always be transported for physician evaluation.
- **Patients who appear unstable and have obvious signs of serious injury, illness, or disease.** The injury or illness is immediately life threatening. These patients require immediate care and transport to a medical facility. Initial on-scene care may include immediate resuscitative measures.

Assessment for Life-Threatening Conditions

To assess for life-threatening conditions, the paramedic should conduct the primary survey to systematically evaluate the patient's level of consciousness, airway, breathing, and circulation.

Level of Consciousness

An early priority with any patient is to assess his or her level of consciousness. The paramedic can usually accomplish this assessment as he or she greets the patient. For example, the paramedic may say, "Hi. My name is _____. I'm a paramedic. How can I help you?" Offering a handshake is useful, if the patient responds in kind. This gesture can provide an immediate sense of a patient's higher level of social functioning, as well as an evaluation of skin temperature. If the patient does not respond to verbal stimuli, the paramedic should assess if the patient responds to painful stimuli. This assessment should begin with gentle tactile stimulation (eg, rubbing the patient's shoulder) along with questions such as "Are you okay?" and "Can you hear me?" If there is no response, firm pressure should be used to elicit a response. An example of an firm pressure is nail bed pressure or sternal or supraorbital pressure. A patient who does not respond to verbal or painful stimuli is considered unresponsive. As described in Chapter 15, *Airway Management, Respiration, and Artificial Ventilation,*

CRITICAL THINKING

What does a patient's level of consciousness tell you about the patient's oxygenation and circulation?

SHOW ME THE EVIDENCE

Nasal flaring decreases airway resistance and is a sign of respiratory distress. Spanish researchers evaluated the relationship of nasal flaring to acidosis in 212 adult patients with severe dyspnea treated in the ED or treated by EMS and transferred to the ED. Of their sample of 212 dyspneic adults, 47 patients (22.2%) presented with nasal flaring. Of the patients with nasal flaring, 55.3% were acidotic versus 11.5% of dyspneic patients without nasal flaring. Nasal flaring was almost 10 times more likely to be associated with acidosis than was any other clinical sign of respiratory distress in their study group. Because of their small sample size, the researchers suggest further studies to confirm these findings in a variety of settings.

Modified from: Zorrilla-Riveiro JG, Arnau-Bartés A, Rafat-Sellarés R, García-Pérez D, Mas-Serra A, Fernández-Fernández R. Nasal flaring as a clinical sign of respiratory acidosis in patients with dyspnea. *Am J Emerg Med.* 2017;35(4):548-553.

the airway of any unconscious patient or any patient without a gag reflex or cough reflex must be managed immediately.

Airway Status

The paramedic should assess the airway of any patient to ensure it is patent with good air exchange. If the patient is unresponsive, the airway should be opened and cleared of any obstructions (see Chapter 15, *Airway Management, Respiration, and Artificial Ventilation*).

A responsive patient should be assessed for the ability to speak, noting signs of airway obstruction or respiratory insufficiency. These signs could include body position (eg, forward flexion of the neck), stridor, retractions, accessory muscle use, snoring, drooling, or gurgling. Any condition that compromises the delivery of oxygen to body tissues is potentially life threatening and must be managed immediately. Factors that may compromise the airway include the following:

- Tongue obstructing the airway in an unconscious patient
- Loose teeth or foreign objects in the patient's airway
- Epiglottitis
- Upper airway obstruction from any cause
- Facial and oral bleeding
- Vomitus
- Soft-tissue trauma to the patient's face and neck
- Facial fractures

A compromised airway must be made patent, initially using manual measures (eg, using a modified jaw-thrust or chin-lift maneuver), airway suctioning, and bag-mask ventilation (**FIGURE 18-10**). If these interventions do not provide adequate ventilation, more invasive measures using adjunct equipment may be needed (eg, oral or nasal airways, suction apparatus, advanced airway device, or continuous positive airway pressure [CPAP], described in Chapter 15, *Airway Management, Respiration, and Artificial Ventilation*). When performing an airway procedure for patients who potentially have a cervical spine injury, the paramedic should minimize manipulation of the cervical spine and stabilize the head and neck in a neutral position. All patients must have a patent airway established and maintained during the primary survey.

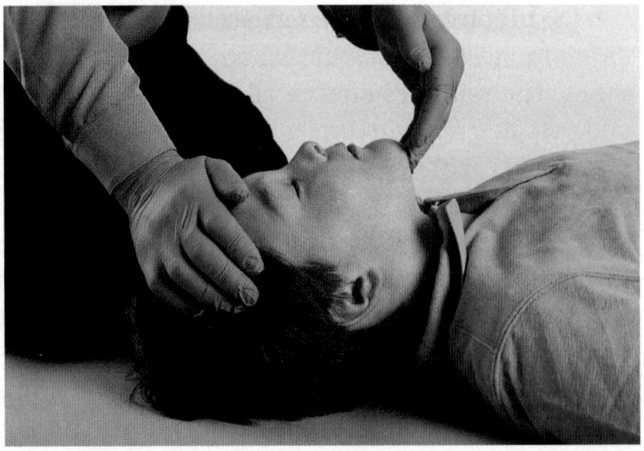

FIGURE 18-10 Paramedic opening an airway with head tilt–chin lift maneuver.

> **NOTE**
>
> The American Heart Association recommends treating patients who are in obvious cardiac arrest first with chest compressions. This step is followed by an assessment of airway and breathing (ie, CAB sequence). For further discussion of cardiac arrest management, see Chapter 21, *Cardiology*.
>
> *Modified from:* American Heart Association, American Red Cross. Web-based integrated 2010 and 2015 American Heart Association and American Red Cross Guidelines for First Aid. Part 15: first aid. American Heart Association website. https://eccguidelines.heart.org/index.php/circulation/aha-red-cross-first-aid-guidelines/part-15-first-aid/. Accessed January 1, 2018.

> **NOTE**
>
> The patient whose airway is obstructed by a foreign object should be managed using the guidelines currently recommended by the American Heart Association. If these maneuvers fail, medical direction may recommend direct laryngoscopy or cricothyrotomy. For further discussion of management of an obstructed airway, see Chapter 15, *Airway Management, Respiration, and Artificial Ventilation*.

Breathing Status

The breathing of a responsive patient can be assessed as adequate rate and quality, too fast (greater than 24 breaths/min), too slow (less than 8 breaths/min), or absent (eg, choking from airway obstruction). The breathing of an unresponsive patient can be assessed as adequate rate and quality, inadequate, or absent.

Breathing can be assessed by evaluating the rate, depth (tidal volume), and symmetry of chest movement. The patient's chest wall should be exposed and palpated for structural integrity, tenderness, and crepitus. Use of muscles of respiration (accessory muscles) in the neck, chest, and abdomen should be observed and noted. The paramedic should auscultate the lungs for the presence of bilateral breath sounds and should listen to the patient's speech. A patient who has difficulty speaking without pain or who cannot talk without gasping for air may need ventilatory support. Respiratory abnormalities discovered during the primary survey that may indicate a potentially life-threatening condition include the following:[1]

- Cyanosis
- Nasal flaring
- Accessory muscle use
- Stridor
- Respiratory distress with dyspnea or hypoxia
- Asymmetrical chest wall movement
- Chest injury (eg, tension pneumothorax, flail segment, open chest wound)
- Tracheal deviation
- Distended neck veins

Ill or injured patients with ineffective respirations need ventilatory support. These patients may require supplemental oxygen to maintain adequate oxygen saturations. The exact target oxygen saturation level is further discussed in Chapter 15, *Airway Management, Respiration, and Artificial Ventilation*, but 94% is considered the minimum acceptable level without supplementation.[5] If the respiratory rate of a critically ill or injured patient is less than 8 or more than 24 respirations per minute, ventilatory assistance may be needed.[1] The paramedic may coordinate assisted ventilation with the patient's respiratory efforts. Or the paramedic may intersperse assisted ventilation between the patient's own respiratory efforts as needed to maintain adequate oxygenation.

CRITICAL THINKING

Why do some patients with adequate breathing rate require assisted ventilation?

If respirations are absent, the paramedic should initiate rescue breathing with a pocket face mask or positive-pressure ventilation via a bag-mask device with supplemental oxygen. Endotracheal intubation or other advanced airway devices may be indicated. The paramedic also should consider spinal precautions if the situation warrants it (see Chapter 15, *Airway Management, Respiration, and Artificial Ventilation*).

Circulatory Status

Except in patients where there is obvious and severe uncontrolled bleeding, the patient's circulatory status should be evaluated after assessing airway and breathing. The paramedic should assess the patient's skin color, moisture, and temperature quickly. The pulse should be evaluated for location, quality, rate, and regularity.

Pulse. A quick evaluation of the patient's radial or carotid pulse may reveal any of the following: a normal rate of 60 to 100 beats/min, tachycardia (a fast rate, greater than 100 beats/min), bradycardia (a slow rate, less than 60 beats/min), an absent rate (asystole), or an irregular heart rate. The site of an obtainable pulse also may offer critical details about a patient's approximate systolic blood pressure and tissue perfusion.[6] For example, if a radial pulse is not palpable in an uninjured extremity, the patient may be in a decompensated state of shock (hypoperfusion). A patient who lacks a palpable femoral or carotid pulse is either severely hypotensive or in cardiac arrest.

Capillary Refill Time. The capillary filling time may offer crucial details about the patient's cardiovascular status. The capillary refill test is most reliable in children younger than 12 years.[7] This test is performed by blanching the patient's nail bed or the fleshy eminence at the base of the thumb, and then measuring the time it takes for normal color to return. A filling time of more than 2 seconds is a sign of shunting and capillary closure to peripheral capillary beds. It indicates inadequate circulation and impaired cardiovascular function. Factors such as the patient's age and sex and the environment may affect the filling time. Capillary refill is one possible indicator of circulatory and perfusion status.[8] Other signs and symptoms of inadequate circulation and impaired cardiovascular function include the following:

- Altered or decreased level of consciousness
- Distended neck veins
- Increased respiratory rate

- Pale, cool, diaphoretic skin
- Distant heart sounds
- Restlessness
- Thirst

CRITICAL THINKING

Why do the patient's age and sex and the environment affect capillary refill time?

NOTE

When an unconscious patient lacks a palpable femoral or carotid pulse, chest compressions should be initiated and cardiac arrest protocols should be followed (see Chapter 21, *Cardiology*). In cases of severe external hemorrhage, bleeding should be controlled using direct pressure. If arterial bleeding is not rapidly controlled with direct pressure, a tourniquet should be applied (see Chapter 37, *Bleeding and Soft-Tissue Trauma*). In most cases, these procedures to control bleeding also are effective during transport. Regardless of the cause, all patients with circulatory compromise need rapid stabilization. Stabilization may involve intravenous administration of fluids and medications and rapid transport to an appropriate medical facility.

Modified from: American Heart Association, American Red Cross. Web-based integrated 2010 and 2015 American Heart Association and American Red Cross Guidelines for First Aid. Part 15: first aid. American Heart Association website. https://eccguidelines.heart.org/index.php/circulation/aha-red-cross-first-aid-guidelines/part-15-first-aid/. Accessed January 1, 2018.

Disability—Brief Neurologic Evaluation

If time permits, a brief neurologic evaluation should be performed on all patients during the primary survey. The brief neurologic examination assesses level of consciousness, pupil size and reactivity, speech, and motor function. The purpose of this brief examination is to gather information about any level of altered consciousness. (The neurologic examination is described in detail in Chapter 19, *Secondary Assessment and Reassessment*.)

- **Level of consciousness.** The initial assessment of level of consciousness performed early in the primary survey classifies a patient as responsive or unresponsive. The brief neurologic examination goes further by establishing that a patient is alert; is oriented to person, place, and date; and is aware of his or her surroundings. A patient who does not "pass" this test is assumed to be disoriented. Any deviations from a "normal" test should be recorded and reported to personnel at the receiving hospital. Other assessments, such as the Glasgow Coma Scale and stroke assessments, also may be indicated when evaluating the patient's level of consciousness (see Chapter 19, *Secondary Assessment and Reassessment*).
- **Pupil size and reactivity.** As a rule, healthy people have pupils that are equal in size and react in concert to light. That is, both pupils should constrict at the same time when exposed to light. Causes of unequal pupils and impaired reactivity include ocular prostheses, eye trauma, head trauma, drug toxicity, stroke, and conditions that may impair oxygenation.
- **Speech.** A healthy person's speech should be clear and easy to understand. Slurred speech, difficulties with speech, or nonsensical speech can result from stroke, seizure, head or facial injury, medical conditions that cause speech impairment, and alcohol or other drug use.
- **Motor function.** An uninjured patient should be able to move all extremities on command and without difficulty. The patient's walk and gait should be smooth and fluid. Conditions that may affect motor function and movement include extremity injury, stroke, head injury, alcohol or other drug use, and medical conditions such as Parkinson disease, multiple sclerosis, and arthritis.

NOTE

A primary purpose of the brief neurologic examination is to form a baseline assessment for future evaluations. This baseline can then be compared with assessments performed by hospital staff after the patient has been delivered to the ED. Baseline assessments help identify negative and positive trends that may occur during the course of a patient's care.

Exposure

Some trauma patients require only minimal care and do not need to have their bodies fully exposed at the scene. Examples include stable patients with minor injuries that are isolated to a specific body part. Other patients with significant injury and those patients who are potentially unstable should be completely undressed as part of the primary survey. Exposure of the body may reveal other injuries that are not easily visible when the patient is clothed. Examples include bullet wounds, stab wounds, hidden fractures, and large areas of bruising or hematoma formation. When full-body exposure is indicated, every effort should be made to ensure the patient's privacy. Ideally, a paramedic of the same sex should remove the patient's clothing, make a visual inspection, and then appropriately cover the patient for privacy and warmth.

Assessment of Vital Functions

The paramedic should obtain a baseline set of vital signs for every patient. Vital functions to be assessed include pulse rate, respiratory rate, and blood pressure. Other assessments may be indicated, such as monitoring the patient's oxygen saturation using pulse oximetry and electrocardiogram monitoring. These baseline measurements of vital functions help to identify positive and negative trends in the course of the patient's care. They also help to identify priority patients. As a rule, vital signs should be measured and recorded every 15 minutes for stable patients and at least every 5 minutes for patients who are unstable or potentially unstable.

Identifying Patients Who Need Priority Care and Transport

The paramedic uses the findings from the primary survey to identify life threats and priority patients. **Priority patients** are unstable patients or potentially unstable patients who need stabilization and rapid transport to an emergency facility. Examples of priority patients include patients with the following presentations/conditions:

- Poor general impression
- Decreased level of consciousness (depressed or absent gag or cough reflex)
- ST-elevation myocardial infarction
- Difficulty breathing
- Shock (hypoperfusion)
- Sepsis
- Complicated childbirth
- Chest pain with a systolic pressure of less than 100 mm Hg
- Uncontrolled bleeding
- Signs of stroke
- Multiple injuries

> NOTE
>
> For patients with stroke, myocardial infarction, sepsis, or internal hemorrhage, life-saving care can begin at the scene, but simultaneous and rapid transport is also needed. The combination of initial on-scene care and rapid transport allows for time-sensitive and definitive treatment to be delivered at the hospital.

Integration of Treatment/Procedures Needed to Preserve Life

In some cases, definitive care for medical patients can be initiated in the prehospital setting. For example, patients who have altered consciousness related to hypoglycemia or narcotic overdose should receive immediate interventions that may completely reverse their life-threatening signs and symptoms. In the case of severe respiratory emergencies, prehospital care can relieve severe hypoxic signs and symptoms before arrival at the hospital. Thus, the time spent on scene with medical patients may be slightly longer.

In contrast, most seriously injured trauma patients require short scene times and rapid transport. These patients should be taken to an appropriate trauma center or other medical facility for definitive care. Patients with internal bleeding, major fractures, head injury, and multiple-system trauma need life-saving care. This care can be provided only by specially trained physicians and support staff. Minimal time should be spent at the scene with these patients. Most trauma life support training programs (eg, International Trauma Life Support, Prehospital Trauma Life Support, and Advanced Trauma Life Support) recommend that patients needing immediate transport be stabilized and prepared for transport ("packaged") within 10 minutes after arrival of EMS.[8] Field management should be limited to stopping external hemorrhage, airway control and ventilatory support, spinal immobilization, and major fracture stabilization. Intravenous fluid therapy should be initiated en route to the hospital. (Trauma management is addressed further in this text in Section 9, *Trauma*.)

Summary

- Scene size-up is a quick assessment of an emergency scene. It is designed to determine resources needed to manage the scene safely and effectively.
- Dispatch information that assists with scene size-up includes location, type of location, type of situation, possible hazards, and unique issues.
- Special rescue, transport, fire, or other public safety resources may need to be dispatched to help manage the scene.
- Many factors can contribute to an unsafe scene. These may include environmental hazards, hazardous substances, violence, and rescue-related hazards.
- Scene assessment should always begin by asking, "Is the scene safe?" If it is not, identify measures that eliminate or reduce the risk to permit safe entry.
- Perform an initial scene survey. On medical calls, attempt to determine the nature of illness. On trauma calls, gather information related to the mechanism of injury.
- If hazards cannot be corrected, remove the patient from the scene as quickly and as safely possible.
- Standard precautions should be used for all patients to minimize the risk of exposure to blood or bloody body fluids.
- Other specialized personal protective equipment may be needed based on the nature of the hazard and the training and role of the paramedic on the scene.
- Multiple-patient situations require many resources. Priorities should always be scene safety with protection of the patient and bystanders. Incident command should be established.
- The primary assessment includes the paramedic's general impression of the patient, the assessment for life-threatening conditions, and the identification of priority patients requiring immediate care and transport.
- Assessment of life-threatening conditions entails a systematic evaluation of the patient's level of consciousness, airway, breathing, circulation, and disability. The patient should also be appropriately exposed during the primary survey to detect life threats.
- Information from the primary survey is used to identify life threats and prioritize patients.
- The paramedic begins resuscitative measures, such as control of exsanguinating hemorrhage, airway maintenance, ventilatory assistance, and cardiopulmonary resuscitation, immediately after recognizing the life-threatening condition that necessitates each respective maneuver.

References

1. National Highway Traffic Safety Administration. *The National Emergency Medical Services Education Standards. Paramedic Instructional Guidelines*. Washington, DC: US Department of Transportation/National Highway Traffic Safety Administration; 2009.
2. Moffatt SE. Hypothermia in trauma. *Emerg Med J*. 2013; 30(12):989-996.
3. Kupas DF. Scene safety best practices. *Domestic Preparedness*. 2015. https://www.nasemso.org/Projects/DomesticPreparedness/documents/Scene-Safety-Best-Practices.pdf. Accessed December 29, 2017.
4. Centers for Disease Control and Prevention, National Center for Emerging and Zoonotic Infectious Diseases, Division of Healthcare Quality Promotion. Infection control. Isolation precautions. Centers for Disease Control and Prevention website. https://www.cdc.gov/infectioncontrol/guidelines/isolation/index.html. Updated October 31, 2017. Accessed December 29, 2017.
5. Majumdar SR, Eurich DT, Gamble JM, Senthilselvan A, Marrie TJ. Oxygen saturations less than 92% are associated with major adverse events in outpatients with pneumonia: a population-based cohort study. *Clin Infect Dis*. 2011;52(3):325-331.
6. National Association of Emergency Medical Technicians. *PHTLS: Prehospital Trauma Life Support*. 8th ed. St. Louis, MO: Mosby; 2016.
7. Fleming S, Gill P, Jones C, et al. Validity and reliability of measurement of capillary refill time in children: a systematic review. *Arch Dis Child*. 2015;100(3):239-249.
8. Torrey S, Fleisher G, Wiley J. Assessment of perfusion in pediatric resuscitation. UpToDate website. https://www.uptodate.com/contents/assessment-of-perfusion-in-pediatric-resuscitation?source=search_result&search=capillary%20refill&selectedTitle=1~94. Updated April 10, 2017. Accessed January 1, 2018.

Suggested Readings

Dries DJ. Initial evaluation of the trauma patient. Medscape website. https://emedicine.medscape.com/article/434707-overview? Updated April 21, 2017. Accessed January 1, 2018.

McDonald W. Eight tips for safer scenes. EMS World website. http://www.emsworld.com/article/10653367/eight-tips-safer-scenes. Published March 8, 2012. Accessed January 1, 2018.

Parker M, Magnusson C. Assessment of trauma patients. *Int J Orthop Trauma Nurs*. 2016:21:21-30.

Thim T, Krarup NH, Grove EL, Rohde CV, Løfgren B. Initial assessment and treatment with the Airway, Breathing, Circulation, Disability, Exposure (ABCDE) approach. *Int J Gen Med*. 2012;5:117-121.

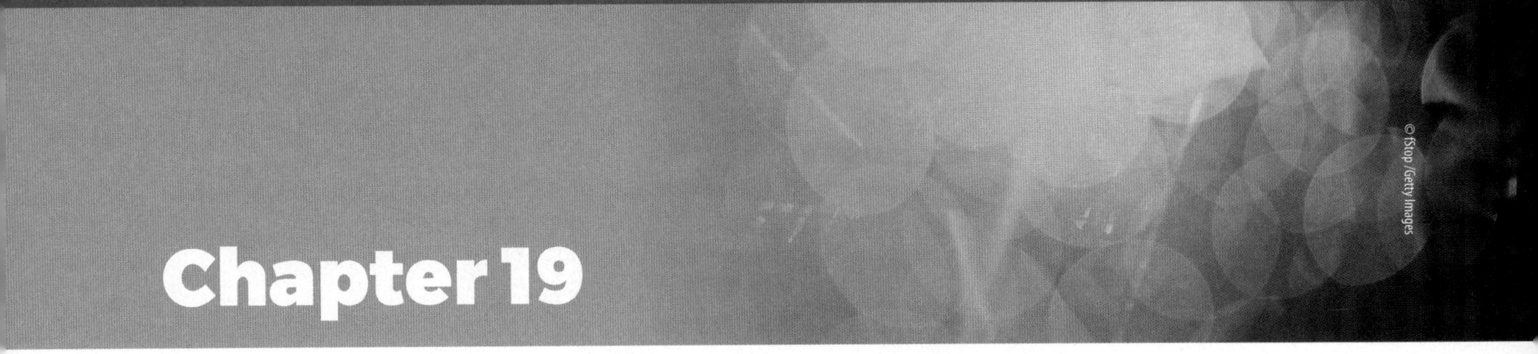

© fStop/Getty Images

Chapter 19

Secondary Assessment and Reassessment

NATIONAL EMS EDUCATION STANDARD COMPETENCIES

Assessment

Integrate scene and patient assessment findings with your knowledge of epidemiology and pathophysiology to form a field impression. Use clinical reasoning to develop a list of differential diagnoses, modify the assessment, and formulate a treatment plan.

Secondary Assessment

- Performing a rapid full-body scan (see Chapter 18, *Scene Size-up and Primary Assessment*)
- Focused assessment of pain (pp 646–650)
- Assessment of vital signs (pp 646–650)
- Techniques of physical examination (pp 632–633)
- Respiratory system (pp 633, 636, 646–647, 656–662)
  - Presence of breath sounds (pp 658–661)

Cardiovascular system (pp 646–648, 662–663)
Neurologic system (pp 671–676)
Musculoskeletal system (pp 667–671)
Techniques of physical examination for all major

- Body systems (pp 632–633)
- Anatomic regions (pp 650–677)

Assessment of

- Lung sounds (pp 658–661)

Monitoring Devices

Obtaining and using information from patient monitoring devices including (but not limited to)

- Pulse oximetry (see Chapter 15, *Airway*, and Chapter 23, *Respiratory*)
- Noninvasive blood pressure (pp 647–648)
- Blood glucose determination (see Chapter 25, *Endocrinology*)
- Continuous ECG monitoring (see Chapter 21, *Cardiology*)
- 12-lead ECG interpretation (see Chapter 21, *Cardiology*)
- Carbon dioxide monitoring (p 635)
- Basic blood chemistry (see Chapter 14, *Medication Administration*)

Reassessment

- How and when to reassess patients (p 677)
- How and when to perform a reassessment for all patient situations (p 677)

OBJECTIVES

Upon completion of this chapter, the paramedic student will be able to:

1. Define the purpose of the secondary assessment. (pp 631–632)
2. Describe physical examination techniques commonly used in the prehospital setting. (pp 632–633)
3. Describe the examination equipment commonly used in the prehospital setting. (pp 634–635)
4. Describe the general approach to physical examination. (p 635)
5. Outline the steps of a comprehensive physical examination. (pp 636–676)
6. Detail the components of the mental status examination. (pp 636–637)
7. Distinguish between normal and abnormal findings in the mental status examination. (pp 636–637)
8. Outline the steps in the general patient survey. (pp 637–650)
9. Distinguish between normal and abnormal findings in the general patient survey. (pp 637–650)

10. Describe physical examination techniques used for assessment of specific body regions. (pp 650–677)
11. Distinguish between normal and abnormal findings when assessing specific body regions. (pp 650–677)
12. Outline the process of patient reassessment. (p 677)
13. State modifications to the physical examination that are necessary when assessing children. (pp 677–680)
14. State modifications to the physical examination that are necessary when assessing the older adult. (pp 680–681)

KEY TERMS

anisocoria A condition characterized by unequal pupil size; may be congenital or indicative of pathology.

aphasia Loss of the ability to understand or express speech.

apical impulse A pulsation of the left ventricle of the heart that is palpable and sometimes visible at the fifth intercostal space to the left of the midline.

ataxia Failure of muscle coordination.

auscultation A technique that requires the use of a stethoscope and is used to assess body sounds produced by the movement of various fluids or gases in organs or tissues.

bronchial breath sounds Breath sounds heard only over the trachea. They are the highest in pitch.

bronchovesicular breath sounds Normal breath sounds heard over the major bronchi or in the posterior chest between the scapula.

bruit An abnormal sound or murmur heard while auscultating an artery, organ, or gland.

crackle A fine, bubbling sound heard on auscultation of the lung. It is produced by air entering distal airways and alveoli that contain serous secretions.

crepitus A grating sound or sensation that may be caused by bone fragments rubbing or other sources, such as a joint with inflammation.

deep tendon reflexes Reflexes that examine the sensory and motor pathways of a nerve; often associated with muscle stretching.

diastolic blood pressure The minimum level of blood pressure measured between contractions of the heart.

dysarthria Difficult and poorly articulated speech resulting from poor control over the muscles of speech.

dysconjugate gaze Failure of the eyes to move with synchronized motion; may be diagnostic of a neurologic injury.

dysphonia An abnormality in the speaking voice, such as hoarseness.

epistaxis Bleeding from the nose.

heart murmurs Abnormal heart sounds caused by altered blood flow into a chamber or through a valve.

inspection A visual assessment of the patient and surroundings.

nystagmus Involuntary jerking movements of the eyes.

palpation A technique in which an examiner uses the hands and fingers to gather information from a patient by touch.

percussion A surface tapping technique used to evaluate the presence of air or fluid in body tissues.

pericardial friction rub A dry, grating sound heard with a stethoscope during auscultation; suggestive of pericarditis.

PERRL Acronym that indicates that the Pupils are Equal and Round, and Reactive to Light.

physical examination An assessment of a patient that includes examination techniques, measurement of vital signs, an assessment of height and weight, and the skillful use of examination equipment.

pleural friction rub A rubbing or grating sound that occurs as one layer of the pleural membrane slides over the other during breathing.

pronator drift test A test to evaluate balance and upper extremity weakness; performed by having the patient close the eyes and hold both arms out from the body.

pulse deficit A condition that exists when the radial pulse is less than the ventricular rate; it indicates a lack of peripheral perfusion.

reassessment The ongoing assessment that follows the paramedic's initial evaluation of the patient.

rhonchi Abnormal, coarse, rattling respiratory sounds, usually caused by secretions in bronchial airways, muscular spasm, neoplasm, or external pressure.

Romberg test A test to evaluate stance and balance; performed by having the patient stand erect with eyes closed, feet together, and arms at the sides.

secondary assessment An assessment that consists of physical examination techniques, measurement of vital signs, an assessment of body systems, and the skillful use of examination equipment.

six cardinal fields of gaze A test to evaluate extraocular muscle function; performed by having the patient visually track an object in six visual fields in an H pattern.

stridor An abnormal, high-pitched musical sound caused by obstruction in the trachea or larynx.

subcutaneous emphysema The presence of air in the subcutaneous tissues.

superficial reflexes Reflexes elicited by sensory afferents from skin.

systolic blood pressure The blood pressure measured during the period of ventricular contraction.

thrills Fine vibrations felt by an examiner's hands over the site of an aneurysm or on the pericardium.

tidal volume The volume of air inspired or expired in a single, resting breath.

tympany A hollow drumlike sound produced when a gas-containing cavity is percussed.

vesicular breath sounds Breath sounds heard over most of the lung fields; the major normal breath sound.

wheeze A form of rhonchus characterized by a high-pitched, musical quality. It is caused by high-velocity airflow through narrowed airways.

The paramedic must have a wide range of knowledge and skills to perform a comprehensive physical examination and to make effective clinical care decisions. This chapter presents the techniques of the basic physical examination. Some of the techniques presented will have application to examinations more likely to be performed in expanded scope of practice activities. The goal of this chapter is to prepare the paramedic with the tools and skills needed to perform a thorough physical examination in any patient care setting.

NOTE

Chapter 18, *Scene Size-up and Primary Assessment*, addresses the components of the primary survey by focusing on recognizing and managing life-threatening conditions in the initial patient care encounter. This chapter is devoted to the techniques of the detailed physical examination—the examination performed in the secondary assessment. Like the primary survey, the secondary assessment integrates patient assessment findings with knowledge of pathophysiology. This comprehensive approach helps to form a final impression and to identify an appropriate treatment plan.

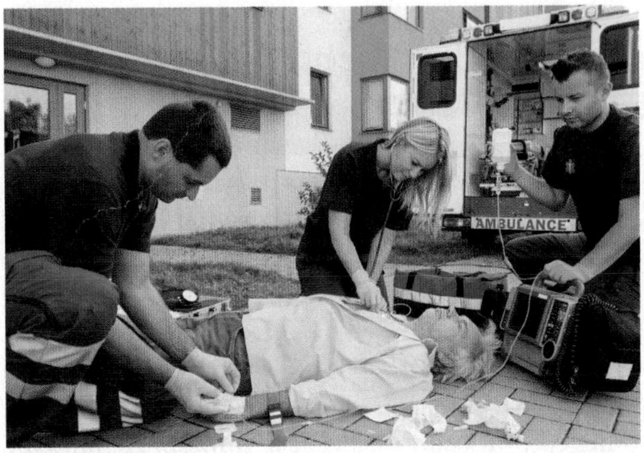

Secondary Assessment: Approach and Overview

The **secondary assessment** consists of physical examination techniques, measurement of vital signs, an assessment of body systems, and the skillful use of examination equipment (BOX 19-1). Physical examination techniques will vary by patient, depending on the chief complaint, present illness, and history. The appropriate assessment of the patient depends on:

- The stability of the patient
- The complaint and history
- The patient's ability to communicate
- The potential for unrecognized illness

NOTE

Some aspects of the physical assessment may not be appropriate for all patients. For example, if the patient has a life-threatening injury or illness, a primary survey and rapid transport with a focused secondary assessment may be all that is provided in the prehospital phase of care. However, if the patient is stable and has a significant history, a more thorough secondary assessment may be indicated. The order of care for this group of patients is as follows:

1. Scene size-up
2. Primary assessment
3. Secondary assessment
4. Reassessment

BOX 19-1 Components of the Physical Examination

Examination Techniques
Inspection
Palpation
Percussion
Auscultation

Measurement of Vital Signs
Pulse
Respirations
Blood pressure
Temperature (especially in children)

Manual Assessment Equipment
Blood pressure cuff
Ophthalmoscope (limited use in the prehospital environment)
Otoscope (limited use in the prehospital environment)
Stethoscope

Examination Techniques

Four techniques commonly are used in the **physical examination**: inspection, palpation, percussion, and auscultation. These terms are referred to often in this text because they relate to the evaluation of specific body systems. Depending on the situation, these techniques may be the sole method for evaluating a patient. For example, this may be the case with an unconscious trauma patient. In other cases, these techniques may be integrated with history taking and other care procedures. If time permits, the paramedic should explain to the patient each technique that requires touch before performing it.

CRITICAL THINKING
You arrive at the scene of a motor vehicle crash. What will you look for during your initial patient inspection?

Inspection

Inspection is the visual assessment of the patient and the surroundings. This technique can alert the paramedic to the patient's mental status. Inspection also can alert the paramedic to possible injury or underlying illness. Patient hygiene, clothing, eye gaze, body language and position, skin color, and odor are significant inspection findings. The emergency medical services (EMS) response may be to the patient's home. In this case, the paramedic should make a visual inspection for cleanliness, prescription medicines, illegal drug paraphernalia, weapons, and signs of alcohol use. These and other items seen by EMS personnel can play a key role in determining patient care activities.

Palpation

Palpation is a technique in which the paramedic uses the hands and fingers to gather information by touch. Generally, the paramedic uses the palmar surface of the fingers and the finger pads to palpate for texture, masses, fluid, and **crepitus** and to assess skin temperature (**FIGURE 19-1**). The dorsal and ulnar hand surfaces may also be used. Palpation may be either superficial or deep; the applications for each type are addressed throughout this chapter. Examining a patient by palpation involves close contact with the patient's body. Therefore, the approach should be gentle and should be initiated with respect.

Percussion

Percussion is used to evaluate the presence of air or fluid in body tissues. This technique is performed by the paramedic striking one finger against another to produce vibrations and sound waves of underlying tissue. Sound waves are heard as percussion tones (resonance) and are determined by the density of the tissue being examined. The denser the body area, the lower the pitch of the percussion tone. To percuss, the paramedic places the distal interphalangeal joint

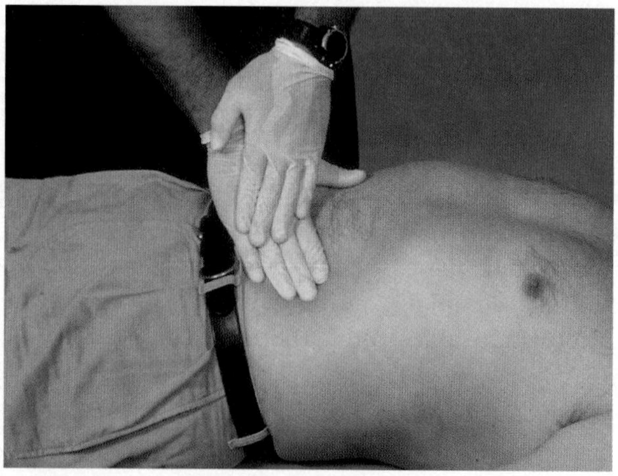

FIGURE 19-1 Deep bimanual palpation.

of the middle finger of the nondominant hand on the patient, keeping the rest of the hand poised above the skin. The fingers of the other hand should be flexed and the wrist action loose. The paramedic then snaps the wrist of the dominant hand downward, with the tip of the middle finger tapping the joint of the finger that is on the body surface. The tap should be sharp and rigid, percussing the same area several times to interpret the tone (**FIGURE 19-2**). **BOX 19-2** describes percussion tones and examples of each. As with any other examination technique, percussion requires practice to obtain the skill needed for the physical examination.

Auscultation

Auscultation calls for the use of a stethoscope. This technique is used to assess body sounds made by the movement of various fluids or gases in the patient's organs or tissues. Auscultation is best performed in a quiet environment to focus on each body sound being assessed. The paramedic should isolate an area to note characteristics of intensity, pitch, duration, and quality. In the prehospital setting, auscultation most often is used to assess blood pressure and to evaluate breath sounds, heart sounds, and bowel sounds. To auscultate, the paramedic should place the diaphragm of the stethoscope firmly against the patient's skin for stabilization (**FIGURE 19-3**). If a bell end piece is used, it should be positioned lightly on the body surface to prevent the damping of vibrations.

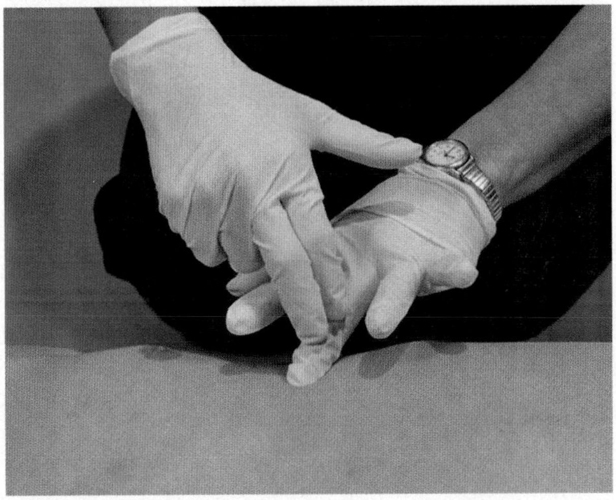

FIGURE 19-2 Percussion technique.

BOX 19-2 Percussion Tones and Examples

Percussion Tone	Example
Tympany (the loudest)	Gastric bubble
Hyperresonance	Air-filled lungs (eg, chronic obstructive pulmonary disease, pneumothorax)
Resonance	Healthy lungs
Dullness	Liver
Flat (the quietest)	Muscle

NOTE

The bell and diaphragm end pieces of a stethoscope selectively emphasize sounds of different frequencies. The bell is central for listening to low-pitched sounds (eg, certain heart sounds). In contrast, the diaphragm filters out low-pitched sounds and therefore emphasizes high-pitched ones. Examples of high-pitched sounds include breath sounds and bowel sounds.

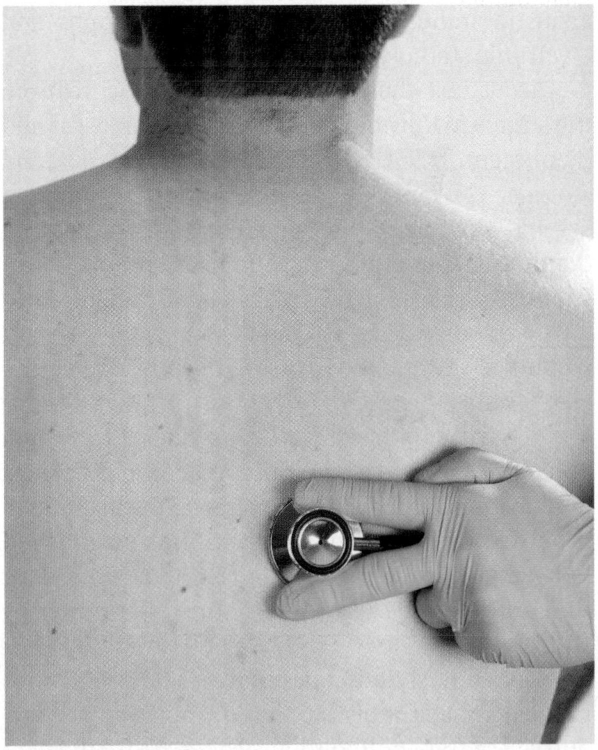

FIGURE 19-3 Position of the stethoscope between the index and middle fingers.

Examination Equipment

Basic equipment used during the comprehensive physical examination includes the stethoscope, ophthalmoscope, otoscope, and blood pressure cuff. The ophthalmoscope and otoscope are nontraditional EMS tools that are being introduced to some paramedics with expanded scope of practice. The knowledge necessary to interpret the findings obtained with the use of these devices is not generally covered in paramedic programs.

> NOTE
>
> Monitoring devices such as capnography, electrocardiography (ECG), and devices used to test blood chemistry are also frequently used in the prehospital setting. These devices will be described throughout this text by subject matter.

Stethoscope

The stethoscope is used to evaluate sounds created by the cardiovascular, respiratory, and gastrointestinal systems. The three major types of stethoscopes are acoustic stethoscopes, magnetic stethoscopes, and electronic stethoscopes (**FIGURE 19-4**).

Acoustic stethoscopes transmit sound waves from the source to the paramedic's ears. Most have a rigid diaphragm. This diaphragm transmits high-pitched sounds. The bell end piece transmits low-pitched sounds. Tunable stethoscopes combine the bell and diaphragm into one surface. To hear low-frequency sounds, the chest piece is placed lightly on the chest for auscultation. High-frequency sounds can be heard when the chest piece is pressed firmly against the chest wall.[1]

Magnetic stethoscopes have a single diaphragm end piece. The end piece contains an iron disk and a permanent magnet. The air column of the diaphragm is activated as magnetic attraction is established between the iron disk and the magnet. A frequency dial adjusts for high-, low-, and full-frequency sounds.

Electronic stethoscopes convert sound vibrations into electrical impulses that are amplified. The impulses are transmitted to a speaker where they are converted to sound. These devices can compensate for environmental noise; therefore, they may be beneficial for use in the prehospital setting. Some of these devices can provide audio or serial data output, wireless Bluetooth transmission, and recording of sound clips. Some also offer visual output of the heart rate and ECG waves detected directly on the device.

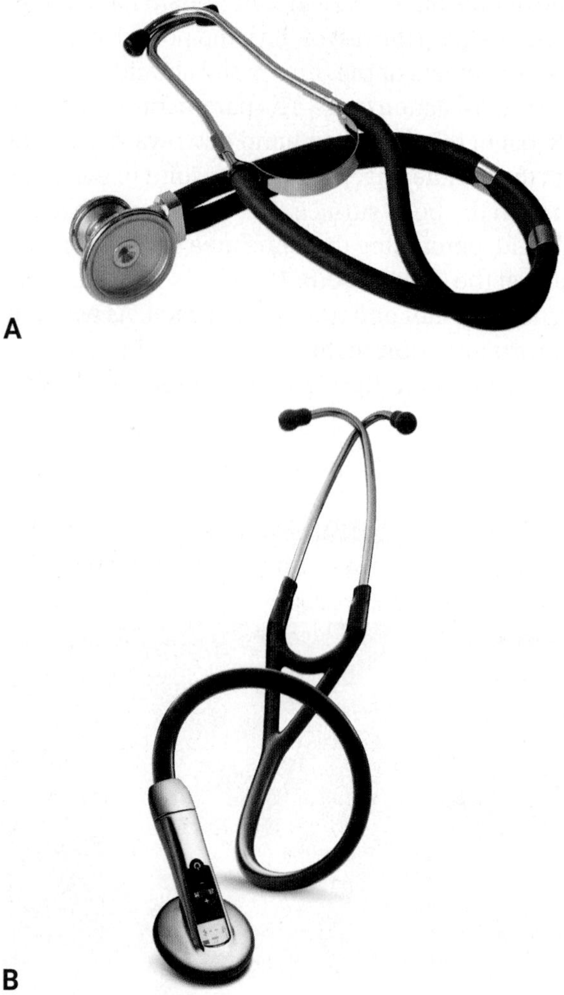

FIGURE 19-4 Stethoscope types. **A.** Acoustic. **B.** Electronic.

Ophthalmoscope

The ophthalmoscope is used to inspect structures of the eye, including the retina, choroid, optic nerve disk, macula (an oval, yellow spot at the center of the retina), and retinal vessels. This device has a battery light source, two dials, and a viewer (**FIGURE 19-5**). The dial at the top of the battery changes the light image. The dial at the top of the viewer allows for the selection of lenses. (Five lenses are available, but the large white light generally is used.)

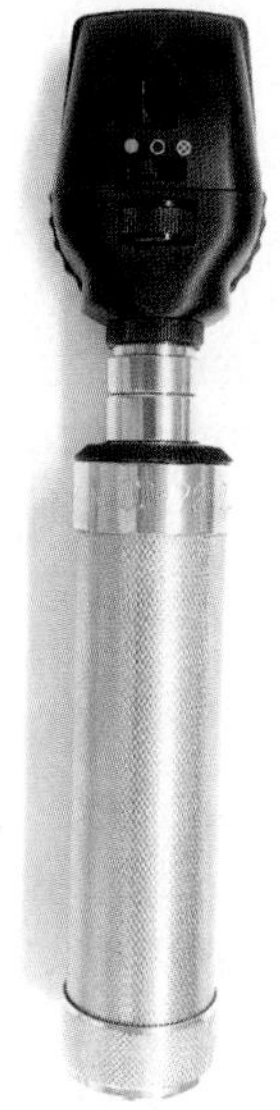

FIGURE 19-5 Ophthalmoscope.

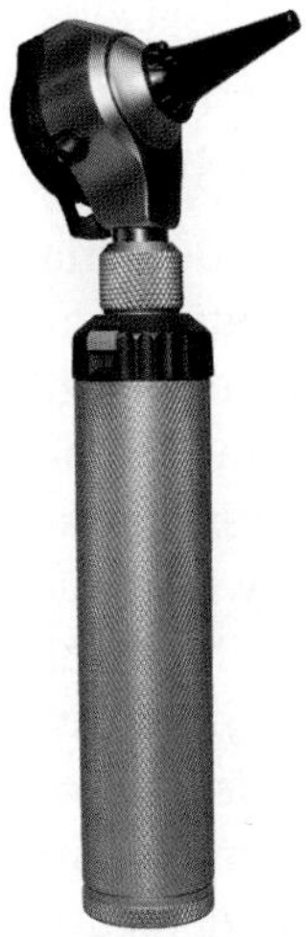

FIGURE 19-6 Otoscope.

Otoscope

The otoscope is used to examine deep structures of the external and middle ear. This device is basically an ophthalmoscope with a special ear speculum attached to the battery tube (**FIGURE 19-6**). Ear specula are available in several sizes to conform to various ear canals. The paramedic should choose the largest one that fits comfortably in the patient's ear. The light from the otoscope allows visualization of the tympanic membrane.

Blood Pressure Cuff

The blood pressure cuff (sphygmomanometer) most commonly is used along with the stethoscope to measure systolic and diastolic blood pressure. The common blood pressure cuff used in the prehospital setting consists of a pressure gauge that registers millimeter calibrations, a synthetic cuff with Velcro closures that encloses an inflatable rubber bladder, and a pressure bulb with a release valve. Blood pressure cuffs are available in several sizes. Adult widths should be one-third to one-half the circumference of the limb. For children, the width should cover about two-thirds of the upper arm or thigh. (Blood pressure cuffs that are too large give a falsely low reading; cuffs that are too small give a falsely high reading.)

Most ECG monitors automatically measure a patient's vital signs. These devices monitor the patient's blood pressure, pulse rate, body temperature, end-tidal carbon dioxide concentration, and oxygen saturation level at regular intervals (**FIGURE 19-7**). Some models also measure carboxyhemoglobin, which permits detection of carbon monoxide toxicity.

General Approach to the Physical Examination

The physical examination is performed as a step-by-step process. Special emphasis is placed on the patient's present illness and chief complaint. The paramedic should know that most patients view a physical examination with some anxiety because they often feel vulnerable and exposed. Therefore, it is important to establish a professional trust early in the encounter, in addition to ensuring the patient's privacy and comfort when possible.

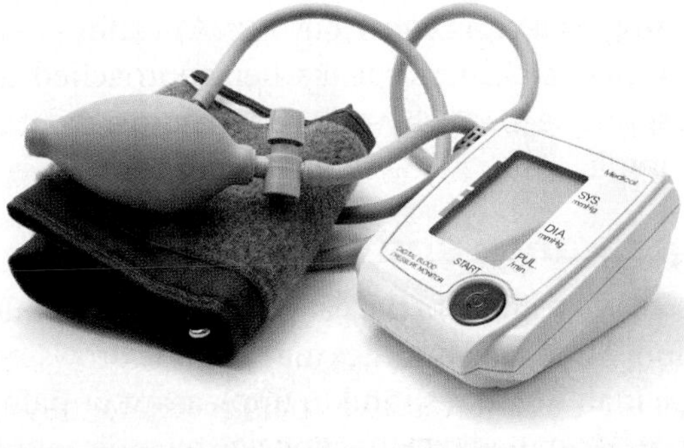

FIGURE 19-7 Electronic blood pressure device.

Overview of a Comprehensive Physical Examination

The physical examination is a systematic assessment of the body that includes the following components:

- Mental status
- General survey
- Vital signs
- Skin
- Head, eyes, ears, nose, and throat
- Chest
- Abdomen
- Posterior body
- Extremities (peripheral vascular and musculoskeletal)
- Neurologic examination

NOTE

The Centers for Disease Control and Prevention and the Occupational Safety and Health Administration have recommended that health care workers wear gloves "when handling blood-soiled items, body fluids, excretions and secretions, as well as surfaces, materials, and objects exposed to them." This text assumes that all paramedics are appropriately gloved for patient care procedures. Personal protective measures are addressed in Chapter 14, *Medication Administration*, and Chapter 27, *Infectious and Communicable Diseases*.

Modified from: Centers for Disease Control and Prevention. Current trends acquired immune deficiency syndrome (AIDS): precautions for clinical and laboratory staffs. *Morbid Mortal Wkly Rep.* 1982;31(43):577-580. Accessed February 16, 2018.

Mental Status

The first step in any encounter with a patient is to note the patient's appearance and behavior, in addition to assessing for level of consciousness. A healthy patient is expected to be alert, speak when approached, and be responsive to touch, verbal instruction, and painful stimuli.

Appearance and Behavior

A visual assessment of the patient can yield key information. Abnormal findings may include drowsiness or the inability to respond to unpleasant or painful stimuli. Most medical direction agencies discourage the use of vague terms to describe a patient's mental status. It is best to describe the patient's reactions and verbal and motor responses with indexes, such as the AVPU (Awake and alert, responsive to Verbal stimuli, responsive to Pain, Unresponsive) scale or the Glasgow Coma Scale. These measurements provide more precise patient information. Coma is a state of profound unconsciousness. A patient in a coma has no spontaneous eye movements. These patients do not respond to verbal or painful stimuli and cannot be aroused.

Posture, Gait, and Motor Activity

The paramedic should observe the patient's posture, gait, and motor activity. This involves assessing pace, range, character, and appropriateness of movement. For example, most patients without physical disabilities can walk with good balance and without a limp, discomfort, or fear of falling. Abnormal findings may include **ataxia** (uncoordinated movement), paralysis, restlessness, agitation, bizarre body posture, immobility, and involuntary movements.

Dress, Grooming, Personal Hygiene, and Breath or Body Odors

Dress, grooming, and personal hygiene should be appropriate for the patient's age, lifestyle, and occupation. A person's dress should be appropriate for environmental temperature and weather conditions. Older adults and children who are improperly dressed for temperatures or who have poor hygiene may be victims of neglect. Medical jewelry (eg, copper bracelets for arthritis, medical insignias) should be noted. Hair, fingernails, and cosmetics may reflect the patient's lifestyle, mood, and personality. These findings can point to a decreased interest in appearance (eg, unkempt hair, faded nail polish), which may help to estimate the length of an illness.

Breath or body odors can point to underlying conditions or illness. Examples of breath odors include alcohol, acetone (seen with some diabetic conditions), feces (seen with bowel obstruction), and halitosis from throat infections, dental caries, and poor dental and oral hygiene. Renal and liver disease and poor hygiene also may result in body odor.

Facial Expression

Facial expressions may reveal anxiety, depression, elation, anger, or withdrawal. They may also show fear, sadness, or pain. The paramedic should be alert to changes in facial expression while the patient is at rest, during conversation, during the examination, and when asking questions. Facial expressions should be appropriate to the situation.

Mood, Affect, and Relation to People and Things

Like facial expression, the patient's mood and affect also should be appropriate to the event. Mood and affect describe the patient's emotional state and the outward display of feelings and emotions; they are expressed verbally and nonverbally. Examples of abnormal findings include unusual happiness in the presence of major illness, indifference, thoughts of suicide, responses to imaginary people or objects, and unpredictable mood swings.

> CRITICAL THINKING
> What physical clues do you look for in your friends or your partner that tell you about their mood?

Speech and Language

The patient's speech should be understandable and of a moderate pace. The paramedic should assess the quantity, rate, loudness, and fluency of the patient's speech patterns. Abnormal findings include **aphasia** (loss of the ability to understand or express speech), **dysphonia** (abnormal speaking voice), **dysarthria** (poorly articulated speech), and speech and language that changes with mood.

Thoughts and Perceptions

A healthy person's thoughts and perceptions are logical, relevant, organized, and coherent. Patients should have an insight into their illness or injury. They also should be able to show a level of judgment in making decisions or plans about their situation and their care. Although accurately assessing a person's thoughts and perceptions is difficult, the following findings usually are considered abnormal:

- Abnormal thought processes
  - Flight of ideas
  - Incoherence
  - Confabulation
  - Blocking
  - Transference
- Abnormal thought content
  - Obsessions
  - Compulsions
  - Delusions
  - Suicidal ideations
  - Homicidal thoughts
  - Feelings of unreality
- Abnormal perceptions
  - Illusions
  - Visual/auditory hallucinations

Memory and Attention

Healthy people normally are alert and oriented to person, place, and date (often documented as "AO × 3"). They also are usually aware of the event that initiated the EMS response ("AO × 4"). The paramedic can use several other methods to assess a patient's memory and attention. One method is to ask the patient to count from 1 to 10 using only even or odd numbers (digit span). Another is to ask the patient to count down from one hundred by sevens (serial sevens). A third method is to ask the patient to spell simple words backward (eg, "Spell *world* backwards"). The paramedic also should assess the patient's remote memory (eg, birthdays) and recent memory (eg, events of the day), and the patient's new learning ability. New learning ability can be evaluated by giving the patient new information (eg, your name, the year and model of the ambulance). Later, the paramedic would ask the patient to recall that information.

General Survey

After assessing a patient's level of consciousness and mental status, the paramedic performs a general survey of the patient. In addition to the assessments described previously, the patient should be evaluated for signs of distress, apparent state of health, skin color and obvious lesions, height and build, sexual development, and weight. Vital signs also are assessed during the general survey.

Signs of Distress

Obvious signs of distress include those that result from cardiorespiratory insufficiency, pain, and anxiety. Examples of these signs and symptoms include the following:

- Cardiorespiratory insufficiency
  - Labored breathing

    - Wheezing
    - Cough
- Pain
    - Wincing
    - Sweating
    - Protectiveness of a painful body part or area
- Anxiety
    - Restlessness
    - Anxious expression
    - Fidgety movement
    - Cold, moist palms

CRITICAL THINKING

Combine one symptom from each of the groups of distress, and imagine how a patient with these symptoms might look and act.

Apparent State of Health

A patient's apparent state of health can be assessed by observation. Elements of general appearance include physical characteristics, such as sex, race, body build, and state of development in relation to chronologic age. The paramedic should also note the patient's basic appearance as being acutely or chronically ill, frail, robust, or vigorous. Although these are subjective assessments, chronically ill patients often "look sick" and may have poor skin color, physical wasting, and loss of weight and muscle mass because of disease. *Frail* describes a patient with a heightened vulnerability to functional dependence, often referring to older patients who have low physical activity, muscle weakness, and slowed performance. *Robust* describes a patient who appears strong and healthy. *Vigorous* patients appear full of energy.

Skin Color and Obvious Lesions

Skin color can vary by body part and from person to person. A patient's normal skin color depends on race and can range from pink or ivory to deep brown, yellow, or olive. Skin color is best assessed by evaluating skin that usually is not exposed to the sun (eg, the palms) or skin that has less pigmentation (eg, lips and nail beds). BOX 19-3 describes abnormal skin colors and their possible causes. Obvious skin lesions that can indicate illness or injury include rashes, bruises, scars, and discoloration (**FIGURE 19-8**, **TABLE 19-1**, and **TABLE 19-2**).

BOX 19-3 Abnormal Skin Color and Possible Causes

Color	Possible Causes
Pallor (decrease in color)	Shock, dehydration, fright
Cyanosis (blue color)	Cardiorespiratory insufficiency, cold environment
Jaundice (yellow-orange color)	Liver disease, red blood cell destruction
Red	Fever, inflammation, carbon monoxide poisoning

NOTE

Skin color, texture, and appearance can be affected by a person's age. For example, the skin color of a pediatric patient with light skin may be milky white and rose, to a deep hue of pink. A child with dark skin may have various brown, yellow, or olive-green or blue tones. In addition, the skin of a child is usually smooth, slightly dry, and not oily or clammy. By comparison, the skin of a geriatric patient is often dry and wrinkly, with uneven pigmentation. The older patient often has thinning of the epidermal skin layers and decreased collagen production and may have various proliferative lesions associated with aging.

Height and Build

Patients generally can be described as average, tall, or short, with a slender, lanky, muscular, or stocky build. These factors can reflect overall health. For example, a patient can be excessively thin (as seen with some eating disorders) or trim and muscular. Age and lifestyle also may affect height and body build.

Sexual Development

Sexual characteristics should be appropriate for the patient's age and sex. Normal changes associated with puberty include facial hair and deepening of the voice in men, increased breast size in women, and hair growth in the axillary and groin areas in both sexes. As a rule, healthy men are taller, heavier, and more muscular than are healthy women.

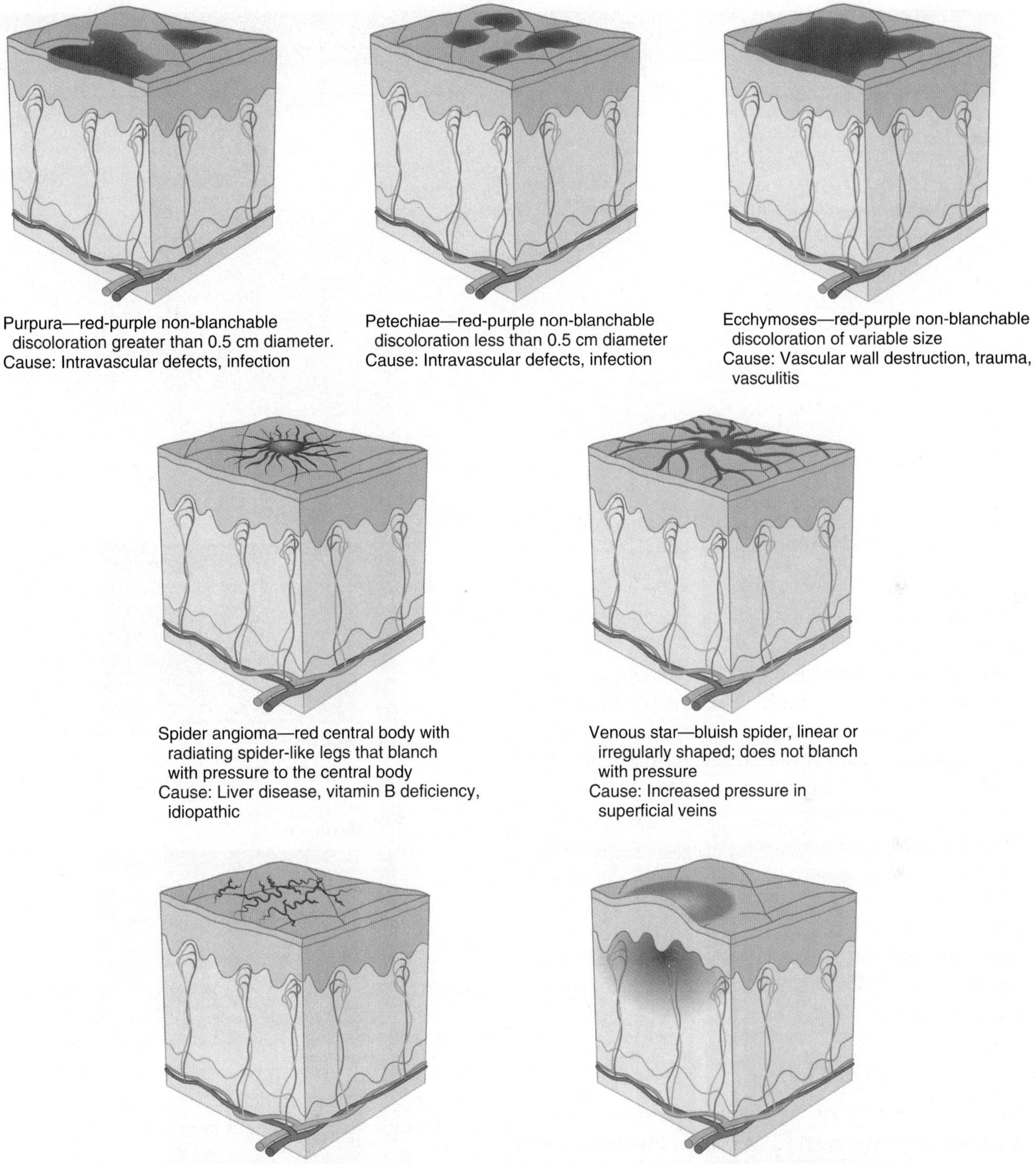

Purpura—red-purple non-blanchable discoloration greater than 0.5 cm diameter.
Cause: Intravascular defects, infection
Petechiae—red-purple non-blanchable discoloration less than 0.5 cm diameter
Cause: Intravascular defects, infection
Ecchymoses—red-purple non-blanchable discoloration of variable size
Cause: Vascular wall destruction, trauma, vasculitis
Spider angioma—red central body with radiating spider-like legs that blanch with pressure to the central body
Cause: Liver disease, vitamin B deficiency, idiopathic
Venous star—bluish spider, linear or irregularly shaped; does not blanch with pressure
Cause: Increased pressure in superficial veins
Telangiectasia—fine, irregular red line
Cause: Dilation of capillaries
Capillary hemangioma (nevus flammeus) —red irregular macular patches
Cause: Dilation of dermal capillaries

FIGURE 19-8 Characteristics and causes of vascular skin lesions.

TABLE 19-1 Primary Skin Lesions

Description (Examples)	
Macule	
A flat, circumscribed area that is a change in color of the skin; <0.4inch (1 cm) in diameter (freckles, flat moles [nevi], petechiae, measles, scarlet fever)	Freckles. 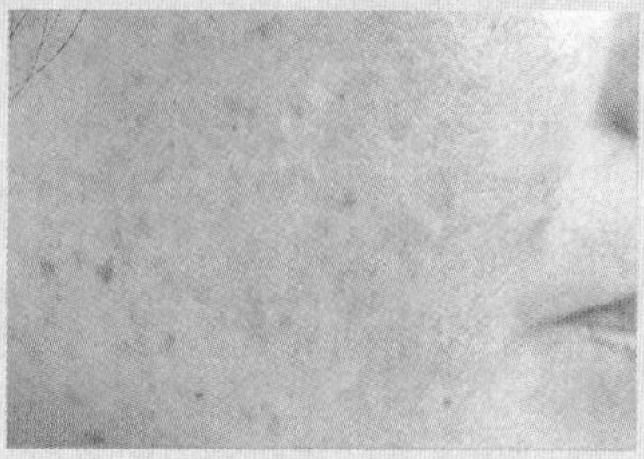 © Srisakorn wonglakorn/Shutterstock
Papule	
An elevated, firm, circumscribed area; <0.4 inch (1 cm) in diameter (wart [verruca], elevated moles, lichen planus)	Lichen planus. 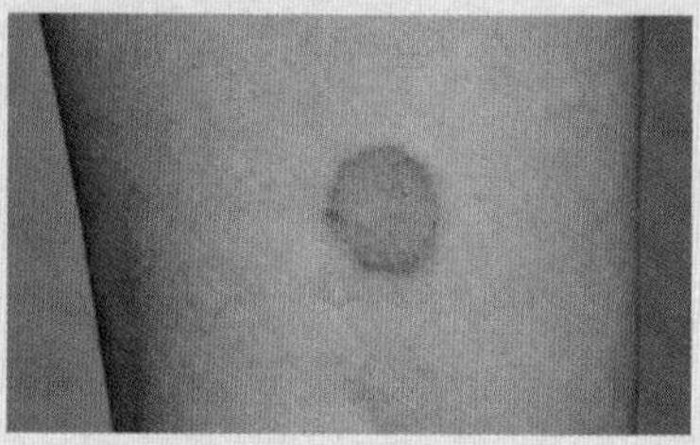 © Elena Stepanova/Shutterstock
Patch	
A flat, nonpalpable, irregular-shaped macule >0.4 inch (1 cm) in diameter (vitiligo, port-wine stains, congenital dermal melanocytosis, café-au-lait patch)	Vitiligo. 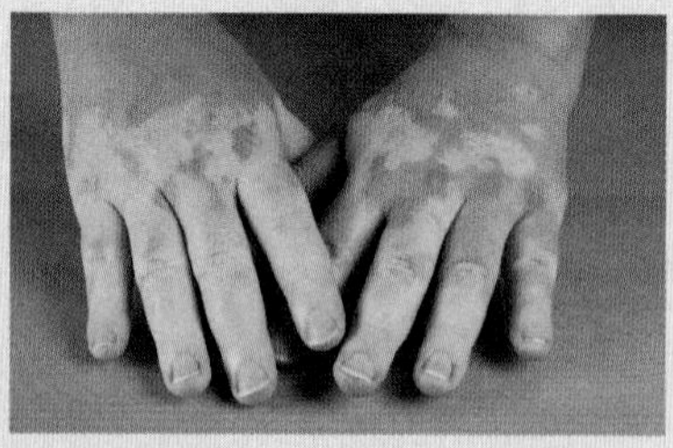 © Axel Bueckert/Shutterstock
Plaque	
Elevated, firm, and rough lesion with flat top surface >0.4 inch (1 cm) in diameter (psoriasis, seborrheic and actinic keratosis)	Plaque. 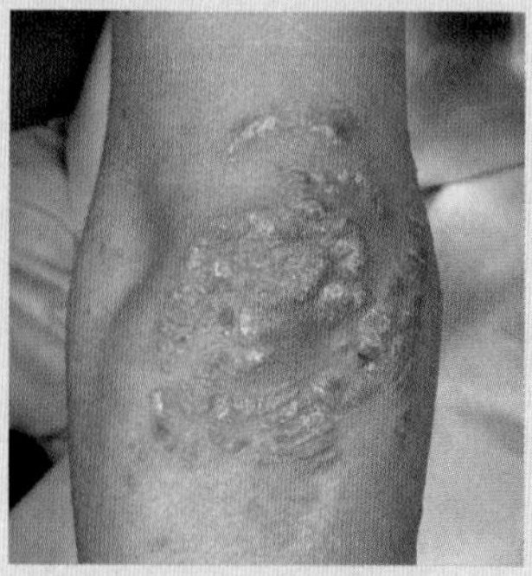 © Mediscan/Alamy Stock Photo.

TABLE 19-1 Primary Skin Lesions *(continued)*

Description (Examples)

Wheal

Elevated, irregular-shaped area of cutaneous edema; solid, transient, variable diameter (insect bites, urticaria, allergic reaction)

Wheal.

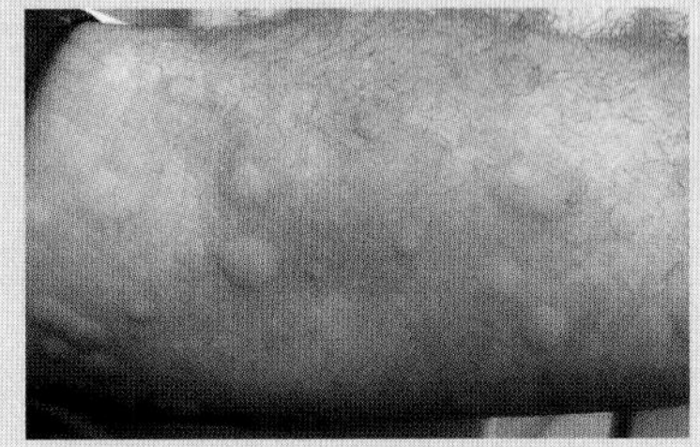

Nodule

Elevated, firm, circumscribed lesion; deeper in dermis than a papule; 0.4–0.8 inch (1–2 cm) in diameter (erythema nodosum, lipomas)

Nodules.

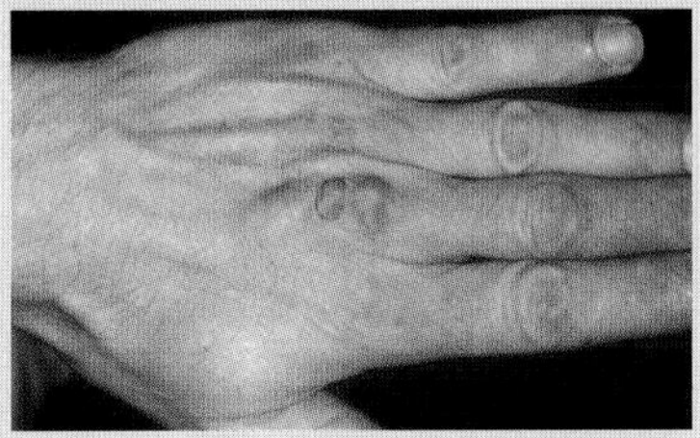

Tumor

Elevated and solid lesion; may or may not be clearly demarcated; deeper in dermis; >0.8 inch (2 cm) in diameter (neoplasms, benign tumor, lipoma, hemangioma)

Tumor.

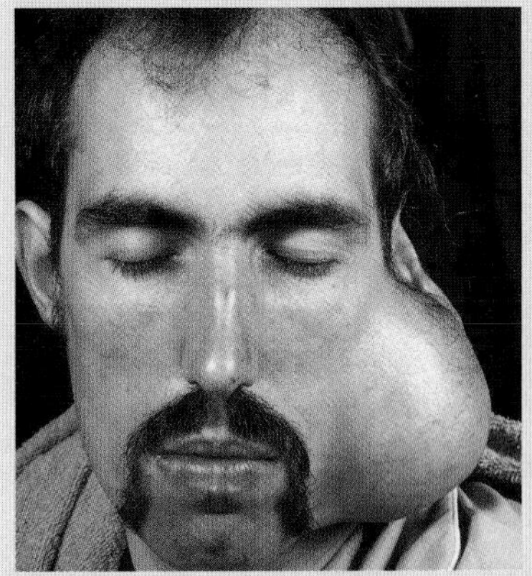

Vesicle

Elevated, circumscribed, superficial, not into the dermis; filled with serous fluid; <0.4 inch (1 cm) in diameter (varicella [chickenpox], herpes zoster [shingles])

Vesicles caused by herpes zoster.

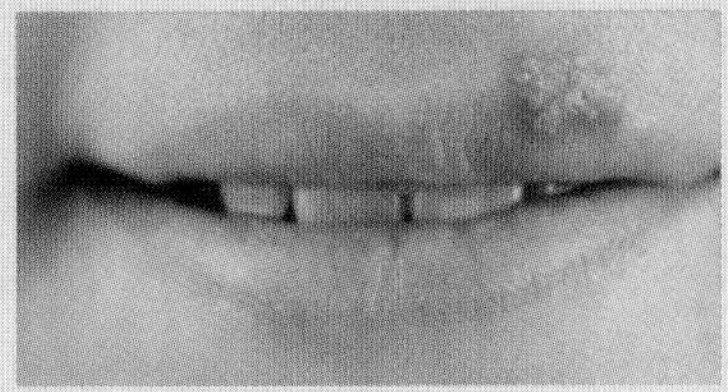

(continued)

TABLE 19-1 Primary Skin Lesions *(continued)*

Description (Examples)

Bulla

Vesicle >0.4 inch (1 cm) in diameter (blister, pemphigus vulgaris)

Bullous pemphigoid.

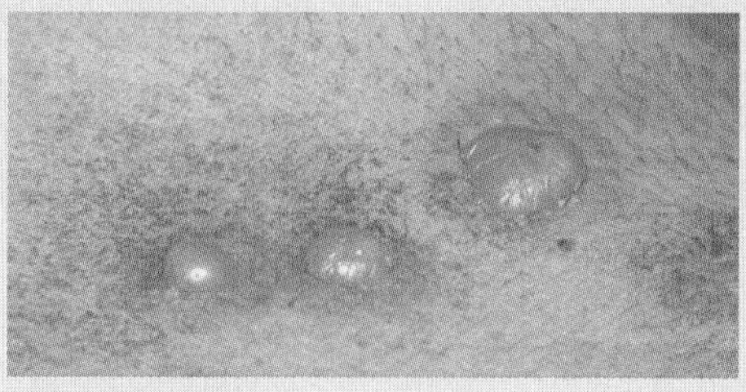

Pustule

Elevated, superficial lesion; similar to a vesicle but filled with purulent fluid (impetigo, acne)

Acne.

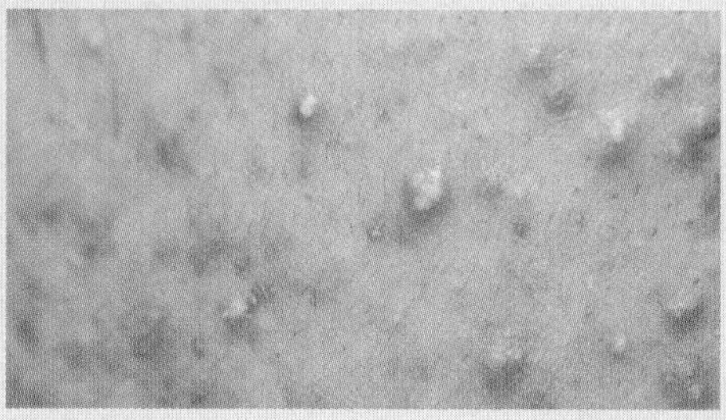

Cyst

Elevated, circumscribed, encapsulated lesion; in dermis or subcutaneous layer; filled with liquid or semisolid material (sebaceous cyst, cystic acne)

Sebaceous cyst.

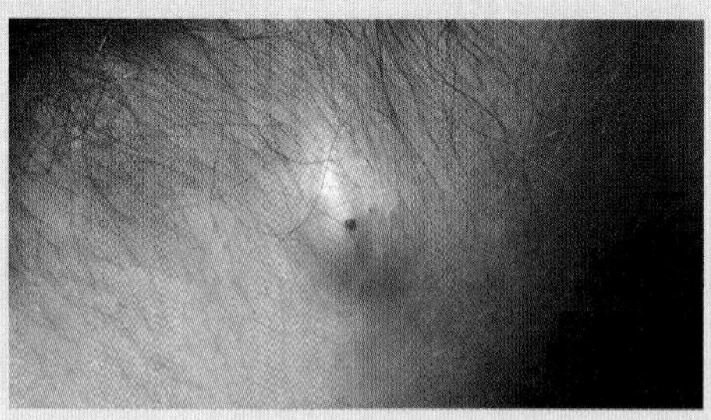

Telangiectasia

Fine, irregular, red lines produced by capillary dilation (telangiectasia in rosacea)

Telangiectasia.

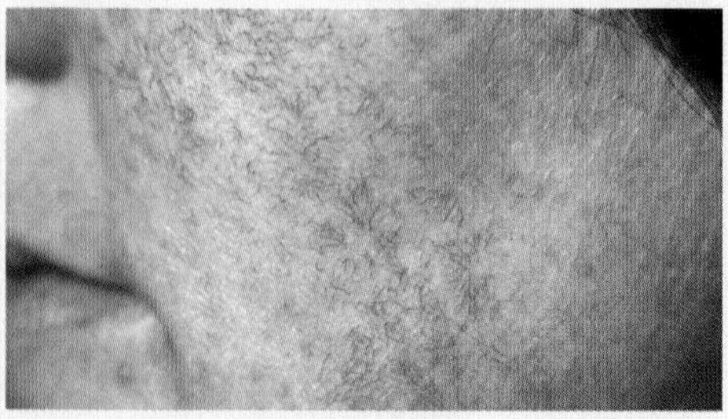

Modified from: Thompson JM, Wilson SF. *Health Assessment for Nursing Practice*. 2nd ed. St. Louis, MO: Mosby; 2001.

TABLE 19-2 Secondary Skin Lesions

Description (Examples)

Scale

Heaped up, keratinized cells, flaky skin; irregular; thick or thin; dry or oily; variation in size (flaking of skin with seborrheic dermatitis following scarlet fever, or flaking of skin following a drug reaction; dry skin)

Scale.

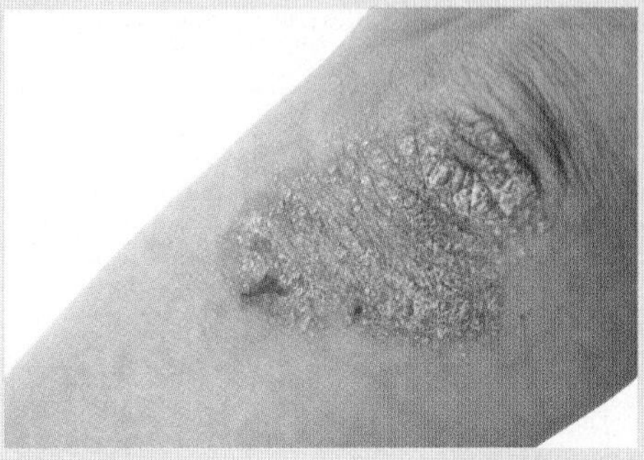

Lichenification

Rough, thickened epidermis secondary to persistent rubbing, itching, or skin irritation; often involves flexor surface of extremity (chronic dermatitis)

Atopic dermatitis.

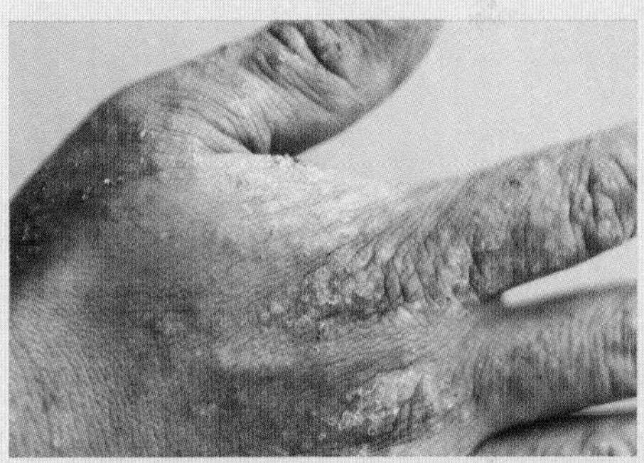

Keloid

Irregular-shaped, elevated, progressively enlarging scar; grows beyond boundaries of wound; caused by excessive collagen formation during healing (keloid formation following surgery)

Keloid.

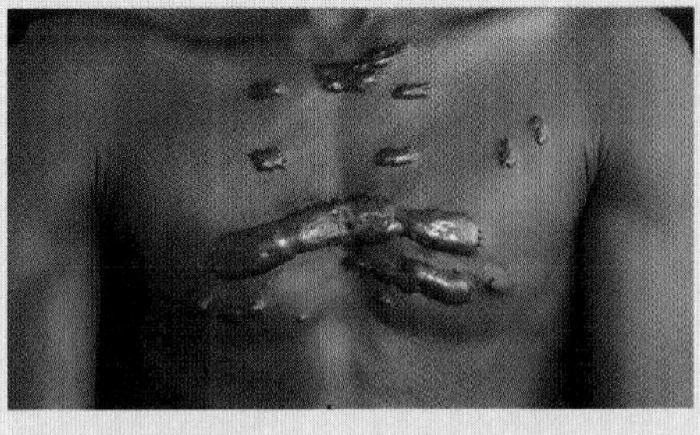

(continued)

TABLE 19-2 Secondary Skin Lesions *(continued)*

Description (Examples)

Scar

Thin to thick fibrous tissue that replaces normal skin following injury or laceration to dermis (healed wound or surgical incision)

Hypertrophic scar.

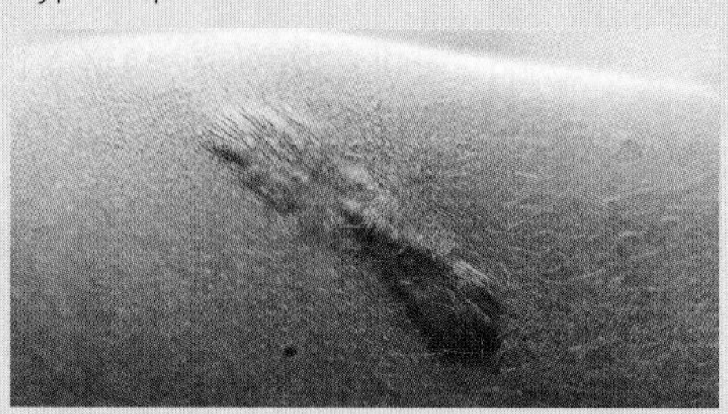

Excoriation

Loss of epidermis; linear hollowed-out, crusted area (abrasion or scratch, scabies)

Scabies.

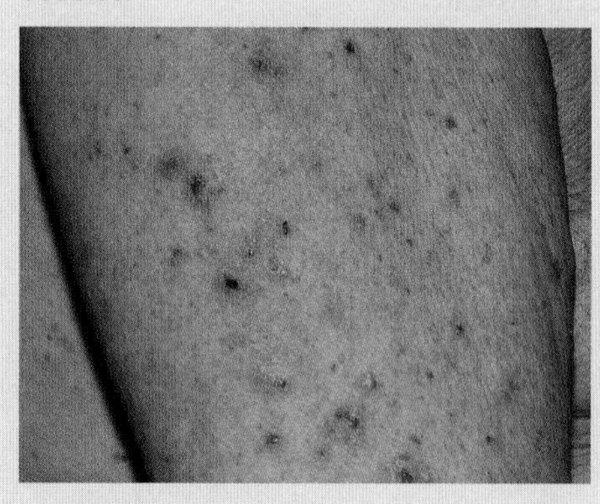

Fissure

Linear crack or break from epidermis to dermis; may be moist or dry (athlete's foot, cracks at the corner of the mouth)

Fissure.

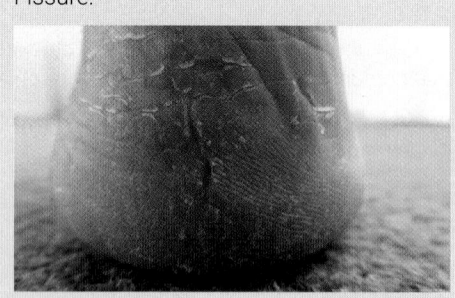

Erosion

Loss of part of the epidermis; depressed, moist, glistening; follows rupture of vesicle or bulla (varicella, variola after rupture)

Erosion.

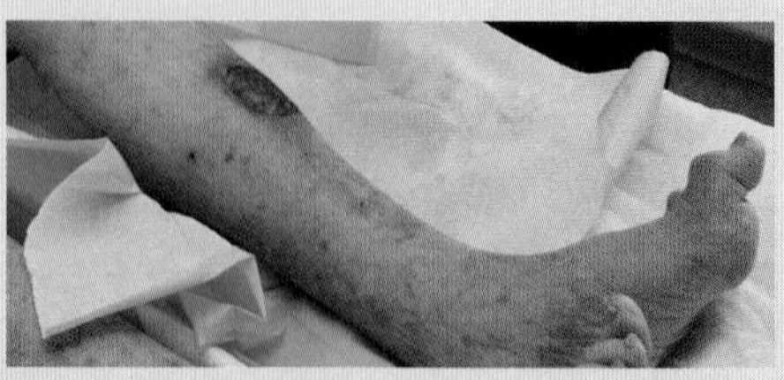

TABLE 19-2 Secondary Skin Lesions *(continued)*

Description (Examples)	
Ulcer	
Loss of the epidermis and dermis; concave; varies in size (decubiti, stasis ulcers)	Stasis ulcer. 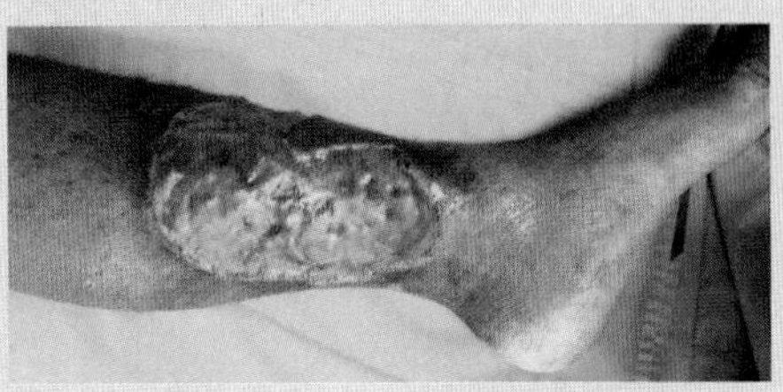 © Casa nayafana/Shutterstock
Crust	
Dried serum, blood, or purulent exudates; slightly elevated; size varies; brown, red, tan, or straw-colored (scab on abrasion, eczema)	Scab. 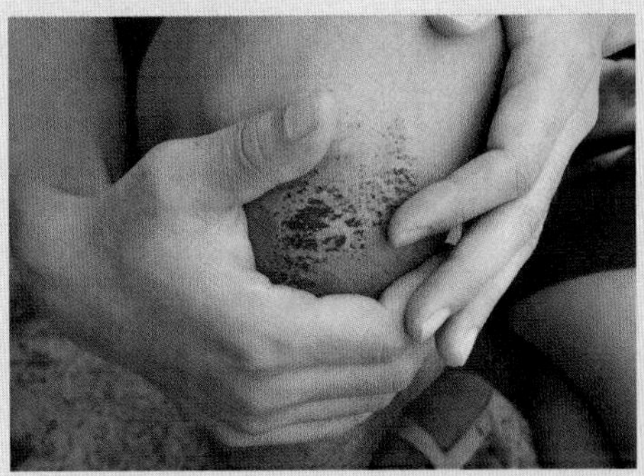 © Choke_AG/Shutterstock
Atrophy	
Thinning of skin surface and loss of skin markings; skin translucent and paperlike (striae; aged skin)	Striae. 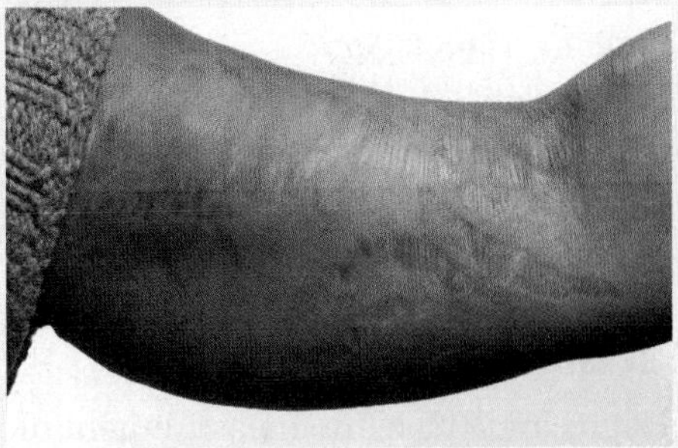 © SPL/Science Source.

Modified from: Thompson JM, Wilson SF. *Health Assessment for Nursing Practice*. 2nd ed. St. Louis, MO: Mosby; 2001.

Weight

Ideally a patient's body weight should be proportionate to height and sex (**FIGURE 19-9**). Weight conditions that are easily observed in the general survey include patients who are emaciated (extremely lean from lack of nutrition), plump, or obese (body weight that is 20% greater than the desirable body weight for a person's age, sex, height, and body build). A recent weight gain or loss is a key finding and may be clinically important. Like body height and build, body weight can reflect the patient's health, age, and lifestyle.

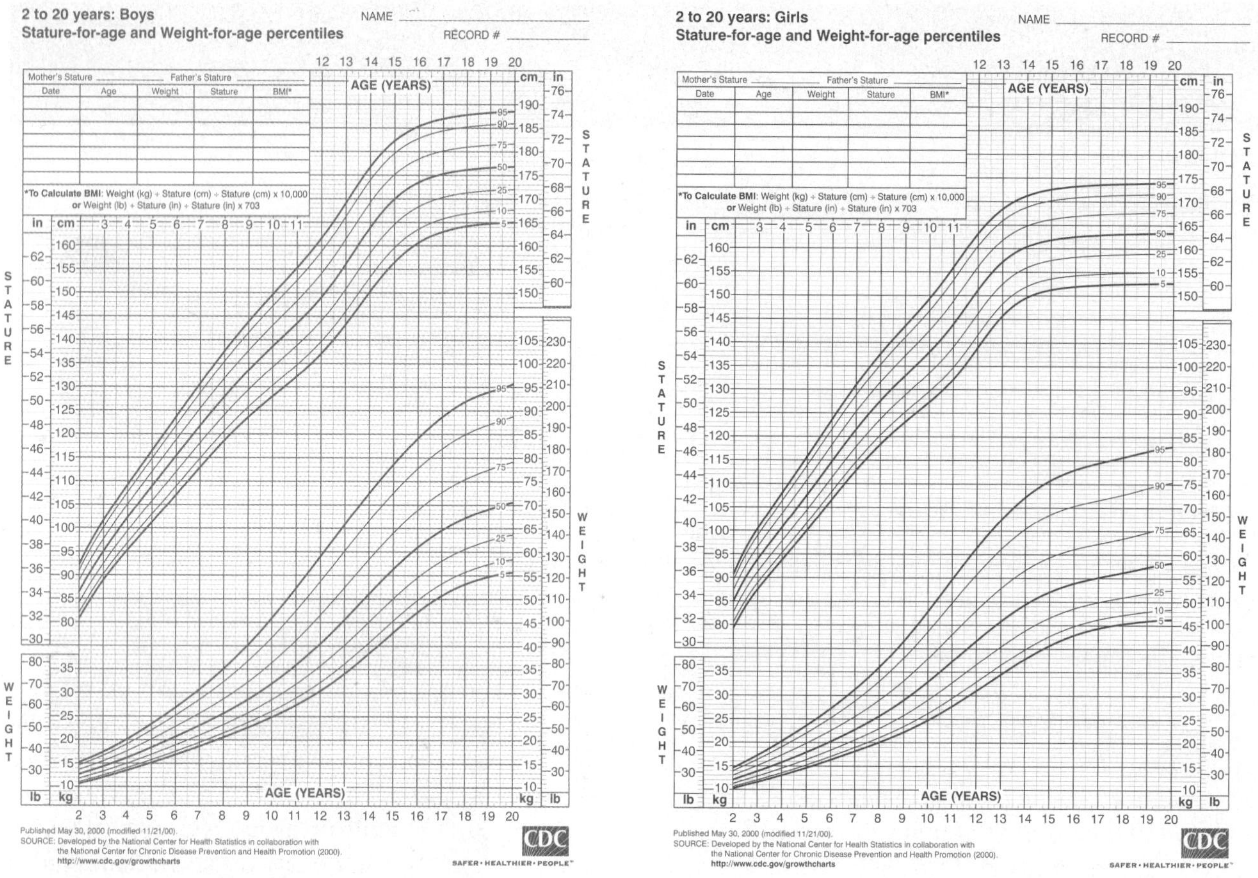

A

B

FIGURE 19-9 Physical growth curves and National Center for Health Statistics percentiles for children, ages 2 through 20 years, for height and weight. **A.** Boys. **B.** Girls.

Courtesy of Centers for Disease Control and Prevention.

> CRITICAL THINKING
>
> Think about three medical conditions that might result in significant weight loss. Now, think about three conditions that might cause a significant weight gain.

Vital Signs

Vital signs are a baseline measurement of function. They are used to assess respiration, pulse (circulation), and blood pressure (perfusion). The following is a brief overview of assessment of vital signs.

Respiration

The normal respiratory rate for adults is between 12 and 24 breaths/min.[2] The respiratory rate is assessed by watching the patient breathe, by feeling for chest movement, or by auscultating the lungs. Respirations are counted for 30 seconds and then multiplied by 2 to measure breaths per minute. Rhythm and depth of respirations are assessed by visualization and auscultation of the thorax. Abnormal findings include shallow, rapid, noisy, or deep breathing; asymmetrical chest wall movement; use of accessory muscles of respiration; or congested, unequal, or diminished breath sounds.

Pulse

A normal resting pulse rate for an adult is usually between 60 and 100 beats/min; it may be affected by the patient's age and physical condition (**TABLE 19-3**). For example, a child's awake pulse rate may be 80 to 205 beats/min. A well-trained athlete's pulse rate may be 45 to 60 beats/min. Factors such as pregnancy, anxiety, and fear also may produce an increased pulse rate in healthy people. In the literature, there is considerable variability in normal vital sign ranges for infants and children.

Pulse rates may be obtained at the carotid artery in the neck or at any site where the artery lies close to

TABLE 19-3 Average Vital Signs by Age

Age	Pulse (beats/min)	Respirations (breaths/min)	Blood Pressure, Systolic/ Diastolic (mm Hg)
Newborn	100–205	30–60	67–84/35–53
1 month to 1 year	100–190	30–53	72–104/37–56
1 to 2 years	98–140	22–37	86–106/42–63
3 to 5 years	80–120	20–28	89–112/46–72
6 to 12 years	75–118	18–25	97–120/57–80
12 to 15 years	70–90	12–20	110–131/64–83
Adult	60–100	12–20	<120/80

the skin. To evaluate the radial pulse, the paramedic places the pads of the index and middle fingers at the distal end of the patient's wrist, just medial to the radial styloid. If pulsations are regular, the paramedic should count for 15 seconds and multiply that number by 4 to determine the number of beats per minute. In addition to the number of times the heart beats per minute, the regularity and strength of the pulse also are important. For example, the pulse can be regular or irregular, weak or strong. Application of an ECG monitor is useful in evaluating cardiovascular status after initial assessment of the pulse.

Blood Pressure

The **systolic blood pressure** is the pressure exerted against the arterial walls when the heart contracts. The **diastolic blood pressure** is the pressure exerted against the arterial walls when the heart relaxes. For all age groups, ideal systolic blood pressure should be less than 120 mm Hg; diastolic pressure should be less than 80 mm Hg.[3] However, treatment usually does not begin until a person's blood pressure is well beyond these numbers: For adults older than 59 years, blood pressure typically exceeds 150/90 mm Hg before treatment is started; for adults 30 to 59 years, blood pressure exceeds 130/80 mm Hg.[4]

Blood pressure is best measured by auscultation or by an electronic device. As a general rule, measure by auscultation once to ensure concordance with the electronic method. The blood pressure cuff is placed on the patient's arm with the lower end of the cuff positioned 1 to 2 inches (3 to 5 cm) above the antecubital space. If measured manually, the cuff is inflated to a point about 30 mm Hg above where the brachial pulse can no longer be palpated. The stethoscope is placed over the brachial artery, and the cuff is slowly deflated at a rate of 2 to 3 mm Hg/sec. As the pressure falls, the paramedic should observe the gauge and note where the first sound or pulsation is heard. This point is the patient's systolic pressure. The point at which the sounds change in quality or become muffled is noted as the patient's diastolic pressure.

> **NOTE**
> At times, determining the correct diastolic pressure is difficult. The difference between the point of muffled tones and the complete disappearance of pulsations varies by person. In some people, the difference is a few millimeters of mercury; however, in others, pulsations never totally disappear. The ability to accurately measure diastolic pressures comes from experience and requires careful listening in a quiet setting.

Blood pressure may be estimated by palpation when vascular sounds are difficult to hear with a stethoscope because of environmental noise. However, this method is less accurate than auscultation is, and it allows only estimation of the systolic pressure. To estimate blood pressure by palpation, the paramedic should locate the brachial or radial pulse and apply the blood pressure cuff as described before. Finger contact should be maintained at the pulse site as the cuff slowly deflates. When the pulse becomes palpable, the gauge reading denotes the systolic pressure. Like pulse rates, a patient's blood pressure may be unusually high because of fear or anxiety. Other factors, such as a patient's age and normal level of physical activity, may be the cause of unusual blood pressure readings.

Alternate sites may be used to assess blood pressure when use of the patient's upper arm is not possible. Blood pressure readings in these alternate sites vary from those taken in the arm (**FIGURE 19-10**). Other methods used to assess oxygenation and perfusion include oxygen saturation, capnography (described in Chapter 15, *Airway Management, Respiration, and Artificial Ventilation*), and capillary refill (described in Chapter 18, *Scene Size-up and Primary Assessment*).

Examination of the Skin

The skin can reveal much information about a patient's status. Assessment includes evaluation of skin color, temperature, and moisture. A patient's skin color and the presence of bruises, lesions, or rashes may indicate serious illness or injury.

Skin temperature may be normal (warm), hot, or cold. Evaluations of temperature may have specific applications in some patient situations. Examples of such situations are febrile seizures and hyperthermic and hypothermic emergencies. Skin that is hot to the touch indicates a possible fever or heat-related

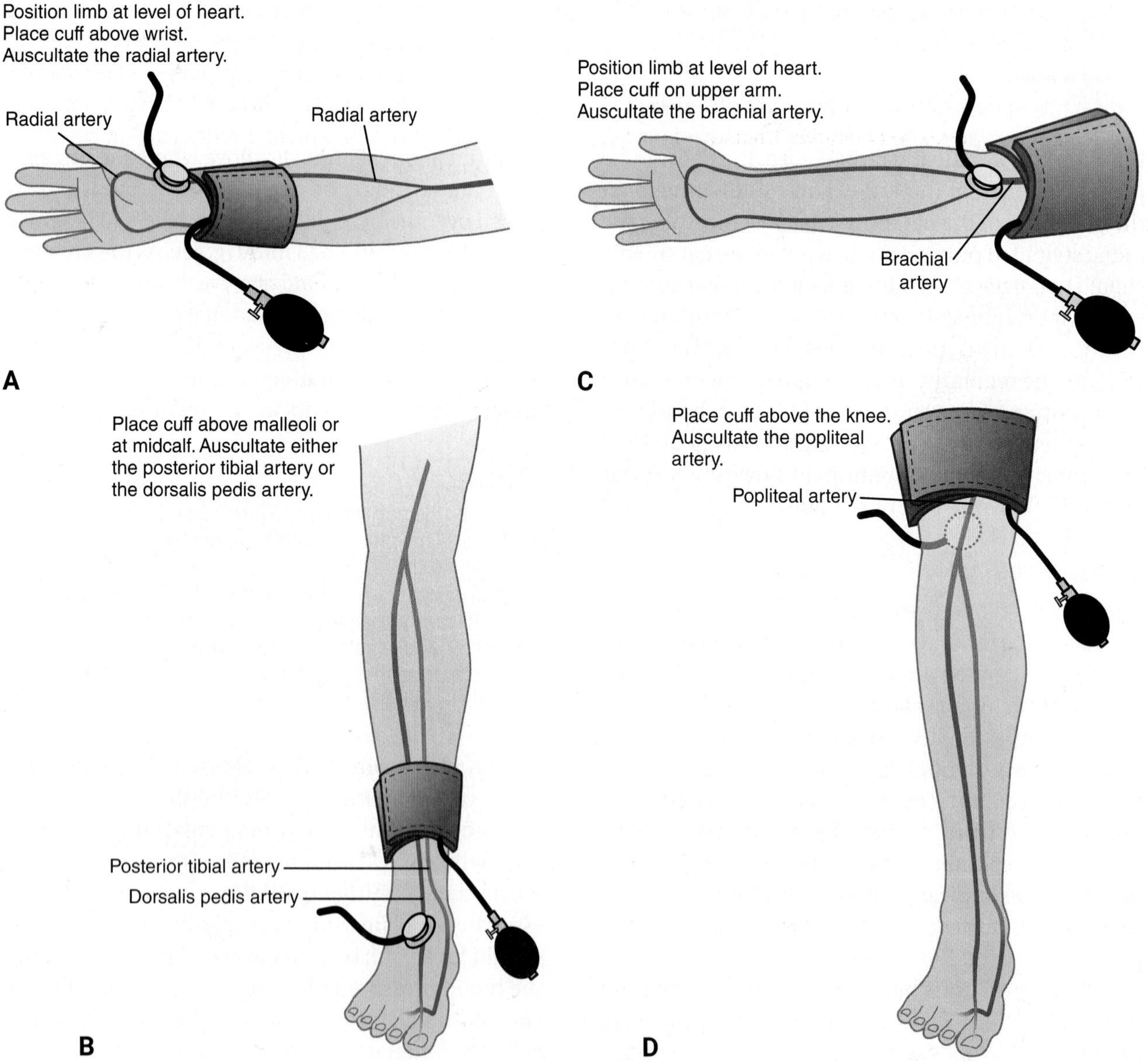

FIGURE 19-10 Blood pressure measurement sites. **A.** Radial artery. **B.** Dorsalis pedis and posterior tibial arteries. **C.** Brachial artery. **D.** Popliteal artery.

illness or injury. Cold skin may indicate decreased tissue perfusion and cold-related illness or injury. The dorsal surface of the hand is more sensitive than the palmar surface is and should be used to estimate body temperature. Normal body temperature is 37°C (98.6°F). Oral, axillary, tympanic, or rectal temperatures can be measured using electronic, digital, temporal (artery), digital dot, or tympanic-membrane thermometers (**FIGURE 19-11**). The temperature probe should be covered by a disposable sheath to help prevent cross-contamination. Temperatures obtained from each site will vary. In general, rectal temperatures are 0.5°C (0.9°F) higher than oral temperatures. Axillary and tympanic temperatures are generally 0.5°C (0.9°F) lower than oral temperatures.[5]

- **Oral measurement.** In patients older than 6 years, temperature is usually measured orally. The readings may be affected by crying, eating, drinking, smoking, oxygen administration by mask, or nebulizer treatments, and by the position of the thermometer in the patient's mouth. When using electronic devices, a brief tone will alert the paramedic when the measurement is complete. Children can be told to hold the thermometer in a "kiss" position and not to bite on the probe.
- **Axillary measurement.** The axillary site often is used to take the temperature in children younger than 6 years. The axilla also is used in children who are uncooperative or have diseases that suppress the immune system and in patients who have an altered level of consciousness. Axillary temperature is measured by placing the electronic probe firmly in the center of the patient's axillary space. The patient's arm should be held against the side of the chest. A tone will sound when the measurement is complete.
- **Tympanic measurement.** The tympanic membrane is close to the hypothalamus. This position

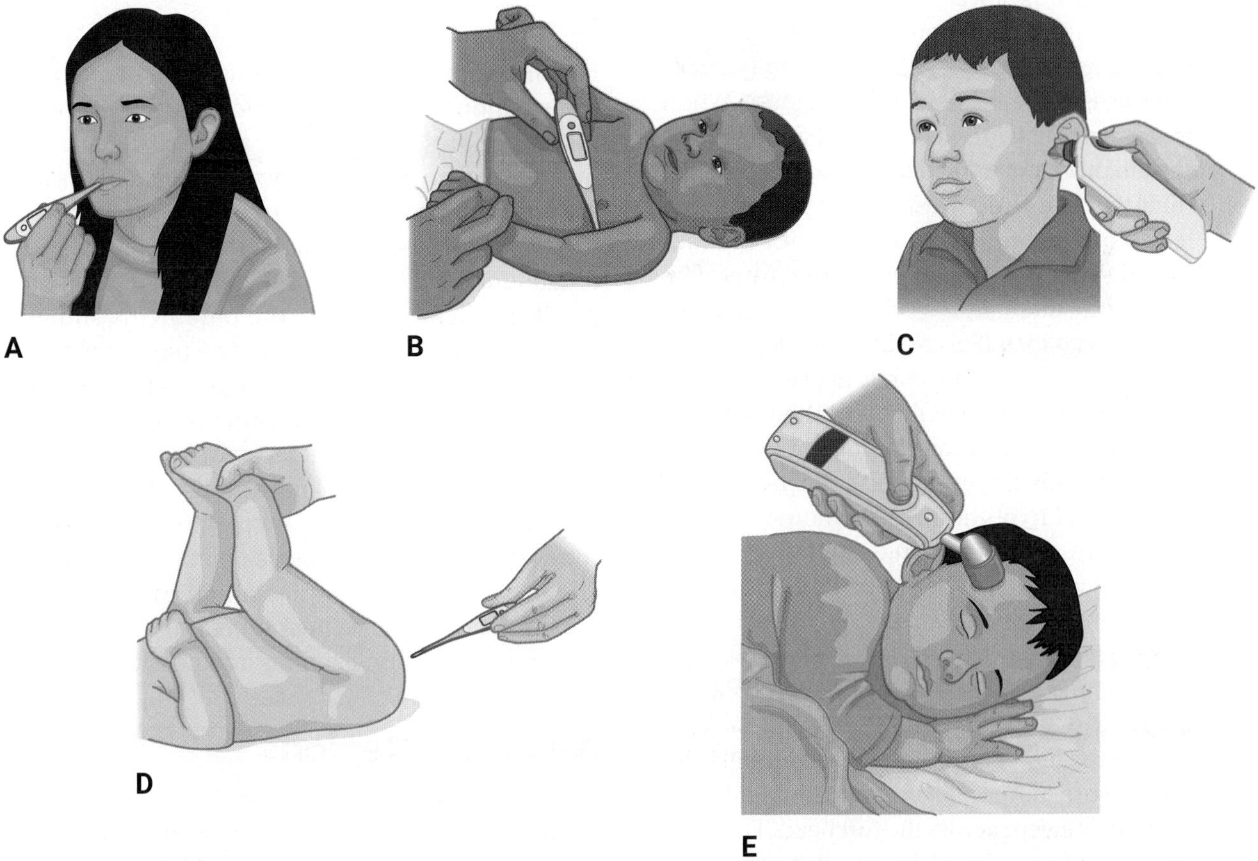

A B C D E

FIGURE 19-11 Temperature assessment. **A.** Oral temperature measurement. **B.** Axillary temperature measurement. **C.** Tympanic temperature measurement. **D.** Rectal temperature measurement. **E.** Temporal temperature assessment.

makes the tympanic membrane an ideal place to measure core temperature. The paramedic takes this measurement by placing the tip of the probe into the patient's ear canal. To obtain the most accurate reading, the ear canal should be straightened by gently pulling the pinna of the ear down and back in children younger than 3 years or up and back in patients older than 3 years. When the thermometer is in the correct position and is activated per the manufacturer's instructions, a temperature reading is obtained within seconds. Tympanic measurement is associated with significant variability in measurements. Readings can be inaccurate in patients who have had ear surgery, have otitis media or excessive cerumen (earwax), have recently exercised, are in situations involving extremes of temperature (eg, incubators, wind, fans), and are younger than 3 years.[4]

- **Rectal measurement.** Measuring a patient's temperature by the rectal route poses a risk of perforation. In addition, the method can be distressing for the patient. This route generally is reserved for young children and patients who have an altered level of consciousness. When measuring rectal temperature, the paramedic should place the patient in the supine position (infants). The patient also can be placed in the left lateral recumbent position with the legs raised. This position exposes the anus. The paramedic inserts a lubricated probe no more than 0.5 to 1 inch (2.5 cm) into the rectum. The probe should be held securely in place until the electronic device sounds the alert. Although rectal readings provide the most accurate assessment, they generally are impractical for prehospital use. Special hypothermic thermometers may be used to measure the rectal temperature of patients with hypothermia (see Chapter 44, *Environmental Conditions*).
- **Temporal measurement.** Temporal temperature measurement can be obtained quickly without discomfort to the patient. It can easily be used to measure temperature in infants and children. To measure temporal temperature, an infrared scanner is swept across the forehead. Then it is lifted and placed behind the ear. The temperature displays within seconds.[5] Hair, head coverings, diaphoresis, and sweating can interfere with the accuracy of readings.

NOTE

An esophageal temperature probe can provide a continuous assessment of core temperature in patients older than 16 years. The procedure is most often used in emergency care to support therapeutic hypothermia after cardiac arrest and when there are concerns for significant hyperthermia or significant hypothermia. The use of these devices requires special training and authorization from medical direction.

Modified from: Makic MB, Lovett K, Azam MF. Placement of an esophageal temperature probe by nurses. *AACN Adv Crit Care*. 2012;23(1):24-31.

Skin moisture usually is classified as dry or wet. Dry skin is normal. Wet skin is clammy or diaphoretic. Diaphoretic skin may indicate a volume problem such as hypovolemia. It may also indicate other illness or injury that results in decreased tissue perfusion or increased sweat gland activity. Examples are cardiovascular and heat-related emergencies, respectively.

Pupils

Examining the pupils for response to light may yield information on the neurologic status of some patients. Unequal pupils (**anisocoria**) may be a normal finding in some patients. However, the pupils usually are equal and constrict when exposed to light. The acronym **PERRL** indicates that the Pupils are Equal and Round, and Reactive to Light. When testing the pupils for light response, the paramedic shines a penlight directly into one eye. The normal reaction is for the pupil exposed to the light to constrict. This occurs with a consensual constriction of the opposite eye. The paramedic should test for accommodation by asking the patient to look at a distant object. The pupils should dilate. The paramedic should then ask the patient to focus on a close object about 3 inches (7 to 8 cm) away. The pupils should constrict as the patient focuses on the near object. **TABLE 19-4** lists abnormal pupillary reactions and possible causes.

Anatomic Regions

The remainder of this chapter discusses techniques of the physical examination as they relate to anatomic regions of the body. The paramedic should recall that anatomic and physiologic aspects of the human body are age-related and vary by person. An examination of the anatomic regions should be guided by a patient's

TABLE 19-4 Abnormal Pupil Reactions

Pupil Size	Possible Causes
Equal	
Dilated or unresponsive	Cardiac arrest, central nervous system injury, hypoxia or anoxia, drug use (LSD [lysergic acid diethylamide], atropine, amphetamines)
Constricted or unresponsive	Central nervous system injury or disease, narcotic drug use (heroin, fentanyl), eye medications
Unequal	
One dilated or unresponsive	Cerebrovascular accident, head injury, direct trauma to eye, eye medications

chief complaint. A full examination of all regions often is not necessary in the emergency setting, but will be described here for a complete discussion. Chapter 10, *Review of Human Systems*, serves as a review of anatomic regions of the body.

Skin

The general assessment of the skin was described previously. In addition, the comprehensive physical examination should include an evaluation of the texture of the skin, hair, and nails (all parts of the integumentary system), as well as the turgor of the skin.[2]

Texture and Turgor

The texture of the skin normally is smooth, soft, and flexible. However, in older adults the skin may be wrinkled and leathery from decreased amounts of collagen and subcutaneous fat as well as reduced secretion from sweat glands. Abnormal skin texture may result from lesions, rashes, tumors, endocrine disorders, and localized trauma.

Turgor refers to the elasticity of the skin (which normally decreases with age). To test skin turgor, the paramedic should pinch ("tent") a fold of skin and assess how quickly and easily the skin returns to its normal position. Skin on the forehead is the most reliable area to look for loss of skin turgor as it is less affected by age-dependent changes. Tented skin that does not quickly return to its normal position may indicate dehydration (**FIGURE 19-12**).

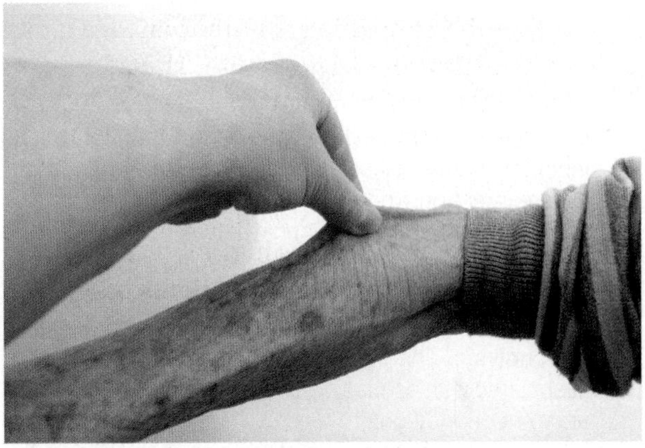

FIGURE 19-12 Assessing skin turgor.

Hair

As part of the examination, the paramedic should inspect and palpate the patient's hair. The paramedic should note quantity, distribution, and texture. Key findings include a recent change in the growth or loss of hair. These changes may result from poor nutrition, chemotherapy, or hormonal changes (eg, hypothyroidism, menopause), or be related to the use of hair products. Thinning hair is common in older men and women.

Fingernails and Toenails

The paramedic should note the color and shape of the patient's fingernails and toenails and assess for the presence or absence of lesions. Uncolored nails usually are transparent. Healthy nails are smooth and firm on palpation. BOX 19-4 describes abnormal findings in the nails. With age, nails often develop longitudinal striations and may have a yellow tint because of insufficient calcium.

Head, Ears, Eyes, Nose, and Throat

An examination of the structures of the head and neck involves inspection, palpation, and auscultation.

Head and Face

To examine the head, the paramedic should inspect the skull for shape and symmetry, keeping in mind that hair can hide abnormalities. The hair should be parted in several places to assess for scaliness, lumps, or other lesions. The assessment should use a systematic palpation, moving from front to back, noting any swelling, tenderness, indentations, or depressions.

BOX 19-4 Abnormal Nail Findings

- **Beau lines.** Transverse deprssions in the nail that inhibit nail growth; associated with systemic illness, severe infection, and nail injury.
- **Clubbing.** A change in the angle between the nail and nail base that approaches or exceeds 180°; associated with flattening and often enlargement of the fingertips; may indicate chronic cardiac or respiratory disease.
- **Onycholysis.** The separation of a nail from its bed; associated with psoriasis, dermatitis, fungal infection, and other conditions.
- **Paronychia.** Inflammation of the skin at the base of the nail; may result from local infection or trauma.
- **Psoriasis.** Pitting, discoloration, and subungual thickening of the nail plate; may lead to splinter hemorrhages.
- **Splinter hemorrhages.** Red or brown linear streaks in the nail bed; associated with minor nail trauma, bacterial endocarditis, and trichinosis.
- **Terry's nails.** The presence of transverse white bands that cover the nail except for a narrow zone at the distal tip; associated with cirrhosis.
- **Transverse white lines.** Longitudinal white streaks in the nail plate; may indicate a systemic disorder.
- **White spots.** The presence of white spots that appear in the nail plate; usually result from minor injury or cuticle manipulation.

The scalp should move freely over the skull, and the patient should be free of pain or discomfort during the examination.

The face should be inspected for symmetry, expression, and contour, noting any asymmetry, involuntary movements, masses, or edema. The paramedic should evaluate facial skin for color, pigmentation, texture, thickness, hair distribution, and any lesions.

Eyes

The paramedic should verify that vision is present in both eyes. Basic information is gathered during the patient history and by asking the patient about any visual disturbances. Visual acuity can be assessed by asking the patient to read printed material or count fingers at a distance and by checking the patient's ability to distinguish light from dark using various eye charts (eg, Snellen chart) (**FIGURE 19-13**).

Both eyes should move equally well in the **six cardinal fields of gaze** (**FIGURE 19-14**). To evaluate a patient's gaze, the paramedic should hold the patient's chin. The patient's eyes should be observed as they track a penlight or finger (or a toy, in the case of a child) when it moves through the six visual fields in an H pattern. Any **nystagmus** (involuntary jerking movements of the eyes) or **dysconjugate gaze** failure of the eyes to move with synchronized motion should be noted. Another method to check visual fields is to ask the patient to look at his or her nose. The paramedic then extends his or her arms with elbows at right angles and wiggles both index fingers at the same time to test peripheral vision. Asking the patient to identify finger movements and to track a moving object can demonstrate if visual fields are grossly normal. This test should be performed in four quadrants (up, down, right, and left). The eyes should also be assessed for normal position and alignment.

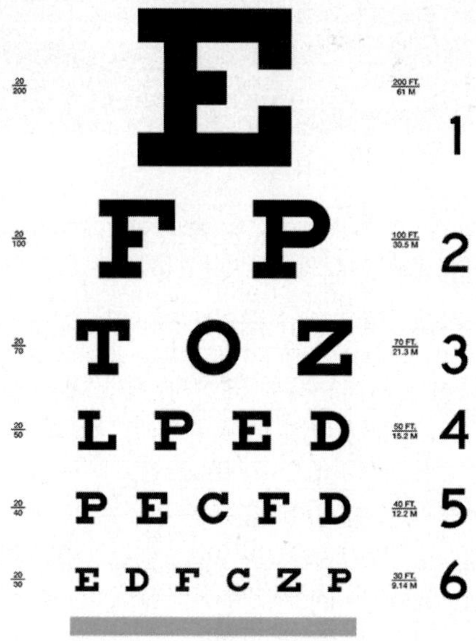

FIGURE 19-13 Snellen chart.

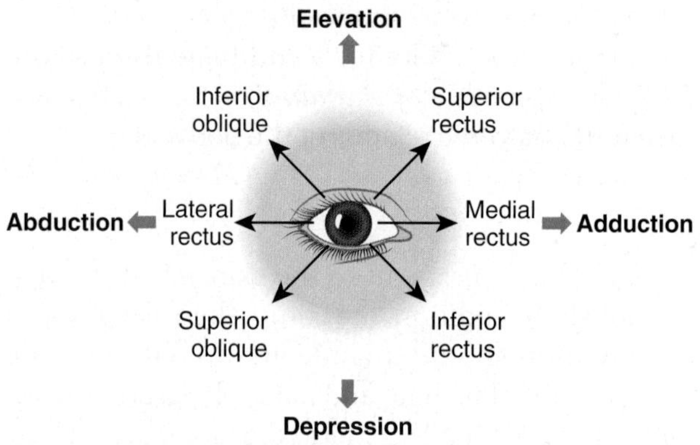

FIGURE 19-14 Six cardinal fields of gaze. Cranial nerves and extraocular muscles associated with the six cardinal fields of gaze.

CRITICAL THINKING

When you perform an examination of the eyes, you are evaluating components of at least four body systems. What are they?

The patient's orbital area should be assessed for edema and puffiness. The eyebrows should be free of scaliness. Inspection of the eyelids consists of noting the width of palpebral fissures (the elliptical opening between the upper and lower lids), edema, color, lesions, condition and direction of the eyelashes, adequacy of lid closure, and drainage. The paramedic also should inspect the regions of the lacrimal gland and lacrimal sac for swelling. Excessive tearing or dryness of the eye should be noted (see Chapter 10, *Review of Human Systems*).

The patient's conjunctiva and sclera are examined by asking the patient to look up while the paramedic depresses both lower lids with the thumbs (**FIGURE 19-15**). The sclera should be white; the cornea and the iris should be clearly visible; and the pupils should be of equal size, round, and reactive to light. Palpating the patient's lower orbital rim determines structural integrity. The paramedic should be alert to the presence of contact lenses and ocular prostheses when examining a patient's eyes.

The ophthalmoscope is used to assess the cornea for foreign bodies, lacerations, abrasions, and infection; the anterior chamber for the presence of blood or pus; and under the eyelid for the presence of foreign bodies. In addition, the retinal vessels, the optic nerve, and the retina of the fundus can be examined along with the vitreous. Ophthalmoscopic examinations should be performed in a darkened room so that the pupils are dilated. Contact lenses do not need to be removed.

To perform an examination with an ophthalmoscope, the paramedic should follow these steps for each eye:

1. Ask the patient to fixate on a distant object.
2. Sit facing the patient at the same seat height.
3. Turn on the ophthalmoscope light and select the 0 lens setting.
4. Use the right hand and eye to examine the patient's right eye and the left hand and eye to examine the patient's left eye.
5. Direct the patient to look over your shoulder, keeping both eyes open.
6. Hold the scope against your face and shine the light on the patient's pupil at a distance of about 10 inches (25 cm) from the face and at a 45° angle. A bright orange glow in the pupil ("red reflex") normally is visible (**FIGURE 19-16**).
7. Move the light slowly toward the pupil to see the structures of the fundus. Rotate the lens to improve focus as needed.
8. Inspect the size, color, and clarity of the disk and the integrity of vessels; assess for retinal lesions and the appearance of the macula. A normal examination will reveal the following (**FIGURE 19-17**):[5]
   - A clear, yellow optic nerve disk
   - Yellow to creamy-pink retina (depending on patient's race)
   - Light red arteries and dark red veins

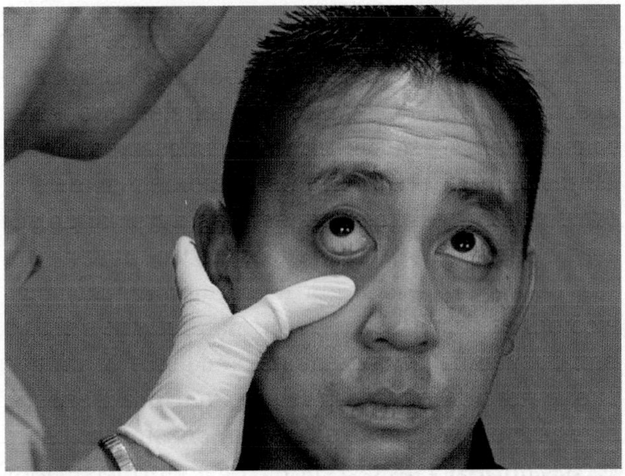

FIGURE 19-15 Examining the cornea and sclera.

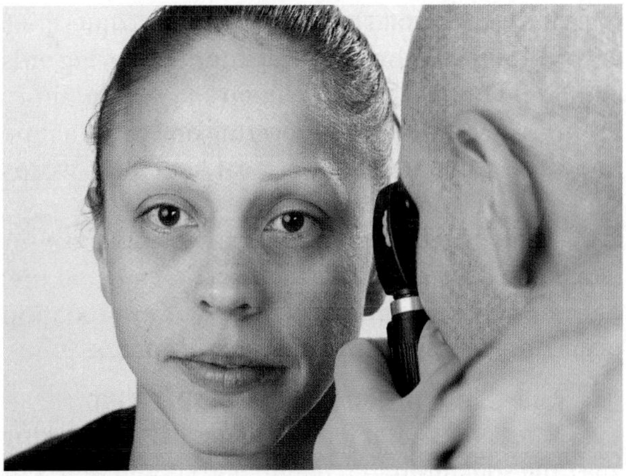

FIGURE 19-16 Paramedic using an ophthalmoscope.

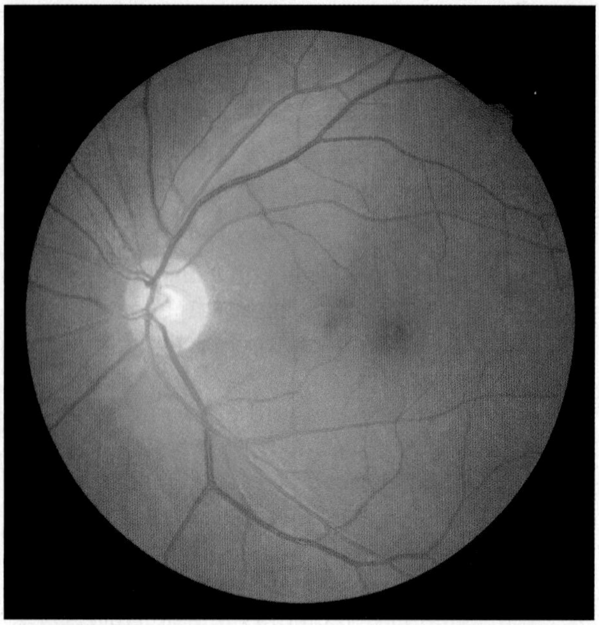

FIGURE 19-17 Normal fundus examination.

- A 3:2 vein-to-artery ratio in size proportion
- The avascular macula

Ears

The paramedic should inspect the external ear and surrounding tissues for signs of bruising, deformity, or discoloration. No discharge should be present in either ear canal. Pulling gently on the earlobes should not produce pain or discomfort. The patient's skull and facial bones surrounding the ear should be palpated. The mastoid area should be inspected for tenderness or discoloration. A patient who is alert and able to hear and who speaks the same language as the paramedic should be able to respond to questions without many requests for repetition. Hearing aids should be noted. An assessment of gross auditory keenness can be made by covering one ear at a time and asking the patient to repeat short test words spoken in soft and loud tones.

An otoscope is used to evaluate the inner ear for discharge and foreign bodies and to assess the eardrum. The paramedic performs an otoscopic examination using the following steps for each ear (**FIGURE 19-18**):

1. Select the appropriate size of speculum.
2. Check the ear for foreign bodies before inserting the speculum.
3. Instruct the patient not to move during the examination to avoid injury to the canal and tympanic membrane. (Infants and young children may need to be restrained.)

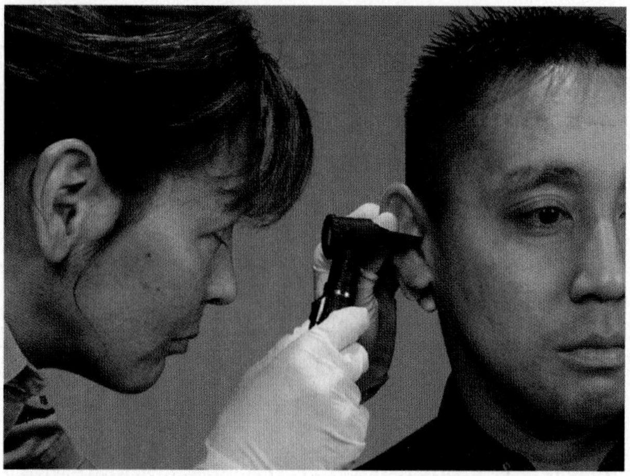

FIGURE 19-18 Paramedic performing an otoscopic exam.

4. Turn on the otoscope and insert the speculum into the ear canal, slightly down and forward. To ease insertion, pull the auricle up and backward in adults; pull back and downward in infants.
5. Identify cerumen and look for foreign bodies, lesions, or discharge.
6. Visualize and inspect the tympanic membrane for tears or breaks. A normal examination will reveal the following:
   - Cerumen will be dry (tan or light yellow) or moist (dark yellow or brown).
   - The ear canal should not be inflamed (a sign of infection).
   - The tympanic membrane should be translucent or pearly gray (pink or red indicates inflammation).

Nose

The patient's nose should be inspected for shape, size, color, and stability. The column of the nose should be midline with the face and the nares positioned symmetrically. (Slight asymmetry of nares is considered normal.) The paramedic should palpate the column of the nose and surrounding soft tissues for pain, tenderness, or deformity. The frontal and maxillary sinuses may be inspected for the presence of swelling. They may also be palpated for tenderness along the bony brow on each side of the nose and the zygomatic processes.

Discharge from the nose can have several causes. For example, cerebrospinal fluid may be present as a result of head trauma; a bloody discharge (**epistaxis**) may result from trauma or from mucosal erosions involving blood vessels, hypertension, or bleeding disorders. A discharge of mucus commonly results from allergy, upper respiratory tract infection, sinusitis, or cold exposure.

Mouth and Pharynx

The paramedic should inspect the lips for symmetry, color, edema, and skin surface irregularities. The lips should be pink. Pallor of the lips is associated with anemia; cyanosis is associated with cardiorespiratory insufficiency; red lips sometimes are a late finding in carbon monoxide poisoning (see Chapter 33, *Toxicology*). The lips should show no swelling, deformity, or pain on palpation.

Healthy gums in the oral cavity are pink and free of lesions and swelling. Patchy areas of pigmentation in the mouths of African Americans are not uncommon. Enlarged gums may indicate pregnancy, leukemia, poor oral hygiene, puberty, or use of some medications (eg, phenytoin). The mouth should be free of loose or broken teeth. Dental appliances may be present.

The patient's tongue should be inspected for size and color. The tongue should be positioned in the midline of the oral cavity and appear nonswollen, dull red, moist, and glistening. To inspect the oropharynx, a tongue blade is used to depress the patient's tongue. The normal palate is white or pink. If the oral cavity is inflamed or covered with exudate, an infection may be present. (Specific breath odors may indicate alcohol or other drug consumption or illness.) The tonsils normally are pink and smooth without edema, ulceration, or inflammation. A patient with a typical sore throat often has a reddened and edematous uvula and tonsillar pillars. A yellow exudate sometimes is present.

Neck

The paramedic should inspect the neck in the patient's normal anatomic position. If trauma is suspected, spinal precautions should be used. The trachea should be midline. No use of accessory muscles or tracheal tugging should occur during respiration. To palpate the neck, the paramedic places both thumbs along the sides of the distal trachea and systematically moves the hands toward the head (**FIGURE 19-19**). Care should be taken not to apply bilateral pressure to the carotid arteries because syncope or bradycardia may result.

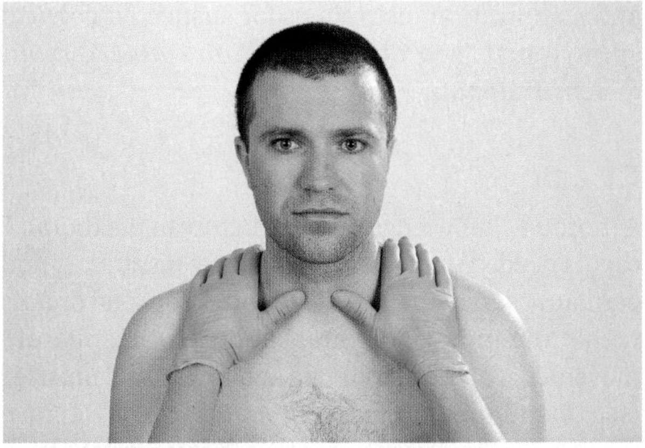

FIGURE 19-19 Position of the thumbs to evaluate the midline position of the trachea.

The lymph nodes should not be tender. Tender or swollen lymph nodes usually are the result of inflammation. The thyroid and cricoid cartilages should be free of pain and should move when the patient swallows. Bubbling or crackling sensations observed during palpation of the soft tissues of the neck may indicate the presence of **subcutaneous emphysema** (the presence of air in the subcutaneous tissues). The paramedic should note distended neck veins or prominent carotid arteries (see Chapter 21, *Cardiology*).

Head and Cervical Spine

The temporomandibular joint connects the mandible of the jaw to the temporal bone of the skull. The joint sometimes can become painful or dislocated. Normally the patient should be able to open and close the mouth without pain or limitation in movement. Temporomandibular joint dysfunction is a common complaint.

For the patient who has not undergone trauma, the paramedic should inspect the cervical spine by palpating for tenderness or deformities. Range of motion can be tested in the following manner:

- **Flexion.** Touching the chin to the chest
- **Rotation.** Touching the chin to each shoulder
- **Lateral bending.** Touching each ear to each shoulder
- **Extension.** Tilting the head backward

The neck of a trauma patient may need to be moved for a general or neurologic examination. Any such movement may be implemented only after ruling out the need for continuous manual protection and stabilization techniques for suspected cervical spine injury (see Chapter 40, *Spine and Nervous System Trauma*).

Chest

A thorough knowledge of the structure of the thoracic cage is needed to perform an adequate respiratory and cardiac assessment. The ribs protect the vital organs within the thorax and offer support for respiratory movements of the diaphragm and intercostal muscles (see Chapter 10, *Review of Human Systems*). Damage to the actual bony structure of the thoracic cavity, such as a flail chest, can prevent or limit respiratory function. The ribs of the thorax also are used as anatomic landmarks in locating specific areas for examination. **FIGURE 19-20** shows the landmarks of the chest. The thorax can be evaluated by using imaginary lines to help describe the location of examination findings (**FIGURE 19-21**). The thorax is assessed through inspection, palpation, percussion, and auscultation.

Inspection

The patient's chest wall should be inspected for symmetry on the anterior and posterior surfaces. The thorax is not completely symmetrical. However, a visual inspection of one side should offer a reasonable comparison with the other side. Chest wall diameter often is increased in patients with obstructive pulmonary disease, resulting in a barrel-shaped appearance of the thorax. Other causes for chest wall deformities or asymmetry include the following (**FIGURE 19-22**):

- **Funnel chest.** An indentation of the lower sternum above the xiphoid process
- **Pigeon chest.** A prominent sternal protrusion
- **Thoracic kyphosis.** Concave curvature of the thoracic segment of the vertebral column
- **Scoliosis.** A lateral deviation of the spine that results in an abnormal curvature

> CRITICAL THINKING
> Evaluate breathing in a supine patient or friend while standing to the person's side, then at the head, and finally at the feet. Which position provides the best view of the symmetry of the thorax?

The paramedic should inspect the skin and nipples for cyanosis and pallor. The presence of suture lines from chest wall surgery, skin pockets enclosing implanted pacemaker devices, implanted central venous lines or ports, and dermal medication patches (eg, nitroglycerin, fentanyl) should be noted. The pattern or rhythm of the patient's respirations should be assessed, noting any use of accessory respiratory muscles (eg, intercostal or supraclavicular retractions or both). In addition, observing the rise and fall of the patient's chest during breathing provides a rough measurement of **tidal volume** (see Chapter 15, *Airway Management, Respiration, and Artificial Ventilation*).

Palpation

The paramedic should palpate the thorax for pulsations, tenderness, bulges, depressions, crepitus, subcutaneous emphysema, and unusual movement and position. The examination begins by noting the position of the patient's trachea, which should be midline and directly above the sternal notch. Starting with the patient's clavicles, both sides of the patient's chest wall are firmly palpated at the same time, front to back and right side to left side. The examination should proceed systematically without pain or discomfort.

To evaluate the anterior chest wall for equal expansion during inspiration, the paramedic places both thumbs along the patient's costal margin and the xiphoid process. The palms should be lying flat on the chest wall. Equal movement should occur as the patient inhales and exhales. The posterior chest

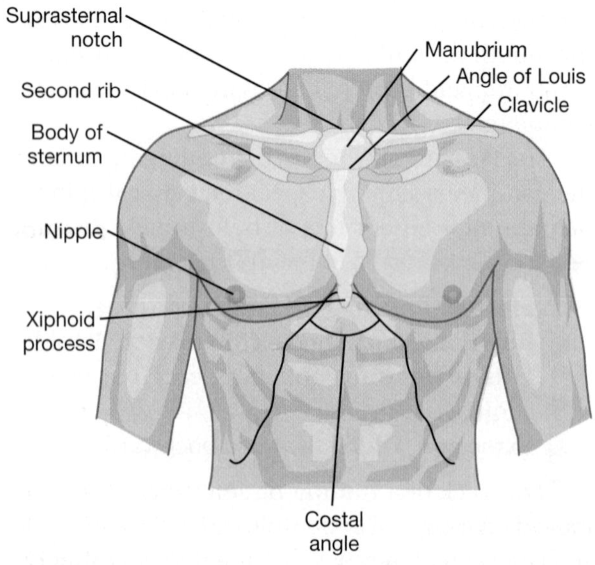

FIGURE 19-20 Topographic landmarks of the chest.

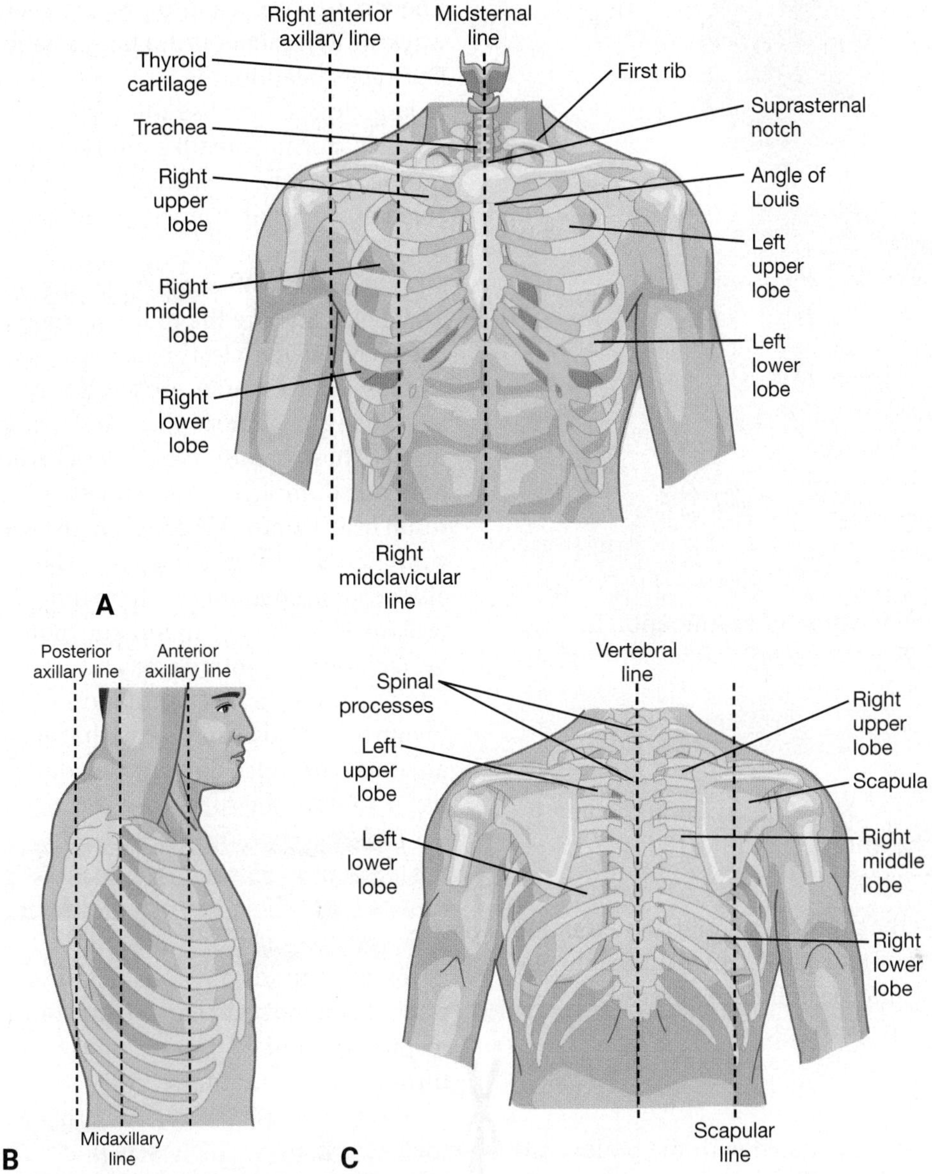

FIGURE 19-21 Thoracic landmarks. **A.** Anterior thorax. **B.** Right lateral thorax. **C.** Posterior thorax.

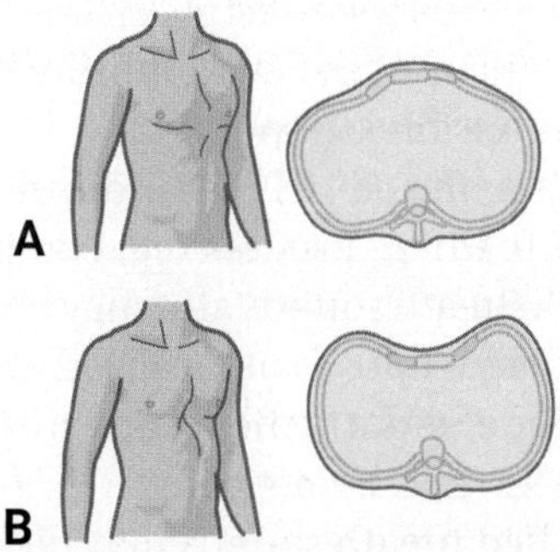

FIGURE 19-22 Chest wall deformities. **A.** Pigeon chest. **B.** Funnel chest.

wall should be examined for symmetrical respiratory movement by placing the thumbs along the spinous processes at the level of the 10th ribs (**FIGURE 19-23**).

Percussion

The paramedic should perform percussion in symmetrical locations from side to side to compare the percussion note (**FIGURE 19-24**). Resonance usually is heard over all areas of healthy lungs. Hyperresonance is associated with overinflation, or hyperinflation, of the lungs. Hyperresonance may indicate pulmonary disease, pneumothorax, or asthma. Dullness or

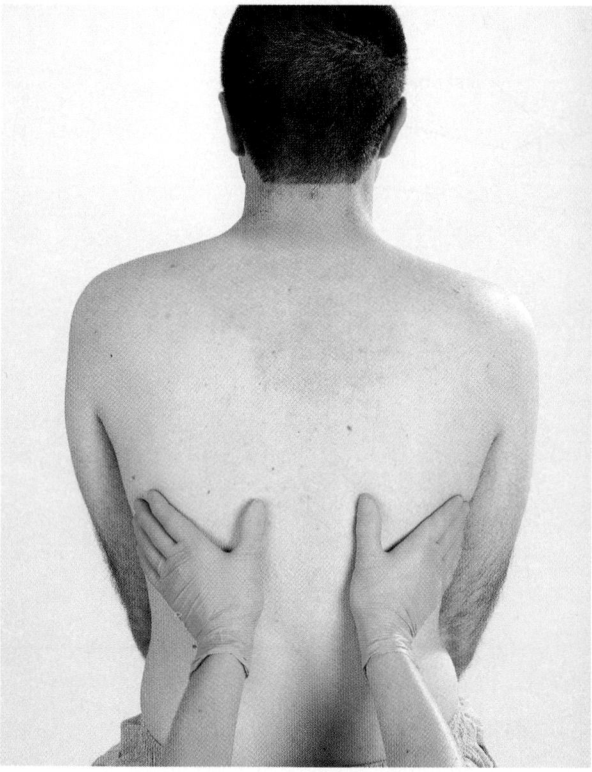

FIGURE 19-23 Palpating the thoracic expansion. The thumbs are at the level of the 10th ribs.

flatness suggests the presence of fluid or pulmonary congestion. The level and movement of the diaphragm during breathing may be limited by disease (eg, emphysema, tumor) or pain (eg, rib fracture).

Auscultation

The thorax is best auscultated with the patient sitting upright (if possible). The patient should breathe deeply and slowly through an open mouth during the examination. The paramedic should be alert to the chance of resulting hyperventilation and fatigue that may occur in ill and older patients.

The diaphragm of the stethoscope is used to auscultate the high-pitched sounds of the patient's lungs. The paramedic holds the stethoscope firmly on the patient's skin and listens carefully as the patient breathes. The chest auscultation should be systematic and thorough. Auscultation should allow evaluation of the anterior and the posterior lung fields.

The movement of air through the respiratory tract creates turbulence, producing breath sounds during inhalation and exhalation. During inhalation, air moves first into the trachea and major bronchi. The air then moves into progressively smaller airways until it reaches its final destination, the alveoli. During exhalation, the air flows from small airways to larger ones. Because this airflow creates less turbulence, normal breath sounds generally are louder during inspiration. Normal breath sounds are classified as vesicular, bronchovesicular, and bronchial (**FIGURE 19-25**).

Vesicular breath sounds are heard over most of the lung fields and are the major normal breath sound. Lungs considered "clear" make normal vesicular breath sounds. These sounds are low pitched and soft and have a long inspiratory phase and a shorter expiratory phase. These breath sounds are classified further as harsh or diminished. Harsh vesicular sounds may result from vigorous exercise. With vigorous exercise, ventilations are rapid and deep. These harsh sounds also occur in children who have thin and elastic chest walls in which breath sounds are more easily audible. Vesicular breath sounds may be diminished in older adults who have less ventilation volume. Vesicular breath sounds also may be diminished in people who are obese or muscular, whose additional overlying tissue muffles the sound.

Bronchovesicular breath sounds are heard over the major bronchi and in the posterior chest between the scapula. These sounds are louder and harsher than are vesicular breath sounds. Bronchovesicular breath sounds are considered to be of medium pitch. Bronchovesicular breath sounds have equal inspiration and expiration phases. They are heard throughout respiration.

Bronchial breath sounds are heard only over the trachea and are the highest in pitch. They are coarse, harsh, loud sounds with a short inspiratory phase and a long expiration. A bronchial sound heard anywhere but over the trachea is considered an abnormal breath sound.

Abnormal breath sounds are classified as absent, diminished, incorrectly located bronchial sounds, and adventitious breath sounds.

Absent breath sounds may indicate total cessation of the breathing process (eg, complete airway obstruction). Breath sounds also may be absent only in a specific area. Causes of localized absent breath sounds include endotracheal tube misplacement, pneumothorax, and hemothorax.

Diminished breath sounds may result from any condition that lessens the airflow. Examples include endotracheal tube misplacement, pneumothorax,

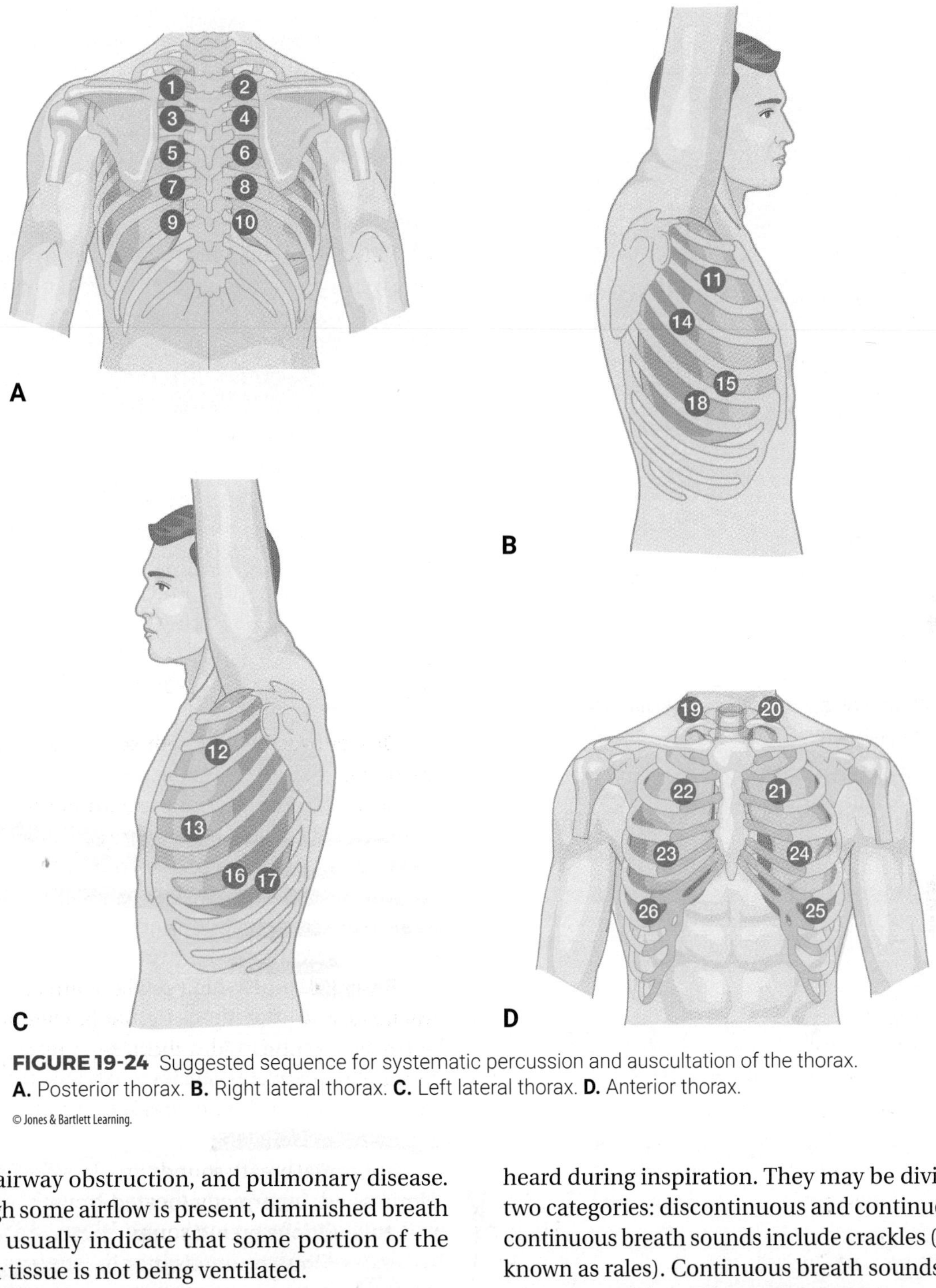

FIGURE 19-24 Suggested sequence for systematic percussion and auscultation of the thorax. **A.** Posterior thorax. **B.** Right lateral thorax. **C.** Left lateral thorax. **D.** Anterior thorax.

partial airway obstruction, and pulmonary disease. Although some airflow is present, diminished breath sounds usually indicate that some portion of the alveolar tissue is not being ventilated.

Bronchial breath sounds auscultated in the peripheral lung field indicate the presence of fluid or exudate in the alveoli. Either of these conditions may block airflow. Diseases that contribute to this condition are tumors, pneumonia, and pulmonary edema.

Adventitious breath sounds result from obstruction of the large or small airways, are heard in addition to normal breath sounds, and are most commonly heard during inspiration. They may be divided into two categories: discontinuous and continuous. Discontinuous breath sounds include crackles (formerly known as rales). Continuous breath sounds include wheezes and rhonchi (**FIGURE 19-26**).

A **crackle** is the high-pitched, discontinuous sound that usually is heard during the end of inspiration. The sound is similar to the sound of hair being rubbed between the fingers. Crackles are caused by the disruptive passage of air in the small airways or alveoli, or both, and may be heard anywhere in the peripheral lung field.

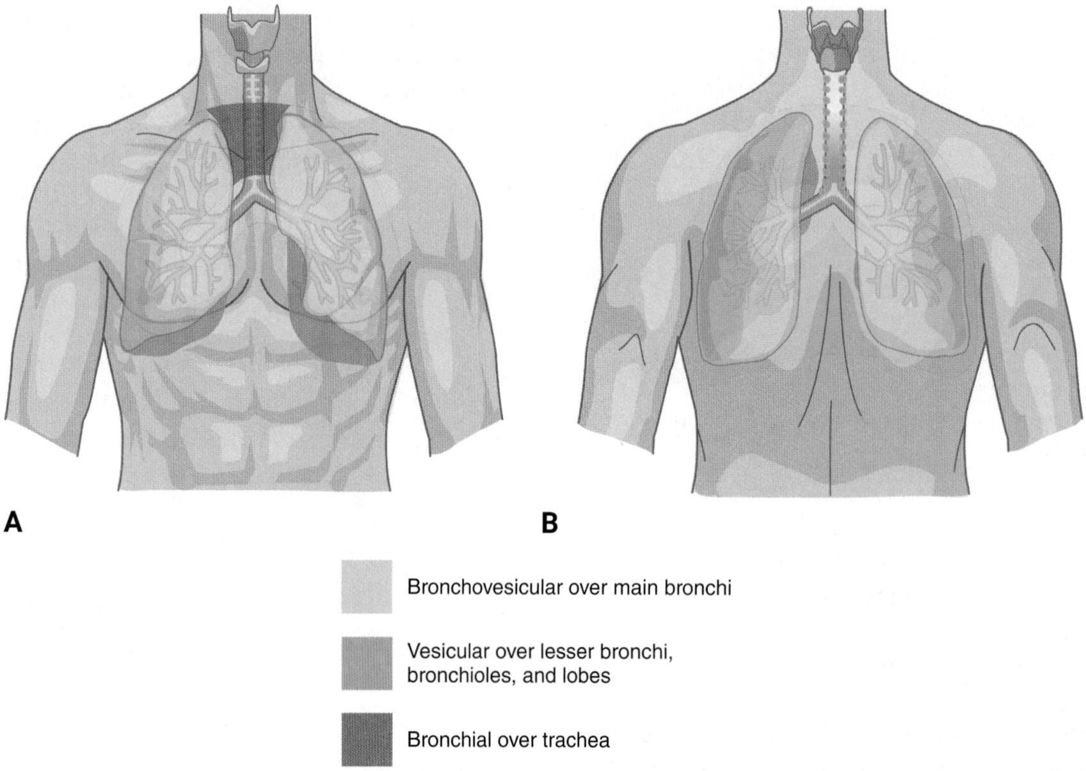

FIGURE 19-25 Expected auscultatory sounds. **A.** Anterior view. **B.** Posterior view.

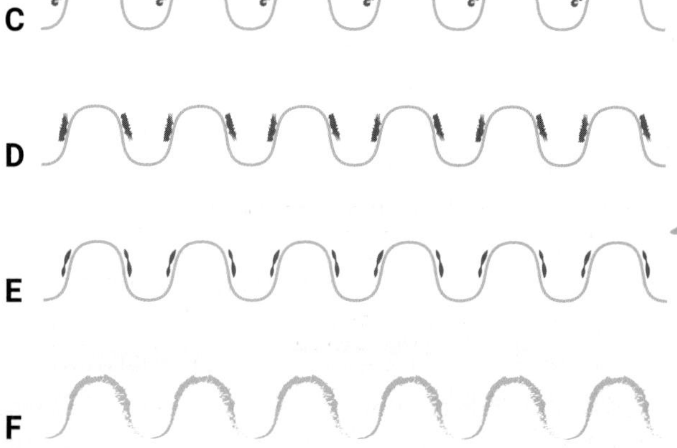

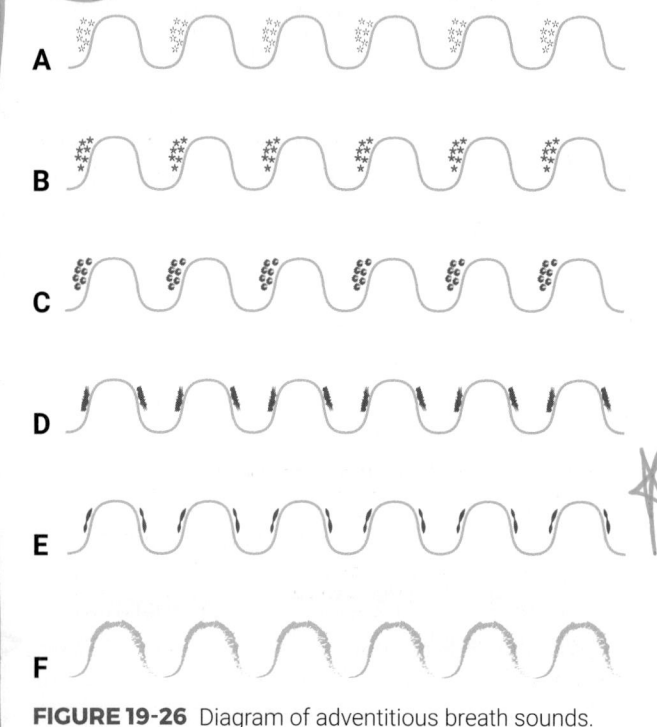

FIGURE 19-26 Diagram of adventitious breath sounds. **A.** Fine crackles. **B.** Medium crackles. **C.** Coarse crackles. **D.** Rhonchi. **E.** Wheeze. **F.** Pleural friction rub.

The most typical causes of crackles are pulmonary edema and pneumonia in its early stages. Because gravity draws fluid downward, crackles often start in the bases of the lungs. Crackles may be classified further as coarse crackles (wet, low-pitched sounds) and fine crackles (dry, high-pitched sounds). Crackles are subtle and sometimes difficult to hear and may be overridden by louder respiratory sounds. If the paramedic suspects crackles when auscultating the chest, the patient should be asked to cough. A cough may clear fine crackles.

A **wheeze** is also known as a sibilant wheeze. Wheezes are high-pitched musical noises that usually are louder during expiration. Wheezes are caused by high-velocity air traveling through narrowed airways. They may occur because of asthma and other constrictive diseases and heart failure. When wheezing occurs in a localized area, the paramedic should suspect a foreign body obstruction, tumor, or mucus plug. Wheezes are classified as mild, moderate, and severe. They should be described as occurring on inspiration or expiration or both. They are often easier to hear over the posterior lung fields.

CRITICAL THINKING

Breathe in and out through an open mouth. Gradually purse your lips until only a small opening is present while you continue to inhale and exhale. How do the sounds change? As you narrow the opening, is the noise louder on inspiration or expiration?

Rhonchi are also known as sonorous wheezes. They are continuous, low-pitched, rumbling sounds usually heard on expiration. Although rhonchi sound similar to wheezes, they do not involve the small airways. They are heard over the trachea and bronchi. Rhonchi are less discrete than crackles and are auscultated easily. Rhonchi are caused by the passage of air through an airway obstructed by thick secretions, muscular spasm, new tissue growth, or external pressure collapsing the airway lumen. These breath sounds may result from any condition that increases secretions, such as pneumonia or drug overdose.

Stridor usually is an inspiratory, crowing-type sound that can be heard without the aid of a stethoscope. It indicates significant narrowing or obstruction of the larynx or trachea and may be caused by epiglottitis, viral croup, anaphylaxis, foreign body aspiration, or more than one of these factors. Stridor is heard best over the site of origin, usually the larynx or trachea. This breath sound often indicates airway compromise that may be life threatening, especially in children. Its presence calls for careful observation for ventilatory failure and hypoxia.

Although a pleural friction rub occurs outside the respiratory tree, it also may be considered an adventitious breath sound. **Pleural friction rub** is a low-pitched, dry, rubbing or grating sound. It is caused by the movement of inflamed pleural surfaces as they slide on one another during breathing. The friction rub may be auscultated on inspiration and expiration and usually is loudest over the lower lateral anterior surface of the chest wall. Presence of a pleural friction rub may indicate pleurisy, viral infection, tuberculosis, or pulmonary embolism (see Chapter 23, *Respiratory*). **FIGURE 19-27** compares breath sounds in ill and well patients.

SHOW ME THE EVIDENCE

Australian researchers evaluated whether undergraduate paramedic students could accurately interpret lung sounds. They had 96 paramedic students evaluate six audio files. Students were found to most accurately assess wheezing and least accurately assess coarse crackles. The researchers concluded that there should be more focus on teaching breath sounds interpretation in paramedic programs.

Modified from: Williams B, Boyle M, O'Meara P. Can undergraduate paramedic students accurately identify lung sounds? *Emerg Med J*. 2009;26(8):580-582.

Vocal Resonance

As part of the respiratory examination, vocal sounds heard on auscultation (vocal resonance) should be

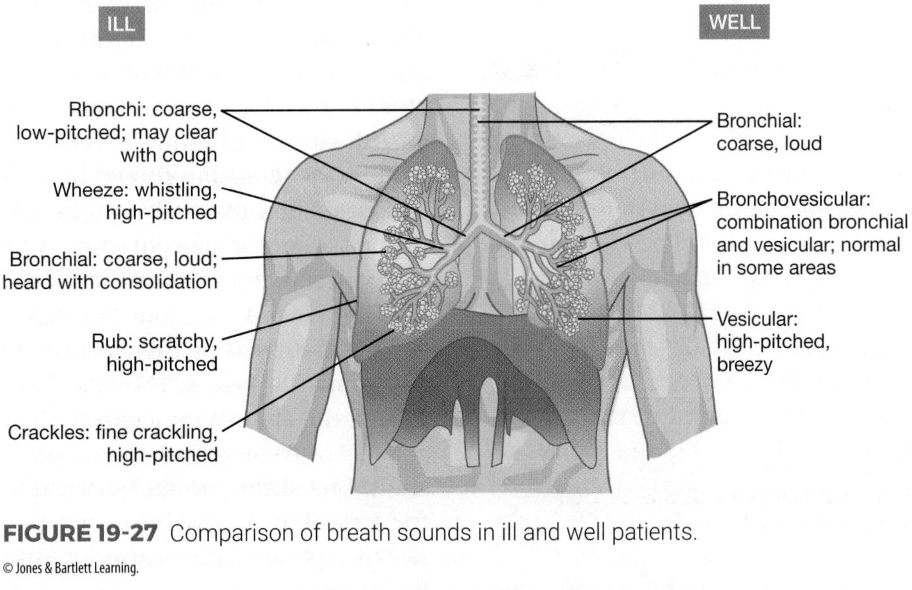

FIGURE 19-27 Comparison of breath sounds in ill and well patients.

assessed to evaluate the presence of lung consolidation. This consolidation usually indicates pneumonia or pleural effusion. Any change in the character of the spoken voice that is higher pitched and less muffled than normal during auscultation should be noted. Normally, the sound of the patient's voice becomes less distinct as the auscultation moves peripherally. Vocal sounds may remain loud at the periphery of the lungs or sound louder than usual over a distinct area when consolidation is present. The following tests can be used to assess vocal resonance:

- In the bronchophony test, the patient is asked to whisper "toy boat" or "blue balloons" while the lungs are auscultated. Vocal sounds will be louder where the consolidation is present.
- In the egophony test, the patient is asked to say the letter "e-e-e." If the vocal sounds more closely resemble the letter "a," lung consolidation may be present.
- In the whispered pectoriloquy test, the patient is asked to whisper as the posterior lungs are auscultated. If vocal sounds are transmitted clearly or there is an increased loudness of whispering during auscultation, it is often a sign of lung consolidation.

Heart

In the prehospital setting, the heart must be examined indirectly; however, a skilled assessment can collect information about the size and effectiveness of the pumping action of the heart. This assessment includes palpation and auscultation.

Palpation

The **apical impulse** is a visible and palpable force. It is produced by the contraction of the left ventricle. Palpation of this impulse may be useful to compare the relationship of peripheral pulses with the pulse produced by ventricular contraction. For example, the hearts of some patients with cardiac irregularities do not always produce a peripheral pulse with every ventricular contraction. By palpating or auscultating the apical impulse and the carotid pulse at the same time, the paramedic can note a **pulse deficit** (**FIGURE 19-28**). Factors such as obesity, large breasts, and muscularity may make this landmark hard to see or palpate.

Auscultation

Heart sounds may be auscultated for frequency (pitch), intensity (loudness), duration, and timing in the cardiac cycle (**FIGURE 19-29**). A full evaluation of heart sounds calls for a high level of skill and experience, a quiet environment, and ample time to listen closely. However, the paramedic may assess two basic heart sounds quickly. These sounds may help to improve understanding of the patient's condition. The basic heart sounds S_1 and S_2 ("lub-dub") are normal sounds that occur when the heart contracts. S_1 (the "lub sound") is caused by the closure of the mitral (M_1) and tricuspid (T_1) valves. S_2 (the "dub" sound) is caused by the closure of aortic (A_2) and pulmonic (P_2) valves. These sounds are best heard toward the apex of the heart at the fifth intercostal space. For evaluation of heart sounds, the patient should be sitting up and leaning slightly forward for auscultating the front and back of the chest (**FIGURE 19-30A** and **FIGURE 19-30B**) or lying in the left lateral recumbent position (**FIGURE 19-30C**). These positions bring the heart closer to the left anterior

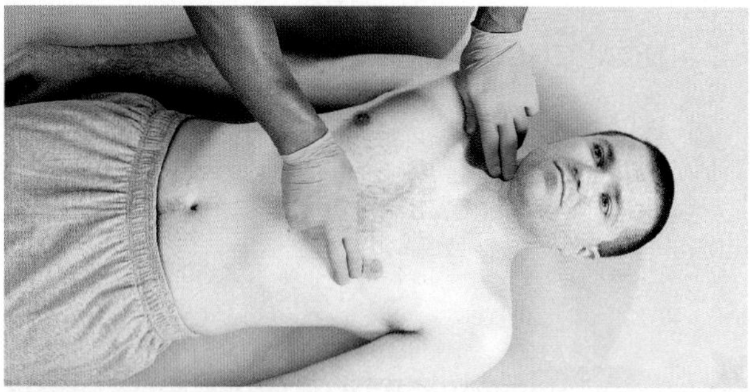

FIGURE 19-28 Simultaneous palpation of the carotoid artery and either palpation or auscultation of the apical impulse.

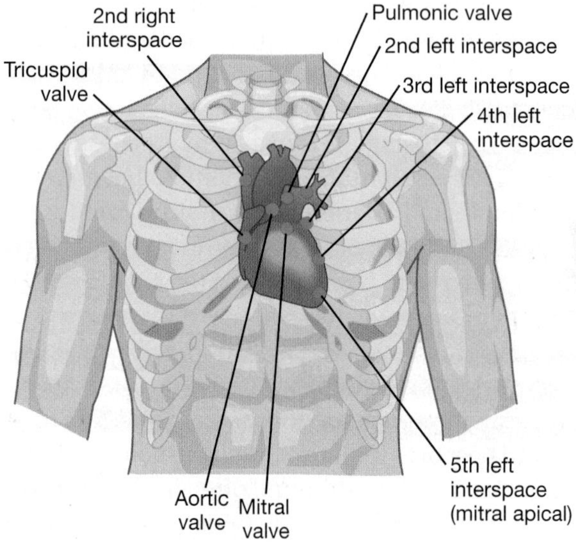

FIGURE 19-29 Areas for auscultation of the heart.

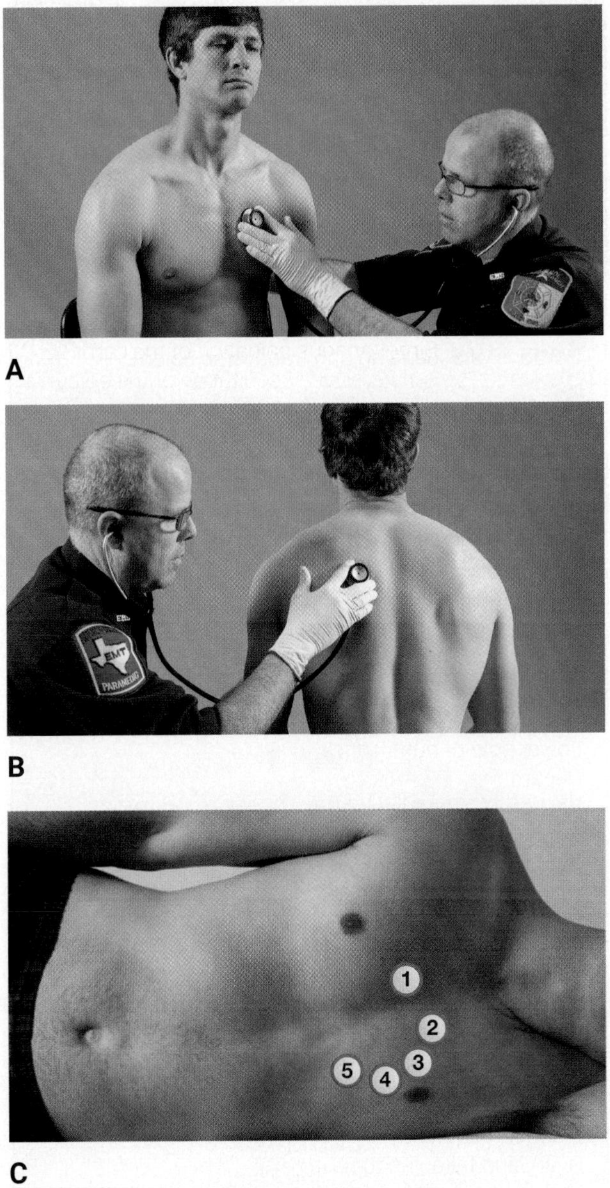

FIGURE 19-30 Patient positions for auscultation. Stethoscope positioning for auscultating the front **(A)** and back **(B)** of the chest while sitting up and leaning slightly forward; stethoscope positioning for a patient in the left lateral recumbent position **(C)**.

chest wall. To listen for S_1, the paramedic should ask the patient to breathe normally and hold the breath in expiration. To listen for S_2, the paramedic should ask the patient to breathe normally again and hold the breath in inspiration.

Heart sounds may be muffled or diminished by obesity or obstructive lung disease. Muffling also may occur because of the presence of fluid in the pericardial sac surrounding the heart muscle. The accumulation of fluid usually is the result of penetrating or severe blunt chest trauma, cardiac tamponade, or cardiac rupture and is considered a true emergency. Other causes of muffled or diminished heart sounds include infectious uremic pericarditis and malignancy. (See Chapter 21, *Cardiology*, for further discussion of abnormal heart sounds.)

Inflammation of the pericardial sac may cause a rubbing sound, called a **pericardial friction rub**, that is audible with a stethoscope. The rub may result from infectious pericarditis, myocardial infarction, uremia, trauma, and autoimmune pericarditis. These rubs have a scratching, grating, or squeaking quality and tend to be louder on inspiration. They can be differentiated from pleural friction rubs by their continued presence when the patient holds his or her breath.

Extra Sounds

Extra sounds that sometimes can be heard during auscultation or can be felt by palpation include heart murmurs, bruits, and thrills. **Heart murmurs** are prolonged sounds caused by a disruption in the flow of blood into, through, or out of the heart. Most murmurs are caused by valvular defects. Although some heart murmurs are serious, others (eg, some that occur in children and adolescents) are benign and have no apparent cause. Heart murmurs can be detected during auscultation of the heart.

A **bruit** is an abnormal sound or murmur that may be heard during auscultation of the carotid artery or another organ or gland. A bruit may indicate local obstruction. Bruits usually are low pitched and difficult to hear. To assess blood flow in the carotid artery, the paramedic should place the bell of the stethoscope over the carotid artery at the medial aspect of the clavicle. The patient is then asked to hold his or her breath (**FIGURE 19-31**).

Thrills are like bruits but are described as fine vibrations or tremors that may indicate blood flow obstruction. Thrills may be palpable over the site of an aneurysm or on the precordium (the area of the chest wall that overlies the heart and epigastrium). Like murmurs and bruits, thrills may be serious or benign.

Abdomen

The abdomen is divided by two imaginary lines that separate the abdominal region into four quadrants. The quadrants are the upper right, lower right, upper left, and lower left (**FIGURE 19-32**). These quadrants and their contents provide the basis for inspection, auscultation, percussion, and palpation (BOX 19-5).

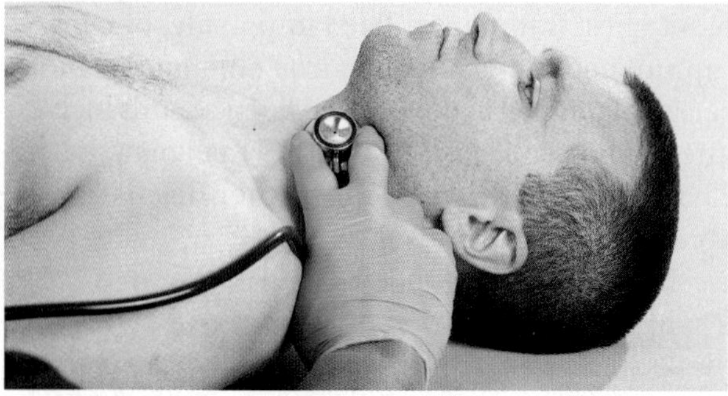

FIGURE 19-31 Evaluation of carotid bruit.

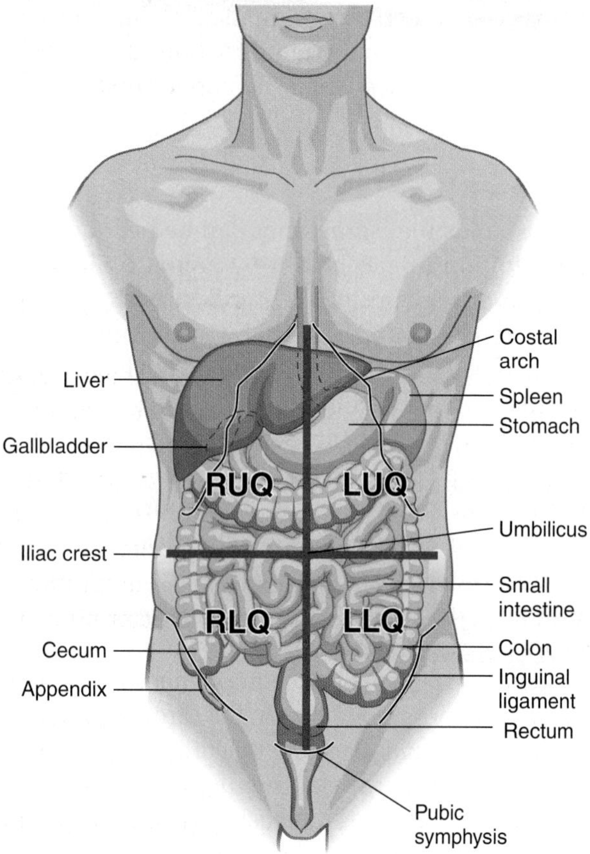

FIGURE 19-32 Four quadrants of the abdomen. RUQ, Right upper quadrant; LUQ, left upper quadrant; RLQ, right lower quadrant; LLQ, left lower quadrant.

When examining a patient's abdomen, the paramedic should ensure that the patient is comfortable (with an empty bladder, if possible) and in a supine position. The paramedic's hands and stethoscope should be warm. The patient should be approached slowly and respectfully. Any painful area should be examined last to avoid "patient guarding" that occurs when the painful area is examined first. Discoloration found in the flank (Grey Turner sign) or around the umbilicus (Cullen sign) may indicate possible injury or disease (see Chapter 28, *Abdominal and Gastrointestinal Disorders*).

BOX 19-5 Abdominal Quadrants

Right Upper Quadrant

Liver and gallbladder
Pylorus
Duodenum
Head of pancreas
Right adrenal gland
Portion of right kidney
Hepatic flexure of colon
Portions of ascending and transverse colon

Left Upper Quadrant

Left lobe of liver
Spleen
Stomach
Body of pancreas
Left adrenal gland
Portion of left kidney
Splenic flexure of colon
Portions of transverse and descending colon

Right Lower Quadrant

Lower pole of right kidney
Cecum
Portion of ascending colon
Appendix
Bladder (if distended)
Ovary and fallopian tube
Uterus (if enlarged)
Right ureter

Left Lower Quadrant

Lower pole of left kidney
Sigmoid colon
Portion of descending colon
Bladder (if distended)
Ovary and fallopian tube
Uterus (if enlarged)
Left ureter

Inspection

The paramedic should inspect the abdomen visually for signs of cyanosis, pallor, jaundice, bruising, discoloration, ascites (swelling of abdomen due to fluid accumulation), masses, and aortic pulsations. Surgical scars and implanted medical devices should also be noted (see Chapter 21, *Cardiology*). The

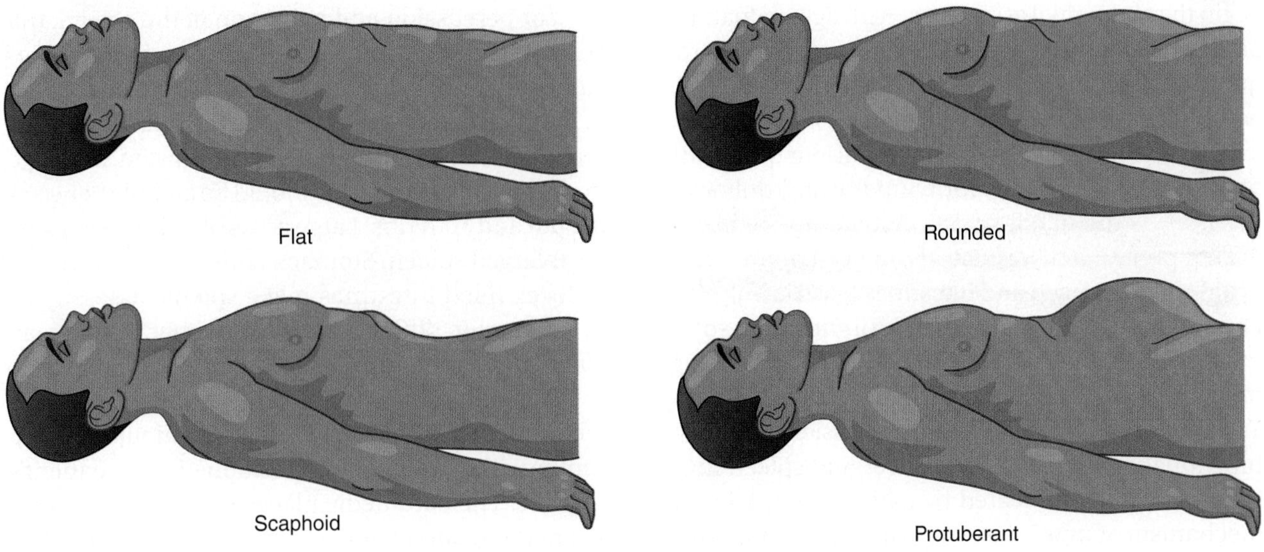

FIGURE 19-33 Shape of the abdomen.

abdomen should be evenly round and symmetrical (**FIGURE 19-33**). Symmetrical distention of the abdomen may result from obesity, enlarged organs, fluid, or gas. Asymmetrical distention may result from hernias, tumor, bowel obstruction, or enlarged abdominal organs. A flat abdomen is common in adults who are athletic. Convex abdomens are common in children and in adults who have poor exercise habits. The umbilicus should be free of swelling, bulges, and signs of inflammation. The normal umbilicus usually is inverted, or it may protrude slightly.

Abdominal movement during respiration should be smooth and even. As a rule, males have more abdominal involvement than do females during respiration, so limited abdominal movement in the male patient with symptoms may indicate a pathologic abdominal condition. Visible pulsations produced by blood flow through the aorta in the upper abdomen may be normal in thin adults. However, marked pulsations may indicate an abdominal aortic aneurysm (see Chapter 21, *Cardiology*).

Auscultation

Noting the presence or absence of bowel sounds to assess motility and to discover vascular sounds has limited value in the prehospital setting. Such findings do not affect or determine the approach to patient care. Moreover, the time needed for complete bowel sound assessment (about 5 minutes per quadrant) far exceeds the justifiable scene time for most patients. However, if auscultation is to be performed, it should always precede palpation. (Palpation may alter the intensity of bowel sounds.)

To auscultate bowel sounds, the paramedic holds the diaphragm of the stethoscope on the abdomen with light pressure. If bowel sounds are present, they usually are heard as rumblings or gurgles. These sounds should occur irregularly and may range in frequency from 5 to 35 per minute. Auscultation should be performed in all four quadrants. A minimum of 5 minutes per quadrant is needed to determine that normal bowel sounds are absent. Increased bowel sounds may indicate gastroenteritis or intestinal obstruction. Decreased or absent bowel sounds may indicate peritonitis (inflammation of the lining of the abdominal cavity) or ileus (inactive peristaltic activity resulting from one of several causes) (see Chapter 29, *Genitourinary and Renal Disorders*).

Percussion and Palpation

Percussion and palpation of the abdomen may help to detect the presence of fluid, air, and solid masses. The paramedic should use a systematic approach, moving from side to side or clockwise and noting any rigidity, tenderness, or abnormal skin temperature or color. The patient's face should be observed for signs of pain or discomfort. If the patient is reporting abdominal pain, the painful quadrant should be examined last so that the patient will not unnecessarily tighten or guard the abdominal area. The paramedic should begin the abdominal assessment with light palpation, using an even pressing motion and avoiding sharp, quick jabs. Palpation may be done simultaneously with percussion.

Percussion begins by evaluating all four quadrants of the abdomen in turn for tympany and dullness. **Tympany** is the major sound that should be noted during percussion because of the normal presence of air in the stomach and intestines (gastric bubble). Dullness should be heard over organs and solid masses. When percussing the abdomen, proceeding from an area of tympany to an area of dullness is best. That way, the change in sound is easier to detect. Individual assessments of the liver and spleen may be performed if indicated by patient complaint or mechanism of injury. Patients who may require surgery for abdominal illness or injury are best served by rapid assessment, stabilization, and transport to an appropriate medical facility.

For percussion and palpation of the liver, percussion begins by starting just above the umbilicus in the right midclavicular line in an area of tympany. Percussion should continue in an upward direction until the change from tympany to dullness occurs. This change usually occurs slightly below the costal margin. It indicates the lower border of the liver. To determine the upper border of the liver, the percussion should begin in the same midclavicular line at the midsternal level, proceeding downward until the tympany from the lung area changes to dullness (usually between the fifth and seventh intercostal spaces). Liver size and span (usually 2.4 to 4.7 inches [6 to 12 cm]) are related to age and sex. The liver usually is proportionately larger in adults than in children and larger in males than in females.

For palpation of the liver, the patient should be supine and comfortable and should have a relaxed abdomen. The paramedic should perform the examination from the patient's right side and should begin by placing the left hand under the patient at the 11th and 12th ribs (**FIGURE 19-34**). The right hand should be placed on the abdomen, with the fingers pointing toward the patient's head and extended, resting just below the edge of the costal margin. The conscious patient should be instructed to breathe deeply through the mouth. During exhalation, the paramedic presses upward with the hand under the patient and gently pushes in and up with the right hand. If the liver is felt, it should be firm and nontender. (A healthy liver usually cannot be palpated unless the patient is thin.)

For percussion and palpation of the spleen, the patient must be lying supine or in a right lateral recumbent position. Percussion should begin at the area of lung tympany, just posterior to the midaxillary line on the left side. When percussing downward, a change from tympany to dullness should be audible between the 6th and 10th ribs. Large areas of dullness suggest an enlarged spleen. Stomach contents and air-filled or feces-filled intestines make splenic assessment by percussion difficult. These and other factors may affect percussion tones of dullness and tympany.

Palpation is a more useful assessment technique for evaluating the spleen. The patient should be lying supine with the paramedic positioned at the patient's left side. The paramedic places the left hand under the patient, supporting the lower left rib cage. The paramedic places the right hand just below the patient's lower left costal margin (**FIGURE 19-35**). The area should be gently palpated by lifting up the left hand and pressing down with the right hand. (A normal spleen usually cannot be palpated in an adult. A palpable spleen is most likely enlarged three times its normal size.) Palpation of the spleen can produce

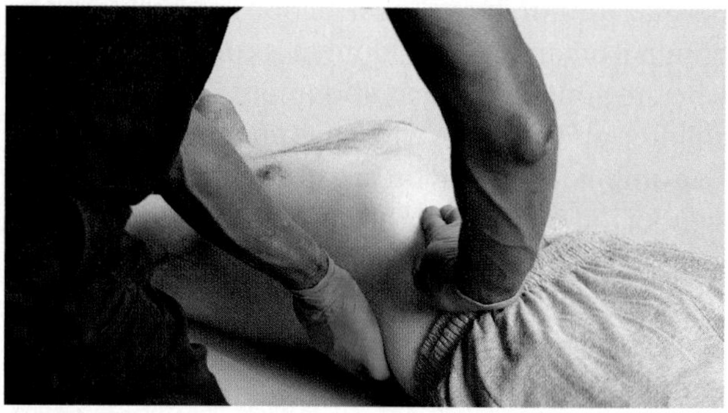

FIGURE 19-34 Palpation of the liver.

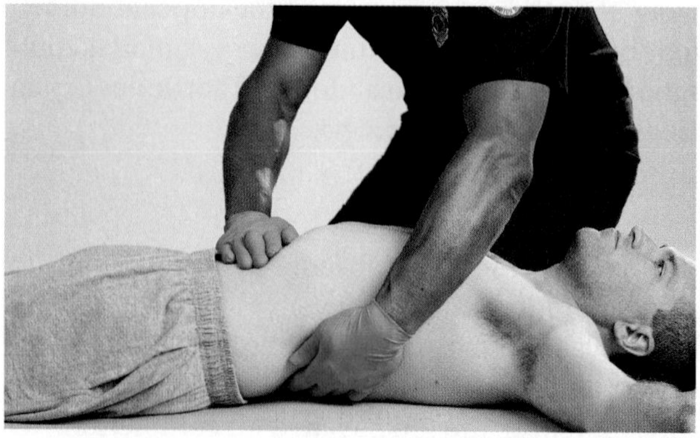

FIGURE 19-35 Palpation of the spleen.

rupture of the organ. Palpation should be performed with caution and only in very rare circumstances.

Female Genitalia

Examination of the genitalia of either sex of patient can be awkward. The patient and the paramedic may feel uncomfortable. When possible, paramedics of the same sex as the patient should perform these examinations. If that is not possible, a second person who acts as a chaperone should be present during the examination.

> NOTE
> Examination of the genitalia of both men and women should be performed in the prehospital setting only if indicated by patient complaint, pregnancy with imminent delivery in women, or the mechanism of injury.

The external genitalia should be inspected visually to note any swelling, redness, discharge, bleeding, or evidence of trauma. Discoloration or tenderness of the genital tissue may be the result of traumatic bruising. Ulcers, vesicles, and discharges (with or without pain) indicate sexually transmitted disease. If touching the anal area is necessary, the paramedic should change the examination gloves afterward to avoid introducing bacteria into the vaginal area.

> CRITICAL THINKING
> When a patient's genitalia must be examined, it is advisable to have another care provider present. Why might this be important?

Male Genitalia

When examining the male genitalia, the paramedic should inspect the area visually. Bleeding or signs of trauma should be noted. The shaft of the penis should be nontender and flaccid. Rarely, patients with leukemia, sickle cell disease, or spinal injury may have a persistent painful erection (priapism). The urethral opening should be free of blood, which is a possible result of pelvic trauma. The opening also should be free of discharge, which is a sign of sexually transmitted disease. The scrotum should be nontender and slightly asymmetrical. A swollen or painful scrotum may result from infection, herniation, testicular torsion, or trauma. Discoloration of the genitals is called Coopernail sign; such discoloration can occur in men or women, and may indicate peritoneal bleeding.

Anus

Examination of the anus is indicated in the presence of rectal bleeding or trauma to the area. Examination can be performed with the patient in one of several positions. Most patients will find the side-lying position to be most comfortable. The paramedic should protect the patient's privacy and use proper drapes. Inspection of the sacrococcygeal and perineal areas should consider abnormal findings, which may include pressure sores, lumps, ulcers, inflammation, rashes, and excoriations (surface injuries caused by scratching or abrasions). Inflamed external hemorrhoids are common in adults and pregnant women.

Extremities

When examining the upper and lower extremities, the paramedic should pay attention to function and structure (see Chapter 10, *Review of Human Systems*). The patient's general appearance, body proportions, and ease of movement are key. Any limitation in the range of motion or an unusual increase in the mobility of a joint should be noted. Abnormal findings include the following:

- Signs of inflammation
  - Swelling
  - Tenderness
  - Increased heat
  - Redness
  - Decreased function
- Asymmetry
- Crepitus
- Deformities
- Decreased muscular strength
- Atrophy

Examining the Upper and Lower Extremities

A full assessment of the upper and lower extremities includes an evaluation of the skin and tissue overlying the muscles, cartilage, and bones. It also includes an examination of the joints. Each extremity should be assessed for soft-tissue injury, discoloration, swelling, and masses. The upper and lower extremities should be symmetrical in structure and muscularity. The paramedic should assess the circulatory status of each extremity by determining skin color, temperature, sensation, and the presence of distal pulses. The bones, joints, and surrounding tissues of the extremities

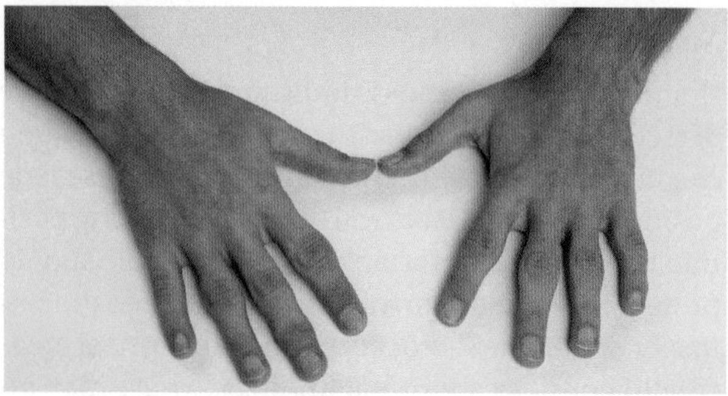

FIGURE 19-36 Hands and wrists.

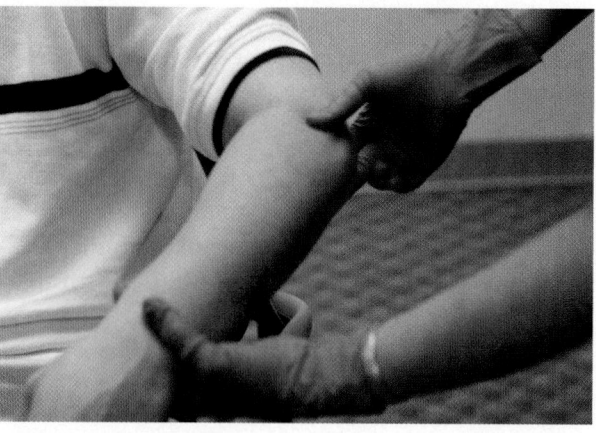

FIGURE 19-37 Palpation of the lateral and medial epicondyles.

are assessed for structural integrity and continuity. Muscle tone should be firm and nontender. Joints are assessed for function by moving each joint through its full range of motion (see Chapter 10, *Review of Human Systems*). A normal range of motion occurs without pain, deformity, limitation, or instability.

The paramedic should inspect both hands and wrists for contour and positional alignment (**FIGURE 19-36**). The wrists, hands, and joints of each finger should be palpated for tenderness, swelling, or deformity. To determine range of motion, the patient should be asked to flex and extend the wrists, make a fist, and touch the thumb to each fingertip. All movements should be performed without pain or discomfort.

The patient's elbows should be inspected and palpated in the flexed and extended positions. To determine the range of motion of the elbow, the patient should be asked to extend the arm and then touch the fingertips to the same shoulder. The paramedic should inspect the grooves between the epicondyle and olecranon by palpation. Pain and tenderness should not be present when pressing on the lateral or medial epicondyle (**FIGURE 19-37**).

The patient's shoulders should be inspected and palpated for symmetry and integrity of the clavicles, scapulae, and humeri. Pain, tenderness, or asymmetrical contour may indicate a fracture or dislocation. The paramedic should ask the patient to shrug the shoulders and raise and extend both arms. These movements should be made without pain or discomfort. The following regions should be palpated, noting any tenderness or swelling (**FIGURE 19-38**):

- Sternoclavicular joint
- Acromioclavicular joint
- Subacromial area
- Bicipital groove

The paramedic should inspect the patient's feet and ankles for contour, position, and size. Tenderness, swelling, and deformity are abnormal findings on palpation. The toes should be straight and aligned with each other. Range of motion can be determined by asking the patient to bend the toes, point the toes, and rotate the feet inward and outward from the ankle. These movements should be possible without pain or discomfort. The paramedic should inspect all surfaces of the ankles and feet for deformities, nodules, swelling, calluses, corns, and skin integrity.

The structural integrity of the pelvis should be verified. To palpate the iliac crest and the symphysis pubis, the paramedic places both hands on each anterior iliac crest and presses downward and outward (**FIGURE 19-39**). To determine stability, the heel of the hand should be placed on the patient's symphysis pubis, pressing downward. If instability is evident, the examination should end to prevent additional injury. Deformity and point tenderness of the pelvis may be signs of fracture. These signs may mask major structural and vascular injury.

The hips should be inspected for instability, tenderness, and crepitus. The paramedic can examine the supine or unconscious patient by assessing the structural integrity of the iliac crest. A mobile patient should be able to walk without discomfort. A supine patient should be able to raise the legs and knees and rotate the legs inward and outward.

The knees should be inspected and palpated for swelling and tenderness. The patella should be smooth, firm, nontender, and midline in position. The patient should be able to bend and straighten each knee without pain.

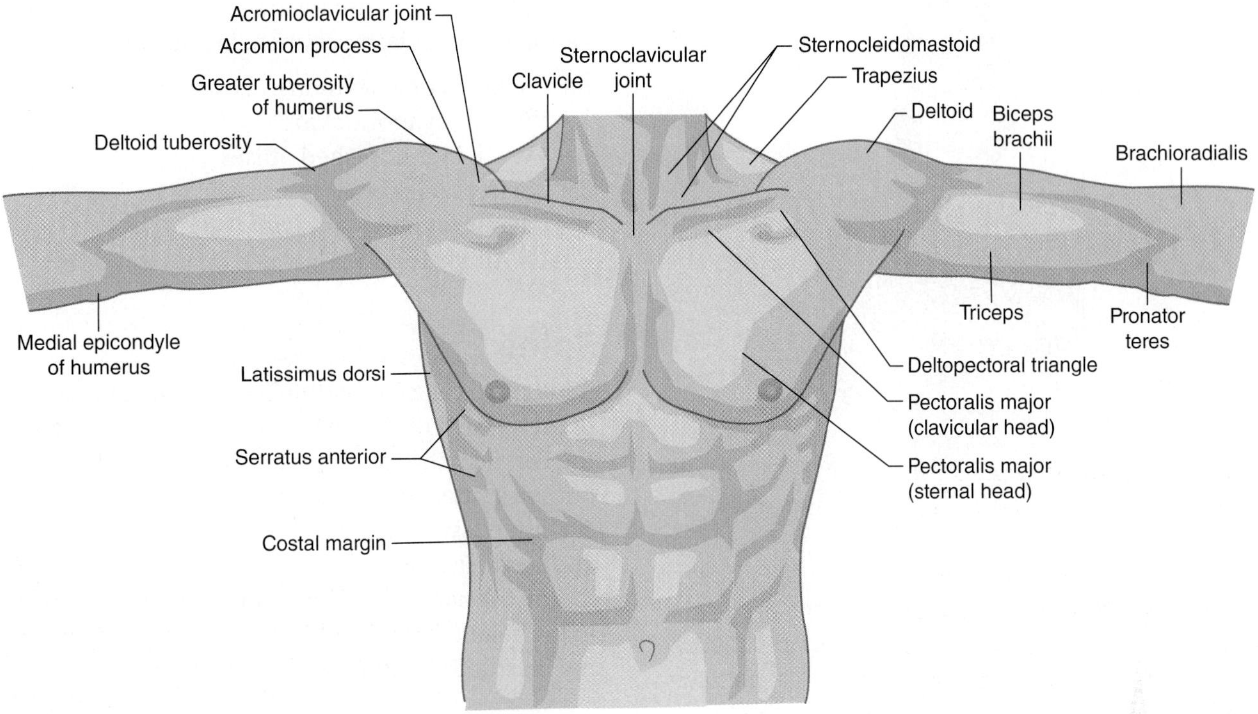

FIGURE 19-38 Anatomy of the shoulder and related structures.

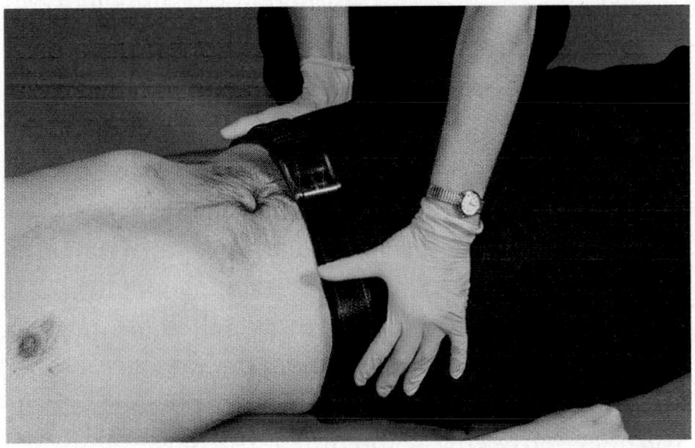

FIGURE 19-39 Palpating the pelvis for stability.

Peripheral Vascular System

The peripheral vascular system includes arteries, veins, the lymphatic system, and lymph nodes (**FIGURE 19-40**). It also includes the fluids exchanged in the capillary bed. This system can be evaluated during the physical examination of the upper and lower extremities.

When evaluating the arms, the paramedic should inspect from the fingertips to the shoulders, noting size, symmetry, swelling, venous pattern, color of the skin and nail beds, and texture of the skin. If arterial insufficiency is noted because of a weak radial pulse, the brachial pulse should be palpated. Epitrochlear nodes and brachial nodes should be nonswollen and nontender. A fine venous network on upper and lower extremities often is visible. The paramedic should be alert for enlargement of superficial veins during the examination.

During examination of the lower extremities, the patient should be supine and draped for privacy. (Shoes, socks, and hosiery should be removed for a full examination.) The paramedic should inspect visually from the groin and buttocks to the feet, noting the following:

- Size and symmetry
- Swelling
- Venous pattern and venous enlargement
- Pigmentation
- Rashes, scars, or ulcers
- Color and texture of the skin
- Presence or absence of hair growth (indicating compromised arterial circulation)

The superficial inguinal nodes in the groin should be palpated to assess for swelling and tenderness. The paramedic should assess all lower extremity pulse sites for circulation, strength, and regularity. These sites include the femoral pulse, the popliteal

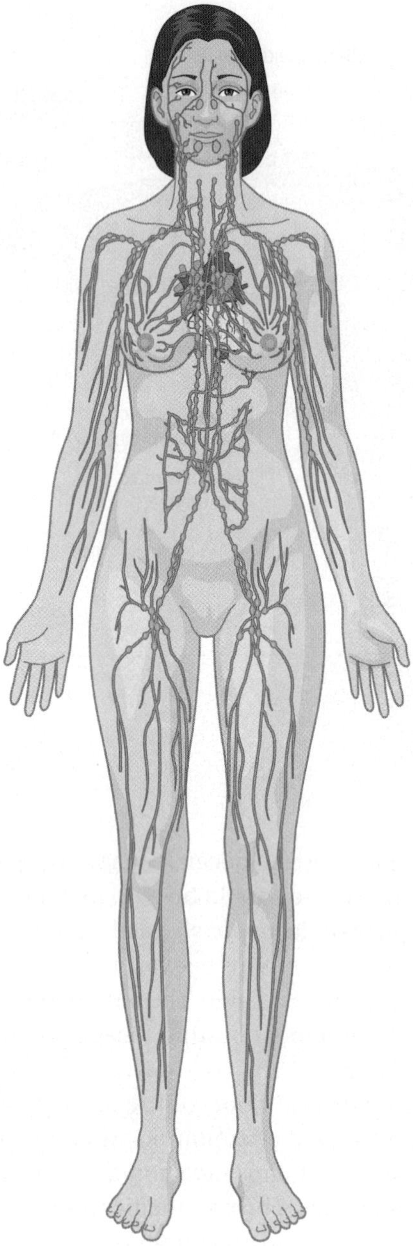

FIGURE 19-40 Lymphatic system including lymph nodes of the body.

pulse, the dorsalis pedis pulse, and the posterior tibial pulse (see Chapter 10, *Review of Human Systems*). The temperature of the feet and legs should be warm, indicating adequate circulation. The paramedic can evaluate for pitting edema over the dorsum of each foot, behind each medial malleolus, and over the shins. This evaluation can be done by pressing firmly on the skin with the thumb for at least 5 seconds. Edema is said to be "pitting" when depression of the tissue remains after removal of pressure.

Findings that are considered abnormal during a peripheral vascular assessment include the following:

- Swollen or asymmetrical extremities
- Pale or cyanotic skin
- Weak or diminished pulses
- Skin that is cold to the touch
- Absence of hair growth
- Pitting edema

Spine

A full physical examination includes an assessment of the spine. This begins with a visual assessment of the cervical, thoracic, and lumbar curves. From the patient's side, any curvature of the spine, including curvature associated with abnormal lordosis, kyphosis, and scoliosis, should be noted (**FIGURE 19-41**). In addition, the paramedic should look for any differences in the height of the shoulders or iliac crests (hips) that may result from abnormal spinal curvature.

> CRITICAL THINKING
>
> Consider a case in which no deformity of the spine is found during an examination. Can spine fracture or dislocation be ruled out?

Cervical Spine

The patient's neck should be in a midline position. If the patient is alert and denies neck pain, the paramedic should palpate the posterior aspect for point tenderness and swelling. The only palpable landmark should be the spinous process of the seventh cervical vertebra at the base of the neck (**FIGURE 19-42**). In the absence of suspected injury, the paramedic tests range of motion by directing the patient to bend the head forward, backward, and from side to side. These movements should not cause pain or discomfort.

> NOTE
>
> The paramedic will need to test range of motion. However, the paramedic should never attempt to move the neck of a person who is unconscious. The paramedic also should never attempt to move the neck of a person who is unable or unwilling to do so on his or her own. Spontaneous cervical muscle spasm frequently is associated with significant cervical spine injury in the trauma victim.

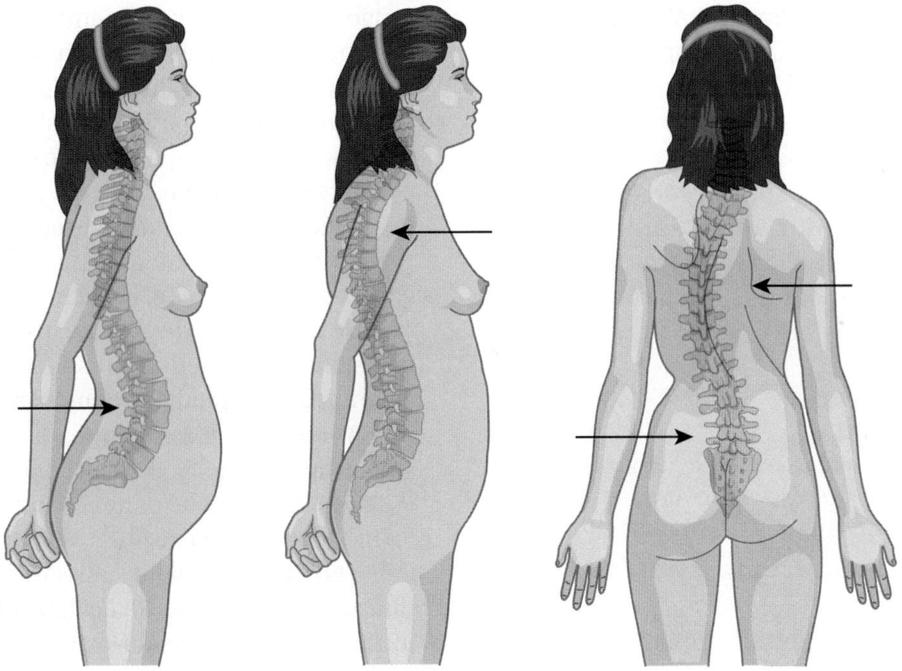

FIGURE 19-41 Spinal curvatures of lordosis, kyphosis, and scoliosis. **A.** Lordosis. **B.** Kyphosis. **C.** Scoliosis.

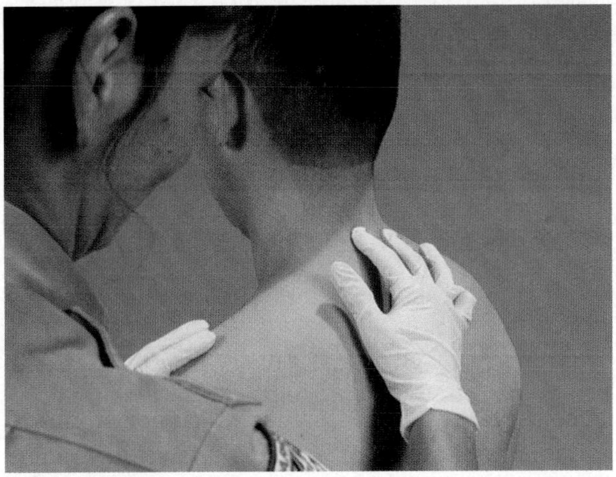

FIGURE 19-42 Palpation of the seventh cervical spinous process.

Thoracic and Lumbar Spine

The thoracic and lumbar areas should be inspected for signs of injury, swelling, and discoloration. Palpation should begin at the first thoracic vertebra and move downward to the sacrum. Under normal conditions, the spine is nontender to palpation. The paramedic can evaluate range of motion by asking the patient to bend at the waist forward and backward and to each side and also to rotate the upper trunk from side to side in a circular motion.

Nervous System

The details of an appropriate neurologic examination vary greatly. The examination usually depends on the origin of the patient's complaint. For example, the examination may depend on whether the complaint refers to the peripheral nervous system or the central nervous system. The assessment and examination of the nervous system may be performed separately. However, neurologic assessment often is completed during other assessments. A neurologic examination may be organized into five categories:

- Mental status and speech
- Cranial nerves
- Motor system
- Sensory system
- Reflexes

Mental Status and Speech

A healthy patient should be oriented to person, place, and date. Patients also should be able to organize their thoughts and converse freely (provided they have no hearing or speech impediments). Abnormal findings include unconsciousness, confusion, slurred speech, aphasia, dysphonia, and dysarthria.

Cranial Nerves

The 12 cranial nerves can be categorized as sensory, somatomotor, proprioceptive, and parasympathetic (see Chapter 10, *Review of Human Systems*). **TABLE 19-5** lists methods that can be used to assess each of the cranial nerves.

> CRITICAL THINKING
> Why should abnormal findings in examination of one or more of the cranial nerves concern you?

Motor System

An evaluation of a patient's motor system includes observing the patient during movement and at rest. The paramedic should evaluate abnormal involuntary movements for quality, rate, rhythm, and fullness of range. Other body movement assessments include posture, level of activity, fatigue, and emotion.

Muscle strength should be bilaterally symmetrical. In addition, the patient should be able to provide reasonable resistance to opposition. One way to evaluate muscle strength in the upper extremities is to ask the patient to extend the elbow. The paramedic then instructs the patient to pull the arm toward the chest against opposing resistance (**FIGURE 19-43A**). Muscle strength in the lower extremities is assessed by asking the patient to push the soles of the feet against the paramedic's palms. Next, the paramedic directs the patient to pull the toes toward the head while the paramedic provides opposing resistance (**FIGURE 19-43B**). The patient should be able to perform these actions easily without evident fatigue. Other methods to evaluate muscle strength and agility (illustrated in Chapter 10, *Review of Human Systems*) include testing for flexion, extension, and abduction of the upper and lower extremities.

To evaluate a patient's coordination, the paramedic should assess the patient's ability to perform rapid

TABLE 19-5 Assessment of the Cranial Nerves

Nerve	Nerve Function and Test
Cranial nerve I	Olfactory: Test sense of smell with aromatic substance.
Cranial nerve II	Optic: Test for visual acuity (described previously).
Cranial nerve III	Oculomotor: Inspect the size and shape of the pupils; test the pupil response to light.
Cranial nerves III, IV, and VI	Oculomotor, trochlear, abducens: Test extraocular movements by asking the patient to look up and down, to the left and right, and diagonally up and down to the left and right (the six cardinal directions of gaze).
Cranial nerve V	Trigeminal: Test motor movement by asking the patient to clench the teeth while you palpate the temporal and masseter muscles. Test sensation by touching the forehead, cheeks, and jaw on each side.
Cranial nerve VII	Facial: Inspect the face at rest and during conversation, noting symmetry, involuntary muscle movements (tics), or abnormal movements. Ask the patient to raise the eyebrows, frown, show upper and lower teeth, smile, and puff out both cheeks. The paramedic can assess strength of the facial muscles by asking the patient to close the eyes tightly so they cannot be opened and gently attempting to raise the eyelids. Observe for weakness or asymmetry.
Cranial nerve VIII	Vestibulocochlear: Assess hearing acuity (described previously).
Cranial nerves IX and X	Glossopharyngeal and vagus: Assess the patient's ability to swallow with ease; to produce saliva; and to produce normal voice sounds. Instruct the patient to hold the breath, and assess for normal slowing of the heart rate. Testing for the gag reflex also will test the cranial nerves.
Cranial nerve XI	Spinal accessory: Ask the patient to raise and lower the shoulders and to turn the head.
Cranial nerve XII	Hypoglossal: Ask the patient to stick out the tongue and to move it in several directions.

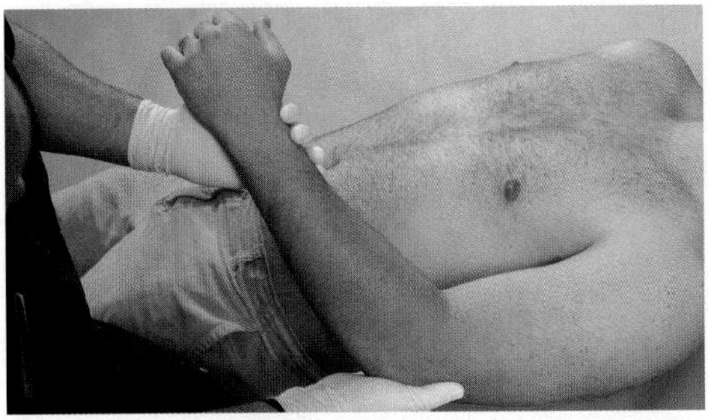

A

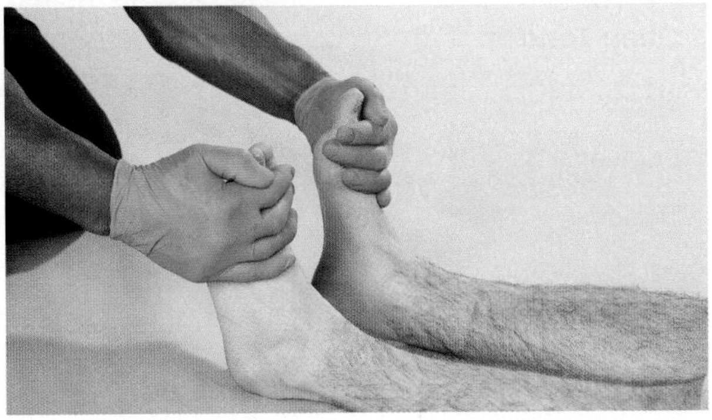

B

FIGURE 19-43 Evaluating muscle strength of the upper **(A)** and lower **(B)** extremities.

alternating movements. These include point-to-point movements, gait, and stance. One point-to-point movement that the patient can perform easily is to touch the finger to the nose, alternating hands. Another test is to ask the patient to touch each heel to the opposite shin. Both movements should be done numerous times and quickly to assess coordination, which should be smooth, rapid, and accurate. Gait can be evaluated in many ways. Depending on age, agility, and general health, most patients should be able to perform each of the following tasks without discomfort or losing balance:

- Walk heel to toe
- Walk on the toes
- Walk on the heels
- Hop in place
- Do a shallow knee bend
- Rise from a sitting position without assistance

Stance and balance can be evaluated by using the **Romberg test** and the **pronator drift test**. To perform the Romberg test, the paramedic asks the patient to stand erect with the feet together and arms at the sides (**FIGURE 19-44**). The patient's eyes initially should

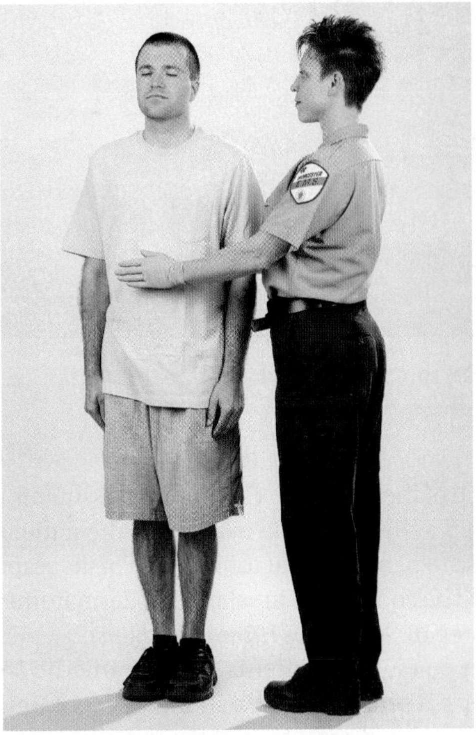

FIGURE 19-44 Romberg test.

be open and then closed. Although slight swaying is normal, a loss of balance is abnormal (a positive Romberg sign).

> **NOTE**
> The paramedic should stay close to the patient being tested for gait, stance, and balance. That way, the paramedic can help to prevent injury from a fall or loss of balance. The paramedic also should consider the patient's age and physical condition when deciding on the appropriateness of these examinations.

The pronator drift test (also known as an arm drift test) is performed by having the patient close the eyes and hold both arms out from the body (**FIGURE 19-45**). A normal test will reveal that both arms move the same or both arms do not move at all. Abnormal findings include one arm that does not move in concert with the other or one arm that drifts down compared with the other arm.

Sensory System

The sensory pathways of the nervous system conduct sensations of pain, temperature, position, vibration, and touch. A healthy patient is expected to be responsive

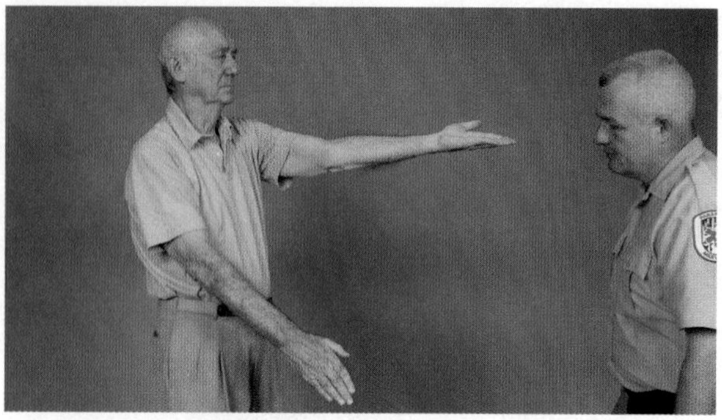

FIGURE 19-45 Pronator drift test.

to each of these stimuli. Common assessments of the sensory system include evaluating the patient's response to pain and light touch. Each of the responses should be considered in relation to dermatomes (see Chapter 10, *Review of Human Systems*).

In conscious patients, the paramedic should perform a sensory examination with light touch on each hand and each foot. If the patient cannot feel light touch or is unconscious, the sensation may be evaluated by gently pricking the hands and soles of the feet with a sharp object. The paramedic should use an object that will not penetrate the skin (eg, a paper clip or cotton swab). The sensory examination should proceed from head to toe. The examination should compare symmetrical areas on each side of the body and the distal and proximal areas of the body. A lack of sensory response may indicate spinal cord or peripheral nerve damage (see Chapter 40, *Spine and Nervous System Trauma*).

Reflexes

Testing a patient's reflexes can evaluate the function of certain areas of the nervous system as they relate to sensory impulses and motor neurons. Reflexes may be categorized as superficial reflexes and deep tendon reflexes (**TABLE 19-6**). Both types of reflexes should be tested as part of a thorough neurologic examination.

Superficial Reflexes

Superficial reflexes are elicited by sensory afferents from the skin. These include the upper abdominal, lower abdominal, cremasteric (for men), and plantar reflexes. All superficial reflexes are tested using the edge of a tongue blade (or similar object) or the end of a reflex hammer. An absent reflex may indicate an upper or lower motor neuron disorder.

TABLE 19-6 Superficial and Deep Tendon Reflexes

Reflex	Spinal Level Evaluated
Superficial	
Upper abdominal	T7, T8, and T9
Lower abdominal	T10 and T11
Cremasteric	T12, L1, and L2
Plantar	L4, L5, S1, and S2
Deep Tendon	
Biceps	C5 and C6
Brachioradial	C5 and C6
Triceps	C6, C7, and C8
Patellar	L2, L3, and L4
Achilles	S1 and S2

Modified from: Rudy EB. *Advanced Neurological and Neurosurgical Nursing*. St. Louis, MO: Mosby; 1984.

- **Upper and lower abdominal reflex.** Place the patient supine. Gently stroke each quadrant of the abdomen with the tongue blade. A normal reflex is a slight movement of the umbilicus toward each area that is stroked.
- **Cremasteric reflex.** Place the patient supine. Gently stroke the inner thigh (proximal to distal). The testicle and scrotum should rise on the side that is stroked.
- **Plantar reflex.** Place the patient with the legs extended. Gently stroke the lateral side of the foot from heel to the ball and then across the foot to the medial side. In the healthy adult, the plantar reflex presents as a downward flexion of the toes toward the source of the stimulus (**FIGURE 19-46**). The Babinski sign is present when there is dorsiflexion of the great toe with or without fanning of the other toes. It should be noted that the Babinski sign is an abnormal finding in older children and adults, but its absence does not rule out a neurologic deficit. It is a normal response in children younger than 2 years. Other reflexes for infants and children are described in Chapter 12, *Life Span Development*.

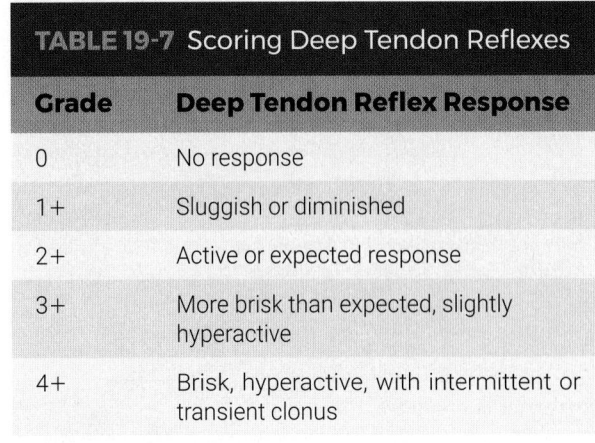

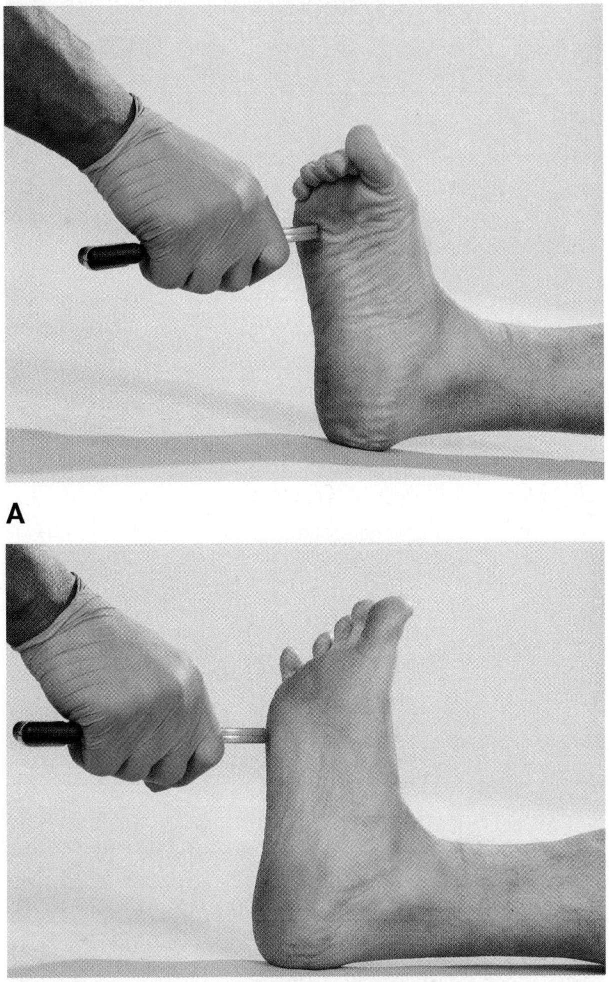

FIGURE 19-46 **A.** Plantar reflex. **B.** The Babinski sign—dorsiflexion of the great toe with or without fanning of the toes.

Deep Tendon Reflexes

Deep tendon reflexes examine the sensory and motor pathways of a nerve. They are often associated with muscle stretching. They include the biceps reflex, brachioradialis reflex, triceps reflex, patellar reflex, and Achilles reflex. These reflexes should be tested on each extremity with a reflex hammer, and a comparison should be made for visible and palpable responses. Deep tendon reflexes are graded using the scoring system in **TABLE 19-7** and are recorded on a stick figure. Diminished or absent reflexes may indicate damage to lower motor neurons or the spinal cord. Hyperactive reflexes may suggest an upper motor neuron disorder such as a brain injury or spinal cord injury. All reflexes are tested with the

TABLE 19-7 Scoring Deep Tendon Reflexes

Grade	Deep Tendon Reflex Response
0	No response
1+	Sluggish or diminished
2+	Active or expected response
3+	More brisk than expected, slightly hyperactive
4+	Brisk, hyperactive, with intermittent or transient clonus

patient in a sitting position in the following manner (**FIGURE 19-47**):

- **Biceps reflex.** Flex the patient's arm to 45° at the elbow. Palpate the biceps tendon in the antecubital fossa. Place your thumb over the tendon and your fingers under the elbow. Strike your thumb with the reflex hammer. Contraction of the biceps muscle should cause visible or palpable flexion of the elbow.
- **Brachioradialis reflex.** Flex the patient's arm up to 45°. Rest the patient's forearm on your arm with the hand slightly pronated. Strike the brachioradialis tendon (about 1 to 2 inches [3–5 cm] above the wrist) with the reflex hammer. Pronation of the forearm and flexion of the elbow should occur.
- **Triceps reflex.** Flex the patient's arm at the elbow up to 90° and rest the patient's hand against the side of the body. Palpate the triceps tendon and strike it with the reflex hammer, just above the elbow. Contraction of the triceps muscle should cause visible or palpable extension of the elbow.
- **Patellar reflex.** Flex the patient's knee to 90°, allowing the lower leg to hang loosely. Support the leg with your hand. Strike the patellar tendon just below the patella. Contraction of the quadriceps muscle should cause extension of the lower leg at the knee.
- **Achilles reflex.** Flex the patient's knee to 90°. Keep the ankle in a neutral position and hold the heel of the patient's foot in your hand. Strike the Achilles tendon at the level of the ankle malleoli. Contraction of the gastrocnemius muscle should cause plantar flexion of the foot.

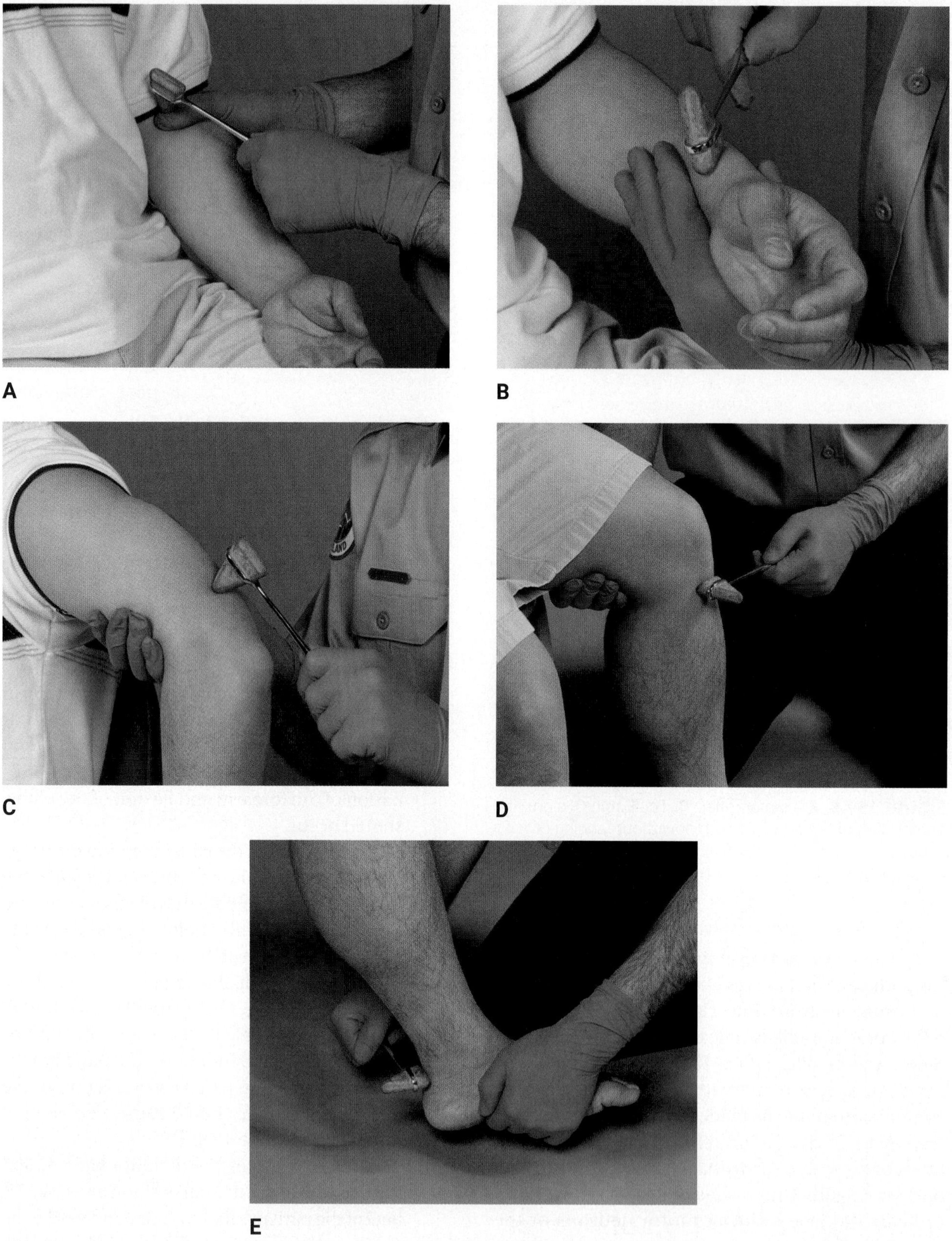

FIGURE 19-47 Location of tendons for evaluation of deep tendon reflexes. **A.** Biceps. **B.** Brachioradialis. **C.** Triceps. **D.** Patellar. **E.** Achilles.

Reassessment

Reassessment refers to the ongoing assessment that follows the paramedic's initial evaluation of the patient. The purpose of reassessment is twofold: (1) It refocuses the primary assessment to ensure that the patient continues to be stable and that initial interventions continue to be successful; (2) it also allows the paramedic to "trend" the patient's condition. That is, is the patient's condition improving or is it deteriorating while at the scene and during transport? Reassessment includes a second look at the following:

- The patient's level of consciousness
- The patient's vital signs
- The patient's response to initial care and treatment
- Positive or negative trends in the patient's condition
- Care interventions that may need to be changed or altered

Other examples of reassessment include reevaluating pulse and sensation in an extremity that has been splinted, verifying lung sounds before and after moving a patient who has been intubated, monitoring the ECG after administering drugs, and monitoring pulse oximetry readings in a patient receiving airway support.

Reassessment also allows the paramedic to verify that nothing was missed or overlooked in the primary or secondary assessments in which the focus of patient care was on identifying and managing life-threatening conditions. Reassessment is an important aspect of providing good patient care.

SHOW ME THE EVIDENCE

Army researchers evaluated the value of vital sign trends in trauma patients. They retrospectively assessed vital signs of patients being transported to a level I trauma center in two time periods: 0–7 minutes and 14–21 minutes. They concluded that vital sign trends over 21 minutes or less are unlikely to be diagnostically useful. Higher acuity patients' vital signs were much more variable and had periodic episodes of instability rather than a steady decline.

Modified from: Chen L, Reisner AT, Gribok A, Reifman J. Exploration of prehospital vital sign trends for the prediction of trauma outcomes. *Prehosp Emerg Care*. 2009;13(3):286-294.

Physical Examination of Infants and Children

Examining the ill or injured child requires special assessment skills. Because children differ physiologically, psychologically, and anatomically from adults, assessment of a pediatric patient must consider age and development.

Approaching the Pediatric Patient

The assessment and management objectives in caring for critically ill or injured children are similar to those for any other patient. However, the approach to the pediatric patient must differ. Because the initial encounter with the sick or injured child sets the tone for the entire patient care episode, the paramedic must consider the patient's age. The paramedic also must be sensitive to how the child perceives the emergency environment. The following six guidelines should be considered when approaching the pediatric patient:[6]

1. Remain calm and confident. The parent's anxiety is infectious. Stay under control and take charge of the situation in a gentle but firm manner.
2. Do not separate the child from the parent unless absolutely necessary. In fact, once parents are reassured, encourage them to touch, hold, or cuddle the child when such actions are practical. This comforts the parents and the child.
3. Establish rapport with the parents and the child. Much of a child's fear and anxiety reflects the parent's behavior. When the family is calm, the child is reassured and is less fearful.
4. Be honest with the child and parent. In simple, direct, nonmedical language, explain to the parent and the child what is happening as it occurs. When a procedure is going to hurt, inform the child. Never lie. Do not give the impression that there are options when none exist. For example, do not say, "Would you like to go for a ride in the ambulance?" The child may answer "No."
5. Whenever possible, assign one paramedic to stay with the child. This person should obtain the history and be the primary person to initiate therapy. Even in a few moments, one person who remains on the child's level can establish a trusting relationship.
6. Observe the patient before the physical examination. If possible, the paramedic should initially assess the alert child with no touching. After the physical examination begins, the child's behavior may change radically, and it may be difficult to assess whether the behavior is a reaction to a physical state or to the perceived intrusion. The paramedic usually can assess the patient's general appearance, skin signs, level of consciousness,

respiratory rate, and behavior easily before approaching the patient. During this observation, the paramedic also should note any area of the body that looks painful and avoid manipulating this area until the end of the examination. The paramedic should inform the child that he or she will give warning before touching the area.

CRITICAL THINKING

The next time you are in a room with an infant or small child, try this "across the room" assessment technique. What can you tell about the level of distress and cardiopulmonary function by doing this?

General Appearance

A child's general appearance is assessed best at a distance. While the patient is in safe, familiar surroundings (eg, a parent's arms), the paramedic visually should assess the child's level of consciousness, spontaneous movement, respiratory effort, and skin color. The child's body position also can offer helpful information. For example, the child may be lying limp or sitting upright to aid breathing. Other clues may help determine the child's willingness to cooperate during the examination. These clues may include crying, eye contact, concentration, and distractibility.

A visual inspection of the child's general appearance can be helpful. Appearance is a reasonably reliable indicator of the patient's need for emergency care. Children who are seriously ill or injured usually do not attempt to hide their state. Their actions generally reflect the severity of the situation; therefore, the patient's appearance is a valuable tool for the paramedic. **TABLE 19-8** provides the key aspects of general appearance in the initial assessment of the pediatric patient.

Physical Examination

A physical examination is best conducted with knowledge of the development of children and changes that occur within age groups (see Chapter 12, *Life Span Development*). The guidelines that follow vary according to the child's development. However, these guidelines may be used as a reference during the examination. Parents and family members also may be a source of information. The paramedic may direct

TABLE 19-8 Components of General Appearance for Assessment

Assessment Finding	Evaluation Considerations
Alertness	How perceptive is the child, and how responsive is the child to the presence of a stranger or to other aspects of the environment?
Distractibility	How readily does a person, object, or sound draw the child's attention? For example, drawing a child's attention to a toy when the child initially appeared disinterested in the surroundings is a positive sign.
Consolability	Can a distressed child be comforted? For example, stopping a child from crying by speaking softly or offering a pacifier or a toy is an encouraging sign.
Speech or cry	Is the speech or cry strong and spontaneous? Weak and muffled? Hoarse? Absent unless stimulated? Absent altogether?
Spontaneous activity	Does the child appear flaccid? Do the extremities move only in response to stimuli, or are movements spontaneous?
Color	Is there pallor, a flushed appearance, cyanosis, or mottling? Does the skin coloring of the trunk differ from that of the extremities?
Respiratory efforts	Are there intercostal, supraclavicular, or suprasternal retractions in the resting state? Nasal flaring indicates respiratory difficulty.
Eye contact	Does the child appear to gaze aimlessly, or does the child maintain eye contact with objects or people? Even small infants, when well, preferentially fix their gaze on a face rather than on other objects.

questions regarding "normal" behavior and activity levels to the parents.

Birth to 6 Months

Children younger than 6 months typically are not frightened by the approach of a stranger; therefore, the physical examination is fairly easy. During the examination, the paramedic should maintain the child's body temperature with a light cover.

Healthy and alert infants usually are in constant motion. They may have a lusty cry. If the patient is younger than 3 months, poor head control is normal. Infants primarily use the diaphragm to breathe and are therefore referred to as "abdominal breathers" or "belly breathers." This diaphragmatic involvement causes the stomach to protrude and the infant's chest wall to retract during inspiration, which may give the impression of labored breathing. Skin color, nasal flaring, and intercostal muscle retraction are the best indicators of respiratory insufficiency.

In the infant, assessing the fontanels is particularly important (**FIGURE 19-48**). These sutures between the flat bones of the skull are wide enough to allow a "give" in the skull during the birth process. (The anterior fontanel, known as the soft spot, usually is present up to the age of 18 months.) The anterior fontanel should be level with the skull or slightly depressed and soft. The fontanel usually bulges during crying and may feel firm if the child is lying down. In the absence of injury, the fontanel is best examined with the child in an upright position. A sunken fontanel may indicate dehydration, and a bulging fontanel in the noncrying upright infant may indicate an increase in intracranial pressure.

7 Months to 3 Years

Patients from 7 months to 3 years of age often are difficult to evaluate. They have little capacity to understand the emergency event. In addition, they are likely to experience emotional reactions as a result of illness, injury, or hospitalization. Children of this age fear strangers and may show separation anxiety. If possible, parents should be present and allowed to hold the child during the examination (**FIGURE 19-49**). The paramedic should approach the child with a quiet, reassuring voice. If time permits, the paramedic should allow the patient to become accustomed to the examination environment.

During the physical assessment, each activity should be explained in short, simple sentences. The paramedic should give this explanation even though it may not improve cooperation. The best approach is to be gentle and firm and to complete the examination as quickly as possible. If physical restraint is necessary and if patient care activities will not be hindered, the paramedic should restrain the child with hands rather than mechanical devices, such as a pediatric immobilization device.

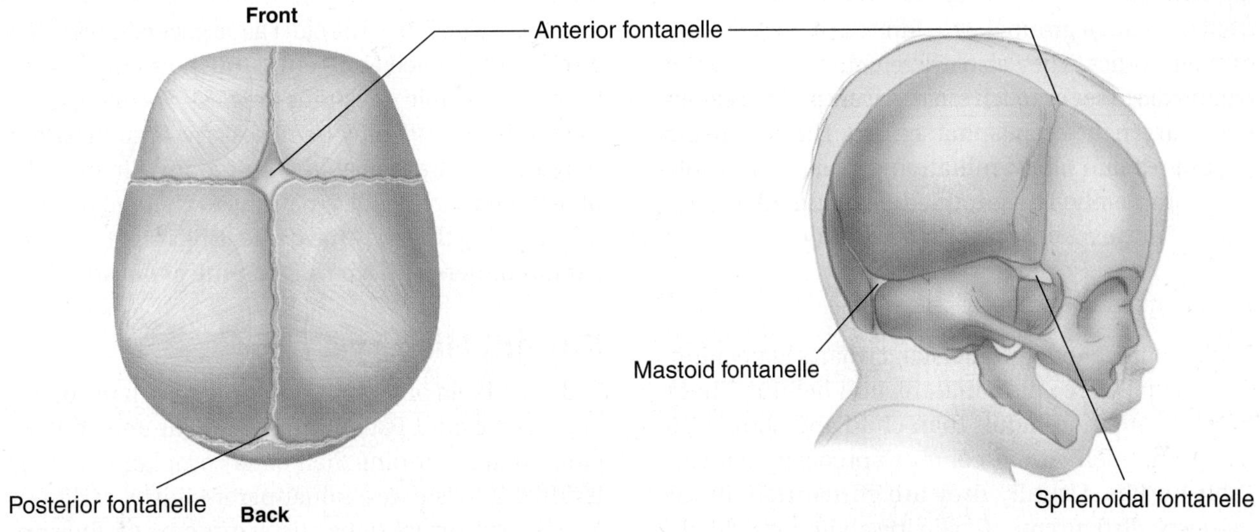

FIGURE 19-48 Palpation of the anterior fontanel.

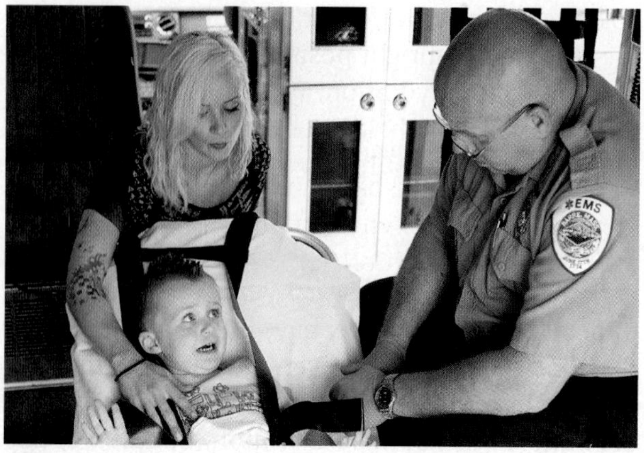

FIGURE 19-49 Examining a child.

4 Years to 11 Years

Children in the 4- to 11-year age group are developing a capacity for rational thought. They may be cooperative during the physical examination. Depending on the child's age and the emergency scenario, the child may be able to provide a limited history of the event. These children also may experience separation anxiety and may view their illness or injury as punishment. Therefore, the paramedic should approach the child slowly and speak in quiet and reassuring tones. Questions should be simple and direct.

During the examination, the paramedic should allow the child to take part by holding the stethoscope, penlight, or other pieces of equipment. This "helping" activity may lessen the child's fear. Helping also may improve the paramedic–patient relationship. Children of this age group have a limited understanding of their bodies. They also are reluctant to allow the paramedic to see or touch their "private parts" (seldom necessary in the prehospital setting). The paramedic should explain all examination procedures simply and completely. The paramedic should advise the child of any expected pain or discomfort.

12 to 18 Years

Adolescents generally understand what is happening. They usually are calm, mature, and helpful. These patients are more adult than child and should be treated as such. Adolescents are preoccupied with their bodies. Usually they are concerned about modesty, disfigurement, pain, disability, and death. If appropriate, reassurance should be provided about these concerns during the examination.

During the patient interview, the paramedic should respect the patient's need for privacy. Some adolescents may hesitate to reveal relevant history in the presence of family and friends. If the adolescent gives vague answers or seems uncomfortable, the parents and patient should be interviewed privately. The possibility of alcohol or other drug use should be considered, as well as the possibility of pregnancy (for postpubescent girls).

Physical Examination of Older Adults

As with pediatric patients, age-related physiologic and psychological variations may create special challenges in patient assessment of older adults. The paramedic should not assume that all older adults are victims of age-related disorders. Individual differences in knowledge, mental reasoning, experience, and personality influence how these patients respond to examination.

Communicating With the Older Adult

Some older adults have sensory losses that may make communications more difficult. For example, hearing and visual impairments are not uncommon. In addition, some older adults experience some memory loss and may become easily confused. Extra time may be needed to communicate effectively with these patients.

The paramedic should remain close to the patient during the interview and face the patient when asking questions, if possible. The older adult generally perceives a reassuring voice and gentle touch as comforting. Short and simple questions are best. Speaking more loudly than usual may be necessary, and questions may need to be repeated. The paramedic must be patient and careful not to patronize or offend patients by assuming that they have a hearing impairment or cannot understand a particular line of questioning.

Patient History

Older patients often have multiple health problems at the same time. Patients may be vague and nonspecific when describing their chief complaint, making it difficult to isolate a nonapparent injury or illness. Moreover, normal signs and symptoms of illness or injury may be absent because of decreased sensory function in some older adult patients.

Older patients with many health problems often take several medications. These medications increase the risk of illness from use and misuse. The paramedic should try to gather a full medication history and must be alert to the relationship among drug interactions, disease, and the aging process (see Chapter 48, *Geriatrics*).

As part of the history, the paramedic should assess the patient's functional abilities and any recent changes in activities of daily living (ADLs). Many older adults attribute these changes to age and may not mention them unless asked. These details may help indicate patient conditions that are not readily observable and may also reveal the need for other pertinent lines of questioning. Examples of functional abilities and ADLs to be discussed with the patient include the following:

- Walking
- Getting out of bed
- Dressing
- Driving a car
- Using public transportation
- Preparing meals
- Taking medications
- Sleeping habits
- Bathroom habits

Physical Examination

During examination, the paramedic should ensure comfort for the older adult patient. All examination procedures should be explained clearly and all questions should be answered sensitively. Many older patients with chronic illness may have lived with pain or discomfort for a long time; therefore, their perception of what is painful may be different from that of other patients. The paramedic should observe for signs such as grimacing or wincing during the examination. These signs may indicate pain or a possible injury site. If the situation permits, the paramedic should perform the examination slowly and gently with consideration to the patient's feelings and needs.

Many older adults believe they will die in a hospital. If transport is needed, patients may become fearful and anxious. The paramedic should be sensitive to these concerns. If appropriate, the patient should be reassured that his or her condition is not serious. The paramedic should attempt to calm these patients and advise them that they will be well treated in the hospital. All examination findings should be carefully recorded (see Chapter 4, *Documentation*).

Summary

- The secondary assessment integrates patient assessment findings with knowledge of epidemiology and pathophysiology to form a field impression and to identify an appropriate treatment plan.
- The examination techniques commonly used in the physical examination are inspection, palpation, percussion, and auscultation.
- Equipment used during the comprehensive physical examination includes the stethoscope and blood pressure cuff. An ophthalmoscope and otoscope may be used, but have limited use in the paramedic scope of practice.
- The physical examination is performed in a systematic manner. The examination is a step-by-step process. Emphasis is placed on the patient's present illness and chief complaint.
- The physical examination includes assessment of mental status; general survey; assessment of vital signs; examination of the body components, including the skin, head, eyes, ears, nose, throat, chest, abdomen, posterior body, and extremities; and neurologic examination.
- The first step in any patient care encounter is to note the patient's appearance and behavior. To do so, the paramedic must assess the patient's level of consciousness, which may include assessment of the following: posture, gait, and motor activity; dress, grooming, hygiene, and breath or body odors; facial expression; mood, affect, and relation to person and things; speech and language; thought and perceptions; and memory and attention.
- During the general survey, the paramedic should evaluate the patient for signs of distress, apparent state of health, skin color and obvious lesions, height and build, sexual development, and weight. The paramedic also should assess vital signs.
- The comprehensive physical examination should include an evaluation of the texture and turgor of the skin, hair, and fingernails and toenails.
- Examination of the structures of the head and neck involves inspection, palpation, and auscultation.
- The paramedic must possess a full knowledge of the structure of the thoracic cage. This knowledge aids in performing a good respiratory and cardiac assessment.
- Air movement creates turbulence as it passes through the respiratory tree. Air movement produces breath sounds during inhalation and exhalation.
- In the prehospital setting the paramedic must examine the heart indirectly. However, the paramedic can obtain

details about the size and effectiveness of pumping action through a skilled assessment that includes palpation and auscultation.

- The four quadrants of the abdomen and their contents provide the basis for inspection, auscultation, percussion, and palpation of this body region.
- An examination of the genitalia of either sex can be awkward for the patient and the paramedic. The paramedic should inspect the genitalia for bleeding and signs of trauma (if indicated).
- Examination of the anus is indicated in the presence of rectal bleeding or specific trauma to the area.
- When examining the upper and lower extremities, the paramedic should direct his or her attention to function. The paramedic also should pay attention to structure.
- Assessment of the spine begins with a visual assessment of the cervical, thoracic, and lumbar curves. The assessment continues with a region-by-region examination for pain, swelling, and range of motion.
- A neurologic examination may be organized into five categories: mental status and speech, cranial nerves, motor system, sensory system, and reflexes.
- Reassessment is the ongoing assessment of the patient to determine changes in condition and response to treatment.
- When approaching the pediatric patient, the paramedic should remain calm and confident. The paramedic should observe the child before beginning the physical examination. The paramedic also should make sure to avoid separation of the child and parent. Moreover, the paramedic must establish a rapport with the parents and child and must be honest. One caregiver should be assigned to the child.
- The paramedic should not assume that all older adults are victims of disorders related to aging. Individual differences in knowledge, mental reasoning, experience, and personality influence how these patients respond to examination.

References

1. 3M Littman Stethoscopes using tunable technology. 3M website. https://www.3m.co.uk/3M/en_GB/Littmann-UK/my-stethoscope/using-your-stethoscope/using-tunable-technology/. Accessed February 18, 2018.
2. National Highway Traffic Safety Administration. *The National EMS Education Standards. Paramedic Instructional Guidelines*. Washington, DC: US Department of Transportation/National Highway Traffic Safety Administration; 2009.
3. Understanding blood pressure readings. American Heart Association website. http://www.heart.org/HEARTORG/Conditions/HighBloodPressure/KnowYourNumbers/Understanding-Blood-Pressure-Readings_UCM_301764_Article.jsp#.WaHjVq2ZPOQ. Accessed February 18, 2018.
4. James PA, Oparil S, Carter BL, et al. 2014 Evidence-based guidelines for the management of high blood pressure in adults: report from the panel members appointed to the Eighth Joint National Committee (JNC 8). *JAMA*. 2014;311(5):507-520.
5. Perry AG, Potter P, Ostendorf WR, Laplante N. *Clinical Nursing Skills and Techniques*. 9th ed. St. Louis, MO: Elsevier; 2018.
6. Seidel J, Henderson D, eds. *Prehospital Care of Pediatric Patients. Paramedic Training Institute*. California EMSC Project. Los Angeles, CA: American Academy of Pediatrics; 1987.

Suggested Readings

Arendts G, Burkett E, Hullick C, Carpenter CR, Nagaraj G, Visvanathan R. Frailty, thy name is . . .. *Emerg Med Aust*. 2017;29(6):712-716.

Ball JW, Dains JE, Flynn JA, Solomon BS, Stewart RW. *Seidel's Guide to Physical Examination*. 8th ed. St. Louis, MO: Mosby; 2018.

Bickley LS. *Bates' Guide to Physical Examination and History Taking*. 11th ed. Philadelphia, PA: Wolters Kluwer, Lippincott Williams & Wilkins; 2013.

Walton J, Robinson T, Zieman S, et al. Integrating frailty research into the medical specialties—report from a U13 conference. *J Am Geriatr Soc*. 2017;65(10):2134-2139.

Zitelli B, McIntire S, Norwalk A. *Zitelli and Davis' Atlas of Pediatric Physical Diagnosis*. 7th ed. St. Louis, MO: Elsevier; 2018.

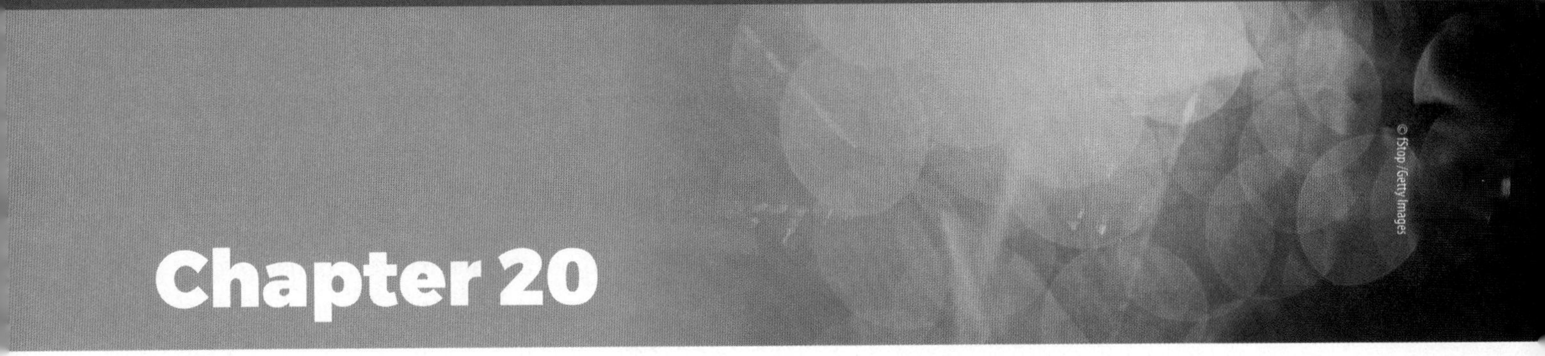

Chapter 20

Assessment-Based Management and Clinical Decision Making

NATIONAL EMS EDUCATION STANDARD COMPETENCIES

Assessment

Integrate scene and patient assessment findings with knowledge of epidemiology and pathophysiology to form a field impression. This includes developing a list of differential diagnoses through clinical reasoning to modify the assessment and formulate a treatment plan.

OBJECTIVES

Upon completion of this chapter, the paramedic student will be able to:

1. Discuss how assessment-based management contributes to effective patient and scene assessment. (p 684)
2. List the key elements of paramedic practice. (pp 684–686)
3. Describe factors that affect assessment and decision making in the prehospital setting. (pp 686–687)
4. Outline effective techniques for scene and patient assessment and choreography. (pp 687–688)
5. Identify essential take-in equipment for general and selected patient situations. (pp 689–690)
6. Outline strategies for patient approach that promote an effective patient encounter. (pp 690–691)
7. Discuss the limitations of protocols, standing orders, and patient care algorithms. (p 691)
8. Outline the key components of the critical-thinking process for paramedics. (pp 691–695)
9. Describe situations that may necessitate the use of the critical-thinking process while delivering prehospital patient care. (pp 693–695)
10. Identify elements necessary for an effective critical-thinking process. (p 695)
11. Describe the six elements required for effective clinical decision making in the prehospital setting. (pp 696–697)
12. Describe techniques to permit efficient and accurate presentation of the patient. (pp 697–698)

KEY TERMS

action plan A plan of action based on the patient's condition and the environment.

application of principles A component of critical thinking in which the examiner makes patient care decisions based on conceptual understanding of the situation and interpretation of data gathered from the patient.

assessment-based management Comprehensive care that is based on patient assessment, the patient's history, and the physical examination.

bias The tendency to make conclusions or decisions based on a preformed idea, assumption, or prejudice.

clinical decision making (clinical reasoning) The process of determining, preventing, or managing patient problems.

clinical judgment The outcome or conclusion a paramedic arrives at based on critical thinking and clinical decision making.

concept formation A component of critical thinking that refers to all elements that are gathered to form a general impression of the patient.

contemplative approach An approach to patient care in which a history is obtained and a physical examination is performed before providing patient care.

critical thinking The ability to quickly focus thinking to get the desired results depending on the situation.

data interpretation A component of critical thinking in which the examiner gathers the necessary data to form a field impression and working diagnosis.

evaluation A component of critical thinking in which the examiner assesses the patient's response to care.

field impression An impression of the patient's condition that the paramedic makes based on pattern recognition that results from experience.

multitasking As it relates to interviewing, the ability to ask questions, take notes, and perform tasks while listening to the patient's answers.

patient handoff The effective communication and transfer of patient information from one health care provider to another as patient care is transferred.

patient management plan A plan of care that is based on principles and applications of findings in the patient assessment.

pattern recognition The process of comparing gathered information with the paramedic's knowledge base of medical illness and disease.

reflection on action A component of critical thinking (usually performed after the event) in which the examiner evaluates a patient care episode for possible improvement in similar future responses.

resuscitative approach An approach to patient care that recognizes the need for immediate intervention for patients with life-threatening illness or injury.

tunnel vision A narrow outlook; the focusing of attention on a particular problem without proper regard for possible consequences or alternative approaches.

Unique to the EMS profession is the uncertainty of the prehospital environment, which is influenced heavily by factors that do not exist in other medical settings. In this challenging environment, paramedics must be able to develop and apply an appropriate **patient management plan**. *To do so, they must gather, evaluate, and synthesize information; formulate a field impression based on pathophysiologic principles and physical findings; and implement a treatment plan for patients with common complaints. To accomplish these objectives, they must apply judgment, exercise independent decision making, and work effectively under pressure. These are the cornerstones of effective paramedic practice.*

Effective Assessment

Assessment-based management describes comprehensive care that is based on patient assessment. Effective assessment depends on the patient's history and the physical examination. The paramedic's knowledge of disease allows him or her to hold a high degree of suspicion for possible illness. This knowledge also helps the paramedic to focus the history toward the patient's complaint and associated problems. Likewise, the paramedic must focus the physical examination toward body systems associated with the complaint. Some field situations may impair the thoroughness of the examination. For example, unsafe scenes or entrapment may hinder this process. Still, the paramedic must not overlook the importance of the physical examination or perform it hastily.

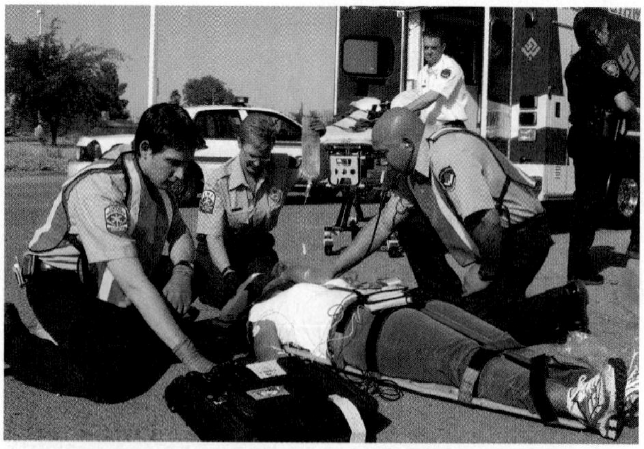

Pattern Recognition

Once paramedics obtain the patient's history and perform the physical examination, they can compare the information gathered with their knowledge base of medical illness and disease. They must consider whether the history and physical examination match a recognized pattern of illness, a process known as **pattern recognition**. For example, a 55-year-old man with chest pain and shortness of breath "matches" a recognized pattern for acute myocardial infarction. However, a 20-year-old woman with similar complaints and no family history of early myocardial events would not match this pattern. Other examples include a 2-year-old child who is in respiratory distress and has a barking cough (matching a pattern for croup) and a 75-year-old woman with distended neck veins and crackles who produces a pink, frothy sputum when she coughs (matching a pattern for heart failure). Pattern recognition makes it possible for the paramedic to form a field impression and to begin a treatment plan. Thus the greater the paramedic's knowledge base and quality of assessment, the greater the probability of appropriate decision making and quality patient care.

CRITICAL THINKING

How can pattern recognition lead you down the wrong path?

Field Impression and Action Plan

The paramedic forms a **field impression** of the patient's condition from pattern recognition that comes from experience and from analytic thinking (**FIGURE 20-1**). The field impression must be confirmed through the patient history and physical examination. Then, the paramedic can formulate an **action plan**. This plan is based on the patient's condition and the environment. Using the previous example of the two patients with chest pain, the field impression of the 55-year-old patient most likely leads to an action plan that includes electrocardiographic (ECG) monitoring, pulse oximetry, intravenous therapy, aspirin administration, and nitroglycerin. The 20-year-old patient's action plan most likely includes ECG monitoring to evaluate for supraventricular tachycardia, pulse oximetry, and a more thorough assessment to detect a recent respiratory illness to rule out the possibility of injury, pleurisy, or pneumonia.

NOTE

The paramedic should not ignore a gut instinct. If something seems wrong, the paramedic should keep looking. Gut instincts often help the paramedic to identify subtle physical findings that are difficult to quantify (eg, patient affect or dull and lackluster eyes).

Following the field impression and the action plan, the paramedic provides basic and advanced life support treatment (**FIGURE 20-2**). These treatments are based on knowledge of the protocols and on judgment—that is, knowing when and how to apply the protocols. Judgment also involves knowing when it is appropriate to deviate from the protocols. For example, consider the administration of nitroglycerin to a 58-year-old man complaining of ischemic chest pain. His blood

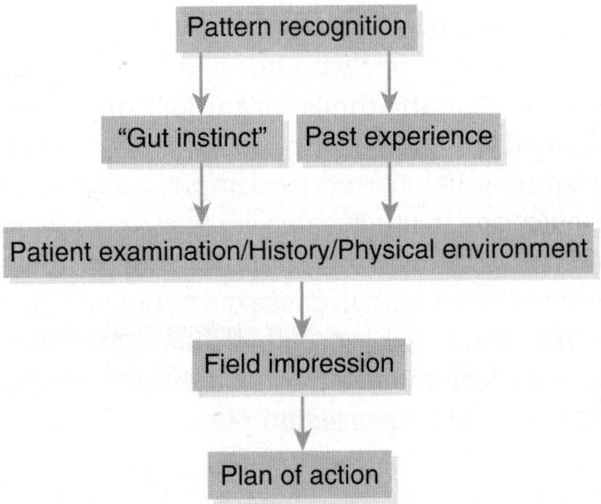

FIGURE 20-1 Matrix pattern.

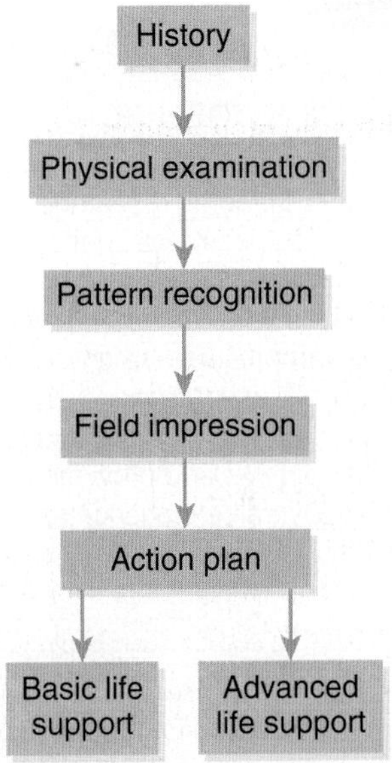

FIGURE 20-2 Effective assessment.

pressure measurement is within normal range, but during the patient history he reveals he has taken Viagra within the past 18 hours. The administration of nitroglycerin can cause a lethal drop in blood pressure in these patients (see Chapter 13, *Principles of Pharmacology and Emergency Medications*). Good judgment in this case would lead the paramedic to deviate from a common protocol used to manage normotensive patients with ischemic chest pain.

CRITICAL THINKING

How can you continue to improve your patient care judgment?

Factors That Affect Assessment and Decision Making

Many factors can affect the quality of assessment and decision making by the paramedic. The following factors are discussed in this section:

- Paramedic's attitude
- Patient's willingness to cooperate
- Distracting injuries
- Bias and tunnel vision
- Environment
- Patient compliance
- Crew considerations

CRITICAL THINKING

Have you ever seen any of these factors affect patient care?

SHOW ME THE EVIDENCE

In a study conducted to observe paramedics' ability to manage difficult situations, researchers evaluated six experienced and four less experienced paramedics as they managed two complex simulated emergency medical services (EMS) calls. They found that more experienced paramedics made more assessments, considered more differential diagnoses, and identified pulmonary embolism earlier. In addition, experienced paramedics made better use of their EMT partner and provided more advanced life support care. Overall, experienced paramedics used more inferential reasoning and more functional and strategic thinking.

Modified from: Smith MW, Bentley MA, Fernandez A, Gibson G, Schweikhart SB, Woods DD. Performance of experienced versus less experienced paramedics in managing challenging scenarios: a cognitive task analysis study. *Ann Emerg Med.* 2013;62(4):367-379.

Paramedic's Attitude

The paramedic must be professional and nonjudgmental in all actions. These traits are required to perform an effective assessment. A biased or judgmental attitude can "short-circuit" the information-gathering process, causing the paramedic to overlook important patient data. For example, a paramedic who assumes that an indigent patient is intoxicated may not consider complications from diabetes or drug use, head injury or hypoxia, or hypovolemia that may have resulted from an internal injury.

Patient's Willingness to Cooperate

Patient cooperation is important in providing patient care. Patients who do not cooperate can complicate the patient assessment required to formulate an action plan. As discussed throughout this text, the paramedic should evaluate patients who are uncooperative, restless, or belligerent for underlying trauma or illness.

Distracting Injuries

Obvious but non–life-threatening injuries can distract the paramedic from performing a thorough assessment for more serious problems. Examples include open fractures and facial bleeding that is profuse. If necessary, these wounds should be covered with dressings during the assessment, which will help the paramedic to focus on the more serious problems.

Bias and Tunnel Vision

Bias and **tunnel vision** can lead to an inaccurate assessment and an incorrect field impression. For example, labeling a patient as "just another drunk" can lead to a biased assessment. Another example is labeling someone who has been transported by ambulance many times for minor complaints or imagined illness as a "frequent flyer." Tunnel vision is assuming an incorrect field impression based on a misplaced or an uneducated gut instinct, or focusing on only a portion of the presenting illness. Either of these assumptions can cause the paramedic to miss the "big picture." Like labeling, tunnel vision can result in a rushed judgment early in the patient assessment and an inappropriate action plan.

Environment

Factors in the environment can adversely affect assessment techniques and decision making at the scene. Examples include scene chaos, violent or dangerous situations, crowds of bystanders or other emergency workers, severe weather, and high noise levels. After ensuring personal safety, the paramedic should quickly establish control of the environment, which may involve requesting the help of law enforcement personnel to control the scene so that appropriate assessment and care can be delivered without distraction.

Patient Compliance

The patient's willingness to cooperate and comply with the assessment may depend on his or her trust in the paramedic crew. For example, the patient who perceives the paramedic as competent and professional often provides a thorough history. The patient also often will agree to a complete physical examination. Other factors that can affect compliance are language/communication difficulties, cultural and ethnic barriers, and other factors (see Chapter 16, *Therapeutic Communications*, and Chapter 17, *History Taking*).

Crew Considerations

Depending on the EMS agency, crews may consist of a single paramedic and an emergency medical technician (EMT), two paramedics, or several types or groups of responders (eg, EMS, fire and rescue, and police). In cases in which only EMS is involved and only one paramedic is at the scene, the paramedic will work with the EMT to develop a proper sequence for gathering information and providing care. If two paramedics are available, the information gathering and treatment often can occur simultaneously, with each paramedic assuming specific duties. If multiple responders and agencies are at the scene, roles and duties should be defined in advance. For example, one paramedic may be in charge of history taking and conferring with medical direction. Another paramedic may be in charge of treatment. The fire-rescue members may be in charge of extrication and gathering of equipment. Finally, law enforcement personnel may be in charge of securing the scene.

CRITICAL THINKING

How can too many paramedics on the scene have a negative influence on patient assessment and care?

Assessment and Management Choreography

In cases where multiple responders are at the scene of an emergency, a coherent assessment can be difficult. A large emergency response may occur with multiple-tier response systems (eg, EMS, fire, and police). The situation often is made more complex if the responders are trained at the same level (eg, paramedic) without a clear direction for individual duties. Therefore, members of the response team must have a preplan for deciding roles. The team can predesignate roles by shift or crew, or roles can rotate among team members.

An example of a preplan for two paramedics is to assign one as the team leader and one as the patient care person. This type of plan must be flexible in rapidly changing field situations. However, the basic "game plan" allows others to participate and is important in preventing confusion at the scene. The following are sample responsibilities for each of the paramedics in this type of preplan:

1. Team leader responsibilities
   - Accompanies the patient to definitive care
   - Establishes contact and a dialogue with the patient
   - Obtains the history
   - Performs the physical examination
   - Presents the patient and gives verbal reports over the radio or after definitive care
   - Completes all documentation
   - Tries to maintain the overall patient perspective and provides leadership to the team by designating tasks and coordinating transport
   - Designates and actively participates in critical interventions during the resuscitative phase of the primary survey
   - Acts as initial EMS command in multiple-casualty situations (see Chapter 53, *Medical Incident Command*)
   - Interprets the ECG, communicates with medical direction and relays drug orders, controls access to bags, and documents drug administration and effects during advanced cardiac life support
2. Patient care person responsibilities
   - Provides scene cover (watches the team leader's back)
   - Gathers scene information and talks to family members and bystanders
   - Obtains vital signs

- Performs skills and interventions as requested by the team leader (eg, attaches monitor leads, provides oxygen, initiates intravenous access, administers drugs, and obtains transport equipment)
- Acts as triage group leader in multiple-casualty situations
- Administers drugs; monitors endotracheal tube placement, pulse oximetry, and basic life support interventions during advanced cardiac life support

Crew Resource Management

Human factors (environmental, organizational, job, and individual) are central to high performance in EMS systems. They are also the cause of many errors within those systems. Crew resource management (CRM) is a process that focuses on communication, teamwork, situational awareness, workload management and decision making as a means to reduce errors and adverse events in high-risk, high-consequence industries such as EMS.[1] The airline industry introduced CRM in 1979 after several major crashes. Its success there led to wider application of the principles in health care and public safety.

The philosophy in CRM is that the responsibility for the care of the patient belongs to everyone on the EMS call—not just the team leader, the paramedic, or the most senior person. Each responder must share accountability for the safety and well-being of the patient while respecting the knowledge and authority of the team leader. The power of the team is central to the success of CRM.[2]

The CRM model begins with establishing a clear leader who can share the vision of the mission and properly delegate tasks so the right person is given the right job and no person is overloaded. The team leader establishes goals, delegates or assumes responsibility, motivates the team, maintains situational awareness, adapts to changing conditions, recognizes team strengths and limitations, listens openly, and sets clear expectations.[3] All team members should acknowledge the role they have been assigned by the team leader and report out when they have achieved their assigned task. Everyone maintains situational awareness to recognize if a hazard to the crew, the patient, or the public develops and notify the team leader clearly of that perceived risk.

The core of CRM involves creating an environment that promotes clear and honest communication. Each team member should be empowered to raise any concerns immediately and directly to the team leader. If team members feel intimidated, they are less likely to speak out about safety issues, which could lead to negative outcomes for the patient, the crew, or the community. Team members must share their concerns early and clearly.

A useful model for resolving concerns about a decision or its effects is the CRM circle of success, developed by LeSage, Dyar, and Evans[2] (**FIGURE 20-3**). The CRM circle of success involves several stages, beginning with inquiry. At this stage, several things can happen. The leader may state the mission objective or give an order to a team member based on the mission objective. Alternately someone on the team might perform an action that catches the attention of other team members or exhibit a behavior thought to be inappropriate to the situation. During this stage, communication can be misunderstood if the message is not clear to the receiver or if people are confused about the situation. In such cases, team members may express discomfort by making vague statements that indicate discomfort with the situation. It is important for the leader to recognize this discomfort and seek clarification with statements such as "tell me what you are concerned about."

FIGURE 20-3 The crew resource management circle of success.

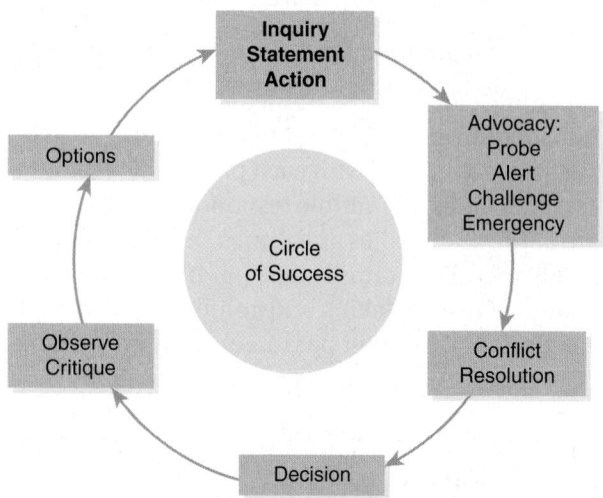

During the advocacy stage, team members should affirm their agreement with an action or statement by verbally stating their agreement or by remaining silent (which should be used sparingly). A team member who is uncomfortable with the situation or needs to make better sense of the situation should challenge the team leader in a respectful manner by following the PACE acronym:

- **Probe.** Probe for better understanding to make sense of the situation. Inquiries should be specific and directed to one person to avoid confusion. For example, "The patient's blood pressure is 84/50 mm Hg. You asked me to give nitroglycerin. Is this what you intended?"
- **Alert.** Alert the leader of specific concerns or abnormal findings that would immediately help the team. For example, "Are you aware that the patient took Viagra 4 hours ago? We may want to wait on the nitroglycerin."
- **Challenge.** Challenge the proposed action or strategy. This approach is used after the alert has failed. The challenge should be direct and include the following elements:
    - An appeal to the leader, addressing him or her by name and rank
    - A statement of what was seen or heard that is believed to be a threat
    - An explanation of why this is thought to be a threat
    - A description of what could occur if the threat is not handled
    - A suggestion of what the team leader could do to mitigate the threat

  The challenge phase may involve moving into the action area to prepare to take additional steps if needed.
- **Emergency.** Intervene if continuing down the proposed path will cause harm. This type of action is rarely needed. It should be employed only when there is imminent and serious danger if the present actions continue. It is used when communications have failed completely or when there is no time to escalate the communication. It may involve physical action and should be employed only in extreme circumstances.

The conflict resolution stage comes next. To resolve conflict in a safety-sensitive situation, crew members must remain open to input from others and remain curious. This attitude will allow members to get to the heart of *what* is right, not *who* is right.[2]

In the decision stage, team leaders must acknowledge the emotions that come with a challenge to their orders, set their ego aside, and try to understand why the concern was raised, and whether it is valid. The leader should reflect on whether the information the team member provided will help successfully complete the mission. Ultimately, the leader is the one who must make the decisions for the team. He or she will also take responsibility for the decisions and how the actions of the team are carried out. The leader who listens carefully to the input and concerns of the team often makes better decisions.

The final stages of the CRM circle of success are more reflective in nature. As the plan identified by the leader is executed, the team should continuously evaluate how well it is working. Asking what is going well—or not going on—and how the plan can be changed based on how things are going will often lead to the best outcome possible given the circumstances. This process is a type of reflection in action that should occur throughout the entire cycle of an EMS call. Locking into a plan without making changes needed based on the patient, the team, or the environment can lead to failure. The process should continue even after the incident has been resolved; often, a full exploration of the situation is not possible until after the call.

The "Right Stuff"

Having the right stuff means carrying the right equipment to the patient's side. Not having the right stuff can compromise care and also can cause panic and confusion. The paramedic crew should always be prepared for the worst event. They should carry essential equipment to manage every aspect of patient care, including cardiac monitoring and defibrillation (BOX 20-1). The concept of having the right stuff can be compared with backpacking. A person who is backpacking must have essential items that are downsized to facilitate rapid movement with minimum weight and bulk.

Specialty "Take-In" Equipment

In addition to essential equipment for the EMS crew, other equipment may be needed based on the nature of the call. For example, many agencies have

BOX 20-1 Essential Items for All Aspects of Patient Care

Personal Protection

- Safety glasses
- Gloves
- Gowns
- Masks

Airway Control

- Endotracheal tubes and supplies
- Supraglottic airway
- Nasal and oral airways
- Suction equipment

Breathing

- Large-bore catheter for thoracic decompression
- Bag-mask device
- Occlusive dressings
- Oxygen masks, cannulae, and extension tubing
- Pulse oximetry and end-tidal carbon dioxide equipment
- Oxygen tank and regulator

Circulation

- Bandages and tape
- Blood pressure cuff and stethoscope
- Dressings
- Tourniquets
- Vascular access equipment and fluids

Disability and Dysrhythmia

- Cardiac monitor and defibrillator
- Flashlight
- Rigid collar

Exposure

- Scissors
- Blanket to cover and protect the patient

a pediatric bag with equipment of appropriate size for infants and children. A mass-casualty kit will be needed for situations involving multiple patients.

Paramedics must carry patient care reports, or an electronic documentation device, on every call. They will also need certain personal items, such as pens or pencils, wristwatches, flashlights, and portable radios or cell phones.

CRITICAL THINKING

Have you been on ambulance calls when you did not have the right equipment? How did it affect patient care?

General Approach to the Patient

A calm and orderly manner is important for the paramedic when approaching a patient. The paramedic must look and act the part of a professional (see Chapter 1, *EMS Systems: Roles, Responsibilities, and Professionalism*). Treatment starts by calming and reassuring the patient at first contact. This, in addition to a caring and confident bedside manner, will help gain the patient's trust and cooperation. Patients may not be able to rate medical performance, but they generally are very good at rating "people skills" and service.

As previously described, a preplan should be in effect to prevent confusion at the scene and improve the accuracy of patient assessment. The team leader is responsible for talking to the patient and directing actions on the call and should employ an active and concerned communication style that allows for careful listening. An initial survey of the scene can offer important clues to help the paramedic formulate an impression.

Setting the Tone for the Patient Encounter

Two approaches in the primary survey set the tone for the patient encounter. The first is the resuscitative approach. The second is the contemplative approach. The **resuscitative approach** recognizes the need for immediate intervention for patients who have life-threatening illness or injury such as the following conditions:

- Cardiorespiratory arrest
- Coma or altered level of consciousness
- Major trauma
- Respiratory distress or failure
- Seizures
- Sepsis
- Shock or hypotension
- ST elevation myocardial infarction
- Stroke
- Unstable cardiac rhythms

If a life-threatening problem is present, the paramedic crew must take resuscitative action. History taking and other details should be delayed until immediate resuscitation measures have been provided. If immediate intervention to manage life threats is not required, the paramedic can use the **contemplative approach**. With this approach, the patient history is obtained and physical examination is performed before providing patient care.

In any patient care encounter, certain conditions, such as the following, may require the paramedic to move the patient immediately to the emergency vehicle:

- The paramedic cannot provide lifesaving interventions at the patient's side.
- The scene is too unstable or unsafe.
- The scene is too chaotic to allow thorough assessment.
- Inclement weather hinders assessment and care.

"Looking to Find"

Paramedics must find something before they can treat or report it. To find something, it must be suspected. Therefore during the primary survey, the paramedic must actively look for any problems that pose a threat to life. The assessment must be systematic so that the patient's chief complaint can be rapidly determined. The paramedic must then assess the degree of distress, obtain baseline vital signs, and stay focused on the patient's history and physical findings. Forming a mental "rule-out list" often is a good approach in "looking to find." This list considers the most serious problems *first* that could cause the patient's signs and symptoms.

Experience assists the paramedic in developing the ability for multitasking. In relation to health care, **multitasking** is the ability to ask questions, take notes, and perform tasks while listening to the patient's answers. In time, the paramedic will gain the level of experience required for multitasking. Until then, it is best to ask direct questions and then carefully listen to the patient's response. Important clues can be lost by not listening. If a particular task is required while the paramedic is obtaining a patient history, a team member should provide the patient care measure if possible.

The patient's ability to describe symptoms and the paramedic's ability to listen may greatly influence the assessment. The paramedic should remember that the chief complaint may not always correlate well with some potentially life-threatening conditions. For example, a patient with myocardial infarction may at first complain of pain only in the arm or shoulder or some other minor discomfort (eg, indigestion). The paramedic's role is to rapidly assess and provide treatment for the worst-case scenario.

The Spectrum of Prehospital Care

The paramedic must have a wide base of knowledge and skills to make good patient care decisions in the prehospital setting (see Chapter 18, *Scene Size-up and Primary Assessment*, and Chapter 19, *Secondary Assessment and Reassessment*). On any given workday, the paramedic may be exposed to obvious critical life threats, potential life threats, and non–life-threatening situations. On each call, the paramedic also is expected to provide proper care and treatment. Protocols, standing orders, and patient care algorithms help to promote a standardized approach to patient care for "classic" presentations. These presentations clearly define and outline performance parameters. However, these standards have some limitations. First, they may not apply to nonspecific patient complaints that do not fit the "model." Second, these standards do not address multiple disease etiologies or multiple treatment modalities. Third, they promote linear thinking, such as standardized care is appropriate for all patients ("cookbook medicine"). The paramedic must develop critical-thinking skills to assist in unique patient care situations.

Critical Thinking, Clinical Decision Making, and Clinical Judgment

Critical thinking is the ability to quickly focus thinking to get the desired results depending on the situation. To think critically, the paramedic must clarify goals, examine assumptions, uncover hidden values, evaluate evidence, accomplish actions, and assess conclusions. Effective critical thinking is more than just memorizing facts, although content knowledge is a prerequisite to this skill. Good critical thinking requires creative, reflective and analytic thinking. It also involves other skills, such as questioning, probing, and judging.[4]

Clinical decision making (clinical reasoning) refers to the process of determining, preventing, or managing patient problems. The paramedic's decision making must be correct to reach the proper clinical judgment about the patient.

Clinical judgment is the outcome or conclusion a paramedic arrives at based on critical thinking and clinical decision making. It can lead the paramedic to a working field diagnosis. Selecting the correct field diagnosis forms the basis for choosing a particular protocol that leads to improved patient condition.

DID YOU KNOW?

The Critical Thinker

A critical thinker is objective during patient analysis and has an open mind to debate alternatives and look for proof. A critical thinker displays the following traits:

- Asks pertinent questions
- Assesses statements and arguments
- Is able to admit a lack of understanding or information
- Has a sense of curiosity and creativity
- Is interested in finding new solutions
- Is able to clearly define a set of criteria for analyzing ideas
- Is willing to examine beliefs, assumptions, and opinions and weigh them against facts
- Listens carefully to others and is able to give feedback
- Suspends judgment until all facts have been gathered and considered
- Looks for evidence to support assumptions and beliefs
- Is able to adjust opinions when new facts are found
- Looks for proof
- Examines problems closely
- Is able to reject information that is incorrect or irrelevant

Modified from: Ferrett S. *Peak Performance: Success in College and Beyond*. 7th ed. New York, NY: McGraw-Hill; 2009.

During the Canadian Patient Safety in EMS Summit, 95% of participants ranked clinical judgment and decision making as highly important to patient safety.[5] They felt that, at times, protocols and standing orders limit the paramedic's ability to use these skills. One of their nine summit recommendations was to support the concept that paramedics are capable of decision making and judgment. Protocols should have a flexible structure to permit them to do so.

Clinical Decision Making for Paramedics

Paramedics and other health care providers make decisions using intuitive (system 1) or analytic (system 2) processes. Intuitive processing is mostly automatic and is said to be made in the blink of an eye.[6] An experienced paramedic often makes decisions in this manner based on patterns observed from earlier calls. While system 1 clinical reasoning is fast, it is more likely to lead to an incorrect decision when used as the only diagnostic method. The intuitive process is subject to error when bias or thinking failure get in the way. An example would be thinking that a patient who is staggering and smells strongly of alcohol is drunk without considering alternative diagnoses such as head injury or stroke. System 2 (analytic) thinking takes longer but is less susceptible to error. A failure of analytic decision making is more likely to occur when cognitive overload, fatigue, or emotional stressors exist.

As a paramedic becomes more experienced and uses the intuitive mode of decision making more often, it is important to develop strategies that can override intuitive thinking to catch errors. Such strategies include considering at least three differential diagnoses, performing a thorough history and

DID YOU KNOW?

Clinical Decision Rules

A key element in clinical decision making is to determine risk. Risk is the "probability that a particular adverse event occurs." Increasingly, the medical community is devising clinical decision rules and tools that help assign the risk or probability that a patient has a particular injury or illness. These rules are based on key examination findings. The Nexus low-risk clinical screening criteria for cervical spine injury is an example of a clinical decision-making tool. Patients who have blunt trauma are considered low risk for cervical spine injury if they do not have tenderness over the spine, altered alertness, distracting injury, intoxication, or focal neurologic changes. This tool has a sensitivity of 99% for cervical spine injury and almost 100% for clinically significant cervical spine injury. In other words, there is little chance that cervical spine injury will be missed in patients who are examined using this criterion. On the other hand, the test is not very specific. A significant number of patients who have one or more positive findings also will not have cervical spine injury.

Researchers are continually searching for evidence-based reliable decision-making tools—tools to help guide clinical practice and evaluate patient risk in emergency care. Areas of focus have been chest pain, syncope, triage, extremity injuries, and others. Each EMS system should evaluate the applicability of a given decision rule to their patient population before it is adopted.

Modified from: Thompson C, Dowding D. *Clinical Decision and Judgment in Nursing*. Edinburgh, Scotland: Churchill Livingstone; 2002; and Panacek EA, Mower WR, Holmes JF, et al. Test performance of the individual NEXUS low-risk clinical screening criteria for cervical spine injury. *Ann Emerg Med*. 2001;38(1):22-25.

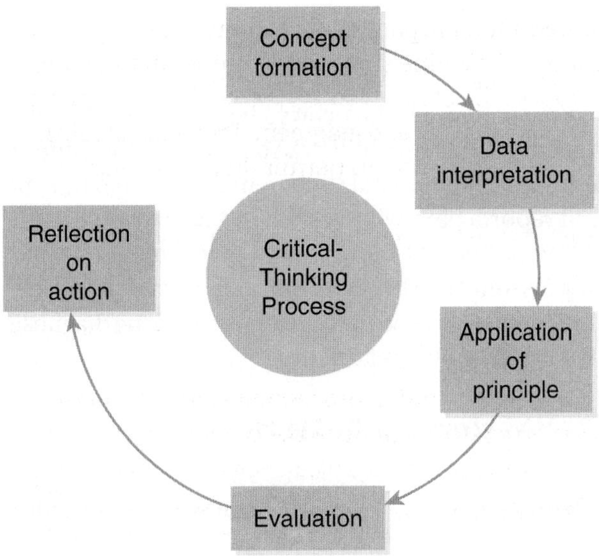

FIGURE 20-4 Critical-thinking process.

examination that not only rules in the paramedic's primary field diagnosis but rules out other potential diagnoses, and reflecting on actions taken.

Specific stages are linked with the critical-thinking process. These stages include concept formation, data interpretation, application of principles, evaluation, and reflection on action[7] (**FIGURE 20-4**).

Concept Formation

Concept formation refers to all elements gathered to form a general impression of the patient. Concept formation is the "what" of the patient story. These elements include the following (see Chapter 18, *Scene Size-up and Primary Assessment*, and Chapter 19, *Secondary Assessment and Reassessment*):

- Scene assessment (mechanism of injury, social setting)
- Chief complaint
- Patient history
- Patient affect
- Initial assessment and physical examination
- Diagnostic tests

Scenario Part 1

Your crew has been dispatched to a local park for a person with "difficulty breathing." On your arrival at the scene, you find an 18-year-old woman sitting on a park bench surrounded by her friends. The scene is safe. She is crying and tells you that she cannot catch her breath. You attempt to calm the patient and provide her with supplemental oxygen. You obtain a history from the patient and her friends that she and her boyfriend had quarreled after a long car ride and that she became emotional during the argument. She has no allergies and has no medical history other than sickle cell disease. She denies any injury but notes pain when taking a deep breath. Aside from her increased respiratory rate, her vital signs on oxygen are within normal range. Consider your concept formation for this patient.

> CRITICAL THINKING
>
> What effect would wrong or incomplete concept formation have on your critical-thinking process during patient care? How can you enhance your concept formation skills while in your paramedic program?

Data Interpretation

Following concept formation, the paramedic must gather the needed data to form a field impression. This process, known as **data interpretation**, is a component of critical thinking that helps the paramedic to form a working diagnosis. This is the "working phase" of patient care.

The quality of data interpretation rests on a few elements: the paramedic's knowledge of anatomy and physiology, pathophysiology, intuition, and previous experience in providing patient care. During the interpretation of data, the paramedic attempts to obtain a complete "picture" of the patient's situation. The success of this phase of critical thinking can be greatly affected by the paramedic's attitude. It can also be affected by the way in which the paramedic–patient encounter proceeds (see Chapter 16, *Therapeutic Communications*). In some cases, the paramedic must condense and convey these data to the online physician, who can help determine appropriate actions.

Scenario Part 2

While assessing this patient, you recall a similar patient encounter. A few years earlier, you provided care to a boy with difficulty breathing. He had just lost a big tennis match. At first you assumed the patient was having breathing difficulty because of emotions that resulted from his loss. This male patient had no allergies and no significant medical history and denied any recent injury. His vital signs were within normal range. However, lung sounds were diminished slightly on the patient's left side. The patient also complained of mild pain on inspiration. You administered supplemental oxygen. Then you rapidly transported the patient to the emergency department. After obtaining a chest radiograph, the emergency physician confirmed your suspicion of a spontaneous pneumothorax (which resolved during the patient's hospitalization). Compare this interpretation of data to that of the female patient you are caring for now.

Application of Principles

The next step in the critical-thinking process is the **application of principles** of proper patient care. These principles are based on the paramedic's conceptual understanding of the situation. They also are based on the interpretation of the data gathered from the patient. Once the paramedic establishes the field impression and working diagnosis, treatment can often be initiated through protocols and standing orders. If necessary, consultation can be made with direct/online medical direction.

Scenario Part 3

Based on your experience, your knowledge of patient care, and your interpretation of the data gathered from your patient, you decide that she may have a pulmonary embolism. You continue the oxygen and monitor breath sounds and vital signs every 5 minutes. Although the female patient you are caring for presented much like the male patient you recall, your working diagnosis is different. You reach this conclusion of pulmonary embolism because of her increased respiratory rate, her medical history, and report of pain when breathing.

Evaluation

The **evaluation** component of critical thinking requires an ongoing assessment of the patient's response to the care provided. Evaluation includes the following:

- Reassessment of the patient (ongoing assessment)
- Reflection on action (effectiveness of the intervention)
- Revision of field impression if needed
- Review of the appropriateness of the protocol, standing orders, or direct orders for the patient
- Revision of the treatment or intervention as needed

Scenario Part 4

After you have provided calming measures and oxygen to your patient, she has slowed her breathing. She also appears to be more relaxed. You reassess the patient. You find that her vital signs remain normal, but she still reports pain when asked to take a deep breath. Based on these findings, you suspect that your field impression of pulmonary embolism was correct and that there is no need to change your working diagnosis or to revise your treatment.

Reflection on Action

Reflection on action happens "after the event." It usually occurs through a formal or informal after-action

DID YOU KNOW?

Avoiding Errors in Clinical Judgment

Assessing and managing patients in the prehospital environment is a difficult task, and paramedics must take steps to avoid errors in decision making. To avoid errors, consider using the following strategies:

1. Consciously think about your thinking and question your decision making. Ask yourself, "Is this the right decision?" or "Does this make sense?" If the answer is no, reexamine your data, consult medical direction, or gather more information.
2. Recognize situations in which errors are more likely, and use extra caution in those instances. For example, it is known that a significant number of patients who refuse care will seek emergency care soon after the refusal. Be especially careful in those situations. Always ensure the patient knows that he or she can call again for help, even after refusing care.
3. Recognize your biases, and use extreme caution when making decisions in situations that involve those biases. For example, you may be frustrated when caring for a patient who is intoxicated with alcohol. This frustration may lead you to immediately attribute the patient's signs and symptoms to the intoxication. A personal bias such as this could lead you to overlook a serious head injury or other medical problem that might be the cause of the patient's presentation. Bias is a known cause of cognitive errors in medicine.

Modified from: Gallagher EJ. The intrinsic fallibility of clinical judgment. *Ann Emerg Med.* 2003;42(3):403-404; Dawson BG, Brewer JGK. EMS "no transports": an evaluation of emergency department presentation and admission rates following patient initiated "no transports." *Ann Emerg Med.* 2008;52(4, suppl):S71; and Croskerry P. Cognitive forcing strategies in clinical decision making. *Ann Emerg Med.* 2003;41(1):110-120.

review, whereby the call is evaluated for improvement in similar future responses. Reflection on action provides paramedics with an avenue to add to or alter their experience base.

SHOW ME THE EVIDENCE

Canadian researchers surveyed paramedics and paramedic students to identify whether their predominant decision-making process was intuitive or rational. Both groups scored their preference for and ability to use rational thinking significantly higher than for intuitive thinking. The paramedic students were more likely to choose the rational style than were the graduate paramedics.

Modified from: Jensen JL, Bienkowski A, Travers AH, et al. A survey to determine decision-making styles of working paramedics and student paramedics. *Can J Emerg Med.* 2016;18(3):213-222.

Scenario Part 5

En route back to quarters, you discuss the call with a paramedic student. This student has just begun her field internship. Like you, she instantly thought that the patient was having breathing difficulty because of the fight she had with her boyfriend. The student admitted that although she had read about pulmonary embolism in her initial EMT training, she had never actually seen a patient who had one. Moreover, she would not have considered this possibility when caring for this patient. You discuss the pathology of pulmonary embolism with her and the importance of considering the history in a patient who is having difficulty breathing. This reflection on action reinforces your data interpretation skills. It also adds to the student's experience base.

Fundamental Elements of Critical Thinking for Paramedics

For an effective critical-thinking process, some basic elements must be present. These elements include adequate knowledge and the ability to do the following:

- Focus on specific and multiple elements of data at the same time.
- Gather and organize data and form concepts.
- Identify and deal with medical ambiguity (patients who do not "fit" the model).
- Differentiate between relevant and irrelevant data.
- Analyze and compare similar situations from past experience.
- Recall cases in which the working diagnosis was wrong.
- Articulate decision-making reasoning and construct arguments to support or discount the decision.

All of these elements were present in the previous scenario. At the scene, the paramedic dealt with the patient's symptoms and the input of friends. In addition, he focused on assessment and history findings. At the same time, he offered initial emergency care. The paramedic did this all within moments of arriving at the patient's side. He gathered and organized the data. He then concluded that the patient might fit the model for pulmonary embolism. The paramedic also decided that the patient's history of sickle cell disease was not likely related to her present respiratory distress. He recalled a previous case in which he had mistakenly attributed a patient's breathing difficulty to emotional stress in his initial working diagnosis, and he avoided making the same assumption in this scenario. The paramedic used clinical decision making to support the diagnosis of pulmonary embolism for this patient. His decision making was based on his experience and on his assessment findings.

Field Application of Assessment-Based Patient Management

Assessment-based patient management places huge responsibility on the paramedic. The paramedic must have a systematic means of analyzing a patient's problems, determining how to solve them, carrying out a plan of action, and evaluating effectiveness of the treatment. The success of assessment-based patient management in the prehospital setting depends on an integration of interpersonal skills, scientific knowledge, and physical activities (skills).

The Patient Crisis Severity Spectrum

EMS is set into action daily for many reasons. Yet few prehospital calls present true threats to life.[8] Minor medical and trauma events require little critical thinking. They result in fairly easy decision making for the paramedic. Likewise, patients with clear life threats pose limited critical thinking challenges because they often fit the "model" for standardized treatment (eg, cardiac arrest). However, many patients fall in the spectrum between minor and life-threatening events. These patients pose the most critical-thinking challenges for the paramedic. An example is a patient with mild to moderate respiratory distress. Another is a patient with diffuse abdominal pain. Either of these situations could be minor or could have life-threatening consequences.

Thinking Under Pressure

Hormonal influences from the fight-or-flight response (described in Chapter 2, *Well-Being of the Paramedic*) can have positive and negative effects on critical decision making. The response may offer greater visual acuity and auditory keenness and improved reflexes and muscle strength. This response can be positive when critical decisions must be made and action must be taken. The negative aspects of the response may include reduced critical-thinking skills, which may result from a decrease in concentration and assessment ability. The key to strong performance under pressure is mental conditioning. Mental conditioning results in "instinctive performance" and "automatic responses" for technical procedures.

Mental Checklist for Thinking Under Pressure

Mental conditioning takes a good deal of practice. A checklist for thinking under pressure may help the paramedic to concentrate during stressful events. The paramedic should use the following mental checklist:

- Stop and think.
- Scan the situation.
- Decide and act.
- Maintain clear and effective control.
- Regularly and continually reevaluate the patient.

> CRITICAL THINKING
>
> Do you think you can improve your performance under pressure by practicing imaginary critical situations in your head? Why or why not?

Practicing this checklist when under pressure will result in behaviors that improve clinical decision making. One of these positive behaviors is staying calm (not panicking). Another is assuming a plan for the worst case (erring on the side of caution). A third is maintaining a systematic assessment pattern. In addition, the paramedic can learn to balance the various styles of situation analysis, data processing, and decision making. Applying the styles of situational analysis (reflective versus impulsive), data processing (divergent versus convergent), and decision making (anticipatory versus reactive) allows the paramedic to provide the best possible care in most situations. In time, paramedics are able to apply all of these approaches with skill.

Putting It All Together: The Six Rs

To put all components required for effective clinical decision making into action, the paramedic can think in terms of the six Rs (**FIGURE 20-5**):

1. **Read the patient.** The paramedic should observe the patient's level of consciousness and skin color. Position of the patient should be noted along with any obvious deformity or asymmetry. Talking to the patient will reveal the chief complaint. This will also identify the presence of a worsening or preexisting condition. Skin temperature and moisture should be evaluated. Pulses should be assessed for rate, strength, and regularity. Auscultation of the lungs will reveal upper or lower airway problems. The paramedic should identify all life threats and obtain an accurate set of vital signs.
2. **Read the scene.** As a part of scene size-up, the paramedic should assess general environmental conditions. The paramedic should evaluate the immediate surroundings and attempt to identify any mechanism of injury or clinical clues of illness.
3. **React.** All life threats should be managed when they are found. The paramedic should determine the most common and likely cause of the life threat that fits the patient's initial presentation. If a clearly defined and recognizable presentation of medical illness cannot be defined in a priority patient, treatment should be based on presenting signs and symptoms.
4. **Reevaluate.** Reevaluation includes a focused and detailed assessment. This assessment analyzes the patient's response to management and interventions and may lead the paramedic to find other problems. These problems may not have been evident during the primary assessment.

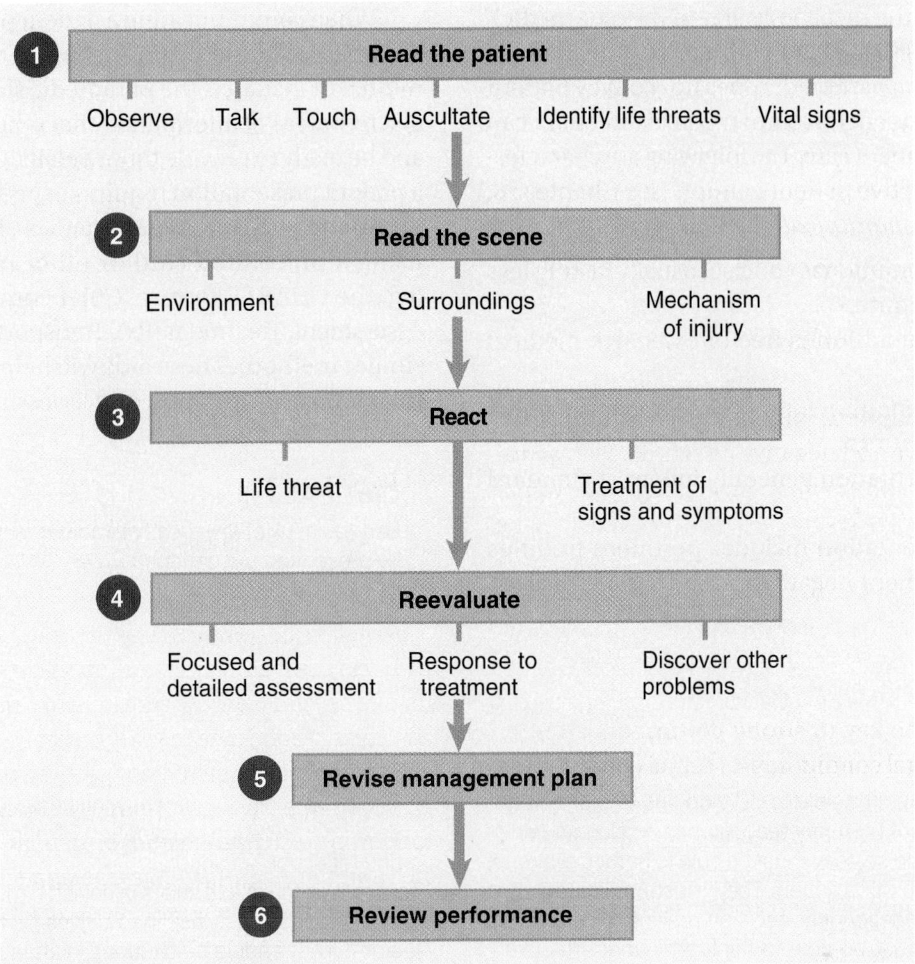

FIGURE 20-5 The six Rs.

5. **Revise the management plan.** Findings obtained during reevaluation may require the paramedic to revise the management plan. This revision will more clearly address the needs of the patient. The facts that patient conditions change and that patients do not respond in the same way to identical treatment interventions highlight the importance of ongoing assessment and reassessment.
6. **Review performance through a run critique.** Reviewing the details of the call through a run critique allows for improvements to be made to similar calls in the future. The interest and investment of paramedics in the outcome of their personal cases often is the strongest stimulus to change their practice patterns favorably. This process also enhances the paramedic's experience base and in turn leads to improvement of data interpretation skills.

CRITICAL THINKING

Consider a negative or punitive after-action call review. How do you think this would influence your ability to perform under a similar circumstance in the future?

Presenting the Patient

The purpose of the **patient handoff** in the course of prehospital and hospital care is twofold. It refers to the skills of effective communication and to the effective transfer of patient information. Patient handoffs or transitions of care are frequently the source of medical errors.

The paramedic may complete the patient handoff face to face, over the phone or radio, or in writing. Good communication during this process helps the paramedic to establish trust and credibility with coworkers and other members of the health care teams.

It helps assure the receiving party of the paramedic's skill and professionalism. Poor communication, as occurs when the paramedic does not convey patient needs and status effectively to medical direction, can compromise patient care. The following are characteristics of an effective patient handoff (see Chapter 16, *Therapeutic Communications*):

- The presentation is concise, usually lasting less than 1 minute.
- The presentation is free of extensive medical jargon.
- The presentation follows the same basic information pattern.
- The presentation generally follows a standard format.
- The presentation includes pertinent findings and pertinent negatives.

When communicating a patient presentation, the paramedic should begin the report with the end in mind. For instance, the paramedic should anticipate discrete areas of information that others will question and be ready to provide those details. Communicating a patient presentation requires experience. Until this experience is gained, paramedics should consider using a preprinted card or other memory device (eg, the CHARTE format [Chief complaint, History, Assessment, Treatment (Rx), Transport, Exceptions] or similar method). These aids will help the paramedic to organize information and assessment findings.

CRITICAL THINKING

Can you think of any areas of improvement for your skills in "presenting the patient"?

Summary

- Paramedics must be able to develop and implement appropriate patient management plans in challenging environments. To do so, they must be able to gather, evaluate, and synthesize information. They must apply judgment and exercise independent decision making as well. Last, paramedics must be able to think and work effectively under pressure.
- Factors that can affect the quality of assessment and decision making include the paramedic's attitude, the patient's willingness to cooperate, distracting injuries, labeling and tunnel vision, the environment, patient compliance, and considerations of personnel availability.
- Promoting a coherent assessment is the goal. Thus members of the response team should have a preplan for determining roles and responsibilities.
- The paramedic crew should always be prepared for the worst event. They should carry the essential equipment necessary to manage every aspect of patient care.
- The paramedic must maintain a calm and orderly manner. This demeanor is especially important when approaching a patient.
- During the initial assessment, the paramedic must look actively for problems that pose a threat to life.
- Protocols, standing orders, and patient care algorithms have several limitations. They may not apply to nonspecific patient complaints that do not fit the model. They also often do not address multiple disease etiologies or multiple treatment plans. Moreover, they may promote linear thinking. Clinical decision rules may help determine risk when evaluating patients.
- The critical-thinking process includes concept formation, data interpretation, application of principles, evaluation, and reflection on action.
- To reduce the risk of errors in decision making, paramedics should consciously ask themselves, "Is this the right decision?" They should be cautious in situations where errors are more likely to occur. They should recognize their own biases and use care when making decisions in cases that involve those biases.
- For effective critical thinking, a paramedic must have a solid knowledge base. The paramedic must be able to organize a large amount of data, deal with ambiguity, and relate the situation to similar past experience. The paramedic also must be able to reason and construct arguments to support or discount a decision.
- When using assessment-based patient management, the paramedic must analyze a patient's problems, determine how to solve them, carry out a plan of action, and evaluate its effectiveness.
- Effective clinical decision making requires the paramedic to read the patient and the scene. The paramedic also must be able to react, reevaluate, and revise the management plan. Then the paramedic must be able to review performance at a run critique.
- To ensure an effective patient handoff, the paramedic, and all other members involved, must communicate thoroughly and thoughtfully.

References

1. Carhart E. Origins and application of crew resource management. EMS Reference website. https://www.emsreference.com/articles/article/origins-and-application-crew-resource-management?category=4. Updated January 5, 2017. Accessed January 5, 2018.
2. LeSage P, Dyar JT, Evans B. *Crew Resource Management: Principles and Practice*. Sudbury, MA: Jones & Bartlett Learning; 2011.
3. National Association of Emergency Medical Technicians. *EMS Safety.* 2nd ed. Burlington, MA: Jones & Bartlett Learning; 2017.
4. Alfaro-LeFevre R. *Critical Thinking, Clinical Reasoning, and Clinical Judgment: A Practical Approach*. 5th ed. St. Louis, MO: Elsevier Saunders; 2013.
5. Bigham BL, Bull E, Morrison M, et al; Pan-Canadian Patient Safety in EMS Advisory Group. Patient safety in emergency medical services: executive summary and recommendations from the Niagra Summit. *Can J Emerg Med.* 2011;13(1):13-18.
6. Croskerry P. From mindless to mindful practice—cognitive bias and clinical decision making. *N Engl J Med.* 2013;368(26):2445-2448.
7. National Highway Traffic Safety Administration, US Department of Transportation. *EMT-Paramedic National Standard Curriculum*. Washington, DC: National Highway Traffic Safety Administration; 1998.
8. National Highway Traffic Safety Administration, US Department of Transportation. *The National EMS Education Standards*. Washington, DC: National Highway Traffic Safety Administration; 2009.

Suggested Readings

Benner P, Kyriakidis PH, Stannard D. *Clinical Wisdom and Interventions in Critical Care: A Thinking-in-Action Approach*. Philadelphia, PA: WB Saunders; 1999.

Croskerry P. Achieving quality in clinical decision making: cognitive strategies and detection of bias. *Acad Emerg Med.* 2002;9(11):1184-1204.

Croskerry P. Cognitive forcing strategies in clinical decision making. *Ann Emerg Med.* 2003;41(1):110-120.

Croskerry P. Diagnostic failure: a cognitive and affective approach. *Adv Patient Safety.* 2008;2:241-254.

Epstein RM. Mindful practice. *JAMA.* 1999;282(9):833-839.

Gladwell M. *Blink: The Power of Thinking Without Thinking*. New York, NY: Little, Brown and Company; 2005.

Jensen JL, Croskerry P, Ah T. Paramedic clinical decision making during high acuity emergency calls: design and methodology of a Delphi study. *BMC Emerg Med.* 2009;9:17.

Krupat E, Sprague J, Wolpaw D, Haidet P, Hatem D, O'Brien B. Thinking critically about critical thinking: ability, disposition or both? *Med Educ.* 2011;45:625-635.

Maggiore WA. How to minimize the influence of bias in patient assessment. *JEMS.* 2008;33(11):116-118.

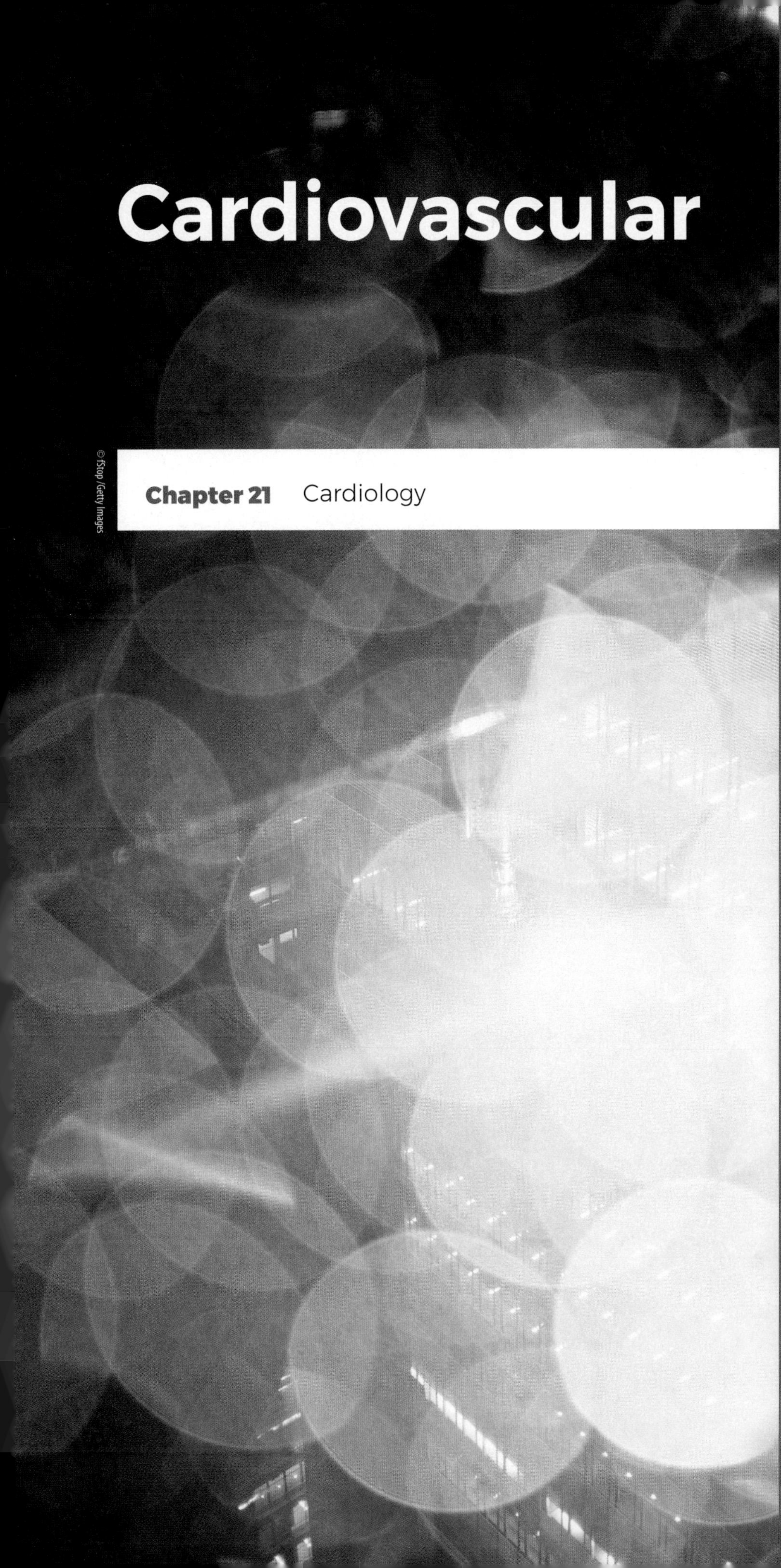

© fStop/Getty Images

Cardiovascular

PART

6

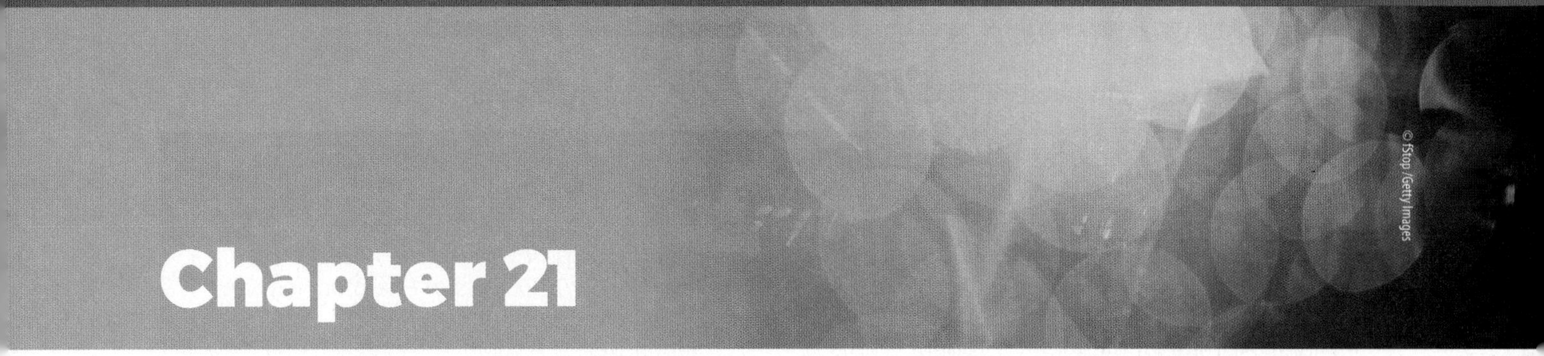

Chapter 21

Cardiology

NATIONAL EMS EDUCATION STANDARD COMPETENCIES

Medicine

Integrates assessment findings with principles of epidemiology and pathophysiology to formulate a field impression and implement a comprehensive treatment/disposition plan for a patient with a medical complaint.

Cardiovascular

Anatomy, signs, symptoms, and management of

- Chest pain (pp 747–817, 820–823, 825–827)
- Cardiac arrest (pp 744–748, 784–792, 852–867)

Anatomy, physiology, epidemiology, pathophysiology, psychosocial impact, presentations, prognosis, and management of

- Acute coronary syndrome (p 827)
  - Angina pectoris (pp 828–829)
  - Myocardial infarction (pp 829–834)
- Heart failure (pp 834–839)
- Nontraumatic cardiac tamponade (pp 840–841)
- Hypertensive emergencies (pp 847–849)
- Cardiogenic shock (p 840)
- Vascular disorders (pp 748–805, 827–847)
  - Abdominal aortic aneurysm (pp 841–843)
  - Arterial occlusion (pp 845–846)
  - Venous thrombosis (pp 846–847)
- Aortic aneurysm/dissection (pp 843–845)
- Thromboembolism (see Chapter 13, *Principles of Pharmacology and Emergency Medications*)
- Cardiac rhythm disturbances (p 744–792)
- Infectious diseases of the heart (pp 850–851)
  - Endocarditis (p 850)
  - Pericarditis (pp 850–851)
- Congenital abnormalities (pp 803–805, 834–836, 843–845, and see Chapter 46, *Neonatal Care*)

Shock and Resuscitation

Integrates comprehensive knowledge of causes and pathophysiology into the management of cardiac arrest and peri-arrest states.

Integrates a comprehensive knowledge of the causes and pathophysiology into the management of shock, respiratory failure, or arrest with an emphasis on early intervention to prevent arrest.

OBJECTIVES

Upon completion of this chapter, the paramedic student will be able to:

1. Identify risk factors and prevention strategies associated with cardiovascular disease. (pp 709–710)
2. Describe the normal anatomy and physiology of the heart. (pp 710–717)
3. Discuss electrophysiology as it relates to the normal electrical and mechanical events in the cardiac cycle. (pp 717–725)
4. Outline the activity of each component of the electrical conduction system of the heart. (pp 722–725)
5. Describe basic monitoring techniques that permit interpretation of an electrocardiogram (ECG). (pp 725–731)
6. Explain the relationship of the ECG tracing to the electrical activity of the heart. (pp 731–736)
7. Describe in sequence the steps in ECG interpretation. (pp 736–744)
8. Identify the characteristics of normal sinus rhythm. (pp 736–747)
9. When shown an ECG tracing, identify the rhythm, site of origin, possible causes, and clinical significance and the prehospital management indicated. (pp 736–748)
10. Outline the appropriate assessment of a patient who may be experiencing a cardiovascular disorder. (pp 744–748)
11. Describe prehospital assessment and management of patients with selected cardiovascular disorders based on knowledge of the pathophysiology of the illness. (pp 748–805)

12. Describe the cause and nature of selected congenital cardiovascular defects. (pp 803–805, 834–836, 843–845, and see Chapter 46, *Neonatal Care*)
13. List indications, contraindications, and prehospital considerations when using selected cardiac interventions, including basic life support, monitor-defibrillators, defibrillation, implantable cardioverter-defibrillators, synchronized cardioversion, and transcutaneous cardiac pacing. (pp 853–854, 856–861, 863–866)
14. List indications, contraindications, dose, and mechanism of action for pharmacologic agents used to manage cardiovascular disorders. (pp 764, 785, 829, 839, and see Chapter 13, *Principles of Pharmacology and Emergency Medications*)
15. Identify clinical scenarios in which prehospital termination of resuscitation is appropriate. (pp 868–869)

KEY TERMS

abdominal aortic aneurysm (AAA) A localized dilation and weakness of the wall of the abdominal aorta.

aberration The abnormal conduction of impulses through cardiac conduction pathways.

absolute refractory period The portion of the action potential during which the membrane is insensitive to subsequent electrical stimuli.

accelerated junctional rhythm A dysrhythmia that results from increased automaticity of the atrioventricular junction.

acute arterial occlusion A sudden blockage of arterial flow, most commonly caused by embolization or thrombosis.

acute coronary syndrome (ACS) A spectrum of clinical disease that is the result of compromise of blood flow through the coronary arteries; includes acute myocardial infarction and unstable angina.

acute myocardial infarction (AMI) Blockage of blood flow within one or more of the coronary arteries causing tissue hypoxia and death of cardiac tissue.

afterload The total resistance against which blood must be pumped; also known as systemic vascular resistance.

algorithm A process or set of rules to be followed during a clinical scenario; commonly used format for clinical guidelines.

amyloidosis The accumulation of amyloid protein in tissues and organs of the body.

aneurysm A weakening and localized dilation of a blood vessel wall.

angina pectoris Ischemic chest pain caused by insufficient blood flow to the myocardium usually as a result of atherosclerosis of the coronary arteries.

angioplasty A procedure to relieve blockage from a blood vessel.

anterior hemiblock Failure in conduction of the cardiac impulse in the anterior fascicle of the left bundle branch.

aortic dissection Separation of layers within the wall of the aorta.

artifact An abnormality in the electrocardiogram tracing produced by factors other than the electrical activity of the heart.

artificial pacemaker A rhythm that is generated by electrical stimulation of the heart through an electrode implanted in the heart.

asystole The absence of electrical and mechanical activity of the heart.

atherosclerosis A common arterial disorder characterized by yellow plaques of cholesterol, lipids, and cellular debris in the inner layers of the walls of large- and medium-size arteries.

atrial fibrillation (AF) An irregularly irregular heart rhythm that results from disorganized and rapid ectopic electrical impulses from the atria.

atrial flutter A dysrhythmia resulting from rapid atrial reentry of electrical impulses over a large, anatomically fixed circuit; characterized by rapid, regular activity at a rate of 180 to 350 beats/min.

atrial kick The priming force contributed by atrial contraction immediately before ventricular systole that acts to improve ventricular filling during diastole.

atrial tachycardia (AT) A rapid heart rhythm that originates in the atria.

atrioventricular (AV) dissociation Any situation in which the atria and the ventricles beat independently.

atrioventricular (AV) junction An area formed by the atrioventricular node and the bundle of His; serves as the normal electrical link between the atria and ventricles in a normal heart.

atrioventricular nodal reentrant tachycardia (AVNRT) A type of reentry supraventricular tachycardia in which the reentrant loop is formed by fast and slow pathways within the atrioventricular node. The most common cause of paroxysmal supraventricular tachycardia in adults.

atrioventricular (AV) node An area of specialized cardiac muscle that receives the cardiac impulse from the sinoatrial node and conducts it to the bundle of His.

atrioventricular reentrant tachycardia (AVRT) A type of reentry supraventricular tachycardia in which one limb of the reentrant loop is constituted by a bypass tract rather than separate fast and slow pathways within the atrioventricular node.

augmented limb leads Unipolar leads that record the difference in electrical potential in cardiac muscle.

automaticity A property of specialized excitable tissue that allows self-activation through spontaneous development of an action potential.

axis The major direction of the overall electrical activity of the heart.

bifascicular block The blockage of two of three pathways (fascicles) for ventricular conduction.

bigeminy A cardiac rhythm disturbance characterized by a premature ventricular complex every other beat.

bipolar leads Leads composed of two electrodes of opposite polarity.

bradycardia A heart rate of less than 60 beats/min.

bruit An abnormal sound or murmur heard while auscultating an artery caused by narrowing of the vessel.

bundle of His A band of fibers in the myocardium through which the cardiac impulse is rapidly transmitted from the atrioventricular node to the ventricles.

bundle of Kent Pathologic fibers that connect atrial muscle to ventricular muscle, bypassing the atrioventricular node; also known as Kent fibers.

cannon A waves Waves of pulse pressure that are visible in the jugular veins of a patient in ventricular tachycardia.

cardiac ejection fraction The percentage of blood volume ejected from the ventricle during a contraction.

cardiogenic shock Shock that results when cardiac action is unable to deliver sufficient circulating blood volume for tissue perfusion.

cardiomyopathy Any disease that affects the myocardium.

coarse ventricular fibrillation (VF) Fibrillatory waves that are greater than 3 mm in amplitude; precedes fine ventricular fibrillation.

compensatory pause A pause following a premature ventricular complex.

contiguous leads Two or more electrocardiograph leads that are anatomically close together and that view the same general area of the heart.

deep vein thrombosis (DVT) Occlusion in any portion of the deep venous system by a thrombus; can be acute or chronic.

defibrillation The delivery of electrical current through the myocardium to terminate ventricular fibrillation and pulseless ventricular tachycardia.

delta wave A slurring or notching of the onset of the QRS complex that is a diagnostic finding in Wolff-Parkinson-White syndrome.

depolarization A change in electrical charge difference across the cell membrane that causes the difference to be smaller or closer to 0 mV; a phase of the action potential in which the membrane potential moves toward zero or becomes positive.

diastole The phase of the heartbeat in which the heart muscle relaxes and allows the chamber to fill with blood; separated into ventricular diastole and atrial diastole.

diastolic heart failure Failure of the ventricles to relax properly during diastole; also known as diastolic dysfunction.

dyspnea The sensation of shortness of breath.

dysrhythmias Variations from a normal rhythm.

ectopic focus An excitable group of cells outside the normally functioning sinus node of the heart that initiates myocardial depolarization.

ejection The forceful expulsion of blood from the ventricle of the heart.

electrical capture Pacing capture in which a pacing stimulus precipitates a ventricular contraction.

electrocardiogram (ECG) A graphic representation of the electrical activity of the heart.

end-diastolic volume The volume of blood in either the left or the right ventricle at the end of ventricular filling (diastole).

endocarditis An inflammation of the endocardium (inner layer of the heart) typically caused by infection.

enhanced automaticity An increase in the firing rate of myocardial cells beyond their inherent rate.

fine ventricular fibrillation (VF) Fibrillatory waves less than 3 mm in amplitude.

first-degree atrioventricular (AV) block A benign dysrhythmia in which there is a delay in conduction, usually at the level of the atrioventricular node; seen as prolongation of the PR interval on an electrocardiogram to greater than 200 milliseconds.

fusion beat A beat that occurs when supraventricular and ventricular electrical impulses act on the same region of the heart at the same time, producing a hybrid complex of intermediate width and morphology.

heart failure An abnormal condition that reflects impaired ventricular filling (diastolic dysfunction) or blood volume ejection (systolic dysfunction); usually a result of myocardial infarction, ischemic heart disease, long-standing hypertension, or cardiomyopathy.

hexaxial reference system The system of intersecting lines of the standard limb leads and three other intersecting lines of reference: aV_R, aV_L, and aV_F leads.

high-grade atrioventricular (AV) block Second-degree heart block with a P-to-QRS ratio of at least 3:1 or higher; distinguished from third-degree block because a conductive relationship between the atria and the ventricles still exists.

high-output heart failure A type of heart failure in which cardiac output remains high but is unable to meet the metabolic needs of the body because of increased demand.

hypertension A disorder characterized by elevated blood pressure that persistently exceeds 130/80 mm Hg.

hypertensive encephalopathy A clinical syndrome of neurologic symptoms including headache, convulsions, and coma resulting from severe blood pressure elevation.

interventricular septum The tissue that separates the right and left ventricles of the heart.

joule A measurement of electrical energy. One joule is the product of 1 volt (potential) multiplied by 1 amp (current) multiplied by 1 second.

jugular venous distention (JVD) Engorgement of jugular veins caused by an increase in central venous pressure. It is estimated by positioning the head of a supine patient at a 45° angle and observing the neck veins.

junctional escape rhythm A rhythm that originates from the atrioventricular junction, usually at a rate of 40 to 60 bpm. Complexes are narrow in morphology and are not related to any preceding atrial activity (P waves).

junctional tachycardia A type of supraventricular tachycardia caused by a reentry mechanism in the junction of the atrioventricular node.

left axis deviation When the mean electrical axis of ventricular contraction is within the quadrant of −30° and −90°.

left bundle branch A division in the bundle of His originating in the septum and extending into the left ventricle that provides pathways for impulse conduction.

left bundle branch block (LBBB) A conduction disturbance in the left bundle branch that alters normal septal activation and sends it in the opposite direction.

left-side heart failure A condition that occurs when the left ventricle fails to work as an effective forward pump, causing a back pressure of blood into the pulmonary circulation; also known as left ventricular failure.

left ventricular assist device (LVAD) A battery-operated mechanical device implanted into the left ventricle that augments blood flow in patients with severe systolic heart failure.

mechanical capture Pacing capture that occurs when an associated pulse is generated with the electrical capture of an artificial pacemaker.

monomorphic ventricular tachycardia (VT) Ventricular tachycardia in which the QRS complex has the same morphology or fixed shape.

multifocal atrial tachycardia (MAT) An atrial tachycardia in which there are P waves of at least three different morphologies. Rates are often in the range of 120 to 150 beats/min.

multifocal premature ventricular complex (PVC) Premature ventricular complexes that originate from multiple sites in the ventricles.

myocardial contractility The intrinsic ability of the heart to contract.

myocarditis Inflammation of the heart muscle.

non–ST-segment elevation myocardial infarction (non-STEMI) A myocardial infarction in which there is no ST-segment elevation.

P wave The first complex of the electrocardiogram, representing depolarization of the atria.

palpitations The sensation of irregular or forceful beating of the heart.

paroxysmal atrial tachycardia (PAT) Atrial tachycardia that begins and ends abruptly.

paroxysmal nocturnal dyspnea Shortness of breath that awakens a person from sleep. It often is associated with left ventricular failure and pulmonary edema.

paroxysmal supraventricular tachycardia (PSVT) An ectopic rhythm usually faster than 170 beats/min that begins abruptly with a premature atrial or junctional beat and is supported by an atrioventricular nodal reentrant mechanism or by an atrioventricular reentry involving an accessory pathway.

pericarditis Inflammation of the pericardium.

point of maximum impulse The location or area where the apical pulse is palpated the strongest, often in the fifth intercostal space of the thorax just medial to the left midclavicular line.

polymorphic ventricular tachycardia (VT) Ventricular tachycardia in which the QRS complex has varying morphology or shape.

posterior hemiblock Failure in conduction of the cardiac impulse in the posterior fascicle of the left bundle branch.

potassium ion channels Electrical channels in the cell membrane that allow for selective flow of potassium ions across the cell membrane.

PR interval The time that elapses between the beginning of the P wave and the beginning of the QRS complex in the electrocardiogram.

precordial leads Unipolar chest leads used in 12-lead electrocardiographic monitoring that record the electrical activity of the heart in the horizontal plane.

precordial thump A technique to restore circulation in monitored, witnessed ventricular fibrillation or unstable ventricular tachycardia.

preexcitation syndrome Anomalous or accelerated atrioventricular conduction associated with an abnormal conduction pathway between the atria and ventricles.

preload The volume of blood returning to the heart.

premature atrial complex (PAC) A cardiac dysrhythmia characterized by an atrial beat occurring before the expected excitation and indicated on the electrocardiogram as an early P wave of a different morphology.

premature junctional complex (PJC) An ectopic beat originating from the atrioventricular junction that occurs earlier than the next expected sinus beat.

premature ventricular complex (PVC) A ventricular beat preceding the next expected electrical impulse. It has an early, wide QRS complex without a preceding related P wave.

proarrhythmia A new or worsened rhythm disturbance seemingly generated by antidysrhythmic therapy.

pulmonary edema The accumulation of extravascular fluid in lung tissues and alveoli.

pulse deficit A condition that exists when the radial pulse is less than the ventricular rate. It indicates a lack of peripheral perfusion.

pulseless electrical activity (PEA) The absence of a detectable pulse in the presence of some type of organized electrical activity other than ventricular tachycardia; also known as electromechanical dissociation.

Purkinje fibers Myocardial fibers that are a continuation of the bundle of His and that extend into the muscle walls of the ventricles.

QRS complex The principal deflection in the electrocardiogram, representing ventricular depolarization.

QT interval The time elapsing from the beginning of the QRS complex to the end of the T wave, representing the total duration of electrical activity of the ventricles.

R-on-T phenomenon The occurrence of a ventricular depolarization during a vulnerable period of ventricular repolarization.

reentry The reactivation of tissue by a returning impulse; the sustaining mechanism in some cases of ventricular tachycardia and paroxysmal supraventricular tachycardia.

refractory period The period after effective stimulation during which excitable tissue will not respond to a stimulus of threshold intensity.

relative refractory period The portion of the action potential after the absolute refractory period during which another action potential can be produced with a greater-than-threshold stimulus strength.

repolarization The phase of the action potential in which the membrane potential moves from its maximum degree of depolarization toward the value of the resting membrane potential.

resting membrane potential The electrical charge difference inside a cell membrane measured relative to just outside the cell membrane.

return of spontaneous circulation (ROSC) Restoration of spontaneous circulation following a cardiac arrest that provides evidence of more than an occasional gasp, occasional fleeting palpable pulse, or arterial waveform.

right axis deviation When the mean electrical axis of ventricular contraction falls between $+90°$ and $\pm180°$.

right bundle branch A division in the bundle of His responsible for depolarization of the right side of the heart.

right bundle branch block (RBBB) A conduction abnormality that occurs when transmission of the electrical impulse is delayed or not conducted along the right bundle branch.

right-side heart failure Failure of the right ventricle to serve as an effective forward pump; also known as right ventricular failure.

second-degree atrioventricular (AV) block type I A conduction block that gradually prolongs the PR interval until a P wave is blocked from initiating a QRS complex; also known as Wenckebach.

second-degree atrioventricular (AV) block type II A conduction block with a constant PR interval where a P wave is blocked from initiating a QRS complex in a fixed or variable pattern.

Sgarbossa criteria A set of electrocardiographic findings that can be used to identify myocardial infarction in the presence of a left bundle branch block or a ventricular paced rhythm.

sinoatrial (SA) node An area of specialized heart tissue within the atria that serves as the endogenous cardiac pacemaker.

sinus arrest The failure of the sinus node, causing short periods of cardiac standstill.

sinus bradycardia Decreased heart rate that results from slowing of the pacemaker rate of the sinoatrial node to less than 60 beats/min in the typical adult.

sinus dysrhythmia A cardiac rhythm disturbance that often is related to the respiratory cycle and to changes in intrathoracic pressure.

sinus tachycardia Increased heart rate of greater than 100 beats/min in the adult that results from an increase in the rate of the sinus node discharge.

sodium ion channels Protein-lined channels in the cell membrane that allow sodium to enter the cell during rapid depolarization.

ST segment The early part of repolarization in the electrocardiogram of the right and left ventricles measured from the end of the S wave to the beginning of the T wave.

standard limb leads Bipolar electrocardiograph leads that record the difference in electrical potential between the left arm, the right arm, and the left leg electrodes.

Starling law of the heart A rule that the stroke volume of the heart increases in response to an increase in end-diastolic volume.

ST-segment elevation myocardial infarction (STEMI) A myocardial infarction in which there is ST-segment elevation.

stroke volume The volume of blood ejected from one ventricle in a single heartbeat.

sudden cardiac death A death that occurs within the first 2 hours after the onset of illness or injury.

supraventricular tachycardia (SVT) A complex group of dysrhythmias that can be broadly defined as any tachycardia that originates above the level of the bundle of His.

synchronized cardioversion An electrical countershock used to terminate dysrhythmias that is timed with the QRS complex. Synchronization is timed with the R wave of the cardiac cycle to avoid shock delivery during the relative refractory period of the cardiac cycle, which could cause ventricular fibrillation.

syncope A brief lapse in consciousness caused by transient cerebral hypoxia.

systemic vascular resistance The total resistance against which blood must be pumped; also known as afterload.

systole Contraction of the atria and ventricles.

systolic heart failure Failure of the ventricles to contract properly during systole; also known as systolic dysfunction.

T wave A deflection in the electrocardiogram after the QRS complex, representing ventricular repolarization.

tachycardia A heart rate equal to or greater than 100 beats/min in an adult.

third-degree atrioventricular (AV) block A condition that results from complete electrical block at or below the atrioventricular node; also known as complete heart block.

threshold potential The value of the membrane potential at which an action potential is produced as a result of depolarization in response to a stimulus.

torsades de pointes A type of polymorphic ventricular tachycardia occurring in the context of QT prolongation.

transcutaneous cardiac pacing (TCP) The delivery of repetitive electrical currents to the heart through an external artificial pacemaker; also known as external cardiac pacing.

trigeminy An underlying rhythm that is interrupted by a ventricular complex after every two beats.

U wave A small deflection after the T wave in the electrocardiogram, seen in pathologic states such as hypokalemia.

unifocal premature ventricular complex (PVC) A premature ventricular complex that originates from a single ectopic ventricular pacemaker site.

unipolar leads Augmented limb leads that record the difference in electrical potential, using one electrode for a positive pole, but having no distinct negative pole.

unstable angina An acute coronary syndrome associated with a pattern of ischemic chest pain that has changed in its ease of onset, frequency, intensity, duration, or quality.

unsynchronized cardioversion An electrical countershock used to terminate ventricular fibrillation and pulseless ventricular tachycardia, given without regard to where the shock occurs in the cardiac cycle; also known as defibrillation.

Valsalva maneuver A vagal maneuver used to slow the heart by stimulating postganglionic parasympathetic nerve fibers in the wall of the atria and specialized tissues of the sinoatrial and atrioventricular nodes via the vagus nerve.

valvular heart disease Any disease process that affects one or more valves of the heart: the mitral, aortic, tricuspid, or pulmonary valves.

vasovagal syncope A brief loss of consciousness that results from overstimulation of the vagus nerve.

ventricular assist device An electromechanical pump to assist ventricular heart function and improve cardiac output.

ventricular escape complex A wide-complex beat originating in the ventricle that occurs when impulses from higher pacemakers fail to fire or to reach the ventricles. When firing at a rate of 30 to 40 beats/min, it is known as an idioventricular rhythm.

ventricular fibrillation (VF) A cardiac dysrhythmia marked by rapid, disorganized depolarization of the ventricular myocardium.

ventricular tachycardia (VT) A tachycardia that usually originates in the Purkinje fibers.

wandering pacemaker An atrial arrhythmia that results from shifting of the pacemaker site between the sinoatrial node, atrioventricular node, and latent pacemaker sites within the atria.

Wolff-Parkinson-White (WPW) syndrome A syndrome of preexcitation of the ventricles of the heart; caused by an accessory pathway (bundle of Kent) that permits abnormal electrical communication from the atria to the ventricles.

Cardiovascular disease accounts for more than 600,000 deaths in the United States each year. Almost one-half of the cases of sudden cardiac death take place outside the hospital.[1] Of those deaths, 70% occur in the home and about one-half are not witnessed.[2] Many of these deaths can be prevented by rapid entry into the EMS system, prompt and ongoing provision of effective cardiopulmonary resuscitation (CPR), and early defibrillation.

CRITICAL THINKING

How many of your friends or family have had a heart attack or stroke? How has that illness affected their lives and the lives of their families?

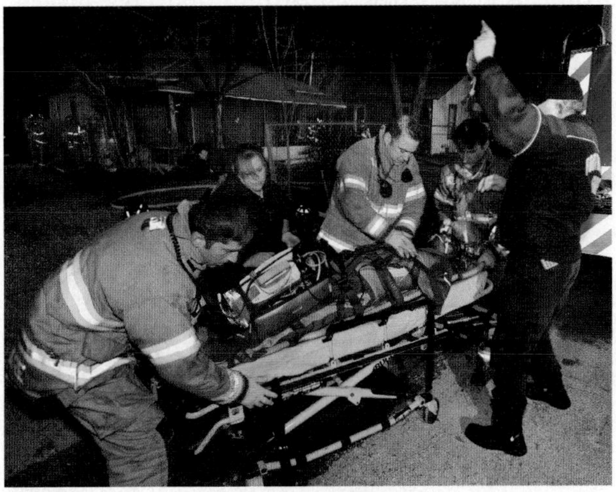

Risk Factors and Prevention Strategies for Cardiovascular Disease

Although death rates from myocardial infarction (MI) have declined over the past several decades, coronary artery disease with resultant sudden death is still a major cause of morbidity and mortality in the United States today.[1] The decline in death rates from sudden death related to coronary heart disease may be related to increased preventive measures such as statins, aspirin, beta blockers, and lifestyle changes.[3] Other factors may include heightened public awareness, the increased availability of automated external defibrillators (AEDs), improved cardiovascular diagnosis and therapy, the use of cardiovascular drugs by people at high risk, improved revascularization techniques, and improved and more aggressive risk factor modification. However, for patients who have experienced an out-of-hospital cardiac arrest, the rate of survival to hospital discharge remains low nationally. In 2016, the Cardiac Arrest Registry to Enhance Survival (CARES) report found a survival to hospital discharge rate of only 10.8% for nontraumatic arrests. Even fewer patients (about 8.9%) went home from the hospital with near normal neurologic function.[4] Jurisdictional variations in treatment and transport practices, such as initiation and quality of basic life support (BLS) and time spent on scene. These variations can affect reported difference in survival rates.[5]

Risk Factors and Risk Factor Modifications

Factors that pose a high risk for cardiovascular disease include advanced age, male sex, and hereditary factors. Having a parent with heart disease increases the risk, as do some racial factors. African Americans, Mexican Americans, American Indians, native Hawaiians, and some Asian Americans have a higher tendency to have heart disease than do Caucasians. Although these factors cannot be controlled, some risk factors are modifiable. These factors include smoking, diabetes mellitus, hypertension, hypercholesterolemia, hyperlipidemia, obesity, and a sedentary lifestyle.[6] Lifestyle modifications that can reduce cardiac risk include the following:

- Cessation of smoking or smoke exposure
- Medical management and control of blood pressure, diabetes mellitus, cholesterol, and lipid disorders
- Exercise
- Weight loss
- Diet

Modifying cardiovascular risk factors can slow the rate of development of arterial disease. It also can reduce the incidence of acute myocardial infarction (AMI), sudden death, renal failure, and stroke.

DID YOU KNOW?

Cocaine: The "Perfect Heart-Attack Drug"

Cocaine use can have adverse cardiac effects, ranging from serious dysrhythmias to MI and sudden death. Therefore, cocaine is known as the perfect heart-attack drug. The National Surveys on Drug Use and Health reported that in 2015, 968,000 people aged 12 years and older (0.4% of the population) initiated cocaine use in the prior year, and 1.7 million young adults aged 18 to 25 years had used cocaine in the prior 12 months.

The incidence of respiratory arrest leading to cardiac arrest and death associated with opiate overdose is well known but not well publicized. Studies by the American Heart Association (AHA) have shown that using cocaine as little as once a month can lead to increased blood pressure and stiffening of both the aorta and left ventricle, thereby increasing the risk for heart attack and stroke. Other drugs known to have adverse effects on the heart are amphetamines and ecstasy (See Chapter 33, *Toxicology*).

Modified from: National Survey on Drug Use and Health. State Estimates of Past Year Cocaine Use Among Young Adults: 2014 and 2015. https://www.samhsa.gov/data/sites/default/files/report_2736/ShortReport-2736.html. Accessed January 21, 2018; and American Heart Association. Illegal Drugs and Heart Disease. www.heart.org/HEARTORG/Conditions/More/MyHeartandStrokeNews/Illegal-Drugs-and-Heart-Disease_UCM_428537_Article.jsp#.WmpmVzGWxes. Accessed January 21, 2018.

Prevention and Community Education Strategies

Paramedics can support activities that help detect or prevent cardiovascular disease. These strategies include community educational programs about nutrition, cessation of smoking (smoking prevention for children), and screening for diabetes and hypertension. Teaching CPR and early use of an AED is an important role of the paramedic. These interventions may have an impact on risk factor modification (see Chapter 3, *Injury Prevention, Health Promotion, and Public Health*).

Anatomy Review of the Heart

The anatomy of the heart is described and illustrated in Chapter 10, *Review of Human Systems*. The following is a brief review.

The human heart is a muscular organ with four chambers (**FIGURE 21-1**). It is cone shaped and about the size of a closed fist. It lies just to the left of the midline in the thorax. The heart is enclosed in a pericardial sac. This sac is lined with three parietal layers of serous membrane that form the wall of the heart. These three layers of tissue are the outer layer (the fibrous pericardium), the middle layer (the parietal pericardium), and the inner layer (visceral pericardium). The four chambers of the heart are the right atrium, right ventricle, left atrium, and left ventricle. The right atrium receives deoxygenated blood from the systemic veins. The left atrium receives oxygenated blood from the pulmonary veins. The heart has two types of valves that keep the blood flowing in the right direction. The valves between the atria and ventricles are the atrioventricular (AV) valves (also called cuspid

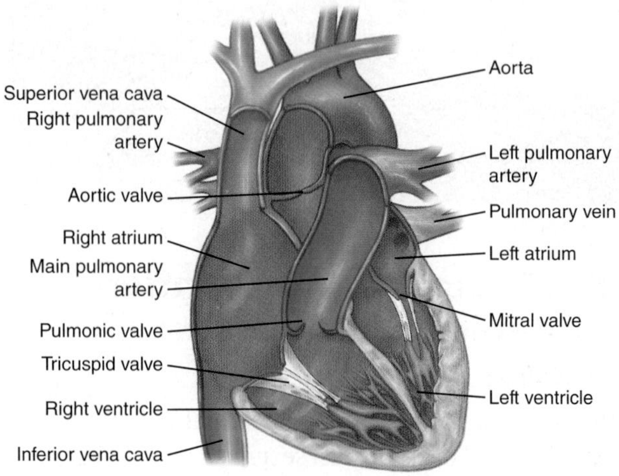

FIGURE 21-1 Internal view of the heart showing the four valves.

valves); the valves at the bases of the large vessels leaving the ventricles are the semilunar valves. The right AV valve is the tricuspid valve. The left AV valve is the bicuspid (or mitral) valve. The valve between the right ventricle and the pulmonary trunk is the pulmonary semilunar valve. The valve between the left ventricle and the aorta is the aortic semilunar valve. When the ventricles contract, AV valves close to prevent blood from flowing back into the atria. When the ventricles relax, semilunar valves close to prevent blood from flowing back into the ventricles.

Blood Supply to the Heart

The coronary arteries are the sole suppliers of arterial blood to the heart. They deliver blood to the myocardium during diastole at a rate of 200 to 250 mL/min (**FIGURE 21-2**). The left coronary artery carries about

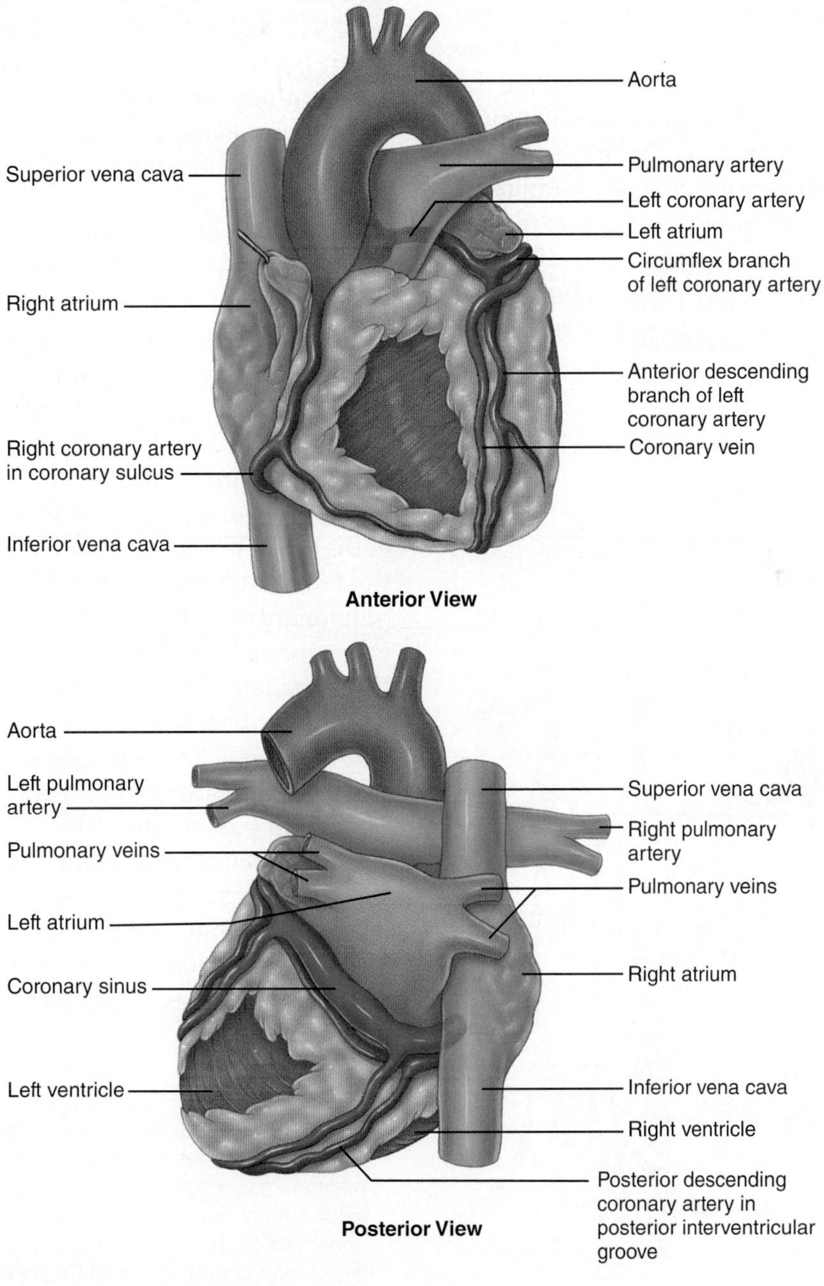

FIGURE 21-2 Blood supply to the myocardium: coronary blood vessels.

85% of the blood supply to the myocardium. The right coronary artery carries the rest. The coronary arteries begin just above the aortic valve where the aorta exits the heart. These arteries run along the epicardial surface. They divide into smaller vessels as they penetrate the myocardium and the endocardial (inner) surface.

The left main coronary artery supplies the left ventricle, the interventricular septum, and part of the right ventricle. Its two main branches are the left anterior descending artery and the circumflex artery. The right coronary artery supplies the right atrium and ventricle, part of the left ventricle, and the conduction system. Its two major branches are the right anterior descending branch and the marginal branch. In addition to the blood supply provided by these arteries, many connections (anastomoses) exist between arterioles to provide backup (collateral) circulation. These anastomoses play a key role in providing alternative routes of blood flow in the event one or more of the coronary vessels become blocked (**FIGURE 21-3**).

CRITICAL THINKING

How does increased heart rate affect the volume of blood supply to the heart and myocardial oxygen demand?

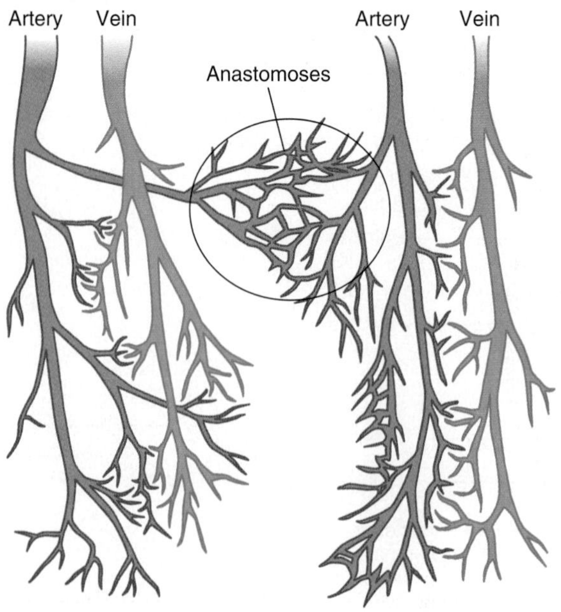

FIGURE 21-3 Minute anastomoses in the normal coronary arterial system.

Coronary capillaries allow for the exchange of nutrients and metabolic wastes. The capillaries merge to form coronary veins. These veins deliver most of the blood to the coronary sinus. The coronary sinus empties directly into the right atrium. The coronary sinus is the major vein draining the myocardium.

Physiology of the Heart

The heart can be thought of as two pumps in one. One is a low-pressure pump (right atrium and right ventricle). This pump supplies blood to the lungs. The other is a high-pressure pump (left atrium and left ventricle). This pump supplies blood to the body. The right atrium receives venous blood from the systemic circulation and from the coronary veins. Most of this deoxygenated blood in the right atrium then passes to the right ventricle as the ventricle relaxes from the previous contraction. Once the right ventricle has received about 70% of its volume, the right atrium contracts. The blood remaining in the atrium is pushed into the ventricle. Contraction of the right ventricle pushes blood against the tricuspid valve (forcing it closed) and through the pulmonic valve (forcing it open). This process allows the blood to enter the lungs via the pulmonary arteries. From the pulmonary arteries, the deoxygenated blood enters the capillaries in the lungs, where gas exchange takes place.

From the lungs the blood travels through four pulmonary veins back to the left atrium. The mitral valve opens, and blood flows to the left ventricle. Once the left ventricle has received about 70% of its volume, the left atrium contracts. The remaining 20% to 30% of the blood is pushed into the ventricles during atrial contraction (known as the **atrial kick**). The blood passing from the left atrium to the left ventricle opens the bicuspid valve when the ventricle relaxes to complete left ventricular filling. As the left ventricle contracts, blood is pushed against the bicuspid valve (closing it) and against the aortic valve (opening it). This process allows blood to enter the

NOTE

The atria work mainly as "primer pumps." Under most conditions, the ventricles can pump enough blood to maintain adequate blood flow to the body without the extra 30% of blood squeezed in by the atria. However, under stress, the heart may pump 300% to 400% more blood than during rest. In such conditions, the priming action of the atria becomes a key factor in maintaining pumping efficiency.

aorta. From the aorta, blood is distributed throughout the systemic arterial circulation and to the coronary arteries during the diastolic phase when the ventricle is relaxed.

Cardiac Cycle

The pumping action of the heart is a product of rhythmic, alternate contraction (**systole**) and relaxation (**diastole**) of the atria and ventricles. (When systole and diastole are used without reference to specific chambers, they mean ventricular systole or diastole.) These heartbeats occur about 70 times per minute (every 0.8 second) in resting adults. These rhythmic contractions of the heart chambers are responsible for the movement of blood (**FIGURE 21-4**).

> NOTE
>
> The cardiac cycle has three phases: phase 1, ventricular filling (middle to late diastole); phase 2, ventricular systole; and phase 3, isovolumetric relaxation (early diastole). In phase 2, ventricular systole, the atria relax and the ventricles begin contracting. Their walls close in on the blood in their chambers and ventricular pressure rises, closing the AV valves. For a split second (0.02 to 0.03 sec), the ventricles are completely closed chambers and blood volume in the chambers remains constant. This moment is called the isovolumetric contraction phase.
>
> *Modified from:* Marieb E, Hoehn K. *Human Anatomy and Physiology.* 8th ed. San Francisco, CA: Benjamin Cummings/Pearson Education; 2009.

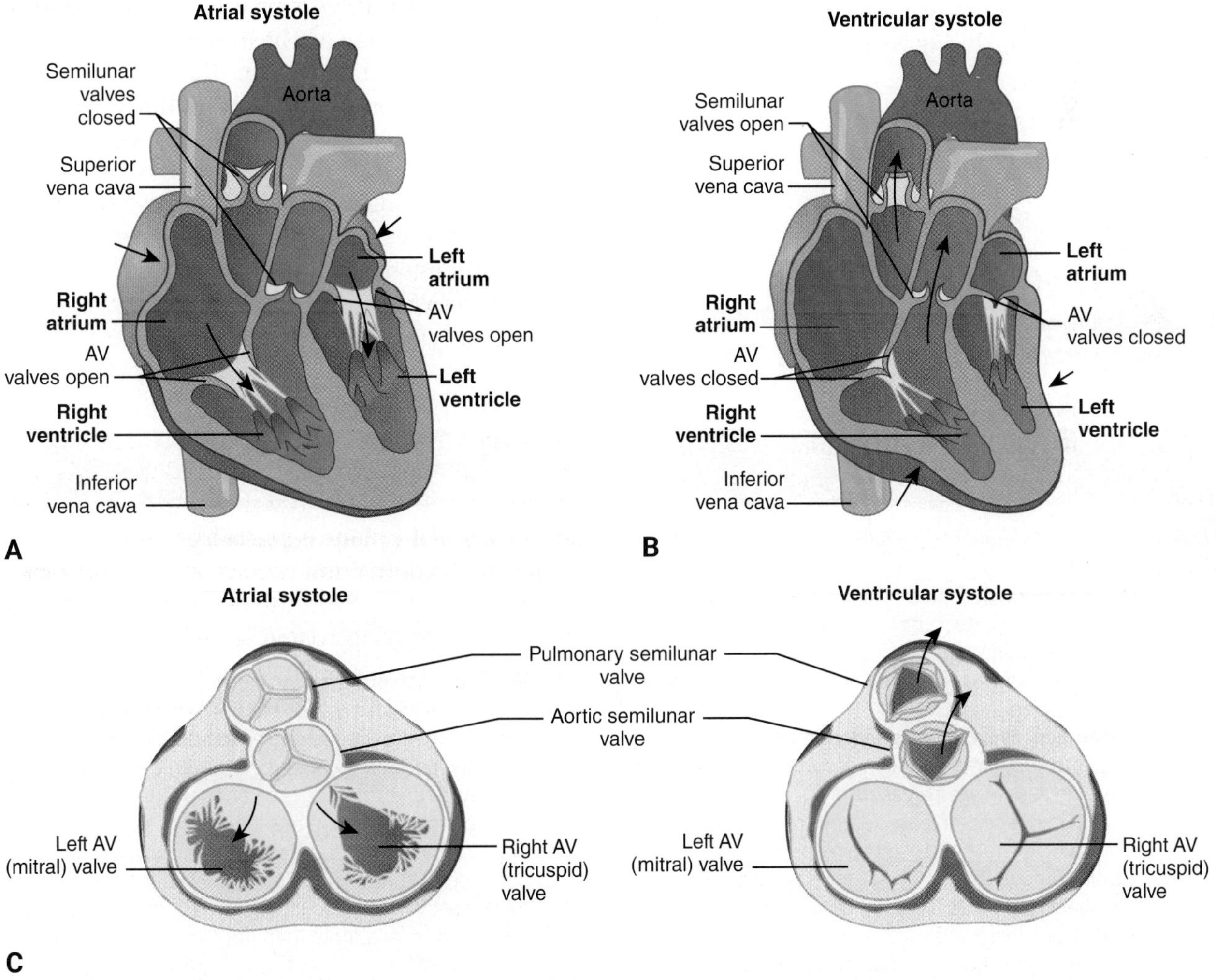

FIGURE 21-4 Heart action. **A.** During atrial systole (contraction), cardiac muscle in the atrial wall contracts, forcing blood through the atrioventricular (AV) valves and into the ventricles. **B.** During the ventricular systole that follows, the AV valves close and blood is forced out of the ventricles through the semilunar valves into the arteries. **C.** The four valves as seen from above (superior) during atrial and ventricular systole.

Ventricular Systole and Diastole

As the ventricles begin to contract, ventricular pressure exceeds atrial pressure, which causes the AV valves to close. As the contraction proceeds, ventricular pressure continues to rise. Pressure rises until it exceeds that in the pulmonary artery on the right side of the heart and in the aorta on the left side. At that time, the pulmonary and aortic valves open. Blood then flows from the ventricles into those arteries (**ejection**).

After ventricular contraction, ventricular relaxation begins. Ventricular pressure falls rapidly. When the pressure falls below the pressure in the aorta or the pulmonary trunk, blood is forced back toward the ventricles. This process closes the pulmonic and aortic valves. As the ventricular pressure drops below the atrial pressure, the tricuspid and mitral valves open. Blood then flows from the atria into the ventricles. Atrial systole occurs during ventricular diastole.

CRITICAL THINKING

What would happen if the valves were scarred and became stiff?

Stroke Volume

The **stroke volume** is the amount of blood ejected from the heart with each ventricular contraction. The stroke volume depends on three factors: **preload** (the volume of blood returning to the heart) (BOX 21-1), **afterload** (the resistance against which the heart muscle must pump), and **myocardial contractility** (the performance of cardiac muscle).

Preload

During diastole, blood flows from the atria into the ventricles. The volume of blood returning to each ventricle is the **end-diastolic volume**. This volume normally reaches 120 to 130 mL. As the ventricles empty during systole, their volume decreases to 50 to 60 mL (end-systolic volume). Therefore, the amount of blood ejected during each cardiac cycle (stroke volume) in the average adult is about 70 mL.

In a patient with a healthy heart, the capacity to increase the stroke volume is great. For example, the strong contraction of a heart during exercise can reduce the end-systolic volume to as little as 10 to 30 mL. If large amounts of blood flow into the ventricles during diastole, their end-diastolic volume can

CRITICAL THINKING

When you blow up a balloon, how does the balloon act like the heart muscle?

BOX 21-1 Venous Return

Venous return is influenced by several factors, including the following:

1. **Muscle contraction (skeletal muscle pump).** Rhythmic contraction of limb muscles, such as occurs during normal exercise (eg, walking, running, swimming), promotes venous return by compressing and decompressing the veins.
2. **Respiratory cycle (thoracoabdominal pump).** During respiratory inspiration, the negative pressure in the chest increases. This increase in pressure reduces right atrial pressure and increases venous return. Therefore, increasing the rate and depth of respiration increases cardiac output. Conversely, when negative pressure in the chest is reduced (eg, from positive pressure ventilation, positive end-expiratory pressure, continuous positive airway pressure, and bilevel positive airway pressure), venous return and cardiac output decrease.
3. **Decreased venous compliance.** Sympathetic activation of veins decreases venous compliance, which increases central venous pressure. The result is an increase in the total blood flow through the circulatory system.
4. **Vena cava compression.** An increase in the resistance of the vena cava, such as occurs when the thoracic vena cava becomes compressed during a Valsalva maneuver or during late pregnancy, reduces return.
5. **Gravity.** The effects of gravity can reduce venous return. When a person stands from a supine position, cardiac output and arterial pressure decrease because right atrial pressure falls. The flow through the entire systemic circulation falls because the arterial pressure falls more than the right atrial pressure does. Therefore, the pressure gradient driving flow throughout the entire circulatory system is decreased.

Modified from: Klabunde R. *Cardiovascular Physiology Concepts*. 2nd ed. Philadelphia, PA: Lippincott Williams & Wilkins; 2012.

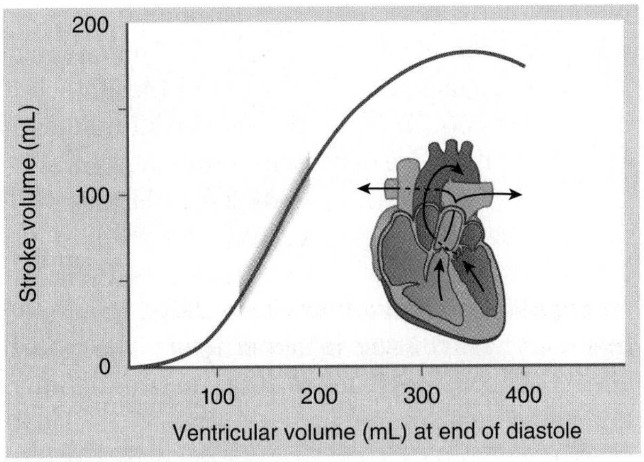

FIGURE 21-5 Starling law of the heart.

be as much as 200 to 250 mL. In this way, the stroke volume can increase to more than double the normal amount. The ability of the heart to pump more strongly when it has a larger preload is explained by the **Starling law of the heart**.

According to the Starling law (**FIGURE 21-5**), myocardial fibers contract more forcefully when they are stretched. (This ability of stretched muscle to contract with increased force is a quality of all striated muscle, not just cardiac muscle.) When the ventricles are filled with larger-than-normal volumes of blood (increased preload), they contract with greater than normal force to deliver all the blood to the systemic circulation.

The Starling law and its effect on stroke volume can be applied only to a certain limit of muscle fiber stretching. Beyond that limit, muscle fiber stretch actually diminishes the strength of the contraction. At that point, the heart begins to fail.

NOTE

Preload is more important in determining cardiac output than is afterload.

Afterload

Afterload is the pressure within the aorta before ventricular contraction. It is a result of **systemic vascular resistance** (the total resistance against which blood must be pumped). The greater the afterload, the more difficult it is for the left ventricle to pump blood to the body. In addition, the amount of blood ejected with ventricular contraction (stroke volume) is reduced. (The decrease in stroke volume is the result of the increased pressure in the aorta that the ventricular muscle must overcome to open the aortic valve and push blood through.) As afterload is reduced (eg, by lowering blood pressure, vasodilators), stroke volume increases, provided there is enough blood in the system.

NOTE

Although the term *afterload* generally is used to refer to the left ventricle, it also can refer to the right ventricle. For example, pulmonary hypertension increases afterload and can cause right ventricular failure.

CRITICAL THINKING

What condition would increase the afterload?

Myocardial Contractility

The unique function of the myocardial muscle fibers and the influence of the autonomic nervous system play a major role in the function of the heart. Ischemia or various drugs can decrease myocardial contractility. Ischemia can reduce the total number of working myocardial cells (as occurs in MI). Hypoxia or beta blockers can decrease the ability of the myocardial cells to contract.

Cardiac Output

Cardiac output is the amount of blood pumped by the ventricles in 1 minute. It can be increased by increasing the heart rate, the stroke volume, or both. Cardiac output is calculated as follows:

$$\text{Cardiac output} = \text{Stroke volume} \times \text{Heart rate}$$

Systemic vascular resistance changes cardiac output by affecting the stroke volume. Vasodilation of the arteries, for example, reduces afterload. This produces an increase in cardiac output. In contrast, vasoconstriction increases afterload. In turn, this tends to reduce cardiac output. However, the body responds to the decrease by constricting the venous circulation. This action increases the amount of blood returning to the heart (preload) and causes the heart to contract more forcefully (Starling law). These actions help maintain or increase cardiac output.

Nervous System Control of the Heart

In addition to the heart itself, the autonomic nervous system controls the behavior of the heart (described in Chapter 10, *Review of Human Systems*). It greatly influences the heart rate, conductivity, and contractility. The autonomic nervous system innervates the atria and ventricles. The atria are well supplied with large numbers of sympathetic and parasympathetic nerve fibers. The ventricles mainly are supplied by sympathetic nerves.

The parasympathetic nervous system is concerned mainly with vegetative functions (eg, digestion, bowel and bladder function). In contrast, the sympathetic nervous system helps prepare the body to respond to stress. These sympathetic and parasympathetic control systems work in a checks-and-balances manner. They stimulate the heart to increase or decrease cardiac output according to the metabolic demands of the body.

CRITICAL THINKING

Consider how you regulate the hot and cold taps in a shower. How is the behavior of the autonomic nervous system similar?

Parasympathetic Control

Parasympathetic control of the heart is accomplished through the vagus nerve. Control by these nerve fibers has a continuous restraining influence on the heart, primarily by reducing the heart rate and, to a lesser extent, contractility. The vagus nerve may be stimulated in several ways, such as the Valsalva maneuver, carotid sinus massage (described later in this chapter), pain, and distention of the urinary bladder. Acetylcholine is the chemical mediator of the parasympathetic nervous system.

Strong parasympathetic stimulation can decrease the heart rate to 20 or 30 beats/min; however, such stimulation generally has little effect on stroke volume. In fact, stroke volume may increase with a decreased heart rate. This response occurs because the longer interval between heartbeats allows the heart to fill with a larger amount of blood and thus contract more forcefully (Starling law).

Sympathetic Control

Sympathetic nerve fibers originate in the thoracic region of the spinal cord. They form groups of nerve fibers called ganglia. Their postganglionic fibers release the chemical norepinephrine. This chemical stimulates an increase in the heart rate (positive chronotropic effect). Norepinephrine also stimulates an increase in the force of muscle contraction (positive inotropic effect). Sympathetic stimulation of the heart causes the coronary arteries to dilate. It also causes constriction of peripheral vessels. These two effects, dilation and constriction, help increase the blood and oxygen supply to the heart. The cardiac effects of norepinephrine result from stimulation of alpha and beta adrenergic receptors.

NOTE

As described in Chapter 13, *Principles of Pharmacology and Emergency Medications*, the term *inotropic* refers to the force of energy of muscular contractions; chronotropic refers to the regularity and rate of the heartbeat; and dromotropic refers to conduction velocity. The effects are classified as positive or negative. For example, a positive inotropic effect would increase the strength of contraction. However, a negative dromotropic effect would decrease the speed of conduction.

Strong sympathetic stimulation of the heart may notably increase the heart rate. When rates are significantly high (>150 beats/min), the time available for the heart to fill is decreased, producing a decrease in stroke volume.

Hormonal Regulation of the Heart

Impulses from the sympathetic nerves are sent to the adrenal medulla at the same time they are sent to all blood vessels. In response, the adrenal medulla secretes the hormones epinephrine and norepinephrine into the circulating blood in response to increased physical activity, emotional excitement, or stress.

Epinephrine has basically the same effect on cardiac muscles as norepinephrine. Epinephrine increases the rate and force of contraction. In addition, it causes blood vessels to constrict in the skin, kidneys, gastrointestinal tract, and other organs (viscera). Epinephrine also causes dilation of skeletal and coronary blood vessels. Epinephrine from the adrenal glands takes longer to act on the heart than does direct sympathetic innervation; however, the effect lasts longer. Norepinephrine causes constriction of peripheral blood vessels in most areas of the body and stimulates cardiac muscle.

Role of Electrolytes

Myocardial cells are bathed in an electrolyte solution, as are all other cells of the human body. The major electrolytes that affect cardiac function (described in the next section) are calcium, potassium, and sodium. Magnesium is a major intracellular cation that also plays an important role. Changes in electrolytes can affect depolarization, repolarization, and myocardial contractility.

CRITICAL THINKING

What drugs can alter the normal balance of electrolytes in the body?

Electrophysiology of the Heart

To provide appropriate care for patients with cardiac disease, the paramedic must understand the mechanical and electrical functions of the heart. Understanding why and how the electrical conduction system can malfunction is crucial. The paramedic also must understand the effect that lack of oxygen to the cells (myocardial ischemia) has on cardiac rhythms. Two basic groups of cells in the myocardium are vital for cardiac function. One group is the specialized cells of the electrical conduction system. These cells are responsible for the formation and conduction of electrical current. The second group is the working myocardial cells. These cells have the property of contractility and perform the actual pumping of blood.

Electrical Activity of Cardiac Cells and Membrane Potentials

As described in Chapter 11, *General Principles of Pathophysiology*, ions are particles that are positively or negatively charged. The charge depends on the ability of the ion to accept or donate electrons. In solutions containing electrolytes, particles with unlike (opposite) charges attract each other, and the particles with like charges push away from each other. This property results in a tendency to produce ion pairs. These ion pairs help keep the solution neutral.

Electrically charged particles may be thought of as small magnets. They require energy to pull them apart if they have opposite charges. They also require energy to push them together if they have like electrical charges. Therefore, separated particles with opposite charges have a force of attraction similar to that of an electrical magnetic, giving them potential energy (**FIGURE 21-6**). The electrical charge creates a membrane potential between the inside and the outside of the cell. The electrical charge (potential difference) between the inside and outside of cells is expressed in millivolts (1 mV equals 0.001 volt). This potential energy is released when the cell membrane separating the ions becomes permeable.

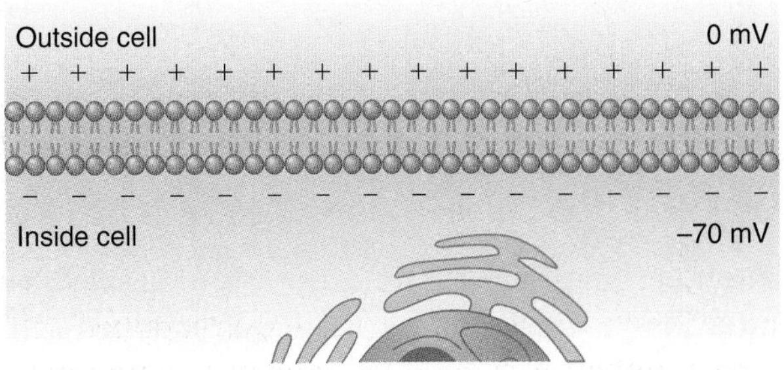

FIGURE 21-6 Electrical activity of cardiac cells and membrane potentials.

Resting Membrane Potential

When the cell is in its resting state, the electrical charge difference is the **resting membrane potential**. The term *potential* is used in the electrical sense as a synonym for voltage. The inside of the cell is negative compared with the outside of the cell membrane. Also, the resting membrane potential is recorded from the inside of the cell. Therefore, the resting membrane potential is reported as a negative number (about –70 to –90 mV).

The resting membrane potential is a result of the balance between two opposing forces. One of these forces is the concentration gradient of ions (mainly potassium) across a permeable cell membrane. The other is the electrical forces produced by the separation of positively charged ions from their negative ion pair. The resting membrane potential mainly is established by the difference between the intracellular potassium ion level and the extracellular potassium ion level. The ratio of 148:5 produces a large chemical gradient for potassium ions to leave the cell. However, the negative intracellular charge relative to the extracellular charge tends to keep potassium ions in the cell (**FIGURE 21-7**).

Sodium ions are positively charged ions on the outside of the cell. These ions have a chemical and electrical gradient. The gradients tend to cause sodium ions to move intracellularly, making the cell more positive on the inside compared with the outside.

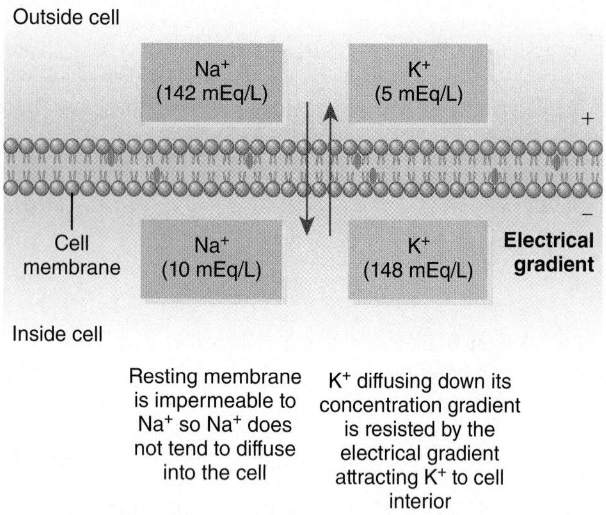

FIGURE 21-7 At equilibrium (resting conditions), the tendency for potassium ions to diffuse out of the cell is opposed by the potential difference (electrical gradient) across the cell membrane. Because the resting membrane is not permeable to sodium ions, sodium ions do not tend to diffuse into the cell.

Diffusion Through Ion Channels

The cell membrane is relatively permeable to potassium, somewhat less permeable to calcium chloride, and minimally permeable to sodium. The cell membrane appears to have individual protein-lined channels: **potassium ion channels** and **sodium ion channels**. These channels allow passage of a specific ion or group of ions. Permeability is influenced by electrical charge, size, and the proteins that open and close the channels (gating proteins).

Because potassium ion channels are smaller than sodium ion channels, they prevent sodium from passing into the cell. Potassium ions are small enough to pass through sodium ion channels, but the cell favors sodium ions entering the cell during rapid depolarization. Rapid depolarization (the rapid entry of sodium ions into cells) creates a local area of current known as the action potential. After one patch of membrane is depolarized, the electrical charge spreads along the cell surface, opening more channels (**FIGURE 21-8**).

> NOTE
>
> **Depolarization** occurs when the resting membrane potential changes from being more negatively charged on the inside of the cell to being more positively charged on the inside of the cell.

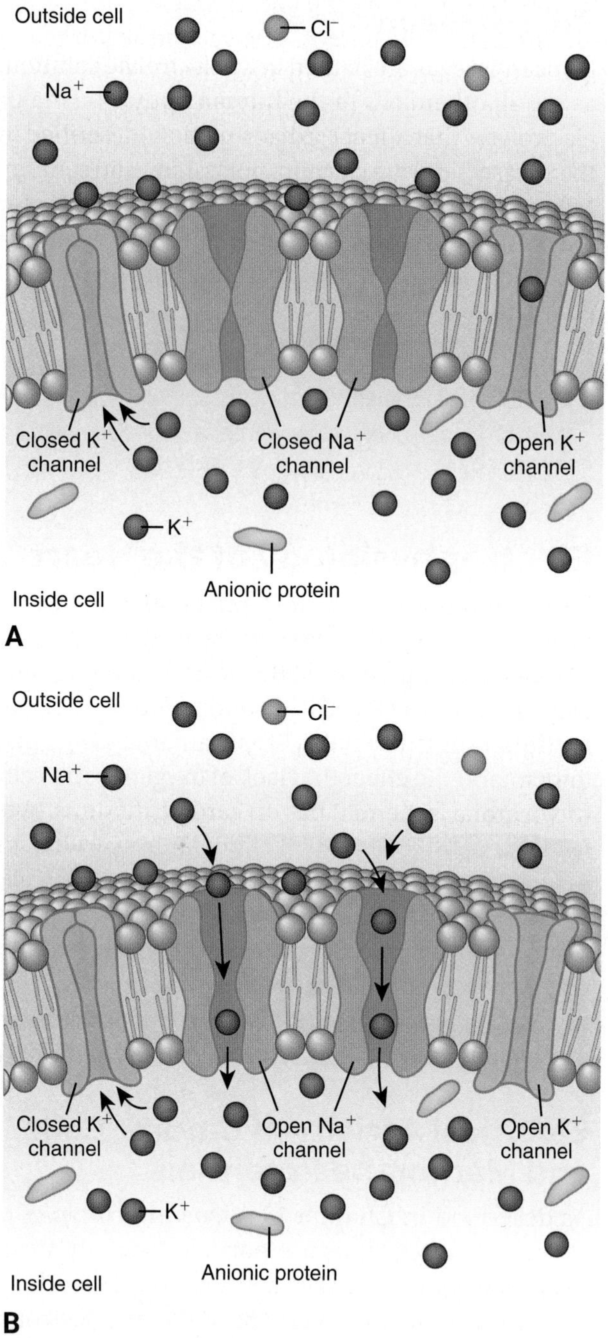

FIGURE 21-8 Effect of a stimulus that causes a voltage change across the cell membrane on the permeability of the cell membrane. **A.** Sodium channels remain closed in a resting (unstimulated) cell membrane. **B.** Depolarization of the cell membrane causes sodium channels to open. Sodium ions then diffuse down their concentration gradient into the cell.

The contribution of unpaired ions to the resting membrane potential depends on two factors. The first factor is the diffusion of ions through the membrane by way of the ion channels. This creates an imbalance of charges. The second factor is the active transport of ions through the membrane by way of the sodium–potassium exchange pump. This also creates an imbalance of charges.

> CRITICAL THINKING
> Which of these processes of electrolyte transfer requires energy to occur?

Sodium–Potassium Exchange Pump

Because the specialized sodium–potassium exchange pump actively pumps sodium ions out of the cell and potassium ions into the cell, this pump separates the ions across the membrane against their concentration gradients. Potassium ions are transported into the cell, increasing their concentration in the cell. Sodium ions are transported out of the cell, increasing their concentration outside the cell (**FIGURE 21-9**).

The sodium–potassium exchange pump normally transports three sodium ions out for every two potassium ions taken in. Therefore, more positively charged ions are transferred outward than inward.

> NOTE
> **Repolarization** occurs when charges inside the cell return to normal (become more negatively charged on the inside), allowing the cell to return to its normal resting state.

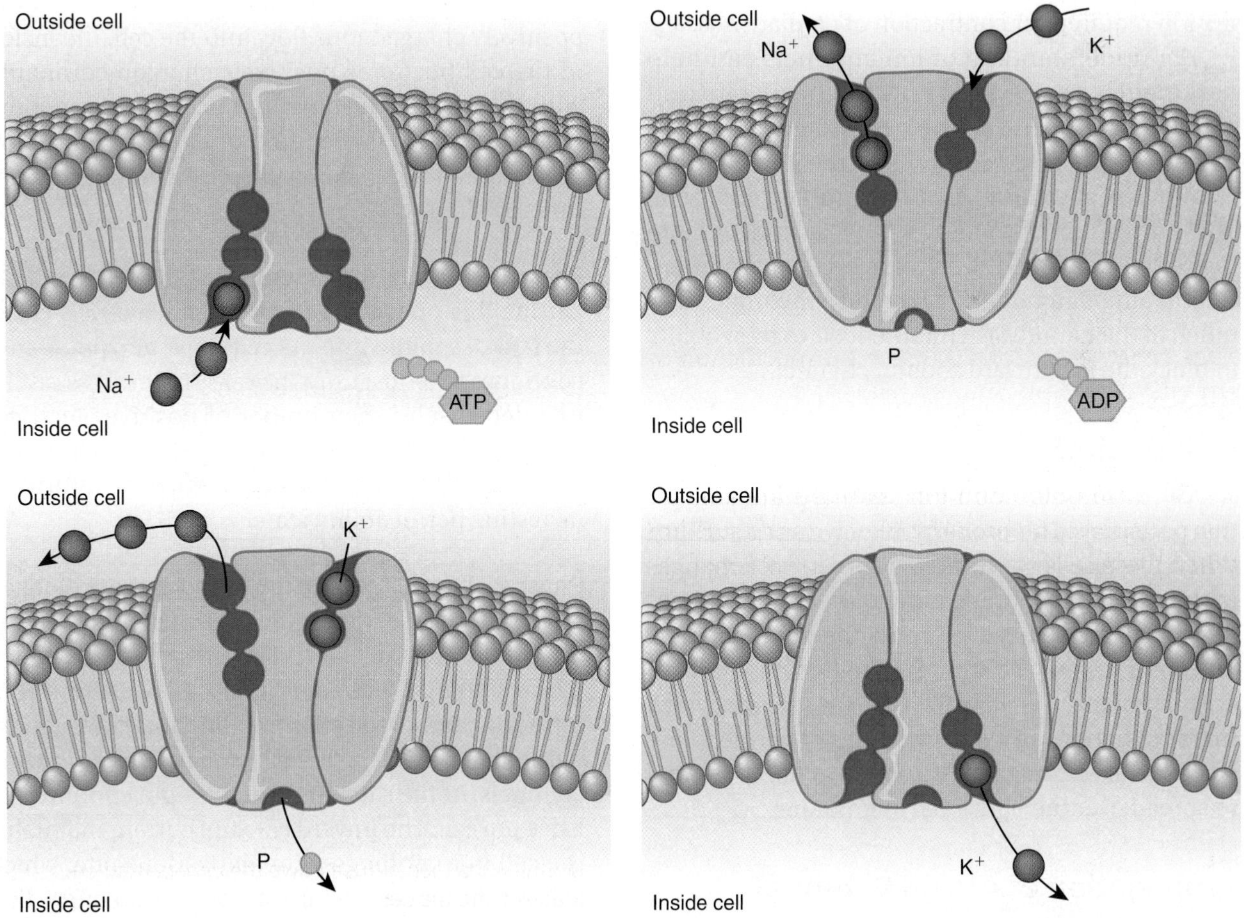

Abbreviations: ADP, adenosine diphosphate; ATP, adenosine triphosphate

FIGURE 21-9 The sodium–potassium exchange pump actively transports sodium ions out of the cell across the cell membrane and potassium ions into the cell across the cell membrane. Adenosine triphosphate is used as the energy source. The pump transports three sodium ions for every two potassium ions transported.

This action repolarizes the cell and returns it to its resting state. In the cell's resting state, the number of negative charges inside the cell is equal to the number of positive charges outside the cell.

Pharmacologic Actions

In cardiac muscle, sodium and calcium ions can enter the cell through two separate channel systems in the cell membrane known as the fast channels and the slow channels. Fast channels are sensitive to small changes in membrane potential. As the cell drifts toward threshold level (the point at which a cell depolarizes), fast sodium channels open. This opening results in a rush of sodium ions into the cell and rapid depolarization. The slow channel has selective permeability to calcium and, to a lesser extent, to sodium. Calcium plays an electrical role by contributing to the number of positive charges in the cell. Calcium also plays a contractile role. Calcium is the ion required for contraction of cardiac muscle.

An understanding of ion channels can help paramedics understand how the heart rate and contractility respond to drugs. For example, calcium channel blockers selectively block the slow channel. Examples of such drugs are verapamil and diltiazem. These drugs limit the movement of calcium ions into the cell without altering its voltage. Other examples, such as amiodarone (a type III antidysrhythmic), owe much of their antidysrhythmic effects to their ability to block the fast inward sodium channel.

Cell Excitability

Nerve and muscle cells are capable of producing action potentials. This property is known as excitability. When these cells are stimulated, a series of changes in the resting membrane potential normally causes depolarization of a small region of the cell membrane. The stimulus may be strong enough to depolarize a cell membrane to a level called the **threshold potential**. In this situation, an explosive series of permeability changes takes place that causes an action potential to spread over the entire cell membrane.

Propagation of Action Potential

An action potential at any point on the cell membrane acts as a stimulus to adjacent regions of the cell membrane. Thus, the excitation process, once started, is spread along the length of the cell and onto the next cell and so on. A stimulus strong enough to cause a cell to reach threshold and depolarize spreads quickly from one cell to another. Regardless of the strength of the stimulus, if such stimulus reaches the threshold potential, the nerve or muscle cell will give a complete response; otherwise, there is no response. This is known as the all-or-none principle. The cardiac action potential can be divided into five phases (phases 0 to 4). Phase 4, which marks the beginning and end of the process, is the period between action potentials when the cell is repolarized and ready to fire again (**FIGURE 21-10**).

Phase 0. At phase 4 the cell has returned to resting membrane potential. However, it will soon be stimulated to begin rapid depolarization again (phase 0). During this phase, the fast sodium channels open momentarily. In this moment, the sodium channels permit rapid entry of sodium into the cell. As the positively charged ions flow into the cell, the inside of the cell becomes positively charged compared with the outside, leading to muscular contraction. Phase 0 represents the rapid upstroke of the action potential and occurs when the cell membrane reaches threshold potential.

Phase 1. Phase 1 is the early rapid repolarization phase. During this phase, the fast sodium channels close, the flow of sodium into the cell stops, and potassium continues to be lost from the cell. This process results in a decrease in the number of positive electrical charges inside the cell and a drop in the membrane potential. As a result, the cell membrane returns to its resting permeability state.

Phase 2. Phase 2 (the plateau phase) is the prolonged phase of repolarization of the action potential. During this phase, calcium enters the myocardial cells, which triggers a large secondary release of calcium from intracellular storage sites and initiates contraction. Calcium slowly enters the cell through the slow calcium channels. At the same time, potassium continues to leave the cell. The inward calcium current maintains the cell in a prolonged depolarization state, which allows time for completion of one muscle contraction before another depolarization begins. This phase also stimulates the release of intracellular stores of calcium and aids in the contraction process.

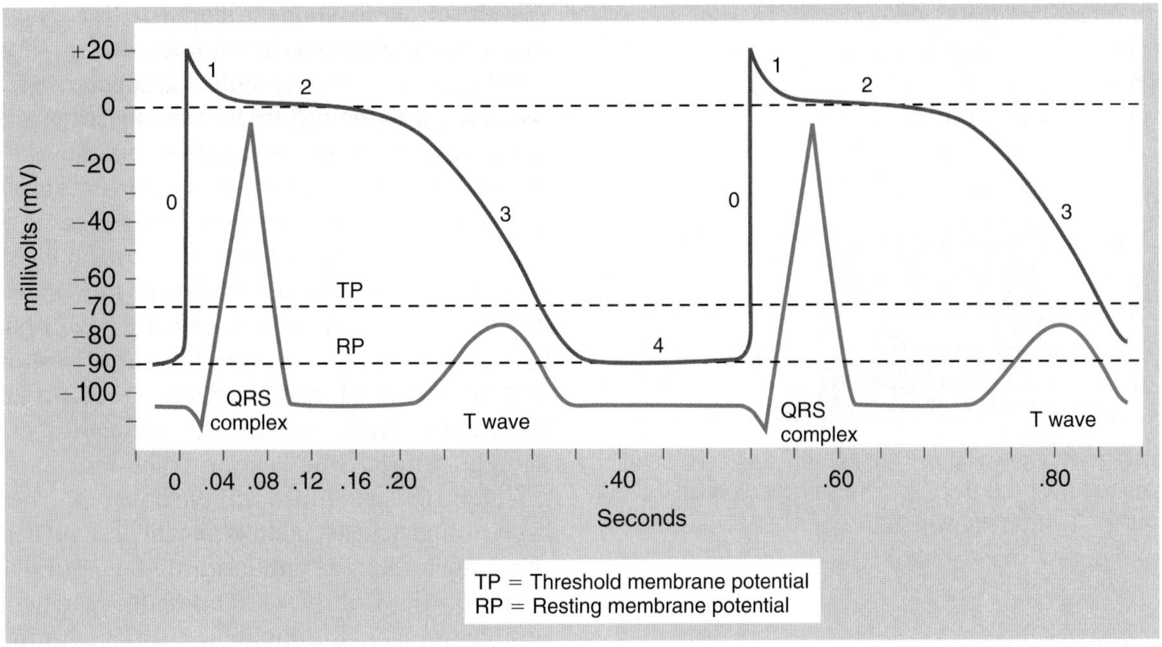

FIGURE 21-10 A cardiac action potential (red tracing) versus an electrocardiographic recording of cardiac electrical activity (green tracing).

Phase 3. Phase 3 is the terminal phase of rapid repolarization. It results in the inside of the cell becoming negatively charged. The membrane potential also returns to its resting state. This phase is initiated by closing of the slow calcium channels and by an increase in permeability with an outflow of potassium. Repolarization is completed by the end of this phase.

Phase 4. Phase 4 represents the period between action potentials, when the membrane has returned to its resting membrane potential. During this phase, the inside of the cell is negatively charged with respect to the outside. However, the cell still has an excess of sodium inside and an excess of potassium outside. This activates the sodium–potassium exchange pump. The excess sodium is transported out of the cell, and the potassium is transported back into the cell. During phase 4, pacemaker cells have a slow depolarization from their most negative membrane potential to a level at which threshold is reached, and phase 0 begins all over again.

Refractory Period of Cardiac Muscle

As does all excitable tissue, cardiac muscle has a **refractory period**, or resting period, in which cells are incapable of repeating a particular action. The refractory period can be further defined in two ways:

- The **absolute refractory period**, in which the cardiac muscle cell cannot respond to any stimulation, regardless of how long the stimulus is applied
- The **relative refractory period**, in which the cardiac muscle cell is more difficult than normal to excite, but the cell still can be stimulated

The refractory period ensures that the cardiac muscle is fully relaxed before another contraction begins. The refractory period of the ventricles lasts about as long as that of the action potential. The refractory period of the atrial muscle is much shorter than that of the ventricles. As a result, the rate of atrial contraction is much faster than that of the ventricles. If the depolarization phase of cardiac muscle is prolonged, the refractory period also is prolonged (**FIGURE 21-11**).

CRITICAL THINKING

How are the relative and absolute refractory periods of the heart similar to the flushing mechanism of your toilet?

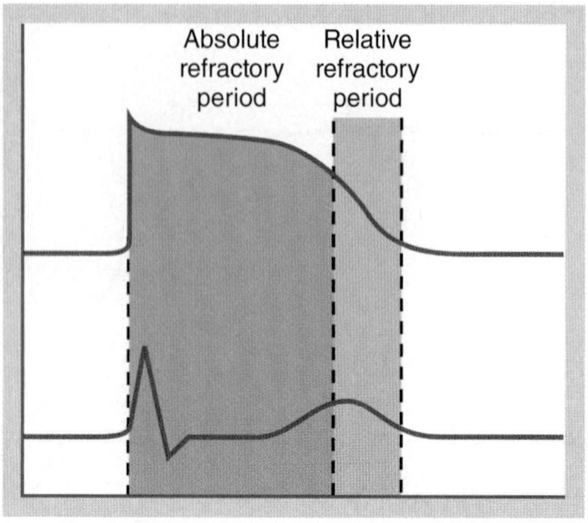

FIGURE 21-11 Absolute and relative refractory periods correlated with the cardiac muscle's action potential and with an electrocardiogram tracing.

Electrical Conduction System of the Heart

The conduction system of the heart is composed of two nodes and a conducting branch (**FIGURE 21-12**). The two nodes are located in the walls of the right atrium and are named according to their location. The **sinoatrial (SA) node** is medial to the opening of the superior vena cava. The **atrioventricular (AV) node** is medial to the right AV valve. The AV node and the **bundle of His** form the **atrioventricular (AV) junction**. In a normal heart, the AV junction serves as the only electrical link between the atria and ventricles. The bundle of His passes through a small opening in the heart and reaches the **interventricular septum**. At that location, the bundle of His divides into the **right bundle branch** and the **left bundle branch**. The left bundle branch then subdivides into the anterior-superior and posterior-inferior fascicles. These structures provide pathways for impulse conduction. A third fascicle of the left bundle branch also innervates the interventricular septum and the base of the heart.

The right and left bundle branches extend beneath the endocardium on either side of the septum to the apical portions of the right and left ventricles. The bundle branches subdivide into smaller branches. The smallest branches are called **Purkinje fibers**. The terminal Purkinje fibers spread electrical impulses from cell to cell through the myocardial fibers. This action results in contraction of the heart muscle. The rapid conduction along these fibers causes depolarization of all right and left ventricular cells. These cells

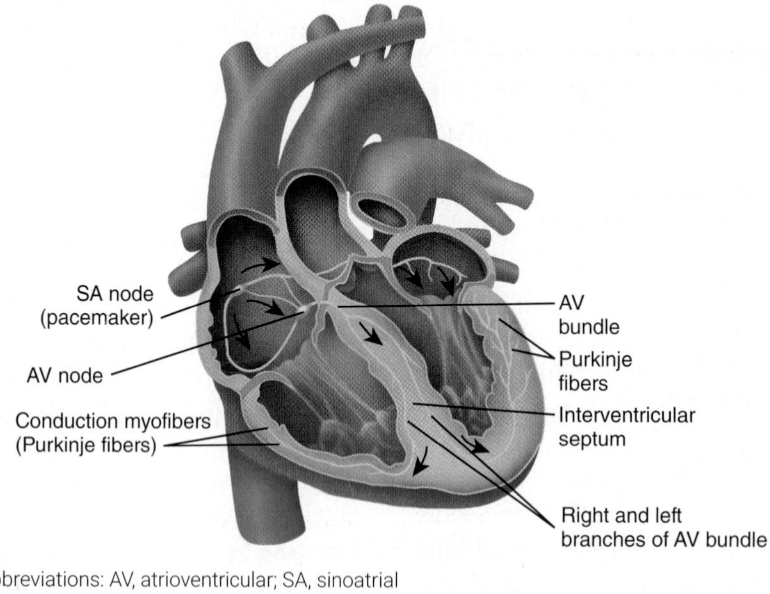

Abbreviations: AV, atrioventricular; SA, sinoatrial

FIGURE 21-12 Conduction system of the heart. Impulses (arrows) travel across the wall of the right atrium from the sinoatrial node to the atrioventricular (AV) node. The AV bundle extends from the AV node through the fibrous skeleton and into the intervertebral septum, where it divides into right and left bundle branches. The bundle branches descend to the apex of the ventricle and then branch repeatedly for distribution throughout the ventricular walls.

contract at about the same time, ensuring a single, coordinated contraction.

Pacemaker Activity

In skeletal and most smooth muscle, the individual cells contract only in response to hormones or nerve impulses from the central nervous system (CNS). However, unlike most other muscle cells, cardiac fibers have specialized cells known as pacemaker cells. These cells can generate electrical impulses spontaneously (**automaticity**). Pacemaker cells can depolarize in a repetitive manner. This rhythmic activity occurs because these tissues do not have a stable resting membrane potential. Instead, the resting membrane potential gradually decreases from its maximum repolarization potential. This continues until the resting membrane potential reaches a critical threshold, leading to depolarization. Sometimes the SA node may fail to generate an electrical impulse. If this occurs, other pacemaker cells take over. These pacemaker cells are capable of spontaneous depolarization and subsequent spread of an action potential; however, their rate is usually slower.

Sequence of Excitation in Cardiac Muscle

Under normal conditions, the chief pacemaker of the heart is the SA node because the SA node reaches its threshold for depolarization more quickly than other pacemaker cells do. The rapid rate of the SA node normally prevents the discharge of slower pacemakers from becoming dominant. If impulses from the SA node do not develop normally, however, the next pacemaker to reach its threshold level would take over the pacemaker duties.

Because of automaticity, cardiac cells can act as a "fail-safe" means of initiating electrical impulses. The backup cells (intrinsic pacemakers) are arranged in cascade fashion: the farther from the SA node, the slower the intrinsic firing rate. In order, the location of cells with pacemaker capabilities and the rates of spontaneous discharge are the SA node (60 to 100 discharges/min); AV junction tissue (40 to 60 discharges/min); and the ventricles, including the bundle branches and Purkinje fibers (20 to 40 discharges/min) (**FIGURE 21-13**).

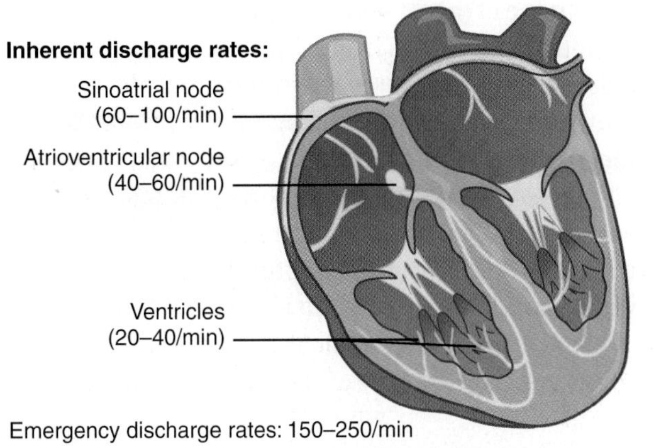

FIGURE 21-13 Intrinsic pacemakers in the atria, atrioventricular node, and ventricles can discharge at their own inherent rate when normal pacemaking fails.

From the SA node, the excitation spreads throughout the right atrium. This is made possible through four conduction tracks that make up the atrial conduction system: the AV node, Bachmann bundle (in the left atrium), Wenckebach tract (in the middle internodal tract), and Thorel tract (in the posterior internodal tract). Through these tracts, impulses travel directly from the right to the left atrium and to the base of the right atrium, resulting in virtually simultaneous contraction of the two atria. About 0.04 second is required for the impulse of the SA node to spread to the AV node. From there, propagation of the action potentials in the AV node is slow compared with the rate in the rest of the conducting system. As a result, a delay of 0.11 second occurs from the time the action potentials reach the AV node until they pass to the AV bundle. The total delay of 0.15 second allows atrial contraction to be completed before ventricular contraction begins.

After leaving the AV node, the impulse picks up speed. It travels rapidly through the bundle of His and the left and right bundle branches. The action potential passes quickly through the individual Purkinje fibers. The impulse ends in near simultaneous stimulation and contraction of the left and right ventricles. Ventricular contraction begins at the apex. Once stimulated, the special arrangement of muscle layers in the wall of the heart produces a wringing action that proceeds toward the base of the heart.

Autonomic Nervous System Effects on Pacemaker Cells

The effects of autonomic nervous system stimulation on the heart rate are mediated by acetylcholine and norepinephrine. Acetylcholine causes the cell membrane of the SA node to become more permeable to potassium ions. This increase in potassium ions delays the pacemaker in reaching threshold and thus reduces the heart rate. Parasympathetic effects also may result from stimulation of the cardiac branch of the vagus nerve, causing the heart rate to slow. An example of vagal stimulation is carotid sinus massage, described later in this chapter. Because excessive vagal stimulation may result in **asystole** (the absence of electrical and mechanical activity in the heart), it sometimes is referred to as the "ultimate bradycardia."

> CRITICAL THINKING
>
> What else can cause vagal stimulation?

Norepinephrine increases the heart rate by increasing the rate of depolarization. The result is an increase in the pacemaker discharge rate in the SA node. Norepinephrine increases the flow of potassium and calcium ions into the cell during depolarization of the action potential. As a result, sympathetic stimulation leads to an increase in the heart rate. The force of cardiac contractions also increases.

Mechanisms of Ectopic Electrical Impulse Formation

When the heart contracts as a result of stimulation by cells other than those in the SA node, the contraction is known as an ectopic beat. These isolated events sometimes are called premature beats because they occur early in the cycle, before the SA node normally would discharge. The new pacemaker is called an **ectopic focus**. Depending on the location of the ectopic focus, these premature complexes may be of atrial origin (premature atrial complexes [PACs]), junctional origin (premature junctional complexes [PJCs]), or ventricular origin (premature ventricular complexes [PVCs]). The ectopic focus may be intermittent or may be sustained and may assume the pacemaker duties of the heart (ie, the pacemaker site that fires the fastest controls the heart).

The two basic means by which ectopic impulses are generated are enhanced automaticity and reentry.

Enhanced Automaticity. **Enhanced automaticity** is caused by an acceleration in depolarization. This condition commonly results from an abnormally high leakage of sodium ions into the cells, causing

> NOTE
>
> An ectopic beat should not be confused with aberrant conduction (aberrancy). An ectopic beat is one that originates in the wrong part of the heart (away from normal). Aberrancy is abnormal conduction. **Aberration** can result from several causes, including PACs, blocks in the bundle branches, and electrolyte abnormalities.

the cells to reach threshold prematurely. As a result, the rate of electrical impulse formation in potential pacemakers increases beyond their inherent rate.

Enhanced automaticity is responsible for **dysrhythmias** (abnormal rhythms) in Purkinje fibers and other myocardial cells. This condition may occur after the release of excess catecholamines (ie, norepinephrine and epinephrine) or as a result of digitalis toxicity, hypoxia, hypercapnia, myocardial ischemia or infarction, increased venous return (preload), hypokalemia or other electrolyte abnormalities, or atropine administration.

Reentry. **Reentry** is the reactivation of myocardial tissue for the second or subsequent time by the same impulse (**FIGURE 21-14**). Reentry occurs when the progression of an electrical impulse is delayed or blocked (or both) in one or more segments of the electrical conduction system of the heart. A delayed or blocked impulse can enter cardiac cells that have just become repolarized. Reentry may produce single or repetitive ectopic beats. Reentry dysrhythmias can occur in the SA node, atria, AV junction, bundle branches, or Purkinje fibers. Reentry is the most common mechanism for producing ectopic beats, including cases of PVCs, ventricular tachycardia (VT), ventricular fibrillation (VF), atrial fibrillation (AF), atrial flutter, and paroxysmal supraventricular tachycardia (PSVT). These and other dysrhythmias are described later in the chapter.

The reentry mechanism requires that conduction through the heart take parallel pathways at some point. Each pathway has different conduction speeds and refractory characteristics. For example, a premature impulse may find one branch of a conducting pathway still refractory from the passage of the last normal impulse. If this occurs, the impulse may pass (somewhat slowly) along a parallel conducting pathway. By the time the impulse reaches the previously blocked pathway, the blocked pathway may have had time to recover its ability to conduct. If the two parallel paths

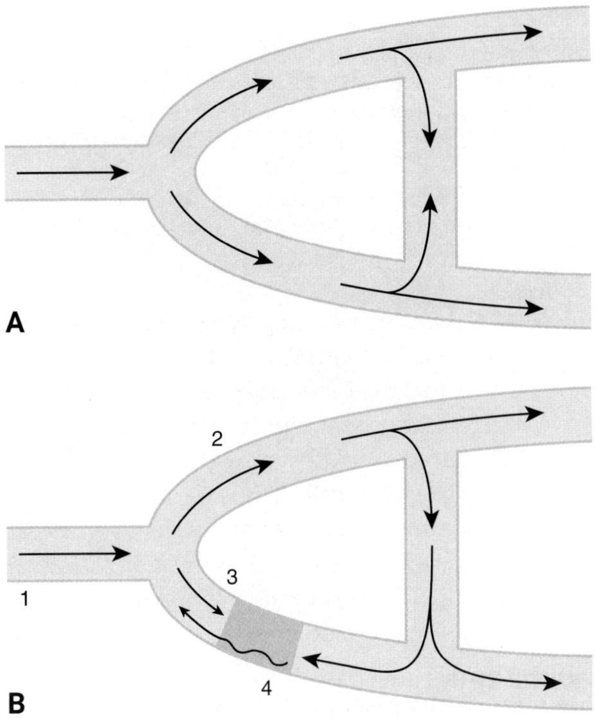

FIGURE 21-14 Reentry in terminal Purkinje fibers. **A.** Conduction through normal Purkinje fibers. The conduction velocity is uniform. **B.** Conduction through a severely depressed segment of terminal Purkinje fibers. The impulse (1) travels normally through normal tissue (2) and is blocked at the severely depressed tissue (3) but returns, with delay, through this tissue from the opposite direction (4).

connect at an area of excitable myocardial tissue, the depolarization process from the slower path may enter the now repolarized tissue. This situation can give rise to a new impulse spawned from the original impulse. Common causes of delayed or blocked electrical impulses include myocardial ischemia, certain drugs, and hyperkalemia.

Basic Concepts of Electrocardiogram Monitoring

An **electrocardiogram (ECG)** is a graphic representation of the electrical activity of the heart. It is produced by the electrical events in the atria and ventricles and is an important diagnostic tool. This graphic reading can help identify several cardiac abnormalities, such as abnormal heart rates and rhythms, abnormal conduction pathways, hypertrophy or atrophy of portions of the heart, and the approximate location of ischemic or infarcted cardiac muscle.

Evaluation of the ECG requires a systematic approach. The paramedic analyzes the ECG and then relates it to the clinical assessment of the patient. The ECG tracing is only a reflection of the electrical activity of the heart. It does not provide information on mechanical events such as force of contraction or blood pressure.

CRITICAL THINKING

Aside from blood pressure, how do you evaluate the mechanical activity of the heart?

The summation of all the action potentials transmitted through the heart during the cardiac cycle can be measured on the surface of the body. This measurement is obtained by applying electrodes connected to an ECG machine to the patient's skin. The voltage changes are fed to the machine, amplified, and displayed visually on the oscilloscope screen, graphically on ECG paper, or both. The voltage may be positive (seen as an upward deflection on the ECG tracing), negative (seen as a downward deflection on the ECG tracing), or isoelectric, when no electrical current is detected (seen as a straight baseline on the ECG tracing) (**FIGURE 21-15**).

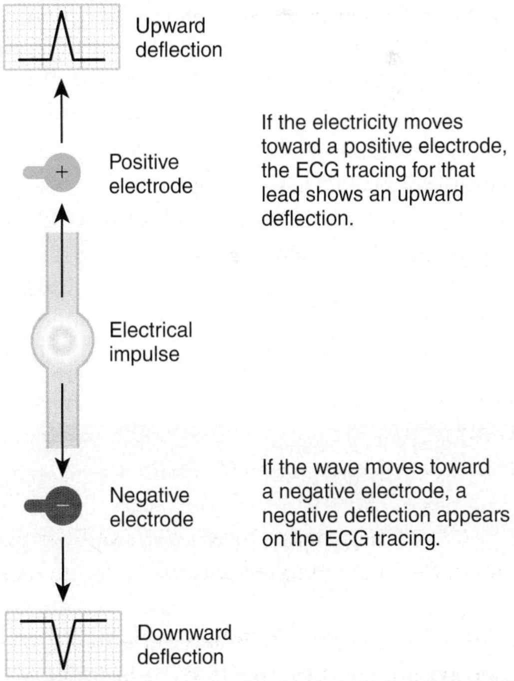

FIGURE 21-15 Rule of electrical flow.

ECG Leads

ECG machines offer many views of the electrical activity of the heart by monitoring voltage changes between the electrodes (leads) applied to the body. A modern ECG views the electrical activity of the heart from 12 leads: 3 standard limb leads; 3 augmented limb leads, and 6 precordial (chest) leads. The standard limb leads are I, II, III; the augmented limb leads are aV_R, aV_L, and aV_F; and the precordial leads are V_1 through V_6. Each lead assesses the electrical activity of the heart from a slightly different view and produces different ECG tracings (**TABLE 21-1**).

NOTE

The various views of electrical activity of the heart provided by the ECG are always from the perspective of the positive electrode. If the net force of electrical activity moves toward the positive electrode, the waveform seen on the ECG is "up." If the net force of electrical activity moves away from the positive electrode, the waveform seen on the ECG is "down."

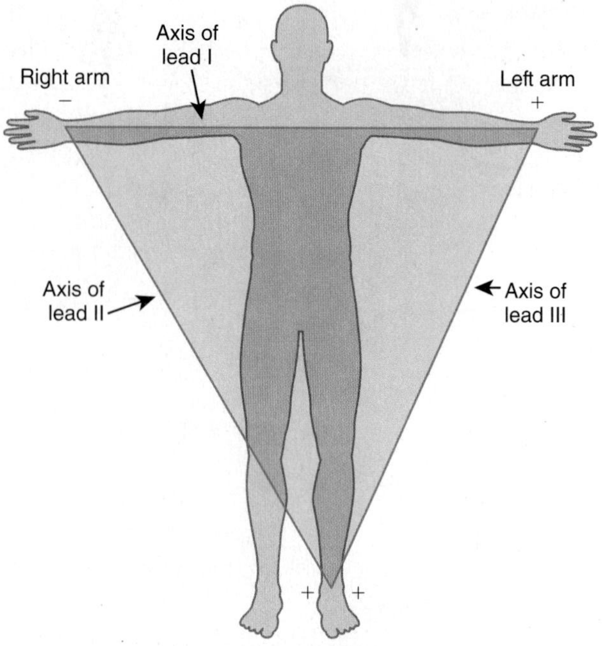

FIGURE 21-16 Leads I, II, and III make up the standard limb leads. An imaginary line joining the positive and negative electrodes of a lead is called the axis of the lead. The axes of these three limb leads form an equilateral triangle with the heart at the center (Einthoven triangle).

Standard Limb Leads

Standard limb leads are **bipolar leads**. That means they use two electrodes of opposite polarity (one pole is positive, the other is negative) to form the lead. Standard limb leads record the difference in electrical potential between the left arm, the right arm, and the left leg electrodes. Lead I records the difference in electrical potential between the left arm (+) and right arm (−) electrodes. Lead II records the difference in electrical potential between the left leg (+) and right arm (−) electrodes. Lead III records the difference in electrical potential between the left leg (+) and left arm (−) electrodes. Imaginary lines (axes) join the positive and negative electrodes of each lead, forming a straight line between the positive and negative poles. These lines form an equilateral triangle with the heart at the center (Einthoven triangle) (**FIGURE 21-16**).

The electrodes of the standard bipolar leads are placed on the following areas of the body:

Lead	Positive Electrode	Negative Electrode
I	Left arm	Right arm
II	Left leg	Right arm
III	Left leg	Left arm

TABLE 21-1 Comparison of Various Leads

Leads	Type	Polarity
I, II, III	Limb leads	Bipolar
aV_R, aV_L, aV_F	Limb leads	Unipolar
V_1 through V_6	Chest leads	Unipolar

Modified from: Phalen T. *The 12-Lead ECG in Acute Myocardial Infarction*. St. Louis, MO: Mosby; 1996.

Augmented Limb Leads

As do standard limb leads, **augmented limb leads** record the difference in electrical potential. However, unlike the standard limb leads, which are bipolar leads, the augmented limb leads are **unipolar leads**. This means that they have one electrode for a positive pole, but they have no distinct negative pole. The negative pole of the augmented limb leads is made by combining two of the negative electrodes. (Augmented limb leads use three electrodes to provide their view of the heart.) Augmented limb leads "augment," or magnify, the voltage of the positive lead (which usually is small). This increases the size of the complexes seen on the ECG so that they are approximately the same size as seen in the standard limb leads. Augmented limb leads use the same set of electrodes as the standard limb leads and are placed on the following areas of the body:

Lead	Positive Electrode	Negative Electrode
aV_L	Left arm	Right arm, left leg
aV_R	Right arm	Left arm, left leg
aV_F	Left leg	Right arm, left arm

The aV_R, aV_L, and aV_F leads intersect at angles different from those of the standard limb leads and produce three other intersecting lines of reference. When these lines of reference are combined with the lines of reference of standard limb leads, they form six lines of reference known as the **hexaxial reference system** (**FIGURE 21-17**). The hexaxial reference system is important for advanced ECG interpretation, described later in this chapter.

> CRITICAL THINKING
> Why is aV_R seldom used in ECG analysis? What view of the heart does it provide?

Precordial Leads

The six **precordial leads**, or chest leads, are unipolar leads that record the electrical activity of the heart in the horizontal plane. These leads, which are used in 12-lead ECG monitoring, measure the amplitude of the heart's electrical current. The precordial leads are projected through the anterior chest wall (through the AV node) toward the patient's back. The projection of the leads separates the body into upper and lower halves, providing the transverse or horizontal plane (**FIGURE 21-18**). The electrodes on the patient's chest are considered positive, but they are considered negative posteriorly (ie, the patient's chest is positive; the patient's back is negative). The chest leads are numbered V_1 to V_6.

When properly positioned on the chest, the chest leads surround the heart from the right to left side (**FIGURE 21-19**). Leads V_1 and V_2 are positioned over the right side of the heart and look at the septum. Leads V_5 and V_6 are positioned over the left side of the heart and look at the lateral wall of the left ventricle. Leads and V_3 and V_4 are positioned over the interventricular septum (right and left ventricle, AV bundle, and right and left bundle branches). These leads look at the anterior wall of the left ventricle.

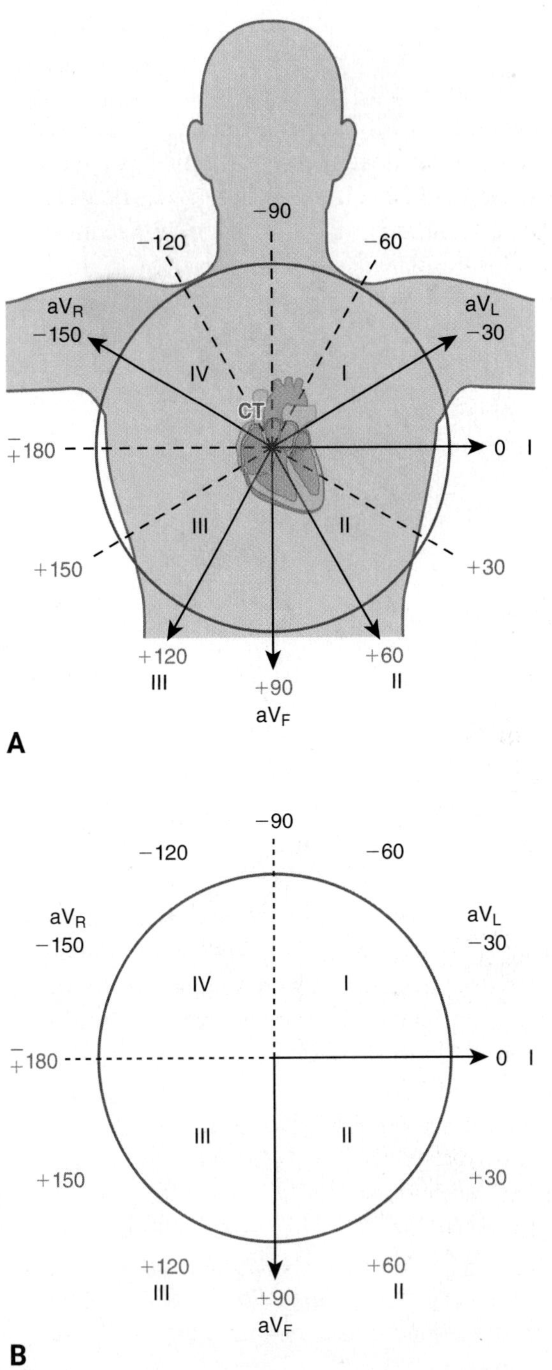

FIGURE 21-17 A. The hexaxial reference figure. **B.** The four quadrants of the hexaxial reference figure.

The precordial leads are placed on the chest in reference to the thoracic landmarks. Proper placement of the chest leads at specific intercostal spaces

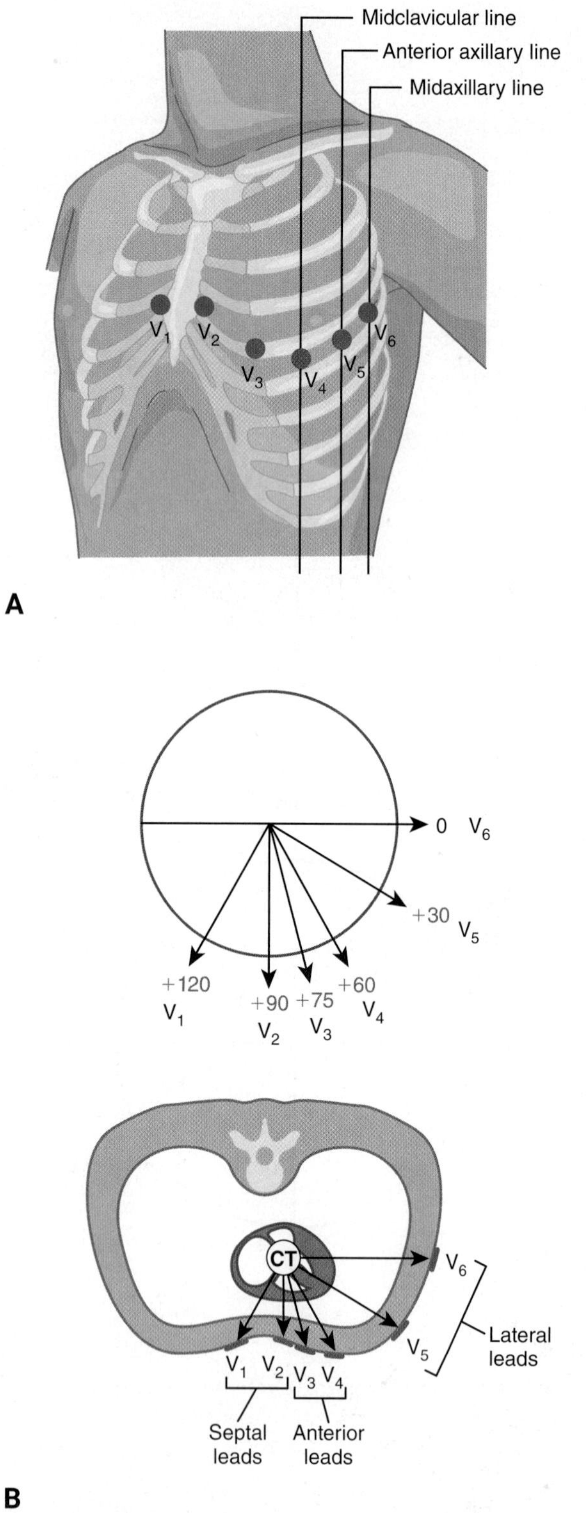

FIGURE 21-18 A. Placement of the precordial electrodes. **B.** Precordial reference figure and lead axes.

is essential for an accurate reading. The following is one method of locating the appropriate intercostal spaces (Figure 21-19):[7]

1. Locate the jugular notch and move downward until the sternal angle is found.
2. Follow the articulation to the right sternal border to locate the second rib. Just below the second rib is the second intercostal space.
3. Move down two intercostal spaces and position the V_1 electrode in the fourth intercostal space, just to the right of the patient's sternum.
4. Move across the sternum to the corresponding intercostal space and position V_2 to the left of the patient's sternum.
5. From V_2, palpate down one intercostal space and follow the fifth intercostal space to the midclavicular line to place the V_4 electrode.
6. Place lead V_3 midway between V_2 and V_4.
7. Place V_5 in the anterior axillary line in a straight line with V_4 (where the arm joins the chest).
8. Place V_6 in the midaxillary line, level with V_4 and V_5. (It may be more convenient to place V_6 first and then V_5.) For women, place the V_4 to V_6 electrodes under the left breast to avoid any errors in the ECG tracing that may occur from breast tissue. Lift the breast away using the back of the hand (Figure 21-19).

> CRITICAL THINKING
>
> Consider that your patient is female. You are performing a 12-lead ECG tracing. What measures can you take to reduce her potential discomfort or embarrassment?

Routine ECG Monitoring

Routine monitoring of cardiac rhythm in the prehospital setting, emergency department (ED), or coronary care unit usually is obtained in lead II or V_1. These are the best leads to monitor for dysrhythmias because of their ability to display P waves (atrial depolarization) on the ECG tracing. Much information can be gathered from a single monitoring lead, and in many cases cardiac monitoring by a single lead is sufficient. For example, monitoring a single lead can determine how fast the heart is beating and how regular the heartbeat is. The paramedic also can determine how long conduction lasts in different parts of the heart.

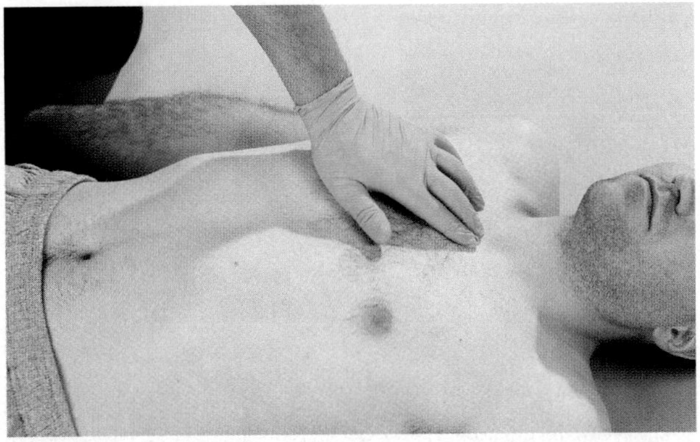

A

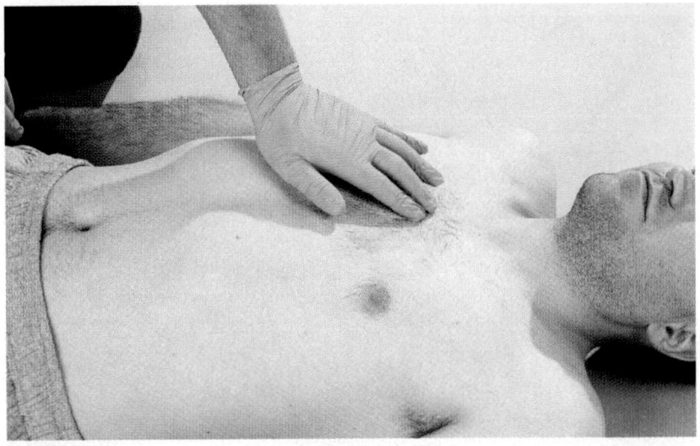

B

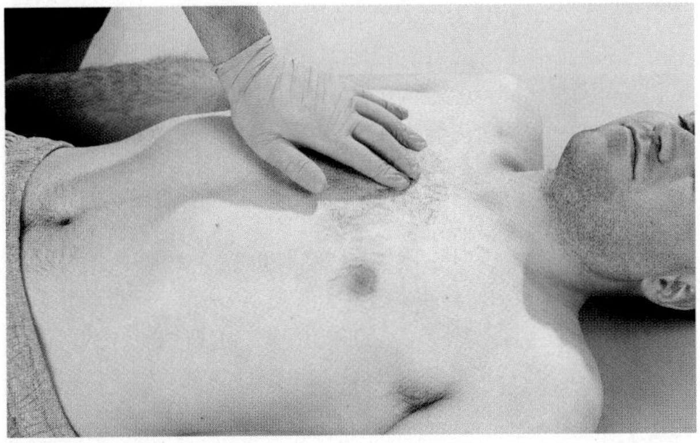

C

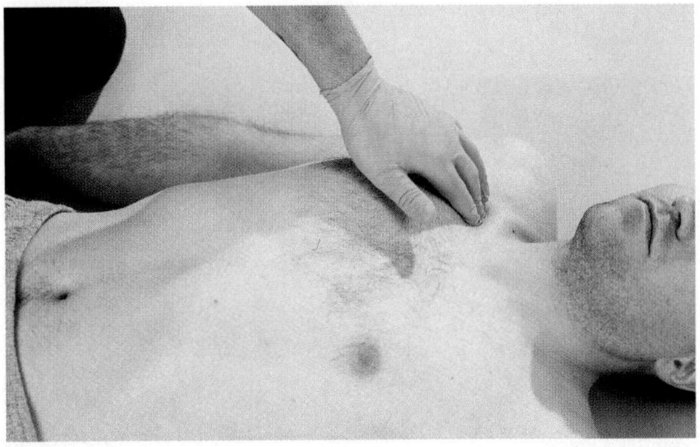

D

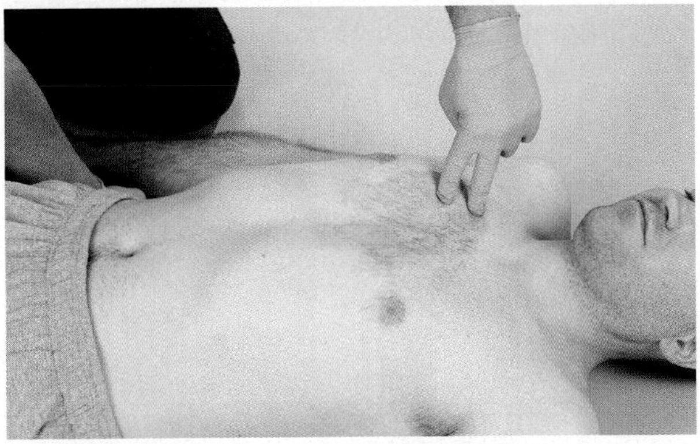

E

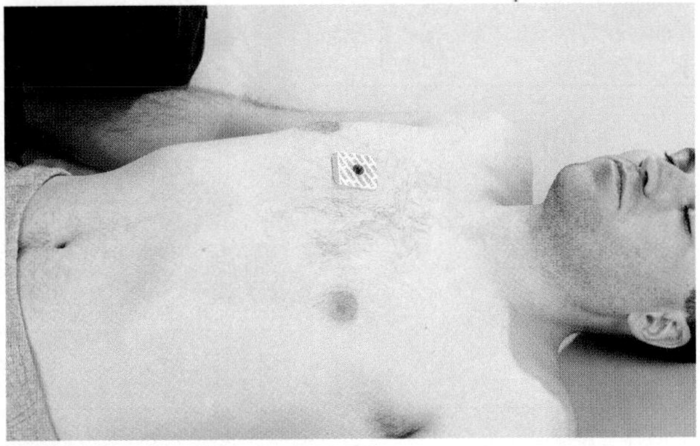

F

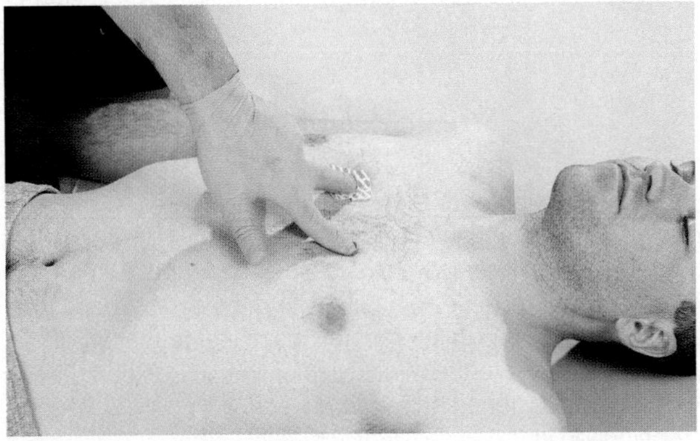

G

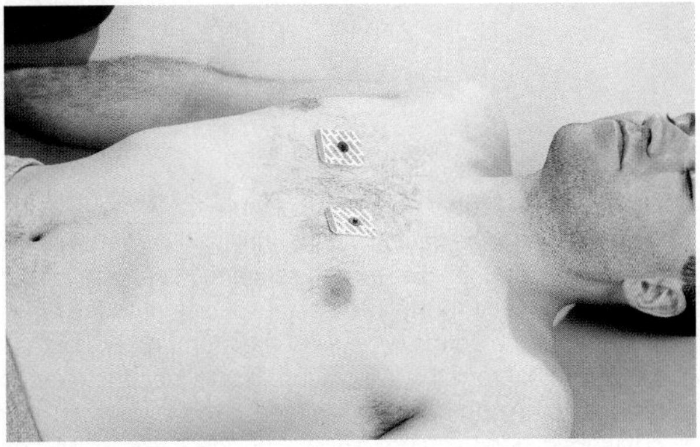

H

(continued)

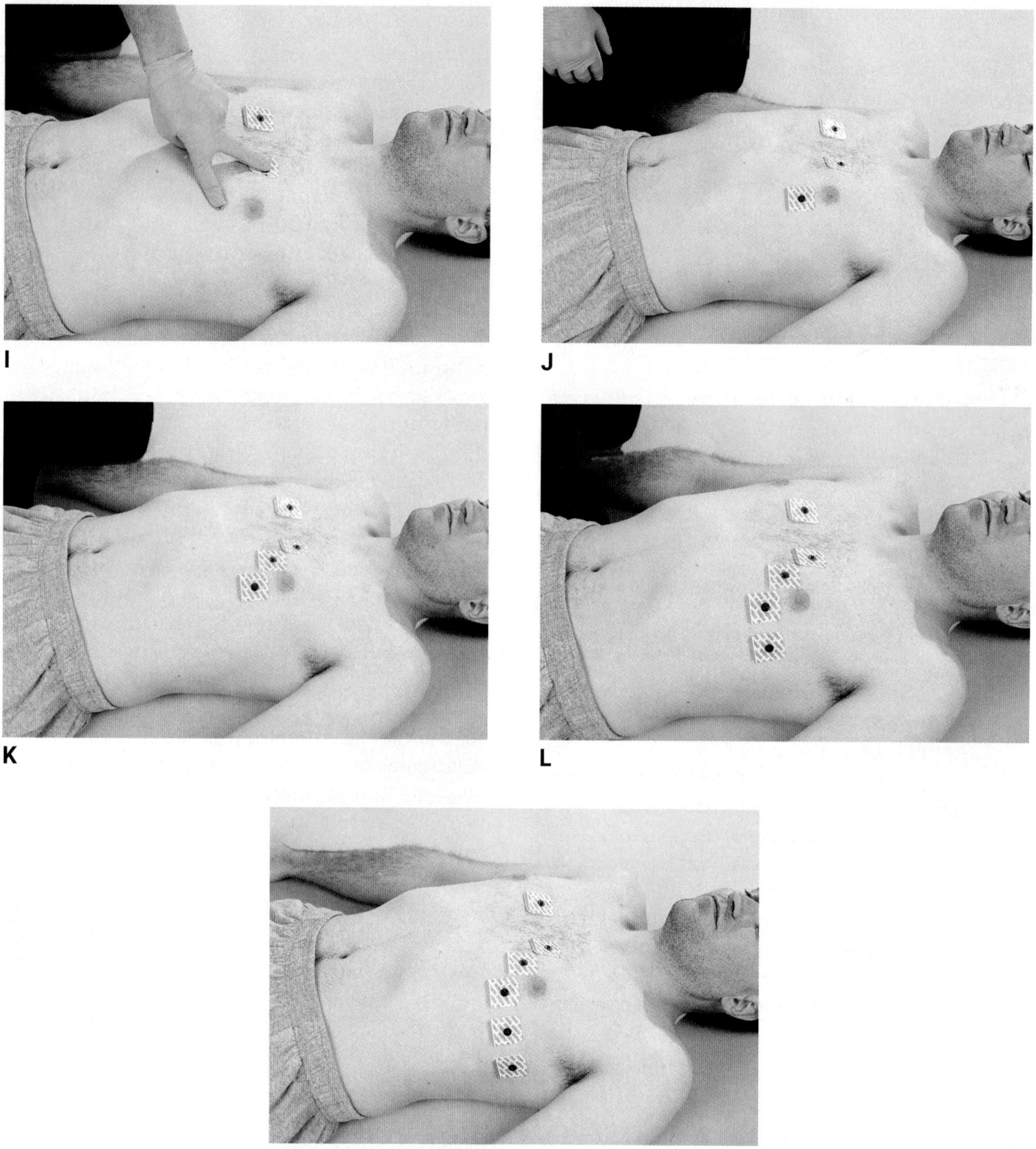

I J K L M

FIGURE 21-19 Proper chest lead placement. **A.** Locate the jugular notch. **B.** Palpate for the angle of Louis. **C.** Follow the angle of Louis to the patient's right until it articulates with the second rib. **D.** Locate the second intercostal space (immediately below the second rib). **E.** From the second intercostal space, the third and fourth intercostal spaces can be found. **F.** Lead V_1 is positioned in the fourth intercostal space just to the right of the sternum. **G.** From the V_1 position, find the corresponding intercostal space on the left side of the sternum. **H.** Place the V_2 electrode in the fourth intercostal space just to the left of the sternum. **I.** From the V_2 position, locate the fifth intercostal space and follow it to the midclavicular line. **J.** Position the V_4 electrode in the fifth intercostal space in the midclavicular line. **K.** Lead V_3 is positioned halfway between V_2 and V_4. **L.** Lead V_5 is positioned in the anterior axillary line, level with V_4. **M.** Lead V_6 is positioned in the midaxillary line, level with V_4.

Single-lead monitoring does have limitations and may fail to reveal various cardiac abnormalities. In most EMS systems that provide advanced life support, the 12-lead ECG is the standard for evaluating patients with chest pain of suspected cardiac origin.

CRITICAL THINKING

What effect does improper lead placement have on the view of the heart and the analysis of the ECG tracing?

Application of Monitoring Electrodes

The most commonly used electrodes for continuous ECG monitoring are pregelled, stick-on disks. These disks can be applied easily to the chest wall. The paramedic should observe the following guidelines to minimize artifacts in the signal and to make effective contact between the electrode and the skin:

1. Choose an appropriate area of skin, avoiding large muscle masses and large amounts of hair, which may prevent the electrode from lying flat against the skin.
2. Cleanse the area with alcohol to remove dirt and body oil. When attaching electrodes to the extremities, use the inner surfaces of the arms and legs. If necessary, trim excess body hair before placing the electrodes. If the patient is extremely diaphoretic, use tincture of benzoin to help secure application or use diaphoretic electrodes.
3. Attach the electrodes to the prepared site.
4. Attach the ECG cables to the electrodes. Most cables are marked for right arm, left arm, right leg, and left leg application.
5. Turn on the ECG monitor and obtain a baseline tracing.

CRITICAL THINKING

Why should alcohol or benzoin not be used under defibrillator pads?

If the signal is poor, the paramedic should recheck the cable connections and the effectiveness of the patient's skin contact with the electrodes. Other common causes of a poor signal include body hair, dried conductive gel, poor electrode placement, and diaphoresis.

ECG Graph Paper

The paper used in recording ECGs is standardized to allow comparative analysis of an ECG wave. The graph paper is divided into squares 1 mm in height and width. The paper is divided further by darker lines every fifth square vertically and horizontally. Each large square is 5 mm high and 5 mm wide (**FIGURE 21-20**).

As the graph paper moves past the needle or pen of the ECG machine, it measures time and amplitude. Time is measured on the horizontal plane (side to side). When the ECG is recorded at the standard paper speed of 25 mm/s, each small square is equal to 1 mm (0.04 second) and each large square (the dark vertical lines) is equal to 5 mm (0.20 second). These squares measure the time it takes an electrical impulse to pass through a specific part of the heart.

Amplitude is measured on the vertical axis (top to bottom) of the graph paper. Each small square of the graph paper is equal to 0.1 mV. Each large square (five small squares) is equal to 0.5 mV. The sensitivity of the 12-lead ECG machine is standardized. When properly calibrated, a 1-mV electrical signal produces a 10-mm deflection (two large squares) on the ECG tracing. ECG machines equipped with calibration buttons should have a calibration curve placed at the beginning of the first tracing (generally a 1-mV burst, represented by a 10-mm "block" wave).

Time interval markings are denoted by short vertical lines and usually are located on the top of the ECG graph paper. When the ECG is recorded at the standard paper speed of 25 mm/s, the distance between each short vertical line is 75 mm (3 seconds). Each 3-second interval contains 15 large squares (0.2 second $\times$ 15 squares = 3 seconds). These markings are used as a method of heart rate calculation (ie, counting the number of QRS complexes in 6 seconds and multiplying by 10).

Relationship of the ECG to Electrical Activity

Each waveform seen on the screen or recorded on the ECG graph paper represents the conduction of an electrical impulse through a certain part of the heart. All waveforms begin and end at the isoelectric line. This line represents the absence of an electrical potential difference between the positive and negative electrode. A deflection above the baseline is

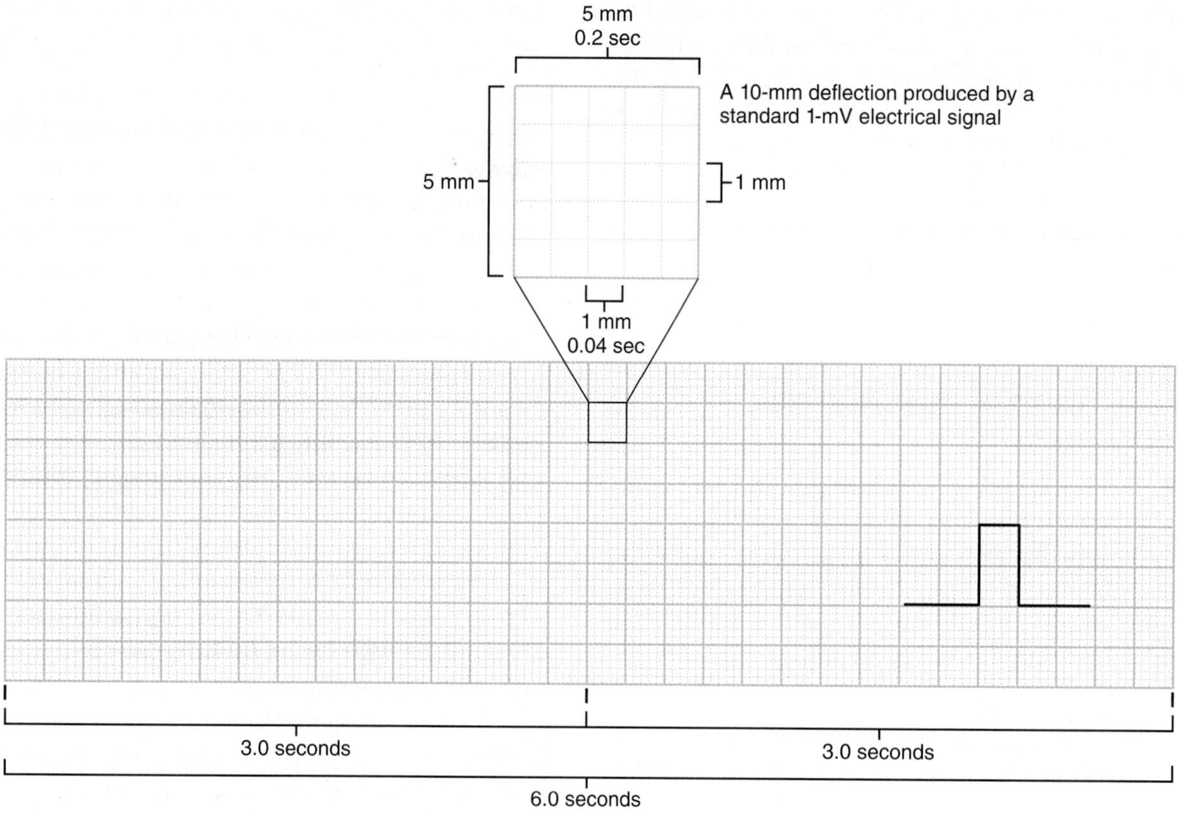

FIGURE 21-20 Electrocardiogram graph paper.

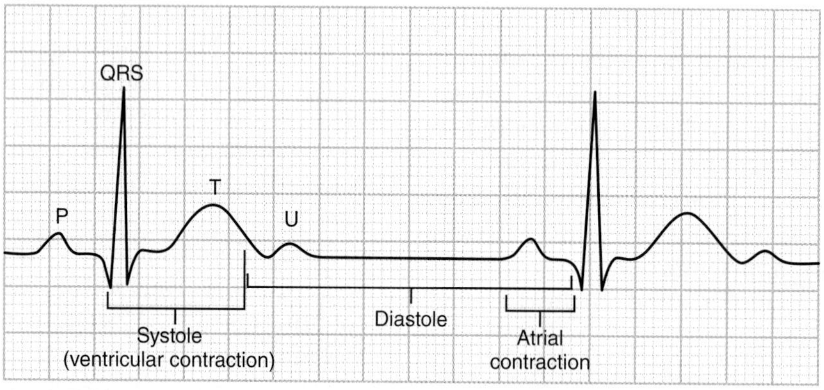

FIGURE 21-21 Summary of the electrical basis of the electrocardiogram.

positive and indicates an electrical flow toward the positive electrode. A deflection below the baseline is negative and indicates an electrical flow away from the positive electrode.

The normal ECG consists of a P wave, QRS complex, and T wave. A U wave sometimes may be seen after the T wave. The **U wave** is thought to represent delayed repolarization of the Purkinje fibers. It also may be associated with electrolyte abnormalities. If present, the U wave usually is a positive deflection. Other key parts of the ECG that should be evaluated include the PR interval, ST segment, and QT interval. The combination of these waves represents a single heartbeat, or one complete cardiac cycle (**FIGURE 21-21**). The electrical events of the cardiac cycle are followed by their mechanical counterparts. The descriptions of ECG waveform components refer to those that would be seen in lead II monitoring (**BOX 21-2**).

BOX 21-2 ECG Waves and Mechanical Counterparts

P wave: Atrial depolarization
QRS complex: Ventricular depolarization
T wave: Ventricular repolarization

NOTE

A segment on an ECG is the region between two waves. For example, the PR segment begins at the end of the P wave and ends at the onset of the QRS complex (see **FIGURE 21-22**). An interval on an ECG includes one segment and one or more waves. For example, the PR interval starts at the beginning of the P wave and ends at the onset of the QRS complex (see **FIGURE 21-23**).

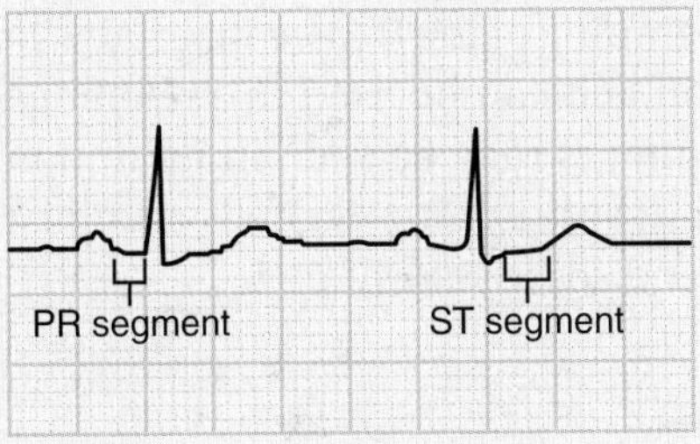

FIGURE 21-22 PR segment and ST segment.

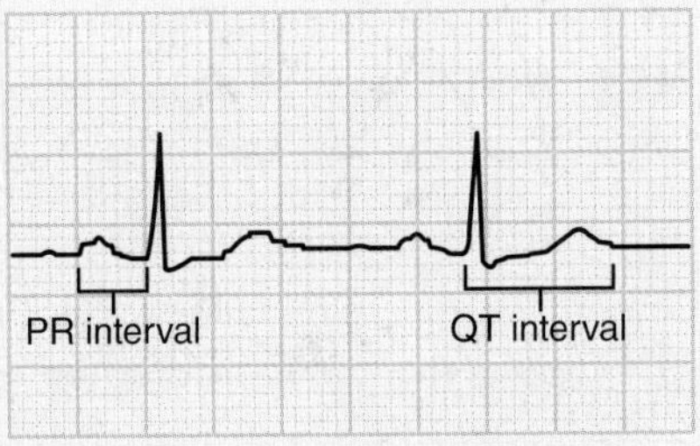

FIGURE 21-23 PR interval and QT interval.

P Wave

The **P wave** is the first positive (upward) deflection on the ECG. It represents atrial depolarization. It usually is rounded and precedes the QRS complex. The P wave begins with the first positive deflection from the baseline and ends at the point where the wave returns to the baseline. The duration of the P wave normally is 0.10 second or less, and its amplitude is 0.5 to 2.5 mm. The P wave usually is followed by a QRS complex. However, if conduction disturbances are present, a QRS complex does not always follow each P wave.

PR Interval

The **PR interval** is the time required for an electrical impulse to be conducted through the atria and the AV node up to the instant of ventricular depolarization. The PR interval is measured from the beginning of the P wave to the beginning of the next deflection on the baseline (the onset of the QRS complex). The normal PR interval duration ranges from 0.12 to 0.20 second (three to five small squares on the graph paper). The PR interval depends on the heart rate and the conduction characteristics of the AV node. When the heart rate is fast, the PR interval normally is shorter than when the heart rate is slow. A normal PR interval indicates that the electrical impulse has been conducted from the atria through the AV node normally.

QRS Complex

The **QRS complex** represents ventricular depolarization and is generally composed of three individual waves: the Q, R, and S waves. (All waves may not be visible in all leads.) The QRS complex begins at the point where the first wave of the complex deviates from the baseline. It ends where the last wave of the complex begins to flatten at, above, or below the baseline. The direction of the QRS complex may be predominantly positive (upright), predominantly negative (inverted), or biphasic (partly positive, partly negative). Because

NOTE

What About a QRS Complex That Is 0.11 Second in Duration?

Question: A normal QRS complex is defined as 0.08 to 0.10 second, and a bundle branch block is suspected when the QRS reaches or exceeds 0.12 second. What does it mean when the QRS is 0.11 second?

Answer: A QRS complex that is 0.10 to 0.11 second indicates a partial or incomplete bundle branch block (IBBB) where there is an intraventricular conduction delay. Although a QRS complex between 0.10 and 0.11 second is considered abnormal, it is not always pathologic. IBBB can be seen in healthy people or as a normal variation between beats. It can also be seen in congenital heart disease (especially atrial septal defects), myocarditis, pulmonary emboli, and right ventricular hypertrophy, and as an induced syndrome following cardiac surgery.

normal ventricular depolarization is rapidly transmitted through the bundle of His, the normal QRS complex is narrow with a duration of 0.08 to 0.10 second (two to two-and-a-half small squares on the graph paper) or less, and its amplitude normally varies from less than 5 mm to more than 15 mm.

The Q wave is the first negative (downward) deflection of the QRS complex on the ECG. However, it may not be present in all leads. The Q wave represents the normal left-to-right depolarization of the interventricular septum and thus, small "septal" Q waves ($<$1 mm $\times$ 1 mm) are typically seen in left-side leads (I, aV_L, V_5, V_6). Deeper Q waves ($>$2 mm deep) may also be seen in leads III and aV_R in a normal ECG. The R wave is the first positive deflection after the P wave. A subsequent positive deflection in the QRS complex that extends above the baseline is called R prime (R′). The S wave is the negative deflection that follows the R wave. The R and S waves represent the sum of electrical forces resulting from depolarization of the right and left ventricles (**FIGURE 21-24**).

CRITICAL THINKING

What is the importance of a QRS complex duration of 0.12 second?

The QRS complex follows the P wave. The QRS complex marks the approximate beginning of mechanical contraction of the ventricles, which continues through the onset of the T wave. The QRS complex represents ventricular depolarization. This includes the conduction of an electrical impulse from the AV node through the bundle of His, Purkinje fibers, and the right and left bundle branches. This impulse results in ventricular depolarization.

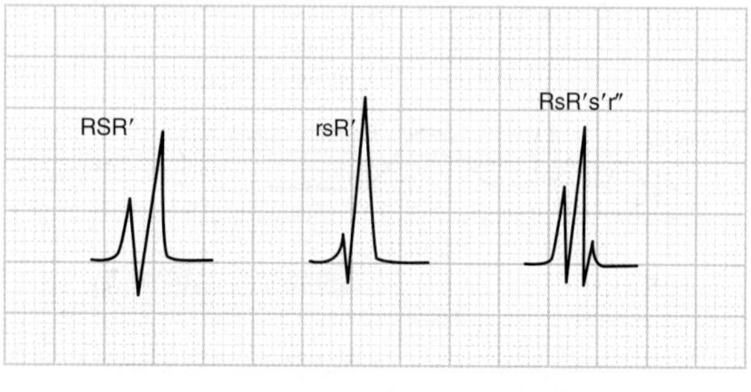

FIGURE 21-24 QRS complexes with more than one positive or negative deflection.

ST Segment

The **ST segment** represents the early phase of repolarization of the right and left ventricles. It immediately follows the QRS complex and ends with the onset of the T wave. The point at which it takes off from the QRS complex is called the J point. In a normal ECG, the ST segment begins at baseline and has a slight upward slope.

The position of the ST segment commonly is judged as normal or abnormal using the baseline of the PR or TP interval as a reference. Deviations above this baseline are referred to as ST-segment elevation. Deviations below baseline are referred to as ST-segment depression (**FIGURE 21-25**). Certain conditions can cause depression or elevation of the PR interval, affecting the reference for ST-segment abnormalities. Usually the baseline from the end of the T wave to the beginning of the P wave maintains its isoelectric position and can be used as a reference. Abnormal ST segments may be seen in infarction, ischemia, and pericarditis; after digitalis administration; and in other disease states.

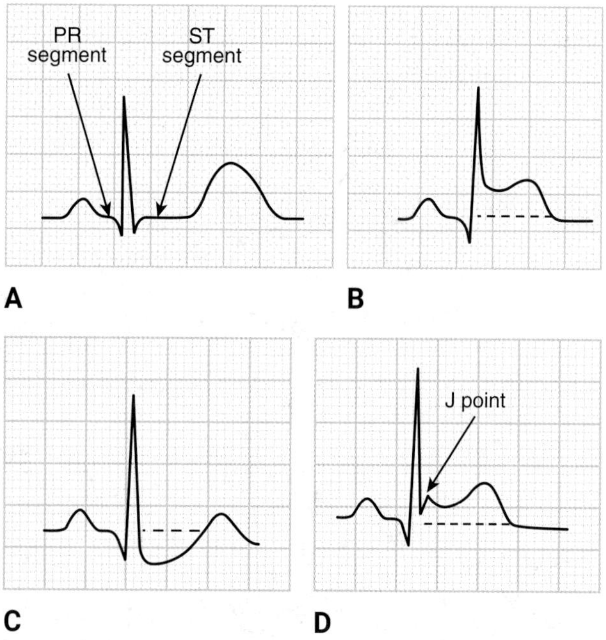

FIGURE 21-25 ST-segment deviations. **A.** Use of the PR segment as a baseline. **B.** The ST segment is elevated with respect to the PR baseline. **C.** The ST segment is depressed with respect to the PR baseline. **D.** J point (ST-segment elevation). A prominent notch marks the takeoff of the ST segment.

T Wave

The **T wave** represents repolarization of the ventricular myocardial cells. The wave occurs during the last part of ventricular contraction. The T wave is identified as the first deviation from the ST segment and ends where the T wave returns to the baseline (**FIGURE 21-26**). This wave may be above or below the isoelectric line. The T wave usually is slightly rounded and slightly asymmetrical.

> NOTE
>
> Deep and symmetrically inverted T waves may indicate cardiac ischemia. A T wave elevated more than one-half the height of the QRS complex (peaked T wave) may indicate new onset of ischemia of the myocardium or hyperkalemia.

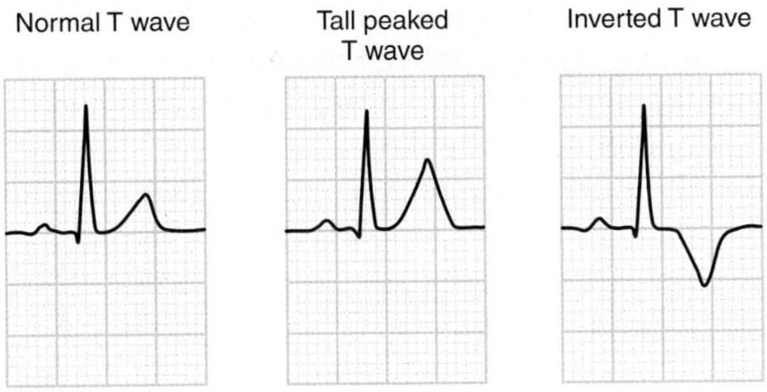

FIGURE 21-26 T waves.

QT Interval

The **QT interval** is measured from the beginning of the QRS complex to the end of the T wave (**FIGURE 21-27**). It represents the time from the beginning of ventricular depolarization until the end of ventricular repolarization. During the initial phase of the QT interval, the heart is completely unable to respond to electrical stimuli. (This is the absolute refractory period described earlier.) During the latter portion of this interval (from the peak of the T wave onward),

> NOTE
>
> The duration of the QT interval depends on the heart rate. This interval usually is somewhat less than one-half of the preceding R-R interval. In general, a QT interval less than one-half the R-R interval is normal, one that is greater than one-half is abnormal, and one that is about one-half is considered borderline. Regardless of the heart rate, a QT interval greater than 440 milliseconds in males and greater than 460 milliseconds in females is considered abnormal.
>
> Commonly prescribed medications that may prolong the QT interval include quinidine, procainamide, amiodarone, and disopyramide. These antidysrhythmics, by virtue of their effect on the QT interval, may lead to potentially lethal dysrhythmias, including VT, VF, and an unusual bidirectional ventricular dysrhythmia called torsades de pointes (described later in this chapter).
>
> *Modified from:* Huszar RJ. *Basic Dysrhythmias: Interpretation and Management*. 3rd ed. St. Louis, MO: Mosby; 2006.

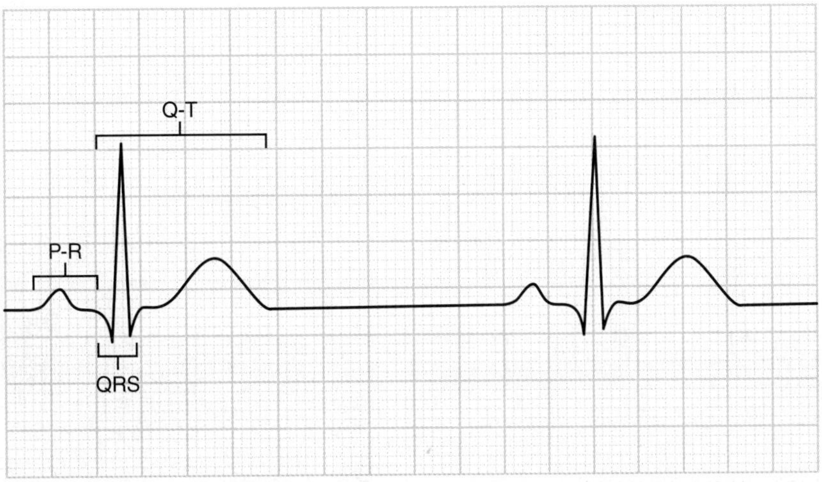

FIGURE 21-27 PR, QT, and QRS intervals.

the heart may be able to respond to premature stimuli (the relative refractory period). During this period, premature impulses may depolarize the heart.

Artifacts

An **artifact** is a mark on the ECG display or tracing caused by activities other than the electrical activity of the heart (**FIGURE 21-28**). Common causes of artifacts are improper grounding of the ECG machine, patient movement, loss of electrode contact with the patient's skin, patient shivering or tremors, implanted medical devices, and external chest compression. Two types of artifacts deserve special mention: alternating current interference (60-cycle interference) and biotelemetry-related interference.

Alternating current interference may occur in a poorly grounded ECG machine. Interference also may occur when an ECG is obtained near high-tension wires, transformers, and some household appliances. This interference results in a thick baseline made up of 60-cycle waves. The P waves may not be discernible because of the interference, but the QRS complex usually is visible. Alternating current interference also may result if the patient or the lead cable touches a metal object, such as a bed rail. Placing a blanket between the metal object and the patient may correct the interference.

Biotelemetry-related interference results in poor reception of biotelemetry ECG signals. This interference may result from weak batteries or from ECG transmission in areas with poor signaling conditions. Interference also may result if the transmitter is located a distance from a base station receiver. Biotelemetry-related interference may produce sharp spikes and waves with a jagged appearance.

ECG Interpretation: Steps in Rhythm Analysis

Evaluation of an ECG requires a systematic approach to analyzing a given rhythm. Numerous methods can be used for rhythm interpretation. This text uses a method that first looks at the rate, the rhythm, and QRS complex (the most important observation in life-threatening dysrhythmias); then the P waves and the relationship between the P waves and the QRS complex; and finally the PR interval. Regardless of the method chosen to analyze a given rhythm, the paramedic should use a consistent format. This section of the text discusses rhythm interpretation as

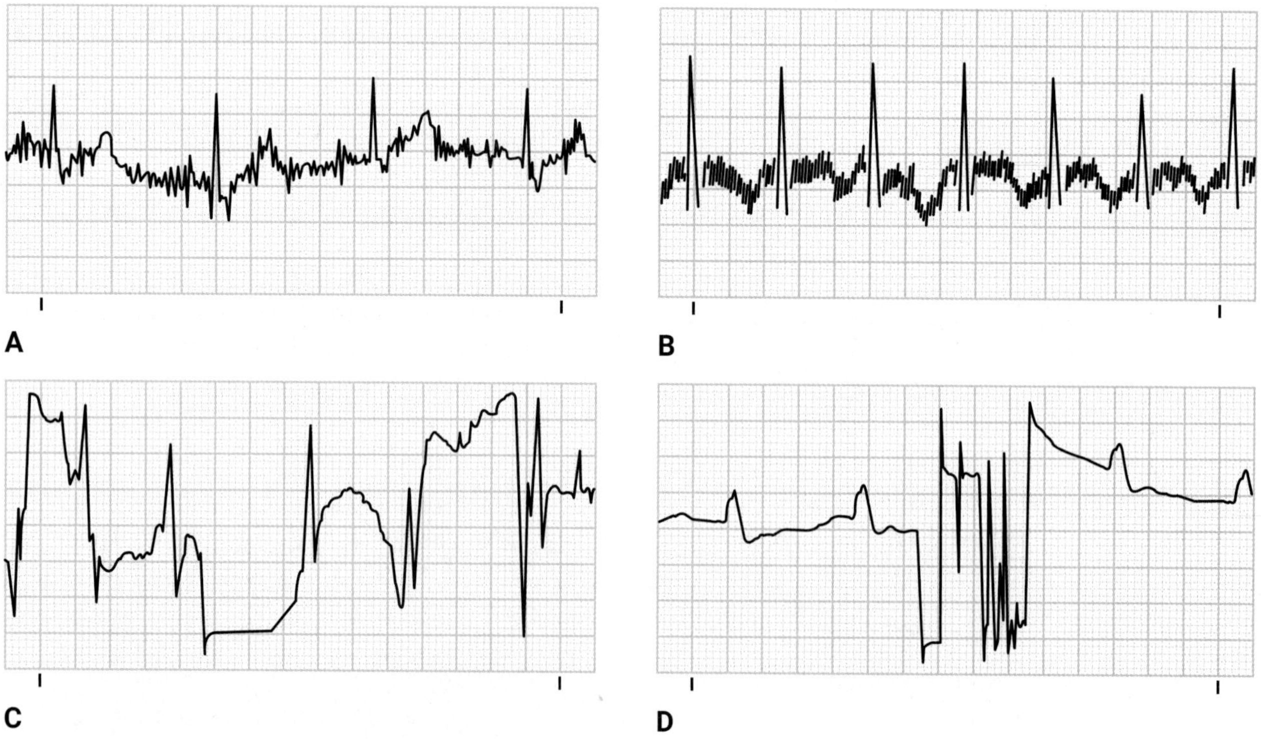

FIGURE 21-28 Artifacts. **A.** Muscle tremors. **B.** Alternating current (60-cycle) interference. **C.** Loose electrodes. **D.** Biotelemetry.

it pertains to standard three-lead ECG monitoring. Evaluation of 12-lead ECG monitoring is presented later in this chapter.

Five questions the paramedic must ask in any rhythm analysis to detect the presence of or potential for life-threatening rhythm disturbances are as follows:

1. Is the patient sick?
2. What is the heart rate?
3. Are there normal-looking QRS complexes?
4. Are there normal-looking P waves?
5. What is the relationship between the P waves and the QRS complexes?

> CRITICAL THINKING
>
> What does the ECG tell you about perfusion?

Step 1: Analyze the Rate

The heart rate can be analyzed in a number of ways. The methods for calculating the heart rate presented in this text are heart rate calculator rulers, the triplicate method, the R-R method, and the 6-second count method. The heart rate is determined by analyzing the ventricular rate (the QRS complex). The normal adult heart rate is 60 to 99 beats/min. A ventricular rate of less than 60 beats/min is considered **bradycardia**; a rate equal to or greater than 100 beats/min is considered **tachycardia**.

> NOTE
>
> In patients with healthy hearts, the atrial and ventricular rates are the same. This is because of the near simultaneous depolarization of the four chambers. If the atrial and ventricular rates are different (as may occur in certain dysrhythmias), the rates should be calculated separately.

Heart Rate Calculator Rulers

Heart rate calculator rulers (**FIGURE 21-29**) are available from several manufacturers. The paramedic should follow the directions that come with the ruler. Heart rate calculator rulers are reasonably accurate if the rhythm is regular. However, the paramedic should not rely solely on a mechanical device or tool to determine the heart rate. Sometimes, a device or tool is not readily available.

Triplicate Method

The triplicate method of determining the heart rate (**FIGURE 21-30**) is accurate only under two circumstances: when the rhythm is regular and when the heart rate is greater than 50 beats/min. To use this method, the paramedic must memorize two sets of numbers: 300-150-100 and 75-60-50. These numbers are derived from the distance between the heavy black lines (each representing $\frac{1}{300}$ minute). Therefore, two $\frac{1}{300}$-minute units are equal to $\frac{2}{300}$ minute, which is equal to $\frac{1}{150}$ minute, or a heart rate of 150 beats/min; three $\frac{1}{300}$-minute units are equal to $\frac{3}{300}$ minute, which is equal to $\frac{1}{100}$ minute, or a heart rate of 100 beats/min. Using these triplicates, the paramedic can calculate heart rate as follows:

1. Select an R wave that lines up with a dark vertical line.
2. Number the next six dark vertical lines consecutively from left to right as 300-150-100 and 75-60-50.
3. Identify where the next R wave falls with reference to the six dark vertical lines. If the R wave falls on 75, the heart rate is 75 beats/min. If the R wave falls halfway between 100 and 150, the heart rate is about 125 beats/min.

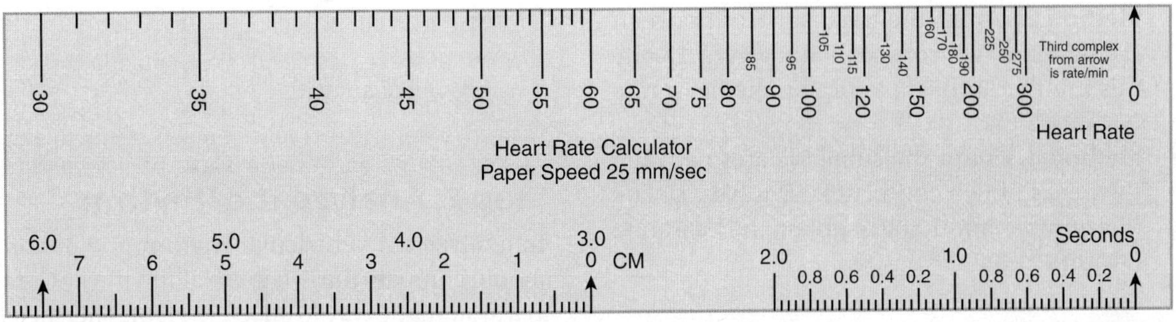

FIGURE 21-29 Heart rate calculator ruler.

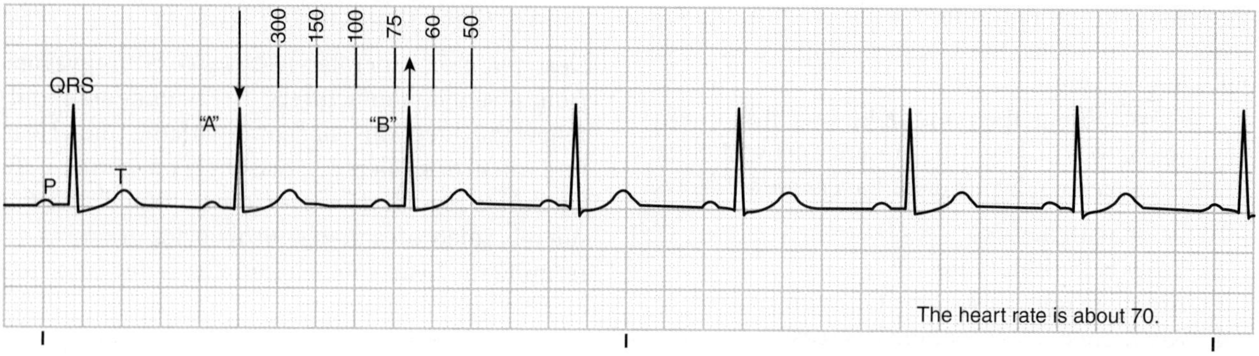

FIGURE 21-30 Triplicate method.

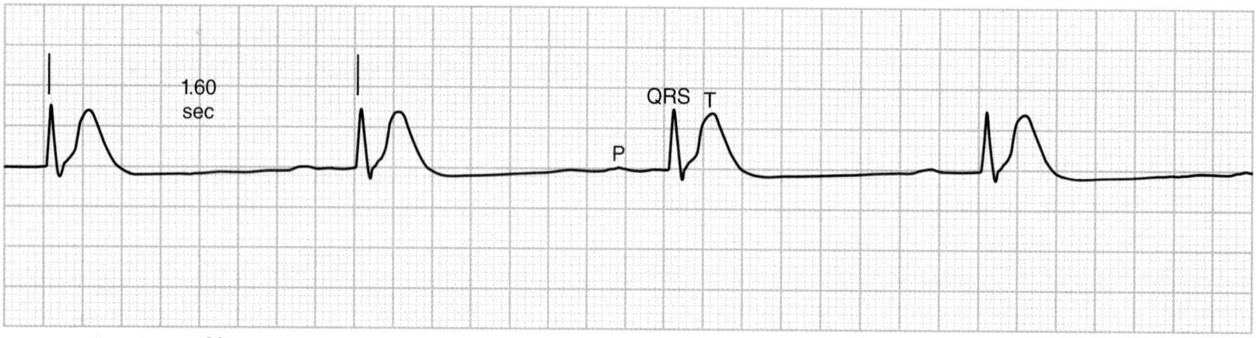

The heart rate $= \frac{60}{1.60 \text{ sec}} = 37.5$ or, rounded off, 38.

FIGURE 21-31 R-R interval, method 1.

R-R Method

The R-R method may be used several different ways to calculate the heart rate. As with the triplicate method, the rhythm must be regular to obtain an accurate reading. However, the R-R method works equally well for slow rates. The three methods are as follows:

- **Method 1.** Measure the distance in seconds between the peaks of two consecutive R waves. Then divide this number into 60 to obtain the heart rate (**FIGURE 21-31**).
- **Method 2.** Count the large squares between the peaks of two consecutive R waves. Divide this number into 300 to obtain the heart rate (**FIGURE 21-32**).
- **Method 3.** Count the small squares between the peaks of two consecutive R waves. Divide this number into 1,500 to obtain the heart rate (**FIGURE 21-33**).

Six-Second Count Method

The 6-second count method (**FIGURE 21-34**) is the least accurate method of determining the heart rate. However, it is useful for quickly obtaining an approximate rate in both regular and irregular rhythms.

As previously stated, the short vertical lines at the top of most ECG graph paper are divided into 3-second intervals when run at a standard speed of 25 mm/s. Two of these intervals are equal to 6 seconds. The heart rate is calculated by counting the number of QRS complexes in a 6-second interval. This number is multiplied by 10.

CRITICAL THINKING

Which of these rate calculation methods is fastest? Which is most accurate?

Step 2: Analyze the Rhythm

To analyze the ventricular rhythm, the paramedic should compare the R-R intervals on the ECG tracing in a systematic way from left to right. This measurement may be taken using ECG calipers or pen and paper. Using calipers, the paramedic should place one tip of the caliper on the peak of one R wave and

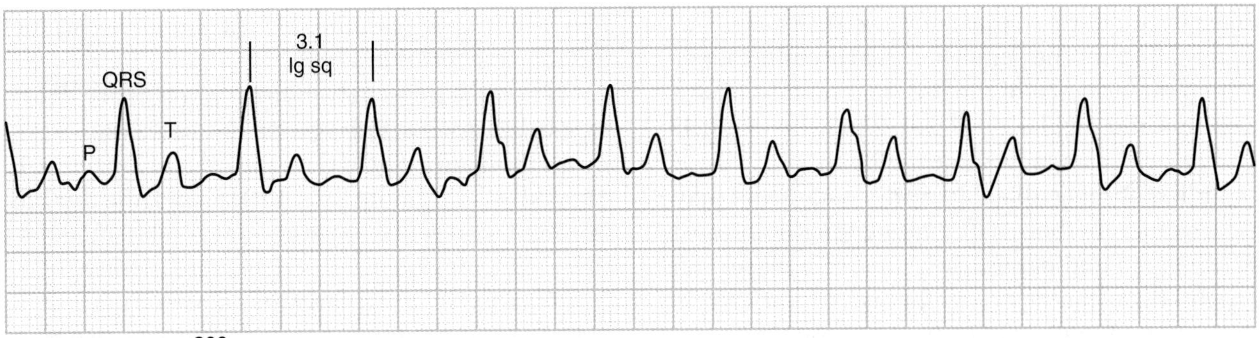

The heart rate = $\frac{300}{3.1 \text{ lg sq}}$ = 97.

FIGURE 21-32 R-R interval, method 2.

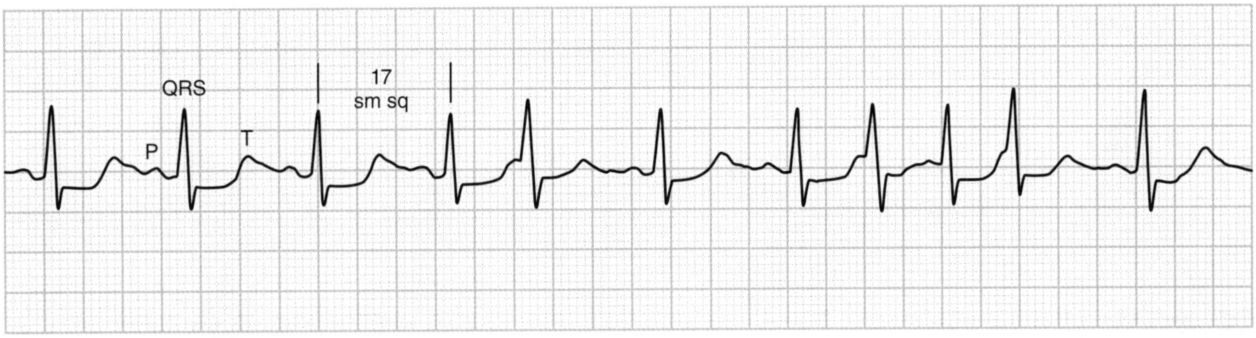

The heart rate = $\frac{1{,}500}{17 \text{ sm sq}}$ = 88.

FIGURE 21-33 R-R interval, method 3.

The heart rate is about 80. (Actual heart rate is 72.)

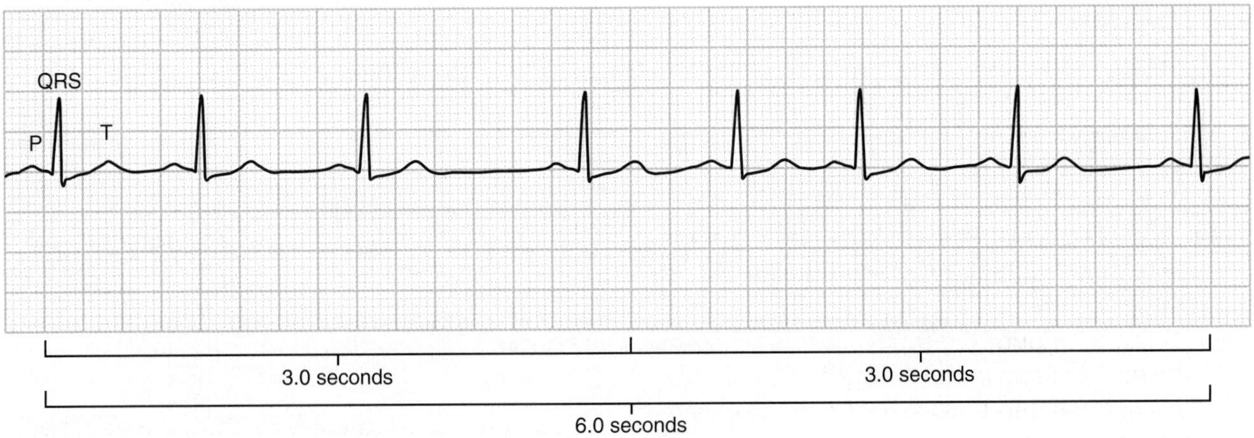

FIGURE 21-34 Six-second count method.

adjust the other tip so that it rests on the peak of the adjacent R wave. The paramedic then uses the caliper to map the distance of the R-R interval to evaluate evenness and regularity. (P waves may be mapped for regularity using this same method.)

In the absence of calipers, the paramedic may use a similar method of evaluating the R-R interval by using pen and paper. The paramedic places the straight edge of the paper near the peaks of the R waves and marks off the distance between the two other consecutive R waves. The paramedic then compares this R-R interval with the other R-R intervals in the ECG tracing (**FIGURE 21-35**).

If the distances between the R waves are equal or vary by less than 0.16 second (four small squares), the rhythm is regular. If the shortest and longest R-R intervals vary by more than 0.16 second, the rhythm is irregular. Irregular rhythms may be classified further. They may be classified as regularly irregular. In this case, the irregularity has a pattern; it is also called "group beating." Irregular rhythms also may be occasionally irregular. In this case, only one or

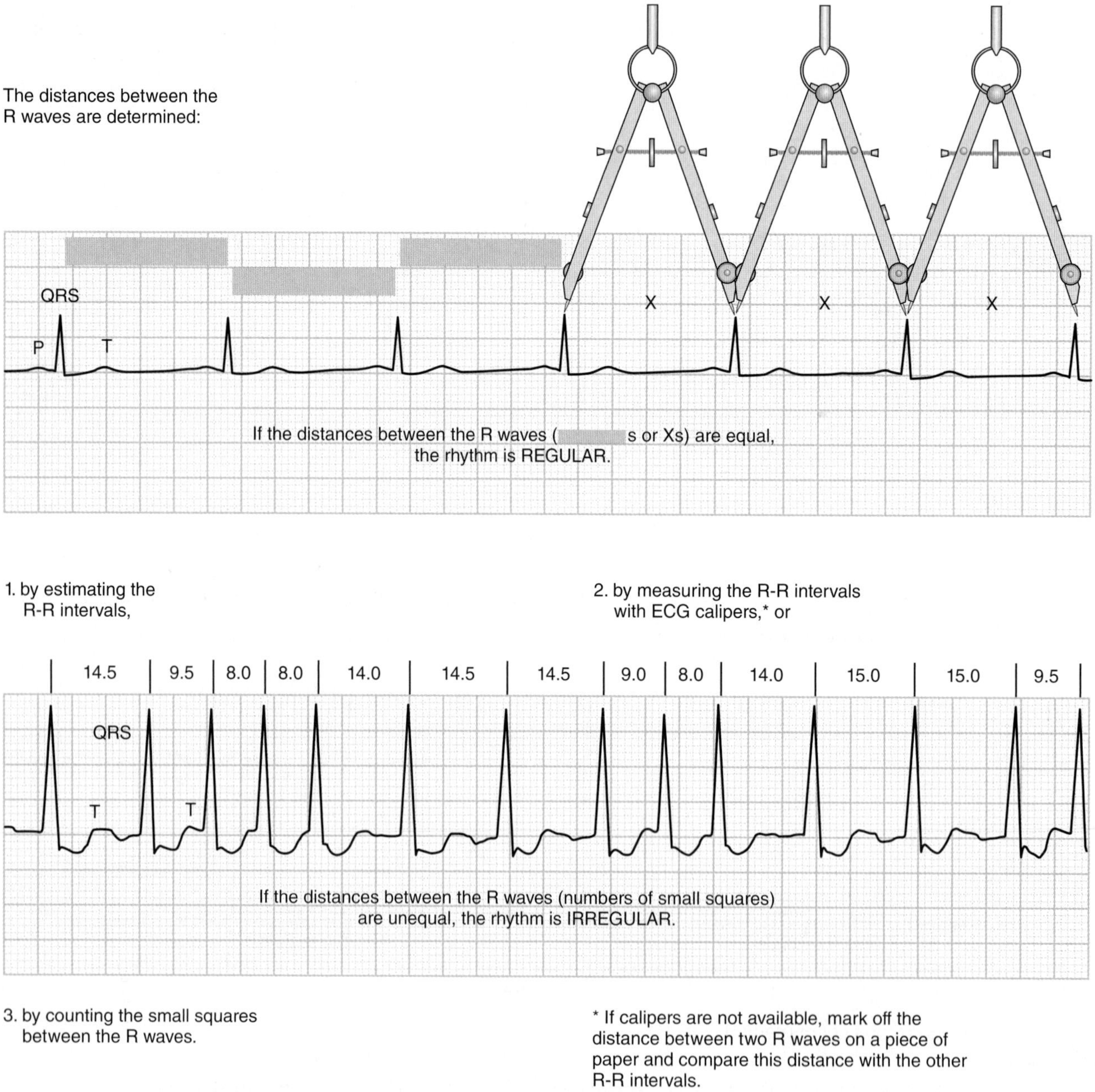

The distances between the R waves are determined:
QRS
P
T
X
If the distances between the R waves (s or Xs) are equal, the rhythm is REGULAR.
1. by estimating the R-R intervals,
2. by measuring the R-R intervals with ECG calipers,* or
14.5
9.5
8.0
8.0
14.0
14.5
14.5
9.0
8.0
14.0
15.0
15.0
9.5
QRS
T
T
If the distances between the R waves (numbers of small squares) are unequal, the rhythm is IRREGULAR.
3. by counting the small squares between the R waves.
* If calipers are not available, mark off the distance between two R waves on a piece of paper and compare this distance with the other R-R intervals.

FIGURE 21-35 Determining the rhythm.

two R-R intervals are unequal. Finally, irregular rhythms may be irregularly irregular. In this case, the rhythm is totally irregular. No relationship is seen between the R-R intervals (**FIGURE 21-36**). Note: The paramedic should always remember that the most common cause of an irregularly irregular rhythm is AF.

Step 3: Analyze the QRS Complex

The paramedic should analyze the QRS complex for regularity and width. QRS complexes less than or equal to 0.10-second wide (fewer than three small squares) are supraventricular in origin and have been transmitted through the bundle of His. Complexes

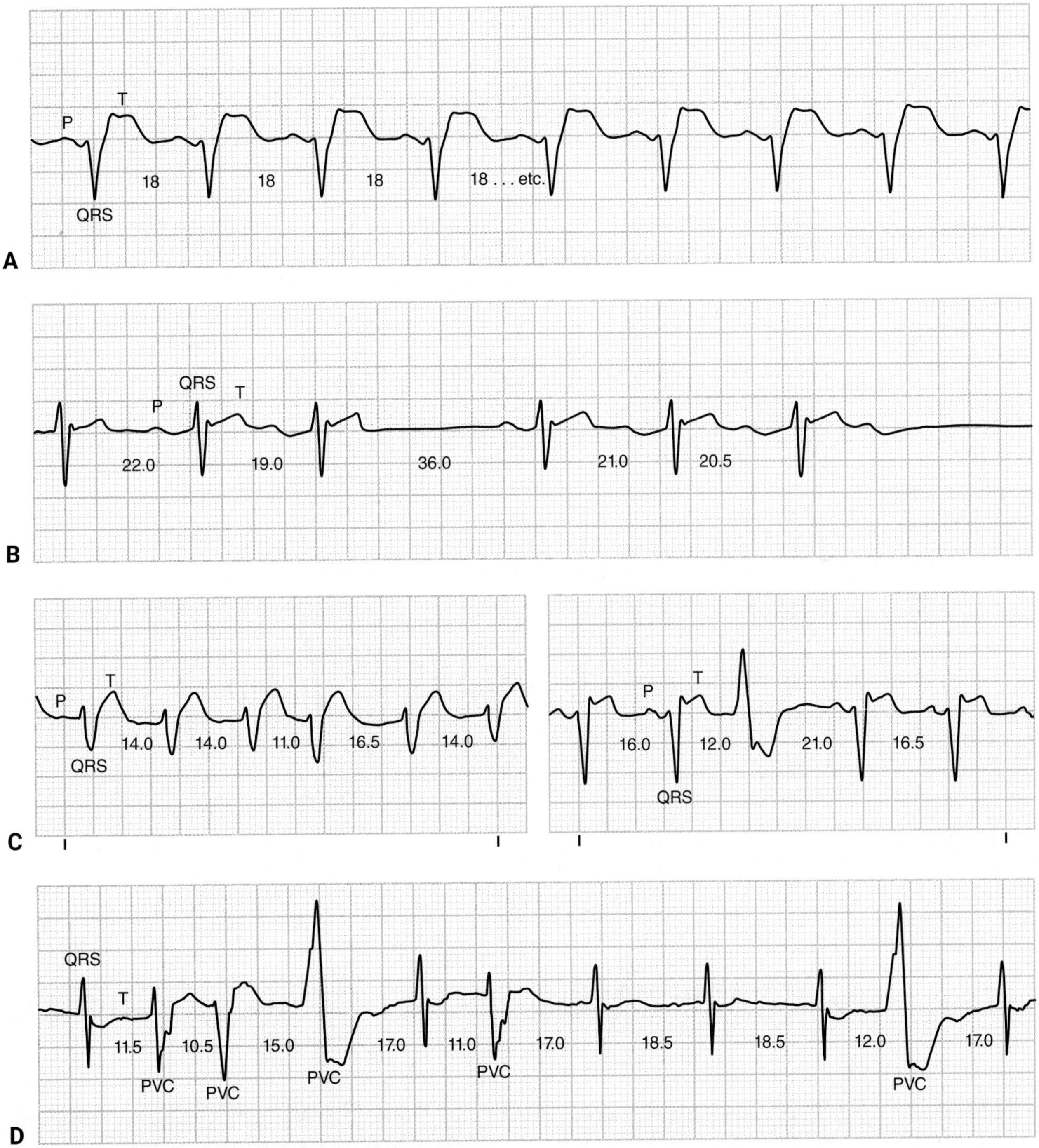

FIGURE 21-36 **A.** Regular rhythm. **B.** Regularly irregular rhythm. **C.** Occasionally irregular rhythm. **D.** Irregularly irregular rhythm.

equal to or greater than 0.12-second wide are abnormal. They indicate either a conduction abnormality in the ventricles or that the electrical depolarization originates in the ventricles (**FIGURE 21-37**). When evaluating an abnormal QRS width, the paramedic should identify the lead with the widest QRS complex because a portion of the QRS complex may be hidden or difficult to see in some leads.

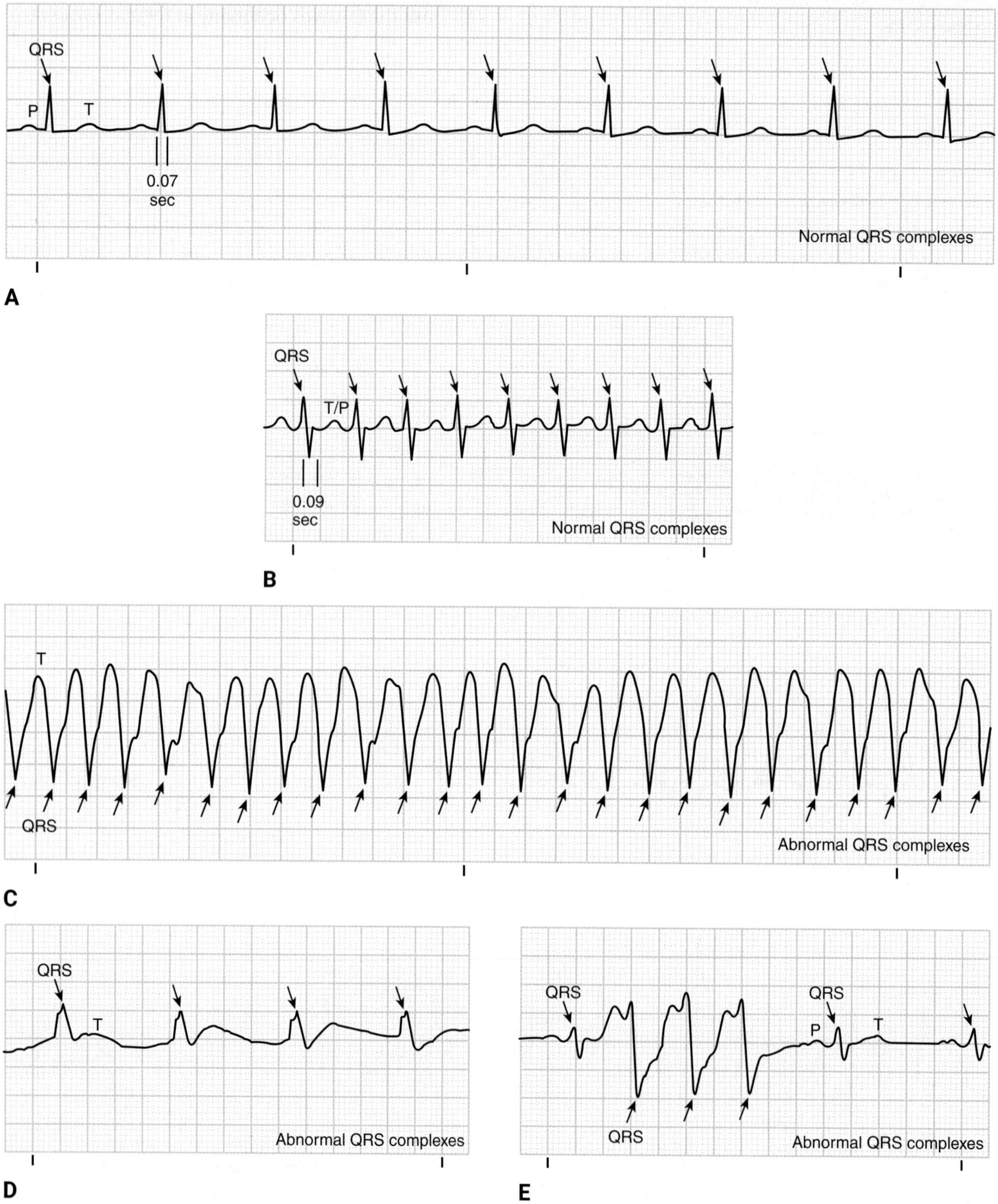

FIGURE 21-37 **A** and **B.** Normal QRS complexes. **C** to **E.** Abnormal QRS complexes.

Step 4: Analyze the P Waves

For a rhythm to be called sinus rhythm, it must meet two criteria. First, there should be a 1:1 relationship between P waves and QRS complexes, with a P wave preceding every QRS complex. Second, the P wave should have a morphology indicating that it originates at the SA node. This means that it should be positive in lead II and biphasic (up, then down) in lead V_1 (**FIGURE 21-38**). Therefore, the paramedic should observe the following five components when evaluating P waves:

1. Are P waves present?
2. Are the P waves occurring at regular intervals?

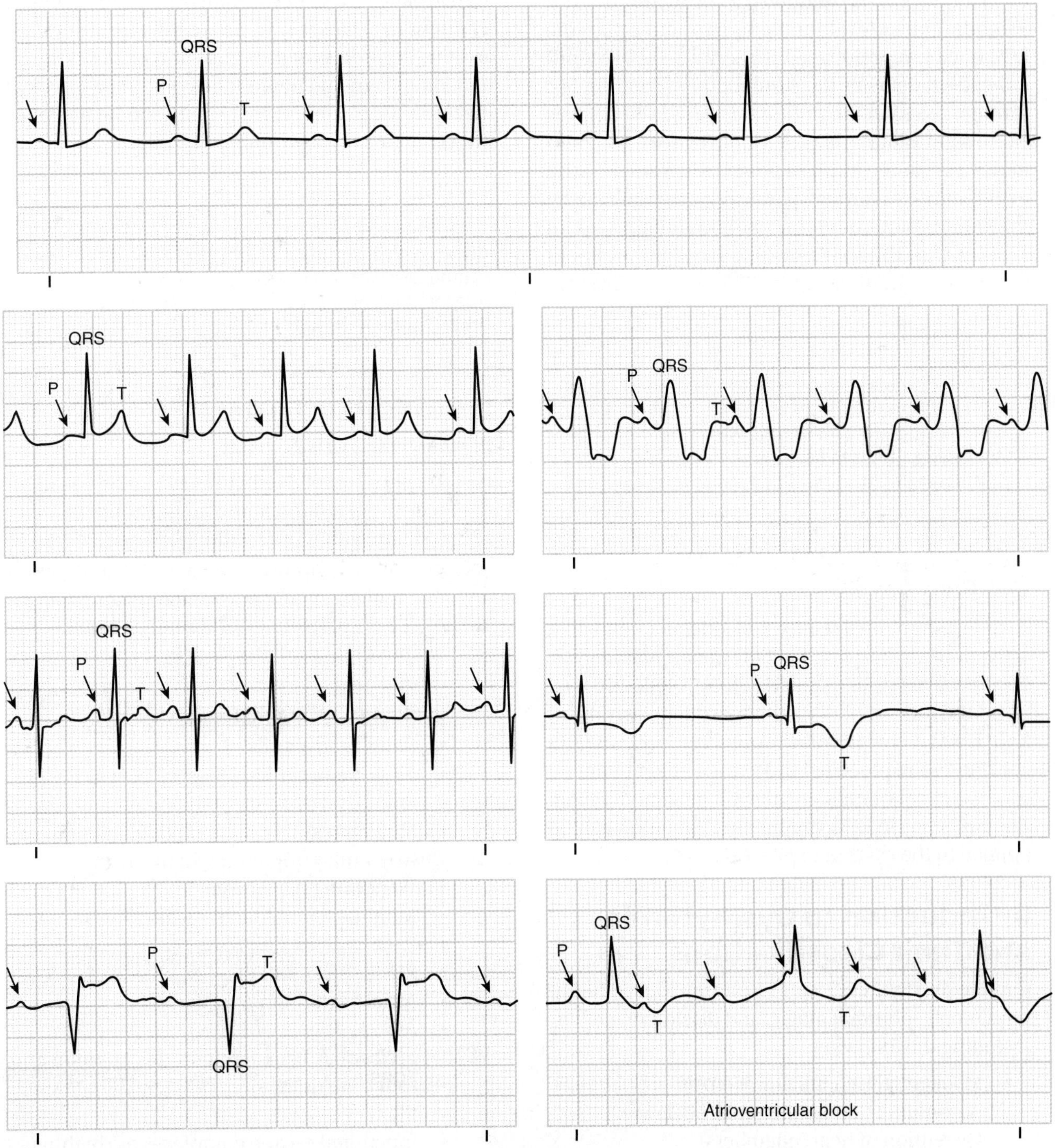

FIGURE 21-38 Normal P waves.

3. Is there one P wave for each QRS complex, and is there a QRS complex after each P wave?
4. Are the P waves upright or inverted?
5. Do they all look alike? (P waves that look alike and are regular are likely from the same pacemaker.)

Step 5: Analyze the PR Interval

The PR interval indicates the time required for an electrical impulse to be conducted through the atria and AV node. The interval should be constant across the ECG tracing. A prolonged PR interval (>0.20 second) indicates a delay in the conduction of the impulse through the AV node or bundle of His. The delay is called an AV block. A short PR interval (<0.12 second) indicates that the impulse progressed from the atria to the ventricles through pathways other than the AV node (**FIGURE 21-39**). This condition is known as an accessory pathway syndrome, the most common of which is **Wolff-Parkinson-White (WPW) syndrome**.

> NOTE
>
> WPW syndrome is a genetic heart abnormality associated with early activation of the ventricles. In the presence of tachycardia, this preexcitation syndrome can be life threatening. (The syndrome is described later in this chapter.)

Analyzing a Rhythm Using the Five Steps

To review, the normal sequence of atrial and ventricular activation as it relates to the ECG tracing is as follows: Each P wave (atrial depolarization) is followed by a normal QRS complex (ventricular depolarization) and T wave (ventricular repolarization); all QRS complexes are preceded by P waves, the PR interval is within normal limits, and the R-R interval is regular. The five steps in ECG rhythm interpretation can be applied to the rhythm in **FIGURE 21-40**.

Introduction to Dysrhythmias and Their Classifications

Cardiac dysrhythmias can result from a number of physiologic, pharmacologic, and disease processes, including the following:

- Myocardial ischemia or necrosis
- Autonomic nervous system imbalance
- Distention of heart chambers
- Acid–base abnormalities
- Hypoxemia
- Electrolyte imbalance
- Drug effects or toxicity
- Electrical injury
- Hypothermia
- CNS injury

In addition to these potential causes of dysrhythmias, some cardiac rhythm disturbances are normal, even in patients who have healthy hearts. For example, a patient may have sinus tachycardia from stress or anxiety. Regardless of the cause or type of dysrhythmia, management should focus on the patient and the underlying cause. Management should not focus merely on the dysrhythmia.

> NOTE
>
> Special considerations regarding cardiac rhythm disturbances and resuscitation in infant and pediatric patients are addressed in Chapter 46, *Neonatal Care*, and Chapter 47, *Pediatrics*.

Classification by Rate and Pacemaker Site

The classification of dysrhythmias can be based on several factors. These include changes in automaticity versus disturbances in conduction, cardiac arrest (lethal) rhythms and noncardiac arrest (nonlethal) rhythms, and site of origin. For learning purposes, this text classifies rhythms by rate and pacemaker site (eg, VT, sinus bradycardia) and includes the following seven groups:

1. Dysrhythmias originating in the SA node
   - Sinus bradycardia
   - Sinus tachycardia
   - Sinus dysrhythmia
   - Sinus arrest
2. Dysrhythmias originating in the atria
   - Wandering pacemaker
   - Multifocal atrial tachycardia (MAT)
   - PAC
   - PSVT
   - Atrial flutter
   - AF
3. Dysrhythmias originating in the AV node and surrounding tissues
   - PJC
   - Junctional escape complexes or rhythms
   - Accelerated junctional rhythm

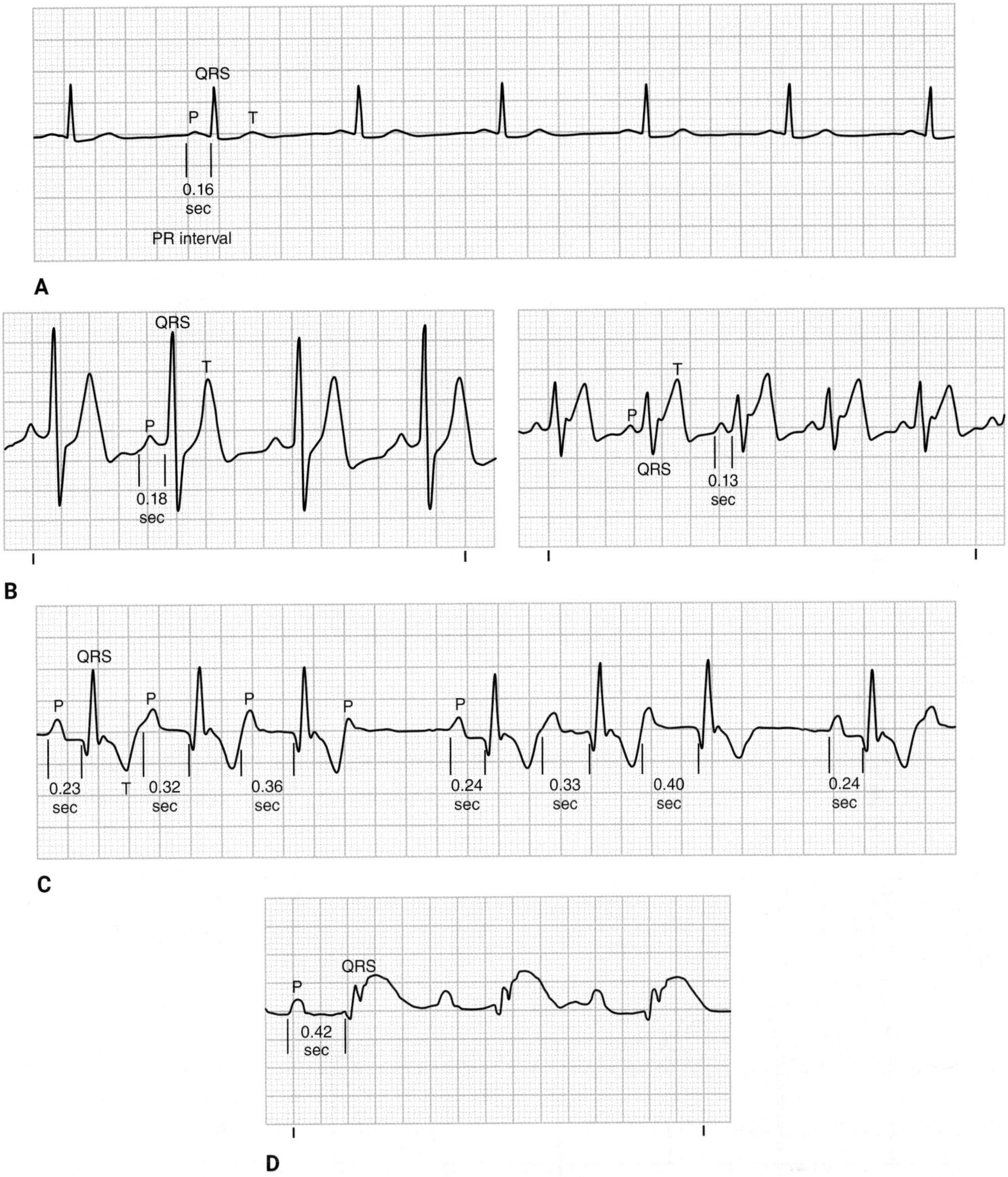

FIGURE 21-39 **A** and **B.** Normal PR intervals. **C** and **D.** Abnormal PR intervals.

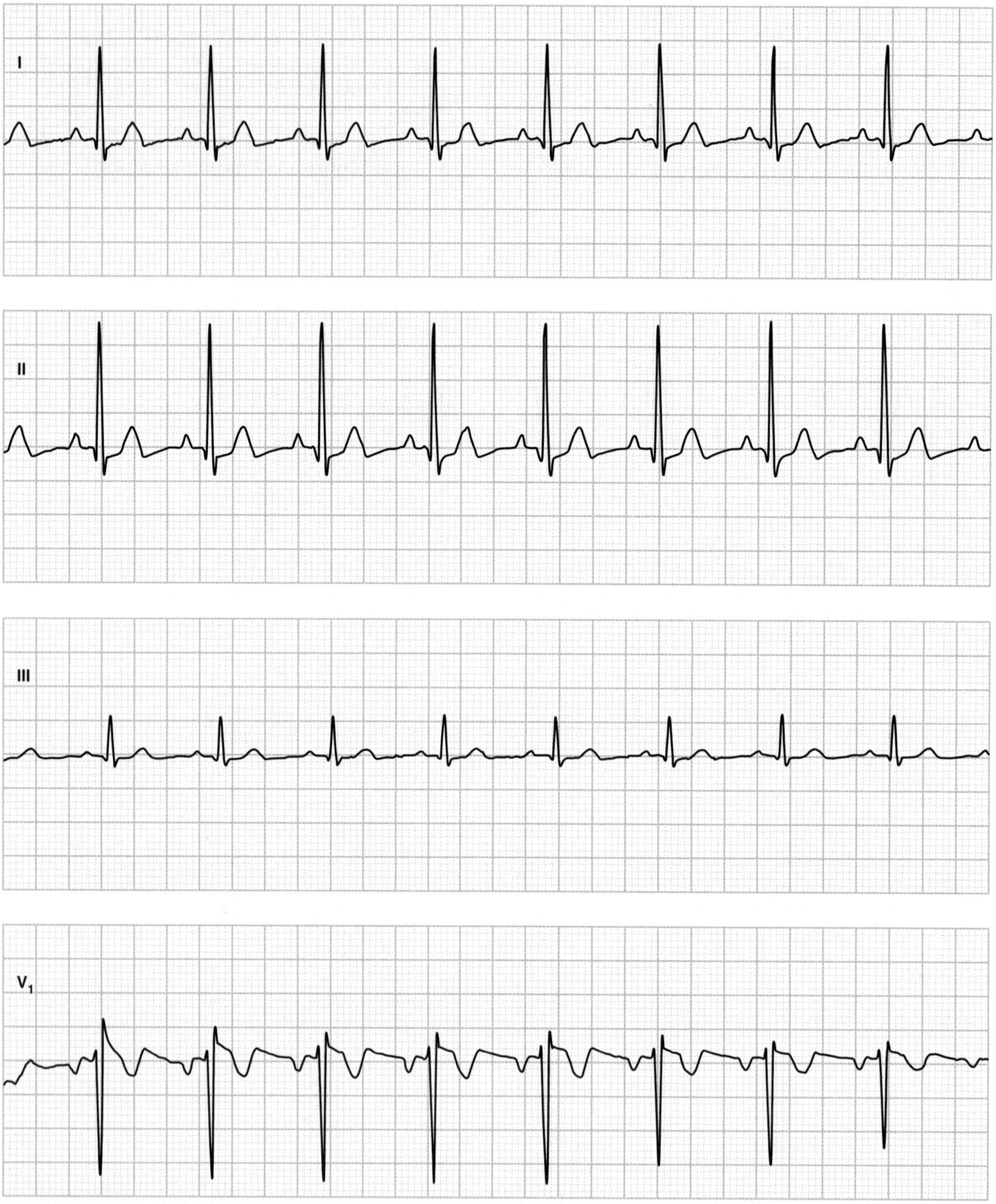

FIGURE 21-40 Normal sinus rhythm.

4. Dysrhythmias originating in the ventricles
   - Ventricular escape complexes or rhythms
   - PVC
   - VT
   - VF
   - Artificial pacemaker rhythms
5. Dysrhythmias that are disorders of conduction
   - AV blocks
     - First-degree AV block
     - Second-degree AV block type I (or Wenckebach)
     - Second-degree AV block type II
     - Third-degree AV block
   - Disturbances of ventricular conduction
   - Preexcitation syndrome (WPW syndrome and Lown-Ganong-Levine [LGL] syndrome)
6. Pulseless electrical activity (PEA)
7. Asystole

NOTE

Broadly speaking, there are only four cardiac arrest rhythms: VF, pulseless VT, asystole, and assorted PEA rhythms.

The text presents each dysrhythmia in lead II. For comparison, the same dysrhythmia also is shown as it would appear in leads I, III, and V_1. In addition, the text discusses how to recognize the dysrhythmia and the emergency treatment of patients with each dysrhythmia. All treatments in this chapter follow the recommendations of the AHA. All treatments are referenced to the AHA algorithms.

Use of Algorithms for Classification

An **algorithm** is a process that can be used to solve a problem and guide decision making. Clinical algorithms contain prehospital and in-hospital management recommendations. The following guidelines apply to the use of all algorithms:[8]

1. Manage the patient, not the monitor.
2. Algorithms for cardiac arrest presume that the condition under discussion continually persists, that the patient remains in cardiac arrest, and that CPR is always performed.
3. Apply different interventions when appropriate indications exist.
4. The algorithms are designed to outline the most common assessments and actions performed for most patients, but they are not designed to be all-inclusive or restrictive.[9] The flow diagrams present treatments mostly in sequential order of priority. Next to a treatment or pharmacologic agent may be a class recommendation (BOX 21-3). The footnotes to the algorithm contain additional important information related to assessment, treatment, and evaluation.

BOX 21-3 Application of Class of Recommendations for CPR and Emergency Cardiovascular Care

Class I (Strong[a])

Benefit significantly outweighs risk.
Treatment is indicated and beneficial.
Treatment should be performed/administered.

Class IIa (Moderate)

Benefit outweighs risk.
Treatment is reasonable.
Treatment is considered effective and useful.

Class IIb (Weak)

Benefit equals or is greater than the risk.
Treatment might be reasonable.
Therapy may be considered.

Class III: No Benefit (Moderate)

Therapy is not recommended.
Treatment is not useful or beneficial.
Treatment should not be administered/performed.

Class III: Harm (Strong)

Risk is greater than benefit.
Therapy is not indicated.
Treatment is associated with excess morbidity/mortality.
Treatment may harm the patient.

---

[a]Qualifiers (moderate, weak, and strong) refer to the level of scientific evidence supporting the recommendation to either perform or withhold the treatment.

Modified from: Applying class of recommendations and level of evidence to clinical strategies, interventions, treatments, or diagnostic testing in patient care. Emergency Cardiovascular Care, American Heart Association, website. https://eccguidelines.heart.org/index.php/tables/applying-class-of-recommendations-and-level-of-evidence-to-clinical-strategies-interventions-treatments-or-diagnostic-testing-in-patient-care/. Accessed April 1, 2018.

5. Effective, minimally interrupted chest compressions and defibrillation, followed by adequate ventilation and oxygenation, are more important than is administration of medications. These measures take precedence over initiating an intravenous (IV) line or injecting pharmacologic agents.
6. In the unlikely event that IV or intraosseous (IO) access is not available, some medications (naloxone, atropine, vasopressin, epinephrine, lidocaine [NAVEL]) can be administered via an endotracheal (ET) tube. For adults, the ET dose is 2 to 2.5 times the IV dose. The ET tube route is the least preferred method of drug administration.
7. As a rule, IV medications are given by the bolus method during cardiac arrest.
8. After each IV medication, a 20- to 30-mL bolus of IV fluid should be given to enhance the delivery of drugs to the central circulation. This delivery may take 1 to 2 minutes.
9. Last, manage the patient, not the monitor.

Dysrhythmias Originating in the SA Node

Most sinus dysrhythmias result from increases or decreases in vagal tone (parasympathetic nervous system). The SA node generally receives sufficient inhibitory parasympathetic impulses from the vagus nerve to keep the SA node in the normal rate of 60 to 100 beats/min. However, if vagus nerve activity increases, the heart rate slows and sinus bradycardia results. If the vagus nerve is slowed or blocked, the heart rate increases and sinus tachycardia results. Dysrhythmias that originate in the SA node include sinus bradycardia, sinus tachycardia, sinus dysrhythmia, and sinus arrest. ECG features common to all SA node dysrhythmias include the following:

- Normal duration of QRS complex (in the absence of bundle branch block)
- Upright P waves in lead II
- Similar appearance of all P waves
- Normal duration of PR interval (in the absence of AV block)

Sinus Bradycardia

Description

Sinus bradycardia results from slowing of the pacemaker rate of the SA node (**FIGURE 21-41**).

Etiology

Possible causes of sinus bradycardia include the following:

- Intrinsic sinus node disease
- Increased parasympathetic vagal tone
- Hypothermia
- Hypoxia
- Hypothyroidism
- Drug effects (eg, digitalis, beta blockers, calcium channel blockers)
- MI

Rules for Interpretation (Lead II Monitoring)

Sinus bradycardia has the following characteristics on the ECG:

- **Rate.** Less than 60 beats/min
- **Rhythm.** Regular
- **QRS complex.** Typically less than 0.12 second, provided no ventricular conduction abnormality is present
- **P waves.** Normal and upright; one P wave before each QRS complex
- **PR interval.** 0.12 to 0.20 second and constant (normal), provided no AV block is present

Clinical Significance

Sinus bradycardia may be normal, pathologic, or iatrogenic (induced by medications). Athletes may have sinus bradycardia because their well-exercised myocardium has a sufficient stroke volume to maintain adequate cardiac output with a lower heart rate (remember: Cardiac output = Stroke volume × Heart rate). However, in some cases a decreased heart rate may compromise cardiac output. It may result in hypotension or other signs of shock, angina pectoris, or CNS symptoms (eg, light-headedness, vertigo, syncope). Sinus bradycardia can result from nausea and vomiting. The dysrhythmia is associated with overstimulation of the vagus nerve that can result in fainting (vasovagal syncope). Sinus bradycardia also may occur after the application of carotid sinus pressure (carotid sinus massage, described later in this chapter). Patients whose home medicines include beta blockers, such as metoprolol or a cardiac glycoside, such as digoxin, will also often have a heart rate between 50 and 60 beats/min.

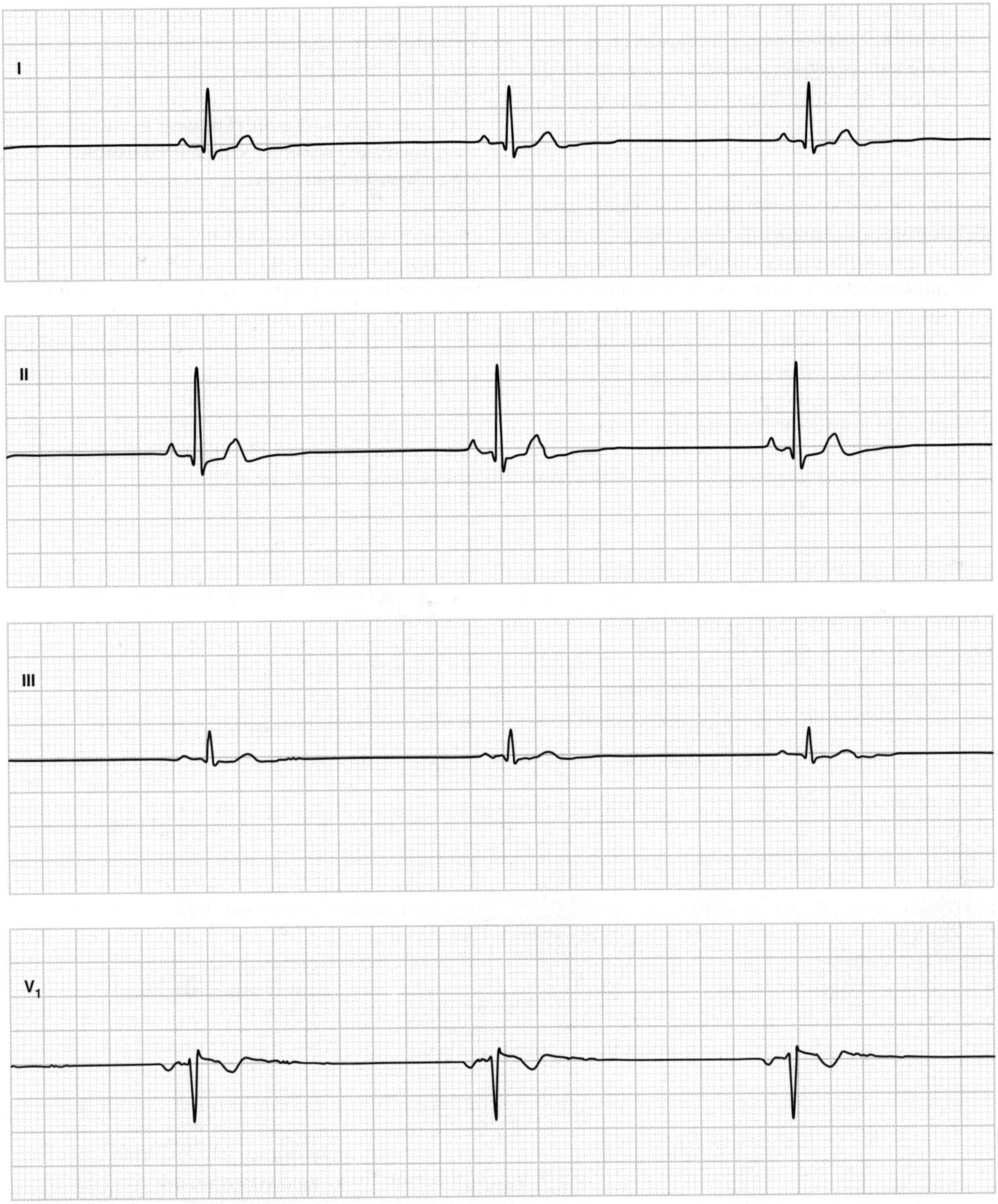

FIGURE 21-41 Sinus bradycardia.

> **CRITICAL THINKING**
> Take a poll of your classmates. How many have a resting heart rate of 60 beats/min?

Management

Prehospital intervention usually is unnecessary unless hypotension, altered mental status caused by inadequate perfusion, acute heart failure, or ventricular irritability is present (these are more common with rates below 50 beats/min). Management of symptomatic bradycardia is aimed at treating the underlying cause and increasing the heart rate to improve cardiac output. Inotropic support also may be required (**FIGURE 21-42**). Treatment options for symptomatic bradycardia include oxygen if hypoxia or dyspnea is present or suspected, ventilation if respirations are inadequate, atropine, patient rewarming for hypothermia, transcutaneous pacing (the use of an external artificial pacemaker, described later in this chapter), a dopamine infusion, or an epinephrine infusion. Transcutaneous pacing is considered a class IIa intervention for symptomatic bradycardias unresponsive to atropine. Immediate pacing might be considered in unstable patients with high-degree AV block when IV access is not available.[1] Because atropine works on the AV node, it will likely not be effective for infranodal (second-degree type II) or third-degree heart block. In these cases, only two to three doses of atropine should be administered prior to initiating another treatment. Transcutaneous pacing or use of beta adrenergic drugs, such as dopamine or epinephrine, is preferred to stabilize this type of patient until a transvenous pacemaker can be inserted at the hospital.[10]

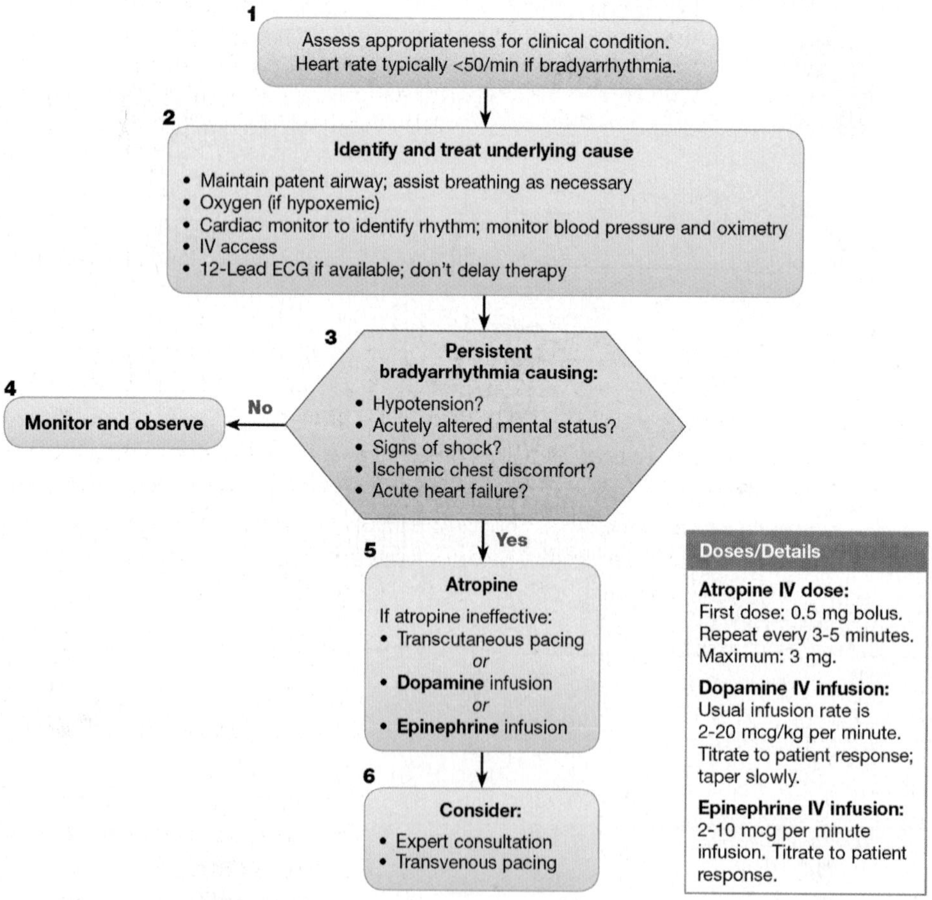

Abbreviations: ECG, electrocardiogram; IV, intravenous

FIGURE 21-42 Bradycardia algorithm.

Note: Sinus bradycardia should prompt the paramedic to build a differential diagnosis. The goal of patient management is to identify and correct (if possible) the most likely cause of the slow rhythm. Examples include acute hypoglycemia, hypoxia, hypothermia, and hyperkalemia.

NOTE

Blocks in electrical conduction may be classified as nodal or infranodal. A nodal block is one that occurs in the AV node. An infranodal block is one that occurs below the AV node. A complete heart block is one in which all electrical signals are blocked from the upper to lower chambers. (See conduction disorders later in this chapter.)

NOTE

Atropine should be used with caution in a patient with an AMI. The drug can increase the heart rate, increasing myocardial oxygen demand. This in turn can worsen ischemia or increase the size of the infarction. Atropine may be beneficial for the treatment of nodal blocks. The drug should be avoided for infranodal blocks and complete heart block with a wide QRS complex because it may worsen the rhythm.

Modified from: American Heart Association. *Advanced Cardiac Life Support Provider Manual*. Dallas, TX: American Heart Association; 2016.

Atropine is administered IV for symptomatic bradycardia. Administration may be repeated every 3 to 5 minutes as needed. The frequency of atropine administration is based on the patient's condition. Atropine should be administered at shorter intervals (every 3 minutes) for severely unstable patients.

If symptoms persist after atropine administration, and external pacing is not effective or available, a pressor infusion such as dopamine or epinephrine may be needed (BOX 21-4). Evaluate the need for fluid bolus infusion in hypotensive bradycardic patients before pressor infusion begins.[1]

An epinephrine infusion can be used for symptomatic bradycardia (BOX 21-5). Generally, this infusion is given after atropine and transcutaneous pacing fail to improve the patient's condition. However, an epinephrine infusion may be administered earlier if the patient displays severe symptoms and is deteriorating quickly.

CRITICAL THINKING

What effect does the excitement and commotion of the arrival of your ambulance likely have on the heart rate and blood pressure of a conscious, alert patient?

BOX 21-4 Dopamine Infusion

- **Initial-dose dopamine.** Begin at 2 mcg/kg per minute, increasing until the desired response is achieved. As the dose of dopamine increases, different effects should be anticipated.
- **Moderate-dose dopamine.** At moderate doses (5 to 10 mcg/kg per minute), dopamine improves contractility, cardiac output, and blood pressure through $alpha_1$ and $beta_1$ receptor stimulation.
- **High-dose dopamine.** Higher doses (10 to 20 mcg/kg per minute) of dopamine have an alpha adrenergic effect, producing peripheral arterial and venous vasoconstriction.

See Chapter 14, *Medication Administration*, for the calculation of dopamine infusions.

BOX 21-5 Epinephrine Infusion

Epinephrine infusions are used for critically unstable patients with bradycardia who have not responded to atropine or pacing. An epinephrine infusion is prepared by mixing 1 mg of epinephrine (1 mg/mL) into 500 mL of 5% dextrose in water or 0.9% normal saline. The concentration is 2 mcg/mL. The recommended rate of infusion is 2 to 10 mcg/minute.

Sinus Tachycardia

Description

Sinus tachycardia results from an increase in the rate of sinus node discharge (**FIGURE 21-43**).

Etiology

Sinus tachycardia is common and may result from multiple factors, including the following:

- Exercise
- Fever
- Infection/sepsis
- Pain
- Ingestion of caffeine or alcohol
- Hypovolemia
- Hyperthyroidism
- Anemia

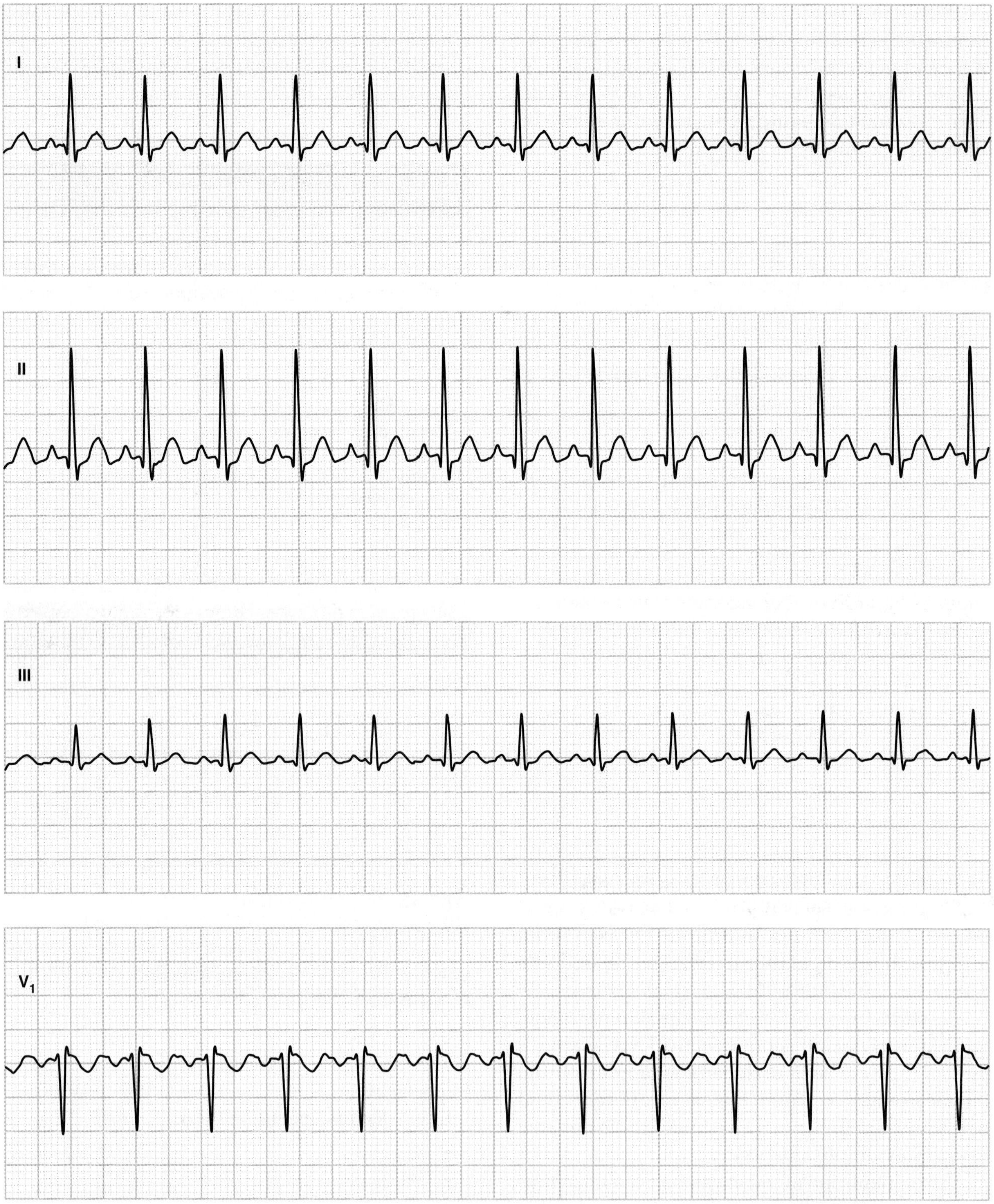

FIGURE 21-43 Sinus tachycardia.

- Heart failure
- Administration of atropine or any sympathomimetic drug (eg, cocaine, phencyclidine, epinephrine)
- Pulmonary embolism

Rules for Interpretation (Lead II Monitoring)

Sinus tachycardia has the following characteristics on the ECG:

- **Rate.** Equal to or greater than 100 beats/min
- **Rhythm.** Regular
- **QRS complex.** Less than 0.12 second, provided no ventricular conduction disturbance is present
- **P waves.** Normal and upright; one before each QRS complex
- **PR interval.** 0.12 to 0.20 second (normal), provided no AV conduction block is present

Clinical Significance

Sinus tachycardia is often a compensatory response to maintain cardiac output and end-organ perfusion in the face of increased myocardial oxygen demand, including hypermetabolic states (eg, exercise, sepsis, hyperthyroidism), hypovolemia, or reduced oxygen-carrying capacity (eg, anemia). It is also commonly seen in situations that stimulate a sympathetic nervous system response, such as pain, anxiety, or toxins.

Management

Because sinus tachycardia is usually a compensatory response to a physiologic insult, the treatment is not to control the heart rate, but to treat the underlying cause, such as poor perfusion, oxygenation, or pain. When the underlying cause is treated or removed, the tachycardia usually resolves gradually and spontaneously. Treating the rate instead of the underlying cause can have disastrous consequences for the patient, including cardiovascular collapse.

Sinus Dysrhythmia

Description

Sinus dysrhythmia is a term used to describe beat-to-beat variation in the P-P interval, leading to an irregular ventricular rate. It is present when the difference between the longest and shortest R-R intervals is greater than 0.16 second (**FIGURE 21-44**). To meet criteria for sinus dysrhythmia, the P waves must be of constant, sinus morphology and the PR interval must remain constant between beats.

Etiology

Sinus dysrhythmia is a normal variant that is the result of changes in intrathoracic pressure during the respiratory cycle. Inspiration decreases vagal tone, leading to a heart rate increase. Conversely, vagal tone is restored during expiration, leading to a heart rate decrease. Sinus dysrhythmia is typically seen in young, healthy people.

Rules for Interpretation (Lead II Monitoring)

Sinus dysrhythmia has the following characteristics on the ECG:

- **Rate.** Usually 60 to 99 beats/min (varies with respiration)
- **Rhythm.** Irregular (changes occur in cycles and usually follow the patient's respiratory pattern)
- **QRS complex.** Less than 0.12 second, provided no ventricular conduction disturbance is present
- **P waves.** Normal and upright; one P wave before each QRS complex
- **PR interval.** 0.12 to 0.20 second and constant (normal)

Clinical Significance

Sinus dysrhythmia is common, especially in young, healthy patients. Nonrespiratory causes of sinus dysrhythmia are far less common. It is typically seen in older adults and is associated with underlying heart disease or certain drugs (eg, digoxin).

Management

Sinus dysrhythmia does not require any prehospital intervention.

Sinus Arrest

Description

Sinus arrest results from a depression in automaticity of the SA node (**FIGURE 21-45**). The failure of the sinus node causes short periods of cardiac standstill. This standstill occurs until lower-level pacemakers

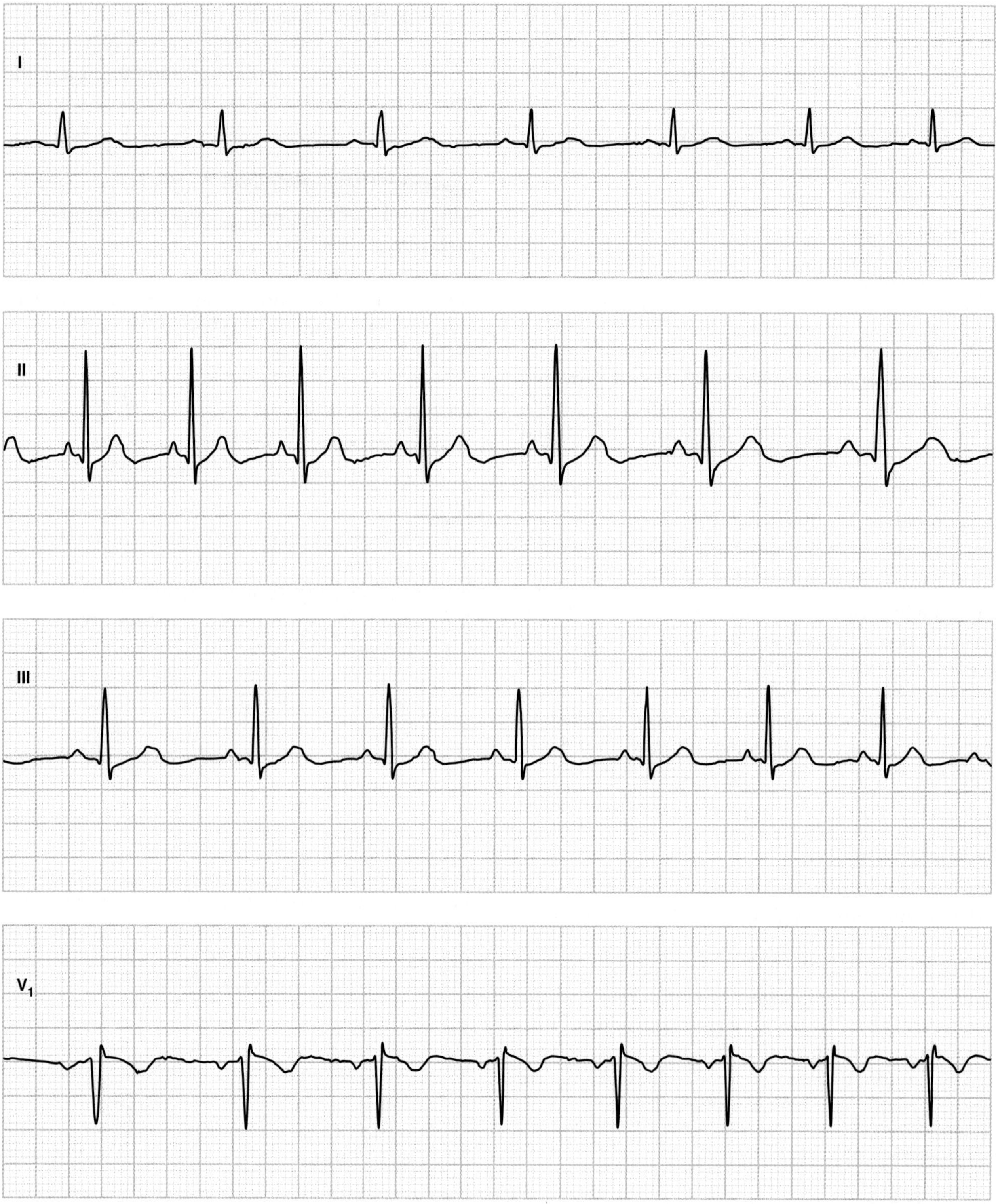

FIGURE 21-44 Sinus dysrhythmia.

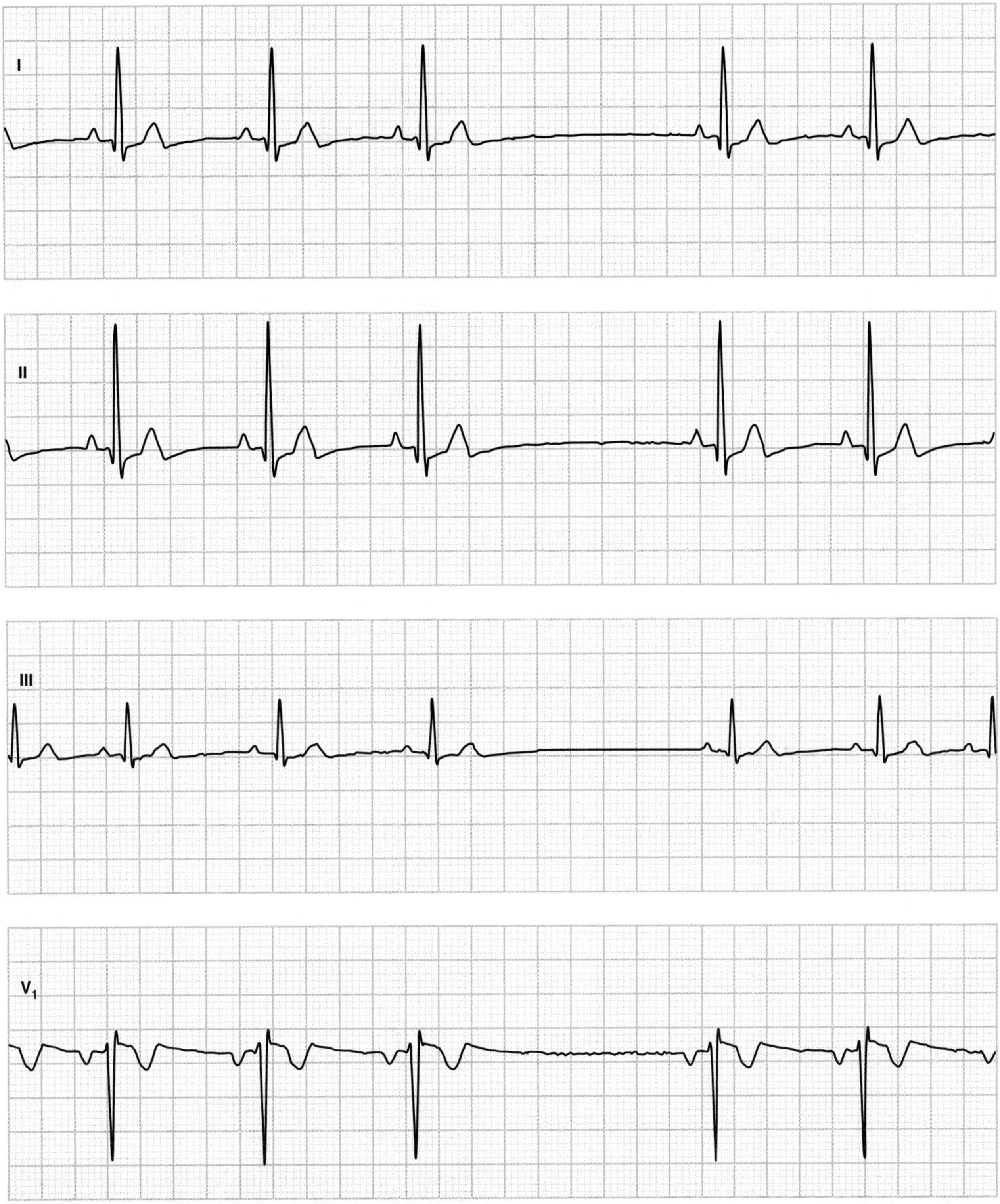

FIGURE 21-45 Sinus arrest.

discharge (escape beats) or the sinus node resumes its normal function.

Etiology

Sinus arrest may be precipitated by an increase in parasympathetic tone on the SA node, hypoxia or ischemia, excessive administration of digitalis, calcium channel blockers (diltiazem, verapamil) or beta blockers (metoprolol), hyperkalemia, or damage to the SA node (eg, AMI, degenerative fibrotic disease that affects the heart).

Rules for Interpretation (Lead II Monitoring)

Sinus arrest has the following characteristics on the ECG:

- **Rate.** Normal to slow, depending on the frequency and duration of sinus arrest.
- **Rhythm.** Irregular when sinus arrest is present.
- **QRS complex.** Less than 0.12 second, provided no bundle branch conduction disturbance is present.
- **P waves.** Normal and upright. If the electrical impulse is not generated by the SA node or blocked from entering the atria, atrial depolarization does not occur and the P wave is dropped.
- **PR interval.** PR intervals (when the P wave is present) of the underlying rhythm are normal (0.12 to 0.20 second) in the absence of AV block. Junctional escape beats may occur with no P waves.

Clinical Significance

Frequent or prolonged episodes of sinus arrest may reduce cardiac output. The overall heart rate slows and the atria do not contract; consequently, ventricular filling is reduced. If an escape pacemaker does not take over, ventricular asystole may result. This condition would cause light-headedness followed by syncope. With this dysrhythmia, the danger exists that sinus node activity will stop completely. Another danger is that an escape pacemaker may not take over pacing, leading to asystole.

Management

If the patient is asymptomatic, close observation is all that is required. In patients with bradycardia that produces symptoms, management may include the administration of atropine or transcutaneous cardiac pacing (TCP) (see Figure 21-42).

Dysrhythmias Originating in the Atria

Atrial dysrhythmias may begin in the tissues of the atria or in the AV junction. Common causes of atrial dysrhythmias are ischemia, hypoxia, and atrial dilation caused by heart failure, mitral valve abnormalities, or increased pulmonary artery pressures. Atrial dysrhythmias include wandering pacemaker, PACs, PSVT, atrial flutter, and AF. ECG features common to all atrial dysrhythmias include the following:

- Normal QRS complexes, in the absence of a ventricular conduction defect
- P waves (if present) that differ in appearance from sinus P waves
- Abnormal, shortened, or prolonged PR intervals

Wandering Pacemaker

Description

Wandering pacemaker (or wandering atrial pacemaker) occurs when the pacemaker shifts from the sinus node to another pacemaker site in the atria or the AV junction (**FIGURE 21-46**). The shift in the site usually is transient, back and forth along the SA node, atria, and AV junction.

Etiology

Wandering pacemaker is a type of sinus dysrhythmia. It may be normal in the very young, in older adults, and in well-conditioned athletes. The dysrhythmia generally is caused by the inhibitory vagal effect on the SA node and AV junction (often related to respiration). Vagal stimulation can cause pacemaker rates to slow. Other causes include associated underlying heart disease and digoxin.

Rules for Interpretation (Lead II Monitoring)

Wandering pacemaker has the following characteristics on the ECG:

- **Rate.** Usually 60 to 99 beats/min. The rate may slow gradually when the pacemaker site shifts from the SA node to the atria or AV junction and may increase when the pacemaker site shifts back to the SA node.

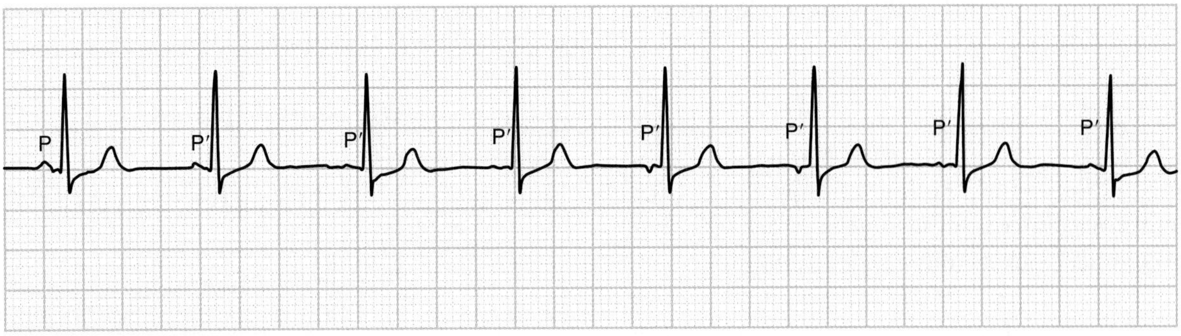

FIGURE 21-46 Wandering atrial pacemaker.

NOTE

Another type of wandering atrial pacemaker is **multifocal atrial tachycardia (MAT)** (**FIGURE 21-47**). MAT resembles wandering pacemaker but is associated with rates often in the range of 120 to 150 beats/min. MAT is always considered pathologic. This atrial tachycardia most often is found in patients with severe chronic obstructive pulmonary disease and may respond to management of the underlying disease. MAT often is mistaken for AF with rapid ventricular response (described later in this chapter).

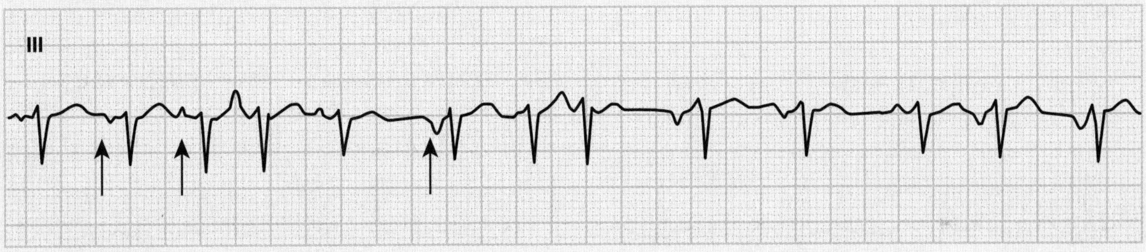

FIGURE 21-47 Multifocal atrial tachycardia.

- **Rhythm.** Usually the underlying rhythm is regular with minor variability when the pacemaker site shifts as noted above.
- **QRS complex.** Usually less than 0.12 second, provided no conduction block is present in the bundle branches.
- **P waves.** Change in P-wave morphology from beat to beat. In lead II, the P waves may be upright, rounded, notched, inverted, biphasic, or buried in the QRS complex.
- **PR interval.** Varies.

Clinical Significance

A wandering pacemaker usually does not produce serious signs and symptoms. Other atrial dysrhythmias (eg, AF) occasionally are associated with this dysrhythmia.

Management

Sometimes a wandering pacemaker is a benign rhythm. In those instances, no treatment is needed. However, MAT may be triggered by acute worsening of chronic obstructive pulmonary disease, heart failure, or mitral valve regurgitation. Management is aimed at the underlying cause.

Premature Atrial Complex

Description

A **premature atrial complex (PAC)** is a single electrical impulse originating in the atria, outside the sinus node (**FIGURE 21-48**). The impulse creates a PAC (P wave). If conducted through the AV node, the impulse also causes a QRS complex before the next expected sinus beat. Because the PAC usually depolarizes the SA

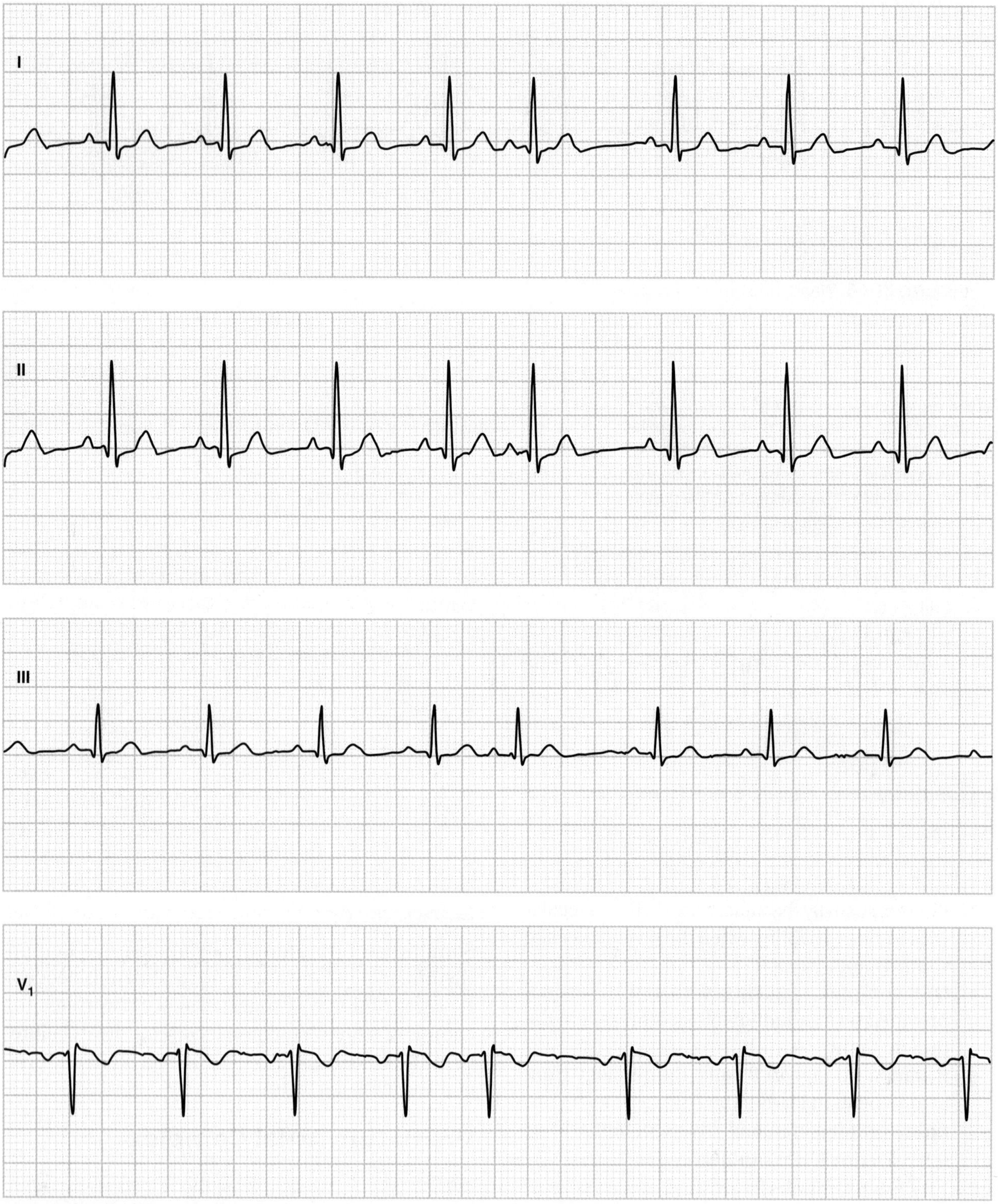

FIGURE 21-48 Premature atrial complex.

node prematurely, the timing of the SA node is reset. The next expected P wave of the underlying rhythm appears earlier than it would have if the SA node had not been disturbed. PACs may originate from a single ectopic pacemaker site or from multiple sites in the atria. PACs are thought to result from enhanced automaticity.

> CRITICAL THINKING
> What do you feel when you palpate the pulse of a patient with PACs?

Etiology

PACs may have no apparent cause or may result from the following:

- Increase in catecholamines and sympathetic tone
- Use of caffeine, tobacco, or alcohol
- Use of sympathomimetic drugs (epinephrine, albuterol, norepinephrine, cocaine, amphetamines)
- Electrolyte imbalance
- Hypoxia
- Digitalis toxicity
- Cardiovascular disease

Rules for Interpretation (Lead II Monitoring)

PACs have the following characteristics on the ECG:

- **Rate.** Depends on the underlying rhythm.
- **Rhythm.** Usually the underlying rhythm is sinus and regular with irregular premature beats when the PACs occur.
- **QRS complex.** Usually less than 0.12 second. The QRS complex may be greater than 0.12 second and appear bizarre if the PAC is conducted abnormally. The QRS complex may be absent as a result of a temporary complete AV block (nonconducted PAC) that occurs during the refractory period of the AV node or ventricles.
- **P waves.** The P wave of a PAC differs in shape from a sinus P wave. It occurs earlier than the next expected sinus P wave and may be so early that it is superimposed or hidden in the preceding T wave. The paramedic should evaluate the preceding T wave to see whether its shape is altered by the presence of a P wave.
- **PR interval.** Usually in the normal range but differs from those of the underlying rhythm.

  The PR interval of a PAC varies from 0.20 second when the pacemaker site is near the SA node to 0.12 second when the pacemaker site is near the AV junction.

> NOTE
> A PAC that looks different from other PACs (PAC with aberrancy) on the ECG may resemble a PVC.

Clinical Significance

Isolated PACs in healthy patients are not significant. Frequent PACs that occur in patients with heart disease may lead to supraventricular dysrhythmias, such as MAT, atrial tachycardia, atrial flutter, AF, or PSVT.

Management

Prehospital care usually requires only observation. PACs that are frequent or that do not produce ventricular contraction (nonconducted PACs) may cause symptomatic bradycardia. In these rare cases, TCP or atropine may be indicated (see Figure 21-42).

Supraventricular Tachycardias

Description

Supraventricular tachycardia (SVT) is a complex group of dysrhythmias. SVT can be broadly defined as any tachycardia that directly or indirectly involves the atria or AV node (above the bundle of His). SVTs described in this section include AV nodal reentrant tachycardia, AV reentrant tachycardia, and atrial tachycardia. SVTs result from rapid atrial or junctional depolarization that overrides the rate of the SA node. (AF and atrial flutter are also SVTs and are discussed later in this chapter.)

Atrioventricular nodal reentrant tachycardia (AVNRT) is the most common type of reentry SVT. AVNRT usually is caused by a PAC. When the dysrhythmia begins and ends abruptly, it is known as **paroxysmal supraventricular tachycardia (PSVT)** (**FIGURE 21-49**). Most SVTs are thought to result from a reentry mechanism that involves abnormal pathways in the AV node. In patients prone to reentry SVTs, the AV node is functionally divided into two pathways: a slow (alpha) pathway with a longer refractory period and a fast (beta) pathway with a shorter refractory period (**FIGURE 21-50**). These pathways permit

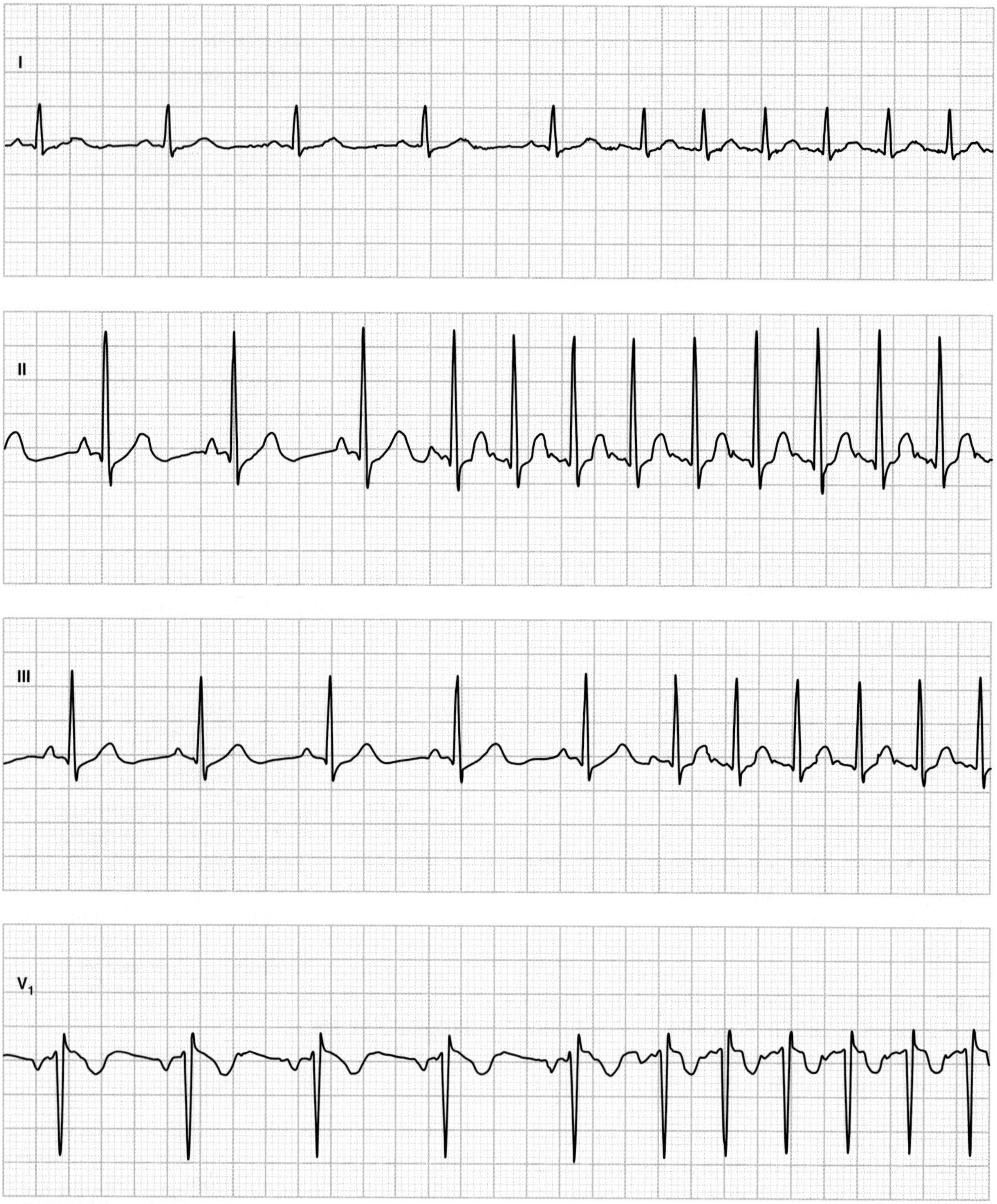

FIGURE 21-49 Paroxysmal supraventricular tachycardia.

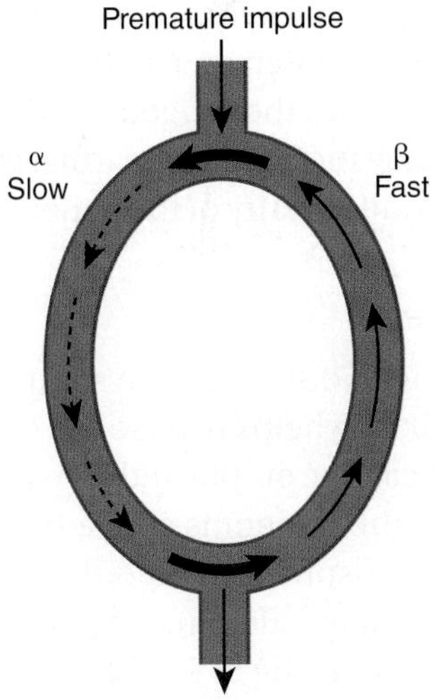

FIGURE 21-50 Pathways of atrioventricular nodal reentrant tachycardia.

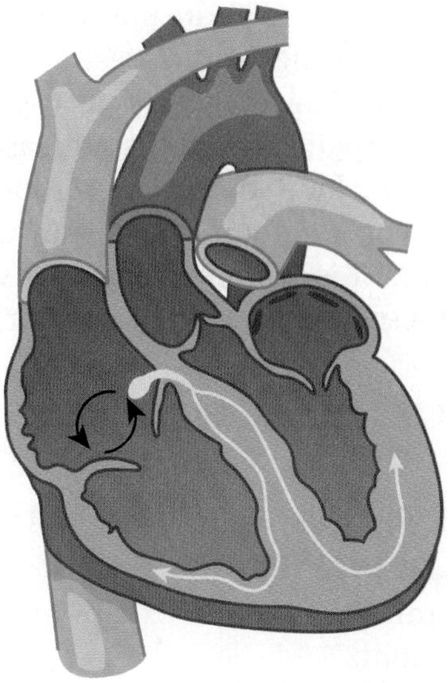

FIGURE 21-51 Atrioventricular nodal reentrant tachycardia.

impulses to be conducted from the atrium to the ventricle (antegrade conduction) or from the ventricle to the atrium (retrograde conduction). Reentry SVTs occur when a premature impulse becomes blocked in the fast pathway and then travels the slow pathway. During this process, the fast pathway recovers while the slow pathway is firing. This produces a reentry circuit in which the electrical impulses are caught in a cycle that continuously circulates around the AV node (**FIGURE 21-51**). The cycle and the tachycardia continue until the reentry pathway is interrupted. Most SVTs are characterized by repeated episodes (paroxysms) of atrial tachycardia. These episodes have a sudden onset (lasting minutes to hours) and an abrupt termination.

Atrioventricular reentrant tachycardia (AVRT) is the second most common type of reentry SVT. AVRT is similar to AVNRT in that the reentry circuit involves the AV node. However, it differs from AVNRT in that one limb of the reentrant loop is formed by abnormal conductive tissue outside of the AV node (called an accessory pathway or bypass tract). This accessory pathway bridges the atrium and ventricles outside of the AV node (**FIGURE 21-52**). The accessory pathways can conduct impulses either antegrade, retrograde, or in both directions.

Atrial tachycardia (AT) is a rhythm disturbance that arises from an irritable site in the atria. The ectopic focus overrides the SA node, producing tachycardia. AT does not require the AV junction, accessory pathways, or ventricular tissue to sustain

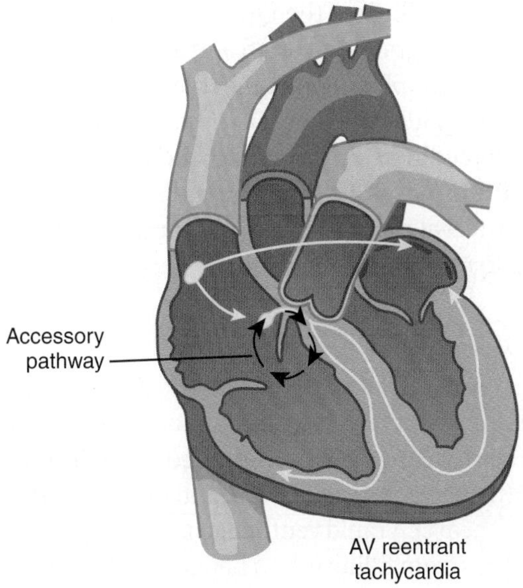

FIGURE 21-52 Atrioventricular nodal tachycardia.

the fast rate. The dysrhythmia presents very similar to sinus tachycardia; however, the P waves differ in shape. The morphology of the P wave in AT depends on the location in the atrium that is responsible for the fast rate. AT that begins and ends abruptly is known as **paroxysmal atrial tachycardia (PAT)**.

Etiology

SVTs may occur at any age. These dysrhythmias are common in young adults and are more common in women than in men. SVTs are not commonly associated with underlying heart disease and are rare in patients with MI. (However, SVTs can trigger angina pectoris or MI in patients with heart disease.) Precipitating factors include stress, overexertion, tobacco use, caffeine consumption, and illicit drug use (eg, cocaine use). SVT is common in patients with WPW syndrome (described later in this chapter).

Rules for Interpretation (Lead II Monitoring)

SVT has the following characteristics on the ECG:

- **Rate.** 150 to 250 beats/min.
- **Rhythm.** Very regular except at onset and termination.
- **QRS complex.** Less than 0.12 second, provided no ventricular conduction disturbance is present.
- **P waves.** May vary based on the atrial tachycardia. For example, in AVNRT and AVRT, there are no P waves before the QRS, but the P waves may be retrograde (inverted and appearing after the QRS complex). Sometimes the P waves cannot be clearly identified because they may be buried in preceding T or U waves or the QRS complexes.
- **PR interval.** If P waves are discernible, the PR interval often is shortened but may be normal or, rarely, prolonged.

Clinical Significance

SVT may occur in patients with healthy hearts. Patients may tolerate it well for short periods. Often the dysrhythmia is accompanied by palpitations, nervousness, and anxiety. The patient often reports a "racing heart." A rapid ventricular rate may prevent the ventricles from filling fully. Therefore, SVT can reduce cardiac output in patients with existing heart disease. Decreased perfusion may cause confusion, vertigo, light-headedness, and syncope and may precipitate angina pectoris, hypotension, or heart failure. In addition, SVT increases the oxygen requirement of the heart, which may increase myocardial ischemia and the frequency and severity of the patient's chest pain.

> NOTE
>
> The distinctions among the various SVTs and VT (a lethal rhythm) may be difficult to make. In the prehospital setting, it is more important for the paramedic to recognize an unstable tachydysrhythmia and perform immediate synchronized cardioversion. Serious signs and symptoms include, but are not limited to, severe chest pain, respiratory distress, altered level of consciousness (especially with hypotension), pulmonary edema, or AMI.

Management

The paramedic should manage symptomatic SVT promptly. Doing so helps reverse the consequences of the reduced cardiac output and increased workload of the heart. If the patient is stable (conscious with normal blood pressure and without chest pain, heart failure, or pulmonary edema), the paramedic should attempt to terminate the SVT using vagal maneuvers and pharmacologic therapies (**FIGURE 21-53**).

Vagal Maneuvers. Vagal maneuvers can slow the heart and reduce the force of atrial contraction. These maneuvers stimulate the parasympathetic nerve fibers in the wall of the atria and in specialized tissues of the SA and AV nodes. They can interrupt and terminate some SVTs. To attempt vagal maneuvers, the patient must be relatively stable and cooperative. Continuous ECG monitoring and an IV line must be in place before beginning these procedures. Atropine and airway equipment should be readily available. Vagal maneuvers include the **Valsalva maneuver** and the ice pack maneuver in children. Unilateral carotid sinus pressure is another procedure that is used in the hospital but is not routinely recommended in the prehospital setting.

- **Valsalva maneuver.** To be effective, the Valsalva maneuver generally requires that the patient generate an intrathoracic pressure of 40 mm Hg.[11] To achieve this, the paramedic places the patient in a semi-sitting position with the head tilted forward. The patient is instructed to take in a deep breath and to bear down as if to have a bowel movement. Another procedure shown to generate 40 mm Hg of pressure for adults involves having the patient blow into the tip of a 10-mL syringe hard enough to force the plunger out.[12] This pressure should be sustained for 15 seconds. (Children can be instructed to blow through a straw.) The forced expiration against a closed glottis stimulates the vagus nerve and may terminate the tachycardia. The procedure may be repeated if unsuccessful. A 2015 study found the success of the Valsalva procedure

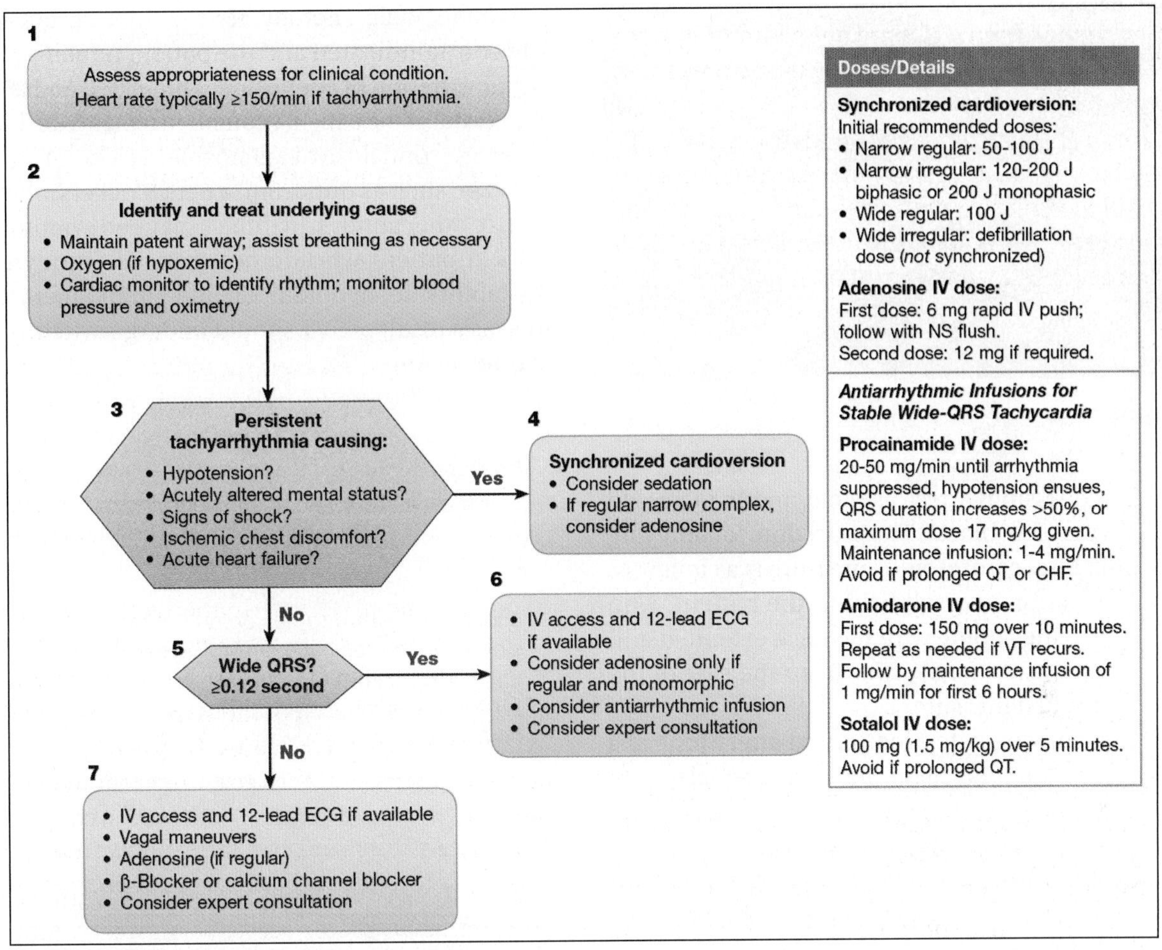
1
Assess appropriateness for clinical condition.
Heart rate typically ≥150/min if tachyarrhythmia.
2
Identify and treat underlying cause
• Maintain patent airway; assist breathing as necessary
• Oxygen (if hypoxemic)
• Cardiac monitor to identify rhythm; monitor blood pressure and oximetry
3
Persistent tachyarrhythmia causing:
• Hypotension?
• Acutely altered mental status?
• Signs of shock?
• Ischemic chest discomfort?
• Acute heart failure?
Yes
4
Synchronized cardioversion
• Consider sedation
• If regular narrow complex, consider adenosine
No
5
Wide QRS? ≥0.12 second
Yes
6
• IV access and 12-lead ECG if available
• Consider adenosine only if regular and monomorphic
• Consider antiarrhythmic infusion
• Consider expert consultation
No
7
• IV access and 12-lead ECG if available
• Vagal maneuvers
• Adenosine (if regular)
• β-Blocker or calcium channel blocker
• Consider expert consultation
Doses/Details
Synchronized cardioversion:
Initial recommended doses:
• Narrow regular: 50-100 J
• Narrow irregular: 120-200 J biphasic or 200 J monophasic
• Wide regular: 100 J
• Wide irregular: defibrillation dose (not synchronized)
Adenosine IV dose:
First dose: 6 mg rapid IV push; follow with NS flush.
Second dose: 12 mg if required.
Antiarrhythmic Infusions for Stable Wide-QRS Tachycardia
Procainamide IV dose:
20-50 mg/min until arrhythmia suppressed, hypotension ensues, QRS duration increases >50%, or maximum dose 17 mg/kg given.
Maintenance infusion: 1-4 mg/min.
Avoid if prolonged QT or CHF.
Amiodarone IV dose:
First dose: 150 mg over 10 minutes.
Repeat as needed if VT recurs.
Follow by maintenance infusion of 1 mg/min for first 6 hours.
Sotalol IV dose:
100 mg (1.5 mg/kg) over 5 minutes.
Avoid if prolonged QT.

Abbreviations: CHF, congestive heart failure; ECG, electrocardiogram; IV, intravenous; NS, normal saline

FIGURE 21-53 Tachycardia algorithm.

could be increased from 17% to 43% by laying the patient supine and passively raising the legs immediately after the Valsalva strain was completed.[13]

- **Ice pack maneuver.** When using the ice pack maneuver, an ice pack is placed over the face or the anterior neck of an infant or young child; this action may stimulate the vagus nerve because of the mammalian diving reflex (see Chapter 44, *Environmental Conditions*). (In the pediatric patient, this technique is performed with a washcloth soaked in ice water. The washcloth is placed across the patient's face, about to nostril level.) The paramedic should not attempt the ice pack maneuver if ischemic heart disease is present or suspected. The procedure may be repeated (per medical direction) if unsuccessful.[14]
- **Unilateral carotid sinus pressure.** Carotid sinus pressure (carotid sinus massage) stimulates the carotid sinus located in the carotid arteries. The carotid sinus is a baroreceptor and interprets this localized pressure as an increase in blood pressure (**FIGURE 21-54**). This response activates the autonomic nervous system and stimulates the vagus nerve. The heart rate slows in an attempt to lower blood pressure. The paramedic should auscultate the carotid arteries for the presence of a bruit (described in Chapter 19, *Secondary Assessment and Reassessment*) before applying carotid sinus pressure. This vagal maneuver should not be used if bruits are present, if the patient is an older adult, or if the patient is known to have carotid artery disease or cerebral vascular disease. Possible complications from the procedure include cerebral emboli, stroke,

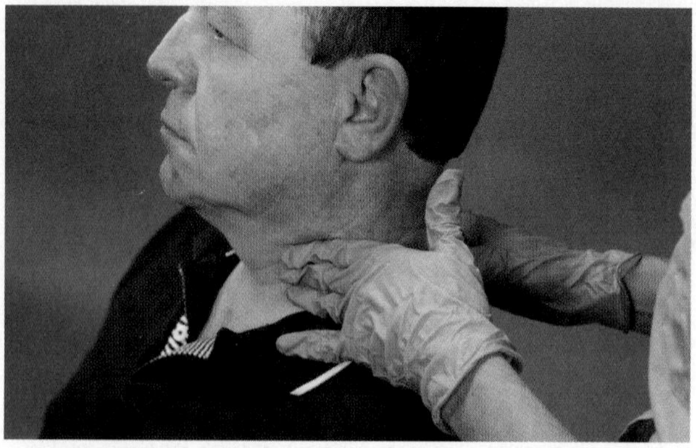

FIGURE 21-54 Carotid sinus massage.

syncope, sinus arrest, asystole, and an increased degree of AV block.[1] The procedure for applying unilateral carotid sinus pressure is as follows:

1. Position yourself behind the patient, who is lying supine with the neck extended and the head turned away from the side of the applied pressure.
2. Gently palpate each carotid artery (one at a time) to confirm the presence of equal pulses. If pulses are unequal or if one is absent, do not apply carotid sinus pressure.
3. While the patient holds his or her breath for 4 to 5 seconds, auscultate for the presence of bruits.
4. To apply carotid sinus pressure, place the index and middle fingers over the artery on the neck just below the angle of the jaw. Compress the artery firmly against the vertebral column while massaging the area. (Inform the patient that he or she may experience some pain or discomfort.) Maintain pressure for no longer than 5 to 10 seconds. Discontinue the massage immediately if bradycardia or signs of heart block develop or if the tachycardia breaks. Apply pressure to only one carotid sinus at a time. Applying bilateral carotid sinus pressure may interfere with cerebral circulation.
5. Observe the ECG monitor, and run a strip during the procedure and obtain a tracing. Repeat the procedure in 2 to 3 minutes if it is ineffective.

CRITICAL THINKING

You perform carotid sinus massage on a patient with bruits or known carotid artery disease. What might occur?

Pharmacologic Therapy. If vagal maneuvers fail or are contraindicated and the patient remains stable, administration of adenosine is indicated and is often successful. If the patient's condition remains unchanged after a second dose of adenosine, a calcium channel blocker, such as diltiazem, a beta blocker (metoprolol), or other antidysrhythmics may end symptomatic SVT. A patient who demonstrates hemodynamic instability (ie, hypotension and altered mental status) as a result of SVT should undergo synchronized cardioversion.

NOTE

SVT may be the result of an underlying rhythm (eg, AF with a rapid ventricular response). The prudent course is to monitor the ECG continuously and run a strip while administering adenosine. Doing so allows the underlying rhythm to be captured once the heart rate slows. Other medications may be needed to treat the underlying rhythm (eg, diltiazem). It is not uncommon for the underlying rhythm to revert to SVT, requiring additional drug therapy.

NOTE

Administration of a drug that blocks electrical transmission at the AV node (eg, adenosine, diltiazem, metoprolol) in a patient with VT can be lethal. The paramedic must carefully evaluate the patient's ECG to distinguish between SVT with aberrant conduction and VT. In general, if the complexes are wide, the paramedic should manage the rhythm as a VT. Synchronized cardioversion is the preferred method of managing a patient who presents with an unstable tachydysrhythmia.

CRITICAL THINKING

What are some of the side effects of diltiazem?

For simplicity, in symptomatic narrow-complex SVT, vagal maneuvers and adenosine should be used first to end the tachydysrhythmia. If adenosine is not effective and if the patient is hemodynamically stable and has no evidence of heart failure, secondary drug treatment options include calcium channel blockers or beta blockers. These agents most likely will be used after diagnosis and evaluation by a physician (**FIGURE 21-55**).

Consecutive use of calcium channel blockers, beta blockers, and primary antidysrhythmics is

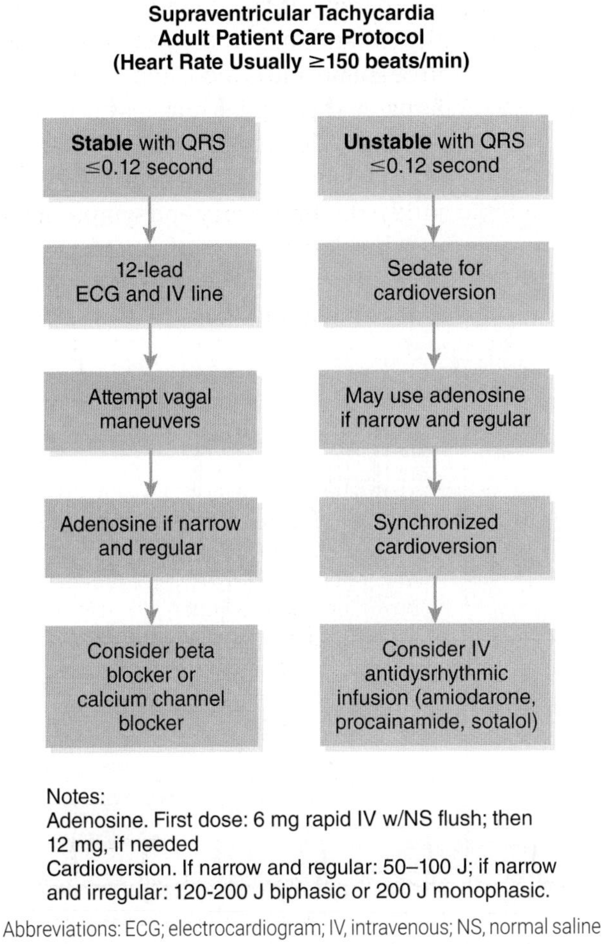
Supraventricular Tachycardia
Adult Patient Care Protocol
(Heart Rate Usually ≥150 beats/min)
Stable with QRS ≤0.12 second
12-lead ECG and IV line
Attempt vagal maneuvers
Adenosine if narrow and regular
Consider beta blocker or calcium channel blocker
Unstable with QRS ≤0.12 second
Sedate for cardioversion
May use adenosine if narrow and regular
Synchronized cardioversion
Consider IV antidysrhythmic infusion (amiodarone, procainamide, sotalol)
Notes:
Adenosine. First dose: 6 mg rapid IV w/NS flush; then 12 mg, if needed
Cardioversion. If narrow and regular: 50–100 J; if narrow and irregular: 120-200 J biphasic or 200 J monophasic.
Abbreviations: ECG; electrocardiogram; IV, intravenous; NS, normal saline

FIGURE 21-55 New supraventricular tachycardia protocol.

discouraged. The general rule is to use only one antidysrhythmic agent; using several can result in hypotension. Furthermore, the paramedic should avoid negative inotropic drugs (eg, diltiazem, beta blockers) in hemodynamically unstable patients and those with underlying heart failure.

Serious signs and symptoms in a patient with narrow-complex SVT point to poor perfusion and clinical instability. In this case, synchronized electrical cardioversion is the treatment of choice to terminate the rhythm. (Cardioversion is presented later in this chapter.) Cardioversion should begin with a synchronized shock of 50 to 100 J.[15] (AF should first be managed with a shock of 120 to 200 J biphasic.[15]) If this energy level fails, the energy may be increased in a stepwise manner per the manufacturer's recommendation. Sedation should be considered before cardioversion if time permits.

CRITICAL THINKING

Why is the drug etomidate an ideal sedative to administer before cardioversion?

Atrial Flutter

Description

Atrial flutter is almost always a result of a rapid atrial reentry focus (**FIGURE 21-56**). Atrial flutter that is not slowed by preexisting AV block usually manifests a 2:1 AV conduction ratio and may look like SVT. (A 2:1 AV conduction ratio means that 50% of the atrial impulses are conducted through the ventricles.) However, 3:1, 4:1, and greater conduction ratios are not uncommon. These ratios produce a discrepancy between atrial and ventricular rates. The conduction ratios may be constant or variable. Atrial flutter may be seen with AF (atrial fib-flutter). In rare cases, atrial flutter may conduct at a 1:1 ratio, resulting in extremely fast ventricular rates with rapid hemodynamic deterioration. Atrial flutter should be considered in any patient who presents with a nonvariable heart rate between 140 and 160 beats/min.

Etiology

Atrial flutter usually is seen in middle-aged or older patients who have heart disease. At times, atrial flutter also occurs in patients with healthy hearts. The dysrhythmia commonly is associated with the following:

- Coronary artery disease
- Hypertensive heart disease
- Cardiomyopathy
- Digitalis toxicity (rare)
- Hypoxia
- Heart failure
- Pericarditis
- Myocarditis

Rules for Interpretation (Lead II Monitoring)

Atrial flutter has the following characteristics on the ECG:

- **Rate.** The atrial rate is 250 to 300 beats/min; the ventricular rate is regular and usually 150 beats/min in a patient with a 2:1 block (most common).
- **Rhythm.** The atrial rhythm is regular; the ventricular rate is usually regular. However,

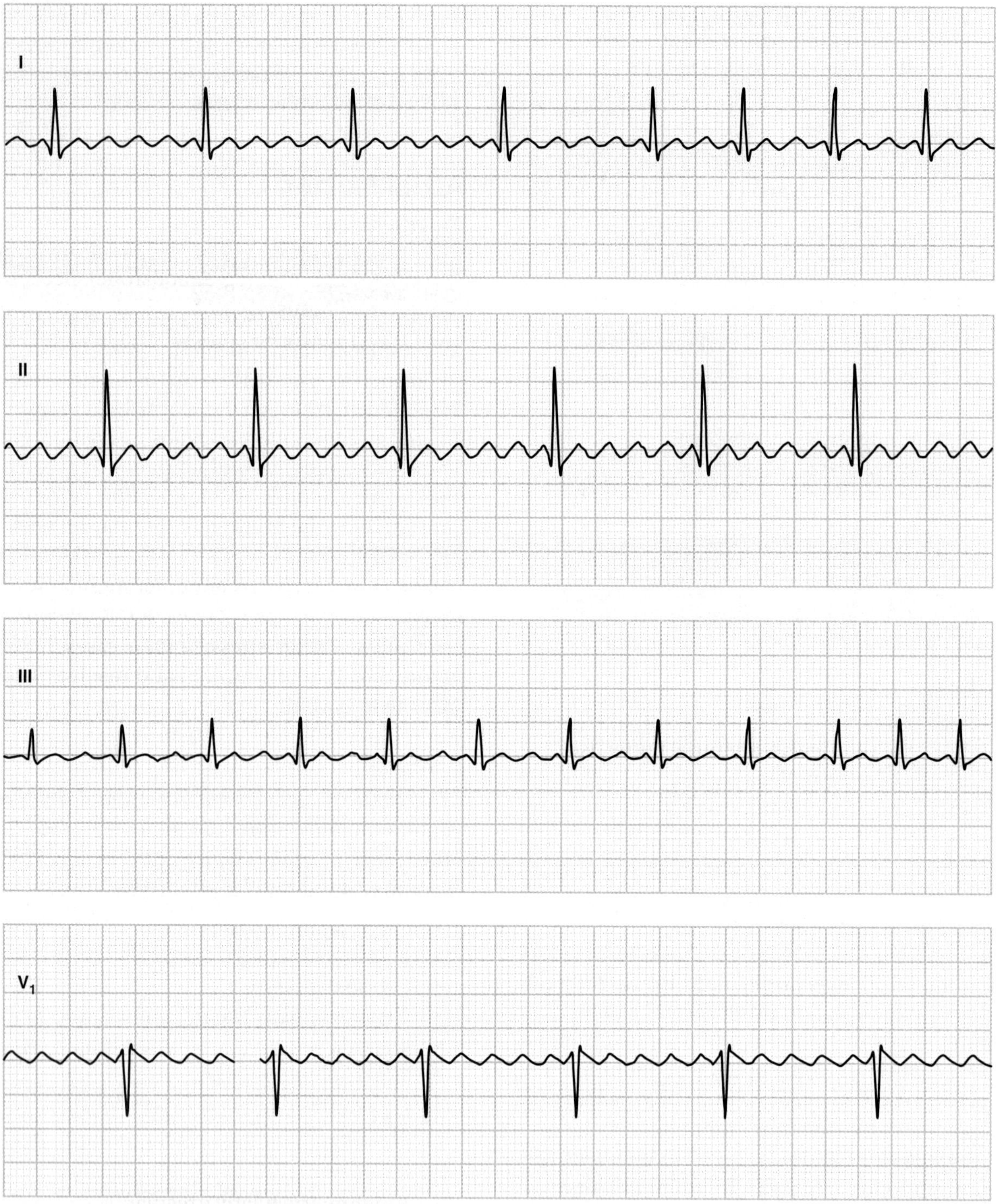

FIGURE 21-56 Atrial flutter.

the ventricular rate may be irregular if the AV conduction ratio varies (variable block).

- **QRS complex.** Less than 0.12 second, unless ventricular conduction disturbance (aberrancy) is present.
- **P waves.** Flutter P waves (F waves) usually resemble a sawtooth or picket fence pattern. They usually appear as inverted P waves in inferior leads (II, III). The flutter waves represent atrial depolarization in an abnormal direction that is followed by atrial repolarization.
- **PR interval.** Usually constant but may vary.

NOTE

Flutter waves may be difficult to identify with a 2:1 ratio of atrial to ventricular complexes because there will be a single P wave prior to every QRS complex. The paramedic should suspect 2:1 flutter when the rhythm is regular and the ventricular rate is 150 beats/min. In this case, a 12-lead ECG should be obtained and P-wave morphology should be carefully examined because flutter P waves do not have normal P-wave morphology (and are usually inverted in lead II).

Clinical Significance

With a normal ventricular rate, atrial flutter usually is well tolerated by the patient. A rapid ventricular rate produces the same signs and symptoms of decreased cardiac output that are seen in patients with SVT. In addition, in some flutter rhythms (particularly a 2:1 atrial flutter), the atria do not contract regularly and empty before each ventricular contraction. The loss of the "atrial kick" results in incomplete filling of the ventricles, which may further reduce cardiac output.

Management

See Management of AF and Atrial Flutter, discussed next.

NOTE

The pulse rate of a patient with this dysrhythmia (and other tachycardias) might not reflect the true heart rate. This is because not all heart contractions produce enough output of blood to create a palpable pulse.

Atrial Fibrillation

Description

Atrial fibrillation (AF) results from multiple areas of reentry within the atria (**FIGURE 21-57**). It also can result from ectopic atrial pacemakers. (The activity of the SA node is suppressed completely by AF.) AF produces chaotic impulses too numerous for all to be conducted by the AV node through the ventricles. AV conduction is random, resulting in an irregularly irregular but usually rapid ventricular response. Medications such as digoxin, beta blockers, or calcium channel blockers often are prescribed to slow the ventricular rate. Patients may also be taking medications to control the rhythm (eg, amiodarone). Because the risk of emboli causing stroke is high in AF, patients often take antiplatelets and anticoagulants (warfarin). A new class of medications called direct oral anticoagulants (DOACs) include dabigatran, rivaroxaban, and apixaban. These drugs do not require the usual monthly blood tests and dietary restrictions typically associated with traditional anticoagulants.[16,17]

Etiology

Sudden-onset (paroxysmal) AF may occur in young adults after heavy alcohol ingestion ("holiday heart" syndrome) or acute stress. In these cases, the fibrillation usually is self-limited and resolves without treatment. Chronic AF may be intermittent. It often is associated with age older than 40 years, underlying heart disease, chronic hypertension, obesity, family history, and sleep apnea. Middle-aged endurance athletes are susceptible to AF, as are people who have other chronic health problems such as diabetes mellitus, hyperthyroidism, and asthma.

Rules for Interpretation (Lead II Monitoring)

AF has the following characteristics on the ECG:

- **Rate.** The atrial rate is 350 to 700 beats/min (cannot be counted); the ventricular rate varies greatly, depending on conduction through the AV node (average 150 to 180 beats/min if uncontrolled).
- **Rhythm:** Irregularly irregular.
- **QRS complex.** Less than 0.12 second, provided no ventricular conduction disturbance is present.
- **P waves.** P waves are absent. Fibrillation waves (F waves) may be fine (<1 mm) or coarse (>1 mm). Fine F waves may be so small that they appear as a wavy or flat (isoelectric) line or are absent. The F waves are irregularly shaped, rounded (or pointed), and dissimilar.
- **PR interval.** None.

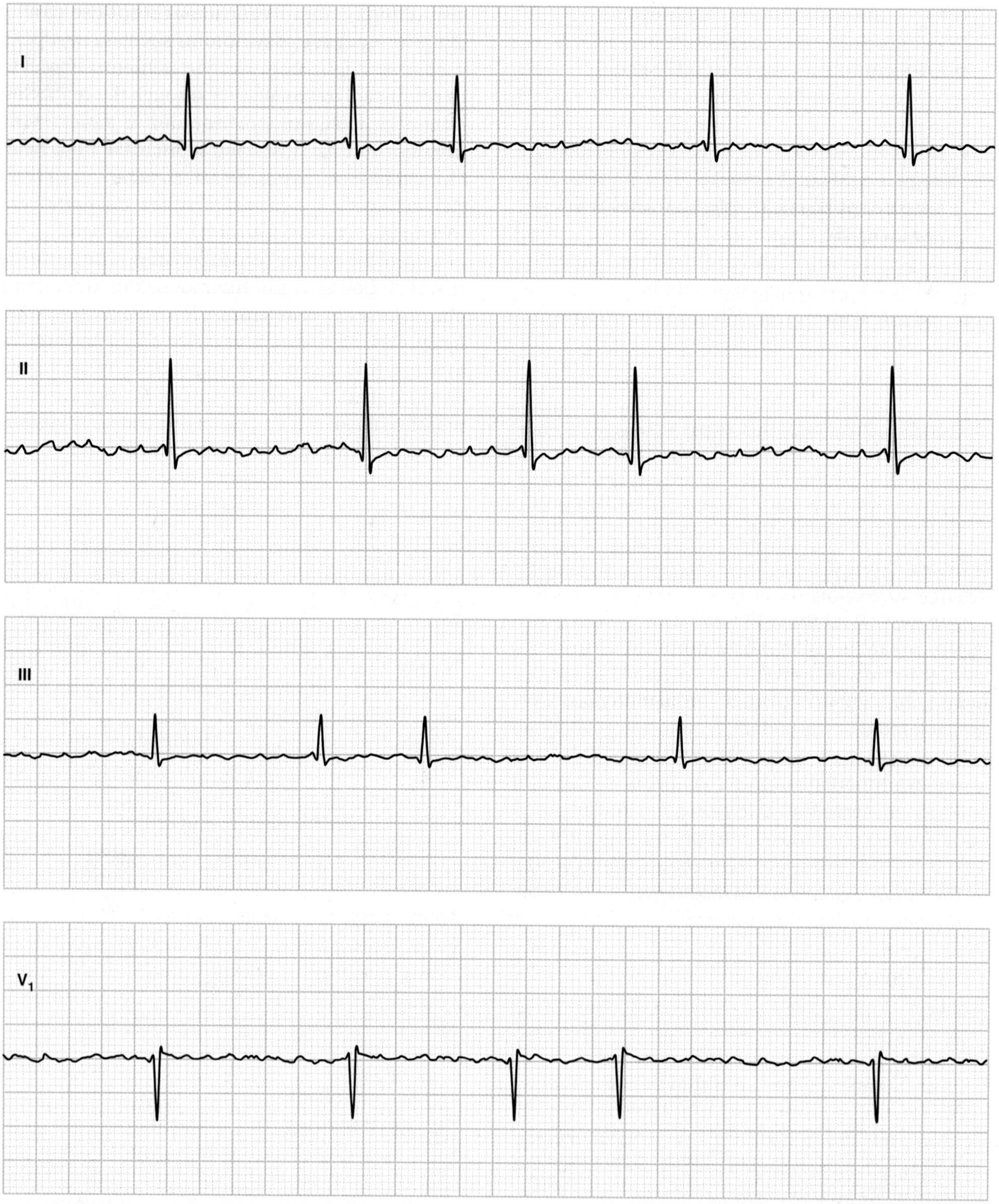

FIGURE 21-57 Atrial fibrillation.

AF w/ RVR

> NOTE
> Irregularly irregular rhythms are almost always AF.

Clinical Significance

The atrial kick is lost in AF. This loss can reduce cardiac output by as much as 15%. This reduced cardiac output, coupled with a rapid ventricular response, may cause cardiovascular decompensation (angina pectoris, MI, heart failure, or cardiogenic shock).

Management of AF and Atrial Flutter

A risk of emboli formation exists when AF or atrial flutter has been present for longer than 48 hours. Formation of emboli in the heart increases the risk of "throwing a clot" or systemic embolization. This condition most often occurs when the AF is converted suddenly to a sinus rhythm. The algorithm cautions against converting AF or atrial flutter without first giving the patient drugs that prevent blood clotting. Electrical cardioversion and the use of antidysrhythmic agents that may convert the rhythm should be avoided unless the patient is unstable or hemodynamically compromised.[7]

Using drugs to control the heart rate is the recommended initial treatment for stable, rapid AF or atrial flutter regardless of how long the patient has had it. Specific drug treatment depends on the patient's condition and how stable the patient is. Using several different drugs can cause a dysrhythmia to develop (a **proarrhythmia**). The paramedic should use only one drug from the list of suggested drug treatments.

In patients with a rapid AF or atrial flutter with a rapid ventricular response, the rate may be controlled with diltiazem or beta blockers. Amiodarone has a potential for rhythm conversion. Therefore, amiodarone should be reserved for use within the first 48 hours of dysrhythmia onset when other medications for rate control have failed. The use of calcium channel blocking agents and beta blocking agents warrants caution in the presence of heart failure because of their negative inotropic properties. Beta blocking agents also should be used with caution in patients with asthma and chronic obstructive pulmonary disease. Another drug that may be effective for converting the rhythm is digoxin. Digoxin should be used only if AF developed within 48 hours or less.

AF with a rapid ventricular response can be the primary cause of symptoms such as chest pain, shortness of breath, or light-headedness. However, as discussed previously, it may also be a symptom of an underlying process. For example, patients who have chronic AF who need to increase their heart rate because of infection or hypovolemia will be at risk for the development of AF with rapid ventricular response instead of sinus tachycardia. Treating the heart rate in these patients rather than addressing the underlying cause can be harmful and have disastrous consequences.[18] Therefore, prior to pharmacologic treatment of a supraventricular dysrhythmia, the paramedic must think carefully about whether the dysrhythmia is likely to be the cause of the symptoms or an effect of an underlying process based on the patient history and physical examination. For example, the sudden onset of signs and symptoms of heart failure with impaired cardiac function (eg, dyspnea, crackles, tachycardia, chest pain, decreased level of consciousness) coinciding with the dysrhythmia suggest that the dysrhythmia is more likely to be the cause; however, this is not absolute (eg, acute pulmonary embolism).

If the patient reports a history of WPW syndrome or if the paramedic forms that impression in the field before the AF developed, alternative treatment is indicated.

If the patient has WPW syndrome, paramedics should not give adenosine, diltiazem, verapamil, digoxin, or, in most cases, beta blockers. These drugs may cause a dangerous increase in the heart rate. If the patient has had the dysrhythmia for longer than 48 hours and is stable, the paramedic should avoid elective cardioversion until anticoagulant drugs have been given. However, when serious signs or symptoms occur, such as chest pain, shortness of breath, pulmonary congestion, a decreased level of consciousness, or hypotension, the paramedic should cardiovert the patient immediately. The initial attempt at cardioversion for atrial flutter should consist of a synchronized shock of 50 to 100 J.[15] If needed, the energy may be increased in a stepwise manner according to the manufacturer's recommendations. Because AF is a more difficult rhythm to convert and lower joule settings have been known to cause asystole, recommendations are to use a synchronized shock of 120 to 200 J biphasic initially, followed by stepwise increases as recommended by the manufacturer if necessary (BOX 21-6).[15]

BOX 21-6 Atrial Fibrillation/Flutter

With or without heart failure:

Rate control. Administer calcium channel blocker (diltiazem) or beta blocker (metoprolol).

Rhythm conversion. Perform synchronized cardioversion when clinical instability is present, such as if the patient has hypotension or alteration in mental status.

DID YOU KNOW?

Catheter Ablation Therapy

Catheter ablation is an in-hospital procedure performed in an electrophysiology or cardiac catheterization laboratory. During the procedure, three to five catheters are inserted into the heart through an artery or vein (or both) in the groin, neck, or arm. A transducer is inserted through one of the catheters so that intracardiac ultrasonography can be performed during the procedure. The ablation catheter is moved from spot to spot to identify the origin of a dysrhythmia. A pacemakerlike device is then used to send electrical impulses to the heart to induce tachycardia. Once the area of the heart responsible for the dysrhythmia has been identified, a radiofrequency impulse is delivered to the area through the catheter. The goal is to "disconnect" the pathway of the abnormal rhythm. Catheter ablation can be used to treat the following conditions:

- AV node reentrant tachycardia
- Accessory pathway disturbances
- Atrial flutter
- VT

CRITICAL THINKING

What signs or symptoms would make you think these patients are unstable?

Dysrhythmias Sustained or Originating in the AV Junction

When the SA node and the atria cannot generate the electrical impulses needed to begin depolarization because of factors such as hypoxia, ischemia, MI, and drug toxicity, the AV node or the area surrounding the AV node may assume the role of the secondary pacemaker. Rhythms that start in the AV node or AV junctional area are junctional rhythms. This type of rhythm usually is a benign dysrhythmia. The paramedic must assess the rhythm to determine the patient's tolerance of the rhythm disturbance. Dysrhythmias that originate in the AV junction include PJCs, junctional escape complexes or junctional escape rhythms, and accelerated junctional rhythm.

In junctional rhythms, electrical impulses travel in a normal pathway from the AV junction through the bundle of His and bundle branches to the Purkinje fibers. The pathway ends in the ventricular muscle. Conduction through the ventricles proceeds normally. The QRS complex, therefore, usually is within normal limits (0.04 to 0.10 second). However, the impulse that depolarizes the atria travels in a backward or retrograde motion. The retrograde depolarization of the atria results in one of three P-wave characteristics: (1) inverted P waves in lead II with a short PR interval, (2) absent P waves, or (3) P waves after the QRS complex.

Premature Junctional Complex

Description

A **premature junctional complex (PJC)** results from a single electrical impulse from the AV junction (**FIGURE 21-58**). The impulse occurs before the next expected sinus impulse. A PJC may occur as an isolated impulse or as a series of impulses (**junctional escape rhythm**) (**FIGURE 21-59**). It is a compensatory response to slowing of the AV node that occurs when the rate of the SA node falls below that of the AV junction. The escape complex or rhythm provided by the AV junction serves as a safety mechanism to prevent cardiac standstill. The AV junction begins firing at an inherent rate of 40 to 60 beats/min within about 1 to 1.5 seconds of not receiving an impulse from the SA node.

Etiology

Isolated PJCs may occur in a healthy person without apparent cause; however, more often they are a result of heart disease or drug toxicity. Usually PJCs result from enhanced automaticity or a reentry mechanism. PJCs have several causes:

- Digitalis toxicity
- Other cardiac medications (quinidine, procainamide)
- Increased vagal tone on the SA node
- Sympathomimetic drugs (eg, cocaine, methamphetamines)
- Hypoxia

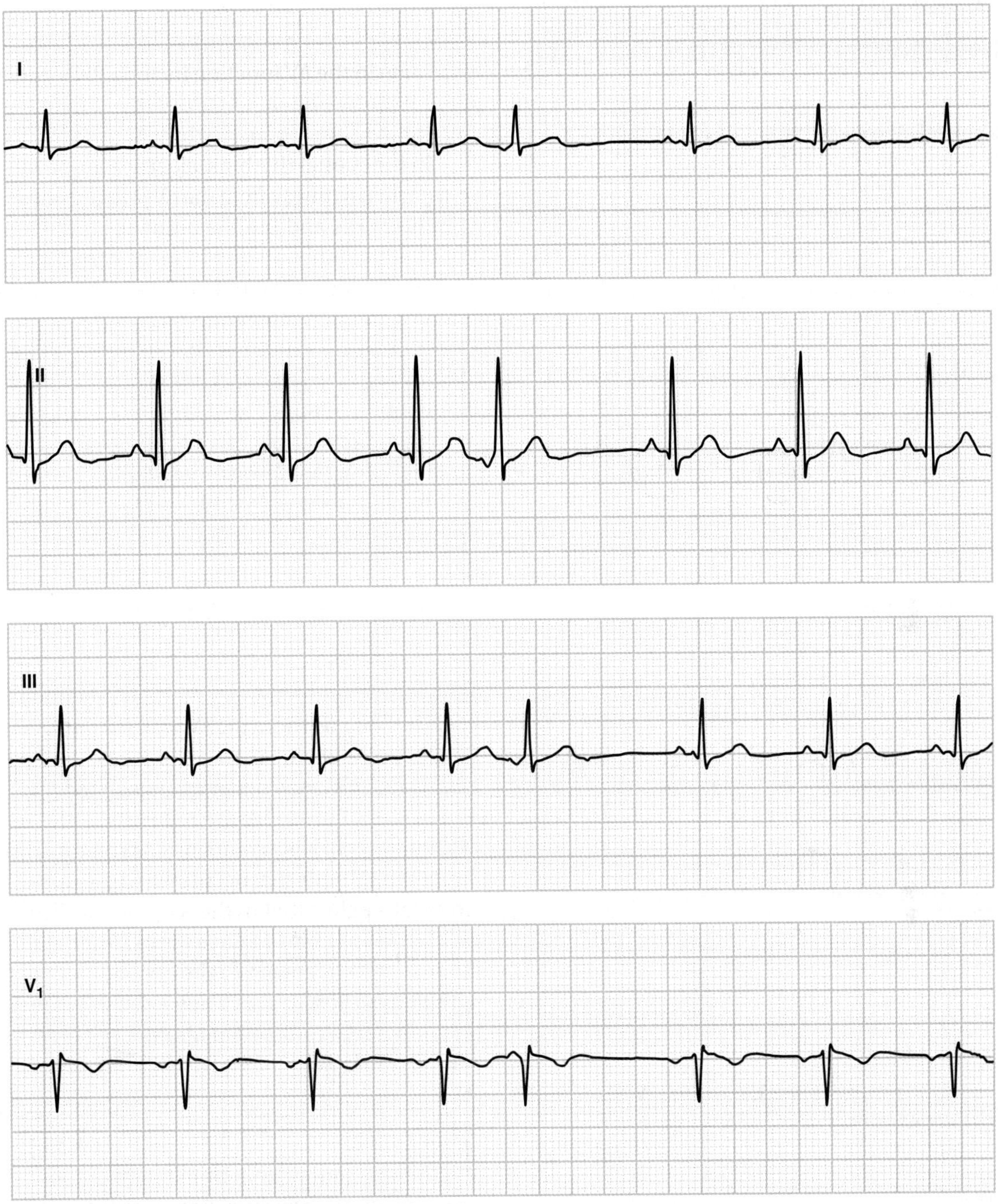

FIGURE 21-58 Premature junctional complexes.

- Heart failure
- Damage to the AV junction

CRITICAL THINKING

Would the P wave be visible if it occurred during the QRS wave?

Rules for Interpretation (Lead II Monitoring)

PJCs have the following characteristics on the ECG:

- **Rate.** The heart rate is that of the underlying rhythm.
- **Rhythm.** Usually regular, except when PJCs are present.

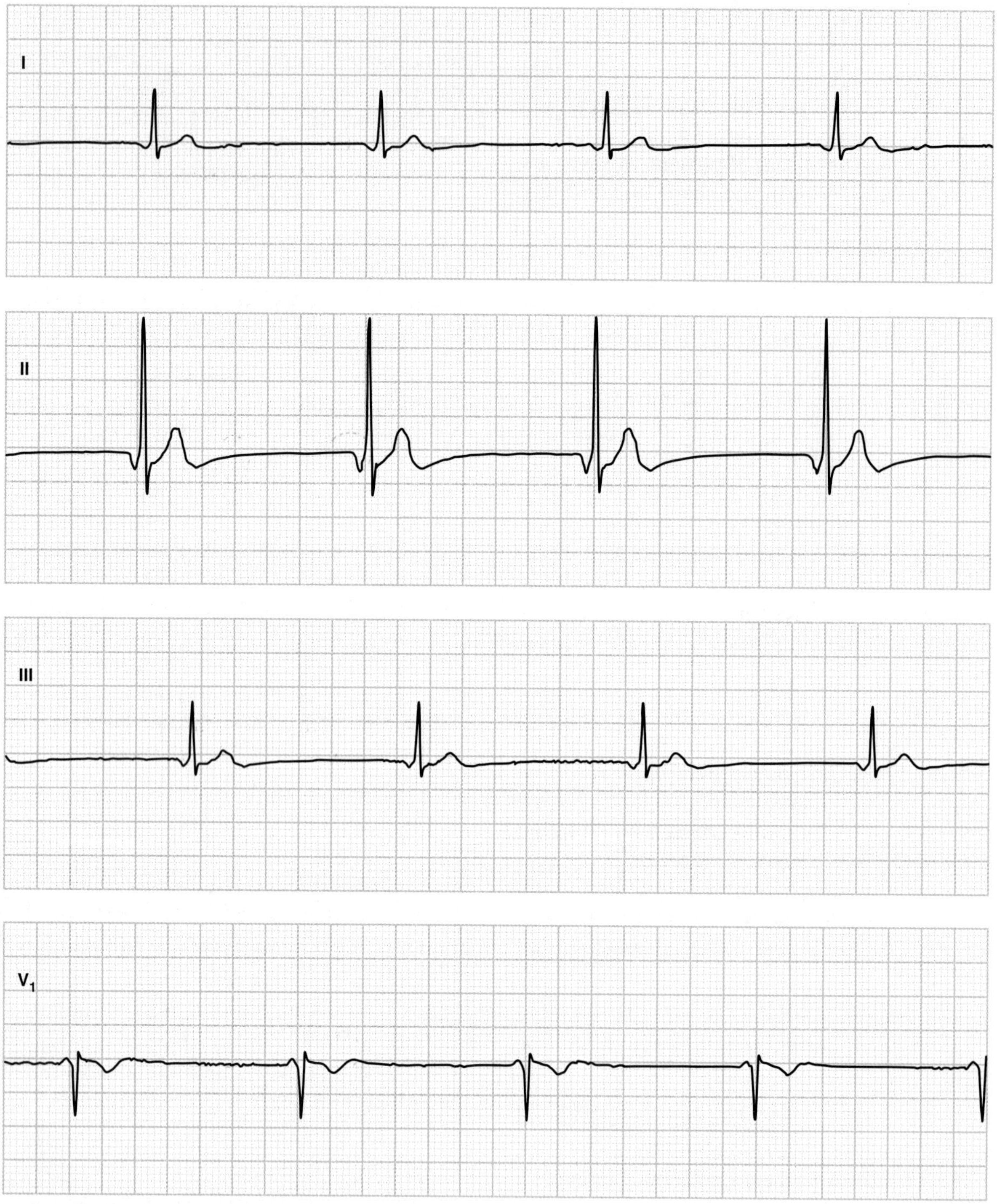

FIGURE 21-59 Junctional escape complex or rhythm.

- **QRS complex.** Usually less than 0.12 second, provided no ventricular conduction disturbance is present.
- **P waves.** May be associated with PJCs. P waves may occur before, during, or after the QRS complex or may be absent. If present, P waves are abnormal, differing in size, shape, and direction from normal P waves.
- **PR interval.** If retrograde P waves precede the QRS complex, the PR interval commonly is shortened (<0.12 second) and constant. If there is no relationship between the P and R waves, consider the presence of a coexisting heart block, one of the causes of junctional escape rhythms.

Clinical Significance

Occasional PJCs usually are not significant. Junctional bradycardias can cause decreased cardiac output. Therefore, patients can have signs and symptoms similar to those of other bradycardias (eg, light-headedness, hypotension, syncope). As a rule, patients usually tolerate junctional rhythms of 50 beats/min or greater.

Management

Patients who are stable do not need to be treated. If the patient is symptomatic or if ventricular irritability is present, drug therapy (beginning with atropine) may be indicated. In severe cases, and in patients unresponsive to atropine, external pacing may be necessary. If the SA node is diseased or damaged, the patient may need a permanent pacemaker (see Figure 21-42).

Accelerated Junctional Rhythm

Description

Accelerated junctional rhythm results from increased automaticity of the AV junction (**FIGURE 21-60**). This increase causes it to discharge faster than its intrinsic rate. (The intrinsic rate is 40 to 60 beats/min.) This rate, in turn, overrides the main (SA node) pacemaker. The rate of this dysrhythmia (usually 60 to 99 beats/min) does not truly constitute a tachycardia. Therefore, the dysrhythmia is called accelerated junctional rhythm. In this text, rapid junctional rhythms equal to or greater than 100 beats/min (**junctional tachycardia** caused by a reentry mechanism) are discussed with other SVTs.

Etiology

An accelerated junctional rhythm commonly is a result of digitalis toxicity. Other causes of this rhythm include excessive catecholamine administration, damage to the AV junction, inferior wall MI (described later in this chapter), and rheumatic fever.

Rules for Interpretation (Lead II Monitoring)

Accelerated junctional rhythm has the following characteristics on the ECG:

- **Rate.** Usually 60 to 99 beats/min.
- **Rhythm.** Regular.
- **QRS complex.** Usually less than 0.12 second, provided no preexisting bundle branch block is present.
- **P waves.** Retrograde P waves may be present (with or without relationship to the QRS complex), absent (retrograde AV block), or buried in the QRS complex. If present, P waves usually are inverted and appear before or after the QRS complex.
- **PR interval.** If the P wave occurs before the QRS complex, the PR interval will be less than 0.12 second. If the P wave follows the QRS complex, it technically is an RP interval and usually is less than 0.20 second.

Clinical Significance

Accelerated junctional rhythm usually is well tolerated by the patient. However, heart disease and lack of oxygen to the heart muscle may cause more serious dysrhythmias.

Management

Accelerated junctional rhythm generally requires no immediate treatment.

> CRITICAL THINKING
>
> Because no drug therapy is indicated, do you need to start an IV line for these patients?

Dysrhythmias Originating in the Ventricles

Ventricular dysrhythmias usually are considered a threat to life. Ventricular rhythm disturbances generally result from enhanced automaticity or reentry

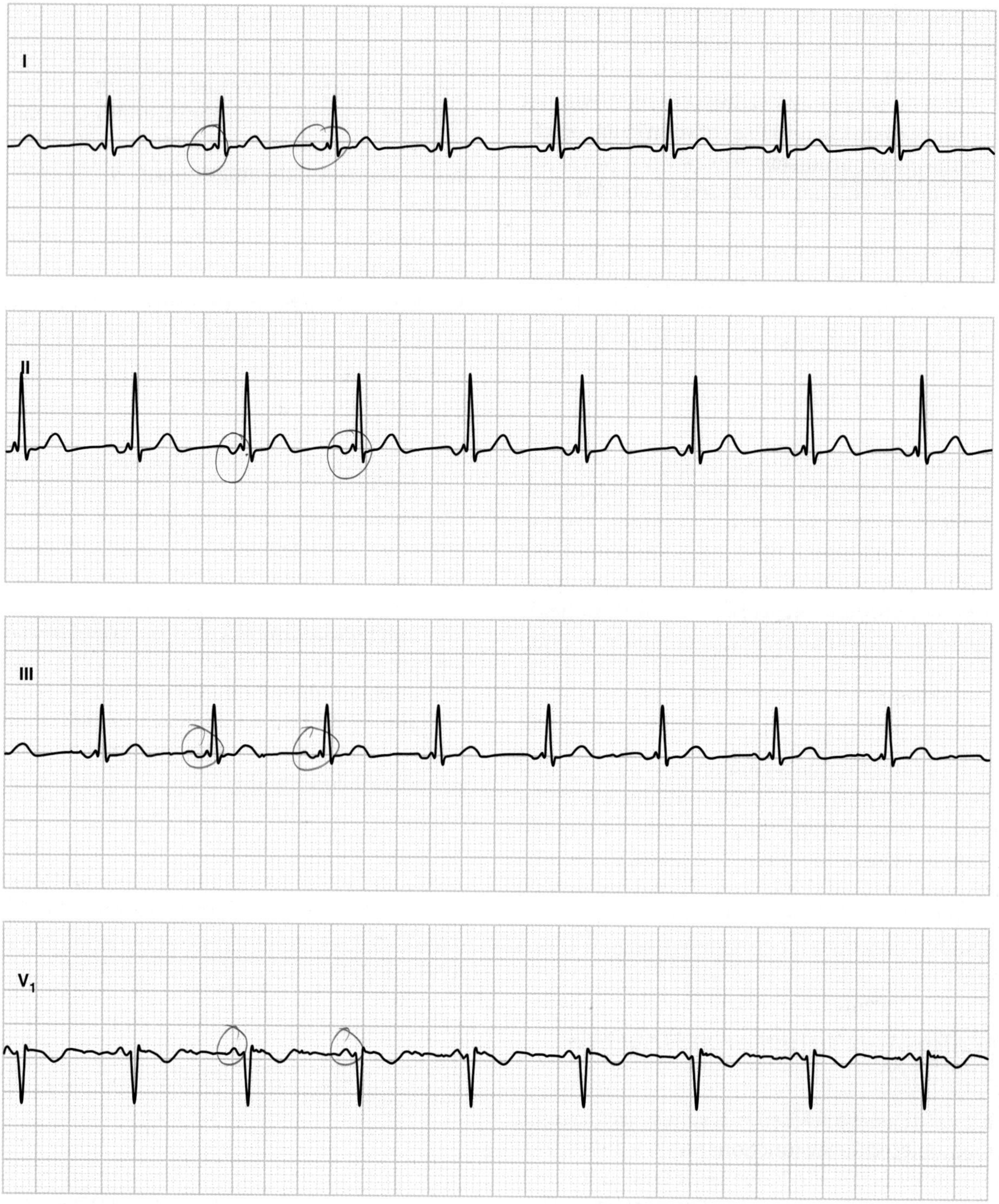

FIGURE 21-60 Accelerated junctional rhythm.

pathways in the ventricles. Enhanced automaticity and reentry can lead to PVCs, VT, and even VF. Ventricular dysrhythmias often are associated with myocardial ischemia or infarction.

The ventricle is the least efficient pacemaker of the heart. It usually generates only 20 to 40 impulses per minute. However, it may discharge at rates of up to 99 impulses per minute (accelerated idioventricular rhythm) or even faster (VT) because of increased automaticity. Dysrhythmias originating in the ventricles include ventricular escape complexes or rhythms, PVCs, VT, VF, and artificial pacemaker rhythm.

Because electrical impulses of ventricular origin start in the lower portion of the heart (the ventricular muscle, bundle branches, or Purkinje fibers), the electrical impulse must travel in a retrograde conduction pathway to depolarize the atria. The impulse may travel in an antegrade direction to depolarize the ventricles, depending on the site of initiation of the impulse. Regardless of the direction of depolarization, the normal, rapid conducting pathways are bypassed, producing three ECG features:

- QRS complexes are wide and bizarre in appearance. They are 0.12 second or greater in duration.
- P waves may be hidden in the QRS complex (which occurs because the atria are depolarized at about the same time as the ventricles). Alternatively, they may be superimposed on every second or third QRS complex when VT with **atrioventricular (AV) dissociation** (P waves that have no set relation to the QRS complexes) is present.
- ST segments usually deviate from baseline. T waves frequently are sloped off in the opposite direction from the QRS complex.

Ventricular Escape Complexes or Rhythms

Description

A **ventricular escape complex** or rhythm is also known as idioventricular rhythm (**FIGURE 21-61** and **FIGURE 21-62**). The dysrhythmia results when impulses from higher pacemakers fail to fire or to reach the ventricles. It also results when the rate of discharge of higher pacemaker sites falls to less than that of the ventricles. Like the junctional escape complex or rhythm, this dysrhythmia serves as a compensatory mechanism to prevent cardiac standstill.

Etiology

Ventricular escape rhythms occur when the rate of impulse formation of the dominant pacemaker (usually the SA node) falls below that of the ventricles and the pacemaker in the AV junction fails or falls below that of the pacemaker in the ventricles. This dysrhythmia often is seen as the first rhythm after defibrillation.

Rules for Interpretation (Lead II Monitoring)

Ventricular escape complexes or rhythms have the following characteristics on the ECG:

- **Rate.** Usually 20 to 40 beats/min; may be lower.
- **Rhythm.** The ventricular rhythm usually is regular but may be irregular.
- **QRS complex.** Generally exceeds 0.12 second and is bizarre in appearance. The shape of the QRS complex may vary in any given lead.
- **P waves.** May be absent. If they are present and have no set relationship to the QRS complex, a third-degree AV block should be suspected.
- **PR interval.** If P waves are present, the PR interval is variable and irregular.

Clinical Significance

A ventricular escape rhythm generally produces symptoms. This dysrhythmia is manifested by hypotension, decreased cardiac output, and decreased perfusion of the brain and other vital organs, often resulting in syncope and shock. Patient assessment is essential because the escape rhythm may have a pulse or (commonly) be nonperfusing (PEA).

Management

If the rhythm is perfusing, management is directed at increasing the heart rate by administering oxygen (if hypoxia is possible), TCP, and/or dopamine. Managing the escape rhythm with lidocaine likely would be lethal and, therefore, is contraindicated. If the rhythm is nonperfusing, BLS measures should be initiated and the protocol for pulseless arrest should be followed (**FIGURE 21-63**).

> CRITICAL THINKING
> Why might procainamide be harmful in this situation?

Premature Ventricular Complex

Description

A **premature ventricular complex (PVC)** is a single ectopic impulse arising from an irritable focus in either ventricle (bundle branches, Purkinje fibers, or

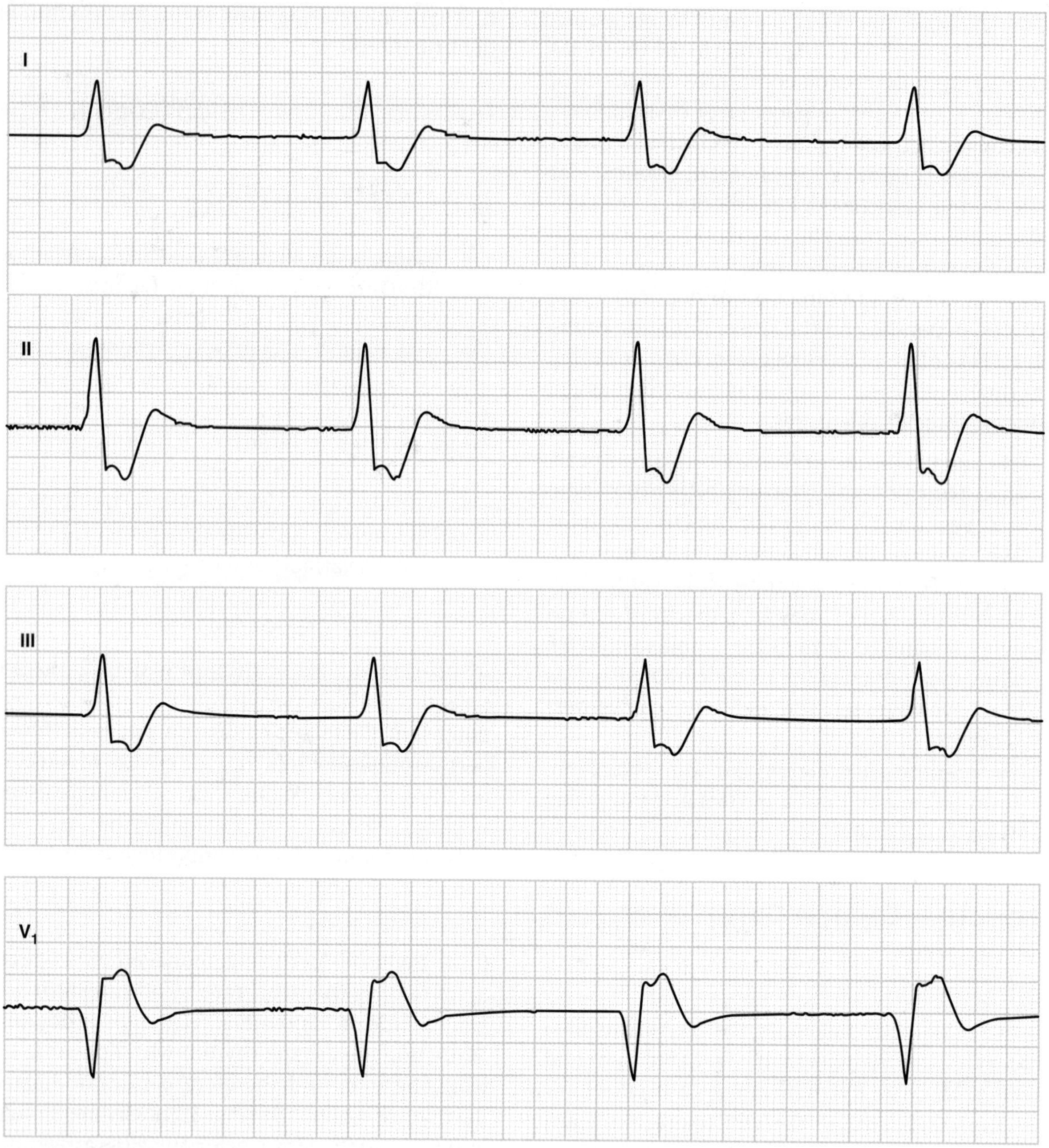

FIGURE 21-61 Ventricular escape rhythm.

ventricular muscle) that occurs earlier than the next expected sinus beat (**FIGURE 21-64**). This dysrhythmia is common and can occur with any underlying cardiac rhythm. The dysrhythmia results from enhanced automaticity or a reentry mechanism.

When the ventricles initiate a PVC, the atria may or may not respond and depolarize. If atrial depolarization does not occur, a P wave is seen on the ECG. If atrial depolarization does occur, the P wave occurs but often is hidden in the QRS complex. This happens because the timing and large electrical force of ventricular depolarization block out the electrical activity from the atrial depolarization. The altered sequence of ventricular depolarization results in a wide, bizarre QRS complex. Depolarization may be deflected in the opposite direction from the QRS complex in the underlying rhythm, or it may be deflected in the same direction (this depends on the location of the focus and the lead selected). The T wave that immediately follows the PVC usually is deflected in the opposite

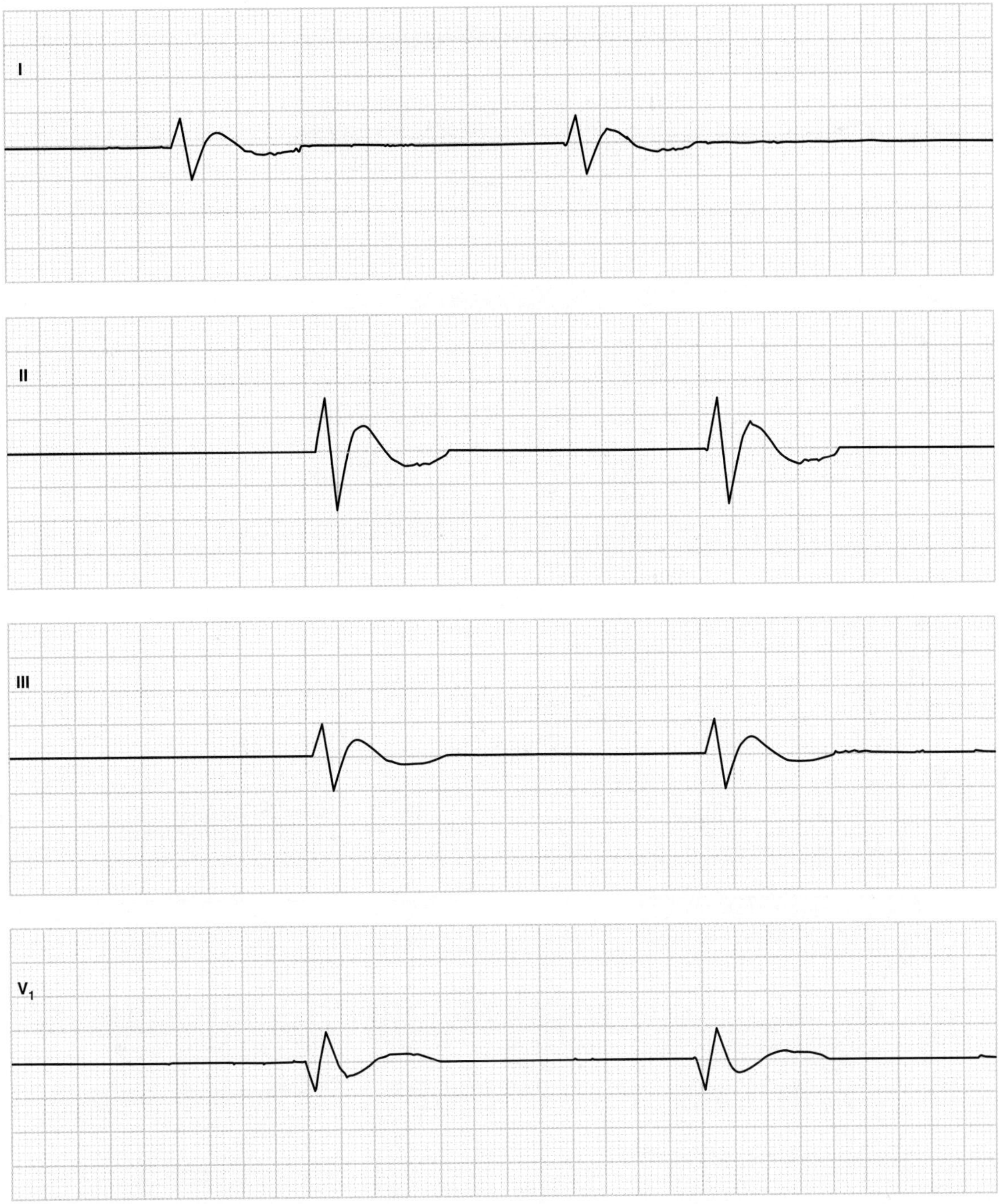

FIGURE 21-62 "Dying heart" (agonal) rhythm.

direction from the QRS complex of the PVC because of the altered sequence of repolarization.

A PVC usually does not depolarize the SA node or interrupt its rhythm (eg, the P wave of the underlying rhythm that follows the PVC occurs at its expected time but is obstructed by the PVC and finds the ventricles refractory). Therefore, the ectopic impulse usually is followed by a full **compensatory pause**. Compensatory pauses are confirmed by measuring the interval between the R wave before the PVC and the R wave after it. If the pause is compensatory, the distance is at least two times that of the R-R interval of the

CRITICAL THINKING

Why is the QRS deflection opposite the underlying rhythm?

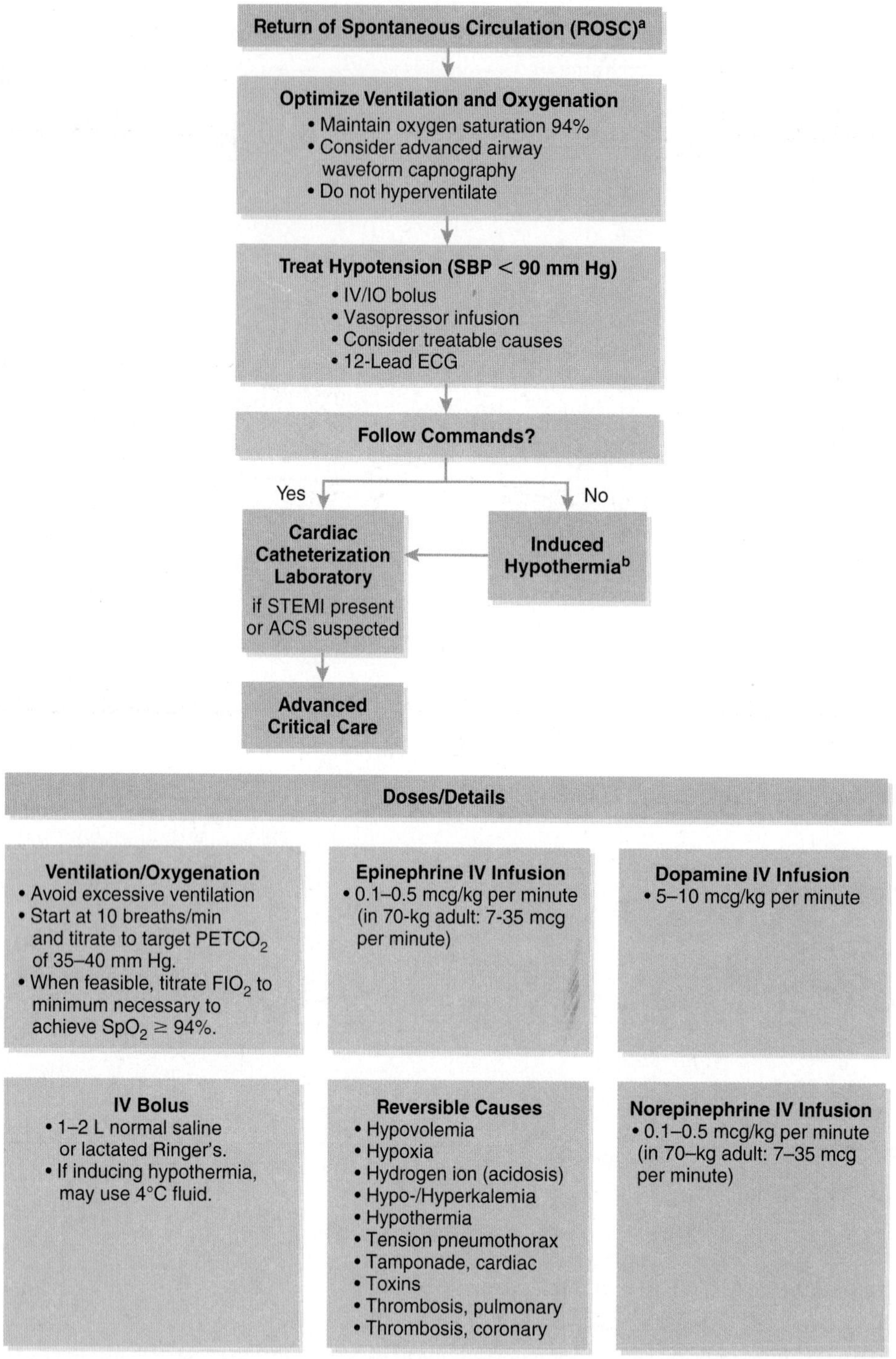
Return of Spontaneous Circulation (ROSC)[a]
Optimize Ventilation and Oxygenation
• Maintain oxygen saturation 94%
• Consider advanced airway waveform capnography
• Do not hyperventilate
Treat Hypotension (SBP < 90 mm Hg)
• IV/IO bolus
• Vasopressor infusion
• Consider treatable causes
• 12-Lead ECG
Follow Commands?
Yes
No
Cardiac Catheterization Laboratory
if STEMI present or ACS suspected
Induced Hypothermia[b]
Advanced Critical Care
Doses/Details
Ventilation/Oxygenation
• Avoid excessive ventilation
• Start at 10 breaths/min and titrate to target PETCO2 of 35–40 mm Hg.
• When feasible, titrate FIO2 to minimum necessary to achieve SpO2 ≥ 94%.
Epinephrine IV Infusion
• 0.1–0.5 mcg/kg per minute (in 70-kg adult: 7-35 mcg per minute)
Dopamine IV Infusion
• 5–10 mcg/kg per minute
IV Bolus
• 1–2 L normal saline or lactated Ringer's.
• If inducing hypothermia, may use 4°C fluid.
Reversible Causes
• Hypovolemia
• Hypoxia
• Hydrogen ion (acidosis)
• Hypo-/Hyperkalemia
• Hypothermia
• Tension pneumothorax
• Tamponade, cardiac
• Toxins
• Thrombosis, pulmonary
• Thrombosis, coronary
Norepinephrine IV Infusion
• 0.1–0.5 mcg/kg per minute (in 70–kg adult: 7–35 mcg per minute)

[a] *Sasson C, Rogers MA, Dahl J, Kellermann AL. Predictors of survival from out of hospital cardiac arrest: a systematic review and metanalysis Circ Cardiovasc Qual Outcomes. 2010;3:63-81.*
[b] *Bruel C, Parienti JJ, Marie W, Arrot X, Mild hypothermia during advanced life support, a preliminary study in out of hospital cardiac arrest. Crit Care. 2008;12: R31.*
**** Callaway CW, Donnino MW, Fink EL, Geocadin RG, Golan E, Kern KB, Leary M, Meurer WJ, Peberdy MA, Thompson TM, Zimmerman JL. Part 8: post-cardiac arrest care: 2015 American Heart Association Guidelines Update for Cardiopulmonary Resuscitation and Emergency Cardiovascular Care. Circulation 2015;132(suppl2):S465-S482.*

Abbreviations: ACS, acute coronary syndrome; ECG, electrocardiogram; F_{IO_2}, fraction of inspired oxygen; IO, intraosseous; IV, intravenous; P_{ETCO_2}, postapneic end-tidal carbon dioxide; SBP, systolic blood pressure; Sp_{O_2}, oxygen saturation as measured by a pulse oximeter; STEMI, ST-segment elevation myocardial infarction

FIGURE 21-63 Advanced cardiac life support pulseless arrest algorithm.

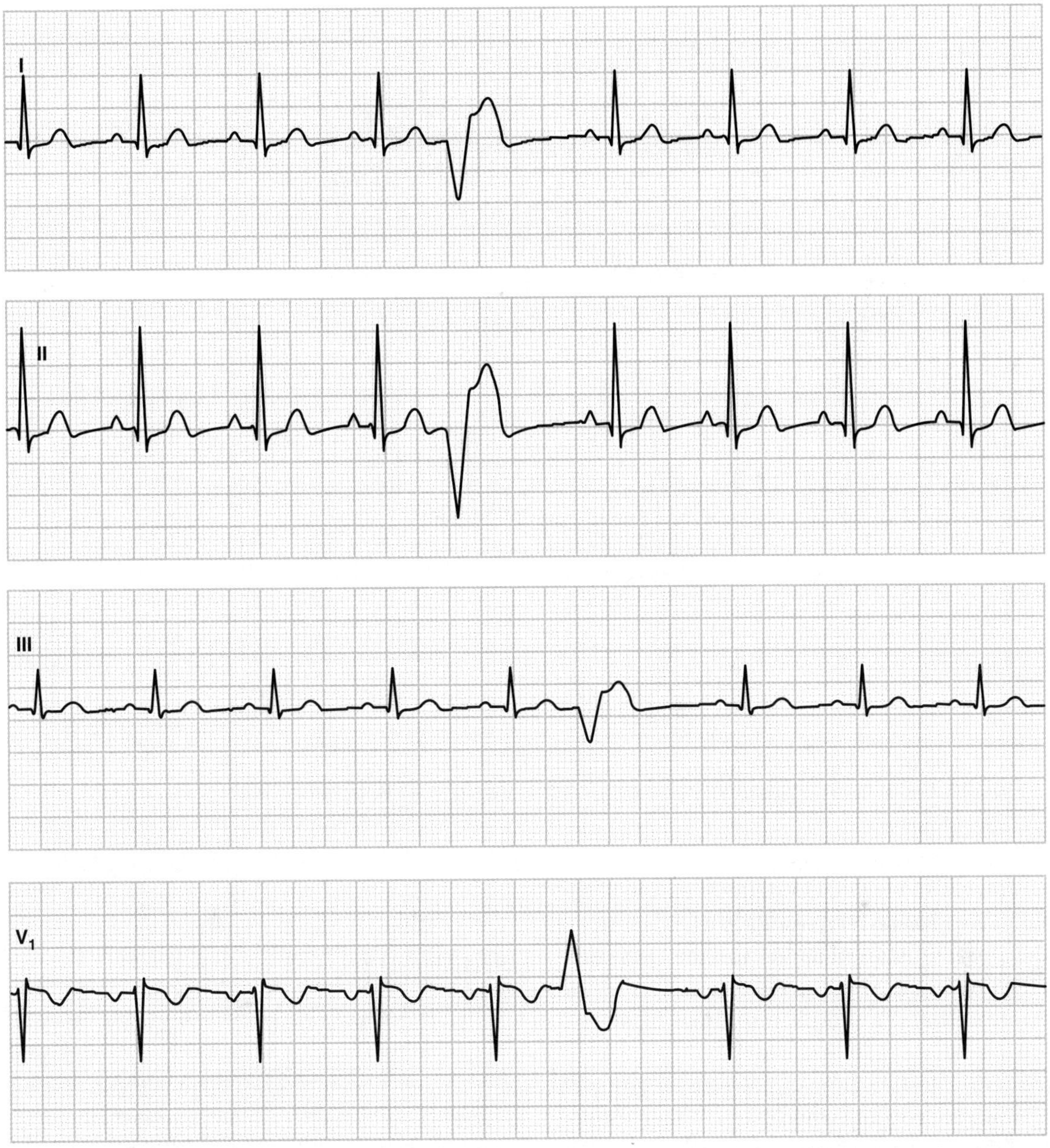

FIGURE 21-64 Premature ventricular complex.

underlying rhythm. At times, a PVC falls between two sinus beats without interrupting the rhythm; this is called an interpolated PVC (**FIGURE 21-65**).

PVCs may originate from a single ectopic pacemaker site (**unifocal premature ventricular complex [PVC]**) or from multiple sites in the ventricles (**multifocal premature ventricular complex [MVC]**) (**FIGURE 21-66**). Unifocal PVCs look alike. Multifocal PVCs have varying shapes and sizes.

Multifocal PVCs are considered higher risk than are unifocal PVCs because they result from increased myocardial irritability. A PVC that occurs at about the same time as ventricular activation by a normal

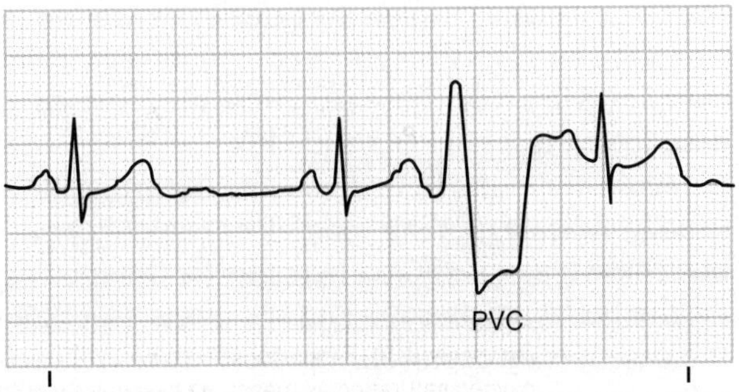

FIGURE 21-65 Interpolated premature ventricular complex.

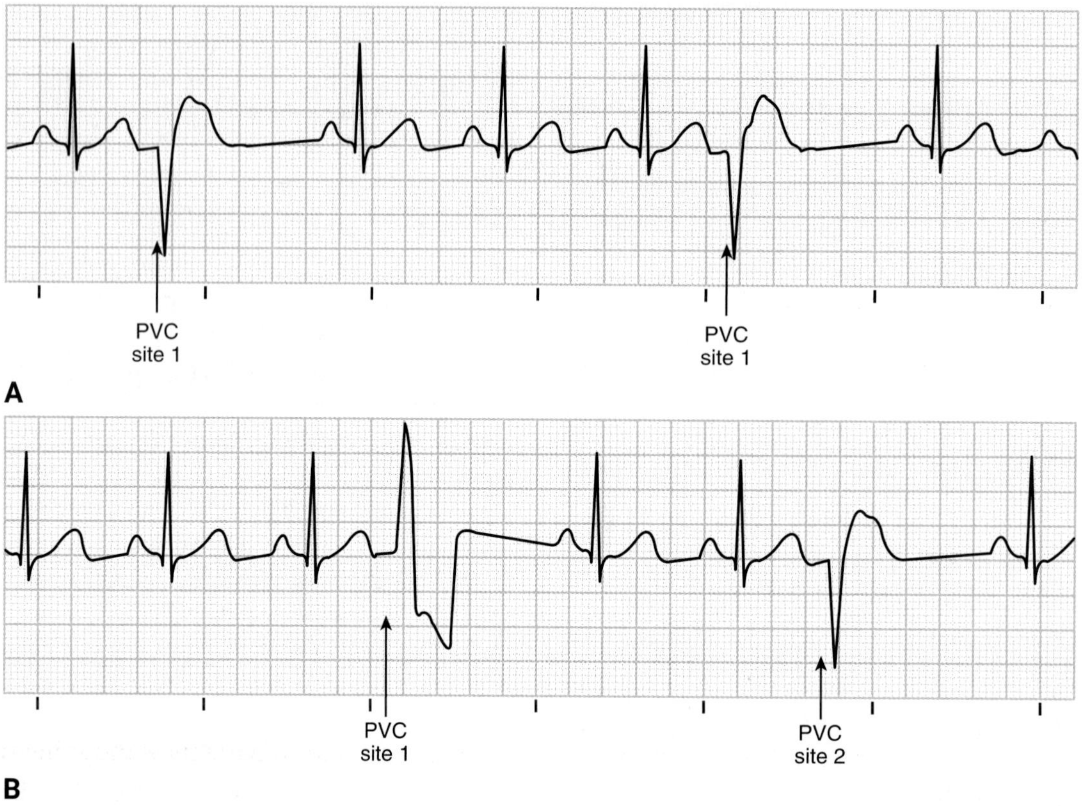

FIGURE 21-66 **A.** Unifocal premature ventricular complexes (PVCs). **B.** Multifocal PVCs.

impulse can cause ventricular depolarization at the same time. This **fusion beat** results in a QRS complex with the characteristics of a PVC and the QRS complex of the underlying rhythm (**FIGURE 21-67**). Fusion beats confirm that the ectopic impulse is located in the ventricle rather than in the atria.

Frequently, PVCs occur in patterns of grouped beating. **Bigeminy** occurs when every other complex is a PVC. **Trigeminy** occurs when every third complex is a PVC (**FIGURE 21-68**). Quadrigeminy occurs when every fourth complex is a PVC. Consecutive PVCs that are not separated by a complex of the underlying rhythm also can occur on the ECG: couplets are two PVCs in a row; triplets are three PVCs in a row (a definition for VT); salvos are three or more ventricular complexes in a row. These terms also may be used to describe patterns of PACs and PJCs.

As do multifocal PVCs, frequently occurring PVCs usually indicate that the ventricles are highly irritable. These types of PVCs can trigger life-threatening dysrhythmias, such as VT and VF. This is especially the case if they occur during the T wave (relative refractory phase) of the cardiac cycle. During this period, the heart muscle is at its greatest electrical instability because in the relative refractory period, some of the ventricular muscle fibers may be partly repolarized, others may be completely repolarized, and still others may be completely refractory. Stimulation of the ventricles in the vulnerable period by an electrical impulse, such as a PVC, cardiac pacemaker, or cardioversion, may cause VF or VT. The occurrence of a ventricular depolarization during the relative refractory period is known as the **R-on-T phenomenon** (**FIGURE 21-69**).

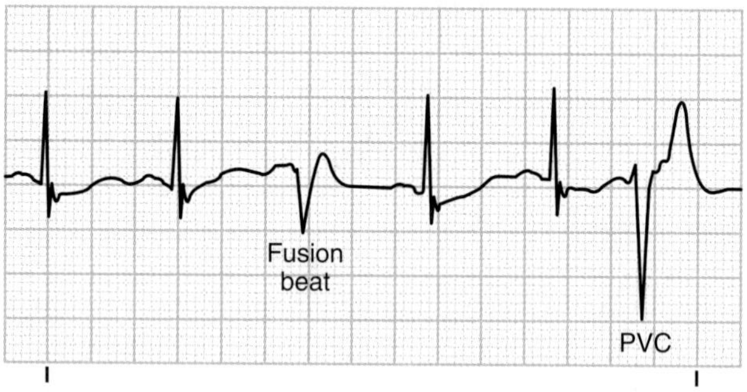

FIGURE 21-67 Fusion beat with premature ventricular complex.

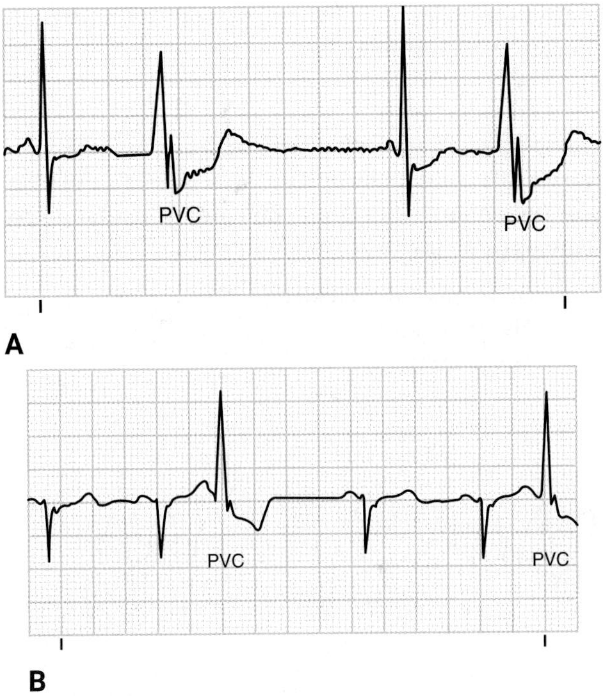

FIGURE 21-68 **A.** Bigeminy (unifocal premature ventricular complexes [PVCs]). **B.** Trigeminy (unifocal PVCs).

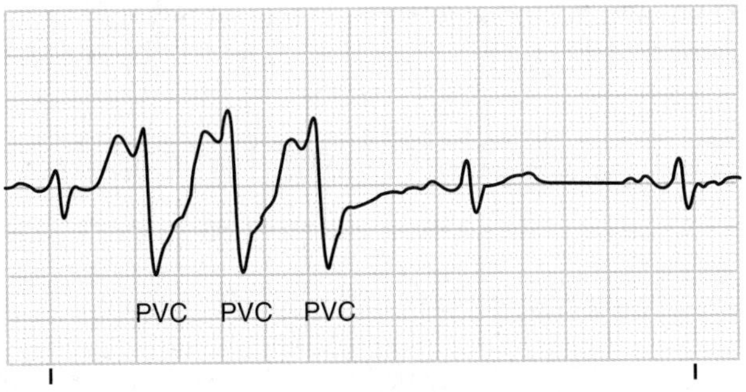

FIGURE 21-69 R-on-T phenomenon (unifocal premature ventricular complexes).

Etiology

Isolated PVCs do occur in healthy people without apparent cause. They usually have no significance. Pathologic PVCs usually are a result of one or more of the following:

- Myocardial ischemia
- Hypoxia
- Acid–base and electrolyte imbalance
- Hypokalemia
- Heart failure
- Increased catecholamine and sympathetic tone (as in emotional stress)
- Ingestion of stimulants (alcohol, caffeine, tobacco)
- Drug toxicity
- Sympathomimetic drugs (cocaine; stimulants such as phencyclidine, epinephrine, and methamphetamine)

Rules for Interpretation (Lead II Monitoring)

PVCs have the following characteristics on the ECG:

- **Rate.** Depends on the underlying rhythm and the number of PVCs.
- **Rhythm.** PVCs interrupt the regularity of the underlying rhythm.
- **QRS complex.** Equal to or greater than 0.12 second.
- **P waves.** Frequently distorted and bizarre P waves may be present or absent. If present, they usually are of the underlying rhythm and have no relationship to the PVC.
- **PR interval.** None.

Clinical Significance

PVCs that occur in patients without heart disease usually do not produce serious signs and symptoms, although these patients may complain of "skipped beats." PVCs that occur with heart disease (myocardial ischemia) may result from enhanced automaticity, a reentry mechanism, or both. These PVCs may trigger lethal ventricular dysrhythmias. PVCs do not permit complete ventricular filling. Also, they may produce a diminished or nonpalpable pulse (nonperfusing PVC). If the PVCs occur often enough and early enough in the cardiac cycle, cardiac output drops.

Warning signs of serious ventricular dysrhythmias in patients with myocardial ischemia include frequent PVCs, multifocal PVCs, early PVCs (R-on-T phenomenon), and patterns of grouped beating.

Management

PVCs that occur in patients without symptoms and without known heart disease seldom require treatment. In patients with myocardial ischemia, frequent PVCs must be treated promptly with oxygen and beta blockers.[19] At the hospital, the serum potassium level should be checked immediately. Hypokalemia, if present, should be treated promptly.

Ventricular Tachycardia

Description

Ventricular tachycardia (VT) is a dysrhythmia defined by three or more consecutive ventricular complexes that occur at a rate of more than 100 beats/min (**FIGURE 21-70**). This dysrhythmia overrides the primary pacemaker. It starts suddenly and is triggered by a PVC. During VT, the atria and ventricles are not beating in step with each other. If VT continues, the patient's condition may become unstable. VT can produce unconsciousness, and occasionally it can lead to loss of a perfusing pulse. However, some patients in VT may be able to walk and talk. The misconception that VT cannot be associated with a reasonable blood pressure may result in inappropriate patient management. The origin of VT is enhanced automaticity or reentry.

Etiology

Like PVCs, VT usually occurs in the presence of myocardial ischemia or significant cardiac disease. Other causes of VT include the following:

- Acid–base and electrolyte imbalance
- Hypokalemia
- Heart failure

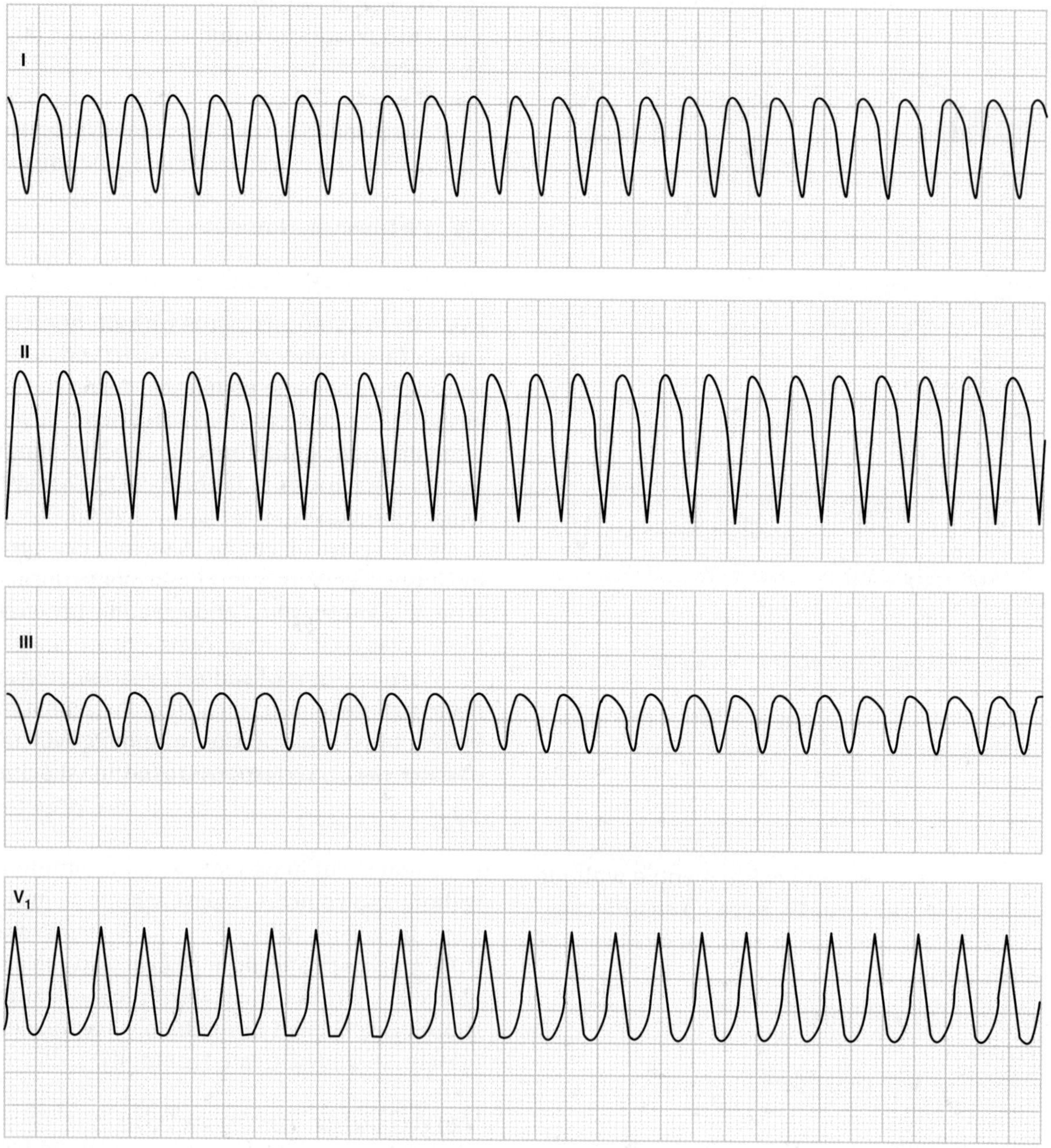

FIGURE 21-70 Ventricular tachycardia.

- Increased catecholamine and sympathetic tone (as in emotional stress)
- Ingestion of stimulants (alcohol, caffeine, tobacco)
- Drug toxicity (digitalis, tricyclic antidepressants)
- Sympathomimetic drugs (cocaine, methamphetamines)
- Prolonged QT interval (may be caused by drugs or metabolic problems or may be congenital)

NOTE

Patients who have had a previous MI with subsequent tachycardias and who are now experiencing a wide-complex tachycardia very likely are in VT.

Rules for Interpretation (Lead II Monitoring)

VT has the following characteristics on the ECG:

- **Rate.** Usually between 100 and 250 beats/min.
- **Rhythm.** Usually regular (unless drug induced) but may be slightly irregular.
- **QRS complex.** Equal to or greater than 0.12 second and usually distorted and bizarre. The QRS complexes generally are identical, but if fusion beats are present, one or more QRS complexes may differ in size, shape, and direction.
- **P waves.** May be absent. If present, P waves have no set relation to the QRS complex (AV dissociation). P waves occur at a slower rate than the ventricular focus and are superimposed on the QRS complexes.
- **PR interval.** If P waves are present, the PR interval varies widely.

NOTE

AV dissociation may precipitate **cannon A waves**. These are waves of pulse pressure that are visible in the jugular veins of a patient in VT. Cannon A waves result when the right atrium pumps against a closed tricuspid valve; the waves of pressure consequently are directed into the jugular veins. AV dissociation is diagnostic of VT. The lack of AV dissociation, however, does not exclude VT.

Modified from: Vereckei A. Current algorithms for the diagnosis of wide QRS complex tachycardias. *Curr Cardio Rev.* 2014;10(3):262-276.

Clinical Significance

VT usually indicates significant heart disease. The rapid rate and the loss of atrial kick cause a drop in cardiac output and decreased coronary artery and cerebral perfusion. The severity of symptoms varies with the rate of the VT and how much heart disease is present. VT may be perfusing or nonperfusing; that is, it may produce a pulse or it may not. VT also may lead to VF.

Management

The treatment of patients with VT is based on their signs and symptoms and whether torsades de pointes is present. **Torsades de pointes** is a type of polymorphic VT (**FIGURE 21-71**). As with other SVTs, the paramedic should obtain a history and identify the rhythm (see Figure 21-53). If the patient is stable, a 12-lead ECG should be obtained.

Treatment of VT depends on whether the QRS complex is monomorphic (having the same shape) or polymorphic (having varying morphology). The paramedic should remember, however, that any wide-complex tachycardia that occurs with serious signs and symptoms (eg, chest pain, dyspnea, decreased level of consciousness, hypotension or other signs of shock) requires immediate cardioversion. In addition, patients who have VT without a pulse should be treated as if the rhythm were VF.

Treatment guidelines for **monomorphic ventricular tachycardia (VT)** are based on clinical signs and symptoms. Signs and symptoms of failing heart function, such as acute heart failure, signs of shock, ischemic chest discomfort, and an acute decreased level of consciousness, indicate clinical instability. Monomorphic VT in a stable patient is managed with procainamide, amiodarone, or sotalol. Unstable patients with monomorphic VT should receive immediate synchronized cardioversion, beginning with an initial shock of 100 J. If no response to the first shock is seen, the dose should be increased (in stepwise fashion)

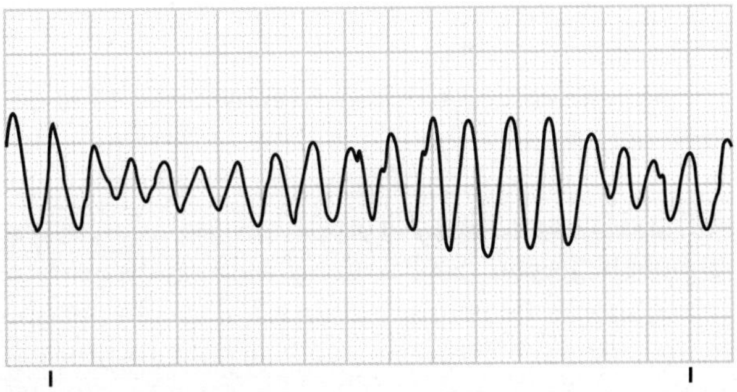

FIGURE 21-71 Torsades de pointes.

according to manufacturer recommendations.[9] When unstable VT is witnessed, a **precordial thump** may be performed while cardioversion is being immediately prepared.

Precordial Thump

Monitored adult patients whose rhythm is observed to be unstable VT may be treated with a single precordial thump provided that a defibrillator is readily available and immediately being prepared for use. (A precordial thump may cause VT to deteriorate to asystole, VF, or PEA.) A precordial thump may terminate a dysrhythmia by causing ventricular depolarization and the resumption of an organized rhythm. To deliver a precordial thump, the paramedic's arm and wrist should be parallel to the long axis of the sternum to avoid rib fractures and other injury. The thump is delivered to the midsternum with the heel of the fist from a height of 10 to 12 inches (25 to 30 cm). A conscious patient should be advised of the procedure.

> DID YOU KNOW?
>
> **Cardiac Ejection Fraction**
>
> The **cardiac ejection fraction** is the percentage of ventricular blood volume released during a contraction. This measurement most often refers to the left ventricle (left ventricular ejection fraction [LVEF]). The LVEF is obtained through echocardiography, cardiac catheterization, or heart scans with magnetic resonance imaging, computed tomography, and nuclear medicine (nuclear stress test).
>
> A normal LVEF ranges from 50% to 70%. The LVEF may be lower if the heart muscle has been damaged by a heart attack, heart muscle disease (cardiomyopathy), or other causes. An LVEF of 35% to 40% may confirm a diagnosis of systolic heart failure. An LVEF below 25% increases the risk of life-threatening dysrhythmias that can cause sudden cardiac arrest and sudden cardiac death. An implantable cardioverter-defibrillator (ICD) often is recommended for these patients.

Polymorphic ventricular tachycardia (VT) can degenerate into VF quickly and therefore requires immediate intervention. If the patient has polymorphic VT and is unstable (as is often the case), the rhythm should be treated as VF with high-energy unsynchronized shocks. (Synchronization is not usually possible with irregular wave forms, such as polymorphic VT.) If the rhythm is torsades de pointes, it may be the result of a prolonged QT interval. Medications, such as procainamide or amiodarone, that prolong the QT interval should be discontinued and IV magnesium sulfate should be given.

> NOTE
>
> Drugs given to treat dysrhythmias also can cause dysrhythmias (proarrhythmic). Sequential use of two or more antidysrhythmic drugs increases the incidence of bradycardias, hypotension, and torsades de pointes. Avoiding the use of more than one antidysrhythmic agent in treating narrow or wide QRS complex tachydysrhythmias is strongly recommended. In most cases, if an adequate dose of a single drug is unsuccessful in ending the dysrhythmia, synchronized cardioversion is the next treatment.

Ventricular Fibrillation

Description

Ventricular fibrillation (VF) is a chaotic ventricular rhythm that results in pulselessness (**FIGURE 21-72**). The cause of VF is multifocal reentry in the ventricles. The electrical impulses initiated by the multiple ectopic ventricular sites do not allow the heart to fully depolarize and repolarize. As a result, organized ventricular contraction does not occur. VF is the most common initial rhythm disturbance in sudden cardiac arrest.

Etiology

VF may be precipitated by PVCs, R-on-T phenomenon (in rare cases), or a sustained VT. Other causes include the following:

- Myocardial ischemia
- AMI
- Third-degree AV block with a slow ventricular escape rhythm
- Cardiomyopathy
- Digitalis toxicity
- Hypoxia
- Acidosis
- Electrolyte imbalance (hypokalemia, hyperkalemia, submersion)
- Electrical injury
- Drug overdose or toxicity (cocaine, tricyclic antidepressants)

Rules for Interpretation (All Leads)

VF has the following characteristics on the ECG:

- **Rate.** No coordinated ventricular contractions are present. The unsynchronized ventricular impulses occur at rates of 300 to 500 beats/min.

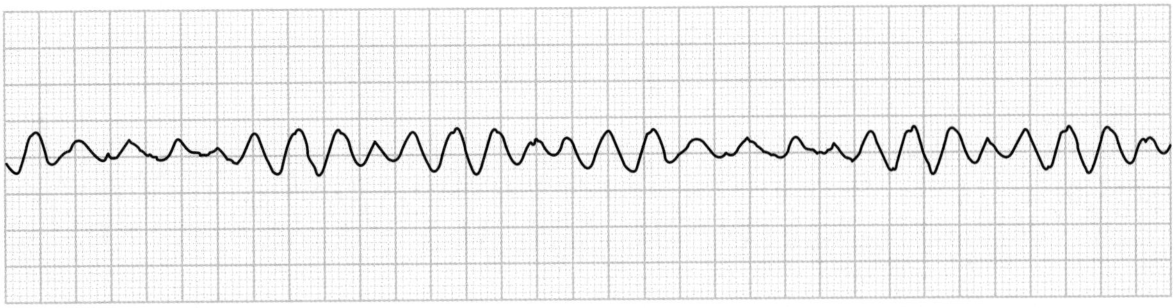

FIGURE 21-72 Ventricular fibrillation.

- **Rhythm.** No organized rhythm.
- **QRS complex.** Absent.
- **P waves.** Absent.
- **PR interval.** Absent.

Because organized depolarizations of the atria and ventricles are absent, P waves, QRS complexes, ST segments, and T waves are absent. Ventricular fibrillatory waves are seen on the ECG screen as bizarre, rounded, or pointed. They also appear considerably different in shape. They also vary at random from positive to negative. These waves represent twitching of small individual groups of muscle fibers. Fibrillatory waves of less than 3 mm in amplitude are called **fine ventricular fibrillation (VF)**. Those greater than 3 mm are called **coarse ventricular fibrillation (VF)** (**FIGURE 21-73**). The fibrillatory waves may be so fine they appear as a flat line, resembling asystole.

NOTE

Coarse VF usually indicates the recent onset of VF. It can be more readily converted by prompt defibrillation. The presence of fine VF that approaches asystole often means that a considerable delay has occurred since collapse. Successful defibrillation is more difficult in these cases.

Clinical Significance

VF results in cessation of circulating blood flow. The dysrhythmia initially may result in light-headedness. VF is followed within seconds by loss of consciousness, apnea, and, if left untreated, death.

Management

For adult resuscitation, management of VF and pulseless VT is the most important sequence because most adult cardiac arrests result from these two rhythm disturbances. Also, most successful resuscitations result from the appropriate management of these two dysrhythmias (see Figure 21-63).[9] VF and nonperfusing VT are managed alike: BLS (if a defibrillator is not immediately available), effective and uninterrupted chest compressions with minimal pre- and post-shock pauses, early defibrillation, IV/IO access, and delivery of these interventions in an organized and choreographed "pit crew" management style. Pharmacologic therapy may also be initiated but is now understood to play a less important role compared with excellent chest compressions and early defibrillation.[20] An advanced airway with capnographic monitoring should be inserted after initial CPR, defibrillation, and drug administration.[9] Other interventions may be performed to treat any identified underlying cause of arrest.

Artificial Pacemaker Rhythms

Description

An **artificial pacemaker** generates a rhythm by regular electrical stimulation of the heart through an electrode implanted in the heart (**FIGURE 21-74**). The electrode is connected to a pulse generator with power source (a battery cell implanted subcutaneously, typically in the right or left side of the chest). The tip of the pacemaker wire is at the apex of the right ventricle (ventricular pacemaker), in the right atrium (atrial pacemaker), or in both locations (dual-chamber pacemaker). One brand of pacemaker is leadless and has no wires. These devices are placed in patients with complete heart block. Pacemakers also are used by patients who have episodes of severe symptomatic bradycardia. Triple-chamber (biventricular) pacemakers have one lead in the right atrium and a lead in each ventricle. They are used in patients with heart failure and improve synchronized contraction of the ventricles to enhance cardiac output.

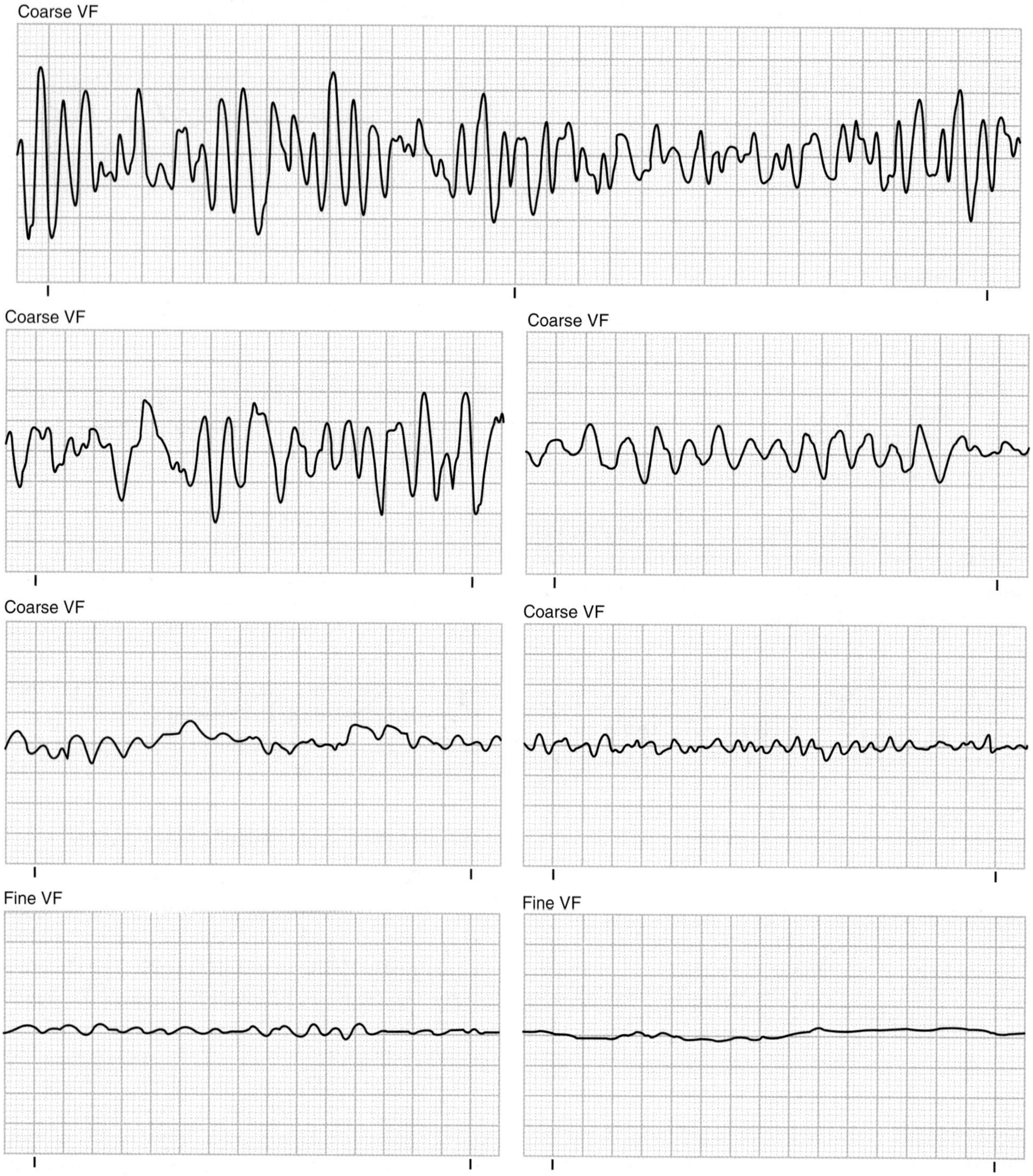

FIGURE 21-73 Coarse and fine ventricular fibrillation.

Modern pacemakers fire only if the patient's own rate drops below the preset rate of the pacemaker (they thereby act as an escape rhythm). These are known as demand pacemakers. Atrial and ventricular demand pacemakers pace the atria and ventricles when the intrinsic rate of the paced chamber drops dangerously low. Atrial synchronous ventricular pacemakers are synchronized with the patient's atrial rhythm. This type of pacemaker paces the ventricle after the patient's atria contract. This pacemaker is useful in patients who have normal sinus node activity but have various degrees of AV block. AV sequential

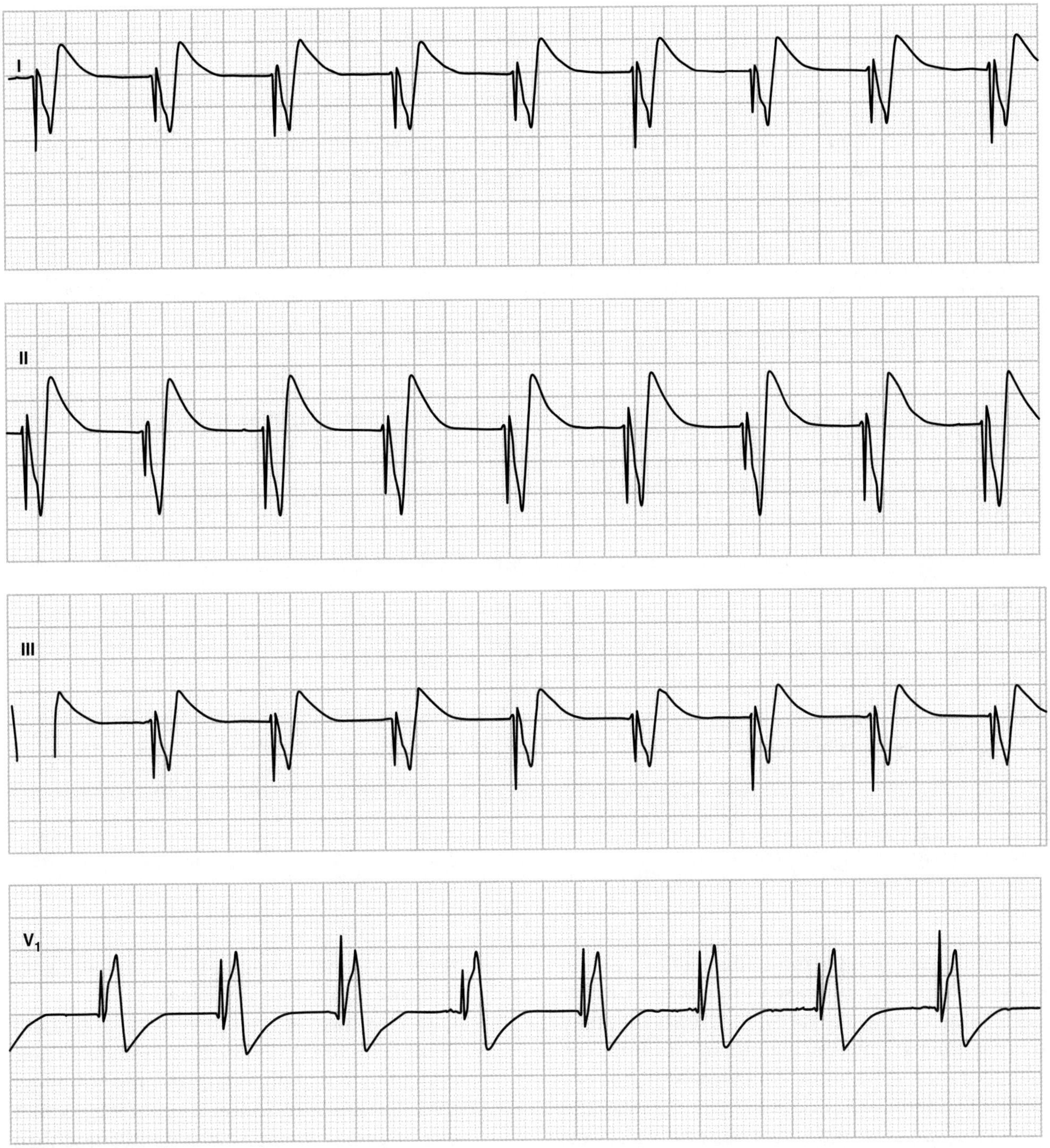

FIGURE 21-74 Artificial pacemaker rhythms.

pacemakers pace the atria first and then the ventricles when normal impulses are absent or slowed in either or both chambers. If regular atrial activity is too slow, for example, the two chambers are paced sequentially to maintain the atrial kick. If the atrial rate is adequate, the atrial pacer does not fire. The ventricular pacemaker still fires if the ventricular rate is below a preset rate. This pacemaker is ideal for sick sinus syndrome and sinus arrest.

Almost all pacemakers are rate-responsive. They can adjust their pacing rates to a patient's needs by sensing when cardiac output should be increased. Several methods of sensing metabolic activity are used. However, most detect patient movement or

NOTE

With cardiac arrest, blood flow stops. Chest compressions create a small amount of blood flow to the vital organs, such as the brain and heart. The better the compressions, the more blood flow they produce. Chest compression depth is one of the main determinants of coronary perfusion pressure (CPP), which in turn is a primary predictor of survival. The AHA recommends that chest compressions be "hard and fast" and at a rate of 100 to 120 per minute and a depth of at least 2 inches (5 cm). The upstroke of the compression must permit full chest recoil to allow the heart to refill before the next compression. When possible, direct feedback regarding depth and rate of chest compressions should be used to ensure quality CPR during the resuscitation. Rescuers should minimize interruptions in chest compressions. Pauses for defibrillation, airway placement, and other tasks are limited to less than 10 seconds. Compressions should resume immediately after defibrillation. Changing compressors every 2 minutes maximizes CPR quality. Continuous chest compressions should be performed after an advanced airway is in place when two or more rescuers are present. After the advanced airway is placed, one breath is given every 6 seconds. (When chest compressions are interrupted, blood flow stops and CPP is reduced.)

The EMS crew should not interrupt CPR while preparing for defibrillation. If the rhythm is shockable, one shock should be delivered, and then CPR should be resumed immediately, beginning with chest compressions. Perishock pauses are less than 10 seconds. CPR should be continued for another five cycles (or about 2 minutes), before the rhythm is checked again. Even when a shock restores an organized ECG, several minutes are required for a normal rhythm to return and for the heart to create more blood flow. A brief period of chest compressions can deliver oxygen and sources of energy to the heart, increasing the likelihood that the heart will be able to pump blood effectively after the defibrillatory shock. In addition, chest compressions should not be interrupted to charge a defibrillator or to "clear" the patient for shock delivery while the defibrillator is charging. (The patient should be cleared immediately before the shock is delivered, with no time wasted in between.)

Rhythm checks should be brief, and pulse checks should be performed only if an organized rhythm is observed (see Figure 21-63).

Postevent monitoring should be performed to ensure that the chest compression fraction (CCF) (proportion of CPR time when chest compressions are performed) is optimal. Research findings regarding the effects of CCF on survival vary. One study found that greater CCF is associated with up to a threefold increase in survival to hospital discharge in patients in VF and an upward trend in survival in non-VF out-of-hospital arrests.

Modified from: American Heart Association. *2015 Handbook of Emergency Cardiovascular Care for Healthcare Providers*. Dallas, TX: American Heart Association; 2015; American Heart Association Guidelines for Cardiopulmonary Resuscitation and Emergency Cardiovascular Care. *Circulation*. 2015;132:S313-S314; Christenson J, Andrusiek D, Everson-Stewart S, et al. Chest compression fraction determines survival in patients with out-of-hospital ventricular fibrillation. *Circulation*. 2009;120(13):1241-1247; Vaillancourt C, Everson-Stewart S, Christenson J, et al. The impact of increased chest compression fraction on return of spontaneous circulation for out-of-hospital cardiac arrest patients not in ventricular fibrillation. *Resuscitation*. 2011;82(12):1501-1507; and Sutton RM, Friess SH, Maltese MR, et al. Hemodynamic-directed cardiopulmonary resuscitation during in-hospital cardiac arrest. *Resuscitation*. 2014;85(8):983-986.

respiratory rate to determine the best firing rate. These devices can increase both cardiac output and tolerance of physical activity. At times they may increase the patient's pacing rate inappropriately, such as if they sense muscle movement that is not caused by increased patient activity. Because the pacemaker spikes are difficult to visualize in all leads, fast pacemaker rates can easily be misinterpreted as VT. Perform a 12-lead ECG if time permits.

Rules for Interpretation (Lead II Monitoring)

Artificial pacemaker rhythms have the following characteristics on the ECG:

- **Rate.** Varies according to the preset rate of the pacemaker. Typically the rate is 60 to 80 beats/min.
- **Rhythm.** Regular if pacing is constant; irregular if pacing occurs only on demand.
- **QRS complex.** If pacemaker-induced QRS complexes are 0.12 second or greater. Their appearance usually is bizarre, resembling a PVC. The most common morphology is that of a left bundle branch block (LBBB; described later in the chapter) because the pacemaker lead usually resides within the right ventricle. The pacemaker is said to have electrical capture if each pacemaker spike elicits a QRS complex. If only the atria are paced, the QRS complexes usually are normal, provided no bundle branch block is present. With demand pacemakers, some of the patient's own QRS complexes may be present. These normal QRS complexes occur without pacemaker spikes.

- **P waves.** May be present or absent, normal, or abnormal. The relationship of the P waves to the pacemaker (QRS) complex varies by type of artificial pacemaker. Pacemaker spikes precede QRS complexes induced by ventricular pacemakers, whereas dual-chamber pacemakers also produce an atrial spike followed by a P wave. The pacemaker spike is a narrow deflection that represents the electrical discharge of the pacemaker. Pacemaker spikes indicate only that a pacemaker is discharging. They provide no information about ventricular contraction or perfusion.
- **PR interval.** The presence and duration of PR intervals depend on the underlying rhythm and vary by the type of artificial pacemaker.

CRITICAL THINKING

If a pacemaker fails, what rhythms might you see on the monitor?

Clinical Significance

Pacemaker spikes indicate that the patient's heart rate is regulated by an artificial pacemaker. Pacemaker spikes followed by QRS complexes indicate electrical capture. If spikes do not elicit a QRS complex, the pacemaker is not capturing the ventricle electrically. Therefore, no ventricular contraction occurs. A large percentage of pacemaker failures occur within the first month after implantation (BOX 21-7).

Management

Pacemaker failure is a true emergency. It requires immediate recognition and rapid transport for definitive care (which may include battery replacement or temporary pacemaker insertion). Paramedics should not delay transport to attempt to stabilize these patients. Five principles apply to the treatment of patients with pacemakers:

1. When examining an unconscious patient, be alert for battery packs implanted under the skin. Also be alert for any medical alert information.
2. Manage all dysrhythmias following the appropriate algorithm.
3. Manage ventricular irritability with appropriate drug therapy without fear of suppressing ventricular response to a pacemaker rhythm if pacemaker failure is not a factor.

BOX 21-7 Four Possible Causes of Pacemaker Malfunction

1. **Battery failure.** Currently most implanted pacemakers use a lithium-iodine cell power source. This source provides stable voltage output for about 80% to 90% of the life of the battery. (The battery life runs 10 years or longer.) Battery failure usually slows the pacemaker rate. It also usually reduces the spike amplitude. If the battery fails, the patient may have bradycardia or asystole.
2. **Runaway pacemaker.** In this condition, the pacemaker develops rapid discharge rates that may reach 300 beats/min. The problem occurs as the batteries reduce their voltage output. This type of failure rarely is seen in pacemakers used today because the newer power sources provide a gradual increase in rate as the batteries run low.
3. **Failure of the sensing device in demand pacemakers.** Demand pacemakers may fail to shut off when patients have an adequate rate of their own. When this occurs, a competition develops between the natural and artificial pacemakers of the heart. The pacemaker may discharge during the vulnerable period of the cardiac cycle, which may result in dysrhythmias.
4. **Failure to capture.** Failure of the pacemaker to capture may have a variety of causes, including battery failure, loose or broken catheter electrode wires, inoperable electrodes, and a shift in the location of the catheter tip. In such cases, pacemaker spikes usually are present. However, they are not followed by P waves or QRS complexes.

4. For patients with artificial pacemakers, defibrillate in the usual manner. However, do not place defibrillation pads directly over the implanted battery pack.
5. TCP, if indicated, may be used in the usual manner.

Asystole

Description

Asystole (cardiac standstill) refers to the absence of all ventricular activity (**FIGURE 21-75**).

Etiology

Asystole is the final common pathway of cardiac arrest. It refers to the absence of all electrical activity. Untreated VF and PEA will eventually become ventricular asystole in the absence of **return of spontaneous circulation (ROSC)**.

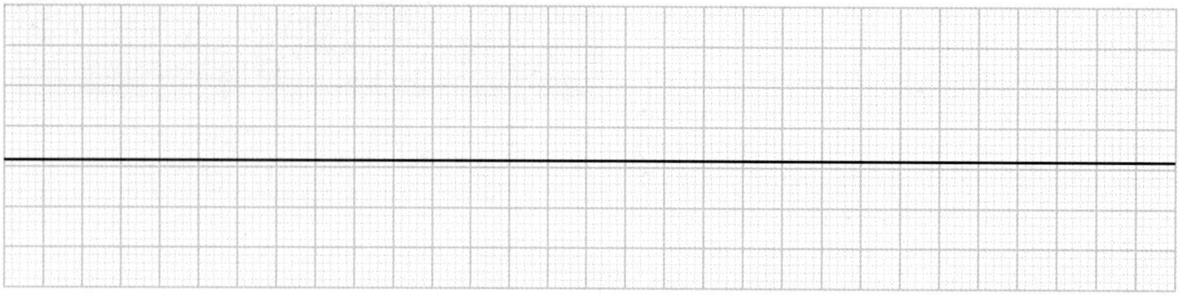

FIGURE 21-75 Ventricular asystole.

Rules for Interpretation (All Leads)

Asystole has the following characteristics on the ECG:

- **Rate.** Absent
- **Rhythm.** Absent
- **QRS complexes.** Absent
- **P waves.** Absent
- **PR interval.** Absent

Clinical Significance

Asystole is the absence of endogenous cardiac activity and is a poor prognostic factor in a patient with cardiac arrest. In the course of a prolonged resuscitation, it often confirms death.

Management

The management of asystole is BLS with effective CPR, and epinephrine administration. The paramedic must establish an advanced airway with an ET tube or supraglottic airway with capnographic monitoring when possible (see Figure 21-63). If fine VF is suspected, defibrillation is indicated. However, defibrillating asystole "just in case" is not recommended. Termination of resuscitation efforts in the prehospital setting, after meeting medical protocol (described later in this chapter), is indicated in this situation. Potential reversible causes of asystole should be considered before cessation of resuscitative efforts. These causes include hypoxia, hypovolemia, hyperkalemia, hypokalemia, hypothermia, tension pneumothorax, cardiac tamponade, **ST-segment elevation myocardial infarction (STEMI)**, pulmonary edema, drug overdose, and acidosis.[9]

> CRITICAL THINKING
>
> What is the benefit to the community and to the patient's family if resuscitation is halted in the field after all appropriate guidelines have been followed?

Pulseless Electrical Activity

The term **pulseless electrical activity (PEA)** (also known as electromechanical dissociation) (**FIGURE 21-76**) is defined as the absence of a detectable pulse and the presence of electrical activity other than VT or VF.[7] The outcome of PEA almost always is poor unless an underlying cause can be identified and corrected. The paramedic must maintain circulation for the patient with basic and advanced life support techniques while searching for a correctable cause.

> CRITICAL THINKING
>
> What rhythms might you see on the monitor when a patient is in PEA?

Patients who are clinically in PEA can have mechanical cardiac activity with minimal perfusion (pseudo-PEA) and may be more amenable to resuscitation. This is especially true for younger patients with higher CPP.[21] Correctable causes of PEA are cardiac tamponade, tension pneumothorax, pulmonary embolism, MI, hypoxemia, acidosis, hypokalemia, hyperkalemia, hypothermia, and overdoses (eg, narcotics, cyclic antidepressants, beta blockers, digitalis). Other, less correctable causes include massive myocardial damage from infarction, prolonged ischemia during resuscitation, profound hypovolemia, and massive pulmonary embolism. Patients in profound shock of any type (including anaphylactic, septic, neurogenic, obstructive, and hypovolemic shock) may have PEA. It should be noted that cardiac ultrasound can help determine reversible causes of cardiac arrest, especially in evaluating the presence or absence of cardiac movements.[22]

The paramedic should manage tension pneumothorax with needle decompression. If the patient is hypoxic, the paramedic should manage the

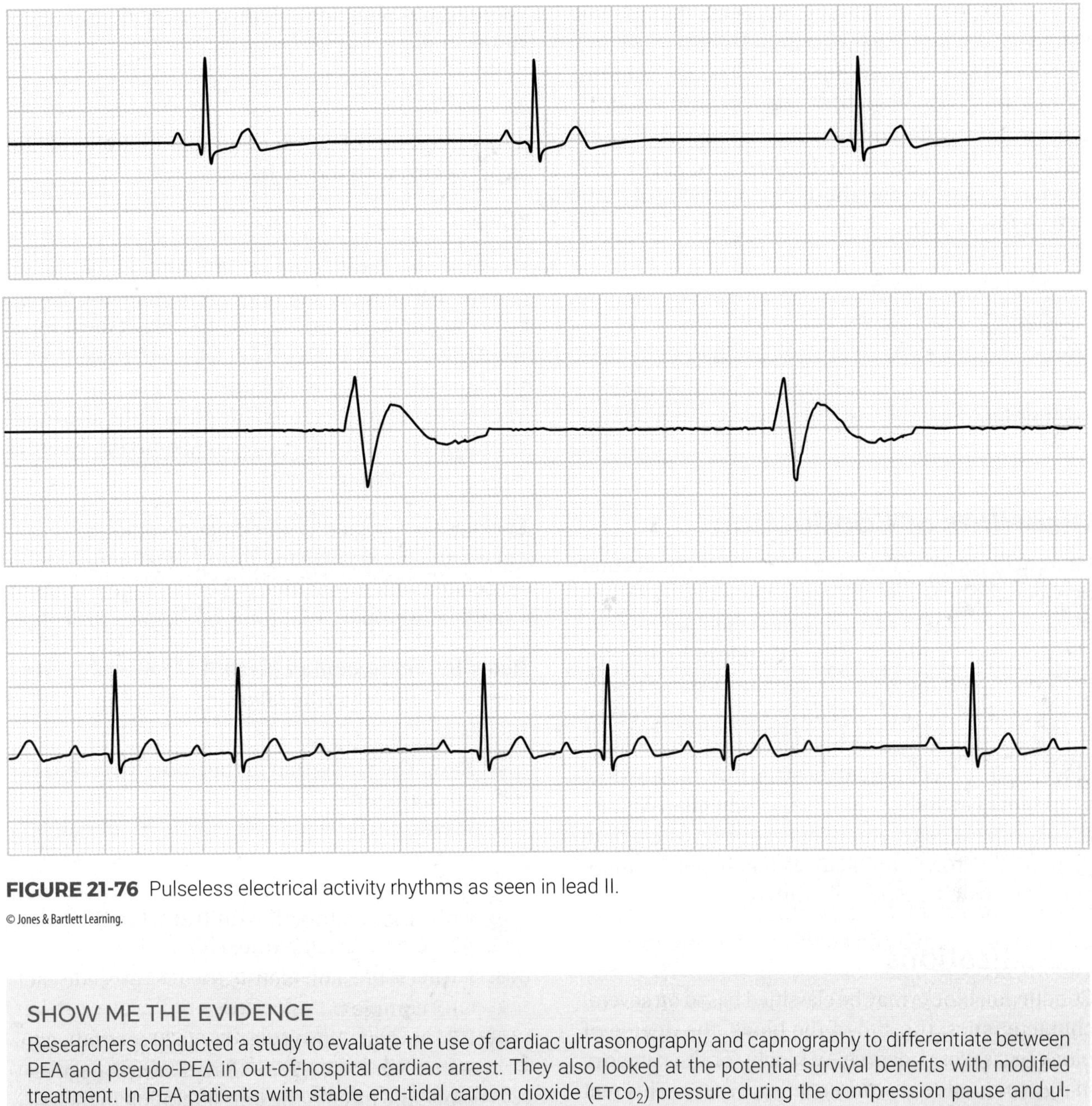

FIGURE 21-76 Pulseless electrical activity rhythms as seen in lead II.

SHOW ME THE EVIDENCE

Researchers conducted a study to evaluate the use of cardiac ultrasonography and capnography to differentiate between PEA and pseudo-PEA in out-of-hospital cardiac arrest. They also looked at the potential survival benefits with modified treatment. In PEA patients with stable end-tidal carbon dioxide ($ETCO_2$) pressure during the compression pause and ultrasonography showing cardiac activity, the compression pause was prolonged for 15 seconds and an additional 20 IU vasopressin was administered. If pulselessness persisted, compressions were continued. Fifteen of 16 patients studied (94%) achieved ROSC; 8 patients (50%) attained a good neurologic outcome. The researchers concluded that pseudo-PEA verified by cardiac ultrasonography enabled additional vasopressor treatment and cessation of chest compressions and was associated with significantly higher rates of ROSC, survival to discharge, and good neurologic outcome.

Modified from: Prosen G, Križmarić M, Završnik J, Grmec Š. Impact of modified treatment in echocardiographically confirmed pseudo-pulseless electrical activity in out-of-hospital cardiac arrest patients with constant end-tidal carbon dioxide pressure during compression pauses. *J Int Med Res*. 2010;38(4):1458-1467.

patient by improving oxygenation and ventilation. If acute hypovolemia is present, the paramedic should begin fluid resuscitation. The paramedic should manage acidosis by ensuring adequate fluid resuscitation and hyperventilation. If preexisting acidosis (eg, diabetic ketoacidosis), cyclic antidepressant overdose, or hyperkalemia is suspected (eg, a patient on home dialysis), use of sodium bicarbonate may be indicated. Calcium is a specific therapy for hyperkalemia and calcium channel blocker toxicity. Both conditions can produce PEA. Besides calcium channel blockers, other drugs taken in toxic amounts can produce wide-complex PEA. These overdoses can be managed with specific therapy. The therapy may be effective in reestablishing a perfusing rhythm (see Figure 21-63).

> CRITICAL THINKING
>
> Why are patients in cardiac arrest from opioid overdose more likely to have PEA or asystole than they are to have VF?

Disorders of Conduction

Delay or blockage of the electrical impulse conduction between the atria and the ventricles is called a heart block. Heart blocks can occur anywhere in the atria between the SA node and the AV node or in the ventricles between the AV node and the Purkinje fibers. These conduction defects can be caused by diseased tissue in the conduction system or by a physiologic block, such as occurs in AF or atrial flutter. Causes of heart blocks include AV junctional ischemia, AV junctional necrosis, degenerative disease of the conduction system, electrolyte imbalances (eg, hyperkalemia), and drug toxicity, especially with digitalis.

Classifications

Conduction blocks may be classified based on several characteristics: the site of the block, the degree of block (eg, second-degree AV block), or the category of AV conduction disturbance (eg, type I). This text presents the conduction disturbance by degree and location. However, the term degree does not reflect directly the gradients of severity when applied to the classification of heart blocks. Any evaluation of heart block must consider the specific rates of the atria and ventricles, the patient's clinical presentation, and the findings of a complete history and physical examination before the clinical severity of AV conduction disturbances can be determined. The conduction disturbances discussed in this section include first-degree AV block, second-degree AV block type I (or Wenckebach), second-degree AV block type II, third-degree AV block (complete heart block), and ventricular conduction disturbances, including bundle branch blocks and hemiblocks.

AV Blocks

The discussion of conduction disturbances of the heart begins with the AV blocks.

First-Degree AV Block

Description. **First-degree atrioventricular (AV) block** is not a true block (**FIGURE 21-77**). Rather, the disturbance is a delay in conduction, usually at the level of the AV node. First-degree AV block is not considered a rhythm in itself because it usually is superimposed on another rhythm. Therefore, the paramedic also must identify the underlying rhythm (eg, sinus bradycardia with first-degree AV block).

Etiology. First-degree AV block may occur for no apparent reason. The conduction disturbance sometimes is associated with myocardial ischemia, AMI, increased vagal (parasympathetic) tone, or digitalis toxicity.

Rules for Interpretation (Lead II Monitoring). First-degree AV block has the following characteristics on the ECG:

- **Rate.** The rate is that of the underlying sinus or atrial rhythm.
- **Rhythm.** The rhythm is that of the underlying rhythm.
- **QRS complex.** Typically normal (<0.12 second), with an AV conduction ratio of 1:1 (a QRS complex follows each P wave).
- **P waves.** Present; identical waves precede each QRS complex.
- **PR interval.** A prolonged (>0.20 second), constant PR interval is the hallmark of first-degree AV block and often is the only alteration in the ECG.

Clinical Significance. As a general rule, first-degree AV block has little or no clinical significance because all the impulses are conducted to the ventricles. In rare cases, however, a newly developed first-degree AV block progresses to a more serious AV block. The presence of first-degree AV block with a right bundle branch block (RBBB) and a hemiblock represents a trifascicular block and can signal the risk of complete heart block.[23]

Management. This conduction disturbance usually does not require treatment.

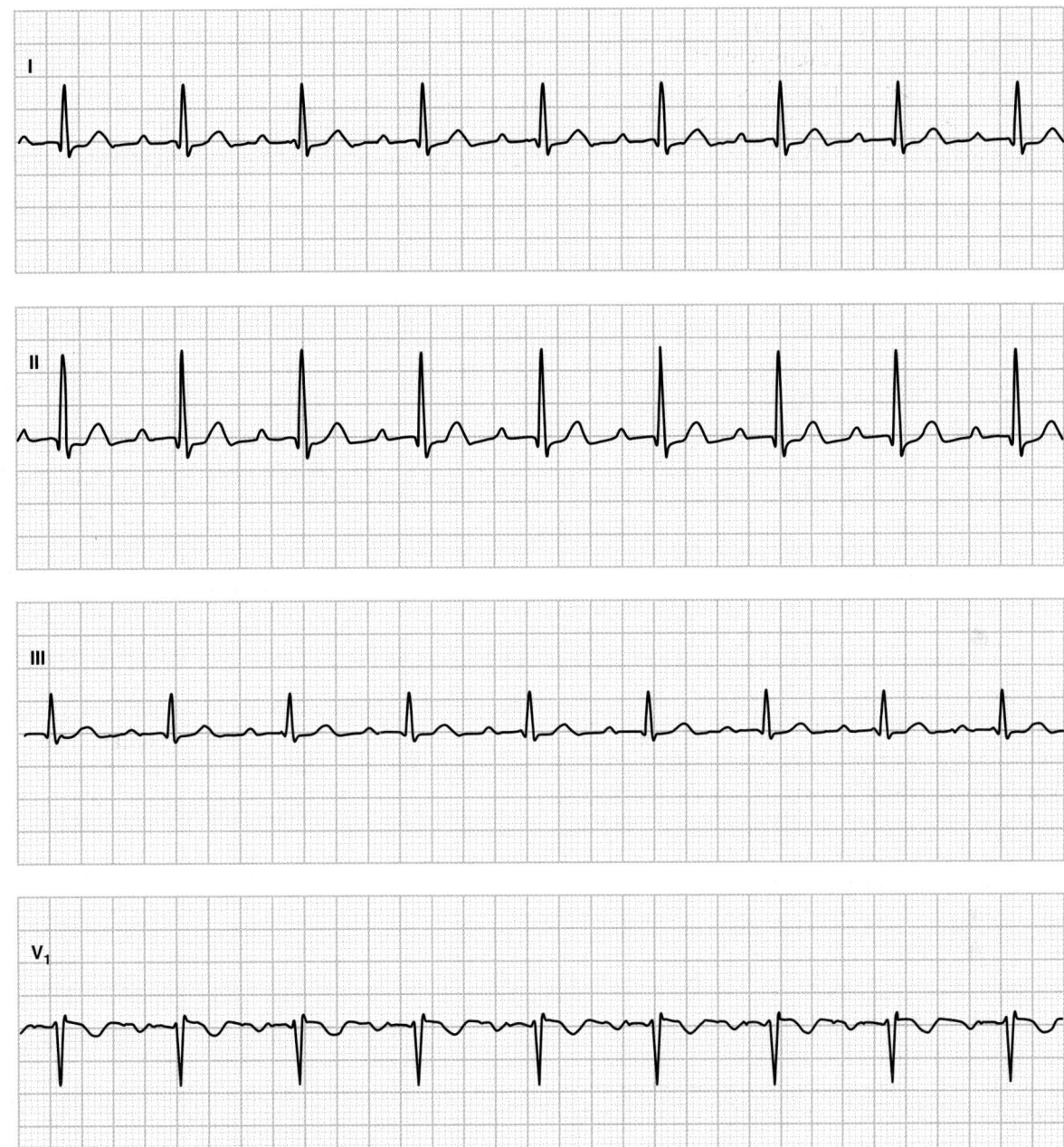

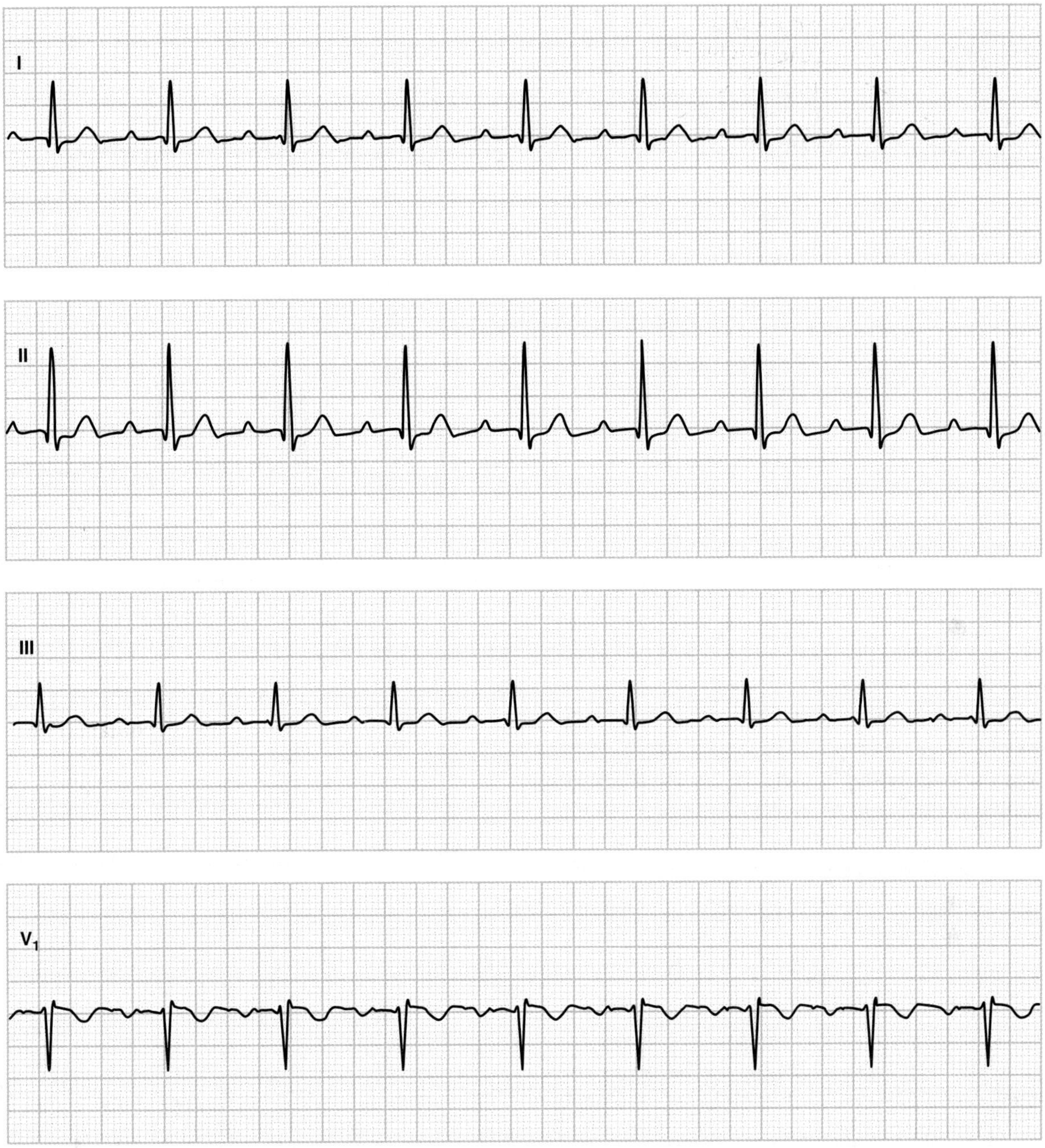

FIGURE 21-77 First-degree atrioventricular block.

Second-Degree AV Block Type I (Wenckebach)

Description. **Second-degree atrioventricular (AV) block type I** is an intermittent block (**FIGURE 21-78**). It usually occurs at the level of the AV node. The conduction delay progressively increases from beat to beat until conduction to the ventricle is blocked. This dysrhythmia produces a characteristic cyclical pattern in which the PR intervals become progressively longer until a P wave occurs that is not followed by a QRS complex. By the time the SA node fires again, AV conduction has had time to recover. The sequence then starts over.

Etiology. Second-degree AV block type I often occurs in AMI or acute myocarditis. Other causes include increased vagal tone, ischemia, drug toxicity (digitalis, propranolol, verapamil), head injury, and electrolyte imbalance.

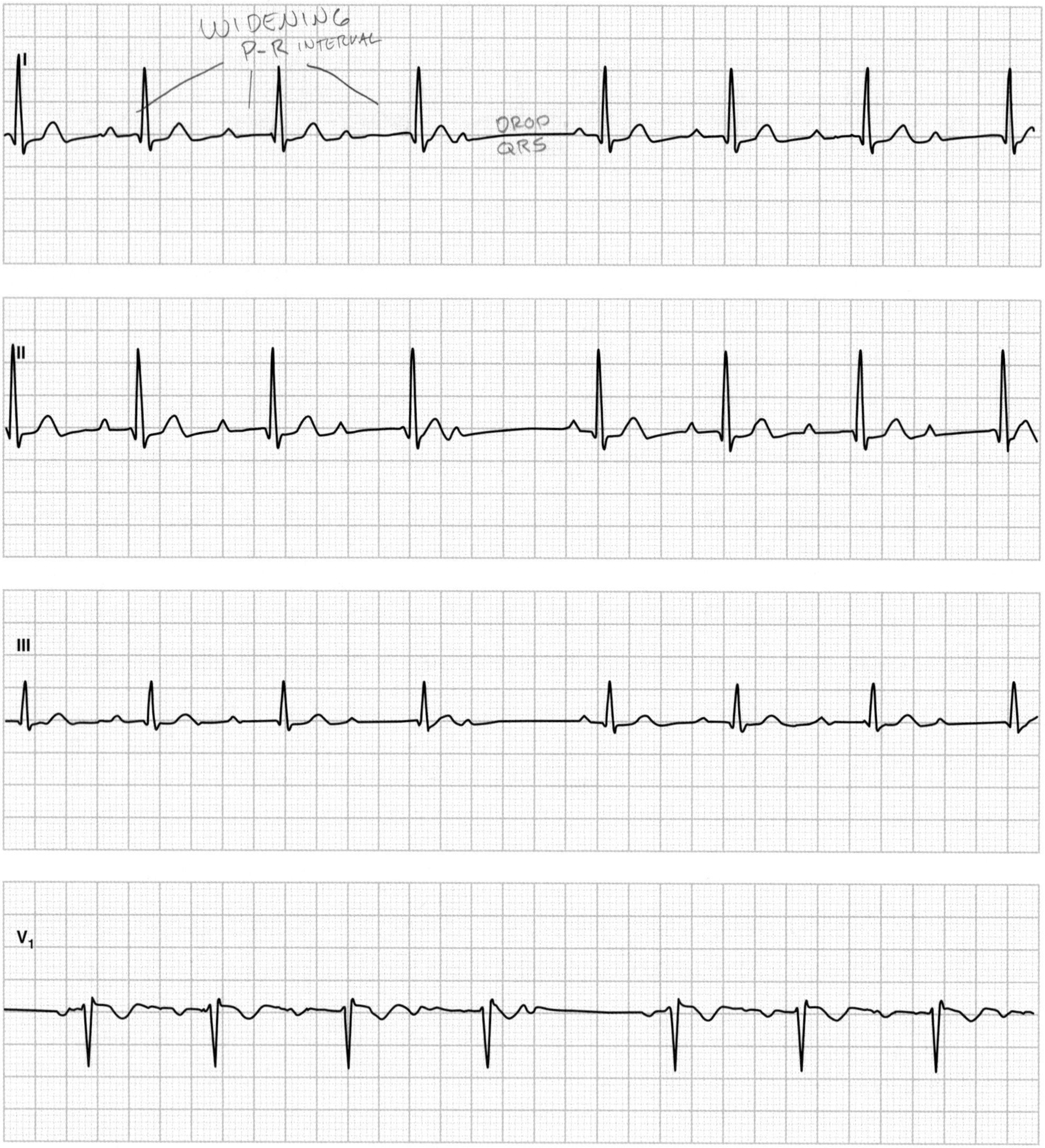

FIGURE 21-78 Second-degree atrioventricular block type I.

Rules for Interpretation (Lead II Monitoring). Second-degree AV block type I has the following characteristics on the ECG:

- **Rate.** The atrial rate is that of the underlying sinus or atrial rhythm. The ventricular rate may be normal or slow but always is slightly less than the atrial rate.
- **Rhythm.** The atrial rhythm is regular; the ventricular rhythm is irregular (characteristic group beating).
- **QRS complex.** Usually less than 0.12 second. Commonly, the AV conduction ratio (P waves to QRS complexes) is 5:4, 4:3, 3:2, or 2:1; the pattern may be constant or variable.

- **P waves.** Upright, uniform, and preceding the QRS complex when the QRS complex occurs.
- **PR interval.** Progressively lengthens before the nonconducted P wave. The P-P interval is constant, but the R-R interval decreases until the dropped beat (producing grouping of QRS complexes).

Clinical Significance. Second-degree AV block type I is usually a benign rhythm disturbance that does not cause hemodynamic compromise. Very rarely, it can progress to a more serious AV block.

Management. No management is required if the patient is asymptomatic. If the dropped beats compromise the heart rate and cardiac output, administration of atropine, TCP, or both may be indicated (see Figure 21-42).

Second-Degree AV Block Type II

Description. **Second-degree atrioventricular block type II** is an intermittent block (**FIGURE 21-79**). This conduction disturbance occurs when atrial impulses are not conducted to the ventricles. Unlike type I, this block is characterized by consecutive P waves that

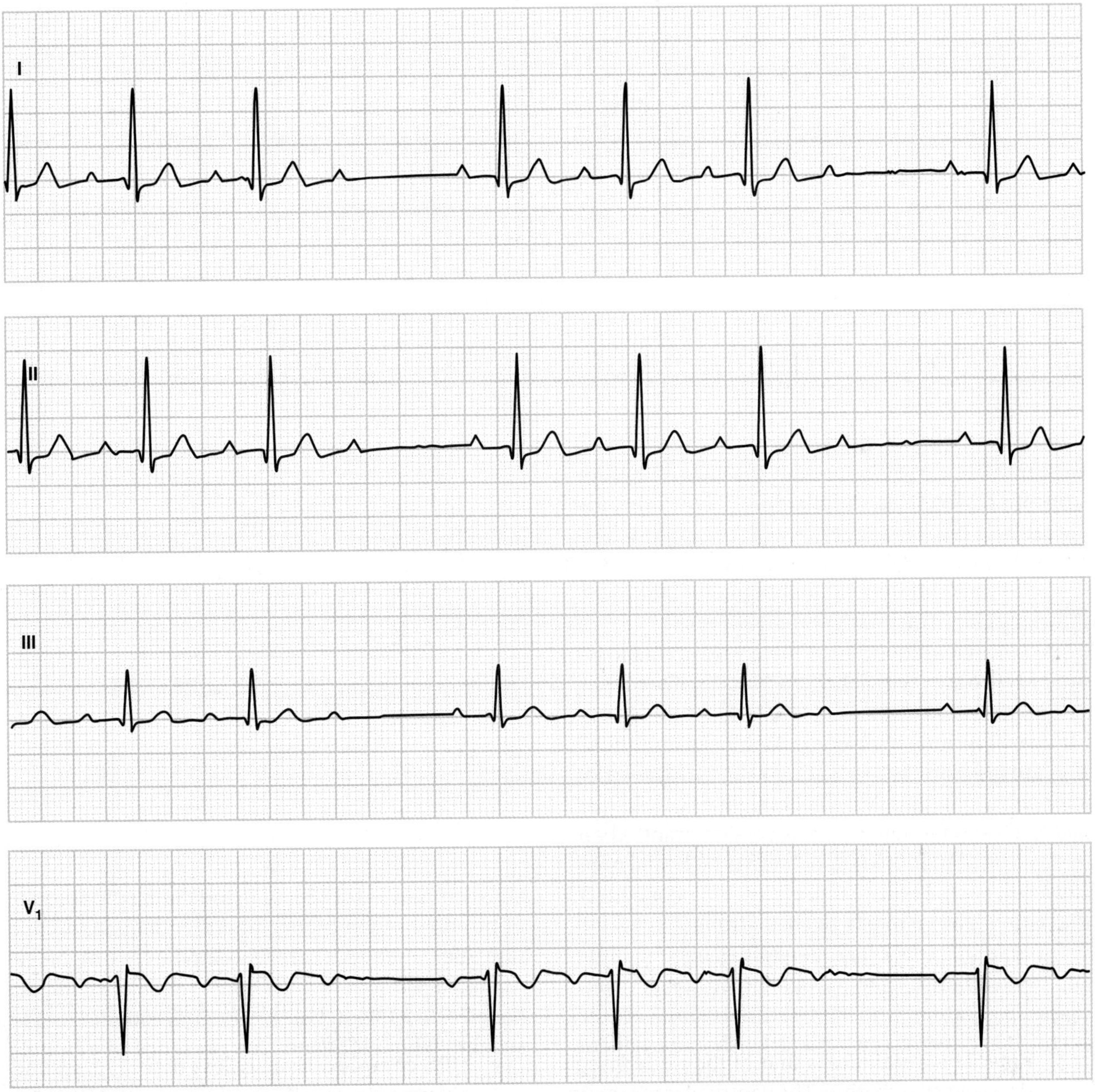

FIGURE 21-79 Second-degree atrioventricular block type II.

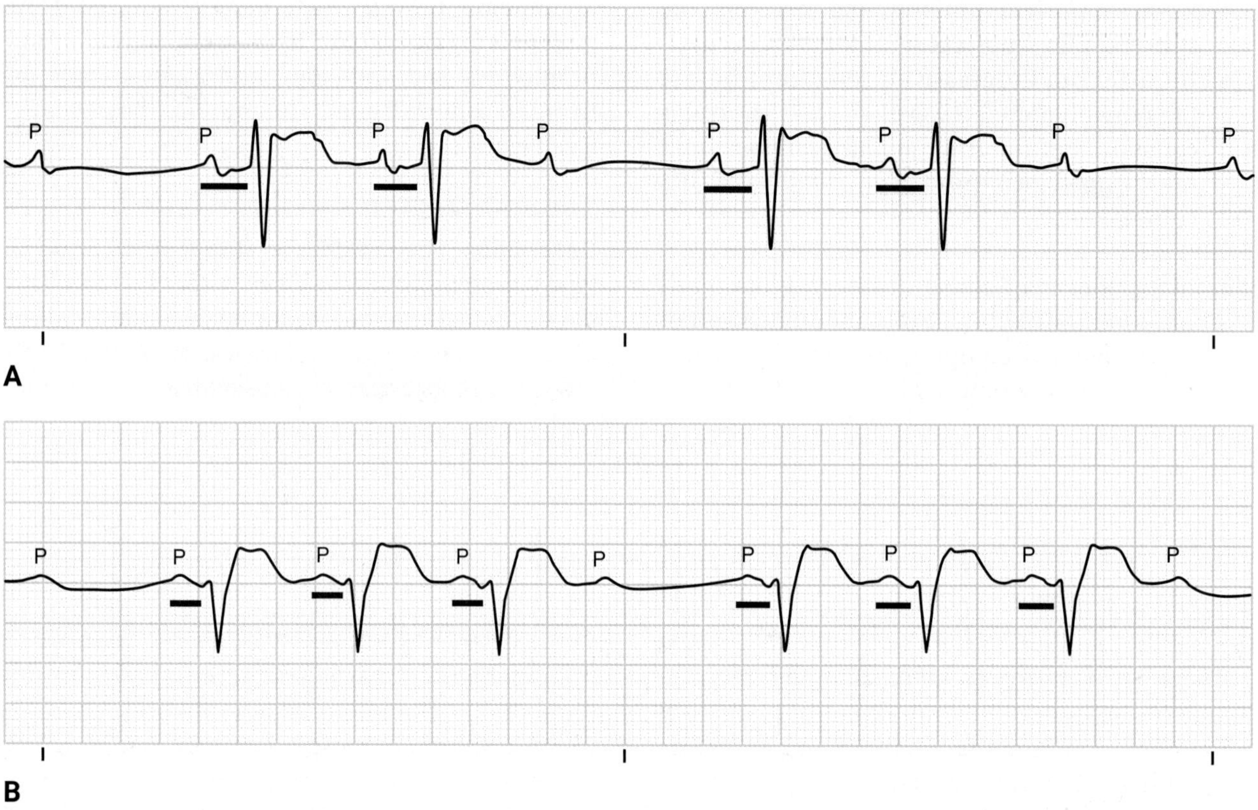

FIGURE 21-80 **A.** A 3:2 atrioventricular block. **B.** A 4:3 atrioventricular block.

are conducted with a constant PR interval before a dropped beat. This variation of AV block usually occurs in a regular sequence with the conduction ratios (P waves to QRS complexes), such as 2:1, 3:2, and 4:3 (**FIGURE 21-80**). Second-degree AV block type II usually occurs below the bundle of His.

When at least two consecutive P waves fail to be conducted to the ventricles, the AV block is referred to as a **high-grade atrioventricular (AV) block** (**FIGURE 21-81**). Clinically, serious high-grade AV blocks and those that are less serious are distinguished by the atrial and ventricular rates. A 2:1 block might be considered high grade (and certainly is clinically significant) when the patient's underlying atrial rate is 60 beats/min. However, such a block is much less of a concern if the patient's atrial rate is 120 beats/min.

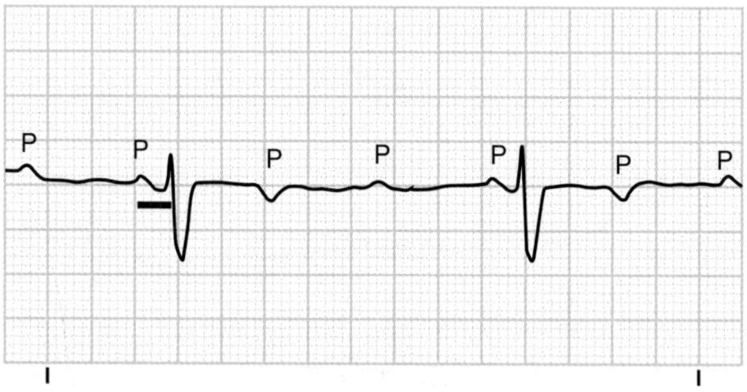

FIGURE 21-81 A 3:1 high-grade atrioventricular block.

A type II 2:1 AV block sometimes may be difficult to distinguish from a type I 2:1 AV block. When assessing a patient who has two atrial complexes for each QRS complex, the paramedic should evaluate the normal cycle. If the normally conducted cycle has a prolonged PR interval (>0.20 second), a narrow QRS complex (<0.12 second, indicating the absence of bundle branch block), and an adequate escape rate, the patient probably has a type I 2:1 AV block. As stated previously, if the conducted QRS complex has a normal PR interval, a wide QRS complex (>0.12 second, which indicates the presence of a bundle branch block), and an adequate escape rate, a type II 2:1 AV block is most likely (**FIGURE 21-82**).

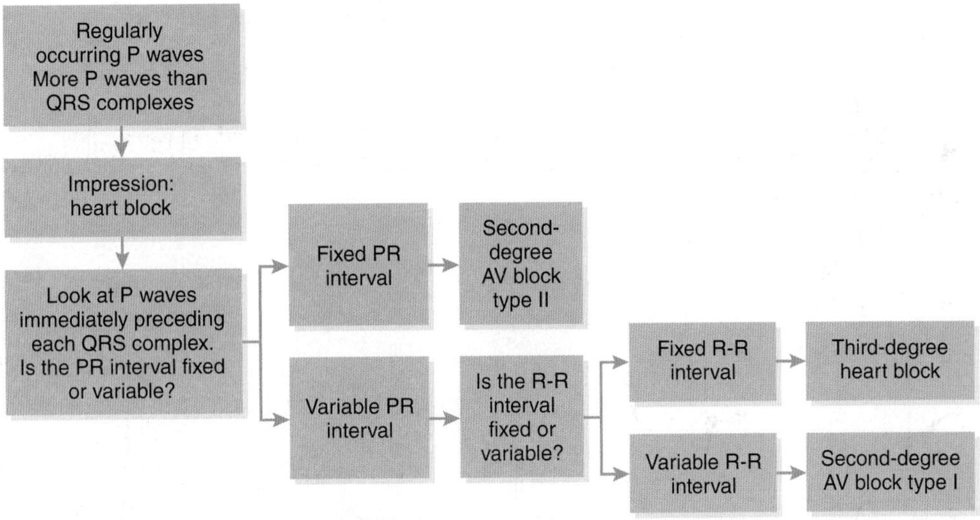

FIGURE 21-82 Identifying heart blocks.

Etiology. Second-degree AV block type II may be associated with an MI involving the septum. Unlike second-degree AV block type I, type II normally does not result solely from increased parasympathetic tone or drug toxicity.

Rules for Interpretation (Lead II Monitoring). Second-degree AV block type II has the following characteristics on the ECG:

- **Rate.** The atrial rate is unaffected and is that of the underlying sinus, atrial, or junctional rhythm. The ventricular rate is less than that of the atrial rate and often is bradycardic.
- **Rhythm.** Regular or irregular, depending on whether the conduction ratio is constant or variable.
- **QRS complex.** May be abnormal (≥0.12 second) because of bundle branch block.
- **P waves.** Upright and uniform. Some P waves are not followed by QRS complexes.
- **PR interval.** Usually constant for conducted beats and may be greater than 0.20 second.

Clinical Significance. Second-degree AV block type II is a serious conduction disturbance. It usually is considered malignant in the emergency setting (unlike type I AV blocks, which usually are considered benign). Slow ventricular rates may result in signs and symptoms of hypoperfusion. This conduction disturbance may progress to a more severe heart block or even to asystole.

Management. Regardless of the patient's initial condition, definitive treatment involves insertion of a pacemaker. Prehospital care for symptomatic patients may consist of atropine, although it may not be effective for this rhythm. Prepare for TCP and possibly the administration of beta adrenergic drugs (see Figure 21-42).[9]

Third-Degree Heart Block

Description. **Third-degree atrioventricular (AV) block** is also known as complete heart block. It results from complete electrical block at or below the AV node (infranodal) (**FIGURE 21-83**). The conduction disturbance produces a serious dysrhythmia that is said to be present when none of the atrial impulses are conducted through the AV node to the ventricles. The only electrical link between the atria and the ventricles is the AV node and bundle of His.

> NOTE
>
> Because atropine acts by increasing firing through the SA node, it may not be effective in patients with complete heart block and wide-complex ventricular escape beats and also in patients with second-degree type II heart block. Preparation should be made for immediate transcutaneous pacing.
>
> *Modified from:* 2015 American Heart Association Guidelines for Cardiopulmonary Resuscitation and Emergency Cardiovascular Care. *Circulation*. 2015;132:S313-S314.

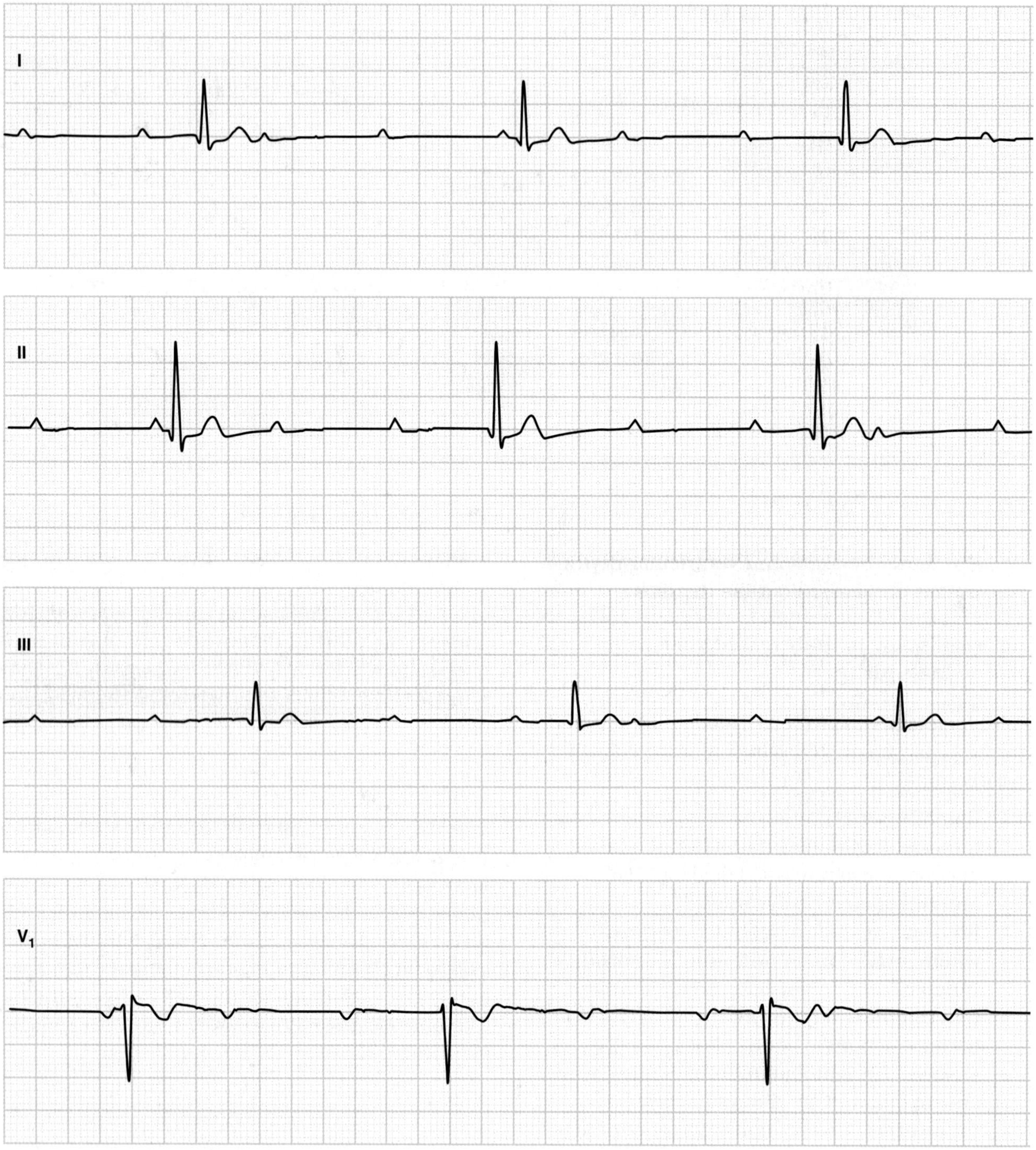

FIGURE 21-83 Third-degree atrioventricular block.

In this condition, the SA node or an ectopic atrial site serves as the pacemaker for the atria. An ectopic focus in the AV node, bundle branches, or Purkinje fibers serves as a pacemaker for the ventricles. P waves and QRS complexes occur rhythmically, yet the rhythms are unrelated to each other (AV dissociation).

Etiology. Common causes of third-degree AV block include inferior MI, drugs that block the AV node (digitalis, beta blocker, or calcium channel blocker), chronic degeneration of the conduction system, and electrolyte imbalance.

NOTE

Third-degree heart block is not the only rhythm with AV dissociation. The term means there is a rhythm that produces independent atrial and ventricular contractions. AV dissociation also occurs in accelerated idioventricular rhythms and VT.

Rules for Interpretation (Lead II Monitoring). Third-degree heart block has the following characteristics on the ECG:

- **Rate.** The atrial rate is that of the underlying sinus or atrial rhythm. The ventricular rate typically is 40 to 60 beats/min if the escape focus is junctional and less than 40 beats/min if the escape focus is in the ventricles.
- **Rhythm.** The atrial and ventricular rhythms usually are regular, but the rhythms are independent of each other.
- **QRS complex.** May be less than 0.12 second if the escape focus is below the AV node and above the bifurcation of the bundle branches or 0.12 second or greater if the escape focus is ventricular. A narrow QRS complex in third-degree heart block is much less common than is a wide QRS complex.
- **P waves.** Present but with no relationship to the QRS complexes. In cases of atrial flutter or fibrillation, complete heart block is manifested by a slow, regular ventricular response.
- **PR interval.** Variable and random because there is no relation between atrial and ventricular activity (**FIGURE 21-84**).

Clinical Significance. The patient often has signs and symptoms of severe bradycardia and decreased cardiac output. These are the result of the slow ventricular rate and asynchronous action of the atria and ventricles. Third-degree AV block associated with wide QRS complexes is an ominous sign. The dysrhythmia potentially is lethal. Patients with this rhythm are often unstable.

NOTE

Complete AV block in the presence of AF often is caused by drug toxicity (usually digitalis). Some AV block almost always occurs with AF or atrial flutter; however, complete AV block is recognized by a slow, regular ventricular response. (The response usually is slower than 60 beats/min.) The QRS complex may be normal if the escape focus is from above the bifurcation of the bundle branches.

Management. Insertion of a pacemaker is the definitive treatment for symptomatic third-degree AV block and for asymptomatic third-degree heart block with bundle branch block. Initial prehospital care includes atropine, although it is often not effective for this rhythm. Preparation should be made for immediate TCP or administration of a dopamine or epinephrine infusion to increase the ventricular rate, if needed.

CRITICAL THINKING

What should you tell the patient before starting TCP?

Ventricular Conduction Disturbances

Ventricular conduction disturbances (bundle branch blocks and hemiblocks) are delays or interruptions in the transmission of electrical impulses. These

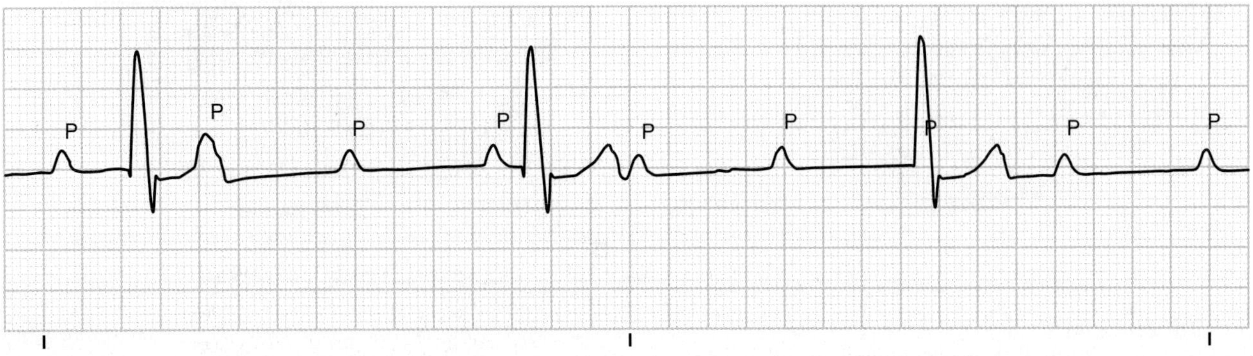

FIGURE 21-84 Third-degree block demonstrating P waves superimposed on the QRS complex.

disturbances occur below the level of bifurcation of the bundle of His. Detection of these blocks is important because it helps to identify the patient who is at increased risk of severe bradycardia and third-degree heart block. This detection is especially important when the patient has other forms of AV block. Common causes of bundle branch block include the following:

- Dilated cardiomyopathy
- Ventricular hypertrophy
- Anterior MI
- Aortic stenosis
- Cardiomyopathy
- Hyperkalemia
- Digoxin toxicity
- Myocarditis
- Toxins (sodium channel blockers)

Bundle Branch Anatomy

To review, the bundle of His begins at the AV node and divides to form the left and right bundle branches (**FIGURE 21-85**). The right bundle branch continues toward the apex and spreads throughout the right ventricle. The left bundle branch subdivides into the anterior and posterior fascicles and spreads throughout the left ventricle. Conduction of electrical impulses through the Purkinje fibers stimulates the ventricles to contract.

With normal conduction, the first part of the ventricle to be stimulated is the left side of the septum. The electrical impulse then traverses the septum to stimulate the other side. Shortly thereafter, the left and right ventricles are stimulated at the same time. The left ventricle normally is much larger and thicker than the right ventricle; therefore, its electrical activity predominates over that of the right ventricle.

Common ECG Findings

When an electrical impulse is blocked from passing through the right or left bundle branch, abnormal conduction occurs and one ventricle depolarizes and contracts before the other. Ventricular activation no longer occurs at the same time. As a result, the QRS complex widens (often with a slurred or notched appearance known as rabbit ears). The hallmark of bundle branch block is a QRS complex equal to or greater than 0.12 second. There are two criteria for recognizing bundle branch block:

- A QRS complex equal to or greater than 0.12 second
- QRS complexes produced by supraventricular activity

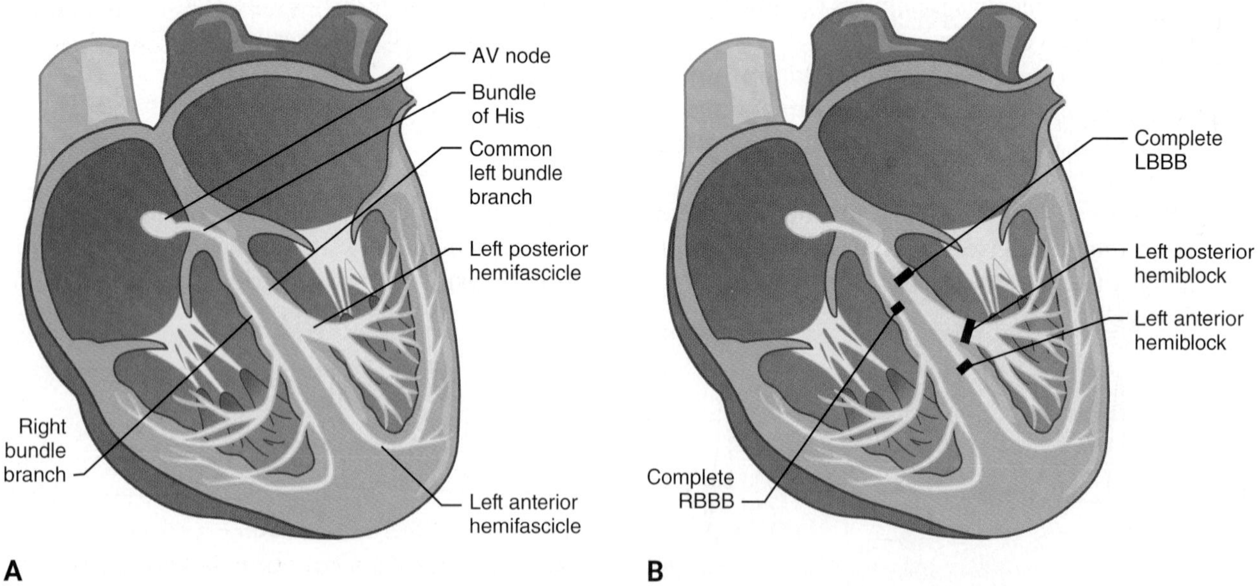

Abbreviations: AV, atrioventricular; LBBB, left bundle branch block; RBBB, right bundle branch block

FIGURE 21-85 A. Simplified illustration of the major divisions of the ventricular conduction system. After passing through the atrioventricular node and the bundle of His, the electrical impulse is carried to the right and common left bundle branches. The latter structure divides into the anterior and posterior hemifascicles. **B.** Possible sites of block and the conduction deficits that may be produced.

> NOTE
> Bundle branch block and hemiblock (fascicular block) are terms used to describe abnormal conduction or the interruption of impulses from above the bundle branches to the ventricles. The interruption may occur in either the anterior (superior) or the posterior (inferior) division. These patterns of abnormal or aberrant conduction must be recognized as different from beats of ventricular origin. Beats of ventricular origin can have similar QRS complex shapes.

Ventricular conduction disturbances are identified best by monitoring leads V_1 and V_6 with a 12-lead machine. These leads permit the easiest differentiation of the right and LBBBs. Lead V_1 looks at right and left bundle branches and should be monitored during transport of these patients.

Normal Conduction. In normal ventricular stimulation, the electrical impulse reaches the septum first. It then travels from the left endocardium to the right endocardium of the septum (**FIGURE 21-86**). This impulse generates a small R wave in V_1. The rest of the impulses mainly are conducted away from the V_1 electrode, yielding a negative deflection. Therefore, during normal conduction, V_1 mainly is negative. The QRS complex also is usually 0.08 to 0.10 second wide (the same as any other narrow QRS complex).

Right Bundle Branch Block. In **right bundle branch block (RBBB)**, the left bundle branch performs normally.

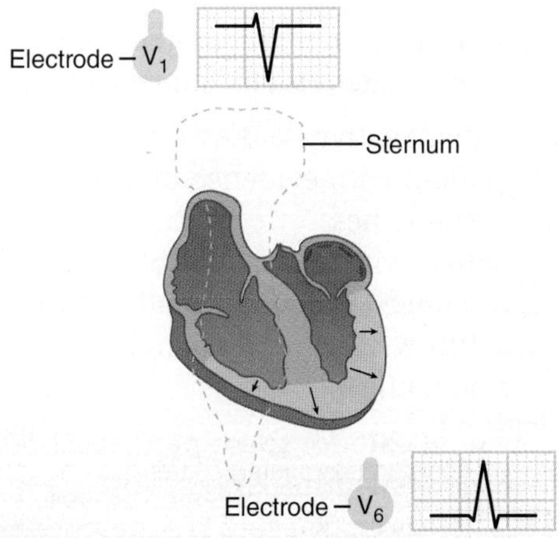

FIGURE 21-86 Normal ventricular conduction.

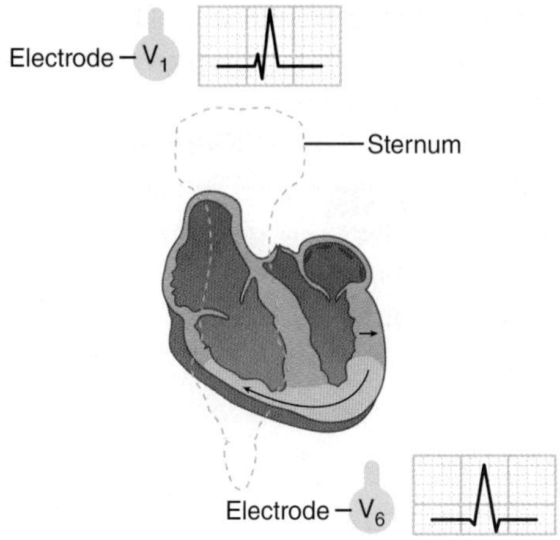

FIGURE 21-87 Right bundle branch block.

Therefore, the left branch activates the left side of the heart before the right (**FIGURE 21-87**). When the left ventricle is activated initially, the impulse travels away from the V_1 electrode, yielding a negative deflection (S wave). The electrical impulse then travels across the interventricular septum and activates the right ventricle. Because the impulse is coming back toward the V_1 electrode, a large positive deflection (R wave) occurs. This results in the RSR pattern seen in V_1 in patients with RBBB. The QRS (or in this case, RSR) complex is at least 0.12 second. Whenever the two criteria for bundle branch block are met and V_1 displays an RSR pattern, RBBB should be suspected.

> NOTE
> In PEA, the left ventricle receives the electrical impulse first. In LBBB, the opposite occurs. Because one ventricle contracts slightly later than the other, two QRS complexes are produced that often appear joined.

Left Bundle Branch Block. When a **left bundle branch block (LBBB)** is present, the fibers that usually stimulate the interventricular septum are blocked. This blockage alters normal septal activation and sends it in the opposite direction (**FIGURE 21-88**). The septum is depolarized by the right bundle branch, and the right ventricle then is activated. Because the impulse is leading away from V_1, the lead shows a deep, wide S wave (QS pattern). As with RBBB, the activation takes at least 0.12 second. Whenever the two criteria for bundle branch block are met and a QS pattern is seen in V_1, LBBB should be suspected.

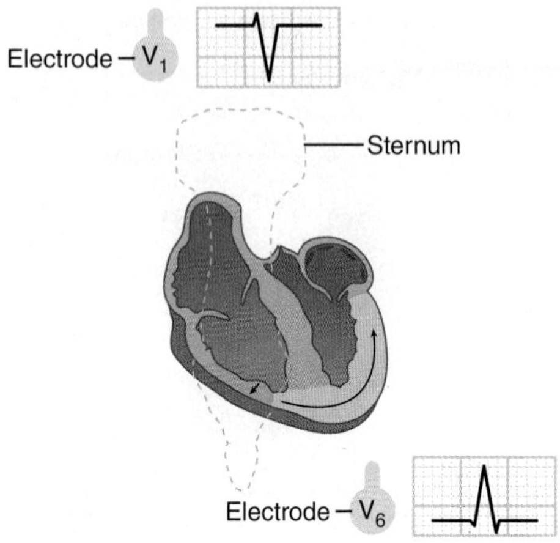

FIGURE 21-88 Left bundle branch block.

© Jones & Bartlett Learning.

NOTE

A clear RSR' or QS pattern in V_1 cannot always be identified. The turn signal method is another means of determining which bundle is blocked. Using this method to evaluate the ECG can help the paramedic identify which ventricle was depolarized last.

The turn signal method (BOX 21-8) is a means of differentiating right and LBBBs.

Management of Bundle Branch Blocks and Hemiblocks

No specific treatment is necessary for persistent bundle branch blocks or hemiblocks. New-onset LBBB with chest pain may be acute coronary syndrome (ACS). In the field, however, it is often not possible to know if a patient's LBBB is new or old. Thus, LBBB is no longer considered a STEMI equivalent. In these cases, field treatment is the same as for ACS unless the **Sgarbossa criteria** are present (BOX 21-9). Patients with LBBB meeting the Sgarbossa criteria are treated as a STEMI equivalent in many EMS systems. If other conditions (eg, hypoxia, ischemia, electrolyte imbalance, drug toxicity) are causing a block, these conditions should be treated. Some emergency medications (eg, procainamide, digoxin, metoprolol, verapamil, diltiazem) administered to patients with cardiac disease can slow electrical impulse conduction through the AV node. To administer these medications safely, the paramedic must make sure the patient is not at a high

BOX 21-8 Turn Signal Method of Determining RBBB or LBBB

As a shortcut for identifying right or LBBB, the paramedic should envision the turn signal mechanism in a vehicle. The turn signal is pushed "up" to turn right and pushed "down" to turn left.

When lead V_1 is monitored, the bundle branch block may be determined by the following procedure:

1. Find a QRS complex that is at least 0.12 second wide.
2. Find the J point of the QRS complex (the junction between the termination of the QRS complex and the beginning of the ST segment) (**FIGURE 21-89**).
3. Draw a line backward from the J point into the QRS complex.
4. Fill in the triangle created by this line and the last portion of the QRS complex.
5. If the triangle points up, it is an RBBB.
6. If the triangle points down, it is LBBB.

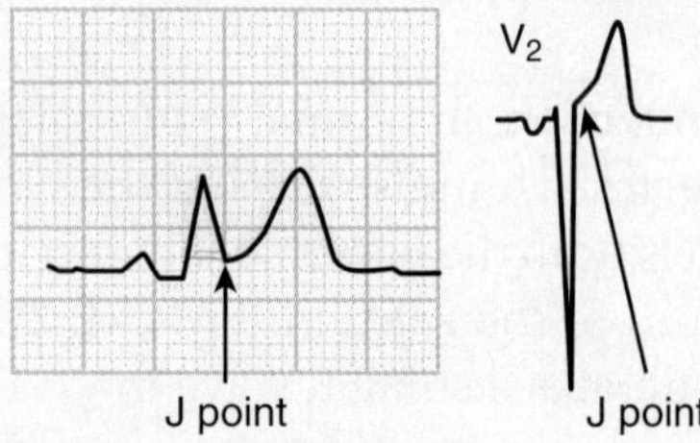

FIGURE 21-89 To distinguish left from right bundle branch blocks, find the J point of the QRS complex, draw a line backward into the QRS complex, and fill in the triangle created by this line and the last portion of the QRS complex. The direction the triangle points distinguishes the two types of blocks.

Reproduced from: Brownfield J, Herbert M. EKG criteria for fibrinolysis: what's up with the J Point? *West J Emerg Med.* 2008;9(1):40-42. Accessed at http://westjem.com/case-report/ekg-criteria-for-fibrinolysis-whats-up-with-the-j-point.html. Accessed May 30, 2018.

risk for the development of complete heart block. Those patients at such risk include the following:

- Any patient with type II AV block
- Any patient with evidence of disease in both bundle branches
- Any patient with two or more blocks of any kind (eg, prolonged PR interval and anterior hemiblock, RBBB and anterior hemiblock, type I AV block, and LBBB)

Prehospital care for these patients should include management of any accompanying signs and symptoms, transport, constant ECG monitoring, and anticipation of the possible need for external pacing.

BOX 21-9 Modified Sgarbossa Criteria

The Sgarbossa criteria are a set of ECG findings that can be used to identify MI in the presence of LBBB or a ventricular paced rhythm (**FIGURE 21-90**). MI is often difficult to detect when LBBB is present. Any one of the following Sgarbossa criteria may suggest a STEMI equivalent in the presence of a LBBB or pacemaker, and a score of 3 or more should prompt activation of the cardiac catheterization lab. A lower score is not considered diagnostic of an AMI, but it does not rule it out and warrants constant patient reassessment (in an effort to improve the sensitivity of the third criterion, Smith et al. modified it to measure a ratio of ST-segment elevation measured at the J point to the S wave). The modified Smith criteria, if positive, are sufficient to diagnose the patient with an AMI worthy of cardiac catheterization lab activation (**FIGURE 21-91**):

1. ST elevation of 1 mm or greater in a lead with a positive QRS complex (concordance).
2. Concordant ST depression of 1 mm or greater in lead V_1, V_2, or V_3.
3. Proportionally excessively discordant ST elevation in V_1 through V_4, as defined by an ST:S ratio no greater than or equal to 0.25 and at least 2 mm of ST elevation. (This replaces the third Sgarbossa criterion, which uses an absolute of 5 mm.) Anything greater than 0.20 is probably STEMI.

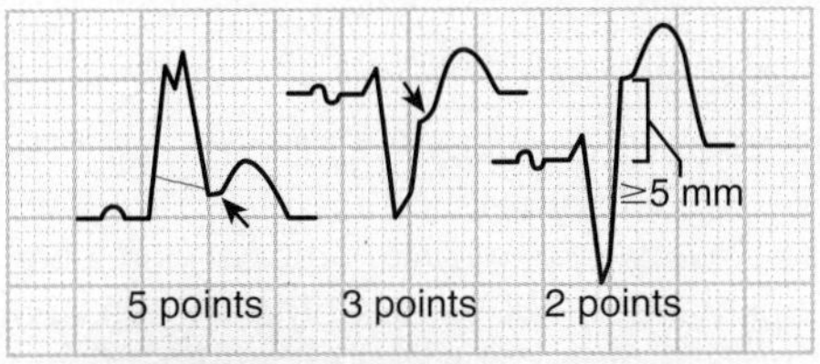

Sgarbossa ECG Criteria for LBBB	
Concordant STE ≥1 mm	5 points
Concordant STD ≥1 mm in V_1–V_3	3 points
Discordant STE ≥5 mm	2 points

FIGURE 21-90 Original Sgarbossa criteria.

Modified from: Cai Q, Mehta N, Sgarbossa E, et al. The left bundle branch block puzzle in the 2013 ST-elevation myocardial infarction guideline: from falsely declaring emergency to denying reperfusion in a high-risk population. Are the Sgarbossa Criteria ready for prime time? *Am Heart J.* 2013;166(3):409-413.

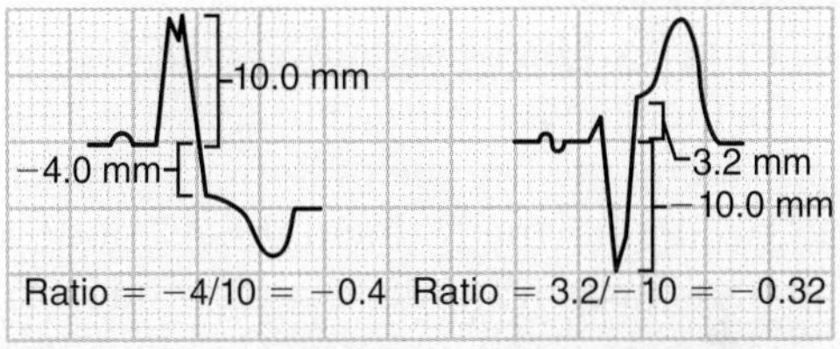

Third Criteria Modified by Smith

Ratio of ST-segment elevation measured at the J point to the R or S wave, whichever was most prominent

FIGURE 21-91 ST/S ratio.

Modified from: Cai Q, Mehta N, Sgarbossa E, et al. The left bundle branch block puzzle in the 2013 ST-elevation myocardial infarction guideline: from falsely declaring emergency to denying reperfusion in a high-risk population. Are the Sgarbossa Criteria ready for prime time? *Am Heart J.* 2013;166(3):409-413.

Modified from: Sgarbossa E, Pinski S, Barbagelata A, et al. Electrocardiographic diagnosis of evolving acute myocardial infarction in the presence of left bundle-branch block. *N Engl J Med.* 1996;334(8):481-487; and Smith S, Dodd K, Henry T, Dvorak D, Pearce L. Diagnosis of ST-elevation myocardial infarction in the presence of left bundle branch block with the ST-elevation to S-wave ratio in a modified Sgarbossa Rule. *Ann Emerg Med.* 2012;60(6):766-776.

Preexcitation Syndromes

Preexcitation syndrome (anomalous or accelerated AV conduction) is associated with an accessory conduction pathway (bypass tract) between the atria and ventricles. This pathway bypasses the AV node or the bundle of His or both and allows the electrical impulses to initiate depolarization of the ventricles earlier than usual. The most common preexcitation syndrome is WPW.

WPW Syndrome

Description. In some hearts, a congenital accessory muscle bundle (the **bundle of Kent** or Kent fibers) connects the lateral wall of the atrium and the ventricle, bypassing the AV node. This condition produces an

NOTE

Another preexcitation syndrome grouped with WPW syndrome is LGL syndrome. As in WPW syndrome, the accessory pathway in LGL syndrome does not share the rate-slowing properties of the AV node and may conduct electrical activity at a significantly higher rate than does the AV node. Proposed theories to explain LGL syndrome are the possible presence of intranodal fibers (James fibers, Mahaim fibers) that bypass all or part of the AV node and run from the atrium to the bundle of His.

Modified from: Derejko P, Szumowski LJ, Sanders P, et al. Atrial fibrillation in patients with Wolff-Parkinson-White syndrome: role of pulmonary veins. *J Cardiovasc Electrophysiol.* 2012;23(3):280-286.

early activation of the ventricle (WPW syndrome). WPW syndrome is thought to be of minor clinical significance unless a tachycardia is present. In that case, the syndrome can become life threatening (see the following Clinical Significance section).

Etiology. WPW syndrome may occur in young, healthy people (mainly men) without apparent cause. It also may occur in multiple members of a family. It may be present in successive generations.

Rules for Interpretation (Lead II Monitoring). WPW syndrome has the following characteristics on the ECG:

- **Rate.** Normal unless associated with SVT.
- **Rhythm.** Regular.
- **QRS complex.** May be normal or wide (depending on whether conduction is retrograde or anterograde along the bundle of Kent). Conduction that occurs normally down the AV node and simultaneously in an anterograde fashion along the accessory pathway results in a meeting of the two waves of depolarization that forms a fusion (delta wave). A **delta wave** is evidenced by slurring or notching of the onset of the QRS complex and is a diagnostic finding in WPW syndrome. (Not all leads show the delta wave.)
- **P waves.** Normal.
- **PR interval.** Less than 0.12 second because the normal delay at the AV node does not occur.

The three characteristic ECG findings in WPW syndrome are a short PR interval, a delta wave, and QRS widening (**FIGURE 21-92**).

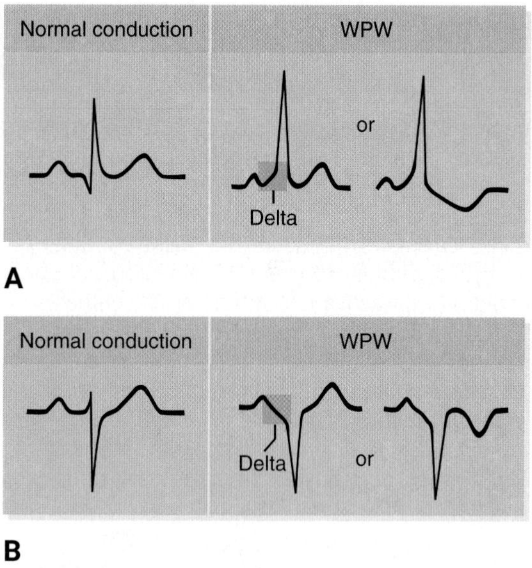

FIGURE 21-92 Characteristic findings in Wolff-Parkinson-White (WPW) syndrome (short PR interval, QRS widening, and delta wave) compared with normal conduction. **A.** Usual appearance of WPW syndrome in leads where the QRS complex is predominantly upright. **B.** Appearance of WPW syndrome; the RS complex is predominantly negative.

> **NOTE**
>
> The QRS complexes in LGL syndrome are normal because ventricular contraction is initiated in the normal manner. The broad complexes seen in an asymptomatic patient with WPW syndrome are not a feature of LGL syndrome. The delta waves seen in WPW syndrome are not seen in LGL syndrome because the accessory pathway does not connect to the ventricles; therefore, ventricular contraction does not start early.

Clinical Significance. Patients with WPW are susceptible to the development of AVRT. The reason is that the accessory pathway provides a ready-made reentry circuit between the atria and the ventricles. AVRTs can take one of two forms. In orthodromic AVRT, a wave of depolarization progresses in an anterograde fashion from the AV node to the bundle of His and back up the accessory pathway to the atria. Because the ventricles are depolarized using the rapid pathway of the bundle of His, orthodromic AVRT appears as a narrow-complex SVT. In antidromic AVRT, the impulse travels in an anterograde fashion down the accessory pathway and back up the AV node to the atria. In this case, the bundle of His is not used for rapid depolarization of the ventricles, and the QRS is wide. Antidromic AVRT will appear on the ECG as a wide-complex tachyarrhythmia that may be difficult to distinguish from VT.

WPW becomes life threatening in the presence of AF. If AF or atrial flutter is present, the tachycardia may be conducted directly through the bundle of Kent, bypassing the AV node completely. Because this accessory pathway may have a much shorter refractory period than does the AV node, an extremely high ventricular rate that can rapidly deteriorate into VF because inadequate cardiac perfusion results. On the ECG and rhythm strip, WPW with AF appears as an irregular, bizarre-appearing wide-complex tachycardia.

Management. AV nodal blocking agents such as adenosine, beta blockers, and calcium channel blockers are contraindicated in patients with AF and WPW syndrome because they can cause a paradoxical increase in the ventricular response to the rapid atrial impulses of AF as they divert conduction from the AV node to the accessory pathway.

The safest course of action is to manage patients with a wide-complex tachycardia as if the rhythm is VT. Patients who are unstable should undergo synchronized cardioversion. In patients who are stable but symptomatic, antiarrhythmic therapy can be considered. The recommended antiarrhythmic treatment of tachydysrhythmias in patients with WPW is procainamide. Because of reported adverse events, amiodarone is considered relatively contraindicated in patients with AF and WPW.[24,25]

Twelve-Lead ECG Monitoring

As stated previously, the 12-lead ECG has become standard in most EMS systems that provide advanced life support. Twelve-lead acquisition and interpretation now are recognized as key skills for paramedics.[26] The ability to interpret a 12-lead ECG can affect transport decisions and medication and treatment selections. In addition, this skill can help paramedics predict the likelihood that a patient will become unstable. Twelve-lead ECG monitoring can be used to do the following:

- Determine the presence and location of bundle branch blocks
- Determine the electrical axis and the presence of fascicular blocks
- Identify ST-segment and T-wave changes relative to myocardial ischemia, injury, and infarction
- Identify VT in wide-complex tachycardia

Lead Review

As explained earlier, ECG machines provide many views of the electrical activity of the heart by monitoring voltage changes between electrodes applied to the body. To review, the modern ECG uses 12 leads: 3 standard limb leads, 3 augmented limb leads, and 6 precordial (chest) leads. The standard limb leads are I, II, and III. The augmented limb leads are aV_R, aV_L, and aV_F. The precordial leads are V_1 through V_6.

NOTE

Leads should not be confused with electrodes. The 12-lead ECG uses only 10 electrodes. However, the machine interprets 12 leads, or "views," of the heart using computerized calculations.

The imaginary lines join the positive and negative electrodes of each lead, forming a straight line between the positive and negative poles. This straight line is known as the axis of the ECG lead. The axes of the standard limb leads represent the average direction of the electrical activity of the heart. If these axes are moved so that they cross a common midpoint without changing their orientation, they form a triaxial reference system (three intersecting lines of reference). Lead I is a lateral (leftward) lead. It assesses the electrical activity of the heart from a vantage point that is defined as 0° on a circle. This circle is divided into an upper negative 180° and a lower positive 180°. Leads II and III are inferior leads. They assess the electrical activity of the heart from vantage points of +60° and +120°, respectively.

The augmented limb leads (**FIGURE 21-93**) record the difference in electrical potential between the positive electrode of an extremity lead and a vantage point. The vantage point of zero electrical potential is at the center of the electrical field of the heart. As a result, the axis of each lead is formed by the line from the electrode site (on the right arm, left arm, or left leg) to the center of the heart. The aV_R, aV_L, and aV_F leads intersect at angles different from the standard limb leads and produce three other intersecting lines of reference. When these six lines of reference are combined (one every 30°), they form the hexaxial reference system (**FIGURE 21-94**). Lead aV_L acts as a lateral (leftward) lead. It records the electrical activity of the heart from a vantage point that looks down from the left arm. Lead aV_F acts as an inferior lead. It records the electrical activity of the heart from a vantage point that looks up from the left lower extremity. Lead aV_R is a distant recording electrode. It looks down at the heart from the right arm. Based on these lead descriptions, the lateral, or left-side, limb leads are I and aV_L. The inferior leads are II, III, and aV_F.

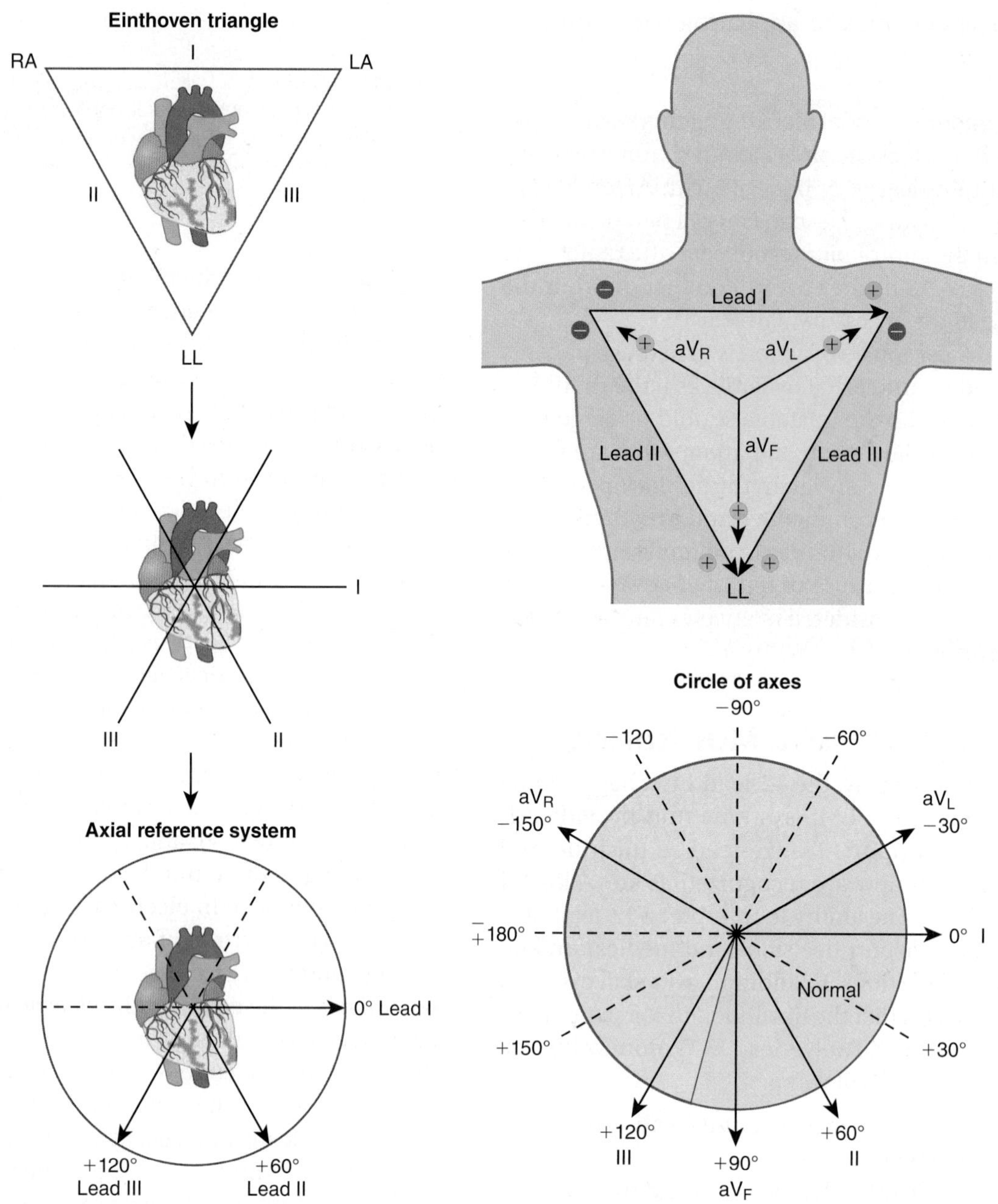

FIGURE 21-93 Augmented limb leads.

NOTE

Each of the six limb leads (three standard limb leads and three augmented limb leads) records the same cardiac activity from a different angle.

The six precordial leads (**FIGURE 21-95**) are projected through the AV node toward the patient's back. In this view, the anterior chest wall is considered positive, and the patient's back is considered negative. This horizontal plane separates the body into top and bottom halves. The chest leads monitor electrical current in successive steps from the patient's right to left side. Leads V_1 and V_2 are right chest leads that view the septum of the heart (septal leads). Leads V_3 and V_4 view the anterior wall of the left ventricle (anterior leads). Leads V_5 and V_6 view the lateral wall of the left ventricle (lateral leads) (**FIGURE 21-96**).

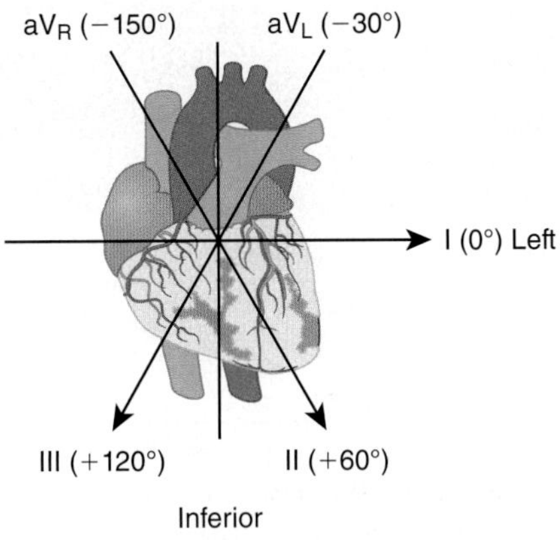

FIGURE 21-94 Hexaxial reference system.

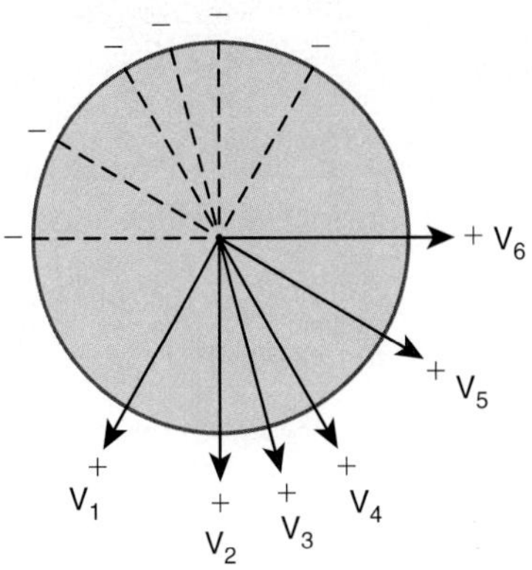

FIGURE 21-95 The precordial leads. The positive poles of the chest leads point anteriorly, and the negative poles (dashed lines) point posteriorly.

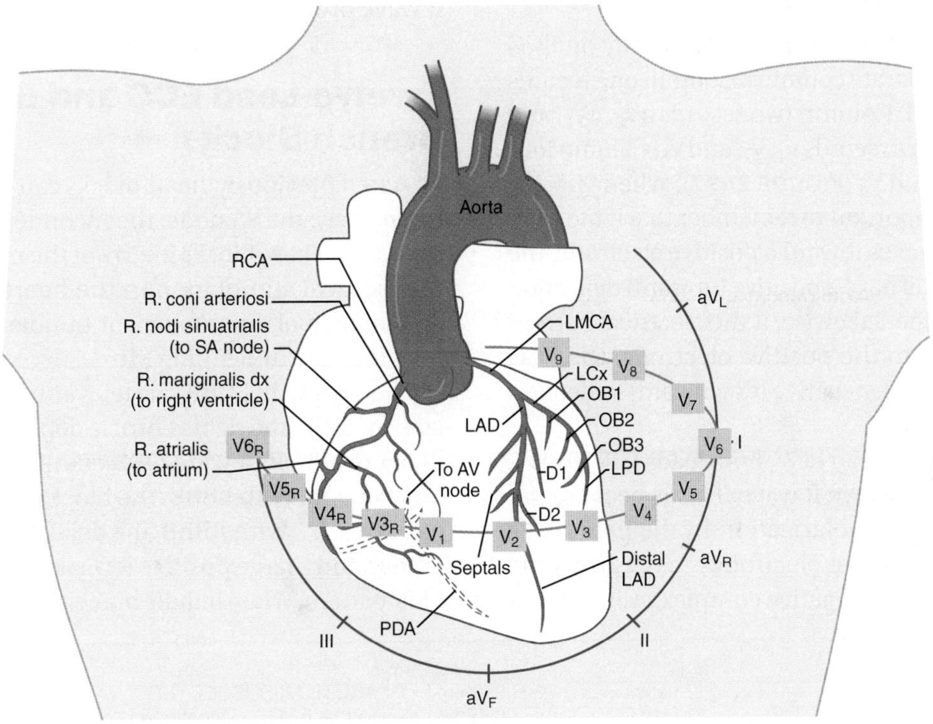

Abbreviations: D, diagonal branches (D1, D2); LAD, left anterior descending artery; LCx, left circumflex artery; LMCA, left main coronary artery; LPD, left posterior descending artery; OB, obtuse marginal (OB1, OB2, OB3; PDA, posterior descending artery; RCA, right coronary artery; septals, septal branches

FIGURE 21-96 Coronary arteries and their relation to the ECG leads.

Modified from: ECGwaves. https://ecgwaves.com/localization-localize-myocardial-infarction-ischemia-coronary-artery-occlusion-culprit-stemi/

NOTE

Lead aV_R is the only limb lead on the right side of the body. It looks at the upper side of the heart. A finding of ST elevation in lead aV_R coupled with diffuse ST depressions in other leads is associated with occlusion of the left main coronary artery, the proximal portion of the left anterior descending artery, or severe three-vessel coronary artery disease.

The aV_R lead may also be useful in patients with acute pericarditis, in tricyclic antidepressant poisoning, and in WPW syndrome.

Modified from: George A, Arumugham PS, Figueredo VM. aVR—the forgotten lead. *Exp Clin Cardiol.* 2010;15(2):e36-e44; and Williamson K, Mattu A, Plautz CU, Binder A, Brady WJ. Electrocardiographic applications of lead aVR. *Am J Emerg Med.* 2006;24(7):864-874.

TABLE 21-2 Lead Views of the Heart

Lead	Area of the Heart
II, III, aV_F	Inferior wall of the left ventricle
V_1, V_2	Septum
V_3, V_4	Anterior wall of the left ventricle
I, V_5, V_6, aV_L	Lateral wall of the left ventricle

TABLE 21-3 Lead Deflections in a Normal 12-Lead ECG

Upward (Positive)	Downward (Negative)
I, II, III, aV_F, aV_L	aV_R
V_2 through V_6	V_1

TABLE 21-2 shows the area of the heart viewed by each of the 12 leads.

Normal 12-Lead ECG

The 12-lead ECG is recorded electronically on ECG paper in four separate columns. Column one records leads I, II, and III. Column two records aV_R, aV_L, and aV_F. Column three records V_1, V_2, and V_3. Column four records V_4, V_5, and V_6 (**FIGURE 21-97**). When viewing any ECG, it is important to remember that if the electrical current moves toward a positive electrode, the ECG complex will have a positive (upward) deflection from the baseline. Likewise, if the electrical current moves away from the positive electrode, the ECG complex will have a negative (downward) deflection from the baseline.

In a normal 12-lead ECG, limb leads I, II, III, aV_F, and aV_L have a positive R wave. This is because the positive wave of depolarization in the heart cells moves toward positive electrodes (aV_R is the only limb lead that has a negative complex). Chest leads are also always positive. However, leads V_1 through V_6 display the progressive nature of ventricular depolarization. As such, chest lead V_1 normally is negative (at or below baseline), V_2 is more positive, V_3 is progressively upright, and V_4 through V_6 are directly upright. This positive movement is called the normal R wave progression (**TABLE 21-3**).

Twelve-Lead ECG and Bundle Branch Blocks

As stated previously, heart blocks can occur in any of three areas: the SA node, the AV node, or the bundle branches. These blocks interrupt the normal passage of electrical stimulation in the heart. The sudden appearance of an AV block or bundle branch block may indicate impending MI.

To review, in LBBB, the left ventricle depolarizes late. In RBBB, the right ventricle depolarizes late. This delay results in a wide QRS complex greater than 0.12 second. With LBBB, the block often yields a QS pattern in V_1. With RBBB, the delay yields a negative S wave and a large positive R wave. This results in an RSR′ pattern. When bundle branch block is suspected,

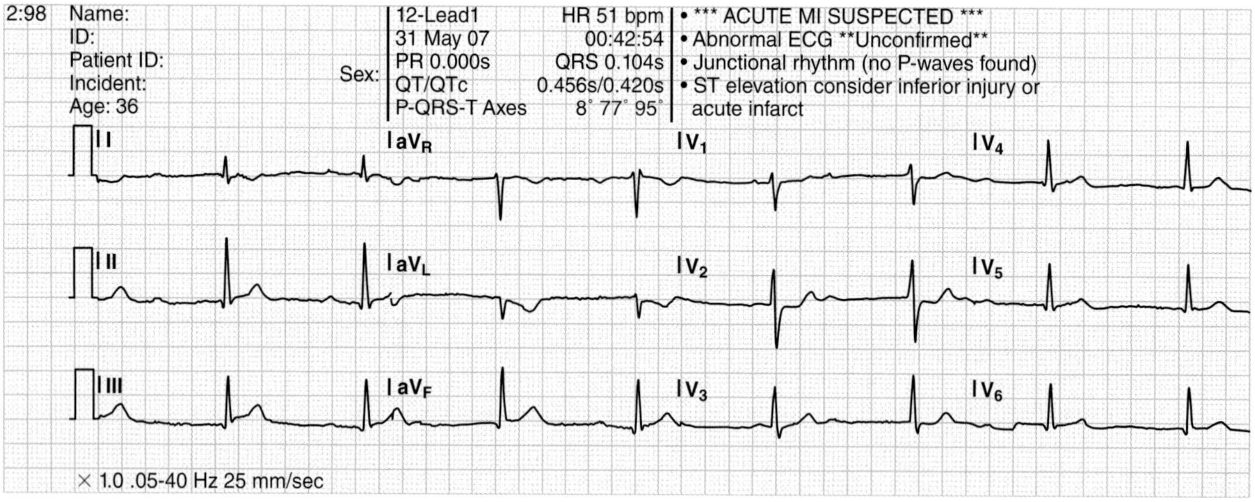

FIGURE 21-97 A 12-lead electrocardiogram strip.

> NOTE
>
> The paramedic should always measure the PR interval and the QRS complex of any ECG. A prolonged PR interval indicates AV node block. A shortened PR interval is associated with ventricular preexcitation such as in WPW. A wide QRS complex indicates either ventricular origin of the depolarization or a block in the bundle branches. Most commonly, preexisting bundle branch block is continuously present (fixed bundle branch block). The patient shows a wide QRS independent of the heart rate. However, as the heart rate increases, the QRS shape may change as a result of changes in the pattern of ventricular activation called aberrancy. This condition can lead to misdiagnosis of VT in these patients. Thorough evaluation of the patient, the ECG, and the electrical axis (described later in the chapter) is important to correctly manage these patients.

the paramedic should look at chest leads V_1 and V_2 (right chest) and leads V_5 and V_6 (left chest). If the QRS complex is wide with an RSR′ pattern in V_1 or V_2, RBBB may be present. If the wide QRS complex has a QS pattern in V_5 or V_6, LBBB may be present (**FIGURE 21-98**).

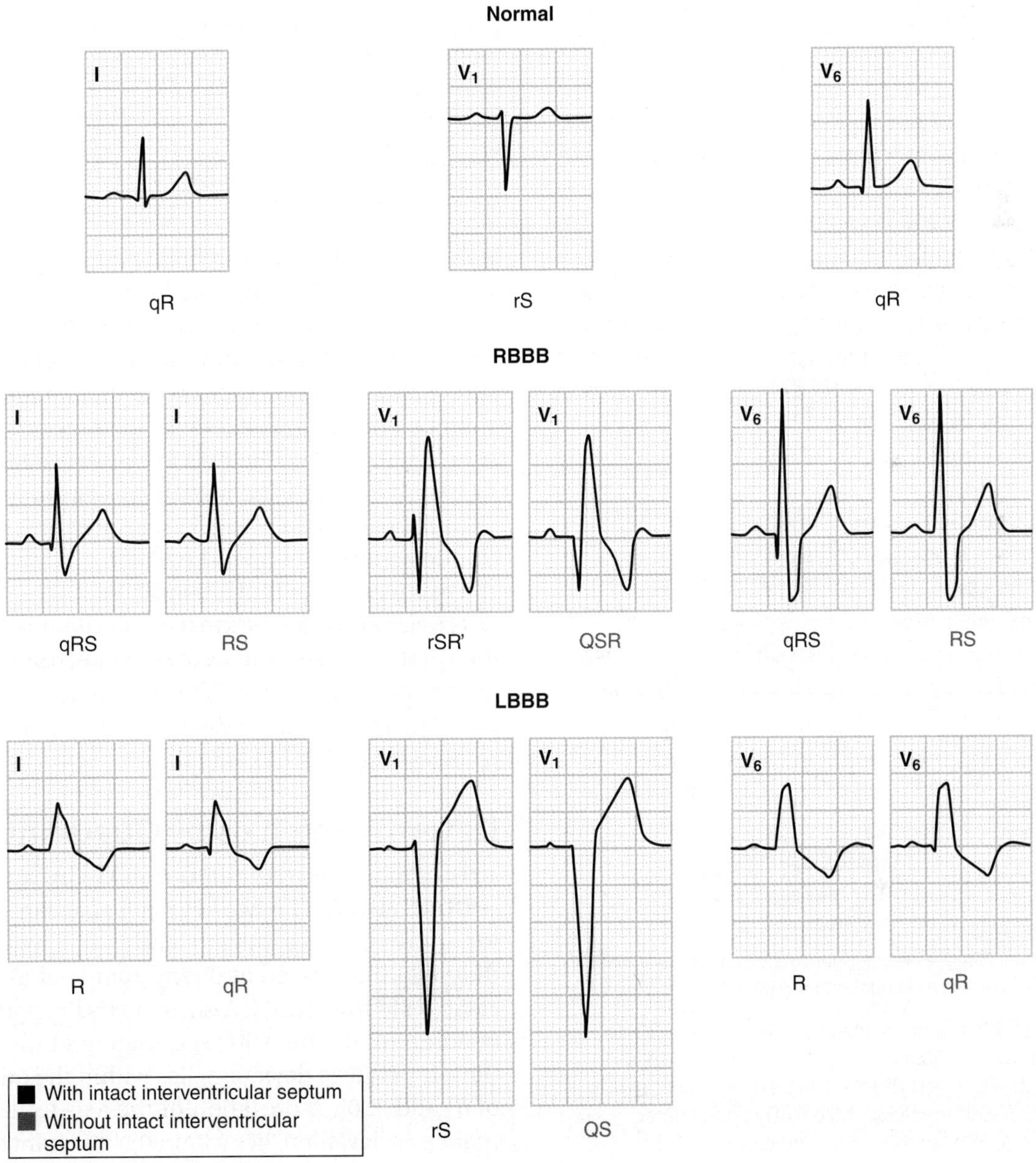

Abbreviations: LBBB, left bundle branch block; RBBB, right bundle branch block

FIGURE 21-98 Comparison of leads I, V_1, and V_6 with normal conduction, right bundle branch block, and left bundle branch block.

Determination of the Axis

As stated previously, the electrical **axis** is the direction of electrical impulse flow in the heart that stimulates contraction. This general direction of ventricular depolarization is known as the mean QRS vector. Generally, the current travels down from the AV node and to the left side of the heart. Therefore, the mean QRS vector points downward and toward the patient's left side. The position of the QRS vector can be visualized in a circle that lies on top of the patient's chest. The circle is divided into degrees, with the AV node at the center. The normal QRS vector is 0° to +90° (**FIGURE 21-99**).

The QRS vector flows slightly to the left of the ventricular septum. This is because the left ventricle has more and larger cardiac cells. Generally, most adults have a unique QRS vector that remains constant throughout life. However, if a person's cardiac status changes, the electrical axis and position of the heart can deviate from normal to right or left of its normal position. **BOX 21-10** lists common causes of axis deviation.

> NOTE
>
> The QRS vector is a representation of the electrical properties of the heart. A 12-lead ECG views the vector from 12 different angles. If the heart is displaced, the QRS vector is displaced in the same direction (right or left of normal). For example, if a patient's left ventricle is enlarged as a result of heart failure, the heart and the QRS vector are pulled to the left.

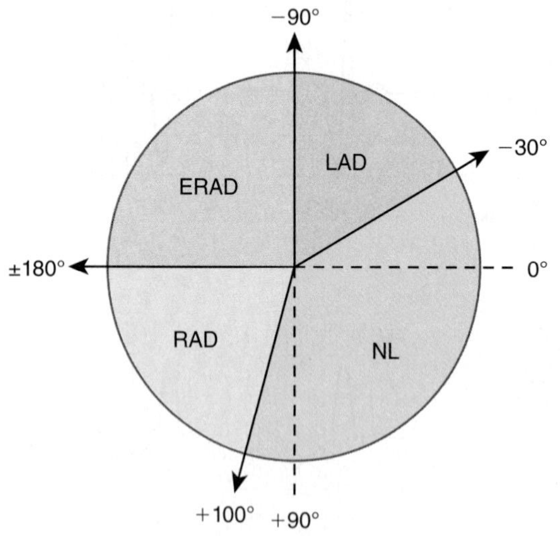

Abbreviations: ERAD, extreme right axis deviation; LAD, left axis deviation; NL, normal; RAD, right axis deviation

FIGURE 21-99 Frontal plane axes. Normal = −30° to +100°; left axis deviation = −30° to −90°; right axis deviation (RAD) = +100° to +180°; extreme right axis deviation = −90° to ±180°. Mild RAD is considered normal in children, adolescents, and young adults.

BOX 21-10 Common Causes of Axis Deviation

Right Axis Deviation

Lateral MI
Chronic lung disease
Posterior hemiblock
Left-side tension pneumothorax
Pulmonary embolism
Right ventricular hypertrophy
WPW syndrome
Sodium channel blocker toxicity
(May be a normal finding in children and tall, thin adults)

Left Axis Deviation

Left ventricular hypertrophy
Anterior hemiblock
LBBB
Mitral regurgitation
Inferior MI
Right-side tension pneumothorax
Ventricular pacemaker
Ventricular ectopy
WPW syndrome

Axis is calculated automatically by modern 12-lead ECG machines (**FIGURE 21-100**). The paramedic then interprets the degree of axis by memorization or by referring to an axis chart. If the ECG machine cannot calculate axis, it can be determined by quadrant or by assessing leads I, II, and III.

Determining Axis by Quadrant

Axis can be approximated quickly by quadrant (**FIGURE 21-101**). The two key leads that can be used for approximating axis are leads I and aV_F. Recall that lead I is located at 0° and that lead aV_F is located +90° from lead I. A normal axis lies within the quadrant of 0° and +90°. A deviation of the axis to the left (**left axis deviation**) lies within the quadrant of 0° and –90°. A deviation of the axis to the right (**right axis deviation**) lies within the quadrant of +90° and ±180°. An indeterminate axis exists when the axis

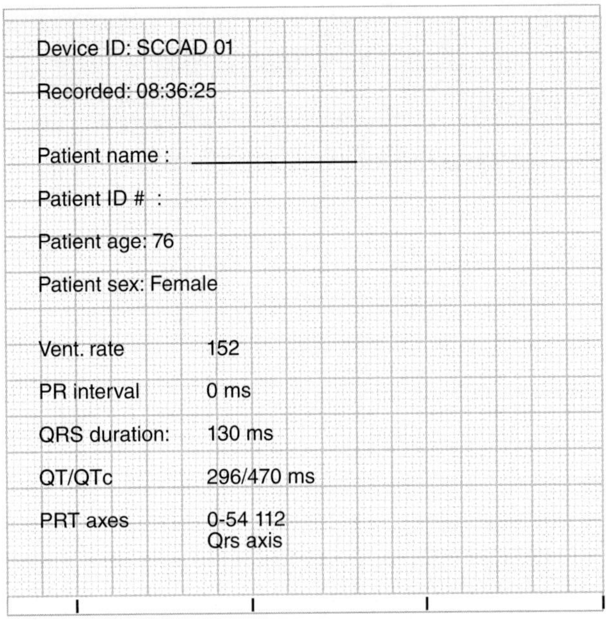

FIGURE 21-100 Axis display on electrocardiogram.

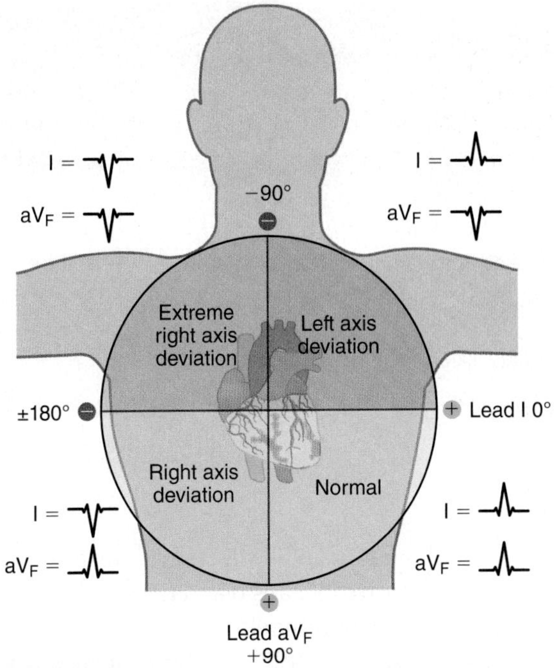

FIGURE 21-101 Approximating axis by quadrant.

> NOTE
>
> If the QRS complex in lead I is upright, then the vector is flowing right to left. If the QRS complex in lead aV_F is upright, the vector is directed top to bottom. If the QRS complex is upright in both lead I and aV_F, the electrical axis must fall into the lower left or normal quadrant (see Table 21-4).

lies within the quadrant of −90° and ±180°. By looking at the net deflection of the mean QRS vector in leads I and aV_F, the paramedic can make an approximate determination of axis (**TABLE 21-4**).

Determining Axis by Leads I, II, and III

Axis can be evaluated by looking at the QRS complexes in leads I, II, and III or aV_F. Using leads I and aV_F is often preferred because they are perpendicular to each other (**TABLE 21-5**):

- **Normal.** QRS deflection is positive (upright) in all bipolar leads.
- **Physiologic left (may be normal in some patients).** QRS deflection is positive in leads I and II but negative (inverted) in lead III/aV_F.

TABLE 21-4 Axis Deviation

	Net QRS Deflection		
Axis	**Lead I**	**aV_F**	**Axis Degrees**
Normal	Positive	Positive	0 to +90
RAD	Negative	Positive	+90 to ±180
LAD	Positive	Negative	0 to −90
Indeterminate	Negative	Negative	−90 to ±180

Abbreviations: LAD, left axis deviation; RAD, right axis deviation

TABLE 21-5 Identifying the Axis by the QRS Complex

Axis	QRS Complex Lead I	Lead II	Lead III/aV$_F$	Indications
Normal	Upright	Upright	Upright	May be normal
Physiologic left	Upright	Upright	Inverted	May be normal
Pathologic left	Upright	Inverted	Inverted	Anterior hemiblock
Right axis	Inverted	Inverted or upright	Upright	Posterior hemiblock[a]
Extreme right	Inverted	Inverted	Inverted	Ventricular in origin

[a]Chronic obstructive pulmonary disease and right ventricular hypertrophy must first be ruled out.

- **Pathologic left.** QRS deflection is positive in lead I and negative in leads II and III/aV$_F$ (indicating an anterior hemiblock).
- **Right axis.** QRS deflection is negative in lead I, negative or positive in lead II, and positive in lead III/aV$_F$. (This condition is pathologic in any adult and may indicate a posterior hemiblock.)
- **Indeterminate ("no man's land").** QRS deflection is negative in all three leads (indicating that the rhythm is ventricular in origin).

Axis and Hemiblocks

As described previously, a hemiblock is a failure in conduction of the cardiac impulse in either of two main divisions of the left bundle branch of the bundle of His. The interruption may occur in either the anterior (superior) or the posterior (inferior) division. Identifying the axis can be useful in determining the presence of hemiblocks.

Anterior Hemiblock

Anterior hemiblock occurs more often than **posterior hemiblock**. The anterior fascicle of the left bundle branch is a longer and thinner structure. Its blood supply comes mainly from the left anterior descending coronary artery. Anterior hemiblock is characterized by left axis deviation in a patient who has a supraventricular rhythm (**FIGURE 21-102**). Other ECG findings associated with an anterior hemiblock include a normal QRS complex (<0.12 second) or

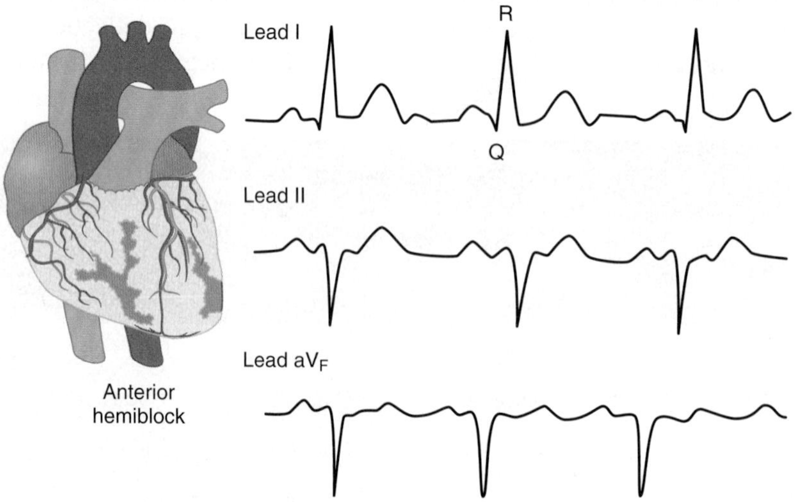

FIGURE 21-102 Anterior hemiblock.

RBBB, a small Q wave followed by a tall R wave in lead I, and a small R wave followed by a deep S wave in lead III. In a patient who has an anterior hemiblock with RBBB, impulses can be conducted only through the ventricles by way of the posterior fascicle of the left bundle branch. These patients are at high risk for the development of complete heart block.

> CRITICAL THINKING
> What rhythms are produced by supraventricular activity?

Posterior Hemiblock

The posterior fascicle of the left bundle branch is not blocked as easily as the anterior fascicle is. This is because the bundle is much thicker and has a double blood supply (left and right coronary arteries). As a result, posterior hemiblock occurs less often. This conduction disturbance is not commonly seen alone, but rather is more often associated with RBBB. For practical purposes, posterior hemiblock can be assumed in patients with right axis deviation and a QRS complex of normal width or with RBBB (**FIGURE 21-103**). Other ECG findings that indicate the presence of a posterior hemiblock include a small R wave followed by a deep S wave in lead I and a small Q wave followed by a tall R wave in lead III.

Bifascicular Block

Bifascicular block refers to the blockage of two of three pathways (fascicles) for ventricular conduction. This condition generally refers to RBBB with block of either the anterior or posterior division of the left bundle branch. (This distinction is because anterior hemiblock combined with posterior hemiblock is difficult to distinguish from LBBB.) Bifascicular block reduces myocardial contractility and cardiac output. Complete heart block may develop suddenly and without warning in patients with this condition. As a rule, the more branches with impaired conduction, the greater the chance the patient will be at risk for the development of complete AV block (especially in patients with AMI).

Twelve-Lead Strategies for Wide-Complex Tachycardias

If an unstable patient's QRS complex is wide (>0.12 second) and fast (>150 beats/min), immediate cardioversion may be indicated. If the patient is stable, however, the following steps in 12-lead assessment may help to distinguish between VT and other wide-complex tachycardias:[27]

1. Assess leads I, II, III, V_1, and V_6. If the QRS complex is negative in leads I, II, and III and positive in V_1, the rhythm indicates VT (**FIGURE 21-104**). If these criteria are not met, proceed to step 2.
2. Assess the QRS deflection in V_1 and V_6. Regardless of the QRS deflection in leads I, II, and III, positive QRS deflections with a single peak, a taller left "rabbit ear," or an RS complex with a fat R wave or slurred S wave in V_1 indicates VT. A negative QS complex, a negative RS complex, or any wide Q wave in V_6 also indicates VT (**FIGURE 21-105**).

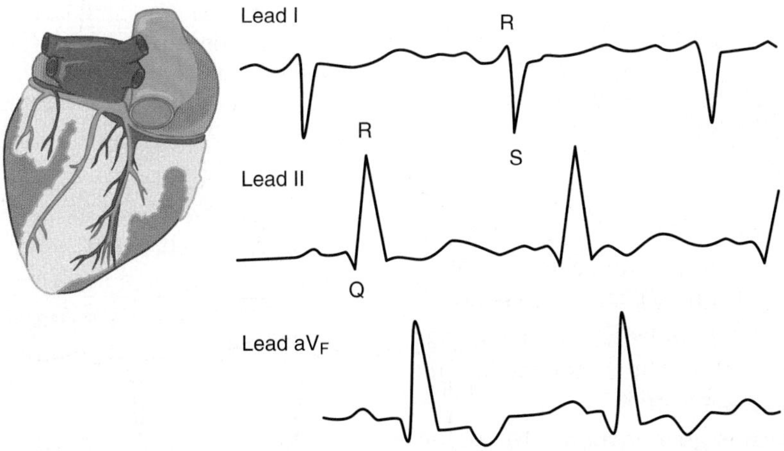

FIGURE 21-103 Posterior hemiblock.

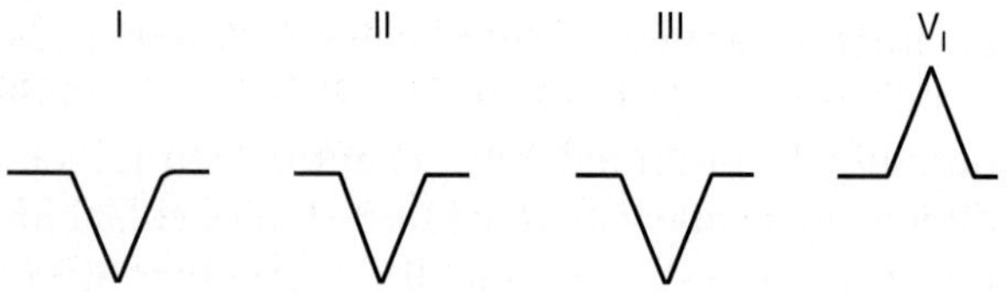

FIGURE 21-104 Criteria for ventricular tachycardia.

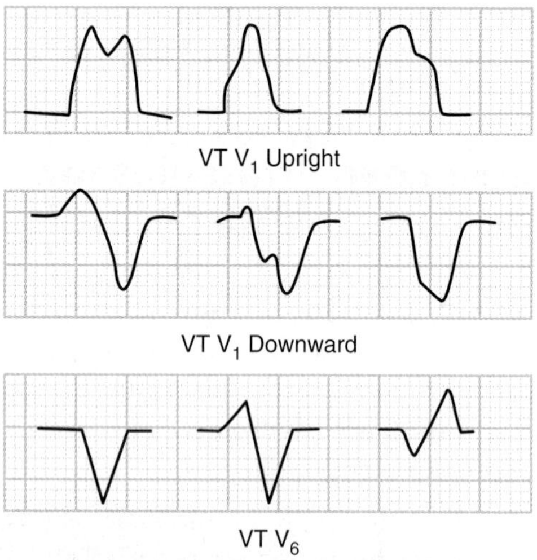

FIGURE 21-105 Step 1: A QRS complex that is negative in leads I, II, and III and positive in V_1 indicates ventricular tachycardia (VT). Step 2: Assess the QRS complex in V_1 and V_6. Step 3: Assess the QRS complex in leads I, II, III, and V_1.

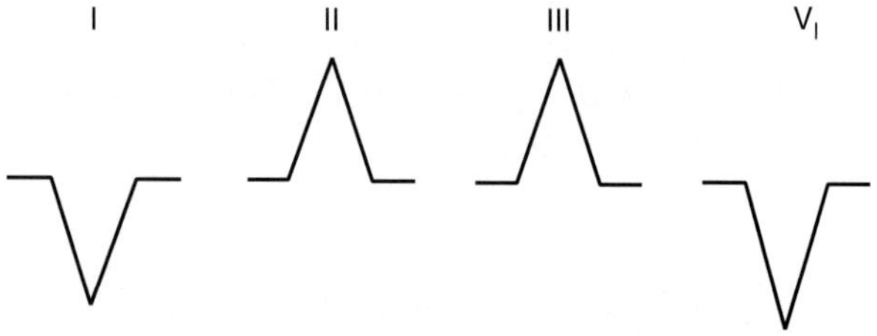

FIGURE 21-106 Right axis deviation with a downward V_1 indicates ventricular tachycardia.

3. A negative QRS complex in lead I, a positive QRS complex in leads II and III, and a negative QRS complex in V_1 indicates VT (**FIGURE 21-106**).
4. If all precordial leads (V leads) are positive or negative (precordial concordance), the rhythm indicates VT (**FIGURE 21-107**).
5. If the RS interval is greater than 0.10 second in any V lead (increased ventricular activation time), the rhythm indicates VT (**FIGURE 21-108**).

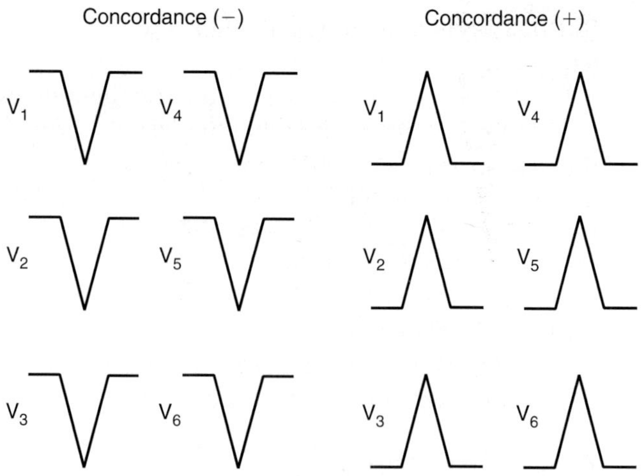

FIGURE 21-107 Ventricular tachycardia concordance.

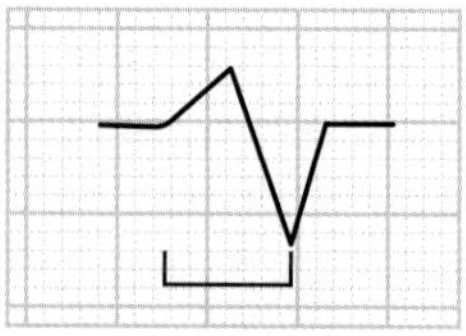

FIGURE 21-108 Ventricular tachycardia (RS interval is 0.16 second).

NOTE

Non-VT precordial concordance may occur in patients who have WPW syndrome and associated LBBB.

NOTE

ECG clues to VT are not 100% reliable. Although certain clues on the ECG tracing may favor VT, there is no absolute way to reliably distinguish VT from SVT with aberrant conduction. When in doubt, assume all regular wide-complex tachycardias are VT (unless the QRS complex is >0.20 second, in which case think toxic and/or metabolic conditions).

CRITICAL THINKING

Why is it important to distinguish between VT and wide-complex tachycardias caused by toxic or metabolic conditions?

CRITICAL THINKING

How would you manage a patient with VT and chest pain, or difficulty breathing, if you could not establish an IV line?

ST-Segment and T-Wave Changes

When the heart muscle is damaged, the damaged area is unable to contract effectively. The area remains in a constant depolarized state. The flow of current between the pathologically depolarized and normally repolarized areas can produce ST-segment elevation (**FIGURE 21-109**), ischemic ST-segment depression, or normal or nondiagnostic changes in the ST segment or T waves. Using these ECG findings, the paramedic can classify the patient into one of three groups:[28]

1. **STEMI.** ST-segment elevation is characterized by new ST-segment elevation at the J point equal to 2 mm or greater in men or 1.5 mm

or greater in women in leads V_2 to V_3 or 1 mm (0.1 mV) or greater in two or more limb leads or two other contiguous chest leads (**BOX 21-11** and **FIGURE 21-110**). A STEMI equivalent is said to exist in patients with LBBB and positive Sgarbossa criteria.

> **NOTE**
>
> Numerous methods have been proposed for measuring ST-segment elevation. Some begin the measurement at the J point. Others begin the measurement at one small box (0.04 second) after the J point. In this case, more than 1 mm of ST-segment elevation in a standard limb lead or chest lead is an abnormal finding that indicates injury.

2. **High-risk** non–ST-segment elevation myocardial infarction (non-STEMI). This group is characterized by ischemic ST-segment depression equal to or greater than 0.5 mm (0.05 mV) or dynamic

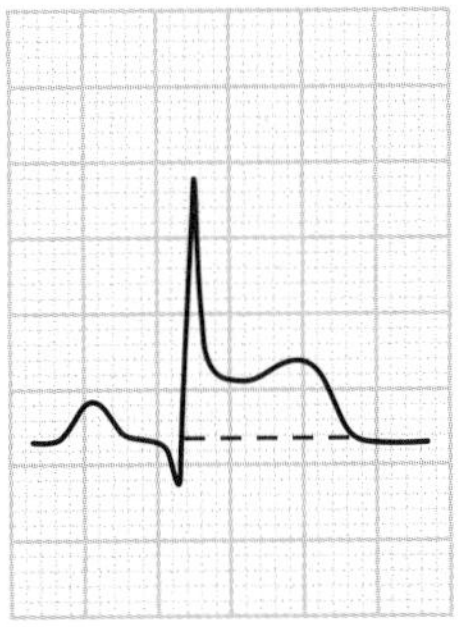

FIGURE 21-109 ST-segment elevation likely to present with acute injury.

© Jones & Bartlett Learning.

> **BOX 21-11** Contiguous Leads
>
> **Contiguous leads** are leads that are anatomically close together and that view the same general area of the heart (specifically, the walls of the left ventricle). Lead aV_R is the only lead that is not considered contiguous with another lead.

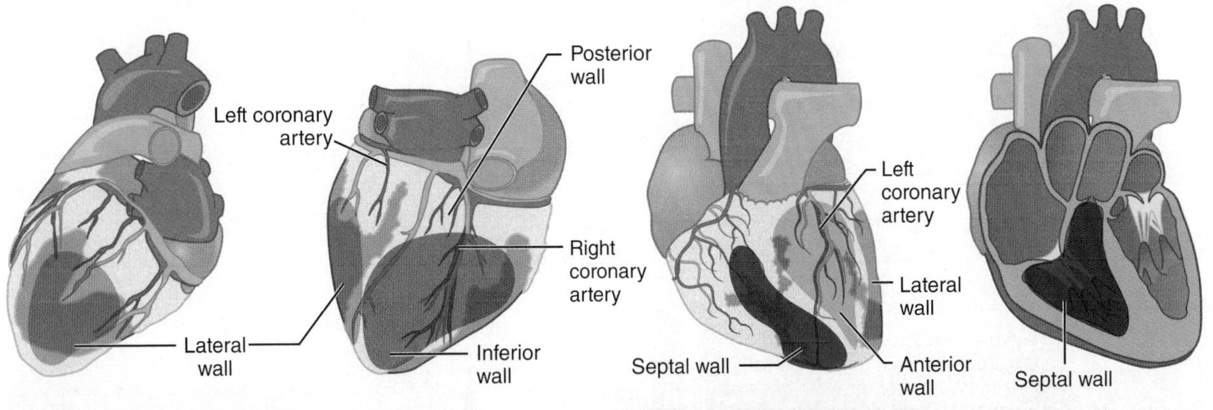

I	Lateral	aV_R	---------	V_1	Septal	V_4	Anterior
II	Inferior	aV_L	Lateral	V_2	Septal	V_5	Lateral
III	Inferior	aV_F	Inferior	V_3	Anterior	V_6	Lateral

■ Lateral I, aV_L, V_5, V_6 ■ Anterior V_3, V_4
■ Inferior II, III, aV_F ■ Septal V_1, V_2

FIGURE 21-110 Localizing electrocardiographic changes by lead with corresponding affected areas of the heart.

© Jones & Bartlett Learning.

T-wave inversion with pain or discomfort. Nonpersistent or transient ST-segment elevation equal to or greater than 0.5 mm (0.05 mV) for longer than 20 minutes is included in this category. Hyperacute T waves are broad-based, tall, and symmetrical and most evident in the anterior precordial leads. They may be the earliest sign of acute ischemia and often evolve rapidly into a STEMI. MI is a dynamic process by which one or more regions of the heart experience a decrease in oxygen supply as a result of atherothrombosis and occlusion. **FIGURE 21-111** shows the typical course of STEMI.

3. **Normal or nondiagnostic changes in ST segment or T wave.** These findings are inconclusive. This classification includes patients with normal ECG findings and those with ST-segment deviation of less than 0.5 mm (0.05 mV) or T-wave inversion less than or equal to 0.2 mV. Special cardiac studies and testing are needed for these patients.

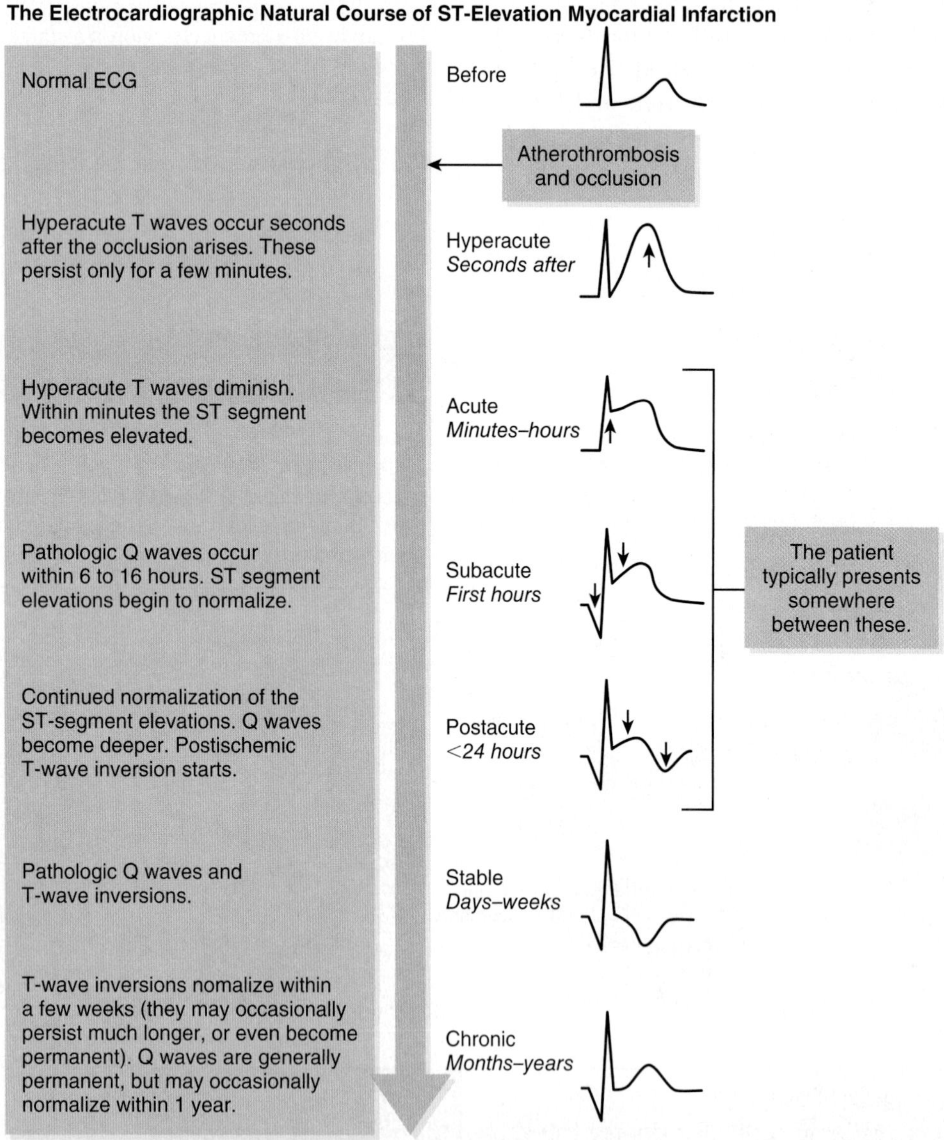

The Electrocardiographic Natural Course of ST-Elevation Myocardial Infarction
Normal ECG
Before
Atherothrombosis and occlusion
Hyperacute T waves occur seconds after the occlusion arises. These persist only for a few minutes.
Hyperacute
Seconds after
Hyperacute T waves diminish. Within minutes the ST segment becomes elevated.
Acute
Minutes–hours
Pathologic Q waves occur within 6 to 16 hours. ST segment elevations begin to normalize.
Subacute
First hours
The patient typically presents somewhere between these.
Continued normalization of the ST-segment elevations. Q waves become deeper. Postischemic T-wave inversion starts.
Postacute
<24 hours
Pathologic Q waves and T-wave inversions.
Stable
Days–weeks
T-wave inversions nomalize within a few weeks (they may occasionally persist much longer, or even become permanent). Q waves are generally permanent, but may occasionally normalize within 1 year.
Chronic
Months–years

Abbreviation: ECG, electrocardiogram

FIGURE 21-111 Normalization of ST-segment elevation and T-wave changes during myocardial infarction. The electrocardiogram shows hyperacute T waves following resolution of ST-segment elevation, followed by pathologic Q waves and ischemic T-wave inversion.

Modified from: ECGwaves. https://ecgwaves.com/the-ecg-in-assessment-of-reperfusion/

NOTE

ST-segment elevation is best measured by drawing a baseline from the end of the T wave to the start of the P wave using either of the methods described previously. The ST segment then is compared with the isoelectric baseline. However, ST-segment elevation is not always present on an initial ECG tracing. This is true even when a patient is experiencing an MI. When ST-segment elevation is present in a symptomatic patient, the paramedic should notify medical direction and transmit an ECG for evaluation (per protocol). Even if infarction is present, ST-segment elevation is a poor indicator of the type or cause of infarction. In addition, ST-segment elevation can be caused by conditions other than AMI, including the following:

- LBBB
- Some ventricular rhythms
- Left ventricular hypertrophy
- Pericarditis
- Ventricular aneurysm
- Early repolarization

Use of a 12-Lead ECG to Assess Infarcts

Early recognition and management of AMI sometimes can salvage a damaged myocardium ("time is muscle"). The current STEMI treatment guidelines recommend that EMS personnel perform a 12-lead ECG at the site of first medical contact if the patient's symptoms are consistent with STEMI (class I).[28] Paramedics can use the following five-step analysis for infarct recognition:[7]

1. **Identify the rate and rhythm.** Manage any life-threatening dysrhythmias.

NOTE

LBBB that impairs repolarization may "look like" STEMI. If LBBB is present, ST-segment elevation measurements will not be diagnostic for infarction. The paramedic should use the Sgarbossa criteria (described previously) to help identify MI in the presence of LBBB.

2. **Identify the area of infarct.** ST-segment elevation is the most reliable indicator during the first hours of infarction. ST-segment elevation can be present before permanent tissue damage has occurred. If ST-segment elevation is present in a patient with chest pain, the paramedic should identify the degree of elevation and visualize the cardiac anatomy to predict which coronary artery is occluded (**FIGURE 21-112**). The paramedic should use a systematic approach for 12-lead assessment. One method is to begin by assessing the inferior leads (II, III, aV_F), followed by the septal leads (V_1, V_2), anterior leads (V_3, V_4), and lateral leads (V_5, V_6, I, aV_L). The paramedic evaluates each lead for ST-segment elevation (the most important sign of injury), deep symmetrically inverted T waves (a sign of ischemia), ST-segment depression (a reciprocal change to ST elevation), and pathologic Q waves (**TABLE 21-6**, **TABLE 21-7**, and **FIGURE 21-113**).

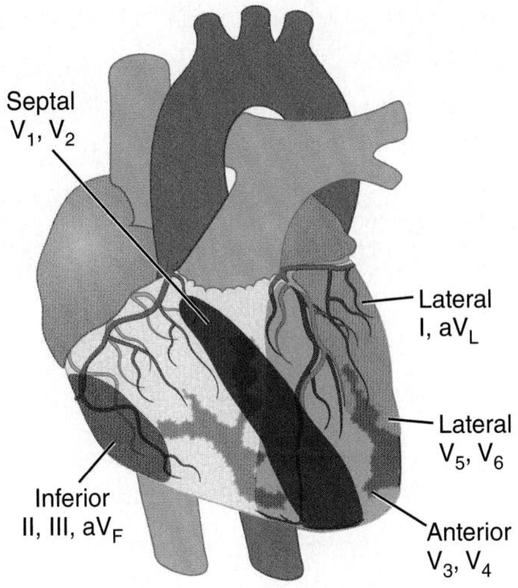

FIGURE 21-112 Multilead assessment of the heart.

NOTE

Within the first 30 minutes after a coronary occlusion, the T-wave amplitude increases and becomes more prominent, symmetrical, and pointed (most evident in the anterior chest leads). T waves that become proportionally large when compared with the QRS are known as hyperacute T waves. The T-wave amplitude is short-lived and is quickly followed by ST-segment elevation and a loss of R-wave amplitude (evident in the precordial leads when advancing from V_1 to V_6). This finding is known as reverse R-wave progression and can indicate ischemia or ventricular dysfunction. (It also can occur with lead placement reversal.) Hyperacute T waves and reverse R-wave progression are suggestive of early anterior wall MI.

Modified from: Dressler W, Roesler H. High T waves in the earliest stage of myocardial infarction. *Am Heart J*. 1947;34(5):627-645.

TABLE 21-6 ST-Segment Elevation and Location of Infarct

Lead	Location of Infarct	Coronary Artery Involved
II, III, aV_F	Inferior wall (most common)	Right
V_1, V_2	Septal wall	Left
V_3, V_4	Anterior wall (most lethal)	Left
I, aV_L, V_5, V_6	Lateral wall	Left
V_{4R}-V_{6R}	Right ventricle	Right

TABLE 21-7 Reciprocal Changes Seen With ST-Segment Elevation Myocardial Infarction

Injury Site	ST Elevation	Reciprocal ST Depression
Septal	V_1, V_2	None
Anterior	V_3, V_4	None
Anteroseptal	V_1, V_2, V_3, V_4	None
Lateral	I, aV_L, V_5, V_6	II, III, aV_F
Anterolateral	I, aV_L, V_3, V_4, V_5, V_6	II, III, aV_F
Inferior	II, III, aV_F	I, aV_L
Posterior	V_7, V_8, V_9	V_1, V_2, V_3, V_4

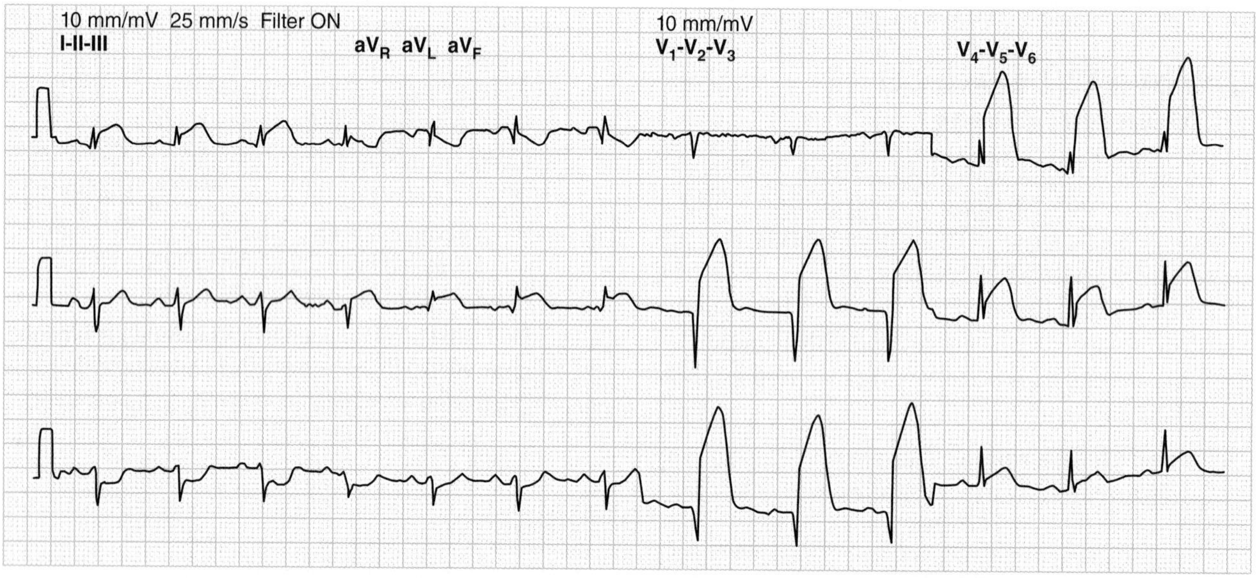

FIGURE 21-113 Twelve-lead electrocardiogram showing ST-segment elevation myocardial infarction and reciprocal ST-segment depression.

In an acute STEMI, reciprocal changes may be seen between leads that face the acute injury and leads that face the lateral boundary of the injury (between ischemic and healthy tissue). Leads that face the injury often show ST-segment elevation. Leads that face the boundary often show ST-segment depression.[29] Reciprocal changes are not always visible on the 12-lead ECG during acute STEMI. However, if they are visible, this confirms the diagnosis.

At times, the extent of the infarction can be gauged by the number of leads showing ST-segment elevation. The degree of ST-segment elevation also is important. For example, large infarcts often show an ST elevation of 7 mm or more in inferior leads and 12 mm or more in anterior leads. ST-segment elevation or new or presumably new LBBB is suspicious for injury and should be assessed using the Sgarbossa criteria.

3. **Consider other conditions** that could be responsible for ST-segment changes (as described previously). These "infarct impostors" also may be present in a patient experiencing AMI. Ventricular rhythms often produce Q waves and ST-segment elevation. Ventricular rhythms also do not have reciprocal ST depression. In addition, early repolarization produces no clinical symptoms.
4. **Assess the patient's clinical presentation** because this is just as crucial as the ECG findings. The findings of a thorough patient history and a physical examination should be incorporated into the ECG interpretation. Not all patients with AMI have classic signs and symptoms. Therefore, the paramedic should maintain a high degree of suspicion in the absence of pain (especially if the patient is diabetic, an older adult, or a postmenopausal woman). As many as 50% of patients with AMI have no early ECG changes. The clinical picture, therefore, is important.
5. **Recognize the infarction and initiate care.** When all indications point to AMI, current guidelines recommend that EMS transport directly to a hospital capable of percutaneous coronary intervention (PCI), with a goal of 90 minutes or less from first medical contact to revascularization device (class I).[28]

SHOW ME THE EVIDENCE

In Ohio, researchers conducted a cross-sectional retrospective review of 200 prehospital 12-lead ECGs transmitted by over 200 EMS agencies to one hospital over 3 years. They compared them with a random control group of 100 ECGs from patients who did not have a STEMI. Computer interpretation of "acute MI suspected" was counted as accurate, whereas other interpretations were scored as misses. None of the control (non-STEMI) ECGs were incorrectly labeled as "acute MI suspected." The specificity was 100% (100/100; 95% confidence interval [CI], 0.96–1.0); however, the sensitivity was 58% (58/100; 95% CI, 0.48–0.67). Thus, there would have been no inappropriate activations of the cardiac catheter lab. However, in 42 cases, the cardiac catheter lab was not activated when it should have been. The researchers concluded that paramedics should not rely on the computer interpretation only.

Modified from: Bhalla MC, Mencl F, Gist MA, Wilber S, Zalewski J. Prehospital electrocardiographic computer identification of ST-segment elevation myocardial infarction. *Prehosp Emerg Care.* 2013;17(2):211-216.

Right-Side and Posterior ECGs

The wall of the right ventricle and the posterior wall of the left ventricle are areas of the heart that are difficult to evaluate with standard precordial leads. For adult patients, right-side and posterior ECGs increase sensitivity for MIs that occur in these areas. The more leads that reveal acute changes in the heart, the larger the area of infarct is presumed to be.

Right-Side ECG (Leads V_{3R} Through V_{6R})

A right-side ECG is useful in detecting right ventricular STEMI associated with occlusion of the right coronary artery. Indications of a right ventricular wall infarction may include the following:[30]

- ST elevation in the inferior leads, II, III, and aV_F (ST elevation that is greatest in lead III is especially significant.)
- ST elevation in lead V_1 (considered to be the only precordial lead that faces the right ventricle on the standard 12-lead ECG)
- Other findings, which may include RBBB, second- and third-degree AV blocks, ST-segment elevation in lead V_2 50% greater than the magnitude of ST-segment depression in lead aV_F
- Hypotension and clear lung fields

When configuring right-side ECG lead placement, V_1 should be labeled V_{1R} (which is the same lead as V_2), V_2 should be labeled V_{2R} (which is the same lead as V_1), V_3 is labeled V_{3R}, V_4 is labeled V_{4R}, V_5 is labeled V_{5R}, and V_6 is labeled V_{6R}. ST elevation across the right-side leads (V_{3R} to V_{6R}) are diagnostic of right ventricular STEMI.

NOTE

It has been reported that an ST-segment elevation in lead V_{4R} that is greater than 1.0 mm has 100% sensitivity, 87% specificity, and 92% predictive accuracy for infarction of the right ventricular wall. Therefore, many EMS systems will move just the V_4 lead to the V_{4R} position for an initial assessment of ST elevation.

Modified from: Somers MP, Brady WJ, Bateman DC, et al. Additional electrocardiographic leads in the ED chest pain patient: right ventricular and posterior leads. *Am J Emerg Med.* 2003;21:563-73; and Robalino BD, Whitlow PL, Underwood DA, et al. Electrocardiographic manifestations of right ventricular infarction. *Am Heart J.* 1989;118(1):138-44.

Posterior ECG (Leads V_7 Through V_9)

A posterior ECG is useful in detecting posterior STEMI associated with occlusion of the circumflex artery or dominant right coronary artery. Indications for a posterior wall infarction include changes in leads V_1 through V_3 on the standard 12-lead ECG predominantly, which include the following:[31]

- Horizontal ST depression
- A tall, upright T wave
- A tall, wide R wave
- R:S wave ratio greater than 1 mm
- Inferior or lateral wall MI, especially if accompanied by ST depression or prominent R waves in leads V_1 through V_3

Lead Placements

Right-side ECG leads (V_{3R} through V_{6R}) are positioned in a mirror image fashion from the standard 12-lead precordial leads. Posterior ECG leads (V_7 through V_9) are applied by moving V_4 through V_6 in the posterior positions (**FIGURE 21-114** and **FIGURE 21-115**).

Assessment of the Patient With Cardiac Disease

A focused evaluation of any patient should identify a chief complaint. It also should cover the history of the event and any significant medical history, and it should include a physical examination. These elements are crucial in determining the cause of the

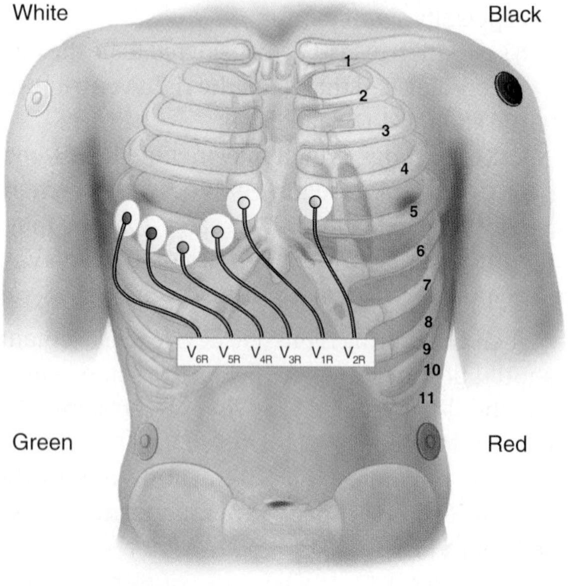

Lead	Location	View
V_{1R}	Left of sternum, 4th intercostal space (ICS)	Ventricular septum
V_{2R}	Right of sternum, 4th ICS	Ventricular septum
V_{3R}	Precisely between V_{2R} and V_{4R}	Right ventricle
V_{4R}	Right midclavicular, 5th ICS	Right ventricle
V_{5R}	Precisely between V_{4R} and V_{6R}	Right ventricle
V_{6R}	Right midaxillary, 5th ICS	Right ventricle

A

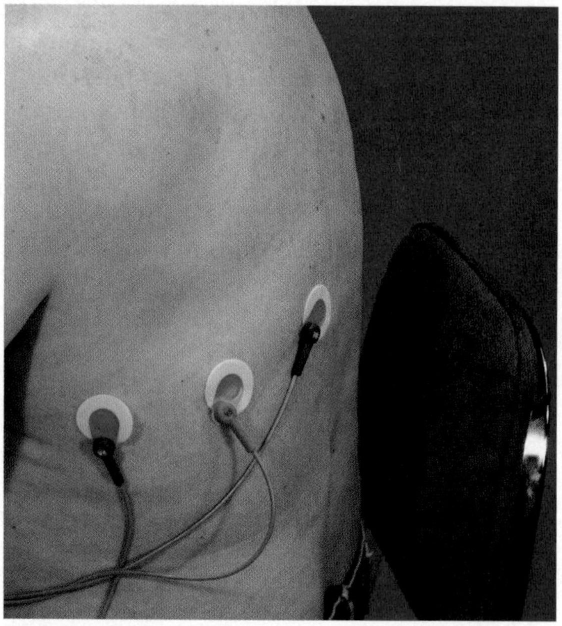

Lead	Location	View
V_7	Posterior axillary line 5th intercostal space	Posterior wall of left ventricle
V_8	Midscapular, 5th intercostal space	Posterior wall of left ventricle
V_9	Just to the left of the spine, 5th intercostal space	Posterior wall of left ventricle

B

FIGURE 21-114 A. Right-side lead placement. Right-side electrocardiographic (ECG) leads (V_{1R} through V_{6R}) are positioned in a mirror image fashion from the standard 12-lead precordial leads. Arm and leg electrodes remain unchanged from the standard 12-lead ECG. **B.** Posterior lead placement. Posterior ECG leads (V_7 through V_9) are applied by moving leads V_4 through V_6 in the posterior positions. Leads V_1 through V_3 remain unchanged from the standard 12-lead ECG. Note: Right-side and posterior leads may need to be hand-labeled on the ECG printout, if such labeling is not done by the ECG machine.

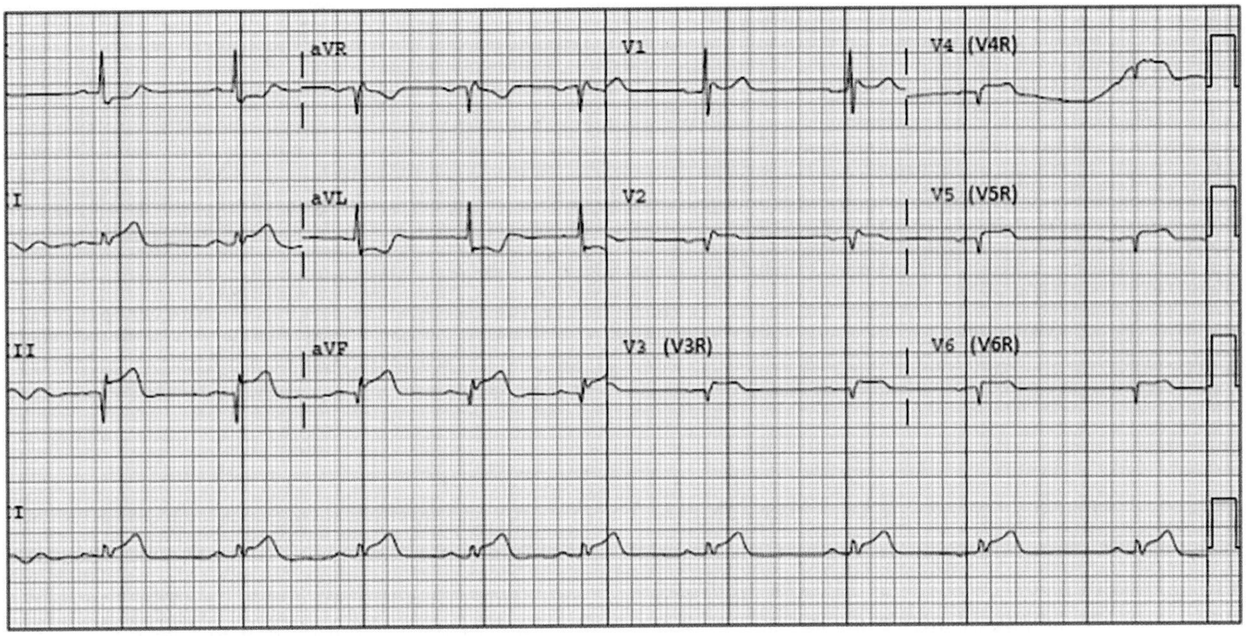

A

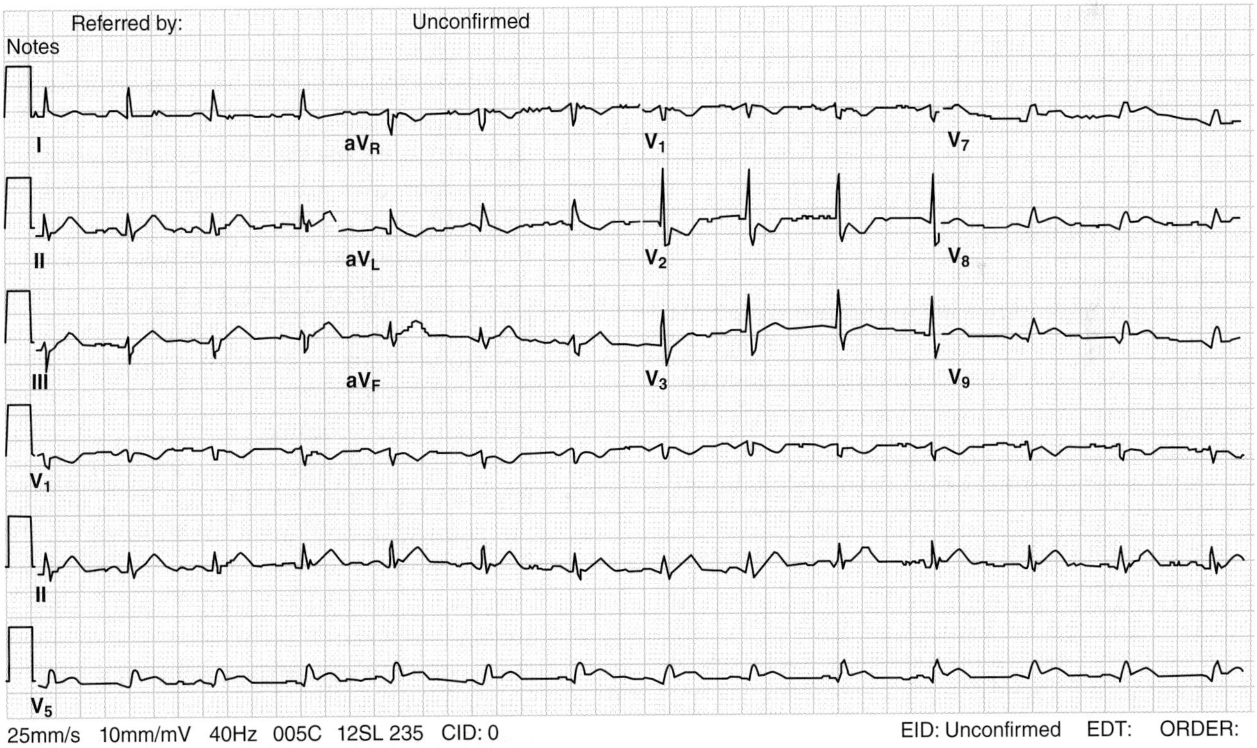

B

FIGURE 21-115 **A.** Right-side electrocardiogram (ECG). Look for ST elevation in lead V_{4R} of 1.0 mm. **B.** Posterior ECG. Look for ST elevation greater than 0.5 to 1.0 mm in leads V_8 through V_9.

A: The Permanente Journal, 21, 16–105, Nagam, M. R., Vinson, D. R., & Levis, J. T., ECG Diagnosis: Right Ventricular Myocardial Infarction, 2017, with permission from The Permanente Press; **B:** Reprinted with permission from SLACK Incorporated.

NOTE

Right ventricular infarction or ischemia may occur in up to 50% of patients with inferior wall MI. Right ventricular infarction should be suspected in patients with inferior wall infarction, hypotension, and clear lung fields. In these cases, a right-side ECG should be obtained to confirm the field impression. ST-segment elevation (>1 mm) in lead V_{4R} is sensitive for right ventricular infarction (sensitivity, 88%; specificity, 78%; diagnostic accuracy, 83%). These findings also are a strong predictor of increased in-hospital complications and mortality. If right ventricular infarction is identified, nitroglycerin may be given with caution based on local protocols.

Modified from: Goldstein JA. Acute right ventricular infarction. *Cardiol Clin*. 2012;30(2):219-232; O'Connor RE, Brady W, Brooks SC, et al. Part 10: acute coronary syndromes: 2010 American Heart Association Guidelines for Cardiopulmonary Resuscitation and Emergency Cardiovascular Care. *Circulation*. 2010;122(18)(suppl 3):S787-S817; 2015; and American Heart Association Guidelines for Cardiopulmonary Resuscitation and Emergency Cardiovascular Care. *Circulation*. 2015;132:S313-S314.

emergency. They also help paramedics determine the initial patient care and anticipate potential problems during transport to a medical facility. The following discussion of patient assessment explains the approach to the patient with a cardiovascular emergency.

CRITICAL THINKING

A patient has made an EMS call about a cardiovascular problem. What emotions might the patient be feeling?

Chief Complaint

Cardiovascular disease may cause a variety of symptoms. Obtaining an appropriate history of each symptom is important to form a field diagnosis of any patient with a possible coronary event. Common chief complaints include chest pain or discomfort, including shoulder, arm, neck, or jaw pain or discomfort; dyspnea; syncope; and abnormal heartbeat or palpitations.

In some patients (eg, some women, older adults, patients with diabetes mellitus), cardiovascular problems commonly have atypical symptoms. These symptoms include mental status changes, abdominal or gastrointestinal symptoms (including persistent heartburn), and vague complaints of feeling ill.

Chest Pain or Discomfort

Chest pain or discomfort is the most common chief complaint of patients with MI. However, many causes of chest pain are not related to cardiac disease (eg, pulmonary embolus, pleurisy, reflux esophagitis). Therefore, a history of chest pain is a key factor. The OPQRST method (or a similar method) should be used to obtain the following information when possible:

- **Onset.** Ask the patient to describe the pain or discomfort: What does it feel like? What were you doing when the pain began? Have you ever had this type of pain before? Is it the same as or different from the last time?
- **Provocation/palliation.** Try to determine the events surrounding the patient's symptoms: What do you think might have caused this pain? Does anything you do make the pain better or worse? Does the pain go away when you rest? Have you taken nitroglycerin for the pain, and if so, did it help? Does the pain get worse when you exercise or walk or when you eat certain foods?
- **Quality.** Ask the patient to describe the pain or discomfort in his or her own words. Common descriptions for the quality of chest pain associated with a coronary event include sharp, tearing, burning, heavy, and squeezing.
- **Region/radiation.** Ask the patient to localize the pain: With one finger, point to where the pain is the most intense. Does the pain move (radiate) to another area of the body or does it stay in one place? If the pain moves, to where does it move? (Cardiac chest pain often radiates to the arms, neck, jaw, and back.)
- **Severity.** Ask the patient to rate the pain or discomfort to establish a baseline: On a scale of 0 to 10, with 10 being the worst pain you have ever had, what number would you use to describe this pain? If you have had pain like this before, is this pain worse than the last time or not as bad as the last time?

- **Timing.** Try to determine the duration of the pain episode and document it. How long have you had this pain? Is the pain better or worse than it was when you called for help? Is the pain constant or does it come and go?

CRITICAL THINKING

What factors may influence a person's perception and description of pain?

NOTE

Chest pain is a common complaint of cocaine users. Cocaine can cause serious cardiac toxicity because of the effect of the drug on the heart. It also stimulates the CNS, which in turn also stimulates the cardiovascular system. Although rare, AMI can occur in these patients, even in the absence of risk factors for ischemic heart disease.

Modified from: 2015 American Heart Association Guidelines for Cardiopulmonary Resuscitation and Emergency Cardiovascular Care. *Circulation.* 2015;132:S313-S314.

Dyspnea

Dyspnea (difficulty breathing) often is associated with MI. It is a main symptom of pulmonary congestion caused by heart failure. Other common causes of dyspnea that may be unrelated to heart disease include chronic obstructive pulmonary disease, respiratory infection, pulmonary embolus, and asthma. Historical factors important in differentiating breathing difficulties include the following:

- Duration and circumstances of onset of dyspnea
- Anything that aggravates or relieves the dyspnea, including medications
- Previous episodes
- Associated symptoms
- Orthopnea
- Previous cardiac problems

Syncope

Syncope is a brief loss of consciousness often caused by a sudden decrease in oxygenated blood to the brain. Initial signs include loss of muscle control, eyelid closure, eye fixation or upward eye deviation and, in some cases, muscle twitching.[31] Cardiac causes of syncope result from events that reduce cardiac output. Risk factors for recurrent syncope in older adults are aortic stenosis, impaired renal function, AV block, LBBB, male sex, chronic obstructive pulmonary disease, heart failure, AF, advancing age, and medications that lower blood pressure.[32] The most common cardiac disorders associated with syncope are dysrhythmias. Other causes of syncope include subarachnoid hemorrhage, ectopic pregnancy, drug or alcohol intoxication, aortic stenosis or dissection, pulmonary embolism, hemorrhage, orthostatic syndromes, transient ischemic attack, and anxiety or panic disorder. In older patients, syncope may be the only symptom of a cardiac problem. Young, healthy people may have a syncopal episode. This episode is often caused by prolonged standing in a hot location or by stimulation of the vagus nerve (**vasovagal syncope**), which can produce hypotension and bradycardia. These types of syncope pose a much lower risk of death than do cardiovascular causes. The history of a syncopal event should include the following:

- Presyncope aura (nausea, weakness, lightheadedness)
- Circumstances of occurrence (eg, patient's position before the event, severe pain, or emotional stress)
- Duration of syncopal episode
- Symptoms before syncopal episode (palpitation, seizure, incontinence)
- Other associated symptoms
- Previous episodes of syncope

NOTE

Cardiac syncope often occurs without warning or with palpitations. By comparison, vasovagal syncope often is preceded by a minute or two of nausea and weakness before the loss of consciousness.

Physical examination after syncope should include assessment of orthostatic vital signs. A 12-lead ECG should also be obtained.

CRITICAL THINKING

Syncopal events often occur in public places, such as a church. How can you ease the feelings of embarrassment the patient may have in this situation?

Abnormal Heartbeat and Palpitations

Many patients are aware of their own heartbeat, particularly if it is irregular (skipping beats) or rapid (fluttering). Abnormal heartbeats may be felt by the patient as **palpitations** (the sensation of irregular or forceful beating of the heart) and often are a benign occurrence. However, they may indicate a serious dysrhythmia. Important information to obtain with these patients includes the following:

- Pulse rate
- Regular versus irregular rhythm
- Circumstances of occurrence
- Duration
- Associated symptoms (chest pain, diaphoresis, syncope, confusion, dyspnea)
- Previous episodes and frequency
- Medication (drug stimulant) or alcohol use

Significant Medical History

The medical history is a vital part of any patient assessment. If possible, the paramedic should determine the following information.

- Is the patient taking prescription medications, particularly cardiac medications? Common medications that should alert the paramedic to a possible coronary event include nitroglycerin, atenolol, metoprolol, and other beta blockers; digoxin; furosemide and other diuretics; antihypertensives; and antihyperlipidemic agents. The paramedic also should ask the patient about his or her compliance in taking medications. The use of any erectile dysfunction drugs or nonprescription drugs, such as over-the-counter medications and herbal supplements, should also be ascertained. Alcohol use or illicit drug use may be a contributing factor in the patient's chief complaint.
- Is the patient being treated for any other illness? A medical history that includes angina pectoris, previous MI, or treatment for coronary artery disease, including coronary artery bypass (**BOX 21-12**) or PCI and stent placement (**angioplasty**) (described later in the chapter), increases the likelihood of a significant coronary event. Chronic illness such as heart failure, valvular disease, renal disease, hypertension, aneurysms, diabetes mellitus, inflammatory cardiac disease (eg, endocarditis, myocarditis), and lung disease also are indicators that heart disease may be present.
- Does the patient have any allergies? Medication allergies (eg, an allergy to aspirin or radiographic dye) may be important in the course of the patient's

BOX 21-12 Coronary Bypass Surgery

During coronary bypass surgery, blood vessels from another part of the body are used to "bypass" diseased coronary arteries. This procedure improves blood flow in the heart. The goal of improved blood flow is to reduce chest pain and to reduce the risk of MI. This surgical procedure is sometimes referred to as coronary artery bypass grafting (CABG; sometimes pronounced cabbage). A patient may have one, two, three, or more bypass grafts, depending on how many coronary arteries are blocked, how significantly they are blocked, and the functional status of the heart muscle those arteries are supplying. Three-vessel and four-vessel coronary bypass surgery is common.

Coronary bypass surgery may be performed with or without a heart-lung machine ("on-pump" or "off-pump" surgery). During surgery, an artery is removed from the patient's chest wall or arm (internal mammary artery or radial artery) and is sewn to the coronary artery below the site of the blockage. If a vein is used (usually the saphenous vein, taken from the patient's leg), it is attached to the aorta and then grafted to the coronary artery below the blocked area. In either case, the surgery allows blood to flow more freely through the grafts to nourish the heart muscle. Grafts normally remain open and function well for 10 to 15 years.

Several alternatives to CABG have made this procedure less common. The preferred treatment in acute situations is generally PCI (formerly called angioplasty with stent). During PCI, several procedures may be achieved. Most often a balloon catheter is placed over a guide wire (balloon angioplasty). The catheter is used to insert a meshlike stent into a narrowed section of a coronary artery. Once positioned, the balloon is inflated, which opens the stent and pushes it against the arterial wall. The balloon then is deflated and removed, leaving the stent permanently in place to keep the artery open. Most modern stents are coated with a medication (drug-eluting stents) that prevents the growth of cells around the stent, thus reducing the chance of the artery closing again (restenosis). Stents also may be placed without angioplasty. Other procedures performed during PCI include atherectomy (removal of atherosclerotic plaque) and use of radiation to prevent restenosis. If PCI is contraindicated or otherwise unavailable, fibrinolytic therapy can be used.

care. The paramedic should document these allergies and report them to medical direction.
- Does the patient have risk factors for a heart attack? Examples of risk factors include older age, tobacco use, diabetes mellitus, a family history of heart disease, obesity, an increased serum cholesterol level (hypercholesterolemia), and illicit drug use.
- Does the patient have an implanted pacemaker, **ventricular assist device**, or ICD? The presence of these devices (described later in the chapter) indicates a significant coronary history.

Physical Examination

The classic presentation of MI is pain or discomfort beneath the sternum or of the left arm that lasts longer than 30 minutes. The pain often is described as crushing, pressure, squeezing, or burning. Associated signs and symptoms may include apprehension, diaphoresis, dyspnea, nausea and vomiting, and a sense of impending doom (eg, patients feel that they are going to die). However, at times the presentation is atypical. The paramedic's skill in gathering a relevant medical history and performing a focused physical examination directs the patient care. For example, patients with myocardial ischemia may deny that they have chest pain. They may need to be asked specifically about tightness or squeezing in the chest.

> CRITICAL THINKING
>
> Think of a way to ask a patient a question about chest pain that cannot be answered with a simple yes or no.

When caring for a patient who has chest pain caused by heart problems, the paramedic should understand that the patient is frightened. Chest pain is associated with life-threatening consequences. These patients should be calmed and reassured to reduce their anxiety.

Primary Survey

The primary survey for a patient with a possible coronary event should include a more in-depth evaluation of the patient's level of consciousness, respirations, pulse, and blood pressure.

A change in the patient's level of consciousness (eg, light-headedness or confusion) may indicate decreased cerebral perfusion caused by poor cardiac output. If possible, the paramedic should determine the patient's normal level of functioning by interviewing the patient, family members, or others who are familiar with the patient (eg, neighbors, nursing staff). In addition, the paramedic should evaluate the patient's baseline vital signs. These findings are important during reassessment to identify trending and to guide patient care.

Physical Examination

The physical examination of a patient with cardiac disease should be organized and complete. The paramedic should use the following look-listen-feel approach. (Chapter 19, *Secondary Assessment and Reassessment*, presents a more detailed discussion of the physical examination.)

Look

- **Skin.** Pale and diaphoretic skin may indicate peripheral vasoconstriction and sympathetic stimulation. Cyanosis is an indicator of poor oxygenation. Pulse oximetry is assessed to determine the need for oxygen application.
- **Jugular veins.** An increase in central venous pressure from heart failure and cardiac tamponade can produce distention of internal jugular veins. **Jugular venous distention (JVD)** is best evaluated with the patient's head elevated to 45°. Distention may be difficult to assess in patients with obesity.
- **Peripheral and presacral edema.** Edema can result from chronic back pressure in the systemic venous circulation. It may be related to right heart failure. Edema is most obvious in dependent areas. (These areas may include the ankles and the sacral region in bedridden patients.) Edema can be classified as nonpitting (minimal or no depression of tissue after removal of finger pressure) or pitting (depression of tissue remains after removal of finger pressure).
- **Additional indicators of cardiac disease.** Other signs of cardiac disease that may be found on a visual inspection include a midsternal scar from coronary surgery (**FIGURE 21-116**), a nitroglycerin patch on the skin, an implanted pacemaker or ventricular assist device or ICD in the left upper chest or abdominal wall, a defibrillator vest, and a medical alert identification necklace or bracelet.

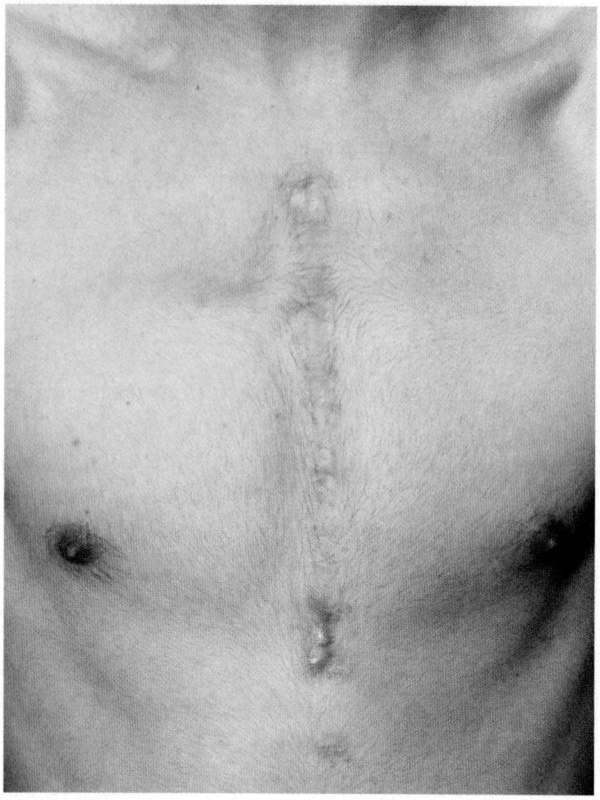

FIGURE 21-116 Midsternal scar suggesting implanted device and/or previous cardiac surgery.

Listen

- **Lung sounds.** The paramedic should assess the patient's chest visually for accessory muscle use in breathing before listening to lung sounds. Lung sounds should be clear and equal bilaterally. As described in Chapter 19, *Secondary Assessment and Reassessment*, crackles may indicate pulmonary congestion or edema.

> CRITICAL THINKING
> What might the presence of wheezing indicate?

- **Heart sounds.** Abnormal heart sounds may indicate heart failure in adult patients (BOX 21-13). Heart sounds are best heard at the **point of maximum impulse**. The point of maximum impulse is the location where the apical impulse is most readily visible or palpable. This often is in the fifth intercostal space, just medial to the left midclavicular line. Although abnormal heart sounds are difficult to detect in the prehospital setting, they can be useful for confirming the paramedic's field impression. Even so, abnormal heart sounds do not alter prehospital care. This evaluation should never delay other patient care measures or transport.
- **Carotid artery bruit.** A **bruit** is a murmur that indicates turbulent blood flow through a vessel. (This is most commonly caused by atherosclerosis.) The presence of a bruit in a patient with cardiac disease is evaluated at the carotid artery with a stethoscope and should always be assessed before carotid sinus massage (described later in this chapter) is performed. If a carotid artery bruit is present, carotid sinus massage is contraindicated. The procedure may dislodge plaque in the artery and cause a stroke.

BOX 21-13 Heart Sounds

Heart sounds typically can be auscultated with a stethoscope during ventricular systole and diastole. When the ventricles contract, both AV valves close at nearly the same time. This closure causes a vibration of the valves and surrounding fluid. Vibration results in a low-pitched sound (often described as a "lub"). Closing of the aortic and pulmonary semilunar valves at the end of ventricular systole produces a higher pitched sound (described as "dub"). These normal heart sounds are referred to as S_1 and S_2, respectively.

In rare cases, a third heart sound can be heard near the end of the first third of diastole (S_3). The third heart sound is caused by turbulent blood flow into the ventricles. It may be normal, but it also may be an indicator of heart failure. A fourth heart sound (S_4) may be heard during the end of diastole. This sound is thought to result from turbulence and chamber stretching caused by the atrial contraction during this part of the cardiac cycle. S_4 often is a sign of a stiffening of the left ventricle and heart failure in adults. S_3 and S_4 contribute to "gallop" rhythms, which are useful clinical indicators of heart failure. Although heart sounds can help define the clinical picture, evaluation of these sounds should never delay emergency care or transport. To summarize:

S_1. First heart sound, which occurs with closure of the AV valves during ventricular systole.
S_2. Second heart sound, which occurs with closure of the aortic and pulmonic valves. It signifies the beginning of ventricular diastole.
S_3. Extra heart sound heard after S_2 (although it is not always present). It may be a normal finding in some patients, or it may indicate heart failure.
S_4. Extra heart sound heard in late diastole (just before S_1). It is associated with atrial contractions and may be heard in patients with heart failure.

Feel

- **Skin.** The paramedic should assess the patient's skin with the back of the hand for diaphoresis or fever. Normal skin is warm and dry.
- **Pulse.** The paramedic should assess the pulse for rate, regularity, and equality. A **pulse deficit** is a radial pulse that is less than the ventricular rate. A pulse deficit in peripheral and apical pulse sites may indicate a rhythm disturbance or vascular disease. The paramedic should note any pulse deficit and report it to medical direction.
- **Thorax and abdomen.** The paramedic should check the thorax and abdomen of a patient with cardiac disease for chest wall tenderness and pulsating masses. Chest wall tenderness is not common in patients with AMI. A pulsating mass or distention in the abdomen or epigastric area may indicate an abdominal aneurysm (described later in this chapter).

Pathophysiology and Management of Cardiovascular Disease

Many medical emergencies are cardiovascular. Cardiovascular emergencies often result from atherosclerosis of the coronary arteries or peripheral arteries. The following specific medical conditions are discussed in this section:

- ACS
- Atherosclerosis
- Angina pectoris
- MI
- Heart failure
- Cardiogenic shock
- Cardiac tamponade
- Thoracic aneurysm and abdominal aortic aneurysm (AAA)
- Acute arterial occlusion
- Noncritical peripheral vascular disorders
- Hypertension

Acute Coronary Syndromes

AMI and unstable angina are part of a spectrum of clinical diseases, collectively known as **acute coronary syndrome (ACS)**. ACS is the most common cause of sudden cardiac death. The pathophysiology of both AMI and is a ruptured or eroded atheromatous plaque. ECG findings common to ACS include ST-segment elevation, ST-segment depression, and T-wave abnormalities. As with other life-threatening conditions, time is of the essence in managing these patients. Rapid transport to a PCI center is indicated for any patient with chest pain of cardiac origin. Other indications for rapid transport include a sense of urgency for reperfusion; no relief of pain with medications; hypotension or hypoperfusion with CNS involvement; and significant changes in the patient's ECG.[9]

The primary goals of therapy for patients with ACS include the following:[9]

- Reducing the amount of myocardial necrosis that occurs in patients with MI, preserving left ventricular function, and preventing heart failure
- Preventing major adverse cardiac events (death, nonfatal MI, the need for urgent revascularization)
- Treating acute, life-threatening complications of ACS (eg, VF, pulseless VT, symptomatic bradycardias, unstable tachycardias)

Atherosclerosis

Atherosclerosis is a disease process characterized by progressive narrowing of the lumina of medium and large arteries (eg, the aorta and its branches, cerebral arteries, coronary arteries). The process results in the development of thick, hard atherosclerotic plaque. This plaque is referred to as atheromata or atheromatous lesions. These lesions most often are found in areas of turbulent blood flow. Such areas include vessel bifurcations or occur in vessels with a decreased lumen diameter.

Atherosclerosis is thought to result from damage to the endothelial cells from mechanical or chemical injury and perhaps inflammation (BOX 21-14). This response includes platelet adhesion and clotting. Smooth muscle cells may move from the middle muscle layer into the lining of the artery. In the lining, the muscle cells form an atheroma. Over time, the atheromata become fibrous and hardened, and eventually, they partly or fully obstruct the opening of the arteries. In most cases, some collateral circulation develops to make up for the narrowed vessels.

Major Risk Factors

Atherosclerosis occurs to some extent in all middle-aged and older people. The disease also occurs in some young people. Atherosclerosis is thought to have a heritable component. It usually is seen at a younger age in men than in women. Associated risk

BOX 21-14 Role of Inflammation in Heart Attack

Studies have suggested that painless inflammation deep in the body plays an important role in triggering heart attacks. The inflammation may arise from such sources as chronic gum disease, lingering urinary tract infections, and others. Inflammation may weaken the walls of the blood vessels, allowing fatty buildups to burst. Inflammation can be assessed in those people at risk for heart disease by testing the blood for an elevated white blood cell count and by measuring the C-reactive protein level. C-reactive protein is a chemical in the blood that plays a role in immunity and infection. It can be lowered with cholesterol-lowering drugs, aspirin, and other medications and through diet and exercise. It is possible that administration of antibodies to attack interleukin-1 beta, a key protein in the inflammatory process, can reduce the risk of cardiovascular events.

Modified from: Rock KL, Latz E, Ontiveros F, Kono H. The sterile inflammatory response. *Annu Rev Immunol.* 2010;28:321-342; and Ridker PM, Everett BM, Thuren T, et al. Antiinflammatory therapy with canakinumab for atherosclerotic disease. *N Engl J Med.* 2017;377(12):1119-1131.

BOX 21-15 Conditions That May Mimic ACS

Acromioclavicular disease
Chest wall pain syndrome
Chest wall trauma
Chest wall tumors
Cholecystitis
Costochondritis
Dyspepsia
Esophageal disease
Gastric reflux
Herpes zoster
Hiatal hernia
Pancreatitis
Peptic ulcer disease
Pericarditis
Pleural irritation
Pneumothorax
Pulmonary embolism
Respiratory infection
Thoracic aortic dissection

factors include age, a family history of heart disease, and diabetes mellitus. Some other risk factors can be reduced or eliminated. These include cigarette smoking, obesity, hypertension, lack of physical activity, and hypercholesterolemia. Some research has shown that plaque formation is not only preventable but also reversible.[33]

Effects

Atherosclerosis has two major effects on blood vessels. First, it disrupts the innermost lining of the vessels. This causes loss of vessel elasticity and an increase in the formation of clots. Second, the atheroma reduces the diameter of the vessel lumen. This reduces the blood supply to tissues. Both effects result in an insufficient supply of nutrients to the tissue, particularly under conditions of increased tissue demand for nutrients and oxygen.

The severity of this insufficiency is related to the extent of narrowing (stenosis) of the blocked artery. The severity also depends on how long the atheroma took to develop and the body's ability to develop collateral circulation around the obstruction. For example, a patient who gradually experiences the development of an atherosclerotic occlusion in an artery of a lower extremity may compensate well through collateral circulation and experience only mild, intermittent pain during periods of exercise. In contrast, sudden-onset occlusion in a coronary artery (after an acute thrombus) almost always results in ischemia, injury, and necrosis to the area of the myocardium supplied by the affected artery.

Angina Pectoris

Angina pectoris is a symptom of myocardial ischemia; the term literally means "choking pain in the chest." Angina is caused by an imbalance between myocardial oxygen supply and demand. The result is a buildup of lactic acid and carbon dioxide in ischemic tissues of the myocardium. These metabolites irritate nerve endings that produce anginal pain. The most common cause of angina pectoris is atherosclerotic disease of the coronary arteries. A temporary occlusion caused by spasm of a coronary artery with or without atherosclerosis (Prinzmetal angina) also can cause angina pectoris (BOX 21-15). Emotional stress and any activity that increases myocardial oxygen demand may cause anginal pain, particularly in patients with atherosclerosis. Myocardial ischemia puts the patient at risk for cardiac dysrhythmias.

NOTE

A number of conditions can mimic the signs and symptoms of heart disease and angina pectoris (see Box 21-15). These include cholecystitis, peptic ulcer disease, aneurysm, hiatal hernia, pulmonary embolism, pancreatitis, pleural irritation, respiratory infection, and others. These conditions should be considered as part of the differential diagnosis when a patient presents with signs and symptoms of an ACS.

Stable Angina

Angina pectoris generally is classified as stable or unstable. Stable angina usually is precipitated by the increased myocardial demand of physical exertion. The pain usually lasts 1 to 5 minutes but may last as long as 15 minutes. Angina is relieved by rest, nitroglycerin, or oxygen. Stable angina attacks usually are similar and are always relieved by the same mode of therapy.

Unstable Angina

Unstable angina (preinfarction angina) is a type of ACS. It denotes an anginal pattern that has changed in its ease of onset, frequency, intensity, duration, or quality. (This includes any new-onset anginal chest pain.) Unstable angina may occur during periods of light exercise or at rest. The pain usually lasts longer than it does in stable angina. The pain is usually not relieved by cessation of activity or nitroglycerin as it is in stable angina. Unstable angina mimics AMI. The two sometimes are difficult to differentiate in the prehospital setting. Patients with unstable angina are at increased risk of AMI and sudden death.

The pain of angina usually is described by the patient as a pressure, squeezing, heaviness, or tightness in the chest. Although many patients with angina feel pain only in the chest, others describe the pain as radiating to the shoulders, arms, neck, and jaw and through the chest to the back. Associated signs and symptoms include anxiety, shortness of breath, nausea or vomiting, and diaphoresis. The patient history often reveals previous attacks of angina. Often, the patient will have taken nitroglycerin before EMS arrival. If so, the paramedic should determine the age of the nitroglycerin prescription (nitroglycerin is unstable and quickly loses its strength), the amount of nitroglycerin taken, and its effect. If the pain is not relieved by rest and medication, the paramedic should suspect an MI.

Management

All patients with chest pain and signs and symptoms of myocardial ischemia should be managed as though an AMI were evolving (**TABLE 21-8**). The goal of management is to increase the coronary blood supply, reduce the myocardial oxygen demand, or both.

Management guidelines include the following:

1. Place the patient at rest physically and emotionally.
2. Administer oxygen if the patient is dyspneic, has signs of heart failure, or has an oxygen saturation level, as measured by an arterial blood gas sampling (Sao_2), of less than 90%.[7]
3. Administer aspirin: 160 to 325 mg, non-enteric coated.
4. Initiate IV therapy.
5. If the patient reports pain, use pharmacologic therapy. This may include sublingual nitroglycerin followed by morphine.
6. Monitor the ECG for dysrhythmias. Monitor a three-lead ECG continuously. Obtain a 12-lead ECG at first medical contact, and record serial 12-lead ECGs during transport. Also measure, record, and communicate any ST-segment changes.
7. Transport the patient to a PCI-capable hospital for evaluation by a physician.

Myocardial Infarction

Acute myocardial infarction (AMI) occurs with a sudden and total blockage or near blockage of blood flowing through an affected coronary artery to an area of heart muscle. This blockage results in ischemia, injury, and necrosis to the area of the myocardium distal to the occlusion. AMI most often is associated with atherosclerotic heart disease.

Precipitating Events

The process of MI is complex. It generally begins with the formation of an atherosclerotic plaque involving the intimal layer of a coronary artery. The plaque disrupts the smooth arterial lining and results in an uneven surface that creates turbulent blood flow. The plaque may rupture. If rupture occurs, the

TABLE 21-8 TIMI Risk Score for Patients With Unstable Angina and Non-STEMI: Predictor Variables

Predictor Variable	Point Value of Variable	Definition
Age ≥65 years	1	
≥3 risk factors for CAD	1	Risk factors: • Family history of CAD • Hypertension • Hypercholesterolemia • Diabetes • Current smoker
Aspirin use in last 7 days	1	
Recent, severe symptoms of angina	1	≥2 anginal events in last 24 hours
Elevated cardiac markers	1	CK-MB or cardiac-specific troponin level
ST deviation ≥0.5 mm	1	ST depression ≥0.5 mm is significant; transient ST elevation ≥0.5 mm for <20 minutes is treated as ST-segment depression and is high risk; ST elevation >1 mm for >20 minutes places these patients in the STEMI treatment category.
Prior coronary artery stenosis ≥50%	1	Risk predictor remains valid even if this information is unknown.

Calculated TIMI Risk Score	Risk of ≥1 Primary End Point[a] in ≤14 days	Risk Status
0 or 1	5%	Low
2	8%	
3	13%	Intermediate
4	20%	
5	26%	High

[a]Primary end points: death, new or recurrent myocardial infarction, or need for urgent revascularization.

Abbreviations: CAD, coronary artery disease; CK-MB, creatine kinase-myocardial band isoenzyme; STEMI, ST-segment elevation myocardial infarction; TIMI, Thrombolysis in Myocardial Infarction trial

Modified from: Antman EM, Cohen M, Bernink PJLM, et al. The TIMI risk score for unstable angina/non-ST elevation MI: a method for prognostication and therapeutic decision making. *JAMA*. 2000;284(7):835-842.

injured tissue is exposed to circulating platelets. This results in the formation of a thrombus that occludes the artery. As the thrombus enlarges, it further reduces blood flow in the coronary vessel.

Acute thrombotic occlusion generally is accepted as the cause of most MIs. Other factors that may lead to AMI include coronary spasm, coronary embolism, severe hypoxia, hemorrhage into a diseased arterial wall, and reduced blood flow after any form of shock. All of these conditions may result in an inadequate amount of blood reaching the myocardium.

Types and Locations of Infarcts

The myocardial cells beyond the occluded artery die (infarct) from lack of oxygen. The size of the infarct is determined by the needs of the tissue supplied by the occluded vessel, by the presence of collateral circulation, and by the time required to reestablish blood flow. Therefore, emergency care is directed at the following:

- If the patient is hypoxic, increasing the oxygen supply by administering supplemental oxygen
- Decreasing the metabolic needs and providing collateral circulation
- Reestablishing perfusion to the ischemic myocardium as quickly as possible after the onset of symptoms

Most AMIs involve the left ventricle or interventricular septum. These areas are supplied by either of the two major coronary arteries. (However, some patients sustain damage to the right ventricle.) If the occlusion is in the left coronary artery, the result is an anterior, lateral, or septal wall infarction. Inferior wall infarction (of the inferior–posterior wall of the left ventricle) usually is a result of right coronary artery occlusion.

ACS can be classified into one of three ischemic syndromes based on the rupture of an unstable plaque in an epicardial artery: unstable angina, non-STEMI, and STEMI.[9] These three types of ACS share common risk factors, and their management overlaps substantially. Sudden cardiac death may occur with any of these syndromes.

- In unstable angina, the early thrombus has not obstructed coronary blood flow completely. This partial occlusion produces symptoms of ischemia. The blockage eventually may result in complete occlusion and produce a non-STEMI. Fibrinolytic therapy (described later in this chapter) is not effective in unstable angina. In fact, such therapy may accelerate the occlusion. Therapy with antiplatelet agents is most effective at this time because the thrombus is rich in platelets.
- Non-STEMI occurs as microemboli from the thrombus become lodged in the coronary arteries, causing ischemia. Cardiac biomarkers, such as troponin, are elevated. This condition produces less damage to the myocardium. Non-STEMIs may have no ECG changes or ST-segment depression or T-wave abnormalities.
- STEMI occurs when the thrombus occludes the coronary vessel for a prolonged period. The infarct is diagnosed by the development of elevated ST segments in two or more contiguous (adjacent) leads (**FIGURE 21-117**). The clot is rich in thrombin; therefore, if rapid PCI is not available, early management with fibrinolytics may help limit the size of the infarct.

Death of Myocardium

When blood flow to the myocardium stops, a series of events begins. Cells switch from aerobic to anaerobic metabolism, resulting in the release of lactic acid and an increase in tissue carbon dioxide levels. These changes contribute to ischemic pain (angina). As cells lose their ability to maintain their electrochemical gradients, they begin to swell and depolarize. These initial changes are reversible. However, within a few hours, if collateral flow and reperfusion are inadequate, much of the muscle distal to the occlusion dies. The area surrounding the necrotic tissue may survive because of collateral circulation. However, surviving tissue may become the origin of dysrhythmias (**FIGURE 21-118**).

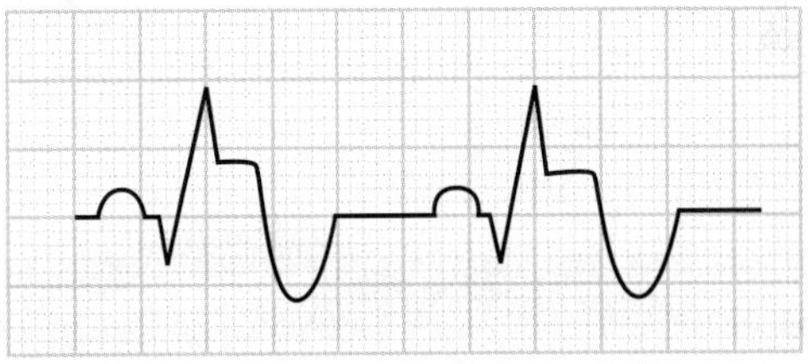

FIGURE 21-117 ST elevation and pathologic Q waves.

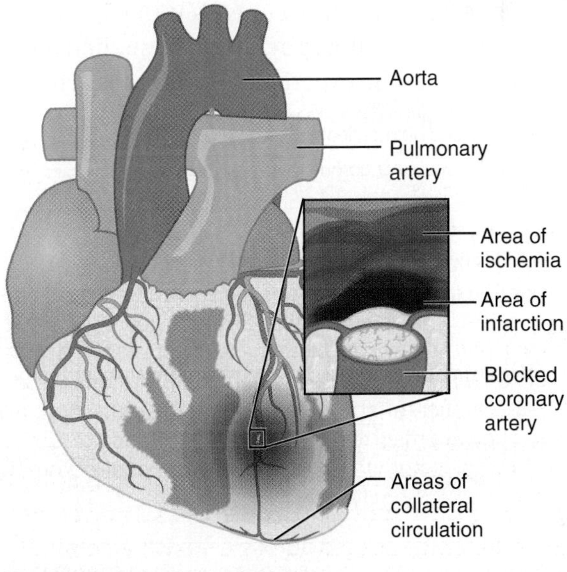

FIGURE 21-118 Areas of infarct.

Scar tissue replaces the infarcted area in a process that takes about 8 weeks. The process starts with deposits of connective tissue on about the 12th day. Scar tissue is durable; however, it lacks elasticity, does not contract, and conducts electrical impulses poorly in the damaged area of the myocardium. The left ventricle can lose as much as 25% of its muscle and still function as an effective pump. Areas with poor perfusion after a large MI may not develop strong scar tissue. This may result in an aneurysm. Such an aneurysm can greatly reduce the effective ventricular contractility. An aneurysm also may lead to the development of serious dysrhythmias.

The damaged myocardium is most susceptible to rupture during the first 1 to 2 weeks after an MI because the scar tissue has not reached adequate strength. Prevention of hypertension and excitement during this period is usually necessary. Even so, the hospital stay of patients with uncomplicated MIs has been shortened, often because early intervention with PCI limits the muscle damage. Currently, most patients leave the hospital within 3 to 5 days.

Death Following MI

Death within the first week or two after MI usually results from lethal dysrhythmias (VT, VF, and cardiac standstill), pump failure (cardiogenic shock and heart failure), or myocardial tissue rupture (rupture of the ventricle, septum, or papillary muscle). Fatal dysrhythmias are the most common cause of death from MI. Deaths that occur within the first 2 hours after the onset of illness or injury are sudden deaths. Most patients who experience sudden death have no immediate warning symptoms.

NOTE

Sudden cardiac death is defined as a sudden dysrhythmic death that occurs within the first 2 hours of cardiac ischemic symptoms. More than 50% of cardiac deaths occur with no evidence of infarction on autopsy when resuscitation attempts fail. Sudden death without infarction is a main reason for the widespread availability of AEDs. (Another reason is that the most common death-producing dysrhythmia is VF.)

Modified from: 2015 American Heart Association Guidelines for Cardiopulmonary Resuscitation and Emergency Cardiovascular Care. *Circulation*. 2015;132:S313-S314.

Signs and Symptoms

Some patients with AMI—particularly patients with diabetes, some women, and those in the older age groups—may have only symptoms of dyspnea, syncope, or confusion. However, substernal chest pain is present in 70% to 90% of patients with AMI. The pain generally has the same characteristics and locations as anginal pain. The pain also may radiate to the arms, neck, jaw, or back. The following signs and symptoms may accompany the pain and occasionally are present even in the absence of pain (silent MI):

- Agitation
- Anxiety
- Cyanosis
- Diaphoresis
- Dyspnea
- Nausea and vomiting
- Palpitations
- Syncope
- Sense of impending doom
- Weakness

CRITICAL THINKING

How can prehospital recognition of an AMI affect the care of the patient at the hospital?

The chest pain associated with AMI often is constant. Also, the pain often is not altered or alleviated by nitroglycerin or other cardiac medications, rest, changes in body position, or breathing patterns. With angina pectoris, the onset often occurs during periods of activity. In contrast, the onset of pain in more than half of all patients with AMI occurs during rest. Some patients may not be able to describe their pain but will present with a clenched fist in the center of the chest. This presentation is known as the Levine sign.[34] Most patients have had warning anginal pains (preinfarction angina) hours or days before the attack. Many patients deny the possibility of an evolving MI. They may blame the chest pain or discomfort on unrelated causes, such as fatigue or indigestion. Denial delays the request for EMS assistance during the most critical phase of the illness. According to the AHA, more than 50% of deaths from ischemic heart disease occur outside the hospital within the first 4 hours after the onset of pain.[9]

CRITICAL THINKING

Why do you think patients deny that their signs and symptoms may be due to a heart attack?

Vital signs vary with an AMI. They depend on the extent of damage to the heart muscle and conduction system. They also depend on the degree and type of autonomic nervous system response. For example, the patient's blood pressure may be normal, elevated (sympathetic discharge), or low (parasympathetic discharge or pump failure). The pulse rate depends on the presence or absence of dysrhythmias. It may be normal, tachycardic, bradycardic, regular, or irregular. Respirations may be normal or increased.

NOTE

Sulfonylurea drugs (drugs for treating diabetes mellitus), such as glyburide or glipizide, may lessen the magnitude of ST-segment elevation in the presence of an infarct. Therefore, it is crucial that paramedics obtain a diabetes history for all patients with a cardiac event.

Modified from: Abdelmoneim AS, Welsh RC, Eurich DT, Simpson SH. Sulfonylurea use is associated with larger infarct size in patients with diabetes and ST-elevation myocardial infarction. *Int J Cardiol.* 2016;202:126-130.

Management of an Uncomplicated AMI

All patients with anginal chest pain are assumed to have an AMI until it is proved otherwise (BOX 21-16). Any patient with chest pain should be transported to a medical facility for evaluation by a physician, regardless of the apparent severity on the arrival of EMS providers or the patient's age, sex, or associated complaints. The primary goals of prehospital care are to identify possible MI, obtain a 12-lead ECG as early as possible, notify the receiving hospital, and provide transport to a PCI center (if possible) in a timely manner.[9] Additional goals are to relieve pain and apprehension, prevent the development of serious dysrhythmias, and limit the size of the infarct. The paramedic should obtain a full patient history while performing the physical examination and during initial patient care. Because time is of the essence, the following aspects of patient care are a high priority:

BOX 21-16 Management of Patients With Symptoms of Ischemia or Infarction

- Monitor and support the ABCs (airway, breathing, and circulation). Be prepared to provide CPR and defibrillation.
- Administer aspirin and consider oxygen, nitroglycerin, and morphine as necessary.
- Obtain a 12-lead ECG; if ST elevation is shown, notify the receiving hospital with the transmission or interpretation with the time of onset and first medical contact.
- The notified hospital will prepare to respond to STEMI.
- If considering prehospital fibrinolysis, use a fibrinolytic checklist.

Modified from: 2015 American Heart Association Guidelines for Cardiopulmonary Resuscitation and Emergency Cardiovascular Care. *Circulation.* 2015;132:S313-S314.

1. Place the patient at rest or in a comfortable position. This helps reduce anxiety and the heart rate and thus oxygen demand.
2. Monitor pulse oximetry.
3. Administer low-concentration oxygen (4 L/min) via the nasal cannula if the Sao_2 level is less than 90%. Patients with respiratory compromise need a higher oxygen concentration.
4. Initiate transport quickly. (If the patient is stable, do not use audible or visual warning devices to help reduce the patient's anxiety.)
5. Administer aspirin (per protocol).
6. Attach ECG electrodes, obtain and interpret a 12-lead ECG (repeat if possible during transport), document the initial rhythm, and monitor for dysrhythmias.
7. Establish an IV line with normal saline or lactated Ringer solution to keep the vein open or to supply fluid boluses (if needed).
8. Obtain baseline vital signs. Repeat the assessment often. Vital sign assessment should include auscultation of the lungs for heart failure indicators (eg, presence of crackles).
9. Administer medications (per protocol) to relieve pain and manage dysrhythmias as follows:
   - Medications that may be used for analgesia and to reduce preload and afterload include nitroglycerin followed by morphine.
   - Medications may be used to manage the various dysrhythmias.

- If a system has been carrying unfractionated heparin or enoxaparin (as an alternative), the medication may be administered to the STEMI patient if PCI treatment is planned, although clear benefit has not been demonstrated.[35]

NOTE

Nitroglycerin is a vasodilating agent that has beneficial hemodynamic effects. These effects include dilation of arterioles and veins in the periphery (thereby reducing preload) and dilation of the coronary arteries. These actions reduce the workload of the heart, lower myocardial oxygen demand, and may relieve ischemic chest pain. Because of these hemodynamic effects, nitroglycerin should not be used in patients with the following conditions:

- Hypotension (systolic blood pressure <90 mm Hg or >30 mm Hg below baseline)
- Extreme bradycardia (heart rate <50 beats/min)
- Tachycardia (heart rate >100 beats/min) unless the patient has heart failure

Nitroglycerin is contraindicated in right ventricular infarction (patients who require adequate right ventricular preload). In these patients, nitroglycerin can cause profound hypotension. Nitroglycerin also is contraindicated in patients who have taken medication for erectile dysfunction within the previous 24 hours (longer for some preparations).

Modified from: American Heart Association. *2015 Handbook of Emergency Cardiovascular Care for Healthcare Providers*. Dallas, TX: American Heart Association; 2015; 2015 American Heart Association Guidelines for Cardiopulmonary Resuscitation and Emergency Cardiovascular Care. *Circulation*. 2015;132:S313-S314.

Fibrinolytic Therapy

Studies performed more than 20 years ago showed that mortality improved with prehospital administration of a fibrinolytic agent when transport times were more than 30 to 60 minutes.[7] Some EMS systems are authorized by medical direction to administer these agents in the prehospital setting. Newer research showed no mortality benefit from direct transport for PCI compared with prehospital fibrinolytic therapy. However, there was a higher risk of intracranial hemorrhage in the fibrinolytic group.[36] The AHA recommends that prehospital systems focus on early diagnosis; the field administration of fibrinolytics *may* be considered when it is available as part of a STEMI system of care, when in-hospital fibrinolysis is the other available treatment option, and when transport times are more than 30 minutes.[9] If, however, primary transport to a PCI center is available, direct transport without prehospital fibrinolytic treatment *may* be preferred. The AHA strongly recommends the following for EMS systems that administer fibrinolytics in the prehospital setting:[9]

- Protocols using fibrinolytic checklists
- Twelve-lead ECG acquisition, transmission, and interpretation
- Experience in advanced life support
- Communication with the receiving institution
- Medical director with training and experience in STEMI management
- Continuous quality improvement

Common fibrinolytic agents include streptokinase, tissue plasminogen activator, tenecteplase, anistreplase, and reteplase. Because of its relative ease of administration, reteplase is typically preferred in the prehospital setting. All these agents work through activation of the plasma protein plasminogen to dissolve the coronary thrombus. Plasminogen is converted to plasmin (the active form). Plasmin degrades fibrin, the basic component of a clot (thrombus). Aspirin and heparin are part of the "fibrinolytic package."

A fibrinolytic agent can dissolve both beneficial and pathologic thrombi. Therefore, the drug is administered selectively. It may be considered if symptom onset was less than 24 hours prior. Most EMS systems that use fibrinolytic agents establish inclusion/exclusion criteria similar to those listed in BOX 21-17.[15]

Heart Failure

Heart failure is a chronic condition that affects the chambers of the heart, making the heart unable to pump blood at a rate that meets the metabolic needs of the tissues. The condition can occur in all age groups (usually a result of congenital heart disease in children) but more commonly is associated with **high-output heart failure** in older adults. Heart failure is often associated with heart disease, hypertension, MI, heart valve abnormalities, cardiomyopathy, congenital heart disease, and severe lung disease. Nearly 5 million Americans are currently living with heart failure, and 500,000 new cases are diagnosed in the United States each year. Heart failure is the most common diagnosis in hospital patients aged

BOX 21-17 Contraindications for Fibrinolytic Therapy

Absolute Contraindications

- History of structural CNS disease
- History of structural vascular brain lesion (eg, AV malformation)
- History of intracranial cancer (primary or metastatic)
- Significant closed head or facial trauma within the previous 3 months
- Stroke onset more than 3 hours before EMS arrival
- Stroke within 3 months of this occurrence
- Recent (within 2 to 4 weeks) major trauma, surgery (including laser eye surgery), gastrointestinal/genitourinary bleed
- Any history of intracranial hemorrhage
- Bleeding, clotting problem
- Possible aortic dissection

Relative Contraindications

- Systolic blood pressure greater than 180 to 200 mm Hg *or* diastolic blood pressure greater than 100 to 110 mm Hg
- History of long-term, severe, poorly controlled hypertension
- Pregnant female
- History of ischemic stroke greater than 3 months, dementia, or other brain pathology not otherwise mentioned
- Surgery within the past 3 weeks
- Traumatic or prolonged CPR for longer than 10 minutes
- Internal bleeding within the past 2 to 4 weeks
- Uncontrolled bleeding from a blood vessel
- Allery to fibrinolytic agent
- Active peptic ulcer
- Use of anticoagulants; risk increases with higher international normalized ratio (a measure of bleeding time)

Modified from: 2015 American Heart Association Guidelines for Cardiopulmonary Resuscitation and Emergency Cardiovascular Care. *Circulation*. 2015;132:S313-S314.

65 years and older. Heart failure has a wide spectrum of severity, ranging from fatigue, peripheral edema, ascites, dyspnea, and tachycardia, to pulmonary edema, respiratory failure, and death. Heart failure can be classified as left-side heart failure (systolic and diastolic failure) and right-side heart failure. It is possible to have left-side and right-side heart failure at the same time. Usually, the disease starts in the left side and then travels to the right when left untreated.

Left-Side Heart Failure

Left-side heart failure (left ventricular failure) occurs when the left ventricle fails to work as an effective forward pump. Left-side heart failure is further classified as heart failure with reduced ejection fraction, also called **systolic heart failure** (often a form of low-output failure), and heart failure with preserved ejection fraction, also called **diastolic heart failure** or diastolic dysfunction. Systolic heart failure leads to manifestations of impaired peripheral circulation and vasoconstriction as the left ventricle loses its ability to contract normally from dilation and weakening of the muscle. This causes a back pressure of blood into the pulmonary circulation. The accumulation of fluid in the lungs leads to pulmonary edema (**FIGURE 21-119**).

With diastolic failure, the left ventricle becomes stiff and loses its ability to relax normally and to properly fill with blood between each beat. In diastolic failure, cardiac output remains high but is unable to meet the metabolic needs of the body. This type of heart failure is associated with hyperthyroidism, anemia, pregnancy, Paget disease, arteriovenous fistulas, beriberi, and sepsis. In practice, differentiating between the types of heart failure is sometimes difficult and does not often affect prehospital care. BOX 21-18 lists the signs and symptoms of left ventricular failure.

Right-Side Heart Failure

Right-side heart failure (right ventricular heart failure) usually occurs as a result of left-side failure. With left ventricular failure, there is an increase in left atrial pressure that is transmitted to the pulmonary veins and capillaries. As pulmonary capillary hydrostatic pressure increases, the plasma portion of blood is forced into the alveoli. At that point, plasma mixes with air, causing the typical finding in pulmonary edema: foamy, blood-tinged sputum (**FIGURE 21-120**). Ultimately the right ventricle is unable to overcome the high pressure in the pulmonary circulation, damaging the heart's right side. As the right side of the heart fails and loses its ability to pump, blood backs up in the veins and tissues of the body and leads to an acute exacerbation of heart failure. Right ventricular failure can result from several diseases,

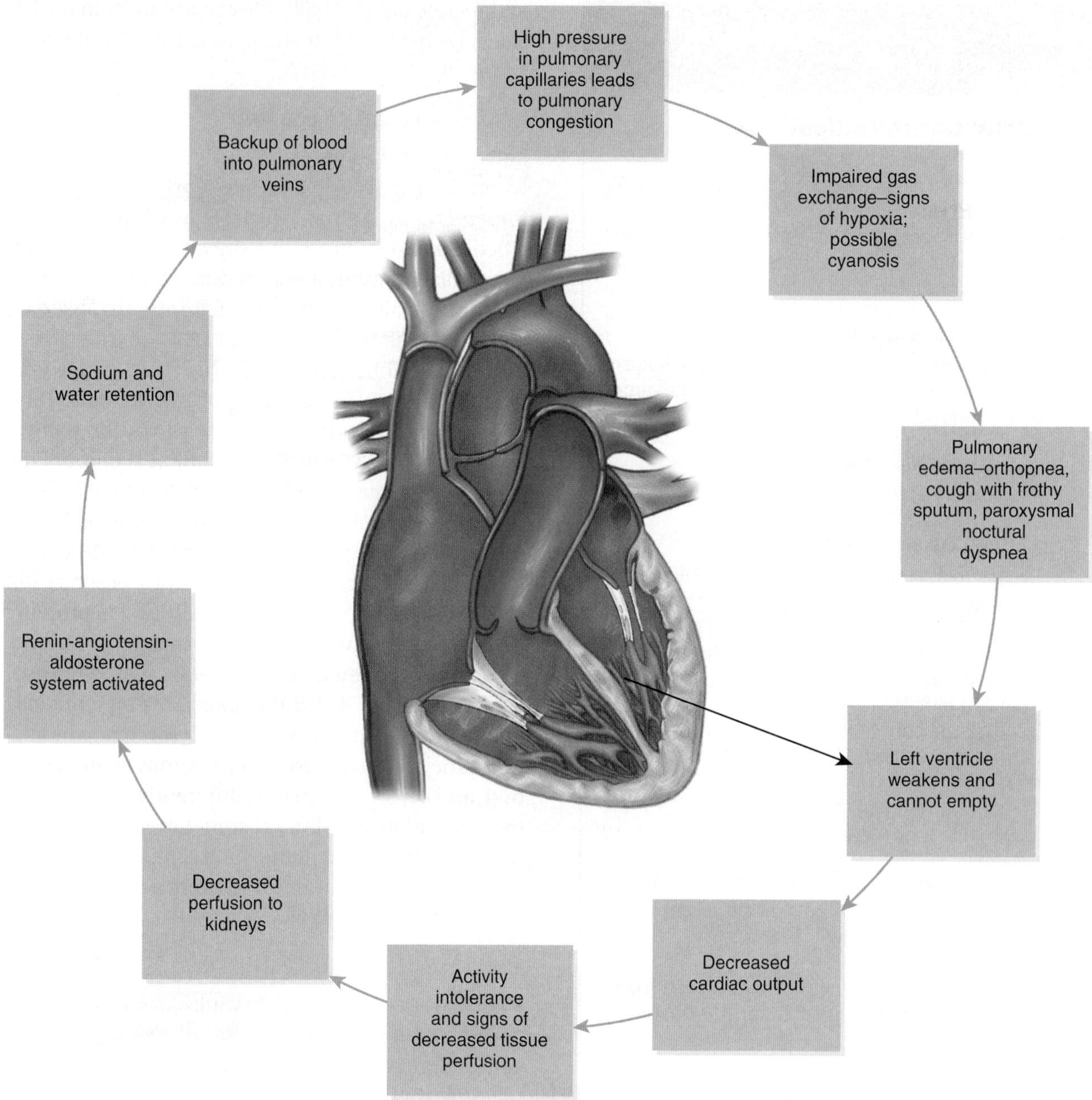

FIGURE 21-119 Left-side heart failure.

including chronic hypertension (in which left ventricular failure usually precedes right ventricular failure), chronic obstructive pulmonary disease, pulmonary hypertension, pulmonary embolism, valvular heart disease, and infarction of the right ventricle. BOX 21-19 lists the signs and symptoms of right ventricular failure. When left and right ventricular failure occur at the same time, the signs and symptoms of each may be present. **TABLE 21-9** can help the paramedic differentiate between the two.

Pulmonary Edema

Pulmonary edema is a condition caused by excess fluid in the lungs. It can occur from pneumonia, following exposure to certain toxins and drugs, and from being

BOX 21-18 Signs and Symptoms of Left Ventricular Failure

- Severe respiratory distress
  - Orthopnea
  - Spasmodic cough that may produce foamy, blood-tinged sputum
  - History of paroxysmal nocturnal dyspnea (a sudden episode of dyspnea that occurs after lying down)
- Severe apprehension, agitation, confusion
- Cyanosis (if severe)
- Diaphoresis
- Adventitious lung sounds
  - Bilateral crackles that do not clear with coughing (usually present at the base of the lungs and up to the level of the scapulae)
  - Rhonchi (fluid in the upper airways)
  - Wheezes (reflex airway spasm, sometimes referred to as cardiac asthma)
- JVD (indicates back pressure through the right heart and into the venous system)
- Abnormal vital signs
  - Blood pressure: Possibly elevated
  - Pulse rate: Rapid to compensate for low stroke volume; possibly irregular if dysrhythmias are present
- Regular alterations of weak and strong beats without changes in the length of the cycle (pulsus alternans); rapid, labored respirations
- Altered level of consciousness (patient may be anxious, agitated, uncooperative, or obtunded because of poor cerebral perfusion or hypoxia)
- Chest pain
  - Presence or absence of pain
  - May be masked by respiratory distress

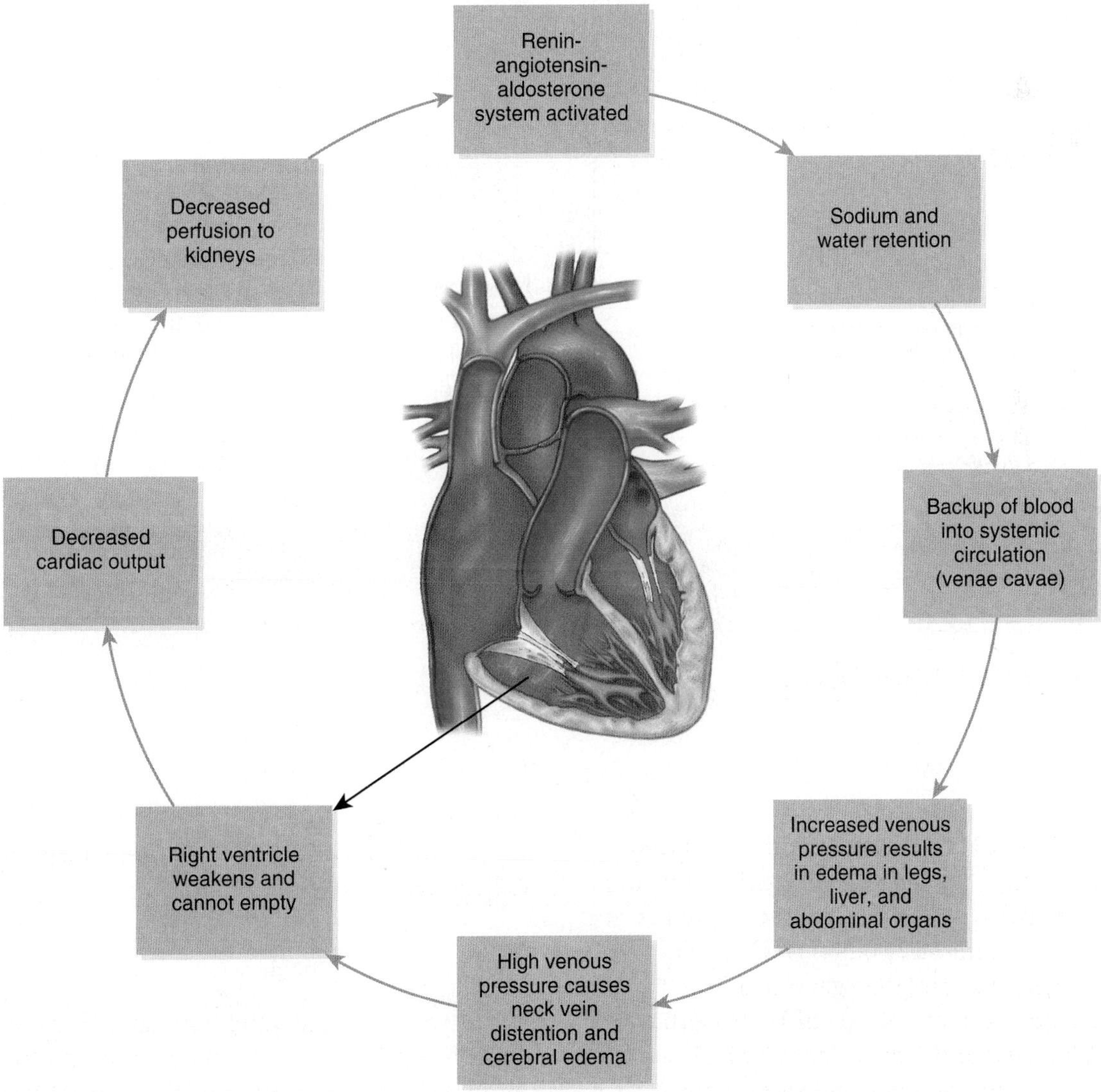

FIGURE 21-120 Right-side heart failure.

at high altitudes. However, the most common cause of pulmonary edema is left ventricular failure. With this condition, there is a compromise of forward flow through the left ventricle, resulting in a reduction of stroke volume. This process initiates several compensatory mechanisms that restore cardiac output and organ perfusion (tachycardia, vasoconstriction, and activation of the renin-angiotensin-aldosterone system). These mechanisms often increase myocardial oxygen demand and further decrease the myocardium's ability to contract. The resultant increase in atrial pressure is transmitted to the pulmonary veins and capillaries. As pulmonary capillary hydrostatic pressure increases, the plasma portion of blood is forced into the alveoli where plasma mixes with air, resulting in the typical finding in pulmonary edema: foamy, blood-tinged sputum. If left unmanaged, the progressive fluid buildup can result in death from hypoxia. MI is a common cause of left ventricular failure and heart failure. Therefore, in all patients with pulmonary edema, particularly those with an abrupt onset with severe dyspnea and hypoxia (flash pulmonary edema), an AMI should be suspected and a 12-lead ECG should be acquired.

BOX 21-19 Signs and Symptoms of Right Ventricular Failure

- Tachycardia
- Venous congestion
  - Engorged liver or spleen, or both
  - Venous distention: distention and pulsation of the neck veins
- Peripheral edema
  - Lower extremities or entire body (anasarca)
  - Sacral region in bedridden patients
  - Pitting edema
- Fluid accumulation in serous cavities
  - Abdominal cavity (ascites)
  - Pericardium (pericardial effusion[a])
- History
  - Often previous MI in patients with chronic heart failure
  - Frequent medication history of digitalis and diuretics to control heart failure

[a]Patients often can tolerate large amounts of effusion without compromise when the effusion develops over an extended period.

NOTE

Paroxysmal nocturnal dyspnea is an abnormal condition of the respiratory system. It is characterized by sudden attacks of shortness of breath, profuse sweating, tachycardia, and wheezing that awaken a person from sleep. The condition often is associated with left ventricular failure and pulmonary edema.

Management. Pulmonary edema is an acute and critical emergency that can lead to death unless it is treated rapidly. Emergency management is directed at reducing the venous return to the heart, improving myocardial contractility, decreasing myocardial oxygen demand, improving ventilation and oxygenation, and

TABLE 21-9 Symptoms and Signs of Chronic Heart Failure

Right Ventricular Dysfunction		Left Ventricular Dysfunction		Nonspecific Findings	
Symptoms	**Signs**	**Symptoms**	**Signs**	**Symptoms**	**Signs**
Abdominal pain	Peripheral edema	Dyspnea on exertion	Bibasilar crackles	Exercise intolerance	Tachycardia
Anorexia	Jugular venous distention	Paroxysmal nocturnal dyspnea	Pulmonary edema	Fatigue	Pallor
Nausea	Engorged liver	Orthopnea	S_3 gallop	Weakness	Cyanosis of digits
Bloating	Engorged spleen	Tachypnea	Pleural effusion	Nocturia	Cardiomegaly
Constipation		Cough	Chest pain	Central nervous system symptoms	Agitation
Ascites		Hemoptysis	Diaphoresis		

rapidly transporting the patient to a medical facility (**FIGURE 21-121**). Pulmonary edema in the setting of severe hypertension should prompt the paramedic to consider rapid afterload reduction with high-dose nitroglycerin in accordance with local protocol or online medical control.

Emergency care entails patient positioning, oxygenation, continuous positive airway pressure (CPAP) or bilevel positive airway pressure (BPAP), ventilatory support as needed, and pharmacologic therapy. As in any other true emergency, the paramedic should perform a full but focused patient history and physical examination while initiating treatment. No characteristic ECG changes are associated with pulmonary edema. However, the paramedic should obtain an initial tracing. The paramedic also should monitor the patient's rhythm continuously for evidence of myocardial irritability and dysrhythmias.

The paramedic should place the patient in a sitting position with the legs dependent. This position increases lung volume and vital capacity. It also diminishes the work of respiration and reduces venous return to the heart.

The paramedic should administer oxygen using noninvasive positive pressure ventilation (CPAP or BPAP). Positive pressure assistance is one of the highest priorities in caring for these patients, and it reduces the need for high levels of inspired oxygen. A pulse oximeter should be used to ensure an Sao_2 level of at least 94%. If an arterial oxygen saturation level of at least 90% cannot be achieved with 100% oxygen or if signs of cerebral hypoxia or progressive hypercapnia are seen, tracheal intubation and assisted ventilations may be indicated.

Nitroglycerin may be used to reduce venous return, enhance contractile function of the myocardium, and reduce dyspnea. It should be noted that nitroglycerin can lower blood pressure. Therefore, care must be taken in patients with pulmonary edema and hypotension (a systolic blood pressure <100 mm Hg).

The effects of nitroglycerin include induction of peripheral vasodilation and reduction of preload and afterload, thereby reducing the myocardial workload and improving cardiac function.

Management of Acute Pulmonary Edema

↓

Perform primary and secondary survey
If feasible, position patient sitting upright (feet dependent)
Administer O_2, place patient on CPAP, BPAP (maintain 94%-98% saturation)
Establish IV access, obtain 12-lead ECG

↓

Systolic BP >100 mm Hg
SL nitroglycerin (1 tab or 1-2 sprays q 5 min; max 3 doses)
Consider morphine (2-4 mg IV)

↓

Consider additional medications for preload/afterload reduction:
- IV nitroglycerin[a] or IV nitroprusside[b]

↓

Consider reversible causes:
- Cardiac dysrhythmias, tamponade, myocardial ischemia, infarction

↓

If refractory to above therapies, hypotensive, or in cardiogenic shock, consult with medical direction
- Consider IV fluids IV inotropics and/or IV vasopressors[c]

Abbreviations: BP, blood pressure; BPAP, bilevel positive airway pressure; CPAP, continuous positive airway pressure; ECG, electrocardiogram; IV, intravenous; SBP, systolic blood pressure; SL, sublingual

FIGURE 21-121 Acute pulmonary edema/hypotension/shock algorithm.

[a]Nitroglycerin: begin at 5 mcg/min; increase gradually until mean systolic pressure falls by 10% to 15%; avoid hypotension (SBP <90 mm Hg)
[b]Nitroprusside: 0.1 to 5 mcg/kg per minute if SBP is >100 mm Hg
[c]Norepinephrine: 0.05 to 0.5 mcg/kg per minute (titrated to effect); dopamine: 2 to 20 mcg/kg per minute; epinephrine: 0.05 to 0.5 mcg/min (titrated to effect)

Note: Use of furosemide is not recommended to manage pulmonary edema in the prehospital setting, unless transport times are long (consult with medical direction).

Data source: National Model EMS Clinical Guidelines Version 2.0. National Association of State EMS Officials website. www.nasemso.org. Revised September 18, 2017. Accessed April 5, 2018. Pg. 99.

CRITICAL THINKING

What happens to the diffusion of oxygen and carbon dioxide in the lungs during this process?

NOTE

Hypotension caused by right ventricular failure (often seen in right ventricular infarction) can mimic cardiogenic shock. In this case, fluid administration helps normalize left ventricular filling. Administration of fluids is crucial and helps restore a normal blood pressure. (This situation is just the opposite of the hypotension associated with cardiogenic shock, in which administration of fluids worsens the condition.) Management may include 250-mL IV boluses of normal saline over 5 to 10 minutes. This intervention helps increase myocardial contractility (Starling law). Fluid administration also improves contractility. Close observation of the patient and the vital signs is crucial.

Cardiogenic Shock

Cardiogenic shock is the most extreme form of pump failure. It occurs when left ventricular function is so compromised that the heart cannot meet the metabolic needs of the body. The result is a significant decrease in stroke volume (resulting from ineffective myocardial contraction), cardiac output, and blood pressure; these decreases produce an inadequate supply of blood to the organs. Cardiogenic shock occurs in 5% to 10% of patients with AMI.[37] It may be the result of acute left- or right-side heart failure.

By definition, cardiogenic shock is present when shock persists after correction of existing dysrhythmias, volume deficit, or decreased vascular tone. Cardiogenic shock usually is caused by extensive MI (often involving more than 40% of the left ventricle) or by diffuse ischemia. Even with aggressive therapy, cardiogenic shock has a mortality rate of 70% or higher.[37]

In addition to the signs and symptoms of MI, patients in cardiogenic shock show clinical evidence of hypoperfusion to vital organs and significant systemic hypotension lasting more than 30 minutes with signs of poor organ perfusion and low cardiac output. Because the signs and symptoms are similar to those of other types of shock, it is sometimes difficult to distinguish the cause. This evidence includes the following:

- Acidosis (elevated serum lactate; >2.0 mmol/L is abnormal)
- Altered level of consciousness
- Cool, clammy, cyanotic, or ashen skin
- Hypoxemia
- Hypotension (systolic blood pressure <80 mm Hg)
- Pulmonary congestion (crackles)
- Sinus tachycardia or other dysrhythmias
- Tachypnea

In the early stages of cardiogenic shock, the patient's heart tries to compensate. The heart rate increases. If possible, the heart also increases contractility and cardiac output. As the condition worsens, the heart progresses toward hypodynamic failure with depressed contractility, reduced stroke volume, and subsequent hypoperfusion (see Chapter 35, *Shock*).

Management

Patients in cardiogenic shock are ill (see Figure 21-121). These patients need rapid transport to a medical facility. Transport should not be delayed by attempting field treatment. Prehospital care should include the following:

- Airway management and ventilatory support with high-concentration oxygen to maintain an oxygen saturation level, as measured using a pulse oximeter (Spo_2), of greater than 94%
- Placement of the patient in a supine position (or semi-Fowler position, if the patient is dyspneic)
- Insertion of an IV line with normal saline or lactated Ringer solution and infusion of fluids at 30 mL/kg, up to 1 L (unless crackles develop, in which case infusion should be at a to-keep-open rate)[38]
- Monitoring of $ETCO_2$ (<25 mm Hg may indicate poor perfusion)
- ECG monitoring
- Correction of dysrhythmias
- Assessment of blood glucose level and correction if less than 60 mg/dL
- Frequent evaluation of vital signs (including auscultation of the lungs and observation for JVD)

A patient in respiratory failure may require intubation and ventilatory support.

> CRITICAL THINKING
>
> You have an unstable patient with signs and symptoms indicating cardiogenic shock. How should you respond when the patient asks, "Am I going to die?"

Drug therapy may include drugs that strengthen the force of contraction (inotropic agents) to improve cardiac output. Such agents include norepinephrine, epinephrine, or dopamine. The use of vasodilator drugs to reduce afterload generally is reserved for in-hospital coronary care. In such settings, the blood pressure and other hemodynamic parameters can be evaluated more accurately. Treatment of pulmonary edema is complicated in the presence of cardiogenic shock because CPAP and nitroglycerin, the mainstays of care, are contraindicated in the presence of hypotension.

> CRITICAL THINKING
>
> What dose of each of these drugs should be given for this condition?

Cardiac Tamponade

Cardiac tamponade (described in Chapter 41, *Chest Trauma*) is defined as impaired diastolic filling of the heart caused by increased intrapericardial pressure and volume. As the pressure of the buildup in pericardial fluid compresses the atria and ventricles, they are unable to fill adequately. This results in a decrease in ventricular filling, which decreases stroke volume. The condition may have a gradual onset. It may result from a cancerous growth or infection. In the out-of-hospital setting, the condition is more often acute, resulting from blunt or penetrating trauma to the chest. Other causes of cardiac tamponade include renal disease, dissecting aneurysm, invasive procedures, or hypothyroidism. Signs and symptoms of cardiac tamponade include the following:

- Chest pain that increases with deep breathing or coughing
- Decreased systolic pressure (a late sign)
- Palpitations
- Elevated venous pressure (an early sign) with associated JVD
- Faint or muffled heart sounds
- Shortness of breath
- Low-voltage QRS complexes and T waves
- Alternating amplitude and vector of P waves, QRS complexes, and T waves (electrical alternans)
- Pulsus paradoxus
- Tachycardia

As described in Chapter 41, *Chest Trauma*, the most important reliable signs of cardiac tamponade are JVD, hypotension, and distant heart sounds (Beck triad).

Management

First, the paramedic must obtain a thorough history to attempt to identify the cause of the cardiac tamponade. Then the paramedic should perform a physical examination. Prehospital care is directed at ensuring an adequate airway, administering oxygen to maintain an Spo_2 of greater than 94%, providing ventilatory support, providing rapid transport for evaluation by a physician, and possibly draining the pericardial sac (pericardiocentesis). A fluid bolus of 30 mL/kg isotonic solution (to a maximum of 1 L) may help support the circulatory system temporarily if the patient becomes hypotensive. This intervention may be repeated twice if indicated. However, definitive management requires drainage of the pericardial sac. Cardiac tamponade may result in death if the condition is not relieved.

> CRITICAL THINKING
>
> Why is drainage of the pericardial sac not done routinely in the prehospital setting?

Thoracic Aneurysms and AAAs

Aneurysm is a nonspecific term that means "dilation of a vessel." An aneurysm may result from atherosclerotic disease (most common), infectious disease (primarily syphilis), traumatic injury, or certain genetic disorders (eg, Marfan syndrome). **FIGURE 21-122** shows the branches of the aorta. AAA and dissecting aneurysm of the aorta are presented here.

Most aneurysms develop at a weak point in the wall of an artery. This weak point results from degenerative changes in the medial layer. Weakening of the supportive elements of the vessel wall allows dilation. This causes turbulence and increasing lateral pressure. The aneurysm tends to enlarge over time as the lateral pressure increases in the dilated segment. Eventually the aneurysm may rupture, possibly producing a life-threatening hemorrhage.

Abdominal Aortic Aneurysm

Abdominal aortic aneurysm (AAA) affects about 2% of the population.[39] The most common site for an AAA is below the renal arteries and above the branching of the common iliac arteries. AAAs are 10 times more common in men. They also are most prevalent in people older than 60 years. The risk of AAA is higher in people who smoke, are male, are white, have a history of other vascular disease, or have a family history of AAA. An abdominal aneurysm usually is asymptomatic as long as it is stable. A small pulsation near the umbilicus is present in about one-third of patients. Clots may form in the enlarged aorta and cause obstructed blood vessels in the legs. Rupture is often sudden; however, if the aneurysm begins to expand or leak, the patient may have abdominal or back pain or tenderness, signaling impending rupture (**BOX 21-20**).

Rupture of an AAA may begin with a small tear in the intima. This small tear allows blood to leak into the wall of the aorta. As the process continues with increasing pressure, the tear may extend through the outer layer of the vessel and cause bleeding into the retroperitoneal space. If bleeding is tamponaded by the retroperitoneal tissues, the patient may be

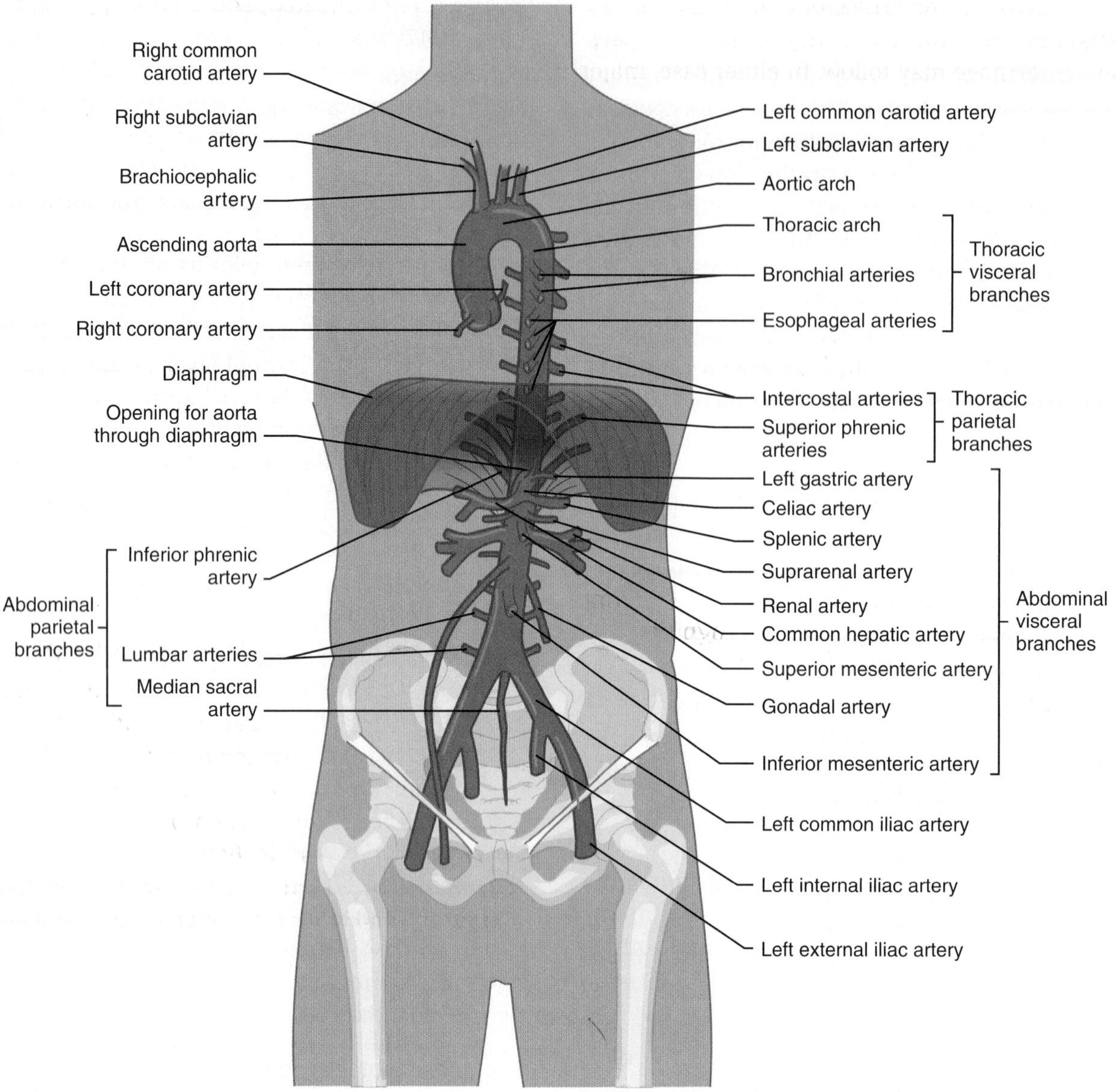

FIGURE 21-122 Branches of the aorta: aortic arch, thoracic aorta, abdominal aorta, and their branches.

BOX 21-20 Signs and Symptoms of a Leaking or Ruptured AAA

- Unexplained hypotension (resulting from hemorrhage or a compensatory vasovagal response mechanism)
- Unexplained syncope (as the aneurysm ruptures, blood pressure drops transiently to zero, producing sudden cerebral hypoperfusion and syncope)
- Sudden onset of abdominal or back pain (described as "tearing" or "ripping") from the physical trauma itself or from inflammation
- Low back or flank pain (radiating to the thigh, groin, testicle, or perineum) that is unrelieved by rest or changes in position
- Signs of peritoneal irritation
- Urge to defecate (caused by retroperitoneal leakage of blood)
- Pulsatile, tender mass (may be palpated when greater than 5 cm), usually located above the umbilicus, left of the midline
- Presence or absence of distal pulses (femoral artery and below), depending on the patient's blood pressure, the occurrence of a dissection, and the degree of peripheral vascular disease

normotensive on the arrival of EMS. If the rupture opens into the peritoneal cavity, however, massive fatal hemorrhage may follow. In either case, major blood loss results and hypovolemic shock ensues.

Often, a patient with a rupturing aneurysm has syncope followed by hypotension with bradycardia despite the loss of a large amount of blood. The reason for bradycardia is stimulation of the vagus nerve. Fibers of the vagus nerve wrap around the aorta. When the aorta tears, the tear stretches these fibers, causing bradycardia. The bradycardia is present despite the hemorrhagic shock condition, which usually causes hypotension and tachycardia in the patient.

Management. Patients with a leaking or ruptured abdominal aneurysm appear ill. They usually need immediate surgery to repair the vessel. About 65% of patients with a ruptured AAA die before arriving at the hospital.[40] Therefore, early recognition and rapid transport to a hospital with vascular surgical capability can reduce the mortality for these patients.

In most cases, prehospital care should be limited to gentle handling, oxygen administration if hypoxemic, cardiac monitoring (including a 12-lead ECG), initiation of two IV lines (18-gauge or larger) en route to the receiving hospital, and alerting the receiving facility to prepare for imminent surgery.

Pulsatile masses (if present) are fragile and in most cases are membrane thin. The paramedic should avoid aggressive examination or deep palpation of the mass. Palpation may cause the mass to rupture. Examination, if needed, can be done by auscultation. Auscultation may reveal a sound similar to that of a systolic murmur or bruit.

The management of blood pressure varies and depends on whether the aneurysm is leaking or ruptured. If rupture has occurred, hypotension, tachycardia, and loss of the pulsating mass may develop suddenly. The patient also may become unresponsive. This state often is followed by full cardiac and respiratory arrest. These patients require rapid and aggressive resuscitation (intubation, ventilation, fluid replacement) and rapid transport for surgery.

Acute Dissecting Aortic Aneurysm

Acute dissecting aortic aneurysm (separation of the arterial wall) is the most common aortic catastrophe. It affects three times as many people as a ruptured AAA.[41] If left untreated, about 33% of patients die within 24 hours and 50% within 48 hours.[41] Factors that can lead to the development of dissecting aneurysm are systemic hypertension, atherosclerosis, cocaine use, congenital abnormalities that affect connective tissue (Marfan syndrome), degenerative changes in the connective tissue of the aortic media (cystic medial necrosis), trauma, and pregnancy. The syndrome affects men twice as often as women. It also is more common in African Americans.

A dissecting aneurysm of the aorta results from a small tear in the intimal layer of the vessel wall (**FIGURE 21-123**). After the tear, the process of dissection begins. The tear in the inner wall allows blood to move between the inner and outer layers. This creates a false passage between the layers of the vessel wall. Blood that enters the false passage results in the formation of a hematoma. This hematoma can rupture through the outer wall (adventitia) at any time, usually into the pericardial or pleural cavity.

Any area of the aorta may be involved. However, in most cases the dissecting aneurysm occurs in the ascending aorta. Once begun, the dissection may extend distally or proximally to involve all of the thoracic and abdominal aorta and tributaries, the coronary arteries, the aortic valve, and the carotid and subclavian vessels. Blood flow is reduced in any vessels bypassed by the dissection, including the carotid and other aortic arch vessels. As a result, **aortic dissection** may cause the following:

- Syncope
- Stroke
- Absent or reduced pulses
- Unequal blood pressure readings (right side compared with left side)
- Heart failure resulting from sudden aortic valve regurgitation
- Pericardial tamponade
- AMI

Signs and Symptoms. The signs and symptoms of a dissecting aortic aneurysm depend on the site of the intimal tear (ascending or descending aorta). They also depend on the extent of dissection. Most patients with acute dissecting aneurysm of the aorta complain of severe pain in the back, epigastrium, abdomen, or extremities. The pain usually is sudden in onset. It may be characterized by the patient as "ripping," "tearing," or "sharp and cutting, like a knife." Pain

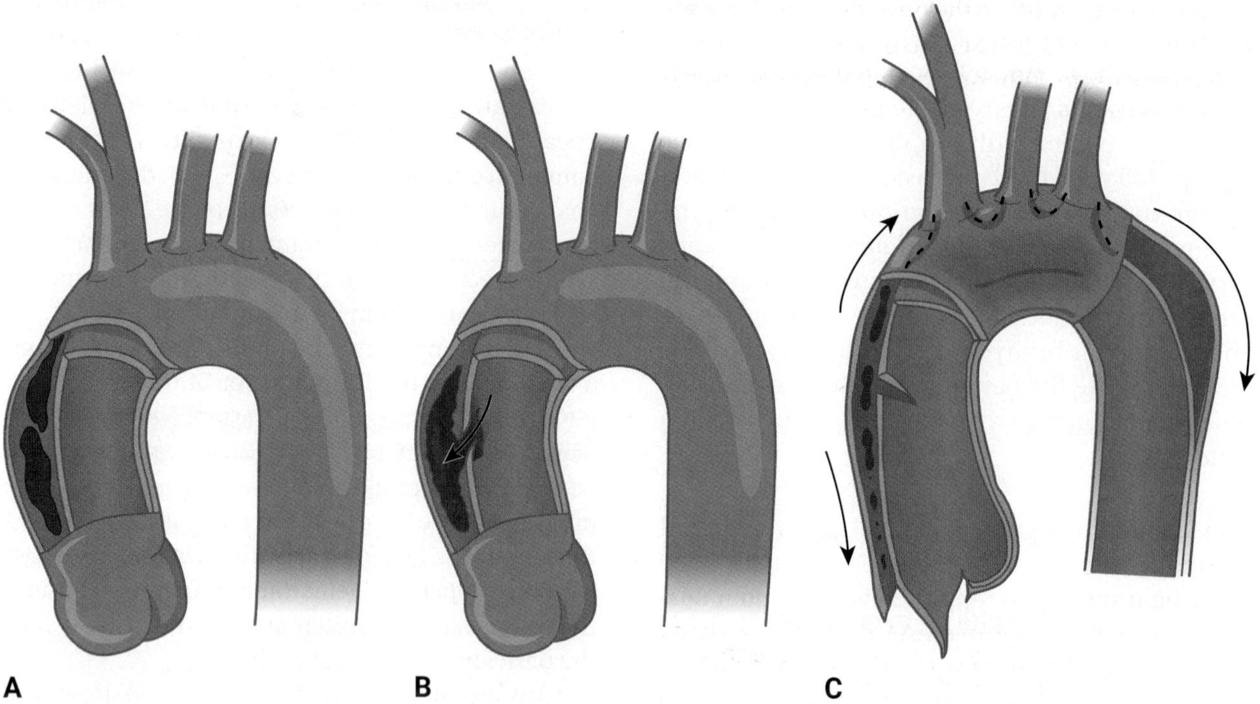

FIGURE 21-123 Pathogenesis of a dissecting aneurysm. **A.** Medial and intimal degeneration of the aortic wall sets the stage. **B.** Hemodynamic forces acting on the aortic wall produce an intimal tear, directing the bloodstream into the middle layer of the wall of the aorta. **C.** The resulting dissecting hematoma is propagated in both directions by a pulse wave produced by each myocardial contraction.

often originates in the back (between the scapulae). The pain possibly extends down into the legs. A patient with acute dissection may appear "shocky" and have pallor, sweating, and peripheral cyanosis (from impaired perfusion), even when the blood pressure is normal or elevated. If the patient is hypotensive, the paramedic should suspect cardiac tamponade or aortic rupture.

CRITICAL THINKING

What condition has signs and symptoms similar to those of an AAA?

Differentiating the pain of aortic dissection from that of MI or pulmonary embolism can be difficult in the prehospital setting. Although no one sign or symptom can positively identify acute aortic dissection, the following distinctive features may help:[42]

- Sudden, severe chest or upper back pain, often described as a tearing, ripping or shearing sensation, that radiates to the neck or down the back
- Sudden severe abdominal pain
- Loss of consciousness
- Shortness of breath
- Sudden difficulty speaking, loss of vision,
- Stroke-like weakness or paralysis of one side of the body
- Weak pulse in one arm or thigh compared with the other
- Leg pain
- Difficulty walking

NOTE

Blood pressure may differ significantly in the two arms if the dissection occludes either subclavian artery, leading to a decreased blood pressure in the affected upper extremity.

Management. The goals of managing suspected aortic dissection in the prehospital setting are relieving pain and providing prompt transport to a medical facility. Transport should not be delayed; analgesics should be administered en route to the hospital. The EMS crew should be ready to resuscitate if the patient begins to decompensate. Other prehospital care measures include the following:

- Handling the patient gently
- Reducing anxiety
- Treating nausea and vomiting with antiemetics
- Administering high-concentration oxygen
- Beginning a large-bore IV line of crystalloid solution (fluids should be infused to maintain a systolic blood pressure that supports adequate perfusion of vital organs)
- Administering a beta blocker to maintain a heart rate of 60 to 80 beats/min
- Giving analgesia (eg, morphine, fentanyl) per medical direction if the diagnosis is strongly suspected

Definitive in-hospital care generally includes reduction of myocardial contractile force to stop progressive dissection (with antihypertensives and beta blockers), monitoring of intra-arterial pressure, and possibly surgical repair.

Acute Arterial Occlusion

Acute arterial occlusion is a sudden blockage of arterial flow. It most commonly is caused by trauma, embolus, or thrombosis. The severity of the ischemic episode depends on the site of occlusion and the extent of collateral circulation around the blockage. Vascular occlusion caused by thrombosis is a complication of atherosclerosis. Occlusions caused by emboli may indicate an abnormal cardiac rhythm, particularly AF.

> CRITICAL THINKING
> Why does AF put the patient at increased risk for emboli?

Arterial occlusion may follow blunt or penetrating trauma; it often is associated with long bone fractures. These injuries vary from injuries to the lining of a vessel to complete severing of a vessel. The occlusion usually is evident because no signs of circulation are seen in the tissue or limb.

An embolism occurs when a blood clot breaks away and enters the arterial system. The clot travels until it reaches a narrow point in a vessel, which is often at a branching site of an artery. Ninety percent of peripheral emboli originate in the heart. Therefore, a history of cardiac disease (eg, dysrhythmia, MI, recent arterial procedure, valvular heart disease) favors a diagnosis of embolic occlusion, particularly if the patient has an asymptomatic opposite extremity with normal pulses. The most common sites of embolic occlusion are the abdominal aorta, common femoral artery, popliteal artery, carotid artery, brachial artery, and mesenteric artery (**FIGURE 21-124**).

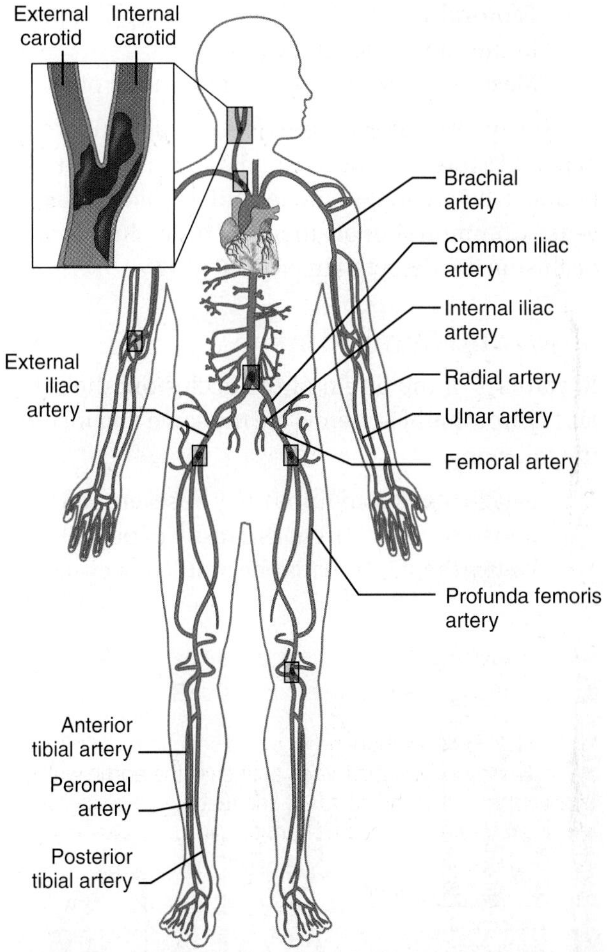

FIGURE 21-124 Common sites of embolic arterial occlusion.

Thrombosis usually results from atherosclerotic disease and usually occurs at a site of severe narrowing of a vessel. Unlike an embolus, a thrombus usually develops over time. As the thrombus enlarges, the collateral blood supply also can become occluded, causing progressive ischemia. The location of the ischemic pain often is related to the site of occlusion:

- **Terminal portion of the abdominal aorta.** Pain in both hips or lower limbs
- **Iliac artery.** Pain in the buttocks or hip on the involved side

- **Femoral artery.** Claudication (cramp-like pain) in the calf of the involved leg
- **Mesenteric artery.** Severe abdominal pain

If severe ischemia persists, muscle necrosis occurs. Thrombotic occlusion is seen most often in people who are male, smoke, and are older than 60 years. Common sites of atherosclerotic (thrombotic) occlusion are depicted in **FIGURE 21-125**.

Signs and Symptoms

Regardless of the origin of the occlusion, the signs and symptoms of ischemia are the same and include the following:

- Pain in the extremity that may be severe and sudden in onset or absent as a result of paresthesia
- Pallor (the skin also may be mottled or cyanotic)
- Lowered skin temperature distal to the occlusion
- Changes in sensory and motor function
- Diminished or absent pulse distal to the injury
- Bruit over the affected vessel
- Slow capillary filling
- Sometimes shock (particularly with mesenteric occlusion)

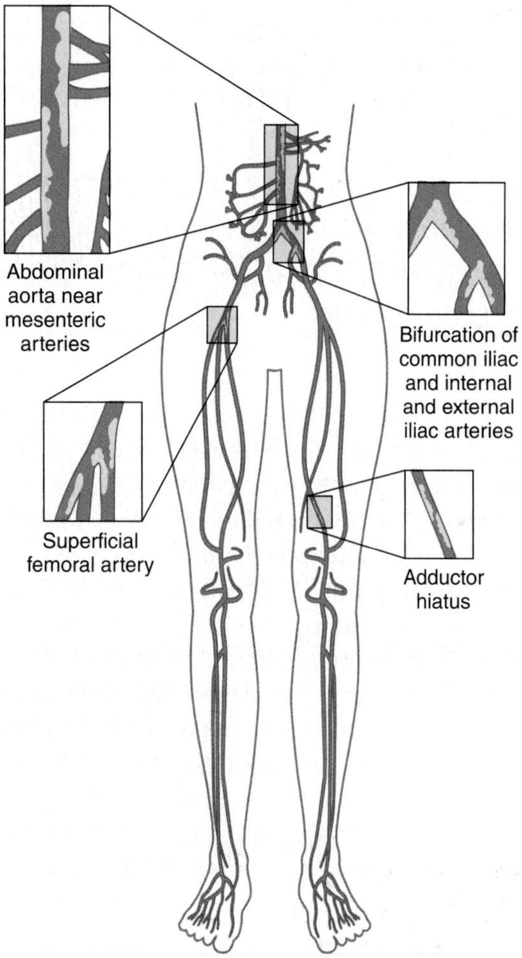

FIGURE 21-125 Common sites of atherosclerotic occlusive disease.

NOTE

Some patients with vascular occlusion have unequal blood pressure readings in the arms. Systolic readings in the arms that differ by 15 mm Hg or more suggest vascular disease. (Normally, the difference between the arms is 5 to 10 mm Hg.)

Management

Acute arterial occlusion in an extremity is serious and painful. The occlusion may be limb threatening if blood flow is not reestablished within 4 to 8 hours. The affected limb should be immobilized and protected. In addition, the patient should be transported for evaluation by a physician. Patients with mesenteric occlusion should be managed for shock with oxygen and IV fluids. Analgesics also may be prescribed by medical direction to relieve pain. In-hospital, definitive care may include anticoagulant or fibrinolytic therapy, transluminal arterial dilation using a balloon catheter, embolectomy, vascular reconstruction, bowel resection, or amputation.

Noncritical Peripheral Vascular Conditions

Noncritical peripheral vascular conditions include varicose veins, superficial thrombophlebitis (described in Chapter 11, *General Principles of Pathophysiology*), and acute deep vein thrombosis (DVT). Of these conditions, DVT is the only one that can cause life-threatening pulmonary embolism. Predisposing factors to venous thrombosis include the following:[43]

- Primary
  - Paralysis after spinal cord injury
  - Fractures of hip, pelvis, or long bones
  - Coagulopathies
  - Multisystem trauma
  - Cancer (especially metastatic)
  - Major general or orthopaedic surgery

- Other
  - Pregnancy or immediate postpartum period
  - Birth control pills or menopausal estrogen treatment
  - Age older than 50 years
  - Obesity (doubles risk)
  - Immobility
  - Family history
  - Genetic blood clotting disorders
  - Physical inactivity (such as a long flight)

Acute Deep Vein Thrombosis

Acute **deep vein thrombosis (DVT)** is a serious, common problem. Occlusion may involve any portion of the deep venous system. However, occlusion is much more common in the lower extremities. Risk factors for DVT include recent lower extremity trauma, recent surgery, advanced age, recent MI, inactivity, confinement to bed, heart failure, cancer, previous thrombosis, oral contraceptive therapy, sickle cell disease, and obesity. Signs and symptoms of acute DVT include the following:

- Pain
- Edema
- Warmth
- Erythema or blue discoloration
- Tenderness

Management

Patients with acute DVT who are at a low risk for pulmonary embolism may be treated at home. Prehospital care usually is limited to immobilization and elevation of the extremity and transport for evaluation by a physician. DVT in the calf of the leg usually is much less serious than is DVT in the thigh or pelvis. The latter has a higher incidence of associated pulmonary embolus. Definitive care includes bed rest, administration of anticoagulants or, rarely, fibrinolytic agents, or thrombectomy.

Hypertension

Hypertension is a common disorder. It afflicts about 30% of the US population, and just over half have it under control.[44] Hypertension is defined by a resting blood pressure consistently greater than 120/80 mm Hg (120-130 mm Hg).[45] The several categories of hypertension are based on the level of blood pressure, symptomatology, and urgency of need for intervention (**TABLE 21-10** and **BOX 21-21**). For the purpose of this text, two general categories are presented: chronic hypertension and hypertensive emergencies. (These emergencies include **hypertensive encephalopathy**.) A common cause of hypertension is discontinuing medication or other therapy prescribed by the physician.

TABLE 21-10 Blood Pressure Categories for Adults (18 Years or Older)[a]

	Blood Pressure (mm Hg)		
Category	**Systolic**		**Diastolic**
Normal	<120	and	<80
Elevated	120–129	and	<80
Hypertension, stage 1	130–139	or	80–89
Hypertension, stage 2	>140	or	>90
Hypertensive crisis	>180	and/or	>120

[a]For those not taking medicine for high blood pressure and not having a short-term serious illness.

Modified from: The facts about high blood pressure. American Heart Association website. https://www.heart.org/HEARTORG/Conditions/HighBloodPressure/GettheFactsAboutHighBloodPressure/The-Facts-About-High-Blood-Pressure_UCM_002050_Article.jsp. Updated March 14, 2018. Accessed April 4, 2018.

BOX 21-21 Signs and Symptoms of Hypertensive Emergencies

Altered mental status
Changes in visual acuity
ECG changes
Epistaxis
Headache
Nausea and vomiting
Paroxysmal nocturnal dyspnea
Seizures
Shortness of breath

CRITICAL THINKING

Why do patients fail to take medicines prescribed for hypertension?

Chronic Hypertension

Chronic hypertension has an adverse effect on the function of the heart and blood vessels. It requires the heart to perform more work than normal, which leads to hypertrophy of the cardiac muscle and left ventricular failure. Because chronic hypertension increases the rate at which atherosclerosis develops, the probability of cardiovascular, cerebrovascular, and peripheral vascular disease and the risk of aneurysm formation is increased. Along with heart failure, conditions commonly associated with chronic, uncontrolled hypertension are cerebral hemorrhage and stroke, MI, renal failure (caused by vascular changes in the kidney), and development of thoracic aneurysm or AAA.

Chronic hypertension leads to an increase in cardiac afterload. The heart responds to the increased workload that results from high systemic vascular resistance by becoming enlarged. Although an enlarged heart may be able to work fine for many years, over time it is no longer able to maintain adequate blood flow. The patient is then at risk for the development of symptoms of pump failure.

Any hypertension-related illness, such as pulmonary edema, dissecting aortic aneurysm, preeclampsia and eclampsia of pregnancy (described in Chapter 45, *Obstetrics*), or stroke, requires stabilization and prompt, appropriate management. The hypertension associated with these situations often is a result of a primary problem. Managing the primary problem often makes controlling the patient's blood pressure easier. However, the primary cause may not be easily correctable. In situations such as dissecting aortic aneurysm, controlling the blood pressure also is a key to managing the primary problem. A life-threatening condition that develops from unmanaged or partially managed hypertension may lead to a hypertensive emergency.

Hypertensive Crisis

Hypertensive crisis is an umbrella term for conditions in which an increase in blood pressure, usually greater than 180/120 mm Hg, can lead to significant, irreversible damage to organs. In some cases, it occurs without a reported history of hypertension. Hypertensive crisis is more practically divided into two categories: emergency and urgency. In hypertensive urgency, the blood pressure does not seem to be causing clinical or laboratory evidence of end-organ damage. However, in hypertensive emergency, end-organ damage is evident, and permanent damage can occur within hours if the blood pressure is not immediately lowered in a carefully controlled manner. The organs most likely to be at risk are the brain, heart, and kidneys. This now uncommon condition is experienced by about 1% to 2% of all hypertensive patients.[46]

In many cases, the patient in hypertensive crisis experiences nonspecific signs and symptoms that may include headache, dizziness, or vomiting. When the heart is impacted, dyspnea, chest pain, arrhythmias, or syncope may occur.

Hypertensive emergencies may cause or worsen the following clinical conditions: (1) myocardial ischemia with hypertension, (2) aortic dissection with hypertension, (3) pulmonary edema with hypertension, (4) hypertensive intracranial hemorrhage, (5) toxemia, (6) hypertensive encephalopathy, and (7) renal failure. Hypertensive encephalopathy results solely from elevated blood pressure, causing elevated intracranial pressure.

Persistent hypertension causes brain damage (hypertensive encephalopathy). It results in a decrease in blood and oxygen to the brain (cerebral hypoperfusion). It also damages the tissues that make up the blood–brain barrier. This damage results in fluid leak into the brain tissue. Hypertensive encephalopathy may progress over several hours from initial symptoms of severe headache, nausea, vomiting, aphasia, and transient blindness to seizures, stupor, coma, and death. The condition is a true emergency. It requires immediate transport to a medical facility for definitive care. The goal of therapy is controlled but rapid lowering of the blood pressure to normalize cerebral blood flow. If the blood pressure is lowered too quickly, infarction of end organs (heart, kidney, brain) may occur.

NOTE

Lateralizing neurologic signs, such as hemiparesis or hemiplegia, are uncommon in hypertensive emergencies. Their presence is suggestive of stroke.

Modified from: Sharma S, Anderson C, Sharma P, Frey D. Management of hypertensive urgency in an urgent care setting. *Journal of Urgent Care Medicine* website. https://www.jucm.com/management-of-hypertensive-urgency-in-an-urgent-care-setting/. Accessed April 6, 2018.

CRITICAL THINKING

How does fluid leakage into the brain affect the intracranial pressure and cerebral perfusion pressure?

Prehospital management of patients with a hypertensive emergency includes the following:

- Supportive care
- Calming the patient
- Oxygen therapy if indicated
- IV line to keep the vein open
- ECG monitoring
- Rapid transport

In most cases, drug therapy for hypertensive emergencies is not initiated in the prehospital setting. However, in severe cases of hypertensive encephalopathy or if transport is delayed, medical direction may recommend the administration of antihypertensives such as labetalol. This drug induces arteriolar vasodilation and may lower the blood pressure.

Specific Heart Diseases

In addition to atherosclerosis that results in coronary artery disease, numerous other diseases affect the heart. These include valvular heart disease, infectious heart disease, and congenital heart disease (see Chapter 46, *Neonatal Care*).

Valvular Heart Disease

Valvular heart disease refers to any disease process that affects one or more valves of the heart: the mitral, aortic, tricuspid, or pulmonary valves. When one or more of these valves become narrowed, hardened, or thickened (stenotic), the valves do not open or close completely. As a result, blood does not flow with proper force or direction. A stenotic valve forces blood back up into the adjacent chamber of the heart. A valve that is unable to close properly allows blood to "leak" back (regurgitate) into the previous chamber (**FIGURE 21-126**). The defects in the pumping action of the valves can cause the heart to enlarge and thicken. This can result in a loss of elasticity and an increased risk of pulmonary embolism or stroke.

> NOTE
>
> Valve leaflets normally are very thin and flexible. However, they can become thickened, rigid, or dysfunctional in response to a disease process, such as coronary artery disease or cardiac hypertrophy. Stenosis often is accompanied by calcification and atherosclerosis-type lesions (valvular lesion).

Valvular heart disease can be congenital. In other cases, it can develop slowly, or it may be acute. Depending on the valve and the course of the disease, signs and symptoms may be similar to those seen in heart failure. They may include palpitations with or without chest pain, fatigue, dizziness or syncope, and weight gain. If the cause of the valvular heart disease is a bacterial infection (eg, endocarditis, described later in the chapter), fever may be present. After evaluation by a physician, treatment may include antibiotics to manage infection, anticoagulants to prevent clot formation, balloon dilation to widen a stenotic valve, clip insertion, and sometimes surgical valve replacement. Prehospital care is primarily

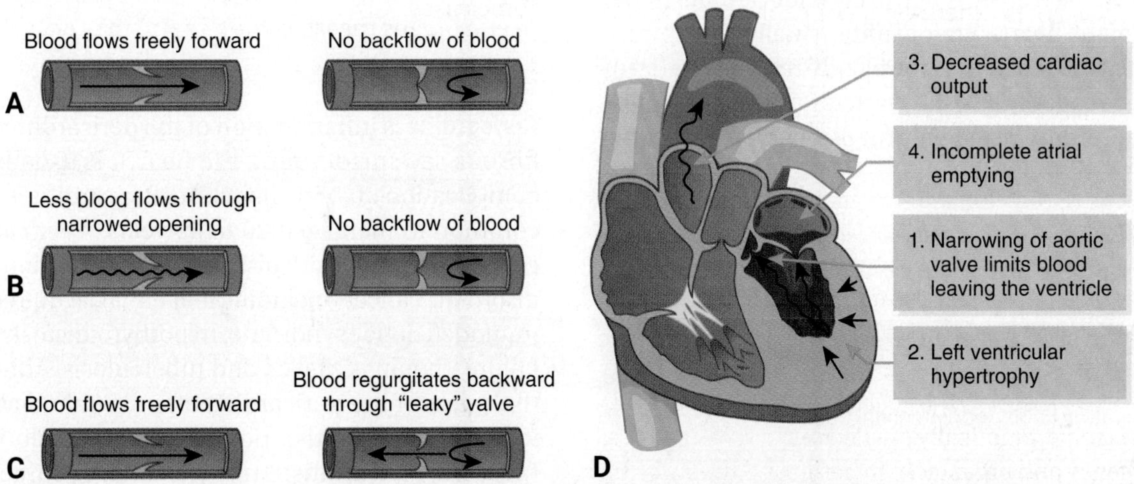

FIGURE 21-126 Effects of heart valve defects. **A.** Normal valve. **B.** Stenosis. **C.** Incompetent valve. **D.** Effect of aortic stenosis.

supportive and may include oxygen administration if the patient is dyspneic or hypoxic, ECG monitoring, vascular access, and transport for evaluation by a physician.

Infectious Heart Disease

Infectious heart disease is caused by intravascular contamination by pathogens. The infections can damage the muscles and valves of the heart. Infections also may lead to the formation of emboli, which can travel to the brain, kidneys, lungs, or abdomen. Three common forms of infectious heart disease are endocarditis, pericarditis, and myocarditis. Most patients with infectious heart disease also have underlying heart disease or problems with the heart valves. Prehospital care for infectious heart disease is primarily supportive.

> NOTE
>
> Rheumatic fever can lead to inflammation of the heart (carditis) and damage to the heart valves (rheumatic heart disease). Rheumatic fever follows infection by group A *Streptococcus* (GAS) bacteria, such as strep throat or scarlet fever. Proper diagnosis and adequate antibiotic treatment of GAS infections can prevent acute rheumatic fever in most cases. Most patients with a GAS infection respond well to antibiotic therapy.
>
> *Modified from:* Cunningham MW. Pathogenesis of group A streptococcal infections. *Clin Microbiol Rev.* 2000;13(3):470-511.

Endocarditis

Endocarditis is an infection of the endocardium (inner layer of the heart). Endocarditis usually results from a bacterium that enters the bloodstream (bacterial or infective endocarditis). Risk factors for the development of endocarditis include IV drug use, permanent central venous access lines, previous valve surgery, recent dental surgery, and weakened heart valves. The incidence of infectious endocarditis has increased along with the increase in IV opioid use.[47] Patients with a history of valvular heart disease or rheumatic fever also are at higher risk for endocarditis. Complications of the disease include AF, blood clots, brain abscess, CNS changes, heart failure, glomerulonephritis, jaundice, severe heart valve damage, and stroke.

> NOTE
>
> *Streptococcus viridans*, a bacterium commonly found in the mouth, is responsible for about 50% of all cases of bacterial endocarditis. For this reason, prophylactic antibiotics often are prescribed for high-risk patients undergoing dental procedures or surgery involving the respiratory, urinary, or intestinal tract.
>
> *Modified from:* Ashley EA, Niebauer J. *Cardiology Explained.* London, England: Remedica; 2004.

Endocarditis may develop slowly or may be sudden in onset. Signs and symptoms include:

- Abnormal urine color
- Chills (common)
- Excessive sweating (common)
- Fatigue
- Fever (common)
- Joint pain
- Muscle aches and pains
- Night sweats
- Nail abnormalities (splinter hemorrhages under the nails)
- Paleness
- Red, painless skin spots on the palms and soles (Janeway lesions)
- Red, painful nodes in the pads of the fingers and toes (Osler nodes)
- Shortness of breath with activity
- Swelling of the feet, legs, abdomen
- Weakness
- Weight loss

Treatment consists of blood cultures to identify the bacterium causing the disease and long-term IV antibiotics. Valve replacement may be necessary in some cases.

Pericarditis

Pericarditis is inflammation of the pericardium (the fibrous sac surrounding the heart). It usually is a complication of a viral infection. Pericarditis is most common in men aged 20 to 50 years.[48] Pericarditis can be associated with diseases such as autoimmune disorders, cancer (including leukemia), acquired immunodeficiency syndrome, hypothyroidism, kidney failure, rheumatic fever, and tuberculosis. Although the cause of the pericarditis often is unknown (idiopathic pericarditis), possible causes include MI (post-MI pericarditis); injury, including surgery or trauma to the chest, esophagus, or heart; medications that suppress the immune system; myocarditis; and radiation therapy to the chest. Signs and symptoms include the following:

- Swelling of the ankles, feet, and legs (occasionally)
- Anxiety
- Difficulty breathing when lying down
  - Crackles
  - Decreased breath sounds
- Chest pain caused by the inflamed pericardium rubbing against the heart
  - May radiate to the neck, shoulders, back, or abdomen
  - Often increases with deep breathing and lying flat; may increase with coughing and swallowing
  - Pleuritic chest pain (often relieved by sitting up and leaning forward)
- Pericardial friction rub
- Dry cough
- Fatigue
- Fever
- Twelve-lead ECG changes
  - Diffuse ST elevation
  - PR-segment depression
  - Notched J point

NOTE

These 12-lead ECG changes are one of the "MI imposters." Pericarditis is suggested by ST elevation in all leads but can be difficult to diagnose with certainty both in the hospital and in the field.

Pericarditis is assessed with diagnostic imaging (echocardiogram). Pericarditis is managed with analgesics, antibiotics, nonsteroidal anti-inflammatory drugs, corticosteroids, and diuretics. With decreased cardiac function or cardiac tamponade (rare), pericardiocentesis may be needed. Most patients recover completely within 2 to 3 months. However, the condition may reoccur.

Myocarditis

Myocarditis is inflammation of the heart muscle. It is an uncommon disorder caused by a viral, bacterial, or fungal infection that reaches the heart. (Myocarditis also can be caused by chemical exposure, allergic reactions, or an inflammatory disease, such as rheumatoid arthritis or sarcoidosis.) The immune response associated with myocarditis can damage the heart muscle and cause the heart to become thick, swollen, and weak, leading to symptoms of heart failure. Some patients with myocarditis are asymptomatic. In other patients, signs and symptoms that may occur with the disease include the following:

- Abnormal heartbeat, sometimes leading to syncope
- Chest pain that may be severe
- Fever and other signs of infection (headache, muscle aches, sore throat, diarrhea, rashes)
- Joint pain or swelling
- Leg swelling
- Shortness of breath
- Decreased urine output

Myocarditis may lead to heart muscle damage, and the patient may need to be treated for heart failure. Dysrhythmias may need to be managed with antidysrhythmics and insertion of a pacemaker or an ICD. Depending on the severity of the damage to the heart, the patient may recover completely or may have permanent heart failure.

Cardiomyopathy

Cardiomyopathy is a weakening of the heart muscle or a change in heart muscle structure. It often is associated with inadequate heart pumping or other heart function problems. Common causes of the disease are alcoholism and cocaine use, chemotherapy drugs, pregnancy, genetic defects, amyloidosis, end-stage kidney disease, viral infection, long-term hypertension, nutritional deficiencies, and lupus. Cardiomyopathy can be classified into three main types:[49]

- Dilated cardiomyopathy (the most common type) is a condition in which the heart becomes weakened and enlarged. It cannot pump blood efficiently. Many different medical problems can cause this type of cardiomyopathy, including coronary artery disease, rheumatoid arthritis, muscular dystrophy, and human immunodeficiency virus infection.
- Restrictive cardiomyopathy refers to a group of disorders in which the heart chambers are unable to properly fill with blood because of stiffness of the heart. The most common causes of restrictive cardiomyopathy are **amyloidosis** (deposits of abnormal protein in heart tissue) and scarring of the heart muscle. This type of cardiomyopathy frequently occurs after heart transplantation.

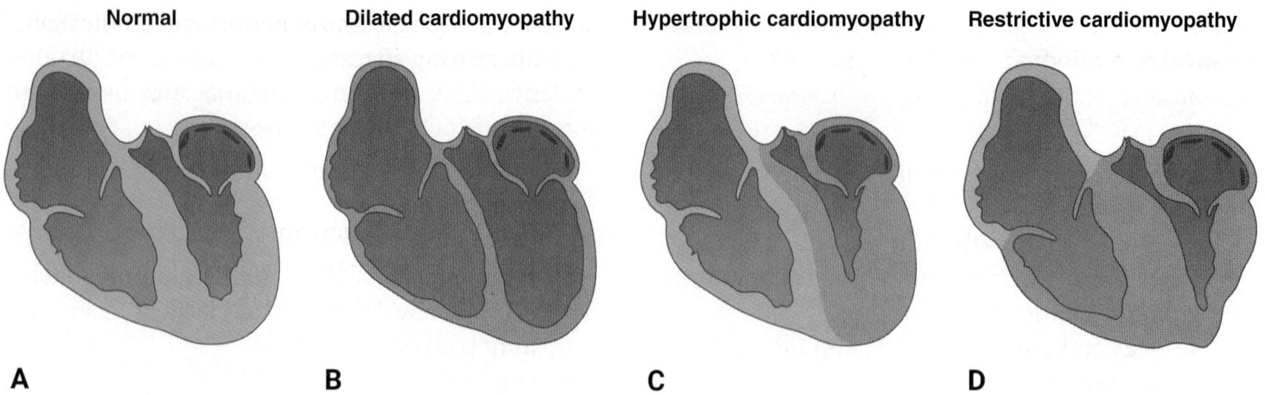

FIGURE 21-127 The three types of cardiomyopathy. **A.** Normal heart. **B.** Dilated cardiomyopathy demonstrating enlargement of all four chambers. **C.** Hypertrophic cardiomyopathy showing a thickened left ventricle. **D.** Restrictive cardiomyopathy characterized by a small left ventricular volume.

- Hypertrophic cardiomyopathy is a condition in which parts of the heart muscle become thicker than other parts. This thickening makes it more difficult for blood to leave the heart and forces the heart to work harder to pump blood. This type of cardiomyopathy is inherited. The first symptom of the disease among many young patients is sudden collapse, and possibly death, caused by dysrhythmias (arrhythmogenic right ventricular dysplasia). Hypertrophic cardiomyopathy is an important cause of death in young athletes who seem completely healthy but who die during heavy exercise (**FIGURE 21-127**).[50]

Signs and Symptoms

Some patients with cardiomyopathy have no signs and symptoms in the early stage of the disease. However, as the disease progresses, signs and symptoms usually appear. These may include:

- Breathlessness with exertion or even at rest
- Swelling of the legs, ankles, and feet
- Bloating (distention) of the abdomen with fluid
- Fatigue
- Irregular heartbeats that feel rapid, pounding, or fluttering
- Dizziness, light-headedness, and fainting

The treatment of cardiomyopathy is based on the patient's age and general health and the specific type and severity of the disease. Drugs often are prescribed to improve heart function and to prevent clot formation and fluid retention. These drugs include vasodilators, digitalis, angiotensin-converting enzyme inhibitors, anticoagulants, and diuretics. Dilated cardiomyopathies usually respond well to medication, at least initially. Treatment of some cardiomyopathies that result from viral infections may not be effective. Therapy for those patients with restrictive cardiomyopathy may be particularly limited. If end-stage heart failure develops, a heart transplant may be necessary.

Techniques for Managing Cardiac Emergencies

This section addresses the various procedures, techniques, and types of equipment used to manage cardiac emergencies. These include basic cardiac life support (BCLS), mechanical CPR devices, monitor-defibrillators (manual, fully automated, and semiautomated), defibrillation, automatic ICDs, synchronized cardioversion, and TCP. This section also offers an overview of the management of a cardiac arrest as it applies to working within an advanced cardiac life support system. The reader is encouraged to review the dysrhythmias and drug therapy protocols presented previously in this text.

Team Approach to Cardiocerebral Resuscitation

The team-based resuscitation approach to cardiocerebral resuscitation (CCR) focuses on more than just ROSC. The overarching goal of CCR is to have patients discharged from the hospital neurologically intact and able to resume a good quality of life. Many EMS systems have adopted a modification of the AHA team-based resuscitation known as Pit Crew CPR or Pit Crew CCR.[51] This approach blends elements of high-quality CPR known to improve survival from cardiac arrest with closed-loop communication and a structured team-based approach to resuscitation.

Essential to this approach are implementation of and quality review of the elements of high-performance CPR:

1. Maximizing the CCF during resuscitation
2. Maintaining chest compression rate at 100 to 120 compressions/min
3. Sustaining depth of chest compressions at a depth of at least 2 inches (5 cm)
4. Allowing for rapid and full chest recoil during compression release
5. Avoiding excessive ventilation

The pit crew approach is modeled after the high-performance teams that have evolved in NASCAR racing. The NASCAR pit crews have just seconds to perform their job and maximize their team's chance to win the race. Each team member has a specific role, with special tools, and is trained and positioned to maximize the efficiency of his or her performance. Prehospital cardiac arrest pit crew teams are similar in many ways but have to be more flexible because the team configuration can change throughout a call. The CCR pit crew roles vary based on how units arrive on the scene and may involve two or more members. Generally, the CCR pit crew has team members performing the following roles:

- **Team leader.** Person who coordinates the resuscitation and monitors team member performance.
- **Airway.** Person who establishes and maintains airway, oxygenation, and ventilation.
- **Compressor.** Person who performs maximally effective chest compressions with real-time feedback.
- **Monitor/electrical therapy.** Person who defibrillates and monitors ECG. (The monitor/compressor positions alternate every 2 minutes to prevent fatigue and maximize quality of chest compressions.)
- **Vascular access medication administration.** Person who establishes IV or IO access; administers medications.

Each person has a job, a position, and a specific role on the scene so noise and confusion are reduced. This cohesive strategy maximizes performance, efficiency, and resuscitation success.

The CCR crew must constantly evaluate performance. Team debriefings held immediately after the call help to identify areas in which care can be improved on future calls. These debriefings should avoid individual criticism and instead focus on enhancing team performance. Later, quality improvement analysis of monitor data can provide objective data to the team related to compression fraction and other quality indicators of CPR. High-performance teams using this approach have reported improved patient outcomes.[51,52]

Basic Cardiac Life Support

The AHA reported more than 350,000 out-of-hospital cardiac arrests in 2016. Of these patients, 12% survived to hospital discharge and 46.1% received bystander CPR.[53] BCLS provides circulation and respiration for a victim of cardiac arrest until advanced cardiac life support (ACLS) is available. The role of high-quality chest compressions is increasingly recognized as a key element influencing survival from sudden cardiac arrest.[54,55] Early CPR can double or triple survival from cardiac arrest.[10] Elements of high-quality CPR include the following:

- Beginning CPR with chest compressions
- Providing chest compressions at a rate of 100 to 120 compressions/min
- Providing chest compressions at a depth of at least 2 inches (5 cm)
- Ensuring full chest recoil between chest compressions
- Minimizing interruptions in chest compressions (maintaining a high compression fraction)
- Avoiding excessive ventilation[2]

Evidence is mixed on the use of continuous compressions. Several studies showed better survival with good neurologic outcome when continuous compressions without ventilation was performed for the first few minutes in patients with witnessed arrest or shockable rhythm.[56-58] Some literature indicates better outcomes with a traditional compression-to-ventilation ratio of 30:2 versus continuous chest compression CPR.[59] It is clear however that any bystander CPR is linked to improved patient outcomes.[60] CCF should be at least 60% with no interruption in chest compressions for more than 10 seconds. The 2015 AHA guidelines state that for witnessed out-of-hospital cardiac arrest with a shockable rhythm it is acceptable to perform up to three cycles of 200 continuous compressions with passive oxygen insufflation and airway adjuncts (class IIb).[2] Cardiac arrest most often is associated with cardiovascular disease and is precipitated by VF or ventricular asystole. Cardiac arrest also may result from noncardiac causes, such as poisoning, drug overdose, toxic inhalation, trauma, and foreign body airway obstruction. For adult cardiac arrest in these cases, the standard 30:2 CPR is indicated.

Physiology of Circulation Provided by External Chest Compression

Two mechanisms are thought to be responsible for blood flow during CPR. The first is direct compression of the heart between the sternum and the spine. This increases pressure within the ventricles enough to provide blood flow to the lungs and through the aorta to other organs. The second mechanism (which is thought to play a more important role than does direct compression of the heart) is the generalized increase in intrathoracic pressure that occurs during CPR. This thoracic pump allows the left heart to act as a conduit for the passage of blood. Complete chest recoil is an essential element of the mechanics of effective CPR. Incomplete chest recoil reduces venous return, CPP, and myocardial blood flow by increasing intrathoracic pressure. Other mechanisms not currently known may be involved as well. Artificial circulation generates only about 20% to 30% of the normal output of the heart.[61]

Research has been conducted for many years on ways to improve CPR. These methods include simultaneous chest compressions and ventilation, abdominal compression with synchronized ventilation, CPR augmented by pneumatic antishock garments, interposed abdominal compression, continuous abdominal binding, and plunger mechanisms for chest compression that cause active compression and active expansion. However, thus far, no alternative method has been shown to improve survival or circulation unequivocally.[62] **FIGURE 21-128** presents the standards of CPR as recommended by the AHA.

Mechanical CPR Devices

A number of mechanical devices (eg, load-distributing band devices, piston devices) have been designed to produce external chest compressions. Most function to reduce intrathoracic pressure during decompression of the chest, thereby improving venous return to the heart. Some devices provide chest compression and synchronized ventilation in the patient with cardiac arrest (**FIGURE 21-129**). These devices may be helpful in systems with limited personnel, during prolonged CPR (such as hypothermic cardiac arrest), and in a moving ambulance (AHA class IIb). It is imperative that teams be properly trained to use these devices to minimize interruptions in chest compressions during their application. These devices are designed for adult patients.

Impedance threshold devices (ITDs) have a pressure-sensitive valve that limits the amount of air that enters the chest during the upstroke (recoil) during chest compressions. This function enhances negative pressure inside the chest without impeding inhalation or exhalation. The ITD can be used with an advanced airway or face mask with a tight seal. It can be used with conventional CPR or as an adjunct to active compression–decompression CPR (ACD-CPR). An ITD produces the following net effects:

- Blood flow to the heart is increased.
- Blood flow to the brain is enhanced.
- Systolic blood pressure doubles.
- Survival to the hospital may be increased.
- Chance of successful defibrillation may be increased.

The AHA has classified ITDs as a class III intervention that does not benefit or harm patients when used with conventional CPR alone.[62]

Active Compression–Decompression CPR and ITDs

ACD-CPR is performed with a handheld suction cup device placed over the sternum. The rescuer pushes the device down to compress the chest and then actively pulls the plunger up during the decompression phase. This action generates negative pressure during chest recoil and increases venous return to the heart, thereby increasing cardiac output. The combination of ACD-CPR with the ITD is thought to improve blood flow. Some research suggests that neurologically favorable survival with this technique may be greater than with conventional CPR, but more study is needed to provide conclusive evidence. Because of this limited research, the 2015 AHA recommendations state this may be a reasonable alternative to

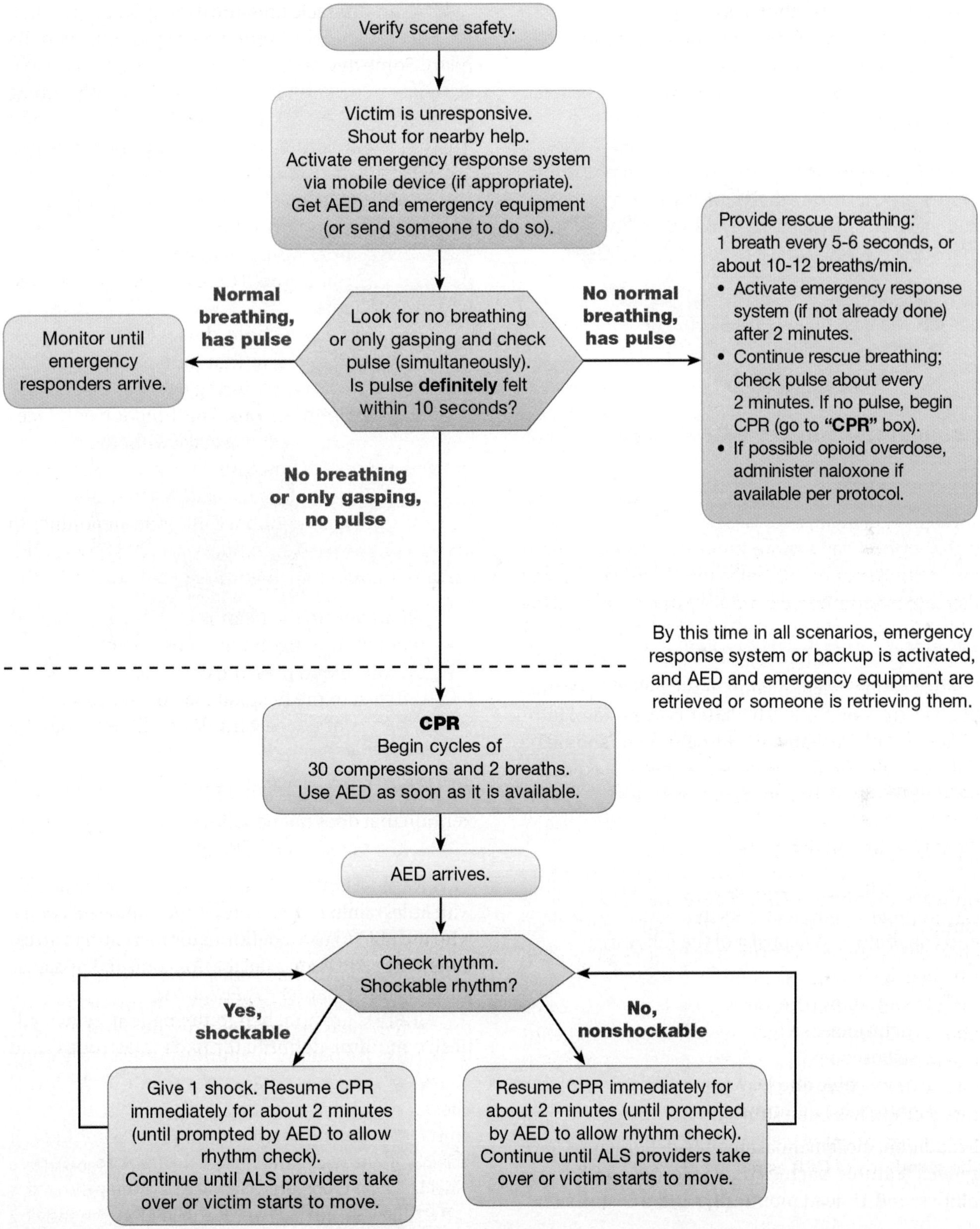

Abbreviations: AED, automated external defibrillator; ALS, advanced life support; BLS; basic life support; CPR, cardiopulmonary resuscitation

FIGURE 21-128 Health care provider algorithm for adult basic life support.

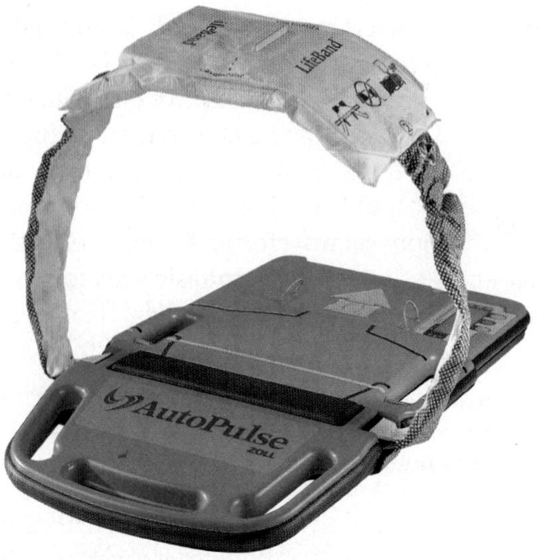

FIGURE 21-129 Mechanical cardiopulmonary resuscitation device.

Provided with permission by ZOLL Medical.

conventional CPR if the appropriate equipment and training are available (Class IIb).[62]

Monitor-Defibrillators

Cardiac monitor-defibrillators are classified as manual defibrillators or AEDs. The latter may be semiautomated or fully automated. The paramedic should be familiar with the monitor-defibrillators used in the local EMS system or community settings.

Manual Monitor-Defibrillators

Monitor-defibrillators are available from a number of equipment manufacturers in a variety of designs and capabilities. All consist of the following:

- Patch electrodes
- Defibrillator controls
- Synchronizer switch
- Oscilloscope
- Patient cable and lead wires
- Controls for monitoring

In addition, most manual monitor-defibrillators have special features, such as data recorders, TCP capabilities, and 12-lead monitoring and transmission.

Automated External Defibrillators

AEDs (**FIGURE 21-130**) analyze the ECG signal. They evaluate the frequency, amplitude, and shape of the ECG waves. They are designed to be used by people with little training. They increase the number of people who are able to use a defibrillator in a cardiac arrest emergency. AEDs are available for adult and pediatric patients (see Chapter 47, *Pediatrics*).

All AEDs are attached to the patient by two adhesive monitor-defibrillator pads (electrodes) and

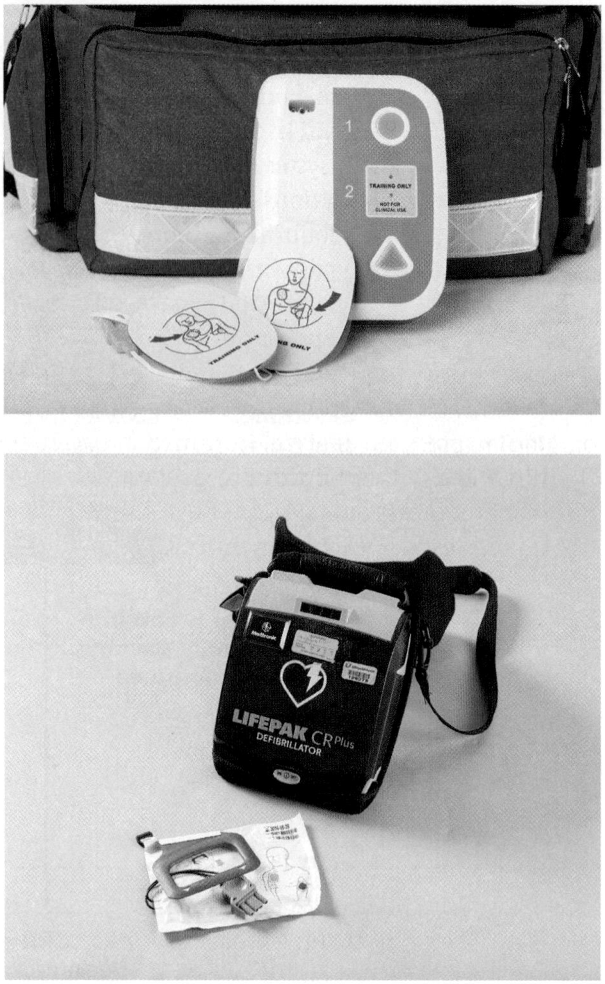

FIGURE 21-130 Automated external defibrillators.

NOTE

There are many community-based first-responder defibrillation programs using AEDs. These programs and others (eg, AEDs located in airports, businesses, and schools, and on public airlines) are supported by the AHA and other groups. The Food and Drug Administration approved nonprescription sales of some AEDs for home use.

connecting cables. AEDs are available from a number of manufacturers. Most units provide programmable modules, data recorders, and voice messages to the operator. All users should become familiar with the AED device used in their system. Moreover, they should follow the recommendations of the manufacturer.

A fully automated defibrillator requires only that the operator attach the defibrillation pads and turn on the device. The rhythm is analyzed in the internal circuitry of the AED. If a shockable rhythm is detected, the AED charges capacitors and delivers a shock.

A semiautomated defibrillator requires the operator to press an "analyze" button to interpret the rhythm and a "shock" button to deliver the shock. The operator presses the shock control only when the AED identifies a shockable rhythm and "advises" the operator to press the "shock" button.

CRITICAL THINKING

What safety measure is still the duty of the person who operates the AED?

AEDs have four safety features:

1. They can analyze ECG waves.
2. They have built-in filters that check for QRS-like signals, radio transmission waves, 60-cycle interference, and loose or poor electrode contact.
3. Most are programmed to detect spontaneous patient movements, continued heartbeat and blood flow, and movement of the patient by others.
4. They make multiple evaluations of the rhythm before making a shock advisory or delivering a shock.

Biphasic Technology

In the past, defibrillation used monophasic waveforms, in which the current travels in only one direction, from the positive pad to the negative pad. These defibrillators require high energy to defibrillate a patient effectively. These machines also require large batteries, energy storage capacitors, inductors, and large, high-voltage mechanical devices.

AEDs and implantable defibrillators use biphasic waveform technology. This technology predicts a patient's energy requirements by determining chest wall impedance. The shock then is delivered by a current that travels in one direction, is stopped, and then is reversed to travel in the opposite direction. This technology allows for effective defibrillation to occur with lower energy for most patients. (Biphasic defibrillation of 115 and 130 J appears to be as effective as 200 and 360 J delivered with monophasic shocks.[63]) Biphasic waveforms are more effective at lower energy than are monophasic waveforms. As a result, AEDs (using smaller batteries) have become smaller, lighter, and more durable. They also have become less expensive to manufacture.

Defibrillation

Defibrillation is the delivery of electrical current through the chest wall. The purpose is to terminate VF and pulseless VT. The shock depolarizes a large mass of myocardial cells at once. If about 75% of these cells are in the resting state (depolarized) after the shock is delivered, a normal pacemaker may resume discharging. Early defibrillation is supported by the following rationales:[9]

- The most frequent initial rhythm in sudden cardiac arrest is VF.
- The most effective management for VF is electrical defibrillation.
- The probability of successful defibrillation decreases rapidly over time.
- VF tends to convert to asystole within a few minutes.

The modern defibrillator is designed to deliver an electrical shock via patches or pads to the patient's chest. The defibrillator accepts the electrical charge from the battery source. It stores the charge in the capacitor and then releases the current into the patient in a short, controlled burst (within 5 to 30 milliseconds).

NOTE

Older defibrillators used "quick look" paddles instead of the modern pads or patches. If paddles are used, they should be coated with electrode paste or gel to reduce resistance and should be held firmly on the patient's chest with about 20 to 25 pounds of pressure.

Patch Electrodes

The electrode patches of the defibrillator (**FIGURE 21-131**) should be placed so that the heart (mainly the ventricles)

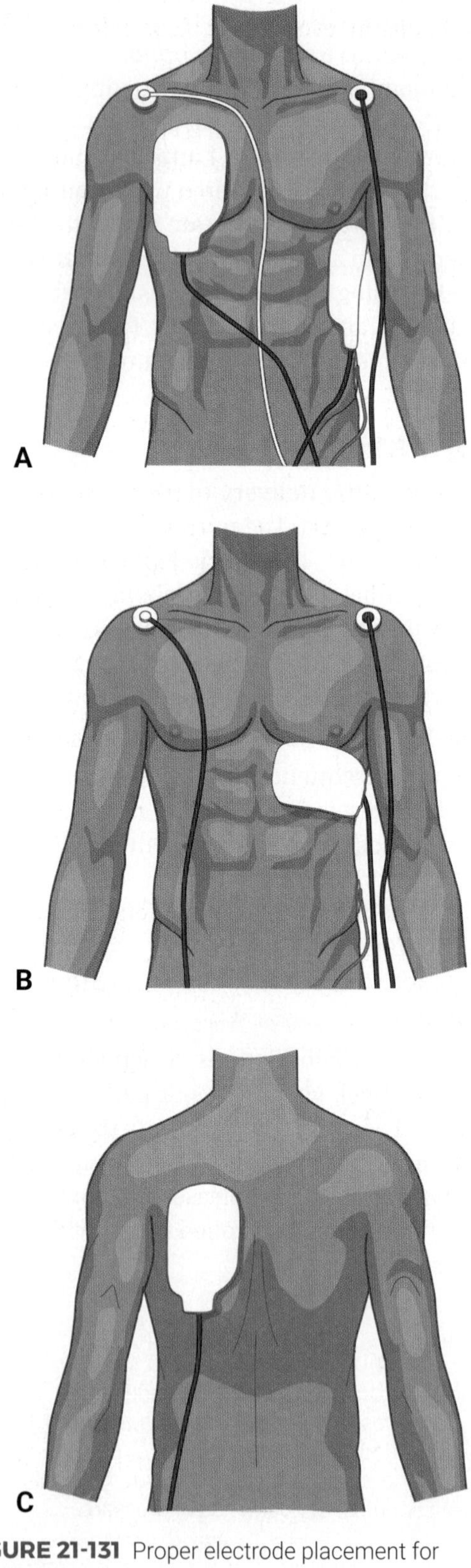

FIGURE 21-131 Proper electrode placement for defibrillation. **A.** Demonstrates anterior-anterior placement. **B.** and **C.** Demonstrate anterior-posterior placement.

is in the path of the current and the distance between the electrodes and the heart is minimized. This placement helps ensure adequate delivery of current through the heart. Bone is not a good conductor. For that reason, the patches should not be placed over the sternum. As recommended by the AHA, one patch should be placed to the right of the upper sternum below the right clavicle and the other patch should be placed to the left of the nipple in the midaxillary line.[9] (The anterior–posterior anterolateral, anterior–left infrascapular, and anterior–right infrascapular positions also are acceptable.) Most manufacturers have adult and pediatric patches available. Adult patches usually are 8 to 12 cm in diameter. Pediatric patches are 4.5 cm in diameter. They are used for children younger than 1 year.

The resistance to current by the chest wall is called impedance. Impedance is determined by body size, bone structure, skin properties, underlying health conditions, and other variables. The greater the resistance, the less current delivered. Dry, unprepared skin has high impedance. To reduce resistance, the electrode patches are gelled. Care must be taken to prevent contact (bridging) between the two conductive areas on the chest wall. If contact between the two areas is made, superficial burns of the skin may result. The effective current also may bypass the heart. Even with proper technique and equipment, minor skin damage may still occur.

Stored and Delivered Energy

The unit commonly used to measure electrical energy is the **joule** (watt second). One joule of electrical energy is the product of 1 volt (potential) multiplied by 1 ampere (current) multiplied by 1 second. Delivered energy is about 80% of stored energy because of losses within the circuitry of the defibrillator and resistance to the flow of current across the chest wall. As a rule, 80% of stored energy approximates the number of joules delivered to the patient. The AHA currently recommends that one initial defibrillation be attempted at 120 to 200 J biphasic (follow manufacturer's instructions) or 360 J monophasic (BOX 21-22).[9] Second and subsequent shocks may be the same or higher. Initial defibrillation in pediatric patients generally is 2 J/kg (acceptable range 2 to 4 J/kg). Subsequent doses of 4 J/kg or higher, to a maximum of 10 J/kg, not exceeding the adult dose, can be delivered if needed.[64]

BOX 21-22 Double Sequential Defibrillation

Double sequential defibrillation has been studied as a novel alternative to traditional defibrillation in cases of refractory VF. With this intervention, the defibrillator operator attaches a second set of pads to the patient, leaving the first set of pads in place, and delivers a shock in a different vector. If that shock does not convert the patient out of VF, then a second monitor/defibrillator is attached to that first set of pads and the patient is defibrillated at maximum joules simultaneously using both machines. Although the technique shows promise, it is not without controversy. Local protocols should be followed. Note: To prevent possible damage to the defibrillator from simultaneous shocks, some EMS programs recommend a one-second pause between shocks delivered by the first and second defibrillators.

Modified from: Cortez E, Krebs W, Davis J, Keseq DP, Panchal AR. Use of double sequential external defibrillation for refractory ventricular fibrillation during out-of-hospital cardiac arrest. *Resuscitation*. 2016;108:82-86.

Procedure for Defibrillation

The steps for defibrillation vary based on the number of rescuers present and whether the patient was being monitored prior to arrest. Chest compressions should be performed until the shock is delivered and should resume immediately after defibrillation.

1. Detect a shockable rhythm.
2. Turn on the defibrillator.
3. Ensure the environment does not pose a risk of sparks, does not contain combustible materials, and is not oxygen enriched.
4. Apply the defibrillation pads to the patient's chest and select pads if limb leads are not yet attached.
5. Select the energy level at 120 to 200 J biphasic (based on manufacturer's recommendation) or 360 J for monophasic defibrillators.
6. Press the "charge" button on the defibrillator controls.
7. Continue CPR while the defibrillator is charging.
8. When the defibrillator is fully charged, state the following (or some suitable equivalent) firmly and quickly before each shock:
   - "I am going to shock on three."
   - "One, two, three, all clear." (Visually check to ensure everyone is clear before pressing the "shock" button.)
9. Press the "shock" button.
10. Resume CPR beginning with chest compressions.
11. Perform five cycles (2 minutes) of CPR.
12. Check the rhythm. If VF/VT remains, recharge the defibrillator at once.
13. Shock at the same or higher biphasic energy (per manufacturer) or 360 J for monophasic defibrillators, repeating the verbal statements in step 8.

Operator and Personnel Safety

The following guidelines will help to ensure safe use of a defibrillator.

1. Make sure all personnel are clear of the patient, the bed, and the defibrillator before defibrillation.
2. Do not touch the patient during discharge.
3. Do not discharge current over a pacemaker or ICD generator or nitroglycerin paste. Remove nitroglycerin patches before defibrillation.

NOTE

Chest compressions and defibrillation are the only therapies proven to increase survival in cardiac arrest. The "hands-off" pauses during defibrillation result in a zero blood flow state that is associated with poorer neurologic recovery. Hands-on defibrillation (HOD) allows for uninterrupted chest compression during defibrillation and may improve resuscitation success. Recent studies have shown that the leakage of current during defibrillation to medical personnel wearing electrical-insulating gloves is low and below several recommended safety standards. Although current guidelines still recommend withholding chest compression during defibrillation as a safety measure, HOD may have future application in cardiac resuscitation.

Modified from: Wampler D, Kharod C, Bolleter S, Burkett A, Gabehart C, Manifold C. A randomized control hands-on defibrillation study—barrier use evaluation. *Resuscitation*. 2016;103:37-40; Deakin CD, Thomsen JE, Lofgren B, Petley GW. Achieving safe hands-on defibrillation using electrical safety gloves—a clinical evaluation. *Resuscitation*. 2015;90:163-167; and Lloyd MS, Heeke B, Walter PF, Langberg JJ. Hands-on defibrillation: an analysis of electrical current flow through rescuers in direct contact with patients during biphasic external defibrillation. *Circulation*. 2008;117(19):2510-2514.

4. Routinely check the defibrillator (including the batteries) to make sure the equipment is functioning properly. Follow the manufacturer's recommendations.

Defibrillator Use in Special Environments

Occasionally, a patient requires defibrillation in a special environment (eg, inclement weather). The guidelines in operator and personnel safety always apply. However, additional precautions are taken in special situations.

A patient can be defibrillated in wet conditions, such as near water, in rain, or in snowy weather. The patient's chest should be kept dry between the defibrillator electrode sites. The operator's hands should be kept as dry as possible. In a rainstorm, the safest course is to find shelter.

Depending on the defibrillator and its equipment specifications, the device may not be guaranteed to work properly in nonpressurized aircraft. In addition, some electrical interference may occur between the radio equipment in the aircraft and the monitor-defibrillator, or vice versa. This interference is affected by the distance and angle between the defibrillator and the radio equipment. Studies have demonstrated that defibrillation with current equipment would be expected to be safe in all types of rotary aircraft used for emergency medical transport.[65] Nonetheless, the medical crew should always inform the pilot when electrical therapy is being used. In addition, the paramedic should consult with the pilot to make sure the flight instruments are well shielded from electromagnetic interference.

Implantable Cardioverter-Defibrillators

ICDs commonly are used in patients at risk for recurrent, sustained VT or VF (**FIGURE 21-132**). During implantation, the various leads of the ICD are fed through a vessel (usually the subclavian vein) into the right ventricle or placed on the epicardium. The leads are tunneled to a pulse generator in the biphasic defibrillator device. The device is placed surgically in the left upper quadrant of the abdomen. (An outline of the generator usually can be felt or seen under the patient's skin.) The leads are used to deliver shocks, monitor cardiac rhythm, and sometimes pace the heart as needed if bradycardia occurs.

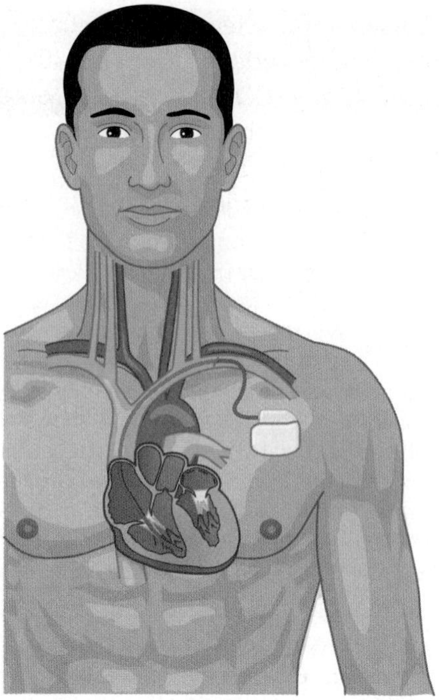

FIGURE 21-132 Implantable cardioverter-defibrillator.

The ICD is a battery-powered device that monitors the patient's cardiac rhythm, rate, and QRS complex morphology. When a monitored ventricular rate exceeds the preprogrammed rate, the ICD delivers a shock of about 6 to 30 J through the patches to restore a normal sinus rhythm. The device requires 10 to 30 seconds to sense VT or VF and to charge the capacitor before delivering the shock. If defibrillation does not restore a normal sinus rhythm, the ICD charges again. It then delivers up to four shocks. A complete sequence of five shocks, if required, may take up to 2 minutes. If the VT or VF persists after five shocks, no further shocks are delivered. Once a slower rhythm (ie, sinus or idioventricular rhythm)

CRITICAL THINKING

These devices are used by what type of patients?

CRITICAL THINKING

A conscious patient has a device that is firing repeatedly in response to the presence of a ventricular rhythm. How can you lessen the patient's discomfort and anxiety?

has been restored for at least 35 seconds, the device can deliver another series of up to five shocks if VT or VF recurs. Many ICDs also provide emergency pacing if bradycardic rhythms occur. A newer type of ICD has multiple pacing leads that help synchronize ventricular contraction in patients with severe heart failure.[66]

The paramedic must manage patients with ICDs as if they did not have a device. The paramedic should follow standard ACLS protocols if the patient is in cardiac arrest or in any other way medically unstable. The AHA recommends the following four guidelines for caring for a patient with an ICD:[9]

1. If the ICD discharges while the rescuer is touching the victim, the rescuer may feel the shock. However, the shock will not be dangerous. Personnel shocked by ICDs report sensations similar to contact with an electrical current.
2. ICDs are protected against damage from traditional transchest defibrillation shocks. However, they require an ICD readiness check after external defibrillation.
3. If VF or VT is present despite an ICD, an external shock should be given immediately because the ICD likely has failed to defibrillate the heart. After an initial series of shocks, the ICD becomes operative again only if a period of nonfibrillatory rhythm occurs to reset the unit.
4. Older ICD units use patch electrodes instead of leads. These electrodes cover a portion of the epicardial surface. They may reduce the amount of current delivered to the heart from transthoracic shocks. Therefore, if transthoracic shocks of up to 360 J fail to defibrillate a patient with an ICD, the chest electrode positions should be changed immediately (eg, anterior–apex to anteroposterior). The transthoracic shocks should be repeated. The different electrode positions could increase transthoracic current flow, thus possibly facilitating defibrillation.

Because the ICD can be deactivated and activated with a magnet, patients with ICDs should be kept away from strong magnets. This precaution prevents accidental deactivation or reactivation of the device. The ability to use a magnet to deactivate and reactivate many of these devices can be useful when the unit is not working properly. However, use of a handheld magnet to turn the unit off or back on should be considered only under the direction of a physician.

Wearable Cardioverter-Defibrillator

When the need for an ICD is not yet clear or contraindicated in a high-risk patient, a wearable external cardioverter-defibrillator (WCD) may be prescribed. The external defibrillator is worn next to the skin as a vest and is removed only to bathe. Electrodes in the vest continuously monitor the ECG. If a life-threatening rhythm is detected, audible, visual, and tactile signals alert the patient that a shock will be delivered. The conscious patient can press two buttons on the battery pack to delay the shock. If the patient is unconscious, or does not delay the shock, blue conductive gel is released over the posterior therapy electrodes and the patient is defibrillated with 75 to 150 J biphasic within 25 to 60 seconds. An audible command stating "do not touch the patient" indicates a defibrillation is imminent and the crew must stay clear to avoid being shocked by the device. The device can deliver up to five shocks. Defibrillation success is reported to be between 69% and 99%.[67] Unlike the ICD, the WCD neither detects nor treats bradycardias. It is approved for use in children as well as adults.

If an EMS crew arrives and the patient is conscious and has been shocked (there will be blue gel on the chest), leave the vest on if it does not interfere with care. If defibrillation with the EMS monitor is needed, pull the battery pack out of the monitoring pack before delivering the shock. The EMS crew should transport the device, battery, and charger to the hospital with the patient.

Mechanical Circulatory Support Devices

Mechanical circulatory support devices are now commonly used in the treatment of severe heart failure as bridges to cardiac transplantation ("bridge to transplant"), as destination therapy for patients who are not transplant candidates, and as bridges to recovery. These devices, which can be used to support the left or right ventricles, or both, restore circulation to the tissues, thereby improving organ function.[68] Two common devices are the left ventricular assist device and the total artificial heart.

Left Ventricular Assist Device

A **left ventricular assist device (LVAD)** is a battery-operated implantable pump that is increasingly being used as a destination therapy for patients not eligible for or awaiting transplant. The LVAD enhances, rather than replaces, the left ventricular contractility. The device is surgically placed. A tube in the pump pulls blood from the weakened left ventricle and then directs the blood into the aorta. A cable called the driveline is brought out of the abdominal wall to the outside of the body, where it can be attached to the pump's battery and control system (**FIGURE 21-133**).

Common complications are power disconnection and driveline failure. Both will stop the pump. For this reason, patients have backup controllers and batteries with them. Even when the pump stops, most patients have some residual cardiac output to sustain life until the problem is remedied. Other possible complications from the device include infection, internal bleeding, blood clots, tachyarrhythmias, stroke, and heart failure (see Chapter 51, *Acute Interventions for Home Care*).

Special Care Considerations

Because the LVAD assumes the pumping function of the left ventricle but provides flow in a continuous manner, patients who have newer devices have no palpable pulse or measurable blood pressure. (This depends on the pulsatility of the specific device and on the patient's own left ventricular function. A Doppler probe may be required for blood pressure readings.) Noninvasive blood pressure readings can be obtained in only about 50% of patients because of decreased pulse pressure in continuous-flow LVADs.[69] Skin color, end-tidal capnography, temperature, and capillary refill may also be used to assess tissue perfusion. Abnormal or undetectable pulse oximetry readings are unreliable in these patients. However, if an Spo_2 level within normal limits is measured, it should be considered reliable.[69]

Some patients with an LVAD do not lose consciousness if VF or VT develops because their pump maintains enough flow to perfuse the brain. The decision to cardiovert or defibrillate is based on whether the patient's perfusion can maintain consciousness and perfusion to other tissues. Some patients who have an LVAD also have an ICD implanted that will defibrillate in the event of VF or VT. $ETCO_2$ should be used to assess perfusion. Chest compressions should be started on an unconscious patient with an LVAD, a mean arterial pressure (MAP) of less than 50 mm Hg, an $ETCO_2$ level of less than 20 mm Hg (in an intubated patient), and no palpable pulse. The AHA consensus recommendation states that "if an LVAD is definitely confirmed by a trained person and there are no signs of life, bystander CPR, including chest compressions should be performed."[69] If available, echocardiography can also be used to determine perfusion.

The patient and family usually are quite knowledgeable about the LVAD and often are a valuable resource. If you are called to care for a patient with an LVAD, proceed as follows:[70]

1. Check the power source. Then assess the level of consciousness, airway, and breathing.
2. Auscultate heart sounds. If it is a continuous-flow device, a whirring sound will be heard.
3. Monitor the ECG rhythm.
4. Assess the device for alarms.
5. The controller (usually around the patient's waist) will have a colored tag to indicate the type of device and a resource number to call in an emergency. Some agencies carry a color-coded resource guide to assist with troubleshooting.
6. Start a large-bore IV line.
7. Attempt to assess noninvasive MAP. A Doppler (if available) can also be used to measure MAP. The first sound heard by the Doppler when deflating the blood pressure cuff is the MAP. Use MAP to

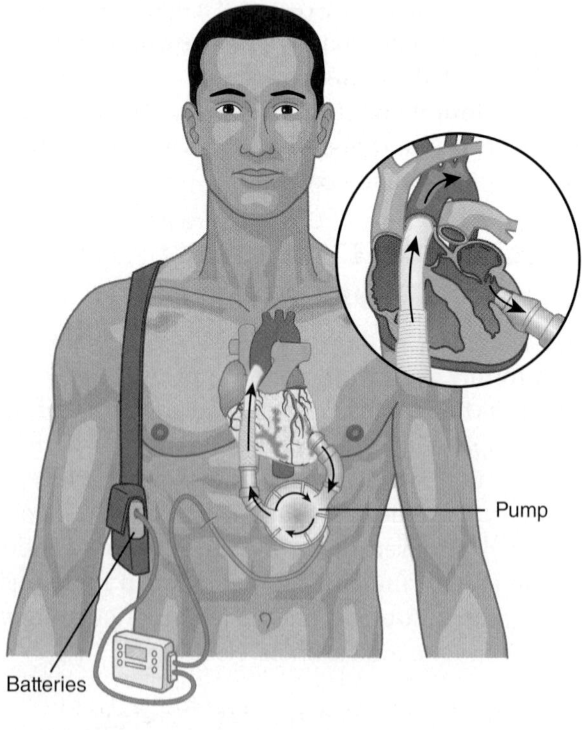

FIGURE 21-133 Left ventricular assist device.

assess adequacy of perfusion. Acceptable MAP varies by device and ranges from 65 to 85 mm Hg.
8. Transport to the closest LVAD center.
9. Bring any LVAD equipment with the patient to the hospital.
10. Transport the patient's significant other to help troubleshoot problems with the device en route.

Total Artificial Heart

A total artificial heart (TAH) replaces both ventricles. The ventricles are removed when the device is implanted. The right pump is joined to the right atrium and pulmonary artery, and the left pump is connected to the left atrium and aorta. An external pneumatic driver powers the pumps. At present, only one of the three approved devices is suitable for patient discharge to their home. The TAH is used in end-stage heart failure. If you are transporting a patient with this device, there are several differences from the LVAD. The patient's ECG tracing will be a flat line because there are no ventricles; however, there should be a palpable pulse. You should be able to auscultate a systolic and diastolic blood (drive) pressure. Two heart sounds will be heard and are often loud enough to be detected without a stethoscope. Because there is no ECG tracing, it is recommended that ECG monitoring not be applied on these patients to avoid misinterpretation of the rhythm for asystole. Suggested emergency care for these patients is seen in **FIGURE 21-134**.

Synchronized Cardioversion

Synchronized cardioversion (or countershock) is used to terminate dysrhythmias other than VF and pulseless VT. Defibrillation (**unsynchronized cardioversion**) delivers the shock on the operator's command and with no regard to where the shock occurs in the cardiac cycle. In contrast, synchronized cardioversion is designed to deliver the shock about 10 milliseconds after the peak of the R wave of the cardiac cycle. This timing avoids the vulnerable relative refractory period of the ventricles. Synchronization may reduce the energy required to end the dysrhythmia. It also may decrease the chance of causing VF.

When the defibrillator is placed in the synchronized mode, the ECG displayed on the oscilloscope shows a marker denoting where in the cardiac cycle the energy will be discharged. This marker should appear on the R wave; if it does not, the paramedic should select another lead. Adjustment of the ECG size may be needed if the marker does not appear. The procedure for synchronized cardioversion is as follows:

1. Consider sedation.
2. Turn on the defibrillator (monophasic or biphasic).
3. Attach monitor leads to the patient ("white to right, red to ribs, what's left over to the left shoulder"), and ensure proper display of the patient's rhythm.
4. Engage the synchronization mode by pressing the "sync" control button.
5. Look for markers on R waves indicating the sync mode.
6. If necessary, adjust the monitor gain until the sync markers occur with each R wave.
7. Select the appropriate energy level.
8. Position the electrode patches on the patient (sternum–apex).
9. Announce to the team members: "Charging defibrillator."
10. Press the "charge" button on defibrillator.
11. When the defibrillator is charged, firmly state the following:
    - "I am going to shock on three. One, I'm clear." (Check to make sure you are clear of contact with the patient, the stretcher, and the equipment.)
    - "Two, you're clear." (Make a visual check to ensure that no one continues to touch the patient or stretcher. In particular, do not forget about the person providing ventilations. That person's hands should not be touching the ventilatory adjuncts, including the tracheal tube. Turn off oxygen or direct the flow away from the patient's chest.)
    - "Three, everybody's clear." (Check yourself one more time before pressing the "shock" button.)
12. Press the "discharge" button.
13. Check the monitor. If tachycardia persists, increase the joules according to the electrical cardioversion algorithm.
14. Reset the sync mode after each synchronized cardioversion because most defibrillators default back to the unsynchronized mode. This default allows an immediate shock if the cardioversion produces VF.

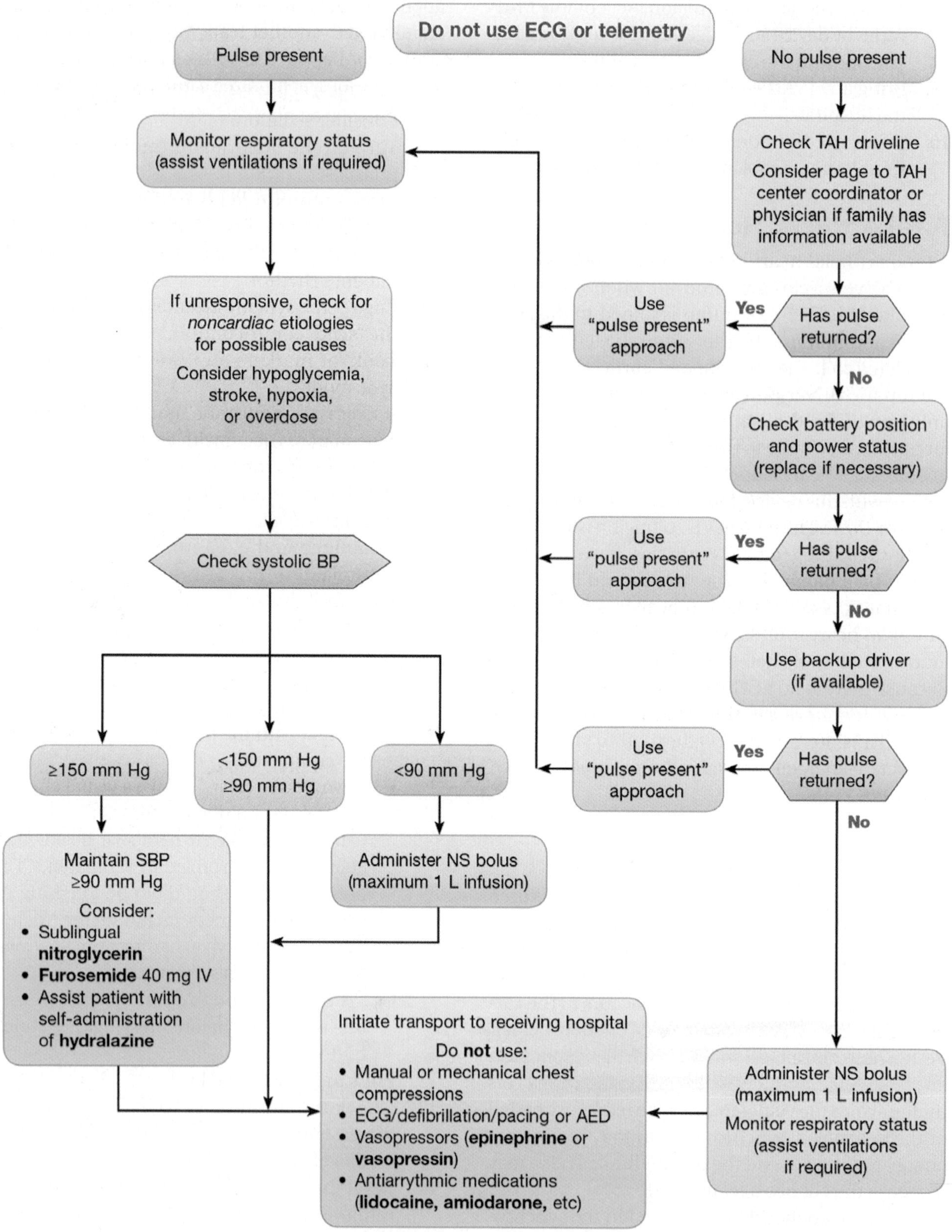

Abbreviations: AED, automated external defibrillator; BP, blood pressure; ECG, electrocardiogram; IV, intravenous; NS, normal saline; SBP, systolic blood pressure; TAH, total artificial heart

FIGURE 21-134 Algorithm showing response to a patient with a total artificial heart with altered mental status.

Transcutaneous Cardiac Pacing

Transcutaneous cardiac pacing (TCP), also known as external cardiac pacing, is an effective emergency therapy for bradycardia. TCP devices have been recognized by the AHA for emergency use until a transvenous pacemaker can be inserted.

Artificial Pacing

Artificial pacemakers deliver repetitive electrical currents to the heart (**FIGURE 21-135**). They can act as a substitute for a natural pacemaker. The natural pacemaker may have become blocked or dysfunctional. Transcutaneous pacing is indicated for patients with unstable bradycardia (<50 beats/min) who are unresponsive to drug therapy, such as atropine. It is contraindicated in hypothermia and not recommended to treat asystole.[7]

The two modes of TCP are nondemand (asynchronous) pacing and demand pacing. Most devices provide both modes. An asynchronous pacemaker delivers timed electrical stimuli at a selected rate. These stimuli occur regardless of the patient's own cardiac activity. These pacing devices are used less often than are demand pacers because they may discharge during the vulnerable period of the cardiac cycle (producing the R-on-T phenomenon). The asynchronous mode generally is used only as a last resort when artifact on the ECG interferes with the machine's ability to sense the patient's own heartbeat. Asynchronous pacing also can be used to override the high heart rates of tachydysrhythmias (eg, torsades de pointes). This intervention is typically done only in the electrophysiology lab of the hospital.

Demand pacing senses the patient's QRS complex. The pacemaker delivers electrical stimuli only when needed. Demand pacing is much safer to apply than is the nondemand mode. When the pacemaker senses an intrinsic beat, it is inhibited. If no beats are sensed, the pacemaker delivers pacing stimuli at a selected rate. The limb leads and defibrillation pads must be attached for pacing to work properly. The device initially is set to discharge at a rate of 60 to 70 mA and may be increased to 80 or 90 beats/min based on the patient's needs. The current is increased in increments, beginning at 0 mA of electricity, until electrical and mechanical capture is achieved, typically not before 50 mA. The current should be set at 2 mA above the value where consistent capture occurred.[9] Generally, the patient's clinical condition (blood pressure, level of consciousness, skin color, and temperature) improves at this point.

> NOTE
>
> **Electrical capture** means that every pacer stimulus is followed by a wide QRS complex, which indicates ventricular contraction. **Mechanical capture** occurs when an associated pulse is generated with the electrical capture.

When capture is achieved, each pacemaker spike on the oscilloscope is followed by a wide QRS complex and a broad T wave. If not, the current should be increased gradually until consistent capture is achieved. Unfortunately, motion artifact often makes ECG confirmation of electrical capture difficult. The only accurate method of monitoring mechanical function of the heart produced by the pacing device is the presence of a pulse with each QRS complex. Therefore, the paramedic must monitor the patient's pulse constantly. The paramedic should assess the patient's pulse rate and blood pressure on the patient's right side, avoiding the carotid pulse. This helps minimize interference from muscle artifact.

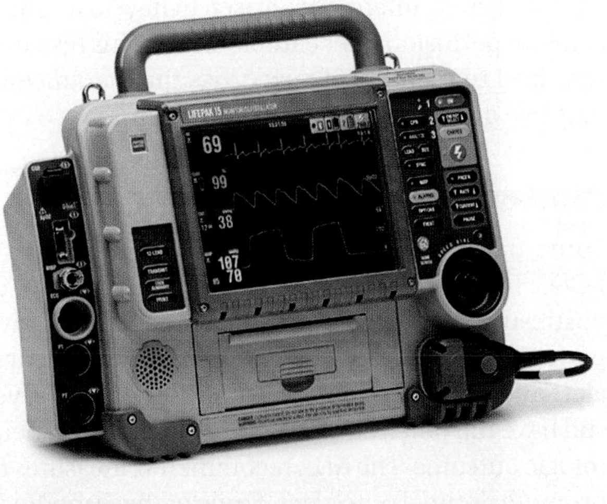

FIGURE 21-135 LifePak 15 defibrillator monitor pacer.

The LIFEPAK® 15 defibrillator monitor courtesy of Physio-Control. Used with permission of Physio-Control, Inc., and according to the Material Release Form provided by Physio-Control.

Procedure for Transcutaneous Pacing

The procedure for transcutaneous pacing is as follows:

1. Consider sedation.
2. Gather the required equipment.

3. Explain the procedure to the patient.
4. Connect the patient to a cardiac monitor and obtain a rhythm strip.
5. Obtain baseline vital signs.
6. Attach the limb leads and apply the pacing electrodes. Often the defibrillation position is used when the same pads can be used for defibrillation and pacing. The pads can also be placed in the anterior–posterior position (left of the lower sternum and just below the left scapula).
7. Select the pacing mode.
8. Select the pacing rate (usually 60 to 80 beats/min); set the current (begin with 0 mA and increase the current until ventricular capture is obtained).
9. Activate the pacemaker, observing the patient and the ECG.
10. Obtain rhythm strips as appropriate.
11. Continue monitoring the patient and anticipate further therapy.

NOTE

As with synchronized cardioversion, selecting the "pacing mode" should result in the appearance of light markers on intrinsic beats. Paramedics should make sure this happens so that they know the demand mode is activated and working properly.

Indications and Contraindications

The primary indications for TCP in the prehospital setting are unstable bradycardia that is unresponsive to atropine and pacemaker failure. As stated previously, cardiac pacing is not indicated in cardiac arrest. Cardiac pacing is not advised for patients with open wounds or burns on the chest or for patients in a wet environment.[7]

CRITICAL THINKING

Why should patient movement be minimized during TCP?

Electrode Placement

Proper placement of the electrodes is one of the keys to effective external pacing. As stated previously, the defibrillation position often is used when the same pads can be used for defibrillation and pacing. Alternatively, the paramedic can apply the negative (anterior) electrode to the left of the sternum. The electrode should be centered as close as possible to the point of maximum cardiac impulse. The positive (posterior) electrode is placed directly behind the anterior electrode, just below the left scapula. When posterior placement cannot be used, the positive electrode can be placed in line with the patient's left nipple at the midaxillary line. (Anterior–anterior placement may produce pronounced chest muscle twitching.) The electrodes should be applied to clean, dry skin free of localized trauma or infection.

A conscious patient most likely will experience some pain and discomfort during TCP. This is related directly to the intensity of muscle contractions and the amount of applied current. Ideally, analgesia or sedation of the patient should be provided.

Cardiac Arrest and Sudden Cardiac Death

It is becoming increasingly evident that patients who cannot be resuscitated in the prehospital setting rarely survive. This is the case even if the patient is resuscitated temporarily in the ED (BOX 21-23). The patient's best chance for survival is rapid recognition and appropriate treatment in the field. The priorities in cardiac arrest are effective CPR and rapid defibrillation (if indicated). Vascular access and advanced airway management are of secondary importance to the initial priorities and should never delay them.

Much research is underway in the area of emergency cardiac care. Some of the research investigates various drugs to improve cardiac and neurologic outcomes after resuscitation. Because a substantial number of patients regain cardiac function but never regain consciousness, interest has arisen in how to improve cerebral perfusion after cardiac arrest. This research may lead to a variety of new drugs that paramedics may use during resuscitation in the future.

Care of the Patient After ROSC

Some patients survive cardiac arrest and have a ROSC. In these situations, the principal objective of postresuscitation care is reestablishment of effective perfusion of organs and tissues. Ideally, the patient is alert and awake. Patients also may be comatose, yet still have full potential for recovery with a good neurologic outcome. The AHA recommends measures to promote optimal outcomes. Some of these methods include hemodynamic and ventilation optimization, immediate coronary reperfusion with PCI, and therapeutic hypothermia.[1]

BOX 21-23 The Utstein Style of Reporting

The Utstein Style is a set of guidelines for uniform reporting of data from out-of-hospital cardiac arrest. (The name derives from a 1990 conference of the European Society of Cardiology and related national societies, held at the Utstein Abbey in Norway.) The purpose of these guidelines (introduced to EMS in 1991) is to develop a uniform and worldwide nomenclature and language used in standard reports. Reporting definitions and templates were updated in 2004 to include dispatch/recognition, patient variables, process variables, and outcomes. Important resuscitation terminology defined in the Utstein guidelines includes the following:

- **Resuscitation.** The technique of providing efforts to return spontaneous pulse and breathing to a patient in full cardiac arrest.
- **Survival.** Resuscitation of a patient who survives to hospital discharge.
- **ROSC.** Restoration of spontaneous circulation that provides evidence of more than an occasional gasp, occasional fleeting palpable pulse, or arterial waveform; the patient may or may not survive.

Modified from: Cummins RO, Chamberlain DA, Abramson NS, et al. Recommended guidelines for uniform reporting of data from out-of-hospital cardiac arrest: the Utstein Style. A statement for health professionals from a task force of the American Heart Association, the European Resuscitation Council, the Heart and Stroke Foundation of Canada, and the Australian Resuscitation Council. *Circulation*. 1991;84:960-975; and Perkins GD, Jacobs IG, Nadkarni VM, et al. ILCOR consensus statement. Cardiac arrest and cardiopulmonary resuscitation outcome reports: Update of the Utstein resuscitation registry templates for out-of-hospital cardiac arrest. *Circulation*. 2014.

Hemodynamic and Ventilation Optimization

To avoid hypoxia in adults with ROSC after cardiac arrest, it is reasonable to use the highest available oxygen concentration until the arterial oxyhemoglobin saturation or the partial pressure of arterial oxygen can be measured. The AHA recommends that ventilations begin at 10 to 12 breaths/min, titrated to achieve an $ETCO_2$ level of 30 to 40 mm Hg or a partial pressure of carbon dioxide ($PacO_2$) level of 35 to 45 mm Hg.[9]

IV fluids and vasoactive and inotropic drugs should be titrated to optimize blood pressure, cardiac output, and systemic perfusion. If post–cardiac arrest systolic blood pressure is less than 90 mm Hg in the context of evidence of inadequate end-organ perfusion such as a decreased level of consciousness, an IV fluid bolus of 1 to 2 L normal saline should be

NOTE

When resources are available to titrate the fraction of inspired oxygen (FIO_2) and to monitor oxyhemoglobin saturation, it is reasonable to decrease the FIO_2 when oxyhemoglobin saturation is 100%, provided the oxyhemoglobin saturation can be maintained at 94% or greater. Shortly after ROSC, patients may have peripheral vasoconstriction that makes measurement of oxyhemoglobin saturation by pulse oximetry difficult or unreliable. In those situations, in-hospital arterial blood sampling may be required before titration of FIO_2.

Modified from: 2015 American Heart Association Guidelines for Cardiopulmonary Resuscitation and Emergency Cardiovascular Care. *Circulation*. 2015;132:S313-S314.

considered. If the patient is not responding to fluid infusion, medications such as norepinephrine, epinephrine, or dopamine should be administered.[10]

Immediate Coronary Reperfusion With PCI

As described earlier, all patients with ROSC should be transported to an appropriate facility that can provide effective postresuscitation care. A 12-lead ECG should be acquired as soon as possible. These therapies include immediate coronary reperfusion (eg, PCI), therapeutic hypothermia, and other treatment modalities to improve post-cardiac arrest survival.

Therapeutic Hypothermia

The 2015 AHA guidelines recommend inducing targeted temperature management in survivors of cardiac arrest who are unable to follow commands. When a patient is resuscitated, reperfusion sets off a series of chemical reactions that can continue for up to 24 hours, possibly causing significant inflammation in the brain. Maintaining the body temperature between 32°C (89.6°F) and 36°C (96.8°F) reduces the intracranial pressure, the cerebral metabolic rate, and the brain's demand for oxygen consumption. In addition, it is thought to suppress many of the chemical reactions associated with reperfusion injury, including free radical production, excitatory amino acid release, and calcium shifts.[71] The AHA specifically recommends *against* routine cooling of prehospital patients after ROSC with rapid infusion of cold IV fluids. In this setting, pulmonary edema and rearrest may occur. It is unknown if other measures to cool patients prehospital are safe.[10]

Termination of Resuscitation

Health care professionals are expected to provide BLS and ACLS as part of their professional duty to respond, with the following exceptions:

- When a person lies dead and has obvious clinical signs of irreversible death
- When attempts to perform CPR would place the rescuer at risk of physical injury
- When the patient or surrogate has indicated that resuscitation is not desired

The termination of resuscitative efforts in the prehospital setting should follow rules established by the local EMS system and medical direction. The rules should include consideration for advance directives and orders specifying no CPR. If at any time paramedics are presented with an advance directive (eg, a written directive, living will, durable power of attorney, or POLST form) that indicates a patient should not be resuscitated, they should follow established protocol or immediately consult with medical direction (see Chapter 6, *Medical and Legal Issues*).

In some cases involving adult patients, resuscitation can be appropriately terminated in the prehospital setting. The National Association of EMS Physicians supports this practice and has published an official position statement outlining criteria and rationale for field termination of resuscitation.[72]

The AHA recommends considering terminating resuscitation when *all* of the following criteria apply:[9]

1. Arrest was not witnessed by EMS personnel.
2. No shocks have been delivered.
3. There has been no ROSC prior to transport.

Finally, unusual clinical features (eg, drowning, profound hypothermia, young age, toxins, electrolyte abnormalities, drug overdose) may be indicators that continued resuscitation is appropriate. Termination of resuscitation in the prehospital setting should be guided by medical direction.

Procedure for Termination of Resuscitation

The process for terminating resuscitation in the field varies by protocol. The paramedic must follow the guidelines set by medical direction. When termination is considered appropriate, the paramedic should contact medical direction to convey the following information:

- Patient's medical condition
- Time from collapse to CPR
- Time from collapse to first defibrillation attempt
- Initial arrest rhythm
- Known causes of the arrest
- Response to resuscitation
- $ETCO_2$ level less than 10 mm Hg after 20 minutes of CPR
- Family's appraisal of the situation and any resistance or uncertainty

While gathering and giving this information to medical direction, the paramedic should maintain ongoing documentation of the event. This documentation should include continuous ECG monitoring. Documentation aids the review of the call. The review usually is performed for quality assurance in most EMS systems. Throughout this process, one rescuer should provide frank, caring updates to the family or significant others informing them of the patient's condition.

SHOW ME THE EVIDENCE

Japanese researchers examined over 250,000 cases of bystander-witnessed cardiac arrest between 2005 and 2012 to determine resuscitation duration. They calculated the minimum prehospital duration to achieve neurologically intact resuscitation in four groups (shockable versus nonshockable rhythm and presence or absence of bystander CPR). They found small statistically significant differences in the groups. Their primary finding, however, was that in the shockable arrest groups, resuscitation should continue for 40 minutes in witnessed out-of-hospital cardiac arrest.

Modified from: Nagao K, Nonogi H, Yonemoto N, et al. Duration of prehospital resuscitation efforts after out-of-hospital cardiac arrest. *Circulation*. 2016;133(14):1386-1396.

CRITICAL THINKING

You have just terminated resuscitation in the home. What resources can you contact to help the family?

Special Considerations

In addition to attending to the needs of the patient, paramedics must consider grief support for the family.

Support services vary by agency. When possible, a paramedic (or other EMS personnel) is assigned to stay with the family for a time. At times a community agency referral is arranged.

Law enforcement officers may have additional duties at the scene as part of their professional role. These duties may include an on-scene determination that the patient be assigned to a medical examiner. This determination may occur when the death or event is suspicious or when a patient's private physician refuses or hesitates to sign the death certificate. The paramedic must be familiar with local and state laws regarding reporting an out-of-hospital death and the disposition of the patient's remains under such circumstances.

DID YOU KNOW?

Helping a Grieving Person

Conveying the news of a death to family members, friends, and loved ones at the scene is difficult. In addition to ensuring the family's privacy, the following guidelines may be helpful in this situation.

What to Say

- Acknowledge the situation (eg, "I'm sorry to say that [patient's name] has died").
- Express your concern (eg, "I'm sorry this has happened to you").
- Offer your support (eg, "Tell me what I can do to help you").

What Not to Say

- "I know how you feel."
- "Look at what you have to be thankful for."
- "It's part of God's plan."
- "He's in a better place now."
- "It's over, and it's all behind you now."

Listen With Compassion

- Accept and acknowledge the feelings of the bereaved.
- Be willing to sit in silence.
- Let the bereaved talk about how their loved one died.
- Offer comfort without minimizing the loss.

Offer Practical Assistance

- Contact a neighbor or other family member.
- Make sure the bereaved has a means of transportation if needed.

Modified from: Segal J, Smith M. Coping with grief and loss: understanding the grieving process. Helpguide.org website. https://www.helpguide.org/. Accessed April 5, 2018.

Summary

- People at high risk for cardiovascular disease include males, older adults, and those with diabetes mellitus, hypertension, a family history of premature cardiovascular disease, and prior myocardial infarction (MI). Prevention strategies include community educational programs in nutrition, cessation of smoking (smoking prevention for children), and screening for hypertension and high cholesterol.
- The left coronary artery carries about 85% of the blood supply to the myocardium. The right coronary artery carries the rest. The pumping action of the heart is a product of rhythmic, alternate contraction and relaxation of the atria and ventricles. The stroke volume is the amount of blood ejected from each ventricle with one contraction. The stroke volume depends on the preload, afterload, and myocardial contractility. Cardiac output is the amount of blood pumped by each ventricle per minute.
- In addition to the intrinsic control of the body in regulating the heart, extrinsic control by the parasympathetic and sympathetic nerves of the autonomic nervous system is a major factor influencing the heart rate, conductivity, and contractility. Sympathetic impulses cause the adrenal medulla to secrete epinephrine and norepinephrine into the blood.
- The major electrolytes that influence cardiac function are calcium, potassium, sodium, and magnesium. The electrical charge (potential difference) between the inside and the outside of cells is expressed in millivolts. When the cell is in a resting state, the electrical charge difference is referred to as a resting membrane potential. The specialized sodium–potassium exchange pump actively pumps sodium ions out of the cell. It also pumps potassium ions into the cell. The cell membrane appears to have individual

protein-lined channels. These channels allow for passage of a specific ion or group of ions.

- Nerve and muscle cells are capable of producing action potentials. This property is known as excitability. An action potential at any point on the cell membrane stimulates an excitation process. This process is spread down the length of the cell and is conducted across synapses from cell to cell.
- The contraction of cardiac and skeletal muscle is believed to be activated by calcium ions. This process results in binding between myosin and actin myofilaments.
- The conduction system of the heart is composed of two nodes and a conducting bundle. One of the nodes is the sinoatrial (SA) node. The other is the atrioventricular (AV) node.
- Parasympathetic stimulation by the vagus nerve affects primarily the SA node and the AV node, causing the heart to slow. Sympathetic stimulation increases the heart rate and contractility.
- The electrocardiogram (ECG) represents the electrical activity of the heart. It is generated by depolarization and repolarization of the atria and ventricles.
- Routine monitoring of cardiac rhythm in the prehospital setting usually is obtained in lead II or V_1. These are the best leads to monitor for dysrhythmias because they allow visualization of P waves. The paper used to record ECGs is standardized, which allows comparative analysis of an ECG wave.
- A normal ECG consists of a P wave, QRS complex, and T wave. The P wave is the first positive deflection on the ECG. The P wave represents atrial depolarization. The PR interval is the time required for an electrical impulse to be conducted through the atria and the AV node up to the instant of ventricular depolarization. The QRS complex represents ventricular depolarization. The ST segment represents the early part of repolarization of the right and left ventricles. The T wave represents repolarization of the ventricular myocardial cells. Repolarization occurs during the last part of ventricular systole. The QT interval is the period from the beginning of ventricular depolarization (onset of the QRS complex) until the end of ventricular repolarization or the end of the T wave.
- The steps in ECG analysis include analyzing the QRS complex, P waves, rate, rhythm, and PR interval.
- Dysrhythmias originating in the SA node include sinus bradycardia, sinus tachycardia, sinus dysrhythmia, and sinus arrest. Most sinus dysrhythmias are the result of increases or decreases in vagal tone.
- Dysrhythmias originating in the atria include wandering pacemaker, premature atrial complexes, paroxysmal supraventricular tachycardia (SVT), atrial flutter, and AF. Common causes of atrial dysrhythmias are ischemia, hypoxia, and atrial dilation caused by heart failure or mitral valve abnormalities.
- When the SA node and the atria cannot generate the electrical impulses needed to begin depolarization because of factors such as hypoxia, ischemia, MI, and drug toxicity, the AV node or the area surrounding it may assume the role of the secondary pacemaker. Dysrhythmias originating in the AV junction include premature junctional complexes, junctional escape complexes or rhythms, and accelerated junctional rhythm.
- Ventricular dysrhythmias pose a threat to life. Ventricular rhythm disturbances generally result from failure of the atria, AV junction, or both to initiate an electrical impulse. They also may result from enhanced automaticity or reentry phenomena in the ventricles. Dysrhythmias originating in the ventricles include ventricular escape complexes or rhythms, premature ventricular complexes, ventricular tachycardia (VT), ventricular fibrillation (VF), asystole, and artificial pacemaker rhythm.
- A 12-lead ECG can be used to help identify changes relative to myocardial ischemia, injury, and infarction; distinguish VT from SVT; determine the electrical axis and the presence of fascicular blocks; and determine the presence of bundle branch blocks.
- Partial delays or full interruptions in cardiac electrical conduction are called heart blocks. Causes of heart blocks include AV junctional ischemia, AV junctional necrosis, degenerative disease of the conduction system, and drug toxicity. Disorders of conduction are first-degree AV block, second-degree AV block type I (Wenckebach), second-degree AV block type II, third-degree AV block, disturbances of ventricular conduction, pulseless electrical activity, and preexcitation (Wolff-Parkinson-White syndrome).
- Common chief complaints of the patient with cardiovascular disease include chest pain or discomfort, including shoulder, arm, neck, or jaw pain or discomfort; dyspnea; syncope; and abnormal heartbeat or palpitations. Paramedics should ask patients suspected of having a cardiovascular disorder whether they take prescription medications, especially cardiac drugs. Paramedics also should ask whether patients are being treated for any serious illness. They should ask whether patients have a history of MI, angina, heart failure, hypertension, diabetes mellitus, or chronic lung disease. In addition, paramedics should ask whether patients have any allergies or other risk factors for heart disease.
- After performing the initial assessment of the patient with cardiovascular disease, the paramedic should look for skin color, jugular venous distention, and the presence of edema or other signs of heart disease. The paramedic should listen for lung sounds, heart sounds, and carotid artery bruit. The paramedic should feel for edema, pulses, skin temperature, and moisture.
- Atherosclerosis is a disease process characterized by progressive narrowing of the lumen of medium and large arteries. It has two major effects on blood vessels. First, it disrupts the intimal surface. This causes a loss of vessel elasticity and an increase in thrombogenesis. Second, the atheroma reduces the diameter of the vessel lumen. This reduces the blood supply to tissues.
- Angina pectoris is a symptom of myocardial ischemia. Angina is caused by an imbalance between myocardial

oxygen supply and demand. Prehospital management includes placing the patient at rest, administering oxygen if the arterial oxygen saturation (Sao_2) level is less than 94%, initiating intravenous (IV) therapy, administering nitroglycerin and possibly morphine, monitoring the patient for dysrhythmias, and transporting the patient for evaluation by a physician.

- Acute MI (AMI) occurs when a coronary artery is blocked and blood does not reach an area of heart muscle. This condition results in ischemia, injury, and necrosis to the area of myocardium supplied by the affected artery. Death caused by MI usually results from lethal dysrhythmias (VT, VF, and cardiac standstill), pump failure (cardiogenic shock and heart failure), or myocardial tissue rupture (rupture of the ventricle, septum, or papillary muscle). Some patients with AMI, particularly those in the older age groups, have only symptoms of dyspnea, syncope, or confusion. However, substernal chest pain is usually present in patients with AMI (70% to 90% of patients). ST-segment elevation greater than or equal to 1 mV in at least two side-by-side ECG leads indicates an AMI. However, some patients experience an infarct without ST-segment elevation. Other conditions also can produce ST-segment elevation. Prehospital management of the patient with a suspected MI should include placing the patient at rest; administering oxygen if the Sao_2 level is less than 94%; frequently assessing vital signs and breath sounds; initiating an IV line with normal saline or lactated Ringer solution to keep the vein open; monitoring for dysrhythmias; administering medications such as nitroglycerin, morphine, and aspirin; screening for risk factors for fibrinolytic therapy; and providing transport to an appropriate hospital.
- Left ventricular failure occurs when the left ventricle fails to function as an effective forward pump. This causes a back pressure of blood into the pulmonary circulation, which in turn may lead to pulmonary edema. Emergency management is directed at reducing the venous return to the heart, improving myocardial contractility, decreasing myocardial oxygen demand, improving ventilation and oxygenation, and rapidly transporting the patient to a medical facility. Systolic and diastolic heart failure may present differently.
- Right ventricular failure occurs when the right ventricle fails as a pump. This causes back pressure of blood into the systemic venous circulation. Right ventricular failure is not usually a medical emergency in itself unless it is associated with pulmonary edema or hypotension.
- Cardiogenic shock is the most extreme form of pump failure. It usually is caused by extensive MI. Even with aggressive therapy, cardiogenic shock has a mortality rate of 70% or higher. Patients in cardiogenic shock require rapid transport to a medical facility.
- Cardiac tamponade is defined as impaired filling of the heart caused by increased pressure in the pericardial sac.
- Abdominal aortic aneurysms usually are asymptomatic. However, signs and symptoms signal impending or active rupture. If the vessel tears, bleeding initially may be stopped by the retroperitoneal tissues. The patient may be normotensive on the arrival of EMS. If the rupture opens into the peritoneal cavity, however, massive fatal hemorrhage may follow.
- Acute dissection is the most common aortic catastrophe. Any area of the aorta may be involved. However, in 60% to 70% of cases, the site of a dissecting aneurysm is in the ascending aorta, just beyond the takeoff of the left subclavian artery. The signs and symptoms depend on the site of the intimal tear. They also depend on the extent of dissection. The goals of managing suspected aortic dissection in the prehospital setting are relief of pain and immediate transport to a medical facility.
- Acute arterial occlusion is a sudden blockage of arterial flow. Occlusion most commonly is caused by trauma, an embolus, or thrombosis. The most common sites of embolic occlusion are the abdominal aorta, common femoral artery, popliteal artery, carotid artery, brachial artery, and mesenteric artery. The location of ischemic pain is related to the site of occlusion.
- Noncritical peripheral vascular conditions include varicose veins, superficial thrombophlebitis, and acute deep vein thrombosis (DVT). Of these conditions, DVT is the only one that can cause the life-threatening problem of a pulmonary embolism.
- Hypertension often is defined by a resting blood pressure that is consistently greater than 130/80 mm Hg. Chronic hypertension has an adverse effect on the heart and blood vessels. It requires the heart to perform more work than normal. This leads to hypertrophy of the cardiac muscle and left ventricular failure. Conditions associated with chronic, uncontrolled hypertension are cerebral hemorrhage and stroke, MI, and renal failure.
- Hypertensive emergencies are conditions in which a blood pressure increase leads to significant, irreversible end-organ damage within hours if not treated. The organs most likely to be at risk are the brain, heart, and kidneys. As a rule, the diagnosis is based on altered end-organ function and the rate of the rise in blood pressure, not the blood pressure level itself.
- Valvular heart disease may occur as a result of infection, or it may be related to heart disease. When one or more of these valves become narrowed, hardened, or thickened (stenotic), the valves do not open or close completely. As a result, blood does not flow with proper force or direction.
- Infectious heart disease includes endocarditis, pericarditis, and myocarditis. Complications can be severe and may include heart failure.
- Cardiomyopathy is an alteration in or weakness of the heart muscle. It can cause heart failure or sudden death. Basic cardiac life support (BCLS) helps maintain the circulation and respiration of a victim of cardiac arrest. BCLS is continued until advanced cardiac life support is available. Two mechanisms are thought to be responsible for blood flow during cardiopulmonary resuscitation. One is direct compression of the heart between the sternum and the spine.

This increases pressure within the ventricles to provide a small but critical amount of blood flow to the lungs and body organs. The second mechanism is increased intrathoracic pressure transmitted to all intrathoracic vascular structures. This creates an intrathoracic-to-extrathoracic pressure gradient. This gradient causes blood to flow out of the thorax. A number of mechanical devices provide external chest compression. Others provide chest compression with ventilation in a cardiac arrest patient.

- Cardiac monitor-defibrillators are classified as manual defibrillators or automated external defibrillators. Defibrillation is the delivery of electrical current through the chest wall. Its purpose is to terminate VF and certain other nonperfusing rhythms.
- Implantable cardioverter-defibrillators (ICDs) monitor the patient's cardiac rhythm. When a monitored ventricular rate exceeds the preprogrammed rate, the ICD delivers a shock of about 6 to 30 J through patches. This shock is an attempt to restore a normal sinus rhythm.
- Synchronized cardioversion is designed to deliver a shock about 10 milliseconds after the peak of the R wave of the cardiac cycle. (Therefore, the device avoids the relative refractory period.) Synchronization may reduce the amount of energy needed to end the dysrhythmia. It also may decrease the chances of causing another dysrhythmia.
- Transcutaneous cardiac pacing is an effective emergency therapy for bradycardia, complete heart block, and suppression of some malignant ventricular dysrhythmias. Proper electrode placement is important for effective external pacing.
- It is becoming increasingly evident that patients who cannot be resuscitated in the prehospital setting rarely survive. This is the case even if they are resuscitated temporarily in the emergency department. Cessation of resuscitative efforts in the prehospital setting should follow system-specific criteria established by medical direction.

References

1. National Center for Chronic Disease Prevention and Health Promotion, Division for Heart Disease and Stroke Prevention. Heart disease facts. Centers for Disease Control and Prevention website. https://www.cdc.gov/heartdisease/facts.htm. Updated November 28, 2017. Accessed April 5, 2018.
2. Kleinman ME, Brennan EE, Goldberger ZD, et al. Part 5: Adult basic life support and cardiopulmonary resuscitation quality: 2015 American Heart Association Guidelines Update for Cardiopulmonary Resuscitation and Emergency Cardiovascular Care. *Circulation.* 2015;132(18)(suppl 2):S414-S435.
3. Dalen JE, Alpert JS, Goldberg RJ, Weinstein RS. The epidemic of the 20th century: coronary heart disease. *Am J Med.* 2014;127:807-812.
4. CARES survival report: all agencies/national data. myCARES website. https://mycares.net/sitepages/uploads/2017/2013-2016%20Non-Traumatic%20National%20Survival%20Report.pdf. Published April 18, 2017. Accessed April 5, 2018.
5. Zive D, Koprowicz K, Schmidt T, et al. Variation in out-of-hospital cardiac arrest resuscitation and transport practices in the Resuscitation Outcomes Consortium: ROC Epistry–Cardiac Arrest. *Resuscitation.* 2011;82(3):277-284.
6. Understand your risks to prevent a heart attack. American Heart Association website. http://www.heart.org/HEARTORG/Conditions/HeartAttack/UnderstandYourRiskstoPreventaHeartAttack/Understand-Your-Risks-to-Prevent-a-Heart-Attack_UCM_002040_Article.jsp#.WbRhwq2ZPOQ. Accessed April 5, 2018.
7. Phalen T, Aehlert B. *The 12-Lead ECG in AMI.* 3rd ed. St. Louis, MO: Elsevier; 2012.
8. ECG Guidelines. Part 6: Advanced Cardiac Life Support: Section 7: Algorithm Approach to ACLS Emergencies. *Circulation.* 2000;102(suppl I):I-140–I-141.
9. 2015 American Heart Association Guidelines for Cardiopulmonary Resuscitation and Emergency Cardiovascular Care. *Circulation.* 2015;132.
10. American Heart Association. *Advanced Cardiac Life Support Provider Manual.* Dallas, TX: American Heart Association; 2016.
11. Junqueira LF. Teaching cardiac autonomic function dynamics employing the Valsalva (Valsalva-Weber) maneuver. *Adv Physiol Educ.* 2008;32(1):100-106.
12. Smith G, Boyle MJ. The 10-mL syringe is useful in generating the recommended standard of 40 mmHg intrathoracic pressure for the Valsalva manoevre. *Emerg Med Australas.* 2009;21(6):449-454.
13. Appelboam A, Reuben A, Mann C, et al. Postural modification to the standard Valsalva manoeuvre for emergency treatment of supraventricular tachycardias (REVERT): a randomised controlled trial. *Lancet.* 2015;386(10005):1747-1753.
14. de Caen AR, Maconochie IK, Aickin R, et al. 2015 International Consensus on Cardiopulmonary Resuscitation and Emergency Cardiovascular Care Science With Treatment Recommendations. *Circulation.* 2015;132(16)(suppl 1):S177-S203.
15. American Heart Association. *2015 Handbook of Emergency Cardiovascular Care for Healthcare Providers.* Dallas, TX: American Heart Association; 2015.
16. What are direct-acting oral anticoagulants (DOACs)? American Heart Association website. https://www.heart.org/idc/groups/heart-public/@wcm/@hcm/documents/downloadable/ucm_494807.pdf. Accessed April 5, 2018.
17. NOAC, DOAC, or TSOAC: What should we call novel oral anticoagulants? Pharmacy Times website. http://www.pharmacytimes.com/contributor/sean-kane-pharmd/2016/09/noac-doac-or-tsoac-what-should-we-call-novel-oral-anticoagulants. Published September 19, 2016. Accessed April 5, 2018.
18. Scheuermeyer FX, Pourvali R, Rowe BH, et al. Emergency department patients with AF or flutter and an acute underlying medical illness may not benefit from attempts to control rate or rhythm. *Ann Emerg Med.* 2015;65(5):511-522.
19. Hine LK, Laird NM, Hewitt P, Chalmers TC. Meta-analysis of empirical long-term antiarrhythmic therapy after myocardial infarction. *JAMA.* 1989;262(21):3037-3040.
20. Ewy GA. Cardiocerebral and cardiopulmonary resuscitation—2017 update. *Acute Med Surg.* 2017;4:227-234.

21. Mehta C, Brady W. Pulseless electrical activity in cardiac arrest: electrocardiographic presentations and management considerations based on the electrocardiogram. *Am J Emerg Med*. 2012;1(30):236-239.
22. Bolvardi E, Pouryaghobi SM, Farzane R, Chokan NM, Ahmadi K, Reihani H. The prognostic value of using ultrasonography in cardiac resuscitation of patients with cardiac arrest. *Int J Biomed Sci*. 2016;12(3):110-114.
23. Huszar RJ. *Basic Dysrhythmias: Interpretation and Management*. 4th ed. St. Louis, MO: Elsevier; 2012.
24. January CT, Wann LS, Alpert JS, et al. 2014 AHA/ACC/HRS guideline for the management of patients with atrial fibrillation. *Am J Coll Cardiol*. 2014;130(23):2071-2104.
25. Safaie A. Management of dysrhythmia in emergency department. *Emergency*. 2014;2(3):147-149.
26. National Highway Traffic Safety Administration. *National EMS Education Standards*. Washington, DC: Department of Transportation; 2009. DOT HS 811 077A.
27. Page B. *Twelve-Lead ECG for Acute and Critical Care Providers*. St. Louis, MO: Brady; 2005.
28. O'Gara PT, Kushner FG, Ascheim DD, et al. ACCF/AHA guideline for the management of ST-elevation myocardial infarction: a report of the American College of Cardiology Foundation/American Heart Association Task Force on Practice Guidelines. *Circulation*. 2013;127(4):e362-e425.
29. Klabunde R. *Cardiovascular Physiology Concepts*. 2nd ed. Philadelphia, PA: Lippincott Williams & Wilkins; 2012.
30. 2012 ENA Clinical Practice Committee. Right-sided and posterior electrocardiograms (ECGs). Emergency Nurses Association website. https://www.ena.org/docs/default-source/resource-library/practice-resources/tips/right-side-ecg.pdf?sfvrsn=836f00e6_8. Updated September 16, 2013. Accessed April 5, 2018.
31. Whinnery T, Forster EM. The first sign of loss of consciousness. *Physiol Behav*. 2017;179:494-503.
32. Shen WK, Sheldon RS, Benditt DG, et al. ACC/AHA/HRS guidelines for the evaluation and management of patients with syncope: a report of the American College of Cardiology/American Heart Association Task Force on Clinical Practice Guidelines and the Heart Rhythm Society. *Circulation*. 2017;136(5):e60-e122.
33. Kalanuria AA, Nyquist P, Ling G. The prevention and regression of atherosclerotic plaques: emerging treatments. *Vasc Health Risk Manag*. 2012;8:549-561.
34. Marcus GM, Cohen J, Varosy PD, et al. The utility of gestures in patients with chest discomfort. *Am J Med*. 2007 Jan;120(1):83-89.
35. O'Connor RE, Ali AS, Brady WJ, et al. Part 9: acute coronary syndromes. *Circulation*. 2015;132:S483-S500.
36. Roule V, Ardouin P, Blanchart K, et al. Prehospital fibrinolysis versus primary percutaneous coronary intervention in ST-elevation myocardial infarction: a systematic review and meta-analysis of randomized controlled trials. *Crit Care*. 2016;20(1):359.
37. Kolte D, Khera S, Aronow WS, et al. Trends in incidence, management, and outcomes of cardiogenic shock complicating ST-elevation myocardial infarction in the United States. *J Am Heart Assoc*. 2014;3(1):e000590.
38. National Model EMS Clinical Guidelines Version 2.0. National Association of State EMS Officials website. www.nasemso.org. Revised September 18, 2017. Accessed April 5, 2018. Pg. 98.
39. Rosen P, Barkin R. *Emergency Medicine: Concepts and Clinical Practice*. 8th ed. St. Louis, MO: Mosby; 2014.
40. Rahimi SA. Abdominal aortic aneurysm. Medscape website. http://emedicine.medscape.com/article/1979501-overview. Updated August 16, 2017. Accessed April 5, 2018.
41. Wiesenfarth JM. Acute aortic dissection. Medscape website. http://emedicine.medscape.com/article/756835-overview#a5. Updated December 28, 2017. Accessed April 5, 2018.
42. Kim HJ, Lee H-K, Cho B. A case of acute aortic dissection presenting with chest pain relieved by sublingual nitroglycerin. *Korean J Fam Med*. 2013;34(6):429-433.
43. Risk factors for venous thromboembolism (VTE). American Heart Association website. http://www.heart.org/HEARTORG/Conditions/VascularHealth/VenousThromboembolism/Risk-Factors-for-Venous-Thromboembolism-VTE_UCM_479059_Article.jsp#.WchbdkyZPOQ. Updated February 7, 2018. Accessed April 5, 2018.
44. National Center for Chronic Disease Prevention and Health Promotion, Division for Heart Disease and Stroke Prevention. High blood pressure. Centers for Disease Control and Prevention website. https://www.cdc.gov/bloodpressure/index.htm. Updated February 16, 2018. Accessed April 5, 2018.
45. The facts about high blood pressure. American Heart Association website. https://www.heart.org/HEARTORG/Conditions/HighBloodPressure/GettheFactsAboutHighBloodPressure/The-Facts-About-High-Blood-Pressure_UCM_002050_Article.jsp. Updated March 14, 2018. Accessed April 5, 2018.
46. Varounis C, Katsi V, Nihoyannopoulos P, Lekakis J, Tousoulis D. Cardiovascular hypertensive crisis: recent evidence and review of the literature. *Front Cardiovasc Med*. 2017;3:51.
47. Sexton DJ, Chu VH. Infective endocarditis in injection drug users. UpToDate website. https://www.uptodate.com/contents/infective-endocarditis-in-injection-drug-users. Updated August 28, 2017. Accessed April 5, 2018.
48. What is pericarditis? American Heart Association website. http://www.heart.org/HEARTORG/Conditions/More/What-is-Pericarditis_UCM_444931_Article.jsp#.Wcm7RkyZOgQ. Updated December 12, 2017. Accessed April 5, 2018.
49. Cardiomyopathy. National Heart, Lung, and Blood Institute website. https://www.nhlbi.nih.gov/health-topics/cardiomyopathy. Accessed April 5, 2018.
50. Sharma GK. Arrhythmogenic right ventricular dysplasia (ARVD). Medscape website. https://emedicine.medscape.com/article/163856-overview. Updated September 23, 2014. Accessed April 5, 2018.
51. Hopkins CL, Burk C, Moser S, Meersman J, Baldwin C, Youngquist ST. Implementation of pit crew approach and cardiopulmonary resuscitation metrics for out-of-hospital cardiac arrest improves patient survival and neurological outcome. *J Am Heart Assoc*. 2016;5(1):pii:e002892.
52. Pearson DA, Darrell Nelson R, Monk L, et al. Comparison of team-focused CPR vs standard CPR in resuscitation from out-of-hospital cardiac arrest: results from a statewide quality improvement initiative. *Resuscitation*. 2016;105:165-172.
53. Statistical update: out-of-hospital cardiac arrest. CPR & First Aid, Emergency Cardiovascular Care website. http://cpr.heart.org/AHAECC/CPRAndECC/General/UCM_477263_Cardiac-Arrest-Statistics.jsp. Accessed April 5, 2018.
54. Bobrow BJ, Spaite DW, Berg RA, et al. Chest compression–only CPR by lay rescuers and survival from out-of-hospital cardiac arrest. *JAMA*. 2010;304(13):1447-1454.
55. Sasson C, Rogers AM, Dahl J, Kellerman AL. Predictors of survival from out-of-hospital cardiac arrest. *Circulation Cardiovasc Qual Outcomes*. 2010;3(1):63-81.

56. Bobrow BJ, Clark LL, Ewy GA. Minimally interrupted cardiac resuscitation by emergency medical services for out-of-hospital cardiac arrest. *JAMA.* 2008;299(10):1158-1165.
57. Bobrow BJ, Ewy GA, Clark L, et al. Passive oxygen insufflation is superior to bag-valve-mask ventilation for witnessed ventricular fibrillation out-of-hospital cardiac arrest. *Ann Emerg Med.* 2009;54(5):656-662.
58. Kellum MJ, Kennedy KW, Barney R, et al. Cardiocerebral resuscitation improves neurologically intact survival of patients with out-of-hospital cardiac arrest. *Ann Emerg Med.* 2008;52(3):244-252.
59. Zhan L, Yang LJ, Huang Y, He Q, Liu GJ. Continuous chest compression versus interrupted chest compression for cardiopulmonary resuscitation of non-asphyxial out-of-hospital cardiac arrest. *Cochrane Database Syst Rev.* 2017;3:CD010134.
60. Ashoor HM, Lillie E, Zarin W, et al. Effectiveness of different compression-to-ventilation methods for cardiopulmonary resuscitation: a systematic review. *Resuscitation.* 2017;118:112-125.
61. Georgiou M, Papathanassoglou E, Xanthos T. Systematic review of the mechanisms driving effective blood flow during adult CPR. *Resuscitation.* 2014;85(11):1586-1593.
62. Brooks SC, Anderson ML, Bruder E, et al. Part 6: alternative techniques and ancillary devices for cardiopulmonary resuscitation. *Circulation.* 2015;132(18)(suppl 2):S436.
63. Phillips Medical Systems. HeartStart defibrillators: biphasic defibrillation. AED Brands website. https://www.aedbrands.com/philips-biphasic-energy.pdf. Accessed April 5, 2018.
64. de Caen AR, Berg MD, Chameides L, et al. Part 12: pediatric advanced life support. *Circulation.* 2015;132(18)(suppl 2):S526.
65. Daly S, Milne HJ, Holmes DP, Corfield AR. Defibrillation and external pacing in flight: incidence and implications. *Emerg Med J.* 2014;31(1):69-71.
66. Knight BP. Patient education: implantable cardioverter-defibrillators (beyond the basics). UpToDate website. https://www.uptodate.com/contents/implantable-cardioverter-defibrillators-beyond-the-basics. Updated September 22, 2017. Accessed April 5, 2018.
67. Piccini JP, Allen LA, Kudenchuk PJ, Page RL, Patel MR, Turakhia MP. Wearable cardioverter-defibrillator therapy for the prevention of sudden cardiac death. *Circulation.* 2016;133(17):1715.
68. Sen A, Larson JS, Kashani KB, et al. Mechanical circulatory assist devices: a primer for critical care and emergency physicians. *Crit Care.* 2016;20:153.
69. Peberdy MA, Gluck JA, Ornato JP, et al. Cardiopulmonary resuscitation in adults and children with mechanical circulatory support: a scientific statement from the American Heart Association. *Circulation.* 2017;135(24):e1115-e1134.
70. Mechanical Circulatory Support Organization. EMS guide: January 2016/17. MyLVAD website. https://www.mylvad.com/ems/field_guides/emergency-medical-services-field-guides-full-document. Accessed April 5, 2018.
71. Vaity C, Al-Subaie N, Cecconi M. Cooling techniques for targeted temperature management post-cardiac arrest. *Crit Care.* 2015;19(1):103.
72. Millin MG, Galvagno SM, Khandker SR, et al. Withholding and termination of resuscitation of adult cardiopulmonary arrest secondary to trauma: resource document to the joint NAEMSP-ACSCOT position statements. *J Trauma Acute Care Surg.* 2013;3(75):459-467.

Suggested Readings

Anile G, Pradeep AS, Figueredo VM. aVR—the forgotten lead. *Exp Clin Cardiol.* 2010;15(2):e36-e44.

Audebert H, Fassbender K, Hussain MS. The PRE-hospital Stroke Treatment Organization. *Int J Stroke.* 2017;12(9):932-940.

Bosson N, Sanko S, Stickney RE, et al. Causes of prehospital misinterpretations of ST elevation myocardial infarction. *Prehosp Emerg Care.* 2017;21(3):283-290.

DeSantis A, Landis P, Alrawashdeh M, Martin-Gill C, Callaway C, Al-Zaiti SA. Abstract 18641: predictors of emergency medical personnel's decision to transmit or not to transmit the prehospital 12-lead ECG of patients with suspected AMI. *Circulation.* 2017;136:A18641.

Fakhri Y, Schoos MM, Sejersten M, et al. Prehospital electrocardiographic acuteness score of ischemia is inversely associated with neurohormonal activation in STEMI patients with severe ischemia. *J Electrocardiol.* 2017;50(1):90-96.

Fassbender K, Grotta JC, Walter S, Grunwald IQ, Ragoschke-Schumm A, Saver JL. Mobile stroke units for prehospital thrombolysis, triage, and beyond: benefits and challenges. *Lancet Neurol.* 2017;16(3):227-237.

Hansen R, Frydland M, Møller-Helgestad OK, et al. Data on association between QRS duration on prehospital ECG and mortality in patients with suspected STEMI. *Int J Cardiol.* 2017;249:55-60.

Johnson B, Runyon M, Weekes A, Pearson D. Team-focused cardiopulmonary resuscitation: prehospital principles adapted for emergency department cardiac arrest resuscitation. *J Emerg Med.* 2018 Jan;54(1):54-63.

Kragholm DL, Chiswell K, Al-Khalidi HR, et al. Improvement in care and outcomes for emergency medical service–transported patients with ST elevation myocardial infarction (STEMI) with and without prehospital cardiac arrest: a mission: Lifeline STEMI Accelerator Study. *JAHA* website. http://jaha.ahajournals.org/content/6/10/e005717. Published October 11, 2017. Accessed April 5, 2018.

Nolte CH, Ebinger M, Scheitz JF, et al. Effects of prehospital thrombolysis in stroke patients with prestroke dependency. *Stroke.* 2018;49:646-651.

Sanello A, Gausche-Hill M, Mulkerin W, et al. Altered mental status: current evidence-based recommendations for prehospital care. *West J Emerg Med Integrat Emerg Care Popul Health.* eScholarship website. Published March 8, 2018. Accessed April 5, 2018.

Vora N, Jung J, Govindarajan P. Abstract WP219: decision analysis tool for prehospital stroke triage in the era of endovascular therapy. *Stroke.* 2018;49:AWP219.

Walker GB, Zhelev Z, Handler JF, Henschke N, Yip S. Abstract TP252: prehospital stroke scales as a tool for early identification of stroke and transient ischemic attacks: a Cochrane systematic review. *Stroke.* 2017;48:ATP252.

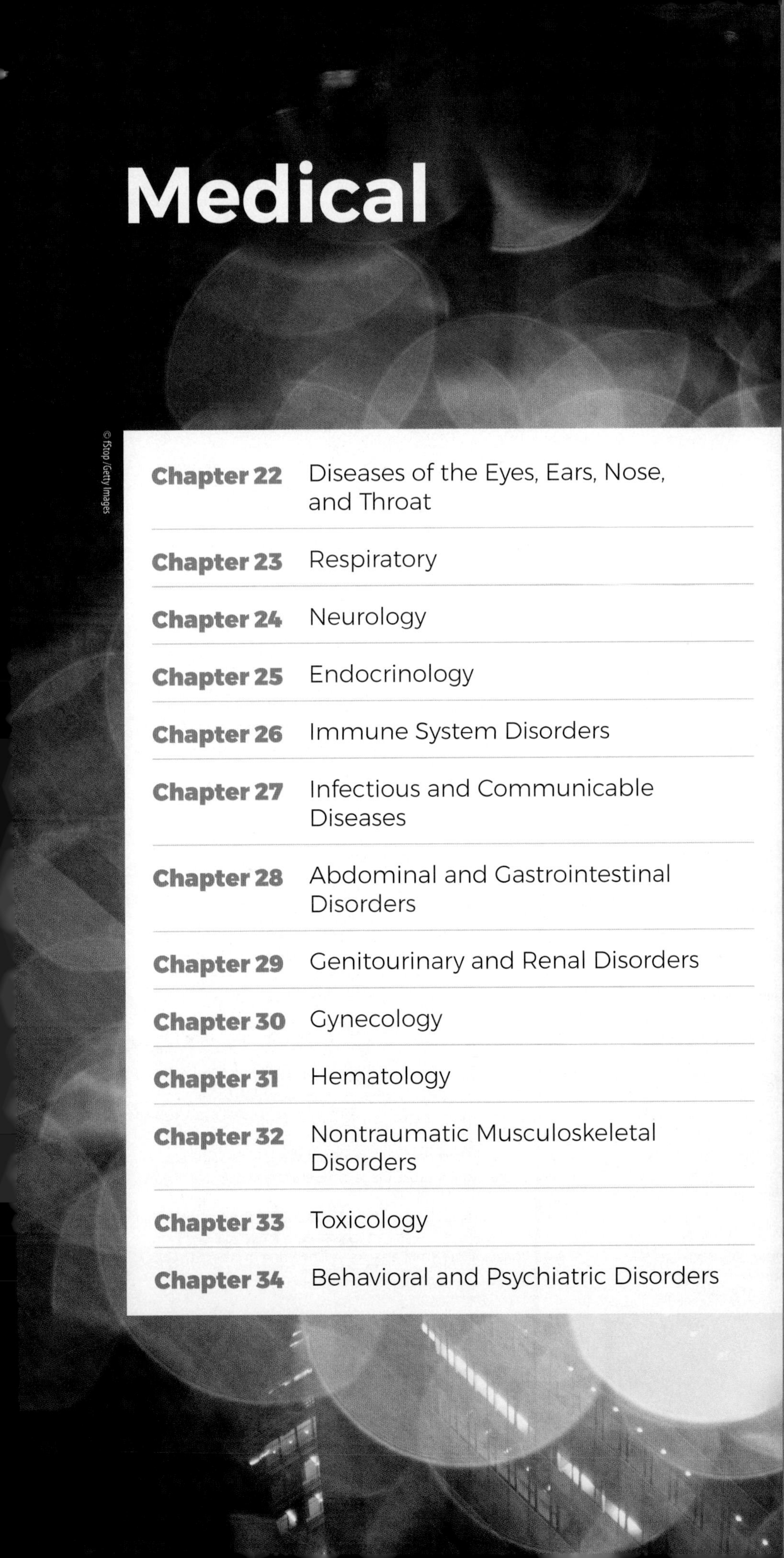

PART 7

Medical

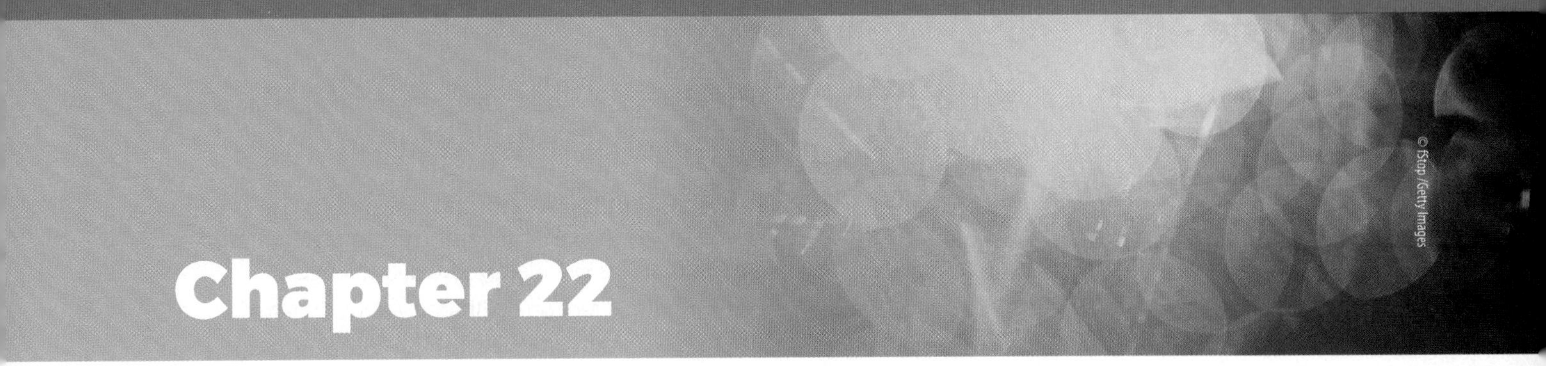
© iStop /Getty Images

Chapter 22

Diseases of the Eyes, Ears, Nose, and Throat

NATIONAL EMS EDUCATION STANDARD COMPETENCIES

Medicine

Integrates assessment findings with principles of epidemiology and pathophysiology to formulate a field impression and implement a comprehensive treatment/disposition plan for a patient with a medical complaint.

Diseases of the Eyes, Ears, Nose, and Throat

Knowledge of the anatomy, physiology, epidemiology, pathophysiology, psychosocial impact, presentations, prognosis, and management of

- Common or major diseases of the eyes, ears, nose, and throat, including nose bleed (pp 879–898)

OBJECTIVES

Upon completion of this chapter, the paramedic student will be able to:

1. Label a diagram of the eye. (p 879)
2. Describe the pathophysiology, signs and symptoms, and specific management techniques for each of the following disorders of the eye: conjunctivitis, corneal abrasion, foreign body, inflammation (chalazion and hordeolum), glaucoma, iritis, papilledema, retinal detachment, central retinal vein occlusion, central retinal artery occlusion, and orbital cellulitis. (pp 879–885)
3. Label a diagram of the ear. (p 886)
4. Describe the pathophysiology, signs and symptoms, and specific management techniques for each of the following conditions that affect the ear: foreign body, impacted cerumen, labyrinthitis, Ménière disease, benign paroxysmal positional vertigo, otitis media, perforated tympanic membrane. (pp 886–890)
5. Label a diagram of the nose. (p 890)
6. Describe the pathophysiology, signs and symptoms, and specific management techniques for each of the following conditions that affect the nose: epistaxis, foreign body, rhinitis, and sinusitis. (pp 890–893)
7. Label a diagram of the oropharynx. (p 894)
8. Describe the pathophysiology, signs and symptoms, and specific management techniques for each of the following conditions that affect the oropharynx and throat: toothache and dental abscess, Ludwig angina, epiglottitis, laryngitis, tracheitis, oral candidiasis, peritonsillar abscess, pharyngitis/tonsillitis, and temporomandibular joint disorders. (pp 893–898)

KEY TERMS

angle-closure glaucoma (also called acute glaucoma, chronic angle-closure glaucoma, or narrow-angle glaucoma) A form of glaucoma associated with a physically obstructed anterior chamber angle; may be chronic or acute.

benign paroxysmal positional vertigo (BPPV) A condition in which calcium carbonate crystals enter one (or several) of the semicircular canals of the ear and disturb the normal fluid movement, causing nystagmus and vertigo.

central retinal artery occlusion (CRAO) The blockage of blood supply to the arteries of the retina.

central retinal vein occlusion (CRVO) The blockage of blood supply to the main vein of the retina.

cerumen A yellow or brown waxy secretion produced in the external ear canal; also known as earwax.

chalazion A small bump in the eyelid caused by the blockage of a tiny oil gland in the upper or lower eyelid.

conjunctivitis Inflammation of the conjunctiva caused by bacterial or viral infection, allergy, or environmental factors.

corneal abrasion A disruption or loss of cells in the top layer of the corneal epithelium.

dental abscess A collection of pus in, around, or underneath a tooth.

dentalgia The medical term for toothache.

epiglottitis Inflammation of the epiglottis; a severe form of the condition that primarily affects children and is characterized by fever, sore throat, stridor, croupy cough, and an erythematous epiglottis.

epistaxis Bleeding from the nose.

glaucoma A condition in which intraocular pressure increases and causes damage to the optic nerve.

hordeolum An acute infection of the oil gland; commonly known as a sty.

iritis Inflammation of the iris of the eye.

labyrinthitis An ear disorder that involves irritation and swelling of the inner ear structure called the labyrinth.

laryngitis Inflammation of the larynx.

Ludwig angina A type of cellulitis that involves inflammation of the tissues of the floor of the mouth, under the tongue.

Ménière disease An abnormality of the inner ear that causes vertigo and tinnitus; associated with fluctuations in hearing loss and a sensation of pressure or pain in the affected ear.

mononucleosis A viral infection that causes fever, sore throat, and swollen lymph glands, especially in the neck.

open-angle glaucoma (also called wide-angle glaucoma) is the most common type of glaucoma. The structures of the eye appear normal, but fluid in the eye does not flow properly through the trabecular meshwork.

oral candidiasis An infection of yeast fungi of the genus *Candida* on the mucous membranes of the mouth; also known as thrush.

orbital cellulitis An acute infection in the tissues posterior to the orbital septum often manifested as swelling of the eyelids, eyebrow, and cheek.

otitis media Infection or inflammation of the middle ear.

papilledema Swelling of the head of the optic disc caused by a rise in intracranial pressure.

perforated tympanic membrane A hole or rupture in the eardrum; usually caused by trauma or infection.

peritonsillar abscess A collection of pus in and around one or both tonsils; often caused by tonsillitis.

pharyngitis Inflammation or infection of the pharynx.

retinal detachment A separation of the light-sensitive retina from its supporting layers.

retinal vascular occlusion Blockage of a vessel in the retina of the eye.

rhinitis Inflammation of the mucous membranes of the nose.

sinusitis Inflammation of one or more paranasal sinuses.

strep throat An infection of the throat caused by streptococcal bacteria.

temporomandibular (TM) joint disorders A set of conditions that cause pain in the area of the TM joint. A TM joint is located on each side of the head in front of the ears where the mandible meets the temporal bones.

tinnitus A ringing sound in the ears.

tonsillitis Inflammation of the tonsils.

tracheitis A bacterial infection of the upper airway and subglottic trachea.

trismus Limited jaw range of motion commonly caused by muscle spasms of the jaw.

vertigo A sensation in which the patient feels as if he or she, or the objects around him or her, are moving in a circular or spinning motion, which causes difficulty in maintaining normal balance in a standing or seated position.

Medical conditions that affect the ears, eyes, nose, and throat are a common occurrence in the prehospital setting.[1] *This chapter will review the anatomy of these structures and discuss the specific findings, symptoms, and management considerations for common diseases.*

NOTE

Many disorders of the eyes, ears, nose, and throat can be benign and will not require emergency transport for physician evaluation; however, serious and life-threatening disorders often masquerade as minor problems. Keeping a high index of suspicion for serious conditions is essential for quality patient care.

Conditions of the Eye

As described in Chapter 10, *Review of Human Systems,* the eye is composed of three layers: the fibrous tunic, consisting of the sclera and cornea; the vascular tunic, consisting of the choroid, ciliary body, and the iris; and the nervous tunic, consisting of the retina (**FIGURE 22-1**). In addition, there are accessory structures that protect, lubricate, move, and aid in the function of the eye. These structures include the eyebrows, eyelids, conjunctiva, and lacrimal gland. BOX 22-1 lists conditions of the eyes that are described in this chapter.

BOX 22-1 Conditions That Affect the Eye

- Conjunctivitis
- Corneal abrasion
- Foreign body
- Inflammation (chalazion and hordeolum)
- Glaucoma
- Iritis
- Papilledema
- Retinal detachment
- Central retinal artery occlusion
- Orbital cellulitis

NOTE

Eye movement is controlled by cranial nerves III, IV, and VI. The paramedic should remember that visual disturbances of the eyes may be an early indication of stroke, tumor, or other central nervous system disease. These possibilities must always be considered when caring for a patient with an eye movement disorder.

CRITICAL THINKING

Which assessment will you perform on an unconscious patient to determine if there is pressure on cranial nerve III?

Conjunctivitis

Conjunctivitis refers to inflammation or infection of the conjunctiva (the membrane lining of the eyes). The condition is commonly called pink eye or Madras eye. Two common causes of conjunctivitis are infection

NOTE

Conjunctivitis can also be caused by agents that irritate the eye, such as an accidental exposure to chemicals or a foreign body in the eye (see Chapter 38, *Burns*, and Chapter 39, *Head, Face, and Neck Trauma*).

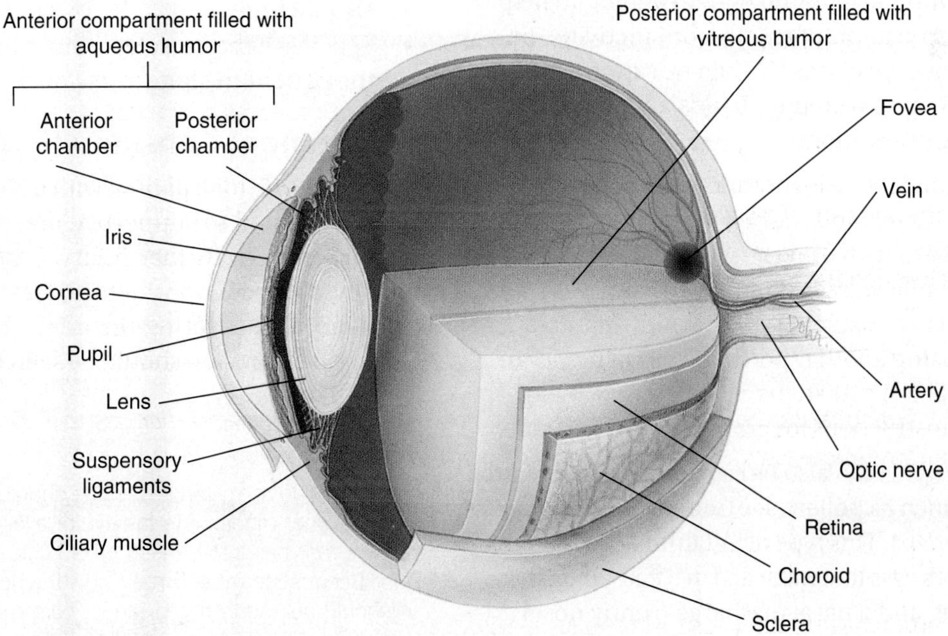

FIGURE 22-1 Anatomy of the eye.

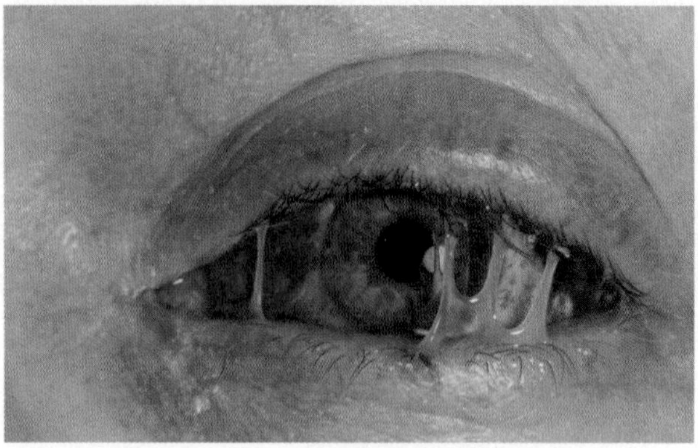

FIGURE 22-2 Gonococcal conjunctivitis, caused by *Neisseria gonorrhoeae*, showing redness and copious discharge in the eye.

(bacterial or, most commonly, viral) and an allergic reaction (**FIGURE 22-2**). In newborns, conjunctivitis can result from an incompletely opened tear duct.

Conjunctivitis caused by viral or bacterial infection is very contagious. Therefore, early diagnosis and treatment can prevent the spread of the disease. This type of conjunctivitis can affect both eyes and is often associated with a cold. If the cause is viral, there may be a discharge of watery mucus. If the cause is bacterial, the discharge may be thick and yellow-green. Most bacterial infections are associated with a respiratory tract infection or sore throat. Bacterial conjunctivitis is more common in children than in adults. To help prevent the spread of infectious conjunctivitis, patients who have the disease should be cautioned not to touch their eyes with their hands and to practice the following precautions:

- Wash hands thoroughly and frequently.
- Change towels and washcloths daily and do not share them with others.
- Change pillowcases often.
- Discard eye cosmetics, particularly mascara.
- Avoid using another person's eye cosmetics or personal eye care items.
- Follow instructions for proper contact lens care.

Conjunctivitis can also be caused by exposure to an allergen such as pollen (see Chapter 26, *Immune System Disorders*). This type of inflammation is often associated with eyes that water and itch and sometimes with sneezing and a nasal discharge (runny nose).

Management Considerations

Although conjunctivitis is irritating to the eye, it rarely affects vision. Bacterial causes of the condition are usually managed with antibiotic eye drops or eye ointment.[2] Symptoms generally improve within 1 to 2 days. Viral and allergic forms of conjunctivitis are usually managed with over-the-counter medicines (eg, antihistamines, decongestants) to relieve symptoms. If the condition is severe, corticosteroids and anti-inflammatory drugs may be prescribed. The symptoms of viral and allergic conjunctivitis may take several days to a week or more to subside.

Corneal Abrasion

A **corneal abrasion** is a painful scrape or scratch on the cornea of the eye. It most often occurs from trauma, such as from being struck in the eye by a tree branch or limb. It is also frequently caused by foreign bodies in the eye that lodge under the upper lid (eg, dust, paint chips, wind debris). Corneal abrasions can also be caused by wearing contact lenses longer than recommended or by allowing the contact lens, fingers, or nails to scratch the eye during insertion or removal of contact lenses. Signs and symptoms of a corneal abrasion include the following:[3]

- Pain (which can be severe with opening or closing the eye)
- A sensation of a foreign body in the eye
- Tearing and redness
- Photophobia (sensitivity to light)
- Blurred vision
- Headache
- Spasms of the muscles around the eye, causing the patient to squint

Management Considerations

Prehospital care for a patient with a corneal abrasion is usually limited to supportive measures to relieve pain and prevent further injury. Care may include applying a topical ophthalmic anesthetic, such as tetracaine, and covering the affected eye. Patients with corneal abrasion should be seen by a physician.

> **NOTE**
>
> Patients who are given tetracaine should be cautioned not to rub or manipulate the eye or eyelid. Doing so to an eye that has been anesthetized can worsen the injury. Because tetracaine may slow the healing process, it should be used only for acute pain management to facilitate an examination and not given as a mode of regular pain relief. Well-meaning providers have given the patient the tetracaine bottle only to find themselves trying to manage complications a few days later.

Foreign Body

As previously discussed, small foreign bodies in the eye are common. They are often irritating to the patient but seldom affect vision. Common complaints are pain, tearing, and a sensation of fullness in the eye.

Management Considerations

Small foreign bodies can be washed or irrigated from the eye using eye cups or saline solution attached to intravenous (IV) tubing. The patient should be instructed not to rub the lid of the affected eye, which could lead to a corneal abrasion. Large or penetrating foreign bodies in the eye are serious in nature and should be managed as described in Chapter 39, *Head, Face, and Neck Trauma.*

Inflammation of the Eyelid

Inflammation of the eyelid usually results from blockage of a gland or from bacterial infection. Two common conditions are chalazion and hordeolum.

Chalazion is a small bump in the eyelid caused by the blockage of a tiny oil gland in the upper or lower eyelid. These oil glands normally secrete oil into tears (**FIGURE 22-3**). The lump appears as localized and hard and may increase in size over days to weeks. Symptoms include tenderness, tearing, painful swelling, and sensitivity to light (photophobia).[4]

> DID YOU KNOW?
> There are about 40 oil glands (meibomian glands) within each upper and lower eyelid. The glands secrete oil into tears through a tiny opening located just behind the eyelashes.

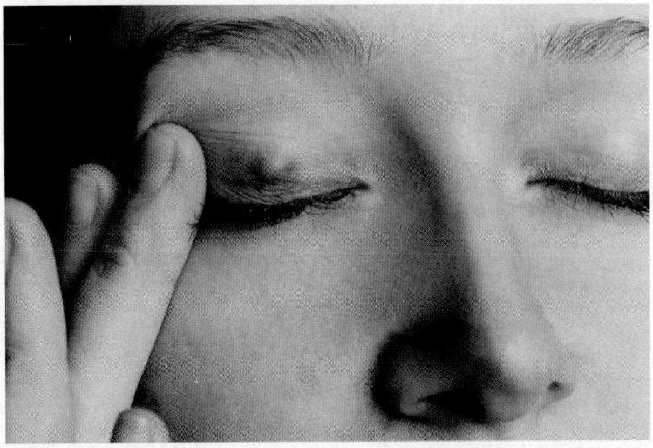

FIGURE 22-3 Chalazion on the upper eyelid.

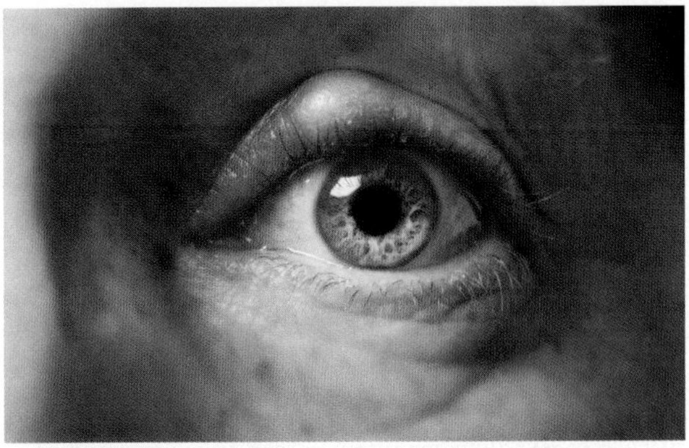

FIGURE 22-4 Acute hordeolum of upper eyelid.

A **hordeolum** is commonly known as a sty. It represents an acute infection of the oil gland. A sty is usually more painful than a chalazion because of inflammation and may look infected (**FIGURE 22-4**). The pain of a sty can cause redness around the eye, the eyelid, and cheek tissue. A sty can be limited to one eyelid or can occur on both eyelids simultaneously.

Management Considerations

Inflammation of the eyelids from either of these conditions usually subsides without treatment within 5 to 7 days.[5] Home care may include applying warm compresses three to four times per day and gentle scrubbing of the affected eyelid with warm water and a mild soap or shampoo. Patients should be advised not to squeeze or puncture the inflamed area because it can result in serious infection. Eye makeup and eye lotions and creams should be avoided until the inflammation clears. If fever or headache develops, the patient should seek physician evaluation.

Glaucoma

Glaucoma refers to a group of diseases that affect the optic nerve (BOX 22-2). It develops when too much aqueous humor accumulates in the anterior chamber of the eye between the cornea and the iris. This fluid normally flows out of the eye through a meshlike channel (trabecular channel) (**FIGURE 22-5**). If this channel becomes blocked, the increase in intraocular pressure damages the optic nerve and can lead to a loss of vision. Without treatment, the condition can lead to permanent blindness. The disease usually occurs in both eyes but affects one more than the other. The direct cause of the blockage is unknown but seems to have a heritable component.[6] Other

BOX 22-2 Two Common Types of Glaucoma

Open-angle glaucoma (also called wide-angle glaucoma) is the most common type of glaucoma. The structures of the eye appear normal, but fluid in the eye does not flow properly through the trabecular meshwork.

Angle-closure glaucoma (also called acute glaucoma, chronic angle-closure glaucoma, or narrow-angle glaucoma) is a less common type of glaucoma. Drainage may be poor because the angle between the iris and the cornea (where the trabecular meshwork is located) is too narrow. Another cause is a pupil that opens too wide, narrowing the angle and blocking the flow of the fluid through that channel (**FIGURE 22-6**).

risk factors for developing the disease include the following:

- African American or Hispanic ethnicity
- Age older than 40 years
- Severe nearsightedness (myopia) or farsightedness (hyperopia)
- Diabetes
- Migraines
- Eye injury
- Use of systemic corticosteroid drugs (eg, prednisone)

Glaucoma can occur at any age (including in children and infants), but occurs most often after age 40 years (see Chapter 48, *Geriatrics*). There may be

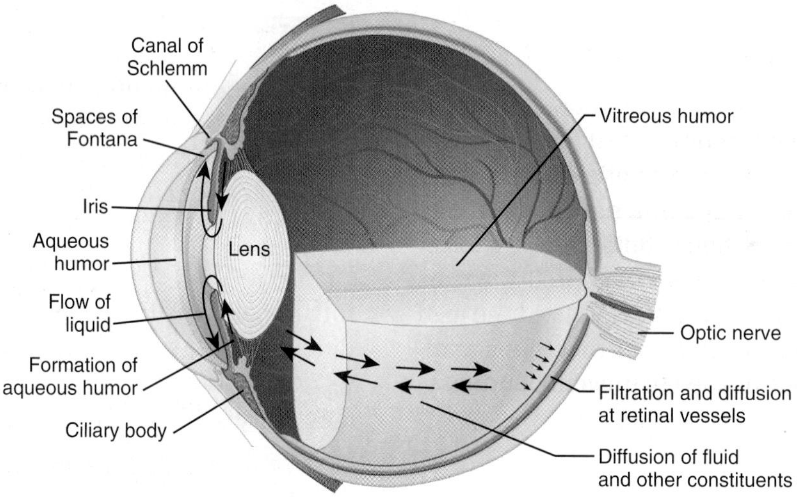

FIGURE 22-5 Formation and flow of fluid in the eye.

Modified from: Hall J. *Guyton and Hall Textbook of Medical Physiology*. 12th ed. Philadelphia, PA: Saunders; 2011.

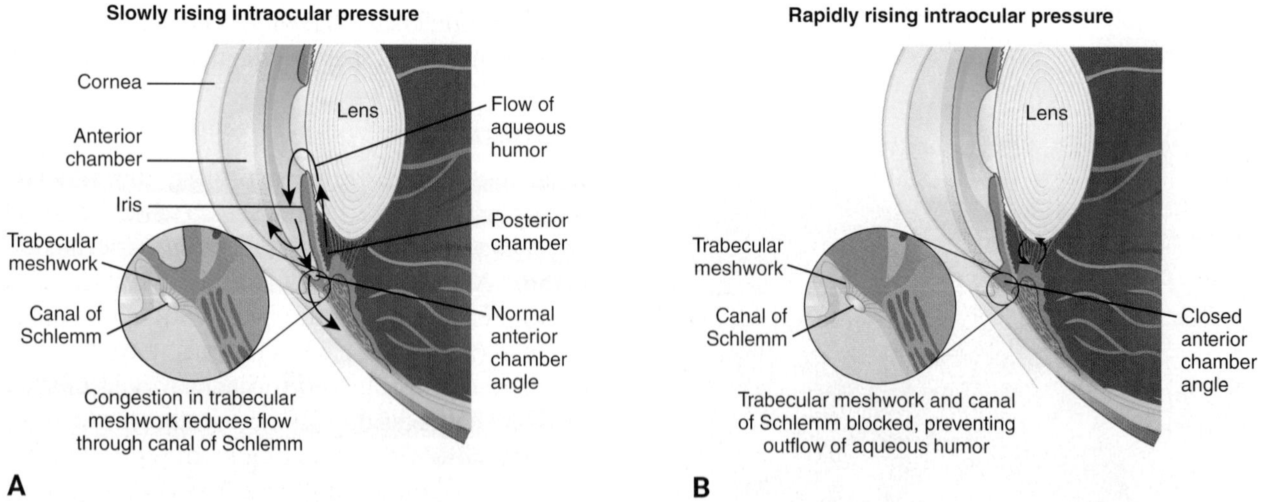

FIGURE 22-6 A. Primary open-angle glaucoma. Congestion in the trabecular meshwork reduces the outflow of aqueous humor. **B.** Primary closed-angle glaucoma (acute). The angle between the iris and the anterior chamber narrows, obstructing the outflow of aqueous humor.

Modified from: Christensen BL, et al. *Adult Health Nursing*. 6th ed. St Louis, MO: Mosby; 2010.

no symptoms of the disease, making early screening every 1 to 2 years important. The first sign of glaucoma is usually a loss of peripheral vision, which can remain unnoticed until the disease has progressed. If the rise in intraocular pressure is severe, the patient may have sudden eye pain, headache, vomiting, and blurred vision. The patient may also complain of seeing halos around lights, which is caused by swelling of the cornea.

CRITICAL THINKING

If a patient presents with these signs and symptoms, what other conditions should you consider in your differential diagnosis?

Management Considerations

Prehospital care for patients with glaucoma is primarily supportive. If symptoms are sudden in onset, rapid transport for physician evaluation is indicated. Physician care to treat glaucoma may include eye drops to reduce the formation of fluid in the eye, laser surgery to increase the outflow of fluid in the eye, or microsurgery to create a new channel to drain the fluid from the eye. In some cases, a combination of these therapies will be needed to prevent blindness.

Iritis

Iritis (anterior uveitis) is inflammation of the iris of the eye. It is a serious disease that can infrequently cause blindness if not treated (**FIGURE 22-7**). Causes of iritis include eye trauma, inflammatory and autoimmune disorders, infection, and cancer. Examples of medical causes of the inflammation include rheumatoid arthritis, lupus, Crohn disease, Lyme disease, herpes, syphilis, tuberculosis, ankylosing spondylitis, and leukemia.[7]

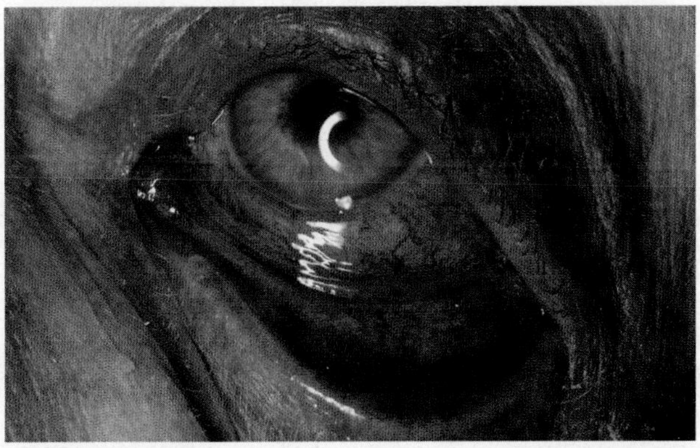

FIGURE 22-7 Iritis.

Iritis can be classified as acute or chronic. The acute form of the disease develops suddenly and usually heals within a few weeks with treatment. Chronic iritis can exist for months or years and is associated with a higher risk of vision impairment or blindness. Iritis can affect one or both eyes. Signs and symptoms of iritis include a reddened eye, ocular or periorbital pain, photophobia, and blurred or cloudy vision.

Management Considerations

Prehospital care is primarily supportive. Physician care may include a variety of steroidal anti-inflammatory eye drops, pressure-reducing eye drops, and oral and injectable steroids to reduce inflammation.

Papilledema

Papilledema is swelling of the head of the optic disc caused by a rise in intracranial pressure (ICP). There are numerous causes of elevated ICP, including cerebral edema, bleeding within the skull, tumors, encephalitis, and increased production of cerebrospinal fluid (CSF), among others (see Chapter 24, *Neurology*, and Chapter 39, *Head, Face, and Neck Trauma*). The swelling of the optic disc is usually bilateral and may be more severe in one eye than in the other. The condition is diagnosed using an ophthalmoscope (described in Chapter 19, *Secondary Assessment and Reassessment*). Visible signs may include the following (**FIGURE 22-8**):

- Venous engorgement (usually the first sign)
- Loss of venous pulsation

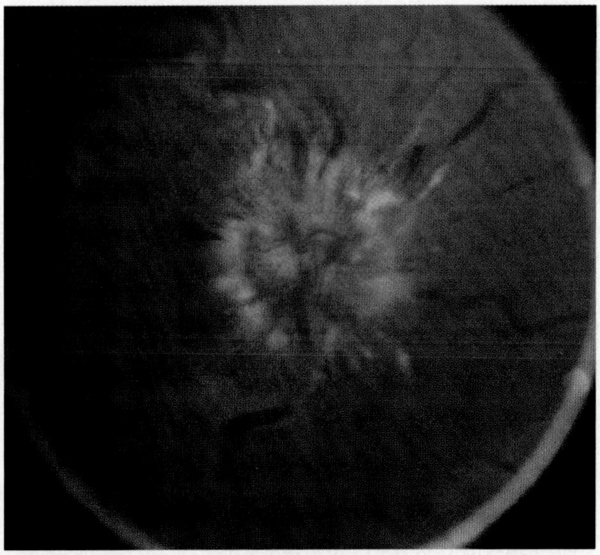

FIGURE 22-8 Severe papilledema.

Reproduced from: Bababeygy SR, Repka MX, Subramanian PS, Minocycline-associated pseudotumor cerebri with severe papilledema. *J Ophthalmol.* 2009;(10):203583.

- Hemorrhages over and/or adjacent to the optic disc
- Blurring of optic margins
- Elevation of the optic disc
- Paton lines (radial retinal lines cascading from the optic disc)

Patient complaints may include a headache that is usually worse on awakening and made worse by coughing, holding the breath, or straining. Other complaints may include nausea and vomiting and vision disturbances (double vision and vision that temporarily flickers or grays).

NOTE

Infants who are victims of shaken baby syndrome may be unconscious with papilledema. Therefore, shaken baby syndrome should be suspected with this presentation. External signs of abuse may or may not be present (see Chapter 49, *Abuse and Neglect*).

Management Considerations

Prehospital care is primarily supportive. Physician care will depend on the cause of the disease. After the underlying cause is determined and treated, medical care may include efforts to reduce increased CSF and corticosteroids to reduce inflammation. If papilledema is diagnosed and managed early, permanent vision damage can often be prevented.

Retinal Detachment

As described in Chapter 10, *Review of Human Systems*, the retina is the light-sensitive tissue that lines the inside of the eye and sends visual messages through the optic nerve to the brain. If the retina detaches, it is lifted or pulled from its normal position, which separates the retinal cells from the blood vessels that supply them with oxygen and nutrients.[8] Small areas of the retina can also be torn. These retinal tears, breaks, or defects can lead to retinal detachment.

Retinal detachment is a true emergency and can lead to permanent vision loss. The condition can occur at any age but is more likely in the following situations:[9]

- Person is extremely nearsighted.
- Person has had a retinal detachment in the other eye.
- Person has a family history of retinal detachment.
- Person has had cataract surgery.
- Person has other eye diseases or disorders.
- Person has had an eye injury.

Signs and symptoms of retinal detachment include a sudden or gradual increase in the number of floaters, which are little cobwebs or specks that float in the field of vision, and/or the number of light flashes in the eye. Another symptom is the appearance of a curtain over the field of vision.

CRITICAL THINKING

How would your life change if you were to lose your sight next week?

Management Considerations

Like most eye conditions, prehospital care for a patient with retinal detachment is primarily supportive. Because the condition is a true emergency, rapid transport for physician evaluation is key. Small tears in the retina may be repaired with laser surgery or a freeze treatment to reattach the retina. Full retinal detachment requires surgery and usually hospitalization. About 90% of patients can be successfully treated if managed early, with varying degrees of visual outcome. Visual results are best if the retinal detachment is repaired before the macula (the center region of the retina responsible for fine, detailed vision) detaches.[9]

Retinal Vascular Occlusion

Retinal vascular occlusion is blockage of a vessel in the retina of the eye. It is a common cause of blindness,[10–12] and can lead to loss of vision. **Central retinal vein occlusion (CRVO)** and **central retinal artery occlusion (CRAO)** are included in this grouping. CRVO is estimated to occur in 0.7% to 1.6% of the general population; CRAO is less common.[13]

Central Retinal Vein Occlusion

CRVO is the blockage of blood supply to the main vein of the retina; the light-sensitive nerve layer at the back of the eye. The obstruction causes the walls of the vein to leak blood and excess fluid into the retina. When fluid collects in the macula (macular edema), vision becomes blurry and may produce "floaters" in the field of vision. In severe cases, the patient experiences painful pressure in the eye and loss of vision in all or part of one eye. Macular edema is one of the main causes of vision loss in CRVO.[14] Central retinal vein occlusions commonly occur with glaucoma, diabetes, age-related vascular disease, high blood pressure, and blood disorders.[15]

A physician will evaluate the patient with CRVO to identify the ischemic or nonischemic source of occlusion and to establish a treatment plan. Treatment for the complications of CRVO may include focal laser treatment, if macular edema is present; injections of antivascular endothelial growth factor (anti-VEGF) drugs into the eye (investigational); laser treatment to prevent the growth of new, abnormal blood vessels that leads to glaucoma; and management of modifiable risk factors. The outcome varies. Patients with CRVO often regain useful vision.

Central Retinal Artery Occlusion

CRAO is the blockage of blood supply to the arteries of the retina. It is essentially a stroke of the eye.[16,17] CRAO produces sudden, painless loss of vision in one eye. This condition is a true ocular emergency and should be treated with the urgency of an acute ischemic stroke. Retinal circulation must be reestablished as soon as possible, ideally within 100 minutes, to prevent permanent loss of vision. Irreversible vision loss typically occurs after 4 hours of occlusion. Occasionally, before total occlusion occurs, the patient may experience transient episodes of blindness called amaurosis fugax. This can be equated to a transient ischemic attack of the retinal artery. Patients usually describe the episode as a shade coming down over the eye. Causes of CRAO include embolus (carotid and cardiac), thrombosis, hypertension, or simple angiospasm (rare) associated with a migraine or atrial fibrillation. Therefore, the patient will need to be thoroughly evaluated to rule out other systemic problems.

To prevent permanent damage, retinal perfusion needs to be reestablished as rapidly as possible. In-hospital care may include vasodilation techniques, ocular massage, and administration of intraocular pressure–lowering drugs, none of which have been shown to be extremely beneficial.[16]

Management Considerations

Prehospital care for retinal vascular occlusion is primarily supportive. The patient requires rapid transport to an appropriate medical facility for evaluation.

Orbital Cellulitis

Orbital cellulitis is an acute infection of the tissues that surround the eye, specifically, the tissues posterior to the orbital septum. Infections anterior to the orbital septum are deemed preseptal cellulitis and are less ominous than is orbital cellulitis. Orbital cellulitis may manifest as swelling of the eyelids, eyebrow, and cheek (**FIGURE 22-9**). Orbital cellulitis is a dangerous infection that can have serious consequences if not treated and can quickly lead to blindness, especially in children. Other complications of the disease include hearing loss, septicemia, sinus thrombosis, and meningitis.

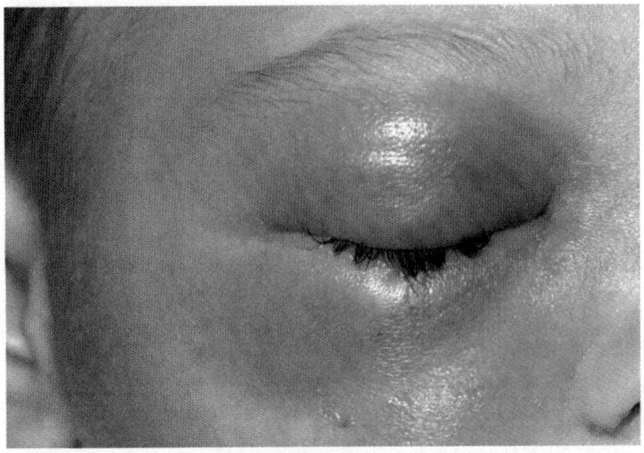

FIGURE 22-9 Orbital cellulitis.

Orbital cellulitis is often caused by bacteria from a sinus infection. The bacteria *Staphylococcus aureus, Streptococcus pneumoniae*, and *Haemophilus influenzae* are the most frequent causes of orbital cellulitis.[18] Other causes of orbital cellulitis include styes and eyelid injuries accompanied by inflammation. Signs and symptoms of the disease include the following:

- Fever, with temperature generally less than 102°F (38.9°C)
- Painful swelling of upper and lower eyelids
- Shiny, red or purple eyelid
- Eye pain
- Weakened eye muscles, causing double vision
- Bulging eyes
- General malaise
- Painful or difficult eye movements

Management Considerations

Prehospital care is focused on recognition of the signs and symptoms and rapid transport for physician evaluation. Patients will usually be hospitalized for diagnostic tests. Physician care may include IV antibiotics and sometimes surgery to drain any abscess associated with the illness. With prompt treatment, most patients will make a full recovery.

CRITICAL THINKING

If a patient with orbital cellulitis has developed sepsis, what additional signs and symptoms should you anticipate?

Conditions of the Ear

As described in Chapter 10, *Review of Human Systems*, the ear can be divided into three portions: the external ear, middle ear, and inner ear. The external ear and middle ear are involved in hearing only. The inner ear functions in both hearing and balance (**FIGURE 22-10**). Common medical conditions that affect the ear are listed in **BOX 22-3**.

Foreign Body

A foreign body in the ear is a fairly common occurrence, especially in toddlers. Most foreign bodies are lodged in the ear canal. Common objects found in the ears of young children include food material and toys that awre usually inserted voluntarily. Children and adults, whether they are awake or asleep, are also subject to insects that enter the ear canal. Foreign bodies in the ear are often easily detected by complaints of pressure, discomfort, and decreased hearing in the affected ear. (If the foreign body stays undetected, serious infection can result.) Bleeding from the ear can also occur if the foreign body is sharp or is manipulated during attempts to remove it.

NOTE

It is not uncommon for young children to have multiple foreign bodies inserted in both ears and the nose. The paramedic should be alert for this possibility. All children should be reminded not to put anything smaller than an elbow in the ear or nose. Live bugs have been known to crawl into the ear canal. This can be particularly distressing if movement of the bug can be felt. The paramedic can place mineral oil or alcohol in the ear canal to kill the insect and thus decrease the patient's distress. The ears will need to be irrigated.

Foreign bodies in the ear are seldom a serious medical condition that requires emergency care. Most objects can be easily removed at a physician's office

BOX 22-3 Conditions That Affect the Ear

- Foreign body
- Impacted cerumen
- Labyrinthitis
- Ménière disease
- Otitis media
- Perforated tympanic membrane

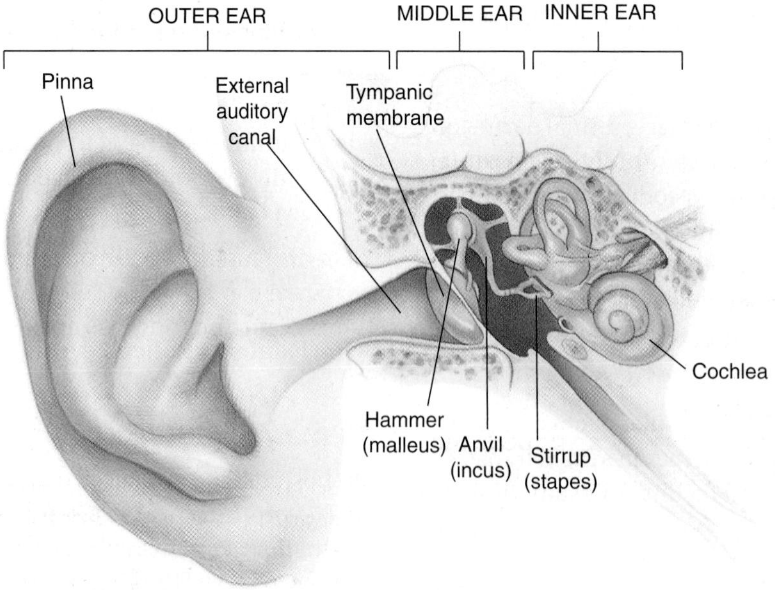

FIGURE 22-10 Anatomy of the ear.

or clinic. Some foreign bodies do require immediate removal in the emergency department (ED). These objects include button-type batteries that can cause chemical burns and food and plant material that can swell when moistened. If the patient complains of significant pain or discomfort, immediate evaluation by a physician is also indicated.

Management Considerations

Prehospital care for foreign bodies in the ear is limited to gentle examination of the external auditory canal. This can be done by gently pulling back on the ear's pinna (changing the shape of the ear canal) and viewing the canal with a penlight or ear speculum. Objects that are visible may sometimes be easily removed with alligator forceps. Care should be taken not to push the object deeper into the canal, which can make the object more difficult to retrieve and may also damage the eardrum. Patients who require physician evaluation should be advised not to eat or drink before their examination because sedation may be needed to safely remove the foreign body. In-hospital care may include diagnostic imaging, irrigation of the ear canal, suction, surgical removal of the foreign body, and prescribed antibiotics.

> CRITICAL THINKING
> What additional signs and symptoms might your patient experience if there is a live insect in his or her ear?

Impacted Cerumen

As described in Chapter 10, *Review of Human Systems*, **cerumen** (earwax) is produced normally by the ceruminous glands that are located in the external auditory canal. Cerumen protects and lubricates the skin of the ear canal and provides some protection from bacteria, fungi, insects, and water. Cerumen is a yellow waxy substance that has the consistency of toothpaste. Excess cerumen can become impacted, pressing up against the eardrum and creating a foreign body in the ear. Excessive cerumen can impede the passage of sound in the ear canal, causing hearing loss. Signs and symptoms of impacted cerumen include the following:

- Earache, fullness in the ear, or a sensation that the ear is plugged
- Partial hearing loss, which may be progressive
- Tinnitus, ringing, or noises in the ear
- Itching, odor, or discharge
- Coughing

Many patients regularly clean their ears of excess cerumen with cotton-tipped swabs. This is a dangerous practice that can push the cerumen deeper into the ear. It is recommended that cerumen not be removed from the ear canal, unless the cerumen is impacted.[19] Most forms of ear blockage respond well to home treatments to soften the wax. These treatments include irrigation and syringing with warm water or saline and wax-dissolving drops (eg, mineral oil, baby oil, glycerin, other commercial drops). Ear candles may cause injury and are not recommended.[19]

> NOTE
> Ears should not be irrigated if a person has diabetes, a perforated eardrum, a tube in the eardrum, or a weakened immune system.
>
> *Modified from*: Schwartz SR, Magit AE, Rosenfield RM, et al. Clinical practice guideline (update): earwax (cerumen impaction). *Otolaryngol Head Neck Surg*. 2017;156(suppl 1):S1-S29.

Management Considerations

Prehospital care for a patient with impacted cerumen is primarily supportive. Patients should be encouraged to see a physician for wax removal. This is most often performed by an otolaryngologist using special equipment and techniques.

Labyrinthitis

Labyrinthitis is an ear disorder that involves irritation and swelling of the inner ear structure called the labyrinth (described in Chapter 10, *Review of Human Systems*). Inflammation of this balance-control area in the ear can cause sudden **vertigo**. It may also cause a temporary hearing loss and a ringing sound in the

> NOTE
> Vertigo is an uncomfortable feeling when there is no actual movement. It is commonly described as spinning or whirling. It may also include the sensations of falling or tilting. Vertigo may cause nausea and vomiting and may impair the patient's ability to walk or stand. Vertigo and ataxia (failure of muscle coordination) also can signal stroke (see Chapter 25, *Endocrinology*).

ears (**tinnitus**). Labyrinthitis can result from a viral infection or, more rarely, a bacterial infection. Common triggers are an upper respiratory tract infection and middle ear infection.

Management Considerations

Prehospital care for patients with labyrinthitis is primarily supportive. Patients should be advised to be careful of falling and to have assistance when walking. Most cases of labyrinthitis resolve without treatment. If infection is to blame, antibiotics may be prescribed. Antiemetics may be prescribed for symptoms of nausea and vomiting.

Ménière Disease

Ménière disease is an abnormality of the inner ear. Like labyrinthitis, this disease causes vertigo and tinnitus and is associated with fluctuations in hearing loss and a sensation of pressure or pain in the affected ear. The symptoms of Ménière disease are associated with a change in fluid volume in the labyrinth. Causes of the disease may include environmental factors, such as noise pollution, viral infection, and biologic factors. It is estimated that about 615,000 Americans have been diagnosed with the disease and that 45,500 new cases are diagnosed each year.[20]

The classic presentation of Ménière disease is a combination of vertigo, tinnitus, and hearing loss that lasts several hours. The symptoms occur suddenly. Episodes can be as frequent as once per day or as infrequent as once per year. The vertigo is often debilitating and can lead to severe nausea and vomiting. Other symptoms of the disease may include headache, abdominal discomfort, and diarrhea.

Management Considerations

Like most other conditions that affect the ear, prehospital care for a patient with Ménière disease is primarily supportive. There is no cure for the illness. Physician care may include medications and diet restrictions to reduce fluid retention. Drug therapy to improve blood circulation in the inner ear may also be prescribed. Eliminating tobacco use and reducing stress may help with the severity of the symptoms.

CRITICAL THINKING

What other conditions in addition to labyrinthitis and Ménière disease can cause vertigo?

Benign Paroxysmal Positional Vertigo

Benign paroxysmal positional vertigo (BPPV) is the most common cause of vertigo. The condition accounts for at least 20% of patients in the United States who present with vertigo (about 200,000 cases each year).[21] It is considered rare in children but can occur in adults, especially those over age 60.[22] The condition occurs when calcium carbonate crystals normally in the utricle become dislodged, allowing them to move into one (or several) of the semicircular canals. The accumulation and movement of these particles within the canal or canals interferes with normal fluid movement for sensing motion of the head, causing nystagmus and vertigo. The nystagmus and vertigo end when the crystals stop moving. BPPV is frequently misdiagnosed. It can also be accompanied by other inner ear diseases (for example, Ménière disease). The effects of BPPV usually have a limited duration (less than 20 seconds) and subside when the head is moved out of the position that produced it.

Management Considerations

Prehospital care is primarily supportive. Following physician evaluation, treatment options for BPPV include monitoring the condition, vestibulosuppressant medication, vestibular rehabilitation, head maneuvers to move the crystals out of the semicircular canals, and in severe cases, surgery. Treatment for BPPV is about 90% effective.[23]

Otitis Media

Otitis media is infection or inflammation of the middle ear. It most commonly affects infants and young children but can also occur in adults. The condition is the most common affliction requiring medical therapy for children younger than 5 years of age.[24]

Otitis media occurs between the eardrum and inner ear and involves the eustachian tube (**FIGURE 22-11**). Otitis often begins with viral or bacterial infections that cause sore throats, colds, or other respiratory problems that spread to the middle ear. Otitis media can be acute or chronic. Signs and symptoms of otitis media include the following:

- Chills
- Diarrhea
- Drainage from the ear
- Earache

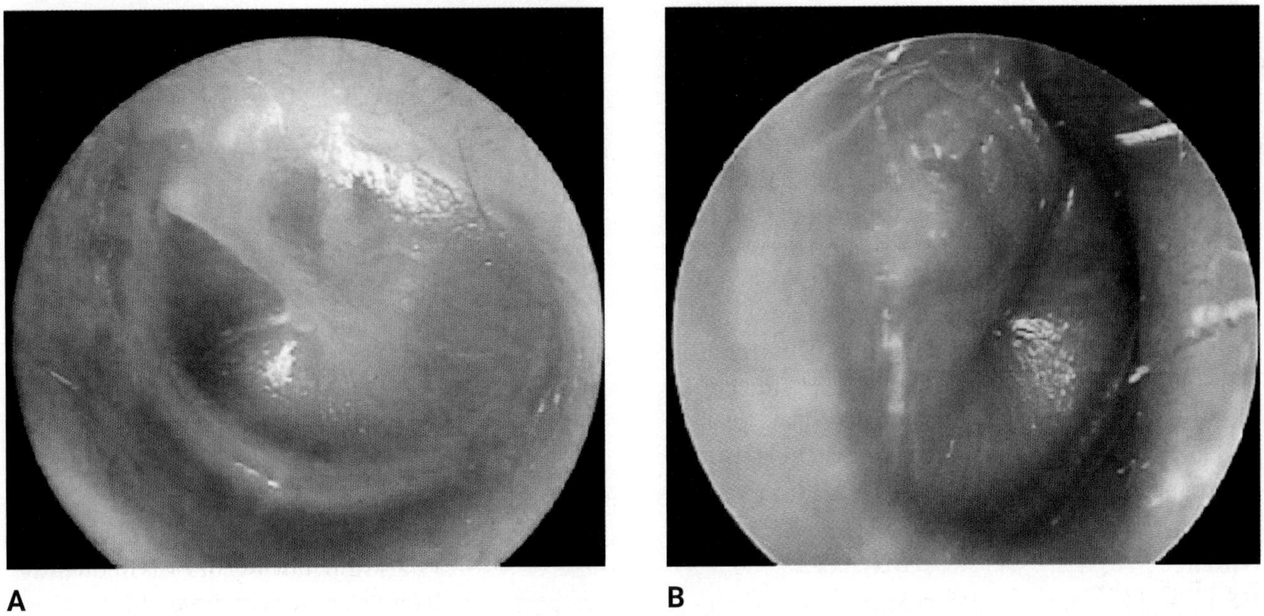

FIGURE 22-11 **A.** Normal tympanic membrane. **B.** Tympanic membrane with otitis media.

Reproduced from: Kuruvilla A, Shaikh N, Hoberman A, and Kovačević J, Automated diagnosis of otitis media: vocabulary and grammar. *Int J Biomed Imaging*. 2013(1):1-15.

- Ear noise or buzzing
- Fever
- Hearing loss
- Discomfort in the ear or ear canal
- Irritability
- General malaise
- Nausea
- Vomiting

Otitis media causes severe pain and can have serious consequences. If untreated, the infection can travel from the middle ear to the brain and may lead to permanent hearing loss. Because the illness often strikes small children with limited speech and communication skills, the paramedic should be attuned to subtle signs and symptoms such as irritability, tugging at the ear, fever, and drainage from the ear. Parents or other caregivers may notice a loss of balance, sleeplessness, and signs of hearing difficulty.

NOTE

Infants and children are more prone to ear infections than are adults. This susceptibility is due in part to the immature immune system of children. It is also related to a child's straighter and shorter eustachian tube that allows bacteria to reach the middle ear and larger adenoids that lie close to the eustachian tube. Enlarged adenoids can interfere with eustachian tube opening and, if infected, can spread the infection through the tube. It is estimated that 75% of children have at least one episode of otitis media by their third birthday. One-half of these children will have three or more ear infections during their first 3 years.

Modified from: Ear infections in children. National Institute on Deafness and Other Communication Disorders website. https://www.nidcd.nih.gov/health/ear-infections-children. Updated May 12, 2017. Accessed October 7, 2017.

Management Considerations

Children with otitis media need to be evaluated by a physician. Until such time, the child should avoid contact with other children who are sick; the child should not be exposed to environmental smoke, which may aggravate the condition. Physician assessment will include an otoscope examination of the outer ear and eardrum. Various tests may also be used to assess middle ear fluid, eardrum movement, and hearing. Prescribed medications may include antibiotics for a bacterial infection and agents to reduce pain and fever. Once the infection is eradicated, fluid may remain in the middle ear for several months. Follow-up with a physician is required. Other treatments may include surgical removal of the adenoids and the placement of tubes in the affected ears (myringotomy) to equalize the pressure in the middle ear. These procedures often are done at the same time.

Perforated Tympanic Membrane

Perforated tympanic membrane is a hole or rupture in the eardrum. The cause of perforation is usually trauma or infection. Examples of traumatic causes of perforated tympanic membrane include blunt trauma to the ear, barotrauma, skull fracture, explosion or blast injury, and foreign bodies in the ear (see section on Trauma). Otitis media is an example of an infection that can cause a perforated tympanic membrane (otitis media with perforation). Signs and symptoms of perforation caused by infection are those of middle ear infections (described previously) and include decreased hearing and an occasional bloody discharge. Pain is usually not persistent with perforation.

Management Considerations

Perforations of the tympanic membrane often cause a patient to be anxious, especially if the perforation is related to trauma. However, prehospital care is primarily supportive. Most perforations of the eardrum heal without treatment within weeks of the rupture, although some perforations may take several months to heal. During the healing process, the affected ear should be protected from water and trauma. Perforations that do not heal on their own require advanced technologies and/or surgical intervention to close the tympanic membrane. These techniques often will restore or improve hearing.

The amount of hearing loss associated with perforations is related to the size and location of the hole in the tympanic membrane. A large hole that is close to inner ear structures will cause a greater hearing loss that may be severe. Chronic infection that results from perforation may also lead to progressive loss of hearing. Patients must be evaluated by a physician to determine the underlying cause.

Conditions of the Nose

As described in Chapter 10, *Review of Human Systems*, the nose is the organ of smell (**FIGURE 22-12**). The nose is composed of several components:

- **External meatus.** The triangular projection in the center of the face
- **External nostrils.** Two chambers divided by the septum
- **Septum.** A structure composed primarily of cartilage and bone and covered by mucous membranes

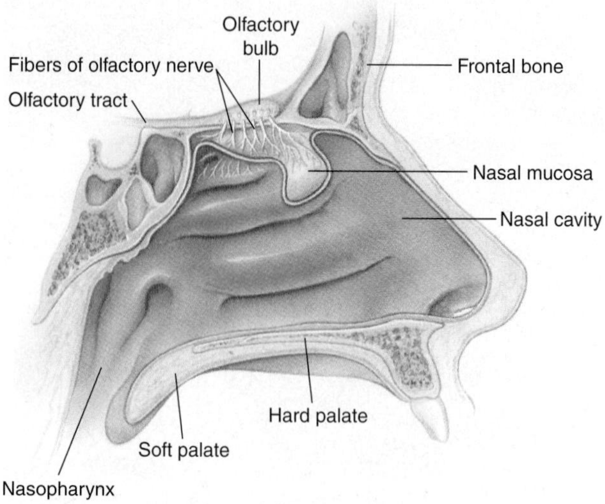

FIGURE 22-12 Anatomy of the nasal cavity.

Modified from: Shade BR. *Mosby's EMT-Intermediate for the 1999 National Standard Curriculum*. 3rd ed. St. Louis, MO: Mosby; 2007.

BOX 22-4 Conditions That Affect the Nose

Epistaxis
Foreign body
Rhinitis
Sinusitis

- **Nasal passages.** Passages that are lined with mucous membranes and cilia
- **Sinuses.** Four pairs of air-filled cavities, also lined with mucous membranes

Common conditions that affect the nose are listed in BOX 22-4.

Epistaxis

Epistaxis is acute hemorrhage from the nostril, nasal cavity, or nasopharynx (**FIGURE 22-13**). It occurs in about 60% of the population.[25] Bleeding from epistaxis is most commonly anterior, originating from the nasal septum. Less common is posterior bleeding, originating from the posterior nasal cavity or nasopharynx. Local trauma (nose picking) is the most common cause of epistaxis. This cause is followed by facial trauma, foreign bodies, nasal or sinus infection, and prolonged breathing of dry air. Less common causes of or risk factors for epistaxis include the following:[26]

- Nasogastric and nasotracheal intubation
- Topical nasal drugs

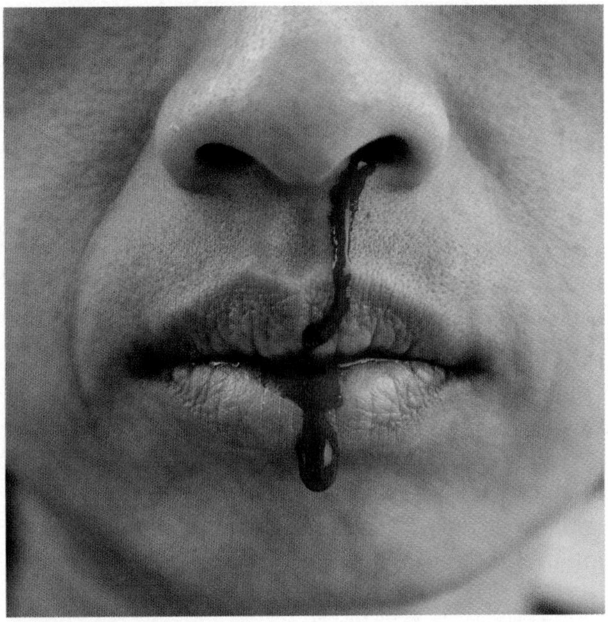

FIGURE 22-13 Epistaxis.

© Phathn Sakdi Skul Phanthu/EyeEm/Getty Images.

SHOW ME THE EVIDENCE

Ambulances in one region of the Netherlands were equipped with HemCon nasal plugs, a type of nasal tampon. The tampon is a sponge that expands on contact with fluid, swelling to fill the nasal cavity and applying pressure over the bleeding area. The study objective was to determine the effectiveness of the nasal plugs to stop bleeding in severe epistaxis. The nasal plugs were inserted when the patient's nosebleed did not stop within 15 minutes of applying standard treatment. The device was used 33 times within 2.5 years. The nasal plugs stopped bleeding in 25 patients. In all instances where the device failed, the emergency medical services personnel stated it was too short to reach the location of bleeding. They found the device to be effective and well-tolerated by patients.

Modified from: Te Grotenhuis R, van Grunsven PM, Heutz WMJM, Tan, ECTH. Use of hemostatic nasal plugs in emergency medical services in the Netherlands: a prospective study of 33 cases. *Prehosp Emerg Care.* 2018;22(1):91-98.

- Upper respiratory tract infection (especially in children)
- Oral anticoagulants
- Medical conditions that affect coagulation, such as splenomegaly, thrombocytopenia, hemophilia, platelet disorders, liver disease, renal failure, chronic alcohol use, or conditions relating ot acquired immunodeficiency syndrome (AIDS)
- Dry climates
- Vascular abnormalities (eg, sclerosis, neoplasm, aneurysm, endometriosis)
- Use of cocaine or other drugs that are inhaled

NOTE

Epistaxis (nosebleeding) can occur at any age but is most common in children ages 2 to 10 years and in adults ages 45 to 65 years. For unknown reasons, nosebleeds most commonly occur in the morning hours.

Modified from: Approach to the adult with epistaxis. UpToDate website. https://www.uptodate.com/contents/approach-to-the-adult-with-epistaxis. Updated July 26, 2017. Accessed February 10, 2018.

Management Considerations

Most nosebleeds can be visualized in the anterior portion of the nasal cavity. If not, the source of bleeding is likely posterior. This is especially true if the bleeding is coming from both nares or if blood is draining into the posterior pharynx. Significant blood can be lost during a posterior nosebleed. Complications such as hypovolemia, myocardial infarction, stroke, respiratory distress, or aspiration can occur, particular in older adults or in patients who take anticoagulants.[27] If time permits, the patient should be questioned about previous nosebleeds, medication use that may cause or worsen epistaxis (eg, aspirin, nonsteroidal anti-inflammatory drugs, dabigatran [Pradaxa], rivaroxaban [Xarelto], apixaban [Eliquis] or warfarin [Coumadin]), hypertension, family history, and preexisting disease.

NOTE

Hypertension is rarely a direct cause of epistaxis. Patients with epistaxis usually have an elevated blood pressure because of their anxiety. However, nosebleeds in hypertensive patients are more often caused by long-standing disease and not the hypertension. Management should focus on controlling hemorrhage and reducing anxiety as the primary means of blood pressure reduction.

Prehospital care for epistaxis consists of controlling the hemorrhage and calming the patient (**FIGURE 22-14**). To control bleeding, the conscious patient should be positioned upright and leaning forward. (An unconscious patient should be positioned

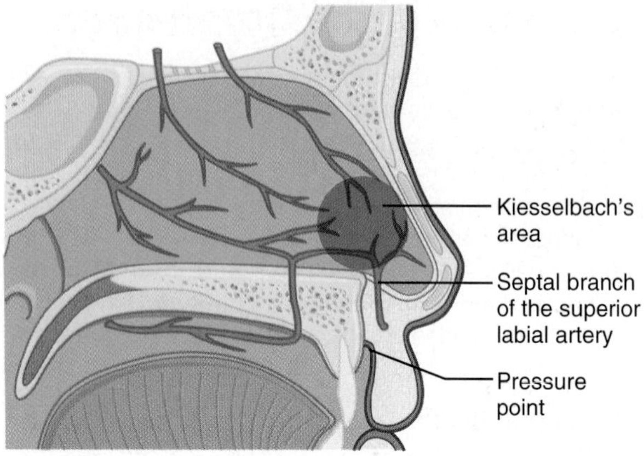

FIGURE 22-14 Blood vessels involved in epistaxis, and pressure point.

Modified from: Kulig K. Epistaxis. In: Rosen P, et al. *Emergency Medicine: Concepts and Clinical Practice.* St. Louis, MO: Mosby; 1983.

on the side, if doing so is not complicated by injury.) Direct pressure should be applied midway on the nose for about 5 minutes or until bleeding subsides. These measures are often unsuccessful if there is a posterior bleed. An emesis basin should be nearby to catch any blood or drainage. Packing the nose to control bleeding should not be attempted in the prehospital setting. If bleeding is severe or prolonged, the patient should be treated for shock and transported for physician evaluation.

Foreign Body

A foreign body placed in the ear or nose is a common occurrence. Beans or other foodstuffs, beads, paper wads, and eraser tips are frequently found in the noses of young children. The foreign bodies usually lodge on the floor of the anterior or middle third of the nasal cavity. Most cases are not serious, and most foreign bodies can be easily removed by a physician. Signs and symptoms of a foreign body in the nose include obstruction to airflow in the affected nostril, nasal discomfort, tearing, and unilateral nasal discharge (sometimes foul smelling). Objects that make it to the mouth become a risk for aspiration.

> NOTE
>
> If a child has inserted a foreign body in the nose, suspect that more than one object has been placed. The ears of the child should also be inspected for foreign bodies.

Management Considerations

Prehospital care for foreign bodies in the nose is limited to gentle examination of the nares. A cooperative patient may be coached to blow his or her nose to try to expel the foreign body. Foreign bodies that are easily visible may be removed with alligator forceps. The patient must be cooperative, and special care must be taken not to push the object deeper into the nasal cavity. Most likely, the patient will require physician evaluation and topical anesthesia. Small children may need to be restrained or sedated for the examination. Methods to remove foreign bodies in the nose include removal by forceps and irrigation or use of an indwelling urinary catheter. After the catheter is passed beyond the foreign body, the balloon is inflated and the object is pulled out through the nose.

Rhinitis

Rhinitis is commonly known as a runny nose. The term is used to describe irritation and inflammation of the mucous membranes of the nose, often caused by a virus, bacteria, or allergens (allergic rhinitis). A foreign body in the nose can also cause rhinitis. The hallmark feature of rhinitis is nasal drip caused by an increase in histamine production. The increase in the amount of histamine increases the production of mucus. Other symptoms of rhinitis include nasal congestion and itchy eyes and nose.

Management Considerations

Prehospital care for a patient with rhinitis is primarily supportive. Emergency care or transport is seldom needed. Patients should be advised to follow up with their physicians if symptoms persist. Treatment for rhinitis usually consists of the use of antihistamines, avoidance of exposure to suspected allergens or irritants, and sometimes administration of antibiotics if the cause is bacterial.

Sinusitis

Sinusitis (sinus infection) is inflammation of the sinuses and nasal passages. The condition can be caused by a viral, bacterial, or fungal infection. Symptoms of sinusitis include headache and pressure in the eyes, nose, or cheek area. Often the discomfort is limited to one side of the head. Sinusitis may also be associated with a cough, fever, bad breath (halitosis), and nasal congestion. The nasal congestion can produce thick nasal secretions. Sinusitis affects 37 million people each year, making it a common health condition in the United States.[28]

As described in Chapter 10, *Review of Human Systems*, the paranasal sinuses are four pairs of air-filled sacs that connect the space between the nostrils and the nasal passages. These include the frontal sinuses (in the forehead), the maxillary sinuses (behind the cheekbones), the ethmoid sinuses (between the eyes), and the sphenoid sinuses (midline within the sphenoid bone). Normally, mucus that collects in the sinuses drains into the nasal passages and is eliminated from the body. When a patient has a cold or allergy, the sinuses can become inflamed and unable to drain, leading to congestion and infection. Sinusitis can be acute or chronic (lasting 3 months or more). Chronic sinusitis can damage the sinuses and cheekbones and can sometimes require surgical intervention.

Management Considerations

Prehospital care for patients with sinusitis is primarily supportive. Because the signs and symptoms are easily confused with those of a cold or allergy, the chart in BOX 22-5 can aid in a differential diagnosis. Patients should be encouraged to follow up with their physicians, who may prescribe antibiotics for bacterial infection, antihistamines, and decongestants.

Conditions of the Oropharynx and Throat

As described in Chapter 10, *Review of Human Systems*, the oropharynx begins at the level of the uvula and extends down to the level of the epiglottis. The oropharynx opens into the oral cavity. This cavity contains the lips, cheeks, teeth, tongue, hard and soft palates, and palatine tonsils. The throat is the anterior portion of the neck, located in front of the vertebral column. The throat consists of the pharynx and larynx. It also contains the epiglottis, which separates the esophagus from the trachea (**FIGURE 22-15**). BOX 22-6 lists common conditions that affect these structures.

Toothache and Dental Abscess

The medical term for toothache is **dentalgia**. Toothache usually refers to pain around the teeth or jaws. Common causes of toothache include dental cavities, **dental abscess** (a bacterial infection in the center of the tooth), a cracked tooth, an exposed tooth root, and gum disease. The most common cause of toothache is a dental cavity; the second most common cause is gum disease.

The normal adult mouth has 32 teeth. Each tooth consists of two sections: the crown and the root. The crown projects above the oral mucosa around the

BOX 22-5 Signs and Symptoms of Sinusitis, Allergy, and Cold

Sign/Symptom	Sinusitis	Allergy	Cold
Facial pressure/pain	Yes	Sometimes	Sometimes
Duration of illness	More than 10 days	Varies	Less than 10 days
Nasal discharge	White or colored	Clear, thin, watery	Thick, white, or thin
Fever	Sometimes	No	Sometimes
Headache	Sometimes	Sometimes	Sometimes
Pain in upper teeth	Sometimes	No	No
Bad breath	Sometimes	No	No
Coughing	Sometimes	Sometimes	Yes
Nasal congestion	Yes	Sometimes	Yes
Sneezing	No	Sometimes	Yes

Modified from: Sinusitis—more than just a cold or allergy. Ear, Nose, and Throat SpecialtyCare website. http://www.entsc.com/patient-corner/educational-brochures/sinusitis-more-than-just-a-cold-or-allery/. Accessed February 10, 2018.

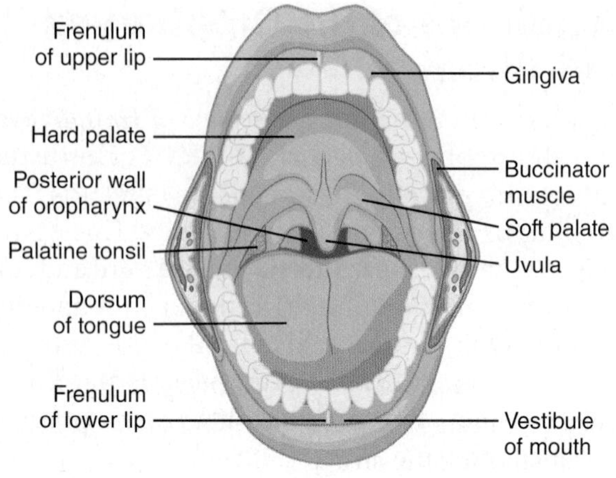

FIGURE 22-15 Anatomic structures of the oral cavity.

BOX 22-6 Conditions That Affect the Oropharynx and Throat

Toothache and dental abscess
Ludwig angina
Foreign body[a]
Epiglottitis
Laryngitis
Tracheitis
Oral candidiasis
Peritonsillar abscess
Pharyngitis/tonsillitis
Temporomandibular joint disorders

[a]Foreign body airway obstruction is described in Chapter 15, *Airway Management, Respiration, and Artificial Ventilation.*

tooth. The root fits into the bony socket of the maxilla or mandible. There are three layers that comprise the hard tissues of the teeth. They are the enamel, the dentin (ivory), and the cementum. The soft tissues of the teeth include the pulp and periodontal membrane (**FIGURE 22-16**). Symptoms of toothache include the following:

- Sharp, throbbing, or constant pain in the tooth
- Swelling around the tooth
- Fever or headache
- Foul-tasting drainage from infection of the tooth

Management Considerations

Prehospital care for a patient with a toothache is primarily supportive. Follow-up with a private dentist or oral surgeon should be recommended. Dental care will vary by the nature of the problem and may include cavity fill, tooth extraction, root canal, radiograph,

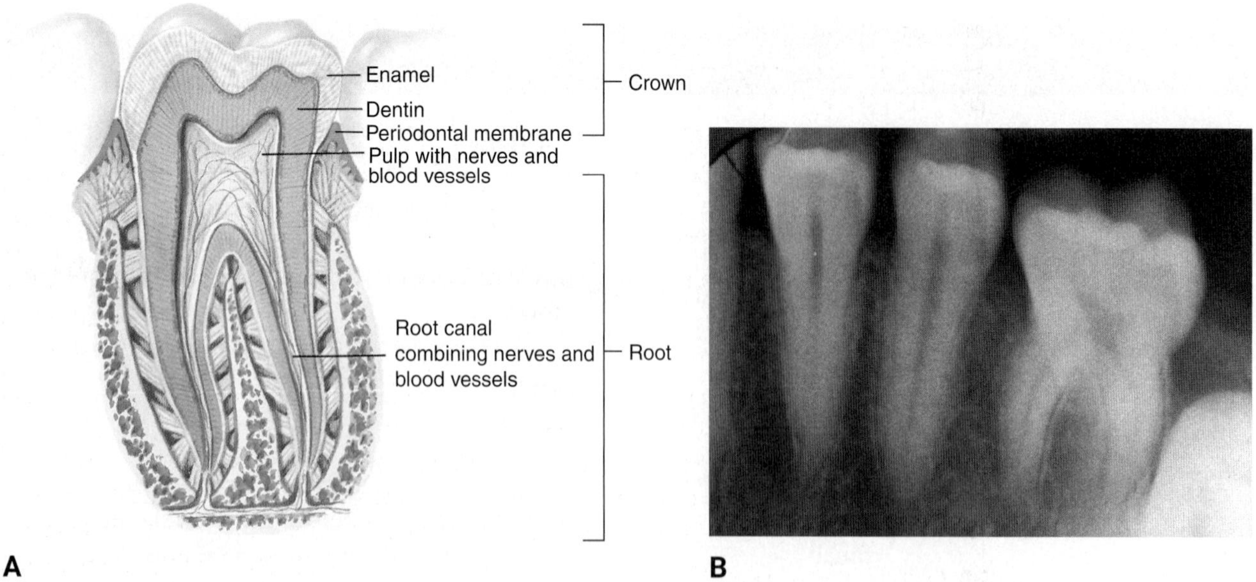

FIGURE 22-16 Tooth anatomy. **A.** Sagittal section of a lower molar. **B.** Radiograph of a healthy tooth.

phototherapy to reduce pain, and antibiotics to treat bacterial infection. Proper identification and treatment of dental infections are important. An infection that is not treated can spread to other parts of the face and skull and may even enter the bloodstream (sepsis). Prehospital care for the patient who has suffered dental trauma is addressed in Chapter 39, *Head, Face, and Neck Trauma.*

CRITICAL THINKING

What serious medical condition should be ruled out in high-risk patients who complain of tooth or jaw pain?

Ludwig Angina

Ludwig angina is a type of cellulitis that involves inflammation of the tissues of the floor of the mouth, under the tongue. It can occur following infection of the second or third mandibular molar or after peritonsillar abscess or infection of the parotid gland. Ludwig angina is most common in adults. The disease can cause bilateral swelling of the tissues that can occur rapidly. The swelling may block the airway or prevent swallowing of saliva. Signs and symptoms of Ludwig angina may include the following:[29]

- Breathing difficulty
- Dysphagia
- Fever and chills
- Stiff neck
- Neck swelling
- Redness of the neck
- Weakness, fatigue
- Drooling
- Earache
- Muffled voice
- Stridor

Management Considerations

Ludwig angina is a medical emergency that can be life threatening. Prehospital care may include airway and ventilatory support. Rapid transport to an ED is indicated. Physician care may include airway maintenance, computed tomography scan, blood cultures to identify the bacteria, IV antibiotics, and surgery to drain fluids that are causing the swelling. Although Ludwig angina can be successfully treated, possible complications include complete airway obstruction, sepsis, and septic shock. Intubation is often difficult, and a cricothyrotomy may be needed if intubation or ventilation of the patient is not possible.[30]

Epiglottitis

As the name implies, **epiglottitis** is inflammation of the epiglottis. The disease is caused by a bacterial infection that can lead to life-threatening airway obstruction. It can occur at any age. The bacterial infection causes edema and swelling of the epiglottis and supraglottic structures. The disease usually begins suddenly in children and frequently occurs after a child goes to bed. Signs and symptoms include dyspnea, sore throat, pain on swallowing, drooling, fever, and a muffled hot potato voice (as if speaking with a hot potato in the mouth), followed by stridor.[31]

NOTE

The HiB vaccine has greatly reduced the number of cases of epiglottitis in children.

Modified from: Epidemiology and prevention of vaccine-preventable diseases: *Haemophilus influenzae* type b. Centers for Disease Control and Prevention website. https://www.cdc.gov/vaccines/pubs/pinkbook/hib.html. Updated September 29, 2015. Accessed February 10, 2018.

Management Considerations

Epiglottitis is a serious emergency that requires prompt recognition and immediate transport for definitive care (see Chapter 47, *Pediatrics*). Airway occlusion can occur suddenly. This can be precipitated by minor irritation of the throat, aggravation, and anxiety. It is, therefore, important that these patients be handled gently. Patients with suspected epiglottitis should not lie down. They should be transported in a position of comfort that helps them breathe and facilitate drainage of oral fluids. IV access should not be attempted in the field to avoid creating anxiety and agitation in the child. High-concentration oxygen should be applied by mask unless it provokes anxiety. If respiratory arrest occurs before ED arrival, ventilation with a bag-mask device should be attempted, and the patient should be intubated by the most experienced paramedic because intubation will likely be difficult. In-hospital care may include airway and circulatory support, placement of a surgical airway, and IV antibiotic therapy.

Laryngitis

Laryngitis is swelling and irritation of the larynx that inflames the vocal cords. It is usually associated with hoarseness or loss of voice and swollen glands and lymph nodes in the neck. The most common form of laryngitis is caused by a virus and often occurs along with an upper respiratory tract infection. Other causes include allergies, bacterial infection, bronchitis, pneumonia, influenza, and exposure to irritants or chemicals.

Management Considerations

Laryngitis is usually not a serious condition and typically improves without treatment. (Only rarely does respiratory distress develop.) Prehospital care is primarily supportive. Patients should be encouraged to follow up with their physician if symptoms persist. Recommendations may include resting the voice and humidifying the air at home. Drug therapy may include analgesics, decongestants, and antibiotics if the infection is bacterial. Young children with laryngitis may need to be seen by a specialist for further evaluation.

Tracheitis

Tracheitis is a bacterial infection of the upper airway and subglottic trachea. The major site of the disease is at the level of the cricoid cartilage, the narrowest part of the trachea. The disease generally occurs in infants and toddlers (1 to 5 years of age), but it can also occur in older children. It frequently follows a viral upper respiratory tract infection (see Chapter 47, *Pediatrics*). Signs and symptoms are those of respiratory distress or respiratory failure (depending on severity). They include agitation, high-grade fever, inspiratory and expiratory stridor, productive cough, hoarseness, and throat pain.

> NOTE
>
> Tracheitis is an uncommon infectious cause of upper airway obstruction but is more prevalent than acute epiglottitis.
>
> *Modified from:* Virbalas J, Smith L. Upper airway obstruction. *Pediatr Rev.* 2015;36(2):62-73.

Management Considerations

Emergency care is focused on providing airway, ventilatory, and circulatory support, and rapid transport to an appropriate medical facility. If respiratory failure or arrest develops in the field, tracheal intubation and tracheal suction are indicated. (High-pressure bag-mask ventilation may be needed because of airway swelling and accumulation of mucus or pus.) In-hospital care will include IV antibiotics after the child's airway has been stabilized.

Oral Candidiasis

Oral candidiasis (also known as *thrush*) is an infection of yeast fungi of the genus *Candida*. It affects the mucous membranes of the mouth. The infection usually appears as thick white or cream-colored deposits on the mucosal membranes (**FIGURE 22-17**). The area may appear inflamed and can be painful. Bleeding can occur from irritation of the area. Oral candidiasis most commonly affects infants and toddlers, and those with impaired immune function. The disease is contagious but is seldom passed from person to person if immune systems are healthy. People at risk for oral candidiasis include the following:

- Newborns
- Those with diabetes
- Those taking antibiotics or inhaled corticosteroids
- Those with immune deficiencies (human immunodeficiency virus [HIV], AIDS, cancer)
- Those with oral piercings
- Denture wearers

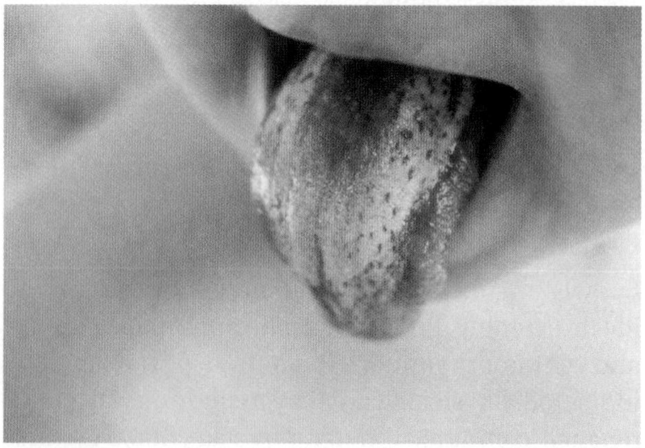

FIGURE 22-17 White, curdlike plaques of thrush (oral candidiasis, oral moniliasis), a common fungal infection in infants.

Management Considerations

Emergency care is seldom required for patients with oral candidiasis. Physician care generally includes the use of topical or oral antifungal drugs. In severe cases, IV antifungal drugs may be needed.

Peritonsillar Abscess

Peritonsillar abscess (also called PTA or quinsy) is a collection of pus in and around one or both tonsils. The abscesses form in the area between the palatine tonsil and its capsule. It is a complication of tonsillitis (infection of the tonsils) and is the most common deep infection of the head and neck in adults. It is most common in people 20 to 40 years of age who have chronic tonsillitis.[32] Presenting symptoms include fever, throat pain, dysphagia, voice changes, drooling, bad breath, swollen lymph nodes in the neck, deviation of the uvula to one side, erythema of the tonsil, and **trismus** (muscle spasms of the jaw).

Management Considerations

Prehospital care for the patient with peritonsillar abscess is primarily supportive. Physician care may include ultrasound, antibiotics, and procedures to remove the abscess material. These procedures may include needle aspiration or incision and drainage. Tonsillectomy may also be indicated.

Pharyngitis and Tonsillitis

Pharyngitis and **tonsillitis** are infections in the throat that cause inflammation. If the tonsils are primarily affected, it is called tonsillitis. If the throat is primarily affected, it is called pharyngitis. Inflammation of the throat usually is associated with an underlying illness. The most common cause of inflammation is a virus, but the inflammation may also be caused by bacteria (especially streptococci), resulting in **strep throat**. Signs and symptoms that accompany pharyngitis and tonsillitis depend on underlying illness, such as the common cold, influenza, and **mononucleosis**:[33]

- Sore throat with common cold:
  - Sneezing
  - Cough
  - Low-grade fever (temperature less than 102°F [38.9°C])
  - Mild headache
- Sore throat with flu:
  - Fatigue
  - Body aches
  - Chills
  - Fever (temperature higher than 102°F [38.9°C])
- Sore throat with mononucleosis:
  - Extreme fatigue
  - Enlarged lymph nodes in the neck and armpits
  - Swollen tonsils
  - Headache and body aches
  - Loss of appetite
  - Swollen spleen, liver, or both
  - Rash

> NOTE
>
> Tonsillitis may be caused by a bacterial or a viral infection. The condition may be acute, recurrent, or chronic.
>
> Nearly all children in the United States have at least one episode of tonsillitis. Complications associated with the disease are rare. The herpes simplex virus, *Streptococcus pyogenes* (GABHS), Epstein-Barr virus (EBV), cytomegalovirus, adenovirus, and the measles virus cause most cases of acute pharyngitis and acute tonsillitis.
>
> *Modified from*: Tonsillitis. American Academy of Otolaryngology—Head and Neck Surgery website. http://www.entnet.org/content/tonsillitis. Accessed February 11, 2018.

Management Considerations

Prehospital care for a patient with pharyngitis or tonsillitis is primarily supportive. Emergency care is seldom needed. Physician care may include antihistamines, cough suppressants, and antipyretics. Throat cultures and blood analyses may be needed if a bacterial infection requiring antibiotics or mononucleosis is suspected. Severe or recurrent tonsillitis may require tonsillectomy.

> CRITICAL THINKING
>
> What complications may occur if a patient's pharyngitis is related to strep throat and is not treated?

Temporomandibular Joint Disorders

The temporomandibular joint (TM joint) is the joint on each side of the head in front of the ears where the mandible meets the temporal bones (**FIGURE 22-18**).

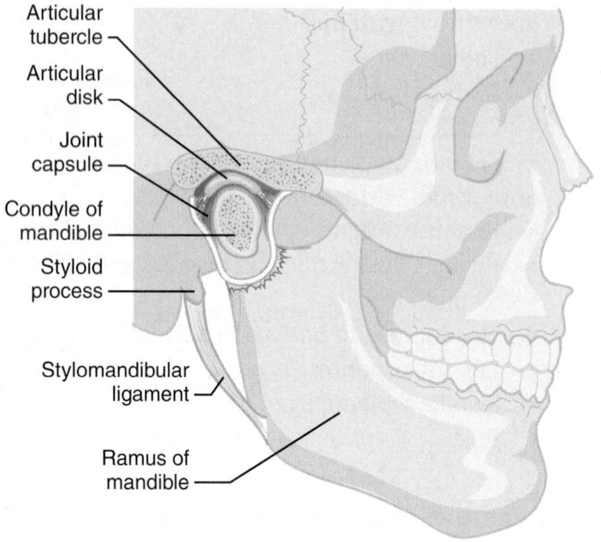

FIGURE 22-18 Structures of the temporomandibular joint.

Modified from: From Seidel H, et al. *Mosby's Guide to Physical Examination*. 6th ed. St. Louis, MO: Mosby; Figure 21-4, page 695.

Temporomandibular (TM) joint disorders are a set of conditions that cause pain in the area of the joint. They may also involve associated muscles and can cause problems using the jaw. One or both of the TM joints may be affected. The disorders can influence a person's ability to speak, eat, chew, swallow, and make facial expressions. In severe cases, TM joint disorders can affect a person's ability to breathe. TM joint disorders affect about 35 million people in the United States. Most who seek treatment are women in their childbearing years.[34]

Some of the causes of TM joint disorders are not clearly understood. Risk factors for developing the disorders include jaw injury, arthritis, dental procedures, infection, autoimmune disease, endotracheal intubation where the jaw is stretched to visualize the airway, and clenching or grinding of the teeth. TM joint disorders may also be a symptom of other diseases such as sinus or ear infection, periodontal disease, headaches, and facial neuralgia. Poor diet, stress, and lack of sleep may also contribute to the disease. Common complaints associated with TM joint disorders include the following:

- Pain in the neck and shoulders
- Headache
- Jaw muscle stiffness
- Limited movement or locking of the jaw
- Painful clicking, popping, or grating in the jaw joint when opening or closing the mouth
- A change in the way the upper and lower teeth fit together or a bite that feels off
- Ringing in the ears
- Ear pain
- Decreased hearing
- Dizziness and vision problems

Management Considerations

The symptoms of TM joint disorders are usually temporary but may be painful. In addition, patients experiencing discomfort will often be anxious. Prehospital care should be focused on calming the patient and providing comfort measures. Physician care may include diagnostic tests of the head, neck, face, and jaw. A complete medical history will also be obtained to rule out other possible causes for the disorder. Health care professionals who may be involved in the patient's treatment and recovery include dentists, sleep specialists, ear, nose, and throat specialists, neurologists, endocrinologists, rheumatologists, and pain specialists.

Summary

- The eye is composed of both primary vision structures and accessory structures, which protect, lubricate, move, and aid in the function of the eye. Cranial nerves control vision, pupil constriction, and movement of the eyes. Consider nervous system disease if these functions are impaired.
- Conjunctivitis is inflammation or infection of the eye and is sometimes called pink eye. Infectious conjunctivitis is contagious.
- A corneal abrasion is a scrape or scratch of the cornea. It is very painful and may cause tearing, redness, and blurred vision. Patch the eye and administer a topical ophthalmic anesthetic if permitted by protocol.
- Foreign bodies in the eye are very painful and cause pain and tearing. Irrigation of the eye may be indicated to remove small foreign bodies.
- Two types of eyelid inflammation are chalazion (obstructed oil gland) and hordeolum (sty).
- Glaucoma is caused by an increase in intraocular pressure related to excess aqueous humor. This condition results in pressure on the optic nerve and can lead to blindness

if untreated. Signs and symptoms include loss of peripheral vision, eye pain, headache, vomiting, or blurred vision.

- Iritis is inflammation of the iris. It can cause blindness if untreated.
- Papilledema is swelling of the optic disc caused by an increase in intracranial pressure (ICP). The increased ICP may be related to illness or injury.
- The retina is the eye structure central to vision. Tears, breaks, or defects in the retina can cause retinal detachment. Without treatment, retinal detachment leads to blindness. Signs and symptoms include an increase in floaters, light flashes in the eye, or the appearance of a curtain over the field of vision.
- Retinal vascular occlusion refers to blockage of a vessel in the retina of the eye. It is a common cause of blindness, and can lead to loss of vision. Central retinal vein occlusion and central retinal artery occlusion are included in this grouping.
- Central retinal vein occlusion is blockage of blood supply to the main vein of the retina. Vision becomes blurry and may produce "floaters" in the field of vision. In severe cases, the patient experiences painful pressure in the eye and loss of vision in all or part of one eye. The outcome varies; patients often regain useful vision.
- Central retinal artery occlusion occurs when blood supply to the retina is blocked. If circulation is not reestablished within 4 hours of occlusion, permanent loss of vision occurs. Onset is marked by sudden, painless loss of vision or the sense that a shade has been pulled down over the eye.
- Orbital cellulitis is an infection of the tissue around the eye that can lead to blindness and other serious complications, such as hearing loss, septicemia, sinus thrombosis, and meningitis. Signs and symptoms include fever; pain and swelling of the eyelids; shiny, red or purple eyelid; eye pain; double vision; bulging eyes; malaise; and painful or difficult eye movement. Immediate treatment with IV antibiotics is essential.
- A foreign body in the ear is a fairly common occurrence, especially in toddlers. Both children and adults are subject to insects that enter the ear canal during sleep. Foreign bodies can be detected by complaints of pressure, discomfort, and decreased hearing in the affected ear. If the foreign body stays undetected, serious infection can result.
- When excess earwax (cerumen) accumulates in the ear, it can cause earache; hearing loss; tinnitus; itching, odor, or discharge; or coughing. Removal of the wax usually resolves the symptoms.
- Swelling of the inner ear causes labyrinthitis, which results in vertigo and tinnitus.
- Ménière disease causes vertigo, tinnitus, and hearing loss. It can lead to nausea and vomiting.
- Benign paroxysmal positional vertigo is a condition in which nystagmus and vertigo occur when calcium carbonate crystals normally in the utricle become dislodged, allowing them to move into one (or several) of the semicircular canals. Prehospital care is primarily supportive.
- Otitis media is an infection or inflammation of the middle ear. In addition to earache, it can produce a number of signs and symptoms.
- Infection or trauma can cause perforation of the tympanic membrane. Signs and symptoms of perforation caused by infection are those of middle ear infections and include decreased hearing and drainage from the affected ear.
- Epistaxis is bleeding from the structures of the nose or nasopharynx. Attempt to control epistaxis by positioning the patient upright, leaning forward. Apply direct pressure on the nose until bleeding is controlled. Treat for shock if indicated.
- It is common for children to place foreign bodies in their nose. Transport for physician examination and removal.
- Rhinitis is a runny nose. Common causes are infection, allergy, or foreign body in the nose.
- Sinusitis is inflammation of sinuses and nasal passages. Signs and symptoms include cough, fever, halitosis, nasal congestion, headache, and pressure sensation over the eyes, nose, or cheek.
- Toothache is frequently caused by tooth decay, abscess, cracked tooth, exposed root, or gum disease. Transport for definitive care and pain management.
- Ludwig angina is cellulitis of the tissues under the tongue. It can cause rapid tissue swelling and airway obstruction. Signs and symptoms include breathing difficulty; dysphagia; fever and chills; neck pain, stiffness, redness, or swelling; earache; muffled voice; weakness; or drooling. Urgent transport is needed.
- Epiglottitis is inflammation of the epiglottis caused by bacterial infection. It can lead to airway obstruction. Signs and symptoms include dyspnea, sore throat, pain on swallowing, fever, drooling, and muffled voice, followed by stridor. Airway obstruction is possible. Perform minimal interventions unless airway obstruction occurs.
- Laryngitis is a hoarse voice and swollen lymph nodes associated with inflamed vocal cords.
- Tracheitis is a bacterial infection of the upper airway and subglottic trachea. It can cause respiratory failure and arrest. Be prepared to manage the airway and assist with ventilation if needed.
- Oral candidiasis is a yeast fungal infection of the mouth. It covers the tongue and mucous membranes with a thick, white or cream-colored coating.

References

1. National Highway Traffic Safety Administration. *The National EMS Education Standards*. Washington, DC: US Department of Transportation/National Highway Traffic Safety Administration; 2009.
2. Facts about pink eye. National Eye Institute (NEI) website. https://nei.nih.gov/health/pinkeye/pink_facts. Accessed February 11, 2018.

3. Corneal abrasion symptoms. American Academy of Ophthalmology website. https://www.aao.org/eye-health/diseases/corneal-abrasion-symptoms. Published July 3, 2012. Accessed February 11, 2018.
4. Chalazion. MedlinePlus website. https://medlineplus.gov/ency/article/001006.htm. Updated December 21, 2017. Accessed February 11, 2018.
5. Chalazion. American Optometric Association website. https://www.aoa.org/patients-and-public/eye-and-vision-problems/glossary-of-eye-and-vision-conditions/chalazion. Accessed February 11, 2018.
6. The genetics of glaucoma. Glaucoma Research Foundation website. https://www.glaucoma.org/glaucoma/the-genetics-of-glaucoma-what-is-new.php. Accessed February 11, 2018.
7. Iritis overview. Iritis Organization website. http://www.iritis.org. Accessed February 11, 2018.
8. Retinal detachment. Mayo Clinic website. www.mayoclinic.com/health/retinal-detachment/DS00254. Accessed February 11, 2018.
9. Retinal detachment. National Eye Institute website. www.nei.nih.gov/health/retinaldetach. Accessed February 11, 2018.
10. Cheung N, Klein R, Wang JJ, et al. Traditional and novel cardiovascular risk factors for retinal vein occlusion: the multiethnic study of atherosclerosis. *Invest Ophthalmol Vis Sci.* 2008;49(10):4297-4302.
11. Klein R, Klein BE, Moss SE, et al. The epidemiology of retinal vein occlusion: the Beaver Dam Eye Study. *Trans Am Ophthalmol Soc.* 2000;98:133–141.
12. Rogers SL, McIntosh RL, Lim L, et al. Natural history of branch retinal vein occlusion: an evidence-based systematic review. *Ophthalmology*. 2010;117(6):1094-1101.
13. Woo SCY, Lip GYH, Lip PL. Associations of retinal artery occlusion and retinal vein occlusion to mortality, stroke, and myocardial infarction: a systematic review. *Eye.* 2016;30(8):1031-1038.
14. London NJ, Brown G. Update and review of central retinal vein occlusion. *Curr Opin Ophthalmol.* 2011;22(3):159-165.
15. Krzystolik MG, Greenberg PB. Retinal diseases and treatments. Southern New England Retinal Associates website. http://www.sneretina.com/retinal-diseases-and-treatments/retinal-vein-and-retinal-artery-occlusion.asp. Accessed March 23, 2018.
16. Varma DD, Cugati S, Lee AW, Chen CS. A review of central retinal artery occlusion: clinical presentation and management. *Eye*. 2013;27(6):688-697.
17. Dattilo M, Biousse V, Newman NJ. Update on the management of central retinal artery occlusion. *Neurol Clin.* 2017;35(1):83-100.
18. Sadaka A. Orbital cellulitis organism-specific therapy. Medscape website. https://emedicine.medscape.com/article/2017176-overview. Updated July 12, 2016. Accessed February 11, 2018.
19. Earwax and care. American Academy of Otolaryngology—Head and Neck Surgery website. http://www.entnet.org/content/earwax-and-care. Accessed February 11, 2018.
20. Ménière disease. National Institute on Deafness and Other Communication Disorders website. https://www.nidcd.nih.gov/health/menieres-disease. Accessed February 11, 2018.
21. Li JC. Benign paroxysmal positional vertigo. Medscape website. https://emedicine.medscape.com/article/884261-overview. Updated February 15, 2018.
22. Woodhouse S. Benign paroxysmal positional vertigo (BPPV). VEDA website. http://vestibular.org/understanding-vestibular-disorders/types-vestibular-disorders/benign-paroxysmal-positional-vertigo.
23. Parnes LS, Agrawal SK, Atlas J. Diagnosis and management of benign paroxysmal positional vertigo (BPPV). *CMAJ*. 2003;169(7):681-693.
24. Minovi A, Dazert S. Diseases of the middle ear in childhood. *J GMS Curr Top Otorhinolaryngol Head Neck Surg.* 2014;13:Doc11.
25. Alter H. Approach to the adult with epistaxis. UpToDate website. https://www.uptodate.com/contents/approach-to-the-adult-with-epistaxis. Updated July 26, 2017. Accessed February 11, 2018.
26. Suh JD, Garg R. Epistaxis (nosebleeds). American Rhinologic Society website. http://care.american-rhinologic.org/epistaxis. Accessed February 11, 2018.
27. Te Grotenhuis R, van Grunsven PM, Heutz WMJM, Tan ECTH. Use of hemostatic nasal plugs in emergency medical services in the Netherlands: a prospective study of 33 cases. *Prehosp Emerg Care*. 2018;22(1):91-98.
28. Sinusitis. American Academy of Otolaryngology—Head and Neck Surgery website. http://www.entnet.org/content/sinusitis. Accessed February 11, 2018.
29. Costain N, Marrie TJ. Ludwig's angina. *Am J Med.* 2011;124(2):115-117.
30. Chow AW. Submandibular space infections (Ludwig's angina). UpToDate website. https://www.uptodate.com/contents/submandibular-space-infections-ludwigs-angina. Updated July 26, 2017. Accessed February 11, 2018.
31. Epiglottitis (supraglottitis): clinical features and diagnosis. UpToDate website. https://www.uptodate.com/contents/epiglottitis-supraglottitis-clinical-features-and-diagnosis. Updated May 3, 2017. Accessed February 11, 2018.
32. Flores J. Peritonsillar abscess in emergency medicine. Medscape website. http://emedicine.medscape.com/article/764188-overview#showall. Updated February 1, 2017. Accessed February 11, 2018.
33. National Center for Immunization and Respiratory Diseases. Epstein-Barr virus and infectious mononucleosis: about infectious mononucleosis. Centers for Disease Control and Prevention website. https://www.cdc.gov/epstein-barr/about-mono.html. Updated September 14, 2016. Accessed February 11, 2018.
34. TMJD basics. The TMJ Association website. http://www.tmj.org/site/content/tmd-basics. Accessed February 11, 2018.

Suggested Readings

Gibson AM, Benko KR, eds. *Head, Eyes, Ears, Nose, and Throat Emergencies. An Issue of Emergency Medicine Clinics*. Vol 31-2. St. Louis, MO: Elsevier; 2013.

Leong P. *ENT Emergencies Handbook: Community ENT Presents ENT Emergencies Handbook*. Lazy Ink Publishing; 2014.

Ludman HS, Bradley PJ, eds. *ABC of Ear, Nose and Throat*. 6th ed. West Sussex, UK: Wiley-Blackwell; 2013.

Ragge N. *Immediate Eye Care*. London, UK: Wolfe; 1990.

Tillotson J, Whittingham E. *Eye Emergencies: A Practitioner's Guide*. 2nd ed. Cumbria, UK: M&K Publishers; 2015.

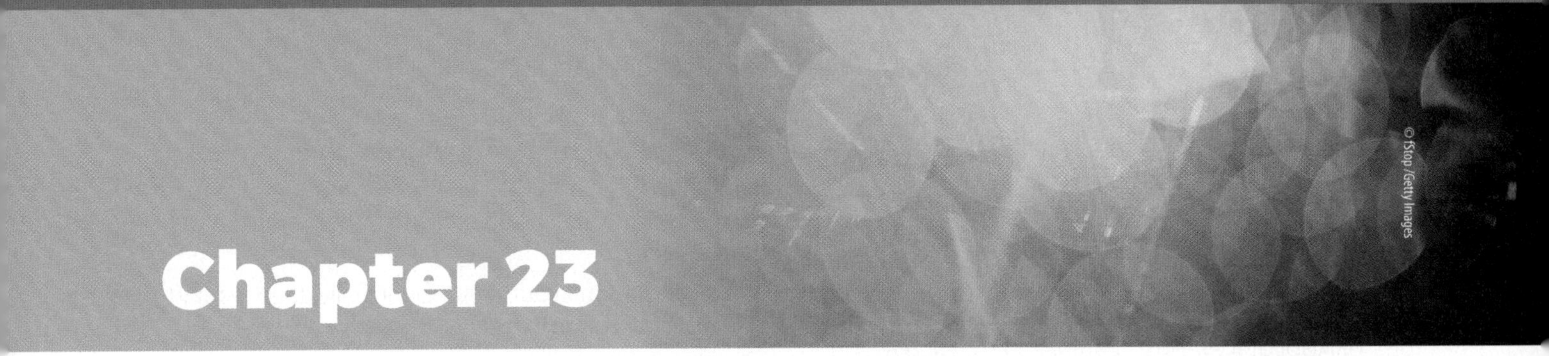
© fStop/Getty Images

Chapter 23

Respiratory

NATIONAL EMS EDUCATION STANDARD COMPETENCIES

Medicine

Integrates assessment findings with principles of epidemiology and pathophysiology to formulate a field impression and implement a comprehensive treatment/disposition plan for a patient with a medical complaint.

Respiratory

Anatomy, signs, symptoms, and management of respiratory emergencies, including those that affect the
- Upper airway (pp 903–904, 907–911, 925–926)
- Lower airway (pp 903–904, 907–911)

Anatomy, physiology, pathophysiology, assessment, and management of
- Epiglottitis (see Chapter 47, *Pediatrics*)
- Spontaneous pneumothorax (p 926)
- Pulmonary edema (pp 923–925)
- Asthma (pp 915–919)
- Chronic obstructive pulmonary disease (pp 911–914)
- Environmental/industrial exposure (p 911 and Chapter 33, *Toxicology*)
- Toxic gas (pp 907, 919, and Chapter 33, *Toxicology*)
- Pertussis (see Chapter 47, *Pediatrics*)
- Cystic fibrosis (see Chapter 50, *Patients With Special Challenges*)
- Pulmonary embolism (pp 923–925)
- Pneumonia (pp 919–922)
- Viral respiratory infections (pp 920–923, 925–926)
- Obstructive/restrictive disease (pp 911–919)

Anatomy, physiology, epidemiology, pathophysiology, psychosocial impact, presentations, prognosis, and management of
- Acute upper airway infections (pp 925–926)
- Spontaneous pneumothorax (p 926)
- Obstructive/restrictive lung diseases (pp 911–919)
- Pulmonary infections (pp 919–922)
- Neoplasm (pp 927–929)
- Pertussis (see Chapter 47, *Pediatrics*)
- Cystic fibrosis (see Chapter 50, *Patients With Special Challenges*)

Shock and Resuscitation

Integrates comprehensive knowledge of causes and pathophysiology into the management of cardiac arrest and pre-arrest states.

Integrates a comprehensive knowledge of the causes and pathophysiology into the management of shock, respiratory failure, or arrest, with an emphasis on early intervention to prevent arrest.

OBJECTIVES

Upon completion of this chapter, the paramedic student will be able to:

1. Distinguish the pathophysiology of respiratory emergencies related to ventilation, diffusion, and perfusion. (pp 904–906)
2. Outline the assessment process for the patient who has a respiratory emergency. (pp 907–909)
3. Describe the causes, complications, signs and symptoms, and prehospital management of patients diagnosed with obstructive airway disease, pneumonia, acute respiratory distress syndrome, pulmonary embolism, upper respiratory tract infection, spontaneous pneumothorax, hyperventilation syndrome, and lung cancer. (pp 911–929)

KEY TERMS

acute lung injury (ALI) Acute onset of pulmonary inflammation with impaired gas exchange and radiologic appearance of pulmonary edema without evidence of heart failure; similar pathology to acute respiratory distress syndrome with less mortality.

acute respiratory distress syndrome (ARDS) A fulminant form of respiratory failure characterized by acute lung inflammation and diffuse alveolar–capillary injury.

aspiration pneumonia Inflammation of the lung tissue from foreign material entering the tracheobronchial tree.

asterixis Hand flapping during hand extension related to pathologic conditions such as hypercapnia, liver failure, or renal failure.

asthma A respiratory disorder characterized by recurring episodes of paroxysmal dyspnea, coughing, and wheezing caused by constriction of the bronchi and viscous mucoid bronchial secretions.

bacterial pneumonia A type of pneumonia associated with a bacterial infection.

bilevel positive airway pressure (BPAP) Airway support that combines partial ventilatory support and continuous positive airway pressure; allows the pressure to vary during each breath cycle.

blebs A small, thin-walled collection of air between the lung and visceral pleura that, when ruptured, results in a spontaneous pneumothorax.

bronchiectasis An abnormal dilation of the bronchi caused by congenital or acquired damage.

bullae Dilated air-filled spaces within the lung parenchyma; most commonly caused by chronic obstructive pulmonary disease.

chronic bronchitis Obstructive airway disease of the trachea and bronchi.

continuous positive airway pressure (CPAP) Airway support that transmits positive pressure into the airways of a spontaneously breathing patient throughout the respiratory cycle at a constant pressure.

deficient ambient oxygen An oxygen concentration in the environment that is less than 21%.

diffusion The process in which solid, particulate matter in a fluid moves from an area of higher concentration to an area of lower concentration, resulting in an even distribution of the particles in the fluid.

emphysema An abnormal condition of the pulmonary system characterized by overinflation and destructive changes in the alveolar walls, resulting in a loss of lung elasticity, impaired gas exchange, and incomplete emptying of the alveoli during exhalation.

glottic opening The vocal cords and the space between them.

hemoptysis Coughing up of blood from the respiratory tract.

hyperventilation syndrome Abnormally deep or rapid breathing that leads to excessive loss of carbon dioxide, resulting in respiratory alkalosis.

lung cancer A disease of uncontrolled cell growth in tissues of the lung.

metastasis The movement or spreading of cancer cells from one organ or tissue to distant locations in the body.

mycoplasmal pneumonia A type of atypical pneumonia. It is caused by the bacterium *Mycoplasma pneumoniae*.

near-fatal asthma Acute asthma associated with respiratory arrest, a drop in blood pressure, and reduced cardiac output.

noninvasive positive pressure ventilation (NIPPV) Nonintubated application of positive airway pressure using either continuous positive airway pressure or bilevel positive airway pressure.

peak expiratory flow rate (PEFR) A measurement of how fast a person can exhale air.

perfusion The circulation of blood to the tissues.

pneumonia An acute inflammation of the lungs, usually caused by infection with bacteria, virus, or fungus.

positive end-expiratory pressure (PEEP) Airway support that maintains a degree of positive pressure at the end of exhalation.

pulmonary embolism The blockage of an artery in the lungs by a substance such as fat, air, tumor tissue, or a thrombus that has moved from elsewhere in the body through the bloodstream

respiration The exchange of oxygen and carbon dioxide between an organism and the environment.

respiratory failure A syndrome in which the respiratory system fails in one or both of its gas exchange functions: oxygenation and carbon dioxide elimination.

spontaneous pneumothorax A condition that results when a subpleural bleb ruptures, allowing air to enter the pleural space from within the lung.

status asthmaticus A severe, prolonged asthma attack that has not been broken with repeated doses of bronchodilators.

upper respiratory tract infection Infection of the upper airway, affecting the nose, throat, sinuses, and larynx.

ventilation The mechanical movement of air into and out of the lungs that makes respiration possible.

Respiratory emergencies are common in the prehospital setting, accounting for more than 3.7 million emergency department visits annually.[1] Each year in the United States, more than 400,000 people die as a result of respiratory emergencies.[2] Chronic lower respiratory diseases remain the third-leading cause of death in the United States. Therefore, patients with respiratory emergencies require the highest priority of care. The paramedic must be able to quickly assess a patient with respiratory distress, identify the cause, initiate management, and provide appropriate care en route to the hospital.

NOTE

Age-related variations in disease and methods of patient assessment are described throughout this textbook by subject matter. Respiratory diseases specific to children are addressed in Chapter 47, *Pediatrics*; those unique to older adults are presented in Chapter 48, *Geriatrics*; and those associated with infectious disease (eg, tuberculosis) are presented in Chapter 27, *Infectious and Communicable Diseases*. Respiratory emergencies related to trauma are presented in the section on Trauma.

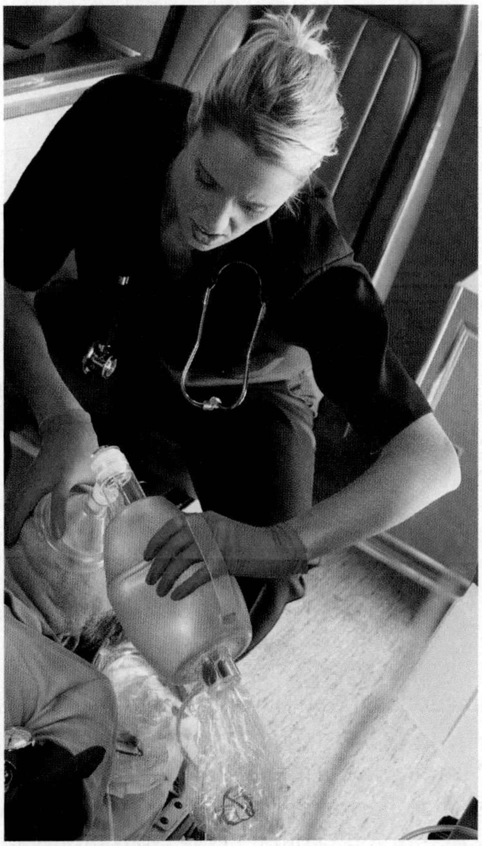

Anatomy and Physiology Review

The structures of the respiratory system are divided into upper and lower airways. The location of each structure is assigned in relation to the **glottic opening** (the vocal cords and the space between them). For the purposes of this chapter, upper airway structures are those located above the glottis, and lower airway structures are those located below the glottis. The upper and lower airway structures include the following (**FIGURE 23-1**):

- Upper airway structures
  - Nasopharynx
  - Oropharynx
  - Laryngopharynx
  - Larynx
- Lower airway structures
  - Trachea
  - Bronchial tree
  - Alveoli
  - Lungs

Physiology

The exchange of gases between the cells of the body and the outside environment is the essence of respiratory physiology. As described in Chapter 15, *Airway Management, Respiration, and Artificial Ventilation*, for gas exchange to occur, air must move freely into and out of the lungs. This process, known as **ventilation**, brings oxygen to the lungs and removes carbon dioxide, which enables external or internal **respiration**.

- **External respiration.** The transfer of oxygen and carbon dioxide between inspired air and pulmonary capillaries.
- **Internal respiration.** The transfer of oxygen and carbon dioxide between the capillary red blood cells and the tissue cells.

Many other factors are essential elements of pulmonary respiration. One of these factors is the structure

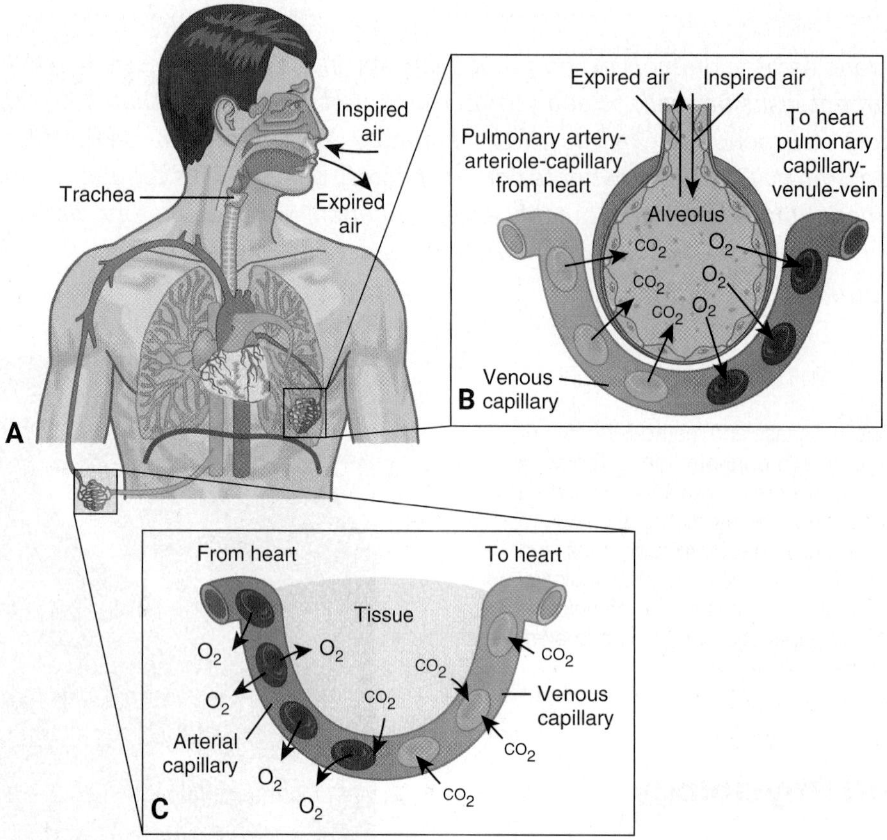

FIGURE 23-1 Structures of the pulmonary system. **A.** The location of the respiratory structures in the body. **B.** An enlarged view of the airways, alveoli (air sacs), and capillaries (tiny blood vessels). **C.** A close-up view of gas exchange between the capillaries and the tissues.

Modified from: How the Lungs Work. U.S. Department of Health & Human Services website. www.nhlbi.nih.gov/health-topics/how-lungs-work. Accessed March 16, 2018.

and function of the chest wall (ie, diaphragm, ribs, intercostal muscles, and accessory muscles). Another factor is the control of breathing by the central nervous system (ie, medulla, phrenic nerve innervation of the diaphragm, spinal nerves that innervate intercostal muscles, and reflexes that prevent overinflation). Acid–base balance mediated by the buffer systems also plays an important role in respiration (see Chapter 11, *General Principles of Pathophysiology*).

Pathophysiology

A variety of problems can affect the pulmonary system's ability to achieve gas exchange. Gas exchange must occur to provide for cellular needs and the excretion of wastes (see Chapter 10, *Review of Human Systems*, and Chapter 15, *Airway Management, Respiration, and Artificial Ventilation*). Specific disorders responsible for respiratory emergencies include those related to ventilation, diffusion, and perfusion. Risk factors associated with the development of respiratory disease are listed in BOX 23-1. The following discussion of pulmonary physiology serves as a review.

Ventilation

As mentioned, ventilation is the process of air movement into and out of the lungs. For ventilation to occur, the following must be intact:

- Neurologic control (to initiate ventilation)
- Nerves between the brainstem and the muscles of respiration
- Functional diaphragm and intercostal muscles
- Patent upper airway
- Functional lower airway
- Alveoli that are functional and have not collapsed

Specific pathophysiologies associated with ventilation include upper and lower airway obstruction, chest wall impairment, lung tissue disease, and

BOX 23-1 Risk Factors Associated With the Development of Respiratory Disease

Intrinsic Factors

Genetic predisposition may influence the development of these conditions:

- Asthma
- Obstructive lung disease
- Cancer

Cardiac or circulatory disorders may influence the development of these conditions:

- Pulmonary edema
- Pulmonary emboli

Stress may increase the following:

- Severity of respiratory complaints
- Frequency of attacks of asthma and chronic obstructive pulmonary disease (COPD)

Extrinsic Factors

Smoking increases the following:

- Prevalence of COPD and cancer
- Severity of virtually all respiratory disorders

Indoor and outdoor environmental pollutants increase the following:

- Prevalence of COPD
- Severity of all obstructive airway disorders

Modified from: Peres J. No clear link between passive smoking and lung cancer. *J Natl Cancer Inst.* 2013;105(24):1844-1846.

BOX 23-2 Causes of Ventilation Problems

Upper Airway Obstruction

Anaphylaxis or angioedema
Trauma
Epiglottitis
Laryngotracheobronchitis
Abscess
Foreign body obstruction
Inflammation of the tonsils

Lower Airway Obstruction

Trauma
Obstructive/restrictive lung disease
Emphysema
Chronic bronchitis
Mucus accumulation
Reactive airway disease
Smooth muscle spasm, including asthma
Airway edema

Central Nervous System Impairment

Toxicity/overdose
Brain injury
Stroke or intracerebral bleed
Spinal cord injury

Chest Wall Impairment

Spontaneous pneumothorax
Pleural inflammation
Pleural effusion
Neuromuscular diseases
Muscular sclerosis
Muscular dystrophy

problems in neurologic control. Emergency treatments for ventilation problems include ensuring the upper and lower airways are open and clear and providing assisted ventilations (BOX 23-2).

Diffusion

Diffusion is the process of gas exchange. This gas exchange occurs between the air-filled alveoli and the pulmonary capillary bed and is driven by the tendency of gases to move from areas of high concentration to areas of low concentration. This exchange occurs until the concentrations are equal. For diffusion to occur, the following must be intact:

- Alveolar and capillary walls that are not thickened
- Interstitial space between the alveoli and the capillary wall that is not enlarged or filled with fluid

Specific pathophysiologies associated with diffusion include inadequate oxygen concentration in ambient air, alveolar disorders, interstitial space disorders, and capillary bed disorders (BOX 23-3). Emergency treatment for diffusion problems includes providing high-concentration oxygen. Treatment is also directed at reducing inflammation in the interstitial space.

Perfusion

Perfusion is the circulation of blood through the lung tissues (capillary bed). For this process to occur, the following must be intact:

- Adequate blood volume
- Adequate hemoglobin in the blood
- Pulmonary capillaries that are not occluded
- Efficient pumping by the heart that provides a smooth flow of blood through the pulmonary capillary bed

BOX 23-3 Causes of Diffusion Problems

Inadequate oxygen concentration in ambient air
Alveolar pathology
Asbestosis; other environmental lung diseases
Blebs/bullae associated with COPD
Inhalation injuries
Interstitial space pathology
Pulmonary edema
Acute lung injury
Acute respiratory distress syndrome
Submersion/drowning

BOX 23-4 Causes of Perfusion Problems

Inadequate blood volume or hemoglobin levels
Hypovolemia
Anemia
Impaired blood flow
Pulmonary embolus

Specific pathophysiologies associated with perfusion include inadequate blood volume, impaired circulatory blood flow, and capillary wall disorders (BOX 23-4). Emergency treatment for perfusion problems includes ensuring that circulating blood volume and hemoglobin levels are adequate. Treatment also may be needed to optimize left-side heart function (see Chapter 21, *Cardiology*).

Unknown Pulmonary Diagnosis

If the patient's diagnosis is unknown, paramedics should try to determine whether it is primarily related to ventilation, diffusion, or perfusion, or to a combination of defects. Care for a patient with an unknown pulmonary diagnosis should be focused on the specific disorder responsible for the respiratory emergency.

Ventilation disorders are managed by assisting the patient's airway using mechanical means (eg, opening the airway, relieving airway obstructions, clearing the airway of secretions, using airway adjuncts); these steps are followed by manual or mechanical ventilation. In a reversible drug overdose, medication, such as naloxone, will also improve ventilation. The medication is administered after initial steps have been taken to open the airway and ventilation of the patient has been implemented.

Diffusion disorders are treated to improve gas exchange between the alveoli and the pulmonary capillary bed. For example, medications may improve breathing and reduce inflammation in the airways, or **noninvasive positive pressure ventilation (NIPPV)**, such as **bilevel positive airway pressure (BPAP)** or **continuous positive airway pressure (CPAP)**, may provide the necessary airway support. Perfusion disorders are managed by improving the circulation of blood through the lung tissues (eg, intravenous [IV] fluids, medications to improve cardiac function). Regardless of the specific disorder, all patients with respiratory compromise should receive high-concentration oxygen and ventilatory support as needed.

Respiratory Failure

Paramedics see many patients who have respiratory distress. Most have illnesses that are not life threatening or that respond quickly to initial interventions. In a small number of cases, patients either present with or decline into respiratory failure. **Respiratory failure** is a syndrome in which the respiratory system fails in one or both of its gas exchange functions: oxygenation and carbon dioxide elimination. It is crucial to recognize and intervene quickly when faced with respiratory failure because mortality for these patients can exceed 30%.[3] In fact, patients admitted to the hospital with respiratory failure are about four times less likely to be discharged alive than are those with cancer or heart disease.[1] The patient may have one of the following conditions:

- **Hypoxemic respiratory failure.** An arterial partial pressure of oxygen (Pao_2) level of less than 60 mm Hg (generally an arterial oxygen saturation [Sao_2] level of less than 90%).
- **Ventilatory failure.** Partial pressure of carbon dioxide (Pco_2) level of greater than 50 mm Hg.
- **Both hypoxemic respiratory failure and ventilatory failure, with a declining pH value.**

Some patients will be in respiratory failure at the outset of the call, whereas others decline during prehospital care as the patient becomes fatigued and increasingly hypoxic or hypercarbic. Along with the features of the patient's underlying illness, key signs of impending respiratory failure include, but are not limited to, the following:

- Decreasing Sao_2 level despite oxygen therapy
- Increasing end-tidal carbon dioxide ($ETCO_2$) level
- Evidence of fatigue
- Decreasing consciousness

- Nasal flaring
- Seesaw ventilation
- Arrhythmias
- Cyanosis

Failure to intervene during respiratory failure will typically lead to respiratory or cardiac arrest. NIPPV is indicated to treat respiratory failure associated with obstructive pulmonary disease and heart failure (see Chapter 15, *Airway Management, Respiration, and Artificial Ventilation*).[4] Increased mortality typically may be expected in patients who fail NIPPV and require emergent intubation.

> NOTE
>
> Pulmonary complaints may be associated with exposure to environments that have deficient ambient oxygen. During the scene size-up, it is crucial to ensure a safe environment for all emergency medical services (EMS) personnel before initiating patient contact. Rescue personnel with special training and equipment should be used as needed to ensure scene safety. **Deficient ambient oxygen** is defined as oxygen concentration in an environment that is less than 21%. (An oxygen concentration less than 16% is immediately dangerous.) Oxygen can be consumed or displaced by toxic or inert gas (eg, carbon monoxide, methane gas). This risk is usually associated with confined or enclosed spaces. Poison gases are hazardous because they can harm lower airways, cause bronchospasm, or interfere with the blood's ability to carry oxygen or the cell's ability to use oxygen (eg, exposure to hydrogen cyanide) (see Chapter 33, *Toxicology*). Inert gases are harmful because they displace oxygen from a space, thus lowering its concentration.

Assessment Findings

Primary Survey

A general impression of the patient can be made in the primary survey. The major focus of the primary survey is to detect and manage any life-threatening conditions that affect airway, breathing, and circulation. This action and initiating resuscitation measures take priority over a detailed assessment. Signs of life-threatening respiratory distress in adults include the following:[3]

- Alterations in mental status
- Severe cyanosis
- Stridor
- Inability to speak one or two words without dyspnea
- Tachycardia (>130 beats/min)
- Pallor and diaphoresis
- Retractions and/or the use of accessory muscles to assist breathing

A quick assessment of lung sounds may be indicated in the primary survey for a patient in respiratory distress. Abnormal breath sounds include absent or diminished breath sounds, crackles, wheezes, and rhonchi. The patient position should be noted as well. Tripod positioning is associated with respiratory distress.

Focused History

The paramedic should ascertain the patient's chief complaint. A chief complaint may include dyspnea, chest pain, productive or nonproductive cough, **hemoptysis** (coughing up blood from the respiratory tract), wheezing, and signs of respiratory tract infection (eg, fever, increased sputum production). The history should focus on the patient's previous experiences with similar or identical symptoms. The patient's objective description of severity often is an accurate indicator of the severity of the current episode if the condition is chronic.

Asking the patient, "What happened the last time you had an attack this severe?" is very useful for predicting what will happen with this episode. The following list offers sample questions, applying the OPQRST mnemonic, that the paramedic might ask to obtain a focused history for a patient with respiratory distress:

Onset. What were you doing when the breathing difficulty began? Do you think anything might have triggered it? Did your breathing difficulty begin gradually, or was it sudden in onset? Did you experience any pain when the breathing difficulty began?

Provocation/palliation. Does lying down or sitting up make your breathing better or worse? Do you have any pain when you breathe? If so, does the pain increase when you take a deep breath, or does it stay the same?

Quality. Is it more difficult to breathe when you inhale or when you exhale? If you have pain when you breathe, would you describe it as sharp or dull?

Region/radiation. What area of the chest has the most discomfort? Can you point with your finger to the specific area that hurts? Does the pain move anywhere, or does it stay in the same place?

Severity. On a scale of 0 to 10 (with 10 being the worst), how would you rate the difficulty of your breathing?

Timing. What time did the breathing difficulty start? Has it been constant since it began? If you have had this type of difficulty before, how long did it last?

NOTE

It is important to ask patients if intubation was ever required to manage their respiratory disease. A history of previous intubation indicates severe pulmonary disease. It also suggests that intubation may be required again.

After obtaining a history of the present illness, the paramedic should obtain a medication history, which may help determine the nature of the respiratory emergency. A medication history includes current medications, medication allergies, cardiac medications, and pulmonary medications (eg, in-home oxygen therapy; inhaled, oral, or parenteral sympathomimetics; inhaled or oral corticosteroids; cromolyn sodium; methylxanthines; leukotriene inhibitors; antibiotics). As part of the medication history, the paramedic should determine when and why the patient takes these medications.

Secondary Assessment

The secondary assessment should be guided by the paramedic's general impression of the patient and by the patient's chief complaint. As part of the secondary assessment, the paramedic should note the patient's position, mental status, ability to speak, respiratory effort, and skin color. Vital signs should be assessed with the following considerations:[3]

- **Pulse rate.** Tachycardia may be a sign of hypoxemia. Bradycardia caused by respiratory problems is a warning sign of severe hypoxemia and imminent cardiac arrest.
- **Blood pressure.** Hypertension may result from the use of medications the patient takes to manage cardiac and respiratory disorders. (Patients with heart failure often are hypertensive.) Hypertension also may result from the patient's fear and anxiety. Like hypertension, hypotension can be caused by medication therapy. It may also result from fluid loss and dehydration in some respiratory illnesses. (Patients with pneumonia often are dehydrated.)
- **Respiratory rate.** The respiratory rate is not an accurate sign of respiratory status unless it is very slow. Trends are essential in evaluating a patient with chronic respiratory disease. A slowing rate in a patient who is not improving suggests exhaustion and impending respiratory insufficiency. Abnormal patterns that may be seen in patients with severe illness or injury include tachypnea, Cheyne-Stokes respirations, central neurogenic hyperventilation, Kussmaul respirations, ataxic respirations, apneustic respirations, and apnea.

The patient's face and neck should be assessed for pursed-lip breathing, grunting, nasal flaring, and use of accessory muscles. (Visible head bobbing in infants indicates they are using the accessory muscles to breathe.) Pursed-lip breathing and grunting help maintain pressure in the airways (even during exhalation). This pressure helps to support the bronchial walls internally that have lost their external support as a result of disease. The use of accessory muscles can quickly result in respiratory fatigue. The patient should be questioned about sputum production. An increasing amount of sputum suggests infection. Thick green or brown sputum may indicate pneumonia; yellow or pale gray sputum may be related to allergic or inflammatory causes; pink, frothy sputum is associated with severe and late stages of pulmonary edema (described in Chapter 21, *Cardiology*, and Chapter 44, *Environmental Conditions*). The patient's neck should be evaluated for jugular vein distention. Jugular vein distention may be a sign of right-side heart failure resulting from severe pulmonary congestion.

The patient's chest should be inspected for injury or for any indicators of chronic disease, such as a barrel chest from long-standing emphysema. Other components of the chest examination include noting accessory muscle use or retractions to facilitate breathing, evaluating chest wall symmetry, and auscultating the patient's lungs for normal and abnormal breath sounds.

The patient's extremities should be assessed for peripheral cyanosis, pitting edema, clubbing of the fingers, asterixis, and carpopedal spasm. Peripheral cyanosis is caused when a large amount of the hemoglobin in the blood is not carrying oxygen. Pitting edema is an indication of heart failure. Clubbing is an abnormal enlargement of the ends of the fingers (**FIGURE 23-2**). It indicates long-standing chronic hypoxemia. **Asterixis** (flapping tremor), when found in respiratory failure, occurs from an elevated carbon dioxide level. If the patient has asterixis, his or her hands

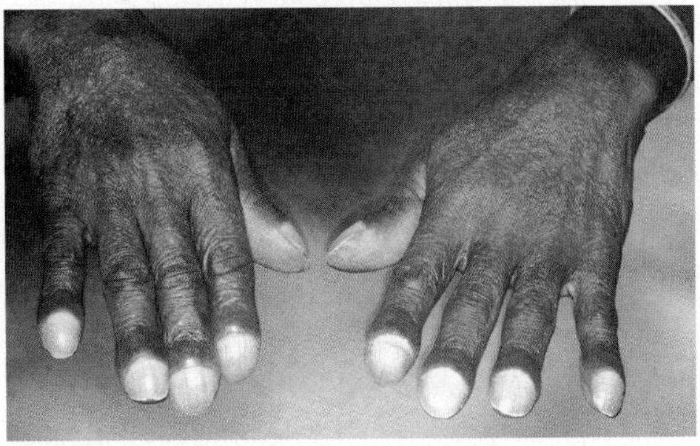

FIGURE 23-2 Severe finger clubbing in a patient with cyanotic congenital heart disease.

will pulse (flap) when attempting to hold them in a flexed position. Carpopedal spasms are spasms of the hands, thumbs, feet, or toes. They often are associated with hypocapnia that results from hyperventilation.

Physical findings in a patient with respiratory disease should be documented on the patient care report. They also should be communicated to the receiving facility.

Diagnostic Testing

Diagnostic testing that may be appropriate for some patients with respiratory disease includes pulse oximetry, capnometry, and the use of peak flow meters. As described in Chapter 15, *Airway Management, Respiration, and Artificial Ventilation*, pulse oximeters measure oxygen saturation. Capnography monitors $ETCO_2$ level. Peak flow meters provide a baseline assessment of airflow for patients with obstructive lung disease.

> NOTE
>
> Other respiratory monitors are available in some EMS and fire service agencies. These devices (eg, Rad57) measure levels of carboxyhemoglobin (Spco), hemoglobin (SpHB), and methemoglobin (SpMET) as well as total arterial oxygen content (Spoc).

Pulse Oximetry

Pulse oximetry helps determine how well the patient is being oxygenated. The device measures the transmission of red and near-infrared light through arterial beds using a probe placed on a finger, toe, or earlobe. Hemoglobin that is bound with oxygen (oxyhemoglobin) absorbs more infrared than red light; reduced hemoglobin absorbs more red than infrared light. The pulse oximeter measures this difference and calculates the Sao_2 level. The low range of normal Sao_2 is 93% to 95%. The upper range is 99% to 100%. An Sao_2 reading below 90% indicates a Pao_2 value of 60 mm Hg or less. An Sao_2 reading of 75% indicates a Pao_2 value of 40 mm Hg. An Sao_2 reading of 50% indicates a Pao_2 value of 27 mm Hg.

Capnography

Capnography is a noninvasive monitoring technique that is used in the prehospital setting to confirm correct tracheal tube placement. When used in conjunction with pulse oximetry and electrocardiographic (ECG) monitoring, capnography also provides insight into ventilation and indirectly to circulation and metabolism. It is a useful indicator of efficient cardiopulmonary resuscitation and also can help confirm the diagnosis of pulmonary embolism. In patients with hemorrhage, continuous capnography provides indirect information about tissue perfusion, and an indication of fluid resuscitation effectiveness for patients in shock (see Chapter 35, *Shock*).[5]

> NOTE
>
> Although capnography is a direct measurement of ventilation in the lungs, it also indirectly measures metabolism and circulation. For example, an increased metabolism will increase the production of carbon dioxide, which increases the $ETCO_2$ level. A decrease in cardiac output will reduce the delivery of carbon dioxide to the lungs, thus decreasing the $ETCO_2$ level.

Use of Capnography in Medical Patients With Spontaneous Respirations

Capnography is the numeric and graphical representation of carbon dioxide concentration exhaled through the breath. The measurements are taken by a capnography adapter attached to a bag mask, nasal cannula, or endotracheal tube. The graphic representation is displayed as a waveform (measured in millimeters of mercury) on a capnograph throughout the respiratory cycle. (A capnometer displays only the numerical value of an indirect measure of $Paco_2$, not the waveform.) Each waveform on the capnograph consists of four phases (**FIGURE 23-3**). Phase 1 (A–B) represents air that is exhaled from the conducting airways with little to no detectable carbon dioxide, because this air did not participate in gas exchange.

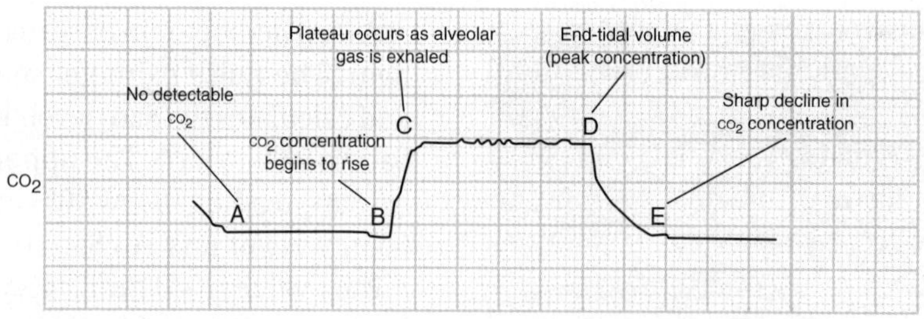

FIGURE 23-3 Capnography waveform.

BOX 23-5 Three Important Waveforms for Monitoring Medical Patients

1. Decreased carbon dioxide

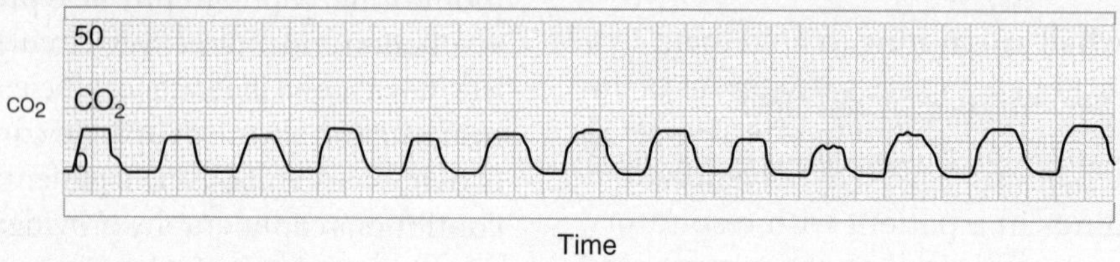

   Possible causes: Anxiety, hyperventilation, bronchospasm, pulmonary embolus, decreased cardiac output, hypotension, pulmonary edema

2. Increased carbon dioxide

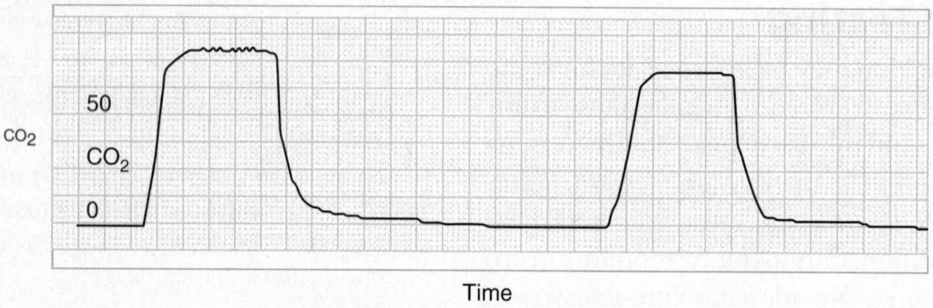

   Possible causes: Sedation, overdose, hypoventilation, chronic hypercapnia

3. Long expiratory phase shown by "shark-fin" waveform

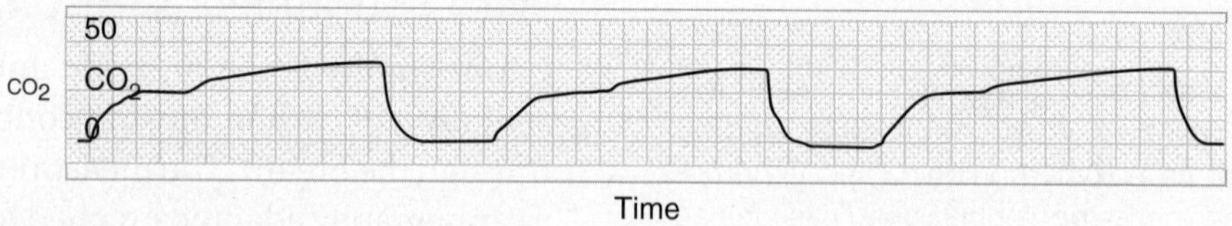

   Possible causes:Asthma, bronchospasm, bronchoconstriction, uneven emptying of the alveoli, breath struggle

$ETCO_2$ Values

Normal: 35–45 mm Hg
Hypoventilation/hypercapnia: >45 mm Hg
Hyperventilation/hypocapnia: <35 mm Hg

Phase 2 (B–C) represents the mixture of air from the anatomic dead space and alveolar gas. It is here that carbon dioxide concentration begins to rise. Phase 3 (C–D) represents a plateau as alveolar gas is exhaled (alveolar plateau). Phase 4 (D–E) represents inspiration (inspiration washout), where D is the end-tidal volume (the peak concentration) and E is the sharp decline in carbon dioxide concentration. BOX 23-5 shows three primary waveforms that are important in monitoring medical patients in the prehospital setting.

The waveform helps to detect any rebreathing of carbon dioxide and is useful in diagnosing problems associated with increased dead space. For example, patients with obstructive lung disease or a pulmonary embolism often have a decreased angle for phase 2, and the slope of the curve during phase 3 often will not reach the alveolar plateau. This presentation is associated with unequal flow rates (ventilation/perfusion mismatch) and the uneven emptying of obstructed alveoli. Ventilation/perfusion mismatch can be caused by blood shunting, as seen with atelectasis. It also can be caused by dead space in the lungs, such as occurs with pulmonary embolism. All of these conditions result in a continuous increase in carbon dioxide concentration. A waveform that plateaus late in the expiration phase can indicate heart failure, COPD, or pulmonary embolus (**FIGURE 23-4**).

Peak Flow Meters

Peak flow meters are used in pulmonary function tests to measure a patient's **peak expiratory flow rate (PEFR)** (**FIGURE 23-5**). PEFR is a measurement of how fast a person can exhale air. These tests most often are used to help determine the severity of an asthma attack. They also can help assess the effectiveness of treatment. Use of peak flow meters requires a cooperative patient who can achieve a maximal respiratory effort. It also requires coaching by the paramedic.

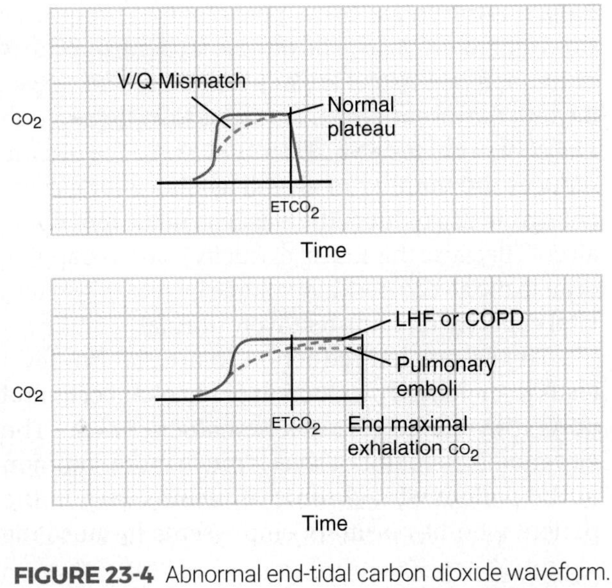

FIGURE 23-4 Abnormal end-tidal carbon dioxide waveform.

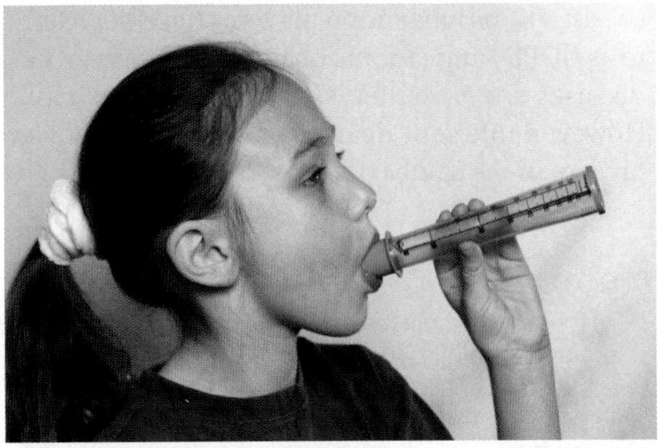

FIGURE 23-5 Peak flow meter.

To determine baseline airflow (before drug administration), the paramedic should instruct the patient to inflate the lungs fully, place the peak flow meter in the mouth with the tongue under the mouthpiece, seal the lips firmly around it, and forcefully exhale as quickly as possible into the flow meter. (Children should be reminded to breathe out as if they were blowing out candles or blowing up a balloon.) The reading is recorded in liters per minute. This measurement should be taken two more times. The highest of the three readings is chosen as the peak value flow. This measurement is then compared with standard tables based on height, sex, and race. A PEFR measurement with variability of less than 20% is considered mild, 20% to 30% is moderate, and more than 30% is severe.[6] Peak flow measurements should be repeated throughout the course of management to evaluate the patient's response to drug therapy.

> **NOTE**
>
> Most children younger than 5 years cannot adequately perform PEFR tests. In addition, this test should not be used when a patient has severe respiratory distress. Drug therapy to reverse the bronchospasm is the priority.

Obstructive Airway Disease

Obstructive airway disease is a major health problem affecting nearly 32 million people in the United States.[7] Predisposing factors that contribute to some forms of obstructive pulmonary disease include smoking, environmental pollution, industrial exposures, and various pulmonary infectious processes. Obstructive airway disease is a triad of distinct diseases that often coexist—bronchitis and emphysema (together referred to as COPD) and chronic obstructive asthma. These diseases are presented separately in this chapter. However, different degrees of each frequently are present in the same patient.

NOTE

Pulmonary function tests are used by many physicians and other health care professionals to diagnose COPD. The tests also allow them to stage the severity of the illness. The mantra advocated by many respiratory support groups is "test your lungs and know your numbers"; doing so provides a way for patients with COPD to assess how well they are responding to treatment and if their disease is progressing. Normal values and steps on how to use the peak expiratory flow meter are widely available.

Modified from: Peak expiratory flow (PEF) meter demonstration for health centers. Public Health Resources website. https://publichealthresources.blogspot.com/2014/03/peak-expiratory-flow-pef-meter.html. Accessed on March 16, 2018.

CRITICAL THINKING

Will patients with COPD always be able to "name" their disease when you ask about their history?

Chronic Bronchitis

Chronic bronchitis is a condition involving inflammatory changes and excessive mucus production in the bronchial tree (**FIGURE 23-6**). Although preventable, over 9.3 million people in the United States were diagnosed with the disease in 2015.[8] Chronic bronchitis is characterized by an increase in the number and size of mucus-producing glands. This increase results from prolonged exposure to irritants (most often cigarette smoke). The condition is diagnosed clinically by the presence of cough with mucus production that is present on most days for at least 3 months for at least 2 consecutive years without another identified cause.[9] The alveoli are not seriously affected, and diffusion remains relatively normal.

Patients with severe chronic bronchitis have a low partial pressure of oxygen (Po_2) level because of changes in the ventilation/perfusion relationships in the lung and hypoventilation. (These patients sometimes are called "blue bloaters" because of their

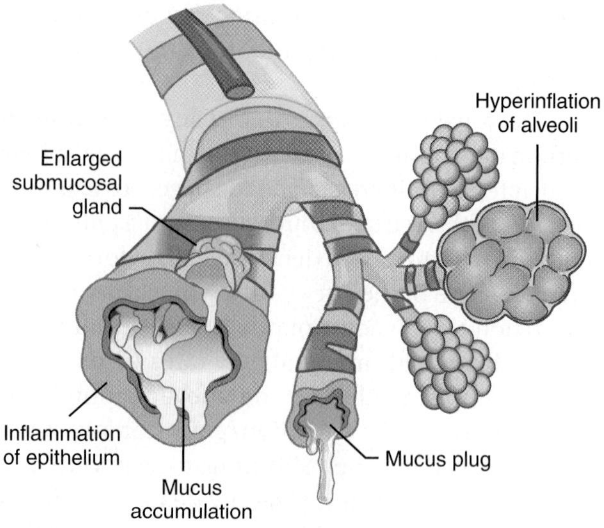

FIGURE 23-6 Chronic bronchitis. Bronchi are filled with excess mucus.

hypoxia and fluid retention.) The hypoventilation leads to hypercapnia (high levels of carbon dioxide), hypoxemia (low levels of oxygen), and increases in Pco_2 level. Patients with chronic bronchitis have frequent respiratory tract infections, which eventually cause scarring of lung tissue. In time, irreversible changes occur in the lung. These changes may lead to emphysema or bronchiectasis. **Bronchiectasis** is an abnormal dilation of the bronchi. It is caused by congenital factors or can be acquired, such as after a purulent infection of the bronchial wall.

Emphysema

Emphysema results from pathologic changes in the lung. It is the end stage of a process that progresses slowly for many years. The disease is characterized by permanent abnormal enlargement of the air spaces beyond the terminal bronchioles and by destruction and collapse of the alveoli (**FIGURE 23-7**). The disease reduces the number of alveoli available for gas exchange. It also reduces the elasticity of the remaining alveoli. Because this loss of elasticity leads to trapping of air in the alveoli, residual volume increases, whereas vital capacity remains relatively normal.

The associated reduction in arterial Po_2 level leads to increased production of red blood cells and polycythemia (an elevated hematocrit value). The elevation in hematocrit level is much more common in the patient with chronic bronchitis than in the patient who has primary emphysema because the

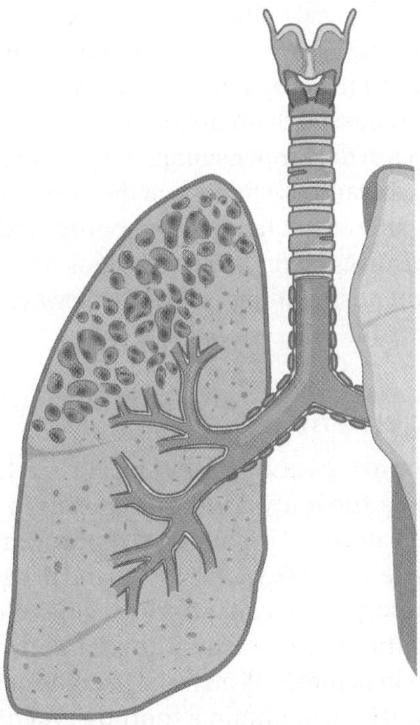

FIGURE 23-7 Cystic changes of lobar emphysema resulting from destruction of alveoli.

© Jones & Bartlett Learning.

Air movement during inspiration Air movement during expiration

Muscle

Alveolar wall

A

Normal expiration Impaired expiration

Reduced airway patency

Easy expiration due to normal elastic recoil of alveolus and open bronchiole

Difficult expiration due to decreased elastic recoil of alveolus and narrowed bronchiole

B

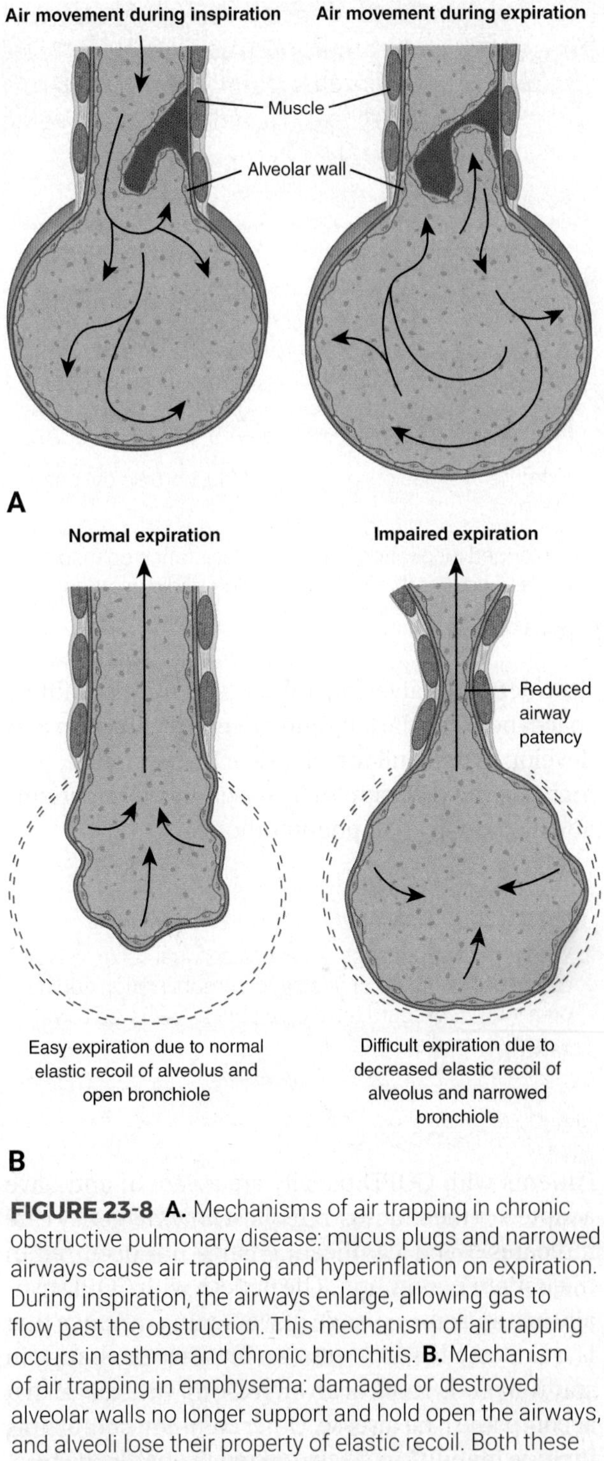

FIGURE 23-8 A. Mechanisms of air trapping in chronic obstructive pulmonary disease: mucus plugs and narrowed airways cause air trapping and hyperinflation on expiration. During inspiration, the airways enlarge, allowing gas to flow past the obstruction. This mechanism of air trapping occurs in asthma and chronic bronchitis. **B.** Mechanism of air trapping in emphysema: damaged or destroyed alveolar walls no longer support and hold open the airways, and alveoli lose their property of elastic recoil. Both these factors contribute to airway collapse during expiration.

© Jones & Bartlett Learning.

patient with chronic bronchitis is more often chronically hypoxemic. Decreases in alveolar membrane surface area and in the number of pulmonary capillaries in the lung reduce the area for gas exchange. These factors are also responsible for an increased resistance to pulmonary blood flow.

Patients with emphysema have some resistance to airflow into and out of the lungs. Yet most of the hyperexpansion is caused by air trapping secondary to loss of elastic recoil (**FIGURE 23-8**). Patients with chronic bronchitis have increased airway resistance during both inspiration and expiration. In contrast, patients with emphysema have increased airway resistance only on expiration. Normally a passive, involuntary act, expiration becomes a muscular act in patients with COPD. (These patients are sometimes called "pink puffers" because of their increased respiratory effort during forced exhalation and higher oxygen level compared with the person with chronic bronchitis, who is more hypoxic.) Over time, the chest becomes barrel-shaped from the trapping of air. The patient must then use the accessory muscles of the neck, chest, and abdomen to move air into and out of the lungs. Full deflation of the lungs becomes more and more difficult, and eventually it becomes impossible.

Often the patient with emphysema is thin because of poor dietary intake and increased caloric consumption required by the work of breathing (**TABLE 23-1**). **Bullae** (dilated, air-filled spaces within the lung parenchyma) often develop in patients with emphysema from the

TABLE 23-1 Comparison of Signs and Symptoms of Emphysema and Chronic Bronchitis

Emphysema	Chronic Bronchitis
Thin, barrel-chest appearance	Typically overweight
Nonproductive cough	Productive cough with sputum
Wheezing and rhonchi	Coarse rhonchi
Pink complexion	Chronic cyanosis
Extreme dyspnea on exertion	Mild, chronic dyspnea
Prolonged inspiration (pursed-lip breathing)	Resistance on inspiration and expiration

destruction of alveolar walls. **Blebs** (air-containing spaces between the lung and visceral pleura) also may develop. When bullae collapse or blebs rupture, they increase the diffusion defect seen in these patients and also can lead to pneumothorax.

CRITICAL THINKING

What effect might application of a cervical collar, use of a short spine board or vest, and immobilization supine on a long backboard have on a patient with COPD who has sustained trauma?

Assessment of COPD

Patients with COPD usually are aware of and have adapted to their illness. A request for emergency care indicates that a significant change has occurred in the patient's condition. The patient with COPD usually has an acute episode of worsening dyspnea that is manifested even at rest, an increase or change in sputum production, or an increase in the malaise that accompanies the disease. Other common complaints include inability to sleep and recurrent headaches.

On EMS arrival, the patient with COPD will likely be in respiratory distress. Often the patient is sitting upright and leaning forward to aid in breathing. The patient frequently is using pursed-lip breathing to maintain positive airway pressures, in addition to using accessory muscles. Increased hypoxemia and hypercapnia may be indicated by tachypnea, diaphoresis, cyanosis, confusion, irritability, and drowsiness.

Other physical findings include wheezes, rhonchi, and crackles. Breath sounds and heart sounds also may be diminished because of reduced air exchange and the increased diameter of the thoracic cavity. In late stages of decompensation, the patient may have peripheral cyanosis, clubbing of the fingers, and signs of right-side heart failure. The patient's ECG may reveal cardiac dysrhythmias or signs of right atrial enlargement, including tall, peaked P waves in leads II, III, and aVF.

Management

The primary goal of prehospital care for these patients is the correction of hypoxemia through improved airflow. Airflow can be improved through administration of oxygen, NIPPV, and drug therapy. Drug therapy may cause serious side effects and complications, especially if the patient has used medication before EMS arrival. Therefore, it is crucial for paramedics to obtain a thorough medical history regarding medication use, home oxygen use, and drug allergies.

An IV line should be established in most patients in respiratory distress. A cardiac monitor also should be applied. If the patient has a productive cough, clearing the airway of phlegm and mucus should be encouraged. Any sputum should be collected and delivered with the patient for laboratory analysis.

Some patients with COPD rely on a hypoxic drive for ventilatory effort. However, the paramedic should never withhold oxygen because of fear of decreasing the hypoxic drive while providing emergency care in the prehospital setting. Oxygen should be titrated based on oxygen saturation. Some of these patients will require ventilatory assistance. In addition, their breathing may require augmentation with CPAP or BPAP) (**FIGURE 23-9**). Both methods can improve oxygenation, reduce the work of breathing, prevent atelectasis, and allow for drug administration. NIPPV may prevent the need for intubation and the risks and complications associated with invasive airway procedures.

The medications used in the prehospital setting to relieve bronchospasm and reduce constricted airways are the beta agonists (eg, levalbuterol, albuterol). A nebulized anticholinergic (eg, ipratropium) is often administered with the beta agonist to promote bronchodilation and inhibit mucus production. In some cases, steroids such as methylprednisolone are given to reduce inflammation.

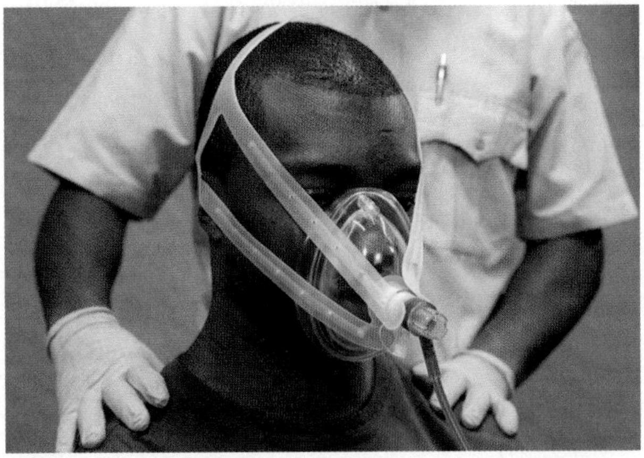

FIGURE 23-9 Patient being treated with continuous positive airway pressure.

Asthma

Asthma, or reactive airway disease, is a common disorder that affects over 18 million American adults and 6.2 million children.[10] It is the most common chronic disease of childhood.[11] Asthma is responsible for over 3,600 deaths each year and is most common in children and young adults.[10] However, asthma can occur in any decade of life. Exacerbating factors tend to be extrinsic (external) in children. In contrast, they tend to be intrinsic (internal) in adults (**FIGURE 23-10**). Childhood asthma often improves or resolves with age. Adult asthma usually is persistent.

Asthma is a broad term that is usually characterized by chronic airway inflammation.[11] It is diagnosed by respiratory symptoms such as wheezing, shortness

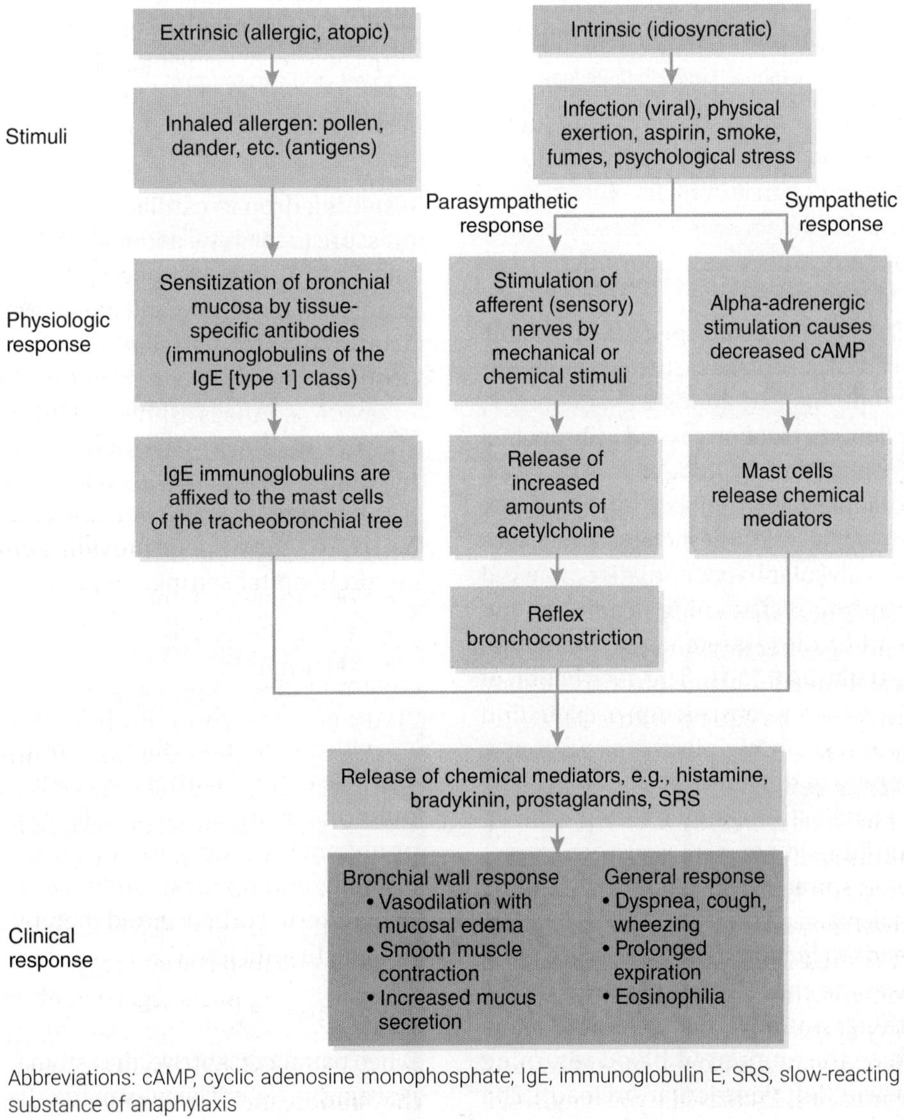

FIGURE 23-10 Extrinsic and intrinsic bronchial asthma.

of breath, prolonged exhalation, chest tightness, and cough that vary over time and in intensity.

SHOW ME THE EVIDENCE

Researchers in Perth, Australia, compared the paramedic diagnosis of asthma and COPD to each patient's diagnosis upon hospital discharge. They wanted to determine the accuracy of paramedic diagnosis of these conditions because the treatment is different for each condition. The positive predictive value of the paramedics' asthma diagnosis (those diagnosed with asthma whose discharge diagnosis was asthma) was 41% (95% confidence interval [CI], 38%–44%). The paramedics' COPD diagnosis had a positive predictive value of 57% (95% CI, 54%–60%). The researchers concluded that owing to the low accuracy in distinguishing between these conditions, it would be helpful to have one protocol that would appropriately treat either condition.

Modified from: Williams TA, Finn J, Fatovich D, Perkins GD, Summers Q, Jacobs I. Paramedic differentiation of asthma and COPD in the prehospital setting is difficult. *Prehosp Emerg Care.* 2015;19(4):535-543.

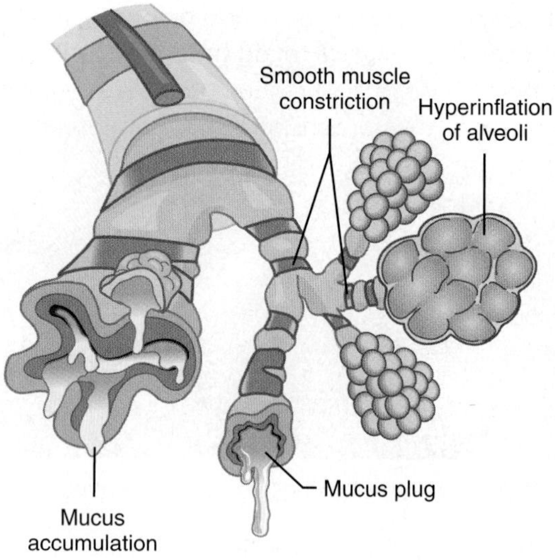

FIGURE 23-11 With bronchial asthma, thick mucus accumulation, mucosal edema, and smooth muscle spasm obstruct the small airways. Breathing becomes labored, and expiration is difficult.

Pathophysiology of an Asthma Attack

Asthma generally occurs in acute episodes of variable duration. Between these episodes, the patient is relatively free of symptoms. The attack is characterized by reversible airflow obstruction caused by bronchial smooth muscle contraction; hypersecretion of mucus, resulting in bronchial plugging; and inflammatory changes in the bronchial walls. The increased resistance to airflow leads to alveolar hypoventilation, marked ventilation/perfusion mismatching (leading to hypoxemia), and carbon dioxide retention (stimulating hyperventilation) (**FIGURE 23-11**). The obstruction of inspiration and the marked obstruction of expiration cause pressure to remain high in the airways as a result of air trapping in the lungs.

During an acute asthma attack (often called a flare-up), the combination of increased airway resistance, increased respiratory drive, and air trapping creates excessive demand on the muscles of respiration. This demand leads to greater use of accessory muscles and increases the chance of respiratory fatigue. If labored breathing continues, high pressures in the thorax can reduce the amount of blood returning to the left ventricle (left ventricular preload). The result is a drop in cardiac output and systolic blood pressure (**near-fatal asthma**). Pulsus paradoxus also may be seen. If the episode continues, hypoxemia and changes in blood flow and blood pressure may lead to death. Most asthma-related deaths occur outside the hospital. The most common cause of death related to severe asthma is asphyxia. Other factors that may contribute to arrest are hypercapnia and acidosis, hypotension related to decreased venous return, and decreased mental status. Complications in patients with severe asthma include the following:[12]

- Pulmonary edema
- Lobar atelectasis
- Pneumonia
- Tension pneumothorax (often bilateral)

Other conditions that may be present in patients with near-fatal asthma include cardiac disease, pulmonary disease, acute allergic bronchospasm or anaphylaxis, drug use or misuse (beta blockers, cocaine, and opiates), and recent discontinuation of long-term corticosteroid therapy (associated with adrenal insufficiency).

Assessment

When paramedics arrive, the asthmatic patient usually is sitting upright. The person may be leaning forward with hands on the knees (tripod position) and using the accessory muscles to aid breathing. The typical asthmatic patient is in obvious respiratory distress. Respirations are rapid and loud, and audible wheezing may be present.

> **NOTE**
> The severity of wheezing does not correlate with the degree of airway obstruction. The absence of wheezing may indicate critical airway obstruction, whereas increased wheezing may indicate a positive response to bronchodilator therapy.

The patient's mental status should be noted and monitored carefully. Lethargy, exhaustion, agitation, nasal flaring, and confusion are serious signs of impending respiratory failure. An initial history must be obtained quickly. Questions about the onset of the current episode, its relative severity, the precipitating cause, medication use, and allergies should be specific and to the point. It is crucial to find out whether the patient has needed intubation previously to manage his or her asthma.

On auscultation, a prolonged expiratory phase may be noted. Usually wheezing is heard from the movement of air through the narrowed airways. Inspiratory wheezing (unlike inspiratory stridor) does not indicate upper airway occlusion. It suggests that the large and medium-sized muscular airways are obstructed, indicating a greater degree of obstruction than if only expiratory wheezes are heard. Inspiratory wheezes also may suggest that the large airways are filled with secretions. A silent chest (ie, no audible wheezing or air movement) may indicate such severe obstruction that the flow of air is too low to generate breath sounds. Other signs of severe asthma include the following:

- Reduced level of consciousness
- Diaphoresis and pallor
- Retractions
- Inability to speak after only one or two words
- Poor, floppy muscle tone
- Pulse rate greater than 130 beats/min
- Respirations greater than 30 breaths/min
- Pulsus paradoxus greater than 20 mm Hg
- Altered mental status or severe agitation
- $ETCO_2$ value greater than 45 mm Hg

L HIGH ETCO2

* HEART = LOW ETCO2

> **NOTE**
> Asthma attacks are serious medical emergencies. Paramedics should manage these episodes aggressively. Deterioration of the patient's condition can be expected, rapid, and fatal. Therefore, the paramedic must monitor the patient carefully and continuously. Initial patient management should be directed at ensuring an adequate airway, providing supplemental oxygen, and reversing the bronchospasm.

Management

Oxygen therapy should be targeted to an Spo_2 reading of 93% to 95% (94% to 98% for children aged 6 to 11 years).[11] Drug therapy is based on the patient's age and severity. Nebulized albuterol is the current cornerstone of asthma treatment in the United States (BOX 23-6). This fast-acting $beta_2$ agonist stimulates beta-adrenergic receptors and thus acts as a rapid bronchodilator. Side effects include transient tachycardia and tremor. Other nebulized drugs used to manage asthma include levalbuterol, ipratropium, or a combination of albuterol and ipratropium. Corticosteroids (typically methylprednisolone or dexamethasone) can be given IV, intramuscularly, or orally in the prehospital setting. Nebulized magnesium sulfate can be considered in children 2 years or older or administered IV in cases of severe bronchospasm.[11]

BOX 23-6 Common Asthma Medications

Nebulized $Beta_2$ Agonists

Albuterol, levalbuterol, pirbuterol, salmeterol
Inhaled anticholinergics
Ipratropium

Corticosteroids (IV)

Methylprednisolone
Dexamethasone

Corticosteroids (Inhaled)

Triamcinolone

Leukotriene Modifiers

Montelukast, zafirlukast, zileuton
Magnesium sulfate (IV)
Epinephrine or terbutaline (subcutaneous or intramuscular)

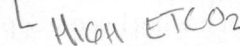

If the severely ill asthma patient does not respond to initial medications, intramuscular epinephrine can be administered. NIPPV can be beneficial in managing reactive airway disease with impending respiratory failure and in some cases prevents the need to intubate if the patient has adequate spontaneous respirations.[12]

IV fluids may be indicated for rehydration. All patients with acute asthma should be transported in a position of comfort to help maximize the use of respiratory muscles. In addition, these patients should be monitored for cardiac rhythm disturbances.

> CRITICAL THINKING
>
> Consider that the patient is unable to hold the nebulizer mouthpiece or needs to be ventilated using a bag-mask device. What can you do to promote bronchodilation?

In rare cases, advanced airway management is required for a patient having a severe asthma attack. Although there are no absolute criteria other than respiratory arrest and coma, the following are indications for acute airway intervention:[13]

- Worsening pulmonary function tests despite vigorous bronchodilator therapy
- Decreasing Pao_2 level
- Increasing $Paco_2$ level
- Progressive respiratory acidosis
- Declining mental status
- Increasing agitation

If a conscious patient requires intubation and the paramedic is trained and authorized to perform rapid sequence induction, it is the preferred method. To manage the airway, the paramedic should perform the following key actions:[12]

- Provide adequate sedation with ketamine or etomidate.
- Paralyze the patient with succinylcholine or vecuronium (if the paramedic is credentialed and authorized in his or her state).
- Select the largest endotracheal tube appropriate for the patient's size to decrease airway resistance.[12]
- Immediately after intubation and confirmation of tube placement, nebulize 2.5 to 5 mg of albuterol via the endotracheal tube.
- Verify endotracheal tube placement with clinical examination and waveform capnography.
- Ventilate the patient's lungs at 6 to 10 breaths/min and with smaller tidal volumes (6 to 8 mL/kg). Deliver breaths with a shorter inspiratory time, and prolong the expiratory time to allow for the escape of air and to avoid sudden hypotension (especially in older adult patients with emphysema).

Even after intubation, ventilating the patient's lungs may be difficult. When positive pressure ventilation is performed, breath stacking can cause intrinsic **positive end-expiratory pressure (PEEP)** (or auto-PEEP) with high airway pressures. This condition can lead to hyperinflation, tension pneumothorax, and hypotension. To avoid this outcome, a slower respiratory rate is delivered with shorter inspiratory time (adult, 80–100 L/min) and a longer expiratory time (inspiratory-to-expiratory ratio of 1:4 or 1:5). Mild hypercapnia is expected. The patient should be sedated after intubation to promote maximal ventilation. Inhaled bronchodilators can be administered through the ventilation circuit.

If the intubated asthma patient deteriorates acutely after intubation, possible causes should be assessed and corrected by using the DOPE mnemonic, which stands for Displacement of tube, Obstruction of tube, Pneumothorax (or auto-PEEP), and Equipment failure (see Chapter 15, *Airway Management, Respiration, and Artificial Ventilation*).[12]

If cardiac arrest develops in the asthmatic patient, the American Heart Association recommends several considerations. Ventilation with low respiratory rate and tidal volume is reasonable (Class IIa) to minimize the effects of auto-PEEP. In addition, a brief pause to disconnect the patient from the bag-mask device or ventilator followed by chest compression may be effective to relieve air trapping (Class IIa). The asthma patient in cardiac arrest should be assessed for the presence of a tension pneumothorax (Class I).

> NOTE
>
> The absence of any significant obstruction to airflow immediately after tracheal intubation suggests that the diagnosis of acute asthma may have been incorrect, and the problem may be in the upper airway.

Status Asthmaticus

Status asthmaticus is a severe, prolonged asthma attack that has not been stopped with repeated doses of bronchodilators. It may be of sudden onset resulting from spasm of the airways. It can also be subtle in onset, resulting from a viral respiratory tract infection or prolonged exposure to one or more allergens. Status asthmaticus is a true emergency. It calls for early recognition and immediate transport of the patient. These patients are in danger of respiratory arrest.

The treatment of patients with status asthmaticus is the same as that for acute asthma attacks; however, the urgency of rapid transport is more important. In addition, these patients usually are dehydrated and typically require IV fluid administration. The patient's respiratory status should be monitored closely, and high-concentration oxygen should be administered. The need for intubation and aggressive ventilatory support should be anticipated. Continuous bronchodilator therapy with nebulized and parenteral drugs may be indicated.

CRITICAL THINKING
When a patient treated for status asthmaticus is reassessed, would decreasing respiratory and heart rates indicate a good outcome or a bad outcome? Why?

Differential Considerations

Wheezing commonly is associated with asthma. However, it may be present in many diseases that cause dyspnea (**TABLE 23-2**). For example, tachypnea, wheezing, and respiratory distress may indicate heart failure, pneumonia, pulmonary edema, pulmonary embolism, pneumothorax, toxic inhalation, foreign body aspiration, and various other pathologic states. Appropriate emergency care is based on the patient assessment and an accurate history.

Pneumonia

Pneumonia is a group of specific infections (not a single disease) that cause an acute inflammatory process of the respiratory bronchioles and the alveoli. The disease kills more than 50,000 Americans each year (**FIGURE 23-12**).[14] Pneumonia can be caused by bacterial, viral, or fungal infection. Associated risk factors include cigarette smoking, immune suppression, alcoholism, exposure to cold, asthma, COPD, and extremes of age (the very young and very old). These diseases may be spread by respiratory droplets through contact with infected people. They also may

TABLE 23-2 Diseases and Signs/Symptoms Associated With Wheezing

Disease	Symptoms
Asthma	Nonproductive cough, tightness in chest
Bacterial pneumonia	Productive cough, pleuritic pain, fever
Chronic bronchitis	Chronic productive cough
Emphysema	Cough
Foreign body aspiration	Cough, wheezing, stridor
Heart failure	Cough, orthopnea, nocturnal dyspnea
Pneumothorax	Sudden, sharp pleuritic pain, dyspnea
Pulmonary disease	Tachypnea, cough, congestion
Pulmonary embolism	Sudden, sharp pleuritic pain, tachycardia, hypoxia
Toxic inhalation	Cough, pain, altered mental status

© Jones & Bartlett Learning.

Lobar pneumonia
(Right upper lobe)

Pneumococcal
pneumonia

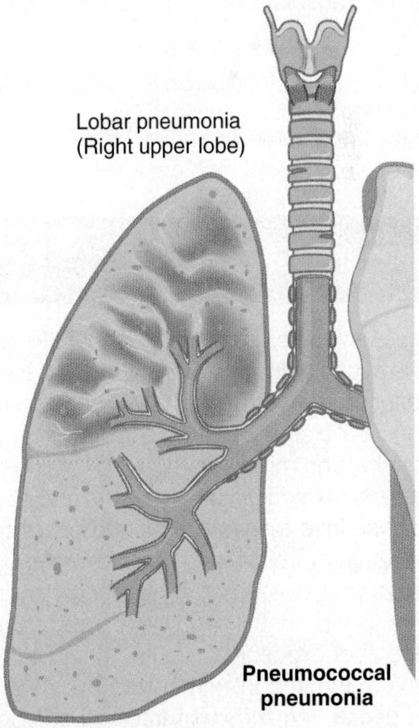

FIGURE 23-12 Pneumonia is an inflammatory process of the respiratory bronchioles and alveoli. It is caused by infection.

© Jones & Bartlett Learning.

be spread by inhaling or aspirating bacteria from one's own nose and mouth.

Pneumonia may be classified as the viral, bacterial, mycoplasmal, or aspiration type. It generally manifests with classic signs and symptoms (typical pneumonia). These include a productive cough, pleuritic chest pain, tachypnea, adventitious breath sounds (wheezing, crackles, or rhonchi), and fever that produces "shaking chills" (usually associated with the bacterial infection). It also may cause nonspecific complaints, particularly in children, older adults, and debilitated patients. Nonspecific complaints may include abdominal pain (children), a nonproductive cough, headache, fatigue, and sore throat (atypical pneumonia).

NOTE

Community-acquired pneumonia is an infection that is acquired from the environment. This category includes infections acquired indirectly as a result of using medications that change the body's ability to fight disease. The occurrence of these infections has risen in recent years because of the increased percentage of the population who are aged 65 years or older and an increasing number of patients taking immunosuppressive drugs for malignancy, transplantation, or autoimmune disease.

Modified from: Walls R, Hockberger R, Gausche-Hill M. *Rosen's Emergency Medicine: Concepts and Clinical Practice*. 9th ed. Philadelphia, PA: Elsevier; 2017.

Viral Pneumonia

Influenza viruses are the most common causes of viral pneumonia (BOX 23-7). In infants and young children, respiratory syncytial virus is a frequent cause of the disease. Influenza often occurs as epidemics in populations of small groups such as schoolchildren, army recruits, and nursing home residents. The interstitial infection caused by the virus predisposes the patient to secondary bacterial pneumonia.

Bacterial Pneumonia

Until 2000, the pneumococcus bacillus (*Streptococcus pneumoniae*) accounted for 90% of incidences of **bacterial pneumonia**. It affected 1 in 500 people each year. The decline in cases is related to vaccination of infants against the pneumococcus bacteria. The peak incidence is in winter and early spring. In 2012, a vaccine effective against this type of pneumonia in adults was introduced and has resulted in further declines in this disease.[15]

Bacterial pneumonia also can be caused by aspiration of mucus or saliva. Therefore, patients in a coma or with seizures, suppressed cough reflex, and increased secretions are at risk for the development of the disease. Other predisposing risk factors that may contribute to the development of bacterial pneumonia include the following:

- Infection
  - Upper respiratory tract infection (influenza)
  - Postoperative infection

BOX 23-7 Influenza

Influenza is an acute, febrile disease that affects the entire body. It is associated with viral infection of the upper and lower respiratory tracts. It usually is characterized by the abrupt onset of a severe protracted cough, fever, headache, muscle ache, and mild sore throat. Of all the viruses, the influenza and parainfluenza viruses are the most common causes of serious respiratory tract infections. Moreover, they have high morbidity and mortality rates.

Influenza viruses A, B, and C (and their many strains) are known for their potential to quickly cause respiratory tract infections after exposure (usually within 24 to 48 hours). The virus is inhaled in respiratory droplets spread by infected people (eg, when an infected person sneezes). The droplets penetrate the surface of upper respiratory tract mucosal cells. The virus eventually spreads to the lower respiratory tract, where it causes cell inflammation and destruction of the cilia. Without the cilia, clearing the airways of infected mucus is more difficult. Consequently, a secondary bacterial infection often develops. This secondary infection may result in pneumonia or acute respiratory failure, particularly in patients with chronic lung disease.

Influenza has the potential for widespread epidemics in high-risk populations.[a] These populations include adults and children with chronic cardiorespiratory or metabolic disorders, residents of nursing homes and other institutions, and health care workers. Current vaccines are effective against some strains of the virus. These vaccines have minimal side effects. If uncomplicated, influenza is self-limiting. Acute symptoms last 2 to 7 days and are followed by a convalescent period of about 1 week.

[a]The H1N1 outbreak of 2009 disproportionally affected healthy young people and pregnant women compared with other influenza viruses.

DID YOU KNOW?

Pneumococcal Polysaccharide Vaccine (PPSV)

Pneumococcal disease is a leading cause of vaccine-preventable disease and death in the United States. The disease can lead to serious infections of the lungs (pneumonia), blood (bacteremia), and brain (meningitis). Pneumococcal pneumonia kills about 1 out of 20 people who contract the disease; both pneumococcal bacteremia and pneumococcal meningitis kill about 1 person in 6.

Pneumococcal conjugate vaccine 13 (PCV13) protects against 13 pneumococcal bacteria. Adults older than 65 years and adults older than 19 years with certain medical conditions should get the PCV13 vaccine before getting the PPSV23 vaccine.

PPSV23 protects against 23 types of pneumococcal bacteria, including those most likely to cause serious disease. In most healthy adults who are vaccinated, protection develops for most or all of these types within 2 to 3 weeks of vaccination. One to three doses are given to adults based on age, time of first dose, and other medical conditions. The vaccine is recommended for the following people:

- All adults age 65 years and older
- Adults 19 years and older with certain health conditions
- Adults 19 years and older who smoke cigarettes

People to whom the vaccine should not be given include those who are allergic to the vaccine or a component of the vaccine. Another type of pneumococcal vaccine (PCV) is routinely recommended for children younger than 5 years.

Modified from: Pneumococcal vaccines (PCV13 and PPSV23): addressing common questions about pneumococcal vaccination for adults. Centers for Disease Control and Prevention website. https://www.cdc.gov/vaccines/hcp/adults/downloads/fs-pneumo-hcp.pdf. Updated May 2016. Accessed March 14, 2018.

- Foreign body aspiration
- Alcohol or other drug addiction
- Cardiac failure
- Stroke
- Syncope
- Pulmonary embolism
- Chronic illness
  - Chronic respiratory disease
  - Diabetes mellitus
  - Heart failure
- Prolonged immobilization
- Compromised immune status

Mycoplasmal Pneumonia

Mycoplasmal pneumonia is caused by infection with *Mycoplasma pneumoniae.* It causes a mild upper respiratory tract infection in school-age children and young adults. Transmission is believed to occur by means of infected respiratory secretions. Therefore, the condition spreads quickly among family members. This form of pneumonia can be treated effectively with antibiotics.

Aspiration Pneumonia

Aspiration pneumonia is an inflammation of the lung tissue (parenchyma). It results when foreign material enters the tracheobronchial tree. The syndrome is common in patients who have an altered level of consciousness (eg, from head injury, seizure activity, stroke, use of alcohol or other drugs, anesthesia, infection, shock), patients who are intubated, and patients who have aspirated foreign bodies. Factors common to victims of aspiration include depression of the cough or gag reflex, inability of the patient to handle secretions or gastric contents, and inability to protect the airway.

Aspiration pneumonia may be nonbacterial. For example, it may develop after aspiration of stomach contents, toxic materials, or inert substances. This nonbacterial type typically is called pneumonitis to distinguish it from infectious pneumonia or bacterial pneumonia (as a secondary complication). Bacterial aspiration pneumonia has a poor prognosis, even with antibiotic therapy.

Management of Pneumonia

The pathophysiology of pneumonia depends on the agent that caused the disease. In viral and mycoplasmal pneumonias, the inflammatory response in the bronchi damages the cilia and the epithelium. This causes congestion, and in some cases it causes hemorrhage. Signs and symptoms include chest pain, cough, fever, dyspnea, and occasionally hemoptysis. Patients usually complain of general malaise. They also complain of upper respiratory and gastrointestinal tract symptoms. Auscultation of the chest may reveal wheezing and fine crackles. In uncomplicated cases, the symptoms usually resolve in 7 to 10 days.

Bacterial pneumonia begins with infection in the alveoli. In time, this infection fills the alveoli with fluid and purulent sputum. The infection spreads from alveolus to alveolus. As this occurs, large areas of the lung, even entire lobes, may become consolidated (filled with fluid and cellular debris). Consolidation reduces the available surface area of respiratory membranes and decreases the ventilation/perfusion ratio. These effects may lead to hypoxemia. Patients with bacterial pneumonia usually have acute shaking chills, fever, tachypnea, tachycardia, cough, and sputum production. The sputum may be rust colored (classic for pneumococcus). More often, though, it is yellow, green, or gray. Additional symptoms include anorexia, malaise, flank or back pain, and vomiting. If the disease is uncomplicated and treated with antibiotics, the patient begins to recover within 3 to 5 days. Antibiotics usually are continued for a total of 7 to 10 days.

The physiologic effects of aspiration pneumonia are based on the volume and pH of the aspirated substances. If the pH level is less than 2.5 (as may occur in the aspiration of stomach contents), atelectasis, pulmonary edema, hemorrhage, and cell necrosis may occur. The alveolar–capillary membrane may be damaged as well, which, in turn, may lead to the accumulation of fluid in the alveoli. In severe cases, it may lead to acute respiratory distress syndrome (described in the next section). The patient's signs and symptoms vary with the scenario and the severity of the insult (eg, drowning, foreign body aspiration, aspiration of gastric contents). Clinical features may include dyspnea, cough, bronchospasm, wheezes, rhonchi, crackles, cyanosis, and pulmonary and cardiac insufficiency. Of these patients, a good percentage are at risk for the development of pulmonary infection.

CRITICAL THINKING

What measures can the paramedic take to reduce a patient's risk of aspiration?

Prehospital care for patients with pneumonia includes airway support, oxygen administration, ventilatory assistance as needed, IV fluids to support blood pressure and to thin and loosen mucus, cardiac monitoring, and transport for evaluation by a physician. (Bronchodilator drugs may also be used if the patient is wheezing.) In cases of aspiration, suctioning of the airway may be required. General patient management usually includes bed rest, analgesics, decongestants, expectorants, antipyretics, and antibiotic therapy. In severe cases, bronchoscopy, intubation, and mechanical ventilation may be required.

Acute Respiratory Distress Syndrome

Acute respiratory distress syndrome (ARDS) is a form of hypoxemic respiratory failure. ARDS is the culmination of a spectrum of disease that begins with direct or indirect **acute lung injury (ALI)**. It is characterized by acute lung inflammation and diffuse alveolar–capillary injury.[16] All disorders that result in ARDS cause severe noncardiogenic pulmonary edema. Each year nearly 200,000 patients are admitted to hospitals with ALI or ARDS.[4] The syndrome develops as a complication of injury or illness, such as trauma, gastric aspiration, cardiopulmonary bypass surgery, gram-negative sepsis, multiple blood transfusions, oxygen toxicity, toxic inhalation, drug overdose, pneumonia, sepsis, and infections. Regardless of the specific cause, increased capillary permeability (high-permeability noncardiogenic pulmonary edema) results in a clinical condition in which the lungs are wet and heavy, congested, hemorrhagic, and stiff, with decreased diffusion capacity across alveolar membranes leading to severe ventilation/perfusion mismatch[4] (**FIGURE 23-13**). The lungs become noncompliant, requiring the patient to increase the pressure in the airways to breathe.

The pulmonary edema associated with ARDS leads to severe hypoxemia, intrapulmonary shunting,

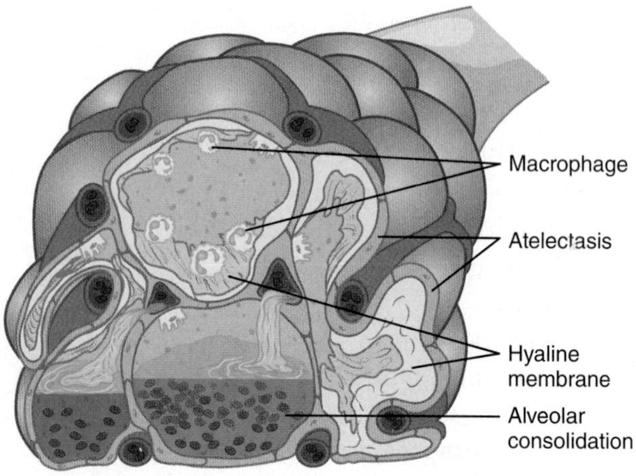

FIGURE 23-13 Cross-sectional view of alveoli in acute respiratory distress syndrome.

reduced lung compliance, and, in some cases, irreversible damage to lung tissue. Unique to this syndrome is that in most instances, ARDS develops in patients who have healthy lungs before the event that caused the disease; that is, the patients have no history of recent respiratory illness or disease. ARDS is generally more common in men than in women, affecting approximately 190,000 people in the United States each year.[17] The death rate is greater than 65%. Complications include respiratory failure, cardiac dysrhythmias, disseminated intravascular coagulation, barotrauma, heart failure, and renal failure.

Management

Depending on the underlying cause and severity of ARDS, prehospital management may include fluid replacement to maintain cardiac output and peripheral perfusion; drug therapy to support mechanical ventilation; the use of pharmacologic agents (eg, corticosteroids) to stabilize pulmonary, capillary, and alveolar walls; and the administration of diuretics.[18,19]

Patients with ARDS usually have tachypnea, labored breathing, and impaired gas exchange 12 to 72 hours after the initial injury or medical crisis. The syndrome often results from another illness or injury. Therefore, paramedics should consider the cause of the underlying problem. They also should provide high-flow nasal oxygen and ventilatory support, including NIPPV, to improve arterial oxygenation (assessed by pulse oximetry). Most patients with moderate to severe respiratory distress require mechanical ventilation. This ventilation includes the use of lung-protective ventilation strategies and should include the following:[4]

- Low tidal volumes (6 mL/kg predicted body weight)
- Limiting of plateau pressure (<30 cm H_20)
- Use of PEEP (starting at 5–8 cm H_20) to avoid oxygen toxicity (fraction of inspired oxygen <0.6)
- Respiratory rate of 12 to 15 breaths/min

When possible, volume-targeted modes of ventilation such as assist control, synchronized intermittent mandatory ventilation, or pressure-regulated volume control should be used (see Appendix B, *Advanced Practice Procedures for Critical Care Paramedics*).

Other strategies employed at the hospital include specialized forms of ventilation (airway pressure release), neuromuscular blockade, nitric oxide inhalation, prone positioning, and extracorporeal membrane oxygenation.

Pulmonary Embolism

Pulmonary embolism is a blockage of a pulmonary artery by a clot or other foreign material that has traveled there from another part of the body (**FIGURE 23-14**). Usually pulmonary embolisms originate in the lower extremities or pelvis. Pulmonary embolism is a relatively common disorder that is estimated to affect up to 900,000 people per year. Of this number, 60,000 to 100,000 people die.[20] Sudden death is the first symptom in about a quarter of patients who have a pulmonary embolism. In cases of severe pulmonary embolism, where shock and heart failure occur, the death rate may be as high as 30%.[21] Pulmonary embolism is

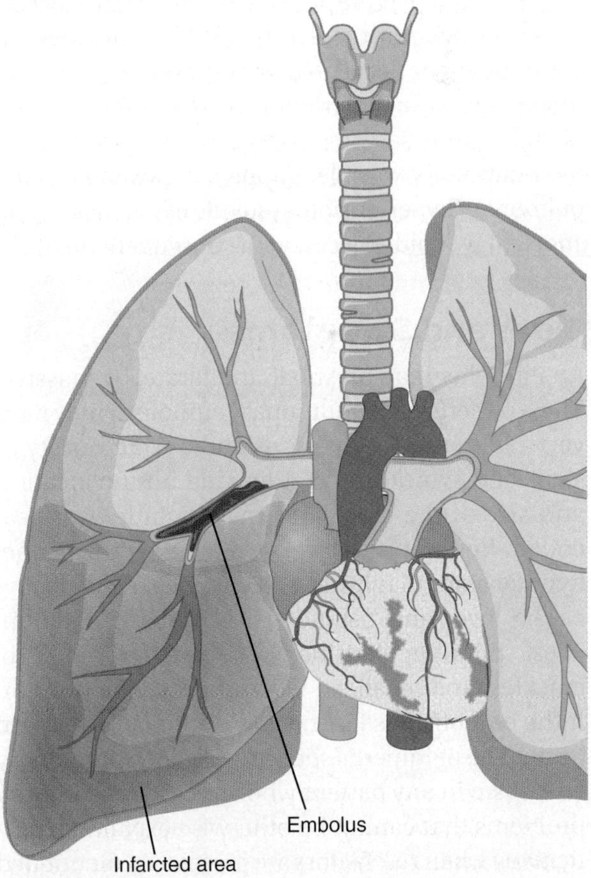

FIGURE 23-14 Pulmonary embolism is the blockage of a pulmonary artery by foreign matter, such as a thrombus. The blockage usually arises from a peripheral vein, fat, air, or tumor tissue. The result is obstruction of the blood supply to the lung tissue.

responsible for 5% of all sudden deaths.[22] However, less than 5% of patients with acute pulmonary embolism have cardiac arrest.[12]

Pulmonary embolism usually begins as a venous disease. It most often is caused by migration of a thrombus from the large veins of the lower extremities, but it also can occur as a result of fat, air, sheared venous catheters, amniotic fluid, or tumor tissue. The clot or embolus dislodges and travels through the venous system to the right side of the heart. From there it travels to the pulmonary arteries, obstructing the blood supply to a section of lung. The most common sites of thrombus formation are the deep veins of the legs and pelvis. There are three factors, known as the Virchow triad, that contribute to clot formation: hypercoagulability, stasis, and vessel injury. Factors that contribute to the development of venous thrombosis are listed in BOX 23-8.

When one or more pulmonary arteries are blocked, an area does not receive blood flow; however, it continues to be ventilated. In response to the lack of blood flow, vasoconstriction occurs. If the vascular obstruction is severe (blockage of 60% or more of the pulmonary vascular supply), hypoxemia, acute pulmonary hypertension, systemic hypotension, and shock may rapidly occur, with subsequent death.[23]

BOX 23-8 Contributing Factors in the Development of Venous Thrombosis

Stasis

Extended travel
Prolonged bed rest
Obesity
Advanced age
Varicose veins

Venous Injury/Trauma

Surgery of the thorax, abdomen, pelvis, or legs
Burns
Long bone fractures
Fractures of the pelvis or legs

Hypercoagulability

Malignancy (especially with metastasis)
Use of oral contraceptives
Pregnancy
Autoimmune disorders
Congenital or acquired coagulation disorders

Disease

Chronic lung disease with polycythemia
Heart failure
Sickle cell anemia
Cancer
Atrial fibrillation
Myocardial infarction
Previous pulmonary embolism
Previous deep vein thrombosis
Infection
Diabetes mellitus

Modified from: Risk factors for venous thromboembolism (VTE). American Heart Association website. http://www.heart.org/HEARTORG/Conditions/VascularHealth/VenousThromboembolism/Risk-Factors-for-Venous-Thromboembolism-VTE_UCM_479059_Article.jsp. Updated February 7, 2018. Accessed March 14, 2018.

Signs and Symptoms

An embolus may be small, moderate, or massive. Thus, patients with pulmonary embolism may have very different presentations and a wide variety of signs and symptoms that depend on the location and size of the clot. They may include dyspnea, cough, hemoptysis (rare), pain, anxiety, syncope, hypotension, diaphoresis, tachypnea, sinus tachycardia, fever, and distended neck veins. In addition, chest splinting, pleuritic pain, pleural friction rub, crackles, and localized wheezing may be present. If the embolism is large, sudden cardiac arrest can occur. The paramedic should consider a pulmonary embolism in any patient who has cardiorespiratory problems that cannot be otherwise explained, particularly when risk factors are present. As mentioned earlier, continuous capnography may be useful in identifying a patient with pulmonary embolism. Shockable rhythms are not common in cardiac arrest related to pulmonary embolism. During cardiac arrest, about 36% to 53% of these patients will be in pulseless electrical activity.[12]

CRITICAL THINKING

Consider that you need to distinguish a pulmonary embolism from other conditions with similar signs and symptoms. What information in the patient assessment may help?

Management

Prehospital care mainly is supportive. The paramedic should administer supplemental high-concentration oxygen, apply a cardiac monitor and pulse oximeter,

NOTE

The ECG may show variable findings in a patient with pulmonary embolism (**FIGURE 23-15**). These findings may include the following:

- Sinus tachycardia (not shown)
- Right bundle branch block
- T-wave inversion in V_1-V_4 and/or the inferior leads (because of high pulmonary pressures)
- Right axis deviation (or extreme right axis deviation) (not shown)
- Dominant R wave in V_2 (because of right ventricular dilation)
- Peaked P wave in lead II greater than 2.5 mm (because of right atrial enlargement) (not shown)
- An S1Q3T3 pattern (a prominent S wave in lead I, a Q wave in lead III, and an inverted T wave in lead III)

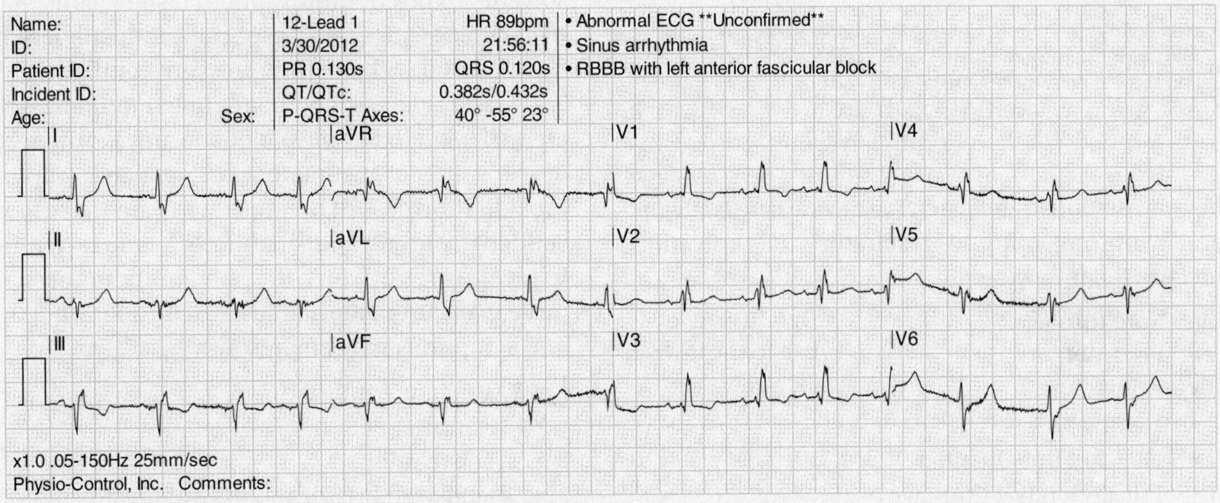

ST measurements are measured at the J point and are expressed in mm.

I	II	III	aVR	aVL	aVF	V1	V2	V3	V4	V5	V6
0.18	0.12	-0.06	-0.15	0.12	0.03	-0.18	0.05	-0.10	0.04	0.02	0.15

FIGURE 23-15

Courtesy of Christopher Touzeau, MS, FNP-C, NRP.

Modified from: Ferrari E, Imbert A, Chevalier T, Mihoubi A, Morand P, Baudouy M. The ECG in pulmonary embolism: predictive value of negative T waves in precordial leads. *Chest*. 1997;111(3):537-543.

and establish an IV line. The patient should be transported in a position of comfort. Definitive care requires hospitalization and in-hospital treatment with fibrinolytic, surgical, or percutaneous embolectomy and, in cases of cardiac arrest, extracorporeal cardiopulmonary resuscitation.[12]

Upper Respiratory Tract Infection

An **upper respiratory tract infection** can affect the nose, throat, sinuses, and larynx. It is among the most common of all illnesses. Adults average two to three colds per year.[24] These illnesses include the common cold, pharyngitis, tonsillitis, sinusitis, and laryngitis. They rarely are life threatening. However, they often exacerbate underlying pulmonary conditions. They also may lead to significant infections in patients with suppressed immune function. A key action for preventing the spread of respiratory tract infections is handwashing. Another crucial action is covering the mouth when sneezing or coughing.

A variety of bacteria and viruses can cause an upper respiratory tract infection. Group A streptococci are responsible for 15% to 30% of cases; 50% of cases

NOTE

Cover Your Cough

- Cover your mouth and nose with a tissue when you cough or sneeze. Put your used tissue in the waste basket.
- If you do not have a tissue, cough or sneeze into your upper sleeve or elbow, not your hands.
- Wash hands often with soap and warm water for 20 seconds. If soap and water are not available, use an alcohol-based hand rub.

Modified from: Cover your cough: stop the spread of germs that can make you and others sick! Centers for Disease Control and Prevention website. https://www.cdc.gov/flu/pdf/protect/cdc_cough.pdf. Accessed March 14, 2018.

have no demonstrated bacterial or viral cause.[25] Signs and symptoms of upper respiratory tract infection include the following:

- Sore throat
- Fever
- Chills
- Headache
- Facial pain (sinusitis)
- Purulent nasal drainage
- Halitosis (bad breath)
- Cervical adenopathy (enlarged cervical lymph nodes)
- Erythematous pharynx (pharyngeal inflammation/irritation)

CRITICAL THINKING

When might an upper respiratory infection become life threatening? Give two or three examples.

Management

Most upper respiratory tract infections are self-limiting and require little or no prehospital treatment. Prehospital care is aimed at relieving the symptoms. Follow-up by a physician is also recommended. The paramedic should follow local protocol.

Spontaneous Pneumothorax

A primary **spontaneous pneumothorax** usually results when a bleb ruptures, allowing air to enter the pleural space from within the lung. This type of pneumothorax may occur in seemingly healthy people aged 20 to 40 years. Often these patients are tall, thin men with long, narrow chests. (In contrast, a secondary spontaneous pneumothorax sometimes may develop from an underlying disease, such as COPD.) The number of spontaneous pneumothoraces is higher in some populations, including people with acquired immunodeficiency syndrome (AIDS) who have pneumonia, and drug abusers who free-base cocaine, smoke marijuana, or huff inhalants (eg, glue, solvents). The condition should also be considered in a patient with COPD, especially if the patient has been treated with positive pressure ventilation.

Most primary spontaneous pneumothoraces that are well tolerated by the patient occupy less than 20% of a lung (partial pneumothorax). Signs and symptoms include shortness of breath, chest pain that often is sudden in onset, pallor, diaphoresis, and tachypnea. In severe cases in which the pneumothorax occupies more than 20% of the hemithorax, the following signs and symptoms may be present:[26]

- Altered mental status
- Cyanosis
- Tachycardia
- Decreased breath sounds on the affected side
- Local hyperresonance to percussion
- Subcutaneous emphysema

Management

Prehospital care is based on the patient's symptoms and degree of respiratory distress. Administration of high-concentration oxygen is indicated, and airway, ventilatory, and circulatory support may be required in severe cases. These patients should be transported in a position of comfort for evaluation by a physician and possible decompression of the pleural space. Surgery is occasionally but rarely necessary. This may be done to allow for lung reexpansion or to prevent recurrence. Rarely do symptoms of tension pneumothorax develop. In these cases, needle chest decompression should be performed.

NOTE

In severe cases, a spontaneous pneumothorax may generate a tension pneumothorax. When this occurs, venous return to the heart is impaired, which can lead to total cardiovascular collapse. Tension pneumothorax is further described in Chapter 41, *Chest Trauma*.

Hyperventilation Syndrome

Hyperventilation syndrome is abnormally deep or rapid breathing that results in an excessive loss of carbon dioxide (which, in turn, produces respiratory alkalosis). As a result, the syndrome produces hypocapnia. The hypocapnia leads to cerebrovascular constriction, reduced cerebral perfusion, paresthesia, dizziness, or even feelings of euphoria. Several conditions can cause hyperventilation syndrome, including the following:

- Anxiety
- Hypoxia
- Pulmonary disease
- Cardiovascular disorders
- Metabolic disorders
- Neurologic disorders
- Fever
- Infection
- Pain
- Pregnancy
- Drug use

CRITICAL THINKING

How can you distinguish between hyperventilation caused by anxiety and hyperventilation caused by a serious medical illness or toxic ingestion?

Signs and symptoms of hyperventilation syndrome include dyspnea with rapid breathing and a high minute volume, chest pain, facial tingling, and carpopedal spasm. Other assessment findings vary, based on the cause of the syndrome. A low $ETCO_2$ measurement is less than 35 mm Hg.

Management

Supportive care is provided if a thorough history and physical examination rule out life threats and it is believed the syndrome is caused by anxiety (psychogenic dyspnea, which is a diagnosis of exclusion). It consists of calming measures and reassurance. Paramedics may suspect that the syndrome is a result of illness (eg, diabetes mellitus, renal disease). They also may suspect drug ingestion. In either case, care includes both oxygen administration and airway/ventilatory support. All patients who are hyperventilating should be calmed, and the paramedic should coach the patient's ventilations. Attempts should not be made to slow ventilations if patients are compensating for hypoxia or metabolic acidosis. If the hyperventilation is severe or complicated by illness or drug ingestion, transport for evaluation by a physician is indicated.

Lung Cancer

Lung cancer (bronchogenic carcinoma) is an epidemic in the United States. An estimated 225,000 new cases are reported each year.[27] Most cases of lung cancer develop in people aged 55 to 65 years. Of the new cases reported, most patients die of the disease within 1 year; 20% have local lung involvement, 25% have metastasis to the lymph system, and 55% have distant metastatic cancer.[28] The most common cause of lung cancer is cigarette smoking. Heavy smokers (more than 1 pack per day) have a 20 times greater chance for the development of lung cancer than do nonsmokers.[27] Other possible risk factors include passive smoking (exposure to someone else's cigarette smoke); exposure to asbestos, radon gas, dust, or coal products; radiation therapy (usually in patients treated for other cancers); pulmonary fibrosis; human immunodeficiency virus infection; genetic factors; alcohol consumption; and exposure to other toxins.

Pathophysiology

Like other cancers, lung cancer is the uncontrolled growth of abnormal cells. At least a dozen different cell types of tumors (neoplasms) are associated with primary lung cancer (**FIGURE 23-16**). The two major cell types of lung cancer are small cell lung cancer and non–small cell lung cancer (which is subcategorized as squamous cell carcinoma, adenocarcinoma, and large cell carcinoma). Each cell type has a different growth pattern. Each also has a different response to treatment. Most abnormal cell growth begins in the bronchi or bronchioles. The lung also is a fairly common site of **metastasis** (the spread of cancer) from other primary sites (eg, breast cancer).

Signs and Symptoms

The signs and symptoms of early-stage disease often are nonspecific. Smokers often attribute them to the effects of smoking. They include coughing, sputum production, lower airway obstruction (noted by wheezing), and respiratory illness (eg, bronchitis). As the disease progresses (when most patients are

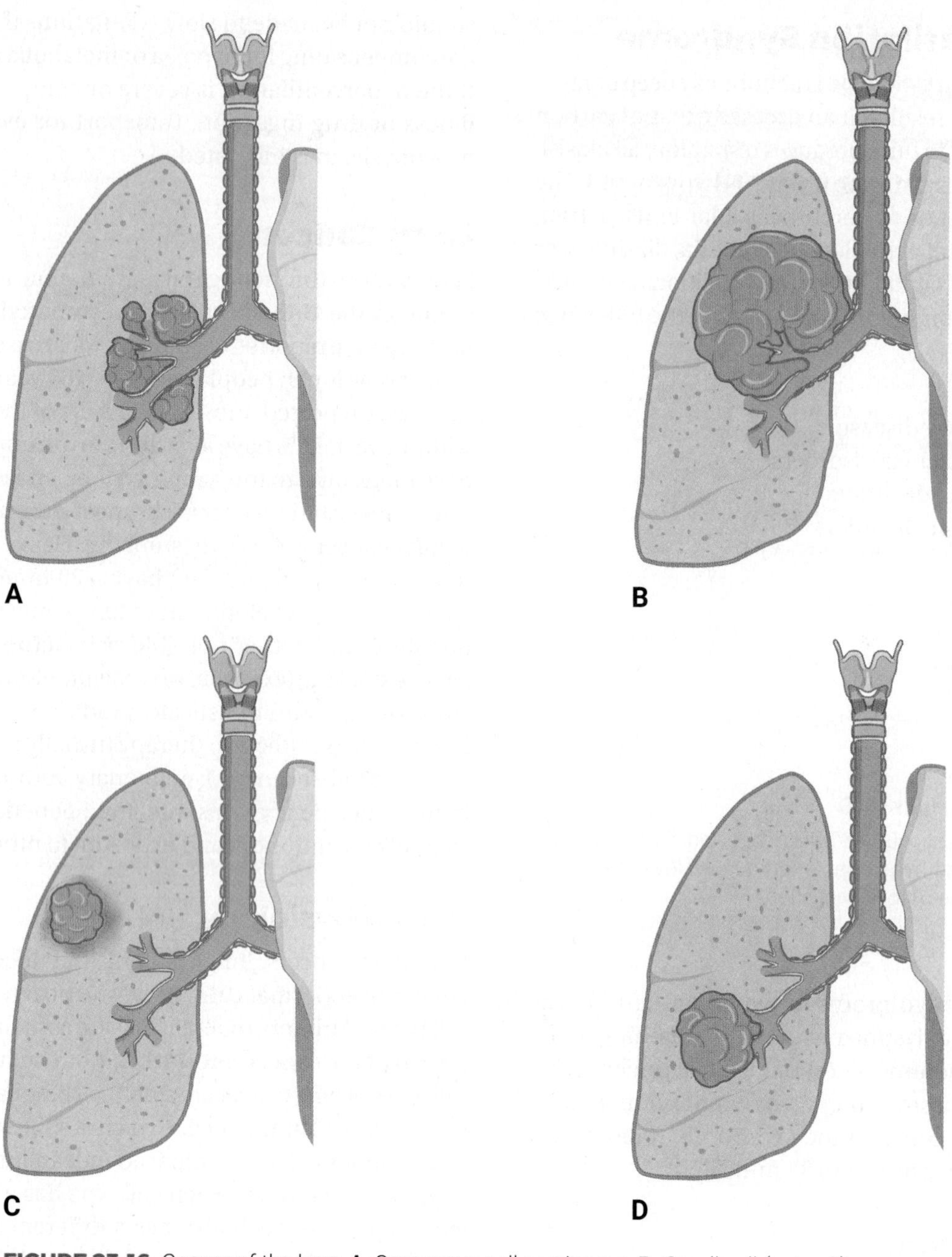

FIGURE 23-16 Cancer of the lung. **A.** Squamous cell carcinoma. **B.** Small cell (oat cell) carcinoma. **C.** Adenocarcinoma. **D.** Large cell carcinoma.

diagnosed), signs and symptoms may include the following:

- Cough
- Hemoptysis (which may be severe)
- Dyspnea
- Hoarseness or voice change
- Dysphagia
- Weight loss/anorexia
- Weakness
- Chest pain

Patients with cancer may call paramedics because of respiratory distress or because of complications resulting from chemotherapy or radiation therapy. Such therapy is toxic to both normal body cells and malignant cells. Associated complaints often include nausea and vomiting, fatigue, and dehydration. These patients should be offered emotional and psychological support.

Management

Most patients with lung cancer are aware of their disease. Prehospital management includes airway, ventilatory, and circulatory support; oxygen administration if indicated; and transport for evaluation by a physician. Depending on the severity of the patient's condition, IV fluids may be needed to improve hydration and to thin sputum. Drug therapy (eg, bronchodilators, corticosteroids) may be needed to improve breathing. Analgesics may be required to relieve pain. End-stage patients may have advance directives or do not resuscitate orders. In these cases, emotional support should also be offered to the family and loved ones.

> CRITICAL THINKING
>
> Should you assume that patients who have been diagnosed with lung cancer want to be managed on a do not resuscitate basis?

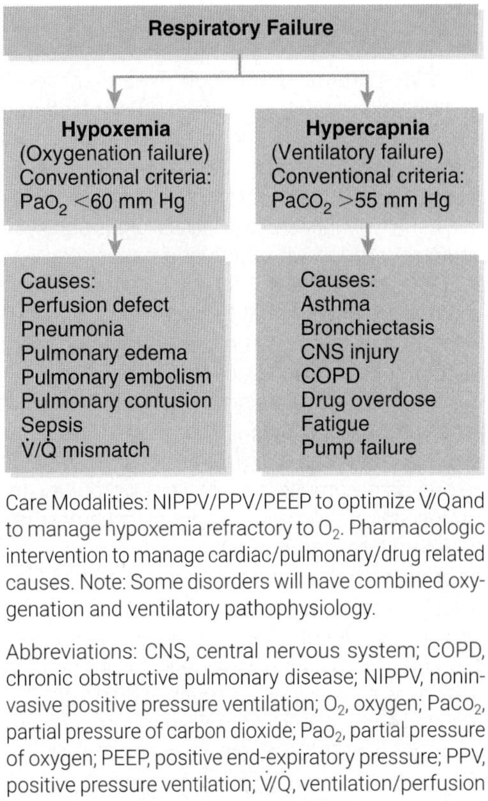

Respiratory Failure
Hypoxemia
(Oxygenation failure)
Conventional criteria:
PaO2 <60 mm Hg
Hypercapnia
(Ventilatory failure)
Conventional criteria:
PaCO2 >55 mm Hg
Causes:
Perfusion defect
Pneumonia
Pulmonary edema
Pulmonary embolism
Pulmonary contusion
Sepsis
V̇/Q̇ mismatch
Causes:
Asthma
Bronchiectasis
CNS injury
COPD
Drug overdose
Fatigue
Pump failure
Care Modalities: NIPPV/PPV/PEEP to optimize V̇/Q̇ and to manage hypoxemia refractory to O2. Pharmacologic intervention to manage cardiac/pulmonary/drug related causes. Note: Some disorders will have combined oxygenation and ventilatory pathophysiology.
Abbreviations: CNS, central nervous system; COPD, chronic obstructive pulmonary disease; NIPPV, noninvasive positive pressure ventilation; O2, oxygen; Paco2, partial pressure of carbon dioxide; Pao2, partial pressure of oxygen; PEEP, positive end-expiratory pressure; PPV, positive pressure ventilation; V̇/Q̇, ventilation/perfusion

FIGURE 23-17 Algorithm of etiologies and treatments of respiratory failure.

Modified from: Mosier JM, Hypes C, Joshi R, Whitmore S, Parthasarathy S, Cairns CB. Ventilator strategies and rescue therapies for management of acute respiratory failure in the emergency department. *Ann Emerg Med.* 2015;66(5):529-541. Art located at https://ars.els-cdn.com/content/image/1-s2.0-S0196064415003790-gr1_lrg.jpg.

Respiratory Failure

As described in this chapter, respiratory emergencies can result from many disease states, including ventilatory failure, oxygenation failure, and shock. Respiratory failure occurs when pulmonary gas exchange is sufficiently impaired to cause hypoxemia (oxygenation failure) with or without hypercapnia (ventilatory failure). **FIGURE 23-17** provides a summary of the various etiologies and care of respiratory failure.

Summary

- Diseases responsible for respiratory emergencies include those related to ventilation, diffusion, and perfusion. Ventilation moves air into and out of the lungs. Diffusion is the process of gas exchange. Perfusion is circulation of blood through the tissues.
- Patients should be assessed for chief complaint, signs and symptoms of respiratory distress, and past medical history. The physical examination should determine vital signs, indicators of increased work of breathing, breath sounds, and peripheral edema or cyanosis. Capnometry, oximetry, and peak flow measurements supplement the physical examination findings.
- Obstructive airway disease is a triad of distinct diseases that often coexist: chronic bronchitis, emphysema, and asthma. The main goal of prehospital care for these patients is the correction of hypoxemia through improved airflow.
- Chronic bronchitis is characterized by inflammatory changes and excessive mucus production in the alveoli. These patients often have low blood oxygen levels and excess carbon dioxide levels.
- Emphysema causes abnormal enlargement of air spaces beyond the terminal bronchioles and destruction and collapse of the alveoli.
- Asthma, or reactive airway disease, is characterized by reversible airflow obstruction caused by bronchial smooth muscle contraction; hypersecretion of mucus, resulting in bronchial plugging; and inflammatory changes in the bronchial walls. The typical patient with asthma is in obvious distress.

Respirations are rapid and loud. Treatment focuses on bronchodilation, hydration, and reduction of inflammation.

- Pneumonia is a group of specific infections (bacterial, viral, or fungal). These infections cause an acute inflammatory process of the respiratory bronchioles and the alveoli. Pneumonia usually manifests with classic signs and symptoms, including a productive cough and associated fever that produces "shaking chills." Prehospital care of patients with pneumonia includes airway support, oxygen administration, ventilatory assistance as needed, intravenous (IV) fluids, cardiac monitoring, and transport.
- Acute respiratory distress syndrome (ARDS) is a fulminant form of respiratory failure. It is characterized by acute lung inflammation and diffuse alveolar–capillary injury. It develops as a complication of illness or injury. In ARDS, the lungs are wet and heavy, congested, hemorrhagic, and stiff, with decreased perfusion capacity across alveolar membranes. Prehospital management includes airway and ventilatory support.
- Positive end-expiratory pressure (PEEP) maintains pressure at the end of exhalation. Adding PEEP in the respiratory circuit keeps alveoli open and pushes fluid from the alveoli back into the interstitium or capillaries. Continuous positive airway pressure (CPAP) maintains constant airway pressure throughout the entire respiratory cycle. CPAP improves diffusion and helps reexpand collapsed alveoli. Bilevel positive airway pressure (BPAP) delivers variable airway pressure throughout the respiratory cycle.
- Pulmonary embolism is a blockage of a pulmonary artery by a clot or other foreign material. When one or more pulmonary arteries are blocked by an embolism, a section of lung is ventilated but hypoperfused. Hypotension, shock, and death can occur. Prehospital care is mainly supportive and includes oxygen administration, IV access, and transport for definitive care.
- Upper respiratory infections affect the nose, throat, sinuses, and larynx. Signs and symptoms of an upper respiratory infection include sore throat, fever, chills, headache, cervical adenopathy, and an erythematous pharynx. Prehospital care is based on the patient's symptoms.
- A primary spontaneous pneumothorax usually results when a subpleural bleb ruptures, allowing air to enter the pleural space from within the lung. Signs and symptoms include shortness of breath and chest pain that often are sudden in onset, pallor, diaphoresis, and tachypnea. Prehospital care is based on the patient's symptoms and degree of distress.
- Hyperventilation syndrome is abnormally deep or rapid breathing. This type of breathing results in an excessive loss of carbon dioxide. If the syndrome clearly is caused by anxiety, prehospital care is mainly supportive (ie, calming measures and reassurance). The paramedic may suspect that the syndrome is a result of illness or drug ingestion. If this is the case, care may include oxygen administration and airway and ventilatory support.
- Lung cancer is an expression of the uncontrolled growth of abnormal cells. As the disease progresses, signs and symptoms may include cough, hemoptysis, dyspnea, hoarseness, and dysphagia. Prehospital management includes airway, ventilatory, and circulatory support.

References

1. Prekker ME, Feemster LC, Hough CL, et al. The epidemiology and outcome of prehospital respiratory distress. *Acad Emerg Med*. 2014;21(5):543-550.
2. Kochanek KD, Murphy SL, Xu J, Arias E. Mortality in the United States. *NCHS Data Brief.* 2014 December;(178):1-8.
3. Wilkins RL, Stoller JK, Kacmarek RM, Shelledy DC, Kester L. *Egans' Fundamentals of Respiratory Care*. 9th ed. St. Louis, MO: Mosby; 2009.
4. Mosier JM, Hypes C, Joshi R, Whitmore S, Parthasarathy S, Cairns CB. Ventilator strategies and rescue therapies for management of acute respiratory failure in the emergency department. *Ann Emerg Med.* 2015;66(5):529-541.
5. Kheng CP, Rahman NH. The use of end-tidal carbon dioxide monitoring in patients with hypotension in the emergency department. *Int J Emerg Med.* 2012;5:31.
6. Bhatt N, Allen B. Pulmonary function testing and asthma. Ohio Asthma Coalition website. http://www.ohioasthmacoalition.org/professionals/documents/oacpfttalkallan.bhatt.pdf. Accessed March 14, 2018.
7. Mosenifar Z. Chronic obstructive pulmonary disease (COPD). Medscape website. https://emedicine.medscape.com/article/297664-overview. Updated September 25, 2017. Accessed March 14, 2018.
8. Centers for Disease Control and Prevention/National Center for Health Statistics. Chronic obstructive pulmonary disease (COPD) includes: chronic bronchitis and emphysema. Centers for Disease Control and Prevention website. https://www.cdc.gov/nchs/fastats/copd.htm. Updated May 3, 2017. Accessed March 14, 2018.
9. Han MK, Dransfield MT, Martinez FJ. Chronic obstructive pulmonary disease: definition, clinical manifestations, diagnosis, and staging. UpToDate website. https://www.uptodate.com/contents/chronic-obstructive-pulmonary-disease-definition-clinical-manifestations-diagnosis-and-staging. Updated January 11, 2018. Accessed March 14, 2018.
10. Centers for Disease Control and Prevention/National Center for Health Statistics. Asthma. Centers for Disease Control and Prevention website. https://www.cdc.gov/nchs/fastats/asthma.htm. Updated March 31, 2017. Accessed March 14, 2018.
11. Reddel HK, Bateman ED, Becker A, et al. A summary of the new GINA strategy: a roadmap to asthma control. *Eur Respir J.* 2015;46(3):622-639.
12. Part 10: special circumstances of resuscitation. *Web-based Integrated 2010 and 2015 American Heart Association Guidelines for Cardiopulmonary Resuscitation and Emergence Cardiovascular Care.* American Heart Association website. https://eccguidelines.heart.org/index.php/circulation/cpr-ecc-guidelines-2/part-10-special-circumstances-of-resuscitation/. Accessed March 14, 2018.

13. Asthma: an evidence-based management update; airway management. EB Medicine website. https://www.ebmedicine.net/topics.php?paction=showTopicSeg&topic_id=59&seg_id=1860. Accessed March 14, 2018.
14. Centers for Disease Control and Prevention/National Center for Health Statistics. Pneumonia. Centers for Disease Control and Prevention website. https://www.cdc.gov/nchs/fastats/pneumonia.htm. Updated January 20, 2017. Accessed March 14, 2018.
15. Yildirim I, Shea KM, Pelton SI. Pneumococcal disease in the era of pneumococcal conjugate vaccine. *Infec Dis Clin North Am*. 2015;29(4):679-697.
16. McCance L, Huether S. *Pathophysiology: The Biologic Basis for Disease in Adults and Children*. 7th ed. St. Louis, MO: Mosby; 2014.
17. Modrykamien AM, Gupta P. The acute respiratory distress syndrome. *Proc (Bayl Univ Med Cent)*. 2015;28(2):163-171.
18. Miyakawa L, Love A, Seijo L, et al. The role of high flow nasal oxygen in patients with acute respiratory distress syndrome. *Am J Resp Crit Care Med*. 2017;195:A3681.
19. Frat JP, Thille AW, Mercat A, et al. High flow oxygen through nasal cannula in acute hypoxemic respiratory failure. *N Engl J Med*. 2015;372(23):2185-2196.
20. Division of Blood Disorders National Center on Birth Defects and Developmental Disabilities, Centers for Disease Control and Prevention. Venous thromboembolism (blood clots): data and statistics. Centers for Disease Control and Prevention website. https://www.cdc.gov/ncbddd/dvt/data.html. Updated June 22, 2015. Accessed March 14, 2018.
21. Bělohlávek J, Dytrych V, Linhart A. Pulmonary embolism, part I: epidemiology, risk factors and risk stratification, pathophysiology, clinical presentation, diagnosis and nonthrombotic pulmonary embolism. *Exp Clin Cardiol*. 2013;18(2):129-138.
22. Goldhaber SZ. Pulmonary thromboembolism. Kasper DL, Braunwald E, Fauci AS, et al., eds. *Harrison's Principles of Internal Medicine*. 16th ed. New York, NY: McGraw-Hill; 2005.
23. Ireland R. Danger, diagnosis and treatment of pulmonary embolisms. *JEMS* website. http://www.jems.com/articles/print/volume-39/issue-7/features/danger-diagnosis-treatment-pulmonary-emb.html. Published July 11, 2014. Accessed March 14, 2018.
24. National Center for Immunizations and Respiratory Diseases, Division of Viral Diseases. Common colds: protect yourself and others. Centers for Disease Control and Prevention website. https://www.cdc.gov/features/rhinoviruses/index.html. Published February 12, 2018. Accessed March 14, 2018.
25. Reglinski M, Sriskandan S. *Molecular Medical Microbiology*. 2nd ed. Philadelphia, PA: Elsevier; 2015.
26. Hess DR, MacIntyre R, Galvin WF, Moshoe SC. *Respiratory Care: Principles and Practice*. 3rd ed. Jones & Bartlett Learning; 2016.
27. Midthun DE. Overview of the risk factors, pathology, and clinical manifestations of lung cancer. UpToDate website. https://www.uptodate.com/contents/overview-of-the-risk-factors-pathology-and-clinical-manifestations-of-lung-cancer?source=search_result&search=lung%20cancer%20incidence%20usa&selectedTitle=9~150. Updated February 3, 2017. Accessed March 14, 2018.
28. Walls R, Hockberger R, Gausche-Hill M. *Rosen's Emergency Medicine: Concepts and Clinical Practice*. 9th ed. Philadelphia, PA: Elsevier; 2017.

Suggested Readings

Beachey W. *Respiratory Care Anatomy and Physiology*. 4th ed. Philadelphia, PA: Elsevier; 2018.

DiPrima PA. *EMS Respiratory Emergency Management Demystified*. New York, NY: McGraw-Hill; 2014.

Hsieh A. EMS use of CPAP for respiratory emergencies: CPAP for emergency management of congestive heart failure and other respiratory emergencies has become the standard of care. EMS1.com website. https://www.ems1.com/ems-products/medical-equipment/airway-management/articles/1349608-EMS-use-of-CPAP-for-respiratory-emergencies/. Published October 24, 2016. Accessed March 14, 2018.

McEvoy M. How to assess and treat acute respiratory distress: a rapid and thorough assessment is critical for patients with acute respiratory distress. *JEMS* website. http://www.jems.com/articles/print/volume-38/issue-8/patient-care/how-assess-and-treat-acute-respiratory-d.html. Published July 19, 2013. Accessed March 14, 2018.

Peres J. No clear link between passive smoking and lung cancer. *J Natl Cancer Inst*. 2013;105(24):1844-1846.

Prekker ME, Feemster LC, Hough CL, et al. The epidemiology and outcome of prehospital respiratory distress. *Acad Emerg Med*. 2014;21(5):543-550.

Walsh BK. *Neonatal and Pediatric Respiratory Care*. 4th ed. Philadelphia, PA: Elsevier; 2015.

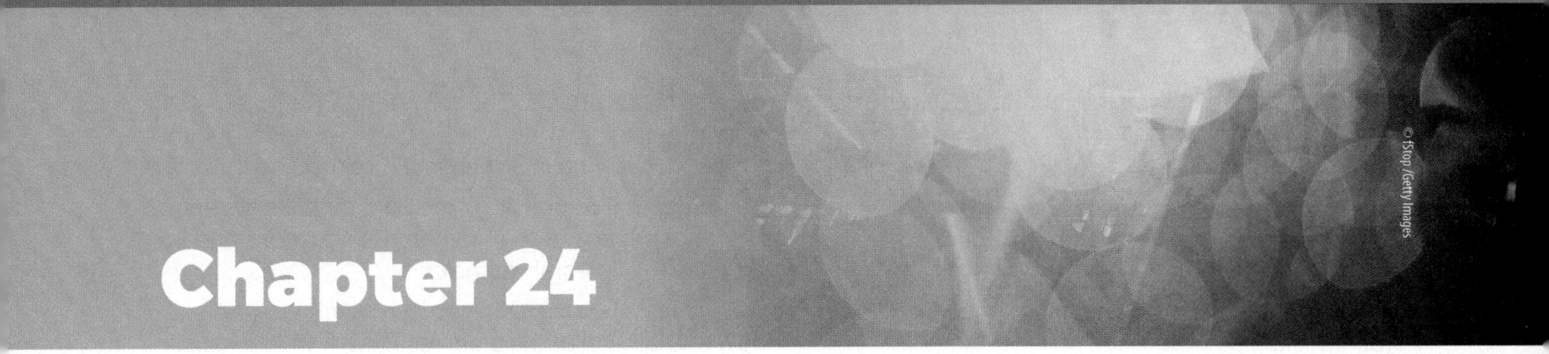

Chapter 24

Neurology

NATIONAL EMS EDUCATION STANDARD COMPETENCIES

Medicine

Integrates assessment findings with principles of epidemiology and pathophysiology to formulate a field impression and implement a comprehensive treatment/disposition plan for a patient with a medical complaint.

Neurology

Anatomy, presentations, and management of
- Decreased level of responsiveness (pp 945–950)

Anatomy, physiology, pathophysiology, assessment, and management of
- Stroke/transient ischemic attack (pp 951–959)
- Seizure (pp 959–964)
- Status epilepticus (pp 964–965)
- Headache (pp 965–966)

Anatomy, physiology, epidemiology, pathophysiology, psychosocial impact, presentations, prognosis, and management of
- Stroke/intracranial hemorrhage/transient ischemic attack (pp 951–959)
- Seizure (pp 959–964)
- Status epilepticus (pp 964–965)
- Headache (pp 965–966)
- Dementia (pp 970–971)
- Neoplasms (pp 968–969)
- Demyelinating disorders (pp 971–972)
- Parkinson disease (pp 973–974)
- Cranial nerve disorders (pp 974–975)
- Movement disorders (pp 973–974)
- Neurologic inflammation/infection (pp 967–968)
- Spinal cord compression (pp 968–969)
- Hydrocephalus (see Chapter 47, *Pediatrics*)
- Wernicke encephalopathy (see Chapter 33, *Toxicology*)

OBJECTIVES

Upon completion of this chapter, the paramedic student will be able to:

1. Describe the anatomy and physiology of the nervous system. (pp 936–941)
2. Outline pathophysiologic changes in the nervous system that may alter the cerebral perfusion pressure. (p 943)
3. Describe the assessment of a patient with a neurologic disorder. (pp 943–949)
4. Describe the pathophysiology, signs and symptoms, and specific management techniques for each of the following neurologic disorders: coma, stroke and intracranial hemorrhage, seizure disorders, headaches, brain neoplasm and brain abscess, and degenerative neurologic diseases. (pp 949–976)

KEY TERMS

absence seizures Seizures characterized by brief lapses of consciousness without loss of posture; also known as petit mal seizures.

action potential A change in membrane potential in an excitable tissue that acts as an electrical signal and is propagated in an all-or-none fashion.

Alzheimer disease A disease characterized by confusion, memory failure, disorientation, speech disturbances, and inability to carry out purposeful movements.

amnesia Memory loss.

amyotrophic lateral sclerosis (ALS) One of a group of rare disorders in which the nerves that control muscular activity degenerate in the brain and spinal cord; also called Lou Gehrig disease.

arteriovenous malformation An abnormal connection between veins and arteries. It is believed to arise during fetal development or soon after birth.

atonic seizures Seizures that cause an abrupt loss of muscle tone, loss of posture, or sudden collapse ("drop attacks").

aura A sensation that may precede a migraine or seizure activity.

automatism Abnormal repetitive motor behavior (eg, lip smacking, chewing, swallowing) during which the patient is amnestic.

axon The main process of a neuron that normally conducts action potentials away from the cell body of the neuron.

Babinski reflex A reflex movement in which the great toe bends upward when the outer edge of the sole is stroked.

Bell palsy A paralysis of the facial muscles caused by inflammation of the facial nerve (cranial nerve VII). The condition usually is one-sided and time-limited. It often develops suddenly.

brain abscess An accumulation of purulent material (pus) surrounded by a capsule within the brain.

brain tumors Masses, benign or malignant, in the cranial cavity.

cell body The part of the cell that contains the nucleus and surrounding cytoplasm, exclusive of any projections or processes. It is concerned more with metabolism of the cell than with a specific function.

central nervous system (CNS) The system composed of the brain and spinal cord.

cerebral aneurysm A weak area in the wall of a blood vessel in the brain that dilates and is at risk of rupture, particularly with hypertension.

cerebral blood flow (CBF) The volume of blood passing through a given amount of brain tissue per unit of time; a function of the cerebral perfusion pressure and the resistance of the cerebral vascular bed.

cerebral embolism An obstruction in a cerebral artery by an embolus, usually resulting in transient or permanent ischemic damage to brain tissue. As a result, it may cause impairment of cognitive, motor, or sensory function.

cerebral perfusion pressure (CPP) The pressure gradient between the systemic blood pressure and the pressure in the cranial compartment that drives cerebral blood flow; calculated by subtracting the intracranial pressure from the mean systemic arterial blood pressure.

cerebral thrombosis The formation of a blood clot (thrombus) in an artery or vein that supplies blood to the brain, resulting in ischemia to brain tissue.

cerebrospinal fluid (CSF) The fluid that fills the subarachnoid space in the brain and spinal cord and is found in the cerebral ventricles.

cerebrovascular accident A sudden interruption in blood flow to a portion of the brain resulting from occlusion of a cerebral artery by an embolus or thrombus, or a cerebral hemorrhage caused by vessel rupture; also called a stroke.

circle of Willis The circle of interconnected blood vessels at the base of the brain that allows for collateral blood flow to both hemispheres.

coma An abnormally deep state of unconsciousness from which the patient cannot be aroused by external stimuli.

complex partial seizure A seizure that originates in the temporal lobe. It usually begins with an aura and is followed by repetitive motor behavior.

confabulation The invention of stories to make up for gaps in memory.

Cushing reflex An attempt by the body to compensate for a decline in cerebral perfusion pressure by increasing the mean arterial pressure.

decerebrate posturing A position in which a comatose patient's arms are extended and internally rotated and the legs are extended with the feet in forced plantar flexion. It usually is seen with compression of the brainstem.

decorticate posturing A position in which a comatose patient's upper extremities are flexed at the elbows and at the wrists. It usually is seen with a lesion in the mesencephalic region of the brain.

dementia A slow, progressive loss of awareness of time and place. It usually involves an inability to learn new things or recall recent events.

dendrites The branching processes of a neuron that receive stimuli and conduct potentials toward the cell body.

dystonia A condition characterized by local or diffuse changes in muscle tone, resulting in painful muscle spasms, unusually fixed postures, and strange movement patterns.

effector organ A muscle or gland that responds to nerve impulses from the central nervous system.

encephalitis Inflammation of the brain.

epilepsy A condition characterized by the tendency to have recurrent seizures (excluding those that arise from correctable or avoidable circumstances).

focal aware seizure A seizure during which the patient is aware of his or her surroundings.

focal impaired awareness seizure A seizure during which there is a change in the patient's level of awareness.

focal onset seizure A seizure that begins within networks of one hemisphere of the brain (previously referred to as a partial seizure). These seizures usually arise from identifiable lesions in the motor or sensory cortex and may spread in an orderly way to surrounding areas (jacksonian march).

gaze palsy Symmetric limitation of the movements of both eyes in the same direction (conjugate gaze).

generalized onset seizure A seizure that begins within networks of both hemispheres of the brain.

Glasgow Coma Scale (GCS) A standardized system for assessing the degree of impairment of consciousness in a critically ill patient and for predicting the duration and ultimate outcome of coma.

glossopharyngeal neuralgia Irritation of the glossopharyngeal nerve (cranial nerve IX).

Guillain-Barré syndrome (GBS) A rare disease associated with a viral infection or immunization that affects the peripheral nervous system, especially the spinal nerves, but also the cranial nerves.

hemifacial spasm A neuromuscular disorder characterized by frequent involuntary contractions of the muscles on one side of the face.

hemiparesis One-sided weakness; a possible complication of stroke.

hemorrhagic stroke A stroke caused by a rupture of weakened blood vessels in the brain.

homeostasis A state of equilibrium in the body with respect to functions and composition of fluids and tissues.

Huntington disease (HD) A rare, hereditary disease characterized by quick, involuntary movements, speech disturbances, and mental deterioration. It is caused by degenerative changes in the cerebral cortex and basal ganglia. Also known as Huntington chorea.

interneurons Neurons that transmit impulses between other neurons, enabling communication between sensory or motor neurons and the central nervous system.

intracerebral hemorrhage A type of intracranial bleed that occurs within the brain tissue or ventricles.

intracranial pressure (ICP) The pressure within the cranial vault.

ischemic stroke A stroke caused by blockage of a cerebral blood vessel; may be thrombotic or embolic in origin; also called an occlusive stroke or dry stroke.

jacksonian march A transitory disturbance in motor, sensory, or autonomic function resulting from abnormal neuronal discharges in a localized part of the brain; also known as a focal seizure.

large vessel occlusion (LVO) Acute ischemic stroke that involves a large blood vessel, such as vertebral, basilar, carotid, or middle and anterior cerebral arteries. LVO is often associated with worse prognosis.

Los Angeles Motor Scale (LAMS) A brief stroke score derived from the Los Angeles Prehospital Stroke Screen that helps distinguish patients that have a large vessel occlusion.

Los Angeles Prehospital Stroke Screen (LAPSS) A prehospital stroke screening tool that enables the examiner to identify indications of a possible stroke and to rule out other causes of altered level of consciousness.

mean arterial pressure (MAP) The average blood pressure in the arterial portion of the circulation; a measurement of perfusion. It is calculated as MAP = [(Diastolic blood pressure × 2) + Systolic blood pressure]/3.

meningitis Inflammation of the membranes (meninges) surrounding the brain and spinal cord.

migraine A severe headache that often is associated with nausea and photophobia, and may be preceded by visual auras.

motor neurons Neurons that innervate muscle fibers.

motor onset seizure A seizure that produces a change in muscle activity, such as weakness, twitching, and stiffening of body parts.

multiple sclerosis (MS) A progressive disease of the central nervous system in which scattered patches of myelin in the brain and spinal cord are destroyed.

muscular dystrophy An inherited muscle disorder of unknown cause marked by a slow but progressive degeneration of muscle fibers.

myoclonic seizures Seizures that cause brief muscle contractions, which usually occur at the same time and on both sides of the body.

neoplasm An abnormal growth; may be malignant or benign.

neuroglia The supporting or nonneuronal tissue cells of the central and peripheral nervous system.

neurons The functional units of the nervous system, consisting of the nerve cell body, the dendrites, and the axon.

nodes of Ranvier The short spaces in the myelin sheath of a nerve fiber between adjacent Schwann cells that allow rapid action potential conduction from one node to the next.

nonepileptic seizure A seizure that stems from psychological causes rather than from electrical disturbances in the brain. This type of seizure does not benefit from antiepileptic medication therapy.

non-motor onset seizure A seizure that can affect any of the senses, causing changes in sensations of smell, taste, and hearing. The patient may also experience visual and/or auditory hallucinations.

normal pressure hydrocephalus (NPH) Obstruction to flow or absorption of cerebrospinal fluid (CSF), resulting in increased CSF volume and potentially increased intracranial pressure.

nuchal rigidity Neck stiffness with flexion, which suggests meningeal irritation and possibly meningitis.

nystagmus Involuntary rhythmic movements of the eyes.

Parkinson disease A degenerative neurologic disease affecting dopaminergic neurons in the brain causing motor function deterioration. Manifestations include resting tremor, rigidity, slowed movements, and gait abnormality.

peripheral nervous system (PNS) The part of the nervous system that lies outside the brain and spinal cord; comprised of the somatic nervous system and the autonomic nervous system.

peripheral neuropathy Diseases and disorders that affect the peripheral nervous system, causing pain and unpleasant sensations in affected areas (often extremities).

postictal phase The period following a seizure in which the patient experiences drowsiness or unconsciousness. On regaining consciousness, the patient may be confused and fatigued.

reflex An automatic response to a stimulus that occurs without conscious thought; produced by a reflex arc.

Schwann cells Cells that form a myelin sheath around each nerve fiber of the peripheral nervous system.

seizure A temporary change in behavior or consciousness caused by abnormal electrical activity in one or more groups of neurons in the brain.

sensory neurons Afferent neurons that transmit impulses to the spinal cord and brain from all parts of the body.

sinus headache A headache characterized by pain in the forehead, nasal area, and eyes.

spinal cord tumors Benign or malignant tumors that originate in the cells within or next to the spinal cord.

status epilepticus Continuous seizure activity lasting 4 to 5 minutes or longer, or consecutive seizures without a return to consciousness between seizures.

subarachnoid hemorrhage Bleeding within the subarachnoid space.

synapse Any junction between nerve cells and other nerve cells, muscle cells, gland cells, or sensory receptors. It serves to transmit action potentials from one cell to another.

tension headache A headache caused by muscle contraction in the face, neck, and scalp.

Todd paralysis Temporary paralysis or weakness following a seizure that resolves within 48 hours. Typically involves one side of the body.

tonic–clonic seizures Generalized seizures involving the entire body; also known as grand mal seizures.

transient ischemic attack (TIA) An acute episode of temporary neurologic dysfunction resulting from focal cerebral ischemia.

trigeminal neuralgia Infection or disease of the trigeminal nerve (cranial nerve V).

Certain acute dysfunctions of the nervous system require rapid assessment and management. These actions can help reduce mortality and morbidity. Early recognition, appropriate assessment, and awareness of hospital destination protocols for acute management of urgent diagnoses, such as acute stroke, are the foundations to limit morbidity and mortality and maximize the patient's potential for rehabilitation and recovery.

Anatomy and Physiology of the Nervous System

The nervous system is divided into two parts: the **central nervous system (CNS)** and the **peripheral nervous system (PNS)** (**FIGURE 24-1**). The ability of the human body to maintain a state of balance (**homeostasis**) is chiefly the result of the nervous system's ability to coordinate and regulate the body's activities. The CNS is encased in and protected by the bony skull and spine. A total of 43 pairs of nerves originate from the CNS to form the PNS, including 12 pairs of cranial nerves originating from the brain and 31 pairs of spinal nerves originating from the spinal cord. (See Chapter 10, *Review of Human Systems*, for review of the nervous system.)

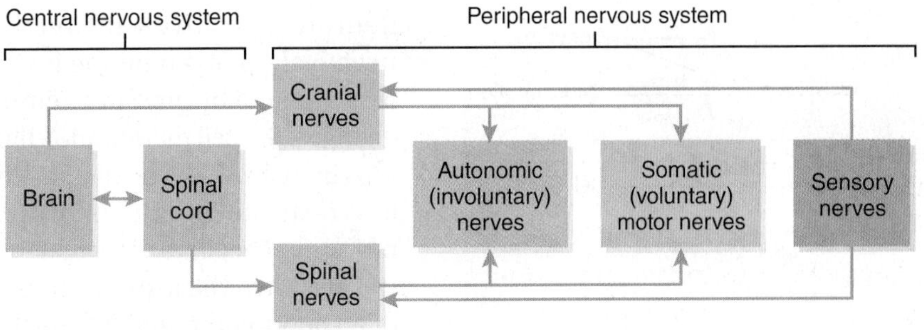

FIGURE 24-1 Divisions of the nervous system.

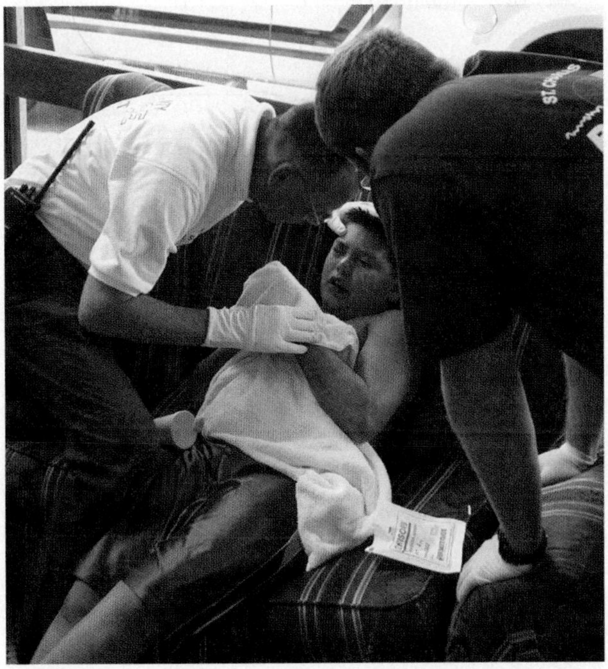

Courtesy of Ray Kemp, St. Charles, MO

Cells of the Nervous System

The cells of the nervous system include **neurons** and connective tissue cells known as **neuroglia**. Each neuron has three main parts: (1) the **cell body**, which has a single, relatively large nucleus with a prominent nucleolus; (2) one or more branching projections, called **dendrites**; and (3) a single, elongated projection, known as an **axon** (**FIGURE 24-2**). Synapses connect neurons and allow the impulses to be transmitted. Axons are surrounded by supportive and protective sheaths formed by the cytoplasmic extensions of neuroglial cells in the CNS (unmyelinated axons). Axons are also surrounded by **Schwann cells** in the PNS.

Bundles of parallel axons with their associated sheaths are white and therefore are called white matter. The **action potential**, which is initiated in the neuron body, is propagated through the axons via conduction pathways or nerve tracts to transmit information from neurons to other body tissues, such as muscles and glands. In the PNS, bundles of axons and their sheaths are called nerves. Collections of nerve cells are grayer and are called gray matter. Gray matter is the site of integration in the nervous system. The outer surface of the cerebrum and the cerebellum consists of gray matter, which forms the cerebral cortex and the cerebellar cortex.

Types of Neurons

Neurons are classified according to their structure, shape, and function, and the direction in which they transmit impulses. **Sensory neurons** (also called afferent neurons) transmit impulses to the spinal cord and brain from all parts of the body. Sensory neurons respond to stimuli such as touch, sound, or light and all other stimuli that affect the cells of the sensory organs.

Motor neurons (also called efferent neurons) transmit impulses in the opposite direction, away from the brain and spinal cord. They transmit impulses only to muscle and glandular epithelial tissue and work to stimulate muscle contraction and to modify proprioceptive sensitivity.

Interneurons (also called central or connecting neurons) conduct impulses from sensory neurons to motor neurons. They connect neurons to other neurons within the same region of the brain or spinal cord in neural networks. There are more than 100 billion interneurons in the human body, which makes them the most abundant of the three major neuron types.

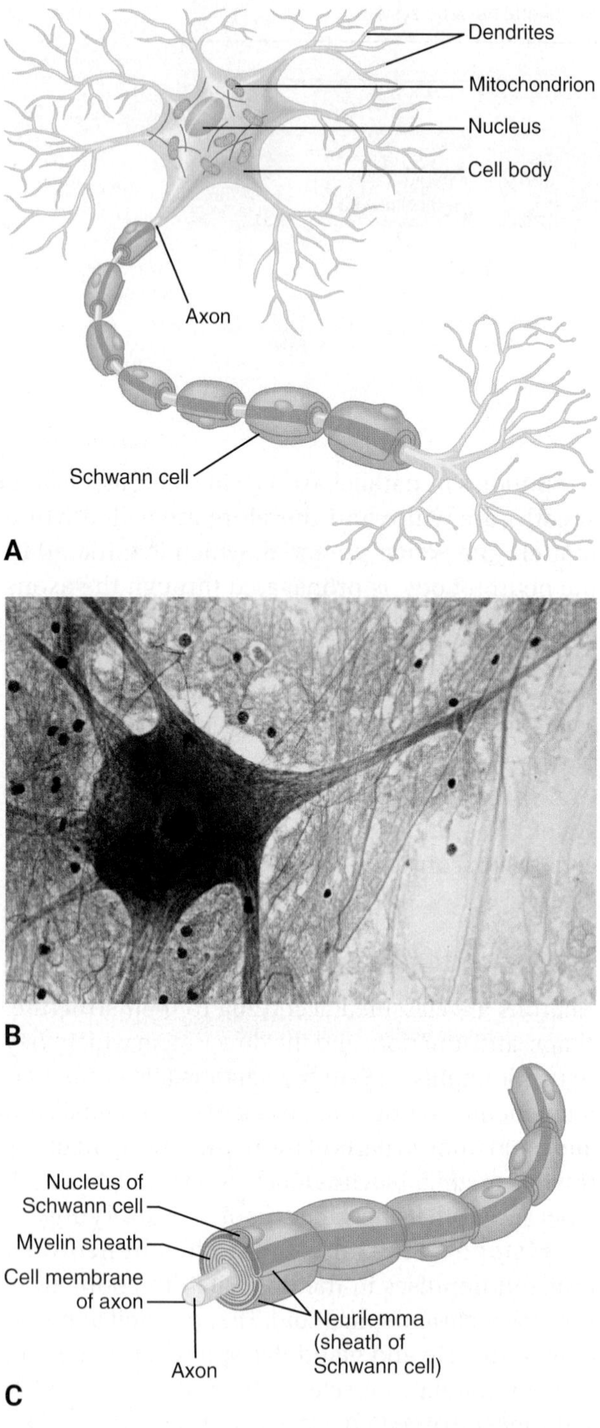

FIGURE 24-2 **A.** Typical neuron showing dendrites, a cell body, and an axon. **B.** Photomicrograph of a neuron. **C.** Segment of a myelinated axon cut to show details of the concentric layers of the Schwann cell filled with myelin.

Impulse Transmission

The transmission of nerve impulses in the nervous system is similar to the conduction of electrical impulses through the heart. In its resting state, the neuron is positively charged on the outside and negatively charged on the inside. When the neuron is stimulated by pressure, temperature, or chemical changes, the cell membrane's permeability to sodium ions increases. As a result, positively charged sodium ions rush into the interior of the neuron. This inward movement begins a wave of depolarization. The wave travels down the axon, resulting in the propagation of an action potential (**FIGURE 24-3**).

> CRITICAL THINKING
> Think of examples of a pressure, a temperature, and a chemical stimulus to a nerve.

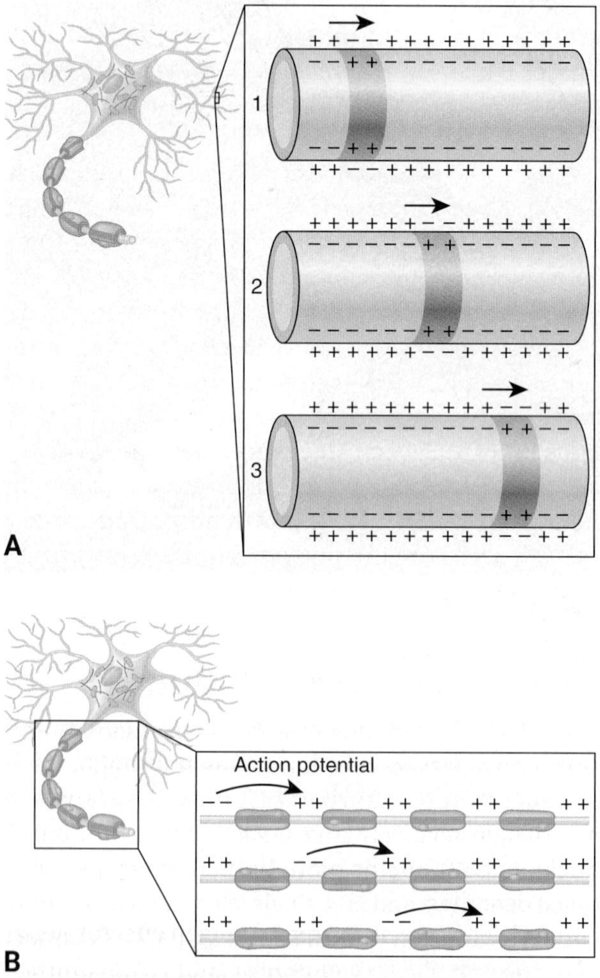

FIGURE 24-3 Conduction of nerve impulses. **A.** In unmyelinated fiber, a nerve impulse (action potential) is a self-propagating wave of electrical disturbance.
B. In myelinated fiber, the action potential "jumps" around the insulating myelin in a rapid type of conduction called saltatory conduction.

In unmyelinated axons, action potentials are spread along the entire axon membrane. Myelinated axons, however, have interruptions in the myelin sheaths. These interruptions, known as **nodes of Ranvier**, allow nerve impulses to "jump" from one node to the next without spreading along the entire length of the cell (saltatory conduction). Myelinated axons, therefore, conduct action potentials faster than do unmyelinated axons.

Synapses

The membrane-to-membrane point of contact between the axon endings of one neuron (presynaptic neuron) and the dendrites of another neuron (postsynaptic neuron) is known as a **synapse**. The structures that compose a synapse are the presynaptic terminal, the synaptic cleft, and the plasma membrane of the postsynaptic neuron. Within each presynaptic terminal are synaptic vesicles that contain neurotransmitter chemicals (**FIGURE 24-4**).

Each action potential arriving at the presynaptic terminal initiates a series of specific events. These events result in the release of the neurotransmitter. The neurotransmitter rapidly diffuses the short distance across the synaptic cleft. It then binds to specific receptor molecules on the postsynaptic membrane. After an impulse has been generated and conducted by the postsynaptic neurons, neurotransmitter activity ends quickly. Several substances have been identified as neurotransmitters; others are thought to be neurotransmitters. Well-known neurotransmitters include acetylcholine, norepinephrine, epinephrine, and dopamine (**TABLE 24-1**).

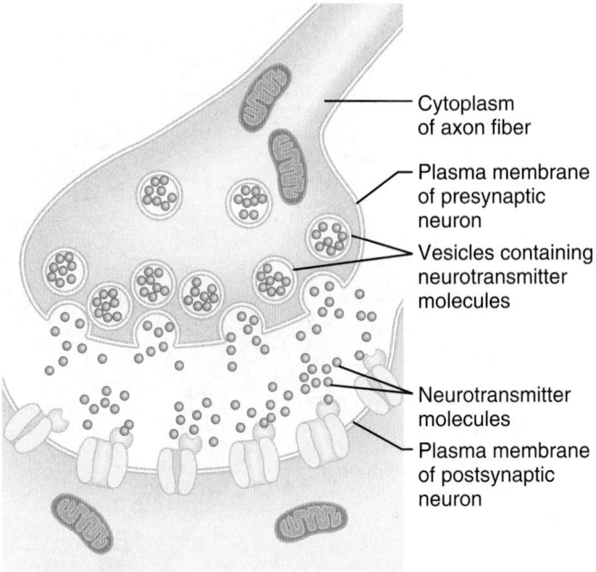

FIGURE 24-4 Components of a synapse. The diagram shows an axon terminal of a presynaptic neuron and a synaptic cleft. When an action potential arrives at the axon terminal of a presynaptic neuron, neurotransmitter molecules are released from vesicles in the axon terminal into the synaptic cleft. The combining of neurotransmitter and receptor molecules in the plasma membrane of the postsynaptic neuron initiates impulse conduction in the postsynaptic neuron.

TABLE 24-1 Major Neurotransmitters

Neurotransmitter	Postsynaptic Effect
Acetylcholine	Excitatory
Norepinephrine	Excitatory
Epinephrine	Excitatory
Dopamine	Excitatory

Reflexes

One type of route traveled by nerve impulses is a reflex, or reflex arc. A **reflex** is the basic unit of the nervous system capable of receiving a stimulus and generating a response. Reflexes allow conduction of impulses over a short arc. They have several basic components: a sensory receptor, a sensory neuron, interneurons, a motor neuron, and an effector organ. (An **effector organ** is a muscle or gland that contracts or secretes, respectively, in direct response to nerve impulses.) Individual reflexes vary in complexity. Some act to remove the body from painful stimuli. Some prevent the body from suddenly falling or moving as a result of external forces. Others are responsible for maintaining a relatively constant blood pressure, body fluid pH, blood carbon dioxide level, and water intake. All reflexes are homeostatic; that is, they function to maintain healthy survival.

Action potentials initiated in sensory receptors spread along sensory axons in the PNS to the CNS. There they synapse with interneurons. Interneurons synapse with motor neurons in the spinal cord; the motor neurons send their axons out of the spinal cord and through the PNS to muscles or glands. This action causes the effector organ to respond. **FIGURE 24-5**

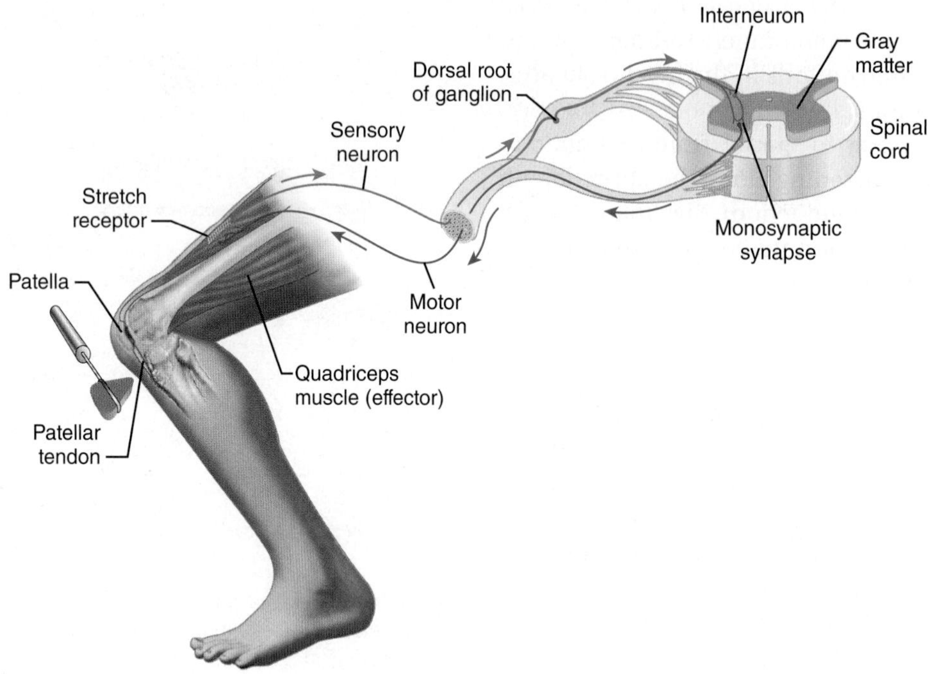

FIGURE 24-5 Neural pathway involved in the patellar (knee jerk) reflex.

shows the transmission of nerve impulses that result in the patellar (knee jerk) reflex.

Blood Supply

The arterial blood supply to the brain comes from the vertebral arteries and the internal carotid arteries (**FIGURE 24-6**). The right and left vertebral arteries (supplying the cerebellum) enter the cranial vault through the foramen magnum. They unite to form the midline basilar artery. The basilar artery branches to supply the pons and the cerebellum. It divides again to form the posterior cerebral arteries, which supply the posterior portion of the cerebrum.

The internal carotid arteries enter the cranial vault through the carotid canals. These vessels give rise to the anterior cerebral arteries. The anterior cerebral arteries supply blood to the frontal lobes of the brain. They end by forming the middle cerebral arteries. These supply a large portion of the lateral cerebral cortex. A posterior communicating artery branches off each internal carotid artery and connects with the ipsilateral posterior cerebral artery. The two posterior cerebral arteries are connected at their common origin from the basilar artery. The anterior cerebral arteries are connected by an anterior communicating artery. Thus, they complete a circle around the pituitary gland and the brain. This circle, called the **circle of Willis**, provides an important safeguard. It helps to ensure the supply of blood to all parts of the brain in the event of a blockage in one of the vertebral or internal carotid arteries.

The veins that drain blood from the head form the venous sinuses. (These sinuses are the spaces in the dura mater surrounding the brain.) Eventually they drain into the internal jugular veins (**FIGURE 24-7**). These veins exit the cranial vault and join with several other veins that drain the external head and face. The internal jugular veins join the subclavian veins on each side of the body.

Ventricles

Each cerebral hemisphere contains a large space filled with **cerebrospinal fluid (CSF)**. This space is known as a lateral ventricle. The lateral ventricles are connected posteriorly. A third ventricle is located in the center of the diencephalon between the two halves of the thalamus. The two lateral ventricles communicate with the third ventricle through two interventricular

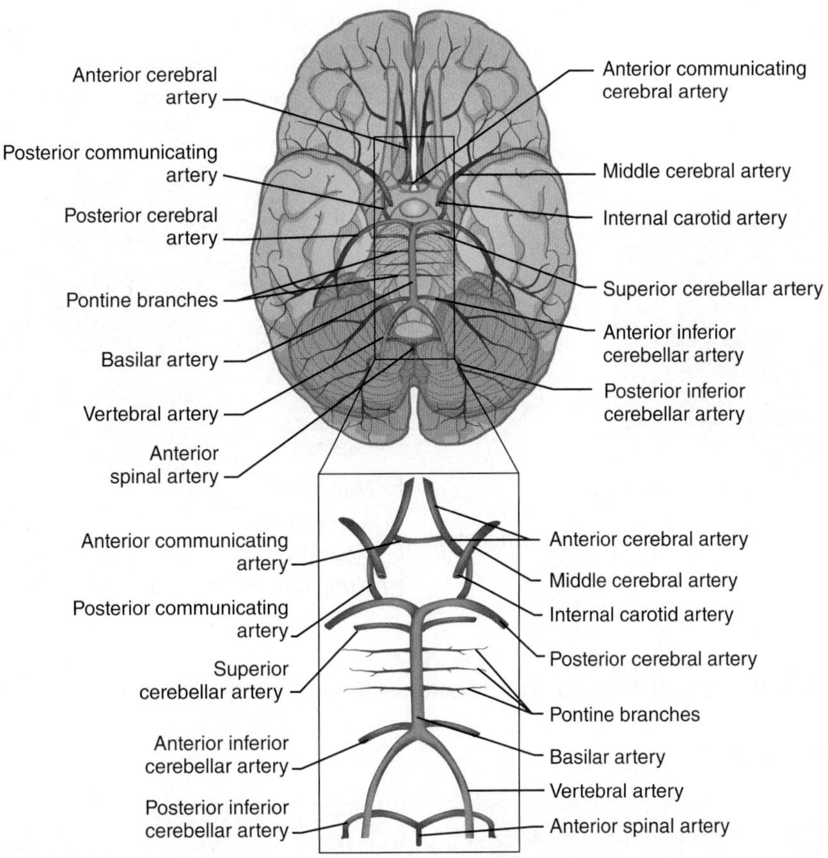

FIGURE 24-6 Inferior view of the brain showing vertebral, basilar, and internal carotid arteries and their branches.

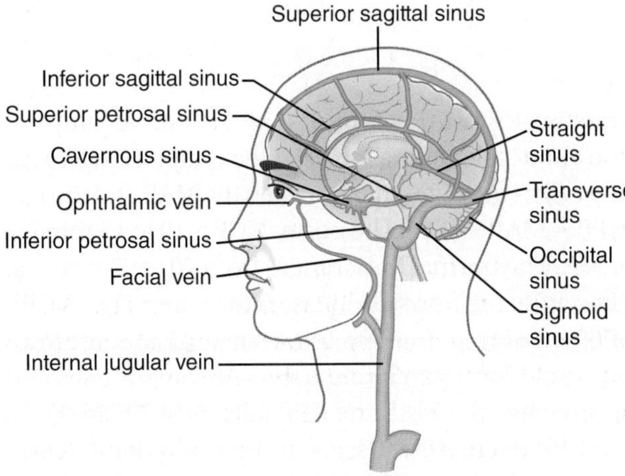

FIGURE 24-7 Venous sinuses associated with the brain.

foramina. The third ventricle communicates with the fourth ventricle (located in the superior region of the medulla) by way of a narrow canal. This canal is known as the cerebral aqueduct. The fourth ventricle is continuous with the central canal of the spinal cord.

CRITICAL THINKING

What happens if the flow in one of these canals becomes obstructed?

Divisions of the Brain

The major divisions of the adult brain are the brainstem (medulla, pons, midbrain, and site of the reticular formation), cerebellum, diencephalon (hypothalamus and thalamus), and cerebrum (**FIGURE 24-8**). (See Chapter 10, *Review of Human Systems*, to review these structures.)

Neurologic Pathophysiology

Some neurologic emergencies are a consequence of structural changes or damage, circulatory changes, or alterations in **intracranial pressure (ICP)** that affect **cerebral blood flow (CBF)**. Three structures occupy the intracranial space: brain tissue (80%), blood (10%), and CSF (10%). Brain tissue contains mostly

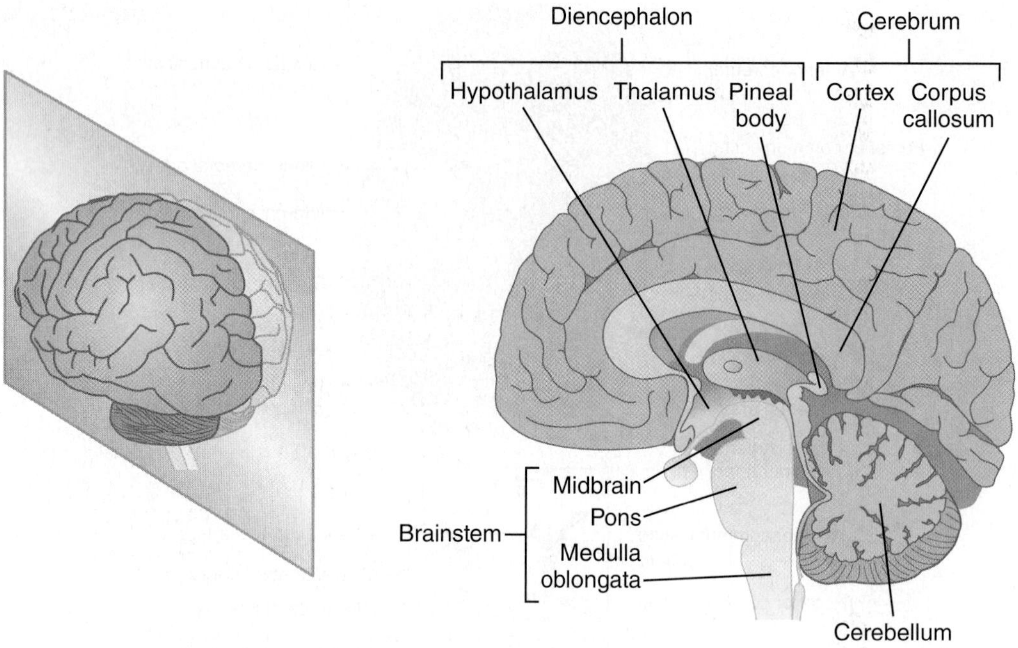

FIGURE 24-8 Divisions of the brain. A midsagittal section of the brain reveals features of its major divisions.

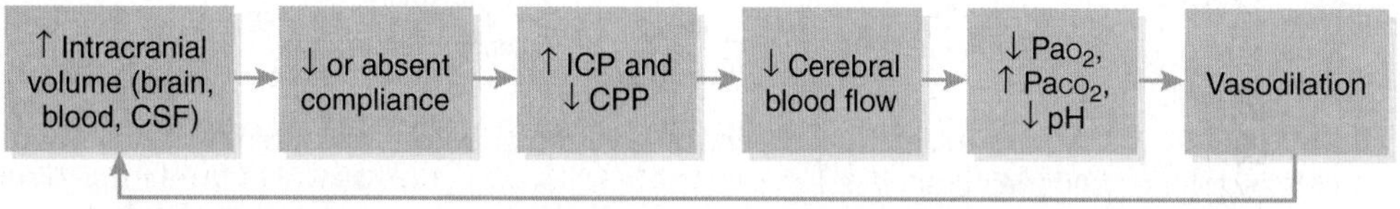

Abbreviations: CPP, cerebral perfusion pressure; CSF, cerebrospinal fluid; ICP, intracranial pressure; $Paco_2$, partial pressure of carbon dioxide, arterial; Pao_2, partial pressure of oxygen, arterial

FIGURE 24-9 Pathophysiology flow diagram for increased intracranial pressure.

water, both intracellular and extracellular. Blood is contained in the major arteries in the base of the brain; in arterial branches, arterioles, capillaries, venules, and veins in the substance of the brain; and in the cortical veins and dural sinuses. Water is located in the ventricles of the brain, in the CSF, and in extracellular and intracellular fluid.

Cerebral Blood Flow

Although the brain accounts for only 2% of adult weight, 20% of total body oxygen use and 25% of total body glucose use are devoted to brain metabolism.[1] Oxygen and glucose delivery is controlled by CBF.

CBF is a function of the **cerebral perfusion pressure (CPP)** and the resistance of the cerebral vascular bed. To measure the CPP, the ICP is subtracted from the **mean arterial pressure (MAP)**. (The MAP is the diastolic blood pressure [DBP] plus one-third of the pulse pressure [PP]: MAP = DBP + 1/3PP. For more information about calculating the MAP, see Chapter 35, *Shock*.) The CBF is the difference between the MAP and the ICP (CPP = MAP − ICP). The normal ICP is 10 to 15 mm Hg or less. The normal MAP ranges from 70 to 95 mm Hg. Therefore, the normal CPP is 60 to 80 mm Hg. (A CPP of 60 mm Hg is thought to be the critical minimum threshold for organ blood flow.[2]) As the ICP rises and approaches the MAP, the CPP falls (**FIGURE 24-9**). As the CPP decreases, vessels in the brain dilate (cerebral vasodilation). This dilation results in increased cerebral blood volume (increasing the ICP) and further cerebral vasodilation. In most emergency medical services (EMS) systems, the CPP is not calculated because the ICP is not measured in the prehospital setting. Maintaining a systolic blood pressure greater than 90 mm Hg may help maintain an adequate MAP in a patient with a potential brain injury.[3]

NOTE

Vascular tone in the normal brain is regulated by the partial pressure of arterial carbon dioxide ($Paco_2$) and the partial pressure of arterial oxygen (Pao_2), and by autonomic and neurohumoral control. The $Paco_2$ has the greatest effect on intracerebral vascular diameter and subsequent resistance. The CBF increases as carbon dioxide increases, resulting in increased CBF and ICP. When autoregulation is impaired, decreases in CPP result in decreases in CBF; in moderate/severe traumatic brain injury, such decreases in CBF may reach ischemic levels, further exacerbating secondary injury. For this reason, hyperventilation with hypocapnia should be strictly avoided. Oxygen delivery should be titrated to avoid episodes of hypoxemia.

Modified from: Kacmarek RM, Stoller JK, Heuer AJ. *Egan's Fundamentals of Respiratory Care*. 11th ed. St. Louis, MO: Elsevier; 2017; Armstead WM. Cerebral blood flow autoregulation and dysautoregulation. *Anesthesiol Clin*. 2016;34(3):465-477; and Tameem A, Krovvidi H. Cerebral physiology. *Contin Educ Anaesth Crit Care Pain*. 2013;13(4):113-118.

Cerebral Perfusion Pressure

As stated previously, CBF depends on the CPP, which is the pressure gradient across the brain. The CBF remains constant when the CPP is 50 to 160 mm Hg. If the CPP falls below 40 mm Hg, CBF declines. This critically affects cerebral metabolism. With mild to moderate elevation of the ICP, the MAP usually rises. The rise in the MAP causes cerebral blood vessels to constrict and prevents the increase in blood volume and CBF that normally would occur.

CRITICAL THINKING

Relate the difficulty created for CBF by increased ICP to having a person push against a door as you try to open it in the opposite direction. How much more difficult is it for you to open the door?

In contrast, if the MAP falls, the cerebral arteries dilate, increasing the CBF. Therefore, with a MAP of 60 to 150 mm Hg, CBF may be maintained in a constant state. However, when ICP elevations are increased (greater than 22 mm Hg), perfusion of brain tissue often decreases despite a rise in the systemic arterial pressure. Therefore, if mass or cerebral edema develops, an immediate reduction in the volume of one or more of these components (brain tissue, blood, or water) must occur to prevent the ICP from rising and compressing brain tissue.

Assessment of the Nervous System

As with all patient encounters, care of a patient with a nontraumatic neurologic emergency begins with a consistent, systematic primary survey. This survey helps to ensure that signs and symptoms that may indicate an urgent condition are not missed. The goals of emergency care are (1) patency of the airway, (2) adequate ventilation, (3) stabilization and support of the cardiovascular system, (4) intervention to limit further cerebral injury, and (5) protection of the patient from further harm while at the scene and during transport to an appropriate medical facility for definitive care.

Primary Survey

The paramedic should begin the primary survey by evaluating scene safety and exsanguinating hemorrhage, airway, breathing, circulation, disability, and exposure (the XABCDEs). This primary survey should include determining the patient's level of consciousness. A patent airway also must be ensured. If the patient is unconscious when paramedics arrive and there is reason to suspect a cervical spine injury, the patient's airway should be opened with spinal precautions and cervical spine movement should be restricted. It is important to remember that an unconscious patient may be unable to maintain his or her airway without assistance. Therefore, airway assessment should include considering whether airway adjuncts are needed to maintain a patent airway. The patient's respiratory rate and minute ventilation also should be closely monitored for changes because increased ICP may result in abnormal breathing patterns and potentially respiratory arrest. The patient should be monitored for vomiting (and related aspiration), which may also be associated with increased ICP. Suction should be readily available.

NOTE

The mantra of the cardiologist is "time is muscle." Many neurologists consider that "time is brain." Rapid stabilization of the patient's condition and transport to an appropriate facility for definitive care and possible intervention represent the most appropriate management in a neurologic emergency.

Adequate ventilation and appropriate supplemental oxygen for hypoxia should be ensured for patients experiencing a neurologic emergency. Hypoxia, even in short episodes, is extremely dangerous for the patient with a brain injury. An increase in the $Paco_2$ level or a decrease in the Pao_2 level results in dilation of the blood vessels. This response occurs presumably because of an increase in cerebral metabolic needs. As the $Paco_2$ level drops, blood volume and blood flow to the brain are reduced. Because of these actions, waveform capnography (when available) and pulse oximetry should be part of routine monitoring of a patient with altered mental status so that inadequate ventilation or changes in end-tidal carbon dioxide ($ETCO_2$) level or minute ventilation are quickly apparent.

Patient Assessment

A patient with a neurologic illness may be difficult to assess, especially if the patient's mental status is impaired. Key elements of the assessment may offer clues to the cause of the neurologic emergency. These elements include the patient history, the history of the event, vital signs, respiratory patterns, and neurologic examination.

History. After any life-threatening problems have been identified and managed in the primary survey, the paramedic should obtain a thorough history. This information can be obtained from the patient (when possible) or from family members or bystanders if the patient is unable to communicate clearly. The following are important elements of the patient history.

1. Details of the presenting illness, including time course of the complaint. The last known normal time is a critical history element for potential stroke patients.
2. Pertinent underlying medical problems:
    - Known neurologic disease (eg, multiple sclerosis [MS])
    - Previous stroke
    - Chronic seizures
    - Diabetes mellitus
    - Hypertension
3. Alcohol or other substance use
4. Previous history of similar symptoms
5. Prescribed medications
6. Recent injury (particularly head trauma)

If a loss of consciousness was involved, the paramedic should ascertain the events that led up to the unconscious state. This information may include the patient's position (sitting, standing, lying down), whether the person complained of a headache, and whether seizure activity or a fall occurred. At times, no history is available. In such cases, paramedics should assume that the onset of unconsciousness was acute. They also should maintain a high level of suspicion for an intracranial hemorrhage. Environmental clues may be very helpful, including current prescribed medications, medical alert identification, alcohol, or drug paraphernalia.

> **CRITICAL THINKING**
> How could having one of the conditions listed in the important elements of the patient history result in a change in the patient's neurologic status?

Vital Signs. The patient's vital signs should be checked and recorded frequently, just as in any critical patient. This monitoring is important because changes in vital signs can indicate deterioration and the need for additional intervention in patients with neurologic emergencies. In a patient with altered mental status, the electrocardiogram (ECG) should be monitored for dysrhythmias, pulse oximetry and continuous waveform capnography should be used, and blood glucose should be measured.

When the ICP begins to rise, a conscious patient may complain of headache, nausea, and vomiting. Progressive hypertension associated with bradycardia and respiratory depression is a late response to critical increases in the ICP.[3] This condition is known as the **Cushing reflex** (also called the Cushing triad or Cushing response). The late stages of increased ICP are marked by an increase in systolic pressure, a widened pulse pressure, and a decrease in the pulse and respiratory rate (**FIGURE 24-10**). In the terminal stages, as the ICP continues to rise and brain tissue and the third (oculomotor) cranial nerve are compressed, the pupils become unequal. The pulse rate generally decreases and the blood pressure falls, particularly after cerebral herniation. Hypotension is a late and ominous sign in these patients.

Respiratory Patterns. The respiratory pattern of a patient with a neurologic emergency may be abnormal. Even without damage to the lower respiratory centers in

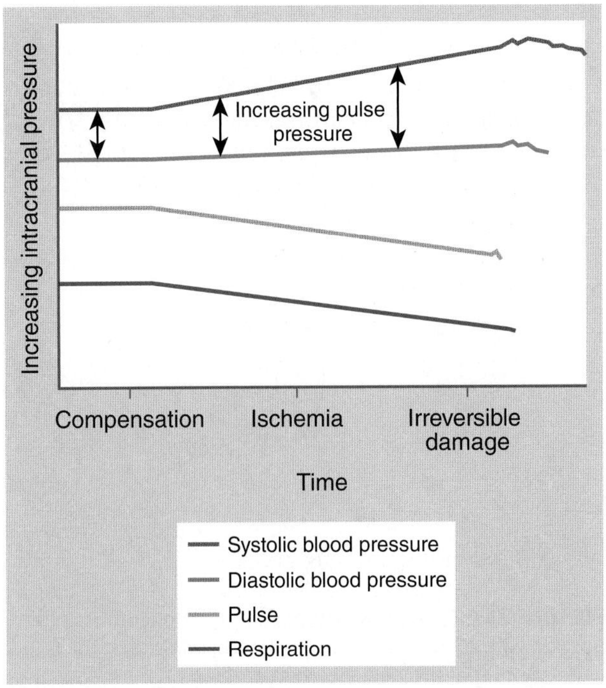

FIGURE 24-10 Vital signs with increased intracranial pressure.

the medulla causing respiratory arrest, abnormalities of the respiratory rate and rhythm may occur. When present, these specific breathing patterns can provide clues to which area of the brain is involved or give a clue to the severity of the neurologic problem. Apnea can occur with loss of consciousness even with relatively minor head trauma. However, acute respiratory arrest usually results from involvement of the medullary respiratory center (brainstem compression or infarct). Damage to neural pathways (anywhere from the cortex down to the medulla) produces problems with the respiratory rhythm more often than it produces respiratory arrest. As described in Chapter 15, *Airway Management, Respiration, and Artificial Ventilation*, abnormal respiratory patterns include the following:

- Cheyne-Stokes respiration
- Central neurogenic hyperventilation
- Ataxic respiration
- Apneustic respiration
- Diaphragmatic breathing

CRITICAL THINKING

Consider a patient who has ataxic or apneustic respirations. Which respiratory control center likely is affected?

Neurologic Evaluation

Some neurologic complications are obvious (eg, hemiparesis). Others may be subtle (eg, a decreasing level of awareness). A sudden or progressively decreasing level of consciousness is highly suggestive of a serious neurologic condition.

The mnemonic AVPU (Awake and alert, responsive to Verbal stimuli, responsive to Pain, Unresponsive) can help determine the patient's baseline neurologic status. The **Glasgow Coma Scale (GCS)** (BOX 24-1) should also be calculated during the initial assessment. These evaluations should be repeated and recorded with any change in patient status.

When evaluating a patient's neurologic status, the paramedic should report and record patient information with descriptive terms. These terms should be specific to responses to certain stimuli. For example, "The patient is amnestic to the event"; "The patient follows commands"; and "The patient does not open his eyes to noxious stimuli." Clear descriptions of the patient's response allow others involved in the patient's care to follow the progression of the condition.

Posturing, Muscle Tone, and Paralysis

Significant neurologic emergencies may be associated with abnormal posturing (**FIGURE 24-11**), weakness or paralysis of limb or limbs, or both. Generally, disturbances of posture result from flexor spasms, extensor spasms, or flaccidity. Abnormal flexion of the elbows with extension of the legs is called

BOX 24-1 Glasgow Coma Scale

The GCS evaluates eye opening, verbal and motor responses, and brainstem reflex function. The GCS scale ranges from a low of 3 to a high of 15. A GCS score of 9 to 12 indicates moderate brain injury; a score of 8 or lower indicates severe brain injury. Hypoxemia and hypotension have been shown to cause falsely low GCS scores. Therefore, the GCS score should be measured after the primary survey and after a patent airway and adequate ventilation have been established.

Modified from: McSwain NE, ed. *Prehospital Trauma Life Support*. Burlington, MA: Jones & Bartlett Learning; 2016.

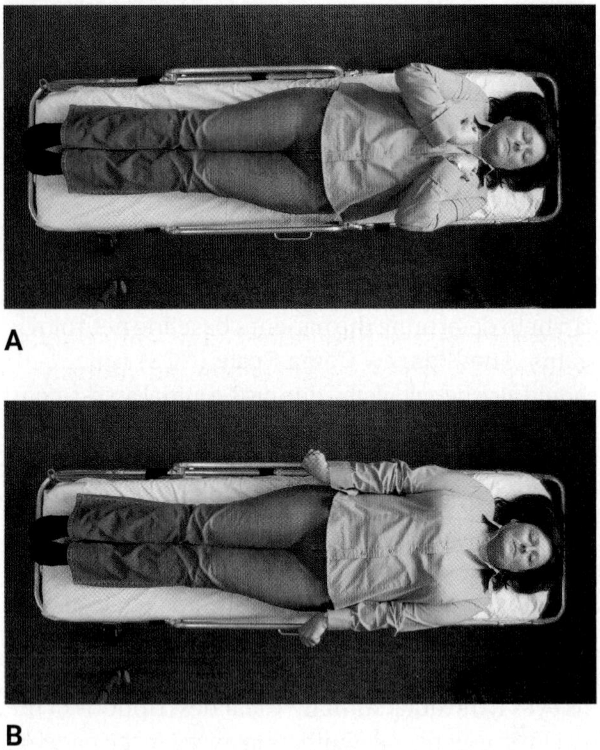

FIGURE 24-11 **A.** Abnormal flexion. **B.** Extension.

Reproduced from: Chuck Sowerbrower, MED, NREMT-P

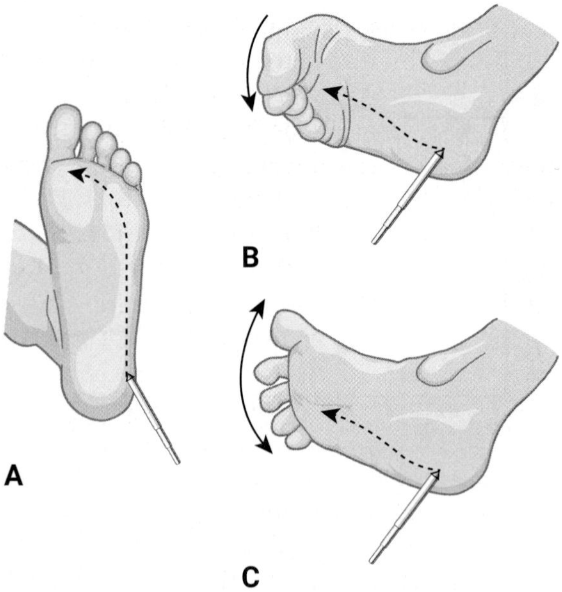

FIGURE 24-12 Babinski reflex. **A.** Light pressure is applied with a hard object to the lateral surface of the sole, starting at the heel, going over the ball of the foot, and ending beneath the great toe. **B.** The normal response is flexion of all the toes. **C.** Babinski reflex is seen as dorsiflexion or extension of the great toe, with or without fanning or abduction of the other toes.

decorticate posturing. This abnormal posturing is thought to result from damage to the thalamus or cerebral hemispheres. Abnormal extension at the elbow with internal rotation of the shoulders and leg extension is called **decerebrate posturing**. It has a worse prognosis than decorticate posturing because it implies both cerebral and midbrain dysfunction. Flaccidity usually is caused by brainstem or cord dysfunction and has a dismal prognosis.

Abnormal reflexes may be associated with decorticate or decerebrate posturing. Babinski reflex (known also as Babinski sign) may be present with such posturing. **Babinski reflex** is an abnormal extensor reflex in adults. (It may be normal in children in the first few years of life but normally disappears by 12 months of age. The reflex is considered abnormal after 2 years of age.) It is characterized by dorsiflexion or extension of the great toe, with or without fanning or abduction of the other toes, when the outer edge of the foot is scratched. It indicates neurologic injury (**FIGURE 24-12**). A patient with a severe injury may also have relaxation of sphincter tone and may be incontinent of urine or feces, or both.

NOTE

There is no "positive" or "negative" Babinski sign. The presence of this response indicates the existence of a pathologic condition.

Pupillary Reflexes

Examination of the pupils can be helpful in an unconscious patient. Illicit substance use may be suspected based on the appearance and reaction of the pupils. If deviations from normal (in relative symmetry, size, and prompt reaction to light) are observed, it is crucial to note whether these deviations are unilateral or bilateral. If both pupils are dilated and do not react to light, the brainstem may be affected. An alert patient with dilated pupils does not have acute intracranial pathology. Pinpoint pupils can be seen with opioid overdose, eye drop use, or pontine stroke (a type of stroke that occurs when blood flow in the brainstem is disrupted). This sign also may occur with severe cerebral anoxia or as a result of toxicity. A history of anisocoria (unequal pupil size) or eye surgery may also explain abnormal pupil findings. **Nystagmus** may be noted with illicit substance use or toxic levels of certain medications.

Pupillary constriction is controlled by parasympathetic fibers. These fibers originate in the midbrain and accompany the oculomotor nerve (cranial nerve III) (**FIGURE 24-13**). Pupillary dilation involves fibers that travel the entire brainstem and return in the cervical sympathetic nerves. Midbrain injury interrupts both pathways. Generally, it results in fixed, midsize pupils. Compression of cranial nerve III interrupts parasympathetic nerve actions, causing a unilateral, fixed, dilated pupil on the affected side. The sudden development of a fixed, dilated pupil in an unconscious patient is an ominous sign and indicates that the patient most likely has sustained a significant neurologic insult.[3] This finding requires immediate transport to a designated trauma or stroke center, depending on the suspected etiology. **TABLE 24-2** serves as a review of cranial nerve assessment.

Extraocular Movements

The evaluation of extraocular movements may identify abnormalities in cranial nerves (oculomotor, trochlear, or abducens) in their course from the brainstem to the orbit, in the brainstem nuclei, or finally, in the higher-order centers and pathways in the cortex and brainstem that control eye movements. A conscious patient should be able to move the eyes in six directions without moving the head. For this test, the paramedic moves a finger to the extreme left and then up and down and to the extreme right and then up and down, making the shape of a large *H*.

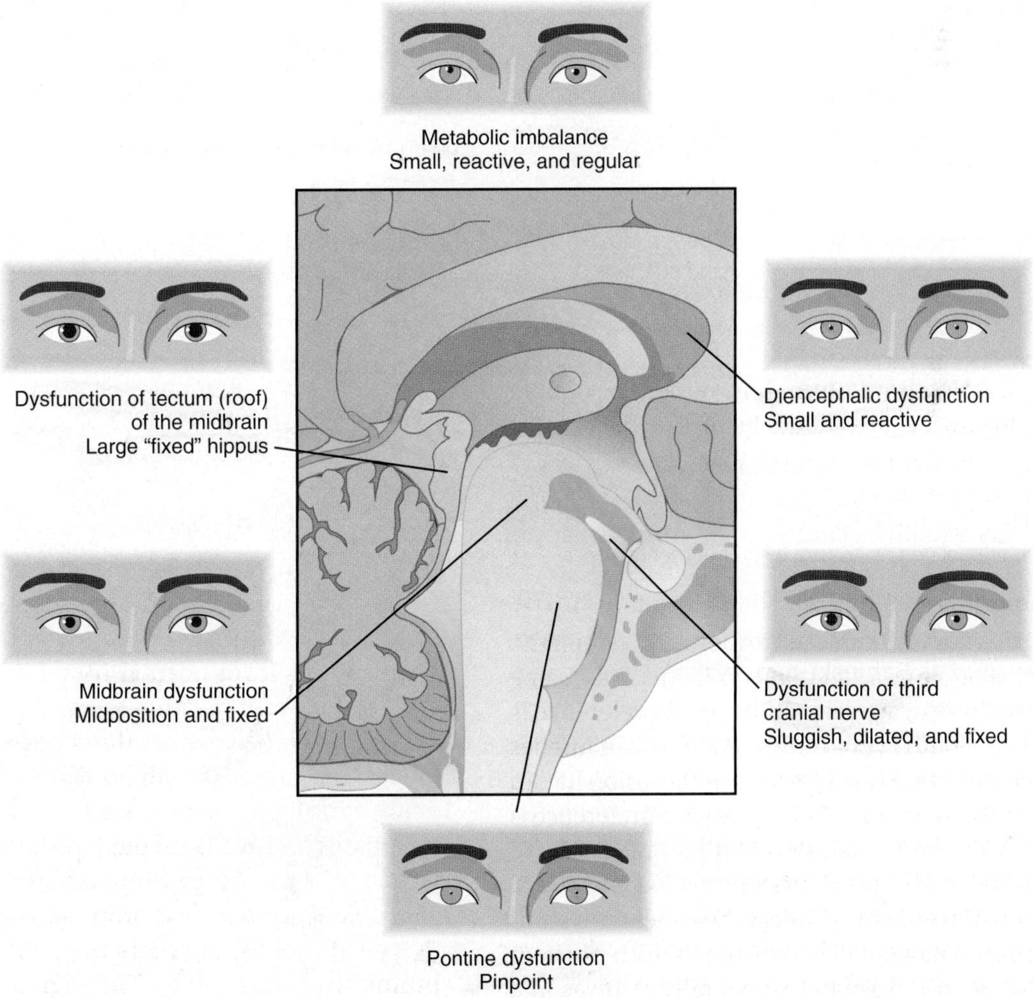

FIGURE 24-13 Pupils at different levels of consciousness.

TABLE 24-2 Cranial Nerve Assessment

Nerve	Name	Function	Test
I	Olfactory	Smell	Have patient smell a familiar odor.
II	Optic	Visual acuity	Have patient identify the number of fingers being held up.
		Visual field	Check peripheral vision.
III	Oculomotor	Pupillary reaction	Shine a light in patient's eye.
IV	Trochlear	Eye movement	Have patient follow finger without moving the head.
V	Trigeminal	Facial sensation	Touch patient's face and ask patient to report sensation.
		Motor function	Have patient hold the mouth open.
VI	Abducens	Motor function	Check lateral eye movements.
VII	Facial	Motor function	Have patient smile, wrinkle the face, and puff the cheeks.
		Sensory	Check different tastes.
VIII	Vestibulocochlear (Acoustic)	Hearing	Snap fingers by patient's ear.
		Balance	Perform Romberg test.
IX	Glossopharyngeal	Swallowing and voice	Have patient swallow and say "Ah."
X	Vagus	Gag reflex	Check for reflex with tongue depressor.
XI	Spinal accessory	Neck motion	Have patient shrug the shoulders.
XII	Hypoglossal	Tongue movement and strength	Have patient stick out the tongue or exert resistance with a tongue depressor.

Any deviations from normal movement or double vision during this test should be recorded.

CRITICAL THINKING

Which cranial nerves control eye movements?

Gaze palsy is a term used to indicate a symmetric limitation of the movements of both eyes in the same direction (conjugate gaze). If the gaze preference is deviation of both eyes to either side at rest, it implies damage to brain tissue (a lesion). If the lesion has an irritative focus (seizure focus), the gaze preference is to look away from the lesion. If it has a destructive focus (stroke), the gaze preference is to look toward the lesion. Uncoupling of the eye movements (dysconjugate gaze) may indicate damage to the brainstem (**FIGURE 24-14**).[4] Gaze palsy generally resolves in a few days, although some gaze impairment may remain. The larger the lesion, the more persistent the

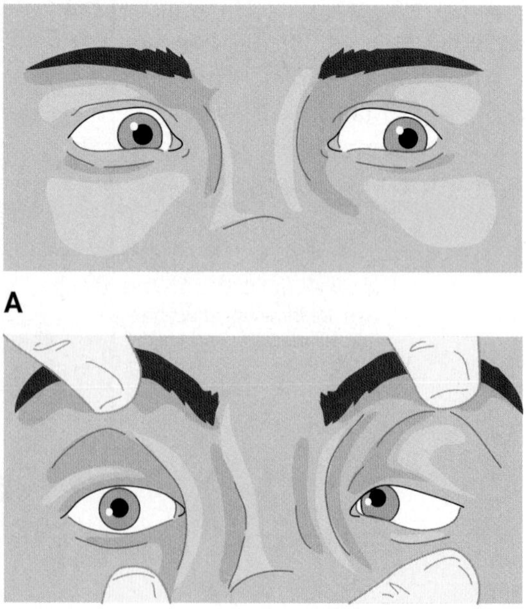

A

B

FIGURE 24-14 **A.** Conjugate gaze. **B.** Dysconjugate gaze.

deviation.[5] In the acute phase of injury, gaze deviation may be a good predictor of large artery occlusion, and if present may aid in interventions. Incorporating their use in prehospital care and increasing their weightage in modified stroke scale scores can be a useful strategy to reduce "the time of onset of symptoms to treatment" in hyperacute stroke. Prehospital stroke scales that include the gaze deviation sign may be useful in clinical practice.[6]

Pathophysiology and Management of Specific CNS Disorders

Disorders of the nervous system have many etiologies. Paramedics must avoid tunnel vision and consider a wide range of causes. They must also perform a complete history and physical assessment to find clues to the nature of the patient's signs and symptoms. Specific disorders discussed in this chapter include weakness and fatigue, structural and metabolic coma, stroke and intracranial hemorrhage (including transient ischemic attack [TIA]), seizure disorders, headaches, and brain neoplasm and brain abscess. Several degenerative neurologic diseases are also discussed.

Coma

Coma is an abnormally deep state of unconsciousness from which the patient cannot be aroused by external verbal or physical stimuli. In general terms, two mechanisms produce coma: structural lesions and toxic/metabolic states. Structural lesions (eg, a tumor or an abscess) depress consciousness by affecting the reticular activating system in the brainstem. Toxic/metabolic conditions involve the presence of toxins or the lack of oxygen or glucose. Either mechanism may result in depression of the cerebrum, with or without depression of the reticular activating system. Within these two primary mechanisms are six general causes of coma (BOX 24-2). A mnemonic that may be helpful for remembering the common causes of coma is AEIOUTIPS (BOX 24-3).

Differentiation of Structural and Toxic/Metabolic Causes of Coma

Structural and toxic/metabolic causes of coma differ in two primary ways. In coma of structural origin, the neurologic signs often are one-sided, or asymmetrical.

BOX 24-2 Six General Causes of Coma

Structural Origin
Intracranial bleeding
Head trauma
Brain tumor or other space-occupying lesion

Metabolic System
Anoxia
Hypoglycemia
Diabetic ketoacidosis
Thiamine deficiency
Kidney and liver failure
Postictal phase of seizure

Toxidromes
Anticholinergic
Cholinergic
Opiate
Hallucinogenic
Sedative-hypnotic
Sympathomimetic

Cardiovascular System
Hypertensive encephalopathy
Shock
Dysrhythmias
Stroke

Respiratory System
Chronic obstructive pulmonary disease
Toxic inhalation (eg, carbon monoxide poisoning)

Infection
Meningitis
Sepsis

BOX 24-3 Mnemonic for Common Causes of Coma: AEIOUTIPS

Alcohol (or acidosis)
Epilepsy, endocrine, electrolytes
Insulin
Opiates and other drugs (overdose)
Uremia (kidney failure)
Trauma, temperature
Infection
Poisoning, psychogenic causes
Shock, stroke, seizure, syncope, space-occupying lesion, subarachnoid hemorrhage

In toxic/metabolic coma, the neurologic findings often are the same on the two sides of the body. In addition, coma of toxic/metabolic origin often is slow in onset, whereas structural lesions occur acutely. Changes in pupil responses are the most important physical sign in distinguishing between structural and toxic/metabolic causes of coma. Equal pupil responses suggest that the coma has a toxic/metabolic cause. Unresponsive or asymmetrical pupils suggest a structural cause.

> NOTE
>
> Some psychiatric conditions can mimic comalike states. In these conditions, the state of unconsciousness has no physical cause. Patients who appear unconscious as a result of a psychiatric condition may respond to annoying physical or verbal stimuli. In contrast, patients with organic sources of coma are unresponsive.

Unlike toxic/metabolic coma, structural coma follows a progressive pattern of deterioration. This pattern is caused by focal pressure or compression in the brain. The syndrome often is sudden in onset, and the examination results are asymmetrical, such as flaccidity on one side of the body (**hemiparesis**). As a rule, when structural lesions damage the reticular activating system, it is a result of increased ICP and herniation of the brain. This type of injury requires rapid surgical intervention. Knowledge of the difference between toxic/metabolic coma and structural coma can help the paramedic anticipate the course of the patient's condition and provide the appropriate prehospital interventions.

Assessment and Management

Regardless of the cause of the coma, prehospital care is directed at supporting vital functions, preventing further deterioration of the patient's condition, establishing vascular access to administer medications and intravenous (IV) fluids if needed, and managing potentially reversible causes of coma. As always, airway maintenance and ventilatory support with supplemental oxygen when needed are the first priorities in patient care. Rapid transport to an appropriate facility for definitive care may be indicated.

If respirations are abnormally slow or shallow, and minute ventilation is inadequate as demonstrated by an elevated $ETCO_2$ level, ventilations should be assisted. If the patient is unconscious and has no gag reflex, invasive airway management should be considered. After securing the airway, the paramedic should take the following steps to treat a patient in a coma of unknown origin. Transport should not be delayed for IV access in a critical patient or patient with acute stroke.

1. Establish an IV line to administer medication or to infuse fluids to manage hypotension (if present).
2. Monitor the ECG, oxygen saturation, and waveform capnograph in a patient with altered mental status.
3. Measure the serum glucose level (see Chapter 25, *Endocrinology*). Administer dextrose if indicated.
4. Administer naloxone if opiate overdose is suspected.
5. If the patient remains comatose, consider transporting in a lateral recumbent position to aid in drainage of secretions and to minimize the possibility of aspiration of stomach contents. Closely monitor the patient's airway and have suction readily available. If the patient's eyes are open, protect them from corneal drying by gently closing them and covering the lids with moist gauze pads.

> NOTE
>
> Narcotic reversal with naloxone should be administered only for patients with inadequate ventilation and altered level of consciousness who are suspected of using narcotics. Patients who are dependent on narcotics may have significant withdrawal symptoms including severe nausea, vomiting, agitation, and abdominal pain. The paramedic should be prepared to manage a patient who becomes agitated or violent following narcotic reversal. The incidence of agitation after reversal appears to be more frequent when naloxone is administered by the IV route rather than the intranasal route. The naloxone dose may need to be repeated if respiratory depression recurs, as the duration of action of some narcotics (particularly with oral sustained-release formulations) may be longer than that of naloxone. Initial and repeat doses should be titrated to patient response required to maintain adequate ventilation.
>
> *Modified from*: Sabzghabaee AM, Eizadi-Mood N, Yaraghi A, Zandifar S. Naloxone therapy in opioid overdose patients: intranasal or intravenous? A randomized clinical trial. *Arch Med Sci.* 2014;10(2):309-314.

Stroke and Intracranial Hemorrhage

A stroke, or **cerebrovascular accident**, is a sudden interruption in blood flow to a portion of the brain, resulting in a neurologic deficit. Stroke is a serious disease that affects almost 800,000 Americans each year.[7] It is the fifth-leading cause of death in the United States, killing about 140,000 patients each year. Stroke is a significant problem because it has potentially devastating permanent neurologic consequences. According to the American Stroke Association, people who are more likely to suffer a stroke have prior risk factors that can be classified as modifiable or nonmodifiable.

Modifiable stroke risk factors include the following:[8]

- Hypertension
- Cigarette smoking
- Heart disease (cardiomyopathy, decreased ejection fraction)
- Atrial fibrillation
- Diabetes mellitus
- Hypercoagulopathic states, including polycythemia, and oral contraceptive use
- Carotid artery disease
- Peripheral artery disease
- Sickle cell disease
- Diet
- Obesity
- Hypercholesterolemia

Nonmodifiable risk factors include the following:

- Age (stroke risk doubles every 10 years after age 55 years)
- Sex (women are at greater risk than are men)
- Race (African Americans are at much greater risk than are Caucasians)
- Previous stroke, TIA, or heart attack
- Heredity

The following factors also may play a role in stroke risk:

- Geographic location (stroke risk is higher in the southeastern United States, in the "stroke belt," where there is a high prevalence of hypertension in the population)
- Low income
- Alcohol or drug abuse
- Poor sleep quality

The best way to prevent strokes is to identify people who are at risk and then to control as many risk factors as possible. Effective prevention methods include good control of hypertension, modification of behavioral risks (listed previously), and drug therapy.

Pathophysiology

As described previously, blood reaches the brain through four major vessels: the two carotid arteries and the two vertebral arteries. (The two carotid arteries provide about 80% of CBF.) The two vertebral arteries combine to form the single basilar artery (supplying the remaining 20% of CBF). These two systems are interconnected at various levels. The principal level is the circle of Willis. In addition, collateral blood flow can be supplied to the brain through connections from blood vessels in the face and scalp to the dura and arachnoid coverings of the brain. The amount of collateral circulation varies from person to person. Beyond this, however, there is no collateral circulation in the depths of the brain.[9] Therefore, occlusion of any one of the more distal vessels may result in ischemia and infarction.

Normally, the CBF is maintained through autoregulation of cerebral vessels. These vessels constrict or dilate to preserve CPP even when the patient is hypotensive. Arterial cerebral perfusion is regulated by the level of oxygen and glucose supplied (ischemia and acidosis are profound vasodilators). Vessel occlusion or hemorrhage causes a sudden cessation of circulation to a portion of the brain. Autoregulatory mechanisms cannot readily correct this problem. The uncorrected ischemia that results within a short period leads to neuronal dysfunction and death. The onset and symptoms of the stroke depend on the area of the brain involved. It is important to note that although some ischemic tissue will not recover, there is a surrounding area that can be preserved with appropriate management and rapid intervention when indicated.

> CRITICAL THINKING
> How much oxygen and glucose can the brain store for emergency situations?

Types of Stroke

Stroke is a general term that refers to the neurologic manifestations of a critical decrease in blood flow to a portion of the brain, regardless of the cause. The American Heart Association has defined two primary categories of stroke: **ischemic stroke**, also called occlusive stroke, and **hemorrhagic stroke**. Each of these categories is subdivided into two classes. For ischemic stroke, these classes are **cerebral thrombosis** (clot forms in the cerebral vessel) and **cerebral embolism** (clot forms elsewhere and lodges in the cerebral vessel—ie, from atrial fibrillation). For hemorrhagic stroke, the classes are **intracerebral hemorrhage** and **subarachnoid hemorrhage**.

> **NOTE**
>
> Ischemic strokes are caused by blood clots. This type of stroke accounts for 85% of all strokes. It is the only type of stroke for which fibrinolytics are administered.
>
> ---
>
> *Modified from*: National Center for Chronic Disease Prevention and Health Promotion, Division for Heart Disease and Stroke Prevention. Stroke facts. Centers for Disease Control and Prevention website. https://www.cdc.gov/stroke/facts.htm. Updated September 6, 2017. Accessed March 25, 2018.

Determining the origin of a stroke frequently is difficult and is generally unnecessary in the prehospital setting. (The best care for all stroke patients is support of ventilation and cerebral perfusion and rapid transport to an appropriate facility for definitive care.) However, a paramedic who understands the various signs and symptoms of each type of stroke is better equipped to anticipate the course of patient care (**TABLE 24-3**). Documentation of a thorough history and physical examination also helps others involved in the patient's care.

Ischemic Stroke. About 85% of strokes are the ischemic type. Some of these strokes are caused by cerebral thrombosis. The thrombosis occurs as a result of atherosclerotic plaques or pressure from a mass in the brain itself. Stroke caused by cerebral thrombosis usually is associated with a long history of blood vessel disease. Therefore, most of these patients are older and have evidence of atherosclerotic disease in other areas of the body (angina pectoris, claudication, previous strokes). The signs and symptoms of thrombotic stroke include the following:[10]

- Hemiparesis or hemiplegia on the side of the body opposite the lesion
- Numbness (decreased sensation) on the side of the body opposite the lesion

TABLE 24-3 Differentiation of Ischemic and Hemorrhagic Stroke

Ischemic Stroke	Hemorrhagic Stroke
Most common	Least common
Usually the result of atherosclerosis or embolism caused by a cardiac dysrhythmia, such as atrial fibrillation	Usually the result of cerebral aneurysms, arteriovenous malformations, hypertension
Disease develops over time, symptoms develop abruptly	Develops abruptly
Long history of vessel disease	Can occur during stress or exertion, or other causes of abrupt increase in blood pressure
May be associated with valvular heart disease and atrial fibrillation	May be associated with use of cocaine and other sympathomimetic amines
History of angina, previous strokes	May be asymptomatic before rupture

© Jones & Bartlett Learning.

- Aphasia
- Confusion or coma
- Convulsions
- Incontinence
- Diplopia (double vision)
- Monocular blindness (painless visual loss in one eye)
- Numbness of the face
- Dysarthria (slurred speech)
- Headache
- Dizziness or vertigo
- Ataxia

A stroke caused by cerebral embolism occurs when an intracranial vessel is blocked by a foreign substance. The vessel is occluded by a fragment of a foreign substance originating outside the CNS. Common sources of cerebral emboli include atherosclerotic plaques (originating from large vessels of the head, neck, or heart). Thrombi that develop on the valves or in the chambers of the heart are very common in patients with heart valve disease and atrial fibrillation. Other, rare causes include air embolism from a chest injury and fat embolism after long bone injury. Bacterial and fungal infections of the heart also can produce emboli. Women taking oral contraceptives and patients with sickle cell disease have an increased risk of stroke, by both thrombotic and embolic origins. Signs and symptoms of a cerebral embolus are similar to those of thrombotic stroke. However, embolic signs and symptoms develop more quickly. Also, they often are associated with an identifiable cause (eg, atrial fibrillation).

Large vessel occlusion (LVO) ischemic strokes involve major cerebral blood vessels and are associated with higher mortality and a poor functional outcome. Blood vessels involved in LVO include vertebral, basilar, carotid, or middle and anterior cerebral arteries. This type of stroke is best treated at a comprehensive stroke center with the ability to perform endovascular treatment (mechanical thrombectomy).[11] The Joint Commission offers the following advanced levels of certification for stroke programs in Joint Commission–accredited hospitals: Acute Stroke Ready Hospital, Primary Stroke Center, Thrombectomy-Capable Stroke Center, and Comprehensive Stroke Center.[12] Paramedics must be knowledgeable of stroke center capabilities in their service area and protocols for which patients should be transported to which center to provide patients the best opportunity for a good outcome.

Strokes affecting the posterior circulation may have more subtle signs and symptoms. They are less common, and their diagnosis is easier to miss. Signs and symptoms vary widely in posterior stroke and may include the following:[13]

- Visual disturbances, which may include partial loss of the visual fields; seeing objects that are not present; inability to see, but ability to respond to movement or changes in environmental lighting; inability to recognize or understand familiar objects; altered color perception or recognition; nystagmus; abnormal gaze or Horner syndrome (miosis, ptosis, anhydrosis)
- Ataxia, which may consist of a staggering gait or loss of eye–hand coordination
- Difficulty sitting without support
- Dysphagia
- Dysarthria
- Memory impairment or confusion
- Posterior headache or pain in the face
- Dizziness, swaying, tilting, or leaning
- Hemiplegia or hemiparesis

Hemorrhagic Stroke. Cerebral hemorrhage accounts for about 13% of all strokes.[14] A hemorrhage may occur anywhere in the brain and its structures. This includes the epidural, subdural, subarachnoid, intraparenchymal, and intraventricular spaces. The most common causes are cerebral aneurysms, arteriovenous malformations, and hypertension. Cerebral aneurysms and arteriovenous malformations are congenital anomalies. They can run in families. They often are asymptomatic until they rupture. Unlike thrombotic and embolic strokes, which have relatively high survival rates, cerebral hemorrhages are fatal in 50% to 80% of cases.[15]

NOTE

A **cerebral aneurysm** is a weak or thin spot on a blood vessel in the brain that balloons and fills with blood. This bulging can put pressure on a nerve or brain tissue. The aneurysm also can rupture or leak, spilling blood into surrounding tissue. Cerebral aneurysms can occur anywhere in the brain, but most are located along a loop of arteries that run between the underside of the brain and the base of the skull.

An **arteriovenous malformation** is an abnormal connection between veins and arteries. These defects in the circulatory system are believed to arise during fetal development or soon after birth. Arteriovenous malformations can develop in many sites in the body. Those in the brain or spinal cord can result in hemorrhage and stroke.

Modified from: Arteriovenous malformations and other vascular lesions of the central nervous system fact sheet. National Institute of Neurological Disorders and Stroke website. https://www.ninds.nih.gov/Disorders/Patient-Caregiver-Education/Fact-Sheets/Arteriovenous-Malformation-Fact-Sheet. Accessed March 25, 2018.

Hemorrhagic strokes often occur during stress or exertion. Cocaine and other sympathomimetic-type drugs also may contribute to intracranial hemorrhage by a drug-induced rapid elevation of blood pressure. The onset of the stroke is sudden. It often begins with a headache (sometimes described as a "thunderclap headache" or the worst headache of the patient's life). The patient is frequently sensitive to light and may have visual changes. The headache can be accompanied by significant nausea and vomiting, and progressive deterioration in mental status. Some patients complain of a stiff neck. Often the patient loses consciousness or experiences a seizure at the time of the initial hemorrhage. As the hemorrhage expands, the ICP rises. As this occurs, the patient becomes comatose, with increasing hypertension, bradycardia, and diminished respiratory effort (Cushing reflex).

CRITICAL THINKING

Why do you think mortality is higher for hemorrhagic stroke than for embolic stroke?

Transient Ischemic Attacks

A **transient ischemic attack (TIA)** is an episode of cerebral dysfunction that appears to last minutes to several hours. A TIA is thought to be the most important indicator of impending stroke; more than 5% of TIA patients have a completed stroke within 7 days.[16] Fifteen percent of major strokes are preceded by a TIA.[17] About one-third of patients who have a TIA have a stroke within a year.[18] A TIA should be taken very seriously because of the risk of progression to a completed stroke.

The signs and symptoms of a TIA are the same as those that characterize stroke: weakness, paralysis, numbness of the face, and speech disturbances. All of these signs and symptoms correspond to vascular occlusion of a specific cerebral artery. Most patients who experience a TIA are hospitalized for close observation, evaluation, and treatment of vascular disease.

DID YOU KNOW?

Stroke Mimics

A small number of patients are diagnosed with stroke when their signs and symptoms actually result from other causes. Conditions that can mimic stroke include drug toxicity, hypoglycemia, and encephalitis, among others. Misdiagnosing these conditions as stroke can lead to harmful interventions for the patient and fail to correct the actual cause of illness.

Todd paralysis (or Todd paresis) is a very convincing stroke mimic. In patients with Todd paralysis, paralysis or weakness (usually unilateral) develops after a generalized motor seizure and usually subsides over several days. If the patient has a history of onset of paralysis after a seizure, this stroke mimic should be considered in the differential diagnosis.

Modified from: Onder H. Todd's paralysis: a crucial entity masquerading stroke in the emergency department. *J Emerg Med.* 2017;52(4):e153-e155.

Role of Paramedics in Stroke Care

In stroke care, the paramedic's role is to identify a stroke event quickly, determine how much time has elapsed since the stroke symptoms began or since the patient was last seen to be in his or her normal state so transport to the appropriate destination can be initiated, notify medical direction, and transport the

DID YOU KNOW?

Primary Stroke Centers

The Joint Commission certifies hospitals as stroke centers to promote improved outcomes for stroke care. Stroke center certification indicates that a center has been deemed to provide specialized care for stroke patients. The Acute Stroke Ready Hospital has access to stroke expertise 24 hours a day and can administer thrombolytics and transfer patients. A Primary Stroke Center has personnel trained in stroke management and a dedicated stroke unit. Thrombectomy-Capable Stroke Centers are equipped to perform endovascular thrombectomy to treat stroke. The Comprehensive Stroke Center has dedicated intensive care unit beds for stroke patients and advanced personnel and equipment. These centers have advanced imaging and interventions to manage stroke patients.

Modified from: Facts about Joint Commission stroke certification. The Joint Commission website. https://www.jointcommission.org/facts_about_joint_commission_stroke_certification/. Published April 21, 2017. Accessed March 25, 2018.

NOTE

About 85% of strokes occur at home. Public education programs focused on people at risk for stroke, their friends, and family members have been shown to reduce the time to arrival at the emergency department (ED; see Chapter 3, *Injury Prevention, Health Promotion, and Public Health*). The American Heart Association and the American Stroke Association have described a "chain of survival" to improve stroke survival. This chain is made up of four links:

1. Rapid recognition and reaction to stroke warning signs
2. Rapid EMS dispatch
3. Rapid EMS transport and hospital prenotification
4. Rapid diagnosis and treatment in the hospital

Modified from: Barbour V, Thakore S. Improving door to CT scanner times for potential stroke thrombolysis candidates—the emergency department's role. *BMJ Qual Improv Rep.* 2017;6(1).

BOX 24-4 Eight Ds of Stroke Management

The first three Ds are the responsibility of the public and EMS providers. The fourth and fifth Ds are the responsibility of EMS, and the last three Ds are performed in the hospital.

Detection. A patient, family member, or bystander recognizes the signs and symptoms of a stroke or TIA.

Dispatch. Someone calls 9-1-1, and EMS dispatchers dispatch the appropriate EMS team with high transport priority.

Delivery. EMS providers respond rapidly, confirm the signs and symptoms of stroke, and transport the patient.

Door. The patient is transported to a stroke center that can provide fibrinolytic therapy within 1 hour of arrival at the ED door for eligible patients.

Data. A computed tomographic scan and appropriate laboratory work are obtained.

Decision. The center determines whether the patient is a candidate for fibrinolytic therapy or other interventions.

Drug. Eligible patients are treated with fibrinolytic therapy or endovascular treatment.

Disposition. The patient is rapidly transferred to a stroke or critical care unit.

Modified from: American Heart Association. *2015 Handbook of Emergency Cardiovascular Care for Healthcare Providers.* Dallas, TX: American Heart Association; 2015.

patient rapidly to a proper facility for hospital-based evaluation and treatment. Key points in the timely management of stroke include the eight Ds: detection, dispatch, delivery, door, data, decision, drug, and disposition (BOX 24-4). (The first three Ds are the responsibility of the public and EMS personnel.)

Assessment

The primary survey of a patient who may have suffered a stroke or TIA follows the same sequence as that for any other ill or injured patient in the emergency setting. The priorities are to maintain a patent airway and to provide adequate ventilatory support with appropriate supplemental oxygen. If the patient is conscious and able to speak, a thorough history should be obtained. The following are important components of the patient history for these patients:

- Last known normal (a specific time when the patient was last known to be at his or her neurologic baseline)
- Previous neurologic symptoms (eg, TIAs)
- Previous neurologi
- Initial symptoms
- Alterations in lev
- Precipitating fac
- Dizziness
- Palpitations
- Significant past medical his include the following:
  - Hypertension
  - Diabetes mellitus
  - Cigarette smoking
  - Oral contraceptive use
  - Cardiac disease
  - Sickle cell disease
  - Previous stroke

Cincinnati Prehospital Stroke Scale. In addition to the abnormal neurologic signs and symptoms described previously, other methods can be used to diagnose stroke. One such method is the Cincinnati Prehospital Stroke Scale (CPSS). This scale evaluates three major physical findings: facial droop, arm drift, and speech (BOX 24-5). The paramedic can use this scale to help identify a patient who may be having a stroke and who needs rapid transport to a hospital. It also allows for prearrival notification of the receiving hospital.

BOX 24-5 Cincinnati Prehospital Stroke Scale

Facial Droop (have the patient show the teeth or smile)

- **Normal.** The two sides of the face move equally well.
- **Abnormal.** One side of the face does not move as well as the other side.

Arm Drift (have the patient close the eyes and hold out both arms, palms up)

- **Normal.** Both arms move the same or both arms do not move at all (other findings, such as pronator, may be helpful).
- **Abnormal.** One arm does not move or one arm drifts down and may pronate compared with the other.

Speech (have the patient say, "You can't teach an old dog new tricks.")

- **Normal.** The patient uses the correct words with no slurring.
- **Abnormal.** The patient slurs words, uses inappropriate words, or is unable to speak.

S has a sensitivity of 59% and a specificity of hen scored by prehospital personnel.[19]

s Angeles Prehospital Stroke Screen. The Los ngeles Prehospital Stroke Screen (LAPSS) is another means of detecting possible stroke. This screening tool requires the examiner to rule out other causes of altered level of consciousness (eg, hypoglycemia, seizure). The examiner then must identify asymmetry (right versus left) in facial smile/grimace, grip, and arm strength (**BOX 24-6**). Asymmetry in any category indicates a possible stroke. Like the CPSS, the LAPSS can be used quickly in the prehospital setting. The LAPSS has a specificity of 97% and a sensitivity of 93%.[20]

Los Angeles Motor Scale. The Los Angeles Motor Scale (LAMS) is a brief stroke score derived from the LAPSS that is easy to perform in the prehospital setting (**TABLE 24-4**). It can be assessed in conjunction with the CPSS by adding one step. The LAMS can help distinguish patients who have an LVO, although its effectiveness in detecting LVO has not been tested in prehospital providers.[21] These patients may benefit from endovascular recanalization treatment and, if available locally, should be transported to a Comprehensive Stroke Center.[22] A patient with a LAMS score of 4 or greater is seven times more likely to have an LVO.

Face-Arm-Speech-Time Test (FAST Test). FAST is a mnemonic to help patients, family members, and

BOX 24-6 Los Angeles Prehospital Stroke Screen

The LAPSS is used to evaluate patients who may have an acute, noncomatose, nontraumatic neurologic condition. If items 1 through 6 are all checked Yes (or Unknown), notify the receiving hospital before arrival of the potential stroke patient. If any are checked No, follow the appropriate treatment protocol.

Interpretation: Ninety-three percent of patients with stroke have positive findings (all items checked Yes or Unknown [sensitivity, 93%]). Of those with positive findings, 97% have a stroke (specificity, 97%). A patient may be having a stroke even if LAPSS criteria are not met.

	Yes	Unknown	No
1. Age >45 years	❑	❑	❑
2. History of seizures or epilepsy absent	❑	❑	❑
3. Symptom duration >24 hours	❑	❑	❑
4. At baseline, patient is not wheelchair bound or bedridden	❑	❑	❑
5. Blood glucose level is 60–400 mg/dL	❑	❑	❑
6. Obvious asymmetry (right versus left) in any of the following three categories (must be unilateral):	❑	❑	❑

	Equal	Right Weak	Left Weak
Facial smile/grimace	❑	❑ Droop	❑ Droop
Grip	❑	❑ Weak grip	❑ Weak grip
	❑	❑ No grip	❑ No grip
Arm strength	❑	❑ Drifts down	❑ Drifts down
	❑	❑ Falls rapidly	❑ Falls rapidly

Modified from: Kidwell CS, Saver JL, Schubert GB, Eckstein M, Starkman S. Design and retrospective analysis of the Los Angeles Prehospital Stroke Screen (LAPSS). *Prehosp Emerg Care.* 1998;2(4):267-273.

TABLE 24-4 The Los Angeles Motor Scale

Facial Droop	
Absent	0
Present	1
Arm Drift	
Absent	0
Drifts down	1
Falls rapidly	2
Grip Strength	
Normal	0
Weak grip	1
No grip	2

the general public identify suspected stroke patients and the need to activate the EMS system:

- **Facial drooping.** A section of the face, usually only on one side, is drooping and hard to move. This can be recognized by a crooked smile.
- **Arm weakness.** The patient is unable to raise the arm fully.
- **Speech difficulties.** The patient cannot understand or produce speech, or has difficulty doing so.
- **Time.** If any of the preceding symptoms are present, time is of the essence; call 9-1-1.

Other Signs and Symptoms. In addition to the stroke scales, other signs and symptoms may be noted in patients who are having a stroke. Paramedics should be on the lookout for signs of the following:

- **Neglect.** The patient seems to be unaware of the affected side of the body; for example, if the left side is paralyzed, the paramedic may find the patient with the head turned to the right.
- **Visual problems.** The patient has a change or loss of vision in one eye, bumps into objects, or sees only half of a printed page when reading.

Management

Once the diagnosis of stroke is suspected, time in the field must be reduced because limited time is available to begin therapy (**FIGURE 24-15**). Fibrinolytics should be given less than 4.5 hours from the onset (some centers have expanded this time frame to 6 hours or more in certain cases).[23,24] This treatment is recommended even when the patient is being transferred for endovascular therapy. Endovascular treatment for clot retrieval is ideally done within 6 hours from symptom onset when the internal or middle cerebral artery is causing the stroke (Class 1); however, that time window may be extended up to 24 hours in some patients with LVO.[25] Whenever possible, the paramedic should establish the last known normal (ie, time of onset of the stroke signs and symptoms). If the patient awoke with the symptoms, the time of onset should be recorded as the last time the patient was known to be normal. It is important that this information be documented as an actual time, rather than using vague terms such as "3 hours ago," to help determine whether the patient is eligible for fibrinolytic or endovascular treatment. The risk of complications, such as intracerebral hemorrhage versus benefit to the patient, increases as time elapses. In addition to the primary survey and management, the most important care a paramedic can provide a stroke victim is quick identification of the possible stroke and early notification followed by rapid transport to the appropriate facility for definitive care.

Airway. Paralysis of the muscles of the throat, tongue, and mouth can lead to partial or complete airway obstruction. (This can be a significant problem in acute stroke.) Frequent suctioning of the oropharynx and nasopharynx may be needed to prevent aspiration. If needed and possible, the patient can be positioned to aid drainage of oral secretions. The paramedic should avoid administering anything by mouth until the patient is assessed for risk of aspiration.

> CRITICAL THINKING
> How can you detect paralysis of the muscles of the throat, tongue, and mouth on your physical examination?

Breathing. Inadequate ventilation should be managed with supplemental oxygen and positive pressure ventilation. Hypoxia and hypercapnia can occur as a result of inadequate ventilation, contributing to cardiac and respiratory instability. Supplemental

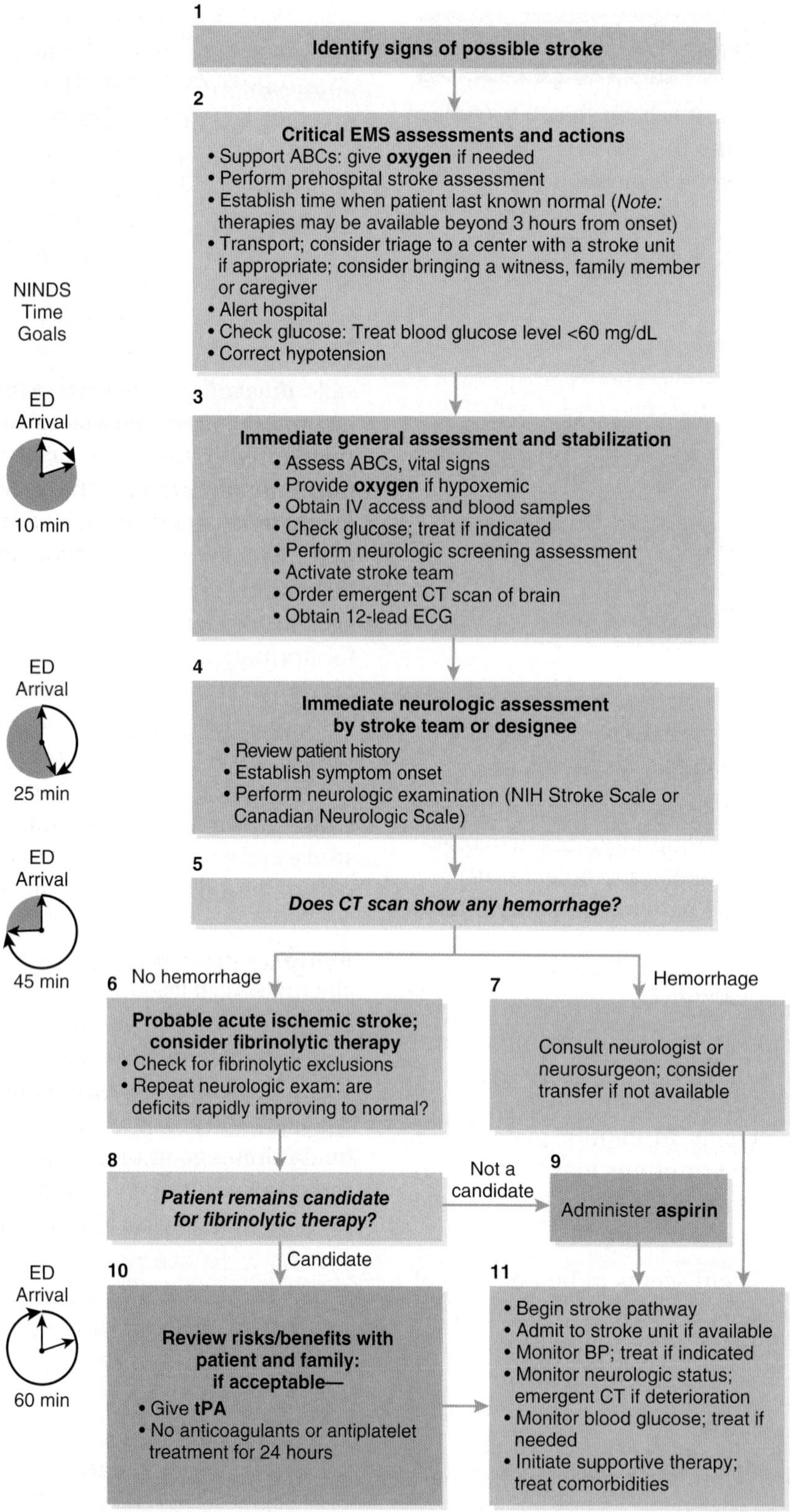

1
Identify signs of possible stroke
2
Critical EMS assessments and actions
• Support ABCs: give oxygen if needed
• Perform prehospital stroke assessment
• Establish time when patient last known normal (Note: therapies may be available beyond 3 hours from onset)
• Transport; consider triage to a center with a stroke unit if appropriate; consider bringing a witness, family member or caregiver
• Alert hospital
• Check glucose: Treat blood glucose level <60 mg/dL
• Correct hypotension
NINDS Time Goals
ED Arrival
10 min
3
Immediate general assessment and stabilization
• Assess ABCs, vital signs
• Provide oxygen if hypoxemic
• Obtain IV access and blood samples
• Check glucose; treat if indicated
• Perform neurologic screening assessment
• Activate stroke team
• Order emergent CT scan of brain
• Obtain 12-lead ECG
ED Arrival
25 min
4
Immediate neurologic assessment by stroke team or designee
• Review patient history
• Establish symptom onset
• Perform neurologic examination (NIH Stroke Scale or Canadian Neurologic Scale)
ED Arrival
45 min
5
Does CT scan show any hemorrhage?
6 No hemorrhage
Probable acute ischemic stroke; consider fibrinolytic therapy
• Check for fibrinolytic exclusions
• Repeat neurologic exam: are deficits rapidly improving to normal?
7 Hemorrhage
Consult neurologist or neurosurgeon; consider transfer if not available
8
Patient remains candidate for fibrinolytic therapy?
Not a candidate
9
Administer aspirin
Candidate
ED Arrival
60 min
10
Review risks/benefits with patient and family: if acceptable—
• Give tPA
• No anticoagulants or antiplatelet treatment for 24 hours
11
• Begin stroke pathway
• Admit to stroke unit if available
• Monitor BP; treat if indicated
• Monitor neurologic status; emergent CT if deterioration
• Monitor blood glucose; treat if needed
• Initiate supportive therapy; treat comorbidities

Abbreviations: ABCs, airway, breathing, circulation; BP, blood pressure; CT, computed tomography; ECG, electrocardiogram; EMS, emergency medical services; IV, intravenous; NIH, National Institutes of Health; NINDS, National Institute of Neurological Disorders and Stroke; tPA, tissue plasminogen activator

FIGURE 24-15 Goals for management of suspected cases of stroke.

oxygen should be given to stroke patients who are hypoxic (oxygen saturation less than 94%) to bring their oxygen saturation to above 94%.[26] Although hyperoxia (excess oxygen) has been shown to worsen patient outcomes during in-hospital treatment,[27] prehospital treatment with supplemental oxygen for hypoxia should not err on the side of being cautious because of the possibility of the patient experiencing short-duration hyperoxia.

Circulation. Cardiac arrest is uncommon. However, it may result from a respiratory arrest. Cardiac dysrhythmias occur frequently; therefore, the patient's ECG and blood pressure require constant monitoring. A difference in blood pressure readings in the upper extremities of 10 mm Hg or more may indicate aortic dissection and compromise of the brain's blood supply. Hypotension associated with stroke symptoms should raise concerns for either vascular dissection (carotid, aorta) or a non-neurologic etiology.

NOTE

Hypertension can be a risk for many patients following a stroke. However, this hypertension usually does not require emergency treatment. Elevated blood pressure after a stroke is not considered a hypertensive emergency unless the patient has other conditions, such as acute myocardial infarction or left ventricular failure. Management of hypertension in the prehospital setting is not recommended in cases of suspected stroke. This is because acutely lowering blood pressure can actually extend the area of ischemia. The paramedic should notify the receiving facility and transfer the patient to a stroke center if available.

Modified from: Ovbiagele B, Turan N, eds. *Ischemic Stroke Therapeutics: A Comprehensive Guide*. New York, NY: Springer International Publishing; 2016.

Other Supportive Measures. If the airway is patent and the patient's condition permits, the person should be kept supine. The head should be elevated 15° to aid venous drainage. Other patient care measures the paramedic can provide while en route to the receiving hospital include the following:

1. Notify the hospital to activate a code stroke (if there is an established stroke protocol).
2. Initiate IV access and draw blood samples (if within local protocol). Correct hypotension and hypovolemia if present.
3. Monitor ECG rhythm and obtain a 12-lead ECG.
4. Perform serum glucose analysis (treat if blood glucose level is <60 mg/dL).
5. If possible, transport a witness to confirm the time of onset. If that is not possible, obtain the most reliable information and a name and contact number of a person who can attest to the time the patient was last known well.
6. Protect paralyzed extremities.
7. Maintain normal body temperature.
8. Control any seizure activity with benzodiazepines.
9. Provide comfort measures and reassurance.

Paramedics must keep in mind that a stroke patient has experienced a catastrophic event, one that may seriously affect the person's independence and quality of life. These patients often are frightened, embarrassed, confused, and frustrated with their inability to move or communicate. They have special physical and emotional needs. As do all other patients, they deserve a compassionate, caring approach.

In-Hospital Treatment

On arrival at the ED, a patient suspected of having a nonhemorrhagic stroke is evaluated as a possible candidate for fibrinolytic therapy. This evaluation includes an emergency neurologic stroke assessment that identifies the patient's level of consciousness. It also identifies the type, location, and severity of the stroke. This assessment is aided by use of the GCS and other standardized scales. These scales and other in-hospital diagnostic studies help measure neurologic function. This function correlates with the severity of the stroke and the long-term outcome. These studies also help identify stroke patients who would benefit from fibrinolytic therapy. Rapid evaluation of the computed tomography scan is crucial to rule out an intracranial hemorrhage. An intracranial hemorrhage is one of the contraindications to fibrinolytic therapy. Fibrinolytics have potential adverse effects. Patients must be evaluated by a physician with inclusion/exclusion criteria to make sure they are candidates for fibrinolytic therapy.

Seizure Disorders

A **seizure** is a brief alteration in behavior or consciousness. It is caused by abnormal electrical activity of one or more groups of neurons in the brain. It is estimated that 300,000 people in the United States experience a first-time seizure each year. Of these people, 120,000 are younger than 18 years—75,000 to 100,000 of whom are children younger than 5 years who are experiencing febrile seizures.[28] A tendency to have recurrent seizures is called **epilepsy** (BOX 24-7). Epilepsy does not include seizures that arise from correctable or avoidable causes, such as alcohol withdrawal.

> CRITICAL THINKING
> What feelings may parents experience after seeing their child have a febrile seizure? How should you respond to those feelings?

The underlying cause of seizures is not well understood. However, a seizure generally is believed to result from a structural lesion or problems with brain metabolism that result in changes in the brain cell's permeability to sodium and potassium ions. When such changes occur, the neurons' ability to depolarize and emit an electrical impulse sometimes results in seizure activity. Seizures may be caused by several factors, including the following:[3]

- Stroke
- Head trauma
- Toxins (including alcohol or other drug withdrawal)
- Hypoxia
- Hypoperfusion
- Hypoglycemia
- Infection
- Metabolic abnormalities
- Brain tumor or abscess
- Vascular disorders
- Eclampsia
- Drug overdose

Note: In the prehospital setting, determining the cause of a seizure is less important than managing the complications and recognizing whether the seizure is reversible with therapy (eg, resulting from hypoglycemia).

BOX 24-7 Epilepsy Statistics

- 2.2 million people in the United States and more than 65 million people worldwide have epilepsy.
- Each year, an estimated 150,000 new cases of epilepsy are diagnosed in the United States.
- Epilepsy will develop in 1 in 26 people in the United States at some point in their lifetime.
- The incidence is highest in infants younger than 2 years and in adults older than 65 years.
- Epilepsy is the fourth most common neurologic disorder in the United States after migraine, stroke, and Alzheimer disease.
- Males are slightly more likely to be at risk for the development of epilepsy than are females.
- The incidence is higher in African Americans and the socially disadvantaged.
- No cause is apparent in 70% of new cases.

Modified from: Shafer PO, Sirven JI. Epilepsy statistics. Epilepsy Foundation website. https://www.epilepsy.com/learn/about-epilepsy-basics/epilepsy-statistics. Published October 2013. Accessed March 25, 2018.

Types of Seizures

All seizures are pathologic; they are never normal. They may arise from almost any region of the brain and therefore have many clinical manifestations. In 2017, the International League Against Epilepsy revised its classification of seizures. The intent of the new classification was to make the diagnosis and identification of seizures easier and more accurate. Seizures are now classified into three basic groups based on where the seizure began in the brain, the patient's level of awareness during the seizure, and other features of seizures. The three basic classifications are focal onset seizures, generalized onset seizures, and unknown onset seizures (**FIGURE 24-16**).[29]

Focal Onset Seizure. A **focal onset seizure** (previously referred to as a partial seizure) is a seizure that begins within networks of one hemisphere of the brain. These seizures usually arise from identifiable lesions in the motor or sensory cortex and may spread in an orderly way to surrounding areas (**jacksonian march**). They can be divided into different categories by the types of symptoms a patient experiences. If the patient is aware of his or her surroundings during the seizure, it is called a **focal aware seizure** (previously referred to as simple partial seizure). Patients who are focal aware remain aware of their surroundings, even if they cannot talk or respond during the seizure. If there is a change in the patient's level of awareness during the seizure, it is considered a **focal impaired awareness seizure** (previously referred to as a **complex partial seizure**). This type of seizure usually arises from the temporal lobe. In some cases, awareness cannot be determined (eg, a patient who lives alone or has a seizure while sleeping). This type of seizure is referred to as

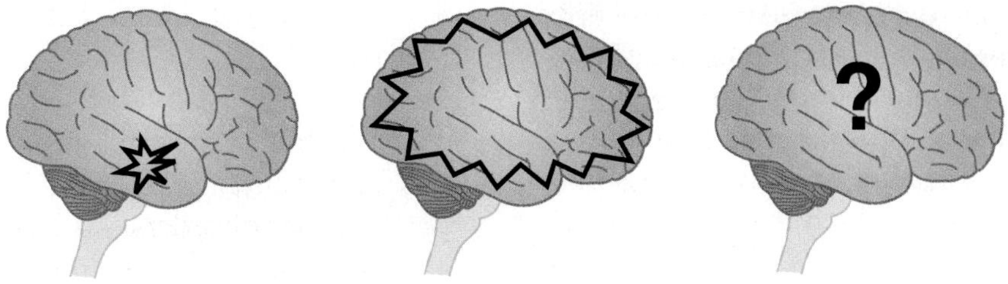

FIGURE 24-16 Seizure types and classifications. Aware indicates awareness during the seizure, knowledge of self and environment, and intact consciousness. Motor indicates movement or motion. Unclassified indicates seizures with patterns that do not fit the other categories or insufficient information to classify the seizure.

Modified from: Epilepsia, a journal of the International League Against Epilepsy.

awareness unknown. In these situations, the focal onset seizure can be classified by movement as motor onset or non–motor onset.

NOTE

Some focal onset seizures may begin in one hemisphere and spread to involve both hemispheres exhibiting motor activity. These seizures are called focal to bilateral tonic–clonic seizures. Focal to bilateral tonic–clonic reflects a propagation pattern of a seizure, rather than a specific seizure type. This characteristic is important in distinguishing a focal onset seizure that begins in one hemisphere from a generalized onset seizure that engages both hemispheres simultaneously.

Modified from: Focal seizure by feature: aura. International League Against Epilepsy website. https://www.epilepsydiagnosis.org/seizure/aura-overview.html. Accessed March 26, 2018.

Motor Onset Seizure. **Motor onset seizures** produce a change in muscle activity, such as weakness, twitching, and stiffening of body parts. These movements may affect the muscles on one or both sides of the body, affect speech, and may include coordinated actions (**automatisms**) such as lip smacking and repetitive hand movements. **Non–motor onset seizures** can affect the senses, resulting in changes in smell, taste, and hearing. Visual and/or auditory hallucinations may also arise. These **auras** (warnings) can occur with or without altered awareness and are thought to reflect the initial seizure discharge. An aura may be an isolated event, or it may progress to a focal onset seizure or a tonic–clonic seizure (described in the following section).[30] Other types of non–motor focal onset seizures include autonomic seizures (eg, odd sensations in the stomach, chest, or head; changes in the heart rate or breathing; sweating; or goose bumps) and emotional/cognitive seizures (eg, problems with memory and speech; unexplained fear or depression; out-of-body experiences; feelings of déjà vu).

NOTE

Seizures should be classified by the earliest prominent motor onset or non–motor onset feature. Classification according to onset has an anatomic basis, whereas classification by level of awareness has a behavioral basis, justified by the practical importance of impaired awareness. Both methods of classification can be used in concert.

Modified from: Fisher RS, Cross JH, French JA, et al. Operational classification of seizure types by the International League Against Epilepsy: Position Paper of the ILAE Commission for Classification and Terminology. *Epilepsia*. 2017;58:522-530.

Generalized Onset Seizure. A **generalized onset seizure** (previously referred to as grand mal) begins within both hemispheres of the brain. Like focal onset seizures, generalized onset seizures are divided into motor and nonmotor (absence) seizures. With generalized seizures, awareness is presumed to be affected in some way. Therefore, no special terms are used to describe awareness in generalized seizures. Motor seizures combine the characteristics of stiffening (tonic) and jerking (clonic) movement and may include the following:

- **Absence seizures** (previously referred to as petit mal seizures) occur most often in children age 4 to 12 years. They are associated with brief lapses of consciousness without loss of posture. However, some children have eye blinking, lip smacking, or isolated contraction of muscles. These seizures usually last less than 15 seconds, during which the patient is unaware of the surroundings. The seizures are followed by the patient's immediate return to normal. Most patients have remission by age 20 years, but later generalized onset seizures may develop.

- **Atonic seizures** produce an abrupt loss of muscle tone, loss of posture, or sudden collapse ("drop attacks"). These seizures can result in physical injury from falls. Patients with atonic seizures sometimes wear protective headgear. These seizures tend to be resistant to drug therapy.
- **Myoclonic seizures** cause brief muscle contractions in a single event or in a series. They often occur on both sides of the body at the same time. (Occasionally they involve one arm or one foot.) People with this disorder often compare the sensation to an abrupt shoulder shrug or the sudden jerk of a foot during sleep.
- **Tonic–clonic seizures** are common and are associated with significant morbidity and mortality.[31] They may be preceded by an aura as a warning of the imminent seizure. The seizure itself is characterized by a sudden loss of consciousness with loss of organized muscle tone. The tonic phase involves extensor muscle tone activity (sometimes flexion) and apnea. Tongue biting and bladder or bowel incontinence may occur. The tonic phase lasts only seconds and is followed by a bilateral clonic phase (rigidity alternating with relaxation). This phase usually lasts 1 to 3 minutes during which a massive autonomic discharge occurs, resulting in hyperventilation, salivation, and tachycardia. After the seizure, the patient usually experiences a period of drowsiness or unconsciousness that resolves over minutes to hours. On regaining consciousness, the patient often is confused and fatigued and have a transient interruption of normal brain function. This part of the seizure is known as the **postictal phase**. Tonic–clonic seizures may be prolonged or may recur before the patient regains consciousness. When this state occurs, the patient is said to be in status epilepticus (described later in this chapter).

> NOTE
>
> The most common cause of death from epilepsy is sudden unexpected death in epilepsy (SUDEP). This diagnosis is made on autopsy when no other cause is identified. Only about one-third of these patients have evidence of a seizure prior to death. The patient is often found prone.
>
> *Modified from*: SUDEP. Epilepsy Foundation website. https://www.epilepsy.com/learn/early-death-and-sudep/sudep. Accessed March 26, 2018.

> NOTE
>
> A **nonepileptic seizure** (a hysterical seizure or pseudoseizure) can mimic a true seizure. However, its cause is psychological; it does not result from an electrical disturbance in the brain. This type of seizure does not respond to the usual treatments. Nonepileptic seizures sometimes can be ended by sharp commands or annoying stimuli (eg, a sternal rub). These maneuvers may help the paramedic distinguish between pathologic and psychogenic seizures. It should be noted that some nonepileptic diseases can cause life-threatening seizures. Paramedics should remember that a seizure is never normal; any seizure should be taken seriously.

Assessment

The assessment process is determined by the patient's seizure state. In most cases, the patient's seizure has ended before paramedics arrive. If possible, the assessment should include a thorough history and physical examination, including a neurologic evaluation.

History. If the patient is in the postictal phase of the seizure, information can be gathered from family members or bystanders who witnessed the event. The following are important components of the patient history:

1. History of seizures
   a. Frequency
   b. Compliance in taking prescribed medications (eg, carbamazepine, levetiracetam, phenobarbital), any recent changes in medication
   c. Use of nonprescribed medications, supplements, alcohol, or illicit drugs
2. Description of seizure activity
   a. Duration of seizure
   b. Typical or atypical pattern of seizure for the patient
   c. Presence of aura
   d. Generalized or focal

   e. Incontinence
   f. Tongue biting
   g. Time to return to baseline mental status
3. Recent or past history of head trauma
4. Recent history of fever, headache, nuchal rigidity (neck stiffness with flexion, suggesting meningeal irritation)
5. Past significant medical history
   a. Diabetes mellitus
   b. Heart disease
   c. Stroke

Physical Examination. During the physical examination, maintaining a patent airway is always of prime importance. The paramedic also should be alert for signs of trauma (head and neck trauma, tongue injury, oral lacerations). These injuries may have occurred before or during the seizure. Other components of the physical examination include the following:

- Level of sensorium, including the presence or absence of **amnesia**
- Cranial nerve evaluation, particularly pupillary findings
- Motor and sensory evaluation, including coordination (abnormalities may be caused by metabolic disturbances, meningitis, intracranial hemorrhage, and drug use)
- Evaluation for hypotension, hypoxia, and hypoglycemia
- Presence of urine or feces (suggesting bladder or bowel incontinence)
- Automatisms
- Cardiac dysrhythmias

CRITICAL THINKING

What are signs and symptoms of valproate toxicity?

NOTE

A vagal nerve stimulator (VNS) is used to treat some patients who have frequent focal onset seizures that are unresponsive to drug therapy. (The device also is used to manage some forms of depression.) The VNS usually is implanted in the left chest; lead wires are fed through the neck and tethered to the vagus nerve (cranial nerve X). The VNS sends electrical impulses regularly to the vagus nerve, causing the widespread release of gamma aminobutyric acid and glycine in the brain. The device also can be activated and deactivated manually by the patient. Although the precise mode of action is unknown, a VNS can be effective in controlling seizures in some patients.

Modified from: Alonso-Vanegas MA. Vagus nerve stimulation for intractable seizures. In: Rocha L, Cavalheiro E, eds. *Pharmacoresistance in Epilepsy*. New York, NY: Springer; 2013.

Differentiation of Syncope and Seizure. Syncope is a complete loss of consciousness caused by a temporary reduction in CBF. Because syncope and seizure have similar presentations, determining whether a patient has experienced a syncopal episode or a seizure can be difficult. The main difference is in the symptoms the patient experiences before and after the event. The factors listed in **TABLE 24-5** may aid differentiation of these two conditions.

TABLE 24-5 Differentiation of Syncope and Seizure

Characteristic	Syncope	Seizure
Position	Syncope usually starts when patient is in a standing position.	Seizure may start with patient in any position.
Warning	Patient usually has a warning period of light-headedness.	Patient has little or no warning.
Level of consciousness	Patient usually regains consciousness immediately on becoming supine; fatigue, confusion, and headache last less than 15 minutes.	Patient may remain unconscious for minutes to hours; fatigue, confusion, and headache last longer than 15 minutes.
Clonic–tonic activity	Clonic movements (if present) are of short duration.	Tonic–clonic movements occur during unconscious state.
Electrocardiographic analysis	Bradycardia is caused by increased vagal tone associated with syncope in some cases.	Tachycardia is caused by muscular exertion associated with seizure activity.

Management

The first step in the management of a patient with seizure activity is to protect the patient from injury. This is best achieved by removing obstacles in the patient's immediate area. If necessary, the patient can be moved to a safe environment, such as a carpeted or soft, grassy area. At no time should a patient with seizure activity be restrained, nor should objects be forced between the patient's teeth to maintain an airway. Restraining activity may harm the patient or paramedic crew. Forcing objects into the oral cavity in an effort to secure an airway or prevent the patient from biting the tongue may evoke vomiting, aspiration, or spasm of the larynx. Placement of a nasopharyngeal airway, along with $ETCO_2$ monitoring should be considered.

Most patients with an isolated seizure can be properly managed in the postictal phase by being placed in a lateral recumbent position. This position allows drainage of oral secretions and aids suctioning (if needed). Supplemental oxygen should be administered via a nonrebreather mask if the patient is hypoxic. When possible, the patient should be moved to a quiet place (away from onlookers) to ensure the patient's privacy. These patients are often embarrassed or self-conscious after a seizure if incontinence has occurred.

All seizure patients should be encouraged to seek care. Some patients should be transported to the ED, including patients who have a history of seizures but who experienced a seizure that is different from the usual one, and patients with a seizure that is complicated by an unusual event (eg, trauma). All patients who have experienced a seizure for the first time should be transported to the ED. Depending on the patient's status and seizure history, an IV line may be necessary to administer drug therapy. However, few patients who experience an isolated seizure require drug therapy in the prehospital setting.

Status Epilepticus

Status epilepticus is defined by the International League Against Epilepsy as a condition resulting either from (1) the failure of the mechanisms responsible for seizure termination or (2) the initiation of mechanisms that lead to continuous tonic–colonic seizures lasting 4 to 5 minutes or longer.[32] Continuous seizure activity that lasts 30 minutes or longer may have long-term consequences, including irreversible brain damage.

Status epilepticus is a serious emergency that requires immediate treatment to stop the seizure activity. In addition to neurologic injury, the condition can lead to pulmonary edema, acidosis, and death. Associated complications of status epilepticus include aspiration and fracture of the long bones and the spine. A common cause of status epilepticus in adults is failure to take prescribed anticonvulsant medications.

Management priorities for patients with status epilepticus include protecting them from injury, securing the airway with oral or nasal adjuncts, and providing supplemental oxygenation and ventilatory support, if needed. All patients with continuous seizures should be transported to a medical facility for physician evaluation. Anticonvulsant medications used to stop the seizure activity include lorazepam or midazolam (intranasal, intramuscular [IM], buccal), or if the others are not available, diazepam (IV).[33] If hypoglycemia is present, dextrose (10%, 25%, or 50%) may be given by slow IV infusion. In patients in the third trimester of pregnancy or immediately postpartum, magnesium sulfate should be considered if eclampsia is the suspected cause of the seizure. While administering these drugs, paramedics should closely

SHOW ME THE EVIDENCE

Researchers compared the effectiveness of IM midazolam to lorazepam to terminate pediatric status epilepticus safely, using a double-blind, randomized noninferiority study. Children seizing for more than 5 minutes were randomized to receive either IM midazolam or IV lorazepam. On arrival in the ED, seizures were absent in 73.4% of the IM midazolam group and in 64% of the IV lorazepam patients (10% absolute difference; 95% confidence interval, 4.0–16.1; $P < 0.001$ for both noninferiority and superiority). Although the seizures stopped more quickly after administration of the IV lorazepam (median 1.6 minutes) versus IM midazolam (3.3 minutes), the time to cessation of the seizure was superior (less) in the midazolam group because there was no delay to establish an IV. Complication rates were not significantly different between the groups. Fewer children in the IM midazolam group were admitted to the hospital ($P = 0.01$). The researchers concluded that IM midazolam is at least as safe and effective as IV lorazepam to stop seizures in the prehospital setting.

Modified from: Silbergleit R, Durkalski V, Lowenstein DH, et al. Intramuscular versus intravenous therapy for status epilepticus. *N Engl J Med*. 2012;366(7):591-600.

monitor the patient's blood pressure and respiratory status, including continuous waveform capnography. They should be prepared for respiratory depression or arrest. If the patient's blood pressure begins to fall or if the respiratory rate or effort decreases or the $ETCO_2$ level rises, paramedics should stop the drug therapy and consult with medical direction.

Headache

Headaches are painful and bothersome. However, most are minor health concerns and are easily managed with analgesics. Headaches are categorized according to their underlying cause. The types of headaches are tension headache, migraine, and sinus headache. Therapies that may be useful in managing these headaches include prescription and over-the-counter medications, herbal remedies, meditation, acupressure, aromatherapy, and others. Headache is an extremely common medical complaint; 14% of American adults report having had a migraine or severe headache within the past 3 months.[34] The pain associated with headaches can arise from the meninges, or from the scalp, its blood vessels, and muscles.

> NOTE
>
> The paramedic should always first consider that a severe headache could be a sign of serious illness. Life-threatening causes of headache include hypertension, stroke, tumor, and toxic exposure (eg, carbon monoxide poisoning), among others. A thorough history and assessment are crucial.

A **tension headache** is caused by muscle contractions of the face, neck, and scalp. This type of headache has a variety of causes, including stress, persistent noise, eyestrain, and poor posture. The pain of tension headaches (usually described as dull, persistent, and nonthrobbing) may last for days or weeks. The pain can cause variable degrees of discomfort. These headaches can be short-lived and infrequent or chronic. Most tension headaches can be managed effectively with over-the-counter analgesics.

A **migraine** is a severe, incapacitating headache. These headaches often are preceded by visual or gastrointestinal (GI) disturbances, or both. They usually begin with an intense, throbbing pain on one side of the head that may spread. They often are accompanied by nausea and vomiting. Complex migraines may be associated with neurologic deficits and can be stroke mimics. The symptoms of migraines are associated with constriction and dilation of blood vessels, which may be brought on by an imbalance of serotonin or hormone fluctuations.[35] Migraines also can be triggered by excessive caffeine use, various foods, changes in altitude, and extremes of emotions. A wide range of medications are prescribed for migraines. These include beta blockers, calcium channel blockers, antidepressants, antiemetics, anticonvulsants, and nonsteroidal anti-inflammatory and serotonin-inhibiting drugs.

A **sinus headache** is characterized by pain in the forehead, nasal area, and eyes. These headaches often produce a feeling of pressure behind the face. Allergies, inflammation, or infection of the membranes lining the sinus cavities usually is responsible for the discomfort. Sinus headaches are managed with medications such as analgesics, decongestants, and potentially antibiotics to treat infection.

Management

Many causes of headaches can be prevented. For example, triggers can be identified, such as irregular meals, prolonged travel, noisy environments, and food additives (in susceptible people). Headaches, such as those described previously, seldom require prehospital emergency care. However, a full history of the headache should be obtained. This history helps identify a more serious cause of the headache, should one be present. For example, the headache may be a sign of an aneurysm or a stroke.

Important assessment findings include the following:

- The patient's general health
- Previous medical conditions
- Medications used
- Previous experience with headaches
- The time course of onset (gradual, sudden)
- Associated symptoms and neurologic findings

After a patient history has been obtained and a neurologic examination has been performed, prehospital care for patients with tension headaches, migraines, and sinus headaches is mainly supportive. Transport of the patient for evaluation by a physician may be indicated. These patients often have light sensitivity. Lights in the ambulance should be dimmed. Antiemetics may be useful for symptom relief. Narcotic medications should be avoided in headache patients because of the risk of more severe rebound headaches (headaches caused by the overuse of pain medications in patients who regularly use them to treat headaches).

Weakness and Fatigue

It is challenging when a patient presents with a chief complaint of weakness or fatigue because there are many potential neurologic and non-neurologic etiologies.[36] In addition, weakness and fatigue may be the result of multiple causes, or a specific cause may not be initially apparent (BOX 24-8). Weakness and fatigue must never be dismissed lightly, because they are of significance to the patient and may represent the first vague warning of disease or a life-threatening illness.

NOTE

Generalized weakness and fatigue has been reported as the fifth most common chief complaint of ED visits among older patients; of those patients, 50% were found to have an acute medical problem. Particularly in the older adult population, it is important to quickly rule out cardiovascular causes of weakness. Atypical presentations, including generalized weakness, may be the only initial sign of an acute coronary syndrome. Other cardiac causes include dysrhythmias.

Modified from: Bhalla MC. Generalized weakness in the elderly. In: Kahn JH, Magauran BG Jr, Olshaker JS, eds. *Geriatric Emergency Medicine: Principles and Practice.* Cambridge, England: Cambridge University Press; 2014:51-58; and Carro A, Kaski JC. Myocardial infarction in the elderly. *Aging Dis.* 2011;2(2):116-137.

BOX 24-8 Possible Causes of Weakness and Fatigue

Cardiac
Acute myocardial infarction
Dysrhythmias

Endocrine/Metabolic
Addison disease
Hyperparathyroidism
Electrolyte imbalance
Thyrotoxicosis
Hypoglycemia
Infection

Nervous System
Stroke
Amyotrophic lateral sclerosis
GBS
MS
Myasthenia gravis
Nerve injury

Muscle Diseases
Muscular dystrophy (Duchenne)

Poisoning
Botulism
Insecticides, nerve gas exposure

Other
Anemia
Psychiatric problems
Medications
Nutritional deficiencies

During the assessment, the paramedic should determine if the weakness is unilateral or generalized, symmetric or asymmetric, and proximal or distal. Unilateral weakness is associated with stroke, intracerebral or subarachnoid hemorrhage, and Todd paralysis (a focal weakness after seizure). When the weakness affects both sides of the body, neurologic causes, such as brainstem stroke and spinal cord diseases caused by inflammation or compression, should be considered. Peripheral nerve diseases causing bilateral weakness include Guillain-Barré syndrome (GBS) and tick paralysis. Neuromuscular diseases, such as myasthenia gravis, can cause weakness in any muscle group.

The paramedic should obtain a history by encouraging the patient to "tell the story" of the problem in an unstructured format and to determine what the patient means by "weakness." For example, if the patient describes the weakness as having shortness of breath and needing to rest while climbing stairs, the initial impression will be quite different than if the patient describes the weakness as "feeling tired all over." A thorough history should include time course of onset, distribution (localized or general), exacerbating and relieving factors, associated signs and symptoms, the setting in which the problem developed, and the impact on daily activities. Identifying the past medical history and current medications may provide essential clues.

The physical examination should include a vital sign assessment and a neuromuscular examination, checking for muscle atrophy, tenderness, and sensory deficits. The physical examination will determine whether there is objective evidence of weakness. Finally, diagnostic assessments are important to rule out treatable causes of weakness, such as hypoglycemia or ST segment elevation myocardial infarction. In many patients, a prehospital diagnosis of the cause of weakness cannot be made. Paramedics must address life threats and transport the patient to an appropriate facility for a more thorough evaluation.

Infections of the CNS

Infections of the CNS can be quite serious and difficult to treat. The most common CNS infections involve meningitis, encephalitis, and brain abscesses. These infections tend to cause more morbidity and mortality than do infections involving other organ systems, especially in people with a weakened immune system.[37] Bacteria and viruses are the most common causes of CNS infections. Viruses that cause CNS infection include herpesviruses, arboviruses, coxsackieviruses, echoviruses, and enteroviruses. Streptococcus and staphylococcus are usually the agents that cause bacterial infections.

Meningitis and Encephalitis

Meningitis is inflammation of the membranes (meninges) surrounding the brain and spinal cord. Myelitis refers to inflammation of the spinal cord. When both the brain and the spinal cord are involved, the condition is called encephalomyelitis. Most cases of meningitis are caused by a viral infection, but bacterial and fungal infections can also be responsible. The swelling from meningitis typically triggers symptoms such as headache, fever, and **nuchal rigidity** (pain with neck flexion). Some cases of meningitis improve without treatment over a period of weeks. Others can be life threatening and require emergent antibiotic intervention. Viral infections are most common (viral or aseptic meningitis). Forms of bacterial meningitis include *Streptococcus pneumoniae* (pneumococcus), *Neisseria meningitidis* (meningococcus), *Haemophilus influenzae* (haemophilus), and *Listeria monocytogenes* (listeria). Some forms of bacterial infections may be associated with kidney and adrenal gland failure and shock.

Encephalitis is inflammation of the brain. Like meningitis, encephalitis results from the same viral or bacterial infections. Other causes of encephalitis can include rabies, fungus, parasites, autoimmune diseases, and certain medications. Most diagnosed cases of encephalitis in the United States are caused by enteroviruses, herpes simplex virus types 1 and 2, rabies virus (this can occur even without a known animal bite, such as exposure to bats), or arboviruses such as West Nile virus, which are transmitted from infected animals to humans through the bite of an infected tick, mosquito, or other blood-sucking insect. Several thousand cases of encephalitis are reported each year, but many more may actually occur because the symptoms may be mild to nonexistent in most patients.[38]

Some forms of bacterial meningitis and encephalitis are contagious and can be spread through contact with saliva, nasal discharge, feces, or respiratory and throat secretions (often spread through kissing, coughing, or sharing drinking glasses, eating utensils, or such personal items as toothbrushes, lipstick, or cigarettes). Meningococcal outbreaks are rare but can occur in communities, schools, colleges, prisons, and other populations. Children who have not been given routine vaccines are at increased risk for the development of certain types of the disease. The Centers for Disease Control and Prevention also recommends meningococcal vaccines for all teens and young adults.[39] Early signs and symptoms of both viral and bacterial meningitis and encephalitis may

> NOTE
>
> Bacterial meningitis is a rare but potentially fatal disease. It can be caused by several types of bacteria that initially cause an upper respiratory tract infection and then travel through the bloodstream to the brain. The disease can also occur when certain bacteria invade the meninges directly (eg, ear or sinus infection, skull fracture). The disease can cause stroke, hearing loss, and permanent brain damage. Approximately 600 to 1,000 people contract the disease in the United States each year. Of these people, 10% to 15% die and one in five will live with permanent disabilities.
>
> *Modified from*: Meningitis and encephalitis fact sheet. National Institute of Neurological Disorders and Stroke website. https://www.ninds.nih.gov/Disorders/Patient-Caregiver-Education/Fact-Sheets/Meningitis-and-Encephalitis-Fact-Sheet. Accessed March 26, 2018; Statistics and disease facts. National Meningitis Association website. http://www.nmaus.org/disease-prevention-information/statistics-and-disease-facts/. Accessed March 26, 2018.

mimic influenza and can develop over 1 to 2 days. Possible signs and symptoms include the following:

- Sudden high fever
- Nuchal rigidity
- Severe headache that seems different than normal
- Headache with nausea or vomiting
- Confusion, disorientation
- Seizures
- Sleepiness or difficulty waking
- Sensitivity to light
- No appetite or thirst
- Skin rash (with meningococcal meningitis)

Important signs of meningitis or encephalitis in infants include fever, lethargy, not waking for feeding, vomiting, body stiffness, unexplained or unusual irritability, and a full or bulging fontanel. Infants with meningitis may be difficult to comfort and may even cry harder when held.

Prehospital care for these patients is mainly supportive. Most will need physician evaluation for appropriate care and follow-up. As a safety measure to prevent exposure to a contagious form of the disease, the EMS crew and the patient should wear masks, and the crew should employ standard precautions. (See Chapter 27, *Infectious and Communicable Diseases.*)

Brain Abscess

A **brain abscess** is an accumulation of purulent material (pus) surrounded by a capsule within the brain. It develops from a bacterial infection that often begins in the nasal cavity, middle ear, teeth, or mastoid cells. The condition also may develop after surgery or penetrating cranial trauma, especially when bone fragments are retained in cranial tissue. Clinical manifestations of a brain abscess are often nonspecific and may be associated with intracranial infection (eg, fever). They also are associated with an expanding intracranial mass (eg, nausea, vomiting, seizures, changes in mental status). Headache is the most common early symptom. Removal of fluid from the abscess or excision, accompanied by antibiotic therapy, generally is recommended to manage this disorder. The incidence of brain abscess is about 1 per 100,000 hospital admissions. The condition is twice as common in males as in females. The mean age for abscess formation ranges from 24 to 57 years.[40]

CNS Tumors

CNS tumors include **brain tumors** and **spinal cord tumors**. The incidence of these tumors tends to increase up to age 70 years and then decrease. CNS tumors are the second most common group of tumors in children and the most common solid organ tumors in pediatric patients.[41]

A brain tumor, or **neoplasm**, is a mass in the cranial cavity. This mass may be either malignant or benign. Heredity may play a role in the development of brain tumors. They also are associated with several risk factors, including exposure to radiation, tobacco use, dietary habits, some viruses, and the use of some medications. The effects of the tumor depend on its size, location, and growth rate and whether any evidence of hemorrhage or edema exists. Brain tumors may cause local and generalized manifestations. Local effects are caused by the destructive action of the tumor on a particular site in the brain and by compression, which reduces CBF (**FIGURE 24-17**). These effects are varied and may include the following:[42]

- Headache (approximately 50%)
- Seizures
- Weakness
- Sensory loss
- Visual disturbances
- Aphasia
- Cognitive dysfunction
- Vomiting (often triggered by sudden position change)

Lesions inside the cranial vault produce pain by distending or stretching the arteries and other pain-sensitive structures of the head and neck. Headache may be present but often is a late finding in the absence of hemorrhage, which may cause a sudden onset of pain.[3] The main treatment for a cerebral tumor is surgical or radiosurgical excision. Surgical decompression may be used if total excision is not possible. Chemotherapy and radiation also may be used to decrease mass size.

Like the brain, the spinal cord can become compressed. In the absence of trauma, compression of the spinal cord can be caused by bone, blood, abscesses, tumors, or a ruptured disk. (Compression of the spinal cord that results from trauma and associated spinal cord syndromes is discussed in Chapter 40, *Spine and Nervous System Trauma.*) Compression of the cord can disrupt normal functions because of pressure on

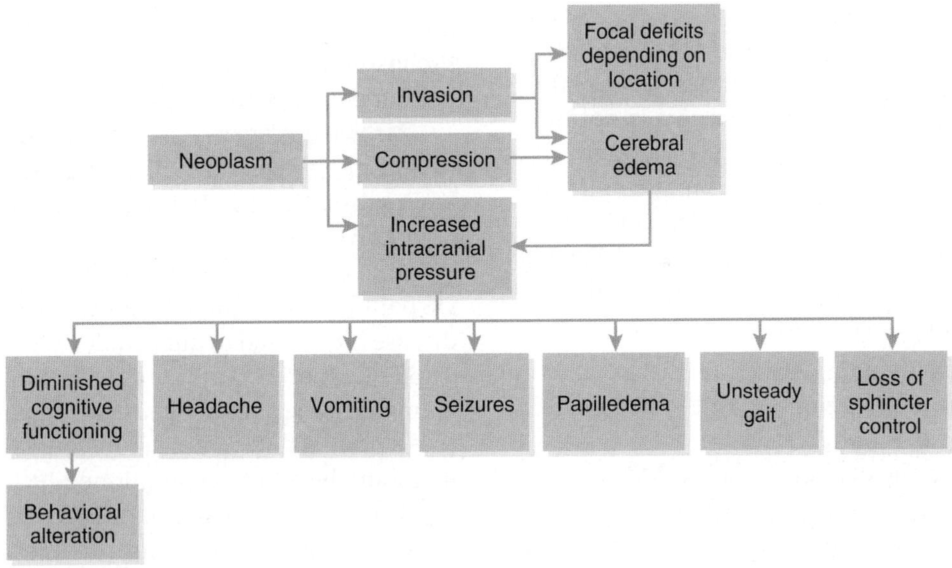

FIGURE 24-17 Origin of signs and symptoms associated with an intracranial neoplasm.

© Jones & Bartlett Learning.

the roots of spinal nerves. Spinal cord compression can occur suddenly, causing immediate symptoms. It also may occur gradually, over weeks to months. Slight compression may cause mild symptoms, such as back pain (that may or may not radiate to the leg or foot), slight muscle weakness, and tingling in the extremities. In men, difficulty urinating, urinary retention, and erectile dysfunction may occur. If the cause of compression is cancer, an abscess, or a hematoma, the back may be tender to the touch in the affected area. Significant compression of the cord may block nerve impulses, which can result in severe muscle weakness, numbness, retention of urine, and loss of bladder and bowel control. If all nerve impulses are blocked, paralysis and complete loss of sensation may result. Definitive care is determined by the cause of the compression. Treatment by a physician will depend on the cause of the cord compression, and in some cases surgery may be required to relieve the compression and prevent permanent nerve damage.

Management

Prehospital care of a patient with a CNS tumor may range from providing comfort and emotional support during patient transport to managing seizure activity and providing airway, ventilatory, and circulatory resuscitation. If the patient's condition permits, a focused history should be obtained and a neurologic evaluation should be performed. Elements of the focused history for these patients should include the following:

- Past significant medical history (eg, surgical removal of a tumor, radiation therapy)
- History and description of any headache
- Dizziness or loss of consciousness
- Seizure activity
- GI disturbances (vomiting, diarrhea)
- New onset of incoordination, difficulty walking or maintaining balance
- Behavioral or cognitive changes
- Weakness or paralysis
- Vision disturbances

> **NOTE**
>
> Spinal epidural abscess is suspected in patients with a recent history of spinal surgery or epidural catheter placement, or in patients who are diabetic or IV drug users. Patients often present with back pain, fever, and progressive neurologic deficit. If untreated, this condition can lead to significant disability with permanent weakness or paraplegia.
>
> ---
>
> *Modified from:* Davis DP, Wold RM, Patel RJ, et al. The clinical presentation and impact of diagnostic delays on emergency department patients with spinal epidural abscess. *J Emerg Med.* 2004;26(3):285-291.

Other Neurologic Diseases

There are many other neurologic diseases. The pathophysiology of many of these disorders is not fully understood. Some diseases may involve Schwann cells, the CSF, or axons of the CNS. Others may result from circulatory and immunologic disorders and exposure to bacterial toxins and chemicals. The following specific neurologic diseases and categories of disease are discussed in this chapter:[33]

- Dementia, including Alzheimer disease
- Huntington disease
- Muscular dystrophy
- Demyelinating disorders, such as MS
- Peripheral neuropathies, such as GBS
- Movement disorders, such as Parkinson disease and dystonia
- Cranial nerve disorders, including Bell palsy
- Motor neuron disorders, such as amyotrophic lateral sclerosis

Dementia

Dementia is a slow, progressive loss of awareness of time and place. It usually involves an inability to learn new things or recall recent events. It often is a result of brain disease caused by strokes, genetic or viral factors, and Alzheimer disease. Dementia generally is considered irreversible. It eventually results in full dependence on others because of progressive loss of cognitive functioning. During the course of the disease, patients often try to conceal their memory loss by **confabulation** (inventing stories to fill gaps in memory). Sudden outbursts or embarrassing conduct may be the first obvious signs of dementia. Some patients eventually regress to a "second childhood." At that point, they need full-time care for feeding, toileting, and physical activity. About 50% of nursing home residents have dementia. Between the years 2000 and 2013, death rates from dementia increased 21% for men and 31% for women older than 75 years.[43] Prehospital care is primarily supportive unless the patient becomes severely agitated.

Alzheimer disease is a type of dementia condition in which nerve cells in the cerebral cortex die and the brain substance shrinks. The disease is the single most common cause of dementia and is the sixth-leading cause of death in the United States.[44] Because the US population is aging, the prevalence of Alzheimer disease is expected to quadruple by 2050. More than 5 million Americans are living with the disease.[45] Alzheimer disease does not cause death directly; rather, these patients ultimately stop eating and become malnourished and deconditioned (BOX 24-9).

The cause of Alzheimer disease is not known. Possible causes include abnormalities in glutamate metabolism, chronic infection, toxic poisoning by metals, reduction in brain chemicals (eg, acetylcholine), and genetics. Early symptoms of Alzheimer disease mainly are related to memory loss, especially the ability to make and recall new memories. As the disease progresses, agitation, violence, and impairment of abstract thinking occur. Judgment and cognitive disabilities begin to interfere with work and social relations. In the advanced stages of Alzheimer disease,

NOTE

Any patient with new onset of altered mental status (eg, confusion, lethargy) should be assessed for organic causes of these symptoms, including infections. Infections that irritate and inflame the membranes of the CNS can cause neurologic disorders, such as encephalitis and meningitis. These diseases are presented in Chapter 27, *Infectious and Communicable Diseases*.

BOX 24-9 Early Signs and Symptoms of Alzheimer Disease

1. Memory loss that disrupts daily life
2. Challenges in planning or solving problems
3. Difficulty completing familiar tasks at home, work, or leisure
4. Confusion with events, time, or place
5. Difficulty understanding visual imagery or spatial relationships
6. New problems with words in speaking or writing
7. Misplacing things and losing the ability to retrace steps
8. Diminished or poor judgment
9. Unfounded suspicions about family, friends, caregivers
10. Withdrawal from work or social activities
11. Changes in mood or personality
12. Difficulty speaking, swallowing, or walking

Modified from: Ten early signs and symptoms of Alzheimer's. Alzheimer's Association website. https://www.alz.org/10-signs-symptoms-alzheimers-dementia.asp. Accessed March 26, 2018.

patients often become bedridden and totally unaware of their surroundings. Once the patient is bedridden, bedsores, feeding problems, and pneumonia shorten the person's life. Currently Alzheimer disease has no cure. Treatment consists mainly of medications to help slow the progression of the disease and nursing and social care for the patient and relatives.

Dementia is also considered a symptom of Parkinson disease, which is discussed later in this chapter.

Huntington Disease

Huntington disease (HD) (also known as Huntington chorea) results from genetically programmed degeneration of neurons in the brain. This degeneration causes uncontrolled movements, loss of intellectual faculties, and emotional disturbance. HD is a rare, inherited disease that is passed from parent to child.[46] Early symptoms of HD are mood swings, depression, irritability, memory loss, and inability to make decisions. As the disease progresses, concentration on intellectual and personal tasks becomes increasingly difficult. Patients may become unable to feed themselves or swallow food or water. The rate of disease progression and the age of onset vary from person to person. A number of medications are used to manage the symptoms of HD, but the course of the disease cannot be altered. Prehospital care is primarily supportive.

NOTE

Approximately 30,000 Americans have HD, and each child of a parent with HD has a 50% chance of inheriting the HD gene. If a child does not inherit the HD gene, there is no risk for development of the disease and it cannot be passed to subsequent generations. The disease will develop in a person who inherits the HD gene. Genetic counseling and testing are available for people who carry the gene.

Modified from: Life with Huntington's disease. Huntington's Disease Foundation website. http://www.huntingtonsdiseasefoundation.org/life-with-hd-1. Accessed March 26, 2018.

Muscular Dystrophy

Muscular dystrophy is an inherited muscle disorder. The disease is marked by a slow but progressive degeneration of muscle fibers. Different forms of the disease are classified by the age at which the symptoms appear, the rate at which the disease progresses, and the way in which it is inherited. Duchenne muscular dystrophy is the most common type. It is caused by an absence of dystrophin, a protein that helps keep muscle cells intact. The disease affects about 1 in 7,250 male children.[47] It is inherited through a recessive sex-linked gene; therefore, only males are affected, and only females can pass on the disease.

Muscular dystrophy often is first diagnosed by the child's physician, who notices that the child is slow in learning to sit up and walk. The disease is confirmed through blood tests that reveal high levels of enzymes released from damaged muscle cells, through nerve conduction studies, and sometimes with muscle biopsy. Muscular dystrophy rarely is diagnosed before age 3 years. As the disease progresses, the child tends to walk with a waddle and has difficulty climbing stairs. Muscles (especially those in the calves) become bulky as wasted muscle is replaced by fat. By about age 12 years, affected children are no longer able to walk. In 2007, just over one-half of patients with muscular dystrophy lived into their 20s; however, it is now more common to survive into their 30s.[48] Death usually results from pulmonary infections and heart failure.

CRITICAL THINKING

How can you determine a child's baseline level of functioning?

No effective treatment exists for muscular dystrophy. Parents or siblings of an affected child should receive genetic counseling. Some types of muscular dystrophy can be diagnosed before birth through blood analysis and amniocentesis (testing of amniotic fluid).

Demyelinating Disorders

Demyelinating disorders have in common the degeneration and destruction of the myelin sheaths on nerve fibers in the CNS. The loss of myelin prevents orderly and rapid conduction of nerve impulses, while other elements of nervous tissue are largely spared. The most important of this group of progressive diseases is **multiple sclerosis (MS)**. (Other demyelinating disorders can be found in BOX 24-10.) Although the etiology is not clear, MS is thought to be an autoimmune disease in which the body's defense system begins to treat the myelin in the CNS

BOX 24-10 Other Demyelinating Disorders

- **Neuromyelitis optica (Devic disease).** A genetic condition consisting of the simultaneous inflammation and demyelination of the optic nerve (optic neuritis) and the spinal cord (myelitis, progressive necrotic myelopathy).
- **Acute disseminated encephalomyelitis.** An immune-mediated inflammatory demyelinating condition that predominately affects the white matter of the brain and spinal cord; often manifests as acute hemorrhagic encephalitis (Weston-Hurst syndrome).
- **Demyelination in association with autoimmune disease** (systemic lupus, Sjögren disease, and related conditions) that affects the entire body.
- **Sarcoid-related demyelination.** Destruction of the myelin sheaths or nerve fibers related to multisystem inflammation in which granulomas, or clumps of inflammatory cells, form in various organs (sarcoidosis).
- **Graft-versus-host disease.** A complication of bone marrow transplants in which T cells in the donor bone marrow graft attack the recipient's tissues.

as foreign, gradually destroying it (demyelination), causing scarring and nerve fiber damage.

MS is the most common acquired disease of the nervous system in young adults, affecting an estimated 2.3 million people worldwide.[49] The ratio of women to men affected is 3:2.[50] The symptoms, which may be active briefly in early adult life and resume years later, vary according to the parts of the brain and spinal cord affected. MS lesions are primarily in the white matter of the brain, either in multiple small foci or in several large foci. Symptoms may be subtle and variable early in the course of the disease and range from numbness and tingling to paralysis and incontinence that may last several weeks to several months during disease flares. Damage to the white matter in the brain may lead to fatigue, vertigo, clumsiness, unsteady gait, slurred speech, blurred or double vision, incontinence, and facial numbness or pain. In most cases, it begins with a relapsing–remitting pattern, with symptom-free periods between MS flares. Other people follow a progressive course and become increasingly disabled from the first attack and are severely debilitated from that point on (BOX 24-11).

The diagnosis of MS is based on clinical criteria and magnetic resonance imaging findings consistent with MS. Patients are managed with medications (eg, corticosteroids, immune-modulating medications) that help control the symptoms of an acute episode and prevent exacerbation. The disease also is managed with physical therapy to help maintain mobility and independence. Currently, no cure exists.

BOX 24-11 Types of MS[a]

- **Clinically isolated syndrome (CIS).** The first episode of neurologic symptoms that last for at least 24 hours; MS may or may not develop in the patient.
- **Relapsing–remitting MS (RRMS).** The most common disease course, characterized by clearly defined acute or subacute attacks of new or increasing neurologic symptoms, followed by periods of partial or complete recovery (remissions).
- **Primary progressive MS (PPMS).** Characterized by worsening neurologic function (accumulation of disability) from the onset of symptoms, without early relapses or remissions.
- **Secondary progressive MS (SPMS).** May follow PPMS in some patients; associated with progressive worsening of neurologic function over time, without signs of remission.

[a]There are variants of MS that are considered borderline MS diseases. These variants include tumefactive MS, Marburg variant, Balo concentric sclerosis, myelinoclastic diffuse sclerosis (Schilder disease), and neuromyelitis optica spectrum disorders. Discriminating these disorders is not always possible at first presentation, but treatment of the acute episode should not be delayed.

Modified from: Types of MS. National Multiple Sclerosis Society website. https://www.nationalmssociety.org/What-is-MS/Types-of-MS. Accessed March 26, 2018; Rahmlow MR, Kantarci O. Fulminant demyelinating diseases. *The Neurohospitalist*. 2013;3(2):81-91.

CRITICAL THINKING

Consider the patient who has been receiving long-term steroid therapy. This person is at risk for what conditions?

Peripheral Neuropathies

As the name implies, **peripheral neuropathy** refers to diseases and disorders that affect the PNS, including the spinal nerve roots, cranial nerves, and peripheral nerves. Most neuropathies arise from damage to or irritation of either the axons or their myelin sheaths. This damage slows or fully blocks the passage of electrical signals. The various types of peripheral neuropathy are classified according to the site and distribution of damage. For example, damage to sensory nerve fibers may cause numbness and tingling, sensations of cold, or pain that often starts in the hands and feet and spreads toward the central body. Damage to motor nerve fibers may cause muscle weakness and muscle wasting. Damage to the nerves of the autonomic nervous system may result in blurred vision, impaired or absent sweating, fluctuations in blood pressure (and associated syncope), GI disorders, incontinence, and impotence.

Some peripheral neuropathies have no identifiable cause. Others may be related to specific causes, including the following:

- Diabetes mellitus
- Dietary deficiencies (especially of the B vitamins)
- Alcoholism
- Uremia
- Lead poisoning
- Drug intoxication
- Viral infection (eg, post-herpetic infection, GBS)
- Rheumatoid arthritis
- Peripheral vascular disease
- Systemic lupus erythematosus
- Malignant tumors (eg, lung cancer)
- Lymphomas
- Leukemias
- Inherited neuropathies (eg, peroneal muscular atrophy)

When possible, management is aimed at the underlying cause (eg, blood glucose control in a patient with diabetes, improved nutrition). If management is successful and the cell bodies of the damaged nerves have not been destroyed, full recovery from the neuropathy is possible.[51]

Guillain-Barré syndrome (GBS) is also an acute or subacute type of progressive polyneuropathy affecting the PNS, likely with an autoimmune component. The disease afflicts about 1 person in 100,000 and can strike at any age.[52] Initial symptoms of the syndrome include prominent weakness with some sensory changes, beginning in the legs and possibly spreading to the arms and upper body. These symptoms can increase in intensity until the muscles can no longer be used, causing total or near-total paralysis, which is clearly life threatening. Patients often require mechanical ventilation to breathe. However, most patients recover from GBS, although some have persistent weakness.

Usually GBS occurs a few days or weeks after the patient has had symptoms of a respiratory or GI viral infection.[52] Occasionally, surgery and very rarely vaccination increase the risk of the syndrome. Recently several cases were found following Zika virus infection.[53] The disorder can develop over the course of hours or days, or it may take up to 3 to 4 weeks. The syndrome is managed by supporting the patient's vital functions. Some patients are treated with plasmapheresis (the removal and replacement of plasma fluids) and high-dose immunoglobulin therapy.

Movement Disorders

The term **dystonia** refers to local or diffuse changes in muscle tone (usually abnormal muscle rigidity) that affects up to 250,000 men, women, and children in the United States each year.[54] These changes cause painful muscle spasms, unusually fixed postures, and strange movement patterns. Localized dystonia may result from torticollis (a painful neck spasm) or scoliosis (an abnormal curvature of the spine). More generalized dystonia results from various neurologic disorders, including Parkinson disease and stroke. It also may be a feature of schizophrenia or a side effect of some antipsychotic drugs. Specific types of dystonia may be managed with medications such as benztropine or diphenhydramine, which help reverse the symptoms.

Parkinson disease is caused by degeneration of nerve cells in the basal ganglia in the brain or damage of unknown origin to those cells. The degeneration causes a lack of dopamine, which prevents the basal ganglia from modifying nerve pathways that control muscle contraction. The result is muscles that are overly tense, causing tremor, joint rigidity, and slow movement. Parkinson disease affects about one million people, and 60,000 new cases are diagnosed in the United States each year.[55] Left untreated, the disease progresses over 10 to 15 years to severe weakness and incapacity. Parkinson disease is the leading cause of neurologic disability in people older than 60 years.

Parkinson disease usually begins as a slight tremor in one hand, arm, or leg. In the early stages, the tremor is worse while the limb is at rest. In the later stages, the disease affects both sides of the body. It causes stiffness, weakness, and trembling of the muscles. Other symptoms include an unusual walking pattern (shuffling) that may break into uncontrollable, tiny running steps; constant trembling of the hands, sometimes accompanied by shaking of the head; a permanent rigid stoop; and an unblinking, fixed facial expression. Speech becomes slow and hesitant as the muscle dysfunction worsens. Balance deteriorates over time in these patients, increasing their risk for falls and serious injury. As Parkinson disease progresses, patients have increasing difficulty swallowing, which can lead to foreign body airway obstruction or aspiration. Aspiration of food or liquids into the lungs may lead to pneumonia. Late in the disease, intellect may be affected and dementia can be a feature of the disease.

At first, Parkinson disease is managed with counseling, exercise, and special assistive aids in the home. As the disease progresses, management may include various combinations of drugs that either mimic or replace dopamine (eg, levodopa and carbidopa). These drugs provide relief from specific symptoms but can cause significant dyskinesias and other side effects. Other management measures may include deep brain stimulation to block electrical signals from affected areas of the brain or brain surgery to reduce tremor and rigidity if medication therapy fails.

NOTE

Normal pressure hydrocephalus (NPH) is a syndrome that affects some older adults. It is caused by an abnormal increase in CSF in the ventricles of the brain. It may result from a subarachnoid hemorrhage, head trauma, infection, tumor, or complications of surgery. Often the cause is unknown. NPH can resemble Parkinson disease, Alzheimer disease, and other degenerative neurologic diseases. Patients may present with a gait disorder, psychomotor slowing, incontinence, progressive dementia, and memory loss. NPH is diagnosed with a computed tomography scan or magnetic resonance imaging studies, or both. The disease is treated by surgical placement of a shunt in the brain to drain excess CSF.

Modified from: Normal Pressure Hydrocephalus Information Page. National Institute of Neurological Disorders and Stroke website. https://www.ninds.nih.gov/disorders/all-disorders/normal-pressure-hydrocephalus-information-page. Updated May 24, 2017. Accessed May 16, 2018.

Cranial Nerve Disorders

Cranial nerve disorders can affect the connections between cranial nerve centers in the brain. These disorders may lead to dysfunction of smell, vision, facial sensation or expression, taste, hearing, and balance, among others. Cranial nerve disorders discussed in this section include trigeminal neuralgia, **glossopharyngeal neuralgia**, and hemifacial spasm. Because the cause of the cranial nerve disorders often is unclear, management sometimes is difficult. Treatment includes drugs to inhibit nerve impulses and sometimes surgery if the cause is a tumor or lesion. Prehospital care for patients with cranial nerve disorders is primarily supportive.

Trigeminal neuralgia refers to infection or disease of the trigeminal nerve (cranial nerve V). Patients with trigeminal neuralgia report paroxysmal episodes of excruciating pain (often described as recurrent bursts of an electric shock) that affect the cheek, lips, gums, or chin on one side of the face. The episode usually is very brief, lasting only a few seconds to minutes, but it may be so intense that the person is unable to function during the attack. The pain of trigeminal neuralgia usually begins from a trigger point on the face. It can be brought on by touching, washing, shaving, eating, drinking, or talking. Trigeminal neuralgia is unusual in people younger than 50 years but may be associated with MS in younger people. Attacks occur in bouts that may last weeks at a time. Treatment typically begins with carbamazepine.

Hemifacial spasm is a neuromuscular disorder characterized by frequent involuntary contractions of the muscles on one side of the face. It most often is caused by a blood vessel that presses on the facial nerve (cranial nerve VII), but it also can be caused by an injury or a tumor. The disorder occurs in both men and women, although it more frequently affects middle aged or older women. The first symptom usually is an intermittent twitching of the eyelid muscle that can lead to forced closure of the eye. The spasm may then gradually spread to involve the muscles of the lower face, which may cause the mouth to be pulled to one side. Eventually the spasms involve all the muscles on one side of the face almost continuously.

Bell palsy (facial palsy) is a unilateral paralysis of the facial muscles caused by inflammation of the facial nerve (cranial nerve VII) (**FIGURE 24-18**). It usually is one-sided and temporary. It often develops suddenly. Bell palsy is the most common cause of facial paralysis; it affects 1 in 60 people in a lifetime.[56] The cause of the inflammation is unclear. However, it has been associated with many past or present infectious processes, including Lyme disease, herpes viruses, mumps, and infection with the human immunodeficiency virus (HIV). Stroke should also be part of the paramedic's differential diagnosis. When

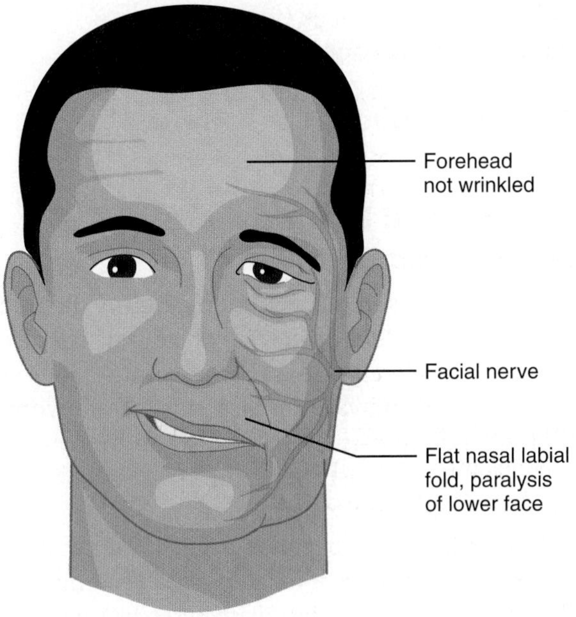

FIGURE 24-18 Bell palsy.

weakness and droop are evident in only the lower face, a central cause, such as stroke, is more likely. In contrast, when all the muscles (including those of the forehead) are affected on one side of the face, the entire facial (peripheral) nerve is likely affected, indicating Bell palsy (BOX 24-12).

CRITICAL THINKING

In the field, should you diagnose and release a patient who has Bell palsy?

Bell palsy usually causes the eyelid and corner of the mouth to droop on one side of the face. It sometimes is associated with numbness and pain. Depending on which branches of the nerve are affected, taste may be impaired, or sounds may seem oddly loud. Management may involve the use of antiviral and anti-inflammatory drugs to reduce inflammation of the nerve, along with analgesics. Recovery usually is complete within 2 weeks to 2 months. A key component of therapy is to protect the affected eye from corneal drying and injury that may result because the paralysis prevents the eyelid from closing. These conditions are best prevented by using lubricating ointments and eye patches.

BOX 24-12 Bell Palsy or Stroke?

To determine if the patient's facial weakness is more likely an indication of Bell palsy or of stroke, the paramedic should first assess the following:

- How fast did the signs and symptoms appear? Stroke is more likely to present within minutes, whereas the signs and symptoms of Bell palsy may develop in hours or days.
- What is the patient's neurologic status?
  - Inspect the mouth. See if the nasolabial fold is still evident or has disappeared. (Bell palsy causes flattening or loss of the nasolabial fold.) Have the patient smile, and look for asymmetry.
  - Inspect the eyes. Look at the space between them (the palpebral fissure) to see whether one eye is open more widely than the other. Then have the patient close his or her eyes tightly until the eyelashes are no longer visible. If one eye does not completely close, suspect facial nerve palsy.
  - Ask the patient to wrinkle the forehead or raise the eyebrows as if he or she were surprised. If the problem is within the brain, the forehead will wrinkle equally on both sides. If the problem is with the peripheral nerves, the affected side will be flaccid or have fewer wrinkles.
- Are any other neurologic signs present? If the patient fails any other element of the neurologic examination (CPSS, slurred speech, double vision, difficulty swallowing, ataxia, vertigo, or other tests), suspect stroke or other neurologic emergency.

Modified from: Loomis C, Mullen MT. Differentiating facial weakness caused by Bell's palsy vs. acute stroke. *JEMS* website. http://www.jems.com/articles/print/volume-39/issue-5/features/differentiating-facial-weakness-caused-b.html?c=1. Published May 7, 2014. Accessed March 26, 2018.

Motor Neuron Diseases

Amyotrophic lateral sclerosis (ALS), also called Lou Gehrig disease, is one of a group of rare disorders known as motor neuron diseases. In these disorders, the nerves that control muscular activity degenerate in the brain and spinal cord. ALS usually affects people older than 50 years and is more common in men than in women. Approximately 6,000 people in the United States are diagnosed with ALS each year, and more than 20,000 Americans have the disease at any given time.[57] About 10% of ALS cases are familial.

Motor neuron diseases may involve deterioration of both the upper and the lower neuron tracts. When only muscles of the tongue, jaw, face, and larynx are involved, the term progressive bulbar palsy is used. When only corticospinal processes are affected, the term primary lateral sclerosis is used. When only lower motor neurons are affected, the term progressive late-onset spinal muscular atrophy is used. The term ALS is used for neuron signs that predominate in the extremities and trunk.

Patients with ALS often first notice weakness in the hands and arms. This symptom is accompanied by involuntary quivering (fasciculations). The disease progresses to involve the muscles of all four extremities and those involved in respiration and swallowing. In the final stages of the disease, patients often are unable to speak, swallow, or move. However, awareness and intellect are maintained. Death usually occurs 2 to 4 years after the diagnosis because of involvement of the respiratory muscles, aspiration pneumonia, and general inanition (starvation, failure to thrive). In some cases, life can be prolonged through the use of feeding tubes and ventilators. Care generally is aimed at airway support when needed and providing emotional support and easing discomfort.

CRITICAL THINKING

Why is there a tendency to treat patients with amyotrophic lateral sclerosis as if they have impaired intelligence?

Differential Diagnosis of Neurologic Disorders

The key process in differentiating among the many neurologic disorders is first to consider which disorders are most likely and most dangerous. Signs and symptoms of the various disorders often overlap, making a diagnosis difficult. Also, in many cases, little correlation exists between a patient's pain and the seriousness of the condition.

The differential diagnosis begins with a thorough patient history and a detailed physical examination. This assessment, combined with personal experience, can help the paramedic identify signs and symptoms of the primary illness.

Summary

- The body's ability to maintain a state of balance (homeostasis) results from the nervous system's regulatory and coordinating activities. The vertebral arteries and the internal carotid arteries supply blood to the brain.
- Neurologic emergencies may be related to structural changes or damage, circulatory changes, or alterations in intracranial pressure (ICP) that affect cerebral blood flow (CBF).
- CBF depends on the cerebral perfusion pressure (CPP). The CPP decreases when the mean arterial pressure (MAP) drops or when the ICP rises (CPP = MAP − ICP).
- The primary survey begins by determining the patient's level of consciousness and by ensuring an open and patent airway. Key elements of the physical examination that may provide clues to the nature of the neurologic emergency include the patient history, the history of the event, vital signs, and respiratory patterns.
- The neurologic examination may include assessment of AVPU (Awake and alert, responsive to Verbal stimuli, responsive to Pain, Unresponsive), the Glasgow Coma Scale score, posturing or paralysis, reflexes, pupil size and response, and extraocular movements.
- Coma is an abnormally deep state of unconsciousness. The patient cannot be aroused from this state by external stimuli. In general, two mechanisms produce coma: structural lesions and toxic/metabolic states.
- Stroke is a sudden interruption in blood flow to the brain that results in a neurologic deficit. Strokes can be classified as ischemic strokes or hemorrhagic strokes. A stroke scale is used to assess for the presence of stroke. Rapid transport to a stroke resource center (if available) is indicated.
- A seizure is a brief alteration in behavior or consciousness. It is caused by abnormal electrical activity of one or more groups of neurons in the brain. In the prehospital setting, determining the cause of a seizure is not as important as other measures, including managing the complications and recognizing whether the seizure is reversible with therapy (eg, it is caused by hypoglycemia).
- The most common types of headaches are tension headaches, migraines, and sinus headaches.
- A CNS tumor, or neoplasm, is a mass in the cranial cavity or spinal cord. This mass can be either malignant or benign. Heredity may play a role in the development of brain tumors. They also are associated with several risk factors, including exposure to radiation, tobacco use, dietary habits, some viruses, and the use of some medications.
- A brain abscess is a buildup of purulent material (pus) surrounded by a capsule within the brain. It develops from a bacterial infection. The infection often starts in the nasal cavity, middle ear, or mastoid bone.
- Dementia is a slow, progressive loss of awareness of time and place. Alzheimer disease is the most common cause of dementia.
- Huntington disease causes degeneration of neurons in the brain. This condition causes uncontrolled movements and intellectual and emotional impairment.

- Muscular dystrophy is an inherited muscle disorder. The cause is unknown. The disease is marked by a slow but progressive degeneration of muscle fibers.
- Damage to the white matter of the brain in multiple sclerosis may lead to fatigue, vertigo, clumsiness, unsteady gait, slurred speech, blurred or double vision, and facial numbness or pain.
- Guillain-Barré syndrome is an autoimmune polyneuropathy. It causes lower extremity muscle weakness, which can ascend to full paralysis that may include the muscles of respiration.
- The term *dystonia* refers to local or diffuse changes in muscle tone. These changes may cause painful muscle spasms, unusually fixed postures, and strange movement patterns.
- Parkinson disease is a type of movement disorder with dementia as a feature. It usually begins as a slight tremor in one hand, arm, or leg. In the later stages, the disease affects both sides of the body, causing stiffness, weakness, and trembling of the muscles with a characteristic flat facial expression.
- The term *trigeminal neuralgia* refers to infection or disease of the trigeminal nerve. This condition causes intense pain of the face.
- Hemifacial spasm results in involuntary contractions of muscles on one side of the face.
- Peripheral neuropathies usually arise from damage to or irritation of either the axons or their myelin sheaths. This damage slows or fully blocks the passage of electrical signals.
- Bell palsy is paralysis of the facial muscles. It is caused by inflammation of the facial nerve (cranial nerve VII). The condition usually is one-sided and temporary. It often develops suddenly.
- Amyotrophic lateral sclerosis is also called Lou Gehrig disease. It is one of a group of rare nervous system disorders of the motor neurons. In these disorders, the nerves that control muscular activity degenerate in the brain and spinal cord.

References

1. Magistretti P, Pellerin L, Martin JL. Brain energy metabolism: an integrated cellular perspective. In: Bloom FE, Kupfer DJ, eds. *Psychopharmacology: The Fourth Generation of Progress.* New York, NY: Raven Press; 1995:657-670.
2. Smith ER, Amin-Hanjani S. Evaluation and management of elevated intracranial pressure. UpToDate website. https://www.uptodate.com/contents/evaluation-and-management-of-elevated-intracranial-pressure-in-adults. Updated June 21, 2017. Accessed March 27, 2018.
3. National Association of Emergency Technicians. *PHTLS: Prehospital Trauma Life Support*. 8th ed. Burlington, MA: Jones & Bartlett Learning; 2014.
4. Bader K, ed. *AANN Core Curriculum for Neuroscience Nursing*. 6th ed. Chicago, IL: American Association of Neuroscience Nurses; 2016.
5. Brazis PW, Masdeu JC. *Localization in Clinical Neurology*. 6th ed. Philadelphia, PA: Wolters Kluwer, Lippincott Williams & Wilkins; 2011.
6. Mahdi Z, Kumar A, Kumar TA, Bhattacharya P, Madhavan R. Gaze deviation and acute stroke care strategies. *Neurology* website. http://n.neurology.org/content/86/16_Supplement/I6.001.short. Published April 4, 2016. Accessed March 27, 2018.
7. National Center for Chronic Disease Prevention and Health Promotion, Division for Heart Disease and Stroke Prevention. Stroke facts. Centers for Disease Control and Prevention website. https://www.cdc.gov/stroke/facts.htm. Updated September 6, 2017. Accessed March 25, 2018.
8. Stroke risks. American Stroke Association website. http://www.strokeassociation.org/STROKEORG/AboutStroke/UnderstandingRisk/Understanding-Stroke-Risk_UCM_308539_SubHomePage.jsp. Accessed March 27, 2018.
9. Grotta JC, Albers GW, Broderick JP, et al. *Stroke: Pathophysiology, Diagnosis, and Management.* 6th ed. New York, NY: Elsevier; 2016.
10. Jauch EC. Ischemic stroke clinical presentation. Medscape website. https://emedicine.medscape.com/article/1916852-clinical?pa=GUiOzIRVPS7%2BOpibj9rMoVNgHEq7rF%2BpN%2FuyexPZaYzTddREJA2YdYwvtgNBulZ%2B%2F%2BDiMdbwX%2FCudkoN5FTRmXum7wC6L3C41M8%2BukeCQMU%3D. Updated February 15, 2018. Accessed March 27, 2018.
11. Lima FO, Furie KL, Silva GS, et al. Prognosis of untreated strokes due to anterior circulation proximal intracranial arterial occlusions detected by use of computed tomography angiography. *JAMA Neurol.* 2014;71(2):151-157.
12. Facts about Joint Commission stroke certification. The Joint Commission website. https://www.jointcommission.org/facts_about_joint_commission_stroke_certification/. Published April 21, 2017. Accessed March 27, 2018.
13. Helseth EK. Posterior cerebral artery stroke clinical presentation. Medscape website. https://emedicine.medscape.com/article/2128100-clinical. Updated July 13, 2017. Accessed March 27, 2018.
14. Hemorrhagic strokes (bleeds). American Stroke Association website. http://www.strokeassociation.org/STROKEORG/AboutStroke/TypesofStroke/HemorrhagicBleeds/Hemorrhagic-Strokes-Bleeds_UCM_310940_Article.jsp#.We3ndHZrz1I. Accessed March 27, 2018.
15. Birenbaum D. Emergency neurological care of strokes and bleeds. *J Emerg Trauma Shock*. 2010;3(1):52-61.
16. Koenig KL. Who's at risk for stroke after TIA? *NEJM* Journal Watch website. https://www.jwatch.org/em200702230000002/2007/02/23/who-s-risk-stroke-after-tia. Published February 23, 2007. Accessed March 27, 2018.
17. Stroke, TIA and warning signs. American Stroke Association website. https://www.strokeassociation.org/idc/groups/stroke-public/@wcm/@hcm/@sta/documents/downloadable/ucm_309532.pdf. Accessed March 27, 2018.
18. TIA (transient ischemic attack). American Stroke Association website. http://www.strokeassociation.org/STROKEORG/AboutStroke/TypesofStroke/TIA/Transient-Ischemic-Attack-TIA_UCM_492003_SubHomePage.jsp. Accessed March 27, 2018.
19. American Heart Association. *Advanced Cardiac Life Support Provider Manual*. Dallas, TX: American Heart Association; 2010.
20. Nentwich LM, Magauran BG, Kahn JH. Acute ischemic stroke. *Emerg Med Clin North Am*. 2012;30(3):15-16.

21. Krebs W, Sharkey-Toppen TP, Cheek F, et al. Prehospital stroke assessment for large vessel occlusions: a systematic review. *Prehosp Emerg Care.* 2018;22(2):180-188.
22. Nazliel B, Starkman S, Liebeskind DS, et al. A brief prehospital stroke severity scale identifies ischemic stroke patients harboring persisting large arterial occlusions. *Stroke.* 2008;39(8):2264-2267.
23. American Heart Association. *2015 Handbook of Emergency Cardiovascular Care for Healthcare Providers*. Dallas, TX: American Heart Association; 2015.
24. Powers WJ, Derdeyn CP, Biller J, et al. 2015 American Heart Association/American Stroke Association focused update of the 2013 guidelines for the early management of patients with acute ischemic stroke regarding endovascular treatment. *Stroke.* 2015;46(10):3020-3035.
25. Powers WJ, Rabinstein AA, Ackerson T, Adeoye OM, Bambakidis NC, Becker K, Biller J, Brown M, Demaerschalk BM, Hoh B, Jauch EC, Kidwell CS, Leslie-Mazwi TM, Ovbiagele B, Scott PA, Sheth KN, Southerland AM, Summers DV, Tirschwell DL; on behalf of the American Heart Association Stroke Council. 2018 Guidelines for the early management of patients with acute ischemic stroke: a guideline for healthcare professionals from the American Heart Association/American Stroke Association. *Stroke.* 2018;49:e46-e99.
26. American Heart Association. *Advanced Cardiac Life Support*. Dallas, TX: American Heart Association; 2016.
27. Rincon F, Kang J, Maltenfort M, et al. Association between hyperoxia and mortality after stroke: a multicenter cohort study. *Crit Care Med.* 2014;42(2):387-396.
28. Goldenberg MM. Overview of drugs used for epilepsy and seizures: etiology, diagnosis, and treatment. *Pharm Ther.* 2010;35(7):392-415.
29. Fisher RS, Shafer PO, D'Souza C. 2017 revised classification of seizures. Epilepsy Foundation website. https://www.epilepsy.com/article/2016/12/2017-revised-classification-seizures. Published December 2016. Accessed March 27, 2018.
30. Focal seizure by feature: aura. International League Against Epilepsy website. https://www.epilepsydiagnosis.org/seizure/aura-overview.html. Accessed March 26, 2018.
31. Devinsky O, Spruill T, Thurman D, et al. Recognizing and preventing epilepsy-related mortality: A call for action. *Neurology.* 2016;86(8):779-786.
32. Trinka E, Cock H, Hesdorffer D, et al. A definition and classification of status epilepticus—report of the ILAE Task Force on Classification of Status Epilepticus. *Epilepsia.* 2015;56(10):1515-1523.
33. National Association of EMS Officials. *National Model EMS Clinical Guidelines*. Version 2.0. National Association of EMS Officials website. https://www.nasemso.org/documents/National-Model-EMS-Clinical-Guidelines-Version2-Sept2017.pdf. Published September 2017. Accessed March 27, 2018.
34. Burch R, Loder S, Loder E, Smitherman T. The prevalence and burden of migraine and severe headache in the United States: updated statistics from government health surveillance studies. *Headache.* 2015;55(1):21-23.
35. Warnock JK, Cohen LJ, Blumenthal H, et al. Hormone-related migraine headaches and mood disorders: treatment with estrogen stabilization. *Pharmacotherapy.* 2017;37(1):120-128.
36. Asimos AW. Evaluation of the patient with acute weakness in the emergency department. UpToDate website. https://www.uptodate.com/contents/evaluation-of-the-adult-with-acute-weakness-in-the-emergency-department. Updated April 26, 2017. Accessed March 5, 2018.
37. Parikh V, Tucci V, Galwankar S. Infections of the nervous system. *Int J Crit Illn Inj Sci.* 2012;2(2):82-97.
38. Meningitis and encephalitis fact sheet. National Institute of Neurological Disorders and Stroke website. https://www.ninds.nih.gov/Disorders/Patient-Caregiver-Education/Fact-Sheets/Meningitis-and-Encephalitis-Fact-Sheet. Accessed March 27, 2018.
39. National Center for Immunization and Respiratory Diseases, Division of Bacterial Diseases. Meningococcal vaccines for preteens, teens. Centers for Disease Control and Prevention website. https://www.cdc.gov/features/meningococcal/. Updated April 24, 2017. Accessed March 27, 2018.
40. Patel K, Clifford DB. Bacterial brain abscess. *Neurohospitalist.* 2014;4(4):196-204.
41. Lau C, Teo W-Y. Epidemiology of central nervous system tumors in children. UpToDate website. https://www.uptodate.com/contents/epidemiology-of-central-nervous-system-tumors-in-children. Updated September 1, 2017. Accessed March 27, 2018.
42. Wong ET. Overview of the clinical features and diagnosis of brain tumors in adults. UpToDate website. www.uptodate.com/contents/overview-of-the-clinical-features-and-diagnosis-of-brain-tumors-in-adults?source=search_result&search=brain%20tumor%20signs%20and%20symptoms&selectedTitle=1~150. Updated July 19, 2017. Accessed March 5, 2018.
43. Centers for Disease Control and Prevention. QuickStats: death rates from dementia among persons aged ≥75 years, by sex and age group—United States, 2000–2013. *Morb Mortal Wkly Rep.* 2015;64(20):561.
44. Taylor C, Greenlund S, McGuire L, Lu H, Croft J. Deaths from Alzheimer's disease—United States, 1999–2014. *Morb Mortal Wkly Rep.* 2017;66(20):521-526.
45. 2018 Alzheimer's disease facts and figures. Alzheimer's Association website. https://www.alz.org/facts/. Accessed March 27, 2018.
46. Huntington disease. National Library of Medicine, National Institutes of Health website. https://ghr.nlm.nih.gov/condition/huntington-disease. Accessed March 27, 2018.
47. Romitti PA, Zhu Y, Puzhankara S, et al. Prevalence of Duchenne and Becker muscular dystrophies in the United States. *Pediatrics.* 2015;135(3):513-521.
48. Duchenne muscular dystrophy (DMD). Muscular Dystrophy Association website. https://www.mda.org/disease/duchenne-muscular-dystrophy. Accessed March 27, 2018.
49. Multiple sclerosis FAQs. National Multiple Sclerosis Society website. https://www.nationalmssociety.org/What-is-MS/MS-FAQ-s. Accessed March 27, 2018.
50. About MS. National Multiple Sclerosis Society website. https://www.nationalmssociety.org/For-Professionals/Clinical-Care/About-MS. Accessed March 27, 2018.
51. Menorca RMG, Fussell TS, Elfar JC. Peripheral nerve trauma: mechanisms of injury and recovery. *Hand Clin.* 2013;29(3):317-330.
52. Guillain-Barré syndrome fact sheet. National Institute of Neurological Disorders and Stroke website. https://www.ninds.nih.gov/Disorders/Patient-Caregiver-Education/Fact-Sheets/Guillain-Barr%C3%A9-Syndrome-Fact-Sheet. Accessed March 5, 2018.
53. Centers for Disease Control and Prevention, National Center for Emerging and Zoonotic Infectious Diseases, Division of Vector-Borne Diseases. Zika and Guillain-Barré syndrome. Centers for Disease Control and Prevention website. https://www.cdc.gov/zika/healtheffects/gbs-qa.html. Updated August 9, 2016. Accessed March 27, 2018.

54. Dystonia. American Association of Neurological Surgeons website. http://www.aans.org/Patients/Neurosurgical-Conditions-and-Treatments/Dystonia. Accessed March 27, 2018.
55. Statistics. Parkinson's Foundation website. http://www.parkinson.org/Understanding-Parkinsons/Causes-and-Statistics/Statistics. Accessed March 5, 2018.
56. Cirpaciu D, Goanta CM, Cirpaciu MD. Recurrences of Bell's palsy. *J Med Life*. 2014;7(Spec No. 3):68-77.
57. Who gets ALS? ALS Association website. http://www.alsa.org/about-als/facts-you-should-know.html. Updated June 2016. Accessed March 27, 2018.

Suggested Readings

Brandler ES, Sharma M, Sinert RH, Levine SR. Prehospital stroke scales in urban environments: a systematic review. *Neurology*. 2014;82(24):2241-2249.

Jagoda AS, Quint DJ, Henry GL, Little N, Pellegrino TR. *Neurologic Emergencies*. 3rd ed. New York, NY: McGraw-Hill; 2010.

Loomis C, Mullen MT. Differentiating facial weakness caused by Bell's palsy vs. acute stroke. *JEMS* website. http://www.jems.com/articles/print/volume-39/issue-5/features/differentiating-facial-weakness-caused-b.html?c=1. Published May 7, 2014. Accessed March 26, 2018.

Pellock JM. *Neurologic Emergencies in Infancy and Childhood*. 2nd ed. St. Louis, MO: Elsevier; 2013.

Rudd M, Buck D, Ford GA, Price CI. A systematic review of stroke recognition instruments in hospital and prehospital settings. *Emerg Med J*. 2016;33(11):818-822.

Sullivan B. Stroke scales: 10 things you need to know to save lives. EMS1.com website. https://www.ems1.com/mobile-healthcare/articles/3014604-Stroke-scales-10-things-you-need-to-know-to-save-lives/. Published July 23, 2015. Accessed March 5, 2018.

Weiner WJ, Shulman LM. *Emergent and Urgent Neurology*. 2nd ed. Lippincott Williams & Wilkins; 1998.

Chapter 25

Endocrinology

NATIONAL EMS EDUCATION STANDARD COMPETENCIES

Medicine

Integrates assessment findings with principles of epidemiology and pathophysiology to formulate a field impression and implement a comprehensive treatment/disposition plan for a patient with a medical complaint.

Endocrine Disorders

Awareness that

- Diabetic emergencies cause altered mental status (p 990)

Anatomy, physiology, pathophysiology, assessment, and management of

- Acute diabetic emergencies (pp 997–1004)

Anatomy, physiology, epidemiology, pathophysiology, psychosocial impact, presentations, prognosis, and management of

- Acute diabetic emergencies (pp 997–1004)
- Diabetes (pp 987–997)
- Adrenal disease (pp 1008–1010)
- Pituitary and thyroid disorders (pp 1004–1008)

OBJECTIVES

Upon completion of this chapter, the paramedic student will be able to:

1. Describe how hormones secreted from endocrine glands help the body maintain homeostasis. (pp 983–987)
2. Describe the anatomy and physiology of the pancreas and the ways hormones maintain normal glucose metabolism. (pp 987–992)
3. Discuss pathophysiology as a basis for key signs and symptoms, patient assessment, and patient management for diabetes and diabetic emergencies of hypoglycemia, diabetic ketoacidosis, and hyperosmolar hyperglycemic nonketotic syndrome. (pp 992–1004)
4. Discuss pathophysiology as a basis for key signs and symptoms, patient assessment, and patient management for disorders of the thyroid gland. (pp 1004–1008)
5. Discuss pathophysiology as a basis for key signs and symptoms, patient assessment, and management of emergencies related to Cushing syndrome and Addison disease. (pp 1008–1010)

KEY TERMS

acetate A by-product of fatty acids in the liver.

Addison disease A rare and potentially life-threatening disorder caused by a deficiency of the corticosteroid hormones normally produced by the adrenal cortex.

Cushing syndrome A condition caused by an abnormally high circulating level of corticosteroid hormones produced naturally by the adrenal glands.

diabetes insipidus (DI) A metabolic disorder characterized by extreme polyuria and polydipsia that is caused by deficient production or secretion of antidiuretic hormone or inability of the kidney tubules to respond to antidiuretic hormone.

diabetes mellitus A complex disorder of carbohydrate, fat, and protein metabolism that primarily results from partial or complete lack of insulin secretion by the beta cells of the pancreas or occurs because of defects in the insulin receptors.

diabetic ketoacidosis (DKA) An acute, life-threatening complication of uncontrolled diabetes characterized by hyperglycemia, hypovolemia, electrolyte imbalance, and a breakdown of free fatty acids, causing acidosis.

endocrine glands Glands that secrete hormones directly into the blood rather than through a duct.

exocrine glands Glands that secrete chemicals and enzymes into a duct.

gestational diabetes mellitus A disorder characterized by impaired ability to metabolize carbohydrates, usually caused by a deficiency of insulin. It occurs in pregnancy and disappears after delivery but in some cases returns years later.

glucagon A hormone produced by the alpha cells in the islets of Langerhans that stimulates the conversion of glycogen to glucose in the liver.

gluconeogenesis The formation of glucose from fatty acids and proteins rather than carbohydrates.

glycogenolysis The breakdown of glycogen to glucose.

Graves disease A type of excessive thyroid activity characterized by generalized enlargement of the gland (goiter) that leads to a swollen neck and often to protruding eyes (exophthalmos).

growth hormone (GH) A polypeptide hormone produced and secreted by the anterior pituitary gland. It acts as an insulin antagonist.

hormone receptors Receptors on target organs and body tissues that are able to respond to a particular hormone.

hormones Substances, usually peptides or a steroids, produced by one tissue and conveyed by the bloodstream to another to effect physiologic activity, such as growth or metabolism.

hyperglycemia A greater-than-normal amount of glucose in the blood.

hyperosmolar hyperglycemic nonketotic syndrome (HHNS) A diabetic state in which the level of ketone bodies is normal. It is caused by hyperosmolarity of extracellular fluid and results in dehydration of intracellular fluid.

hypoglycemia A lower-than-normal amount of glucose in the blood.

insulin A hormone secreted by the pancreatic islets.

ketogenesis The formation or production of ketone bodies.

ketone bodies The normal metabolic products of lipid and pyruvate within the liver. Excessive production leads to their excretion in the urine.

myxedema A condition that results from a deficiency of thyroid hormone.

nonsteroid hormones Hormones synthesized chiefly from amino acids, such as insulin, parathyroid hormone, and others.

steroid hormones Hormones synthesized by endocrine cells from cholesterol. They include cortisol, aldosterone, estrogen, progesterone, and testosterone.

thyroid storm An acute life-threatening form of hyperthyroidism.

thyrotoxicosis Any toxic condition that results from thyroid hyperfunction.

type 1 diabetes Diabetes characterized by inadequate production of insulin by the pancreas. It may occur any time after birth and requires lifelong treatment with insulin.

type 2 diabetes Diabetes usually characterized by a decrease in the production of insulin by the pancreatic beta cells and diminished tissue sensitivity to insulin (insulin resistance).

The endocrine system and the nervous system allow the body to regulate many functions and to communicate among millions of cells. Paramedics encounter many patients with endocrine system disorders. These disorders can range from minor changes in functioning to life-threatening conditions.

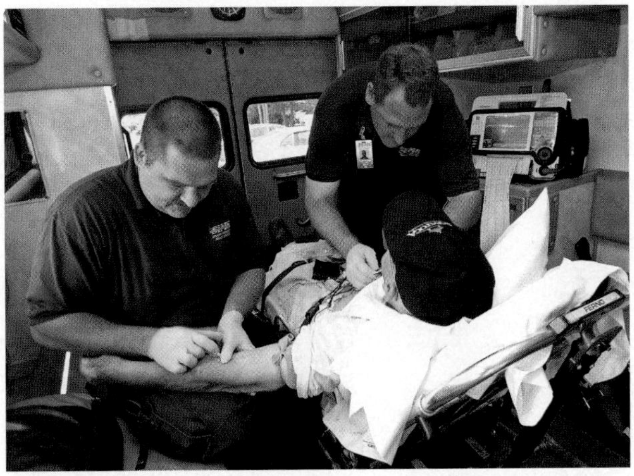

Courtesy of Ray Kemp, St Charles, MO

Anatomy and Physiology of the Endocrine System

The endocrine system is composed of ductless glands and tissues that produce and secrete **hormones**. The major endocrine glands are the pituitary, thyroid, and parathyroid glands; the adrenal cortex and medulla; the pancreatic islets; and the ovaries and testes (**FIGURE 25-1** and **TABLE 25-1**). Other specialized groups of cells that secrete hormones are found in the kidneys and the mucosa of the gastrointestinal (GI) tract.

Endocrine glands secrete hormones directly into the bloodstream and regulate various metabolic functions. Because the products of endocrine glands travel throughout the body via the blood (or tissue fluids), they are able to exert their effects at widespread sites, often distant from their source. The endocrine hormones are released in response to a change in the cellular environment, to maintain a normal level (ie, homeostasis) of hormones or other substances, or to stimulate or inhibit organ functions. This integrated chemical and coordination system enables reproduction, growth and development, and the regulation of energy.

Most hormones can be categorized as proteins, polypeptides, derivatives of amino acids, or lipids. Hormones also may be classified as steroid or nonsteroid. **Steroid hormones** are synthesized by endocrine cells from cholesterol; they include cortisol, aldosterone, estrogen, progesterone, and testosterone. **Nonsteroid hormones** are synthesized chiefly from amino acids; these hormones include insulin and parathyroid hormone, among others.

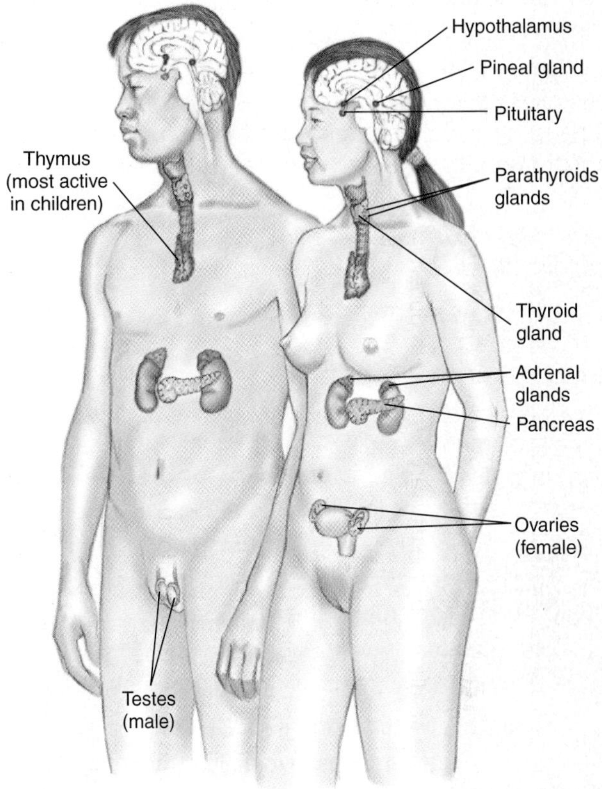

FIGURE 25-1 Major endocrine glands.

© Jones & Bartlett Learning.

Hormone Receptors

As shown in Table 25-1, each hormone may affect a specific organ or tissue, or it can have a general effect on the entire body. In the former case, the hormone's target organs and body tissues have **hormone receptors** and are able to respond to that particular hormone. Hormones act on cells with appropriate receptors to initiate specific cell functions or activities.

Hormone receptor sites may be present on the outside of the cell membrane or in the interior of the cell. Cells with fewer receptor sites bind with less hormone than do cells with many receptor sites (**FIGURE 25-2**). Abnormalities in the presence or absence of specific hormone receptors can result in endocrine disorders.

> CRITICAL THINKING
>
> How are hormones and their target organs like a lock and key?

TABLE 25-1 Review of Endocrine Glands, Hormones, and Effects of Improper Function

Endocrine Gland	Location/ Description	Hormones Produced	Gland/Hormone Function	Effects of Improper Function
Hypothalamus	Lower middle of the brain; communicates with both nervous and endocrine systems	GHRH	Stimulates GH production by the pituitary	Early puberty Thyroid diseases Diabetes insipidus
		TRH	Stimulates TSH production in the pituitary	
		CRH	Stimulates ACTH production by the pituitary	
		GnRH	Stimulates LH and FSH production by the pituitary	
		PIH (dopamine)	Inhibits prolactin production	
		Oxytocin; produced by the hypothalamus; stored and secreted by the pituitary	Stimulates uterine contraction during labor	
		AVP, also called ADH; produced by the hypothalamus; stored and secreted by the pituitary	Maintains water balance	
		Somatostatin	Inhibits GH release from pituitary and also may have some effects on TSH and ACTH release	
Pituitary	Below hypothalamus, behind sinus cavity	PRL	Enables milk production	Hypopituitarism Galactorrhea (milk production outside of pregnancy and normal breastfeeding because of high PRL level) Acromegaly or gigantism GH deficiency Cushing disease Hyperthyroidism/hypothyroidism Loss of menstrual period Loss of sex drive Infertility
		GH	Stimulates childhood growth, cell production, helps maintain muscle and bone mass in adults	
		ACTH	Stimulates hormone production (cortisol, androgens, and, to a smaller degree, aldosterone) by the adrenal glands	
		TSH	Stimulates thyroid hormone production	
		LH, FSH	Regulate testosterone and estrogen, fertility	

Thyroid	Butterfly-shaped; lies flat against trachea in the throat	T_3, T_4	Help regulate the rate of metabolism	Thyroid diseases (including hypo-thyroidism and hyperthyroidism) Myxedema Thyroid storm Thyrotoxicosis
		Calcitonin	Helps regulate bone status, blood calcium	
Parathyroid	Four tiny glands located behind, next to, or below the thyroid	PTH	Regulates blood calcium	Hyperparathyroidism Hypoparathyroidism
Adrenal	Two triangular organs, on top of each kidney	Epinephrine (adrenaline) Norepinephrine (catecholamines)	Regulates blood pressure, stress reaction, heart rate	Pheochromocytoma (adrenal tumor results in elevated levels of epinephrine and norepinephrine) Cushing syndrome Addison disease
		Aldosterone	Maintains salt, water balance	
		Cortisol	Controls stress reaction	
		DHEA-S	Controls body hair development at puberty	
Ovaries (females only)	Two, located in the pelvis	Estrogen Progesterone	Controls female sex characteristics	Polycystic ovary syndrome
Testes (males only)	Two, located in the scrotum	Testosterone	Controls male sex characteristics	Hypogonadism
Endocrine pancreas	Large, gourd-shaped gland, located behind the stomach	Insulin Glucagon Somatostatin	Regulates glucose[a]	Diabetes mellitus (types 1 and 2) Hyperosmolar hyperglycemic non-ketotic syndrome Zollinger-Ellison syndrome
Pineal	Lower side of the brain	Melatonin	Not well understood; helps control sleep patterns, affects reproduction	

Abbreviations: ACTH, adrenocorticotropic hormone; ADH, antidiuretic hormone; AVP, arginine vasopressin; CRH, corticotropin-releasing hormone; DHEA-S, dehydroepiandrosterone sulfate; FSH, follicle-stimulating hormone; GH, growth hormone; GHRH, growth hormone-releasing hormone; GnRH, gonadotropin-releasing hormone; LH, luteinizing hormone; PIH, prolactin inhibitory hormone; PRL, prolactin; PTH, parathyroid hormone; T_3, triiodothyronine; T_4, thyroxine; TRH, thyrotropin-releasing hormone; TSH, thyroid-stimulating hormone

[a]In the gastrointestinal tract, somatostatin inhibits the release of gastrointestinal hormones such as secretin and gastrin.

Modified from: Endocrine system and syndromes. Lab Tests Online website. https://labtestsonline.org/conditions/endocrine-system-and-syndromes. Updated January 24, 2018. Accessed February 13, 2018.

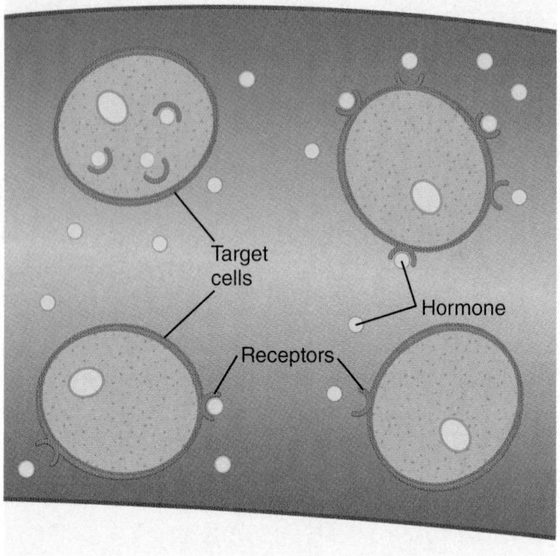

FIGURE 25-2 Target cell concept. Cells with fewer receptor sites bind with less of a particular hormone than do cells with many receptor sites.

Regulation of Hormone Secretion

All hormones operate with feedback systems, which are classified as either positive or negative. Collectively, these feedback systems help maintain the optimal internal environment within the body.

An example of positive feedback can be found in childbirth. The hormone oxytocin stimulates and enhances uterine contractions during labor. As the baby moves toward the birth canal, pressure receptors in the cervix send messages to the brain to secrete oxytocin. Oxytocin travels through the bloodstream to the uterus, where it stimulates the muscles in the uterine wall to contract more strongly. The contractions intensify and increase in frequency until the baby is delivered. When the stimulus to the pressure receptors in the cervix ends, both oxytocin secretion and uterine contractions stop.

Negative feedback (**FIGURE 25-3**) is the mechanism most commonly used to maintain homeostasis.

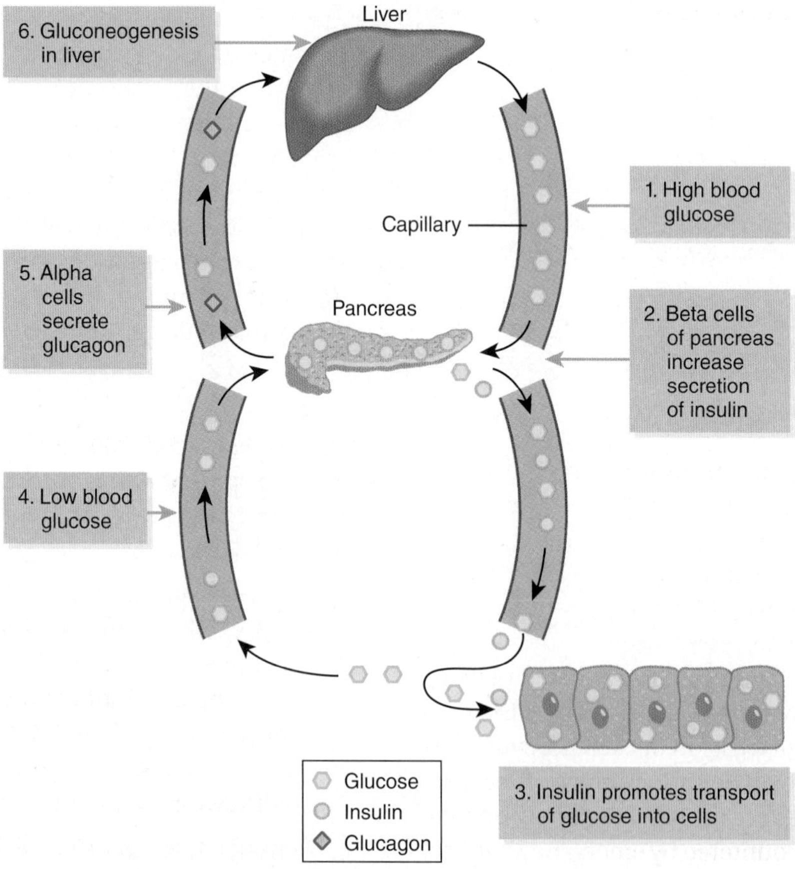

FIGURE 25-3 Negative feedback.

Modified from: Gould BE. *Pathophysiology for the Health Professions*. 3rd ed. St. Louis, MO: Saunders; 2006.

For example, after a person eats a candy bar, the following feedback pathway is activated:

1. Glucose from the ingested lactose or sucrose is absorbed in the intestine. Consequently, the level of glucose in the blood rises.
2. The increase in the blood glucose concentration stimulates the pancreas to release insulin. Insulin facilitates the entry of glucose into the cells, so the blood glucose level falls.
3. When the blood glucose level has dropped sufficiently, the endocrine cells in the pancreas stop producing and releasing insulin.

Another example of negative feedback is seen with the hypothalamus receptors that monitor blood levels of thyroid hormones. Neurons in the hypothalamus secrete thyrotropin-releasing hormone (TRH), which stimulates cells in the anterior pituitary to secrete thyroid-stimulating hormone (TSH). TSH binds to receptors on epithelial cells in the thyroid gland, stimulating synthesis and secretion of thyroid hormones, which affect most cells in the body. When blood concentrations of thyroid hormones increase above a certain threshold, TRH-secreting neurons in the hypothalamus are inhibited and stop secreting TRH.

NOTE

Negative feedback loops can be distinguished from positive feedback loops in a relatively simple way:

1. Negative feedback typically attempts to bring the system/body back toward its normal state (ie, homeostasis).
2. Positive feedback tends to push the system/body away from normal.

Disorders of the Endocrine System

Disorders of the endocrine system arise from the effects of an imbalance in the production of one or more hormones. They also arise from the effects of a change in the body's ability to use the hormones produced. The clinical effects of endocrine gland disorders are determined by the degree of dysfunction as well as by the age and sex of the affected person.

There are many types of endocrine disorders and diseases, but a discussion of each is beyond the scope of this textbook. The endocrine disorders presented in this chapter are the most common, and the most likely to be encountered by emergency medical systems (EMS) personnel. The paramedic should remember that most endocrine disorders are related to hormone imbalance or nutritional deficiencies. After diagnosis, most patients require lifelong treatment.

Disorders of the Pancreas: Diabetes Mellitus

Diabetes mellitus is a systemic disease of the endocrine system that usually results from a dysfunction of the pancreas. This complex disorder of fat, carbohydrate, and protein metabolism affects more than 30 million adults in the United States; another 84 million people are believed to have prediabetes (described later).[1] Diabetes mellitus is potentially lethal. It can put the patient at risk for several kinds of medical emergencies.

Anatomy and Physiology of the Pancreas

The pancreas is important in the absorption and use of carbohydrates, fat, and protein; it is the chief regulator of glucose levels in the blood. The pancreas is located retroperitoneally, adjacent to the duodenum on the right and extending to the spleen on the left. A healthy pancreas has both exocrine and endocrine functions. Recall that **exocrine glands** secrete substances through a duct onto the inner surface of an organ or the outer surface of the body, whereas **endocrine glands** secrete chemicals directly (not through a duct) into the bloodstream. The exocrine portion of the pancreas consists of acini (glands that produce pancreatic juice) and a duct system, which carries the pancreatic fluids to the small intestine. The endocrine portion consists of pancreatic islets (islets of Langerhans) that produce hormones (**FIGURE 25-4**).

Islets of Langerhans

Approximately 500,000 to 1 million pancreatic islets are dispersed among the ducts and acini of the pancreas. Each islet is composed of beta cells, alpha cells, and delta cells:

- Beta cells produce and secrete insulin.
- Alpha cells produce and secrete glucagon.
- Delta cells produce and secrete somatostatin, a hormone that inhibits the secretion of growth hormone and TSH and also inhibits the secretion of insulin and glucagon, thereby preventing rapid swings in blood glucose levels.

Nerves from both divisions of the autonomic nervous system innervate the pancreatic islets, and each islet is surrounded by a well-developed capillary network.

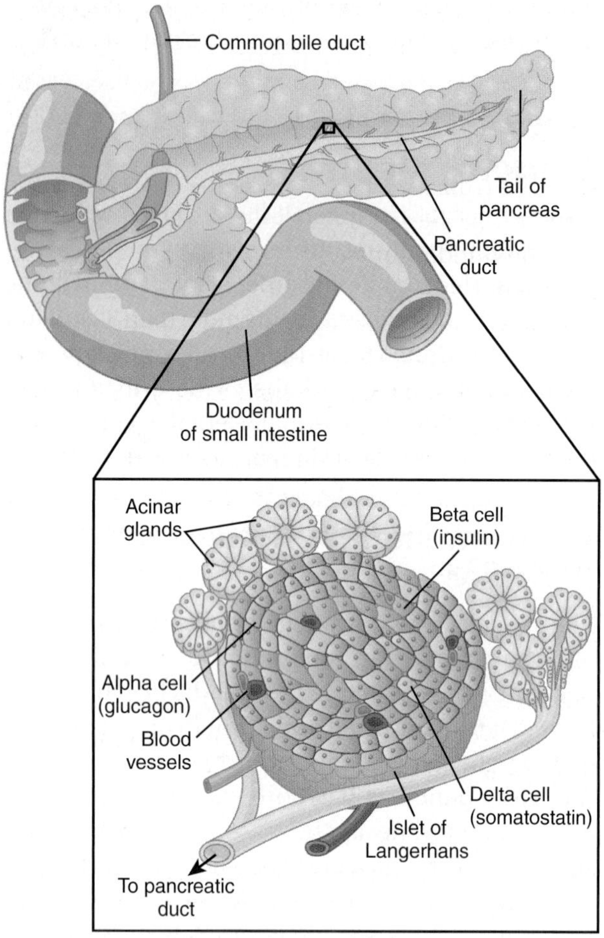

FIGURE 25-4 Pancreatic islets (islets of Langerhans), or hormone-producing areas, are evident among the pancreatic cells that produce the pancreatic digestive juice.

> CRITICAL THINKING
>
> Suppose that part of a patient's pancreas must be removed as a result of traumatic injury. Will the patient still be able to produce insulin and glucagon?

Pancreatic Hormones

Insulin. **Insulin** is a small protein that is released by the beta cells when blood glucose levels rise. The main functions of insulin are as follows:

- Increase glucose transport into cells
- Increase glucose metabolism by cells
- Increase liver glycogen levels
- Decrease the blood glucose concentration toward normal levels

Many of the functions of insulin antagonize the effects of glucagon.

Glucagon. **Glucagon** is a protein that is released by the alpha cells when blood glucose levels fall. Glucagon has two major effects:

- It increases blood glucose levels by stimulating the liver to release glucose stores from glycogen and other glucose storage sites—a process called **glycogenolysis**.
- It stimulates **gluconeogenesis** (glucose formation) through the breakdown of fats and fatty acids, thereby maintaining a normal blood glucose level (**FIGURE 25-5**).

> NOTE
>
> Glycogenolysis and gluconeogenesis can be confusing terms. Glycogenolysis is the breakdown of glycogen to form glucose. Gluconeogenesis generates "new" glucose. (*Lysis* means to break or lyse; *neo* means new.)

Sympathetic stimulation and decreasing concentrations of glucose increase the secretion of glucagon, which acts primarily on liver cells to increase the rate of glycogen breakdown and the secretion of glucose from the liver. The release of glucose from the liver helps maintain blood glucose levels. Increasing blood glucose levels have an inhibitory effect on glucagon secretion. In addition, increasing concentrations of glucose and amino acids stimulate the beta cells of the pancreatic islets to secrete insulin. Parasympathetic stimulation also causes insulin secretion. Insulin acts on most tissues to increase the uptake of glucose and amino acids. As the blood levels of glucose and amino acids decrease, the rate of insulin secretion also decreases.

Growth Hormone. **Growth hormone (GH)** is a polypeptide hormone that is produced and secreted by the anterior pituitary gland. GH secretion is triggered by many physiologic stimuli, including exercise, stress, sleep, and hypoglycemia. GH acts as an insulin antagonist and therefore decreases insulin's actions on cell membranes, which reduces the ability of muscles and adipose and liver cells to absorb glucose.

Regulation of Glucose Metabolism

Under normal conditions, the body maintains the serum glucose level in the range of 60 to 120 mg/dL.

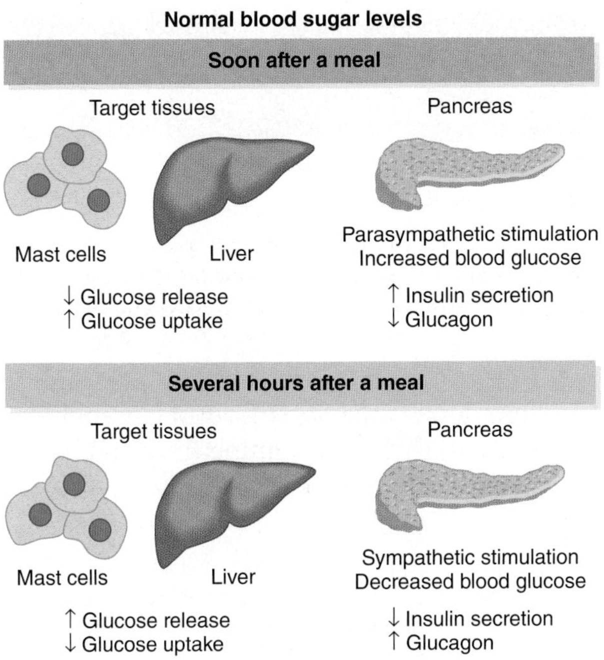

FIGURE 25-5 Regulation of insulin and glucagon secretion.

Normal fasting blood glucose is less than 100 mg/dL.[2] A knowledge of food intake and digestion is required to understand glucose metabolism.

Dietary Intake

The three main organic components of food are carbohydrates, fats, and proteins. (Food also contains minerals and vitamins.) Carbohydrates, which are found in all sugary, starchy foods, are a ready source of near-instant energy. They are the first food substances to enter the bloodstream after a meal is ingested. Breakdown of carbohydrates yields the simple sugar glucose. If not "burned" for immediate energy, glucose is stored in the liver and muscles as glycogen for short-term energy needs, or it is stored in adipose tissue for intermediate and long-term needs.

Digestion Process

Before food compounds can be used by body cells, they must be digested and absorbed into the bloodstream. Digestion begins in the mouth, where both physical forces (chewing) and chemical (enzymatic) forces are applied to the food. These actions begin the process that reduces the food to soluble molecules and particles small enough to be absorbed.

After food has been swallowed, it enters the stomach. There, various nutrients are absorbed into the circulatory system—namely, glucose, salts, water, and some other substances (alcohol and certain other drugs). The remaining material (chyme) is shunted from the stomach into the intestine for further digestion.

The duodenum sends signals that trigger the release of hormones that mobilize the pancreas to contribute its molecule-splitting enzymes and the gallbladder to release bile salts. These enzymes and salts neutralize acids and help emulsify fats. After undergoing this breakdown process, carbohydrates are absorbed into the bloodstream in the form of simple sugars, fats are absorbed as fatty acids and glycerol, and proteins are absorbed as amino acids. These nutrients are then carried from the intestine to the liver by way of the portal vein. (Water and the remaining salts are absorbed from food residues in the colon.) The liver synthesizes glycogen from the absorbed glucose, lipoproteins from the absorbed fatty acids, and many proteins required for health from absorbed amino acids.

Carbohydrate Metabolism. The secretion of insulin is controlled by chemical, neural, and hormonal means. An increased blood glucose concentration, parasympathetic stimulation, and GI hormones involved in the regulation of digestion cause the beta cells of the pancreas to release insulin after dietary intake of carbohydrates. This insulin then travels through the blood to its target tissues, where it combines with specific chemical receptors on the surface of the cell membrane to permit glucose to enter the cell (**TABLE 25-2**). This process both allows the cells to use glucose for energy and ensures that the body does not have to resort to alternative energy sources (proteins and fat cells). In addition, insulin promotes the uptake of glucose into the liver, where it is converted to glycogen for storage. This rapid uptake and storage of glucose normally prevents a large increase in blood glucose levels, which might otherwise occur even after eating just a normal meal. When the blood

> **CRITICAL THINKING**
> Why do people with diabetes eat carbohydrates instead of protein or fat when they sense that their glucose level is too low?

TABLE 25-2 Effects of Insulin and Glucagon on Target Tissues

Target Tissue	Response to Insulin	Response to Glucagon
Skeletal muscle, cardiac muscle, cartilage, bone, fibroblasts, leukocytes, and mammary glands	Increased glucose uptake and glycogen synthesis; increased uptake of certain amino acids	Little effect
Liver	Increased glycogen synthesis; increased use of glucose for energy (glycolysis)	Rapid increase in the breakdown of glycogen to glucose (glycogenolysis) and release of glucose into the blood Increased formation of glucose (gluconeogenesis) from amino acids and, to some degree, from fats Increased metabolism of fatty acids, resulting in increased ketones in the blood
Adipose cells	Increased glucose uptake, glycogen synthesis, fat synthesis, and fatty acid uptake; increased glycolysis	High concentrations cause breakdown of fats (lipolysis); probably unimportant under most conditions
Nervous system	Little effect except to increase glucose uptake in the satiety center	No effect

Modified from: Seeley R. *Anatomy and Physiology.* 11th ed. St. Louis, MO: Mosby; 2017.

glucose level later begins to fall, the liver releases glucose back into the circulating blood.

Thus, the liver removes excess glucose from the blood after a meal, and it returns the glucose to the blood when it is needed between meals. Under normal circumstances, approximately 60% of the glucose in a meal is stored in the liver as glycogen and released later.

If the muscles are not exercised after a meal, much of the glucose transported into the muscle cells by insulin is stored as muscle glycogen. Muscle glycogen differs from liver glycogen and cannot be reconverted into glucose and released into the circulation. Instead, this stored glycogen is used by the muscle for energy.

The brain is recognized as an insulin-sensitive organ that is responsible for physiologic changes in altered metabolic disorders such as obesity and Alzheimer disease.[3] However, the brain is quite different from other body tissues with regard to glucose uptake. The cells of the brain do not have adequate storage capacity to maintain their own supplies of glucose. Also, because the brain normally uses only glucose for energy, it cannot depend on stored supplies of glycogen to meet its energy demands. Therefore, it is essential that the serum glucose be maintained at a level that provides adequate energy to the brain tissues. If the serum glucose level falls too low, signs and symptoms of hypoglycemia—including progressive irritability, altered mental status, fainting, convulsions, and even coma—can develop quickly.

Fat Metabolism. Only a limited amount of glycogen can be stored in the liver and skeletal muscles. Indeed, an estimated one-third of all glucose that passes through the liver is converted to fatty acids. Under the influence of insulin, fatty acids are converted to triglycerides (storable fats), which are then stored in adipose tissue. In the absence of insulin, these stored fats are broken down, so that the plasma concentration of free fatty acids increases rapidly. Thus, a low level of insulin in the blood can result in high levels of triglycerides and cholesterol (in the form of lipoproteins) in the plasma. This process is thought to contribute to the development of atherosclerosis in patients with serious diabetes.[1]

If needed (such as when levels of insulin are low), fatty acids in the liver can be metabolized and used for energy. A by-product of the breakdown of fatty acids in the liver is **acetate**, which is converted to acetoacetic acid and beta-hydroxybutyric acid. These products are released into the circulating blood as **ketone bodies** and may cause acidosis and coma (diabetic ketoacidosis [DKA]) in a patient with diabetes.

NOTE

Coma is relatively rare in patients with diagnosed diabetes. For paramedics, however, it is essential to be aware of the situations that increase risk of coma. The three most common causes of coma in people with diabetes are severe hypoglycemia, severe DKA, and hyperglycemic hyperosmolar state. Coma associated with severe hypoglycemia is more likely to occur from low blood glucose levels if the patient takes a large insulin overdose, if alcohol is in the body during hypoglycemia, or when exercise has depleted the body's glycogen supply.

Modified from: Diabetic coma. Diabetes.co.uk website. https://www.diabetes.co.uk/diabetes-complications/diabetic-coma.html. Accessed February 15, 2018.

Protein Metabolism. Insulin influences the metabolism of protein in addition to the metabolism of carbohydrates and fats. Through the actions of GH and insulin, amino acids are actively transported into the various cells of the body. Most amino acids are used as building blocks to form new proteins—a process called protein synthesis. However, some amino acids enter the metabolic cycle by being converted to glucose after their initial breakdown in the liver.

In the absence of insulin, protein storage stops and protein breakdown (particularly in muscle) begins. This breakdown releases large amounts of amino acids into the circulation. The excess amino acids are used directly for energy or as substrates for gluconeogenesis. Degradation of the amino acids leads to increased excretion of urea in the urine. This "protein wasting" has serious effects in diabetes mellitus, causing extreme weakness and dysfunction of many organs.

Glucagon and Its Functions

Glucagon has several functions that are the opposite of the functions of insulin. Its most important function is to increase the blood glucose concentration. Glucagon has two major effects on glucose metabolism: It promotes the breakdown of liver glycogen (glycogenolysis), and it stimulates the production of glucose (gluconeogenesis).

As the serum glucose returns to its normal level several hours after dietary intake, insulin secretion decreases with continued fasting. The blood sugar level then begins to drop. As a result, glucagon, cortisol, GH, and epinephrine (from sympathetic stimulation) are secreted. These substances initiate the release of glucose from glycogen and other glucose-storage sites. Glycogen is converted back to glucose and released into the blood. Uptake of glucose by most tissues helps maintain the blood glucose at levels necessary for normal function (**FIGURE 25-6**).

In summary, there are four mechanisms for achieving adequate blood glucose regulation:

1. The liver functions as a blood glucose buffer system. It removes excess glucose from the blood and stores it as glycogen. It also returns glucose to the blood when the glucose concentration and insulin secretion decline.
2. Insulin and glucagon function as a negative feedback control system. They work to maintain normal serum glucose concentrations. When the serum glucose level rises, insulin is secreted to lower this level toward normal. Conversely, when the serum glucose level falls, glucagon is secreted to raise this level toward normal.
3. Low serum glucose levels stimulate the sympathetic nervous system to secrete epinephrine. Epinephrine, and to a lesser degree norepinephrine, have a glucagon like effect that promotes liver glycogenolysis.
4. GH and cortisol play roles in less immediate regulation of serum glucose levels. They are secreted in response to more prolonged hypoglycemic episodes, such as a late overnight fast. They also increase the rate of glucose production and decrease the rate of glucose use.

CRITICAL THINKING

Which signs and symptoms will a patient have in response to the release of epinephrine that occurs when the blood glucose level falls?

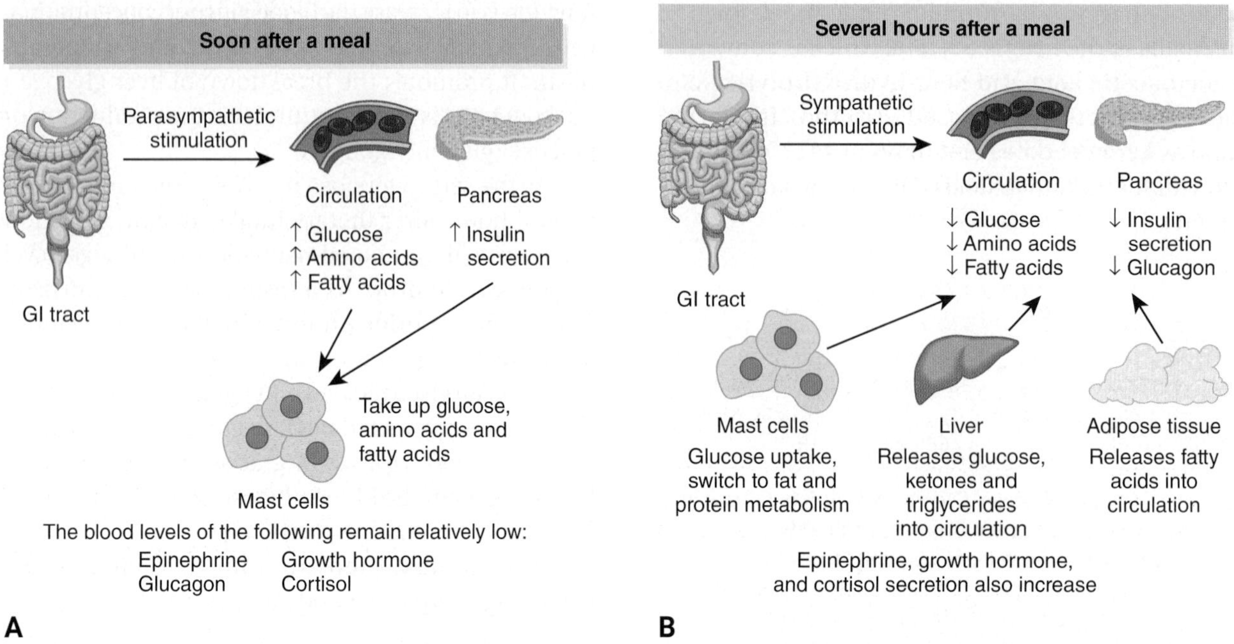

FIGURE 25-6 **A.** Soon after a meal, glucose, amino acids, and fatty acids enter the bloodstream from the intestinal tract. Glucose and amino acids stimulate insulin secretion. Cells take up the glucose and amino acids and use them in their metabolism. **B.** Several hours after a meal, absorption from the intestinal tract decreases, and the blood levels of glucose, amino acids, and fatty acids decrease. As a result, insulin secretion decreases, and glucagon, epinephrine, and growth hormone secretion increases. Cell uptake of glucose decreases, and the use of fats and proteins increases.

Pathophysiology of Diabetes Mellitus

Diabetes is the seventh-leading cause of death in the United States.[4] This disease is characterized by a deficiency of insulin or by an inability of the body to respond to insulin. Diabetes often is associated with excretion of large amounts of urine that contains glucose (polyuria, glucosuria), a resulting excessive thirst (polydipsia) with an increased intake of fluid, and weight loss.

> NOTE
>
> **Diabetes insipidus (DI)** is a disorder marked by an abnormal increase in urine output, fluid intake, and often thirst. DI ("water diabetes") is not the same as or even related to diabetes mellitus ("sugar diabetes"), even though the symptoms of both diseases include increased urination and thirst. DI has a variety of causes, the most common of which is a lack of vasopressin. Vasopressin normally acts on the kidney to reduce urine output by increasing the concentration of the urine.
>
> Most patients with DI are aware of their disease. The paramedic should consider DI as a differential diagnosis in a patient who presents with increased urination and thirst.

Diabetes mellitus generally is classified as type 1 or type 2. Type 1 diabetes previously was called insulin-dependent diabetes mellitus (IDDM) or juvenile diabetes. Type 2 previously was called noninsulin-dependent diabetes mellitus (NIDDM) or adult-onset diabetes. The current classification system endorsed by the American Diabetes Association identifies four types of diabetes—type 1, type 2, gestational diabetes mellitus, and "specific types of diabetes due to other causes"—to address the continuum of **hyperglycemia** (elevated blood glucose) and insulin requirements.[5]

Type 1 Diabetes

Type 1 diabetes is characterized by inadequate production of insulin by the pancreas. Only 5% to 10% of people with diabetes have this form of the disease.[6] Although type 1 diabetes may occur at any age, the incidence in children typically "peaks" in adolescents from 10 to 14 years of age.[7] About one-half of type 1 diabetes cases occur in adulthood[7]—an onset that is termed latent autoimmune diabetes of adulthood.

Type 1 diabetes results from a genetic abnormality or susceptibility that causes the body to destroy its own insulin-producing cells; thus the disease can be inherited. A person with a parent or sibling with type 1 diabetes has a 10% chance of developing the disease.[8] The disease appears to be an autoimmune phenomenon. The incidence of type 1 diabetes onset is higher in the autumn and winter seasons. Although some evidence links it to viral, hygiene, or dietary factors, no single factor has been clearly identified as its etiology.[9]

The symptoms of type 1 diabetes, which usually appear suddenly, include polyuria, polydipsia, dizziness, blurred vision, and rapid, unexplained weight loss. The disease requires lifelong treatment with insulin, exercise, and dietary regulation.

Type 2 Diabetes

Type 2 diabetes begins with diminished tissue sensitivity to insulin (insulin resistance). Later in their illness, many patients with type 2 diabetes experience a decrease in the production of insulin by the pancreatic beta cells. Most people with type 2 diabetes are insulin resistant, meaning they have either too few insulin receptors or faulty insulin receptors. As a result, the circulating insulin cannot be used in the normal way.

Type 2 diabetes accounts for 90% to 95% of all diagnosed cases of diabetes.[10] This disease occurs most often in adults older than 45 years; in women with a history of gestational diabetes; in people of African American, Alaskan Native, American Indian, Hispanic/Latino, or Pacific Islander American race or ethnicity; in people who are overweight; and in people with metabolic syndrome (BOX 25-1).[11] Obesity predisposes a person to this form of diabetes, because larger amounts of insulin are needed for metabolic control in people with obesity than in people of normal weight. Because of the increase in childhood obesity, a growing number of children and young adults are being diagnosed with type 2 diabetes.

BOX 25-1 Metabolic Syndrome

Many people with insulin resistance and high blood glucose levels have other conditions that increase their risk of developing type 2 diabetes and cardiovascular disease. These conditions include excess weight around the waist, high blood pressure, and abnormal blood levels of cholesterol and triglycerides. A person with several of these conditions is said to have metabolic syndrome. Metabolic syndrome is defined as the presence of any three of the following:

- Waist measurement of 40 inches (102 cm) or more for men or 35 inches (89 cm) or more for women
- Triglyceride level of 150 mg/dL or greater or treatment with medication for elevated triglycerides
- High-density lipoprotein (HDL; "good" cholesterol) level below 40 mg/dL for men or below 50 mg/dL for women or treatment with medication for low HDL levels
- Blood pressure of 130/85 mm Hg or greater or treatment with medication for elevated blood pressure
- Fasting blood glucose level of 100 mg/dL or greater or treatment with medication for elevated blood glucose levels

Modified from: About metabolic syndrome. American Heart Association website. http://www.heart.org/HEARTORG/Conditions/More/MetabolicSyndrome/About-Metabolic-Syndrome_UCM_301920_Article.jsp#.WeybXUyZPOQ. Updated October 20, 2017. Accessed February 14, 2018.

NOTE

Prediabetes is a condition that is becoming common in the United States. People with prediabetes have blood glucose levels that are higher than normal but not high enough to make a diagnosis of diabetes. This condition increases the risk that the person will develop type 2 diabetes, heart disease, and stroke. The Centers for Disease Control and Prevention estimates that 84 million adults age 18 years and older have prediabetes. People with prediabetes are likely to develop type 2 diabetes within 10 years unless steps are taken to prevent or delay diabetes. Preventive measures include weight loss, diet modification, and exercise.

Modified from: Centers for Disease Control and Prevention. National diabetes statistics report, 2017. Centers for Disease Control and Prevention website. https://www.cdc.gov/diabetes/data/statistics/statistics-report.html. Updated July 17, 2017. Accessed February 14, 2018.

Most patients with type 2 diabetes require oral hypoglycemic medications, exercise, and dietary regulation to control their illness. A small number of patients require insulin. Warning signs of type 2 diabetes, if present, develop gradually. They include all of those associated with type 1 diabetes, plus fatigue, hunger, slow-healing wounds, and tingling, numbness, and pain in the extremities.

CRITICAL THINKING

Would patients with type 1 or type 2 diabetes have a greater risk of complications related to this disease?

Gestational Diabetes Mellitus

Gestational diabetes mellitus develops in some women during late pregnancy. Although this type of diabetes usually resolves with childbirth, some women go on to develop type 2 diabetes within 5 to 10 years.[12] Gestational diabetes is addressed further in Chapter 45, *Obstetrics.*

Other Types of Diabetes

Although less common than type 1 and type 2 diabetes, a number of other types of diabetes exist. These types are caused by the following conditions:[11]

- Genetic defects of the pancreatic beta cells, insulin, and insulin action
- Diseases of the pancreas or conditions that damage the pancreas, such as pancreatitis, trauma, and cystic fibrosis
- Excess amounts of certain hormones as a result of some medical conditions that work against the action of insulin (eg, cortisol in Cushing syndrome)
- Medications that reduce the action of insulin (eg, glucocorticoids) or chemicals that destroy beta cells (eg, dioxin)
- Infections, such as congenital rubella and cytomegalovirus
- Rare immune-mediated disorders (eg, lupus erythematosus)
- Genetic syndromes associated with diabetes, such as Down syndrome

A person may show characteristics of more than one type.

Effects of Diabetes

Most of the effects of diabetes can be attributed to one of three outcomes of decreased insulin levels:[13]

- Decreased use of glucose by the body cells, which results in an increase in the serum glucose level
- Markedly increased mobilization of fats from the fat-storage areas, causing abnormal fat metabolism, which may result in DKA in the short term and severe atherosclerosis in the long term
- Depletion of protein in body tissues and muscle wasting

Loss of Glucose in the Urine

When the amount of glucose entering the kidneys exceeds the kidneys' ability to reabsorb it, a significant portion of the glucose "spills" into the urine. The loss of glucose in the urine causes diuresis, as the osmotic effect of glucose prevents the kidneys from reabsorbing water (osmotic diuresis). The effect is dehydration. If left untreated, this dehydration can lead to hypovolemic shock.

Acidosis in Diabetes

The shift from carbohydrate metabolism to fat metabolism results in the formation of ketone bodies (*ketoacids*). Ketone bodies are acids, so their continuous production leads to a metabolic acidosis. Often the respiratory system at least partly compensates for the acidosis; this compensation often takes the form of Kussmaul respirations—that is, deep, rapid, labored breathing. The kidneys' ability to clear the acid is overwhelmed by the continuous production of ketone bodies, such that profound acidosis eventually occurs. This acidosis, along with the usually severe dehydration that occurs as a result of the osmotic diuresis, can lead to death. Hyperkalemia, secondary to acidosis, also leads to cardiac dysrhythmias, some of which may be lethal. Treatment of this condition can be lifesaving.

Chronic Complications of Diabetes

Diabetes mellitus is a systemic disease with many long-term complications, including the following:[14]

- **Blindness.** Diabetes is the leading cause of blindness in adults.[15]
- **Kidney disease.** Approximately 36% of patients older than 20 years with diabetes develop some

form of kidney disease, including end-stage kidney failure.

- **Peripheral neuropathy.** This disease results in nerve damage to the hands and feet and an increased incidence of foot infections.
- **Autonomic neuropathy.** This disease damages the nerves controlling voluntary and involuntary functions. It may also affect sexual function, bladder and bowel control, blood pressure, and the ability to recognize signs of hypoglycemia.
- **Heart disease and stroke.** People with diabetes are two to four times as likely to die from heart disease as are those without the disease[16] and are two to four times as likely to have a stroke.[17]
- **High blood glucose and blood fat levels.** These complications contribute to atherosclerosis.
- **Peripheral vascular disease.** This disease, which is also secondary to atherosclerosis, results in the need for amputations.

Patients with diabetes also suffer from decreased immune function as a long-term complication of the disease, placing them at higher risk for increased morbidity and mortality from infectious diseases, such as influenza. These patients also are prone to infection-related complications from surgeries and other invasive procedures (eg, intravenous [IV] therapy, bladder catheterization).

DID YOU KNOW?

Diabetic Foot

Approximately 25% of patients hospitalized with diabetes have foot problems. These problems result from sensory neuropathy, ischemia, and infection. The loss of sensation leads to pressure necrosis from poorly fitting footwear. In addition, small wounds on the feet frequently go unnoticed by the patient, leading to foot ulcers and infection. The most common cause of foot injury is pressure on the plantar bony prominences.

Care should always be taken to assess the feet of any patient with diabetes. Findings may include infected ulcerations, foreign bodies in the foot tissue, and bone abnormalities. Full-thickness ulcerations and cellulitis can be limb-threatening and can lead to sepsis. Patients with a diabetic foot should not be permitted to put weight or pressure on the affected area. Wounds should be dressed. Treatment by a physician may include debridement of devitalized tissue, advanced wound care, and antibiotic therapy. Some patients must be hospitalized.

Modified from: Thewjitcharoen Y, Krittiyawong S, Porramatikul S, et al. Outcomes of hospitalized diabetic foot patients in a multi-disciplinary team setting: Thailand's experience. *J Clin Transl Endocrinol.* 2014;1(4):187-191.

Management of Diabetes

The treatment of diabetes consists of drug therapy (insulin or oral hypoglycemic agents), dietary regulation, and exercise. These therapies both allow patients to control their serum glucose levels and help restore normal metabolism.

Pancreatic transplantation remains an experimental treatment for diabetes mellitus. In a promising technique that is being investigated, pancreatic islet cells are harvested from a donor and implanted into the portal vein of the liver of a person with diabetes.[18] Over time, the new islet cells attach to blood vessels and release insulin. As with other transplants, the patient must take immunosuppressant drugs to prevent rejection of the foreign cells; these drugs have significant side effects.

NOTE

The hemoglobin A1c (Hgb A1c) test is a general measure of diabetes care, which is often performed two to four times per year. It measures the amount of glucose attached to hemoglobin A proteins, thereby providing an average of the person's blood glucose levels for the past 2 to 3 months. The test result is reported as a percentage. For a person without diabetes, a typical Hgb A1c level is about 5%. The American Association of Clinical Endocrinologists recommends a level of 6.5% or lower. Many patients with diabetes know their Hgb A1c number. Maintaining tight glycemic control with a low Hgb A1c level reduces chronic complications but may increase the patient's risk of hypoglycemic episodes.

Modified from: Garber AJ, Abrahamson MJ, Barzilay JI, et al. Consensus statement by the American Association of Clinical Endocrinologists and American College of Endocrinology on the comprehensive type 2 diabetes management algorithm: 2017 executive summary. *Endocr Pract.* 2017;23(2):207-238.

Insulin

Genetically engineered human insulin is available in regular, rapid-, intermediate-, and long-acting preparations (**TABLE 25-3**). Often several types are premixed in a vial for ease of use. Insulin is typically administered by injection rather than as an oral medication because it is a protein that would be broken

TABLE 25-3 Types of Insulin

Insulin Type	Names	Onset[a]	Peak[a]	Duration[a]
Rapid-acting	Insulin glulisine (Apidra), insulin aspart (NovoLog), insulin lispro (Humalog)	15 minutes	1 hour	2–4 hours
Regular (short-acting)	Humulin R, Novolin R	30 minutes	2–3 hours	3–6 hours
Intermediate-acting	Humulin N, Novolin N	2–4 hours	4–12 hours	12–18 hours
Long-acting	Insulin detemir (Levemir), insulin glargine (Lantus)	Several hours	Evenly over 24 hours	24 hours

[a]The values for these parameters are approximate.

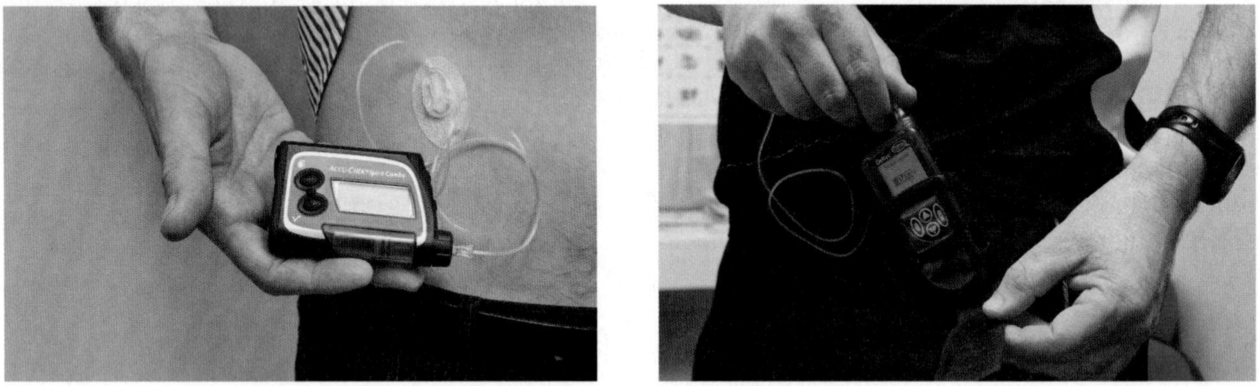

A B

FIGURE 25-7 Insulin pump. **A.** Device and insertion site. **B.** Paramedic with diabetes using an insulin pump.

down during the process of digestion. A patient with type 1 diabetes usually takes one or two doses of a long-acting insulin preparation each day. At meal times, the patient also takes a rapid-acting insulin (which lasts only a few hours).[19]

An inhaled rapid-acting insulin (insulin human, Afrezza) has been available since 2015 and can be used by patients with either type 1 or 2 diabetes. The patient inhales the medicine orally through a small device at the beginning of a meal. This medication is taken in combination with injectable long-acting insulin.[20]

An insulin infusion pump (**FIGURE 25-7**) is another means by which patients may self-administer insulin. The pump delivers a continuous "basal" level of insulin through a plastic catheter inserted in the subcutaneous tissue through a needle; this needle is left in with some devices and discarded with others. The patient inserts a new catheter every 2 to 3 days. The patient supplements the basal level with a bolus dose after eating, which is calculated based on his or her caloric intake. The glucose level must be monitored regularly to ensure adequate medication control. The medication balance is a delicate one: The dosage of insulin that appears correct at one time may be too much or too little at another time. The dosage depends on various factors, such as exercise or the presence of infection. Some insulin pumps also have continuous glucose monitoring capability.

Oral Hypoglycemic Agents

Some oral hypoglycemic agents stimulate the release of insulin from the pancreas. These medications are effective only in patients who have functioning beta cells that produce some insulin (type 2 diabetes). Other agents help the body better use insulin or prevent the body from manufacturing or absorbing glucose (**TABLE 25-4**). Oral hypoglycemic drugs can have important side effects, so their use requires careful patient monitoring (eg, periodic tests of liver and kidney function).

Diabetic Emergencies

Three life-threatening conditions may result from diabetes mellitus: hypoglycemia (insulin shock), hyperglycemia (DKA), and hyperosmolar hyperglycemic nonketotic syndrome.

NOTE

Patients with type 2 diabetes who have an episode of hypoglycemia should be transported for evaluation by a physician. A patient who refuses transport should be advised of the associated risks and should be encouraged to call again for help if needed. These patients should not be left alone if possible.

Hypoglycemia

Hypoglycemia is a syndrome related to blood glucose levels less than 70 mg/dL.[21] Symptoms usually occur at levels less than 60 mg/dL or at slightly higher blood

TABLE 25-4 Medications Used in the Treatment of Diabetes

Generic Name	Brand Name	Effect
Biguanides		
Metformin	Glucophage	Decreases glucose production in liver. Increases tissue sensitivity to insulin.
Sulfonylureas (Second-Generation)		
Glimepiride	Amaryl	Stimulate release of insulin from pancreas.
Glipizide	Glucotrol	
Glyburide	DiaBeta, Glynase, Micronase	
Meglitinides		
Repaglinide	Prandin	Stimulate release of insulin from pancreas.
Nateglinide	Starlix	
Thiazolidinediones		
Pioglitazone	Actos	Help the body use insulin more effectively.
Rosiglitazone	Avandia	
Alpha-Glucosidase Inhibitors		
Acarbose	Precose	Slow the digestion of sugar and block the breakdown of starches.
Miglitol	Glyset	
Dipeptidyl Peptidase 4 (DPP-4) Inhibitors		
Sitagliptin	Januvia	Improve Hgb A1c without causing hypoglycemia. Prevent breakdown of a compound that reduces blood glucose. Must be given with other treatments to be effective.
Saxagliptin	Onglyza	
Linagliptin	Tradjenta	
Alogliptin	Nesina	

(continued)

TABLE 25-4 Medications Used in the Treatment of Diabetes *(continued)*

Generic Name	Brand Name	Effect
Sodium–Glucose Co-transporter 2 (SGLT2) Inhibitors		
Canagliflozin	Invokana	Block reabsorption of glucose in kidneys, allowing excess glucose to be excreted.
Dapagliflozin	Farxiga	
Empagliflozin	Jardiance	
Bile Acid Sequestrants		
Colesevelam	Welchol	Lowers cholesterol and blood glucose.
Glucagon-like Peptide-1 (GLP-1) Agonists		
Dulaglutide	Trulicity	Lower blood glucose by enhancing insulin secretion, slowing gastric emptying, and reducing postprandial glucagon levels.[a]
Liraglutide	Victoza	
Exenatide	Byetta, Bydureon	

[a]Sanjay K, Baruah MP, Sahay RK, et al. Glucagon-like peptide-1 receptor agonists in the treatment of type 2 diabetes: past, present, and future. *Indian J Endocrinol Metab.* 2016;20(2):254-267.

Modified from: American Diabetes Association. What are my options? American Diabetes Association website. http://www.diabetes.org/living-with-diabetes/treatment-and-care/medication/oral-medications/what-are-my-options.html. Updated March 3, 2015. Accessed February 14, 2018.

glucose levels if the decrease in glucose concentration has been rapid.

In patients with diabetes, hypoglycemic reactions usually are caused by the following:

- Too much insulin (or some types of oral hypoglycemic medication)
- Decreased dietary intake (a delayed or missed meal)
- Unusual or vigorous physical activity
- Administration of specific combinations of antibiotics (with oral hypoglycemic agents) (BOX 25-2)

Some patients who have type 2 diabetes are at higher risk for hypoglycemia. This group includes those who take insulin or sulfonylurea oral hypoglycemic agents; have severe kidney disease; are 77 years of age or older; and have had an emergency department visit related to hypoglycemia within the year.[22]

Hypoglycemia may also occur in patients who do not have diabetes. In such cases, it is usually a result of an excessive response to glucose absorption, physical exertion, alcohol or drug effects, pregnancy and lactation, or decreased dietary intake. Less common causes and predisposing factors include the following:

- Chronic alcoholism (alcohol depletes liver glycogen stores)
- Adrenal gland dysfunction
- Liver disease (ie, hepatic insufficiency or failure)
- Malnutrition
- Pancreatic tumor
- Cancer
- Hypothermia
- Sepsis
- Administration of beta blockers (eg, propranolol)

BOX 25-2 Antibiotics Associated With Hypoglycemia

Compared with noninteracting antimicrobials, the following antibiotics were associated with higher rates of hypoglycemia in patients taking concomitant sulfonylureas: clarithromycin (odds ratio [OR]: 3.96), levofloxacin (OR: 2.60), sulfamethoxazole-trimethoprim (OR: 2.56), metronidazole (OR: 2.11), and ciprofloxacin (OR: 1.62). The study data demonstrated that 13.2% of hypoglycemic events occurred when patients were taking one of these five interacting antibiotics.

Modified from: Parekh TM, Raji M, Lin Y, et al. Hypoglycemia after antimicrobial drug prescription for older patients using sulfonylureas. *JAMA Intern Med.* 2014;174(10):1605–1612.

- Administration of salicylates (eg, aspirin) in ill infants or children
- Intentional overdose with insulin, oral hypoglycemic agents, or salicylates

> NOTE
> Relative hypoglycemia can occur when glucose levels fall rapidly below normal fasting levels for a particular person. This condition commonly is overlooked in patients with diabetes who have elevated fasting levels, as these patients may be symptomatic even with near-normal glucose readings. In addition, relative hypoglycemia is common in a newborn whose mother has diabetes.

Signs and Symptoms. The signs and symptoms of hypoglycemia usually appear quickly, often within minutes. They are related to the release of epinephrine that occurs as the body tries to compensate for the drop in blood sugar. In the early stages, the patient may complain of extreme hunger. He or she may then demonstrate one or more of the following signs and symptoms because of the decreased availability of glucose to the brain:

- Nervousness or trembling
- Irritability
- Psychotic (combative) behavior
- Weakness and incoordination
- Confusion
- Appearance of intoxication
- Weak, rapid pulse
- Cold, clammy skin
- Drowsiness
- Seizures
- Coma (in severe cases)
- Cardiac arrest

Hypoglycemia should be suspected in any patient with diabetes who shows behavioral changes, confusion, abnormal neurologic signs, or unconsciousness. This condition is a true emergency: It requires immediate administration of glucose to prevent permanent brain damage or death.

Most patients with diabetes recognize the signs and symptoms of hypoglycemia and can take steps to correct it or alert someone that they are in trouble. A small percentage of these patients have reduced autonomic responses and develop hypoglycemic unawareness—that is, the onset of low levels of glucose in the central nervous system (CNS) before autonomic warning symptoms, such as palpations, sweating, shaking, and anxiety, appear. These patients are susceptible to severe hypoglycemia.[23]

> CRITICAL THINKING
> Why might a call for a patient with hypoglycemia be dispatched as a behavioral emergency?

Diabetic Ketoacidosis

Diabetic ketoacidosis (DKA) results from an absence of or resistance to insulin (BOX 25-3). The low insulin level prevents glucose from entering the cells, so glucose accumulates in the blood. Consequently, the cells become starved for glucose and begin to use other sources of energy, principally fat. The metabolism of fat generates fatty acids and glycerol. The glycerol provides some energy to the cells, but the fatty acids are further metabolized to form ketoacids, resulting in acidosis.

Acidosis increases the transport of potassium from the intracellular space into the intravascular space. The subsequent diuresis results in a high potassium concentration in the urine and a total body potassium deficit. In addition, the sodium concentration in the extracellular fluid usually decreases through osmotic dilution. The sodium is replaced by increased hydrogen ions—a condition that adds greatly to the acidosis. As the blood sugar level rises, the patient undergoes massive osmotic diuresis. This, combined with vomiting, causes dehydration and shock. Although an overall loss of potassium occurs, the patient is still

> **BOX 25-3** Common Causes of Diabetic Ketoacidosis
>
> Infection
> Undiagnosed diabetes
> Inadequate insulin dose
> Failure to take insulin
> Increased stress (trauma, surgery)
> Increased dietary intake
> Decreased metabolic rate
> Other, less common predisposing factors, including significant emotional stress, alcohol consumption (often associated with hypoglycemia), and pregnancy
>
> *Modified from*: Umpierrez GE, Murphy MB, Kitabchi AE. Diabetic ketoacidosis and hyperglycemic hyperosmolar syndrome. *Diab Spectrum.* 2002;15(1):28.

hyperkalemic, which can lead to cardiac dysrhythmias and cardiac abnormalities (eg, peaked T waves, a prolonged PR interval, and widening of the QRS complex). Electrolyte imbalances may also cause altered neuromuscular activity, including seizures.

NOTE

Patients may present with DKA without knowing that they have diabetes (ie, their diabetes has not yet been diagnosed). This is especially true in children.

Modified from: Chumięcki M, Prokopowicz Z, Deja R, Jarosz-Chobot P. Frequency and clinical manifestation of diabetic ketoacidosis in children with newly diagnosed type 1 diabetes [in Polish]. *Pediatr Endocrinol Diab Metab.* 2013;19(4):143-147.

Signs and Symptoms. The signs and symptoms of DKA usually are related to hypovolemia and acidosis. They typically have a slow onset (over 12 to 48 hours) and include the following:

- Diuresis
- Increased blood glucose level

NOTE

An elevation in blood glucose is common in the early phase of stroke. It is estimated that as many as one-third of patients with acute stroke have either diagnosed or newly diagnosed diabetes. A significant proportion of these patients are likely to have stress hyperglycemia, mediated partly by the release of cortisol and norepinephrine. This form of hyperglycemia is associated with poor outcomes, such as a dependent state or intracerebral hemorrhage. If a transient ischemic attack (TIA) or stroke is suspected in a patient older than 50 years, administration of a concentrated glucose solution may worsen cerebral damage. However, glucose should not be withheld if the patient is hypoglycemic.

Modified from: Snarska KK, Bachórzewska-Gajewska H, Kapica-Topczewska K, et al. Hyperglycemia and diabetes have different impacts on outcome of ischemic and hemorrhagic stroke. *Arch Med Sci.* 2017;13(1):100-108.

CRITICAL THINKING

How can you distinguish Kussmaul respirations from hyperventilation?

- Warm, dry skin
- Dry mucous membranes
- Tachycardia and thready pulse
- Postural hypotension
- Weight loss
- Polyuria
- Polydipsia
- Polyphagia
- Acidosis
- Abdominal pain (usually generalized)
- Anorexia, nausea, and vomiting
- Acetone breath odor (fruity odor)
- Kussmaul respirations (as the body attempts to reduce carbon dioxide levels)
- Diminished level of consciousness

Patients with DKA seldom are deeply comatose. Patients who are unresponsive with normal or elevated blood glucose levels should be assessed for another cause, such as head injury, stroke, or drug overdose.

Hyperosmolar Hyperglycemic Nonketotic Syndrome

Hyperosmolar hyperglycemic nonketotic syndrome (HHNS) is a condition of acute diabetic decompensation. It is a life-threatening emergency characterized by marked hyperglycemia, hyperosmolarity, dehydration, and decreased mental functioning. In fewer than 20% of patients with HHNS, it may lead to coma.[24] HHNS often occurs in older patients with type 2 diabetes and in patients with undiagnosed diabetes (**BOX 25-4**). The syndrome is easily mistaken for DKA, but differs from DKA in that enough insulin may be present to prevent the metabolism of fats (**ketogenesis**) and the development of DKA. However, the amount of insulin may not be enough to prevent hyperglycemia or to reduce gluconeogenesis by the liver.

HHNS develops from sustained hyperglycemia that produces a hyperosmolar state. This condition causes an osmotic diuresis that results in marked dehydration and electrolyte losses. In HHNS, protein and fats are not used to create new supplies of glucose to the same degree as in DKA, and the ketotic cycle is either never started or does not occur until the glucose is extremely elevated.[25] These patients usually have blood glucose levels greater than 600 mg/dL. They also have less ketone formation, resulting in less acidemia than in patients with DKA (**FIGURE 25-8**).

BOX 25-4 Causes of Hyperglycemic Hyperosmolar Nonketotic Syndrome

External Insult
Trauma
Burns
Dialysis
Hyperalimentation

Disease Process
Cushing syndrome and other endocrinopathies
Hemorrhage
Myocardial infarction
Renal disease
Subdural hematoma
Cerebrovascular accident
Infection
Down syndrome

Drugs
Antimetabolites
L-asparaginase
Chlorpromazine
Chlorpropamide
Cimetidine
Diazoxide
Didanosine
Ethacrynic acid
Furosemide
Glucocorticoids
Immunosuppressants
Phenytoin
Propranolol
Thiazides

Modified from: Marx J, Hockberger R, Walls R. *Rosen's Emergency Medicine: Concepts and Clinical Practice*. 8th ed. St. Louis, MO: Mosby; 2014.

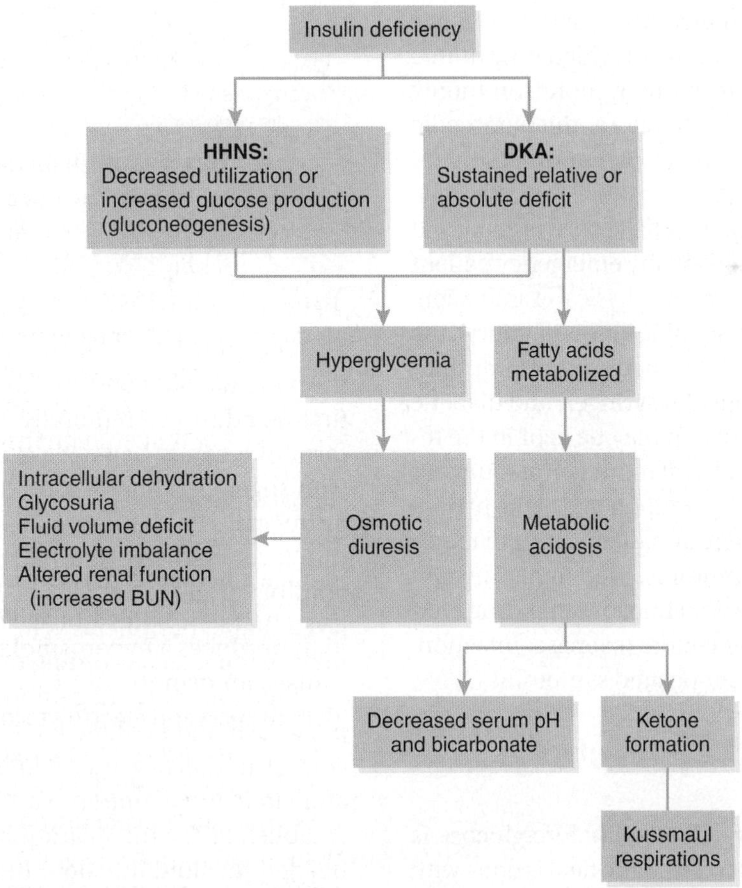

Abbreviations: BUN, blood urea nitrogen; DKA, diabetic ketoacidosis; HHNS, hyperosmolar hyperglycemic nonketotic syndrome

FIGURE 25-8 Pathophysiology of hyperosmolar hyperglycemic nonketotic syndrome.

Modified from: Sole ML. *Introduction to Critical Care Nursing*. 5th ed. St. Louis, MO: Saunders; 2009.

NOTE

HHNS can occur when a diabetic (or nondiabetic) patient is unable to drink sufficient fluids to offset urinary losses. This situation can result from stroke, Alzheimer disease, and other diseases that can lead to dehydration. It also can occur as a result of drug use, trauma, burns, and dialysis.

HHNS tends to develop slowly, often over several days. It has a high mortality rate. Early signs and symptoms are mostly related to volume depletion—namely, polyuria and polydipsia. Associated signs and symptoms may include orthostatic hypotension, dry mucous membranes, and tachycardia. CNS dysfunction may result in lethargy, confusion, and coma.

Assessment of the Patient With Diabetes

A patient with a diabetic emergency may have a range of signs and symptoms, many of which may mimic the signs and symptoms of other, more commonly encountered conditions. Therefore, the paramedic must have a high degree of suspicion for illness related to diabetes.

In addition to performing a patient assessment and the measures appropriate for any emergency patient encounter (primary assessment, physical examination, and treatment of life-threatening illness or injury), the paramedic should search for medical alert information, an insulin pump, insulin syringes, and diabetic medications. Notably, insulin may be kept in the refrigerator, though it is stable at room temperature for about a month. Important components of the patient history in the assessment of patients with diabetes include the onset of symptoms, food intake, insulin or oral hypoglycemic use, alcohol or other drug consumption, predisposing factors (exercise, infection, illness, stress), and any associated symptoms.

Management of the Hypoglycemic Diabetic Patient

Blood glucose is always assessed before glucose is administered. Glucose testing in the field is done with a glucometer (**FIGURE 25-9**). Patients who have a glucose reading less than 60 mg/dL (varies by protocol) *and* who have signs and symptoms consistent with hypoglycemia generally should be given glucose.[26]

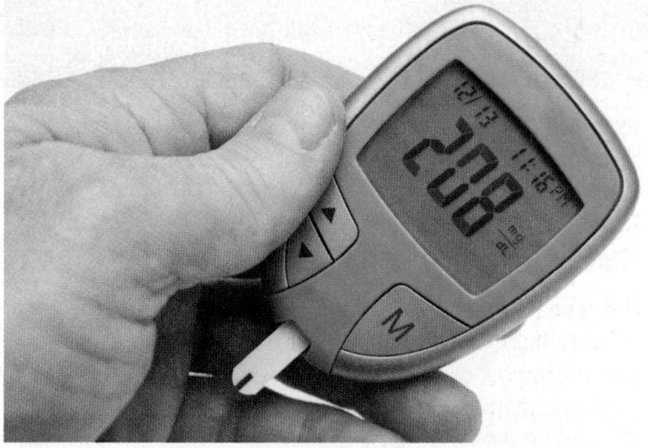

FIGURE 25-9 Glucometer for measuring serum glucose levels.

NOTE

A patient who may have taken an unintentional overdose of insulin always requires evaluation by a physician. These patients can develop delayed, profound, and protracted hypoglycemia. This is especially true with long-acting insulin preparations.

Modified from: Hoffman RS, Howland MA, Lewin NA, Nelson LS, Goldfrank LR. *Goldfrank's Toxicologic Emergencies*. 10th ed. New York, NY: McGraw-Hill; 2015.

The methods of glucose administration vary. If the patient is alert and able to swallow, sugar should first be administered orally. It can be given in the form of a candy bar, a glass of orange juice mixed with sugar, or a nondiet soft drink, or by sublingual or buccal administration of a glucose gel preparation (preferred). An alternative method is to slowly administer dextrose (50%, 25%, or 10%) through a large, stable peripheral vein (**BOX 25-5**). This dose may be repeated according to protocol (**BOX 25-6**).

Prehospital management of any unconscious patient should be directed at airway management, administration of oxygen if indicated, and ventilatory and circulatory support. Vascular access should be established for medication administration and if needed for fluid infusion. Before glucose is given, the patient's blood glucose level should be measured. If alcoholism or other drug abuse is suspected, the administration of thiamine or naloxone, or both, may be indicated.

If an IV line cannot be established, glucagon may be given by the intramuscular route or intranasally[27] via mucosal atomization (per protocol[26]). Glucagon can help raise the serum glucose level by stimulating the breakdown of liver glycogen, but it is not effective in any patient with decreased liver glycogen. Examples of such patients include patients with chronic alcoholism or liver disease, patients who are malnourished or on certain diets, and endurance athletes.

If the patient has an insulin pump, the paramedic should leave it running if prompt treatment with dextrose or glucagon can be administered. If the patient's Glasgow Coma Scale score is less than 15 and the patient cannot ingest oral glucose or advanced life support (ALS) care is not possible, stop or disable the pump (remove the batteries or disconnect the unit[26]).

Some patients with diabetes who have experienced a hypoglycemic reaction may be treated at the scene and released; others may need to be transported for evaluation by a physician (BOX 25-7). The paramedic should consult with medical direction or follow

BOX 25-5 Cautions for Intravenous Administration of Glucose

- Fifty percent dextrose should not be administered to infants or young children or to patients with suspected stroke.
- It was once thought that administration of 50% dextrose might lead to neurologic complications in alcoholics and other patients with thiamine deficiency. However, a mounting body of evidence shows that administration of thiamine before or during administration of dextrose is not necessary in these patients to prevent Wernicke encephalopathy. Paramedics should not delay glucose administration in hypoglycemic patients, although prompt thiamine supplementation after or concurrent with a return to normal glucose levels is recommended.
- IV dextrose may raise Hgb A1c levels.

BOX 25-6 Glucose Preparations

Concentrated dextrose in water is designed for IV administration and is available in several concentrations. High-concentration dextrose solutions may infiltrate tissues, causing sloughing and necrosis of the vein. Therefore, concentrated dextrose must be given through a large, stable vein. It may also be given by the intraosseous route.

The following concentrations are used most often in prehospital care:

- **50% dextrose in water.** Recommended for adults and children older than 8 years only
- **25% dextrose in water.** Can be used for adults and children
- **10% dextrose in water.** Can be safely used for all patients; recommended for neonates)

Note that 50% dextrose is very acidic and has a high osmolarity. If given through an IV line that has infiltrated, it is considered a vesicant and can cause compartment syndrome or tissue necrosis. It quickly elevates blood glucose—often to levels that are higher than desirable. For these reasons, many EMS systems are using 10% dextrose infusions preferentially to correct hypoglycemia.

Modified from: Hern HG, Kiefer M, Louie D, Barger J, Alter HJ. D10 in the treatment of prehospital hypoglycemia: a 24 month observational cohort study. *Prehosp Emerg Care.* 2017;21(1):63-67; Chinn M, Colella MR. Prehospital dextrose extravasation causing forearm compartment syndrome: a case report. *Prehosp Emerg Care.* 2017;21(1):79-82; and Moore C, Woollard M. Dextrose 10% or 50% in the treatment of hypoglycaemia out of hospital? A randomized controlled trial. *Emerg Med J.* 2005;22:512-515.

BOX 25-7 Patient Disposition After Hypoglycemic Episode

A patient who is asymptomatic after treatment for hypoglycemia may be released without transport if the following criteria are met:

1. The patient did not have a seizure.
2. The repeat blood glucose level is greater than 80 mg/dL.
3. The patient takes only insulin or metformin to control diabetes. Sulfonylureas (glimepiride, glyburide, glipizide) have long half-lives, which increases the risk of recurrent hypoglycemia.
4. The patient can promptly obtain and eat a carbohydrate-based meal.
5. The patient, legal guardian (if any), medical control, and EMS agree transport is not needed.

established protocol. If a patient who received glucose refuses transport, the paramedic should ensure the patient has been advised of the possibility of recurrent hypoglycemia before leaving the scene. In addition, the paramedic should make sure the patient has a "meal" available that is high in complex carbohydrates and protein. The meal should be consumed within 30 minutes of receiving the glucose, ideally before EMS providers leave the scene.

SHOW ME THE EVIDENCE

In one study, researchers sought to describe the variability in treatment of prehospital hypoglycemia in the United States. They evaluated prehospital protocols published on the EMS Protocols website (www.emsprotocols.org) and manually searched the protocols in the 50 most populous cities in the United States. They evaluated protocols from 185 EMS agencies. Of those, 70% used only 50% dextrose to treat adult hypoglycemia, 8% used only 10% dextrose, and 22% used either 10% or 50% dextrose. Of the agencies, 97% allowed glucagon use when vascular access was not possible. The researchers concluded that there are major differences in the treatment provided for hypoglycemia.

Modified from: Rostykus P, Kennel J, Adair K, et al. Variability in the treatment of prehospital hypoglycemia: a structured review of EMS protocols in the United States. *Prehosp Emerg Care.* 2016;20(4):524-530.

Management of the Hyperglycemic Diabetic Patient

Definitive treatment for patients with DKA or HHNS requires administration of insulin, fluid replacement, electrolyte monitoring, treatment of underlying causes, and in-hospital observation. If signs of hyperkalemia are present, the patient should be monitored closely for serious dysrhythmias, which can lead to cardiac arrest. They result from electrolyte abnormalities (hyperkalemia) and may require drug therapy—for example, albuterol, calcium (gluconate or chloride), furosemide, insulin, and sodium bicarbonate (see Chapter 21, *Cardiology*). If the blood glucose level is higher than 250 mg/dL, the paramedic should infuse IV normal saline: 1-L bolus for the adult, and repeat with a second 1-L bolus if needed. Fluid resuscitation for pediatric patients is a 10- to 20-mL/kg bolus, repeated to a total of 40 mL/kg.[26]

Assessment for signs of dehydration is performed after completing the primary survey and determining

NOTE

Administration of one dose of dextrose only minimally worsens DKA or HHNS. This drug can be lifesaving therapy for patients who are hypoglycemic. Thus, in the rare event that the blood glucose cannot be measured rapidly in an unconscious patient, dextrose may still be given.

Modified from: Marx J, Hockberger R, Walls R. *Rosen's Emergency Medicine: Concepts and Clinical Practice.* 8th ed. St. Louis, MO: Mosby; 2014.

that the patient is hyperglycemic. Sepsis should be suspected and the patient assessed to identify a possible source of infection. The paramedic should evaluate a 12-lead electrocardiogram (ECG) for peaked T waves or other indicators of hyperkalemia.

Differential Diagnosis

The signs and symptoms of diabetic emergencies can sometimes overlap, making the exact cause of the patient's condition difficult to identify. Although blood glucose monitoring is a standard of care, **TABLE 25-5** may help in making a differential diagnosis in difficult cases.

Disorders of the Thyroid Gland

Common disorders of the thyroid gland include hyperthyroidism and hypothyroidism. Hyperthyroidism is an excess of thyroid hormones in the blood, which may result in thyrotoxicosis. Hypothyroidism is an insufficiency of thyroid hormones in the blood, which may result in myxedema.

Anatomy and Physiology of the Thyroid Gland

The thyroid gland is situated in the front of the neck just below the larynx. It consists of two lobes, one on each side of the trachea, which are joined by a narrower portion of tissue called the isthmus (**FIGURE 25-10**).

Thyroid tissue is composed of two types of secretory cells: follicular cells and parafollicular cells (or C cells). Follicular cells, which make up most of the gland, are arranged in the form of hollow, spherical follicles. They secrete the iodine-containing hormones thyroxine (T_4) and triiodothyronine (T_3). Parafollicular cells occur singly or in small groups in the spaces between the follicles. They secrete the hormone calcitonin, which helps regulate the level of calcium in the body.

TABLE 25-5 Differential Diagnosis Considerations in Diabetic Emergencies

Findings	Hypoglycemia	DKA	HHNS
History			
Food intake	Insufficient	Excessive	Excessive
Insulin dosage	Excessive	Insufficient	Insufficient
Onset	Rapid	Gradual	Gradual
Infection	Uncommon	Common	Common
Gastrointestinal Tract			
Thirst	Absent	Intense	Intense
Hunger	Intense	Absent	Intense
Vomiting	Uncommon	Common	Uncommon
Respiratory System			
Breathing	Variable	Deep and rapid	Shallow/rapid
Breath odor	Normal	Acetone smell	Normal
Cardiovascular System			
Blood pressure	Normal	Low	Low
Pulse	Normal, rapid, or full	Rapid and weak	Rapid and weak
Skin	Pale and moist	Warm and dry	Warm and dry
Nervous System			
Headache	Present	Absent	Irritable
Consciousness	Irritable	Restless	Seizure or coma
	Seizure or coma	Coma (rare)	Irritable
Urine			
Glucosuria	Absent	Present	Present
Acetone	Usually absent	Usually present	Absent
Serum glucose levels	<60 mg/dL	>300 mg/dL	>600 mg/dL
Treatment response	Immediate (after glucose administration[a]); response is slower after oral glucose or glucagon administration	Gradual (within 6–12 hours after medication and fluid replacement)	Gradual (within 6–12 hours after medication and fluid replacement)

[a]If the hypoglycemic episode is prolonged or severe, response may be delayed and may require more than one dose.

Abbreviations: DKA, diabetic ketoacidosis; HHNS, hyperosmolar hyperglycemic nonketotic syndrome

Modified from: Freeman Clark JB, Queener SF, Karb VB. *Pharmacological Basis of Nursing.* 4th ed. St. Louis, MO: Mosby; 1993.

Thyroid hormones play a key role in controlling body metabolism. They are essential in children for normal physical growth and mental development. The secretion of T_3 and T_4 is controlled by a feedback system involving the pituitary gland and the hypothalamus. (The secretion of calcitonin is regulated directly by the level of calcium in the blood, independent of the pituitary gland or hypothalamus.)

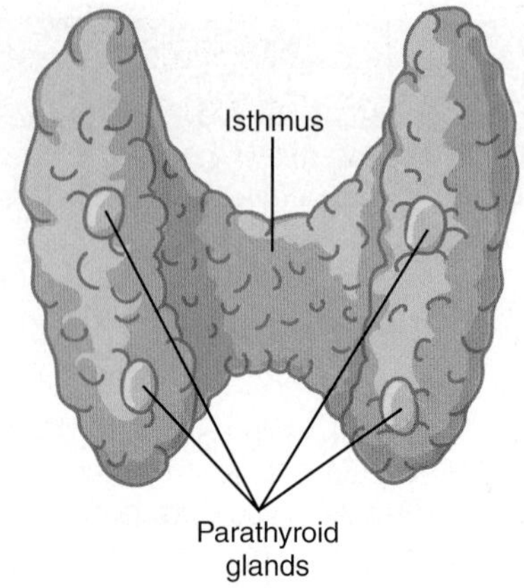

FIGURE 25-10 Thyroid gland, as viewed from behind.

Causes of Thyroid Disorders

Disorders of the thyroid gland may result from defects in the gland itself or from disruption of the hypothalamic–pituitary hormonal control system (BOX 25-8).

Thyroid diseases tend to advance slowly and may produce nonspecific signs and symptoms over months to years. Hyperthyroidism also may culminate in an acute episode (thyroid storm). Nonspecific signs and symptoms of thyroid hyperactivity include fatigue, anxiety, palpitations, sweating, weight loss, diarrhea, and heat intolerance. **TABLE 25-6** lists the signs and symptoms of hyperthyroidism and hypothyroidism.

Thyrotoxicosis

Thyrotoxicosis is a mild form of hyperthyroidism; it is fairly common and develops over time. **Thyroid storm** is an acute, life-threatening form of hyperthyroidism that may occur spontaneously. This rare condition may be brought on by infection, stress, or a surgical manipulation of the thyroid gland in patients with hyperthyroidism.

Most cases of hyperthyroidism occur as a consequence of toxic diffuse goiter, called Graves disease.[28] **Graves disease** is a type of excessive thyroid activity characterized by generalized enlargement of the gland (goiter), which leads to a swollen neck and, often, protruding eyes (exophthalmos) (**FIGURE 25-11**). Graves disease most often occurs in young women. It may arise as a result of an autoimmune process in which an antibody stimulates the thyroid cells.

In acute episodes of thyroid storm, the signs and symptoms are those related to adrenergic hyperactivity:

- Severe tachycardia
- Heart failure
- Cardiac dysrhythmias
- Shock
- Hyperthermia
- Restlessness
- Agitation and paranoia
- Abdominal pain
- Delirium
- Coma

The paramedic should consider other causes of symptoms related to adrenergic hyperactivity, most notably hypoglycemia, use of cocaine and amphetamines, and withdrawal from alcohol and other drugs.

BOX 25-8 Causes of Thyroid Gland Disorders

Congenital defects
Genetic disorders
Infection (thyroiditis)
Tumors (benign or malignant)
Autoimmune disorders
Hormonal disorders during puberty or pregnancy
Nutritional disorders

TABLE 25-6 Signs, Symptoms, and Medications Used in Hyperthyroidism and Hypothyroidism

Hyperthyroidism	Hypothyroidism
Exophthalmos	Facial edema
Goiter	Jugular venous distention (sometimes goiter)
Warm, flushed skin	Cool skin
Sensitivity to heat	Sensitivity to cold
Fever	Hypothermia
Agitation/psychosis	Coma
Hyperactivity	Weakness
Weight loss	Weight gain
Common Medications Used in Treatment	
Iodine	Levothyroxine (Synthroid, Levoxyl)
Methimazole (Tapazole)	Liothyronine (Cytomel)
Propylthiouracil (Propacil)	Liotrix (Euthroid)
Propranolol (Inderal)	

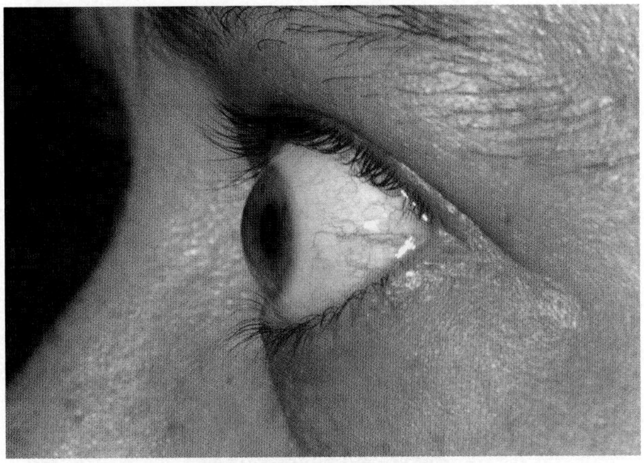

FIGURE 25-11 Protrusion of the eyes (exophthalmos) in a patient with Graves disease.

CRITICAL THINKING

What medical emergencies could produce signs and symptoms similar to those of thyroid storm?

Management

Mild hyperthyroidism requires no emergency therapy, but rather is best managed with physician follow-up. Thyroid storm, however, is a true emergency that requires immediate treatment. Emergency care efforts are directed at providing airway, ventilatory, and circulatory support and rapid transport to an appropriate medical facility. In-hospital care focuses on inhibiting hormone synthesis, blocking hormone release and the peripheral effects of thyroid hormone with antithyroid drugs, and providing general support of the patient's vital functions. Beta blockers also are given to control the heart rate, tremors, and anxiety.

NOTE

All patients with disorders related to the thyroid gland should be closely monitored for cardiac dysrhythmias. Atrial fibrillation and supraventricular tachycardia are common in these patients. Efforts to control the heart rate may not be effective until the thyroid disorder has been treated.

Myxedema

Myxedema is a condition that results from hypothyroidism. It may be associated with inflammation of the thyroid gland (eg, Hashimoto thyroiditis) or atrophy of the thyroid gland; it also may be a consequence of treatment for hyperthyroidism. Myxedema causes an accumulation of mucinous material in the skin, which in turn results in thickening and coarsening of the skin and other body tissues—most notably the lips, nose, and throat (**FIGURE 25-12**). The condition is most common in adults older than 40 years, especially women.

NOTE

Symptoms of hypothyroidism in children and adolescents differ from those in adults. In newborns, hypothyroidism causes cretinism (neonatal hypothyroidism). This condition is characterized by jaundice, poor appetite, constipation, a hoarse cry, outpouching of the navel (umbilical hernia), and slowed bone growth. If not diagnosed and treated within a few months of birth, hypothyroidism can lead to intellectual impairment. Hypothyroidism that begins in childhood (juvenile hypothyroidism) slows growth. This condition sometimes results in disproportionately short limbs and delays tooth development.

Myxedema coma is a rare illness. In addition to myxedema, it is characterized by hypothermia and a reduced level of consciousness. Myxedema coma is a medical emergency that may be precipitated by the following factors:

- Exposure to cold
- Infection (usually pulmonary)
- Heart failure

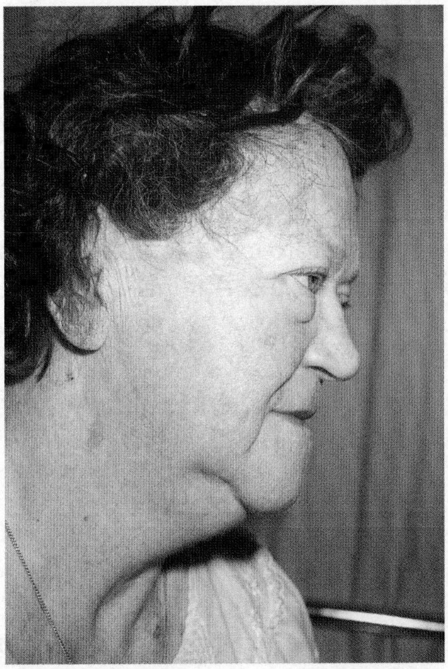

FIGURE 25-12 Myxedema characteristics—facial puffiness, including periorbital edema, lateral eyebrow thinning, and sparse dry, course hair.

- Trauma
- Drugs (sedatives, hypnotics, anesthetics)
- Stroke
- Internal hemorrhage
- Hypoxia
- Hypercapnia
- Hyponatremia
- Hypoglycemia

Management

Prehospital care of myxedema coma is directed toward managing life-threatening conditions (airway, ventilatory, and circulatory compromise) and providing rapid transport to an appropriate medical facility for evaluation by a physician. En route, the patient's body temperature should be maintained and the ECG should be monitored closely for cardiac dysrhythmias. Once other causes of the coma have been ruled out and the patient's condition has been stabilized, treatment of myxedema can begin with oral administration of T_4. This treatment must be continued for life.

NOTE

The goiter associated with thyroid disease affects the patient's neck and throat. It may make for a difficult airway if intubation is required.

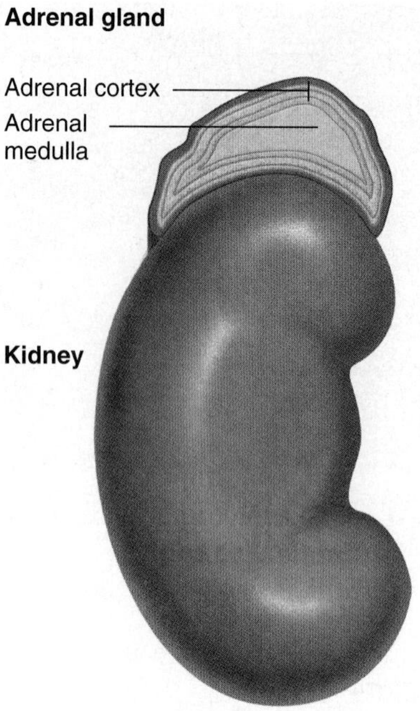

FIGURE 25-13 Adrenal gland.

Disorders of the Adrenal Glands

Two disorders of the adrenal gland are Cushing syndrome and Addison disease. Cushing syndrome is caused by excessive activity of the adrenal cortex. Addison disease is caused by inactivity of the adrenal cortex.

Anatomy and Physiology of the Adrenal Glands

The adrenal glands are triangular-shaped endocrine glands located on top of both kidneys (**FIGURE 25-13**). Each gland consists of a medulla, the center of the gland, which is surrounded by the cortex. The medulla is responsible for producing epinephrine and norepinephrine. The adrenal cortex produces other hormones necessary for fluid and electrolyte balance in the body (eg, cortisone and aldosterone).

Cushing Syndrome

Cushing syndrome is a rare condition caused by an abnormally high circulating level of corticosteroid hormones. It mainly affects women 30 to 50 years of age.[29] The syndrome may be produced directly by an adrenal gland tumor, which causes excessive secretion of corticosteroids. It also may be produced by long-term administration of corticosteroid drugs, such as prednisone, dexamethasone, or methylprednisolone. These drugs are used to treat conditions such as rheumatoid arthritis, inflammatory bowel disease, chronic obstructive pulmonary disease, and asthma. Finally, it may be produced by enlargement of both adrenal glands as a result of a pituitary tumor. The pituitary gland controls the activity of the adrenal gland by producing adrenocorticotropic hormone, which in turn stimulates growth of the adrenal cortex.

People with Cushing syndrome have a characteristic appearance (**FIGURE 25-14**). The face appears round ("moon face") and red (**FIGURE 25-15**). Also, the trunk tends to become obese from disturbances in fat metabolism, whereas the limbs become wasted from muscle atrophy. Acne develops, and purple stretch marks may appear on the abdomen, thighs, and breasts. The skin often thins and bruises easily.

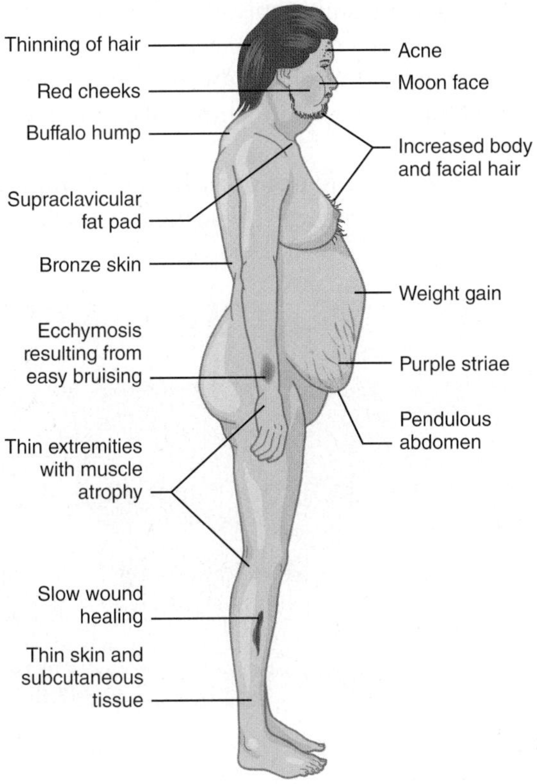

FIGURE 25-14 Characteristic body features associated with Cushing syndrome.

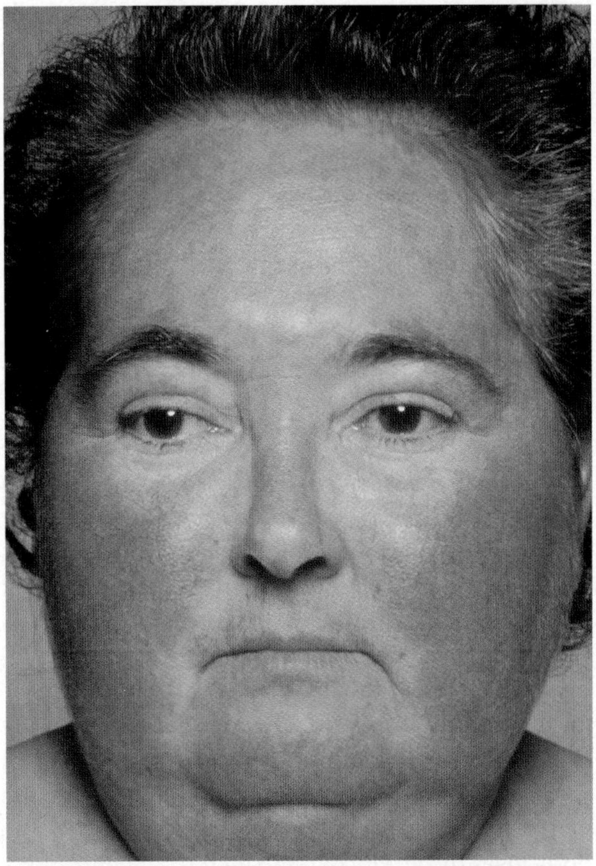

FIGURE 25-15 Moon-faced appearance in a patient with Cushing syndrome.

Weakened bones are at increased risk of fracture. Other features of the disease include the following:

- Increased body and facial hair
- Hump on the back of neck ("buffalo hump")
- Supraclavicular fat pads
- Weight gain
- Hypertension
- Psychiatric disturbances (depression, paranoia)
- Insomnia
- Diabetes mellitus

CRITICAL THINKING

How do you think patients who suffer from Cushing syndrome feel about their body image?

Management

Prehospital care for patients with Cushing syndrome is mainly supportive. The disease is diagnosed through measurement of hormone levels in the blood and urine and by radiologic imaging (eg, computed tomography [CT]). If the cause of the syndrome is overtreatment with corticosteroid drugs, the condition usually is reversible when the drug dosages are adjusted. If the cause is a tumor or overgrowth of the adrenal gland, the gland may require surgical removal. If the tumor is in the pituitary gland, the usual treatment involves surgery, radiation, and medication. Treatment usually is successful, but lifelong hormone replacement therapy is required.

Addison Disease

Addison disease is a rare, sometimes life-threatening disorder caused by a deficiency of the corticosteroid hormones cortisol and aldosterone. Because these hormones normally are produced by the adrenal cortex, Addison disease can be caused by any disease process that destroys the adrenal cortices. Such disease processes may include adrenal hemorrhage or infarction, infections (tuberculosis, fungi, viruses), and autoimmune diseases. However, the most common cause of Addison disease is shrinking of the adrenal tissue. When this occurs, production of corticosteroid hormones is inadequate to meet the body's metabolic requirements. Signs and symptoms associated with this disease include the following:

- Progressive weakness
- Progressive weight loss
- Progressive anorexia
- Skin hyperpigmentation (caused by increased hormone production by the pituitary gland, which stimulates melanin) (**FIGURE 25-16**)
- Hypotension
- Hyponatremia
- Hyperkalemia
- GI disturbances (nausea, vomiting, diarrhea)

Addison disease usually has a slow onset and a chronic course. The symptoms develop gradually over months to years. However, acute episodes (Addisonian crisis) may be brought on by emotional and physiologic stress. Examples of such stressors include surgery, alcohol intoxication, hypothermia, myocardial infarction, severe illness, trauma, hypoglycemia, and infection. During these events, the adrenal glands cannot increase the production of the corticosteroid hormones to help the body cope with stress. As a result, blood glucose levels drop; the body loses the ability to regulate the concentrations of sodium, potassium, and water in body fluids, causing dehydration and extreme muscle weakness; blood volume and blood pressure fall; and the body may not be able to maintain circulation efficiently. In the prehospital setting, airway, ventilatory, and circulatory support are required as immediate treatments. The serum glucose level should be monitored closely. ECG findings as a result of hyperkalemia may include an increase in T-wave amplitude, flattened P waves, and widening of the QRS complex. Some EMS systems carry hydrocortisone (Solu-Cortef) to manage adrenal insufficiency.

NOTE

Many patients with Addison disease carry injectable hydrocortisone in case of crisis. The paramedic may need to contact medical direction for an order to administer the drug to an unstable patient.

Management

In-hospital treatment for Addison disease focuses on maintaining the patient's vital functions and correcting the sodium deficiency and dehydration. After the life-threatening episode has been managed, treatment consists of administration of corticosteroids. The patient often is advised to increase the dosage of these drugs during times of emotional and physiologic stress.

TABLE 25-7 compares the signs and symptoms of Cushing syndrome with those of Addison disease.

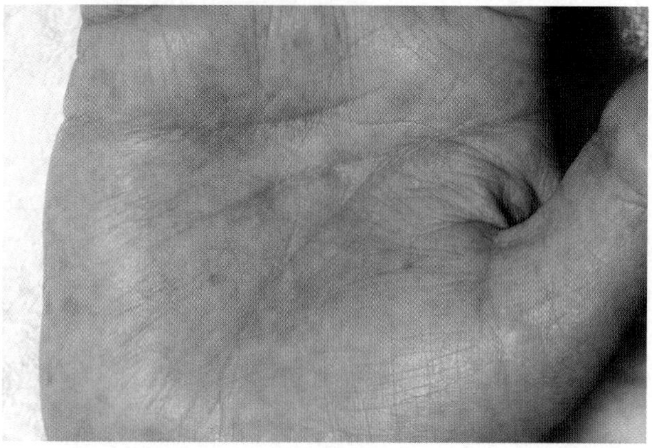

FIGURE 25-16 Hyperpigmentation in a patient with Addison disease.

TABLE 25-7 Signs, Symptoms, and Medications Used in Adrenal Gland Disorders

Corticosteroid Excess (Cushing Syndrome)	Adrenal Insufficiency (Addison Disease)
Weight gain	Weight loss
Weakness	Weakness
Hump on back of neck	Hypotension
Slow healing	Gastrointestinal disorders
Increased body and facial hair	Skin hyperpigmentation (even in areas never exposed to the sun)
Common Medications Used in Treatment	
Pasireotide (Signifor)	Dexamethasone (Decadron)
Metyrapone (Metopirone)	Hydrocortisone (Solu-Cortef)
Ketoconazole	

Summary

- The endocrine system consists of ductless glands and tissues, which produce and secrete a variety of hormones directly into the bloodstream. Hormones, which exert regulatory effects on various metabolic functions, operate within either positive or negative feedback systems that work to maintain the optimal internal environment.
- The pancreatic islets are composed of beta cells (which secrete insulin), alpha cells (which secrete glucagon), and other cells.
- The chief functions of insulin are to increase glucose transport into cells, increase glucose metabolism by cells, increase the liver glycogen level, and decrease the blood glucose concentration toward normal.
- Glucagon has two major effects: (1) It increases blood glucose levels by stimulating the liver to release glucose stores from glycogen and other glucose storage sites (glycogenosis), and (2) it stimulates gluconeogenesis through the breakdown of fats and fatty acids, thereby maintaining a normal blood glucose level.
- Diabetes mellitus is characterized by a deficiency of insulin production or an inability of the body to respond to insulin.
- Type 1 diabetes is caused by inadequate insulin production. Its treatment consists of insulin administration, exercise, and dietary regulation.
- Type 2 diabetes is caused by cellular resistance to insulin and, ultimately, decreased insulin production. Most patients with type 2 diabetes require oral hypoglycemic medications, exercise, and dietary regulation to control the illness, and some require insulin administration.
- Hypoglycemia is a syndrome in which blood glucose levels are less than 70 mg/dL. A patient with diabetes who exhibits behavioral changes or unconsciousness should be treated for hypoglycemia; immediate administration of glucose or glucagon is required to prevent permanent brain damage or death.
- Diabetic ketoacidosis results from an absence of or a resistance to insulin; its signs and symptoms reflect the presence of hypovolemia and usually have a slow onset.
- Hyperosmolar hyperglycemic nonketotic syndrome is a life-threatening emergency that often occurs in older patients with type 2 diabetes and in people with undiagnosed diabetes. The hyperglycemia produces a hyperosmolar state, which causes osmotic diuresis, dehydration, and electrolyte imbalances.
- Important components of the patient history in the assessment of patients with diabetes include the onset of symptoms, food intake, insulin or oral hypoglycemic use, alcohol or other drug consumption, predisposing factors, and any associated symptoms.
- Any patient with a glucose reading less than 70 mg/dL (varies by protocol) and signs and symptoms consistent with hypoglycemia generally should be given glucose.
- Thyroid hormones play a key role in controlling body metabolism and are essential in children to ensure normal physical growth and development.
- Hyperthyroidism is an excess of thyroid hormones in the blood, which may result in thyrotoxicosis. Thyroid storm is a life-threatening condition resulting from an overactive thyroid gland.
- Hypothyroidism is an insufficiency of thyroid hormones in the blood, which may result in myxedema. Myxedema coma is a rare, life-threatening illness that is characterized by hypothermia and altered mental status.
- Cushing syndrome is caused by an abnormally high circulating level of corticosteroid hormones, which are produced naturally by the adrenal glands.
- Addison disease is a rare but life-threatening disorder caused by a deficiency of the corticosteroid hormones cortisol and aldosterone, which are normally produced by the adrenal cortex.

References

1. Statistics about diabetes. American Diabetes Association website. http://www.diabetes.org/diabetes-basics/statistics/. Published 2017. Accessed February 15, 2018.
2. Diagnosing diabetes and learning about prediabetes. American Diabetes Association website. http://www.diabetes.org/diabetes-basics/diagnosis/. Updated November 21, 2016. Accessed February 15, 2018.
3. Lee SH, Zabolotny JM, Huang H, et al. Insulin in the nervous system and the mind: Functions in metabolism, memory, and mood. *Molecular Metabolism.* 2016;5(8):589-601.
4. Centers for Disease Control and Prevention/National Center for Health Statistics. Leading causes of death. Centers for Disease Control and Prevention website. https://www.cdc.gov/nchs/fastats/leading-causes-of-death.htm. Updated March 17, 2017. Accessed February 15, 2018.
5. American Diabetes Association. Classification and diagnosis of diabetes. *Diab Care.* 2015;38(suppl 1):S8-S16.
6. Type 1 diabetes. American Diabetes Association website. http://www.diabetes.org/diabetes-basics/type-1/. Accessed February 15, 2018.
7. Imperatore G, Mayer-Davis E, Orchard TJ, Zhong VW. Prevalence and incidence of type 1 diabetes among children and adults in the United States and comparison with non-US countries. In: Cowie C, Casagrande S, Menke A, et al., eds. *Diabetes in America.* 3rd ed. Bethesda, MD: National Institutes of Health; 2016.
8. Rewers M, Stene LC, Norris JM. Risk factors for type 1 diabetes. In: Cowie C, Casagrande S, Menke A, et al., eds. *Diabetes in America.* 3rd ed. Bethesda, MD: National Institutes of Health; 2016.
9. Nelsen D, Krych L, Buschard K, Hansen CHF, Hansen AK. Beyond genetics: influence of dietary factors and gut microbiota on type 1 diabetes. *FEBS Lett.* 2014;588(22):4234-4243.

10. McCance K, Heuther S. *Pathophysiology: The Biologic Basis for Disease in Adults and Children.* 5th ed. St. Louis, MO: Mosby; 2006.
11. National Institute of Diabetes and Digestive and Kidney Diseases. *Causes of Diabetes* (14-5164). Bethesda, MD: National Institutes of Health; 2014.
12. Herath H, Herath R, Wickremasinghe R. Gestational diabetes mellitus and risk of type 2 diabetes 10 years after the index pregnancy in Sri Lankan women: a community based retrospective cohort study. *PLoS One.* 2017;12(6):e0179647. doi:10.1371/journal.pone.0179647.
13. McCance K, Heuther S. *Pathophysiology: The Biologic Basis for Disease in Adults and Children.* 7th ed. St. Louis, MO: Mosby; 2014.
14. Centers for Disease Control and Prevention. National diabetes statistics report, 2017. Centers for Disease Control and Prevention website. https://www.cdc.gov/diabetes/data/statistics/statistics-report.html. Updated July 17, 2017. Accessed February 14, 2018.
15. National Center for Chronic Disease Prevention and Health Promotion, Centers for Disease Control and Prevention. Diabetic retinopathy. Centers for Disease Control and Prevention website. https://www.cdc.gov/visionhealth/pdf/factsheet.pdf. Accessed February 14, 2018.
16. Cardiovascular disease and diabetes. American Heart Association website. http://www.heart.org/HEARTORG/Conditions/More/Diabetes/WhyDiabetesMatters/Cardiovascular-Disease-Diabetes_UCM_313865_Article.jsp/#.We0DhEyZPOQ. Published August 2015. Accessed February 15, 2018.
17. Diabetes and stroke. National Stroke Association website. http://www.stroke.org/sites/default/files/resources/DiabetesBrochure.pdf. Published 2013. Accessed February 15, 2018.
18. Pancreatic islet transplantation. National Institute of Diabetes and Digestive and Kidney Diseases website. https://www.niddk.nih.gov/health-information/diabetes/overview/insulin-medicines-treatments/pancreatic-islet-transplantation. Published September 2013. Accessed February 15, 2018.
19. Insulin basics. American Diabetes Association website. http://www.diabetes.org/living-with-diabetes/treatment-and-care/medication/insulin/insulin-basics.html. Published July 16, 2015. Accessed February 15, 2018.
20. MannKind Corporation. Afrezza how-to guide. Afrezza website. https://www.afrezza.com/afrezza-how-to-guide/. Published November 2017. Accessed February 15, 2018.
21. Hypoglycemia (low blood glucose). American Diabetes Association website. http://www.diabetes.org/living-with-diabetes/treatment-and-care/blood-glucose-control/hypoglycemia-low-blood.html. Updated July 1, 2015. Accessed February 15, 2018.
22. Karter AJ, Warton EM, Lipska KJ, et al. Development and validation of a tool to identify patients with type 2 diabetes at high risk of hypoglycemia-related emergency department or hospital use. *JAMA Intern Med.* 2017;177(10):1461-1470.
23. Martín-Timón I, del Cañizo-Gómez FJ. Mechanisms of hypoglycemia unawareness and implications in diabetic patients. *World J Diab.* 2015;6(7):912-926.
24. Avichal D. Hyperosmolar hyperglycemic state. Medscape website. https://emedicine.medscape.com/article/1914705-overview. Published March 27, 2017. Accessed February 15, 2018.
25. Gosmanov AR, Gosmanova EO, Kitabchi AE. Hyperglycemic crises: diabetic ketoacidosis (DKA), and hyperglycemic hyperosmolar state (HHS). In: De Groot LJ, Chrousos G, Dungan K, et al., eds. *Endotext* [Internet]. National Center for Biotechnology Information website. https://www.ncbi.nlm.nih.gov/books/NBK279052/. Updated May 19, 2015. Accessed February 15, 2018.
26. National Association of EMS Officials. *National Model EMS Clinical Guidelines*. Version 2.0. National Association of EMS Officials website. https://www.nasemso.org/documents/National-Model-EMS-Clinical-Guidelines-Version2-Sept2017.pdf. Published September 2017. Accessed February 15, 2018.
27. Rickels MR, Ruedy KJ, Foster NC, et al. Intranasal glucagon for treatment of insulin-induced hypoglycemia in adults with type 1 diabetes: a randomized crossover noninferiority study. *Diab Care*. 2015;39(2):264-270.
28. Goldman L, Schafer A. *Goldman-Cecil Medicine.* 25th ed. Philadelphia, PA: Elsevier Saunders; 2016.
29. Endocrine facts and figures: adrenal. Endocrine Society website. http://endocrinefacts.org/health-conditions/adrenal/3-cushings/. Published 2016. Accessed February 15, 2018.

Suggested Readings

Gardner DG, Shoback D. *Greenspan's Basic and Clinical Endocrinology.* 10th ed. New York, NY: McGraw-Hill Education; 2018.

Hsieh A. Four endocrine emergencies EMS providers need to know. EMS1.com website. https://www.ems1.com/ems-products/Medical-Monitoring/articles/3019584-4-endocrine-emergencies-EMS-providers-need-to-know/. August 4, 2015. Accessed February 15, 2018.

Matfin G, ed. *Endocrine and Metabolic Medical Emergencies: A Clinician's Guide.* Washington, DC: Endocrine Press, Endocrine Society; 2014.

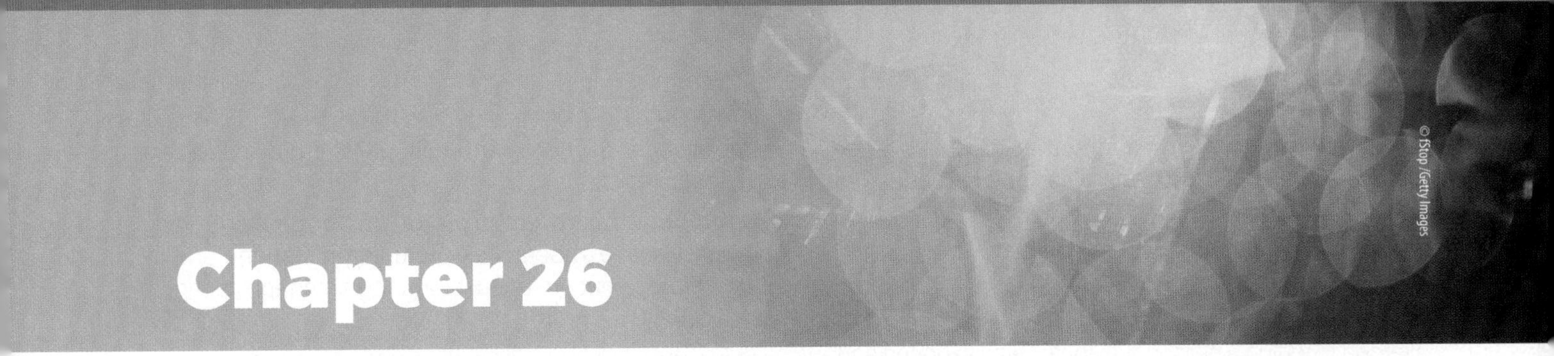

© IStop/Getty Images

Chapter 26

Immune System Disorders

NATIONAL EMS EDUCATION STANDARD COMPETENCIES

Medicine

Integrate assessment findings with principles of epidemiology and pathophysiology to formulate a field impression and implement a comprehensive treatment/disposition plan for a patient with a medical complaint.

Immunology

Recognition and management of shock and difficulty breathing related to
- Anaphylactic reactions (pp 1023–1024, 1026–1027, 1029)

Anatomy, physiology, pathophysiology, assessment, and management of hypersensitivity disorders and/or emergencies
- Allergic and anaphylactic reactions (pp 1019–1029)

Anatomy, physiology, epidemiology, pathophysiology, psychosocial impact, presentations, prognosis, and management of common or major immunologic system disorders and/or emergencies
- Hypersensitivity (pp 1019–1021)
- Allergic and anaphylactic reactions (pp 1019–1029)
- Anaphylactoid reactions (p 1022)
- Collagen vascular diseases (pp 1029–1032)
- Transplant-related problems (pp 1032–1035)

OBJECTIVES

Upon completion of this chapter, the paramedic student will be able to:

1. Outline the structure of the immune system. (pp 1015–1016)
2. Distinguish between natural and acquired immunity. (pp 1017–1018)
3. Differentiate between a normal immune response and an allergic reaction. (pp 1018–1021)
4. Describe the antigen–antibody response. (p 1019)
5. Distinguish among the four types of hypersensitivity reaction. (p 1021)
6. Describe the signs, symptoms, and management of local allergic reactions based on an understanding of the pathophysiology associated with this condition. (p 1022)
7. Identify allergens associated with anaphylaxis. (p 1022)
8. Describe the pathophysiology, signs and symptoms, and management of anaphylaxis. (pp 1022–1029)
9. Describe the pathophysiology, signs and symptoms, and management of anaphylactoid reaction. (pp 1022–1029)
10. Define collagen vascular disease and explain its relationship to autoimmune disease. (pp 1029–1030)
11. Describe the pathophysiology, signs and symptoms, and prehospital considerations for patients who have systemic lupus erythematosus. (pp 1030–1031)
12. Describe the pathophysiology, signs and symptoms, and prehospital considerations for patients who have scleroderma. (pp 1031–1032)
13. Identify major complications associated with organ transplantation. (pp 1032–1035)
14. Identify infections associated with organ transplantation. (pp 1032–1034)
15. Identify characteristics of organ rejection. (p 1034)
16. Recognize side effects associated with antirejection medications. (pp 1034–1035)

KEY TERMS

acquired immunity Immunity that develops after exposure to specific antigens; also known as adaptive immunity.

allergens Antigens that can produce hypersensitivity reactions in the body.

allergic reaction A hypersensitivity response to an allergen to which a person previously was exposed and to which the person has developed antibodies.

allografting The transplantation of cells, tissues, or organs between nonidentical (genetically unrelated) people.

anaphylactoid reaction An allergic reaction that is not mediated by an antigen–antibody reaction. It presents exactly like anaphylaxis but does not require previous exposure.

anaphylaxis An exaggerated, life-threatening hypersensitivity reaction to an antigen.

angioedema A localized edematous reaction of the deep dermal or subcutaneous or submucosal tissues that appears as giant wheals.

antibodies Substances produced by the body that destroy or inactivate a specific substance (antigen) that has entered the body.

antigen–antibody reaction The binding of an antibody with an antigen of the type that stimulated the formation of the antibody. This binding makes the antigen more susceptible to ingestion and destruction by phagocytes or neutralization of an exotoxin.

antigens Substances (usually proteins) that are capable of generating an immune response causing the formation of an antibody that reacts specifically with that antigen.

autoimmune disease A condition that occurs when the immune system mistakenly attacks and destroys healthy body tissue.

B lymphocytes The lymphocytes responsible for antibody-mediated immunity.

basophils White blood cells that promote inflammation.

biphasic reaction An anaphylactic reaction that resolves and then recurs hours later without further exposure to the trigger.

cell-mediated immunity Immunity characterized by the formation of a population of lymphocytes that attack and destroy foreign material.

collagen vascular disease An autoimmune disease characterized by inflammation in the connective tissues. It results in the accumulation of extra antibodies in the circulation.

degranulation A cellular process that releases antimicrobial substances from secretory vesicles (granules) found inside mast cells and basophils. It plays a role in allergic reactions.

eosinophil chemotactic factor of anaphylaxis A group of active substances, including histamine and leukotrienes, that are released during an anaphylactic reaction.

eosinophils White blood cells that act as a cell mediator of inflammation. They are thought to release leukotrienes.

erythema Redness of the skin, caused by hyperemia of the capillaries in the lower layers of the skin.

Fc receptors Proteins found on the surface of certain cells that contribute to the protective functions of the immune system. These receptors bind to antibodies that are attached to infected cells or invading pathogens.

histamine An amine released by mast cells and basophils that promotes inflammation.

humoral immunity One of the two forms of immunity that respond to antigens such as bacteria and foreign tissue.

immune system A complex network of cells, tissues, and organs that work together to protect the body against "attacks" by foreign substances.

immunoglobulin A (IgA) An antibody that plays a crucial role in mucosal immunity.

immunoglobulin D (IgD) An antibody present on the surface of most, but not all, B cells early in their development. It signals B cells to activate.

immunoglobulin E (IgE) An antibody that plays an important role in allergies. It is especially associated with type I anaphylactic reactions.

immunoglobulin G (IgG) The most abundant antibody. It is equally distributed in blood and tissue liquids.

immunoglobulin M (IgM) A basic antibody that produces B cells; the first antibody to appear in response to initial exposure to an antigen.

immunologic memory The body's ability to rapidly produce large numbers of specific immune cells after subsequent exposure to a previously encountered antigen.

immunology A broad branch of medical science that covers the study of the immune system.

immunosuppression Reduction in the activation or efficiency of the immune system. It often is caused by drugs or radiation administered to prevent the rejection of grafts or transplanted tissues or to control autoimmune disease.

isografting The transplantation of cells, tissues, or organs between identical twins.

leukotrienes A class of biologically active compounds that occur naturally in leukocytes and that produce allergic and inflammatory reactions.

lymphocyte A type of white blood cell formed in the lymphoid tissue.

macrophages Phagocytic cells in the immune system.

mast cells Specialized cells of the inflammatory response.

memory cells Cells that remember a pathogen so that antibody production to the same pathogen can occur more rapidly with future exposures. They are produced by the division of B cells.

natural immunity Non–antigen-specific immunity that is present at birth; also known as innate immunity or nonspecific immunity.

neutrophils Small, phagocytic white blood cells with a lobed nucleus and small granules in the cytoplasm.

organ transplantation The replacement of a failing organ with a healthy one from a donor.

pathogen A disease-causing agent.

pathogenic microbe A microscopic pathogen, such as a bacterium, parasite, fungus, or virus, that can cause infection.

phagocytosis The process by which cells ingest solid substances such as other cells, bacteria, bits of necrosed tissue, and foreign particles.

pruritus A sensation that causes the desire or reflex to scratch.

Raynaud phenomenon A condition in which cold temperatures or strong emotions cause blood vessel spasms that block blood flow to the fingers, toes, ears, and nose.

scleroderma A collagen vascular disease thought to arise when the immune system stimulates certain cells (fibroblasts) that cause increased production of collagen.

sensitization An acquired reaction in which specific antibodies develop in response to an antigen.

systemic lupus erythematosus (SLE) A chronic inflammatory autoimmune disease that affects many systems of the body. It is characterized by severe vasculitis, renal involvement, and lesions of the skin and nervous system.

T lymphocytes The lymphocytes responsible for cell-mediated immunity.

thromboxanes Antagonistic prostaglandin derivatives that are synthesized and released by degranulating platelets, causing vasoconstriction and promoting the degranulation of other platelets.

urticaria A pruritic skin eruption characterized by transient wheals of various shapes and sizes that have well-defined margins and pale centers; also known as hives.

wheals Small areas of swelling of the skin that result from an allergic reaction.

Immunology *is a broad branch of medical science that covers the study of the immune system. A healthy immune system is the body's best defense against disease. However, sometimes the immune system goes awry, and the body begins to attack its own tissues and organs. People with immune system disorders are susceptible to a number of diseases, some of which can be life threatening. This chapter reviews the immune system and some of the more common immune disorders that may be encountered in the prehospital setting. These disorders include allergic reaction and anaphylaxis, collagen vascular disease, and transplant disorders.*

Overview of the Immune System

The **immune system** is a complex network of cells, tissues, and organs that work together to protect the body against "attacks" by foreign substances. Most of these foreign substances come in the form of a **pathogenic microbe**, which is a microscopic **pathogen**. Examples include bacteria, parasites, fungi, and viruses that can cause infection. The primary role of the immune system is to prevent these foreign substances from entering the body. If that fails, the immune system launches an attack so that these foreign bodies are found and destroyed.

Immune System Structure

The organs of the immune system include the spleen, tonsils, adenoids, lymph nodes, and thymus (**FIGURE 26-1**). These organs are positioned throughout the body and are important outposts for lymphocytes, the key players in the immune system.

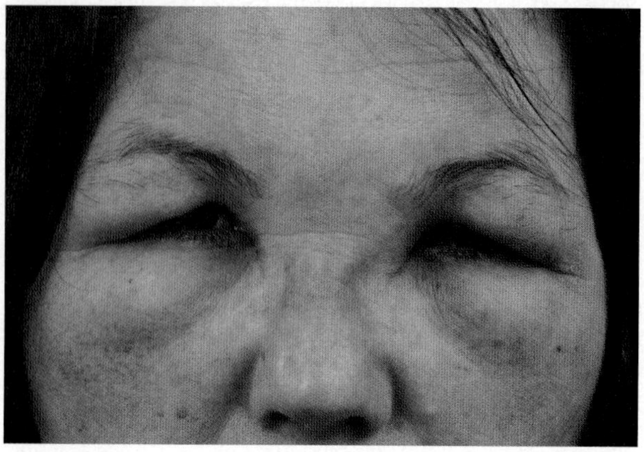

© SPL/Science Source

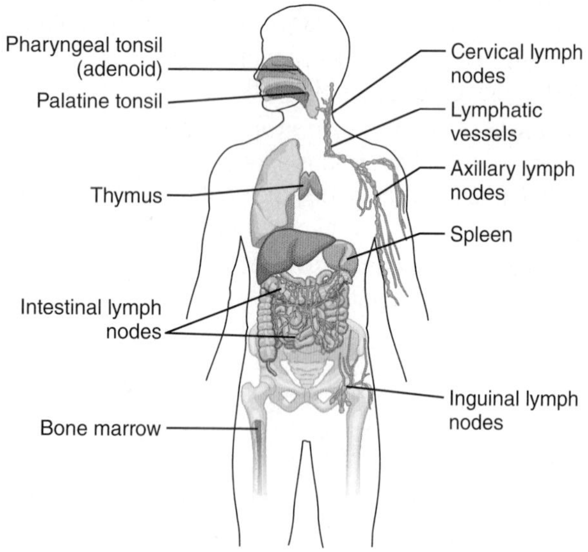

FIGURE 26-1 Structures of the immune system.

© Jones & Bartlett Learning.

Lymphocytes

The **lymphocyte** is the fundamental cellular unit of the immune system. Approximately 25% of circulating white blood cells are lymphocytes. Lymphocytes are divided into two major classes that have different and complementary roles: **B lymphocytes** (B cells) and **T lymphocytes** (T cells).

B cells produce **antibodies**—proteins that act as "magic bullets" by seeking out specific invaders, or antigens. **Antigens** have marker molecules that identify them as foreign. When antibodies find these antigens, they trigger a process that destroys the invaders. The antibodies in blood and lymph make up the body's **humoral immunity**—that is, the form of immunity that responds to antigens, such as bacteria and foreign tissue.

NOTE

The process by which leukocytes destroy and digest pathogens is called **phagocytosis**. Circulating **macrophages** are specialized white cells that are responsible for clearing the area of the resulting dead cells and debris.

Like B cells, T cells also respond only to specific organisms, but instead of producing antibodies, they perform other tasks. The work of T cells, called **cell-mediated immunity**, activates lymphocytes that attack and destroy foreign material. There are three varieties of T cells:

- Killer T cells attack the invading organism with chemicals.
- Helper T cells encourage B cells to produce antibodies.
- Suppressor T cells help regulate the immune response to protect the body from its own defense.

DID YOU KNOW?

Anatomy of an Antibody

There are five varieties of antibodies: **immunoglobulin A (IgA)**, **immunoglobulin D (IgD)**, **immunoglobulin E (IgE)**, **immunoglobulin G (IgG)**, and **immunoglobulin M (IgM)**. IgA is found mainly in the body's mucous membranes, where it intercepts antigens in the nose and throat. IgE binds to certain antigens to cause allergic reactions. The exact function of IgD is largely unknown, but it is thought to bind to basophils and mast cells, activating the cells to produce antimicrobial factors that participate in the respiratory immune defense. The largest antibody is IgM, while the most common antibody is IgG. Together, these two play the major role in attacking many bacteria and other antigens.

Each antibody consists of chains of amino acids (the building blocks of protein). In the antibody, two long, thick amino chains join to form a Y, with two smaller, thin chains positioned along each branch of the Y (**FIGURE 26-2**). At the end of these four chains, the antibody binds with a specific antigen, similar to a lock and key arrangement. The *class* of immunoglobulin (eg, IgG or IgM) determines whether the antibody is able to destroy antigens through an enzymatic chain reaction in the bloodstream.

Modified from: Kato A, Hulse KE, Tan BK, Schleimer RP. B lymphocyte lineage cells and the respiratory system. *J Allergy Clin Immunol.* 2013;131(4):933-957.

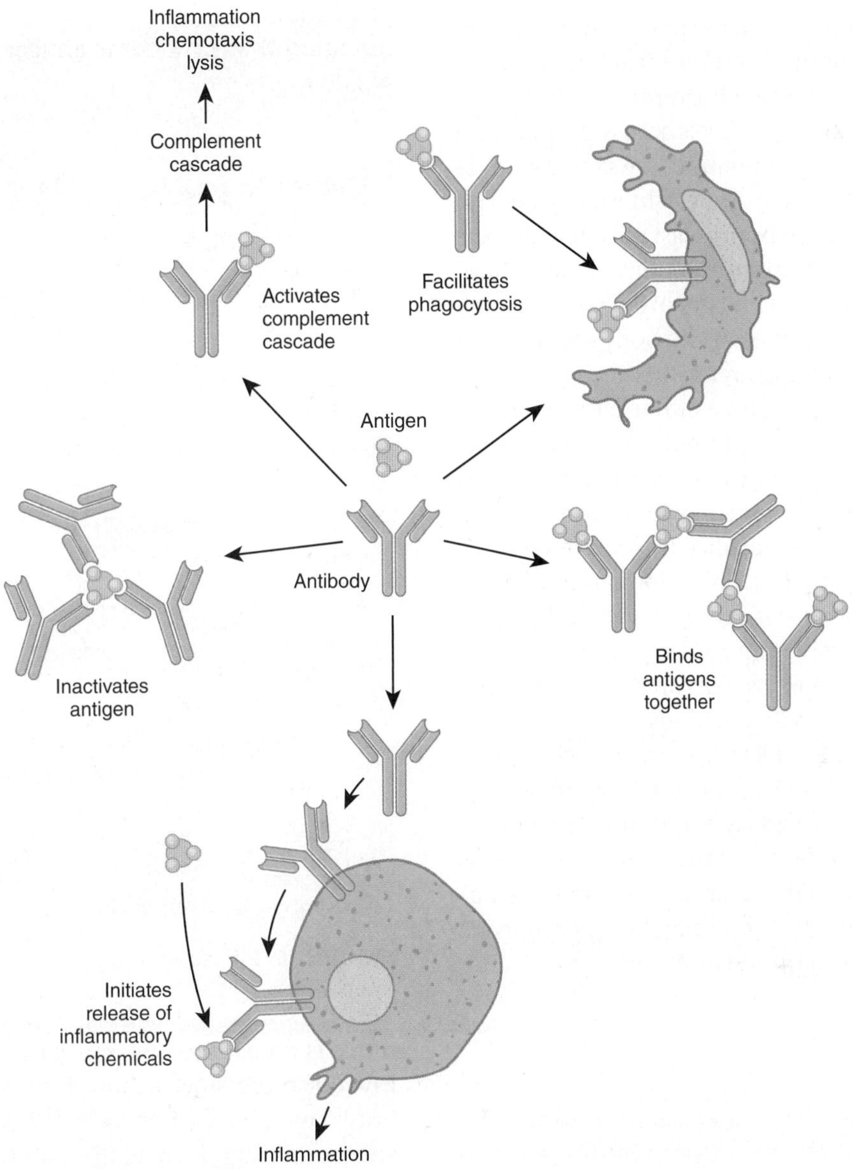

FIGURE 26-2 Antibodies act on antigens by inactivating and binding them together to facilitate phagocytosis and by initiating inflammation and activating the complement cascade.

Natural and Acquired Immunity

Once B cells and T cells have been activated by an antigen, some of these cells become **memory cells**. Many of the memory cells take up permanent residence in the lymph nodes, the gastrointestinal (GI) tract, and the spleen. Other memory cells travel through the lymphatic system and bloodstream. There, they join with other lymphocytes and remain on guard for their chosen antigen. Memory cells ensure that the next time the body is exposed to the same antigen that produced the memory cell, the immune system is set into motion to destroy it. This memory is known as **immunologic memory**, and the process by which it occurs is known as immunity. Immunity can be either natural or acquired.

Natural Immunity

Natural immunity, also known as innate immunity or nonspecific immunity, is immunity that exists "naturally." This type of immunity is not antigen-specific and does not require previous exposure to an antigen. Instead, natural immunity is present at birth because of antibodies that the newborn receives from the mother. For example, IgG travels across the placenta and makes the newborn immune to the same microbes to which the mother is immune, while children who are breastfed receive IgA from breast milk that protects the infant's stomach. Natural immunity also may have a heritable component. This type of immunity, which is quick to respond, serves as the body's first line of defense against invading organisms.

Natural immunity can be either passive or active. The natural immunity present at birth is passive. Passive immunity also can be conveyed through serum obtained from a person who is immune to a specific infectious agent (artificially acquired passive immunity). For example, gamma globulin sometimes is given to travelers who visit countries where hepatitis is widespread. Passive immunity usually provides protection for only a few weeks and also carries the risk of causing sensitivity reactions.

Active immunity can be triggered by infection and vaccination. For example, exposure to a person with an illness can provide active immunity. The person exposed to the specific agent that caused the illness becomes immune to that specific disease. Vaccinations given with inactive (noninfectious) pathogens also provide active acquired immunity.

TABLE 26-1 Characteristics of Natural and Acquired Immunity

Natural Immunity	Acquired Immunity
Is not antigen dependent	Is antigen dependent
Results in immediate response	Requires time between exposure and response
Results in no immunologic memory	Results in immunologic memory

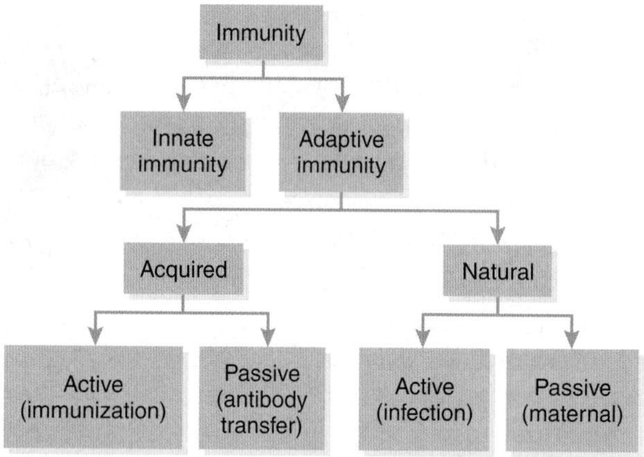

FIGURE 26-3 Passive versus active immunity.

NOTE

Passive natural immunity is achieved by the transfer of antibodies produced by one person to another person. Active natural immunity is achieved by the production of antibodies against a specific agent by the immune system. Natural immunity provides short-term protection for immediate threats but does not change or prepare the immune system for future challenges.

Acquired Immunity

Acquired immunity, also known as adaptive immunity, is immunity that develops after exposure to specific antigens. This type of immunity is "acquired" after the activation of B cells and T cells, which creates immunologic memory. Acquired immunity also may occur through immunization with a vaccine that contains a weak form of a specific antigen. Acquired immunity generally is a long-term immunity and often is considered permanent. It responds to an invader more slowly than does natural immunity, but it significantly improves the rate of response to subsequent exposure to the same antigen. Acquired immunity acts as the body's second line of defense against invading organisms (**TABLE 26-1**). Like natural immunity, acquired immunity can be passive (acquired by the transfer of antibodies) or active (through immunization) (**FIGURE 26-3**).

NOTE

Acquired immunity is obtained deliberately. It changes and prepares the immune system to respond to future challenges.

Immune Response

The first two lines of defense against infection use the same mechanism to respond to all pathogens, though the immune response is specific to individual pathogens (see Chapter 27, *Infectious and Communicable Diseases*). The immune system that makes up the immune response has four unique characteristics:

1. It can distinguish between "self" and "nonself" molecules; therefore, it usually responds only to foreign antigens.
2. It produces antigen-specific antibodies; that is, new antibodies can be produced in response to new antigens.
3. The memory cells produced by some of the antibody-producing lymphocytes allow for a more rapid response to repeat invasions by the same antigen.
4. The immune system is self-regulated, becoming activated only when a pathogen invades. This ability prevents healthy tissues from being destroyed. When this function goes awry, allergic reactions and autoimmune disease can occur. The immune system also may require extrinsic regulation with drugs in patients with transplanted organs or severe autoimmune diseases.

CRITICAL THINKING

Which major immune disorder causes life-threatening airway, breathing, and circulation problems?

Allergic Reactions

Antigens can enter the body exogenously (from the outside) by injection, ingestion, inhalation, or absorption (see Chapter 33, *Toxicology*). Once in the body, antigens stimulate the immune system to produce antibodies, which then help neutralize the antigens and remove them from the body. This normal **antigen–antibody reaction** protects the body from disease by activating the immune response.

The immune responses usually are protective, but sometimes they may become oversensitive to harmless antigens to which people are routinely exposed (eg, ragweed, pollen). Such responses are termed allergic. Antigens or substances that cause an allergic response are called **allergens**. Common allergens include drugs, insect bites or stings, foods, latex (**BOX 26-1**), animals, pollens, and mold. The healthy body responds to an antigen challenge by activating its immunity defenses.

An **allergic reaction** (also known as a hypersensitivity reaction) is marked by an increased physiologic response to an antigen after a previous exposure to the same antigen—a process known as **sensitization**. The allergic reaction starts when a circulating antibody combines with a specific foreign antigen, resulting in hypersensitivity reactions, or with antibodies bound to mast cells or basophils. To review, **mast cells**, which are found in several types of tissues, contain granules that are rich in histamine and heparin. Mast cells are similar to **basophils**, a class of white blood cells that promote inflammation through the release of chemical mediators (described later in the chapter). Mast cells and basophils and the release of these chemicals play an important role in allergic reactions (**FIGURE 26-4**).

Allergic reactions can be mild, moderate, or severe, including anaphylaxis. Mild and moderate reactions usually are localized, affecting the skin, upper and lower airways, and GI tract. They are not

BOX 26-1 Latex Allergies

Latex allergy was relatively unknown until the acquired immunodeficiency syndrome (AIDS) epidemic in the mid-1980s, which resulted in a tremendous increase in glove use. In addition to gloves, health care workers and latex-sensitive patients can be exposed to latex on medical instruments, surgical equipment, and other medical appliances.

The symptoms of latex allergy can range from mild discomfort to life-threatening anaphylaxis. Most often the first manifestation of a latex allergy is urticaria, which typically is localized to the hands but may be widespread. A type I hypersensitivity to latex can manifest in symptoms that include rash, lacrimation, rhinitis, wheezing, bronchospasm, laryngeal edema, hypotension, dysrhythmia, and, in rare cases, respiratory or cardiac arrest.

Health care facilities, EMS agencies, and other public services agencies have addressed this issue by developing "latex-safe" environments and by using latex-free gloves and equipment. Most health care workers wear low-protein, powder-free gloves when latex gloves are necessary and latex-free synthetic gloves (neoprene, polyisoprene, or vinyl gloves) when the risk of exposure to bloodborne pathogens is low. All patients should be questioned about latex allergy; people with latex allergy should wear appropriate medical-alert identification. Sensitivity to latex should be documented on the patient care report, and this information should be conveyed to medical direction.

Modified from: Gad SC, McCord MG. *Safety Evaluation in the Development of Medical Devices and Combination Products*. 3rd ed. Boca Raton, FL: CRC Press; 2008.

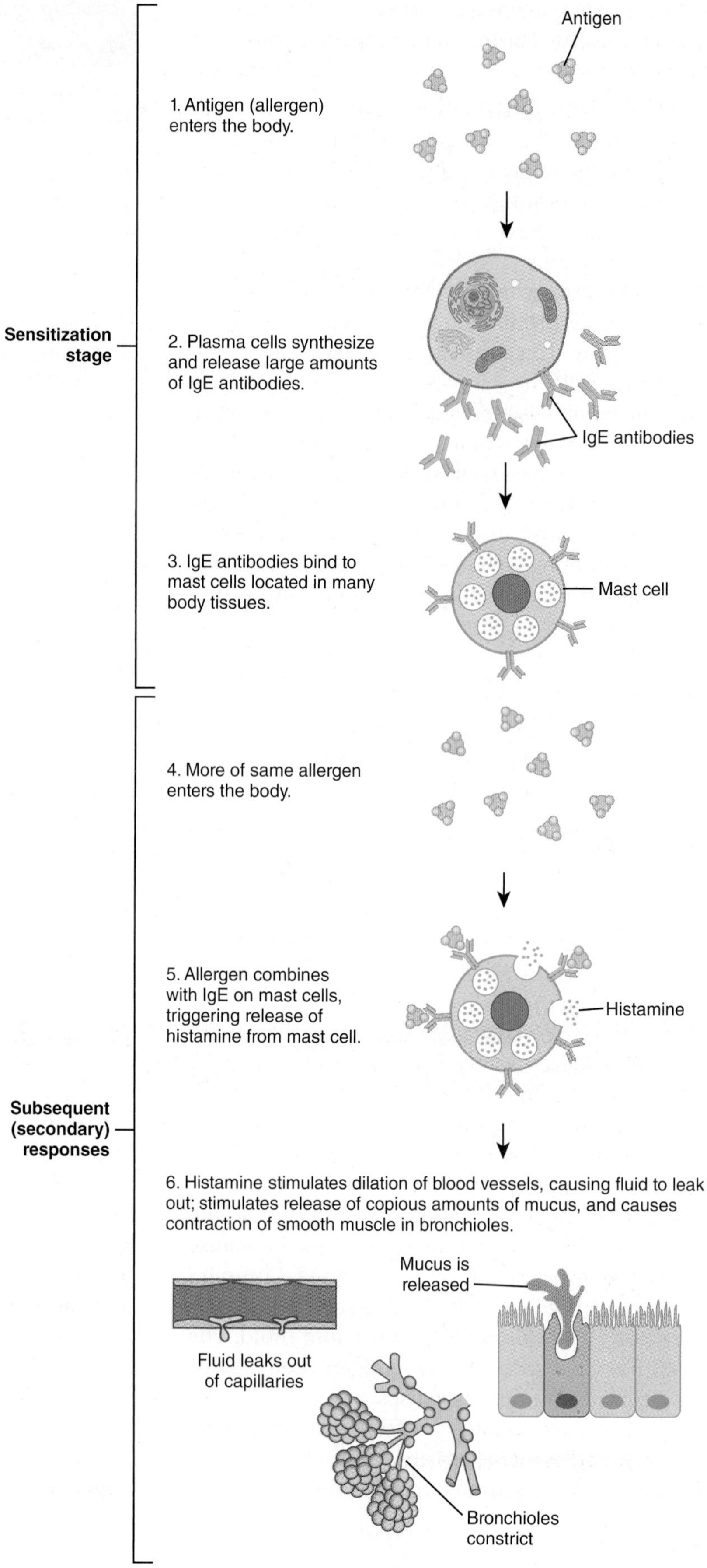
Antigen
1. Antigen (allergen) enters the body.
Sensitization stage
2. Plasma cells synthesize and release large amounts of IgE antibodies.
IgE antibodies
3. IgE antibodies bind to mast cells located in many body tissues.
Mast cell
4. More of same allergen enters the body.
5. Allergen combines with IgE on mast cells, triggering release of histamine from mast cell.
Histamine
Subsequent (secondary) responses
6. Histamine stimulates dilation of blood vessels, causing fluid to leak out; stimulates release of copious amounts of mucus, and causes contraction of smooth muscle in bronchioles.
Mucus is released
Fluid leaks out of capillaries
Bronchioles constrict

Abbreviation: IgE, immunoglobulin E

FIGURE 26-4 In an allergic reaction, antigen stimulates the production of massive amounts of immunoglobulin E (IgE), a type of antibody produced by plasma cells. IgE attaches to mast cells. This is the sensitization stage. When the antigen enters again, it binds to the IgE antibodies on the mast cells, triggering a massive release of histamine and other chemicals. Histamine, in turn, causes blood vessels to dilate and become leaky, which triggers the production of mucus in the respiratory tract. In some people, the chemicals released by the mast cells cause the small air-carrying ducts in the lungs to constrict, making breathing difficult.

life threatening. Severe allergic reactions affect the same body systems but may be life threatening.

Types of Hypersensitivity Reactions

Hypersensitivity reactions are divided into four distinct types (**TABLE 26-2**):

- **Type I.** Immediate (IgE-mediated) reactions
- **Type II.** Cytotoxic (tissue-specific) reactions
- **Type III.** Immune complex–mediated reactions
- **Type IV.** Delayed (cell-mediated) reactions

A type I (immediate) reaction is the most dramatic; it may lead to life-threatening anaphylaxis (described later).

BOX 26-2 presents examples of antigens that may cause hypersensitivity reactions. Patients who have a known sensitivity to these or other agents should avoid exposure.

TABLE 26-2 Comparison of Hypersensitivity Types

Characteristics	Type I (Immediate)	Type II (Cytotoxic)	Type III (Immune Complex)	Type IV (Delayed)
Antibody	IgE	IgG, IgM	IgG, IgM	None
Antigen	Exogenous	Cell surface	Viral (soluble)	Tissues and organs
Onset	Within minutes	Minutes to hours	3–8 hours	48–72 hours
Appearance	Wheal and flare	Lysis and necrosis	Erythema, edema, necrosis	Erythema and sclerosis
Cell type (histology)	Basophils and eosinophils	Antibody and complement	Complement and neutrophils	Monocytes and lymphocytes
Initiated by	Antibody	Antibody	Antibody	T cells
Examples	Urticaria, hay fever	Hemolytic anemia, glomerulonephritis	Systemic lupus erythematosus, serum sickness	Contact dermatitis, transplant rejection

Abbreviations: IgE, immunoglobulin E; IgG, immunoglobulin G; IgM, immunoglobulin M

BOX 26-2 Agents That May Commonly Cause Allergies and Anaphylaxis

Drugs and Biologic Agents

Antibiotics
Anticancer agents
Aspirin
Cephalosporins
Chemotherapeutics
Insulin
Local anesthetics
Muscle relaxants
Nonsteroidal anti-inflammatory agents
Opiates
Vaccines

Insect Bites and Stings

Bees
Fire ants
Hornets
Wasps

Food

Cod, halibut, shellfish (eg, shrimp)
Cottonseed
Egg white
Food additives
Mango
Milk
Peanuts, soybeans
Sesame and sunflower seeds
Strawberries
Tree-grown nuts
Wheat and buckwheat

Other

Intravenous (IV) contrast agents

CRITICAL THINKING

Consider the list of antigens in Box 26-2. Based on this list, what are some likely locations to which you may be dispatched to care for a patient experiencing an anaphylactic reaction?

Localized Allergic Reactions

Contact with an allergen bridges adjacent antibodies. Each antibody binds with the invading organism at a different site, which in turn changes the alignment of the antibodies on the surface of the mast cell. As a result, the mast cell bursts and releases active chemical mediators into the surrounding fluid. Localized allergic reactions do not involve the entire body; that is, the sites of mast cell and basophil mediator release are limited. Common signs and symptoms of localized allergic reactions include the following:

- Conjunctivitis (inflammation of the conjunctiva of the eyes)
- Rhinitis (runny nose)
- Angioedema (swelling)
- Urticaria (hives)
- Pruritus (itching)

Localized allergic reactions are best managed with drugs that compete with histamine for receptor sites. This competition prevents histamine from performing its physiologic actions (described later). Common antihistamines include over-the-counter oral and nasal decongestants and prescription and nonprescription diphenhydramine. Other medications that may be helpful for some local reactions include steroids and topical creams.

Anaphylaxis

Anaphylaxis is an immediate, systemic, life-threatening allergic reaction that is associated with major changes in the cardiovascular, respiratory, GI, and/or cutaneous systems. Prompt recognition and appropriate drug therapy in the prehospital phase are vital to the patient's survival. Although deaths are rare due to prompt treatment, anaphylactic reactions are not. Anaphylaxis, a term derived from Greek words meaning "against or opposite of protection," is the most extreme form of an allergic reaction, accounting for 63 to 99 deaths each year in the United States.[1] Rapid recognition and aggressive therapy are essential in treating this disorder, as most deaths from anaphylaxis occur within 1 hour of onset of symptoms.[2]

Causative Agents

Almost any substance can cause anaphylaxis. The antigenic agents most frequently associated with anaphylaxis are foods (especially nuts and shellfish), followed by drugs such as penicillin (by ingestion or injection).[2] Regardless of the offending antigen, in people with sensitivity, the risk of anaphylaxis increases with each exposure. To a lesser extent, the risk increases with the length of exposure or site of inoculation.

Pathophysiology of Anaphylaxis

A person first must be exposed to a specific antigen to develop hypersensitivity. In the first exposure, the antigen enters the body by injection, ingestion, inhalation, or absorption, whereupon it activates the immune system. In susceptible people, large amounts of IgE antibody are produced during this response. These IgE antibodies leave the lymphatic system and bind to IgE-specific **Fc receptors** on the cell membranes of basophils that are circulating in the blood and to mast cells that are in tissues surrounding the blood vessels. The antibodies remain there in an inactive state until the same antigen is introduced into the body a second time (**FIGURE 26-5**). With the next exposure to the specific antigen, the allergen cross-links at least two of the cell-bound IgE molecules, resulting in **degranulation** (release of internal substances) of the mast cells and basophils and the onset of anaphylaxis (**BOX 26-3**).

NOTE

An **anaphylactoid reaction** is an allergic reaction that is not mediated by an antigen–antibody reaction. These reactions present exactly as anaphylaxis does but do not require previous exposure to occur. For example, an anaphylactoid reaction can be caused by an IV medication that produces an excessive release of histamine in some patients. The distinction is not crucial with regard to treatment of an acute reaction; the two conditions are treated in the same way.

Modified from: Walls RM, Hockberger RS, Gausche-Hill M. *Rosen's Emergency Medicine: Concepts and Clinical Practice.* 9th ed. St. Louis, MO: Elsevier; 2018.

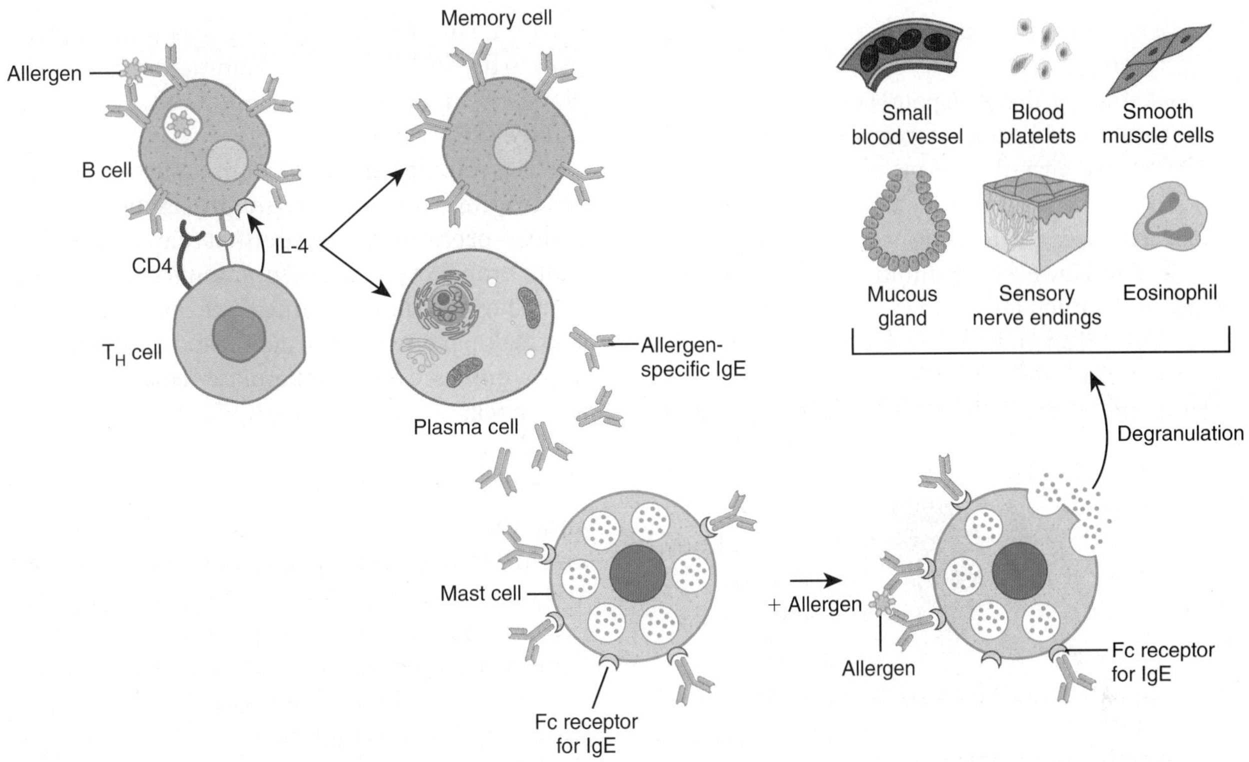

Abbreviations: CD4, cluster of differentiation 4; IgE, immunoglobulin E; IL-4, interleukin 4

FIGURE 26-5 General mechanism underlying an allergic reaction. Exposure to an allergen activates B cells to form immunoglobulin E (IgE)-secreting plasma cells. The secreted IgE molecules bind to IgE-specific Fc receptors on mast cells and basophils. After a second exposure to the allergen, the bound IgE is cross-linked, which triggers the release of pharmacologically active mediators from mast cells and basophils. The mediators cause smooth muscle contraction, increased vascular permeability, and vasodilation.

BOX 26-3 Anaphylaxis

Three conditions must be met for sensitization of a person and generation of an anaphylactic response:

1. Antigen-induced stimulation of the immune system must occur, with specific IgE antibody formation.
2. A latent period must follow the initial antigenic exposure, to allow for sensitization of mast cells and basophils.
3. The person must subsequently be exposed to the same specific antigen.

Degranulation of the target cell is associated with the release of pharmacologically active chemical mediators from inside the affected basophils and mast cells. These chemicals include histamine, leukotrienes, eosinophil chemotactic factor of anaphylaxis, **neutrophils**, heparin, kinins, prostaglandins, and **thromboxanes**. All of these chemicals mediate or trigger an internal systemic response.

Histamine is a protein released by mast cells and basophils. It promotes vascular permeability and causes dilation of capillaries and venules and contraction of smooth muscle in the GI tract and bronchial tree. An associated increase in gastric, nasal, and lacrimal secretions also occurs, resulting in tearing and rhinorrhea. The increased capillary permeability allows plasma to leak into the interstitial space, thereby reducing the amount of intravascular volume available for the heart to pump. The profound body-wide vasodilation further reduces cardiac preload, which in turn decreases stroke volume and cardiac output. Collectively, these responses lead to flushing, urticaria, angioedema, and hypotension (**FIGURE 26-6**). Although the onset of action for histamine is rapid, its effects are short-lived, because they are quickly broken down by plasma enzymes.

FIGURE 26-7 illustrates the pathophysiology of anaphylactic shock.

Leukotrienes, the most potent of the bronchoconstrictors, cause wheezing, coronary vasoconstriction, and increased vascular permeability. Leukotrienes formerly were known as slow-reacting substances of anaphylaxis, because their effects were delayed relative to histamine. However, the duration of action of these chemicals is much longer than that of histamine.

Eosinophil chemotactic factor of anaphylaxis is a group of active substances, including histamine and leukotrienes, that are released during an anaphylactic reaction. The process of anaphylaxis attracts **eosinophils** to the site of allergic inflammation; these white blood cells are thought to contain an enzyme that can release leukotrienes.

The remaining chemical mediators—heparin, neutrophils, thromboxanes, prostaglandins, and kinins—exert varying effects that may include fever, chills, bronchospasm, and pulmonary vasoconstriction. These complex chemical processes can rapidly lead to upper airway obstruction and bronchospasm, dysrhythmias, cardiac ischemia, circulatory collapse, and shock.

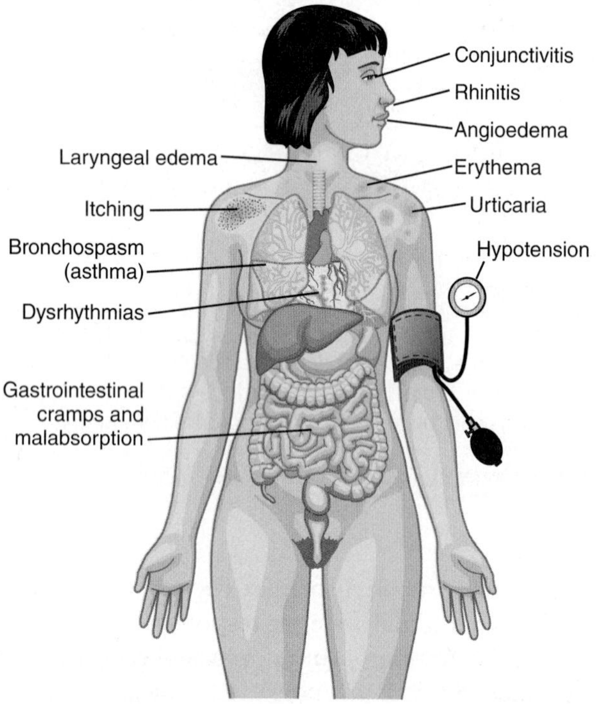

FIGURE 26-6 Manifestation of allergic reactions as a result of type I hypersensitivity includes itching, angioedema (swelling of the face, hands, feet, or genitals), edema of the larynx, urticaria (hives), bronchospasm, hypotension, dysrhythmias, and gastrointestinal cramping caused by inflammation of the gastrointestinal mucosa.

Assessment Findings

An accurate history and physical assessment are necessary to differentiate between severe allergic reactions and other conditions that may mimic anaphylaxis (BOX 26-4). A flawed prehospital assessment in patients with these conditions can have life-threatening consequences. Disease entities that may present similar signs and symptoms of anaphylaxis include the following:

- Severe asthma with respiratory failure
- Upper airway obstruction
- Toxic or septic shock
- Pulmonary edema (with or without myocardial infarction)
- Drug overdose
- Dystonic reaction to antipsychotics
- Scombroid poisoning
- Angiotensin-converting enzyme (ACE) inhibitor angioedema
- Hypovolemic shock

Respiratory Effects

The initial signs of respiratory involvement associated with anaphylaxis may vary (BOX 26-5). Signs may range from sneezing and coughing to complete airway obstruction, caused by laryngeal and epiglottic edema. The patient may complain of throat tightness

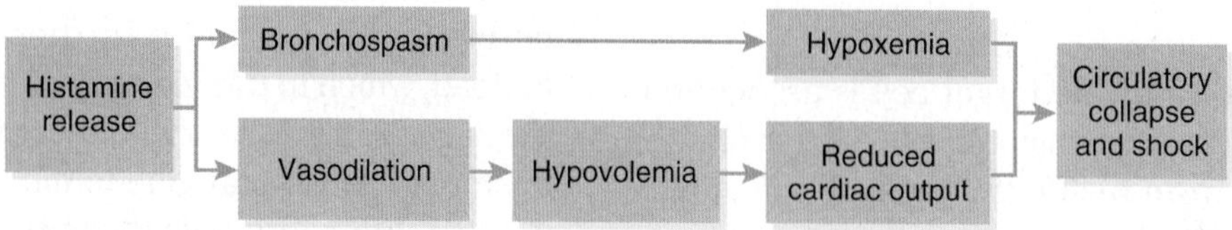

FIGURE 26-7 Pathophysiology of anaphylactic shock.

BOX 26-4 Clinical Criteria for Diagnosing Anaphylaxis

Anaphylaxis is highly likely when any one of the following three criteria are fulfilled:

1. Acute onset of an illness (minutes to several hours) with involvement of the skin, mucosal tissue, or both (eg, generalized urticaria, pruritus or erythema, angioedema) and at least one of the following:
   - Respiratory compromise (eg, dyspnea, wheezing and bronchospasm, stridor, reduced peak expiratory flow, hypoxemia)
   - Reduced blood pressure or associated symptoms of end-organ dysfunction (eg, hypotonia [collapse], syncope, incontinence)
2. Two or more of the following that occur rapidly after exposure to a likely allergen for that patient (minutes to several hours):
   - Involvement of the skin and mucosal tissue (eg, generalized urticaria, pruritus, erythema, angioedema)
   - Respiratory compromise (eg, dyspnea, wheeze–bronchospasm, stridor, reduced peak expiratory flow, hypoxemia)
   - Reduced blood pressure or associated symptoms (eg, hypotonia [collapse], syncope, incontinence)
   - Persistent GI symptoms (eg, crampy abdominal pain, vomiting)
3. Reduced blood pressure after exposure to a known allergen for that patient (minutes to several hours):
   - **Infants and children.** Low systolic blood pressure (age-specific) or greater than 30% decrease in systolic blood pressure[a]
   - **Adults.** Systolic blood pressure of less than 90 mm Hg or greater than 30% decrease from that person's baseline

[a]Low systolic blood pressure for children is defined as less than 70 mm Hg from 1 month to 1 year; less than 70 mm Hg + (2 × Age) from 1 to 10 years; and less than 90 mm Hg from 11 to 17 years.

Modified from: Russell WS, Farrar JR, Nowak R, et al. Evaluating the management of anaphylaxis in US emergency departments: guidelines vs practice. *World J Emerg Med.* 2013;4(2):98-106.

BOX 26-5 Signs and Symptoms of Anaphylaxis

Upper Airway
Hoarseness or muffled voice
Laryngeal or epiglottic edema
Rhinorrhea
Stridor

Lower Airway
Accessory muscle use
Bronchospasm
Decreased breath sounds
Increased mucus production
Wheezing

Cardiovascular System
Chest tightness
Dysrhythmias
Hypotension
Tachycardia

GI System
Abdominal cramps
Diarrhea
Nausea
Vomiting

Neurologic System
Anxiety
Coma
Dizziness
Headache
Seizure
Syncope
Weakness

Cutaneous System
Angioedema
Edema
Erythema
Pallor
Pruritus
Tearing of the eyes
Urticaria

and dyspnea. Stridor or voice changes also may be evident. Lower airway bronchospasm and associated hypersecretion of mucus caused by the actions of histamine, leukotrienes, and prostaglandins may produce wheezing and significant respiratory distress. Symptoms can develop with startling rapidity.

Cardiovascular Effects

The cardiovascular manifestations of allergic reactions range from mild hypotension to vascular collapse and profound shock. Dysrhythmias (including severe bradycardia) are common and may be related to the severe hypoxia and loss of circulating fluid volume that occurs. The patient may complain of chest pain if myocardial ischemia is present.

GI Effects

Nausea, vomiting, diarrhea, and severe abdominal cramping may occur in a patient having an anaphylactic reaction. The increased GI activity is related to smooth muscle contraction, increased production of mucus, and outpouring of fluid from the gut wall into the intestinal lumen initiated by the chemical mediators.

Nervous System Effects

The nervous system responses are caused in large part by the impaired gas exchange and shock associated with anaphylaxis. Initially, the patient may be agitated and speak of a sense of impending doom. As hypoxia and shock worsen, brain functions deteriorate, which may result in confusion, weakness, headache, syncope, seizures, and coma.

Cutaneous Effects

The most visible signs that distinguish anaphylaxis from other medical conditions relate to the skin. These signs are caused by the vasodilation induced by histamine release from the mast cells. Initially, the patient may complain of warmth and **pruritus** (itching). Physical examination often reveals diffuse **erythema** (redness) and **urticaria** (hives). The hives are well-circumscribed **wheals** of 0.4 to 2.4 inches (1 to 6 cm), which may be either redder or more pallid than the surrounding skin. Often they are accompanied by severe pruritus (**FIGURE 26-8**). Significant swelling of the face, tongue, and deep tissues (**angioedema**) also may be present, owing to involvement of deeper capillaries of the skin and mucous membranes. As hypoxia and shock continue, cyanosis may be evident.

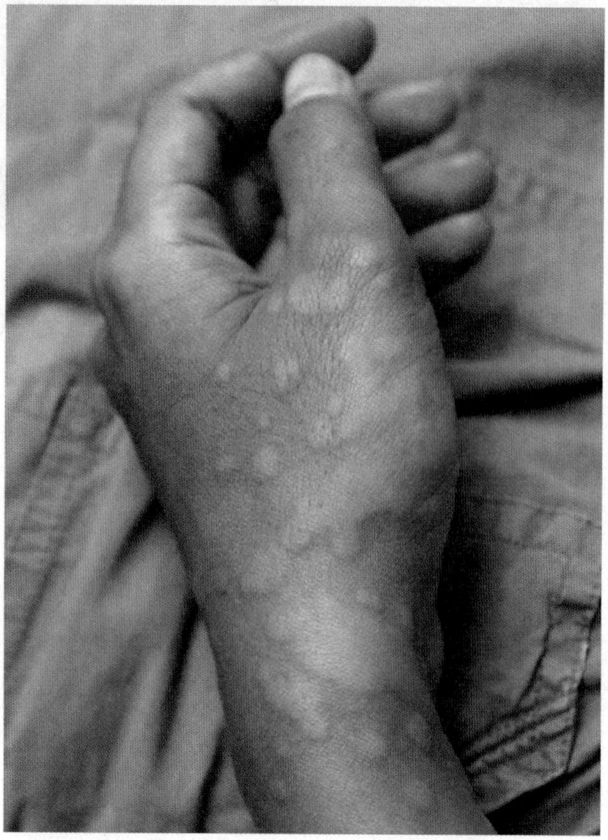

FIGURE 26-8 Urticaria as a result of an allergic reaction.

> NOTE
>
> Angioedema is a localized swelling of the deep dermis or subcutaneous or submucosal tissues that is caused by swelling under the skin. Angioedema is of most concern when it occurs in the face, tongue, and larynx, but it can also be found in the arms and legs. Patients with angioedema are at high risk for rapid deterioration.
>
> *Modified from:* Lavonas EJ, Drennan IR, Gabrielli A, et al. Part 10: special circumstances of resuscitation. 2015 American Heart Association guidelines update for cardiopulmonary resuscitation and emergency cardiovascular care. *Circulation.* 2015;132:S501-S518.

Primary Survey

As in any emergency, initial patient care is directed at providing adequate support for the airway, ventilation, and circulation. Drug therapy (described later in this chapter) often is the definitive treatment in anaphylaxis and should be initiated as quickly as possible.

Airway assessment is crucial, because most deaths from anaphylaxis are related directly to upper airway obstruction. A conscious patient should be evaluated for voice changes, stridor, or a barking cough. Complaints of tightness in the neck and dyspnea should alert the paramedic to impending airway obstruction. While epinephrine is being administered, the airway of an unconscious patient should be assessed and secured. If air movement is blocked, an advanced airway should be placed. If laryngeal and epiglottic edema is severe, surgical or needle cricothyrotomy may be indicated to provide airway access. Early, elective intubation is indicated for patients with hoarseness, lingual edema, and posterior or oropharyngeal swelling. If respiratory function deteriorates, medical direction may recommend tracheal intubation (with sedation).

The paramedic should monitor the patient closely for signs of respiratory distress, as indicated by pulse oximetry, capnography, skin color, accessory muscle use, wheezing, diminished breath sounds, and abnormal respiratory rates. Circulatory status also may deteriorate quickly. Therefore, the pulse quality, rate, and location should be assessed frequently.

History

A history may be difficult to obtain. However, ruling out other medical emergencies that may mimic anaphylaxis can be crucial. The patient should be questioned about the chief complaint and the rapidity of the onset of symptoms. The signs and symptoms of anaphylaxis usually appear within 5 to 30 minutes of introduction of the antigen.[3] The onset of a reaction can be delayed if the exposure occurs by the oral route.

Important medical history includes previous exposure and response to the suspected antigen. In addition, the paramedic should identify the method of exposure to the antigen: Injection of an antigen often produces the most rapid and severe response. Other significant history includes chronic or concurrent illness and medication use. Preexisting cardiac disease or bronchial asthma should alert the paramedic to anticipate severe complications as a result of the allergic reaction. Beta blocker drugs may diminish the patient's response to epinephrine and may necessitate the administration of other medications. The paramedic also should determine whether the patient has an emergency epinephrine drug kit (eg, EpiPen [BOX 26-6]) and whether the medication was administered before the paramedic crew arrived. Some patients with a history of allergic reaction may have taken an oral antihistamine (eg, diphenhydramine) or used aerosolized epinephrine. Although the paramedic should try to determine whether the patient has taken these drugs, appropriate intervention should not be delayed for this history.

BOX 26-6 Epinephrine Autoinjectors

Epinephrine autoinjectors (eg, EpiPen, Adrenaclick, Anapen) are prescribed for people with a history of severe allergic reactions or anaphylaxis. EpiPen, which has the largest market share, contains a single dose of 0.3 mg epinephrine. This dose is appropriate for people who weigh 66 pounds (29.7 kg) or more. EpiPen Junior contains 0.15 mg epinephrine. This dose is appropriate for children who weigh 33 to 66 pounds (14.9 to 29.7 kg). The drug is administered by pushing the autoinjector against the anterolateral thigh and holding it in place for 10 seconds. (The EpiPen self-injects through clothing.) The EpiPen is available as a single-unit package or a double-unit package (2-Pak), for instances when a second dose of the drug is needed to manage an allergic reaction.

Modified from: Rice C. Despite woes, EpiPen still dominates the market. Athena Insight website. https://www.athenahealth.com/insight/despite-woes-epipen-still-dominates-market. Published September 12, 2017. Accessed April 20, 2018.

SHOW ME THE EVIDENCE

Jacobsen and colleagues conducted a blinded cross-sectional nationwide survey of paramedics to determine their ability to recognize and appropriately treat classic and atypical anaphylactic presentations. Of their 3,537 (36.6%) responses, 98.9% correctly identified a typical anaphylaxis presentation, but only 2.9% correctly identified the atypical presentation. Only 46.2% identified epinephrine as the first drug to treat anaphylaxis. Of those who chose epinephrine, only 38.9% correctly identified the intramuscular (IM) route for administration, and only 11.6% selected the thigh as the preferred site. The researchers concluded that improved education is needed regarding this topic.

Modified from: Jacobsen RC, Toy S, Bonham AJ, et al. Anaphylaxis knowledge among paramedics: results of a national survey. *Prehosp Emerg Care*. 2012;16(4):527-534.

Physical Examination

In patients with anaphylaxis, vital signs should be assessed often. In severe reactions, most patients initially are tachycardic, tachypneic, and hypotensive if deterioration to cardiac arrest has not occurred. The paramedic should inspect the patient's face and neck for angioedema, urticaria, tearing, and rhinorrhea, and should note the presence of erythema or urticaria in other body regions. Along with vital signs, the paramedic should assess airway and lung sounds often to evaluate the patient's clinical progress. Such assessment also helps the paramedic monitor the effectiveness of interventions. Cardiac monitoring should be instituted as soon as possible to aid in evaluation of the patient.

Key Interventions to Prevent Arrest

Organ involvement in anaphylaxis varies, which makes a standardized approach to patient management difficult. The following key interventions commonly are used to manage anaphylaxis:[2,4]

1. Give epinephrine to all patients who are suspected of having anaphylaxis (may repeat every 5 to 15 minutes). Epinephrine is given by the IM route in the anterolateral thigh.
2. Place the patient supine unless he or she is unable to tolerate it due to dyspnea.[2]
3. Administer high-concentration oxygen if the patient is dyspneic or hypoxic. Early recognition of the potential for a difficult airway in anaphylaxis is paramount in patients who develop hoarseness, lingual edema, stridor, or oropharyngeal swelling. Planning for advanced airway management, including a surgical airway, is recommended.
4. Initiate IV therapy with normal saline solution if hypotension is present and does not respond rapidly to epinephrine. Repeat 1,000-mL IV boluses (up to 4 L) to maintain a systolic pressure greater than 90 mm Hg. Rapid infusion of 1 to 2 L (up to 4 L) may be needed initially.
5. If hypotension with altered mental status, pallor, and poor perfusion persists despite IM epinephrine and IV fluids, consider an epinephrine IV drip (0.5 mcg/kg per minute).
6. If wheezing persists after administration of epinephrine, administer albuterol 2.5 to 5 mg nebulized (or epinephrine 1 mg/mL, 5 mL nebulized).
7. To treat urticaria or pruritus, administer diphenhydramine 1 mg/kg (maximum dose 50 mg) IM or IV (IV is preferred if severe shock is present).
   a. Histamine-2 (H_2)–blocking antihistamines (eg, famotidine, cimetidine) may be given IV or orally with diphenhydramine.
8. Steroids such as methylprednisolone or dexamethasone may be considered, though their onset of action is slow.
9. Transport the patient for evaluation by a physician. Most patients are observed carefully in the hospital for up to 24 hours. Some patients without complete resolution of symptoms and/or where there is concern that symptoms might recur may be kept in the hospital for 24 hours (**biphasic reaction**)[5] (BOX 26-7).

BOX 26-7 Biphasic Reactions

As many as 25% of patients who have an anaphylactic reaction experience a recurrence in the hours after the beginning of the reaction and will require further medical treatment. This type of delayed reaction is called biphasic, meaning it involves two phases. The second phase usually occurs after an asymptomatic period of 1 to 8 hours, but a delay of up to 24 hours is possible. Epinephrine is again the treatment of choice, and the drug should be administered immediately. Posttreatment observation of these patients is necessary, and they should remain within ready access of emergency care for the next 48 hours.

Modified from: Sreevastava D, Tarneja V. Anaphylactic reaction: an overview. *Med J Armed Forces India.* 2003;59(1):53-56.

NOTE

Complications of IV administration of epinephrine are significant and include the development of uncontrolled systolic hypertension, vomiting, seizures, dysrhythmias, and myocardial ischemia. This route should be used only in patients with profound hypotension or imminent cardiovascular collapse. IV administration of epinephrine rarely is performed in conscious patients; it is performed with extreme caution in rare circumstances and only with authorization from medical direction. Epinephrine 1 mg/mL should never be given undiluted as an IV bolus. The paramedic should follow local protocol.

Modified from: 2015 American Heart Association guidelines update for cardiopulmonary resuscitation and emergency cardiovascular care. *Circulation.* 2015;132:S313-S314.

CRITICAL THINKING

How does epinephrine reverse the signs and symptoms of anaphylaxis?

Other Drug Therapy

Epinephrine is the only drug that can reverse the life-threatening complications of anaphylaxis immediately and is the drug of choice. Several other drugs may be used after epinephrine, however (BOX 26-8). For example, antihistamine (diphenhydramine) may be administered to antagonize the effects of histamine, beta agonists (albuterol) may be given for bronchodilation, and steroids (methylprednisolone or dexamethasone) may be used to reduce inflammation. In rare cases, glucagon is given for patients taking beta blockers who are unresponsive to epinephrine. Vasopressors can be given to manage protracted hypotension. Some protocols recommend that H_2 antagonists such as cimetidine or ranitidine be given in cases of hypotension that are unresponsive to epinephrine or to patients with GI symptoms or to reduce the incidence of biphasic reactions. Nevertheless, administering repeated doses of epinephrine is more appropriate than is adding other drugs in the initial stabilization of refractory anaphylaxis.

BOX 26-8 Additional Drug Therapy for Anaphylaxis

Antihistamines
Diphenhydramine
Hydroxyzine
Promethazine
Cimetidine
Ranitidine
Famotidine

Corticosteroids
Methylprednisolone
Hydrocortisone
Dexamethasone

Beta Agonists
Albuterol
Levalbuterol

Anticholinergic Bronchodilator
Ipratropium

Vasopressors
Dopamine
Norepinephrine

Glucagon

Key Interventions During Arrest

Cardiac arrest from anaphylaxis may be associated with profound vasodilation, intravascular collapse, tissue hypoxia, and asystole. Special considerations for resuscitation of these patients are described next.[5,6]

Airway, Oxygenation, and Ventilation

Swelling of the airway can make bag-mask ventilation and endotracheal intubation difficult or impossible in patients with anaphylaxis. In addition, landmarks may not be visible because of severe swelling in the soft tissues of the neck. Video laryngoscopy, fiberoptic intubation, and digital intubation are alternative methods to consider in these situations. Endotracheal tubes that are slightly smaller than normal may be needed because of associated edema.

Support of Circulation

Cardiac arrest from anaphylaxis requires rapid, aggressive volume replacement (2 to 4 L) to support circulation and the use of vasopressor drugs to support blood pressure. Epinephrine IV (including immediate use of epinephrine autoinjectors, if available) is the drug of choice for the treatment of anaphylaxis accompanied by vasodilation and hypotension in cardiac arrest.

Asystole and pulseless electrical activity with a heart rate less than 60 beats/min are the most common arrest rhythms in anaphylaxis. Cardiac arrest from anaphylaxis may respond to prolonged periods of cardiopulmonary resuscitation, especially when the patient is young and has a healthy heart and cardiovascular system.

Collagen Vascular Disease

Collagen vascular disease is also known as connective tissue disease. Collagen is the principal structural protein of most body tissues. Many connective tissue diseases feature abnormal immune system activity accompanied by inflammation in the tissues, resulting from the immune system being directed against the patient's own body tissues (**autoimmune disease**). Collagen vascular disease may have both genetic and environmental causes. The immune system disorder results in the accumulation of extra antibodies in the circulation.

Two "classic" collagen vascular diseases described in this chapter are systemic lupus erythematosus and scleroderma. Some patients have a combination

LOW AMPS LOOK LIKE MI IN ALL LEADS

of these diseases, known as mixed connective tissue disease.[7] Other autoimmune diseases, such as rheumatoid arthritis, are discussed in Chapter 32, *Nontraumatic Musculoskeletal Disorders.*

NOTE

Physician care for patients with collagen vascular disease often is multidisciplinary because of the nature of the disease and the affected organs and body systems. Specialists involved in this care may include rheumatologists, clinical immunologists, dermatologists, neurologists, nephrologists, cardiologists, psychologists, social workers, and others. Prehospital care is primarily supportive. When possible, these patients should be transported to their primary hospital for their specialized care.

Systemic Lupus Erythematosus

Systemic lupus erythematosus (SLE), often referred to as lupus, is one of many disorders of the immune system. Although SLE usually first affects people between 15 and 45 years of age, it also can occur in childhood or later in life.

NOTE

SLE primarily is a disease of young women, beginning mainly between the ages of 15 and 40 years. Women are about nine times more likely to have SLE than are men. SLE can be common in families, but the risk that a child or a brother or sister of a patient will also have SLE is still quite low. SLE occurs in both siblings in approximately 25% to 50% of identical twins and 5% of fraternal twins.

Modified from: Aldridge B, Corelli R, Ernst ME, et al., eds. *Koda-Kimble and Young's Applied Therapeutics: The Clinical Use of Drugs.* 10th ed. Baltimore, MD: Lippincott Williams & Wilkins; 2013; Unlocking the reasons why lupus is more common in women. National Resource Center on Lupus website. https://resources.lupus.org/entry/why-lupus-more-common-in-women. Accessed April 20, 2018.

In all autoimmune diseases, the immune system produces antibodies against the body's healthy cells and tissues. With SLE, these antibodies, called autoantibodies, contribute to the inflammation of various parts of the body and can damage organs and tissues. The most common type of autoantibody that develops in people with SLE is antinuclear antibody, so named because it reacts with parts of the cell's nucleus. SLE can affect many parts of the body, including the joints, skin, kidneys, heart, lungs, blood vessels, and brain. Patients with SLE frequently develop inflammatory heart disease (pericarditis) and may experience early-onset atherosclerosis as a complication of the disease.

People with SLE can have many different symptoms (**BOX 26-9**).[8] Among the most common are extreme fatigue, painful or swollen joints (arthritis), unexplained fever, and skin rashes. Patients with renal and neurologic involvement will have more serious signs and symptoms. A common finding in a patient with SLE is a characteristic reddish skin rash, called the butterfly or malar rash, that typically appears across the nose and cheeks (**FIGURE 26-9**). Systemic effects of SLE may include the following:[9]

- GI ulceration or hemorrhage, abdominal pain, pancreatitis, cholecystitis, bowel infarction

BOX 26-9 Signs and Symptoms of SLE

Painful or swollen joints and muscle pain
Unexplained fever
Red rash, most commonly on the face
Chest pain on deep breathing
Unusual loss of hair
Pale or purple fingers or toes from cold or stress (Raynaud phenomenon)
Sensitivity to the sun
Swelling (edema) in legs or around eyes
Mouth ulcers
Swollen glands
Extreme fatigue

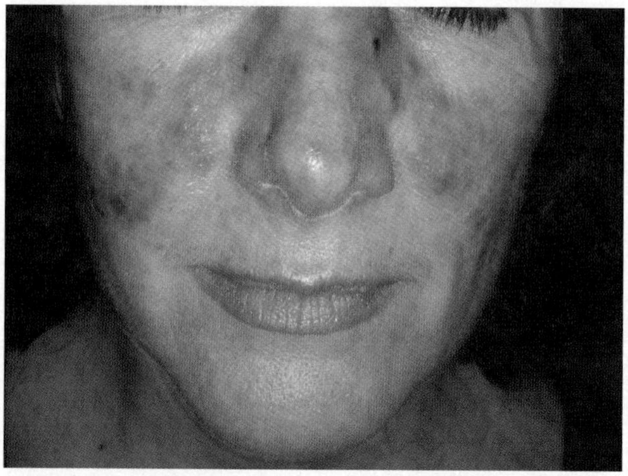

FIGURE 26-9 Systemic lupus erythematosus flare. The classic butterfly rash occurs in 10% to 50% of patients with acute cutaneous lupus erythematosus. The rash appears over the nose and cheeks.

- Renal failure
- Anemia and clotting abnormalities
- Pericarditis
- Pleurisy or pleural effusions
- Skin rash
- Behavioral changes, seizures, headaches, stroke

Management

The symptoms of SLE may be either mild or serious. The goal of treatment is to prevent disease flares, organ damage, and complications. Physician care may include nonsteroidal anti-inflammatory drugs and corticosteroids to decrease inflammation, and antimalarial agents to treat fatigue, joint pain, skin rashes, and lung inflammation. Other therapies may include immunosuppressants. Currently, no cure is available for the disease.

If the patient complains of chest pain, a 12-lead electrocardiogram should be obtained. Pericarditis is common in these patients.[10]

Scleroderma

Scleroderma is derived from the Greek words *sklerosis*, meaning "hardness," and *derma*, meaning "skin." This "hard skin" disease is thought to occur when the immune system stimulates certain cells (fibroblasts) to increase their production of collagen. The excess collagen collects in the skin and internal organs, interfering with their function. Blood vessels and joints also can be affected.

Scleroderma is more common in women than in men. Because it can be difficult to diagnose, only rough estimates of its prevalence are available. Currently, the number of people in the United States with systemic sclerosis is estimated at 58,000.[11]

This disease can be either localized or systemic, and both groups have subgroups. The localized forms of the disease are limited to the skin and related tissues and may involve underlying muscle; internal organs are not affected. Localized scleroderma does not progress to systemic forms. Although localized conditions often subside, the skin changes and damage from the event can be permanent (**FIGURE 26-10**). Two types of the localized conditions are recognized:[12]

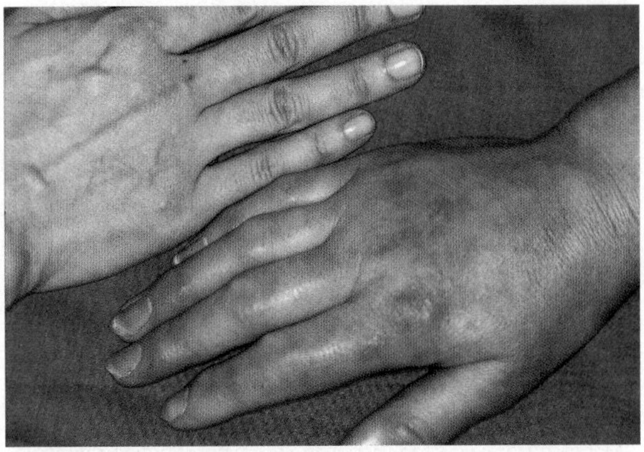

FIGURE 26-10 Scleroderma (acrosclerosis). Note the inflammation and shiny skin.

- **Morphea** is marked by local patches of hardened skin, which may occur at any site. Red patches of skin develop white centers with purplish borders, and lesions remain active for weeks to several years. Spontaneous softening that leaves a darkened area of skin often occurs. In localized morphea, one or a few patches are seen. In generalized morphea, the patches may grow over large areas of the body.
- **Linear scleroderma** is characterized by a single line or band of thickened, discolored skin. The line usually runs down an arm or leg but sometimes runs down the forehead. When the band runs down the forehead, it may be called *en coup de sabre* (French for "sword stroke").

Systemic scleroderma (systemic sclerosis) affects the skin, blood vessels, and major organs. Two types of systemic disease are recognized:[13]

- **Limited systemic sclerosis.** Skin thickening generally is limited to the fingers, forearms, legs, face, and neck. Raynaud phenomenon may be present for years before any other symptoms develop. People with this form are less likely to develop severe organ involvement than are people with diffuse disease.
- **Diffuse systemic sclerosis.** Skin thickening may occur anywhere on the body, including the trunk. Only a short period elapses between the onset of Raynaud phenomenon and significant organ involvement. Damage typically occurs over the first 3 to 5 years, after which most patients enter a stable phase that varies in length. Organ involvement may lead to diseases and dysfunction of the esophagus, GI tract, kidneys, heart, and lungs.

NOTE

In a person with **Raynaud phenomenon**, cold temperatures or emotional distress can cause the arteries feeding the hands or feet (or both) to constrict. This constriction causes the hands and feet to feel cold, turn white, and then turn blue. After the vessels reopen (usually within 10 to 15 minutes), the hands turn red or mottled. More than 90% of people with scleroderma have Raynaud phenomenon. Often presenting as the first symptom of the disease, this condition is found in patients with SLE as well.

Modified from: Hansen-Dispenza H. Raynaud phenomenon. Medscape website. https://emedicine.medscape.com/article/331197-overview. Published September 6, 2017. Accessed April 20, 2018.

CRITICAL THINKING

How might Raynaud phenomenon affect your assessment of a patient who is hypoxic?

Management

No one treatment for the complicated process that causes scleroderma has proved effective, but evidence does support treatment and management of specific organ manifestations.[14] Treatment decisions are made on a symptom-by-symptom and an organ-by-organ basis.

Pulse oximetry readings are often difficult to obtain in the fingers of patients with Raynaud phenomenon. If a forehead probe is available, it can be used to obtain an accurate reading.[15] Low oxygen saturation readings, as measured by pulse oximeter, may also be related to pulmonary fibrosis associated with the patient's scleroderma. If that is the case, the oxygen saturation may not increase significantly when oxygen is administered.

Vascular access also is often difficult in these patients. Using a smaller-gauge catheter and, if possible, warming the site prior to attempting placement of the IV may be helpful.

If the patient is receiving medication via an infusion pump, the infusion should not be interrupted during care. The infusion must run continuously to effectively treat pulmonary arterial hypertension.

Patients with systemic scleroderma can suffer serious organ failure as a result of their disease. Thickening of vessels can lead to significant hypertension and pulmonary, cardiovascular, and renal failure. As a result, these patients can present with hypertensive crisis, renal failure, and heart failure. Drug therapy that may be needed to manage these disorders includes nitrates and calcium channel blockers to lower blood pressure, and ACE inhibitors to reverse renal crisis. If patients are being treated with immune suppressants, their risk of infection will be high. Prehospital care may include both basic and advanced life support.

Transplantation Complications

Every 10 minutes, a new name is added to the national organ transplant waiting list in the United States.[16] Many of these people are waiting for a solid-organ transplant—that is, a kidney, liver, pancreas, heart, or lungs. In 2016, 33,600 Americans received an organ transplant.[17] Recently, there has been an increase in viable organs for transplantation because of the number of young, otherwise healthy adults dying from opioid overdose.[18] In the face of this trend, the likelihood of EMS personnel caring for a patient who has undergone **organ transplantation** is great.

Common complications in patients who have received an organ transplant are related to **immunosuppression**, including infection, rejection, and drug toxicity.[10]

NOTE

Two major complications associated with solid-organ transplantation are infection and malignancy, which result from the lifelong immunosuppressive therapy that must be endured by transplant recipients to maintain function. The organisms most commonly associated with posttransplantation infection represent a reactivation of latent infection carried by the donor organ or the recipient. They also may be acquired through new exposures in the community or in the hospital.

Modified from: Fishman JA, Ramos E. *Infection in Renal Transplant Recipients in Chronic Kidney Disease, Dialysis and Transplantation.* 2nd ed. Philadelphia, PA: W. B. Saunders; 2005.

Infection

Infection is the most common life-threatening complication of long-term immunosuppressive therapy in patients who have received an organ transplant.[10] Some patients taking immunosuppressant therapy develop neutropenia—that is, a low concentration of neutrophils. Neutrophils account for 50% to 70% of white blood cells and are essential to fight infection; thus, neutropenic patients are at high risk for infection and sepsis. Any patient who is neutropenic with a fever requires immediate transport.

Infection after transplantation of a solid organ can have many causes (BOX 26-10), including the following:[10]

- Community-acquired bacterial and viral diseases
- Opportunistic infections
- Health care–acquired infections
- Travel-related infections
- Infections related to the patient's work, sexuality, or pets

After a patient has been infected, the inflammatory responses associated with the invasion of microbes are impaired by immunosuppressive therapy. As a result, the signs and symptoms of infection that normally would be evident are masked. Consequently, infections often are advanced or have spread by the time of the patient complaint or clinical presentation. Established infection is difficult to treat in immunocompromised transplant recipients.[19] Significant

BOX 26-10 Possible Causes of Infection After Organ Transplantation

Infections in transplant recipients usually are categorized according to three phases that follow transplantation: early posttransplantation (month 1), months 2 to 6, and late posttransplantation (after 6 months). Certain infections are more likely to occur during a specific phase.

- **Month 1 (early posttransplantation).** The immune system usually is most suppressed in the first month after transplantation. Most infections during this period result from surgical- or hospital-acquired infections, including infections caused by bacteria or *Candida* organisms. Infections may present as a urinary tract infection, wound infection, pneumonia, or bloodstream infection. Herpes simplex virus (HSV) may reactivate (eg, as cold sores). Many transplant recipients are prescribed medications to prevent the reactivation of HSV.
- **Months 2 to 6.** During this period, transplant recipients are at risk for unusual or opportunistic infections, such as *Pneumocystis jirovecii* pneumonia (formerly called *Pneumocystis carinii* pneumonia) or tuberculosis. During this phase, the transplant recipient also is at highest risk for reactivation of certain viruses, including cytomegalovirus, varicella zoster virus, Epstein-Barr virus, and the hepatitis viruses (see Chapter 27, *Infectious and Communicable Diseases*).
  - **Cytomegalovirus (CMV).** CMV infection occurs in 44% to 85% of patients who have received a kidney, heart, or liver transplant. Symptomatic CMV disease occurs in 8% to 29% of kidney and liver transplant recipients. This disease can occur if a transplant recipient without a history of CMV receives an organ transplant from a donor with a history of CMV (primary infection). CMV disease also can reactivate after transplantation in a recipient who has a history of a previous CMV infection. This infection can present in a variety of ways, such as a flulike illness with fever, muscle aches, and fatigue, or as hepatitis. CMV is both preventable and treatable with antiviral medications such as ganciclovir, valganciclovir, and foscarnet.
  - **Varicella zoster virus (VZV).** VZV is the virus that causes chickenpox. Ninety percent of adult transplant recipients were exposed to VZV during childhood, and they are at risk for reactivation of VZV in a form called shingles. Shingles is a painful, blisterlike rash.
  - **Epstein-Barr virus (EBV).** EBV is the virus that causes mononucleosis (also called mono). Transplant recipients who are not immune to EBV may get mononucleosis. Symptoms include fever, fatigue, muscle aches, and pains. EBV also may reactivate and cause posttransplantation lymphoproliferative disease in 1% of patients with kidney transplants and 2% of patients with liver transplants. Symptoms can include fever, sore throat, abdominal pain, jaundice, or kidney and liver dysfunction. Treatment depends on the level of disease.
  - **Hepatitis B virus (HBV) and hepatitis C virus (HCV).** Viral hepatitis can recur in transplant recipients who receive their transplants because of chronic hepatitis. HBV recurs in 5% to 10% of patients; HCV recurs in 80% to 90% of recipients.
- **After 6 months (late posttransplantation).** Most transplant recipients do well 6 months after transplantation. They are at risk for community-acquired infections, such as urinary tract infections, influenza, and pneumococcal (bacterial) pneumonia.

Modified from: Fishman JA, Rubin RH. Changing timeline of infection after organ transplantation. *N Engl J Med.* 2007;357(25):2601-2614; Infections in solid organ transplants. Lahey Hospital and Medical Center website. http://www.lahey.org/Departments_and_Locations/Departments/Infectious_Diseases/Infection_Prevention/Infections_in_Solid_Organ_Transplants.aspx. Accessed April 20, 2018.

antimicrobial toxicities are common, often as a result of diminished renal or hepatic function and drug interactions (described later).

NOTE

Paramedics should observe strict aseptic technique when caring for transplant recipients to avoid introducing infection. Hand hygiene is essential. Vascular access should be avoided unless the need is clear.

CRITICAL THINKING

Which signs and symptoms of infection may be masked by immunosuppressive treatment?

Rejection

Tissues or cells from another person (except an identical twin) carry nonself markers and may be recognized by the body as foreign—which explains why some tissue transplants (grafts) are rejected. Most solid-organ transplants are donated by nonidentical (genetically unrelated) people, in which case the procedure is known as **allografting.**[20] If the transplanted tissue is donated by an identical twin, the procedure is termed **isografting**. Because allografts are more common than isografts, organ rejection is a major complication for recipients of solid-organ transplants. Rejection can be classified as hyperacute, acute, or chronic (BOX 26-11).[21]

Signs and symptoms of transplant rejection vary, depending on the transplanted organ and the recipient's general health. General signs and symptoms include the following:

- Pain at the site of the transplant
- General malaise
- Irritability (in children)
- Flulike symptoms
- Fever
- Weight changes
- Swelling and edema
- Change in the heart rate or blood pressure

BOX 26-11 Classes of Rejection

- **Hyperacute rejection** is a complement-mediated response in transplant recipients with preexisting antibodies to the donor (eg, ABO blood type antibodies). Hyperacute rejection occurs within minutes. The transplant must be removed immediately to prevent a severe systemic inflammatory response.
- **Acute rejection** usually begins 1 week after transplantation. The risk of acute rejection is highest in the first 3 months after transplantation. Acute rejection occurs to some degree in all transplant recipients (except in isografts between identical twins). This type of rejection can be successfully managed if recognized quickly.
- **Chronic rejection** refers to cases of transplant rejection in which the rejection is due to a poorly understood chronic inflammatory and immune response against the transplanted tissue.

Drug Toxicity

Many drugs are necessary to manage a patient who has received a solid-organ transplant. Most of the medications are required for life to ensure the patient's survival and the success of the graft. The primary goals of drug therapy are to prevent organ rejection and infection. A major complication of the drug therapy is drug toxicity and adverse effects.

A variety of immunosuppressant drugs are used in the United States:[22]

- Antibody therapies prevent T cell multiplication and movement of B and T cells from blood into transplanted organs. Example: basiliximab
- Calcineurin inhibitors prevent T cells from being activated and attacking the transplanted organ. Examples: tacrolimus, cyclosporine

NOTE

Other medications and some foods may interact with posttransplantation medications. Complications can arise from the following:

- Some prescription medicines, such as erythromycin, clarithromycin (Biaxin), diltiazem (Cardizem, Tiazac), and verapamil (Calan, Verelan)
- Over-the-counter products, such as cimetidine (Tagamet) or herbal products or natural remedies, including St. John's wort, echinacea, black cohosh, and others
- Eating grapefruit or drinking grapefruit juice, which can alter drug metabolism

Modified from: Moore LW. Food, food components, and botanicals affecting drug metabolism in transplantation. *J Ren Nutr.* 2013;23(3):e71-e73.

- MTOR (mammalian target of rapamycin) inhibitors stop T cells from multiplying. Examples: sirolimus, everolimus
- Antiproliferative agents block deoxyribonucleic acid (DNA) in B and T cells to prevent them from multiplying. Examples: mycophenolate mofetil (MMF), azathioprine, mycophenolate sodium
- Corticosteroids suppress the immune system. Examples: prednisone, methylprednisolone

Three drugs commonly associated with drug toxicity and adverse drug interactions in transplant recipients are cyclosporine, azathioprine, and corticosteroids.

Management of Patients With Transplant Disorders

Prehospital care for a patient who has received a solid-organ transplant may vary from providing only comfort measures to supporting vital functions. Infection control measures are essential. If the patient is neutropenic, extra precautions should be taken to prevent spreading infection to the patient. The paramedic should wear a gown, mask, and gloves. These patients often have a long and complex medical history, and most require transport directly to their primary care facility when possible.

Summary

- The immune system is designed to prevent foreign substances from entering the body. If that effort fails, this system launches an attack to find and destroy these foreign substances.
- Lymphocytes are the primary units of the immune system. B lymphocytes produce antibodies, which provide humoral immunity. T lymphocytes provide cell-mediated immunity with three types of cells: Killer T cells attack invading organisms, helper T cells encourage B cell antibody production, and suppressor T cells regulate the immune response so that it does not attack the body.
- Natural immunity is present at birth and is not antigen-specific. Acquired immunity develops after exposure to specific antigens.
- Antigens are substances that trigger antibody formation. Antibodies bind to the antigens that produced them, thereby helping neutralize the antigens and remove them from the body.
- An allergic reaction is an increased physiologic response to an antigen after a previous exposure to the same antigen.
- Localized allergic reactions do not affect the entire body. They affect the skin, nasal passages, or eyes, but not the lungs or cardiovascular system. They are treated with antihistamines (eg, diphenhydramine).
- Anaphylaxis is a type I hypersensitivity reaction and a life-threatening event. Rapid recognition and aggressive therapy are needed for patient survival.
- Almost any substance can cause anaphylaxis. The risk of anaphylaxis increases with the frequency of exposure.
- Chemical substances released by basophils and mast cells cause signs and symptoms of anaphylaxis; these chemicals include histamine, leukotrienes, and other substances.
- Symptoms of anaphylaxis may include a sudden onset of hives, angioedema, and pruritus; sneezing and coughing; airway obstruction; wheezing; hypotension or vascular collapse; chest pain; nausea, vomiting, or diarrhea; and weakness, headache, syncope, seizures, or coma. The paramedic should know the criteria for diagnosing anaphylaxis.
- The paramedic should determine whether the patient experiencing an allergic reaction or anaphylaxis has used an epinephrine autoinjector or taken diphenhydramine before arrival of the paramedic crew.
- Treatment of anaphylaxis includes administration of epinephrine and, if the patient is hypotensive, 1 to 2 L of normal saline. (1 to 2 L is typical, but in certain situations much more fluid may be needed.) Additional interventions may include antihistamines, inhaled beta agonists, corticosteroids, glucagon, and vasopressors.
- Autoimmune disease occurs when the body's immune system attacks normal body cells, causing harm. One type of autoimmune disease is collagen vascular disease, also called connective tissue disease.
- Systemic lupus erythematosus is a disease that can cause severe damage to the gastrointestinal (GI) organs, kidneys, lungs, and central nervous system. Typically presenting in young women, it often causes a butterfly rash on the nose and cheeks.
- Scleroderma is caused by increased collagen production. Systemic scleroderma may cause Raynaud phenomenon and dysfunction of the esophagus, GI tract, kidneys, heart, and lungs.
- Solid organs that may be transplanted include the kidneys, liver, pancreas, heart, and lungs.
- Infection, rejection, and drug toxicity are the key complications seen after organ transplant.
- Infection after transplantation of a solid organ can have many causes, including community-acquired bacterial or viral diseases, opportunistic infections, and others. Normal signs and symptoms of infection may be masked by the immunosuppressive therapy.
- When the body recognizes the transplanted tissue as "nonself," it begins to reject it. Rejection may be hyperacute (occurring within minutes), acute (occurring within 1 week), or chronic (occurring after 1 week).
- Immunosuppressive drugs have many side effects. Three drug groups known to cause many adverse effects are cyclosporine, azathioprine, and corticosteroids.

References

1. Greenberger PA, Wallace DV, Lieberman PL, Gregory SM. Contemporary issues in anaphylaxis and the evolution of epinephrine autoinjectors. *Ann Allergy Asthma Immunol.* 2017;119(4):333-338.
2. Lieberman P, Nicklas R, Randolph C, et al. Anaphylaxis: a practice parameter update 2015. *Ann Allergy Asthma Immunol.* 2015;115:341-384.
3. Mustafa SS. Anaphylaxis clinical presentation. Medscape website. https://emedicine.medscape.com/article/135065-clinical. Updated February 22, 2017. Accessed April 20, 2018.
4. National Association of EMS Officials. *National Model EMS Clinical Guidelines*. Version 2.0. National Association of EMS Officials website. https://www.nasemso.org/documents/National-Model-EMS-Clinical-Guidelines-Version2-Sept2017.pdf. Published September 2017. Accessed April 20, 2018.
5. Walls RM, Hockberger RS, Gausche-Hill M. *Rosen's Emergency Medicine: Concepts and Clinical Practice.* 9th ed. St. Louis, MO: Elsevier; 2018.
6. Lavonas EJ, Drennan IR, Gabrielli A, et al. Part 10: special circumstances of resuscitation. 2015 American Heart Association guidelines update for cardiopulmonary resuscitation and emergency cardiovascular care. *Circulation.* 2015;132:S501-S518.
7. Fogo AB, Kashgarian M. *Diagnostic Atlas of Renal Pathology.* 3rd ed. Philadelphia, PA: Elsevier; 2017.
8. Lupus symptoms. Arthritis Foundation website. https://www.arthritis.org/about-arthritis/types/lupus/symptoms.php. Accessed April 20, 2018.
9. Bartels CM. Systemic lupus erythematosus (SLE) clinical presentation. Medscape website. https://emedicine.medscape.com/article/332244-clinical. Updated November 14, 2017. Accessed April 20, 2018.
10. Collopy KT. The impaired immune system. EMS World website. https://www.emsworld.com/article/11227096/impaired-immune-system. Published November 8, 2013. Accessed April 20, 2018.
11. Prevalence and incidence of systemic scleroderma in the US. Scleroderma Education Project website. http://sclerodermainfo.org/prevalence-and-incidence-of-systemic-scleroderma-in-the-us/. Published November 29, 2016. Accessed April 20, 2018.
12. Genetic and Rare Disease Information Center. Localized scleroderma. National Institutes of Health website. https://rarediseases.info.nih.gov/diseases/7058/localized-scleroderma/cases/21751. Accessed April 20, 2018.
13. Varga J, Hinchcliff M. Systemic sclerosis: beyond limited and diffuse subsets? *Nat Rev Rheumatol.* 2014;10(4):200-202.
14. Shah AA, Wigley FM. My approach to the treatment of scleroderma. *Mayo Clinic Proc.* 2013;88(4):377-393.
15. Attention: emergency medical responders. Scleroderma Foundation website. http://www.scleroderma.org/site/DocServer/Scleroderma_Emergency_Information_Kit.pdf. Accessed April 20, 2018.
16. Data. United Network for Organ Sharing website. https://unos.org/data/. Accessed April 20, 2018.
17. *Statistics.* Donate Life America website. http://donatelife.net/understanding-donation/statistics/. Accessed April 20, 2018.
18. Mulvania P. The impact of increased opioid overdose on donation. Gift of Life Institute website. http://www.giftoflifeinstitute.org/impact-increased-opioid-overdose-donation/. Published November 29, 2017. Accessed April 20, 2018.
19. Ljungman P, Snydman D, Boeckh M, eds. *Transplant Infections.* 4th ed. New York, NY: Springer; 2018.
20. Ahmed N, Dawson M, Smith C, Wood E. *The Biology of Disease.* New York, NY: Taylor and Francis Group; 2007.
21. Moreau A, Varey E, Anegon I, Cuturi M-C. Effector mechanisms of rejection. *Cold Spring Harbor Persp Med.* 2013;3(11):a015461.
22. Anti-rejection drugs: types of anti-rejection drugs. Transplant 360 website. https://transplant360.com/patient-home/your-medication/anti-rejection-drugs/types-of-anti-rejection-drugs.aspx. Published August 2016. Accessed April 20, 2018.

Suggested Readings

Brasted ID. Anaphylaxis and its treatment. EMS World website. https://www.emsworld.com/article/12239445/anaphylaxis-and-its-treatment. Published August 2, 2016. Accessed April 20, 2018.

Cohen J, Powderly WG, Opal SM. *Infectious Diseases.* 4th ed. Philadelphia, PA: Elsevier; 2017.

Gangaram P, Alinier G, Menacho AM. Crisis resource management in emergency medical settings in Qatar. *Int Paramedic Pract.* August 18, 2017. https://doi.org/10.12968/ippr.2017.7.2.18.

Li XC, Anthony MJ. *Transplant Immunology.* Hoboken, NJ: Wiley-Blackwell; 2015.

Maddux AB, Hiller TD, Overdier KH, et al. Innate immune function and organ failure recovery in adults with sepsis. *J Intens Care Med.* April 4, 2017.

Mund E. Second life for lungs. EMS World website. https://www.emsworld.com/article/10915193/second-lives-lungs. Published April 4, 2013. Accessed April 20, 2018.

Mustafa SS. Anaphylaxis treatment and management. Medscape website. https://emedicine.medscape.com/article/135065-treatment. Updated February 22, 2017. Accessed April 20, 2018.

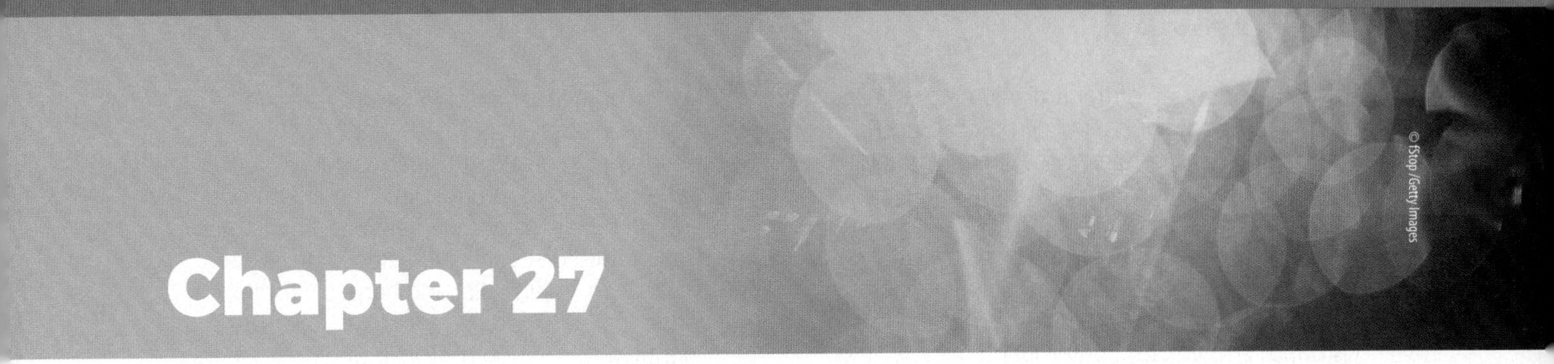

Chapter 27

Infectious and Communicable Diseases

NATIONAL EMS EDUCATION STANDARD COMPETENCIES

Medicine

Integrates assessment findings with principles of epidemiology and pathophysiology to formulate a field impression and implement a comprehensive treatment/disposition plan for a patient with a medical complaint.

Infectious Diseases

Awareness, assessment, and management of
- A patient who may have an infectious disease (pp 1041–1045)
- How to decontaminate equipment after treating a patient (pp 1044–1045)

Assessment and management of
- How to decontaminate the ambulance and equipment after treating a patient (pp 1044–1045)
- A patient who may be infected with a bloodborne pathogen (pp 1042–1045, 1057–1058, 1087)
  - Human immunodeficiency virus (HIV) (pp 1053–1058)
  - Hepatitis B (pp 1058–1061)
- Antibiotic-resistant infections (pp 1071–1073)
- Current infectious diseases prevalent in the community (p 1072)

Anatomy, physiology, epidemiology, pathophysiology, psychosocial impact, presentations, prognosis, and management of
- HIV-related disease (pp 1053–1058)
- Hepatitis (pp 1058–1061)
- Pneumonia (pp 1067–1068, and Chapter 23, *Respiratory*)
- Meningococcal meningitis (pp 1064–1066)
- Tuberculosis (pp 1061–1064)
- Tetanus (pp 1068–1069)
- Viral diseases (pp 1047, 1053–1061, 1065, 1067–1071, 1073–1080, 1082–1083; see also Chapter 23, *Respiratory*, and Chapter 47, *Pediatrics*)
- Sexually transmitted diseases (pp 1080–1083)
- Gastroenteritis (see Chapter 28, *Abdominal and Gastrointestinal Disorders*)
- Fungal infections (p 1054)
- Rabies (pp 1069–1070)
- Scabies and lice (pp 1083–1085)
- Lyme disease (see Chapter 33, *Toxicology*)
- Rocky Mountain spotted fever (see Chapter 33, *Toxicology*)
- Antibiotic-resistant infections (pp 1071–1073)

OBJECTIVES

Upon completion of this chapter, the paramedic student will be able to:
1. Identify general public health principles related to infectious disease. (pp 1041–1047)
2. Describe the chain of elements necessary for an infectious disease to occur. (pp 1047–1049)
3. Explain how internal and external barriers affect susceptibility to infection. (pp 1049–1052)
4. Differentiate the four stages of infectious disease: the latent period, the incubation period, the communicability period, and the disease period. (pp 1052–1053)
5. Describe the mode of transmission, pathophysiology, prehospital considerations, and personal protective measures to be taken for human immunodeficiency virus, hepatitis, tuberculosis, bacterial meningitis, bacterial endocarditis, and pneumonia. (pp 1053–1068)

6. Describe the mode of transmission, pathophysiology, signs and symptoms, and prehospital considerations for patients who have tetanus, rabies, hantavirus infection, or mosquito-borne illness. (pp 1068–1071)
7. List the signs, symptoms, and possible secondary complications of antibiotic-resistant infections, including *Clostridium difficile*, carbapenem-resistant Enterobacteriaceae, and *Neisseria gonorrhoeae*. (pp 1071–1073)
8. List the signs, symptoms, and possible secondary complications of selected childhood viral diseases, including rubella, rubeola, mumps, chickenpox, and pertussis. (pp 1073–1076)
9. List the signs, symptoms, and possible secondary complications of influenza, severe acute respiratory syndrome, and mononucleosis. (pp 1077–1080)
10. Describe the mode of transmission, pathophysiology, prehospital considerations, and personal protective measures for sexually transmitted diseases, including syphilis, gonorrhea, chlamydia, and herpes simplex virus. (pp 1080–1083)
11. Identify the signs, symptoms, and prehospital considerations for lice and scabies. (pp 1083–1085)
12. Describe the reporting process for exposure to infectious or communicable diseases. (pp 1085–1087)
13. Discuss the paramedic's role in preventing disease transmission. (p 1087)

KEY TERMS

airborne precautions Steps taken to avoid infection spread by airborne droplet nuclei (typically 5 microns or smaller in size). Such steps include wearing an N95 respirator or powered air-purifying respirator.

asplenia Congenital absence or surgical removal of the spleen.

bacterial endocarditis Inflammation and infection of the endocardium and one or more heart valves; also known as infective endocarditis.

bacterial meningitis A life-threatening illness that results from bacterial infection of the meninges.

body lice Tiny parasites that concentrate around the waist, shoulders, axillae, and neck.

***C diff* colitis** Inflammation of the colon caused by colonization and infection with the bacterium *Clostridium difficile*.

chancre A painless ulcer, particularly one developing on the genitals as a result of a sexually transmitted disease.

chemotactic factors Biochemical mediators that are important in activating the inflammatory response.

chickenpox An acute, highly contagious viral disease caused by a herpesvirus, varicella-zoster virus. It occurs primarily during childhood and is characterized by crops of pruritic vesicular eruptions on the skin. Also known as varicella.

Chikungunya virus A viral illness spread by mosquitoes that causes fever and joint pain, which is often severe and debilitating.

chlamydia A sexually transmitted disease caused by infection with the bacterium *Chlamydia trachomatis* that frequently causes of sterility.

Clostridium difficile A bacterium that normally is present in small numbers in the intestines that may cause symptoms ranging from diarrhea to life-threatening inflammation of the colon when present in high numbers.

communicability period A stage of infection that begins when the latent period ends and continues as long as the agent is present and can spread to other hosts.

communicable disease An infectious disease that can be transmitted from one person to another.

complement system A group of proteins that coat bacteria. The proteins then either help kill the bacteria directly or assist neutrophils (in the blood) and macrophages (in the tissues) to engulf and destroy the bacteria.

congenital rubella syndrome A serious disease that affects approximately 25% of infants born to women infected with rubella during the first trimester of pregnancy. It is associated with multiple congenital anomalies, mental retardation, and an increased risk of death.

contact precautions Steps taken to avoid infection spread by contact with a patient or contaminated items in a patient's room or surroundings. Such steps include wearing a gown and gloves while caring for a patient or while in the patient's room/surroundings.

croup A childhood infection of the upper airways (larynx, trachea, bronchial tubes) that causes a distinctive "seallike" barking cough. It is usually caused by a virus (most commonly parainfluenza) but rarely can be bacterial. Also known as laryngotracheobronchitis.

dengue fever A mosquito-borne illness caused by dengue virus in tropical and subtropical areas. Symptoms include high fever, joint pain, and rash. Severe cases may result in hemorrhage and shock. Also known as breakbone fever.

designated infection control officer (DICO) A person who serves as a liaison between the public safety agency and community health agencies involved in monitoring and responding to communicable diseases.

disease period A stage of infection that follows the incubation period. The duration of this stage varies with the disease.

droplet precautions Steps taken to avoid infection spread in tiny droplets (typically greater than 5 microns in size and traveling no more than approximately 3 feet [1 m]). Such steps include wearing a surgical mask with face shield, gown, and gloves.

epidemic A widespread occurrence of an infectious disease in a community at a particular time (eg, influenza in the winter).

epiglottitis Inflammation of the epiglottis; a severe form of the condition that primarily affects children and is characterized by fever, sore throat, stridor, croupy cough, and an erythematous epiglottis.

exposure incident Any specific contact of the eyes, the mouth, other mucous membranes, or nonintact skin, or any parenteral contact, with blood, blood products, bloody body fluids, or other potentially infectious materials.

external barriers The surface of the body that is exposed to the environment, including the skin and the mucous membranes of the digestive, respiratory, and genitourinary tracts. The body's first line of defense against infection.

gonorrhea A sexually transmitted disease that results from contact with the causative organism *Neisseria gonorrhoeae*.

hantavirus A virus that is carried by rodents and spread to humans through body fluids of rodents. Several strains can cause different forms of severe illness, such as hemorrhagic fever with renal syndrome and hantavirus pulmonary syndrome.

head lice Tiny parasites that concentrate around the scalp (sometimes including the eyebrows and eyelashes).

hepatitis Inflammation of the liver caused by viruses, trauma, toxins, autoimmune or metabolic disorders, genetic diseases, or fat deposits.

herpes simplex virus type 1 (HSV-1) An infection caused by the herpes simplex virus that tends to occur above the waist, particularly in the facial area, such as around the mouth and nose.

herpes simplex virus type 2 (HSV-2) An infection caused by the herpes simplex virus that usually is limited to the genital region.

host The human or animal exposed to an infectious agent.

host susceptibility Factors of the host that contribute to prevention or continuation of infection.

human immunodeficiency virus (HIV) The viral agent responsible for acquired immunodeficiency syndrome.

incubation period The stage of infection during which an organism reproduces. It begins with invasion of the agent and ends when the disease process begins. The host is asymptomatic during this period.

indigenous flora Agents normally found on various sites of the body that could produce disease if allowed access to the interior of the body.

infectious disease Any illness caused by a specific microorganism.

influenza A highly contagious infection of the respiratory tract transmitted by droplet spread. Researchers have identified three main types of the virus (types A, B, and C).

internal barriers Protection against germs provided by the inflammatory response and the immune response; the body's second line of defense against infection.

latent period A stage of infection that begins when a pathogenic agent invades the body and ends when the agent can be shed or communicated.

latent TB infection Tuberculosis that is not symptomatic or infectious. It must be treated to prevent active TB disease.

malaria An infection spread by mosquitoes and caused by *Plasmodium* parasites. It results in fever, vomiting, headache.

meningitis Inflammation of the membranes (meninges) surrounding the brain and spinal cord.

meningococcal meningitis Meningitis caused by the bacterium *Neisseria meningitidis*; the deadliest form of meningitis, which is spread by respiratory droplets.

methicillin-resistant *Staphylococcus aureus* (MRSA) A *Staphylococcus* infection that is resistant to multiple antibiotics. It is spread by person-to-person contact.

mode of transmission The way in which diseases are transmitted; may be direct or indirect contact.

mononucleosis A viral infection causing fever, sore throat, and swollen lymph glands, especially in the neck.

mumps An acute viral disease characterized by swelling of the parotid glands.

opportunistic infections Infections that are pathogenic (disease-causing) only in immunocompromised hosts (eg, HIV-infected patients, patients receiving chemotherapy, patients following transplantation).

pandemic An infectious disease outbreak that affects large numbers of people worldwide.

pathogen A disease-causing agent.

pertussis An acute, highly contagious respiratory disease characterized by paroxysmal coughing that often ends in a loud, whooping inspiration; also known as whooping cough.

pneumonia An acute inflammation of the lungs, usually caused by infection with bacteria, virus, or fungus.

portal of entry The means by which the pathogenic agent enters a new host.

portal of exit The method by which a pathogenic agent leaves one host to invade another.

pubic lice Tiny parasites that concentrate in the pubic area.

rabies An acute, usually fatal viral disease of the central nervous system of animals. It is transmitted from animals to human beings by infected blood, tissue, or, most commonly, saliva.

reservoir Any person, animal, plant, soil, or substance in which an infectious agent normally lives and multiplies. It typically harbors the infectious agent without injury to itself and serves as a source from which other people can be infected.

resistance The immune status of the host; the ability to ward off infection.

respiratory syncytial virus A viral infection of the lower respiratory tract that causes cold symptoms in most cases but can be severe with bronchiolitis. Premature babies and infants younger than 1 year are at risk of severe infection.

reticuloendothelial system Part of the immune system composed of immune cells in the spleen, lymph nodes, liver, bone marrow, lungs, and intestines. It stores mature B and T cells until the immune system is activated.

rubella A contagious viral disease characterized by fever, symptoms of mild upper respiratory tract infection, lymph node enlargement, and a diffuse, fine, red maculopapular rash. It is spread by droplet infection. It results in congenital rubella syndrome in unborn babies of pregnant women infected with the disease. Also known as German measles.

rubeola An acute, highly contagious viral disease involving the respiratory tract. It is characterized by a spreading, maculopapular, cutaneous rash and occurs primarily in young children who have not been immunized. Complications include pneumonia, encephalitis, neurologic damage, and death. In pregnant women, this disease, also known as measles, can result in premature delivery and/or low birth weight of their unborn babies.

scabies A contagious parasitic skin infection characterized by superficial burrows and intense pruritus; caused by the mite *Sarcoptes scabiei*.

severe acute respiratory syndrome (SARS) An infection caused by coronavirus, which resulted in a pandemic in 2003 with high mortality rates.

sexually transmitted disease (STD) Any of a group of infections that are passed from one person to another through sexual contact.

sexually transmitted infection (STI) An infection (without symptoms) that has not yet developed into a disease.

sexually transmitted nonspecific urethritis A sexually transmitted disease characterized by inflammation or infection of the urethra in which the cause is not defined; also known as nongonococcal urethritis.

shingles An acute infection caused by reactivation of the latent varicella-zoster virus. It is characterized by painful vesicular eruptions that follow a dermatome from a spinal root. Also known as herpes zoster.

standard precautions Protective measures that have traditionally been developed by the Centers for Disease Control and Prevention for use in dealing with objects, blood, body fluids, or other potential exposure risks of communicable disease; considers all body fluids, except sweat, to present a possible risk.

syphilis A sexually transmitted disease characterized by distinct stages of effects over a period of years; may involve any organ system.

tabes dorsalis An abnormal condition characterized by the slow degeneration of all or part of the body and the progressive loss of peripheral reflexes; results from untreated syphilis infection that has spread to the spinal cord.

TB disease Active tuberculosis.

tetanus An acute, potentially fatal infection of the central nervous system caused by the tetanus bacillus *Clostridium tetani*. It is characterized by muscle spasms and convulsions.

tuberculosis (TB) A chronic granulomatous infection caused by *Mycobacterium tuberculosis*. It usually affects the lungs and generally is transmitted by airborne spread.

vancomycin-resistant enterococcus (VRE) A type of bacteria that commonly live in the bowel and have become resistant to many antibiotics.

viral meningitis Meningitis caused by viral infection (eg, enteroviral infection, herpesvirus infection, mumps, and, less commonly, influenza); also known as aseptic meningitis.

virulence The relative harmfulness or severity of a pathogen.

West Nile virus A virus spread by mosquitoes that can cause fever, headache, body aches, vomiting, diarrhea, and rash.

Zika A viral infection acquired from the bite of an infected mosquito or through blood or sexual contact with an infected person. Zika can spread from a pregnant woman to her fetus, which can result in microcephaly, severe brain malformations, and other birth defects.

Emergencies that involve infectious and communicable diseases are common in the prehospital setting. They can pose a significant health risk to both the public and EMS personnel. This chapter addresses the duties of the paramedic and EMS agencies in ensuring personal protection. It also presents the causes of infectious and communicable diseases, as well as special aspects of providing care for these conditions.

Public Health Principles Related to Infectious Diseases

An **infectious disease** is any illness caused by a specific microorganism. A **communicable disease** is an infectious disease that can be passed from one person to another. Not all infectious diseases are communicable.

Infectious diseases can affect entire populations of people. These populations or groups of people may be defined by location, age, socioeconomic status, and the relationships between the groups. Groups display varying susceptibilities to infection and varying degrees of susceptibility. In addition to demographics, several other factors can affect the life cycle of an infectious agent within a population:

- International travel
- Age distributions
- Population settling and migration
- Genetic factors
- The effectiveness of treatment once the infection has been established (BOX 27-1)

When a disease outbreak occurs, local, state, private, and federal health agencies and other organizations become involved in prevention and management. Local agencies usually are the first line of defense in disease surveillance and outbreak. They include municipal, city, and county agencies such as health departments, fire departments, and EMS agencies. Local public health agencies can also play an important role during a disease outbreak in a community by providing education to public service agencies, distributing vaccines through immunization clinics, and performing outbreak surveillance and tracking of infectious agents.

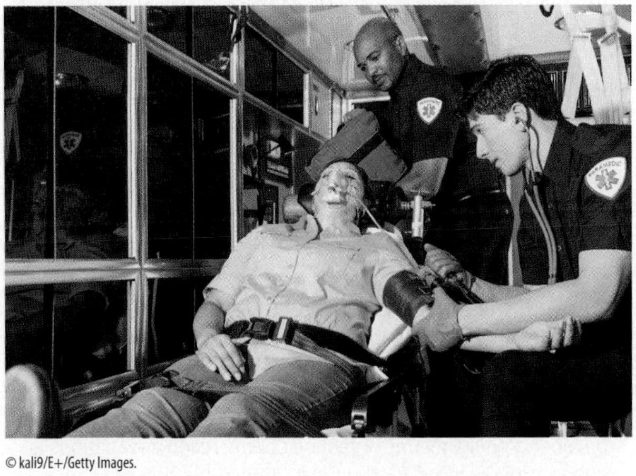

BOX 27-1 The Emergence of Acquired Immunodeficiency Syndrome (AIDS): An Outbreak of Disease

Human immunodeficiency virus (HIV) first appeared in humans in 1959 in the Democratic Republic of Congo. Within 20 to 30 years, it became an **epidemic** as poor and young sexually active people migrated from rural areas to urban centers in developing countries.

Acquired immunodeficiency syndrome (AIDS) was first identified in the United States in 1981 when young, healthy homosexual men in New York and California were found to have an unusual clustering of rare diseases (most notably Kaposi sarcoma, *Pneumocystis jirovecii* pneumonia [previously called *Pneumocystis carinii*, a term that is no longer used for human infections], and unexplained persistent lymphadenopathy). Blood tests taken at that time found antibodies to HIV, suggesting that the virus entered the US population in the late 1970s. In 2016, an estimated 36.7 million people worldwide were living with HIV infection. Since the pandemic began in 1981, more than 35 million people have died of AIDS-related illnesses.

Modified from: Division of HIV/AIDS Prevention, National Center for HIV/AIDS, Viral Hepatitis, STD, and TB Prevention, Centers for Disease Control and Prevention. HIV/AIDS: basic statistics. Centers for Disease Control and Prevention website. https://www.cdc.gov/hiv/basics/statistics.html. Updated December 18, 2017. Accessed April 8, 2018; and Global HIV and AIDS statistics. Avert website. https://www.avert.org/global-hiv-and-aids-statistics. Updated September 1, 2017. Accessed April 8, 2018.

State agencies may be involved in the enforcement of federal guidelines. They frequently are required by statute or public law to meet or exceed federal guidelines and recommendations for prevention and management of disease outbreaks.

The private sector is composed of regional and national health care providers, local and national health maintenance organizations, laboratories (hospital and private), infection control and disease specialists, and others. These groups influence the development of protocols and guidelines for tracking diseases and responding to outbreaks.

Federal and national organizations include the US Congress, which plays an integral role in national health policy by passing public laws and drafting the federal budget; the US Department of Labor's Occupational Safety and Health Administration (OSHA); and agencies under the US Department of Health and Human Services, such as the Centers for Disease Control and Prevention (CDC) and the National Institute for Occupational Safety and Health (NIOSH). Other federal and national organizations involved in the prevention and management of disease outbreaks include the US Department of Defense, the Federal Emergency Management Agency (FEMA), the National Fire Protection Association (NFPA), the US Fire Administration (USFA), the Department of Homeland Security (DHS), the Federal Interagency Committee on EMS (FICEMS), and the International Association of Fire Fighters (IAFF).

> CRITICAL THINKING
> Have you had an outbreak of a communicable disease in your region? How was it controlled?

Agency Responsibility in Infectious Agent Exposure

National concerns regarding communicable disease and infection control have resulted in public laws, guidelines, standards, and recommendations to protect health care personnel and emergency responders from infectious diseases (see Chapter 2, *Well-Being of the Paramedic*). Every health care agency's exposure control plan should include at least the following components:[1]

- Health maintenance and surveillance
- Appointment by the agency of a **designated infection control officer (DICO)** to serve as a liaison between the agency and community health agencies involved in monitoring and responding to communicable diseases
- Identification of job classifications and, in some cases, specific tasks when exposure to bloodborne pathogens is possible
- A schedule detailing when and how the provisions of bloodborne pathogen standards will be implemented
- Personal protective equipment (PPE)
- **Standard precautions**
- Procedures for evaluating exposure and post-exposure counseling
- Procedures for notifying EMS agency of potential exposure (Ryan White Act)
- Procedures for notifying and working with local health authorities and state and federal agencies regarding exposures
- Personal, building, vehicle, and equipment disinfection and storage
- Education of employees regarding disinfection agents
- After-action analysis of the agency's response
- Correct disposal of needles and sharps in appropriate containers
- Correct handling of linens and supplies that become contaminated with body fluids during patient care
- Identification of agency and/or contracted personnel for counseling, authorization of acute medical care, and documentation

> SHOW ME THE EVIDENCE
> Researchers in Las Vegas, Nevada, conducted a prospective observational study to determine the use of standard precautions by EMS providers. Research assistants in one adult emergency department (ED) observed crews' infection control practices as they arrived at the hospital and restocked and cleaned the ambulance. During the study period, 423 observations were made (96.5% ground transports, 3.5% air transports). Only 59% of EMS providers arrived wearing gloves. Even fewer (27.8%) were observed to wash their hands either in the patient's room or prior to leaving the ED. The stretcher was disinfected in 55% of cases, whereas other reusable equipment such as backboards, electrocardiogram (ECG) monitors and cables, stethoscopes, and ambulances were disinfected less than 31.6% of the time. The researchers concluded that EMS provider adherence to standard precautions is not optimal.
>
> *Modified from*: Bledsoe BE, Sweeney RJ, Berkeley RP, et al. EMS provider compliance with infection control recommendations is suboptimal. *Prehosp Emerg Care*. 2014;18(2):290-294.

Guidelines, Recommendations, Standards, and Laws

To protect health care workers against the spread of infection, OSHA requires that PPE be made available to all employees considered at high risk for exposure to infectious diseases. It also requires that all employees be offered preexposure prophylaxis against hepatitis B virus (HBV) through inoculation with the hepatitis B vaccine.[1] The CDC and NFPA have established similar guidelines, recommendations, and standards regarding the protection of health care workers and emergency personnel from communicable disease. These guidelines include regular testing for tuberculosis (TB) as well as vaccination for measles in people who do not have immunity (BOX 27-2).

BOX 27-2 Recommended Immunizations for EMS Personnel

- **HBV.** Vaccination is required by the federal OSHA.
- **Tdap (tetanus, diphtheria, pertussis).** Once every 10 years; once during each pregnancy.
- **Influenza.** Annually.
- **MMR (measles, mumps, rubella).** Varies by age, prior illness, and immunizations.
- **Varicella.** If no prior chickenpox or varicella vaccine.
- **Meningococcal.** If routinely exposed to *Neisseria meningitidis*.

Testing for TB is often required at the time of initial employment and annually thereafter. Additional vaccinations are recommended for EMS personnel involved in disaster services, military employment, or international work.

Modified from: National Center for Immunization and Respiratory Diseases. Vaccine information for adults: recommended vaccines for healthcare workers. Centers for Disease Control and Prevention website. https://www.cdc.gov/vaccines/adults/rec-vac/hcw.html. Updated April 20, 2017. Accessed April 8, 2018.

DID YOU KNOW?

Ryan White Act

The Ryan White Comprehensive AIDS Resources Emergency Act (PL 101-381), was signed into law in 1990. The Act required that emergency responders be notified if they have been exposed to infectious diseases. Employers were also required to name a DICO to direct communications between the hospital and emergency service in case of an exposure. Notification must be made within 48 hours of determination of the presence of the disease.

In December 2006, the Ryan White Treatment Modernization Act of 2006 (PL 109-415) became law. The portion of the law in the original act that addressed notification of disease exposure to first responders was removed from the legislation but was later restored. In addition, many states have laws in place that require emergency responders to be notified if they have been exposed to infectious disease.

Modified from: Public Health Service Act, Title XXI—HIV Health Care Services Program, 42 USC, Pub L No. 114-113 § 2602 1351-1445 (December 18, 2015). https://hab.hrsa.gov/sites/default/files/hab/About/RyanWhite/legislationtitlexxvi.pdf. Accessed April 8, 2018.

Currently, medical facilities are not required to test patients for any infectious disease. If paramedics have a significant exposure to blood or body fluids, they may submit a written notice to the DICO. The DICO, in turn, must submit a written request for a determination to the medical facility that treated the patient. The medical facility must try to identify the source patient and review any signs and symptoms shown by the patient that may correspond to the CDC list of infectious diseases. After determining whether a paramedic may have been exposed to an infectious disease, the medical facility must notify the DICO within 48 hours of receiving the request. If it is a significant exposure and the source patient is known, the medical facility will usually ask for patient consent to test for HIV, HBV, and hepatitis C virus (HCV) infection. (Some states permit unconsented HIV testing in cases of occupational exposure.[2]) In addition, the paramedic will be counseled about the need for postexposure prophylaxis (PEP) based on the patient's risk factors as well as the need for safe sex practices until follow-up results are known. If the patient refuses to be tested or if the source patient is unknown, follow-up monitoring for the paramedic is arranged. Follow-up monitoring for the development of HIV, HBV, and HCV is important because PEP is most effective if started immediately.

NOTE

Immediate testing of the paramedic will reveal infection only from a previous exposure—not from the exposure that prompted the immediate testing. In other words, a paramedic who tests positive for an infectious disease through an immediate test has had a previous exposure to the disease. Conversely, a paramedic who tests negative for an infectious disease through an immediate test may still become infected from the exposure that prompted the test.

> CRITICAL THINKING
> Which rights do you think paramedics had to obtain infectious disease information before the Ryan White law was passed?

Personal Responsibilities in Infectious Agent Exposure

Paramedics should familiarize themselves with the laws, regulations, and national standards regarding infectious disease, and they should take personal protective measures against exposure to these pathogens (BOX 27-3). At some point, all paramedics will provide patient care to a person with an infectious disease, so they must be aware of the potential consequences of the disease for public health and through contact with family members and friends. The CDC guidelines are designed to help prevent the spread of infectious disease to public safety and emergency response workers (see Chapter 2, *Well-Being of the Paramedic*). These guidelines include universal and standard precautions as well as **airborne precautions, droplet precautions**, and **contact precautions**. Paramedics should follow their local protocols regarding similar or additional precautions for personal protection and should be aware of their individual responsibilities, including the following:

- A proactive attitude toward infection control
- Maintenance of personal hygiene
- Attention to wounds and maintenance of the skin (the external barrier to infection)
- Effective handwashing after every patient contact using warm water and antiseptic cleanser or waterless antiseptic cleanser when water is unavailable
- Washing or disposing of work garments before entering the home
- Handling uniforms in accordance with the agency's definition of PPE
- Proper handling and laundering of work clothes soiled with body fluids, with consideration for bathing and showering after the work shift and before returning home
- Preparing food and eating in appropriate areas
- Maintenance of general physiologic and psychological health to prevent stress, which can compromise the immune system of a healthy person
- Use of needleless or safe needle devices if available
- Proper disposal of needles and sharps in appropriate containers
- Proper disposal of body fluid–tinged linens and supplies
- Regular disinfection/decontamination of work surfaces such as stretcher, radios, and handrails
- Awareness and avoidance of tendencies to wipe the face and/or rub the eyes, nose, or mouth with gloved hands
- Knowledge of general classifications of exposure to determine the extent of infection control measures applied to the health care worker

Decontamination Methods and Procedures

Guidelines for cleaning, disinfecting, and sterilizing patient care equipment have been established by the CDC, OSHA, the Environmental Protection Agency (EPA), USFA, and other agencies and organizations. These guidelines are part of an EMS agency's protocols and standard operating procedures. The following is a brief description of these decontamination methods and procedures.[3]

Sterilization destroys all forms of microbial life. It is used for instruments that penetrate the skin or come in contact with normally sterile parts of the body (eg, scalpels, needles). Methods that may be used for sterilization include steam under pressure (autoclave), gas (ethylene oxide), dry heat, and immersion in an EPA-approved chemical sterilant.

High-level disinfection destroys all forms of microbial life *except* high numbers of bacterial spores. This procedure is used for reusable instruments that have contact with mucous membranes (eg, laryngoscope blades, endotracheal tubes). Methods that may be used for high-level disinfection include hot water pressurization and exposure to an EPA-registered chemical sterilant.

Intermediate-level disinfection destroys *Mycobacterium tuberculosis*, most viruses, vegetative bacteria, and most fungi, but not bacterial spores. It is used for surfaces that come in contact with intact skin (eg, stethoscopes, blood pressure cuffs, splints) and for surfaces that have been visibly contaminated with blood or body fluids. (Surfaces must be cleaned of visible material before disinfection.) Methods that may be used for intermediate-level disinfection include use of EPA-registered "hospital disinfectant" chemical germicides that claim to be tuberculocidal

BOX 27-3 Guidelines for Prevention of Transmission of HIV and HBV to Health Care and Public Safety Workers

Employees must be protected from exposure to blood and other potentially infectious body fluids. The following guidelines can assist rescue personnel in making decisions about the use of PPE and resuscitation equipment, documentation, disinfection, and disposal procedures.

PPE should be made available by the employer to reduce the risk of exposure. If the chance of exposure is high (eg, responses involving cardiopulmonary resuscitation, vascular access, trauma, or childbirth), the worker should take protective measure before beginning patient care.

Gloves

All personnel should have ready access to disposable gloves before giving any care that involves any exposure to possible infection to which standard precautions apply. The choice of disposable gloves should consider dexterity, durability, fit, and the task to be performed. If exposure to large amounts of blood is likely, the gloves should fit tightly to prevent contamination. Gloves should be changed between patients, when possible.

Other protective measures are indicated when broken glass and sharp edges are encountered. Examples include vehicle extrication when structural firefighting gloves[a] should be worn to protect against sharp or rough surfaces.

While wearing gloves, paramedics should avoid handling personal items (eg, phones, pens) that could become soiled or contaminated. Gloves that have become contaminated with blood or other body fluids should be removed as soon as possible and placed and transported for proper disposal or disinfection in containers that prevent leakage.

Mask, Eyewear, and Gowns

Masks, eyewear, and gowns should be readily available and used when appropriate, based on the level of possible exposure. In the absence of visible blood or body fluids do not routine require the use of barrier precautions. An extra change of work clothing should be available at all times.

Resuscitation Equipment

The transmission of HBV or HIV infection while providing artificial ventilation has not been documented. However, because of the risk of transmission of other infectious diseases through saliva, disposable airway equipment or resuscitation bags should be used. Diseases that can be spread in saliva include herpes simplex infection and *N meningitidis*. Theoretically, a risk exists of HIV and HBV transmission during artificial ventilation of trauma victims.

Disposable resuscitation equipment and devices should be discarded after use. Reusable equipment should be thoroughly cleaned and disinfected after each use according to the manufacturer's recommendations.

[a]Standards are presented in 29 Code of Federal Register (CFR) 1910.156 and in NFPA Standard 1581, Standard on Fire Department Infection Control Program (2015 edition).

Modified from: US Department of Health and Human Services, Centers for Disease Control and Prevention, National Institute of Occupational Safety and Health. *Guidelines for Prevention of Transmission of Human Immunodeficiency Virus and Hepatitis B Virus to Health-Care and Public-Safety Workers.* Washington, DC: US Department of Health and Human Services; 1989.

on the label, hard-surface germicides, and solutions containing at least 550 parts per million (ppm) free available chlorine (1:100 dilution of common household bleach: approximately 1 cup of bleach per 1 gallon of water).

Low-level disinfection destroys some viruses, most bacteria, and some fungi, but not *M tuberculosis* or bacterial spores. It is used for routine housekeeping and to clean up soiled surfaces when no blood is visible. Methods that may be used for low-level disinfection include use of EPA-registered "hospital disinfectants." (The label carries no claim of tuberculocidal activity.)

Environmental disinfection cleans soiled surfaces in the environment, such as floors, ambulance seats, and countertops. Such surfaces should be disinfected with cleaners or disinfectant agents.

Exposure and the Risk of Infection

As described in Chapter 26, *Immune System Disorders*, the body's immune response to an invading pathogen depends on the size of the pathogen and the pathogen's ability to stimulate production of an antibody. Often, peripheral phagocytic cells encounter a pathogen first, but circulating B and T cells also are scouting for pathogens (BOX 27-4). Complex interactions occur among neutrophils, macrophages, and B and T cells. These cells assist each other in processing antigens that allow them to recognize and destroy the invading pathogens.

The B cells' role is to produce antibodies (humoral immunity). When the B cell encounters a foreign invader, an antibody coats the pathogen and facilitates

BOX 27-4 Types of T Cells

Sensitized T cells develop into distinct groups, with each group having its own specific set of functions that coordinate the activity of other components of the immune system.

- Killer T cells (like B cells) are sensitized and stimulated to multiply by the presence of antigens on abnormal body cells. Unlike B cells, killer T cells do not produce antibodies.
- Helper T cells "turn on" the activities of killer (cytotoxic) cells. They also control other aspects of the immune response.
- Suppressor T cells "turn off" the action of the helper and killer T cells, preventing them from causing harmful immune reactions.

phagocytosis. Antibodies can also fix complement. The **complement system** is a group of proteins that coat bacteria and help to kill them directly. Alternatively, the proteins can ensure that the bacteria are taken up by neutrophils in the blood or by macrophages in the tissues.

T cells not only process antigens for the B cells but also include a subpopulation of "killer cells." These cells play a major role in cell-mediated immunity (**FIGURE 27-1**).

Both the humoral and the cell-mediated types of immunity take time to work, and both also require previous exposure to a pathogen or antigen to mobilize specialized white cells. In time, these white cells learn to differentiate between antibodies and can organize

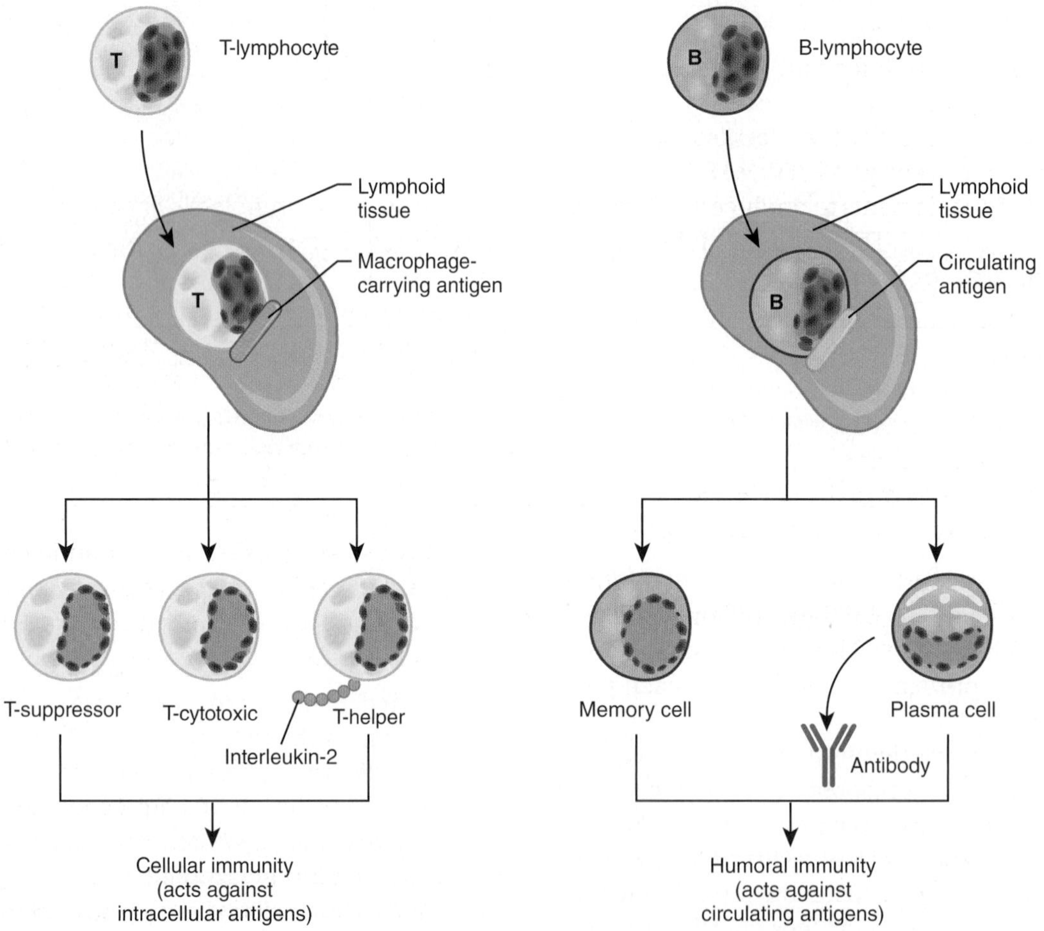

FIGURE 27-1 Cellular and humoral immunity. Cellular immunity results from activation of T cells through contact with intracellular organisms. Activated T cells differentiate and proliferate. Humoral (antibody-mediated) immunity results from the activation of B cells.

an attack on the foreign material. By comparison, the complement system recognizes and kills invaders on first sight; it does not take repeated exposure or extra time to mobilize specialized responses.

The **reticuloendothelial system** works with the lymphatic system to dispose of the debris left in the wake of the immune system's attack on invading organisms. The reticuloendothelial system is composed of immune cells in the spleen, lymph nodes, liver, bone marrow, lungs, and intestines. These structures store mature B and T cells until the immune system is activated.

Pathophysiology of Infectious Disease

The development and/or manifestations of clinical disease depend on several factors, including the **virulence** (degree of pathogenicity) of the infectious agent, the number of infectious agents (dose), the **resistance** (immune status) of the **host** (the human or animal who is exposed to the infectious agent), and the correct mode of entry.[4] All of these factors rely on an intact chain of elements to produce an infectious disease (**FIGURE 27-2**). The elements of the chain of infection include the following:[5]

- The pathogenic agent
- A reservoir
- A portal of exit from the reservoir
- An environment conducive to transmission of the pathogenic agent
- A portal of entry into the new host
- Susceptibility of the new host to the infectious disease

Even if all these elements are present, exposure does not necessarily mean that a person will become infected.

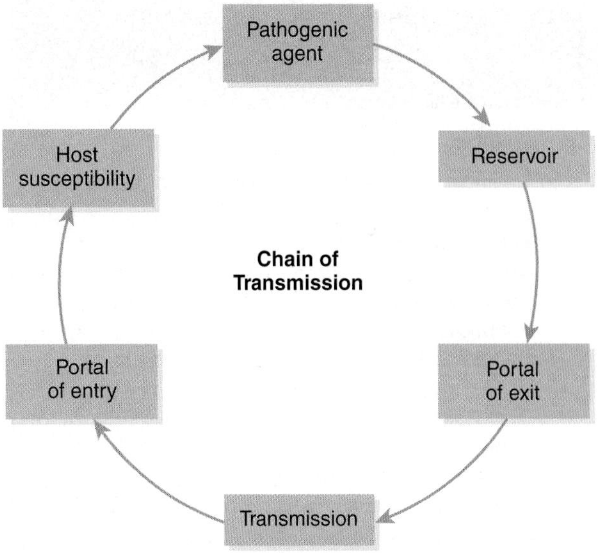

FIGURE 27-2 Chain of transmission for infection. The chain must be intact for an infection to be transmitted to another host. Transmission can be controlled by breaking any link in the chain.

CRITICAL THINKING

Describe a precaution or intervention that could break each of the links in the chain of disease transmission.

Pathogenic Agent

A **pathogen** is an organism that can cause disease in the human host. Pathogens are classified according to their shape (morphology), chemical composition, growth requirements, and viability. They rely on a host to supply their nutritional needs.

Some pathogens (eg, certain bacteria) are metabolically equipped to survive outside a host. In contrast, others (eg, certain viruses) can survive only in the human cell (**BOX 27-5**). Some viruses, such as HIV and HBV, can survive for several hours outside a host—a factor that explains why blood products can be infectious.

Most bacteria are susceptible to antibiotics. These drugs either kill the bacteria or inhibit their growth. Viruses, however, are more difficult to eradicate because they reside in cells for most of their life cycle and become intricately enmeshed in the host cell's deoxyribonucleic acid (DNA). The following factors affect a pathogen's ability to cause disease:

- The ability to invade and reproduce in a host, and the mode by which the pathogen does so
- The speed of reproduction, the ability to produce a toxin, and the degree of tissue damage that results
- Pathogenicity and virulence
- The ability to induce or evade an immune response in the host

BOX 27-5 Review of Infectious Agents and Their Properties

Bacteria

- Bacteria are prokaryotic, meaning that the nuclear material is not contained within a distinctive envelope known as a nucleus.
- They can self-reproduce without a host cell.
- Signs and symptoms depend on the cells and tissues affected.
- Bacteria produce toxins, which are often more lethal than the bacterium itself.
- Endotoxins (chemicals, usually proteins), also known as lipopolysaccharides, are integral parts of a bacterium's outer membrane and are constantly shed from living bacteria. They are found only in gram-negative bacteria. The endotoxins are released when bacteria are lysed; if they enter the bloodstream, sepsis may result.
- Exotoxins (proteins) are released by bacteria and can cause disease symptoms by damaging specific cells. Examples include neurotoxins (nerve cells) and enterotoxins in intestinal cells.
- Bacteria can cause localized or systemic infection.

Viruses

- Viruses are neither prokaryotic nor eukaryotic; rather, they are living organisms without a nucleus.
- Viruses must invade host cells to reproduce.
- Many cannot survive outside a host cell.

Fungi

- Fungi are eukaryotic, meaning the nuclear material is contained within a distinct envelope known as a nucleus.
- A protective capsule surrounds the cell wall to protect the organism from phagocytes.

Protozoa

- Protozoa are eukaryotic.
- Protozoa are single-celled microorganisms but are more complex than bacteria.

Helminths (Worms [Including Tapeworms], Roundworms)

- Helminths are eukaryotic.
- Helminths are pathogenic parasites but are not necessarily microorganisms.

Reservoir

Pathogens live and reproduce within a **reservoir**, which may be humans or other animal hosts (including arthropods), plants, soil, water, food, or some other organic substance, or a combination of these reservoirs. When infected, the human host may either show signs of clinical illness or be an asymptomatic carrier (ie, a person who can pass the pathogen to others without showing signs of illness). As stated previously, the life cycle of the infectious agent depends on three factors: the demographics of the host, genetic factors, and the efficacy of therapeutic interventions once infection has been established.

Portal of Exit

The method by which a pathogenic agent leaves one host to invade another involves a **portal of exit**. The portal of exit from the human host depends on the agent. It may be single or multiple, involving the genitourinary (GU) tract, intestinal tract, oral cavity, respiratory tract, an open lesion, or any wound through which blood escapes. The time during which an actively infectious pathogen escapes to produce disease in another host coincides with the period of communicability (described later in this chapter); this period varies with each disease.

Mode of Transmission

The portal of exit and the portal of entry determine the **mode of transmission**. This mode may be either direct or indirect. Direct transmission results from physical contact between the source and the victim. Examples of direct transmission include direct physical contact (handshake), oral contact, droplet spread, airborne spread, fecal contamination, and sexual contact. In indirect transmission, the organism survives on animate or inanimate objects for a time without a human host. Diseases can be transmitted indirectly by air, food, water, soil, or biologic matter.

Portal of Entry

The **portal of entry** is the means by which the pathogenic agent enters a new host. It may be by ingestion, inhalation, percutaneous injection, crossing of a mucous membrane, or crossing of the placenta. The time it takes for the infectious process to begin in a new host varies with the disease and host susceptibility. The duration of the exposure to the pathogen and the number of organisms required to initiate the infectious process also vary. Exposure to an infectious agent does not always produce infection.

SHOW ME THE EVIDENCE

Prevalence of Methicillin-Resistant *Staphylococcus aureus* Among EMS Personnel

Researchers performed a cross-sectional research study to determine the rate and prevalence of methicillin-resistant *S aureus* (MRSA) cultured from the noses of Ohio EMS providers. They surveyed and tested 280 EMS personnel from 84 agencies representing all 10 EMS regions in the state. EMS workers with an open wound (including lesions, boils, infections) were 6.75 times more likely (95% confidence interval [CI], 1.25–36.36; $P = 0.262$) to have a positive MRSA culture than were those who did not. Providers who reported washing their hands fewer than eight times per shift or those reporting less frequent handwashing after glove use were also significantly more likely to have positive MRSA cultures than were those who washed their hands more frequently. The researchers estimated that the prevalence of MRSA carriage in EMS personnel in Ohio was two to three times higher than that of the general population. Their results support CDC guidelines for frequent handwashing.

Modified from: Orellana RC, Hoet AE, Bell C, et al. Methicillin-resistant *Staphylococcus aureus* in Ohio EMS providers: a statewide cross-sectional study. *Prehosp Emerg Care.* 2016;20(2): 184-190.

Host Susceptibility

Host susceptibility is influenced by a person's immune response. It also is influenced by several other factors:

1. Human characteristics
   - Age
   - Sex
   - Ethnic group
   - Heredity
2. General health status
   - Nutrition
   - Hormonal balance
   - Presence of concurrent disease
   - History of previous disease
3. Immune status
   - Prior exposure to disease (conferring resistance)
   - Effective immunization against disease (conferring host immunity)
4. Geographic and environmental conditions
5. Cultural behaviors
   - Eating habits
   - Personal hygiene
   - Sexual behaviors

Physiology of the Human Response to Infection

The human body is regularly exposed to pathogens that can cause illness. Even so, most people do not succumb to infectious disease because of the protection conferred by the body's external and internal barriers, which act as lines of defense against infection.

External Barriers

The first line of defense against infection is the surface of the body, which is exposed to the environment. The body's **external barriers** include the skin and the mucous membranes of the digestive, respiratory, and GU tracts. These areas are inhabited by **indigenous flora** (agents that could produce disease if allowed access to the interior of the body). The surface of the body forms a continuous closed barrier between the internal organs and the environment (**FIGURE 27-3**).

Flora

Nearly the whole body surface is inhabited by normal microbial flora. Flora enhances the effectiveness of the

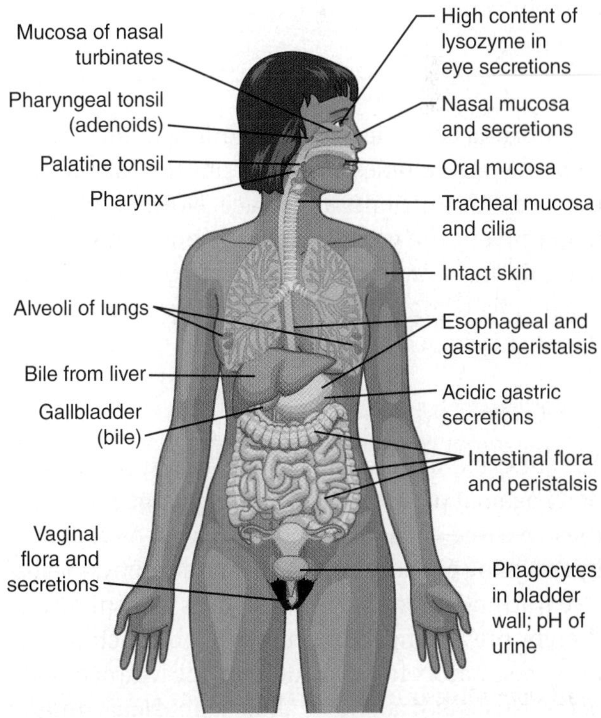

FIGURE 27-3 First line of defense: external barriers.

surface barrier by interfering with the establishment of pathogenic agents in several ways. Indigenous flora competes with pathogens for space and nutrients and also maintains a pH optimal for its own growth, which can be incompatible with the pH needed for many pathogenic agents to survive. In addition, some flora secretes germicidal substances and is thought to stimulate the immune system.

Although normal flora plays a key role in the body's defense, some indigenous flora can be pathogenic under certain conditions. For example, these organisms can cause infection when the skin or mucous membranes are interrupted (eg, in cellulitis). They also can cause infection when flora is displaced from its natural habitat to another area of the body (eg, in urinary tract infection). Finally, an overgrowth of flora may result in disease (eg, in *Clostridium difficile* colitis).

Skin

Intact skin defends the body against infection in two ways. First, it prevents penetration of the pathogens into the internal environment of the body. Second, it maintains an acidic pH level that inhibits the growth of pathogenic bacteria. In addition, microbes are sloughed from the skin's surface with dead skin cells, and oil and sweat wash microorganisms from the skin's pores.

Gastrointestinal System

The normal bacteria in the gastrointestinal system compete with colonies of microorganisms that invade the body for nutrients and space. Normal bacteria help prevent the growth of pathogenic organisms. In addition, stomach acid may destroy some microorganisms or deactivate their toxic products. The digestive system eliminates pathogens through feces.

Upper Respiratory Tract

The sticky membranes of the upper airway protect the body against pathogens by trapping large particles; these particles may then be swallowed or expelled by coughing or sneezing. Coarse nasal hairs and cilia also trap and filter foreign substances in inspired air, thereby preventing the pathogens from reaching the lower respiratory tract. In addition, the lymph tissues of the tonsils and adenoids allow a rapid local immunologic response to pathogenic organisms that may enter the respiratory tract.

GU Tract

The natural process of urination and urine's ability to kill bacteria help prevent infections in the GU tract. Antibacterial substances in prostatic fluid and the vagina also help prevent infection in the GU system.

> NOTE
>
> Enterococci are bacteria that are normally present in the human intestines, the female genital tract, and the environment. These bacteria may cause infections. Vancomycin is an antibiotic that is often used to treat infections caused by enterococci. In some instances, enterococci have become resistant to this drug and thus are called **vancomycin-resistant enterococci (VRE)**. Most VRE infections occur in hospitals. Enterococci also may become resistant to most or all other standard drug therapies (multidrug-resistant enterococci).

Internal Barriers

Internal barriers protect the body against microorganisms when the external lines of defense cannot. Internal barriers include the inflammatory response and the immune response, which share many of the same processes and cellular components.

Inflammatory Response

Inflammation (described in Chapter 11, *General Principles of Pathophysiology*, and Chapter 26, *Immune System Disorders*) is a local reaction to cellular injury. It occurs in response to a microbial infection and is activated when an invasion of a pathogen occurs. It works to prevent further incursion of the pathogen by isolating, destroying, or neutralizing the microorganism (**FIGURE 27-4**).

The inflammatory response usually is protective and beneficial, but sometimes it may initiate destruction of the body's own tissue. In particular, it may prove damaging if the response is sustained or directed against the host's own antigens. To review, the inflammatory response may be divided into three separate stages: (1) cellular response to injury, (2) vascular response to injury, and (3) phagocytosis.

Cellular Response to Injury. The body mounts various types of cellular responses to injury. Some cells are the targets of specific inflammatory mediators (eg, leukotrienes, histamine). When these cells are injured,

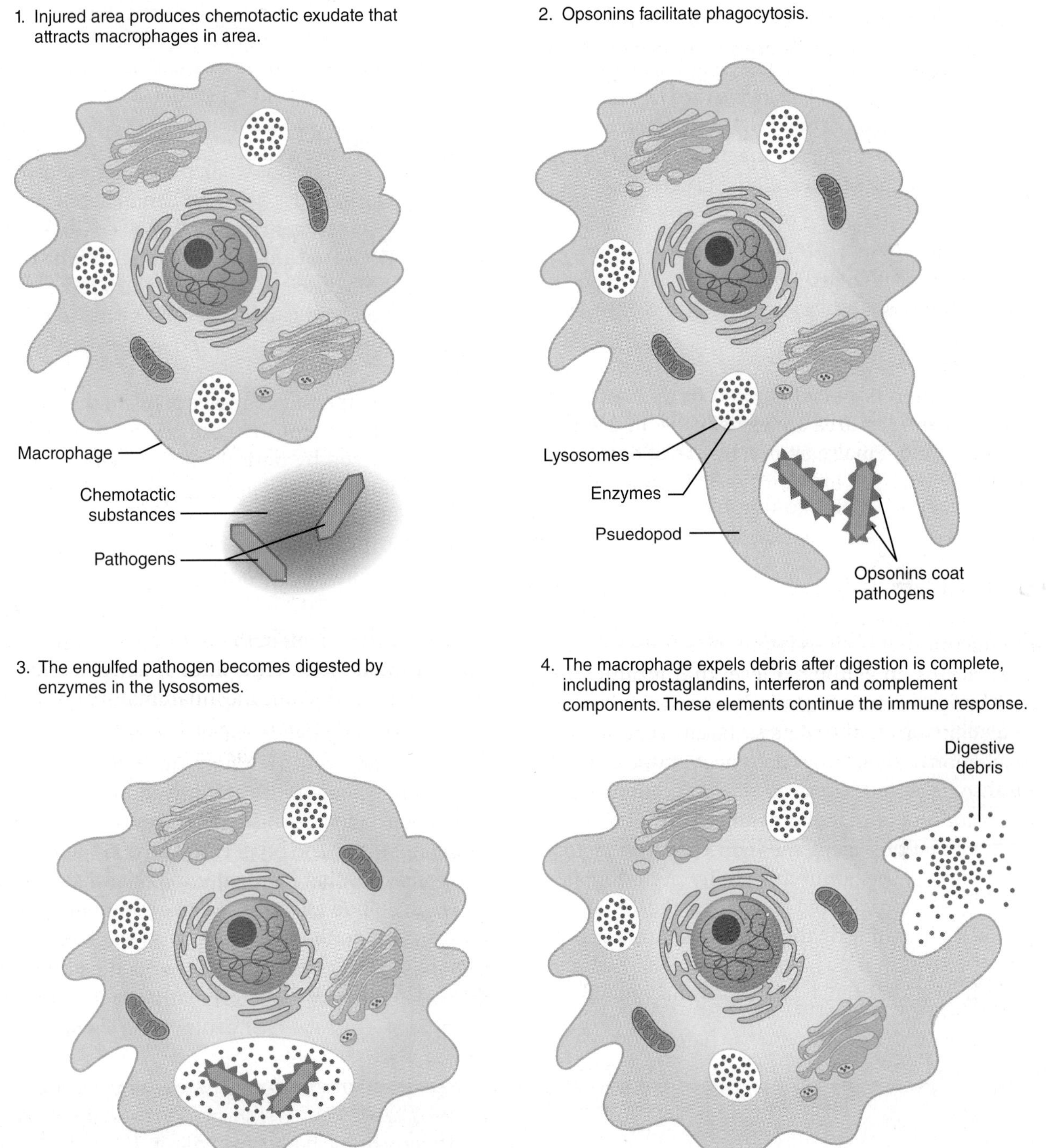
1. Injured area produces chemotactic exudate that attracts macrophages in area.
Macrophage
Chemotactic substances
Pathogens
2. Opsonins facilitate phagocytosis.
Lysosomes
Enzymes
Psuedopod
Opsonins coat pathogens
3. The engulfed pathogen becomes digested by enzymes in the lysosomes.
4. The macrophage expels debris after digestion is complete, including prostaglandins, interferon and complement components. These elements continue the immune response.
Digestive debris

FIGURE 27-4 Second line of defense: inflammatory response.

the cell's metabolism is damaged, which decreases the energy reserves available in the cell. The depletion of energy reserves results in an accumulation of sodium ions which causes the cell to swell. The increasing acidosis and swelling further impairs the cell's ability to function and leads to deterioration of the cell membranes. Eventually, the cell membranes begin to leak, which contributes to cellular destruction, autolysis, and stimulation of the inflammatory response in surrounding tissues.

Vascular Response to Injury. Localized hyperemia (an increase in blood flow in the area) develops after cellular injury and produces edema. During this process, leukocytes collect inside the vessels, where they release **chemotactic factors** (chemicals that attract more leukocytes to the area). These factors eventually migrate to the injured tissue.

> CRITICAL THINKING
> Which physical examination finding is related to this infection-fighting property?

Phagocytosis. Through phagocytosis, leukocytes engulf, digest, and destroy the invading pathogens. Circulating macrophages clear the area of dead cells and other debris. The ingestion of bacteria and dead cells (internal phagocytosis) releases chemicals that destroy leukocytes.

Stages of Infectious Disease

The progression from exposure to an infectious agent to the onset of clinical disease progresses in a series of specific stages, described as the latent period, the incubation period, the communicability period, and the disease period (**TABLE 27-1**). The duration of each stage and the potential outcomes vary, depending on the infectious agent and individual host factors. For example, the communicability period may or may not overlap with the incubation and/or disease periods, depending on the agent. In some cases, the risk of infection may be theoretical; that is, transmission is acknowledged to be possible but has not actually occurred. The risk of infection is considered measurable when infection is confirmed or deduced from reported data.

Latent Period

The **latent period** begins when the pathogen invades the body. During this period, infection has occurred but the infectious agent cannot be passed (or "shed") to someone else or cause clinically significant symptoms. In some diseases (eg, HIV), the latent period is quite stable and can last several years. In others (eg, influenza), the latent period may last only 24 to 72 hours.

The latent period as a stage of infectious disease differs from a latent infection. A latent infection is characterized by periods of inactivity between attacks. Herpesviruses are examples of pathogens that readily enter a latent stage. During this stage, symptoms disappear but may reappear when the latent infection is reactivated.

Incubation Period

The **incubation period** is the interval between exposure to the pathogen and the first onset of symptoms. Like the latent period, the incubation period varies in length, ranging from a few hours to 15 years or longer (eg, in some people with HIV infection). During the incubation period, the infectious organism reproduces in the host, and the body is stimulated to produce antibodies specific for the disease or antigen. Thus, a person's blood may test positive (seroconversion) for exposure to the disease. A window phase, however, follows infection. In this phase, the antigen is present but there is no detectable antibody. A person

TABLE 27-1 Stages of Infectious Disease

Stage	Begins	Ends
Latent period	With invasion	When the agent can be shed
Incubation period	With invasion	When the disease process begins
Communicability period	When the latent period ends	Continues as long as the agent is present and can spread to others
Disease period	After the incubation period	Variable duration

whose blood is tested for disease-specific antibodies in the window phase may test negative, even when infection is present.

Communicability Period

The **communicability period** follows the latent period. It lasts as long as the agent is present and can spread to other hosts. (Clinically significant symptoms from the infection may manifest during this period.) This stage is variable and may occur during the incubation and/or disease periods. It often is the major determining factor in ease of transmission. The communicability period and the method of transmission can vary in some diseases (eg, TB, syphilis, gonorrhea), depending on the stage of the disease and the primary site of infection.

Disease Period

The **disease period** follows the incubation period. It varies in duration, depending on the specific disease. This stage may be free of symptoms or may be characterized by overt symptoms. These symptoms can arise directly from the invading organism or from the body's response to the disease. During the disease period, the body may sometimes be able to rid itself of the disease entirely. In other cases, the organism may become incorporated and lie inactive inside certain cells (a latent disease); HIV infection and hepatitis are examples of this disease process. Thus, the resolution of symptoms does not always mean the infectious agent has been destroyed.

> CRITICAL THINKING
>
> Which of the four stages of infectious disease can overlap? Which problems can the overlap (or overlaps) pose?

Human Immunodeficiency Virus

Human immunodeficiency virus (HIV) is present in the blood and serum-derived body fluids (semen, breast milk, vaginal or cervical secretions) of people infected with the virus. The pathogen is directly transmitted from person to person; that is, it is passed through anal or vaginal intercourse, across the placenta, or by contact between infected blood or body fluids and mucous membranes or open wounds. The virus also can be transmitted indirectly, through transfusion with contaminated blood or blood products, transplantation of tissues and organs, and the use of contaminated needles or syringes. The incidence of HIV is highest in men having sex with men. In all people, it is associated with the following risk factors:[6]

Highest risk:
- High-risk sexual behavior (unprotected vaginal or anal sex)
- Sharing intravenous (IV) needles with an HIV-positive person (HIV can live on a contaminated needle for up to 42 days)

Less often:
- Needlestick from HIV-contaminated needle or sharp object
- Infant born to or breastfed by an HIV-positive mother

Rarely:
- Oral sex
- Blood transfusion recipient (this risk was high between 1978 and 1985)
- Eating prechewed food (mother to infant)
- Bite from an HIV-positive person
- Direct contact between broken skin or mucous membranes with HIV-infected blood or body fluids
- Deep open-mouthed kissing when both partners have openings in the mucous membranes

Other factors that may affect susceptibility to HIV infection include a concurrent sexually transmitted disease (STD) or **sexually transmitted infection (STI)**, especially with STDs or STIs that cause skin ulcerations.

Pathophysiology

HIV infection results from one of two retroviruses, HIV-1 and HIV-2, which convert genetic ribonucleic acid (RNA) to DNA after entering the host cell. Once the retrovirus is inside the cell, the cell's genetic material is altered into a hybrid of part virus and part cell. The virus basically takes over the cell's machinery to manufacture more viral particles. When enough of the viral particles have been produced, the host cell ruptures, destroying the cell and releasing the virus into the blood to seek new target cells. The cell receptors sought by HIV are CD4 molecules located on the surface of T cells (CD4 T cells). T cells, as mentioned earlier, play an important role in the immune system. When HIV attaches itself to the CD4 molecule, the virus is able to enter and infect the cell, damaging the cell in the process. The CD4 T-cell count is used to determine how active the disease is; a very low count suggests severe disease. CD4 molecules are also found on the surface of certain nerve cells, and on monocytes and phagocytes, which probably carry the disease to other parts of the body.

Even though the body develops antigen-specific antibodies to HIV, these antibodies do not protect against HIV. Secondary complications generally are caused by **opportunistic infections** that develop as the immune system deteriorates. These infections include the following:[7]

- Pulmonary TB
- Recurrent pneumonia
- Fungal infections (candidiasis and others)
- *Pneumocystis jirovecii* pneumonia
- Cancers (Kaposi sarcoma, cervical cancer, lymphoma)
- Wasting syndrome
- HIV encephalitis
- Viral infections (herpes simplex, cytomegalovirus)
- Parasitic infections causing diarrhea (cryptosporidiosis and others)
- Toxoplasmosis of the central nervous system (CNS)

NOTE

The two types of HIV (HIV-1 and HIV-2) are serologically and geographically distinct, but share similar epidemiologic characteristics. HIV-1 is much more pathogenic than is HIV-2. Most cases worldwide and in the United States are caused by HIV-1. HIV-2 seems to be more restricted to West Africa.

Modified from: HIV strains and types. Avert website. https://www.avert.org/professionals/hiv-science/types-strains. Updated January 23, 2018. Accessed April 9, 2018.

Classification and Categories

The average interval from transmission of HIV to the development of serious complications is approximately 10 years if the condition is untreated.[8] However, this time frame can vary greatly (**TABLE 27-2**).

The CDC has devised a classification system for HIV (revised in 2014) with three categories based on the CD4+ T-lymphocyte count or CD4+ T-lymphocyte percentage of total lymphocytes.[9] For people 6 years or older, these categories are as follows:

- **Category 1.** Cell count of 500/mcL or higher ($\geq$26%)
- **Category 2.** Cell count of 200 to 499/mcL (14% to 25%)
- **Category 3.** Cell count below 200/mcL ($<$14%)

As the number of CD4 T cells decreases, the risk and severity of opportunistic illness increase.

After viral transmission, the progression of HIV in adolescents and adults can be divided into three clinical stages, labeled 1, 2, and 3. These stages should not be confused with the three categories mentioned earlier. The categories refer to the specific cell count, whereas the stages indicate the clinical stage—that is, the patient's signs and symptoms and severity of disease.

Stage 1: Acute HIV Infection

The stage 1 syndrome generally occurs 2 to 4 weeks after exposure. Clinical features include a flulike illness with fever, adenopathy, and sore throat. The febrile illness is self-limited and usually lasts 1 to 2 weeks. During this stage, a transient decrease is observed in the CD4 T-cell count. During this period, specific antigen testing or advanced antibody testing is needed to detect the disease in the blood, as the serologic response with antigen-specific antibodies to HIV generally occurs 6 to 12 weeks after transmission. During this stage, the CD4 T-cell count returns to normal.

CRITICAL THINKING

What is the likely result of a rapid HIV test purchased from the pharmacy during the third week after exposure?

Stage 2: Clinical Latency (Asymptomatic HIV Infection or Chronic HIV Infection)

In stage 2, the patient may not have symptoms, but the virus is still reproducing slowly. People taking HIV antiretroviral therapy diligently during this stage may have very low viral loads and are less likely to transmit the disease. As this phase ends, the patient's

TABLE 27-2 Incubation and Communicability Periods of Various Infectious Diseases

Incubation Period	Communicability Period
Childhood Diseases	
Chickenpox	
2–3 weeks (average: 13–17 days)	Occurs 1 or 2 days before onset of rash and until lesions have crusted over, and not more than 6 days after appearance of vesicles
Mumps	
2–3 weeks (average: 18 days)	Occurs 6 days before parotid symptoms to 9 days after; disease is most communicable 48 hours after parotid swelling develops
Pertussis	
7–14 days, commonly 7–10 days	Occurs 7 days after exposure and lasts 3 weeks after disease stage onset; highly communicable in early stage before cough; not communicable after 3 weeks, although cough may be present
Rubella (German Measles)	
14–23 days (average: 16–18 days)	Occurs from 1 week before to 4 days after appearance of rash; infants with congenital rubella syndrome may shed virus for months after birth
Rubeola (Measles)	
Commonly 10 days, 8–13 days until fever, 14 days until rash	Occurs a few days before fever to 5–7 days after appearance of rash
Hantavirus	
3 days to 6 weeks	No known human-to-human transmission
Hepatitis Virus	
Hepatitis A Virus	
15–50 days (average: 28–30 days)	Usually occurs in the latter half of the incubation period and continues for several days after onset of jaundice
Hepatitis B Virus	
45–180 days (average: 60–90 days)	Occurs during the incubation period and lasts throughout the clinical course (carrier state may persist for years)
Hepatitis C Virus	
2 weeks to 6 months (average 6–9 weeks)	Occurs 1 or more weeks before onset of symptoms; indefinitely during chronic and carrier states
HIV	
Varies: 6–12 weeks from exposure to seropositivity, up to 10 years (variable) for symptomatic immune suppression and to diagnosis of AIDS	Is lifelong, from the presence of HIV in serum until death; degree of communicability may vary during the course of HIV infection
Influenza	
24–72 hours	Occurs 3 days after onset of symptoms; infection produces immunity to specific strain of virus, but duration of immunity varies

(continued)

TABLE 27-2 Incubation and Communicability Periods of Various Infectious Diseases *(continued)*

Incubation Period	Communicability Period
Meningitis	
2–10 days	Varies; lasts as long as infectious agents remain in nasal and oral secretions; microorganisms disappear from the upper respiratory tract within 24 hours of antibiotic therapy
Mononucleosis	
4–6 weeks	Prolonged; pharyngeal excretion may last for years; 15–20% of adults are carriers
Pneumonia	
1–3 days	Occurs until organisms have been eliminated from respiratory discharges (24–48 hours after antibiotic treatment)
Rabies	
Usually 2–16 weeks (may be shorter depending on the dose of exposure)	Human-to-human transmission by bite, scratch, or aerosolization has not been documented; theoretical transmission from contact with secretions of infected person
Severe Acute Respiratory Syndrome	
10 days	Information to date suggests that people are most likely to be infectious when they have symptoms, such as fever or cough; however, it is not known how long before or after symptoms appear that disease can be transmitted
Sexually Transmitted Diseases	
Chlamydia	
5–10 days	Unknown; may extend for months or longer if untreated, especially in asymptomatic persons; reinfections are common; effective treatment ends infectivity
Gonorrhea	
2–7 days	Occurs for months if disease is untreated
HSV	
HSV-1: 2–12 days	Occurs when lesions are present; transmission can also occur when visible lesions are not present; virus is found in saliva as long as 7 weeks after recovery from lesions; transient shedding of virus is common
HSV-2: 2–12 days (average 6 days)	Occurs when lesions are present; transient shedding of virus in the absence of lesions probably occurs
Syphilis	
10 days to 10 weeks (average 3 weeks)	Varies; occurs during primary and secondary stages and in mucocutaneous recurrences (2–4 years if disease is untreated)
Tetanus	
3–21 days, commonly 10 days	Not directly transmitted; recovery from tetanus does not confer permanent immunity
Tuberculosis	
4–12 weeks after exposure or anytime disease is in a latent stage	Occurs as long as bacilli are present in sputum, sometimes intermittently for years

Abbreviations: AIDS, acquired immunodeficiency virus; HIV, human immunodeficiency virus; HSV, herpes simplex virus viral load increases and the CD4+ cell count drops, predisposing the patient to opportunistic infections.

Stage 3: AIDS

When patients enter the AIDS phase, they develop chills, fever, sweats, swollen lymph glands, weakness, and weight loss. Without treatment, patients who progress to AIDS typically survive about 3 years. Antiretroviral treatment can be helpful for patients with AIDS and is likely to benefit patients with HIV no matter when it is started. AIDS is defined as a CD4 count of less than 200/mcL or the presence of an AIDS-defining illness (opportunistic infection). During stage 3, the immune system is severely compromised and the patient develops opportunistic infections such as bacterial pneumonia with *P jirovecii*; pulmonary TB; debilitating diarrhea; tumors in any body system, including Kaposi sarcoma (**FIGURE 27-5**); HIV-associated dementia; and neurologic manifestations.

Aging With HIV

Since the advent of highly active antiretroviral treatment (HAART), survival of patients diagnosed with HIV has markedly improved, such that HIV infection is now considered a chronic disease.[10] It appears, though, that the aging process is accelerated in people infected with HIV. It is not understood whether this effect relates to the disease itself or to the treatment for the disease. Other chronic illnesses such as heart, liver, and kidney disease; cancer; and diabetes are also more prevalent in aging HIV-positive patients. In fact, in developed countries, death is more likely to be related to one of these chronic illnesses than to HIV or AIDs.[11] Bone density decreases in HIV-infected patients, putting them at increased risk for fractures. Neurocognitive impairment is another frequent finding in these patients as they age. Thus, it is important to recognize these risk factors for disease in the HIV-infected patient population.

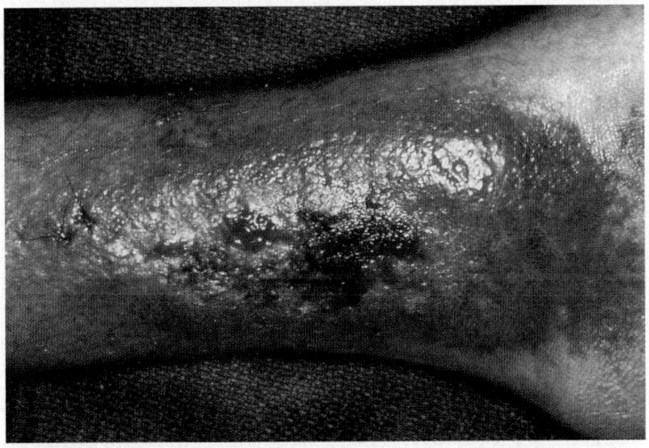

FIGURE 27-5 Kaposi sarcoma of the distal leg and ankle.

Courtesy of Centers for Disease Control and Prevention.

Personal Protection

Strict compliance with standard precautions is the only preventive measure that health care workers can take to protect themselves against all bloodborne communicable diseases, including HIV. In reality, the chance of EMS personnel acquiring HIV infection through exposure to infected blood is low. The CDC reports 58 confirmed and 150 possible cases of occupationally acquired HIV among health care workers since 1985.[12] There have been no confirmed cases in emergency medical technicians (EMTs) or paramedics, although 13 possible cases have been recorded. The risk to health care workers increases under the following circumstances:

- The exposure involves a large amount of blood. This situation can occur when a piece of equipment is visibly contaminated with blood, when care of the patient involves placing a needle in a vein or an artery, and when the exposure involves a deep injury.
- The exposure involves an HIV-infected patient with a terminal illness, possibly reflecting a higher viral load in the late course of AIDS.
- Patients have a high HIV count (viral load) in their blood.

The overall risk of HIV transmission with a needlestick is estimated at 0.04% to 5%, depending on these factors.[13] In any case, the risk of exposure must be understood in terms of how the exposure occurred and which factors were involved. Although the potential for disease transmission may appear high, the actual probability may be quite low. Paramedics should follow agency protocol for notification and reporting of significant exposures to any infectious disease.

CRITICAL THINKING

Why would testing within 2 to 3 weeks of exposure be needed?

NOTE

Several types of tests are available to diagnose HIV. Home tests and rapid tests detect antibodies to HIV in the blood or oral fluid. If one of these tests is positive, follow-up with additional lab testing is needed to confirm the disease.

A combination HIV antibody and antigen blood test can detect antibodies to both types of HIV. The HIV antigen (p24) is a viral protein that can be detected prior to antibody development with a standard or rapid test. The p24 antigen test can detect p24 protein, on average, 10 to 14 days after HIV infection. A positive p24 test means that someone is HIV-positive. However, a negative p24 test alone does not completely rule out HIV infection. For example, the test may not detect the p24 protein because the person was infected more than 4 to 6 weeks earlier, or the levels of p24 antigen are too low to be detectable with current technologies.

The HIV nucleic amplification test assesses for the presence and amount of the actual virus. Unlike the p24 test, this test always gives a positive result as long as there is HIV in a person's blood.

Modified from: Tooley L. Detecting HIV earlier: advances in HIV testing. CATIE website. http://www.catie.ca/en/pif/fall-2010/detecting-hiv-earlier-advances-hiv-testing. Published Fall 2010. Accessed April 9, 2018.

Postexposure Prophylaxis

If exposure is confirmed or suspected, the paramedic should immediately notify the DICO (per protocol). When possible, the source patient should be tested to confirm HIV infection. Information on primary HIV indicates that systemic infection does not occur immediately; thus, there exists a narrow window of opportunity in which postexposure antiretroviral intervention may modify viral replication.[14]

PEP should begin as soon as possible after exposure to HIV and continue for 4 weeks.[15] The PEP regimen should include three or more antiretroviral drugs. The exposed EMS worker should have close follow-up beginning in 72 hours and be provided with counseling, baseline and follow-up HIV testing, and monitoring for PEP drug toxicity (liver toxicity). Follow-up HIV testing may end at 4 months after exposure if a p24 antigen–HIV antibody test is used. In other cases, testing should continue for 6 months. The preferred 4-week treatment PEP for HIV exposure is a combination of raltegravir (Isentress) plus tenofovir disoproxil fumarate (Viread) plus emtricitabine (Emtriva).[16]

NOTE

An important goal of PEP is to encourage and facilitate compliance with the 4-week PEP regimen of three drugs used for most HIV exposures. All antiretroviral drugs have been associated with side effects, although these side effects are less common with the newer generation of antiviral agents. Monitoring for and treatment of side effects will help ensure the exposed provider completes the 4-week PEP treatment.

Hepatitis

Hepatitis is an inflammation of the liver that can have many causes, including infection, drugs, and alcohol. Several types of viruses can cause hepatitis, but the most common are hepatitis A virus (HAV), HBV, and HCV (**TABLE 27-3**).

NOTE

Several other types of hepatitis viruses exist:

- Hepatitis D (delta) virus (HDV) cannot sustain infection without the help of HBV.
- Hepatitis E virus (HEV) and hepatitis G virus (HGV, also known as GBV-C) are rare. HEV is spread by contaminated food and water (like HAV). The routes of transmission for HEV and HGV are thought to be similar to those for HCV.

Hepatitis A Virus

HAV is a vaccine-preventable infection. The incidence of infection has declined in the United States due to immunization, but the incidence of this disease is much higher in developing countries.[17] This infection may be acquired by ingesting HAV-contaminated food or drink or by the fecal–oral route. The virus becomes localized in the liver, reproduces, enters the bile, and is carried to the intestinal tract. From there, it is shed in the feces. (Fecal shedding usually occurs before the onset of clinical symptoms.) Antibodies (anti-HAV) develop during acute disease as well as late in convalescence. Once infected, the person is immune to HAV for life.

Notably, HAV does not have a carrier state and does not lead to chronic liver disease or a chronic carrier state. Many HAV infections are subclinical, but others may manifest with flulike symptoms. Death from HAV is unusual except in patients with existing liver disease.

TABLE 27-3 The ABCs of Hepatitis

	HAV	HBV	HCV	HDV	HEV
What is it?	HAV causes inflammation of the liver. It does not lead to chronic disease.	HBV causes inflammation of the liver. It can cause liver cell damage, leading to chronic infection, cirrhosis, and cancer.	HCV causes inflammation of the liver. It can cause liver cell damage, leading to chronic infection, cirrhosis and cancer.	HDV causes inflammation of the liver. It infects only people with HBV.	HEV causes inflammation of the liver. It is rare in the United States. In rare cases, it can cause chronic disease.
Incubation period	2–7 weeks; average: 4 weeks	6–23 weeks; average: 17 weeks	2–25 weeks; average: 7–9 weeks	2–8 weeks	2–9 weeks; average: 40 days
How is it spread?	Transmitted by fecal–oral (anal/oral sex) route, close person-to-person contact, ingestion of contaminated food and water, or hand-to-mouth contact after contact with feces, such as changing diapers.	Transmitted through contact with infected blood, seminal fluid, vaginal secretions, or contaminated needles, including tattoo and body-piercing tools; by infected mother to newborn; or through human bite or sexual contact.	Transmitted through contact with infected blood, contaminated intravenous needles, razors, or tattoo and body-piercing tools; or by infected mother to newborn. Not easily spread through sex.	Transmitted through contact with infected blood or contaminated needles; or through sexual contact with HDV-infected person.	Transmitted through fecal–oral route (like HAV). Outbreaks associated with contaminated water supply in other countries.
Symptoms	Children may have none. Adults usually have light stools, dark urine, fatigue, fever, nausea, vomiting, abdominal pain, and jaundice.	May have none. Some people have mild flulike symptoms, dark urine, light stools, jaundice, fatigue, and fever.	Same as HBV; often asymptomatic for years.	Same as HBV.	Same as HAV.
Vaccine	Two doses of vaccine to anyone older than 1 year.	Three doses may be given to people of any age.	None for HCV. Should receive HAV and HBV vaccines.	HBV vaccine prevents HDV infection.	None commercially available.
Who is at risk?	People have household or sexual contact with an infected person or living in an area with HAV outbreak, travelers to developing countries, people engaging in anal/oral sex, and injection-drug users.	Infants born to an infected mother, person having sex with an infected person or multiple partners, injection-drug users, emergency responders, health care workers, people engaging in anal/oral sex, and hemodialysis patients.	Blood transfusion recipients before 1992, health care workers, injection-drug users, hemodialysis patients, infants born to an infected mother, and people with multiple sex partners.	Injection-drug users, people engaging in anal/oral sex, and people having sex with an HDV-infected patient.	Travelers to developing countries, especially pregnant women.
Prevention	Vaccination or immune globulin within 2 weeks of exposure. Washing hands with soap and water after going to the toilet. Use household bleach (10 parts water to 1 part bleach) to clean surfaces contaminated with feces, such as changing tables. Safer sex.	Vaccination provides protection for 20-plus years. Clean up blood with household bleach and wear protective gloves. Do not share razors, toothbrushes, or needles. Safer sex. Hepatitis B immune globulin for vaccine nonresponders after exposure.	Clean up spilled blood with household bleach. Wear gloves when touching blood. Do not share razors, toothbrushes, or needles with anyone. Safer sex.	Hepatitis B vaccine to prevent HBV/HDV infection, Safer sex.	Avoid drinking or using potentially contaminated water.

Abbreviations: HAV, hepatitis A virus; HBV, hepatitis B virus; HCV, hepatitis C virus; HDV, hepatitis D virus; HEV, hepatitis E virus

Modified from: Hepatitis Foundation website. http://www.hepatitisfoundation.org/ABOUT/contact.html. Accessed April 9, 2018.

Administration of immune globulin (IG) can provide temporary immunity to the virus (ie, 2 to 3 months), though it must be given before exposure to HAV or within 2 weeks after contact. The hepatitis A vaccine is recommended for all children at age 1 year. Adults not previously immunized should consider vaccination if they meet any of the following criteria:[18]

- Live in a community with a high incidence of HAV infection
- Work or travel to countries with a high rate of HAV infection
- If male, have sex with other men
- Use illicit drugs
- Work with HAV-infected animals or with HAV in a research center
- Have chronic liver disease or clotting factor disorders

Some employers require proof of HAV vaccination. The safety of the vaccine during pregnancy has not been determined.[19]

Hepatitis B Virus

Infectious HBV particles are found in blood and in secretions containing serum (eg, oozing, cutaneous lesions) as well as in secretions derived from serum (eg, saliva, semen, vaginal secretions). Like other viral types of hepatitis, HBV affects the liver and causes the signs and symptoms described previously. The virus may produce chronic infection, which may potentially lead to cirrhosis and other complications such as liver cancer (hepatocellular carcinoma). Although HBV usually lasts less than 6 months, the carrier state may persist for years.

> **NOTE**
>
> HBV is 100 times more infectious than HIV. In 2015, there were an estimated 21,900 new cases of HBV infection in the United States. An estimated 257 million people have this disease worldwide.
>
> *Modified from*: Hepatitis B. World Health Organization website. http://www.who.int/mediacentre/factsheets/fs204/en/. Reviewed July 2017. Accessed April 9, 2018.

The effects of HBV vary. Some people may experience only a low-grade fever and malaise (flulike illness), with complete resolution of their symptoms. In other patients, extensive liver necrosis may develop that can lead to death. Other complications associated with HBV include coagulation defects, impaired protein production, impaired bilirubin elimination, pancreatitis, and hepatic cancer. Exposure generally occurs in one of five ways:[20]

1. Direct percutaneous inoculation of infectious serum or plasma by needle or transfusion of infected blood or blood products. Risk of transmission with needlestick is as high as 30%.[21]
2. Indirect percutaneous introduction of infective serum or plasma (eg, skin cuts or abrasions, tattoo/body piercing).
3. Absorption of infective serum or plasma through mucosal surfaces (eg, the eyes or mouth), transplacentally, or through contamination from the mother's infected blood at birth.
4. Absorption of infective secretions (eg, saliva or semen) through mucosal surfaces, as might occur during vaginal, anal, or oral sexual contact (but never fecal transmission), or when sharing straws to snort drugs.
5. Transfer of infective serum or plasma via inanimate environmental surfaces. HBV is stable on environmental surfaces and can remain infective in visible blood for longer than 7 days.[22]

> **CRITICAL THINKING**
>
> Why is information about exposure risks important to paramedics?

Preexposure Prophylaxis

With regulatory and legislative efforts and the publication of OSHA's *Bloodborne Pathogen Standard*, the number of cases of HBV in health care workers has decreased dramatically. Health care workers who have developed antibodies to the virus after immunization are at almost no risk of acquiring the disease. (The exposure risk for unvaccinated health care providers working with HBV-positive patients is estimated to be 6% to 30% with needlestick exposure.[23]) The CDC recommends, and OSHA requires, that HBV vaccines be offered to all health care workers.

Children should have their first hepatitis vaccine at birth and complete the series before age 18 months. The vaccine is also recommended for adults who engage in high-risk sex practices, inject drugs, need dialysis, have HIV, have chronic liver disease, are older than 60 years and have diabetes, live or travel in countries where HBV infection is common, or work in certain high-risk settings.[24]

Blood is the most important potential source of HBV exposure in the workplace. The risk of infection is directly proportional to the probability that the blood contains HBV, the recipient's immunity status, and the efficacy of transmission. If the entire series is complete, HBV vaccinations do not need to be repeated following an exposure.[25] The HBV vaccination schedule generally requires three intramuscular doses over 6 months. For the best protection against HBV, the series should be completed before an exposure occurs.

Postexposure Prophylaxis

PEP in health care workers may be indicated if an unvaccinated person (ie, a person who signed a declination form) or a person who has not completed the vaccination schedule is exposed to HBV. Before treatment, a blood test is performed to determine whether the health care worker has sufficient antibodies against hepatitis B (anti-HBs). Those with a known exposure who have no or insufficient anti-HBs receive the HBV vaccine and hepatitis B immune globulin; the latter is an antibody used in postexposure treatment to provide passive immunity to HBV. If the exposed person has sufficient anti-HBs, no further care is needed.

Hepatitis C Virus

HCV is a bloodborne virus that causes a disease similar to that caused by HBV. Between 2010 and 2015, there was more than a 2.9-fold increase in reported HCV infections, most likely due to more case detection and the increased use of IV drugs.[26] Currently, approximately 3.5 million Americans are believed to be infected with the virus. HCV is the infection that most often results from injection-drug use, needlestick injuries, and inadequate infection control in health care settings.[26] Much less frequently, it is acquired through sexual contact (especially men having sex with men), from unregulated tattoos, and in infants born to HCV-positive mothers. Of health care workers who become infected, 70% to 85% become chronic carriers.[27] Approximately one-half to two-thirds of those infected with HCV develop chronic hepatitis; one in five suffers severe liver disease, such as cirrhosis and liver cancer.

No vaccine is available for HCV. Antiviral and immunologic treatments for HCV are more than 90% effective in controlling the virus, with the treatments employed being based on the specific genotype of the virus. The national goal is to reduce cases of chronic HCV infection by 90% by 2030.[28] In some cases, HCV can be permanently cleared.[29]

Signs and symptoms of HCV, when they occur, are similar to those of other types of hepatitis. Most people infected with HCV are asymptomatic.

Signs and Symptoms

On the one hand, infection with any of the viruses that cause hepatitis may not produce any symptoms. On the other hand, it may cause a typical hepatitis with an abrupt onset of flulike illness (fever, fatigue, nausea, vomiting) that is followed by abdominal pain, jaundice, dark urine, and clay-colored stools. A patient is most infectious during the first week of symptoms (see Table 27-2). Within 2 to 3 months of infection, the patient usually develops nonspecific symptoms—for example, anorexia, nausea and vomiting, fever, joint pain, and generalized rashes. Approximately 1% of patients hospitalized with HBV develop full-blown liver crisis and die.[30]

Patient Management and Protective Measures

The management of patients with hepatitis in the prehospital setting is mainly supportive. The goal is to maintain circulatory status and prevent shock. All health care workers involved in the patient's care must follow standard precautions.

Tuberculosis

In 2015, 10.5 million new cases of **tuberculosis (TB)** occurred worldwide, and 1.8 million people died of the disease.[31] Reports of TB in the United States have declined continually since the turn of the 20th century. In 1985, this trend temporarily reversed (attributed to the HIV epidemic), and in 2016 9,272 cases were reported, representing a 2.9% decline from the prior year.[32]

The incidence of TB is much higher among patients with HIV and in people with weakened immune systems. Other risk factors for developing the TB disease include the following:

- Close contact with a person with infectious TB
- Immigration from an area with a high prevalence of TB
- Age younger than 5 years[33]
- Living or working in high-risk environments, such as in correctional facilities, homeless shelters, hospitals, and nursing homes, or with IV drug users

Susceptibility to mycobacterial infection generally is highest in children younger than 3 years; in adults older than 65 years; and in chronically ill, malnourished, and immunosuppressed or immunocompromised people.

Pathophysiology

TB is a chronic pulmonary disease that is acquired through inhalation of a dried-droplet nucleus containing tubercle bacilli (*M tuberculosis, Mycobacterium bovis,* or a variety of atypical mycobacteria). Although the pathogen is spread mainly by infected people coughing or sneezing the bacteria into the air, it can also be passed through contact with the sputum of an infected person. People who share the same air space as those who have infectious TB are at highest risk for infection.[34] Transmission also may occur by ingestion or through the skin or mucous membranes, though this means is less common.

The pathology of TB is related to the production of inflammatory lesions throughout the body as well as the ability of the TB bacillus to break through the body's natural defenses. The caseating granulomas (necrotic inflammatory cells), known as TB cavitary lesions, that are formed may cause chronic and debilitating lung disease.

The infection may remain dormant for an indefinite time (latent), or it may lead to active, contagious disease. Thus, two TB-related conditions are distinguished: **latent TB infection** and **TB disease** (**TABLE 27-4**).

Signs and symptoms of TB include cough, fever, night sweats, weight loss, fatigue, and hemoptysis. Organ systems outside the lungs can also be infected with TB (known as Pott disease). The organ systems affected and the associated complications include the following:

1. Cardiovascular system
   - Pericardial effusions
   - Lymphadenopathy (cervical lymph nodes are usually involved)

TABLE 27-4 Tuberculosis: The Difference Between Latent TB Infection and TB Disease

A Person With Latent TB Infection	A Person With TB Disease
Has no symptoms	Has symptoms that may include: • A bad cough that lasts ≥3 weeks • Pain in the chest • Coughing up blood or sputum • Weakness or fatigue • Weight loss • No appetite • Chills • Fever • Sweating at night
Does not feel sick	Usually feels sick
Cannot spread TB bacteria to others	May spread TB bacteria to others
Usually has a skin test or blood test result indicating TB infection	Usually has a skin test or blood test result indicating TB infection
Has a normal chest radiograph and a negative sputum smear	May have an abnormal chest radiograph or a positive sputum smear or culture
Needs treatment for latent TB infection to prevent active TB disease	Needs treatment to treat active TB disease
Health care workers who have latent TB who are receiving treatment can still work with patients.	Health care workers with TB disease need to be removed from patient care until no longer contagious.

Abbreviation: TB, tuberculosis

Modified from: Division of Tuberculosis Elimination. Tuberculosis (TB): fact sheets. Centers for Disease Control and Prevention website. https://www.cdc.gov/tb/publications/factsheets/general/tb.htm. Updated October 28, 2011. Accessed April 9, 2018.

2. Skeletal system
   - Intervertebral disk deterioration
   - Chronic arthritis of one joint
3. CNS
   - Subacute meningitis
   - Brain granulomas
4. Systemic TB (extensive dissemination by the bloodstream of tubercle bacilli)

Paramedics should maintain a high degree of suspicion for TB in people with undiagnosed lung disease, especially patients who are HIV positive.

TB Testing

The signs and symptoms of initial TB infection may be minimal. Early infection can be detected using the Mantoux tuberculin skin test (purified protein derivative [PPD]) or a TB blood test. A positive reaction to the PPD test indicates a person may be infected with TB; further testing, however, needs to be done to establish a definitive diagnosis. Patients with positive test results usually have a chest radiograph and an acid-fast bacilli (AFB) sputum culture to confirm that they have the disease before treatment begins. By law, every state is required to report cases of TB.

A negative TB skin test result does not fully rule out TB infection, especially in people with TB-like symptoms, HIV, or AIDS. In these cases, a repeat skin test may be warranted 10 weeks after exposure.

Because identification and early treatment of TB are important, all health care workers should receive a routine evaluation consisting of PPD test and, if indicated, a chest radiograph and AFB culture. A negative immune response does not preclude reinfection with subsequent exposure.

Patient Care and Protective Measures

Paramedics should be aware of areas with a high incidence of active TB in their service region; this information is reported by the local health authorities. Prehospital care for patients with infectious TB is mainly supportive.

Airborne precautions need to be followed whenever TB is suspected. Surgical masks are insufficient for preventing inhalation of TB bacteria, although they do reduce the number of droplet nuclei escaping from the patient. Thus, such a mask should be placed on the patient during transport if an oxygen mask has not been applied. NIOSH recommends that health care workers use particulate filter respirators that filter at least 95% (N-95 mask or respirator) of airborne particles when caring for patients with TB (**FIGURE 27-6** and BOX 27-6). Ambulance ventilation systems that include high-efficiency particulate air (HEPA) filtration and a nonrecirculating ventilation cycle are another means of preventing exposure to TB during patient transport.

Hospitals should be advised when EMS providers are bringing in a patient suspected to have TB. This warning allows them to prepare and follow appropriate airborne precautions, including placing the patient in a negative pressure room. After each call, all patient care equipment should be disinfected.

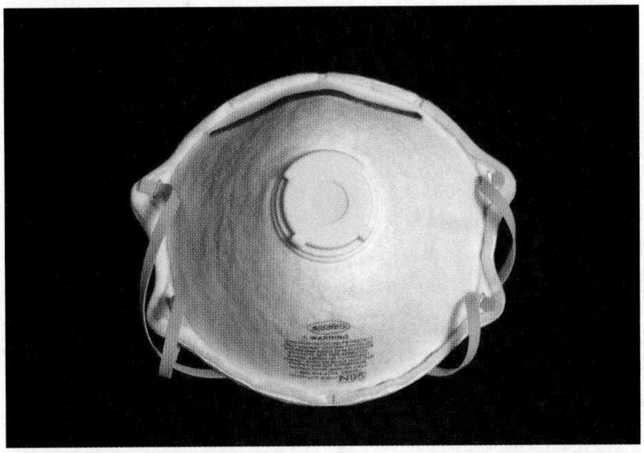

FIGURE 27-6 High-efficiency particulate air respirator.

BOX 27-6 TB-Protective Respirators

OSHA, in conjunction with guidelines established by the CDC, currently requires the use of respirators when patients have, or are suspected of having, TB. OSHA is enforcing the use of these devices while developing specific standards for preventing the exposure of health care workers to TB. The required respirator certified by NIOSH must have a disposable (or replaceable) HEPA filter capable of trapping airborne particles.

Whenever respirators (including disposables) are required, a complete respiratory protection program must be implemented in accordance with federal regulations.[a] Elements of the required respiratory protection program include the following:

1. Permissible practices for respirator use
2. Respirator program administration
3. Selection of respirators
4. Inspection of respirators
5. Cleaning and maintenance of respirators
6. Storage of respirators
7. Training in respiratory protection
8. Fit testing of respirators (to ensure accurate sizing)
9. Respirator program evaluation
10. Medical surveillance of respirator users

[a]These specifications are found in 29 CFR 1910.134.

Modified from: US Department of Health and Human Services, National Institute of Occupational Safety and Health. *NIOSH Guide to the Selection and Use of Particulate Respirators, Certified Under 42 CFR 84.* Washington, DC: US Department of Health and Human Services; 1996. Publication No. 96-101.

CRITICAL THINKING

Can a patient with latent TB transmit the disease to a health worker through droplet exposure?

Treatment

If effective treatment is begun without delay and taken as prescribed to completion, TB is usually curable. Multidrug-resistant TB (MDR-TB) is on the rise, however (BOX 27-7). Most patients with TB are started on a 6- to 9-month drug regimen that may include isoniazid, rifampin, pyrazinamide, and ethambutol.[35] Patients should be monitored for drug side effects. Sputum and cultures usually become negative 3 to 8 weeks after the start of therapy.

Bacterial Meningitis

Bacterial meningitis is a rapidly progressing disease that affects the meninges of the brain and spinal cord, and can cause death within hours. The usual mode of transmission is prolonged, direct contact with upper respiratory tract secretions from an infected person or carrier. Once inhaled, the bacteria invade the respiratory passages and travel through the blood to the brain and spinal cord. With the spread of infection, bacterial meningitis causes toxic effects in the involved organ system. Droplet precautions should be followed with any patient suspected of having **meningitis**, including use of a surgical mask and eye protection.

Bacterial meningitis strikes an estimated 4,100 Americans each year and causes 500 deaths.[36] The incidence of bacterial meningitis has declined in the United States because of the availability of vaccines to prevent the disease resulting from three types of bacteria: *N meningitides, Streptococcus pneumoniae,* and *Haemophilus influenzae* type b (Hib).

BOX 27-7 Multidrug-Resistant TB

MDR-TB is resistant to isoniazid and rifampin and one first-line anti-TB drug. It is a serious form of TB with limited preventive therapy. Patients who have extensively drug-resistant TB are resistant to even more antibiotics. People at high risk for MDR-TB include the following:

- People recently exposed to MDR-TB (especially if they are immunocompromised)
- Patients with TB who fail to take medications as prescribed
- Patients who come from a country where MDR-TB is common
- Patients previously treated for TB

A major cause of treatment failure and drug-resistant TB is failure of the patient to follow the treatment regimen. This noncompliance threatens the health of TB patients and poses a serious public health risk. It also leads to prolonged infectivity and the spread of TB in the community.

Modified from: Division of Tuberculosis Elimination. Tuberculosis (TB): treatment for TB disease. Centers for Disease Control and Prevention website. https://www.cdc.gov/tb/topic/treatment/tbdisease.htm. Updated August 11, 2016. Accessed April 9, 2018.

Bacterial Agents Known to Cause Meningitis

Meningococcal meningitis is caused by *N meningitidis*—the most common cause of bacterial meningitis in teens and young adults, as well as the deadliest cause of bacterial meningitis. An estimated 5% to 10% of the population may carry these meningococci at any point in time.[37] The throat's epithelial lining generally prevents the pathogens from invading the meninges and the cerebrospinal fluid. Outbreaks of disease in the United States have decreased since the 1990s. Transmission is prevented by following droplet precautions, including wearing a surgical mask and eye protection. If paramedics suspect a patient has meningitis, they should suspect the causative agent is *N meningitidis* until proven otherwise. They should also notify their DICO, because exposure to this form of meningitis requires PEP.

Other bacteria that cause meningitis include *S pneumoniae*, Hib, group B *Streptococcus* (GBS), and *Listeria monocytogenes*. Fortunately, none of the bacteria that cause meningitis are as contagious as the common cold or flu. In addition, they are not spread by casual contact or by simply breathing the air where a person with meningitis has been. Regardless, droplet precautions should be followed. PEP is needed in case of exposure to *N meningitidis*.

S pneumoniae is the most common cause of bacterial meningitis in infants, children, and older adults; the second most common cause of bacterial meningitis in teens and young adults; the most common cause of pneumonia in adults; and the most common cause of otitis media (middle ear infection) in children.[37] Meningitis from *S pneumoniae* is usually caused by untreated otitis media resulting in infection spread to the meninges. Droplet precautions should be followed with this type of infection.

Meningitis from *H influenzae* has decreased thanks to vaccinations. Vaccines for children were introduced in 1981. Before that time, *H influenzae* was the leading cause of bacterial meningitis in children 6 months to 3 years of age.

L monocytogenes comes from contaminated food. Meningitis from this bacterium usually occurs in people who are immunocompromised.[37]

GBS is the most common cause of bacterial meningitis in newborns secondary to exposure to this pathogen in the birth canal of GBS-positive mothers.[37] Mothers get tested for these bacteria in the third trimester; if they are positive, they are treated with antibiotics during labor to prevent this infection in the newborn.

Viral Meningitis

Viral meningitis (aseptic meningitis) is a syndrome generally associated with an existing systemic viral disease (eg, enteroviral infection, herpesvirus infection, mumps, measles, influenza). Symptoms are similar to those of bacterial meningitis but are usually less severe. In most cases, viral meningitis is self-limited, and the patient recovers fully. The patient may experience muscle weakness and malaise during prolonged convalescence.

> NOTE
>
> Viral meningitis that is caused by enteroviruses can be spread by direct contact with an infected person's stool. Examples of possible exposures include small children who are toilet training and adults who handle soiled diapers of infected infants. Enteroviruses and other viruses (such as mumps and varicella-zoster virus) can also be spread through direct or indirect contact with respiratory secretions. Although there are risks for infection through exposure, it is unlikely such exposure would lead to meningitis as a complication of the illness.
>
> *Modified from:* National Center for Immunization and Respiratory Diseases. Meningitis: viral meningitis. Centers for Disease Control and Prevention website. https://www.cdc.gov/meningitis/viral.html. Updated June 15, 2016. Accessed April 9, 2018.

Signs and Symptoms

The signs and symptoms of meningitis depend on the patient's age and general health. In infants, signs of meningeal irritation may be absent. If present, however, they may include fever, irritability, poor feeding or vomiting, a high-pitched cry, and fullness of the fontanel. In older infants and children, signs of meningitis may include malaise, low-grade fever, projectile vomiting, petechial and purpuric rash (a hallmark; **FIGURE 27-7**), headache, and stiff neck from meningeal irritation (nuchal rigidity). Adults and older children may experience headache, nausea, vomiting, photophobia, nuchal rigidity, and altered mental status. Diagnostic signs of meningitis in adults and older children include the Brudzinski sign (involuntary flexion of the arm, hip, and knee when the neck is passively flexed), the Kernig sign (loss of the ability in a seated or supine patient to completely extend the knee due to pain when the thigh is flexed on the abdomen), and nuchal rigidity.

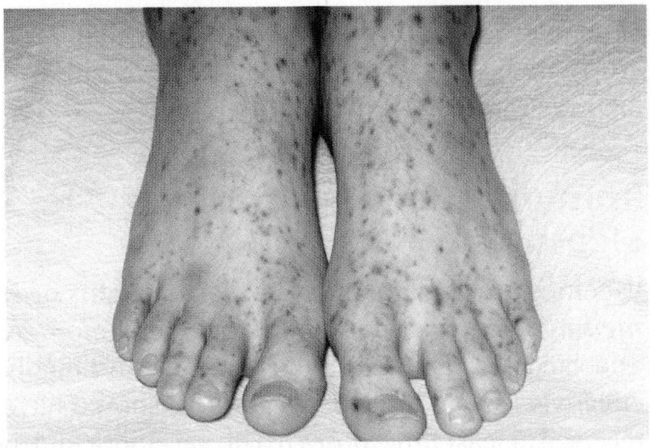

FIGURE 27-7 Petechial rash in meningococcal infection.

> CRITICAL THINKING
>
> Does a petechial rash blanch after compression?

The risk of bacterial meningitis is most significant in neonates and infants, but infection should be suspected in any patient with fever, headache, and stiff neck. Additional symptoms that should increase suspicion of meningitis include altered mental status, petechiae and/or purpura (meningococcal meningitis), and underlying health problems (eg, recent neurosurgery, trauma, immunocompromise).

With meningococcal meningitis, death can occur in 6 to 8 hours. Other conditions and long-term complications associated with severe meningitis include blindness and deafness (from cranial nerve damage), arthritis, myocarditis, and pericarditis. Death can follow overwhelming infection.

Immunization and Control Measures

Vaccines are available for Hib, some strains of *N meningitidis*, and many types of *S pneumoniae*. The vaccines against Hib are very safe and highly effective. By 6 months of age, infants should have received at least three doses of Hib vaccine; a fourth dose ("booster") is recommended between 12 and 15 months of age.

Vaccination against some strains of *N meningitidis* is recommended for children 11 to 12 years of age, with a booster at 16 years. This vaccine is indicated only for infants 2 months and children up to 10 years with specific medical or environmental conditions.[38]

Pneumococcal vaccines to prevent meningitis caused by *S pneumoniae* also can prevent other forms of infection arising from the bacterium, such as pneumonia and otitis media. The pneumococcal conjugate vaccine is recommended for babies and children younger than 2 years, adults 65 years and older, and people aged 2 to 64 years with some medical conditions.[39] The pneumococcal polysaccharide vaccine is indicated for adults 65 years and older, people 2 through 64 years with some medical conditions, and adults 19 to 64 years who smoke cigarettes.

Patient Management and Protective Measures

Patient management of meningitis focuses on ensuring an adequate airway and providing ventilatory and circulatory support. Sepsis protocols are often followed to manage these patients.

The paramedic must take protective measures when caring for patients who have signs and symptoms of meningitis. Droplet precautions (with surgical masks on both patient and provider, and eye protection for the paramedic) should be used during care and transport. The EMS agency should have an exposure control plan for meningitis.

Early diagnosis and treatment of bacterial meningitis are essential. The diagnosis usually is confirmed by finding the bacteria in a sample of the patient's spinal fluid obtained through a lumbar puncture. The disease is then treated using several antibiotics. PEP for meningococcal meningitis exposure to prevent the disease is available for those who may have had intimate contact with the patient (eg, family members, EMS providers).

NOTE

Meningitis is a true medical emergency. A chief goal of emergency care is administration of a bacterium-specific antibiotic. The drug should be given as soon as possible after arriving at the ED. Delay in antibiotic administration is associated with increased mortality and poorer outcome on discharge.

Modified from: Bodilsen J, Dalager-Pedersen M, Schønheyder HC, Nielsen H. Time to antibiotic therapy and outcome in bacterial meningitis: a Danish population-based cohort study. *BMC Infect Dis.* 2016;16:392.

Bacterial Endocarditis

Bacterial endocarditis (also known as infective endocarditis) is infection of the endocardium and one or more heart valves. This condition can be caused by any of a variety of structural heart abnormalities that render the heart susceptible to this infection. The pathogenic bacteria settle in the heart and grow on the valves of the heart in structures called vegetation.

Over time, the infection damages the heart valves and may cause them to leak. In severe cases, heart failure develops. If the bacteria dislodge from the valves and enter the bloodstream, they can cause vascular occlusion, resulting in stroke, vision impairment, and severe damage to other organ systems. They can also result in infection in other locations of the body.

Bacterial endocarditis is most common in men older than 60 years.[40] Other factors associated with the development of endocarditis include IV drug use and dental infection. Approximately three-fourths of patients with infectious endocarditis have a structural heart problem that leaves them susceptible to endocarditis—for example, valvular disease, prosthetic heart valve, congenital heart disease, prior infective endocarditis, intravascular device, chronic hemodialysis, or HIV infection.[41]

Signs and symptoms of endocarditis may develop slowly or have an acute onset. The disease can be difficult to diagnose, as early symptoms may resemble the flu or other illnesses. These signs and symptoms include the following:[42]

- Fatigue
- Weakness
- Fever
- Chills
- Night sweats
- Weight loss
- Muscle aches and pains
- Excessive sweating
- Joint pain

Other signs and symptoms of endocarditis include red, painless skin spots located on the palms and soles (Janeway lesions); red, painful nodes in the pads of the fingers and toes (Osler nodes); jaundice; and splinter hemorrhages under the nails. If the patient's heart valves are seriously affected, a heart murmur, shortness of breath, chest discomfort, and dysrhythmias may be present. Other findings during the physical examination may include retinal hemorrhages, petechiae in the conjunctiva, and an enlarged spleen.

Diagnosis of endocarditis is made through blood cultures to identify the bacteria and transesophageal echocardiograms. Hospitalization is usually required, along with long-term antibiotic therapy (4 to 6 weeks) and sometimes heart valve replacement. Following recovery, prophylactic antibiotic therapy is often prescribed for these patients before dental procedures and surgeries. Those who have had endocarditis are at a higher risk of contracting the disease again. Some patients will carry an endocarditis wallet card issued by the American Heart Association or other organizations to provide information about their condition to health care personnel.

Pneumonia

Pneumonia is an acute inflammation of the bronchioles and alveoli. It can be spread by droplets and by direct and indirect contact with respiratory secretions. Etiologic agents responsible for this disease may be bacterial (*S pneumoniae, Mycoplasma pneumoniae, S aureus, H influenzae, Klebsiella pneumoniae, Moraxella catarrhalis, Legionella* sp), viral (influenza), or fungal. These organisms may affect several body systems, including the respiratory system (pneumonia); the CNS (meningitis); and the ears, nose, and throat (otitis media, pharyngitis). The signs and symptoms of pneumonia include the following:

- Sudden onset of chills, high-grade fever, chest pain with respirations, and dyspnea
- Tachypnea and chest retractions (an ominous sign in children)
- Congestion caused by the development of purulent alveolar exudates in one or more lobes
- A productive cough with yellow-green phlegm

Susceptibility and Resistance

Susceptibility to pneumonia is increased by processes such as smoking, pulmonary edema, influenza, exposure to inhaled toxins, chronic lung disease, and aspiration of any form (following alcohol ingestion, near drowning, regurgitation caused by gastric distention from bag-mask ventilation). Extremes of age also appear to increase susceptibility to the disease (eg, older adults, infants with a low birth weight and/or malnourishment). Other high-risk groups for pneumonia include those with the following conditions:

- Sickle cell disease
- Cardiovascular disease
- Chronic respiratory disease (eg, chronic obstructive pulmonary disease, asthma, cystic fibrosis)
- **Asplenia** (congenital absence or surgical removal of the spleen)
- Diabetes
- Chronic renal failure (or other kidney disease)
- HIV
- Organ transplantation
- Multiple myeloma, lymphoma, Hodgkin disease, lung cancer

Patient Management and Protective Measures

Prehospital care for patients with pneumonia includes providing airway support, oxygen, ventilatory assistance (as needed), bronchodilators if wheezing is present, IV fluids, cardiac monitoring, and transport for evaluation by a physician. Bacterial pneumonia is usually managed with analgesics, decongestants, expectorants, and antibiotic therapy. In hospitals, patients with pneumonia may be isolated from other patients who may be more susceptible to infection.

Measures for protecting health care workers include droplet precautions and effective handwashing.

Airborne precautions should be used if TB is suspected. Immunizations exist for some causes of pneumonia.

Tetanus

Tetanus is a rare, sometimes fatal, noncommunicable disease of the CNS. It is caused by infection of a wound with spores of *Clostridium tetani*. Tetanus spores live mainly in soil and manure but are also occasionally found in the human intestine. If the spores enter the body's tissues (eg, through a puncture wound or burn), they multiply and produce a toxin that acts on the nerves controlling muscular activity. (Dead or necrotic tissue is a favorable environment for *C tetani*.) Patient deaths can occur from wounds that appear too trivial for medical evaluation.

Death from tetanus occurs often secondary to severe spasms of the respiratory muscles resulting in respiratory failure. In an 8-year period, only 233 cases and 26 deaths were reported in the United States. The small number of tetanus cases in the United States is a result of widespread immunization of the general population with tetanus vaccines.[43]

Signs and Symptoms

The most common symptom of tetanus is trismus (stiffness of the jaw). Trismus is also known as lockjaw because of the accompanying difficulty in opening the mouth. Other symptoms include the following:

- Muscular tetany (muscle spasms and twitching)
- Painful muscular contractions in the neck, moving to the trunk
- Abdominal rigidity (often the first sign in pediatric patients)
- Painful spasms (contortions) of the face (*risus sardonicus*), which produce a grotesque smile
- Respiratory failure

Patient Management and Protective Measures

The prehospital care goals for patients with tetanus are to support vital functions, which may require aggressive airway management (intubation and surgical or needle cricothyrotomy). Muscle spasms should be treated with guidance from medical direction, and medications administered may include diazepam,

NOTE

In 1992 (and as revised in 2016), a definition for systemic inflammatory response syndrome (SIRS) was introduced to identify patients with a high probability of suspected infection who are at risk for complications (eg, intensive care unit admission, in-hospital mortality), sepsis, and septic shock. Defining SIRS allows for the identification of the best clinical response to nonspecific illness of infectious or noninfectious origin. The criteria for SIRS were established as a patient with a suspected or confirmed source of infection and with two or more of the following variables:

- Fever or hypothermia more than 38°C (100.4°F) or less than 36°C (96.8°F)
- Heart rate of more than 90 beats/min
- Respiratory rate of more than 20 breaths/min or arterial carbon dioxide pressure of less than 32 mm Hg
- Abnormal white blood cell count (leukocytosis, leukopenia, or bandemia)

The SIRS criteria, along with other screening tools (sequential organ failure assessments [SOFA, qSOFA] and logistical organ dysfunction system [LODS]), attempt to identify patients with an increased risk for sepsis, septic shock, or a severe outcome.

Some EMS systems provide a SIRS alert notification to the receiving facility so appropriate resources are ready for the patient's arrival. In some cases, the prehospital SIRS protocol includes drawing blood for culture and antibiotic administration prior to arrival at the ED.

Modified from: Bone RC, Balk RA, Cerra FB, et al. Definitions for sepsis and organ failure and guidelines for the use of innovative therapies in sepsis. The ACCP/SCCM Consensus Conference Committee. American College of Chest Physicians/Society of Critical Care Medicine. *Chest.* 1992;101(6):1644-1655; Kaplan LJ. Systemic inflammatory response syndrome. Medscape website. https://emedicine.medscape.com/article/168943-overview. Updated September 13, 2017. Accessed April 9, 2018; Tusgul S, Carron P-N, Yersin B, Calandra T, Dami F. Low sensitivity of qSOFA, SIRS criteria and sepsis definition to identify infected patients at risk of complication in the prehospital setting and at the emergency department triage. *Scand J Trauma Resusc Emerg Med.* 2017;25:108; and Willoughby J, Damodaran A, Belvitch P. Critical care: SIRS, qSOFA, sepsis: what's in a name? Diagnostic differences between SOFA scores and SIRS criteria in an ICU cohort. *Am J Respir Crit Care Med.* 2017;195:A1918. http://www.atsjournals.org/doi/abs/10.1164/ajrccm-conference.2017.195.1_MeetingAbstracts.A1918. Accessed April 9, 2018.

midazolam, or lorazepam (ie, benzodiazepines) or paralytic agents (per medical direction). Other treatments that may be indicated include IV fluids, magnesium sulfate, narcotics, and antidysrhythmics.

After evaluation by a physician and stabilization of the patient's condition, care for people with tetanus includes administration of antitoxin (tetanus immune globulin) to provide postexposure passive immunity, treatment to eliminate the toxin, active immunization with tetanus toxoid, and wound care. The case fatality rate is between 12% and 53%.

CRITICAL THINKING

When a patient with an open skin wound refuses care, should you explain the risks of tetanus infection?

Immunization

Immunization against tetanus usually is started in childhood. It is achieved using diphtheria, tetanus, and pertussis (DTaP) vaccination—a combined immunization against diphtheria (laryngitis, pharyngitis with discharge), pertussis (whooping cough), and tetanus. After the initial immunization, children receive a DTaP booster shot before starting elementary school. After that, a tetanus and diphtheria booster shot is recommended every 10 years.

Patients who have a recent wound should be counseled about postinjury tetanus prophylaxis and effective wound care. If it is suspected that a wound could carry tetanus, the tetanus vaccination will not adequately prevent infection; the patient will need tetanus immunoglobulin. The "tetanus shot" (tetanus immunization) prevents only tetanus exposure in future wounds; thus, all patients should be questioned about their tetanus immunization status. Recovery from infection does not confer immunity.

Rabies

Rabies (hydrophobia) is an acute viral infection of the CNS. This disease mainly affects animals, but it can be transmitted from an infected animal to a human through virus-laden saliva (eg, by a bite or scratch). (Transmission from person to person is theoretical but has never been documented.[44,45]) In the United States, wildlife rabies is found in skunks, raccoons, bats, foxes, dogs, wolves, jackals, woodchucks, groundhogs, mongooses, and coyotes. Because healthy wild animals (eg, skunks) are seldom seen by casual observance, a high degree of suspicion for rabies is indicated for all animals found outside their natural habitat. Hawaii is the only rabies-free state in the United States.

Humans are highly susceptible to the rabies virus after exposure to saliva in a bite or scratch from an infected animal. Several factors govern the severity of infection, including the following:

- Severity of the wound
- Richness of nerve supply close to the wound
- Distance from the wound to the CNS
- Amount and strain of the virus
- Degree of protection provided by clothing

Signs and Symptoms

The incubation period between a bite and the appearance of symptoms ranges from 9 days to 7 years. Initial symptoms include low-grade fever, headache, loss of appetite, hyperactivity, disorientation, and, in some cases, seizures. Often the patient has an intense thirst, but attempts to drink result in violent, painful spasms in the throat (hence the name "hydrophobia"). Eye and facial muscles may become paralyzed as the disease progresses. Once a person begins to exhibit signs of the disease, survival is rare. Without medical intervention, the disease lasts 2 to 6 days, often resulting in death secondary to respiratory failure.

Patient Management and Protective Measures

Physicians treat the signs and symptoms of the disease and provide respiratory and cardiovascular support (as needed). Patients also are treated with sedatives and analgesics. Thorough debridement of the wound without sutures (if possible) is indicated to allow for free bleeding and drainage.

PEP can be given to patients with high-risk animal bites or exposures. Human rabies immune globulin may be given to provide passive immunization. Also, a rabies vaccine (human diploid rabies vaccine, rabies vaccine) is given by injections spread over several weeks. Tetanus prophylaxis and antibiotics may be indicated for treatment of the bite wound.

If given within 2 days of the bite, immunizations almost always prevent development of rabies. Immunizations should be given for contact with open wounds or for exposure of mucous membranes to saliva. In addition, they should be given to people with a high probability of contact with animal reservoirs (eg, animal care workers, animal shelter personnel, and outdoor workers). If an animal is suspected of being rabid, it should be destroyed by the proper authorities, and its brain should be examined for rabies inclusion bodies. If no inclusion bodies are found, the patient's rabies treatment is stopped.

In the United States, most cases of rabies in humans are not directly attributable to an animal bite. Of the ones that are, exposure to a bat is the primary mode of transmission.[46] However, the possibility of rabies must be considered with *all* mammal bites. Scene safety and use of standard precautions during wound management are paramount. Law enforcement personnel and animal control authorities should be contacted to assist in scene control.

> CRITICAL THINKING
> Has a case of rabies ever occurred in your community? How was it identified? Which type of animal was implicated?

Hantavirus

Hantavirus was previously known to be associated with a type of hemorrhagic fever with renal syndrome that occurs in Asia. Hantaviruses also are associated with a syndrome of severe respiratory distress and shock that has occurred in several areas of the United States.[47] The virus is carried by rodents and is transmitted by inhalation of aerosol material contaminated with rodent urine and feces (see Table 27-2). Many forms of this disease occur in specific geographic areas, although more than 96% of US cases have occurred in states west of the Mississippi River.[48]

Hantavirus can cause significant disease in humans. Patients are usually healthy adults who experience an onset of fever and malaise, which are followed several days later by respiratory distress. Other signs and symptoms may include fever, chills, headache, gastrointestinal upset, and capillary hemorrhage. The severity of the illness is determined by the strain of the virus. With severe infection, oliguria, kidney failure, and hypotension occur. Death typically results from decreased cardiac output and eventual cardiovascular collapse.

Treatment is supportive and guided by medical direction. Body substance isolation precautions are indicated because of the infectious nature of these viruses.

Mosquito-Borne Illness

Several mosquito-borne illnesses have been reported in the United States, including Chikungunya virus, dengue, West Nile virus, Zika, and malaria. Prevention has the highest impact on these diseases. Using personal protection and minimizing mosquito habitats are key measures to diminish the risk of transmission. In communities at risk, use of insect repellents containing EPA-recommended active ingredients is advised. Sources of standing water should be eliminated, as they serve as breeding grounds for mosquitos. Currently, no vaccines are available that can prevent these diseases.[49]

In the United States, **Chikungunya virus** has been reported in most states; however, all reported cases of the virus occurred in travelers returning from affected areas. To date, no locally transmitted cases have been reported in the continental United States.[50] Most patients experience fever and joint pain when infected. Headache, myalgias, joint swelling, and rash are also possible. There is no vaccine to protect against this disease.

Flavivirus can cause **dengue fever**. Outbreaks in the continental United States have been rare, but this disease is common in the US territories and may be acquired elsewhere by travelers or immigrants. Patients who have dengue will have a high fever and at least two of the following signs or symptoms:[51]

- Severe headache
- Severe pain behind the eyes
- Joint pain
- Muscle and/or bone pain
- Rash
- Mild bleeding (from nose, gums, or petechiae or bruising)
- Low white blood cell count

Three to 7 days after the onset of symptoms, the patient is at high risk for serious illness that can include ascites, pleural effusions, thrombocytopenia with bleeding, and shock. Warning signs that these life-threatening symptoms may occur include severe abdominal pain, petechiae, bleeding from the nose or gums, melena, mental status changes, dyspnea, and signs of shock. Treatment is symptomatic.

In the United States, **West Nile virus** infection of people, birds, or mosquitoes has been reported in 47 states and the District of Columbia. In 2017, 1,622 cases were reported to the CDC. Most people who acquire the disease are asymptomatic.[52] In approximately

20% of patients, a fever, headache, myalgias, vomiting, diarrhea, or rash develops. Only about 1 in 150 infected patients experiences encephalitis or meningitis. Treatment is symptomatic.

Zika is a virus that is spread by the bites of specific types of mosquitos (*Aedes aegypti* and *Aedes albopictus*) and through the blood. Infected women can transmit the viral infection to their unborn children, in whom the virus leads to serious birth defects such as microcephaly. Additionally, the virus is spread through sex from an infected partner—even when that person has no symptoms. Prior to 2016, the Zika virus had been reported only south of the United States, but in 2016 several areas in Florida and one county in Texas were put on alert for risk of Zika after infected mosquitoes were found in those areas. In 2017, more than 300 cases of symptomatic Zika infection were reported in the United States through October, although most of them were acquired during travel to high-risk areas of the world. Three of the cases were acquired through sexual transmission, and only one presumed case was from local mosquito infection.[53]

Many of those infected with Zika have only mild symptoms, or no symptoms. Approximately 20% of Zika-infected people have signs and symptoms that include the following:[54]

- Fever
- Maculopapular rash
- Headache
- Joint pain
- Myalgias
- Conjunctivitis (without pus)

There is no known treatment for patients diagnosed with Zika infection; instead, treatment is primarily supportive. People who are symptomatic and have visited an area known to be at high risk for Zika should see a physician. The provider should assess the patient for dehydration and infuse fluids if needed. The patient may take acetaminophen to reduce fever and discomfort. Because dengue is also found in areas at high risk for Zika, the patient should not take aspirin or other nonsteroidal anti-inflammatory drugs without a physician's assessment to reduce the risk of bleeding.

Malaria (*Plasmodium* infection) is caused by a mosquito-borne parasite, rather than a virus, as with other mosquito-borne illnesses. Worldwide, almost 500,000 people die of this disease each year.[55] In the United States, nearly 1,700 cases are diagnosed annually, mostly in patients who have returned from countries with a high incidence of the disease.[56] Signs and symptoms may not appear for several weeks or even months after a person has been infected. The patient may experience fever, chills, malaise, sweats, headaches, myalgias, and nausea and vomiting. On physical examination, sweating, tachypnea, weakness, splenomegaly, jaundice, or liver enlargement may be found.

Severe malaria can cause impaired brain function, severe anemia, hemoglobinuria, acute respiratory distress syndrome, coagulopathies, kidney failure, metabolic acidosis, hypoglycemia, and shock. Prehospital care will be based on the patient's presenting signs and symptoms. Drugs used to treat malaria are based on the species of parasite infecting the patient and the patient's condition and medical history.

Antibiotic-Resistant Infections

For more than 70 years, antimicrobial drugs have had an important impact against illness and death worldwide. However, the widespread use and overuse of these drugs has caused some forms of bacteria to become resistant to the effects of these agents.[57] It has been reported that at least 2 million people become infected with bacteria that are resistant to antibiotics, and at least 23,000 people die each year as a direct result of these infections. Most of these deaths occur in health care settings such as hospitals and nursing homes.[58]

The CDC has identified 18 drug-resistant threats to the United States and categorized them as urgent (high-consequence threats), serious (may become urgent; requires careful monitoring), and concerning (low antibiotic resistance; multiple treatment options) (BOX 27-8). The three urgent threats discussed in this chapter are *C difficile*, carbapenem-resistant Enterobacteriaceae, and *Neisseria gonorrhoeae.*

Clostridium difficile

Clostridium difficile causes life-threatening diarrhea. A 2015 CDC study found that this bacterium caused almost 500,000 infections among patients in the United States in a single year. An estimated 15,000 deaths annually are directly attributable to *C difficile* infections, making it a substantial cause of infectious disease death in the United States.[58]

The "*C diff*" bacterium normally is present in small numbers in the intestines. It can overpopulate

BOX 27-8 Serious and Concerning Threats as Defined by the CDC

Serious

- Multidrug-resistant *Acinetobacter*
- Drug-resistant *Campylobacter*
- Fluconazole-resistant *Candida*
- Extended spectrum Enterobacteriaceae (ESBL)
- Vancomycin-resistant *Enterococcus* (VRE)
- Multidrug-resistant *Pseudomonas aeruginosa*
- Drug-resistant non-typhoidal *Salmonella*
- Drug-resistant *Salmonella* serotype *typhi*
- Drug-resistant *Shigella*
- MRSA (BOX 27-9)
- Drug-resistant *S pneumoniae*
- Drug-resistant TB

Concerning Threats

- Vancomycin-resistant *S aureus*
- Erythromycin-resistant group A *Streptococcus*
- Clindamycin-resistant GBS

Modified from: Antibiotic/antimicrobial resistance: biggest threats. Centers for Disease Control and Prevention website. https://www.cdc.gov/drugresistance/biggest_threats.html. Accessed April 14, 2018.

the colon, especially after extended antibiotic therapy, leading to ***C diff* colitis**. The toxins invade the intestinal wall and cause ulcerations. Initially, diarrhea and cramping occur, followed by flulike symptoms, weakness, abdominal pain, fever, nausea, vomiting, dehydration, and bloody stools. In late stages of the disease, life-threatening inflammation of the colon can occur, resulting in sepsis and, rarely, death. Illness from *C diff* most commonly affects older adults in hospitals or in long-term care facilities. The disease can be spread through the fecal–oral route. Contact precautions are indicated; hand sanitizers do not clear these spores. Health care personnel must wash their hands after contact with these patients.

BOX 27-9 Methicillin-Resistant *S aureus*

S aureus (often referred to as "staph") is a bacterium that can cause a number of illnesses, ranging from minor skin infections (eg, pimples, boils) to life-threatening illness such as pneumonia and sepsis. Some of the infections may be resistant to penicillin-related antibiotics.

Methicillin-resistant *Staphylococcus aureus* (MRSA) is a type of staph that is resistant to methicillin and other antibiotics. MRSA occurs more often in older adults or very ill patients in hospitals and other health care facilities. Patients often have an open wound (eg, bed sore) or an indwelling urinary catheter or are receiving IV therapy. Staphylococci and MRSA most often are spread by direct physical contact but can also be transmitted through indirect contact. Examples include touching items (eg, towels, sheets, wound dressings, clothes) contaminated by the skin of a person with MRSA or staph bacterial infection. To avoid spreading these pathogens, health care providers should be diligent to use contact precautions, wash hands before and after each patient encounter (including after glove removal), and avoid contact with open wounds or contaminated materials.

Staph and MRSA also cause illness in people outside of hospitals and health care facilities. These infections are known as community-associated MRSA (CA-MRSA) infections. Staph or MRSA infections in the community are usually manifested as skin infections, such as pimples and boils, and occur in otherwise healthy people. Clusters of CA-MRSA skin infections have been noted among athletes, military recruits, children, and prisoners. Factors that have been associated with the spread of MRSA skin infections include close skin-to-skin contact, dermal cuts or abrasions, contaminated items and surfaces, crowded living conditions, and poor hygiene.

Modified from: Centers for Disease Control and Prevention, National Center for Emerging and Zoonotic Infectious Diseases, Division of Healthcare Quality Promotion. General information about MRSA in the community. Centers for Disease Control and Prevention website. https://www.cdc.gov/mrsa/community/index.html. Updated March 25, 2016. Accessed April 9, 2018; and MDRO—multidrug-resistant organisms: MRSA. Occupational Safety and Health Administration website. https://www.osha.gov/SLTC/etools/hospital/hazards/mro/mrsa/mrsa.html. Accessed April 9, 2018.

Carbapenem-Resistant Enterobacteriaceae

CRE are a group of untreatable and hard-to-treat infections caused by bacteria. They have become resistant to all, or nearly all, of the current antibiotics. Almost one-half of hospitalized patients who get sepsis from CRE bacteria die from the infection. Altogether, these pathogens are responsible for approximately 9,000 infections per year and 600 deaths.[58]

Klebsiella species and *Escherichia coli* are strains of bacteria (Enterobacteriaceae) that normally reside in flora of the human intestines. Some Enterobacteriaceae have become highly resistant to the carbapenem class of antibiotics, making CRE infections outside of the gut quite serious and difficult to treat.

Like *C difficile* infections, CRE infections primarily affect patients who are hospitalized or living in other facilities providing care, such as people living in nursing homes, patients receiving long-term antibiotic therapy, and patients receiving support from invasive devices such as IV catheters.[59] Contact precautions are indicated when caring for these patients.

Neisseria gonorrhoeae

N gonorrhoeae causes gonorrhea, an STD that can result in discharge and inflammation at the urethra, cervix, pharynx, or rectum. Each year, there are about 820,000 gonorrhea infections, of which 246,000 are drug-resistant infections.[58] Gonorrhea is discussed later in this chapter along with other STDs.

Infectious Diseases of Childhood

The childhood infectious diseases presented in this chapter include rubella (German measles), rubeola (red measles or hard measles), mumps (parotitis), chickenpox (varicella), and pertussis (whooping cough). These infectious diseases are preventable with immunization for chickenpox; with the triple immunization of the measles, mumps, and rubella (MMR) vaccine; and as part of the DTaP vaccine for pertussis. The incidence of these childhood diseases has declined because of widespread immunization of children; immunization provides long-lasting immunity.

All health care workers should use personal protective measures when caring for children with infections. Protective immunization, effective handwashing, appropriate level of precautions, and careful handling of linens, supplies, and equipment that may be contaminated are important in preventing the spread of these diseases.

Rubella (German Measles)

Rubella is a mild, febrile, and highly communicable viral disease caused by the rubella virus. The disease usually is transmitted by direct contact with nasopharyngeal secretions or droplet spray from an infected person, but it may also be passed transplacentally (producing active infection in the fetus) and by contact with articles contaminated with blood, urine, or feces. It is characterized by a diffuse, punctate, macular rash (**FIGURE 27-8**). This rash spreads from the forehead to the face to the torso to the extremities (lasting 3 days). (A rash that lasts longer than 3 days indicates the presence of rubeola.) Maximal communicability appears to be the first few days before and 5 to 7 days after the onset of the rash. Although complications from the disease are rare, self-limiting arthritis sometimes develops in young females. Droplet precautions should be followed by those not immunized against rubella.

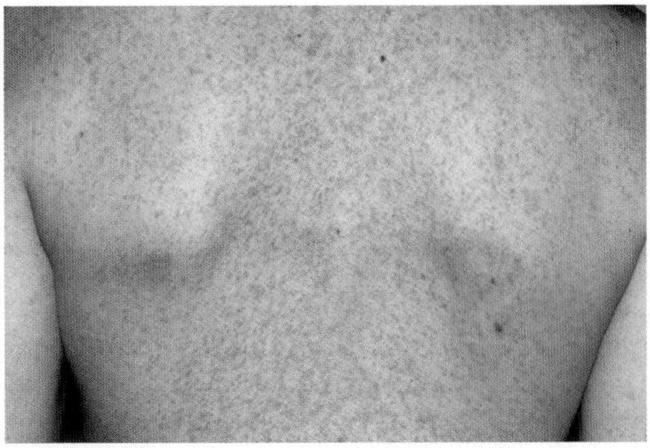

FIGURE 27-8 Rash related to rubella (German measles).

> CRITICAL THINKING
>
> Is there any way a paramedic can avoid rubella other than being immunized for it?

Congenital rubella syndrome is acquired when an infected pregnant woman passes the disease to her unborn child.[60] The risk of the baby developing congenital defects is highest in the first trimester of pregnancy but is low after 20 weeks' gestation. The disease is associated with cataracts, developmental delay, deafness, and congenital heart disease. In 2004, a panel of experts declared that rubella was eliminated from the United States. There are, however, rare cases reported in people traveling from other countries. As a precaution, pregnant EMS workers should not be exposed to patients with rubella. Droplet precautions should be followed by those not immunized against this disease.

Rubeola (Measles)

Rubeola is an acute, highly communicable viral disease that is caused by the measles virus. It is characterized by fever, conjunctivitis, upper respiratory infection symptoms, cough, bronchitis, and a blotchy red rash (**FIGURE 27-9**). The virus is found in the blood, urine, and pharyngeal secretions. It usually is passed directly or indirectly through contact with infected respiratory secretions. Airborne precautions should be followed by those not immunized against rubeola.

With exposure, the virus invades the respiratory epithelium, then spreads via the lymph system. Rubeola may predispose a person to secondary bacterial complications such as otitis media, pneumonia, and myocarditis. The most serious life-threatening complication is subacute sclerosing panencephalitis, a slowly progressing neurologic disease that is marked by loss of mental capacity and muscle coordination.

Early (prodromal) symptoms that mark the onset of rubeola include high fever, nasal discharge, conjunctivitis, photophobia, and cough. About 1 or 2 days before the rash emerges, white spots are usually noted on the inside of the cheek (Koplik spots). The dermal rash begins a few days after respiratory tract involvement, coinciding with the production of serum antibodies. This red, maculopapular rash spreads from the forehead to the face, neck, and torso and eventually to the feet, usually by the third day (centripetal spread). Uncomplicated cases of rubeola usually last 6 days. Recovery from the illness confers lifelong immunity.

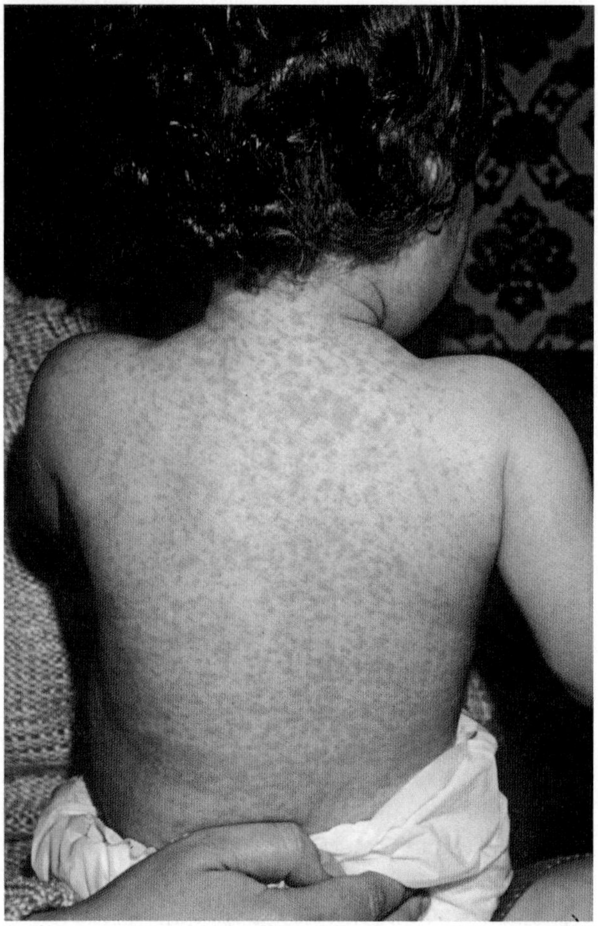

FIGURE 27-9 Rubeola (measles) rash on the third day.

Mumps

Mumps is an acute, communicable systemic viral disease caused by the mumps virus. It is characterized by localized edema of one or more of the salivary glands (usually the parotid). The swelling may affect both sides or only one side of the neck (**FIGURE 27-10**). In some cases, involvement of other glands also occurs. The virus is passed through direct contact with the saliva droplets of an infected person, so droplet precautions should be followed by those not immunized against mumps.

The virus invades and multiplies in the parotid gland or the upper respiratory tract passages. From there, it enters the bloodstream and localizes in

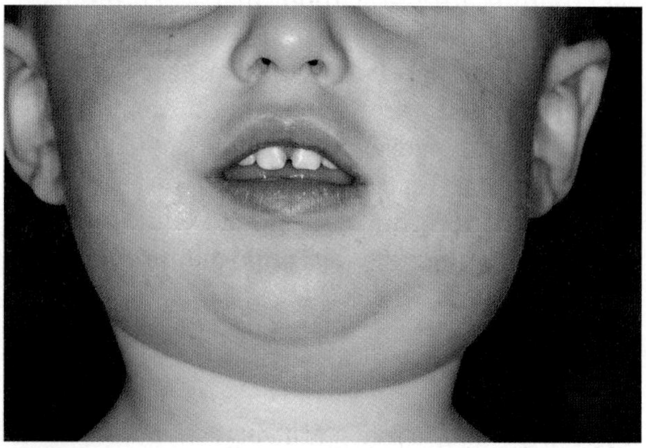

FIGURE 27-10 Mumps in a young child.

glandular or nervous tissue. The parotid glands, testes, and pancreas may be affected. When mumps occurs after the onset of puberty, it may cause a painful inflammation of the testicle (orchitis) and testicular atrophy; however, sterility is rare. The intensity of symptoms in mumps varies; 30% of infections are asymptomatic.

Immunity after recovery is lifelong. Placental transfer of antibodies sometimes occurs.

> CRITICAL THINKING
> Why are some viral diseases of childhood still seen despite widespread immunization?

Chickenpox

Chickenpox is a common childhood disease caused by the varicella-zoster virus, a member of the herpesvirus family. Chickenpox is highly communicable. The virus is passed by direct and indirect contact with droplets (mainly airborne) from the respiratory passages of an infected person. Exposure to linen tainted with vesicular or mucous membrane discharges of infected people has been implicated in spread of the disease. Airborne and contact precautions should be followed by those not immunized against the disease.

Chickenpox is characterized by a sudden onset of low-grade fever, mild malaise, and a skin eruption that is maculopapular for a few hours and vesicular for 3 to 4 days, leaving a granular scab (**FIGURE 27-11**). The skin lesions appear first on the trunk, then usually progress to the extremities. The crops of skin eruptions (each associated with itching) usually are more abundant on areas of the body that are covered with clothing. The scalp, conjunctivae, and upper respiratory tract may also be affected. The appearance of crops of vesicles (fresh vesicles appearing while other lesions are scabbed) differentiates chickenpox from smallpox; smallpox has skin lesions of the same age. Children with chickenpox should be isolated from schools, medical offices, EDs, and public places until all lesions are crusted and dry.

Treatment is symptomatic. Complications may include secondary bacterial infections of the skin, pneumonia, encephalitis, meningitis, sepsis, bleeding problems, and dehydration.[61]

After recovery, the virus is thought to remain in the body in an asymptomatic latent stage, and possibly may be localized in the dorsal root ganglia. The virus may reactivate during periods of stress or immunosuppression. During these periods, it may produce an illness known as **shingles**. The vesicles associated with shingles appear on the skin area supplied by the sensory nerves of a single group or associated groups of dorsal root ganglia known as dermatomes (**FIGURE 27-12**). Unlike chickenpox, shingles is not passed through respiratory droplets unless it is spread to other areas of the body. However, it can cause chickenpox in susceptible people who come in contact with open skin lesions. Contact precautions need to be followed in those not immunized against chickenpox. If the shingles is disseminated, then airborne and contact precautions should be followed.

Antiviral drugs may shorten the length and severity of symptoms of shingles as well as prevent a complication known as postherpetic neuralgia, a long-term neuropathic pain that persists even after the rash is long gone.

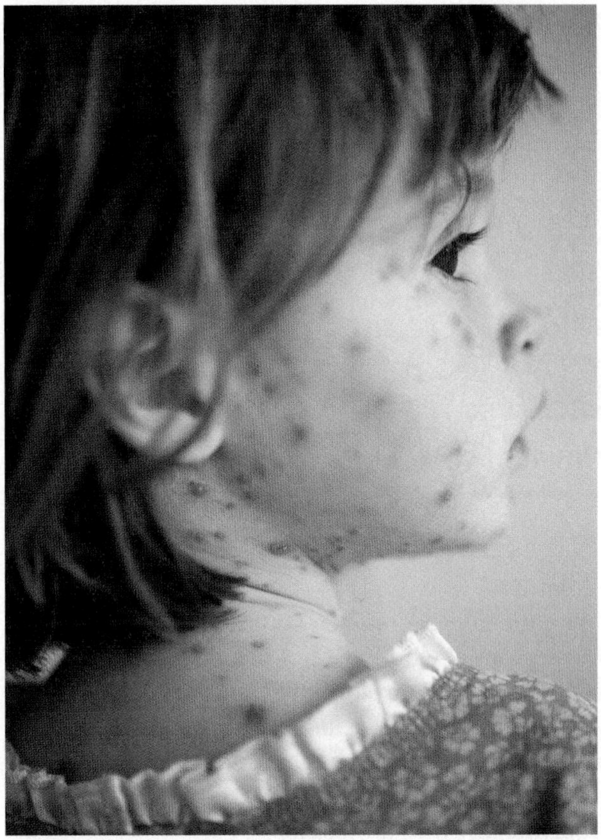

FIGURE 27-11 Chickenpox skin lesions.

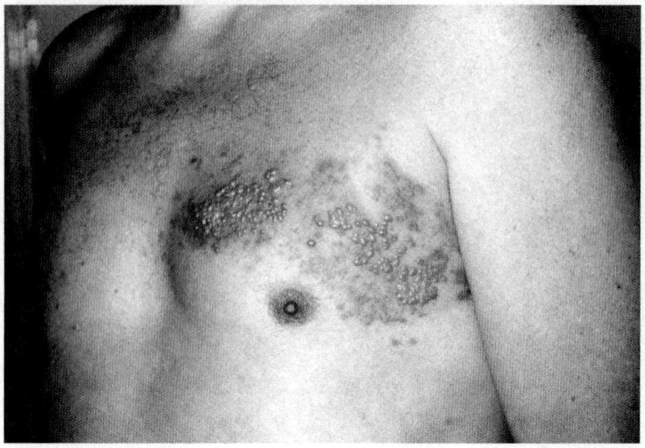

FIGURE 27-12 Vesicles associated with shingles.

Varicella vaccine is recommended by the CDC for personnel who have not been vaccinated, have not had chickenpox, or have undetectable varicella antibody titers.[62] Varicella-zoster immune globulin is recommended for pregnant women with exposure to chickenpox who are not immunized (either naturally or artificially with a vaccine).

Pertussis

Pertussis is an infectious disease that mainly affects infants and young children. It is caused by *Bordetella pertussis* bacteria and is spread by direct contact with discharges from mucous membranes contained in droplets. Thus, droplet precautions need to be followed when this disease is present or suspected.

Pertussis causes inflammation of the entire respiratory tract as well as a subtle onset of cough that becomes paroxysmal in 1 to 2 weeks and can last 1 to 2 months.[63] The coughing episodes are violent (sometimes without an intervening inhalation, causing the high-pitched inspiratory "whoop") and end with expulsion of clear mucus and vomiting. The whoop often is not present in children younger than 6 months.

Before the introduction of a vaccine against pertussis in the 1950s, this disease killed more children in the United States than did all other infectious diseases combined.[64] The incidence of the disease has increased since 1980, reaching a peak in 2012. Pertussis vaccine usually is given in combination with DTaP vaccines to children at 2, 4, and 6 months of age; a booster dose is given at age 5 years. The pertussis vaccine is 80% to 90% effective, but after 2 years its protection declines, so it is still possible to acquire pertussis after immunization, although the course of the disease is shorter and not as severe.

Pertussis is infectious from the onset of symptoms (runny nose, fever) until the third week after the onset of the paroxysmal coughing or until 5 days of antibiotic treatment.[65] Paramedics exposed to pertussis should be evaluated for the need of postexposure treatment with antibiotics.

Other Childhood Diseases

Other common childhood diseases include respiratory syncytial virus, croup (laryngotracheobronchitis), and epiglottitis. For more information, see Chapter 47, *Pediatrics*.

Respiratory Syncytial Virus

Respiratory syncytial virus is a very common respiratory illness that infects the lower respiratory tract. It usually occurs during the winter months. It typically causes a mild cold-like illness that resolves within a week or two, but it can also cause serious illness especially in infants younger than 1 year, premature babies, and older adults. In the latter cases, bronchiolitis (inflammation of the small airways) and pneumonia may occur with wheezing, hypoxia, cyanosis, and tachypnea. Treatment includes oxygen and nebulized albuterol. Droplet precautions need to be followed.

Croup (Laryngotracheobronchitis)

Croup is an infection of the upper airways (larynx, trachea, bronchi) in young children. It most commonly affects children between 6 months and 5 years of age and is most often caused by viruses, with the most common agent being parainfluenza. Croup typically causes a gradual onset of coldlike illness with low-grade fever, rhinorrhea, and cough. The cough develops into a characteristic "seallike," barking cough. In severe cases, the inflammation of the upper airway can cause significant obstruction with respiratory distress (retractions and tachypnea) and stridor.

Treatment includes keeping the child as calm as possible. Children have narrow upper airways, and agitating them can turn a partial obstruction into a complete one. Other treatment for severe croup includes nebulized racemic epinephrine and steroids (dexamethasone); these medications decrease the swelling in the upper airways. Droplet precautions should be followed when caring for a child with suspected croup.

Epiglottitis

Epiglottitis is an infection of the epiglottis. In the past, it most often occurred in children younger than 5 years, and the most common cause was Hib. Today, vaccinations against Hib have greatly reduced the frequency of epiglottitis.

Signs and symptoms include the rapidly progressive (unlike croup) development of high fever, sore throat, hoarseness, respiratory distress, and drooling. Prehospital treatment should focus on minimizing child anxiety to avoid progression to complete airway obstruction. These children often need advanced airway management in the operating room.

Other Important Infectious Diseases

Other diseases easily transmitted during the course of patient care include influenza, severe acute respiratory syndrome, mononucleosis, and herpes simplex type 1 (HSV-1) infection (described later in this chapter).

Influenza

Influenza ("the flu") is a respiratory infection that is caused by influenza viruses A, B, and C. It is spread by virus-infected droplets that are coughed or sneezed into the air; thus, droplet precautions should be followed. Influenza usually occurs in small outbreaks or, every few years, in epidemics and occasionally pandemics. Resistance is normally conferred after recovery, although this resistance is only to the specific strain or variant (BOX 27-10). The influenza virus mutates rapidly, creating new strains every

NOTE

For more than half a century, global influenza virologic surveillance has been conducted by the World Health Organization (WHO) through its Global Influenza Surveillance and Response System. Surveillance tracks the location of the influenza activity, its related illnesses, and the types of viruses involved. The CDC's Influenza Division, which also provides international influenza surveillance, has collaborated with the WHO since 1956 to support in the preparation and planning of public health interventions based on the surveillance findings.

Modified from: Centers for Disease Control and Prevention, National Center for Immunization and Respiratory Diseases. Influenza (flu): monitoring for influenza viruses. Centers for Disease Control and Prevention website. https://www.cdc.gov/flu/pandemic-resources/monitoring/index.html. Updated November 3, 2016. Accessed April 9, 2018.

BOX 27-10 Human Influenza Virus Types A, B, C

People infected with certain strains of A or type B influenza acquire immunity to that strain. However, these strains occasionally mutate to produce new strains, which in turn can lead to a new infection. Type B virus is relatively stable. However, it occasionally mutates to overcome resistance that can lead to small outbreaks of infection. Type A virus is highly unstable (mutates often) and has caused worldwide flu epidemics. These variants are named for the geographic site and year of isolation (eg, the Spanish flu in 1918, Asian flu in 1957, and Hong Kong flu in 1968) and the culture number (eg, A/Japan/305/57). Seasonal influenza vaccines protect against specific influenza A and B subtypes predicted to be common during that period, which explains why occasionally people who have had the influenza vaccine still acquire the disease.

Type C virus stimulates antibodies that provide immunity for life.

Modified from: Epidemiology and prevention of vaccine-preventable diseases, influenza. Centers for Disease Control and Prevention website. https://www.cdc.gov/vaccines/pubs/pinkbook/flu.html. Accessed May 18, 2018.

DID YOU KNOW?

CDC Recommendations for EMS and Medical First Responder Personnel, Including Firefighter and Law Enforcement First Responders, During an Outbreak of Influenza (H1N1)

Patient Assessment: Interim Recommendations

These recommendations were developed following the H1N1 influenza pandemic in 2009 and 2010. There has been no update.

If there has *not* been swine-origin influenza reported in the geographic area, EMS personnel should assess all patients as follows:

1. Remain at least 6 feet (2 m) away from patients and bystanders with symptoms. They should use appropriate respiratory precautions while assessing all patients for suspected cases of swine-origin influenza.
2. Assess all patients for symptoms of acute febrile respiratory illness (fever with nasal congestion/rhinorrhea, sore throat, or cough).
   - If no acute febrile respiratory illness, proceed with normal EMS care.
     - If symptoms of acute febrile respiratory illness are present, question all patients about travel to geographic areas within the last week where cases of swine-origin influenza have been confirmed. Question the patient about close contact with someone with recent travel to these areas.
   - If travel exposure has occurred, don appropriate PPE for influenza.
   - If no travel exposure exists, place a surgical mask on the patient and use appropriate PPE for cases of acute febrile respiratory illness described in the PPE section).

If the CDC confirmed swine-origin influenza in the geographic area:

1. Address scene safety.
   - If the public safety answering point (PSAP), advises of a potential for acute febrile respiratory illness EMS personnel should don appropriate before the entering scene.
   - If the PSAP has not identified people with symptoms of acute febrile respiratory illness on scene, EMS personnel should stay at least than 6 feet (2 m) away from patients and bystanders with symptoms and use appropriate respiratory precautions during patient assessment.
2. Assess all patients for symptoms of acute febrile respiratory illness.
   - If no symptoms of acute febrile respiratory illness, provide routine EMS care.
   - If symptoms of acute febrile respiratory illness, don appropriate PPE for a suspected case of swine-origin influenza.

PPE: Interim Recommendations

- When treating a patient with a suspected case of swine-origin influenza as defined above, the following PPE should be worn:
  - Fit-tested disposable N95 respirator and eye protection (eg, goggles, eye shield), and disposable nonsterile gloves and gown, when coming into close contact with the patient.
- When treating a patient who is not suspected to have swine-origin influenza but who has symptoms of acute febrile respiratory illness, the following precautions should be taken:
  - Place a surgical mask on the patient, if tolerated. If not tolerated, EMS personnel may wear a standard surgical mask.
  - Practice good respiratory hygiene: Use nonsterile gloves for contact with the patient, patient secretions, or surfaces that may have been contaminated. Follow hand hygiene, including handwashing or cleansing with alcohol-based hand disinfectant after contact.
- Encourage good patient compartment vehicle airflow and ventilation to reduce the concentration of aerosol accumulation.

Modified from: Centers for Disease Control and Prevention. Interim guidance for emergency medical services (EMS) systems and 9-1-1 public safety answering points (PSAPs) for management of patients with confirmed or suspected swine-origin influenza A (AN1) infection. Centers for Disease Control and Prevention website. https://www.cdc.gov/h1n1flu/guidance_ems.htm. Updated August 5, 2009. Accessed April 9, 2018.

CRITICAL THINKING

Which locations in your area are at high risk for influenza outbreaks?

year. Influenza vaccine has variable effectiveness every year depending on how well it matches with the strain of that year.

Influenza signs and symptoms typically include chills, fever, headache, muscular aches, loss of appetite, and fatigue. These symptoms are followed by upper respiratory tract infection and a cough (often severe and drawn out) that lasts for 2 to 7 days. Patient management is mainly supportive. Mild cases of viral infection usually are not treated.

Severe cases (especially in older adults and those with lung or heart disease) may result in secondary bacterial infection (eg, *S pneumoniae*); these cases can be fatal. Other viral respiratory diseases that can lead to bacterial complications include acute afebrile viral respiratory disease (excluding influenza) and acute febrile respiratory disease. Both diseases may cause illnesses in the upper and lower respiratory tracts, including pharyngitis, laryngitis, croup, bronchitis, and bronchiolitis (BOX 27-11).

Flu vaccines contain killed strains of type A and type B virus that are known to be currently in circulation. In the past, a nasal spray flu vaccine was also approved for protection against influenza A and B viruses in healthy people between 5 and 49 years of age. However, the effectiveness of the nasal vaccine has been questioned and for several years the CDC has not recommended its use.[66] The vaccine must be repeated each year just before the start of the flu season (by the end of October in the United States). Health care workers should be immunized in the fall of each year with the current vaccine.

The vaccines may help prevent infection. In contrast, treatment with antiviral drugs early in the course of illness may reduce the duration and severity of influenza.

CRITICAL THINKING

Will you get the influenza vaccine? What influenced your decision?

Severe Acute Respiratory Syndrome

Severe acute respiratory syndrome (SARS) is a viral respiratory illness caused by coronavirus that created a pandemic in 2003. It results in high fever, muscles

BOX 27-11 Bird Flu: The Next Pandemic?

A **pandemic** is an infectious disease outbreak that infects large numbers of people in a large geographic region and may occur worldwide. These outbreaks occur three to four times each century when new subtypes of viruses are easily transmitted from person to person. Any infectious disease may become a pandemic, but influenza is of great concern because it can be fatal and spreads easily and rapidly. WHO has predicted that the next pandemic influenza could kill between 2 million and 8 million people worldwide.

Avian influenza (bird flu) is an infectious disease of birds, and less commonly pigs. It is caused by the influenza type A strain most likely to become the next pandemic. The virus is similar in makeup to the 1918 variety and can mutate rapidly, causing severe disease in infected persons. The mortality in humans who get this form of flu approaches 60%. There is concern that as the virus continues to spread among migratory birds, it may mutate or merge with human strains of another virus, and enabler the disease to be spread in human throughout the world and could persist for years.

Because the virus has not spread easily to humans, a vaccine specific for Avian flu has not been developed Antiviral drugs, including oseltamivir (Tamiflu), peramivir (Rapivab), and zanamivir (Relenza), are clinically effective in interrupting the ability of the influenza A virus to replicate in humans. However, the prophylactic use of these drugs to prevent avian flu is not recommended, as it may result in the development of a resistant strain. Annual flu vaccinations are not effective against bird flu but are effective against other flu viruses that may complicate the avian flu should an outbreak occur.

Modified from: Influenza. World Health Organization website. http://www.who.int/mediacentre/factsheets/2003/fs211/en/. Revised March 2003. Accessed April 9, 2018; Centers for Disease Control and Prevention. H1N1 flu: CDC estimates of 2009 H1N1 influenza cases, hospitalizations and deaths in the United States. Centers for Disease Control and Prevention website. https://www.cdc.gov/h1n1flu/estimates_2009_h1n1.htm. Updated June 24, 2014. Accessed April 9, 2018; Cheng M. *WHO Outbreak Communication*. WHO/CDS/2005.37. World Health Organization website. http://www.who.int/csr/don/Handbook_influenza_pandemic_dec05.pdf. Updated December 2005. Accessed April 9, 2018; and Centers for Disease Control and Prevention, National Center for Immunization and Respiratory Diseases. Influenza (flu): first human avian influenza A (H5N1) virus infection reported in Americas. Centers for Disease Control and Prevention website. https://www.cdc.gov/flu/news/first-human-h5n1-americas.htm. Updated January 8, 2014. Accessed April 10, 2018.

aches, cough, and pneumonia. In the 2003 pandemic, the mortality rate was almost 10%.[67] There have been no known cases since 2004.

Poor prehospital and hospital preparation for the SARS outbreak resulted in several lessons learned. For example, almost half of Toronto's paramedics had to be quarantined because they failed to take proper precautions when exposed to SARS patients.[68] Other lessons learned included the need for an emergency plan in place before an outbreak occurs, communication and education early about potential outbreaks and appropriate levels of PPE and disinfection to prevent spread, and early communication with frontline staff.

Mononucleosis

Mononucleosis (often referred to as "mono") is usually caused by the Epstein-Barr virus (EBV), though other organisms such as cytomegalovirus (CMV) occasionally cause a mononucleosislike syndrome (BOX 27-12). Both EBV and CMV are members of the herpesvirus family. Mononucleosis is spread from person to person via the oropharyngeal route and saliva (hence the nickname *kissing disease*). Blood transfusions, organ transplant, or contact with semen or blood during sexual intercourse also can be modes of transmission. Most people with a healthy immune system are able to fend off the infection even after significant exposure. Transmission from caregivers to young children is common. Approximately 90% of people older than 35 years have antibodies to CMV or EBV,[69] probably as the result of mild childhood infection, which is often erroneously attributed to a common cold or the flu. Previous infection with EBV generally confers a high degree of resistance to future exposures.

Signs and symptoms of mononucleosis appear gradually. They include fever (which may last for weeks), sore throat, oropharyngeal discharges, lymphadenopathy (especially posterior cervical), and splenomegaly with abdominal tenderness. Some patients experience a generalized rash or darkened areas in the mouth that resemble bruises. Although recovery usually occurs in a few weeks, some patients take months to regain their former level of energy. Patients may remain carriers for several months after symptoms disappear. No immunization is available for mononucleosis.

BOX 27-12 Facts About CMV

General Information

- The majority of adults in the United States are infected with CMV by 40 years of age.
- Approximately 1 in 200 infants is born with congenital CMV infection.
- Only about 20% of infants born with CMV will develop health problems related to it.

About the Virus

- CMV is a member of the herpesvirus family (the herpes simplex viruses and the varicella-zoster virus and EBV.
- CMV is found in body fluids
- Most CMV infections cause no signs or symptoms in an infected person (a silent infection).
- CMV can cause disease in unborn babies and in people with a weakened immune system.

Transmission and Prevention

- Transmission of CMV occurs from person to person, through close contact with body fluids.
- The overall risk of contracting CMV infection from casual contact is small.

Modified from: National Center for Immunization and Respiratory Diseases, Division of Viral Diseases. Cytomegalovirus (CMV) and congenital CMV infection: about CMV. Centers for Disease Control and Prevention website. https://www.cdc.gov/cmv/overview.html. Updated December 5, 2017. Accessed April 9, 2018.

Complications of EBV infection include peritonsillar abscesses, bacterial sinusitis, mastoiditis, swelling of salivary glands, and, rarely, airway obstruction. Several cancers are linked to EBV infection, including lymphoma and nasopharyngeal carcinoma.[70]

Sexually Transmitted Diseases

A **sexually transmitted disease (STD)** is a disease that can be passed from person to person through sexual activity. A sexually transmitted infection may be transmitted to another person even when the infected person has no symptoms. More than 20 pathogens have been identified as belonging to this group of diseases, including HBV, HCV, and HIV.[71] Other common STDs are syphilis, gonorrhea, chlamydia, and herpesvirus infections. Patients with STD syndromes often have multiple STDs.

Syphilis

Syphilis is a systemic disease that can have serious, long-term complications. The disease results from penetration of the skin, whether intact or broken, by the bacterium *Treponema pallidum*. Common modes of transmission include direct contact with fluid or pus from lesions on the skin and mucous membranes, blood transfusions or needlesticks (rare), and congenital transmission. After penetration, the organisms travel (within hours) to the lymph nodes. From there, they are carried throughout the body. After the initial infection, syphilis follows four well-defined stages of disease unless it is treated with antibiotic therapy.[72] No immunization is available. It is estimated that 30% of exposures result in infection.[73]

Primary Stage

Within 10 to 90 days of exposure to syphilis, a primary lesion, or **chancre**, develops at the site of initial invasion by the pathogen (**FIGURE 27-13**). The surface of the chancre is usually crusted or ulcerated. The lesion is usually painless, varies in size from about 0.5 to 1 inch (1 to 2 cm) in diameter. It generally heals spontaneously within 1 to 5 weeks. Syphilis is highly communicable during this stage.

Secondary Stage

If the patient does not receive antibiotics during the primary stage, the condition will progress to the secondary stage of syphilis. The secondary stage begins about 2 to 10 weeks after the appearance of the primary lesion and lasts for 2 to 6 weeks. Systemic symptoms include headache, malaise, anorexia, fever, sore throat, lymphadenopathy, and bald spots in the area of infection. In addition, the patient may develop a rash on the palms and soles which is usually bilateral and symmetrical. Painless, wart-like lesions (condylomata lata), which are extremely infectious, may also be found in moist, warm sites (eg, the inguinal area). The CNS, eyes, bones, joints, or kidneys may be affected during this stage.

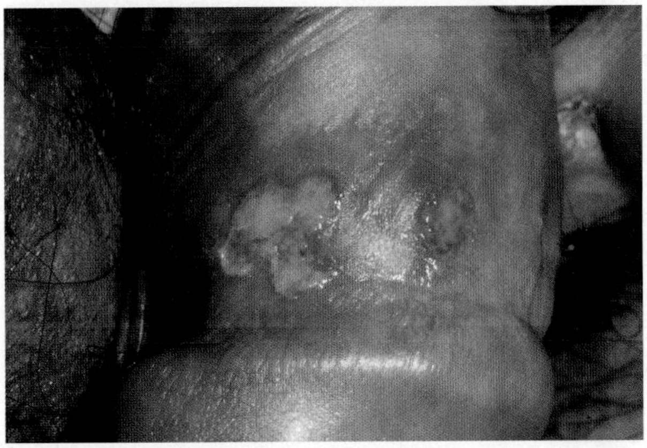

FIGURE 27-13 Primary syphilis chancre.

> CRITICAL THINKING
> Why do you think a patient in the secondary stage of syphilis would call EMS?

Latency

A latency period follows the secondary stage in untreated people; it may range from 1 year to several decades. During this period, recurrent episodes of secondary stage symptoms with subclinical infection may occur. Tertiary syphilis, or neurosyphilis, can occur at any time following infection and may include the following manifestations:[74,75]

1. Skin
   - Granulomatous lesions (gummas) on skin (painless) and bone (painful)
2. CNS
   - Paresis
   - **Tabes dorsalis**—spinal column degeneration characterized by a wide gait and ataxia ("syphilitic shuffle")
   - Loss of reflexes, pain, and temperature sensation
   - Meningitis
   - Psychosis
3. Cardiovascular
   - Cerebrovascular occlusion
   - Dissecting aneurysm of the ascending aorta
   - Myocardial insufficiency; aortic necrosis, which can lead to aortic rupture and death

Gonorrhea

Gonorrhea is caused by the bacterium *N gonorrhoeae*. It is transmitted between people by fluids and pus from infected mucous membranes; it can also be spread from an infected mother to her baby during pregnancy and delivery. The course and severity of the disease differ in men and women as do the signs and symptoms. Gonorrhea often is treatable with antibiotics, but some strains are now resistant to all antibiotic therapy. Immunization is not available. Antibodies develop after exposure, but the antibodies are specific to the strain of gonorrhea that caused the infection. This allows for future reinfection with other strains.

Affected areas of the male anatomy are the urethra, Littre gland, Cowper gland, prostate gland, seminal vesicles, and epididymis. A sudden onset of dysuria and urinary urgency and frequency is seen several days after exposure. The associated urethral discharge rapidly becomes purulent and profuse. Direct spread of the infection may result in prostatitis, epididymitis, and seminal vesiculitis. Primary gonorrheal infections may also affect the pharynx, conjunctivae, and anus.

Affected areas of the female anatomy are the Bartholin glands, Skene glands, urethra, cervix, and fallopian tubes. More than 50% of infected women remain free of symptoms; others have a mucopurulent discharge that ranges from scant to profuse.[76] Contiguous spread of the disease may lead to endometritis, salpingitis, and pelvic inflammatory disease. The formation of tubo-ovarian abscesses and tubal obstruction may result in infertility.

Between 1% and 3% of gonococcal infections become disseminated in the blood.[77] This extension of the disease may produce septicemia, septic arthritis, endocarditis, meningitis, and skin lesions. In the bacteremic stage, the patient may complain of fever, chills, and malaise. Erythematous lesions are common, especially on the extremities. They may occur in clusters or singly.

Chlamydia

Chlamydia, which is spread by the bacterium *Chlamydia trachomatis,* is a major cause of **sexually transmitted nonspecific urethritis** or nongonococcal genital infection. It is the most common sexually transmitted disease in the United States[78] and is a leading cause of preventable blindness.[79] The signs and symptoms of chlamydia are similar to those of gonorrhea, which makes differentiation between the two diseases difficult. No immunization for chlamydia is available.

In men, chlamydia may cause a penile discharge as well as complications such as swelling of the testes, which, if untreated, may lead to infertility. In women, chlamydia usually is asymptomatic, though it may also cause a vaginal discharge or pain with urination, salpingitis, and cervicitis. Like gonorrhea, chlamydia can progress to pelvic inflammatory disease and tubo-ovarian abscess and long-term complications such as sterility and ectopic pregnancy. Transmission occurs secondary to direct contact with exudates, either sexually or during birth (**FIGURE 27-14**). Chlamydial infections are treated with antibiotics.

Herpesvirus Infections

Many herpesviruses have been identified, but only a few infect humans: the herpes simplex virus; CMV, which is associated with mononucleosis, hepatitis, and severe systemic disease; EBV, which causes mononucleosis; and the varicella-zoster virus, which causes chickenpox and shingles. This section addresses only the herpesviruses associated with STDs.

The two antigenically distinct herpes simplex viruses responsible for STDs are **herpes simplex virus type 1 (HSV-1)** and **herpes simplex virus type 2 (HSV-2)**. Both pathogens can cause herpes infection, with the infection occurring anywhere in the body. As a rule, HSV-1 most often is associated with herpes above the waist, whereas HSV-2 generally is associated with genital herpes. However, either type can cause disease in the genital area. Immunization is not available for either virus.

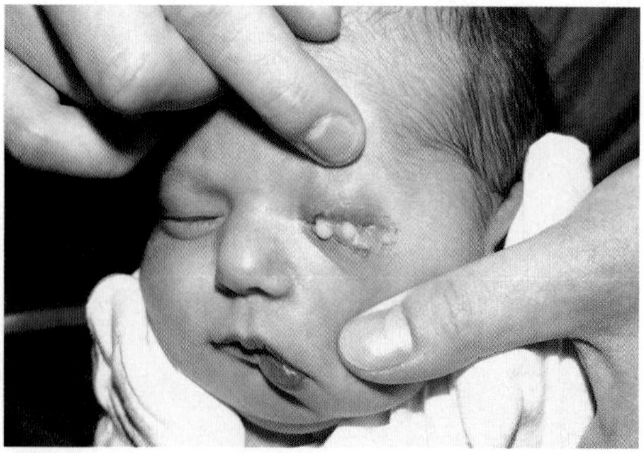

FIGURE 27-14 Conjunctivitis from a chlamydial infection in an 8-day-old infant.

HSV is common in the United States, causing 300,000 to 500,000 new infections each year; approximately 50 million Americans are thought to carry the virus.[80] It is estimated that 70% to 90% of adults have antibodies against HSV-1.

The mode of transmission for HSV is strictly skin-to-skin contact with an infected area of the body through a break in the skin or through mucous membranes. Sexual contact is not required for transmission. Touching the herpesvirus may result in finger infection (herpetic whitlow). Young children who develop HSV-1 probably contract the virus through a casual kiss from a parent or relative. The virus also may be spread to other body sites by autoinoculation (eg, from lip to finger to genitalia).

CRITICAL THINKING

Why do you think the incidence of herpetic whitlow in health care workers has declined over the last 20 years?

The initial HSV-1 transmission usually occurs by 5 years of age.[81] It is manifested by gingivostomatitis ("cold sores" or "fever blisters") (**FIGURE 27-15**). Initial HSV-2 infection generally results from sexual activity. It is manifested by painful vesicular lesions of the cervix, vulva, penis, rectum, anus, and mouth.

Once present in tissue, HSV produces an acute infection and an isolated vesicular lesion (blister). The lesion heals spontaneously without scarring. However, the virus remains active in the body despite circulating antibodies.

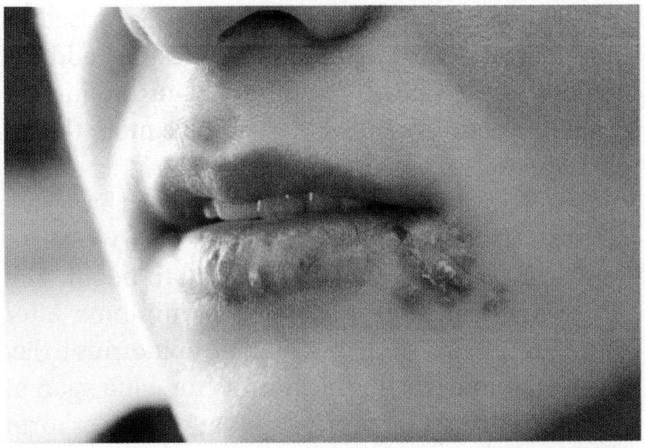

FIGURE 27-15 "Fever blisters" caused by the herpes simplex virus.

After the primary infection, HSV enters the CNS nearest to the site of initial infection. It travels along sensory nerve pathways to a sensory nerve ganglion, where it remains in a latent stage until reactivated. When triggered by another infectious disease, menstruation, emotional stress, or immunosuppression, the virus reaches the epidermis by way of peripheral nerves. It then produces a recurrent infectious disease state, which usually lasts 4 to 10 days. In most cases, the lesions appear in the area of initial inoculation. The number of lesions a person might experience during any given episode varies.

HSV can remain inactive in some people without future outbreaks. Others may experience periodic outbreaks. Antiviral agents such as acyclovir may shorten the duration of an outbreak and may be prescribed as a prophylactic agent.

Lice and Scabies

Lice and scabies are potential health hazards for all health care providers. Both can transmit communicable skin diseases and systemic illness, as well as dermatitis and discomfort. (Other vector-borne illnesses [eg, Lyme disease] are described in Chapter 33, *Toxicology*.)

Lice

Lice are small, wingless insects that are ectoparasites of birds and mammals. Most are host specific. Two of the species are human parasites (**FIGURE 27-16**):

- *Phthirus pubis*—the pubic, or crab, louse.
- *Pediculus humanus*, which has two forms—*Pediculus capitis* (the head louse) and *Pediculus corporis* (the body louse). The latter was involved in outbreaks of epidemic typhus and trench fever in World War I.

Lice have a three-stage life cycle. The eggs hatch in 7 to 10 days, the nymph stage lasts 7 to 13 days, and the egg-to-egg cycle lasts about 3 weeks. Lice spread through close personal contact, and sharing of clothing and bedding may result in outbreaks (eg, at schools, in day care facilities, in families). Lice subsist on blood from the host and have mouths modified for piercing and sucking. During biting and feeding, secretions from the louse cause a small, red macule and pruritus. Long infestation periods may

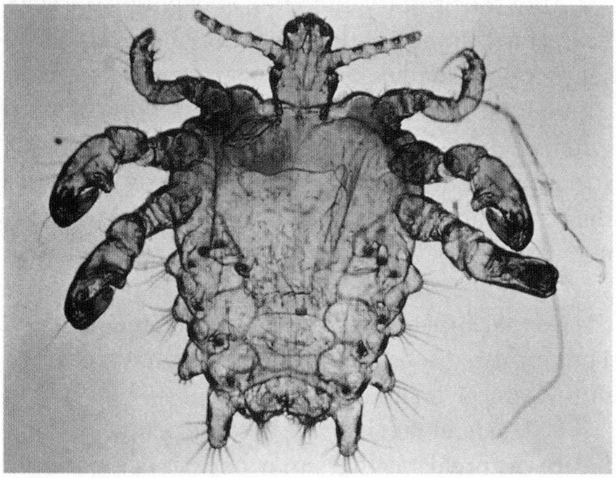

A

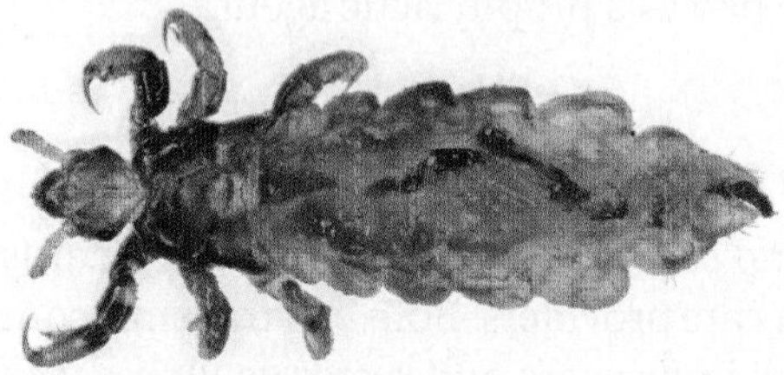

B

FIGURE 27-16 **A.** The pubic, or crab, louse. **B.** Male of the human head louse.

A: Courtesy of Centers for Disease Control and Prevention; B: © Tomasz Klejdysz/Shutterstock.

result in a decrease in pruritus and often a thick, dry, scaly appearance to the skin. In severe cases, oozing and crusting may be present. If sensitization to lice saliva and feces occurs, inflammation may develop. Secondary infection may result from scratching of lesions.

Pubic lice have a distinctive appearance, suggestive of miniature crabs and may be observed as gray-blue spots on the abdomen and thighs of infested patients. The eggs (nits or ova) often are evident on the shaft of pubic hairs. They are sometimes seen in the eyelashes, eyebrows, and axillary hairs. Pubic lice usually are acquired during sexual activity or from unchanged bedding in which egg-infested pubic hairs have been shed. Although primary bite lesions seldom are evident, the patient normally complains of intense pruritus and pubic scratching.

Head lice have an elongated body with a head that is slightly narrower than the thorax. Each louse has three pairs of legs with delicate hooks at the distal extremities. The nits of head lice tend to be white and oval in shape (usually with one nit to a hair shaft). They are easily mistaken for dandruff, but cannot be brushed out. These parasites most frequently affect children.

Body lice are slightly larger than head lice and concentrate around the waist, shoulders, axillae, and neck. Body lice and their nits usually are found in seams and on the fibers of clothing. The lesions from their bites begin as small, noninflammatory red spots, which quickly become papular wheals that resemble linear scratch marks (parallel scratch marks on the shoulders are a common finding). Head lice and body lice interbreed.

The treatment for all types of lice is designed to eradicate the parasites and nits and to prevent re-infestation. Patients usually are advised to wash all clothing, bedding, and personal articles thoroughly in hot water. They also are advised to wash the infected body area with gamma benzene hexachloride shampoo (Kwell), crotamiton (Eurax), Rid, or Nix. (Overtreatment should be avoided to prevent toxicity.)

Scabies

The human **scabies** mite (*Sarcoptes scabiei* var *hominis*) is a parasite. It completes its entire life cycle in and on the epidermis of its host. Scabies infestation resembles a lice infestation, but scabies bites generally are concentrated around the hands and feet, especially in the webs of the fingers and toes (**FIGURE 27-17**). Other common infestation areas include the face and scalp of children, the nipples in females, and the penis in males. The scabies mite usually is passed by intimate contact or acquired from infested bedding, furniture, and clothing. The mite can burrow into the skin within minutes. It will not survive more than 2 to 3 days away from its human host.[82]

Scabies infestation often is manifested by severe nocturnal pruritus. However, it takes 2 to 6 weeks for sensitization to develop and itching to begin. The adult female mite is responsible for symptoms. After impregnation, she burrows into the epidermis to lay her eggs, remaining in this burrow for a life span of about 1 month. Although vesicles and papules form at the surface, they often go unnoticed by the results of scratching. In severe cases (eg, Norwegian scabies), oozing, crusting, and secondary infection may result. Although all people are susceptible to scabies, people with a previous exposure usually develop fewer mites

DID YOU KNOW?

Bed Bugs

Bed bug infestations were common in the United States before World War II but were mostly eradicated in the 1940s and 1950s from the widespread use of DDT (dichlorodiphenyltrichloroethane). In recent years, the common bed bug, *Cimex lectularius*, has become more prevalent. It can be encountered in homes, apartments, hotels, motels, health care facilities, dormitories, shelters, schools, and modes of transportation. This resurgence may be the result of international travel.

The most common place to find bed bugs is in bedding, where they often hide within seams and crevices of a mattress, box spring, bed frame, and headboard. They can also conceal themselves behind baseboards, wallpaper, upholstery, picture frames, and electrical switch plates. The adult bed bug is red-brown, has a flattened body, and is easily visible. They can move quickly, but do not fly, and are often mistaken for ticks.

Bed bugs usually bite at night while people are sleeping. The bites may cause an itchy welt or localized swelling, similar to a mosquito bite, and can occur in clusters. These reactions may be immediate or delayed for several days after the bite. Scratching the bites can lead to skin infections. Although bed bugs can harbor pathogens in and on their bodies, transmission of disease to humans is considered unlikely.

Visible signs of bed bugs include blood stains or fecal spots on bedding, furniture, and walls. If infestation is severe, there may be a sweet and musty odor in the room. Bed bug infestations require professional extermination.

EMS personnel should take the following precautions:

- Tuck pant legs inside socks or boots and seal with adhesive tape. Take similar precautions with gloves and other clothing to prevent exposure.
- Wear disposable shoe covers while at the scene and dispose of them in a sealed, plastic bag. Inspect work shoes before entering the ambulance or EMS base. Infested gear should not be taken into living quarters.
- Place any clothing item with visible bed bugs in a plastic, sealed bag. Do not use the clothing again until it has been placed in a hot clothes dryer for at least 15 minutes to destroy the bed bugs.

Modified from: Potter MF. Bed bugs. University of Kentucky, College of Agriculture, Food and Environment website. https://entomology.ca.uky.edu/ef636. Revised May 2012. Accessed April 9, 2018.

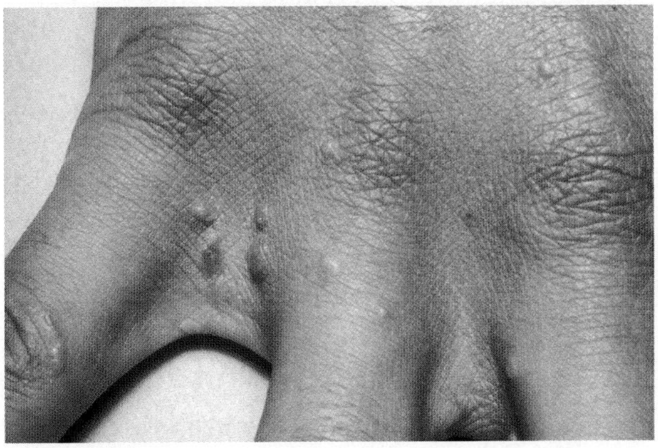

FIGURE 27-17 Common site of burrows in scabies.

on later exposures and experience symptoms earlier (within 1 to 4 days).

The treatment for scabies is similar to that prescribed for lice infestation. Symptoms may persist for longer than 1 month, until the mite and mite products are shed with the epidermis. (Mites are communicable until all mites and eggs have been destroyed.) Reinfestation is common; therefore the patient should be reexamined if the itching has not abated after several weeks. Antibiotic therapy may be needed to treat secondary bacterial infection.

Immunization against scabies is not available. Protective measures against lice and scabies infestation are presented in BOX 27-13.

Reporting an Exposure to an Infectious or a Communicable Disease

An **exposure incident** (significant exposure) is any specific contact of the eyes, the mouth, other mucous membranes, or nonintact skin, or parenteral contact, with blood, blood products, bloody body fluids, or other potentially infectious materials.[83] Exposures and all suspected exposures to an infectious or communicable disease must be reported to the DICO. Reporting a possible exposure is important for the following reasons:

1. It permits immediate medical follow-up. This allows identification of infection and immediate intervention.

BOX 27-13 Protective Measures Against Scabies

Personal Protection

Because scabies can be contagious, especially when the patient's skin is crusted, contact precautions should be observed and personal protective garments should be worn when providing care. Thorough hand washing after care is essential. Treatment for health care providers who become infected includes permethrin cream or ivermectin.

Environmental Disinfection

Contaminated linens and clothing need to be transported in plastic bags and machine washed in hot water and dried with high heat. Vacuum and clean any areas where patients have received treatment.

Modified from: Global Health, Division of Parasitic Diseases. Parasites: crusted scabies cases (single or multiple). Centers for Disease Control and Prevention website. https://www.cdc.gov/parasites/scabies/health_professionals/crusted.html. Updated November 2, 2010. Accessed April 10, 2018.

2. It enables the DICO to evaluate the circumstances of the incident. It also allows the DICO to determine what changes to make to prevent future exposures.
3. It aids follow-up testing of the source person if permission for testing can be obtained.

Reporting also ensures that if the health care worker is infected, it has been documented that the disease occurred from a work-related exposure.

Submitting the Report

As described earlier, the Ryan White Act requires employers to appoint a DICO. That person or officer follows the exposure control plan. The plan must comply with standards and guidelines relative to the exposure and must meet any local reporting requirements.

Medical Evaluation and Follow-up

By law, employers must provide free medical evaluation and treatment to exposed employees, including the following elements:[84]

- Counseling regarding the risks, signs and symptoms, probability of developing clinical disease, and ways to prevent future spread of the potential infection
- Appropriate treatment in line with current US Public Health Service recommendations
- A discussion of medications offered and their side effects and contraindications
- Evaluation of any reported illness to determine whether the symptoms are related to HIV or hepatitis

Steps Involved

Blood tests of exposed employees are always contingent on employee agreement. Employees have the option to provide blood samples, but they can refuse permission for HIV testing at the time the sample is drawn. The employer must maintain the blood samples for 90 days in case employees change their mind regarding testing if HIV-like or hepatitislike symptoms develop.

CRITICAL THINKING

How would you feel if you were stuck by a contaminated needle and the patient refused HIV testing?

In addition, the law requires the employer to take the following steps: (1) provide counseling to the employee based on test results, (2) provide informed consent regarding prophylaxis and therapeutic regimens, and (3) implement those regimens after receiving approval from the employee. Vaccines also should be made available to all employees who are exposed to blood and other potentially infectious materials during their work.

Written Report and Confidentiality

The agent of the employer will send a written report to the DICO of the employer, indicating whether vaccination was offered to the exposed employee. The report should also state whether the employee received this vaccination. The written report must note that the employee was informed of the results of the evaluation and told of any medical conditions resulting from the exposure that may require further evaluation or treatment. A copy of this report must be provided to the employee and to the DICO for the agency's files.

All other elements of the employee's medical record are confidential and cannot be supplied to the employer. The employee must give written consent for anyone to view the records. To comply with OSHA standards regarding access to employee exposure and medical records, the records must be maintained for the duration of employment plus 30 years. (States that are not governed by OSHA must also follow these guidelines.)

The Paramedic's Role in Preventing Disease Transmission

Paramedics will inevitably deal with patients who have infectious diseases. Given this reality, it is important for them to be vigilant about the consequences of transmitting such diseases to themselves, to their patients, and to their coworkers. Part of this professional duty in preventing the spread of disease is knowing when *not* to go to work. A health care worker should not go to work if any of the following are present:

- Fever
- Diarrhea
- Draining wound or any type of wet lesion
- Jaundice
- Mononucleosis
- Treatment with a medication and/or shampoo for lice or scabies
- Strep throat (unless antibiotics have been taken for longer than 24 hours)
- Cold with productive cough (unless the paramedic wears a surgical mask)

Health care workers also should ensure that their personal immunization status is current for MMR, HBV, DTaP, polio, chickenpox, and influenza.

CRITICAL THINKING

Have you come to school or work with any of these conditions?

Other Considerations in Disease Prevention

When called to provide emergency care, paramedics should always approach the scene with caution, keeping in mind that an uncontrolled scene increases the likelihood of transmission of body fluids. Appropriate precautions (contact, droplet, airborne, and bloodborne precautions) should be observed at all times. Measures necessary to maintain these precautions may include wearing gloves, protective eyewear, a face shield, and a gown (if splash or spray is possible) and wearing an appropriate particulate mask when airborne disease is suspected. Regardless of the patient's infectious status, the paramedic should do the following:

- Provide the same level of care to all patients.
- Disinfect equipment and the patient compartment with the proper disinfectant solution.
- Practice effective handwashing.
- Report any infectious exposure to the agency's DICO.

CRITICAL THINKING

Imagine that you are on a call and get a small splash of blood in your eyes. What do you think would prevent you from reporting it immediately so that your postexposure care could begin?

Summary

- National concerns about communicable disease and infection control have resulted in public laws, standards, guidelines, and recommendations to protect health care providers and emergency responders against infectious diseases. Paramedics must be familiar with these guidelines. They also must take personal protective measures against exposure to these pathogens.
- The chain of elements needed to transmit an infectious disease includes the pathogenic agent, a reservoir, a portal of exit from the reservoir, an environment conducive to transmission of the pathogenic agent, a portal of entry into the new host, and susceptibility of the new host to the infectious disease.
- The human body is protected from infectious disease by both external and internal barriers, which serve as lines of defense against infection. External barriers include the skin, gastrointestinal system, upper respiratory tract, and genitourinary tract. Internal barriers include the inflammatory response and the immune response.
- The progression of infectious disease from exposure to the onset of symptoms occurs in four stages: the latent period, the incubation period, the communicability period, and the disease period.
- The human immunodeficiency virus (HIV) may be transmitted directly from person to person (eg, through anal or vaginal intercourse) or indirectly through blood transfusion

or tissue transplant, or by the use of contaminated needles or syringes. The virus affects the CD4 T cells. Progression of the disease can be divided into stage 1 (acute retroviral infection, seroconversion, and asymptomatic infection), stage 2 (early symptomatic HIV), and stage 3 (late symptomatic HIV and advanced HIV). Secondary complications are usually related to opportunistic infections that arise as the immune system deteriorates. Paramedics should observe strict compliance with universal precautions for protection against HIV, but patient care should also include helping these patients feel that they can obtain acceptance and compassion from health care workers.
- Infectious hepatitis is a viral disease that produces pathologic changes in the liver. The three main classes of hepatitis virus are hepatitis A, hepatitis B, and hepatitis C. Infection with hepatitis may cause mild symptoms, liver failure, or death.
- Tuberculosis (TB) is a chronic pulmonary disease that is acquired through inhalation of tubercle bacilli. The infection is passed mainly when infected people cough or sneeze the bacteria into the air or by contact with sputum that contains virulent TB bacilli. The infection is characterized by stages of early infection (frequently asymptomatic), latency, and a potential for recurrent disease.
- Meningitis is an inflammation of the membranes that surround the spinal cord and brain. It can be caused by bacteria, viruses, and other microorganisms.
- Bacterial endocarditis is inflammation of the endocardium and any one or more heart valves. This disease can be rapidly fatal if left untreated.
- Pneumonia is an acute inflammatory process of the respiratory bronchioles and alveoli. Bacteria, viruses, and fungi can cause this disease.
- Tetanus is a serious, sometimes fatal, disease of the central nervous system (CNS). It is caused by infection of a wound with spores of the bacterium *Clostridium tetani*. The most common symptom is trismus, difficulty opening the mouth (lockjaw).
- Rabies is an acute viral infection of the CNS. Humans are highly susceptible to the rabies virus after exposure to saliva from the bite or scratch of an infected animal.
- Hantaviruses are carried by rodents and are transmitted through inhalation of material contaminated with rodent urine and feces. Many forms of this disease occur in specific geographic areas.
- Several mosquito-borne illnesses have been reported in the United States, including Chikungunya virus, dengue, West Nile virus, Zika, and malaria. Prevention has the highest impact on these diseases, as no vaccines are available that can prevent them.
- The Centers for Disease Control and Prevention (CDC) has identified three antibiotic-resistant infections that are considered urgent (high-consequence threats): *Clostridium difficile*, carbapenem-resistant Enterobacteriaceae, and *Neisseria gonorrhoeae*.
- Rubella is a mild, febrile, highly communicable viral disease that is characterized by a diffuse, punctate, macular rash. The CDC recommends that all health care providers receive immunization if they are not immune as a result of previous rubella infection.
- Rubeola is an acute, highly communicable viral disease caused by the measles virus. It is characterized by fever, conjunctivitis, cough, bronchitis, and a blotchy red rash.
- Mumps is an acute, communicable systemic viral disease that is characterized by localized unilateral or bilateral edema of one or more of the salivary glands. Occasionally other glands are also involved.
- Chickenpox, a highly communicable infection, is characterized by a sudden onset of low-grade fever, mild malaise, and a maculopapular skin eruption that lasts for a few hours. This is followed by a vesicular eruption that lasts for 3 to 4 days, leaving a granular scab. The virus may reactivate during periods of stress or immunosuppression, causing the illness known as shingles.
- Pertussis is an infectious disease that leads to inflammation of the entire respiratory tract. It causes an insidious cough, which becomes paroxysmal in 1 to 2 weeks and lasts 1 to 2 months.
- Influenza is mainly a respiratory tract infection. It is spread by influenza viruses A, B, and C.
- Lessons learned from the severe acute respiratory syndrome (a viral respiratory illness caused by coronavirus) pandemic in 2003 included the need for an emergency plan in place before an outbreak occurs, communication and education early about potential outbreaks and appropriate levels of PPE and disinfection to prevent spread, and early communication with frontline staff.
- Mononucleosis is caused by either the Epstein-Barr virus or the cytomegalovirus. Both of these pathogens are members of the herpesvirus family.
- Syphilis is a systemic disease that is characterized by a primary lesion, a secondary eruption involving skin and mucous membranes, long latency periods, and eventually seriously disabling lesions of the skin, bone, viscera, CNS, and cardiovascular system.
- Gonorrhea is caused by the sexually transmitted bacterium *N gonorrhoeae*. It can be treated with antibiotics, although some strains do not respond to the usual antibiotic therapy.
- Chlamydia is a major cause of sexually transmitted nonspecific urethritis or genital infection. Signs and symptoms are similar to those of gonorrhea.
- Herpes simplex virus is transmitted by skin-to-skin contact with an infected area of the body. The primary infection produces a vesicular lesion (blister), which heals spontaneously. After the primary infection, the virus travels to a sensory nerve ganglion, where it remains in a latent stage until reactivated.
- Lice are small, wingless insects that are ectoparasites of birds and mammals. During biting and feeding, lice secrete a substance that causes small, red macules and pruritus.
- The human scabies mite is a parasite that completes its life cycle in and on the epidermis of the host. Scabies bites are usually concentrated around the hands and feet, especially in the webs of the fingers and toes.

- Reporting a possible communicable disease exposure permits immediate medical follow-up. It also enables the DICO to make changes that might prevent exposures in the future. Moreover, it helps employees to obtain the proper evaluation and testing.
- Part of the paramedic's professional duty with regard to infectious disease transmission is to know when not to go to work. Paramedics also have a duty to use the proper precautions at all times.

References

1. Regulations (Standards–29 CFR): table of contents. US Department of Labor, Occupational Safety and Health Administration website. https://www.osha.gov/pls/oshaweb/owadisp.show_document?p_table=STANDARDS&p_id=10051. Accessed April 10, 2018.
2. Cowan E, Macklin R. Unconsented HIV testing in cases of occupational exposure: ethics, law, and policy. *Acad Emerg Med.* 2012;19(10):1181-1187.
3. Rutala WA, Weber D; Healthcare Infection Control Practices Advisory Committee. Guideline for disinfection and sterilization in healthcare facilities, 2008. Centers for Disease Control and Prevention website. https://www.cdc.gov/infectioncontrol/pdf/guidelines/disinfection-guidelines.pdf. Updated February 15, 2017. Accessed April 10, 2018.
4. McCance K, Huether S. *Pathophysiology: The Biologic Basis for Disease in Adults and Children*. 7th ed. St. Louis, MO: Mosby; 2014.
5. Centers for Disease Control and Prevention, Office of Public Health Scientific Services, Center for Surveillance, Epidemiology, and Laboratory Services, Division of Scientific Education and Professional Development. Principles of epidemiology in public health practice, third edition: an introduction to applied epidemiology and biostatistics. Lesson 1: introduction to epidemiology. Centers for Disease Control and Prevention website. https://www.cdc.gov/ophss/csels/dsepd/ss1978/lesson1/section10.html. Updated May 18, 2012. Accessed April 10, 2018.
6. Division of HIV/AIDS Prevention, National Center for HIV/AIDS, Viral Hepatitis, STD, and TB Prevention, Centers for Disease Control and Prevention. HIV/AIDS: HIV transmission. Centers for Disease Control and Prevention website. https://www.cdc.gov/hiv/basics/transmission.html. Updated March 16, 2018. Accessed April 10, 2018.
7. Division of HIV/AIDS Prevention, National Center for HIV/AIDS, Viral Hepatitis, STD, and TB Prevention, Centers for Disease Control and Prevention. HIV/AIDS: opportunistic infections. Centers for Disease Control and Prevention. https://www.cdc.gov/hiv/basics/livingwithhiv/opportunisticinfections.html. Updated May 30, 2017. Accessed April 10, 2018.
8. Carpenter RJ. Early symptomatic HIV infection. Medscape website. https://reference.medscape.com/article/211873-overview. Updated May 18, 2017. Accessed May 18, 2018.
9. Selik RM, Mokotoff ED, Branson B, et al. Revised surveillance case definition for HIV infection—United States, 2014. *Morb Mortal Wkly Rep.* 2014;63(RR03):1-10.
10. Calcagno A, Nozza S, Muss C, et al. Ageing with HIV: a multidisciplinary review. *Infection.* 2015;43(5):509-522.
11. Deeks SG, Lewin SR, Havlir DV. The end of AIDS: HIV infection as a chronic disease. *Lancet.* 2013;382(9903):1525-1533.
12. Joyce MP, Kuhar D, Brooks JT. Notes from the field: occupationally acquired HIV infection among health care workers—United States, 1985–2013. *Morb Mortal Wkly Rep.* 2015;65(53):1245-1246.
13. Bass RR, Brice JH, Delbridge TR, Gunderson MR. *Emergency Medical Services: Clinical Practice and Systems Oversight Medicine. Volume 2: Medical Oversight of EMS.* Hoboken, NJ: John Wiley & Sons; 2015:369-410.
14. Eohlié S, Anglaret X. Decline of HIV-2 prevalence in West Africa: good news or bad news? *Int J Epidemiol.* 2006;5(5):1329-1330.
15. Kuhar DT, Henderson DK, Struble KA, et al. Updated US Public Health Service guidelines for the management of occupational exposures to human immunodeficiency virus and recommendations for postexposure prophylaxis. *Infect Control Hosp Epidemiol.* 2013;34(9):875-892.
16. Medical Care Criteria Committee. PEP for occupational exposure to HIV guideline. HIV Clinical Resource website. https://www.hivguidelines.org/pep-for-hiv-prevention/occupational/. Published October 2014. Accessed April 10, 2018.
17. Hepatitis A questions and answers for health professionals. Centers for Disease Control and Prevention website. https://www.cdc.gov/hepatitis/hav/havfaq.htm. Accessed May 18, 2018.
18. National Center for Immunization and Respiratory Diseases. Vaccines and preventable diseases: hepatitis A in-short. Centers for Disease Control and Prevention website. https://www.cdc.gov/vaccines/vpd/hepa/public/in-short-adult.html#who. Updated January 11, 2017. Accessed April 10, 2018.
19. National Center for Immunization and Respiratory Diseases. Pregnancy and vaccination: guidelines for vaccinating pregnant women. Centers for Disease Control and Prevention website. https://www.cdc.gov/vaccines/pregnancy/hcp/guidelines.html. Updated October 3, 2017. Accessed April 10, 2018.
20. National Highway Traffic Safety Administration. *The National EMS Education Standards.* Washington, DC: US Department of Transportation; 2009.
21. Cooley L, Sasadeusz J. Clinical and virological aspects of hepatitis B co-infection in individuals infected with human immunodeficiency virus type-1. *J Clin Virol.* 2003;26(2):185-193.
22. Hepatitis B. World Health Organization website. http://www.who.int/mediacentre/factsheets/fs204/en/. Reviewed July 2017. Accessed April 10, 2018.
23. Centers for Disease Control and Prevention, National Center for Infectious Diseases, Division of Healthcare Quality Promotion and Division of Viral Hepatitis. Exposure to blood: what healthcare personnel need to know. Centers for Disease Control and Prevention website. https://www.cdc.gov/hai/pdfs/bbp/exp_to_blood.pdf. Updated July 2003. Accessed April 10, 2018.
24. National Center for Immunization and Respiratory Diseases. Vaccines and preventable diseases: hepatitis B in-short. Centers for Disease Control and Prevention website. https://www.cdc.gov/vaccines/vpd/hepb/public/in-short-adult.html#who. Updated March 1, 2017. Accessed April 10, 2018.
25. Division of Viral Hepatitis, National Center for HIV/AIDS, Viral Hepatitis, STD, and TB Prevention. Viral hepatitis: hepatitis B FAQs for the public. https://www.cdc.gov/hepatitis/hbv/bfaq.htm#bFAQ38. Centers for Disease Control and Prevention website. Updated May 23, 2016. Accessed April 10, 2018.

26. Division of Viral Hepatitis, National Center for HIV/AIDS, Viral Hepatitis, STD, and TB Prevention. Viral hepatitis: surveillance for viral hepatitis—United States, 2015. Centers for Disease Control and Prevention website. https://www.cdc.gov/hepatitis/statistics/2015surveillance/commentary.htm. Updated June 19, 2017. Accessed April 10, 2018.
27. Viral hepatitis. Centers for Disease Control and Prevention website. https://www.cdc.gov/hepatitis/hcv/index.htm. Accessed May 18, 2018.
28. Initial treatment of HCV infection. American Association for the Study of Liver Diseases, Infectious Diseases Society of America website. https://www.hcvguidelines.org/treatment-naïve. Updated September 21, 2017. Accessed April 10, 2018.
29. Pierce JM. Hepatitis C 101: Can Hepatitis C be Cured? HepatitisC.net website. https://hepatitisc.net/living/hepatitis-c-101-can-hepatitis-c-be-cured/. May 13, 2015. Accessed June 19, 2018.
30. Division of Viral Hepatitis, National Center for HIV/AIDS, Viral Hepatitis, STD, and TB Prevention. Viral hepatitis: hepatitis B FAQs for health professionals. Centers for Disease Control and Prevention website. https://www.cdc.gov/hepatitis/hbv/hbvfaq.htm#overview. Updated January 11, 2018. Accessed April 10, 2018.
31. Global tuberculosis report 2017. World Health Organization website. http://www.who.int/tb/publications/global_report/en/. Accessed April 10, 2018.
32. Division of Tuberculosis Elimination. Tuberculosis (TB): trends in tuberculosis, 2016. Centers for Disease Control and Prevention website. https://www.cdc.gov/tb/publications/factsheets/statistics/tbtrends.htm. Updated November 15, 2017. Accessed April 10, 2018.
33. Division of Tuberculosis Elimination. Tuberculosis (TB): children. Centers for Disease Control and Prevention website. https://www.cdc.gov/tb/topic/populations/tbinchildren/default.htm. Updated October 10, 2014. Accessed April 10, 2018.
34. Tuberculosis. Centers for Disease Control and Prevention website. https://www.cdc.gov/niosh/topics/tb/default.html. Accessed May 18, 2018.
35. Division of Tuberculosis Elimination. Tuberculosis (TB): treatment for TB disease. Centers for Disease Control and Prevention website. https://www.cdc.gov/tb/topic/treatment/tbdisease.htm. Updated August 11, 2016. Accessed April 10, 2018.
36. National Center for Immunization and Respiratory Diseases. Meningitis: bacterial meningitis. Centers for Disease Control and Prevention website. https://www.cdc.gov/meningitis/bacterial.html. Updated January 25, 2017. Accessed April 10, 2018.
37. MacNeil J, Patton M; National Center for Immunization and Respiratory Diseases. Manual for the surveillance of vaccine-preventable diseases. Chapter 8: meningococcal disease. Centers for Disease Control and Prevention website. https://www.cdc.gov/vaccines/pubs/surv-manual/chpt08-mening.html. Updated April 2, 2018. Accessed April 10, 2017.
38. Briere EC, Rubin L, Moro PL, et al. Prevention and control of *Haemophilus influenzae* type B disease: recommendations of the Advisory Committee on Immunization Practices (ACIP). *MMWR Recomm Rep.* 2014;63(RR01):1-14.
39. National Center for Immunization and Respiratory Diseases. Vaccines and preventable diseases: pneumococcal vaccination. Centers for Disease Control and Prevention website. https://www.cdc.gov/vaccines/vpd/pneumo/index.html. Updated December 6, 2017. Accessed April 10, 2018.
40. Vilcant V, Hai O. Endocarditis, Bacterial. National Center for Biotechnology website. https://www.ncbi.nlm.nih.gov/books/NBK470547/. Updated November 27, 2017. Accessed May 18, 2018.
41. Sexton DJ, Chu VH. Epidemiology, risk factors, and microbiology of infective endocarditis. UpToDate website. https://www.uptodate.com/contents/epidemiology-risk-factors-and-microbiology-of-infective-endocarditis?source=search_result&search=infective%20endocarditis&selectedTitle=3~150. Updated March 8, 2018. Accessed April 10, 2018.
42. Cabell CH, Abrutyn E, Karchmer AW. Bacterial endocarditis: the disease, treatment, and prevention. *Circulation.* 2003;107(20):e185-e187.
43. Walls R, Hockberger R, Gausche-Hill M. *Rosen's Emergency Medicine: Concepts and Clinical Practice.* 9th ed. Philadelphia, PA: Elsevier; 2018.
44. Centers for Disease Control and Prevention, National Center for Emerging and Zoonotic Infectious Diseases, Division of High-Consequence Pathogens and Pathology. Rabies: how is rabies transmitted? Centers for Disease Control and Prevention website. https://www.cdc.gov/rabies/transmission/index.html. Updated April 22, 2011. Accessed April 10, 2018.
45. World Health Organization. *Current WHO Guide for Rabies Pre- and Post-Exposure Treatment in Humans*. Geneva, Switzerland: World Health Organization; 2002.
46. Wild animals. Centers for Disease Control and Prevention website. https://www.cdc.gov/rabies/location/usa/surveillance/wild_animals.html. Accessed May 18, 2018.
47. Centers for Disease Control and Prevention, National Center for Emerging and Zoonotic Infectious Diseases, Division of High-Consequence Pathogens and Pathology. Hantavirus. Centers for Disease Control and Prevention website. https://www.cdc.gov/hantavirus/index.html. Updated February 9, 2018. Accessed April 10, 2018.
48. Centers for Disease Control and Prevention, National Center for Emerging and Zoonotic Infectious Diseases, Division of High-Consequence Pathogens and Pathology. Hantavirus: reported cases of hantavirus disease. Centers for Disease Control and Prevention website. https://www.cdc.gov/hantavirus/surveillance/index.html. Updated July 19, 2017. Accessed April 10, 2018.
49. WHO factsheet: vector-borne diseases. Factsheet #387. World Health Organization website. http://www.who.int/kobe_centre/mediacentre/vbdfactsheet.pdf. Published March 2014. Accessed April 10, 2018.
50. 2017 provisional data for the United States. Centers for Disease Control and Prevention website. https://www.cdc.gov/chikungunya/geo/united-states-2017.html. Accessed May 18, 2018.
51. Centers for Disease Control and Prevention, National Center for Emerging and Zoonotic Infectious Diseases, Division of Vector-Borne Diseases. Dengue: symptoms and what to do if you think you have dengue. Centers for Disease Control and Prevention website. https://www.cdc.gov/dengue/symptoms/index.html. Updated September 27, 2012. Accessed April 10, 2018.
52. Centers for Disease Control and Prevention, National Center for Emerging and Zoonotic Infectious Diseases, Division of Vector-Borne Diseases. West Nile virus: preliminary maps and data for 2017. Centers for Disease Control and Prevention

website. https://www.cdc.gov/westnile/statsmaps/preliminarymapsdata2017/index.html. Updated January 10, 2018. Accessed April 10, 2018.

53. Centers for Disease Control and Prevention, National Center for Emerging and Zoonotic Infectious Diseases, Division of Vector-Borne Diseases. Zika virus. Centers for Disease Control and Prevention website. https://www.cdc.gov/zika/index.html. Updated April 5, 2018. Accessed April 10, 2018.
54. LaBeaud AD. Zika virus infection: an overview. UpToDate website. https://www.uptodate.com/contents/zika-virus-infection-an-overview. Updated March 9, 2018. Accessed April 10, 2018.
55. Global Health—Division of Parasitic Diseases and Malaria. Malaria: disease. Centers for Disease Control and Prevention website. https://www.cdc.gov/malaria/about/disease.html. Updated October 7, 2015. Accessed April 10, 2018.
56. Global Health—Division of Parasitic Diseases and Malaria. Malaria: frequently asked questions (FAQs). Centers for Disease Control and Prevention website. https://www.cdc.gov/malaria/about/faqs.html. Updated December 20, 2017. Accessed April 10, 2018.
57. Centers for Disease Control and Prevention, National Center for Emerging and Zoonotic Infectious Diseases, Division of Healthcare Quality Promotion. Antibiotic/antimicrobial resistance. Centers for Disease Control and Prevention website. https://www.cdc.gov/drugresistance/index.html. Updated March 29, 2018. Accessed April 10, 2018.
58. Centers for Disease Control and Prevention, National Center for Emerging and Zoonotic Infectious Diseases, Division of Healthcare Quality Promotion. Antibiotic/antimicrobial resistance: antibiotic resistance threats in the United States, 2013. Centers for Disease Control and Prevention website. https://www.cdc.gov/drugresistance/threat-report-2013/index.html. Updated April 10, 2017. Accessed April 10, 2018.
59. Centers for Disease Control and Prevention, National Center for Emerging and Zoonotic Infectious Diseases, Division of Healthcare Quality Promotion. Healthcare-associated infections: carbapenem-resistant Enterobacteriaceae in healthcare settings. Centers for Disease Control and Prevention website. https://www.cdc.gov/hai/organisms/cre/index.html. Updated February 23, 2018. Accessed April 10, 2018.
60. Lanzieri T, Redd S, Abernathy E, Icenogle J; National Center for Immunization and Respiratory Diseases. Manual for the surveillance of vaccine-preventable diseases. Chapter 15: congenital rubella syndrome. Centers for Disease Control and Prevention website. https://www.cdc.gov/vaccines/pubs/surv-manual/chpt15-crs.html. Updated November 17, 2017. Accessed April 10, 2018.
61. National Center for Immunization and Respiratory Diseases, Division of Viral Diseases. Chickenpox (varicella): complications. Centers for Disease Control and Prevention website. https://www.cdc.gov/chickenpox/about/complications.html. Updated April 11, 2016. Accessed April 10, 2018.
62. National Center for Immunization and Respiratory Diseases. Vaccine information for adults: recommended vaccines for healthcare workers. Centers for Disease Control and Prevention website. https://www.cdc.gov/vaccines/adults/rec-vac/hcw.html. Updated April 20, 2017. Accessed April 8, 2018.
63. National Center for Immunization and Respiratory Diseases, Division of Bacterial Diseases. Pertussis (whooping cough): about pertussis. Centers for Disease Control and Prevention website. https://www.cdc.gov/pertussis/about/index.html. Updated June 27, 2016. Accessed April 10, 2018.
64. Chow MYK, Khandaker G, McIntyre P. Global childhood deaths from pertussis: a historical review. *Clin Infect Dis.* 2016;63(suppl 4):S134-S141.
65. National Center for Immunization and Respiratory Diseases, Division of Bacterial Diseases. Pertussis (whooping cough): treatment. Centers for Disease Control and Prevention website. https://www.cdc.gov/pertussis/clinical/treatment.html. Updated August 7, 2017. Accessed April 10, 2018.
66. Centers for Disease Control and Prevention, National Center for Immunization and Respiratory Diseases. Influenza (flu): frequently asked flu questions 2017–2018 influenza season. Centers for Disease Control and Prevention website. https://www.cdc.gov/flu/about/season/flu-season-2017-2018.htm. Updated March 30, 2018. Accessed April 10, 2018.
67. National Center for Immunization and Respiratory Diseases, Division of Viral Diseases. Severe acute respiratory syndrome (SARS): about severe acute respiratory syndrome (SARS). Centers for Disease Control and Prevention website. https://www.cdc.gov/sars/about/index.html. Updated December 6, 2017. Accessed April 10, 2018.
68. Silverman A, Simor A, Loutfy MR. Toronto Emergency Medical Services and SARS. *Emerg Infect Dis.* 2004;10(9):1688-1689.
69. Wang X, Yang K, Wei C, Huang Y, Zhao D. Coinfection with EBV/CMV and other respiratory agents in children with suspected infectious mononucleosis. *Virol J.* 2010;7:247.
70. National Center for Immunization and Respiratory Diseases. Epstein-Barr virus and infectious mononucleosis: for healthcare providers. Centers for Disease Control and Prevention website. https://www.cdc.gov/epstein-barr/hcp.html. Updated September 14, 2016. Accessed April 10, 2018.
71. What are some types of and treatments for sexually transmitted diseases (STDs) or sexually transmitted infections (STIs)? National Institutes of Health, Eunice Kennedy Shriver National Institute of Child Health and Human Development website. https://www.nichd.nih.gov/health/topics/stds/conditioninfo/types. Reviewed January 31, 2017. Accessed April 10, 2018.
72. Division of STD Prevention, National Center for HIV/AIDS, Viral Hepatitis, STD, and TB Prevention, Centers for Disease Control and Prevention. Sexually transmitted diseases (STDs): syphilis: CDC fact sheet (detailed). Centers for Disease Control and Prevention website. https://www.cdc.gov/std/syphilis/stdfact-syphilis-detailed.htm. Updated February 13, 2017. Accessed April 10, 2018.
73. Long SS, Pickering LK, Prober CG, eds. *Principles and Practice of Pediatric Infectious Diseases*. 4th ed. Philadelphia, PA: Elsevier; 2012.
74. Syphilis stages and symptoms. Plush Care website. https://www.plushcare.com/blog/syphilis-stages-and-symptoms/. Published May 19, 2017. Accessed April 10, 2018.
75. Knudsen RP. Neurosyphilis overview of syphilis of the CNS. Medscape website. https://emedicine.medscape.com/article/1169231-overview. Updated August 22, 2017. Accessed April 10, 2018.
76. Hahn AW, Barbee LA. Gonorrhea. National STD Curriculum website. https://www.std.uw.edu/go/pathogen-based/gonorrhea/core-concept/all. Updated November 14, 2017. Accessed April 10, 2018.

77. Klausner JD. Disseminated gonococcal infection. UpToDate website. https://www.uptodate.com/contents/disseminated-gonococcal-infection. Updated February 14, 2018. Accessed April 10, 2018.
78. Centers for Disease Control and Prevention. *Sexually Transmitted Disease Surveillance, 2016*. Atlanta, GA: Department of Health and Human Services; September 2017.
79. Trachoma. World Health Organization website. http://www.who.int/mediacentre/factsheets/fs382/en/. Updated July 2017. Accessed April 10, 2018.
80. Skolnik NS, Clouse AL, Woodward J, eds. *Sexually Transmitted Diseases: A Practical Guide for Primary Care, Current Clinical Practice*. New York, NY: Springer Science+Business Media; 2013.
81. Herpes simplex virus in the newborn. New York State Department of Health website. https://www.health.ny.gov/diseases/communicable/herpes/newborns/fact_sheet.htm. Reviewed October 2011. Accessed April 10, 2018.
82. Global Health—Division of Parasitic Diseases. Parasites: workplace frequently asked questions (FAQs). Centers for Disease Control and Prevention website. https://www.cdc.gov/parasites/scabies/gen_info/faq_workplace.html. Updated July 19, 2013. Accessed April 10, 2018.
83. OSHA fact sheet, bloodborne pathogen exposure incidents, 2011. Occupational Safety and Health Administration website. https://www.osha.gov/OshDoc/data_BloodborneFacts/bbfact04.pdf. Accessed May 18, 2018.
84. The National Institute for Occupational Safety and Health (NIOSH) Ryan White HIV/AIDS Treatment Extension Act of 2009. Centers for Disease Control and Prevention website. https://www.cdc.gov/niosh/topics/ryanwhite/. Accessed May 18, 2018.

Suggested Readings

Barry JM. *The Great Influenza: The Story of the Deadliest Pandemic in History*. London, England: Penguin Books; 2005.

Bennett JE, Dolin R. *Mandell, Douglas, and Bennett's Principles and Practice of Infectious Diseases*. 8th ed. Philadelphia, PA: Elsevier; 2014.

Centers for Disease Control and Prevention. *Sexually Transmitted Diseases Treatment Guidelines, 2015. MMWR Recomm Rep.* June 5, 2015;64(3). https://www.cdc.gov/mmwr/pdf/rr/rr6403.pdf. Accessed April 10, 2018.

Kasper DL, Fauci AS. *Harrison's Infectious Diseases*. 3rd ed. New York, NY: McGraw-Hill; 2016.

Southwick FS. *Infectious Diseases: A Clinical Short Course*. 3rd ed. New York, NY: Lange; 2013.

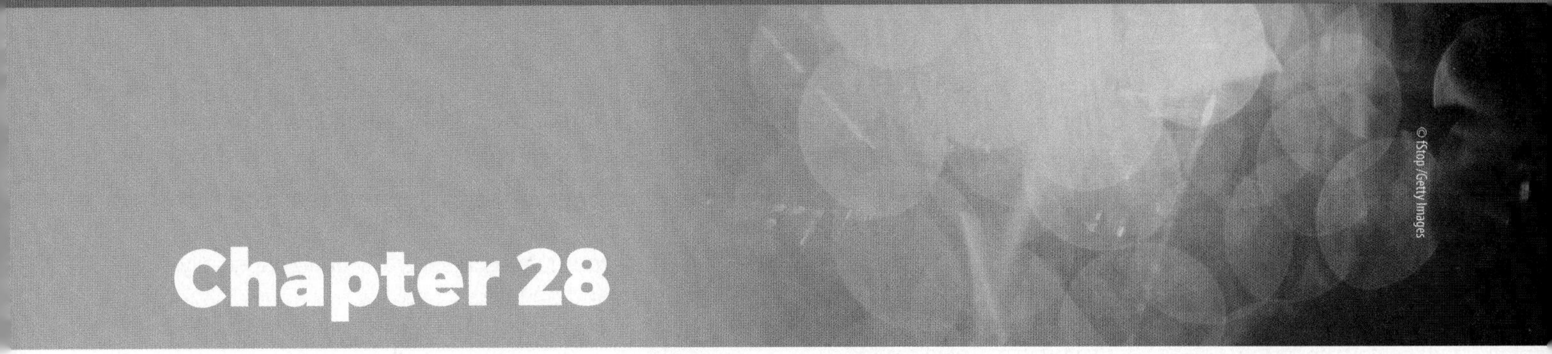

Chapter 28

Abdominal and Gastrointestinal Disorders

NATIONAL EMS EDUCATION STANDARD COMPETENCIES

Medicine

Integrates assessment findings with principles of epidemiology and pathophysiology to formulate a field impression and implement a comprehensive treatment/disposition plan for a patient with a medical complaint.

Abdominal and Gastrointestinal Disorders

Anatomy, presentations, and management of shock associated with abdominal emergencies

- Gastrointestinal bleeding (pp 1095–1096, 1101–1103)

Anatomy, physiology, epidemiology, pathophysiology, psychosocial impact, presentations, prognosis, and management of

- Acute and chronic gastrointestinal hemorrhage (pp 1101–1105, 1110–1111)
- Liver disorders (pp 1112–1114)
- Peritonitis (pp 1097–1099, 1102, 1107, 1109)
- Ulcerative diseases (pp 1105–1106, 1107–1109)
- Irritable bowel syndrome (p 1105)
- Inflammatory disorders (pp 1105–1107)
- Pancreatitis (p 1110)
- Bowel obstruction (pp 1109–1110)
- Hernias (p 1109)
- Infectious disorders (pp 1103–1105)
- Gallbladder and biliary tract disorders (p 1112)
- Rectal abscess (p 1112)
- Rectal foreign body obstruction (p 1112)
- Mesenteric ischemia (p 1110)

OBJECTIVES

Upon completion of this chapter, the paramedic student will be able to:

1. Identify the abdominal organs and describe their function. (pp 1095–1096)
2. Outline the prehospital assessment of a patient complaining of abdominal pain. (pp 1095, 1097–1102)
3. Distinguish between pain characteristics in abdominal pain. (pp 1097–1100)
4. Describe general prehospital management techniques for a patient complaining of abdominal pain. (pp 1100, 1102)
5. Describe signs and symptoms, complications, and prehospital management for the following abdominal and gastrointestinal disorders: gastrointestinal bleeding, acute and chronic gastroenteritis, inflammatory bowel disease (ulcerative colitis and Crohn disease), diverticulosis, appendicitis, peptic ulcer disease, bowel obstruction, pancreatitis, esophageal varices, hemorrhoids, cholecystitis, acute hepatitis, and hereditary hemochromatosis. (pp 1102–1115)
6. Recognize that abdominal conditions may present differently in pediatric and geriatric patients. (p 1115)

KEY TERMS

acute gastroenteritis Inflammation of the stomach and intestines with an associated sudden onset of vomiting and diarrhea.

acute mesenteric ischemia An abrupt interruption of intestinal blood flow. It may result from an embolism, thrombosis, or a low-flow state (decreased perfusion).

anal abscess An infected, pus-filled cavity near the rectum.

anal fistula An abnormal passage between the end of the bowel and the cutaneous surface of the anus.

appendectomy Surgical removal of the appendix.

appendicitis Inflammation of the appendix.

ascites An abnormal intraperitoneal accumulation of fluid containing large amounts of protein and electrolytes.

bowel obstruction An occlusion of the intestinal lumen that results in blockage of normal flow of intestinal contents.

cholecystectomy Surgical removal of the gallbladder.

cholecystitis Inflammation of the gallbladder, most often associated with the presence of gallstones.

chronic gastroenteritis Inflammation of the stomach and intestines that accompanies numerous gastrointestinal disorders.

cirrhosis A chronic and progressive disease in which normal liver cells are replaced by fibrotic scar tissue.

Crohn disease A chronic, inflammatory bowel disease of unknown origin that usually affects the ileum, the proximal colon, or both, but may affect any part of the gastrointestinal tract.

diverticulitis Inflammation of one or more diverticula.

diverticulosis The presence of pouchlike herniations through the muscular layer of the colon.

diverticulum A pouchlike herniation through the muscular wall of a tubular organ. It may be present in the stomach, small intestine, or, most commonly, the colon.

esophagitis Inflammation of the esophagus.

esophageal varices A complex of longitudinal, tortuous veins at the lower end of the esophagus that become enlarged and swollen as a result of portal hypertension.

fecalith A hard, impacted mass of feces in the colon.

gangrene Dead or dying body tissues attributable to blood supply that is lost or inadequate.

gastroesophageal reflux disease (GERD) A condition in which the stomach contents leak backward from the stomach into the esophagus.

hematemesis Vomiting of bright red blood, indicating upper gastrointestinal bleeding.

hematochezia The passage of red blood through the rectum.

hemorrhoids Swollen, distended veins (internal, external, or both) in the rectoanal area.

hepatic encephalopathy A spectrum of neuropsychiatric dysfunction caused by liver disease and commonly associated with ammonia intoxication.

hepatitis Inflammation of the liver caused by viruses, trauma, toxins, autoimmune or metabolic disorders, genetic diseases, or fat deposits.

hereditary hemochromatosis An inherited condition in which the body absorbs and stores too much iron. The extra iron accumulates in several organs, especially the liver, heart, and pancreas.

hernia Protrusion of any organ through an opening in the muscle or tissue holding it in place or where it normally resides.

hiatal hernia Herniation of the stomach through the diaphragm and up into the chest.

ileus Cessation of peristalsis of the intestines, which may be paralytic or mechanical.

inflammatory bowel disease (IBD) A general term that describes two diseases—ulcerative colitis and Crohn disease—that cause chronic inflammation of the digestive tract.

intussusception Telescoping of one portion of the intestine into another, which results in decreased blood supply of the involved segment.

involuntary guarding An unconscious rigid contraction of the abdominal muscles; a sign of peritoneal inflammation.

lactose intolerance A sensitivity disorder that results in the inability to digest lactose because of a deficiency of or defect in the enzyme lactase.

Mallory-Weiss syndrome A condition characterized by bleeding after a tear in the mucous membrane at the junction of the esophagus and the stomach; usually self-limited but may be severe.

melena Abnormal black, tarry stools containing digested blood.

pancreatitis Inflammation of the pancreas, which causes severe epigastric pain.

paralytic ileus A decrease in or the absence of intestinal peristalsis that can closely mimic bowel obstructions.

peptic ulcer disease An illness that results from a complex pathologic interaction among the acidic gastric secretions and proteolytic enzymes and the mucosal barrier.

permissive hypotension A fluid resuscitation strategy in which fluid and blood products are restricted, in spite of lower than normal blood pressures, until bleeding has been controlled.

rebound tenderness Pain caused by the sudden release of fingertip pressure on the abdomen. It is a sign of peritoneal inflammation.

referred pain Pain felt at a site distant from its origin.

somatic pain Pain that arises from skeletal muscles, ligaments, vessels, or joints.

ulcerative colitis An inflammatory condition of the large intestine characterized by severe diarrhea and ulceration of the mucosa of the colon and/or rectum.

visceral pain Deep pain that arises from smooth vasculature or organ systems.

volvulus Twisting of the intestines.

Acute abdominal pain is a common chief complaint in emergency care that may reflect serious illness. This condition accounts for as many as 10% to 20% of all visits to the emergency department each year.[1] *This chapter reviews the gastrointestinal anatomy and disorders that produce gastrointestinal bleeding and abdominal pain. Appropriate evaluation and management in the prehospital setting may prevent the development of life-threatening complications.*

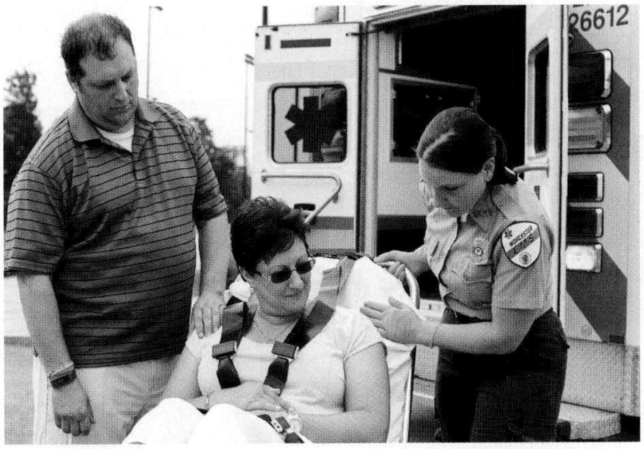

Review of Gastrointestinal Anatomy

The gastrointestinal (GI) system provides the body with water, electrolytes, and other nutrients used by the cells. The major organs of the GI system are the esophagus, stomach, small and large intestines, liver, gallbladder, and pancreas (**FIGURE 28-1** and **BOX 28-1**). The genitourinary system also can produce abdominal pain and bleeding.

Assessment of the Patient With Acute Abdominal Pain

When caring for a patient with abdominal pain, the paramedic should begin the primary survey by ensuring that the scene is safe. The paramedic should then determine whether the patient's abdominal pain is a result of trauma or a medical condition. This distinction may be evident from the initial scene survey. The nature of the pain also may become evident through information obtained from the patient, family, or bystanders. The paramedic should inspect the nearby area for medication bottles and signs of alcohol or other drug use, as they may offer clues to the cause of the patient's condition. If alcohol or other drug use is suspected, it is important to relay this information to the receiving hospital staff.

SHOW ME THE EVIDENCE

Kennedy and colleagues studied the protocols of medical priority dispatch systems to evaluate the protocols' ability to predict patients who needed advanced life support (ALS) skills. Their study included patients with a chief complaint of abdominal pain who were transported to selected study hospitals. Of the 343 patients with a complaint of abdominal pain, 67% met the criteria to be included in the study. In total, 84% of these patients were found not to meet ALS criteria. The researchers concluded that significant overtriage of patients with abdominal pain occurs.

Modified from: Kennedy JD, Sweeney TA, Roberts D, O'Connor RE. Effectiveness of a medical priority dispatch protocol for abdominal pain. *Prehosp Emerg Care.* 2003;7:89-93.

After addressing life threats identified in the primary survey, assessment of the patient with acute abdominal pain begins with a thorough history focused on the chief complaint. The paramedic should assess and document baseline vital signs and perform a systematic physical examination. This examination helps the paramedic identify abdominal emergencies, including those indicating the development of shock or the need for immediate transport for surgical intervention.

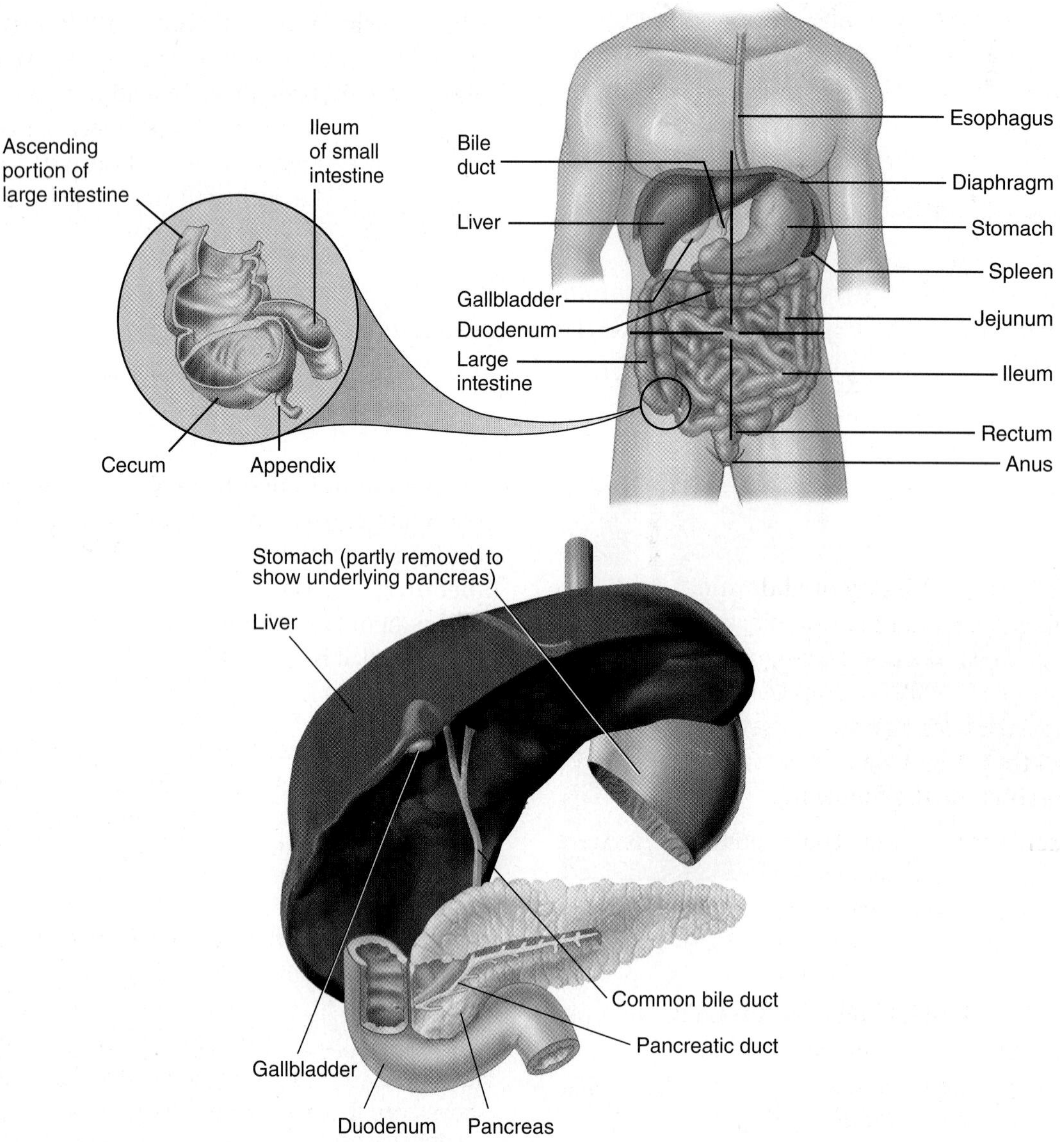

FIGURE 28-1 Location of the gastrointestinal system organs.

BOX 28-1 Organs of the Gastrointestinal System

- **Esophagus.** The muscular canal extending from the pharynx to the stomach.
- **Stomach.** The major organ of digestion, located mostly in the left upper quadrant of the abdomen.
- **Small intestine.** The largest portion of the digestive tract. It is divided into the duodenum, jejunum, and ileum.
- **Large intestine.** The portion of the digestive tract comprising the ascending, transverse, and descending colons; cecum, appendix, and rectum.
- **Liver.** The largest and most complex gland of the body. It is located in the upper right quadrant of the abdomen. It produces and secretes bile, stores glucose as glycogen, synthesizes proteins and fats, stores vitamins, processes hemoglobin, filters harmful substances from the blood, metabolizes drugs, and converts poisonous ammonia to urea.
- **Gallbladder.** A pear-shaped excretory sac on the visceral surface of the right lobe of the liver, which serves as a reservoir for bile.
- **Pancreas.** A fish-shaped, nodular gland located across the posterior abdominal wall in the epigastric region of the body. It secretes various substances, including digestive enzymes and the hormones insulin and glucagon.

NOTE

Abdominal surgery may be necessary for the treatment of many conditions, including inflammatory bowel disease [IBD]; (Crohn disease or ulcerative colitis), diverticulitis, small bowel obstruction, or malignant diseases, such as colon cancer and rectal cancer. Other common types of abdominal surgery include weight-loss surgery; hernia repair; liver, pancreatic, or stomach cancer surgery; **appendectomy**; **cholecystectomy**; and adhesiolysis (removal of scar tissue). Persistent abdominal pain that lasts several hours or longer warrants an increased suspicion for a serious underlying condition, though it should not be the only criterion for transport.

History

When obtaining a history of abdominal pain, the paramedic should attempt to identify the location and type of pain and any associated signs and symptoms. The mnemonic OPQRST or a similar method can help the paramedic organize this information. Sample questions that might be included in the OPQRST evaluation include the following:

- **Onset.** Was the onset of pain sudden? What were you doing when it started?
- **Provocation/palliation.** What makes the pain better? What makes the pain worse? Does a sitting or lying position affect your discomfort? Does a deep breath increase the pain? Does the pain change after you eat or drink?
- **Quality.** What does the pain feel like? Is it sharp, dull, burning, tearing?
- **Region/radiation.** Where is the pain located? Does it travel (radiate) to another area of the body, or does it stay in the same place?
- **Severity.** Is the pain mild, moderate, or severe? What is the degree of discomfort on a scale of 0 to 10 (with 10 being the worst)?
- **Time.** When did the pain begin? Is it constant or intermittent? If intermittent, how long does the pain episode last?

Other key elements of a patient history can be obtained through a SAMPLE history (Signs and symptoms, Allergies, Medications, Pertinent past medical history, Last oral intake, Events leading up to the illness or injury). Also inquire about any recent illness and past significant medical history. Of particular importance are hypertension or cardiac or respiratory disease that may manifest in abdominal pain, medication use, alcohol or other drug use, the last bowel movement and any significant changes in the patient's bowel habits, and previous abdominal surgeries. Women of childbearing age should be questioned about menstrual periods (including regularity and the date of the last menstrual period) and the possibility of pregnancy.

CRITICAL THINKING

Which factors can influence a patient's perception and description of pain?

Location and Type of Abdominal Pain

To assess a specific disorder, the paramedic can seek to relate the anatomic location of GI organs and structures to the origin of the pain. **TABLE 28-1** lists locations of abdominal pain and possible causes of illness associated with them. The types of abdominal pain that may result from chronic or acute episodes may be classified as visceral, somatic, or referred.

Visceral Pain

Visceral pain (or organ pain) is caused by the stimulation of autonomic nerve fibers that surround an organ. It can also be caused by compression and inflammation of solid organs and by distention or stretching of hollow organs or the ligaments. The patient usually describes the pain as cramping or gas-type pain. It may vary in intensity, increasing to severe and then subsiding. Visceral pain generally is diffuse, so it is difficult to localize. Often the pain is centered at the umbilicus or lower in the midline.

Visceral pain often is associated with other symptoms of autonomic nerve involvement, such as tachycardia, diaphoresis, nausea, or vomiting. Common causes of visceral abdominal pain include early appendicitis, pancreatitis, cholecystitis, and intestinal obstruction (described later in this chapter).

Somatic Pain

Somatic pain is produced by bacterial or chemical irritation of nerve fibers in the peritoneum (peritonitis). Unlike visceral pain, somatic pain usually is constant and localized to a specific area. Patients often describe the pain as sharp or stabbing and generally

TABLE 28-1 Common Conditions That Cause Acute Abdominal Pain

Condition	Usual Pain Characteristics	Possible Associated Findings
Appendicitis	Initially periumbilical or epigastric; colicky; later becomes localized to RLQ, often at the McBurney point	Guarding tenderness; positive iliopsoas and obturator signs; RLQ skin hyperesthesia; anorexia, nausea, or vomiting after onset of pain; low-grade fever; positive Aaron, Rovsing, Markle, and McBurney signs
Peritonitis	Sudden or gradual onset; generalized or localized, dull or severe and unrelenting; guarding; pain on deep inspiration	Shallow respirations; positive Blumberg, Markle, and Ballance signs; reduced or absent bowel sounds; nausea and vomiting; positive obturator and iliopsoas tests
Cholecystitis	Severe, unrelenting RUQ or epigastric pain; may be referred to right subscapular area	RUQ tenderness and rigidity; positive Murphy sign; palpable gallbladder; anorexia; vomiting; fever; possible jaundice
Pancreatitis	Dramatic, sudden, excruciating LUQ, epigastric, or umbilical pain; may be present in one or both flanks; may be referred to left shoulder	Epigastric tenderness; vomiting; fever; shock; positive Grey Turner and Cullen signs (both signs occur 2–3 days after onset)
Salpingitis	Lower quadrant; worse on left	Nausea, vomiting, fever, suprapubic tenderness, rigid abdomen, pain on pelvic examination
Pelvic inflammatory disease	Lower quadrant; increases with activity	Tender adnexa and cervix, cervical discharge, dyspareunia
Diverticulitis	Epigastric, radiating down left side of abdomen, especially after eating; may be referred to back	Flatulence, borborygmus, diarrhea, dysuria, tenderness on palpation
Perforated gastric or duodenal ulcer	Abrupt onset in RUQ; may be referred to shoulders	Abdominal free air and distention with increased resonance over liver; tenderness in epigastrium or RUQ; rigid abdominal wall; rebound tenderness
Intestinal obstruction	Abrupt, severe, spasmodic; referred to epigastrium, umbilicus	Distention, minimal rebound tenderness, vomiting, localized tenderness, visible peristalsis; bowel sounds absent (with paralytic obstruction) or hyperactive high pitched (with mechanical obstruction)
Volvulus	Referred to hypogastrium and umbilicus	Distention, nausea, vomiting, guarding; sigmoid loop volvulus may be palpable
Leaking abdominal aneurysm	Steady throbbing midline over aneurysm; may radiate to back, flank	Nausea, vomiting, abdominal mass, bruit
Biliary stones, colic	Episodic, severe, RUQ, or epigastrium lasting 15 minutes to several hours; may be referred to subscapular area, especially right	RUQ tenderness, soft abdominal wall, anorexia, vomiting, jaundice, subnormal temperature
Renal calculi	Intense; flank, extending to groin and genitals; may be episodic	Hematuria; nausea, vomiting, frequency, urgency
Ectopic pregnancy	Lower quadrant; referred to shoulder; agonizing with rupture	Hypogastric tenderness, symptoms of pregnancy, spotting, irregular menses, soft abdominal wall; ruptured: shock, rigid abdominal wall, distention; positive Kehr and Cullen signs
Ruptured ovarian cyst	Lower quadrant, steady, increases with cough or motion	Vomiting, low-grade fever, anorexia, tenderness on pelvic examination, significant bleeding
Splenic rupture	Intense; LUQ, radiating to left shoulder; may worsen with elevation of foot of bed	Shock, pallor, pleuritic pain, positive Kehr sign

Abbreviations: LUQ, left upper quadrant; RLQ, right lower quadrant; RUQ, right upper quadrant

Modified from: Seidel H, Ball JW, Dains JE, Flynn JA, Solomon BS, Stewart RW. *Mosby's Guide to Physical Examination*. 7th ed. St. Louis, MO: Mosby; 2011.

are hesitant to move about. They may lie on the back or side with the legs flexed to prevent additional pain stemming from stimulation of the peritoneal area. These patients often show **involuntary guarding** of the abdomen during the physical examination and **rebound tenderness** (signs of peritoneal inflammation). Other physical signs in patients with acute abdominal pain are presented in **TABLE 28-2**.[2] Common causes of somatic pain are appendicitis and an inflamed or perforated viscus (ulcer, gallbladder, or small or large intestine).

> NOTE
>
> Ask the patient to take a deep breath as you palpate the right upper quadrant of the abdomen. An inflamed gallbladder descends during inspiration and causes discomfort—a reaction known as the Murphy sign.

Referred Pain

Referred pain is pain in a part of the body considerably removed from the tissues that cause the pain. This type of pain arises when branches of visceral fibers synapse in the spinal cord with the same second-order neurons that receive pain fibers from the skin. When these pain fibers are stimulated intensely, pain sensations spread. The patient experiences the pain in areas distant from the source.

A knowledge of referred pain is important because many visceral ailments cause no symptoms except referred pain (**FIGURE 28-2**). For example, cardiac pain may be referred to the neck and jaw, shoulders, and pectoral muscles and down the arms; biliary pain to the right subscapular area; renal colic to the genitalia and flank area; uterine and rectal pain to the lower back; and a leaking aortic aneurysm to the lower back or buttocks.

TABLE 28-2 Physical Signs in Patients With Acute Abdominal Pain

Sign	Characteristics/Significance
Aaron sign	Pain in chest or epigastrium when the McBurney point is palpated; possible sign of appendicitis
Cullen sign	Periumbilical blue discoloration; may indicate retroperitoneal hemorrhage, pancreatic hemorrhage, or rupture of an AAA
Grey Turner sign	Blue discoloration of the flanks; may indicate retroperitoneal hemorrhage, pancreatic hemorrhage, or AAA rupture
Kehr sign	Severe left shoulder pain; may indicate splenic rupture or rupture of an ectopic pregnancy
Markle sign	Pain when dropping from standing on the toes to the heels with a jarring landing; may indicate localized peritonitis due to acute appendicitis
McBurney sign	Tenderness midway between the anterior–superior iliac spine and the umbilicus; may indicate acute appendicitis
Murphy sign	Cessation of inspiration during examination of the right upper quadrant; may indicate acute cholecystitis
Obturator sign	Pain with flexed right hip rotation; may indicate appendicitis
Psoas (iliopsoas) sign	Pain when raising a straight leg against resistance; may indicate appendicitis, right-side AAA
Rovsing sign	Pain in right lower quadrant of the abdomen when the left lower quadrant is palpated; possible sign of appendicitis

Abbreviation: AAA, abdominal aortic aneurysm

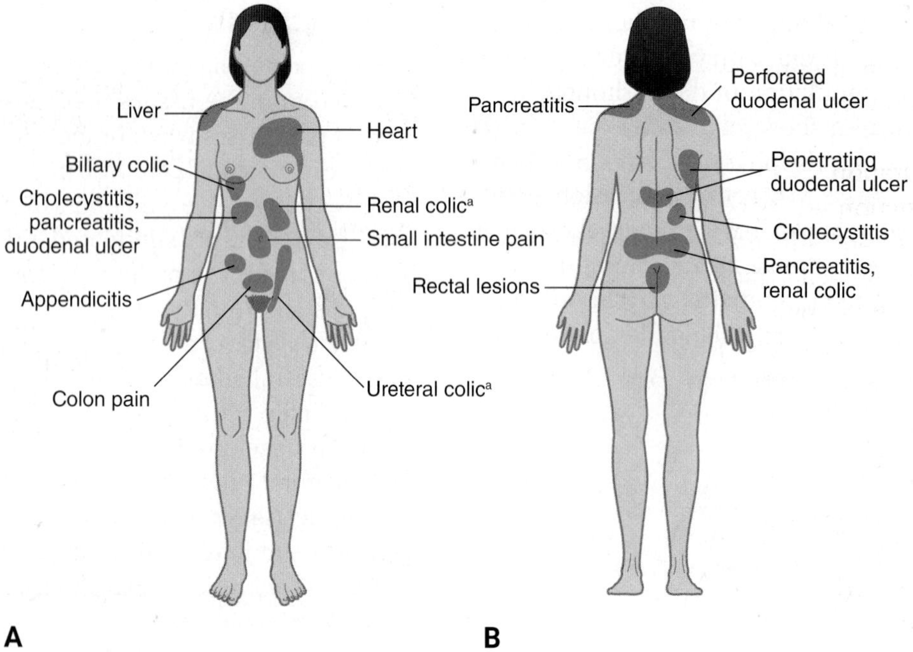

[a]Can occur on either the right or left.

FIGURE 28-2 Referred pain. **A.** Anterior view. **B.** Posterior view.

NOTE

In the past, providing analgesics to manage abdominal pain in the prehospital setting was controversial. Some medical experts believed the drugs might mask serious signs and symptoms. An American College of Emergency Physicians policy document states, "EMS personnel should not withhold narcotic analgesia from patients with abdominal pain because of a misplaced fear of clouding the ultimate diagnosis."

Modified from: American College of Emergency Physicians Board of Directors. Out-of-hospital use of analgesia and sedation. *Ann Emerg Med*. 2016;67(2):305-306.

Signs and Symptoms

Although numerous signs and symptoms may be associated with acute abdominal pain, the following, along with possible causes, are commonly noted:

1. Nausea, vomiting, anorexia
   - Appendicitis
   - Biliary tract disease
   - Gastritis
   - Gastroenteritis
   - High intestinal obstruction
   - Pancreatitis

DID YOU KNOW?

There are several mnemonics that can be used to remember possible, common causes of acute abdominal pain. One such method is BAD-GUT-PAINS.

Bowel obstruction
Appendicitis
Diverticulitis, diabetic ketoacidosis, diarrhea drug withdrawal

Gastroenteritis, gallbladder disease/stones/obstruction/infection
Urinary tract obstruction (stone), infection (pyelonephritis/cystitis)
Testicular torsion, toxins

Pneumonia, pleurisy, pancreatitis, perforated bowel/ulcer
Abdominal aneurysm
INfarcted bowel, infarcted myocardium, incarcerated hernia, IBD
Splenic rupture/infarction, sickle cell crisis

Note: Another mnemonic specific for female patients is ECTOPIC: Ectopic pregnancy, endometriosis; Cystic rupture; Torsion of ovary; Ovulation; Pelvic inflammatory disease; Incomplete abortion; Cystitis.

Modified from: Platt A. A differential diagnosis mnemonics handbook—and the parts of the medical history. Emory University School of Medicine website. https://med.emory.edu/pa/documents/mnemonicdoc.pdf. Accessed February 21, 2018.

2. Diarrhea
   - Inflammatory process (gastroenteritis, ulcerative colitis)
3. Constipation
   - Dehydration
   - Obstruction
   - Medication-induced decreased intestinal motility (codeine, morphine)
4. Change in stool color
   - Biliary tract obstruction (clay-colored stools)
   - Lower intestinal bleeding (black, tarry stools)
   - Infectious diarrhea
5. Chills and fever
   - Appendicitis
   - Bacterial infection
   - Cholecystitis
   - Pyelonephritis

Vital Signs

Vital sign assessment should include evaluation and documentation of the patient's blood pressure, pulse rate (including electrocardiographic assessment), respiratory rate, temperature, and skin condition (color, moisture, temperature, and turgor). The presence or absence of orthostatic pulse and blood pressure changes should be noted if possible. Rising from a recumbent position to a sitting or standing position, with an associated fall in systolic pressure (after 1 minute) of 10 to 15 mm Hg and/or a concurrent rise in the pulse rate (after 1 minute) of 10 to 15 beats/min, indicates significant volume depletion and a decrease in perfusion status. The paramedic also should assess the blood pressure, pulses, and capillary refill in each extremity to evaluate the patient for aortic dissection.

Physical Examination

The physical examination of a patient with acute abdominal pain involves the skills of inspection, auscultation, percussion, and palpation—in that order. If a life-threatening illness is suspected, rapid stabilization and transport of the patient are the first priorities. Further examination can be completed en route to the receiving hospital. The physical examination of a patient's abdomen is described in Chapter 19, *Secondary Assessment and Reassessment.* The following discussion serves as a review. (Female physical examinations to evaluate genitourinary complaints are discussed in Chapter 30, *Gynecology.*)

Inspection

In the initial patient encounter, the paramedic should note the position in which the patient is lying. As stated previously, many patients with abdominal peritoneal irritation lie on the side. The knees often are flexed and pulled in toward the chest. Other visual clues that may indicate abdominal pain are skin color, facial expressions (eg, grimacing), and the presence or absence of voluntary movement. The paramedic should remove the patient's clothing (while ensuring privacy) and inspect the abdominal wall for bruises, scars, ascites (**FIGURE 28-3**), abdominal distention, or abdominal masses.

> NOTE
>
> **Ascites** is an abnormal accumulation of fluid—which contains large amounts of protein and electrolytes—in the peritoneal cavity. It is caused by high pressure in the blood vessels of the liver (portal hypertension) and low albumin levels. Individuals with ascites usually have severe liver disease, but some may have congestive heart failure or pancreatitis.

Auscultation

Determining the presence or absence of bowel sounds by auscultation usually is performed as part of the assessment in the emergency department. However, if auscultation is to be done in the field, the paramedic should auscultate the abdomen as appropriate given the time and noise level of the surroundings to determine whether bowel sounds are absent. Note that it can be difficult to hear these sounds in the

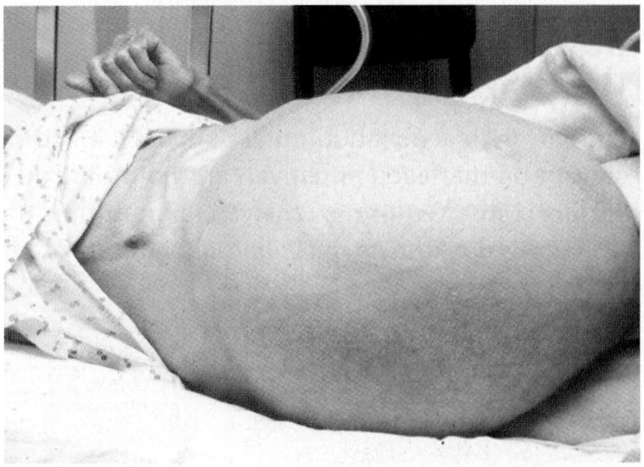

FIGURE 28-3 Gross ascites in a patient.
Courtesy of Leonard V. Crowley, MD

often noisy field or ambulance setting. Auscultation should always precede palpation and percussion, because these procedures may alter the intensity of bowel sounds.

An increase in the number, duration, or intensity of bowel sounds indicates the possibility of gastroenteritis or intestinal obstruction. A considerable decrease in the number and intensity of bowel sounds (or their absence) may indicate peritonitis or ileus (with obstruction of the intestine).

Percussion

If time permits, a general assessment of tympany and dullness by percussion may be performed. This evaluation is intended to detect the presence of fluid, air, or solid masses in the abdomen. The paramedic should use a systematic approach and move from side to side or clockwise. Tenderness and the temperature and color of the abdominal skin should be noted. Tympany is the major sound that should be noted during percussion because of the normal presence of air in the stomach and intestines; dullness should be heard over organs and solid masses.

Palpation

The paramedic should begin palpation of the abdomen gently and avoid the painful area until the remainder of the abdomen has been examined. The paramedic should note signs of rigidity or spasm, tenderness or masses, and the patient's facial expressions, as they may provide clues to the severity of the pain. In addition, the paramedic should identify the abdomen as soft or rigid.

Management of the Patient With an Abdominal Emergency

Patients with acute abdominal pain or GI bleeding cannot be managed effectively in the prehospital setting. Most require extensive evaluation in the emergency department, including laboratory analysis, radiologic imaging, fluid and medication therapy, and perhaps surgical intervention. The role of the paramedic, therefore, is to support the patient's airway and ventilatory status; to perform and document an initial patient assessment, including a thorough history; to monitor vital signs and cardiac rhythm; to initiate intravenous (IV) therapy for fluid replacement or fluid resuscitation; to administer analgesics and antiemetics per protocol; and to transport the patient for evaluation by a physician (**FIGURE 28-4**).

Specific Abdominal Emergencies

Abdominal emergencies can result from inflammation, infection, and obstruction. Some disorders may be associated with upper GI bleeding—for example, lesions, peptic ulceration, and esophageal varices. Other disorders may be associated with lower GI bleeding—for example, colonic lesions, diverticulosis, and hemorrhoids. Still other disorders, such as pancreatitis and cholecystitis, more often are associated with acute abdominal pain in the absence of bleeding. The specific GI disorders discussed in this chapter include GI bleeding, acute and chronic gastroenteritis, IBD (ulcerative colitis and Crohn disease), diverticulosis, appendicitis, peptic ulcer disease, bowel obstruction, pancreatitis, esophageal varices, hemorrhoids, cholecystitis, acute hepatitis, and hereditary hemochromatosis.[3]

GI Bleeding

GI bleeding is a common clinical problem seen by paramedics, and one that often requires hospitalization. It can range from chronic blood loss to a massive, life-threatening hemorrhage, which may be difficult to control. Although many bleeding episodes resolve spontaneously, evaluation by a physician to identify the bleeding site is crucial to help prevent a recurrence. Bleeding from the GI tract can be classified by site of origin as *upper* or *lower* GI bleeding.

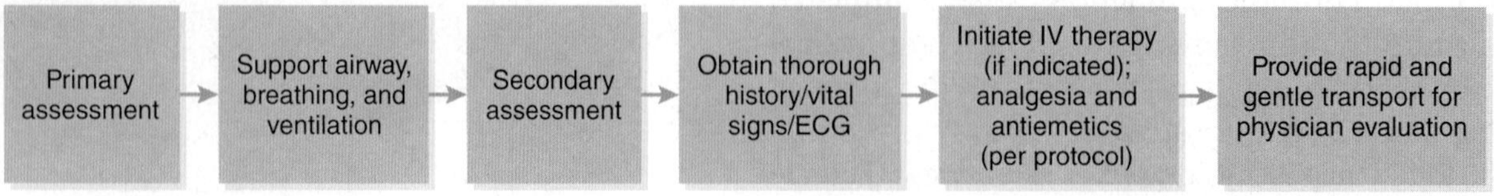

FIGURE 28-4 Abdominal pain algorithm.

The most common causes of upper GI bleeding are gastric or duodenal ulcers and variceal rupture (eg, esophageal varices that result from underlying chronic liver disease, such as cirrhosis).[4] Other causes of upper GI bleeding are esophagitis, gastritis, or **Mallory-Weiss syndrome** (an esophageal laceration that usually results from repeated vomiting or retching). Tumors or cancers of the esophagus or stomach may also cause bleeding. Factors that may aggravate upper GI bleeding include use of nonsteroidal anti-inflammatory drugs (NSAIDs) such as aspirin and other antiarthritic drugs, chronic liver disease, blood-thinning medications (eg, dabigatran [Pradaxa], rivaroxaban [Xarelto], apixaban [Eliquis], warfarin), and underlying medical conditions such as renal disease, hypertension, and cardiorespiratory diseases. Upper GI bleeding accounts for more than 20,000 deaths per year in the United States.[5] Risk factors include advancing age, alcohol and tobacco use, and coexisting illnesses, such as hypertension, diabetes, and cardiorespiratory disease.

The most common cause of lower GI (colon) bleeding is diverticulosis. Other causes include colon cancers, colon polyps, and IBDs, such as ulcerative colitis and Crohn disease. Like upper GI bleeding, lower GI bleeding may be either mild or brisk and difficult to control. Complaints often associated with such bleeding include cramping abdominal pain, diarrhea (which may be bloody), nausea, vomiting, and changes in the patient's stool and bowel habits.

The seriousness of GI bleeding depends on the acuity and the source of the blood loss. Mild chronic GI blood loss may present without any noticeable bleeding but result in an iron-deficiency anemia. Affected patients often are unaware that they are bleeding and may or may not notice small amounts of blood with their bowel movements. Patients with severe cases of chronic or acute bleeding can have signs of anemia, such as weakness, pallor, dizziness, shortness of breath, or angina. Note that the hematocrit level of these patients may be within normal range in the early phase of the hemorrhage.

More serious GI bleeding may be accompanied by **hematemesis** (bloody vomitus). This vomit may be red or may have a dark, coffee ground–like appearance. Blood in the stool could present as bright red, dark and clotted, or black and tarry; the presentation depends on the location of the bleeding source. A black, tarry stool (**melena**) often indicates an upper GI source of bleeding, such that blood has been partially digested. Alternatively, bleeding could originate from the small intestine or right colon. Bright red blood from the rectum (**hematochezia**) after a bowel movement usually signifies a bleeding source close to the rectal opening. Although such bleeding often results from hemorrhoids, conditions such as rectal cancers, polyps, ulcerations, arteriovenous malformations, and infections also can cause this type of bleeding.

GI bleeding that is active or severe usually requires transport of the patient. In the hospital, the patient's hypovolemia can be managed with IV fluids or blood transfusions if needed. To identify and stop the source of hemorrhage, practitioners may use medications, diagnostic tests (eg, barium GI studies, nuclear scans, angiography, endoscopy, and colonoscopy), and other therapeutic measures, such as gastric lavage, placement of a Sengstaken-Blakemore tube (to tamponade bleeding in the esophagus), and, in some cases, surgery.

Prehospital care for patients with active and severe GI bleeding includes airway monitoring and management, provision of emotional support, administration of high-concentration oxygen, measurement of serum lactate (greater than 2 mmol/L is abnormal), blood glucose measurement, and assessment of end-tidal carbon dioxide (less than 25 mm Hg indicates poor perfusion). IV fluid resuscitation should begin with IV fluids (30 mL/kg isotonic fluid; maximum of 1 L) over less than 15 minutes.[6]

NOTE

In the prehospital setting, GI bleeding often cannot be controlled by the paramedic. In some cases hypotension can be protective, because a reduced blood pressure can minimize blood loss. Medical direction may recommend that the patient's systolic blood pressure be maintained between 80 and 90 mm Hg (**permissive hypotension**) until the patient has been delivered to the emergency department for definitive care.

Modified from: Chatrath V, Khetarpal R, Ahuja J. Fluid management in patients with trauma: restrictive versus liberal approach. *J Anaesthesiol Clin Pharmacol.* 2015;31(3):308-316; and National Association of Emergency Medical Technicians. *PHTLS: Prehospital Trauma Life Support.* 8th ed. Burlington, MA: Jones & Bartlett Learning; 2014.

Acute Gastroenteritis

Acute gastroenteritis is inflammation of the stomach and intestines accompanied by the sudden onset of vomiting and diarrhea. As many as 179 million episodes occur yearly in the United States, most of which are transmitted by person-to-person contact.[7] Between 2009 and 2013, 459 deaths from gastroenteritis were reported in the United States.[7] The top three organisms responsible for US outbreaks are norovirus (more than one-half), followed by *Shigella* and *Salmonella.* Acute gastroenteritis may be caused by bacterial or viral infection, parasites (eg, organisms that cause "traveler's diarrhea," *Giardia lamblia* and *Cyclospora cayetanensis,* which are reported to be transmitted through ingestion of contaminated water), chemical toxins, and other conditions such as allergies, lactose intolerance, and immune disorders. The inflammation causes hemorrhage and erosion of the mucosal layers of the GI tract and can alter the way water and nutrients are absorbed.

DID YOU KNOW?

Lactose Intolerance

Lactose intolerance is the inability or insufficient ability to digest lactose, a sugar found in milk and milk products. (Lactose intolerance should not be confused with cow's milk allergy.) Lactose intolerance is caused by a deficiency of the enzyme lactase, which is produced by the cells lining the small intestine. Lactase breaks down lactose into two simpler forms of sugar called glucose and galactose, which then are absorbed into the bloodstream.

People with lactose intolerance may feel uncomfortable 30 minutes to 2 hours after consuming milk and milk products. Symptoms range from mild to severe, based on the amount of lactose consumed and the person's level of tolerance. Common symptoms include abdominal pain and bloating, gas, diarrhea, and nausea. Although the body's ability to produce lactase cannot be changed, the symptoms of lactose intolerance can be managed with dietary changes. The *2015–2020 Dietary Guidelines for Americans* recommend that people with lactose intolerance choose dairy products with lower levels of lactose or products that are lactose-free.

Modified from: US Department of Health and Human Services, US Department of Agriculture. *Dietary Guidelines for Americans: 2015–2020.* 8th ed. Health.gov website. https://health.gov/dietaryguidelines/2015/guidelines/. Published December 2015. Accessed February 21, 2018.

Infectious forms of acute gastroenteritis usually are caused by exposure to norovirus (Norwalk virus) or rotavirus. (The often-used term "stomach flu" for these diseases is a misnomer, as the infections are not caused by influenza viruses.) Children between 6 months and 2 years of age are most vulnerable to rotaviruses,[8] though the incidence of rotoviral infection has decreased markedly since the introduction of vaccines for these pathogens. Adenoviruses and astroviruses cause diarrhea mostly in young children, although older children and adults can be affected as well. Noroviruses infect people of all ages.

Infectious acute gastroenteritis usually is transmitted through the fecal–oral route and by ingestion of infected food or contaminated water. It often arises in institutional settings (eg, long-term care facilities, schools, child care centers, hospitals) and other group settings (eg, banquet halls, cruise ships, dormitories, campgrounds), where it can spread quickly.

Infectious acute gastroenteritis also can arise among travelers in endemic areas (native populations generally are resistant) and in populations in disaster areas where water supplies are contaminated. Bacteria that may be responsible for acute gastroenteritis include *Salmonella* species, *Escherichia coli, Campylobacter* species, and *Staphylococcus* species. Contamination generally results from poor sanitation, a lack of safe drinking water, or contaminated food.

As the name implies, acute gastroenteritis often is abrupt and violent in onset. Patients rapidly lose fluids and electrolytes through constant vomiting and diarrhea. The resulting fluid loss and dehydration may be especially severe in children, older adults, and immunosuppressed people. Hypokalemia, hyponatremia, acidosis (from prolonged diarrhea), or alkalosis (from prolonged vomiting) may develop. Treatment mainly is supportive, consisting of IV fluid replacement, sedation, bed rest, and medications to control vomiting and diarrhea. Bacterial causes of gastroenteritis can be treated with antibiotic therapy.

NOTE

Loss of gastric contents by vomiting results in alkalosis because of loss of hydrochloric acid. Diarrhea results in acidosis because of loss of bicarbonate.

Emergency medical services (EMS) personnel working in disaster areas should observe the following guidelines:

- If ill, avoid patient contact.
- Know the source of water supplies, or drink hot beverages that have been boiled or disinfected.
- Avoid habits that aid fecal–oral or mucous membrane transmission.

- Observe body substance isolation precautions. Also observe good handwashing procedures.
- Disinfect EMS equipment and ambulance surfaces with appropriate cleansers. Alcohol and bleach will not be adequate to destroy some of these pathogens.

CRITICAL THINKING
What would be your main concern for a patient with a history of severe gastroenteritis?

Chronic Gastroenteritis

Chronic gastroenteritis results from inflammation of the stomach and intestines, which can produce long-term changes or damage to the gastric mucosa. This condition usually is due to microbial infection, hyperacidity, or chronic use of alcohol, aspirin, and NSAIDs. Chronic gastroenteritis commonly results from *Helicobacter pylori* infection but also may be caused by infection with other bacteria, such as *E coli, Klebsiella pneumoniae, Enterobacter* species, *Campylobacter jejuni, Vibrio cholerae, Shigella* species, and *Salmonella* species. Many of the bacteria responsible for chronic gastroenteritis are part of the normal intestinal flora, so effective vaccination against these strains is not possible. Other causes of chronic gastroenteritis include Norwalk virus and rotavirus infection and parasitic infection from protozoa such as *G lamblia* and *Cryptosporidium parvum*. The pathogenic agents responsible for the disease may be contracted through fecal–oral transmission and from contaminated food and water. EMS personnel should follow the same guidelines for personal safety as described previously.

Signs and symptoms of chronic gastroenteritis include epigastric pain, nausea and vomiting (which may be severe), fever, anorexia, mucosal bleeding (erosive gastritis), and epigastric tenderness on palpation. In severe cases, patients may be experiencing hypovolemia and shock. The condition is treated with dietary regulation, medications (antibiotics, antacids), and fluid replacement or fluid resuscitation if hypovolemia or dehydration occurs.

Inflammatory Bowel Disease

Inflammatory bowel disease (IBD) is a general term that describes two conditions—ulcerative colitis and Crohn disease—that cause chronic inflammation of the digestive tract. In the United States, IBD affects more than 1 million people.[9] Over time, the inflammation found in both diseases causes permanent damage to the GI tract.

NOTE
The term *irritable bowel syndrome (IBS)* is used to describe abnormally increased motility of the small and large intestines. Unlike IBD, IBS is a syndrome rather than a disease. Another important difference is that IBS does not permanently damage the GI tract, whereas IBD does. The symptoms of IBS include abdominal pain, constipation, and/or diarrhea. The pain generally is temporarily relieved after a bowel movement.

Modified from: Inflammatory bowel disease and irritable bowel syndrome: similarities and differences. Crohn's and Colitis Foundation of America website. http://www.crohnscolitisfoundation.org/assets/pdfs/ibd-and-irritable-bowel.pdf. Published July 2014. Accessed February 21, 2018.

Ulcerative Colitis

Ulcerative colitis is an IBD affecting the large intestine. It is characterized by ulceration of the mucosa of the intestine, usually in the rectum and lower part of the colon but sometimes over the entire colon. The inflammation makes the colon empty often (causing diarrhea). In addition, the ulceration causes bleeding and produces pus. Ulcerative colitis can occur at any age, although it most often starts between ages 15 and 30 years or, less often, between ages 50 and 70 years.[10] The condition affects men and women equally, and a family history of the disease is present in 20% of cases.[10] Approximately 700,000 people in the United States are affected by ulcerative colitis.[10] Although the cause of ulcerative colitis is unknown, the disorder may be related to the way the immune system reacts to a virus or bacterium that causes chronic inflammation in the intestinal wall. Other possible causes include allergies to certain foods (eg, lactose intolerance) and environmental and psychological factors.

The most common signs and symptoms of ulcerative colitis are abdominal pain, fatigue, weight loss, anorexia, and bloody diarrhea with or without mucus.[11] Symptoms may be mild or more severe. Some patients with the disease have remissions that last for months or years, though the symptoms eventually return in most individuals.

After evaluation by a physician and stabilization of the condition, ulcerative colitis usually is managed with steroids, electrolytes, antibiotics, immunotherapy, and dietary regulation. Few patients require surgery, although surgical removal of the diseased colon may be indicated in severe cases. Prehospital care is dictated by the severity of the patient's condition. The care may vary from providing only emotional support and transport for evaluation by a physician, to providing airway, ventilatory, and circulatory support to manage hypovolemia and shock.

NOTE

In patients with acquired immunodeficiency syndrome (AIDS), the chronic diarrhea and diffuse colonic involvement of Kaposi sarcoma (see Chapter 27, *Infectious and Communicable Diseases*) may mimic chronic ulcerative colitis. Undiagnosed signs of human immunodeficiency virus (HIV) infection also may be the cause. In some cases, surgical bowel resection may be required in these patients.

Modified from: Kumar V, Soni P, Garg M, et al. Kaposi sarcoma mimicking acute flare of ulcerative colitis. *J Investig Med High Impact Case Rep*. 2017;5(2):2324709617713510.

Crohn Disease

Crohn disease is a chronic IBD that usually affects the ileum, the colon, or both, but may occur anywhere in the GI tract from the mouth to the anus. Crohn disease may occur in individuals of all ages but is primarily a disease of young adults. (Most cases are diagnosed between ages 15 and 35 years.) The disease is thought to be autoimmune in origin and tends to run in families and in certain ethnic groups. Like ulcerative colitis, Crohn disease affects approximately 700,000 people in the United States.[12]

The inflammation associated with Crohn disease may cause blockage of the intestine: The disease tends to thicken the intestinal wall with swelling and scar tissue, narrowing the passage. It also may cause ulcers that tunnel through the affected area into surrounding tissues, such as the bladder, vagina, or skin. The areas around the anus and rectum often are involved. The tunnels, called fistulae, are a common complication of Crohn disease, but are less common with ulcerative colitis. They often become infected and may require surgery. Other complications associated with Crohn disease include arthritis, skin problems, inflammation of the eyes or mouth, kidney stones, gallstones, and other diseases of the liver and biliary system.

Crohn disease can be difficult to diagnose, because its symptoms are similar to those of ulcerative colitis. Crohn disease is characterized by frequent attacks of diarrhea, severe abdominal pain, nausea, fever, chills, weakness, anorexia, and weight loss. In addition, patients with Crohn disease and similar disorders often develop depression because of the relentless and painful characteristics of these conditions. The paramedic should suspect this disease in any patient with chronic inflammatory colitis and a history of rectal fistulae or abscesses.

Patients with Crohn disease are frequently hospitalized. Once their condition has been stabilized, the disease may be managed with antibiotics, steroids, and antimotility agents in an attempt to induce remission, as well as dietary regulation.

Diverticulosis

A **diverticulum** is a sac or pouch that develops in the wall of the colon (**FIGURE 28-5**). Diverticula are a common development with older age and are associated with diets low in fiber. Diverticular outpouchings (a condition known as **diverticulosis**) tend to develop because of the high pressure in the contracting sigmoid colon that regulates movement of stool into the rectum. The outpouchings are most common at the weakest point in the colon wall—on the left side, just above the rectum. As a diverticulum expands, it develops a thin wall compared to the rest of the colon. Subsequently, bacteria may seep through and cause

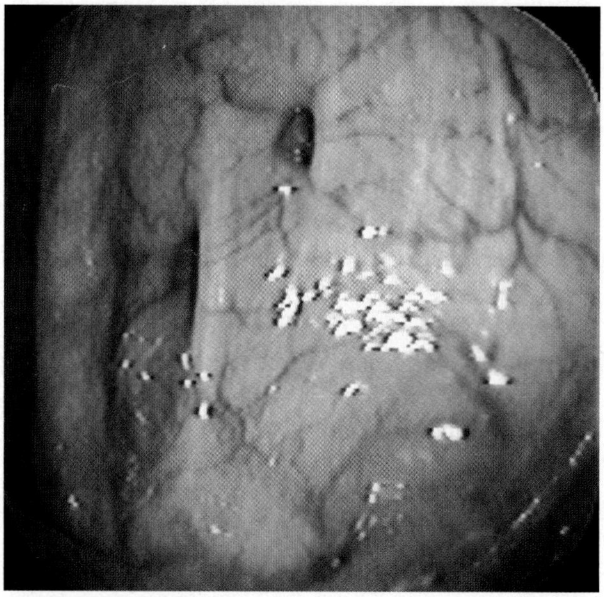

FIGURE 28-5 Diverticular disease. The outpouchings of mucosa in the sigmoid colon appear as slitlike openings from the mucosal surface of the opened bowel.

infection. Often a small artery or arteriole is present in the neck of the diverticulum from which subsequent bleeding may occur.

Most patients with diverticula are completely symptom-free, but as many as 25% experience **diverticulitis** when one or more diverticula become obstructed with fecal matter.[13] Mild complications of diverticulitis include irregular bowel habits (alternating constipation and diarrhea), fever, and lower left quadrant pain. Diverticulitis tends to recur within the first 5 years after the onset of symptoms. Definitive care for these patients includes dietary regulation, a high-fiber diet to stimulate daily bowel movements, antibiotic therapy, and, in some cases, surgical repair.

Serious complications of diverticular disease are associated with lower GI bleeding, inflammation, abscess formation, fistulae, strictures, and perforation of the bowel. These complications include massive bright red rectal bleeding (or dark stools if bleeding is from a diverticulum in the right colon). Hemorrhage from a diverticulum can occur rapidly, is often painless, and is the most common cause of massive rectal bleeding in older adults. If bacteria escape into the abdomen, peritonitis or an abscess may develop. The hemorrhage often stops spontaneously. However, if the bleeding does not stop, emergency surgery may be necessary.

Appendicitis

Appendicitis is a common abdominal emergency, affecting 7% of the US population.[14] Although this condition may present at any age, most patients are 10 to 19 years old.[15]

In some cases, appendicitis occurs when the passageway between the appendix and the cecum becomes obstructed by fecal matter (**fecalith**). Alternatively, it may be due to inflammation of the area caused by a viral or bacterial infection. Obstruction of the passageway leads to distention of the appendix, and poor lymphatic and venous drainage allows bacterial infection to develop. If the condition continues, the inflamed organ eventually develops **gangrene** and ruptures into the peritoneal cavity. The spilling of its contents typically results in peritonitis (which may progress to shock) or the development of abscesses.

Because of variations in the position of the appendix, the patient's age, and the degree of inflammation, the clinical presentation of appendicitis can vary dramatically (BOX 28-2). In addition, many other disorders have similar signs and symptoms. Notably, young children and older adults may have atypical illness because of a reduced inflammatory response associated with extremes of age—which in turn makes appendicitis more difficult to diagnose in these age groups. The classic presentation of appendicitis is abdominal pain or cramping, nausea, vomiting, chills, low-grade fever, flatulence, and anorexia. At first the pain is periumbilical and diffuse. Later it becomes intense and localized to the right lower quadrant just medial to the iliac crest about one-third the distance from the anterior superior iliac spine to the umbilicus (McBurney point). The location of the pain can vary, however, based on the location of the tip of the appendix. If the appendix ruptures, the patient's pain diminishes before peritoneal signs become evident. The goal of definitive care for appendicitis is surgical removal of the appendix (appendectomy) before the organ ruptures.

BOX 28-2 Abdominal Signs of Appendicitis

- **Rebound tenderness.** Exert pressure in the right lower quadrant at McBurney point and then release. Sharp abdominal pain when the pressure is released suggests appendicitis.
- **Iliopsoas muscle test.** With the patient supine, ask the patient to raise the right leg and flex at the hip as you press down on the lower thigh. Lower quadrant pain—that is, a positive psoas sign—may indicate appendicitis.
- **Obturator muscle test.** With the patient supine, flex the right leg at the hip and knee, then rotate the leg laterally and medially. Pain in the hypogastric region may indicate a ruptured appendix.

CRITICAL THINKING

Which other illnesses present with similar signs or symptoms as appendicitis?

Peptic Ulcer Disease

Peptic ulcer disease results from a complex pathologic interaction among the various acidic gastric secretions and proteolytic enzymes and the mucosal barrier in the digestive tract. As part of digestion, the stomach produces hydrochloric acid and an enzyme called pepsin. From the stomach, food passes into the duodenum, where digestion and nutrient absorption continue. The stomach normally protects itself from the corrosive nature of the digestive fluids by producing

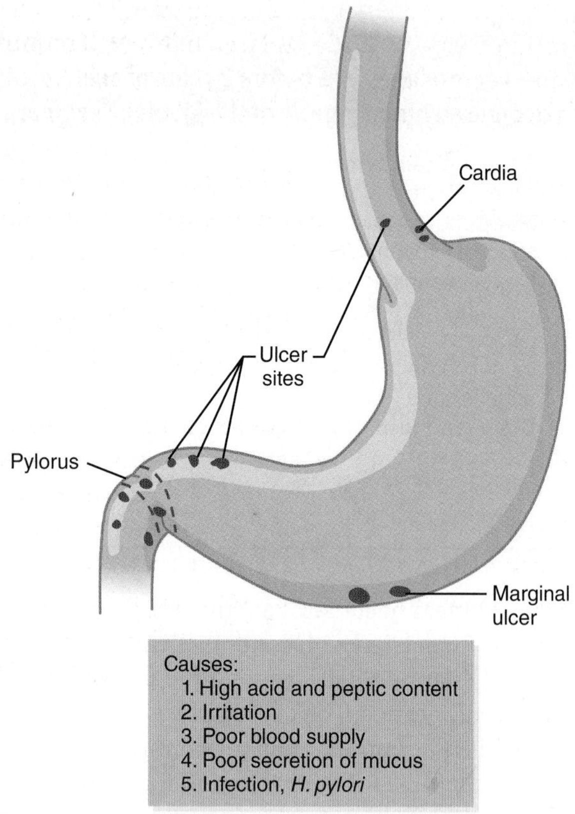

FIGURE 28-6 Peptic ulcer disease.

mucus to shield stomach tissues. Blood circulation to the stomach lining, cell renewal, and cell repair also help protect the stomach (**FIGURE 28-6**).

Ulcers can form in the lining of the stomach or the duodenum, where acid and pepsin are present. These sores cause the disintegration and death of tissue as they erode the mucosal layers in the affected areas. If the sores are left untreated, massive hemorrhage or perforation may result. Ulcers can develop at any age but are rare among teenagers and even more uncommon in children. Duodenal ulcers usually occur for the first time between the ages of 30 and 50 years and are more common in men than in women.

The two main causes of peptic ulcer disease are *H. pylori* infection and the use of NSAIDs. Another, less common cause is increased circulatory gastrin from gastrin-secreting tumors in the duodenum or pancreas (Zollinger-Ellison syndrome).[16]

A patient with a peptic ulcer usually is aware of the condition and may use over-the-counter antacids in an effort to relieve the discomfort. The ulcer pain often is described as a burning or gnawing discomfort in the epigastric region or left upper quadrant (in the case of gastric ulcer). The discomfort develops before meals (classically, in the early morning) or during stressful periods, when the production of gastric acids increases. The pain usually has a sudden onset and is

NOTE

The bacterium *H. pylori* resides between the epithelial surface and the overlying mucosa in the human stomach. It is believed to cause mucosal inflammation, which then disrupts the normal defense mechanism of the stomach and can lead to ulceration. *H. pylori* infection is more prevalent in developing countries with contaminated water and may be spread in adults and children through the fecal–oral route.

DID YOU KNOW?

Gastroesophageal Reflux Disease Versus Peptic Ulcer Disease

Gastroesophageal reflux disease (GERD) is a condition in which food or liquid travels backward from the stomach to the esophagus. This action can irritate the esophagus, causing heartburn and other symptoms. The classic symptoms of GERD are heartburn, regurgitation, or both. If a patient complains of a burning sensation rising from the stomach into the chest or toward the neck, it is most likely due to GERD. **Hiatal hernia**—an anatomic abnormality in which part of the stomach protrudes through the diaphragm and up into the chest—increases the likelihood of GERD. Classically, GERD symptoms (eg, heartburn, regurgitation) may be worsened by consumption of alcohol and certain foods, including fatty foods and foods containing caffeine, garlic, or peppermint. These foods and alcohol can cause relaxation of the lower esophageal sphincter, allowing the refluxate to enter the esophagus from the stomach, causing heartburn or regurgitation.

In contrast, peptic ulcer disease typically is characterized by symptoms such as pain or discomfort localized in the center of the abdomen. The symptoms often improve when a patient either has an empty stomach or consumes enough food to be satisfied and fill the stomach.

Proton pump inhibitors often are recommended to inhibit production of acid in the stomach. These over-the-counter medications include Prevacid, Prilosec, and others.

Modified from: Fass R. Epidemiology and pathophysiology of symptomatic gastroesophageal reflux disease. *Am J Gastroenterol.* 2003;98:S2-S7.

often relieved by eating, taking antacids, or vomiting. In addition to pain and vomiting of blood, the patient may experience melena as a result of blood passing through the GI tract.

Prehospital care for patients with peptic ulcer disease includes obtaining a pertinent history, evaluating for hypotension, and providing circulatory support as needed. After evaluation by a physician, definitive care may involve antibiotics, antacids, histamine-2 receptor antagonists or other medications, and, occasionally, dietary regulation (though its benefits remain controversial). Some patients with acute peptic ulcer disease require hospitalization for fluid or blood replacement or for surgery if medications are not effective or blood loss continues.

Bowel Obstruction

Bowel obstruction is an occlusion of the intestinal lumen that results in blockage of normal flow of intestinal contents. Bowel obstruction may be caused by an **ileus**, a condition in which the bowel does not work properly. More commonly, however, it results from mechanical obstruction, such as adhesions, **hernia** (BOX 28-3), fecal impaction, polyps, and tumors. Other causes of bowel obstruction include **intussusception** (telescoping of one portion of the intestine into another, which occurs mostly in children between 3 months and 3 years of age [75% before 2 years of age], results in decreased blood supply of the involved segment), **volvulus** (twisting of the intestines), ingested foreign bodies, and foreign bodies introduced from the anus (sexual or intentional insertion). Most bowel obstructions occur in the small bowel (accounting for 20% of all hospital admissions for abdominal complaints) and are caused by adhesions or hernias.[17] Large bowel obstructions most often result from tumors or fecal impactions.

Signs and symptoms of intestinal obstruction include nausea and vomiting, abdominal pain, diarrhea, constipation (a late finding), and abdominal distention. The speed of onset and degree of symptoms depend on the anatomic site of obstruction—that is, small versus large bowel. The most significant danger is perforation of the bowel, which may lead to generalized peritonitis and sepsis. An elevated lactate level may signal the onset of sepsis.

BOX 28-3 Hernia

A hernia is the protrusion of an organ from its normal position through a congenital or acquired opening. Herniation most often occurs through the musculature of the groin or abdominal wall. Increases in intra-abdominal pressure—for example, with straining, coughing, or lifting—can cause the peritoneum to push outward through such an opening. When this occurs, a sac forms, into which various organs in the peritoneal cavity may enter.

Most hernias are uncomplicated and can be placed back into the peritoneal cavity by a physician. If the hernia cannot be returned to its proper position, the trapped contents of the peritoneal sac (usually a portion of bowel) can become strangulated. Patients with this condition often have acute abdominal pain and systemic signs, such as fever and tachycardia. Incarcerated or strangulated hernias can lead to serious complications, including intestinal ischemia, intestinal obstruction, perforation, and peritonitis. Definitive care for complicated hernias is in-hospital observation, IV rehydration, pain medication, and surgical repair.

NOTE

Paralytic ileus—a decrease in or the absence of intestinal peristalsis—can closely mimic bowel obstructions. This pseudo-obstruction may result from a number of localized or systemic conditions, such as medications (especially narcotics), intraperitoneal infection, complications of abdominal surgery, and metabolic disturbances (eg, decreased potassium levels).

A patient with bowel obstruction often has abdominal pain; dehydration may result from vomiting, decreased intestinal absorption, and fluid loss into the lumen and interstitium (bowel wall edema). As the affected portion of the bowel distends, its blood supply is decreased and the segment becomes ischemic (BOX 28-4). The wall is weakened and perforates, producing peritonitis. If the intestine becomes strangulated, blood or plasma also may be lost from the affected intestinal segment. Definitive care involves

CRITICAL THINKING

Have you ever responded to a call for "constipation"? Which differential diagnoses did the paramedics consider? What was their attitude toward the patient?

BOX 28-4 Acute Mesenteric Ischemia

Acute mesenteric ischemia is the abrupt interruption of intestinal blood flow. It may result from an embolism, a thrombosis, or a low-flow state (decreased perfusion). The ischemia disrupts the mucosal barrier, allowing the release of bacteria, toxins, and vasoactive mediators. This, in turn, leads to myocardial depression and a systemic inflammatory response. If the condition goes unrecognized and untreated, the ischemia can result in multisystem organ failure and death.

Suspect acute mesenteric ischemia whenever a patient presents with abdominal pain that is out of proportion to the physical findings (especially in patients older than 50 years). Definitive care may include surgery (embolectomy, revascularization, resection), infusion of vasodilators, and long-term therapy with anticoagulation and antiplatelet drugs.

Modified from: Tilsed J, Casamassima A, Kurihara H, et al. ESTES guidelines: acute mesenteric ischaemia. *Eur J Trauma Emerg Surg*. 2016;42:253-270.

fluid replacement, antibiotics, placement of a nasogastric tube for decompression and, frequently, surgery to correct the obstructing lesion.

Pancreatitis

The pancreas, which lies behind the stomach, secretes digestive enzymes into the duodenum to help break down food into small molecules that can then be absorbed by the body. In addition, the pancreas secretes insulin and glucagon into the bloodstream; these hormones help maintain an adequate glucose concentration. When the pancreas becomes inflamed—a condition called **pancreatitis**—this gland releases pancreatic enzymes into the blood, the pancreatic duct, and the pancreas itself. These enzymes cause further inflammation and autodigestion of the gland. Pancreatitis occurs in two stages, acute and chronic.

Acute pancreatitis has a sudden onset, occurring soon after the pancreas becomes damaged or irritated by its own enzymes. It usually results from obstruction by gallstones in the bile duct or from alcohol abuse. Other, less common causes of acute pancreatitis include elevated serum lipids, thromboembolism, drug toxicity, infection, and some surgeries. Acute pancreatitis affects approximately 80,000 Americans each year.[18]

Chronic pancreatitis begins as acute pancreatitis but becomes chronic when the pancreas becomes scarred. Although this condition usually results from long-term and excessive alcohol consumption or from gallstones, it may also develop from other causes of pancreatitis. Chronic pancreatitis can lead to exocrine and endocrine failure and, in rare cases, to pancreatic cancer.

Pancreatitis may cause severe epigastric pain as well as nausea, vomiting, and abdominal tenderness and distention. The abdominal pain usually is described as severe, radiating from the patient's mid-umbilicus to the back and shoulders. In severe cases, patients may develop fever, tachycardia, and signs of generalized sepsis and shock. These patients are hospitalized and treated with IV fluids, pain medication, and placement of a nasogastric tube if they are vomiting.

Esophageal Varices

Esophageal varices are a complex of longitudinal, tortuous veins at the lower end of the esophagus that become enlarged and swollen as a result of a pathologic elevation in portal venous pressures (portal hypertension). These tangles of veins are common in patients with liver disease and often result from portal hypertension caused by cirrhosis of the liver. Obstruction to blood flow in the liver, as a result of the fibrosis in the liver, increases pressure. Obstruction also dilates vessels that drain into the liver, which then leads to dilation of thin-walled veins around the lower esophagus and upper end of the stomach (**FIGURE 28-7**). Approximately one-half of all patients with alcoholic cirrhosis develop these types of esophageal varices. Of those with varices, about one-third will develop bleeding, sometimes resulting in life-threatening hemorrhage.[19] Other causes of esophageal bleeding include **esophagitis** (associated with chronic use of alcohol and NSAIDs), malignancy, and episodes of prolonged, violent vomiting that produce a tear or laceration in the mucosa of the upper esophagus (Mallory-Weiss syndrome).

Clinically, a patient with esophageal bleeding has bright red hematemesis, which is sometimes severe. If bleeding is profuse, melena or even frankly bloody stools may be evident and the patient may manifest

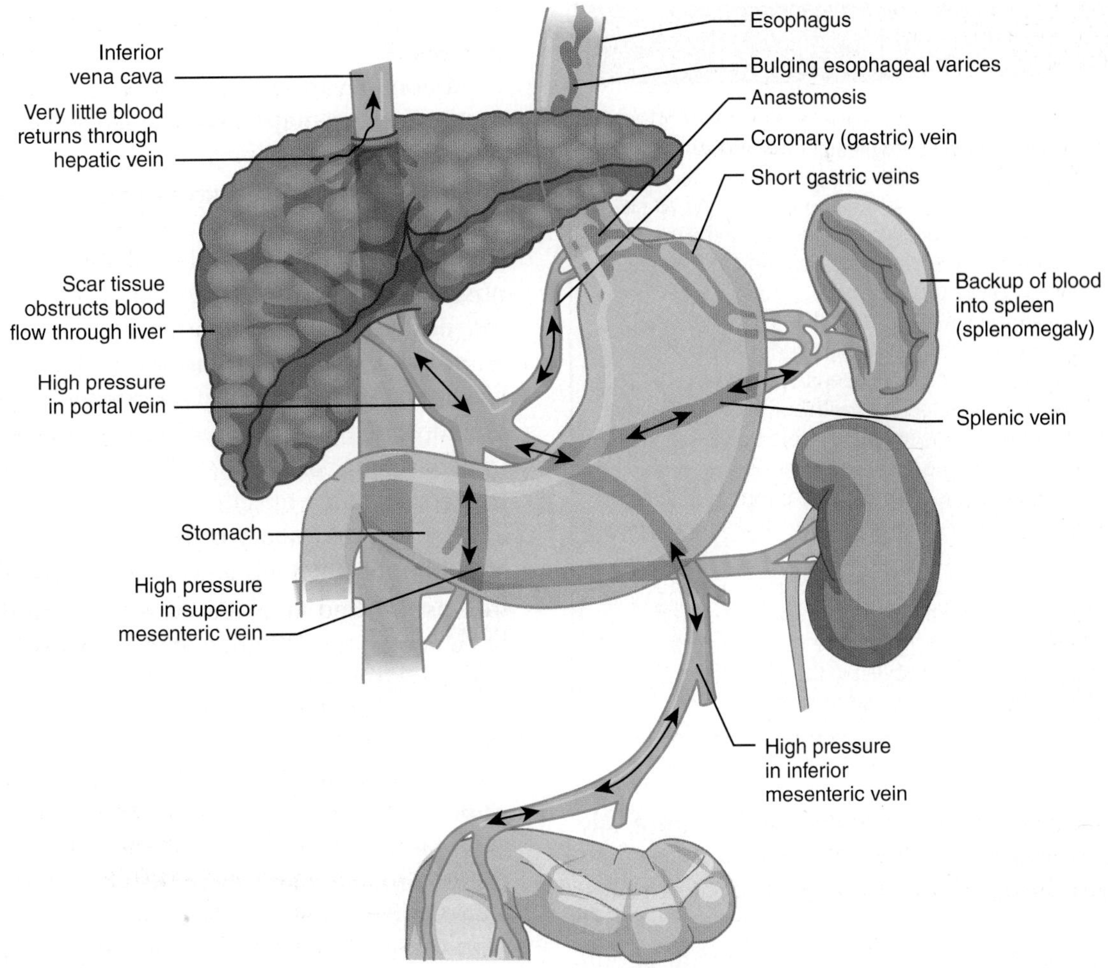

FIGURE 28-7 Development of esophageal varices secondary to liver disease.

the classic signs of shock. Variceal bleeding, which is usually massive and generally difficult to control, has a mortality rate of about 20% to 30%.[19]

Emergency interventions include ensuring a patent airway and fluid resuscitation. The patient should be turned to one side and the bed elevated to a high Fowler position. A hard-tip suction should be available and used to suction the oropharynx if needed. Patients with massive hemorrhage may need intubation for airway control. Blood transfusion is usually needed at the hospital. Definitive care may include strategies to improve blood clotting (vitamin K and fresh frozen plasma), medicine to reduce portal pressure, placement of a Sengstaken-Blakemore tube to tamponade bleeding vessels, and endoscopic ligation of or injection of a sclerosing agent into the bleeding varices.

Hemorrhoids

Hemorrhoids are swollen, distended veins inside the anus (internal) or under the skin around the anus (external). Hemorrhoids are common during pregnancy; in pregnant women, they result from fetal pressure in the abdomen and hormonal changes that cause hemorrhoidal vessels to enlarge. In the general population, hemorrhoids are present in 50% of all people by age 50 years.[20] Irritation of the distended veins is worsened by straining during bowel movements and by rubbing or cleaning around the anus, which

BOX 28-5 Rectal Pain

Pain in the rectal area also may result from a rectal abscess, anal fistula, or foreign body. An **anal abscess**—a pus-filled, infected cavity near the anus—arises when the anal glands just inside the anus become blocked. Treatment consists of surgical drainage of the pus from the infected cavity. An incision also may be made near the anus to relieve pressure.

An **anal fistula** is an abnormal passage between the anal canal or rectum and the skin surface. Most fistulae begin as an abscess that opens spontaneously. This condition also is associated with some diseases, such as tuberculosis, cancer, and irritable bowel disorders. Pain occurs when the fistula becomes blocked, leading to recurrence of an abscess. Symptoms include discharge of pus and fecal material. The fistula requires surgical removal.

Foreign bodies placed in the rectum may result from self-exploration, sexual practices, or abuse. If a foreign body has been inserted in the rectum, no attempt should be made to remove it in the prehospital setting. Treatment by a physician is required.

may produce itching, bleeding, or both. As a rule, hemorrhoidal symptoms subside within a few days.

Pain from hemorrhoids is infrequent unless thrombosis, ulceration, or infection is present. If the patient has rectal pain, the paramedic should consider other possible causes (BOX 28-5). Slight bleeding is the most common symptom; rarely do hemorrhoids cause significant hemorrhage. The bleeding usually occurs during or after defecation, with patients noting blood dripping into the toilet after defecation or blood-streaked toilet paper after wiping. In some cases, however, recurrent episodes of bleeding may be significant enough to produce anemia. Definitive care includes dietary modification, stool softeners, tissue fixation techniques, and operative hemorrhoidectomy for severe cases.

Cholecystitis

Cholecystitis is inflammation of the gallbladder. This disease, which is common in the United States, affects 15% to 20% of the population and is more frequently noted in women 30 to 50 years of age than in men.[21] Risk factors for cholecystitis include female sex, oral contraceptive use, older age, obesity, diabetes mellitus, chronic alcohol ingestion, recent bariatric surgery, and African American, Asian, or Latin American with significant Amerindian heritage ethnicity. The condition may be chronic, with recurrent subacute symptoms, or it may be acute as a result of gallstone obstruction.

In 90% of cases, acute cholecystitis is caused by gallstones (composed mainly of cholesterol) in the gallbladder. On occasion, the gallstones completely obstruct the neck or cystic duct of the gallbladder; this outlet leads to the common bile duct, which empties into the small intestine. As the trapped bile becomes concentrated, it causes irritation and pressure buildup in the gallbladder, which can lead to bacterial infection and perforation. The increased pressure triggers a sudden onset of right upper quadrant or epigastric pain (biliary colic) that lasts more than 4 to 6 hours. The pain usually radiates to the right upper quadrant or right scapula. The patient will likely have fever, guarding, a positive Murphy sign, and an elevated white blood cell count. Associated signs and symptoms include nausea, vomiting that may be bile stained and described as bitter (variable), and pain and tenderness on palpation in the right upper quadrant. Patients with gallbladder disease commonly experience episodes of pain at night, with these episodes typically being associated with recent ingestion of fried or fatty foods. Severe illness, alcohol abuse, and, in rare cases, tumors of the gallbladder also can cause cholecystitis.

Other hallmarks of cholecystitis include previous episodes and a family history of gallbladder disease. Passage of stones into the common bile duct, with subsequent obstruction of this duct, may cause shaking chills, high fever, jaundice, and acute pancreatitis.

Prehospital care for cholecystitis includes vascular access and IV fluids if there are signs of dehydration, administration of an antiemetic if nausea or vomiting is present, and pain management with NSAIDs or narcotics. Treatment may include hospitalization, IV fluid therapy, antibiotics, and placement of a nasogastric tube. Definitive treatment is surgical removal of the gallbladder.

Acute Hepatitis

Hepatitis is inflammation of the liver (see Chapter 27, *Infectious and Communicable Diseases*). It is the single most important cause of liver disease in the United States and worldwide (BOX 28-6).

BOX 28-6 Hepatitis and Liver Disease in the United States

- Approximately 30 million Americans (1 in 10) are or have been affected by some form of liver disease. As many as 50% of these individuals have no symptoms.
- There are six known kinds of viral hepatitis: A, B, C, D, E, and G. Hepatitis B (HBV) and hepatitis C (HCV) have the greatest potential for long-term liver damage. A vaccine is available for the prevention of hepatitis A (HAV) and HBV, but not for HCV.
- Approximately 1.2 million people in the United States have HBV. One in 250 people is a carrier of HBV and can pass it on to others, often unknowingly, through contact with blood or body fluids.
- The HBV virus is 100 times more infectious than is the HIV, the virus that causes AIDS. A teaspoonful of blood holds 500 million hepatitis viral particles, but only 5 to 10 HIV particles.
- More than 4 million people (1.9% of the population) have been exposed to HCV, and most do not know they are infected. The virus is spread through infected human blood and blood products.
- Approximately 15,000 Americans die each year from liver cancer or chronic liver disease associated with viral hepatitis.
- The estimated medical and work loss costs per year from viral hepatitis are greater than $500 million.
- Currently, approximately 16,000 adults and children are on the national waiting list for liver transplants.

Modified from: Liver disease facts. SLUCare Physician Group website. https://www.slucare.edu/gastroenterology-hepatology/liver-center/liver-disease-facts.php. Accessed February 22, 2018; Your liver. American Liver Foundation website. https://www.liverfoundation.org/for-patients/about-the-liver/. Accessed February 22, 2018.

BOX 28-7 Risk Factors for Hepatitis

Hepatitis A (spread by fecal–oral route)

- Health care practice without body substance isolation precautions
- Household or sexual contact with an infected person
- Living in an area with an HAV virus outbreak
- Travel to developing countries
- Engaging in sex with infected partners or multiple partners
- Drug use by injection
- Ingesting contaminated food, typically from an infected food handler

Hepatitis B (spread by infectious blood)

- Health care practice without body substance isolation precautions
- Infant born to mother infected with HBV virus
- Engaging in sex with infected partners or multiple partners
- Drug use by injection
- Receiving hemodialysis

Hepatitis C (spread by infectious blood)

- Health care practice without body substance isolation precautions
- Receiving a blood transfusion before July 1992
- Infant born to mother infected with the HCV virus
- Engaging in sex with infected partners or multiple partners
- Drug use by injection; blood-contaminated straws used to snort drugs
- Receiving hemodialysis

Acute hepatitis is associated with the sudden onset of malaise, weakness, anorexia, intermittent nausea and vomiting, and dull right upper quadrant pain. These signs usually are followed within 1 week by the onset of jaundice, dark urine, or both.

Many viruses can infect the liver. However, the three classes of viruses that are of main concern as causes of acute infectious hepatitis are HAV, HBV, and HCV. All types produce similar pathologic changes in the liver. These viruses also stimulate an antibody response that is specific to the type of virus causing the disease (BOX 28-7). Many hepatitis infections are subclinical (nearly or completely asymptomatic); they often present with influenza-like symptoms. Serious conditions associated with hepatitis are **cirrhosis** (scarring of the liver; **FIGURE 28-8**), **hepatic encephalopathy** (brain and nervous system sequelae that occur as a complication of liver disease), and liver cancer. These conditions are discussed in Chapter 27, *Infectious and Communicable Diseases*, and Chapter 33, *Toxicology*.

The inflammation of hepatitis has many possible causes, including alcohol or other drug use, autoimmune disorders, and toxic bacterial, fungal, parasitic,

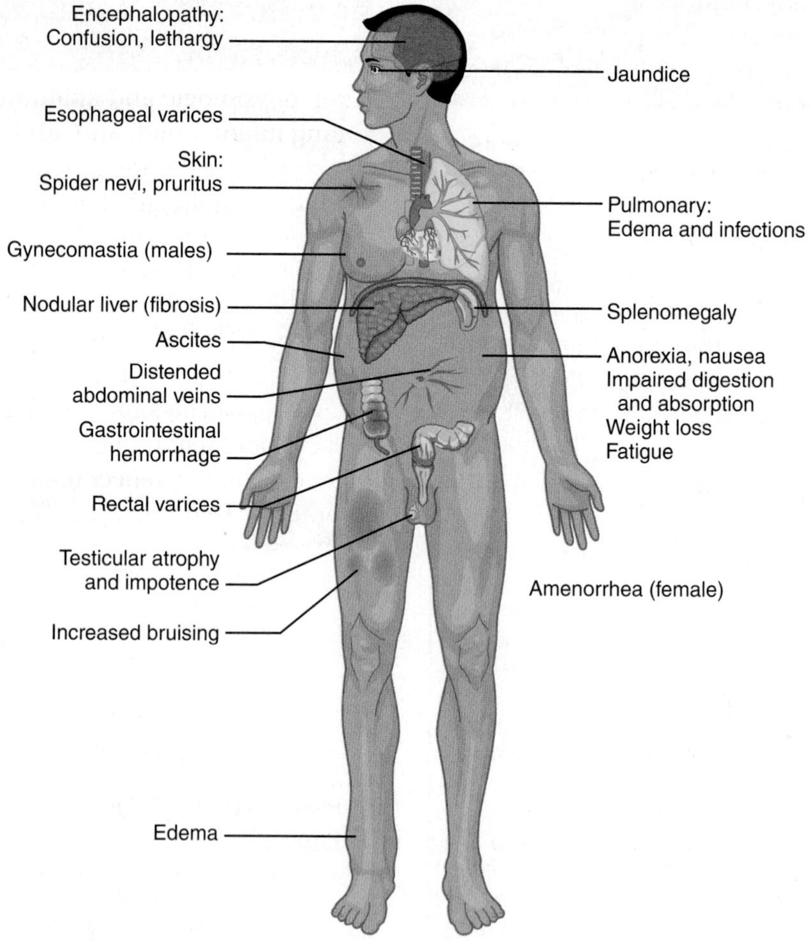

FIGURE 28-8 Effects of advanced cirrhosis.

and viral infections. Patients with hepatitis require a physician's evaluation and care. Proper immunization of paramedics against HAV and HBV is important. In addition, it is crucial that paramedics strictly adhere to body substance isolation procedures when caring for these patients.

Hereditary Hemochromatosis

Hereditary hemochromatosis is one of the most common genetic disorders in the United States.[22] In this inherited condition, the body absorbs and stores too much iron. The extra iron accumulates in several organs, but especially the liver, heart, and pancreas. Many people with hemochromatosis have no symptoms, even in advanced stages. When symptoms do appear, joint pain is the most common complaint. Other common symptoms include fatigue, abdominal pain, decreased libido, and heart problems. Symptoms tend to occur in men between the ages of 30 and 50 years and in women older than 50 years. If the disease is not detected early and treated by ridding the body of excess iron with regular phlebotomy, serious illness (including death) may result. Systemic illness that develops from hemochromatosis includes the following conditions:[23]

- Arthritis
- Liver disease, including an enlarged liver, cirrhosis, cancer, and liver failure
- Damage to the pancreas, possibly causing diabetes mellitus
- Heart abnormalities, such as irregular heart rhythms or congestive heart failure

- Testicular atrophy; impotence
- Early menopause
- Abnormal pigmentation of the skin, making it look gray or bronze
- Pituitary damage
- Damage to the adrenal gland

Life expectancy is normal if the disease is diagnosed before these secondary disorders develop.

To develop hemochromatosis, a person must inherit the defective gene from both parents. Those who inherit the defective gene from only one parent are carriers of the disease but usually do not develop it. Siblings, parents, children, and other close relatives of people who have the disease should consider being tested.[22]

Age-Related Variations in Abdominal Pain

Many physiologic and anatomic differences exist among infant, child, and adult patients. The way in which these groups experience abdominal pain may also be quite different. For example, causes of abdominal pain in the older adult population are more likely to be diseases that require surgical treatment, a vascular catastrophe, ischemic heart disease, or sepsis. Infants and young children are unable to communicate their history or degree of pain; as a result, they can become dehydrated and septic more quickly than adults do. Vital signs in these groups often do not accurately reflect their degree of illness (see Chapter 47, *Pediatrics*, and Chapter 48, *Geriatrics*).[24]

Summary

- The major organs associated with the gastrointestinal (GI) system include the esophagus, stomach, small and large intestines, liver, gallbladder, and pancreas.
- After the scene survey and primary assessment of a patient with abdominal pain, the paramedic should obtain a thorough history. The physical examination may help determine whether the pain is visceral, somatic, or referred.
- The type and location of the pain may help narrow the differential diagnosis.
- Important signs and symptoms associated with abdominal pain include nausea, vomiting, anorexia, diarrhea, constipation, stool color, and fever.
- The most common treatment for abdominal pain is provided at the hospital. The paramedic should provide supportive treatment, manage life threats, and transport the patient to an appropriate facility.
- GI bleeding can be slow and chronic or rapid and life threatening. Causes of GI bleeding include esophageal varices, Mallory-Weiss syndrome, cancer, medication use, and other systemic diseases.
- Gastroenteritis is inflammation of the stomach and intestines caused by infectious agents, chemicals, or other conditions.
- Gastritis is acute or chronic inflammation of the gastric mucosa. It commonly results from hyperacidity, alcohol or other drug ingestion, bile reflux, and *Helicobacter pylori* infection.
- Ulcerative colitis is an inflammatory condition of the large intestine. Colitis is characterized by severe diarrhea and ulceration of the mucosa of the intestine (ulcerative colitis).
- Crohn disease is a chronic inflammatory bowel disease of unknown origin.
- Diverticulosis may result in bright red rectal bleeding if perforation occurs.
- Diverticulitis results when a diverticulum becomes obstructed with fecal matter.
- Appendicitis occurs when the passageway between the appendix and the cecum is obstructed, such as by fecal material, by inflammation caused by infection, or by a swallowed foreign body.
- Peptic ulcer disease occurs when open wounds or sores develop in the stomach or duodenum.
- Bowel obstruction is an occlusion of the intestinal lumen that results in blockage of the normal flow of intestinal contents.
- Inflammation of the pancreas, a condition called pancreatitis, causes severe abdominal pain.
- Esophageal varices arise from increased esophageal venous pressures attributable to obstruction of blood flow to the liver as a result of liver disease. Rupture of the varices can cause hemorrhage and death.
- Hemorrhoids are distended veins in the rectoanal area.
- Cholecystitis is inflammation of the gallbladder. It most often is associated with the presence of gallstones.
- Acute hepatitis is characterized by the sudden onset of malaise, weakness, anorexia, intermittent nausea and vomiting, and dull right upper quadrant pain. These signs usually are followed within 1 week by the onset of jaundice, dark urine, or both.
- Hereditary hemochromatosis is a condition in which the body absorbs and stores too much iron. It can cause severe damage when the iron collects in the liver, heart, and pancreas.
- The way in which infants, children, adults, and older adults experience abdominal pain may be quite different. Vital signs in children and older adults often do not accurately reflect their degree of illness.

References

1. Kendall JL, Moreira ME. Evaluation of the adult with abdominal pain in the emergency department. UpToDate website. https://www.uptodate.com/contents/evaluation-of-the-adult-with-abdominal-pain-in-the-emergency-department. Updated November 6, 2017. Accessed February 22, 2018.
2. Goldman L, Shafer A. *Goldman–Cecil Medicine*. 25th ed. Philadelphia, PA: Elsevier; 2016.
3. National Highway Traffic Safety Administration. *The National EMS Education Standards*. Washington, DC: US Department of Transportation/National Highway Traffic Safety Administration; 2009.
4. Rockey DC. Causes of upper gastrointestinal bleeding in adults. UpToDate website. https://www.uptodate.com/contents/causes-of-upper-gastrointestinal-bleeding-in-adults. Updated January 12, 2016. Accessed February 22, 2018.
5. El-Tawil AM. Trends on gastrointestinal bleeding and mortality: where are we standing? *World J Gastroenterol.* 2012;18(11):1154-1158.
6. National Association of EMS Officials. *National Model EMS Clinical Guidelines*. Version 2.0. National Association of EMS Officials website. https://www.nasemso.org/documents/National-Model-EMS-Clinical-Guidelines-Version2-Sept2017.pdf. Published September 2017. Accessed February 22, 2018.
7. Wikswo ME, Kambhampati A, Shioda K, Walsh KA, Bown A, Hall A. Outbreaks of acute gastroenteritis transmitted by person-to-person contact, environmental contamination, and unknown modes of transmission—United States, 2009–2013. *Morb Mortal Wkly Rep.* 2015;64(SS12):1-16.
8. Matson DO. Acute viral gastroenteritis in children in resource-rich countries: clinical features and diagnosis. UpToDate website. https://www.uptodate.com/contents/acute-viral-gastroenteritis-in-children-in-resource-rich-countries-clinical-features-and-diagnosis. Updated October 24, 2017. Accessed February 22, 2018.
9. National Center for Chronic Disease Prevention and Health Promotion, Centers for Disease Control and Prevention. Inflammatory bowel disease (IBD). Centers for Disease Control and Prevention website. https://www.cdc.gov/ibd/ibd-epidemiology.htm. Updated March 31, 2015. Accessed February 22, 2018.
10. Understanding ulcerative colitis. Crohn's and Colitis website. https://www.crohnsandcolitis.com/ulcerative-colitis. Accessed February 22, 2018.
11. Danese S, Fiocchi C. Ulcerative colitis. *New Engl J Med.* 2011;365(18):1713-1725.
12. Understanding Crohn's disease. Crohn's and Colitis website. https://www.crohnsandcolitis.com/crohns. Accessed February 22, 2018.
13. Weizman AV, Nguyen GC. Diverticular disease: epidemiology and management. *Can J Gastroenterol.* 2011;25(7):385-389.
14. Craig S. Appendicitis. Medscape website. https://emedicine.medscape.com/article/773895-overview#a6. Updated January 19, 2017. Accessed February 22, 2018.
15. Martin RF. Acute appendicitis in adults: clinical manifestations and differential diagnosis. UpToDate website. https://www.uptodate.com/contents/acute-appendicitis-in-adults-clinical-manifestations-and-differential-diagnosis. Updated July 12, 2017. Accessed February 22, 2018.
16. Rosen P, Barkin R. *Emergency Medicine: Concepts and Clinical Practice.* 9th ed. St. Louis, MO: Elsevier; 2018.
17. Ramnarine M. Small-bowel obstruction. Medscape website. https://emedicine.medscape.com/article/774140-overview. Updated April 28, 2017. Accessed February 22, 2017.
18. Pancreatitis. National Institute of Diabetes and Digestive and Kidney Diseases, US Department of Health and Human Services website. https://www.niddk.nih.gov/health-information/digestive-diseases/pancreatitis. Accessed February 22, 2017.
19. Smith M. Emergency: variceal hemorrhage from esophageal varices associated with alcoholic liver disease. *Am J Nurs.* 2010;110(2):32-39.
20. Lohsiriwat V. Hemorrhoids: from basic pathophysiology to clinical management. *World J Gastroenterol.* 2012;18(17):2009-2017.
21. Rakel RE, Rakel D, eds. *Textbook of Family Medicine*. 8th ed. Philadelphia, PA: Elsevier/Saunders; 2011.
22. Hemochromatosis. National Institute of Diabetes and Digestive and Kidney Diseases, US Department of Health and Human Services website. https://www.niddk.nih.gov/health-information/liver-disease/hemochromatosis. Published March 2014. Accessed February 22, 2017.
23. Hemochromatosis. American Liver Foundation website. https://www.liverfoundation.org/for-patients/about-the-liver/diseases-of-the-liver/hemochromatosis/. Accessed February 22, 2017.
24. Kliegman RM, Stanton BMD, St. Geme J, Schor NF. *Nelson Textbook of Pediatrics*. 20th ed. Philadelphia, PA: Elsevier; 2016.

Suggested Readings

Feldman M, Friedman LS, Brandt LJ. *Sleisenger and Fordtran's Gastrointestinal and Liver Disease E-Book: Pathophysiology, Diagnosis, Management*. 10th ed. Philadelphia, PA: Elsevier Health Sciences; 2015.

Locarnini S, Chen D-S, Shibuya K. No more excuses: viral hepatitis can be eliminated. *Lancet*. 2016;387:1703-1704.

Ng SC, Bernstein CN, Vatn MH, et al. Geographical variability and environmental risk factors in inflammatory bowel disease. *Gut.* 2013;62:630-649.

Peery AF, Crockett SD, Barritt AS, et al. Burden of gastrointestinal, liver, and pancreatic diseases in the United States. *Gastroenterology.* 2015;149:1731-1741.

Srinivasan S, Friedman LS. *Essentials of Gastroenterology.* Hoboken, NJ: John Wiley & Sons; 2011.

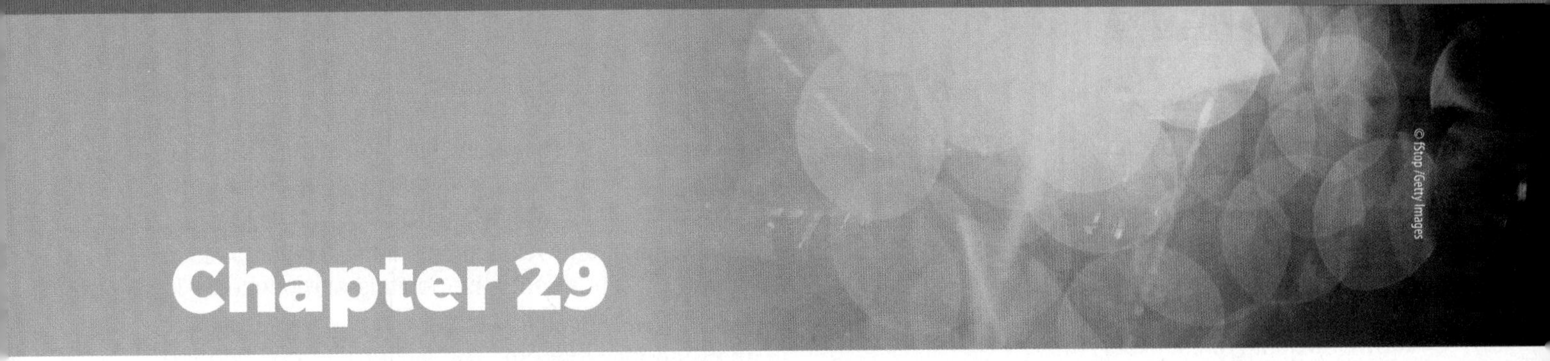

Chapter 29

Genitourinary and Renal Disorders

NATIONAL EMS EDUCATION STANDARD COMPETENCIES

Medicine

Integrates assessment findings with principles of epidemiology and pathophysiology to formulate a field impression and implement a comprehensive treatment/disposition plan for a patient with a medical complaint.

Genitourinary/Renal

- Blood pressure assessment in hemodialysis patients (p 1129)

Anatomy, physiology, pathophysiology, assessment, and management of

- Complications related to
  - Renal dialysis (pp 1126–1131)
  - Urinary catheter management (not insertion) (p 1131)
- Kidney stones (pp 1133–1134)

Anatomy, physiology, epidemiology, pathophysiology, psychosocial impact, presentations, prognosis, and management of

- Complications of
  - Acute renal failure (pp 1121–1125)
  - Chronic renal failure (pp 1125–1126)
  - Dialysis (pp 1126–1131)
- Renal calculi (pp 1133–1134)
- Acid–base disturbances (p 1126)
- Fluid and electrolytes (pp 1126–1127)
- Infection (pp 1131–1132)
- Male genital tract conditions (pp 1134–1140)

OBJECTIVES

Upon completion of this chapter, the paramedic student will be able to:

1. Label a diagram of the urinary system. (p 1121)
2. Distinguish between acute and chronic renal failure. (pp 1121–1126)
3. Outline the pathophysiology of renal failure. (pp 1121–1126)
4. Identify the signs and symptoms of renal failure. (pp 1121–1126)
5. Describe the process of hemodialysis and peritoneal dialysis. (p 1127)
6. Describe the signs and symptoms and care of emergency conditions associated with dialysis. (pp 1126–1131)
7. Describe the pathophysiology, signs and symptoms, assessment, and prehospital management of a patient with urinary retention, urinary tract infection, pyelonephritis, urinary calculus, epididymitis, Fournier gangrene, phimosis, paraphimosis, priapism, benign prostatic hypertrophy, testicular masses, and testicular torsion. (pp 1131–1140)
8. Outline the physical examination of patients with genitourinary disorders. (p 1140)
9. Discuss the general prehospital management of a patient with a genitourinary disorder. (p 1140)

KEY TERMS

acute prostatitis Inflammation of the prostate gland that develops suddenly.

acute kidney injury (AKI) A clinical syndrome that results from a sudden, significant decrease in filtration through the glomeruli, leading to the accumulation of salt, water, and nitrogenous wastes in the body. Also known as acute renal failure.

acute tubular necrosis The death of tubular cells, which form the tubule that transports urine to the ureters.

anuria The inability to urinate; the cessation of urine production; a diminished urinary output of less than 100 to 250 mL/d.

arteriovenous fistula An internal anastomosis between an artery and a vein.

arteriovenous graft A synthetic material grafted between the patient's artery and vein.

autonomic hyperreflexia Overactivity of the autonomic nervous system that causes an abrupt onset of extremely high blood pressure.

azotemia A condition marked by retention of excessive amounts of nitrogenous compounds in the blood.

benign prostatic hypertrophy (BPH) Enlargement of the prostate gland.

chronic kidney disease (CKD) A progressive, irreversible systemic disease, caused by kidney dysfunction, that leads to abnormalities in blood counts and blood chemistry levels. Formerly known as chronic renal failure.

circumcision Surgical removal of the penile foreskin.

creatinine A chemical waste molecule generated by muscle metabolism.

cystitis Inflammation of the urinary bladder and ureters.

dialysate A solution used in dialysis.

dialysis A technique used to normalize blood chemistry in patients with acute or chronic renal failure and to remove blood toxins in some patients who have taken a drug overdose.

disequilibrium syndrome A group of neurologic findings that sometimes occur during or immediately after dialysis. They are thought to result from a disproportionate decrease in the osmolality of the extracellular fluid compared with that of the intracellular compartment in the brain or cerebrospinal fluid.

dysuria Difficult or painful urination.

end-stage renal disease Complete or near-complete failure of the kidneys to function.

epididymitis Inflammation of the epididymis, a tubular section of the male reproductive system that carries sperm from the testicle to the seminal vesicles.

Fournier gangrene A life-threatening bacterial infection of the skin that affects the genitals and perineum in both men and women.

genitourinary system The system comprising the genital and reproductive organs.

hematuria The presence of blood in the urine.

hemodialysis A procedure in which impurities or wastes are removed from the blood. It is used to treat renal insufficiency and various toxic conditions.

hydrocele A fluid-filled sac along the spermatic cord in the scrotum.

intrarenal disease Disease or damage within the kidney.

nephron The functional unit of the kidney.

nocturia Excessive urination at night.

oliguria A condition marked by diminished capacity to form or pass urine.

orchitis Painful inflammation of the testicle.

overflow incontinence A form of urinary incontinence in which urine is released from an overfull urinary bladder. The patient may or may not have the urge to urinate.

paraphimosis A condition in uncircumcised men marked by the inability to pull the retracted foreskin back over the head of the penis.

peritoneal dialysis A dialysis procedure that uses the peritoneum as a diffusible membrane. It is performed to correct an imbalance of fluid or electrolytes in the blood or to remove toxins, drugs, or other wastes normally excreted by the kidney.

phimosis Tightness of the prepuce (foreskin) of the penis that is unable to be retracted off the head of the penis.

postrenal disease Disease that blocks the system that collects urine. It usually is caused by urinary tract obstruction.

prepuce In males, the free fold of skin that covers the glans penis; the foreskin. In females, the external fold of the labia minora that covers the clitoris.

prerenal disease Disease that compromises renal perfusion.

priapism Painful, persistent erection of the penis.

pseudoaneurysm A condition resembling an aneurysm that is caused by enlargement and tortuosity of a vessel.

pyelonephritis Inflammation of the kidney parenchyma caused by microbial infection.

spermatocele A benign cystic accumulation of sperm that arises from the head of the epididymis.

testicular mass An enlargement or growth on one or both testicles.

testicular torsion The twisting of a testicle on its spermatic cord, disrupting its blood supply.

urea A nitrogen-containing waste product.

uremia A condition marked by an excess of urea and other nitrogenous wastes in the blood.

urethritis Inflammation of the urethra.

urinary calculi Solid particles in the urinary system, commonly known as kidney stones.

urinary retention Inability to empty the bladder.

urinary tract infection (UTI) Infection of one or more structures of the urinary tract.

varicocele An abnormal enlargement of the veins that drain the testicle.

Like gastrointestinal disorders, many genitourinary and renal disorders can produce acute abdominal pain and systemic illness. Treatment for these patients frequently begins in the prehospital setting. Successful outcomes often are determined in large part by the assessment skills of the paramedic.

Anatomy and Physiology Review

The genitourinary and renal systems work with other body systems to maintain homeostasis. The **genitourinary system** refers to two different body systems. *Genito* refers to genital organs and the reproductive system. This system is responsible for perpetuation of our species. The genital system is composed of the male and female reproductive organs (**FIGURE 29-1**, **FIGURE 29-2**, and **BOX 29-1**). *Urinary* refers to the system responsible for the removal of metabolic waste products from the blood, the removal of concentrated urine, and the conservation of water.

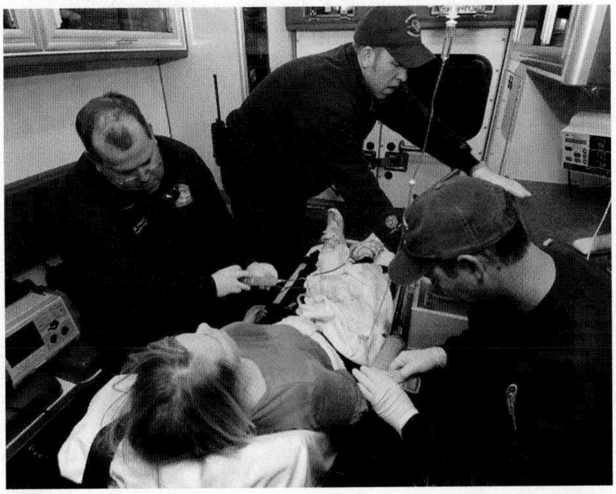

Courtesy Ray Kemp, St. Charles, MO.

This system plays a primary role in the following processes:[1]

- Regulation of water and electrolytes
- Regulation of the acid–base balance
- Excretion of waste products and foreign chemicals
- Regulation of the arterial blood pressure
- Production of red blood cells
- Stimulation of glucose production

BOX 29-1 Reproductive Organs

Male Reproductive Organs

Testes
Epididymis
Ductus deferens
Seminal vesicles
Prostate gland
Bulbourethral glands
Scrotum
Penis

Female Reproductive Organs

Ovaries
Uterine (fallopian) tubes
Uterus
Vagina
External genital organs
Internal reproductive organs
Mammary glands

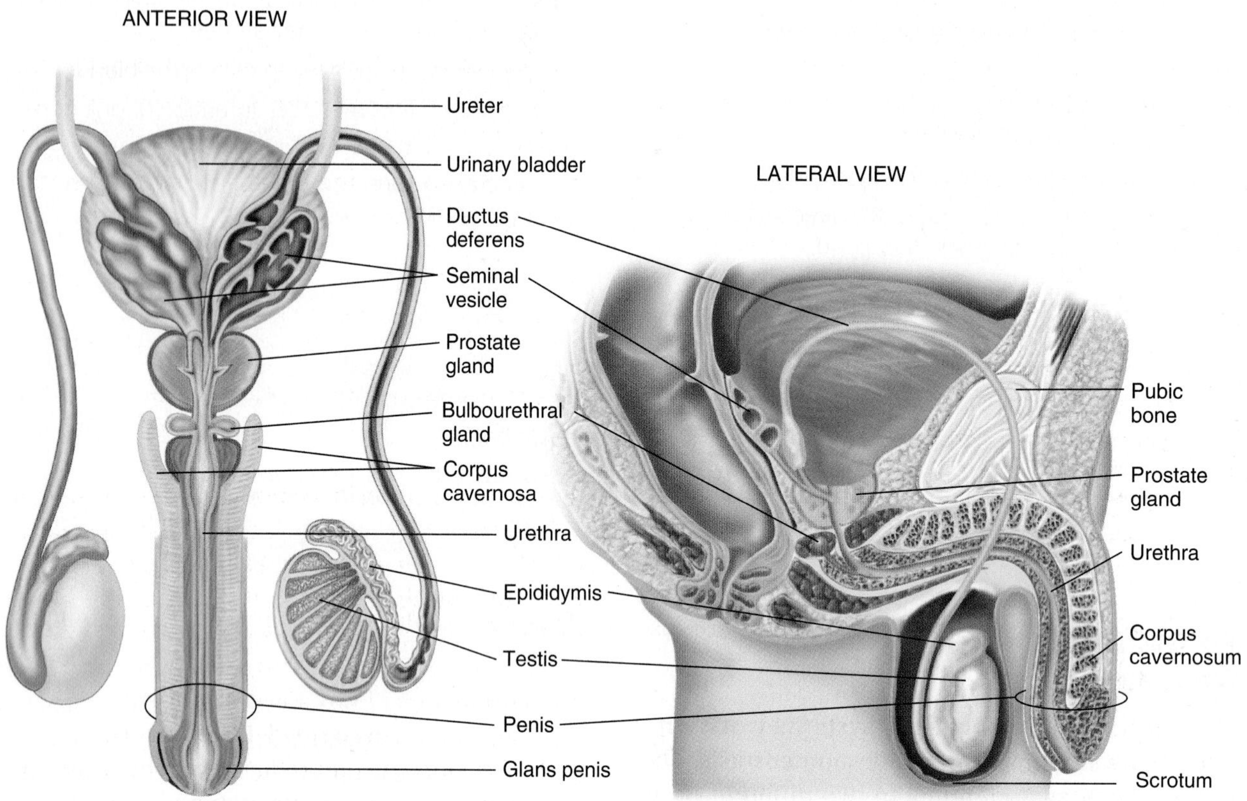

FIGURE 29-1 Male reproductive organs.

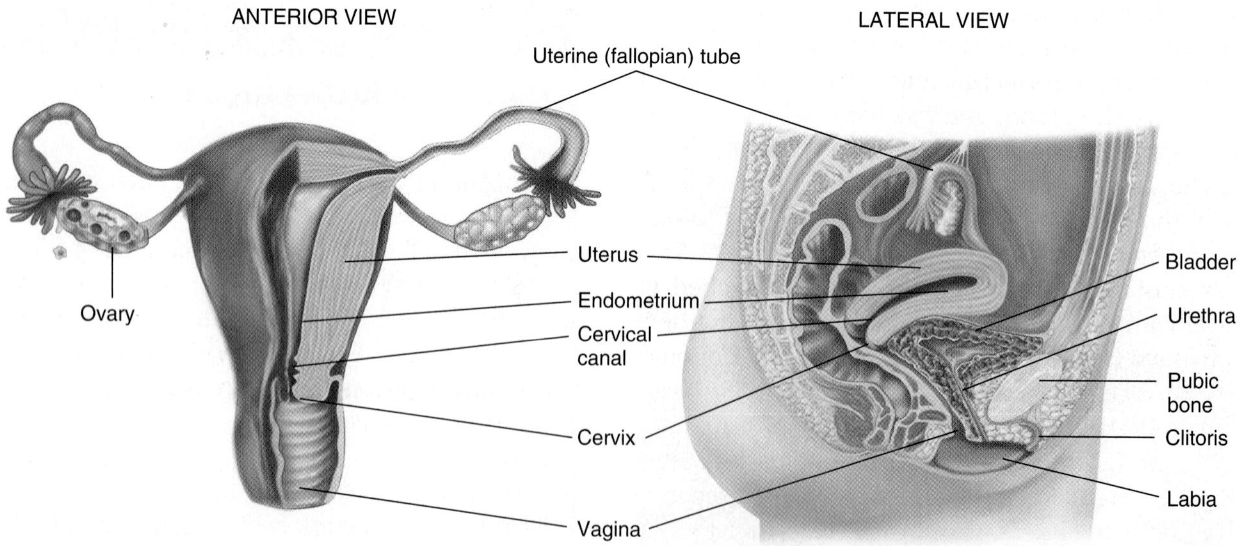

FIGURE 29-2 Female reproductive organs.

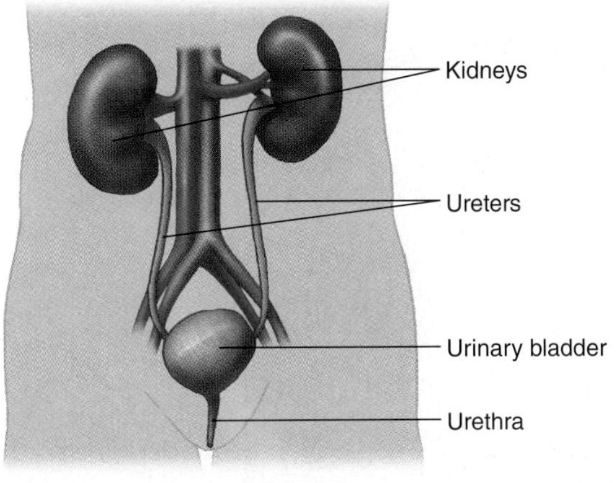

FIGURE 29-3 Components of the urinary system.

The urinary system is made up of two kidneys, two ureters, the urinary bladder, and the urethra (**FIGURE 29-3**). The renal structures are the kidneys and their related structures (**FIGURE 29-4**). This chapter addresses renal diseases, urinary system conditions, and male genital tract conditions. Conditions that affect the female reproductive system are presented in Chapter 30, *Gynecology*.

Renal Diseases

The kidneys are two bean-shaped organs about the size of a person's fist. They lie on the posterior abdominal wall behind the peritoneum. The superior border of the kidney reaches the level of the 12th thoracic vertebra. The inferior border lies just above the horizontal plane of the umbilicus, typically level with the third lumbar vertebra. The inferior border is one finger breadth superior to the iliac crest. The center of the kidney, where the ureter is attached, is level with the intervertebral disk between the first and the second lumbar vertebrae. The superior pole of each kidney is protected by the rib cage. The basic functional unit of the kidney is the **nephron**. Millions of nephrons are inside each kidney. The roles of the nephron are to filter blood, remove waste products, and produce urine. Damage to the nephrons results in renal (kidney) disease.

The causes of renal failure can be classified as prerenal, intrarenal, and postrenal (**TABLE 29-1**). **Prerenal disease** is characterized by inadequate blood flow (perfusion) to the kidneys as a consequence of renal hypoperfusion in relation to events "outside" the kidney. **Intrarenal disease** (intrinsic disease) refers to disease or damage within the kidney. **Postrenal disease** refers to disease that blocks the system that collects urine. All these conditions can result in acute or chronic renal failure (CRF), leading to end-stage renal disease. The classification of disease depends on the duration of renal failure and the potential for reversibility. Assessment findings and symptoms of renal failure are listed in **TABLE 29-2**.

> NOTE
>
> About 14% of Americans have chronic kidney disease (CKD), and more than 600,000 have kidney failure. Of these patients, just under 500,000 are on dialysis, and approximately 190,000 have a transplanted kidney. About one-half of the patients with CKD have diabetes mellitus and cardiovascular disease.
>
> *Modified from*: Kidney disease statistics for the United States. Health Statistics. National Institute of Diabetes and Digestive and Kidney Diseases website. https://www.niddk.nih.gov/health-information/health-statistics/kidney-disease. Published December 2016. Accessed February 11, 2018.

> CRITICAL THINKING
>
> Think about why complications would develop in the patient who has end-stage renal disease.

Acute Kidney Injury

Acute kidney injury (AKI) (also known as acute renal failure [ARF]) is a clinical syndrome that results from a sudden, significant decrease in filtration through the glomeruli. This action leads to the buildup of high levels of uremic toxins in the blood. AKI occurs when the kidneys are unable to excrete the daily load of toxins in the urine. Patients with AKI are divided into two groups, based on the amount of urine excreted in 24 hours. One group is oliguric; these patients excrete less than 500 mL/d. The other group is nonoliguric; these patients excrete greater than 500 mL/d. AKI is a life-threatening condition. The mortality rate for patients hospitalized for the disease is as high as 62%.[2] However, if AKI is recognized early and treated appropriately, it may be reversible. A variety of conditions can cause AKI, such as trauma, shock, infection, urinary obstruction, and multisystem diseases.

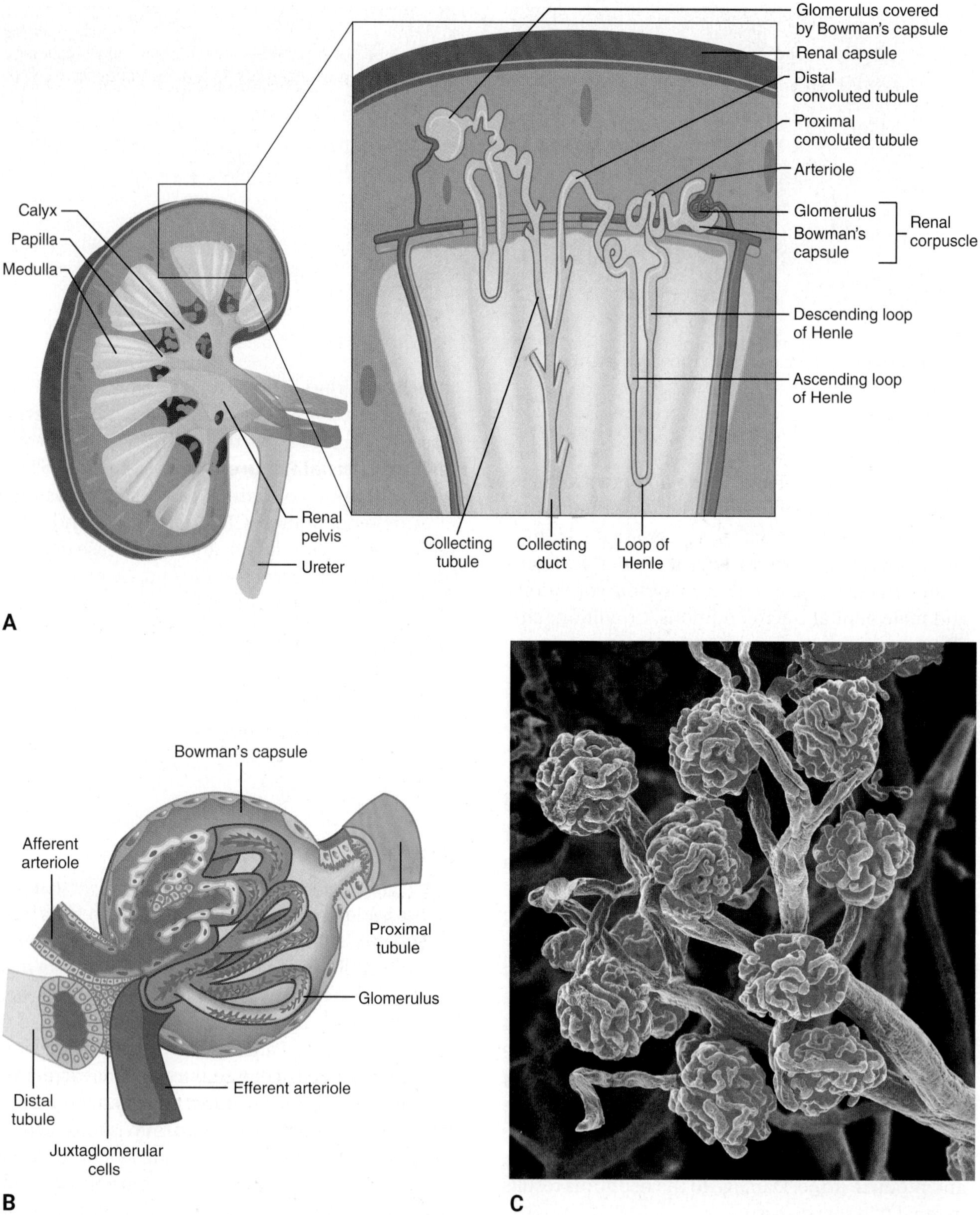

FIGURE 29-4 Location and components of the nephron. **A.** Magnified wedge cut from a renal pyramid. **B.** Schematic showing relationship of glomerulus to the Bowman capsule and adjacent structures. **C.** Scanning electron micrograph showing several glomeruli and their associated blood vessels.

TABLE 29-1 Classification of Acute Renal Failure

Area of Dysfunction	Possible Causes

Prerenal	• Hypovolemia
	  • Hemorrhagic blood loss (trauma, gastrointestinal bleeding, complications of childbirth)
	  • Loss of plasma volume (burns, peritonitis)
	  • Water and electrolyte losses (severe vomiting or diarrhea, intestinal obstruction, uncontrolled diabetes mellitus, inappropriate use of diuretics)
	• Hypotension or hypoperfusion
	• Septic shock
	• Cardiac failure or shock
	• Massive pulmonary embolism
	• Stenosis or clamping of renal artery

Intrarenal	• Acute tubular necrosis (postischemic or nephrotoxic) • Glomerulopathies • Malignant hypertension • Coagulation defects
Postrenal	• Obstructive uropathies (usually bilateral) • Ureteral obstruction (edema, tumors, stones, clots) • Bladder neck obstruction (enlarged prostate)

Modified from: McCance KL, Huether SE. *Pathophysiology: The Biologic Basis for Disease in Adults and Children*. 4th ed. St. Louis, MO: Mosby; 2010.

The onset of AKI can occur within hours. As normal kidney function rapidly deteriorates, urine output frequently decreases (**oliguria**) or stops completely (**anuria**), resulting in **uremia**. Uremia is an excess of **urea** and other nitrogenous wastes in the blood. The condition generally results from kidney malfunction. Uremia may be associated with the following findings (**TABLE 29-3**):

- Generalized edema from water and salt retention
- Acidosis from failure of the kidneys to rid the body of normal acidic products
- High concentrations of nonprotein nitrogens (especially urea) from failure of the body to secrete metabolic end products
- High concentrations of other products of renal excretion (eg, uric acid, potassium)

TABLE 29-2 Assessment Findings and Symptoms of Renal Failure

Acute Renal Failure
• Reduced or no urinary output • Excessive urinary output at night • Lower extremity swelling • Neuropathy of the hands and feet • Anorexia • Altered mental status • Metallic taste in mouth • Tremors or seizures • Easy bruising or prolonged bleeding • Flank pain • Tinnitus • Hypertension • Abdominal pain or discomfort
Chronic Renal Failure
• Headache • Weakness • Anorexia • Vomiting • Increased urination • Rust-colored or brown urine • Increased thirst • Hypertension • Pruritus
End-Stage Renal Disease
• Confusion • Altered level of consciousness • Shortness of breath • Chest pain • Bone pain • Pruritus • Nausea, vomiting, diarrhea • Bruising • Muscle twitching, tremors, seizures • Hallucinations

If uremia is not recognized early and treated appropriately, renal dysfunction leads to the development of heart failure, volume overload, hyperkalemia, and metabolic acidosis.

Prerenal AKI

Prerenal AKI results from inadequate perfusion of the kidneys. The damaged kidneys are unable to rid the blood of waste products, such as urea and **creatinine**. This condition may be caused by

TABLE 29-3 Systemic Effects of Uremia

System	Manifestations	Mechanisms	Treatment
Skeletal	Spontaneous fracture and bone pain, deformities of long bones	Bone inflammation with fibrous degeneration related to hyperparathyroidism, bone resorption associated with vitamin D and calcium deficiency	Control of hyperphosphatemia to reduce hyperparathyroidism; administration of calcium and aluminum hydroxide antacids, together with a phosphate-restricted diet; vitamin D replacement; avoidance of magnesium antacids
Cardiopulmonary	Hypertension, pericarditis with fever, chest pain, ischemic heart disease, pericardial friction rub, pulmonary edema, Kussmaul respirations	Extracellular volume expansion as a cause of hypertension, hypersecretion of renin also associated with hypertension, fluid overload associated with pulmonary edema, acidosis leading to Kussmaul respirations	Volume reduction with diuretics that are not potassium sparing (to avoid hyperkalemia); ACE inhibitors; combination of propranolol, hydralazine, and minoxidil for those patients with high levels of renin; dialysis or successful kidney transplantation
Neurologic	Encephalopathy (fatigue, loss of attention, difficulty problem solving); peripheral neuropathy (pain and burning in the legs and feet, loss of vibration sense and deep tendon reflexes); loss of motor coordination, twitching	Uremic toxins associated with end-stage renal disease, stroke or intracerebral hemorrhage associated with chronic dialysis	Dialysis or successful kidney transplantation
Endocrine	Retarded growth in children, higher incidence of goiter, osteomalacia	Elevated parathyroid hormone levels, decreased growth hormone	Exogenous recombinant human growth hormone; thyroid hormone replacement; same as skeletal above
Hematologic	Anemia, platelet disorders with prolonged bleeding times	Reduced erythropoietin and reduced red cell production, uremic toxins associated with shortened red cell survival and altered platelet function, retention of metabolic acids and waste products	Dialysis; recombinant human erythropoietin (controversial) and iron supplementation; conjugated estrogens; desmopressin; transfusion
Gastrointestinal	Anorexia, nausea, vomiting, mouth ulcers, stomatitis, ruinous breath (uremic fetor), hiccups, peptic ulcers, gastrointestinal bleeding, pancreatitis associated with end-stage renal failure	Retention of urea, metabolic acids, and other metabolic waste products	Protein-restricted diet for relief of nausea and vomiting; Na^+-based alkali or alkali-inducing food
Integumentary	Abnormal pigmentation, pruritus	Retention of urochromes, high plasma calcium levels, neuropathy associated with pruritus	Dialysis with control of serum calcium and phosphate levels
Immunologic	Increased risk of infection that can cause death, increased risk of cancer	Suppression of cell-mediated immunity, reduction in number and function of lymphocytes, diminished phagocytosis	Routine dialysis
Reproductive	Sexual dysfunction: menorrhagia, amenorrhea, decreased testosterone levels, infertility, decreased libido in both sexes	Dysfunction of ovaries and testes, presence of neuropathies	No specific treatment

Abbreviation: ACE, angiotensin-converting enzyme; Na^+, sodium ion

Modified from: McCance KL, Huether SE. *Pathophysiology: The Biologic Basis for Disease in Adults and Children*. 7th ed. St. Louis, MO: Mosby; 2014.

hypovolemia or impaired cardiac output. Obstruction of renal arteries results in decreased blood flow to the kidneys. It also causes an increase in renal vascular resistance that effectively shunts blood away from the kidneys. Many patients with prerenal AKI are critically ill. They may have several preexisting medical conditions, such as atherosclerosis, chronic liver disease, and heart failure. (Dehydration caused by use of diuretics in patients with heart failure is a major cause of prerenal AKI.) In addition, perfusion often is poor in many organs, possibly leading to multiple organ failure.

Signs and symptoms of prerenal AKI include dizziness, dry mouth, thirst, hypotension, tachycardia, and weight loss. The goal of treatment is to improve kidney perfusion and function by treating the underlying condition (eg, infection, heart failure, liver failure). Fluids are administered intravenously to most patients to treat dehydration. With this intervention, urine output generally increases and renal function improves.

Intrarenal AKI

Intrarenal AKI is also known as intrinsic AKI. It results from conditions that damage or injure one or both kidneys. Examples include glomerular and other microvascular diseases, tubular diseases, and interstitial diseases that directly damage the kidney parenchyma. Nearly 90% of cases are caused by ischemia or toxins. Both these causes can lead to **acute tubular necrosis** (death of tubular cells).[3] Nephrotoxic causes of intrarenal ARF occur most often in older adult patients and in those who have CRF. Drugs and other compounds that can trigger intrarenal AKI include antibiotics, nonsteroidal anti-inflammatory drugs, anticancer drugs, radiocontrast dyes, alcohol, and other drugs (eg, cocaine). The condition also is associated with hypertension, autoimmune diseases (eg, systemic lupus erythematosus), and pyelonephritis (described later in this chapter).

Signs and symptoms of intrarenal AKI include fever, flank pain, joint pain, headache, hypertension, confusion, seizure, and oliguria. The goal of treatment is to maintain adequate renal blood flow and address the underlying cause and its complications. In severe cases, renal dialysis (described later in the chapter) or kidney transplantation may be needed to manage the disease.

Postrenal AKI

Postrenal AKI is caused by obstruction to urine flow from both kidneys. This form of renal failure may be caused by ureteral and urethral obstructions (eg, bilateral calculi, prostatic enlargement, urethral strictures). It also can result from obstruction of a urinary catheter. The blockage of urine causes pressure to build in the renal nephrons and ultimately can cause the nephrons to shut down. The degree of renal failure corresponds directly to the degree of obstruction. Signs and symptoms of postrenal AKI include urine retention; a distended bladder; gross **hematuria**; pain in the lower back, abdomen, groin, or genitalia; and peripheral edema. The condition can be reversed by removing the obstruction to urine flow or diverting the flow of urine. Nephrostomy tubes are placed through the patient's back into the kidney and connected to an external urinary collection bag.

Chronic Kidney Failure

Chronic kidney disease (CKD) (formerly known as CRF) is a progressive, irreversible systemic disease. It develops over months to years as internal structures of the kidney are slowly damaged. As renal function steadily declines, CKD leads to **end-stage renal disease**, which eventually requires dialysis or kidney transplantation. CKD may be caused by congenital disorders or prolonged pyelonephritis. However, in the industrialized world, CKD more often results from systemic diseases (eg, diabetes, hypertension) and autoimmune disorders. The kidneys attempt to make up for renal damage by hyperfiltration in the remaining working nephrons. Over time, hyperfiltration causes further nephron damage and loss of kidney function. Chronic loss of function causes generalized wasting and progressive scarring in all parts of the kidney, resulting in a reduction in nephron mass and renal mass.

NOTE

End-stage renal disease affects more than 600,000 people in the United States. More than 89,000 Americans die each year from the disease.

Modified from: End stage renal disease in the United States. National Kidney Foundation website. https://www.kidney.org/news/newsroom/factsheets/End-Stage-Renal-Disease-in-the-US. Updated January 2016. Accessed February 12, 2018.

CKD results in the buildup of fluid and waste products in the body. This buildup causes **azotemia** (the retention of excessive amounts of nitrogenous compounds in the blood) and uremia. Most body systems are affected by CKD. Complications of the disease may include hypertension, heart failure, anemia, electrolyte abnormalities, and other issues. Once CKD has been diagnosed and the cause has been identified, treatments are started to delay or possibly stop the progressive loss of kidney function. In its final stages, CKD often requires treatment with dialysis (hemodialysis or peritoneal dialysis) or kidney transplantation for the patient to survive. In addition to oliguria, a patient with CKD may show the following six systemic manifestations:

1. Gastrointestinal manifestations
   - Anorexia
   - Nausea
   - Vomiting
   - Metallic taste in the mouth
2. Cardiopulmonary manifestations
   - Hypertension
   - Pericarditis
   - Pulmonary edema
   - Peripheral, sacral, and periorbital edema
   - Myocardial ischemia
3. Nervous system manifestations
   - Anxiety
   - Delirium
   - Progressive obtundation
   - Hallucinations
   - Muscle twitching
   - Neuropathies of the hands and feet
   - Tremors or seizures
4. Metabolic or endocrine manifestations
   - Glucose intolerance
   - Electrolyte disturbances
   - Anemia
5. Personality changes
   - Fatigue
   - Mental dullness
   - Confusion
6. Signs of uremia
   - Pasty, yellow skin and thin extremities from protein wasting
   - Uremic frost (**FIGURE 29-5**), caused by the formation of urea crystals on the skin (late finding)

Four treatment options are available for patients who have kidney failure. Three options involve kidney replacement therapy, including kidney transplantation, peritoneal dialysis, and hemodialysis. Supportive care without transplantation or dialysis is the fourth option.[4]

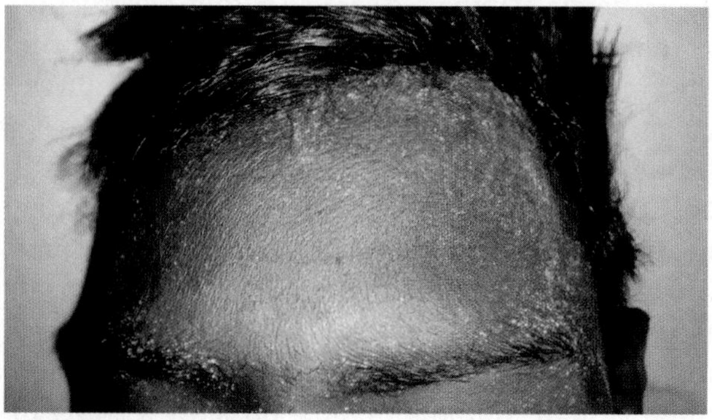

FIGURE 29-5 Uremic frost. Note the fine white powder on the skin of this patient with kidney failure.

Reproduced from: Mathur M, D'Souza A, Malhotra V, Agarwal D, Beniwal P. Uremic frost. *Clin Kidney J.* 2014;7(4):418-419.

Transplantation

For most patients, transplantation can provide the best survival rate and quality of life. A kidney transplant is not appropriate for all patients. Patients must be healthy enough to withstand the surgery, have access to an appropriate kidney donor, and be willing and able to take antirejection drugs. They must also have lifelong routine follow-up. Most transplanted kidneys do not function forever. At 1 year, greater than 90% of living and deceased donor kidneys are likely to be working well. However, 10 years after surgery, approximately 60% of living donor kidneys and just under half of deceased donor kidneys will still be functioning.[5]

Renal Dialysis

Dialysis is a technique used to normalize blood chemistry and remove excess fluid in patients with acute or CRF. Dialysis also removes blood toxins in some patients who have taken a drug overdose. The two types of dialysis are hemodialysis and peritoneal dialysis. Both techniques bring the patient's blood into contact with a semipermeable membrane, across which water-soluble substances diffuse into a dialyzing fluid (**dialysate**). Eventually, electrolytes are balanced between the patient's blood and the dialysis fluid, and waste products are eliminated.

The amount of substance that transfers during dialysis depends on the difference in the concentrations of solutions on the two sides of the semipermeable membrane, the molecular size of the substance, and the length of time the blood and the dialysate remain in contact with the membrane. In patients with end-stage renal disease, hemodialysis usually is performed three times a week. Each session may last 3 to 4 hours.

Hemodialysis

In **hemodialysis**, the patient's heparinized blood is pumped through a surgically constructed **arteriovenous fistula** (an internal anastomosis between an artery and a vein) or an **arteriovenous graft** (a synthetic material grafted between the patient's artery and vein [**FIGURE 29-6**]). These internal shunts usually are located in the inner aspect of the patient's forearm. Less often, they may be located in the upper arm or the medial aspect of the lower extremity (see Chapter 51, *Acute Interventions for Home Care*). Blood is taken from the arm and flows through a dialyzer machine that filters the blood through tiny filaments in a dialysis solution. Waste products diffuse from the blood into the dialysis solution, and the blood is then returned to the body. Hemodialysis must be performed three or more times per week, with each session lasting 3 to 4 hours. It is typically performed at a dialysis center located in an outpatient setting or within a hospital. For convenience, patients are increasingly choosing to undergo home hemodialysis; however, a trained second person generally is required to assist.

Peritoneal Dialysis

In **peritoneal dialysis**, the dialysis membrane is the patient's own peritoneum (**FIGURE 29-7**). Using a temporary or permanently implanted catheter, usually 2 liters of dialysate are infused into the peritoneal cavity over a period of approximately 10 minutes, filling the space around the kidneys, intestines, liver, stomach, and spleen. Fluids move by osmosis, and solutes (creatinine, electrolytes, urea, uric acid) diffuse from the blood in the peritoneal capillaries into the dialysate during the dwell period (the period that the dialysis solution stays in the abdomen). Equilibration occurs after several hours and varies by patient. At this point, the dialysate is drained over a course of approximately 20 minutes.

Two systems are used for peritoneal dialysis. Continuous ambulatory peritoneal dialysis is performed manually and has a dwell time of about 4 hours. Automated peritoneal dialysis uses a machine called a cycler that controls the inflow, dwell, and drainage of the dialysate. This method may perform in a 24-hour cycle or be set to work intermittently at night. Peritoneal dialysis works much more slowly than does hemodialysis. Over time, however, it is just as effective. In addition, peritoneal dialysis does not require chronic blood access.

A major complication of peritoneal dialysis is peritonitis, which is caused by infection. Infection usually results when proper aseptic technique is not used. Signs and symptoms of peritonitis include cloudy drainage; exit-site redness, tenderness, swelling, or pus; abdominal pain; abdominal distention; diarrhea; and in some cases fever. Peritoneal dialysis may be performed regularly in the home by the patient or by the family caregiver.

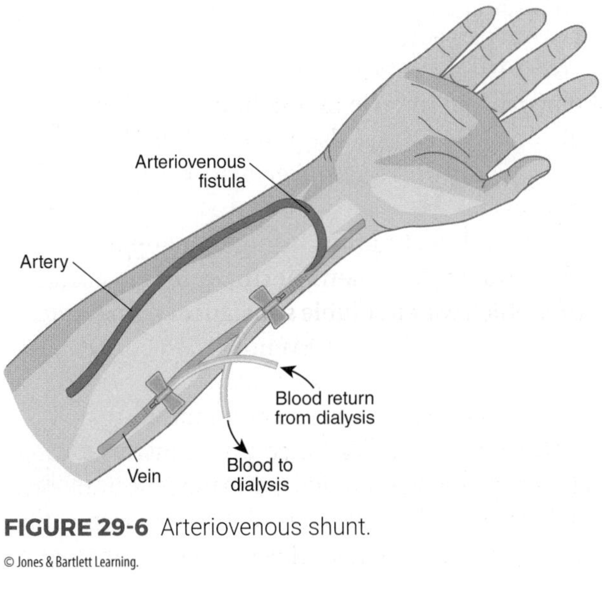

FIGURE 29-6 Arteriovenous shunt.

Dialysis Emergencies

Emergencies the paramedic may encounter when caring for a patient with acute or CRF may result from the disease process itself or from complications of the dialysis. For example, patients may experience problems associated with vascular access, hemorrhage, hypotension, chest pain, severe hyperkalemia, disequilibrium syndrome (described later in the chapter), and the development of an air embolism. In addition, the paramedic should be aware of problems that may result from concurrent medical illness and its treatment. Examples include decreased ability to tolerate the stress of significant illness or trauma, inadvertent overadministration of intravenous (IV) fluid, and altered metabolism and unpredictable action of drugs.

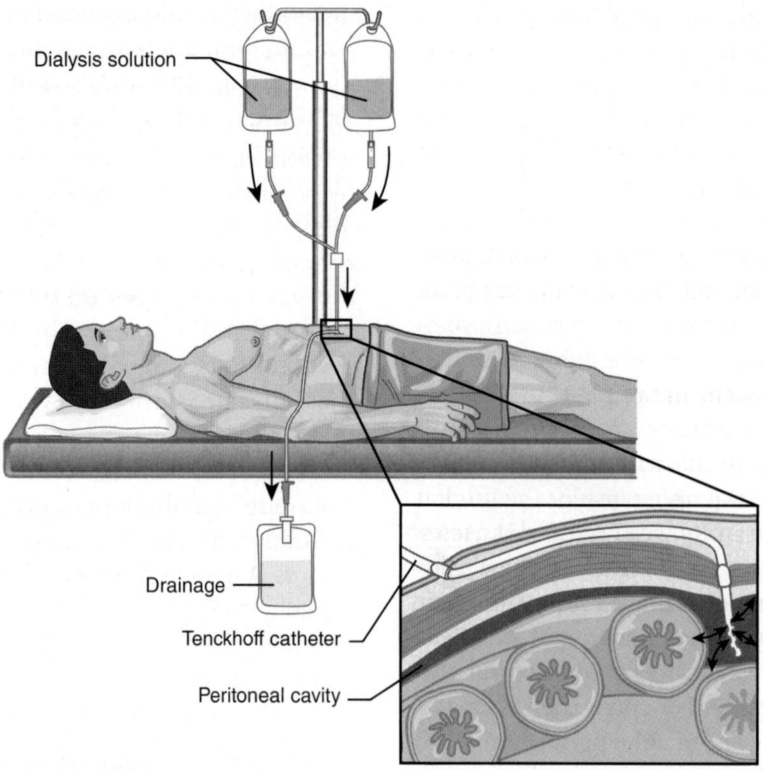

FIGURE 29-7 Peritoneal dialysis.

Vascular Access Problems. Problems associated with vascular access include bleeding at the site of puncture for dialysis, thrombosis, and infection. Bleeding from

NOTE

Renal failure is a cause of pericardial disease, including pericarditis and pericardial effusions. These conditions may result from uremia (uremic pericarditis) and may also occur in patients who are on maintenance dialysis because of inadequate dialysis or fluid overload. The electrocardiographic (ECG) changes typically seen in pericarditis are absent in patients with uremic pericarditis. Most patients with pericardial disease report fever and pleuritic chest pain. The chest pain often is worsened by movement or breathing and may intensify when the patient is lying down. A pericardial friction rub may be audible. Signs of cardiac tamponade may be seen, particularly in patients with rapid accumulation of pericardial fluid.

Modified from: Black RM. Pericarditis in renal failure. UptoDate website. https://www.uptodate.com/contents/pericarditis-in-renal-failure. Updated January 17, 2018. Accessed February 11, 2018; and Singh G, Sabath B. Over-diuresis or cardiac tamponade? An unusual case of acute kidney injury and early closure. *J Community Hosp Intern Med Perspect*. 2016;6(2):31357.

SHOW ME THE EVIDENCE

More than 50% of dialysis patients experience cardiac arrest in the first 5 years of hemodialysis. A study was conducted to describe the outcome of cardiac arrests at hemodialysis centers to which emergency medical services (EMS) responded. The records of 110 patients who had experienced cardiac arrest who had met that criteria between 1990 and 2004 were examined. Of that group, 104 patients experienced an arrest before EMS providers arrived. Four had return of spontaneous circulation before EMS providers arrived after dialysis center personnel used an automatic external defibrillator (AED) to perform defibrillation. Ventricular fibrillation and pulseless ventricular tachycardia were reported in 67% of cases. When an AED was available, it was used in only 53% of arrests.

Modified from: Davis TR, Young BA, Eisenberg MS, Rea TD, Copass MK, Cobb LA. Outcome of cardiac arrests attended by emergency medical services staff at community outpatient dialysis centers. *Kidney Int*. 2008;73(8):933-939.

CRITICAL THINKING

Which of the dialysis complications discussed could pose an immediate threat to life?

the fistula or graft usually is minimal and can often be controlled by direct fingertip pressure over the site. However, excessive pressure can cause thrombosis in the graft or fistula. If severe external hemorrhage from a graft or fistula occurs and cannot be controlled by direct pressure, a tourniquet should be applied. A rare but potential complication of an internal shunt is the development of a **pseudoaneurysm** (a dilation resembling an aneurysm that occurs at the site of the graft). The pseudoaneurysm can rupture and may cause a large hematoma and possible hypovolemia. If this condition occurs, the paramedic should apply direct pressure to the hematoma and assess and treat the patient for significant blood loss. This situation requires immediate transport for care by a physician.

Fistulae and grafts that become occluded as a result of thrombus formation usually require surgical intervention or the administration of a thrombolytic agent to restore flow. Patients with a surgical anastomosis are instructed to check periodically for a bruit or "thrill," which verifies unobstructed circulation. Attempts to clear the graft by irrigation or aspiration generally are not advised. If thrombosis occurs while the patient is undergoing dialysis, the dialysis should be stopped. Fluids then should be given intravenously at an alternate site. Decreased blood flow is a common trigger for thrombosis and is the main reason the blood pressure should not be taken in the arm with a vascular access.

An infection at the site of vascular access usually is the result of the puncture made during dialysis. Therefore, careful sterile technique is the rule when caring for these patients. Routine vascular access using the dialysis route should be discouraged. Vascular access infection should be considered when a dialysis patient has unexplained fever, malaise, or other signs of systemic infection.

NOTE

When drawing blood or infusing IV fluids in a patient with a surgical anastomosis, the paramedic should choose an alternative site. In addition, the paramedic should avoid taking blood pressure measurements and using tourniquets in an extremity with an arteriovenous fistula or graft. The internal shunt is not used to obtain vascular access.

Hemorrhage. Patients undergoing dialysis are at increased risk of hemorrhage. This risk arises from their regular exposure to anticoagulants during hemodialysis and from the decrease in their platelet function. Therefore, a patient who experiences hemorrhage from trauma or a medical condition (eg, gastrointestinal bleeding) should be monitored closely for signs of hypovolemia. Most patients on dialysis have anemia related to a decrease in the production of erythropoietin. This condition lowers their ability to compensate for blood loss when they have acute hemorrhage. Any significant blood loss (whether external or internal) may produce dyspnea or angina.

NOTE

If hemorrhage from trauma occurs in an extremity with a fistula or graft, the paramedic should control the bleeding and immobilize the extremity. Special care must be taken not to obstruct circulation in the anastomosis if at all possible, but if the choice is life versus limb, choose life and apply a tourniquet for uncontrollable hemorrhage.

Hypotension. Hypotension can occur with hemodialysis. It may result from the rapid reduction in intravascular volume, abrupt changes in electrolyte concentrations, or vascular instability that may occur during the procedure. In addition, the patient's mechanisms for coping with these physiologic changes may be impaired, potentially resulting in an inability to maintain normal blood pressure. Patients with hypotension caused by dialysis must be managed cautiously with the administration of volume-expanding fluids. The paramedic should be careful not to produce a fluid overload, which may manifest as hypertension and the classic signs of heart failure (BOX 29-2). Most patients respond to a small fluid challenge (200 to 250 mL).[6] If they do not respond, other potentially serious causes should be considered.

Chest Pain. The episodes of hypotension and mild hypoxemia that often occur during dialysis may result in myocardial ischemia and chest pain. The patient also may report other symptoms associated with decreased oxygen delivery, such as headache and dizziness. These complaints may indicate an evolving myocardial infarction; therefore, a 12-lead ECG should be obtained. The symptoms often are relieved by the administration of oxygen, fluid replacement, and antianginal medications. However, all patients with

BOX 29-2 Classic Signs of Heart Failure

- Crackles
- Engorged neck veins
- Liver congestion and engorgement
- Pitting edema
- Pulmonary edema
- Shortness of breath

chest pain should be treated as though a myocardial infarction has occurred.

Dysrhythmias that result from myocardial ischemia also may be associated with dialysis. The most common ischemic rhythm disturbances are premature ventricular contractions. If dialysis is in progress, the paramedic should stop the procedure and confer with medical direction.

Severe Hyperkalemia. Severe hyperkalemia (potassium >6.5 mmol/L) is an emergency that poses a serious threat to life.[7] It can occur rapidly in patients with AKI. Severe hyperkalemia often results from poor dietary regulation and missed dialysis treatments. Patients with severe hyperkalemia may have weakness, paralysis, paresthesias, impaired deep tendon reflexes, or dyspnea, but often are asymptomatic.[7] Typical ECG changes seen with hyperkalemia initially demonstrate a tall or tented T wave. As the potassium levels rise, conduction slows, resulting in a prolonged PR interval, depressed ST segments, and sometimes the loss of P waves. These patterns may be followed by a widened QRS complex, deep S waves, blended S and T waves, and delayed conduction in the interventricular conducting system. The ECG patterns resemble bundle branch blocks (**FIGURE 29-8**). Hyperkalemic disturbances may not become apparent until dangerous levels of potassium are present. Therefore, any patient with renal failure who is in cardiac arrest should be suspected of having severe hyperkalemia. Based on the patient history, medical direction may recommend separate administration of calcium (to stabilize the myocardial cell membrane) and sodium bicarbonate (to drive potassium from the vascular space into the cell) during resuscitation.[8] Other strategies that may be considered to promote movement of potassium into the cell are high-dose nebulized albuterol to reduce the plasma potassium concentration, and glucose plus insulin to help drive potassium to the intracellular compartment. Treatments to enhance excretion of potassium include administering furosemide or Sodium polystyrene sulfonate (kayexalate; controversial) or performing dialysis.[7]

NOTE

Dialysis patients with CKD tolerate increased potassium levels better than do patients with normal kidney function.

Modified from: Clinical update on hyperkalemia. National Kidney Foundation website. https://www.kidney.org/sites/default/files/02-10-6785_HBE_Hyperkalemia_Bulletin.pdf. Published 2014. Accessed February 12, 2018.

Disequilibrium Syndrome. **Disequilibrium syndrome** refers to a group of neurologic findings that sometimes occur during or immediately after dialysis. These symptoms usually are mild (eg, headache, restlessness, nausea, fatigue), but they may be severe (eg, confusion, seizures, coma). The syndrome is thought to result from a disproportionate decrease in the osmolality of the extracellular fluid compared with

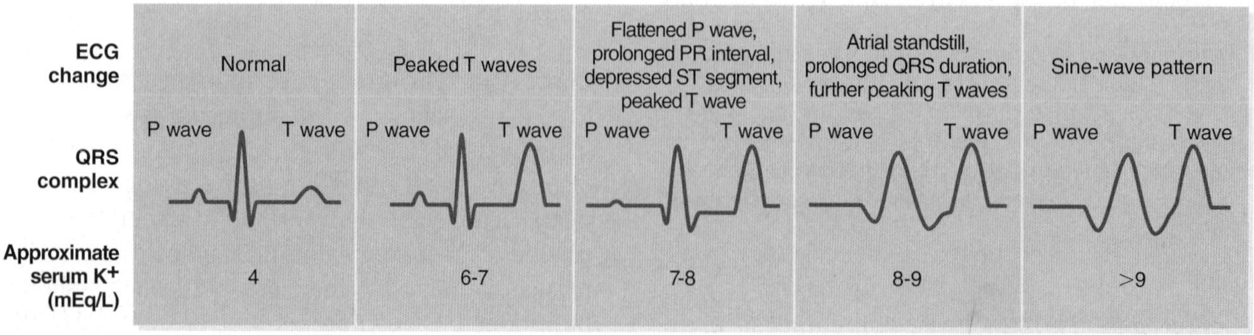

FIGURE 29-8 Electrocardiographic changes seen in hyperkalemia.

that of the intracellular compartment in the brain or cerebrospinal fluid.[9] This results in an osmotic gradient between the blood and the brain, which in turn causes the movement of water into the brain, followed by cerebral edema and increased intracranial pressure. If seizures occur, an anticonvulsant may be indicated.

Air Embolism. Negative pressure on the venous side of the dialysis tubing or a malfunction in the machine can allow an air embolus to enter the patient's bloodstream. This situation is very rare because of safeguards in modern dialysis machines. If air embolism occurs, the embolus may be carried to the right ventricle of the heart where it may block the passage of blood to the left myocardium. The patient may experience severe dyspnea, cyanosis, hypotension, decreased end-tidal carbon dioxide, and respiratory distress. A patient with an air embolus requires high-concentration oxygen, infusion of IV fluid, and rapid transport to a medical facility. To trap the embolus where it will be least likely to obstruct blood flow, the paramedic should position the patient on his or her left side. For transport, the patient should be in the left lateral recumbent position.[8,10]

Management

To review, the prehospital management of patients with chronic or ARF is based on their presenting signs and symptoms and may include the following:

- Airway and ventilatory support with supplemental high-concentration oxygen if hypoxic
- Vascular access for fluid replacement, medication therapy (diuretics, antidysrhythmics, vasopressors), or fluid resuscitation if needed
- ECG and other vital sign monitoring
- Rapid transport to an appropriate medical facility that has access to an emergent hyperbaric chamber

Urinary System Conditions

There are many types of urinary tract diseases, which can range from mild to severe. Urinary system disorders that may cause acute pain include urinary retention, urinary tract infection (cystitis, urethritis), pyelonephritis, and renal calculi. Similar to disorders of the abdomen, urinary system disorders may produce visceral, somatic, and referred pain.

Urinary Retention

Urinary retention is caused by the inability to urinate. Possible causes include urethral stricture, an enlarged prostate (benign or malignant prostatic hypertrophy), central nervous system (CNS) dysfunction, foreign body obstruction, and use of certain drugs, such as parasympatholytic or anticholinergic agents. Urinary retention develops in men more often than in women, most commonly because of an enlarged prostate. However, other common causes can be found in both sexes.

The signs and symptoms of urinary retention include severe abdominal pain associated with an urgent need to urinate and a distended bladder. The distended bladder often is palpable. Patients with a progressive obstruction, such as prostatic hypertrophy, often have a history of urinary hesitancy, a poor urine stream, a sense of incomplete emptying of the bladder, **nocturia** (excessive urination at night), and **overflow incontinence** (an emptying of urine from the bladder often without the urge to urinate). The condition may also cause delirium, especially in older adult patients. In the emergency department, passage of a urethral catheter to empty the bladder often is required. Urinary retention is painful for the patient. Prehospital care for these patients mainly is supportive. If abdominal pain is present, an IV line to keep the vein open may be indicated. If the cause of the retention is not easily correctable after examination by a physician, the patient may require hospitalization. Some EMS systems may permit urinary catheterization in the prehospital setting to empty the patient's bladder (see Chapter 51, *Acute Interventions for Home Care*).

> CRITICAL THINKING
> Have you ever been in a situation in which you needed to urinate urgently but could not because of the circumstances? How did you feel?

Urinary Tract Infection

Urinary tract infection (UTI) accounts for over 10 million visits to physicians' offices each year and 2 to 3 million ED visits.[11] These infections usually develop first in the lower urinary tract (the urethra or bladder). If left untreated, they can progress to the upper urinary tract (the ureters or kidneys). Upper

> **NOTE**
>
> Normal urination is essentially a spinal reflex coordinated by the CNS (brain, brainstem, spinal cord). CNS injury or disease (eg, spinal cord injury or multiple sclerosis) can affect this spinal reflex, resulting in autonomic hyperreflexia (also called autonomic dysreflexia). **Autonomic hyperreflexia** (also known as autonomic dysreflexia) is overstimulation of the autonomic nervous system that results in the abrupt onset of extremely high blood pressure. A common cause of autonomic hyperreflexia in patients with spinal cord injury primarily is urinary retention. Inability to urinate causes overstretching or irritation of the bladder wall. The irritation sends nerve impulses to the spinal cord, in which they travel upward until they are blocked by the area of injury or dysfunction. Because the impulses cannot reach the brain, a reflex is activated that increases the activity of the sympathetic portion of the autonomic nervous system. This activation results in vasoconstriction, causing a rise in the blood pressure. In rare cases, autonomic hyperreflexia can be fatal.

tract infections often are associated with kidney infection (pyelonephritis, described later in this chapter) or abscesses that form in the kidney tissue. These conditions can lead to reduced kidney function. If left untreated, severe cases can be fatal.

Common sites of lower UTI include the urethra (**urethritis**) and the bladder (**cystitis**). These infections occur when enteric flora (particularly *Escherichia coli*, normally found in the bowel) enter the opening of the urethra and colonize the urinary tract. They are more common in women because the urethra is short and close to the vagina and rectum. The infection also occurs in men (as a result of urethritis, prostatitis, and cystitis) and children. However, urethritis and prostatitis in young men most often results from venereal disease rather than a true UTI. Other factors that may contribute to a lower UTI include the use of contraceptive devices (women who use a diaphragm are prone to the development of infections more often; condoms with spermicidal foam may cause the growth of *E coli* in the vagina, which may enter the urethra), unsafe sexual practices, the presence of renal stones, bladder catheterization, and a suppressed immune system. In addition, men and women infected with *Chlamydia trachomatis* or *Mycoplasma hominis* can transmit the bacteria to their partner during sexual intercourse. These bacteria then could cause a UTI.

Signs and symptoms of UTI include painful or difficult urination (**dysuria**), urinary frequency, hematuria, cloudy or rust-colored urine (sometimes with an unusual or foul odor), and flank or suprapubic abdominal pain. Often the patient has a history of UTI episodes. In addition, fever, chills, and malaise may be present. The diagnosis is confirmed in the hospital through urinalysis and microscopic examination for blood cells, sediment, and bacteria. UTIs generally are treated with antibiotic therapy.

> **DID YOU KNOW?**
>
> UTI is the second most common infection diagnosed in the acute hospital setting and accounts for almost 5% of all emergency department visits by adults aged 65 years and older each year. A number of factors predispose older patients to UTIs, including the use of urinary catheters and external urine collection devices, urinary and fecal incontinence, prostate disease, and urinary retention. In addition, some neurologic conditions common in older adults (eg, cerebral vascular disease, Alzheimer disease, Parkinson disease) are associated with impaired bladder emptying. The classic presentation of UTI may not be present in older adults, as they are less likely to present with localized genitourinary symptoms. Instead, older adults may exhibit symptoms such as confusion, agitation, unusual behavioral changes, and altered level of consciousness. UTI in the older adult population is often mistaken for the early stages of dementia or Alzheimer disease. The presence of cognitive impairment in the older patient should alert the paramedic to the possibility of UTI.
>
> *Modified from*: Rowe TA, Juthani-Mehta M. Diagnosis and management of urinary tract infection in older adults. *Infect Dis Clin North Am*. 2014;28(1):75-89; Beveridge LA, Davey PG, Phillips G, McMurdo ME. Optimal management of urinary tract infections in older people. *Clin Intervent Aging*. 2011;6:173-180; Rowe TA, Juthani-Mehta M. Urinary tract infection in older adults. *Aging Health*. 2013;9(5); and *Testimony at Department of Housing and Neighborhood Revitalization Oversight Hearing. Submitted by Marcia Bernbaum, People for Fairness Coalition Downtown Washington DC Public Restroom Initiative. February 16, 2017*. People for Fairness Coalition website. http://pffcdc.org/wp-content/uploads/2017/02/Marcia-Bernbaum-PFFC-testimony-for-February-16-2017-Committee-on-Housing-Neighborhood-Revitalization-Oversight-Hearing-.pdf. Accessed February 12, 2018.

Pyelonephritis

Pyelonephritis is inflammation of the kidney parenchyma (upper urinary tract). This inflammation most often occurs as a result of a lower UTI. The disease is associated with bacterial infection, particularly in cases of occasional or persistent backflow (reflux) of infected urine from the bladder into the ureters or kidney pelvis. The bacterial infections may also be carried to one or both kidneys. They may be carried through the bloodstream or lymph glands from the infection that began in the bladder. Pyelonephritis is more common in adult women, but the condition can affect people of any age and either sex. Acute episodes can be severe in older adults and in people who are immunosuppressed.

The onset of signs and symptoms of pyelonephritis usually is abrupt. Patients often mistake the pain of pyelonephritis for low back strain. The condition may be complicated by systemic infection, with signs and symptoms that include fever, chills, flank pain, cloudy or bloody urine, nausea, and vomiting. Left untreated, pyelonephritis can progress to a chronic condition that can last for months or years. It may lead to scarring and possible loss of kidney function. Therapeutic intervention consists primarily of antibiotics, fluid replacement, and sometimes hospitalization.

CRITICAL THINKING

How would you examine the patient for flank pain?

Urinary Calculus

Urinary calculi (kidney stones) are pathologic concretions that originate in the renal pelvis. They are one of the most painful and most common disorders of the urinary tract, affecting 1 in 11 people in the United States.[12] Kidney stones result from supersaturation of the urine with insoluble salts. When the level of insoluble salts or uric acid in the urine is high, the urine lacks citrate (a chemical that normally inhibits the formation of stones). Kidney stones also can form if insufficient water is present in the kidneys to dissolve waste product. Kidney stones are more common in men than in women; they most often occur in men between the ages of 20 and 50 years, and the disease is recurrent. Associated risk factors for this condition include dehydration, CNS disorders (absent sensory/motor impulses from injury or disease), drug use (anesthetics, opiates, psychotropic agents, some herbal medicines), and surgery (postoperative complication).

The chemical composition of the kidney stones depends on the chemical imbalance in the urine. The four most common types of stones are composed of calcium, uric acid, struvite, and cystine. Calcium stones account for about 85% of all kidney stones.[13] They typically occur in patients with metabolic disorders (eg, gout) or

SHOW ME THE EVIDENCE

A randomized controlled study was conducted to evaluate pain management in 130 patients presumed to have kidney stones. One group was treated with IV morphine, another was treated with IV ketorolac, and the third group received both drugs. The group that received the combination of morphine and ketorolac had better pain relief. This group also experienced less nausea and vomiting than did the morphine group.

Modified from: Safdar B, Degutis LC, Landry K, Vedere SR, Moscovitz HC, D'Ononfrio G. Intravenous morphine plus ketorolac is superior to either drug alone for treatment of acute renal colic. *Ann Emerg Med*. 2006;48(2):173-181.

hormonal disorders (eg, hyperparathyroidism). Stones composed of uric acid account for about 10% of kidney stones; their formation is more common in men, and they may have a heritable component. Struvite stones (also known as infection stones) are more common in women and are often linked to chronic bacterial UTI or frequent bladder catheterization. Cystine stones are the least common and result from a rare congenital condition that results in large amounts of cystine (an amino acid) in the urine. These stones are difficult to treat and may require lifelong therapy.

Signs and symptoms of urinary calculus vary according to the location of the stones. Most stones obstruct the ureters at points where they narrow in their passage from the kidneys to the bladder. This condition produces acute, excruciating pain. The pain originates in the flank area and radiates to the right or left lower abdominal quadrant, groin, and testes (in men). Renal or ureteral colic produces severe cyclical pain. The pain occurs as the ureter tries to use forceful contractions to push the stone into the bladder. This pain often has been described as having the same intensity as labor pain. The pain may be accompanied by restlessness, nausea and vomiting, urinary urgency or frequency, diaphoresis, hematuria, dysuria, and elevated blood pressure (because of the pain). In older patients, abdominal aortic aneurysm can present nearly the same as a urinary calculus, and delays in diagnosis can be deadly. When managing these patients, paramedics should have a high index of suspicion and perform a thorough abdominal and vascular examination.

Prehospital care may include IV fluids, transport in a position of comfort, antiemetics, and pain

BOX 29-3 Strategies for Preventing the Recurrence of Renal Calculi

The composition of a kidney stone determines the strategy used to prevent the formation of more stones. Patients may be advised to do the following:

- Increase water consumption.
- Avoid foods containing calcium oxalate (eg, chocolate, beets, rhubarb, okra, spinach, sweet potatoes).
- Eat food with calcium, but avoid calcium supplements.
- Avoid foods that raise uric acid levels (eg, anchovies, sardines).
- Reduce uric acid by eating a low-protein diet.
- Limit salt intake to reduce the level of calcium oxalate in the urine.

management as needed (nitrous oxide, ketorolac, narcotic analgesics). Care by a physician may include analgesics (anesthetics, opiates, psychotropics), fluid replacement, antiemetics, and possibly hospitalization. If the calculus does not pass spontaneously, lithotripsy (high-energy shock waves to break down the stone) or surgical intervention may be required (BOX 29-3).

NOTE

It is not uncommon for "drug seekers" to feign symptoms of kidney stones to obtain narcotics. Most hospitals check the patient's urine for blood before providing narcotics. Hematuria is a very common finding in patients with renal colic. However, a minority of patients may have ureteral stones without hematuria.

CRITICAL THINKING

Have you cared for or known someone who had a urinary calculus? How did that person describe the pain? What was the level of discomfort?

Male Genital Tract Conditions

Paramedics encounter numerous genital tract conditions in the prehospital setting. Some may be related to disease; others may be the result of trauma (traumatic conditions are presented in Chapter 42, *Abdominal Trauma*). Disorders of the male genital tract discussed in this chapter include epididymitis, Fournier gangrene, and various structural conditions (phimosis, priapism, benign prostatic hypertrophy, testicular masses, and testicular torsion). The anatomy of the male genital tract is presented in Chapter 10, *Review of Human Systems.*

Epididymitis

Epididymitis is inflammation of the epididymis, a tubular section of the male reproductive system that carries sperm from the testicle to the seminal vesicles. Epididymitis often is caused by a bacterial infection associated with other structures of the genitourinary tract. Infection tends to occur in sexually active young men. The most common type of epididymitis in young men results from sexually transmitted disease, such as *Chlamydia trachomatis* or *Neisseria gonorrhoeae*. In men older than 35 years who do not practice anal intercourse, urinary tract outflow obstruction from benign prostatic hypertrophy is a more likely cause.[14]

The signs and symptoms of epididymitis include a gradual onset of unilateral scrotal pain that radiates to the spermatic cord. At times, tender swelling of the scrotum and testicle occurs. This swelling produces inflammation of one or both testes (**orchitis**). The patient may have a recent history of UTI, fever, and malaise, and a urethral discharge may be present. After evaluation by a physician, therapeutic intervention includes antibiotics, bed rest, analgesics, and elevation of the scrotum.

Fournier Gangrene

Fournier gangrene is a bacterial infection of the skin that affects the genitals and perineum in both men and women. It is a urologic surgical emergency that results after a wound or an abrasion becomes infected. A combination of microorganisms (eg, staphylococci) and fungi (eg, yeast) causes the infection to spread. It can lead to necrosis of the skin, subcutaneous tissue, and muscle. Fournier gangrene can be fatal if the infection enters the bloodstream, causing sepsis, shock, and organ failure. The disease is much more likely to develop in men. Men aged 60 to 80 years who have predisposing conditions are the most susceptible. Predisposing factors and conditions include alcoholism, IV drug use, genital piercing, obesity, diabetes mellitus, leukemia, and immune system disorders. The condition also can develop as a complication of surgery. Hallmarks of the disease are intense pain and tenderness in the genitalia (**FIGURE 29-9**). Depending on the stage of disease, assessment findings in the genital area may

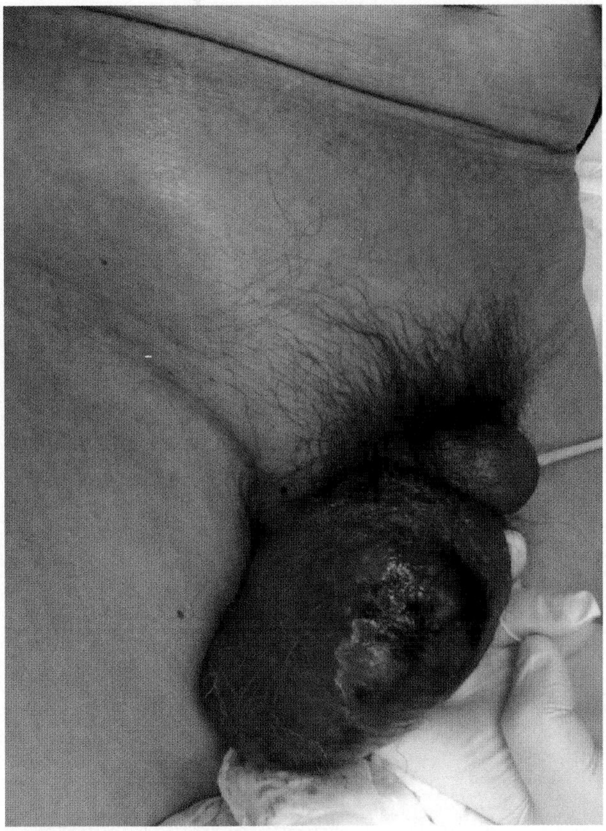

FIGURE 29-9 Fournier gangrene.

Reproduced from: Cheung P, Graham C. Fournier's gangrene. Int J Emerg Med. 2009;2(4):257-257.

include crepitus of the skin, gray-black coloration from decay (gangrene), drainage of pus, and fever. Fournier gangrene usually progresses through five stages:[15]

1. Fever and lethargy, which may be present for 2 to 7 days
2. Intense genital pain and tenderness, usually associated with edema of the overlying skin
3. Increasing genital pain and tenderness with progressive erythema of the overlying skin
4. Dusky appearance of the overlying skin; subcutaneous crepitation
5. Obvious gangrene of a portion of the genitalia; purulent drainage from wounds

Prehospital care may range from providing only emotional support and rapid transport to full resuscitation measures to manage shock. After the patient's condition has been stabilized, care by a physician includes various methods to restore normal organ perfusion and function. These methods may include antibiotic therapy, hyperbaric oxygen therapy, and surgery (including reconstruction).[16]

Phimosis

Phimosis is tightness of the **prepuce** (foreskin) of the penis. The condition prevents retraction of the foreskin over the glans (**FIGURE 29-10**). It can be caused by failure of the foreskin to loosen during growth, infection, genital disease, and trauma. Phimosis usually is a painless condition. However, infection can occur with ineffective cleaning of the penis, resulting in swelling, redness, and discharge. In rare cases, a patient may report problems with urination or intercourse.

Paraphimosis is an inability to pull the retracted foreskin back over the head of the penis. This condition can restrict blood flow and requires emergency

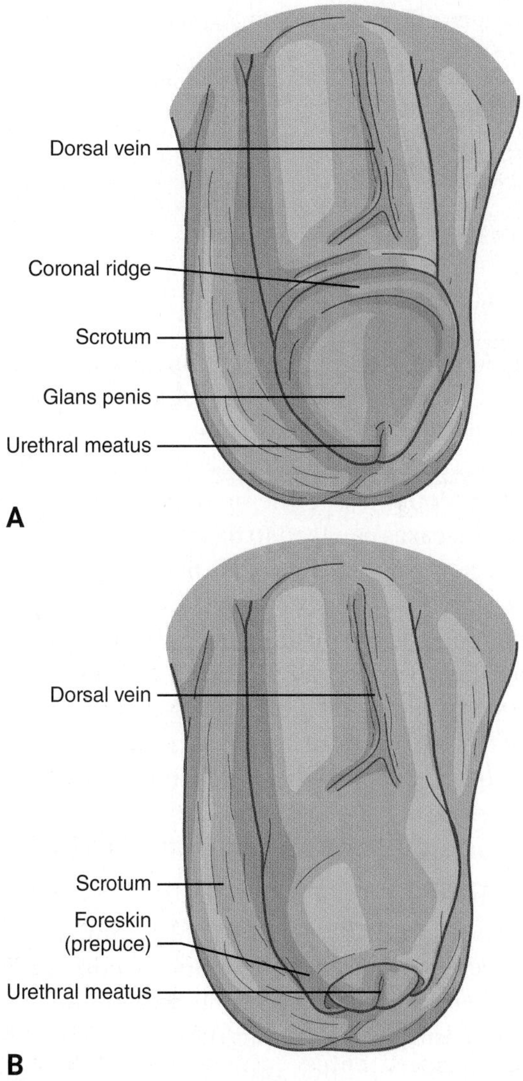

FIGURE 29-10 Appearance of the penis. **A.** Circumcised. **B.** Uncircumcised.

DID YOU KNOW?

Circumcision is the surgical removal of the foreskin. The procedure often is performed on healthy boys for cultural or religious reasons. In the United States, if a newborn is to be circumcised, the procedure usually is done before the infant leaves the hospital. Jewish boys, however, are circumcised when they are 8 days old. In other parts of the world, including Europe, Asia, and South and Central America, circumcision is rare in the general population. The merits of circumcision have been debated. Opinions about the need for circumcision in healthy boys vary among health care professionals. Some believe there is great value to having an intact foreskin, such as allowing for a more natural sexual response during adulthood. According to the American Academy of Pediatrics, current evidence indicates that the health benefits of newborn male circumcision outweigh the risks. The American Academy of Pediatrics recommends that parents make an informed decision based on their religious, ethical, and cultural beliefs to determine if the procedure is in the best interest of their child.

Modified from: Circumcision policy statement. American Academy of Pediatrics, Task Force on Circumcision. *Pediatrics*. 2012;130(3):686.

care. A hallmark sign of paraphimosis is a "doughnut" of swollen skin around the shaft, near the head of the penis. Paraphimosis occurs most often in children and older adults. If left untreated, it can disrupt blood flow to the tip of the penis,[17] which in severe cases can lead to damage of the tip of the penis, gangrene, and loss of the penis tip. Emergency care may include gentle compression of the head of the penis while pushing the foreskin forward or wrapping the penis in plastic and applying ice to reduce swelling, allowing the foreskin to return to its extended position. If these interventions fail, the patient may require hospitalization and surgical circumcision.

Priapism

Priapism is a persistent, usually painful, erection that lasts 4 hours or longer and occurs without sexual stimulation. The condition develops when blood in the penis becomes trapped and unable to drain. If the condition is not treated immediately, it can lead to scarring and permanent erectile dysfunction. Priapism can occur in all age groups, including newborns. However, it usually affects male children aged 5 to 10 years and men aged 20 to 50 years. Priapism is subcategorized into two types, low flow and high flow.[18]

- Low-flow priapism results when blood is trapped in the erection chambers of the penis. It often occurs for unknown reasons in men who are otherwise healthy. This type also affects men with sickle cell disease, leukemia and other cancers, or malaria.
- High-flow priapism is less common than the low-flow type and usually is less painful. The condition results from a ruptured artery, which occurs because of an injury to the penis or the perineum. The rupture prevents blood in the penis from circulating normally.

NOTE

Sickle cell disease is a common cause of priapism in men. Eventually, priapism will develop in approximately 42% of men with the disease.

Modified from: US National Library of Medicine. Priapism in boys and men with sickle cell disease—demographics, characteristics and prevalence. ClinicalTrials.gov website. https://clinicaltrials.gov/ct2/show/NCT00300235. Updated January 28, 2016. Accessed February 12, 2018.

Some medications can cause priapism. Examples include antidepressants (eg, trazodone hydrochloride), antipsychotics (eg, chlorpromazine), injection drugs used to treat erectile dysfunction, and oral erectile dysfunction drugs (eg, sildenafil citrate). Other causes of priapism include trauma to the spinal cord or genital area, black widow spider bites, carbon monoxide poisoning, and illicit drug use (eg, marijuana, cocaine). Prehospital care for a patient with priapism is primarily supportive. All patients should be transported and evaluated by a physician.

Benign Prostatic Hypertrophy

Benign prostatic hypertrophy (BPH) is enlargement of the prostate gland. The prostate gland is the male organ that produces prostatic fluid, a component of semen. It sits beneath the bladder and surrounds the urethra. Most men have a period of prostate growth in their middle to late 40s, when cells in the central portion of the gland reproduce rapidly. As tissues in the area enlarge, they often compress the urethra and may partly block the flow of urine.

NOTE

The prostate gland is assessed during a rectal examination. The physician palpates the gland for size, consistency, nodularity, and tenderness. In benign prostatic hypertrophy, the gland is smooth, symmetrical, and feels slightly rubbery. In contrast, a cancerous prostate may feel asymmetrical and have a stony consistency. Discrete nodules may be palpable. Marked prostatic tenderness suggests **acute prostatitis**. If a patient has signs and symptoms of prostate irregularities, the blood may be tested for prostate-specific antigen; if this value is elevated, the prostate may be biopsied to rule out cancer.

Not all men with BPH are symptomatic. However, some patients report urinary frequency, a weak urine stream, difficulty starting and stopping urination, overflow incontinence, hematuria, and UTI. Treatment of BPH depends on the severity of the signs and symptoms and how they affect daily life. Treatment options include medications, surgery, and nonsurgical therapies. Enlargement of the prostate gland is not related to the development of prostate cancer.[19]

Testicular Masses

A **testicular mass** is an enlargement or growth on one or both testicles (**TABLE 29-4**). Most masses are benign, but some may be malignant. Three of the most common benign testicular masses are hydroceles, spermatoceles, and varicoceles.

TABLE 29-4 Abnormalities in the Scrotum

Disorder	Clinical Findings	Comments
Testicular torsion	*S:* Sudden onset of excruciating pain in testicle, often during sleep or after trauma; patient may also have lower abdominal pain, nausea and vomiting, no fever *O:* Inspection—Red, swollen scrotum, one testis (usually left) higher because of rotation and shortening Palpation—Cord feels thick, swollen, tender; epididymis may be anterior; cremasteric reflex absent on side of torsion *A:* Testicular torsion	Sudden twisting of the spermatic cord usually occurs in late childhood to early adolescence; it is rare after age 20 years. Torsion usually occurs on the left side. Faulty anchoring of the testis on the scrotal wall allows the testis to rotate. The anterior part of the testis rotates medially toward the other testis. Blood supply is cut off, resulting in ischemia and engorgement. This is an emergency that requires surgery; the testis can become gangrenous in a few hours.
Epididymitis	*S:* Sudden onset of severe pain in scrotum that is somewhat relieved by elevation (positive Prehn sign); rapid swelling, fever *O:* Inspection—Enlarged, reddened scrotum Palpation—Exquisitely tender; epididymis enlarged, indurated, and may be difficult to distinguish from testis; overlying scrotal skin may be thick and edematous Laboratory—White blood cells and bacteria in urine *A:* Tender swelling of epididymis	Acute infection of the epididymis commonly occurs as a result of prostatitis; after prostatectomy because of the trauma of urethral instrumentation; or because of a chlamydial, gonorrheal, or other bacterial infection. Differentiating between epididymitis and testicular torsion often is difficult.
Spermatic cord varicocele	*S:* Dull pain; constant pulling or dragging feeling; or may be asymptomatic *O:* Inspection—Usually no sign; may show blue color through light scrotal skin Palpation—When patient is standing, a soft, irregular mass is felt posterior to and above the testis; this mass collapses when the patient is supine and refills when standing upright; mass feels distinctive, like a "bag of worms"; testis on the side of the varicocele may be smaller because of impaired circulation *A:* Soft mass on spermatic cord	A varicocele is dilated, tortuous varicose veins in the spermatic cord resulting from incompetent valves in the vein; this permits the reflux of blood. Varicoceles are found most often on the left side, perhaps because the left spermatic vein is longer and inserts at a right angle into the left renal vein. The condition is common in young men. Screening should be done in early adolescence; early treatment is important to prevent the possibility of infertility in adulthood.

(continued)

TABLE 29-4 Abnormalities in the Scrotum *(continued)*

Disorder	Clinical Findings	Comments
Spermatocele	*S:* Painless, usually found on examination *O:* Inspection—Transilluminates higher in the scrotum than a hydrocele; sperm may fluoresce Palpation—Round, freely movable mass lying above and behind testis; if large, feels like a third testis *A:* Free cystic mass on epididymis	Retention cyst in the epididymis. The cause is unclear but may be obstruction of tubules. Cyst is filled with thin, milky fluid that contains sperm. Most spermatoceles are small (about 1 cm); occasionally they may be larger and sometimes mistaken for a hydrocele.
Diffuse tumor	*S:* Enlarging testis (most common symptom); when enlarged, it has the feel of increased weight *O:* Inspection—Enlarged testis, does not transilluminate Palpation—Enlarged, smooth, ovoid, firm Important—Firm palpation does not cause usual sickening discomfort seen with normal testis *A:* Nontender swelling of testis	Diffuse tumor maintains the shape of the testis.
Hydrocele	*S:* Painless swelling, although the patient may report weight and bulk in the scrotum *O:* Inspection—Enlarged; mass transilluminates with a pink or red glow (in contrast to a hernia) Palpation—Nontender mass; able to get fingers above mass (in contrast to scrotal hernia) *A:* Nontender swelling of testis	Cystic, circumscribed collection of serous fluid in the tunica vaginalis, surrounding the testis. It may occur after epididymitis, trauma, hernia, or tumor of the testis, or spontaneously in the newborn.
Scrotal hernia	*S:* Swelling; may have pain with straining *O:* Inspection—Enlarged; may reduce when patient is supine; does not transilluminate Palpation—Soft, mushy mass; palpating fingers cannot get above mass; mass is distinct from normal testicle *A:* Nontender swelling of scrotum	Scrotal hernia usually is the result of indirect inguinal hernia.
Orchitis	*S:* Sudden onset of acute or moderate pain; swollen testis; feeling of weight; fever *O:* Inspection—Enlarged, edematous, reddened; does not transilluminate Palpation—Swollen, congested, tense, and tender; difficult to distinguish testis from epididymis *A:* Tender swelling of testis	Acute inflammation of testis. Most common cause is mumps, although it can occur with any infectious disease. Patient may have an associated hydrocele that transilluminates.

Abbreviations: S, subjective data; O, objective data; A, assessment

Modified from: Jarvis C. *Physical Examination and Health Assessment*. 7th ed. St. Louis, MO: Elsevier; 2016.

A **hydrocele** is a fluid-filled sac along the spermatic cord in the scrotum (**FIGURE 29-11**). A **spermatocele** is a benign cystic accumulation of sperm that arises from the head of the epididymis (**FIGURE 29-12** and **FIGURE 29-13**). Both conditions result in collections of fluid in the scrotal sac. These masses are generally soft and painless. Their size can change rapidly as fluid enters or leaves the scrotum. A **varicocele** is an enlargement of the veins that drain the testicles (**FIGURE 29-14**). These masses are soft scrotal swellings that often are more prominent when the man is standing or exercising. Varicoceles sometimes may cause a sensation of heaviness or a dull ache in the genital area.

Ultrasonographic and transillumination techniques are used to diagnose testicular masses. Most testicular masses require no treatment. If a hydrocele or spermatocele is large or painful (or both), surgery may be needed to drain fluid. A varicocele may require surgery to tie off the affected veins.

Testicular cancer also may present as a testicular mass, with or without pain. The mass usually feels firm

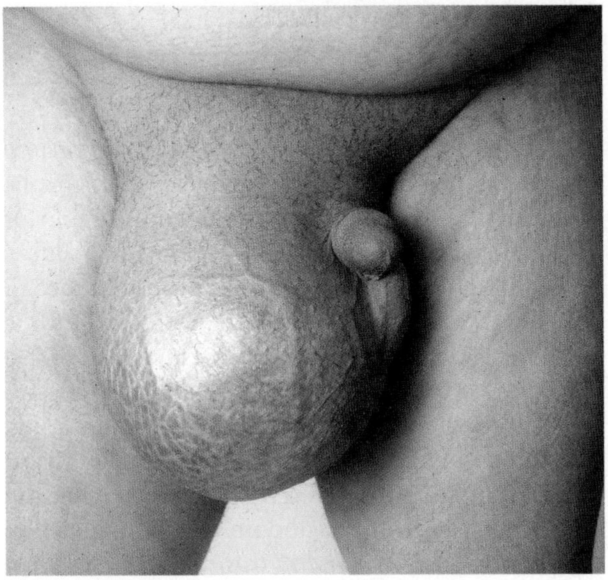

FIGURE 29-11 Hydrocele.

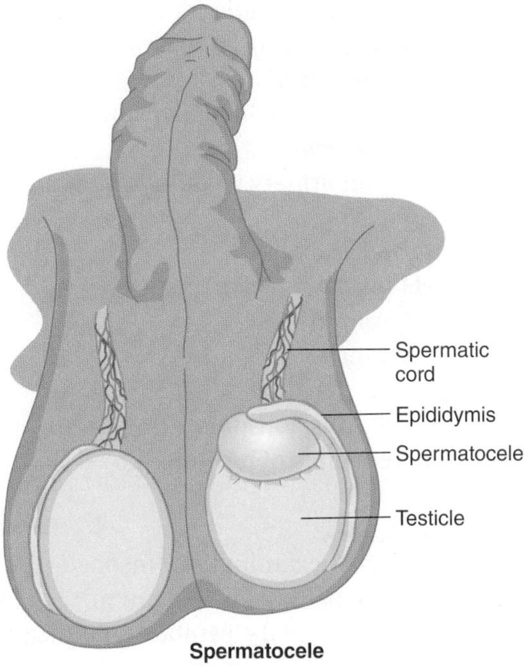

FIGURE 29-12 Spermatocele.

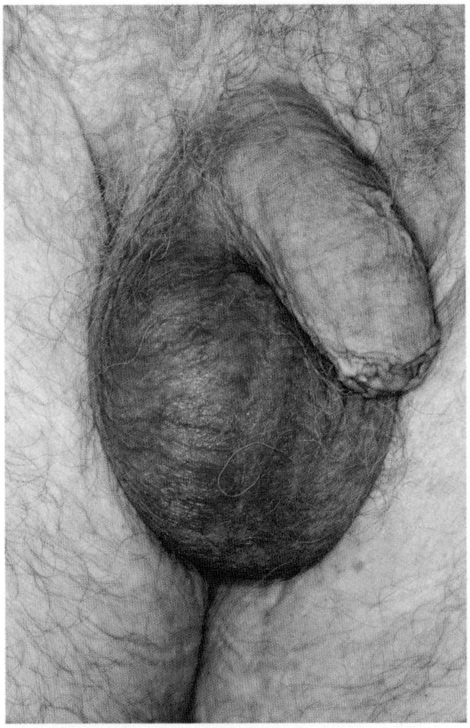

FIGURE 29-13 Epididymitis.

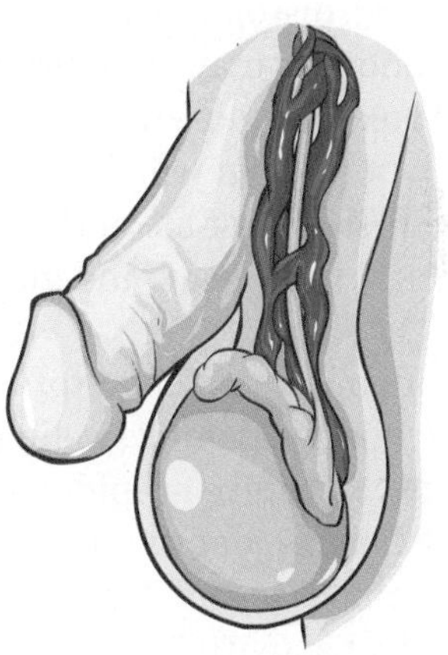

FIGURE 29-14 Varicocele.

and arises from the testicle. The diagnosis is made using blood tests and scrotal ultrasound. Treatment involves surgery to remove the affected testicle, chemotherapy, and/or radiation. The average age for diagnosis is 33 years. About 7% of cases are found in children and teens, and about 7% of cases occur in men older than 55 years. Monthly self-examination of the testicles is recommended for men in this age group. Each year more than 8,800 new cases of testicular cancer are diagnosed in the United States, and about 410 men die of the disease.[20]

Testicular Torsion

Testicular torsion is a true urologic emergency. In this condition, a testicle (usually the left) twists on

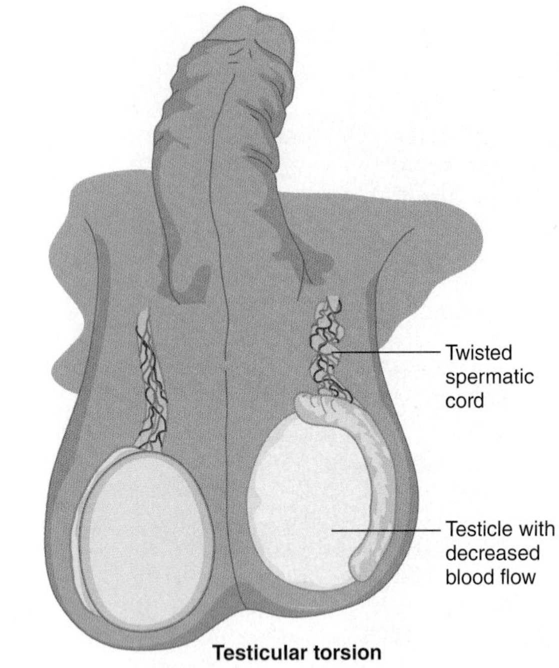

FIGURE 29-15 Left testicular torsion.

its spermatic cord, disrupting the blood supply of the testicle. The condition may result from blunt trauma to the scrotal area, but more often it is spontaneous. The two peak periods in which torsion is likely to occur are the first year of life and puberty (the age range is 5 months to 41 years, and the average age of occurrence is 14 years).[21]

Like epididymitis, testicular torsion results in a tender epididymis and painful swelling of the scrotal sac (**FIGURE 29-15**). Unlike in epididymitis, however, the patient usually is afebrile. The pain is sudden in onset and usually severe. It often is preceded by vigorous physical activity. The pain sometimes radiates to the ipsilateral lower abdominal quadrant, is unrelieved by rest or scrotal elevation, and often is associated with nausea and vomiting. Testicular torsion should be diagnosed and treated within 6 hours to prevent loss of the testis from ischemic infarction.[22] Therapeutic intervention includes the application of ice packs to the scrotum and manual manipulation by a physician to reduce the torsion. The patient must undergo surgical repair within 4 to 6 hours of onset of the torsion. Therefore, rapid transport to the ED and early recognition are crucial for treatment.

Physical Examination of Patients with Genitourinary or Renal Disorders

As described in Chapter 19, *Secondary Assessment and Reassessment*, assessment of the abdomen and genitalia of either sex can be awkward and uncomfortable for the patient and the paramedic. The paramedic should protect the patient's privacy with proper drapes to ensure privacy. When possible, paramedics of the same sex as the patient should perform these examinations. If this is not possible, a chaperone should be present. The paramedic should proceed with a calm, caring, and competent attitude. The patient and significant others should be informed of all actions. As in the care of a patient with an abdominal complaint (see Chapter 28, *Abdominal and Gastrointestinal Disorders*), the examination should include the following:

- Primary assessment
- Focused history
  - OPQRST (Onset, Provocation/palliation, Quality, Region/radiation, Severity, Timing)
  - Previous history of similar event
  - Nausea or vomiting
  - Change in bowel habits or stool (constipation, diarrhea)
  - Change in urinary voiding pattern
  - Weight loss
  - Last oral intake
  - Last bowel movement
- Physical examination
  - Appearance
  - Posture
  - Level of consciousness
  - Apparent state of health
  - Skin color
  - Vital signs
  - Abdominal examination (inspection, auscultation, percussion, palpation)
  - Examination of the genitalia (if indicated)

Management and Treatment Plan

The paramedic should treat patients with genitourinary disorders as they would any other patient with acute pain. This management includes addressing life threats, monitoring ECG and vital signs, and transporting for evaluation by a physician in the patient's position of comfort. Patients should not be permitted to eat or drink because surgery may be indicated.

Summary

- The urinary system removes waste products from the blood. It also helps maintain a constant body fluid volume and composition.
- The nephron is the functional unit of the kidney. It filters blood, removes waste products, and produces urine.
- Renal failure may result in uremia, hyperkalemia, acidosis, hypertension, and volume overload with heart failure.
- Acute kidney injury (AKI) occurs when the kidneys are unable to excrete the daily load of toxins in the urine. Its onset may be within hours.
- Prerenal AKI results from poor perfusion of the kidneys. Intrarenal AKI is caused by conditions that damage the tissues of the kidney. Postrenal AKI is caused by obstruction of urine flow from both kidneys.
- Dialysis is a technique used to normalize blood chemistry in patients with acute or chronic renal failure. It also is used to remove blood toxins. The two dialysis techniques are hemodialysis and peritoneal dialysis. Dialysis emergencies may include problems with vascular access, hemorrhage, hypotension, chest pain, severe hyperkalemia, disequilibrium syndrome, air embolism, or cardiac arrest.
- Urinary retention is the inability to empty the urinary bladder.
- Urinary tract infections can involve the upper or lower urinary tract.
- Pyelonephritis is inflammation of the kidney parenchyma. It can lead to chronic renal problems.
- Urinary calculi are stones that originate in the kidney.
- Epididymitis is inflammation of the epididymis. The epididymis is the tube that carries sperm from the testicle to the seminal vesicles.
- Fournier gangrene is a bacterial infection of the genitals that can lead to death of skin tissue and systemic sepsis.
- Phimosis is tightness of the foreskin of the penis causing an inability to retract it. Paraphimosis occurs when a male is unable to return retracted foreskin back over the head of the penis to the normal anatomic position.
- Priapism is a painful, sustained erection.
- Benign prostatic hypertrophy is enlargement of the prostate gland. It may be associated with urinary difficulty and urinary tract infections.
- Testicular masses may be benign or cancerous.
- In testicular torsion a testicle twists on its spermatic cord, disrupting the blood supply to the testicle. This condition is a true emergency.
- The physical examination for a patient with a urinary tract problem is similar to that for abdominal pain. Patients with genitourinary pain should be managed in the same way as any other patient with acute pain.

References

1. National Highway Traffic Safety Administration. *The National EMS Education Standards*. Washington, DC: US Department of Transportation; 2009.
2. Doyle JF, Forni LG. Acute kidney injury: short-term and long-term effects. *Crit Care*. 2016;20(1):188.
3. Basile DP, Anderson MD, Sutton TA. Pathophysiology of acute kidney injury. *Compr Physiol*. 2012;2(2):1303-1353.
4. Norton JM, Newman EP, Romancito G, Mahooty S, Kuracina T, Narva AS. Improving outcomes for patients with chronic kidney disease: part 2. *Am J Nurs*. 2017;117(3):26-35.
5. United States Renal Data System. *2015 Annual Data Report: Epidemiology of Kidney Disease in the United States*. Ann Arbor, MI: USRDS Coordinating Center; 2015.
6. *Nephrology Book*. Family Practice Notebook website. http://www.fpnotebook.com/Renal/index.htm. Accessed February 12, 2018.
7. American Heart Association. Part 10: special circumstances of resuscitation. In: *Web-Based Integrated 2010 and 2015 American Heart Association Guidelines for Cardiopulmonary Resuscitation and Emergence Cardiovascular Care*. American Heart Association website. https://eccguidelines.heart.org/index.php/circulation/cpr-ecc-guidelines-2/part-10-special-circumstances-of-resuscitation/. Published 2015. Accessed February 12, 2018.
8. National Association of EMS Officials. *National Model EMS Clinical Guidelines*. Version 2. National Association of EMS Officials website. https://www.nasemso.org/documents/National-Model-EMS-Clinical-Guidelines-Version2-Sept2017.pdf. Published 2017. Accessed February 12, 2018.
9. Tuchman S, Khademian ZP, Mistry K. Dialysis disequilibrium syndrome occurring during continuous renal replacement therapy. *Clin Kidney J*. 2013;6(5):526-529.
10. Muth CM, Shank ES. Gas embolism. *New Engl J Med*. 2000;342(7):476-482.
11. Flores-Mireles AL, Walker JN, Caparon M, Hultgren SJ. Urinary tract infections: epidemiology, mechanisms of infection and treatment options. *Nat Rev Microbiol*. 2015;13(5):269-284.
12. Scales CD Jr, Smith AC, Hanley JM, Saigal CS. Prevalence of kidney stones in the United States. *Eur Urol*. 2012;62(1):160-165.
13. Cloutier J, Villa L, Traxer O, Daudon M. Kidney stone analysis: "Give me your stone, I will tell you who you are!" *World J Urol*. 2015;33(2):157-169.
14. Division of STD Prevention, National Center for HIV/AIDS, Viral Hepatitis, STD, and TB Prevention, Centers for Disease Control and Prevention. 2015 sexually transmitted diseases treatment guidelines: epididymitis. Centers for Disease Control and Prevention website. https://www.cdc.gov/std/tg2015/epididymitis.htm. Updated June 4, 2015. Accessed February 12, 2018.
15. Pais VM. Fournier gangrene. Medscape website. https://emedicine.medscape.com/article/2028899-overview. Updated January 10, 2018. Accessed February 12, 2018.
16. Ferretti M, Saji AA, Phillips J. Fournier's gangrene: a review and outcome comparison from 2009 to 2016. *Adv Wound Care*. 2017;6(9):289-295.

17. Jordan GH, Schlossberg SML. Surgery of the penis and urethra. In: Wein AJ, ed. *Campbell-Walsh Urology.* 9th ed. Philadelphia, PA: Saunders; 2007.
18. Al-Qudah HS. Priapsim. Medscape website. https://emedicine.medscape.com/article/437237-overview. Updated November 28, 2016. Accessed February 12, 2018.
19. Understanding prostate changes: a health guide for men. National Cancer Institute, National Institutes of Health, website. https://www.cancer.gov/types/prostate/understanding-prostate-changes. Accessed February 12, 2018.
20. American Cancer Society medical and editorial content team. Key statistics for testicular cancer. American Cancer Society website. https://www.cancer.org/cancer/testicular-cancer/about/key-statistics.html. Updated January 4, 2018. Accessed February 12, 2018.
21. Marx J, Hockberger R, Walls R. *Rosen's Emergency Medicine: Concepts and Clinical Practice.* 7th ed. St. Louis, MO: Mosby; 2010.
22. Rottenstreich M, Glick Y, Gofrit ON. The clinical findings in young adults with acute scrotal pain. *Am J Emerg Med.* 2016;34(10):1931-1933.

Suggested Readings

Borcato C. How to identify, assess and treat renal failure. *JEMS* website. http://www.jems.com/articles/print/volume-38/issue-9/features/how-identify-assess-treat-renal-failure.html. Published August 13, 2013. Accessed February 12, 2018.

Hashim H, Reynard J, Cowan NC, Wood D, Armenakas N, eds. *Urological Emergencies in Clinical Practice*. 2nd ed. London, England: Springer; 2013.

Palka J. Twelve urologic emergencies you need to know. Medscape website. https://reference.medscape.com/slideshow/urologic-emergencies-6008708. Published May 17, 2017. Accessed February 12, 2018.

Pauly R, Eastwood D, Marshall M. Patient safety in home hemodialysis: quality assurance and serious adverse events in the home setting. International Society of Home Dialysis website. http://www.ishd.org/5-patient-safety-in-home-hemodialysis-quality-assurance-and-serious-adverse-events-in-the-home-setting/. Accessed February 12, 2018.

Thurtle D, Biers S, Sut M, Armitage J, eds. *Emergency Urology.* Shropshire, UK: TFM Publishing; March 1, 2016.

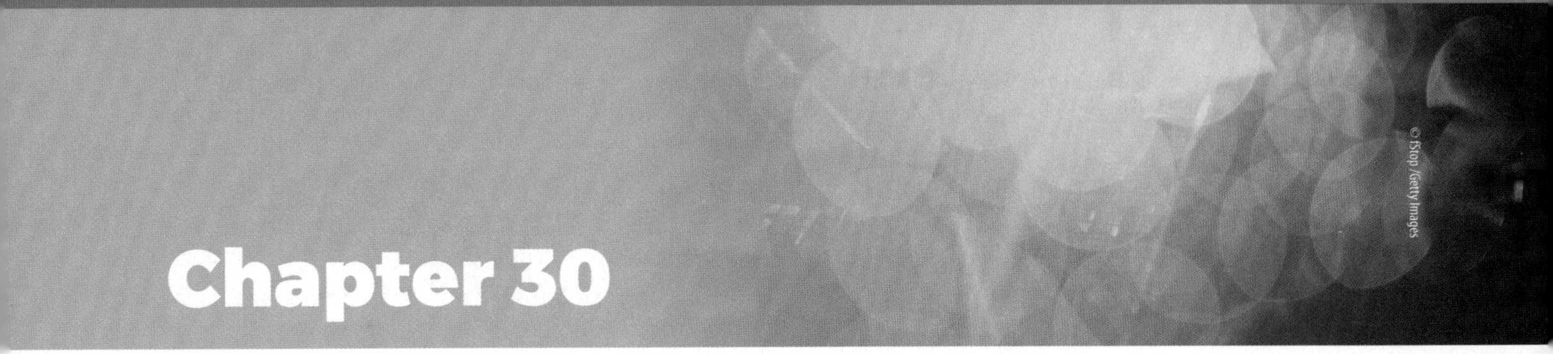

Chapter 30

Gynecology

NATIONAL EMS EDUCATION STANDARD COMPETENCIES

Medicine

Integrates assessment findings with principles of epidemiology and pathophysiology to formulate a field impression and implement a comprehensive treatment/disposition plan for a patient with a medical complaint.

Gynecology

Recognition and management of shock associated with
- Vaginal bleeding (pp 1152–1153, 1156)

Anatomy, physiology, assessment findings, and management of
- Vaginal bleeding (pp 1152–1153, 1156)
- Sexual assault (to include appropriate emotional support) (pp 1156–1157)
- Infections (pp 1149, 1151)

Anatomy, physiology, epidemiology, pathophysiology, psychosocial impact, presentations, prognosis, and management of common or major gynecologic diseases and/or emergencies
- Vaginal bleeding (pp 1152–1153, 1156)
- Sexual assault (pp 1156–1157)
- Infections (pp 1149, 1151)
- Pelvic inflammatory disease (pp 1148–1149)
- Infections (pp 1149, 1151)
- Ovarian cysts (pp 1149–1150)
- Dysfunctional uterine bleeding (p 1153)
- Vaginal foreign body (p 1154)

OBJECTIVES

Upon completion of this chapter, the paramedic student will be able to:

1. Describe the physiologic processes of menstruation and ovulation. (pp 1145–1148)
2. Describe the pathophysiology of the following nontraumatic causes of abdominal pain in females: pelvic inflammatory disease, Bartholin abscess, vaginitis, ruptured ovarian cyst, ovarian torsion, cystitis, dysmenorrhea, mittelschmerz, endometritis, endometriosis, ectopic pregnancy, vaginal bleeding, dysfunctional uterine bleeding, uterine prolapse, and vaginal foreign body. (pp 1148–1154)
3. Outline the prehospital assessment and management of a female with abdominal pain or bleeding. (pp 1154–1155)
4. Outline the specific assessment and management of a patient who has been sexually assaulted. (p 1157)
5. Describe specific prehospital measures to preserve evidence in sexual assault cases. (pp 1156–1157)

KEY TERMS

Bartholin abscess An accumulation of pus that forms a lump in one of the Bartholin glands. It results when blockage of the gland's duct allows infection to develop.

cesarean delivery A surgical procedure in which the abdomen and uterus are incised and the baby is delivered through the abdomen.

cystitis Inflammation of the urinary bladder and ureters.

date rape Nonconsensual sex between people who are already acquainted (eg, friends, acquaintances, or people who are dating).

dilation and curettage (D&C) A gynecologic procedure in which the uterine cervix is widened and the endometrium of the uterus is scraped away.

dysfunctional uterine bleeding (DUB) Abnormal bleeding that occurs because of changes in hormone levels.

dysmenorrhea Pain associated with menstruation.

dyspareunia Pain with intercourse.

ectopic pregnancy An abnormal pregnancy that develops outside the uterus.

endometriosis An abnormal gynecologic condition characterized by ectopic growth and function of endometrial tissue. It is thought to result when fragments of endometrium from the lining of the uterus are regurgitated during menstruation backward through the fallopian tubes into the peritoneal cavity; there, they attach and grow as small cystic structures.

endometritis An inflammatory condition of the endometrium, usually caused by bacterial infection.

endometrium The mucous membrane lining of the uterus, which changes in thickness and structure with the menstrual cycle.

fallopian tubes A pair of ducts that open at one end into the uterus and at the other end into the peritoneal cavity, over the ovaries; also known as uterine tubes.

female external genital organs The outer parts of the female genitalia. They consist of the labia majora, the labia minora, Bartholin glands, and the clitoris. Also known as the vulva.

hysterectomy The surgical removal of the uterus.

mammary glands External accessory sex organs in females; breasts.

menarche The first menstruation and commencement of the cyclic menstrual function.

menopause The cessation of menses.

menstruation The periodic discharge through the vagina of a blood secretion containing tissue debris from the shedding of the endometrium from the nonpregnant uterus.

mittelschmerz Abdominal pain in the region of the ovary during ovulation. It usually occurs midway through the menstrual cycle.

oocytes Incompletely developed ova.

ovarian torsion Twisting of an ovary around its vascular pedicle.

ovaries A pair of female gonads found on each side of the lower abdomen beside the uterus.

ovulation The release of an ovum or secondary oocyte from the vesicular follicle.

pelvic inflammatory disease (PID) Any inflammatory condition of the female pelvic organs, especially one caused by bacterial infection.

rape Nonconsensual sex or an attempt to force another person to have sex against his or her will. It includes intercourse in the vagina, anus, or mouth.

ruptured ovarian cyst A ruptured globular sac filled with fluid or semisolid material that develops in or on the ovary.

sexual assault The forcible perpetration of an act of sexual contact on the body of another person, male or female, without his or her consent.

uterine prolapse The falling or sliding of the uterus from its normal position in the pelvic cavity into the vaginal canal.

uterus The hollow, pear-shaped internal female organ of reproduction.

vagina The part of the female genitalia that forms a canal from the orifice through the vestibule to the uterine cervix.

vaginal bleeding The loss of blood through the vagina where the source of bleeding may be the uterus, the cervix, or the vaginal wall itself.

vaginitis Inflammation of the vaginal tissues.

zygote The developing ovum from the time it is fertilized until it is implanted in the uterus as a blastocyst.

A number of disorders can occur in the female reproductive system. Some of these can lead to gynecologic emergencies. This chapter discusses the causes of and emergency care for problems associated with the female reproductive system and the treatment of victims of sexual assault.

Organs of the Female Reproductive System

The female reproductive organs include the ovaries, fallopian (uterine) tubes, uterus, vagina, external genital organs, and mammary glands (**FIGURE 30-1**; also see Chapter 10, *Review of Human Systems*). The following is a brief review of these structures.

The **ovaries** are small, oval-shaped glands on either side of the uterus. Each ovary consists of a

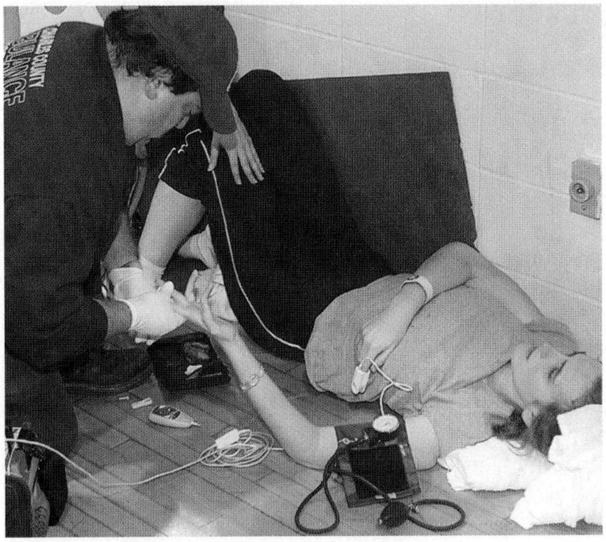

Courtesy Ray Kemp, St. Charles, MO.

dense outer portion (cortex) and a less dense inner portion (medulla). The ovaries produce eggs (ova) and hormones, especially estrogen and progesterone. The **fallopian tubes** are the uterine ducts for the ovaries. An ovum that is fertilized in the fallopian tube normally implants in the lining of the uterus (endometrium). This occurrence is the beginning of a pregnancy.

The **uterus** (womb) is a muscular organ the size and shape of a medium-sized pear. The main function of the uterus is to accept and nourish a fertilized ovum. A fertilized ovum that is not implanted in the uterus is shed from the body through menstruation.

The **vagina** (birth canal) is the female organ of copulation. It is a canal that joins the cervix (the lower portion of the uterus) to the outside of the body. It receives the penis during intercourse.

The **external genital organs** (vulva) are the outer parts of the female genitalia. They also protect the internal organs from infectious disease. The external genital organs consist of the labia majora, the labia minora, Bartholin glands, and the clitoris.

The **mammary glands** are the organs of milk production. They are located in the breasts (mammae). Under the influence of hormones, the glands secrete milk during nursing.

Menstruation and Ovulation

Menstruation

In women of reproductive age, the body prepares for a possible pregnancy about once a month. If pregnancy does not occur (ie, a fertilized ovum does not implant in the uterine wall), menstruation follows. **Menstruation** is the normal, periodic discharge of blood, mucus, and cellular debris from the uterine mucosa. The normal menstrual cycle lasts about 28 days. It occurs at more or less regular intervals from puberty to menopause (except during pregnancy and lactation). The average menstrual flow is 0.8 to 2 ounces (25 to 60 mL). The flow usually lasts 4 to 6 days and is fairly constant from cycle to cycle. The onset of menses (**menarche**) generally begins between

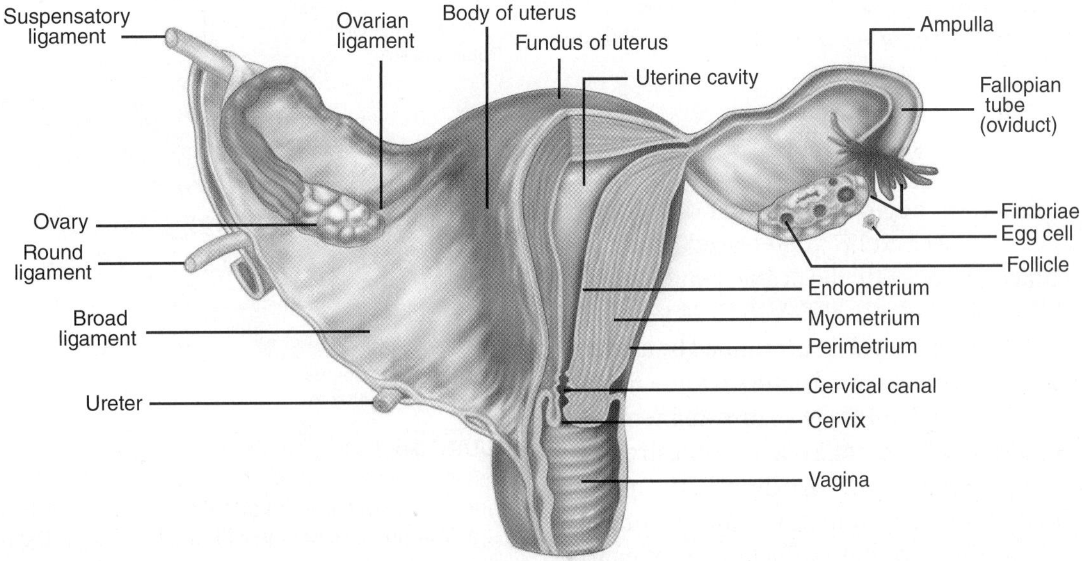

FIGURE 30-1 Female reproductive organs.

BOX 30-1 Hysterectomy

A **hysterectomy** is the surgical removal of the uterus. Hysterectomy is one of the most frequently performed gynecologic surgeries in the United States. It most often is performed to treat fibroid tumors that have caused symptoms and cancer of the uterus or cervix. Other indications for the surgery include heavy menstrual bleeding, endometriosis, pelvic inflammatory disease, and the removal of a prolapsed uterus. Depending on the type of hysterectomy, the surgery may be performed through the abdomen or vagina, laparoscopically or robot-assisted laparoscopically.

In a subtotal hysterectomy, only the upper part of the uterus is removed; the cervix is not. The fallopian tubes and ovaries may or may not be removed. In a total hysterectomy, the body of the uterus and the cervix are removed. The ovaries may or may not be removed. If cancer is present or in an advanced stage, a radical hysterectomy may be required, in which part of the vagina and some ligaments and pelvic lymph nodes also are removed. After a hysterectomy, a woman is unable to bear children, does not menstruate, and needs no contraception.

Serious complications can occur from the surgery, including blood clots, infection, adhesions, postoperative hemorrhage, bowel injury, or injury to the urinary tract. In addition to the direct surgical risks, long-term physical and psychological effects are possible. If the ovaries are removed along with the uterus before menopause, the risk of osteoporosis and heart disease may be increased.

Modified from: Janda M, Armfield NR, Page K, et al. Factors influencing women's decision making in hysterectomy [published online September 7, 2017]. *Patient Educ Couns*. doi:https://doi.org/10.1016/j.pec.2017.09.006; Mann WJ Jr. Radical hysterectomy. UpToDate website. https://www.uptodate.com/contents/radical-hysterectomy?source=see_link. Updated September 28, 2017. Accessed February 9, 2018.

ages 12 and 13 years. Menstruation ends permanently (**menopause**) at an average age of 47 years. However, the normal age for menopause can range from 35 to 60 years (BOX 30-1). Menstruation occurs in three phases: the follicular phase, the ovulatory phase, and the luteal phase.

NOTE

All phases of the menstrual cycle are affected by the release of hormones. These hormones include follicle-stimulating hormone (FSH), luteinizing hormone (LH), estrogen, and progesterone.

Follicular Phase

The follicular phase begins on the first day of the menstrual cycle. FSH and LH are released from the brain and make contact with the ovaries, which stimulates each ovary to release about 15 to 20 **oocytes** (immature ova). Each oocyte is surrounded by a layer of cells (granulosa cells). The structure is known as a primary follicle. FSH and LH also cause an increase in the production of estrogen. The rise in estrogen levels stops the production of FSH, limiting the number of primary follicles that mature into secondary follicles. A mature secondary follicle continues to enlarge and produce estrogen and eventually forms a lump on the surface of the ovary. The fully mature follicle is known as the vesicular (or graafian) follicle (**FIGURE 30-2**).

Ovulatory Phase

Cellular secretions of the graafian follicle cause the follicle to swell more rapidly than can be accommodated by follicular growth. The rise in estrogen

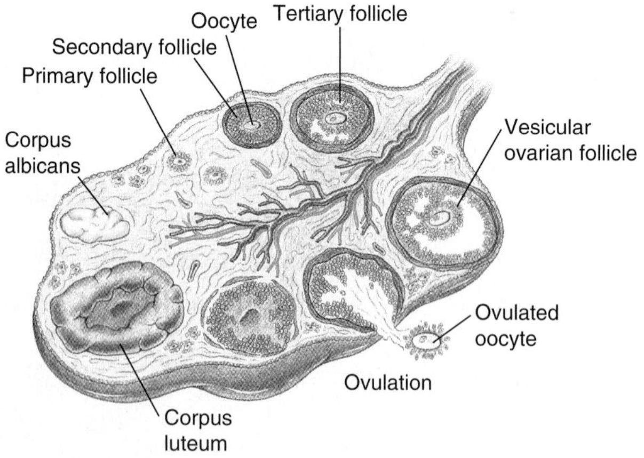

FIGURE 30-2 Diagram of the ovary and oogenesis. A cross section of the mammalian ovary shows successive stages of the ovarian (graafian) follicle and ovum development. The process begins with the first stage, the primary follicle, and (following clockwise) proceeds to the final stage, degeneration of the corpus luteum.

during this phase triggers the release of LH, which causes the follicle to expand and rupture and forces a small amount of blood and follicular fluid out of the vesicle. Shortly after the initial burst of fluid, an oocyte escapes from the follicle. The release of this secondary oocyte is called **ovulation**, which starts about 14 days after the follicular phase. It is the midpoint in the menstrual cycle. The egg is captured in the fallopian tube, where it may or may not be fertilized.

Luteal Phase

After ovulation, the empty follicle is transformed into a yellow glandular structure called the corpus luteum. The cells of this structure secrete large amounts of progesterone and some estrogen. If pregnancy occurs, the fertilized oocyte (**zygote**) travels through the fallopian tube to implant in the uterus. Chorionic gonadotropin is released to prevent the corpus luteum from degenerating. As a result, blood levels of estrogen and progesterone do not decrease and the menstrual period does not occur. If pregnancy does not occur, the corpus luteum degenerates and no longer produces progesterone; the estrogen level decreases, and the top layers of the lining are shed with the menstrual flow.

Hormonal Control of Ovulation and Menses

Hormones released from the hypothalamus and anterior pituitary control ovulation and menses. Under the influence of the ovarian hormones, the **endometrium** (the lining of the uterus) goes through two phases of development: the proliferative phase and the secretory phase (**FIGURE 30-3**).

> CRITICAL THINKING
> What might happen to a woman's menstrual cycle if her hormonal balance were off?

The proliferative phase starts with and is sustained by increasing amounts of estrogen produced by the maturing follicle. Estrogen stimulates the endometrium to grow and increase in thickness and prepares the uterus for implantation of a fertilized ovum. The secretory phase begins after ovulation. During this phase, which is under the combined influence of estrogen and progesterone, the endometrium is prepared for implantation of the fertilized ovum. Within 7 days after ovulation (about day 21 of the menstrual cycle), the endometrium is ready to receive the developing embryo if fertilization has occurred.

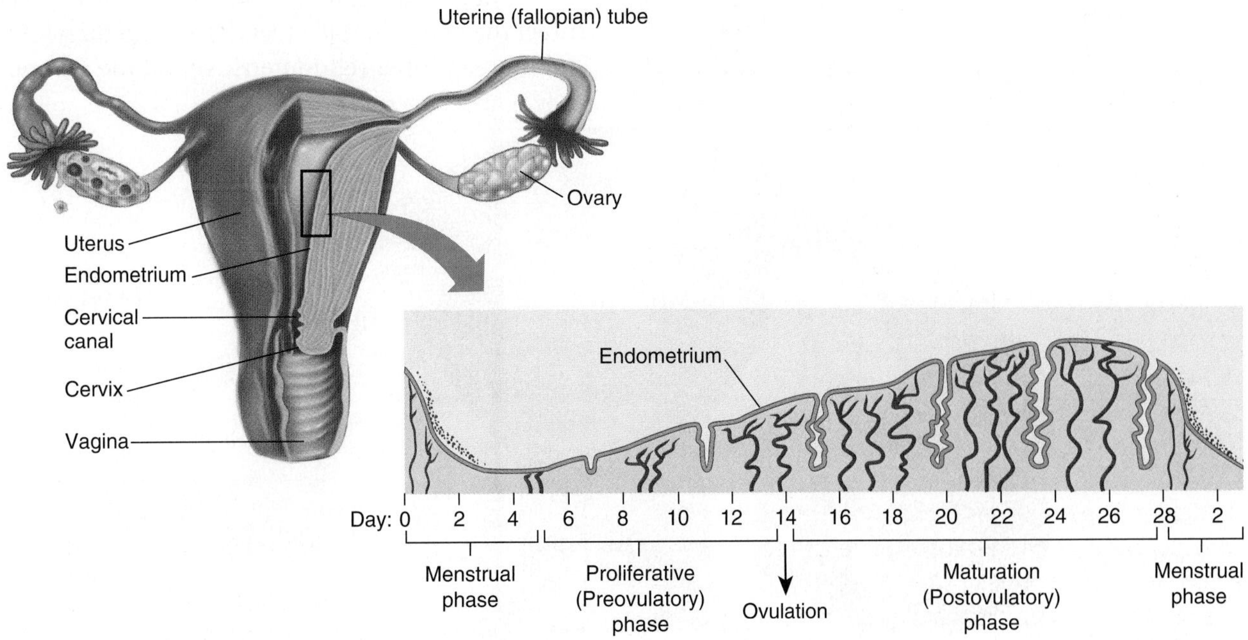

FIGURE 30-3 The female reproductive cycle.

If fertilization does not occur, the ovum can survive only 6 to 24 hours. After this time, the hormone levels drop and the endometrium is shed as menstrual flow. This process usually takes place on day 28 of the cycle (about 14 days after ovulation). The oocyte can be fertilized for up to 24 hours after ovulation (see Chapter 45, *Obstetrics*).

Gynecologic Emergencies

Gynecologic emergencies to be discussed in this chapter are medical conditions and sexual assault (BOX 30-2). (Other traumatic injuries are addressed in Chapter 42, *Abdominal Trauma*; genitourinary causes of abdominal pain are described in Chapter 29, *Genitourinary and Renal Disorders*; and obstetric emergencies are presented in Chapter 45, *Obstetrics*.)

BOX 30-2 Gynecologic Emergencies

- Gynecologic disorders
  - Pelvic inflammatory disease
  - Bartholin abscess
  - Vaginitis
  - Ruptured ovarian cyst
  - Ovarian torsion
  - Cystitis
  - Dysmenorrhea
  - Mittelschmerz
  - Endometritis
  - Endometriosis
  - Ectopic pregnancy
  - Vaginal bleeding
  - Dysfunctional uterine bleeding
  - Uterine prolapse
- Sexual assault

Acute or chronic infection involving a patient's uterus, ovaries, fallopian tubes, and adjacent structures may be a source of severe abdominal pain. Abdominal pain associated with the female reproductive system can indicate a wide range of conditions; it may mark minor episodes of difficult menstruation, or it may indicate potentially life-threatening hemorrhage from a ruptured ovarian cyst or ectopic pregnancy. Regardless of the type of emergency, pregnancy should always be considered in any woman of childbearing age until a physician determines otherwise.

Pelvic Inflammatory Disease

Pelvic inflammatory disease (PID) is a general term for infection of the cervix, uterus, fallopian tubes, and ovaries and their supporting structures (**FIGURE 30-4**). In 2015, PID affected about 68,000 women in the United States.[1] PID usually is caused by sexually transmitted bacteria, most commonly *Neisseria gonorrhoeae* (gonorrhea) and *Chlamydia trachomatis* (chlamydia). Staphylococci, streptococci, and other pathogens also may cause infection. However, these organisms usually are transmitted by instruments used during medical procedures.

Pathogens ascending from the vaginal area may infect the cervix initially (cervicitis) and then infect the uterus proper (endometritis) and the fallopian

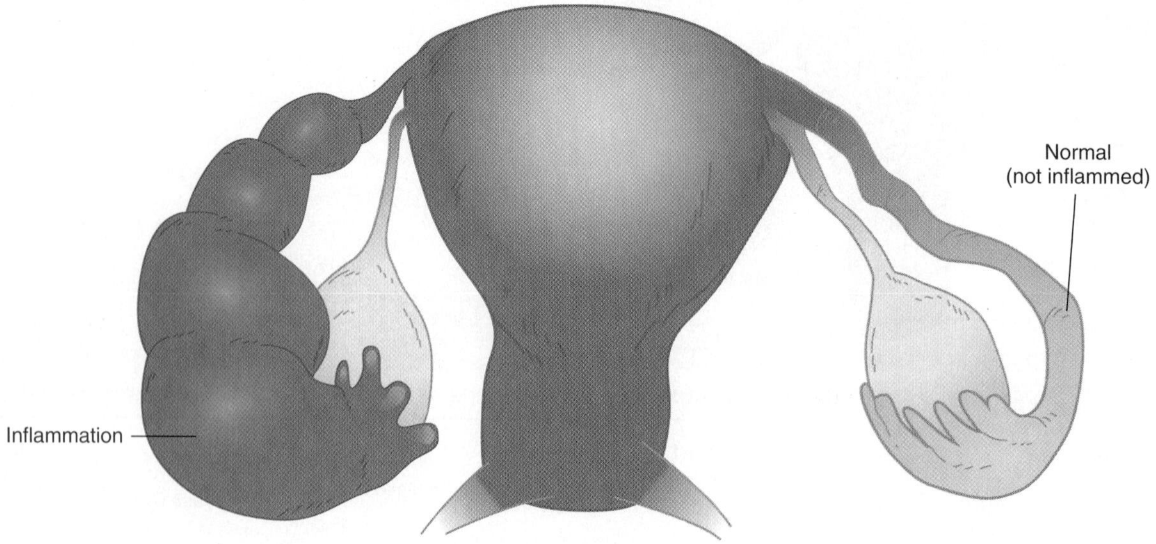

FIGURE 30-4 Pelvic inflammatory disease.

tubes (salpingitis). Finally, the supporting structures around the uterus and fallopian tubes (parametritis) may become infected. Vaginal examination at the health care facility will yield either cervical, uterine, or adnexal tenderness. In addition, the patient will usually have one of the following signs or symptoms: oral temperature greater than 101°F (>38.3°C), purulent vaginal discharge, or abnormal lab values (ie, elevated erythrocyte sedimentation rate, elevated C-reactive protein, or positive cultures for gonorrhea or trichomonas). Many women have mild symptoms or signs such as abnormal bleeding, dyspareunia (pain with sexual intercourse), or vaginal discharge. The inflammation often follows the onset of menstrual bleeding by 7 to 10 days. At that time, the reproductive organs are vulnerable to bacterial infection because the lining of the uterus has been shed during menstruation.

PID often is accompanied by pain on ambulation; the patient bends forward and takes short, slow steps, often guarding the abdomen ("PID shuffle"). Consequences of PID include secondary infertility, ectopic pregnancies, and tubo-ovarian abscesses. In severe cases, the reproductive organs may need to be removed surgically. Definitive treatment usually consists of antibiotic therapy, which helps control the infection and prevent damage to the fallopian tubes.

Prehospital care is primarily supportive for all infections that affect the female reproductive system. In most cases, evaluation and care by a physician are required. Without treatment, abscess, ectopic pregnancy, chronic pain or infertility can occur.[2]

Bartholin Abscess

Bartholin abscess is an accumulation of pus that forms a lump (swelling) in one of the Bartholin glands. It occurs when blockage of the duct of the gland allows an infection to develop. The abscess can take years to form, or it may arise quickly, over several days. Signs and symptoms include swelling and inflammation of the gland and a visible lump on one side of the vaginal opening. Fever also may be present. Any activity that puts pressure on the vulva (including walking, sitting, and sexual intercourse) can cause severe pain and discomfort.

After examination by a physician, treatment may include a biopsy to rule out malignancy, surgical incision to drain the infected gland, and oral antibiotic therapy. In a few cases, infections recur. Surgery sometimes is required for recurrent infections.

Vaginitis

Vaginitis (vulvovaginitis) is inflammation of the vagina that can occur from infectious and noninfectious causes. It can occur in young girls and women of all ages but is most common in postmenopausal and postpartum women secondary to hormonal changes resulting in atrophic vaginitis. It is a very common disease that affects millions of women each year. Many cases of vaginitis result from *Candida* (yeast) infections, bacterial infections (bacterial vaginosis), and the sexually transmitted disease trichomoniasis (see Chapter 27, *Infectious and Communicable Diseases*). Vaginitis also can be caused by parasites, viruses, and poor personal hygiene. Patients with vaginitis often complain of irritation and itchiness of the genital area, in addition to the following:

- Inflammation (redness and swelling) of the labia majora, labia minora, or perineal area
- Vaginal discharge
- Foul vaginal odor
- Discomfort or burning with urination

NOTE
Noninfectious vaginitis usually is caused by an allergic reaction (eg, to detergents, soaps) or irritation from vaginal sprays, douches, and spermicidal products. This form of vaginitis can cause the same signs and symptoms as the infectious form.

Depending on the cause of the infection, treatment for vaginitis may include antiyeast or antifungal creams, vaginal suppositories, and antibiotics. Patients are advised not to engage in sexual activity until the infection has resolved. Vaginitis can be spread to sexual partners, who also may require treatment if the etiology is infectious in nature.

Ruptured Ovarian Cyst

A **ruptured ovarian cyst** can be a gynecologic emergency that may result in significant internal hemorrhage. An ovarian cyst is a thin-walled, fluid-filled sac on the surface of the ovary (**FIGURE 30-5**). The abdominal pain caused by an ovarian cyst may result from rapid expansion, torsion that produces ischemia (described later), or acute rupture. The type of cyst most prone to rupture is the corpus luteum cyst, which forms as a result of hemorrhage in a mature corpus luteum. Because the corpus luteum develops after ovulation

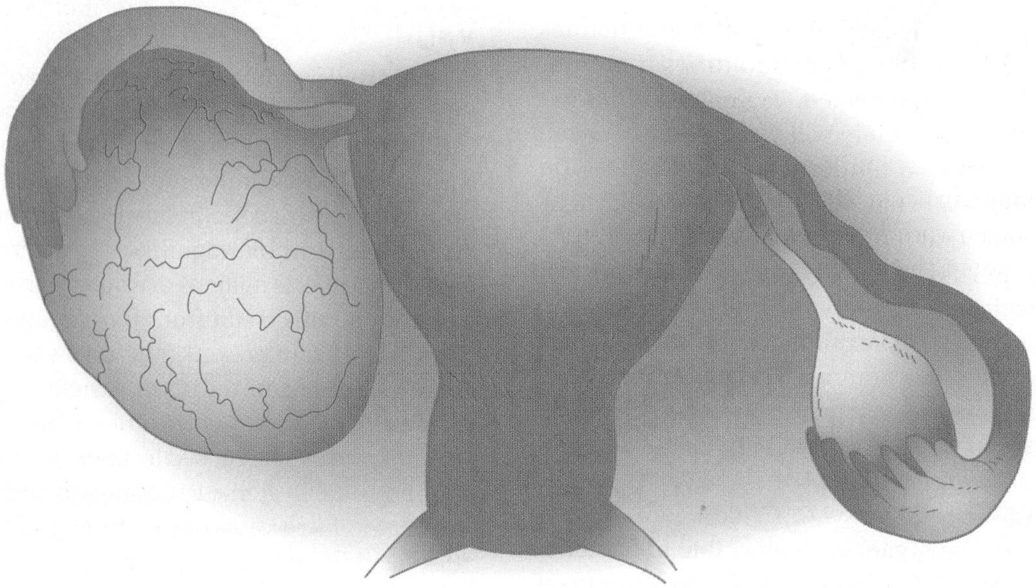

FIGURE 30-5 Ovarian cyst.

(day 14 of the 28-day cycle), most ruptures occur about 1 week before menstrual bleeding is to begin. However, some patients with a ruptured ovarian cyst have vaginal bleeding or report a late or missed period at the time of rupture.

> CRITICAL THINKING
>
> Consider a patient you suspect has a ruptured ovarian cyst. How would you assess for the possibility of bleeding?

A ruptured ovarian cyst can result in localized, one-sided lower abdominal pain. A ruptured cyst also can result in generalized signs of peritonitis if massive hemorrhage has occurred. The onset of pain often is associated with minimal abdominal trauma, sexual intercourse, or exercise.

Ovarian Torsion

Ovarian torsion is the twisting of the ovary. Numerous conditions can cause such torsion, including congenital abnormalities, ovarian cysts or tumors, disease that affects the fallopian tube or ovary, adhesions from previous pelvic surgeries, trauma, and others. As a rule, torsion affects only one ovary and commonly the oviduct (adnexal torsion). Ovarian torsion is the fifth most common gynecologic surgical emergency. Women who are of childbearing age, pregnant, or taking infertility treatment are at highest risk.[3]

Signs and symptoms of ovarian torsion include a sudden onset of lower abdominal pain (usually on the right side) that may radiate to the back, pelvis, or thigh. The pain often begins with exercise. The patient usually describes the pain as sharp or stabbing. Often the patient complains of nausea and vomiting. Fever may be present but is usually a late sign. Care by a physician may include pain management and fluid replacement. Surgery may be indicated to manage vascular compromise, peritonitis, or necrosis.

Cystitis

Cystitis is inflammation of the inner lining of the bladder. It usually is caused by a bacterial infection. Both males and females can develop infection. However, cystitis is more common in women, because the urethra is shorter. The main symptom of cystitis is a frequent urge to pass urine, with only a small amount of urine passed each time. Other signs and symptoms may include painful (burning) urination, fever, chills, and lower abdominal pain. The urine occasionally may be foul smelling or contain blood. Cystitis also can occur as a result of a structural abnormality of the ureters (this is common in children) or compression of the urethra as a result of inflammation. Indwelling urinary catheters are another cause. Prompt treatment of cystitis with a complete course of antibiotics usually settles the infection within 24 hours.

Dysmenorrhea and Mittelschmerz

Dysmenorrhea is pain during menstruation. The condition may include headache, faintness, dizziness, nausea, diarrhea, backache, and leg pain. In severe cases, chills, headache, diarrhea, nausea, vomiting, and syncope can occur. Dysmenorrhea occurs more often in women who are not sexually active and women who have not borne children. The lower abdominal pains associated with dysmenorrhea are thought to be related to muscular contraction of the myometrium (the muscular layer of the uterus). These muscle contractions are mediated by local prostaglandins. Other factors associated with dysmenorrhea include infection, inflammation, and the presence of an intrauterine contraceptive device.

Mittelschmerz is German for "middle pain." This pain may occur from the rupture of the graafian follicle and bleeding from the ovary during the menstrual cycle. Mittelschmerz is characterized by pain in the right or left lower quadrant of the abdomen. The pain occurs in the normal midcycle of a menstrual period (after ovulation) and lasts about 24 to 36 hours. The hormones produced by the ovary also may produce slight endometrial bleeding and low-grade fever. Dysmenorrhea and mittelschmerz do not pose a threat to life. However, evaluation by a physician is required to rule out more serious causes of menstrual pain. Evaluation also is required to differentiate the pain from that of appendicitis and other surgical emergencies.

Endometritis

Endometritis is inflammation of the uterine lining. It usually results from infection. Often, it occurs after childbirth or abortion and usually is caused by retained placental tissue. (The condition also is a feature of PID and other sexually transmitted infections.) Endometritis may affect the uterus and fallopian tubes. If left untreated, endometritis may result in sterility, sepsis, and death. Signs and symptoms of endometritis include fever, purulent vaginal discharge, and lower abdominal pain. Treatment includes removal of any foreign tissue and antibiotic therapy.

Endometriosis

Endometriosis is an abnormal gynecologic condition characterized by the growth of endometrial tissue outside the uterus, usually on the ovaries, fallopian tubes, and other pelvic structures.[4] This condition may occur because fragments of endometrium have been regurgitated backward (during menstruation) through the fallopian tubes into the peritoneal cavity, where the fragments attach and grow as small cystic structures. In a patient with endometriosis, the endometrial tissue functions cyclically and undergoes periodic menstrual breakdown. This process can result in bleeding within cysts, stretching of the cyst wall, and pain.

Endometriosis is more common in women who defer pregnancy. The average age of women found to have endometriosis is 37 years.[5] Characteristic symptoms of endometriosis are pain (particularly dysmenorrhea), painful defecation, and suprapubic soreness. Other common symptoms include vaginal spotting of blood before the start of a period and infertility. After evaluation by a physician, treatment may consist of drug therapy with analgesics or hormones and, in some cases, surgery.

> CRITICAL THINKING
>
> Why do you think patients with endometriosis tend to be infertile?

Ectopic Pregnancy

An **ectopic pregnancy** is a pregnancy that develops outside the uterus (**FIGURE 30-6**). It is the third-leading cause of maternal death and accounts for about 3% to 4% of maternal mortality.[6] The pregnancy most commonly develops in the fallopian tube or ovary. In rare cases, it develops in the abdominal cavity or cervix. An ectopic pregnancy can be a life-threatening emergency. Most ectopic pregnancies are discovered in the first 2 months, often before the woman realizes she is pregnant. Before rupture, the patient may present with nonspecific findings such as vaginal bleeding (usually intermittent and light), which may be accompanied by crampy abdominal or pelvic discomfort. After rupture, signs and symptoms include severe abdominal pain that may radiate to the shoulder (that worsens on inspiration) and vaginal spotting. If rupture occurs, internal hemorrhage, sepsis, and shock may develop.

Once an ectopic pregnancy has been confirmed, surgery is performed to remove the developing fetus, placenta, and any damaged tissue at the site of the pregnancy. Ectopic pregnancy occurs in approximately 1% to 2% of all pregnancies in the United States.[6]

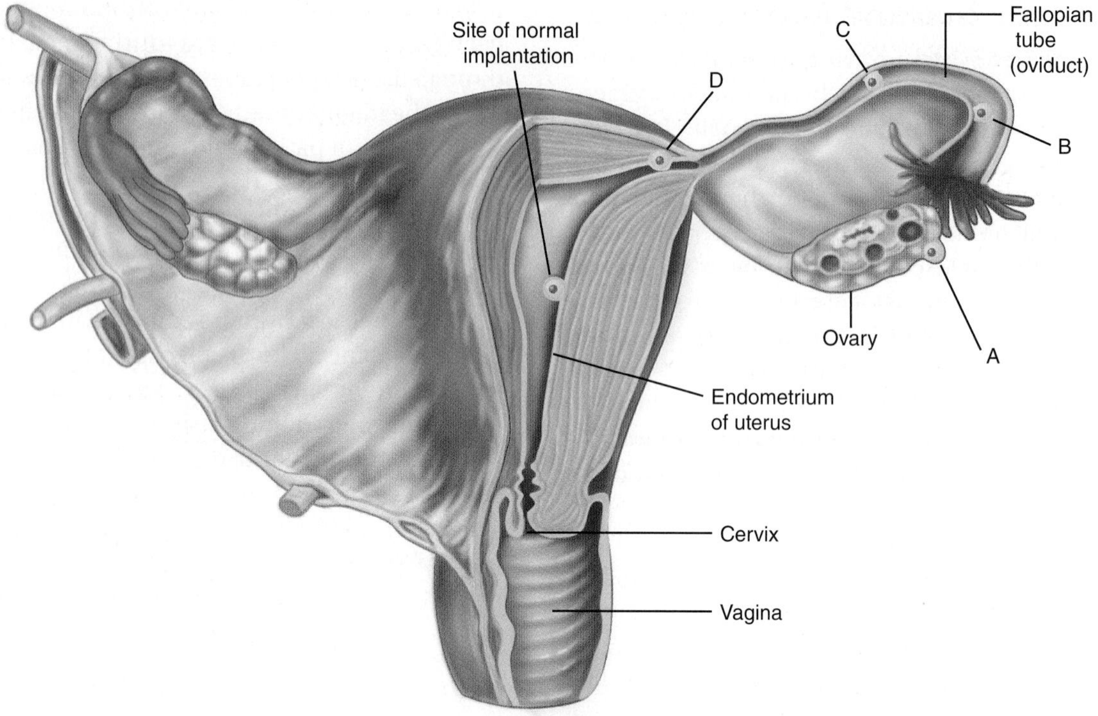

FIGURE 30-6 Ectopic pregnancy. *A*, *B*, *C*, and *D* are potential ectopic sites. The fallopian tube is the most common site for ectopic pregnancies (95%), but they also can occur on the ovary or on the surface of the peritoneum. Normal implantation takes place on the inner lining (endometrium) of the uterus.

Ectopic pregnancy should be considered in any female of reproductive age who has abdominal pain (see Chapter 45, *Obstetrics*). Women at highest risk are those with a history of salpingitis, adhesions related to endometriosis, appendicitis or infection, previous ectopic pregnancy, increasing age, abnormalities of the tube, and cigarette smoking.[7]

Vaginal Bleeding

Vaginal bleeding is the loss of blood through the vagina where the source of bleeding may be the uterus, the cervix, or the vaginal wall itself. The most common source of nontraumatic vaginal bleeding is menstruation. This bleeding rarely results in a request for emergency care. Possible causes of serious nonmenstrual bleeding include the following:

- Spontaneous abortion
- Disorders of the placenta
- Cancer
- Hormonal imbalances (especially menopause)
- Lesions
- PID
- Onset of labor

The paramedic should never assume that vaginal hemorrhage is due to *normal* menstruation. Some causes of vaginal bleeding may be life threatening and can lead to hypovolemic shock and death. (Vaginal

NOTE

Normal menses blood loss is defined as less than 2 ounces (<50 mL); moderate blood loss, 2 to 3 ounces (60 to 80 mL); and heavy blood loss, greater than 3 ounces (>100 mL). Traditionally, patients have been asked to evaluate their blood loss by reporting the number of sanitary pads used in 1 hour. Using the number of sanitary pads to estimate blood loss is unreliable, as different brands and types hold significantly different volumes of fluid. Although patient reports of the number of sanitary pads should be documented, paramedics should use objective measurements (eg, vital signs, oxygen saturation) in assessing and managing these patients.

Modified from: Fraser IS, Warner P, Marantos PA. Estimating menstrual blood loss in women with normal and excessive menstrual fluid volume. *Obstet Gynecol.* 2001 Nov;98(5 Pt 1):806-814; Yahalom S, Gupta A, Dehdashtian S, Scheiner M. Reliability of counting sanitary pads in evaluating severity of vaginal bleeding. *Ann Emerg Med.* 2010;56(3):S314.

passage of clots usually indicates bleeding at a rate greater than menstrual flow.)

Dysfunctional Uterine Bleeding

Dysfunctional uterine bleeding (DUB) is abnormal bleeding that occurs because of changes in hormone levels without any other gynecologic cause. The most common cause of the bleeding is failure of an ovary to release an oocyte (anovulation); consequently, ovulation does not take place. This condition results in continuous, unopposed production of estradiol, which stimulates overgrowth of the endometrium. Without progesterone, the endometrium proliferates and eventually outgrows its blood supply, leading to necrosis. The end result is overproduction of uterine blood flow. With symptoms of DUB, a patient may notice changes in her menstrual cycle, such as the following:[8]

- Vaginal bleeding or spotting that occurs between periods
- Menstrual periods less than 28 days or longer than 35 days apart
- Timing of menstrual periods that changes with each cycle
- Heavier than normal bleeding (passing large clots; changing protection during the night; soaking through a sanitary pad or tampon every hour for 2 to 3 hours in a row)
- Bleeding that lasts for more days than normal or for more than 7 days
- Tenderness and dryness of the vagina

DUB is most common at the extreme ages of a woman's reproductive years, either at the beginning or near the end, but it may occur at any time during reproductive life. Cancer must be ruled out as a cause of bleeding in postmenopausal women. Care by a physician may include a pregnancy test, intravenous hormone therapy, methods to tamponade the bleeding, and sometimes surgery.

Uterine Prolapse

Uterine prolapse is the falling or sliding of the uterus from its normal position in the pelvic cavity into the vaginal canal. The main portion of the uterus (the body) is positioned between the fundus and the cervix (see Chapter 10, *Review of Human Systems*). The uterus is held in place by connective tissue, muscles, and the broad ligament, round ligaments, and uterosacral ligaments. If these muscles and ligaments stretch and weaken, the uterus has inadequate support and descends into the vaginal cavity (**FIGURE 30-7**). Factors that may cause uterine prolapse include the following:[9]

- Trauma during vaginal childbirth
- Large babies and difficult vaginal delivery
- Loss of muscle tone associated with aging
- Menopause and reduced amounts of circulating estrogen
- Pelvic cavity tumors

Obesity, chronic constipation, and chronic obstructive pulmonary disease can put a strain on the muscles and connective tissue in the pelvis. These conditions may also play a role in the development of uterine prolapse.

If the uterine prolapse is mild and the patient is asymptomatic, treatment may not be necessary. In these cases, patients often are advised to make lifestyle changes to slow progression of the prolapse. These

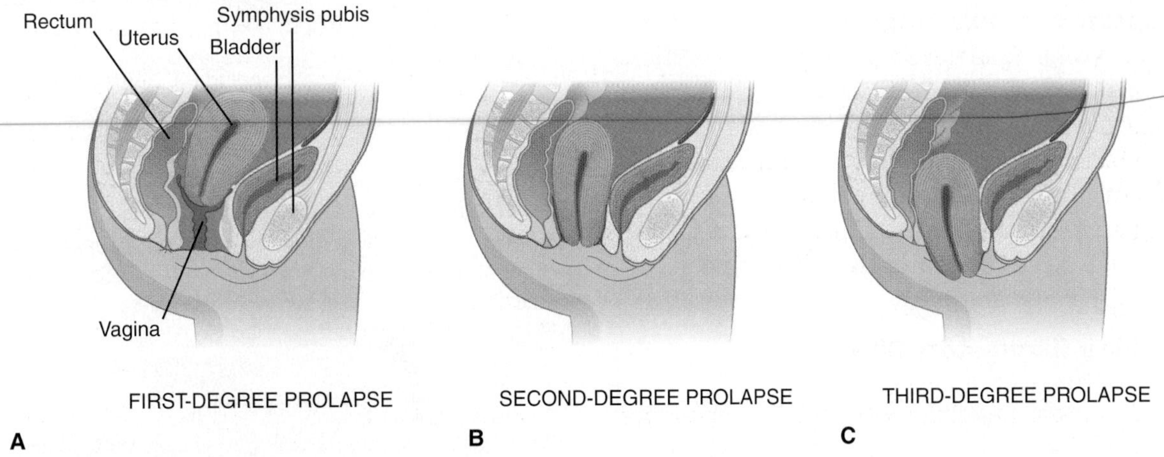

FIGURE 30-7 Degrees of uterine prolapse.

changes may include losing weight, stopping smoking, and preventing coughing. Heavy lifting and straining also should be avoided. Signs and symptoms of a more severe prolapse include patient complaints of feeling like she is "sitting on a small ball," heaviness in the vaginal area, low back pain, difficult or painful intercourse, and vaginal bleeding. In these cases, placement of a vaginal pessary (a device similar to a diaphragm) or surgery may be needed to hold the uterus in place.

Vaginal Foreign Body

It is not uncommon to find a foreign body inserted in the vagina. This is especially true of children, who may insert a foreign body during self-exploration and not tell their parents or caregivers. The foreign body can cause a foul-smelling, purulent discharge with or without vaginal bleeding. Vaginal foreign bodies also may be a result of a psychiatric disorder, unusual sexual practices, or an episode of abuse. Occasionally a tampon, broken portions of condoms, or a pessary is forgotten or lost and causes discomfort and a vaginal discharge. Less common symptoms may include pain or urinary discomfort. No attempt should be made in the prehospital setting to remove a foreign body in the vagina. The patient should be transported for evaluation by a physician.

Assessment and Management of Gynecologic Emergencies

Finding the cause of lower abdominal pain is difficult in both men and women. It can be especially challenging in women, because many gynecologic conditions produce common characteristics. For example, a ruptured ectopic pregnancy, ruptured ovarian cyst, and PID can have identical presentations (**TABLE 30-1**). The goal of prehospital care is to quickly identify the conditions that require aggressive therapy and to rapidly transport the patient for definitive care. Prehospital care includes obtaining a history of the present illness (including a thorough gynecologic history); providing airway, ventilatory, and circulatory support as needed; and transporting the patient for evaluation by a physician.

History of Present Illness and Obstetric History

The paramedic should obtain a history of the present illness to better understand the patient's chief complaint (see Chapter 17, *History Taking*). Important associated symptoms include fever, diaphoresis, syncope, diarrhea, constipation, and abdominal cramping. The interview should include a thorough

TABLE 30-1 Characteristics of Abdominal Pain in Gynecologic Emergencies

Onset	Location	Quality	Radiation	Vaginal Discharge	Menstrual History
Ruptured Ectopic Pregnancy					
Rapid (can become generalized)	Unilateral (can become generalized)	Cramplike, then steady	Shoulder (may indicate intraperitoneal bleeding)	Vaginal bleeding	Amenorrhea, 6 weeks or more since last period
Ruptured Ovarian Cyst					
Sudden	Unilateral (can become generalized)	Steady	Shoulder (may indicate intraperitoneal bleeding)	Possible vaginal bleeding	Usually 1 week before period
Pelvic Inflammatory Disease					
Gradual (can become generalized)	Diffuse, bilateral	Steady ache	Right upper quadrant	Watery, foul-smelling discharge	Usually within 1 week after period

obstetric history. The obstetric history includes the following 10 components:[10]

1. **Pregnancy.** The paramedic should determine the total number of pregnancies the patient has had and the number of pregnancies that were carried to term (see Chapter 45, *Obstetrics*).
2. **Previous cesarean deliveries.** A **cesarean delivery** is a surgical procedure in which the abdomen and uterus are incised and the baby then is delivered through the abdomen. Cesarean delivery usually is done when maternal or fetal conditions might make vaginal delivery risky. A history of a previous cesarean delivery may indicate a high-risk pregnancy.
3. **Last menstrual period.** The paramedic should obtain information about the patient's last menstrual period. Questions to ask include the following:
   - When did it start (the date)? When did it end (the duration)? Have your menstrual periods occurred regularly?
   - Was your last menstrual period normal for you? Was the menstrual flow heavier or lighter than other periods?
   - Did any bleeding occur between periods?
4. **Possibility of pregnancy.** Some patients may hesitate to disclose a possible pregnancy. They may not answer a direct question honestly (eg, "Could you be pregnant?"). If pregnancy is suspected (but not confirmed by the patient), the paramedic should ask specific questions about missed or late periods, breast tenderness, urinary frequency, morning sickness (nausea and/or vomiting), and unprotected sexual activity to determine the likelihood of a pregnancy.

CRITICAL THINKING

Will a patient always give you accurate information about whether she is pregnant? Why?

5. **History of previous gynecologic problems.** The paramedic should identify any previous gynecologic problems. Knowledge of these problems can be helpful to others who may be involved in the patient's care. Examples of important previous gynecologic problems include infections, bleeding, painful intercourse (**dyspareunia**), miscarriage, abortion, **dilation and curettage (D&C)**, and ectopic pregnancy.

NOTE

D&C is a gynecologic procedure that involves widening of the uterine cervix and scraping away of the endometrium of the uterus. The procedure is used for a variety of conditions, including diagnosing disease of the uterus, correcting heavy or prolonged vaginal bleeding, and emptying the uterus of the products of conception after delivery or abortion.

6. **Present blood loss.** If the patient is actively bleeding, the paramedic should ask questions about the color (bright versus dark red blood), the amount of blood loss (estimated by the number of pads or tampons soaked per hour), and the duration of the bleeding episode.
7. **Vaginal discharge.** If the patient has a discharge, the paramedic should question her about the color, amount, and odor of the discharge. These findings may indicate the presence of infection, sexually transmitted disease, or other illness.
8. **Use and type of contraceptive.** The use and type of contraception is a key part of the obstetric history. For example, the use of birth control pills has been associated with hypertension and pulmonary embolus. Also, intrauterine devices can cause intrauterine bleeding and infection. Other methods of contraception include the withdrawal or rhythm method (which may increase the likelihood of pregnancy), the use of spermicides and condoms, implanted contraceptives (eg, Nexplanon), and surgical tubal ligation (a permanent form of female sterilization in which the fallopian tubes are severed and sealed).
9. **History of trauma to the reproductive system.** The paramedic should question all patients about any injury to the reproductive tract. Such an injury may be responsible for vaginal bleeding or discharge. The paramedic should ask a sexually active patient whether pain or bleeding has occurred during or after intercourse.
10. **Degree of emotional distress.** The paramedic should evaluate the patient's emotional distress. Factors that may be responsible for a patient's emotional distress include personal health issues, depression, an unwanted pregnancy, and financial worries.

Physical Examination

The physical examination should be conducted in a comforting, professional manner with consideration shown for the patient's modesty, privacy, and discomfort. When evaluating the potential for serious blood loss, the paramedic should assess the patient's skin and mucous membranes for color, cyanosis, or pallor. Assessment of vital signs should include orthostatic measurements. If indicated, an external vaginal exam may be performed to identify hemorrhage or obvious vaginal discharge, and the color, amount, and presence of clots or tissue (or both) should be noted. Always have a female present when examining the external genitalia (preferably another EMS provider). The patient's abdomen should be palpated to assess for masses, areas of tenderness, guarding, distention, and rebound tenderness.

Patient Management

Management includes support of the patient's vital functions and administration of high-concentration oxygen if indicated during transport. Intravenous access usually is not needed unless the patient is showing signs of impending shock or has excessive vaginal bleeding. Transport in a position of comfort. Vaginal bleeding is managed with application of sanitary pads or trauma dressings. The vagina should never be packed with dressings or tampons. The paramedic should count the number of soaked pads and should record the number on the patient care report.

During transport, the paramedic should monitor the patient for the onset of serious bleeding. If such bleeding occurs, or if the patient's condition begins to deteriorate, the paramedic should establish one or two large-bore intravenous lines with normal saline or lactated Ringer solution and infuse fluid boluses as necessary to maintain mental status. At this point, electrocardiographic and pulse oximetry monitoring are indicated. Analgesics should be considered.

Sexual Assault

Sexual assault is a crime of violence with serious physical and psychological implications. Anyone of either sex at any age can be sexually assaulted (see Chapter 49, *Abuse and Neglect*). Women and girls, however, are most often the victims. Estimates indicate that one in five women will experience a completed or attempted rape during her lifetime and that many of these crimes will go unreported.[11]

Often the paramedic is first to encounter these patients. Tact, kindness, and sensitivity during the patient care episode are essential.

CRITICAL THINKING

How do you feel about rape? How would you manage a patient who has been raped?

DID YOU KNOW?

Rape and Date Rape

Rape occurs when sex is nonconsensual (not agreed upon) or when a person forces or attempts to force another person to have sex against his or her will. Rape includes intercourse in the vagina, anus, or mouth. It is a felony offense that can happen to men, women, and children. Rape can cause physical or emotional harm, or both, to the victim.

Date rape is nonconsensual sex between people who are already acquainted (eg, friends, acquaintances, people who are dating). The difference between rape and date rape is that in cases of date rape, the victim agreed to spend time with the attacker. Date rape often occurs in the context of domestic violence. It sometimes involves the use of illegal "date rape drugs" that produce amnesia and anesthesia in the victim. These drugs include ketamine, gamma hydroxybutyrate (GHB), and flunitrazepam (Rohypnol [roofies]). Date rape is still rape. It is a felony offense. A nationally representative survey found the following:

- In cases involving female victims, perpetrators were reported to be intimate partners (51.1%), family members (12.5%), and acquaintances (40.8%) and strangers (13.8%).
- In cases involving male victims, perpetrators were reported to be acquaintances (52.4%) and strangers (15.1%).

Modified from: National Center for Injury Prevention and Control, Centers for Disease Control and Prevention. Sexual violence: facts at a glance, 2012. Centers for Disease Control and Prevention website. https://www.cdc.gov/violenceprevention/pdf/sv-datasheet-a.pdf. Published 2012. Accessed February 9, 2018.

Initially, paramedics should care for a victim of sexual assault as they would any other injured patient. The first priority is to manage any injury that poses a threat to life. After that, however, the approach should be modified with regard to history taking and the physical examination. Before taking a history or performing an examination, the paramedic should move the patient to a private area. If possible, the patient should be interviewed and examined by a paramedic of the same gender.

> SHOW ME THE EVIDENCE
>
> Feldhaus and colleagues interviewed women who reported to the emergency department of an urban level I trauma center for any cause during random periods in 1997. These women were not critically ill. The patients were asked if they had ever been sexually assaulted at any time in their lives. During that time, 360 patients who were eligible for the researchers' study consented to be enrolled in it. Of that group, 39% said they had been sexually assaulted at some point in their life, and an additional 12% reported an attempted sexual assault. When the sexual assault occurred during adulthood, 70% of the time the victim knew the perpetrator. Another 8% of the assaults involved multiple attackers. A weapon was used or threatened to be used during the assault 40% of the time. Of this adult assault group, only 45% reported the assault to the police. A report was more likely to be filed if the woman did not know her attacker. Those who were assaulted sought medical aid less than one-half the time. This study revealed a high lifetime incidence of sexual assault in this group of women.
>
> *Modified from*: Feldhaus KM, Houry D, Kaminsky R. Lifetime sexual assault prevalence rates and reporting practices in an emergency department population. *Ann Emerg Med*. 2000;36:23-27.

History Taking

As a rule, victims of sexual assault should not be questioned in detail about the incident in the prehospital setting. The history should be limited to the elements needed to provide emergency care. For example, questions about penetration, sexual history, or sexual practices are irrelevant to prehospital care. They only add to the patient's emotional stress. The patient should be allowed to speak openly, and all information should be recorded accurately and thoroughly. Common reactions to sexual assault include anxiety, withdrawal and silence, denial, anger, and fear.

Assessment

The physical examination should identify any physical trauma, including trauma outside the pelvic area, that requires immediate attention. Facial fractures, human bites of the hands and breasts, long bone fractures, broken ribs, and trauma to the abdomen are not unusual. The paramedic should examine the genitalia only if a severe injury is present or suspected. When possible, a paramedic of the same gender should provide care and explain all procedures before initiating them. All examination findings should be documented, including the patient's emotional state, the condition of the patient's clothing, obvious injuries, and any patient care provided. A professional attitude is important. The paramedic's feelings about the victim or the assault should not affect the delivery of care.

Management

After the management of life-threatening injuries, emotional support is the most important patient care procedure paramedics can offer a victim of sexual assault. The paramedic should provide a safe environment for the patient and should respond appropriately to the victim's physical and emotional needs. Paramedics also should be aware of the need to preserve evidence from the crime scene (further described in Chapter 55, *Crime Scene Awareness*). Special considerations include the following:

- Handle clothing as little as possible.
- Do not clean wounds unless absolutely necessary.
- Do not allow the patient to drink or brush the teeth.
- Use paper bags; do not use plastic bags for bloodstained articles.
- Bag each clothing item separately.
- Ask the victim not to change clothes or bathe.
- Disturb the crime scene as little as possible.

Summary

- Menstruation is the normal, periodic discharge of blood, mucus, and cellular debris from the uterine mucosa. Ovulation is the release of a secondary oocyte from the ovary.
- Pelvic inflammatory disease results from infection of the cervix, uterus, fallopian tubes, and ovaries and their supporting structures.
- Bartholin abscess is a buildup of pus in one of the Bartholin glands.
- Vaginitis is inflammation of the vagina that can occur from infectious and noninfectious causes.
- A ruptured ovarian cyst occurs when a thin-walled, fluid-filled sac on the ovary ruptures. This condition can cause internal hemorrhage.

- Ovarian torsion is twisting of the ovary caused by another condition or disease.
- Cystitis is inflammation of the inner lining of the bladder. It usually is caused by a bacterial infection.
- Dysmenorrhea is characterized by painful menses. It may be associated with headache, faintness, dizziness, nausea, diarrhea, backache, and leg pain.
- *Mittelschmerz* is German for "middle pain." This pain may occur from the rupture of the graafian follicle and bleeding from the ovary during the menstrual cycle.
- Endometritis is inflammation of the uterine lining. Endometriosis is characterized by endometrial tissue growing outside the uterus.
- An ectopic pregnancy is a pregnancy that develops outside the uterus. Rupture of an ectopic pregnancy can cause life-threatening hemorrhage.
- Vaginal bleeding is the loss of blood through the vagina where the source of bleeding may be the uterus, the cervix, or the vaginal wall itself.
- Uterine prolapse occurs when the uterus descends into the vagina.
- Vaginal foreign bodies can cause vaginal discharge, pain, and urinary discomfort.
- The history obtained from a patient with a gynecologic emergency should include the pregnancy history, history of cesarean births, last menstrual period, possibility of pregnancy, history of previous gynecologic problems, blood loss, vaginal discharge, contraceptives used, history of trauma to the reproductive system, and degree of emotional distress.
- The goal of prehospital care of lower abdominal pain in the female is to obtain a history (including a gynecologic history); provide airway, ventilatory, and circulatory support as needed; and provide transport for evaluation by a physician.
- Sexual assault is a crime of violence. It can have serious physical and psychological effects.
- Paramedics should be aware of the need to preserve evidence from a sexual assault crime scene.

References

1. Division of STD Prevention, National Center for HIV/AIDS, Viral Hepatitis, STD, and TB Prevention, Centers for Disease Control and Prevention. 2016 sexually transmitted diseases surveillance. Table 44. Selected STDs and complications—initial visits to physicians' offices, national disease and therapeutic index, United States, 1966–2015. Centers for Disease Control and Prevention website. https://www.cdc.gov/std/stats16/tables/44.htm. Updated September 26, 2017. Accessed February 9, 2018.
2. Division of STD Prevention, National Center for HIV/AIDS, Viral Hepatitis, STD, and TB Prevention, Centers for Disease Control and Prevention 2015 sexually transmitted diseases treatment guidelines. Pelvic inflammatory disease (PID). Centers for Disease Control and Prevention website. https://www.cdc.gov/std/tg2015/pid.htm. Updated June 4, 2015. Accessed February 9, 2018.
3. Laufer MR. Ovarian and fallopian tube torsion. UpToDate website. https://www.uptodate.com/contents/ovarian-and-fallopian-tube-torsion. Updated January 14, 2018. Accessed February 9, 2018.
4. Women's Heath Care Physicians. Having a baby after age 35. The American College of Obstetricians and Gynecologists website. https://www.acog.org/Patients/FAQs/Having-a-Baby-After-Age-35. Published September 2017. Accessed February 9, 2018.
5. Senie RT. *Epidemiology of Women's Health*. Burlington, MA: Jones and Bartlett Learning; 2014.
6. Centers for Disease Control and Prevention. Ectopic pregnancy mortality. *Morbidity and Mortality Weekly Report*. Centers for Disease Control and Prevention website. https://www.cdc.gov/mmwr/preview/mmwrhtml/mm6106a2.htm. Updated February 17, 2012. Accessed February 9, 2018.
7. Tillman E. Clinician instructor materials. Centers for Disease Control and Prevention website. https://www.cdc.gov/des/hcp/resources/materials/clinician_ins_materials.pdf. Accessed February 9, 2018.
8. US National Library of Medicine. Abnormal uterine bleeding. MedlinePlus website. https://medlineplus.gov/ency/article/000903.htm. Updated December 21, 2017. Accessed February 9, 2018.
9. Tsikouras P, Dafopoulos A, Vrachnis N, et al. Uterine prolapse in pregnancy: risk factors, complications and management. *J Matern Fetal Neonatal Med*. 2014;27(3):297-302.
10. National Highway Traffic Safety Administration. *The National EMS Education Standards*, Washington, DC: US Department of Transportation/National Highway Traffic Safety Administration; 2009.
11. Black MC, Basile KC, Breiding MJ, et al. *The National Intimate Partner and Sexual Violence Survey: 2010 Summary Report*. Atlanta, GA: National Center for Injury Prevention and Control, Centers for Disease Control and Prevention; 2011.

Suggested Readings

Benrubi GI. *Handbook of Obstetric and Gynecologic Emergencies*. 4th ed. Philadelphia, PA: Lipincott Williams & Wilkins; 2010.

Dantoni SE, Papadakos, PJ, eds. Obstetrics and gynecology emergencies. *Crit Care Clin*. 2016;32(1):xi-xii.

Facts and figures: ending violence against women. UN Women website. http://www.unwomen.org/en/what-we-do/ending-violence-against-women/facts-and-figures. Updated August 2017. Accessed February 9, 2018.

National Center for Injury Prevention and Control, Division of Violence Prevention. Violence prevention: sexual violence. Centers for Disease Control and Prevention website. https://www.cdc.gov/violenceprevention/sexualviolence/index.html. Updated April 14, 2017. Accessed February 9, 2018.

PTSD: National Center for PTSD. Sexual assault against females. US Department of Veterans Affairs website. https://www.ptsd.va.gov/public/ptsd-overview/women/sexual-assault-females.asp. Updated August 13, 2015. Accessed February 9, 2018.

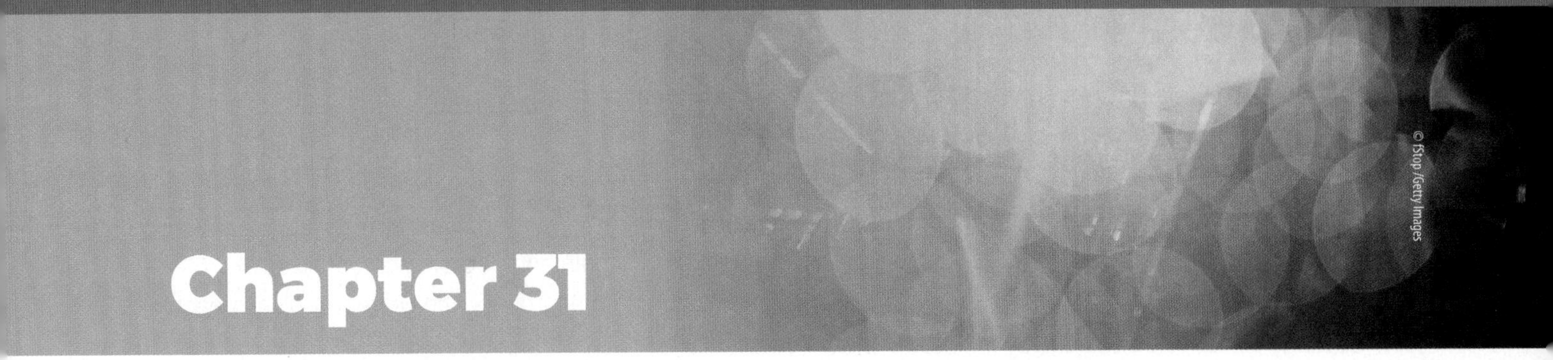

Chapter 31

Hematology

NATIONAL EMS EDUCATION STANDARD COMPETENCIES

Medicine

Integrates assessment findings with principles of epidemiology and pathophysiology to formulate a field impression and implement a comprehensive treatment/disposition plan for a patient with a medical complaint.

Hematology

Anatomy, physiology, pathophysiology, assessment, and management of
- Sickle cell crisis (pp 1176–1179)
- Clotting disorders (pp 1164–1165, 1173–1176)

Anatomy, physiology, epidemiology, pathophysiology, psychosocial impact, presentations, prognosis, and management of common or major hematological diseases and/or emergencies
- Sickle cell crisis (pp 1176–1179)
- Blood transfusion complications (p 1171)
- Hemostatic disorders (pp 1164–1165, 1173–1176)
- Lymphomas (pp 1170–1173)
- Red blood cell disorders (pp 1166–1168, 1173, 1176–1179)
- White blood cell disorders (pp 1168–1173, 1179)
- Coagulopathies (pp 1173–1174)

OBJECTIVES

Upon completion of this chapter, the paramedic student will be able to:
1. Describe the physiology of blood and its components. (pp 1161–1164)
2. Discuss the pathophysiology and signs and symptoms of specific hematologic disorders. (pp 1165–1179)
3. Outline the general assessment and management of patients with hematologic disorders. (pp 1179–1180)

KEY TERMS

acute chest syndrome A serious vaso-occlusive crisis in the pulmonary vasculature that often presents as an abnormal consolidation on a chest radiograph in a patient with sickle cell disease.

albumin A water-soluble protein containing carbon, hydrogen, oxygen, nitrogen, and sulfur.

anemia A decrease in the blood hemoglobin level.

basophils White blood cells that promote inflammation.

bilirubin The orange-yellow pigment of bile, formed principally from the breakdown of hemoglobin in red blood cells after termination of their normal life span.

blood clot The end result of the clotting process in blood. It normally consists of red blood cells, white blood cells, and platelets enmeshed in an insoluble fibrin network.

clotting cascade The blood clotting system or coagulation pathway.

clotting factors Substances in the blood that act in sequence to stop bleeding by forming a clot.

differential count A laboratory test that identifies the different types of leukocytes present in blood; also called the diff.

disseminated intravascular coagulopathy (DIC) A grave coagulopathy that results from the overstimulation of the clotting and anticlotting processes in response to disease or injury.

eosinophils White blood cells that act as cellular mediators of inflammation; thought to play a key role in asthma and allergy as well as parasitic infections.

fibrinogen A soluble blood protein that is converted into insoluble fibrin during clotting.

globulins Simple proteins classified based on their solubility, mobility, and size.

hematology The scientific study of blood and blood-forming organs.

hemoglobin A complex protein–iron compound in the blood that carries oxygen to the cells from the lungs and carbon dioxide away from the cells to the lungs.

hemolysis The breakdown of red blood cells and the release of hemoglobin.

hemolytic anemia A condition in which delivery of oxygen to tissues is reduced because of an increase in hemolysis of erythrocytes.

hemophilia A group of hereditary bleeding disorders in which one of the factors necessary for blood coagulation is deficient.

hemophilia A A condition caused by a deficiency of coagulation factor VIII. It is considered the classic type of hemophilia.

hemophilia B A condition caused by a deficiency of coagulation factor IX.

hemostasis The cessation of bleeding by mechanical or chemical means or by substances that arrest the blood flow.

Hodgkin lymphoma A malignant disorder of the lymphatic system characterized by the presence of Reed-Sternberg cells at biopsy. It is associated with pain and progressive enlargement of lymphoid tissue.

iron-deficiency anemia Anemia caused by inadequate supplies of iron needed to synthesize hemoglobin.

leukemia A type of cancer in which an abnormal proliferation of white blood cells occurs, usually in the bone marrow.

leukopenia A decrease in the number of white blood cells (most commonly neutrophils).

lymphocytes White blood cells formed in lymphoid tissue; the primary cells found in lymph fluid.

lymphoma A group of cancers of the immune system and white blood cells. The two main categories are Hodgkin lymphoma and non-Hodgkin lymphoma.

macrophages Phagocytic cells in the immune system created from monocytes in the tissue.

malignant Very dangerous or virulent; likely to cause death; a cancerous tumor that tends to metastasize.

monocytes White blood cells found in lymph nodes, spleen, bone marrow, and loose connective tissue. These can differentiate into a macrophages.

multiple myeloma A malignant neoplasm of plasma cells that tend to accumulate in the bone marrow, causing bone pain and pathologic fractures.

neutrophils Small, phagocytic white blood cells, each of which has a lobed nucleus and small granules in the cytoplasm; the most abundant leukocytes in circulating blood.

non-Hodgkin lymphoma Cancer of the lymphocytes, which can accumulate in any tissue but particularly collect in the lymph nodes, spleen, and other organs of the immune system.

pernicious anemia Anemia that results from a vitamin B_{12} deficiency.

plasma The fluid portion of blood.

platelet plug A plug consisting of a mass of linked platelets that seals an injured vessel; part of the clotting process.

platelets Fragments of cells. These initiate the clotting process.

polycythemia A condition characterized by an unusually large number of red blood cells in the blood as a result of their increased production by the bone marrow.

primary polycythemia A rare disorder of the bone marrow in which increased production of red blood cells causes the blood to thicken; also known as polycythemia vera.

prothrombin A chemical that is part of the clotting cascade; the precursor of thrombin.

prothrombin activator A substance that combines with an enzyme to increase its catalytic activity. It converts prothrombin to thrombin.

red bone marrow Specialized soft tissue found in many bones of infants and children, in the spongy bone of the proximal epiphyses of the humerus and femur. In adults, it is mostly found in the sternum, ribs, and vertebral bodies. It is essential in the manufacture of red blood cells. Also known as red marrow.

secondary polycythemia A condition of increased production of red blood cells caused by reduced air pressure and low oxygen concentration. It may be a natural response to chronic hypoxia.

sickle cell anemia Low hemoglobin as a result of sickle cell disease.

sickle cell crisis An acute, episodic, vaso-occlusive condition causing severe pain. It occurs in people with sickle cell disease.

sickle cell disease A debilitating and unpredictable recessive genetic illness that produces an abnormal type of hemoglobin with an inferior oxygen-carrying capacity.

thrombin An enzyme formed in plasma as part of the clotting process. It causes fibrinogen to change to fibrin, which is essential in the formation of a clot.

thrombocytopenia An abnormal hematologic condition in which the number of platelets is reduced.

tumor lysis syndrome A group of metabolic complications that can occur after treatment of cancer, usually non-Hodgkin lymphomas and acute leukemias. It results from the breakdown products of dying cancer cells being released into the bloodstream.

yellow marrow Specialized soft tissue (mainly adipose) found in the compact bone of most adult epiphyses.

Hematology *is the study of blood and blood-forming organs. Dysfunction in the hematologic system can affect other body systems, resulting in the variety of clinical manifestations that characterize hematologic disorders. Prehospital care for most patients with hematologic disorders is mainly supportive, but the paramedic's knowledge of these diseases enhances assessment skills. It also provides an understanding of the treatments that these patients need.*

Blood and Blood Components

As described in Chapter 10, *Review of Human Systems*, blood is composed of cells and formed elements surrounded by plasma. Approximately 95% of the volume of formed elements consists of red blood cells (RBCs; erythrocytes); the remaining 5% consists of white blood cells (WBCs; leukocytes) and cell fragments (platelets) (**FIGURE 31-1** and **TABLE 31-1**). The continuous movement of blood keeps the formed elements dispersed throughout the plasma, where they are available to carry out their chief functions:[1] (1) delivery of substances needed for cellular metabolism in the tissues, (2) defense against invading microorganisms and injury, and (3) maintenance of acid–base balance.

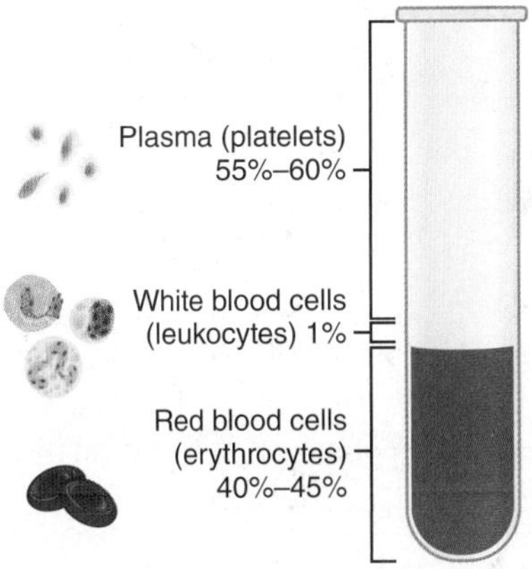

FIGURE 31-1 Blood settles into three distinct, proportional layers when treated with salt. The transparent yellow layer at the top is plasma—the liquid portion of blood through which solid elements travel. White blood cells (WBCs) settle in the narrow white band in the center, and red blood cells (RBCs), which give blood its crimson color, fall to the bottom of the flask. RBCs outnumber WBCs 600 to 1.

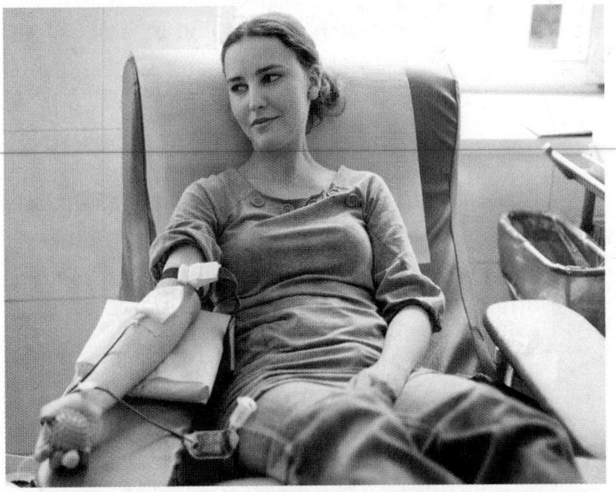

All types of blood cells are formed within the red bone marrow, which is present in all tissues at birth. In adults, the **red bone marrow** is primarily found in membranous bone such as the vertebrae, pelvis, sternum, and ribs. **Yellow marrow** produces some WBCs but is composed mainly of connective tissue and fat. Other blood-forming organs include the following:

- The spleen, which stores large quantities of blood and produces lymphocytes, specifically plasma cells, which produce antibodies

TABLE 31-1 Cellular Components of the Blood

Cell	Structural Characteristics	Normal Amounts in Circulating Blood	Function	Life Span
Erythrocyte (red blood cell)	Nonnucleated cytoplasmic disk containing hemoglobin	4.2–6.2 million/mm^3	Gas transport to and from tissue cells and lungs	80–120 days
Leukocyte (white blood cell)	Nucleated cell	5,000–10,000/mm^3	Body defense mechanisms	Described below
Lymphocyte	Mononuclear immunocyte	25%–33% of leukocyte count (leukocyte differential)	Humoral and cell-mediated immunity	Days or years depending on type
Monocyte and macrophage	Large mononuclear phagocyte	3%–7% of leukocyte differential	Phagocytosis; mononuclear phagocyte system	Months or years
Eosinophil	Segmented polymorphonuclear granulocyte	1%–4% of leukocyte differential	Phagocytosis, antibody-mediated defense against parasites, allergic reactions, associated with Hodgkin lymphoma, recovery phase of infection	2–5 days
Neutrophil	Segmented polymorphonuclear granulocyte	57%–67% of leukocyte differential	Phagocytosis, particularly during early phase of inflammation	4 days
Basophil	Segmented polymorphonuclear granulocyte	0–0.75% of leukocyte differential	Unknown, but associated with allergic reactions and mechanical irritation	2–3 days
Platelet	Irregularly shaped cytoplasmic fragment (not a cell)	140,000–340,000/mm^3	Hemostasis after vascular injury; normal coagulation and clot formation/retraction	8–11 days

Modified from: McCance KL, Huether SE. *Pathophysiology: The Biologic Basis for Disease in Adults and Children.* 7th ed. St. Louis, MO: Mosby; 2014.

- The liver, a blood-forming organ only during intrauterine life, which plays an important role in the coagulation process

Plasma

Plasma, the clear portion of blood, is approximately 92% water. In addition to salts, metals, and inorganic compounds, plasma contains three important proteins:

- **Albumin**—the most plentiful protein—is similar to egg white and gives blood its gummy texture. The presence of these large proteins keeps the water concentration of blood low so that water diffuses readily from tissues into the blood.
- **Globulins** (alpha, beta, and gamma) transport other proteins and provide the body with immunity to disease.
- **Fibrinogen** is essential for blood clotting.

Plasma proteins perform various functions, including maintaining blood pH (acting as either an acid or a base); transporting fat-soluble vitamins, hormones, and carbohydrates; and allowing the body to digest them temporarily for food.

Red Blood Cells

RBCs, the most abundant cells in the body, are primarily responsible for tissue oxygenation. They are composed mainly of water and the red-colored protein **hemoglobin**. RBC production occurs in the bone marrow and continues throughout life to replace blood cells that grow old and die, are killed by disease, or are lost through bleeding. During RBC production, the cells produce hemoglobin until the concentration of this protein accounts for 95% of the dry weight of the cell. At this point, the cell expels its nucleus, giving the cell its characteristic pinched look (**FIGURE 31-2**). The new shape of the RBC increases the surface area of the cell and, therefore, its oxygen-carrying potential. RBCs have a life span of about 120 days. As the cells age, their internal chemical machinery weakens, they lose elasticity, and they become trapped in small blood vessels in the bone marrow, liver, and spleen. They then are destroyed by specialized WBCs (**macrophages**). Although most of the components of destroyed hemoglobin molecules are used again, some are broken down to the waste product **bilirubin**.

Each RBC contains approximately 270 million hemoglobin molecules. Each hemoglobin molecule carries four oxygen molecules. The normal amount of hemoglobin in blood is about 15 g per 100 mL, although it is usually a little higher in males than in females. The number of RBCs is about 4.2 to 6.2 million cells/mm^2.

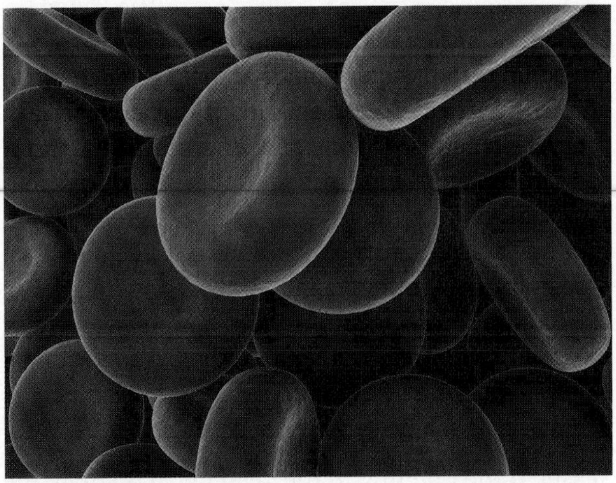

FIGURE 31-2 Mature erythrocytes appear as small rounded disks with nearly hollowed-out centers.

BOX 31-1 Laboratory Tests

Hematocrit is the fraction of the total volume of blood that consists of RBCs. For example, a value of 45% (the normal level) implies that there is 45 mL of RBCs in 100 mL of blood. The normal hematocrit for males is 40% to 54%. In females, a normal hematocrit is 38% to 47%. A low hematocrit value often indicates anemia, which may result from trauma, surgery, internal bleeding, nutritional deficiency (eg, iron or vitamin B_{12}), bone marrow disease, or sickle cell disease. Because hematocrit measures the percentage of formed elements in blood, a low hematocrit may also indicate relative volume overload. A high hematocrit value may be caused by dehydration, lung disease, certain tumors, polycythemia, and disorders of the bone marrow.

Hemoglobin is reported in grams per 100 mL of blood. The normal hemoglobin level for males is 13.5 to 18 g/100 mL. In women, a normal hemoglobin measurement is 12 to 16 g/100 mL.

The reticulocyte count offers details about the rate of RBC production. A reticulocyte count of less than 0.5% of the RBC count usually indicates a deceleration in the process of RBC formation. A reticulocyte count greater than 1.5% usually indicates an acceleration of RBC formation.

BOX 31-1 describes the various laboratory tests used to quantify the components of blood.

White Blood Cells

As described in Chapter 10, *Review of Human Systems*, WBCs arise from the bone marrow and are released into the bloodstream. WBCs destroy foreign substances (eg, bacteria, viruses) and clear the bloodstream of debris. Leukocyte production increases in response to infection, which in turn causes an elevated WBC count in the blood. Chapter 26, *Immune System Disorders*, and Chapter 27, *Infectious and Communicable Diseases*, discuss blood groups, the inflammatory process, and the immune response.

The bone marrow and lymph glands continually produce and maintain a reserve of WBCs. However, there are not many WBCs in the bloodstream of a healthy person—only 5,000 to 10,000 cells/mm^2. **Monocytes** make up about 5% of the total WBC count, though their concentration increases with chronic infections. **Lymphocytes** account for about 27.5%, **neutrophils** about 65%, and **eosinophils** and **basophils** together about 2.5% of the total WBC count. A rise in the number of WBCs aids in the diagnosis of some diseases. For example, an increased WBC count is suggestive of illnesses such as bacterial infection, inflammation, leukemia, trauma, and stress.

The **differential count** (also called the diff) identifies the different types of leukocytes (WBCs) present in blood. This test is performed by spreading a drop of blood on a microscope slide, staining the slide, and examining it under a microscope. Cells are identified by the shape and appearance of the nucleus, the color of cytoplasm (the background of the cell), and the presence and color of granules. The percentage of each cell type is reported. At the same time, RBCs and platelets are examined for abnormalities in appearance.

CRITICAL THINKING

Which body functions are impaired if the number or function of the WBCs is diminished?

Platelets

Platelets (thrombocytes) are small, sticky cell fragments of megakaryocytes (large bone marrow cells that produce platelets). They play an important role in blood clotting. When a blood vessel is cut, platelets travel to the site, where they swell into odd, irregular shapes and adhere to the damaged vessel wall. In this way, platelets plug the leak and allow other cells to stick to them and to form a clot. However, if the damage to the vessel is too great, the platelets chemically signal for the complex clotting process or **clotting cascade** (described later) to begin. Platelets repair millions of ruptured capillaries each day and often render the rest of the clotting cascade unnecessary (BOX 31-2).

BOX 31-2 Clotting Measurements

Clotting time is normally 7 to 10 minutes. The patient bleeds if the clotting time is prolonged; he or she develops intravascular clots if the clotting time is less than normal. Prothrombin time (PT) measures the clotting time of plasma—specifically, the extrinsic clotting cascade (tissue factor pathway). The PT test is used to monitor patients taking certain medications (eg, warfarin), to monitor patients with liver failure, and to diagnose clotting disorders. It specifically evaluates the presence of factors I (fibrinogen), II (prothrombin), V, VIIa, and X. A drop in the concentration of any of these factors will cause the blood to take longer to clot, so a prolonged PT time is considered abnormal. The PT test is used in combination with the partial thromboplastin time (PTT) to screen for hemophilia and other hereditary clotting disorders.

The PTT uses blood to which a chemical has been added to prevent clotting before the test begins. This test measures the integrity of the intrinsic clotting cascade (contact activation pathway), which is affected by some blood-thinning medications (eg, heparin, dabigatran). The PTT can help determine a possible cause of abnormal bleeding or bruising. Increased PTT in a person with a bleeding disorder may indicate that a clotting factor is missing or defective.

The international normalized ratio (INR) helps to standardize the PT, which varies from lab to lab. It is determined by dividing the patient's PT by the mean normal PT of the healthy adult population. The INR is expressed as a number to one decimal place with no unit of measure.

Hemostasis

Hemostasis is the initial physiologic response to wounding that causes bleeding to cease. Hemostasis is initiated when there is a break in the integrity of the vascular endothelium. The vascular reaction or physiology of hemostasis involves vasoconstriction, formation of a platelet plug, coagulation, and the growth of fibrous tissue into the blood clot that permanently closes and seals the injured vessel.

Vasoconstriction resulting from injury is rapid but temporary. In response to injury, severed blood vessels constrict and retract with the aid of the surrounding subcutaneous tissues. This vessel spasm slows blood loss immediately. Vasoconstriction may close the ends of the injured vessels completely. This response usually is sustained for as long as 10 minutes, during which time blood coagulation mechanisms are activated to produce a blood clot.

Platelets adhere to injured blood vessels and to collagen in the connective tissue that surrounds the injured vessel. When the platelets come in contact with the collagen, they swell, become sticky, and secrete chemicals that activate other surrounding platelets. This process, which causes the platelets to adhere to one another, creates a **platelet plug** in the injured vessel. If the opening in the vessel wall is small, the plug may be sufficient to stop blood loss completely. If the opening in the vessel is large, however, a **blood clot** is necessary to arrest the flow of blood.

Blood coagulation occurs as a result of a chemical process that begins within seconds of a severe vessel injury. Coagulation progresses rapidly: Within 3 to 6 minutes after the rupture of a vessel, the entire end of the vessel is filled with a clot. Within 30 minutes, the clot retracts and the vessel is sealed further. The blood-clotting mechanism is a complex process that includes three mechanisms (**FIGURE 31-3**):

1. **Prothrombin activator** is formed in response to rupture or damage of the blood vessel.
2. Prothrombin activator stimulates the conversion of **prothrombin** to **thrombin**.
3. Thrombin, in the presence of calcium ions, acts as an enzyme to convert fibrinogen into fibrin threads. These threads entrap platelets, blood cells, and plasma to form the clot.

The process of hemostasis usually is protective and is required for survival. In some instances, though, hemostasis can result in responses that threaten life and function. Examples include myocardial infarction or stroke.

NOTE

Certain diseases or genetic factors that interrupt the clotting cascade can impair hemostasis, thereby retarding the process of clot formation. Examples include hemophilia, thrombocytopenia (low platelet count), and liver disease, which affects the production of some **clotting factors** (substances in the blood that act in sequence to stop bleeding by forming a clot). Various drugs also can impair coagulation. For example, aspirin decreases platelet activity, and warfarin suppresses the ability of the liver to make certain clotting factors. In any patient with impaired hemostasis, even minor trauma can result in uncontrollable and life-threatening hemorrhage.

Specific Hematologic Disorders

The hematologic disorders presented in this chapter are anemia, leukemia, lymphomas, polycythemia, disseminated intravascular coagulopathy, hemophilia, thrombocytopenia, sickle cell disease, and multiple myeloma (BOX 31-3).

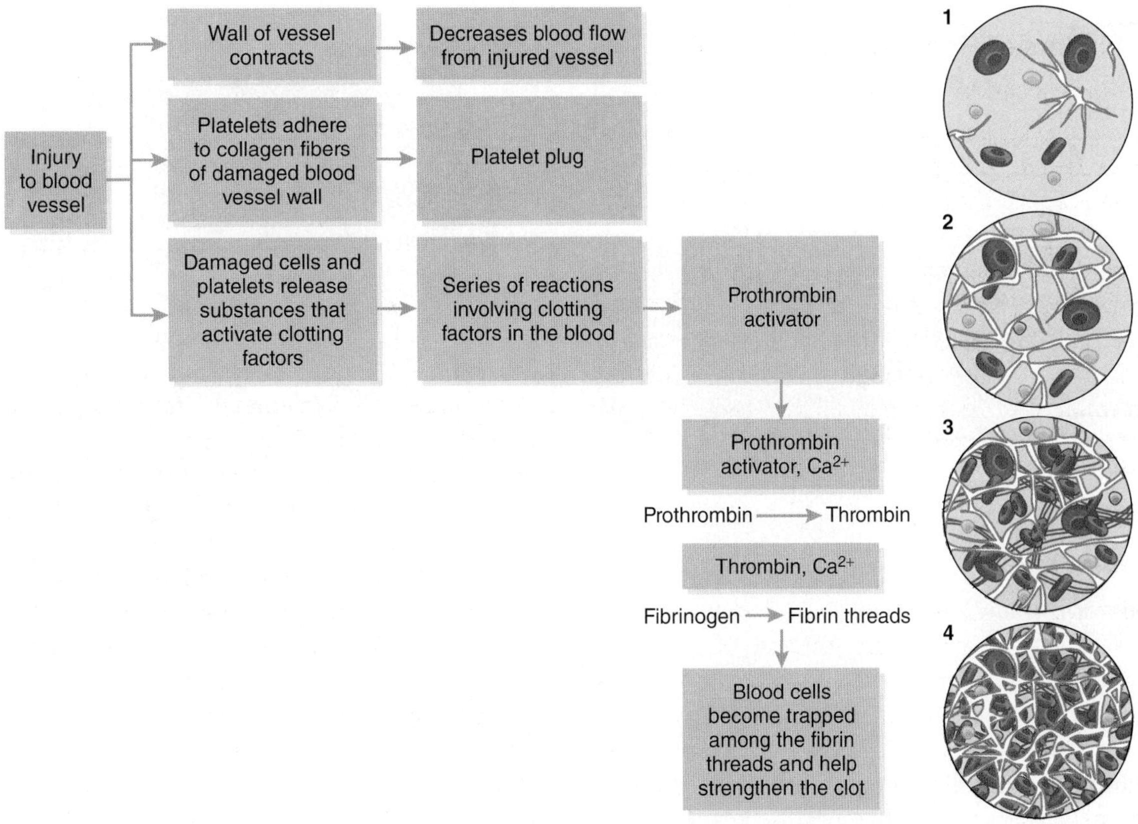

FIGURE 31-3 Overview of blood clotting. Fibrin threads form the webbing of the clot. Blood cells, platelets, and plasma become trapped among the fibrin threads and help strengthen the clot.

Anemia

Anemia is a condition in which the concentration of hemoglobin or erythrocytes in the blood is lower than normal (**TABLE 31-2**). Anemia is not a disease itself, but rather a symptom of a disease. Precipitating causes of anemia may include chronic or acute blood loss, decreased production of erythrocytes, and increased destruction of erythrocytes. Those at greatest risk are people with chronic kidney disease, diabetes, heart disease, and cancer; chronic inflammatory conditions such as rheumatoid arthritis or inflammatory bowel disease; and persistent infections such as human immunodeficiency virus (HIV). These conditions can cause anemia by interfering with the production of oxygen-carrying RBCs. In the case of cancer and chemotherapy, anemia sometimes can be caused by the treatment itself. Two common forms of anemia are **iron-deficiency anemia** and **hemolytic anemia**.

BOX 31-3 Hematologic Disorders by Cell Type

Disorders of RBCs

Anemia
Polycythemia
Sickle cell disease

Disorders of WBCs

Hodgkin lymphoma
Non-Hodgkin lymphomas
Leukemia
Leukopenia
Multiple myelomas

Disorders of Hemostasis

Disseminated intravascular coagulation
Hemophilia
Thrombocytopenia

TABLE 31-2 Normal Hemoglobin and Hematocrit Values

Age/Sex	Hemoglobin (g/dL)	Hematocrit (%)
At birth	17	52
Childhood	12	36
Adolescence	13	40
Adult man	16 (±2)	47 (±6)
Adult woman (menstruating)	13 (±2)	40 (±6)
Adult woman (postmenopausal)	14 (±2)	42 (±6)
During pregnancy	12 (±2)	37 (±6)

Modified from: Hillman RS, Ault KA, Leporrier M, Rinder HM. *Hematology in Clinical Practice*. 5th ed. New York, NY: McGraw-Hill; 2010.

CRITICAL THINKING

Can you predict the signs and symptoms of anemia?

Iron-Deficiency Anemia

Iron is the crucial part of a hemoglobin molecule, giving it the ability to bind oxygen (**FIGURE 31-4**). The lack of iron associated with iron-deficiency anemia prevents

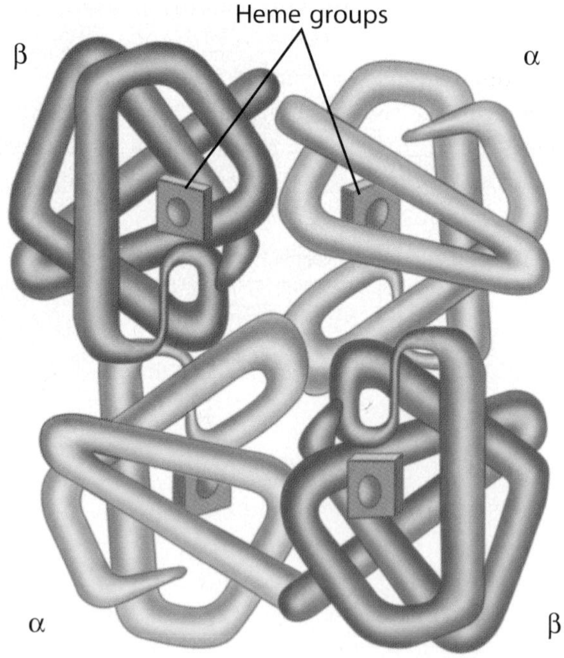

FIGURE 31-4 The hemoglobin molecule is made up of two alpha and two beta polypeptide chains. Each heme group contains an iron atom that is able to bind to one oxygen molecule. Because hemoglobin contains four heme groups, each hemoglobin protein can bind four oxygen molecules. Each red blood cell holds 270 million of these vital protein molecules.

BOX 31-4 Pernicious Anemia

Pernicious anemia results from a vitamin B_{12} deficiency. It has several causes, including surgery, infection, medication use, and poor diet. This condition can also result from a lack of intrinsic factor (a protein in the stomach), which is needed for the absorption of vitamin B_{12} from food. The deficiency of vitamin B_{12} prevents the body from making an adequate number of healthy RBCs. Severe vitamin B_{12} deficiency can cause neurologic problems, such as confusion, dementia, depression, and memory loss. The condition is usually treated with vitamin B_{12} oral supplements or injections.

Modified from: Pernicious anemia. National Heart, Lung, and Blood Institute, National Institutes of Health website. https://www.nhlbi.nih.gov/health-topics/pernicious-anemia. Accessed March 5, 2018.

the bone marrow from making enough hemoglobin for the RBCs. The RBCs produced are small, have a pale center, and have a reduced oxygen-carrying capacity. (BOX 31-4 describes pernicious anemia, another type of anemia in which the body fails to make an adequate number of healthy RBCs.) Common factors linked to iron-deficiency anemia are heavy menstrual bleeding, pregnancy or breastfeeding, inflammatory bowel or peptic ulcer disease, bariatric surgery, a vegetarian or vegan diet that does not include iron-rich foods, and daily consumption of more than 16 to 24 ounces (473–710 mL) of cow's milk in children younger than 1 year. Cow's milk not only contains little iron, but also can decrease absorption of iron and irritate the intestinal lining, causing chronic blood loss.[2]

Hemolytic Anemia

Premature destruction of RBCs in the blood (**hemolysis**) causes hemolytic anemia. This destruction can result from an inherited disorder inside the RBC, or it can result from a disorder outside the cell, which is usually acquired later in life.

Inherited Disorders. Hemolysis can occur because of abnormal rigidity of the cell membrane. This rigidity causes the cell to become trapped at an early stage of its life span in smaller blood vessels (usually within the spleen). In these smaller blood vessels, the RBC is destroyed by macrophages. This type of anemia can occur from a genetic defect in the hemoglobin within the cell (eg, sickle cell anemia, thalassemia). It also can occur from a defect in one of the enzymes in the cell that helps protect the cell from chemical damage during infectious illness. A deficiency of one of the enzymes, glucose-6-phosphate dehydrogenase (G6PD), is common in people from parts of Asia, Africa, the Middle East, and the Mediterranean.[3]

Acquired Disorders. Acquired hemolytic anemia results from one of three conditions:

1. Disorders in which normal RBCs are disrupted from mechanical forces (eg, abnormal blood vessel linings or blood clots)
2. Autoimmune disorders, which can destroy RBCs with antibodies that are produced by the immune system (eg, drug-induced hemolytic anemia or an incompatible blood transfusion; described in Chapter 11, *General Principles of Pathophysiology*)
3. Conditions that can cause hemolytic anemia when RBCs are destroyed by microorganisms in the blood (eg, malaria)

NOTE

Drug-induced hemolytic anemia is a blood disorder that occurs from an autoimmune response. This autoimmune response can be triggered by a number of drugs, including cephalosporin antibiotics, fludarabine (an anticancer agent), lorazepam and its derivatives, nonsteroidal anti-inflammatory drugs (eg, diclofenac), and others. The immune system attacks RBCs and causes their early breakdown and destruction. This condition usually resolves with a good outcome when the drug responsible for the disorder is discontinued.

Signs and Symptoms of Anemia

All forms of anemia share common signs and symptoms, including fatigue and headaches, sometimes a sore mouth or tongue, brittle nails, and, in severe cases, breathlessness and chest pain (**TABLE 31-3**). Other patient complaints are related to an abnormal decrease in the number of WBCs (leukopenia) or a reduction in platelets (thrombocytopenia) and may include the following:

- Bleeding from mucous membranes
- Cutaneous bleeding
- Fatigue
- Fever
- Lethargy

TABLE 31-3 Causes, Signs and Symptoms, and Treatment for Specific Forms of Anemia

Form of Anemia	Causes	Signs and Symptoms	Treatment
Iron-deficiency anemia	Insufficient intake of iron Gastrointestinal disorders (eg, ulcer disease) External and/or internal bleeding Prolonged aspirin or NSAID therapy Gastrectomy (surgical removal of part or all of stomach)	Those related to the underlying cause (eg, bleeding) Those common to all forms of anemia	Correction of the underlying cause Supplemental iron tablets or injections
Hemolytic anemia	Genetic red blood cell disorder Autoimmune disorders Malaria and other infections	Jaundice Those common to all forms of anemia	Splenectomy Immunosuppressant drugs Avoidance of drugs or foods that precipitate hemolysis Antimalarial drugs Blood transfusions

Abbreviation: NSAID, nonsteroidal anti-inflammatory drug

Diagnosis and Treatment

The patient's signs and symptoms, history, and blood, as examined through blood tests and bone marrow biopsy, indicate a diagnosis of most forms of anemia. For example, in iron-deficiency anemia, laboratory examination usually reveals RBCs that are smaller than normal. In hemolytic anemia, the examination shows immature and abnormally shaped RBCs. After diagnosis, treatment is begun to correct, modify, or diminish the mechanism or process that is leading to defective RBC production or reduced RBC survival.

NOTE

A bone marrow biopsy specimen taken from the sternum or the pelvis offers details about the various parts of blood. The specimen also provides information about the presence of cells foreign to the marrow. Bone marrow biopsy is useful in diagnosing many hematologic disorders, such as anemia, leukemia, and certain infections. A bone marrow transplant sometimes is used as part of the treatment of these and other diseases.

Leukemia

Leukemia refers to any of several types of cancer in which an abnormal proliferation of WBCs occurs, usually in the bone marrow (**FIGURE 31-5**). The excess production of leukemic cells crowds and impairs the normal production of RBCs, WBCs, and platelets. Leukemia is more common in males than in females, and is more common in Caucasians than in African Americans. The estimated number of new cases in 2017 was 62,130, with approximately 24,500 deaths projected to occur from this cause. In 2014, there were about 387,728 people living with leukemia in the United States.[4]

The exact cause of leukemia is not known; however, genetics may play a role. Abnormal chromosomes associated with congenital disorders (eg, Down syndrome) and HIV-type viruses are associated with certain forms of this disease. Other factors that may play a role in the development of leukemia include exposure to radiation, viral infections, immune

NOTE

Leukopenia is a decrease in the number of WBCs (most commonly neutrophils). When WBCs are depleted, the immune system is weakened, which places the person at risk for developing infection. Leukopenia has many causes, including chemotherapy, radiation therapy, post-transplant medications, leukemia, various anemias, and other diseases. The condition is diagnosed with blood testing (complete blood count).

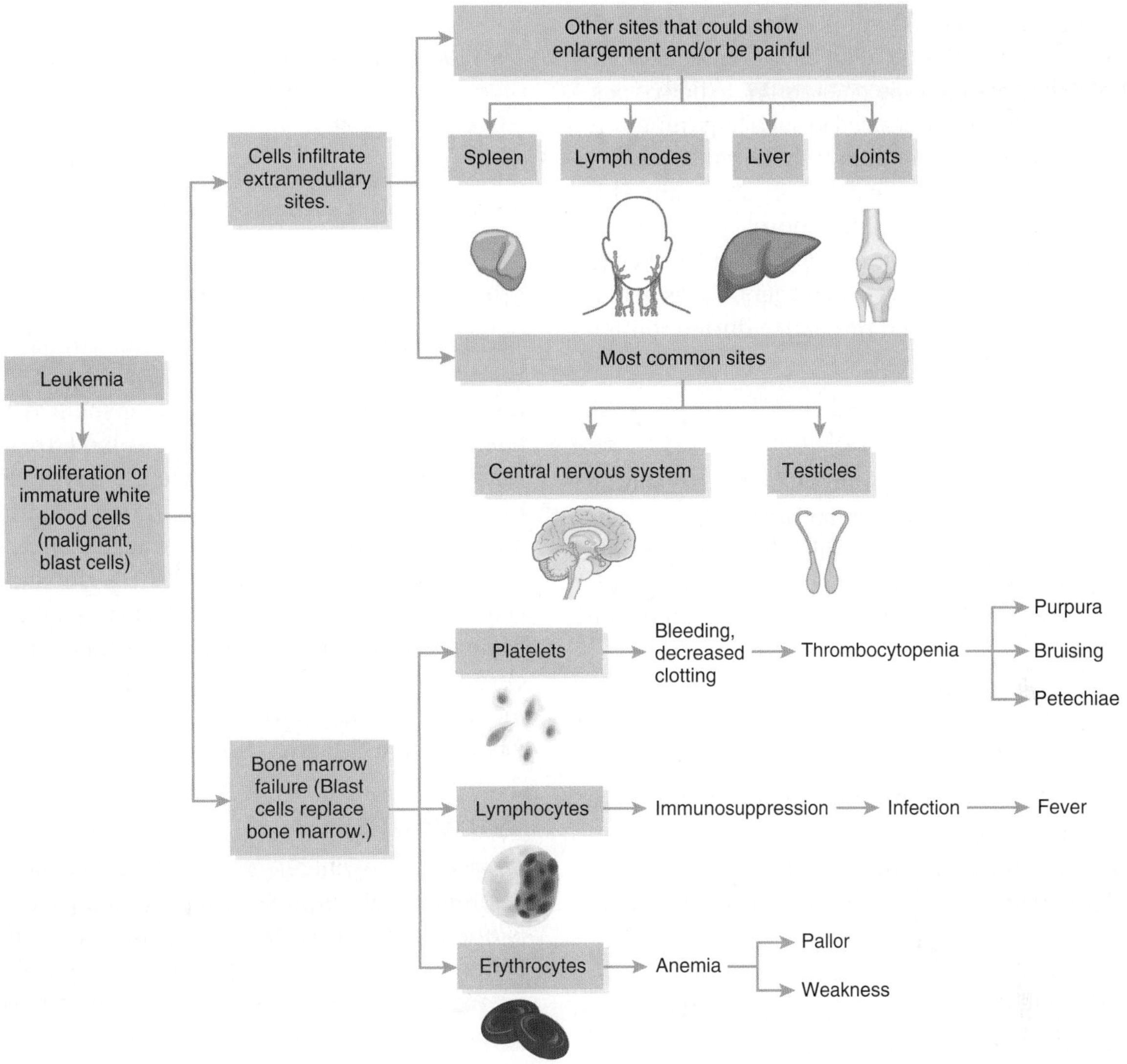

FIGURE 31-5 Pathophysiology of leukemia.

defects, and exposure to various chemicals in home and work environments.

Classifications

Leukemia is classified as either acute or chronic. Cancer cells in acute leukemia begin proliferating at an early stage of their development; that is, their development is arrested when they are immature cells. Chronic leukemia implies an abnormal proliferation of more mature but not fully differentiated cells.

Leukemias are classified further according to the type of WBC involved (BOX 31-5). Two common forms of leukemia are acute lymphocytic leukemia (ALL) and acute myelogenous leukemia (AML). ALL

BOX 31-5 Types of Leukemia

The terms *lymphocytic* and *lymphoblastic* indicate that the cancerous change takes place in a type of marrow cell that forms lymphocytes. The terms *myelogenous* and *myeloid* indicate that the cell change takes place in a type of marrow cell that normally matures to form RBCs, some types of WBCs, and platelets.

ALL and AML are each composed of blast cells, known as lymphoblasts and myeloblasts, respectively. Acute leukemias progress rapidly without treatment.

Chronic leukemias have few or no blast cells. Chronic lymphocytic leukemia and chronic myelogenous leukemia usually progress slowly compared to acute leukemias.

affects mostly children younger than 15 years and, therefore, is sometimes called childhood leukemia. AML affects mostly middle-aged adults. In both types, abnormal WBCs are produced in such large amounts that they eventually accumulate in the vital organs—for example, the liver, spleen, lymph, and brain. This accumulation impedes the function of these organs and leads to death. Chronic forms of leukemia can develop slowly, often over many years. Cases of disease often are discovered by chance during routine blood analysis.

Signs and Symptoms

The proliferation of leukemic cells or the resulting inadequate production of other normal blood cells makes the patient with leukemia highly susceptible to serious infections, anemia, and bleeding episodes. Signs and symptoms of leukemia include the following:[5]

- Abdominal fullness
- Bleeding
- Bone pain
- Elevated body temperature and diaphoresis (ie, sweating)
- Enlargement of lymph nodes
- Enlargement of the liver, spleen, and testes
- Fatigue
- Frequent bruising
- Headache
- Heat intolerance
- Night sweats
- Weight loss

> CRITICAL THINKING
> If a child has a lot of odd bruises, what would you suspect if a diagnosis of leukemia is not known?

Diagnosis and Treatment

The diagnosis of leukemia is confirmed by bone marrow biopsy. The severity of the disease is assessed by the degree of liver and spleen enlargement, extent of anemia, and lack of platelets in the blood. Treatment for acute leukemia can include the transfusion of blood and platelets, antibiotic therapy to manage anemia and infection, and the use of anticancer drugs and sometimes radiation to destroy the leukemic cells. In some cases, the leukemia is treated with a bone marrow transplant (BOX 31-6). Patients with chronic leukemia can be managed effectively with medication. Many patients require no treatment in its preliminary stages.

Lymphomas

Lymphoma is a general term applied to any neoplastic disorder of the lymphoid tissue. Hodgkin lymphoma is one type; all others, despite their diversity, are called non-Hodgkin lymphomas. All lymphomas are **malignant**—that is, cancerous tumors that tend to metastasize.

BOX 31-6 Blood and Marrow Stem Cell Transplantation

A stem cell is a cell whose daughter cells may develop into other cell types. Some cells can develop into several distinct types of mature cells, including lymphocytes, granulocytes, thrombocytes, and erythrocytes. Stem cells reside in marrow and also circulate in the blood. They also circulate in large numbers in fetal blood; thus, they can be recovered from umbilical cord and placental blood after childbirth. Stem cells can be harvested, frozen, and stored for future transplantation.

Stem cell transplantation is standard therapy for selected patients with leukemia, lymphoma, and myeloma. The two major types of stem cell transplants are autologous and allogenic. An autologous transplant uses the patient's own marrow. The marrow is collected while the patient is in remission. Before it is given back to the patient, the marrow may be treated with chemotherapeutic agents or antibodies to cleanse it of cancer cells that may be present in the marrow. An allogenic transplant uses marrow from a donor—usually a relative with the same tissue type, often a sibling. If a familial match is not available, a search of bone marrow registries for tissue-typed volunteers can be made for an unrelated donor. In addition to treating some cancers and other blood disorders, stem cells may play a key role in the future in treating diseases such as Alzheimer disease, Parkinson disease, and heart disease.

Modified from: Leukemia and Lymphoma Society. *Blood and Marrow Stem Cell Transplantation.* White Plains, NY: Leukemia and Lymphoma Society; 2013.

DID YOU KNOW?

Blood Transfusion Complications

Each year, almost 5 million Americans receive a blood transfusion. The transfusion may be of whole blood (containing RBCs, WBCs, platelets, and plasma) or, more commonly, an individual component of whole blood—that is, RBCs (most common), plasma, or platelets and clotting factors. Blood for transfusions is usually obtained through blood banks, which collect, test, and store the blood to ensure its safety and availability. The blood is typed as A, B, AB, or O, and its Rh status (negative or positive) is determined (described in Chapter 11, *General Principles of Pathophysiology*). The blood is also tested for viral or bacterial infection (HIV, hepatitis B and C, variant Creutzfeldt-Jakob disease).

Complications of blood transfusions (if any) are usually mild. Some, however, can be serious and life threatening. Possible complications include the following:

- **Allergic reaction.** May be mild or severe. Signs and symptoms include anxiety, nausea, pain in the chest or back, dyspnea, fever and chills, tachycardia, and hypotension.
- **Viral or infectious disease from tainted blood.** Extremely rare.
- **Fever.** May occur within 24 hours of the transfusion. Fever is usually a response to the WBCs.
- **Volume overload.** Primary signs and symptoms are dyspnea, orthopnea, peripheral edema, and a rapid rise in blood pressure.
- **Hemochromatosis.** Iron overload resulting from frequent blood transfusions or a genetic disorder. The iron may accumulate and damage the heart, lung, and other organs.
- **Transfusion-related acute lung injury (TRALI).** Usually a complication only in very ill patients. Although rare, injury usually occurs within 6 hours of the transfusion. The cause is unknown but may be related to proteins found in the donated plasma of women who have been pregnant. The donated plasma of men is sometimes preferred.
- **Acute immune hemolytic reaction.** A rare and serious complication that results from error in type matching or cross-matching of patient and donor blood. Signs and symptoms of the reaction are usually sudden in onset and include fever, chills, chest pain, nausea, and dark urine. Hemolytic reactions attack new RBCs and can lead to kidney damage.
- **Delayed hemolytic reaction.** A slower version of the acute immune hemolytic reaction that may not be noticed until the patient's RBC count is quite low.
- **Graft-versus-host disease (GVHD).** An often-fatal illness caused by WBCs in donated blood. The disease causes destruction of host tissue. Symptoms usually begin within 1 month of the transfusion and include fever, rash, and diarrhea. GVHD is most common in patients with immune suppression.

Signs and symptoms of these reactions and complications require that the transfusion be stopped immediately. In-hospital care for these patients will be determined by the severity and cause of the adverse reaction.

Modified from: Blood transfusion. National Heart, Lung, and Blood Institute, National Institutes of Health website. https://www.nhlbi.nih.gov/health-topics/blood-transfusion. Accessed March 6, 2018.

NOTE

Blood cancers such as leukemia, Hodgkin lymphoma, non-Hodgkin lymphoma, myeloma, and myelodysplastic syndromes are cancers that originate in the bone marrow or lymphatic tissues. They are considered to be related cancers because they involve the uncontrolled growth of cells with similar functions and origins. These diseases result from an acquired genetic injury to the deoxyribonucleic acid (DNA) of a single cell, which becomes abnormal (malignant) and multiplies continuously. The accumulation of malignant cells interferes with the body's production of healthy blood cells.

Every 4 minutes, one person is diagnosed with a blood cancer. An estimated 139,860 people in the United States were diagnosed with leukemia, lymphoma, or myeloma in 2009. New cases of leukemia, Hodgkin lymphoma, non-Hodgkin lymphoma, and myeloma account for 9.5% of the more than 1.4 million new cancer cases diagnosed in the United States each year.

Modified from: Facts 2016–2017. Leukemia and Lymphoma Society website. https://www.lls.org/sites/default/files/file_assets/PS80_Facts_2016-2017_FINAL.pdf. Accessed March 6, 2018.

Hodgkin Lymphoma

Hodgkin lymphoma (formerly known as Hodgkin disease) is characterized by painless, progressive enlargement of lymphoid tissue found mainly in the lymph nodes and spleen (**FIGURE 31-6**). Left unchecked, these cancer cells multiply and eventually displace healthy lymphocytes, suppressing the immune system. Signs and symptoms include swollen lymph nodes in the neck, axillae, or groin; fatigue; chills; and night sweats. Some patients also experience severe itching, persistent cough, weight loss, shortness of breath, and chest discomfort.

Hodgkin lymphoma is a rare cancer of unknown cause that may have a heritable component; the risk of developing this disease is higher when a young sibling has the disease. People who have had mononucleosis caused by the Epstein-Barr virus are at greater risk of developing this type of lymphoma. The disease is more common in males than in females, with two peak incidences—first in the 20s and later in people older than 55 years. Those from a higher socioeconomic background and patients with HIV infection are also at increased risk of developing Hodgkin lymphoma.[6]

The disease is confirmed by the identification of Reed-Sternberg cells in lymph nodes or organs affected by the cancer. Treatment depends on the level of lymph node and organ system involvement (the stage of the disease) and can consist of radiation and chemotherapy with anticancer drugs. Hodgkin lymphoma is one of the most curable cancers.

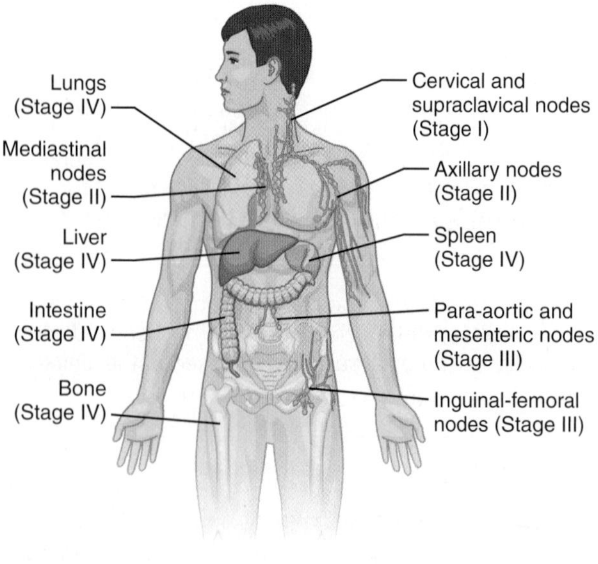

FIGURE 31-6 Pathophysiology of Hodgkin lymphoma.

Non-Hodgkin Lymphomas

Non-Hodgkin lymphoma includes numerous lymphomas that vary in their malignancy according to the nature and activity of the abnormal cells. At least 10 types of non-Hodgkin lymphomas have been identified, each of which is graded as low, intermediate, or high based on how aggressively the disease behaves. Low-grade diseases usually progress slowly and tend not to spread beyond the lymphatic system. By comparison, high-grade diseases can spread to distant organs within a few months. Signs and symptoms include painless swelling of one or more

DID YOU KNOW?

Tumor Lysis Syndrome

Tumor lysis syndrome is a group of metabolic disturbances that can occur after treatment of cancer, usually non-Hodgkin lymphomas and acute leukemias. These complications are caused by the breakdown products of dying cancer cells and the release of their intracellular components into the bloodstream. Complications include hyperkalemia, hyperphosphatemia, hyperuricemia and hyperuricosuria, hypocalcemia, and consequent acute uric acid nephropathy and acute renal failure. A constellation of clinical symptoms may develop before initiation of chemotherapy or more commonly within 72 hours after administration of cytotoxic therapy. Signs and symptoms may include the following:

- Nausea and vomiting
- Lethargy
- Edema
- Fluid overload
- Heart failure
- Cardiac dysrhythmias
- Seizures
- Muscle cramps
- Tetany
- Syncope
- Sudden death

Because of the array of complications that may be associated with tumor lysis syndrome, prehospital care can range from providing only comfort measures to full cardiac life support. In-hospital care may include the control of hyperuricemia to lower the uric acid level, hydration to correct electrolyte imbalances, and administration of sodium bicarbonate to alkalinize the urine. In severe cases, dialysis may be needed.

Modified from: Larson RA, Pui C-H. Tumor lysis syndrome: prevention and treatment. UpToDate website. https://www.uptodate.com/contents/tumor-lysis-syndrome-prevention-and-treatment. Updated January 4, 2018. Accessed March 6, 2018; and Ikeda AK. Tumor lysis syndrome: practice essentials. Medscape website. https://emedicine.medscape.com/article/282171-overview. Updated November 14, 2017. Accessed March 6, 2018.

groups of lymph nodes, enlargement of the liver and spleen, fever, and, in rare cases, abdominal pain and gastrointestinal bleeding.

The causes of these cancers are largely unknown.[7] They are typically found in patients older than 60 years. These lymphomas have been linked to acute and chronic infections (viral infections such as herpes, HIV, and others), some breast implants, some autoimmune conditions (eg, Sjögren disease, lupus, rheumatoid arthritis), exposure to radiation, and some chemical exposures.[8] Treatment consists of radiation therapy, administration of anticancer drugs, and sometimes bone marrow transplantation.

Polycythemia

Polycythemia is an increase in the total RBC mass of the blood. The condition may occur for unknown reasons (primary polycythemia) or be a natural response to chronic hypoxia (secondary polycythemia). Polycythemia also can result from dehydration (apparent polycythemia), in which case the RBC production does not exceed the upper limits of normal.

Primary Polycythemia

Primary polycythemia, also known as polycythemia vera, is a rare disorder of the bone marrow in which increased production of RBCs causes the blood to thicken. This condition primarily develops in people older than 50 years and can lead to several physiologic problems, such as the following:

- Blurred vision
- Dizziness
- Generalized itching
- Headache
- Hypertension
- Red hands and feet; red-purple complexion
- Splenomegaly

Other complications associated with primary polycythemia include platelet disorders, which cause bleeding or clot formation; stroke; and the development of other bone marrow diseases (eg, leukemias). Treatment consists of phlebotomy—the slow removal of blood through a vein—as well as anticancer drug therapy to control the overproduction of RBCs in the marrow.

Secondary Polycythemia

Secondary polycythemia can be naturally present in people who live in or visit areas of high altitude. Polycythemia in such instances is due to reduced air pressure and low oxygen concentration. When the oxygen supply to the blood is reduced, the kidneys produce the hormone erythropoietin, which stimulates RBC production in the bone marrow to compensate for the reduced oxygen supply. The result is an increase in the oxygen-carrying efficiency of the blood. The RBC numbers return to normal when the person returns to sea level.

Secondary polycythemia also can be present in heavy smokers. The disease can be caused by chronic bronchitis and conditions that increase erythropoietin production (eg, liver cancer, some kidney disorders).

Disseminated Intravascular Coagulopathy

Disseminated intravascular coagulopathy (DIC) is an abnormal clotting disorder that arises as a complication of severe injury, trauma, pregnancy, or disease. It is most often seen in the critical care setting. DIC disrupts the balance among procoagulants, inhibitors, thrombus formation, and lysis. Signs and symptoms of DIC include dyspnea and bleeding and symptoms associated with hypotension and hypoperfusion.

DIC occurs in two phases.[9] The first phase is characterized by free thrombin in the blood, fibrin deposits, and the aggregation of platelets. The second phase is characterized by hemorrhage caused by the depletion of clotting factors. The clinical consequences of these processes predispose the patient to multiple-system organ failure from bleeding and coagulation disorders caused by the following factors (**FIGURE 31-7**):

- Loss of platelets and clotting factors
- Fibrinolysis
- Fibrin degradation interference
- Small vessel obstruction, tissue ischemia, RBC injury, and anemia from fibrin deposits

DIC is confirmed through laboratory tests, with treatment then being aimed at reversing the underlying illness or injury that triggered the event. In an effort to control the depletion of clotting factors, in-hospital care includes the replacement of platelets, coagulation factors, and blood. At the same time, attempts are made to manage the primary process.

Hemophilia

Hemophilia is a medical condition that causes uncontrolled bleeding and that involves the loss of bleeding control mechanisms; it comprises a group of inherited

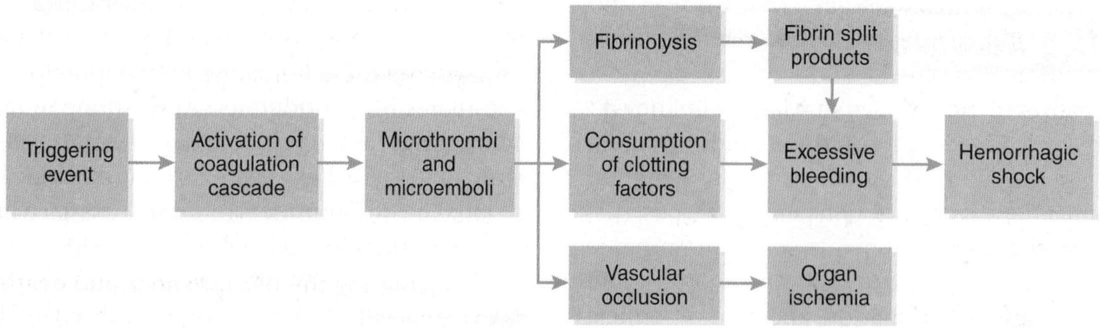

FIGURE 31-7 Pathophysiology of disseminated intravascular coagulation. Clotting and bleeding occur simultaneously, resulting in organ ischemia and hemorrhagic shock.

BOX 31-7 Hereditary Characteristics of Hemophilia

During human reproduction, chromosomes contributed by the mother link with an equal number of chromosomes contributed by the father, and each pair determines the type of information that the offspring's genes carry. Females have two X chromosomes, while males have an X and a Y chromosome. The mother passes on the X chromosome to her child, and the father passes on either an X or a Y. Two X chromosomes produce a female child; an X and a Y produce a male child.

Hemophilia stems from an abnormal gene on the X chromosome. A female with an abnormal X chromosome usually is spared the disease because, although she received one abnormal X chromosome from one parent, the normal X chromosome passed on from her other parent counteracts the abnormal gene. However, she is a carrier of the disease and can pass it on to her children. A woman can have hemophilia only if her mother is a carrier and her father has hemophilia, which is rare. Affected males do not pass the defective gene to their sons, but they do pass it on to their daughters. A male, however, receives only one X chromosome. If his mother is a carrier, a male child will have a 50% chance of having hemophilia; that is, he will receive either the mother's abnormal X chromosome or her normal X chromosome.

Modified from: If a genetic disorder runs in my family, what are the chances that my children will have the condition? Genetics Home Reference, US National Library of Medicine, National Institutes of Health website. https://ghr.nlm.nih.gov/primer/inheritance/riskassessment. Published February 27, 2018. Accessed March 6, 2018.

bleeding disorders (BOX 31-7). **Hemophilia A** is caused by a deficiency in factor VIII, which is essential to the process of blood clotting (**TABLE 31-4**). Another, less common form of hemophilia, caused by a deficiency of factor IX, is known as **hemophilia B** or Christmas disease (named for the 5-year-old boy in whom the disease was first described in 1952). All types of hemophilia present with similar problems, but the specific factor involved determines the severity of bleeding. Approximately 20,000 people in the United States have hemophilia; about 400 are born with the disorder each year.[10]

Bleeding from hemophilia can occur even after minor injury and during some medical procedures (eg, tooth extraction). Although hemorrhage can occur anywhere in the body, bleeding into joints, deep muscles, the urinary tract, and intracranial sites is the most common. Head trauma is potentially life threatening in these patients. Central nervous system bleeding is the major cause of death for patients with hemophilia in all age groups.[11]

Hemophilia is controlled by infusions of concentrates of factor VIII (or factor IX for people with type B hemophilia). These infusions can be administered by the patient. However, serious or unusual bleeding often requires hospitalization. People with hemophilia are advised to avoid activities that may increase their risk of injury (eg, contact sports). Most patients with hemophilia are knowledgeable about their disease and seek emergency care only when complicated problems and trauma-related issues arise.

TABLE 31-4 Clotting Factors and Synonyms

Factor	Synonyms
I	Fibrinogen
II	Prothrombin
III	Thromboplastin
IV	Calcium
V	Proaccelerin
VI	None in use
VII	Serum prothrombin conversion accelerator
VIII	Antihemophilic globulin, antihemophilic factor
IX	Plasma thromboplastin component, Christmas factor
X	Stuart factor
XI	Plasma thromboplastin antecedent
XII	Hageman factor
XIII	Fibrin-stabilizing factor

CRITICAL THINKING

Imagine that you are caring for a patient with hemophilia who has fallen 15 feet (5 m) from a ladder. This patient refuses care and transport. What should you do?

NOTE

Factor VIII is made from large pools of donor blood. During the first few years of the acquired immunodeficiency syndrome (AIDS) epidemic, many people with hemophilia and their sexual partners became infected with HIV through factor VIII infusions. Careful screening protocols for blood are now in place, but infusions still carry a minute risk of transmitting hepatitis B virus, hepatitis C virus, and HIV to factor VIII recipients. Another factor VIII product, recombinant factor VIII, is produced by inserting cloned factor VIII into animal tissues. Recombinant factor VIII is not made from human plasma, is the purest form of factor VIII, does not transmit viral contamination, and is as effective as plasma-derived factor VIII.

Modified from: Franchini M. Plasma-derived versus recombinant factor VIII concentrates for the treatment of haemophilia A: recombinant is better. *Blood Transfus.* 2010;8(4):292-296.

Thrombocytopenia

Thrombocytopenia is a low platelet count. In healthy people, blood normally contains 150,000 to 450,000 platelets/mcL of blood. At levels of 20,000 to 30,000 platelets/mcL of blood, bleeding can occur with relatively minor trauma. At levels below 20,000 platelets/mcL of blood, spontaneous bleeding can occur, increasing the risk for shock and death. This risk is especially dire if bleeding occurs in the brain. Bleeding on the skin is usually the first sign of a low platelet count and may have the following appearance:

- Small red or purple spots on the skin (petechiae), often on the lower legs
- Purple, brown, and red bruises (purpura) that happen easily and often
- Prolonged bleeding, even from minor cuts
- Bleeding or oozing from the mouth or nose, especially nosebleeds or bleeding from brushing teeth
- Unusually heavy menstrual flow

Thrombocytopenia can occur if the body does not produce enough platelets or destroys too many platelets, or if the spleen retains too many platelets. This disease is often associated with leukemia or lymphoma, aplastic anemia, vitamin B_{12} or folic acid deficiency anemias, an enlarged spleen, infectious diseases such as HIV/AIDS, and massive blood transfusions. Increased destruction of platelets may result in the following two conditions:[12]

- **Idiopathic thrombocytopenic purpura (ITP).** ITP occurs when antibodies attack and destroy the body's platelets for unknown reasons. In children, ITP can be an acute condition that occurs after infection. There is a female preponderance in the incidence of ITP throughout adulthood until around age 60 years, after which the overall incidence increases in both sexes, and the ratio of affected women to men is about equal.
- **Thrombotic thrombocytopenic purpura (TTP).** TTP is a life-threatening disease that occurs when small blood clots form suddenly throughout the body. It can result in cardiac hemorrhage and death. TTP occurs more often in women and is associated with pregnancy, metastatic cancer, chemotherapy, HIV/AIDS, and some prescription drugs. Patients with TTP experience kidney failure or decreased kidney function, fever, and neurologic complications.

Treatment for thrombocytopenia depends on the disease's cause and severity. Some patients will require only careful monitoring of their platelet counts. Other, more serious cases may be treated with administration of corticosteroids (prednisone), transfusion of platelets, and, rarely, surgical removal of the spleen.

Sickle Cell Disease

Sickle cell disease is an inherited blood disorder that affects RBCs. Of the various types of sickle cell disease, the most common is **sickle cell anemia**. Sickle cell disease is a debilitating and unpredictable genetic illness that affects people who have ancestors from sub-Saharan Africa, South America, the Caribbean, Central America, Saudi Arabia, or India, and, less commonly, people of Mediterranean origin. One in 365 African American births and more than 100,000 Americans of different ethnic origins are estimated to have sickle cell disease. It is estimated that 1 in 13 black or African American babies is born with sickle cell trait (**BOX 31-8**).[13]

BOX 31-8 Characteristics of Sickle Cell Trait

A person must inherit two sickle cell genes—one from each parent—to develop sickle cell disease. When only one gene is present, the condition is known as a sickle cell trait. People with sickle cell trait usually do not experience symptoms, except occasionally under low-oxygen conditions (eg, scuba diving or traveling at high altitudes). However, these people can pass the gene, and possibly the disease, on to their children. If both parents have sickle cell trait, the child has a 25% chance of developing the disease, a 50% chance of having sickle cell trait, and a 25% chance of having neither. Genetic counseling should be considered for carriers of the disease who plan to become parents. All 50 states require sickle cell screening of newborns. Some colleges and universities also screen young athletes for the sickle cell trait as part of the athlete's health assessment. People with the sickle cell trait are more susceptible to heatstroke and muscle breakdown (rhabdomyolysis) when performing vigorous exercise in high heat and humidity conditions.

Modified from: Keltz E, Khan FY, Mann G. Rhabdomyolysis: the role of diagnostic and prognostic factors. *Muscles Ligaments Tendons J.* 2013;3(4):303-312; and Nelson A, Deuster P, Carter R, et al. Sickle cell trait, rhabdomyolysis, and mortality among US Army soldiers. *N Engl J Med.* 2016;375:435-442.

Acute emergencies related to sickle cell disease are vaso-occlusive crisis, acute chest syndrome, splenic sequestration syndrome, and anemia. Other serious complications of sickle cell disease include the following:

- Delayed growth, development, and sexual maturation in children
- Jaundice
- Priapism in adolescent and adult males
- Splenomegaly
- Acute renal failure
- Central retinal artery occlusion
- Stroke

Pathophysiology

Sickle cell disease produces an abnormal type of hemoglobin, called hemoglobin S, that has an inferior oxygen-carrying capacity. When hemoglobin S is exposed to low oxygen states, it crystallizes, which distorts the RBCs into a sickle shape (**FIGURE 31-8**). The sickle-shaped cells are fragile and easily destroyed. They are unable to pass easily through the tiny blood vessels and consequently block flow to various organs and tissues, most commonly in bones and bone marrow.[14] The resulting vaso-occlusive **sickle cell crisis** can be life threatening. As fewer RBCs pass through congested vessels, tissues and joints become starved for oxygen and other nutrients, causing excruciating pain, most frequently in the back or extremities. Other signs and symptoms of sickle cell disease include increased weakness, aching, chest pain with shortness of breath, sudden and severe abdominal pain, bony deformities, icterus (jaundice) of the sclera (**FIGURE 31-9**), fever, and arthralgia (joint pain) (**FIGURE 31-10**).

Sickle cell crisis can occur in any part of the body and can vary in intensity from one person to the next, and from one crisis to the next. Over time, the crises can destroy the spleen, kidneys, gallbladder,

FIGURE 31-8 Sickle cell versus normal erythrocyte.

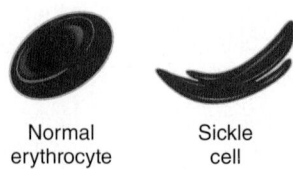

NOTE

Acute chest syndrome is defined as a new, abnormal consolidation on a chest radiograph accompanied by fever and/or respiratory symptoms in a patient with sickle cell disease. This condition is caused by vaso-occlusion of the pulmonary vasculature, leading to pulmonary infarction from a sickle crisis in adults, and infection in children. The syndrome may be associated with acute pleuritic chest pain, fever, hypoxia, and respiratory findings such as cough, wheezing, crackles, or tachypnea. Approximately one-third of these patients have infection. Acute chest syndrome is a common medical emergency for patients with sickle cell disease and is their leading cause of death. Administration of oxygen and bronchodilators is often indicated for these patients.

Modified from: Ballas SK, Lieff S, Benjamin LJ, et al. Definitions of the phenotypic manifestations of sickle cell disease. *Am J Hematol.* 2010;85(1):6-13; and Raam R, Mallemat H, Jhun P, Herbert M. Sickle cell crisis and you: a how-to guide. *Ann Emerg Med.* 2016;67(6):787-790.

CRITICAL THINKING

How do you think a patient with such chronic pain must feel at the beginning of a sickle cell crisis?

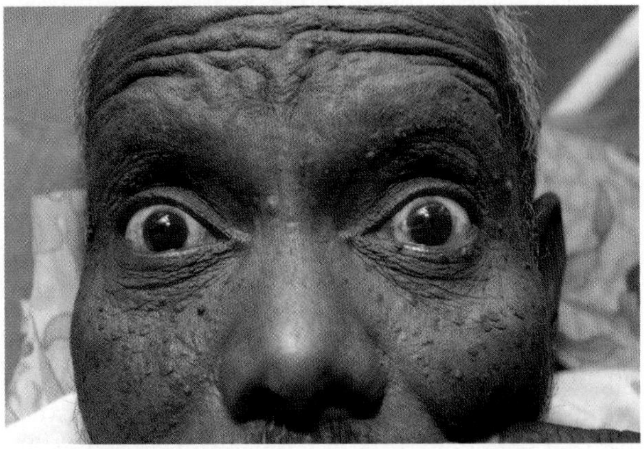

FIGURE 31-9 Jaundice of the sclera.

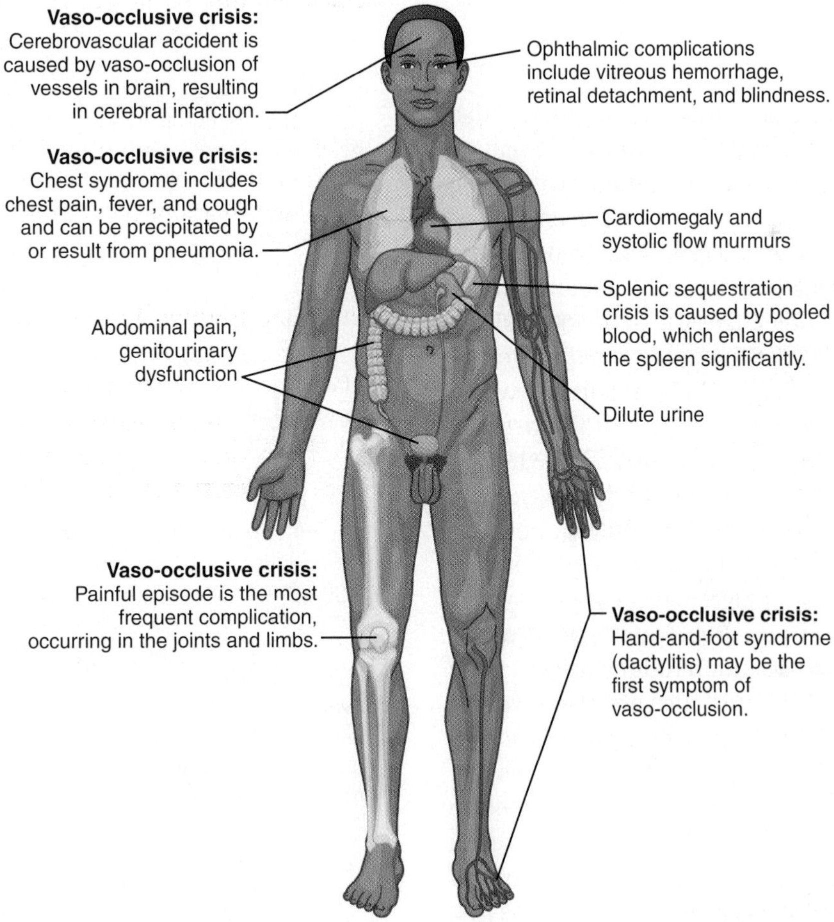
Vaso-occlusive crisis: Cerebrovascular accident is caused by vaso-occlusion of vessels in brain, resulting in cerebral infarction.
Ophthalmic complications include vitreous hemorrhage, retinal detachment, and blindness.
Vaso-occlusive crisis: Chest syndrome includes chest pain, fever, and cough and can be precipitated by or result from pneumonia.
Cardiomegaly and systolic flow murmurs
Splenic sequestration crisis is caused by pooled blood, which enlarges the spleen significantly.
Abdominal pain, genitourinary dysfunction
Dilute urine
Vaso-occlusive crisis: Painful episode is the most frequent complication, occurring in the joints and limbs.
Vaso-occlusive crisis: Hand-and-foot syndrome (dactylitis) may be the first symptom of vaso-occlusion.

FIGURE 31-10 Pathophysiology of sickle cell disease.

and other organs. Sickle cell crisis may occur for no apparent reason, or it may be triggered by conditions such as the following:

- Dehydration
- Exposure to extremes in temperature
- Infection
- Lack of oxygen
- Strenuous physical activity
- Stress
- Trauma

Three less common types of sickle cell crisis are aplastic, hemolytic, and splenic sequestration. In aplastic crisis, the bone marrow temporarily stops producing RBCs. In hemolytic crisis, the RBCs break down too rapidly to be replaced adequately. In splenic sequestration, which usually affects children between 1 and 4 years of age, RBCs become trapped in the spleen. This causes the organ to enlarge, lowers the hemoglobin level, and leads to shock and, in some cases, death.

Management

In some cases, sickle cell disease can be cured with a bone marrow transplantation. Because of the eventual damage that occurs to the spleen, patients with sickle cell disease are at increased risk for septicemia if infected by certain types of bacteria. Children with the disease should be kept current with all immunizations.

The main care objectives for patients in sickle cell crisis are to provide (1) supplemental oxygen by face mask or nasal cannula to help counter tissue hypoxia and reduce cell clumping if the arterial blood gas is less than 95%; (2) maintenance hydration (intravenous [IV] therapy if unable to tolerate oral liquids); (3) electrolyte replacement, because hypoxia results in metabolic acidosis, which also promotes sickling; (4) analgesics for the severe pain from vaso-occlusion; and (5) blood replacement as needed to treat anemia and to reduce the viscosity of the sickled blood.[15] Antibiotics are also given to manage infection. While patients may receive either non-narcotic (ketorolac) or narcotic analgesics (eg, morphine, fentanyl) to manage pain, they may require higher doses of medication to achieve adequate relief. BOX 31-9 describes a new pharmacologic treatment for complications of sickle cell disease that has just reached the US market.

NOTE

Fluid boluses should be reserved for patients who are hypovolemic (eg, sepsis, diarrheal illness, vomiting). While it is thought that dehydration may precipitate pain crisis, overhydration—especially with isotonic crystalloid—does not help resolve a pain crisis and may have detrimental effects.

Modified from: Grewal K, Helman, A, eds. Episode 68: emergency management of sickle cell disease. Emergency Medicine Cases website. https://emergencymedicinecases.com/wp-content/uploads/filebase/pdf/Episode%20068%20Aug2015%20Sickle%20Cell%20Disease.pdf. Published August 2015. Accessed March 6, 2018.

SHOW ME THE EVIDENCE

In a study published in 2013, researchers surveyed a cross-sectional convenience sample of attendees at a national emergency physicians conference. Their goal was to identify factors for self-reported nonadherence to national guidelines for treatment of patients with sickle cell disease with vaso-occlusive pain in the emergency department. They hypothesized that physicians' negative attitudes toward patients with sickle cell disease and patient demographics might lessen the likelihood of adhering to national treatment guidelines for this condition.

A total of 671 responses were included in the analysis. A large number of the respondents (67.9%) worked at teaching hospitals, and most (83.2%) practiced in the United States. The researchers found that pediatric providers had more positive attitudes toward patients with sickle cell disease, whereas adult providers had more negative attitudes. Providers treating greater numbers of these patients per week had more negative attitudes, and black providers had more positive attitudes than did providers of other races/ethnicities. Other variables (age, sex, ethnicity, level of practice, hospital teaching status, institutions with comprehensive sickle cell clinics) did not affect physicians' attitudes.

Providers with the highest negative attitudes were significantly less likely to provide repeat doses of opioids within 30 minutes for inadequate pain relief. The researchers also found other gaps in use of national guidelines to manage vaso-occlusive crisis within the overall group. On the basis of their findings, they suggested that national organizations should issue papers promoting adherence to national treatment guidelines for these patients.

Modified from: Glassberg JA, Tanabe P, Chow A, et al. Emergency provider analgesic practices and attitudes toward patients with sickle cell disease. *Ann Emerg Med.* 2013;62(4):293-302.

BOX 31-9 New Treatment Approved for Sickle Cell Disease

In 2017, the US Food and Drug Administration approved the drug Endari (L-glutamine oral powder) to lower the risk of sickle cell complications in patients 5 years of age and older. In clinical trials, the drug decreased the incidence of vaso-occlusive crisis in these patients. In situations when the patient had a crisis, patients taking Endari also had significantly fewer episodes of acute chest syndrome than did those given placebo. It has been 20 years since a new drug was approved to treat this disease.

For sickle cell pain, some centers are using IV lidocaine in a setting that monitors the patient for cardiac changes with good results.

Modified from: FDA approves new treatment for sickle cell disease [FDA news release]. US Food and Drug Administration website. https://www.fda.gov/newsevents/newsroom/pressannouncements/ucm566084.htm. Updated July 18, 2017. Accessed March 6, 2018; and Nguyen NL, Kome AM, Lowe DK, et al. Intravenous lidocaine as an adjuvant for pain associated with sickle cell disease. *J Pain Palliat Care Pharmacother*. 2015;29(4):359-364.

Multiple Myeloma

Multiple myeloma is a malignant neoplasm of plasma cells that tend to accumulate in the bone marrow. The cells destroy bone tissue (especially in flat bones), which causes pain, fractures, hypercalcemia, and skeletal deformities. In myeloma, the neoplastic cells produce large amounts of protein (M protein) that affect the viscosity of the blood. Masses of coagulated protein can accumulate within the tissues and impair function. Some patients with this disease die of kidney failure—a condition that develops from the buildup of proteins that infiltrate the kidneys and block the renal tubules. In many ways, multiple myeloma resembles leukemia, but the plasma cell proliferation generally is confined to the bone marrow.

CRITICAL THINKING
Which are the flat bones?

Other disorders associated with multiple myeloma include proteinuria, anemia, weight loss, pulmonary complications from rib fracture, and recurrent infections from suppression of the immune system. Patient complaints associated with multiple myeloma may include weakness, skeletal pain, hemorrhage, hematuria, lethargy, weight loss, and frequent fractures.

Multiple myeloma occurs only rarely in people younger than 40 years, but its incidence then increases with age. The disease is more common in males than in females and may have a heritable component.[1]

Multiple myeloma is diagnosed through radiography, blood studies, urine testing, and tumor biopsy. Treatment consists of chemotherapy with anticancer drugs, radiation therapy, plasma exchange, and bone marrow transplantation.

General Assessment and Management of Patients With Hematologic Disorders

Most patients with diagnosed hematologic disorders are knowledgeable about their disease. Often, they call emergency medical services to help manage a "change" in their condition. They also may call to arrange for transport to an emergency department for physician evaluation. The situations that invoke a call for emergency care vary by patient and disease. Common chief complaints can be classified by body system (**TABLE 31-5**).

Prehospital Care

In many cases, the prehospital care for a patient with a hematologic disorder will be mainly supportive. As with any other patient care encounter, however, the paramedic should perform a general assessment, a focused history, and a focused physical examination. These measures will guide patient care and help determine the urgency of emergency transport. Some patients with hematologic disorders will have complex medical histories. When possible, these patients should be transported to the primary hospital where they usually receive their medical care.

As referenced in Table 31-5, a patient with a hematologic disorder may have a variety of complaints and physical findings. Some patient complaints may be vague (eg, fever, fatigue, headache), which can further complicate the paramedic's assessment. After ensuring adequate airway, ventilatory, and circulatory status, the paramedic should assess vital signs and perform a physical examination. The patient's skin should be assessed for color and turgor, noting any

TABLE 31-5 Chief Complaints of Patients With Nonmalignant Hematologic Disorders Classified by Body System

Body System	Complaints	Possible Causes
Central nervous system	Altered level of consciousness, stroke	Anemia, sickle cell disease
	Increased weakness, numbness	Autoimmune disease
	Visual disturbances/loss of vision	Unilateral sensory deficits
Cardiorespiratory	Dyspnea/crackles	Heart failure, acute chest syndrome
	Anemia	Bleeding disorders
	Pulmonary edema	Hemoptysis
	Chest pain	Tachycardia, acute chest syndrome
Integumentary	Prolonged bleeding Bruising Itching/petechiae Pallor	Hemolytic anemia, polycythemia Sickle cell disease, liver disease Jaundice
Musculoskeletal	Bone or joint pain	Autoimmune disease
	Fracture	Hemophilia
Gastrointestinal	Abdominal pain Bleeding of gums/gingivitis Epistaxis	Hemolytic anemia, viral disease Blood-clotting abnormalities Autoimmune disease
		Generalized sepsis
	Ulceration	Melena/hematemesis
Genitourinary	Hematuria	Sickle cell disease, bleeding disorders
	Menorrhagia/amenorrhagia	
	Priapism	Infection
		Sexually transmitted disease

cyanosis or jaundice, warmth or coolness, bruising, edema, or ulcerations. The paramedic also should ascertain any new onset of fever, weakness, cough, rash, spontaneous bleeding (eg, bleeding gums, epistaxis), vomiting, or diarrhea. In some hematologic disorders, the blood's ability to deliver enough oxygen to tissues is altered. Thus, the paramedic should question all patients with hematologic disorders specifically about recent dizziness, syncope, difficulty breathing, and heartbeat irregularities.

Other key elements of the patient assessment and history include identifying existing hematologic disease (including any family history of hematologic disease), any significant medical history or recent injury, the patient's medication use (prescriptions, over-the-counter medications, herbal supplements), allergies, and alcohol or illicit drug use.

Based on the patient's condition, prehospital care measures may include oxygen administration, IV fluid replacement, administration of antidysrhythmics, and administration of analgesics for pain management. Some of these patients will be gravely ill; calming and comfort measures for the patient and family should be provided.

Summary

- Blood is composed of cells and formed elements surrounded by plasma. Approximately 95% of the volume of formed elements consists of red blood cells (RBCs; erythrocytes); the remaining 5% consists of white blood cells (WBCs; leukocytes) and cell fragments (platelets).
- Anemia is a condition in which the amount of hemoglobin or erythrocytes in the blood is less than normal; two common forms are iron-deficiency anemia and hemolytic anemia. Signs and symptoms of anemia include fatigue and headaches, sometimes a sore mouth or tongue, brittle nails, and, in severe cases, breathlessness and chest pain.
- Leukemia comprises several types of cancer in which an abnormal proliferation of WBCs occurs, usually in the bone marrow. These cells crowd out and impair the normal production of RBCs, WBCs, and platelets, rendering the patient highly susceptible to serious infections, anemia, and bleeding episodes.
- Lymphoma refers to a group of diseases that range from slowly growing chronic disorders to rapidly evolving acute conditions. Hodgkin lymphoma is one type; all others are called non-Hodgkin lymphomas.
- Polycythemia is characterized by an unusually large number of RBCs in the blood as a result of these cells' increased production by the bone marrow. It may occur for unknown reasons (primary polycythemia) or be a natural response to hypoxia (secondary polycythemia).
- Disseminated intravascular coagulopathy (DIC) is a complication of severe injury, trauma, or disease that disrupts the balance among procoagulants, thrombin formation, inhibitors, and lysis. Signs and symptoms of DIC include dyspnea, bleeding, and symptoms associated with hypotension and hypoperfusion. Treatment is aimed at reversing the underlying illness or injury that triggered the event.
- Hemophilia A is caused by a deficiency of the blood protein called factor VIII; hemophilia B is caused by a deficiency of factor IX. Bleeding from hemophilia can occur spontaneously, after even minor injury, or during some medical procedures.
- Thrombocytopenia is a low platelet count. It can occur when the body does not produce enough platelets or destroys too many platelets, or if the spleen retains too many platelets. Bleeding is the chief complication of thrombocytopenia.
- Sickle cell disease is a debilitating and unpredictable recessive genetic illness. It affects mostly people of African descent, but occasionally people of Mediterranean origin. Sickle cell disease occurs when the body produces hemoglobin S, an abnormal type of hemoglobin with an inferior oxygen-carrying capacity. Complications of sickle cell disease may include episodes of severe pain, fatigue, pallor, jaundice, stroke, delayed growth, hematuria, priapism, and splenomegaly.
- Multiple myeloma is a malignant neoplasm of plasma cells that tend to accumulate in the bone marrow. The tumor destroys bone tissue (especially flat bones), which causes pain, fractures, hypercalcemia, and skeletal deformities.
- In many cases of hematologic disorders, the prehospital treatment is supportive. Treatment includes ensuring adequate airway, ventilatory, and circulatory support.

References

1. McCance KL, Huether SE. *Pathophysiology: The Biologic Basis for Disease in Adults and Children*. 7th ed. St. Louis, MO: Mosby; 2014.
2. Iron-deficiency anemia. American Society of Hematology website. http://www.hematology.org/Patients/Anemia/Iron-Deficiency.aspx. Accessed March 6, 2018.
3. Glucose-6-phosphate dehydrogenase deficiency. Genetics Home Reference, US National Library of Medicine, National Institutes of Health website. https://ghr.nlm.nih.gov/condition/glucose-6-phosphate-dehydrogenase-deficiency. Published March 6, 2018. Accessed March 6, 2018.
4. Cancer stat facts: leukemia. National Cancer Institute, National Institutes of Health website. https://seer.cancer.gov/statfacts/html/leuks.html. Accessed March 6, 2018.
5. Leukemia. American Society of Hematology website. http://www.hematology.org/Patients/Cancers/Leukemia.aspx. Accessed March 6, 2018.
6. Hodgkin lymphoma risk factors. American Cancer Society website. https://www.cancer.org/cancer/hodgkin-lymphoma/causes-risks-prevention/risk-factors.html. Updated March 28, 2017. Accessed March 6, 2018.
7. Hodgkin lymphoma. Cancer Council NSW website. https://www.cancercouncil.com.au/hodgkin-lymphoma/. Reviewed June 2017. Accessed March 6, 2018.
8. Non-Hodgkin lymphoma: causes, risk factors, and prevention. American Cancer Society website. https://www.cancer.org/cancer/non-hodgkin-lymphoma/causes-risks-prevention. Accessed March 6, 2018.
9. Kaneko T, Wada H. Diagnostic criteria and laboratory tests for disseminated intravascular coagulation. *J Clin Exp Hematopathol*. 2011;51(2):67-76.
10. National Center on Birth Defects and Developmental Disabilities, Centers for Disease Control and Prevention. Hemophilia: data and statistics. Centers for Disease Control and Prevention website. https://www.cdc.gov/ncbddd/hemophilia/data.html. Updated July 11, 2016. Accessed March 6, 2018.
11. Walls R, Hockberger R, Gausche-Hill M. *Rosen's Emergency Medicine: Concepts and Clinical Practice*. 9th ed. Philadelphia, PA: Elsevier; 2017.
12. Izak M, Bussel JB. Management of thrombocytopenia. *F1000 Prime Rep*. 2014;6:45.
13. Centers for Disease Control and Prevention. Sickle cell disease: data and statistics. Centers for Disease Control and Prevention website. https://www.cdc.gov/ncbddd/sicklecell/data.html. Updated August 31, 2017. Accessed March 6, 2018.
14. Evidence-based management of sickle cell disease: expert panel report, 2014. National Heart, Lung, and Blood Institute, National Institutes of Health website. https://www.nhlbi.nih

.gov/health-topics/evidence-based-management-sickle-cell-disease. Published September 2014. Accessed March 6, 2018.

15. National Association of EMS Officials. *National Model EMS Clinical Guidelines*. Version 2.0. National Association of EMS Officials website. https://www.nasemso.org/documents/National-Model-EMS-Clinical-Guidelines-Version2-Sept2017.pdf. Published September 2017. Accessed March 6, 2018.

Suggested Readings

Blood disorders: why should I know about blood conditions? American Society of Hematology website. http://www.hematology.org/Patients/Blood-Disorders.aspx. Accessed March 6, 2018.

Blanchette V, Branado L, Breakey VR, Revel-Vilk S, eds. *SickKids Handbook of Pediatric Thrombosis and Hemostasis*. 2nd ed. Basel, Switzerland: Karger; 2017.

Chen TH, Farooq AV, Shah HA. Pediatric patient with T-cell lymphoblastic lymphoma and acute vision loss. *JAMA Ophthalmol*. 2018;136(2):213-214.

Glassburg JA. Improving emergency department-based care of sickle cell pain. *Hematol Am Soc Hematol Educ Program.* 2017 Dec 8;2017(1):412-417.

Hoffman R, Benz E, Silberstein LE, Heslop H, Weitz J, Anastasi J. *Hematology: Basic Principles and Practice*. 7th ed. Philadelphia, PA: Elsevier; 2018.

Ishii E. *Hematological Disorders in Children: Pathogenesis and Treatment*. New York, NY: Springer; 2017.

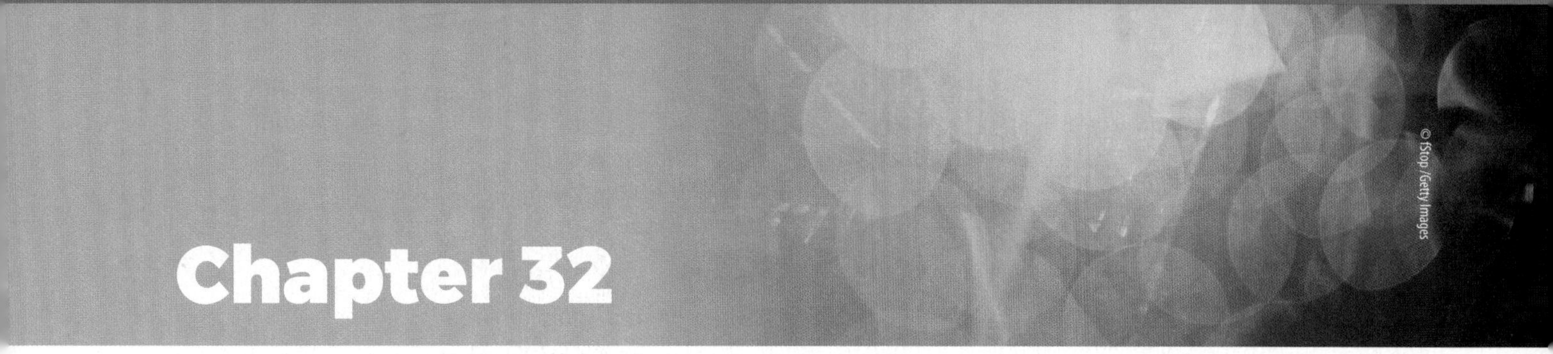

Chapter 32

Nontraumatic Musculoskeletal Disorders

NATIONAL EMS EDUCATION STANDARD COMPETENCIES

Trauma

Integrates assessment findings with principles of epidemiology and pathophysiology to formulate a field impression to implement a comprehensive treatment/disposition plan for an acutely injured patient.

Orthopaedic Trauma

Recognition and management of
- Open fractures (see Chapter 43, *Orthopaedic Trauma*)
- Closed fractures (see Chapter 43, *Orthopaedic Trauma*)
- Dislocations (see Chapter 43, *Orthopaedic Trauma*)
- Amputations (see Chapter 37, *Bleeding and Soft-Tissue Trauma*)

Pathophysiology, assessment, and management of
- Upper and lower extremity orthopaedic trauma (see Chapter 43, *Orthopaedic Trauma*)
- Open fractures (see Chapter 43, *Orthopaedic Trauma*)
- Closed fractures (see Chapter 43, *Orthopaedic Trauma*)
- Dislocations (see Chapter 43, *Orthopaedic Trauma*)
- Sprains/strains (see Chapter 43, *Orthopaedic Trauma*)
- Pelvic fractures (see Chapter 43, *Orthopaedic Trauma*)
- Amputations/replantation (see Chapter 37, *Bleeding and Soft-Tissue Trauma*)
- Compartment syndrome (see Chapter 43, *Orthopaedic Trauma*)
- Pediatric fractures (see Chapter 47, *Pediatrics*)
- Tendon laceration/transection/rupture (Achilles and patellar) (see Chapter 43, *Orthopaedic Trauma*)

Medicine

Integrates assessment findings with principles of epidemiology and pathophysiology to formulate a field impression and implement a comprehensive treatment/disposition plan for a patient with a medical complaint.

Nontraumatic Musculoskeletal Disorders

Anatomy, physiology, pathophysiology, assessment, and management of
- Nontraumatic fracture (pp 1190, 1192, 1193, 1195)

Anatomy, physiology, epidemiology, pathophysiology, psychosocial impact, presentations, prognosis, and management of common or major nontraumatic musculoskeletal disorders, including
- Disorders of the spine (pp 1189, 1192–1194, 1200)
- Joint abnormalities (pp 1194–1197)
- Muscle abnormalities (pp 1197–1199)
- Overuse syndromes (pp 1199–1201)

OBJECTIVES

Upon completion of this chapter, the paramedic student will be able to:

1. Outline musculoskeletal structure and function. (pp 1186–1187)

2. Describe how to perform a detailed assessment of the extremities and spine. (p 1189)
3. Specify questions in the patient history that help identify musculoskeletal problems. (p 1190)
4. Describe assessment and management of specific nontraumatic musculoskeletal disorders based on an understanding of the pathophysiology. (pp 1187–1190)

KEY TERMS

ankylosing spondylitis (AS) A form of arthritis that primarily affects the spine, although other joints can become involved.

appendicular skeleton The bones of the upper and lower extremities.

arthritis An inflammatory condition of the joints, characterized by pain and swelling.

atrophy Decrease in size (shrinkage) of a cell, which adversely affects cell function.

axial skeleton The bones of the head, neck, and torso.

benign Nonmalignant; generally considered less harmful.

bone spurs Bony growths formed on normal bone.

bone tumor An abnormal growth of cells within a bone. It may be malignant or benign.

bursa A small sac containing synovial fluid that helps ease friction between a tendon and skin or between a tendon and bone.

bursitis An inflammation of the bursa, the connective tissue structure surrounding a joint.

carpal tunnel syndrome An entrapment neuropathy that occurs when the median nerve becomes pressed or squeezed at the wrist in the carpal tunnel.

cartilaginous joints Joints that are slightly movable.

cauda equina syndrome A rare disorder of the lumbar spine that affects the bundle of nerve roots at the lower end of the spinal cord. It is a surgical emergency.

chronic fatigue syndrome (CFS) A debilitating and complex disorder, characterized by profound fatigue that is not improved by bed rest and that may be worsened by physical or mental activity.

dermatomyositis An inflammatory myopathy characterized by a skin rash that precedes or accompanies progressive muscle weakness.

epiphyseal plate The site of bone elongation; also known as the growth plate.

fascia The loose areolar connective tissue found beneath the skin or dense connective tissue that encloses and separates muscle.

fasciitis Inflammation of the fascia.

fibromyalgia A disorder that causes extreme fatigue; associated with "tender points" on the neck, shoulders, back, hips, arms, and legs.

fibrous joints Joints that are immovable.

flexor tenosynovitis A pathologic state that causes a disruption of tendon function in the hand; usually the result of infection.

gait A manner of walking or moving on foot.

gangrene Dead or dying body tissues attributable to blood supply that is lost or inadequate.

gout A disease associated with an inborn error of uric acid metabolism that increases production of or interferes with excretion of uric acid; also known as hyperuricemia.

herniated disk An injury in which all or part of a spinal disk is forced through a weakened part of the disk.

inflammatory myopathies A group of diseases that involve chronic muscle inflammation accompanied by muscle weakness.

joint Any one of the connections between bones that are classified according to structure and mobility as fibrous, cartilaginous, or synovial. Fibrous joints are immovable, cartilaginous joints are slightly movable, and synovial joints are freely movable.

joint disorder Any disease or injury that affects human joints.

kyphosis An abnormal condition of the vertebral column characterized by increased convexity in the curvature of the thoracic spine as viewed from the side.

laminectomy Surgery to remove a portion of a lamina of one or more vertebrae that is compressing the nerve in a herniated disk.

ligaments Bands of white, fibrous tissue that connect bones.

lordosis An inward curvature in the lumbar spine that is normally present to some degree.

malignant Having the ability to metastacize; very dangerous or virulent; likely to cause death.

metastasis The movement or spreading of cancer cells from one organ or tissue to other locations in the body.

microdiskectomy The surgical removal of a disk using minimally invasive techniques.

muscle strains Slight tears in a muscle or tendon.

muscle tone The constant tension produced by muscles of the body for long periods of time.

muscular system The body system responsible for execution of movement and postural maintenance.

musculoskeletal system The body system that comprises bones, muscles, tendons and ligaments, and articulating surfaces (eg, joints, bursae, disks).

myalgia Diffuse muscle pain, usually accompanied by malaise. It occurs in many infectious diseases.

myositis Inflammation of the muscles; also known as inclusion body myositis.

necrotizing fasciitis A rare but critical rapidly progressive inflammatory infection of the fascia with secondary necrosis of skin and subcutaneous tissues; requires urgent surgical intervention.

osteoarthritis A form of arthritis in which one or many joints undergo degenerative changes.

osteomyelitis Local or generalized infection of bone and bone marrow, usually caused by bacteria introduced by trauma or surgery.

paronychia A common skin infection that occurs around the nails and that allows for an invasion of bacteria, yeast, or fungus.

pathologic fracture A fracture through abnormally weak bone from a force that would not fracture a normal bone.

point-to-point movements Methods used to evaluate a patient's coordination.

polymyositis Slow but progressive muscle weakness that affects skeletal muscle on both sides of the body.

postural maintenance The result of muscle tone responsible for keeping the back and legs straight, the head in an upright position, and the abdomen from bulging; also balances the distribution of body weight.

primary tumor A malignant tumor in the original site where it first arose.

pseudogout Inflammation caused by calcium pyrophosphate crystals; often clinically indistinguishable from gout.

rheumatoid arthritis (RA) A chronic, sometimes deforming destructive collagen disease that has an autoimmune component.

sciatica Pain that radiates along the path of the sciatic nerve.

scoliosis A lateral curvature of the spine.

secondary tumor A malignant tumor that originates in one area of the body and spreads to another area of the body.

septic arthritis A condition that results from direct invasion of the joint space by various microorganisms; also known as infectious arthritis.

skeletal muscle Muscle tissue that appears microscopically to consist of striped myofibrils; also known as striated muscle and voluntary muscle.

skeletal system The bony structures that provide support and protection for the body. It also provides a system of levers on which muscles act to produce body movement.

slipped capital femoral epiphysis A separation of the ball of the hip joint from the femur at the upper, growing end (growth plate) of the bone.

spinal stenosis Narrowing of the spinal canal.

sprain A partial tearing of a ligament caused by a sudden twisting or stretching of a joint beyond its normal range of motion.

stance The position of the body while standing.

strain An injury to the muscle or its tendon from overexertion or overextension.

synovial joints Joints that are freely movable.

tendons Bands or cords of dense connective tissue that connect muscle to bone or other structures; characterized by strength and nonstretchability.

tendonitis An inflammatory condition of a tendon, usually caused by a sprain.

ulnar nerve entrapment An injury that occurs when the ulnar nerve in the arm becomes compressed.

Nontraumatic musculoskeletal disorders are common afflictions. These diseases cause pain in the bones, joints, muscles, and surrounding structures. Although the disorders are often associated with aging, they can affect all age groups and frequently cause impairments, disabilities, and handicaps. Nontraumatic musculoskeletal disorders are rarely life threatening. Paramedics, however, should be familiar with these common ailments and the supportive care required for these patients. BOX 32-1 *lists the musculoskeletal disorders discussed in this chapter.*[1]

BOX 32-1 Musculoskeletal Disorders

Osteomyelitis
Bone tumors
Low back pain
Joint disorders
Muscle disorders
Overuse syndromes
Peripheral nerve syndromes
Soft-tissue infections

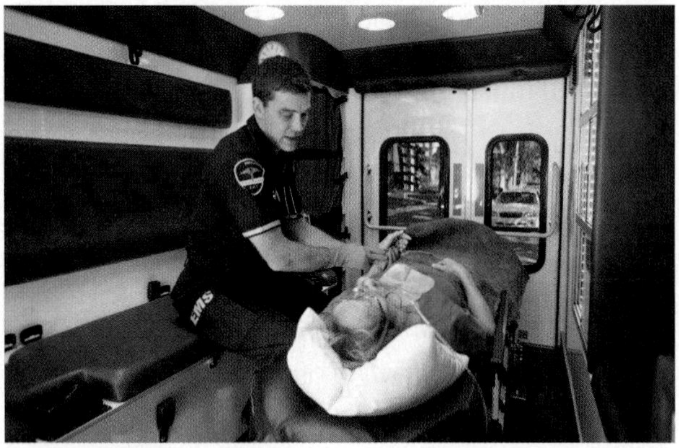

NOTE

Approximately 126.6 million Americans (one in two adults) are affected by musculoskeletal disorders that limit range of motion or cause pain in a joint or an extremity.

Modified from: American Academy of Orthopaedic Surgeons. One in two Americans have a musculoskeletal condition: new report outlines the prevalence, scope, cost and projected growth of musculoskeletal disorders in the US. ScienceDaily website. https://www.sciencedaily.com/releases/2016/03/160301114116.htm. Published March 1, 2016. Accessed February 15, 2018.

Anatomy and Physiology Review

The **musculoskeletal system** comprises bones, muscles, tendons and ligaments, and articulating surfaces (eg, joints, bursae, disks). This discussion will provide a brief review of the skeletal system and the muscular system.

The Skeletal System

The **skeletal system** contains the bony structures that provide support and protection for the body. It also provides a system of levers on which muscles act to produce body movement. The skeletal system contains 206 individual bones. These bones are divided into two categories: the **axial skeleton** and the **appendicular skeleton**. The axial skeleton contains the skull, hyoid bone, vertebral column, and thoracic cage. The appendicular skeleton contains the bones of the upper and lower extremities and their girdles, by which they are attached to the body (**FIGURE 32-1**).

Body movement is made possible by bones that are connected to other bones. With the exception of the hyoid bone, each bone in the body connects to at least one other bone by way of a **joint**. The three major classes of joints are fibrous, cartilaginous, and synovial. **Fibrous joints** consist of two bones that have little or no movement and are united by fibrous tissue. An example of a fibrous joint is the suture in skull bones. **Cartilaginous joints** unite two bones by means of hyaline cartilage and fibrocartilage. These types of joints are slightly movable. Examples of cartilaginous joints are the **epiphyseal plate** of a growing bone and junctions of the intervertebral disks. **Synovial joints** contain synovial fluid that allows for considerable movement. Most joints that unite the bones of the appendicular skeleton are synovial. Examples of synovial joints are the hinge joint of the elbow and knee and the ball-and-socket joints of the shoulder and hip. **FIGURE 32-2** illustrates the movement found in different kinds of joints.

The Muscular System

The **muscular system** is responsible for execution of movement and postural maintenance. The major types of muscles are skeletal, cardiac, and smooth muscle. Of the three types, skeletal muscle is most common and is the focus of this chapter. It is also the muscle type most involved in musculoskeletal disorders. Skeletal muscles are attached to bones by **tendons**. **Ligaments** connect bone or cartilage and help strengthen and support joints.

Skeletal muscle has specialized contractile cells known as muscle fibers. When a nerve impulse passes through the muscle fiber, specialized chemicals cause the muscle to contract. Most skeletal muscles extend from one bone to another and cross at least one joint. The contraction of some muscles and the

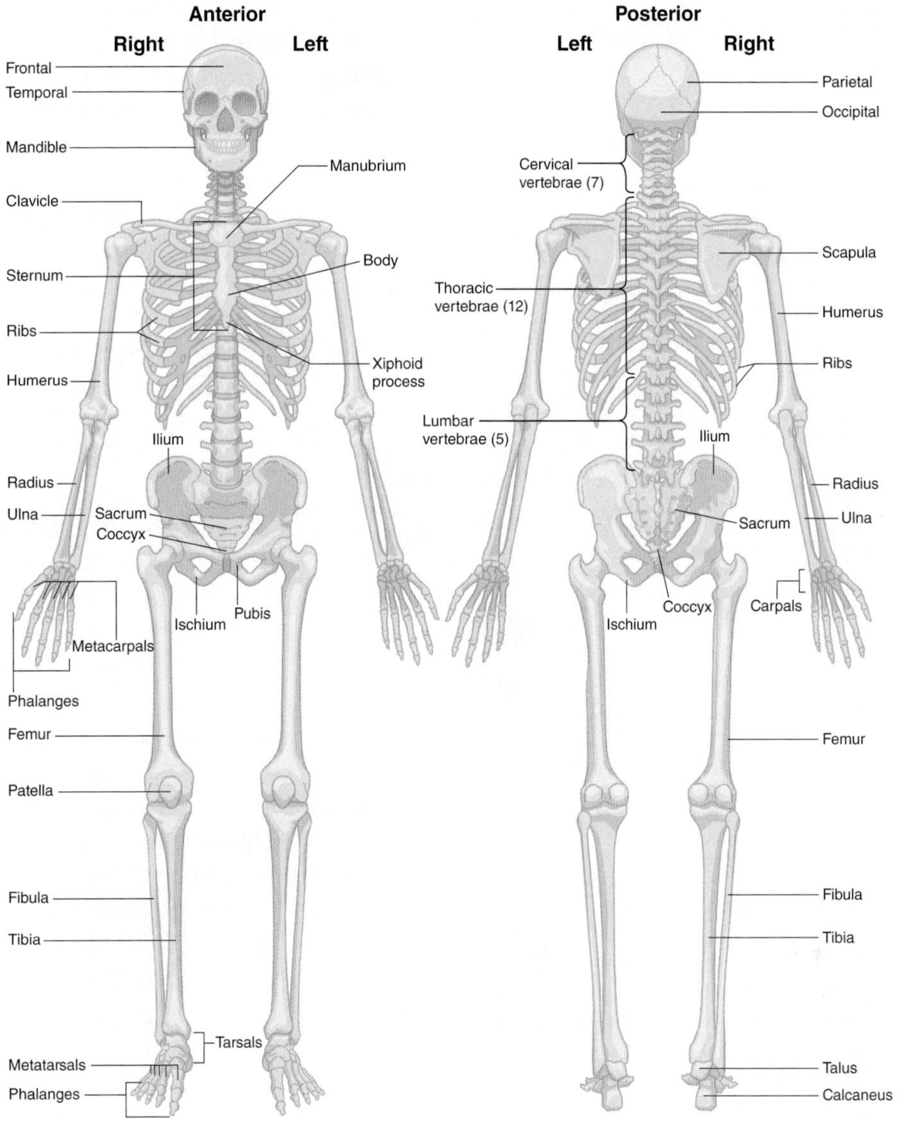

FIGURE 32-1 Skeleton.

simultaneous relaxation of other muscles combine to produce body movement. These movements are made possible by pulling one of the bones toward the other across a movable joint.

Postural maintenance is the result of muscle tone. **Muscle tone** is the constant tension produced by muscles of the body for long periods of time and is responsible for keeping the back and legs straight, the head in an upright position, and the abdomen from bulging. Postural maintenance also balances the distribution of body weight, which places less strain on muscles, tendons, ligaments, and bones.

General Assessment Strategies

The general assessment of a patient's musculoskeletal system includes an examination of the extremities, spine, vascular system, and motor system. The purpose of the assessment is to identify abnormal findings, which may include the following:[1]

- Pain or tenderness
- Swelling
- Abnormal or loss of movement
- Decreased sensation
- Circulatory changes
- Deformity

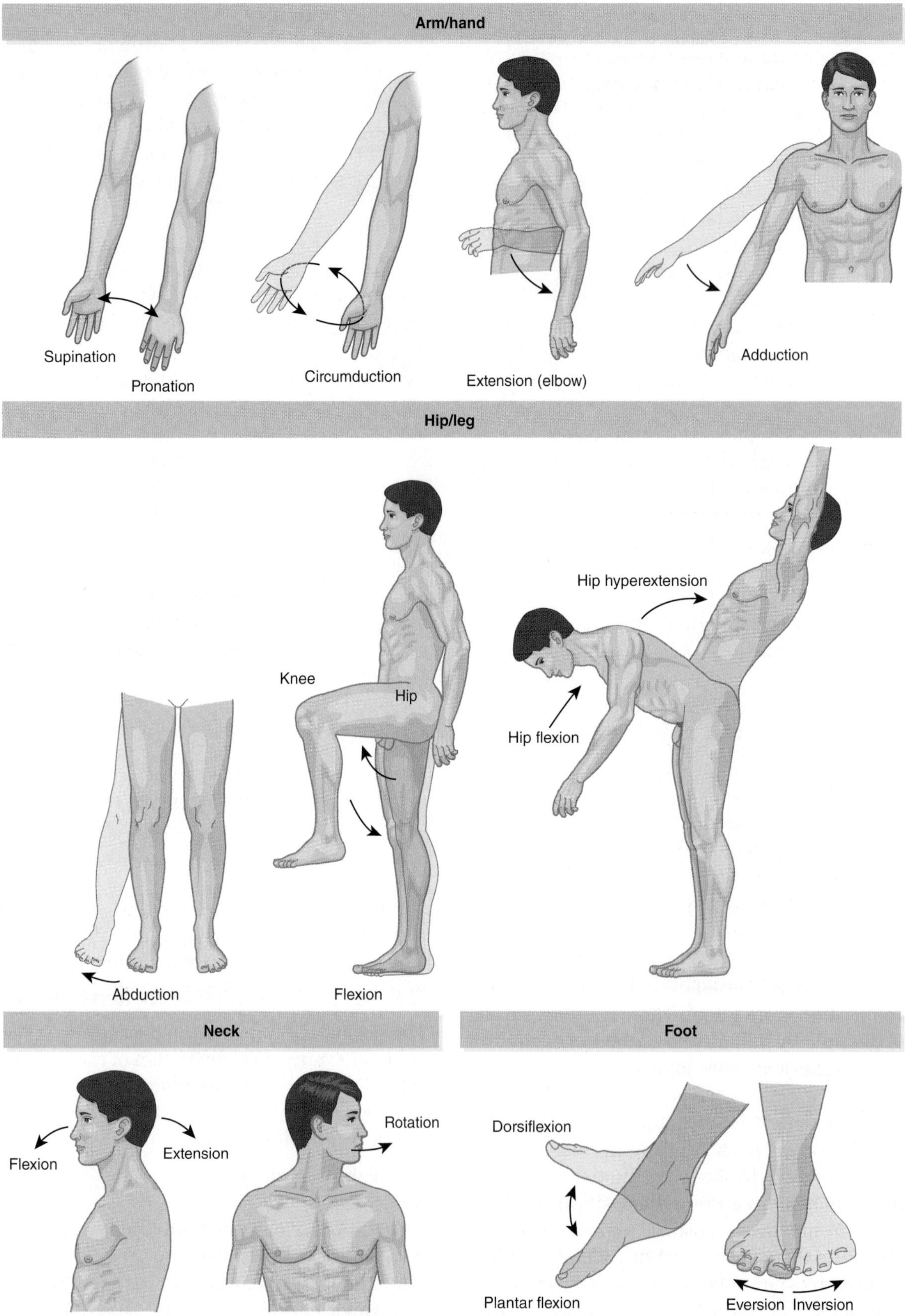

FIGURE 32-2 Joints.

Extremity Examination

The patient's extremities should be examined for function and structure. General appearance, body proportions, and ease of movement should be noted. Another important observation is limitation in the range of motion, or an unusual increase in the mobility of a joint. Abnormal findings may include signs of inflammation (swelling, tenderness, increased heat, redness, decreased function), asymmetry, crepitus, deformities, decreased muscular strength, and **atrophy** (muscle wasting).

An assessment of the upper and lower extremities should include an evaluation of the skin and tissue overlying the muscles, cartilage, and bones. It should also include an assessment of the joints for soft-tissue injury, discoloration, and swelling. The upper and lower extremities should be reasonably symmetrical in structure and muscularity. Skin color, temperature, sensation, and the presence of distal pulses will help determine the circulatory status of each extremity. The patient's joints should be assessed for full range of motion. All movement should be made without pain, deformity, limitation, or instability. Specific components of the extremities should be assessed as follows:

- **Hands and wrists.** The patient's hands and wrists should be inspected for contour and positional alignment. The hands, wrists, and joints of each finger should be assessed for tenderness, swelling, and deformity.
- **Elbows.** The patient's elbows should be assessed and palpated in both flexed and extended positions. All movement should be made without pain or discomfort.
- **Shoulders.** Both shoulders should be symmetrical and should be palpated for integrity of the clavicles, scapulae, and humeri. In addition, the patient should be able to shrug the shoulders and raise and extend both arms without pain or discomfort.
- **Pelvis and hips.** Structural integrity of the patient's iliac crest and symphysis pubis should be assessed to determine stability. There should be no deformity or point tenderness during palpation.
- **Knees.** The knees should be inspected and palpated for swelling and tenderness. The patella should be nontender and in midline position. The patient should be able to bend and straighten each knee without pain.
- **Ankles and feet.** The ankles and feet should be inspected for contour, position, and size. Tenderness, swelling, and deformity are abnormal findings. The patient's toes should be straight and aligned with each other. The surface of the ankles and feet should be free of deformities, nodules, swelling, and calluses.

Spine Examination

A visual assessment should be made of the patient's cervical, thoracic, and lumbar curves. Abnormal findings may include curvature of the spine from abnormal **lordosis**, **kyphosis**, and **scoliosis**. In addition, there should be no major differences in the height of the shoulders or iliac crest that might result from abnormal spinal curvature.

The patient's neck should be in a midline position. The posterior neck should be free of point tenderness and swelling. In addition, the patient should be able to bend the head forward, backward, and from side to side without pain or discomfort.

The patient's thoracic and lumbar (thoracolumbar) spine should be inspected for signs of injury, swelling, or discoloration. In a normal examination, the spine is not tender to palpation.

Vascular Examination

The peripheral vascular system includes arteries, veins, the lymphatic system, and the fluids exchanged in the capillary beds. An assessment of the vascular system should be part of the general assessment strategy. The patient's upper and lower extremities should be assessed for color and texture and for arterial insufficiency. Lymph nodes should not be swollen or tender. Abnormal findings in a vascular examination include the following:

- Pale or cyanotic skin
- Weak or diminished pulses
- Skin that is cold to the touch
- Absence of hair growth
- Pitting edema

Motor Examination

The patient should be observed while moving and while at rest. Any abnormal or involuntary movements should be noted, as well as the patient's posture, level of activity, and fatigue. Muscle strength should be equal on both sides of the body. Patients should be assessed for agility and tested for flexion, extension, and abduction of the upper and lower extremities.

Coordination can be evaluated for point-to-point movements, gait, and stance. Examples of **point-to-point movements** include touching the finger to the nose and touching each heel to the opposite shin. Methods to evaluate **gait** include asking the patient to walk toe to toe, walk on the toes, and walk on the heels. **Stance** and balance can be evaluated through the Romberg test and the pronator drift test (see Chapter 19, *Secondary Assessment and Reassessment*).

Finally, a healthy patient should be responsive to sensations of pain, temperature, position, vibration, and touch. These sensations are conducted by the sensory pathways of the nervous system. Sensory examinations can be performed on conscious patients by using light touch on each hand and each foot. The examination should proceed from head to toe and be symmetrical on both sides of the body.

BOX 32-2 Questions to Ask for Musculoskeletal Disorders

Complaint: Joint Pain

Where is the specific site of pain?
Does the pain change during the course of the day?
Have you had a recent injury?
How long has there been pain in the joint?
Does the pain get better or worse with movement?

Complaint: Muscle Weakness

Is the weakness widespread or isolated to one area?
Is the weakness related to a painful extremity?
Does the weakness fluctuate or is it constant?
Is the weakness increasing in severity?
Is the weakness associated with sensory changes?
Is there a family history of muscle disease?
Is the weakness the same on both sides of the body?

Complaint: Back Pain

Is the pain confined to the back or does it radiate to the upper or lower limbs?
Is the pain made worse by coughing or sneezing?
Was the pain sudden or gradual in onset?

Complaint: Gait or Balance Issues

Do you trip when walking?
Do you stagger to one particular side?
Do you ever injure yourself when walking?

General Management Strategies

General management strategies for a patient with a musculoskeletal disorder are the same as those for most other patient care encounters. Prehospital care will be guided by the patient's chief complaint and the severity of the patient's condition. General management strategies include the following:

- Scene size-up to ensure personal safety
- A primary survey to ensure airway, ventilation, and circulation
- Secondary assessment and reassessment
- Pharmacologic and nonpharmacologic measures to ensure comfort
- Transport considerations
- Effective therapeutic communications

The Patient History

The patient history should be thorough and focused on the patient's chief complaint. In addition to the general medical history described in Chapter 17, *History Taking*, specific questions to ask a patient with a musculoskeletal disorder are listed in BOX 32-2.

Management Guidelines

Prehospital care for most musculoskeletal disorders will be primarily supportive. Management most often is limited to immobilization of the affected area or body part, application of ice and/or elevation of an extremity to reduce pain and swelling, administration of analgesics to relieve pain, and gentle transport for physician evaluation.

Osteomyelitis

Osteomyelitis is an acute or chronic bone infection. The infection can be caused by a number of microbial agents, most commonly *Staphylococcus aureus.* Osteomyelitis also can develop from a puncture wound, an open fracture, or a minor wound infection, or following bone or joint surgery. It can also result from systemic infection (eg, urinary tract infection, pneumonia) that allows bacteria to spread in the bloodstream and enter the bone. If left untreated, the infection can become chronic, resulting in a decreased blood supply to the bone and eventual death of the bone tissue. Osteomyelitis affects both children and adults and can affect any bone. In adults, the vertebrae are most often affected by the disease; in children, the long bones are most often involved.

BOX 32-3 Signs and Symptoms of Osteomyelitis

Pain and/or tenderness in the infected area
Swelling and warmth in the infected area
Fever, chills
General malaise
Drainage of pus through the skin
Excessive sweating
Back or neck pain (if the spine is involved)
Swelling of the ankles, feet, and legs
Walking that is painful or with a limp

The following populations are at increased risk for developing osteomyelitis:

- People who have undergone recent orthopedic surgery
- Older adults
- Intravenous (IV) drug abusers
- People with sickle cell disease
- People receiving hemodialysis
- People with diabetes
- People with compromised immune systems

Signs, Symptoms, and Patient Care

Signs and symptoms of osteomyelitis are listed in BOX 32-3. The disease is diagnosed using blood tests to confirm infection, and blood cultures to identify the bacteria. Other diagnostic tools include needle aspiration, biopsy, radiography, magnetic resonance imaging (MRI), computed tomography (CT), and bone scans. Once the diagnosis has been made, patients are treated with oral or IV antibiotics to manage the infection and to prevent reinfection. Other care may include surgical drainage of a wound or abscess, immobilization of the affected bone or surrounding joints, and sometimes surgery to scrape the infection from the affected bone. In rare cases, amputation of an affected limb may be required.

Bone Tumors

A **bone tumor** is an abnormal growth of cells within a bone. The tumor can be **malignant** (cancerous) or **benign** (noncancerous). Most bone tumors are benign and not life threatening. Common bone tumors that are benign include nonossifying fibroma, unicameral bone cyst, osteochondroma, giant cell tumor, enchondroma, and fibrous dysplasia.

Malignant tumors can spread cancer cells throughout the body (**metastasis**) via blood or the lymphatic system. Cancers of the breast, lung, thyroid, renal cells, and prostate often metastasize to the bone. A **primary tumor** is a malignant tumor that is in the original site where it first arose. A **secondary tumor** is a malignant tumor that originates in another area of the body and spreads to the bone. The four most common types of primary bone tumors are described as follows:[2]

- **Multiple myeloma.** Multiple myeloma is the most common primary bone cancer. It is a malignant tumor of bone marrow (**FIGURE 32-3**). Multiple myeloma affects approximately 6 people per 100,000 each year.[3] Most cases are seen in patients between the ages of 50 and 70 years. Any bone can be involved.
- **Osteosarcoma.** Osteosarcoma is the second most common bone cancer. It occurs in 2 to 5 people per 1 million each year. Most cases occur in teenagers or children. Most tumors occur around the knee in the tibia or femur. Other common locations include the hip and shoulder.
- **Ewing sarcoma.** Ewing sarcoma most commonly occurs between 5 and 20 years of age. The most common locations are the upper and lower leg, pelvis, upper arm, and ribs.
- **Chondrosarcoma.** Chondrosarcoma occurs most commonly in patients between 40 and 70 years of age. Most cases occur around the hip and pelvis or the shoulder.

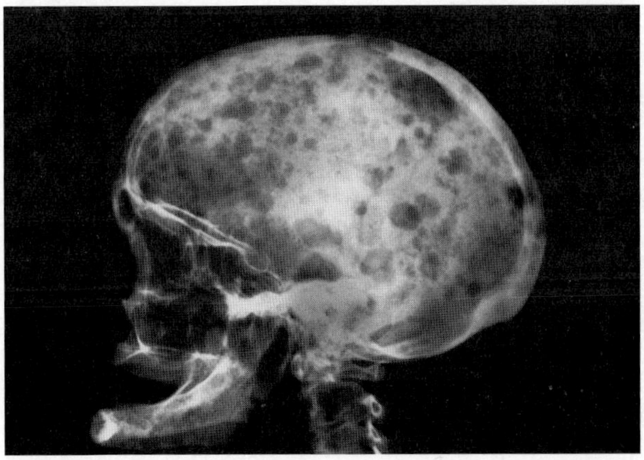

FIGURE 32-3 Multiple myeloma of the skull. Radiograph shows punched-out bone lesions filled with soft tumor.

Signs, Symptoms, and Patient Care

Most patients with a bone tumor experience a dull or aching pain in the area of the tumor. The pain is sometimes made worse with physical activity and often awakes the patient at night. Other patients will not complain of pain but will have discovered a painless mass on self-examination. Pathologic fractures are common in these patients. These fractures result from trauma or a metabolic disease, such as osteoporosis, in which the bone weakened by the tumor breaks.

Benign tumors may or may not require treatment (depending on the specific tumor). Some benign tumors can be aggressive and quickly destroy bone. Malignant tumors may require medication therapy or surgical removal. Still other tumors resolve on their own (especially some bone tumors in children). Most malignant tumors are surgically removed and treated with radiation. If the cancer has metastasized, other treatment may include additional radiation, chemotherapy, and cryosurgery (the freezing and killing of cancer cells with liquid nitrogen). In some patients, a bone implant or amputation of an affected limb will be needed. Patient follow-up with regular blood tests and radiography is required because bone cancer can recur. People who have had bone cancer, particularly children and adolescents, have an increased likelihood of developing another type of cancer later in life.[4]

NOTE

A **pathologic fracture** is a fracture through abnormally weak bone from a force that would not fracture a normal bone. Any disease process that weakens a bone (especially the cortex) predisposes the bone to pathologic fracture. Pathologic fractures are commonly associated with tumors, osteoporosis, infections, and metabolic bone disorders. In some of these patients, very minor trauma or even no apparent trauma (eg, turning over in bed) can cause a pathologic fracture.

Modified from: Patel AA, Ramanathan R, Kuban J, Willis MH. Imaging findings and evaluation of metabolic bone disease. *Advances in Radiology.* Hindawi website. https://www.hindawi.com/journals/ara/2015/812794/. Published February 24, 2015. Accessed February 15, 2018.

Low Back Pain

Most everyone at some point has back pain that interferes with work, routine daily activities, or recreation. Americans visit the emergency department (ED) 2.7 million times annually because of low back pain.[5] Three months after their ED visit, 20% to 35% of these patients continue to report pain and impaired function. Back pain is one of the primary reasons older adults call emergency medical services (EMS) within 30 days of a prior transport.[6]

The vertebral column consists of 33 bones that are divided into 5 regions: 7 cervical vertebrae, 12 thoracic vertebrae, 5 lumbar vertebrae, 5 sacral vertebrae, and 4 (the number of bones can range from 3 to 5) coccygeal vertebrae (fused). Together, the vertebrae protect the spinal cord, the rootlets, and the 31 pairs of spinal nerves that convey sensation. The weight-bearing portion of the vertebra is a bony vertebral body. Intervertebral disks are located between the bodies of adjacent vertebrae and serve as shock absorbers (**FIGURE 32-4**). The disks allow for flexibility of the back. They also prevent the vertebral bodies from rubbing against each other.

Low back pain may be classified as *acute* or *chronic*. Acute back pain is usually of short duration, lasting only a few days to a few weeks. Most acute back pain is caused by trauma to the low back (eg, a sports injury or heavy lifting). It can also be caused by arthritis or other degenerative joint disease of the spine, viral infections, and congenital abnormalities. Chronic back pain is back pain that persists for 3 or more months. Although the cause of chronic back pain can be difficult to determine, it can be progressive and debilitating. The conditions discussed in this chapter are disorders of the intervertebral disks, cauda equina syndrome, and sprains and strains of the muscles and supporting structures of the back.

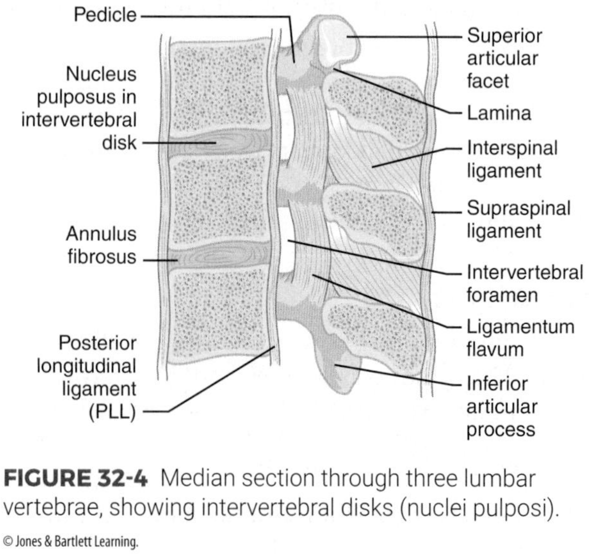

FIGURE 32-4 Median section through three lumbar vertebrae, showing intervertebral disks (nuclei pulposi).

NOTE

Prehospital care for patients with low back pain is primarily supportive. Most care is focused on obtaining a thorough history and providing comfort measures and gentle transport for physician evaluation. Physicians investigate most cases of low back pain through radiography, MRIs, and CT scans. A nonsteroidal anti-inflammatory drug (NSAID) such as ketorolac may be administered if local protocol permits.

Disorders of the Intervertebral Disks

As stated previously, the intervertebral disks are found between the bodies of the vertebrae. They act as shock absorbers, prevent the bones of the spine from grinding against each other, and allow for flexibility of the back. Each disk has a central area composed of a jellylike substance, called the nucleus pulposus, which is surrounded by concentric rings of fibrous tissue (annulus fibrosus). Undue stress (along with degenerative disease) on a disk can force the gel against the inner ring and crack it. From there, the gel pushes outward, cracking successive rings in its path. If stress on the back is severe enough, the vertebral disks and fibrous tissues can be damaged, causing the disk to bulge or protrude. If the gel eventually breaks through the outer ring, it can pinch the nerve root leading from the vertebra, resulting in a **herniated disk**, often referred to as a "slipped disk" (**FIGURE 32-5**).

Disk injury most often affects the lumbar spine (most commonly L4-L5, L5-S1) in patients 30 to 50 years of age.[7] The most common risk factor for developing lumbar disk disease is lack of exercise that allows the muscles of the back to weaken. Symptoms of a herniated disk vary greatly depending on the position of the herniated disk and the size of the herniation. Common signs and symptoms may include the following:

- Low back ache
- Numbness or weakness in the lower extremities
- Deep muscle pain and muscle spasms
- Acute or gradual leg pain (usually in only one leg)
- "Shooting" pain in the leg when sneezing, coughing, or straining; may be aggravated by sitting, prolonged standing, bending, or twisting
- Nerve-related symptoms, including muscle weakness in one or both legs, pain in the front of the thigh, and sciatica (**BOX 32-4**)

The goal of treatment for a herniated disk is to relieve pain, weakness, or numbness in the leg caused by pressure on the spinal nerve root or spinal cord. Most patients are first treated with bed rest, analgesics, anti-inflammatories, muscle relaxants, and corticosteroids, either orally or by injection directly into the epidural space surrounding the affected nerve root. Physical therapy and exercise programs can help strengthen the back and prevent recurrent injury. Most herniated disks heal without

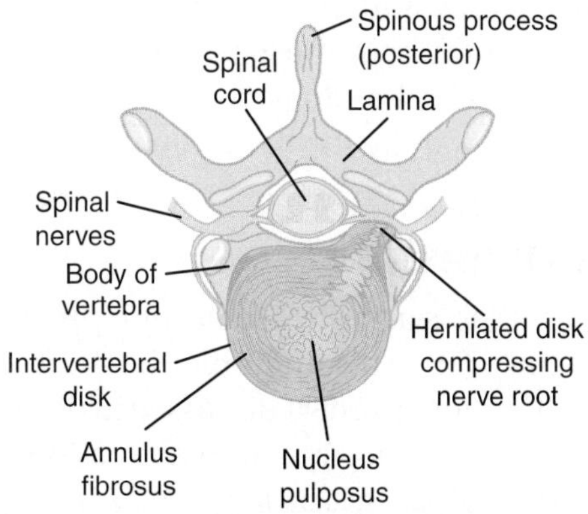

FIGURE 32-5 Herniated intervertebral disk.

BOX 32-4 Sciatica

Sciatica (sciatic neuralgia) is a symptom of compression or inflammation of the sciatic nerve. The sciatic nerve is the largest nerve in the body. It runs from the spinal cord to the buttock and hip area and down the back of each leg. This nerve innervates muscles in the back of the knee and lower leg. It also provides sensation to the back of the thigh, lower leg, and sole of the foot. Inflammation of the sciatic nerve causes pain, weakness, numbness, and tingling along its path. Sciatica usually affects only one leg.

Sciatica is a common condition that occurs in about 40% of adults at some point in their lives. It is often caused by a herniated disk or spinal stenosis. It can also be caused by injury (eg, pelvic fracture). Although the discomfort of sciatica can be severe and debilitating, it usually resolves without treatment or surgery in 4 to 8 weeks.

Modified from: Ergun T, Lakadamyali H. CT and MRI in the evaluation of extraspinal sciatica. *Br J Radiol*. 2010;83(993):791-803.

surgery to remove the herniated portion of the disk (**microdiskectomy**) or to remove part of the bone or tissue that is compressing the nerve (**laminectomy**).

Cauda Equina Syndrome

Cauda equina syndrome is a rare disorder of the lumbar spine that affects the bundle of nerve roots at the lower end of the spinal cord. It is a surgical emergency that occurs when the nerve compression leads to muscle paralysis, cutting off sensation and movement. If not treated, the syndrome can result in permanent paralysis, impaired bladder and bowel function, and loss of sexual sensation. Even with surgery to relieve the pressure on nerve roots, nerve damage may be irreversible.

Cauda equina syndrome can be caused by a herniated disk, spinal tumor, infection, and **spinal stenosis** (narrowing of the spinal canal). It can also result from spinal trauma, including direct trauma, falls, gunshot wounds, and stabbings. (Children born with spinal abnormalities also can develop the syndrome.) Signs and symptoms of cauda equina syndrome vary in intensity and may evolve slowly over time. They include the following:

- Bladder and/or bowel dysfunction (loss of control; inability to urinate or defecate)
- Severe or progressive weakness in the lower extremities
- Loss of sensation or an altered sensation between the legs, in the perineum and genital areas, over the buttocks, in the inner thighs and back of the legs (saddle area), and in the feet and heels
- Pain, numbness, or weakness that spreads to one or both legs and may cause a stumbling gait or difficulty rising from a sitting position

Sprains and Strains of the Lower Back

The lower back carries much of the body's weight during walking, running, lifting, and other activities. Because muscles, ligaments, and bones of the spine provide control and strength for many movements, sprains and strains of the lower back (especially the lumbar spine) are common injuries. They are often caused by twisting or pulling and from improper lifting that puts the back at risk for injury. More than 50% of EMS personnel responding to a large national survey reported back pain within the prior two weeks.[8]

SHOW ME THE EVIDENCE

Researchers sought to identify nonmechanical factors associated with back pain among EMS workers. They conducted a cross-sectional study, sending a survey to a sample of 3,359 participants enrolled in the Longitudinal EMT Attributes and Demographics Study (LEADS) who had previously reported a back problem. In addition, they randomly sampled 1,050 participants with no report of back problems. Half of the respondents reported one or more days of recent pain (within 2 weeks). Odds of having back pain were greater in those who had a prior back problem than in those who did not (odds ratio [OR], 3.56; 95% confidence interval [CI], 2.72–4.68). Fair or poor health was much more often cited (OR, 5.22; 95% CI, 2.17–8.61) in those with back pain compared to those without pain. In addition, those who were dissatisfied or very dissatisfied with their job were more likely to have back pain than were those who were satisfied with their job (OR, 3.23; 95% CI, 2.00–5.22).

Modified from: Studnek JR, Crawford M, Wilkins RL, Pennell M. Back problems among emergency medical services. *Am J Ind Med*. 2010;53(1):12-22.

A **strain** is an injury to a muscle or tendon. A **sprain** is the stretching or tearing of a ligament beyond its normal range of movement. Differentiating a sprain from a strain is difficult and unnecessary in the prehospital setting. The signs, symptoms, treatment, and prognosis for both conditions are the same. Signs and symptoms include pain, warmth, muscle spasms, and swelling of the affected area. Most muscle sprains and strains of the lower back are successfully treated with bed rest for 24 to 48 hours to allow the back to heal. Analgesics, muscle relaxants, and anti-inflammatories may be prescribed. Physical therapy and exercise programs can help to strengthen the back muscles and prevent future injury. Back pain that does not resolve with these measures will require further evaluation.

Joint Disorders

A **joint disorder** is any disease or injury that affects human joints. These disorders may be short-lived or chronic. The joint disorders discussed in this chapter are those that produce inflammation as a result of disease, including various forms of arthritis. Joint disorders that result from trauma are discussed in Chapter 43, *Orthopaedic Trauma*.

Arthritis

Arthritis is an inflammatory condition of the joint, characterized by pain and swelling. The disease has been diagnosed in about 54 million adults and is a leading cause of disability in the United States.[9] Although there are many kinds of arthritis, the disease can be grouped into several general categories: osteoarthritis, rheumatoid arthritis (RA), septic arthritis, and gout. Systemic lupus (described in Chapter 26, *Immune System Disorders*) is associated with severe joint pain and is sometimes classified with arthritic conditions.

NOTE

Prehospital care for joint disorders is primarily supportive, as it is for most other nontraumatic musculoskeletal disorders. Care is often limited to providing comfort measures and gentle transport for physician evaluation. Physician care for most joint disorders includes a combination of patient education, physical therapy, weight control, and medications to reduce pain and inflammation. In some cases, surgery or joint replacement may be indicated.

Osteoarthritis

Osteoarthritis is a chronic, degenerative joint disease most often seen in people older than 50 years, especially those who are obese.[10] The onset of the disease is gradual and affects women more often than it does men. Osteoarthritis is mechanical in nature, resulting from normal wear and tear on joints over the course of a person's life. It is marked by the breakdown of cartilage that covers the surfaces of joints and by the formation of **bone spurs** (bony growths formed on normal bone). The wearing away of cartilage and the overgrowth of bone lead to pain and stiffness. As the disease progresses, bone rubs against bone, causing severe pain and reduced mobility. The joints most commonly affected are those in the knees, hips, hands, and the cervical and lumbar spine (BOX 32-5).

NOTE

Osteoarthritis and *osteoporosis* have similar names but are very different conditions. Osteoporosis is a disease characterized by the loss of bone tissue, causing the bones to weaken and easily fracture. Osteoarthritis is primarily a disease of the joint cartilage (see Chapter 48, *Geriatrics*).

Rheumatoid Arthritis

Rheumatoid arthritis (RA) is an inflammatory disease of the joints that causes pain, swelling, stiffness, and loss of function. It is estimated that about 1.3 million people in the United States have the disease.[11] It occurs in all races and ethnic groups. Symptoms of the disease usually become apparent in middle and later life but can also develop in young adults and children (BOX 32-6).

RA develops when lymphocytes travel to the synovium in the joints, causing inflammation (synovitis). During this process, the normally thin synovium becomes thick and makes the joint swollen and puffy to the touch. As the disease progresses, the inflamed synovium invades and damages the cartilage and bone of the joint. Surrounding muscles, ligaments, and tendons become weakened. RA also can cause more generalized bone loss that may lead to osteoporosis. Unlike some other forms of arthritis, where only a specific joint is affected, RA generally occurs in a symmetrical pattern (eg, both hands, both knees). A hallmark of the disease is visible swelling and inflammation of the finger joints closest to the affected hand (**FIGURE 32-6**). RA may also affect other areas of the body (neck, shoulder, elbows, feet) and is often associated with fatigue, occasional fever, and general malaise.

BOX 32-5 Slipped Capital Femoral Epiphysis

Slipped capital femoral epiphysis is a separation of the ball of the hip joint from the femur at the upper, growing end (growth plate) of the bone. It occurs in about 2 out of every 100,000 children. It is most common in boys 11 to 15 years of age, in children who are obese, in those who have hormone imbalances, and in those having growth spurts. The condition may affect one or both hips and can occur after even minor trauma (eg, jumping from a small height). Signs and symptoms include pain and tenderness in the thigh and hip or knee. The affected limb may be slightly rotated in an outward position. This external rotation deformity is more pronounced as the hip is flexed. Patients with this condition should not bear weight on the affected leg. A slipped capital femoral epiphysis most often requires surgery to stabilize the hip joint. The condition is associated with early arthritis of the hip joint and a greater risk for osteoarthritis later in life.

Modified from: US National Library of Medicine. Slipped capital femoral epiphysis. MedlinePlus website. https://medlineplus.gov/ency/article/000972.htm. Updated February 7, 2018. Accessed February 15, 2018.

BOX 32-6 Ankylosing Spondylitis

Ankylosing spondylitis (AS) is a form of arthritis that primarily affects the spine, although other joints can become involved. It causes inflammation of the vertebrae that can lead to severe, chronic pain and discomfort. In the most advanced cases, this inflammation can lead to new bone formation on the spine, causing the spine to fuse in a fixed, immobile position. This condition sometimes creates a forward-stooped posture (kyphosis). AS can cause inflammation, pain, and stiffness in other areas of the body (eg, the shoulders, hips, ribs, heels, and small joints of the hands and feet). The eyes can also be involved. Rarely, the lungs and heart can be affected. Unlike other forms of arthritis and rheumatic diseases, general onset of AS commonly occurs in younger people, before age 30 years. Symptoms begin after age 45 years in only 5% of people with AS. The disease is more common in men than in women. The severity of the disease varies from person to person and may lead to permanent disability.

Paramedics and other emergency personnel must remember that patients with AS have inflexible spines that cannot be moved. EMS procedures must be modified to accommodate these patients to prevent further injury. Modifications may be needed for splinting procedures, airway procedures, and transport considerations. For example, patients with AS will require additional padding with splinting techniques. Airway procedures must be performed without flexing the neck. If possible, advanced airway devices that do not require visualization of the airway (eg, King L&D, laryngeal mask airway [LMA]) should be used instead of endotracheal intubation. Padding with pillows to support the patient's head, neck, and upper back will need to be applied during transport. Special training is available to EMS personnel for managing patients with this condition.

Modified from: National Institute of Arthritis and Musculoskeletal and Skin Diseases. What is ankylosing spondylitis? National Institutes of Health website. https://www.niams.nih.gov/sites/default/files/catalog/files/ankylosing_spondylitis_ff.pdf. Published November 2014. Accessed February 15, 2018; Overview of ankylosing spondylitis. Spondylitis Association of America website. www.spondylitis.org/about/as.aspx. Accessed February 15, 2018.

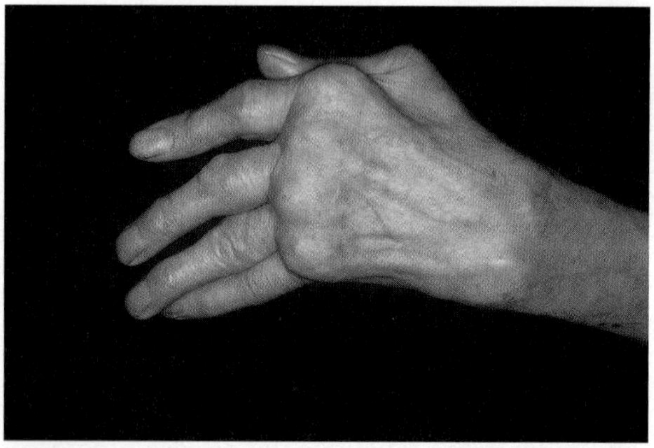

FIGURE 32-6 Rheumatoid arthritis of the hands.

NOTE

Juvenile rheumatoid arthritis (JRA), also known as juvenile idiopathic arthritis (JIA), is a classification system for chronic arthritis in children. Most forms of juvenile arthritis are autoimmune disorders. Children with the disease are thought to have a genetic predisposition to it. Development of the disease is then triggered by an environmental factor, such as a virus. The most common symptoms of all types of juvenile arthritis are persistent joint swelling, fatigue, pain, and stiffness that is typically worse in the morning or after a nap. The pain may limit movement of the affected joint, although many children, especially younger ones, will not complain of pain. Other symptoms include high fever and rash. Children with RA require multidisciplinary treatment and specialty care.

Patients with RA have varying degrees of the disease. Some patients have only limited bouts, followed by remission and little damage. In other patients, the disease is regularly active, lasting many years to a lifetime. This form of RA often leads to severe joint damage and disability. Physician care may include anti-inflammatories to reduce pain and inflammation, disease-modifying antirheumatic drugs to slow the course of the disease, analgesics, and physical therapy. Some patients have secondary treatment with biologic response modifiers (biologicals). Commonly performed surgical procedures include joint replacement, tendon reconstruction, and synovectomy.

NOTE

Biologic response modifiers are a class of drugs used for the treatment of RA. They help reduce inflammation and damage to the joints by blocking the action of cytokines (proteins of the body's immune system that trigger inflammation during normal immune responses). Examples of these drugs include etanercept (Enbrel), certolizumab (Cimzia), infliximab (Remicade), adalimumab (Humira), sarilumab (Kevzara), rituximab (Rituxan), abatacept (Orencia), tofacitinib (Xeljanz), and anakinra (Kineret). All biologics increase the patient's risk for serious infections.

Modified from: Biologics overview. Arthritis Association website. http://www.arthritis.org/living-with-arthritis/treatments/medication/drug-types/biologics/drug-guide-biologics.php. Accessed February 15, 2018; Saux NL. Biologic response modifiers to decrease inflammation: focus on infection risks. *Paediatr Child Health*. 2012;17(3):147-150.

CRITICAL THINKING

When caring for a patient with severe RA, how might you have to modify your care if you suspect spine injury?

Septic Arthritis

Septic arthritis is also known as infectious arthritis. The condition results from direct invasion of the joint space by microorganisms. These microorganisms include bacteria (most common), viruses, mycobacteria, and fungi. The incidence of septic arthritis in the United States appears to be increasing.[12] It can occur in both children and adults.

The disease process begins when the infectious agent (most commonly, *aureus*) enters the joint. This situation usually occurs from active infection elsewhere in the body, such as a respiratory tract infection or urinary tract infection. Infection also can occur from direct invasion (eg, an open wound near the joint, joint surgery). When the bacterium reaches the synovium in the joint, the immune system is activated, and cartilage begins to be destroyed. This process results in inflammation and reduced blood flow to the joint and surrounding structures. Previously damaged joints, especially from RA, are the most susceptible to infection. The most commonly involved joint is the knee, followed by the hip, shoulder, ankle, and wrist. Signs and symptoms of septic arthritis include fever; shaking chills; and severe pain, warmth, and swelling in the affected joint. Septic arthritis is treated with surgical drainage and irrigation followed by antibiotics to resolve the infection. In severe cases, the joint may require surgical reconstruction or replacement.

Gout

Gout is a form of arthritis marked by the deposit of uric acid crystals in and around a joint. Gout affects mostly men and is thought to be hereditary. For unknown reasons, gout surfaces most often in the metatarsophalangeal joint of the big toe. It usually appears in only one joint at a time. Other joints often affected are the other toe joints, the ankle, and the knee. The disease is associated with an increased risk for developing kidney stones.[13]

NOTE

Pseudogout is inflammation caused by calcium pyrophosphate crystals. It is often clinically indistinguishable from gout. Both conditions are treated the same. Like gout, pseudogout is associated with a variety of metabolic disorders. However, unlike gout, there is no specific therapeutic regimen to treat the underlying cause of the disease. The most common sites for pseudogout are the knees, wrists, and shoulders. The symptoms often occur gradually over several days.

In acute gout, the affected joint and surrounding tissues appear hot, red, and swollen. The pain is usually intense and made worse by stimulation or light touch (eg, covering the toe with a blanket). Gout may remit for long periods, followed by flares that last days to weeks. Chronic gout can lead to a degenerative form of arthritis called gouty arthritis. Risk factors for gout include joint injury, obesity, heart failure, hypertension, alcohol use, diuretics that lead to hyperuricemia, and diets that are rich in meat and seafood.[13] Of the forms of arthritis discussed here, gout is the most treatable form of the disease. It is managed with anti-inflammatories (colchicine and corticosteroids). An acute episode usually subsides within 24 hours after treatment begins. Some patients are prescribed allopurinol to reduce uric acid production and prevent recurrence.

Muscle Disorders

The muscles of the body fulfill many purposes, such as movement, postural maintenance, and heat production. Inflammation of skeletal muscle can result from injury, infection, or autoimmune disease. Skeletal muscle disorders discussed in this chapter include myalgia and chronic fatigue syndrome (CFS). Trauma-related causes of muscle weakness, such as rhabdomyolysis and compartment syndrome, are described in Chapter 37, *Bleeding and Soft-Tissue Trauma.*

Myalgia

Myalgia means muscle pain or pain in multiple muscles. There are many causes and various types of myalgia. The condition can be acute and temporary, or it can be chronic. Myalgia most often results from overuse, muscle injury, or stress (described later in this chapter) and can also result from a virus, an infection, or an autoimmune disorder. Myalgia can be an indication of serious illness, including inflammatory myopathies and CFS.

Inflammatory Myopathies

Inflammatory myopathies refer to a group of diseases that involve chronic muscle inflammation accompanied by muscle weakness. Causes of these disorders may include injury, infection, autoimmune disease, alcohol and illicit drug use (eg, cocaine), and some prescribed medications (eg, some statins). The three main types of inflammatory myopathies are polymyositis, dermatomyositis, and myositis. These are rare disorders that can affect both children and adults. General symptoms that are common to these disorders include the following:[14]

- Slow and progressive muscle weakness that begins in the muscles closest to the trunk of the body
- Fatigue after walking or standing
- Frequent trips and falls
- Difficulty swallowing or breathing

Dermatomyositis is characterized by a skin rash that precedes or accompanies progressive muscle weakness. The rash looks patchy, with blue-purple or red discolorations. It characteristically develops on the eyelids and on muscles used to extend or straighten joints, including knuckles, elbows, heels, and toes. Red rashes and swelling may also occur on the face, neck, shoulders, upper chest, back, and other locations. The rash sometimes occurs without obvious muscle involvement. Dermatomyositis may be associated with collagen-vascular or autoimmune diseases, such as lupus.

Polymyositis causes muscle weakness affecting both sides of the body. It is rarely seen in people younger than 20 years; most cases are in adults between the ages of 30 and 60 years.[15] Slow but progressive muscle weakness leads to difficulties climbing stairs, rising from a sitting position, lifting objects, or reaching overhead. People with polymyositis may also experience arthritis, shortness of breath, difficulty swallowing and speaking, and cardiac dysrhythmias. In some cases of polymyositis, muscles farther from the trunk of the body, such as those in the forearms and around the ankles and wrists, may be affected as the disease progresses. Polymyositis may be associated with collagen-vascular or autoimmune diseases (eg, lupus) and with infectious disorders, such as human immunodeficiency virus/acquired immunodeficiency syndrome (HIV/AIDS).

Myositis is also known as inclusion body myositis and is an inflammatory muscle disease characterized by progressive muscle weakness and wasting. The disorder is characterized by progressive muscle weakness and wasting. Myositis often begins with weakness in the wrists and fingers that causes difficulty with pinching, buttoning, and gripping objects. There may be weakness of the wrist and finger muscles and atrophy of the muscles in the forearms and legs. Difficulty swallowing occurs in about one-half of patients.[14] Symptoms of the disease usually begin after the age of 50 years, although the disease can occur much earlier.

Management

There is no cure for inflammatory myopathies. Options for dermatomyositis and polymyositis include medications to reduce inflammation, physical therapy, exercise, heat therapy, orthotics, assistive devices, and rest. The standard treatment for these conditions includes oral or IV corticosteroid drugs and immunosuppressant drugs. Periodic treatment using IV immunoglobulin may also improve recovery.

There is no standard course of treatment for myositis. The disease is generally unresponsive to corticosteroids and immunosuppressive drugs. Physical therapy may be helpful in maintaining mobility. Other therapy is symptomatic and supportive.

Chronic Fatigue Syndrome

Chronic fatigue syndrome (CFS) is also known as myalgic encephalomyelitis (ME); thus the condition is often referred to as ME/CFS. It is a debilitating and complex disorder that is characterized by profound fatigue that is not improved by bed rest and that may be worsened by physical or mental activity. ME/CFS affects between 836,000 and 2.5 million Americans, although it is estimated up to 90% of those with the disorder have not been diagnosed.[16] About 25% of those who have ME/CFS are bed- or housebound because of the illness. The exact etiology of ME/CFS is unknown, but infection, immune system changes, stress, changes in energy production, and genetics are being studied as possible causes (BOX 32-7).[17]

NOTE

Fibromyalgia is another disorder that causes extreme fatigue. In addition to fatigue, fibromyalgia is associated with increased sensitivity to pain. The most common symptoms are generalized pain or stiffness; fatigue; depression; sleep problems; impaired memory, thinking, and concentration; and headaches. Some patients also experience paresthesias in the hands or feet, temporomandibular joint syndrome, and digestive problems.

Modified from: Bennett R. Clinical features of fibromyalgia. Fibromyalgia Information Foundation website. http://www.myalgia.com/Clinical_features_RB.htm. Accessed February 15, 2018.

BOX 32-7 Facts About Myalgic Encephalomyelitis/Chronic Fatigue Syndrome

- ME/CFS affects women more often than it does men.
- Most patients currently diagnosed with ME/CFS are Caucasian, but some studies suggest that ME/CFS is more common in minority groups of the US population.
- The average age of onset is 33 years, although ME/CFS has been reported in patients younger than 10 years and older than 70 years.
- At least one-fourth of ME/CFS patients are bed- or housebound at some point in their illness.
- Symptoms can persist for years, and most patients never regain their predisease level of health or functioning.
- ME/CFS patients experience loss of productivity and high medical costs that contribute to a total economic burden in the United States of $17 to $24 billion annually.

Modified from: Institute of Medicine of the National Academies. Myalgic encephalomyelitis/chronic fatigue syndrome (ME/CFS): key facts. National Academies Press website. https://www.nap.edu/resource/19012/MECFS_KeyFacts.pdf. Published February 2015. Accessed February 15, 2018.

Signs and Symptoms of ME/CFS

There are three core indicators of ME/CFS:

1. Marked decline in the ability to perform normal activities. This decline is accompanied by fatigue and persists at least 6 months.
2. Worsening of ME/CFS symptoms after physical or mental activities that would not have caused a problem before the illness.
3. Sleep disturbances, including fatigue even after adequate sleep, and difficulty falling asleep or remaining asleep.

In addition, difficulties with memory and concentration, and worsening symptoms when standing or sitting upright (orthostatic intolerance) must be present to diagnose ME/CFS. Other symptoms may include the following:[18]

- Irritable bowel or other digestive problems
- Pain
  - Muscle aches or pains
  - Joint pain without swelling or redness
  - Headaches
- Lymph node tenderness in the neck or axilla
- Chills and night sweats
- Frequent sore throat
- Allergies or sensitivities to foods, odors, chemicals, medications, or noise

ME/CFS often follows a cyclical course, alternating between periods of illness and relative well-being. Some patients experience partial or complete remission of symptoms during the course of the illness, but symptoms often reoccur.

Management

Prehospital care is primarily supportive. Diagnosis of ME/CFS and fibromyalgia is based on history and clinical signs and symptoms; there is no laboratory marker to confirm the disorders. Most patients are managed with a combination of therapies tailored to the severity of the illness. These methods may include counseling and behavioral therapy, drug therapy to relieve symptoms, relaxation therapy to reduce anxiety, and support groups with others who have the illness. There is no cure for the illness.

Overuse Syndromes

The overuse of muscles, tendons, ligaments, and supporting structures can result in numerous injuries and ailments (overuse syndromes). The specific disorders discussed in this chapter are bursitis, muscle strain, and tendonitis.

Bursitis

Bursitis is an inflammation of one or more bursae often caused by excessive use of a joint. A **bursa** is a small sac containing synovial fluid that helps ease friction between a tendon and skin or between a tendon and bone (**FIGURE 32-7**). Inflammation from injury, compression, overuse, or infection is the most common cause of bursitis. Bursitis is also associated with diseases such as gout, RA, and scleroderma. Areas most commonly affected include the elbow, shoulder, hip, knee, and Achilles tendon. Risk factors for developing bursitis include the following:[19]

- **Repetitive stress (overuse) injury.** This injury can occur when running, stair climbing, bicycling, or standing for long periods.
- **Hip injury.** An injury to the point of the hip can occur by falling onto the hip, bumping the hip, or lying on one side of the body for an extended period.
- **Spine disease.** Diseases of the spine include scoliosis, arthritis of the lumbar (lower) spine, and other spine problems.
- **Leg-length inequality.** When one leg is significantly shorter than the other, it affects the way a person walks and can lead to irritation of a hip bursa.
- **RA.** This disease makes the bursa more likely to become inflamed.
- **Previous surgery.** Surgery around the hip or prosthetic implants in the hip can irritate the bursa and cause bursitis.
- **Bone spurs or calcium deposits.** These can develop within the tendons that attach muscles to the trochanter. They can irritate the bursa and cause inflammation.

Bursitis most commonly affects people older than 40 years. The primary symptom of bursitis is pain, which may be sudden and severe. Loss of motion in a joint caused by crystal deposits can also indicate bursitis. Initial self-care for bursitis is described in **BOX 32-8**. Other treatment options may include corticosteroids (orally or by injection), antibiotics, physical therapy, needle aspiration of bursal fluid, and surgical removal or drainage of an infected bursal sac.

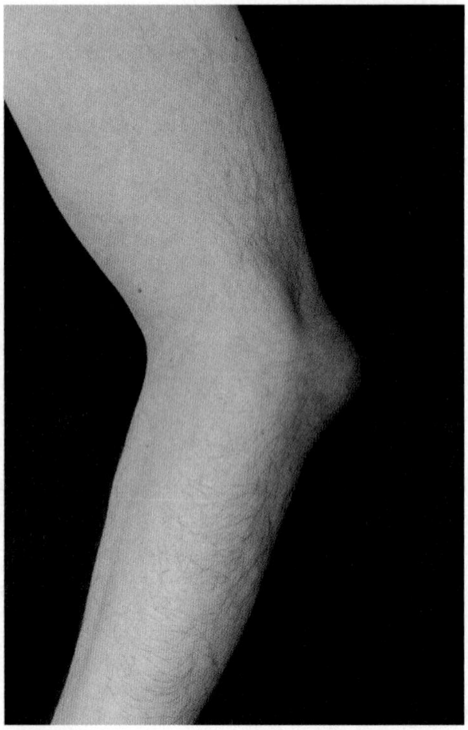

FIGURE 32-7 Bursitis.

BOX 32-8 Self-Care for Overuse Injuries

A self-care management approach for bursitis and other injuries, such as muscle strains, can be remembered using the acronym PRICEM:

- **Protection.** Protect the bursae that are close to the skin with padding.
- **Rest.** The affected body part must be given rest until the symptoms improve. Avoid any activities that cause additional pain.
- **Ice.** Ice packs can be effectively used in reducing the symptoms of inflammation and pain.
- **Compression.** Affected joints can be compressed by using elastic bandages or dressings to relieve pain.
- **Elevation.** Elevating the affected body part above the level of the heart may stop the blood from collecting in the bursae and help reduce inflammation.
- **Medication.** NSAIDs or over-the-counter pain medications such as ibuprofen can be effective in relieving the pain and reducing inflammation.

Modified from: Shiel WC Jr. Bursitis. MedicineNet.com website. https://www.medicinenet.com/acute_and_chronic_bursitis/article.htm. Accessed February 15, 2018.

Muscle Strains

Muscle strains, or "pulled muscles," are slight tears in muscles or tendons. They usually result from excessive stretching or use. The tiny tears in the damaged muscle cause muscle fibers to spasm, resulting in pain that can last for days to weeks. When strained muscles heal, scar tissue replaces the injured muscle fibers. The scar tissue may cause some weakening of the muscle and may allow muscle injury to recur. Two commonly injured muscles in athletes are the hamstring and quadriceps, both of which cross the hip and knee joints. Other common sites for muscle strains are the thigh and lower back.

NOTE

A person who experiences a muscle strain in the thigh will frequently describe a "popping" or "snapping" sensation as the muscle tears. Pain is sudden and may be severe. The area around the injury may be tender to the touch, with visible bruising.

Muscle strains are graded according to their severity. A grade 1 strain is mild and usually heals readily, whereas a grade 3 strain is a severe tear of the muscle that may take months to heal.[20] Most muscle strains can be successfully treated using the PRICEM acronym, described in Box 32-8. More severe injury may require surgical repair of torn ligaments, muscles, and tendons.

Tendonitis

Tendonitis is inflammation of a tendon. A tendon is a tough, flexible band of fibrous tissue that connects muscles to bones. Tendons most often become inflamed from overuse. This inflammation may result in the tendon and surrounding tissues becoming swollen and tender. Movement may be painful or limited. Almost any tendon can become inflamed. The most common areas affected by tendonitis are the wrist, ankle and heel, knee, and rotator cuff of the shoulder. Risk factors associated with tendonitis include older age; occupations that involve repetitive motions, forceful exertion, or awkward positions; and certain sports, such as bowling, swimming, tennis, baseball, and basketball.

Tendonitis is usually diagnosed by a history and physical examination. As a rule, radiography or other imaging tests are not needed unless there is suspicion of fracture or underlying illness. Treatment usually consists of PRICEM (see Box 32-8). Some patients (eg, those with arthritis and gout) may be prescribed exercise and physical therapy to prevent recurrent injury.

Peripheral Nerve Syndromes

The peripheral nervous system consists of all the nerves that exit the brain and spinal cord. Two common peripheral nerve syndromes are carpal tunnel syndrome and ulnar nerve entrapment. Both of these conditions can cause pain, tingling, and numbness in the arms, wrists, and fingers.

Carpal Tunnel Syndrome

Carpal tunnel syndrome is an entrapment neuropathy that occurs when the median nerve becomes pressed or squeezed at the wrist in the carpal tunnel. The carpal tunnel is a narrow, rigid passageway of ligament and bones at the base of the hand. This tunnel houses the median nerve and tendons (**FIGURE 32-8**). The median nerve controls sensations to the palm

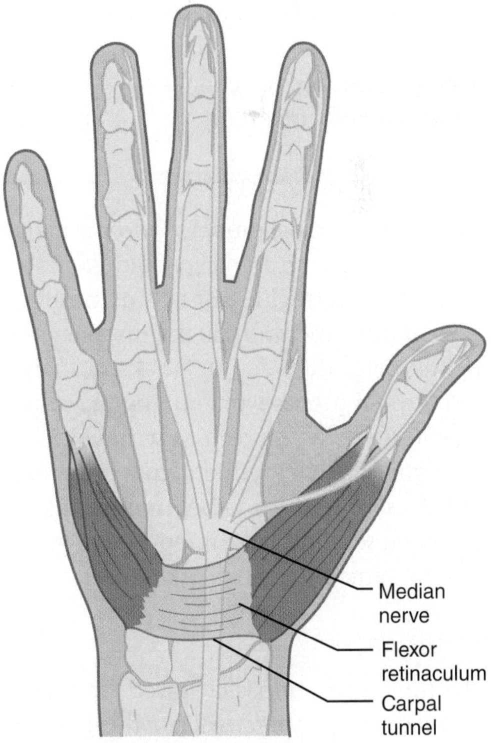

FIGURE 32-8 Carpal tunnel.

side of the thumb and fingers (although not the little finger). This nerve also provides impulses to small muscles in the hand that allow the fingers and thumb to move. Compression of the median nerve can cause pain, weakness, or numbness in the hand and wrist, radiating up the arm. Compression can be caused by any condition that decreases the space in the carpal tunnel (eg, irritated tendons or other swelling).

There are few clinical data to prove whether repetitive and forceful movements of the hand and wrist during work or leisure activities can cause carpal tunnel syndrome.[21] The condition is most likely due to a congenital predisposition; that is, the carpal tunnel is simply smaller in some people than in others. Women are three times more likely than men are to develop carpal tunnel syndrome. This is perhaps because the carpal tunnel itself may be smaller in women than in men. Other contributing factors include the following:

- Trauma or injury to the wrist that causes swelling (eg, sprain or fracture)
- Overactivity of the pituitary gland
- Hypothyroidism
- RA
- Mechanical problems in the wrist joint
- Repeated use of vibrating hand tools
- Fluid retention during pregnancy or menopause
- Cyst or tumor in the canal
- Elevated body mass index

Signs and Symptoms

The symptoms of carpal tunnel syndrome usually begin gradually, often during sleep. Complaints include frequent burning, tingling, or itching numbness in the palm of the hand and the fingers. Sleep is often interrupted with the need to "shake out" the wrist or hand. As symptoms worsen, tingling may occur during the day. The patient may have decreased grip strength, making it difficult to form a fist, grasp small objects, or perform other manual tasks. Early diagnosis and treatment are important in preventing permanent damage to the median nerve.

Management

Carpal tunnel syndrome is diagnosed through various tests that may include percussion of the median nerve (Tinel sign), wrist-flexion tests (Phalen test), compression tests, and nerve conduction studies.[22] Treatment may include drug therapy to control pain, decrease swelling, and reduce inflammation; wrist splinting to maintain correct wrist position; exercise and physical therapy to restore wrist strength; and sometimes surgery to release pressure in the carpal tunnel.

Ulnar Nerve Entrapment

Ulnar nerve entrapment occurs when the ulnar nerve in the arm becomes compressed. The ulnar nerve (the point at the elbow where it passes over the humerus is often called the "funny bone") travels from under the clavicle and along the inside of the upper arm. It passes through the cubital tunnel, behind the inside of the elbow, where it can be palpated. Beyond the elbow, the nerve travels under muscles on the inside of the arm and into the hand on the side of the palm with the little finger (**FIGURE 32-9**). The ulnar nerve provides sensation to the little finger and the palm half of the ring finger. It also controls most of the small muscles in the hand that help with fine movements and some larger muscles in the forearm that help a person make strong grips. Entrapment of the ulnar nerve most commonly occurs behind the elbow. The syndrome may be associated with previous injury to the elbow, bone spurs, and swelling. Cysts may also be a cause of the entrapment.

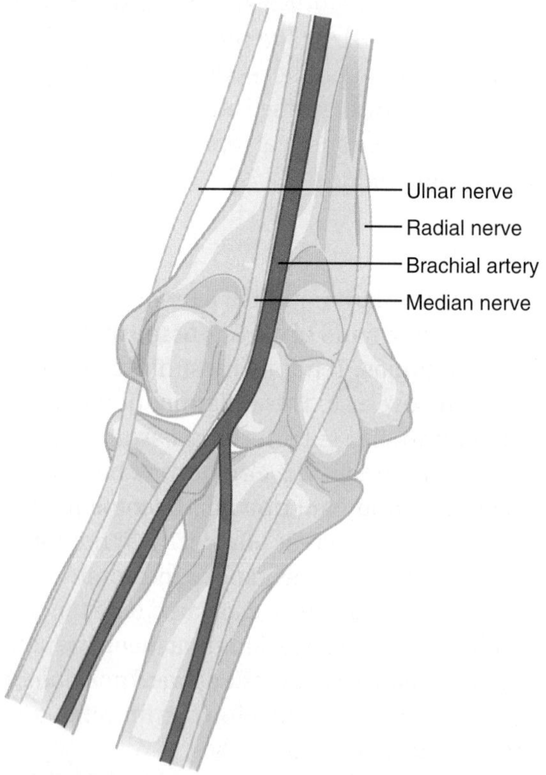

FIGURE 32-9 Ulnar nerve, median nerve, and radial nerve locations about the elbow.

Signs and symptoms of ulnar nerve entrapment are similar to those caused by compression of the median nerve. They include numbness, pain, and tingling in the elbow, forearm, wrist, and fingers. Often the patient complains that the hand has "fallen asleep." Symptoms frequently occur during sleep when the elbows are commonly flexed and during daytime activities that involve bending of the elbow. Ulnar nerve entrapment is diagnosed and treated with tests and therapies similar to those for carpal tunnel syndrome. Surgery is sometimes used to decompress the ulnar nerve.

Soft-Tissue Infections

There are soft-tissue infections that can destroy muscles, skin, and underlying tissue. Most are rare and are caused by a bacterial infection. Soft-tissue infections specific to nontraumatic musculoskeletal disorders discussed in this chapter include fasciitis, gangrene, paronychia, and flexor tenosynovitis of the hand.

NOTE

The occurrence of serious and rare skin infections is on the rise. This rise is attributed to an increase in immunocompromised patients with diabetes, cancer, alcoholism, vascular insufficiencies, organ transplants, and HIV.

Modified from: Chandrasekar PH, ed. *Infections in the Immunosuppressed Patient: An Illustrated Case-Based Approach*. Oxford, UK: Oxford Press; 2016:461-490.

Fasciitis

Fasciitis refers to inflammation of the fascia. **Fascia** is a strong connective tissue that forms under the skin. The tissue performs a number of functions. It envelops and isolates muscles, and sometimes groups of muscles, in the body. It also provides support and protection for body organs and structures.

Necrotizing fasciitis (also called "flesh-eating bacteria") is a rare , critical, rapidly progressive inflammatory infection of the fascia. It quickly spreads in the deep fascial plane with secondary necrosis (tissue death) in the skin and subcutaneous tissue. The area of tenderness may exceed the area of abnormal skin. Necrotizing fasciitis is most likely to occur in people with compromised immune systems. Many bacteria can cause the disease, some of which are resistant to antibiotics (BOX 32-9).

BOX 32-9 Bacteria That Cause Necrotizing Fasciitis[a]

Group A *Streptococcus pyogenes*
S. aureus
Klebsiella
Clostridium perfringens
Escherichia coli
Aeromonas hydrophila

[a]The term *flesh-eating bacteria* is a misnomer. The bacteria do not actually eat the tissue. Skin and muscle are destroyed by the release of toxins, which causes the overproduction of cytokines.

Modified from: National Center for Immunization and Respiratory Diseases, Division of Bacterial Diseases. Necrotizing fasciitis. Centers for Disease Control and Prevention website. https://www.cdc.gov/features/necrotizingfasciitis/index.html. Updated July 3, 2017. Accessed February 15, 2018.

The infection usually begins at a site of broken skin (minor or major trauma or surgery) and spreads quickly. Often the patient will complain of intense pain that is out of proportion to the appearance of the injury. As the disease progresses, the affected area quickly becomes red, hot, and swollen. The skin color may become violet-purple, and blisters may form as necrosis develops in the subcutaneous tissues. Fever, chills, diarrhea, and vomiting are common. If left untreated, the infection may become systemic, leading to death.

NOTE

Since 2010, about 600 to 1,200 cases of necrotizing fasciitis have been reported in the United States each year. Overall morbidity and mortality is reported between 20% and 80%. The mean age of survivors is 35 years. The mean age of nonsurvivors is 49 years. The disease rarely occurs in children.

Modified from: National Center for Immunization and Respiratory Diseases, Division of Bacterial Diseases. Necrotizing fasciitis. Centers for Disease Control and Prevention website. https://www.cdc.gov/features/necrotizingfasciitis/index.html. Updated July 3, 2017. Accessed February 15, 2018.

Patients with necrotizing fasciitis require emergent surgical intervention. This condition is managed with surgical debridement of the affected area, IV antibiotics, and support of vital functions. The need for skin grafts is not uncommon. Most patients require intensive care monitoring. Hyperbaric oxygen therapy (HBOT) may be an adjunct to surgical debridement. Hyperbaric oxygen can increase the oxygen within the body's tissues, force oxygen into hypoxic tissue, decrease edema, destroy anaerobic bacteria, and promote the growth of new blood vessels within soft tissue.

Gangrene

Gangrene is a complication of tissue necrosis. It is characterized by the decay and death of body tissue, which becomes black (and/or green) and malodorous (foul smelling) (**FIGURE 32-10**). Gangrene results from decreased blood supply to a body part or organ, most commonly the toes, fingers, feet, and hands. It can also result from infection, disease, frostbite, and other soft-tissue injury. Two major types of gangrene exist:

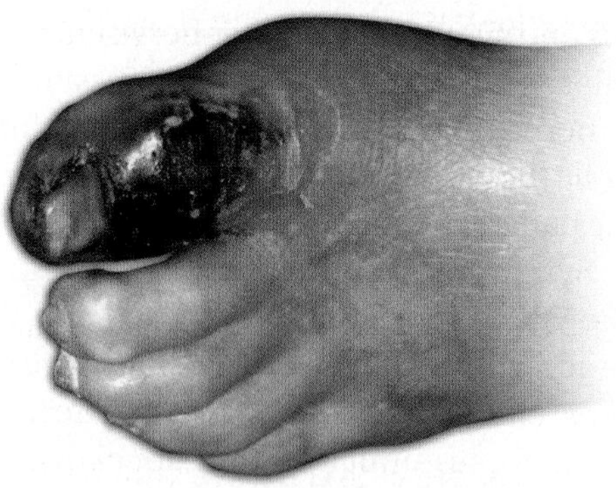

FIGURE 32-10 Gangrene of toes—dry gangrene.

- **Dry gangrene.** This type of gangrene is caused by a reduction of blood flow through the arteries (not infection). It appears gradually and progresses slowly. Dry gangrene is associated with arteriosclerosis, diabetes, cigarette smoking, genetics, and other factors. In dry gangrene, tissues appear dry and discolored and will eventually slough away.
- **Wet gangrene (moist gangrene).** This type of gangrene develops as a complication of an untreated, infected wound. Swelling results from the bacterial infection that causes a sudden decrease in blood flow. (Gas gangrene is a type of wet gangrene caused most commonly by the bacteria *Clostridia*, which produce poisonous toxins and gas.) In wet gangrene, tissues appear moist and produce oozing fluid or pus.

Management

Treatment of gangrene depends on the type of gangrene (dry versus wet) and on how much tissue is compromised. Immediate treatment is needed in all cases of wet gangrene and in some cases of dry gangrene. Treatment for both types of gangrene usually involves surgery, antibiotic therapy, anticoagulant therapy, pain management, supportive care, and rehabilitation (especially with surgical amputation or

DID YOU KNOW?

Hyperbaric Oxygen Therapy

Altering the surrounding air pressure for medical treatment is a practice that dates back to the 1600s. At that time, "fevers and inflammations" were treated in crude chambers that were pressurized using hand bellows. Today, HBOT is carried out in single-person chambers called monoplace chambers. The treatment also can be done in larger multiplace chambers, which can house several patients and the attending hyperbaric health care workers (see Chapter 44, *Environmental Conditions*.)

HBOT has proved to be effective in the treatment of a wide variety of medical disorders, including air embolism and decompression sickness; carbon monoxide poisoning and smoke inhalation; carbon monoxide poisoning complicated by cyanide poisoning (controversial); clostridial myonecrosis (gas gangrene); crush injury, compartment syndrome, and other acute traumatic ischemias; intracranial abscesses; and thermal burns. It also has been shown to enhance the healing of certain problem wounds, including tissue necrosis. HBOT accomplishes the following:

- Greatly increases oxygen concentration in all body tissues, even with reduced or blocked blood flow
- Stimulates the growth of new blood vessels to locations with reduced circulation, thereby improving blood flow to areas with arterial blockage
- Causes a rebound arterial dilation after HBOT, resulting in a blood vessel diameter that is greater than that before therapy, improving blood flow to compromised organs
- Aids in the treatment of infection by enhancing white blood cell action and potentiating germ-killing antibiotics

Modified from: Levett D, Bennett MH, Millar I. Adjunctive hyperbaric oxygen for necrotizing fasciitis [published online January 15, 2015]. *Cochrane Database Syst Rev.* Hyperbaric oxygen. Pacific Medical Center of Hope website. http://www.theregenerativemedicine.com/Hyperbaric_Oxygen.html. Accessed January 17, 2018.

autoamputation). If available, HBOT may be indicated as additional therapy for gas gangrene.

Paronychia

Paronychia is a common skin infection that occurs in the lateral fold around the nails. It is usually caused by an injury (eg, nail-biting, pulling a hangnail, trimming a cuticle) that allows for an invasion of bacteria, yeast, or fungus (**FIGURE 32-11**). The condition is also common in people with diabetes and in those who have their hands submerged in water for long periods. Symptoms include the following:

- Pain and redness around the nail
- Pus-filled blisters (especially with bacterial infection)
- Nails that are abnormally shaped or have an unusual color

Management

Physician care for patients with paronychia may include incision and drainage of the infection, nail removal, and antibiotic therapy. Warm hand soaks may also relieve discomfort. The condition usually

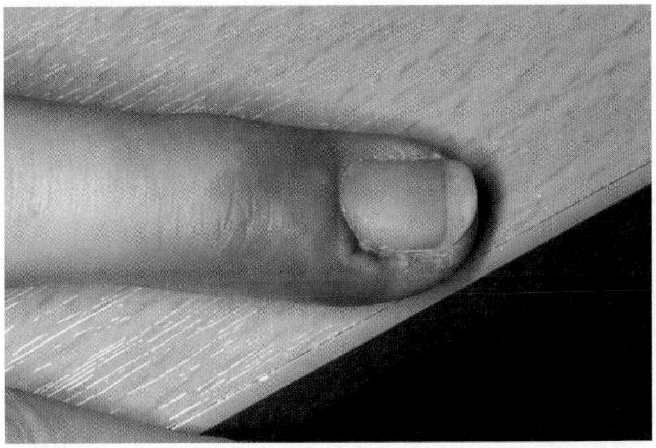

FIGURE 32-11 Paronychia.
© Hercules Robinson/Alamy Stock Photo.

responds well to treatment. Rarely, some infections can be prolonged, requiring additional therapy. Signs of systemic infection from paronychia include chills, red streaks proximal to the infection, fever, malaise, joint pain, and muscle spasm.[23]

Flexor Tenosynovitis

Flexor tenosynovitis is a pathologic state that causes a disruption of tendon function in the hand. Most cases are the result of infection. The condition can also be secondary to acute or chronic inflammation as a result of overuse or disease (eg, diabetes, arthritis). When infectious agents enter the closed space of a tendon sheath, the immune response causes swelling. This swelling interferes with the gliding mechanism of the wrist, hand, and fingers, and can result in disruption of the tendon sheath. It may also lead to tendon necrosis. Flexor tenosynovitis is considered an orthopedic emergency. If left untreated, the infection may result in tendon rupture, permanent contracture, fingertip vascular compromise, or spread to fascia, synovial joint spaces, and skin. Subsequent osteomyelitis may result.[24]

The primary cause of infectious flexor tenosynovitis is penetrating trauma that allows native skin flora (both *Staphylococcus* and *Streptococcus*) to invade the tendon sheath. The patient may present with fever and chills. Other signs and symptoms include the Kanavel's cardinal signs:

- Severe pain on passive range of motion
- Swollen digits ("sausage links")
- Fingers that are held slightly flexed
- Swelling and tenderness along the flexor sheath

Management

In most cases of infectious flexor tenosynovitis, surgical drainage is required. Other treatment may include prescribing antibiotics, splinting, and elevating the hand. All patients require physician care and follow-up. Prehospital care may include elevating the extremity and applying ice for comfort.

Summary

- Although more common in advanced age, nontraumatic musculoskeletal disorders affect patients of all ages.
- The musculoskeletal system comprises bones, muscles, tendons, ligaments, and articulating surfaces. Three types of joints are fibrous, cartilaginous, and synovial. Muscles are responsible for movement, posture, and heat production.
- The extremities and spine should be examined to determine structure and function. Specific assessments include range of motion, vascular evaluation, and a motor and sensory examination.
- Prehospital management of nontraumatic musculoskeletal disorders includes routine care and pain management.
- Important historical data to gather on a patient with this type of disorder should relate to onset of signs and symptoms, nature and location of pain, presence of weakness or other alteration in motor function, and presence of sensory abnormalities.
- Osteomyelitis is a bone infection. It may result from an open fracture, wound infection, or systemic infection. Signs and symptoms include pain, signs of inflammation, fever, pus, and other functional alterations.
- Bone tumors are benign or malignant abnormal cell growths within a bone. Multiple myeloma is the most common type of primary bone cancer. This disorder is characterized by pain and fractures.
- Acute or chronic low back pain is common. It may be caused by trauma, arthritis, infections, or congenital abnormalities.
- Intervertebral disks can herniate and compress adjacent nerves, causing severe pain and weakness.
- Cauda equina syndrome is caused by compression of the nerve roots at the distal end of the spine. If the compression is not relieved promptly, permanent paralysis and incontinence can occur.
- A strain is an injury to a muscle or tendon. A sprain is stretching or tearing of a ligament. Both conditions cause pain.
- Arthritis is an inflammatory condition of a joint characterized by pain and swelling. There are several general categories of arthritis:
  - Osteoarthritis is a chronic degenerative joint disease that has a gradual onset.
  - Rheumatoid arthritis is an autoimmune disease that affects synovial joints. It causes severe pain, disability, and deformity.
  - Ankylosing spondylitis primarily affects the spine. It requires modifications in prehospital care.
  - Septic arthritis is infection of a joint.
  - Gout is a type of arthritis caused by deposits of uric acid in the joint space. Gout is marked by the deposit of uric acid crystals in and around a joint, causing painful swelling of the joint.
- Myalgia is pain in one or more muscles. It can be caused by an autoimmune disorder, overuse, or infection.
- Inflammatory myopathies are a group of diseases characterized by muscle inflammation and weakness. They can be caused by autoimmune disease, injury, infection, or drugs.
- Chronic fatigue syndrome is characterized by severe fatigue not improved by rest.
- Fibromyalgia causes fatigue and "tender points" on the neck, shoulders, back, hips, arms, and legs.
- Bursitis is inflammation of one or more bursae. It is often caused by overuse.
- Muscle strains are slight tears in the muscle caused by overuse or by injury.
- Tendonitis is inflammation of a tendon.
- Carpal tunnel syndrome is a type of neuropathy caused by entrapment of the median nerve at the wrist. It causes pain, numbness, and weakness.
- Ulnar nerve entrapment occurs when the ulnar nerve (funny bone) is compressed.
- Fasciitis is inflammation of the connective tissue that lies under the skin. Necrotizing fasciitis ("flesh-eating bacteria") is a rare, critical, rapidly progressive inflammatory infection that begins in the fascia and can rapidly become systemic.
- Gangrene is a complication of tissue necrosis. It occurs when tissue decays.
- Paronychia is a skin infection around the nails.
- Flexor tenosynovitis is often caused by infection. It can lead to dysfunction, necrosis, and systemic infection.

References

1. National Highway Traffic Safety Administration. *The National EMS Education Standards*, Washington, DC: US Department of Transportation/National Highway Traffic Safety Administration; 2009.
2. American Academy of Orthopaedic Surgeons. Bone tumor. OrthoInfo website. https://orthoinfo.aaos.org/en/diseases--conditions/bone-tumor. Accessed February 16, 2018.
3. American Cancer Society. *Cancer Facts and Figures, 2017*. Atlanta, GA: American Cancer Society; 2017.
4. National Cancer Institute. Bone cancer. National Institutes of Health website. https://www.cancer.gov/types/bone/bone-fact-sheet. Accessed February 16, 2018.
5. Rothberg S, Friedman B. Complementary therapies in addition to medication for patients with nonchronic, nonradicular low back pain: a systematic review. *Am J Emerg Med*. 2017;35(1):55-61.
6. Evans CS, Platts-Mills TF, Fernandez AR, et al. Repeated emergency medical services use by older adults: analysis of a comprehensive statewide database. *Ann Emerg Med*. 2017;70(4):506-515.
7. Marx JA, Hockberger RS, Walls RM. *Rosen's Emergency Medicine: Concepts and Clinical Practice*. 8th ed. St. Louis, MO: Elsevier; 2013:643-655.
8. Studnek JR, Crawford M, Wilkins RL, et al. Back problems among emergency medical services. *Am J Ind Med*. 2010;53(1):12-22.

9. Centers for Disease Control and Prevention, National Center for Chronic Disease Prevention and Health Promotion, Division of Population Health. Arthritis. Centers for Disease Control and Prevention website. https://www.cdc.gov/arthritis/index.htm. Updated January 29, 2018. Accessed February 16, 2018.
10. Kane A. How fat affects arthritis. Arthritis Foundation website. http://www.arthritis.org/living-with-arthritis/comorbidities/obesity-arthritis/fat-and-arthritis.php. Accessed February 16, 2018.
11. Rheumatoid arthritis facts and statistics. Rheumatoid Arthritis Support Network website. https://www.rheumatoidarthritis.org/ra/facts-and-statistics/. Updated August 3, 2016. Accessed February 16, 2018.
12. Sharff KA, Richards EP, Townes JM. Clinical management of septic arthritis. *Curr Rheumatol Rep*. 2013;15(6):332.
13. Centers for Disease Control and Prevention, National Center for Chronic Disease Prevention and Health Promotion, Division of Population Health. Gout. Centers for Disease Control and Prevention website. https://www.cdc.gov/arthritis/basics/gout.html. Updated April 14, 2017. Accessed February 16, 2018.
14. National Institute of Neurological Disorders and Stroke. Inclusion body myositis information page. National Institutes of Health website. https://www.ninds.nih.gov/Disorders/All-Disorders/Inclusion-Body-Myositis-Information-Page. Accessed February 16, 2018.
15. National Institute of Neurologic Disorders and Stroke. Inflammatory myopathies fact sheet. National Institutes of Health website. https://www.ninds.nih.gov/Disorders/Patient-Caregiver-Education/Fact-Sheets/Inflammatory-Myopathies-Fact-Sheet. Updated December 4, 2017. Accessed February 16, 2018.
16. Institute of Medicine. *Beyond Myalgic Encephalomyelitis/Chronic Fatigue Syndrome: Redefining an Illness*. Washington, DC: The National Academies Press; 2015.
17. Centers for Disease Control and Prevention; National Center for Emerging and Zoonotic Infectious Diseases (NCEZID); Division of High-Consequence Pathogens and Pathology (DHCPP). Myalgic encephalomyelitis/chronic fatigue syndrome. Centers for Disease Control and Prevention website. https://www.cdc.gov/me-cfs/index.html. Updated February 16, 2017. Accessed January 17, 2018.
18. Centers for Disease Control and Prevention; National Center for Emerging and Zoonotic Infectious Diseases (NCEZID); Division of High-Consequence Pathogens and Pathology (DHCPP). Myalgic encephalomyelitis/chronic fatigue syndrome: symptoms. Centers for Disease Control and Prevention website. https://www.cdc.gov/me-cfs/index.html. Updated December 15, 2017. Accessed February 16, 2018.
19. American Academy of Orthopaedic Surgeons. Hip bursitis. OrthoInfo website. https://orthoinfo.aaos.org/en/diseases--conditions/hip-bursitis. Accessed February 16, 2018.
20. American Academy of Orthopaedic Surgeons. Diseases and conditions: muscle strains in the thigh. OrthoInfo website. https://orthoinfo.aaos.org/en/diseases--conditions/muscle-strains-in-the-thigh. Accessed February 16, 2018.
21. National Institute of Neurological Disorders and Stroke. Carpal tunnel syndrome fact sheet. National Institutes of Health website. https://www.ninds.nih.gov/Disorders/Patient-Caregiver-Education/Fact-Sheets/Carpal-Tunnel-Syndrome-Fact-Sheet. Accessed February 16, 2018.
22. Schulz SA. Necrotizing fasciitis. Medscape website. https://emedicine.medscape.com/article/2051157-overview#a6. Updated November 21, 2017. Accessed February 16, 2018.
23. Rabarin F, Jeudy J, Cesari B, et al. Acute finger-tip infection: management and treatment. A 103-case series. *Orthop Traumatol Surg Res*. 2017;103(6):933-936.
24. Barry RL, Adams NS, Martin MD. Pyogenic (suppurative) flexor tenosynovitis: assessment and management. *Eplasty*. 2016;16:ic7.

Suggested Readings

Bellan M, Molinari R, Castello L, et al. Profiling the patients visiting the emergency room for musculoskeletal complaints: characteristics and outcomes. *Clin Rheumatol*. 2016;35:2835.

Edwards J, Hayden J, Asbridge M, et al. Prevalence of low back pain in emergency settings: a systematic review and meta-analysis. *BMC Musculoskelet Disord*. 2017;18:143.

Spondylitis Association of America. Ankylosing spondylitis: managing patients in an emergency setting—a primer for first responders. Spondylitis Association of America website. http://www.spondylitis.org/Spondylitis-Plus/Spondylitis-Plus-Articles/Summer-2009. Published summer 2009. Accessed February 16, 2018.

Swash M, Schwartz MS. *Neuromuscular Diseases: A Practical Approach to Diagnosis and Management*. 3rd ed. London, UK: Springer; 2013.

Layon J, ed. *Civetta, Taylor, and Kirby's Critical Care Medicine*. 5th ed. Philadelphia, PA: Wolters Kluwer; 2018.

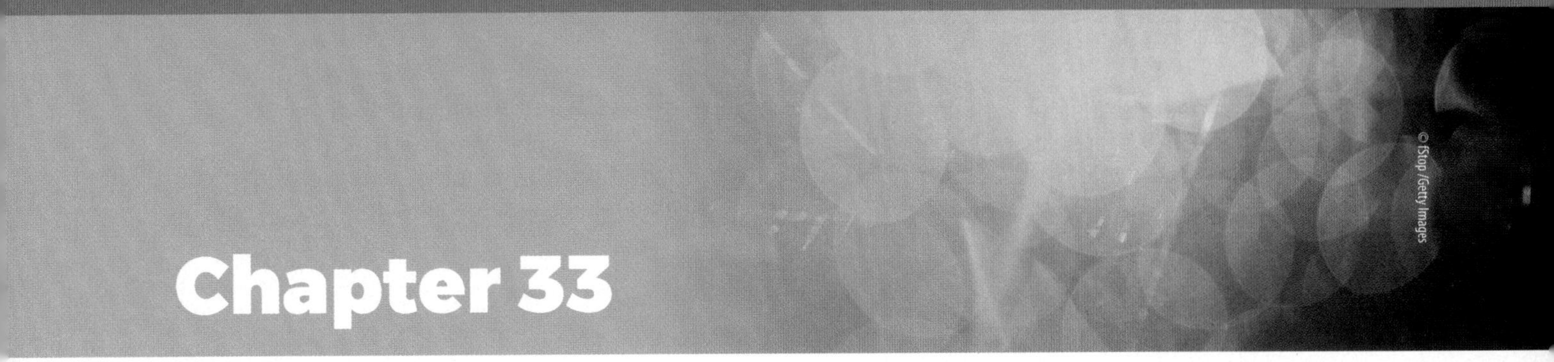
© fStop /Getty Images

Chapter 33

Toxicology

NATIONAL EMS EDUCATION STANDARD COMPETENCIES

Medicine

Integrates assessment findings with principles of epidemiology and pathophysiology to formulate a field impression and implement a comprehensive treatment/disposition plan for a patient with a medical complaint.

Toxicology

Recognition and management of
- Carbon monoxide poisoning (p 1225)
- Nerve agent poisoning (pp 1212, 1213, 1238, 1239)

How and when to contact a poison control center (pp 1121–1122)

Anatomy, physiology, pathophysiology, assessment, and management of
- Inhaled poisons (pp 1224–1228)
- Ingested poisons (pp 1214–1224)
- Injected poisons (pp 1228–1237)
- Absorbed poisons (pp 1237–1240)
- Alcohol intoxication and withdrawal (pp 1257–1263)
- Opiate toxidrome (pp 1245–1248)

Anatomy, physiology, epidemiology, pathophysiology, psychosocial impact, presentations, prognosis, and management of the following toxidromes and poisonings:
- Cholinergics (p 1212)
- Anticholinergics (p 1212)
- Sympathomimetics (p 1213)
- Sedative-hypnotics (p 1248)
- Opiates (p XX)
- Alcohol intoxication and withdrawal (pp 1257–1263)
- Over-the-counter and prescription medications (pp 1255–1257)
- Carbon monoxide (pp 1225, 1226)
- Illegal drugs (p 1249)
- Herbal preparations (p 1251)

OBJECTIVES

Upon completion of this chapter, the paramedic student will be able to:
1. Define poisoning. (p 1211)
2. Identify management principles for the most common toxic syndromes (toxidromes) based on a knowledge of the characteristic physical findings associated with each. (pp 1212–1213)
3. Describe the principles for assessment and management of the patient who has ingested poison. (pp 1213–1214)
4. Describe the causative agents and pathophysiology of selected ingested poisons and the management of patients who have taken them. (pp 1214–1224)
5. Distinguish among the three categories of inhaled toxins: simple asphyxiants, chemical asphyxiants and systemic poisons, and irritants or corrosives. (p 1225)
6. Describe how physical and chemical properties influence the effects of inhaled toxins. (p 1225)
7. Describe the principles of managing the patient who has inhaled poison. (p 1225)
8. Describe the signs, symptoms, and management of patients who have inhaled cyanide, ammonia, or hydrocarbon. (pp 1225–1228)
9. Describe the signs, symptoms, and management of patients injected with venom by insects, reptiles, and hazardous aquatic creatures. (pp 1129–1137)
10. Describe the signs, symptoms, and management of patients with organophosphate or carbamate poisoning. (pp 1237–1240)
11. Outline the principles of managing patients with a drug overdose. (p 1245)

12. Describe the effects, signs and symptoms, and specific management for selected therapeutic and illegal drug overdoses. (pp 1240–1257)
13. Describe the short- and long-term physiologic effects of ethanol ingestion. (p 1262)
14. Describe signs, symptoms, and management of alcohol-related emergencies. (pp 1261–1262)

KEY TERMS

adsorb To accumulate on a surface in a condensed layer.

alcohol dependence A disorder characterized by chronic, excessive consumption of alcohol that results in injury to health or in inadequate social function and the development of withdrawal symptoms when the person suddenly stops drinking.

antidote A drug or other substance that opposes the action of a poison.

botulism A rare but life-threatening form of food poisoning caused by the bacillus *Clostridium botulinum*.

cathartic A substance that accelerates defecation.

cirrhosis A chronic and progressive disease in which normal liver cells are replaced by fibrotic scar tissue.

delirium tremens An acute and sometimes fatal psychotic reaction caused by cessation of excessive intake of alcohol over a long period of time; also known as DTs.

disulfiram-ethanol reaction A potentially life-threatening physiologic response caused by co-ingestion of disulfiram and ethanol that produces ill effects on the gastrointestinal, cardiovascular, and autonomic nervous systems; disulfiram is prescribed to some patients with alcohol use disorder to help them maintain abstinence.

drug abuse Self-medication or self-administration of a drug in chronically excessive amounts, resulting in psychological or physical dependence (or both), functional impairment, and deviation from approved social norms.

envenomation The injection of snake, arachnid, or insect venom into the body.

food poisoning Poisoning that results from food contaminated by toxic substances or by bacteria containing toxins.

gastric lavage Irrigation of the stomach with sterile water or normal saline.

gastrointestinal decontamination The use of medical methods to empty the stomach of ingested toxins to prevent absorption.

Korsakoff psychosis A form of amnesia often seen in patients with alcohol use disorder, characterized by a loss of short-term memory and an inability to learn new skills.

liquefaction Conversion of solid tissues to a fluid or semifluid state.

Lyme disease An acute, recurrent inflammatory infection transmitted by a tick.

mediastinitis Inflammation of the mediastinum.

methemoglobin Hemoglobin with ferrous iron in the oxidized (Fe^{3+}) state.

methemoglobinemia The presence of methemoglobin in the blood, causing cyanosis as a result of the inability of the red blood cells to release oxygen.

nematocysts Capsules containing threadlike, venomous stinging cells found in some coelenterates.

nystagmus Involuntary jerking movements of the eyes.

phencyclidine psychosis A psychiatric emergency that may mimic schizophrenia.

pneumoperitoneum The presence of air or gas within the peritoneal cavity of the abdomen.

poison Any substance that produces harmful physiologic or psychological effects.

Rocky Mountain spotted fever A serious tick-borne infectious disease, characterized by chills, fever, severe headache, mental confusion, and rash.

serotonin syndrome A potentially life-threatening drug reaction; most often occurs when two or more drugs that affect serotonin levels are taken together.

surface tension The tendency of the surface of a liquid to minimize the area of its surface by contracting.

tick paralysis A rare, progressive, reversible disorder caused by several species of ticks that release a neurotoxin that causes weakness, incoordination, and paralysis.

toxidromes Clinical syndromes grouped together for the successful recognition of poisoning patterns.

toxin A poison that is produced by a living organism.

venom A toxin that is injected from one living organism into another.

viscosity The resistance of a liquid to flow.

volatility The ability of a liquid to vaporize.

Wernicke encephalopathy A stage of Wernicke-Korsakoff syndrome that usually develops suddenly, with the clinical manifestations of ataxia, nystagmus, disturbances of speech and gait, signs of neuropathy, stupor, or coma.

Wernicke-Korsakoff syndrome A disease that results from chronic thiamine deficiency combined with an inability to use thiamine because of a heritable disorder or because of a reduction in intestinal absorption and metabolism of thiamine by alcohol.

Our environment contains a large number of potentially harmful substances that are both natural and synthetic. These substances can be accidentally or deliberately introduced into the body. Harmful substances include animal and plant toxins, industrial and household chemicals, prescription medications, and drugs of abuse. Early identification of these agents and rapid transport for definitive care are crucial in managing patients with toxicologic emergencies.

Poisoning

A **poison** can be defined as any substance that produces harmful physiologic or psychological effects. Emergencies that involve poisons are a major cause of morbidity and mortality in the United States. In 2015, there were 1,482,121 unintentional nonfatal poisonings reported.[1] There were 52,404 drug poisoning deaths that year (84% unintentional, 10% suicides, and 6% undetermined).[2] According to the National Safety Council, poisoning was the leading cause of unintentional injury in the United States in 2014.[3]

NOTE

Unintentional poisoning is poisoning that occurs when a person takes or gives a substance without the intent to harm. Intentional poisoning results when there is intent to cause harm.

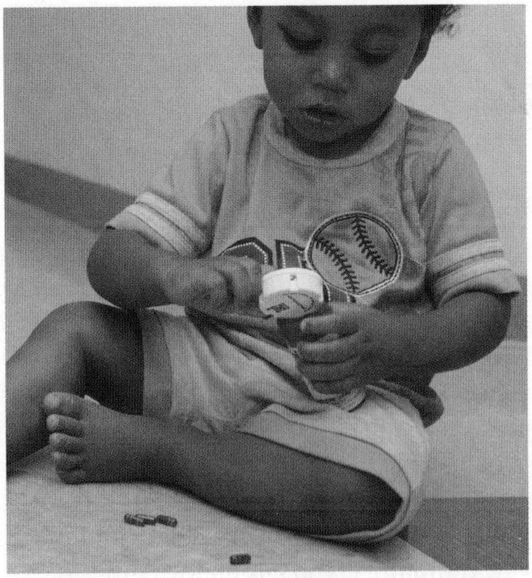

CRITICAL THINKING

How many substances that fit the definition of a poison are there in or around your home?

Poison Control Centers

There are 55 poison control centers in the United States to help treat poisoning emergencies.[4] Most centers are based in major medical centers or teaching hospitals. Each one belongs to regional centers designated by the American Association of Poison Control Centers. Medical professionals staff regional centers. They offer 24-hour telephone access (1-800-222-1222) to population bases of at least 1 million. In 2015, an estimated 2.8 million poisonings were reported to poison control centers throughout the United States. More than 90% of these poisonings happen in a residence; just under one-half of the people who have been poisoned are children younger than 6 years.[5] By helping people manage emergencies outside the health care system, these centers save more than $1.8 billion each year.

Information and treatment advice are given immediately by the poison control center on request. The center provides this information through a large database of references on more than 427,000 toxic substances.[5] These substances include drugs (legal, illicit, foreign, and veterinary), chemicals, plants, animals, insects, fish, snakes, cosmetics, and hazardous materials. Each request for information is followed up to determine the effectiveness and outcome of the treatment. In addition, the centers are responsible for the following elements of an organized poison system:[6,7]

1. Treatment information and toxicologic consultation with health care providers (eg, hospitals, physicians, emergency medical services [EMS] agencies) and the public, using a toll-free number with linkage into various 9-1-1 systems
2. Professional education to train those involved in the care of patients who have been poisoned
3. Data collection on all poisonings in the region for epidemiologic and evaluation purposes
4. Public education and prevention
5. Research

6. Regional EMS poison system development (eg, patient classification criteria, triage and management protocols, and regional transfer agreements)

Regional poison control centers are a ready source of information for any toxicologic emergency. Depending on local communications protocol, poison control centers may be contacted directly by EMS and other public service agencies by phone, dispatching center, or medical direction. The immediate determination of potential toxicity is based on the specific agent or agents. It also is based on the amount ingested, the time of exposure, the patient's weight and medical condition, and any treatment given before EMS arrival. The poison center also can coordinate treatment protocol by notifying the receiving hospital while the patient is en route to the emergency department (ED).

Management Principles for Toxic Syndromes

Grouping toxic agents and physical findings into toxic syndromes, or **toxidromes**, provides a tool for rapid detection of the suspected cause and can focus the differential diagnosis to consideration of only a few chemicals with similar toxic effects. Toxidromes aid the paramedic in remembering assessment and management strategies (**TABLE 33-1**). The most important toxidromes to recognize are as follows:[8]

1. Cholinergic
2. Anticholinergic
3. Hallucinogenic
4. Opioid
5. Sympathomimetic

> NOTE
> Toxic syndrome classification does not consider how or why the toxin was introduced into the body. Thus the paramedic should consider route of entry in addition to specific treatments.

Cholinergics

Exposure to cholinergics is uncommon. However, it is important to recognize cholinergic poisoning so that lifesaving care can be initiated. Causative agents include pesticides (organophosphates, carbamates) and nerve agents (eg, sarin, soman). Assessment findings include headache, dizziness, weakness, bradycardia, nausea, and a wet presentation manifested by profound Salivation, Lacrimation, Urination, Defecation, Gastrointestinal upset, and Emesis (SLUDGE). In severe cases, coma and convulsions may be present. In addition to airway, ventilatory, and circulatory support and decontamination, drug therapy may include administration of atropine, pralidoxime, diazepam or lorazepam, and activated charcoal.

Anticholinergics

Exposure to anticholinergics is fairly common because so many medications and plants have anticholinergic properties. Examples include drugs such as antihistamines, antipsychotics, antispasmodics, and tricyclic antidepressants and plants such as jimsonweed, night blooming jessamine, panther mushroom, and angel's trumpet. The signs and symptoms include tachycardia; dry, flushed skin; dilated pupils; and facial flushing. This dry patient presentation usually is managed with airway, ventilatory, and circulatory support. Physostigmine may be given as an antidote in rare cases, in the absence of tricyclic antidepressant overdose.

> NOTE
> Jimsonweed and angel's trumpet are sometimes ingested in search of recreational high, while panther mushrooms are sometimes mistaken for edible mushrooms.
>
> *Modified from*: Dewitt MS, Swain R, Gibson LB Jr. The dangers of jimson weed and its abuse by teenagers in the Kanawha Valley of West Virginia. *W V Med J*. 1997;93(4):182-185.

Hallucinogens

Common hallucinogens include lysergic acid diethylamide (LSD), phencyclidine (PCP), peyote, psilocybin mushrooms, and mescaline. Depending on the agent and dose, signs and symptoms may include central nervous system (CNS) stimulation and/or depression, behavioral disturbances, delusions, hypertension, chest pain, tachycardia, seizures, and respiratory and cardiac arrest. Prehospital care for these patients is focused on ensuring personal safety and providing airway, ventilatory, and circulatory support.

Opioids

The opioid syndrome carries a hallmark triad of depressed level of consciousness, respiratory depression, and pinpoint pupils. Common causative agents include heroin, morphine, codeine, meperidine,

TABLE 33-1 Toxicologic Syndromes

Common Signs	Causative Agents	Specific Treatment
Cholinergic (Wet Patient Presentation)		
Confusion, CNS depression, weakness, SLUDGE, bradycardia, wheezing, bronchoconstriction, miosis, coma, convulsions, diaphoresis, seizures	Organophosphate and carbamate insecticides, nerve agents, some mushrooms	Atropine, pralidoxime (2-PAM chloride), diazepam or lorazepam
Anticholinergic (Dry Patient Presentation)		
Delirium, tachycardia, dry and flushed skin, dilated pupils (mydriasis), seizures, and dysrhythmias (in severe cases)	Antihistamines, antiparkinson medications, atropine, antipsychotic agents, antidepressants, skeletal muscle relaxants, many plants (eg, jimsonweed and *Amanita muscaria*)	Midazolam, diazepam or lorazepam, activated charcoal, rarely physostigmine (Antilirium)
Hallucinogens		
Visual hallucinations, delusions, bizarre behavior, flashbacks, respiratory and CNS depression	LSD, PCP, mescaline, some mushrooms, marijuana, jimsonweed, nutmeg, mace, some amphetamines	Minimal sensory stimulation, calming measures, midazolam, diazepam, or lorazepam if necessary
Opioids		
Euphoria, hypotension, respiratory depression/arrest, nausea, pinpoint pupils,[a] pupil dilation (meperidine [Demerol]), seizures, coma	Heroin, morphine, codeine, meperidine, propoxyphene, fentanyl	Naloxone (Narcan)
Sympathomimetics		
Delusions, paranoia, tachycardia or bradycardia, hypertension, diaphoresis; seizures, hypotension, and dysrhythmias in severe cases	Cocaine, amphetamine, methamphetamine, over-the-counter decongestants	Minimal sensory stimulation, calming measures, midazolam, diazepam, or lorazepam if necessary; management of dysrhythmias

[a]Meperidine overdose often causes mydriasis instead of miosis.

Abbreviations: CNS, central nervous system; LSD, lysergic acid diethylamide; PCP, phencyclidine; SLUDGE, salivation, lacrimation, urination, defecation, gastrointestinal upset, emesis.

oxycodone, hydrocodone, and fentanyl. Drugs in this class often are mixed with alcohol or other drugs (eg, benzodiazepines), which leads to increased respiratory depression, hypotension, and bradycardia. Other signs and symptoms may include euphoria, nausea, pinpoint pupils, and seizures. In addition to ensuring airway, ventilatory, and circulatory support, drug therapy may include the administration of naloxone or another opioid-specific antidote agent.

CRITICAL THINKING

Why is it important to be able to identify these toxic syndromes?

Sympathomimetics

The sympathomimetic syndrome usually results from acute overdose of amphetamines or cocaine. Signs and symptoms include elevated blood pressure, tachycardia, dilated pupils, and altered mental status, including paranoid delusions. In severe cases, cardiovascular collapse can occur. Management consists of ensuring personal safety and providing airway, ventilatory, and circulatory support.

Guidelines for Managing a Poisoned Patient

Poisons may enter the body through ingestion, inhalation, injection, and absorption. BOX 33-1 lists three

BOX 33-1 Types of Toxicologic Emergencies

Unintentional Poisoning

Childhood poisoning
Dosage errors
Environmental exposure
Idiosyncratic reactions
Occupational exposure

Drug and Alcohol Abuse

Intentional Poisoning/Overdose

Assault/homicide
Chemical warfare
Suicide attempts

types of toxicologic emergencies that may result in poisoning. With the exception of administering life-saving antidotes for specific poisons, as described later in this chapter, most poisoned patients require only supportive therapy to recover (BOX 33-2).

When caring for a patient who has been poisoned, the paramedic's personal safety remains the top priority. A toxicologic emergency response may involve hazardous materials. It also may involve patient behavior that is unpredictable or violent. If the scene is not safe, the paramedic crew should retreat to a safe staging area and wait there until the scene has been secured by the proper personnel. Most poisonings occur in the home and usually involve ingestions that do not pose a risk to rescuers, but safety must be confirmed in each case.

Situations in a residence related to drug labs, suicides, or homicides may involve highly toxic chemicals. Patients exposed to gases do not generally pose a risk to the rescuers once they are safely out of the toxic environment. Their clothing may off-gas poisons, so they should be removed and placed in a plastic bag in an outside compartment of the ambulance to prevent any secondary exposure. When a cutaneous exposure occurs, the type of chemical, amount of chemical, and location of exposure determine whether a crew can approach and decontaminate the patient or whether a hazardous materials team should respond. For example, small exposures of caustic household materials in a person's eye may require only standard personal protective equipment (PPE) to decontaminate by flushing the tissue. A skin exposure with a poison such as cyanide or hydrofluoric acid would require specialized PPE and equipment. When in doubt, rescuers should not approach. Conferring with poison control and local hazardous materials officials prior to entry is prudent if unsure of the situation.

BOX 33-2 Guidelines for Poisoning Management

Management of the poisoned patient in the prehospital setting typically follows these guidelines:

1. Wear appropriate PPE and approach the patient if there is no obvious risk to rescuer safety. If poison gases are suspected, use an environmental monitor. Remove the patient from the hazardous environment as soon and as safely as possible. Remove the patient's clothing and decontaminate them with the help of appropriate resources if indicated.
2. Ensure adequate airway, ventilation, and circulation. Take action to prevent or reduce the risk of aspiration by carefully monitoring the patient's airway.
3. Assess blood glucose, arterial blood gas, and end-tidal carbon dioxide levels.
4. Attempt to identify the toxic agent by toxidrome, using formal or informal methods. Call poison control if specific information is needed.
5. Assess the impact or risk of harm to vital organs.
6. Determine if there is an antidote or other therapy to minimize harm or treat complications.
7. Consider and assess for other causes of the patient's signs and symptoms.
8. Look for signs of prior drug use (eg, track marks, drug paraphernalia)
9. When possible, identify the substance taken and, if safe to do so, transport the medication container with the patient.
10. Consult with medical direction or a poison control center for specific management to prevent further absorption of the toxin or antidote therapy.
11. Frequently reassess the patient; monitor vital signs and the electrocardiogram (ECG).
12. Transport the patient for physician examination.

Modified from: National Association of EMS Officials. *National Model EMS Clinical Guidelines*. Version 2.0. National Association of EMS Officials website. https://www.nasemso.org/documents/National-Model-EMS-Clinical-Guidelines-Version2-Sept2017.pdf. Published September 2017. Accessed February 28, 2018.

Poisoning by Ingestion

Ingestion of poisons was the route of exposure in 83.6% of cases reported to American poison control centers in 2015.[5] The most common poison exposures in this group result from analgesics, followed by household cleaning products and cosmetics or personal care products. Intentional poisonings may occur from the following:

- Attempts at suicide
- Recreational or experimental drug use or abuse
- Chemical warfare or acts of terrorism
- Assault and homicide

The toxic effects of ingested poisons may be immediate or delayed, depending on the substance that was ingested. For example, corrosive substances such as strong acids and alkalis may produce immediate tissue damage, as evidenced by burns to the lips, tongue, throat, and upper gastrointestinal (GI) tract. Other substances, such as medications and toxic plants, usually require absorption and distribution through the bloodstream. They also may require alterations by different organs to produce toxic effects. Because only minimal absorption occurs in the stomach, poisons enter the bloodstream through the small intestine in minutes to hours depending on many factors, including gastric emptying, solubility of the poison, underlying and preexisting diseases, and intestinal motility. Therefore, early management of the ingested poisoning is focused on treating the patient's symptoms and providing supportive care.

Assessment and Management

The primary survey and initial management of a poisoned patient begin with ensuring scene safety. Then the paramedic should manage immediate threats to the patient's life. During scene size-up, the paramedic crew should be alert for specific clues or details that suggest a toxicologic emergency. Examples include open medication bottles, scattered pills, vomitus, and open containers of household products. Patient findings that may suggest poisoning include a decreased level of consciousness, airway compromise/injury (eg, vomitus or pills in the mouth, burns in the oral cavity), abnormal respiratory patterns, and dysrhythmias (eg, tachycardia, bradycardia, premature atrial contractions, premature ventricular contractions).

> **NOTE**
> The paramedic must consider the possibility of poisoning whenever the patient's signs and symptoms cannot be attributed to other explainable conditions (eg, hypoglycemia/hyperglycemia, cardiac dysfunction).

The primary goal of physical assessment of poisoned patients is to identify effects on the three vital organ systems most likely to produce morbidity or death. These organ systems are the respiratory system, the cardiovascular system, and the CNS. Obtaining a detailed history of the event and any significant medical or psychiatric history also is important. This information may help to direct treatment in the field or in the ED. For example, preexisting cardiac, liver, or renal disease and some psychiatric illnesses may be worsened by a toxic ingestion. These conditions may require care in addition to managing the toxic ingestion.

Respiratory Complications

The first priority in managing a poisoned patient after ensuring scene safety is to secure a patent airway. The paramedic should provide adequate ventilatory support as needed. This support includes monitoring pulse oximetry and end-tidal carbon dioxide, administering oxygen if the patient is hypoxic, and possibly implementing advanced airway management to protect the airway and prevent aspiration. Other respiratory complications that may be associated with poisoning include the early development of noncardiogenic pulmonary edema or the later development of acute respiratory distress syndrome (see Chapter 23, *Respiratory*). Bronchospasm may result from direct or indirect toxic effects.

Cardiovascular Complications

The most common cardiovascular complication of poisoning by ingestion is the development of cardiac dysrhythmias. Thus, the paramedic should assess the patient's circulatory status and continually monitor it by ECG and frequent blood pressure measurements. The presence of tachydysrhythmias or bradydysrhythmias may indicate serious metabolic disorders such as hypoxia and acidosis. Acute conduction disturbances such as widened QRS complexes and QT-interval prolongation may signal ion-channel toxicity. Another cardiovascular complication is the development of hypotension associated with decreased vascular tone.

Neurologic Complications

The paramedic should perform and document a baseline neurologic examination. Deviations from a normal level of consciousness may range from mild drowsiness and agitation to hallucinations, seizures, coma, and death. Neurologic complications may result from the poison itself, such as lead poisoning in children who have ingested paint chips. Alternatively, the complications may result from a metabolic or perfusion disorder, such as poor cardiac output from dysrhythmias.

History

A thorough history of the exposure and any significant medical history should be obtained from the patient, family members, or bystanders. Although this information may be unreliable (as in cases involving pediatric patients, drug abuse, or suicide attempts), the following should be ascertained if possible:

- What was ingested or inhaled? Obtain the poison container and remaining contents unless doing so poses a threat to rescuer safety.
- When was (were) the substance or substances ingested? This timing may affect the decision to use activated charcoal or gastric lavage or to administer an antidote.
- How much of the substance was ingested?
- Was alcohol or any other substance taken?
- Was an attempt made to induce vomiting? Did the patient vomit?
- Has an antidote or activated charcoal been administered?
- Does the patient have a psychiatric history pertinent to suicide attempts? Has the patient had episodes of recent depression?

Gastrointestinal Decontamination

Gastrointestinal decontamination is the use of medical methods to empty the stomach of an ingested **toxin** to prevent absorption. These methods include the administration of activated charcoal, **gastric lavage**, and whole-bowel irrigation. Before attempting to remove poison from the GI tract, the paramedic should consult with medical direction or a poison control center. Although once a mainstay in the management of ingested toxins, GI decontamination plays a less important role in poison treatment today. With rare exceptions, gastric lavage and whole-bowel irrigation are no longer recommended.[9]

Activated Charcoal

Activated charcoal is an inert, nontoxic product of wood material that has been heated to an extremely high temperature. Single-dose activated charcoal is generally recommended for patients who have ingested a life-threatening poison when no antidotes are available and when the charcoal can be administered within 1 hour of poisoning. The surface characteristics of activated charcoal enable it to **adsorb** (collect in a condensed form) molecules of chemical toxins while it is in the intestinal tract. Activated charcoal is indicated for some toxic ingestions, or for drugs that have delayed emptying. It should not be given in cases where strong acid, strong alkali, or ethanol is the toxicant. BOX 33-3 lists the agents for which activated charcoal generally should and should not be given.[10]

Activated charcoal comes mixed in an aqueous solution with or without a **cathartic** (most commonly sorbitol). A cathartic is an agent that causes bowel evacuation. It decreases the transit time and expels the charcoal within a short period (BOX 33-4). Complications of activated charcoal are poor patient acceptance in consuming the charcoal and vomiting with risk of aspiration. It should not be given to patients with declining consciousness or those unable to protect their airway unless intubated.[11] EMS personnel should protect themselves, the patient, and the immediate area from the staining properties of the charcoal. Personal protective measures also should be taken when administering this agent.

> **NOTE**
>
> It should be noted that GI decontamination rarely affects the clinical outcome of poisoned patients. GI decontamination is useful only for patients who have ingested a poison within 1 hour of being seen. After 1 hour, the toxin most likely will have passed from the stomach into the small intestine, where it will be absorbed. Therefore, care for most poisoned patients is primarily supportive. Decisions regarding the use of GI decontamination are made by medical direction or a poison control center on a case-by-case and drug-by-drug basis.
>
> *Modified from*: Part 1: executive summary: 2010 American Heart Association Guidelines for Cardiopulmonary Resuscitation and Emergency Cardiovascular Care. *Circulation.* 2010;122(18)(suppl 3):S840.

> **CRITICAL THINKING**
>
> Why might a patient be reluctant to take activated charcoal?

BOX 33-3 Activated Charcoal: Indications and Contraindications

Agents for Which Activated Charcoal May Be Given[a]

Carbamazepine
Dapsone
Drugs with anticholinergic effects
Opioids
Phenobarbital
Quinine
Sustained-release drugs
Theophylline
Drug packets ingested to avoid detection by law enforcement

Agents for Which Activated Charcoal Should Not Be Given[b]

Cyanide
Hydrocarbons
Ethanol intoxication
Ferrous sulfate or other iron salts
Lithium
Mineral acid ingestion
Methanol
Strong acids or alkalis

[a]When drugs have a delayed emptying.
[b]When specific antidotes are available.

NOTE

Syrup of ipecac is an over-the-counter liquid medication used to induce vomiting. It was once the treatment of choice in preventing the absorption of poisons. However, studies showed that ipecac-induced emesis reduced drug absorption by only about 30%. The drug also may interfere with the effectiveness of other methods of decontamination and can increase the risk of aspiration. In 2004, the Federal Drug Administration withdrew approval of syrup of ipecac. Although the drug may be found in a patient's home, it should not be administered to manage an ingested poison. Patients should be advised to remove syrup of ipecac from their home and to call 9-1-1 or a poison control center if needed.

Modified from: Murff S. *Safety and Health Handbook for Cytotoxic Drugs*. Lanham, MD: Government Institutes; 2012.

Antidotes

An **antidote** is an agent used to neutralize or counteract the effects of a specific poison. Some antidotes work by aiding the elimination of the toxin. Others reactivate enzymes that have been altered by the poison. With a few exceptions described in this chapter, most antidotes are given under physician supervision in the hospital setting (**TABLE 33-2**).

BOX 33-4 Dosage of Activated Charcoal

- 1 to 2 g/kg of body mass
- Adults: 30 to 100 g
- Children: 15 to 30 g
- Prepared in a slurry and administered orally or by gastric tube

TABLE 33-2 Antidotes to Common Toxins[a]

Toxin	Antidote
Acetaminophen	*N*-Acetylcysteine
Anticholinergic agents	Physostigmine
Benzodiazepines	Flumazenil
Beta blockers	Glucagon[a]
Calcium channel blockers	Calcium
Cyanide	Hydroxocobalamin[a]
Digoxin tricyclic antidepressants	Digoxin immune Fab, bicarbonate
Ethylene glycol	Fomepizole
Iron	Deferoxamine
Isoniazid	Pyridoxine
Methanol	Fomepizole
Methemoglobinemia	Methylene blue
Opioids	Naloxone[a]
Organophosphates	Atropine,[a] pralidoxime[a]
Sulfonylureas	Glucose,[a] octreotide

[a]Often available to EMS crews.

Modified from: Murphy CM. Principles of toxicology. In: Cone D, Brice JH, Delbridge TR, Myers JB, eds. *Emergency Medical Services: Clinical Practice and Systems Oversight*. Vol 2. 2nd ed. West Sussex, England: John Wiley & Sons; 2015:333-340.

Management of Specific Ingested Poisons

Specific ingested poisons discussed in this section include strong acids and alkalis, hydrocarbons, methanol, ethylene glycol, isopropanol, metals (iron, lead, and mercury), and poisons from food and plants. Few effective antidotes are available for ingested poisons. Thus managing the patient's symptoms is the main goal in caring for the poisoned patient.

Strong Acids and Alkalis

Caustics are typically acids and bases and are defined by their ability to burn or corrode organic tissue by chemical action. Caustic substances include those found in toilet bowl cleaners, rust remover, ammonia, and most liquid drain cleaners (BOX 33-5). These acids and alkalis may cause burns to the mouth, pharynx, esophagus, and sometimes the upper respiratory and GI tracts. The severity of injury is related to the concentration of the product, time in contact with body tissues, and the body tissue affected. Perforation of the esophagus or stomach may result in vascular collapse, **mediastinitis** (inflammation of the mediastinum), or **pneumoperitoneum** (air or gas in the peritoneal cavity of the abdomen). The frequency of caustic ingestions (most commonly lye) is highest in small children, accounting for 5,000 to 8,000 accidental exposures each year.[12]

BOX 33-5 Common Acid and Alkali Substances

Acids	Alkalis
Acetic acid	Ammonia
Automotive battery acid	Bleach
Citric acid	Disk (button) batteries
Hydrochloric acid	Drain cleaners
Metal cleaners	Hair dyes and tints
Phenol	Jewelry cleaners
Sulfuric acid	Metal cleaners or polishes
Swimming pool cleaners	Paint removers
Toilet bowl cleaners	Sodium or potassium hydroxide (lye)
Glass etching chemicals	Laundry and dishwasher detergents

The ingestion of caustic and corrosive substances generally produces immediate damage to the mucous membrane and the intestinal tract. Acids generally cause coagulation necrosis and complete their damage within 1 to 2 minutes. Alkalis, however, may continue to cause **liquefaction** of tissue and damage for minutes to hours. (Liquefaction is the conversion of solid tissue to a fluid or semifluid state.) Thus, the prehospital care usually is limited to airway and ventilatory support, intravenous (IV) fluid replacement, and rapid transport to an appropriate medical facility. For ocular exposures, however, prehospital care should include copious irrigation of the affected eye on scene and en route, especially with alkaline injuries.

In some cases, medical direction or poison control may recommend diluting the acid or alkali if the patient is conscious. Dilution is done with the oral administration of milk or water: 200 to 300 mL for an adult, and 15 mL/kg maximum for a child.[13] Efforts to neutralize the ingested agent with other fluids such as fruit juice, lemon juice, or vinegar are contraindicated. These fluids have the potential to induce intense heat-releasing reactions that can cause severe thermal burns.

NOTE

The American Association of Poison Control Centers reported almost 10,000 exposures of children younger than 5 years to single-load laundry packets ("pods") in a 10-month period in 2017. Children who have ingested these products experience profuse vomiting and respiratory symptoms that include wheezing. In some cases, intubation is required. In cases where the detergent contacts the child's eyes, corneal abrasions have been reported.

Modified from: Laundry detergent packets and children. American Association of Poison Control Centers website. http://www.aapcc.org/alerts/laundry-detergent-packets/. Accessed February 28, 2018.

CRITICAL THINKING

What is a risk of administering milk or water to a patient with this type of ingestion?

Hydrocarbons

Hydrocarbons are a group of compounds that are derived mainly from crude oil, coal, or plant sources. Mixtures vary in their viscosity, surface tension, and volatility. **Viscosity** is the resistance of a liquid to flow;

surface tension is the ability of a liquid to minimize the area of its surface by contracting; **volatility** is the ability of a liquid to vaporize. These attributes determine the toxic effects of these agents. Other contributing factors include the presence of other chemicals in the product, total amount of product, and route of exposure. There are three primary methods of hydrocarbon exposure:[14]

1. Unintentional ingestion by children
2. Industrial exposures on the skin or by inhalation
3. Intentional inhalational abuse

Hydrocarbons are found in many household products. Examples include cleaning and polishing agents, spot removers, paints, cosmetics, pesticides, and hobby and craft materials. Hydrocarbons also are found in petroleum distillates, such as turpentine, kerosene, gasoline, lighter fluids, and pine oil products. In addition, a large group of halogenated hydrocarbons and aromatic hydrocarbons exists. Examples of halogenated hydrocarbons include carbon tetrachloride, trichloromethane, trichloroethylene, and methyl chloride. Examples of aromatic hydrocarbons are toluene, xylene, and benzene. Hydrocarbon poisonings are common, accounting for 7% of all ingestions in children younger than 5 years.[3] Most ingestions occur between May and September. A wide variety of petroleum products (eg, cleaning products, fuels for lawn and garden tools) are used during these months, increasing children's opportunities for exposure.

The most important physical characteristic in the potential toxicity of ingested hydrocarbons is its viscosity. The lower the viscosity, the higher the risk of aspiration and associated complications.[15] For example, an ingested hydrocarbon product with a low viscosity, such as gasoline, turpentine, or mineral spirits (such as baby oil), rapidly spreads over the surface of the mouth and throat. The more volatile components become gases on contact with the warm mucous membranes. This exposure causes irritation, coughing, and possible aspiration. If aspiration occurs, it may allow a toxic amount of hydrocarbons to enter the lungs. Aspiration destroys surfactant and causes a general inflammatory response, resulting in ventilation–perfusion mismatch and bronchospasm.

The signs and symptoms after acute inhalation typically advance through several stages, beginning with euphoria and followed by excitability, disinhibition, and finally impulsive behavior. Freon inhalation intoxication starts with symptoms of headache, dizziness, and nausea, which is followed by slurred speech, confusion, hallucinations, double vision, tremors, ataxia, visual changes, and weakness. In the final stage, the patient's level of consciousness declines, leading to coma, seizures, and, in some cases, death.[15] Hydrocarbons with high viscosity (eg, asphalt, grease, tar) are not aspirated or absorbed in the GI tract and therefore do not have significant toxicity.

NOTE

A mnemonic for remembering hydrocarbons is CHAMP: Camphor, Halogenated hydrocarbons, Aromatic hydrocarbons, (heavy) Metal-containing hydrocarbons, and Pesticide-containing hydrocarbons.

The clinical features of hydrocarbon ingestion vary widely, depending on the type of agent involved (BOX 33-6). Their effects are most prominent in the CNS, and most are CNS depressants. Liphophilic hydrocarbons pass through the blood brain barrier more easily and have a greater effect on the CNS.

If the patient is not displaying symptoms on EMS arrival, the chances of serious complications usually are low. These patients generally are observed in the ED for several hours. They often require no treatment. However, any patient suspected of hydrocarbon ingestion who coughs, chokes, cries, or has spontaneous emesis on swallowing should be assumed to have aspirated the hydrocarbon until proven otherwise. Follow the guidelines for management of poisoned patients (see Box 33-2). In addition, when caring for symptomatic patients who have ingested hydrocarbon products, paramedics should avoid decontamination of the stomach; decontamination of the stomach increases the risk of aspiration.[15] The use of activated charcoal or diluents has not been shown to be effective in managing hydrocarbon ingestion.[12]

CRITICAL THINKING

Will the potential lethal effects of this ingestion always be visible on the scene?

Methanol

Methanol (wood alcohol) is a poisonous alcohol found in a variety of products, including windshield washer fluid, gas line antifreeze, paints, paint removers, varnishes, canned fuels such as Sterno, embalming fluids,

BOX 33-6 Clinical Features of Hydrocarbon Ingestion

Immediate: Up to 6 Hours

Gastrointestinal System
Abdominal pain
Belching
Irritation
Mucous membrane hyperemia
Nausea and vomiting

Respiratory System
Cough and choking
Cyanosis
Dyspnea
Inspiratory stridor
Tachypnea

Neurologic System
Coma
Fever
Lethargy
Malaise
Seizures
Systemic factors

Delayed: Days to Weeks

Gastrointestinal System
Diarrhea
Hepatic toxicity

Respiratory System
Atelectasis
Bacterial pneumonia
Dyspnea
Hemolytic and aplastic anemias
Pulmonary edema
Spontaneous hemorrhage
Sputum production
Systemic factors

and many shellacs. Methanol is a colorless liquid. It has an odor that is distinct from that of ethanol, the form of alcohol in alcoholic beverages. Poisonings may result from intentional or unintentional ingestions, absorption through the skin, or inhalation. Examples include deliberate use of the agent by patients with severe alcohol use disorder to maintain an inebriated state, unintentional ingestion resulting from misuse or distribution of methanol in place of ethanol (as in contraband liquor), and accidental ingestions in children.

The metabolites of methanol are extremely toxic. As methanol is absorbed, it rapidly is converted in the liver to formaldehyde and then to formic acid. The accumulation of formic acid in the blood affects the CNS (lethargy, confusion, seizure) and the GI tract (abdominal pain, nausea and vomiting) and leads to the development of metabolic acidosis (shock, multisystem failure, death). The patient's vision also may be affected (blurred vision, photophobia). Ingestion of 10 to 15 mL of methanol can cause severe systemic toxic effects, in particular irreversible blindness and central nervous system depression concomitant with metabolic acidosis. A dosage of approximately 1 mL of methanol per kilogram of body weight may result in death.[16] The symptoms of methanol poisoning correlate with the degree of acidosis. The onset of symptoms after ingestion ranges from 40 minutes to 72 hours. If methanol poisoning is not treated, as many as 28% of patients die and 30% of survivors sustain visual problems or blindness.[17]

CRITICAL THINKING

Do you think the risk of blindness associated with methanol could have been the origin of the expression "blind drunk"?

Paramedics should follow the guidelines for management of poisoned patients (see Box 33-2) in addition to the following emergency care for methanol poisoning:[17]

1. **Adequate ventilation.** Adequate ventilation is essential to ensure adequate oxygenation to help correct the profound metabolic acidosis and to maximize respiratory excretion.
2. **GI decontamination.** Activated charcoal is ineffective and should not be given.
3. **Correction of metabolic acidosis.** Medical direction may recommend an attempt to correct the metabolic acidosis (if known) with sodium bicarbonate. Large or repeated doses may be necessary.
4. **Prevention of the conversion of methanol to formic acid.** The conversion of methanol to formic acid may be prevented by the administration of fomepizole. In the past, ethanol was used to accomplish this, but ethanol administration is associated with more adverse effects.[18] Ethanol has 10 to 20 times greater affinity for the enzyme that converts methanol to formic acid.[19]
5. **Hemodialysis.** Hemodialysis may be necessary to remove toxic levels of methanol and formate. It is often needed if ethanol is used to treat the patient.

Ethylene Glycol

Ethylene glycol is a colorless, odorless, water-soluble liquid. It is commonly used in windshield deicers, detergents, paints, radiator antifreeze, and coolants. The accidental ingestion of ethylene glycol is common in young children because of the brilliant colors added to these preparations as well as their naturally sweet taste. The agent also is sometimes consumed by patients with alcohol use disorder as a substitute for ethanol. Without treatment, ingestion of as little as 0.2 mL/kg has been reported to be lethal to an adult.[20]

Early signs and symptoms of CNS depression usually are caused by the ethanollike effects of ethylene glycol. However, toxicity from ethylene glycol, as from methanol, is caused by the accumulation of glycolic and oxalic acids after metabolism and occurs primarily in the liver and kidneys. The metabolic molecules may affect the CNS and cardiopulmonary and renal systems. The initial signs and symptoms of ethylene glycol poisoning may include slurred speech, nausea and vomiting, hallucinations, seizure, stupor, and coma, which can be followed by pulmonary edema and cardiac failure.

Emergency care for ethylene glycol poisoning is similar to that used for methanol poisoning. In addition, the paramedic should anticipate orders from medical direction or a poison control center for the following medications:[21]

- Thiamine to degrade glycolic acid to nontoxic metabolites
- Midazolam, diazepam, or lorazepam to control seizure activity

> **CRITICAL THINKING**
>
> The effects in the first stage of ethylene glycol poisoning could be mistaken for what condition?

Isopropanol

Isopropanol (isopropyl alcohol) is a volatile, flammable, colorless liquid. It has a characteristic odor and bittersweet taste. Rubbing alcohol is the most common household source of this agent. It also is used in disinfectants, degreasers, cosmetics, industrial solvents, and cleaning agents. Common routes of toxic exposure to isopropanol include intentional ingestion as a substitute for ethanol, accidental ingestion, and inhalation of high concentrations of local vapor. Isopropanol is more toxic than ethanol, but less toxic than methanol or ethylene glycol. A lethal dose in adults is rare.[13] In children, any amount of ingestion should be considered potentially toxic.

Isopropanol poisoning affects several body systems, including the central nervous, GI, and renal systems. The signs and symptoms often occur within 30 minutes after ingestion. They include vomiting, ataxia, CNS and respiratory depression, abdominal pain, gastritis, hematemesis, and hypovolemia.[22] Isopropanol poisoning causes acids to accumulate in the blood (acetonemia) and ketones to accumulate in the urine (ketonuria). However, associated metabolic acidosis usually does not occur unless the patient develops hypotension.

Paramedics should follow the principles for management of poisoned patients (Box 33-2) in addition to the following emergency care for isopropanol poisoning, which is mainly supportive.[13] Care includes airway and ventilatory support to ensure adequate respiratory elimination of acetone, fluid resuscitation as needed, and rapid transport to an appropriate medical facility, where dialysis may be necessary. Gastric lavage and activated charcoal are not effective.[8] Administration of ethanol has not proven to inhibit the toxic metabolite to the same degree as in methanol or ethylene glycol poisoning.

> **NOTE**
>
> Most hand sanitizers contain 60% ethyl alcohol, but the concentration may be as high as 95%. By comparison, concentrations of ethyl alcohol in wine and beer range from 5% to 15%. These sanitizer products look and smell very attractive to children. Ingestion of more than a sip can cause alcohol poisoning. Signs and symptoms include confusion, vomiting, drowsiness, and possibly respiratory arrest and death. The National Poison Control Center recorded over 15,000 exposures to hand sanitizer in the 10 months through the end of October 2017.
>
> *Modified from*: Hand sanitizer. The American Association of Poison Control Centers website. http://www.aapcc.org/alerts/hand-sanitizer/. Accessed February 28, 2018.

Metals

Infants and children are high-risk groups for unintentional iron, lead, and mercury poisoning. Their immature immune systems and increased absorption as a function of age contribute to this risk.

Iron Poisoning. About 10% of ingested iron (mainly ferrous sulfate) is absorbed each day from the small intestine. After absorption, the iron is converted and is stored in iron storage protein. Then, the iron is transported to the liver, spleen, and bone marrow for incorporation into hemoglobin. When ingested iron exceeds the ability of the body to store it, the free iron circulates in the blood. The iron then is deposited into other tissues. Most iron poisonings result from the ingestion of iron-containing pediatric multivitamins by children younger than 6 years.[23]

Unintentional or intentional ingestion of iron may be fatal. Ingested iron is corrosive to the lining of the GI tract. Iron may produce GI hemorrhage, bloody vomitus, painless bloody diarrhea, and dark stools. Severe cases involve the ingestion of more than 20 mg/kg. Ingestion of more than 60 mg/kg can produce seizures, liver failure, cardiovascular collapse, and death.[24] Prehospital care includes supportive measures and rapid transport for physician evaluation and possible GI decontamination to prevent further absorption. The use of activated charcoal generally is not recommended because it adsorbs iron poorly. Most patients with iron poisoning survive the episode. The long-term prognosis is favorable.

Lead Poisoning. Metallic lead has been used by humans for thousands of years. In 1978, lead-based paint was recognized as a major health hazard and was banned from household paints in the United States (BOX 33-7). Children are the most common group to be found with lead poisoning; an estimated 500,000 children in the United States ages 1 to 5 years have levels of lead in their bloodstream of 5 mcg/dL or greater.[25] Most pediatric poisonings result from ingestion of lead-based paint chips and contaminated house dust. Lead toxicity in adults most commonly results from exposure by inhalation. If exposure is not detected early, children with high levels of lead in their bodies can suffer from damage to the brain and nervous system. This damage can result in behavioral and learning problems, hyperactivity, slowed growth, hearing problems, and headaches. Even children who appear healthy can have dangerous levels of lead in their bodies. Adults with high levels of lead in their systems can experience difficult pregnancies, reproductive problems, hypertension, nerve disorders, muscle and joint pain, and problems with memory and concentration.

BOX 33-7 Places Where Lead Can Be Found

- Homes in the city, country, or suburbs
- Apartments, single-family homes, and private and public housing painted before 1978
- Soil around a home (soil contaminated from exterior paint or other sources such as past use of leaded gasoline in cars)
- Painted windows and window sills
- Doors and door frames
- Stairs, railings, and banisters
- Porches and fences
- Paint surfaces that have been scraped, dry-sanded, or heated (lead dust)
- Old painted toys and furniture
- The air after vacuuming or sweeping contaminated surfaces
- Food and liquid stored in lead crystal or lead-glazed pottery or porcelain
- Lead smelters or other industries
- Hobbies that use lead (eg, making pottery or stained glass)
- Folk remedies (greta or azarcon used to treat an upset stomach)

Most lead poisoning is slow in onset and results from chronic ingestion or inhalation, eventually resulting in toxicity. The metal is excreted by the body slowly and tends to accumulate in body tissues (mainly bone). Lead exposure that results in acute intoxication may lead to paralysis, seizures, coma, and death. Patients who survive are likely to sustain brain damage. Prehospital care is focused on recognizing the potential for lead poisoning and transporting the patient for physician evaluation. If lead poisoning is confirmed through radiograph and laboratory testing, care may include GI decontamination or whole-bowel irrigation. Following treatment, all patients must be discharged to a lead-free environment. Outpatient chelation therapy may be indicated to detoxify the lead and excrete the metal from the body.

CRITICAL THINKING

Paramedics play a key role in the emergency management of lead poisoning. What other role can they play in the management of this problem?

Mercury Poisoning. Mercury is the only metal that is liquid at room temperature. It has been used in thermometers, sphygmomanometers, and dental fillings that contain elemental mercury (Hg) as their main component.[26] Various compounds of mercury also are used in some energy-saving light bulbs, paints, pesticides, cosmetics, and drugs, and in certain industrial processes. Some seafood contains mercury. There are three forms of mercury: elemental, organic, and inorganic salts. Toxicity largely depends on the form of mercury that the patient was exposed to, but all forms of mercury are poisonous.

Inhalation of mercury vapor is the most common route of mercury poisoning. It may cause shortness of breath and lung damage. Mercury also may be absorbed through the skin, causing severe inflammation, and through the intestines after ingestion. After mercury enters the body, it passes into the bloodstream. It later accumulates in various organs, mainly the brain (where it remains for years) and kidneys. This accumulation causes a wide range of symptoms that may include the following:

- Malaise
- Incoordination
- Excitability
- Tremors
- Numbness in the limbs
- Vision impairment
- Nausea and emesis (symptoms of renal failure)
- Mental status changes

Prehospital care mainly is supportive. Following physician evaluation, patients are managed with GI decontamination, if the ingestion was recent, and with chelating agents. In severe cases, hemodialysis may be indicated.

Food Poisoning

Food poisoning is a term used for any illness of sudden onset suspected of being caused by food eaten within the previous 48 hours. It is usually associated with stomach pain, vomiting, and diarrhea. Food poisoning can be classified as infectious (bacterial and viral) or noninfectious.

Infectious (Bacterial) Types. One of the common types of bacteria responsible for food poisoning is *Salmonella.* This organism is found in many animals (especially poultry) and in humans. *Salmonella* bacteria also may be transferred to food from the excrement of infected animals or humans, and by an infected person handling food. Other bacteria (eg, strains of staphylococcal bacteria) cause formation of toxins. These toxins may be difficult to destroy even with thorough cooking of the food. Other bacteria that commonly cause diarrhea are certain strains of *Escherichia coli* (traveler's diarrhea) and *Campylobacter* and *Shigella* organisms.

Botulism is a rare but life-threatening form of food poisoning. It may result from eating improperly canned or preserved food that is contaminated with the bacterium *Clostridium botulinum.* This organism is found in soil and untreated water in most parts of the world. It also is harmlessly present in the intestinal tracts of many animals, including fish. Its spore-forming properties resist boiling, salting, smoking, and some forms of pickling, allowing the bacterium to thrive in improperly preserved or canned foods. Although foodborne botulism is rare, the disease is more common in the United States because of the popularity of preserving food in the home. Botulism is associated with severe CNS symptoms. These symptoms appear in a characteristic head-to-toe progression: headache, blurred or double vision, dysphagia, respiratory paralysis, and quadriplegia. Respiratory failure occurs in 50% of patients.[4] Death, however, is rare with treatment.

> NOTE
>
> Infant botulism is the most common form of the illness in the United States, accounting for 72% of all cases. It occurs in children younger than 1 year, with a peak incidence between 2 and 6 months of age. The illness often is caused by consuming infected spores from honey and, to a lesser degree, corn syrup.
>
> *Modified from:* Dodd C, Aldsworth T, Stein RA, Cliver D, Riemann H. *Foodborne Diseases.* 3rd ed. Amsterdam, Netherlands: Elsevier; 2017.

Infectious (Viral) Types. The viruses that most often cause food poisoning are the norovirus (Norwalk) virus (a common contaminant of shellfish) and rotavirus. Both agents may be responsible for illness when raw or partly cooked foodstuffs have been in contact with water contaminated by human excrement.

Noninfectious Types. Noninfectious types of food poisoning may result from consuming mushrooms and toadstools. Food poisoning also can result from eating fresh foods and vegetables that are accidentally contaminated with large amounts of insecticide. Chemical food poisoning may result from eating food stored in a contaminated container (eg, a container that previously was used to store poison). It also can result from improperly preparing and cooking various exotic foods.

Management Guidelines. The onset of signs and symptoms from food poisoning varies by cause and by how heavily the food was contaminated. As a rule, symptoms usually develop within 30 minutes in the case of chemical poisoning, in 1 to 12 hours in the case of bacterial toxins, and in 12 to 48 hours with viral and bacterial infections.[14] Principles of the management for patients with suspected food poisoning include the following:

- Use precautions to avoid contamination of self and equipment. Wear gloves, a gown, or both, if appropriate.
- Ensure adequate airway, ventilatory, and circulatory support.
- Gather a complete history. The history should include time and onset of symptoms, recent travel, the relation of symptoms to ingestion of a particular food, and effects on others who ate the same food. In addition, the paramedic should obtain information on the consistency, frequency, and odor of stool (including the presence of mucus or blood). Fever should be noted as well. Any patient history also should include significant medical history, allergies, and use of medications.
- Initiate IV therapy with a crystalloid solution. This will help to manage dehydration and electrolyte disturbances resulting from vomiting and diarrhea.
- Transport the patient for physician evaluation.

Plant Poisoning

Toxic plant ingestion is in the top 10 pediatric toxic exposures reported to poison control centers.[5] This type of toxin accounts for 2.7% of poisonings reported in 2015.[5] While most of these poisonings relate to children who ingest plants in and around their homes, adolescent experimentation with hallucinogenic plants and misidentification by hikers or foragers who think they are edible also account for illness.[27] Poison control should be consulted to identify the plant. When possible, transport the plant (including any flowers, berries, leaves) along with the patient.

> CRITICAL THINKING
> What features of a plant would make it attractive for children to eat?

Signs and Symptoms. The signs of toxicity following the ingestion of major poisonous plants are predictable. They are categorized by the chemical and physical properties of the plant and described as plant toxidromes. Most signs and symptoms tend to be consistent with the type of major toxic chemical component in the plant. They usually appear within several hours after ingestion but may be delayed 1 to 3 days. **TABLE 33-3** lists plant toxidromes, common plants in these groups, and the signs and symptoms of poisonings from these toxidromes. Paramedics should be familiar with common poisonous plant life in their response area.

Management. Several hundred species of green plants and more than 100 varieties of mushrooms in the United States contain toxic compounds. These plants and mushrooms have widely varying potencies and combinations of toxins. In addition, such factors as the age of the plant and soil conditions may influence the severity of toxic symptoms. Thus, management guidelines should be customized to the patient's symptoms rather than to one type of ingestion. Identification of the plant is important if possible. However, the inability to do so should not delay patient care. The paramedic should consult with medical direction or a poison control center regarding appropriate management. Emergency care for toxic plant ingestion includes the administration of activated charcoal in conscious patients, IV fluids, and ensuring adequate airway, ventilatory, and circulatory support. Most patients are hospitalized for observation and treatment as indicated for the toxin involved. Dialysis has not been shown to be effective in removing most plant toxins.[28]

Poisoning by Inhalation

The unintentional or intentional inhalation of poisons can lead to a life-threatening emergency. The type and location of injury caused by toxic inhalation

TABLE 33-3 Plant Toxidromes

Plant Toxidromes	Signs and Symptoms	Common Plants in This Group
Cardiotoxic poisonings	Nausea, vomiting, abdominal pain, bradycardia, atrioventricular blocks, ventricular dysrhythmias, hyperkalemia	Foxglove, oleander, Japanese yews, hellebores
Neurotoxic poisonings	Dry skin, tachycardia, fever, dilated pupils, blurred vision, ileus, urinary retention, agitation, vertigo, aggression, confusion, dysarthria, hallucinations, coma or fasciculations, seizures, ventricular dysrhythmias	Angel's trumpet, jimsonweed, thorn apples, poison hemlock, smoking tobacco, blue cohosh, water hemlock, *Salvia* (herb diviner's sage), morning glory seeds
Cytotoxic poisonings	Vomiting, diarrhea, dehydration, hypovolemic shock, oral pain, neuropathy, seizures	Castor bean (ricin), cyanogenics (pits or seeds of apples, apricots, cherries, peaches, plums), jequirity, rosary pea, vinca, mayapple
Gastrointestinal toxins and hepatotoxins	Intense oral pain, eye pain if ocular exposure upper right quadrant abdominal pain, acute hepatitis	Species of *Caladium*, *Dieffenbachia*, *Philodendron*, *Schefflera*, and *Spathiphyllum*

Modified from: Diaz JH. (2016). Poisoning by herbs and plants: rapid toxidromic classification and diagnosis. *Wilderness Environ Med.* 2016;27(1):136-152.

depend on the specific actions and behaviors of the chemical involved.[29] Respiratory difficulty may not appear for several hours after exposure to toxic fumes and smoke. All patients should be encouraged to seek physician evaluation. This includes even those who are asymptomatic.

CRITICAL THINKING

Do you think that situations involving toxic gas inhalation are likely to involve one patient or multiple patients? Why?

Classifications

Toxic gases can be classified in three categories: simple asphyxiants, chemical asphyxiants, and irritants/corrosives. Simple asphyxiants (eg, methane, propane, inert gases) cause toxicity by displacing or lowering the amount of oxygen in the air. Chemical asphyxiants (eg, carbon monoxide, cyanide) can cause a number of local and pulmonary reactions when inhaled. Their toxic systemic effects prevent the uptake of oxygen by the blood and can interfere with tissue oxygenation. Irritants/corrosives (eg, chlorine, ammonia) cause cellular destruction and inflammation as they come into contact with moisture. **TABLE 33-4** provides an overview of toxic gases and their clinical features.

General Management

To treat patients who have inhaled toxins, follow the guidelines for management of poisoned patients (see Box 33-2). In addition, irrigation of the eyes may be needed if indicated. Other care is based on the mechanism of action of the specific toxin.

Management of Specific Inhaled Poisons

The specific inhaled poisons discussed in this section include cyanide, ammonia, and hydrocarbons. Carbon monoxide poisoning is described in Chapter 38, *Burns*. Other gases associated with atmospheres with low oxygen levels and chemical and biologic warfare are discussed in Chapter 56, *Hazardous Materials Awareness*, and Chapter 57, *Bioterrorism and Weapons of Mass Destruction*.

Cyanide

Cyanide refers to any number of highly toxic substances that contain the cyanogen chemical group.

TABLE 33-4 Clinical Features of Toxic Gases and Fumes

Class of Toxin	Toxin	Source	Clinical Features	Management
Simple asphyxiants	Propane Methane Carbon dioxide Inert gases (nitrogen, argon)	Cooking gas Cooking gas All fires Industry (especially welding)	Displacement of normal air and lower fractional inspired oxygen concentration, symptoms of hypoxemia without airway irritation	Remove patient from source; give oxygen.
Chemical asphyxiants	Carbon monoxide	Fires	Formation of carboxyhemoglobin; inhibition of oxygen transport (headache is earliest symptom)	Give 100% oxygen.
	Hydrocyanic acid	Industry, burning plastics, furniture, fabrics	Highly toxic cellular asphyxiant	Give hydroxocobalamin.
	Hydrogen sulfide	Liquid manure pits, decaying organic materials	Highly toxic cellular asphyxiant similar to cyanide; sudden collapse; ability to smell characteristic odor of rotten eggs; rapid fatigue	Use sodium nitrite for cyanide (makes sulfmethemoglobin). Do not use thiosulfate.
Irritants: high solubility in water	Chlorine gas Hydrochloric acid	Industry, swimming pool chemicals, bleach mixed with acid at home	Early onset of lacrimation, sore throat, stridor, tracheobronchitis; with heavy exposure, pulmonary edema in 26 hours	Use humidified oxygen, bronchodilators, and airway management.
Irritants: low solubility in water	Ammonia Nitrogen dioxide	Industry, burning fabrics Burning cellulose, fabrics	Sweet electric smell; delayed onset (12–24 hours) of tracheobronchitis, pneumonitis, and pulmonary edema; late chronic bronchitis	Give oxygen and observe for 24–48 hours; give steroids (controversial).
	Ozone	Grain silos (acrid red gas) Inert gas arc welding, industry	Coughing, shortness of breath, throat irritation	Provide supportive care.
	Phosgene	Burning of chlorinated organic material	Coughing, burning sensation in eyes/throat, lacrimation, dyspnea, nausea; late signs include pulmonary edema	Provide airway support, and observe for at least 48 hours.
Allergenic	Toluene diisocyanate	Manufacture of polyurethanes	Reactive bronchoconstriction; possible long-term effects (chronic obstructive pulmonary disease) in susceptible people	Use bronchodilators.
Metal fumes	Zinc Copper Tin Teflon	Welding (especially galvanized metal welding)	Metal fumes fever; chills, fever, myalgias, headache, nonproductive cough, leukocytosis 4–8 hours after exposure	Condition is self-limited (12–24 hours).
	Arsine	Burning arsenic-containing ores, electronics industry	Highly toxic effect; hemolysis, pulmonary edema, renal failure; chronic arsenic toxicity	Perform exchange transfusion; use dimercaprol (BAL) for chronic arsenic toxicity only.
	Mercury Lead	Industry, welding	See specific metals	

Modified from: Ho MT. *Current Emergency Diagnosis and Treatment.* 3rd ed. Norwalk, CT: Appleton & Lange; 1990; National Center for Emerging and Zoonotic Infectious Diseases (NCEZID). Phosgene. Centers for Disease Control and Prevention website. https://emergency.cdc.gov/agent/phosgene/basics/facts.asp. Updated April 12, 2013. Accessed February 28, 2018.

Because of its toxicity, cyanide has few applications. The agent sometimes is used in industry in electroplating ore extraction, fumigation of buildings, and fertilization. Cyanide has been used in gas chambers as a means of execution. It is one of the by-products of combustion from burning many substances, including nylon and polyurethane. Thus, cyanide is a hazard in fire environments.

Cyanide poisoning may result from the inhalation of cyanide gas; the ingestion of cyanide salts, nitriles, or cyanogenic glycosides (eg, amygdalin, a substance found in the seeds of cherries, apples, pears, and apricots, and the principal constituent of Laetrile); or the infusion of nitroprusside. Cyanide also can be absorbed across the skin. Regardless of the route of entry, cyanide is a rapidly acting poison. It combines and reacts with ferric ions (Fe^{3+}) of the respiratory enzyme cytochrome oxidase to prevent the cellular mitochondria from using oxygen to make energy in the form of adenosine triphosphate. The cytotoxic hypoxia produces a rapid progression of symptoms from dyspnea to paralysis, unconsciousness, and death (BOX 33-8). Large doses usually are fatal within minutes from respiratory arrest.

After ensuring personal safety and removing the patient from the toxic environment, emergency care for a patient with cyanide poisoning begins with securing an open airway and providing adequate ventilatory support with high-concentration oxygen. Appropriate PPE is needed for treating patients with cyanide ingestion. When stomach acids mix with cyanide, hydrogen cyanide gases may be produced and expelled if the patient vomits or belches.[9] Oxygen displaces cyanide from cytochrome oxidase and increases the effectiveness of drug administration. Older cyanide antidotes (BOX 33-9), such as those

BOX 33-8 Early and Advanced Signs and Symptoms of Cyanide Poisoning

Early Effects

Agitation
Anxiety
Confusion
Tachypnea/hyperpnea (early)
Hypertension with reflex bradycardia
Pupil dilation
Nausea

Late Effects

Acidosis
Dysrhythmias
Bradypnea/apnea (late)
Hypotension
Seizures

DID YOU KNOW?

Methemoglobin is a dysfunctional form of hemoglobin that cannot transport oxygen. An increased level of methemoglobin in the blood is known as methemoglobinemia. This condition reduces blood oxygenation and produces a functional anemia. **Methemoglobinemia** causes a leftward shift of the oxyhemoglobin dissociation curve. This impedes the unloading of oxygen from normal hemoglobin, reduces the amount of oxygen available to tissues, and leads to tissue hypoxia.

Methemoglobinemia may be congenital. It also may be acquired from exposure to industrial toxins (eg, nitrites in grain silos) and the ingestion and overuse of some medications, such as nitrates, nitrites, and sulfonamides. Signs and symptoms of methemoglobinemia include shortness of breath, cyanosis, mental status changes, headache, fatigue, dizziness, and loss of consciousness. The Rad 57 is an oximetry device that can be used in the prehospital setting to measure arterial blood gas, carboxyhemoglobin levels, and, in some cases, methemoglobin levels. In the emergency setting, methemoglobinemia is treated with oxygen and in-hospital administration of methylene blue. Methylene blue restores the iron in hemoglobin to its normal (reduced) oxygen-carrying state.

BOX 33-9 Cyanide Antidotes

Hydroxocobalamin (preferred antidote)

- Adults: 5 g IV
- Children: 70 mg/kg IV (do not exceed adult dose)
- Dilute in 200 mL normal saline, lactated Ringer solution, or 5% dextrose in water; infuse over 15 minutes; may follow with sodium thiosulfate (separate IV line)

25% Sodium Thiosulfate

- Adults: 12.5 g (50 mL of 25% solution) IV over 10 minutes
- Children: 500 mg/kg (1.65 mL/kg of 25% solution) IV over 10 minutes (do not exceed adult dose)

Modified from: National Association of EMS Officials. *National Model EMS Clinical Guidelines*. Version 2.0. National Association of EMS Officials website. https://www.nasemso.org/documents/National-Model-EMS-Clinical-Guidelines-Version2-Sept2017.pdf. Published September 2017. Accessed February 28, 2018.

found in the Pasadena cyanide antidote kit (also known as the Lilly Cyanide Poison Kit and the Taylor Kit), induced **methemoglobin** production. They are no longer manufactured. Hydroxocobalamin (Cyanokit) is a vitamin B_{12} precursor that can be used to treat cyanide poisoning. It has a central cobalt atom that binds to cyanide in the blood and forms cyanocobalamin (vitamin B_{12}). Detoxification with hydroxocobalamin does not create methemoglobin, so it does not lower the oxygen-carrying capacity of the blood. Rare cases of allergic reaction have been reported. Hydroxocobalamin does not cause hypotension,[30] which makes it possible to use to treat all types of cyanide poisoning, including smoke inhalation.

Cyanide poisoning is treated by giving IV hydroxocobalamin, with or without sodium thiosulfate (See the Appendix, *Emergency Drug Index*).[31] These drugs help detoxify cyanide so that it can be eliminated by the kidneys.[13] It should be noted that hydroxocobalamin and sodium thiosulfate are incompatible and should not be infused through the same IV line. Prehospital care for patients with cyanide poisoning includes the guidelines for management of poisoned patients (see Box 33-2) as well as administration of high-concentration oxygen, despite normal oxygen saturation (pulse oximetry prior to treatment is not a reliable indicator of tissue oxygenation) and hydroxocobalamin IV infusion. Paramedics should anticipate hypertension as a side effect. In addition, the patient should be observed closely for signs of anaphylaxis.

Ammonia Inhalation

Ammonia is a toxic irritant that causes local pulmonary complications after inhalation. These complications include inflammation and irritation and, in severe cases, destruction of the mucosal tissue of all respiratory structures. Injury occurs as the ammonia vapor combines with water, producing a highly caustic alkaline compound. Patients usually develop coughing, choking, congestion, burning, and tightness in the chest and a feeling of suffocation. These respiratory symptoms often are associated with burning eyes and tearing. In severe cases, bronchospasm and pulmonary edema may develop. In addition to the guidelines for management in Box 33-2, emergency care may include positive pressure ventilation and the administration of diuretics and bronchodilators.

Hydrocarbon Inhalation

The hydrocarbons that pose the greatest risk for injury have low viscosity, high volatility, and high surface tension (ie, adhesion of molecules along a surface). These characteristics allow hydrocarbons to enter the pulmonary tree, which causes aspiration pneumonitis and creates the potential for systemic effects as well. Examples of such effects include CNS depression and liver, kidney, or bone marrow toxicity.

Most hydrocarbon inhalations result from recreational use of halogenated hydrocarbons (eg, carbon tetrachloride, methylene chloride) or aromatic hydrocarbons (eg, benzene, toluene). These agents may produce a state of inebriation or euphoria through sniffing (inhaling vapor directly from a container), huffing (inhaling vapor from a cloth soaked in the hydrocarbon that is held over the nose and mouth), or bagging (inhaling vapor from a paper or plastic bag containing a rag soaked in solvent). The onset of these effects usually is rapid, typically occurring within seconds. It may be followed by CNS depression, respiratory failure, or cardiac dysrhythmias. Other signs and symptoms of hydrocarbon inhalation include the following:

- Burning sensation on swallowing
- Nausea and vomiting
- Abdominal cramps
- Weakness
- Anesthesia
- Hallucinations
- Changes in color perception
- Blindness
- Seizures
- Coma

Paramedics should follow the guidelines for management of poisoned patients (Box 33-2). Emergency care for hydrocarbon inhalation generally is supportive.

Poisoning by Injection

In addition to poisoning from injection drug misuse or abuse, poisoning by injection also may result from bites and stings from arthropods, reptiles, and hazardous aquatic life. In contrast to most chemical compounds described previously, poisons from **envenomation** are mixtures of many different substances. These mixtures may produce several different toxic reactions in humans; thus, the paramedic must be prepared to manage reactions in many organ systems at the same time. Management guidelines for most envenomations from bites and stings include the following:

1. Ensure personal safety.
2. Provide adequate airway, ventilatory, and circulatory support as needed. Watch for signs of a serious allergic reaction.
3. Clean the affected area with saline. Cover it with a sterile or clean dressing. Obstruction tourniquets or suction devices do not help to delay absorption and should not be used. Commercially prepared antivenin (if available) sometimes is given in the ED after appropriate sensitivity testing.
4. Moderate to severe symptoms may require aggressive management. According to medical direction, muscle spasm, severe headache, vomiting, and may be managed with benzodiazepines, antiemetics, and pain medication.
5. Transport the patient for physician evaluation. Most patients recover fully. Those at greatest risk for morbidity are the very young, older adults, and people with underlying hypertension or other medical conditions.

Arthropod Bites and Stings

Arthropods are invertebrates with segmented bodies and jointed limbs. Some arthropods bite, some sting, and a few bite and sting. Arthropod **venom** is complex and diverse in chemistry and pharmacology and has the highest need for emergency care of any type of bite or sting injury. These venoms may produce major toxic reactions in sensitized people. Such reactions include anaphylaxis and upper airway obstruction. The various reactions to venoms are classified as local, toxic, systemic, and delayed (BOX 33-10).[32]

BOX 33-10 Types of Reactions to Venoms

Local Reaction

Marked and prolonged edema at the sting site
Possible involvement of one or more neighboring joints
Possible occurrence in the mouth or throat, producing airway obstruction
Severe local reactions that may increase the likelihood of future systemic reactions
Symptoms that usually subside within 24 hours

Toxic Reaction[a]

GI disturbances
- Diarrhea
- Light-headedness
- Vomiting

Other symptoms
- Convulsions (rare)
- Edema without urticaria (hives)
- Fever
- Headache
- Involuntary muscle spasms
- Symptoms that usually subside within 48 hours
- Syncope (common finding)

Systemic (Anaphylactic) Reaction[b]

Reactions that can progress to death within minutes

Immediate symptoms
- Facial flushing
- Generalized urticaria
- Itching eyes or generalized itching

Subsequent symptoms
- Angioedema
- Chest or throat constriction, or both
- Chills and fever
- Cyanosis
- Dyspnea
- Hypotension
- Laryngeal stridor
- Loss of bowel or bladder control
- Loss of consciousness
- Nausea and vomiting with or without abdominal pain
- Respiratory failure, cardiovascular collapse, or both
- Shock
- Wheezing

Delayed Reaction[c]

Serum sickness symptoms
- Fever
- Headache
- Malaise
- Polyarthritis
- Urticaria

[a]Should be considered with a history of 10 or more stings.
[b]May occur in response to single or multiple stings.
[c]Usually occurs 10 to 14 days after a sting.

Hymenoptera (Wasps, Bees, Ants)

Hymenoptera is the name of a large, highly specialized order of insects that includes wasps, bees, and ants. Their venom contains mixtures of toxins, enzymes, and other compounds such as histamines, serotonin, acetylcholine, and dopamine. A single wasp, bee, or ant sting in an unsensitized person usually causes instant pain. This pain is followed by a wheal-and-flare reaction with variable edema. Anaphylaxis is the most serious complication of Hymenoptera stings. An estimated 0.4% of the US population has some degree of chemical allergy to insect venoms; 90 to 100 deaths caused by anaphylaxis from insect stings occur each year.[33] People with a history of allergic reactions to stings often wear medical alert identification. They also often carry an emergency kit that contains a preloaded syringe of epinephrine (EpiPen). The ant species of greatest concern in the United States is the imported fire ant. Stings or bites from fire ants may produce systemic reactions, including anaphylaxis.

Honey bees (and other Hymenoptera) often leave their stingers in the wound. If a stinger is present, it should be scraped or brushed off the skin. Stingers should not be removed with forceps; squeezing the attached venom sac may worsen the injury. Anaphylaxis should be managed as described in Chapter 26, *Immune System Disorders*.

Arachnida (Spiders, Scorpions, Ticks)

Arachnida is a large class of arthropods. These organisms usually have four pairs of legs and a body divided into a cephalothorax (a combined head and thorax) and abdomen. This discussion will be limited to spiders, scorpions, and ticks.

Spider Bites. Most spiders have venom glands. Two major types of reactions occur from spider venom: neurotoxic reactions resulting from the black widow bite and local tissue necrosis resulting from the bites of most other spiders—most notably in the United States, the brown recluse spider.

- **Black widow spider.** The female black widow spider is shiny and black with a red hourglass marking on the undersurface of the abdomen (**FIGURE 33-1**). The male is about half the size of the female, brown, and nonvenomous to humans. The spider generally is found in undisturbed areas (under stones, logs, and clumps of vegetation). They rarely inhabit occupied dwellings.

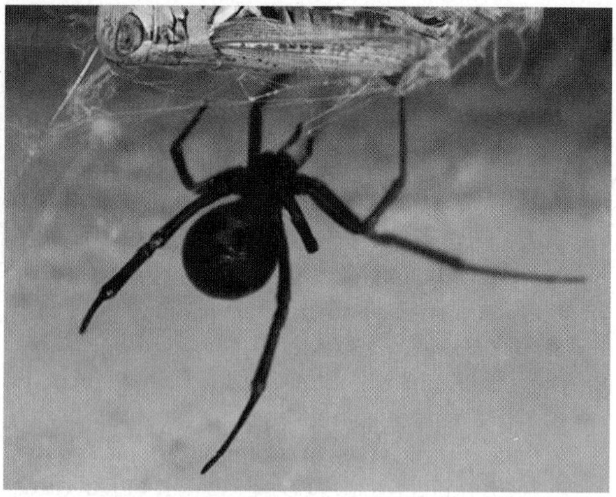

FIGURE 33-1 Black widow spider.

In the United States, most black widow bites occur in rural and suburban areas of southern and western states between April and October.

The bite of a black widow usually is described by patients as a slight pinprick that is initially painless. As a rule, the only physical findings are two small fang marks that are about 1 mm apart and surrounded by a small papule. Multiple bites usually rule out any type of spider envenomation because spiders rarely bite more than once. Within 1 hour of envenomation, the neurotoxin produces characteristic muscle spasms and cramps, which may result in abdominal rigidity and intense pain. Associated symptoms include paresthesia (frequently described as a burning sensation in the soles of the feet or entire body); pain in the muscles of the shoulders, back, and chest; headache; dizziness; nausea and vomiting; edema of the eyelids; and increased perspiration and salivation. Most patients recover fully within 36 to 72 hours.

NOTE

Abdominal rigidity in the absence of palpable tenderness is a crucial finding. This finding helps to distinguish envenomation from an acute abdominal condition.

- **Brown recluse spider.** The brown recluse spider is also known as the fiddle-back spider. This species of spider prefers hot, dry, and abandoned environments such as vacant buildings and is most prevalent in the Mississippi-Ohio-Missouri

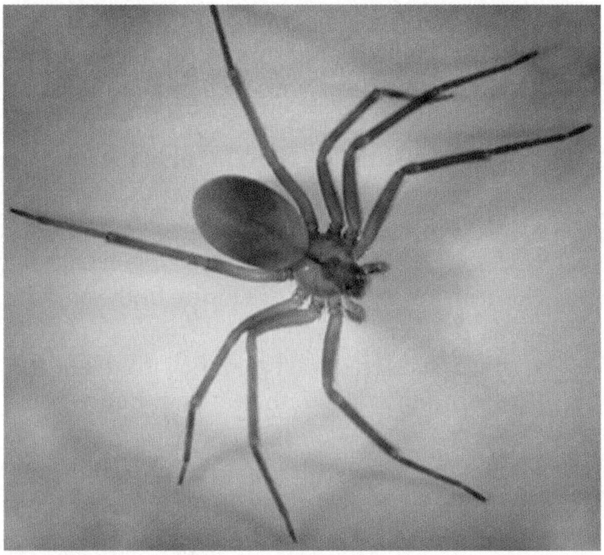

FIGURE 33-2 Brown recluse spider.

Courtesy of Kenneth Cramer, Monmouth College.

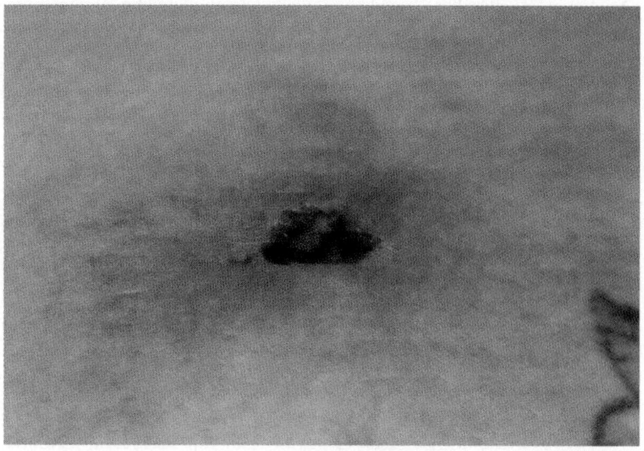

FIGURE 33-3 Brown recluse spider bite.

© Robert D Brozek/Shutterstock.

river basin and the southwestern United States. It often is found in clothing closets. The spider is fawn to dark brown and is between 0.4 and 0.8 inch (1–2 cm) long (**FIGURE 33-2**). Identifying characteristics of the brown recluse are six white eyes arranged in a semicircle on the head (versus the usual eight eyes of most other spiders) and the presence of a dark, violin-shaped marking on the top of the cephalothorax. The brown recluse is considered shy. It generally does not attack unless threatened. Like black widows, these spiders are most active from April to October.

The venom of the brown recluse initially causes little pain and often is overlooked by the person who has been bitten. Approximately 1 to 2 hours later, localized pain and erythema develop (**FIGURE 33-3**). This often is followed within 2 days by a blister or vesicle. The lesion may be surrounded by an ischemic ring that is outlined further by an irregular red halo, producing the classic bull's-eye appearance seen with this bite. Over the next 72 hours, the area often becomes larger and the center of the lesion may become purple or develop a black eschar (dead tissue). The eschar eventually sloughs, leaving an ulcer of variable size and depth. The wound typically is slow to heal and may be visible for months to years after the bite. Occasionally, excision and skin grafting are necessary. Systemic involvement is uncommon. It presents with signs and symptoms that include fever, chills, malaise, nausea and vomiting, generalized rash, and the development of hemolytic anemia, disseminated intravascular coagulation, and acute renal failure.[34] Death occasionally occurs, usually from disturbance of the coagulation system or hepatic injury.

> CRITICAL THINKING
>
> For which type of spider bite is a patient most likely to call an ambulance? Why?

Scorpion Stings. Only a few of the more than 650 species of scorpions produce human envenomation. In North America, the sculptured or bark scorpion is the only species that is dangerous to humans. This scorpion is found in the southwestern United States and Mexico. It is nocturnal and favors wooded areas along the edges of desert washes. Occasionally the scorpion invades homes, especially adobe houses. The sculptured scorpion is small and yellow to brown, and some have tail stripes (**FIGURE 33-4**). The species is most active from April to August, and hibernates during the winter.

The venom of the scorpion is delivered by a stinger on the telson. The venom is a mixture of proteins that causes the release of acetylcholine. It also stimulates sympathetic nerves and directly stimulates the CNS, causing hyperactivity. The sculpture scorpion's venom does not contain enzymes that cause tissue destruction. Thus, local inflammation is not a feature. If swelling, ecchymosis, or redness is present, the scorpion was not of the neurotoxic type. BOX 33-11 lists the signs and symptoms of sculptured scorpion stings. Despite

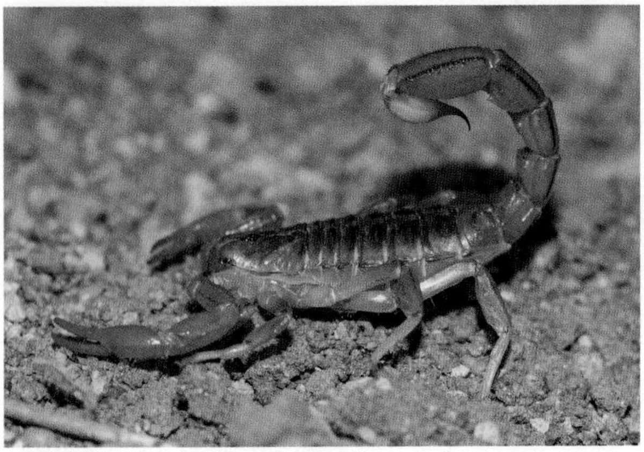

FIGURE 33-4 The sculptured scorpion commonly found in the deserts of Arizona, New Mexico, and California.

BOX 33-11 Signs and Symptoms of Scorpion Envenomation

Hyperesthesia at the site of the bite
Pain, tingling, and a burning sensation radiating along the nerves at the location of the bite
SLUDGE
Cardiac dysrhythmias
Muscle twitching
Convulsions
Roving eye movements (cranial nerve dysfunction)

the potential for life-threatening systemic effects, mild analgesics, cool compresses, and in-hospital observation are all that are required for these patients.

Tick Bites. Tick bites seldom require emergency care. However, they are capable of causing human disease. They can transmit microorganisms or secrete toxins or venoms. In North America, hard ticks are the most familiar type, although soft ticks also are common to western states. Local reactions to tick bites vary from the formation of a small pruritic nodule to the development of extensive areas of ulceration. Some of the more important diseases for which ticks are vectors include Rocky Mountain spotted fever, Lyme disease, and tick paralysis.

- **Rocky Mountain spotted fever.** Rocky Mountain spotted fever is an infectious disease transmitted from rabbits and other small mammals to humans by the bites of the wood tick and dog tick. The disease occurs more commonly on the Atlantic seaboard and accounts for about 40 deaths in the United States each year.[13] Signs and symptoms usually develop within 1 week of the tick bite and include headache, high fever, and loss of appetite. These signs and symptoms may be followed by small pink spots that appear on the wrists and ankles. Eventually the rash spreads over the entire body, and the spots darken, enlarge, and become petechial. In mild cases, recovery occurs within 20 days. The mortality rate, if untreated, is between 8% and 25%.[32]
- **Lyme disease.** Lyme disease is the most commonly reported tick-borne disease in the United States. The disease is caused by the bite of an *Ixodes* tick known to infect deer and dogs. The course of the disease follows several stages. Initially a red dot appears at the site of the tick bite that gradually expands into a reddened rash. During this stage, fever, lethargy, muscle pain, and general malaise may develop. These signs and symptoms may be followed by a second stage that is manifested by cardiac abnormalities (including various atrioventricular blocks) and neurologic effects such as cranial nerve palsies. Still later, a third stage may develop, with arthritis as the primary symptom. Unless the disease is diagnosed and treated, symptoms may continue for several years, gradually declining in severity.
- **Tick paralysis.** Tick paralysis results from a prolonged bite by a female wood tick. The disease occurs sporadically during the spring and summer months. The paralysis is caused by a neurotoxin secreted from the salivary glands of the tick after the tick attaches to the host. At first the patient is restless and complains of paresthesia in the hands and feet. Over the next 48 hours, a flaccid paralysis may develop with loss of deep tendon reflexes. The paralysis begins at the feet and travels upward, affecting both sides of the body. In severe cases, death may result from respiratory paralysis. Removal of the tick usually results in rapid improvement and complete resolution within several days. If undiagnosed, the disease may be fatal, especially in young and older patients.

The principal treatment of tick bites is proper removal of the tick. The paramedic should grasp

CRITICAL THINKING

How can you distinguish tick paralysis from other conditions that cause progressive paralysis?

the tick as close to the skin surface as possible with forceps, tweezers, or protected fingers and pull it out with steady pressure. Care should be taken not to crush or squeeze the body of the tick, which can transmit disease from infective tick fluid. Other methods of tick removal, such as applying fingernail polish, isopropanol, or a hot match head, should be avoided. These traditional methods are ineffective and may induce the tick to salivate or regurgitate into the wound. After removal, the bite should be disinfected with soap and water and covered with a sterile or clean dressing.

Reptile Bites

The National Institute of Occupational Safety and Health (NIOSH) estimates 7,000 to 8,000 people are bitten by venomous snakes each year.[35] Of these envenomations, about five people die. This reflects the high morbidity and low mortality associated with snake venom poisoning. Of the 115 species of snakes in the United States, only 19 are venomous. The two main families of venomous snakes indigenous to the United States are pit vipers and coral snakes.

Pit Vipers

The pit viper family that inhabits the United States consists of rattlesnakes, the cottonmouth or water moccasin, the copperhead, the pigmy rattlesnake, and the Massasauga rattlesnake. The vast majority of snakebites in the United States are caused by the rattlesnake family. The identifying features of pit vipers are vertical elliptical pupils and a triangular head that is distinct from the rest of the body. The rattlesnake is characterized further by interlocking horny segments (rattles) formed on the tail that sometimes vibrate in direct relation to environmental temperatures (**FIGURE 33-5**).

The venom apparatus of pit vipers is connected to one or more elongated hollow fangs on each side of the head. The venom is designed to immobilize, kill, and digest prey. Depending on the species and the amount of venom injected, the venom may be capable of producing various toxic effects on blood and other tissues, including hemolysis, intravascular coagulation, convulsions, and acute renal failure (BOX 33-12). Bleeding caused by coagulation defects and massive swelling can lead to hypovolemic shock. On any given strike, the snake may release a quantity of venom varying from little or none to almost the entire contents of the glands.

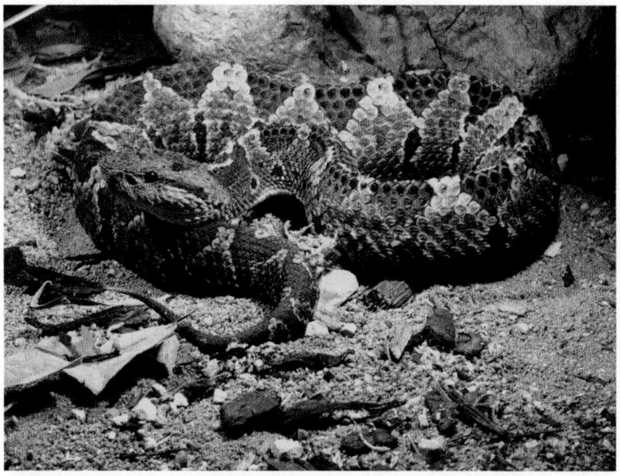

FIGURE 33-5 A Central American jumping pit viper, also called a ground rattlesnake.

BOX 33-12 Signs and Symptoms of Pit Viper Envenomation

Mild Envenomation

Presence of one or more fang marks
Local swelling and pain
Lack of systemic symptoms

Moderate Envenomation

Presence of one or more fang marks
Pain and edema beyond the site
Systemic signs and symptoms
Weakness
Diaphoresis
Nausea and vomiting
Paresthesias

Severe Envenomation

Presence of one or more fang marks
Massive edema
Subcutaneous ecchymosis
Severe systemic symptoms
Shock

Coral Snakes

Two members of the coral snake family are found in the United States: the Arizona coral snake and the Eastern coral snake. In contrast to the pit viper, the coral snake has round pupils and small, fixed fangs located near the anterior end of the maxilla. Most coral snakes have a three-color pattern with red, black, and yellow or white bands that completely encircle the body, along with a black snout (**FIGURE 33-6**). Many nonvenomous snakes in the United States mimic the appearance of the coral snake. The coral snake is identified by the sequence of colors: Red bands bordered by yellow indicate a venomous species. Thus, there is a mnemonic: "Red on yellow, kill a fellow; red on black, venom lack."

Most coral snakes are shy and docile and seldom bite unless threatened. The small mouth and fangs of the snake make it difficult to bite anything larger than a finger, toe, or fold of skin. The coral snake tends to hang on and chew rather than to strike and release like the pit viper. The venom of the coral snake mainly is neurotoxic, and the bite generally produces little or no pain and no necrosis or edema. Early signs and symptoms of a coral snakebite are slurred speech, dilated pupils, and dysphagia (usually delayed several hours after the bite). If untreated, the venom produces flaccid paralysis and death within 24 hours. Death is caused by respiratory failure, following nervous system dysfunction.

Management of Snake Envenomation

Venom, like any drug or toxin, has absorption, distribution, and elimination phases. Tissue damage increases as venom spreads into the lymphatics and blood. Thus, emergency care is directed at retarding the systemic spread of the venom. Prehospital management of snakebites includes the following:

1. Stay clear of the striking range of the snake (about the length of the snake) and move the patient to a safe area. If the snake is dead before EMS arrival, a digital picture of the snake should be taken to the ED with the patient. EMS personnel should make no attempt to capture or kill the snake; doing so may result in a paramedic being bitten. Identification of the snake is not necessary to manage the patient appropriately.
2. Provide adequate airway, ventilatory, and circulatory support to the patient as needed. Continually monitor vital signs and the ECG. Establish an IV line in an unaffected extremity with a volume-expanding fluid.
3. Medical direction may recommend that a bitten extremity be immobilized in a neutral position. Immobilization by splinting may delay systemic absorption and may diminish local tissue necrosis. Every effort should be made to keep the patient at rest. Application of ice or chemical cold packs, incision and suction devices, pressure bandages, and tourniquets should be avoided. Their use may further damage tissue.[35]
4. Prepare the patient for immediate transport to a proper medical facility.
5. In severe cases, administration of antivenin to neutralize the venom may be required. Antivenin is provided in the hospital after the patient has been tested for allergies to it.

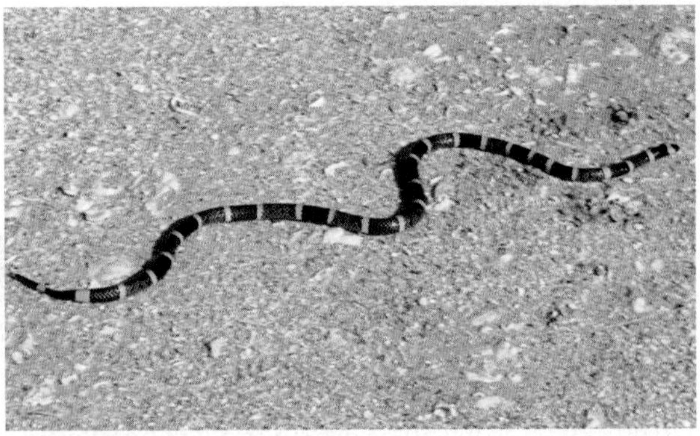

FIGURE 33-6 Coral snake.

Courtesy of Luther C. Goldman/U.S. Fish & Wildlife Service.

NOTE

If transport time is long or delayed, the leading edge of swelling on a bitten extremity should be marked with pen or marker every 15 minutes with a time notation. As an alternative, digital pictures taken every 15 minutes can indicate progression of swelling and can be added to the patient's medical record. Pain should be treated per protocol, avoiding nonsteroidal anti-inflammatory drugs (NSAIDs) due to potential coagulation effects.

CRITICAL THINKING

What strategies can you use to calm the emotional state of a patient who has sustained a snakebite?

Hazardous Aquatic Life

The marine animals most likely to be involved in human poisonings in US coastal waters are the coelenterates, echinoderms, and stingrays. The specialized venom apparatuses of these animals are used for defense and for capturing prey. In addition to venom produced by the animal, aquatic life may contain other poisonous substances as a result of toxic ingestions. Exposures to hazardous aquatic life result from recreational, industrial, scientific, and military oceanic activities.

After stabilizing the patient with adequate airway, ventilatory, and circulatory support, the two primary goals of managing all envenomations from hazardous aquatic life are preventing further venom discharge and relieving pain by neutralizing the effects of the venom.[33,36]

Coelenterates (Jellyfish, Sea Anemones, Fire Coral)

Coelenterates are a group of species that may be encountered in the ocean (**FIGURE 33-7**). Some of these species carry venomous stinging cells (**nematocysts**). The nematocyst is venom filled and contains a long, coiled, hollow, threadlike tube that serves as a tiny hypodermic needle. The severity of envenomation is related to the type and toxicity of the venom, the number of nematocysts discharged, and the physical condition of the person.

Jellyfish occur throughout the Atlantic and Pacific oceans. The Portuguese man-of-war is the largest jellyfish. The nematocyst-bearing tentacles of this jellyfish may be up to 100 feet (30 m) long, and a single envenomation may involve several hundred thousand nematocysts. A swimmer who comes in contact with these tentacles may suffer enough envenomation to produce systemic signs and symptoms. Nematocysts often remain embedded in the tissues of the envenomated person. Detached tentacle fragments can retain their potency for months.

Sea anemones are colorful bottom dwellers; they are sometimes found in tidal pools. They have a flowerlike appearance and possess slender projections that are used to sting and paralyze passing fish. These nematocyst-type projections are capable of producing mild to moderate pain in humans.

Fire corals are not true, stony corals, but rather ocean-bottom dwellers. They often are mistaken for seaweed because they commonly are attached to rocks, shells, and corals. These stinging corals may grow up to 7 feet (2 m) high and have a razor-sharp exoskeleton with thousands of protruding nematocyst-bearing tentacles.

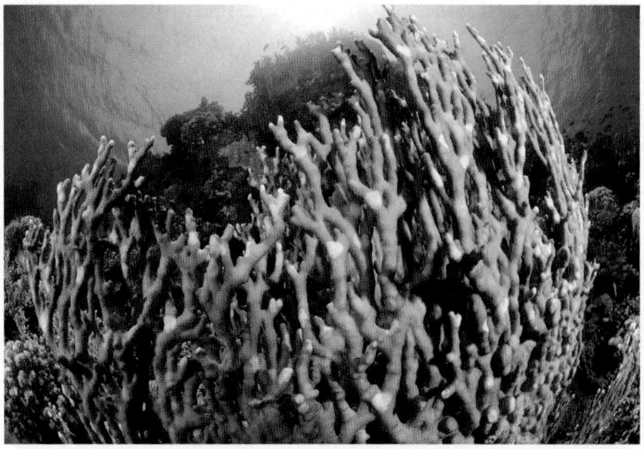

A

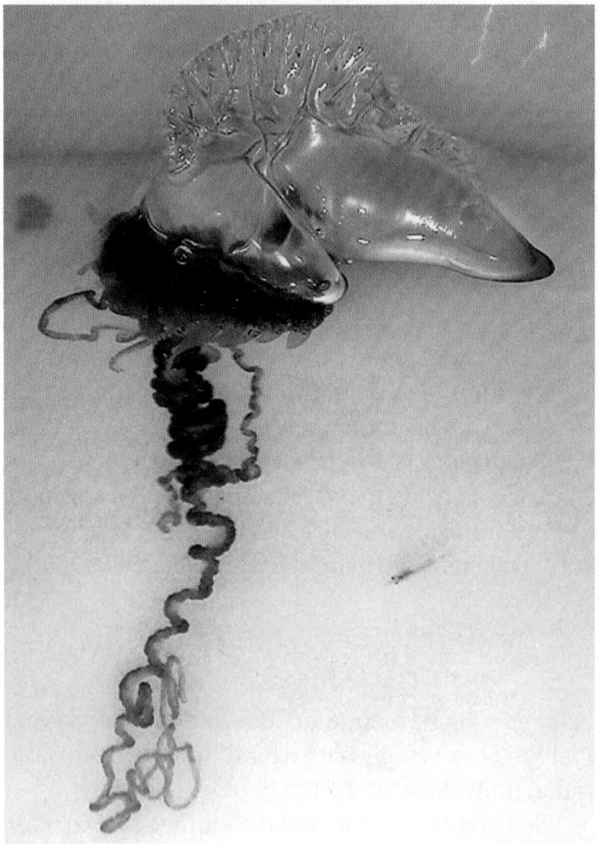

B

FIGURE 33-7 Coelenterates. **A.** Fire coral. **B.** Portuguese man-of-war.

A: © Borut Furlan/WaterFrame/Getty Images; B: Courtesy of NOAA.

Management. Coelenterate envenomation ranges in severity from irritant dermatitis to excruciating pain, respiratory depression, anaphylaxis, and life-threatening cardiovascular collapse. Envenomation most often is mild and usually is characterized by a stinging sensation, paresthesias, pruritus, and red-brown linear wheals or tentacle prints. If a potent venom or a large body surface area is involved, systemic symptoms may include nausea, vomiting, abdominal pain, headache, bronchospasm, pulmonary edema, hypotension, and respiratory arrest. Emergency care includes the following:

- Remove visible tentacle fragments with forceps. Avoid touching the tentacles.
- Immediately wash the stings with liberal amounts of vinegar (4% to 6% acetic acid solution) or a baking soda slurry for at least 30 seconds. Do not apply wet sand or freshwater; these substance usually cause the nematocysts to discharge their venom. Vinegar should not be used on stings from *Physalia* (Australian) jellyfish and sea nettles, because it may increase pain.[9]
- Instruct the patient to take a hot shower or immerse the affected body part in hot water when possible. The water should be as hot as can be tolerated without scalding, but no warmer than 113°F (45°C). The immersion should last for as long as pain persists. If hot water is not available, dry hot or cold packs may be helpful in decreasing pain.
- Administer analgesics as needed.
- Transport the patient for physician evaluation.

Echinoderms (Sea Urchins, Starfish, Sea Cucumbers)

Echinoderms are marine animals with a water-vascular system. They usually have a hard, spiny skeleton and radial body (**FIGURE 33-8**).

Sea urchins have a globular, dome-shaped body and are found on rocky bottoms or burrowed in sand or crevices. These animals have tiny spines, some of which are venomous. Some also have small pincerlike organs that are thought to discharge a poisonous substance. The spines are dangerous to handle and may break off easily in the flesh, lodging deeply and making removal difficult.

Some starfish are covered with thorny spines that secrete toxins. As the spine enters the skin, it carries venom into the wound, causing immediate pain,

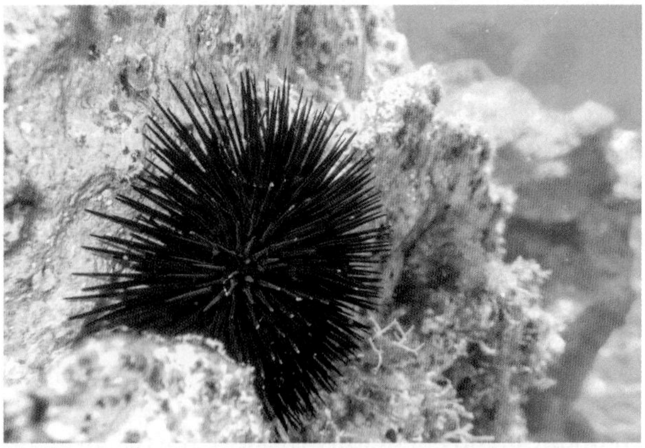

A

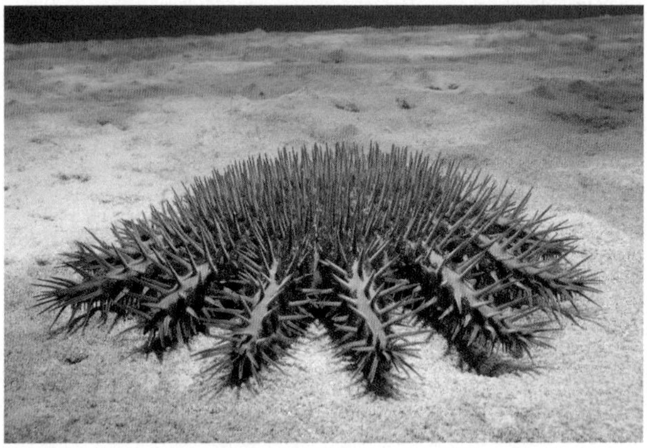

B

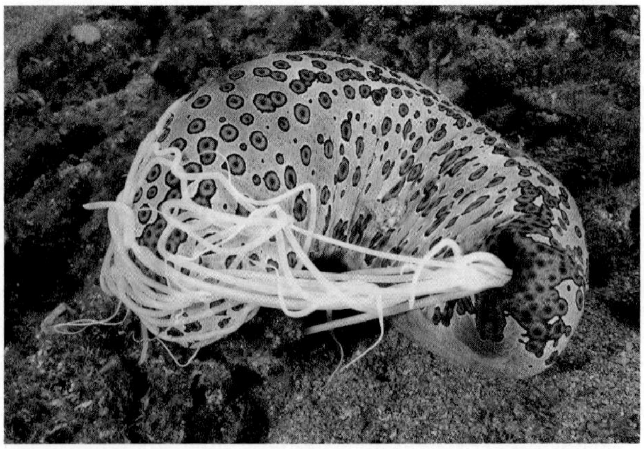

C

FIGURE 33-8 Echinoderms. **A.** Black sea urchin. **B.** Crown-of-thorns starfish. **C.** Sea cucumber.

copious bleeding, and mild edema. Multiple puncture wounds may result in acute systemic reactions.

Sea cucumbers are sausage-shaped animals found in shallow and deep water. They produce a liquid toxin in a tentacle-shaped organ. This organ can be projected and extended anally. Generally the liquid is secreted into the surrounding ocean. It usually produces only a minor dermatitis or conjunctivitis in swimmers and divers.

Management. Emergency management for echinoderm envenomation usually involves caring for puncture wounds caused by spines and inactivating the venom. The paramedic should remove embedded spines with forceps. Protective gloves should be worn to avoid self-contamination. Larger spines may require surgical removal by a physician.

Echinoderm toxins may cause immediate intense pain, swelling, redness, aching in the affected extremity, and nausea. Delayed toxic effects may include respiratory distress, paresthesia of the lips and face, and, in severe cases, respiratory paralysis and complete atonia. The paramedic must be prepared to deal with a variety of physical reactions.

Most marine venoms lose their toxicity when exposed to changes in temperature or humidity. The recommended management for stable patients is to immerse the affected area (usually the foot or hand) in hot water before and during transport. As a safety precaution, it generally is recommended that both hands or feet not be immersed at the same time. This precaution protects against thermal injury that may be unnoticed by the patient because of numbness or pain in the affected part.

Stingrays

Stingrays are responsible for about 1,800 injuries each year in the United States.[34] These marine animals vary in size from 2 inches (5 cm) to 14 feet (4 m). They often are found half-buried in mud or sand in shallow water (**FIGURE 33-9**). The venom organ of stingrays consists of two to four venomous barbs on the dorsum of a whiplike tail. Envenomation generally occurs from stepping on the sand-buried ray. In response, the ray's tail thrusts up and forward, driving the barb into the person's leg or foot. The defensive barb produces a large, severe laceration that may be more than 6 to 8 inches (15–20 cm) long. In addition to injecting venom into the wound, the entire barb tip of the venom apparatus sometimes is detached and embedded in the tissue.

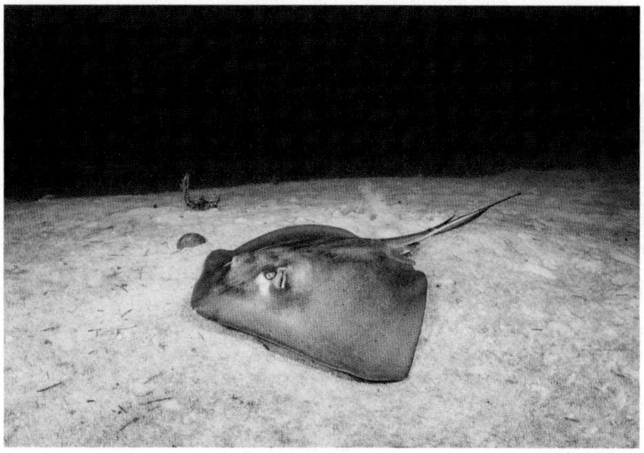

FIGURE 33-9 Stingray.

Stingray venom has local and systemic complications. Locally, the venom produces a traumatic injury that causes immediate, intense pain; edema; variable bleeding; and necrosis. Systemic manifestations include weakness, nausea, vomiting, diarrhea, vertigo, seizures, cardiac conduction abnormalities, paralysis, hypotension, and death.

Management. Prehospital care is directed to life support, alleviation of pain, inactivation of venom, and prevention of infection. The wound should be irrigated with normal saline or tap water. If the venom apparatus is visible, it should be carefully removed. The affected part should be immersed in hot (but not scalding) water and remain there until pain subsides or until the patient reaches the ED.[9] Analgesics may be needed to manage pain.

Poisoning by Absorption

Many poisons can be absorbed through the skin. Two compounds, organophosphates and carbamates, are responsible for a large number of skin-absorbed poisonings each year. Organophosphates and carbamates are commonly available for commercial and public use in the form of pet, home, and commercial insecticides. Because of the widespread availability of insecticides that contain organophosphate/carbamate compounds, paramedics must be aware of the nature of these chemicals, the necessary precautions for personal safety, and the immediate management that may be required before signs or symptoms of illness occur.

Organophosphates and carbamates are highly toxic. In addition, they are well absorbed by ingestion, inhalation, and dermal routes. Both classes have similar pharmacologic actions, inhibiting the effects of acetylcholinesterase, an enzyme that degrades acetylcholine at nerve terminals. To review, acetylcholine is a cholinergic neurotransmitter for preganglionic autonomic fibers, somatic nerves to skeletal muscle, and many synapses in the CNS. When acetylcholinesterase is inhibited, acetylcholine accumulates at the synapses, resulting in a cholinergic overdrive. The signs and symptoms resulting from cholinergic overdrive are seen in organophosphate and carbamate poisoning.

NOTE

The nerve agents sarin (GB), soman (GD), tabun (GA), cyclosarin (GF), and VX are chemical warfare agents. These agents produce signs and symptoms similar to, but more potent than, those of organophosphate pesticides. They may be inhaled or absorbed through skin or mucous membranes. Treatment for nerve agent toxicity is the same as for organophosphate poisoning (see Chapter 57, *Bioterrorism and Weapons of Mass Destruction*).

Signs and Symptoms

Early signs and symptoms of organophosphate or carbamate poisoning may be nonspecific, including headache, dizziness, weakness, and nausea. As overstimulation and disruption of transmission in the central and peripheral nervous systems occur, signs and symptoms begin to develop. These signs and symptoms result from a wide range of physiologic and metabolic derangements (BOX 33-13).

The rapidity and sequence in which these signs and symptoms develop depend on the particular compound and on the amount and route of exposure. The onset of symptoms is probably quickest after inhalation. Onset is slowest after a primary skin exposure and may be delayed for several hours. There are helpful mnemonics to recognize the signs of poisoning. One is SLUDGE. Another is DUMBBELLS—Diarrhea; Urination; Miosis (constriction of the pupils), muscle weakness; Bradycardia, bronchospasm, bronchorrhea (discharge of mucus from the lungs); Emesis; Lacrimation; Seizures, salivation, sweating. Rapidly changing pupils with miosis are common with vapor exposure of organophosphates. Muscle twitching (fasciculations) can follow rapidly. Individual muscle twitching can result from liquid contact and local skin absorption at the site.

BOX 33-13 Signs and Symptoms of Organophosphate or Carbamate Poisoning

Cardiovascular System
Bradycardia
Variable blood pressure (usually hypotensive)

Respiratory System
Bronchoconstriction
Dyspnea
Rhinorrhea
Wheezing

Gastrointestinal System
Blurred vision
Cramps
Defecation
Emesis
Increased bowel sounds

Central Nervous System
Anxiety
Coma
Dizziness
Respiratory depression
Seizures

Musculoskeletal System
Fasciculations
Flaccid paralysis

Skin
Diaphoresis

Other Signs and Symptoms
Lacrimation
Miosis
Rapidly changing pupil size
Salivation
Urination

CRITICAL THINKING

Consider a person who does not suspect poisoning. What condition might that person think he or she is suffering from at the beginning of this clinical presentation?

Management

Emergency care begins by following the guidelines for management of poisoned patients (see Box 33-2). Clothing is removed and the skin is washed with soap and water. Organophosphates and carbamates produce similar physiologic effects. However, carbamates have a shorter duration of action, and therefore their effects decrease more rapidly than do those of organophosphates.

Respiratory Support

Respiratory tract symptoms usually are first to appear after exposure to organophosphates or carbamates. In addition, respiratory paralysis may occur suddenly without warning. The need for advanced airway management and ventilatory support should be anticipated. Copious bronchial secretions may require suctioning. Bronchoconstriction also may necessitate positive pressure ventilation and positive end-expiratory pressure. Administer oxygen to maintain oxygen saturation, as measured by a pulse oximeter, of 94% to 98%.

Drug Administration

Drug therapy in organophosphate or carbamate poisoning is directed at blocking the effects of acetylcholine, separating cholinesterase from the chemical compound, and suppressing seizure activity if present. Atropine is the primary antidote for organophosphate, carbamate or nerve agent poisoning. Pralidoxime chloride is administered to reactivate acetylcholinesterase. It may be given concurrently with atropine by an auto-injector (DuoDote). Benzodiazepines (midazolam, lorazepam, or diazepam) are indicated to treat seizure activity.

> **NOTE**
> Drug therapy should be initiated only if the patient has two or more signs or symptoms of poisoning and/or respiratory distress is present. Drug therapy should be initiated only after consulting with medical direction or a poison control center.

Atropine reverses the muscarinic effects (bradycardia, bronchoconstriction, increased respiratory secretions, and miosis) of moderate to severe organophosphate or carbamate poisoning. The drug competitively antagonizes the actions of acetylcholine, resulting in a decrease in the hyperactivity of smooth muscles and glands. The drug is indicated to dry the patient's secretions. It also helps to decrease pulmonary resistance to ventilation. Patients poisoned with these substances often require the administration of large doses of atropine (see the Appendix, *Emergency Drug Index*). Atropine is the drug of choice for carbamate poisonings.[9] The dose range for a normal adult begins at 2 mg intramuscularly (IM) for mild exposures and can be doubled every 3 to 5 minutes by IV or intraosseous (IO) route as needed in severe exposures (frequent repeated doses of atropine are often needed). These doses may be administered by autoinjector. However, the combination autoinjector with pralidoxime (2-PAM) chloride should not be given past the recommended dose; this is the maximum dose unless otherwise specified by medical direction.

> **NOTE**
> As a rule, cholinergic poisoning causes the patient to be wet. This is manifested by profuse sweating, lacrimation, salivation, vomiting, diarrhea, and incontinence. Anticholinergic poisoning generally causes the patient to be dry. This is manifested by dry, flushed skin; elevated temperature; and urinary retention. Being cognizant of this wet versus dry symptomatology can be lifesaving for the poisoned patient. The wet-appearing patient will require atropine.

Pralidoxime is the treatment of choice for organophosphate poisoning after (or with) the administration of atropine. Pralidoxime is indicated for nearly all patients with significant exposures, particularly those with muscular twitching and weakness. Pralidoxime reactivates acetylcholinesterase. It should be administered as soon as possible after the exposure to be effective. The adult and pediatric doses for pralidoxime can be found in the Appendix, *Emergency Drug Index*.

Midazolam or diazepam are preferred if seizure activity is present because their onset of action is faster than that of lorazepam.[9] The need for seizure control may arise before decontamination is complete. In this case, the drugs can be administered by the IM route to control seizure activity (see the Appendix, *Emergency Drug Index*). As a safety precaution, IV therapy usually is not initiated until a patient is decontaminated. Because the onset of symptoms is rapid, the IM route of administration is preferred to avoid the delays associated with establishing IO or IV access. The paramedic should be alert to the risk for respiratory and CNS depression.

CRITICAL THINKING

Consider that you give midazolam or diazepam for seizures in this case. Will that eliminate the need for atropine?

ECG Monitoring

ECG monitoring may reveal a variety of abnormalities, including idioventricular rhythms, multifocal premature ventricular contractions, ventricular tachycardia, torsades de pointes, ventricular fibrillation, complete heart block, and asystole. These dysrhythmias usually occur in two phases. The first phase begins with a transient episode of intense sympathetic tone that results in sinus tachycardia. This phase is followed by a period of extreme parasympathetic tone that may manifest as sinus bradycardia, atrioventricular block, and ST segment and T-wave abnormalities.

Drugs of Abuse

The term **drug abuse** refers to the use of prescription drugs for nonprescribed purposes. It also refers to the use of drugs that have no prescribed medical use (BOX 33-14). Emergencies that result from drug abuse include adverse effects caused by the drug or impurities or contaminants mixed with the drug, life-threatening infections from IV or intradermal injection of drugs with unsterile equipment, injuries during intoxication, and drug dependence or withdrawal syndrome resulting from the habit-forming potential of many drugs (see Chapter 13, *Principles of Pharmacology and Emergency Medications*).

Because of the widespread use and misuse of drugs (BOX 33-15), the paramedic should maintain a high degree of suspicion and consider the possibility for a drug-related problem in any patient of any age who has seizures, behavioral changes, or decreased level of consciousness.

BOX 33-14 Drug Abuse Terminology

- **Physical dependence.** An adaptive physiologic state occurring after prolonged use of many drugs. Discontinuation causes withdrawal syndromes that are relieved by readministering the same drug or a pharmacologically related drug.
- **Psychological dependence.** Emotional reliance on a drug. Manifestations range from a mild desire for a drug to craving and drug-seeking behavior to repeated compulsive use of a drug for its subjectively satisfying or pleasurable effects.
- **Substance use disorder.** A diagnosis that is made when the recurrent use of alcohol and/or drugs causes clinical and functionally significant impairment, including health conditions, disability, or inability to fulfill responsibilities at work, school, or home. The diagnosis is based on evidence of impaired control, social impairment, risky use, and pharmacologic evidence. It is classified as mild, moderate, or severe based on the number of diagnostic criteria that are present and is usually referred to by the drug involved (eg, opioid use disorder or alcohol use disorder).
- **Tolerance.** A tendency to increase drug dosage to experience the same effect formerly produced by a smaller dose.
- **Withdrawal syndrome.** A predictable set of signs and symptoms that occurs after a decrease in the amount of the usual dose of a drug or its sudden cessation.

Modified from: DSM 5 Criteria for Substance Use Disorder. BupPractice.com website. https://www.buppractice.com/node/12351. Updated February 23, 2018. Accessed March 1, 2018.

CRITICAL THINKING

Why might a patient (or his or her friends) delay calling for help in a situation involving a drug overdose?

EMS personnel often encounter people who are suffering from the toxic effects of drugs. Toxicity may be the result of an overdose, a potential suicide attempt, polydrug administration, or an accident (unintentional ingestion, miscalculation, changes in drug strength). BOX 33-16 lists the drugs discussed in this chapter.

Common drugs of abuse, along with their names and uses, vary widely in different geographic areas. Also, the drugs of abuse often change over time. **TABLE 33-5** is a partial list of common drugs of abuse, their street names, and miscellaneous terminology relating to drug use.

BOX 33-15 Substance Use in the United States

- Drug overdose deaths tripled from 1999 to 2015.
- In 2016, health care professionals wrote 66.5 opioid and 25.2 sedative prescriptions for every 100 Americans.
- In 2015, about 47.7 million Americans aged 12 years or older used illegal drugs or misused prescription drugs.
- There were about 418,000 ED visits for nonfatal unintentional drug toxicity in 2014. Of those, opioids accounted for 22%, cocaine for about 2%, and methamphetamines for about 3%.

Modified from: Centers for Disease Control and Prevention, National Center for Injury Prevention and Control. *Annual Surveillance Report of Drug-Related Risks and Outcomes: United States, 2017*. Centers for Disease Control and Prevention website. https://www.cdc.gov/drugoverdose/pdf/pubs/2017-cdc-drug-surveillance-report.pdf. Published August 31, 2017. Accessed March 1, 2018.

BOX 33-16 Common Agents Involved in Poisoning

Acetaminophen
Cardiac medications
Drugs abused for sexual purposes/sexual gratification
Hallucinogens
Lithium
Metals (iron, lead, and mercury)
Monoamine oxidase (MAO) inhibitors
Nonprescription pain medicines
Opioids
PCP
Salicylates
Sedatives-hypnotics
Stimulants
Tricyclic antidepressants

Modified from: Common and dangerous poisons. National Capital Poison Center website. https://www.poison.org/common-and-dangerous-poisons. Accessed March 1, 2018.

TABLE 33-5 Commonly Abused Drugs and Their Street Names[a]

Substances: Category and Name	Examples of Commercial and Street Names	DEA Schedule[b]; Method of Use[c]	Intoxication Effects and Potential Health Consequences
Tobacco			
Nicotine	Found in cigarettes, cigars, bidis, and smokeless tobacco (snuff, spit tobacco, chew, e-cigarettes), drug patches	Not scheduled; smoked, snorted, chewed	Increased blood pressure and heart rate Chronic lung disease; cardiovascular disease; stroke; cancers of mouth, pharynx, larynx, esophagus, stomach, pancreas, cervix, kidney, bladder, and acute myeloid leukemia; adverse pregnancy outcomes; addiction
Alcohol			
Alcohol (ethyl alcohol)	Found in liquor, beer, and wine	Not scheduled; swallowed	In low doses, euphoria, mild stimulation, relaxation, lowered inhibitions; in higher doses, drowsiness, slurred speech, nausea, emotional volatility, loss of coordination, visual distortions, impaired memory, sexual dysfunction, loss of consciousness

(continued)

TABLE 33-5 Commonly Abused Drugs and Their Street Names[a] *(continued)*

Substances: Category and Name	Examples of Commercial and Street Names	DEA Schedule[b]; How Administered[c]	Intoxication Effects and Potential Health Consequences
			Increased risk of injuries, violence, fetal damage (in pregnant women); depression; neurologic deficits; hypertension; liver and heart disease; addiction; fatal overdose
Cannabinoids			
Hashish	Boom, gangster, hash, hemp	I; swallowed, smoked	Euphoria; relaxation; slowed reaction time; distorted sensory perception; impaired balance and coordination; increased heart rate and appetite; impaired learning, memory; anxiety; panic attacks; psychosis Cough, frequent respiratory tract infections; possible mental health decline; addiction
Marijuana	Blunt, bud, ganja, grass, joint, Mary Jane, pot, reefer, green, smoke, sinsemilla, skunk, weed	I; swallowed, smoked	
Opioids			
Heroin Fentanyl Carfentanil Codeine	Diacetylmorphine: Smack, horse, brown sugar, dope, H, junk, skag, skunk, white stuff, China white; Syrup, Purple Drank, Sizzurp ,or Lean (codeine with promethazine cough syrup mixed with soda)	I; injected, smoked, snorted	Euphoria; drowsiness; impaired coordination; dizziness; confusion; nausea; sedation; feeling of heaviness in body; slowed or arrested breathing Constipation; endocarditis; hepatitis; HIV; addiction; fatal overdose
Opium	Laudanum, paregoric: Buddha, Chillum, Chinese molasses, gee, Ze	II, III, V; swallowed, smoked	
Stimulants			
Cocaine	Cocaine hydrochloride: blow, bump, C, candy, Charlie, coke, crack, flake, rock, snow, toot	II; snorted, smoked, injected	Increased heart rate, blood pressure, body temperature, metabolism; feelings of exhilaration; increased energy, mental alertness; tremors; reduced appetite; irritability; anxiety; panic; paranoia; violent behavior; psychosis Weight loss, insomnia; cardiac or cardiovascular complications; stroke; seizures; addiction Also, for cocaine—nasal damage from snorting Also, for methamphetamine—severe dental problems
Amphetamine (Adderall, Dexedrine) Methylphenidate (Ritalin, Concerta)	Biphetamine, Dexedrine: bennies, black beauties, crosses, hearts, LA turnaround, speed, truck drivers, uppers	II; swallowed, snorted, smoked, injected	
Methamphetamine	Desoxyn: meth, ice, crank, chalk, crystal, fire, glass, go fast, speed	II; swallowed, snorted, smoked, injected	

TABLE 33-5 Commonly Abused Drugs and Their Street Names[a] *(continued)*			
Substances: Category and Name	**Examples of Commercial and Street Names**	**DEA Schedule[b]; How Administered[c]**	**Intoxication Effects and Potential Health Consequences**
Club Drugs			
MDMA	Ecstasy, Adam, clarity, Eve, lover's speed, peace, uppers, Molly	I; swallowed, snorted, injected	**MDMA** Mild hallucinogenic effects; increased tactile sensitivity; empathic feelings; lowered inhibition; anxiety; chills; sweating; teeth clenching; muscle cramping Sleep disturbances; depression; impaired memory; hyperthermia; addiction **Flunitrazepam** Sedation; muscle relaxation; confusion; memory loss; dizziness; impaired coordination Addiction **GHB** Drowsiness; nausea; headache; disorientation; loss of coordination; memory loss Unconsciousness; seizures; coma
Flunitrazepam[d]	Rohypnol: forget-me pill, Mexican Valium, R2, roach, Roche, roofies, roofinol, rope, rophies	IV; swallowed, snorted	
GHB[d]	G, Georgia home boy, grievous bodily harm, liquid Ecstasy, soap, scoop, goop, liquid X	I; swallowed	
Dissociative Drugs			
Ketamine	Ketalar SV: cat Valium, K, Special K, vitamin K	III; injected, snorted, smoked	Feelings of being separate from one's body and environment; impaired motor function Anxiety; tremors; numbness; memory loss; nausea Also, for ketamine—analgesia; impaired memory; delirium; respiratory depression and arrest; death Also, for PCP and analogs—analgesia; psychosis; aggression; violence; slurred speech; loss of coordination; hallucinations Also, for DXM—euphoria; slurred speech; confusion; dizziness; distorted visual perceptions
PCP and analogs	Angel dust, boat, hog, love boat, peace pill	I, II; swallowed, smoked, injected	
Salvia divinorum	Salvia, Shepherdess Herb, Maria Pastora, magic mint, Sally-D	Not scheduled; chewed, swallowed, smoked	
DXM	Found in some cough and cold medications: Robotripping, robo, triple C	Not scheduled; swallowed	
Hallucinogens			
LSD	Acid, blotted, cubes, microdot, yellow sunshine, blue heaven, windowpane	I; swallowed, absorbed through mouth tissues	Altered states of perception and feeling; hallucinations; nausea Also, LSD and mescaline—increased body temperature, heart rate, blood pressure; loss of appetite; sweating;
Mescaline	Buttons, cactus, mesc, peyote	I; swallowed, smoked	

(continued)

TABLE 33-5 Commonly Abused Drugs and Their Street Names[a] *(continued)*

Substances: Category and Name	Examples of Commercial and Street Names	DEA Schedule[b]; How Administered[c]	Intoxication Effects and Potential Health Consequences
Psilocybin	Magic mushrooms, purple passion, shrooms, little smoke	I; swallowed	sleeplessness; numbness, dizziness, weakness, tremors; impulsive behavior; rapid shifts in emotion Also, for LSD—flashbacks, hallucinogen persisting perception disorder Also for psilocybin—nervousness; paranoia; panic
Other Compounds			
Anabolic steroids	Anadrol, Oxandrin, Durabolin, Depo-Testosterone, Equipoise: roids, juice, gym candy, pumpers	III; injected, swallowed, applied to skin	No intoxication effects Hypertension; blood clotting and cholesterol changes; liver cysts; hostility and aggression; acne; in adolescents—premature cessation of growth; in males—prostate cancer, reduced sperm production, shrunken testicles, breast enlargement; in females—menstrual irregularities, development of beard and other masculine characteristics
Inhalants	Solvents (paint thinners, gasoline, glues); gases (butane, propane, aerosol propellants, nitrous oxide); nitrites (isoamyl, isobutyl, cyclohexyl): laughing gas, poppers, snappers, whippets	Not scheduled; inhaled through nose or mouth	(varies by chemical) Stimulation; loss of inhibition Headache; nausea or vomiting; slurred speech; loss of motor coordination; wheezing Cramps; muscle weakness; depression; memory impairment; damage to cardiovascular and nervous systems; unconsciousness; sudden death

[a]For more information on prescription medications, visit the websites listed as sources in this table.

[b]Schedule I and II drugs have a high potential for abuse. They require greater storage security and have a quota on manufacturing, among other restrictions. Schedule I drugs are available for research purposes; most have no approved medical use. Schedule II drugs are available by prescription only (unrefillable) and require a form for ordering. Schedule III and IV drugs are available by prescription, may have five refills in 6 months, and may be ordered verbally. Some Schedule V drugs are available over the counter.

[c]Some of the health risks are directly related to the route of drug administration. For example, injection drug use can increase the risk of infection through needle contamination with staphylococci, HIV, hepatitis, and other organisms.

[d]Associated with sexual assaults.

Abbreviations: DEA, Drug Enforcement Administration; DXM, dextromethorphan; GHB, gamma-hydroxybutyrate; HIV, human immunodeficiency virus; LSD, lysergic acid diethylamide; MDMA, methylenedioxymethamphetamine; PCP, phencyclidine

Modified from: Commonly abused drugs charts. National Institute on Drug Abuse website. www.nida.nih.gov/DrugPages/PrescripDrugsChart.html. Updated January 2018. Accessed March 1, 2018; Commonly abused drugs charts. National Institute on Drug Abuse website. https://www.drugabuse.gov/sites/default/files/cadchart.pdf. Updated March 2011. Accessed March 1, 2018.

DID YOU KNOW?

Dextromethorphan (DXM) is an ingredient found in more than 120 over-the-counter cough medicines and cold remedies, such as Robitussin. When consumed in excessive doses, the drug can cause euphoria and dysphoria. It also may cause cardiac irregularities, seizure, loss of consciousness, and brain damage. Each year there are approximately 6,000 ED visits in the United States from the abuse of cough medicines. Paramedics should consider the possibility of DXM abuse in any patient who appears to be high.

Modified from: Linn KA, Long MT, Pagel PS. "Robo-tripping": dextromethorphan abuse and its anesthetic implications. *Anesth Pain Med.* 2014;4(5): e20990; and Dextromethorphan: what's the problem? National Capital Poison Center website. https://www.poison.org/articles/2015-sep/dextromethorphan. Accessed March 1, 2018.

Management Principles

Paramedics should follow the guidelines for management of poisoned patients (see Box 33-2) when caring for patients who have abused drugs or overdosed. In addition to following those guidelines, paramedics need to do the following:

1. Obtain any significant medical or psychiatric history.
2. Recognize that IV drug users are at high risk of harboring infectious disease. The nasal administration of naloxone should be considered if opiate toxicity is suspected.
3. Administer activated charcoal (per protocol) for orally administered drugs taken within the previous hour when the patient is alert and able to swallow.

When examining any patient suspected of abusing drugs, the paramedic should always look for track marks, which may be in the antecubital space, under the tongue, or on the top of the foot. The possibility of body packing (concealing packets of drugs in body cavities of the stomach, rectum, and vagina) and body stuffing (swallowing drugs to avoid arrest) should be considered when a person who abuses drugs appears ill for no apparent reason.

CRITICAL THINKING

For what illnesses is the patient who uses IV narcotics at risk?

Opioid Overdose

Heroin overdose death rates have more than quadrupled since 2010.[37] Pure heroin is a bitter-tasting white powder that usually is adulterated or cut for street distribution. A typical bag is the single-dose unit of heroin and may weigh 100 mg. On average, heroin is only 20% to 30% pure and often is mixed with other drugs such as fentanyl. Other opioid drugs include morphine, hydromorphone, codeine, oxycodone, propoxyphene, hydrocodone, and designer opioids that have been chemically modified such as alpha-methylfentanyl (China white), carfentanil, and U-4770. Patients may also overdose on methadone and buprenorphine (Suboxone). Both of these drugs are used to medically assist patients in recovery from opiate substance use disorder.

NOTE

Vicodin (hydrocodone) is one of the most commonly prescribed and most commonly abused pain medications today. Vicodin and its related medications, Lorcet, Lortab, Percodan, and OxyContin, are opioid-based drugs. Vicodin is a derivative of opium, which is also used to manufacture heroin. Vicodin successfully diminishes pain, but it is highly addictive. The drug can be taken orally in pill form, chewed, or crushed and sniffed like cocaine. Physical effects from misusing these drugs include dizziness, blurred vision, constipation, fluctuations in heart rate, hallucinations, nausea, vomiting, sedation, and respiratory depression. Signs and symptoms of withdrawal from these drugs are similar to those of other opioids. Overdose is not uncommon, and higher doses of naloxone may be required to manage these patients.

Depending on the preparation, these drugs may be taken orally, injected intradermally (skin popping) or intravenously (mainlining), taken intranasally (snorted), or smoked. All opioids are CNS depressants and can cause life-threatening respiratory depression. In severe intoxication, hypotension, profound shock, and pulmonary edema may be present. Signs and symptoms of narcotic/opioid overdose include the following:

- Euphoria
- Arousable somnolence (nodding)
- Nausea
- Pinpoint pupils (except under hypoxic conditions or in combination with other types of drugs)
- Slow and shallow respirations
- Coma
- Seizures

SHOW ME THE EVIDENCE

Researchers reviewed records retrospectively to determine the frequency of repeat naloxone dosing in suspected narcotic overdose. They reviewed records of 2,166 adult patients who had an initial dose of intranasal (IN) naloxone administration and were then cared for by paramedics to determine if an additional dose of naloxone was needed. No patients whose Glasgow Coma Scale score was 15 needed another dose. One hundred ninety-five (9%) received two doses, and 53 (2%) received three doses of naloxone. The authors concluded that IN naloxone is effective to reverse opioid toxicity.

Modified from: Klebacher R, Harris MI, Ariyaprakai N. Incidence of naloxone redosing in the age of the new opioid epidemic. *Prehosp Emerg Care.* 2017;21(6):682-687.

Scene Safety

In 2017, NIOSH issued guidelines for appropriate response to fentanyl overdose in response to fears that first responders could be injured and suffer respiratory depression and other effects of overdose if exposed to fentanyl and carfentanil during patient care.[38] The NIOSH report emphasized that brief skin contact is not likely to lead to overdose unless a very large exposure remains on the skin for an extended time. NIOSH recommends that, when responding to a scene suspected to involve fentanyl, responders observe the following precautions:

- Do not eat, drink, smoke, or use the bathroom in the area where the drug is present.
- Do not touch the eyes, mouth, or nose after contact with surfaces possibly contaminated with fentanyl.
- Never handle fentanyl or its analogs unnecessarily or without appropriate PPE.
- Avoid procedures that might aerosolize fentanyl powder. If aerosolization is suspected, higher levels of PPE, including respiratory protection, is needed.
- Wash hands with soap and water after leaving the scene; do not use hand sanitizers or bleach solutions to clean skin contaminated with fentanyl.

If a first responder has a suspected exposure, the paramedic should observe for standard signs and symptoms of opiate overdose: miosis, decreased level of consciousness, and respiratory depression. If present, the paramedic should follow standard treatment for opiate overdose.

The levels of risk for exposure are as follows:

- **Minimal.** Fentanyl may be present but products are not visible on the scene.
- **Moderate.** Small amounts of fentanyl are visible on the scene.
- **High.** Liquid fentanyl or large amounts of fentanyl products are visible (production or distribution locations) on the scene.

For EMS response where there is minimal risk, only nitrile gloves are recommended for PPE. In a moderate-risk situation, in addition to gloves, EMS responders are advised to have safety goggles or glasses, wrist and arm protection (can be uniform with sleeves, sleeve covers, gowns, or coveralls), and respiratory protection that should be either a disposable N100, R100, or P100 FFR (filtered face-piece respirator) mask. NIOSH recommends that EMS personnel not enter high-risk exposure settings.[38]

Skin contact with fentanyl requires immediate decontamination using soap and water. Hand sanitizers or bleach should not be used to clean the skin. Contaminated clothing should be removed as soon as possible and washed, using care not to disturb powder residue. EMS workers with significant contact to fentanyl should shower immediately.

Antidote Therapy

Naloxone is a pure opioid antagonist effective for virtually all opioid and opioidlike substances. The drug reverses the three major symptoms of opioid overdose: respiratory depression, coma, and miosis. Its use should be considered when opioid intoxication is confirmed or suspected.[37] Naloxone is given by the IV, IM, IN, or endotracheal tube route. The paramedic should determine whether naloxone has been given prior to arrival. Many first responders, patients, and their families have IN naloxone. The EMS crew should be prepared to restrain the patient. The patient's behavior may be unpredictable when the effects of the drug are reversed and the patient experiences withdrawal symptoms. In a small number of cases, the patient may demonstrate aggressive behavior after treatment. Medical direction may recommend that the naloxone be given in an amount that is just enough to restore airway reflexes and adequate breathing, without fully awakening the patient. The patient should be ventilated with a bag-mask device before naloxone administration. If the patient does not respond to treatment with naloxone, intubation should be considered. (Note: In the absence of respiratory depression, the use of naloxone is controversial; seizure activity is a possible side effect of the drug.)

NOTE

Two other pure opioid antagonists are available but rarely used in the prehospital setting. Naltrexone is an oral medication used in long-term programs for opioid addiction. Nalmefene appears to be as effective as naloxone in acute opioid intoxications. Moreover, nalmefene has a longer duration of action (4 to 8 hours) than naloxone has.

Some opioids (eg, methadone) have a prolonged duration of action up to 4 hours, which is longer than naloxone's duration. Thus, the patient must be monitored closely during antidote therapy. Repeated doses of naloxone may be needed as well. In communities where abuse of naloxone-resistant opioids or the use of synthetic opioids is common, larger initial doses of naloxone may be needed. The desired signs of reversal of opioid intoxication are adequate airway reflexes and ventilations, not complete arousal.

Naloxone can cause a withdrawal syndrome in opioid-dependent patients. Paramedics should slowly administer a smaller dose of the drug for these patients. Withdrawal usually can be managed by symptomatic and supportive care. BOX 33-17 lists signs and symptoms of opioid withdrawal.

Some opioids have other toxic effects that can cause life threats. Methadone can prolong the QT interval, placing the patient at risk for polymorphic ventricular tachycardia. Tramadol (Ultram) may cause seizures.[9]

Many prescribed opioids are combination drugs and may contain aspirin, acetaminophen, or other medications. It is important that the medication containers be transported so all possible toxicities can be considered.

Patients who have been resuscitated from opiate overdose often decline transport to the hospital. The EMS system should have a structured protocol for this refusal, which typically should include the following:

- Requirements to ensure the patient has decision-making capacity
- Instructions to a family or friend to remain with the patient and call 9-1-1 should symptoms reappear
- Administration of a dose of IM naloxone

BOX 33-17 Signs and Symptoms of Opioid Withdrawal

Abdominal cramps
Anorexia
Cold sweats or chills
Diaphoresis
Diarrhea
Fever
General malaise
Gooseflesh (cutis anserina)
Insomnia
Irritability
Nausea and vomiting
Pulmonary edema
Severe agitation
Tachycardia
Tremors
Ventricular dysrhythmias

High-Potency Opioids

Compared to heroin and other opioids, some opioids are much stronger and therefore more likely to cause life-threatening respiratory depression. The patient may believe that his or her injected drug was heroin when in fact it was either a stronger synthetic opioid or mixed with one.

Fentanyl is a synthetic opioid increasingly seen in overdose and is 50 to 100 times more potent than morphine. Prescribed forms are available in oral liquids or tablets or transdermal patches. Patients addicted to opioids may repurpose the legal forms to inject them. If a transdermal patch is present, it should be removed with a gloved hand. Overdose from fentanyl can cause chest wall rigidity. Positive end-expiratory pressure may need to be added to adequately ventilate these patients.[9]

Other synthetic opioids include carfentanil and W-18. These drugs are 10,000 times stronger than morphine is. Their formulation may not be detected on a standard drug test.

Pediatric Considerations

Adolescent and teenage children represent a significant number of overdoses related to opioids. From 1997 to 2012, the incidence of hospitalization for opioid toxicity in children 1 to 19 years increased.[39] In children aged 15 to 19 years, admissions caused by heroin and methadone also increased during that time frame.

Due to the rise in opioid overdoses, a significant number of younger pediatric patients are exposed to these drugs in their homes and may have an unintended ingestion. Intoxication and deaths have been reported in children younger than 6 years after ingesting methadone, buprenorphine, or fentanyl patches.[40] Consider the possibility of opioid overdose in children. The same constellation of signs and symptoms will be present: miosis, respiratory depression, and unresponsiveness.

If there is a child present in the home when an adult overdoses on an opioid, the paramedic must consider the potential for risk of harm. Often a state's mandatory reporter laws require that the paramedic report the incident to state child abuse authorities. Malicious use of pharmaceuticals is another type of child abuse that must be reported. It occurs when an adult administers medications or other substances to a child. In a review of the US National Poison System data, 1,439 cases were found. Of these, one-half of exposures and 90% of deaths involved sedating agents such as antihistamines, opioids, or benzodiazepines.[41]

Sedative-Hypnotic Overdose

Sedative-hypnotic agents include benzodiazepines and barbiturates and are usually taken orally, although they may be diluted and injected intravenously. Taking these drugs with alcohol greatly increases their effects. Sedative-hypnotic drugs commonly are known as downers.

Benzodiazepines are among the best-known and most widely prescribed drugs used to control symptoms of anxiety, stress, and insomnia. These drugs sometimes are used to manage alcohol withdrawal and to control seizure disorders. They promote sleep and relieve anxiety by depressing brain function. Often they are abused for their sedative effects. Individually, these drugs are somewhat nontoxic. They may accentuate the effects of other sedative-hypnotic agents. Common benzodiazepines are diazepam (Valium), alprazolam (Xanax), and lorazepam (Ativan).

Barbiturates are general CNS depressants that inhibit impulse conduction in the brainstem. These drugs once were widely used to treat anxiety and insomnia. Their addictive properties, lower therapeutic index, and potential for abuse have led to their replacement by benzodiazepines and other nonbarbiturate drugs. Barbiturates that commonly are abused include phenobarbital, amobarbital, and secobarbital.

Signs and symptoms of sedative-hypnotic overdose chiefly are related to the central nervous and cardiovascular systems. Adverse effects include excessive drowsiness, staggering gait, and, in some cases, paradoxical excitability. In cases of severe toxicity, the patient may become comatose, with respiratory depression, hypotension, and shock. The pupils may be constricted, but more often, they become fixed and dilated even in the absence of significant brain damage. Airway control and ventilatory management are the most important actions in managing significant sedative-hypnotic overdose. Flumazenil is a benzodiazepine antagonist that can be used to reverse the effects of benzodiazepines.[37] The drug, however, can produce seizure activity, dysrhythmias, and hypotension.[37] Flumazenil is contraindicated in patients who are prone to seizures and in those with tricyclic antidepressant overdose. It is generally used only to reverse benzodiazepine effects after procedural sedation.

Stimulant Overdose

Commonly abused stimulant drugs are those of the sympathomimetic family (eg, amphetamine sulfate, dextroamphetamine, cocaine, methamphetamine, PCP, khat, and synthetic cathinones [bath salts]) (BOX 33-18). Bupropion (Wellbutrin) is structurally similar to amphetamine and is abused by snorting or injection. Seizures are very common after use and can appear suddenly without evidence of other toxic effects.

Sympathomimetic drugs often are used to produce general mood elevation, improve task performance, suppress appetite, and prevent sleepiness. Structurally, the amphetamines are similar to the catecholamines epinephrine and norepinephrine, yet they differ in their more pronounced effects on the CNS. Adverse effects include tachycardia, hypertension, tachypnea, agitation, dilated pupils, tremors, and disorganized behavior. In severe intoxication, the patient may exhibit psychosis and paranoia and may experience hallucinations. Sudden withdrawal or cessation of amphetamine use may result in a crash stage. In this stage the patient becomes depressed, suicidal, incoherent, or nearly comatose. As a rule, these drugs are taken orally. They also may be smoked or injected

BOX 33-18 Methamphetamine

Methamphetamine is a synthetically manufactured CNS stimulant. It is legally manufactured for medicinal purposes (eg, Methedrine, Desoxyn), yet illicit production of methamphetamine as a street drug in the United States continues. Common names for methamphetamine include meth, speed, crank, crystal, water, or ice.

Illegal methamphetamine can be produced inexpensively in clandestine meth labs with common chemical methods (hydriodic acid, phenyl-2-propane, sodium ammonia, thionyl chloride). The drug then can be smoked, injected, snorted, or taken orally. Once methamphetamine enters the body, it can produce skeletal muscle tremors, sleeplessness, and euphoria that can last up to 10 days. During these drug-induced sleepless binges, users may become hostile and paranoid. This effect is followed by a crash (an emotionally depressed state) that can last for several days.

In addition to ensuring personal safety when responding to these patients, the paramedic crew should be keenly aware of potential hazards associated with clandestine labs. These hazards include the production of highly explosive toxic gases (eg, phosphine) that can be absorbed readily through the skin in quantities that can be fatal, the presence of an oxygen-depleted environment, the use of toxic solvents that can lead to lab explosions, and exposure to other dangerous chemicals. Any time a meth lab is suspected, the EMS crew should withdraw. Patients and bystanders should be evacuated. Law enforcement and specialized hazardous materials personnel should be summoned to the scene. Drug-making paraphernalia that should alert the paramedic to the presence of a meth lab include the following:

- Unusual, strong odors like cat urine, ether, ammonia, acetone, or other chemicals
- Coffee filters containing a white pasty substance, a dark red paste, or small amounts of shiny white crystals
- Glass cookware or stove pans containing a powdery residue
- Various measuring and funnel devices
- Blacked-out windows
- Amber stains on walls, furniture, and counters
- Open windows vented with fans during the winter
- Excessive trash, including large amounts of items such as antifreeze containers, lantern fuel cans, engine starting fluid cans (including products such as HEET), lithium batteries and empty battery packages, wrappers, red chemically stained coffee filters, drain cleaner, and duct tape
- Unusual amounts of clear glass containers

Modified from: Dangers of meth labs. US Forest Service website. https://www.fs.fed.us/lei/dangers-meth-labs.php. Accessed March 1, 2018.

for a more rapid onset of action. Amphetamines commonly are known as speed or uppers.

In addition to the primary assessment, the temperature should be measured to assess for hyperthermia. Determine whether the patient has chest pain. Continuous cardiac monitoring is indicated, and a 12-lead ECG should be obtained when possible. Paramedics should assess blood glucose and evaluate for trauma or self-inflicted injury. They should ask law enforcement to check the patient for weapons prior to transport.[9]

Cocaine

Cocaine is a popular illegal drug in the United States. Cocaine is a fine, white crystalline powder. Like heroin, street forms of cocaine usually are adulterated. They vary in purity from 25% to 90%; doses vary from near 0 to 200 mg. This form of cocaine generally is taken intranasally by snorting a line containing 10 to 35 mg of the drug (depending on purity). After absorption through the mucous membranes, the effects of the drug begin within minutes. Peak effects occur 15 to 60 minutes after use, with a half-life of 1 to 6 hours.[41] Cocaine also is used by the subcutaneous, IM, and IV routes; the IV route provides immediate absorption and intense stimulation. Taken IV, the peak occurs within 5 minutes and with a half-life of about 50 minutes. Speed-balling refers to an injection of a combination of cocaine and heroin.

Freebase or crack cocaine is a more potent formulation of the drug. Crack is prepared by mixing powdered street cocaine with an alkaline solution and then adding a solvent such as ether. The combination separates into two layers. The top layer contains the dissolved cocaine. Evaporation of the solvent results in pure cocaine crystals, which are smoked and absorbed via the pulmonary route. Cocaine in this form is called rock or crack because of the popping sound produced when the crystals are heated. Freebase cocaine generally is combined with marijuana or tobacco and is smoked in a pipe or a cigarette. The reactions are similar to those experienced in IV use, with equal intensity and effects.

Cocaine is a major CNS stimulant that causes profound sympathetic discharge. The increased levels of circulating catecholamines result in excitement, euphoria, talkativeness, and agitation. The effects of the drug can cause significant cardiovascular and neurologic complications, such as cardiac dysrhythmias, myocardial infarction, seizures, intracranial hemorrhage, hyperthermia, and psychiatric disturbances. Cocaine is a sodium channel blocker and may cause conduction abnormalities and a widened QRS. Cocaine overdose can occur with any form of the drug and any route of administration. The adult fatal dose is thought to be about 1,200 mg (1.2 g), but fatalities from cocaine-induced cardiac dysrhythmias have been reported with single doses of as little as 25 to 30 mg.[42]

Prehospital management of the cocaine-intoxicated patient may be difficult. Cocaine toxicity may range from minor symptoms to life-threatening overdose. Emergency care may require a full spectrum of basic and advanced life support measures, including aggressive airway management, ventilatory and circulatory support, drug therapy, and rapid transport to an appropriate medical facility. Signs of acute coronary syndrome are typically related to vasospasm rather than blood vessel occlusion. Paramedics should administer nitroglycerin as in acute coronary syndrome. In addition, administration of benzodiazepines is indicated in mitigating cocaine-associated chest pain and reducing the sympathetic overdrive.[43]

If signs of cardiac toxicity with widened QRS are present, paramedics should acquire a 12-lead ECG. They should treat with sodium bicarbonate if indicated by medical direction.

Phencyclidine Overdose

PCP is a dissociative analgesic originally used as a veterinary tranquilizer. The drug has sympathomimetic and CNS stimulant and depressant properties. PCP is a potent psychoactive drug illegally sold in liquid, tablet, or powder form to be taken by the oral, IN, IV, or IM route, or with other drugs to be smoked (eg, a Sherman; a marijuana cigarette [with or without tobacco] dipped in liquid PCP or dusted with PCP powder). Most tablets contain about 5 mg of PCP. As a rule, PCP in its powder form is purer (50% to 100% PCP). Chronic use can result in permanent memory impairment and loss of higher brain functions. The pharmacologic effects are dose-related. They can be divided into low-dose and high-dose toxicity.[44] Ketamine is a derivative of PCP and has similar actions.

Low-Dose Toxicity. In low doses that are less than 10 mg, PCP intoxication produces an unpredictable state that can resemble drunkenness. The user may have a sense of euphoria or confusion, disorientation, agitation, or sudden rage. An intoxicated patient often has a blank stare and a stumbling gait. The patient often is in a dissociative state. The patient's pupils generally are reactive. The patient may experience flushing, diaphoresis, facial grimacing, hypersalivation, and vomiting. **Nystagmus** with a burstlike quality is characteristic of low-dose PCP use. In this range of toxicity, death usually is related to behavioral disturbances resulting from spatial disorientation, drug-induced immobility, and insensitivity to pain. Ordinarily, pain limits a person's muscle activity; without this limitation, the person may undertake bold acts of strength.

> **CRITICAL THINKING**
> Why does this type of drug intoxication put the patient at a high risk for injury?

In low-dose toxicity, sensory stimulation should be avoided. Verbal and physical stimuli will likely make the clinical symptoms worse. Violent and combative patients require protection from self-injury. Safeguards also must be provided for the emergency crew and bystanders. The paramedic should monitor the patient's vital signs and level of consciousness closely. The patient should be observed for increasing motor activity and muscle rigidity as well. These signs may precede seizures.

High-Dose Toxicity. Patients with high-dose PCP intoxication from more than 10 mg may be in a coma that can last from hours to several days. These patients often are unresponsive to painful stimuli. Respiratory depression, hypertension, and tachycardia also may be present, depending on the dosage. In severe cases, a hypertensive crisis causing cardiac failure, hypertensive encephalopathy, seizures, and intracerebral hemorrhage may result. Prehospital care is directed at managing respiratory and cardiac arrest, controlling status epilepticus, and rapidly transporting the patient for physician evaluation.

Phencyclidine Psychosis

Phencyclidine psychosis is a psychiatric emergency that may mimic schizophrenia.[45] The psychosis usually is of acute onset. It may not become apparent until several days after drug ingestion. Psychosis can occur after a single low-dose exposure to PCP. Psychosis also may last from several days to weeks. Signs and symptoms may range from a catatonic and unresponsive state to bizarre and violent behavior. The patient often appears agitated and suspicious, and may experience auditory hallucinations and paranoia. Appropriate management usually requires involuntary hospitalization, control of violent behavior, and administration of antipsychotic agents. When interacting with these patients in the prehospital setting, personal safety is of prime importance; law enforcement personnel should be called upon for assistance.

Hallucinogen Overdose

Hallucinogens are substances that cause perceptual distortions. The most common hallucinogen in use today is LSD. Other hallucinogens include mescaline, found in the buttons of peyote cactus, which can be used legally in some religious settings; psilocybin mushrooms, found in the United States and Mexico; marijuana, the active agent of the plant *Cannabis sativa*; morning glory plant; nutmeg; mace; and some amphetamines, such as 3,4-methylenedioxymethamphetamine (MDMA, commonly called Ecstasy).

SHOW ME THE EVIDENCE

Researchers described a series of 21 cases of patients aged 6 to 60 years transported to the ED for illness related to cannabis eaten in a gummy candy. Signs and symptoms included tachycardia, hypertension, elevated lactate, visual changes, dizziness, lethargy, confusion, nausea and vomiting, dry mucous membranes, and abdominal pain. Pediatric patients were more likely to be admitted and had a longer length of stay than did the adults. The authors caution practitioners to anticipate food-related ingestions of cannabis products.

Modified from: Vo KT, Horng H, Li K, et al. Cannabis intoxication case series: the dangers of edibles containing tetrahydrocannabinol. *Ann Emerg Med.* 2018;17(3):306-313.

Depending on the agent, the effects of hallucinogens may range from minor visual to more serious complications associated with LSD use. The more serious effects include respiratory and CNS depression (rare). Prehospital management usually is limited to supportive care, minimal sensory stimulation, calming measures, and transport to a medical facility. After arrival at the ED, these patients generally are placed in a quiet environment for observation.

Tricyclic Antidepressant Overdose

Tricyclic antidepressants often are prescribed to help manage depression and certain pain syndromes. These drugs work by blocking the uptake of norepinephrine and serotonin into the presynaptic neurons. They

NOTE

In recent years, a synthetic substitute for marijuana has been distributed and sold throughout the United States. The product usually is packaged and marketed as an herbal product intended to be burned as incense. It is available under various names, including K2 and Spice. The active ingredient in the synthetic substitute may be a cannabinoid, a class of drug that includes tetrahydrocannabinol (THC; the active ingredient in marijuana), but to be clear, it is *not* marijuana. The effects of the product are widely variable and unpredictable when smoked or inhaled. There is a synthetic THC, dronabinol, that may be legally prescribed for medicinal use (Marinol). The marijuana pill has been found to relieve the nausea and vomiting associated with chemotherapy for cancer patients and to assist with loss of appetite with acquired immunodeficiency syndrome (AIDS) patients.

Bath salts, also sold in the United States, produce effects similar to methamphetamine when snorted, inhaled, or injected. These powders are sold under names such as Ivory Wave, White Lightning, and Hurricane Charlie. They contain mephedrone and methylenedioxypyrovalerone (also known as MDPV) and can cause hallucinations, paranoia, tachycardia, and suicidal thoughts. The Synthetic Drug Control Act of 2015 (HR 3537) listed 300 substances to be classified as Schedule I federally controlled drugs. This list included chemicals used in these products.

Modified from: Synthetic cannabinoids (K2/spice) unpredictable danger. National Institute on Drug Abuse website. https://www.drugabuse.gov/related-topics/trends-statistics/infographics/synthetic-cannabinoids-k2spice-unpredictable-danger. Updated October 2017. Accessed March 1, 2018; *To Amend the Controlled Substances Act to Clarify How Controlled Substance Analogues Are to Be Regulated, and for Other Purposes.* 114th Cong 1st Sess (September 17, 2017), HR 35, 37.

also alter the sensitivity of brain tissue to the actions of these chemicals. Serious tricyclic antidepressant toxicity results in sodium channel blockade in the myocardium. Other toxicities include potassium efflux blockade and blockade of blood vessels, anticholinergic effects, and seizures. Commonly prescribed antidepressant drugs include the tricyclic antidepressants amitriptyline, amoxapine (Asendin), desipramine, doxepin (Silenor), imipramine (Tofranil-PM), nortriptyline (Pamelor), protriptyline, and trimipramine. The newer selective serotonin reuptake inhibitors such as fluoxetine, sertraline, and paroxetine are chemically unrelated to tricyclic antidepressants. These agents are considered safer and as effective compared with tricyclic antidepressants (BOX 33-19).

Early symptoms of tricyclic antidepressant overdose are dry mouth, blurred vision, confusion, inability to concentrate, and occasionally visual hallucinations. More severe symptoms include delirium, depressed respirations, hypertension, hypotension, hyperthermia, hypothermia, seizures, and coma (BOX 33-20). Cardiac effects may range from tachycardia to bradycardia and various dysrhythmias caused by atrioventricular block. A prolonged QRS complex, right bundle branch block, and a Glasgow Coma Scale score less than 8 are characteristic findings that should alert the paramedic to a major toxicity with potentially serious complications. Sudden death from a cardiac arrest may occur several days after an overdose.

Prehospital management for major toxicity of a tricyclic antidepressant overdose is basic supportive care for the patient and rapid transport. About 25% of patients who ultimately die as a result of the overdose are alert and awake, and 75% have normal sinus rhythm when EMS personnel arrive.[5] Tachycardia, especially with a wide QRS complex greater than 100 ms, is an early sign of toxicity. Sodium bicarbonate should be administered if this is observed.[9] Any patient with a history of tricyclic antidepressant ingestion should receive airway, ventilatory, and circulatory support; IV access with fluid challenge of 20 mL/kg if hypotensive[9]; ECG monitoring; and rapid transport for physician evaluation. If the patient is agitated, the paramedic should consider administering a benzodiazepine. Benzodiazepines are indicated for treatment of seizures. The paramedic should ensure transport to the ED without delay on the scene.

BOX 33-19 Serotonin Syndrome

Serotonin syndrome is a potentially life-threatening drug reaction. The reaction most often occurs when two or more drugs that affect serotonin levels are taken together. The drugs then cause too much serotonin to be released or to remain within brain tissue. Drug combinations that are associated with serotonin syndrome include migraine medicines (triptans) together with selective serotonin reuptake inhibitors (SSRIs) and selective serotonin/norepinephrine reuptake inhibitors (SNRIs). Popular SSRIs include Celexa, Zoloft, Prozac, Paxil, and Lexapro. SNRIs include Cymbalta and Effexor. Brand names of triptans include Imitrex, Zomig, Frova, Maxalt, Axert, Amerge, and Relpax. Drugs of abuse, such as Ecstasy and LSD, have also been associated with serotonin syndrome. St. John's wort in high doses or in combination with SSRIs has been linked to serotonin syndrome. Symptoms occur within minutes to hours and may include the following:

- Agitation or restlessness
- Diarrhea
- Tachycardia
- Hallucinations
- Increased body temperature
- Loss of coordination
- Nausea
- Overactive reflexes
- Rapid changes in blood pressure
- Vomiting

Patients with serotonin syndrome usually require hospitalization for close observation and supportive care. Treatment may include benzodiazepines to decrease agitation, seizurelike movements, and muscle stiffness; cyproheptadine (Periactin) to block serotonin production; IV fluids; and the withdrawal of medicines that caused the syndrome.

Modified from: Volpi-Abadie J, Kaye AM, Kaye AD. Serotonin syndrome. *Ochsner J*. 2013;13(4):533-540.

BOX 33-20 Five Signs of Major Tricyclic Antidepressant Toxicity

Cardiac dysrhythmias
Coma and seizures
GI disturbances
Hypotension or hypertension
Respiratory depression

CRITICAL THINKING

What is the most accurate way to measure QRS duration on the ECG?

Lithium

Lithium is a mood-stabilizing drug that is prescribed for the management of bipolar disorder (see Chapter 34, *Behavioral and Psychiatric Disorders*). The drug has a low toxic-to-therapeutic dose ratio. Thus, lithium overdose is common. Patients who are prescribed lithium have frequent blood tests to monitor the level of lithium in the body.

Lithium helps to prevent mood swings. It does this by interfering with hormonal responses to cyclic adenosine monophosphate and by increasing the reuptake of norepinephrine. These actions produce an antiadrenergic effect. As a result of these actions, lithium has many effects on the body, including muscle tremor, thirst, nausea, increased urination, abdominal cramping, and diarrhea. With toxic ingestion, signs and symptoms may include the following:[46]

- Muscle weakness
- Slurred speech
- Severe trembling
- Blurred vision
- Confusion
- Seizure
- Apnea
- Coma

Prehospital care for patients with suspected lithium overdose should focus on airway management, ventilatory and circulatory support, and the control of seizure activity if present. Activated charcoal does not effectively bind lithium and should not be administered. In-hospital care may include restoring intravascular volume, maintaining urine output, correcting hyponatremia, and sometimes undergoing dialysis.

Cardiac Medications

Cardiac drugs are a common cause of poisoning deaths in children and adults. The drugs responsible for the majority of these fatalities are digoxin, beta blockers, and calcium channel blockers (BOX 33-21). As in all other cases of poisoning, patients with toxic ingestion of cardiac drugs require high-concentration oxygen administration, IV access, and careful monitoring of vital signs and ECG.

Digoxin exerts direct and indirect effects on sinoatrial and atrioventricular nodal fibers. At toxic levels, the drug can halt impulses in the sinoatrial node, depress conduction through the atrioventricular node, and increase sensitivity of the sinoatrial and atrioventricular nodes to catecholamines.[13] Digoxin affects the Purkinje fibers as well by decreasing the resting potential and action potential duration of the heart and increasing automaticity. These actions can cause an increase in premature ventricular contraction formation. Unlike most cardiovascular drugs, digoxin can produce almost any dysrhythmia or conduction block. In addition to dysrhythmias, common signs and symptoms of digoxin toxicity include nausea, anorexia, fatigue, visual disturbances, and a variety of disorders of the GI, ophthalmologic, and neurologic systems. Oral overdoses sometimes are managed with activated charcoal (for acute, accidental ingestion) and drugs to treat life-threatening dysrhythmias. Severe overdoses are managed with IV digoxin-specific Fab (Digibind). This drug decreases the morbidity and mortality associated with digoxin overdose.

BOX 33-21 Toxic Effects of Common Cardiac Drugs

Digoxin

Atrial fibrillation
Atrial tachycardia
Bigeminal and multifocal premature ventricular contractions
First- and second-degree atrioventricular block
Sinus bradycardia
Ventricular tachycardia/ventricular fibrillation

Beta Blockers

Bradycardia
Hypotension
Respiratory arrest
Seizure
Unconsciousness
Ventricular tachycardia/ventricular fibrillation (rare)

Calcium Channel Blockers

Acute respiratory distress syndrome
Asystole
Atrioventricular dissociation
Coma
Confusion
Hypotension
Lactic acidosis
Mild hyperglycemia/hyperkalemia
Pulmonary edema
Respiratory depression
Sinus arrest
Sinus bradycardia
Slurred speech

CRITICAL THINKING

Why is it possible that this type of overdose would not be noticed immediately?

Beta Blocker and Calcium Channel Blocker Toxicity

Beta Blockers. The generic names of the beta blockers end in *olol*, such as atenolol (Tenormin) and metoprolol (Lopressor, Toprol XR). These drugs are absorbed rapidly after ingestion. Toxicity impairs sinoatrial and atrioventricular node function, which leads to bradycardias and atrioventricular blocks. The associated depression in ventricular conduction and sodium channel blockade may cause the QRS complex to widen, and occasionally, patients become susceptible to ventricular dysrhythmias. However, rarely will these patients exhibit ventricular tachycardia or ventricular fibrillation. Other signs and symptoms include CNS and respiratory depression, dyspnea, hypotension, and possible seizures.

Treatment for patients with beta blocker overdose may include administration of activated charcoal without sorbitol (especially for extended-release formulations) if the patient's mental status is not declining. Paramedics should prepare for early airway protection because some patients' mental status declines quickly. Paramedics should assess blood glucose. Beta blocker toxicity can cause hypoglycemia in children.[9] Paramedics should consider atropine if the patient has symptomatic bradycardia. A fluid challenge up to 20 mL/kg can be infused if the patient is bradycardic and hypotensive. In addition, glucagon can be administered IV at higher doses than for hypoglycemia. High doses of glucagon can cause vomiting, so paramedics should consider prophylactic administration of ondansetron (Zofran). If hypotension and bradycardia persist, vasopressors or transcutaneous pacing may be indicated. Seizures and widening QRS are more likely after propranolol overdose. Seizures should be treated with benzodiazepines. If the QRS duration is widened (≥100 ms), administration of sodium bicarbonate should be considered.

NOTE

Even one beta blocker or calcium channel blocker tablet may be fatal when ingested by a toddler. Contact poison control early, and transport all medication containers to the ED.

Modified from: National Association of EMS Officials. *National Model EMS Clinical Guidelines*. Version 2.0. National Association of EMS Officials website. https://www.nasemso.org/documents/National-Model-EMS-Clinical-Guidelines-Version2-Sept2017.pdf. Published September 2017. Accessed February 28, 2018.

Calcium Channel Blockers. Calcium channel blockers include drugs such as diltiazem, verapamil, amlodipine (Norvasc), felodipine, isradipine, and others. Toxic ingestion of calcium channel blockers can lead to myocardial depression and peripheral vasodilation with negative inotropic, chronotropic, dromotropic, and vasotropic effects. Hypotension and bradycardia are early signs of toxicity. Overdose may result in serious dysrhythmias that include atrioventricular block of all degrees, sinus arrest, atrioventricular dissociation, junctional rhythm, and asystole. (Calcium channel blockers have little effect on ventricular conduction; ventricular dysrhythmias are uncommon.) Other signs and symptoms of calcium channel toxicity include hyperglycemia and cardiogenic shock.

If the patient's mental status is not decreasing, paramedics should consider administration of activated charcoal without sorbitol. If symptomatic bradycardia is present, they should consider administering atropine sulfate and calcium gluconate or calcium chloride. If the patient is hypotensive, they should consider an IV fluid bolus of normal saline or lactated Ringer solution, 20 mL/kg up to 2 liters. Other vasopressors may be administered if hypotension persists despite initial drug and fluid treatment. Glucagon IV is considered when atropine, calcium, and vasopressors do not correct symptomatic bradycardia. Transcutaneous pacing can be attempted if drug therapy does not correct symptomatic bradycardia.[9]

NOTE

Toxicity from nifedipine and amlodipine may initially cause torsades de pointes. Later, the patient may develop bradycardia.

Monoamine Oxidase Inhibitors

MAO inhibitors block the breakdown of monoamines (norepinephrine, dopamine, serotonin). These CNS transmitters are distributed throughout the body. The highest concentration is in the brain, liver, and kidneys. MAO inhibitors are prescribed as antidepressants,

BOX 33-22 Effects of Monoamine Oxidase Inhibitor Toxicity

Agitation
Bradysystolic rhythms
Cardiovascular system manifestations
CNS depression
Hallucinations
Hyperthermia
Hypertension
Hypotension with vascular collapse
Neuromuscular system manifestations
Nystagmus
Rigidity
Seizure
Sinus tachycardia

antineoplastics, antibiotics, and antihypertensives. They include isocarboxazid (Marplan), phenelzine (Nardil), selegiline (Emsam), and tranylcypromine (Parnate). Some MAO inhibitors (eg, the antidepressants phenelzine and tranylcypromine) have active metabolites. Signs of MAO inhibitor toxicity usually are delayed, presenting 6 to 24 hours after ingestion. The duration of effects also may last for several days (BOX 33-22). These effects include CNS depression and various neuromuscular and cardiovascular system manifestations.

The prehospital care is mainly supportive. Care includes airway, ventilatory, and circulatory support; cardiac medications as needed; and rapid transport for physician evaluation. Activated charcoal may be indicated. Along with routine cooling measures, paramedics should consider administration of midazolam if the patient is hyperthermic.[9]

Nonsteroidal Anti-inflammatory Drugs

NSAIDs are a group of drugs that have an analgesic and antipyretic action. They also reduce inflammation of joints and soft tissues such as muscles and ligaments. They work by blocking the production of prostaglandins, which are chemicals that cause inflammation and trigger transmission of pain signals to the brain. NSAIDs are used widely to relieve symptoms caused by types of arthritis (rheumatoid arthritis, osteoarthritis, gout) and to treat back pain, menstrual pain, headaches, minor postoperative pain, and soft-tissue injuries. Common NSAIDs include diflunisal, fenoprofen, ibuprofen, and naproxen. Ibuprofen and naproxen are available over the counter.

Ibuprofen Overdose

Ibuprofen is one of the most commonly ingested NSAIDs in overdose. The effects usually are reversible and are seldom life threatening. However, significant toxicity may result in coma, seizure, hypotension, and acute renal failure. Chronic and acute ingestion is usually more than 300 mg/kg.[47] In such an ingestion, common symptoms include mild GI and CNS disturbances that usually resolve within 24 hours after ingestion. Other less common effects include mild metabolic acidosis, muscle fasciculations, chills, hyperventilation, hypotension, and asymptomatic bradycardia. Emergency care for patients who have ingested toxic amounts of ibuprofen may consist of GI decontamination. These patients require careful monitoring for secondary complications such as hypotension and dysrhythmias.

Salicylate Overdose

Salicylates are widely available in prescription and over-the-counter products such as acetylsalicylic acid (aspirin), many cold preparations, and oil of wintergreen (methyl salicylate), and in combination with some analgesics such as propoxyphene and oxycodone. **TABLE 33-6** contains guidelines for salicylate toxicity.

NOTE

At one time, the ingestion of colorful and tasty children's aspirin was the most common cause of pediatric poisoning. In response to this problem, the number of tablets in chewable aspirin packaging now is limited to 36 per container. Because of the association of aspirin with Reye syndrome, aspirin is not recommended in children younger than 16 years who have viral symptoms.

The process of toxicity with salicylate poisoning is complex. Toxicity includes direct CNS stimulation, interference with cellular glucose uptake, and inhibition of Krebs cycle enzymes that affect energy production and amino acid metabolism. The volume of distribution is dose-dependent and usually small. With toxic ingestion, however, redistribution of the drug into the CNS occurs. This prolongs elimination

TABLE 33-6 Toxicity Guidelines for Salicylate

Toxicity	Amount Ingested
Mild	<150 mg/kg
Moderate to severe	150–300 mg/kg
Severe	>300 mg/kg
Fatal	>500 mg/kg

Modified from: Lilley LL, Rainforth Collins S, Schneider JS. *Pharmacology and the Nursing Process*. 8th ed. Maryland Heights, MO: Mosby; 2017.

of the drug from the body. Complications that may result from chronic or acute ingestion of salicylates include CNS stimulation, GI irritation, inhibition of glucose metabolism, fluid and electrolyte imbalance, neurologic symptoms, and coagulation defects. Confusion, lethargy, convulsions, respiratory arrest, coma, and brain death can occur in severe salicylate poisoning.

CRITICAL THINKING

Would you predict tachypnea or bradypnea in these patients? Why?

In addition to general supportive measures, prehospital care for salicylate poisoning may include the administration of activated charcoal without sorbitol. Treatment also may include IV glucose if hypoglycemia is detected. Salicylates are weak acids that can be excreted by the kidney. Thus medical direction may recommend the administration of sodium bicarbonate in an effort to produce alkaline urine. Definitive care includes in-hospital intensive care observation, continued support of vital functions, and perhaps hemodialysis.

Acetaminophen Overdose

Acetaminophen is a commonly prescribed analgesic and antipyretic agent. Acetaminophen is available in many prescription and nonprescription preparations (eg, Tylenol, Panadol). The widespread availability of acetaminophen accounts for its high incidence in unintentional and intentional poisoning. Acetaminophen is 1 of the 10 most commonly used drugs for intentional self-poisoning and is associated with significant morbidity and mortality.[48] Acetaminophen overdose can cause life-threatening liver damage from toxic metabolites if it is not managed within 16 to 24 hours of ingestion. As few as 30 standard-size (325-mg) acetaminophen tablets can be toxic in an average adult. Acetaminophen also is present in many drug combinations, including Darvocet-N, Excedrin, and Sinutab.

Acute acetaminophen overdose results from doses of 150 mg/kg or greater. The toxic effects of such an ingestion can be classified in four stages (BOX 33-23).[49] The course of toxicity begins with

BOX 33-23 Stages of Acetaminophen Poisoning

Stage I: Gastrointestinal Irritability (0 to 24 hours)

Anorexia
Diaphoresis
General malaise
Nausea
Pallor
Vomiting

Stage II: Abnormal Laboratory Findings (24 to 48 hours)

Possible abdominal pain and tenderness in the right abdominal quadrant
Resolution of stage I symptoms

Stage III: Hepatic Damage (72 to 96 hours)

Dysrhythmias
Hepatotoxicity with significant increase in hepatic enzymes
Hypoglycemia
Jaundice
Lethargy
Vomiting

Stage IV: Recovery (4 to 14 days) or Progressive Hepatic Failure[a]

Resolution of hepatic dysfunction
Lack of permanent effects in patients who recover

[a]The percentage of patients who recover in stage IV depends on the amount of acetaminophen ingested and whether effective therapy (activated charcoal, acetylcysteine, or both) was given. Patients with serum levels in the hepatotoxic range have mortality rates up to 25% if untreated.

mild symptoms that may be overlooked or masked by more dramatic effects of other agents followed by temporary clinical improvement and finally peak liver damage. (If acetaminophen was the only drug taken and a dangerously high dose was ingested, the first two stages may be asymptomatic.) If antidote management is started within 8 hours of ingestion, full recovery should occur.

> CRITICAL THINKING
> Do you think most laypeople realize that acetaminophen overdose can be fatal?

Emergency care includes respiratory, cardiac, and hemodynamic support in critically ill patients. If ingestion is within 1 hour and the patient is alert, medical direction may recommend the administration of activated charcoal without sorbitol. Patients with progressive acetaminophen toxicity require administration of its antidote, N-acetylcysteine.

Drugs Abused for Sexual Purposes or Sexual Gratification

Some drugs are abused for sexual purposes or for sexual gratification. These drugs commonly are classified by users as uppers, downers, and all-arounders (those that have more than one primary effect). BOX 33-24 gives a sampling of these drugs. These drugs generally are taken alone or in combination to produce one or more of the following effects:

- A sense of euphoria
- Excitation (rush)
- Relaxation (blissed out)
- A loss of inhibition

BOX 33-24 Uppers, Downers, and All-Arounders

Uppers
Anabolic steroids
Coke/crack
Ecstasy
Speed/meth/crystal

Downers
Alcohol
Benzodiazepines (diazepam, temazepam, Rohypnol)
Gamma-hydroxybutyrate (GHB)
Heroin

All-Arounders
Cannabis/skunk
Ketamine
LSD
Poppers (alkyl nitrates)

Each of these drugs has different chemical structures, mechanisms of action, and side effects, so the problems associated with their use can vary greatly. Signs and symptoms of use of these drugs can range from mild nausea and vomiting to life-threatening respiratory depression, hypotension, methemoglobinemia (elevated serum methemoglobin level), coma, and death. The emergency care for these patients mainly is supportive. Paramedics should follow the guidelines for management of poisoned patients (see Box 33-2).

Alcohol Use Disorder

Alcohol and related illness continue to be a major problem in the United States. It is estimated that 16 million Americans have alcohol use disorder (AUD),[50] of whom 9.8 million are men and 5.3 million are women. In 2015, an estimated 623,000 adolescents ages 12 to 17 years had AUD. In addition, the most recent statistics report that alcohol is a key factor in 29% of vehicle fatalities.[51] The economic cost of alcohol-related crashes is $44 billion annually.[3]

> CRITICAL THINKING
> How many calls have you been on that involved patients intoxicated with alcohol? What kinds of calls were they?

Alcohol Dependence

Alcohol dependence, which results from AUD, is characterized by chronic, excessive consumption of alcohol that causes injury to health or inadequate social function and the development of withdrawal symptoms when the patient stops drinking suddenly.[52] AUD is a chronic, progressive, potentially fatal disease characterized by remissions, relapses, and potentially recovery with remission but not cures. The active ingredient in all alcoholic beverages is ethanol, a colorless, flammable liquid produced from the fermentation of carbohydrates by yeast.

DID YOU KNOW?

The development of alcohol dependence can be divided into four main stages that merge imperceptibly. The time frame of these stages may range from 5 to 25 years, but the average is about 10 years. In the first stage, tolerance of the drug develops in the heavy social drinker. This allows a person to consume larger quantities of alcohol before experiencing its ill effects. On entering the second stage, the drinker experiences memory lapses relating to events occurring during the drinking episodes. The third stage is characterized by loss or lack of control over alcohol; the drinker can no longer be certain of discontinuing alcohol consumption at will. The final stage begins with prolonged binges of intoxication. This is associated with mental and physical complications. Some drinkers halt their consumption for a brief time or permanently during one of the first three stages.

Modified from: Jellinek EM. *The Disease Concept of Alcoholism.* Eastford, CT: Martino Fine Books; 2010.

People diagnosed with AUD have met at least 2 of the 11 criteria in the *Diagnostic and Statistical Manual of Mental Disorders* (*DSM-5*) for the disease (**BOX 33-25**).

Metabolism of Ingested Alcohol

About 80% to 90% of ingested alcohol is absorbed within 30 minutes. Twenty percent is absorbed in the stomach, the rest in the small intestine.[53] Once absorbed, the drug is distributed rapidly throughout the vascular space. Alcohol reaches virtually every organ system. About 3% to 5% of alcohol is excreted unchanged via the lungs and kidneys; the rest is metabolized in the liver to carbon dioxide and water. The actual rate at which alcohol is metabolized depends on individual variation (eg, physical and mental state, body weight and size). Metabolism also depends on whether the drinker is alcohol-dependent.

Measurement of Blood Alcohol Content

The alcohol content of blood is measured in terms of mass (milligrams) of alcohol per given volume of blood (deciliter). Blood alcohol content is used widely to evaluate the CNS status of an intoxicated person. In most states,, the legal limit of intoxication is 80 mg/dL. (This is equivalent to 0.08%.) Some states have laws that allow paramedics to assist in conducting breathalyzer or blood tests to detect alcohol or drug intoxication.

BOX 33-25 Criteria for Alcohol Use Disorder[a]

To evaluate the severity of the disease, the patient is asked the following questions.

In the past year, have you:

1. Had times when you ended up drinking more, or longer, than you intended?
2. More than once wanted to cut down or stop drinking, or tried to, but couldn't?
3. Spent a lot of time drinking? Or being sick or getting over the aftereffects?
4. Experienced craving—a strong need, or urge, to drink?
5. Found that drinking—or being sick from drinking—often interfered with taking care of your home or family? Or caused job troubles? Or school problems?
6. Continued to drink even though it was causing trouble with your family or friends?
7. Given up or cut back on activities that were important or interesting to you, or gave you pleasure, in order to drink?
8. More than once gotten into situations while or after drinking that increased your chances of getting hurt (such as driving, swimming, using machinery, walking in a dangerous areas, or having unsafe sex)?
9. Continued to drink even though it was making you feel depressed or anxious or adding to another health problem? Or after having had a memory blackout?
10. Had to drink much more than you once did to get the effect you want? Or found that your usual number of drinks had much less effect than before?
11. Found that when the effects of alcohol were wearing off, you had withdrawal symptoms, such as trouble sleeping, shakiness, irritability, anxiety, depression, restlessness, nausea, or sweating? Or sensed things that were not there?

[a]The severity of the disease (mild, moderate, or severe) is determined by the number of criteria that are met. In mild disease, there is a presence of 2–3 symptoms; 4–5 symptoms are considered moderate; 6 or more symptoms are considered severe.

Modified from: National Institute on Alcohol Abuse and Alcoholism (NIAAA) website. Alcohol Use Disorder. https://www.niaaa.nih.gov/alcohol-health/overview-alcohol-consumption/alcohol-use-disorders. Accessed April 5, 2018.

EMS personnel should be well versed in the laws of their state before assisting with these tests and follow established protocols carefully.

CRITICAL THINKING

Can you use an alcohol prep to prepare the site before drawing a blood alcohol specimen? Why?

Medical Consequences of Chronic Alcohol Ingestion

Alcohol affects nearly every organ system of the body. Thus, people who consume large amounts of alcohol are at risk for a number of physical and mental disorders, including dependence, neurologic disorders, nutritional deficiencies, fluid and electrolyte imbalances, GI disorders, cardiac and skeletal muscle myopathy, and immune suppression. In addition, alcohol may affect a patient's ability to tolerate traumatic injury.

Neurologic Disorders

Alcohol is a potent CNS depressant. When consumed in moderate amounts, the drug reduces anxiety and tension. Alcohol gives most drinkers a feeling of relaxation and confidence. Initial feelings of well-being develop into impaired judgment and discrimination, slowed reflexes, and incoordination and drowsiness. These effects ultimately may progress to stupor and coma. The long-term neurologic effects of chronic alcohol abuse are similar to those of the aging process. They include short-term memory deficit, problems with coordination, and difficulty with concentration and abstraction.

Nutritional Deficiencies

Alcohol can satisfy the caloric requirements of the body for a brief time, but alcohol does not have essential vitamins, proteins, or fats. As a result, people who are alcohol-dependent may have a decreased dietary intake and malabsorption. This condition leads to multiple vitamin and mineral deficiencies that can cause altered immunity, poor wound healing, anorexia, cardiac dysrhythmias, and seizures.

Wernicke-Korsakoff Syndrome. People who are alcohol-dependent are at particular risk of developing **Wernicke-Korsakoff syndrome**, a condition that results from a reduction in intestinal absorption and metabolism of thiamine caused by alcohol. Wernicke-Korsakoff syndrome disrupts central and peripheral nerve function, affecting the brain and nervous system. It may consist of two stages: Wernicke encephalopathy and Korsakoff psychosis, or a combination of the two.

Wernicke encephalopathy usually develops suddenly with the clinical manifestations of ataxia, nystagmus, disturbances of speech and gait, signs of neuropathy (paresthesias, impaired reflexes), stupor, and (rarely) coma.[54] Because the body needs thiamine to metabolize glucose, it was once thought that this syndrome may be caused by the IV administration of glucose or glucose-containing fluids in the malnourished patient. However, there has not been a single documented case of a single dose of dextrose precipitating Wernicke encephalopathy. The malnourished hypoglycemic patient should receive dextrose without delay, and concurrent administration of thiamine should be undertaken if deficiency is suspected.[55]

CRITICAL THINKING

Why do you think recognizing this syndrome is delayed in patients with alcohol use disorder?

Many patients with AUD also display signs of **Korsakoff psychosis**, a mental disorder often found with Wernicke encephalopathy. Signs include apathy, poor retentive memory, retrograde amnesia, confabulation (invention of stories to make up for gaps in memory), and dementia. Korsakoff psychosis usually is considered irreversible. It leaves the patient permanently handicapped by memory loss, requiring continual supervision.

Fluid and Electrolyte Imbalances

Urinary output increases after ingesting alcohol, over and above that expected from the amount of fluid ingested. This diuresis results because alcohol blocks the secretion of antidiuretic hormone. It can lead to dehydration and electrolyte imbalances.

GI Disorders

The effects of alcohol on the GI system can produce several types of alcohol-related illnesses and diseases. The alcohol-related GI disorders most likely to initiate an EMS response include GI hemorrhage, cirrhosis, and acute or chronic pancreatitis.

GI Hemorrhage. Four primary causes of GI hemorrhage in patients who drink alcohol are gastritis, ulcer formation, esophageal tear (Mallory-Weiss syndrome), and variceal hemorrhage (see Chapter 28, *Abdominal and Gastrointestinal Disorders*).

Gastritis results from the toxic effects of ethanol on the gastric mucosa. This leads to diffuse or localized areas of erosion. In the chronic form of gastritis, blood may ooze continually from the mucosal lining, and ulcers may develop.

Esophageal tears of the gastroesophageal junction, stomach, or esophagus usually follow severe or protracted vomiting or retching. The injury results when gastric contents are forced against an unrelaxed gastroesophageal junction. This produces a sudden increase in pressure and a mucosal tear with subsequent bleeding. The bleeding can be worsened by clotting abnormalities. Such abnormalities are common in patients with alcoholic liver disease.

Varices are a result of portal hypertension caused by cirrhosis. Any of these thin-walled, blood-engorged veins are subject to rupture and hemorrhage, but the most common site is the varices of the esophagus. Bleeding esophagogastric varices remain one of the most difficult conditions to manage. Severe blood loss through vomiting requires aggressive supportive care with large-bore IV lines and judicious fluid resuscitation until blood products can be initiated in the ED. Like other forms of GI bleeding described in Chapter 28, *Abdominal and Gastrointestinal Disorders,* permissive hypotension to maintain mental status and/or a systolic blood pressure of 80 to 90 mm Hg may be prudent.[56] The paramedic should consult with medical direction or follow established protocol.

Cirrhosis. Cirrhosis of the liver is caused by chronic damage to liver cells and eventual necrosis. In the disease process, bands of fibrous scar tissue develop and disturb the normal structure of the liver. The distortion and fibrosis of the liver lead to portal hypertension, which results in complications such as ascites, splenomegaly, and bleeding esophageal and gastric varices. In addition, cirrhosis may lead to hepatic encephalopathy, resulting from the accumulation of toxic metabolic waste products that normally would be detoxified by a healthy liver. Cirrhosis and chronic liver disease represent the 16th-leading cause of death by disease, accounting for 38,000 deaths each year.[57]

Acute or Chronic Pancreatitis. Alcohol is the most common cause of acute and chronic pancreatitis. Chronic pancreatitis usually produces the same symptoms as the acute form (described in Chapter 28, *Abdominal and Gastrointestinal Disorders*). The pain, however, may last from several hours to several days. The attacks also become more frequent as the condition progresses. The effects of chronic pancreatitis include malabsorption and electrolyte imbalances. Diabetes mellitus also may develop from insufficient insulin production. Complications of pancreatitis are hemorrhagic pancreatitis, sepsis, and pancreatic abscess. These complications are associated with high mortality.

Cardiac and Skeletal Muscle Myopathy

Cardiac and skeletal muscle damage related to alcohol abuse is thought to result from a direct toxic effect of alcohol or its metabolites. In heart muscle, these toxic effects can result in a decreased force of contraction, dysrhythmias, and a tendency to develop congestive heart failure. In skeletal muscle, the major symptoms are weakness and muscle wasting.

Immune Suppression

Long-term alcohol abuse renders the immune system less effective. Alcohol abuse suppresses bone marrow production of white blood cells. In addition, production of red blood cells and platelets is often decreased. Alcohol has direct, specific effects on lung tissue. These effects may impair macrophage mobilization and protective ciliary function. As a result, the ability of the body to fight pulmonary infection is lowered, making the person with AUD more susceptible to viral and bacterial pneumonia.

CRITICAL THINKING

For what other pulmonary disease is the immune-suppressed patient with alcohol use disorder at risk?

Trauma

Alcohol suppresses clotting factors that are produced in the liver. This blood-clotting deficiency makes the person with AUD prone to bruising and internal hemorrhage. The deficiency also adds to the frequency of subdural bleeding, even after relatively minor head trauma (see Chapter 39, *Head, Face, and Neck Trauma*).[58]

Emergency Care for AUD

Several other conditions caused by consumption or abstinence from alcohol may require emergency care. These conditions include acute alcohol intoxication, alcohol withdrawal syndrome, and disulfiram-ethanol reaction. Alcohol-induced ketoacidosis and hypoglycemia are discussed in Chapter 25, *Endocrinology.*

Acute Alcohol Intoxication

The ingestion of alcohol may cause acute poisoning if consumed in large amounts over a short period. At toxic levels, hypoventilation (including respiratory arrest), hypotension, and hypothermia may develop. The patient who has signs and symptoms of acute alcohol intoxication should be evaluated for hidden trauma and coexisting medical conditions. These conditions include hypoglycemia, cardiac myopathy and dysrhythmias, GI bleeding, polydrug abuse, and ethylene glycol or methanol (toxic alcohols) ingestion. Because the patient is prone to injury and usually has other medical conditions, the paramedic should never assume that an intoxicated patient is merely inebriated.

Management. A patient who is mildly intoxicated may need to be transported for physician evaluation. In most cases, management requires patient observation in the ED only until the patient is sober. The paramedic should monitor the patient's vital signs and level of consciousness carefully en route. A thorough physical examination is warranted to rule out illness or injury masked by alcohol ingestion.

Care of the acutely intoxicated patient is aimed at protecting the patient from further injury and maintaining vital functions. If the patient is conscious and agitated, restraints may be necessary. If physical restraint becomes necessary, the police should be summoned. After scene safety has been established, the primary survey and resuscitation should include the following:

1. Rapidly evaluate airway patency with spinal precautions. Assess the patient's ventilatory and hemodynamic status while obtaining a history. The patient's account of the event may be unreliable because of the alcohol ingestion.
2. Initiate IV therapy. Draw blood samples for laboratory analysis. If hypoglycemia is confirmed, administer dextrose and thiamine (per protocol). Give naloxone if opioid overdose is suspected.
3. Continually monitor the patient's airway, and provide adequate ventilatory and circulatory support as needed. Be prepared to provide suction and aggressive airway management.
4. Monitor the ECG for dysrhythmias.
5. Rapidly transport the patient for physician evaluation.

Alcohol Withdrawal Syndrome

A period of relative or full abstinence from alcohol may cause withdrawal in a person with AUD. Alcohol withdrawal syndrome (AWS) is mediated by several mechanisms that result in CNS hyperexcitability. Biochemical changes such as respiratory alkalosis and hypomagnesemia may also play a role. AWS can be divided into four general categories: initial withdrawal symptoms, alcohol hallucinations, withdrawal seizures, and delirium tremens.[59]

Initial Withdrawal Symptoms. Initial withdrawal symptoms begin about 6 to 8 hours after cessation or reduction of alcohol intake. These symptoms peak within 72 hours and may diminish after 5 to 7 days of abstinence. When alcohol withdrawal is confined to minor reactions, the prognosis for full recovery is excellent with the proper management. Minor reactions include insomnia, anxiety, diaphoresis, nausea and vomiting, headache, palpitations, and generalized tremor made worse by agitation. Mild tachycardia, hypertension, and increased body temperature also may be present.[59]

> CRITICAL THINKING
> What kinds of feelings do you think the patient and the patient's family may be having during withdrawal reactions?

Alcohol-Induced Hallucinations. Alcohol-induced hallucinations, which are experienced in 7% to 8% of patients with AWS, usually occur 12 to 24 hours after the patient stops drinking alcohol.[60] Tactile hallucinations (eg, the sensation of crawling skin) are common, and persecutory auditory hallucinations (eg, hearing threatening voices) are also experienced by some patients. The latter can produce agitation, fear, and panic. The prognosis for hallucinations is the same as that for initial withdrawal symptoms.

Withdrawal Seizures. Withdrawal seizures (or rum fits) usually occur 12 to 48 hours after ethanol cessation and most often are generalized tonic-clonic seizures of short duration; status seizures are rare.[13] This category of withdrawal may be self-limiting. About one-third of patients who have seizures progress to delirium tremens. Because of the high drug tolerance level of the patient with AUD, seizure activity may require IV administration of large doses of midazolam, diazepam, or lorazepam. These drugs may synergistically interact with any ethanol still in the patient's system. Therefore, vital signs, respirations, and mental status should be monitored closely.

Delirium Tremens. Delirium tremens, the most dramatic and serious form of alcohol withdrawal, affects about 3% to 5% of all patients with AUD hospitalized for withdrawal.[59] Delirium tremens usually occurs 72 hours after withdrawal symptoms begin but may appear as early as 8 hours after the last drink. The syndrome is characterized by psychomotor, speech, and autonomic hyperactivity; profound confusion; disorientation; delusion; vivid hallucinations; tremor; agitation; and insomnia. A single episode may last 1 to 8 days and, with multiple recurrences, may last up to 1 month. Delirium tremens is a true medical emergency that has a mortality rate of up to 15%—and is as low as 5% in the context of proper care in an intensive care unit.[61] Associated alcohol-related illnesses such as pneumonia, pancreatitis, and hepatitis are frequent contributing causes of death.

Management. The care for patients with AWS mainly is supportive. The paramedic should carefully monitor the patient's airway, ventilatory, and circulatory status. IV therapy should be initiated with a saline solution for rehydration. Pharmacologic therapy may be indicated for an altered level of consciousness, dysrhythmias, or seizure activity. In addition, these patients need calm reassurance and frequent reorientation. All patients with signs and symptoms of AWS require physician evaluation. Benzodiazepines (eg, midazolam, lorazepam, diazepam) are often prescribed at regular intervals to help control the withdrawal symptoms. The role of ketamine in the treatment of symptoms of AWS is being studied.

Disulfiram-Ethanol Reaction

Disulfiram (tetraethylthiuram disulfide [Antabuse]) is a medication prescribed to some patients with AUD to help them abstain. The drug works by inhibiting ethanol metabolism and by allowing the accumulation of the metabolite acetaldehyde. Acetaldehyde produces ill effects in the GI, cardiovascular, and autonomic nervous systems. Acetaldehyde is the metabolic product that is thought to be responsible for the common hangover. Patients who take disulfiram and then drink alcohol experience an unpleasant and potentially life-threatening physiologic response.

The disulfiram-ethanol reaction begins 15 to 30 minutes after the ingestion of two to five alcoholic drinks. The reaction continues for 1 to 2 hours. It causes the patient to experience vertigo, headache, vomiting, and flushing, which may give the skin a lobster-red appearance. Other effects include dyspnea, diaphoresis, abdominal pain, and sometimes chest pain. More serious reactions include hypotension, shock, and dysrhythmias. Sudden death, myocardial and cerebral infarction, and cerebral hemorrhage also have been reported after as little as one drink of ethanol in patients taking high doses of disulfiram.[62] Acute overdose of disulfiram is now uncommon with current dosing regimens.[13]

Management. Prehospital care for a disulfiram-ethanol reaction involves airway, ventilatory, and circulatory support; administration of IV fluids to manage hypotension; pharmacologic therapy as needed to manage dysrhythmias; and rapid transport for physician evaluation. Most patients recover from these episodes. Supportive care and in-hospital observation are usually all that are required.

Summary

- The most common toxic syndromes are cholinergic, anticholinergic, hallucinogenic, opioid, and sympathomimetic. Using these classifications allows the paramedic to group similar toxic agents together. It allows the paramedic to more easily remember how to assess and treat the poisoned patient.
- A poison is any substance that produces harmful physiologic or psychological effects.
- The toxic effects of ingested poisons may be immediate or delayed, depending on the substance that is ingested. The primary goal is to identify effects on the three vital organ systems most likely to produce immediate morbidity or death—the respiratory system, the cardiovascular system, and the central nervous system (CNS). In some cases, serious poisonings by ingestion are managed by preventing the toxic substance from reaching the small intestine, thus limiting its absorption.
- Strong acids and alkalis may cause burns to the mouth, pharynx, esophagus, and sometimes the upper respiratory and gastrointestinal (GI) tracts. Prehospital care is usually limited to airway and ventilatory support, intravenous (IV) fluid replacement, and rapid transport to the appropriate medical facility.
- The most important physical characteristic in the potential toxicity of ingested hydrocarbons is its viscosity. The lower the viscosity, the higher the risk of aspiration and associated complications. Hydrocarbon ingestion may involve the patient's respiratory, GI, and neurologic systems. The clinical features may be immediate or delayed in onset.
- Methanol is a poisonous alcohol found in a variety of products. Its metabolites (formaldehyde and formic acid) are very toxic. Ingestion can affect the CNS, the GI tract, and the eyes. It also can cause the development of metabolic acidosis.
- Ethylene glycol toxicity is caused by the buildup of toxic metabolites, especially glycolic and oxalic acids after metabolism. This occurs mainly in the liver and kidneys. This toxicity may affect the CNS and cardiopulmonary and renal systems.
- The majority of isopropanol (isopropyl alcohol) is metabolized to acetone after ingestion. Isopropanol poisoning affects several body systems, including the central nervous, GI, and renal systems.
- Infants and children are high-risk groups for accidental iron, lead, and mercury poisoning. This risk is due to their immature immune systems and increased absorption as a function of age. Ingested iron is corrosive to GI tract mucosa. It may produce GI hemorrhage, bloody vomitus, painless bloody diarrhea, and dark stools.
- Food poisoning is a term used for any illness of sudden onset (usually associated with stomach pain, vomiting, and diarrhea) suspected of being caused by food eaten within the previous 48 hours. Food poisoning can be classified as infectious, resulting from a bacterium or virus. It also can be classified as noninfectious, resulting from toxins and pollutants.
- The toxic effects of major poisonous plant ingestions are predictable. They are categorized by the chemical and physical properties of the plant. Most responses are consistent with the type of major toxic chemical component in the plant.
- Simple asphyxiants cause toxicity by lowering ambient oxygen concentration. Chemical asphyxiants possess intrinsic systemic toxicity. This toxicity occurs after absorption into the circulation. Irritants or corrosives cause cellular destruction and inflammation as they come into contact with moisture in the respiratory tract.
- The concentration of a chemical in the air and duration of exposure help to predict the severity of an inhalation injury. Solubility also influences the extent of an inhalation injury. Highly reactive chemicals cause more severe and rapid injury than do less reactive chemicals. Properties that determine chemical reactivity are chemical pH, direct-acting potential of chemicals, indirect-acting potential of chemicals, and allergic potential of chemicals.
- Cyanide refers to any number of highly toxic substances that contain the cyanogen chemical group. Regardless of the route of entry, cyanide is a rapidly acting poison. It combines and reacts with ferric ions of the respiratory enzyme cytochrome oxidase. This action inhibits cellular oxygenation, which can produce a rapid progression from dyspnea to paralysis, unconsciousness, and death.
- Ammonia is a toxic irritant that causes local pulmonary complications after inhalation. In severe cases, bronchospasm and pulmonary edema may develop.
- Hydrocarbon inhalation may cause aspiration pneumonitis. It also has the potential for systemic effects such as CNS depression and liver, kidney, or bone marrow toxicity. Emergency care for hydrocarbon inhalation generally is supportive and includes the principles for management of poisoned patients.
- Arthropod venoms are complex and diverse in their chemistry and pharmacology and have the highest need for emergency care of any type of bite or sting injury. They may produce major toxic reactions in sensitized people. Such reactions include anaphylaxis and upper airway obstruction.
- The two main families of venomous snakes indigenous to the United States are pit vipers and coral snakes. Pit viper venom can produce various toxic effects on blood and other tissues. These effects include hemolysis, intravascular coagulation, convulsions, and acute renal failure. The venom of the coral snake is mainly neurotoxic. Signs and symptoms range from slurred speech, dilated pupils, and dysphagia to flaccid paralysis and death within 24 hours.
- The marine animals most likely to be involved in human envenomations in US coastal waters are coelenterates, echinoderms, and stingrays.
  - Coelenterate envenomation ranges in severity from irritant dermatitis to excruciating pain, respiratory depression, anaphylaxis, and life-threatening cardiovascular collapse.

  - Echinoderm toxins may cause immediate intense pain, swelling, redness, aching in the affected extremity, and nausea. Delayed effects may include respiratory distress, paresthesia of the lips and face, and, in severe cases, respiratory paralysis and complete atonia.
  - Locally, stingray venom produces a painful traumatic injury. It may cause bleeding and necrosis. Systemic manifestations range from weakness and nausea to seizures, paralysis, hypotension, and death.
- Organophosphates and carbamates inhibit the effects of acetylcholinesterase. A mnemonic that may help the paramedic to recognize this type of poisoning is SLUDGE (Salivation; Lacrimation; Urination; Defecation; GI upset; Emesis). The most specific findings, however, are miosis, rapidly changing pupils, and muscle fasciculation.
- Principles for managing drug abuse and overdose include providing scene safety; ensuring adequate airway, breathing, and circulation; obtaining a history; identifying the substance; performing a focused physical examination; initiating an IV; administering an antidote if needed; preventing further absorption; and providing rapid patient transport.
- Narcotics are CNS depressants. They can cause life-threatening respiratory depression. In severe intoxication, hypotension, profound shock, and pulmonary edema may be present. Naloxone is a pure narcotic antagonist effective for virtually all narcotic and narcoticlike substances.
- Sedative-hypnotic agents include benzodiazepines and barbiturates. Signs and symptoms of sedative-hypnotic overdose are chiefly related to the central nervous and cardiovascular systems. Flumazenil (Romazicon) is a benzodiazepine antagonist. It is useful in reversing the effects of these agents if they were given in a clinical setting.
- Commonly used stimulant drugs are those of the amphetamine family. Adverse effects include tachycardia, hypertension, tachypnea, agitation, dilated pupils, tremors, and disorganized behavior. With sudden withdrawal, the patient becomes depressed, suicidal, incoherent, or nearly comatose.
- Phencyclidine (PCP) is a dissociative analgesic with sympathomimetic and CNS stimulant and depressant properties. In low doses, PCP intoxication produces an unpredictable state that can resemble drunkenness (and rage). High-dose intoxication may cause coma. This may last from several hours to days. Respiratory depression, hypertension, and tachycardia may be present. PCP psychosis is a psychiatric emergency that may mimic schizophrenia.
- Hallucinogens are substances that cause distortions of perceptions. Depending on the agent, overdose may range from visual hallucinations to more serious complications, including respiratory and CNS depression.
- Tricyclic antidepressant toxicity is thought to result from central and peripheral, atropinelike anticholinergic effects and direct depressant effects on myocardial function. A prolonged QRS complex, right bundle branch block, and a Glasgow Coma Scale score less than 8 should alert the paramedic to a major toxicity with potentially serious complications.
- Lithium is a mood-stabilizing drug. Toxic ingestion can include CNS effects that can range from blurred vision and confusion to seizure and coma.
- Cardiac drugs are a common cause of poisoning deaths in children and adults. The drugs responsible for the majority of these fatalities are digitalis, beta blockers, and calcium channel blockers.
- Monoamine oxidase inhibitors block or diminish the activity of the monoamines (norepinephrine, dopamine, serotonin). Toxic effects include CNS depression and various neuromuscular and cardiovascular system manifestations.
- Nonsteroidal anti-inflammatory drugs work by blocking the production of prostaglandins. The effects of overdose of ibuprofen are usually reversible, are seldom life threatening, and include mild GI and CNS effects. Salicylate poisoning may cause CNS stimulation, GI irritation, inhibition of glucose metabolism, fluid and electrolyte imbalance, neurologic symptoms, and coagulation defects.
- Acetaminophen overdose may cause life-threatening liver damage. This results from formation of a hepatotoxic intermediate metabolite if the overdose is not managed within 16 to 24 hours of ingestion.
- Some drugs are abused for sexual purposes or for sexual gratification. These are commonly classified by users as uppers, downers, and all-arounders (having more than one primary effect). Problems associated with their use vary widely.
- Alcohol use disorder is characterized by chronic, excessive consumption of alcohol that results in injury to health or in inadequate social function and the development of withdrawal symptoms when the patient stops drinking suddenly. Alcohol causes multiple systemic effects, including neurologic disorders, nutritional deficiencies, fluid and electrolyte imbalances, GI disorders, cardiac and skeletal muscle myopathy, and immune suppression. Several conditions caused by consumption or abstinence from alcohol that may require emergency care are acute alcohol intoxication, alcohol withdrawal syndrome, and disulfiram-ethanol reaction.

References

1. National estimates of the 10 leading causes of nonfatal injuries treated in hospital emergency departments, United States-2015. Centers for Disease Control and Prevention website. https://www.cdc.gov/injury/wisqars/pdf/leading_causes_of_nonfatal_injury_2015-a.pdf. Accessed March 1, 2018.
2. Centers for Disease Control and Prevention, National Center on Health Statistics. NCHS Data on Drug-Poisoning Deaths: fact sheet. Centers for Disease Control and Prevention website. https://www.cdc.gov/nchs/data/factsheets/factsheet_drug_poisoning.htm. Updated April 5, 2016. Accessed March 1, 2018.

3. Injury facts: the source for injury stats. National Safety Council website. http://www.nsc.org/learn/safety-knowledge/Pages/injury-facts.aspx. Accessed March 1, 2018.
4. Poison centers nationwide. Poison Help, Health Resources and Services Administration website. https://poisonhelp.hrsa.gov/poison-centers/. Accessed March 1, 2018.
5. Gummin DD, Mowry JB, Spyker DA, Brooks DE, Fraser MO, Banner W. 2016 Annual Report of the American Association of Poison Control Centers' National Poison Data System (NPDS): 34th annual report. *Clin Toxicol.* 2017;55(10):1072-1254.
6. National Academy of Sciences. *Forging a Poison Prevention and Control System.* Washington, DC: National Academic Press; 2004.
7. Poison centers—an information paper. American College of Emergency Physicians website. https://www.acep.org/Content.aspx?id=70370#sm.0000vyjqgsa95e2uwy91hykef6zea. Accessed March 1, 2018.
8. Toxic syndrome/toxidromes. Chemical Hazards Emergency Medical Management, US Department of Health and Human Services website. https://chemm.nlm.nih.gov/toxicsyndromes.htm. Accessed March 1, 2018.
9. Part 1: executive summary: 2010 American Heart Association Guidelines for Cardiopulmonary Resuscitation and Emergency Cardiovascular Care. *Circulation.* 2010;122(18)(suppl 3):S840.
10. Olson KR. Activated charcoal for acute poisoning: one toxicologist's journey. *J Med Toxicol.* 2010;6(2):190-198.
11. Murphy CM. Principles of toxicology. In: Cone D, Brice JH, Delbridge TR, Myers JB, eds. *Emergency Medical Services: Clinical Practice and Systems Oversight.* Vol 2. 2nd ed. West Sussex, England: John Wiley & Sons; 2015:333-340.
12. Kurowski JA, Kay M. Caustic ingestions and foreign bodies ingestions in pediatric patients. *Pediatr Clin North Am.* 2017;64(3):507-524.
13. Marx JA, Hockberger RS, Walls RM. *Rosen's Emergency Medicine: Concepts and Clinical Practice.* 8th ed. St. Louis, MO: Saunders; 2014.
14. Tormoehlen LM, Tekulve KJ, Nañagas KA. Hydrocarbon toxicity: a review. *Clin Toxicol.* 2014;52(5):479-489.
15. Larson D. *Clinical Chemistry: Fundamentals and Laboratory Techniques.* Amsterdam, Netherlands: Elsevier; 2016.
16. BASF Chemical Emergency Medical Guidelines: Methanol (CH_3OH): Information and recommendations for doctors at hospitals/emergency departments. Code: E021-004. BASF Corporation. https://www.basf.com/documents/corp/en/sustainability/employees-and-society/employees/occupational-medicine/medical-guidelines/Methanol_C_BASF_medGuidelines_E021.pdf. Reviewed 2016. Accessed April 11, 2018.
17. Brent J. Fomepizole for ethylene glycol and methanol poisoning. *N Engl J Med.* 2009;360(21):2216-2223.
18. Thanacoody RH, Gilfillan C, Bradberry SM, et al. Management of poisoning with ethylene glycol and methanol in the UK: a prospective study conducted by the National Poisons Information Service (NPIS). *Clin Toxicol.* 2016;54(2):134-140.
19. Korabathina K. Methanol toxicity treatment and management. Medscape website. https://emedicine.medscape.com/article/1174890-treatment. Updated January 30, 2017. Accessed March 1, 2018.
20. Ethylene glycol: Toxicology Data Network. National Institutes of Health website. https://toxnet.nlm.nih.gov/cgi-bin/sis/search/a?dbs+hsdb:@term+@DOCNO+5012. Updated April 26, 2012. Accessed March 1, 2018.
21. Ethylene glycol and propylene glycol toxicity: how should patients exposed to ethylene glycol be treated? Agency for Toxic Substances and Disease Registry website. https://www.atsdr.cdc.gov/csem/csem.asp?csem=12&po=13. Updated October 3, 2007. Accessed March 1, 2018.
22. Stremski E, Hennes H. Accidental isopropanol ingestion in children. *Pediatr Emerg Care.* 2000;16(4):238-240.
23. Iron poisoning. Poison Control, National Capital Poison Center website. https://www.poison.org/articles/2014-jun/iron-poisoning. Accessed March 1, 2018.
24. Abhilash KPP, Arul JJ, Bala D. Fatal overdose of iron tablets in adults. *Indian J Crit Care Med.* 2013;17(5):311-313.
25. National Center for Environmental Health, Division of Emergency and Environmental Health Services. Lead. Centers for Disease Control and Prevention website. https://www.cdc.gov/nceh/lead/. Updated December 4, 2017. Accessed March 1, 2018.
26. Bjørklund G, Dadar, M, Mutter, J, Aaseth J. The toxicology of mercury: current research and emerging trends. *Environ Res.* 2017;159(suppl C):545-554.
27. Diaz JH. Poisoning by herbs and plants: rapid toxidromic classification and diagnosis. *Wilderness Environ Med.* 2016;27(1):136-152.
28. Stone CK, Humphries RL. *CURRENT Diagnosis and Treatment: Emergency Medicine.* 8th ed. New York, NY: McGraw Hill Education/Medical; 2017.
29. McKay CA Jr. Toxin-induced respiratory distress. *Emerg Med Clin North Am.* 2014;32(1):127-147.
30. Schaider JJ, Barkin RM, Hayden SR, et al. *Rosen and Barkin's 5-Minute Emergency Medicine Consult.* 4th ed. Philadelphia, PA: Lippincott Williams and Wilkins; 2010.
31. Zakharov S, Vaneckova M, Seidl Z, et al. Successful use of hydroxocobalamin and sodium thiosulfate in acute cyanide poisoning: a case report with follow-up. *Basic Clin Pharmacol Toxicol.* 2015;117(3):209-212.
32. Auerbach PS, Cushing TA, Harris NS. *Wilderness Medicine.* 7th ed. Amsterdam, Netherlands: Elsevier; 2016.
33. National Institute for Occupational Safety and Health Education and Information Division. Insects and scorpions. Centers for Disease Control and Prevention website. https://www.cdc.gov/niosh/topics/insects/default.html. Updated July 1, 2016. Accessed March 1, 2018.
34. McDade J, Aygun B, Ware RE. Brown recluse spider (*Loxosceles reclusa*) envenomation leading to acute hemolytic anemia in six adolescents. *J Pediatr.* 2010;156(1):155-157.
35. National Institute for Occupational Safety and Health Education and Information Division. Venomous snakes. Centers for Disease Control and Prevention website. https://www.cdc.gov/niosh/topics/snakes/default.html. Updated July 1, 2016. Accessed March 1, 2018.
36. Part 1: executive summary: 2010 American Heart Association Guidelines for Cardiopulmonary Resuscitation and Emergency Cardiovascular Care. *Circulation.* 2010;122(18)(suppl 3):S639-S946.
37. Centers for Disease Control and Prevention, National Center for Injury Prevention and Control, Division of Unintentional Injury Prevention. Heroin. Centers for Disease Control and Prevention website. https://www.cdc.gov/drugoverdose/opioids/heroin.html. Updated August 29, 2017. Accessed March 1, 2018.
38. The National Institute for Occupational Safety and Health Education and Information Division. Fentanyl: preventing occupational exposure to emergency responders. Centers

for Disease Control and Prevention website. https://www.cdc.gov/niosh/topics/fentanyl/default.html. Accessed March 1, 2018.

39. Gaither JR, Leventhal JM, Ryan SA, Camenga DR. National trends in hospitalizations for opioid poisonings among children and adolescents, 1997 to 2012. *JAMA Pediatr*. 2016 Dec 1;170(12):1195-1201.
40. Fentanyl patch can be deadly to children. US Food and Drug Administration, US Department of Health and Human Services website. https://www.fda.gov/ForConsumers/ConsumerUpdates/ucm300803.htm. Updated January 4, 2018. Accessed March 1, 2018.
41. Yin S. Malicious use of pharmaceuticals in children. *J Pediatr*. 2010;157(5):832-836.
42. Barceloux DG. *Medical Toxicology of Drug Abuse: Synthesized Chemicals and Psychoactive Plants*. Hoboken, NJ: John Wiley & Sons; 2012.
43. Honderick T, Williams D, Seaberg D, Wears R. A prospective, randomized, controlled trial of benzodiazepines and nitroglycerin or nitroglycerin alone in the treatment of cocaine-associated acute coronary syndromes. *Am J Emerg Med*. 2003;21(1):39-42.
44. US Department of Transportation, National Highway Traffic Safety Administration. *EMT-Paramedic: National Standard Curriculum*. EMS.gov website. https://www.ems.gov/pdf/education/Emergency-Medical-Technician-Paramedic/Paramedic_1998.pdf. Accessed March 1, 2018.
45. Forrest JS. Phencyclidine (PCP)-related psychiatric disorders. Medscape website. https://emedicine.medscape.com/article/290476-overview. Updated February 14, 2018. Accessed March 1, 2018.
46. Gitlin M. Lithium side effects and toxicity: prevalence and management strategies. *Int J Bipolar Disord*. 2016;4:27.
47. Ibuprofen—drug summary. Prescribers' Digital Reference website. http://www.pdr.net/drug-summary/Ibuprofen-Tablets-ibuprofen-2618. Accessed March 1, 2018.
48. Yoon E, Babar A, Choudhary M, Kutner M, Pyrsopoulos N. Acetaminophen-induced hepatotoxicity: a comprehensive update. *J Clin Transl Hepatol*. 2016;4(2):131-142.
49. Farrell SE. Acetaminophen toxicity. Medscape website. https://emedicine.medscape.com/article/820200-overview. Updated January 23, 2018. Accessed March 1, 2018.
50. Alcohol use disorder. National Institute on Alcohol Abuse and Alcoholism website. https://www.niaaa.nih.gov/alcohol-health/overview-alcohol-consumption/alcohol-use-disorders. Accessed March 1, 2018.
51. Centers for Disease Control and Prevention, National Center for Injury Prevention and Control, Division of Unintentional Injury Prevention. Impaired driving: get the facts. Centers for Disease Control and Prevention website. https://www.cdc.gov/motorvehiclesafety/impaired_driving/impaired-drv_factsheet.html. Updated June 16, 2017. Accessed March 1, 2018.
52. Alcohol use disorder: a comparison between DSM-IV and DSM-5. National Institute on Alcohol Abuse and Alcoholism website. https://pubs.niaaa.nih.gov/publications/dsmfactsheet/dsmfact.pdf. Accessed March 1, 2018.
53. Aggrawal A. *Forensic Medicine and Toxicology for MBBS*. New Delhi, India: Avichal Publishing Company; 2017.
54. Thomson AD, Marshall EJ. The natural history and pathophysiology of Wernicke's encephalopathy and Korsakoff's psychosis. *Alcohol*. 2006;Mar-Apr41(2):151-158.
55. Donnino MW, Vega J, Miller J, Walsh M. Myths and misconceptions of Wernicke's encephalopathy: what every emergency physician should know. *Ann Emerg Med*. 2007; Dec;50(6):715-721.
56. National Association of Emergency Medical Technicians. *PHTLS: Prehospital Trauma Life Support*. 8th ed. Burlington, MA: Jones & Bartlett Learning; 2014.
57. Centers for Disease Control and Prevention, National Center for Health Statistics. Chronic liver disease and cirrhosis. Centers for Disease Control and Prevention website. https://www.cdc.gov/nchs/fastats/liver-disease.htm. Updated October 6, 2016. Accessed March 1, 2018.
58. Easter JS, Haukoos JS, Claud J, et al. *Traumatic Intracranial Injury in Intoxicated Patients With Minor Head Trauma*. Des Plaines, IL: The Society for Academic Emergency Medicine; 2013.
59. Long D, Long B, Koyfman A. The emergency medicine management of severe alcohol withdrawal. *Am J Emerg Med*. 2017;35(7):1005-1011.
60. National Clinical Guideline Centre (UK). NICE Clinical Guidelines, No. 100. *Alcohol Use Disorders: Diagnosis and Clinical Management of Alcohol-Related Physical Complications* [Internet]. London, England: Royal College of Physicians (UK); 2010.
61. Burns MJ. Delirium tremens (DTs). Medscape website. https://emedicine.medscape.com/article/166032-overview. Updated March 7, 2017. Accessed March 1, 2018.
62. Barker LR, Fiebach NH, Kern DE, Thomas PA, Ziegelstein RC, Zieve PD. *Principles of Ambulatory Medicine*. 7th ed. Philadelphia, PA: Lippincott Williams and Wilkins; 2006.

Suggested Readings

ACMT and AACT position statement: preventing occupational fentanyl and fentanyl analog exposure to emergency responders. American College of Medical Toxicology website. https://www.acmt.net/_Library/Fentanyl_Position/Fentanyl_PPE_Emergency_Responders_.pdf. Accessed March 1, 2018.

DeBoer S, Seaver M. Pediatric toxicology emergencies. *J Emerg Nurs*.

Drugs of abuse. National Institute on Drug Abuse website. https://www.drugabuse.gov/drugs-abuse. Accessed March 1, 2018.

Emergency toxicology: from database to subspecialty. American College of Emergency Physicians website. https://www.acep.org/content.aspx?id=34084#sm.0000vyjqgsa95e2uwy91hykef6zea. Accessed March 1, 2018.

Hoffman RS, Howland MA, Lewin NA, Nelson LS, Goldfrank LR. *Goldfrank's Toxicologic Emergencies*. 10th ed. New York, NY: Appleton & Lange; 2011.

Overview of alcohol consumption. National Institute on Alcohol Abuse and Alcoholism website. https://www.niaaa.nih.gov/alcohol-health/overview-alcohol-consumption. Accessed March 1, 2018.

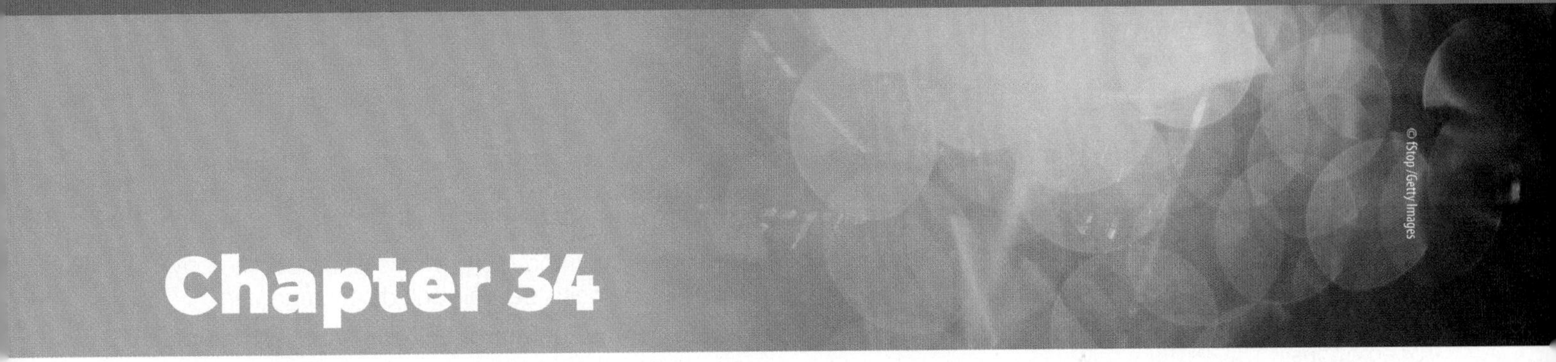
© fStop/Getty Images

Chapter 34

Behavioral and Psychiatric Disorders

NATIONAL EMS EDUCATION STANDARD COMPETENCIES

Medicine

Integrates assessment findings with principles of epidemiology and pathophysiology to formulate a field impression and implement a comprehensive treatment/disposition plan for a patient with a medical complaint.

Psychiatric

Recognition of
- Behaviors that pose a risk to the EMS provider, patient, or others (p 1291)

Assessment and management of
- Basic principles of the mental health system (p 1269)
- Suicidal/risk (pp 1285–1287)

Anatomy, physiology, epidemiology, pathophysiology, psychosocial impact, presentations, assessment, prognosis, and management of
- Acute psychosis (pp 1272–1276, 1286, 1291–1293)
- Agitated delirium (pp 1272–1276, 1278, 1291–1293)
- Cognitive disorders (pp 1277–1279)
- Thought disorders (pp 1280–1281, 1282–1283)
- Mood disorders (pp 1283–1285)
- Neurotic disorders (pp 1281–1282)
- Substance-related disorders/addictive behavior (p 1287)
- Somatoform disorders (pp 1287–1288)
- Factitious disorders (p 1288)
- Personality disorders (p 1290)
- Patterns of violence/abuse/neglect (Chapter 49, *Abuse and Neglect*)
- Organic psychoses (pp 1270–1272)

OBJECTIVES

Upon completion of this chapter, the paramedic student will be able to:

1. List three crucial principles that should be considered in the prehospital care of any patient with a behavioral emergency. (p 1269)
2. Define what constitutes a behavioral emergency. (pp 1269–1270)
3. Identify potential causes for behavioral and psychiatric illnesses. (pp 1270–1272)
4. Describe effective techniques for interviewing a patient during a behavioral emergency. (p 1275)
5. Outline key elements in the prehospital patient examination during a behavioral emergency. (pp 1275–1276)
6. Distinguish between key symptoms and management techniques for selected behavioral and psychiatric disorders. (pp 1276–1290)
7. Identify factors that must be considered when assessing suicide risk. (p 1286)
8. Formulate appropriate interview questions to determine suicidal intent. (p 1287)
9. Explain prehospital management techniques for the patient who has attempted suicide. (p 1287)
10. Explain variations in approach to behavioral emergencies in children. (p 1291)
11. Describe assessment of the potentially violent patient. (p 1291)
12. Outline measures that may be used in an attempt to safely defuse a potentially violent patient situation. (pp 1292–1293)
13. List situations when patient restraints can be used. (pp 1292–1293)
14. Discuss key principles in patient restraint. (pp 1293–1294)
15. Describe safety measures taken when patient violence is anticipated. (pp 1296–1297)

KEY TERMS

acute psychosis A condition that refers to a patient who presents with one or more of the following criteria: a sudden onset of delusions that rapidly change; hallucinations; bizarre behavior and posture; or disorganized speech.

affect An outward manifestation of a person's feelings or emotions.

anhedonia The inability to enjoy what is usually pleasurable.

anorexia nervosa An emotional disturbance concerning body image manifested as an eating disorder characterized by a prolonged refusal to eat, resulting in emaciation, amenorrhea, and an abnormal fear of becoming obese.

anxiety A state or feeling of apprehension, uneasiness, agitation, uncertainty, and fear resulting from the anticipation of some threat or danger.

autism spectrum disorder (ASD) A range of neurodevelopmental disorders characterized by three sets of behavioral features: (1) impairment in social interaction, (2) communication deficits (both verbal and nonverbal), and (3) restricted, repetitive behaviors, including decreased imaginative play, stereotyped behaviors, and inflexible adherence to routines.

behavioral emergency A change in mood or behavior that cannot be tolerated by the involved person or others and that requires immediate attention.

biologic disturbances Disorders that result from a physical rather than a purely psychological cause.

bipolar disorder A disorder marked by alternating periods of mania and depression; formerly known as manic-depressive disorder.

bulimia nervosa A disorder characterized by an insatiable craving for food, often resulting in episodes of binge eating followed by purging (through self-induced vomiting or use of laxatives), depression, and self-deprivation.

chemical restraint The use of drugs to control behavior.

conversion disorder A constellation of neurologic symptoms that are not consciously or deliberately produced and that cannot be explained by a physical examination. These disorders often cause clinically significant disruption in social or occupational functioning. Also referred to as functional neurologic disorder.

delirium A medical emergency characterized by an abrupt disorientation for time and place, usually with delusions and hallucinations; may be reversible if causative etiology is identified.

delusions Persistent beliefs or perceptions held by a person despite evidence that refutes those beliefs (ie, false beliefs).

dementia A slow, progressive, and irreversible loss of awareness of time and place. It usually involves an inability to learn new things or recall recent events.

depression A mood disturbance characterized by feelings of sadness, despair, and discouragement.

disruptive, impulse-control, and conduct disorders A group of psychiatric conditions characterized by the inability to control emotions or to resist an impulse or a temptation to perform some act that is unlawful, socially unacceptable, or self-harmful.

dissociative disorders A group of psychological illnesses in which a particular mental function is separated (dissociated) from the mind as a whole.

dyskinesia A movement disorder characterized by involuntary muscle movements; often an adverse effect of prolonged use of antipsychotic medications.

dysthymia A form of depression that is chronic in nature, lasting as long as 2 years or more.

excited delirium A sudden state of delirium, extreme psychomotor agitation, unusual strength, and hyperadrenergic autonomic dysfunction, typically in the setting of acute or chronic drug abuse or serious mental illness.

factitious disorders A group of disorders in which symptoms are deliberately produced, feigned, or exaggerated to mimic a true illness. There is no motive for personal gain; the goal is merely to assume the role of a patient.

hallucinations The apparent perception of sights, sounds, and other sensory phenomena that are not actually present.

major depression A disabling condition that adversely affects a person's family, work, or school life, sleeping and eating habits, and general health; also known as major depressive disorder and clinical depression.

mania A mood disorder characterized by extreme excitement, hyperactivity, agitation, and sometimes violent and self-destructive behavior.

mental status examination (MSE) An evaluation tool that includes an assessment of appearance and behavior, speech and language, emotional stability, and cognitive abilities.

mood disorders Conditions in which the emotions that a person normally experiences in life (eg, happiness, depression, fear, anxiety) undergo undesirable and possibly distressing changes.

Munchausen syndrome A self-imposed factitious disorder imposed in which the patient makes routine pleas for treatment and hospitalization for a symptomatic, but imaginary, illness to gain sympathy or attention.

Munchausen syndrome by proxy A factitious disorder imposed on another in which a person injures or induces illness in others (usually children) to gain sympathy or attention.

neurocognitive disorder A disorder that results in a disturbance of cognitive functioning.

obsessive-compulsive disorder (OCD) A psychiatric disorder in which a person feels stress or anxiety about thoughts or rituals over which the person has little control.

panic disorder An anxiety disorder characterized by unexpected and repeated episodes of intense fear accompanied by physical symptoms that may include chest pain, heart palpitations, shortness of breath, dizziness, or abdominal distress.

paranoia A condition characterized by an elaborate, overly suspicious system of thinking.

personality disorders A large group of conditions distinguished by a failure to learn from experience or to adapt appropriately to changes; results in personal distress and impairment of social functioning.

phobia An anxiety disorder characterized by an obsessive, irrational, and intense fear of a specific object or activity.

posttraumatic stress disorder (PTSD) An anxiety disorder that can occur following a series of disturbing events or a single, emotionally traumatic incident.

psychotic behavior Maladaptive behavior involving major distortions of reality.

schizophrenia A group of disorders characterized by recurrent episodes of psychotic behavior.

somatic symptom disorders Any of a large group of neurotic disorders characterized by symptoms suggesting physical illness or disease, for which there are no organic or physiologic causes; also known as somatoform disorder.

suicide The act of a human being intentionally causing his or her own death.

Caring for a patient with a behavioral or psychiatric emergency can be challenging, even for the most experienced paramedic. These emergencies call for strong diagnostic skills and a good understanding of pharmacology and toxicology. They also require thorough assessment skills to identify organic illness that can masquerade as a psychiatric condition. Behavioral and psychiatric emergencies demand excellent communication skills, a compassionate and caring approach, and supportive measures to prevent a crisis from escalating.

Understanding Behavioral Emergencies

An estimated 17.9% of Americans aged 18 years and older (1 in 5 adults) have a diagnosable mental disorder in a given year. This number translates to about 43.4 million people. These numbers do not include substance use disorders.[1] The National Institute of Mental Health has estimated that 1 in 25 people have mental illnesses that severely limit their daily activities.[2] Mental health problems are a leading cause of disability in the United States.

There is no clear agreement or ideal model for normal behavior. Normal behavior generally is considered to be adaptive behavior that is accepted by society, which can vary by culture and ethnic group. The concept of abnormal (maladaptive) behavior also is defined by society and involves the following characteristics:

- Deviates from society's norms and expectations
- Interferes with well-being and ability to function
- Harms the person or group

Courtesy Ray Kemp, St. Charles, MO.

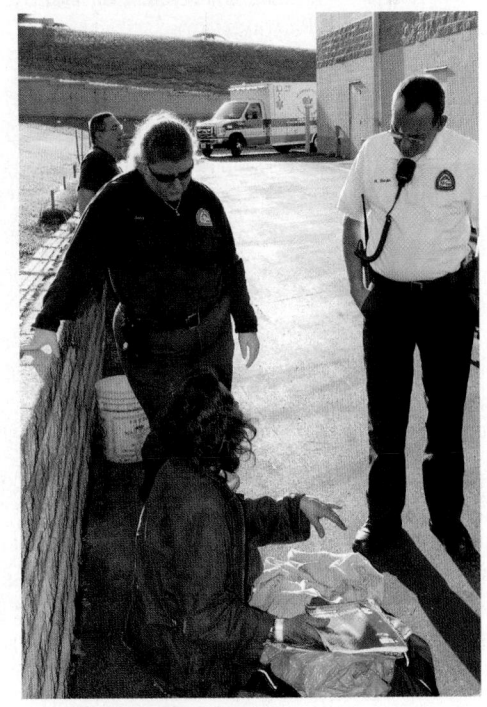

CRITICAL THINKING

Can you think of a time in your life when you, a family member, or a close friend had a behavior that fit the definition of abnormal behavior? How did it make you feel?

A **behavioral emergency** can be defined as a change in mood or behavior that cannot be tolerated by the involved person or others and that requires immediate attention. Behavioral emergencies may range from a brief inability to cope with stress or anxiety to more intense situations in which patients may be dangerous to themselves and others. However, most people with mental illness function well on a daily basis. Common conditions such as depression, anxiety disorders, and mild personality disorders often are effectively managed with medication, therapy, and counseling in outpatient mental health centers. Most behavioral emergencies have a biologic/organic, psychosocial, or sociocultural cause. Mental illness also may be the result of more than one of these factors (**FIGURE 34-1**). Common myths about mental illness are listed in **BOX 34-1**.

Biologic Causes

Physical or biochemical disturbances in the brain can result in significant changes in behavior. In mental health care, **biologic disturbances** are disorders that result from a physical rather than a purely psychological cause that may cause or contribute to a mental problem. Examples of biologic causes include genetic factors, prenatal and postnatal factors (including infection, and endocrine, metabolic, and vascular disorders), an imbalance in brain chemistry (which may have a heritable component), and alterations in neurotransmission. An example of a biologic mental illness is schizophrenia, described later in this chapter. In this illness, specific genes have been identified that may influence the balance of chemicals in the brain. As described in Chapter 13, *Principles*

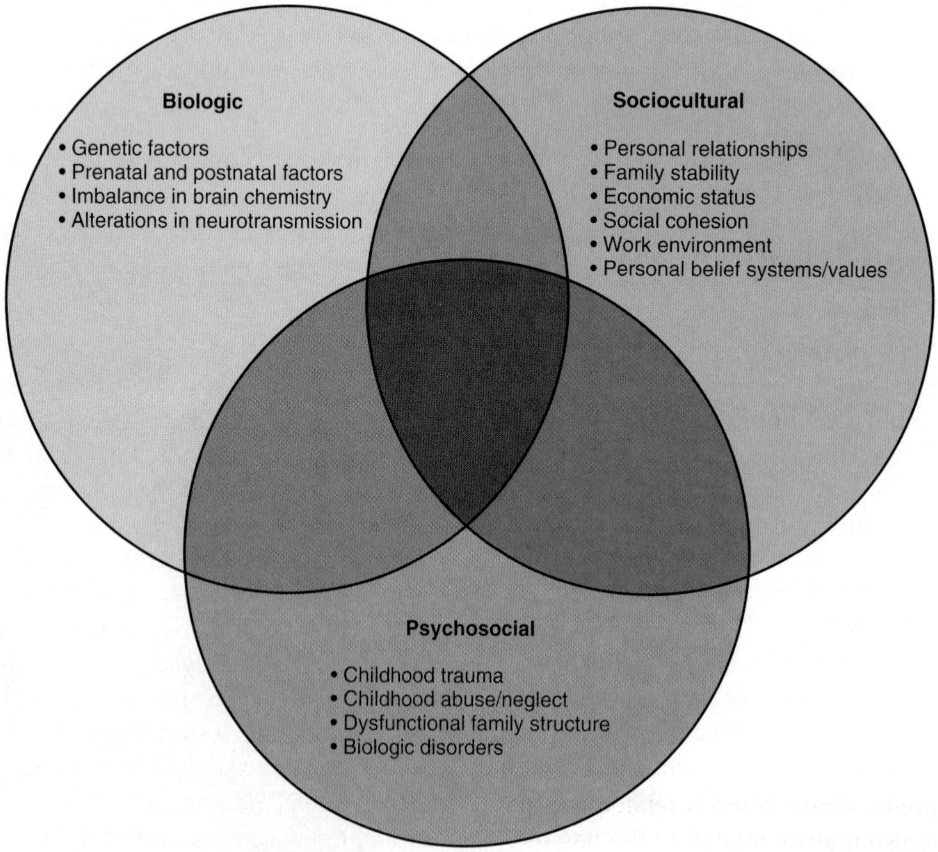

FIGURE 34-1 Common causes of behavioral emergencies.

BOX 34-1 Common Myths About Mental Illness

Myth. Psychiatric disorders are not true medical illnesses like heart disease and diabetes.
Fact. Brain disorders, like heart disease and diabetes, are true medical illnesses. Research shows that psychiatric disorders have genetic and biologic causes. Also, these diseases can be treated effectively.
Myth. People with a severe mental illness are usually dangerous and violent.
Fact. Statistics show that the incidence of violence among people who have a brain disorder is not much higher than it is in the general population. People living with mental illness are more likely to have violence inflicted upon them.
Myth. Mental illness is the result of bad parenting.
Fact. Most experts agree that biologic factors, along with environmental risk factors, lead to psychiatric disorders. In other words, mental illnesses result from a combination of factors. One in five children aged 13 to 18 years have or will develop a mental illness.
Myth. Depression is just sadness. People who are depressed can just snap out of it.
Fact. Depression is not something that can be wished away. It results from changes in brain chemistry or brain function. Medication and/or cognitive therapy often help people with depression to recover.
Myth. Mental illness is caused by personal weakness.
Fact. Like other serious illnesses, mental illness is not a result of personal weakness. It is caused by environmental and biologic factors.
Myth. Some races are more prone to mental illness.
Fact. All races and ethnicities are affected by the same rate of mental illness. There is no single group of people more likely than others to have a mental health condition.
Myth. Addiction is a lifestyle choice and shows a lack of willpower. People with a substance abuse problem are morally weak or "bad."
Fact. Addiction is a disease that generally results from changes in brain chemistry. It has nothing to do with being a bad person.

Modified from: Powell S. Dispelling myths on mental illness. National Alliance on Mental Illness website. https://www.nami.org/Blogs/NAMI-Blog/July-2015/Dispelling-Myths-on-Mental-Illness. Published July 17, 2015. Accessed Janaury 28, 2018.

of Pharmacology and Emergency Medications, neurotransmitters are responsible for communication among the brain cells. To review, the predominant neurotransmitters in the brain include glutamate, gamma-aminobutyric acid (GABA), serotonin, dopamine, and norepinephrine. Most scientists believe that mental illnesses result from problems with communication between these neurotransmitters and the neurons in the brain.

Organic causes of behavioral emergencies that are discussed throughout this text include substance abuse, trauma, illness (eg, diabetes, electrolyte imbalance), infections, tumors, and dementia (BOX 34-2). It is important that the paramedic consider the possibility of these medical conditions as part of a differential diagnosis in all behavioral emergencies.

Psychosocial Causes

Psychosocial mental illness often is related to personality type. It also may be related to the person's ability to resolve situational conflict in life. For example, psychosocial mental illness may result from childhood trauma, child abuse or neglect, or a dysfunctional family structure that affects relationships with parents and siblings. Biologic disorders may contribute to psychosocial causes of mental illness.

Sociocultural Causes

Sociocultural causes of mental illness are related to the way a person balances emotions, thoughts, and interactions in society. When this balance shifts rapidly, a person may experience emotional turmoil that results in crisis. Factors that may be related to sociocultural causes of behavioral emergencies include personal relationships, family stability, economic status, social cohesion, work environment, and personal belief systems and values. Changes in behavior caused by personal or situational stress often are linked to a specific event (eg, the death of a loved one) or a series of events. Examples include environmental violence related to society (eg, war, terrorism, riots), personal violence (eg, rape, assault), ongoing discrimination or prejudice, and economic and employment problems.

BOX 34-2 Common Medical Conditions That Manifest as Behavioral Disorders

Metabolic Disorders
Glucose, sodium, calcium, or magnesium imbalance
Acid–base imbalance
Acute hypoxia
Renal failure
Hepatic failure

Endocrine Disorders
Thyroid disease
Parathyroid disease
Adrenal hormone imbalance

Infectious Diseases
Encephalitis
Meningitis
Brain abscess
Severe systemic infection

Trauma
Concussion
Intracranial hematoma (especially subdural hematoma)

Cardiovascular Disorders
Cardiac dysrhythmia
Hypotension
Transient ischemic attack
Cerebrovascular accident (or stroke)
Hypertensive encephalopathy

Neoplastic Diseases
Central nervous system tumors or metastases

Degenerative Diseases
Alzheimer-type dementia
Other dementias

Drug Abuse
Alcohol
Barbiturates
Narcotics
Sedative-hypnotics
Amphetamines and other stimulants
Hallucinogens

Drug Reactions
Beta adrenergic blockers
Antihypertensives
Cardiac drugs
Bronchodilators
Beta adrenergic agonists
Anticonvulsants

NOTE

The disability-adjusted life year (DALY) is a measure of overall disease burden, expressed as the number of years lost due to ill health, disability, or early death. The World Health Organization estimates that in the United States, 13.6% of DALYs are caused by disorders in the mental and behavioral disorders category.

Modified from: US DALYs contributed by mental and behavioral disorders. National Institute of Mental Health website. https://www.nimh.nih.gov/health/statistics/disability/us-dalys-contributed-by-mental-and-behavioral-disorders.shtml. Accessed February 23, 2018.

Assessment and Management of Behavioral Emergencies

The initial assessment and management of a patient with a behavioral emergency are similar to those used in any other emergency medical services (EMS) response. These steps include ensuring scene safety, containing the crisis, providing proper emergency medical care, and transporting the patient to an appropriate health care facility. In addition, most EMS systems have protocols that call for law enforcement personnel to evaluate the scene for possible danger and to control any acts of aggression by the patient.

Assessment

Paramedics should begin the assessment by creating a rapport with the patient. They can do this while gathering information needed for immediate management of life-threatening conditions. On arrival, paramedics should survey the scene for any relevant details. Such details may include evidence of substance abuse, a suicide attempt, or other clues that may shed light on the state of the patient. The patient should be observed for emotional response, such as fear, anger, confusion, or hostility. While providing patient care, the paramedic should focus the evaluation on the patient's level of cognitive functioning, which includes alertness, orientation, speech patterns, **affect**, and the way in which the patient interacts with friends, loved ones, and family members. When possible, the number of people around the patient should be limited, which helps to control the scene. Anyone who interferes with the scene or the patient assessment or who adversely affects the patient's condition should be asked to leave the area or law enforcement may need to assist.

Other information can be volunteered by the patient, obtained from the patient interview, or provided by family members, bystanders, and first responders. The patient's family or caregiver should be interviewed about the patient's usual level of functioning, recent stress in the patient's life, and approaches that may help the paramedic to gain the patient's trust and cooperation. Information that should be obtained for a full background and history of the event include significant medical history, medications the patient has taken (**TABLE 34-1**), past psychiatric problems, and

TABLE 34-1 Examples of Drugs Used to Treat Psychiatric Disorders

Trade Name(s)	Generic Name	Drug Class
Abilify	Aripiprazole	Antipsychotic
Adderall	Amphetamine/ dextroamphetamine	CNS stimulant used to treat ADHD
Akineton	Biperiden	Antiparkinson agent
Anafranil	Clomipramine	Antidepressant
Asendin	Amoxapine	Antidepressant
Ativan	Lorazepam	Antianxiety
Aventyl	Nortriptyline	Antidepressant
Buspar	Buspirone	Anxiolytic
Celexa	Citalopram	SSRI
Clozaril	Clozapine	Antipsychotic
Cymbalta, Irenka	Duloxetine	Antidepressant
Desyrel	Trazodone	Antidepressant
Elavil, Levate, Amitriptyline, Triptyn	Amitriptyline	Antidepressant
Enlafax XR	Venlafaxine	Antidepressant
Fluanxol	Flupenthixol dihydrochloride	Antipsychotic
Geodon	Ziprasidone	Antipsychotic
Haldol, Haloperidol, Peridol	Haloperidol	Antipsychotic
Lamictal	Lamotrigine	Anticonvulsant
Latuda	Lurasidone	Antipsychotic
Lexapro	Escitalopram	SSRI antidepressant
Lithium, Lithane, Carbolith, Duralith, Lithizine	Lithium carbonate	Antipsychotic
Luvox	Fluvoxamine maleate	Antidepressant
Marplan	Isocarboxazid	Antidepressant
Mellaril, Thioridazine, Ridazine	Thioridazine	Antipsychotic
Modecate, Fluphenazine, Permitil, Moditen	Fluphenazine	Antipsychotic
Nardil	Phenelzine	Antidepressant

(continued)

TABLE 34-1 Examples of Drugs Used to Treat Psychiatric Disorders *(continued)*

Trade Name(s)	Generic Name	Drug Class
Neuleptil	Pericyazine	Antipsychotic
Norpramin, Pertofrane	Desipramine	Antidepressant
Nozinan	Methotrimeprazine	Antipsychotic
Orap	Pimozide	Antipsychotic
Parnate	Tranylcypromine	Antidepressant
Paxil	Paroxetine	SSRI
Piportil L4	Pipotiazine	Antipsychotic
Prozac	Fluoxetine	Antidepressant
Remeron	Mirtazapine	Antidepressant
Risperdal	Risperidone	Antipsychotic
Ritalin	Methylphenidate	Cerebral stimulant
Seroquel	Quetiapine	Antipsychotic
Serentil	Mesoridazine	Antipsychotic
Serzone	Nefazodone	Antidepressant
Sinequan, Doxepin, Triadapin	Doxepin	Antidepressant
Sparine	Promazine	Antipsychotic
Stelazine, Trifluoperazine, Terfluzine, Flurazine, Solazine	Trifluoperazine	Antipsychotic
Stemetil, Prorazin, Prochlorperazine	Prochlorperazine	Antipsychotic
Surmontil, Trimip, Tripramine, Rhotrimine	Trimipramine	Antidepressant
Tegretol, Carbamazepine, Mazepine	Carbamazepine	Antipsychotic
Thorazine, Largactil, Chlorpromanyl, Chlorpromazine	Chlorpromazine	Antipsychotic
Tofranil, Imipramine, Impril, Pramine	Imipramine	Antidepressant
Trilafon, Perphenazine	Perphenazine	Antipsychotic
Trileptal, Oxtellar XR	Oxcarbazepine	Anticonvulsant
Triptil	Protriptyline	Antidepressant
Valium, Diazepam, Diazemuls, Vivol	Diazepam	Antianxiety
Wellbutrin	Bupropion	Antidepressant
Xanax, Alpraz, Alprazol, Nu-Alpraz	Alprazolam	Antianxiety
Zoloft	Sertraline	SSRI antidepressant
Zyprexa	Olanzapine	Antipsychotic

Abbreviations: ADHD, attention-deficit/hyperactivity disorder; CNS, central nervous system; SSRI, selective serotonin reuptake inhibitor any precipitating factors that may have contributed to the behavioral emergency.

Interview Techniques

After managing any life-threatening illness or injury, the patient should be interviewed if possible. The paramedic should not ask for more details than are needed. A limited and supportive interview strengthens the paramedic's rapport with the patient. It also can help to establish and maintain a relationship during the provision of patient care. As described in Chapter 17, *History Taking*, and Chapter 18, *Scene Size-up and Primary Assessment*, effective interview techniques include active listening, showing support and empathy, preventing interruptions, and respecting the patient's personal space by limiting physical touch (BOX 34-3).

Mental Status Examination

A **mental status examination (MSE)** is an evaluation tool that can help the paramedic during the patient assessment. Although many variations of MSEs are available (BOX 34-4), most include an assessment of appearance and behavior, speech and language, cognitive abilities, and emotional stability.[3] The following factors should be assessed in each of these areas.

Appearance and behavior

- How does the patient look? Is the person neatly dressed and well groomed?
- Is the patient pleasant and cooperative, or agitated?
- Is the patient's behavior appropriate for the situation?
- What is the patient's body language?
- Do body movements or posture suggest tension, anxiety, hostility, or aggression?
- Does the patient maintain eye contact during the patient interview?

Speech and language

- Is the patient's speech intelligible and normal in tone, volume, and rate?
- Does the tone of the patient's voice change?

BOX 34-3 Ten Useful Interviewing Skills for Behavioral Emergencies

1. Listen to the patient in a caring, concerned, and receptive manner. Be aware of nonverbal cues, such are eye contact, facial expression, and posture. These cues can reassure the patient that you are responding with empathy.
2. Elicit feelings as well as facts to help develop a more accurate impression of the patient. If the patient is anxious, encourage the person to share details relevant to that feeling.
3. Respond to the patient's feelings by acknowledging and labeling them. (For example, you might say, "You seem angry.") This may help validate and legitimize the patient's intense and sometimes overwhelming feelings.
4. Correct cognitive misconceptions or distortions. If a distorted sense of reality is producing fear or anxiety, offer a simple and correct explanation.
5. Explain to the patient the care he or she can expect to receive upon arrival at the medical facility.
6. Offer honest and realistic reassurance and support. Providing this support helps to calm the patient and establishes rapport.
7. Ask effective questions. Ask closed-ended questions if you are seeking immediate information. For example, "Are you thinking of hurting yourself?" and "What medicines did you take?" Open-ended questions are appropriate after you have identified problems that require immediate attention. Such questions allow the patient to develop answers that usually help the paramedic more fully understand the problem.
8. Avoid leading questions, which may cause the person to say things he or she did not intend.
9. Structure the interview to develop a pattern rather than allowing a nonsequential flow of details. Histories or sequences of events in chronologic order usually allow for a fuller understanding of the patient's problem. (This is particularly true for causal relationships.) This order also helps the patient to organize thoughts. Keep the patient's responses focused; for example, ask questions such as "What happened next?" and "Was that before or after what you were just telling me about?"
10. Conclude the interview. After obtaining the relevant information, encourage the patient to describe other important events or feelings.

Modified from: Bassuk EL. *Behavioral Emergencies: A Field Guide for EMTs and Paramedics*. Boston, MA: Little, Brown and Company; 1983.

BOX 34-4 COASTMAP

A memory aid that may help direct components of the MSE is COASTMAP:
Consciousness
Orientation
Activity
Speech
Thought
Memory
Affect and mood
Perception

Modified from: National Highway Traffic Safety Administration. *The National EMS Education Standards*. Washington, DC: US Department of Transportation/National Highway Traffic Safety Administration; 2009.

- Is speech spontaneous, with ease of expression?
- Do the patient's words and sentences proceed in an orderly fashion?

Cognitive abilities

- Is the patient oriented to person, time, and place?
- Does the patient know who and where he or she is?
- Does the patient know who you are?
- Can the patient remain focused on your questions and conversation?
- Is the patient's attention span appropriate?
- Can the patient follow a series of short commands?
- Does the patient respond to directions appropriately?
- Are the patient's comments logical and presented in an organized fashion?

Emotional stability

- Is the patient aware of his or her environment?
- Can the patient describe or rate his or her mood using a scale of 1 to 10?
- Does the patient appear happy, sad, depressed, or angry?
- Is the patient's mood appropriate for the specific situation?
- Does the patient show mood swings or behaviors that indicate anxiety, depression, anger, or hostility?
- Does the patient stay focused during the interview or stray quickly to related topics?
- Is the patient experiencing perceptual distortions or hallucinations?

CRITICAL THINKING

Think about interviewing techniques that you have seen EMS crews use when caring for patients with behavioral emergencies. Were the techniques effective? Could the paramedics have improved their patient care by using any of the techniques listed in Box 34-3?

Difficult Patient Interviews

Some patients with behavioral or psychiatric disorders are difficult to interview. For example, a patient may refuse to talk to the paramedic, as often happens when the family requested EMS assistance without the patient's consent. If a patient refuses to be interviewed, paramedics should speak to the patient in a quiet voice. They should avoid questions that the patient may interpret as an interrogation. Also, paramedics should allow the patient extra time to respond. In contrast, a patient may be extremely talkative, may have disorganized speech, or may be confrontational. Patients who are too talkative need to have their attention focused on the interview, which the paramedic may accomplish by raising a hand or calling the person's name. With a confrontational patient, additional help may be required to ensure scene safety.

Other Patient Care Measures

After the initial assessment and history taking, the remainder of the examination is determined by the patient's overall condition and the nature of the psychiatric problem. The benefits of a thorough physical examination must be weighed against the risks of a patient who might construe the examination as a physical violation. If there is reason to suspect an organic cause for the patient's condition, a physical examination may prove informative. Otherwise, patient care for a person with a behavioral emergency may be limited to maintaining an effective rapport with the patient during transfer to the medical facility.

Specific Behavioral and Psychiatric Disorders

Nearly 300 psychiatric conditions have been identified by mental health professionals.[4] Some patients may have symptoms that are associated with more than one condition. The following are common classifications of mental disorders discussed in this chapter:[5]

- Neurocognitive disorders
- Schizophrenia
- Anxiety disorders
- Mood disorders
- Substance-related disorders
- Somatoform disorders
- Factitious disorders
- Dissociative disorders
- Eating disorders
- Impulse-control disorders
- Personality disorders

Patient care for most behavioral emergencies in the prehospital environment is primarily supportive.

NOTE

The American Psychiatric Association has identified major classes of psychiatric disorders, which it has defined in the *Diagnostic and Statistical Manual of Mental Disorders*. The fifth edition, published in 2013, is referred to by the abbreviation *DSM-5*. Many mental health professionals use the *DSM-5* classifications for assessment and diagnostic purposes. The chapter represents some of the major categories of mental illnesses as discussed in the *DSM-5*, which include the following:

- Neurodevelopmental disorders
- Schizophrenia spectrum and other psychotic disorders
- Bipolar and related disorders
- Depressive disorders
- Anxiety disorders
- Obsessive-compulsive and related disorders
- Trauma- and stressor-related disorders
- Dissociative disorders
- Somatic symptom and related disorders
- Feeding and eating disorders
- Elimination disorders
- Sleep–wake disorders
- Sexual dysfunctions
- Gender dysphoria
- Disruptive, impulse-control, and conduct disorders
- Substance-related and addictive disorders
- Neurocognitive disorders
- Paraphilic disorders
- Other mental disorders
- Other conditions that may be the focus of clinical attention

Modified from: American Psychiatric Association. *Diagnostic and Statistical Manual of Mental Disorders*. 5th ed. Washington, DC: American Psychiatric Association; 2013.

It usually involves providing emotional support, assessing and managing coexisting emergency medical conditions, and transporting the patient for evaluation by a physician. In some cases, paramedics may need to take measures to protect the patient and others from harm. These measures may include the use of physical and chemical restraint (described later in this chapter).

Neurocognitive Disorders

A **neurocognitive disorder** may have an organic cause (eg, a disease process) or be a result of physical or chemical injury, such as trauma or drug abuse. All neurocognitive disorders result in a disturbance of cognitive functioning, which may manifest as delirium or dementia (described in Chapter 24, *Neurology*).

Delirium

Delirium is an abrupt disorientation of time and place that usually involves delusions and hallucinations. **Delusions** are false beliefs. **Hallucinations** are the perception of sights, sounds, and other sensory phenomena that are not actually present. The symptoms vary according to the person's personality, the environment, and the severity of the illness. Common signs and symptoms of delirium include fluctuating symptoms of inattention, memory impairment, disorientation, clouding of consciousness, delusions, and vivid visual hallucinations. Treatment of delirium is aimed at correcting the underlying physical disorder to reduce anxiety (BOX 34-5) and associated mortality. Sedatives may be required to manage the patient. The exact occurrence rate of delirium is unknown. However, some groups of people are more susceptible to delirium than others are. These groups include the following:

- Older adults
- Children
- Burn patients
- Patients who have had major heart surgery
- Patients who have had a previous brain injury (eg, stroke)
- Patients with acquired immunodeficiency syndrome (AIDS)

Dementia

Dementia, now also known as major neurocognitive disorder, is a clinical state characterized by loss of function in multiple cognitive domains. It is a slow,

BOX 34-5 Excited Delirium Syndrome

Excited delirium is a medical emergency and describes a person with profound psychomotor agitation and delirium. It is characterized by (1) acute onset and fluctuating course, (2) reduced clarity of awareness of the environment, (3) perceptual disturbance, disorientation, or memory disturbance, and (4) an underlying general medical condition. Excited delirium is not currently recognized as a medical or psychiatric condition by the America Psychiatric Association or the World Health Organization. It is a label assigned to the state of acute behavioral disinhibition manifested in a cluster of behaviors that may include bizarreness, aggressiveness, agitation, ranting, hyperactivity, **paranoia**, panic, violence, public disturbance, surprising physical strength, profuse sweating attributable to hyperthermia, respiratory arrest, and death. Excited delirium has been reported to result from substance intoxication, psychiatric illness, alcohol withdrawal, head trauma, or a combination of these factors. The condition has gained public notice because it often is blamed for the deaths of people being restrained by law enforcement personnel or who have died while in custody.

Modified from: Best practice guideline: guidelines for the management of excited delirium/acute behavioural disturbance (ABD). Royal College of Emergency Medicine website. https://www.rcem.ac.uk/docs/College%20Guidelines/5p.%20RCEM%20guidelines%20for%20management%20of%20Acute%20Behavioural%20Disturbance%20(May%202016).pdf. Published May 2016. Accessed February 28, 2018; Pollanen MS, Chiasson DA, Cairns JT, et al. Unexpected death related to restraint for excited delirium: a retrospective study of deaths in police custody and in the community. *CMAJ*. 1998;158(12):1603-1607.

BOX 34-6 Some Causes of Dementia

Degenerative Diseases (60% to 70% of cases)

Alzheimer-type dementia
Huntington disease
Parkinson disease (not in all cases)
Cerebellar degenerations
Amyotrophic lateral sclerosis (not in all cases)
Rare genetic and metabolic diseases
Lewy body disease
Prion disease

Vascular Dementia (15% to 20% of cases)

Multi-infarct dementia
Microinfarct dementia
Large infarct dementia
Cerebral embolic disease

Anoxic Dementia (<5% of cases)

Cardiac arrest
Cardiac failure (severe)
Carbon monoxide poisoning

Traumatic Dementia

Dementia pugilistica (boxer's dementia)
Head injury (open or closed)

Infectious Dementia

AIDS dementia
Opportunistic infection
Postencephalitic dementia
Herpes dementia
Fungal meningitis or encephalitis
Bacterial meningitis or encephalitis
Parasitic encephalitis
Brain abscess
Neurosyphilis (general paresis)

Space-Occupying Lesions

Chronic or acute subdural hematoma
Primary brain tumor
Metastatic tumor

Autoimmune Disorders

Disseminated lupus erythematosus
Vasculitis

Toxic Dementia

Alcohol
Metals (eg, lead, mercury, arsenic)
Organic poisons (eg, solvents, some insecticides)

progressive loss of awareness of time and place that usually involves an inability to learn new things or to remember recent events. About 75 types of dementia have been identified (BOX 34-6); however, most cases result from cerebrovascular disease (including stroke) and Alzheimer disease (described in Chapter 24, *Neurology*). Dementia is a major health problem in the United States because of the long life spans of Americans. The prevalence of dementia rapidly increases from about 2% to 3% among those aged 70 to 75 years to 20% to 25% among those aged 85 years or more.[6] The personal habits of patients with dementia often deteriorate, and their speech may become incoherent. Many patients revert to a second childhood and require total care for feeding, toileting, and physical activities. Treatment of certain illnesses may help to slow the mental decline associated with the disease.

Delirium and dementia may be difficult to differentiate, because both may cause disorientation and impaired memory, thinking, and judgment. Dementia develops slowly and worsens progressively over time. It usually does not cause diminished alertness. Sleeping and waking problems occur less often in people with dementia than in those with delirium. People with dementia may have difficulty with short- and long-term memory, as well as impairment of judgment and abstract thinking. Delirium is acute in onset and sometimes may occur at the same time as dementia, particularly in older adults or people with chronic illnesses.

CRITICAL THINKING

Besides auditory hallucinations, think of other sensory hallucinations that can occur in these patients.

Neurodevelopmental Disorders

Several groups of disorders fall under the neurodevelopmental disorder category in the *DSM-5*, including intellectual disabilities, communication disorders, attention-deficit/hyperactivity disorder, specific learning disorder, motor disorders, and autism spectrum disorder.[4]

Autism Spectrum Disorder

Autism spectrum disorder (ASD) is a range of neurodevelopmental disorders that include autistic disorder (classic autism), Asperger syndrome, and pervasive developmental disorder—not otherwise specified (PDD-NOS, or atypical autism) (BOX 34-7). Each of these disorders is characterized by two behavioral features: (1) impairment in social communication and interaction across multiple contexts and (2) restricted, repetitive behaviors, interests, or activities, including decreased imaginative play, stereotyped behaviors, and inflexible adherence to routines.

BOX 34-7 Forms of Autism

Autistic disorder. Generally classified by impairment in social interactions and communication and includes some restrictive or repetitive behaviors.

Asperger syndrome. A syndrome characterized by impairments in social interactions and the presence of restricted interests and activities, with no clinically significant general delay in language, and testing in the range of average to above-average intelligence.

PDD-NOS. A general category of disorders characterized by severe and pervasive impairment in several areas of development, including communication and social interactions.

The degree to which these behaviors are manifested may vary between the disorders as well as between each person. The symptoms of ASD can usually be observed in infants by 18 months of age but often are unnoticed and therefore undiagnosed (BOX 34-8). ASD is more common in boys, in siblings of those with autism, and in people with certain developmental disorders (eg, inherited intellectual impairment). Social communication disorder is a new diagnosis in the *DSM-5*. It is similar to autism but without the repetitive behaviors.

About 30% of children with autism may engage in self-injurious behaviors such as hitting, biting, or scratching themselves, head-banging, and picking at their skin or sores.[7] In addition, a person with autism may not respond to pain in a normal manner. These characteristics, combined with an impaired ability to communicate, can present the paramedic with challenges in assessment and patient care. The risk for injury is high in these children. They are at risk for running away into dangerous situations, which can lead to outcomes such as being struck by vehicles or drowning. Care for traumatic injuries may be complicated by the patient's communication disorder. Paramedics should employ the therapeutic communications techniques described in Chapter 16, *Therapeutic Communications*. They should also be prepared to provide gentle restraint to ensure personal safety, the safety of the patient, and others. Strategies to help defuse a crisis situation when treating a child with autism include the following:[8]

1. Remain calm and move slowly.
2. Examine from toe to head.

BOX 34-8 Possible Signs and Symptoms of ASD

The child with ASD might exhibit the following signs or symptoms:

- Does not respond to his/her name
- Cannot explain what he or she wants
- Has trouble relating to others
- Is slow to develop language skills or has delayed speech
- Has trouble understanding others' feelings or talking about how he or she feels
- Prefers not to be held or cuddled or might cuddle only when he or she wants to
- Is interested in people but be unable to talk, play, or relate to them
- Appears not to hear when someone talks to him or her but responds to other sounds
- Does not point at objects to show interest
- Repeats (echos) words and phrases
- Has trouble expressing what he or she needs using typical words or communication
- Does not engage in pretend play (eg, does not pretend to feed a doll)
- Does not adapt to a change in routine
- Repeats actions again and again
- Has unusual reactions to the way things smell, taste, look, feel, or sound
- Loses skills he or she once had (stops saying words previously used)
- Avoids eye contact
- Does not look at an object when someone points at it

Modified from: Division of Birth Defects, National Center on Birth Defects and Developmental Disabilities, Centers for Disease Control and Prevention. Facts about ASD. Centers for Disease Control and Prevention website. https://www.cdc.gov/ncbddd/autism/facts.html. Updated March 28, 2016. Accessed January 26, 2018.

NOTE

Recent studies estimate that 1 in every 68 children is diagnosed with ASD. These studies reflect roughly a 30% increase in reported cases since 2012 (1 in 88 children), thought to be the result of changes in reporting practices. The cause of the vast majority of cases is unknown. Possible factors associated with the likelihood of an ASD diagnosis include genetics and environmental and biologic factors.

There is no cure for ASD. Therapies and early behavioral interventions to manage specific symptoms can result in substantial improvement in some patients. There are many different types of treatments available for ASD, which may include auditory training, discrete trial training, and vitamin therapy. Other treatments may include facilitated communication, music therapy, occupational therapy, physical therapy, sensory integration, and applied behavioral analysis.

Modified from: Division of Birth Defects, National Center on Birth Defects and Developmental Disabilities, Centers for Disease Control and Prevention. Autism spectrum disorder (ASD): data and statistics. Centers for Disease Control and Prevention website. https://www.cdc.gov/ncbddd/autism/data.html. Updated July 11, 2016. Accessed February 26, 2018; Division of Birth Defects, National Center on Birth Defects and Developmental Disabilities, Centers for Disease Control and Prevention. Autism spectrum disorder (ASD): facts about ASD. Centers for Disease Control and Prevention website. https://www.cdc.gov/ncbddd/autism/facts.html. Updated March 28, 2016. Accessed February 26, 2018; Centers for Disease Control and Prevention. CDC estimates 1 in 68 children has been identified with autism spectrum disorder. Centers for Disease Control and Prevention website. https://www.cdc.gov/media/releases/2014/p0327-autism-spectrum-disorder.html. Accessed February 26, 2018; and Hansen SN, Schendel DE, Parner ET. Explaining the increase in the prevalence of autism spectrum disorders: the proportion attributable to changes in reporting practices. *JAMA Pediatr*. 2015;169(1):56-62.

3. Remove sensory distractions from the area.
4. Give clear directions and use simple language.
5. Minimize tactile sensations that may cause anxiety or aggression related to bandages or other adhesives.
6. Recognize pain that may be manifested by laughing, singing, or removing clothing.
7. Ask the parents for advice about calming measures.

Schizophrenia

Schizophrenia is a group of disorders characterized by recurrent episodes of **psychotic behavior**. Psychotic behavior can be defined as an inability or unwillingness to recognize and acknowledge reality and to relate with others. Although the exact cause of the disease has not yet been identified, it may result from a combination of genetics (a family history of schizophrenia often exists), chemical and hormonal changes, autoimmune illness, viral infection, and other stress factors.[4] An estimated 3.5 million adult Americans are affected by the disease.[9]

Schizophrenia usually becomes apparent during adolescence or early adulthood, and the signs and symptoms become more pronounced and severe as the disease progresses. Symptoms fall into three categories: positive, negative, and cognitive. Positive symptoms are psychotic behaviors that are not found in healthy people. They include delusions, thought disorders (unusual or dysfunctional ways of thinking), movement disorders, and hallucinations (eg, hearing voices that insult or make demands) (BOX 34-9). These symptoms often manifest themselves in paranoia. Negative symptoms disrupt normal emotions and behaviors and include a flat affect, anhedonia (inability to feel pleasure), difficulty starting and staying with activities, and reduced speaking. Cognitive symptoms vary by patient. They include poor executive functions (ability to understand and use information), difficulty focusing, and problems with working memory.[10]

There is no cure for schizophrenia, but 20% to 25% of patients are successful at managing the disease at a high level; 50% improved over a 10-year period; and 25% do not improve.[11]

Many patients with schizophrenia function quite well with antipsychotic drugs and psychotherapy. These patients require lifelong therapy and compliance with drug therapy to control the symptoms of the disease. Other patients function poorly between frank psychotic episodes that often are the result of failure to comply with drug therapy. Noncompliance with medications is common in these patients, and the drugs may produce side effects, especially **dyskinesia** (abnormal muscular movements) and tremor.

Anxiety Disorders

A certain amount of **anxiety** is useful and necessary for adapting constructively to stress. However, a patient who has an anxiety disorder has a persistent, fearful feeling that cannot be consciously related to reality.[12] This type of illness can be disabling and the patient may withdraw from daily activities, which is usually

BOX 34-9 Responding to Paranoia, Delusions, and Hallucinations

1. First, assess whether the problem is troublesome or frightening to the person experiencing it. If not, ignoring it may be the best approach.
2. If a person seems to be hallucinating, leave the person alone or approach slowly so as not to frighten the person. Respond with caution.
3. Do not try to argue or rationalize. Realize that hallucinations and delusions seem very real to the person who is experiencing them. Arguing does not build trust.
4. Offer reassurance and validation. You might say, "I know this is troubling for you. Let me see if I can help."
5. Check out the reality of the situation; maybe what the person sees or thinks is true.
6. Sometimes things in the environment may be misinterpreted (ie, a glare or shadow in the window, a noisy furnace), and these things may be frightening. Explain the potential or actual misinterpretation (eg, that the noise is the furnace turning on).
7. Modify the environment if necessary. (A mirror may become distracting or confusing; adding more lights may be helpful at night.)
8. Assess whether the person is having problems with hearing or vision. Resolving such problems can reduce the degree of disability.
9. Recall that whispering or laughing around the person may be misinterpreted.
10. Do not take any accusations personally.
11. Use distraction to try to pull the person's focus from the delusion or hallucination.
12. If the person asks you directly whether you see or hear something, be honest. However, do not struggle to convince or reason with the person about what is real.
13. Try to respond to what the person may be feeling: insecurity, fear, and confusion.
14. Rule out any illnesses or the use of any medicines that could be contributing to the problem.
15. Use tact and firmness to persuade the patient to be transported to the medical facility.

Modified from: Robinson A, Spencer B, White L. The Alzheimer's Association handout: *Hallucinations and Delusions and Understanding Difficult Behaviors.* Ypsilanti, MI: Geriatric Education of Michigan University; 1991.

an unsuccessful attempt to avoid the episodes of intense activity. Severe anxiety disorders may manifest in a **panic disorder** (panic attack)—a condition that affects about 6 million Americans each year.[13] As compared to anxiety disorders that may result from acute grief or various phobias, for example, panic disorders often have no precipitating cause of the attack. About 40 million adults aged 18 years and older in the United States have anxiety disorders. Most people have their first episode by 21 years of age; 11 years is the average age of onset.[14]

A panic attack is defined as an episode in which four or more of the following signs and symptoms occur:[15]

- Hyperventilation
- Sweating
- Feeling of breathlessness or smothering
- Nausea or abdominal discomfort
- Feelings of unreality or being detached
- Fear of losing control
- Fear of dying
- Somatic complaints
- Chest discomfort
- Palpitations or tachycardia
- Dyspnea or smothering sensation
- Sensation of choking
- Faintness, dizziness or light-headedness
- Feeling chilled or hot
- Trembling or shaking

At least one of these attacks is followed within a month by feelings of worry about them causing the person to lose control. They are also often accompanied by changes in activity designed to avoid having another panic attack.[15]

Patient treatment is mainly supportive. The paramedic should assure these patients that although they may feel as if they are dying, they are not. Also, the paramedic should assure them that effective treatment is available. Panic attacks may mimic a number of medical emergencies, including myocardial infarction. Therefore, any patient who shows the signs and symptoms of a panic attack should be fully assessed at the scene and transported for evaluation by a physician.

Phobia

A **phobia** is a type of anxiety disorder that affects about 6.8% of the US population.[16] A person with a phobia has transferred anxiety onto a situation or an object in the form of an irrational, intense fear, such as a fear of heights, closed spaces, water, or other people. As the object or situation comes closer, the person's anxiety increases. If the crisis is allowed to continue, the patient's anxiety may escalate into a panic attack. These patients usually recognize that their fear is unreasonable; however, they cannot overcome the phobia. In some cases, the phobia does not initiate the EMS response but becomes a secondary complication in emergency care. An example is a person who is phobic of water (aquaphobia) being trapped in a submerged vehicle. Other common types of phobias include the fear of heights (acrophobia), spiders (arachnophobia), flying (aviophobia), or crowds (enochlophobia or demophobia).

> CRITICAL THINKING
>
> Do you know someone with an intense fear of a situation or object? How does this person behave when subjected to the object of the phobia?

When caring for patients with a phobia, the paramedic should take care to explain each step of an emergency or rescue procedure. The key is a careful rehearsal with the patient, in which the paramedic explains exactly what care will be given and how it will be performed. In addition, the EMS crew should show patience and understanding of the phobia. They should assure the patient that no forceful steps will be taken to place the person in an unwilling position.

Obsessive-Compulsive Disorder and Related Disorders

Obsessive-compulsive disorder (OCD) is categorized with a number of illnesses with similar characteristics, including hoarding disorder, body dysmorphic disorder, trichotillomania (hair-pulling disorder), and excoriation (skin-picking) disorder. OCD is the most common illness found in this category.[17]

Obsessive-Compulsive Disorder

Obsessive-compulsive disorder (OCD) is a psychiatric disorder in which a person feels stress or anxiety about thoughts or rituals over which he or she has little control. Obsessions may manifest as repetitive thoughts, images, or impulses that intrude on the person's thoughts, causing anxiety and stress. Compulsions are the repetitive acts or rituals that the person uses to reduce anxiety. The person believes these actions will prevent the thing that he or she dreads. Obsessions and compulsions can take many forms, including upsetting thoughts (eg, violence, vulgarities, harm to oneself or others) followed by actions such as incessant handwashing or showering. These thoughts and actions are so frequent and time consuming that they interfere with the person's normal activities or even their job. Compulsions also may involve silently repeating special numbers, colors, single words or phrases, and sometimes melodies. About 2.2 million American adults have OCD in a given year. First symptoms often begin in childhood and adolescence; median age of onset is 19 years.[18]

Although most adults realize to some degree that these obsessions and compulsions are without merit, they have great difficulty stopping them. Children with OCD may not realize that their behavior is unusual. OCD affects men and women equally, can start at any age, and may have a heritable component. People with OCD often cleverly hide their condition from family, friends, and coworkers. Medications and behavior therapy are often effective in controlling the symptoms of this disorder.

Trauma- and Stressor-Related Disorders

Trauma- and stressor-related disorders are somewhat related to the anxiety disorders. They include illnesses that require exposure to a specific traumatic event as part of the diagnosis.

Posttraumatic Stress Disorder

Posttraumatic stress disorder (PTSD) is an anxiety reaction to severe psychosocial events (BOX 34-10). These events often are shocking, frightening, or life threatening. Examples include events associated with military or emergency medical service, natural and human-caused disasters, and rape. The events often result in repetitive, intrusive symptoms that persist for at least 1 month. People diagnosed have symptoms from four categories: reexperiencing symptoms, avoidance symptoms, arousal and reactivity symptoms, and cognition or mood symptoms. Manifestations of this illness may include depression, sleep disturbances, nightmares, and survivor guilt. The syndrome often is complicated by substance abuse.[19]

About 7.7 million people in the United States have PTSD during the course of a given year.[20] The disorder can develop at any age, including childhood; median age of onset is 23 years. About 30% of men and women who have spent time in a war zone experience PTSD.[21] The disorder can also occur after violent personal assaults, such as rape, child abuse, mugging, or domestic violence; terrorism; natural or human-caused disasters; and accidents.

EMS personnel and other emergency responders may be subject to PTSD as a result of their work. For example, major incidents with a large number of injured people, the death of a coworker, or a case of sudden infant death syndrome could precipitate this syndrome, as could the cumulative stress associated with responding to emergency calls (see Chapter 2, *Well-Being of the Paramedic*).

BOX 34-10 Symptoms of Posttraumatic Stress Disorder

Reexperiencing Symptoms

Flashbacks
Bad dreams
Frightening thoughts

Avoidance Symptoms

Staying away from places, people, events, and objects that are reminders of the trauma
Avoiding thoughts or feelings about the traumatic event

Arousal and Reactivity Symptoms

Easily startled
Feeling tense or on edge
Difficulty sleeping
Having angry outbursts

Cognition and Mood Symptoms

Difficulty recalling specific features of the traumatic event
Negative thoughts about self or others
Exaggerated feeling of guilt or blame
Loss of interest in enjoyable activities

Mood Disorders

Mood disorders are conditions in which the emotions that a person normally experiences in life (eg, happiness, depression, fear, anxiety) undergo undesirable and possibly distressing changes. Two conditions commonly associated with mood disorders are depression and bipolar disorder, both of which are associated with an increased risk of suicide.[5]

Depression

Depression is a mood disturbance characterized by feelings of sadness, despair, and discouragement. It is one of the most prevalent major psychiatric conditions, affecting more than 16.1 million adult Americans (about 7% of the adult population).[22] Depression is a frequent and serious complication of heart attack, stroke, diabetes, and cancer. Depression is usually episodic (episodes usually last longer than 1 month) with periods of remission. It is known to have either a gradual or a rapid onset, and at times a clustering of episodes occurs. The patient with depression may show feelings of hopelessness, extreme isolation, tenseness, and irritability. In severe cases, the depression may be followed by **anhedonia**, which is the inability to feel pleasure or happiness from experiences that ordinarily are pleasurable. Other effects of severe depression include insomnia or hypersomnia, weight loss from diminished appetite, weight gain from overeating, decreased libido, and deep feelings of worthlessness and guilt. The mnemonic *IN SAD CAGES* identifies the major features of depression:[22,23]

Loss of **in**terest in activities

Sleep disturbance
Appetite change
Depressed mood

difficulty **c**oncentrating
Activity level change
Excessive **g**uilt
Loss of **e**nergy
Suicidal thoughts, plan, or attempt

NOTE

Depression can be classified as dysthymia or clinical (major) depression. **Dysthymia** is a less severe form of depression that is chronic in nature, lasting up to 2 years or more. In contrast to **major depression** (also called major depressive disorder or clinical depression), the symptoms of dysthymia may not always result in clinically significant distress. They are not always associated with impairment in social, occupational, academic, or other major areas of functioning (as is more common with major depression). Both forms of depression share similar symptoms, including depressed mood, disturbed sleep, low energy, and poor concentration. Parallel symptoms include poor appetite, low self-esteem, and hopelessness in dysthymia. The more severe symptoms of weight change, excessive guilt, and thoughts of death or suicide are associated with major depression.

Modified from: Depression. National Institute of Mental Health website. https://www.nimh.nih.gov/health/topics/depression/index.shtml. Revised October 2016. Accessed February 26, 2018.

Depression is common in older adults. It also is associated with an increased risk of suicide for all age groups (described later in this chapter). Care for patients with depression is directed at quietly talking to the patient about things that appear to be of interest and trying to gain responsiveness. Depression may be treated with antidepressant drug therapy, counseling, psychotherapy, and, in a small number of cases, electroconvulsive therapy (ECT).

DID YOU KNOW?

Electroconvulsive Therapy

ECT is provided to an anesthetized patient by passing a small electric current through the brain, producing a seizure. The current is supplied for 1 second or less while monitoring the patient's seizure activity (by electroencephalogram) and cardiac rhythm (by electrocardiogram). ECT is usually given 3 times per week for a total of 6 to 12 treatments. Following the treatment, most patients regain consciousness within 10 to 15 minutes. They often will experience a brief period of confusion, headache, and muscle stiffness. ECT is particularly useful for patients who cannot take antidepressants or for whom antidepressants are ineffective and for suicidal patients. ECT may be considered for pregnant women who have bipolar disorder or severe depression if other therapy is unsuccessful, but its use in these patients is controversial. It can be effective in treating some forms of schizophrenia and other affective disorders. ECT is not a cure but is shown to produce substantial improvement in about 80% of patients.

Modified from: Anderson EL, Reti IM. ECT in pregnancy: a review of the literature from 1941 to 2007. *Psychosom Med.* 2009;71(2):235-242; Leiknes KA, Cooke MJ, Jarosch-von Schweder L, et al. Electroconvulsive therapy during pregnancy: a systematic review of case studies. *Arch Womens Ment Health*. 2015;18:1-39; and What is electroconvulsive therapy (ECT)? American Psychiatric Association website. https://www.psychiatry.org/patients-families/ect. Accessed February 26, 2018.

Bipolar Disorder

Bipolar disorder is a biphasic emotional disorder in which depressive and manic episodes alternate (**FIGURE 34-2**). It affects about 2.6% of the American population.[24] **Mania** is characterized by excessive elation, talkativeness, flight of ideas, motor activity, irritability, accelerated speech, and, often, delusions that center around personal grandeur. Bipolar disorders sometimes develop slowly over time. However, they may occur abruptly and may be instigated by a single event. The manic phase can be very brief or can last weeks to months. Compared with depression, mania

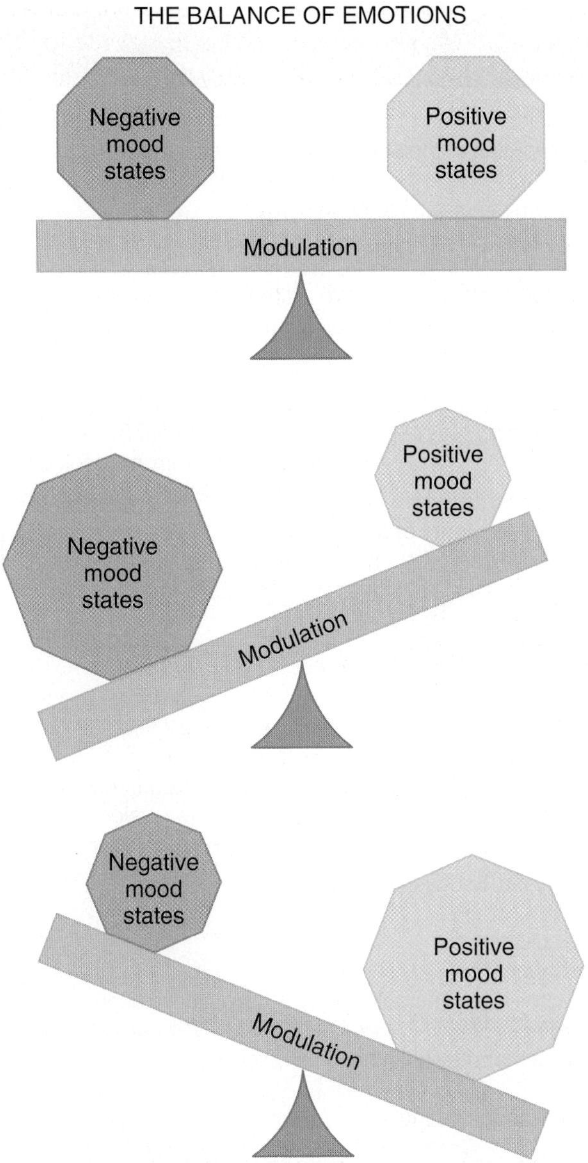

FIGURE 34-2 Bipolar disorder.

© Jones & Bartlett Learning.

BOX 34-11 Types of Bipolar Disorder

Bipolar I Disorder

Manic episodes that last at least 7 days *or*
Severe manic symptoms requiring hospitalization
Often with depressive periods lasting 2 weeks
Episodes with concurrent manic and depressive symptoms possible

Bipolar II Disorder

Pattern of depressive and hypomanic episodes
Lacking the full-blown manic episodes of bipolar I disorder

Cyclothymic Disorder (Cyclothymia)

Numerous episodes of hypomanic symptoms with numerous periods of depressive symptoms lasting 2 years or more (1 year in adolescents)
Symptoms not severe enough to meet diagnostic criteria for hypomanic or depressive episode

Other Specified and Unspecified Bipolar and Related Disorders

Bipolar disorder symptoms that do not match the other categories

Modified from: Bipolar disorder. National Institute of Mental Health website. https://www.nimh.nih.gov/health/topics/bipolar-disorder/index.shtml. Revised April 2016. Accessed January 26, 2018.

CRITICAL THINKING

Do you think patients would be at higher risk for suicide during the depressive or the manic phase of bipolar disorder? Why?

is rare. The most frequent age for initial episodes is 20 to 35 years. There are four general types of bipolar disorder (BOX 34-11).

Many patients with bipolar disorder are treated with lithium. Lithium has a narrow therapeutic index; a common illness, such as influenza with diarrhea and/or vomiting, can result in lithium toxicity.

Emergency care should consist of emotional support and transport for evaluation by a physician. If this is the patient's first manic episode, the paramedic should consider the possibility of drug abuse in the differential diagnoses. Stimulation should be kept to a minimum. When possible, EMS transport should proceed without using emergency lights and audible warning devices.

Suicide and Suicide Threats

A threat of **suicide** is an indication that a patient has a serious crisis that calls for immediate intervention. Suicidal ideation is the presence of thoughts related to ending one's own life. Active suicidal ideation occurs when the person has thoughts of suicide and a plan; this indicates a higher risk.[25] In many cases, suicide attempts are a cry for help. They also may be a form of direct or indirect communication. For example, the patient may be saying, "I do not want to live" or "I am

BOX 34-12 Myths About Suicide

Myth. People who talk about killing themselves rarely commit suicide.
Fact. Most people who commit suicide have given some clue or warning of their intent. Suicidal threats and attempts should always be treated seriously.
Myth. The tendency to commit suicide is inherited. It is passed from generation to generation.
Fact. Suicide does tend to run in families. However, the tendency does not appear to be transmitted genetically.
Myth. All suicidal people are deeply depressed.
Fact. Depression is often associated with suicidal feelings. However, not all people who kill themselves are obviously depressed. In fact, some suicidal people appear to be happier than they have been in quite a while because they have decided to do something that they believe will resolve all their problems at the same time.
Myth. There is a very low correlation between alcoholism and suicide.
Fact. Alcoholism and suicide often go hand in hand. People with alcoholism are prone to suicide. Even people who do not normally drink often ingest alcohol shortly before killing themselves.
Myth. Suicidal people are mentally ill.
Fact. Many suicidal people are depressed and distraught. However, most of them would not be diagnosed as mentally ill.
Myth. If a person attempts suicide, that person will always entertain thoughts of suicide.
Fact: Most people who are suicidal are that way for only a brief period in their lives. An attempter who receives the proper assistance and support probably will never be suicidal again. Only about 10% of attempters later complete the act.
Myth. Asking a person about his or her suicidal intentions encourages the person to act.
Fact. Actually, the opposite is true. Asking a person directly about suicidal intent often lowers the person's anxiety level. In fact, it often acts as a deterrent to suicidal emotions.
Myth. Suicide is more common among the lower classes.
Fact. Suicide occurs in all socioeconomic groups. No one class is more susceptible to it than another.
Myth. Suicidal people rarely seek medical attention.
Fact. Research has consistently shown that about 75% of suicidal people visit a physician within 3 months of killing themselves.
Myth. Suicide is basically a problem limited to young people.
Fact. The suicide rate rises with age and reaches a peak among older Caucasian men.
Myth. Professional people do not kill themselves.
Fact. Physicians, lawyers, dentists, and pharmacists have high suicide rates.
Myth. When a person's depression lifts, the danger of suicide disappears.
Fact. The greatest danger of suicide exists during the first 3 months after a person recovers from a deep depression.
Myth. Suicide is a spontaneous activity that occurs without warning.
Fact. Most people plan their self-destruction. Then they give clues that they have become suicidal.
Myth. Suicide rates rise during the holiday season.
Fact. Suicide rates actually fall during the winter months and peak in the spring.

Modified from: Caruso K. Suicide myths. Suicide.org website. http://www.suicide.org/suicide-myths.html. Accessed February 26, 2018.

angry with you" (BOX 34-12). In assessing the risk of suicide, the paramedic should consider these facts:[25,26]

1. In 2014, suicide was the 10th-leading cause of death. More than 42,000 suicides occurred in the United States.[27]
2. In the United States, Caucasian men older than 65 years have the highest suicide rate.[25]
3. Women attempt suicide more often than men do.
4. Men commit suicide at about four times the rate at which women do.
5. Firearms are the most commonly used method for suicide in men. Poisoning is the most common method for suicide in women.
6. The more specific and detailed the suicide plan, the greater the potential for a completed suicide.

Other factors associated with suicide threats include a history of previous attempts, family history of suicide, recent death of a loved one or loss of a significant relationship, a financial setback or job loss, chronic or debilitating illness, social isolation, alcohol or other drug abuse, major depression, **acute psychosis**, bipolar disorder, and schizophrenia.[25] Suicide ideation is also higher in teens and young adults who identify as lesbian, gay, bisexual, or transgender than in the general population.[28]

If a suicide attempt is suspected, the paramedic should discuss these intentions with the patient. Questions such as the following are appropriate: "Do you have thoughts about killing yourself or others?" "Have you ever tried to kill yourself?" Many depressed patients are willing to discuss their suicidal (or homicidal) thoughts. During the patient interview, the paramedic should try to determine three important factors: (1) whether the patient has a plan (how and when the suicide will be done), (2) whether the plan is intended to be successful, and (3) whether the patient has the means or method to follow through with the plan.

CRITICAL THINKING

How would you feel about asking a patient, "Have you ever thought about killing yourself?"

When responding to a suicide attempt, paramedics should request police protection before approaching the scene. Armed patients must be considered homicidal as well as suicidal. After scene safety has been ensured and paramedics have gained access to the patient, the scene should be surveyed for the presence of dangerous objects.

The first priority in patient management is medical care. Unconscious patients should be managed with airway, ventilatory, and circulatory support and rapid transport. If the patient is conscious, creating rapport as soon as possible is essential. The paramedic should conduct a brief interview to assess the situation and determine the need for and direction of further action. To help reduce the potential for suicide, paramedics can take the following six steps:

1. Provide support and honest assurance about the patient's well-being.
2. Provide for physical safety as well as emotional security. Establish protective limits and measures. Doing so helps to prevent injury to the patient or others. It also conveys to these patients that the paramedic will help them control their behavior until they can gain self-control.
3. Listen to the person, even if the speech seems bizarre, inappropriate, or unrealistic. Do not feel that every statement must be answered or that advice or opinions must be given. During the interview, acknowledge the patient's feelings; do not argue with the patient's wish to die. Explain alternatives to suicide that the patient may not have considered (eg, counseling, support groups, pastoral care).
4. Determine the patient's support system or significant others when possible. Others may be better able to communicate with and calm the patient.
5. Encourage and reassure the patient during the crisis.
6. Transport the patient to the proper facility for emergency intervention.

Substance-Related Disorders

Some patients with a behavioral emergency may also be using alcohol or illegal drugs. The effects of these substances may cause difficulties during the physical examination. (Substance-related disorders are described in Chapter 33, *Toxicology*.) Often these patients are trying to self-medicate to improve their mood or lessen the anxiety associated with mental illness. Other patients self-medicate before receiving a diagnosis for their illness or before seeking professional help. Signs that may indicate alcohol or illicit drug use include a breath odor of alcohol, the presence of drug paraphernalia, and needle tracks on the extremities.

Patients With a Dual Diagnosis

Some people struggle with both serious mental illness and substance abuse. This dual diagnosis may be difficult to identify because one disorder may mimic the symptoms of the other.[29] It therefore is easy to attribute the patient's symptoms to only one of the two afflictions. It is estimated that as many as 7.9 million mentally ill people have a substance use disorder. The drug most often used is alcohol. Other commonly used drugs include marijuana, cocaine, heroin, hallucinogens, inhalants, and prescription pain relievers and depressants.[30,31] Other prescription drugs such as tranquilizers and sleeping medicines may also be abused.

Patients who have a dual diagnosis may alternate between requesting EMS assistance for mental illness and for substance abuse. Most psychiatric and drug counseling organizations agree that integrated treatment for the two disorders should be done at the same time.[32]

Somatic Symptom Disorder

Somatic symptom disorders (also called somatoform disorders) are conditions that suggest a medical disorder lasting 6 months or more when no physical cause can be found for the patient's symptoms. Two of the most common disorders in this group are conversion disorder and factitious disorder. Both are associated with anxiety, depression, and threats of suicide. Patients with these disorders most often complain of neurologic symptoms (double vision, seizure, weakness), gynecologic symptoms (painful menstruation, painful intercourse), and gastrointestinal symptoms (abdominal pain, nausea). No definitive causes for most of the somatic symptom disorders have been established. Treatment often requires psychotherapy, which can address the emotional conflicts that manifest in these illnesses. Contributing factors may include childhood neglect, sexual abuse, and history of alcohol and substance abuse. In addition, somatic symptom disorder has been associated with personality disorders.[33] The prevalence of somatic symptom disorder in the general population is an estimated 5% to 7%, making this one of the most common categories of patient concerns in the primary care setting.[4]

Conversion Disorder

Conversion disorder (also called functional neurologic disorder) is a constellation of neurologic symptoms that are not consciously or deliberately produced and that are unexplained by physical examination or objective data and not better explained by other medical or mental disorders. They often cause clinically significant disruption in social or occupational functioning and typically manifest as neurologic symptoms. A loss of sensory or motor capabilities or of special senses may occur. For example, the person suddenly may not be able to speak, hear, see, or feel, or an arm or a leg may be paralyzed. In many cases, the areas of the body affected do not correspond to the actual arrangement of neural pathways. The symptoms also may be intermittent or may appear at different times and in different areas of the body. Conversion disorder is rare, with an estimated incidence of 2 to 5 people per 100,000 each year.[4]

Factitious Disorders

Factitious disorders are a group of disorders in which symptoms mimic a true illness. However, the symptoms have actually been invented so that the person may assume the role of a patient. The symptoms are under the control of the patient who is attempting to gain attention. The most common disorder in this group is a self-imposed factitious disorder called **Munchausen syndrome**. A patient with this disorder makes routine pleas for treatment and hospitalization for a symptomatic, but imaginary, acute illness. Other complaints that may be associated with factitious disorders include bereavement, Cushing syndrome, dental problems, infection with the human immunodeficiency virus (HIV), hypoglycemia, and stroke. Factitious disorder imposed on another (**Munchausen syndrome by proxy**) is a form of this disorder in which a person injures or induces illness in others (usually children) to gain sympathy. Munchausen syndrome by proxy is often considered to be a form of child abuse.[34]

The symptoms of a factitious disorder are often dramatic but plausible. They usually resolve with treatment. After the treatment, the person seeks treatment for another invented disease. Once the factitious disorder is diagnosed, treatment is aimed at protecting these people from unnecessary surgeries and other treatments they do not need.

Management

Paramedics should manage symptoms of somatic symptom disorders as if they are real because differentiating these disorders from an organic ailment may be difficult. The paramedic should recognize that these patients are not faking; they believe their illness or loss of function to be factual. These patients require evaluation by a physician.

Dissociative Disorders

Dissociative disorders are a group of psychological illnesses in which a particular mental function is separated (dissociated) from the mind as a whole. It is estimated that 2% of people experience dissociative disorders, with women being more likely to be diagnosed than are men. These disorders include the following:[35]

- **Dissociative amnesia.** A disorder characterized by the blocking out of vital personal information, usually of a traumatic or stressful nature. Dissociative amnesia, unlike other types of amnesia, does not result from other medical trauma.
- **Dissociative identity disorder.** A disorder that has been called multiple personality disorder.
- **Depersonalization disorder.** A condition marked by a feeling of detachment or distance from one's own experience, body, or self.

Dissociative disorders usually are associated with emotional conflicts. These conflicts are so repressed that a split in the personality occurs, which results in an altered state of consciousness or confusion in identity. The condition also may be caused by an inability to cope with severe stress or conflict. Dissociation can occur soon after a catastrophic event, such as the traumatic death of a child or spouse. People with dissociative disorders often are unable to remember their names or personal histories. However, they can still speak, read, and learn new material. Treatment may include antianxiety medications, hypnosis, and psychotherapy.

Feeding and Eating Disorders

The two most common feeding and eating disorders considered to be forms of psychiatric illness are anorexia nervosa and bulimia nervosa[36] (BOX 34-13). Both of these eating disorders can lead to serious dehydration, starvation, and electrolyte imbalances and may cause critical illness or death. The disorders are best managed with supervision and regulation of eating habits, psychotherapy, and, sometimes, antidepressants. Many patients require hospitalization.

BOX 34-13 Facts About Eating Disorders

- At least 30 million people of all ages and both sexes have an eating disorder in the United States.
- Every 62 minutes, at least one person dies as a direct result of an eating disorder.
- Eating disorders are associated with the highest mortality rate of any mental illness.
- Of women older than 50 years, 13% engage in eating disorder behaviors.
- In a large national study of college students, 3.5% of sexual minority[a] women and 2.1% of sexual minority men reported having an eating disorder.
- Of transgender college students, 16% reported having an eating disorder.
- In a study following active-duty military personnel over time, 5.5% of women and 4% of men had an eating disorder at the beginning of the study, and within just a few years of continued service, 3.3% more women and 2.6% more men developed an eating disorder.
- Eating disorders affect all races and ethnic groups.
- Genetics, environmental factors, and personality traits all combine to create risk for an eating disorder.

[a]Sexual minority indicates a group whose sexual identity, orientation, or practices differ from the majority of the surrounding society (eg, lesbian, gay, bisexual, transgender).

Modified from: Eating disorders. National Institute of Mental Health website. https://www.nimh.nih.gov/health/topics/eating-disorders/index.shtml. Revised February 2016. Accessed February 26, 2018.

Anorexia Nervosa

Anorexia nervosa is an eating disorder characterized by a distorted body image causing an intense fear of being obese, severe weight loss, malnutrition, and, eventually, amenorrhea (absence of menstrual bleeding). A patient feels intensely hungry, even though hunger pains are denied. Signs and symptoms include weight loss, obsession with exercise, fatigue, binge eating, induced vomiting, and use of laxatives to promote weight loss. The condition primarily is seen in female girls and usually is associated with emotional stress or conflict. It often is difficult to identify an exact underlying cause for this disease.

Bulimia Nervosa

Bulimia nervosa is sometimes considered a form of anorexia. It is an insatiable craving for food. This craving often results in episodes of binge eating, followed by purging (through self-induced vomiting or use of laxatives), depression, and self-deprivation. Like anorexia, bulimia is most common in adolescent girls and young women. Anorexic and bulimic patients often worry about their compulsive behavior. As a result, they may become depressed and suicidal.

NOTE

Binge-eating disorder involves recurrent binge-eating episodes. People with this disorder are unable to limit their impulses to overeat, which often leads to weight gain or obesity. Psychiatric conditions, including anxiety and depression, often accompany the disorder. Because people feel extreme guilt or disgust about overeating, the cycle of binge eating is difficult to break. Treatment with psychotherapy and medications may help reduce bingeing episodes.

Disruptive, Impulse-Control, and Conduct Disorders

Disruptive, impulse-control, and conduct disorders are a group of psychiatric conditions. They are characterized by the inability to control emotions or to resist an impulse or a temptation to perform some act that is unlawful, socially unacceptable, or self-harmful. The prevalence of conduct disorders is estimated at 6% to 9% of the US population and is more commonly diagnosed in men older than 18 years.[37] Disorders in this category include the following:[38]

- **Intermittent explosive disorder.** A condition marked by frequent and often unpredictable episodes of extreme anger or physical outbursts. Between episodes, there is usually no evidence of violence or physical threat.
- **Kleptomania.** The failure to resist impulses to steal things that are not needed either for personal use or for their monetary value.
- **Pathologic gambling.** A persistent and maladaptive pattern of gambling that causes difficulties with interpersonal, financial, and vocational functioning.
- **Pyromania.** Deliberate and purposeful fire-setting for nonmonetary gain. This condition typically is associated with tension or heightened arousal before the act and with gratification or relief afterward.
- **Oppositional defiant disorder.** A pattern of uncooperative, defiant, and hostile behavior toward authority that interferes with normal function.
- **Conduct disorder.** Behaviors that demonstrate aggression or cruelty to other people and to animals; property destruction; lying or stealing; or serious rules violations.
- **Antisocial personality disorder.** Pattern of disregard for, and violation of, the rights of others.

Disruptive, impulse-control, and conduct disorders often are difficult to treat. Most are managed with behavior modification and drug therapy. Failure to control these disorders may result in violent behavior or unlawful activities (eg, road rage). Incarceration is common.

Personality Disorders

Personality disorders are a large group of conditions distinguished by a failure to learn from experience or to adapt appropriately to changes. This failure creates ways of thinking and feeling about oneself and others that adversely affect how the person functions in life, resulting in personal distress and impairment of social functioning. These disorders may have an environmental component or may be genetic. Personality disorders become especially obvious during times of stress.

The symptoms of a personality disorder usually are first recognized in early adolescence. They continue throughout the person's life. The symptoms may vary in frequency and intensity. Generally, however, they are relatively constant. They usually affect most aspects of a patient's life, including thoughts, emotions, relationships and interpersonal skills, and impulse control.

The *DSM-5* lists 10 personality disorders and allocates each to one of three groups or clusters: A (odd, bizarre, eccentric), B (dramatic, erratic), and C (anxious, fearful).[4] Three common personality disorders are as described follows:

- **Antisocial personality disorder.** A long-standing pattern (after the age of 15 years) of disregard for the rights of others. It often is associated with irresponsible behavior and a lack of remorse for wrongdoing.
- **Borderline personality disorder.** A pattern of unstable relationships, poor or negative self-image, mood swings, and poor impulse control. It may be associated with destructive and self-harming behaviors (eg, suicide attempts, self-mutilation), an intense fear of abandonment, and displays of sudden anger.
- **Narcissistic personality disorder.** A pattern of grandiosity, need for admiration, and sense of entitlement. It often is associated with exaggerated achievements and fantasies about unlimited success, power, love, or beauty.

Many factors are associated with the development of a personality disorder, including unstable relationships during childhood, family violence, and childhood abuse or neglect. Treatment involves behavior modification techniques, counseling, drug therapy, and individual psychotherapy.

Special Considerations for Patients With Behavioral Problems

In addition to caring for the immediate needs of patients with behavioral problems, paramedics may have to deal with complications arising from the situation or other factors affecting the patient. Among these factors are the patient's age and the possibility of violent behavior. Special considerations for pediatric patients, older adult patients, and the potentially violent patient are presented in this section.

CRITICAL THINKING

When responding to a behavioral emergency that involves a child or an adolescent, do you use the same safety guidelines that you would use with an adult?

Behavioral Problems in Children

Young children who experience emotional crises need to be managed with different techniques than those used to care for older children and adults. The following suggestions may be helpful to the paramedic in caring for some children:[5]

1. Gain the child's trust and try to convince the child that you are a friend who can help.
2. Make it clear that you are strong enough to be in control but will not hurt the child.
3. Keep the interview questions brief; the child's attention span may be extremely short.
4. Never lie; be honest.
5. Use all available resources to communicate (eg, drawing pictures, telling stories).
6. Involve parents or caregivers in the interview or examination if appropriate.
7. Take any threat of violence seriously.

If the child's behavior or physical condition makes restraint necessary, the paramedic should use only humane and reasonable force (the minimum force necessary to ensure the patient's safety and the safety of the EMS crew). Sufficient personnel should be available. Calming measures may fail to work. If so, follow departmental policy or consult online medical direction. As with any method of restraint, the paramedic should monitor and document the child's airway and circulation and ensure that they are not compromised.

Behavioral Problems in Older Adults

An estimated 20% of people older than 55 years in the United States have a mental illness, and more than 20% of older adults are clinically depressed.[39] Most of these disorders can be diagnosed and treated successfully, but many of these people do not seek care. Problem behavior in an older adult patient can be a sign of a longstanding psychiatric disorder, a newly emerging psychiatric problem, a medical illness, substance abuse, drug noncompliance or drug interactions, or other concerns (see Chapter 48, *Geriatrics*). The following suggestions may be helpful to the paramedic in communicating with some older adult patients:

1. Identify yourself and speak at eye level to make sure the patient can see you.
2. Address the patient by surname (eg, Mr. Jones or Miss [or Mrs.] Smith) unless directed otherwise.
3. Speak slowly, distinctly, and respectfully.
4. Ask one question at a time and allow time for complete answers.
5. Listen closely.
6. Explain what you are doing and why.
7. Provide reassuring physical touch as appropriate by social, cultural, or religious standards.
8. Be patient.
9. Permit family members and caregivers to remain with the patient if appropriate.
10. Preserve the patient's dignity.

Assessing the Potentially Violent Patient

Only a small number of people with mental health problems are potentially violent. Nonetheless, assessment and management of the potentially violent patient should be part of an EMS protocol. The following suggestions may help the paramedic determine the potential for a violent episode:

- **Past history.** Has the patient previously shown hostile, aggressive, or violent behavior?
- **Posture.** Is the patient sitting or standing? Does the patient appear to be tense or rigid?
- **Vocal activity.** Loud, obscene, and erratic speech indicates emotional distress.
- **Physical activity.** Is the patient pacing or agitated or protecting his or her physical boundaries?

If any of these signs of potentially violent behavior are present, paramedics should try to reduce the stress of the situation while avoiding confrontation. Paramedics should prepare a way to cope with the crisis that reduces the potential for a life-threatening incident. It also should reduce the chance for psychologically damaging consequences.

NOTE

Paramedics should retreat from the scene if they anticipate violence that would threaten their personal safety or the safety of the crew. They should wait for law enforcement personnel to ensure that the scene is safe.

Controlling Violent Situations

Severely agitated patients who pose a threat to themselves or others may need to be restrained, transported, and hospitalized against their will. Each state has a law establishing the criteria for involuntary commitment. The paramedic should be familiar with all relevant laws. The premise on which most state laws are based suggests that one person may restrain another to protect life or prevent injury.[5] The four main objectives guiding the care of the agitated patient are as follows:[40]

1. Ensure the safety of the patient, crew, and others.
2. Help the patient manage his or her emotions or distress to either maintain or regain control of his or her behavior.
3. Avoid the use of restraint whenever possible.
4. Avoid interventions that appear coercive and could escalate the patient's agitation.

Strategies for managing the agitated and potentially violent patient vary by setting and the available resources. Some general guidelines include controlling the environment, which includes moving objects that may be used as weapons, maintaining space between the crew and the patient, and ensuring the patient does not block the exit. The crew must monitor their own emotions when approaching the patient. Verbal tone and volume as well as body language should appear calm. Ten domains of deescalation can be used as a guide to communication with the agitated patient:[40]

1. **Respect personal space.** Remain at least two arm lengths from the patient.
2. **Avoid provocation.** Crew body language should appear calm and include unclenched hands that are visible to the patient. Crew members should stand at an angle to the patient with knees slightly bent. Avoid any statements that could embarrass the patient.
3. **Establish verbal contact.** One person should be designated to conduct the deescalation communication initially. That person should introduce himself or herself to the patient and explain that he or she is there to keep the patient safe and to make sure no harm comes to the patient or anyone else on the scene. The patient should be addressed by name and reassured that the crew is there to help regain control of the situation.
4. **Be concise.** Talk to the patient in short sentences using nonclinical words. Repetition is essential to successful deescalation. Repeat key messages to the patient, especially those related to setting limits, offering choices, or proposing alternatives. Actively listen and when possible agree with the patient.
5. **Identify wants and feelings.** Try to determine what the patient's top need or priority is.
6. **Listen closely to what the patient is saying.** Use techniques of active listening. Clarifying statements, such as, "What I hear you saying is . . .," let the patient know you are listening. Try to imagine that the patient's statements are true to get to the root of the emotions.
7. **Agree or agree to disagree.** Try to find something in the patient's statements you can agree with. There are three ways to agree with a patient: (1) agreeing with the truth ("Having to wait for an appointment is frustrating."), (2) agreeing in principle ("I think everyone deserves to be heard."), and (3) agreeing with the odds ("Others would be upset in that situation, too."). Acknowledge the patient's emotions relating to delusions while admitting that you are not experiencing the delusion. Sometimes you will have to agree to disagree.
8. **Lay down the law and set clear limits**. Calmly and in a matter-of-fact manner tell the patient what behavior is and is not acceptable. For example, the paramedic may need to say, "It's not okay for you to hurt yourself or others." Limit setting must be reasonable and respectful. Coach the patient on behaviors to help regain or maintain control.
9. **Offer choice and optimism.** Propose alternatives to violence. Comfort items may delay violent behaviors. Do not make promises that cannot be fulfilled. Offer or tell the patient you are going to give medication to help calm the behaviors.
10. **Debrief the patient and staff.** If involuntary chemical or physical restraint measures are performed, explain the rationale to the patient. Debrief the family or bystanders.

When a psychiatric patient refuses care, EMS personnel should follow specific protocols developed by their EMS system.[41] If violent behavior must be contained, reasonable force should be used to restrain the patient. The safety of EMS personnel, and protection of patients from injury, should be overriding objectives in any restraint situation. Restraint should be used as humanely as possible and with respect for the patient's dignity. In most cases, the restraint duty should be given to law enforcement personnel. As in all other aspects of health care, details of the incident should be carefully documented for future reference. The patient should be assessed and treated for medical conditions associated with violent behavior. When managing a patient who may require restraint, the paramedic should do the following:

1. Provide a safe environment.
2. Gather a significant medical and psychiatric history.
3. Attempt to gain the patient's cooperation.
4. Be confident but not confrontational.

CRITICAL THINKING

Have you ever seen an EMS crew member or a police officer lose control of his or her own behavior when interacting with a violent patient? How did it affect the patient's physical or psychological state?

DID YOU KNOW?

Tasers

Tasers (conducted energy weapons) are electronic control devices designed for self-defense and to subdue unruly or violent people. Tasers are used by many law enforcement, military, and security personnel. In most states, the devices are legal for civilian use (though some states or municipalities restrict or ban them). Tasers deliver a high-voltage, low-amperage electric charge (about 3 milliampere [mA] or 0.3 joule [J]). The charge is delivered through two small dartlike electrodes tethered to the device by conductive wires. The electrodes in most devices can be quickly launched about 15 feet (5 m). The darts are pointed to penetrate clothing and barbed to prevent removal once in place. (Other styles of Taser devices are available and use different methods.) The delivered current disrupts the voluntary control of muscles and produces neuromuscular incapacitation. Once the electricity stops flowing (preset time sequences up to 30 seconds in each cycle), the subject regains immediate control of all muscular activity. The use of Tasers is considered highly controversial by some in the medical community and other groups.

Assessing Patients Prior to Restraint

The *National Model EMS Clinical Guidelines*, published by the National Association of State EMS Officials, suggests that violent or agitated patients be evaluated using a validated risk assessment tool prior to restraint.[42] Such tools include the Richmond Agitation–Sedation Scale (RASS), the Altered Mental Status Score (AMSS), and the Behavioral Activity Rating Scale (BARS).

Richmond Agitation–Sedation Scale. The RASS is used to measure alertness and agitation. Patients with a RASS of 2 to 4 are not sedated enough and should be assessed for pain, anxiety, or delirium. The underlying etiology of the agitation should be investigated and appropriately treated to achieve a RASS of −2 to 0 (**TABLE 34-2**).[43]

Altered Mental Status Scale. The AMSS measures both agitation (+1 to +4) and sedation (−1 to −4).[44] The AMSS has been noted to be difficult to use and perhaps contains too many elements (**TABLE 34-3**).

Behavioral Activity Rating Scale. The BARS measures the degree of agitated behavior. The BARS was designed to assess the effectiveness of the drug ziprasidone (**TABLE 34-4**).[45]

Restraint Guidelines

The following guidelines can help paramedics to use restraint appropriately:[5]

- If the patient is homicidal, do not attempt restraint without assistance from law enforcement personnel. If the patient is armed, move everyone out of range and retreat from the scene. Wait for law enforcement personnel.

TABLE 34-2 Richmond Agitation–Sedation Scale

Combative	+4
Very agitated	+3
Agitated	+2
Restless	+1
Alert and calm	0
Drowsy	−1
Light sedation	−2
Moderate sedation	−3
Deep sedation	−4
Unarousable sedation	−5

Modified from: Sessler C. Richmond Agitation-Sedation Scale (RASS). MDCalc website. https://www.mdcalc.com/richmond-agitation-sedation-scale-rass. Accessed February 27, 2018.

TABLE 34-3 Altered Mental Status Scale

Score	Responsiveness	Speech	Facial Expression	Eyes
4	Combative, violent, out of control	Loud outbursts	Agitated	Normal
3	Very anxious, agitated	Loud outbursts	Agitated	Normal
2	Anxious, agitated	Loud outbursts	Normal	Normal
1	Anxious, restless	Normal	Normal	Normal
0	Responds easily to name, speaks in a normal tone	Normal	Normal	Clear, no ptosis
−1	Lethargic response to name	Mild slowing and thickening	Mild relaxation	Glazed or mild ptosis involving less than one-half of the eye
−2	Responds only if name is called loudly	Slurring or prominent slowing	Marked relaxation	Glazed and marked ptosis involving more than one-half of the eye
−3	Responds only after mild prodding	Few recognizable words	Marked relaxation, slacked jaw	Glazed and marked ptosis involving more than one-half of the eye
−4	Doesn't respond to mild prodding or shaking	Few recognizable words	Marked relaxation, slacked jaw	Glazed and marked ptosis involving more than one-half of the eye

Modified from: Calver LA, Stokes B, Isbister GK. Sedation assessment tool to score acute behavioural disturbance in the emergency department. *Emerg Med Australas*. 2011;23(6):732-740.

TABLE 34-4 The Behavioral Activity Rating Scale

Difficult or unable to arouse	1
Asleep but responds normally to verbal or physical contact	2
Drowsy, appears sedated	3
Quiet and awake	4
Signs of overt (physical or verbal) activity, calms down with instructions	5
Extremely or continuously active, not requiring restraint	6
Violent, requires restraint	7

Modified from: Pfizer Advisory Committee briefing document. Appendix 1: the Behavioural Activity Rating Scale. Food and Drug Administration website. https://www.fda.gov/ohrms/dockets/ac/01/briefing/3685b2_02_pfizer_appendix.pdf. Published January 10, 2011. Accessed February 27, 2018.

- Remember that the patient may not comprehend his or her actions.
- When planning the restraining action, include a backup plan in case the initial attempt fails.
- Make sure adequate help is available. At least four capable people should be available to help restrain an adult patient.
- Keep in mind that the potential for personal injury and legal liability is always present.

Restraint Methods

A number of restraint methods can be used to manage a violent patient. A gentle, nonthreatening, low-profile technique should be attempted first. The approach should move to more direct intervention as needed. The options of physical restraint should always be explained to the patient before force is applied. If still unwilling to cooperate, the patient should be informed that restraint is required to protect against injury and to ensure the safety of others.

SHOW ME THE EVIDENCE

In assessing the use of chemical sedation in EMS, authors presented the cases of two men exhibiting excited delirium. In both cases, law enforcement officers struggled unsuccessfully to control the aggressive behavior and restrain the patient. In the first case, EMS personnel administered 500 mg of ketamine intramuscularly through the patient's clothing. They reported excellent sedation within 4 minutes of drug administration. In the second case, EMS personnel administered 375 mg of ketamine intramuscularly. They reported good effect from the ketamine in 3 minutes. On arrival to the emergency department, both patients were unresponsive to painful stimuli and had an elevated body temperature. Arterial blood gases in both cases showed uncompensated metabolic acidosis. Both patients were intubated and admitted, returning to baseline by day 2 or 3. The authors concluded that in cases where excited delirium is suspected, ketamine can be an appropriate chemical sedative to safely manage the patient and reduce responders' risk of death.

Modified from: Ho JD, Smith SW, Nystrom PC, et al. Successful management of excited delirium syndrome with prehospital ketamine: two case examples. *Prehosp Emerg Care*. 2013;17(2):274-279.

NOTE

The patient should not be restrained prone with or without the hands secured behind the back (hobbling or hog-tying). Sandwiching the patient between backboards or using restraint techniques that constrict the neck or obstruct the airway is considered dangerous, and these are not acceptable means for restraint. EMS personnel should also not use weapons to assist in patient restraint.

Modified from: Patient restraint in emergency medical services. *Prehosp Emerg Care*. 2017;21(3):395-396.

Before approaching a violent patient, the paramedic should be aware of the patient's surroundings. Seemingly harmless items should be noted, such as ashtrays, lighted cigarettes, hot coffee, letter openers, soda bottles, cans, and furniture. No attempt should be made to enter the patient's physical space until the other members involved in the restraint action are ready to proceed. (The patient's physical space usually is considered to be two arm lengths.)

The patient's muscle groups and potential range of motion should be considered before restraint is initiated. The paramedic should plan to position the patient in a way that limits strength and range of motion. Each member of the restraint team should be assigned a specific body part or responsibility before the actual restraint procedure begins.

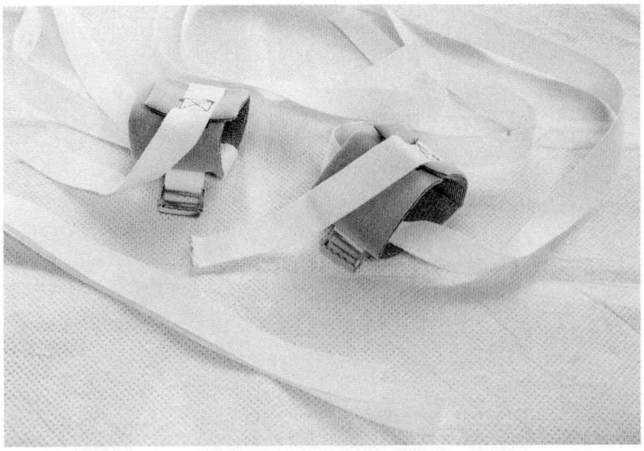

FIGURE 34-3 Restraint devices.

Paramedics must be familiar with the restraint devices available and should be able to improvise if the need arises. The preferred method is to use commercially manufactured wrist/waist/ankle padded leather or Velcro straps, or full jacket restraints (**FIGURE 34-3**). Restraint devices must allow for rapid removal to manage emergency airway or respiratory problems. If the restraint device requires a key to unlock the device, the key must accompany the patient at all times.

Effective restraints also may be improvised using common materials such as the following:[5]

- Small towels that can be wrapped around the patient's wrists and ankles and secured with tape to the stretcher
- Cravats
- Webbed straps ordinarily used to secure patients to spine boards
- Roller bandage
- Blanket roll

Regardless of the types used, restraints should be strong enough to achieve the desired effect. However, they should not compromise circulatory or respiratory status.

Sequence of Restraint Actions

Trained personnel can use many restraint techniques. The following sequence is an example of a restraint action that may be used to contain violent behavior.

1. The paramedic offers the patient one final chance to cooperate.

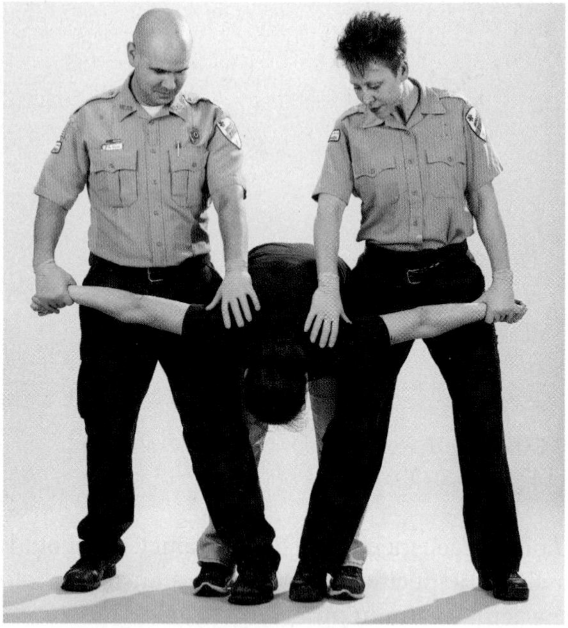

FIGURE 34-4 Control position. Rescuers face the same direction. The rescuers' inside legs are placed in front of the patient. The rescuers' outside hands hold the patient's wrists. The rescuers' inside hands form a "C" on the patient's shoulders.

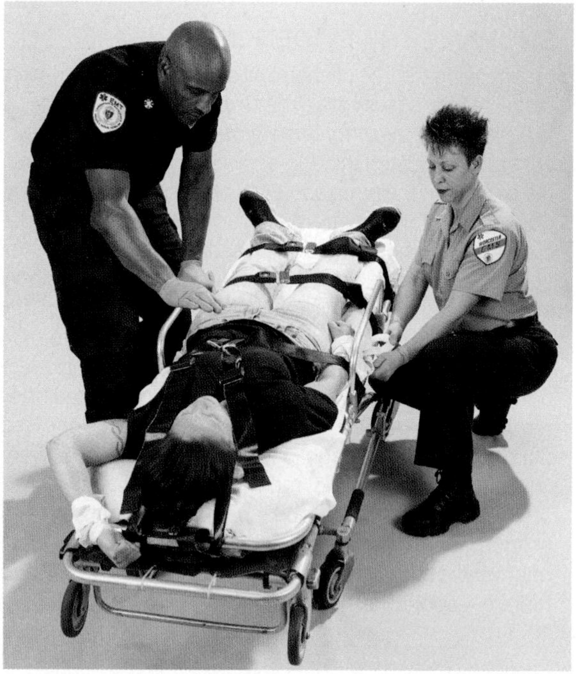

FIGURE 34-5 Patient restrained in supine position.

2. If the patient does not respond, at least four rescuers move swiftly toward the person. They position themselves close to and slightly behind the patient. Two rescuers should then position an inside leg in front of the patient's leg to force the patient to the ground if necessary (**FIGURE 34-4**). Swift movement by several rescuers minimizes the patient's ability to focus on restraint actions. It also reduces the accuracy of kicks or blows. During the restraint procedure, the patient should be continually reassured by a rescuer not involved in the physical maneuver.
3. If the patient calms and agrees to be transported without restraints, the paramedic positions the patient lateral or supine on a stretcher (if not contraindicated by the mechanism of injury or medical condition). The paramedic secures the patient with straps to limit range of motion (**FIGURE 34-5**). If the patient becomes dangerous en route to the medical facility, restraints should be used.
4. Once applied, restraints should not be removed until the patient is delivered to the emergency department or there are adequate resources to control the situation. The patient's respiratory and circulatory status should be assessed frequently and documented. This monitoring ensures that the restraint action has not compromised vital functions. If a change in the restraints is required, additional manpower must be available for assistance. Also, only one limb should be repositioned at a time.
5. If the patient continues to struggle forcefully after the restraint application, the paramedic should consider chemical sedation. Violent struggling can be associated with hyperkalemia and rhabdomyolysis, which can lead to cardiac arrest.[41]

Restraint procedures should be fully documented on the patient care report. Any attempts at negotiation and a description of the patient's behavior before restraint should be clearly described. Paramedics should document that circulatory evaluation and continued monitoring of the patient were performed after restraint. Again, physical restraint is advised only when all verbal and nonverbal techniques have been exhausted and only when a person presents a danger to self or others.

Personal Safety

Paramedics' personal safety should be considered in any emergency response. However, behavioral emergencies are more likely to require that paramedics protect themselves and the crew from hostile injury.

The following measures for preventing personal injury should be considered:

- When possible, remain a safe distance from the patient.
- Do not allow the patient to block the exit.
- Keep large furniture between you and the patient. Do not allow a single paramedic to remain alone with the patient.
- Do not make statements that the patient might perceive as threatening.
- Use folded blankets or cushions to absorb the impact of thrown objects.

Various training programs have been developed to provide safety and security to the rescuer and the violent patient. Paramedics should learn nonviolent personal protection maneuvers and should practice these maneuvers under the supervision of a qualified instructor.

Chemical Restraint

The term **chemical restraint** refers to the use of drugs to control behavior. Drug treatment varies. However, it generally is intended to provide sedation. Several groups of drugs are effective for chemical restraint. They include ketamine or other dissociative agents, benzodiazepines, and antipsychotics (butyrophenones) (see Chapter 13, *Principles of Pharmacology and Emergency Medications*). Paralytics should not be used for chemical restraint unless their use is indicated to manage another underlying clinical condition and concurrent sedation is available.[41] Drugs should be chosen based on availability, patient age, underlying conditions, and route and onset of action.

Ketamine is a dissociative agent that provides both sedation and anesthesia. Ketamine is administered at 2 mg/kg intravenously (onset, 1 minute) or 4 mg/kg intramuscularly (onset, 3 to 5 minutes).[46]

Benzodiazepines bind to specific receptors in the cerebral cortex and limbic system (a major integrating system that governs emotional behavior). These drugs are popular because of their very high therapeutic index. They have four main actions: anxiety reduction, sedative-hypnotic effects, muscle relaxation, and anticonvulsant effects. Benzodiazepines commonly used for chemical restraint include midazolam, lorazepam, or diazepam (**TABLE 34-5**).

Antipsychotics block dopamine receptors in specific areas of the central nervous system. These drugs are primarily used to treat schizophrenia. They also are used to treat other conditions that produce disturbed behavior (eg, Tourette syndrome). Antipsychotics used for chemical restraint include droperidol, haloperidol, olanzapine, and ziprasidone (**TABLE 34-6**). Short-term use of antipsychotics rarely produces extrapyramidal reactions. However, if such reactions occur, administration of diphenhydramine may reverse these side effects.

Benzodiazepines and antipsychotics can be very effective at controlling hostile or combative patients. As with all other restraint methods, paramedics should consult with medical direction, follow protocol, monitor the patient, and carefully document the event.

TABLE 34-5 Benzodiazepines Commonly Used for Chemical Restraint

Drug	Dose/Route	Onset
Diazepam	5 mg IV 10 mg IM	2–5 minutes 15–30 minutes
Lorazepam	2 mg IV 4 mg IM	2–5 minutes 15–30 minutes
Midazolam	5 mg IV 5 mg IM 5 mg IN	3–5 minutes 10–15 minutes 3–5 minutes

Abbreviations: IM, intramuscular; IN, intranasal; IV, intravenous

Modified from: National Association of EMS Officials. *National Model EMS Clinical Guidelines*. Version 2.0. National Association of EMS Officials website. https://www.nasemso.org/documents/National-Model-EMS-Clinical-Guidelines-Version2-Sept2017.pdf. Published September 2017. Accessed February 27, 2018.

TABLE 34-6 Antipsychotics Commonly Used for Chemical Restraint

Drug	Dose/Route	Onset of Action
Droperidol	2.5 mg IV 5 mg IM	10 minutes 20 minutes
Haloperidol	5 mg IV 10 mg	5–10 minutes 10–20 minutes
Olanzapine[a]	10 mg IM	15–30 minutes
Ziprasidone	10 mg IM	10 minutes

[a]Not for use with IM/IV benzodiazepines (fatalities have been reported).

Abbreviations: IM, intramuscular; IV, intravenous

Modified from: National Association of EMS Officials. *National Model EMS Clinical Guidelines*. Version 2.0. National Association of EMS Officials website. https://www.nasemso.org/documents/National-Model-EMS-Clinical-Guidelines-Version2-Sept2017.pdf. Published September 2017. Accessed February 27, 2018.

NOTE

Extrapyramidal reactions are neuromuscular effects that can be caused by some antipsychotic medications. These effects include Parkinson like symptoms (eg, tremor, muscle rigidity, pill-rolling motion, shuffling gait), akathisia (abnormal restlessness, agitation), dystonias (abnormal muscle tone or posturing), and tardive dyskinesia (involuntary, repetitious movement). The occurrence and severity of extrapyramidal reactions frequently are dose related. They often subside when the dose is reduced or the drug is discontinued. However, in some patients, tardive dyskinesia persists even after drug therapy is stopped. This risk is especially high in patients prescribed long-term drug therapy. These rhythmical, involuntary movements are most evident in the tongue, face, mouth, or jaw. They are characterized by protrusion of the tongue, puffing of the cheeks, puckering of the mouth, chewing movements, and sometimes involuntary movements of the extremities.

Summary

- A behavioral emergency is a change in mood or behavior that cannot be tolerated by the involved person or others and that requires immediate attention. Physical or biochemical disturbances can result in significant changes in behavior. Psychosocial mental illness is often the result of childhood trauma, child abuse or neglect, or a dysfunctional family structure. Changes in behavior caused by interpersonal or situational stress are often linked to specific incidents, such as environmental violence, death of a loved one, economic or employment problems, or prejudice and discrimination.
- When managing behavioral emergencies, the paramedic should contain the crisis. This effort begins with establishing a rapport with the patient. The paramedic should provide the proper emergency care and transport the patient to an appropriate health care facility.
- During the patient assessment, the paramedic should attempt to determine the patient's mental state, name and age, significant medical history, medications (and compliance), and past psychiatric problems, as well as the precipitating situation or problem.
- Effective interviewing techniques include employing active listening, being supportive and empathetic, preventing interruptions, and respecting the patient's personal space. A mental status examination includes assessment of appearance and behavior, speech and language, cognitive abilities, and emotional stability.
- All neurocognitive disorders result in a disturbance in thinking that may manifest as delirium or dementia.
- Autism spectrum disorder is a range of neurodevelopmental disorders that include two behavioral features, which include impairment in social communication and interaction and restricted, repetitive behaviors, interests, or activities.
- Schizophrenia is characterized by symptoms that fall into three categories: positive, negative, and cognitive. Positive symptoms (eg, delusions, thought disorders, movement disorders) are psychotic behaviors not found in healthy people. Negative symptoms (eg, flat effect, anhedonia) disrupt normal emotions and behaviors. Cognitive symptoms vary by patient but can include poor executive functions, trouble focusing, and problems with working memory.
- Anxiety disorders may cause a panic attack. Anxiety disorders include phobias, obsessive-compulsive disorders, and posttraumatic stress disorder.
- Depression is a mood disorder. A person with depression may have feelings of hopelessness, loss of appetite, decreased libido, and feelings of worthlessness and guilt. Bipolar disorder is a biphasic emotional disorder in which depressive and manic episodes alternate.
- Suicide threats or attempts indicate the patient has a serious crisis. Certain factors increase the risk of suicide. Patients who express the wish to harm or kill themselves should be transported. Paramedics should ask questions that determine the patient's ideation, plan, intent, and means to commit suicide. After ensuring scene safety, the first priority in patient management after a suicide attempt is medical care. If the patient is conscious, developing rapport as soon as possible is essential.
- Some patients with a behavioral emergency may also be using alcohol or illegal drugs. Signs that may indicate alcohol or illicit drug use include a breath odor of alcohol, the presence of drug paraphernalia, and needle tracks on the extremities.
- Somatic symptom disorders (somatoform disorders) are conditions in which there are physical symptoms for which no physical cause can be found. Patients with these disorders most often complain of neurologic symptoms, gynecologic symptoms, and gastrointestinal symptoms. The cause is thought to be psychological. These disorders include conversion disorder.
- Factitious disorders are disorders in which symptoms mimic a true illness. However, the symptoms have been invented so that the person may assume the role of a patient.
- Dissociative disorders are a group of psychological illnesses. In these disorders, a particular mental function is separated from the mind as a whole.
- The most common feeding and eating disorders considered to be forms of psychiatric illness are anorexia nervosa and bulimia nervosa.
- Disruptive, impulse-control, and conduct disorders are characterized by the inability to control emotions or resist an impulse or temptation to perform an act that is unlawful, socially unacceptable, or self-harmful. Personality disorders are conditions characterized by failing to learn from experience or adapt appropriately to changes. This results in personal distress and impairment of social functioning.

- Children who experience emotional crises need to be managed with different techniques than those used to care for older children and adults. Some techniques include gaining the child's trust, keeping the interview questions brief, being honest, and taking threats of violence seriously.
- Problem behavior in an older adult patient can be a sign of a longstanding psychiatric disorder, a newly emerging psychiatric problem, a medical illness, substance abuse, drug noncompliance or drug interactions, or other concerns. The paramedic must speak slowly, distinctly, and respectfully and allow time for complete answers.
- In assessing whether a patient may become violent, the paramedic should consider the patient's history of violence, posture, vocal activity, and physical activity.
- When trying to defuse a situation involving a potentially violent patient, the paramedic should ensure the safety of the patient, crew, and others, help the patient to manage his or her emotions, avoid the use of restraint whenever possible, and avoid interventions that appear coercive.
- Severely disturbed patients who pose a threat to themselves or others may need to be restrained. Reasonable force to restrain a patient should be used as humanely as possible. An adequate number of personnel are needed to ensure patient and rescuer safety during restraint. The risk of personal injury and legal liability is always present.
- Personal safety measures while responding to a behavioral emergency should include not allowing the patient to block the exit, keeping large furniture between you and the patient, avoiding threatening statements, and using soft objects to absorb the impact of thrown objects.

References

1. Substance Abuse and Mental Health Services Administration (SAMHSA). *Behavioral Health Trends in the United States: Results From the 2014 Survey on Drug Use and Health.* Rockville, MD: Substance Abuse and Mental Health Services Administration (SAMHSA); 2015.
2. US Burden of Disease Collaborators. The state of US health, 1990–2010: burden of diseases, injuries, and risk factors. *JAMA.* 2013;310(6):591-608.
3. Ball JW, Dains JE, Flynn JA, Solomon BS, Stewart RW. *Seidel's Guide to Physical Examination.* 8th ed. St. Louis, MO: Mosby; 2014.
4. American Psychiatric Association. *Diagnostic and Statistical Manual of Mental Disorders.* 5th ed. Washington, DC: American Psychiatric Association Publishing; 2013.
5. National Highway Traffic Safety Administration. *The National EMS Education Standards*, Washington, DC: US Department of Transportation/National Highway Traffic Safety Administration; 2009.
6. Rizzi L, Rosset I, Roriz-Cruz M. Global epidemiology of dementia: Alzheimer's and vascular types. *BioMed Res Int.* 2014;2014:908915.
7. Soke GN, Rosenberg S, Hamman RF. Brief report: prevalence of self-injurious behaviors among children with autism spectrum disorder—a population-based study. *J Autism Dev Disord.* 2016;46(11):3607-3614.
8. Emergency medical services. Autism Speaks website. https://www.autismspeaks.org/family-services/autism-safety-project/first-responders/emergency-services. Accessed February 27, 2018.
9. About schizophrenia. Schizophrenia and Related Disorders Alliance of America website. https://sardaa.org/resources/about-schizophrenia/. Accessed February 27, 2018.
10. Schizophrenia. National Institute of Mental Health website. https://www.nimh.nih.gov/health/topics/schizophrenia/index.shtml. Accessed February 27, 2018.
11. Breier A, Schreiber JL, Dyer J, et al. National Institute of Mental Health longitudinal study of chronic schizophrenia: prognosis and predictors of outcome. *Arch Gen Psychiatry.* 1991;48(3):239-246.
12. National Institute of Mental Health. The numbers count: mental disorders in America. Library of the US Courts of the Seventh Circuit website. http://www.lb7.uscourts.gov/documents/12-cv-1072url2.pdf. Published October 1, 2013. Accessed February 27, 2018.
13. Understanding anxiety disorders: when panic, fear, and worries overwhelm. NIH News in Health website. https://newsinhealth.nih.gov/2016/03/understanding-anxiety-disorders. Published March 2016. Accessed February 27, 2018.
14. Any anxiety disorder. National Institute of Mental Health website. https://www.nimh.nih.gov/health/statistics/any-anxiety-disorder.shtml. Updated November 2017. Accessed February 27, 2018.
15. Locke AB, Kirst N, Shultz CG. Diagnosis and management of generalized anxiety disorder and panic disorder in adults. *Am Fam Physician.* 2015 May 1;91(9):617-624.
16. Social anxiety disorder. National Institute of Mental Health website. https://www.nimh.nih.gov/health/statistics/social-anxiety-disorder.shtml. Updated November 2017. Accessed February 27, 2018.
17. Obsessive-compulsive disorder. National Institute of Mental Health website. https://www.nimh.nih.gov/health/topics/obsessive-compulsive-disorder-ocd/index.shtml. Updated. January 2016. Accessed February 27, 2018.
18. Obsessive-compulsive disorder (OCD). National Institute of Mental Health website. https://www.nimh.nih.gov/health/statistics/obsessive-compulsive-disorder-ocd.shtml. Updated November 2017. Accessed February 27, 2018.
19. Marx JA, Hockberger RS, Walls RM. *Rosen's Emergency Medicine: Concepts and Clinical Practice.* 8th ed. St. Louis, MO: Saunders; 2013.
20. Post-traumatic stress disorder (PTSD). National Institute of Mental Health website. https://www.nimh.nih.gov/health/statistics/post-traumatic-stress-disorder-ptsd.shtml. Updated November 2017. Accessed February 27, 2018.
21. What is PTSD (posttraumatic stress disorder)? Nebraska Department of Veterans' Affairs website. http://www.ptsd.ne.gov/what-is-ptsd.html. Accessed February 27, 2018.
22. Major depression. National Institute of Mental Health website. https://www.nimh.nih.gov/health/statistics/prevalence/major-depression-among-adults.shtml. Updated November 2017. Accessed February 27, 2018.
23. Rund DA. Behavioral disorders: clinical features. In: Tintinalli JE, Kelen GD, Stapczynski JS, eds. *Emergency Medicine: A Comprehensive Study Guide.* 6th ed. Irving, TX: American College of Emergency Physicians; 2004:1810.
24. Bipolar disorder. National Institute of Mental Health website. https://www.nimh.nih.gov/health/statistics//bipolar-disorder.shtml. Updated November 2017. Accessed February 27, 2018.

25. Reich JA, Stinton A. Behavioral health emergencies. In: Brice J, Delbriddge TR, Meyers JB, eds. *Emergency Services: Clinical Practice and Systems Oversight*. 2nd ed. West Sussex, England: John Wiley & Sons Ltd; 2015:412-422.
26. Soreff S. Suicide. Medscape website. https://emedicine.medscape.com/article/2013085-overview?pa=Sf1mhlRyfXrg1%2BnrFDtrbsu%2FmTPGa0hTfzbpbblRwET45yfarDdjumufRdc1nkNaVrJxKJt4DRD8mxYr6kYfOw%3D%3D. Updated December 7, 2017. Accessed February 27, 2018.
27. National Safety Council. *Injury Facts: 2017 Edition*. Itasca, IL: National Safety Council; 2017.
28. Haas AP, Eliason M, Mays VM, et al. Suicide and suicide risk in lesbian, gay, bisexual, and transgender populations: review and recommendations. *J Homosex*. 2011;58(1):10-51.
29. Dual diagnosis. National Alliance on Mental Illness website. https://www.nami.org/Learn-More/Mental-Health-Conditions/Related-Conditions/Dual-Diagnosis. Updated August 2017. Accessed February 27, 2018.
30. Green M. Eight most commonly abused drugs in the US. Absolute Advocacy website. https://www.absoluteadvocacy.org/most-commonly-abused-drugs/. Published July 1, 2014. Accessed February 27, 2018.
31. The Alliance on Mental Illness. Dual diagnosis: mental illness and substance abuse. Dartmouth College website. https://www.dartmouth.edu/~eap/library/dualdiagnosis1.pdf. Accessed February 27, 2018.
32. Co-occurring disorders. Substance Abuse and Mental Health Services Administration website. https://www.samhsa.gov/disorders/co-occurring. Updated March 8, 2016. Accessed February 27, 2018.
33. Greenberg DB. Somatization: epidemiology, pathogenesis, clinical features, medical evaluation, and diagnosis. UpToDate website. http://cursoenarm.net/UPTODATE/contents/mobipreview.htm?18/34/18977?source=see_link. Accessed February 27, 2018.
34. Gehlawat P, Gehlawat VK, Singh P, Gupta R. Munchausen syndrome by proxy: an alarming face of child abuse. *Indian J Psychol Med*. 2015;37(1):90-92.
35. Dissociative disorders. National Alliance on Mental Illness website. https://www.nami.org/Learn-More/Mental-Health-Conditions/Dissociative-Disorders. Accessed February 27, 2018.
36. Eating disorder statistics. National Association of Anorexia Nervosa and Associated Disorders website. http://www.anad.org/get-information/about-eating-disorders/eating-disorders-statistics/. Accessed February 27, 2018.
37. Gathright MM, Tyler LH. Disruptive behaviors in children and adolescents. Little Rock, AR: Psychiatric Research Institute, University of Arkansas for Medical Sciences; 2014.
38. Disruptive, impulse-control, and conduct disorders. American Psychiatric Association website. https://dsm.psychiatryonline.org/doi/10.1176/appi.books.9780890425596.dsm15. Accessed February 27, 2018.
39. Growing mental and behavioral health concerns facing older Americans. American Psychological Association website. http://www.apa.org/advocacy/health/older-americans.aspx. Accessed February 27, 2018.
40. Richmond J, Berlin JS, Fishkind AB, et al. Verbal de-escalation of the agitated patient: consensus statement of the American Association for Emergency Psychiatry Project BETA De-escalation Workgroup. *West J Emerg Med*. 2012;13(1):17-25.
41. Patient restraint in emergency medical services, NAEMSP restraint position statement. The National Association of EMS Physicians website. http://www.naemsp.org/Documents/Restraint%20position%20statement%20Approved%20Version%20for%20PEC.pdf. Accessed February 27, 2018.
42. National Association of EMS Officials. *National Model EMS Clinical Guidelines*. Version 2.0. National Association of EMS Officials website. https://www.nasemso.org/documents/National-Model-EMS-Clinical-Guidelines-Version2-Sept2017.pdf. Published September 2017. Accessed February 27, 2018.
43. Sessler CN, Gosnell MS, Grap M, et al. The Richmond Agitation–Sedation Scale validity and reliability in adult intensive care unit patients. *Am J Respir Crit Care Med*. 2002;166(10):1338-1344.
44. Calver LA, Stokes B, Isbister GK. Sedation assessment tool to score acute behavioural disturbance in the emergency department. *Emerg Med Australas*. 2011;23(6):732-740.
45. Pfizer Advisory Committee briefing document. Appendix 1: The Behavioural Activity Rating Scale. Food and Drug Administration website. https://www.fda.gov/ohrms/dockets/ac/01/briefing/3685b2_02_pfizer_appendix.pdf. Published January 10, 2011. Accessed February 27, 2018.
46. Busti AJ. Sedative hypnotics medications used in anesthesia and procedural sedation. Evidence-Based Medicine Consult website. https://www.ebmconsult.com/articles/sedative-hypnotics-anesthesia-procedural-sedation. Accessed February 27, 2018.

Suggested Readings

American College of Emergency Physicians Excited Delirium Task Force. *White Paper Report on Excited Delirium Syndrome*. Irving, TX: American College of Emergency Physicians; 2009.

American Psychiatric Association. *Diagnostic and Statistical Manual of Mental Disorders*. 5th ed. Washington, DC: American Psychiatric Association Publishing; 2013.

Cuddeback G, Patterson PD, Moore C, et al. Utilization of emergency medical transports and hospital admissions among persons with behavioral health conditions. *Psychiatr Serv*. 2010;61(4):412-415.

Freise G. Expert tips for EMS handling of behavioral emergencies. EMS1.com website. https://www.ems1.com/ems-assaults/articles/57080048-Expert-tips-for-EMS-handling-of-behavioral-emergencies/. Published February 4, 2016. Accessed February 27, 2018.

Ingersoll RE, Rak CF. *Psychopharmacology for Mental Health Professionals: An Integrative Approach*. 2nd ed. Boston, MA: Cengage; 2016.

Kleespies PM. *Behavioral Emergencies: An Evidence-Based Resource for Evaluating and Managing Suicidal Behavior, Violence, and Victimization*. Washington, DC: American Psychiatric Association Publishing; 2008.

Pediatric mental health emergencies in the emergency medical services system. American College of Emergency Physicians website. https://www.acep.org/Clinical---Practice-Management/Pediatric-Mental-Health-Emergencies-in-the-Emergency-Medical-Services-System/#sm.0000vyjqgsa95e2uwy91hykef6zea. Accessed February 27, 2018.

Polk DA; American Academy of Orthopaedic Surgeons. *Prehospital Behavioral Emergencies and Crisis Response*. Sudbury, MA: Jones and Bartlett Publishers; 2008.

Pozgar GD. *Legal and Ethical Issues for Health Professionals*. Burlington, MA: Jones & Bartlett Learning; 2016.

PART

8

Shock and Resuscitation

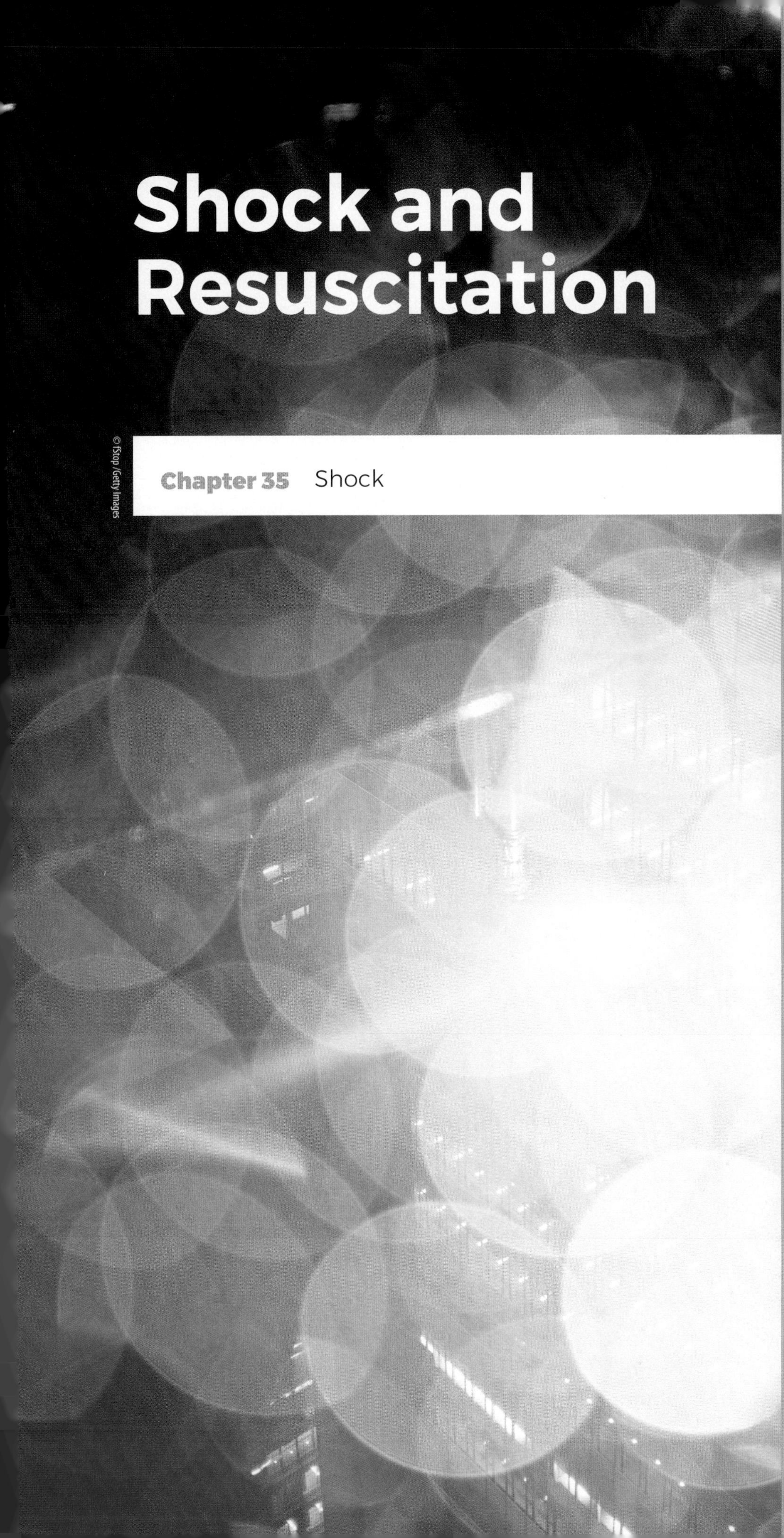

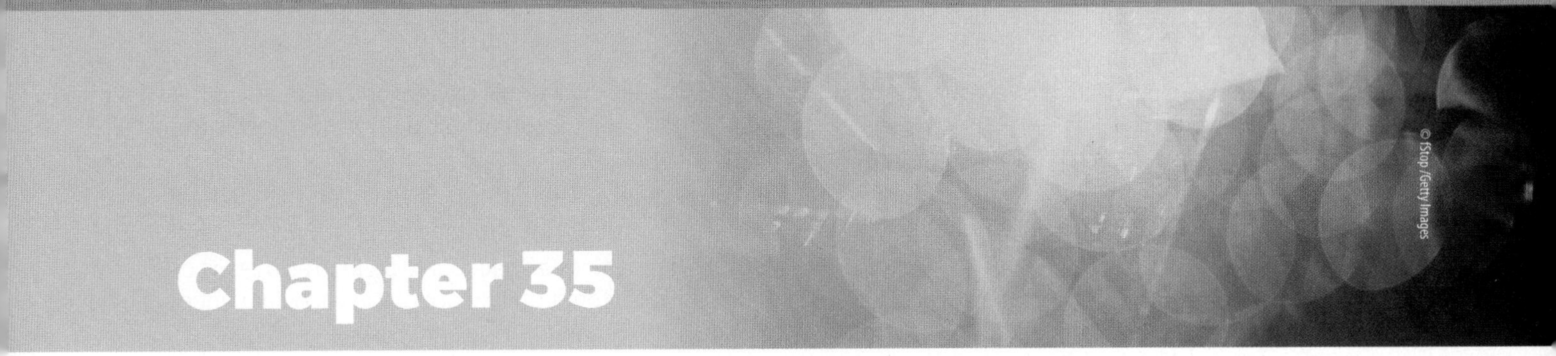

Chapter 35

Shock

NATIONAL EMS EDUCATION STANDARD COMPETENCIES

Shock and Resuscitation

Integrates a comprehensive knowledge of the causes and pathophysiology of shock, respiratory failure, or arrest into the management of these conditions, with an emphasis on early intervention to prevent arrest.

OBJECTIVES

Upon completion of this chapter, the paramedic student will be able to:

1. Define shock. (pp 1304–1305)
2. Outline the factors necessary to achieve adequate tissue oxygenation. (pp 1305–1307)
3. Describe how the diameter of resistance vessels influences preload. (pp 1305–1308)
4. Calculate mean arterial pressure when given a blood pressure. (p 1305)
5. Outline the changes in the microcirculation during the progression of shock. (pp 1308–1309)
6. List the causes of hypovolemic, cardiogenic, obstructive, and distributive shock. (pp 1309–1314)
7. Describe pathophysiology as a basis for signs and symptoms associated with the progression through the stages of shock. (pp 1314–1317)
8. Describe key assessment findings that distinguish the etiology of the shock state. (pp 1317–1322)
9. Outline the prehospital management of the patient in shock based on knowledge of the pathophysiology associated with each type of shock. (pp 1317, 1321–1324, 1325–1329)
10. Discuss how to integrate the assessment and management of the patient in shock. (pp 1317–1322, 1329)
11. Describe principles of fluid administration in shock. (pp 1319–1325)

KEY TERMS

anaphylactic shock A form of distributive shock that occurs when the body is exposed to a substance that produces a severe, exaggerated, life-threatening hypersensitivity reaction to an antigen.

cardiogenic shock A condition caused by loss of 40% or more of the functioning myocardium; the heart is no longer able to circulate sufficient blood to maintain adequate oxygen delivery.

colloid solutions Solutions that contain molecules (usually proteins) that are too large to pass through the capillary membrane.

compensated shock An early stage of shock in which the body is still able to maintain mean arterial blood pressure through compensatory changes in heart rate, stroke volume, or systemic vascular resistance.

crystalloid solutions Solutions created by dissolving crystals such as salts and sugars in water.

disseminated intravascular coagulation (DIC) A grave coagulopathy that results from the overstimulation of the clotting and anticlotting processes in response to disease or injury.

distributive shock Shock that occurs when peripheral vasodilation causes a decrease in systemic vascular resistance or as a result of impaired distribution of blood flow.

hemodilution An increase in the fluid content of the blood that results in a lowered concentration of formed elements and lowered blood viscosity.

hemostasis The cessation of bleeding by mechanical or chemical means or by substances that arrest the blood flow.

hypertonic solutions Solutions that have higher osmotic pressure than body cells have.

hypoperfusion Severely inadequate circulation that results in insufficient delivery of oxygen and nutrients necessary for normal tissue and cellular function; may cause shock.

hypovolemic shock A form of shock that is most frequently caused by inadequate circulating blood volume.

irreversible shock A stage of shock that results in cellular ischemia and necrosis and subsequent organ death, even once oxygenation and perfusion are restored.

mean arterial pressure (MAP) The average blood pressure in the arterial portion of the circulation; a measurement of perfusion. It is calculated as MAP = [(Diastolic blood pressure × 2) + Systolic blood pressure]/3.

microcirculation Circulation of blood in the smallest blood vessels, including arterioles, capillaries, shunts, and venules.

microinfarcts Small infarctst caused by obstruction of circulation in capillaries, arterioles, or small arteries.

neurogenic shock A type of shock in which circulatory failure is caused by disruption of the nerves that control the size of the blood vessels, leading to widespread dilation; seen in patients with spinal cord injuries.

obstructive shock Shock that results from obstruction of forward blood flow.

perfusion The delivery of oxygen and nutrients to the cells, organs, and tissues of the body; also involves the removal of wastes.

pulse pressure The difference between the systolic and diastolic blood pressures.

relative hypovolemia Inadequate preload as a result of vasodilation or shift of fluid out of the vascular space.

sepsis Life-threatening organ dysfunction caused by a dysregulated host response to infection.

septic shock A subset of sepsis in which profound circulatory, cellular, and metabolic abnormalities cause severe compromise of end-organ perfusion. It carries a greater risk of mortality than does sepsis alone.

shock Hypoxia at the cellular level.

shock index A measurement calculated to detect shock by dividing heart rate by systolic blood pressure. Adult scales vary; typically a value of 0.9 or greater suggest shock in an adult; for pediatrics, there is an age-adjusted score.

systemic vascular resistance The total resistance against which blood must be pumped; also known as afterload.

uncompensated shock A stage of shock that occurs when the body is no longer able to maintain systemic blood pressure.

viscosity The physical property of a liquid. It is characterized by the degree of friction between its component molecules.

Severe illnesses and injury can threaten the normal perfusion of the body cells and tissues. During such events, the protective systems of the body try to compensate to maintain cellular oxygenation. The paramedic must be able to integrate pathophysiologic principles and assessment findings to form a field impression and to implement a treatment plan for the patient in shock.

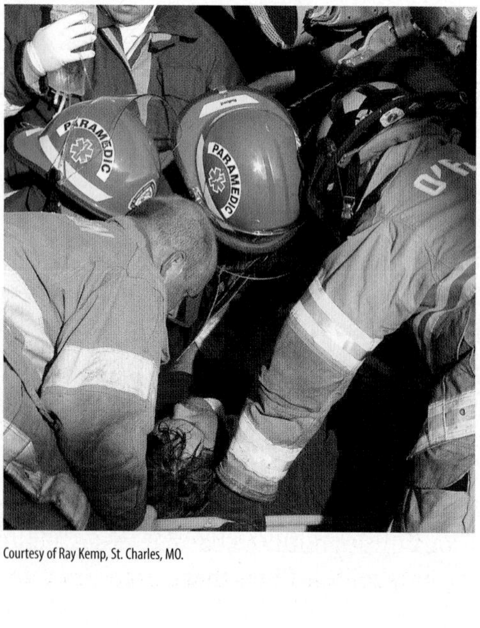

Courtesy of Ray Kemp, St. Charles, MO.

Shock

In 1861, Gross defined **shock** as a "rude unhinging of the machinery of life."[1] Since then, this term has been redefined by many others. Robert M. Hardaway, professor of surgery at Texas Tech University School of Medicine in El Paso, Texas, defines shock this way:[2]

> I believe that the best definition of shock is inadequate capillary perfusion. As a corollary of this broad definition, almost anyone who dies, except one who is instantly destroyed, must go through a stage of shock—a momentary pause in the act of death.

Shock is not a single event, and it does not have one specific cause and treatment. Rather, it is a complex group of physiologic abnormalities that can result from a variety of disease states and injuries.[3] There are many complexities involved in shock: It is not adequately defined by pulse rate, blood pressure, or cardiac function. Moreover, it cannot be reduced to loss of circulating blood or loss of pressure in the vascular system. Shock may affect the entire body, or it may occur at a tissue or cellular level, even with normal hemodynamics.

At its fundamental core, shock is hypoxia at the cellular level. Thus, an understanding of cellular physiology is needed to recognize the more subtle aspects of shock. This understanding also will aid in properly assessing the severity of various stages of shock.

Oxygen Delivery to the Tissues

Cells require oxygen for the production of energy by aerobic metabolism. Systemic oxygen delivery to the tissues depends on two factors: (1) adequate delivery of blood through the capillary bed in tissues (**perfusion**) and (2) adequate oxygen content of the blood. For effective tissue perfusion to occur, oxygen supply and oxygen demand must be in balance. Achieving this balance requires proper functioning of the heart, vasculature, and lungs.

Heart

Systemic oxygen delivery is the product of cardiac output and the arterial oxygen content. Cardiac output depends on several factors, including the strength of the heart's contraction (inotropy), the rate of contraction (chronotropy), and the amount of venous return available to the ventricle (preload). The formula to determine cardiac output is as follows:

$$\text{Cardiac output (CO)} = \text{Heart rate (HR)} \times \text{Stroke volume (SV)}$$

When oxygen delivery is inadequate, the first compensatory response is to increase cardiac output, which is accomplished by increasing heart rate and/or stroke volume.

Preload, Afterload, and MAP

Important terms in understanding cardiac physiology and shock are preload, afterload, and mean arterial pressure. To review, preload is the amount of venous return to the ventricle (the ventricular volume at the end of diastole). Afterload is the total resistance against which blood must be pumped. Total peripheral vascular resistance is determined by the volume of blood in the vascular system and by the diameter of the vessel walls (described later in this section).

Mean arterial pressure (MAP) is a function of total cardiac output (CO) and systemic vascular resistance (SVR):

$$\text{MAP} = \text{CO} \times \text{SVR}$$

MAP represents the average pressure in the vascular system that perfuses the tissues. Because more time is spent in diastole than in systole, MAP is not the average of diastolic blood pressure (DBP) and systolic blood pressure (SBP), but rather reflects the relative time spent in each portion of the cardiac cycle.[4] Because more time is spent in diastole then systole, the formula for MAP is as follows:

$$\text{MAP} = [(\text{DBP} \times 2) + \text{SBP}]/3$$

Example. For a patient whose blood pressure is 120/80 mm Hg, MAP is calculated as follows:

$$\begin{aligned}\text{MAP} &= [(80 \times 2) + 120]/3 \\ &= 280/3 \\ &= 93 \text{ mm Hg}\end{aligned}$$

A systolic pressure of 80 to 90 mm Hg (MAP of 60 to 65 mm Hg) is needed to maintain adequate tissue perfusion. MAP is further discussed later in this chapter and in Chapter 38, *Burns*.

Ejection Fraction

Ejection fraction is a measurement of the percentage of blood volume pumped out of the left ventricle with each contraction. Normally, 50% to 70% of the blood is ejected out of the left ventricle. A borderline ejection fraction is 41% to 49%. At this level, a patient may have shortness of breath on exertion. When the ejection fraction is less than 40%, tissue perfusion may be compromised. Echocardiograms are used to estimate ejection fraction.

Vasculature

The entire vascular system of the body is lined with smooth, low-friction endothelial cells. All vessels larger than capillaries have layers of tissue surrounding the endothelium, known as tunicae. These layers provide supporting connective tissue to counter the pressure of blood contained in the vascular system. They also have elastic properties that enable the blood vessels to dampen pressure pulsations and minimize flow variations throughout the cardiac cycle. Finally, the tunicae have muscle fibers that can contract and relax to control the vessel diameter. The vascular system maintains blood flow by changes in pressure and peripheral vascular resistance.

Systemic Vascular Resistance

Blood flow to an organ is dependent on three factors: arterial pressure, venous pressure, and vascular resistance.

Flow = [Arterial pressure − Venous pressure] / Vascular resistance

Changes in resistance are the primary means by which blood flow is regulated within organs. On a systemic level, afterload (**systemic vascular resistance**) is the total resistance against which blood must be pumped. It is determined primarily by a change in the diameter of the arterioles. Arteriolar constriction raises MAP by preventing the free flow of blood into the capillaries, whereas dilation has the opposite effect. Reflex control of vasoconstriction and vasodilation is mediated by the sympathetic nervous system.[5]

Systemic vascular resistance is a measurement of friction between the vessel walls and fluid, and between the molecules of the fluid themselves, both of which oppose flow. When the resistance to flow increases, blood pressure must increase for the flow to remain constant. Resistance to blood flow increases with increased fluid viscosity or vessel length and decreased vessel diameter. **Viscosity** is a physical property of a liquid that reflects the degree of friction between its component molecules (eg, between the blood cells and between the plasma proteins). Viscosity normally plays a minor role in blood flow regulation because it remains fairly constant in healthy people. Vessel length in the human body also remains fairly constant. Vessel diameter is the main factor affecting the resistance to blood flow.

> **CRITICAL THINKING**
>
> How do firefighters use these principles of viscosity and vessel diameter when fighting a fire?

The major arteries in the body are quite large and, therefore, offer little resistance to flow unless they have an abnormal narrowing (stenosis). By comparison, arterioles have a much smaller diameter than arteries have and offer the major resistance to blood flow. The smooth muscle in the arteriole walls can relax or contract, changing the diameter inside the arteriole by as much as fivefold. Thus the vasoconstriction or vasodilation of these vessels primarily regulates arterial blood pressure.

Fluid flows through any kind of tube—including blood vessels—in response to pressure gradients between the two ends of the tube. The difference in pressure between the two ends, rather than the absolute pressure in the tube, determines flow. In many animals and humans, the two ends of this "tube" are the aorta and the venae cavae.

Systemic pressure (left-sided pressure) and pulmonic pressure (right-sided pressure) are the measurements of pressure in the vascular system. Both types of pressures have two phases: systolic and diastolic. The difference between these two pressures, known as the **pulse pressure**, reflects the tone of the arterial system. This pressure is greatest at its origin (the heart) and is least at its terminating point (the venae cavae). Pulse pressure is more sensitive to changes in perfusion than is the systolic pressure or the diastolic pressure alone.

Microcirculation

Microcirculation refers to circulation of blood through the smallest vessels in the circulatory system (arterioles, venules, shunts, and capillaries). Microcirculation exists in all tissues and organs except the cartilage, epithelia, cornea, and lens of the eye. The microcirculation of the body is divided into pulmonary microcirculation and peripheral microcirculation. Separate pumps—the right side and left side of the heart, respectively—produce pressure in each of these divisions.

At any given moment, approximately 5% of the total circulating blood is flowing through the capillaries, exchanging nutrients and picking up the wastes generated by cellular metabolism.[6] The muscular arterioles are the major resistance vessels; they regulate regional blood flow to the capillary beds. The venules and veins serve as collecting channels and storage vessels; these capacitance vessels normally contain approximately 70% of the blood volume.

The following mechanisms control blood flow to the tissues (as described in Chapter 11, *General Principles of Pathophysiology*):

- Local control of blood flow by the tissues
- Nervous control of blood flow
- Baroreceptor reflexes
- Chemoreceptor reflexes

- Central nervous system ischemia response
- Hormonal mechanisms
- Adrenal–medullary mechanism
- Renin–angiotensin–aldosterone mechanism
- Vasopressin mechanism
- Reabsorption of tissue fluid

Lungs

Tissue cells require adequate oxygen to function. To ensure that they obtain the needed oxygen, adequate oxygen must be available to be picked up by the red blood cells as they pass through the capillary membranes in the lungs. The high partial pressure of oxygen in inspired air, adequate depth and rate of ventilation, and matching of pulmonary ventilation and perfusion make adequate oxygenation possible.

> CRITICAL THINKING
> What might impair each of these components of adequate oxygenation?

The Body as a Container

The healthy body can be viewed as a smooth-flowing fluid delivery system inside a container. This container must be filled to achieve adequate preload and tissue oxygenation. The external size of the container of any human body is relatively constant, yet the volume of the vascular component in the container is related directly to the diameter of the resistance vessels. This diameter can change rapidly. Any change in the diameter of the vessels changes the volume of fluid that the container holds, which in turn affects preload.

As an example of this principle, consider a 5-L container—the normal container size for a 70-kg adult male (**FIGURE 35-1**). If the fluid volume is 5 L, preload is adequate. With a strong heart, cardiac output and perfusion also are adequate. In contrast, if 2 L of this fluid is lost, externally or internally, the 3 L that remains will be inadequate to supply an effective preload. Because cardiac output depends on preload, a decrease in preload notably decreases cardiac output.

If the patient is hypovolemic and the 5-L container remains the same size despite the 3-L volume, the patient becomes hypotensive or loses pressure in the container because of decreased cardiac output. However, if the container is reduced to 3 L by compensatory mechanisms (eg, vasoconstriction), the 3-L container can provide adequate preload to the heart with the 3 L of available fluid—albeit at the expense of certain tissues that are not perfused in this constricted state.

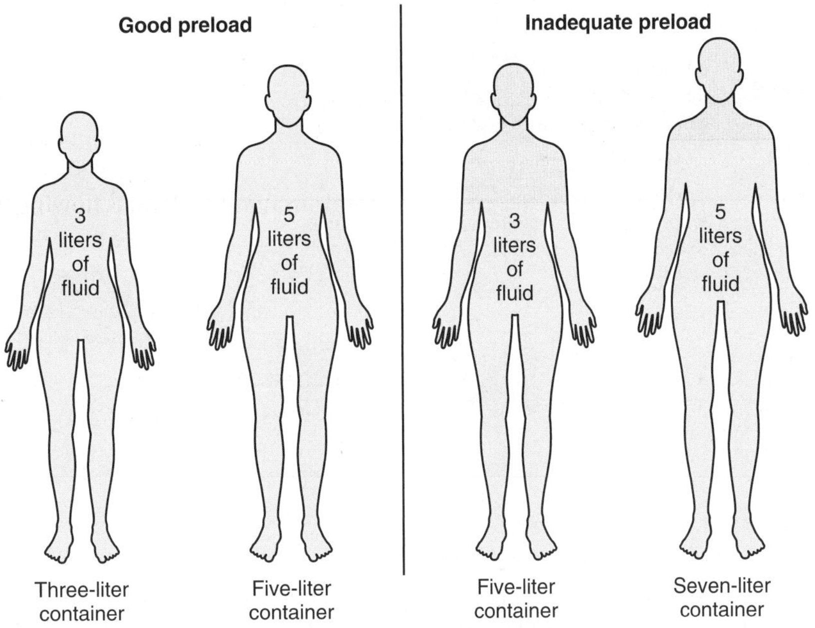

FIGURE 35-1 Fluid volume versus container volume.

If fluid is adequate for a 5-L container but the container size has been enlarged to 7 L by illness or injury that results in vasodilation, the 5 L of fluid does not provide adequate preload for the container (**relative hypovolemia**). Factors that occasionally are responsible for vasodilation include cardiac and blood pressure medications, allergic reaction, heat- and cold-related injuries, and alcohol or other drug use.

Capillary–Cellular Relationship in Shock

No matter what the cause of shock, this condition is characterized by a homeostatic vasoconstrictor response with arteriolar narrowing, a reduction in the number of open capillaries, and a decrease in venous return and cardiac output.[7] Without treatment, anaerobic metabolism develops, leading to an increase in lactic acid and metabolic acidosis (**FIGURE 35-2**). The arteriolar and precapillary sphincter control fails. Capillary engorgement and clumping of red blood cells follow, affecting nutritional flow and the removal of metabolic waste products. Blood begins to coagulate in the microcirculation—a condition known as **disseminated intravascular coagulation (DIC)**. Eventually the cells begin to swell and die. **Microinfarcts** develop in the organs and set the stage for pulmonary edema, respiratory failure, and acute

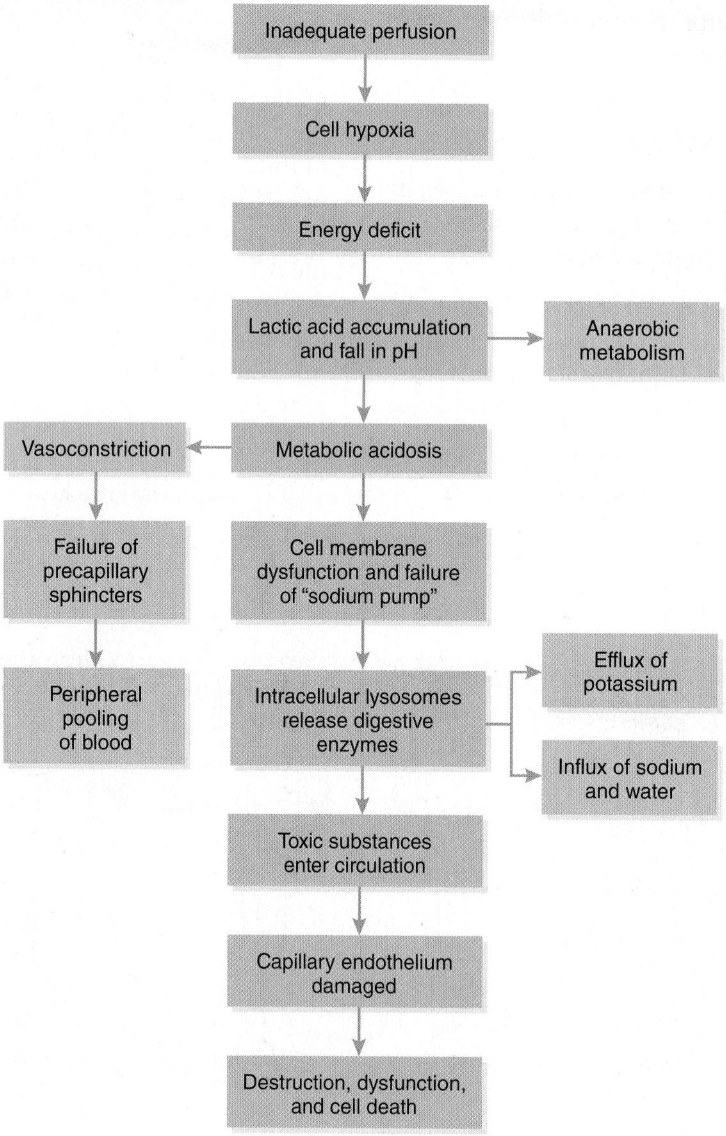

FIGURE 35-2 Cellular shock.

Modified from: Original chart created by User:Panthro, CC0, https://commons.wikimedia.org/w/index.php?curid=18229109.

respiratory distress syndrome to develop. If shock and DIC continue, the patient progresses to multiple-organ failure. If cellular necrosis damages enough of a vital organ, the organ soon fails. Failure of the liver and kidneys is common and often presents early in the final stages of shock.

> CRITICAL THINKING
> What happens to the function of the heart as acidosis increases?

Severe microcirculatory failure cannot be remedied with fluid replacement. Eventual outcomes can include heart failure, gastrointestinal bleeding, sepsis, severe pancreatitis, pulmonary thrombosis, respiratory failure, and death.

Classifications of Shock

The major classifications of shock, which differ by etiology and clinical presentation, are hypovolemic (hemorrhagic), cardiogenic, obstructive, and distributive. Although these classifications are separate and distinct, more than one type of shock can occur simultaneously. Regardless of the classification, the final common defect is hypoxia at the cellular level.

Hypovolemic Shock

Hypovolemic shock is due to an inadequate circulating blood volume (**FIGURE 35-3**). The most common causes of hypovolemic shock are hemorrhage and dehydration. Illnesses and injuries that can lead to hypovolemic shock include trauma, gastrointestinal bleeding, burns, diarrhea, vomiting, endocrine disorders, and internal third-space loss, as in peritonitis.

When the circulating blood volume (preload) decreases, the first response in hypovolemic shock is tachycardia to increase cardiac output (MAP = CO × SVR). As shock becomes more severe, blood pressure is maintained by an increase in systemic vascular resistance, leading to a narrowing of the pulse pressure. Thus, narrowing of pulse pressure is one of the early clinical signs of compensated shock. Finally, the body is unable to use compensatory mechanisms to maintain blood pressure and there is a drop in blood pressure and end-organ perfusion (uncompensated shock). **TABLE 35-1** summarizes the four stages of hypovolemic shock.

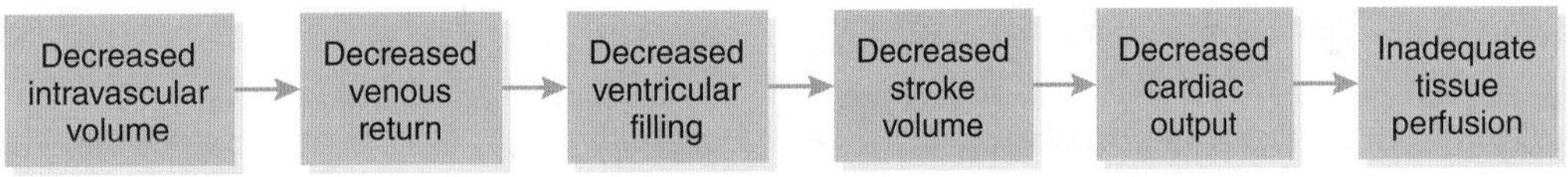

FIGURE 35-3 Pathophysiology of hypovolemic shock.

TABLE 35-1 Stages of Hypovolemic Shock

Parameter	Class I	Class II	Class III	Class IV
Percent loss in circulating volume	Up to 15%	15–30%	30–40%	>40%
Pulse rate	Normal	Mild tachycardia (100–120 beats/min)	Moderate tachycardia (120–140 beats/min)	Severe tachycardia (>140 beats/min)
Pulse pressure	Normal	Decreased	Decreased	Decreased
Blood pressure	Normal	Normal	Decreased	Decreased
Mental status (measurement of end-organ perfusion)	Slightly anxious	Mildly anxious	Anxious, confused	Confused, lethargic

Modified from: American College of Surgeons Committee on Trauma. *Advanced Trauma Life Support for Doctors. Student Course Manual*. 8th ed. Chicago, IL: American College of Surgeons; 2008.

> NOTE
>
> Most patients with shock have hypovolemia. Thus, shock is assumed to be hypovolemic in origin until proven otherwise. Patients with hypovolemia are initially managed with fluid replacement by administering normal saline or lactated Ringer solution (per protocol) to stabilize blood pressure. However, achieving a balance between organ perfusion and **hemostasis** is crucial for optimal fluid resuscitation. The concept of "permissive hypotension" refers to managing trauma patients by restricting the amount of resuscitation fluid and maintaining blood pressure in a lower-than-normal range if there is continuing bleeding during the acute period of injury. This approach is intended to avoid the adverse effects of early and high-dose fluid resuscitation (eg, hemodilution, edema, hypothermia, acidosis). Paramedics should consult with medical direction for fluid resuscitation strategies when caring for trauma patients.
>
> *Modified from*: Kudo D, Yoshida Y, Kushimoto S. Permissive hypotension/hypotensive resuscitation and restricted/controlled resuscitation in patients with severe trauma. *J Intens Care.* 2017;5:11; and National Association of Emergency Medical Technicians. *PHTLS: Basic and Advanced Prehospital Trauma Life Support.* 8th ed. Burlington, MA: Jones & Bartlett Learning; 2014.

Cardiogenic Shock

Cardiogenic shock (described in Chapter 21, *Cardiology*) is the result of a severe compromise in cardiac output such that inadequate tissue perfusion occurs despite an adequate amount of circulating blood volume. Cardiogenic shock can result from pump failure (eg, myocardial infarction, third-degree heart block), depression of cardiac contractility (eg, myocarditis, myocardial contusion), mechanical obstruction to forward blood flow (eg, aortic stenosis), or regurgitation of the left ventricular output (eg, acute aortic insufficiency such as may be seen with aortic dissection) (**FIGURE 35-4**).[8] Myocardial infarction is the most common cause of cardiogenic shock,[9] with this type of shock occurring in approximately 5% to 6% of patients hospitalized for myocardial infarction. The associated mortality rate in these patients ranges from 48% to 74%.[10] Risk factors for death include older age, underlying coronary disease, the source of the decompensation (often myocardial ischemia), decreased ejection fraction, elevated serum lactate levels, and evidence of brain or kidney dysfunction.[11]

> NOTE
>
> Cardiogenic shock is commonly known as "cold shock" because in the face of inability to increase cardiac output, blood pressure is maintained by increasing systemic vascular resistance and shunting blood to the central circulation. Clinically, this process results in cold extremities with delayed capillary refill.

> CRITICAL THINKING
>
> Why does cardiogenic shock develop in a patient who has had a severe myocardial infarction?

Obstructive Shock

Obstructive shock is a form of shock associated with the inability to produce adequate cardiac output despite normal intravascular volume and myocardial function. Causes of obstructive shock include pericardial tamponade, tension pneumothorax, and pulmonary embolism. Pericardial tamponade directly impairs diastolic filling of the right ventricle; tension pneumothorax indirectly impairs right ventricular filling by obstructing venous return; and pulmonary embolism may obstruct lobar arteries and cause impaired systolic contraction (increased ventricular afterload).[12] As discussed later in this chapter, treatment of obstructive shock centers on

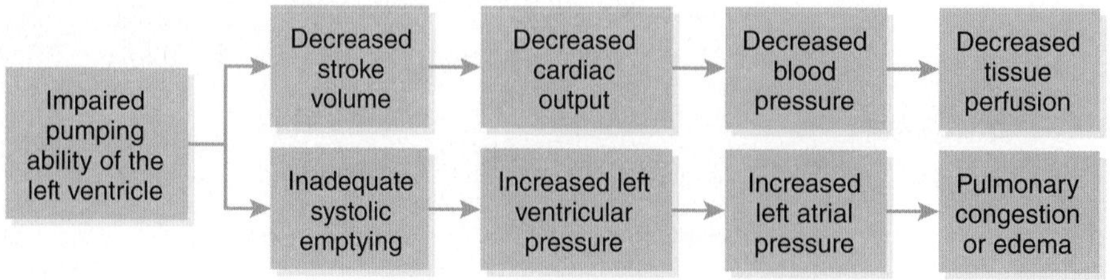

FIGURE 35-4 Cardiogenic shock.

ensuring adequate preload and treating the cause of the obstruction.

Distributive Shock

Distributive shock occurs when peripheral vasodilation causes a decrease in systemic vascular resistance. The most common causes of distributive shock are neurogenic shock, anaphylactic shock, and septic shock. In contrast to hypovolemic and cardiogenic shock, distributive shock is a "warm shock." Because the underlying etiology of inadequate circulating volume and compromised perfusion leads to peripheral vasodilation, patients will tend to have warm extremities, particularly early in the course of disease when the body is able to compensate by significantly increasing the cardiac output.

> NOTE
>
> Neurogenic shock, anaphylactic shock, and septic shock are subsets of spinal cord injury, extreme anaphylaxis, and sepsis, respectively. All of these subsets are forms of distributive shock.

Neurogenic Shock

Neurogenic shock (also known as vasogenic shock) results from loss of normal vasomotor tone due to unopposed parasympathetic response after disruption of the spinal cord at midthoracic levels and above. Because the normal function of the sympathetic nervous system produces peripheral vasoconstriction, the loss of sympathetic impulses causes a drop in systemic vascular resistance and increases the size of the body's "container" (**FIGURE 35-5**). Therefore, even normal intravascular volume is inadequate to fill the enlarged vascular compartment and perfuse the tissues. Moreover, unopposed parasympathetic input to the heart via the vagus nerve leads to bradycardia.

> NOTE
>
> Be careful not to confuse the terms *neurogenic shock* and *spinal shock*. Spinal shock refers to the flaccid areflexia (limb weakness, hypoflexia, bowel/bladder dysfunction) that may occur after spinal cord injury and may last hours to weeks. It is not a true form of shock, but rather a "concussion" of the spinal cord that may resolve as soft-tissue swelling improves. Priapism (persistent, painful erection) may be present with this condition.

Anaphylactic Shock

Anaphylactic shock (described in Chapter 26, *Immune System Disorders*) is the most extreme form of anaphylaxis. Anaphylaxis may occur when the body is exposed to an antigen (eg, antibiotic agent, venom, insect sting) that produces a severe allergic reaction. The body responds by releasing histamine and other mediators that act on receptors in the systemic and pulmonary microcirculation and produce an effect on bronchial smooth muscle. Histamine causes arterioles and capillaries to dilate and increases capillary membrane permeability. Intravascular fluid leaks into the interstitial space, causing edema, thereby decreasing the intravascular volume (**FIGURE 35-6**). In addition, many of the mediators released cause constriction of the upper and lower airways, which creates the potential for complete airway obstruction. When anaphylaxis progresses to the end stage of cardiorespiratory failure, the patient is in anaphylactic shock.

Sepsis and Septic Shock

Sepsis (described in Chapter 11, *General Principles of Pathophysiology*) is a systemic inflammatory response syndrome (SIRS) to a known or presumed infection (**FIGURE 35-7**); it can lead to severe organ dysfunction and death. This syndrome involves altered function in major organs and body processes.

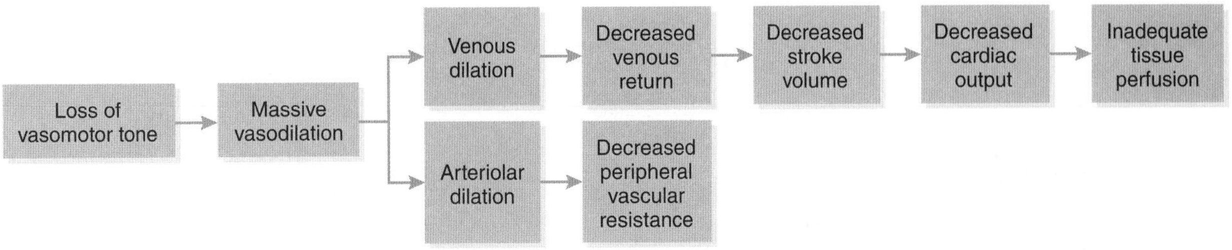

FIGURE 35-5 Pathophysiology of neurogenic shock.

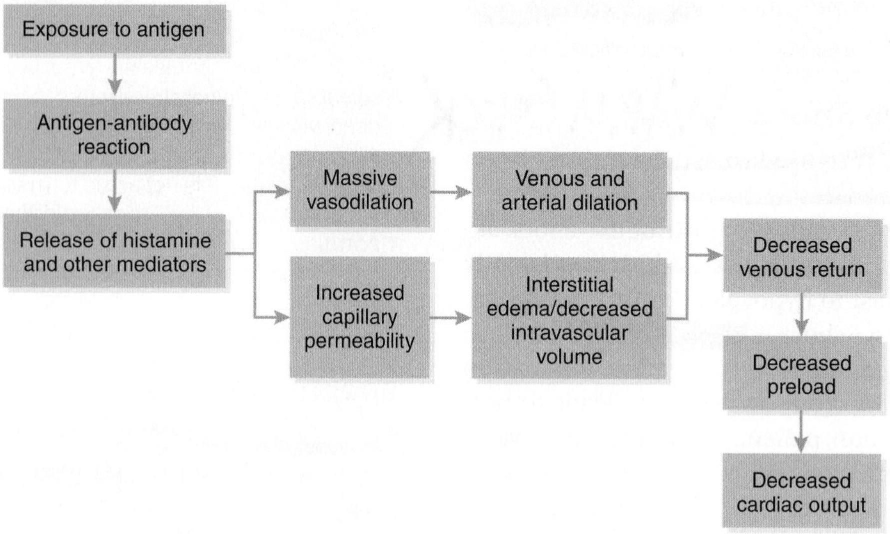

FIGURE 35-6 Pathophysiology of anaphylactic shock.

© Jones & Bartlett Learning.

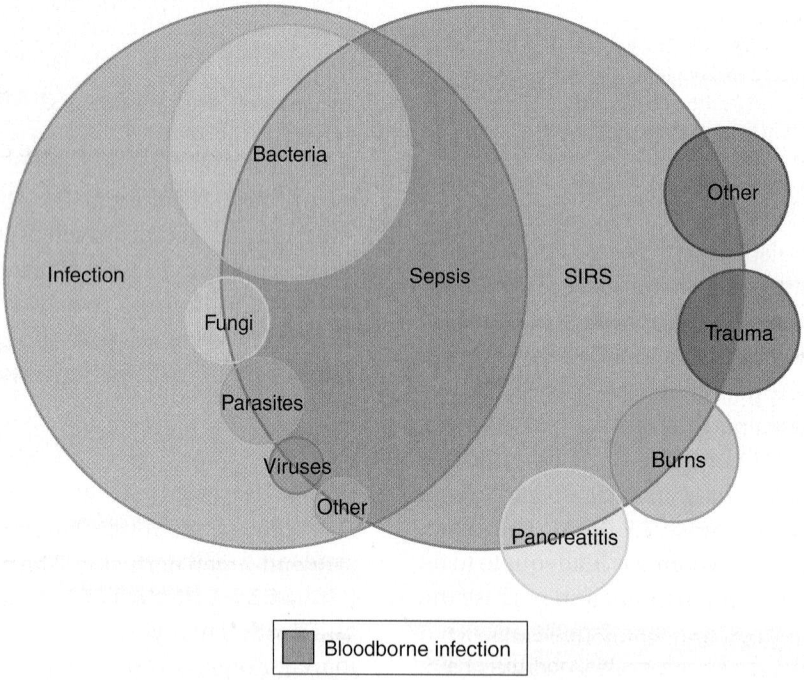

Abbreviation: SIRS, systemic inflammatory response syndrome

FIGURE 35-7 Venn diagram showing the overlap of infection, bacteremia, sepsis, systemic inflammatory response syndrome, and multiorgan dysfunction.

Image reproduced with permission from Septic shock. Medscape Drugs & Diseases (https://emedicine.medscape.com) website. https://emedicine.medscape.com/article/168402-overview#a32018. Published 2018.

Septic shock is a subset of sepsis and a more severe syndrome in which profound circulatory, cellular, and metabolic abnormalities cause a greater risk of mortality than does sepsis alone (**FIGURE 35-8**).[13] It is diagnosed when sepsis criteria are present, vasopressors are needed to elevate the MAP to 65 mm Hg or greater, and serum lactate is greater than 2 mmol/L (18 mg/dL) despite adequate fluid resuscitation. More than 500,000 people develop severe sepsis each year; mortality ranges from 15% to 50%.[14] Septic shock most

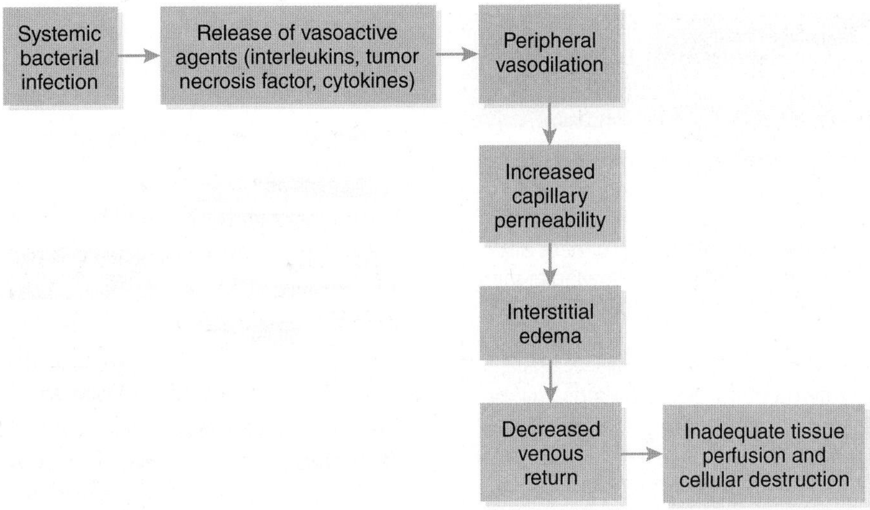

FIGURE 35-8 Pathophysiology of septic shock.

NOTE

Multiple conditions resulting in inadequate oxygen delivery, disproportionate oxygen demand, and diminished oxygen use may lead to elevated lactate levels. Normal serum lactate concentration is 0.5 to 1 mmol/L. Patients with critical illness can be considered to have normal lactate concentrations of less than 2 mmol/L. Hyperlactatemia is a cardinal finding of sepsis and septic shock and is associated with increased mortality in adult patients.

Modified from: Jat KR, Jhamb U, Gupta VK. Serum lactate levels as the predictor of outcome in pediatric septic shock. *Indian J Crit Care Med.* 2011;15(2):102-107; and Nicks BA, Khardori R. Acute lactic acidosis. Medscape website. https://emedicine.medscape.com/article/768159-overview. Updated December 21, 2017. Accessed March 23, 2018.

NOTE

Adrenal insufficiency is a frequent complication of critical illnesses, such as severe sepsis, and may be associated with a worse outcome. This syndrome can occur in critically ill patients who have blood corticosteroid levels that are inadequate to counter the severe stress response they experience. A dangerous drop in the hormone cortisol can also occur secondary to congenital or acquired adrenal insufficiency, or when a patient who is prescribed steroid medications abruptly stops taking them.

Modified from: Annane D, Maxime V, Ibrahim F, Alvarez JC, Abe E, Boudou P. Diagnosis of adrenal insufficiency in severe sepsis and septic shock. *Am J Respir Crit Care Med.* 2006;174(12):1319-1326.

often occurs in older adults (particularly nursing home residents), patients with chronic illness (eg, diabetes, lung disease, cancer, kidney disease), and patients who are immunosuppressed (eg, neonates; patients with alcoholism, cancer, human immunodeficiency virus [HIV] infection, or sickle cell disease).

Approximately 34% of patients diagnosed with sepsis and 60% of those with severe sepsis are transported by ambulance to the hospital.[15] Early recognition in the prehospital setting of a patient with possible sepsis and hospital notification are essential so fluid therapy can begin and antibiotics can be rapidly initiated on arrival.

A number of screening criteria have been developed to support prehospital sepsis identification. The basis of most of these tools is identification of suspected infection, an inflammatory response, and evidence of poor end-organ perfusion. The most common sites of infection include the lungs, urinary tract, and skin.[16] Signs of inflammatory response include the SIRS criteria, described in BOX 35-1 (see also Chapter 11, *General Principles of Pathophysiology*). Signs of poor end-organ perfusion include altered mental status (poor brain perfusion) and metabolic acidosis due to lactate production. The presence of lactic acidosis can be assessed by monitoring for the compensatory respiratory alkalosis and the resultant drop in end-tidal carbon dioxide ($ETCO_2$) level. A prehospital protocol requiring a sepsis alert for patients with suspected infection, two or more SIRS criteria, and an $ETCO_2$ level of less than 25 mm Hg has been shown to be quite sensitive for prehospital identification of patients with sepsis.[17]

BOX 35-1 Systemic Inflammatory Response Syndrome

SIRS occurs when the body responds to an insult such as infection, trauma, burn, organ inflammation, or a variety of other injuries. It is the first step in the sepsis pathway as well as in other destructive pathways. To meet SIRS criteria, patients must have two of the following signs:

1. Temperature greater than 38°C (100.4°F) or less than 36°C (96.8°F)
2. Heart rate greater than 90 beats/min
3. Respiratory rate greater than 20 breaths/min or partial pressure of carbon dioxide, arterial, level of less than 32 mm Hg
4. White blood cell count greater than 12,000 cells/mm^3 or less than 4,000 cells/mm^3, or the presence of greater than 10% immature neutrophils (bands)

The SIRS criteria are extremely useful for emergency medical services (EMS) providers, as three out of the four criteria need no special equipment to assess. The last of these criteria is not typically assessable in the prehospital setting. However, the information may be available when transporting critical patients with laboratory records to or from heath care facilities.

Modified from: Long B, Koyfman A. Clinical mimics: an emergency medicine-focused review of sepsis mimics. *J Emerg Med.* 2017;52(1):34-42.

Progression of Shock

Shock progresses in three phases based on the degree of hypoperfusion and anaerobic metabolism: compensated shock, uncompensated (or decompensated) shock, and irreversible (terminal) shock.[3]

TABLE 35-2 lists the phases of shock and the signs and symptoms of each.

Compensated Shock

Compensated shock (**FIGURE 35-9**) is associated with some decreased blood flow and perfusion to the tissues, but the compensatory responses of the body can overcome the decrease in available fluid. An increase in catecholamine production maintains cardiac output and a normal systolic blood pressure.

The decrease in perfusion and subsequent increase in acidosis lead to a chemoreceptor response that increases the rate and depth of ventilation, thereby helping correct the acidosis by decreasing the partial pressure of carbon dioxide (PCO_2) level. Sympathetic stimulation increases the heart's rate and contractility. In addition, it causes bronchodilation, increases peripheral vascular resistance, and decreases capillary flow in some capillary beds, such as in the gastrointestinal tract. The patient may exhibit delayed capillary refill and cool skin as blood is shunted from the skin to the vital organs. Despite maintaining normal blood pressure and urinary output, some patients may show signs of decreased central nervous system perfusion (lethargy, confusion, combativeness), even at this stage. If the underlying cause of shock is untreated, the compensatory mechanisms will eventually collapse.

Uncompensated Shock

Uncompensated shock (**FIGURE 35-10**) occurs when the body is no longer able to maintain systemic blood pressure. The systolic pressure usually drops

TABLE 35-2 Phases of Shock: Signs and Symptoms of Each

Vital Signs	Compensated Shock	Uncompensated Shock	Irreversible Shock
Heart rate	Mild tachycardia	Moderate tachycardia	Bradycardia, severe dysrhythmias
Level of consciousness	Lethargy, confusion, combativeness	Confusion, unconsciousness	Coma
Skin	Delayed capillary refill, cool skin	Delayed capillary refill, cold extremities, cyanosis	Pale, cold, clammy skin
Blood pressure	Normal or slightly elevated measurement	Decreased systolic and diastolic pressure	Frank hypotension

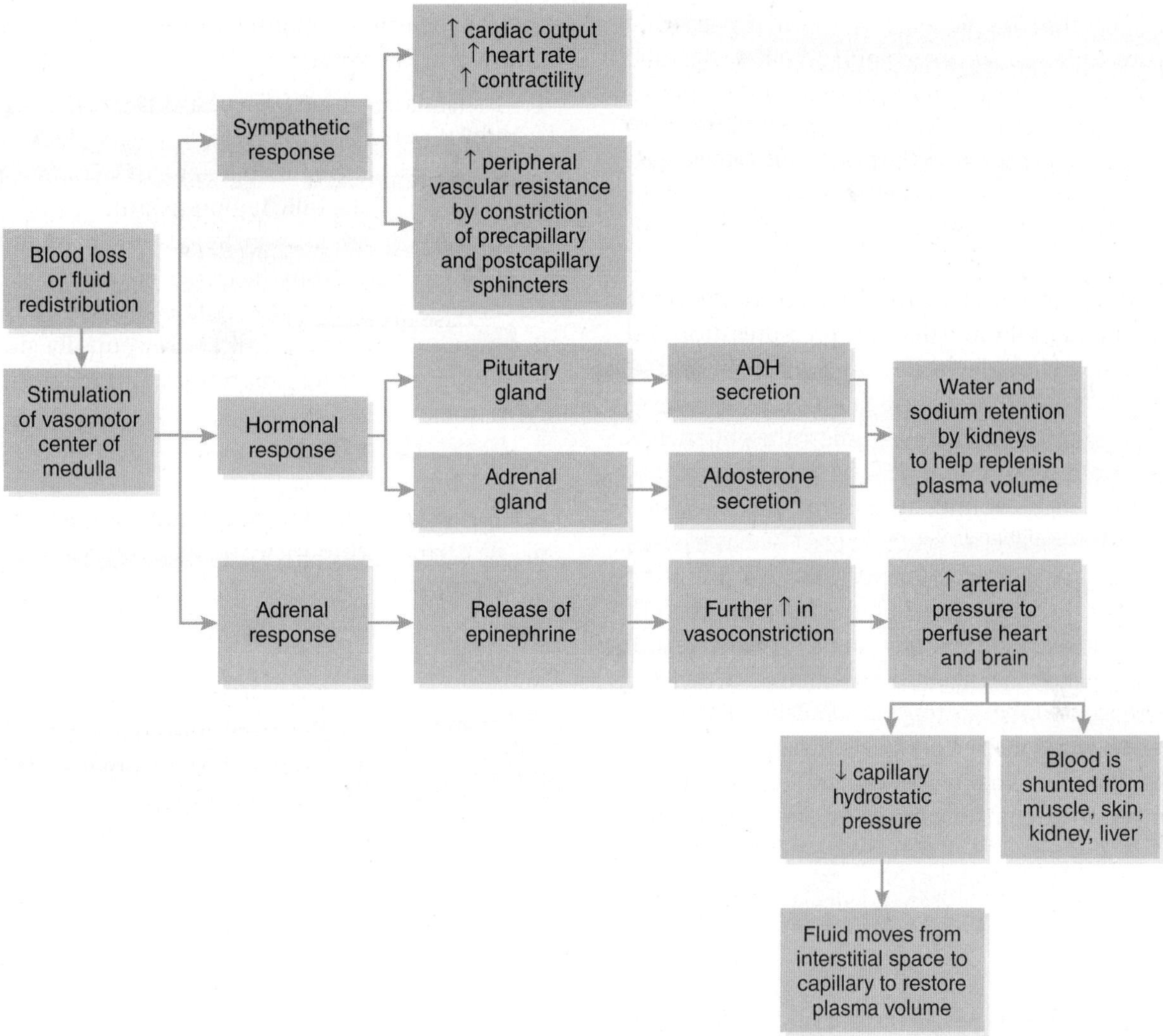

Abbreviation: ADH, antidiuretic hormone

FIGURE 35-9 Compensated shock. This stage of shock is reversible.

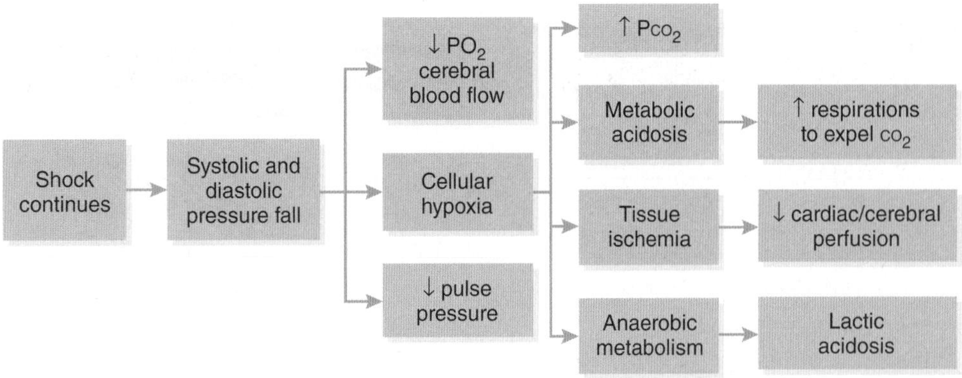

Abbreviations: CO_2, carbon dioxide; PCO_2, partial pressure of carbon dioxide; PO_2, partial pressure of oxygen

FIGURE 35-10 Uncompensated shock.

before the diastolic pressure because the systolic pressure depends more on blood volume. Diastolic pressure may rise at first because of vasoconstriction. The decrease in systolic pressure, along with maintained or increased diastolic pressure, can lead to a narrow pulse pressure—so narrowed, in fact, that the pulse pressure is not detectable with a blood pressure cuff.

As the compensatory mechanisms of the body begin to fail, systolic and diastolic pressures drop and cerebral blood flow decreases. The partial pressure of oxygen (Po_2) level may drop, though the Pco_2 level usually remains normal or low unless the patient has a head or chest injury that leads to hypoventilation. The clinical signs of uncompensated shock include hypotension, tachycardia, tachypnea, delayed capillary refill, and decreased urinary output. Shunting of blood and tissue hypoxia may cause the patient to have cold extremities and cyanosis. Effects on the cardiovascular system include a decreased preload and an increased rate of contraction caused by catecholamine stimulation. Myocardial contractions initially can be stronger as a result of catecholamine release. However, in the latter phases of uncompensated shock, myocardial strength may decrease as a result of the following factors:

1. Ischemia can result from a reduction of circulating red blood cells, a lower Po_2 level, and decreased coronary perfusion because of hypotension (especially diastolic hypotension).
2. Cardiodepressant substances (eg, myocardial toxin released from the ischemic pancreas) can depress heart function in late shock.
3. Injury of the myocardium (essentially simulating myocardial infarction) can result from associated ischemia.
4. Decreased preload can lead to decreased contractility.
5. Acidosis can lead to decreased contractility.
6. Cardiac rhythm disturbances can result from hypoxia.

Irreversible Shock

The progression of cellular ischemia and necrosis and subsequent organ death, even with oxygenation and perfusion restored, indicate **irreversible shock**, the third phase of shock (**FIGURE 35-11**). Despite a return

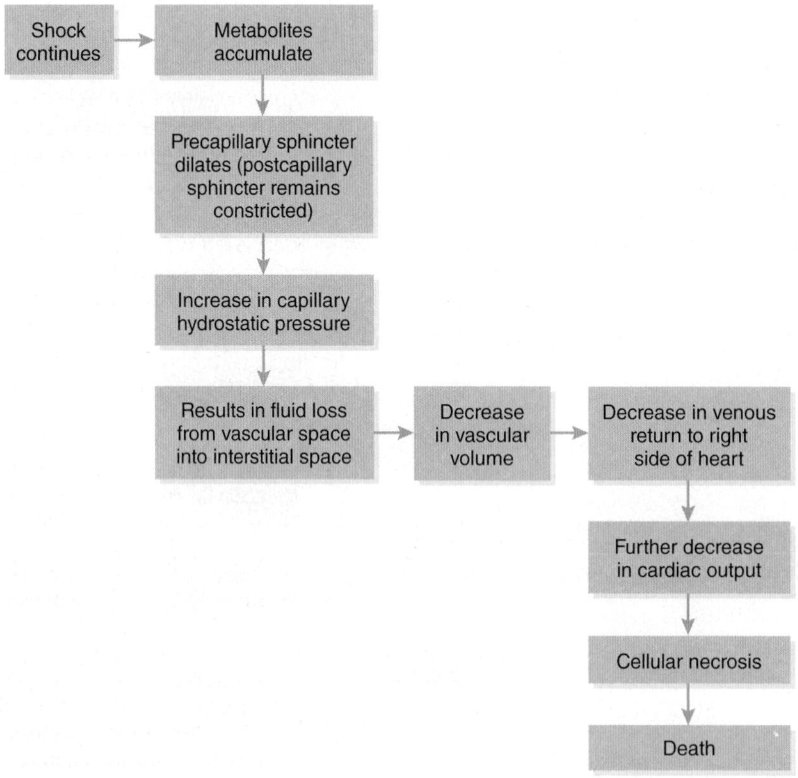

FIGURE 35-11 Irreversible shock.

to normal perfusion, patients with irreversible shock as a result of massive cellular damage do not survive. Cells and the vital organs begin to die from the lack of energy, the membrane pumps fail, and the various organelles in the cells sequentially break down. Thus, necrosis is inevitable even if cell perfusion is restored.

Decompensation may occur suddenly or may be delayed from 1 day to 3 weeks after the onset of shock. The clinical signs of irreversible shock include bradycardia; serious dysrhythmias; frank hypotension; evidence of multiple organ failure; and pale, cold, and clammy skin. Cardiopulmonary collapse usually is imminent in these patients.

NOTE

During the prehospital management of shock, it is impossible to distinguish between uncompensated and irreversible shock, so management of the shock victim should always focus on resuscitation. Because the consequences of irreversible shock become evident over a longer period, rapid resuscitation and transport to an appropriate medical facility may prevent the development of this final stage of shock. Fluid resuscitation in these patients should be guided by medical direction and established protocol.

Variations in Physiologic Response to Shock

Many variations in physiologic response occur among patients who are in shock. Determining factors include the following:

- Age
  - Older adults are less able to compensate.
  - Children compensate for a longer period but deteriorate faster.
- General health
  - Preexisting disease
  - Other injuries
  - Pregnancy
- Ability to activate compensatory mechanisms
- Medications, some of which can interfere with compensatory mechanisms
- Specific organ system(s) affected

CRITICAL THINKING

Which diseases can influence a patient's response to shock?

Assessment and Management of the Patient in Shock

The assessment of the patient in shock focuses on evaluation of oxygenation and perfusion of the body organs and identification of clinical findings that suggest the underlying etiology. **FIGURE 35-12** summarizes the signs and symptoms of shock. The goals of the treatment plan are to ensure adequate oxygenation and ventilation and to restore perfusion by addressing the most likely underlying etiology, keeping mind that many patients will present with more than one form of shock (eg, distributive and cardiogenic).

SHOW ME THE EVIDENCE

The qSOFA (quick Sequential [Sepsis-related] Organ Failure Assessment) score was developed by critical care physicians as a tool to prompt clinicians to consider sepsis as part of the differential diagnosis. The qSOFA score has three components: altered mental status (+1), systolic blood pressure less than 100 mm Hg (+1), and respiratory rate greater than 22 breaths/min (+1). In patients with sepsis, a qSOFA score greater than 2 has been found to be predictive of high mortality.

Washington University researchers conducted a retrospective chart review to evaluate the sensitivity and specificity of a qSOFA score of 2 or greater to identify patients with severe sepsis or septic shock in the prehospital setting. They found that a prehospital qSOFA score of 2 or greater was 16.3% sensitive (95% confidence interval [CI], 6.8–30.7%) and 97.3% specific (95% CI, 92.1–99.4%) for patients later confirmed to have severe sepsis or septic shock in the emergency department. They concluded that the dynamic nature of sepsis as a clinical syndrome makes identification difficult in the prehospital setting.

Modified from: Dorsett M, Kroll M, Smith CS, Asaro P, Liang SY, Moy HP. qSOFA has poor sensitivity for prehospital identification of severe sepsis and septic shock. *Prehosp Emerg Care.* 2017;21(4):489-497; Hunter CL, Silvestri S, Ralls G, Stone A, Walker A, Papa L. A prehospital screening tool utilizing end-tidal carbon dioxide predicts sepsis and severe sepsis. *Am J Emerg Med.* 2016;34(5):813-819; Peltan ID, Rowhani-Rahbar A, Vande Vusse LK, et al. Development and validation of a prehospital prediction model for acute traumatic coagulopathy. *Crit Care.* 2016;20(1):371; and Seymour CW, Liu VX, Iwashyna TJ, et al. Assessment of clinical criteria for sepsis: for the Third International Consensus Definitions for Sepsis and Septic Shock (Sepsis-3). *JAMA.* 2016;315(8):762-774.

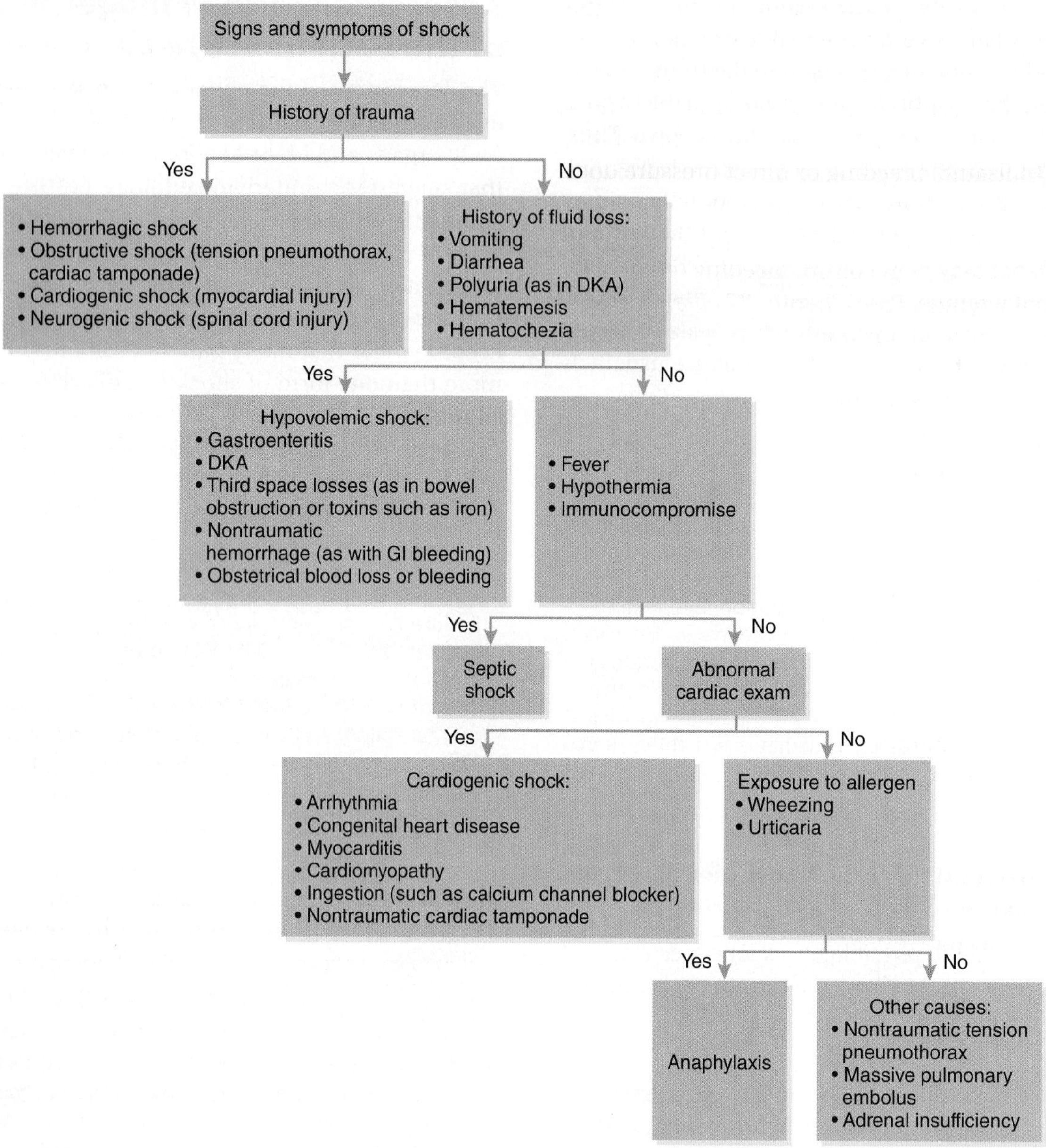

Abbreviation: DKA, diabetic ketoacidosis; GI, gastrointestinal

FIGURE 35-12 Signs and symptoms of different types of shock.

Reproduced with permission from: Waltzman M. Initial evaluation of shock in children. In: UpToDate, Post TW (Ed), UpToDate, Waltham, MA. Copyright © 2018 UpToDate, Inc. For more information visit www.uptodate.com.

Primary Survey

The primary survey can help to identify whether cell perfusion is adequate. The following six-step (XABCDE [eXsanguinating hemorrhage, Airway, Breathing, Circulation, Disability, Exposure]) description of the primary survey focuses on evaluating the patient with shock, but the paramedic should be aware of common objectives in evaluating any patient with other types of serious illness or injury.

Exsanguinating Hemorrhage

Address any exsanguinating hemorrhage with wound packing for truncal injuries or tourniquet application for extremity wounds. In the patient with trauma, in whom hemorrhagic (hypovolemic) shock is the most common type of shock to develop, circulatory assessment begins with identification of uncontrolled hemorrhage. In cases of external hemorrhage, applying direct pressure often controls bleeding. If there is arterial (pulsatile) bleeding or direct pressure does not immediately control vigorous bleeding in an extremity, a tourniquet should be applied. Hemostatic agents may help control bleeding on torso or junctional wounds. (See Chapter 37, *Bleeding and Soft-Tissue Trauma*, for methods to control external bleeding.) Hypotension may mask the site of hemorrhage, so the paramedic should be aware of all injuries, particularly those anatomically likely to involve a major artery.

Airway

Confirm that the airway is open and patent to ensure adequate air movement.

Breathing

The patient's respiratory pattern often reflects the adequacy of ventilation, so it can offer clues to the presence of shock. For example, if the patient is acidotic, the rate and depth of ventilation will increase in an attempt to reduce the carbon dioxide content of the blood and compensate for the metabolic acidosis. Administer high-concentration oxygen as an initial treatment. Pulse oximetry should be closely monitored to maintain an oxygen saturation (Spo_2) level at 94% or greater.

> NOTE
> Crackles and respiratory distress can indicate cardiogenic shock caused by left heart failure. Absent breath sounds and respiratory distress may indicate the presence of obstructive shock caused by tension pneumothorax.

> CRITICAL THINKING
> Consider a patient with early signs and symptoms of shock but a normal oxygen saturation reading. Should you administer oxygen?

Circulation

The paramedic should evaluate the rate, character, and location of the patient's pulses (radial, carotid, femoral) as part of the circulatory assessment. Patients with neurogenic shock or cardiogenic shock caused by heart block may be bradycardic, while pulse rates increase fairly early in patients with hypovolemic shock. The increased heart rate helps to maintain an adequate cardiac output. The strength of contraction also may increase. However, both of these attempts to maintain cardiac output may be negated by the decrease in preload. Tachycardia usually will not occur until the patient has suffered a 10% to 15% volume depletion (relative to container size) as a result of blood loss or an increase in container size.

The character of the pulse can be strong or weak. The strength of the pulse provides an estimate of the filling volume of the artery being palpated and an indirect measurement of systolic pressure. A narrow pulse pressure is an indicator of impending uncompensated hypovolemic shock.

Tissue perfusion sometimes can be estimated by evaluating the color, moisture, and temperature of the skin. These guidelines, however, can be unreliable in older patients and in those who have been exposed to extremes of temperature. They can be unreliable in patients with septicemia and shock caused by neurologic injury, as these patients tend to exhibit peripheral vasodilation. An evaluation of the fingers and toes (the most distal points of circulation) is crucial. These areas can be the first to show signs of inadequate tissue perfusion (cyanosis, cool skin). If ambient temperatures are moderate and tissue perfusion is adequate, these areas will be pink, warm, and dry.

The capillary refill test (described in Chapter 18, *Scene Size-up and Primary Assessment*) can offer useful details on the pediatric patient's tissue perfusion. These measurements should be used only as a guide. The accuracy of this test can be affected by the environment and by the patient's general health, age, and sex.

If the paramedic suspects internal bleeding, rapid transport to a proper facility while ensuring adequate ventilation is the highest priority. Internal bleeding should be suspected in any trauma patient with signs of shock, especially trauma patients without evidence of external blood loss. Intravenous (IV) fluid therapy, if initiated in the field, should be performed en route to avoid a delay in the provision of definitive care. In the absence of concomitant brain injury, fluid administration should be titrated to mental status or to maintain a systolic blood pressure of 80 mm Hg (90 mm Hg in a patient with a head injury), as over-resuscitation with crystalloids may lead to an increase in internal bleeding by promoting coagulopathy.[18,19]

Disability

The evaluation of the patient's level of consciousness is crucial in assessing cerebral oxygenation. The patient can become restless, agitated, and confused as cerebral ischemia develops. In addition to shock, cerebral edema and intracranial hemorrhage from head injury can compromise cerebral perfusion. Any significant change in the patient's sensorium should be considered an indicator of a critical perfusion deficit, whether the decrease in cerebral circulation is from shock or from an increase in intracranial pressure. The paramedic can measure the patient's level of consciousness with the AVPU (Awake and alert, responsive to Verbal stimuli, responsive to Pain, Unresponsive) scale or other evaluation methods (see Chapter 40, *Spine and Nervous System Trauma*).

NOTE

Patients with neurogenic shock will demonstrate a sensorimotor deficit below the level of injury, which is usually T6 or higher.

Modified from: Chin LS. Spinal cord injuries clinical presentation. Medscape website. https://emedicine.medscape.com/article/793582-clinical. Updated August 10, 2017. Accessed March 21, 2018.

NOTE

Some authorities believe that the level of consciousness and other indicators of adequate brain functions are the best way to determine appropriate blood pressure for the trauma patient. They contend that the brain is the organ most sensitive to changes in physiologic state. The goals of this patient-focused method of shock management are to ensure that systolic pressure is at least 80 mm Hg and that the patient has positive peripheral pulses and is awake or responsive to stimuli.

Modified from: National Association of Emergency Medical Technicians. *PHTLS: Basic and Advanced Prehospital Trauma Life Support*. 8th ed. Burlington, MA: Jones & Bartlett Learning; 2014.

Exposure of the Body Surfaces

The paramedic should expose the body surfaces in the primary survey as indicated by scenario or mechanism of injury. A visual inspection can reveal conditions that may be life threatening but that are hidden by clothing.

CRITICAL THINKING

Can blood donation cause a fluid deficit large enough to cause shock? If so, how is that fluid deficit managed?

Secondary Assessment

As discussed, the first action is the primary survey and management of any life-threatening conditions. After completing this step, the paramedic should evaluate the patient further. A systematic approach offers a way to evaluate potentially life-threatening conditions and allows the paramedic to further assess the patient's perfusion status. This assessment should begin with baseline measurements of the patient's vital signs and evaluation of the patient's electrocardiogram.

The paramedic should expect the pulse rate to increase above normal limits after fluid volume drops 10% to 15%. Some patients continue to have normal pulse rates even though a volume deficit of this extent exists. Thus, the patient's pulse rate should be only one factor in evaluating the patient's level of perfusion. Some patients may have a pulse rate within normal limits even with a volume deficit. Examples include patients who are extremely fit and patients on medications such as beta blockers.

Bradycardia, which can result from hypoxemia, existing neurologic injury, increased vagal tone, preexisting illness, or prior medication use, also can indicate severe myocardial ischemia (a primary cause of cardiogenic shock). In some cases involving intra-abdominal bleeding (eg, ruptured aortic aneurysm, ectopic pregnancy), the heart rate may remain relatively slow despite significant blood loss. Bradycardic rhythms often become evident just before cardiac arrest occurs. If the rhythm is bradycardic, the paramedic should optimize oxygenation by increasing the fraction of inspired oxygen and by assisting ventilations if needed.

Serial blood pressure assessments should be obtained, trended, and evaluated in the context of the patient's normal state. Any episode of hypotension in the prehospital setting should be noted in the handoff report, as this condition has been found to be associated with higher in-hospital mortality.[20]

The diastolic pressure at first rises as peripheral vascular resistance increases with increased vascular tone. These changes decrease the container size. Blood also is shunted away selectively from certain portions of the body. When the heart can no longer pump blood to keep the container full on the arterial side, the diastolic pressure begins to drop. The paramedic should expect this finding when blood loss is greater than 20% to 25% of normal circulating blood volume.

The systolic pressure falls when the heart can no longer pump enough blood to fill the container at the end of cardiac contraction. Systolic pressure usually is more sensitive to volume depletion than is diastolic pressure, so it drops first. As the fluid deficit approaches 25%, both systolic and diastolic pressures decrease.

Pulse pressure should be noted. Pulse pressure readings of less than 30 mm Hg or 25% of the systolic blood pressure may indicate early hypovolemic or obstructive shock. A wide pulse pressure suggests distributive shock.[20]

The paramedic should consider evaluation of orthostatic vital signs in conscious patients suspected of having lost circulating blood volume. This evaluation should be performed only in the absence of suspected spinal injury or another condition that precludes this assessment. A change from a recumbent position to a sitting or standing position that is associated with a decrease in systolic pressure (after 1 minute) of 10 to 15 mm Hg and/or a concurrent rise in pulse rate (after 1 minute) of 10 to 15 beats/min indicates a significant (at least 10%) volume depletion (postural hypotension) and a decrease in perfusion status.

A fluid deficit can persist even after the systolic pressure returns to normal following fluid replacement. However, continuing IV fluids after indicators of adequate tissue perfusion are present (eg, improved skin color, capillary refill time of less than 2 seconds in pediatric patients, and normal pulse oximetry readings) is controversial. Aggressive fluid resuscitation can result in **hemodilution** (diluting the blood of elements), the disruption of clots, and renewed hemorrhage.[21] As a rule, patients who have suspected internal hemorrhage in their chest, abdomen, or pelvis should have fluids titrated to maintain a systolic blood pressure of 80 mm Hg (MAP of 60–65 mm Hg). Permissive hypotension can be protective and may prevent further blood loss. The paramedic should follow the local protocol established by medical direction.

If available, serum lactate can be measured using an approved testing device. A value greater than 2.0 mmol/L is abnormal and may signal anaerobic metabolism. Some research suggests that serum lactate elevation can be detected prior to a drop in blood pressure.[22]

NOTE

The **shock index** is another measurement that can be calculated to detect the presence of a shock state before it is otherwise evident. To calculate this index, divide the pulse rate by the systolic blood pressure. When the ratio is greater than 1.0, shock may be present. Additionally, a ratio greater than 1.0 has been shown to predict hemorrhage that may require transfusion. As an example, a patient with a heart rate of 120 beats/min and a systolic blood pressure of 90 mm Hg would have a shock index of 1.33, suggesting the presence of shock.

Modified from: Pottecher J, Ageron F-X, Fauché C, et al. Prehospital shock index and pulse pressure/heart rate ratio to predict massive transfusion after severe trauma: retrospective analysis of a large regional trauma database. *J Trauma Acute Care Surg.* 2016;81(4):713-722.

NOTE

Occasionally, portable ultrasonography is being used in the prehospital setting, particularly by specialty care teams. Ultrasonography can detect bleeding in the abdomen, cardiac tamponade, and heart pumping function. EMS systems considering adoption of this technology should develop procedures for its use so efforts to obtain ultrasonographic imaging do not delay transport to definitive care for patients in shock. (See Chapter 42, *Abdominal Trauma*, for more about use of ultrasonographic equipment.)

Differential Shock Assessment Findings

Shock is assumed to be hypovolemic until proven otherwise. Nevertheless, some assessment findings can help the paramedic to differentiate between hypovolemic shock and other causes of shock.

Cardiogenic Shock

The patient with cardiogenic shock often has a chief complaint of chest pain, dyspnea, or extreme heart rates (tachycardia, bradycardia, and other dysrhythmias). Some patients also show signs of heart failure such as jugular vein distention (described in Chapter 21, *Cardiology*, and Chapter 41, *Chest Trauma*). Jugular venous distention, which must be assessed while the patient is sitting, may be seen in patients with cardiogenic or obstructive shock (pulmonary embolism, cardiac tamponade, tension pneumothorax) and should be considered in combination with the patient's history and clinical findings.

Obstructive Shock

Obstructive shock is caused by obstruction to blood flow. Patients with this type of shock often are the victims of a major chest injury (usually a penetrating type of injury), or they have a history that is consistent with pulmonary embolism (eg, recent surgery, long bone fracture). Patients with cardiac tamponade or tension pneumothorax often have jugular vein distention. Also, patients with tension pneumothorax almost always have decreased breath sounds on the affected side (see Chapter 41, *Chest Trauma*).

Distributive Shock

When the patient has some type of distributive shock (neurogenic shock, anaphylactic shock, septic shock), the history or scene assessment may reveal a mechanism that suggests vasodilation as the cause of the shock state. Signs and symptoms of distributive shock that are unusual in the presence of hypovolemic shock include warm, flushed skin (especially in dependent areas). Those of neurogenic shock include a normal pulse rate (relative bradycardia).

Resuscitation

Resuscitation of a patient who is experiencing shock is aimed at restoring adequate peripheral tissue oxygenation as quickly as possible. To do so, the paramedic must ensure adequate oxygenation, maintain an effective ratio of volume to container size, and rapidly transport the patient to an appropriate medical facility. As previously stated, medical direction and protocol should guide fluid resuscitation strategies.

Red Blood Cell Oxygenation

Adequate oxygenation of red blood cells is required for adequate tissue oxygenation, which in turn means the patient must have a patent airway. Ventilation also must be supported with oxygen to maintain an Spo_2 level of 94% or greater. If hypovolemia is suspected, a fraction of inspired oxygen of 100% should be maintained. An $ETCO_2$ level of less than 25 mm Hg may be a sign of poor perfusion.[17,23] Any abnormality that interferes with adequate ventilation should be corrected if possible. If needed, the paramedic can assist ventilation with positive pressure. Examples include an obstructed airway, pneumothorax, hemothorax, open chest wound, and unstable chest wall (see Chapter 41, *Chest Trauma*).

Ratio of Volume to Container Size

The second requirement in maintaining adequate oxygen-carrying capacity is that the container be full of fluid. To achieve this condition, the paramedic can decrease the size of the container, especially when the shock state is not associated with hemorrhage. In addition, in some cases of distributive shock, the paramedic can administer vasoconstricting drugs to manage the shock when reduction of container size is the main concern. Volume replacement also may be necessary in these patients. Note that vasoconstricting drugs are not recommended to treat patients in hypovolemic shock until fluid volume replacement is complete. Complete volume replacement rarely occurs in the prehospital setting.

Fluid Resuscitation in Shock

Almost every patient in shock requires volume expanders as part of resuscitation. The selection of IV fluids for initial volume replacement varies according

DID YOU KNOW?

What Happened to the Antishock Garment?

Military antishock trousers (MAST), also known as the pneumatic antishock garment (PASG), were used in the Vietnam War to treat severe blood loss and to stabilize pelvic fractures prior to transport. During the 1970s, the PASG was commonly used by civilian EMS providers to stabilize patients with shock due to lower body and obstetric hemorrhage.

Research has since shown that the advantages of PASG were overstated and of questionable benefit in managing hypovolemic shock, and that these patients would be best served by rapid transport for definitive care. It is rarely used in modern EMS systems.

Modified from: Cutler BS, Daggett WM. Application of the "G-suit" to the control of hemorrhage in massive trauma. *Ann Surg*. 1971;173(4):511-514; Miller S, Fathalla MMF, Ojengbede OA, et al. Obstetric hemorrhage and shock management: using the low technology non-pneumatic antishock garment in Nigerian and Egyptian tertiary care facilities. *BMC Pregnancy Childbirth*. 2010;10:64; and O'Connor RE, Domeier R. Use of the pneumatic antishock garment (PASG): NAEMSP Position Paper. *Prehosp Emerg Care*. 1997;1(1):32-35.

to medical direction. In prehospital care, the most common emergency requiring fluid replacement is loss of volume caused by hemorrhage or dehydration. The type of fluid replacement needed depends on the nature and extent of the volume loss. The two main categories of fluids used in resuscitation are crystalloids and colloids. The paramedic should follow the recommendations for fluid resuscitation provided by medical direction.

Crystalloids

Crystalloid Solutions. Crystalloid solutions are created by dissolving crystals such as salts and sugars in water. These solutions do not have as much osmotic pressure as colloid solutions have. They can be expected to equilibrate more quickly between the vascular and extravascular spaces. Two-thirds to three-fourths of the infused crystalloid fluid leaves the vascular space within 30 minutes to 1 hour,[20] so 3 mL of a crystalloid solution is needed to replace 1 mL of blood loss. Infusion of large volumes of crystalloid fluids may result in hypothermia, altered coagulation, and hyperchloremic acidosis.[19]

NOTE

Initial fluid therapy for shock in the prehospital setting should be administered through a single 18-gauge catheter in 250-mL boluses, with recheck of vital signs thereafter and prior to the next bolus (maximum of 2 L, or 20 mL/kg).

Modified from: National Association of Emergency Medical Technicians. *PHTLS: Basic and Advanced Prehospital Trauma Life Support*. 8th ed. Burlington, MA: Jones & Bartlett Learning; 2014.

Hypertonic Solutions. Hypertonic solutions have higher osmotic pressure than do body cells (greater than 300 mOsm/L). They include 5% dextrose in 0.9% sodium chloride, 3% saline, 5% saline, 7.5% saline, 10% dextrose in water, 5% dextrose in lactated Ringer solution, 5% dextrose in 0.9% saline, and 5% dextrose in 0.45% sodium chloride. Hypotonic solutions have a lower osmotic pressure than do body cells. They include 0.225% saline (one-quarter normal saline) and 0.45% sodium chloride. Infusion of 7.5% normal saline (not approved for civilian use in the United States) expands fluid to the equivalent of 2 to 3 L of isotonic crystalloids but has not been shown to improve survival.[20]

Isotonic Solutions. Lactated Ringer solution is a well-balanced solution that contains many of the chemicals found in human blood. It contains sodium chloride, small amounts of potassium and calcium, and 28 mEq of lactate, which can act as a buffer to neutralize acidity when metabolized by the liver. One-third of the infused solution remains in the vascular space after 1 hour.

Normal saline contains 154 mEq/L of sodium; it does not have any buffering capabilities. Although this isotonic solution is preferred by some physicians, the higher chloride content of normal saline makes it less desirable than the more balanced lactated Ringer solution. As with lactated Ringer solution, nearly one-third of the infused normal saline remains in the vascular space after 1 hour. This property makes it an equally effective volume expander. The paramedic should follow the local protocol when choosing IV fluids.

Glucose-containing solutions (eg, 5% dextrose in water) have immediate volume expansion effects, but the glucose leaves the intravascular compartment rapidly, resulting in a free water increase. Because the volume-replacement benefits of glucose solutions last only 5 to 10 minutes while the glucose is metabolized, 5% dextrose in water should not be used to replace a volume deficit. Glucose solutions most often are used to maintain vascular access for administration of IV medications.

NOTE

Five percent dextrose in water is an isotonic solution. When administered, however, the dextrose molecules leave the circulation so rapidly that its effect is that of a hypotonic solution.

Colloids

Colloid solutions contain molecules (usually protein) that are too large to pass through the capillary membrane; thus they exhibit osmotic pressure and remain within the vascular compartment for a considerable time. Examples of colloid solutions include whole blood, packed red blood cells, blood plasma, and plasma substitutes. Synthetic colloids include Gelofusine and Hetastarch, both of which are expensive and have a high risk of allergic reaction.[21] Colloids generally are reserved for in-hospital use and are not recommended for prehospital management of shock.[20]

Whole-blood replacement is rarely given in the United States for management of shock and is usually unavailable in the emergency department. Instead, packed red blood cells are transfused, and other blood components are transfused as necessary. (Packed red blood cells have a volume of hemoglobin per unit that is almost twice that of whole blood.)

A type and cross-match should be obtained when possible before a patient is given blood products to determine the patient's ABO group and Rh type (described in Chapter 11, *General Principles of Pathophysiology*). Typing and cross-matching also will determine whether other antibodies are present that may cause a transfusion reaction. Although type-specific blood should be used for resuscitation when the patient's condition and time permit, blood that is not cross-matched is usually given immediately for patients with hypotension and uncontrolled hemorrhage.[24] Group O universal donor blood cells do not have A or B antigens on their surface; this blood type is not agglutinated by anti-A or anti-B antibodies. O-negative blood is used for women of childbearing age who are at risk for Rh complications with future pregnancies. O-positive blood is used in all other patients.

NOTE

Several types of blood transfusion reactions may occur during or up to 96 hours after infusion. Symptoms may range from mild fever to life-threatening shock. If a reaction is suspected (eg, during an interhospital transfer), the paramedic should stop the transfusion and contact medical direction. The blood bag or tubing should not be discarded.

Modified from: White L, Duncan G, Baumle W. *Medical Surgical Nursing: An Integrated Approach.* 3rd ed. Clifton Park, NY: Cengage Learning; 2013.

Blood plasma may be given without concern for ABO compatibility. Blood plasma contains fibrinogen, albumin, gamma globulins, hemagglutinins (an agglutinin that clumps red blood corpuscles), prothrombin, other clotting factors, sugar, and salts. It is sometimes used to restore effective blood volume in circulatory failure associated with burns, traumatic shock, and hemorrhage, but more commonly is used to correct clotting deficiencies. This product is often supplied as fresh-frozen plasma.

Blood substitutes to improve oxygenation are under development. They include perfluorocarbons. Perfluorocarbons do not contain hemoglobin, but they carry 50 times more oxygen than does plasma. Hemoglobin-based oxygen carriers contain hemoglobin not bound within a cell membrane. Blood substitutes have several advantages: They stay in the intravascular space longer than crystalloid solutions do; they do not carry HIV or hepatitis viruses; and they do not require typing and cross-matching before administration. Such products are currently considered experimental, and their value in prehospital care remains unknown.[19]

Theory of Fluid Flow

The flow of fluid through a catheter is related directly to its diameter (to the fourth power) and inversely related to its length. Therefore, a catheter with a large

NOTE

Tranexamic acid (TXA) is an antifibrinolytic medication that has been used to treat bleeding in a number of clinical situations. This medication can be thought of as a "clot stabilizer," in that it helps to inhibit natural clot breakdown. A number of studies have evaluated the potential usefulness of TXA in the management of trauma patients, with researchers determining that TXA administration within 3 hours to trauma patients with hemorrhage reduces mortality. TXA is administered as an initial bolus dose and subsequent infusion. Several systems have begun to administer prehospital TXA to trauma patients with massive hemorrhage, although this treatment requires collaboration with the local trauma service given the need for prolonged infusion. (For more information on TXA, see Chapter 37, *Bleeding and Soft-Tissue Trauma*.)

Modified from: CRASH-2 Collaborators. The importance of early treatment with tranexamic acid in bleeding trauma patients: an exploratory analysis of the CRASH-2 randomised controlled trial. *Lancet.* 2011;377(9771):1096-1101; Morrison JJ, Dubose JJ, Rasmussen TE, Midwinter MJ. Military Application of Tranexamic Acid in Trauma Emergency Resuscitation (MATTERs) study. *Arch Surg.* 2012;147(2):113-119; and Strosberg DS, Nguyen MC, Mostafavifar L, Mell H, Evans DC. Development of a prehospital tranexamic acid administration protocol. *Prehosp Emerg Care.* 2016;20(4):462-466.

diameter has a much greater flow rate than does a catheter with a small diameter, and a short catheter provides a faster flow rate than does a longer catheter of equal diameter. Other factors that affect the flow of fluid include the diameter and length of the tubing, the size of the patient's vein, the height of the fluid bag, and the viscosity and temperature of the IV fluid. (Temperature affects viscosity; warm fluids generally flow better than cold ones.)

Pressure bags are available that pressurize the IV system to 300 mm Hg to maximize the rate of fluid administration. **TABLE 35-3** lists the maximum rate of fluid flow for various gauges of 2-inch (5-cm) Medicut catheters without pressure on the bag at a height of 3 feet (1 m) above the patient.[25] When aggressive fluid resuscitation is indicated, the paramedic should do the following:

- Use short, large-diameter catheters.
- Use warm fluids of low viscosity (if possible).
- Keep the tubing short, and pressurize the IV system.

TABLE 35-3 Needle Gauges and Maximum Fluid Flow

Needle Gauge[a]	Maximum Fluid Flow
18 gauge	4.81 L/hr or 80 mL/min
16 gauge	7.45 L/hr or 124 mL/min
14 gauge	9.67 L/hr or 161 mL/min

[a]Inside diameter.

CRITICAL THINKING

Aside from improved flow, what benefits do warmed fluids offer for the patient in shock who needs a large-volume fluid bolus?

NOTE

Fluid flow through intraosseous (IO) needles varies according to the site. Higher flow rates are achievable through the proximal humerus than through the tibia. A wide variety of IO fluid flow rates (while under pressure) have been reported, ranging from 200 mL/hr to 9,900 mL/hr. In one randomized controlled study involving volunteer subjects, mean flow rates under 300 mL of pressure were 5 L/hr in the humerus and 1 L/hr through the tibia. Flow rates are improved when a 10-mL normal saline flush with a syringe is performed prior to fluid infusion.

Modified from: Vidacare Corporation. *The Science and Fundamentals of Intraosseous Vascular Access: Including Frequently Asked Questions.* 2nd ed. Teleflex website. https://www.teleflex.com/en/usa/ezioeducation/documents/EZ-IO_SAFIOVA-M-607%20Rev%20B-PrintVersion.pdf. Published 2013. Accessed March 22, 2018.

Key Principles in Managing Shock

The paramedic should follow these key principles as part of the plan for managing shock (**FIGURE 35-13**):

1. Control life-threatening external bleeding.
2. Establish and maintain an open airway.
3. Administer high-concentration oxygen. Assist ventilation as needed.
4. Determine whether early definitive care is needed:
   - Epinephrine intramuscularly (IM) for anaphylaxis

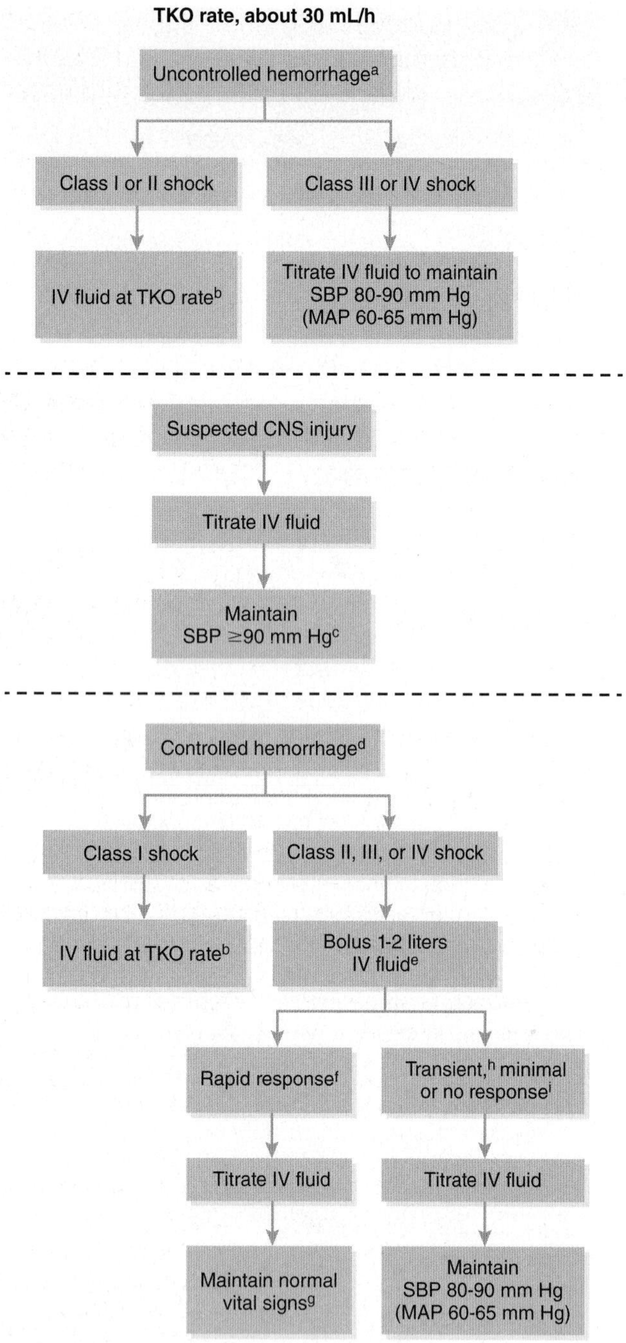

Notes:
[a] Suspected intrathoracic, intra-abdominal or retroperitoneal hemorrhage
[b] TKO rate, about 30 mL/h
[c] Consider MAP 85-90 mm Hg for spinal cord injury
[d] External hemorrhage controlled with pressure dressing, topical hemostatic agent, or, if extremity hemorrhage, tourniquet
[e] Warmed crystalloid solution (102°F, if possible)
[f] Rapid response = vital signs return to normal
[g] HR <120/min; SBP >90 mm Hg for adults
[h] Transient response = vital signs initially improve, then deteriorate
[i] Minimal or no response = little or no change in vital signs

A

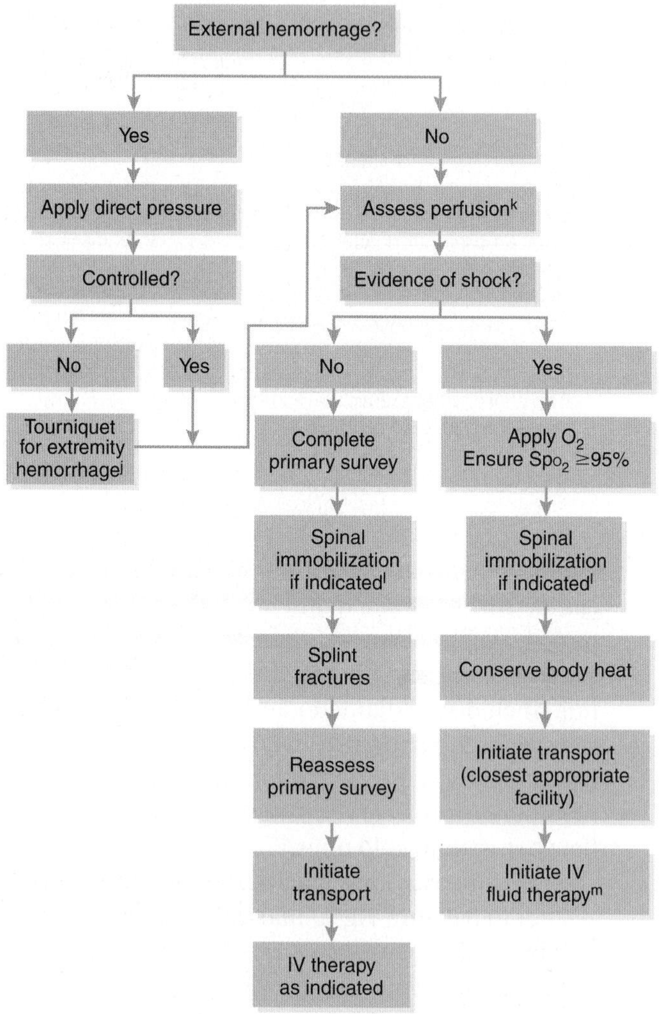

Notes:
[j] A manufactured tourniquet, blood pressure cuff, or cravat should be placed just proximal to the bleeding site and tightened until bleeding stops. The application time is marked on the tourniquet.
[k] Assessment of perfusion includes, presence, quality, and location of pulses; skin color, temperature, and moisture; and capillary refilling time.
[l] See Indications for Spinal Immobilization algorithm.
[m] Initiate two large-bore IV catheters en route.

B

Abbreviations: CNS, central nervous system; HR, heart rate; IV, intravenous; MAP, mean arterial pressure; O_2, oxygen; SBP, systolic blood pressure; Spo_2, oxygen saturation as measured by a pulse oximeter; TKO, to keep open

FIGURE 35-13 **A.** Managing volume resuscitation algorithm. **B.** Shock management algorithm.

Modified from: McSwain NE, ed. Prehospital Trauma Life Support. 8th ed. Burlington, MA: Jones & Bartlett Learning; 2016.

- Electrical therapy or medication for cardiac dysrhythmias
- Chest decompression for tension pneumothorax

5. Initiate IV fluid replacement if appropriate. Obtain vascular access if administering a volume-expanding fluid. The IV administration of fluids in the prehospital setting should not delay patient transport. Crystalloid solutions cannot restore the oxygen-carrying capacity of blood.
6. Determine the cause of the shock and manage it appropriately.
7. Maintain the patient's normal body temperature. Patients in shock often are unable to conserve body heat and can easily become hypothermic.
8. Transport the patient in the supine position; provide spinal motion restriction if indicated.
9. Monitor cardiac rhythm, $ETCO_2$ level, and oxygen saturation.
10. Frequently reassess vital signs en route to the emergency department.

Management of Specific Forms of Shock

In addition to the general management appropriate for all patients in shock, certain management guidelines are specific to each shock classification (BOX 35-2).

BOX 35-2 Categories of Shock According to Primary Treatment

Causes That Require Primarily the Infusion of Volume

Hemorrhagic shock
Traumatic
Gastrointestinal bleeding
Hypovolemia
Gastrointestinal losses
Dehydration from insensible losses (fluid lost through the skin and respiratory tract)
Third-space sequestration from inflammation

Causes That Require Improvement in Pump Function by Either Infusion of Inotropic Support or Reversal of the Cause of Pump Dysfunction

Myocardial ischemia
Coronary artery thrombosis
Arterial hypotension with hypoxemia
Cardiomyopathy
Acute myocarditis
Chronic diseases of heart muscle (ischemic, diabetic, infiltrative, endocrinologic, congenital)
Cardiac rhythm disturbances
Atrial fibrillation with rapid ventricular response
Ventricular tachycardia
Supraventricular tachycardia
Hypodynamic septic shock (late sepsis)
Overdose of negative inotropic drug
Beta blocker
Calcium channel antagonist overdose (eg, verapamil)
Structural cardiac damage
Traumatic (eg, flail mitral valve)
Ventriculoseptal rupture
Papillary muscle rupture

Causes That Require Volume Support and Vasopressor Support

Hyperdynamic sepsis syndrome (early sepsis)
Anaphylactic shock
Central neurogenic shock
Drug overdose (dihydropyridines, alpha$_1$-antagonists)

Problems That Require Immediate Relief From Obstruction to Cardiac Output

Pulmonary embolism
Cardiac tamponade
Pneumothorax
Valvular dysfunction
Acute thrombosis of prosthetic valve
Critical aortic stenosis
Congenital heart defects in newborn (eg, closure of patent ductus arteriosus with critical aortic coarctation)
Critical idiopathic subaortic stenosis

Cellular Poisons That Require Specific Antidotes

Carbon monoxide
Methemoglobinemia
Hydrogen sulfide
Cyanide

Modified from: Marx JA, Walls R, Hockberger RS. *Rosen's Emergency Medicine: Concepts and Clinical Practice.* 8th ed. St. Louis, MO: Saunders/Mosby; 2014:68, Box 6-1.

Hypovolemic Shock

The management of hypovolemic shock is not considered complete until the volume is replaced and the cause or causes of shock are corrected. This care will include crystalloid fluid replacement in cases of simple dehydration or volume replacement because of hemorrhage, definitive surgery, critical care support, and postoperative rehabilitation. The amount of fluid replaced in trauma is controversial and should be guided by medical direction.

Trauma patients who are stable should not receive aggressive fluid resuscitation.[21] The volume of fluid that should be given to trauma patients will depend on the type of trauma and the patient's condition. Fluid resuscitation volume should be titrated to a patient's mental status, which typically correlates to a minimum systolic blood pressure of 80 mm Hg (MAP of 60–65 mm Hg).[26] When external hemorrhage has been controlled and the patient exhibits signs of shock, 250 mL boluses up to a total of 1 to 2 L of warmed crystalloid solution can be infused (20 mL/kg for children).

In nontraumatic hypovolemic shock, infuse crystalloid fluids beginning with 30 mL/kg to a maximum of 1 L over less than 15 minutes. This treatment may be repeated up to three times if indicated.[23]

Cardiogenic Shock

The management of cardiogenic shock focuses on improving the pumping action of the heart and on managing cardiac rhythm irregularities. The paramedic should initiate fluid resuscitation in the adult with 100 to 200 mL of a volume-expanding fluid. Fluid resuscitation should be initiated as long as the patient has no crackles in the lung fields that would indicate pulmonary edema. If the patient improves, fluid therapy should be continued cautiously. Fluid therapy should continue until the blood pressure stabilizes and the pulse rate decreases. The paramedic should assess lung sounds often. If the patient shows signs of increased lung congestion, the paramedic should adjust the rate of infusion to keep the vein open.

Drug therapy for cardiogenic shock varies according to the cause of the shock. It can include vasopressors (norepinephrine, epinephrine, dopamine), inotropic drugs, and antidysrhythmics (usually after fluid infusion) (see Chapter 21, *Cardiology*). Patients with cardiogenic shock caused by myocardial ischemia or infarction require reperfusion strategies (clot-busting drugs or surgery) and possibly circulatory support.

Obstructive Shock

Common causes of obstructive shock include pericardial tamponade, tension pneumothorax, and pulmonary embolism. The goals of prehospital care are to identify and relieve the obstruction to flow. Emergency care for pericardial tamponade includes aggressive fluid replacement to maintain adequate preload. Tension pneumothorax may require needle decompression. Pulmonary embolism requires in-hospital treatment with fibrinolytic, surgical, or percutaneous embolectomy therapy. The specific management for these disorders is described in Chapter 23, *Respiratory*, and Chapter 41, *Chest Trauma*.

Distributive Shock

The most common types of distributive shock are neurogenic shock, anaphylactic shock, and septic shock.

Neurogenic Shock

The management of neurogenic shock is similar to the management of hypovolemia. However, the paramedic must take care during fluid therapy to avoid circulatory overload. Throughout the resuscitation phase, the paramedic should monitor the patient's lung sounds closely for signs of pulmonary congestion. In addition, patients in neurogenic shock may respond to the administration of vasopressors (eg, norepinephrine, epinephrine, dopamine).

Anaphylactic Shock

IM administration of epinephrine is the treatment of choice for patients with acute anaphylactic reactions. Depending on the severity of reaction and the anticipated transport time, other treatment modalities can include administration of antihistamines such as diphenhydramine or corticosteroids. The paramedic can administer bronchodilators to treat bronchospasm that persists after administration of epinephrine and can administer corticosteroids to reduce the inflammatory response.

Crystalloid volume replacement also is indicated. Crystalloids may compensate for the increased container size caused by vasodilation resulting from histamine release during an anaphylactic reaction. Administration of 1 to 3 L of normal saline is indicated in patients who have signs of shock after administration of epinephrine.

Paramedics should anticipate the need for aggressive airway management in any allergic reaction (see Chapter 26, *Immune System Disorders*).

Septic Shock

The management of septic shock in the prehospital setting can include the management of hypovolemia (if present) and the correction of metabolic acid–base imbalance. Depending on the patient's response to the infection, prehospital care may involve fluid resuscitation, respiratory support, and administration of vasopressors to improve cardiac output. If possible, the paramedic should obtain a thorough patient history to help identify the cause of sepsis. Any patient with immunocompromise has an increased risk of septic shock; examples of such patients include those with HIV infection, some cancer patients receiving chemotherapy, and patients with indwelling urinary or vascular catheters.

Patients with adrenal insufficiency associated with sepsis may not respond to fluid resuscitation or sympathomimetic drugs. In such a case, a corticosteroid is administered as part of the shock resuscitation. If the patient has a history of adrenal insufficiency or chronic steroid therapy, medical direction may recommend the administration of either of the following medications:

- Hydrocortisone succinate: 2 mg/kg (maximum 100 mg) IV or IM (preferred) *or*
- Methylprednisolone: 2 mg/kg IV (maximum 125 mg)

Integration of Patient Assessment and the Treatment Plan

Many complications of shock are possible (BOX 35-3). The goals of prehospital care for the patient with severe hemorrhage or shock include rapid recognition of the event, initiation of treatment, prevention of additional injury, rapid transport to an appropriate medical facility by ground or air ambulance, and advanced notification of the receiving facility. The paramedic should follow guidelines established by local protocol and medical direction in determining the appropriate prehospital level of care for patients and in identifying the appropriate medical facility for patient transport.

BOX 35-3 Complications of Shock

Acute renal failure
Acute adult respiratory distress syndrome
Hematologic failure
Multiple organ dysfunction syndrome
Sepsis
Acute respiratory distress syndrome
Death of organs
Death of organism
DIC

Summary

- Shock is hypoxia at the cellular level. It is not a single event, but rather the culmination of a complex group of physiologic abnormalities.
- Perfusion is the passage of fluid through the circulatory system or lymphatic system to an organ or a tissue. The heart, lungs, and blood vessels (and blood volume) must all be working effectively to achieve normal perfusion.
- The blood vessels form the body's container. This container must be able to shrink and grow and must be filled with an adequate volume to achieve normal tissue perfusion.
- Uncorrected shock progresses through a series of stages—namely, vasoconstriction, capillary and venous opening, disseminated intravascular coagulation, and multiple organ failure.

- Hypovolemic shock occurs when excess blood or body fluid is lost.
- Cardiogenic shock results from pump failure related to a heart muscle, valve, or rhythm problem.
- Obstructive shock is associated with physical obstruction of the great vessels or the heart itself. Causes of obstructive shock include pericardial tamponade, tension pneumothorax, and pulmonary embolism.
- Distributive shock occurs when peripheral vasodilation causes a decrease in systemic vascular resistance. The most common causes of distributive shock are neurogenic shock, anaphylactic shock, and septic shock.
- Neurogenic shock occurs when there is vasomotor paralysis high on the spinal cord.
- Anaphylactic shock is an extreme manifestation of anaphylaxis that causes impaired vasomotor tone, fluid volume loss, airway obstruction, and bronchospasm.
- Septic shock occurs as a result of a systemic infection. Chemical toxins released from the infectious agent cause a cascade of events that impair cardiac output.
- The three stages of shock are compensated, uncompensated, and irreversible shock.
- Treatment of the patient in shock aims to ensure a patent airway, provide adequate oxygenation, and restore perfusion. The means to achieve each of those objectives varies according to the type of shock and the condition of the patient.
- Fluid resuscitation in shock varies according to the cause. If the patient has uncorrected internal hemorrhage, an isotonic crystalloid solution should be infused to maintain a systolic blood pressure of 80 mm Hg.
- Treatment of cardiogenic shock aims to normalize the heart rate and improve the pumping action of the heart.
- During neurogenic shock, fluids should be administered cautiously with frequent monitoring of lung sounds.
- Anaphylactic shock is treated with epinephrine, diphenhydramine, and fluid bolus.
- Treatment for patients with septic shock will include fluid resuscitation and possibly administration of vasopressors.

References

1. Mann FC. Systems of surgery. *Bull Johns Hopkins Hosp.* 1914;25:205.
2. Hardaway R, ed. *Shock: The Reversible Stage of Dying.* Littleton, MA: PSG Publishing; 1988.
3. National Highway Traffic Safety Administration. *The National EMS Education Standards.* Washington, DC: US Department of Transportation, National Highway Traffic Safety Administration; 2009.
4. Banasik JL, Copstead-Kirkhorn L-E. *Pathophysiology.* 5th ed. Philadelphia, PA: Elsevier; 2018.
5. McCance KL, Huether S. *Pathophysiology: The Biologic Basis for Disease in Adults and Children.* 6th ed. St. Louis, MO: Mosby; 2010.
6. Patton KT, Thibodeau GA. *Anatomy and Physiology.* 9th ed. St. Louis, MO: Mosby; 2015.
7. Stalker AL. The microcirculation in shock. *J Clin Pathol.* 1970;3-4(suppl):10-15.
8. Peacock W, Weber J. Cardiogenic shock. In: Tintinalli JE, ed. *Emergency Medicine: A Comprehensive Study Guide.* 6th ed. New York, NY: McGraw-Hill; 2004:242-247.
9. Ren X. Cardiogenic shock. Medscape website. https://emedicine.medscape.com/article/152191-overview. Updated January 11, 2017. Accessed March 23, 2018.
10. Hochman J, Reyentovich A. Prognosis and treatment of cardiogenic shock complicating acute myocardial infarction. UpToDate website. https://www.uptodate.com/contents/prognosis-and-treatment-of-cardiogenic-shock-complicating-acute-myocardial-infarction?source=search_result&search=Cardiogenic%20Shock&selectedTitle=1~150. Updated November 20, 2017. Accessed March 23, 2018.
11. Rudiger A. Understanding cardiogenic shock. *Eur J Heart Failure.* 2015;17:466-467.
12. Kumar A, Parrillo JE. Shock: classification, pathophysiology, and approach to management. In: *Critical Care Medicine.* 3rd ed. Philadelphia, PA: Elsevier/ScienceDirect; 2008: 379-422.
13. Singer M, Deutschman CS, Seymour CW. The Third International Consensus Definitions for Sepsis and Septic Shock (Sepsis-3). *JAMA.* 2016;315(8):801-810.
14. Dorsett M, Kroll M, Smith CS, Asaro P, Liang SY, Moy HP. qSOFA has poor sensitivity for prehospital identification of severe sepsis and septic shock. *Prehosp Emerg Care.* 2017:1-9.
15. Wang HE, Weaver MD, Shapiro NI, Yealy DM. Opportunities for emergency medical services care of sepsis. *Resuscitation.* 2010;81(2):193-197.
16. Centers for Disease Control and Prevention, National Center for Emerging and Zoonotic Infectious Diseases, Division of Healthcare Quality Promotion. Sepsis: basic information. Centers for Disease Control and Prevention website. https://www.cdc.gov/sepsis/basic/index.html. Updated January 23, 2018. Accessed March 23, 2018.
17. Hunter CL, Silvestri S, Ralls G, Stone A, Walker A, Papa L. A prehospital screening tool utilizing end-tidal carbon dioxide predicts sepsis and severe sepsis. *Am J Emerg Med.* 2016; 34(5):813-819.
18. Albreiki M, Voegeli D. Permissive hypotensive resuscitation in adult patients with traumatic haemorrhagic shock: a systematic review. *Eur J Trauma Emerg Surg.* 2017:1-12.
19. Hubmann B, Lefering R, Taeger G, et al. Influence of prehospital fluid resuscitation on patients with multiple injuries in hemorrhagic shock in patients from the DGU trauma registry. *J Emerg Trauma Shock.* 2011;4(4):465.
20. Roth RN, Fowler RL, Guyette FX. Hypotension and shock. In: Brice J, Delbriddge TR, Myers JB, eds. *Emergency Services: Clinical Practice and Systems Oversight.* Vol 1. 2nd ed. West Sussex, England: John Wiley & Sons; 2015:69-77.
21. National Association of Emergency Medical Technicians. *PHTLS: Basic and Advanced Prehospital Trauma Life Support.* 8th ed. Burlington, MA: Jones & Bartlett Learning; 2014.
22. Lee SM, An WS. New clinical criteria for septic shock: serum lactate level as new emerging vital sign. *J Thoracic Dis.* 2016;8(7):1388-1390

23. National Association of State EMS Officials website. https://nasemso.org/documents/National-Model-EMS-Clinical-Guidelines-2017-Distribution-Version-05Oct2017.pdf. Published September 2017. Accessed March 23, 2018.
24. Marx JA, Walls R, Hockberger RS. *Rosen's Emergency Medicine: Concepts and Clinical Practice.* 8th ed. St. Louis, MO: Saunders/Mosby; 2014.
25. Haynes BE, Carr FJ, Niemann JT. Catheter introducers for rapid fluid resuscitation. *Ann Emerg Med.* 1983;12(10):606.
26. Jansen JO, Thomas R, Loudon MA, Brooks A. Damage control resuscitation for patients with major trauma. *BMJ.* 2009; 338.

Suggested Readings

Guerra WF, Mayfield TR, Meyers MS, Clouatre AE, Riccio JC. Early detection and treatment of patients with severe sepsis by prehospital personnel. *J Emerg Med.* 2013;44(6):1116-1125.

Lieberman P, Nicklas R, Oppenheimer J, et al. The diagnosis and management of anaphylaxis practice parameter: 2010 update. *J Allergy Clin Immunol.* 2010;126(3):477-480.

Murdock AD, Berséus O, Hervig T, Strandenes G, Lunde TH. Whole blood: the future of traumatic hemorrhagic shock resuscitation. *Shock.* 2014;41(suppl 1):62-69.

Revell M, Greaves I, Porter K. Endpoints for fluid resuscitation in hemorrhagic shock. *J Trauma.* 2003;54(5):S63-S67.

Sampson HA, Muñoz-Furlong A, Campbell RL, et al. Second symposium on the definition and management of anaphylaxis: summary report—Second National Institute of Allergy and Infectious Disease/Food Allergy and Anaphylaxis Network Symposium. *Ann Emerg Med.* 2006;47(4):373-380.

Seymour CW, Kahn JM, Cooke CR, et al. Prediction of critical illness during out-of-hospital emergency care [Research]. *JAMA.* 2010;304(7):747-754.

Wang HE, Yealy D. Assessing critical illness during emergency medical services care [Editorial]. *JAMA.* 2010;304(7):797-798.

PART 9

Trauma

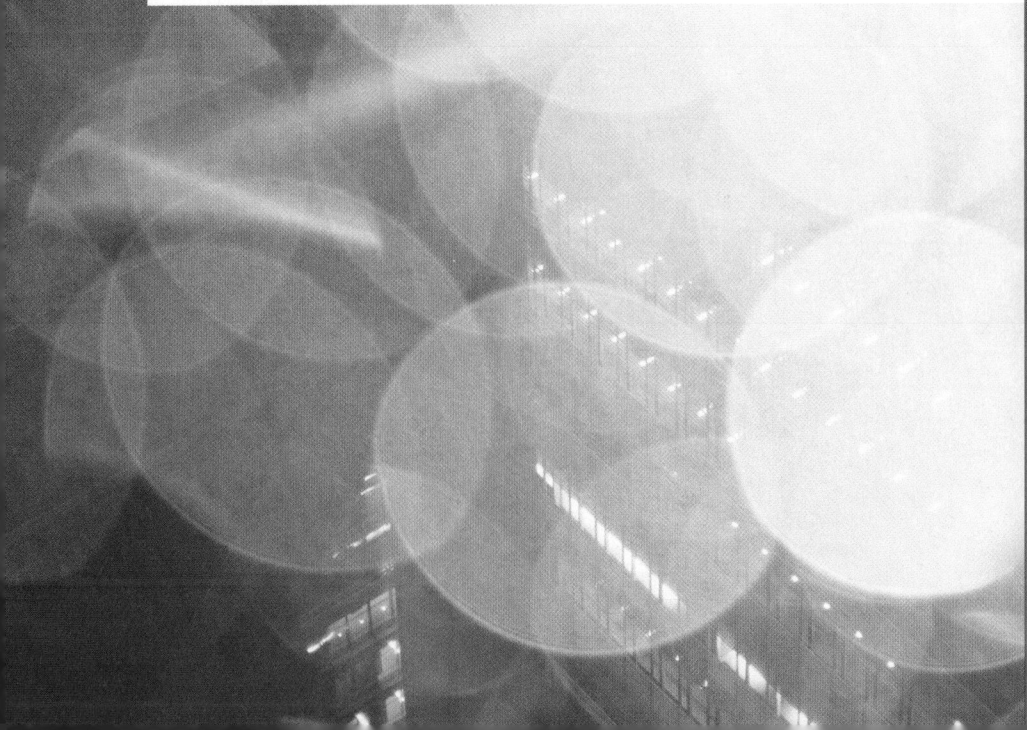

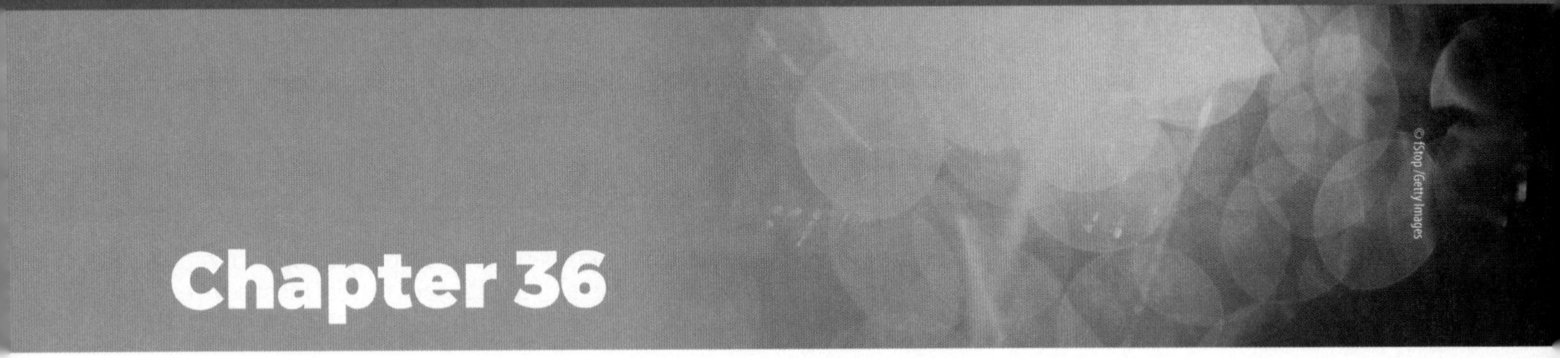

Chapter 36

Trauma Overview and Mechanism of Injury

NATIONAL EMS EDUCATION STANDARD COMPETENCIES

Trauma

Integrates assessment findings with principles of epidemiology and pathophysiology to formulate a field impression to implement a comprehensive treatment/disposition plan for an acutely injured patient.

Trauma Overview

Pathophysiology, assessment, and management of the trauma patient

- Trauma scoring (Chapter 39, *Head, Face, and Neck Trauma*)
- Rapid transport and destination issues (pp 1337, 1339–1341)
- Transport mode (p 1341)

Multisystem Trauma

Recognition, pathophysiology, assessment, and management of

- Multisystem trauma (pp 1345, 1352–1353)

Pathophysiology, assessment, and management of

- Blast injuries (pp 1353–1355)

OBJECTIVES

Upon completion of this chapter, the paramedic student will be able to:

1. Describe the incidence and scope of traumatic injuries and deaths. (pp 1336–1338)
2. Identify the role of each component of the trauma system. (p 1338)
3. Predict injury patterns based on knowledge of the laws of physics related to forces involved in trauma. (pp 1341–1342)
4. Describe injury patterns that should be suspected when injury occurs related to a specific type of blunt trauma. (pp 1342–1345)
5. Describe the role of restraints in injury prevention and injury patterns. (pp 1345–1347)
6. Discuss how organ motion can contribute to injury in each body region depending on the forces applied. (pp 1347–1350)
7. Identify selected injury patterns associated with motorcycle and all-terrain vehicle crashes. (pp 1350–1352)
8. Describe injury patterns associated with motor vehicle–pedestrian collisions. (pp 1352–1353)
9. Identify injury patterns associated with sports injuries, blast injuries, and vertical falls. (pp 1353–1356)
10. Describe factors that influence tissue damage related to penetrating injury. (pp 1356–1361)

KEY TERMS

acceleration An increase in the velocity of a moving object.

blunt trauma An injury produced by the wounding forces of compression and change of speed, both of which can disrupt tissue.

cavitation A temporary or permanent opening produced by a force that pushes body tissues laterally away from the track of a projectile.

deceleration A decrease in the velocity of a moving object.

event phase The phase of trauma that refers to the trauma event.

kinematics The process of predicting injury patterns that can result from the forces and motions of energy.

penetrating trauma An injury produced by crushing and stretching forces of a penetrating object that results in some form of tissue disruption.

postevent phase The phase of trauma in which emergency care is delivered to injured patients.

preevent phase The phase of trauma that refers to the prevention of intentional and unintentional trauma deaths.

trauma centers Specialized medical facilities distinguished by the immediate availability of specialized personnel, equipment, and services to treat most severe and critical injuries.

Trauma is a major cause of morbidity (nonfatal injury), mortality (death), and years of life lost from normal life expectancy. The paramedic must have an appreciation of trauma systems and how they impact patient care. The paramedic also must be able to recognize how mechanisms of injury predict injury patterns and severity. With these two abilities, the paramedic will be able to enhance patient assessment and emergency care. The purpose of this chapter is to provide an overview of trauma. Care considerations are addressed in later chapters by subject matter.

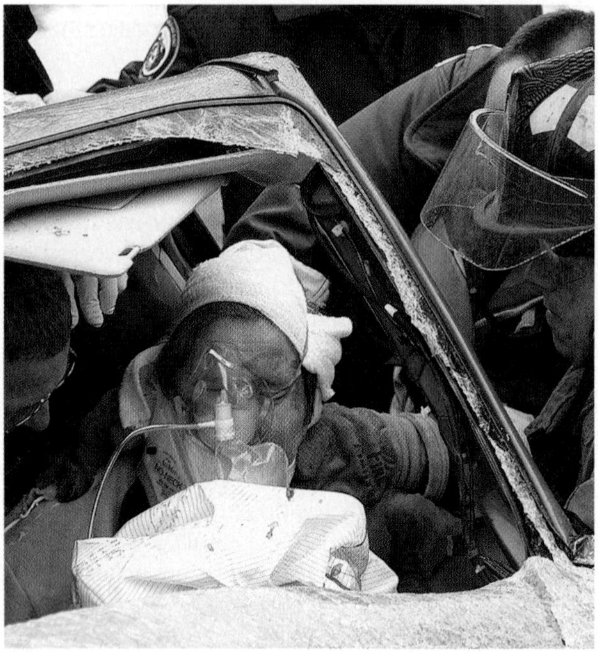

Courtesy of Ray Kemp, St. Charles, MO

Epidemiology of Trauma

Unintentional injury is a devastating medical and social problem. It is the leading cause of death among people 1 to 44 years of age and the fourth-leading cause of death among all Americans.[1] Unintentional deaths in 2015 were exceeded only by deaths attributable to heart disease, cancer, drug overdose involving opioids, and chronic lower respiratory tract diseases. In 2015, about 146,571 unintentional injury deaths occurred in the United States. The National Safety Council estimates that the total number of nonfatal unintentional injuries requiring medical care in the United States approaches 40.6 million annually. The economic effect of unintentional injuries in the United States exceeds $4,424 billion each year.

> NOTE
>
> In any given 10-minute period in the United States, 3 people are killed. In that same time, about 772 people suffer an injury serious enough to seek medical care. Costs in these 10-minute periods amount to more than $16.8 million.
>
> *Modified from*: National Safety Council. *Injury Facts: 2017 Edition*. Itasca, IL: National Safety Council; 2017.

Trends in Trauma Deaths

Deaths from unintentional injury are increasing annually; however, most deaths from trauma can be prevented. The increase in deaths indicates the need for increased safety and health efforts to reverse the trend. Poisoning by solids and liquids, motor vehicle crashes, falls, fire and flames, drowning, and choking have been the leading causes of trauma deaths since 1970 (**FIGURE 36-1**) (BOX 36-1).[1] In recent years, poisonings have replaced motor vehicle crashes at the top position, fueled largely by the opioid crisis.[2]

Phases of Trauma Care

Trauma care is divided into three phases: preevent, event, and postevent.[3] The **preevent phase** refers to the factors and events existing before the injury, such

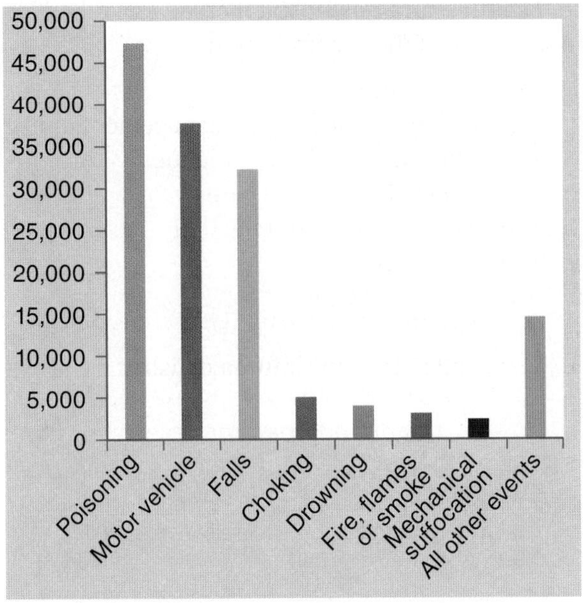

FIGURE 36-1 Deaths from unintentional injury by event.

Data Source: 10 Leading Causes of Injury Deaths by Age Group Highlighting Unintentional Injury Deaths, United States–2016. Centers for Disease Control and Prevention website. https://www.cdc.gov/injury/images/lc-charts/leading_causes_of_death_highlighting_unintentional_2016_1040w800h.gif. Accessed May 30, 2018.

BOX 36-1 Classifications of Deaths Attributable to Trauma in the United States[a]

All external causes of mortality
Motor vehicle crashes
Pedestrian injury
Motorcycle crashes
Falls
Mechanical forces (struck by object or machinery)
Drowning
Electric current
Intentional self-harm
Assaults (firearms)

[a]Poisonings are not included.

Modified from: National Highway Traffic Safety Administration. *The National EMS Education Standards*. Washington, DC: US Department of Transportation/National Highway Traffic Safety Administration; 2009.

as intoxication, heart disease, or poor vision, that may influence the cause of the event or the patient's response to it. Paramedics and other health care professionals play a key role in this phase. A part of this phase includes participating in public education and prevention activities. For example, paramedics may educate the public on the use of personal restraint systems, motorcycle helmets, and the proper use of 9-1-1. Paramedics also promote legislation that supports injury prevention programs (see Chapter 3, *Injury Prevention, Health Promotion, and Public Health*).

The **event phase** is the trauma event. It begins at first contact with the injuring force and ends when the energy causing injury is no longer applied.

The **postevent phase** is when the paramedic uses his or her expertise and skills. This phase is the delivery of emergency care to injured patients. Important responsibilities for the paramedic in this phase include the following:

- Gathering information
- Performing lifesaving maneuvers
- Properly preparing the patient for transport to an appropriate medical facility
- Promptly transporting the patient to the appropriate medical facility (BOX 36-2)

BOX 36-2 Concepts in Urgent Care for Trauma Patients

Concepts that emphasize the urgency of care for major trauma patients have been advocated in medical literature since the early 1970s. The concepts refer to the critical time after severe injury in which interventions can be performed to maximize the patient's chance of a favorable outcome. Two of these concepts are known as the Golden Period (or the Golden Hour) and the Platinum 10 Minutes.

The Golden Period stresses that an injured patients has 60 minutes from the time of injury to receive definitive care, after which morbidity and mortality increases significantly. The Platinum 10 Minutes is a companion to the Golden Hour. Its premise is that seriously injured patients should have no more than 10 minutes of scene-time stabilization prior to transport for definitive care.

Although both of these concepts are controversial and lack conclusive evidence, there *is* an aspect of trauma care that is time dependent. The paramedic must recognize patients who are in this group and ensure that prehospital care does not delay patient transportation. These patients can best served through rapid assessment, stabilization of life-threatening injuries, and rapid transportation to an appropriate medical facility for definitive care.

Modified from: Cowley RA. A total emergency medical system for the state of Maryland. *Md State Med J*. 1975;45:37-45; Daban JL, Falzone E, Boutonnet M, Peigne V, Lenoir B. [Wounded in action: the platinum ten minutes and the golden hour]. *Soins*. 2014;Sept(788):14-15; and Rogers F, Rittenhouse K. The Golden Hour in trauma: dogma or medical folklore? *J Lancaster Gen Hospital*. Spring 2014;9(1).

The factor most important to any severely injured patient's survival is the length of time that elapses between the incident and definitive care (BOX 36-3).[3]

Trauma Systems

A comprehensive trauma system consists of many different components. These components are integrated and coordinated to provide cost-effective services for injury prevention and patient care. At the center of this system is the continuum of care, which includes injury prevention, prehospital care, acute care facilities, and posthospital care.[4] The following is a sampling of these components:

1. Injury prevention
2. Prehospital care, including management, transport, and trauma triage guidelines
3. Emergency department care
4. Interfacility transport if needed
5. Definitive care
6. Trauma critical care
7. Rehabilitation
8. Data collection and trauma registry

BOX 36-3 Prevention of Trauma Deaths

Deaths from trauma occur in three periods: immediate, early, and late. Each period presents its own unique problems.

Immediate

Immediate death occurs within seconds or minutes of the injury. Lacerations of the brain, brainstem, upper spinal cord, heart, aorta, or other large vessels usually cause these deaths. Few if any patients in this category can be saved. Effective injury prevention programs are the only way to reduce the number of these deaths.

Early

The second peak of death occurs within the first 2 to 3 hours after injury. The causes of these deaths usually are major head injury, hemopneumothorax, ruptured spleen, lacerated liver, pelvic fracture, or multiple injuries associated with significant blood loss. Most of these injuries can be treated with available techniques; however, the time lapse between injury and definitive care is crucial.

Late

The third peak of death occurs days or weeks after the injury. These deaths most often result from sepsis, infection, or multiple organ failure. Prehospital emergency care focused on early recognition and management of life-threatening injuries is crucial to the prevention of late deaths from trauma.

Modified from: Baker CC, Oppenheimer L, Stephens B, et al. Epidemiology of trauma deaths. *Am J Surg*. 1980;140:144; and Trunkey DD. Trauma. Accidental and intentional injuries account for more years of life lost in the US than cancer and heart disease. Among the prescribed remedies are improved preventive efforts, speedier surgery and further research. *Sci Am*. 1983;249:28-35.

CRITICAL THINKING

How can you learn more about the components of the trauma system during your career as a paramedic?

The paramedic plays a crucial role in the trauma system. One aspect of this role is being involved in injury prevention programs. Another aspect includes entering appropriate patients into the trauma care system while providing appropriate patient care. Lastly, the paramedic fulfills this role by taking part in data collection and research. This research can influence health care improvements to care for injured patients (BOX 36-4).

Trauma Centers

The US Department of Health and Human Services released the *Position Paper on Trauma Center Designation* in 1980. Since then, states have developed

BOX 36-4 Trauma Registries

Trauma registries allow for the collection of injury data by individual medical facilities or groups of medical facilities on a local, regional, or state level. The American College of Surgeons funded these registries and the data collection software programs. (An example of a registry is the National Trauma Data Bank. An example of a software program is NATIONAL TRACS.) The registries and programs are meant to provide online data management. They also are intended to provide national exchange of injury data for a variety of commercial registry programs. Trauma registries generate periodic standard reports that offer statistical data. The data allow facilities to compare trends and to compare other key details of trauma care.

comprehensive trauma systems. As of 2017, over 2,000 medical facilities have a designated specialty in trauma.[5]

The American Medical Association recommended categorization of medical facility emergency services in the early 1970s.[6] In 1990 (revised in 1999), the Task Force of the American College of Surgeons (ACS) Committee on Trauma published *Resources for Optimal Care of the Injured Patient.* The paper described three levels of **trauma centers**. These levels are based on resources (essential and desired), admissions, staff, research, and education involvement. Since that time, two additional categories of trauma centers have been added.

A level I trauma center has a full range of specialists and equipment available 24 hours a day and is a regional resource for severely injured patients. Additionally, a level I center has a program of research, is a leader in trauma education and injury prevention, and is a referral center for communities in neighboring regions through community outreach.[7] A level I trauma center can provide total care for every aspect of injury. The level I center is followed by levels II through V facilities (**BOX 36-5**).

The assignment of category to a trauma center also enables emergency medical services (EMS) personnel to transport patients rapidly to the most appropriate facility. Other specialized care facilities, such as pediatric trauma centers, burn centers, hyperbaric centers, and poison treatment centers, provide care for critically ill or injured patients with special needs. The ACS Committee on Trauma also established guidelines for field triage, interhospital triage to specialized care facilities, and mass-casualty triage. These criteria are based on the patient's condition, mechanism of injury (MOI), injury severity indexes, and available patient care resources (**FIGURE 36-2**).

CRITICAL THINKING

Where can you find the trauma triage criteria for your area?

Transportation Considerations

Determining the proper level of care and medical facility destination is based on the patient's needs and condition and sometimes the advice of medical

BOX 36-5 Trauma Centers

A trauma center is a specialized medical facility distinguished by the immediate availability of specialized personnel, equipment, and services to treat the most severe and critical injuries. Its resources include ready-to-go teams that perform immediate surgery and other necessary procedures for people with serious or life-threatening injuries. The mission of a trauma center is to ensure continuity and quality of care for injured patients from the scene of injury through treatment at the trauma center and ultimately through physical rehabilitation.

Trauma centers are classified by the following levels based on the amount of equipment, staff, and care provided.

- **Level I.** Has a full range of specialists and equipment available 24 hours per day. Admits a minimum required annual volume of severely injured patients. Has a research program, is a leader in trauma education and injury prevention, and is a referral resource for communities in neighboring regions.
- **Level II.** Usually works in collaboration with a level I center but may be the only resource in a rural community. Provides 24-hour availability of all essential specialties, personnel, and equipment with immediate surgery capability. Provides an injury prevention program but is not required to have an ongoing program of research or a surgical residency program.
- **Level III.** Has resources for the emergency resuscitation, stabilization, emergent surgery, and intensive care of most trauma patients. Has 24-hour emergency medicine physicians and on-call general surgeons and anesthesiologists. Has transfer agreements with level I and/or level II trauma centers. Has an injury prevention program. Does not have the full availability of specialists, except surgery and orthopaedics, in most states.
- **Level IV.** Provides initial evaluation, emergency resuscitation, and stabilization of trauma patients, but most patients will require transfer to higher-level trauma centers. Has 24-hour emergency coverage by a physician and a 24-hour lab.
- **Level V.** Has basic emergency department facilities and transfer agreements with level I or II trauma centers.

Modified from: Trauma center levels explained. American Trauma Society website. http://www.amtrauma.org/?page=traumalevels. Accessed March 7, 2018.

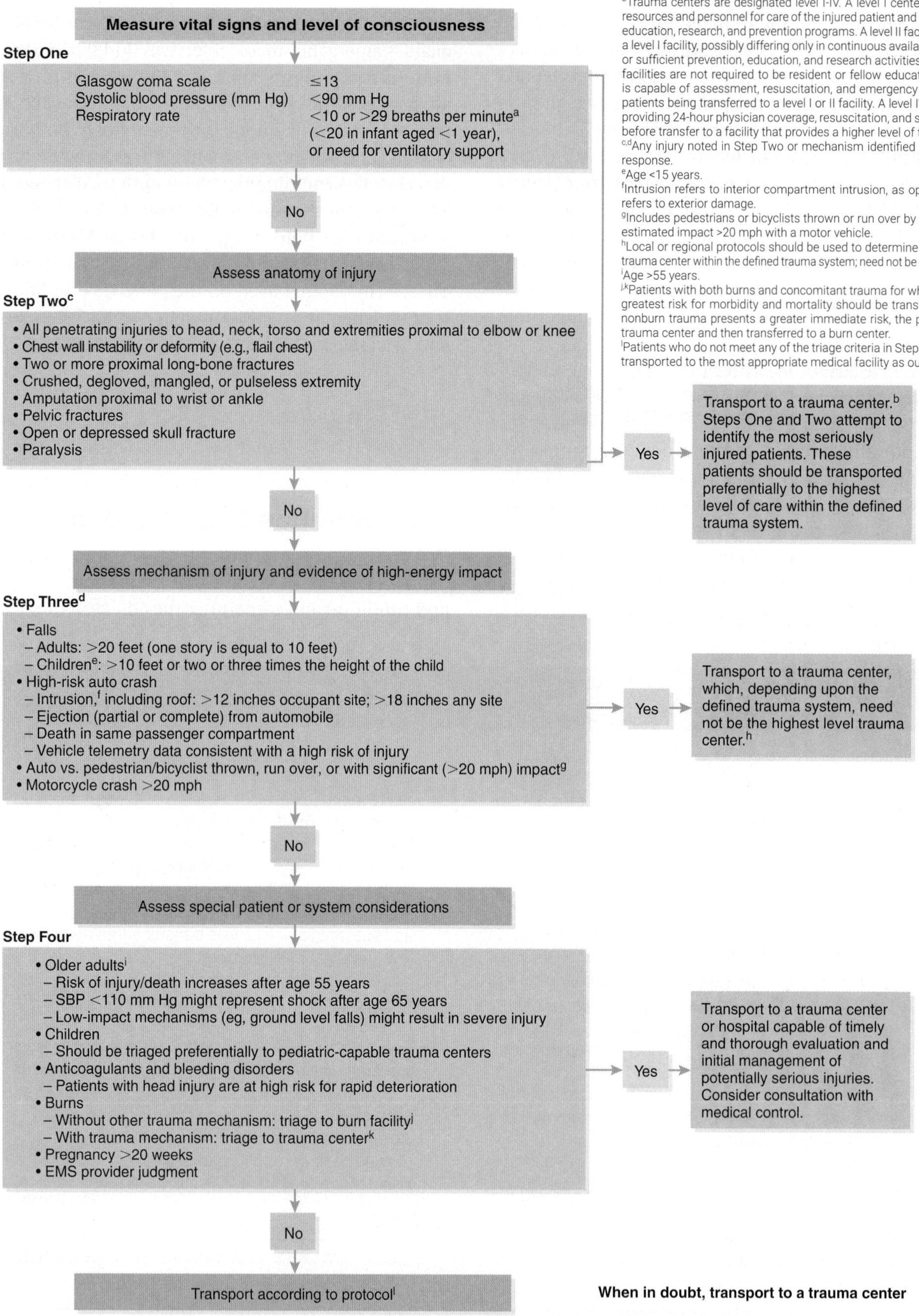

[a]The upper limit of respiratory rate in infants is >29 breaths per minute to maintain a higher level of overtriage for infants.
[b]Trauma centers are designated level I-IV. A level I center has the greatest amount of resources and personnel for care of the injured patient and provides regional leadership in education, research, and prevention programs. A level II facility offers similar resources to a level I facility, possibly differing only in continuous availability of certain subspecialties or sufficient prevention, education, and research activities for level I designation; level II facilities are not required to be resident or fellow education centers. A level III center is capable of assessment, resuscitation, and emergency surgery, with severely injured patients being transferred to a level I or II facility. A level IV trauma center is capable of providing 24-hour physician coverage, resuscitation, and stabilization to injured patients before transfer to a facility that provides a higher level of trauma care.
[c,d]Any injury noted in Step Two or mechanism identified in Step Three triggers a "yes" response.
[e]Age <15 years.
[f]Intrusion refers to interior compartment intrusion, as opposed to deformation which refers to exterior damage.
[g]Includes pedestrians or bicyclists thrown or run over by a motor vehicle or those with estimated impact >20 mph with a motor vehicle.
[h]Local or regional protocols should be used to determine the most appropriate level of trauma center within the defined trauma system; need not be the highest-level trauma center.
[i]Age >55 years.
[j,k]Patients with both burns and concomitant trauma for whom the burn injury poses the greatest risk for morbidity and mortality should be transferred to a burn center. If the nonburn trauma presents a greater immediate risk, the patient may be stabilized in a trauma center and then transferred to a burn center.
[l]Patients who do not meet any of the triage criteria in Steps One through Four should be transported to the most appropriate medical facility as outlined in local EMS protocols.

Abbreviations: EMS, emergency medical services; mph, miles per hour; SBP, systolic blood pressure

FIGURE 36-2 Guidelines for field triage of injured patients: United States, 2011.

Modified from: Sasser SM, Hunt RC, Faul M, et al. Guidelines for Field Triage of Injured Patients: Recommendations of the National Expert Panel on Field Triage, 2011. Centers for Disease Control and Prevention website. https://www.cdc.gov/mmwr/preview/mmwrhtml/rr6101a1.htm. Updated: January 13, 2012. Accessed May 12, 2018.

direction. (The Centers for Disease Control and Prevention along with key experts in trauma care have developed guidelines to assist EMS personnel in identifying and triaging patients who need trauma center care.[8] Other methods of triage are addressed in Chapter 53, *Medical Incident Command.*) Once the paramedic determines the level of care needed and the destination facility, decisions can be made about the mode of transportation. For example, the paramedic chooses between ground or air ambulance.

SHOW ME THE EVIDENCE

Using existing trauma records, researchers calculated actual (observed) trauma undertriage (UT) and overtriage (OT) rates in Ohio compared with the rates of UT and OT that would be achieved using the National Field Triage Decision Scheme (NFTDS) and the existing Ohio state triage guidelines. They found that both NFTDS and state triage guidelines produced lower UT (about 9%) compared to the observed rate (~17%). The OT rates were higher with the NFTDS and state triage guidelines (~85%) compared to the observed rate (~54%). Using a multiple logistic regression model that included factors not in the triage schemes that were evaluated (change in responsiveness, specific body region injury), they found improved triage accuracy. The researchers concluded that adding body region–specific factors to the existing triage schemes will improve accuracy.

Modified from: Parikh PP, Parikh P, Guthrie B, et al. Impact of triage guidelines on prehospital triage: comparison of guidelines with a statistical model. *J Surg Res.* 2017;220:255-260.

Ground Transport

As a rule, the paramedic should use ground transport by ambulance if the appropriate facility can be reached within a reasonable time. Reasonable time is defined by national standards (eg, definitive care within 60 minutes after the injury for severe trauma) and local protocol.[9] Factors that affect the decision to use ground or air transport include geographic location, topographic area, population, weather, availability of resources, traffic conditions, and time of day.

Aeromedical Transport

The availability and use of aeromedical services vary throughout the United States. Aeromedical services can provide rapid response time, high-quality medical care, and rapid transport to appropriate care facilities. Helicopters also can provide aerial surveillance and transport of additional personnel and equipment to the emergency scene. Paramedic crews should consult with medical direction and follow local protocol regarding the use of aeromedical services. The effect of aeromedical transport on the survival of trauma patients is not clear and must take many factors into account, including injury characteristics, injury indexes, and the level of care provided prior to air transport.[10,11] The paramedic should consider air transport in the following situations:

- The time needed to transport a patient by ground to an appropriate facility poses a threat to the patient's survival and recovery.
- Weather, road, or traffic conditions would seriously delay the patient's access to definitive care.
- Critical care personnel and equipment are needed to adequately care for the patient during transport.

Kinematics

Kinematics is the process of predicting injury patterns. Specific types and patterns of injuries are associated with certain mechanisms. In addition to individual factors (such as age) and protective factors (such as restraint systems, helmets, and airbags), the paramedic should consider the following when evaluating the trauma patient:

- MOI
- Force of energy applied
- Anatomy
- Energy (eg, mass, velocity, distance, and thermal, electrical, and chemical forms)

Energy

A transfer of energy from an external source to the human body causes injuries. The extent of injury is determined by (1) the type and amount of energy applied, (2) the speed with which energy is applied, and (3) the part of the body to which energy is applied.

Physical Laws

Knowledge of four basic laws of physics is required to understand the wounding forces of trauma:[2,3]

1. **Newton's first law of motion.** An object, whether at rest or in motion, remains in that state unless acted on by an outside force.

2. **Conservation of energy law.** Energy cannot be created or destroyed; it can only change form. (Energy can take mechanical, thermal, electrical, chemical, and nuclear forms.)
3. **Newton's second law of motion.** Force (F) equals mass (m) multiplied by acceleration (a) or deceleration (d):

$$F = m \times a \quad \text{or} \quad F = m \times d$$

4. **Kinetic energy.** Kinetic energy (KE) equals one-half the mass (m) multiplied by the velocity squared (v^2).

$$KE = \frac{1}{2} m \times v^2$$

As the kinetic energy formula shows, velocity is much more impactful than mass is in determining total kinetic energy. For example, a car and its unrestrained 150-lb driver are traveling 60 miles per hour (mph). According to Newton's first law of motion, the car remains in motion until acted on by an outside force. If the driver gradually applies the brakes, the friction of the brakes slowly converts the mechanical energy of the car to thermal energy (conservation of energy law); the energy transfer occurs gradually through the slow deceleration. If the car strikes a tree, though, and is stopped instantly, the tree absorbs the mechanical energy, the car, and the driver. When the front of the car has stopped, the rear of the car continues forward until all of the energy of its motion is absorbed. The driver is traveling in the same direction and at the same speed as the car before impact. So, like the rear of the car, the driver continues forward. The driver suffers injuries in areas of the body that strike the vehicle.

In this sequence, the tree stops the motion of the front of the car. The steering column continues forward and stops against the dashboard. The driver's sternum stops against the steering column. The driver's chest cavity and its contents hit the sternum and are crushed from behind by the posterior thorax, deforming the entire chest. The kinetic energy in this example is calculated as follows:

KE = one-half of the mass times the velocity squared,

$$\text{or } KE = \frac{1}{2} m \times v^2$$

$$KE = \frac{150}{2} \times 60^2$$

KE = 270,000 units of energy

As shown in this calculation, the 150-lb driver traveling 60 miles per hour (mph) must change 270,000 units of kinetic energy (known as foot-pounds [ft-lb], calculated as pounds multiplied by miles per hour) into another form of energy when he or she stops. In addition, recall that force equals mass multiplied by acceleration (Newton's second law of motion). Thus the 150-lb driver is moving forward in the car with about 9,000 ft-lb of force when stopped by the steering column. The energy of the motion of the body causes tissue destruction as this energy is absorbed into the body cells when the body stops. This example illustrates the principle. However, the actual total force also is determined by the true rate of deceleration, or g-force, and several other factors. Lap and shoulder restraints and airbags increase the distance over which the body stops its movement, which can decrease the deceleration force a great deal. New car construction is also designed to absorb some of this energy and lessen the force transmitted to the vehicle occupants.

> CRITICAL THINKING
>
> Can you apply these same four laws of physics to another traumatic situation, such as a fall onto concrete? What force is applied? What factors influence the kinetic energy?

Blunt Trauma

Blunt trauma is an injury produced by the wounding forces of compression and change of speed (usually deceleration). These forces can disrupt tissue. Direct compression is the pressure on a structure and is the most common type of force applied in blunt trauma. The amount of injury depends on the length of time of compression, the force of compression, and the area compressed. For example, compression of the thorax can lead to rib fracture or pneumothorax. Other compression injuries include contusions and lacerations of solid organs and rupture of hollow (air-filled) organs.

Acceleration is an increase in the velocity of a moving object, while **deceleration** is a decrease in the velocity of a moving object. Both can produce major injury. For example, consider a car that stops abruptly. The occupant's body continues its constant velocity after the impact until it decelerates as a result of striking the steering wheel, restraint system, or dashboard. The external aspect of the body is stopped forcibly. However, the contents of the cranial, thoracic, and peritoneal cavities remain in motion because of inertia. As a result, tissues can be stretched, crushed, ruptured, lacerated, or sheared from their points of attachment. Examples of injuries caused by a change of speed include concussion, cardiac or pulmonary contusion, organ laceration, and aortic tear.

Motor Vehicle Crash

The various injuries produced by blunt trauma are illustrated best through the examination of vehicle crashes. Forces that cause blunt trauma, however, can result from a variety of impacts. As described in the previous example, a vehicle crash involves three separate impacts as the energy is transferred. In the first impact, the vehicle strikes an object. In the second, the occupant collides with the inside of the car. In the third, the internal organs collide inside the body. The injuries that result depend on the type of crash and the position of the occupant inside the vehicle. The injuries also depend on the use or nonuse of active or passive restraint systems.

> NOTE
>
> The Centers for Disease Control and Prevention report that 9 people are killed and more than 1,000 are injured daily in crashes involving a distracted driver. Distraction occurs when drivers take their eyes off the road, their hands off the wheel, or their mind off of driving. Texting and driving is particularly dangerous because it combines all three distractions. A vehicle driving at 55 mph (89 km/h) can travel the length of a football field while the driver takes 5 seconds to send or read a text message.
>
> *Modified from*: Centers for Disease Control and Prevention, National Center for Injury Prevention and Control, Division of Unintentional Injury Prevention. Distracted driving. Centers for Disease Control and Prevention website. https://www.cdc.gov/motorvehiclesafety/distracted_driving/index.html. Updated July 9, 2017. Accessed March 7, 2018.

A vehicle crash is classified by the type of impact: head-on, lateral, rear-end, rotational, and rollover. The forces of compression and change of speed produce predictable injury patterns in each type of crash.

Head-on (Frontal) Impact

Head-on crashes result when forward motion stops abruptly (eg, one vehicle collides with another one traveling in the opposite direction). The first impact occurs when the vehicle hits the second vehicle, resulting in damage to the front of the car. As the vehicle abruptly stops, the occupant continues to move at the speed of the vehicle before impact. The front seat occupant continues forward into the restraint system, steering column, or dashboard, resulting in the second impact. The occupant who is not restrained usually travels in one of two pathways in relationship to the dashboard: a down-and-under pathway or an up-and-over pathway. The precise course of this pathway determines how the organs collide inside the body and the extent of tissue damaged.

In the down-and-under pathway, the occupant travels downward into the vehicle seat and forward into the dashboard or steering column (**FIGURE 36-3**). The knees become the leading part of the body, striking the dashboard. The upper legs absorb most of the impact. Predictable injuries include knee dislocation, patellar fracture, femoral fracture, fracture or posterior dislocation of the hip, fracture of the acetabulum, vascular injury, and hemorrhage. After the initial impact of the knees into the dashboard, the body rotates forward. As the chest wall hits the

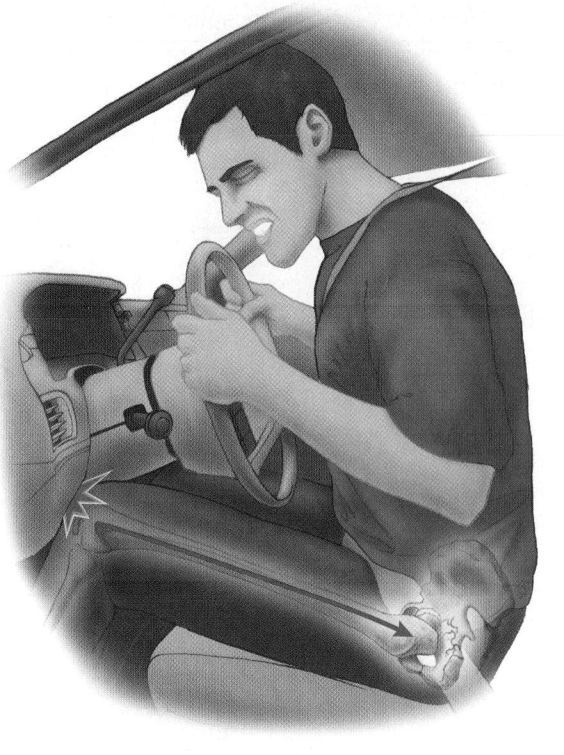

FIGURE 36-3 Down-and-under pathway.

steering column or dashboard, the head and torso absorb energy as indicated in the description of the up-and-over pathway.

> CRITICAL THINKING
> How does the use of lap and shoulder restraints influence the patterns of injury described here?

In the up-and-over pathway, the body in forward motion strikes the steering wheel. As this impact occurs, the ribs and underlying structures absorb the momentum of the thorax (**FIGURE 36-4**). Predictable injuries from this transfer of energy include rib fracture, ruptured diaphragm, hemopneumothorax, pulmonary contusion, cardiac contusion, myocardial rupture, and vascular disruption (most notably aortic rupture).

If the abdomen is the point of impact, compression injuries can occur to the hollow abdominal organs, solid organs, and lumbar vertebrae. The kidneys, liver, and spleen are subject to vascular tears from supporting tissue. Such injuries may include the tearing of renal vessels from their points of attachment to the inferior vena cava and descending aorta. Predictable injuries include liver laceration, spleen rupture, internal hemorrhage, and abdominal organ incursion into the thorax (ruptured diaphragm).

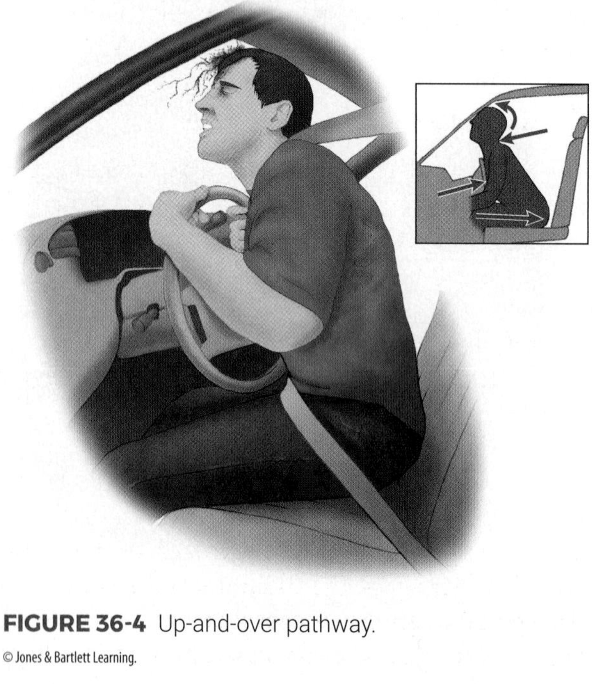

FIGURE 36-4 Up-and-over pathway.

If the head absorbs most of the impact, the cervical vertebrae absorb the continued momentum of the body. Cervical flexion, axial loading, and hyperextension can result in fracture or dislocation of the cervical vertebrae. In addition, severe angulation of the cervical vertebrae can damage the soft tissues of the neck. This mechanism may cause spinal cord injury and spinal instability, even without fracture. Other predictable injuries include trauma to the brain (eg, concussion, contusion, shearing injury, edema) and disruption of vessels inside the head (intracranial vascular disruption), resulting in subdural or epidural hematoma (see Chapter 39, *Head, Face, and Neck Trauma*).

Lateral Impact

Lateral impact occurs when a vehicle is struck from the side. Injury patterns depend on whether the damaged vehicle remains in place or moves away from the point of impact. The external shell of a vehicle that remains in place after impact usually intrudes into the passenger compartment and usually directs force at the lateral aspect of the person's body. Predictable injuries result from compression to the torso, pelvis, and extremities. Examples of these injuries include fracture of the clavicle, ribs, or pelvis; pulmonary contusion; ruptured liver or spleen (depending on the side involved); and head and neck injury. Vehicles that have side-impact airbags can guard against injury in some lateral impacts.

If the damaged vehicle moves away from the point of impact, the occupant accelerates away from the point of impact. The occupant moves laterally with the car. The effects of inertia on the head, neck, and thorax produce lateral flexion and rotation of the cervical spine. This movement can result in neurologic injury. Such movement also can result in tears or strains of the lateral ligaments and supporting structures of the neck. Injuries also can occur on the side of the passenger opposite the impact as the occupant is propelled toward the other side of the car. If other occupants are in the vehicle, secondary impact with other passengers is likely.

Rear-End Impact

A vehicle that is struck from behind rapidly accelerates, causing it to move forward under the occupant. The greater the difference in the forward speed of the two vehicles, the greater the force and damaging energy of the initial impact. For example, consider a vehicle that is traveling 50 mph (80 km/h) and hits a stationary vehicle. The damaging energy is greater than that of a vehicle traveling 50 mph (80 km/h) that hits another vehicle moving in the same direction at 30 mph (48 km/h). In rear-end collisions, the difference between the two speeds is the damaging velocity. In contrast, in forward collisions, the sum of the speeds of both vehicles is the velocity that produces damage.[3]

Predictable injuries in rear-end collisions include back and neck injuries and cervical strain or fracture caused by hyperextension. The cervical portion of the spine is susceptible to secondary hyperextension caused by the rapid forward acceleration of the vehicle and subsequent relative rearward movement of the occupant. If the vehicle collides with an object in front of it, the paramedic should suspect injuries associated with frontal impact.

Rotational Impact

Rotational impacts occur when an off-center portion of the vehicle (usually the front quarter) strikes an immovable object or one that is moving more slowly or in the opposite direction. The part of the vehicle striking the object stops during impact while the rest of the vehicle continues in the forward motion until the energy is transformed completely. The occupant moves inside the vehicle with the forward motion and usually is struck by the side of the vehicle as it rotates around the point of impact. A rotational impact results in the same injuries commonly found in head-on and lateral crashes.

Rollover Crashes

In rollover crashes, the person tumbles inside the vehicle and can be ejected if unrestrained. The occupant is injured wherever his or her body strikes the vehicle. The various impacts occur at many different angles, which can cause multisystem injuries. Predicting injury patterns from rollover crashes is difficult. These crashes can produce any of the injury patterns that are associated with other types of crashes.

Restraints

In recent years, public awareness programs and various state laws have increased the use of personal restraints. According to the National Safety Council, seat belt use hit a record high of 90% in 2016. When used properly, safety belts reduce the risk of fatal injury by 50% and the risk of serious or critical injuries by 65%. Among passenger vehicle occupants older than 4 years, safety belts saved an estimated 13,941 lives in 2015.[1] Another 2,804 lives could have been saved if *all* passengers older than 4 years had worn safety belts. At this time, all states and the District of Columbia have child safety seat laws. Forty-nine states and the District of Columbia have mandatory safety belt use laws in effect. The one exception is New Hampshire, where only drivers and passengers younger than 18 years are required to use them.[12]

A serious hazard to unrestrained occupants is ejection from the vehicle after impact. People who do not wear a seat belt are 30 times more likely to be ejected from their vehicle during a crash, and 75% of ejected people die from their injuries.[13]

> CRITICAL THINKING
>
> How can you apply this knowledge about ejection statistics to your practice in each of the phases of trauma care (preevent, event, and postevent)?

Four restraining systems are available in the United States: lap belts, diagonal shoulder straps, airbags, and child safety seats. All of these restraints significantly reduce injuries. If they are used inappropriately, however, these protective devices can produce injuries.

Lap Belts

The lap belt, used alone or with a shoulder strap, is the most commonly used active restraint system. A person should use the lap belt at a 45° angle to the floor between the anterior-superior iliac spine and the femur (**FIGURE 36-5**). A lap belt worn tightly enough to stay in this position absorbs energy forces. The belt protects the abdominal cavity by transferring energy to the strong, bony pelvis.

However, the lap belt often is worn incorrectly. If the lap belt is worn above the anterior iliac spine, the forward motion of the body during impact is absorbed by vertebrae T12, L1, and L2. As the thorax is propelled forward, the abdominal organs are compressed between the vertebral column and the lap belt. This compression can cause injury to the liver,

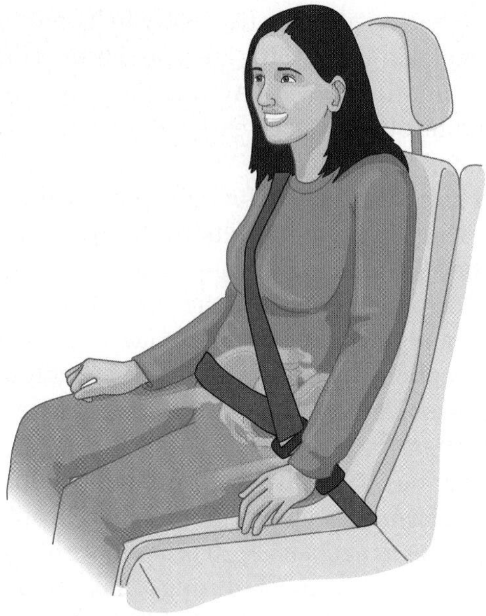

FIGURE 36-5 Properly positioned seat belt.

spleen, duodenum, and pancreas. A sign of these abdominal injuries is abrasions or a lap belt imprint over the abdomen.

Major injury can result even when a person uses a lap belt correctly. These injuries occur from angulation of the lumbar spine, pelvis, thorax, and head around the restraint system. Injuries also occur from failure of the restraint system to decrease the impact forces. Injuries that can occur during high-speed impacts include sternal fractures, chest wall injuries, lumbar vertebral fractures, head injuries, and maxillofacial trauma.

Diagonal Shoulder Straps

Use of a shoulder strap helps absorb the forward motion of the thorax after impact. It should be positioned across the torso and on the shoulder (over the clavicle), avoiding contact with the neck. When a person wears the shoulder strap with the lap belt, the shoulder strap prevents the thorax, face, and head from striking the dashboard, windshield, or steering column. Clavicular fracture can result from the position of the shoulder strap. Organ collision inside the body with resultant internal organ injury, cervical fracture, and spinal cord injury still can occur during high-speed impacts, even when personal restraint systems are used.

NOTE

Pregnant women should wear personal restraints when in traveling in a vehicle. The lap strap should be positioned under the belly, across the hips, and as high as possible on the thighs. The shoulder strap should be placed between the breasts, and off to the side of the belly. Seat belt straps should never be placed directly across the belly. The seat belt should fit snugly and airbags should remain operable.

Modified from: Seat belt use during pregnancy. *Am Fam Physician*. 2004 Oct 1;70(7):1313. https://www.aafp.org/afp/2004/1001/p1313.html. Accessed March 21, 2018.

Airbags

Some vehicles are equipped with side-impact airbags, curtain airbags, knee airbags, safety belt airbags, and rear-curtain airbags to protect against impacts. However, the more common airbag is a frontal airbag that inflates from the center of the steering wheel and from the dashboard during frontal impact. These devices cushion the forward motion of the occupant when used with a lap and shoulder belt. Frontal airbags deflate rapidly. They are effective only with initial frontal and near-frontal crashes. They are ineffective in multiple impacts, rear-impact crashes, and lateral or rollover impacts. These systems do not prevent movement in the down-and-under pathway. Thus the occupant's knees still may be the point of impact, which may result in leg, pelvis, and abdominal injuries.

An airbag can produce significant injury if it is deployed in proximity (10 inches [25 cm] or closer) to the occupant. Deployment in these situations can produce spinal fractures, hand and eye injury, and facial and forearm abrasions. The following groups are at higher risk of injury from airbag deployment:[14]

- Infants and children younger than 13 years
- Adults of short stature (shorter than 4 feet 6 inches [137 cm])
- Older adults
- People with special medical conditions

Most airbag injuries are minor cuts, bruises, or abrasions. Most of these injuries are far less serious than are the head, neck, and chest injuries that airbags prevent. According to the National Highway Traffic Safety Administration, frontal airbags saved more than 39,000 lives between 1987 and 2012.[14] Although deaths do sometimes occur from airbag deployment, most are a result of the occupant being too close to the airbag when it deployed. This problem occurred more commonly from the child not being restrained adequately with lap/shoulder devices or child safety seats during precrash braking. To protect against injury from airbag deployment, the driver of the vehicle should hold the steering wheel in a 9-o'clock and 3-o'clock positions (formerly 10 o'clock and 2 o'clock were recommended) to avoid hand, head, and facial injury should the airbag deploy); be positioned at least 10 inches (25 cm) from the airbag cover; the front seat passenger should be positioned at least 18 inches (46 cm) from the airbag cover; and children younger than 12 years should always ride in the backseat and be in the proper restraint device for their size.

Child Safety Seats

The leading cause of death in children between 1 and 4 years of age is injuries sustained in motor vehicle crashes. Car seats reduce the incidence of death in vehicle crashes by 71% for infants and 54% for toddlers.[15] The Centers for Disease Control and Prevention reports that 266 lives were saved by child restraints in 2015.[15]

Child safety seats are available in several shapes and sizes to accommodate different stages of physical development. These seats include infant carriers, booster seats, and toddler seats. Child safety seats use a combination of lap belts, shoulder belts, full-body harnesses, and harness-and-shield apparatus to protect the child during vehicle crashes. The proper child restraints vary by age (**TABLE 36-1**).

Predictable injuries likely to occur even with the appropriate use of child safety seats include blunt abdominal trauma, change-of-speed injuries from deceleration forces, and neck and spinal injury. Public education on the correct use of child safety seats is a key prevention measure. For information on transport of children in an ambulance, see BOX 36-6.

TABLE 36-1 Child Restraints by Age[a]

Birth to 2 years	Rear-facing car seat in the backseat[b]
2 to 5 years	Forward-facing car seat in the backseat
5 years and older (until seat belts fit properly[c])	Booster seat in the backseat for best protection

[a]Ages are estimates. For best accuracy, refer to the manufacturer's guidelines.

[b]The backseat provides the best protection.

[c]A seat belt fits properly when the lap belt lies across the upper thighs (not abdomen) and the shoulder belt stretches across the chest (not the neck).

Modified from: Child passenger safety. Centers for Disease Control and Prevention website. https://www.cdc.gov/features/passengersafety/index.html. Updated September 18, 2017. Accessed March 7, 2018.

Organ Injuries From Crashes

Organs can be injured as a result of movement caused by deceleration and compression forces. The paramedic must maintain a high degree of suspicion regarding injuries to organs based on the principles of kinematics. (In-depth discussions of these injuries are presented in later chapters by subject matter.)

Deceleration Injuries

When body organs are put into motion after an impact, they continue to move. They move in opposition to the structures that attach them to the body. Thus a risk exists of separation of body organs from their attachments. Injury to the vascular pedicle or mesenteric attachment can lead to brisk or exsanguinating hemorrhage.

Head Injuries

When the head strikes a stationary object, the cranium comes to an abrupt stop. However, brain tissue inside the cranium continues to move. The brain moves until it is compressed against the skull (**FIGURE 36-6**). This movement can cause brain tissue to be concussed, bruised, crushed, or lacerated. Such movement also can cause blood vessels attached to the brain and skull to be torn, producing intracranial hemorrhage. Other injuries associated with deceleration of the head include central nervous system injury, caused by stretching of the spinal cord and its attachments, and cervical fracture.

Thoracic Injuries

The aorta often is injured by severe deceleration forces. The aorta is affixed at several points. Proximally, the aorta is affixed by the aortic valve in the descending portion of the aortic arch by the ligamentum arteriosum.

BOX 36-6 Transport of Children in an Ambulance

Although no formal regulations have been established, it is recommended that child safety seats be available in emergency vehicles. In addition to practicing safe driving in all patient transports, the paramedic should observe the following recommendations for five situations identified by the National Highway Traffic Safety Administration. The goal of these recommendations is to prevent forward motion/ejection, secure the torso, and protect the head, neck, and spine of all children transported in an emergency ground ambulance:

Situation. The child is not ill or injured (ie, is accompanying an ill or injured patient).

Transport the child in a vehicle other than an emergency ground ambulance using a size-appropriate child restraint system. Consult the child restraint manufacturer's guidelines to determine optimal orientation for the child restraint depending on the age and size of the child.

Situation. The child is ill or injured, but the condition does not require continuous or intensive medical monitoring or interventions.

Transport the child in a size-appropriate child restraint system secured appropriately on the cot.

Situation. The child's condition requires continuous or intensive medical monitoring or interventions.

Transport the child in a size-appropriate child restraint system secured appropriately on the cot.

Situation. The child's condition requires spinal immobilization or lying flat.

Secure the child to a size-appropriate backboard and secure the backboard to the cot, headfirst, with a tether at the foot (if possible) to prevent forward movement. Secure the backboard to the cot with three horizontal restraints across the torso (chest, waist, and knees) and a vertical restraint across each shoulder.

Situation. The child or children require transport as part of a multiple-patient transport (eg, newborn with mother or multiple patients).

If possible, for multiple patients, transport each patient as a single patient according to the guidance shown for the previous situations. Transport in a forward-facing captain's chair in a size-appropriate child restraint system.

For the mother and newborn, transport the newborn in an approved size-appropriate child restraint system in the rear-facing captain's chair that prevents both lateral and forward movement, leaving the cot for the mother. Use a convertible seat with a forward-facing belt path. Do not use a rear-facing-only seat in the rear-facing captain's chair. An integrated child restraint system may also be used.

Note: A child passenger, especially a newborn, must never be transported in an adult's lap. Newborns should always be transported in an appropriate child restraint system.

Modified from: National Highway Traffic Safety Administration. *Working Group Best-Practice Recommendations for the Safe Transportation of Children in Emergency Ground Ambulances*. Washington, DC: US Department of Transportation/National Highway Traffic Safety Administration; 2012; NASEMSO Safe Transport of Children Ad Hoc Committee. Safe transport of children by EMS: interim guidance. National Association of EMS Officials website. https://www.nasemso.org/Committees/STC/documents/Safe-Transport-of-Children-by-EMS-InterimGuidance-08Mar2017-FINAL.pdf. Published March 8, 2017. Accessed March 7, 2018.

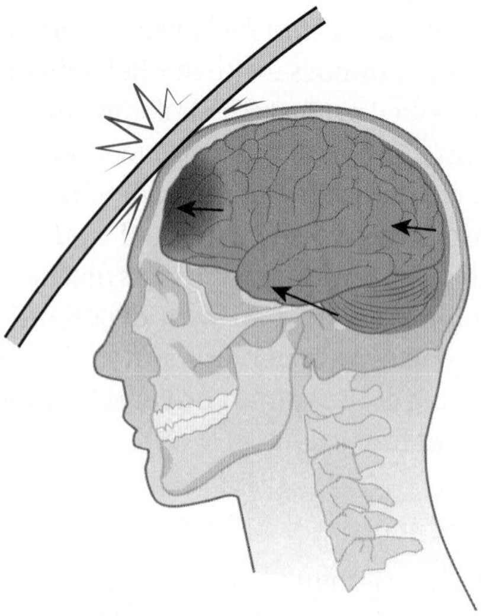

FIGURE 36-6 After cessation of forward motion of the skull, the brain continues its motion, resulting in possible contusion and intracerebral hemorrhage.

The descending aorta also is attached to the thoracic spine. As the thorax hits a stationary object, the heart and aorta continue in motion. This motion is in opposition to their attachment at the lower end of the aortic arch. The aorta usually is sheared at the level of its ligamentum arteriosum attachment (**FIGURE 36-7**). Frank rupture of the aorta leads to rapid exsanguination; however, transection and dissection through to the internal lining (intima and media of the aorta) can result in cardiac tamponade. This condition can allow patients to arrive at an emergency department and survive the injury.

Abdominal Injuries

When deceleration forces are applied to the abdomen, intra-abdominal organs and retroperitoneal structures (most commonly the kidneys) are affected. The forward motion of the kidneys can shear them away from their vascular pedicle attachments (**FIGURE 36-8**).

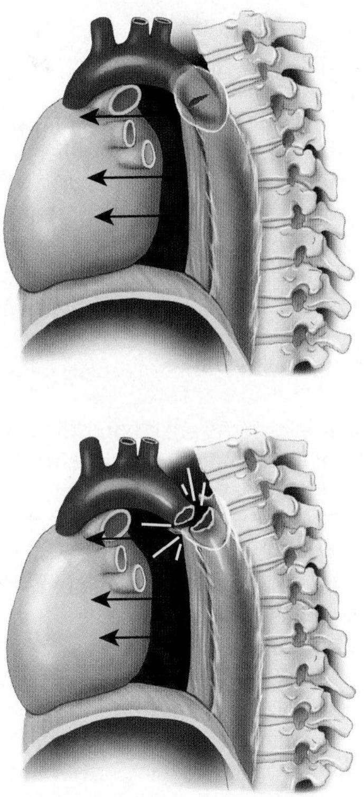

FIGURE 36-7 Shearing forces along the descending aorta move in opposition to the attachments at the lower end of the aortic arch.

Reproduced from: National Association of Emergency Medical Technicians. *PHTLS: Prehospital Trauma Life Support*. 8th ed. Burlington, MA: Jones & Bartlett Learning; 2016.

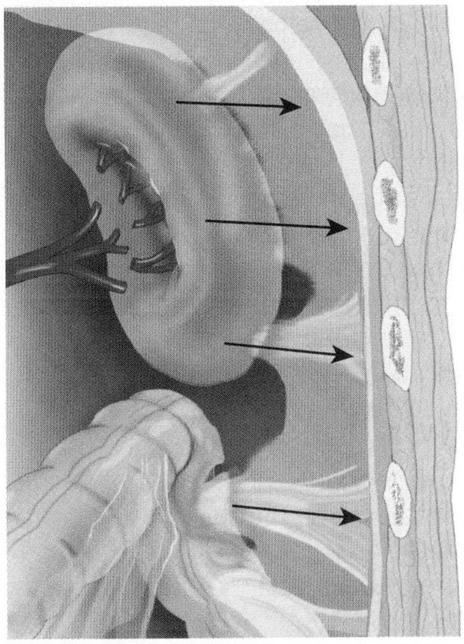

FIGURE 36-8 Forward motion of the spleen can cause separation at its midpoint from its vascular pedicle.

Reproduced from: National Association of Emergency Medical Technicians. *PHTLS: Prehospital Trauma Life Support*. 8th ed. Burlington, MA: Jones & Bartlett Learning; 2016.

The forward motion of the small and large intestines can result in mesenteric tears. The downward and forward motion of the liver can cause separation at its midpoint from its vascular and hepatic duct pedicle. The spleen is restrained by the diaphragm and abdominal wall attachments. The forward motion of the spleen can result in a tear of the splenic capsule.

Compression Injuries

Compressive forces can injure any portion of the body. This discussion is limited to injuries of the head, thorax, and abdomen.

Head Injuries

Compression injuries to the head can result in open fractures, closed fractures, and bone fragment penetration (depressed skull fracture). Associated injuries include brain contusion and lacerations of brain tissue. Compression forces to the skull also can produce hemorrhage from fractured bone, meningeal vessels, or the brain itself. If facial structures are involved in the injury, soft-tissue trauma and facial bone fractures can occur. The paramedic also should consider central nervous system injury and assume cervical fracture when evaluating injuries to the head. Compression injury to the vertebral bodies can result in compression fracture, hyperextension, and hyperflexion injury.

Thoracic Injuries

Compression injury to the thorax often involves the lungs and heart. Associated injuries to external structures include fractured ribs and sternum, which can lead to an unstable chest wall, open pneumothorax, or both.

A serious lung injury that can occur from compression forces is called the paper bag effect. This injury occurs when increased intrathoracic pressure causes the rupture of the lungs. For example, a driver of a car is threatened by an approaching vehicle. The driver notes the potential collision and instinctively takes a deep breath and holds it. This protective inhalation fills the lungs (paper bag) with air against the closed glottis and creates a closed container (**FIGURE 36-9**). As the thorax strikes the steering column, the inward motion of the chest wall causes an increase in lung pressure. This increased pressure results in alveolar rupture (as when a hand strikes the paper bag). This phenomenon is thought to be the cause of most pneumothoraces after vehicle trauma. Penetration of a fractured rib through the pleura and laceration of the lung also contribute to pneumothorax after blunt trauma to the chest.

During compression injury to the thorax, the heart can become trapped between the sternum

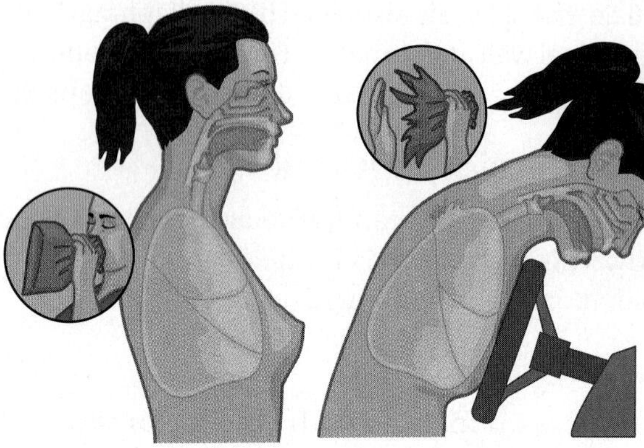

FIGURE 36-9 In a crash, the lungs are similar to an air-filled paper bag held tightly at the neck and compressed with the other hand. Thoracic compression against the closed glottis causes the lungs to pop.

and the thoracic spine. Depending on the amount of energy applied, the compression of the contents of the abdomen, and an increase in the pressure in the aorta, the aortic valve could rupture. Compression of the patient's heart between the sternum and the vertebral column can cause cardiac dysrhythmias, myocardial contusion, or atrial or ventricular rupture.

Abdominal Injuries

Compression injuries to the abdominal cavity can have serious effects. Some of these effects include solid organ rupture, vascular organ hemorrhage, and hollow organ perforation into the peritoneal cavity. Common injuries include rupture of the bladder, especially if it is full, and lacerations to the spleen, liver, and kidneys.

Just as the paper bag effect produces a pneumothorax in thoracic injury, compression of the abdominal cavity can cause increases in intra-abdominal pressure. This increase in pressure can exceed the tensile strength (resistance to lengthwise stretch) of the walls of hollow organs or the diaphragm. Predictable injuries include rupture or herniation of the diaphragm and rupture of hollow organs, such as the gallbladder, urinary bladder, duodenum, colon, stomach, and small bowel.

Other Motorized Vehicular Crashes

Injuries from other motorized vehicular crashes include those involving motorcycles, all-terrain vehicles (ATVs),

DID YOU KNOW?

Farm and Agricultural Injury

The farm as a workplace is dangerous. Farm and agricultural injuries have high morbidity and mortality. Death from injury is more common in the agricultural industry than in any other occupation, with 401 deaths occurring in 2015. Each day about 100 farm workers sustain an injury serious enough to miss work, and every 3 days a child dies in an agriculture-related incident. Motorized vehicles and other machinery that are associated with many of these injuries include the following:

- **Tractors.** Overturns are a common cause of severe injury, including traumatic brain injury, spinal cord injury, and major thoracoabdominal injuries. Deaths from tractor overturns can be prevented with rollover protection structures. These devices are often lacking or removed to provide access in low-clearance situations.
- **Power take-off (PTO).** These devices deliver energy from the tractor to run other machines. The protective housing is often removed or becomes jammed, providing a site for entanglement. Disengaging power to the PTO prior to dismounting is important in avoiding injury caused by entanglement of limb or clothing.
- **ATVs.** These vehicles are often used on farms and are a common cause of injury.

In addition to trauma caused by motorized vehicles and machinery, there are multiple other injury factors common in farm or agricultural settings. Examples include the following:

- **Animals.** Agricultural animals pose a threat because of their size and unpredictable behavior, resulting in a high incidence of injury.
- **Falls.** Farmers often work at heights without the use of protective gear.
- **Weather.** Impaired visibility, cold distraction, and equipment malfunction contribute to trauma in agricultural settings.
- **Suffocation.** Silos and pits present common risks.
- **Delayed discovery.** Farmers often work alone and at a distance from help or traffic.

Injury forces and kinematics for farm and agricultural injuries are the same as those for other injuries and injury patterns described in this chapter. In addition to patient care measures, some of the injuries will require specialized forms of rescue.

Modified from: National Children's Center for Rural and Agricultural Health and Safety. 2017 fact sheet: childhood agricultural injuries in the US. Marshfield Clinic website. https://www.marshfieldresearch.org/Media/Default/NFMC/PDFs/2017%20Child%20Ag%20Injury%20Fact%20Sheet.pdf. Updated March 2017. Accessed March 7, 2018.

motorized personal transportation devices, snowmobiles, motorboats, water bikes, jet skis, and farm machinery. This text discusses only motorcycles and ATVs because of their common recreational use and popularity. According to the National Highway Traffic Safety Administration, about 88,000 motorcycle riders and passengers are injured each year. More than 4,975 die from their injuries.[16]

Small motorized vehicles are thought to be more dangerous than other motor vehicles because they offer little protection to the rider. They offer minimum protection from the transfer of energy associated with crashes. The injuries from small motor vehicle crashes usually are more severe than are those from car crashes. As with other types of motor vehicle crash, predictable injuries depend on the type of crash that occurs.

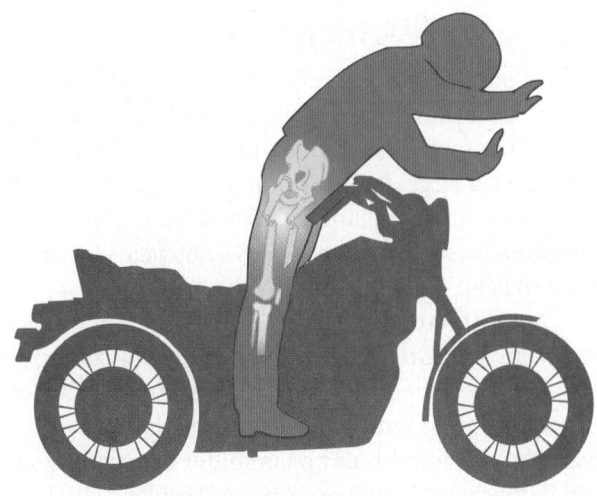

FIGURE 36-10 Head-on impact motorcycle crash.

Modified from: National Association of Emergency Medical Technicians. *PHTLS: Prehospital Trauma Life Support*. 8th ed. Burlington, MA: Jones & Bartlett Learning; 2016.

Motorcycle Crashes

Common motorcycle crashes result from impact that is head-on or at an angle. They also result from laying the motorcycle down.

Head-on Impact

The center of gravity of a motorcycle is above the front axle, forward of the rider's seat. When the motorcycle strikes an object that stops its forward motion, the rest of the bike and the rider continue forward until acted on by an outside force. Usually, the motorcycle tips forward. At that point, the rider is propelled over the handlebars. Secondary impacts with the handlebars or other objects stop the forward motion of the rider. Predictable injuries caused by these secondary impacts include head and neck trauma and compression injuries to the chest and abdomen. If the feet remain on the footrests during impact, the midshaft of the femur absorbs the rider's forward motion (**FIGURE 36-10**). This mechanism can result in bilateral fractures to the femur and lower leg. Severe perineal injuries can result if the rider's groin strikes the tank or handlebars of the motorcycle.

Angular Impact

A motorcycle may strike an object at an angle. When this occurs, the rider often is caught between the motorcycle and the second object. Predictable injuries include crush-type injuries to the patient's affected side, such as open fractures to the femur, tibia, and fibula and fracture and dislocation of the malleolus.

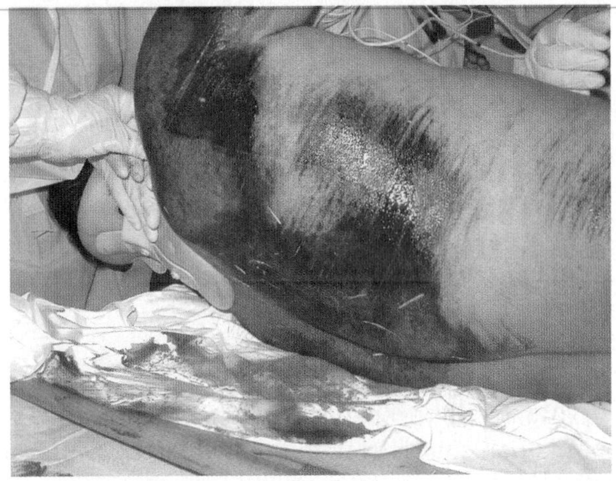

FIGURE 36-11 Road rash (abrasions).

Courtesy of Dr. Jeffrey Guy

Laying the Motorcycle Down

Professional racers and recreational riders often use the strategy of laying the motorcycle down before striking an object. (This is especially true for motorcycles not equipped with antilock braking systems.)[17] This protective maneuver separates the rider from the motorcycle and the object, allowing the rider to slide away from the bike. Predictable injuries include massive abrasions (road rash) and fractures to the affected side as the rider slides on the ground or pavement (**FIGURE 36-11**). These injuries can be severe; however, they usually are less serious than are the injuries that occur from other types of impacts.

All-Terrain Vehicle Crashes

Injuries from crashes involving ATVs are different from those seen in motorcycle crashes. ATVs have a higher center of gravity than motorcycles have. They also have a large, flat front tire that makes them difficult to steer. A specific balance different than that required for riding motorcycles or bicycles is necessary to keep the ATV from overturning.

A natural tendency is for the rider to put a foot down to support the ATV when stopping. Doing so can lead to the rear tire running over the rider's foot, catching the leg, and throwing the rider forward off the vehicle and onto his or her shoulder or crushing the rider. Predictable injuries from ATV crashes include extremity injury and fracture, clavicular fracture, and serious head and neck injuries.

Personal Protective Equipment

Protective equipment for riders of small motor vehicles includes boots, leather clothing, eye protection, and helmets. Helmets are structured to absorb the energy of an impact, thereby reducing injuries to the face, skull, and brain, and are estimated to be 37% effective in preventing fatal injuries to motorcycle operators and 41% effective in preventing injuries to their passengers.[1]

Pedestrian Injuries

In 2015, 160,000 people were injured in motor vehicle–pedestrian collisions in the United States. Of those injuries, 6,700 were fatal.[1] All collisions of this nature can cause serious injuries. They require a high degree of suspicion for multisystem trauma.

Three main mechanisms of injury (multiple impacts) exist in motor vehicle–pedestrian collisions. The first impact occurs when the bumper of the vehicle strikes the body. The second occurs as the pedestrian strikes the hood of the vehicle. The third occurs when the pedestrian strikes the ground or another object.

Predictable injuries depend on whether the pedestrian is an adult or a child. Variations in the height of the pedestrian in relation to the bumper and hood of the car affect the injury pattern. The velocity of the vehicle also is a major factor. However, even low speeds can result in serious trauma because of the mass of the vehicle and the transfer of energy. Another consideration in evaluating a motor vehicle–pedestrian collision is the possibility the patient was hit by another vehicle.

Adult Pedestrian

Most adult pedestrians who are threatened by an oncoming vehicle try to protect themselves by turning away from the vehicle. Therefore, injuries often are a result of lateral or posterior impacts. During the initial impact, the adult usually is struck by the vehicle bumper in the lower legs, which often produces lower-extremity fractures.

The second impact occurs as the pedestrian falls toward the hood of the vehicle. This impact can result in fractures to the femur, pelvis, thorax, and spine and also can produce intra-abdominal or intrathoracic injury. The head and spine can be injured if the pedestrian strikes the hood or windshield.

The third impact occurs as the pedestrian strikes the ground or is thrown against another object. This impact can result in serious damage to the hip and shoulder of the affected side as the body makes contact with the landing surface. Sudden deceleration and compression forces are associated with this impact. These forces can cause fractures, internal hemorrhage, and head and spinal injury.

Child Pedestrian

As noted, adults try to protect themselves from injury before being struck by a vehicle. However, children tend to face the oncoming vehicle; therefore, their injuries often are the result of a frontal impact. Because children are smaller than most adults, the initial impact of the vehicle occurs higher on the body, usually above the knees or pelvis. Predictable injuries from the initial impact include fractures to the femur and pelvic girdle and internal hemorrhage.

The second impact occurs as the front of the hood of the vehicle continues forward, making contact with the child's thorax. The child instantly is thrown backward, forcing the head and neck to flex forward. Depending on the position of the patient in relation to the vehicle, the child's head and neck may contact the hood of the vehicle. Predictable injuries include abdominopelvic and thoracic trauma, facial trauma, and head and neck injury.

The third impact occurs as the child is thrown downward to the ground or another landing surface.

Because of the child's smaller size and weight, the child can fall under the vehicle and be dragged for some distance. The child also can fall to the side of the vehicle and be run over by the front or rear wheels. Predictable injuries consist of those previously described and may include traumatic amputation.

Other Causes of Blunt Trauma

Other causes of blunt trauma include sports injuries, blast injuries, and vertical falls.

Sports Injuries

People of all ages take part in sports. Sports offer a range of health benefits; however, they also can produce severe injury. Sports that often are associated with injuries include contact sports, such as football, basketball, hockey, soccer, and wrestling; high-velocity sports, such as downhill skiing, water skiing, bicycling, rollerblading, and skateboarding; racquet sports; water sports, such as swimming and diving; and recreational and competitive equestrian sports.

Injuries related to sports are caused by forces of acceleration and deceleration, compression, twisting, hyperextension, and hyperflexion. The paramedic can use the general principles of kinematics to predict injuries by determining the following:

- What energy forces were transferred to the patient?
- To what part of the body was the energy transferred?
- What associated injuries should be considered as a result of the energy transfer?
- How sudden was the acceleration or deceleration?
- Was compression, twisting, hyperextension, or hyperflexion involved in the injury?

CRITICAL THINKING

Injuries related to sports often occur outside. What other considerations will you have for patient care based on the environment?

If the patient used protective equipment, the paramedic should evaluate it. The condition of the equipment may help the paramedic determine the MOI. For example, the condition and structural stability of a helmet can provide clues concerning the amount of energy transferred to the patient during the injury. Other examples include broken skis, broken hockey sticks, and structural deformities of bicycles.

Blast Injuries

Blast injury is damage that a patient sustains through exposure to a pressure field that is produced by an explosion of volatile substances. Explosions of this nature mainly have been a wartime concern. However, in recent years the number of blast injuries has increased, largely as a result of homemade bombs used in social protests and terrorist activities. Other causes of blast injury include explosions relating to car batteries, industrial use of volatile substances, chemical reactions in clandestine drug laboratories, mining operations, and transportation incidents or crashes involving hazardous materials.

CRITICAL THINKING

In all incidents related to blast injury, what is your first consideration on the scene?

Blasts release large amounts of energy. This energy is in the form of pressure and heat. If this release of energy is confined in a casing (eg, a bomb), the pressure ruptures the casing and ejects fragments of the housing at a high velocity. The remaining energy is transmitted to the surrounding environment. This energy can severely injure bystanders. Blast injuries are classified as primary, secondary, tertiary, and quaternary (**FIGURE 36-12**).[18]

Primary Blast Injuries

Primary blast (blast wave) injuries result from sudden changes in environmental pressure from a high-order detonation. These injuries usually occur in gas-containing organs. The most severe damage occurs when poorly supported tissue is displaced beyond its elastic limit. The organs and tissues most vulnerable to primary blast injury are the ears, lungs, central nervous system, eyes, and gastrointestinal tract. Predictable damage to these areas includes hearing loss, blast lung injury (BLI) (**BOX 36-7**), pulmonary hemorrhage, concussion, globe rupture, abdominal hemorrhage, and bowel perforation. In closed spaces, because of blast reflection, people farther from the

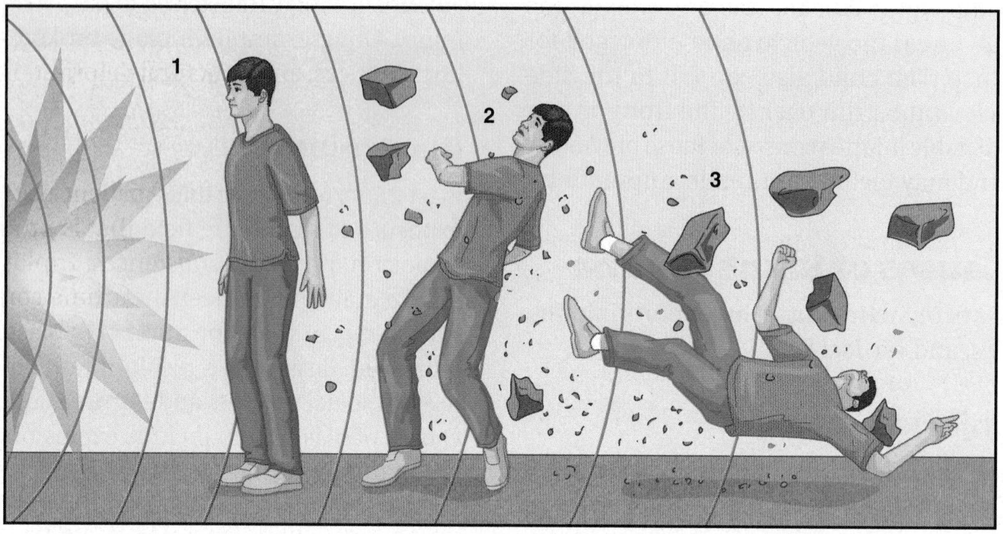

FIGURE 36-12 Three phases of injury occur during a blast. First, the pressure wave strikes the patient. Second, flying debris can produce injury. In the third phase, the patient is thrown and injured by the impact with the ground or other objects.

BOX 36-7 Blast Lung Injury: What Clinicians Need to Know

BLI is caused by the blast wave from high-explosive detonations on the body. BLI is a major cause of death and disability for blast victims. The force of the blast wave causes injury and edema of the lung. This results in ventilation/perfusion mismatch. Patients with BLI have respiratory difficulty and hypoxia, in some cases without obvious external injury to the chest.

Despite the frequency of bombings related to international terrorism, it is unusual for paramedics in the United States to have experience treating patients with these injuries. Optimal prehospital care involves an understanding of the assessment findings and management of BLIs.

Assessment Findings

- Symptoms may include dyspnea, hemoptysis, cough, and chest pain.
- Signs may include tachypnea, hypoxia, cyanosis, apnea, wheezing, decreased breath sounds, and hemodynamic instability.
- Other injuries may include bronchopleural fistula, air emboli, and hemothoraces or pneumothoraces.

Management

- Administer oxygen sufficient to prevent hypoxemia.
- Intubate the airway if there is impending airway compromise, swelling, or massive hemoptysis.
- Monitor breath sounds to detect a hemothorax or pneumothorax.
- Intubation is indicated if the patient develops respiratory failure. Monitor intubated patients for pneumothorax or air embolism related to excessive airway pressure.
- If air embolism is suspected, medical direction may recommend transport to a hyperbaric chamber.

Modified from: Blast injuries: fact sheets for professionals. Centers for Disease Control and Prevention website. https://stacks.cdc.gov/view/cdc/21571. Published March 1, 2012. Accessed May 30, 2018.

explosion may be injured as severely as those close to the explosion. Primary blast injury will only be seen when a detonation occurs resulting from a high-order explosive.

Secondary Blast Injuries

Secondary blast injuries usually result when bystanders are struck by flying debris, such as glass, metal, or falling mortar. Obvious injuries are lacerations and fractures, but flying debris also can cause high-velocity missile-type injuries. This type of injury can result if nails, screws, or casing fragments are part of the debris.

Tertiary Blast Injuries

Tertiary blast injuries occur when people are propelled through space by an explosion or blast wind and strike a stationary object. These injuries are similar to those from vertical falls. They also are similar to those from ejections from cars or small motor vehicles. In most cases, the sudden deceleration from the impact causes more damage than the acceleration through space because the deceleration is more sudden. Injuries from these forces include damage to the abdominal viscera, central nervous system, and musculoskeletal system.

Quaternary Blast Injuries

Quaternary blast injuries are all explosion-related injuries, illnesses, or diseases that are not caused by primary, secondary, or tertiary mechanisms. This classification includes exacerbation or complications of existing conditions. Quaternary blast injuries can affect any body part. Types of injuries include burns (inhalation injury, flash, partial-thickness, and full-thickness burns); radiation injuries; crush injuries; closed and open brain injuries; asthma, chronic obstructive pulmonary disease, or other breathing problems from dust, smoke, or toxic gases (further described in Chapter 57, *Bioterrorism and Weapons of Mass Destruction*); angina; hyperglycemia; and hypertension.

Vertical Falls

Falls accounted for 33,381 deaths in 2015 and were the third-leading cause of accidental death in the United States.[1] One out of five falls causes a serious injury (eg, a fracture).[19] In predicting injuries associated with falls, the paramedic should evaluate three things: the distance fallen, the body position of the patient on impact, and the type of landing surface struck. Injuries associated with vertical falls are a result of deceleration and compression. One in four people 65 years of age or older falls annually.[20]

Falls of short distance are rarely associated with fatal injury. However, falls from distances greater than three times the person's height (15–20 feet [5–6 m]) are more likely to be associated with severe injuries.[21] As a point of reference for these distances, the roof of a one-story house is about 15 feet (5 m) from the ground, and the roof of a two-story house is about 30 feet (9 m) from the ground.

CRITICAL THINKING

What patients may be susceptible to serious injury from a fall that is from a low level?

Adults who have fallen more than 15 feet (5 m) usually land on their feet. A predictable injury from this vertical fall is bilateral calcaneus fractures. As the energy dissipates from the initial impact, the head, torso, and pelvis push downward. The body is forced into flexion. When this type of impact occurs, hip dislocations and compression fractures of the spinal column in the thoracic and lumbar areas are seen. About 10% of patients with calcaneal fracture have associated spinal fractures.[22] If the patient leans forward or tries to break the fall with outstretched hands, distal radius fractures to the wrists (frequently clinically evident by the so-called silver fork deformity) are possible.

DID YOU KNOW?

A distal radius fracture almost always occurs about 1 inch (2.5 cm) from the end of the bone. The break can occur in many different ways, however. One of the most common distal radius fractures is a Colles fracture, in which the broken fragment of the radius tilts upward. This fracture was first described in 1814 by an Irish surgeon and anatomist, Abraham Colles—hence the name "Colles" fracture.

Modified from: Distal radius fractures (broken wrist). American Academy of Orthopaedic Surgeons OrthoInfo website. https://orthoinfo.aaos.org/en/diseases--conditions/distal-radius-fractures-broken-wrist/. Accessed March 21, 2018.

If the distance fallen is less than 15 feet (5 m), most adults land in the position in which they fell. For example, an adult who falls headfirst strikes the landing surface with the head, arms, or both. Predictable injuries depend on the body part that strikes the landing surface and the route of transfer of energy through the body. The paramedic should suspect internal injuries if the trunk of the body is the initial impact area. The ability of the landing surface to absorb energy influences the severity of injury. For example, less damage is expected from a fall on a soft, grassy surface than from a fall on asphalt or concrete.

Children tend to fall headfirst, regardless of distance fallen or body position during the fall. They fall headfirst because their heads are proportionally larger and heavier. For this reason, children who experience a vertical fall usually sustain head injuries. Older adult patients sustain a high number of low-distance falls, often resulting in hip fracture.

Penetrating Trauma

Penetrating trauma is an injury that occurs when an object pierces the skin and enters a tissue of the body, creating an open wound. All penetrating objects, regardless of velocity, cause tissue disruption. This damage occurs as a result of two types of forces: crushing and stretching. The character of the penetrating object, its speed of penetration, and the type of body tissue it passes through or into determine which of the two mechanisms of injury predominates.

Cavitation

Cavitation is an opening produced by a force that pushes body tissues laterally away from the tract of a projectile. The amount of cavitation produced by a projectile is related directly to the density of tissue it strikes. Cavitation also is related directly to the ability of the body tissue to return to its original shape and position. For example, consider a person who receives a high-velocity strike to the abdomen. This person experiences abdominal cavitation at the moment of impact; however, because of the lower density of the abdominal musculature, the cavitation is temporary. (Cavitation lasts only a few microseconds.) Cavitation is temporary even in the presence of severe intra-abdominal injury (**FIGURE 36-13**).

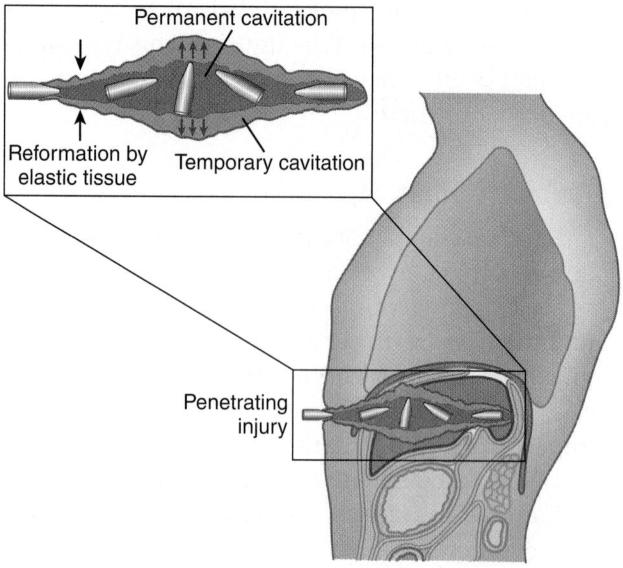

FIGURE 36-13 Permanent and temporary cavitation.

Permanent cavities are produced by penetrating injuries in which the force of the projectile exceeds the tensile strength of the tissue. Tissues with high water density (eg, liver, spleen, muscle) or solid density (eg, bone) are more prone to permanent cavitation. Certain injuries (eg, a stab wound to the abdomen) can produce cavitation as tissues are displaced in frontal and lateral directions.

Ballistics

The energy created and dissipated by the object into surrounding tissues determines the effect of a projectile on the body. The paramedic should consider the principles of kinematics when dealing with injuries from penetrating trauma. To review, kinetic energy equals half the mass of an object multiplied by the square of its velocity. With reference to ballistic trauma, doubling the mass doubles the energy. However, doubling the velocity quadruples the energy; therefore a small-caliber bullet traveling at a high speed can produce more serious injury than a large-caliber bullet traveling at a lower speed. This is the case unless the large-caliber bullet strikes a major vessel or organ.

Damage and Energy Levels of Projectiles

Injuries caused by penetrating trauma result from three energy levels: low, medium, and high. This discussion considers hand-driven weapons as low-energy projectiles and bullets as medium- and high-energy projectiles.

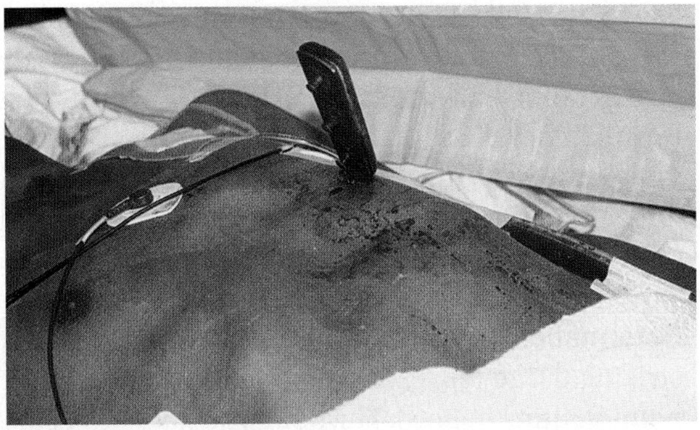

FIGURE 36-14 Stab wound in which a knife penetrated the spleen and pancreas and lacerated the left lung and hemi-diaphragm.

Low-energy projectiles such as knives, needles, and ice picks cause tissue damage by their sharp, cutting edges (**FIGURE 36-14**). The amount of tissue crushed in these injuries usually is minimal because the amount of force applied in the wounding process is small. The more blunt the penetrating object, the more force that must be applied to cause penetration. The more force needed to cause penetration, the more tissue crushed. The damage of tissue from low-energy injuries usually is limited to the pathway of the projectile.

When evaluating a patient with a stab wound, the paramedic should attempt to identify the weapon used to cause the wound. The paramedic also should consider the possibility of multiple wounds, embedded weapons, hidden yet extensive internal damage to organs of the thorax and abdomen, and penetration of multiple body cavities. A high degree of suspicion of serious injury is also indicated for stab wounds to areas of the back and flank. These wounds may be associated with penetrating injuries to hollow organs and injuries to retroperitoneal organs, specifically the kidneys. Penetrating injuries of the thorax can involve the abdomen, just as abdominal injuries can involve the thorax.

CRITICAL THINKING

Your patient has a stab wound in the midaxillary line, lateral to the left nipple. What organs may be affected by this mechanism? What else would you like to know about this injury?

Firearms can be labeled as medium- and high-energy weapons. Medium-energy weapons include handguns and some rifles with a muzzle velocity of 1,000 feet per second (304 m/s). The injury tract (permanent cavity) produced by medium-energy weapons usually is two to three times the diameter of the projectile and is influenced by yaw and fragmentation (described later). Firearms are designed to shoot ammunition of varying velocities and energies. In general, handguns fire ammunition of lower velocities while rifles generally are designed to fire projectiles of much higher velocity with resultant higher energies. These weapons have a muzzle velocity of more than 2,000 feet per second (610 m/s). As with medium-energy injuries, the injury tract produced by high-energy weapons usually is two to three times the diameter of the projectile.[23]

Implications of Soft Body Armor

Some EMS agencies have adopted soft body armor policies. The armor offers extra protection for paramedics against blunt and penetrating trauma. Most agencies follow US Department of Justice guidelines to determine the type of body armor protection for the types of weapons most commonly found in their community. There are six basic classification types of body armor protection, but none offers complete protection.[24] Authorities generally recommend a type III or higher protection level for EMS personnel. These soft vests protect against low-velocity and some medium-velocity and high-velocity weapons. Multiprotection vests are available (usually used by specialty teams, such as SWAT teams), and are rated for edged weapons and/or spiked weapons (see Chapter 55, *Crime Scene Awareness*).

Wounding Forces of Medium- and High-Energy Projectiles

A firearm cartridge is composed of a bullet made of metal, gunpowder to propel the bullet, a primer to explode and ignite the gunpowder, and a cartridge case that surrounds these components. When the trigger is pulled, the metal hammer strikes the firing pin, which ignites the primer. The gunpowder ignites and forces the bullet to exit the cartridge case.

The MOI from firearms is related to the energy created and dissipated by the bullet into the surrounding tissues. When a firearm is discharged, several events affect this dissipation of energy and ultimately the wounding forces of the missile:[25]

1. As the missile travels through air, it experiences wind resistance, or drag. The greater the drag, the greater the slowing effect on the missile. Therefore a firearm discharged at close range usually produces a more severe injury than the same firearm discharged at a greater distance.
2. As the missile travels through air, a sonic pressure wave spreads out behind the missile. Because the speed of sound in tissue is about four times the speed of sound in air, the sonic pressure wave jumps ahead and precedes the missile through the tissue. This pressure wave has the potential to displace tissue and may sometimes stretch it dramatically, but is not thought to be responsible for permanent injury.[26]
3. The localized crush of tissue in the path of the missile and the momentary stretch of the surrounding tissue cause tissue disruption.

When a projectile strikes a body, tissue stretches at the point of impact to allow entry of the penetrating object (temporary cavitation). The energy of the projectile exceeds the tensile strength of the tissue. Thus tissue crush occurs, forcing surrounding tissues outward from the path of the projectile (permanent cavitation). The differences in wounds caused by projectiles vary with the amount and location of crushed and stretched tissue (**FIGURE 36-15**). The wounding forces of a missile depend on the projectile mass, deformation, fragmentation, type of tissue struck, striking velocity, and range.[27]

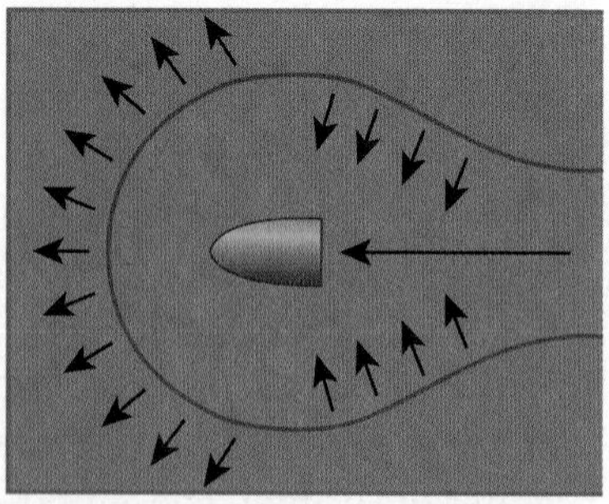

FIGURE 36-15 Bullet passing through tissue. Outward stretching of the permanent cavity as the tissue particles move away from the penetrating missile causes the temporary cavity.

Projectile Mass. Tissue crush is limited by the physical size or profile of the projectile. If the missile strikes point-first, the crushed area is no larger than the diameter of the bullet. If the missile is tilted as it strikes the body, the amount of crushed tissue is no larger than the length and longitudinal cross section of the bullet.

Deformation. Some firearm missiles deform when striking tissue (eg, expanding hollow-point or soft-point hunting bullets). The points of these projectiles typically flatten on impact. The diameter of the bullet expands, creating a larger area of crushed tissue. Military use of these bullets in war is forbidden.

Fragmentation. Each piece of missile crushes its own path through tissue, causing extensive tissue damage. These fragments produce a larger frontal area than does a single, solid bullet and disperse energy into the surrounding tissues rapidly. Tissues weaken from the multiple fragment tracts and increase the subsequent stretch of the temporary cavity. The higher the velocity, the more likely the bullet is to fragment. If a bullet fragments, there may be no exit wound.

Type of Tissue Struck. Tissue disruption varies greatly with tissue type. For example, elastic tissues such as the bowel wall, lung, and muscle tolerate stretch much better than do nonelastic organs such as the liver.

Striking Velocity. The velocity of a missile determines the extent of cavitation and tissue damage. Low-velocity missiles localize injury to a small radius from the center of the injury tract. These missiles have little disruptive effect, pushing the tissue aside. High-velocity missiles produce more serious injuries because they lose more energy to the tissues and produce more cavitation.

Bullet yaw, or tumble, in tissue also contributes to cavitation and tissue damage. The center of gravity of a wedge-shaped bullet is nearer to the base than to the nose. As the missile strikes body tissue, it slows rapidly. Momentum carries the base of the bullet forward; the center of gravity becomes the leading part of the missile. This forward rotation around the center of mass causes an end-over-end motion. This movement in turn produces more energy exchange and more tissue damage.

Range. The distance of the weapon from the target is a key factor in the severity of ballistic trauma. Air resistance (drag) slows the missile significantly; therefore increasing the distance of the projectile from the target decreases the velocity at the time of impact.

If the firearm is discharged at close range (within 3 feet [1 m]), cavitation can occur from the combustion of powder and the forceful expansion of gases. The gas and powder can enter the body cavity and cause internal explosion of tissue. This is common with shotgun wounds. Internal explosion of tissue is less common with handguns because they produce a small amount of gas and create a small entrance wound. The expansion of only gas can cause extensive tissue destruction, especially in an enclosed area (eg, the skull).

> NOTE
>
> Blanks are ammunition without projectiles. The explosion of gas explains how blanks can cause injury or death when fired at short range.

Shotgun Wounds

Shotguns are short-range, low-velocity weapons that fire multiple pellets. These pellets are encased in a larger shell. Each pellet (there may be 9 to 400 or more, depending on pellet size and gauge of gun) is considered a missile capable of producing tissue damage. Each shell contains pellets, gunpowder, and a plastic or paper wad that separates the pellets from the gunpowder. This wad of unsterile material increases the potential for infection in shotgun wounds.

The energy transferred to body tissue and the tissue damage that results depend on several factors: gauge of the gun, size of the pellets, powder charge, and distance from the injured person. For example, a 12-gauge, full-choke shotgun with number 6 shot (275 pellets) concentrates 95% of the pellets into a 7-inch (18-cm) circle at 10 yards. At close range, a shotgun injury can create extensive tissue damage similar to that from a high-velocity missile weapon.

Entrance and Exit Wounds

The presence of entrance and exit wounds is affected by several factors, including range, barrel length, caliber, powder, and weapon (**FIGURE 36-16**). In general, an entrance wound in soft tissue is round or oval and may be surrounded by an abrasion rim or collar. If the firearm is discharged at intermediate range, tattooing may be present (**BOX 36-8**).

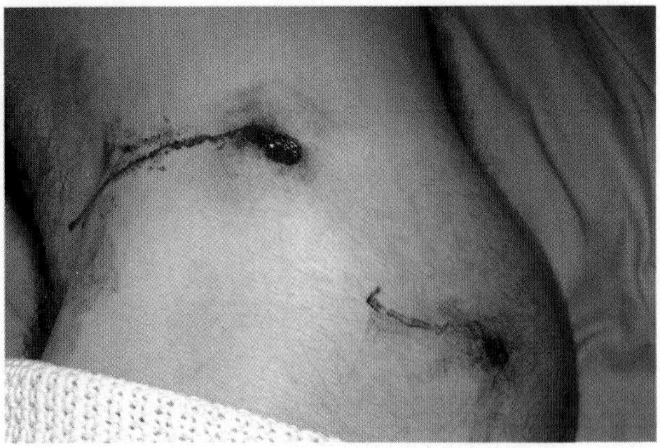

FIGURE 36-16 The powder marks show that this .22-caliber bullet wound was inflicted at close range.

Exit wounds, if present, may be larger than entrance wounds because of the cavitational wave that occurs as the bullet passes through the tissues. As the bullet exits the body, the skin can explode, resulting in ragged and torn tissue.

> CRITICAL THINKING
>
> You locate an entrance wound but no exit wound on a patient who was shot. Does this mean that the injury is not serious?

If the muzzle is in direct contact with the skin at the time of firearm discharge, expanding gases can enter the tissue. These gases can produce crepitus

> NOTE
>
> Determining entrance and exit wounds cannot be done solely by visual inspection, unless there is gunpowder speckling or barrel rim impression. The wound generally requires pathologic microscopic evaluation. The paramedic should describe and document the appearance of all wounds in detail but should refrain from commenting or speculating on which wound is the entry or exit wound. Such speculation can result in the paramedic being subpoenaed to testify in court in an area that is beyond the scope of paramedic practice.

BOX 36-8 Forensic Considerations in Managing Gunshot Wounds

Lifesaving procedures always take precedence over forensic considerations; however, the paramedic should not touch or move weapons or other environmental clues unless it is absolutely necessary for patient care. Other forensic considerations follow:

- Document the exact condition of the patient and wound appearance on arrival at the scene. This description should include the environment of the patient and the body position in relation to objects and doorways.
- Disturb the scene as little as possible.
- If possible, cut or tear clothing along a seam to avoid altering tears made by a penetrating object.
- Avoid cutting through a bullet hole in the clothing.
- Do not shake clothing.
- Keep all clothing in a paper bag rather than a plastic bag, which may alter evidence. Do not give clothing to the injured person's family members.
- Save any avulsed tissue for forensic pathologic examination.
- If the bullet is retrieved, place it in a padded container to prevent marring, and secure the evidence until it is delivered to the authorities (obtain a receipt).

Modified from: National Highway Traffic Safety Administration. *The National EMS Education Standards*. Washington, DC: US Department of Transportation/National Highway Traffic Safety Administration; 2009.

and thermal injury at the entrance site and along the injury tract.

Special Considerations for Specific Injuries

Locating ballistic injuries requires a thorough physical examination of the patient because the resulting trauma from high- and medium-velocity missiles is unpredictable. The impact of any projectile is crucial in determining the type and severity of injury. Fractions of an inch can make a significant difference in the amount of trauma the patient suffers. These differences often are impossible to distinguish in the field.

Head Injuries. Gunshot wounds to the head typically are devastating because of the direct destruction of brain tissue and subsequent swelling. Patients with head wounds often sustain severe face injuries as well. These injuries can result in major blood loss, difficulty in maintaining airway control, and spinal instability.

As a medium-energy projectile penetrates the skull, the energy is absorbed within the closed space of the cranium. The force of the injury compresses brain tissue against the cranial cavity, often fracturing orbital plates and separating the dura from the bone. Depending on the qualities of the missile, the bullet may not have enough force to exit the skull after penetration, as occurs with .22- and .25-caliber handguns. In these injuries, the bullet follows the curvature of the interior of the skull. As it follows this curvature, it produces significant damage.

High-velocity wounds to the skull produce massive destruction. Pieces of the skull and brain typically are destroyed. At close range, high-velocity wounds result in part from the large quantities of gas produced by combustion of the propellant. If the weapon is held in contact with the head, the gas follows the bullet into the cranial cavity, producing an explosive effect.

Thoracic Injuries. Gunshot wounds to the thorax can result in severe injury to the pulmonary and vascular systems. If the lungs are penetrated by a missile, the pleura and pulmonary parenchyma (the tissue of an organ, as distinguished from supporting and connective tissue) are likely to be disrupted, producing a pneumothorax. On occasion, the pulmonary defect allows air that cannot be expelled to continue to flow into the thoracic cavity. The subsequent increase in pressure eventually can cause collapse of the lung and a shift in the mediastinum to the unaffected side (tension pneumothorax).

Vascular trauma from penetrating injuries can result in massive internal and external hemorrhage. For example, if the pulmonary artery or vein, venae cavae, or aorta is injured, the patient can bleed to death within minutes. Other vascular injuries from penetrating trauma to the thorax can result in hemothorax and, if the heart is involved, myocardial rupture or pericardial tamponade.

Penetrating injury can cause thoracic trauma in the absence of visible chest wounds. For example, a bullet can enter the abdomen and travel upward through the diaphragm and into the thorax. The paramedic should suspect abdominal injury in all people with gunshot wounds to the chest and suspect chest trauma in all people with gunshot wounds to the abdomen.

Abdominal Injuries. Gunshot wounds to the abdomen usually require surgery to determine the extent of injury. Penetrating trauma can affect multiple organ systems, causing damage to air-filled and solid organs, vascular injury, trauma to the vertebral column, and spinal cord injury. The paramedic should assume a serious injury when managing people with penetrating abdominal trauma, even if a patient appears to be stable.

Extremity Injuries. At times, gunshot wounds to the extremities are life threatening. Sometimes such wounds can result in lifelong disability. Special considerations with these injuries include vascular injury with bleeding into soft tissues and damage to nerves, muscles, and bones. Nerve injury and nerve laceration can be quite serious, and can result in long-term functional morbidity.[28] The paramedic should evaluate any extremity that has sustained penetrating trauma for bone injury, motor and sensory integrity, and the presence of adequate blood flow (eg, pulses and capillary refill).

Vessels can be injured by being struck by the bullet or by temporary cavitation. Either mechanism can damage the lining of the blood vessel, producing hemorrhage or thrombosis. Penetrating trauma can damage muscle tissue by stretching it as the muscle expands away from the path of the missile. Stretching that exceeds the tensile strength of the muscle produces hemorrhage.

Bone can be deformed and fragmented directly if struck by a penetrating object, or indirectly from the pressure created by the sonic wave of the temporary cavity.[29] If this occurs, the transfer of energy causes pieces of bone to act as secondary missiles, crushing their way through surrounding tissue.

Trauma Assessment

Assessment and management of the trauma patient are presented in depth throughout this textbook by subject matter. For most injury scenes, there are nine major components of assessment for trauma patients. The order of assessment is as follows:[2]

1. Standard precautions
2. Scene size-up
3. General impression
4. MOI
5. Primary survey
6. Baseline vital signs
7. Patient history and history of the event
8. Secondary assessment
9. Reassessment

Assessment Strategies Using MOI

MOI can be used to guide assessment for trauma patients.[2] MOI can be categorized as significant or nonsignificant. Examples of significant and nonsignificant MOIs are provided in BOX 36-9.

Using MOI as a guide for the potential for severe injury allows the paramedic to make decisions about on-scene assessment and care. For example, if the MOI is significant, the patient may be in serious or critical condition. These patients need to be rapidly assessed, stabilized if possible, and quickly transported

BOX 36-9 Mechanism of Injury

Significant MOI–Adult (including injuries to multiple body systems, but not limited to)

- Vehicle crashes with intrusion into the driver/passenger compartments
- Falls from heights >20 feet (6 m)
- Motor vehicle–pedestrian collisions
- Motorcycle crashes >20 mph (32 km/h)
- Death of an occupant in the same vehicle
- Ejection
- Vehicle telemetry system indicates high risk of injury
- Intrusion >12 inches (30 cm) near occupant; intrusion >18 inches (46 cm) anywhere

Significant MOI–Child (including, but not limited to)

- Falls >10 feet (3 m) without loss of consciousness
- Falls <10 feet (3 m) with loss of consciousness
- Bicycle crash
- Medium to high-speed vehicle crash (<25 mph [40 km/h])

Nonsignificant MOI–All Ages (including isolated trauma to a body part, but not limited to)

- Falls without loss of consciousness

to an appropriate facility for definitive care. Scene time should be limited to that required for control of exsanguinating hemorrhage, airway, breathing, and circulatory support, and spinal immobilization.

> NOTE
>
> MOI must be reevaluated during the patient care encounter. For example, the paramedic may initially find the patient to have a nonsignificant MOI. However, findings in the secondary assessment might indicate a more serious injury requiring rapid assessment and transport.

By comparison, on-scene assessment and care for patients with nonsignificant MOI can be modified as needed. After completing the primary survey, it may be appropriate to perform a thorough secondary assessment while at the scene. This assessment is focused on the patient's chief complaint or on findings in the initial assessment. Then the patient is transported for definitive care.

> NOTE
>
> In some cases, even a low-impact MOI can cause injury. For example, a motor vehicle crash in which an infant is improperly restrained in the front seat can result in serious injury even at low speed. A low-speed crash in which the airbag deploys could also produce serious injury. Every patient requires careful evaluation.

Role of Documentation in Trauma

As described in Chapter 4, *Documentation*, findings at the scene and the provision of patient care should be well documented on the patient care report. A thorough written record of the EMS response will help paint a picture or recreate the injury event for others who will be involved in the patient's care. A complete report is essential and will be referred to by medical facility personnel. Documentation should include notations on an anatomic drawing for the location of wounds. It also should include a description of the scene and history of the event.

Summary

- Unintentional injury is the leading cause of death among people 1 to 44 years of age and is the fifth-leading cause of death among all Americans.
- Trauma care is divided into three phases: preevent, event, and postevent.
- Components of the trauma system include injury prevention, prehospital care, emergency department care, interfacility transport (if needed), definitive care, trauma critical care, rehabilitation, data collection, and trauma registry.
- A trauma center is a specialized medical facility distinguished by the immediate availability of specialized personnel, equipment, and services to treat the most severe and critical injuries. There are five levels of trauma centers recognized by the American College of Surgeons, I through V.
- Transport decisions for trauma patients should be made based on structured triage guidelines.
- Injuries are caused by a transfer of energy from some external source to the human body. The extent of injury is determined by the type and amount of energy applied, by how quickly it is applied, and by the part of the body to which the energy is applied.
- Four laws of physics describe energy and forces that produce injury: Newton's first law of motion, the conservation of energy law, Newton's second law of motion, and the formula for kinetic energy.
- Kinematics is the process of predicting injuries based on mechanism of injury, forces involved, anatomy, and energy.
- Blunt trauma is an injury produced by the wounding forces of compression and change of speed, which can disrupt tissues.
- Forces that cause blunt trauma can result from a variety of impacts. A vehicle crash involves three separate impacts as the energy is transferred. In the first impact, the vehicle strikes an object. In the second, the occupant collides with the inside of the vehicle. In the third, the internal organs collide inside the body.
- Four restraining systems are available in the United States: lap belts, diagonal shoulder straps, airbags, and child safety seats. All of these restraints significantly reduce injuries. If they are used inappropriately, however, these protective devices can produce injuries.
- Organ injuries can result from sudden movement caused by deceleration and compression forces. The paramedic must maintain a high degree of suspicion regarding injuries to organs based on the principles of kinematics.
- Compression forces can injure any portion of the body. Injuries to the head can result in open fractures, closed fractures, and bone fragment penetration; injuries to the thorax often involve the lungs and heart; and injuries to the abdominal cavity can result in organ rupture, vascular

organ hemorrhage, and hollow organ perforation into the peritoneal cavity.

- Small motorized vehicles such as motorcycles, all-terrain vehicles, motorized personal transportation devices, snowmobiles, motorboats, water bikes, jet skis, and farm machinery are considered to be more dangerous than other motor vehicles. They are more dangerous because they offer little protection to the rider and offer minimal protection from the transfer of energy associated with crashes.
- All motor vehicle–pedestrian collisions can produce serious injuries. They require a high degree of suspicion for multisystem trauma.
- Sports provide a variety of health benefits; however, they also can produce severe injury. Sports injuries are related to acceleration and deceleration, compression, twisting, hyperextension, and hyperflexion mechanisms of injury.
- Blast injury is damage produced by an explosion of volatile substances. Blasts release large amounts of energy in the form of pressure and heat. Blast injuries are classified as primary, secondary, tertiary, and quaternary.
- Falls from distances greater than three times the person's height (15–20 feet [5–6 m]) are associated with an increased incidence of severe injuries. In predicting injuries associated with falls, the paramedic should evaluate three things: the distance fallen, the body position of the patient on impact, and the type of landing surface struck.
- All penetrating objects, regardless of velocity, cause tissue disruption. The character of the penetrating object, its speed of penetration, and the type of body tissue it passes through or into determine whether crushing or stretching forces will cause injury.
- For most injury scenes, there are nine major components of assessment for trauma patients. The order of assessment is standard precautions, scene size-up, general impression, mechanism of injury, primary survey, baseline vital signs, patient history and history of the event, secondary assessment, reassessment.
- Findings at the scene and the provision of patient care should be well documented on the patient care report. A thorough written record of the EMS response will help paint a picture or recreate the injury event for others who will be involved in the patient's care.

References

1. National Safety Council. *Injury Facts: 2017 Edition*. Itasca, IL: National Safety Council; 2017.
2. National Highway Traffic Safety Administration. *The National EMS Education Standards*. Washington, DC: US Department of Transportation/National Highway Traffic Safety Administration; 2009.
3. National Association of Emergency Medical Technicians. *PHTLS: Prehospital Life Support*. 8th ed. Burlington, MA: Jones and Bartlett Learning; 2016.
4. National Highway Traffic Safety Administration. *Trauma System Agenda for the Future*. Washington, DC: National Highway Traffic Safety Administration; 2002.
5. The Committee on Trauma. Part 4: America's incomplete trauma system. American College of Surgeons website. https://www.facs.org/quality-programs/trauma/trauma-series/part-iv. Accessed March 8, 2018.
6. Mehrotra A, Sklar DP, Tayal VS, Kocher KE, Handel DA, Myles RR. Important historical efforts at emergency department categorization in the United States and implications for regionalization. *Acad Emerg Med.* 2010;17:e154-e160.
7. Trauma center levels explained. American Trauma Society website. http://www.amtrauma.org/?page=traumalevels. Accessed March 8, 2018.
8. Sasser SM, Hunt RC, Faul M, et al. Guidelines for field triage of injured patients: recommendations of the National Expert Panel on Field Triage, 2011. *MMWR Recomm Rep.* 2012;61(RR-1):1-20.
9. Lee E, Wu J, Kang T, Craig M. Estimate of mortality reduction with implementation of advanced automatic collision notification. *Traffic Inj Prev.* 2017;18(suppl 1):S24-S30.
10. Shaw JJ, Psoinos CM, Santry HP. It's all about location, location, location: a new perspective on trauma transport. *Ann Surg.* 2016;263(2):413-418.
11. Ingalls N, Zonies D, Bailey JA, et al. A review of the first 10 years of critical care aeromedical transport during Operation Iraqi Freedom and Operation Enduring Freedom: the importance of evacuation timing. *JAMA Surg.* 2014;149(8):807-813.
12. New Hampshire. Governors Highway Safety Association website. http://www.ghsa.org/state-laws/states/new%20hampshire. Accessed March 8, 2018.
13. Centers for Disease Control and Prevention, National Center for Injury Prevention and Control, Division of Unintentional Injury Prevention. Policy impact: seat belts. Centers for Disease Control and Prevention website. https://www.cdc.gov/motorvehiclesafety/seatbeltbrief/index.html. Updated January 21, 2014. Accessed March 8, 2018.
14. Air bags. National Highway Traffic Safety Association website. https://www.nhtsa.gov/equipment/air-bags. Accessed March 8, 2018.
15. Child passenger safety. Centers for Disease Control and Prevention website. https://www.cdc.gov/features/passengersafety/index.html. Updated September 18, 2017. Accessed March 8, 2018.
16. National Highway Traffic Safety Association, National Center for Statistics and Analysis. *Traffic Safety Facts: 2015 Data Motorcycles*. Washington, DC: US Department of Transportation/National Highway Traffic Safety Association; 2017:DOT HS 812 353.
17. Rizzi M, Strandroth J, Holst J, Tingvall C. Does the improved stability offered by motorcycle antilock brakes (ABS) make sliding crashes less common? In-depth analysis of fatal crashes involving motorcycles fitted with ABS. *Traffic Inj Prev.* 2016;17(6):625-632.
18. Explosions and blast injuries: a primer for clinicians. Centers for Disease Control and Prevention website. https://www.cdc.gov/masstrauma/preparedness/primer.pdf. Accessed March 8, 2018.
19. Centers for Disease Control and Prevention, National Center for Injury Prevention and Control, Division of Unintentional

Injury Prevention. Important facts about falls. Centers for Disease Control and Prevention website. https://www.cdc.gov/homeandrecreationalsafety/falls/adultfalls.html. Updated February 10, 2017. Accessed March 8, 2018.
20. Falls prevention facts. National Council on Aging website. https://www.ncoa.org/news/resources-for-reporters/get-the-facts/falls-prevention-facts/. Accessed March 8, 2018.
21. Hwang HF, Cheng CH, Chien DK, Yu WY, Lin MR. Risk factors for traumatic brain injuries during falls in older persons. *J Head Trauma Rehabil*. 2015;30(6):E9-E17.
22. Worsham JR, Elliott MR, Harris AM. Open calcaneus fractures and associated injuries. *J Foot Ankle Surg*. 2016;55(1):68-71.
23. Lerner A, Soudry M, eds. *Armed Conflict Injuries to the Extremities*. Berlin, Germany: Springer-Verlag; 2011.
24. Tan DK. EMS body armor: what providers need to know. EMS1.com website. https://www.ems1.com/ems-products/Body-Armor/articles/91866048-EMS-body-armor-What-providers-need-to-know/. Published May 18, 2016. Accessed March 8, 2018.
25. Maiden NR. *The Assessment of Bullet Wound Trauma Dynamics and the Potential Role of Anatomical Models*. Adelaide, Australia: The University of Adelaide; 2014.
26. Breeze J, Sedman AJ, James GR, Newbery TW, Hepper AE. Determining the wounding effects of ballistic projectiles to inform future injury models: a systematic review. *J R Army Med Corps*. 2014;160(4):273-278.
27. Penn-Barwell JG, Brown KV, Fries CA. High velocity gunshot injuries to the extremities: management on and off the battlefield. *Curr Rev Musculoskelet Med*. 2015;8(3):312-317.
28. Dicpinigaitis PA, Koval KJ, Tejwani NC, et al. Gunshot wounds to the extremities. *Bull NYU Hosp Jt Dis*. 2006;64(3,4).
29. Dougherty PJ, Sherman D, Dau N, Bir C. Ballistic fractures: indirect fracture to bone. *J Trauma*. 2011;71(5):1381-1384.

Suggested Readings

Birnbaum M, Williams A. Kinematics and mechanisms of injury (MOI). Presented at Paramedic Training Center; October 8, 2014. University of Wisconsin Health website. https://www.uwhealth.org/files/uwhealth/docs/pdf6/EEC_courses/paramedic_training_61/kinematics_and_mechanisms_of_injury.pdf. Accessed March 8, 2018.

Champion HR, Holcomb JB, Young LA. Injuries from explosions: physics, biophysics, pathology, and required research focus. *J Trauma*. 2009;66(5):1468-1477.

Moeng MS, Boffard KD. Ballistics in trauma. In: Velmahos G, Degiannis E, Doll D, eds. *Penetrating Trauma*. Berlin, Germany: Springer; 2017.

Prahlow JA. Forensic autopsy of sharp force injuries. Medscape website. https://emedicine.medscape.com/article/1680082-overview. Updated October 18, 2016. Accessed March 8, 2018.

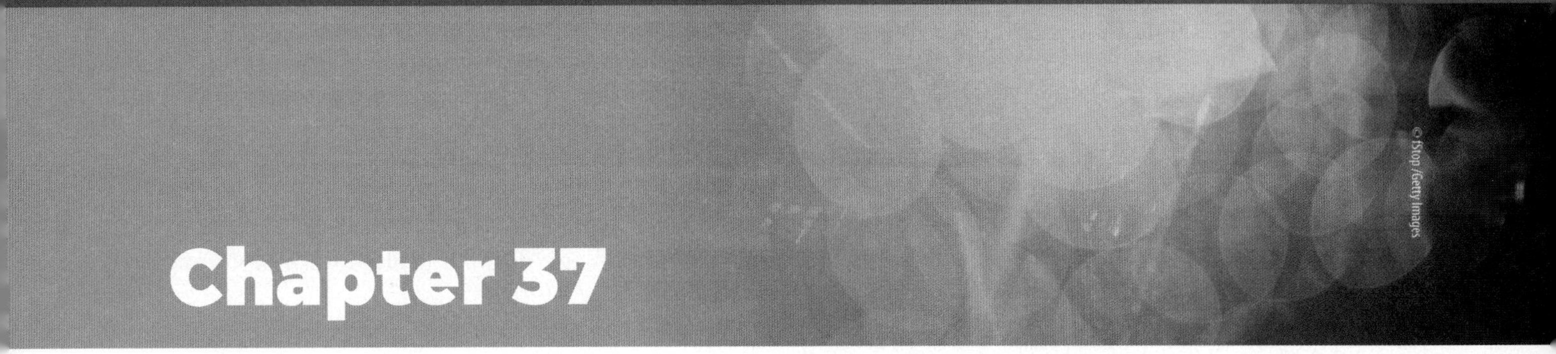

Chapter 37

Bleeding and Soft-Tissue Trauma

NATIONAL EMS EDUCATION STANDARD COMPETENCIES

Trauma

Integrates assessment findings with principles of epidemiology and pathophysiology to formulate a field impression to implement a comprehensive treatment/disposition plan for an acutely injured patient.

Bleeding

Recognition and management of
- Bleeding (pp 1378–1381)

Pathophysiology, assessment, and management of
- Bleeding (pp 1378–1381)
- Fluid resuscitation (pp 1388–1390)

Soft-Tissue Trauma

Recognition and management of
- Wounds (pp 1368–1377)
- Burns (see Chapter 38, *Burns*)
  - Electrical (see Chapter 38, *Burns*)
  - Chemical (see Chapter 38, *Burns*)
  - Thermal (see Chapter 38, *Burns*)
- Chemicals in the eye and on the skin (see Chapter 38, *Burns*, and Chapter 39, *Head, Face, and Neck Trauma*)

Pathophysiology, assessment, and management of
- Wounds
  - Avulsions (pp 1373–1374)
  - Bite wounds (pp 1374–1375)
  - Lacerations (p 1372)
  - Puncture wounds (pp 1372–1373)
  - Incisions (p 1372)
- Burns
  - Electrical (see Chapter 38, *Burns*)
  - Chemical (see Chapter 38, *Burns*)
  - Thermal (see Chapter 38, *Burns*)
  - Radiation (see Chapter 38, *Burns*)
- High-pressure injection (pp 1375–1376)
- Crush syndrome (pp 1388–1390)

OBJECTIVES

Upon completion of this chapter, the paramedic student will be able to:

1. Describe the normal structure and function of the skin. (pp 1367–1368)
2. Describe the pathophysiologic responses to soft-tissue injury. (pp 1368–1371)
3. Discuss pathophysiology as a basis for key signs and symptoms, and describe the mechanism of injury and signs and symptoms of specific soft-tissue injuries. (pp 1371–1377)
4. Outline management principles for prehospital care of soft-tissue injuries. (pp 1377–1378)
5. Describe, in the correct sequence, patient management techniques for control of hemorrhage. (pp 1378–1381)
6. Identify the characteristics of general categories of dressings and bandages. (p 1381)
7. Describe prehospital management of specific soft-tissue injuries not requiring closure. (pp 1381–1386)
8. Discuss factors that increase the potential for wound infection. (pp 1371, 1374–1375, 1386)
9. Describe the prehospital management of selected soft-tissue injuries. (pp 1386–1390)

KEY TERMS

abrasion A partial-thickness injury caused by scraping or rubbing away of a layer or layers of skin.

amputation A complete or partial loss of a limb caused by mechanical force.

avulsion A full-thickness skin loss in which the wound edges cannot be approximated.

compartment syndrome The result of an intolerably high pressure within a body space or cavity causing compromise of blood flow. It most commonly occurs in the extremities due to compressive forces or blunt trauma to muscle groups confined in tight fibrous sheaths, but may also be seen in overuse situations.

contusion A closed, soft-tissue injury characterized by swelling, discoloration, and pain.

crush injury Injury from exposure of tissue to a compressive force sufficient to interfere with the normal structure and metabolic function of the involved cells and tissues.

crush syndrome A life-threatening and sometimes preventable complication of prolonged immobilization or compressive forces; a pathologic process that causes destruction, alteration, or both of muscle tissue.

deep fascia The dense layer of fibrous tissue beneath the dermis. It provides for insulation, cushioning, caloric reserve, and body substance and shape.

degloving injury An injury usually involving the hand or finger, although it can occur anywhere in the body, in which the soft tissue is removed down to the bone.

dermis Dense, irregular connective tissue that forms the deep layer of the skin.

ecchymosis Skin discoloration (bruising) caused by the escape of blood into the tissues from ruptured blood vessels.

epidermis The outer portion of skin. It is formed of epithelial tissue that rests on or covers the dermis.

hematoma A closed injury characterized by blood vessel disruption and swelling beneath the epidermis.

hemorrhage A disruption, or "leak," in the vascular system resulting in the flow of blood.

hypertrophic scar An excess accumulation of scar tissue within the original wound borders.

junctional hemorrhage Compressible bleeding in a location where a tourniquet cannot be placed (axilla, groin, base of neck).

keloid An excessive accumulation of scar tissue that extends beyond the original wound borders.

laceration A torn or jagged wound.

puncture wound A penetrating injury that is deeper than it is long.

rhabdomyolysis An acute, sometimes fatal, disease characterized by destruction of skeletal muscle.

tourniquet A constricting or compressing device used to control venous and arterial bleeding in an extremity.

The skin and its accessory organs are the primary defensive structures of the body and perform many functions that are critical to survival. The paramedic must fully understand hemorrhage and soft-tissue trauma. This knowledge allows the paramedic to quickly assess life-threatening injury and to intervene to promote normal healing and function.

Hemorrhage

Hemorrhage occurs when there is a disruption, or "leak," in the vascular system. Sources of hemorrhage can be external or internal.

External Hemorrhage

External hemorrhage results from soft-tissue injury. Most soft-tissue trauma is accompanied by mild hemorrhage and does not pose a threat to life. However, even mild soft-tissue trauma can carry major risks of

NOTE

The Stop the Bleed campaign is a federally initiated public education project that was launched in 2015. It is designed to reduce preventable deaths related to external hemorrhage. Stop the Bleed training materials aim to teach the public how to use a tourniquet, how to pack a wound, and how to apply pressure until emergency medical services (EMS) personnel arrive.

Modified from: BleedingControl.org website [homepage]. http://www.bleedingcontrol.org. Accessed March 9, 2018.

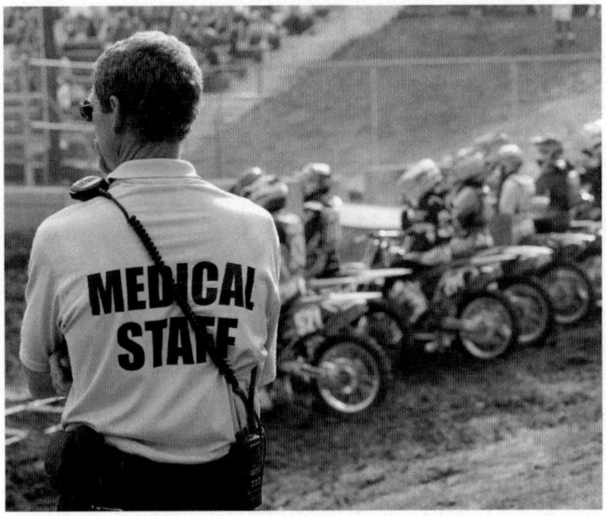

Courtesy of Ray Kemp, St. Charles, MO.

morbidity and disfigurement. The seriousness of the injury depends on three factors: the anatomic source of the hemorrhage (arterial, venous, capillary), the degree of vascular disruption, and the amount of blood loss that the patient can tolerate.

Internal Hemorrhage

Internal hemorrhage can result from either blunt or penetrating trauma, or from acute or chronic illnesses. This type of bleeding may lead to an insufficient amount of circulating blood in one of four body cavities: the chest, abdomen, pelvis/retroperitoneum, and thigh. Compared to external hemorrhage, internal hemorrhage is associated with higher morbidity and mortality rates. The following signs and symptoms may indicate the presence of significant internal hemorrhage:

- Bright red blood from mouth, rectum, or other orifice
- Coffee-ground appearance of vomitus
- Melena (black, tarry stools)
- Hematochezia (passage of red blood through the rectum)
- Dizziness or syncope on sitting or standing
- Orthostatic hypotension

> CRITICAL THINKING
> Internal hemorrhage is associated with an increase in morbidity and mortality rates as compared to external hemorrhage. Why do you think this is the case?

Anatomy and Physiology of the Skin

The anatomy and physiology of the skin are described in Chapter 10, *Review of Human Systems*. The following discussion serves as a review.

The skin is a tough, supple membrane that covers the entire body. It constitutes the largest and most dynamic organ of the body, covering more than 20 square feet (2 m^2) and making up 16% of total body weight. It comprises two distinct layers of tissue: the epidermis (outer layer) and the dermis (inner layer) (**FIGURE 37-1**).

Epidermis

The **epidermis** is a thin, nonvascular epithelial tissue that derives its nourishment from the capillaries of the dermis. Although the epidermis is only as thick as a page of this text, it is composed of five layers:

- Stratum basale, the innermost layer
- Stratum spinosum

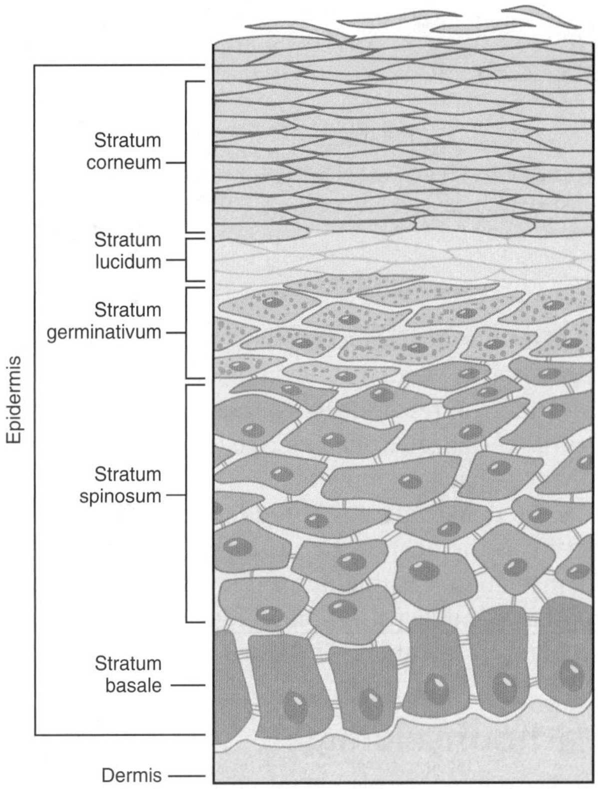

FIGURE 37-1 Tissue layers of the skin.

- Stratum granulosum
- Stratum lucidum
- Stratum corneum, the most superficial layer

The stratum corneum is composed of about 20 layers of dead skin cells that are filled with the waterproofing protein keratin.

Dermis

The **dermis** lies beneath the epidermis. This layer of the skin contains connective tissue, elastic fibers, blood vessels, lymph vessels, and motor and sensory fibers. The dermis also houses other structures of the integumentary system—for example, hair, nails, and sebaceous and sweat glands. The dermis protects the body against bacterial invasion and also helps maintain fluid balance.

Connective tissue and elastic fibers in the dermis give the skin its strength and elasticity. Blood vessels in this tissue layer nourish all skin cells and facilitate body temperature regulation through vasoconstriction or vasodilation. Nerves in the dermis generate impulses to dermal muscles and glands. These nerves also are responsible for carrying impulses away from sensory receptors in the skin in response to pain, touch, heat, and cold.

CRITICAL THINKING

Predict the effects of destruction of a large segment of skin, which includes the dermis, based on your knowledge of its functions.

The dermis has a reservoir of defensive and regenerative elements, which collectively combat infection and repair deep wounds by activating the use of specialized white blood cells, lymphatics, and other cellular components.

The dense layer of fibrous tissue beneath the dermis is the **deep fascia**. This skin layer provides for insulation, cushioning, caloric reserve, and body substance and shape. Its primary function is to support and protect the underlying structures.

Pathophysiology

Surface trauma can disrupt the normal distribution of body fluids and electrolytes and can interfere with the maintenance of body temperature. The two physiologic responses to surface trauma—that is, vascular and inflammatory reactions—can lead to healing, scar formation, or both. The extent and success of these responses are influenced by the amount of tissue that has been disrupted.

Hemostasis of Wound Healing

Hemostasis is the initial physiologic response to wounding. This vascular reaction involves vasoconstriction, formation of a platelet plug, coagulation, and the growth of fibrous tissue into the blood clot that permanently closes and seals the injured vessel. To review, vasoconstriction resulting from injury is rapid but temporary. In response to injury, severed blood vessels constrict and retract with the aid of the surrounding subcutaneous tissues. This vessel spasm slows blood loss immediately and may completely close the ends of the injured vessels. The vasoconstriction usually is sustained for as long as 10 minutes. During this time, blood coagulation mechanisms are activated to produce a blood clot.

Platelets adhere to injured blood vessels and to collagen in the connective tissue that surrounds the injured vessel. As platelets contact collagen, they swell, become sticky, and secrete chemicals that activate other surrounding platelets. This process creates a platelet plug in the injured vessel. If the opening in the vessel wall is small, the plug may be sufficient to completely stop blood loss. For larger wounds, however, a blood clot is necessary to stop the flow of blood (**FIGURE 37-2**).

Blood coagulation occurs as a result of a chemical process that begins within seconds of a severe vessel injury and within 1 to 2 minutes of a minor wound. Coagulation progresses rapidly; within 3 to 6 minutes after the rupture of a vessel, the entire end of the vessel is filled with a clot.[1] Within 30 minutes, the clot retracts and the vessel is sealed further. As described in Chapter 31, *Hematology*, the clotting cascade is a complex process and includes the following three mechanisms:

1. Prothrombin activator is formed in response to rupture or damage of the blood vessel.
2. Prothrombin activator stimulates the conversion of prothrombin to thrombin.
3. Thrombin acts as an enzyme to convert fibrinogen into fibrin threads. These threads entrap platelets, blood cells, and plasma to form the clot.

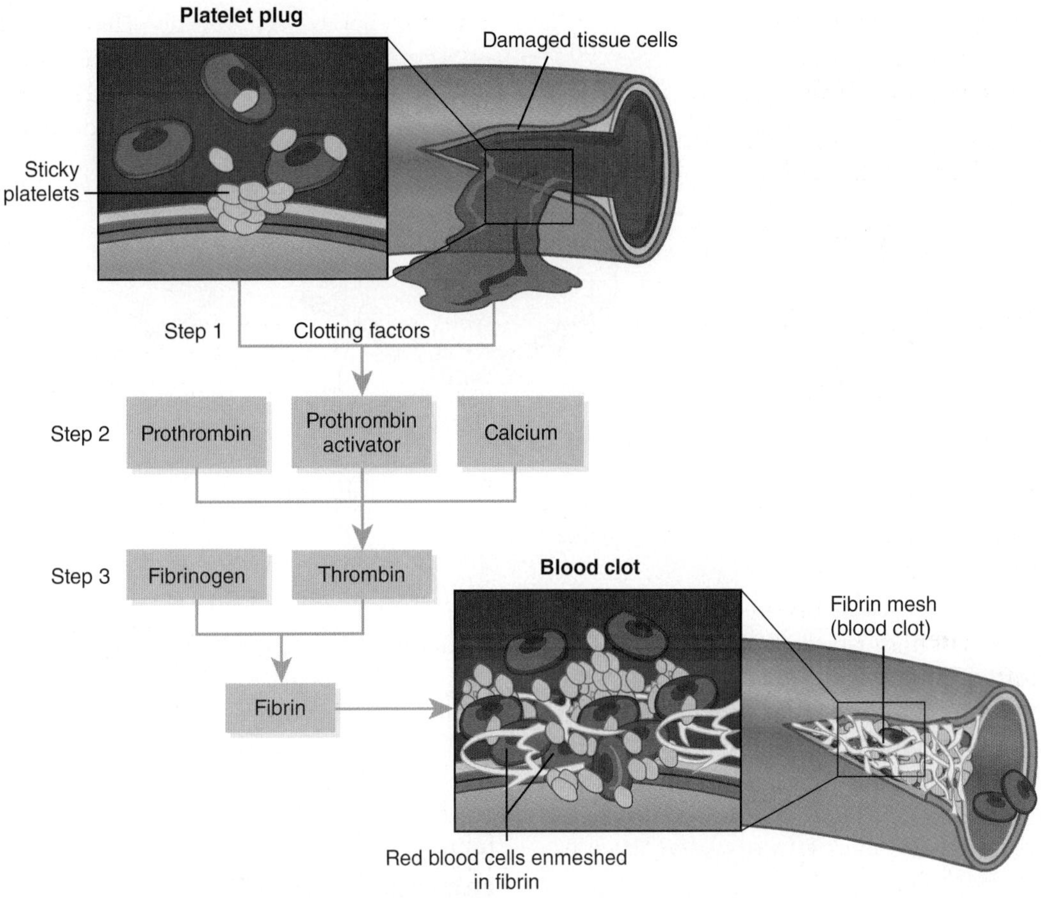

A

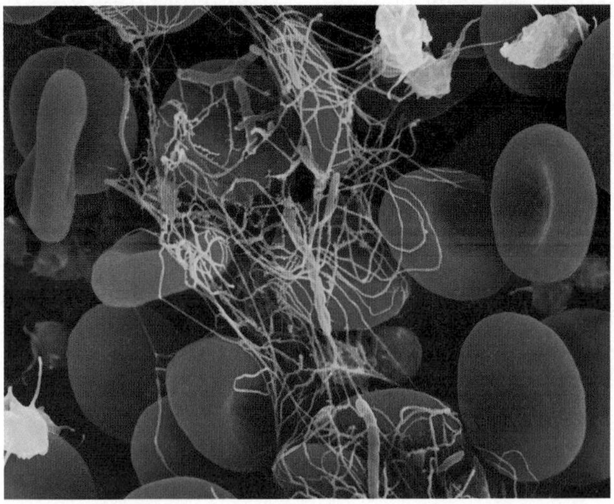

B

FIGURE 37-2 Blood clotting. **A.** The extremely complex clotting mechanism can be condensed into three basic steps: (1) release of clotting factors from both injured tissue cells and sticky platelets at the injury site (which form a temporary platelet plug), (2) a series of chemical reactions that eventually result in the formation of thrombin, and (3) formation of fibrin and trapping of red blood cells to form a clot. **B.** Red blood cells and white blood cells (blue) entrapped in a fibrin (yellow) mesh during clot formation.

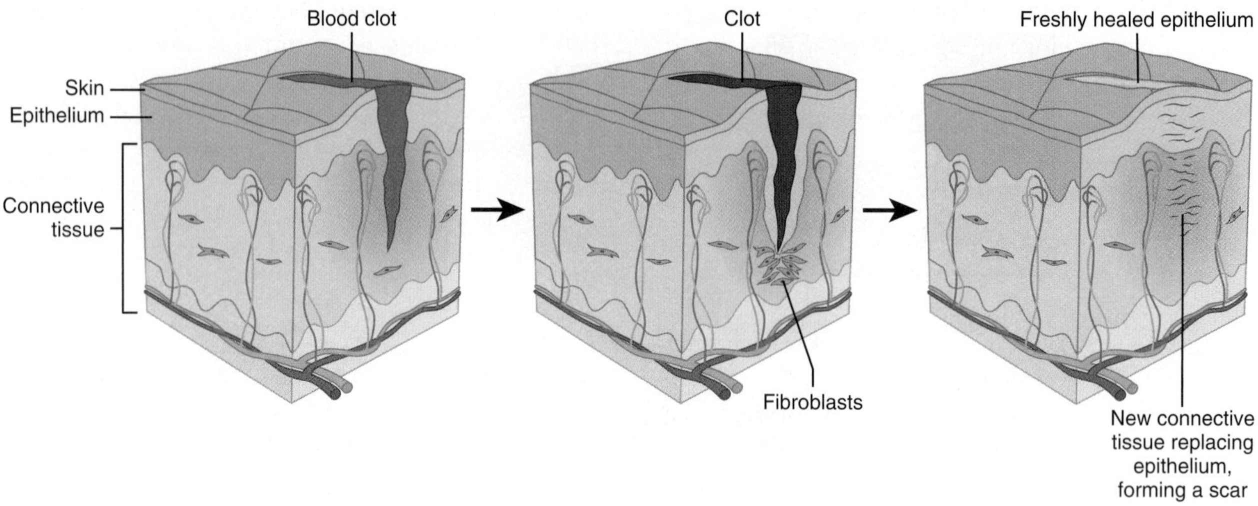

FIGURE 37-3 Healing of a minor wound.

The process of hemostasis usually is protective and is required for survival. However, hemostasis also can result in responses that threaten life and function. Examples include blood clots that form in atherosclerotic vessels that lead to myocardial infarction or stroke.

> CRITICAL THINKING
> List some drugs that may impair the normal clotting functions.

Inflammatory Response

The release of chemicals from the injured vessel and various blood components (platelets, white blood cells) causes localized vasodilation of arterioles, precapillary sphincters, and venules. This response increases the permeability of the affected capillaries and vessels.[2] Plasma, plasma proteins, electrolytes, and chemical substances from the leaking venules accumulate in the extracellular space for approximately 72 hours after the injury. In addition, blood flow increases to the area of injury to supply the metabolic demands of the tissues during healing. These responses result in the redness, swelling, and pain associated with inflammation.

The transport of granulocytes, lymphocytes, and macrophages to the injured area also increases local blood flow. These specialized cells prepare the wound for healing by clearing out foreign bodies and dead tissue, and they trigger new vessel formation as well. Within 12 hours of the injury, new epithelial cells are regenerated in a process called the epithelialization phase. These cells begin the process of healing through the reestablishment of skin layers (**FIGURE 37-3**).

Collagen is the main structural protein of most body tissues. The normal repair of tissues depends on collagen synthesis and deposition. In the healthy body, fibroblasts synthesize and deposit collagen within 48 hours after injury. Collagen increases the tensile strength of the tissue, although most injured tissue will not regain its full strength and function until at least 4 months later.[3]

Alterations of Wound Healing

Many factors can affect or alter wound healing, including anatomic factors, concurrent drug use, medical conditions and diseases, and wounds that are high risk.

Anatomic Factors

Some tissues of the body heal better and faster than others because of the body region in which they are located and the amount of tension on the tissues (lines of tension). The elasticity of the skin and lines of tension vary in different areas of the body. Moreover, they are affected by muscular contraction and the body movements of flexion and extension, which affect wound healing and scar formation. For example, a soft-tissue injury to the forearm generally heals better and faster than does a similar injury over a joint. Other anatomic factors that may adversely affect wound healing and scar formation include oily skin and pigmentation.

Concurrent Drug Use, Existing Medical Conditions, and Diseases

Certain factors can delay or interfere with the normal wound-healing process through various mechanisms. For instance, a patient's concurrent drug use can interfere with or delay this process. Commonly used drugs that can alter wound healing include corticosteroids, nonsteroidal anti-inflammatory drugs such as aspirin, colchicine, anticoagulants, and antineoplastic agents. Existing medical conditions also may have this effect, and some diseases can delay or interfere with the process:[4]

- Advanced age
- Alcoholism and tobacco use
- Acute uremia
- Diabetes
- Immunosuppression
- Hypoxia
- Obesity
- Peripheral vascular disease
- Malnutrition
- Stress
- Advanced cancer
- Hepatic failure
- Cardiovascular disease

High-Risk Wounds

High-risk wounds have an increased potential for infection because of the location of the wound or the nature of the wounding force. Examples of high-risk wounds include those located on or near the hands, feet, and perineal areas. Wounds that are associated with a high risk for infection include those produced by human and animal bites, foreign bodies, and injection (eg, high-pressure grease guns). Other high-risk wounds are those contaminated with organic material or that have a significant amount of dead (devitalized) tissue, crush wounds, and any wounds in patients who are immunocompromised or who have poor peripheral circulation.

Abnormal Scar Formation

Abnormal scar formation can result in a keloid or hypertrophic scar. A **keloid** is the excessive accumulation of scar tissue that extends beyond the original wound borders. Such a scar is more common following injuries to the ears, upper extremities, lower abdomen, or sternum and in darkly pigmented patients. A **hypertrophic scar** features an excess accumulation of scar tissue within the original wound borders. This scar is more common in areas of high tissue stress such as the flexion creases across joints.

Wounds Requiring Closure

Although all serious wounds should be evaluated by a physician, the paramedic should expect the following types of wounds to require closure:

- Wounds to cosmetic regions (eg, face, lips, eyebrows)
- Gaping wounds
- Wounds over tension areas (eg, joints)
- Degloving injuries (described later in this chapter)
- Ring finger injuries
- Skin tearing

Many techniques are used to close a wound, including suture, tape, staples, adhesive strips, and tissue adhesives.

Pathophysiology and Assessment of Soft-Tissue Injuries

Soft-tissue injuries are classified as closed or open depending on the absence or presence, respectively, of a break in the continuity of the epidermis. Soft-tissue wounds often are the most readily evident injuries but are generally considered low-priority injuries unless life-threatening hemorrhage or associated airway compromise is present.

Closed Wounds

Although closed soft-tissue injuries usually are associated with little blood loss, some of these injuries can cause significant hemorrhage in the cavities of the thorax, abdomen, pelvis, or soft tissues of the legs. This text classifies closed wounds as contusions, hematomas, or crush injuries.

Contusions and Hematomas

Blunt trauma causes contusions and hematomas. A **contusion** is characterized by blood vessel disruption

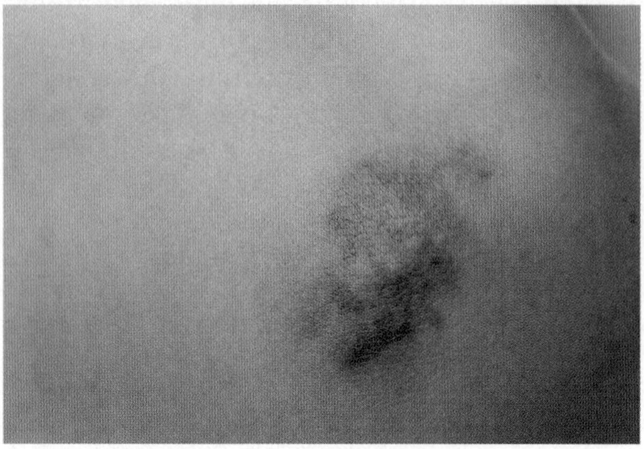

FIGURE 37-4 Spotty bruising in a well-padded part of the shoulder.

© lzf/iStock/Getty Images

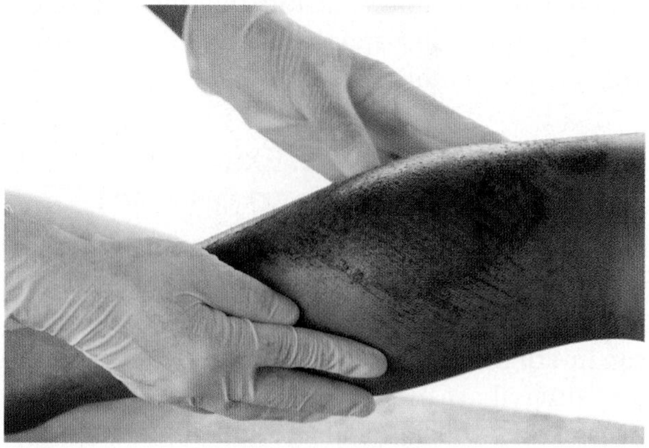

FIGURE 37-5 Deep abrasion caused by a fall from a bicycle.

© Krumanop/Shutterstock

beneath the epidermis. It results in swelling, pain, and **ecchymosis** (bruising) that can occur 24 to 48 hours after the injury. A **hematoma** is a collection of blood beneath the skin. It may occur with a contusion but represents a larger amount of tissue damage and the disruption of larger vessels (**FIGURE 37-4**). Although these wounds are usually superficial, on occasion, they are associated with underlying fractures, vascular involvement, and significant hemorrhage.

Open Wounds

Open soft-tissue injuries are classified as abrasions, lacerations, punctures, avulsions, amputations, and bites. (Burns that include open and closed injury are addressed in Chapter 38, *Burns*.)

Abrasion

An **abrasion** is a partial-thickness skin injury that is caused by the scraping or rubbing away of a layer or layers of skin (**FIGURE 37-5**). This kind of wound usually results from friction with a hard object or surface; for example, abrasions occur in sports injuries and motorcycle crashes. Although these wounds often are superficial, they are painful and are at high risk for infection from contamination.

Laceration

A **laceration** results from a tear, a split, or an incision of the skin (**FIGURE 37-6**). Lacerations most often are caused by a knife or other sharp object, resulting in a linear wound or incision. The sizes and depths of lacerations vary greatly depending on the injury sites and wounding mechanism. Lacerations can be sources of significant bleeding.

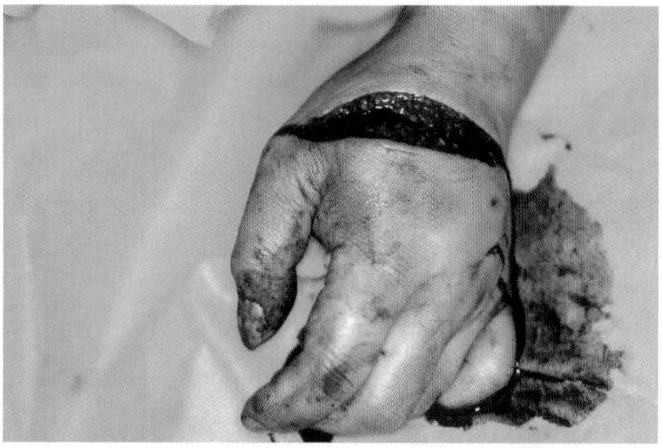

FIGURE 37-6 Large laceration caused by a broken power saw.

© Mediscan/Alamy Stock Photo.

Puncture

Contact with a sharp, pointed object—for example, a wooden splinter, needle, staple, piece of glass, or nail—commonly causes a **puncture wound**. Although the entrance wound generally is small, these injuries often may be associated with deep penetration and injury to underlying tissues. Punctures can be difficult to assess in the prehospital setting. Even an injury that appears to be minor can conceal a considerable amount of internal damage.

In some penetrating injuries, the object remains embedded or impaled in the wound (**FIGURE 37-7**). If the chest or abdomen is involved, severe bleeding

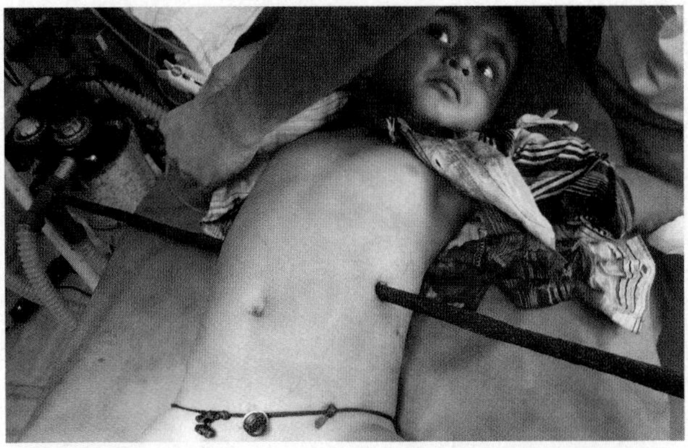

FIGURE 37-7 Piece of metal impaled through abdomen of a child.

© STRDEL/AFP/Getty Images.

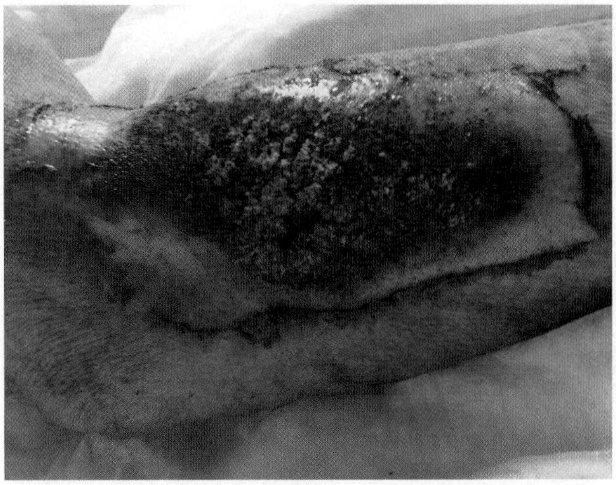

FIGURE 37-8 A burn caused by molten aluminum in the right forearm of 65-year-old male.

Reproduced with permission from McCarthy J, Trigger C. High-pressure injection injury with molten aluminum. Integrating Emergency Care with Population Health. *West J Emerg Med*. 2014:15(2). Accessed at https://westjem.com/diagnostic-acumen/high-pressure-injection-injury-with-molten-aluminum.html.

and major underlying damage to internal organs can occur. Examples include the following:

- Chest injury
- Pneumothorax (simple, open, tension)
- Hemothorax
- Pericardial tamponade
- Penetrating heart wound
- Rupture of the esophagus, aorta, diaphragm, or main stem bronchus
- Abdominal injury
- Hollow and solid organ damage
- Peritonitis (bacterial, chemical)
- Evisceration

CRITICAL THINKING

Why should a person always seek medical care to have a penetrating object removed?

The injection of a substance—for example, grease, paint, turpentine, dry-cleaning fluids, and molten plastics—into the body under high pressure also can cause a puncture wound (**FIGURE 37-8**). These injuries often have life- or limb-threatening potential. They often require rapid surgical decompression and debridement. Such injuries usually are associated with minimal bleeding, and they may not appear serious. Numbness and blanching of the involved area often occur because of increased tissue pressure owing to the presence of the injected substance. Most injection injuries are surgical emergencies. Complications can include infection, contracture, limb dysfunction, and the development of compartment syndrome (described later in this chapter). Amputation may be needed if treatment is delayed.

Avulsion

An **avulsion** is a full-thickness skin loss (**FIGURE 37-9**) in which the wound edges cannot be approximated. Frequently involved body areas are the earlobes, nose tip, and fingertips. Common causes of avulsion injury include industrial equipment, such as meat slicers or sawing devices, and domestic violence, such as human bites.

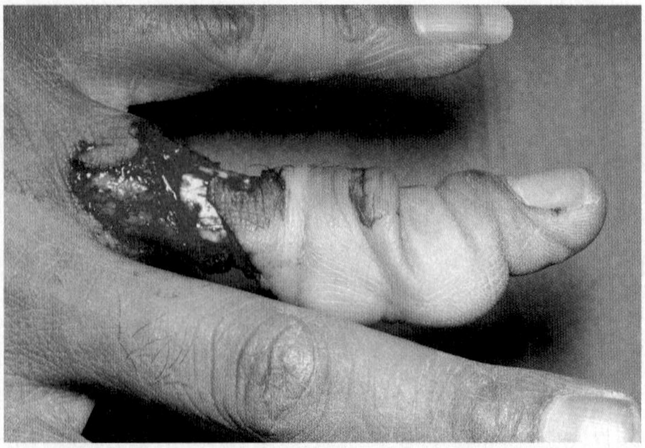

FIGURE 37-9 Ring avulsion injury.

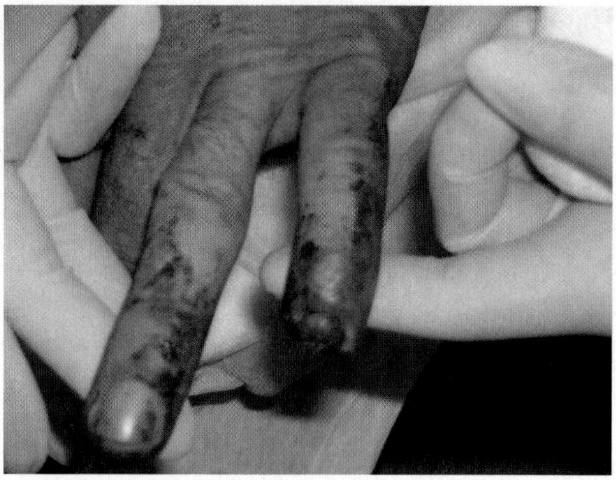

FIGURE 37-11 Amputation of the fingertip.

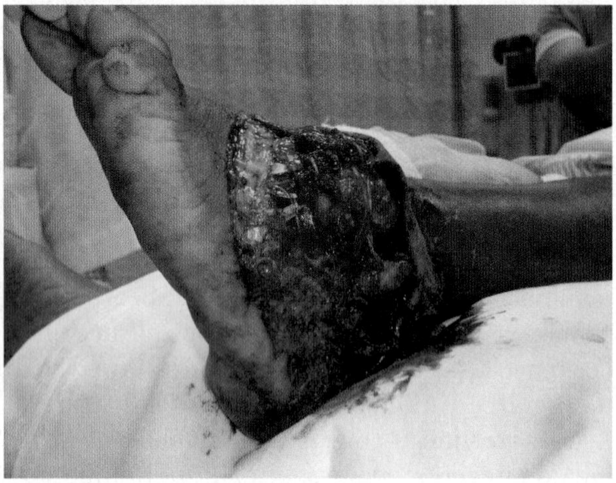

FIGURE 37-10 Degloving injury of the foot.

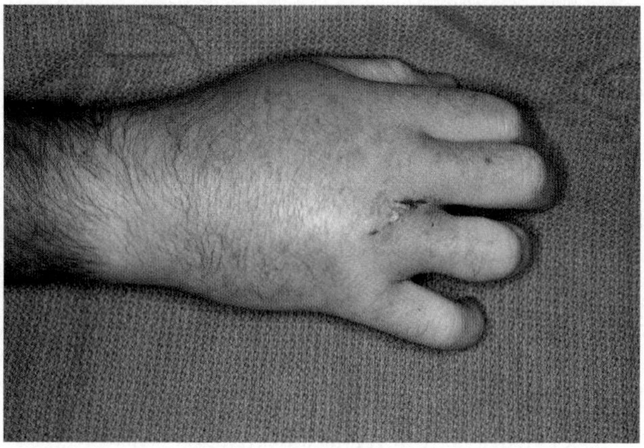

FIGURE 37-12 Human bite to the hand.

A **degloving injury** is a type of avulsion in which shearing forces separate the skin from the underlying tissues (**FIGURE 37-10**). A common cause of such an injury is entanglement of an extremity in industrial machinery, which produces circumferential tearing. Another common cause is finger jewelry that gets caught on a stationary object, which can produce a shearing of the soft tissue and possibly of the bone of the digit. Another common cause is machinery that entraps hair, resulting in scalp avulsion. Degloving injuries sometimes are associated with underlying skeletal damage and massive loss of tissue in the affected area. Bleeding can be significant.

Amputation

Traumatic **amputation** involves a complete or partial loss of a limb by a mechanical force (**FIGURE 37-11**). The digits, lower leg, hand and forearm, and distal portion of the foot are the body parts most often injured in this way. Bleeding is a possibly fatal complication of an amputation injury. In cases in which a complete amputation has occurred, injured arteries often retract, such that hemorrhage may be less severe than in partial amputation injuries.

Bites

An animal or human bite wound frequently is a combination of puncture, laceration, avulsion, and crush injury (**FIGURE 37-12**). (Insect bites and stings, which are also sources of soft-tissue injuries, are addressed in Chapter 33, *Toxicology*.) The pressure from a bite can be as great as 400 pounds per square inch (psi; 2,758 kPa).[4] The bite can involve deep structures such as tendons, muscles, and bones. Complications from bite wounds, particularly human bites, include abscesses, lymphangitis, cellulitis, osteomyelitis, tenosynovitis, tuberculosis, hepatitis B, and tetanus. Although it is theoretically possible for a human bite to transmit human immunodeficiency virus (HIV), the Centers for Disease Control and Prevention suggests that the potential for salivary transmission of the virus is remote.[5] Other, less common complications of mammalian bites include the transmission of diseases such as actinomycosis, syphilis, and, rarely, rabies. All patients who have been bitten should seek physician evaluation.

NOTE

There is a common misperception that dog bites are "clean" bites and that a dog's mouth has fewer germs than a human mouth has. In reality, the mouths of dogs (and cats) are filled with bacteria, many of which can cause disease if they enter broken skin. More than 130 disease-causing microbes have been isolated from dog and cat bite wounds. Animal saliva is heavily contaminated with bacteria. Diseases that can be transmitted to humans through a bite from a dog or cat include pasteurellosis, streptococcal and staphylococcal infections, and *Capnocytophaga* infection, among others.

Modified from: Veterinary Public Health Section, Infectious Diseases Branch, Division of Communicable Disease Control, Center for Infectious Diseases, California Department of Public Health. *Investigation, Management, and Prevention of Animal Bites in California*. 3rd ed. California Department of Public Health website. https://www.cdph.ca.gov/Programs/CID/DCDC/CDPH%20Document%20Library/InvestigationManagementandPreventionofAnimalBitesinCA.pdf. Published 2014. Accessed March 10, 2018.

CRITICAL THINKING

Consider that you are caring for a person who has sustained an animal bite. Aside from caring for the patient's wounds and documenting that care, which other concerns and responsibilities do you have?

Crush Injury

Crush injury is one of the three types of injuries that occur when tissue is exposed to a compression force. This force can be sufficient to interfere with the normal structure and metabolic function of the involved cells and tissues. The degree of injury produced by the crushing force depends on the amount of pressure applied to the body, the amount of time the pressure remains in contact with the body, and the specific body region in which the injury occurs. A massive crush injury to vital organs can cause immediate death.

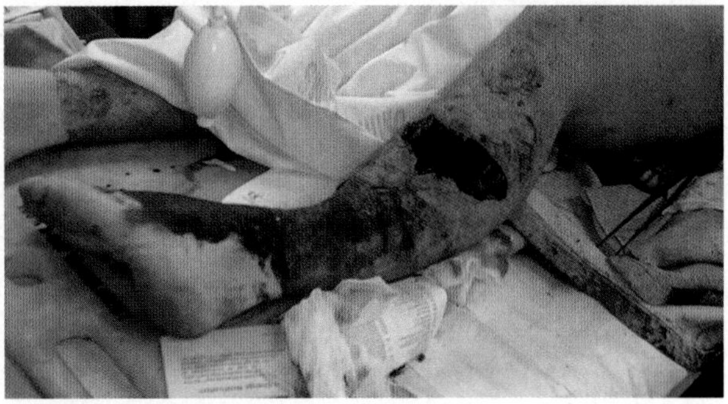

FIGURE 37-13 A crush injury with an open wound.

Courtesy of Andrew N. Pollak, MD, FAAOS. Used with permission.

Crush injury usually involves the upper or lower extremities, torso, or pelvis. It can result from entrapment under a heavy object, as in a foundation collapse, or from some other massive compressive force (**FIGURE 37-13**). Examples of situations that can cause crush injury include the following:

- Collapse of masonry or steel structures
- Collapse of earth (eg, mud slides, earthquakes)
- Motor vehicle crashes
- Warfare injuries
- Industrial incidents
- Swelling under casts

Crush injuries also occur when unresponsive people lie immobile on a hard surface for a prolonged time, as may occur, for example, after a stroke, drug overdose, or alcohol intoxication.[6]

CRITICAL THINKING

What are some mechanisms of crush injury?

Compartment Syndrome

Compartment syndrome, which occurs from increased external or internal pressure, is usually a result of crush injury and is a surgical emergency and a limb-threatening event. Compartment syndrome in the extremities typically results from compressive forces or blunt trauma to muscle groups confined in tight fibrous sheaths with minimal ability to stretch (below the knee, above the elbow). Other less common causes of compartment syndrome include the following:[3]

- Electrical injury
- Hemorrhage into a compartment (eg, coagulopathy among hemophiliacs)
- Circumferential deep burns and electrical burns
- Vascular occlusion
- High-pressure injection injuries
- Immobility with the development of pressure necrosis (eg, from alcohol intoxication, illicit use of drugs, or a stroke)
- Dextrose 50% extravasation[7]

CRITICAL THINKING

Why would alcohol intoxication, the illicit use of drugs, or a stroke create a risk for development of compartment syndrome?

Compartment syndrome develops as associated hemorrhage and edema increase pressure in the closed fascial space (compartment). The resulting ischemia to the muscle causes further muscle cell swelling as the intracompartmental pressure continues to rise. As swelling occurs, pressure will impede outflow (venous drainage) before it occludes inflow (arterial flow) leading to the development of increased pressure. Irreversible tissue damage from lack of oxygen develops within hours (6 or more) after injury.[8] In addition to muscular damage, any nerves that travel through the compartment can undergo necrosis if the condition remains untreated. Signs and symptoms of compartment syndrome in an extremity include those of vascular insufficiency; the classic presentation can be remembered using the six Ps of compartment syndrome mnemonic (BOX 37-1). Other signs and symptoms that can indicate the presence of compartment syndrome include the following:

- Pain seemingly out of proportion to injury
- Swelling (tautness of the compartment with "woodlike" firmness)
- Tenderness to palpation
- Weakness of the involved muscle groups
- Pain on passive stretch (earliest finding)

BOX 37-1 Six Ps of Compartment Syndrome

1. Pain
2. Pallor (pale skin or poor capillary refill)
3. Paresthesia (pins and needles sensation)
4. Pulselessness (diminished or absent)
5. Paralysis (inability to move)
6. Poikilothermia (body part that has normalized its temperature to the surrounding environment)

Note: Several of the Ps occur late in the development of compartment syndrome and should not be used to diagnose the condition. For example, if the patient is pulseless, has paralysis, or has poikolothermia, the damage to the patient may be permanent. *The key signs and symptoms are pain out of proportion and pain on passive stretch, which may have passed if the case is late or the limb has had a regional block.*

The recognition of compartment syndrome calls for a high degree of suspicion based on patient history and mechanism of injury. Compartment syndrome most often is associated with tibial fracture of the lower leg, but it can also occur with crush injury or fracture of the femur, forearm, or upper arm. Delayed treatment can result in nerve death, muscle necrosis, and crush syndrome (described later).

Blast Injuries

Severe injuries—classified as primary, secondary, tertiary, and quaternary injuries (**TABLE 37-1**)—can result from an initial air blast, from flying debris, and from secondary contact with another object as the victim is thrown by the blast. Examples of situations that can result in blast injury include natural gas or gasoline explosions, fireworks explosions, explosions in grain elevators, commercial tire explosion,[9] and terrorist bombings. Ensuring scene and personal safety is of the highest priority when blast injury is suspected. Paramedics should not enter the scene where a blast injury occurred until the scene has been made safe by the authorities—for example, by law enforcement, fire service, specialized rescue teams, hazardous materials teams, or other public service agencies.

Injuries from blasts can be either superficial or deep, with deep injuries potentially damaging internal organs (**FIGURE 37-14**). Compression injuries that occur to air-filled organs can include rupture of the eardrum, sinuses, lungs, stomach, and intestines.

TABLE 37-1 Mechanisms of Blast Injury

Category	Characteristics	Body Part Affected	Types of Injuries
Primary	Unique to high explosives; results from the impact of the overpressurization wave with body surfaces	Gas-filled structures are most susceptible: lungs, gastrointestinal tract, and middle ear may be affected.	Blast lung (pulmonary barotrauma) Tympanic membrane rupture and middle ear damage Abdominal hemorrhage and perforation Globe (eye) rupture Concussion (traumatic brain injury without physical signs of head injury)
Secondary	Results from flying debris and bomb fragments	Any body part may be affected.	Penetrating ballistic (fragmentation) or blunt injuries Eye penetration (can be occult)
Tertiary	Results from the person being thrown by the blast wind	Any body part may be affected.	Fracture and traumatic amputation Closed and open brain injury
Quaternary	All explosion-related injuries, illnesses, or diseases not due to primary, secondary, or tertiary mechanisms; includes exacerbation or complications of existing conditions	Any body part may be affected.	Burns (flash, partial-thickness, and full-thickness) Crush injuries Closed and open brain injury Asthma, chronic obstructive pulmonary disease, or other breathing problems from dust, smoke, or toxic fumes Angina Hyperglycemia Hypertension

Modified from: El Kader SA. Blast injuries. SlidePlayer website. http://slideplayer.com/slide/4701224/. Accessed March 12, 2018.

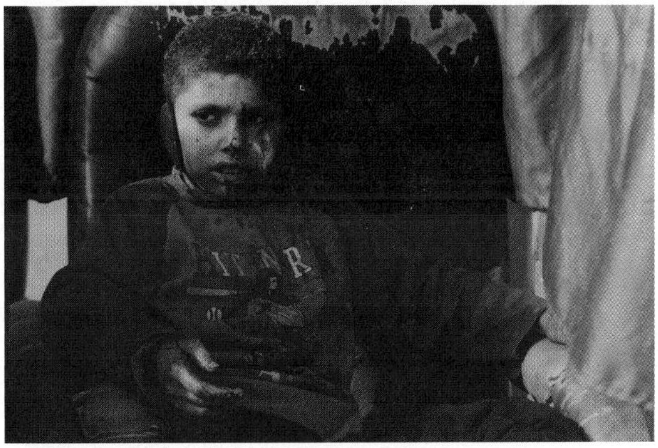

FIGURE 37-14 Blast injury to the face.

Patients who suffer blast injury require rapid stabilization (airway and ventilatory support with spinal precautions; circulatory support) and rapid transport for physician evaluation. Blast injuries and associated trauma can be difficult to identify in the prehospital setting. Patients with these injuries will need extensive evaluation in a trauma center.

CRITICAL THINKING

What injury do you suspect if a patient who has suffered a blast injury has a sudden onset of hearing loss?

Management Principles for Soft-Tissue Injuries

Ensuring personal and scene safety is always the priority in any emergency response. If indicated in the specific circumstances, law enforcement and rescue personnel should advise the EMS crew that the scene is relatively safe to enter and that any perpetrators have been apprehended. Even so, the paramedic must always be alert for possible hazards at the scene (eg, a second perpetrator or secondary explosive device). Help from other public service agencies also may be needed if other types of dangers exist, such as hazardous materials or bombs.

Treatment Priorities

The assessment of life-threatening injuries and resuscitation precede evaluation of, and interventions for, non–life-threatening soft-tissue injuries. Uncontrolled external bleeding is managed first using direct pressure. If direct pressure does not control life-threatening extremity bleeding or if the circumstances warrant immediate evacuation or other priorities, then a tourniquet should be applied.[10] The paramedic should evaluate wounds that do not pose a threat to life later in the physical examination.[11] General wound assessment includes a history of the wounding event and a careful examination of the injury.

Wound History

A wound history should include the following information:

- Time of injury
- Environment where the injury occurred (risk of infection is greater in unclean environments)
- Mechanism of injury and likelihood of concurrent or associated injuries
- Volume of blood loss
- Severity of pain
- Medical history, including use of medications that may impair hemostasis
- Tetanus immunization

Physical Examination

Physical examination of a wound should include the following components:

- Inspection of the wound for bleeding, size, depth, presence of foreign bodies, amount of tissue lost, edema, and deformity
- Inspection of the area surrounding the wound for damage to underlying structures, arteries, nerves, tendons, or muscle
- Assessment of sensory or motor function of the extremity
- Evaluation of the perfusion status of the wound and tissue distal to the wound
- Palpation of the injury and associated structures to evaluate capillary refill, distal pulses, tenderness, temperature, edema, and crepitus (if underlying bony injury is suspected)

> CRITICAL THINKING
> Will you perform this physical examination on every wound in the prehospital setting?

Hemorrhage and Control of Bleeding

Blood loss often is associated with soft-tissue injury and may result from damage to arteries, veins, capillaries, or a combination of these. Generally, arterial bleeding is characterized as bright red and spurting, venous bleeding is dark red-blue and flowing, and capillary bleeding is bright red and oozing. Differentiation among the types of vessel hemorrhage, however, often is difficult. In the prehospital setting, the main concern with a patient who has hemorrhage, regardless of its origin, is to control bleeding.

Methods of hemorrhage control include direct pressure and the use of tourniquets. When there are fractures, immobilization by splinting may reduce bleeding.

Direct Pressure

The paramedic can control external hemorrhage by applying direct pressure over the injury site (**FIGURE 37-15**). Direct pressure controls most types of hemorrhage within 4 to 6 minutes.[4] To maintain control, a pressure dressing can be applied over the site and held in place with an elastic bandage. The paramedic must continue the direct pressure, even when a pressure dressing is applied. Once the dressing has been applied, the paramedic should not remove it because removal can disrupt the fresh blood clot. If bleeding resumes and the dressing becomes soaked with blood, a second dressing should be applied on top of the first and held in place with direct pressure until the bleeding is controlled. If multiple dressings soak through, then more aggressive or alternative measures of hemostasis must be performed.

> CRITICAL THINKING
> Why should the pressure point chosen to control hemorrhage be proximal to the injury?

Tourniquet

The use of a **tourniquet** to control bleeding was once considered a "last resort" in bleeding control. However,

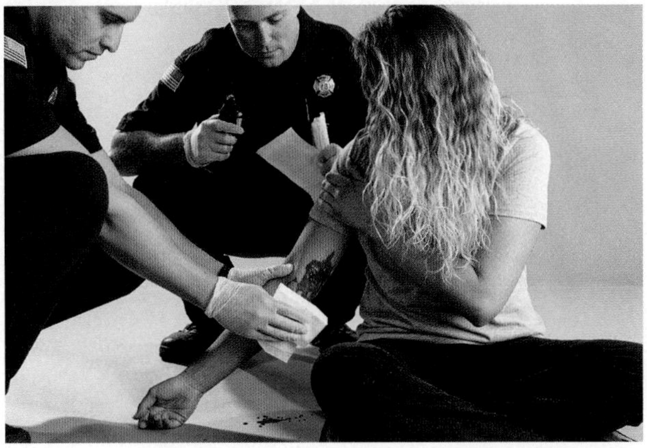

A

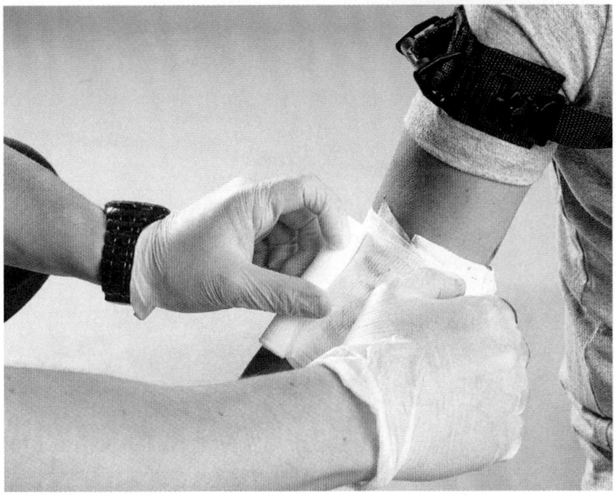

B

FIGURE 37-15 A. Application of direct pressure to control hemorrhage. **B.** Pressure dressing with a tourniquet placed on the upper arm.

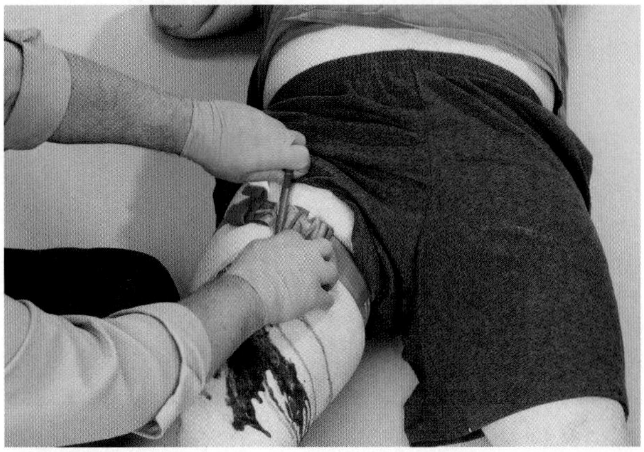

FIGURE 37-16 Application of a tourniquet to control hemorrhage.

studies based on wartime injuries in Iraq and Afghanistan have shown that tourniquets are safe and effective when properly applied.[12] Guidelines for application of a tourniquet are as follows (**FIGURE 37-16**):[13]

1. Select a site for the tourniquet. The site should avoid joints and be about 2 inches (5 cm) proximal to the wound.[14] If the site of actual bleeding is not known or if multiple wounds are present, then applying the tourniquet in a "high and tight" fashion, as proximal on the affected limb as possible, is appropriate. This approach is typically used when under fire or time is limited; the positioning may later be converted to 2 to 3 inches (5–8 cm) above the wound as time allows and if safe to do so.[15] A blood pressure cuff applied over the brachial artery also can act as a tourniquet.
2. Place the commercial tourniquet (eg, Combat Application Tourniquet [CAT], Emergency Military Tourniquet [EMT], Special Operations Forces Tactical Tourniquet [SOFTT]) 2 to 3 inches (5–8 cm) above the wound and over the artery to be compressed.
3. If a commercial tourniquet is not available, then choose a wide (4 inches [10 cm]), flat tourniquet material and place a pad (a roll of gauze or thick folded dressings) over the artery to be compressed. Do not use thin material such as rope or twine because it may damage underlying tissue. If a blood pressure cuff is used as a tourniquet, inflate the cuff until the cuff pressure exceeds the arterial pressure to the point at which the hemorrhage stops in conjunction with obliteration of the distal pulse.
4. Encircle the tourniquet twice around the extremity and pad, and tie it in a half-knot over the pad.
5. Place a windlass (stick, pen, or similar object) on the half-knot, and secure it in place with a square knot.
6. Tighten the windlass by twisting until hemorrhage stops. Assess for a pulse distal to the tourniquet. If a pulse is still palpable, tighten the tourniquet until there is no pulse. Secure the windlass in that position. Never loosen the tourniquet once it is tightened.
7. If the first tourniquet does not adequately control the bleeding, apply a second tourniquet next to the first.

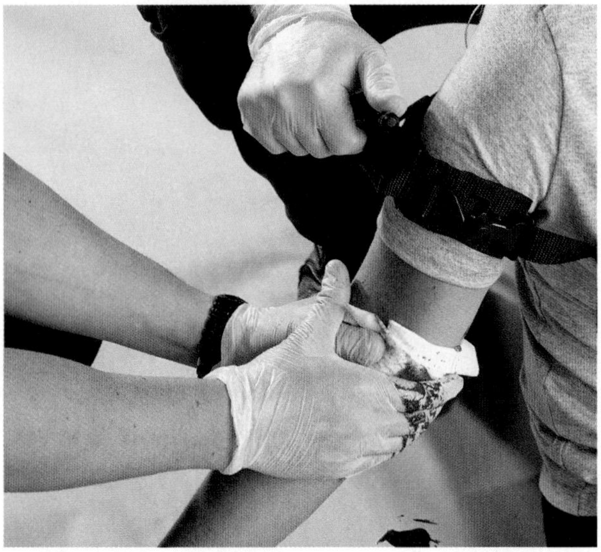

FIGURE 37-17 Commercial tourniquet application.

8. Secure a note to the patient communicating the time of tourniquet application, or clearly mark "TK" on the patient's forehead. Document the tourniquet procedure on the patient care report (**FIGURE 37-17**).

Junctional Hemorrhage Control

Tourniquets effectively control most extremity hemorrhage, but they are not as effective for bleeding that occurs at the junction of an extremity and the torso—for example, at the groin, the axilla, and the base of the neck.[16] Bleeding in each of these areas can be compressed externally. The Department of Defense Committee on Tactical Combat Casualty Care (CoTCCC) currently recommends three devices to control **junctional hemorrhage**: the Combat Ready Clamp (CRoC), the Junctional Emergency Treatment Tool (JETT), and the SAM Junctional Tourniquet (SJT).

The CRoC is a clamp that applies pressure directly over a wound or indirectly over the inguinal or axillary areas to control bleeding (**FIGURE 37-18**). The JETT components include a belt, pads, and a windlass designed to "footprint" at a 30° angle over the femoral vessels just below the inguinal ligament (**FIGURE 37-19**). The SJT consists of a belt and bladders that inflate to compress the wound (**FIGURE 37-20**). Although both the JETT and the SJT have also been used to stabilize pelvic fractures, only the SJT is approved by the Food and Drug Administration (FDA) for that purpose. All of these devices must be removed

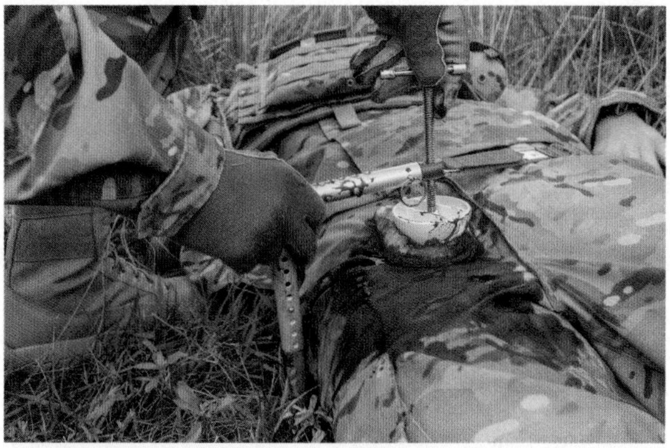

FIGURE 37-18 The Combat Ready Clamp.

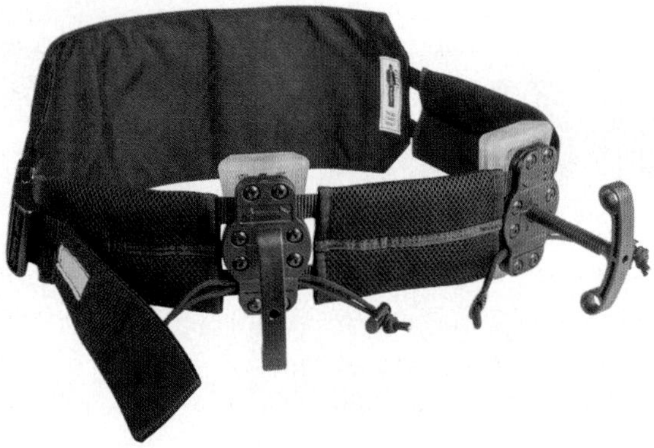

FIGURE 37-19 The Junctional Emergency Treatment Tool.

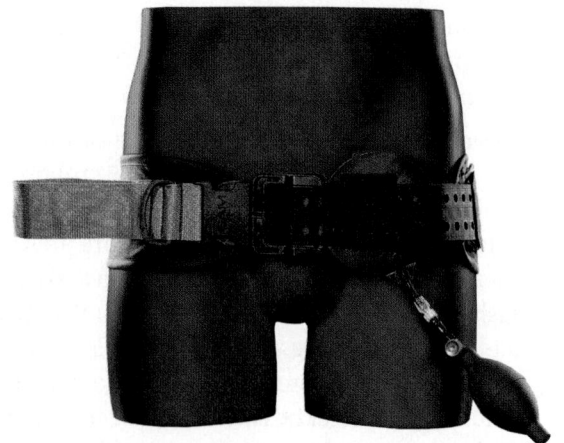

FIGURE 37-20 The SAM Junctional Tourniquet.

within 4 hours. Combat gauze with pressure should be used to attempt bleeding control if there is a delay in applying the junctional device.

NOTE

Bleeding will be more difficult to control if the patient takes an anticoagulant medication such as warfarin (Coumadin), dabigatran (Pradaxa), apixaban (Eliquis), or rivaroxaban (Xarelto).

Immobilization by Splinting

Patient movement promotes the flow of blood. This movement can disrupt the clot or increase vascular injury. After external bleeding is controlled, patients should be immobilized whenever possible as an adjunct to bleeding control.

Dressing Materials Used With Soft-Tissue Trauma

A variety of dressings and bandages are used in trauma care. There are six general categories of dressings:

1. Sterile dressings are processed to eliminate bacteria. They should be used whenever infection of the wound is a concern.
2. Nonsterile dressings are not sterilized. They can be used when infection is not a prime concern.
3. Occlusive dressings do not allow the passage of air through the material. These dressings are useful in treating wounds of the thorax and major vessels where negative pressure can cause air to enter the body, resulting in a pneumothorax or air embolism, respectively (see Chapter 41, *Chest Trauma*).
4. Nonocclusive dressings allow air to pass through the material and are indicated for managing most soft-tissue injuries.
5. Adherent dressings attach to the wound surface by incorporating wound exudate into the dressing mesh. Use of these dressings sometimes can assist in controlling acute bleeding.
6. Nonadherent dressings allow the passage of wound exudate and do not adhere to the wound surface. These dressings do not damage the wound when removed and often are used after wound closure.

Bandages hold dressings in place. They are classified as absorbent, nonabsorbent, adherent, and nonadherent. Like dressings, bandages are sterile or nonsterile.

Complications of Improperly Applied Dressings and Bandages

Improperly applied dressings and bandages can harm the patient and cause discomfort. For example, dressings that are applied too loosely often do not stop bleeding. Bandages that are applied too tightly can cause tissue ischemia and structural damage to vessels, nerves, tendons, muscles, and skin and can potentially precipitate compartment syndrome.

Basic Concepts of Open Wound Dressing

The basic concepts of open wound dressing include the following steps:

1. Assess the wound for size, depth, location, and contamination.
2. Properly prepare the wound for dressing. Prehospital care usually is limited to cleaning the injured surface of gross contaminants by irrigation of the wound with sterile water or normal saline. Do not attempt extensive debridement in the prehospital setting.
3. Apply the appropriate dressing.
4. Secure the dressing in place with bandages or gauze wrappings.
5. Tape the loose ends of the bandage.

Management of Specific Soft-Tissue Injuries Not Requiring Closure

The paramedic will encounter many minor open wounds that do not require closure or evaluation by a physician. In these cases, the paramedic should provide basic first aid and instruct the patient in self-care.

Dressings and Bandages

Depending on the nature and location of the patient's injury, dressings, bandages, and immobilization may be indicated to care for the wound properly. (**FIGURE 37-21** illustrates basic dressing and bandaging

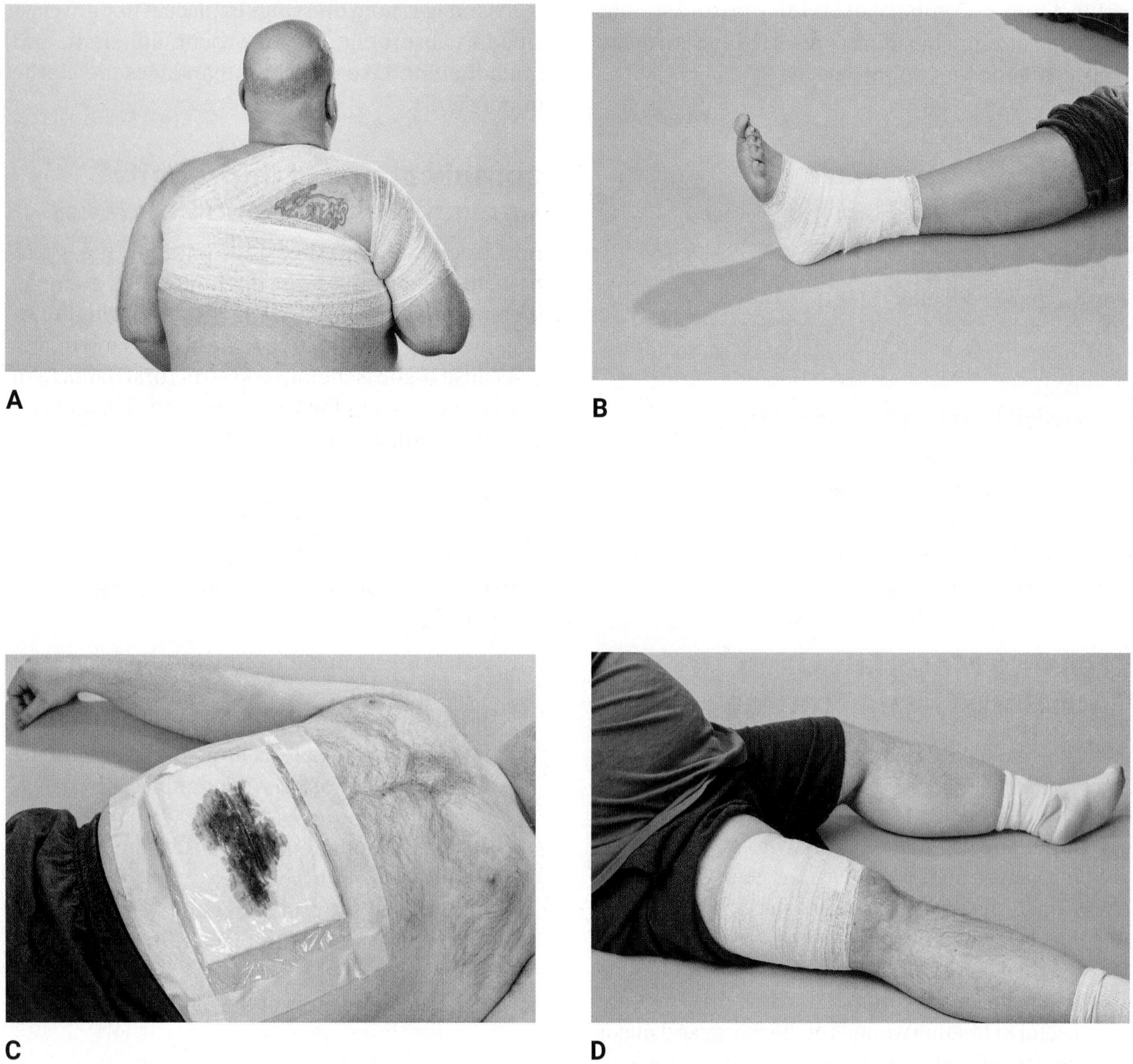

FIGURE 37-21 Types of dressings. **A.** Shoulder dressing. **B.** Ankle dressing. **C.** Abdominal dressing. **D.** Thigh dressing.

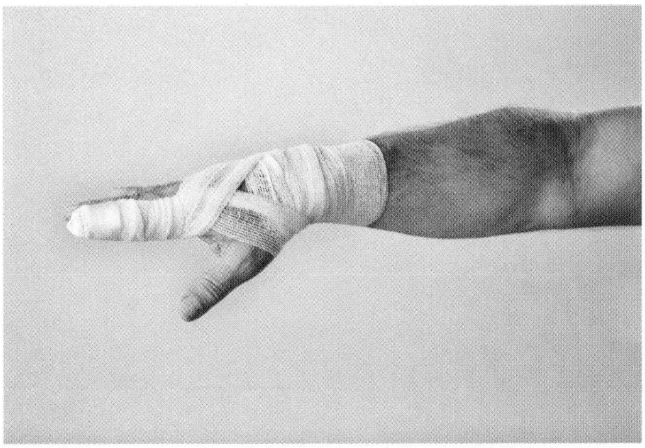

E

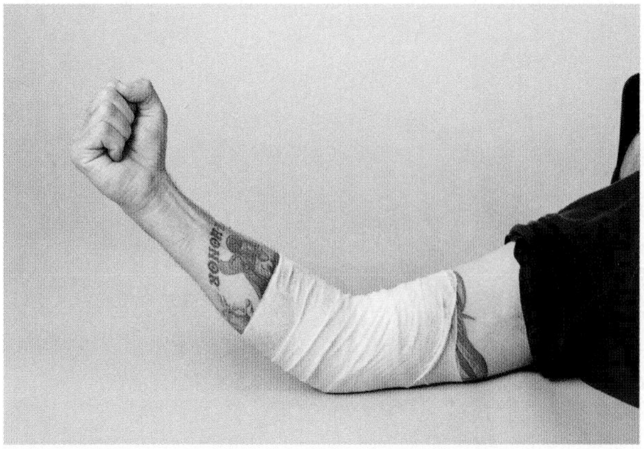

F

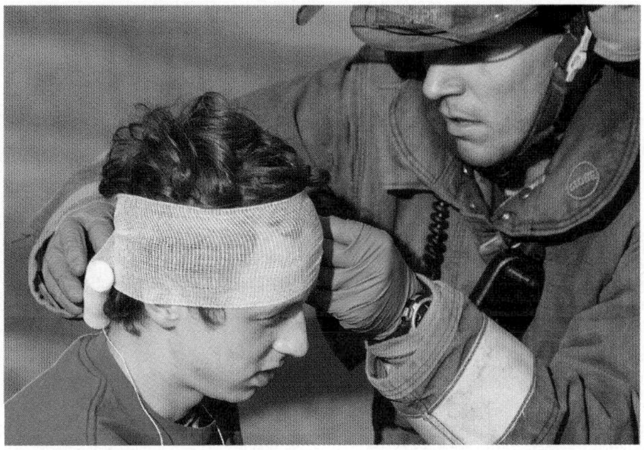

G

FIGURE 37-21 *(continued)* **E.** Finger dressing. **F.** Elbow dressing. **G.** Forehead dressing.

(continued)

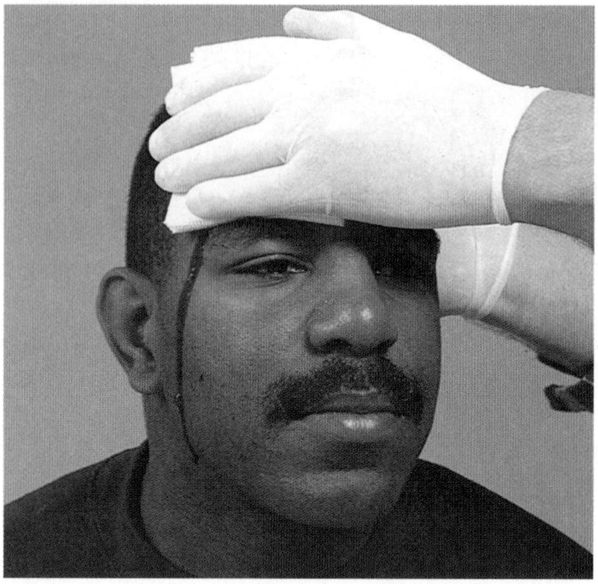

H-1

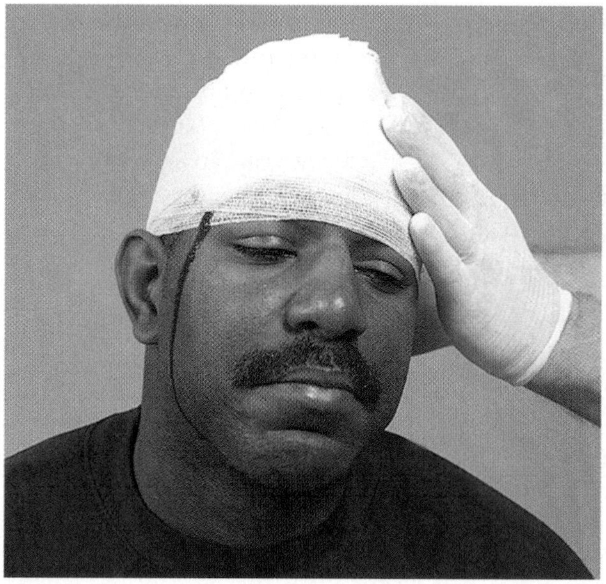

H-2

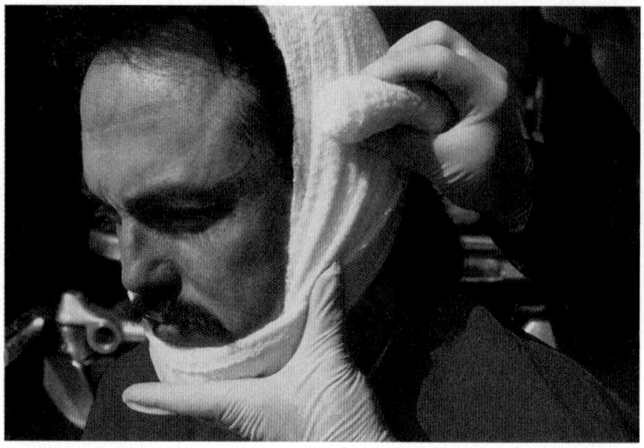

I

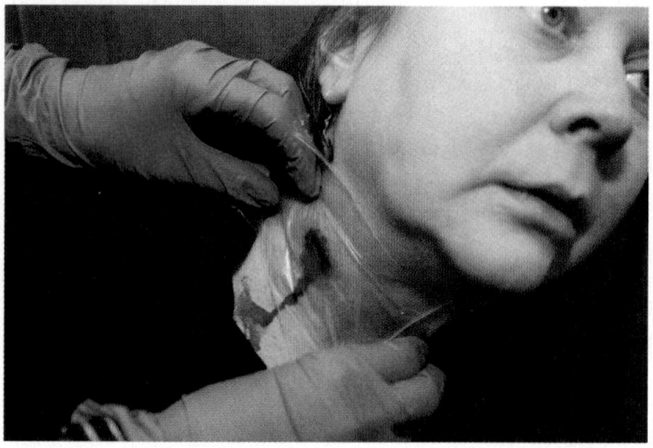

J

FIGURE 37-21 *(continued)* **H.** Scalp dressing. **I.** Ear/mastoid dressing. **J.** Neck dressing.

procedures for various wounds.) Open wounds that usually require physician evaluation include those with the following characteristics:

- Neural, muscular, or vascular compromise
- Tendon or ligament compromise
- Heavy contamination
- Cosmetic complications (eg, facial trauma)
- Foreign bodies
- All animal bites, but especially those associated with deep punctures

Patients with soft-tissue injuries that pose a threat to life or limb require rapid assessment, stabilization, and rapid transport for physician evaluation.

Hemostatic Wound Products

Topical hemostatic wound products are used as an adjunct to other dressings to enhance clotting and decrease bleeding times in severe wounds; for example, these products may be used as adjuncts to extremity or junctional tourniquets or for wounds not suitable for a tourniquet. The products presently recommended for use in the prehospital setting are QuikClot Combat Gauze (top military choice) and Celox Gauze, ChitoGauze Pro, or XStat (best for deep narrow wounds) as alternatives.[17] At least 3 minutes of direct pressure should be applied after application of the hemostatic gauze or dressing.

Tranexamic Acid

Tranexamic acid (TXA) is an antifibrinolytic medication used to reduce or prevent bleeding. It inhibits activation of plasminogen to plasmin, thereby preventing breakdown of clots. Some military and civilian research suggests that prehospital administration of TXA reduces mortality[18] or the amount of blood products needed.[19] Patients who receive TXA may have an increased risk of thromboembolic events. Although the current evidence for or against the use of TXA is not conclusive,[20] it is important that administration of TXA in the field not delay other bleeding control or transport to the appropriate trauma center. The TXA protocol must be developed and implemented collaboratively with local trauma system personnel. Protocols for administration of TXA should be directed toward patients with life-threatening hemorrhage requiring transfusion.[21]

The initial prehospital dose of TXA is 1 g in 50 mL of normal saline administered over 10 minutes. It may not be infused with any solution except normal saline.[21] This agent is not used in patients with clotting disorders, isolated head injuries, or known allergy.

SHOW ME THE EVIDENCE

Boston researchers conducted a retrospective review of prehospital care reports from one EMS agency to describe use of tourniquets and their complications. During the 8-year period reviewed, a prehospital tourniquet was applied 98 times: 67.4% for penetrating injuries, 7.1% for blunt trauma, and 23.5% for hemorrhage from hemodialysis shunt (15%) or wound (chronic wounds or varicose vein) bleeding. In 91.6% of cases, the tourniquet was documented as successful in controlling bleeding. There was one case of forearm numbness and one case with possible vascular complication. The researchers concluded that in this agency, with its short transport time, tourniquet application appears to be safe, with a low incidence of complications.

Modified from: Kue RC, Temin ES, Weiner SG, et al. Tourniquet use in a civilian emergency medical services setting: a descriptive analysis of the Boston EMS experience. *Prehosp Emerg Care.* 2015;19(3):399-404.

Evaluation

Local protocol may permit the paramedic to manage and release the patient with minor soft-tissue injury to the patient's own care. It also may allow the paramedic to manage and refer the patient to the patient's private physician for follow-up care. Paramedics may be permitted to give written and verbal instructions regarding care to patients who will not be transported by ambulance for physician evaluation.

NOTE

Some EMS systems allow paramedics to provide tetanus vaccinations. Tetanus is a serious, sometimes fatal disease of the central nervous system caused by infection of a wound with spores of the bacterium *Clostridium tetani*. The patient can be protected against tetanus by periodic immunization with a tetanus vaccine. In the United States only about 50 or fewer cases are reported each year, all of which occur in nonimmunized people. Tetanus infection occurs most commonly in people older than 50 years, and people at the highest risk of mortality include those 60 years or older and people with diabetes.

Children and adults in the United States routinely receive a combined immunization against diphtheria, tetanus, and pertussis (whooping cough). (Acellular pertussis [TDaP] is given to people older than 7 years; whole-cell pertussis [DTaP] is given to infants and toddlers.) After initial immunization during childhood, children receive booster vaccines every 5 to 10 years. Patients who have not been previously immunized against tetanus receive tetanus immune globulin because it confers instant immunity. During wound care, the paramedic should ascertain the patient's last tetanus immunization. The paramedic also should determine any prior allergic reactions to tetanus preparations. Normal side effects from the vaccine include slight fever, sore injection site, and minor rash. The tetanus vaccine is contraindicated in infants younger than 6 weeks, in pregnant patients, and in those who are hypersensitive to the vaccine.

Data source: Facts about tetanus for adults. National Foundation for Infectious Diseases website. http://www.adultvaccination.org/vpd/tetanus/facts.html. Published January 2012. Accessed March 12, 2018.

CRITICAL THINKING

Why is it crucial for you to be knowledgeable about tetanus and to ask the patient about tetanus vaccination if the vaccine is not carried on your ambulance?

Patient Instructions

Verbal and written instructions sometimes are referred to as a "patient instruction sheet." Paramedics should give instructions to all patients with wounds who are not transported for physician evaluation (**FIGURE 37-22**). These instructions should include information on the following topics:

- Protection and care of the wounded area
- Dressing change and follow-up
- Wound cleansing recommendations
- Signs of wound infection

Wound Infection

One goal of wound care is to prevent infection, as this condition is a common complication of soft-tissue injury. Infection results from a break in the continuity of the skin and subsequent exposure to the nonsterile external environment. Although most infections are minor, some can be serious. Factors that influence the likelihood of infection include unclean wounds and wound mechanisms (eg, wounds contaminated by soil, dirt, or grease) and a patient's poor state of health. These factors can have both local and systemic complications and can affect the patient's general recovery.

Causes of Wound Infection

Many factors can cause wound infection, including the following:[4]

- **Time.** The risk of infection can be reduced greatly if the wound is cleaned and repaired within 8 to 12 hours after injury. Bacterial proliferation to a level that can result in infection can occur as early as 3 hours after injury.
- **Mechanism.** Lacerations caused by fine cutting forces resist infection better than crush injuries do. High-velocity missile injuries can produce internal damage that may not be apparent for several days.
- **Location.** Injuries of the foot, lower extremity, and perineum have a higher-than-normal risk for infection.
- **Severity.** The more tissue damage produced by the injury, the higher the risk for infection.
- **Contamination.** The presence of foreign matter in a wound increases the likelihood of infection. Of particular concern are wounds contaminated by soil, saliva, and feces.
- **Preparation.** Removal of body, facial, and head hair by clipping rather than by shaving reduces the risk of wound infection. Shaving can cause additional injury by abrading the skin and potentially moving skin flora into the larger wound.
- **Cleansing.** Wound cleansing should be performed with normal saline and a high-pressure syringe.
- **Technique of repair.** Wounds at high risk for infection (eg, animal bites) may need to be cleaned, debrided, left open for 4 to 5 days, and then closed through a technique called delayed primary closure.
- **General patient condition.** Older adult patients and patients with concurrent illness or preexisting disease (eg, diabetes) often are less able to ward off infection.

Assessment of Wound Healing

A paramedic can assess a wound for proper healing by doing the following:

- **Examine dressings for excess drainage.** Change saturated dressings to prevent contamination of the wound.
- **Examine wounds for early signs of infection or delayed healing.** Inflammation, edema, and bloody drainage are normal during the first 3 days but should subside gradually as the wound heals.

Signs of wound infection include increasing inflammation or edema, purulent drainage, foul odor, persistent pain, delayed healing, enlarged lymph nodes proximal to the wound, and fever. If any of these signs is present, the paramedic should consult with medical direction. Medical direction may advise patient transport to the emergency department or may direct patient referral to a private physician for follow-up care.

Special Considerations for Soft-Tissue Injuries

As stated earlier, assessment of life-threatening injuries and resuscitation precede evaluation of, and interventions for, non–life-threatening soft-tissue

WOUND CARE INSTRUCTION SHEET

Patient name: ______________________________

1. Call your physician. He/she may have further instructions to offer for your care.
2. Keep the wound and dressing as dry as reasonably possible, since water aids bacterial growth.
3. Remove the dressing applied after 2 days.
4. Check for signs of infection:
   a. Swelling
   b. Excessive redness
   c. Pain
   d. Heat—either locally or systemically as reflected by a fever
   e. Excessive drainage from wounds
5. Reapply a sterile gauze dressing, taping it down at the edges. Repeat this every 2 days until the wound heals.
6. Wounds in areas of high mobility, such as around joints, are subject to excessive tension. Appropriate precautions should be taken to decrease the motion of the affected joint to assist in healing.

Other instructions: ______________________________

____

____

Treatment rendered: ______________________________

Tetanus: Yes / No Type: ______________________________

I hereby acknowledge that I have read the instructions above, that they have been explained to me, that I understand them, and that I have received a copy of them.

I understand that I have had emergency treatment only and that I may be released before all of my medical problems are known and treated. I will arrange for the follow-up care as instructed.

______________________________ ______________________________
Responsible Party's Signature Relationship

______________________________ ______________________________
Witness Title

Original to Patient Care Report
Copy to Patient

____
Date/Time

FIGURE 37-22 Sample instruction sheet for wound care.

injuries. The paramedic can proceed with wound care after ensuring adequate airway, breathing, and circulatory status (with spinal precautions if indicated); controlling severe hemorrhage; and maintaining normal body temperature. Special considerations for specific wounds are described in the following subsections.

Penetrating Chest or Abdominal Injury

Open wounds to the chest and upper abdomen must be covered properly with sterile and occlusive dressings. (Open wounds to the neck must also be covered with occlusive dressings to prevent air embolism, as described in Chapter 39, *Head, Face, and Neck Trauma*.) Open chest wounds can involve severe pulmonary injuries, including pneumothorax and tension pneumothorax (described in Chapter 41, *Chest Trauma*). Major complications of penetrating abdominal injury include hemorrhage from a major vessel or solid organ and perforation of a segment of bowel (see Chapter 42, *Abdominal Trauma*).

The paramedic should observe the following guidelines in managing a penetrating wound to the chest or abdomen in which an impaled object is present:

1. Do not remove the impaled object; severe hemorrhage or damage to underlying structures can occur.
2. Do not manipulate the impaled object unless it is necessary to shorten the object for extrication or for patient transport.
3. Control bleeding with direct pressure applied around the impaled object.
4. Stabilize the object in place with bulky dressings; immobilize the patient to prevent movement.

Avulsion

Prehospital management of avulsed tissue varies by protocol, but two guidelines generally apply:

1. If the tissue is still attached to the body, do the following:
   - Clean the wound surface of gross contaminants with sterile saline.
   - Gently fold the skin back to its normal position.
   - Control bleeding, dress the wound with bulky pressure dressings, and maintain direct pressure.
2. If the tissue is completely separated from the body, do the following:
   - Control the bleeding with application of direct pressure.
   - Retrieve the avulsed tissue, if possible, but do not delay transport to locate amputated body parts.
   - Wrap the tissue in gauze, either dry or moistened with lactated Ringer or saline solution (per protocol).
   - Seal the tissue in a plastic bag.
   - Float the sealed bag in ice water; never place tissue directly on ice.

> CRITICAL THINKING
>
> Why should you use normal saline or lactated Ringer solution instead of sterile water to wrap or clean avulsed tissue?

Amputations

As with other open wounds, hemorrhage control for amputation should initially involve direct pressure, assuming that focused digital pressure can be placed on the source of bleeding. If the bleeding vessel cannot be identified and hemorrhaging continues, the provider should not delay in placing an appropriate tourniquet. An amputated limb should be retrieved and managed in the same manner as avulsed tissue.

Crush Syndrome

Crush syndrome is a life-threatening and sometimes preventable complication of prolonged immobilization or compression of the body. This rare condition is most likely to occur in catastrophic events in which patient rescue and extrication are delayed beyond 4 hours (eg, earthquake, building collapse), but in some circumstances, it can occur within 1 hour. In an earthquake, patient deaths from crush syndrome are second only to those from direct trauma.[22] When large numbers of patients sustain crush injury in a massive earthquake, the health care system often does not have sufficient resources to acutely manage these patients (eg, on-scene expert nephrologists). It has been reported that about 50% of the patients with crush syndrome develop acute renal failure.[23] Early appropriate fluid resuscitation and expert advice may reduce the incidence of acute kidney injury and the need for dialysis in these patients. Thus, the prehospital management of crush syndrome can influence patient outcome.

NOTE

Because of the many variables involved, crush syndrome is complex and often difficult to diagnose and treat. These variables include the extent of tissue damage, duration and force of compression, the patient's general health, and associated injuries.

Crush syndrome is a systemic insult due to crush injury and may not become evident until pressure on musculoskeletal tissue is released during an attempted rescue.[24] The pathologic process disrupts vascular integrity and causes loss of structure of the cell and the cell membranes, thereby disrupting or altering muscle tissue. Patients with crush syndrome may appear stable for hours or days, as long as the compressive forces remain in place. When the patient is released from the entrapment, however, three harmful processes occur at the same time that can lead to death:

1. Oxygen-rich blood returns to the ischemic extremity. This reperfusion produces a pooling of intravascular volume into crushed tissue and reduces total circulating volume, which often leads to shock.
2. With the return of oxygen-rich blood, various toxic substances and waste products of anaerobic metabolism are released into the systemic circulation, which causes metabolic acidosis. High levels of intracellular solutes and water are released from damaged cells, with this flood then leading to hyperkalemia, hyperuricemia, and hyperphosphatemia. Hypocalcemia results from the injured muscles' absorption of water and calcium.
3. Myoglobin is released from the damaged muscle cells (part of **rhabdomyolysis**) of the injured extremity. Myoglobin is typically filtered easily through the kidneys, but large amounts clog the glomerulus and result in acute renal failure.

Acute respiratory distress syndrome is observed in some patients with crush injury. Factors leading to its development may include inflammatory responses, excess fluid administration, or fat emboli if the patient has long bone fractures.

Infection and sepsis are frequent complications of crush syndrome. Their emergence is often associated with wound contamination that the patient's compromised immune system is unable to fight.[25]

Management

The management of crush syndrome is controversial, and a medical direction physician who is familiar with this pathologic process must supervise the prehospital care. The emergency care must be coordinated with rescue efforts so that the timing of the release from entrapment follows medical treatment—a sequence intended to prevent hypovolemic shock and crush syndrome. After ensuring an adequate airway, oxygenation, and ventilatory support, initial prehospital care focuses on aggressive intravenous (IV) hydration to manage hypotension and to prevent renal failure.[26] Normal saline is preferred for resuscitation;[27] fluids that contain potassium, such as lactated Ringer solution, are not recommended. Generally, no more than 3 to 6 L of fluid should be infused in the prehospital setting if the patient cannot be monitored closely.[28] If the ambient temperature is low, and the patient is possibly hypothermic, less fluid is indicated. The paramedic should closely monitor patients at risk for fluid overload and, when possible, consult medical direction regarding infusion volumes. Mannitol (Osmitrol) is included in some protocols, but its effectiveness is controversial.[29]

Tourniquet use is advised only when needed to control life-threatening extremity bleeding. Other care at the scene should be guided by on-scene or online medical direction. BOX 37-2 lists patient care measures for crush syndrome.

BOX 37-2 Patient Care Measures for Crush Syndrome

Initial Management: Prior to Extrication (when possible)

- Administer IV fluids before releasing the crushed body part. This step is especially important in cases of prolonged crush (more than 4 hours); however, crush syndrome can occur in crush scenarios of less than 1 hour.
- Initiate vascular access and infuse 0.9% normal saline 10–15 mL/kg (prior to extrication when possible).
- Acidosis: Administer IV sodium bicarbonate 1 mEq/kg (maximum 50 mEq) and begin a sodium bicarbonate drip (2 ampules, 100 mEq, of sodium bicarbonate in 1 L of 5% dextrose in water infused over 60 minutes). This intervention treats acidosis and hyperkalemia, and reduces myoglobin and uric acid deposition in kidneys.
- Pretreatment: In anticipation of hyperkalemia in crush syndrome, just prior to the release ("the lift") of the patient from a crushing force, start nebulized updraft of albuterol 10 mg, push 10 units of insulin, followed with 25 g of dextrose if the patient was not previously hyperglycemic, and administer 1 g of calcium gluconate over 2 minutes. If, for whatever reason, pretreatment is not possible prior to the lift, then place a tourniquet on the injured extremity to mitigate sudden hyperkalemia when the pressure is released.
- Monitor electrocardiographic (ECG) rhythm and obtain a 12-lead ECG to observe for dysrhythmias and signs of hyperkalemia (before and after release from pressure).

Management After Extrication

- Continue normal saline infusion at 500–1,000 mL per hour for adults, and at 10 mL/kg per hour for pediatric patients.
- If the ECG suggests hyperkalemia, consider administering the following for the adult:
  - Calcium gluconate 10% 2 g IV intraosseously over 5 minutes, or calcium chloride 10% 1 g IV over 5 minutes
  - If not already administered, sodium bicarbonate 1 mEq/kg IV slow push
  - Albuterol 5 mg by nebulizer
- Consider the need for analgesia.

Modified from: National Association of State EMS Officials. *National Model EMS Clinical Guideline*. Version 2.0. National Association of EMS Officials website. https://www.nasemso.org/documents/National-Model-EMS-Clinical-Guidelines-Version2-Sept2017.pdf. Published September 2017. Accessed March 12, 2018; Sever MS, Vanholder R. Management of crush victims in mass disasters: highlights from recently published recommendations. *Clin J Am Soc Nephrol.* 2013;8(2):328-335.

Summary

- Hemorrhage can be internal or external.
- The skin and its accessory organs perform many functions that are crucial to survival. The skin is composed of two distinct layers of tissue: the epidermis (outer layer) and the dermis (inner layer).
- Surface trauma can disrupt the normal distribution of body fluids and electrolytes as well as interfere with the maintenance of body temperature. The two physiologic responses to surface trauma—vascular and inflammatory reactions—can lead to healing, scar formation, or both.
- Soft-tissue injuries are classified as closed or open based on the absence or presence, respectively, of a break in the continuity of the epidermis. Closed wounds include contusions, hematomas, and crush injuries. Open wounds include abrasions, lacerations, punctures, avulsions, amputations, and bites.
- Assessment of life-threatening injuries and resuscitation precede evaluation of, and interventions for, non–life-threatening soft-tissue injuries. General wound assessment should include a history of the event that caused the wound and a careful examination of the injury.
- Methods of hemorrhage control include direct pressure and use of tourniquets. When there are fractures, immobilization by splinting may reduce bleeding.
- The general categories of dressings used in trauma care are sterile and nonsterile, occlusive and nonocclusive, and adherent and nonadherent. The general categories of bandages are absorbent and nonabsorbent, and adherent and nonadherent.
- Depending on the nature and location of the patient's injury, cleansing, dressings, bandages, and immobilization may be indicated to care for a wound properly.
- One goal of wound care is to prevent infection. Factors that influence the likelihood of infection include unclean wounds, certain wound mechanisms, and an otherwise poor state of health.
- Special considerations for specific wounds include penetrating chest or abdominal injury, avulsion, amputation, and crush syndrome.

References

1. Hall JE. *Pocket Companion to Guyton and Hall Textbook of Medical Physiology*. 13th ed. Philadelphia, PA: Elsevier; 2015.
2. Simon PE. Skin wound healing. Medscape website. https://emedicine.medscape.com/article/884594-overview. Updated January 20, 2016. Accessed March 12, 2018.
3. Rosen P, Barkin R. *Emergency Medicine: Concepts and Clinical Practice*. 8th ed. St. Louis, MO: Mosby; 2014.
4. National Highway Traffic Safety Administration. *The National EMS Education Standards*. Washington, DC: US Department of Transportation, National Highway Traffic Safety Administration; 2009.
5. Division of HIV/AIDS Prevention, National Center for HIV/AIDS, Viral Hepatitis, STD, and TB Prevention, Centers for Disease Control and Prevention. HIV risk behaviors. Centers for Disease Control and Prevention website. https://www.cdc.gov/hiv/risk/estimates/riskbehaviors.html. Updated December 4, 2015. Accessed March 12, 2018.
6. Bigham B. Are you considering crush injury in narcotic overdoses? EMS World website. https://www.emsworld.com/article/12317524/are-you-considering-crush-injury-in-narcotic-overdoses. Published March 20, 2017. Accessed March 12, 2018.
7. Chinn M, Colella MR. Prehospital dextrose extravasation causing forearm compartment syndrome: a case report. *Prehosp Emerg Care*. 2016;21(1):79-82.
8. Rasul AT. Acute compartment syndrome. Medscape website. https://emedicine.medscape.com/article/307668-overview#a5. Updated April 3, 2018. Accessed May 29, 2018.
9. Pomara C, D'Errico S, Riezzo I, Perilli G, Volpe U, Fineschi V. Blast overpressure after tire explosion: a fatal case. *Am J Forensic Med Pathol*. 2013;34(4):306-310.
10. Bulger EM, Snyder D, Schoelles K, et al. An evidence-based prehospital guideline for external hemorrhage control: American College of Surgeons Committee on Trauma. *Prehosp Emerg Care*. 2014;18(2):163-173.
11. Spahn DR, Bouillon B, Cerny V, et al. Management of bleeding and coagulopathy following major trauma: an updated European guideline. *Crit Care*. 2013;17(2):R76.
12. Beekley AC, Sebesta JA, Blackborne LH, et al. Prehospital tourniquet use in Operation Iraqi Freedom: effect on hemorrhage control and outcomes. *J Trauma*. 2008;64(2 suppl):S28-S37.
13. National Association of Emergency Medical Technicians. *PHTLS: Prehospital Trauma Life Support*. 8th ed. Burlington, MA: Jones & Bartlett Learning; 2014.
14. Kragh JF Jr, Walters TJ, Baer DG, et al. Practical use of emergency tourniquets to stop bleeding in major limb trauma. *J Trauma*. 2008;64:S38-S50.
15. Shackelford SA, Butler FK Jr, Kragh JF Jr, et al. Optimizing the use of limb tourniquets in tactical combat casualty care: TCCC guidelines change 14-02. *J Spec Oper Med*. 2015;15(1):17-31.
16. Kotwal RS, Butler FK. Junctional hemorrhage control for tactical combat casualty care. *Wilderness Environ Med*. 2017;28(2 suppl):S33-S38.
17. Bennett BL. Bleeding control using hemostatic dressings: lessons learned. *Wilderness Environ Med*. 2017;28(2 suppl):S39-S49.
18. CRASH-2 Trial Collaborators. Effects of tranexamic acid on death, vascular occlusive events, and blood transfusion in trauma patients with significant haemorrhage (CRASH-2): a randomised, placebo-controlled trial. *Lancet*. 2010;376(9734):23-32.
19. Neeki MM, Dong F, Toy J, et al. Efficacy and safety of tranexamic acid in prehospital traumatic hemorrhagic shock: outcomes of the Cal-PAT study. *Western J Emerg Med*. 2017;18(4):673-683.
20. Fischer PE, Bulger EM, Perina DG, et al. Guidance document for the prehospital use of tranexamic acid in injured patients. *Prehosp Emerg Care*. 2016;20(5):557-559.
21. Strosberg DS, Nguyen MC, Mostafavifar L, Mell H, Evans DC. Development of a prehospital tranexamic acid administration protocol. *Prehosp Emerg Care*. 2016;20(4):462-466.
22. Sever MS, Vanholder R. Management of crush victims in mass disasters: highlights from recently published recommendations. *Clin J Am Soc Nephrol*. 2013;8(2):328-335.
23. Vanholder R, Sever MS, Erek E, et al. Acute renal failure related to the crush syndrome: towards an era of seismo-nephrology? *Nephrol Dial Transpl*. 2000;15(10): 1517-1521.
24. Rajagopalan S. Crush injuries and the crush syndrome. *Med J Armed Forces India*. 2010;66(4):317-320.
25. Genthon A, Wilcox SR. Crush syndrome: a case report and review of the literature. *J Emerg Med*. 2014;46(2):313-319.
26. Vanholder R, Sever MS. Crush-related acute kidney injury (acute renal failure). UpToDate website. https://www.uptodate.com/contents/crush-related-acute-kidney-injury-acute-renal-failure?search=Crush-related%20acute%20kidney%20injury&source=search_result&selectedTitle=1~1&usage_type=default&display_rank=1. January 4, 2018. Accessed March 12, 2018.
27. Wise R, Faurie M, Malbrain MLNG, Hodgson E. Strategies for intravenous fluid resuscitation in trauma patients. *World J Surg*. 2017;41(5):1170-1183.
28. Sever MS, Vanholder R. Management of crush victims in mass disasters: highlights from recently published recommendations. *Clin J Am Soc Nephrol*. 2013;8(2):328-335.
29. Sever MS, Vanholder R. Management of crush victims in mass disasters: highlights from recently published recommendations. *CJASN*. 2013;8(2):328-335.

Suggested Readings

Bulger EM, Snyder D, Schoelles K, et al. An evidence-based prehospital guideline for external hemorrhage control: American College of Surgeons Committee on Trauma. *Prehosp Emerg Care*. 2014;18:163-173.

Cervellin G, Comelli I, Benatti M, Sanchis-Gomar F, Bassi A, Lippi G. Non-traumatic rhabdomyolysis: background, laboratory features, and acute clinical management. *Clin Biochem*. 2017;50(12):656-662.

Gulland A. Lessons from the battlefield. *Br Med J*. 2008;336(7653):1098-1100.

Kalish J, Burke P, Feldman J. The return of tourniquets: original research evaluates the effectiveness of prehospital tourniquets for civilian penetrating extremity injuries. *J Emerg Med Serv*. 2008 Aug;33(8):44-6, 49-50, 52, 54.

Zeller J, Fox A, Pryor J. Beyond the battlefield: the use of hemostatic dressings in civilian EMS. *J Emerg Med Serv*. 2008 Mar;33(3):102-109.

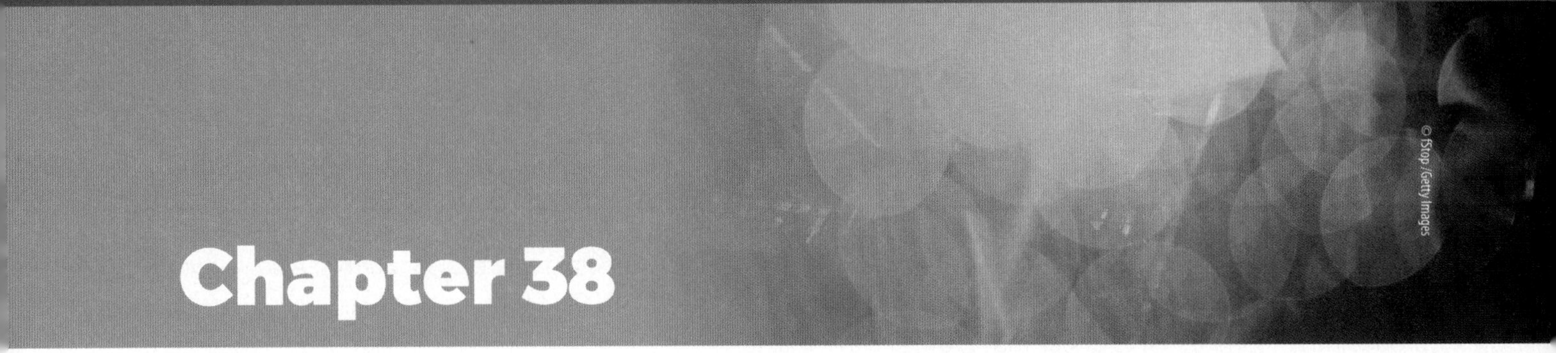

Chapter 38

Burns

NATIONAL EMS EDUCATION STANDARD COMPETENCIES

Trauma

Integrates assessment findings with principles of epidemiology and pathophysiology to formulate a field impression to implement a comprehensive treatment/disposition plan for an acutely injured patient.

Soft-Tissue Trauma

Recognition and management of

- Wounds (Chapter 37, *Bleeding and Soft-Tissue Trauma*)
- Burns
  - Electrical (pp 1396, 1413–1417)
  - Chemical (pp 1395–1396, 1410–1413)
  - Thermal (p 1395)
- Chemicals in the eye and on the skin (pp 1396, 1411)

Pathophysiology, assessment, and management of

- Wounds (Chapter 37, *Bleeding and Soft-Tissue Trauma*)
  - Avulsions (Chapter 37, *Bleeding and Soft-Tissue Trauma*)
  - Bite wounds (Chapter 37, *Bleeding and Soft-Tissue Trauma*)
  - Lacerations (Chapter 37, *Bleeding and Soft-Tissue Trauma*)
  - Puncture wounds (Chapter 37, *Bleeding and Soft-Tissue Trauma*)
  - Incisions (Chapter 37, *Bleeding and Soft-Tissue Trauma*)
- Burns
  - Electrical (pp 1396, 1413–1417)
  - Chemical (pp 1395–1396, 1410–1413)
  - Thermal (pp 1395)
  - Radiation (pp 1396, 1417–1420)
- High-pressure injection (Chapter 37, *Bleeding and Soft-Tissue Trauma*)
- Crush syndrome (Chapter 37, *Bleeding and Soft-Tissue Trauma*)

OBJECTIVES

Upon completion of this chapter, the paramedic student will be able to:

1. Describe the incidence, patterns, and sources of burn injury. (pp 1394–1396)
2. Describe the pathophysiology of local and systemic responses to burn injury. (pp 1396–1397)
3. Classify burn injury according to depth, extent, and severity based on established standards. (pp 1397–1402)
4. Discuss the pathophysiology of burn shock as a basis for key signs and symptoms. (pp 1402–1403)
5. Outline the physical examination of the burned patient. (p 1404)
6. Describe the prehospital management of the patient who has sustained a burn injury. (pp 1404–1407)
7. Discuss pathophysiology as a basis for key signs, symptoms, and management of the patient with an inhalation injury. (pp 1408–1410)
8. Outline the general assessment and management of the patient who has a chemical injury. (pp 1410–1412)
9. Describe specific complications and management techniques for selected chemical injuries. (pp 1412–1413)
10. Describe the physiologic effects of electrical injuries as they relate to each body system based on an understanding of key principles of electricity. (pp 1413–1415)
11. Outline assessment and management of the patient with electrical injury. (pp 1415–1416)
12. Describe the distinguishing features of radiation injury and considerations in the prehospital management of these patients. (pp 1417–1420)

KEY TERMS

burn shock A combination of hypovolemic and distributive shock that results from local and systemic responses to thermal trauma.

carboxyhemoglobin A compound produced by the exposure of hemoglobin to carbon monoxide.

circumferential burns Burns that encircle a body part, producing a tourniquet-like effect that may quickly compromise circulation.

contracture deformity An abnormal, usually permanent condition of a joint characterized by flexion and fixation and caused by atrophy and shortening of muscle fibers or by loss of elasticity of the skin.

eschar A scab or dry crust of dead tissue resulting from a thermal or chemical burn.

escharotomy Surgical incision that splits an eschar to prevent or relieve compartment syndrome.

full-thickness burn A burn injury in which the entire thickness of the epidermis and dermis is destroyed; also known as a third-degree burn.

inhalation injury An upper and/or lower airway injury that results from thermal and/or chemical exposure.

Lund and Browder chart A method to estimate burn injury that assigns specific numbers to each body part and that accounts for developmental changes in percentages of body surface area.

Parkland formula A formula used to calculate the fluid needs of a burn-injured patient over the first 24 hours after injury; also known as the consensus formula.

partial-thickness burn A burn injury that extends through the epidermis to the dermis. It is considered a superficial partial-thickness injury if it involves minimal papillary dermis; it is considered a deep partial-thickness injury if it extends to the reticular dermis. Also known as a second-degree burn.

rule of nines A method to estimate burn injury that divides the total body surface area into segments that are multiples of 9%.

skin graft A portion of skin implanted to cover areas where skin has been lost through burns or injury or by the surgical removal of nonviable tissue.

smoke inhalation injury Inhalation injury caused by the accumulation of toxic by-products of combustion.

superficial burn A burn injury in which only a superficial layer of epidermal cells is destroyed; also known as a first-degree burn.

zone of coagulation In a burn wound, the central area that has sustained the most intense contact with the thermal source. In this area, coagulation necrosis of the cells has occurred and the tissue is nonviable.

zone of hyperemia An area in which blood flow is increased as a result of the normal inflammatory response to injury. It lies at the periphery of the zone of stasis.

zone of stasis The area of burn tissue that surrounds the critically injured area. It consists of tissue that is potentially viable despite the serious thermal injury.

The management of burns often poses a challenge for the paramedic. Understanding the long-term results of a serious burn injury is important. Appropriate prehospital management can reduce morbidity and mortality for burn patients.

Incidence and Patterns of Burn Injury

Burns are a devastating form of trauma. They are associated with high mortality rates, lengthy rehabilitation, cosmetic disfigurement, and permanent physical disabilities. In 2016, about 486,000 Americans sought medical attention for burns. Of these patients, about 3,275 died because of thermal injury or smoke inhalation.[1] BOX 38-1 lists common complications that contribute to thermal injury deaths.

Morbidity and mortality rates from burn injury follow significant patterns regarding sex, age, and socioeconomic status. For example, just over two-thirds of all fire fatalities are men, the death rate from thermal injury is highest among children and older adults, and about 81% of all fire deaths occur in the home.[2] A key part of the professional role of

BOX 38-1 Physiologic and Systemic Complications of Thermal Injuries

Depending on the severity of the thermal injury, physiologic and systemic complications may include the following:

- Acidosis
- Anoxia
- Dysrhythmias
- Electrolyte loss
- Fluid loss
- Heart failure
- Hypothermia
- Hypovolemia
- Hypoxia
- Infection
- Liver failure
- Renal failure

BOX 38-2 Burn Facts: Selected Statistics on Admissions to Burn Centers, 2005–2014

- Survival rate: 97%
- Ethnicity: 59% Caucasian, 20% African American, 14% Hispanic, 7% other
- Burn cause: 43% fire/flame, 34% scald, 9% hot object contact, 4% electrical, 3% chemical, 7% other
- Place of occurrence: 73% home, 8% occupational, 5% street/highway, 5% recreational/sport, 9% other

Modified from: Burn incidence fact sheet. Burn incidence and treatment in the United States: 2016. American Burn Association website. http://ameriburn.org/who-we-are/media/burn-incidence-fact-sheet/. Accessed March 16, 2018.

the paramedic is community education. This education should stress prevention as the most effective management of these injuries (see Chapter 3, *Injury Prevention, Health Promotion, and Public Health*) (BOX 38-2).

Major Sources of Burns

The transfer of energy to living cells causes burn injuries. The source of this energy may be thermal, chemical, electrical, or radiation.

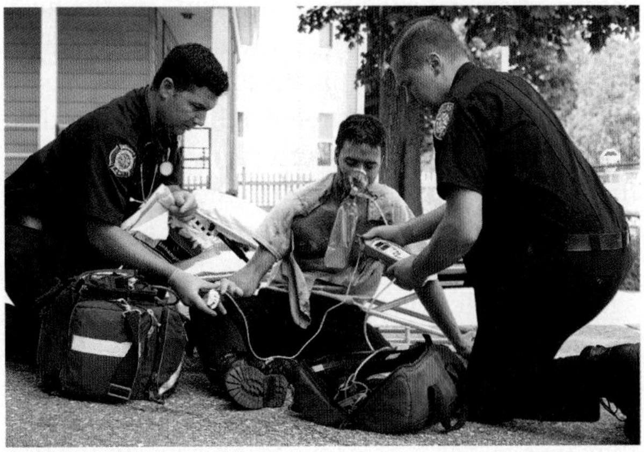

Thermal Burns

The majority of burns are thermal. These burns commonly result from flames, scalds, or contact with hot substances. (Frostbite is also a thermal injury. It is addressed in Chapter 44, *Environmental Conditions.*) Studies have shown that surface temperatures of 111°F (44°C) do not produce burns unless exposure time exceeds 6 hours.[3] At temperatures between 111°F and 124°F (44°C to 51°C), the rate of epidermal necrosis approximately doubles with each degree of temperature increase. At 156°F (69°C) or greater, the exposure time required to cause transepidermal necrosis is less than 1 second.[4] The degree of tissue destruction depends on the temperature and on the duration of exposure. Factors that influence the ability of the body to resist burn injury include the water content of the skin tissue, thickness and pigmentation of the skin, presence or absence of insulating substances such as skin oils or hair, and peripheral circulation of the skin, which affects the dissipation of heat.

CRITICAL THINKING

Based on these facts and your knowledge of life span development, given the same energy source, would you predict a burn to be deeper in an 18-year-old or a 75-year-old patient? Why?

Chemical Burns

Chemical burns are caused by a substance capable of producing chemical changes in the skin. These chemical changes disrupt the protein structure of the skin, with or without the production of heat. Heat may be generated during the burning process, yet the chemical changes in the skin, not the heat, produce the greatest injury. Chemical burns differ from thermal burns in that the topical agent usually adheres to the skin for prolonged periods, producing continuous tissue destruction. The severity of the chemical injury is related to the tissue affected, the type of agent, the concentration and volume of the agent, and the duration of contact. Chemical agents that often cause burn injury include acids and alkalis, which are found in many household cleaning products and organic compounds. Chemical burns are associated with high morbidity, especially when they involve the eyes or the esophagus. Inhalation injury (described later in this chapter) may also result from thermal and/or chemical exposure.

NOTE

There are more than 25,000 chemicals used in industry and farming and in homes that are known to cause burns. These chemicals constitute only about 3% of all burns; however, they have high morbidity (often requiring surgery), often involve cosmetic areas of the body, and have a high mortality (about 30%).

Modified from: Porrett PM, Drebin J. *The Surgical Review: An Integrated Basic and Clinical Science Study Guide*. Philadelphia, PA: Wolters Kluwer; 2016.

Electrical Burns

Electrical injuries (including lightning injuries) result from direct contact with an electric current and can also result from the arcing of electricity between two contact points near the skin. In a direct-contact injury, the current itself is not considered to have any thermal properties; however, the potential energy of the current is changed into thermal energy. This transformation occurs when electricity meets the electrical resistance of biologic tissue interposed between the entrance and exit sites. Arc injuries are localized at the termination of current flow and are caused by the intense heat or flash that occurs when the current jumps and makes contact with the skin. Flame burns also may occur as a result of arcing if the heat generated ignites clothing or another fuel source near the patient.

CRITICAL THINKING

Electrical energy is transformed to heat, causing tissue damage in a human being. Then why does an electrical cord not feel hot when you touch it?

Radiation Burns

Radiation injury is caused by ionizing and nonionizing radiation (described later in this chapter). Burns may result from a high level of radiation exposure to a specific body area; however, radiation injuries make up a very small percentage of burn injuries.

Local Response to Burn Injury

Burn injuries immediately destroy cells or so fully disrupt their metabolic functions that cellular death ensues. Cellular damage is distributed over a spectrum of injury. Some cells are destroyed instantly, while others are irreversibly injured. Some injured cells, though, may survive if rapid and appropriate intervention is provided in the prehospital setting and through in-hospital care.

Major thermal burns have three distinct zones of injury (referred to as the Jackson thermal wound theory).[5] These zones usually appear in a bull's-eye pattern (**FIGURE 38-1**). The central area of the burn wound, which has sustained the most intense contact with the thermal source, is the **zone of coagulation**. In this area, coagulation necrosis of the cells has occurred, and the tissue is nonviable. The **zone of stasis** surrounds the critically injured area and consists of potentially viable tissue despite the serious thermal injury. In this zone, cells are ischemic because of clotting and vasoconstriction. The cells die within 24 to 48 hours after injury if no supportive measures are undertaken. At the periphery of the zone of stasis is the **zone of hyperemia**. This zone has increased blood flow as a result of the normal inflammatory response. The tissues in this area recover in 7 to 10 days if infection or profound shock does not develop.

Tissue damage from burns depends on the degree of heat and on the duration of exposure to the thermal source. As a rule, the burn wound swells rapidly because of the release of chemical mediators. These mediators cause an increase in capillary permeability and a fluid shift from the intravascular space into the injured tissues. The increased permeability is accentuated by injury to the sodium pump in the cell walls. As sodium moves into the injured cells, it causes an increase in osmotic pressure. This increase in osmotic pressure increases the influx of vascular fluid into the wound. Finally, the normal process of evaporative loss of water to the environment is accelerated (5 to 15 times that of normal skin) through the burned tissue. In a small wound, these physiologic alterations

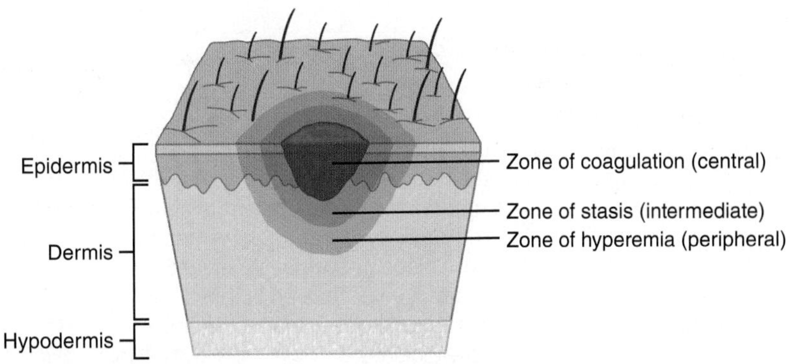

FIGURE 38-1 Three zones of intensity: zone of hyperemia (peripheral), zone of stasis (intermediate), and zone of coagulation (central).

BOX 38-3 Systemic Responses to Major Burn Injury

Pulmonary Response

Hyperventilation to meet increased metabolic needs

Gastrointestinal Response

Decrease in splanchnic perfusion that may lead to mucosal hemorrhage and transient adynamic ileus
Vomiting and aspiration
Stress ulcers

Musculoskeletal Response

Decreased range of motion from immobility and edema
Possible osteoporosis and demineralization (late)

Neuroendocrine Response

Increased amounts of circulating epinephrine and norepinephrine and transient elevation of aldosterone levels

Metabolic Response

Elevated metabolic rate, particularly with infection or surgical stress

Immune Response

Altered immunity, resulting in increased susceptibility to infection
Depressed inflammatory response

Emotional Response

Physical pain
Isolation from loved ones and familiar surroundings
Fear of disfigurement, deformities, and disability
Altered self-image
Depression

produce a classic local inflammatory response (pain, redness, swelling) without major systemic effects. If the wound covers a large area, however, these local tissue responses can produce effects throughout the body and life-threatening hypovolemia.

Systemic Response to Burn Injury

As local events occur at the injury site, other organ systems become involved in a general response to the stress caused by the burn. One of the earliest manifestations of the systemic effects of a large thermal injury is hypovolemic shock. This hypovolemic shock is a component of burn shock (described later in this chapter). Burn shock is associated with a decrease in venous return, decreased cardiac output, and increased vascular resistance. Burn shock can lead to renal failure. BOX 38-3 lists other systemic responses to major burn injury.

Classifications of Burn Injury

The amount of tissue damage may not be evident for hours or even days after a burn injury. However, burns should be assessed and classified as correctly as possible in the field to ensure the proper treatment and transport to an appropriate facility. Early assessment and classification also helps to monitor the progression of tissue damage.

DID YOU KNOW?

Skin Grafts

A skin graft is a patch of skin that is removed via surgery from one area of the body (autografting) and transplanted, or attached, to another area. Healthy skin is taken from an area on the patient's body called the donor site. (Commercial skin substitutes [heterografts] or temporary skin substitutes [cadaver allografts] are used in some patients instead of autografting.) Most grafts are split-thickness skin grafts; that is, the epidermis and part of the dermis are transplanted from the donor site. The donor site can be any area of the body (most often an area that is hidden by clothes, such as the buttock or lateral thigh). The transplanted graft is held in place by special pressure dressings, staples, fibrin glue, synthetic adhesives and/or tapes, or small sutures. The donor site area is covered with a sterile or clean dressing for 3 to 5 days.

Patients with deeper tissue loss may need a full-thickness skin graft; that is, the entire thickness of the skin is transplanted from the donor site. The graft of skin from the donor site includes the epidermis and full thickness of the dermis. It does not contain muscle or a blood supply. A new blood supply is established within 36 hours following transplantation. Common donor sites for full-thickness grafts include skin grafts (used in burns) and muscle flaps (used to fill soft-tissue defects) from the back or the abdominal wall. Full-thickness grafts require a longer recovery period than do split-thickness grafts. Most patients will be hospitalized for at least 7 to 10 days following the procedure. Possible complications of skin grafts include the following:

- Bleeding (which can be severe)
- Infection
- Loss of grafted skin (poor graft take)
- Scarring
- Reduced or lost skin sensation and/or increased sensitivity
- Chronic pain (rarely)
- Uneven skin surface, discoloration, and disfigurement

The process of excising and grafting large areas of burns is stressful. The surgery is tolerated poorly by patients with advanced age, other severe injuries (especially **smoke inhalation injury** and blunt trauma), and preexisting or coexisting medical conditions (especially diabetes or cardiovascular and peripheral vascular disease).

Depth of Burn Injury

Burns are classified in terms of depth as superficial, partial-thickness, and full-thickness.[6] Superficial and partial-thickness burns usually heal without surgery, if the burns are uncomplicated by infection or shock. A full-thickness burn usually requires a **skin graft**. Other depth classifications may be preferred by medical direction.

Superficial Burns

A **superficial burn** is also known as a first-degree burn. These burns characteristically are painful, red, and dry and blanch with pressure (**FIGURE 38-2**). Superficial burns usually occur after prolonged exposure to low-intensity heat or a short-duration flash exposure to a heat source. In these burns, only a superficial layer of epidermal cells is destroyed. The cells slough (peel away from healthy tissue underneath the wound) without residual scarring. Superficial burn injuries usually heal within 2 to 3 days, although some may take longer. An example of a superficial burn is sunburn.

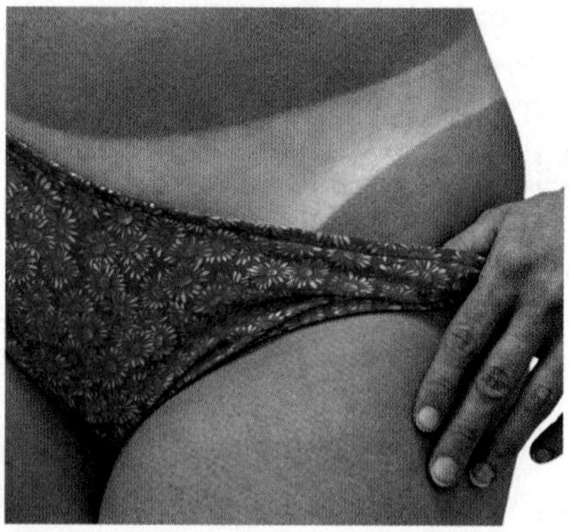

FIGURE 38-2 Superficial burn.

Partial-Thickness Burns

A **partial-thickness burn** is also known as a second-degree burn (**FIGURE 38-3**). These burns may be divided into two groups: superficial partial-thickness and deep partial-thickness wounds. The superficial partial-thickness injury is characterized by blisters and often is caused by skin contact with hot, but not boiling, water or other hot liquids, explosions producing flash burns, hot grease, and flame.

In superficial partial-thickness burns, injury extends through the epidermis to variable levels of the dermis and the basal layers of the skin may be

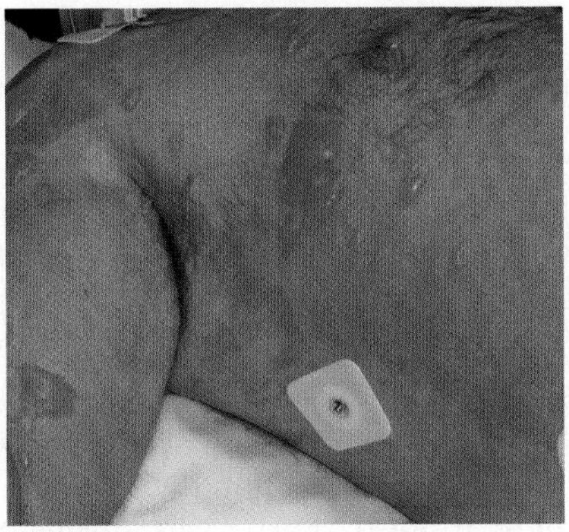

FIGURE 38-3 Partial-thickness burn.

damaged. The skin regenerates within a few days to a week. Edematous fluid infiltrates the dermal–epidermal junction, creating the blisters characteristic of this depth of wound. Intact blisters provide a seal that protects the wound from infection and excessive fluid loss. For this reason, blisters should not be broken in the prehospital setting unless it is a chemical burn. The injured area usually is red, wet, and painful and may blanch when the tissue around the injury is compressed. In the absence of infection, these wounds heal without scarring, usually within 14 days.

NOTE

The dermal layer of skin in children and older adults is significantly thinner than in the average adult. Therefore, a burn that looks like a partial-thickness burn may actually be a more serious full-thickness burn in these patients.

If the depth of the partial-thickness burn involves the reticular layer of the dermis, the burn is considered a deep partial-thickness burn. As in superficial partial-thickness burns, edema forms at the epidermal–dermal junction. Sensation in and around the wound may be diminished because of the destruction of basal layer nerve endings. The injury may appear red and wet or white and dry, but the appearance depends on the degree of vascular injury. Wound infection and subsequent sepsis and fluid loss are major complications of these injuries. If uncomplicated, deep partial-thickness burns generally heal within 3 to 4 weeks. Skin grafting may be needed to promote timely healing and minimize thick scar tissue formation. The formation of thick scar tissue may severely restrict joint movements and may cause persistent pain and disfigurement.

Full-Thickness Burns

In a **full-thickness burn** (also known as a third-degree burn), the entire thickness of the epidermis and dermis is destroyed along with variable amounts of hypodermis (subcutaneous tissue) destruction; thus, a skin graft is necessary for timely and proper healing (**FIGURE 38-4**). The wound is characterized by coagulation necrosis of the cells. The wound appears pearly white, charred, or leathery. A definitive sign of a full-thickness burn is a translucent surface in the depths of which thrombosed veins are visible. **Eschar**, a tough, nonelastic coagulated collagen of the dermis, is present in these injuries.

NOTE

Escharotomy is the surgical incision through the eschar to release constricting tissues. This surgery is sometimes performed to allow body tissue and organs to maintain normal perfusion and function. Escharotomy releases the constriction caused by burns but does not remove the eschar. Additional surgery may be required.

Sensation and capillary refill are absent in full-thickness burns because small blood vessels and nerve endings are destroyed. This often results in large plasma volume loss, infection, and sepsis. Natural wound healing may produce **contracture deformity** (a fixed tightening of the muscles, bones, ligaments, and skin that prevents normal movement). Severe scarring also may develop. Surgical intervention with skin grafting is necessary to close full-thickness wounds, minimize complications, and allow restoration of maximal function.

Some burn classifications also describe a full-thickness injury (sometimes called a fourth-degree burn) that penetrates the subcutaneous tissue, muscle, fascia, periosteum, or bone. These burns often result from incineration-type exposure and electrical burns

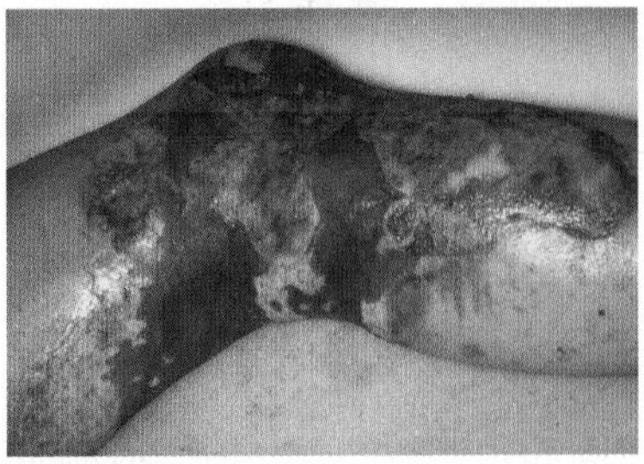

FIGURE 38-4 Full-thickness burn.

in which the heat is great enough to destroy tissues below the skin.

Extent and Severity of Burn Injury

There are several methods to evaluate the extent of burn injury. Two common methods include the **rule of nines** and the **Lund and Browder chart**. The paramedic should use a method for determining the extent of burn injury approved by medical direction. Use of any method to evaluate a burn injury should never delay patient care or transport.

Rule of Nines

The rule of nines commonly is used in the prehospital setting. The measurement divides the total body surface area (TBSA) into segments that are multiples of 9%. This method provides a rough estimate of burn injury size and is most accurate for adults and children older than 10 years. **FIGURE 38-5** explains the rule of nines.

> **CRITICAL THINKING**
> Why is the calculation of body surface area different for children younger than 10 years?

If the burn is irregularly shaped or has a scattered distribution throughout the body, the rule of nines is difficult to apply. In these cases, burn size can be estimated by visualizing the patient's hand as an indicator of percentage. This technique is called the *rule of palms*. The surface of the patient's hand, including fingers, equals about 1% of the TBSA.

> **NOTE**
> Only partial- and full-thickness burns are included when calculating TBSA. For large burns, TBSA may be calculated more easily by subtracting the percentage of unburned area from 100.

Lund and Browder Chart

The Lund and Browder chart (**FIGURE 38-6**) is a more accurate method of determining the area of burn

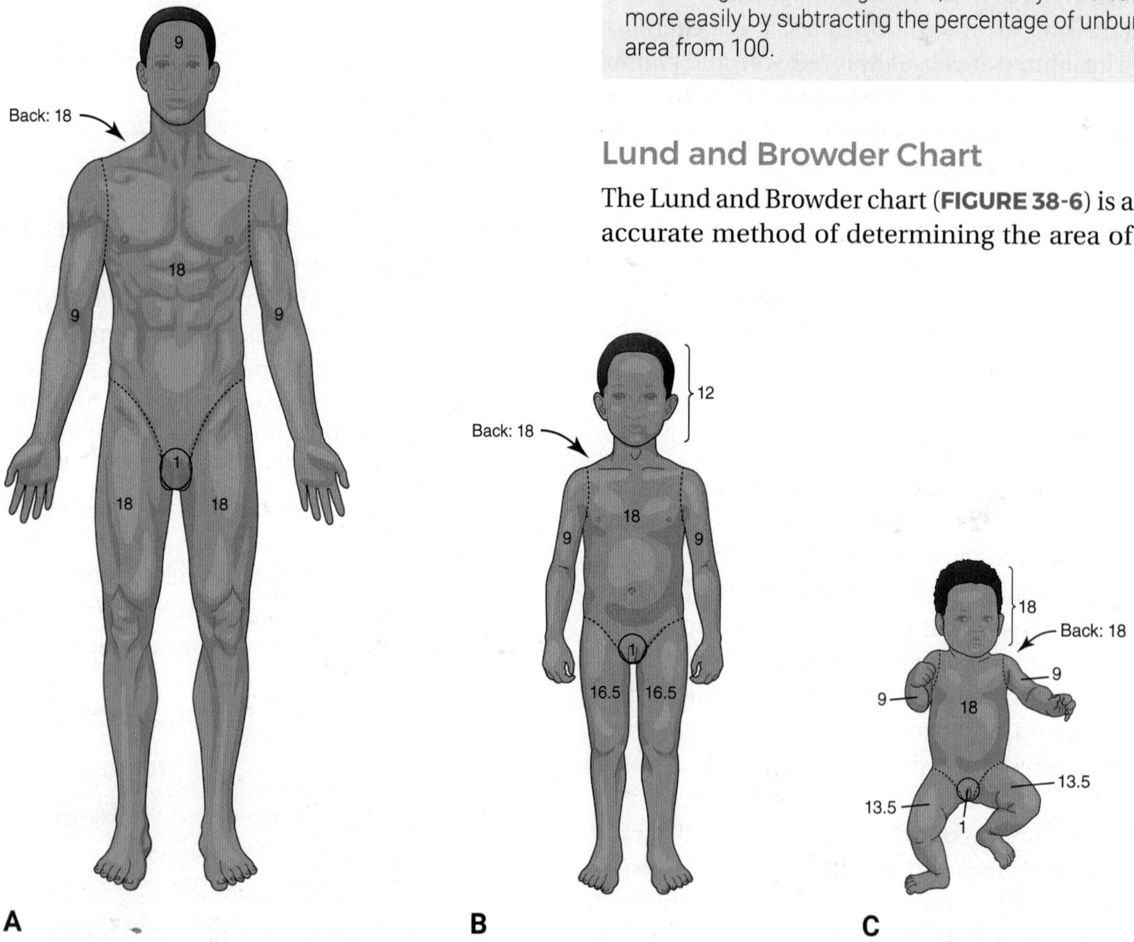

FIGURE 38-5 The rule of nines. **A.** Adult. **B.** Child. **C.** Infant.

Region	%
Head	
Neck	
Ant. Trunk	
Post. Trunk	
Right arm	
Left arm	
Buttocks	
Genitalia	
Right leg	
Left leg	
Total burn	

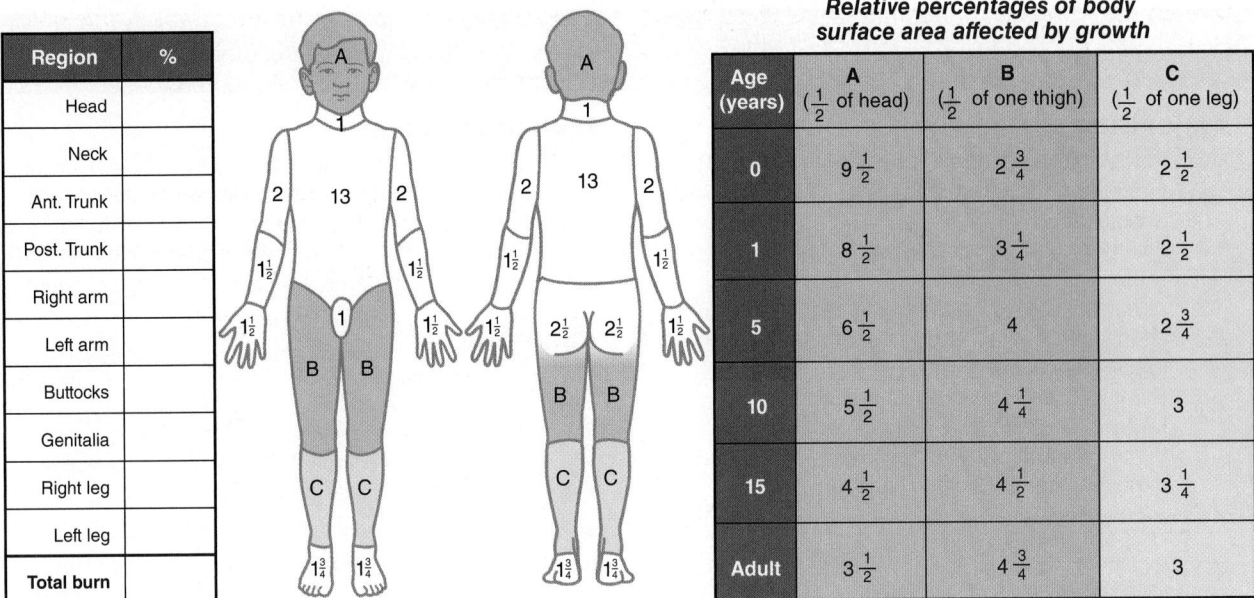

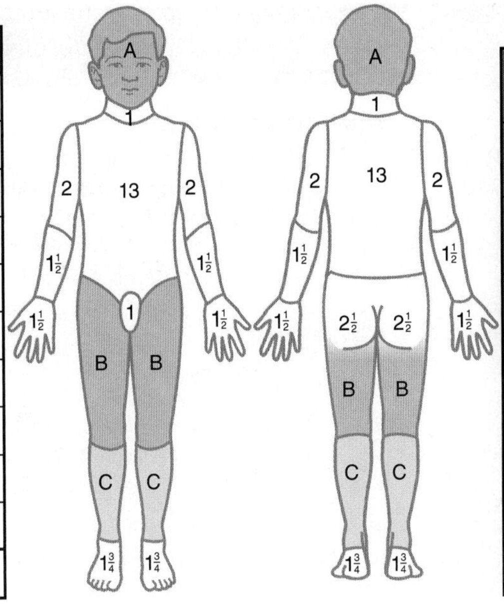

Relative percentages of body surface area affected by growth

Age (years)	A ($\frac{1}{2}$ of head)	B ($\frac{1}{2}$ of one thigh)	C ($\frac{1}{2}$ of one leg)
0	$9\frac{1}{2}$	$2\frac{3}{4}$	$2\frac{1}{2}$
1	$8\frac{1}{2}$	$3\frac{1}{4}$	$2\frac{1}{2}$
5	$6\frac{1}{2}$	4	$2\frac{3}{4}$
10	$5\frac{1}{2}$	$4\frac{1}{4}$	3
15	$4\frac{1}{2}$	$4\frac{1}{2}$	$3\frac{1}{4}$
Adult	$3\frac{1}{2}$	$4\frac{3}{4}$	3

FIGURE 38-6 Lund and Browder chart.

Data from Lund CC, Browder NC. The estimation of areas of burns. *Surg Gynecol Obstet.* 1944;79:352-358.

injury because it assigns specific numbers to each body part and allows for developmental changes in percentages of body surface area. For example, the adult head is 9% of TBSA, but the newborn head is 18% of TBSA.

American Burn Association Categorization

The American Burn Association has devised a method of categorizing burns to determine severity. The method is based on the extent, depth, and location of burn injury; age of the patient; etiologic agents involved; presence of inhalation injury; and coexisting injuries or preexisting illness. Using these criteria, burn injuries are categorized as major, moderate, and minor (BOX 38-4).

In determining severity, the paramedic also must consider factors such as the patient's age, the presence of concurrent medical or surgical problems, and the complications that accompany certain types of burns, such as those of the face and neck, hands and feet, and genitalia. For example, burns of the face and neck may cause respiratory compromise. They also may interfere with the ability to eat or drink. Burns of the hands and feet may interfere with ambulation and activities of daily living. Perineal burns present a high risk of infection because of the contaminants in this region. These burns may disrupt the normal patterns of elimination.

Burn Center Referral Criteria

Many emergency medical services (EMS) systems use categories or other criteria determined by medical direction as the basis for determining which patients need transport to specialized burn centers. (See the triage guidelines described in Chapter 36, *Trauma Overview and Mechanism of Injury.*) According to the Committee on Trauma of the American College of Surgeons and the American Burn Association, burn injuries usually requiring referral to a burn center include the following:[7]

1. Partial-thickness burns greater than 10% of TBSA.
2. Burns that involve the face, hands, feet, genitalia, perineum, or major joints.
3. Third-degree burns in any age group.
4. Electrical burns, including lightning injury.
5. Chemical burns.
6. Inhalation injury.
7. Burn injury in patients with preexisting medical disorders that could complicate management, prolong recovery, or affect mortality.
8. Burns and concomitant trauma (such as fractures) in which the burn injury poses the greatest risk of morbidity or mortality. If the trauma poses

BOX 38-4 Classification of Burn Severity

Major Burns

1. Partial-thickness burns greater than 25% of TBSA in adults or greater than 20% of TBSA in children or older adults
2. Full-thickness burns between 2% and 10% of TBSA
3. All burns involving the face, eyes, ears, hands, feet, or perineum that may result in functional or cosmetic impairment
4. Burns caused by caustic chemical agents
5. High-voltage electrical injury
6. Burns complicated by inhalation injury, major trauma, or patient status as a poor surgical risk

Moderate Burns

1. Partial-thickness burns 15% to 25% of TBSA in adults and 10% to 20% of TBSA in children or older adults
2. Full-thickness burns less than 10% of TBSA
3. Burns not involving risk to areas of specialized function such as the face, eyes, ears, hands, feet, or perineum

Minor Burns

1. Burns less than 15% of TBSA in adults or 10% of TBSA in children or older adults
2. Full-thickness burns less than 2% of TBSA
3. No functional or cosmetic risk to areas of specialized function

Modified from: American Burn Association. American Burn Association Injury Severity Grading System. *J Burn Care Rehabil.* 1990;11:98-104; with additional information from Hartford CE. Care of outpatient burns. In Herndon DN, ed. *Total Burn Care*. Philadelphia, PA: Saunders; 1996:71-80.

the greater immediate risk, the patient may be stabilized initially in a trauma center before transfer to a burn center. Physician judgment will be necessary in such situations and should be in concert with the regional medical control plan and triage protocols.

9. Burns in children. Children with burns should be transferred to a burn center verified to treat children. In the absence of a regional pediatric burn center, an adult burn center may serve as a second option for the management of pediatric burns.
10. Burn injury in patients who will require special social, emotional, or long-term rehabilitative intervention.

NOTE

Verification of burn centers is a joint program of the American Burn Association and the American College of Surgeons. It is a rigorous review program designed to verify that a burn center's resources meet the requirements for the provision of optimal care to burn patients from the time of injury through rehabilitation.

Pathophysiology of Burn Shock

As stated previously, shock can result from burns involving a large body surface area. **Burn shock** results from local and systemic responses to thermal trauma. The trauma leads to edema and accumulation of vascular fluid in the tissues in the area of injury. Locally, a brief initial decrease in blood flow to the area occurs (this is the *emergent phase*). This phase is followed by a considerable increase in arteriolar vasodilation. A concurrent release of vasoactive substances from the burned tissue causes increased capillary permeability, which in turn produces intravascular fluid loss and wound edema (the *fluid shift phase*). The fluid shifts cause cardiovascular changes such as a compromised cardiac output, increased systemic vascular resistance, and reduced peripheral blood flow.

NOTE

Hypovolemia caused by burn trauma usually is not generally seen in the prehospital setting. This is because burn edema develops over the first several hours after the burn. A hypovolemic patient with burns should be evaluated at the scene for other injuries that may be responsible for the volume loss.

Hypovolemia results from fluid loss in the injured tissues and fluid that evaporates from the body because of the loss of the skin. Despite the compensatory effort of the body to retain sodium and water, sodium is lost, and potassium is released into the body's extracellular fluid. The blood becomes concentrated. In severe burns, red blood cells may burst (hemolyze). When combined with hemolysis, rhabdomyolysis, and subsequent hemoglobinuria and myoglobinuria seen with major burns and electrical injury, this hypovolemic state can lead to renal failure (see Chapter 11, *General Principles of Pathophysiology*). Impaired peripheral blood flow can damage tissue further and can result in metabolic acidosis.

The greatest loss of intravascular fluid occurs in the first 8 to 12 hours. This loss is followed by a continued, moderate loss over the next 12 to 16 hours. At some point within 24 hours, the leaking of fluid from the cells greatly diminishes (this is the *resolution phase*). At this point, a balance between the intravascular space and the interstitial space is reached. Peripheral vascular resistance will increase in response to hypovolemia and the resulting decrease in cardiac output. With volume replacement, cardiac output can increase to levels above normal (this is the *hypermetabolic phase* of thermal injury) (**FIGURE 38-7**).

Assessment of the Burn Patient

As with any other trauma patient, emergency care for a burn patient begins with scene safety and the primary survey. In this assessment, the paramedic should recognize and treat injuries that pose a threat to life. In burn patients, however, the dramatic appearance of burns, the patient's intense pain, and the characteristic odor of burnt flesh may distract the paramedic from life-threatening problems. A confident assessment by the paramedic and direction of efforts away from the burn wound and toward the patient as a whole are crucial.

Primary Survey

The evaluation of the patient's airway is a major concern, particularly for the patient with an inhalation injury (described later in this chapter). The paramedic should observe for stridor (an ominous sign of airway narrowing), facial burns, soot in the nose or mouth, singed facial or nasal hair, edema of the lips and oral cavity, coughing, inability to swallow secretions in the pharynx, hoarse voice, and **circumferential burns** around the neck or thorax. Airway management should be aggressive with these patients (**FIGURE 38-8**).

> CRITICAL THINKING
>
> Consider a patient who has a large burn. Your initial assessment reveals that the airway is patent. Why should you perform frequent reassessment of the airway?

The paramedic should evaluate breathing for rate, depth, and the presence of wheezes, crackles, or rhonchi. The patient's circulatory status is evaluated

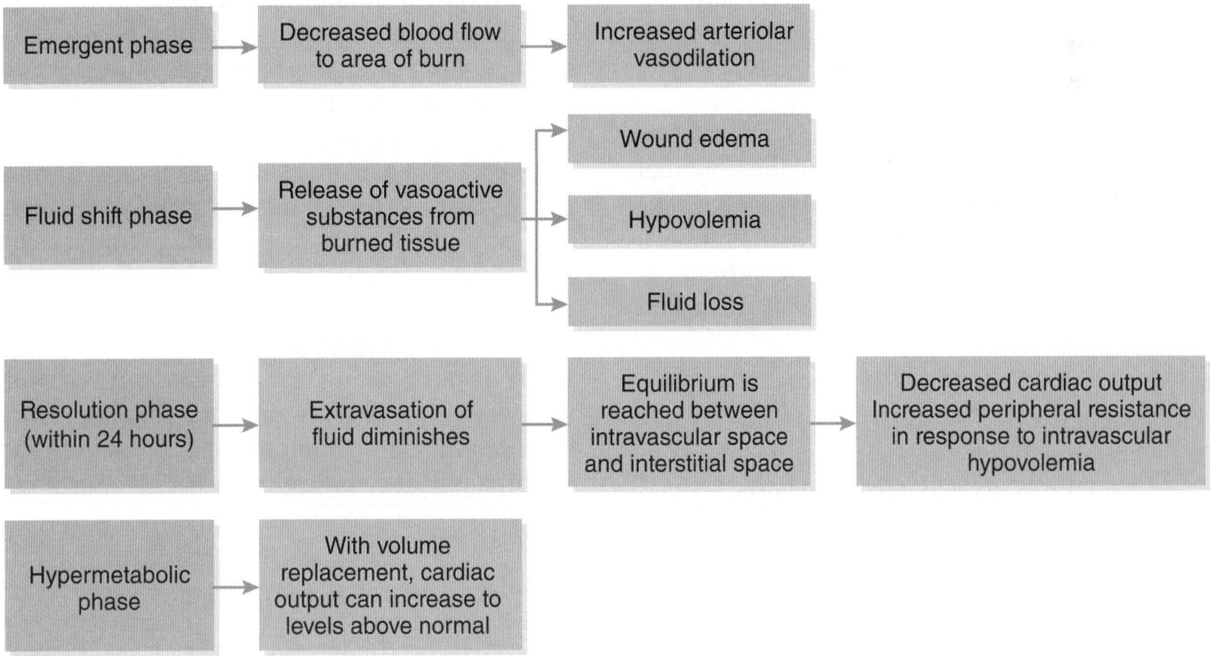

FIGURE 38-7 Phases of burn shock.

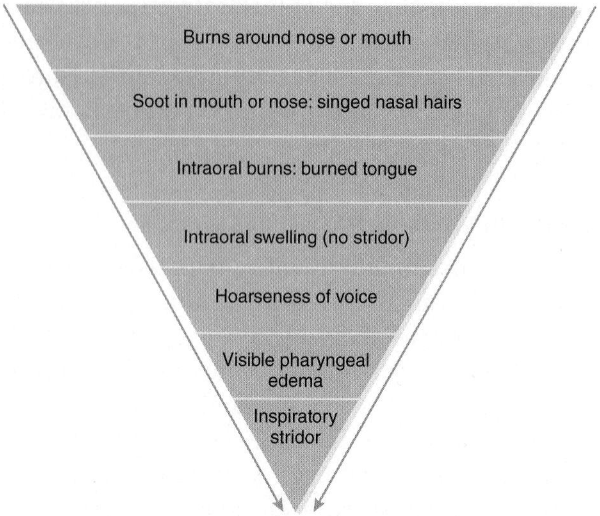

FIGURE 38-8 Indicators of decreasing size of airway (increasing probability of upper airway obstruction).

by assessing the presence, rate, character, and rhythm of pulses; checking capillary refill; assessing skin color and temperature; monitoring pulse oximetry, which may be inaccurate in the presence of carbon monoxide; and looking for obvious arterial bleeding. If there are any deviations from normal neurologic status, causes such as hypoxia, decreased cerebral perfusion from hypovolemia, and cerebral injury resulting from head trauma should be considered. After the primary survey, a history of the event should be obtained while performing the secondary assessment.

An accurate history from the patient or bystanders can help the paramedic to determine the potential for inhalation injury, concomitant trauma, or preexisting conditions that may influence the physical examination or patient outcome. When obtaining the patient history, the paramedic should ascertain the following information:

1. What is the patient's chief complaint (eg, pain, dyspnea)?
2. What were the circumstances of the injury?
   - Did the injury occur in an enclosed space?
   - Were explosive forces involved?
   - Were hazardous chemicals involved?
   - Is there related trauma?
3. What was the source of the burning agent (eg, flame, metal, liquid, chemical)?
4. Does the patient have any significant medical history?
5. What medications does the patient take (including recent ingestion of illegal drugs or alcohol)?
6. Did the patient lose consciousness at any time? (If so, suspect inhalation injury.)
7. What is the patient's status of tetanus immunization?

Physical Examination

At the start of the physical examination, the paramedic should obtain a full set of vital signs. The paramedic should obtain a blood pressure measurement from an unburned extremity, if available. If all extremities are burned, the paramedic may place sterile gauze under the blood pressure cuff and attempt to auscultate a blood pressure. Patients with severe burns or preexisting cardiac or medical illness should be monitored with pulse oximeter, end-tidal carbon dioxide detector, and electrocardiogram. Lead placement may need to be modified to avoid placing electrodes over burned areas (see Chapter 21, *Cardiology*). Field care and medical facility destination are determined by the depth, size, location, and extent of burned tissue and the presence of associated illness or injury.

General Principles in Burn Management

Goals for prehospital management of the severely burned patient include preventing further tissue injury, maintaining the airway, administering oxygen and ventilatory support, managing pain, providing fluid resuscitation, transporting to an appropriate medical facility, using clean technique to minimize the patient's exposure to infectious agents, maintaining body warmth, and providing psychological and emotional support. Patients with burns also should be evaluated for other types of trauma that pose a threat to life. Some will have additional injuries associated with the burn event, including blunt or penetrating trauma sustained in motor vehicle crashes, blast injury, and skeletal or spinal injury from attempts to escape the thermal source or contact with electric current.

> NOTE
>
> Some burns will be very painful for the patient. Medications used to manage pain may include morphine, fentanyl, hydromorphone, and others. Pain management is a crucial aspect of care for the burned patient.

Stopping the Burning Process

The first step in managing any burn is to stop the burning process. This step must be achieved with the safety of the emergency crew in mind because it often occurs in proximity to the source that caused the burn. With superficial burns, the burning process can be terminated by cooling the local area with cool tap water.[8] Ice-cold water, ice, snow, or ointments should not be applied to the burn. These agents may increase the depth and severity of thermal injury. In addition, ointments may impair or delay assessment of the injury when the patient arrives in the emergency department.

In cases of severe burns, the paramedic should move the patient rapidly and safely from the burning source to an area of safety, if possible. A person whose clothing is in flames or smoldering should be placed on the floor or ground and rolled in a blanket to smother the flames or should be doused with large quantities of the cleanest available room-temperature water. (Cool water to decrease skin temperature rapidly is preferred.) Contaminated water sources, such as lakes or rivers, should be avoided. These patients should never be allowed to run or remain standing. Running may fan the flame, and an upright position may increase the likelihood of the patient's hair being ignited.

NOTE

The National Fire Protection Association developed a training program called Stop, Drop, and Roll. The program was designed to teach children and adults that in the event their clothing catches fire, they should stop (do not run), drop (cover their face with their hands and drop to the ground in a prone position), and roll (to smother the fire until the flames are extinguished).

The paramedic should remove the patient's clothing completely while cooling the burn so that heat is not trapped under the smoldering cloth. If pieces of smoldering cloth have adhered to the skin, the paramedic should cut, not pull, the clothing and gently remove it. Melted synthetic fabrics that cannot be removed should be soaked in water to stop the burning process. After the burn is cooled and wet clothing is removed, the patient with a large body surface area injury should be covered with a dry sterile or clean dressing or clean sheet to prevent hypothermia. Local cooling of less than 9% TBSA can be continued longer than 30 minutes to relieve pain.

SHOW ME THE EVIDENCE

In a prospective 11-year study, researchers in Pennsylvania evaluated the incidence of hypothermia in burn patients and the factors associated with hypothermia in these patients. Of burn patients arriving by EMS to the emergency department during that period, 42% were hypothermic (temperature ≤97.7°F [36.5°C]). Factors associated with increased risk of hypothermia were burn of 20% to 39% TBSA (odds ratio [OR], 1.44; 95% confidence interval [CI], 1.17–1.79), burns of 40% or more TBSA (OR, 2.39; 95% CI, 1.57–3.64), age older than 60 years (OR, 1.5; 95% CI, 1.30–1.74), multisystem trauma (OR, 1.58; 95% CI, 1.19–2.09), Glasgow Coma Scale score of less than 8 (OR, 2.01; 95% CI, 1.46–2.78), incidents involving extrication (OR, 1.49; 95% CI, 1.30–1.71), and winter months (OR, 1.54; 95% CI, 1.33–1.79). Patient weight of greater than 198 pounds (90 kg) (OR, 0.63; 95% CI, 0.46–0.88) was associated with decreased risk of hypothermia. The researchers concluded that many burn patients are hypothermic on arrival and that prehospital providers should recognize risk factors and take measures to reduce the incidence.

Modified from: Weaver MD, Rittenberger JC, Patterson PD, et al. Risk factors for hypothermia in EMS-treated burn patients. *Prehosp Emerg Care.* 2014;18(3):335-341.

Airway, Oxygen, and Ventilation

The paramedic should evaluate the adequacy of airway and breathing in all burn patients. Humidified high-concentration oxygen (if available) should be given to any patient with severe burns. Breathing should be assisted as needed. Use of continuous pulse oximetry is indicated in these patients. If inhalation injury is suspected, the paramedic should observe the patient closely for signs of impending airway obstruction. Life-threatening laryngeal edema may be progressive and may make tracheal intubation difficult if not impossible. The decision to intubate these patients should not be delayed. Vocal changes and stridor are key signs of airway narrowing. The paramedic should make every attempt to intubate the patient's trachea with a normal-sized (not smaller) endotracheal tube. The lungs of these patients often are difficult to ventilate, even with an appropriately sized tube. The decision to intubate in the field should be guided by transport time to the receiving medical facility and indications of impending airway obstruction. End-tidal carbon dioxide monitoring is the gold standard in assessing the patient's ventilation status in the EMS setting.

Circulation

The need for fluid resuscitation is based on the severity of the injury, the patient's vital signs, and the transport time to the receiving medical facility. Some authorities contend that prompt intervention of intravenous (IV) therapy in the critically burned patient is essential to prevent long-term complications such as burn shock and renal failure. (The paramedic should consult with medical direction and follow local protocol regarding fluid replacement via the IV or intraosseous route.)

If IV therapy is to be performed, it should be initiated with a large-bore catheter in a peripheral vein in an unburned extremity. (The arm is the preferred site.) If an unburned site is not available, the paramedic may insert the catheter through burned tissue (superficial or partial thickness), although doing so increases the risk of subsequent infection. Care should be taken to secure the catheter with a sterile or clean dressing; tape may not adhere to the injured area as the tissue begins to leak fluid.

The administration of pain medication is an early intervention. Medical direction may recommend that patients with painful burns be given IV morphine or fentanyl, or other analgesic agents (eg, nitrous oxide). Some of these medications can cause vasodilation and respiratory depression. Thus, fluid resuscitation and ventilation support must be adequate. Other pharmacologic therapy that may be given after arrival in the emergency department includes topical applications (eg, silver sulfadiazine, special synthetic dressings), oral analgesics, and tetanus immunization.

CRITICAL THINKING

How should you administer pain medicine to a patient with a large burn? Why did you choose this route?

Sometimes transport of the burn patient is delayed or a lengthy interfacility transport may be anticipated. In either case, other patient care procedures may be required. One such procedure includes the placement of a nasogastric tube to prevent gastric distention or vomiting. Another procedure is the placement of an indwelling urinary catheter that will measure urine output and maintain patency of the urethra in patients with burns to the genitalia (see Chapter 51, *Acute Interventions for Home Care*).

NOTE

Urine output is a means to evaluate the effectiveness of fluid resuscitation. When the Parkland formula is used, the fluid is titrated to maintain urine output of 0.3 to 1.0 mL/kg per hour and a mean arterial pressure of 60 mm Hg or greater.

Modified from: Sole M, Klein DG, Moseley MJ. *Introduction to Critical Care Nursing*. 7th ed. Philadelphia, PA: Elsevier Saunders; 2017.

Fluid Replacement Formulae

Within minutes of a major burn injury, all capillaries in the circulatory system (not just those in the area of the burn) lose the ability to retain fluid. This increase in capillary permeability prevents the creation of an osmotic gradient between the intravascular and extravascular space and allows colloid solutions to equilibrate quickly across the capillaries and into the surrounding tissue. The process of burn shock continues for about 24 hours, at which time the normal capillary permeability is restored.[4] Therefore, therapy for burn shock is aimed at supporting the patient's vital organ function through the period of hypovolemic shock. Crystalloid solution is considered the fluid of choice in initial resuscitation. Because of the large volume of fluid often needed in burn patients, lactated Ringer solution is preferred over normal saline because it is less likely to contribute to acidosis.[9]

NOTE

Fluid resuscitation in patients with burn injury is controversial. As a rule, fluid resuscitation should be initiated in the prehospital setting in patients with burns of more than 20% of TBSA if IV access can be quickly accomplished. Transport should not be delayed to begin IV therapy.

Modified from: Marx JA, Hockberger RS, Walls RM. *Rosen's Emergency Medicine: Concepts and Clinical Practice*. 8th ed. St. Louis, MO: Saunders; 2014.

Several fluid resuscitation formulae consider body size and extent of burned body surface area. These formulae have proved clinically useful in replacing fluids. The two most common formulae for estimating fluid replacement are the Parkland formula and the rule of 10. The **Parkland formula** stipulates that one-half of the total calculated amount of fluid should be infused over the first 8 hours from the time of the injury, and the second half should be infused over the following 16 hours. Fluid resuscitation must be guided by regular monitoring of measures of hemodynamic function, including the patient's vital signs, respiratory rate, lung sounds, capillary refill, and, in some cases, urinary output. *When determining the percentage of burn for fluid resuscitation, the paramedic should calculate only partial- and full-thickness burns.*

Inadequate fluid resuscitation can lead to shock and renal failure. Excessive fluid administration may cause pulmonary and cardiac overload and increased edema.[10]

Parkland Formula

According to the Parkland formula, in the first 24 hours after injury, the paramedic should administer 4 mL/kg lactated Ringer solution or normal saline multiplied by the patient's body weight in kilograms multiplied by the percentage of TBSA burned:

- 50% of the calculated amount infused in the first 8 hours
- 25% of the calculated amount infused in the second 8 hours
- 25% of the calculated amount infused in the third 8 hours

Example: A patient who weighs 100 kg has 30% TBSA burns. Total fluid to be infused in the first 24 hours at 4 mL/kg is calculated as follows: 4 mL × 30% TBSA × 100 kg = 12,000 mL. Of the 12,000 mL, 6,000 mL should be infused in the first 8 hours at a rate of 750 mL/hr. Note that the volume of fluid actually infused may be adjusted according to patient needs as prescribed by medical direction.

The amount and type of fluids required after the first 24 hours are vastly different from those administered during the first 24 hours. Fluid replacement is dictated by the patient's response to the burn and the treatment regimen.

Rule of 10

The rule of 10 can be used to calculate fluid volume resuscitation for patients who weigh at least 40 kg.[11]

1. Calculate the TBSA to the nearest 10%.
2. Multiply the TBSA by 10 to determine the initial fluid rate in mL/hr (for patients 40–80 kg).
3. Add 100 mL/hr for every 10 kg of patient weight over 80 kg.

Example: A patient who weighs 100 kg has 32% TBSA burns. The TBSA is rounded to 30%, and 30% TBSA × 10 = 300 mL/hr initial fluid rate. Add 200 mL (patient weighs 20 kg over 80 kg) for a total hourly fluid rate of 500 mL/hr.

Special Considerations

All burn injuries warrant good patient assessment and care; however, burns of specific body regions require special consideration. These include burns to the face and extremities and circumferential burns.

Burns of the face swell rapidly and may be associated with airway problems. If not contraindicated by potential spinal trauma, the head of the stretcher should be elevated at least 30° to minimize the edema.[12] If the patient's ears are burned, the paramedic should avoid the use of a pillow to minimize additional injury to the area.

If burns involve the extremities or large areas of the body, the paramedic should remove all of the patient's rings, watches, and other jewelry as soon as possible to help to prevent vascular compromise with increased wound edema. Peripheral pulses should be assessed frequently, and burned limbs should be elevated above the patient's heart if possible.

> CRITICAL THINKING
> What life- or limb-threatening problems can develop from this swelling?

Burn injuries that encircle a body region can pose a threat to the patient's life or limbs. Circumferential burns that occur to an extremity may produce a tourniquet-like effect that may quickly compromise circulation and can cause irreversible damage to the limb. Circumferential burns of the chest can severely restrict movement of the thorax and may impair chest wall compliance significantly. If this occurs, the depth of respirations is reduced, tidal volume is decreased, and the patient's lungs may become difficult to ventilate, even by mechanical means. Definitive treatment for circumferential burns involves an in-hospital escharotomy to reduce compartment pressure and allow adequate blood volume to flow to and from the affected limb or thorax.

Inhalation Burn Injuries

Pulmonary complications result in 77% of deaths from residential fires.[13] Many are related to **inhalation injury**. The presence of inhalation injury increases the mortality from burns by 20%, and when combined with pneumonia by 60%.[14] Prehospital considerations in caring for patients with inhalation injury include recognition of the dangers inherent in the fire environment, awareness of the pathophysiologic principles of inhalation injury, and early detection and treatment of impending airway or respiratory problems.

Smoke inhalation most often occurs in a closed environment such as a building, a vehicle, or an airplane. Such injury is caused by the accumulation of toxic by-products of combustion. Inhalation injury also can occur in an open space. Therefore, all burn-injured persons should be evaluated for this injury. The following dangers contribute to inhalation injury in a fire environment:

- Heat
- Consumption of oxygen by the fire
- Production of carbon monoxide
- Production of other toxic gases such as cyanide and hydrogen sulfide

Inhalation injury also may occur in the absence of significant thermal injury from exposure to toxic gases (eg, carbon monoxide).

> NOTE
> Responding to a scene with a possibility of smoke inhalation injury also poses a threat to EMS personnel. Carbon monoxide meters and other testing devices to measure dangerous gases should be used to ensure scene safety.

Pathophysiology

Smoke inhalation and inhalation injury can produce a large number of complications. For this text, these complications are classified as carbon monoxide poisoning, inhalation injury above the glottis (supraglottic), and inhalation injury below the glottis (infraglottic).

Carbon Monoxide Poisoning

Carbon monoxide is a colorless, odorless, tasteless gas produced by incomplete burning of carbon-containing fuels. Carbon monoxide does not harm lung tissue physically; however, it displaces oxygen from the hemoglobin molecule, forming **carboxyhemoglobin**. The result is low circulating volumes of oxygen despite normal partial pressures. In addition, the presence of carboxyhemoglobin requires that tissues be hypoxic before oxygen is released from the hemoglobin to fuel the cells. This condition is reversible.

Carbon monoxide has about 250 times the attraction to hemoglobin that oxygen has. Therefore, small concentrations of carbon monoxide in inspired air can result in severe physiologic impairments, including tissue hypoxia, inadequate cellular oxygenation, inadequate cellular and organ function, and eventually death. The physical effects of carbon monoxide poisoning are related to the level of carboxyhemoglobin in the blood (BOX 38-5).

> NOTE
> The pulse oximeter is unreliable in determining effective oxygenation in a patient with carbon monoxide poisoning. (Pulse oximeters overestimate arterial oxygenation in patients with severe carbon monoxide poisoning.) Noninvasive CO-oximeters are available to assess for carbon monoxide. These devices use multiple-wavelength pulse oximetry to detect and measure carbon monoxide levels in the blood noninvasively and continuously. Measurements are taken by placing a sensor on a patient's fingertip, much the same way a pulse oximeter is used.
>
> *Modified from*: Chan ED, Chan MM, Chan MM. Pulse oximetry: understanding its basic principles facilitates appreciation of its limitations. *Respir Med.* 2013;107(6):789-799.

BOX 38-5 Physical Effects of Carbon Monoxide Blood Levels

Carbon monoxide levels less than 10% usually do not cause symptoms; these levels are common in smokers, traffic police officers, truck drivers, and others who are exposed to carbon monoxide chronically. At carbon monoxide levels of 20%, a healthy patient may complain of headache, nausea, vomiting, and loss of manual dexterity. At 30%, the patient may become confused and lethargic, and electrocardiogram abnormalities may be present. At levels between 40% and 60%, coma may develop. Levels above 60% typically are fatal. Tachypnea and cyanosis usually are not present in these patients because arterial oxygen tension is normal. Patients with high carboxyhemoglobin levels may have a skin appearance that is bright red, but more commonly, the patient has normal or pale skin and lip coloration.

Prehospital care for the patient with carbon monoxide poisoning includes ensuring a patent airway, providing adequate ventilation, and administering high-concentration oxygen. The half-life of carbon monoxide at room air is about 4 hours. This half-life can be reduced to 30 to 90 minutes if 100% oxygen and adequate ventilations are provided.[15] The use of hyperbaric oxygen therapy may be recommended in treating carbon monoxide poisoning. This therapy promotes the elimination of carboxyhemoglobin and improves mitochondrial function. The paramedic should follow local protocol.

In addition to carbon monoxide, other gases (eg, cyanide, hydrogen sulfide) may be released when some materials are burned. The inhalation of these toxic gases can result in inhalation poisoning (eg, thiocyanate intoxication). Inhalation poisoning may require pharmacologic therapy (eg, hydroxocobalamin), as described in Chapter 33, *Toxicology*.

CRITICAL THINKING

Can carbon monoxide poisoning be ruled out if the patient does not have these signs or symptoms?

Inhalation Injury Above the Glottis

The structure and function of the airway superior to the glottis make it susceptible to injury if exposed to high temperatures. The upper airway is vascular and has a large surface area, allowing the upper airway to normalize temperatures of inspired air. Because of this design, actual thermal injury to the lower airway is rare. The upper airway sustains the impact of injury when environmental air is superheated.

Thermal injury to the airway can result in immediate edema of the pharynx and larynx (above the level of the true vocal cords), which can progress rapidly to complete airway obstruction. Signs and symptoms of upper airway inhalation injury include the following (**FIGURE 38-9**):

- Facial burns
- Singed nasal or facial hairs
- Carbonaceous sputum
- Edema of the face, oropharyngeal cavity, or both
- Signs of hypoxemia
- Hoarse voice
- Stridor
- Brassy cough
- Grunting respirations

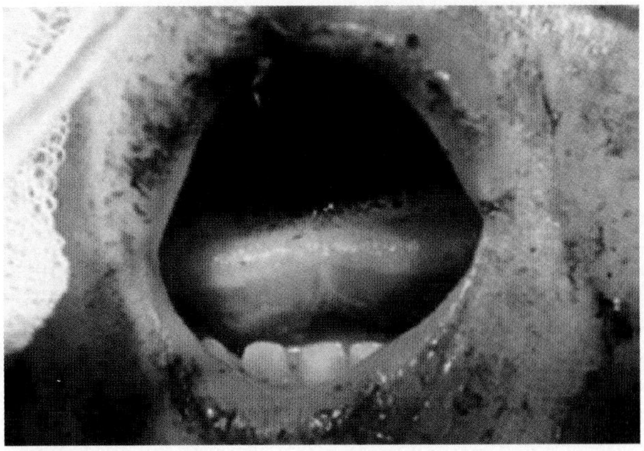

FIGURE 38-9 Signs of inhalation injury.

https://blogs.nejm.org/now/index.php/fire-related-inhalation-injury/2016/08/04/

Prompt assessment of the airway is crucial in these patients. The paramedic must establish and protect the airway. If impending airway obstruction is suspected, early intubation may be warranted; progressive edema can make intubation hazardous if not impossible. If available, video laryngoscopy should be employed to facilitate these difficult procedures. It may be necessary to establish access to the airway at the front of the neck (ie, cricothyrotomy) if there is too much laryngeal edema and the paramedic is unable to oxygenate and ventilate from above the vocal cords (see Chapter 15, *Airway Management, Respiration, and Artificial Ventilation*).

Inhalation Injury Below the Glottis

The two main mechanisms of direct injury to the lung tissue are heat and toxic material inhalation. Thermal injury to the lower airway is rare. One cause of such injury is the inhalation of superheated steam. This steam has 4,000 times the heat-carrying capacity of dry air.[4] Another cause is the aspiration of scalding liquids. Explosions are another cause. These injuries occur as the patient is breathing liquids, and breathing high concentrations of oxygen under pressure during an explosion.

Most lower airway injuries in fires result from the inhalation of toxic chemicals. Such chemicals include the gaseous by-products of burning materials. Signs and symptoms of lower airway injury may be immediate, but more often they are delayed. Signs and symptoms may begin several hours after the exposure and include the following:

- Wheezes
- Crackles or rhonchi

- Productive cough
- Signs of hypoxemia
- Spasm of bronchi and bronchioles

Prehospital care should be directed at maintaining a patent airway and providing high-concentration oxygen and ventilatory support. Specific airway and ventilatory management should be guided by online or direct medical direction. This management may include tracheal intubation and drug therapy with bronchodilators.

SHOW ME THE EVIDENCE

Researchers used data from a trauma registry to compare burn patients injured in incidents relating to methamphetamine production to another group of burn patients. Body surface area burned was similar in both groups. Methamphetamine-injured patients needed endotracheal intubation more often and required a larger fluid volume for resuscitation than did the controls. The methamphetamine group was more likely to have inhalation injury and to develop pneumonia than was the control group.

Modified from: Blostein PA, Plaisier BR, Maltz SB, et al. Methamphetamine production is hazardous to your health. *J Trauma*. 2009;66(6):1712-1717.

Chemical Burn Injuries

Caustic chemicals often are present in the home and workplace, and unintentional exposure is common. Three types of caustic agents often are associated with burn injuries: alkalis, acids, and organic compounds. They often have extreme pH values—less than 3 or greater than 11.[10] Alkalis are strong bases with a high pH and include hydroxides and carbonates of sodium, potassium, ammonium, lithium, barium, and calcium. These compounds commonly are found in oven cleaners, household drain cleaners, fertilizers, heavy industrial cleaners, and the structural bonds of cement and concrete. Strong acids are in many household cleaners, such as rust removers, bathroom cleaners, and swimming pool acidifiers (**FIGURE 38-10**).

Organic compounds are chemicals that contain carbon. Most organic compounds, such as wood and coal, are harmless chemicals; however, several organic compounds produce caustic injury to human tissue. These compounds include phenols and creosote and petroleum products such as gasoline. In

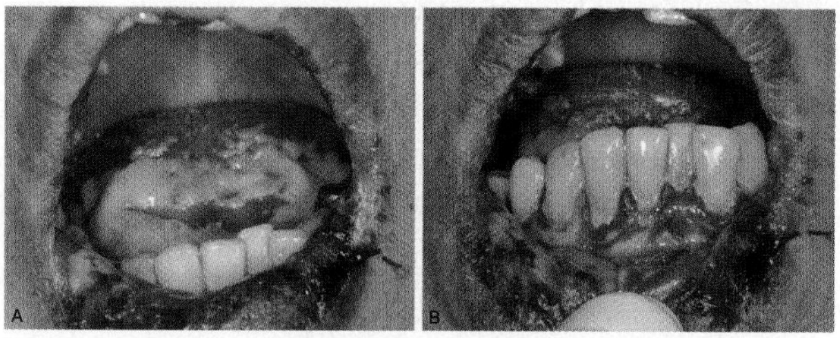

FIGURE 38-10 Intraoral chemical burns from ingesting bleach.

Reproduced with permission from: Naganawa T, Murozumi H, Kumar A, Okuyama A, Okamoto T, Ando T. Intraoral chemical burn in an elderly patient with dementia. *Int J Burns Trauma*. 2015:5(3):79-81.

addition to their role in producing chemical burns, organic compounds may be absorbed by the skin. As described in Chapter 33, *Toxicology*, absorption in turn may cause serious systemic effects. Complications include cellulitis, pneumonia, and respiratory failure. The severity of chemical injury is related to the type of chemical agent, concentration and volume of the chemical, and duration of contact.

Assessment

While obtaining the patient history, the paramedic should collect facts about the exposure. When dealing with a chemical exposure, the paramedic should determine the following:

- Type of chemical substance (If the container is available and can be transported safely, it should be taken to the medical facility.)
- Concentration of chemical substance
- Volume of chemical substance
- Mechanism of injury (eg, local immersion of a body part, injection, splash)
- Time of contamination
- First aid administered before EMS arrival
- Appearance (Chemical burns vary in color.)
- Pain

Management

As with all burn injuries, the safety of the rescuers must be the first priority in managing the patient with chemical injury. Law enforcement, fire service, and special rescue personnel may be needed to secure the scene before entry. The paramedic must consider the use of protective gear before entering the scene. Depending on the scene and the chemical agent or agents, decontamination may be required. Personal protection may include gloves, eye shields, protective garments, and appropriate breathing apparatus. A response to a hazardous materials incident requires special safety considerations and trained rescue personnel (see Chapter 56, *Hazardous Materials Awareness*).

The treatment of chemical injuries varies little from that of thermal burns during the primary survey. Treatment is directed at stopping the burning process, which can best be achieved by the following actions:

1. Remove all of the patient's clothing, including shoes. Clothing can trap concentrated chemicals.
2. Brush off powdered chemicals.
3. Remove blisters that may contain chemicals.
4. Irrigate the affected area with copious amounts of water.[11]
   - In otherwise stable patients, irrigation takes priority over transport. That is the case unless irrigation can be continued en route to the emergency department.
   - If a large body surface area is involved, a shower should be used for irrigation, if available.

Chemical Burn Injury to the Eyes

Chemical exposure to the eyes may cause damage ranging from superficial inflammation (chemical conjunctivitis) to severe burns. Patients with these conditions have local pain, visual disturbance, lacrimation (tearing), edema, and redness of surrounding tissues. After removing patients from the contaminated area, management guidelines include flushing the eyes with water. Flushing can be done by using a mild flow from a hose, IV tubing, or water from a container. The affected eye should be irrigated from the medial to the lateral aspect. This technique will help to avoid flushing the chemical into the unaffected eye. Irrigation should be continued during transport. If contact lenses are present, they should be removed. When retracting the lids to irrigate the eyes, the paramedic should take care to apply pressure only to the bony structures surrounding the eye. Pressure on the globe should be avoided.

Some EMS systems use nasal cannulas to irrigate both eyes simultaneously. The cannula is placed over the bridge of the nose, with the nasal prongs pointing down toward the eyes. The cannula is attached to an IV administration set using normal saline or lactated Ringer solution, and the fluid is run continually into both eyes (**FIGURE 38-11**). Irrigation lenses (eg, Morgan therapeutic lens) may be useful for prolonged eye irrigation in adults provided that edema is absent and there are no lacerations or penetrating wounds of the globe or eyelids (**FIGURE 38-12**). Anesthetic drops such as tetracaine may be considered to relieve pain.[11] A chemical burn to the eye can be frightening for the patient. The patient may fear loss of sight from the injury. The paramedic should attempt to calm the patient and explain the importance of thorough eye irrigation, which may be uncomfortable. This approach often improves the patient's cooperation. Patients who are wheezing should be treated for bronchospasm.

Use of Antidotes or Neutralizing Agents

According to the American Burn Association, no agent has been found to be superior to water for treating

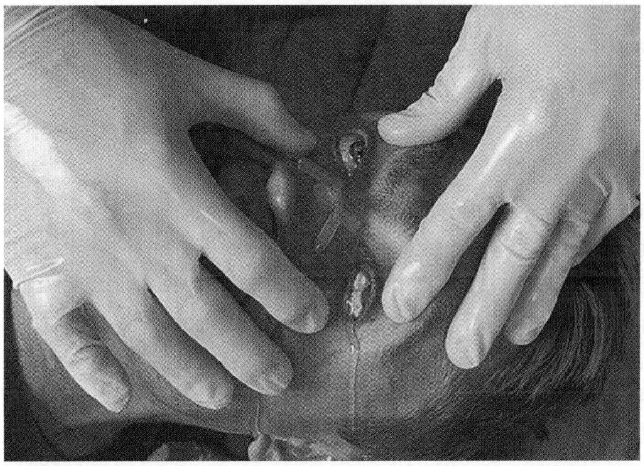

FIGURE 38-11 Use of nasal cannula for eye irrigation.

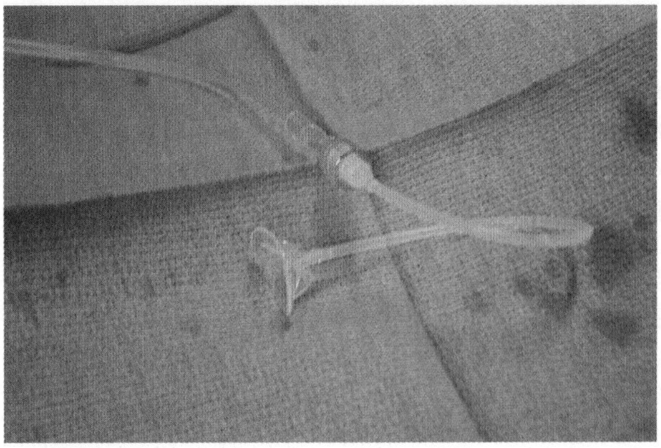

FIGURE 38-12 Commercial irrigation lens.

Courtesy of Dr. Jeffrey Guy

most chemical burns.[16] Thus, the use of antidotes or neutralizing agents should be avoided in initial prehospital management of most burn injuries. Many neutralizing agents produce heat, and they may increase injury when applied to the wound.

In special circumstances, such as when an industrial complex within a response area is known to use a chemical agent with a specific antidote, medical direction may elect to have the EMS stock the neutralizer. In this case, paramedics should receive special training on the indications, contraindications, use, and side effects of these agents.

Specific Chemical Injuries

The main treatment for most chemical burns is copious irrigation with water; however, a number of chemicals produce injuries that necessitate further discussion. These chemicals include petroleum, hydrofluoric acid, phenols, ammonia, chlorine, and alkali metals. Personal safety is a priority when working around any of these chemicals.

Petroleum

In the absence of flame, products such as gasoline and diesel fuel can cause significant chemical burns if prolonged contact occurs. This situation may occur, for example, with entrapment in a vehicle that is surrounded by spilled gasoline. At first, the injury may appear to be only a superficial or partial-thickness burn. In fact, though, it may be a full-thickness injury. Systemic effects such as central nervous system depression, organ failure, and death may result from the absorption of various hydrocarbons.

Hydrofluoric Acid

Hydrofluoric acid is one of the most corrosive materials known. The acid is used in industry for cleaning fabrics and metals, for glass etching, and in the manufacture of silicone chips for electronic equipment. The hydrogen ion and fluoride ion are damaging to tissue. Fluoride hinders several chemical reactions that are required for cell survival. Fluoride also continues to penetrate and kill cells even when it is neutralized by binding to calcium or magnesium. Thus, endogenous or exogenous hydrofluoric acid has the potential to produce deep, painful, and severe injuries. If greater than 20% TBSA is involved, the patient may experience severe hypocalcemia. This condition can develop rapidly and may include muscle spasms, seizure, prolonged QT interval, ventricular dysrhythmias, and even death.[10] Even the most minor-appearing wounds that involve hydrofluoric acid should be evaluated at a proper medical facility.

Irrigation of the exposed area with large amounts of water for 15 minutes should be started immediately. Treatment may include the following interventions, if the resources are available:

1. Apply calcium gluconate gel topically over the wounds for at least 20 minutes. This product is available commercially or can be prepared by mixing calcium gluconate solution with water-soluble gel.
2. If ingested or large skin exposure, consider administration of calcium gluconate after consulting with medical direction.

Phenol

Phenol (carbolic acid) is an aromatic hydrocarbon. Phenol is derived from coal tar and is used widely in industry as a disinfectant in cleaning agents. Phenol also is used in the manufacture of plastics, dyes, fertilizers, and explosives. Skin contact with phenol can result in local tissue coagulation and systemic toxicity if the agent is absorbed. A soft-tissue injury from phenol exposure may be painless because of the anesthetic properties of the agent. Minor exposures may cause central nervous system depression and dysrhythmias. Patients with significant exposures (10% to 15% TBSA) may require systemic support. These patients should be observed carefully for signs of respiratory failure.

Wounds should be irrigated with large volumes of water. After irrigation, medical direction may advise that the wound be swabbed with a suitable solvent such as glycerol, vegetable oil, or soap and water to bind phenol and prevent its systemic absorption.

Ammonia

Ammonia is a noxious, irritating gas. It is a strong alkali that is very soluble in water. Ammonia is hazardous if introduced into the eye and may result in corneal burns, ulcers, tissue necrosis, and blindness. The patient with an ammonia burn to the eye probably will have tears and swelling or spasm of the eyelids. These injuries must be irrigated with water or a balanced salt solution for up to 24 hours.

When exposed, patients may complain of a unique sharp smell and experience irritation and burning in the nasopharynx. Other signs and symptoms include skin or airway burns, sneezing, coughing, altered mental status, dyspnea, chest tightness, wheezing, vocal changes, noncardiogenic pulmonary edema, and possible upper airway obstruction.[11]

> NOTE
> Anhydrous ammonia burns may be encountered as a result of methamphetamine lab explosions (see Chapter 33, *Toxicology*).

Respiratory injury from ammonia vapors depends on two factors: the concentration and the duration of exposure. For example, short-term, high-concentration exposure usually results in upper airway edema. Long-term, low-concentration exposure may damage the lower respiratory tract. The initial care for patients with respiratory injury includes high-concentration oxygen administration, ventilatory support as needed, and rapid transport to an appropriate medical facility.

Chlorine

Patients exposed to chlorine have signs and symptoms similar to those of ammonia exposure; however, they are more likely to have bronchiolar burns and develop wheezing. Noncardiogenic pulmonary edema may develop within 6 to 24 hours after a significant exposure.

Alkali Metals

Sodium and potassium are highly reactive metals, and they can ignite spontaneously. Water generally is contraindicated when these metals are imbedded in the skin because they react with water and produce large amounts of heat. Physically removing the metal or covering it with oil minimizes the thermal injury.

Electrical Burn Injuries

Electrical injuries account for about 3% of admissions to burn centers.[2] Good patient care and personal safety at the scene of an electrical burn injury depend on understanding how electricity flows (current) through the body (**BOX 38-6**).

Types of Electrical Injury

Three basic types of injury may occur as a result of contact with electric current: direct-contact burns, arc injuries, and flash burns. Direct-contact burns occur when electric current directly penetrates the resistance of the skin and underlying tissues. The hand and wrist are common entrance sites, and the foot is a common exit site (**FIGURE 38-13**). Although the skin may initially resist current flow, continued contact with the source lessens resistance and permits increased current flow. The greatest tissue damage occurs directly under and adjacent to the contact points and may include fat, fascia, muscle, and bone. Tissue destruction may be massive at the entrance and exit sites; however, injury to the area between these wounds is what poses the greatest threat to the patient's life.

Arc injuries occur when a person is close enough to a high-voltage source that the current between two contact points near the skin overcomes the resistance in the air, passing the current flow through the air to the bystander. Temperatures generated by these sources can be as high as 3,632°F to 7,232°F (2,000°C to 4,000°C). The arc may jump as far as 10 feet (3 m).[17]

Flame and flash burn injuries can occur when the heat of electric current ignites a nearby combustible source. Common injury sites include the face and eyes (welder's flash). Flash burns also may ignite a person's clothing or cause fire in the surrounding environment. No electric current passes through the body in this type of burn.

Effects of Electrical Injury

Electrical injuries often are unpredictable. They vary based on amps of current, patient, body areas burned, and current pathway, yet certain physiologic effects should be expected by the paramedic crew.

The skin is almost always the first point of contact with electric current. Direct contact and passage of the current through tissue may cause wide areas of coagulation necrosis. The entrance site is often a bull's-eye wound. The site may appear dry, leathery, charred, or depressed. The exit wound may be ulcerated and may appear exploded. Areas of tissue may be missing.

Oral burns often are seen in children younger than 2 years. These wounds usually are caused by chewing or sucking on a low-tension electrical cord. Oral burns

BOX 38-6 Principles of Tissue Damage Caused by Electricity

Tissue damage produced by electric current is a function of the following six factors:

1. **Amperage.** Amperage is a measure of the current flow (intensity) per unit of time. One ampere is a passage of 1 coulomb of charge per second past any point in the circuit; thus, a 10-amp flow means that 10 coulombs of electricity are passing a point per second.
2. **Voltage.** Voltage is a continuous force (tension) applied to any electrical circuit that produces a flow of electricity. Volts are the driving force for electric current. One volt is the force needed to drive 1 amp of current in a circuit with 1 ohm of resistance. High-voltage electrical injuries result from contact with a source of 1,000 volts or greater. High-tension accidents usually range from 7,200 to 19,000 volts, yet they may involve current with as high as 100,000 to 1 million amps.
3. **Resistance.** An ohm is a measure of the resistance of an electrical conductor. Electrical resistance is composed of four factors: (1) resistivity, the capacity of a material to resist current flow; (2) the size of the object pathway; (3) the length of the object pathway; and (4) temperature. Resistance to the flow of electricity varies greatly within the body because various tissues have different resistance to current flow. Tissue resistance to electrical flow in the body is highest in bone and decreases progressively through the fat, skin, muscle, blood, and nerve tissue.
4. **Type of current.** Two basic forms of electric current are in common usage: direct current (DC) and alternating current (AC). The type of current can influence patterns and severity of injury. DC flows in one direction only. It often is used in industry and is the type of current produced by batteries. DC commonly is used in electrosurgical devices and defibrillators and is characterized by high amperage and low voltage.

   AC reverses the direction of flow at regular intervals (60-cycle current has 60 reversals per second). These alterations in current direction can cause tetanic muscle contractions. These contractions may freeze the person to the source until the current is terminated. Household current in the United States generally is AC and either 120 or 220 volts. AC is a more common cause of electrical injury.
5. **Current pathway.** Electricity normally flows along a continuous pathway, which is known as an electrical circuit. The current pathway can be unpredictable; however, as a rule, low-voltage current (less than 1,000 volts) follows the path of least resistance. High-voltage current follows the shortest path. In either case, the greater the current flow, the greater the heat generated.

   The pathway of the current through the body is important because it gives a clue as to what anatomic structures are damaged. For example, if the current travels from one hand to the other, it may flow across the heart and provoke ventricular fibrillation or other dysrhythmias.
6. **Duration of flow.** Tissue injury results from the conversion of electrical energy into heat. The amount of heat produced is directly proportional to the square of the current strength multiplied by the resistance of the tissue multiplied by the duration of the current flow (Joule law). Therefore, injury is directly proportional to the duration of contact with the electrical source.

Modified from: Spies C, Trohman RG. Narrative review: electrocution and life-threatening electrical injuries. *Ann Intern Med.* 2006;145(7):531-537.

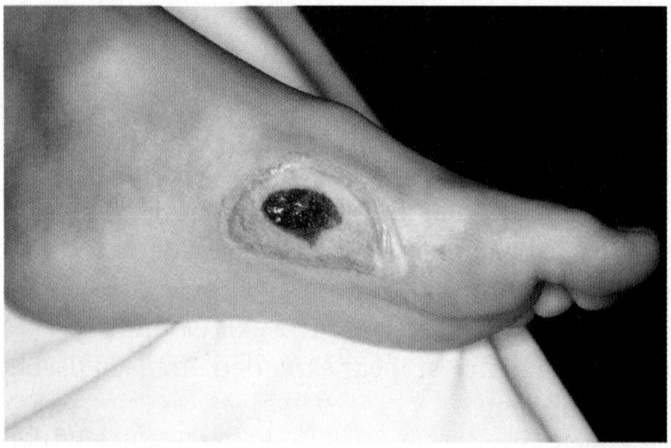

A

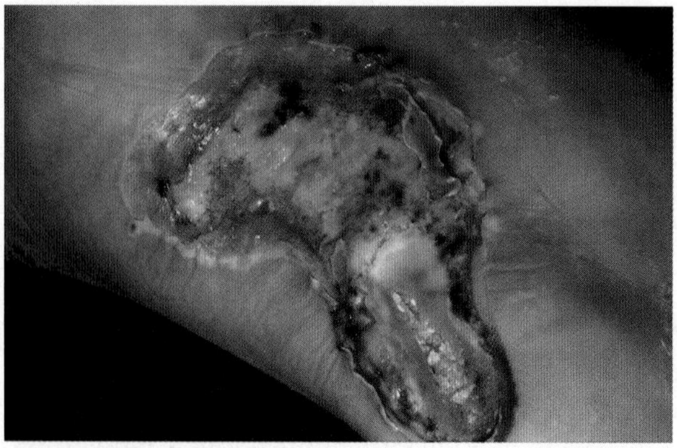

B

FIGURE 38-13 Direct-contact burn of the foot. **A.** Entry wound. **B.** Exit wound. The injuries shown here are several days to a week old.

may be associated with injury to the tongue, palate, and face. These patients should be transported to a burn center.

Hypertension and tachycardia associated with a large release of catecholamines is a common finding in electrical injury. Electric current also may cause significant dysrhythmias (including immediate ventricular fibrillation and asystole) and damage to the myocardium as it passes through the body. The patient may have suffered cardiac arrest. If early rescue and resuscitation can be initiated, success rates are high.

Nerve tissue is a good conductor of electric current. Thus, nerve tissue often may be affected in electrical injuries. Central nervous system damage may result in seizures or coma with or without focal neurologic findings. Peripheral nerve injury may lead to motor or sensory deficits. These deficits may be permanent. If the current passes through the brainstem, respiratory arrest or depression, cerebral edema, or hemorrhage may rapidly lead to death.

Electrical injury can cause extensive necrosis of blood vessels. This damage may not be evident upon the arrival of EMS. However, such injuries can cause immediate or delayed internal hemorrhage or arterial or venous thrombosis and embolism with subsequent complications.

Damage within the extremities after an electrical burn is similar to that sustained by crush injury (described in Chapter 37, *Bleeding and Soft-Tissue Trauma*). Severe muscle necrosis releases myoglobin. Bursting of the red blood cells (hemolysis) releases hemoglobin. Both of these large molecules can precipitate in the renal tubules, producing acute renal failure. Some patients may require amputation of the affected extremity, which results from decreased circulation and compartment syndrome. In the electrocuted patient, severe muscle spasms can produce bony fractures. These spasms also may produce dislocations, even of major joints. A patient may fall after the electrical shock and sustain skeletal trauma (including damage to the cervical spine).

Acute renal failure can be a serious complication from significant direct-contact electrical injuries. Acute renal failure may result from a combination of myoglobin or hemoglobin sludging in the renal tubules, disseminated intravascular coagulation caused by tissue damage, hypovolemic shock, and DC damage. Acute renal failure is not of immediate consequence in the prehospital setting, yet prompt fluid resuscitation and management of shock may have a positive impact on these patients.

Ventilation may be impaired when electrical burns produce central nervous system injury or chest wall dysfunction. If the respiratory center is disrupted, hypoventilation can lead to immediate patient death. Contact with any AC sources also has been known to produce respiratory arrest and death from tetany of the muscles of respiration.

Conjunctival and corneal burns and ruptured tympanic membranes may be found in some electrical injuries. Cataracts and hearing loss also may appear as late as 1 year after the event.

A number of other internal structures may be damaged from electrical injury, including the abdominal organs and urinary bladder. Submucosal hemorrhage may occur in the bowel; various forms of ulceration are possible. Each patient requires a thorough physical assessment and a high degree of suspicion for associated trauma.

Assessment and Management

Patient assessment should begin by ensuring that no hazards exist for the rescuers or bystanders. If the patient is still in contact with the electrical source, the paramedic should summon the electrical company, fire department, or other specially trained personnel before approaching the patient. Patient intervention may not begin until the scene is safe.

> CRITICAL THINKING
>
> What will you do if you respond to a scene and there is a child still in contact with electric current and having tetanic movements? A large crowd has gathered and is screaming at you to help. The fire department is 3 minutes away. How will you feel?

Primary Survey

The primary survey should proceed as it does for all other trauma patients. The paramedic should take care to stabilize the cervical spine. If the patient is not breathing, assisted ventilation should begin immediately. The paramedic should perform intubation as soon as possible because apnea may persist for lengthy periods. A patient who is breathing should have a patent airway maintained. Respirations should be supported with supplemental high-concentration oxygen as well. If the patient is in cardiac arrest, the paramedic should initiate resuscitation efforts according to protocol. If possible, a history of the event should be obtained that includes the following:

- Patient's chief complaint (eg, injury, disorientation)
- Source, voltage, and amperage of the electrical injury
- Duration of contact
- Level of consciousness before and after the injury
- Significant medical history

NOTE

The source, voltage, and type of current (AC versus DC) are essential information for the attending physician to estimate the internal damage from the electric current.

Physical Examination

The physical examination should be thorough. The paramedic should search for entrance and exit wounds, or any associated trauma caused by tetany or a fall. The paramedic should recall that there may have been multiple pathways of current, which would mean multiple wounds. The paramedic should remove all of the patient's clothing and jewelry and examine the areas between the patient's fingers and toes for sites of entry or exit. Distal pulses, motor function, and sensation in all extremities should be assessed and documented to monitor for possible development of compartment syndrome. The paramedic should cover entrance and exit wounds with sterile or clean dressings and should manage any associated trauma appropriately.

Internal damage from electric current may be much more significant than external wounds. Frequent reassessment is necessary because of the progressive nature of electrical injury. In addition, electrocardiogram monitoring should be implemented at the scene and continued during patient transport. As previously discussed, electrical injury may cause a variety of dysrhythmias, some of which can be lethal.

Management

Early administration of fluids is vital for patients with severe electrical injury. Fluid administration helps to prevent hypovolemia and subsequent renal failure. If possible, the paramedic should establish two large-bore IV lines. These lines should be in an extremity without entry or exit wounds. The fluid of choice generally is lactated Ringer solution or normal saline without glucose. The flow rate should be determined by the patient's clinical status.

In the emergency department or during interhospital transfer, the patient's IV fluid rates will be regulated to maintain a urine output of 1 to 1.5 mL/kg per hour.[8] This rate decreases the potential for renal damage caused by myoglobin accumulation. Emergency department management may include the administration of sodium bicarbonate to help maintain an alkaline urine. Alkalinity in turn increases the solubility of hemoglobin and myoglobin and decreases the risk of renal failure.

Apply dry sterile or clean dressings to burn wounds. The patient will often have significant pain, so analgesia should be administered according to local protocol.

Lightning Injury

Lightning strikes the Earth about 8 million times each year and accounts for about 35 deaths each year.[18] Lightning can deliver DC of up to 200,000 amps at a potential of 100 million or more volts, with temperatures up to 50,000°F (27,760°C), which is five times hotter than the surface of the sun.[19] Lightning injuries can occur from a direct strike or by a side flash (splash) between a person and a nearby object that has been struck by lightning. About 10% of those struck by lightning die, leaving 90% with various degrees of disability.[20] Lightning strikes are most common in Florida, Louisiana, and Mississippi.[21]

Lightning strikes produce tissue injuries that differ from other types of electrical injury because the pathway of tissue damage often is *over* rather than *through* the skin (**FIGURE 38-14**). The duration of the lightning is short (0.01–0.001 second); thus, skin burns are less severe than are burns seen with other high-voltage current. Full-thickness burns are rare. Common lightning burns are linear, feathery, and punctate (pinpoint). Depending on the severity of the strike, cardiac and respiratory arrest can occur.

Lightning injuries may be classified as minor, moderate, or severe. The patients with minor lightning injuries usually are conscious. These patients often are confused and amnesic. Burns or other signs of injury are rare. The vital signs of these patients usually are stable.

The patients with moderate injury may be combative or comatose. These patients may have associated injuries from the impact of the lightning strike.

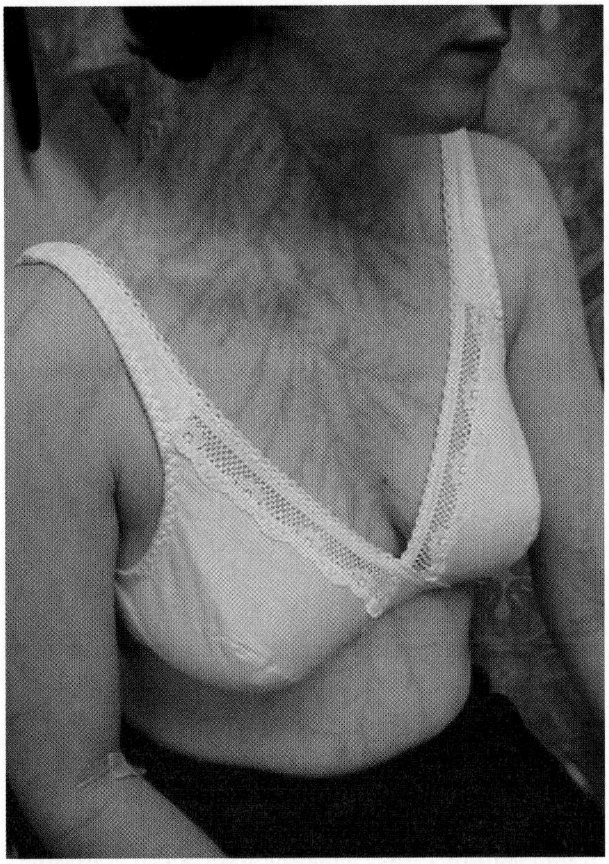

FIGURE 38-14 Lightning injuries may produce linear or feathery burn patterns depending on the severity of the strike.

Superficial and partial-thickness burns are common, as is tympanic membrane rupture. These patients may have serious internal organ damage and should be observed carefully for signs and symptoms of cardiorespiratory dysfunction.

Severe lightning injuries include those that cause immediate brain damage, seizures, respiratory paralysis, and cardiac arrest. The prehospital care is directed at basic and advanced life support measures and rapid transport to a proper facility.

Assessment and Management

Like all other emergency responses, scene safety is the first priority. If the electrical storm is still in progress, all patient care should take place in a sheltered area. To prevent injury from subsequent lightning strikes, the paramedic crew should stay away from objects that project from the ground, such as trees, fences, and high buildings. The crew also should avoid areas of open water. If rescue attempts in an open area are necessary, the paramedic should stay low to the ground.

The prehospital management of lightning injuries is the same as that for other severe electrical injuries. Initial patient care is directed at airway and ventilatory support; basic and advanced life support; patient immobilization; fluid resuscitation to prevent hypovolemia and renal failure; pharmacologic therapy (per protocol) to manage seizures (if present), promote excretion of myoglobin, and treat dysrhythmias; wound care; and rapid transport to a proper facility.

NOTE

Although morbidity and mortality from lightning strike are high, patients who respond to immediate treatment have an excellent chance of recovery. Once the scene is safe, rescuers should provide prompt cardiopulmonary resuscitation and early defibrillation even when the victim appears dead. Triage for multiple patients struck by lightning should follow a *reverse triage method*, whereby cardiac arrest victims are treated first rather than "black tagged," giving them optimal chance of survival.

Modified from: Field JM, Hazinski MF, Sayre MR, et al. Part 1: executive summary; 2010 American Heart Association Guidelines for Cardiopulmonary Resuscitation and Emergency Cardiovascular Care. *Circulation*. 2010;122(18)(suppl 3):S639-S946; and Davis C, Engeln A, Johnson EL, Scott E. Wilderness Medical Society practice guidelines for the prevention and treatment of lightning injuries: 2014 update. *Wilderness Environ Med.* 2014;25:S86-S95.

Radiation Exposure

The most common radiation incidents involve sealed radioactive sources used in industrial radiography and nondestructive testing. People involved in these types of incidents rarely require emergency care. However, EMS may be called to building fires and crashes that involve radioactive materials. Thus, an understanding of the hazards of radiation exposure is important. As with all incidents involving hazardous materials, the paramedic crew should never enter the scene until it has been made safe by the proper authorities.

Generally, safety issues regarding radiation have been minor because of excellent adherence to radiation regulations throughout the world. However, hazards associated with radiation became well known as a result of several incidents. First, the serious potential for disaster occurred at Three Mile Island in Pennsylvania in 1979. Second, a disastrous incident occurred at the Chernobyl Nuclear Power Station in the Soviet Union in 1986. Most recently, the earthquake and tsunami that struck Japan in 2011 caused a serious radiation event when the Fukushima Daiichi Nuclear Power Plant was damaged.

> CRITICAL THINKING
> What industries in your area use radioactive materials? Is there a preplan for incidents at those sites?

Characteristics of Ionizing Radiation

Ionizing radiation results from energy released by atoms and travels in electromagnetic waves.

Radioactive particles generally are classified into three types: alpha, beta, and gamma. Alpha particles are large and travel only a few millimeters. They have little penetrating ability and in fact may be stopped by paper, clothing, or skin. These particles are considered the least dangerous external radiation source; however, if alpha particles enter the body through inhalation, ingestion, or absorption, they can damage internal organs and interfere with the chemical functions of the body. Alpha radiation is the most dangerous form of internal radiation exposure.

Alpha particles are almost 60 times larger than beta particles, yet beta particles have much more energy and penetrating power. Beta particles can penetrate subcutaneous tissue. They usually enter the body through damaged skin, ingestion, or inhalation. Protection from alpha and beta radiation requires full protective clothing, including a positive-pressure self-contained breathing apparatus.

Gamma rays and x-rays are the most dangerous forms of penetrating radiation. They require lead shields for protection. Gamma rays have 10,000 times the penetrating power of alpha particles and have 100 times the penetrating power of beta particles.[22] Protective clothing does not stop gamma rays. Gamma rays pose internal and external hazards and may produce localized skin burns and extensive internal damage.

Harmful Effects From Radiation Exposure

Nonionizing radiation includes radio waves and microwaves. Nonionizing radiation usually is considered safe. Ionizing radiation is produced by nuclear weapons, reactors, radioactive material, and radiograph machines. Although rare, the exposure to ionizing radiation poses a threat to patients and rescue workers when it occurs.

The amount of emitted radiation is expressed in roentgens and indicates the ionization produced in the air by gamma or x-ray radiation. Other units used to measure radiation are the rad (radiation absorbed dose) and the rem (roentgen equivalent man). A rad is a measure of the amount of ionized radiation being emitted and the amount that has been absorbed and is active within the body tissues. A rem is used to assess the biologic effects of the various types of radiation. For emergency purposes, rescue workers should assume that 1 roentgen equals 1 rad equals 1 rem.[23]

Doses of less than 100 rem usually do not cause significant acute problems. Doses from 100 to 200 rem may cause symptoms, yet the doses are not life threatening. When an exposure of 200 rem is neared, nausea, vomiting, and diarrhea begin within 2 to 4 hours. After an exposure of 450 rem, cognitive impairment occurs. Mortality is high with exposures of 600 rem or more.[24] People exposed to radiation rarely show immediate signs or symptoms. Thus, all patients with possible exposure should be presumed to have a radiation injury until proved otherwise (**BOX 38-7**).

> NOTE
> An object or a person who has been exposed to radiation is not radioactive. Only the presence of the radioactive residue poses a threat to rescuers.

Emergency Response to Radiation Accidents

If the EMS crew has been advised that radioactive materials are present at an emergency scene, the team should approach the site with caution. Crew members should not enter the scene until it has been secured by proper authorities (see Chapter 56, *Hazardous Materials Awareness*). Rescue personnel, emergency vehicles, and the command post should be positioned 200 to 300 feet (61–91 m) upwind of the site. Emergency workers should not eat, drink, or smoke at the site or in any rescue vehicle. The proper local authorities should be contacted (state

BOX 38-7 Types of Radiation Injury

The harmful effects from radiation may be classified as external irradiation, contamination by radioactive materials, incorporation of radioactive materials, and combined radiation injury.

External irradiation occurs when all or part of the body is exposed to penetrating radiation from an external source. An example of external irradiation is a medical radiograph. The degree of radiation injury depends on the intensity of radiation, which in turn depends on the duration of exposure. Degree of injury also depends on the distance from the source. A patient who has been exposed to large amounts of radiation may have nausea, vomiting, and diarrhea. In severe cases, additional symptoms may include weight loss, hair loss, fever, bleeding, mouth and throat sores, skin burns, lowered body resistance, vesiculation, and ulceration. The effects from this type of radiation are not contagious; there is little or no risk to the rescuer in providing care.

Contamination occurs when radioactive materials in the form of gases, liquids, or solids are released into the environment. These materials contaminate people internally, externally, or both. When radioactive material remains on the patient's clothing or skin or in open wounds, a potential hazard is present for the rescuer and the patient. Patients who have been contaminated should be considered medical emergencies. They may pose significant risk to emergency providers.

Incorporation refers to the uptake of radioactive materials by body cells, tissues, and target organs such as the bone, liver, thyroid, or kidney. Incorporation is impossible unless contamination has occurred.

A combination radiation injury involves external irradiation, contamination, incorporation, or some combination of these. This type of exposure usually is the result of a major incident. Exposure may be complicated by a patient's physical injury.

After exposure to radiation, a person may be at risk for delayed complications. Such complications include cell and chromosomal changes, subsequent reproductive genetic aberrations, cell death, and sterility. Diseases such as anemia and forms of cancer may develop as well.

Modified from: Bevelacqua AS, Stilp RH. *Terrorism Handbook for Operational Responders.* 3rd ed. Clifton Parks, NJ: Cengage Learning; 2009.

radiologic health office, local specialists). Medical direction should be notified as well. Protective clothing suitable for other hazardous material releases should be worn by all emergency workers. In addition, dose meters should be available for all rescue personnel. Self-contained breathing apparatus should be used if fire, smoke, or gas is present.

Personal Protection From Radiation

The Federal Emergency Management Agency and the Environmental Protection Agency recommend that basic radiation protection for the rescuer and the patient include the following:[24]

1. **Time.** The less time spent in a radiation field, the less radiation exposure. If adequate personnel are available, a rotating team approach can be used to keep individual radiation exposure to a minimum.
2. **Distance.** The farther a person is from the source of radiation, the lower the radiation dose. Even moving several feet away from a radioactive source greatly reduces the level of exposure.
3. **Shielding.** The general principle of shielding is that the denser the material, the greater its ability to stop the passage of radiation. Lead shields provide the best protection from exposure; however, vehicles, mounds of dirt, and pieces of heavy equipment placed between the radiation source and the rescuer and patient also can diminish exposure levels. Protective clothing and self-contained breathing apparatus may provide adequate protection from all alpha and some beta radiation, but protective clothing does not prevent penetration of gamma rays. If adequate shielding is not readily available, rescuers should use the time and distance factors to reduce radiation exposure.
4. **Quantity.** Limiting the amount of radioactive material in a specific area lessens the radiation exposure. Examples include removing contaminated clothing, bagging all contaminated items, and moving containers of radioactive material from the area.

Paramedics should use respiratory protection and consider prophylactic medication (usually potassium iodide) to block the uptake or reduce the retention time of radioactive material that has entered the body.

Emergency Care for Patients With Radiation Exposure

Even though a patient who has been exposed to ionizing radiation is not radioactive, external contamination and radioactive materials can remain on the patient's clothing and skin or in open wounds. If this occurs, the rescuer should consult with medical direction and follow agency protocol. The effects of radiation exposure may be instant (eg, burns) or delayed.

With the exception of dealing with contaminants and containing their spread, there are no emergency care procedures specific to radiation injury. The EMS crew should move the patient away from the source of radiation as soon as possible. Lifesaving care should not be delayed for patient transfer or decontamination procedures. IV fluid replacement should be initiated if indicated. (Strict aseptic technique should be used.) If an IV line is not needed for specific therapy, its use should be avoided to prevent introducing contaminants into the body. An antiemetic should be administered if the patient is nauseated.

Radiation Decontamination Procedures

Radiation emergencies involving patients may be defined in two ways: clean and dirty. *Clean* means that the patient was exposed but not contaminated. *Dirty* means that the patient was contaminated. Only properly trained personnel (eg, hazardous materials teams and qualified county, state, or federal health department personnel) should attempt on-scene decontamination of patients who have been exposed to radiation. A patient who is to be transported to a medical facility for decontamination should be isolated from the environment (described in Chapter 57, *Bioterrorism and Weapons of Mass Destruction*). Also, all patient effects should be transported with the patient.

Summary

- In 2016, about 486,000 Americans sought medical attention for burns. Morbidity and mortality rates from burn injury follow significant patterns regarding sex, age, and socioeconomic status. The transfer of energy to living cells causes burn injuries. The source of this energy may be thermal, chemical, electrical, or radiation.
- Tissue damage from burns depends on the degree of the heat and the duration of exposure to the thermal source. As local events occur at the injury site, other organ systems become involved in a general response to the stress caused by the burn.
- Burns are classified in terms of depth as superficial, partial-thickness, and full-thickness.
- The rule of nines provides a rough estimate of burn injury extent and is most accurate for adults and for children older than 10 years. The Lund and Browder chart is a more accurate method of determining the area of burn injury.
- Severity of burn injury and burn center referral guidelines are based on standards that take into account the extent, depth, and location of burn injury; age of the patient; etiologic agents involved; presence of inhalation injury; and coexisting injuries or preexisting illness.
- Shock after thermal injury results from edema and accumulation of vascular fluid. These tissue changes occur in the area of injury and can produce systemic hypovolemia if the burn area is large.
- Emergency care for a burn patient begins with the initial assessment. The goal is to recognize and treat life-threatening injuries.
- Goals for prehospital management of the severely burned patient include preventing further tissue injury, maintaining the airway, administering oxygen, providing ventilatory support, managing pain, providing fluid resuscitation, transporting to an appropriate medical facility, using clean technique to minimize the patient's exposure to infectious agents, maintaining body warmth, and providing psychological and emotional support.
- Several fluid resuscitation formulae have proved clinically useful in replacing fluids. The two most common formulae are the Parkland formula and the rule of 10. The Parkland formula stipulates that half of the total calculated amount of fluid should be infused over the first 8 hours from the time of the injury, and the second half should be infused over the following 16 hours. The rule of 10 can be used to calculate fluid volume resuscitation for patients who weigh more than 40 kg.
- Prehospital considerations in caring for patients with inhalation injury include recognition of the dangers inherent in the fire environment, awareness of the pathophysiologic principles of inhalation injury, and early detection and treatment of impending airway or respiratory problems.
- The severity of chemical injury is related to three factors: the type of chemical agent, the concentration and volume

of the chemical, and the duration of contact. Treatment is directed at stopping the burning process by brushing off powdered chemicals, removing blisters that may contain chemicals, and using copious irrigation.

- Three types of injury may occur as a result of contact with electric current: direct-contact burns, arc injuries, and flash burns. Once the scene is safe, patient intervention may begin. Internal damage from electric current may be much more significant than are the external wounds.
- People who are injured by radiation rarely require emergency care. Radioactive particles are classified into three types: alpha, beta, and gamma. The Federal Emergency Management Agency and the Environmental Protection Agency recommend that basic radiation protection for the rescuer and the patient include four factors: (1) Minimize time in the radiation field, (2) maintain a safe distance from the source, (3) place shielding between the rescuers and the source, and (4) limit the amount of radioactive material in a specific area.

References

1. Burn incidence fact sheet. Burn incidence and treatment in the United States: 2016. American Burn Association website. http://ameriburn.org/who-we-are/media/burn-incidence-fact-sheet/. Accessed March 16, 2018.
2. National Safety Council. *Injury Facts: 2017 Edition*. Itasca, IL: National Safety Council; 2017.
3. ASTM International. *Standard Guide for Heated System Surface Conditions That Produce Contact Burn Injuries*. West Conshohocken, PA: ASTM International; 2014. ASTM C1055-03(2014).
4. Herndon D. *Total Burn Care*. 4th ed. Philadelphia, PA: Saunders Elsevier; 2012.
5. Jackson DM. The diagnosis of the depth of burning. *Br J Surg*. 1953;40(164):588-596.
6. National Highway Traffic Safety Administration. *The National EMS Education Standards*. Washington, DC: US Department of Transportation/National Highway Traffic Safety Administration; 2009.
7. Committee on Trauma, American College of Surgeons. *Resources for Optimal Care of the Injured Patient*. Chicago, IL: American College of Surgeons; 2014. https://www.facs.org/~/media/files/quality%20programs/trauma/vrc%20resources/resources%20for%20optimal%20care.ashx. Accessed March 16, 2018.
8. Marx JA, Hockberger RS, Walls RM. *Rosen's Emergency Medicine: Concepts and Clinical Practice*. 8th ed. St. Louis, MO: Saunders; 2014.
9. National Association of Emergency Medical Technicians. *PHTLS: Prehospital Trauma Life Support*. 8th ed. Burlington, MA: Jones & Bartlett Learning; 2014.
10. McManus J, Schwartz RB, Braithwaite SA. Thermal and chemical burns. In: Brice J, Delbridge TR, Myers JB, eds. *Emergency Services: Clinical Practice and Systems Oversight*. Vol 1. 2nd ed. West Sussex, England: John Wiley & Sons; 2015:253-260.
11. National Association of EMS Officials. *National Model EMS Clinical Guidelines*. Version 2.0. National Association of EMS Officials website. https://www.nasemso.org/documents/National-Model-EMS-Clinical-Guidelines-Version2-Sept2017.pdf. Published September 2017. Accessed March 16, 2018.
12. Bope ET, Kellerman RD. *Conn's Current Therapy 2016*. Amsterdam, Netherlands: Elsevier; 2015.
13. Mlcak RP. Inhalation injury from heat, smoke, or chemical irritants. UpToDate website. https://www.uptodate.com/contents/inhalation-injury-from-heat-smoke-or-chemical-irritants?source=search_result&search=Smoke%20inhalation&selectedTitle=1~86. Updated February 28, 2018. Accessed March 16, 2018.
14. Sheridan RL. Fire-related inhalation injury. *N Engl J Med*. 2016;375:464-469.
15. Hess DR, MacIntyre NR, Mishoe SC, Galvin WF, Adams AB. *Respiratory Care: Principles and Practice*. 2nd ed. Burlington, MA: Jones & Bartlett Learning; 2012.
16. Rajeev RB, Puri V, Gibran N, et al. ISBI practice guidelines for burn care. *Burns*. 2016;42(5):953-1021.
17. Cambell RB, Dini DA. Occupational injuries from electrical shock and arc flash events. The Fire Protection Research Foundation website. https://www.nfpa.org/~/media/files/news-and-research/resources/research-foundation/research-foundation-reports/electrical/rfarcflashoccdata.pdf?la=en. Published March 2015. Accessed March 16, 2018.
18. National Center for Environmental Health (NCEH)/Agency for Toxic Substances and Disease Registry (ATSDR), National Center for Injury Prevention and Control (NCIPC). Lightning. Centers for Disease and Prevention website. https://www.cdc.gov/disasters/lightning/index.html. Updated February 6, 2014. Accessed March 16, 2018.
19. How hot is lightning? National Weather Service website. http://www.lightningsafety.noaa.gov/temperature.shtml. Accessed March 16, 2018.
20. How dangerous is lightning? National Weather Service website. http://www.lightningsafety.noaa.gov/odds.shtml. Accessed March 16, 2018.
21. Dolce C. Top 5 lightning prone states. The Weather Channel website. https://weather.com/safety/thunderstorms/news/top-5-lightning-prone-states-20120509#/6. Published July 8, 2013. Accessed March 16, 2018.
22. Radiation protection: radiation basics. Environmental Protection Agency website. https://www.epa.gov/radiation/radiation-basics. Accessed March 16, 2018.
23. Measures relative to the biological effect of radiation exposure. NDT Resource Center website. https://www.nde-ed.org/EducationResources/CommunityCollege/RadiationSafety/theory/Measures.htm. Accessed March 16, 2018.
24. Office of Radiation and Indoor Air Radiation Protection Division, US Environmental Protection Agency. *PAG Manual: Protective Action Guides and Planning Guidance for Radiological Incidents*. Washington, DC: US Environmental Protection Agency; 2017.

Suggested Readings

Ainsbury E, Higueras M, Puig P, et al. Uncertainty of fast biological radiation dose assessment for emergency response scenarios. *Int J Radiat Biol*. 2017;93(1):127-135.

Cancio LC, Sheridan RL, Dent R, et al. Guidelines for burn care under austere conditions: special etiologies: blast, radiation, and chemical injuries. *J Burn Care Res*. 2017;38(1):e482-e496.

Jeschke MG, Peck MD. Burn care of the elderly. *J Burn Care Res*. 2017;38(1):e625-e628.

Palao R, Monge I, Ruiz M, et al. Chemical burns: pathophysiology and treatment. *Burns*. 2010;36(3):295-304.

Shih JG, Shahrokhi S, Jeschke MG. Review of adult electrical burn injury outcomes worldwide: an analysis of low-voltage vs high-voltage electrical injury. *J Burn Care Res*. 2017;38(1):e293-e298.

Usatch B. When lightning strikes: bolting down the facts and fiction. *JEMS* website. www.jems.com/news_and_articles/articles/jems/3404/when_lightning_strikes.html. Published March 31, 2009. Accessed March 16, 2018.

Wiechman S, Saxe G, Fauerbach JA. Psychological outcomes following burn injuries. *J Burn Care Res*. 2017;38(3):e629-e631.

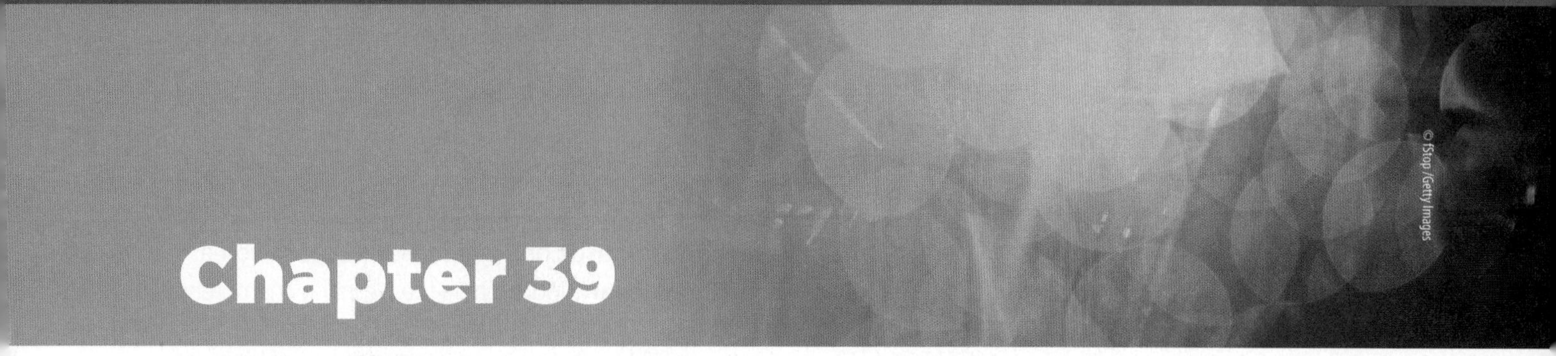
© iStop/Getty Images

Chapter 39

Head, Face, and Neck Trauma

NATIONAL EMS EDUCATION STANDARD COMPETENCIES

Trauma

Integrates assessment findings with principles of epidemiology and pathophysiology to formulate a field impression and implement a comprehensive treatment/disposition plan for an acutely injured patient.

Head, Facial, Neck, and Spine Trauma

Recognition and management of
- Life threats (p 1426)
- Spine trauma (see Chapter 40, *Spine and Nervous System Trauma*)

Pathophysiology, assessment, and management of
- Penetrating neck trauma (pp 1438)
- Laryngotracheal injuries (p 1439)

Spine trauma
- Dislocations/subluxations (see Chapter 40, *Spine and Nervous System Trauma*)
- Fractures (see Chapter 40, *Spine and Nervous System Trauma*)
- Sprains/strains (see Chapter 40, *Spine and Nervous System Trauma*)
- Facial fractures (pp 1426–1429)
- Skull fractures (pp 1440–1443)
- Foreign bodies in the eyes (pp 1432–1435)
- Dental trauma (pp 1435–1436)
- Unstable facial fractures (pp 1426–1429)
- Orbital fractures (p 1429)
- Perforated tympanic membrane (p 1430)
- Mandibular fractures (p 1427)

OBJECTIVES

Upon completion of this chapter, the paramedic student will be able to:

1. Describe the mechanisms of injury, assessment, and management of maxillofacial injuries. (pp 1425–1429)
2. Describe the mechanisms of injury, assessment, and management of ear, eye, and dental injuries. (pp 1430–1436)
3. Describe the mechanisms of injury, assessment, and management of anterior neck trauma. (pp 1436–1440)
4. Describe the mechanisms of injury, assessment, and management of injuries to the scalp, cranial vault, or cranial nerves. (pp 1440–1443)
5. Distinguish between types of traumatic brain injury based on an understanding of pathophysiology and assessment findings. (pp 1443–1453)
6. Describe cardiovascular complications that are common after brain injury. (p 1450)
7. Outline the prehospital management of the patient with cerebral injury. (pp 1451–1453)
8. Calculate a Glasgow Coma Scale score and trauma score when given appropriate patient information. (pp 1453–1455)

KEY TERMS

antegrade amnesia The loss of memory for events that occurred immediately after recovery of consciousness.

barotitis An inflammation of the ear caused by changes in atmospheric pressure.

basilar skull fracture A fracture, usually caused by substantial blunt force trauma, that involves at least one of the bones that compose the base of the skull; most commonly involves the temporal bones but may involve the occipital, sphenoid, ethmoid, and the orbital plate of the frontal bone.

Battle sign Bruising over the mastoid bone behind the ear, which may indicate a basilar skull fracture; also called retroauricular ecchymosis or raccoon eyes.

blowout fracture A fracture of the floor of the orbit caused by a blow that suddenly increases the intraocular pressure.

brain lesion An abnormal area of the brain often reflective of traumatic injury.

central vision The vision that results from images falling on the macula of the retina.

cerebral contusion Bruising of the brain in the area of the cortex or deeper within the frontal (most common), temporal, or occipital lobes.

cerebral perfusion pressure (CPP) A measure of the amount of blood flow to the brain calculated by subtracting the intracranial pressure from the mean systemic arterial blood pressure.

concussion A temporary loss or alteration of part or all of the brain's abilities to function without actual physical damage to the brain.

consensual movement The movement of one eye acting in concert with the other.

contrecoup An injury that occurs at a site opposite the side of impact.

corneal abrasion The rubbing off of the outer layers of the cornea.

coup Local damage that occurs at the site of impact.

Cushing triad Increased systolic blood pressure, bradycardia, and irregular respiratory rates that result from increased intracranial pressure.

decerebrate posturing A position that is also called abnormal extension posturing, in which a comatose patient's arms are extended and internally rotated and the legs are extended with the feet in forced plantar flexion; usually observed in patients who have compression of the brainstem.

decorticate posturing A position that is also called abnormal flexion posturing, in which the comatose patient's upper extremities are rigidly flexed at the elbows and at the wrists; usually observed in patients who have a lesion in the mesencephalic region of the brain.

dental malocclusion A misalignment of the teeth.

depressed skull fracture Any fracture of the skull in which fragments are depressed below the normal surface of the skull.

diffuse axonal injury (DAI) A disease process characterized by diffuse microscopic damage to the brain coupled with focal lesions that are the result of shear forces sustained in head trauma; a type of diffuse brain injury.

epidural hematoma Accumulation of blood between the dura mater and the cranium.

focal injury A specific, grossly observable brain lesion concentrated in one region of the brain.

Glasgow Coma Scale (GCS) A standardized system for assessing the degree of conscious impairment of consciousness in the critically ill patient and for predicting the duration and ultimate outcome of coma.

hemotympanum Blood behind the tympanic membrane often from fractures of the temporal bone.

intracerebral hematoma An accumulation of blood or fluid within the tissue of the brain.

Le Fort fractures Classifications used to describe fracture patterns of the midface.

linear skull fracture A skull fracture that does not displace the bone tissue.

mean arterial pressure (MAP) The arithmetic mean of the blood pressure in the arterial portion of the circulation.

mild DAI A Grade 1 axonal injury with microscopic changes of the cerebral hemispheres, the corpus callosum, the brainstem and, less commonly, the cerebellum; an example is a concussion.

moderate DAI A Grade 2 axonal injury that results in minute petechial bruising of brain tissue.

open vault fracture A fracture that results in direct communication between a scalp laceration and cerebral substance.

peripheral vision The ability to see objects that reflect light waves on areas of the retina other than the macula.

photophobia Abnormal sensitivity to light.

primary brain injury The direct trauma to the brain and the associated vascular injuries that occurred from the initial injury.

raccoon eyes Ecchymosis of one or both orbits with tarsal plate sparing caused by fracture of the base of the sphenoid sinus.

retrograde amnesia The loss of memory for events that occurred before the event that precipitated the amnesia.

secondary brain injury Brain injury that evolves over time from initial impact (primary injury) through intracellular and extracellular derangements contributing to further destruction of brain tissue.

severe DAI A Grade 3 axonal injury that involves severe mechanical shearing of many axons in both cerebral hemispheres extending to the brainstem.

stellate wound A star-shaped wound.

subarachnoid hemorrhage A collection of blood or fluid in the subarachnoid space.

subdural hematoma Accumulation of blood between the dura mater and the arachnoid mater.

subgaleal hematoma Bleeding in the potential space between the skull periosteum and the scalp galea aponeurosis.

traumatic brain injury (TBI) A traumatic insult to the brain capable of producing physical, intellectual, emotional, social, and vocational change.

traumatic hyphema A hemorrhage into the anterior chamber of the eye; usually is a result of blunt trauma.

traumatic perforation A tear or puncture of the tympanic membrane.

visual acuity A measurement of the clarity or sharpness of vision.

vitreous humor The transparent, jellylike material that fills the space between the lens and the retina of the eye.

Each year, an estimated 2.8 million people in the United States visit emergency departments (EDs), are admitted to hospitals, or die because of traumatic brain injury.[1] The categories of head trauma discussed in this chapter include maxillofacial trauma; ear, eye, and dental trauma; anterior neck trauma; and trauma to the skull and brain.

Maxillofacial Injuries

Major causes of maxillofacial trauma are assaults, motor vehicle crashes, falls, sporting injuries, animal bites, and industrial injuries. Maxillofacial trauma may include soft-tissue injuries and facial fractures.

Soft-Tissue Injuries

The face receives its blood supply from the branches of the internal and external carotid arteries. These branches provide a rich vascular supply (**FIGURE 39-1**). As a result, soft-tissue injuries to the face often appear to be serious (**FIGURE 39-2**). With the exception of a compromised upper airway and possible significant

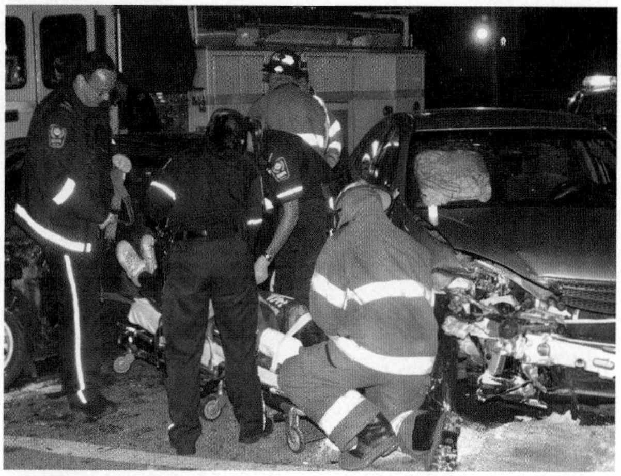

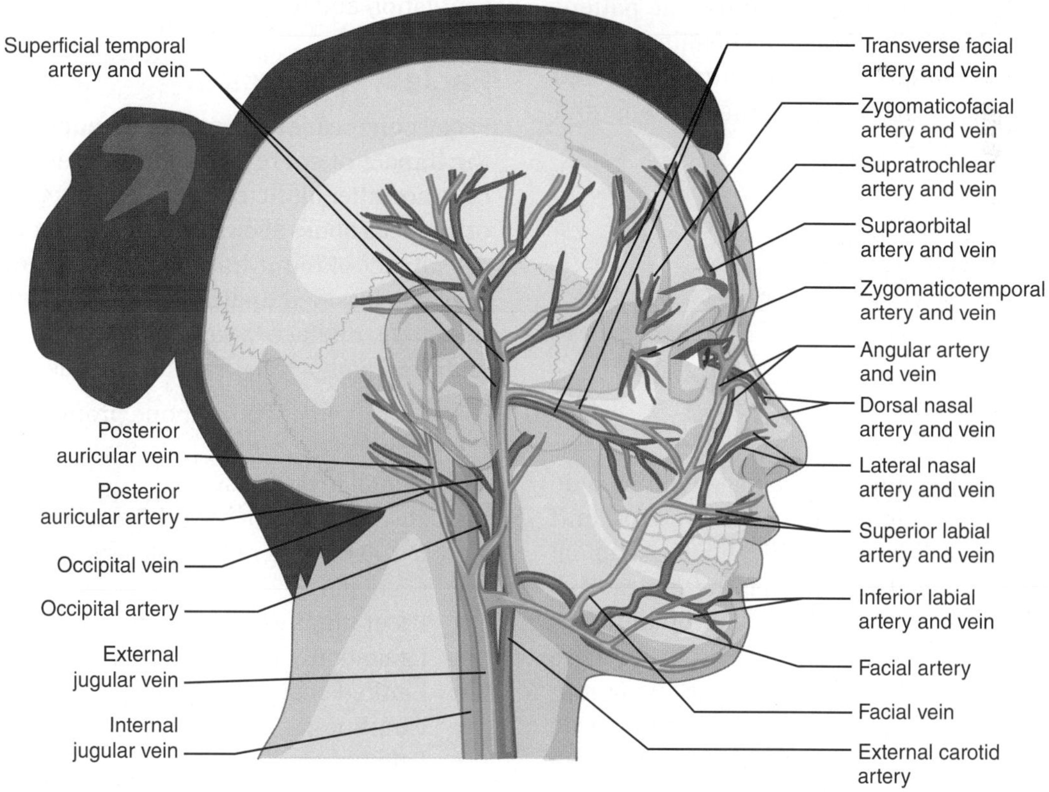

FIGURE 39-1 Arterial blood supply to the face.

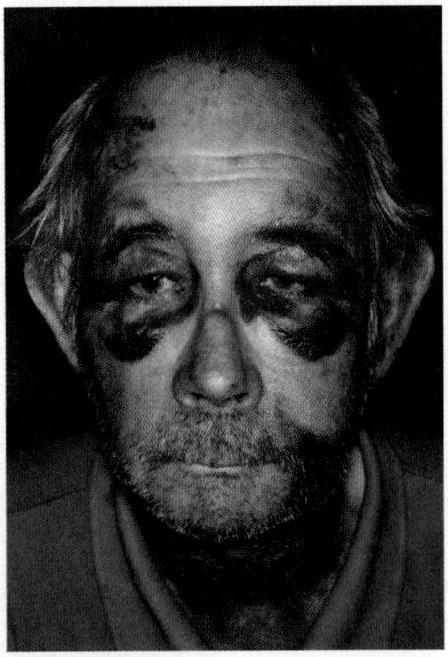

FIGURE 39-2 Appearance of a patient after being attacked.

bleeding, damage to the tissues of the maxillofacial area is seldom life threatening. Depending on the mechanism of injury, facial trauma may range from minor cuts and abrasions to more serious injuries. The more serious injuries may involve extensive soft-tissue lacerations and avulsions. The patient history should include mechanism of injury; events leading up to the injury; time of injury; associated medical problems; and allergies, medications, and last oral intake.

CRITICAL THINKING

Why might it be difficult to obtain a history from a patient with this type of injury?

Management

The key principles of wound management include the control of bleeding with direct pressure and pressure bandages. The paramedic should use spinal precautions if indicated; however, these measures should not inhibit management of the patient's airway, as airway management is a priority for these patients. Soft-tissue injuries to the nose and mouth are common with facial injuries. The paramedic should assess the patient's airway for obstruction caused by blood, vomitus, bone fragments, broken teeth, dentures, and damage to the anterior neck. Suction may be needed to clear the patient's airway. Also, oral or nasal adjuncts, tracheal intubation, or cricothyrotomy may be required to ensure adequate ventilation and oxygenation.

Facial Fractures

Facial bones can withstand tremendous forces from the impact of energy. However, facial fractures are common after blunt trauma. The anatomic structure of the facial bones allows a stepwise fracture to absorb the impact of blunt trauma. Blunt trauma injuries may be classified anatomically as fractures to the mandible, midface, zygoma, orbit, and nose. Signs and symptoms of facial fractures include the following:

- Asymmetry of cheekbone prominences
- Crepitus
- Dental malocclusion
- Discontinuity of the orbital rim
- Displacement of the nasal septum
- Ecchymosis
- Lacerations and bleeding
- Limitation of forward movement of the mandible
- Limited ocular movements
- Numbness
- Pain

- Swelling
- Visual disturbances

Fractures of the Mandible

The mandible is the single facial bone in the lower third of the face. Because of its prominence, fractures to this bone rank second in frequency after nasal fractures. The mandible is a hemicircle of bone. It may break in multiple locations, often distant from the point of impact. Signs and symptoms specific to mandibular fractures include **dental malocclusion** (patients may complain that their teeth do not "feel right" when their mouths are closed), numbness in the chin, and inability to open the mouth. The patient also may have difficulty swallowing and may have excessive salivation.

Anterior dislocation of the mandible in the absence of fracture also may occur as a result of blunt trauma to the face (rare), an abnormally wide yawn, and dental treatment requiring that the jaws remain open for long periods. In these cases, the condylar head advances forward beyond the articular surface of the temporal bone. The jaw-closing muscles spasm. As a result, the mouth becomes locked in a wide-open position. The patient usually feels severe pain from the spasm. The patient also experiences anxiety and discomfort that perpetuate the spasm. Mandibular dislocations are reduced manually in the ED with the aid of a muscle relaxant or sedative, or possibly in the operating room with general anesthesia.

> CRITICAL THINKING
> What will be your patient care priority with these patients?

Fractures of the Midface

The middle third of the face includes the maxilla, zygoma, floor of the orbit, and nose. Fractures to this region result from direct or transmitted force. For example, fractures may result from blunt trauma to the mandible with the energy transmitted to produce fractures to the maxilla. These injuries often are associated with central nervous system (CNS) injury and spinal trauma (**FIGURE 39-3**).

In 1901, a cadaver study done by Le Fort described three patterns of injuries (**Le Fort fractures**).[2] These injuries occur in the midface region (**FIGURE 39-4**). The Le Fort I fracture involves the maxilla up to the level of the nasal fossa. The Le Fort II involves the nasal bones and medial orbits. The fracture line generally is shaped like a pyramid. The Le Fort III is a complex fracture in which the facial bones are separated from the cranial bones. Depending on the severity of injury, different combinations of Le Fort fractures may be present.

Signs and symptoms specific to midface fractures include midfacial edema, unstable maxilla, lengthening of the face (donkey face), epistaxis, numb upper teeth, nasal flattening, and cerebrospinal fluid (CSF) rhinorrhea (CSF leakage from the nose caused by

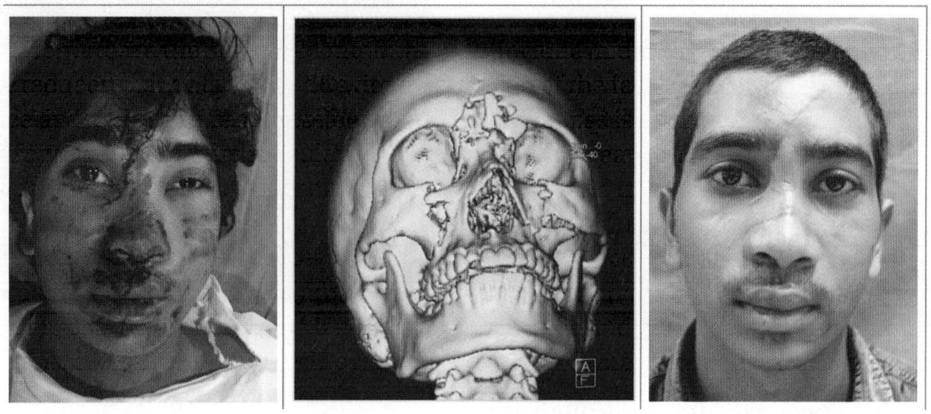

FIGURE 39-3 Fracture of the middle third of the face.

Reproduced from: Short Notes in Plastic Surgery, compiled by Ravin Thatte for the Association of Plastic Surgeons of India. Accessed at,https://shortnotesinplasticsurgery.wordpress.com/2013/08/16/36-fractures-of-the-maxilla/.

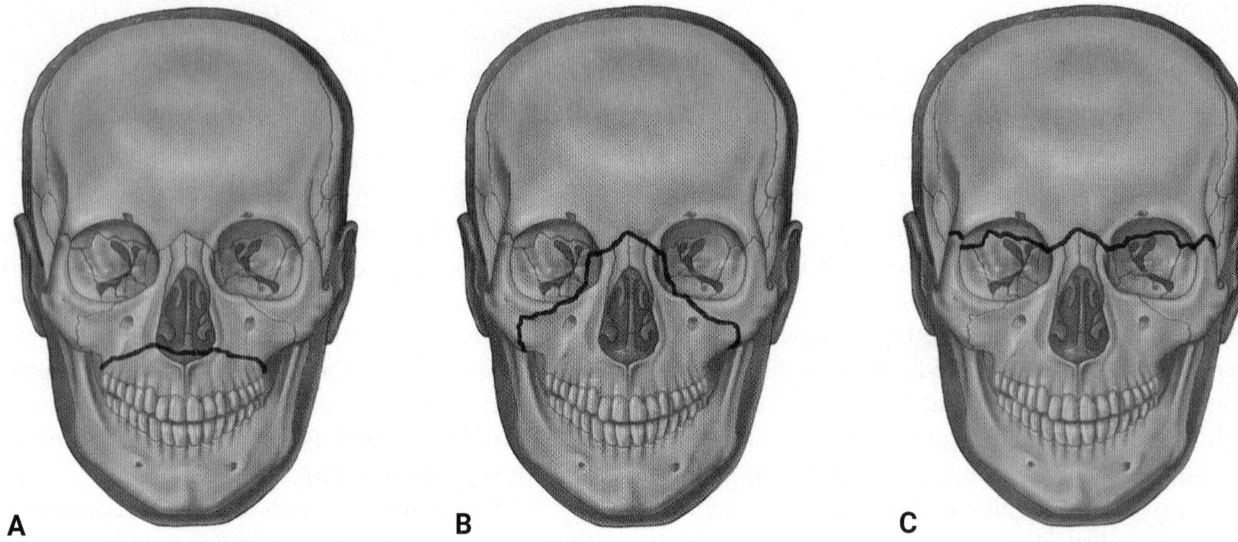

FIGURE 39-4 **A.** Le Fort I facial fracture. **B.** Le Fort II fracture. **C.** Le Fort III fracture.

© Jones & Bartlett Learning.

ethmoid cribriform plate fracture). Patients with midface fractures require hospitalization. These patients (particularly those with Le Fort II and III fractures) are at risk of having serious airway problems related to swelling and bleeding. Because of the extent of the fractures, there is a risk of placing nasogastric or even nasotracheal tubes into the brain tissue.

> **NOTE**
> Nasal airways, nasogastric tubes, and nasotracheal intubation are contraindicated in patients who have fractures of the basal skull or facial bones. CSF leakage from the ear or nose should be allowed to drain freely. The paramedic should not attempt to control CSF leakage with direct pressure.

Fractures of the Zygoma

The zygoma (malar eminence) articulates with the frontal, maxillary, and temporal bones. The zygoma commonly is called the cheekbone. It is rarely fractured because of its sturdy construction. When fractures occur, they usually are a result of physical assaults and vehicle crashes. Zygomatic fractures often are associated with orbital fractures and manifest similar clinical signs (**FIGURE 39-5**). The two types of fractures are distinguished by radiologic examination. Signs and symptoms specific to zygomatic fractures include flatness of a usually rounded cheek area; numbness of the cheek, nose, and upper lip (particularly if an orbital fracture is involved); epistaxis; and altered vision.

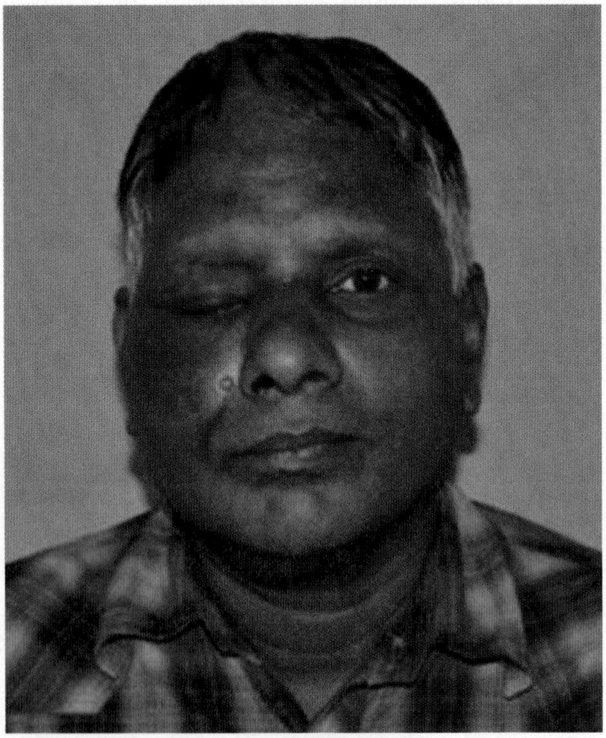

FIGURE 39-5 Fracture of the zygomatic bone.

Reproduced from: Short Notes in Plastic Surgery, compiled by Ravin Thatte for the Association of Plastic Surgeons of India. Accessed at, https://shortnotesinplasticsurgery.wordpress.com/2013/08/16/36-fractures-of-the-maxilla/.

Fractures of the Orbit

The orbital contents are protected by a bony ring. The ring resembles a pyramid, with the apex pointed toward the back of the head. The bones of the walls, floor, and roof of the orbit are thin and are fractured easily by direct blows and transmitted forces. In addition, many orbital fractures are associated with other facial injuries, such as Le Fort II and III fractures.

A **blowout fracture** to the orbit can occur when an object of greater diameter than that of the bony orbital rim strikes the globe of the eye and surrounding soft tissue (**FIGURE 39-6**). This impact pushes the globe into the orbit and in turn compresses the orbital contents. The sudden increase in intraocular pressure is transmitted to the orbital floor. The orbital floor is the weakest part of the orbital structure. If the orbital floor fractures, the orbital contents may be forced into the maxillary sinus, where soft tissue and extraocular muscles may be trapped in the defect. Signs and symptoms of blowout fractures include periorbital edema, subconjunctival ecchymosis, diplopia (double vision), enophthalmos (recessed globe), epistaxis, anesthesia in the region of the infraorbital nerve (anterior cheek), and impaired extraocular movements.

CRITICAL THINKING

How do you assess a patient's eye movement?

Orbital fractures often are associated with other fractures, including the Le Fort II and III injuries and those of the zygomatic complex. In addition, injury to the orbital contents is common. The paramedic should suspect such injury with any facial fracture.

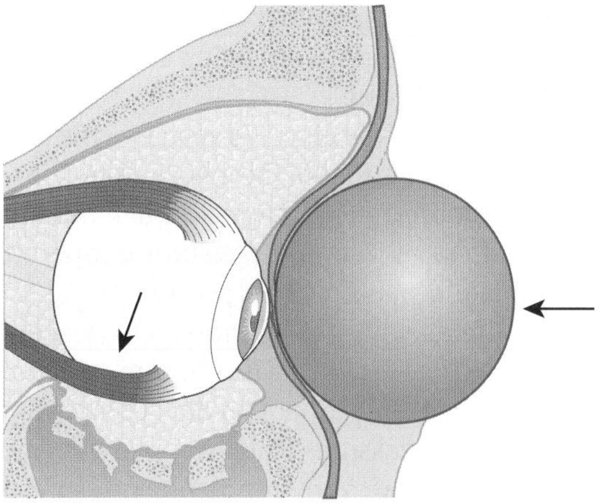

FIGURE 39-6 Representation of a blowout fracture caused by the impact of a ball.

Fractures of the Nose

Of all the facial bones, the nasal bones have the least structural strength. They are fractured most frequently. The external portion of the nose, formed mostly of hyaline cartilage, is supported mainly by the nasal bones and the frontal processes of the maxillary bones. Injuries to the nose may depress the dorsum of the nose, displace it to one side, or result only in epistaxis and swelling without apparent skeletal deformity. Fractures to the orbit also may be present. In children, minimal displacement of nasal bones can result in growth changes and ultimate deformity.

Management of Facial Fractures

When caring for a patient with facial fractures, the paramedic should assess the patient for possible cervical spine injury, and spinal precautions should be considered because facial fractures have been associated with a high percentage of related cervical spine fractures.[3] This approach is particularly important if the injury resulted from a motor vehicle crash or a fall. The paramedic should assess the patient's airway for obstruction caused by blood, vomitus, bone fragments, broken teeth, dentures, and damage to the anterior neck. Suction may be needed to clear the airway of debris and fluid. The paramedic may need to maintain the airway with a nasal (in the absence of suspected midface or basal skull fracture) or oral adjunct, tracheal intubation, or cricothyrotomy if indicated. Unstable facial fractures are also an immediate concern.

Bleeding usually can be controlled by direct pressure and pressure bandages. Epistaxis may be severe and should be controlled by applying external pressure to the anterior nares. To prevent blood from draining down the throat, mild epistaxis is best controlled in the conscious patient by instructing the patient to sit upright or to lean forward (in the absence of spinal injury) while compressing the nares. An unconscious patient should be positioned on the side (if not contraindicated by injury). If bleeding is severe, the paramedic should evaluate the patient for hemorrhagic shock.

CRITICAL THINKING

What issues might arise if the blood drains posteriorly?

Ear, Eye, and Dental Trauma

The ears, eyes, or teeth may be injured separately or along with other forms of head and facial trauma. Injury to these regions may be minor. However, such injuries may result in permanent sensory function loss and disfigurement. Regardless of the severity, the paramedic should evaluate ear, eye, and dental trauma and treat it only after identifying and managing life-threatening problems.

Ear Trauma

Trauma to the ear may include lacerations and contusions, thermal injuries, chemical injuries, traumatic perforations, and barotitis.

Lacerations and Contusions

Lacerations and contusions usually result from blunt trauma. They are particularly common in victims of domestic violence (**FIGURE 39-7**). These injuries are treated by using direct pressure to control bleeding. In addition, the application of ice or cold compresses decreases soft-tissue swelling. If a portion of the outer ear (auricle) has been avulsed, the paramedic should retrieve the avulsed tissue if possible. The tissue should be wrapped in moist gauze for protection, sealed in plastic, placed in ice water, and transported with the patient for surgical repair. Cartilage tears often heal poorly and are easily infected.

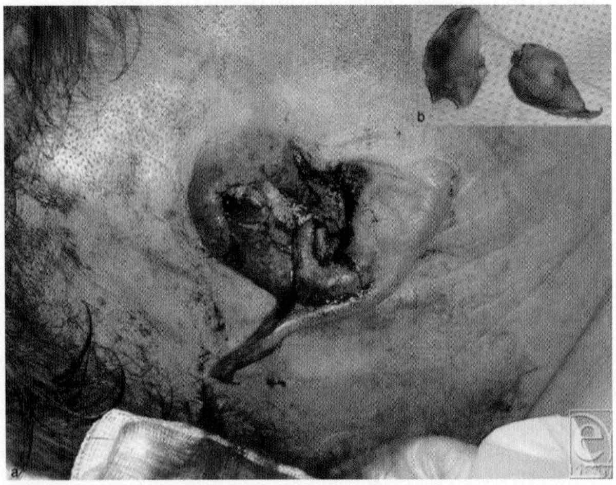

FIGURE 39-7 Partially detached auricle.

Reproduced from: Manoli T, Jaminet P, Kraus A, Schaller H-E, Werdin F, Sinis N. One-stage ear reconstruction after avulsion injury, using the amputated cartilage and a retroauricular transposition flap. *Eplasty*. 2010;10:e13.

Chemical Injuries

Strong acids or alkalis produce burns on contact. Emergency care consists of copious irrigation. After irrigation, the paramedic should bathe the ear and ear canal with saline or sterile water, allowing the irrigation liquid to remain in the ear canal for 2 to 3 minutes. This procedure should be repeated three or four times, after which the ear should be dried and covered to prevent contamination. The patient should be transported for evaluation by a physician.

Traumatic Perforations

The tympanic membrane can be perforated. **Traumatic perforation** can occur by objects such as a cotton-tipped applicator and by changes in pressure. Pressure injuries may result from explosions (blast injuries) or scuba diving (barotrauma). These injuries usually heal spontaneously without treatment. Still, evaluation by a physician is necessary.

If the injury is caused by a penetrating object, the paramedic should stabilize the object in place and cover the ear to prevent further contamination. The inner or middle ear canal may have been contaminated (eg, by swimming water or a foreign object). In that case, antibiotic therapy usually is prescribed. Serious complications that may result from perforations include facial nerve palsy frequently accompanied by temporal bone fractures, hearing loss, and vertigo.

Barotitis

Barotitis occurs when a person is exposed to changes in barometric pressure great enough to produce inflammation and injury to the middle ear. Barotitis can result, for example, from flying at high altitudes and from scuba diving.

Gas pressure in the air-filled spaces of the middle ear normally equals that of the environment. Boyle's law (further described in Chapter 44, *Environmental Conditions*) states that at a constant temperature, the volume of a gas is inversely proportional to the pressure. On ascent, gas expands. On descent, it contracts. Therefore, when gases become trapped or partially trapped, they expand in direct proportion to the decrease in pressure. When trapped gas cannot reach equilibrium with environmental pressure, pain and the sensation of a blocked ear may develop. To equalize the pressure in the middle ear, the patient can be directed to bear down (Valsalva maneuver), yawn, swallow, and move the lower jaw. These methods may cause the eustachian tube to open, which will equalize the pressure in the middle ear cavity.

Eye Trauma

More than 2.5 million eye injuries are estimated to occur each year in the United States, and about 50,000 people lose part or all of their sight.[4] Common causes of eye injury are being struck by an object, falling, fires or burns, motor vehicle crashes, and environmental causes.

Evaluation

Acute eye injuries may be difficult to identify because a patient with normal vision may have a serious underlying injury. Symptoms requiring a high degree of suspicion include the following:

- Obvious trauma with eye injury
- Visual loss or blurred vision that does not improve with blinking, indicating possible damage to the globe, ocular contents, or optic nerve
- Loss of a portion of the visual field, indicating possible detachment of the retina, hemorrhage into the eye, or optic nerve injury

Evaluation of eye injury should include a thorough history and measurement of visual acuity, pupillary reaction, and extraocular movements (see Chapter 19, *Secondary Assessment and Reassessment*). Assessing the patient's vision will be a rough estimation at best. The patient's vision will be reevaluated in the ED under controlled circumstances.

> CRITICAL THINKING
> Aside from trauma, what are some other causes of visual disturbances?

History. A thorough history should include the following information:

- Exact mode of injury
- Previous ocular, medical, and drug history, including cataracts or glaucoma
- Use of eye medications
- Use of corrective glasses or contact lenses
- Presence of ocular prostheses
- Duration of symptoms and treatment interventions that may have been attempted before emergency medical services (EMS) arrival

Visual Acuity. The measurement of **visual acuity** is usually the first step in any examination of the patient's eyes, but should never delay transport. (The exception is a chemical burn to the eye. In this case, irrigation should be performed before measurement of visual acuity.) Visual acuity can be measured with a handheld visual acuity chart (eg, Snellen chart) or any printed material with small, medium, and large point sizes (eg, an intravenous [IV] fluid bag). The paramedic should record the distance that the printed item was held from the patient's face.

The vision of each eye should be assessed separately while covering the other eye. (No pressure should be applied.) The injured eye should be tested first for acuity comparison with the uninjured eye. If the patient wears corrective lenses, acuity should be measured with lenses first and then without lenses. Illiterate or non–English-speaking patients require an alternative method of evaluation. Such methods may include finger counting, hand motion, and presence or absence of light perception. Abnormal responses to any of these methods indicate significant loss of vision.

> CRITICAL THINKING
> The assessment of visual acuity may be difficult on some calls. What factors in the prehospital setting may make it difficult?

> NOTE
> Vision may be categorized as being central or peripheral. **Central vision** results from images falling on the macula of the retina. **Peripheral vision** is the ability to see objects that reflect light waves on areas of the retina other than the macula.

Pupillary Reaction

Pupils should be black, round, and equal in size. The pupils also should react to light in the same way and at the same time. Both eyes should constrict in response to light and dilate in response to dark. (A direct response to light refers to constriction of the illuminated pupil. A consensual response to light refers to constriction of the opposite pupil.) Abnormal pupillary responses after blunt trauma to the eye are common and may be caused by tearing.

More commonly, though, they are caused by direct trauma to the pupillary sphincter muscle. Abnormal responses also may suggest a more serious injury involving the optic nerve or globe. Causes of pupil abnormalities in the absence of recent injury include drug use, cataracts, previous surgical procedures, ocular prosthesis, physiologic anisocoria (normal or congenital unequal pupil size), CNS disease, strokes, and previous injury. The paramedic should document all of the patient's pupil abnormalities.

DID YOU KNOW?

When the eyes are open, the CNS is exposed. This exposure exists nowhere else in the human body. Fortunately, the brain is well wired to provide protection. A sudden movement near the face, a flash of bright light, or a loud noise will cause the eyelids to slam shut, forming a waterproof, airtight shield. Strong tarsal plates shield, support, and protect the eyelids. Eyelashes are rooted in nerve cells that are so sensitive that a particle of grit caught by one lash will close both eyelids automatically.

Extraocular Movements

Extraocular muscles are responsible for movements of the globe, or eyeball. Voluntary muscles are innervated by cranial nerves III, IV, and VI. The muscles are attached to the outside of the eyeball and bones of the orbit and move the globe in any desired direction. Involuntary eye muscles are innervated by sympathetic nerves. These muscles are located within the eye. Examples of involuntary eye muscles are the iris and the ciliary muscle. These muscles dilate and constrict the pupil and change the shape of the lens, respectively.

To evaluate the extraocular movement of the eyes (described in Chapter 19, *Secondary Assessment and Reassessment*), the paramedic should instruct the patient to visually track the movement of an object. (For example, the object may be a finger, pencil, or penlight.) The patient should be asked to track the object to the right, then up, down, and to the left, then up and down—representing an H pattern. Abnormalities in movement may indicate orbital content edema, cranial nerve injury, contusions or lacerations of extraocular muscles, or muscle entrapment in a fracture. Patients with limited or abnormal extraocular movements often report double vision in one or more directions of gaze. The paramedic should document all findings.

Evaluation and Management of Specific Eye Injuries

Few eye injuries are urgent. However, all victims of ocular trauma should be evaluated by a physician. Some patients need specialized care by an ophthalmologist. If the paramedic suspects a serious injury that may require specialized care, medical direction should be advised as soon as possible. That way, services will be ready when the patient arrives in the ED (**FIGURE 39-8**).

Foreign bodies in the cornea, conjunctiva, or eyelid usually cause the patient to report the sensation of something in the eye (especially when opening and closing the eyelids) and to have profuse tearing. If a foreign body is suspected, the inner surface of the upper and lower lids and conjunctivae should be inspected. The paramedic should remove the foreign body by gentle, copious irrigation with clear fluid. For example, tap water, normal saline, or sterile water are appropriate. Medical direction may recommend that an ophthalmic anesthetic, such as tetracaine, be applied for patient comfort. The paramedic should advise and remind the patient not to touch or rub the eye after the administration of tetracaine. Doing so can result in serious eye injury.

Corneal abrasion occurs when the outer layers of the cornea are avulsed. The injury often results from a foreign body scratching the cornea and is common in those who wear some types of contact lenses. Patients with a corneal abrasion usually report pain and a foreign body sensation under the upper eyelid, **photophobia** (abnormal light sensitivity),

DID YOU KNOW?

Routine eye patching for corneal abrasion is no longer recommended. Studies have found that routine patching does not speed healing or affect pain relief and may even hinder the healing process.

Modified from: Lim CHL, Turner A, Lim BX. Eye patches for corneal abrasion. Cochrane website. http://www.cochrane.org/CD004764/EYES_eye-patches-corneal-abrasion. Published July 26, 2016. Accessed April 7, 2018.

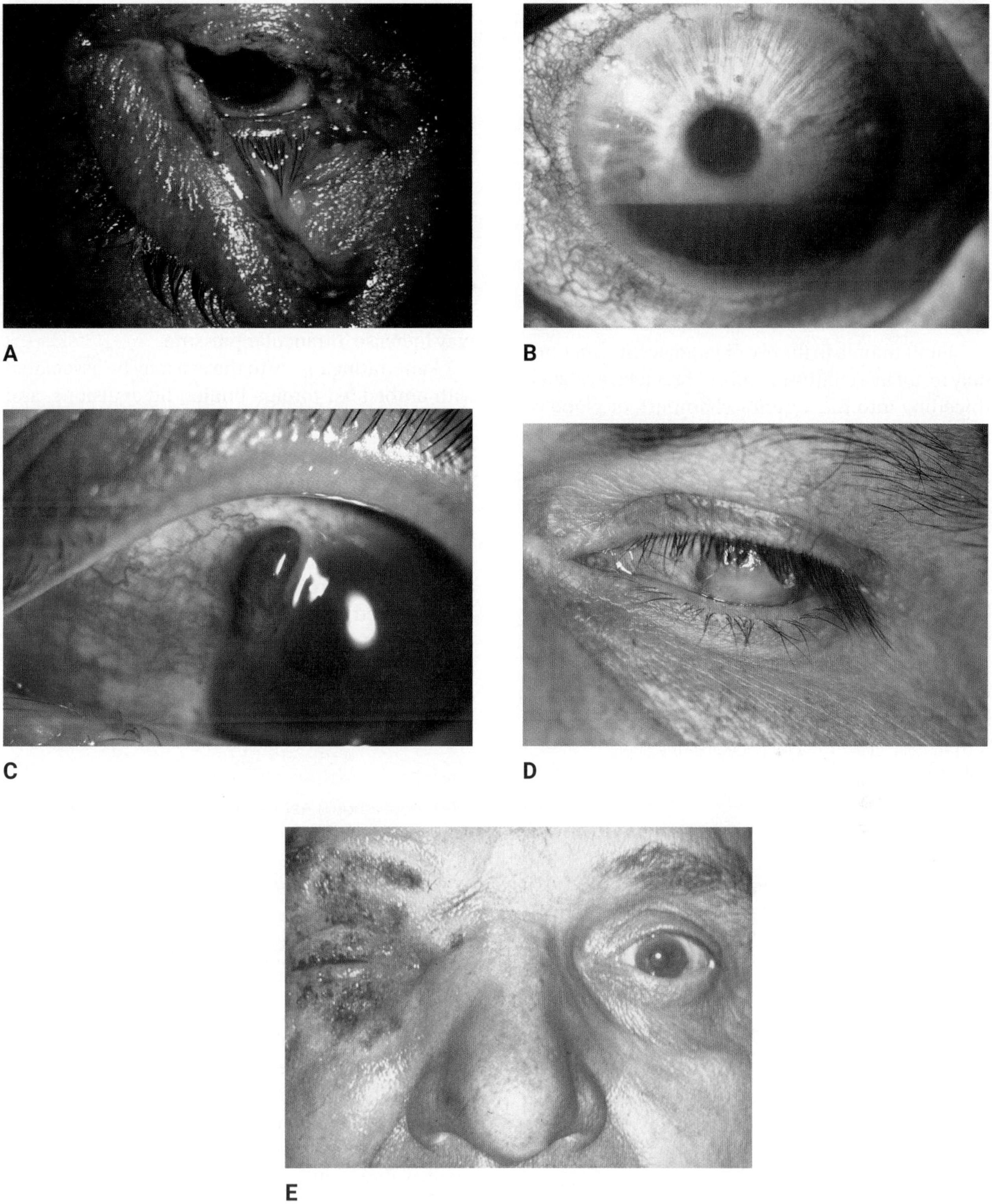

FIGURE 39-8 A. Avulsion of lid. **B.** Hyphema. **C.** Ruptured globe. **D.** Acid burn. **E.** Alkali burn.

A: Reproduced from Agrawal R, Rao G, Naigaonkar R, Ou X, Desai S. Prognostic factors for vision outcome after surgical repair of open globe injuries. *Indian J Ophthalmol*. 2011;59(6):465-470. http://doi.org/10.4103/0301-4738.86314; **B:** © Jones & Bartlett Learning; **C:** © Paul Whitten/Science Source; **D:** © Hercules Robinson/Medical Images; **E:** © Jones & Bartlett Learning.

excessive tearing, and sometimes a decrease in visual acuity. Often these signs and symptoms are delayed. The prehospital management of corneal abrasion is gentle irrigation with clear fluid. Corneal abrasions generally heal within 24 to 48 hours.

CRITICAL THINKING

Why will the patient with a suspected corneal abrasion need to be evaluated by a physician?

Blunt trauma to the eye or its adjacent structures may result in a contusion injury, **traumatic hyphema** (bleeding into the anterior chamber), or globe or scleral rupture. BOX 39-1 lists the signs and symptoms of these injuries.

Blunt injury to the eye may be associated with other serious injuries. Such injuries include orbital fracture, vitreous hemorrhage, and dislocation of the lens. The prehospital care should be limited to the control of any bleeding by application of gentle, direct pressure; protection of the eye with a metal shield or cardboard cup; and rapid transport for physician evaluation. If the paramedic suspects a traumatic hyphema or globe or scleral rupture, the patient's head should be elevated 30° to 45° to decrease intraocular pressure.[5] The patient should also be instructed to avoid any activity that might increase intraocular pressure. Analgesics and antiemetics may be indicated for pain relief and nausea. These drugs can reduce movement, straining, coughing, and retching that may increase intraocular pressure.

BOX 39-1 Signs and Symptoms of Eye Injuries

Contusion Injury

Traumatic dilation or constriction of the pupil
Pain
Photophobia
Blurred vision
Tears of the iris (tear-shaped pupil)

Traumatic Hyphema

Decreased pupil reactivity
Poor visual acuity
Blood in the anterior chamber (may be visible with a penlight)

Globe or Scleral Rupture

Decrease in visual acuity to hand movements or light perception
Lowered intraocular pressure (soft eye)
Pupil irregularity
Hyphema

Modified from: Owens PL, Mutter R. Emergency department visits related to eye injuries, 2008. HCUP Statistical Brief #112. Healthcare Cost and Utilization Project website. https://www.hcup-us.ahrq.gov/reports/statbriefs/sb112.pdf. Published May 2011. Accessed April 8, 2018.

Penetrating injury to the eye may be associated with embedded foreign bodies, lid avulsions, and lacerations to the lids, sclera, or cornea. Penetrating globe injuries can damage retinal structures and can cause a loss of **vitreous humor** (the jellylike fluid in the eye that fills the space between the lens and the retina) and subsequent blindness. The paramedic should control any bleeding around the eye by applying gentle, direct pressure. The globe should be protected from dehydration or contamination from foreign material. One way is to cover the orbital area with plastic or damp, sterile dressings and an eye shield.

NOTE

Eyedrops should not be used when globe rupture is suspected. Aggressive pain management is crucial to prevent or decrease expulsion of intraocular contents. If the patient is nauseated, antiemetics should be given.

The paramedic should stabilize foreign bodies protruding from the eye and should cover these with a cardboard cup and secure the cup with tape. The unaffected eye should also be covered to prevent **consensual movement** (one eye acting in concert with the other). The paramedic should not attempt to remove the object. If needed, the penetrating object may be shortened for transport (after consulting with medical direction).

Chemical injury to the eye (described in Chapter 38, *Burns*) may be associated with loss of corneal epithelial tissue, globe perforation, and scarring and deformation of eyelids and conjunctivae. These injuries are true emergencies and require immediate intervention.

A chemical exposure generally mandates extensive, continuous irrigation of both eyes with a neutral fluid for 20 minutes before patient transport and, if possible, while en route to the ED. Irrigation should be done in consultation with on-line medical direction to limit prolonged scene time and to prevent a delay in specialized ophthalmologic care.

Contact Lenses

Contact lenses are of three general types: hard, soft hydrophilic, and rigid gas-permeable. Hard lenses are microlenses that sometimes are prescribed for astigmatism (these lenses rarely are used today). Soft (hydrophilic) lenses usually are large in diameter (extending onto the conjunctiva). Soft lenses may be designed for daily or extended wear. Rigid gas-permeable lenses are similar in size to microlenses. These lenses have a low water content and high oxygen permeability.

As a rule, paramedics should not attempt to remove contact lenses in patients with eye injuries. To do so may cause more damage and may aggravate the injury. If management of an eye injury is complicated by the presence of contact lenses (eg, chemical burns to the eyes), medical direction may recommend that the lenses be removed. If the patient is unable to remove the lenses, the paramedic may be instructed to do so (BOX 39-2).

Dental Trauma

The adult normally has 32 teeth. Each tooth consists of two sections: the crown, which projects above the gingiva (the portion of the oral mucosa surrounding the tooth), and the root, which fits into the bony socket (alveolus) of the maxilla or mandible. Three layers make up the hard tissues of the teeth: the enamel, the dentin (ivory), and the cementum. The soft tissues of the teeth include the pulp and the periodontal membrane (**FIGURE 39-9**).

The teeth and associated alveolar process may be injured alone or along with fractures of the jaw or facial bones. The two most common types of dental trauma involve fractures and avulsions of the anterior teeth. If a tooth is fractured, the paramedic should examine the oral cavity carefully for tooth fragments. Removal of fragments reduces the risk of aspiration and obstruction of the airway. Lacerations

BOX 39-2 Removal of Contact Lenses

Removal of Hard and Rigid Gas-Permeable Lenses

1. With gloved hands, separate the eyelids so that the margins of the lids are beyond the top and bottom edges of the lens.
2. Gently pass the eyelids down and forward to the edges of the lens.
3. Move the eyelids toward each other, forcing the lens to slide out between them.
4. Store the lens in a container with water or saline, and label the container with the patient's name. If a contact lens container is not available, store each lens in a separate container and label as left or right.
5. If lens removal is difficult, gently move the lens downward from the cornea to the conjunctiva overlying the sclera until arrival in the ED.

Note: Special suction cups are also available for the removal of hard and rigid contact lenses. This device should be moistened with saline or sterile water before contacting the lens.

Removal of Soft Lenses

1. With gloved hands, pull down the lower eyelid.
2. Gently slide the soft lens down onto the conjunctiva.
3. Using a pinching motion, compress the lens between the thumb and index finger.
4. Remove the lens from the eye.
5. Store the lens in a container (marked right or left) with water or saline, and label the container with the patient's name.

FIGURE 39-9 Longitudinal section of a tooth.
© Jones & Bartlett Learning.

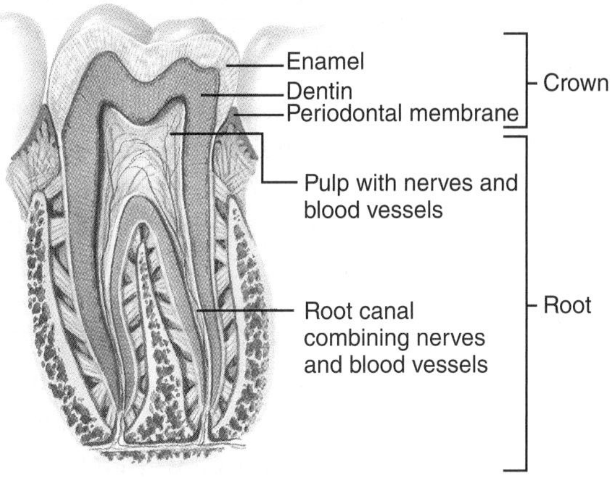

and avulsions to the tongue and surrounding mucous membranes often occur with dental trauma. These injuries often are painful and may bleed profusely. They may compromise the patient's airway as well.

Tooth avulsions are common, and some teeth can be saved with proper emergency treatment.[6] Permanent teeth that have been avulsed have a good survival rate if reimplanted and stabilized within 1 hour. (Deciduous teeth [milk or baby teeth] generally are not reimplanted. They may become fused to the bone, delaying formation and eruption of the permanent tooth.) If the avulsed tooth has been out of the patient's mouth for less than 15 minutes, medical direction may recommend reimplanting the tooth into the original socket. The paramedic should take care not to reimplant the tooth backward and should be alert for possible aspiration. Alternately, an alert cooperative patient may hold the tooth in the mouth where the saliva can keep it moist, although this approach is not recommended in patients with evidence intoxication, nausea or vomiting, decreased level of consciousness, or with any potential to develop any of these conditions. If reimplantation is impossible, the paramedic should follow the guidelines established by the American Dental Association and the American Association of Endodontists:

1. Never place an avulsed tooth in anything that can dry or crush the outside of the tooth.
2. Do not handle the tooth roughly. Do not rinse it off or rub, scrape, or disinfect the outside of the tooth in any way. (Any adherent membrane or fibrous tissue should be left in place to avoid stripping off the periodontal membrane and ligament, which are crucial to the survival of a reimplanted tooth.)
3. Place the tooth in a nurturing, break-resistant storage device (eg, Emergency Tooth Preserving System). This device should have a tightly fitted top and soft inner walls.
4. Store the tooth in a pH-balanced, isotonic, glucose-, calcium-, and magnesium-enriched cell-preserving fluid (eg, Hank solution). Use refrigerated fresh whole milk as the best alternative storage medium. (Powdered milk is not suitable.) For short periods (1 hour or less), use sterile saline. Do not use tap water because it damages the periodontal ligament.
5. Advise medical direction of avulsed teeth so that appropriate services will be available when the patient arrives in the ED.

Anterior Neck Trauma

Anterior neck injuries are caused by blunt and penetrating trauma (**FIGURE 39-10**). These injuries may result in damage to the skeletal structures, vascular structures, nerves, muscles, and glands of the neck. Common mechanisms of injury to the anterior neck are as follows:

- Strangulation from clothing, jewelry, or personal equipment getting caught in machinery
- All-terrain vehicles and other small motor vehicles (clothesline injuries to the neck from running into wires, ropes, or fences)
- Blow to the neck
- Contact sports (boxing, karate, basketball, football, hockey)
- Missile from a firearm
- Hanging
- Horseback riding
- Hyperextension and hyperflexion
- Industrial activities
- Motor vehicle crash (eg, neck striking dashboard or steering column)
- Sport and recreational activities (eg, snow skiing, water skiing)

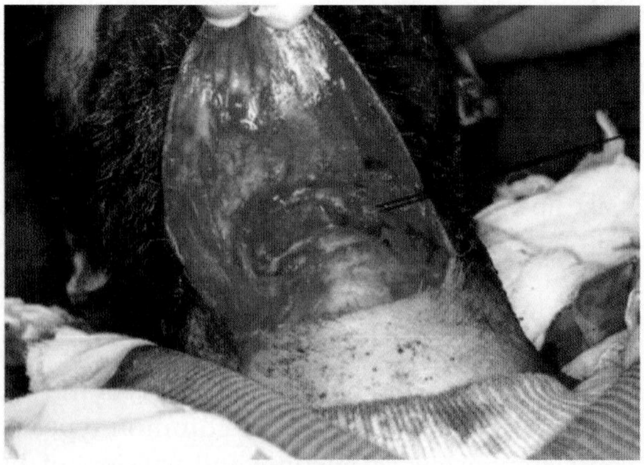

FIGURE 39-10 A stab wound that had entered the pharynx.

Reproduced from: Beigh Z, Ahmad R. Management of cut-throat injuries. *Egypt J Otolaryng*. 2014;30(3):268.

- Stabbing (knives, screwdrivers, or ice pick)
- Violent altercation

NOTE

The forces associated with blunt injury to the neck may cause a spinal injury (see Chapter 40, *Spine and Nervous System Trauma*). Therefore, the paramedic should consider and assess for cervical spine injury in these patients. Routine spine immobilization is not recommended for penetrating trauma to the head, neck, or torso.

Modified from: Haut ER, Kalish BT, Efron DT, et al. Spine immobilization in penetrating trauma: more harm than good? *J Trauma.* 2010;68:115-120; Vanderlan WB, Tew BE, McSwain NE. Increased risk of death with cervical spine immobilisation in penetrating cervical trauma. *Injury.* 2009;40:880-883; and Stuke LE, Pons PT, Guy JS, Chapleau WP, Butler FK, McSwain NE. Prehospital spine immobilization for penetrating trauma: review and recommendations from the Prehospital Trauma Life Support Executive Committee. *J Trauma.* 2011;71:763-769.

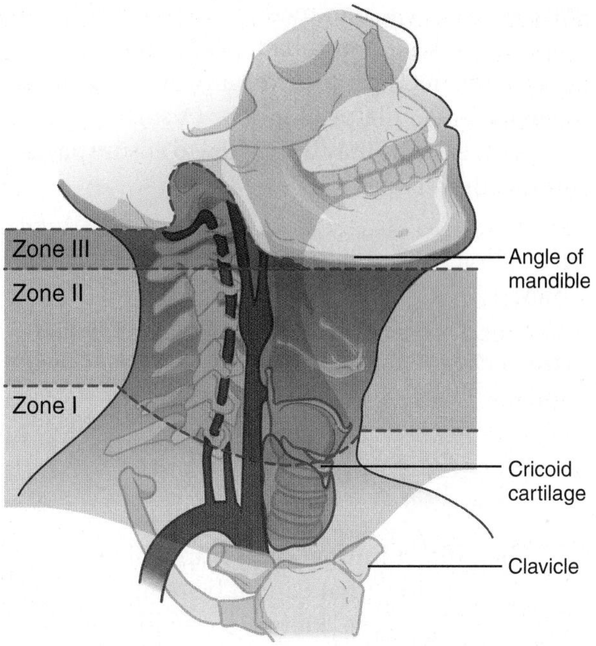

FIGURE 39-11 Zones of the neck. The junction of zone I and zone II is described variously as the cricoid cartilage or top of the clavicles.

Evaluation

For purposes of evaluating the trauma patient, the neck can be divided into three zones defined by horizontal planes (**FIGURE 39-11**).[7] Zone I represents the base of the neck. This zone extends from the sternal notch to the top of the clavicles or the cricoid cartilage. Injuries to this zone have the highest mortality rate because of the risk of injury to major vascular and thoracic structures (subclavian vessels and jugular veins, lungs, esophagus, trachea, cervical spine, cervical nerve roots).

Zone II extends from the clavicles or cricoid cartilage cephalad to the angle of the mandible. The carotid artery, jugular vein, trachea, larynx, esophagus, and cervical spine are the vital structures in this zone. Because of the relative size of zone II, injuries to this zone are the most common. However, they have a lower mortality rate than do zone I injuries.

Zone III is the part of the neck above the angle of the mandible. The risk of injury to the distal carotid artery, salivary glands, and pharynx is greatest in this zone.

Soft-Tissue Injuries

Soft-tissue injuries to the neck from blunt trauma often produce hematoma and associated edema or direct laryngeal or tracheal injury and can result in airway compromise. Penetrating trauma may produce lacerations and puncture wounds with resultant vascular, laryngotracheal, or esophageal injury. Blunt trauma may cause vascular injuries as well; however, this is uncommon. As with all trauma victims, initial evaluation and resuscitation must begin with rapid assessment, control of the airway, and consideration for spinal injury.

CRITICAL THINKING

Is prehospital airway control always possible in patients with anterior neck injuries?

Hematoma and Edema

Edema of the pharynx, larynx, trachea, epiglottis, and vocal cords may produce enough pressure in the neck tissues to obstruct the airway completely. If the airway is compromised (evidenced by dyspnea, inspiratory stridor, cyanosis, or changes in voice quality), the paramedic should consider oral or nasal intubation. Intubation stabilizes damaged areas of the neck, protects the airway, and provides a means for ventilatory support. (A slightly smaller endotracheal tube may be needed to ensure passage through the airway.)

> NOTE
> Crushed or severed airways can be blocked totally or partially by attempts at oral or nasal intubation. In these cases (if the patient is moving air), rapid transport with high-concentration oxygen is perhaps the most prudent course.

When direct intubation is impossible because of blood, vomitus (that cannot be removed by suction), or progressive edema, a cricothyrotomy or translaryngeal cannula ventilation (described in Chapter 15, *Airway Management, Respiration, and Artificial Ventilation*) may be indicated as a last resort in securing the airway, as there are many risks to the procedure. Another measure that may help in treating edematous airways includes the administration of cool, humidified oxygen. Yet another measure is the slight elevation of the patient's head.

Lacerations and Puncture Wounds

Lacerations and puncture wounds may be superficial or deep. Superficial wounds usually can be managed by covering the wound. The covering helps to prevent further contamination. Deep wounds are associated with more serious injuries to underlying structures. These injuries may require aggressive airway therapy and ventilatory support, suction, hemorrhage control by direct pressure, and fluid replacement. Signs and symptoms of significant penetrating neck trauma include the following:

- Active bleeding
- Dysphagia
- Dyspnea
- Hematemesis
- Hemoptysis
- Hoarseness
- Large or expanding hematoma
- Mobility and crepitus
- Neurologic deficit (stroke, brachial plexus injury, spinal cord injury)
- Pulse deficit
- Shock
- Stridor
- Subcutaneous emphysema
- Tenderness to palpation

> CRITICAL THINKING
> Why is rapid transport crucial when caring for a patient who has anterior neck injuries?

Vascular Injury

Blood vessels are the most commonly injured structures in the neck; they may be injured by blunt or penetrating trauma. Vessels at risk of injury include the carotid, vertebral, subclavian, innominate, and internal mammary arteries and the jugular and subclavian veins. Laceration of these major vessels can result in rapid exsanguination (death from extensive blood loss) if bleeding is not controlled.

Control of exsanguinating hemorrhage is the first priority. In the absence of exsanguination, securing the airway to provide adequate ventilatory support is the most important goal. Bleeding control can be achieved with constant, direct pressure. The paramedic should apply pressure only to the affected vessels so as not to completely obstruct blood flow to the brain. If bleeding cannot be controlled in this manner, medical direction may advise applying direct pressure with a gloved finger to the vessel.

> NOTE
> Under no circumstances should cervical vessels be clamped with hemostats in the prehospital setting. Doing so may traumatize vital vascular structures and may produce permanent nerve injury.

If the paramedic suspects a venous injury, the patient should be kept supine or in a slight Trendelenburg position. This position will help to prevent an air embolism (a rare but lethal complication). If the paramedic suspects an air embolism (described in Chapter 14, *Medication Administration*), the paramedic should turn the patient on the left side. The patient's head should be lower than the feet in an attempt to trap the air embolus in the right ventricle. Venous neck wounds should be dressed with an occlusive dressing.

Fluid replacement for hypovolemia should be guided by medical direction. Fluid replacement may include using large-bore catheters and isotonic crystalloid (lactated Ringer solution or normal saline). If penetrating injury to the base of the neck (zone I) has occurred, upper extremity venous drainage may be compromised by the laceration. In this event, placement of at least one IV line in a lower extremity should be considered. Medical direction may advise that a second IV line be placed in the upper extremity on the side opposite the injury.

Laryngeal or Tracheal Injury

Injury from blunt or penetrating trauma to the anterior neck may cause fracture or dislocation of the laryngeal and tracheal cartilages, hemorrhage, or swelling of the air passages. These injuries can compromise the airway and cause respiratory distress. Airway injury can lead to death in head and neck trauma patients. Thus, rapid and judicious control of the airway and prevention of aspiration are crucial. In addition, a high degree of suspicion for associated vascular disruption and esophageal, chest, and intra-abdominal injury is a key aspect of preventing death. Injuries that may be associated with laryngeal and tracheal trauma include the following:

- Fracture of the hyoid bone, resulting in laceration and distortion of the epiglottis
- Separation of the hyoid and thyroid cartilages, resulting in epiglottis dislocation, aspiration, and subcutaneous emphysema
- Fractures of the thyroid cartilage, resulting in epiglottis and vocal cord avulsion, arytenoid dislocation, and aspiration of blood and bone fragments
- Dislocation or fracture of the cricothyroid, resulting in long-term laryngeal stenosis, laryngeal nerve paralysis, and laryngotracheal avulsion
- Fracture to the trachea, resulting in tracheal avulsion, complete airway obstruction, and subcutaneous emphysema

The management of laryngeal and tracheal trauma is controversial. Some medical direction agencies recommend oral or nasal intubation. Other agencies believe that intubation attempts may contribute to the potential for injury resulting from a lack of oxygen during the procedure. These attempts also may further damage the airway structures. Alternative methods of airway management include the use of bag-mask ventilation, cricothyrotomy, and translaryngeal cannula ventilation.

> **NOTE**
>
> Airway procedures that involve entry through the neck generally are avoided in the field because of the associated risks. As a rule, these patients should be well ventilated with a bag-mask device. They should be transported rapidly to the receiving facility for surgical tracheotomy as well. As described in Chapter 15, *Airway Management, Respiration, and Artificial Ventilation*, translaryngeal cannula ventilation is hazardous in the presence of complete airway obstruction. Incorrectly used, this technique does not provide adequate exhalation of gases and air. The technique may result in carbon dioxide retention and significant injury from high pressure developing in the chest and airways (barotrauma). Nevertheless, in a life-threatening situation where tracheal intubation and bag-mask ventilation cannot be performed to restore adequate gas exchange, the maneuver may be considered with authorization from medical direction.
>
> *Modified from*: Jagminas L. Percutaneous transtracheal jet ventilation. Medscape website. https://emedicine.medscape.com/article/1413327-overview. Updated April 02, 2018. Accessed April 14, 2018.

If penetrating trauma causes complete disruption of the laryngotracheal structure, medical direction may recommend dissection through the wound. That way, the exposed distal trachea can be cannulated directly with a cuffed endotracheal tube. Regardless of the method chosen, emergency care is directed at securing the airway, providing adequate ventilatory support, controlling hemorrhage, treating for shock, and providing rapid transport to an appropriate medical facility for definitive surgical care.

Esophageal Injury

Esophageal injuries should be suspected in patients with trauma to the neck or chest. Specific injuries that require a high degree of suspicion for associated esophageal injury include tracheal fractures, penetrating trauma from stab or gunshot wounds, and ingestion of caustic substances.

Esophageal injury is difficult to diagnose. It may be overlooked as the paramedic focuses on more obvious injuries that pose a threat to life. Signs and symptoms may include subcutaneous emphysema, neck hematoma, and bleeding from the mouth and nose.

Esophageal perforation is associated with a high mortality rate. Death results from mediastinitis caused by the release of gastric contents into the thoracic cavity. If not contraindicated, the paramedic should place the patient with a suspected esophageal tear in a semi-Fowler position. (This is an inclined position. The upper half of the body is raised by elevating the head or stretcher about 30°.) This position will help to prevent reflux of gastric contents.

CRITICAL THINKING

Are these signs and symptoms so unique that you will be able to distinguish esophageal injury as the cause, versus other kinds of traumatic conditions?

Head Trauma

The anatomic components of the skull are the scalp, beneath which is the cranial vault, beneath which are the dural membrane, the arachnoid membrane, the pia mater, and brain substance. Injuries to the skull may be classified as soft-tissue injuries to the scalp and as skull fractures.

NOTE

All patients with head or neck trauma must be suspected to have a spinal injury. Appropriate evaluation for cervical spine injury must be performed and spinal precautions taken when needed.

Soft-Tissue Injuries to the Scalp

The most common scalp injury is an irregular linear laceration. Like the face, the scalp is very vascular. Thus, scalp lacerations may bleed heavily (**FIGURE 39-12**).

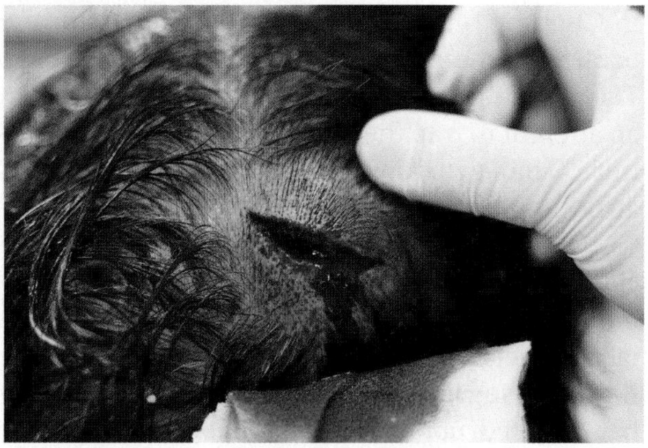

FIGURE 39-12 Even small wounds from the scalp can bleed profusely.

They also may result in hypovolemia, particularly in infants and children. Other, less-frequent scalp injuries include the **stellate wound** (star-shaped wound that can be caused by close contact with a ballistic wound), avulsions, and **subgaleal hematoma** (bleeding in the potential space between the skull and the scalp).

Management of soft-tissue injuries to the scalp includes efforts to prevent contamination of open wounds, use of direct pressure or pressure dressings to decrease blood loss, and replacement of fluids if needed. The potential for underlying skull fracture and brain and spinal trauma also exists with these injuries. Scalp lacerations that are the only injury rarely produce life-threatening complications. However, such lacerations can result in excessive blood loss. If the dressing on a scalp wound continues to saturate with blood, hemostasis has not been achieved. Additional dressings should not be applied until direct pressure or other techniques have provided hemorrhage control. If not contraindicated, the paramedic should position all patients with head or facial trauma on a stretcher with the head elevated 30° (semi-Fowler position).

Skull Fractures

Skull fractures may be classified as linear fractures, basilar fractures, depressed fractures, and open vault fractures (**FIGURE 39-13**). Complications associated with these injuries are cranial nerve injury, vascular involvement (eg, meningeal artery and dural sinuses), infection, underlying brain injury, and dural defects

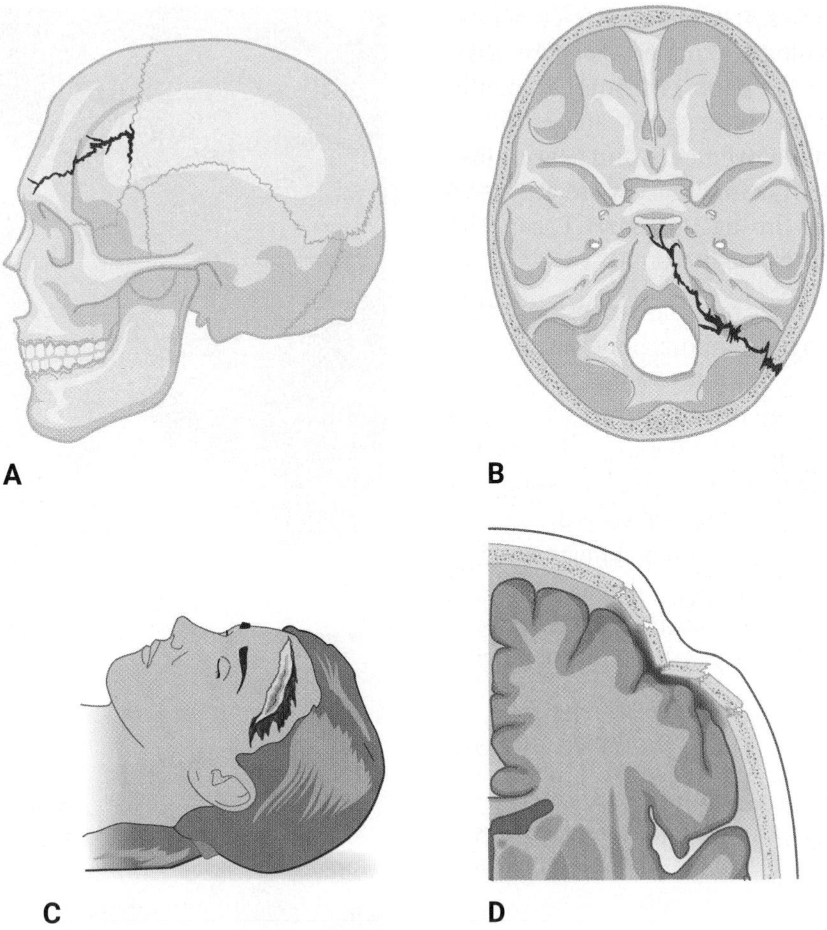

FIGURE 39-13 Skull fractures. **A.** Linear skull fracture. **B.** Basilar skull fracture. **C.** Open vault fracture. **D.** Depressed skull fracture.

caused by depressed bone fragments. As with all injuries to the head, the paramedic should consider the possibility of a spinal injury, and appropriate spinal precautions should be taken when needed.

Linear Skull Fractures

Linear skull fracture (seen as a straight line on the radiograph) accounts for 80% of all fractures to the skull.[8] Such fractures usually are not depressed. Often linear fractures occur without an overlying scalp laceration. As an isolated injury, these fractures usually have a low rate of complication. However, if the fracture is associated with a scalp laceration, infection is possible. Linear fractures that cross the meningeal groove in the temporal–parietal area, midline, or occipital area may lead to epidural bleeding from the middle cerebral artery.

> CRITICAL THINKING
> How will you be able to detect linear skull fractures during a physical examination in the prehospital setting?

Basilar Skull Fractures

A **basilar skull fracture** is usually associated with major-impact trauma. These injuries may occur when the mandibular condyles perforate into the base of the skull. More commonly, though, they result from an extension of a linear fracture into the floor of the anterior and middle fossae. Basilar skull fractures can cause a dural tear leading to a connection between the subarachnoid space, the paranasal sinuses, and the middle ear. Patients may have nausea and vomiting, abnormal extraocular movements, and hearing loss or facial palsies when cranial nerves are affected.[9] These injuries usually are diagnosed by CT scan. The following signs may also be present:

- Ecchymosis over the mastoid process resulting from fracture to the temporal bone or sphenoid bone (**Battle sign**) (**FIGURE 39-14A**)
- Ecchymosis of one or both orbits with tarsal plate sparing that impedes the spread of bruising caused by fracture of the base of the sphenoid sinus (**raccoon eyes**) (**FIGURE 39-14B**)
- Blood behind the tympanic membrane caused by fractures of the temporal bone (**hemotympanum**)
- CSF leakage from the nose (rhinorrhea) or eyes (otorrhea) that can result in bacterial meningitis

NOTE

Battle sign and raccoon eyes usually do not occur until 1 to 3 days after the injury. If they are present on the arrival of EMS, the bruising is most likely the result of a prior injury.

Other complications associated with basilar skull fractures include cranial nerve injuries and massive hemorrhage from vascular involvement of the carotid artery. Treatment for basilar skull fractures includes bed rest, in-hospital observation, and evaluation for hearing loss caused by acoustic nerve injury.

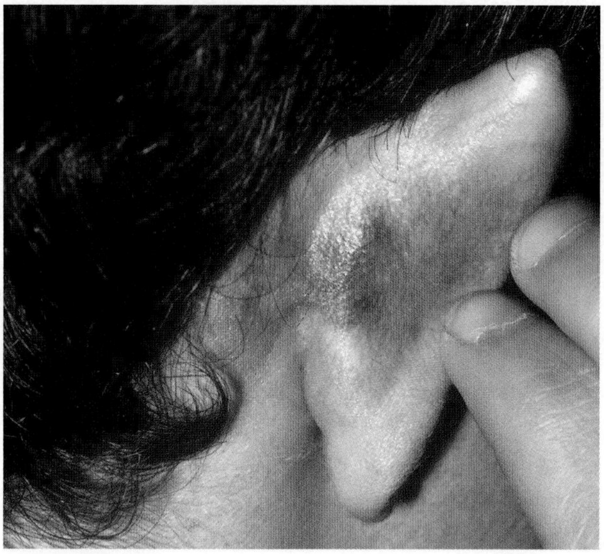

A

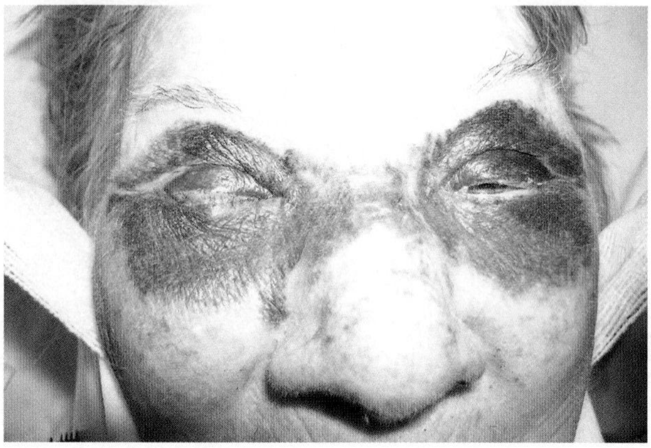

B

FIGURE 39-14 **A.** Battle sign. **B.** Raccoon eyes.

Depressed Skull Fractures

A **depressed skull fracture** is usually resulting from a relatively small object striking the head at high speed. Thus, they commonly are associated with scalp lacerations causing an open fracture. These patients have a risk of infection and seizures. Depressed skull fractures occur when a portion of the skull is pushed below the level of the adjacent skull. The frontal and parietal bones most often are affected by these fractures. Some patients with depressed skull fractures will have associated hematoma and cerebral contusions. If the depression is greater than the thickness of the skull, dural laceration also is likely. Patients with depressed skull fractures often require surgical removal of the bone fragments (craniectomy).

Open Vault Fractures

An **open vault fracture** results when an opening exists between a scalp laceration and brain tissue. Because of the nature of these injuries and the force required to produce them, they often are associated with trauma to other systems. They have a high mortality rate. Exposure of brain tissue to the external environment may lead to infection (meningitis). Open vault fractures require surgical repair. Prehospital management usually is limited to evaluation for the need of spinal precautions, ventilatory support, efforts to prevent contamination, and rapid transport to an appropriate medical facility.

Cranial Nerve Injuries

As described in Chapter 10, *Review of Human Systems*, 12 pairs of cranial nerves leave the brain and pass through openings in the skull called foramina. Injury to cranial nerves usually is associated with skull fractures. Signs and symptoms of common cranial nerve injuries are as follows:

Cranial nerve I (olfactory nerve)
- Loss of smell
- Impaired taste (dependent on food aroma)
- Hallmark of basilar skull fracture

Cranial nerve II (optic nerve)
- Blindness in one or both eyes
- Visual field defects

Cranial nerve III (oculomotor nerve)
- Ipsilateral (same side), dilated, fixed pupil
- Especially compression by the temporal lobe
- Mimics direct ocular trauma

Cranial nerve VII (facial nerve)
- Immediate or delayed facial paralysis
- Basilar skull fracture

Cranial nerve VIII (vestibulocochlear [auditory] nerve)
- Deafness
- Basilar skull fracture

Traumatic Brain Injury

A **traumatic brain injury (TBI)** is defined by the Brain Injury Association of America as "an alteration in brain function, or other evidence of brain pathology, caused by an external force" (BOX 39-3).[10] TBI can be divided into two categories: **primary brain injury** and **secondary brain injury**. Primary brain injury refers to direct trauma to the brain and to the associated vascular injuries that occurred from the initial injury. Secondary brain injury results from intracellular and extracellular derangements that were either initiated at the time of the injury or result from a consequence of the initial injury. These derangements may include hypoxia, hypocapnia, and hypercapnia from airway compromise, aspiration of gastric contents, and thoracic injury; anemia and hypotension from external and internal hemorrhage; and hyperglycemia or hypoglycemia that can further injure ischemic brain tissue. The adverse effects of secondary brain injury can potentially be minimized if they are recognized and properly managed in the prehospital setting. Brain injuries can be classified as diffuse (moderate or severe) or focal. (The two forms are commonly found together.[11])

BOX 39-3 Brain Injury Facts

According to the Centers for Disease Control and Prevention's National Center for Injury Prevention and Control, annually in the United States:
- At least 2.5 million people sustain a TBI.
- Approximately 56,000 people die from a TBI.
- Approximately 329,290 TBIs occur among those 19 years and younger from sports-related injuries.
- Falls are the leading cause of TBI.
- Adults aged 75 years or older have the highest rates of TBI-related hospitalization and death.

Modified from: Centers for Disease Control and Prevention, National Center for Injury Prevention and Control, Division of Unintentional Injury Prevention. Traumatic brain injury and concussion. TBI: get the facts. Centers for Disease Control and Prevention website. https://www.cdc.gov/traumaticbraininjury/get_the_facts.html. Updated April 27, 2017. Accessed April 7, 2018.

Diffuse injuries (usually caused by acceleration–deceleration forces)
- Diffuse axonal injury (DAI)
- Hypoxic–ischemic damage
- Meningitis
- Vascular injury

Focal injuries (generally caused by contact)
- Scalp injury
- Skull fracture
- Surface contusions
- Brain hemorrhage

Diffuse Brain Injuries

Diffuse brain injuries include concussion and **diffuse axonal injury (DAI)**. The major cause of damage in diffuse injury is the disruption of axons—the neural processes that allow one nerve to communicate with another.

NOTE

Diffuse Brain Injury, DAI, and Concussion: How Are They Different?

The term *diffuse axonal injury* was coined by Thomas Gennarelli in the early 1980s. He described DAI as a frequent form of TBI in which a clinical spectrum of increasing injury severity is paralleled by progressively increasing amounts of axonal damage in the brain. He described brain injury as a disease or process, not an event (**TABLE 39-1**). DAI and concussion are subtypes of diffuse brain injury. Less-severe DAI is associated with concussive syndromes. When most severe, DAI causes a prolonged traumatic coma that is not related to lesions, increased intracranial pressure (ICP), or ischemia. Rather, it is related to the increasing numbers of damaged axons. The table provides definitions of diffuse brain injury categories. The categories are commonly determined by using the abbreviated injury scale and the Ommaya-Genneralli scale.

Reproduced from: Gennarelli T, Pintar F, Yoganandan N. Biomechanical Tolerances for Diffuse Brain Injury and a Hypothesis for Genotypic Variability in Response to Trauma. Annual Proceedings/Association for the Advancement of Automotive Medicine. 2003(47):624-628.

Concussion

Concussion is sometimes called a **mild DAI**. Concussion is caused by a mild to moderate impact to the skull, movement of the brain within the cranial vault, or both. It is a syndrome of "biomechanically induced alteration of brain function, typically affecting memory and orientation, which may involve loss of consciousness."[12] Concussion occurs when the function of the brainstem (particularly the reticular activating system) or both cerebral cortices are temporarily disturbed. This results in a brief altered level of consciousness, but not always a loss of consciousness. (If a loss of consciousness occurs, it is usually less than 5 minutes in duration.) A concussion may be a serious injury; no concussion is minor.

The altered level of consciousness or loss of consciousness often is followed by periods of drowsiness, restlessness, and confusion, with a fairly rapid return to normal behavior. The patient may have no recall of the events before the injury (**retrograde amnesia**). In addition, amnesia may exist after recovery of consciousness (**antegrade amnesia**). This inability to create new memories may produce anxiety. The patient may ask repetitive questions (eg, Where am I? What happened?). Other signs and symptoms of concussion are vomiting; combativeness; transient visual disturbances (eg, light flashes, wavy lines); defects in equilibrium and coordination; and changes in blood pressure, pulse rate, and respiration (rare). After physician evaluation, treatment usually consists of in-hospital or home observation by a reliable observer for 24 to 48 hours.

TABLE 39-1 Definitions of Diffuse Brain Injury Categories

Category	Abbreviated Injury Scale	Ommaya-Gennarelli Concussion Grade	Loss of Consciousness
Mild concussion	1	1–3	None
Classical concussion	2	4	<1 hour
Severe concussion	3	4	1–6 hours
Mild DAI	4	5	6–24 hours
Moderate DAI	5	5	>24 hours[a]
Severe DAI	5	5	>24 hours[b]

[a]No brainstem abnormality.

[b]With decerebration, decortication.

Abbreviation: DAI, diffuse axonal injury

Modified from: Gennarelli TA, Pintar FA, Yoganandan N. Biomechanical tolerances for diffuse brain injury and a hypothesis for genotypic variability in response to trauma. *Annual Proceedings/Association for the Advancement of Automotive Medicine*. 2003;47:624-628.

CRITICAL THINKING

Consider the patient with a new onset of retrograde or antegrade amnesia. Why should the patient not be considered a reliable historian?

A concussion injury affects the patient most severely at the time of impact but is followed by improvement. Concussion is the most common type of brain injury. Any patient whose condition worsens over time or whose level of consciousness deteriorates rather than improves must be suspected of having a more serious injury. Therefore, documentation of baseline measurements of level of consciousness, memory status, and neurologic function (eg, Glasgow Coma Scale [GCS] or AVPU [Awake and alert, responsive to Verbal stimuli, responsive to Pain, Unresponsive] scale) in any patient with a head injury is important. If a patient with a concussion has a loss of consciousness lasting more than 5 minutes, the paramedic should suspect a more serious injury caused by a contusion or hemorrhage.

Moderate DAI

A **moderate DAI** is a head injury that results in minute petechial bruising of the brain tissue. The involvement of the brainstem and reticular activating system leads to unconsciousness. These injuries account for 20% of all severe head injuries and 45% of all cases of diffuse injury.[13] These patients will often have a basilar skull fracture. Most patients will survive the injury; however, permanent neurologic impairment is common.

A patient with moderate DAI initially will be unconscious, followed by persistent confusion, disorientation, and amnesia of the event. During recovery, these patients often experience an inability to concentrate, frequent periods of anxiety, uncharacteristic mood swings, and sensorimotor deficits (eg, an altered sense of smell). Patients with moderate DAI are managed similar to those patients with concussion, with frequent reassessments of the level of consciousness and ensuring that the airway and tidal volume are adequate. If possible, patients with a head injury should be moved to a quiet, calm area. Exposure to bright lights should be avoided. (Patients often are photophobic.) In addition, constant reorientation of the patient may be necessary.

Severe DAI

As the name implies, a **severe DAI** is the severest form of brain injury. Severe DAI was once known as a brainstem injury. It involves severe mechanical shearing of many axons in both cerebral hemispheres extending to the brainstem. Severe DAI occurs in approximately 16% of patients with severe head trauma.[14] These patients often are unconscious for prolonged periods. They may exhibit abnormal posturing and other signs of ICP, described later in this chapter. The prehospital care for these patients is focused on ensuring an adequate airway and tidal volume. Hypoxia must be prevented in all patients with head injury. (This helps to avoid secondary injury to brain tissue.)

CRITICAL THINKING

Can a patient with a DAI die as a result of that injury?

Focal Injury

A **focal injury** is a specific, grossly observable **brain lesion** concentrated in one region of the brain. Included in this category are lesions that result from skull fracture (previously described), contusion, edema with associated increased ICP, ischemia, and hemorrhage. The brain occupies 80% of the intracranial space. It is divided into four areas: the brainstem (consisting of the medulla, pons, and midbrain), the diencephalon (including the thalamus and hypothalamus), the cerebrum, and the cerebellum. The intracranial contents consist of brain water (58%), brain solids (25%), CSF (7%), and intracranial blood (10%).

Cerebral Contusion

A **cerebral contusion** is bruising of the brain in the area of the cortex or deeper within the frontal (most common), temporal, or occipital lobes. This bruising produces a structural change in the brain tissue. Bruising results in greater neurologic deficits and abnormalities than are seen with concussions. These abnormalities may include seizures, hemiparesis, aphasia, and personality changes. If the brainstem also is contused, the patient may lose consciousness. In some cases, the comatose state may be prolonged. It may last hours to days or longer.

Of the patients who die from head injury, the majority have cerebral contusions at autopsy.

If applied force is enough to cause the brain to be displaced against the irregular surfaces of the skull, tiny blood vessels in the pia mater may rupture. The brain substance may be damaged locally at the site of impact (**coup**). Or the brain may be damaged on the opposite, or contralateral, side (**contrecoup**). Contrecoup injuries often are caused by deceleration of the head. This injury may occur, for example, in a fall or motor vehicle crash.

The most important complication associated with cerebral contusion is increased ICP manifested by headache, nausea, vomiting, seizures, and a declining level of consciousness. These signs usually are delayed responses to the injury. Therefore, they usually are not seen in the prehospital emergency setting. Treatment is aimed at reducing cerebral swelling.

Edema

Major injuries to the brain often result in swelling of the brain tissue with or without associated hemorrhage. The swelling results from humoral and metabolic responses to injury. Swelling leads to considerable increases in ICP. This increased pressure in turn can lead to decreased cerebral perfusion (described later) or herniation.

Ischemia

Ischemia can result from vascular injuries, secondary vascular spasm, or increased ICP. In any case, focal or more global infarcts can result.

Hemorrhage

The same forces that result in concussion and contusion also may cause serious vascular damage. This damage may result in hemorrhage into or around brain tissue. These injuries may cause an epidural or subdural hematoma. The hematoma compresses the underlying brain tissue, or produces intraparenchymal hemorrhage (bleeding directly into the brain tissue). This bleeding often results from cerebral contusions and skull fractures.

Cerebral Blood Flow. Although the brain accounts for only 2% of adult weight, 20% of total body oxygen use and 25% of total body glucose use are devoted to brain metabolism. Oxygen and glucose delivery are controlled by cerebral blood flow.

Cerebral blood flow is a function of **cerebral perfusion pressure (CPP)** and resistance of the cerebral vascular bed. Cerebral blood flow is determined by the **mean arterial pressure (MAP)** (see Chapter 35, *Shock*) minus the ICP (CPP = MAP − ICP). Normal MAP ranges from 85 to 95 mm Hg. ICP is normally 10 to 15 mm Hg or less. Thus, normal CPP is between 70 and 80 mm Hg. (A CPP of 60 mm Hg is the minimum threshold to adequately perfuse the brain.[15]) As ICP approaches the MAP, the gradient for flow decreases and cerebral blood flow decreases. That is, when ICP increases, CPP decreases. As CPP decreases, vessels in the brain dilate (cerebral vasodilation). This vasodilation results in increased cerebral blood volume (increasing ICP) and further cerebral vasodilation. In most EMS systems, the MAP is calculated by the monitor. However, ICP is not typically measured in the prehospital setting. To compensate, maintaining a systolic blood pressure (SBP) above the recommended level for the patient's age (90 mm Hg for an adult) may help maintain adequate MAP.[16]

CRITICAL THINKING

When ICP is increasing and CPP is decreasing, what happens to the flow of oxygen to the brain and carbon dioxide from the brain to the capillaries?

Vascular tone in the normal brain is regulated by partial pressure of carbon dioxide (P_{CO_2}), partial pressure of oxygen (P_{O_2}), and autonomic and neurohumoral control; P_{CO_2} has the greatest effect on intracerebral vascular diameter and subsequent resistance. For example, if P_{CO_2} is increased from 40 to 80 mm Hg, cerebral blood flow is doubled. This results in increased brain blood volume and ICP.

Intracranial Pressure. The normal range of ICP is 10 to 15 mm Hg or less. When ICP rises above this level, the body has difficulty maintaining adequate CPP, usually because of an expanding mass or diffuse swelling. Cerebral blood flow is diminished when the CPP is not adequate. As the cranial vault continues to fill (because of brain edema or expanding hematoma), the body tries to compensate for the decline in CPP by an increase in MAP (Cushing reflex). However, this increase in cerebral blood flow further elevates the ICP. As pressure continues to increase, CSF is displaced to make up for the expansion (**FIGURE 39-15**). If unresolved, the brain substance may herniate over the edge of the tentorium (**FIGURE 39-16**). (The tentorium is one of three extensions of the dura mater that separates the cerebellum from the occipital lobe of the cerebrum.) Alternatively, it may herniate through the foramen magnum.

Early signs and symptoms of increased ICP include headache, nausea and vomiting, and altered level of consciousness (**BOX 39-4**). These signs and symptoms eventually are followed by increased SBP, bradycardia, and irregular respiratory pattern (**Cushing triad**). Pulse pressure may widen as SBP increases, and irregular respirations may deteriorate into apnea. As the volume continues to expand in the cranial vault, herniation of the temporal lobe of the brain through the tentorium may occur. The herniation causes compression

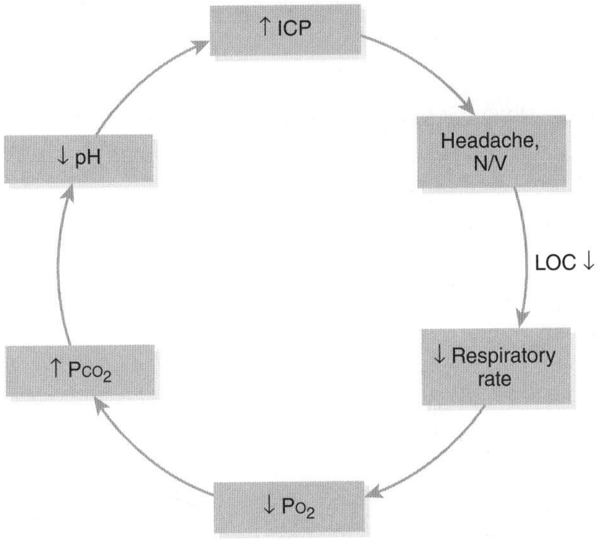

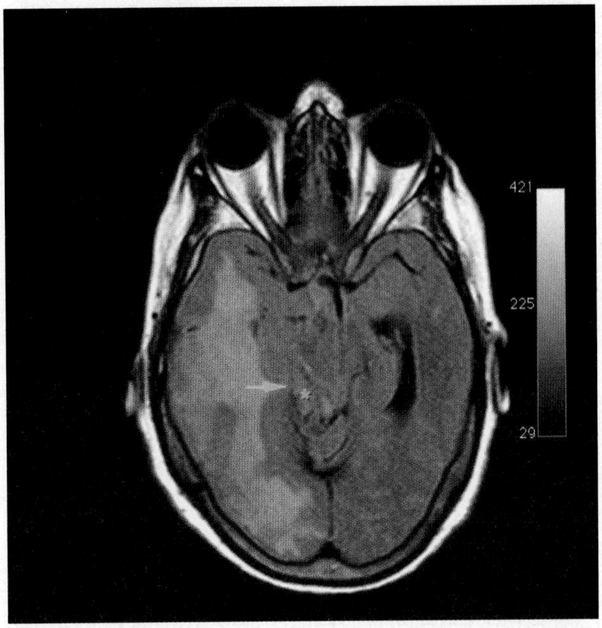

FIGURE 39-16 Medial part of the right temporal lobe is seen to be herniating over the tentorium (arrow), causing compression of the mesencephalon.

Reproduced with permission from Radiopaedia.

Abbreviations: ICP, intracranial pressure; LOC, level of consciousness; N/V, nausea or vomitting; Pco₂, partial pressure of carbon dioxide; Po₂, partial pressure of oxygen

FIGURE 39-15 Effects of increased intracranial pressure.

© Jones & Bartlett Learning.

BOX 39-4 Levels of Increasing ICP

Cortex and Upper Brainstem

Blood pressure rises; pulse rate slows.
Pupils remain reactive.
Cheyne-Stokes respirations may be present.
Patient initially will try to localize and remove painful stimuli (eventually withdraws and flexion occurs).
All effects are reversible at this stage.

Middle Brainstem

Wide pulse pressure and bradycardia are present.
Pupils become nonreactive or sluggish.
Central neurogenic hyperventilation develops.
Abnormal posturing (extension) occurs.
Few patients function normally with injury at this level.

Lower Portion of Brainstem/Medulla

Pupil is "blown" (fixed and dilated) on same side of injury.
Respirations become ataxic.
Patient will be flaccid.
Pulse rate is irregular.
QRS, ST-segment, and T-wave changes will be present.
Blood pressure will fluctuate.
These patients generally do not survive.

of cranial nerve III. This produces a dilated pupil and loss of the light reflex on the side of compression. The patient rapidly becomes unresponsive to verbal and painful stimuli. The patient may exhibit **decorticate posturing**, or abnormal flexion posturing, which is characterized by extension of the legs and flexion of the arms at the elbows. Or the patient may exhibit **decerebrate posturing**, or abnormal extension posturing, which is characterized by extension of all four extremities (**FIGURE 39-17**).

CRITICAL THINKING

Why is cranial nerve III affected by this shift in brain tissue?

Respiratory Patterns. As ICP continues to rise, abnormal respiratory patterns (described in Chapter 15, *Airway Management, Respiration, and Artificial Ventilation*) may develop. Respiratory abnormalities associated with increased ICP and significant brainstem injury include hypoventilation, Cheyne-Stokes breathing (which may accompany decorticate posturing), central neurogenic hyperventilation (which may accompany decerebrate posturing), and ataxic breathing. The presence of decorticate (abnormal flexion) or decerebrate (abnormal extension) posturing and abnormal respiratory patterns indicate a relatively severe injury; abnormal posturing is suggestive of herniation or impending herniation.[17]

NOTE

Some motion of the limbs, albeit abnormal, is better than no motion of the limbs. No motion indicates a worse level of neurologic function.

Types of Brain Hemorrhage

Traditionally, brain hemorrhages are classified according to their location as epidural, subdural, subarachnoid, or cerebral (intraparenchymal) (**FIGURE 39-18**).

Epidural Hematoma. An **epidural hematoma** (accounting for 0.5% to 1% of all head injuries[18]) is a collection of blood between the cranium and the dura in the epidural space (**FIGURE 39-19**). The hematoma usually is a rapidly developing lesion and is commonly associated

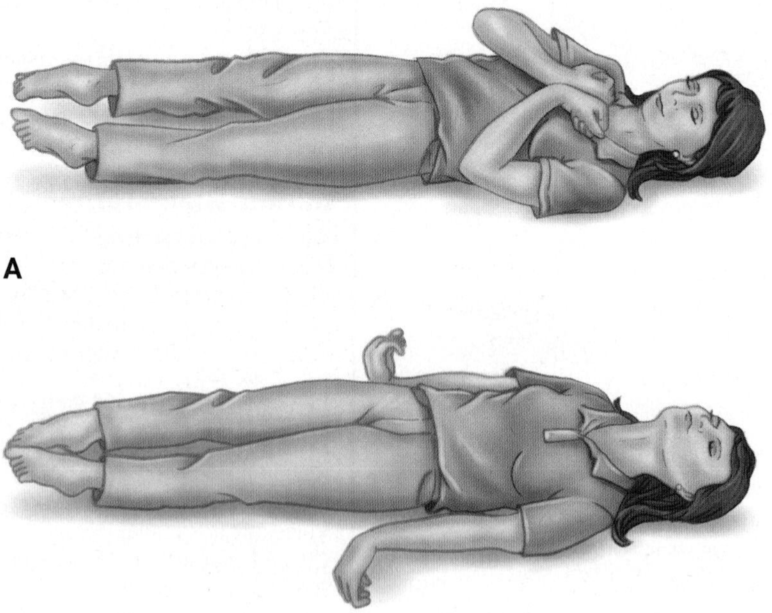

A

B

FIGURE 39-17 A. Abnormal flexion (decorticate posturing). **B.** Abnormal extension (decerebrate posturing).

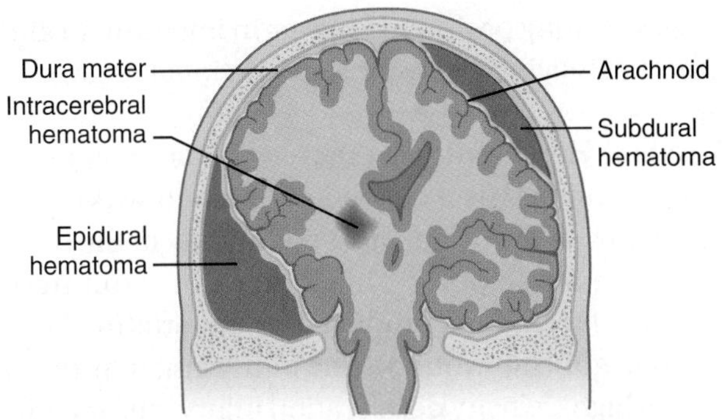

FIGURE 39-18 Varieties of intracranial hemorrhage.

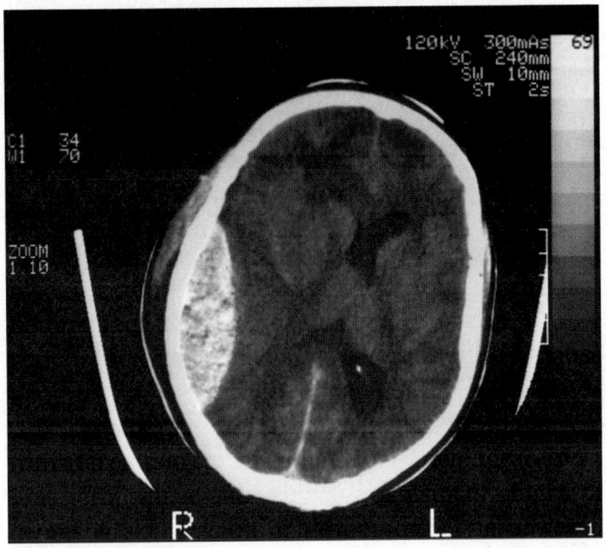

FIGURE 39-19 Computed tomography scan of the head showing an epidural hematoma.

with a laceration or tear of the middle meningeal artery. This hemorrhage often occurs as a result of a linear or depressed skull fracture in the temporal bone; however, bleeding from other sites can also produce epidural hemorrhage. If the source of hemorrhage is mostly venous, deterioration usually is not as rapid because low-pressure vessels bleed more slowly.

Some patients with epidural hematoma have a transient loss of consciousness, followed by a lucid interval in which neurologic status returns to normal; others may have a variable presentation or never regain consciousness. The lucid interval usually lasts between 6 and 18 hours. During this time the hematoma enlarges. As ICP rises, the patient develops a headache and becomes lethargic, with a decreasing level of consciousness and contralateral hemiparesis. In the early stages of an epidural hematoma, the patient may report only a headache and drowsiness. Definitive treatment includes immediate recognition and rapid transport to a proper facility for surgery. Common causes of epidural hematoma include low-velocity blows to the head, violent altercations, and deceleration injuries. About 20% of these patients who are comatose die.[18]

CRITICAL THINKING

What could account for delays in surgical treatment, causing subsequent death, in patients who have an epidural hematoma?

Subdural Hematoma. A **subdural hematoma** is a collection of blood between the dura and the arachnoid mater in the subdural space (**FIGURE 39-20**). This injury usually results from bleeding of the veins that bridge the subdural space. Associated contusion or laceration of the brain often is present. The hematoma often results from blunt head trauma.

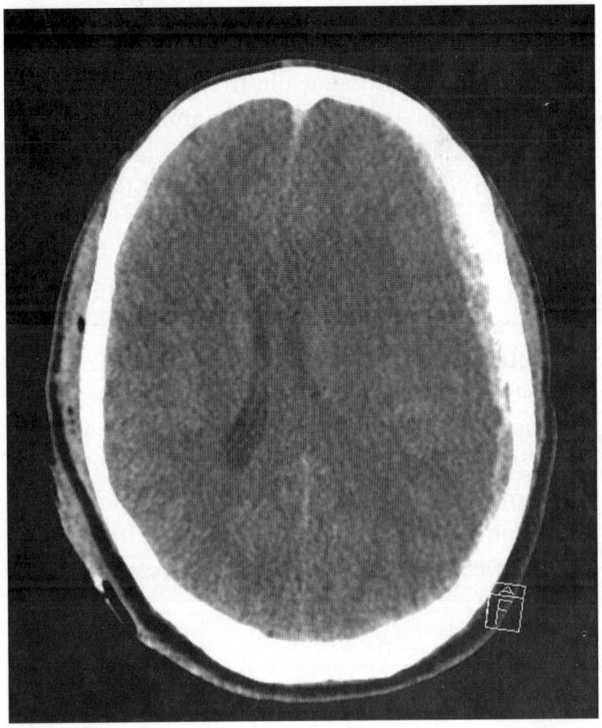

FIGURE 39-20 Computed tomography scan of the head showing an acute subdural hematoma.

Commonly the hematoma is associated with skull fracture. Subdural hematomas are classified as acute, subacute, and chronic. Classification depends on the time lapse between the injury and the development of symptoms. As a general rule, if symptoms occur within 24 hours, the hematoma is considered acute; between 2 and 10 days, subacute; and after 2 weeks, chronic.[18] Subdural hematomas are more common than epidural hematomas.

Signs and symptoms of subdural hematoma are similar to those of epidural hematoma and include headache, nausea and vomiting, decreasing level of consciousness, coma, abnormal posturing, paralysis, and, in infants, bulging fontanelles. These findings may be subtle because of the slow development of the hematoma in the subacute and chronic phases. Definitive care consists of surgery to remove the blood from the hematoma. People at increased risk for the development of subdural hematoma include older adults, patients with clotting deficiencies (eg, people with alcoholism, people with hemophilia, people taking anticoagulants), and patients with cortical atrophy (eg, older adults, people with alcoholism).

Subarachnoid Hemorrhage. A **subarachnoid hemorrhage** refers to intracranial bleeding into the CSF. This condition results in bloody CSF and meningeal irritation. Bleeding that results from trauma, rupture of an aneurysm, or arteriovenous anomaly may extend into the brain if the force of the bleeding from the broken vessel is sudden and severe. Patients with this injury often report a sudden and severe headache. The headache initially may be localized. Then the headache spreads (from meningeal irritation) and becomes dull and throbbing. Other characteristics of a subarachnoid hemorrhage include dizziness, neck stiffness, unequal pupils, vomiting, seizures, and loss of consciousness. Severe hemorrhage may result in coma and death. Permanent brain damage is common in those who survive, although the extent of the damage and the degree of recovery individuals achieve over time is highly variable, with some patients demonstrating profound long-term impairment and others achieving a substantial functional recovery.

> CRITICAL THINKING
>
> What causes the vomiting, seizures, and loss of consciousness in a patient with subarachnoid hemorrhage?

Cerebral Hematoma. An **intracerebral hematoma** may be defined as a collection of blood within the substance of the brain, most commonly in the frontal or temporal lobe.[19] This injury can result from multiple lacerations produced by penetrating head trauma (gunshot wound). The injury also may result from a high-velocity deceleration injury (automobile crash) in which vessels are torn as the brain moves across rough surfaces of the skull. Increased ICP can produce an intracerebral hematoma as the result of the brain being compressed.

Cerebral hematoma often is associated with subdural hemorrhage and skull fracture. Signs and symptoms may be immediate or delayed, depending on the size and location of the hemorrhage. Once symptoms appear, the patient usually deteriorates rapidly. The mortality rate after surgical evacuation of the hematoma (if possible) approaches 45%.[18]

Cardiovascular Complications

Cardiovascular complications are common after brain injury and are associated with increased morbidity and mortality.[20] The spectrum of abnormalities includes hypertension, hypotension, electrocardiographic changes, cardiac dysrhythmias, release of biomarkers of cardiac injury, and left ventricular dysfunction. Most of these complications are related to brain injury–induced catecholamine and neuroinflammatory responses. They are more likely to occur in patients with the severest injuries.[21] Abnormalities are usually reversible; therefore, management should focus on general supportive care and on treatment of the underlying brain injury.[22]

Penetrating Injury

Penetrating injuries to the brain usually are caused by missiles fired from handguns and stab wounds caused by sharp objects. Such objects include knives, scissors, screwdrivers, and nails. Less often, penetrating trauma may result from falls and high-velocity vehicle crashes. Associated injuries include skull fracture; damage to cerebral arteries, veins, or venous sinuses; and intracranial hemorrhage. Complications include infection and posttraumatic epilepsy. Definitive care for these injuries requires neurosurgical intervention.

Assessment and Neurologic Evaluation

Prehospital management of the patient with a head injury is determined by a number of factors, including the mechanism and severity of injury and the patient's level of consciousness. Associated injuries affect the priorities of emergency care.

Airway and Ventilation. The initial step in treating all patients with head trauma is to ensure an open airway while keeping in mind the possible need for spinal precautions. The next step is to provide adequate ventilation with high-concentration oxygen. Airway management may include oral or nasal adjuncts, supraglottic airways, or nasal or tracheal intubation to maintain and protect the airway. Tracheal intubation and ventilatory support usually are recommended in all patients with head injuries who have a GCS score of 8 or less.[23] (GCS is described later in the chapter.)

CRITICAL THINKING

Imagine the appearance of a patient with a GCS score of 8 or less. Why should these patients be intubated? Is intubation needed if the GCS score improves rapidly?

Patients with head injuries are likely to vomit. If the patient has a decreased level of consciousness after the airway is secured, a gastric tube should be inserted to empty the stomach. In the presence of facial fractures, rhinorrhea (CSF discharge from the nose), or otorrhea (CSF discharge from the ear), an orogastric tube rather than a nasogastric tube should be inserted. Use of this tube helps to avoid possible intubation of the cranial cavity through the fracture site. In addition, a long backboard may be used for securing the patient as well as for safe patient movement. Suction equipment with large-bore suction catheters should be available as well.

Ventilatory support should be focused on ensuring that the arterial oxygen saturation (Sao_2) level never drops below 94%.[23-25] (A single episode of hypotension in combination with a decrease in Sao_2 below 90% can double mortality.) Capnography monitoring can be used to ensure adequate ventilation to optimize cerebral perfusion. Aggressive hyperventilation should be avoided because it reduces carbon dioxide concentration; it can lead to secondary brain injury through cerebral vasoconstriction and a decrease in cerebral blood flow. Thus, in the absence of capnography to guide ventilatory support, normal ventilations should be provided at 10 breaths/min for adults, 20 breaths/min for children, and 25 breaths/min for infants. This targets an end-tidal carbon dioxide level of 35 to 40 mm Hg. With evidence of herniation (BOX 39-5), the patient should be hyperventilated at the following rates: 20 breaths/min for adults, 25 breaths/min for children, and 30 breaths/min for infants. These rates should yield a Pco_2 level of about 30 to 35 mm Hg.[23]

BOX 39-5 Indicators of Herniation for Hyperventilation

Cushing triad: increased SBP, bradycardia, and irregular respiratory pattern

Or

An unresponsive patient with bilateral, dilated, unresponsive pupils or asymmetrical pupils (>1 mm)

And

Abnormal extension (decerebrate) posturing or no motor response to painful stimuli

NOTE

When assessing and managing an adult with a severe head injury, remember the "90-90-9 rule":

- A single drop in the patient's Sao_2 level to less than 90% doubles his or her chance of death.
- A single drop in the patient's SBP to less than 90 mm Hg doubles his or her chance of death.
- A single drop in the patient's GCS score to less than 9 doubles his or her chance of death. A drop in the GCS score of 2 or more points, at any time, also doubles mortality.

Modified from: American Academy of Orthopaedic Surgeons. *Advanced Assessment and Treatment of Trauma*. Sudbury, MA: Jones & Bartlett Publishers; 2009.

Circulation. After the airway has been secured, support of the patient's cardiovascular function becomes the next priority. The paramedic should control major external bleeding and should assess the patient's vital signs. Assessment establishes a baseline for future

BOX 39-6 SBP Lower Limit Guidelines in Head-Injured Patients

Age <1 month, maintain SBP >60 mm Hg.
Age 1 to 12 months, maintain SBP >70 mm Hg.
Age 1 to 10 years, maintain SBP >70 + 2 × age in years.
Age >10 years to adult, maintain SBP ≥110 mm Hg.
Age 15 to 49 or >70 years, maintain SBP ≥110 mm Hg.
Age 50 to 69 years, maintain SBP ≥100 mm Hg.

Modified from: Brain Trauma Foundation. *Guidelines for the Management of Severe Traumatic Brain Injury.* 4th ed. Brain Trauma Foundation: New York, NY; 2016. https://braintrauma.org/uploads/03/12/Guidelines_for_Management_of_Severe_TBI_4th_Edition.pdf. Accessed April 7, 2018.

evaluations. A cardiac monitor will detect changes in rhythm (particularly bradycardia and tachycardia) that can occur with increasing ICP and brainstem injury. The blood pressure of every patient should be maintained at normal levels with fluid replacement (per medical direction). A single episode of hypotension doubles mortality and increases morbidity in the patient with TBI.[16] Therefore, the paramedic should administer IV fluids to avoid hypotension or limit it to the shortest duration possible. SBP thresholds that can be used to define hypotension in head-injured patients are listed in BOX 39-6.

Persistent hypotension from an isolated head injury is a rare and terminal event. The exception is head injury in infants and small children. Closed head injury in the adult does not produce hypovolemic shock. Thus, a patient with head injuries who also is hypotensive should be evaluated for other injuries that could cause hemorrhage. The paramedic also should evaluate the patient for the possibility of neurogenic shock from spinal cord trauma. Infusion of isotonic fluids (lactated Ringer solution or normal saline) may be indicated for hemorrhagic shock.

Neurologic Examination. Conscious patients should be interviewed to determine their memory status before and after the injury and establish significant medical history (eg, heart disease, hypertension, diabetes mellitus, epilepsy, medication use, alcohol or other drug use, allergies). The history also should include the mechanism of injury and the events that led up to the injury. For example, the history may detail a loss of consciousness before or after the injury incident.

The paramedic should evaluate the motor skills of conscious patients. Evaluation determines the patient's ability to follow commands and helps the paramedic to note any paralysis. (Hemiparesis or hemiplegia, especially with a sensory deficit on the same side, indicates brain damage rather than spinal trauma.) If the patient is unconscious on EMS arrival, the paramedic should interview bystanders about the history of the event. The paramedic also should ask bystanders about the length of time the patient has been unconscious. The most important indicator of increasing ICP is deterioration in the patient's sensorium. Thus, the paramedic should evaluate the level of consciousness using the GCS every 5 minutes. A decrease of 2 points with a GCS score of 9 or lower is significant; it indicates significant injury.[16]

CRITICAL THINKING

How reliable will the patient be regarding the duration of his or her loss of consciousness?

After the patient has been resuscitated and stabilized, the paramedic should assess the patient's pupils for symmetry, size, and reactivity to light. Abnormal pupillary responses may indicate an increase in ICP and cranial nerve involvement. Asymmetrical pupils differ more than 1 mm in size. Dilated pupils are greater than or equal to 4 mm in adults. A fixed pupil shows less than 1-mm change in response to bright light. (The paramedic should evaluate pupil size every 5 minutes.) Alcohol and

NOTE

The initial pupil evaluation and the GCS score establish the baseline against which all subsequent neurologic evaluations are compared.

Modified from: Brust J. *Current Diagnosis and Treatment: Neurology.* 2nd ed. New York, NY: McGraw-Hill; 2012.

some other drugs can cause abnormal pupillary reactions, but the reactions commonly are bilateral (except for certain eyedrops, if placed in one eye). If the patient is conscious, the paramedic also should evaluate extraocular movement.

Fluid Therapy. In the absence of hypotension, fluid therapy normally should be restricted in a patient with head injury to minimize cerebral edema. If the patient is hemodynamically stable, the paramedic should establish vascular access. If significant hypovolemia is present from another injury, the paramedic should give the patient an isotonic fluid bolus. The patient also should be transported rapidly to a proper facility. In this case, the injury causing hypovolemia usually is more immediately life threatening than is the head injury. Although there is no true consensus, studies suggest that hypotension in the presence of head injury initially should be managed with fluid boluses to maintain a SBP between 90 mm Hg and 120 mm Hg in most adults.[19,26]

Drug Therapy. Prehospital use of drugs for the treatment of head injuries is controversial. If needed, drugs may be prescribed by medical direction to decrease cerebral edema or circulating blood volume.

> NOTE
>
> The administration of glucose (dextrose 50%) is contraindicated in patients with head injuries unless hypoglycemia is confirmed. IV dextrose 50% may worsen cerebral damage.

Anticonvulsant agents, such as lorazepam and diazepam, are used to control seizure activity in head-injured patients. As a rule, these drugs are not used in the initial management of head injuries because of their sedating effects.

In addition, the use of sedatives and paralytics for some patients with head injuries may be indicated for airway management. These drugs also may be used to aid in the transport of combative patients (especially in aeromedical transport). The paramedic should follow local protocol and consult with medical direction regarding the use of these drugs.

Injury Rating Systems

Several injury rating systems are used to triage, guide patient care, predict patient outcome, identify changes in patient status, and evaluate trauma care in epidemiologic studies and quality assurance reviews. These rating systems are important to prehospital personnel. They aid in determining patient care needs with reference to hospital resources. Rating systems commonly used in emergency care include the GCS score and trauma score.

Glasgow Coma Scale

The **Glasgow Coma Scale (GCS)** evaluates eye opening, verbal and motor responses, and brainstem reflex function. The scale is considered one of the best indicators of eventual clinical outcome and should be part of any neurologic examination for patients with head injury (**TABLE 39-2**).[27] The highest possible GCS score is 15, and the lowest possible score is 3. A GCS score of 9 to 13 indicates moderate TBI; a GCS score of 8 or less indicates a severe TBI. Hypoxemia and hypotension have been shown to affect GCS scoring negatively. Thus, GCS should be measured after the primary survey. The score should be measured after a clear airway is established. Also, the GCS should be measured after necessary ventilation and circulatory resuscitation including hemorrhage control have been performed. Unresponsive patients with a GCS score

> SHOW ME THE EVIDENCE
>
> Researchers in Arizona evaluated database records of 7,521 adults and older children with moderate or severe TBI. Using logistic regression, they assessed the relationship between a SBP of less than 90 mm Hg and time of hypotension to determine the impact on odds of death in the hospital. Mortality was 7.8% in patients without a SBP less than 90 mm Hg and 33.4% among hypotensive patients. Mortality was higher as the length of hypotension increased. The researchers concluded that careful ongoing monitoring for hypotension is essential to provide prompt treatment to minimize the time patients are hypotensive.
>
> *Modified from*: Spaite DW, Hu C, Bobrow BJ, et al. Association of out-of-hospital hypotension depth and duration with traumatic brain injury mortality. *Ann Emerg Med.* 2017;70(4):522-530.

TABLE 39-2 Glasgow Coma Scale

Eye Opening		Best Verbal Response		Best Motor Response	
Spontaneous	4	Oriented conversation	5	Follows commands	6
To verbal command	3	Disoriented conversation	4	Localizes pain	5
To pain	2	Nonsensical speech	3	Withdraws to pain	4
No response	1	Unintelligible sounds	2	Abnormal flexion	3
		No response	1	Abnormal extension	2
				No response	1

Scores:
15: Indicates no neurologic disabilities
13–14: Mild dysfunction
9–12: Moderate to severe dysfunction
8 or less: Severe dysfunction (The lowest possible score is 3.)

TABLE 39-3 Revised Trauma Score Calculation

GCS Score	Systolic Blood Pressure (mm Hg)	Respiratory Rate (breaths/min)	Value
13 to 15	>89	10 to 29	4
9 to 12	76 to 89	>29	3
6 to 8	50 to 75	6 to 9	2
4 to 5	1 to 49	1 to 5	1
3	0	0	0

Abbreviation: GCS, Glasgow Coma Scale

Modified from: Table 1, Triage Revised Trauma Score (T-RTS). *Int Journal Emerg Med.* 2008; http://www.ncbi.nlm.nih.gov/pmc/articles/PMC2536180/table/Tab1/. Copyright © Springer-Verlag London Ltd. 2008. Published online March 15, 2008. Accessed April 16, 2018.

of 3 to 8 should be transported to a trauma center with TBI capabilities.[18]

Trauma Score

The trauma score was developed in 1980 to predict outcomes for patients with blunt or penetrating injuries. This score has limited use in the prehospital setting and does not predict adequately the mortality for isolated, severe head injury.

The Revised Trauma Score, published in 1989, uses the GCS with measurements for SBP and respiratory rate that are divided into five intervals (**TABLE 39-3**). A range of values for these physiologic measurements is assigned a number between 0 and 4. These numbers then are added to give a total between 0 and 12. A score of 0 indicates the most critical; a score of 12 indicates the least critical. Usually, this score is calculated after arrival at the ED using initial assessment data from radio reports and the prehospital care report.

NOTE

A newer version of the Revised Trauma Score is the *New Trauma Score* (NTS), which includes the actual GCS score instead of a GCS code, the SBP interval used for the code value, and the incorporation of peripheral oxygen saturation (Spo_2) instead of the respiratory rate. The NTS predicts in-hospital mortality substantially better than the Revised Trauma Score. It is also used as a triage tool during the initial phase of trauma management.

Modified from: Jeong JH, Park YJ, Kim DH, et al. The new trauma score (NTS): a modification of the revised trauma score for better trauma mortality prediction. *BMC Surg*. 2017;17:77.

Summary

- Major causes of maxillofacial trauma are motor vehicle crashes, home accidents, athletic injuries, animal bites, intentional violent acts, and industrial injuries.
- With the exception of a compromised airway and possible significant bleeding, damage to the tissues of the maxillofacial area is seldom life threatening. Some facial fractures are associated with basilar skull fracture. Blunt trauma injuries may be classified as fractures to the mandible, midface, zygoma, orbit, or nose.
- Injury to the ears, eyes, or teeth may be minor or may result in permanent sensory function loss and disfigurement. Trauma to the ear may include lacerations and contusions, thermal injuries, chemical injuries, traumatic perforation, and barotitis. Evaluation of the eye should include a thorough history and measurement of visual acuity, pupillary reaction, and extraocular movements.
- Anterior neck injuries may result in damage to the skeletal structures, vascular structures, nerves, muscles, and glands of the neck. The patient should be assessed for airway compromise, bleeding, and cervical spine injury.
- Injuries to the skull may be classified as soft-tissue injuries to the scalp and skull fractures. Skull fractures may be classified as linear fractures, basilar fractures, depressed fractures, and open vault fractures.
- The categories of brain injury include diffuse axonal injury (DAI) and focal injury. DAI may be mild (concussion), moderate, or severe. Focal injuries are specific, grossly observable brain lesions. Included in this category are lesions that result from skull fracture, contusion, edema with associated increased intracranial pressure, ischemia, and hemorrhage.
- The prehospital management of a patient with head injuries is determined by a number of factors. One factor is the mechanism of injury. A second factor is the severity of injury. A third factor is the patient's level of consciousness. Associated injuries affect the priorities of care.
- Several injury rating systems are used to triage, guide patient care, predict patient outcome, identify changes in patient status, and evaluate trauma care. Rating systems commonly used in emergency care include the Glasgow Coma Scale score and the trauma score.

References

1. Centers for Disease Control and Prevention, National Center for Injury Prevention and Control, Division of Unintentional Injury Prevention. Traumatic brain injury and concussion. TBI: get the facts. Centers for Disease Control and Prevention website. https://www.cdc.gov/traumaticbraininjury/get_the_facts.html. Updated April 27, 2017. Accessed April 7, 2018.
2. Tessier P. The classic reprint: experimental study of fractures of the upper jaw. I and II. Rene Le Fort, MD. *Plast Reconstr Surg*. 1972;50(5):497-506.
3. Mukherjee S, Abhinav K, Revington PJ. A review of cervical spine injury associated with maxillofacial trauma at a UK tertiary referral centre. *Ann R Coll Surg Engl*. 2015;97(1):66-72.
4. Owens PL, Mutter R. Emergency department visits related to eye injuries, 2008. HCUP Statistical Brief #112. Healthcare Cost and Utilization Project website. https://www.hcup-us.ahrq.gov/reports/statbriefs/sb112.pdf. Published May 2011. Accessed April 8, 2018.
5. Hawkins E, Mills MD. Ocular injuries. In: Brice J, Delbridge TR, Myers JB, eds. *Emergency Services: Clinical Practice and Systems Oversight*. Vol 1. West Sussex, England: John Wiley & Sons; 2015:280-283.
6. Endodontics: colleagues for excellence. The treatment of traumatic dental injuries. American Association of Endodontists website. https://www.aae.org/specialty/wp-content/uploads/sites/2/2017/06/ecfe_summer2014-final.pdf. Published Summer 2014. Accessed April 8, 2018.
7. American Academy of Otolaryngology—Head and Neck Surgery Foundation. *Resident Manual of Trauma to the Face, Head, and Neck*. Alexandria, VA: American Academy of Otolaryngology; 2012. https://www.entnet.org/sites/default/files/Trauma-Chapter-7.pdf. Accessed April 8, 2018.

8. American Academy of Orthopaedic Surgeons. *Advanced Assessment and Treatment of Trauma*. Sudbury, MA: Jones and Bartlett Publishers; 2009.
9. Heegaard WG, Biros MH. Skull fracture in adults. UpToDate website. https://www.uptodate.com/contents/skull-fractures-in-adults#H10. Updated July 26, 2017. Accessed April 8, 2018.
10. BIAA adopts new TBI definition. Brain Injury Association of America website. http://www.biausa.org/announcements/biaa-adopts-new-tbi-definition. Published February 6, 2011. Accessed April 8, 2018.
11. National Highway Traffic Safety Administration. *The National EMS Education Standards*. Washington, DC: US Department of Transportation/National Highway Traffic Safety Administration; 2009.
12. Giza CC, Kutcher JS, Ashwal S, et al. Summary of evidence-based guideline update: evaluation and management of concussion in sports: report of the Guideline Development Subcommittee of the American Academy of Neurology. *Neurology*. 2013;80(24):2250-2257.
13. McCance KL, Huethe SE. *Pathophysiology: The Biologic Basis for Disease in Adults and Children*. 7th ed. Philadelphia, PA: Elsevier; 2014.
14. Brust J. *Current Diagnosis and Treatment: Neurology*. 2nd ed. New York, NY: McGraw-Hill; 2012.
15. Carney N, Totten AM, O'Reilly C, et al. Guidelines for the management of severe traumatic brain injury, fourth edition. *Neurosurgery*. 2017;80(1):6-15.
16. Brain Trauma Foundation. *Guidelines for the Management of Severe Traumatic Brain Injury*. 4th ed. Brain Trauma Foundation: New York, NY; 2016. https://braintrauma.org/uploads/03/12/Guidelines_for_Management_of_Severe_TBI_4th_Edition.pdf. Accessed April 7, 2018.
17. Bricolo A, Turazzi S, Alexandre A, Rizzuto N. Decerebrate rigidity in acute head injury. *J Neurosurg*. 1977(Nov);47(5):680-689.
18. Walls RM, Hockberger RS, Gausche-Hill M, et al. *Rosen's Emergency Medicine: Concepts and Clinical Practice*. 9th ed. Philadelphia, PA: Elsevier; 2018.
19. Roach E, Bettermann K, Biller J. Intracerebral hemorrhage. In: *Toole's Cerebrovascular Disorders*. Cambridge, MA: Cambridge University Press; 2010:217-233.
20. van der Bilt IA, Hasan D, Vandertop WP, et al. Impact of cardiac complications on outcome after aneurysmal subarachnoid hemorrhage: a meta-analysis. *Neurology*. 2009;72(7):635-642.
21. Lim HB, Smith M. Systemic complications after head injury: a clinical review. *Anaesthesia*. 2007;62(5):474-482.
22. Gregory T, Smith M. Cardiovascular complications of brain injury. *Contin Educ Anaesthes Crit Care Pain*. 2012;12(2):67-71.
23. National Association of Emergency Medical Technicians. *PHTLS: Prehospital Trauma Life Support*. 8th ed. Burlington, MA: Jones & Bartlett Learning; 2014.
24. Spaite DW, Hu C, Bobrow BJ, et al. The impact of combined prehospital hypotension and hypoxia on mortality in major traumatic brain injury. *Ann Emerg Med*. 2017;69(1):62-72.
25. Spaite DW, Hu C, Bobrow BJ, et al. Mortality and prehospital blood pressure in patients with major traumatic brain injury implications for the hypotension threshold. *JAMA Surg*. 2017;152(4):360–368.
26. National Association of EMS Officials. *National Model EMS Clinical Guidelines*. Version 2. National Association of EMS Officials website. https://www.nasemso.org/documents/National-Model-EMS-Clinical-Guidelines-Version2-Sept2017.pdf. Published September 2017. Accessed April 8, 2018.
27. Traumatic brain injury statistics. Center for Neuroskills website. https://www.neuroskills.com/brain-injury/traumatic-brain-injury-statistics.php. Accessed March 25, 2018.

Suggested Readings

Ball CG. Penetrating nontorso trauma: the head and the neck. *Can J Surg*. 2015;58(4):284-285.

Carrick MM, Leonard J, Slone DS, Mains CW, Bar-Or D. Hypotensive resuscitation among trauma patients. *BioMed Research International*. 2016;8901938.

Centers for Disease Control and Prevention, National Center for Injury Prevention and Control, Division of Unintentional Injury Prevention. Traumatic brain injury and concussion. Severe TBI. Centers for Disease Control and Prevention website. https://www.cdc.gov/traumaticbraininjury/severe.html. Updated March 30, 2017. Accessed April 8, 2018.

Levy DB. Neck trauma. Medscape website. https://emedicine.medscape.com/article/827223-overview. Updated July 12, 2017. Accessed April 8, 2018.

Rajendran CM, Raman M, Sivakumar B. A study on modes of injury, management, and its visual outcome in paediatric ocular trauma. *J Evid Based Med Healthcare*. 2017;4(46);2790-2795.

Shankar KH, Paparajamurthy MHK, Anand K. A clinical analysis of outcome in management of head injury in patients with highway road accidents. *Int J Res Med*. 2016;4(6):2079-2083.

Sharma VK, Rango J, Connaughton AJ, Lombardo DJ, Sabesan VJ. The current state of head and neck injuries in extreme sports. *Orthop J Sports Med*. 2015;3(1):2325967114564358.

Sperry JL, Moore EE, Coimbra R, et al. Western Trauma Association critical decisions in trauma: penetrating neck trauma. *J Trauma Acute Care Surg*. 2013;75(6):936-940.

Van Waes OJ, Cheriex KC, Navsaria PH, van Riet PA, Nicol AJ, Vermeulen J. Management of penetrating neck injuries. *Br J Surg*. 2012;99(suppl 1):149-154.

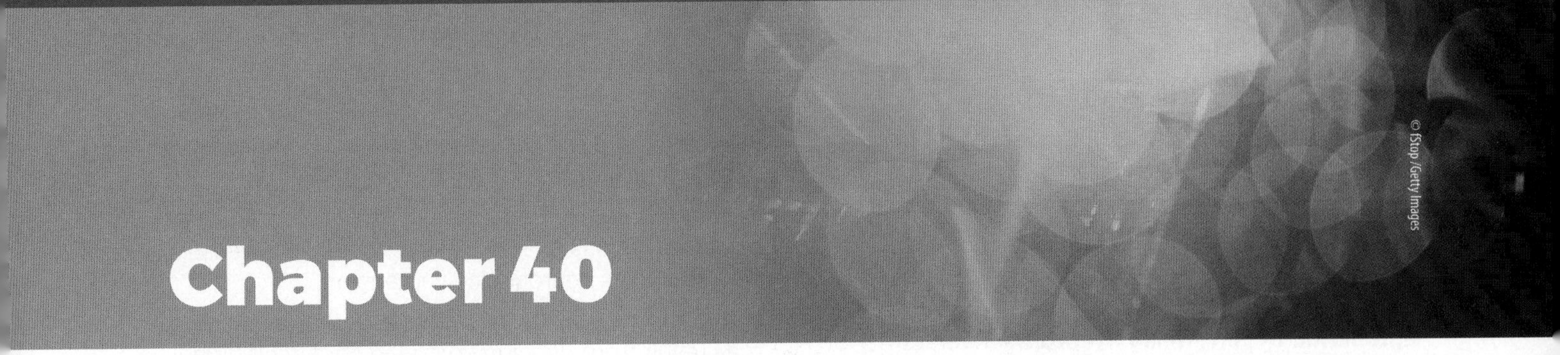

Chapter 40

Spine and Nervous System Trauma

NATIONAL EMS EDUCATION STANDARD COMPETENCIES

Trauma

Integrates assessment findings with principles of epidemiology and pathophysiology to formulate a field impression to implement a comprehensive treatment/disposition plan for an acutely injured patient.

Head, Facial, Neck, and Spine Trauma

Recognition and management of
- Life threats (p 1469)
- Spine trauma (pp 1466–1469)

Pathophysiology, assessment, and management of
- Penetrating neck trauma (see Chapter 39, *Head, Face, and Neck Trauma*)
- Laryngotracheal injuries (see Chapter 39, *Head, Face, and Neck Trauma*)
- Spine trauma
  - Dislocations/subluxations (pp 1461–1463)
  - Fractures (pp 1464–1466)
  - Sprains/strains (pp 1463–1464)
- Facial fractures (see Chapter 39, *Head, Face, and Neck Trauma*)
- Skull fractures (see Chapter 39, *Head, Face, and Neck Trauma*)
- Foreign bodies in the eyes (see Chapter 39, *Head, Face, and Neck Trauma*)
- Dental trauma (see Chapter 39, *Head, Face, and Neck Trauma*)
- Unstable facial fractures (see Chapter 39, *Head, Face, and Neck Trauma*)
- Orbital fractures (see Chapter 39, *Head, Face, and Neck Trauma*)
- Perforated tympanic membrane (see Chapter 39, *Head, Face, and Neck Trauma*)
- Mandibular fractures (see Chapter 39, *Head, Face, and Neck Trauma*)

Nervous System Trauma

Pathophysiology, assessment, and management of
- Traumatic brain injury (see Chapter 39, *Head, Face, and Neck Trauma*)
- Spinal cord injury (pp 1469–1471)
- Spinal shock (p 1483)
- Cauda equina syndrome (see Chapter 32, *Nontraumatic Musculoskeletal Disorders*)
- Nerve root injury (see Chapter 32, *Nontraumatic Musculoskeletal Disorders*)
- Peripheral nerve injury (see Chapter 32, *Nontraumatic Musculoskeletal Disorders*)

OBJECTIVES

Upon completion of this chapter, the paramedic student will be able to:

1. Describe the incidence, morbidity, and mortality related to spinal injury. (p 1458)
2. Describe the anatomy and physiology of the spine and spinal cord. (pp 1459–1461)
3. Predict mechanisms of injury that are likely to cause spinal injury. (pp 1461–1463)
4. Outline the general assessment of a patient with suspected spinal injury. (pp 1466–1469)
5. Distinguish between types of spinal injury. (pp 1463–1466)
6. Describe prehospital evaluation and assessment of spinal cord injury. (pp 1469–1471)
7. Identify prehospital management of the patient with spinal injuries. (pp 1471–1483)
8. Distinguish between spinal shock, neurogenic shock, and autonomic hyperreflexia syndrome. (pp 1483–1485)
9. Describe selected nontraumatic spinal conditions. (p 1485)

KEY TERMS

anterior cord syndrome A spinal cord injury usually seen in flexion injuries; caused by damage to the anterior aspect of the spinal cord by a ruptured intervertebral disk or fragments of the vertebral body extruded posteriorly into the spinal canal or by damage to the anterior spinal artery.

autonomic hyperreflexia syndrome Overactivity of the autonomic nervous system that causes an abrupt onset of extremely high blood pressure.

axial loading Vertical compression of the spine that results when direct forces are transmitted along the length of the spinal column.

Brown-Séquard syndrome A functional hemitransection of the spinal cord resulting in weakness of the upper and lower extremities on the same side and loss of pain and temperature sensation on the opposite side.

central cord syndrome A spinal cord injury commonly seen with hyperextension cervical injuries; less commonly seen with flexion injuries; characterized by greater motor impairment of the upper extremities than of the lower extremities.

dermatome The skin surface area supplied by a single spinal root.

distraction A spinal injury that occurs if spinal motion is stopped suddenly relative to body motion, causing the weight and momentum of the body to shift away from it; a pulling apart.

neurogenic shock Hypotension following spinal injury; caused by a loss of sympathetic tone to the vessels; also known as neurogenic hypotension.

spinal cord injury (SCI) Damage to the spinal cord; may result from direct injury to the cord itself or indirectly from damage to surrounding bones, tissues, or blood vessels.

spinal shock Temporary loss or depression of all or most spinal reflex activity below the level of the injury; may or may not include loss of sympathetic tone that causes hypotension.

spondylosis A condition of the spine characterized by fixation or stiffness of the vertebral joint.

subluxation A partial dislocation.

tetraplegia Weakness or paralysis of all four extremities and the trunk; also known as quadriplegia.

torticollis A twisting of the neck caused by injuries to the cervical spine that generate muscle spasms. This condition causes a painful fixed head tilt that is accompanied by shoulder elevation.

transection A complete or incomplete lesion to the spinal cord.

More than 285,000 people live with spinal cord injury in the United States, and more than 17,500 new spinal cord injuries will occur each year.[1] More than 4,800 of these injured people will die before they are admitted to a medical facility.[2] Education in injury prevention, prehospital assessment, and proper handling and transport of these patients can decrease morbidity and mortality.

Spinal Trauma: Incidence, Morbidity, and Mortality

Spinal cord injury (SCI) most commonly results from motor vehicle crashes (38.4%), falls (30.5%), acts of violence (13.5%), sports (8.9%), medical/surgical (4.7%), and other (4%). In adults older than 45 years, falls are the leading cause of SCI (**FIGURE 40-1**). The average age at which SCI occurs has increased and is now 45 years, with males accounting for about 81% of new cases.[1]

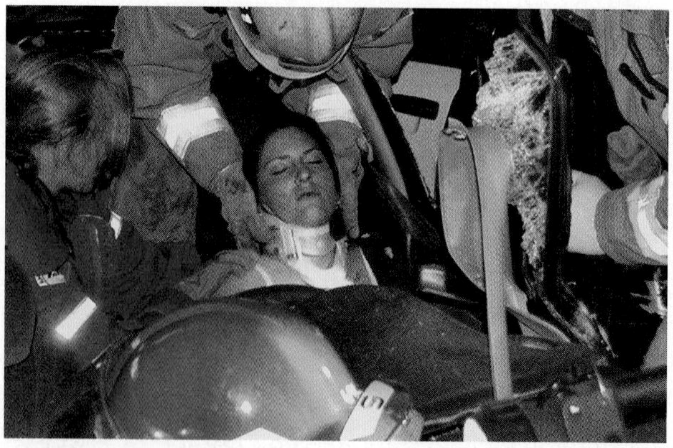

In addition to the devastating emotional and psychological impact on people with SCIs and their families, the annual cost to society exceeds $5 billion. The average yearly costs that can be attributed to SCI vary greatly by the severity of injury. The cost of lifelong care for a 25-year-old person with a permanent and severe SCI is estimated at more than $4.7 million.[1] Injury prevention strategies can have a positive effect on incidence, morbidity, and mortality associated with spinal trauma.

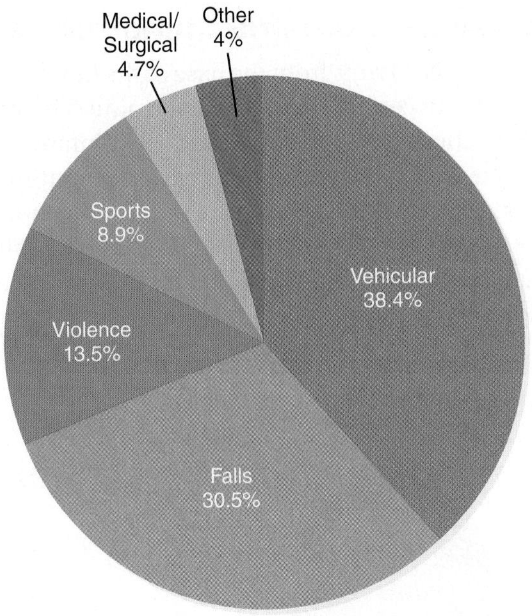

FIGURE 40-1 Mechanism of spinal injury.

> CRITICAL THINKING
> Why do you think males are at increased risk for spinal injuries?

Review of Spinal Anatomy

Anatomy of the spine is presented in Chapter 10, *Review of Human Systems*. The following discussion serves as a brief review.

The Spinal Column

The spinal column is composed of 33 bones (vertebrae) that are divided into five sections. The sections include 7 cervical, 12 thoracic, 5 lumbar, 5 sacral (fused), and 4 coccygeal (fused; the number of bones can range from 3 to 5) vertebrae. The anterior elements of the spine include vertebral bodies, intervertebral disks, and anterior and posterior longitudinal ligaments that connect the vertebral bodies anteriorly and inside the canal (**FIGURE 40-2**).

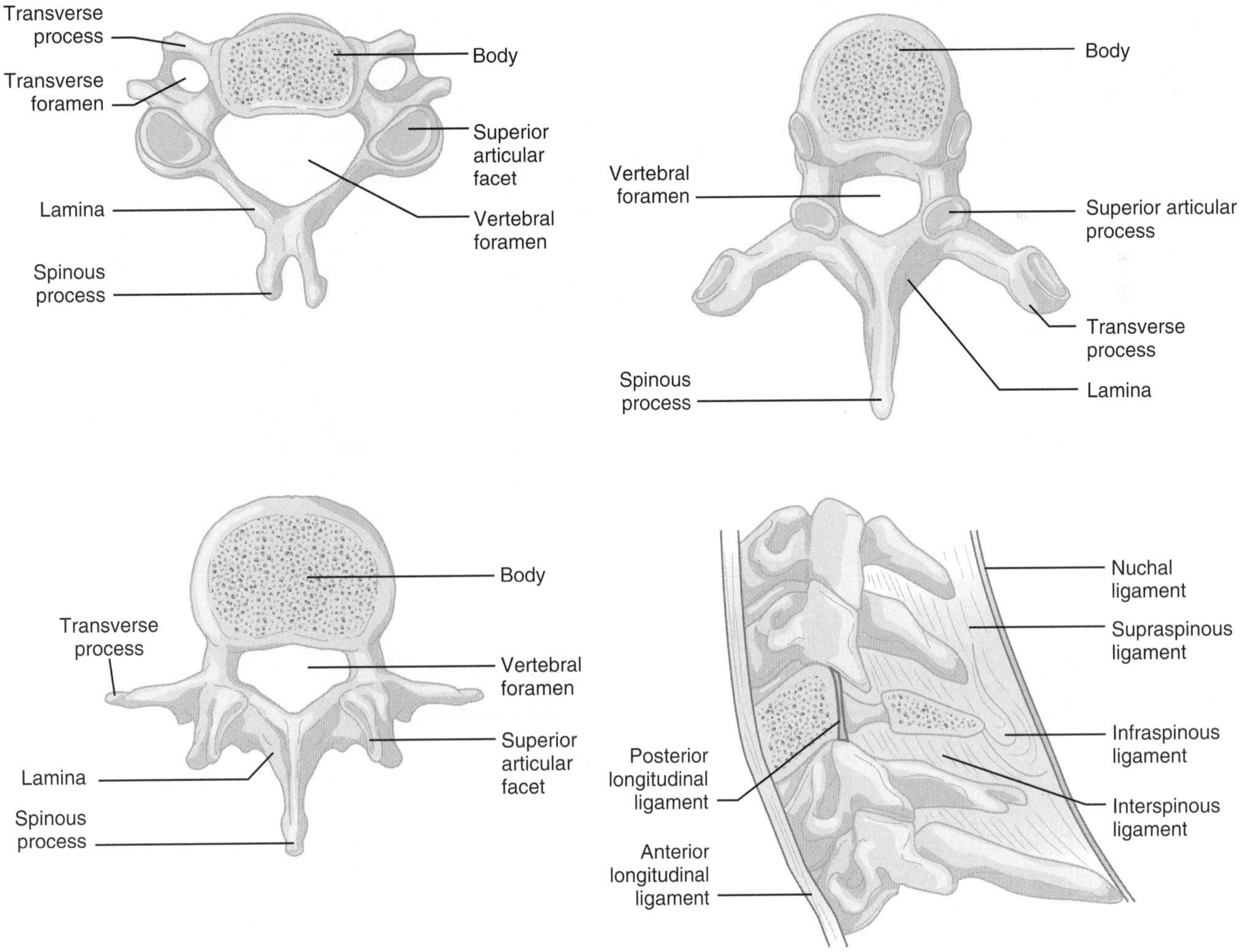

FIGURE 40-2 Vertebral bodies and elements of the spine.

Each vertebra, except for the first (C1) and second (C2) vertebrae (which have no vertebral body), consists of a solid body that bears most of the weight of the vertebral column, a posterior spinous process, and, in some vertebrae, a transverse process. Ligaments between the spinous processes provide support for the movements of flexion and extension, and those between the laminae provide support during lateral flexion. The spinal cord lies in the upper portion of the spinal canal.

The Spinal Cord and Spinal Nerves

The spinal cord runs from the base of the brain down through the cervical and thoracic spine. The cord ends at about L1-L2 in adults and L3 in infants. Below that area, a collection of nerve roots continues, looking somewhat like a horse's tail (cauda equina) (**FIGURE 40-3**). The nerve roots pass out of the spinal canal through the intervertebral foramina. The anterior nerve root is motor while the posterior nerve

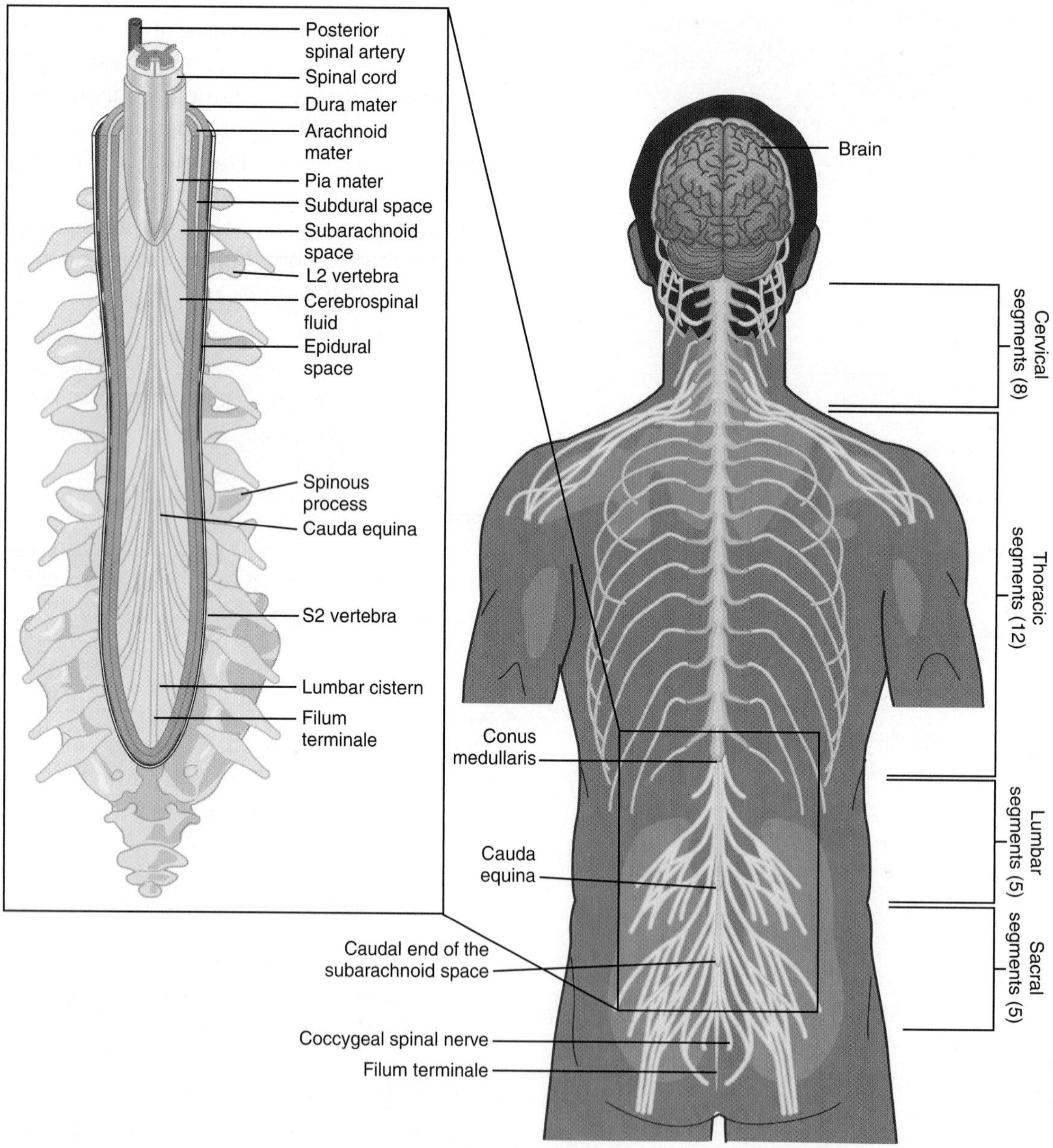

FIGURE 40-3 The spinal cord, spinal nerves, and meninges. Spinal meninges are similar to cranial membranes. Spinal meninges end at S2, creating a cerebrospinal fluid–filled cistern below the spinal cord. The cauda equina (horse's tail) is formed by the lumbar and sacral nerves, which protrude from the end of the spinal cord.

root at each level is sensory. Ascending nerve tracts carry sensory impulses from various parts of the body through the cord up to the brain. Descending nerve tracts carry motor impulses from the brain through the spinal cord and down to the body. Each level of nerve functions in the spinal cord is represented by a **dermatome** (the sensory area on the body innervated by a nerve root). The anterior divisions of the nerves supply the front of the spine including the limbs. The posterior divisions of the nerves are distributed to the muscles behind the spine. The spinal cord provides a means of communication between the brain and peripheral nerves. **FIGURE 40-4** shows the relationship between the spinal column, the spinal nerves, and the areas of the body that can be affected by injury or disease.

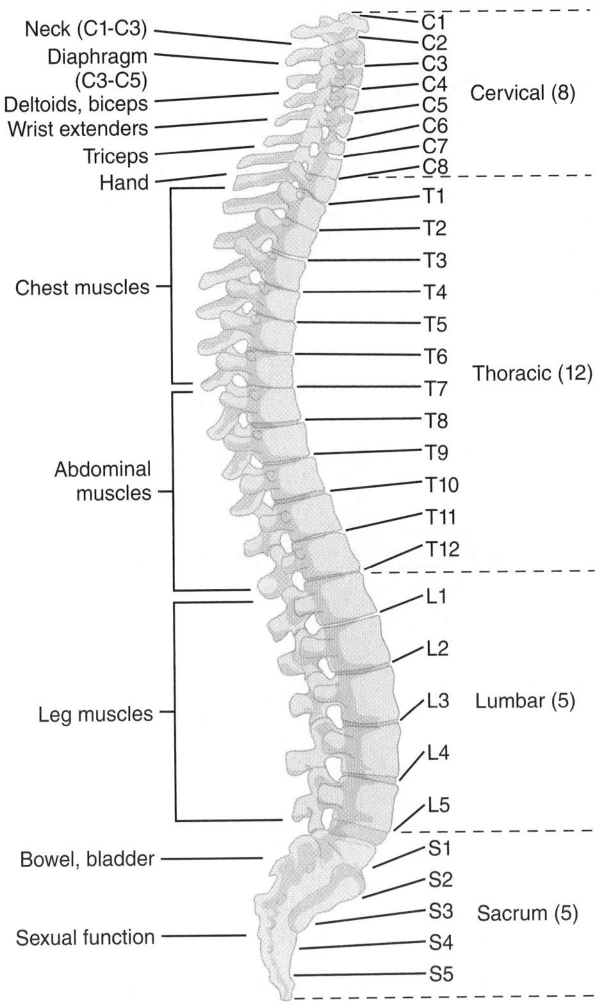

FIGURE 40-4 Nerve tracts.

Mechanisms of Spinal Injury

Spinal injury most often results from the spine being forced beyond its normal range and limits of motion (**FIGURE 40-5**). The adult head weighs approximately 8 to 12 pounds. The skull sits on top of the first cervical vertebra (C1), or the atlas. The second cervical vertebra (C2), or the axis, and its odontoid process allow the head to move with about a 180° range of motion. Because of the weight and position of the head in relation to the thin neck and cervical vertebrae, the cervical spine is particularly susceptible to injury.[3] Other spinal components that affect physiologic limits of motion are the posterior neck muscles and the sacrum. The posterior neck muscles allow up to 60° of flexion and 70° of extension without stretching of the spinal cord. The sacrum is joined to the pelvis by immovable joints.

The specific mechanisms of injury that often cause spinal trauma are axial loading; extremes of flexion, hyperextension, or hyperrotation; excessive lateral bending; and distraction. These mechanisms may result in stable and unstable injuries, depending on the extent of damage to spinal structures and the relative strength of the structures remaining intact.

Axial Loading

Axial loading (vertical compression) of the spine results when direct forces are sent down the length of the spinal column. Examples of these injuries include striking the head against the windshield of a car, shallow diving injuries, vertical falls, and being struck on the head or a helmet with a heavy object. These forces may produce a compression fracture or a crushed vertebral body without SCI and most commonly occur from T12 to L2.[4]

Flexion, Hyperextension, and Hyperrotation

Extremes in flexion, hyperextension, or hyperrotation may result in fracture, ligament injury, or muscle injury. SCI is caused when one or more of the cervical vertebrae dislocate, a process called **subluxation**, and are forced into the spinal canal, which injures the spinal cord. Examples of these motion extremes include rapid acceleration or deceleration forces from motor vehicle crashes, hangings, and midfacial skeletal or soft-tissue trauma. Serious injuries often are the result of a combination of loading and rotational

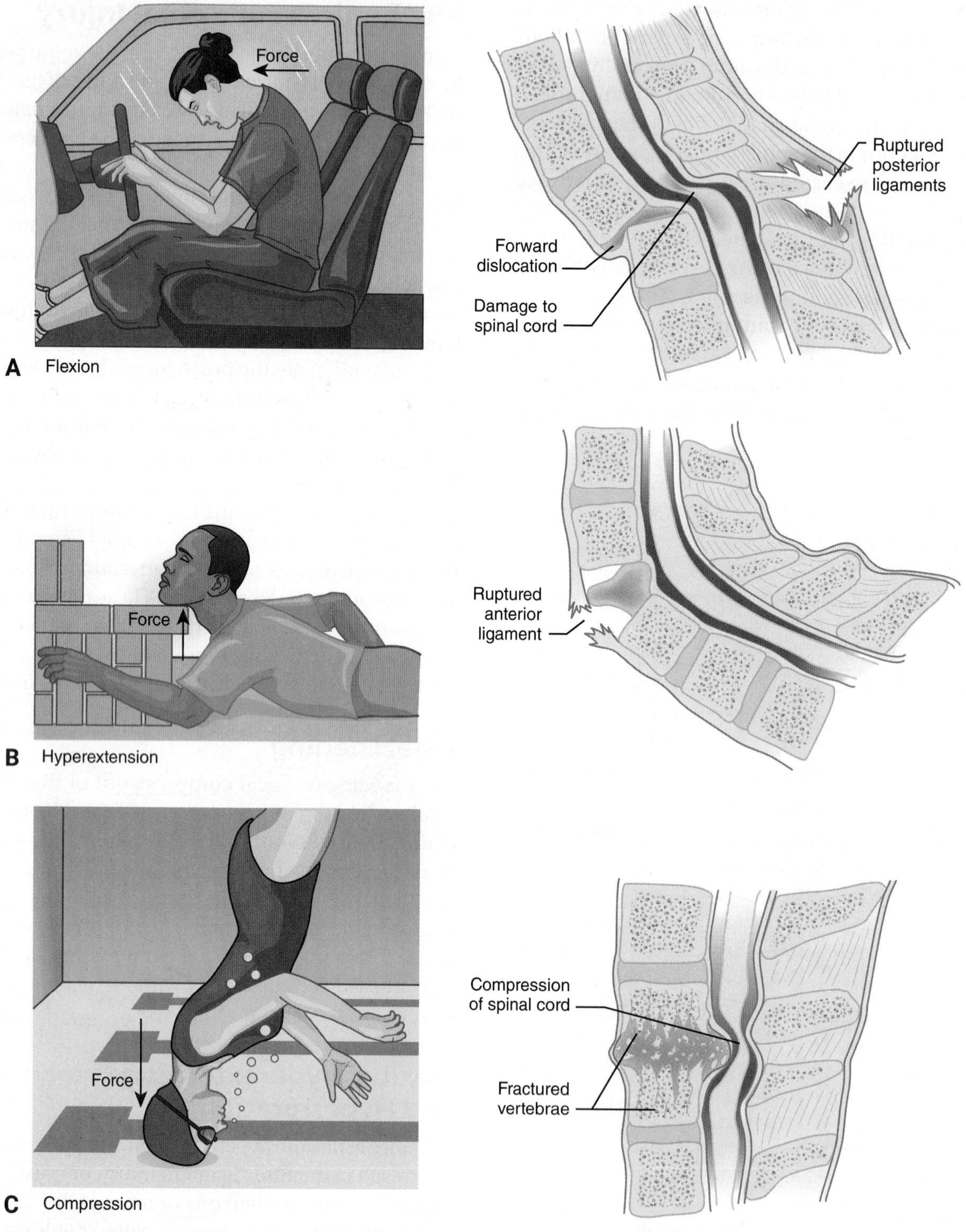

FIGURE 40-5 Mechanisms of spinal cord injury. Many situations may produce these consequences. This figure shows examples only. **A.** Flexion injury of the cervical spine ruptures the posterior ligaments. **B.** Hyperextension injury of the cervical spine ruptures the anterior ligaments. **C.** Compression or axial loading injuries result in burst fractures that crush the vertebrae and force bony fragments into the spinal canal.

forces. These forces produce displacement or fracture of one or more vertebrae.

Lateral Bending

Excessive lateral bending may result in dislocations and bony fractures to the cervical and thoracic spine. The injury occurs when a sudden lateral impact moves the torso sideways. Initially, the head tends to remain in place, and then the head is pulled along by the cervical attachments. Examples of forces that produce lateral bending include side or angular collisions from motor vehicle crashes and injuries from contact sports. The mechanism of this lateral force requires less movement to produce an injury than do flexion or extension forces in frontal or rear impacts.

Distraction

Distraction may occur if the cervical spine is stopped suddenly while the weight and momentum of the body pull away from it. This force or stretching may result in tearing and occasional actual laceration of the spinal cord. Examples of distraction injuries include intentional or unintentional hangings (eg, suicide, school yard or playground injuries).

Other Mechanisms

Other less common mechanisms of spinal injury include blunt and penetrating trauma and electrical injury. The spinal cord, like the brain, may suffer concussions, contusions, and lacerations. It may develop hematomata and edema in response to blunt trauma. Examples include spinal injuries that result from direct blows such as from falling tree limbs or other heavy objects.

Penetrating trauma to the spine may be caused by missile-type injuries or stab wounds to the neck, chest, or abdomen. These forces may result in laceration of the spinal cord or nerve roots over a wide area. At times, penetrating trauma may produce a complete **transection** (lesion). In addition, areas of edema or contusion adjacent to the laceration may disrupt cord tissue.

Spinal trauma may occur from direct electrical injury or from the violent muscle spasms that accompany electrical shock (described in Chapter 38, *Burns*).

Classifications of Spinal Injury

Spinal injuries may be classified as sprains and strains, fractures and dislocations, sacral and coccygeal fractures, and cord injuries. Unnecessary movement should be avoided until injury to the spine or spinal cord can be excluded by clinical examination and radiography. An unstable spine can be ruled out by radiography, by physical examination combined with assessment of symptoms in an awake and reliable patient, or by lack of any potential mechanism for the injury.[5]

Spinal injury (bony or ligamentous injury) can occur with or without SCI. Likewise, a patient may have SCI without bony or ligamentous injury. SCI without radiologic abnormality is a more common finding in children.[6]

The damage produced by the injury forces can be complicated further by the patient's age (calcification from the aging process), preexisting bone diseases (osteoporosis, **spondylosis**, rheumatoid arthritis, Paget disease), and congenital spinal cord anomalies (eg, fusion or narrow spinal canal). Spinal cord neurons do not regenerate to any great extent; thus, any injury to the central nervous system that causes destruction of tissue often results in irreparable damage and permanent loss of function. The role of the paramedic in protecting this vital area cannot be overemphasized.

Sprains and Strains

Sprains and strains usually result from hyperflexion and hyperextension forces. A sprain is an injury to a ligament (tissue that connects two or more bones at a joint). A strain is an injury to a muscle or tendon (fibrous cords of tissue that connect muscle to bone). Although the terms often are used interchangeably, they are two different injuries. A hyperflexion sprain occurs when the posterior ligamentous complex tears at least partially. This sprain also can result in tears of the joint capsules. The sprain may allow partial dislocation (subluxation) of the intervertebral joints. Hyperextension strains are common in low-speed, rear-end car crashes. They are known commonly as whiplash. Injury occurs as the person is thrown backward against the posterior thorax during impact. This action damages anterior soft tissues of the neck. It may also cause a sprain of the anterior longitudinal ligament.

CRITICAL THINKING

How can the paramedic distinguish between a cervical sprain/strain and a spinal fracture in the prehospital setting?

With sprains and strains, local pain may be produced by spasms of the neck muscles and injury to the vertebrae, intervertebral disks, and ligamentous structures. The pain usually is described as a nonradiating, aching soreness of the neck or back muscles. The discomfort often varies in intensity and with changes in posture.

On examination, a deformity of the spine may be palpable if dislocation (subluxation) has occurred. The patient may complain of associated point tenderness and swelling. Until a spinal column injury has been ruled out by radiography, the paramedic should treat these patients as having unstable cervical spine injuries with a potential for damage to the spinal cord. After the diagnosis is confirmed, treatment of cervical sprain or strain usually is symptomatic, but in some cases, management includes surgical intervention. Following physician evaluation, treatment occasionally may include a cervical collar to decrease neck movement, heat application, and analgesics.

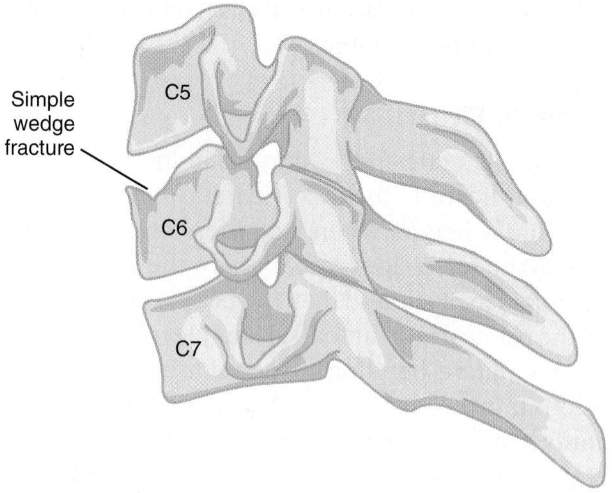

FIGURE 40-6 Lateral view of simple wedge fracture.

Fractures and Dislocations

The most frequently injured spinal regions, in descending order, are C5 through C7, C1 through C2, and T12 through L2.[4] Of these injuries, the most common are wedge-shaped compression fractures and teardrop fractures or dislocations. Neurologic deficits associated with these fractures and dislocations vary with the location and also vary with the extent of injury. In addition, spinal injuries at multiple levels are common.

> CRITICAL THINKING
> Look at an illustration of the spinal column. Why do you think these areas are susceptible to fractures?

Wedge-shaped fractures (**FIGURE 40-6**) are hyperflexion injuries. They usually result from compressive force applied to the anterior portion of the vertebral body. This force results in stretching of the posterior ligaments. (These injuries often result from injuries and falls in industrial settings.) These fractures usually occur in the mid- or lower cervical segments or at T12 and L1. They generally are considered stable because the posterior ligaments rarely are disrupted totally.

Teardrop fractures and dislocations (**FIGURE 40-7**) are unstable injuries that result from a combination of severe hyperflexion and compression forces and often are seen in motor vehicle crashes. During impact, the vertebral body is fractured. The anterior-inferior corner of the vertebral body is pushed forward. Unlike

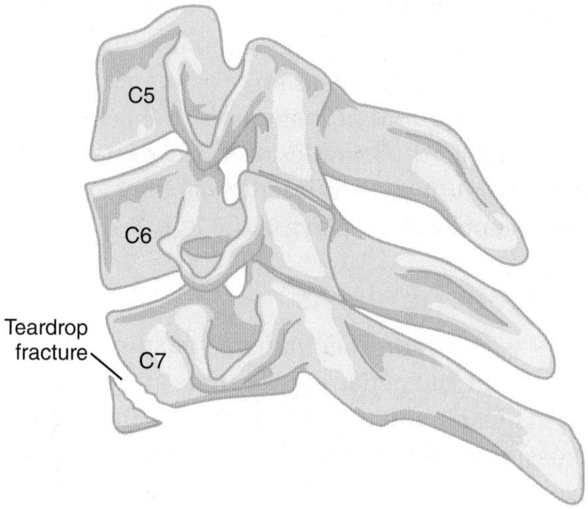

FIGURE 40-7 Lateral view of teardrop fracture.

simple wedge fractures, these fractures may be associated with neurologic damage and are among the most unstable injuries of the spine. A number of other spinal injuries are associated with the mechanisms of flexion, extension, rotation, and axial loading. Most of these injuries are unstable and require careful spinal motion restriction.

Sacral and Coccygeal Fractures

The majority of serious spinal injuries occur in the cervical, thoracic, and lumbar regions. One reason for this is the location of the spinal cord and its termination in the adult spine at about L2. Another reason is the protection provided by the ring structure of the pelvis and the musculature of the buttocks and lower back; however, fractures through the foramina of S1-S2 are fairly common. These fractures may compromise several sacral nerve elements and result in loss of perianal sensory motor function or damage to the bladder and bladder sphincters.

The sacrococcygeal joint also may be injured as a result of direct blows and falls. Patients often complain that they have broken their tailbone. They often experience moderate pain from the mobile coccyx. Diagnosis usually is confirmed by a physician through radiographic evaluation and a rectal examination.

Cord Injuries

SCIs may be classified further as primary or secondary injuries.[7] Primary injuries occur at the time of impact. Secondary injuries occur after the initial injury and can include swelling, ischemia, and movement of bony fragments. Like other tissues, the spinal cord can be concussed, contused, compressed, and lacerated. All of these mechanisms can cause temporary or permanent loss of cord-mediated functions distal to the injury from compression or ischemia. Bleeding from damaged blood vessels also can occur in the tissue of the spinal cord, which can cause an obstruction to spinal blood supply. The severity of these injuries depends on the amount and type of force that produced them and the duration of the injury.

Cord Lesions

Lesions (transections) to the spinal cord are classified as complete or incomplete. Complete lesions usually are associated with penetrating injury, spinal fracture, or dislocation. Patients have total absence of pain, pressure, and joint sensation and complete motor paralysis below the level of the injury (BOX 40-1). Autonomic nervous system dysfunction may be associated with complete cord lesions, depending on the level of cord involvement. Manifestations of autonomic dysfunction include the following:

- Bradycardia caused by loss of sympathetic autonomic activity (T6 and above)
- Hypotension caused by loss of vasomotor control and peripheral vascular resistance
- Priapism (T6 and above)
- Loss of sweating and shivering
- Poikilothermia (impaired regulation of body temperature causing variation with ambient temperature)
- Loss of bowel and bladder control

BOX 40-1 Complete Cord Lesions

C1 through C4 tetraplegia[a] (high tetraplegia). Injuries involving C1 through C4 often result in partial or total loss of movement in the upper and lower extremities (commonly referred to as quadriplegia). Patients with lesions at C1 and C2 may have functional phrenic nerves and may not need long-term ventilatory assistance after the acute phase of care. Patients with C3 lesions may be ventilator dependent. Patients with C1 through C4 tetraplegia will require life-long assistance for all personal care and movement function (eg, wheelchairs, lift devices).

C5-C6 tetraplegia. Injuries involving C5 and C6 will usually leave patients with the ability to flex the elbow and/or extend the wrist, but limited hand function. These patients often will need special devices and orthotics for hand and wrist control. Although many will be able to live independently, some will require assistance for bathing, grooming, and personal hygiene.

C7-C8 tetraplegia. Injuries involving C7 and C8 leave the patient with functional triceps and the ability to bend and extend the elbows and finger and wrist flexion. This functionality allows the patient greater mobility, self-care, and independent living. Many patients are able to drive an automobile with special adaptations. C7 is usually the highest level at which patients can have an injury and still be able to live independently.

Thoracic and lumbar paraplegia (below T1). Injuries below T1 usually spare the innervation and function of all upper extremity muscles and hand and wrist function. With some adaptive and assistive devices, these patients can usually achieve functional independence for most aspect of self-care and activities of daily living.

[a]Tetraplegia is also known as quadriplegia (paralysis of four limbs).

Modified from: McKinley W. Functional outcomes per level of spinal cord injury. Medscape website. https://emedicine.medscape.com/article/322604-overview. Updated July 11, 2017. Accessed March 19, 2018.

NOTE

The 31 pairs of spinal nerves are numbered according to the vertebra at which they exit the spinal column. From the first thoracic vertebra downward, all spinal nerves exit below their equivalently numbered vertebrae. For example, the spinal nerve T4 exits the spinal column through the foramen below the fourth thoracic vertebra (between T4 and T5); the spinal nerve L5 exits the spinal cord below the foramen in the fifth lumbar vertebra (between L5 and S1). In the cervical region of the spinal cord, the spinal nerves exit above the vertebrae. A change occurs at the C7 vertebra, however, where the C8 spinal nerve exits the vertebra below the C7 vertebra (between C7 and T1). Therefore, there is an eighth cervical spinal nerve, even though there is no eighth cervical vertebra. In descending order, the cervical nerves supply feeling and movement to the arms, neck, and upper trunk; thoracic nerves supply the trunk and abdomen; and lumbar and sacral nerves supply the legs, bladder, and sexual organs.

The paramedic should be familiar with signs and symptoms of several incomplete spinal cord syndromes. Knowledge of these rare syndromes helps the paramedic to understand the potential for further injury. The three syndromes associated with incomplete lesions of the spinal cord are as follows:

1. **Central cord syndrome.** Central cord syndrome commonly occurs with hyperextension cervical injuries; less commonly, flexion cervical injuries may result in this syndrome. The syndrome is characterized by greater motor impairment of the upper extremities than of the lower extremities. Signs and symptoms of central cord syndrome are as follows
   - Paralysis of the arms
   - Sacral sparing (the preservation of sensory or voluntary motor function of the perineum, buttocks, scrotum, or anus)
2. **Anterior cord syndrome.** Anterior cord syndrome usually is seen in flexion injuries. The syndrome is caused by injury to the anterior aspect of the spinal cord by a ruptured intervertebral disk or fragments of the vertebral body forced posteriorly into the spinal canal or by compromised blood flow from the anterior spinal artery. Signs and symptoms include the following:
   - Decreased sensation of pain and temperature below the level of the lesion (including lesions of the sacral region)
   - Intact light touch and position sensation
   - Paralysis below the level of the lesion
3. **Brown-Séquard syndrome.** Brown-Séquard syndrome is a functional hemitransection of the spinal cord. This syndrome may result from a ruptured intervertebral disk or the pushing of a fragment of vertebral body on the spinal cord. It also occurs after knife or missile injuries. In the classic presentation, injury to half of the spinal cord results in weakness or paralysis of the extremities on the ipsilateral (same) side with loss of pain and temperature sensation on the contralateral (opposite) side.

CRITICAL THINKING

How will the prehospital care differ for a patient who has signs or symptoms of one of these syndromes?

NOTE

The benefits of pharmacologic agents (glucocorticoids, naloxone, calcium channel blockers, GM-1 ganglioside, and others) in the management of incomplete cord injury are controversial. None is presently recommended for prehospital treatment of patients with SCI.

Modified from: Chin LS. Spinal cord injuries treatment and management. Medscape website. https://emedicine.medscape.com/article/793582-treatment#d11. Updated August 10, 2017. Accessed March 19, 2018.

Spinal Assessment Criteria

Assessment of suspected SCIs traditionally has focused on mechanism of injury (MOI). While it is used as a piece of evidence to help determine the need for immobilization, the clinical examination is key. The paramedic should apply clear clinical guidelines (clinical criteria) for evaluating the possibility of SCI, which includes the following signs and symptoms:[8,9]

- Altered level of consciousness (Glasgow Coma Scale score less than 15)
- Spinal pain or tenderness
- Neurologic deficit or complaint
- Anatomic deformity of the spine
- Unreliable patient

> NOTE
>
> In some situations a patient may be considered "unreliable" to provide an accurate history of an event. Examples include patients who do not understand the questioning, have a speech barrier or an inability to communicate, and those who have a mental or intellectual disability. Other factors that may contribute to a patient being unreliable are alcohol or other drug use. The paramedic should also stay alert for another injury that may distract the patient from complaining about a more serious injury (*distracting injury*).

Mechanism of Injury

Determining MOI in a patient who may have spinal trauma is a crucial element in evaluating the likelihood of spinal injury. MOI combined with the clinical criteria for spinal injury can help the paramedic identify situations in which suspicion for spinal injury should be high. When in doubt, the paramedic should use appropriate spinal precautions (**FIGURE 40-8**).

Positive MOI

In a positive MOI, the forces exerted on the patient are highly suggestive of SCI. A positive MOI with physiologic findings on examination that are suspicious for spinal injury mandates careful movement of the patient during extrication from the scene and transport to the medical facility. Examples of positive MOIs include the following:

- Violent impact to the head, neck, torso, or pelvis
  - Assault
  - Entrapment after structural collapse
- Incidents related to sudden acceleration, deceleration, or lateral bending forces to the neck or torso
  - High-speed motor vehicle crashes
  - Pedestrian struck
  - Explosion
- Falls, especially involving older adults
- Ejection or fall from a motorized or motor-powered transportation device
- Shallow-water diving incidents[5]

In the absence of signs and symptoms of SCI, some medical control authorities may not recommend immobilization. Medical direction bases this decision on the paramedic's assessment, a reliable patient history, and the absence of distracting injuries. Even in the presence of SCI, spinal motion restriction, as opposed to spinal immobilization, is increasingly recognized as a better approach to the overall management of the spine-injured patient.[5]

> NOTE
>
> Two terms are commonly used to describe methods to prevent movement of the spinal column: *spinal immobilization* and *spinal motion restriction*. Although the terms are similar in meaning, spinal immobilization usually refers to the use of equipment to immobilize the spine, such as cervical collars and backboards. Spinal motion restriction has the same goal of preventing spinal movement by maintaining alignment of the spine. However, spinal motion restriction focuses on the judicious use of adjunctive devices.
>
> *Modified from*: National Registry of EMT's Resource Document on Spinal Motion Restriction/Immobilization. National Registry of Emergency Medical Technicians website. https://www.nremt.org/rwd/public/document/news-spinal-11-11-16. Accessed March 22, 2018; and White CC IV, Domeier RM, Millin MG, and the Standards and Clinical Practice Committee, National Association of EMS Physicians. EMS spinal precautions and the use of the long backboard—Resource Document to the Position Statement of the National Association of EMS Physicians and the American College of Surgeons Committee on Trauma. *Prehosp Emerg Care*. 2014;18(2):306-314.

Negative MOIs

A negative MOI includes events in which force or impact does not suggest a likely spinal injury. In the absence of SCI signs and symptoms, negative MOIs do not require spinal immobilization. Examples of negative MOIs include the following:

- Dropping an object on the foot
- Twisting an ankle while running
- Isolated soft-tissue injury

Patient Reliability

When evaluating the need for spinal immobilization, the paramedic must ensure that the patient is reliable. A reliable patient is one who is calm, cooperative, sober, alert, and oriented. Patients who would be considered unreliable present with any of the following characteristics:

- Have a Glasgow Coma Scale score of less than 15
- Are intoxicated with alcohol or drugs

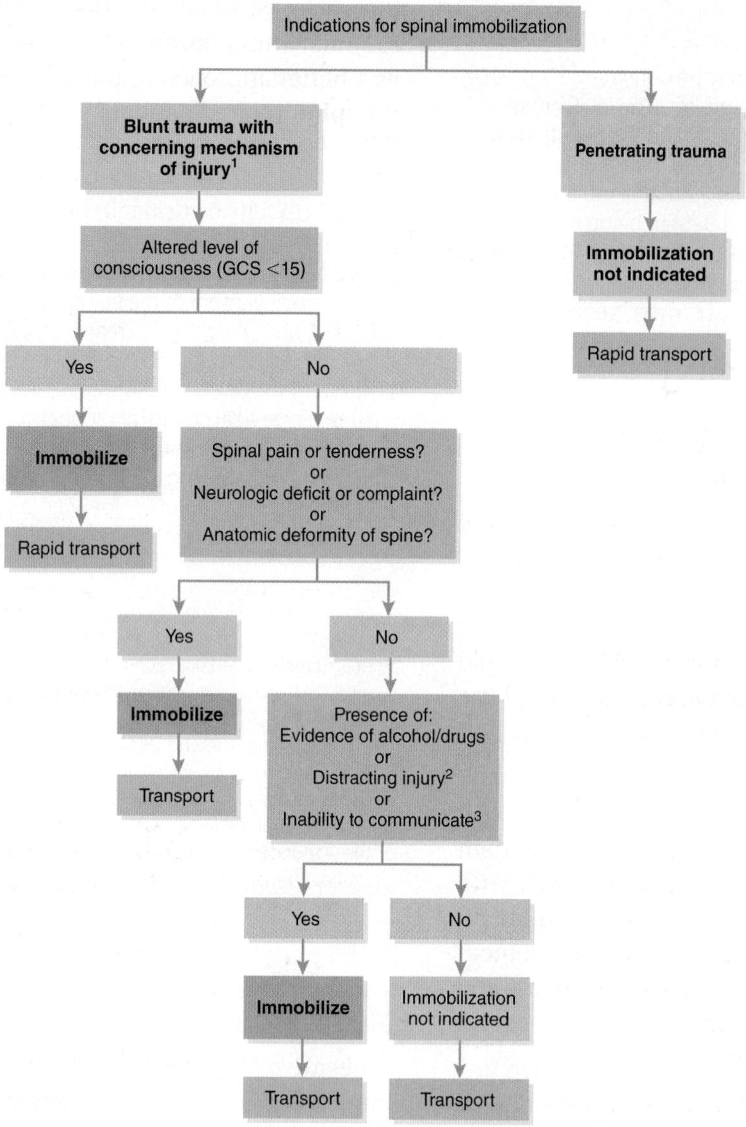

Notes:

[1]Concerning Mechanisms of Injury

- Any mechanism that produced a violent impact to the head, neck, torso, or pelvis (eg, assault, entrapment in structural collapse, etc.)
- Incidents producing sudden acceleration, deceleration, or lateral bending forces to the neck or torso (eg, moderate- to high-speed MVC, pedestrian struck, involvement in an explosion, etc.)
- Any fall, especially in the elderly
- Ejection or fall from any motorized or human-powered transportation device (eg, scooters, skateboards, bicycles, motor vehicles, motorcycles or recreational vehicles)
- Victim of shallow-water diving incident

[2]Distracting Injury

Any injury that may have the potential to impair the patient's ability to appreciate other injuries. Examples of distracting injuries include (a) long bone fracture; (b) a visceral injury requiring surgical consultation; (c) a large laceration, degloving injury, or crush injury; (d) large burns, or (e) any other injury producing acute functional impairment. (Adapted from Hoffman JR, Wolfson AB, Todd K, Mower WR. Selective cervical spine radiography in blunt trauma: methodology of the National Emergency X-Radiography Utilization Study [NEXUS]. *Ann Emerg Med.* 1998 Oct;32(4):461-469.)

[3]Inability to communicate. Any patient who, for reasons not specified above, cannot clearly communicate so as to actively participate in their assessment. Examples: speech or hearing impaired, those who only speak a foreign language, and small children.

Abbreviations: GCS, Glasgow Coma Scale; MVC, motor vehicle crash

FIGURE 40-8 Indications for spinal immobilization.

Modified from: National Association of Emergency Medical Technicians. *PHTLS: Prehospital Trauma Life Support*. 8th ed. Burlington, MA: Jones & Bartlett Learning; 2016.

- Have distracting injuries (ie, injuries that impair their ability to appreciate other injuries)
  - Long bone fractures
  - Serious chest or abdominal injuries
  - Large laceration, degloving injury, or crush injury
  - Large burn
  - Other injuries causing functional impairment
- Have problems communicating
  - Speech or hearing impaired
  - Speak a foreign language
  - Young children[5]

CRITICAL THINKING

The reliability of a patient is not always easy to assess quickly in the prehospital setting. Why is this?

NOTE

Any patient who has altered mental status or altered pain perception should be considered unreliable. Examples include patients with Alzheimer disease, patients with a psychiatric illness, and those under the influence of alcohol or other drugs.

Evaluation of SCI

Spinal cord trauma should be evaluated only after all injuries that pose a threat to life have been assessed and treated. As with any scenario of serious illness or injury, the paramedic's first priority must be scene survey, including ensuring personal safety. The primary survey and assessment and management of exsanguinating hemorrhage, the patient's airway, breathing, and circulation must be performed in a way that minimizes further injury. The second priority is to preserve spinal cord function and avoid secondary injury to the spinal cord.

The primary injury to the spine occurs at impact. Thus, the key role of paramedics is to prevent secondary injury. A secondary injury could result from unnecessary movement of an unstable spinal column, hypoxemia, edema, or shock (which may reduce perfusion of the injured cord). These goals are best met by maintaining a high degree of suspicion for the presence of spinal trauma (based on scene survey, kinematics, and history of the event), providing early spinal motion restriction, providing oxygen and ventilator support (if indicated), and rapidly correcting any volume deficit through fluid replacement.

After any life-threatening problems found in the initial assessment have been treated, the paramedic should perform a neurologic examination. This examination may be done in the field or en route to the receiving medical facility if the patient's condition requires rapid transport. Any movement of the patient for performing a general or neurologic examination must be accompanied by continuous, manual protection and in-line stabilization of the spine. Once the spine has been stabilized, the paramedic should palpate the entire spine. Any report of pain on palpation indicates a higher likelihood of injury to the spine. Full documentation of the paramedic's findings provides an important baseline. This information will be useful for further assessment and evaluation of the patient in the emergency department. The components of the neurologic examination include evaluation of motor and sensory findings and reflex responses.

Motor Findings

The paramedic should question conscious patients about pain in the neck or back with and without palpation. The paramedic also should ask patients about their ability to move their arms and legs. If possible, the paramedic should test the strength and motion of all four extremities, which can be done by asking the patient to flex the elbows (biceps, C6), extend the elbows (triceps, C7), and abduct/adduct the fingers (C8, T1). In unconscious patients, painful stimuli in the hands and lower extremities may initiate an involuntary muscle reflex unless the patient is in profound coma.

Upper Extremity Neurologic Function Assessment

To test voluntary muscle function in the fingers and hands (controlled by the T1 nerve roots), the paramedic should instruct the patient to spread the fingers of both hands. The patient then should be instructed to keep the fingers apart while the paramedic squeezes the second and fourth fingers. Normal resistance should be springlike and equal on both sides.

To test the extensors of the hands and fingers (controlled by the C7 nerve roots), the paramedic should instruct the patient to hold his or her wrists or fingers straight out and to keep them out while the paramedic presses down on the fingers. (The arm should be supported at the wrist to avoid testing arm function and other nerve roots.) Moderate resistance will normally be felt with moderate pressure. Both sides of the patient should be evaluated if not contraindicated by injury.

Lower Extremity Neurologic Function Assessment

To test plantar flexors of the foot (controlled by the S1 and S2 nerve roots), the paramedic should place his or her hands at the sole of each foot and instruct the patient to push against the hands. Both sides should feel equal and strong.

To test dorsal flexors of the foot and great toe (controlled by the L5 nerve roots), the paramedic should hold the patient's foot (with fingers on toes) and instruct the patient to pull the feet back or toward the nose. Both sides should feel equal and strong.

Sensory Findings

In conscious patients, sensory examination should be performed with light touch on each hand and each foot (while the patient's eyes are closed) to evaluate the ability to feel this type of stimulus. (Light touch is carried by more than one nerve tract.) Sensation should be equal on both sides. The paramedic also should question the patient about weakness, numbness, paresthesia, or radicular pain (shooting pain that travels along a nerve).

If the patient cannot feel light touch or is unconscious, the paramedic may evaluate sensation by gently pricking the hands and soles of the feet with a sharp object that will not penetrate the skin (eg, the end of a pen, a broken cotton-tipped applicator). One method of evaluation moves from head to toe, with the paramedic recording the level at which sensation stops or the unconscious patient ceases to respond to a painful stimulus by marking that location on the patient's skin with ink or a marker. Another method is to begin the sensory assessment by moving from an area of no sensation to an area where sensation begins. The paramedic notes the area where sensation begins with ink or a marker. These marks make it possible to compare sensory level accurately after repeated examinations. Lack of response to stimulation in the upper extremities indicates cord damage in the cervical region; failure of only the lower extremities to respond indicates cord injury in the thoracic region, lumbar region, or both.

CRITICAL THINKING

How will you respond to the patient who fearfully asks you, "Why can't I move or feel my arms or legs?"

Dermatomes (described in Chapter 10, *Review of Human Systems*) correspond to spinal nerves (**TABLE 40-1**), so the following four landmarks may be useful for a quick sensory evaluation in the prehospital setting:

1. The C2 through C4 dermatomes provide a collar of sensation around the neck and over the anterior chest to below the clavicles.
2. The T4 dermatome provides sensation to the nipple line.
3. The T10 dermatome provides sensation to the umbilicus.
4. The S1 dermatome provides sensation to the soles of the feet.

Reflex Responses

Reflex responses seldom are evaluated in the prehospital setting. However, some abnormal responses are observed easily and may indicate autonomic nerve injury. These responses include loss of temperature control, hypotension, bradycardia, and priapism. Another pathologic reflex includes the presence of Babinski sign (the plantar reflex, rarely associated with acute injury). The Babinski sign is a reflex movement in which the great toe bends upward when the outer edge of the sole of the foot is scratched (**FIGURE 40-9**). This sign, which may indicate a spinal cord lesion in the older child or adult, is a normal and expected response in children younger than 2 years.

Other Methods of Evaluation

A visual inspection of the spine may reveal the presence of injury and its level. For example, transection of the cord above C3 often results in respiratory arrest. Lesions that occur at C4 may result in paralysis of the diaphragm; however, transections that occur at C5-C6 usually spare the diaphragm, allowing diaphragmatic breathing. This occurs because the intercostal muscles are innervated sequentially between T1 and T12. As a result, intercostal muscle groups may be paralyzed with cervical or thoracic spinal cord lesions below the level where diaphragmatic nerves are located. (The higher the lesion, the greater the loss of intercostal muscle function.)

TABLE 40-1 Common Nerve Root and Motor/Sensory Correlation

Nerve Root	Motor	Sensory
C3, C4	Trapezius (shoulder shrug)	Top of shoulder
C3 through C5	Diaphragm	Top of shoulder
C5	Biceps (elbow flexion)	Thumb
C7	Triceps (elbow extension), wrist/finger extension	Middle finger
C8, T1	Finger abduction/adduction	Little finger
T4	Nipple	
T10	Umbilicus	
L1, L2	Hip flexion	Inguinal crease
L3, L4	Quadriceps	Medial thigh/calf
L5	Great toe/foot dorsiflexion	Lateral calf
S1	Knee flexion	Lateral foot
S1, S2	Foot plantar flexion	
S2 through S4	Anal sphincter tone	Perianal

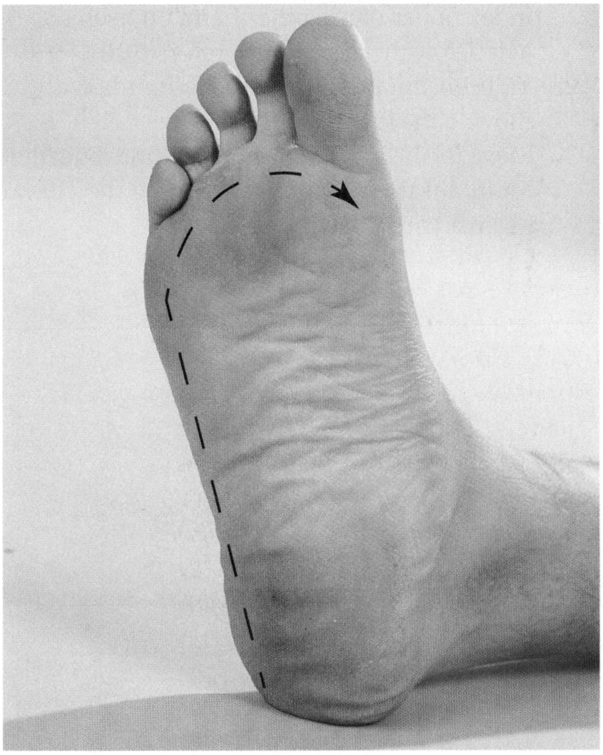

FIGURE 40-9 Babinski sign is assessed by stroking the sole of the foot.

The patient's body position also may offer clues about neurologic injury. For example, a patient with a spinal injury at C6 may lie with the arms flexed at the elbows and wrists (the holdup position).

General Management of Spinal Injuries

A significant spinal injury may be present even if the patient does not show signs of spinal injury.[10] Some patients with cervical spinal injuries have normal responses to motor, sensory, and reflex examinations. Thus, if the paramedic suspects a spinal injury for any reason, the paramedic must protect the patient's spine. In addition, the patient's ability to walk does not always rule out the need for spinal precautions. As previously stated, an unstable spine can be ruled out only by clinical assessment including examination, radiography, and the evaluation of any potential mechanism for spinal injury.

General principles of spinal motion restriction include the following:

1. The primary goal is to prevent further injury.
2. The spine should be treated as a long bone with a joint at either end (the head and pelvis).

3. Spinal motion restriction begins in the initial assessment of blunt trauma and, when indicated, is maintained until the patient is delivered to the emergency department. There is no role for spinal motion restriction in penetrating trauma.[11]
4. The patient's head and neck must be placed in a neutral, in-line position unless contraindicated by condition or MOI. (Neutral positioning allows for the most space for the spinal cord, thereby reducing cord hypoxia and excess pressure.)

Spinal Motion Restriction Techniques

As soon as a potential spinal injury is recognized, the paramedic should manually protect the patient's head and neck if the patient has altered mental status and is unable to follow commands. Conscious, cooperative patients should be instructed to remain still and not move their heads. The basic principle to follow is that the head and neck must be maintained in line with the long axis of the body. If other injuries require treatment, the paramedic must maintain the patient's head and neck position without interruption.

A number of devices for immobilizing the spinal column are designed for prehospital use. When properly applied to patients who are sitting, standing, or lying, these devices can provide adequate spinal protection; however, no device should be considered for use until the head and neck have been stabilized with manual in-line immobilization.

> NOTE
>
> All spinal immobilization techniques discussed in this text follow the guidelines recommended by the Prehospital Trauma Life Support Committee of the National Association of Emergency Medical Technicians in cooperation with the Committee on Trauma of the American College of Surgeons and the National Association of EMS Physicians.
>
> *Modified from*: National Association of Emergency Medical Technicians. *PHTLS: Prehospital Trauma Life Support*. 8th ed. Burlington, MA: Jones & Bartlett Learning; 2014.

Manual In-Line Immobilization

Manual in-line immobilization can be done from almost any patient position, but it should be applied without traction on the head. It is designed to minimize movement of the neck from a neutral position. After manual immobilization has been initiated, it is continued without interruption until the head and spine are immobilized to a proper device (short backboard or vest, long backboard, or stretcher).

Contraindications for moving the patient's head to an in-line position follow. If any of these contraindications exist, all manual movement of the patient's head should stop. At that point, the head and neck should be stabilized in the position found. Contraindications include the following:

- Resistance to movement
- Neck muscle spasm
- Increased pain
- The presence or increase in neurologic deficits during movement (eg, numbness, tingling, loss of motor function)
- Compromise of the airway or ventilation
- Severe misalignment of the head away from the midline of the shoulders and body axis (rare)

Manual Immobilization From the Sitting or Standing Patient's Side.

1. Stand alongside the patient, holding the back of the head with one hand. Place the thumb and index finger of the other hand on each cheek, just below the zygomatic arch (**FIGURE 40-10**).
2. Tighten the position of both hands without moving the head or neck.
3. Move the head to an in-line position if needed. Maintain this position by bracing the elbows against your torso for support.

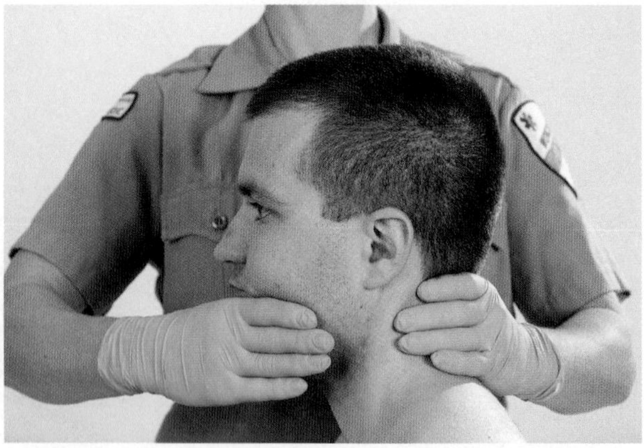

FIGURE 40-10 Manual in-line immobilization from the side.

Manual In-Line Immobilization From the Front of the Sitting or Standing Patient.

1. Stand in front of the patient and place the thumb of each hand on the patient's cheeks, just below the zygomatic arch.
2. Place the little fingers of each hand on the posterior aspect of the patient's skull.
3. Spread the remaining fingers of each hand on the lateral planes of the head and increase the strength of the grip (**FIGURE 40-11**).
4. Move the head to an in-line position if needed. Maintain this position by bracing the elbows against your torso for support.

Manual In-Line Immobilization With a Supine Patient.

1. Kneel or lie at the patient's head and place the thumbs of each hand just below the zygomatic arch of each cheek (**FIGURE 40-12**).
2. Place the little fingers of each hand on the posterior aspect of the patient's skull.

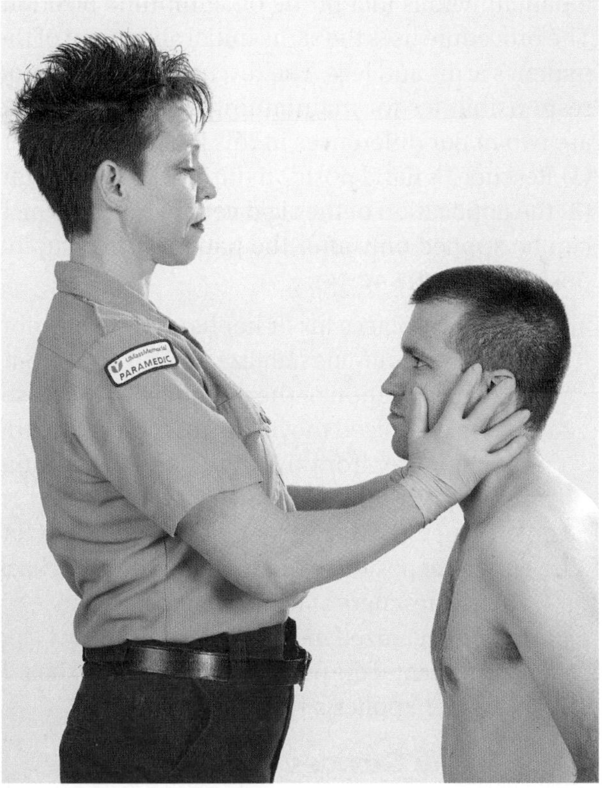

FIGURE 40-11 Manual in-line immobilization from the front.

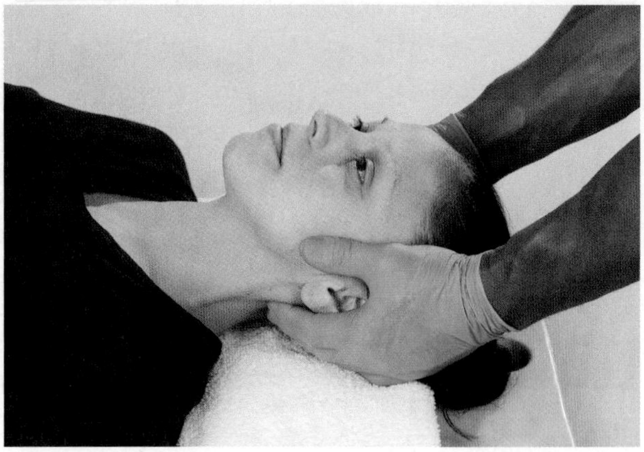

FIGURE 40-12 Manual in-line immobilization with a supine patient.

3. Spread the remaining fingers of each hand on the lateral planes of the head and increase the strength of the grip.
4. Move the head to an in-line position if needed. Maintain this position by bracing the elbows against your torso or ground surface for support.

Log Roll With Spinal Precautions. Log rolling methods are used to move patients with a possible spinal injury. Examples include moving patients onto a mechanical immobilization device and turning patients from a prone to a supine position. Log rolling maneuvers require at least four rescuers for adequate spinal protection. The position of the patient's arms during a log rolling maneuver may affect thoracic-lumbar motion and further compromise the stability of the spine. One method that may minimize lateral motion and help to maintain neutral alignment of the pelvis and legs is to position the patient with arms extended at the side. The patient's palms should be on the lateral thighs.

Log Roll of the Supine Patient. The following steps should be used to log roll patients in the supine position (**FIGURE 40-13**).

1. Rescuer 1 should be positioned at the patient's head. Rescuer 1 should provide in-line manual stabilization. Another rescuer should apply a rigid cervical collar and place a long backboard at the patient's side.
2. Rescuers 2 and 3 should be positioned at the patient's midthorax and knees. The patient's

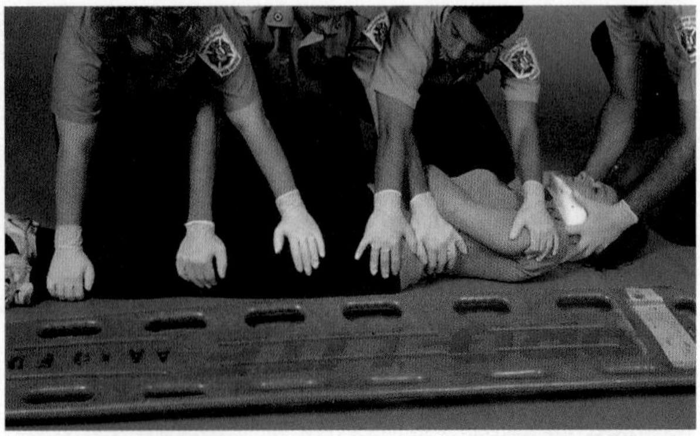

A

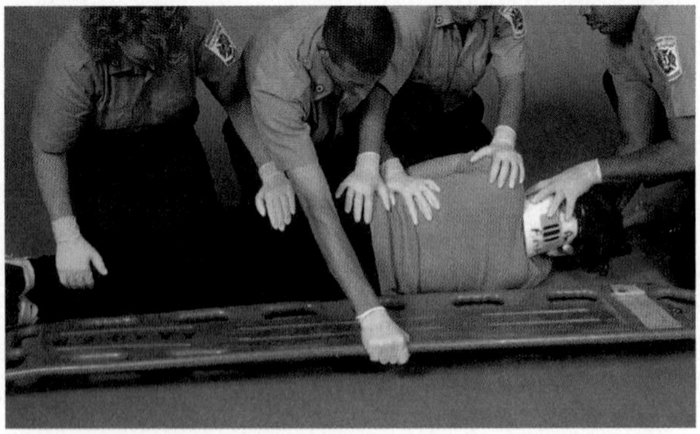

B

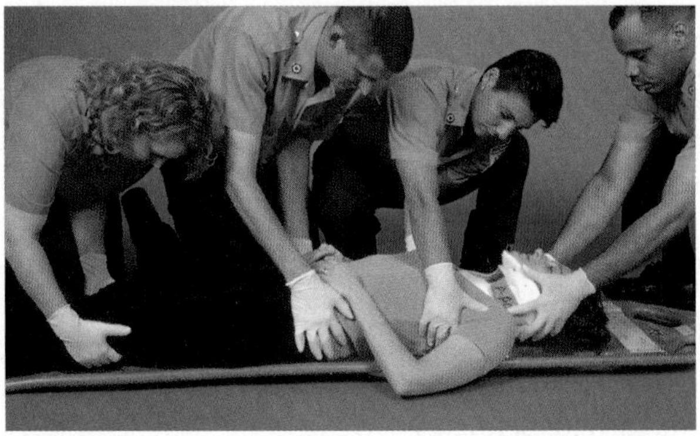

C

FIGURE 40-13 A. To log roll a supine patient, Rescuer 1 is positioned at the patient's head, providing in-line manual stabilization. Rescuers 2 and 3 are positioned at the patient's midthorax and knees. **B.** While maintaining immobilization, the rescuers slowly log roll the patient onto his or her side perpendicular to the ground in one organized move. Rescuer 4 positions the long backboard by placing the device flat on the ground or at a 30° to 40° angle against the patient's back. **C.** In one organized move, the rescuers slowly log roll and center the patient onto the long backboard.

arms should be extended at the sides, palms on lateral thighs. The legs should be brought together for neutral alignment.

3. Rescuer 2 grasps the far side of the patient at the shoulder and wrist. Rescuer 3 grasps the hips (just distal of the wrists) and both lower extremities at the ankles.
4. In one organized move, the rescuers slowly log roll the patient onto his or her side. At the same time, they slide the backboard under the patient. In-line support of the patient's head must be maintained, which is accomplished by rotating the head exactly with the torso to avoid flexion or hyperextension. In addition, the ankles must be elevated slightly to maintain lateral and anterior-posterior alignment.
5. Rescuer 4 positions the long backboard by placing the device flat on the ground or at a 30° to 40° angle against the patient's back.
6. In one organized move, the rescuers slowly log roll and center the patient on the long backboard.

Log Roll of the Prone Patient. The basic principles used in log rolling supine patients can be applied to a patient who is in a prone or semiprone position. The procedure uses the same initial alignment of the patient's arms and legs. The rescuers have the same responsibilities for maintaining alignment. There are two major differences in this log roll maneuver: (1) Rescuer 1's hand position during the log roll and (2) the application of the rigid cervical collar, which can be applied only after the patient is in a supine position (**FIGURE 40-14**).

1. Rescuer 1 places his or her hands in a position that provides in-line stabilization and that accommodates rotation of the patient with the torso.
2. In one organized move, the rescuers rotate the patient away from the direction of the initial prone position.
3. A rescuer places the long backboard on a flat surface or positions it between the patient's back and the rescuers at the patient's side.
4. In one organized move, the rescuers slowly log roll and center the patient on the long backboard.
5. A rescuer applies a rigid cervical collar.

Mechanical Devices

Spinal motion restriction equipment includes rigid cervical collars, short backboards, and long backboards. This text presents only general principles of

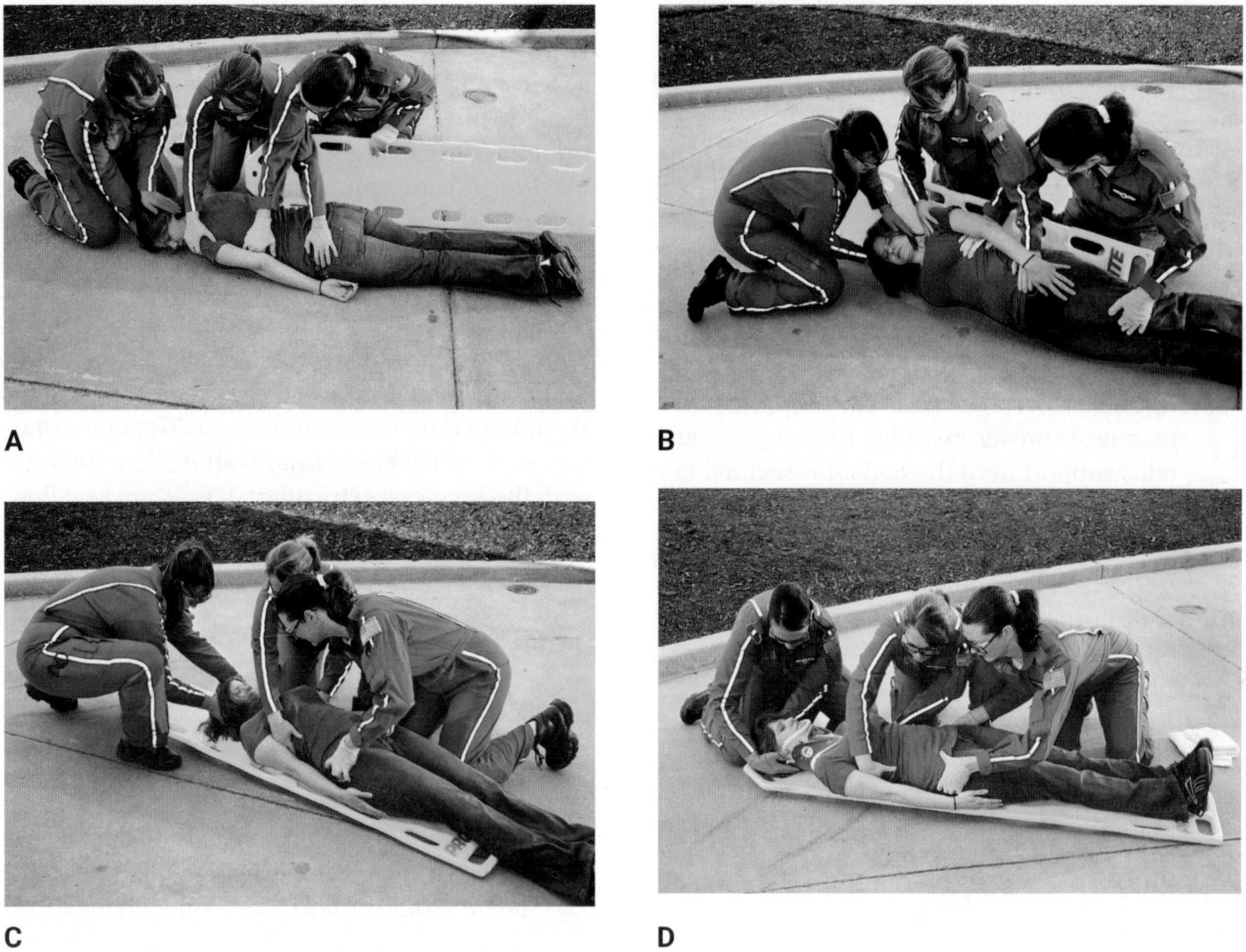

FIGURE 40-14 **A.** Rescuer 1 places his or her hands in a position that provides in-line stabilization and that accommodates the rotation of the patient with the torso. Rescuer 2 positions the long backboard. **B.** In one organized move, the rescuers rotate the patient away from the direction of his or her initial prone position. **C.** In one organized move, the rescuers slowly log roll and center the patient onto the long backboard. **D.** Another rescuer then applies a rigid cervical collar.

spinal motion restriction by mechanical devices. The specific methods of application vary by device. Paramedics should become familiar with the equipment used in their locale and follow the manufacturer's application guidelines.

Rigid Cervical Collars. Rigid cervical collars are designed to protect the cervical spine from compression. These devices may reduce movement and some range of motion of the head; however, they do not by themselves provide adequate immobilization of the spine. These devices must always be used along with manual in-line stabilization or motion restriction by a suitable device (eg, vest, short backboard, long backboard). An effective rigid collar sits on the chest, posterior thoracic spine and clavicle, and trapezius muscles, where tissue movement is at a minimum.[5] The collar also must be correctly sized for the patient. A rigid cervical collar should be applied in the following situations:

- Complaint of midline neck or spine pain
- Tenderness or anatomic deformity on palpation of midline neck or spine
- Unreliable patient
  - Glasgow Coma Scale score of less than 15
  - Alcohol or drug intoxication
  - Distracting injury present
  - Communication barrier
- Focal or neurologic deficit
- **Torticollis** in children

Ambulatory patients can be immobilized on the stretcher with a cervical collar. To apply a rigid cervical collar, the paramedic should follow these general steps (**FIGURE 40-15**):

1. Rescuer 1 applies manual in-line immobilization from behind the patient and maintains this position throughout the procedure.
2. Rescuer 2 properly angles the collar for placement.
3. Rescuer 2 positions the collar bottom.
4. Rescuer 2 sets the collar in place around the patient's neck.
5. Rescuer 2 secures the collar with the Velcro straps.
6. Rescuer 1 spreads his or her fingers and maintains support until the patient is secured to a short or long backboard.

Rigid cervical collars are available in a number of sizes (or they are adjustable). They can accommodate the range of physical characteristics of patients. Choosing the proper size reduces flexion or hyperextension of the neck. These movements may occur during patient extrication and packaging. These movements also may result from acceleration and deceleration forces that normally occur during patient transport. The following guidelines apply to the use of rigid cervical collars:[5]

- They do not adequately immobilize by their use alone.
- They must be properly sized to the patient.
- They must not inhibit the patient's ability to open his or her mouth or the paramedic's ability to open the patient's mouth if vomiting occurs.
- They must not obstruct or hinder ventilation in any way.

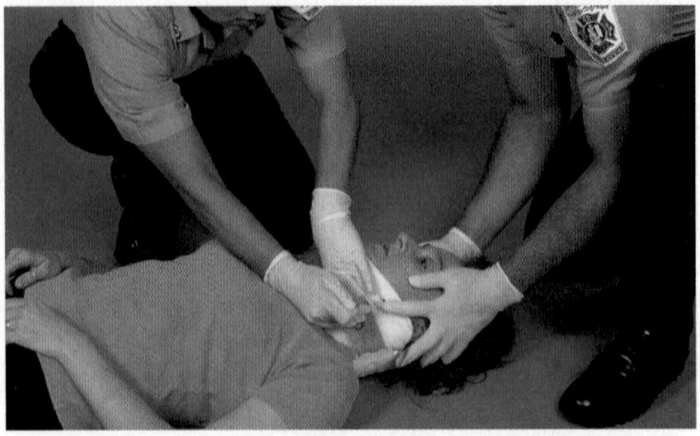

FIGURE 40-15 Rescuer 2 positions the collar and secures it with Velcro straps.

Short Backboards. Short backboards or other short spine extrication devices are used to splint the cervical and thoracic spine. These devices vary in design, and they are available from a number of manufacturers. In general, short backboards are used to provide spinal immobilization when the patient is sitting or is in a confined space. After short backboard immobilization, the patient is moved to a long backboard device to facilitate transfer to the ambulance stretcher. Examples of short backboards include the plastic or synthetic half backboard, the Kendrick extrication device, the Oregon Spine Splint II, and the Hare extrication device. General principles of short backboard application, demonstrated with the Kendrick extrication device, are as follows (**FIGURE 40-16**):

CRITICAL THINKING

When would the use of the short board *not* be indicated for spinal column immobilization?

1. After manual in-line immobilization and the application of a rigid cervical collar, place the short backboard device behind the patient. The board should be positioned snugly beneath the patient's axillae; this will prevent it from moving up the torso.
2. Immobilize the upper and middle torso by fastening the chest straps, starting with the middle chest straps and followed by the lower chest straps. The upper chest strap (if used) should not be so tight that it impedes patient ventilation.[5]

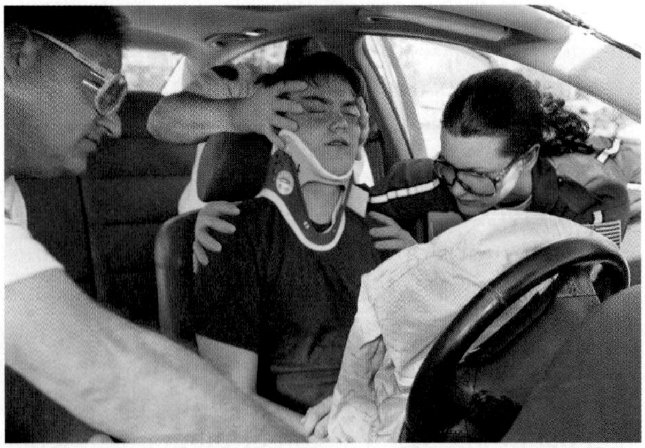

FIGURE 40-16 Application of the Kendrick extrication device.

The middle and lower straps should be snug so that fingers cannot be slipped beneath the straps. Readjust as needed.

3. Position and fasten each groin strap separately, forming a loop. These straps prevent the Kendrick extrication device from moving up and the lower end from moving laterally.
4. Pad the device as needed and secure the head to the short backboard.
5. Carefully move the patient as a unit to a long backboard by rotating the patient and Kendrick extrication device onto the board. Hold the legs proximal to the knees and lift them during the transition.
6. Center the patient on the long backboard, release the leg straps, and slowly lower the patient's legs to an in-line position.
7. Secure the patient and Kendrick extrication device to the long backboard, maintaining a neutral in-line position with the long axis of the body, and then slightly loosen the Kendrick extrication device leg straps.

> NOTE
>
> The use of a short backboard should be considered only if the patient's condition allows. If the patient is unstable because of life-threatening injury or the need for immediate resuscitation, or if the time required to apply the device would jeopardize the patient's life (eg, a patient with a carotid pulse but absent radial pulse), the patient's head and neck should be stabilized with manual, in-line support, and the patient should be moved as a unit to a long backboard.

Rapid Extrication

The steps required for rapid extrication may vary depending on the size and make of the vehicle. They also may vary based on the patient's location inside the vehicle. The following lists offer a general description of the steps required for rapid extrication.

Three or More Rescuers (FIGURE 40-17).

1. Rescuer 1 supports the patient's head and neck and uses manual in-line stabilization from behind the patient or from the patient's side. Rescuer 1 maintains this stabilization throughout the extrication process.
2. After a rapid initial assessment, Rescuer 2 applies a rigid cervical collar and positions a long backboard near the vehicle.

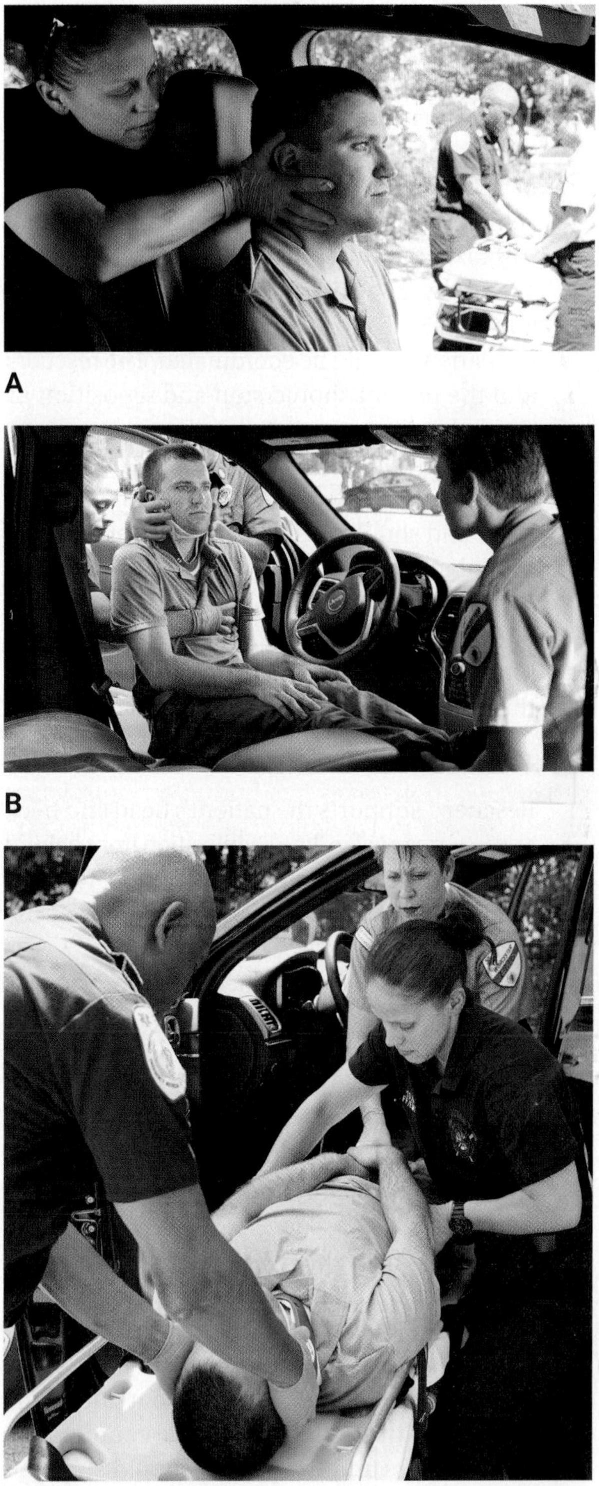

A

B

C

FIGURE 40-17 **A.** Rescuer 1 supports the patient's head and neck and uses manual in-line stabilization throughout the procedure while Rescuer 2 supports the patient's midthorax. **B.** The rescuers carefully lower the patient onto a long backboard. **C.** The rescuers center and prepare to secure the patient on the long backboard.

3. Rescuer 3 manually stabilizes and controls movement of the patient's upper and lower torso and legs during extrication.
4. The rescuers then rotate the patient in a series of short, controlled movements so that the patient's back faces the open doorway. Rescuer 2 exits the vehicle. Rescuer 2 assumes control of manual stabilization from outside the vehicle. Rescuer 1 assumes control of the patient's lower torso and legs. Each movement during the rotation of the patient should be coordinated. The rescuers and the patient should stop and reposition as needed to limit unwanted patient movement.
5. A rescuer should insert the foot end of the long backboard on the car seat at the patient's buttocks and should position the head end on the ambulance stretcher. Rotation of the patient continues until the patient can be positioned onto the long backboard.
6. The rescuers center and secure the patient on the long backboard as described later.

Two Rescuers (FIGURE 40-18).

1. Rescuer 1 supports the patient's head and neck and uses manual in-line stabilization from behind the patient or from the patient's side. Rescuer 1 maintains this stabilization throughout the extrication process.
2. After a rapid initial assessment, Rescuer 2 applies a rigid cervical collar and places a prerolled blanket around the patient. Rescuer 2 places the center of the blanket roll at the patient's midline on the rigid cervical collar. Rescuer 2 then wraps the ends of the blanket roll around the cervical collar and places them under the patient's arms. Rescuer 2 positions a long backboard near the vehicle.
3. Using the ends of the blanket roll, the rescuers rotate the patient in a series of short, controlled movements so that the patient's back faces the open doorway. Each movement during the rotation of the patient should be coordinated. The rescuers and the patient should stop and reposition as needed to limit unwanted patient movement.
4. Rescuer 1 takes control of the blanket ends, moving them under the patient's shoulders, and moves the patient by the blanket while Rescuer 2 controls the patient's lower torso, pelvis, and legs.

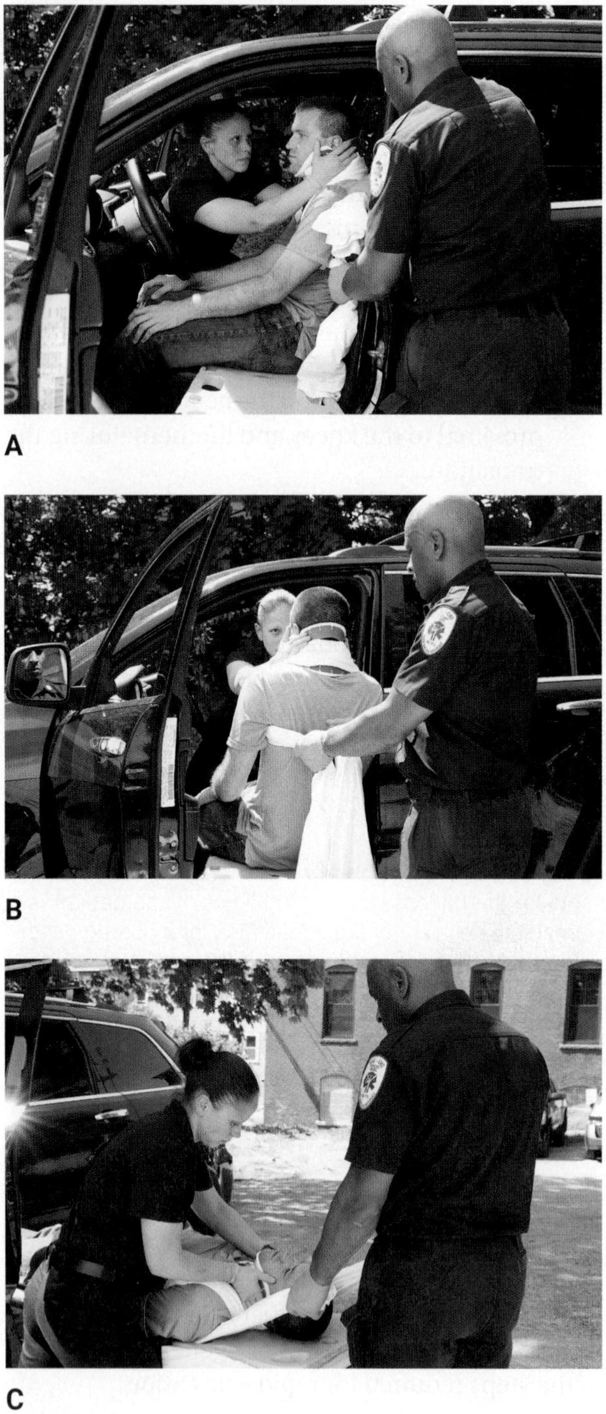

FIGURE 40-18 A. Rescuer 1 supports the patient's head and neck and uses manual in-line stabilization throughout the procedure. **B.** After assessment and application of a cervical collar, a rescuer positions the center of a blanket roll at the patient's midline on the cervical collar. The rescuer wraps the ends of the blanket roll around the cervical collar and places them under the patient's arms. **C.** The rescuers rotate the patient using the ends of the blanket roll until the patient's back faces the open doorway.

5. The rescuers center and secure the patient on the long backboard as described next.

Long Backboard With Supine Patient. Similar to short backboards, long backboards are available in a variety of configurations. Designs include plastic and synthetic backboards, metal alloy backboards, vacuum mattress splints, and split litters (scoop stretchers) that must be used along with a long backboard. Long backboards are not a treatment, and paramedics should avoid transporting patients on a long backboard. The usefulness of long backboards comes in extrication of patients from a scene to the stretcher. The following description of securing patients on a long backboard may be applied to any long spinal immobilization device.

NOTE

Significant evidence suggests that rigid long backboard immobilization for suspected SCI does not improve patient outcome and can be associated with complications. Prolonged immobilization on a backboard is very uncomfortable and can lead to pressure injuries to the skin, pain, aspiration, increased intracranial pressure, and patient agitation. Tight strap application can impair ventilation. Further, the discomfort associated with prolonged immobilization on a backboard can lead to unneeded radiologic testing, and in children, increased admission to the medical facility.

Spinal precautions should include, at a minimum, applying a cervical collar, securing the patient to the stretcher, minimizing movement and transfers, and maintaining in-line stabilization when moving the patient. Because the stretcher is in essence a padded spineboard, when used with a cervical collar it is a more comfortable alternative to the hard long backboard and is associated with fewer complications in low-risk patients.

Some situations warrant the use of long backboards. They may be used to move a patient to the stretcher or immobilize a patient with multiple long bone fractures. In these situations, the board should be padded when possible or a vacuum splint applied.

Modified from: National Association of EMS Physicians and American College of Surgeons Committee on Trauma. EMS spinal precautions and the use of the long backboard. *Prehosp Emerg Care.* 2013;17(3):361-372; White CC, Domeier RM, Millin MG. EMS spinal precautions and the use of the long backboard—resource document to the position statement of the National Association of EMS Physicians and the American College of Surgeons Committee on Trauma. *Prehosp Emerg Care.* 2014;18(2):306-314; and Leonard JC, Mao J, Jaffe DM. Potential adverse effects of spinal immobilization in children. *Prehosp Emerg Care.* 2012;16(4):513-518.

Immobilization of the torso to a long backboard must be done before immobilization of the head. This sequence will prevent angulation of the cervical spine. The torso must not be allowed to move up, down, or to either side. Straps should be placed at the shoulders or upper chest below the axillae to avoid compression and lateral movement of the thorax, around the midtorso, and across the iliac crest to prevent movement of the lower torso. The paramedic should take care not to tighten the straps to the point of reducing chest wall movement.

After immobilization of the torso, the head and neck should be immobilized in a neutral, in-line position. When most adults are placed on a long or short spinal device, a large space is produced between the back of the head and the backboard. Therefore, noncompressible padding (eg, commercial padding, folded towels) should be added (body shims). This padding can be placed before securing the head (**FIGURE 40-19A**). The amount of padding required for in-line immobilization varies by patient and must be evaluated on an individual basis. Too little padding may cause hyperextension of the head, and too much padding may cause flexion; both may increase spinal cord damage. Children have proportionally larger heads than adults have and may require padding under the torso to allow the head to lie in a neutral position on the board (**FIGURE 40-19B**). The padding (if needed) should be firm and should extend the full length and width of the torso from the buttocks to the top of the shoulders to prevent movement and misalignment of the spine. In addition to providing enhanced stabilization, padding improves patient comfort during transport.

The head is secured to the spinal device by placing commercial pads or rolled blankets on both sides of the head and securing them with the included straps, 2- to 3-inch (5- to 8-cm) tape strips, or a self-adhering firm wrap (eg, Coban, Medi-Rip, or Elastoplast). (Elastic or gauze bandages do not prevent movement.) The upper forehead should be secured across the supraorbital ridge. The lower portion of the head should be secured across the anterior portion of the rigid cervical collar. Chin straps, sandbags, and intravenous bags are considered less optimal in immobilizing the head to a spinal device.

The patient's legs should be secured to the long backboard. Two or more straps can be applied above and below the knees. Towels, blankets, or suitable padding may be placed on both sides of the patient's

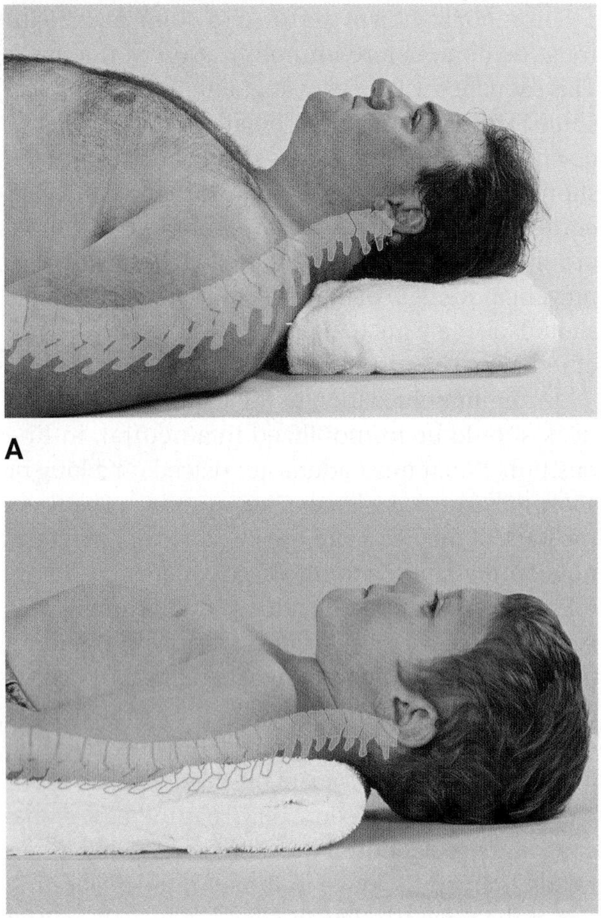

A

B

FIGURE 40-19 Padding requirements for adult **(A)** and pediatric **(B)** patients.

Reproduced from: National Association of Emergency Medical Technicians. *PHTLS: Prehospital Trauma Life Support.* 8th ed. Burlington, MA: Jones & Bartlett Learning; 2016.

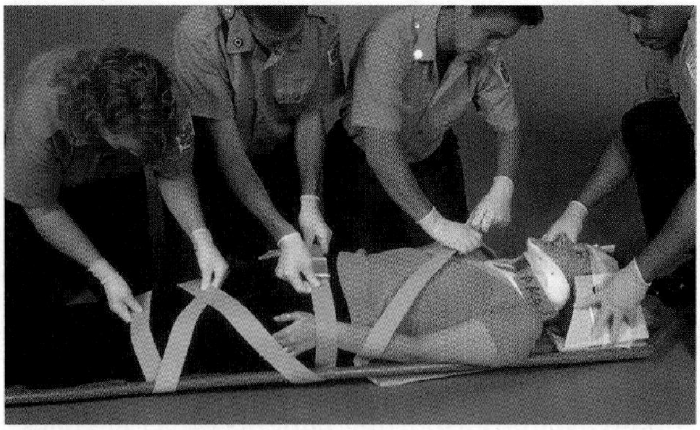

FIGURE 40-20 Long backboard immobilization (supine patient).

© Jones & Bartlett Learning. Courtesy of MIEMSS.

> **NOTE**
>
> The incidence of unstable injuries requiring intervention following penetrating trauma to the spine is very low. In addition, research has shown significantly higher mortality for patients with penetrating trauma who were immobilized. Because of these findings, use of a backboard is no longer recommended for patients who have penetrating trauma without neurologic deficits or complaints.
>
> ---
>
> *Modified from:* National Association of EMS Physicians and American College of Surgeons Committee on Trauma. EMS spinal precautions and the use of the long backboard. *Prehosp Emerg Care.* 2013;17(3):361-372; White CC, Domeier RM, Millin MG. EMS spinal precautions and the use of the long backboard—resource document to the position statement of the National Association of EMS Physicians and the American College of Surgeons Committee on Trauma. *Prehosp Emerg Care.* 2014;18(2):306-314; National Association of Emergency Medical Technicians. *PHTLS: Prehospital Trauma Life Support.* 8th ed. Burlington, MA: Jones & Bartlett Learning; 2014; and EMS management of patients with potential spinal injury. *Ann Emerg Med.* 2015;66(4):445.

lower legs. This padding will minimize movement and will help to maintain the patient's central position on the spinal device (**FIGURE 40-20**).

Before moving the patient, the paramedic should secure the patient's arms to the spinal device for safety. This is best achieved by placing the patient's arms at his or her side, with the patient's palms facing the body. The arms should be secured with a separate strap placed across the forearms and torso.

Once a patient is safely positioned on an ambulance stretcher, transfer or extrication devices may be removed if an adequate number of trained personnel are present to minimize unnecessary movement during the removal process. The risks of patient manipulation must be weighed against the benefits of device removal. If transport time is expected to be short, it may be better to transport a patient on the device and remove it on arrival at the medical facility. If the decision is made to remove the extrication device in the field, spinal motion restriction should be maintained by ensuring that the patient remains securely positioned on the ambulance stretcher with a cervical collar in place.

Immobilizing Pediatric Patients

As with adult patients, prehospital management of a pediatric patient with suspected spinal trauma requires manual in-line immobilization, a rigid cervical collar, and a long spinal immobilization device.

SHOW ME THE EVIDENCE

Researchers performed an interventional study to compare spine movement between the traditional long backboard with the Ferno Scoop Stretcher (FSS) when applied to live subjects. Electromagnetic sensors were placed on the forehead and over the C3 and T12 spinous process of 32 adults. Spinal flexion and rotation were recorded at baseline, application of the device (log roll for long backboard and placement of the FSS around the patient), secured log roll, and lifting. They found 6° to 8° greater motion during application of the long backboard compared to the FSS ($P < 0.001$). During the lift to the FSS, there was more sagittal flexion than with the long backboard ($P < 0.001$). Subjects felt more secure and rated the FSS as more comfortable on all body areas (except the occiput) as compared to the long backboard. The researchers concluded that the FSS was as effective as, and in some cases superior to, the long backboard.

Modified from: Krell JM, McCoy MS, Sparto PJ, et al. Comparison of the Ferno Scoop Stretcher with the long backboard for spinal immobilization. *Prehosp Emerg Care.* 2006;10(1):46-51.

Position statements from major EMS systems do not specifically include or exclude children. The spinal injury assessment criteria have been found to perform well in children older than 8 years. Therefore, it is recommended that traditional spinal precautions are indicated for children younger than 8 years when a significant MOI is present.[9] Many different pediatric immobilization devices are available from manufacturers (**FIGURE 40-21**).[9] If pediatric immobilization devices are not available, children may be secured on an adult long backboard. (A great deal of padding, however, is needed to fill voids and prevent movement.) If extrication from a vehicle is necessary and other injuries do not interfere, infants and toddlers should be managed with in-line immobilization and extricated while strapped into their car seats.

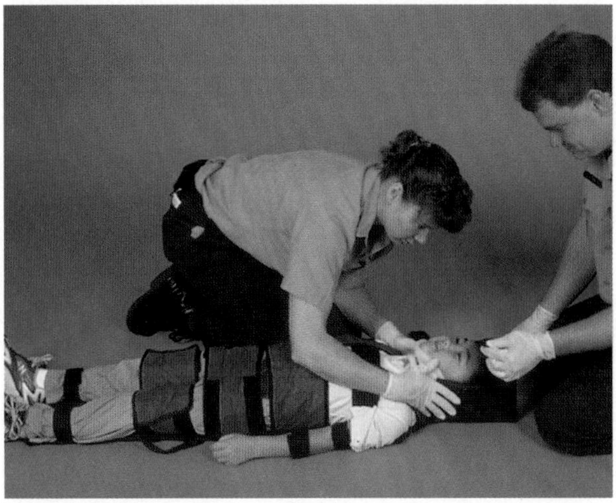

FIGURE 40-21 Infant and pediatric immobilization board.

Helmet Issues

The purpose of helmets is to protect the head and brain. Helmets are not intended to protect the neck, which leaves the cervical spine open to injury. The various types of helmets include full-face or open-face designs (used in motorcycling, bicycling, in-line skating, and other activities) and helmets designed for sports such as football and motocross. Factors that the paramedic should consider when determining the need to remove a helmet from an injured patient who requires airway management and spinal immobilization include the following:

- Athletic trainers may have special equipment (and training) to remove face pieces from sports helmets, allowing easier access to the patient's airway.
- Sports equipment (eg, shoulder pads) could compromise the cervical spine further if only the helmet were removed.
- The firm fit of a helmet may provide firm support for the patient's head.

Helmet Removal

Patients who are wearing full-face helmets must have the helmet removed early in the assessment process. Removing the helmet allows the rescuers to assess and manage a patient's airway and ventilatory status completely. In addition, rescuers can look for bleeding. The bleeding may be hidden by the helmet. They also can move the patient's head (from the flexed position caused by large helmets) into neutral alignment. The paramedic should consult with medical direction if the patient complains of increased pain during removal of the helmet or if the helmet is hard to remove in the field. The following steps in full-face helmet removal are recommended by the American College of Surgeons Committee on Trauma:[5]

1. Rescuer 1 immobilizes the helmet and head in an in-line position (**FIGURE 40-22**). Rescuer 1 presses his or her palms on each side of the

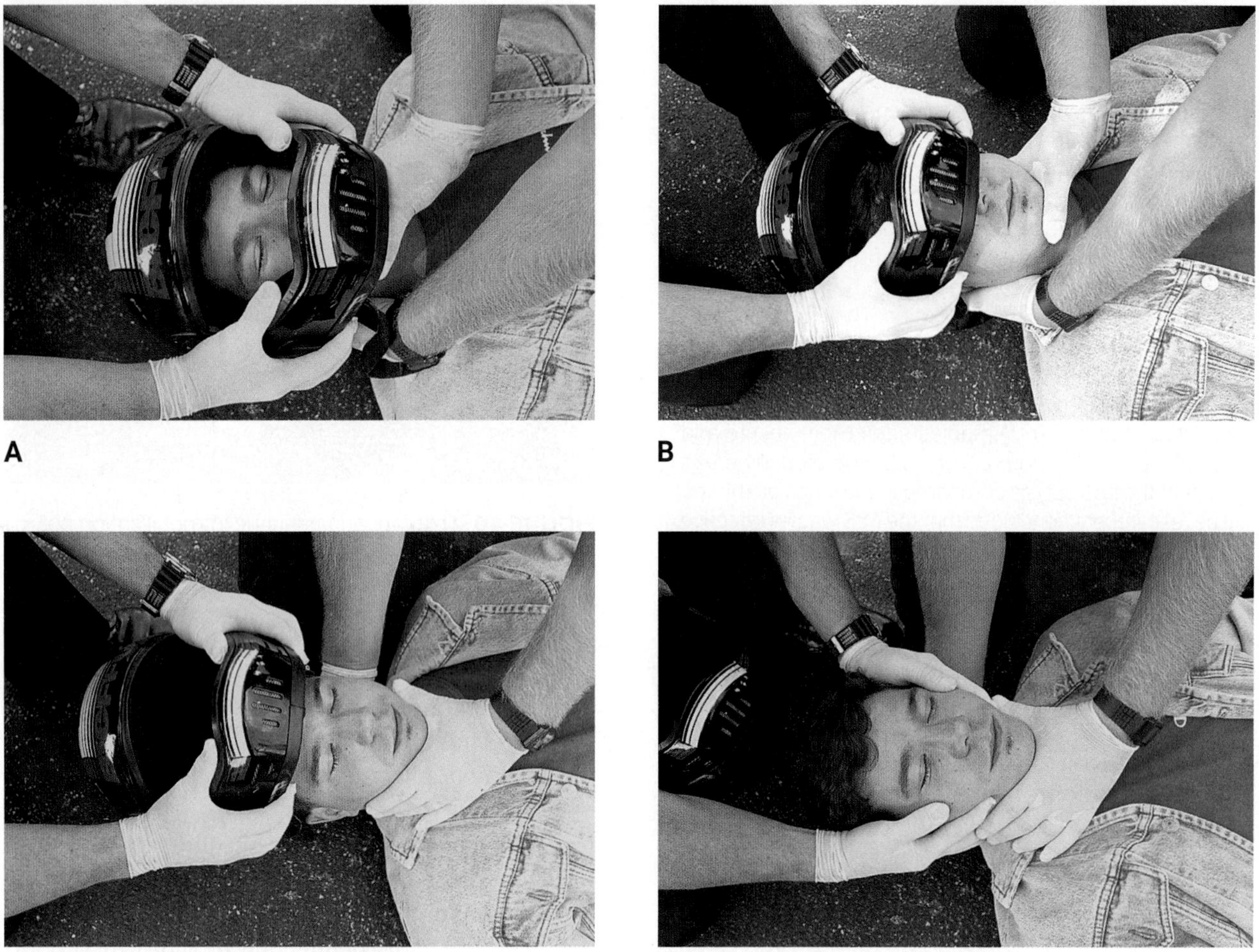

FIGURE 40-22 **A.** Rescuer 1 immobilizes the helmet and head in an in-line position. Rescuer 2 grasps the patient's mandible by placing the thumb at the angle of the mandible on one side and two fingers at the angle on the other side. Rescuer 2 places the other hand under the patient's neck at the base of the skull, producing in-line immobilization of the patient's head. **B.** Rescuer 1 carefully spreads the sides of the helmet away from the patient's head and ears. Rescuer 1 rotates the helmet toward himself or herself and away from Rescuer 2, then partially removes the helmet to clear the nose. **C.**Rescuers pause to reposition hands so that in-line immobilization will be maintained during the next move. Then, Rescuer 1 rotates the helmet approximately 30°, following the curvature of the patient's head, and finishes removing the helmet carefully in a straight line. **D.** After the removal of the helmet, Rescuer 1 applies in-line immobilization. Rescuer 2 applies a rigid cervical collar and places padding under the head.

helmet with the fingertips curled over the lower margin of the helmet.

2. Rescuer 2 removes the face shield and chin strap. Rescuer 2 assesses the patient's airway and ventilatory status.
3. Rescuer 2 grasps the patient's mandible by placing the thumb at the angle of the mandible on one side and two fingers at the angle on the other side. Rescuer 2 places his or her other hand under the neck at the base of the skull, taking over in-line immobilization of the patient's head.
4. Rescuer 1 carefully spreads the sides of the helmet away from the patient's head and ears and then rotates the helmet toward himself or herself and away from Rescuer 2, to clear the patient's nose. Rescuer 1 then partially removes the helmet, until it has cleared the nose.
5. At this point, the rescuers pause in the helmet removal process to adjust as follows. Rescuer 1 assumes in-line immobilization by squeezing the sides of the helmet against the patient's head. Rescuer 2 repositions his or her hands to

support the head and to prevent it from dropping as the helmet is removed. This is accomplished by the rescuer placing a hand farther up on the occipital area of the head and by grasping the maxilla with the thumb and first fingers of the other hand on each side of the nose. After securing this position, Rescuer 2 takes over in-line immobilization.

6. Once this repositioning has occurred, in order for the helmet to clear the occiput, Rescuer 1 rotates the helmet about 30° away from himself or herself and toward Rescuer 2, following the curvature of the patient's head. Rescuer 1 finishes removing the helmet by carefully pulling it in a straight line.
7. After removal of the helmet, Rescuer 1 applies in-line immobilization, and Rescuer 2 applies a rigid cervical collar.

NOTE

A key point to remember during helmet removal is that in-line immobilization must be maintained throughout the procedure. Thus, the rescuers should never remove their hands from the patient at the same time. In addition, the helmet must be rotated in one direction to clear the nose. The helmet must be rotated in the opposite direction to clear the back of the patient's head.

Spinal Immobilization in Diving Incidents

Most diving incidents involve injury to the patient's head, neck, and spine. If the patient is still in the water when EMS arrives, the patient should be managed as follows:

1. Ensure scene and personal safety. Only rescuers trained in water rescue should enter the water.
2. Float a supine patient to a shallow area without unnecessary movement of the spine (**FIGURE 40-23A**).
3. Approach a prone patient from the top of the head. Position one arm under the patient to support the head, neck, and torso. Place the other arm across the patient's head and back, splinting the head and neck between the rescuer's arms. Carefully turn the patient to a supine position and quickly assess airway and breathing. The paramedic may initiate rescue breathing while in the water (**FIGURE 40-23B**).[12]
4. A second rescuer slides a long backboard or other rigid device under the patient's body while the first rescuer continues to support the patient's head and neck without flexion or extension (**FIGURE 40-23C**). Apply a rigid cervical collar. Maintain manual in-line immobilization throughout the rescue.
5. Float the spinal immobilization device to the edge of the water and lift it out (**FIGURE 40-23D**).
6. The patient should be immobilized completely on the long backboard as previously described.

Cord Injury Presentations

Three cord injury presentations deserve special mention: spinal shock, neurogenic shock (described in Chapter 35, *Shock*), and autonomic hyperreflexia syndrome.

Spinal Shock

Spinal shock refers to a temporary loss or depression of all or most spinal reflex activity below the level of the injury. Signs and symptoms of spinal shock include flaccid paralysis distal to the injury site and loss of autonomic function, which may be demonstrated by hypotension, vasodilation, loss of bowel and bladder control, priapism, and loss of thermoregulation. Spinal shock does not always involve permanent, primary injury. The autonomic dysfunction usually resolves within 24 hours. Rarely, though, spinal shock may last a few days to a few weeks. Careful handling of these patients to avoid secondary injury is crucial. Initial management includes spinal motion restriction, high-concentration oxygen administration, and administration of intravenous crystalloids (per protocol).

Neurogenic Shock

Neurogenic shock (neurogenic hypotension) results from the blockade of vasoregulatory fibers, motor fibers, and sensory fibers. This block produces a loss of sympathetic tone to the vessels or vasodilation and is usually associated with injuries at or above the level of T6. Patients with neurogenic hypotension often have relative hypotension (a systolic blood pressure of 80 to 100 mm Hg); warm, dry, and pink skin (from cutaneous vasodilation); and relative bradycardia.

Neurogenic hypotension is rare. Initially, it should not be considered as a cause of hypotension in the patient with a spinal injury. The paramedic should

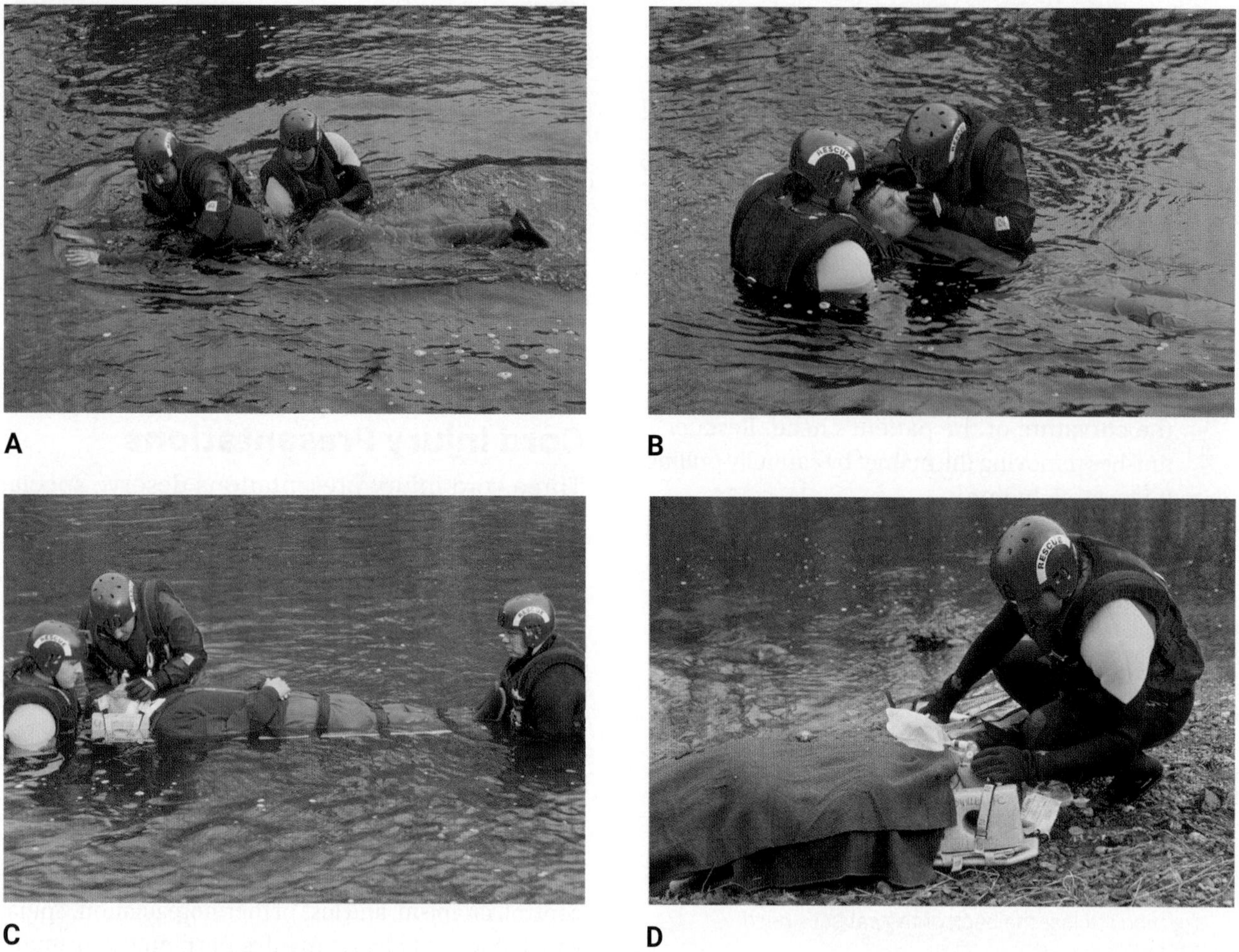

FIGURE 40-23 Stabilizing a suspected spinal injury in the water. **A.** Turning the patient to a supine position in the water. **B.** Providing artificial ventilation. **C.** Securing the patient to a backboard. **D.** Providing care to the patient out of the water.

consider other causes of hypotension, including internal hemorrhage, cardiac tamponade, and tension pneumothorax. If hypotension is severe, the paramedic should initiate shock management (per protocol) and begin fluid resuscitation. Drug therapy to improve blood pressure and heart rate may be indicated as described in Chapter 35, *Shock*.

Autonomic Hyperreflexia Syndrome

Autonomic hyperreflexia syndrome, also known as autonomic dysreflexia, may occur after resolution of spinal shock and is associated with chronic SCI in patients who have injuries at T6 or above.[13] The syndrome often is triggered by an irritating or noxious stimulus distal to the level of injury, such as urinary bladder distention or rectal distention from constipation. The effects of this syndrome result from a massive, uncompensated cardiovascular response that stimulates the sympathetic nervous system. The stimulation of sensory receptors below the level of cord injury causes the intact autonomic nervous system to respond with spasms of the arterioles. These spasms in turn increase blood pressure. The baroreceptors sense the rise in blood pressure and stimulate the parasympathetic nervous system. This response decreases heart rate and sends the message to the peripheral and visceral vessels to dilate. Because of the cord injury, however, vasodilation is not possible.

Thus, blood pressure continues to rise and could pose a threat to life. The characteristics of this syndrome include the following:

- Paroxysmal hypertension (up to 300 mm Hg)
- Pounding headache
- Blurred vision
- Sweating (above the level of injury) with flushing of the skin
- Increased nasal congestion
- Nausea
- Bradycardia (30–40 beats/min)

Removing the noxious stimulus or precipitant, such as emptying of the bladder or bowel, often relieves the syndrome. Blood pressure may need to be controlled with antihypertensive agents. These patients are best managed in the medical facility setting under close physician supervision.

Nontraumatic Spinal Conditions

Nontraumatic spinal conditions include low back pain, degenerative disk disease, spondylosis, herniated intervertebral disk, and spinal cord tumors. These conditions and management strategies are described in Chapter 32, *Nontraumatic Musculoskeletal Disorders.*

Summary

- Most spinal cord injuries (SCIs) are the result of motor vehicle crashes. Other causes include falls, acts of violence, sports, medical/surgical, and other events.
- The spinal column is composed of 33 vertebrae that are divided into five sections. The sections include 7 cervical, 12 thoracic, 5 lumbar, 5 sacral (fused), and 4 coccygeal (fused) vertebrae.
- The specific mechanisms of injury (MOIs) that frequently cause spinal trauma are axial loading; extremes of flexion, hyperextension, or hyperrotation; excessive lateral bending; and distraction. Other mechanisms can include blunt and penetrating trauma and electrical injury.
- Spinal injuries may be classified as sprains and strains, fractures and dislocations, sacral and coccygeal fractures, and cord injuries. The spinal cord may sustain a primary or a secondary injury. Lesions (transections) of the spinal cord are classified as complete or incomplete.
- The paramedic can classify the MOI as positive or negative. This classification is combined with the clinical guidelines for evaluating SCI, which include the following signs and symptoms: altered level of consciousness, spinal pain or tenderness, neurologic deficit or complaint, anatomic deformity of the spine, and unreliable patient. An unreliable patient has evidence of alcohol or other drugs, a distracting injury, or an inability to communicate. This system can help to identify cases in which spinal immobilization is appropriate.
- With spinal injuries, the first priority is to ensure scene safety and to evaluate and manage any threats to life. The second priority is to preserve spinal cord function. This includes avoiding secondary injury to the spinal cord. These goals are best met by maintaining a high degree of suspicion for the presence of spinal trauma, by providing early spinal motion restriction, by rapidly correcting any volume deficit, and by providing oxygen and ventilator support if indicated.
- General principles of spinal motion restriction include prevention of further injury; treating the spine as a long bone with a joint at either end (the head and pelvis); using the appropriate spinal motion restriction based on initial assessment and maintained until patient care is handed off in the emergency department; and placing the patient's head in a neutral, in-line position, unless contraindicated.
- Spinal shock refers to a temporary loss of all or most spinal reflex activity below the level of the injury.
- Neurogenic shock produces a loss of sympathetic tone to the vessels. This causes relative hypotension; warm, dry, and pink skin; and relative bradycardia.
- Autonomic hyperreflexia syndrome results from a massive, uncompensated cardiovascular response that stimulates the sympathetic nervous system. This response in turn causes an increase in blood pressure and other symptoms.

References

1. National Spinal Cord Injury Statistical Center. Spinal cord injury: facts and figures at a glance. *2017 SCI Data Sheet.* https://www.nscisc.uab.edu/Public/Facts%20and%20Figures%20-%202017.pdf. Published 2017. Accessed March 20, 2018.
2. National Spinal Cord Injury Association Resource Center. Factsheets. http://www.makoa.org/nscia/index.html. Accessed March 20, 2018.
3. Le T. *First Aid for the USMLE Step 1 2014*. 24th ed. New York, NY: McGraw-Hill Professional Publishing; 2014.
4. Marx JA, Hockberger RS, Walls RM. *Rosen's Emergency Medicine: Concepts and Clinical Practice*. 8th ed. St. Louis, MO: Saunders; 2014.

5. National Association of Emergency Medical Technicians. *PHTLS: Prehospital Trauma Life Support*. 8th ed. Burlington, MA: Jones & Bartlett Learning; 2014.
6. Szwedowski D, Walecki J. Spinal cord injury without radiographic abnormality (SCIWORA)—clinical and radiological aspects. *Pol J Radiol.* 2014;79:461-464.
7. Hansebout RR, Kachur E. Acute traumatic spinal cord injury. UpToDate website. https://www.uptodate.com/contents/acute-traumatic-spinal-cord-injury?search=spinal%20cord%20injury&source=search_result&selectedTitle=1~150&usage_type=default&display_rank=1. Updated October 20, 2014. Accessed March 20, 2018.
8. National Association of EMS Physicians and American College of Surgeons Committee on Trauma. EMS spinal precautions and the use of the long backboard. *Prehosp Emerg Care.* 2013;17(3):361-372.
9. White CC, Domeier RM, Millin MG. EMS spinal precautions and the use of the long backboard—resource document to the position statement of the National Association of EMS Physicians and the American College of Surgeons Committee on Trauma. *Prehosp Emerg Care.* 2014;18(2):306-314.
10. Benzel E. *The Cervical Spine.* 5th ed. Philadelphia, PA: Lippincott Williams & Wilkins; 2012.
11. Haut ER, Kalish BT, Efron DT, et al. Spinal Immobilization in penetrating trauma: more harm than good? *J Trauma.* 2010;68:115-121.
12. Field JM, Hazinski MF, Sayre MR, et al. Part 1: executive summary: 2010 American Heart Association Guidelines for Cardiopulmonary Resuscitation and Emergency Cardiovascular Care Science. *Circulation.* 2010;122(18)(suppl 3):S640-S456.
13. US Department of Transportation, National Highway Traffic Safety Administration. *EMT-Paramedic National Standard Curriculum.* Washington, DC: US Department of Transportation; 1998.

Suggested Readings

EMS management of patients with potential spinal injury. *Ann Emerg Med.* 2015;66(4):445.

Feller R, Reynolds C. EMS, immobilization (seated and supine). In: *StatPearls* [Internet]. National Center for Biotechnology Information website. https://www.ncbi.nlm.nih.gov/books/NBK459341/. Updated October 6, 2017. Accessed March 20, 2018.

Oteir AO, Smith K, Stoelwinder JU, Middleton J, Jennings PA. Should suspected cervical spinal cord injury be immobilised? A systematic review. *Injury.* 2015;46(4):528-535.

Samuel AM, Bohl DD, Basques BA, et al. Analysis of delays to surgery for cervical spinal cord injuries. *Spine.* 2015;40(13):992-1000.

Selvarajah S, Haider AH, Schneider EB, Sadowsky CL, Becker D, Hammond ER. Traumatic spinal cord injury emergency service triage patterns and the associated emergency department outcomes. *J Neurotrauma.* December 2015;32(24):2008-2016.

Sikka S, Vrooman A, Callender L, et al. Inconsistencies with screening for traumatic brain injury in spinal cord injury across the continuum of care. *J Spinal Cord Med.* 2017 July 31:1-10.

White CC, Domeier RM, Millin MG. EMS spinal precautions and the use of the long backboard—resource document to the position statement of the National Association of EMS Physicians and the American College of Surgeons Committee on Trauma. *Prehosp Emerg Care.* 2014;18(2):306-314.

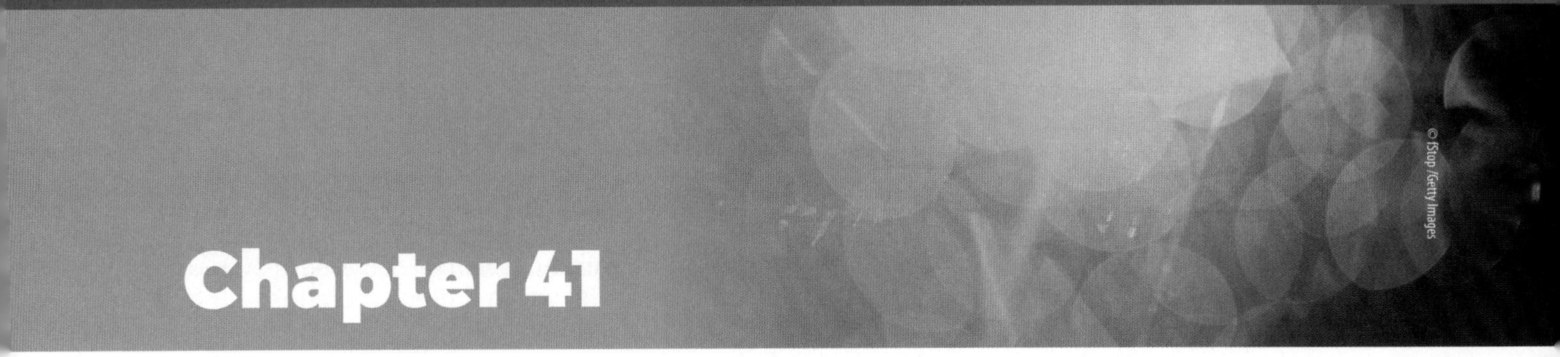

Chapter 41

Chest Trauma

NATIONAL EMS EDUCATION STANDARD COMPETENCIES

Trauma

Integrates assessment findings with principles of epidemiology and pathophysiology to formulate a field impression to implement a comprehensive treatment/disposition plan for an acutely injured patient.

Chest Trauma

Recognition and management of
- Blunt vs. penetrating mechanisms (pp 1489–1504)
- Open chest wound (pp 1493–1495, 1497)
- Impaled object (see Chapter 37, *Bleeding and Soft-Tissue Trauma*)

Pathophysiology, assessment, and management of
- Blunt vs. penetrating mechanisms (pp 1489–1504)
- Hemothorax (pp 1498–1499)
- Pneumothorax (pp 1492–1499)
  - Open (pp 1493–1496)
  - Simple (p 1493)
  - Tension (pp 1496–1498)
- Cardiac tamponade (pp 1500–1501)
- Rib fractures (pp 1489–1490)
- Flail chest (pp 1490–1491)
- Commotio cordis (p 1500)
- Traumatic aortic disruption (pp 1502–1503)
- Pulmonary contusion (p 1492)
- Blunt cardiac injury (pp 1499–1500)
- Tracheobronchial disruption (p 1503)
- Diaphragmatic rupture (p 1504)
- Traumatic asphyxia (p 1499)

OBJECTIVES

Upon completion of this chapter, the paramedic student will be able to:

1. Discuss the mechanism of injury associated with chest trauma. (p 1488)
2. Describe the mechanism of injury, signs and symptoms, and management of skeletal injuries to the chest. (pp 1488–1492)
3. Describe the mechanism of injury, signs and symptoms, and prehospital management of pulmonary contusion. (p 1492)
4. Describe the mechanism of injury, signs and symptoms, and prehospital management of other pulmonary trauma injuries. (pp 1492–1499)
5. Describe the mechanism of injury, signs and symptoms, and prehospital management of injuries to the heart and great vessels. (pp 1499–1503)
6. Outline the mechanism of injury, signs and symptoms, and prehospital care of the patient with esophageal and tracheobronchial injury and diaphragmatic rupture. (pp 1503–1504)

KEY TERMS

atelectasis An abnormal condition characterized by the collapse of lung tissue. It prevents respiratory exchange of oxygen and carbon dioxide.

Beck triad A combination of three signs that suggest the presence of cardiac tamponade: jugular venous distention, muffled heart sounds, and hypotension.

commotio cordis A dysrhythmia resulting from blunt-force chest trauma that often leads to cardiac arrest.

costochondral separation Separation of the costochondral cartilages from either the ribs or the sternum or both.

crepitus A grating sound associated with rubbing of bone fragments together or air bubbles beneath the skin.

diaphragmatic rupture Traumatic rupture of the diaphragm, which often results from sudden compression of the abdomen.

electrical alternans Beat-to-beat variability in the amplitude of a patient's electrocardiographic waveforms. It is a rare finding in cardiac tamponade.

flail chest A chest wall injury in which two or more adjacent ribs are fractured in two or more places.

hemopneumothorax A collection of air and blood in the pleural space; also known as a pneumohemothorax.

hemothorax The accumulation of blood and other fluids in the pleural space caused by bleeding from the lung parenchyma or damaged vessels.

jugular notch The superior margin of the manubrium, which is palpated easily at the anterior base of the neck; also known as the suprasternal notch.

manubrium One of the three bones of the sternum. It has a broad, quadrangular shape that narrows caudally at its articulation with the superior end of the body of the sternum.

mediastinal shift A shift in a patient's mediastinum that moves tissue and organs within the chest cavity to one side.

myocardial contusion Trauma-induced damage to the heart that may range from a localized bruise to a full-thickness injury to the wall of the heart with hemorrhage and edema.

myocardial rupture Traumatic rupture of the myocardium that occurs when blood-filled chambers of the ventricles are compressed with enough force to rupture the chamber wall, septum, or valve.

open pneumothorax A chest wall injury that exposes the pleural space to atmospheric pressure.

paradoxical motion Contrary movement of an injured segment of the chest wall with inspiration and expiration.

pericardial tamponade Compression of the heart produced by the accumulation of fluid or blood in the pericardial sac.

pulmonary contusion Bruising of the lung tissue that results in rupture of the alveoli and interstitial edema.

pulsus paradoxus An abnormal decrease in systolic blood pressure in which it drops more than 10 to 15 mm Hg during inspiration compared with expiration.

simple pneumothorax A collection of air or gas in the pleural space that causes the lung to collapse without exposing the pleural space to atmospheric pressure; also known as closed pneumothorax.

sternal angle The point at which the manubrium joins the body of the sternum; also known as the angle of Louis.

sternal fracture Fracture of the sternum; usually results from a direct blow to the chest or from a massive crush injury.

sternoclavicular joint The double gliding joint between the sternum and the clavicle.

tension pneumothorax An accumulation of air or gas in the pleural cavity that can lead to an increase in intrathoracic pressure to the point of cardiorespiratory compromise or collapse.

tracheal deviation Movement of the trachea from its midline position to the right or left.

traumatic aortic rupture Rupture of the aorta that is thought to be a result of shearing forces.

traumatic asphyxia A severe crushing injury to the chest and abdomen that causes an increase in the intrathoracic pressure. The increased pressure forces blood from the right side of the heart into the veins of the upper thorax, neck, and face.

Chest injuries are directly responsible for more than 20% of all traumatic deaths (regardless of mechanism) and account for about 16,000 deaths per year in the United States.[1] Chest injuries are caused by blunt trauma, penetrating trauma, or both.[2] They often are the result of motor vehicle crashes, falls from heights, blast injuries, blows to the chest, chest compression, gunshot wounds, and stab wounds. Thoracic trauma may be classified as skeletal injury, pulmonary injury, heart and great vessel injury, and diaphragmatic injury.

Skeletal Injuries

Skeletal injuries may be caused by blunt and/or penetrating trauma. The injuries discussed in this chapter include clavicular fractures, rib fractures, flail chest, and sternal fractures. Chest anatomy is presented in Chapter 10, *Review of Human Systems*. To review, the thoracic cage protects vital organs within the chest. It also prevents the collapse of the thorax during breathing. The skeletal components of the thoracic cage include the 12 thoracic vertebrae, 12 ribs (with their associated costal cartilages), the clavicle and the sternum. The superior 7 ribs (the "true ribs") are attached by cartilage to the sternum. The inferior

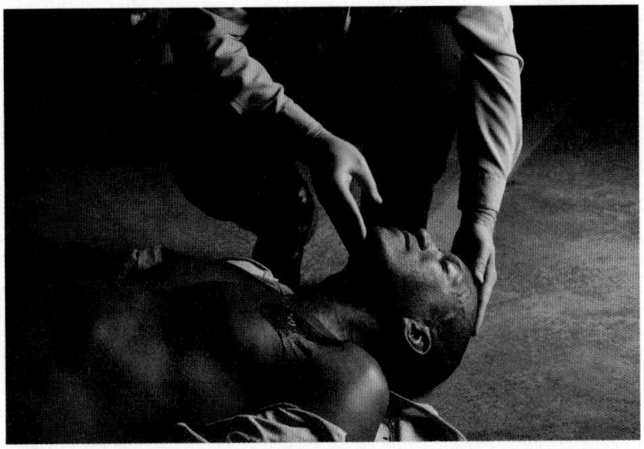

5 ribs (the "false ribs") articulate with the vertebrae, but do not attach directly to the sternum. Ribs 8, 9, and 10 are joined to a common cartilage, which is attached to the sternum. Ribs 11 and 12 are "floating ribs" that have no attachment to the sternum.

The sternum has three parts: the **manubrium**, the body, and the xiphoid process. The **jugular notch** is located at the superior end of the manubrium. The manubrium joins the body of the sternum at the **sternal angle** (also known as the angle of Louis). The clavicles are part of both the chest and the appendicular skeleton and attach the upper limbs to the axial skeleton. This attachment is made at the **sternoclavicular joint** between the clavicles and the sternum (**FIGURE 41-1**).

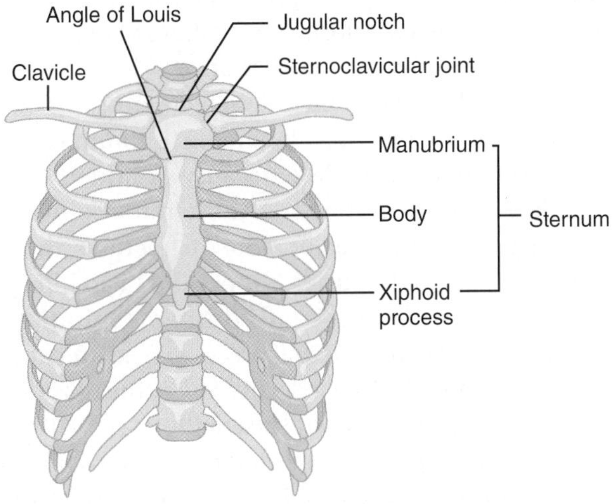

FIGURE 41-1 Thoracic cage.

Clavicular Fractures

The clavicle accounts for 5% of all fractures and is the most frequently fractured bone in children.[1] An isolated clavicular fracture is seldom a significant injury. It is common in children who fall on their shoulders or outstretched arms as well as in athletes involved in contact sports. Treatment usually involves applying a clavicle strap or a sling and swathe that immobilizes the affected shoulder and arm for purposes of pain control (see Chapter 43, *Orthopaedic Trauma*). These injuries usually heal well within 4 to 6 weeks in children. In adults, healing can be somewhat prolonged, and surgery may be recommended.

Signs and symptoms of clavicular fractures include pain, point tenderness, and evident deformity. A very rare complication that may be associated with a clavicular fracture is injury to the subclavian vein or artery. Vascular injury can occur when bony fragments from the fracture puncture a vessel, resulting in a hematoma or venous thrombosis.

Rib Fractures

Rib fractures most often occur on the lateral aspect of the third through eighth ribs, where the ribs are least protected by musculature (**FIGURE 41-2**). Such fractures are more likely to occur in adults than in children, because younger patients have more resilient cartilage that is not fully calcified. Thus, when blunt forces are applied to the ribs of children, the energy is transmitted to the lung, where pulmonary contusion is a more frequent injury than is rib fracture. Morbidity or mortality from rib fractures depends on the patient's age and the number and location of the fractures.[3] Morbidity increases after age 45 years and

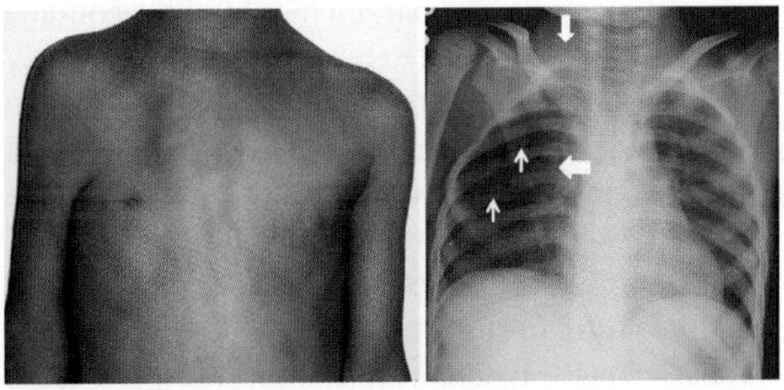

FIGURE 41-2 Chest wall asymmetry caused by rib fractures.

Reproduced from Aliza M, Aggarwal KC. Poland's anomaly. *Indian J Med Res*. 2014;139(3):476.

then again after age 65 years; it also increases when more than three ribs are fractured, when there are bilateral rib fractures, and in the presence of pulmonary contusion.

CRITICAL THINKING

Why would you expect greater underlying pulmonary injury in a child than in an adult with rib fractures?

NOTE

Separation of the costochondral cartilages also can occur from blunt anterior chest trauma. Signs and symptoms are similar to those for rib fracture. In addition, the patient may complain of a "snapping" sensation with deep respiration. These patients should be evaluated by a physician to rule out cardiac contusion. The pain associated with **costochondral separation** can persist for several weeks.

Simple rib fractures are usually very painful, but rarely are life threatening. Most patients can localize the fracture by pointing to the area, and the site of injury may then be confirmed by palpation. Sometimes movement or grating of the bone ends (**crepitus**) can be felt. One complication of rib fracture is respiratory or diaphragmatic splinting, which occurs when the patient holds his or her breath or minimizes chest wall movement to lessen pain. Such splinting can lead to **atelectasis** (the collapse of alveoli). Another complication is ventilation–perfusion mismatch, which occurs when alveoli are perfused but not ventilated.

The goals of treatment for rib fractures are to relieve the pain and maintain pulmonary function to prevent atelectasis. The paramedic should encourage the patient to cough and to breathe deeply. Pain may be relieved by splinting the patient's arm against the chest wall with a sling and swathe; circumferential splinting should *not* be used because it may inhibit complete expansion of the chest wall during inspiration. Administration of analgesics (per protocol) may be helpful in some cases.

Based on the mechanism of injury, the paramedic should consider the possibility of more serious trauma, such as closed pneumothorax and internal bleeding. Fractures to the lower ribs (8 through 12) may be associated with injuries to the spleen, kidneys, or liver. Great force is required to fracture the first and second ribs because of their shape and the protection provided by the scapulae, clavicles, and upper chest musculature. Thus, fractures of the first and second ribs may be associated with myocardial contusion, bronchial tears, and vascular injury.

NOTE

The true danger of a fractured rib is not the injured rib itself, but rather the potential for penetrating injury to the pleura, lung, liver, or spleen. Older adult patients and patients with preexisting respiratory disease are often unable to compensate for even minor trauma to the chest wall. These patients require careful monitoring for respiratory distress or fatigue.

Flail Chest

A **flail chest** may occur when two or more adjacent ribs are fractured in two or more places.[4] This injury may be difficult to detect in the prehospital setting because of the muscle spasm that often accompanies the injury. Within 2 hours after the injury, however, the muscle spasm subsides. At that point, the injured segment of the chest wall may begin to move in a contrary fashion (**paradoxical motion**) with inspiration and expiration (**FIGURE 41-3**). The flail segment moves inward with inspiration and outward with expiration as opposed to the intact portion of the chest wall that moves in exactly the opposite manner. This paradoxical motion interrupts the normal mechanics of breathing and decreases effective ventilation.

Causes of flail chest include vehicle crashes, falls, industrial accidents, assault, and birth trauma. The mortality rate is 8% to 35% because of underlying, associated injuries.[1] The mortality rate increases with advanced age, seven or more rib fractures, three or more associated injuries, shock, and head injury.

The diaphragm descends during inspiration, which lowers the intrapleural pressure. The unstable chest wall is pulled ("sucked") inward by the negative intrathoracic pressure as the rest of the chest wall expands. During expiration, the diaphragm rises, and the intrapleural pressure exceeds atmospheric pressure. The unstable chest wall then moves outward, which decreases the effectiveness of ventilation. Patients with

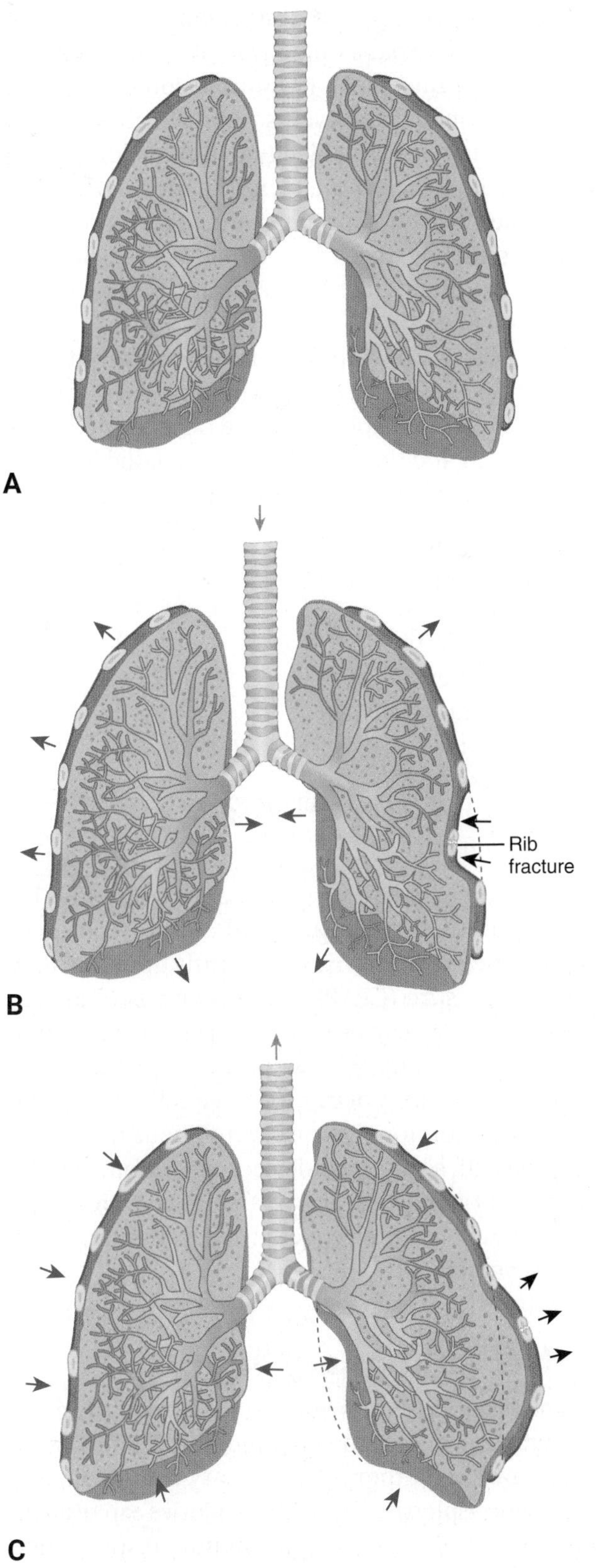

FIGURE 41-3 Paradoxical motion secondary to flail chest. **A.** Normal lungs. **B.** Flail chest during inspiration. **C.** Flail chest during expiration.

flail chest often also develop hypoxia due to ventilator insufficiency and due to the pulmonary contusions that usually accompany this injury. Bleeding from the alveoli and the lung tissue results from the injury and leads to decreased vital capacity and vascular shunting of deoxygenated blood.

Signs and symptoms of flail chest include bruising, tenderness, and bony crepitus on palpation as well as paradoxical motion (a late sign). Oxygen saturation (Spo_2) as measured by a pulse oximeter and possibly capnography should be monitored for changes in respiratory status that can indicate deterioration.

Prehospital management of patients with flail chest includes assisting ventilation with high-concentration supplemental oxygen to maintain Spo_2 of 95% or higher. Vascular access should be established en route if transport time permits. Field stabilization of the flail segment is not recommended.[4] Intubation and positive pressure ventilation are indicated in patients with severe respiratory distress and a flail chest who cannot maintain normal oxygenation and ventilation. A high index of suspicion for concomitant pneumothorax should prompt the paramedic to frequently reassess the patient for the development of tension pneumothorax, especially if the patient requires positive pressure ventilation.[5]

CRITICAL THINKING

Why is positive pressure ventilation the treatment of choice for flail chest?

Sternal Fractures

A **sternal fracture** usually results from a direct blow to the chest (eg, striking a steering column or dashboard) or from a massive crush injury (**FIGURE 41-4**). Sternal fractures, which are very painful, may be associated with an unstable chest wall, myocardial injury, or cardiac tamponade. They occur in only 2% of patients with blunt chest trauma.[6] Signs and symptoms include a history of significant anterior chest trauma, tenderness, and abnormal motion or crepitation over the sternum. Prehospital management includes maintaining a high degree of suspicion for associated injuries.

Most sternal fractures are clinically insignificant, but they may sometimes be associated with other

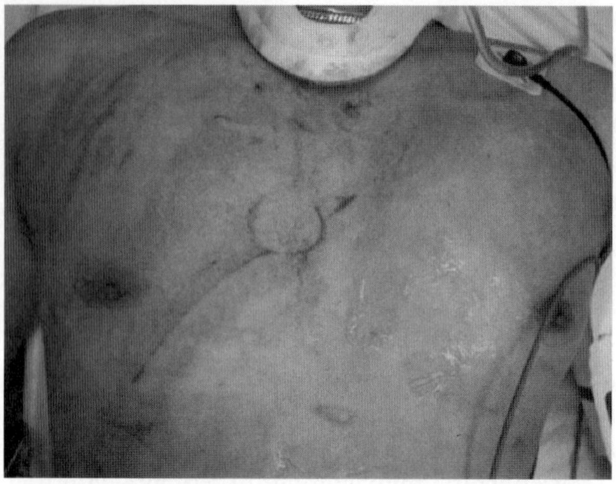

FIGURE 41-4 Injuries related to steering wheel contact.

Reproduced from: Olshaker J, Jackson M, Smock W (Eds.). (2007). Forensic emergency medicine. Lippincott Williams & Wilkins.

serious injuries. For example, the following thoracic injuries may be associated with sternal injury:[7]

- Pulmonary contusion
- Rib fractures
- Pneumothorax or hemothorax
- Thoracic spine or scapular fractures
- Pneumomediastinum or mediastinal hematoma
- Aortic or great vessel injury

Pulmonary Contusion

Pulmonary contusion most often is caused by rapid deceleration forces, like those created by motor vehicle crashes and by injuries that result in a flail chest. These forces push the lung against the chest wall and result in rupture of the alveoli, with subsequent hemorrhage and swelling of the lung tissue. More than 50% of patients with blunt chest trauma have pulmonary contusion.[1]

During sudden inertial deceleration and direct impact, fixed and mobile parts of the lung move at varying speeds. The result is stretching and shearing of alveoli and intravascular structures (the inertial effect). This kinetic shock wave of energy is partly reflected at the alveolar membrane surface because of the different densities of gas and liquid. The shock wave triggers a localized release of energy, causing denser lung tissue to be driven into less dense tissue, disrupting the gas and liquid interface at the level of the alveolus (the spalling effect[7,8]). Overexpansion of air in the lungs occurs after the primary energy wave has passed, with low-pressure rebound shock waves then causing overstretching and damage to lung tissue from overexpansion of gas bubbles, which can also disrupt the alveoli (the implosion effect). The combination of these events results in alveolar and capillary damage with bleeding into the lung tissue and alveoli. Because the contused area of the lung is unable to function properly after injury, profound hypoxemia may develop. The degree of respiratory complication is directly related to the size of the contused area.

The signs and symptoms of pulmonary contusion are subtle at first, but then worsen over 24 hours. They should be suspected based on the kinematics of the event and the presence of associated injuries. Common signs and symptoms include the following:

- Tachypnea
- Tachycardia
- Cough
- Hemoptysis
- Apprehension
- Respiratory distress
- Dyspnea
- Crackles
- Evidence of blunt chest trauma
- Cyanosis

Emergency care for pulmonary contusion includes ventilatory support and administration of high-concentration oxygen. Continuous positive airway pressure (CPAP) or bilevel positive airway pressure (BPAP) can be used to improve oxygenation if needed.[4] Patients with associated injuries or preexisting pulmonary or cardiovascular disease should be closely monitored in case ventilations need to be assisted with a bag-mask device, intubation, or both. Pulmonary contusions may be associated with a major chest injury, but they generally heal spontaneously over several weeks.

Other Pulmonary Injuries

Pulmonary injuries may be classified as simple (closed) pneumothorax, tension pneumothorax, open pneumothorax, hemothorax, pulmonary contusion, and traumatic asphyxia. Any of these injuries can result in difficulty in breathing and respiratory insufficiency. Prehospital treatment must be directed at ensuring an open airway, providing ventilatory support, correcting immediately life-threatening ventilatory problems (eg, tension pneumothorax), and arranging rapid transport for definitive care.

Simple Pneumothorax

A **simple pneumothorax** (closed pneumothorax) is caused by the presence of air in the pleural space. This air causes the lung to partially or totally collapse (**FIGURE 41-5**). A common cause of pneumothorax is a fractured rib that penetrates the pleura and underlying lung, although pneumothoraces also may occur without rib fractures. A pneumothorax may be caused by excessive pressure on the chest wall against a closed glottis (paper bag effect; see Chapter 36, *Trauma Overview and Mechanism of Injury*) or by rupture or tearing of the lung tissue and visceral pleura from no apparent cause (eg, spontaneous pneumothorax). Closed pneumothorax occurs in 15% to 50% of patients with severe blunt chest trauma, and in almost 100% of patients with penetrating chest trauma.[1]

CRITICAL THINKING

How does high-flow oxygen promote faster resolution of a closed pneumothorax?

The signs and symptoms of a closed pneumothorax depend on the severity of hypoxia, the degree of ventilation impairment, and the percentage of the lung that has collapsed. These signs and symptoms may include chest pain, dyspnea, and tachypnea.

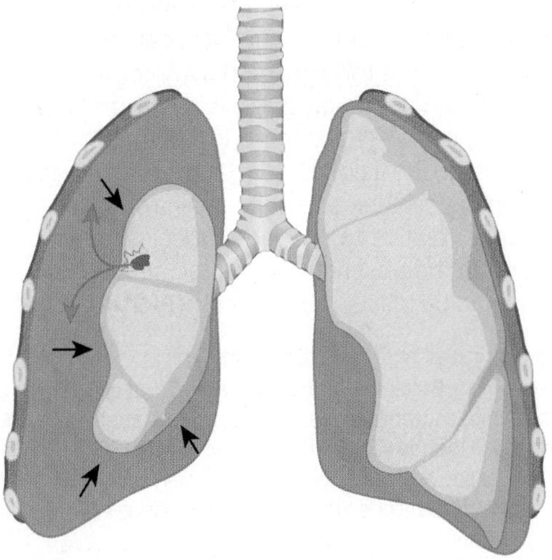

FIGURE 41-5 Closed (simple) pneumothorax.

CRITICAL THINKING

Will you always be able to distinguish between simple pneumothorax and pulmonary contusion in the prehospital setting? Why or why not?

Breath sounds may be diminished or absent on the affected side.

Treatment includes ventilatory support with high-concentration oxygen. Patients should be carefully monitored for signs of a tension pneumothorax (described later). They should be transported in the semi-Fowler position unless this position is contraindicated by the mechanism of injury.

Most healthy patients have large circulatory and ventilatory reserve capacities, so closed pneumothoraces usually do not pose a threat to life. However, life-threatening consequences may develop if the pneumothorax is a tension pneumothorax, if it occupies more than 40% of the hemithorax, or if it occurs in a patient with shock or preexisting pulmonary or cardiovascular diseases.[1]

Open Pneumothorax

An **open pneumothorax** (communicating pneumothorax) develops when a chest injury exposes the pleural space to atmospheric pressure (**FIGURE 41-6**). The severity of the injury is directly proportional to the size of the wound. When a chest wound is only about two-thirds of the diameter of the patient's trachea, given that it is much a shorter distance between the atmospheric air and the chest cavity than via the trachea, air preferentially enters the chest wound instead of the mouth and nose when the patient inhales because resistance to airflow is much less through the chest wound. As the air accumulates in the pleural space, the lung on the injured side collapses and begins to shift toward the uninjured side. Because very little air enters the tracheobronchial tree to be exchanged with intrapulmonary air on the affected side, decreased alveolar ventilation and decreased perfusion develop. The normal side also is adversely affected, because expired air may enter the lung on the collapsed side. This air is then rebreathed into the functioning lung with the next ventilation. Rebreathing of the deoxygenated air may result in severe ventilatory dysfunction, hypoxemia, and death unless the condition is quickly recognized and corrected.

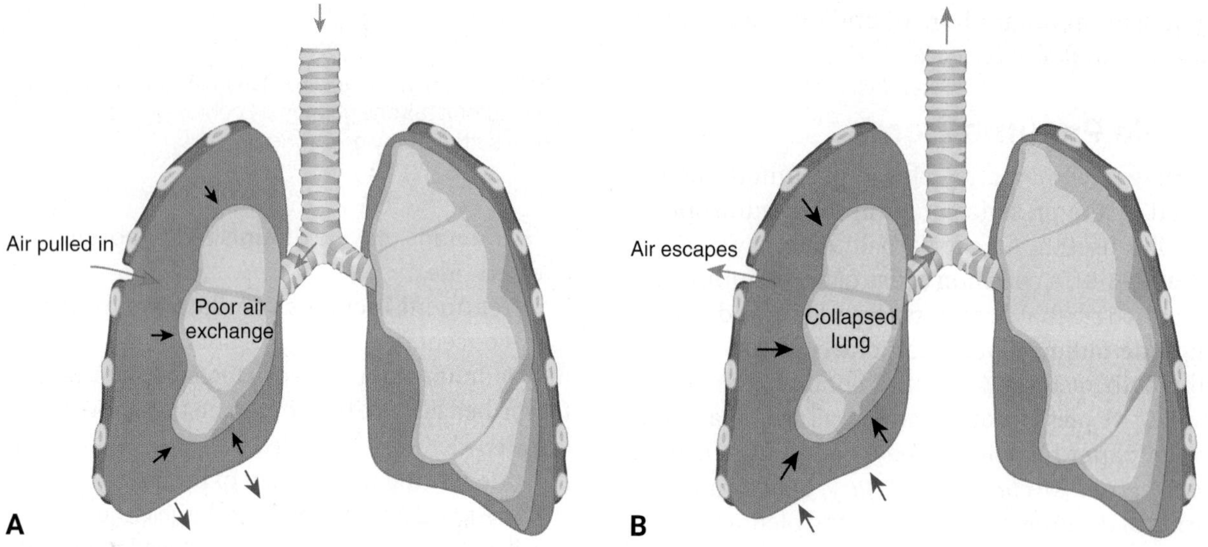

FIGURE 41-6 Open pneumothorax. **A.** Air enters the pleural cavity during inspiration. **B.** Air exits the pleural cavity during expiration.

NOTE

A small open chest wound may function like a ball-valve mechanism, allowing air in but not out. The accumulation of air may result in a shift in the patient's mediastinum, moving the tissue and organs within the chest cavity to one side. A **mediastinal shift** can lead to reduced preload and a reduction in cardiac output (**FIGURE 41-7**).

Signs and symptoms of open pneumothorax include shortness of breath, pain, and a sucking or gurgling sound as air moves into and out of the pleural space through the open chest wound (thus the term *sucking chest wound*). Prehospital treatment of an open pneumothorax proceeds as follows:

1. Close the chest wound by first applying direct pressure with a gloved hand. The chest wound can then be sealed by applying an occlusive dressing or a dressing of foil or plastic, and securing it with tape.[4] If the patient develops severe dyspnea, remove the dressing and assist ventilations if needed. Treat the patient for tension pneumothorax if signs and symptoms appear.
2. Provide ventilatory support as needed with high-concentration oxygen, and monitor oxygen saturation.
3. Establish vascular access en route to the hospital.
4. Rapidly transport the patient to an appropriate medical facility.

NOTE

In theory, a three-sided dressing prevents the development of a tension pneumothorax. However, it is now believed to be more important to simply seal the hole in the chest and expedite transport to a trauma center while monitoring the patient for signs and symptoms consistent with a tension pneumothorax. Specially manufactured vented chest seals (as opposed to three-sided dressings improvised in the field) do exist, and if one is available, it is certainly acceptable and may confer a speed and safety advantage relative to nonvented occlusive dressings; however, in the absence of a vented seal, a nonvented seal should be placed immediately (**FIGURE 41-8**).

Modified from: Butler FK, Dubose JJ, Otten EJ, et al. Management of open pneumothorax in tactical combat casualty care: TCCC Guidelines Change 13-02. *J Spec Oper Med*. 2003;13(3):61-66; National Association of Emergency Medical Technicians. *PHTLS: Prehospital Trauma Life Support*. 8th ed. Burlington, MA: Jones & Bartlett Learning; 2016.

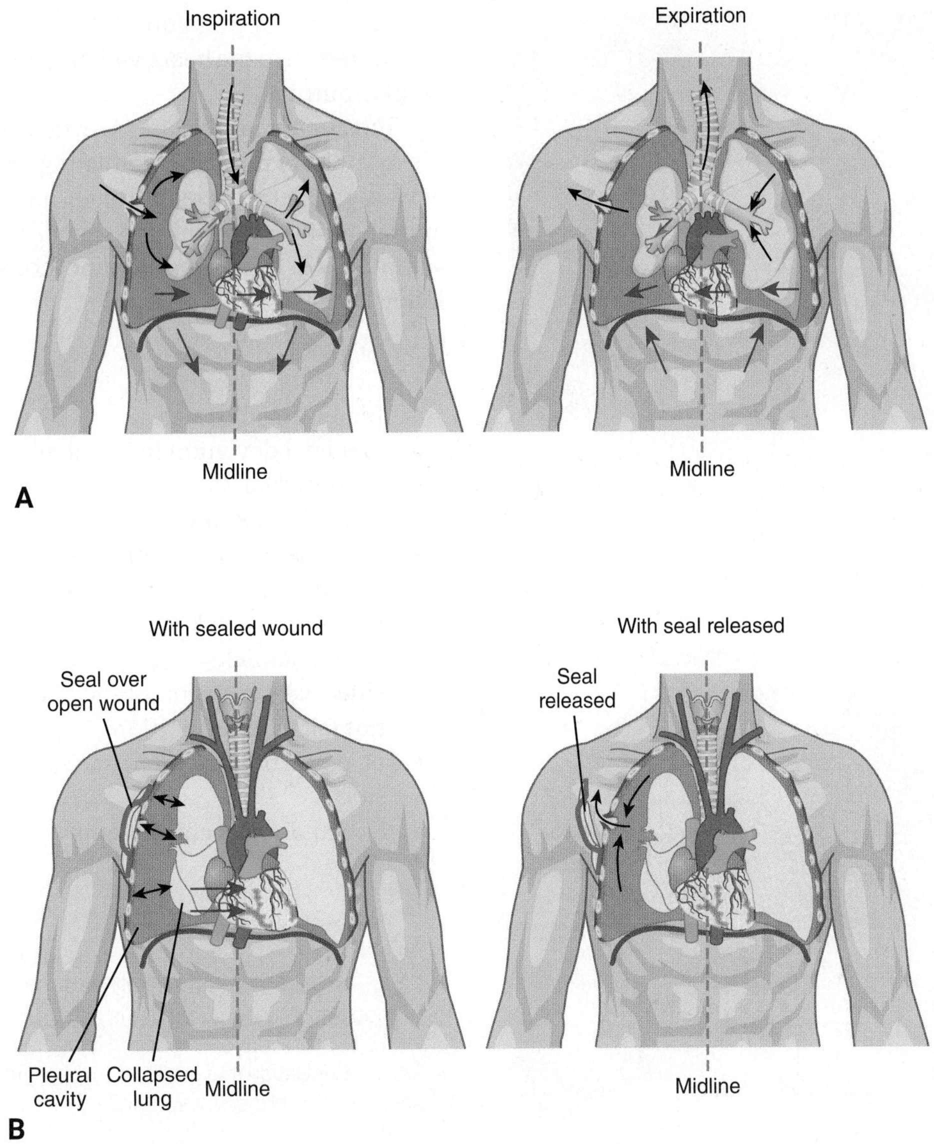

FIGURE 41-7 **A.** Open pneumothorax. Black and green arrows represent tissue and air movement; blue arrows represent structural movement. On inspiration, air is sucked into the pleural space through the open chest wound and the lung on the affected side collapses. Black arrows represent air movement. The mediastinal contents shift toward the unaffected side. On expiration, air exits through the open wound, and the mediastinal contents swing back toward the affected side (mediastinal flutter). **B.** Tension pneumothorax. An airtight dressing can cause a tension pneumothorax when air accumulates in the pleural space through a tear in the lung tissue. The air cannot exit if there is no open chest wound, and pressure builds, shifting the contents of the mediastinum toward the unaffected side and impairing circulatory and respiratory function (mediastinal shift). Release of the seal on the airtight dressing causes air to escape, relieving the symptoms of tension pneumothorax.

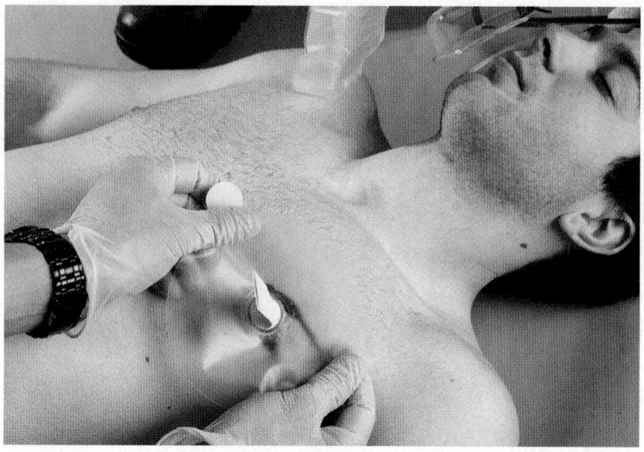

FIGURE 41-8 Vented dressing. In the absence of a vented dressing, a nonvented dressing should be placed immediately.

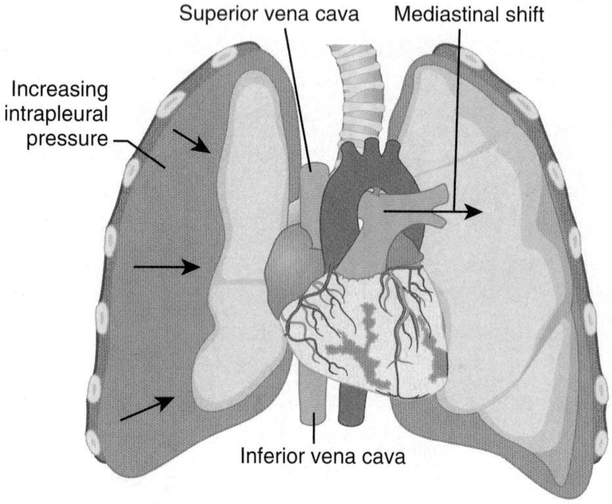

FIGURE 41-9 Tension pneumothorax.

Tension Pneumothorax

When air in the thoracic cavity cannot exit the pleural space, a **tension pneumothorax** may develop (**FIGURE 41-9**). This condition is an emergency that results in profound hypoventilation and impaired perfusion. Tension pneumothorax may result in death if it is not immediately recognized and managed.

When air is allowed to leak into the pleural space during inspiration and becomes trapped during expiration, the pleural pressure increases. The increased pressure produces a shift in the mediastinum that further compresses the lung on the uninjured side. In addition, compression of the vena cava reduces venous return to the heart, which results in decreased cardiac output.

Tension pneumothorax is evidenced by increasing dyspnea or difficulty ventilating with a bag-mask device, unilateral decreased or absent breath sounds, and signs of decompensated shock.[4] Other signs and symptoms of a tension pneumothorax include the following:[9]

- Anxiety
- Cyanosis
- Increasing dyspnea
- Tracheal deviation (a late sign)
- Tachycardia
- Hypotension or unexplained signs of shock
- Diminished or absent breath sounds on the injured side
- Distended neck veins (unless the patient is hypovolemic)
- Unequal expansion of the chest (tension does not fall with respiration)
- Hyperresonance on percussion of the affected side
- Subcutaneous emphysema

NOTE

Tracheal deviation may result from the displacement of mediastinal structures but is an inconsistent finding with pneumothorax. If it occurs, it is often a late finding. Tracheal deviation that results from chest injury is seldom seen in the prehospital setting.

Modified from: Daley BJ. Pneumothorax clinical presentation. Medscape website. https://emedicine.medscape.com/article/424547-clinical#b3. Published December 11, 2017. Accessed March 2, 2018.

CRITICAL THINKING

Why might the neck veins be distended in a patient with a tension pneumothorax?

A suspected tension pneumothorax should be managed aggressively. Emergency care is directed at reducing the pressure in the pleural space—that is, returning the intrapleural pressure to atmospheric or subatmospheric levels.

NOTE

The value of chest percussion in the prehospital setting is questionable. In the field, it should not be the only method used to identify a tension pneumothorax or hemothorax. Generally, hyperresonance on percussion points to the presence of air (pneumothorax), whereas dullness on percussion suggests the presence of blood and other fluids (hemothorax).

Modified from: National Association of Emergency Medical Technicians. *PHTLS: Prehospital Trauma Life Support*. 8th ed. Burlington, MA: Jones & Bartlett Learning; 2016.

SHOW ME THE EVIDENCE

California researchers conducted a retrospective observational study of patients who had prehospital needle thoracostomy (NT) from a large EMS system that included urban, suburban, rural, and wilderness areas. They found 169 patients (61% blunt trauma) who had field NT. No complications related to the NT were reported. Benefit from NT was significantly higher in patients who were unstable but still had vital signs when EMS providers arrived. Clinical change after NT was predictive of survival ($P = 0.02$).

Modified from: Weichenthal L, Crane D, Rond L. Needle thoracostomy in the prehospital setting: a retrospective observational study. *Prehosp Emerg Care*. 2016;20(3):399-403.

Tension Pneumothorax Associated With Penetrating Trauma

As mentioned previously, sealing an open pneumothorax with an occlusive dressing may produce a tension pneumothorax. In such cases, the increased pleural pressure can be relieved by momentarily removing, or "burping," the dressing. When the dressing is lifted from the wound, an audible release of air from the thoracic cavity should be noted. After the pressure has been released, the wound should again be sealed. The dressing may need to be removed more than once to relieve pleural pressure during transport.

If the tension is not relieved with this procedure, needle decompression of the thorax (needle thoracentesis; NT) should be performed. In penetrating chest trauma, needle decompression should be performed when the patient has worsening respiratory distress or providers encounter increasing difficulty in ventilating the patient with a bag-mask device.

Tension Pneumothorax Associated With Closed Trauma

A tension pneumothorax that develops in a patient with closed chest trauma must be relieved through thoracic decompression (NT). This procedure can be done safely in the field using a large-bore needle or a commercially available thoracic decompression kit.[10]

For needle decompression, a large-bore 10- or 14-gauge hollow catheter-over-needle (8 cm or longer)[4] is inserted into the affected pleural space. High failure rates from needle chest decompression have been reported,[11] but failures are believed to be related to inadequate needle length. When an 8-cm needle, rather than a 5-cm needle, is used for NT, success rates are significantly higher, especially for patients with a body mass index greater than 30 kg/m^2.[12] A minimum catheter length of 8 cm (3.25 inches) is recommended by the Committee on Tactical Combat Casualty Care (CoTCCC) to penetrate the pleural space in most patients.[13,14]

The needle can be placed in the fourth or fifth intercostal space laterally on the involved side or inserted anteriorly in the second intercostal space in the midclavicular line (**FIGURE 41-10**).[1] The needle should be inserted just above the rib to avoid the nerve, artery, and vein that lie just beneath each rib. After insertion of the needle, an audible rush of air should be noted, which indicates pressure escaping from the pleural space (confirming the tension pneumothorax). At this point, the patient should show signs of improvement (ie, the patient's lungs will be easier to ventilate or the patient's breathing will be less labored). The needle should be withdrawn and the catheter secured in place with tape. Needle decompression may need to be repeated if the catheter becomes occluded with a blood clot and tension pneumothorax recurs.[4]

CRITICAL THINKING

Put your finger on the point on your chest where a needle would be inserted for decompression of a tension pneumothorax. Is it easy to identify?

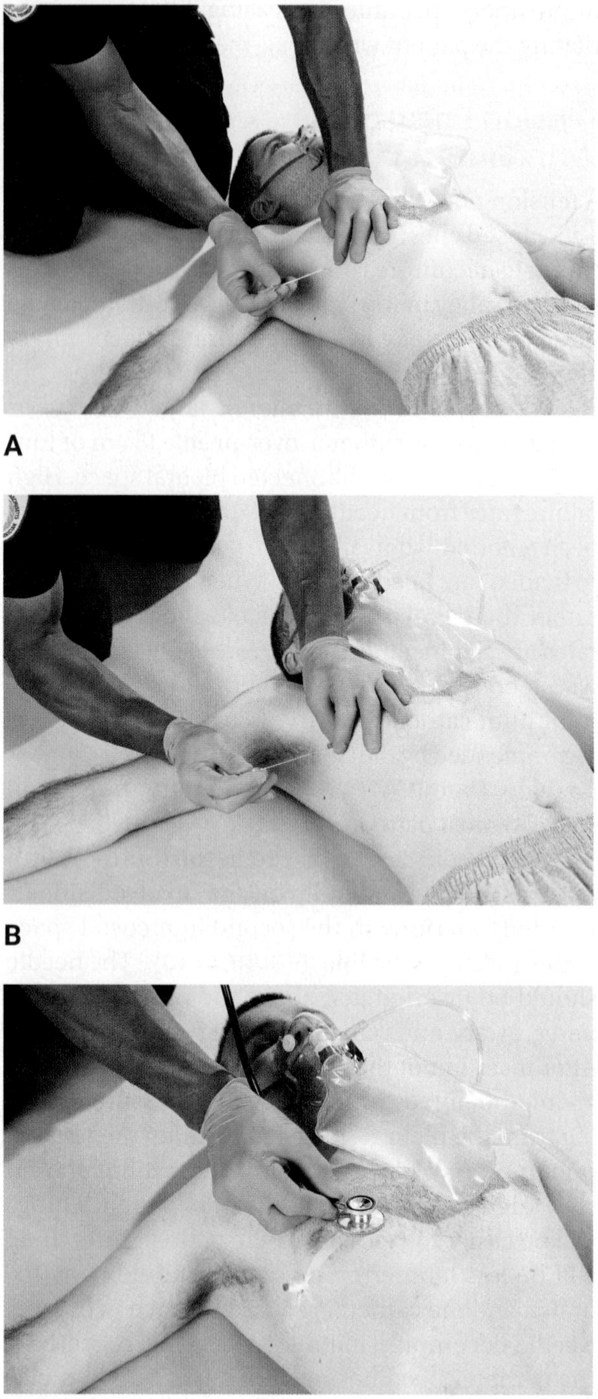

A

B

C

FIGURE 41-10 Needle decompression. **A.** A 3.25-inch (8-cm) long, 10- or 14-gauge hollow needle or catheter is inserted into the fifth intercostal space slightly anterior to the midaxillary line. **B.** After insertion of the needle, an audible rush of air should be noted as pressure escapes from the pleural space. **C.** The catheter is secured in place with tape. Care is taken to prevent reentry of air into the pleural space. The patient's respiratory status is monitored carefully.

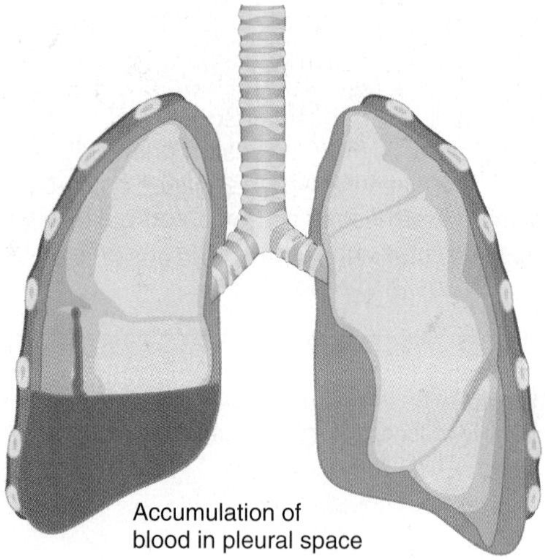

FIGURE 41-11 Hemothorax.

Hemothorax

A **hemothorax** is the accumulation of blood in the pleural space. It is caused by bleeding from the lung parenchyma or damaged vessels (**FIGURE 41-11**). If this condition is associated with a pneumothorax, it is called a **hemopneumothorax**. Blood loss may be massive in these patients; each side of the thorax can hold 30% to 40% (2,000–3,000 mL) of the patient's blood volume.[15] (A severed intercostal artery can easily bleed 50 mL per minute.) Thus patients with a hemothorax often have hypovolemia and hypoxemia. Hemothorax is commonly associated with pneumothorax (25%) and extrathoracic injuries (73%).[1]

As blood continues to fill the pleural space, the lung on the affected side may collapse. In rare cases, the mediastinum may even shift away from the hemothorax and compress the unaffected lung. The resultant effects of respiratory and circulatory compromise are responsible for the following signs and symptoms:

- Tachypnea
- Dyspnea
- Cyanosis (often not evident in hemorrhagic shock)
- Diminished or decreased breath sounds (dullness on percussion)
- Hypovolemic shock
- Narrow pulse pressure
- Tracheal deviation to the unaffected side (rare)

Prehospital care for patients with a hemothorax is directed at correcting ventilatory and circulatory problems. It includes administration of high-concentration oxygen; implementation of ventilatory support with a bag-mask device or intubation, or both; administration of volume-expanding fluids to correct the hypovolemia; and rapid transport to an appropriate medical facility for surgical intervention. Hemothorax associated with great vessel or cardiac injury has a high mortality rate: 50% of these patients die within 1 hour of their injury.[16]

> CRITICAL THINKING
> Hemothorax is associated with a higher mortality rate than a simple (closed) pneumothorax. Why is that the case?

Traumatic Asphyxia

The term **traumatic asphyxia** is used to describe a severe crushing injury to the chest and abdomen that results in an increase in intrathoracic pressure (**FIGURE 41-12**). The increased pressure forces blood from the right side of the heart into the veins of the upper thorax, neck, and face, leading to capillary rupture and giving the patient's head and neck a purple-red appearance. The forces involved in this phenomenon may cause lethal injury, but traumatic asphyxia alone is not life threatening[1] (although brain and eye hemorrhages may occur[4]).

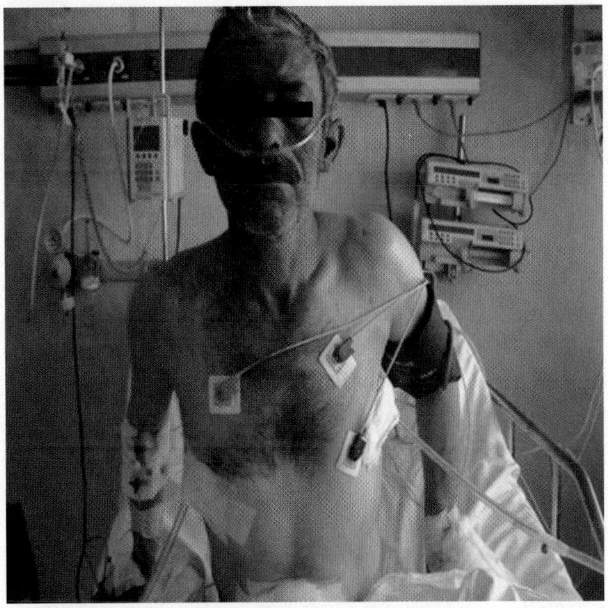

FIGURE 41-12 A patient with traumatic asphyxia.

Reproduced from: Karamustafaoglu Y, Yavasman I, Tiryaki S, Yoruk Y. Traumatic asphyxia. *Int J Emerg Med.* 2010;3(4):379–380. http://doi.org/10.1007/s12245-010-0204-x.

Signs and symptoms of traumatic asphyxia include purple-red discoloration of the face and neck (the skin below the area remains pink), jugular vein distention (JVD), and swelling or hemorrhage of the conjunctiva (subconjunctival petechiae may appear). Emergency care is directed at ensuring an open airway, providing adequate ventilation, and caring for associated injuries. The paramedic should be ready to manage hypovolemia and shock when the compressive force is released.

Heart and Great Vessel Injuries

Trauma to the heart and great vessels—that is, the aorta, pulmonary arteries and veins, and superior and inferior venae cavae—may result from blunt or penetrating trauma and associated forces. The injuries discussed in this section include myocardial contusion, pericardial tamponade, myocardial rupture, and traumatic aortic rupture. These injuries may lead to potentially fatal complications:

- Life-threatening dysrhythmias
- Conduction abnormalities
- Congestive heart failure
- Cardiogenic shock
- Cardiac tamponade
- Cardiac rupture
- Coronary artery occlusion

Myocardial Contusion

A **myocardial contusion** usually is caused by a vehicle collision. In these cases the chest wall strikes the dashboard or steering column, causing blunt-force injury to the heart. (Sternal and multiple rib fractures are common.) Therefore, a deformed dashboard or steering column should alert the paramedic to the possibility of a cardiac injury. Blunt myocardial injury

> NOTE
> The clinical findings in blunt cardiac trauma are often subtle and frequently overlooked for several reasons: (1) Multiple injuries direct attention elsewhere, (2) often, little evidence of thoracic injury is present, and (3) signs of cardiac injury may not be present on initial examination. The goals of prehospital care are to recognize the potential for cardiac trauma (based on the mechanism of injury) and to monitor the patient for potentially fatal complications that may arise.

CRITICAL THINKING

How would you manage a cardiac rhythm disturbance resulting from a myocardial contusion?

occurs in as many as 55% of patients who experience blunt trauma to the chest.[1]

The extent of the myocardial contusion may vary from a localized bruise to a full-thickness injury to the wall of the heart with hemorrhage and edema. Blood may accumulate in the pericardium (hemopericardium) as a result of a tear in the epicardium or endocardium. This, in turn, may result in cardiac rupture or a traumatic myocardial infarction. The fibrinous reaction at the contusion site may lead to delayed rupture or ventricular aneurysm.

Patients with a myocardial contusion may have no symptoms, or they may complain of chest pain similar to that seen with a myocardial infarction. Other signs and symptoms include electrocardiographic (ECG) abnormalities (sinus tachycardia occurs in 70% of patients[1]), ventricular rhythms, ST elevation, right bundle branch block, a new cardiac murmur (indicating valve disruption), signs of heart failure, and palpitations. While rare, blunt cardiac rupture can occur, causing immediate exsanguination and death on the scene.[4] (BOX 41-1 describes another potentially fatal cardiac condition following chest trauma—commotio cordis.)

Emergency care for patients with myocardial contusion is similar to that for patients with myocardial infarction: oxygen administration, ECG monitoring, and pharmacologic therapy for dysrhythmias and hypotension (see Chapter 21, *Cardiology*). Any intervention that increases myocardial oxygen demand should be avoided.

Pericardial Tamponade

Penetrating trauma (and, in rare cases, blunt trauma) may cause tears in the heart chamber walls, allowing blood to leak from the heart. If the pericardium has been torn sufficiently, blood can leak into the thoracic cavity, with the patient then rapidly dying from hemorrhage. Often, however, the pericardium remains intact. In such cases, the blood enters the pericardial space, which causes an increase in pericardial pressure and volume (**pericardial tamponade**). The increased pressure prevents the heart from expanding and refilling with blood; the presence of 60 to 100 mL of blood and clots in the pericardial sac can cause tamponade.[1] The resulting decrease in stroke volume and cardiac output diminishes myocardial perfusion because of pressure effects on the walls of the heart and decreased diastolic pressures. Associated ischemic dysfunction may result in myocardial infarction.

Pericardial tamponade occurs in fewer than 2% of patients who suffer blunt chest trauma. By comparison, tamponade develops in 60% to 80% of patients with stab wounds involving the heart.[17]

BOX 41-1 Commotio Cordis

Commotio cordis is a Latin term that means commotion or disturbance of the heart. The condition describes sudden death that follows a blow to the chest. Cardiac arrest is thought to occur secondary to ventricular fibrillation (VF) when the chest trauma coincides with the cardiac T wave. It may also be associated with coronary vasospasm or changes in myocardial contractility as a result of the chest trauma. Although commotio cordis can happen to anyone, victims are overwhelmingly young male athletes. In sports, it typically occurs as a result of impact with a projectile, most commonly a baseball, but has also been noted in hockey, softball, lacrosse, and karate. Despite the fact that it is very rare, commotio cordis is the second-leading cause of death among young athletes (accounting for 10 to 20 deaths per year).

Commotio cordis is managed in a manner similar to that used for cardiac arrests resulting from myocardial infarction rather than those resulting from trauma. The cardiac rhythm should be determined quickly, and rapid defibrillation with effective minimally interrupted cardiopulmonary resuscitation should be administered if VF is identified.

Modified from: National Association of Emergency Medical Technicians. *PHTLS: Prehospital Trauma Life Support*. 8th ed. Burlington, MA: Jones & Bartlett Learning; 2016; Zipes DP. *Cardiac Electrophysiology: From Cell to Bedside*. 6th ed. Philadelphia, PA: Elsevier; 2013.

NOTE

Penetrating injuries to the heart, such as those caused by some knife and gunshot wounds, may result in death from hemorrhage rather than tamponade. This outcome happens when the wound in the heart is so large that the blood in the pericardial space cannot be contained.

At first, most patients with pericardial tamponade have peripheral vasoconstriction. The diastolic blood pressure rises more than the systolic blood pressure, which leads to a decreased pulse pressure. These patients are also tachycardic. The increase in their heart rate compensates for their decrease in cardiac output.

Up to this point, pericardial tamponade and hemorrhagic shock have similar signs, but a key clinical finding often allows differentiation of the two forms of shock. The trio of clinical findings first described by Beck[18] in 1935, and now known as the **Beck triad**, consists of JVD, muffled heart sounds, and hypotension. The first element of the Beck triad, JVD, is the single best way to distinguish pericardial tamponade from hemorrhagic shock.[1]

> NOTE
>
> There can be many causes of JVD. Examples include tension pneumothorax, right ventricular dysfunction in cardiogenic shock, pulmonary hypertension, tricuspid valve stenosis, superior vena cava obstruction, and constrictive pericarditis.

Other signs and symptoms of pericardial tamponade include the following:

- Tachycardia
- Respiratory distress
- Narrow pulse pressure
- Cyanosis of the head, neck, and upper extremities

Another finding in pericardial tamponade may be **pulsus paradoxus**, an exaggerated decrease in systolic blood pressure—more than 10 to 15 mm Hg—during inspiration compared with expiration.[19] (Normally, this drop is minimal.) The excessive decline in systolic pressure occurs in cardiac tamponade when pleural pressure is reduced during inspiration. The reduction of pleural pressure provides some relief from the tamponade and causes the inspiratory decline in arterial flow and systolic pressure. Pulsus paradoxus is difficult to measure in the prehospital setting, especially if the patient is hypotensive.

Electrical alternans is a rare finding in cardiac tamponade. It comprises a change in the amplitude of a patient's ECG waveforms that varies with every other cardiac cycle (**FIGURE 41-13**).

Pericardial tamponade is a dire emergency. Pericardial blood must be removed in these patients, and the bleeding must be stopped if the patient is to survive the injury. Prehospital management includes careful monitoring, oxygen administration, aggressive fluid replacement to maintain adequate preload (if transport time is short), and rapid transport to an appropriate medical facility. Treatment at the medical facility involves needle pericardiocentesis to remove blood from the pericardial sac. Removal of as little as 20 mL may drastically improve cardiac output.[20] If cardiac arrest occurs, hospital physicians may perform a resuscitative thoracostomy to open the chest and repair the wounds.

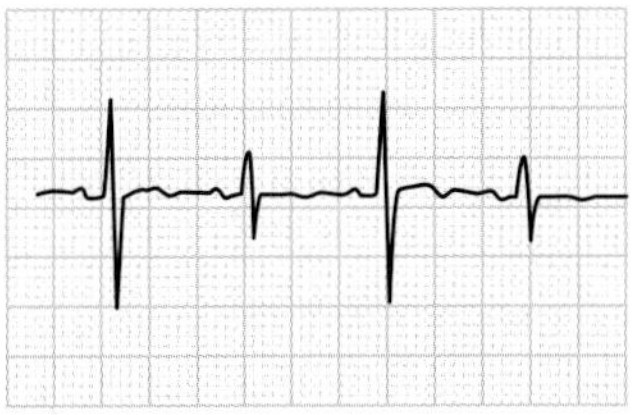

FIGURE 41-13 Lead II rhythm strip taken from a patient with acute pericarditis complicated by a large pericardial effusion and tamponade physiology. Note the resting sinus tachycardia with relatively low voltage and electrical alternans.

Myocardial Rupture

Myocardial rupture occurs when blood-filled chambers of the ventricles are compressed with enough force to rupture the chamber wall, septum, or valve. Although this injury is nearly always immediately fatal, approximately 20% of patients will survive 30 minutes or longer, allowing time for rapid transport and surgical repair.[1]

Motor vehicle crashes are responsible for most cases of myocardial rupture, accounting for 15% of fatal thoracic injuries. Other proposed mechanisms include the following:

- Deceleration or shearing forces that disrupt the inferior and superior venae cavae
- Upward displacement of blood (causing an increase in intracardiac pressure) after abdominal trauma
- Direct compression of the heart between the sternum and the vertebrae
- Laceration from a rib or sternal fracture
- Complications of myocardial contusion

These patients often present with a significant mechanism of injury, and signs and symptoms of congestive heart failure and cardiac tamponade may be present. Patients should be closely monitored for signs of pericardial tamponade. Prehospital care for these patients is mainly supportive, including airway and ventilatory support and rapid transport for definitive care.

It is crucial that paramedics also consider the possibility of a tension pneumothorax in these patients. The signs and symptoms of tension pneumothorax mimic those of myocardial rupture with tamponade.

Traumatic Aortic Rupture

Traumatic aortic rupture is thought to be a result of shearing forces that develop between tissues that decelerate at different rates. Common mechanisms of injury include rapid deceleration in high-speed motor vehicle crashes, falls from great heights, and crushing injuries. Aortic rupture is responsible for 15% of all deaths from motor vehicle collisions.[21] Of patients with aortic rupture, 80% to 90% die at the scene as a result of massive hemorrhage because the tear extends through the full thickness of the aortic wall; only 10% to 20% survive the first hour after such an injury.[1] Survival in these cases occurs because the bleeding is initially tamponaded by the surrounding adventitia of the aorta and intact visceral pleura, though 30% of these patients develop ruptures within 6 hours. For these reasons, rapid and pertinent evaluation and transport to an appropriate medical facility are crucial.

The usual site of damage to the aorta is in the distal arch, which is located just beyond the branching of the left subclavian artery and at the level of the ligamentum arteriosum (**FIGURE 41-14**). The ligamentum arteriosum and descending thoracic arch are somewhat fixed, whereas the transverse portion of the arch is somewhat mobile. If shearing forces exceed the tensile strength of the arch, the junction of the mobile and fixed points of attachment may be partly torn. If the outer layer of tissue around the aorta remains intact, the patient may survive long enough for surgical or endovascular repair to be performed.

Aortic rupture is a severe injury, with approximately 85% of affected patients dying before they reach a hospital.[22] Any trauma patient who has unexplained shock and an appropriate mechanism of injury (rapid deceleration) should be suspected of having a ruptured aorta. Blood pressure may be normal or elevated, with a significant difference in pressures noted between the two arms. In addition, upper extremity hypertension

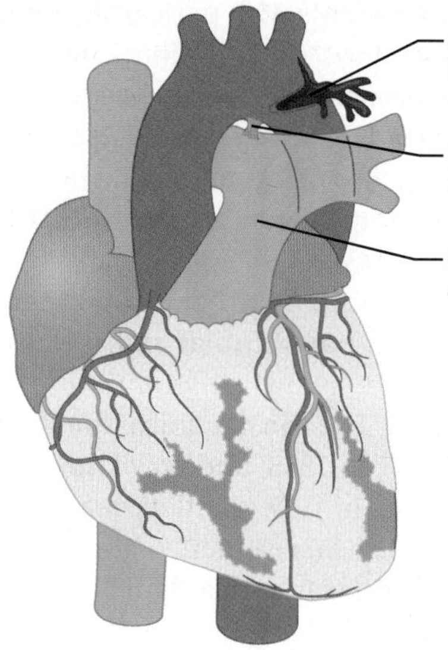

FIGURE 41-14 Aortic rupture.

with absent or weak femoral pulses can occur in these patients, likely as the result of the expanding hematoma's compression of the aorta. Other patients have hypertension because of increased activity of the sympathetic nervous system. Some patients will have a harsh systolic murmur that can be heard over the pericardium or between the scapulae. In rare cases, patients may have paraplegia without a cervical or thoracic spine injury. This condition occurs as a consequence of decreased blood flow through the anterior spinal artery. This artery, which is found in the thoracic region, is composed of branches from the posterior intercostal arteries, which in turn are branches of the thoracic aorta.

> NOTE
> A difference in pulse quality between the arms and the lower torso, or between the left arm and the right arm, is sometimes detected with aortic rupture. For this reason, checking both radial and femoral pulses is important.[4]

Prehospital management of patients with traumatic aortic rupture includes advising medical direction of the suspected rupture, administering high-concentration oxygen, providing ventilatory support with spinal precautions, establishing vascular access without delay in transport (and without fluid infusion if signs of shock are not present), and ensuring rapid transport for surgical repair. If interfacility transfer of these patients is needed, targeted blood pressure control may be achieved with an infusion of medication such as a beta blocker to maintain mean arterial pressure at 70 mm Hg or less.[4]

Penetrating Wounds of the Great Vessels

Penetrating wounds of the great vessels usually involve injury to the chest, abdomen, or neck. These wounds often are accompanied by massive hemothorax, hypovolemic shock, cardiac tamponade, and enlarging hematomas that may cause compression of the vena cava, trachea, esophagus, great vessels, and heart. Prehospital care for patients with penetrating injury to the great vessels is directed at providing airway and ventilatory support, managing hypovolemia with judicious fluid therapy (guided by medical direction), and ensuring rapid transport for definitive care.

Other Thoracic Injuries

Other injuries that may be associated with blunt or penetrating trauma to the thorax include esophageal and tracheobronchial injuries and diaphragmatic rupture.

Esophageal and Tracheobronchial Injuries

Esophageal injuries most often are caused by penetrating trauma—for example, by projectile or knife wounds. They also can result from spontaneous perforation caused by cancer and from anatomic distortions caused by diverticula or gastric reflux, both of which can lead to violent vomiting. Assessment findings may include pain, fever, hoarseness, dysphagia, respiratory distress, and shock. If esophageal perforation occurs in the cervical region, local tenderness, subcutaneous emphysema, and resistance to neck movement may be noted. Esophageal perforation that occurs lower in the thoracic region may result in mediastinal and subcutaneous emphysema, inflammation of the mediastinum, and splinting of the chest wall.

NOTE

Boerhaave syndrome is a full-thickness tear of the esophagus, usually due to repeated episodes of retching and vomiting following recent excessive dietary and alcohol intake. The sudden onset of severe chest pain after episodes of vomiting is worsened by swallowing, and the patient may experience pain in the left shoulder. The mortality of this syndrome is estimated at approximately 35%, making it the most lethal perforation of the gastrointestinal tract. The best outcomes are associated with early diagnosis and definitive surgical management within 12 hours of rupture. If intervention is delayed longer than 24 hours, the mortality rate (even with surgical intervention) rises to higher than 50% and to nearly 90% after 48 hours. Left untreated, the mortality rate is close to 100%.

Modified from: Roy PK. Boerhaave syndrome. Medscape website. https://emedicine.medscape.com/article/171683-overview. Published July 6, 2015. Accessed March 2, 2018.

Tracheobronchial injuries (tracheobronchial disruptions) are rare, occurring in fewer than 3% of victims of blunt or penetrating chest trauma. The mortality rate for these injuries is approximately 10%, depending on associated injuries, early diagnosis, and surgical repair.[1] Although most injuries occur within 3 cm (about 1.5 inches) of the carina, they can occur anywhere along the tracheobronchial tree. Signs and symptoms of tracheobronchial injury include the following:

- Severe hypoxia
- Tachypnea
- Tachycardia
- Massive subcutaneous emphysema
- Dyspnea
- Respiratory distress
- Hemoptysis

Emergency care for patients with an esophageal or a tracheobronchial injury is directed at providing airway, ventilatory, and circulatory support and ensuring rapid transport for definitive care at an appropriate medical facility.

NOTE

A tension pneumothorax that does not improve after needle decompression or the presence of a continuous flow of air from the needle after decompression should alert the paramedic to the possibility of a tracheobronchial injury.

Diaphragmatic Rupture

The diaphragm is a sheet of dome-shaped muscle that separates the abdominal cavity from the thoracic cavity. Sudden compression of the abdomen, such as with blunt trauma to the trunk, results in a sharp increase in intra-abdominal pressure. The pressure differences may then cause abdominal contents to rupture through the thin diaphragmatic wall and enter the chest cavity (**FIGURE 41-15**). **Diaphragmatic rupture** is detected more often on the left side of the diaphragm than on the liver-shielded right side.[23] However, rupture on either side may allow intra-abdominal organs to enter the thoracic cavity where they may compress the lung, resulting in reduced ventilation, decreased venous return, decreased cardiac output, and shock. Because of the mechanical forces involved, patients with diaphragmatic rupture often have multiple injuries.

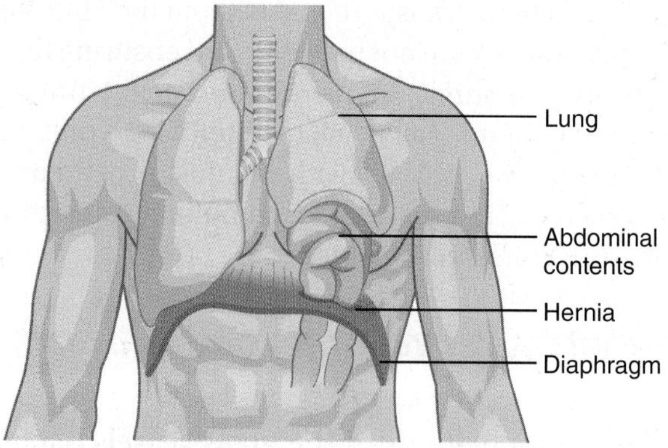

FIGURE 41-15 Diaphragmatic rupture. Sudden compression of the abdomen may increase intra-abdominal pressure, causing the abdominal contents to rupture through the thin diaphragmatic wall and enter the chest cavity.

Signs and symptoms of a ruptured diaphragm include abdominal pain, shortness of breath, and decreased breath sounds. If most of the abdominal contents are forced into the chest, the abdomen may have a hollow or empty appearance. Also, bowel sounds may be heard in the chest.

Prehospital management includes oxygen administration, ventilatory support as needed (positive pressure ventilation may worsen the injury), use of volume-expanding fluids, and rapid transport with the patient in a supine position to an appropriate medical facility for surgical repair. Some medical direction agencies also may recommend that a nasogastric tube be placed to empty the stomach and reduce abdominal pressure.

Summary

- Chest injuries are caused by blunt or penetrating trauma, which often results from motor vehicle crashes, falls from heights, blast injuries, blows to the chest, chest compression, gunshot wounds, and stab wounds.
- Fractures of the clavicle, ribs, or sternum as well as flail chest may be caused by blunt or penetrating trauma. Complications of skeletal trauma of the chest may include cardiac, vascular, or pulmonary injuries.
- Pulmonary contusion results when trauma to the lung causes alveolar and capillary damage. Severe hypoxemia may develop, with the degree of hypoxemia being directly related to the size of the contused area.
- Closed pneumothorax may be life threatening if (1) it is a tension pneumothorax, (2) it occupies more than 40% of the hemithorax, or (3) it occurs in a patient in shock or with a preexisting pulmonary or cardiovascular disease.
- Open pneumothorax may result in severe ventilatory dysfunction, hypoxemia, and death unless it is quickly recognized and corrected.
- Tension pneumothorax is a true emergency. It results in profound hypoventilation and may lead to death if it is not quickly recognized and managed.
- Hemothorax may result in massive blood loss, so patients with this condition often have hypovolemia and hypoxemia.
- Traumatic asphyxia results from forces that cause an increase in intrathoracic pressure. When it occurs alone, it is often not lethal. However, brain hemorrhages, seizures, coma, and death have been reported after these injuries.
- The extent of injury from myocardial contusion may vary from a localized bruise to a full-thickness injury to the wall of the heart. A full-thickness injury may result in cardiac rupture, ventricular aneurysm, or a traumatic myocardial infarction.
- Pericardial tamponade occurs when 150 to 200 mL of blood enters the pericardial space suddenly, which triggers a decrease in stroke volume and cardiac output.
- Myocardial rupture is an acute traumatic perforation of the ventricles or atria. It is nearly always immediately

fatal, though death may be delayed for several weeks after blunt trauma.

- Aortic rupture is a severe injury that has an 80% to 90% mortality rate in the first hour after its occurrence. The paramedic should consider the possibility of aortic rupture in any trauma patient who has unexplained shock after a rapid deceleration injury.
- Esophageal injuries most frequently are caused by penetrating trauma (eg, missile projectile, knife wounds). Tracheobronchial injuries are rare, occurring in fewer than 3% of victims of blunt or penetrating chest trauma, but their mortality rate is more than 30%. A tension pneumothorax that does not improve following needle decompression or the absence of a continuous flow of air from the needle following decompression should alert the paramedic to the possibility of a tracheobronchial injury.
- Diaphragmatic ruptures may allow abdominal organs to enter the thoracic cavity, where they can cause compression of the lung, resulting in a reduction in ventilation, a decrease in venous return, a decrease in cardiac output, and shock.

References

1. Walls RM, Hockbreger RS, Gausche-Hill M, et al., eds. *Rosen's Emergency Medicine: Concepts and Clinical Practice.* 9th ed. St. Louis, MO: Elsevier; 2018.
2. US Department of Transportation, National Highway Traffic Safety Administration. *EMT Paramedic National Standards Curriculum.* Washington, DC: US Department of Transportation; 1998.
3. Pressley CM, Fry WR, Philp AS, Berry SD, Smith RS. Predicting outcome of patients with chest wall injury. *Am J Surg.* 2012;204(6):910-913.
4. National Association of Emergency Medical Technicians. *PHTLS: Prehospital Trauma Life Support.* 8th ed. Burlington, MA: Jones & Bartlett Learning; 2016.
5. Simon B, Ebert J, Bokhari F, et al. Management of pulmonary contusion and flail chest. *J Trauma.* 2012;73(5):S351-S361.
6. Perez MR, Rodriguez RM, Baumann BM, et al. Sternal fracture in the age of pan-scan. *Injury.* 2015;46(7):1324-1327.
7. Costantino M, Gosselin MV, Primack SL. The ABC's of thoracic trauma imaging. *Semin Roentgenol.* 2006;41(3):209-225.
8. Mellor SG. The pathogenesis of blast injury and its management. *Br J Hosp Med.* 1988;39:536-539.
9. Block J, Jordanov MI, Stack LB, Thurman RJ. *The Atlas of Emergency Radiology.* New York, NY: McGraw-Hill; 2013.
10. Weichenthal L, Crane D, Rond L. Needle thoracostomy in the prehospital setting: a retrospective observational study. *Prehosp Emerg Care.* 2016;20(3):399-403.
11. Kaserer A, Stein P, Simmen H-P, Spahn DR, Neuhaus V. Failure rate of prehospital chest decompression after severe thoracic trauma. *Am J Emerg Med.* 2017;35(3):469-474.
12. Lyng J, Pokorney-Colling K, West M, Beilman G. The relationship between adult body mass index and anticipated failure rate of needle decompression using a 5 cm needle for tension pneumothorax. *Ann Emerg Med.* 2017;70(4):S145-S146.
13. *Needle decompression of tension pneumothorax: Tactical Combat Casualty Care Guideline Recommendations 2012-05* [Memo]. Falls Church, VA: Defense Health Board; July 6, 2012.
14. Clemency BM, Tanski CT, Rosenberg M, May PR, Consiglio JD, Lindstrom HA. Sufficient catheter length for pneumothorax needle decompression: a meta-analysis. *Prehosp Disaster Med.* 2015;30(3):249-253.
15. Mancini MC. Hemothorax. Medscape website. https://emedicine.medscape.com/article/2047916-overview. Updated January 15, 2017. Accessed March 2, 2018.
16. Mahoozi HR, Volmerig J, Hecker E. Modern management of traumatic hemothorax. *J Trauma Treat.* 2016;5:326.
17. Gerhardt M, Gravlee G. Anesthesia considerations for cardiothoracic trauma. In: Smith C, ed. *Trauma Anesthesia.* Cambridge, England: Cambridge University Press; 2015:499-525.
18. Beck C. Two cardiac compression triads. *JAMA.* 1935;104:714-716.
19. Roberts JR, Hedges JR. *Roberts and Hedges' Clinical Procedures in Emergency Medicine.* Philadelphia, PA: Elsevier Saunders; 2014.
20. McKean SC, Ross JJ, Dressler DD, Scheurer DB. *Principles and Practice of Hospital Medicine.* 2nd ed. New York, NY: McGraw-Hill; 2017.
21. Benjamin MM, Roberts WC. Fatal aortic rupture from nonpenetrating chest trauma. *Proc Baylor Univ Med Center.* 2012;25(2):121-123.
22. Gwon JG, Kwon T-W, Cho Y-P, Han YJ, Noh MS. Analysis of in hospital mortality and long-term survival excluding in hospital mortality after open surgical repair of ruptured abdominal aortic aneurysm. *Ann Surg Treat Res.* 2016;91(6):303-308.
23. Khan AN. Imaging in diaphragm injury and paresis. Medscape website. https://emedicine.medscape.com/article/355284-overview. Updated October 19, 2015. Accessed March 2, 2018.

Suggested Readings

Candefjord S, Buendia R, Caragounis EC, Oveland NP. Forty-one new methods for diagnosis of thoracic trauma in prehospital care. *BMJ Open.* 2017;7(suppl 3).

Chest trauma: EMS assessment and treatment: the injuries from blunt or penetrating chest trauma can cause life-threatening disruption to perfusion, ventilation or both. EMS1.com website. https://www.ems1.com/ems-products/Bleeding-Control/articles/38224048-Chest-trauma-EMS-assessment-and-treatment/. Published December 10, 2015. Accessed March 2, 2018.

Kaserer A, Stein P, Simmon H-P, Spahn DR, Neuhaus V. Failure rate of prehospital chest decompression after severe thoracic trauma. *Am J Emerg Med.* 2017;35(3):469-474.

Schauer SG, April MD, Naylor JF, et al. Chest seal placement for penetrating chest wounds by prehospital ground forces in Afghanistan. *J Spec Oper Med.* 2017;17(3):85-89.

Van Vleddera MG, Van Waes OJF, Kooij FO, Peters JH, Van Lieshout EMM, Verhofstad MHJ. Out of hospital thoracotomy for cardiac arrest after penetrating thoracic trauma. *Injury.* 2017;48(9):1865-1869.

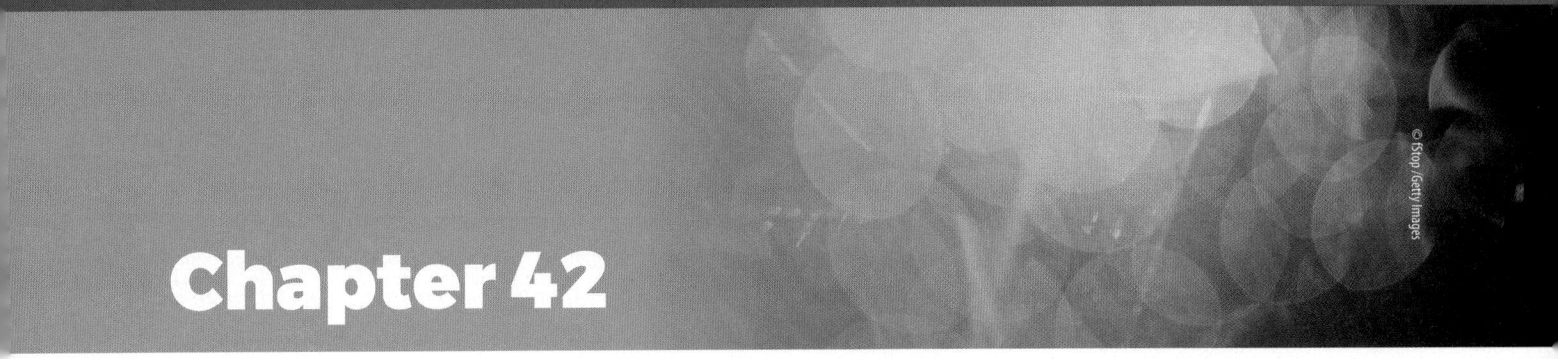

Chapter 42

Abdominal Trauma

NATIONAL EMS EDUCATION STANDARD COMPETENCIES

Trauma

Integrates assessment findings with principles of epidemiology and pathophysiology to formulate a field impression to implement a comprehensive treatment/disposition plan for an acutely injured patient.

Abdominal and Genitourinary Trauma

Recognition and management of
- Blunt versus penetrating mechanisms (pp 1509–1510)
- Evisceration (p 1514)
- Impaled object (pp 1510–1514)

Pathophysiology, assessment, and management of
- Solid and hollow organ injuries (pp 1510–1512)
- Blunt versus penetrating mechanisms (pp 1509–1510)
- Evisceration (p 1514)
- Injuries to the external genitalia (see Chapter 49, *Abuse and Neglect*)
- Vaginal bleeding due to trauma (see Chapter 30, *Gynecology*)
- Sexual assault (see Chapter 30, *Gynecology* and Chapter 49, *Abuse and Neglect*)
- Vascular injury (p 1514)
- Retroperitoneal injuries (pp 1512–1513)

OBJECTIVES

Upon completion of this chapter, the paramedic student will be able to:
1. Identify mechanisms of injury associated with blunt and penetrating abdominal trauma. (pp 1509–1510)
2. Describe mechanisms of injury, signs and symptoms, and complications associated with abdominal injury to a solid organ, hollow organ, retroperitoneal organ, and pelvic organ. (pp 1510–1514)
3. Outline the significance of injury to intra-abdominal vascular structures. (p 1514)
4. Describe the prehospital assessment priorities for the patient suspected of having an abdominal injury. (pp 1514–1515)
5. Outline the prehospital care of the patient with abdominal trauma. (p 1516)

KEY TERMS

Cullen sign The appearance of irregularly formed hemorrhagic patches on the skin around the umbilicus.

evisceration The protrusion of an internal organ or the peritoneal contents through a wound or surgical incision, especially in the abdominal wall.

Grey Turner sign Bruising of the skin of the flanks or loin in retroperitoneal hemorrhage and acute hemorrhagic pancreatitis; also known as Turner sign.

hematuria The presence of blood in the urine.

hemodilution An increase in the fluid content of the blood that results in a lowered concentration of formed elements and lowered blood viscosity.

hemoperitoneum The presence of extravasated blood in the peritoneal cavity.

Kehr sign Pain in the left shoulder thought to be caused by referred pain secondary to irritation of the adjacent diaphragm.

peritonitis Inflammation of the serous membrane that covers the abdominal wall (parietal peritoneum) or the abdominal organs (visceral peritoneum).

ultrasonography A diagnostic test that uses sound waves to make images of internal organs and structures. It is often used in the emergency department to view the peritoneal cavity for the presence of fluid or blood. The resulting image is known as a sonogram.

Abdominal trauma may be difficult to evaluate in the prehospital setting because of the wide spectrum of potential injuries to multiple organs. In addition, physical findings may be absent, minimal, or exaggerated. Patients may also have altered levels of pain perception as a result of preexisting conditions, shock, alcohol or other drug use, head injury, or other factors. For all these reasons, the paramedic must have a high degree of suspicion based on the mechanism of injury and kinematics. Death from abdominal trauma usually is a result of ongoing hemorrhage and the delay of surgical repair.

NOTE

Like most other types of trauma, many abdominal injuries can be prevented. An important prevention strategy is taking part in community programs that promote safety. For example, the paramedic could work to promote proper installation of child safety seats. Another strategy would be stressing the importance of proper seat belt usage.

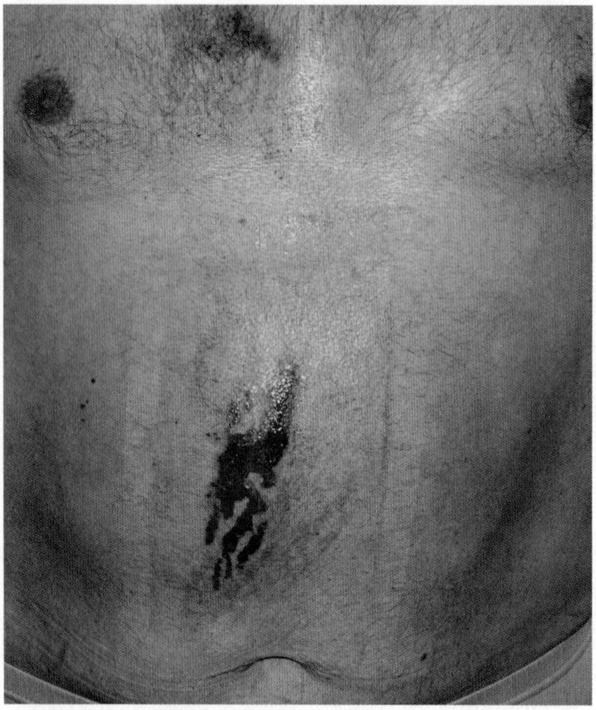

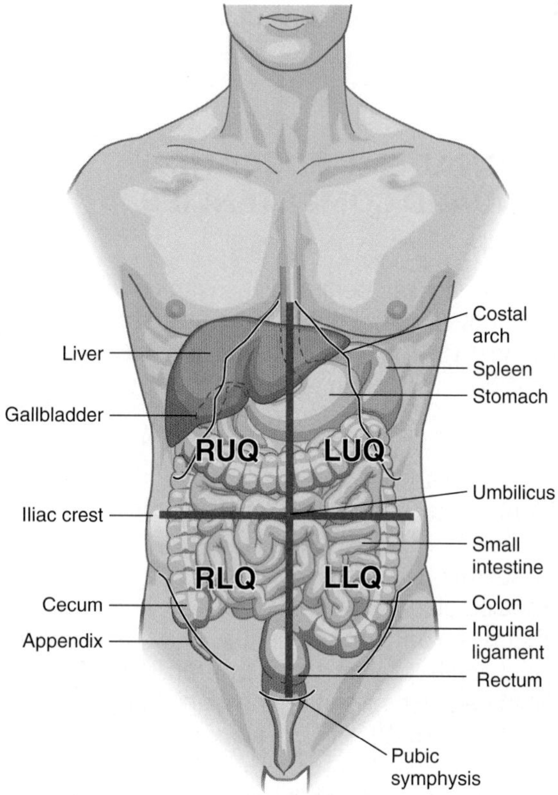

FIGURE 42-1 Abdominal quadrants and the positions of major viscera. Anterior view of a man.

Review of Abdominal Anatomy

Organs in the abdomen include the intestines, kidneys, liver, gallbladder, pancreas, spleen, and stomach (**FIGURE 42-1** and **FIGURE 42-2**). In addition to these organs, the abdomen has many vascular structures, including the following:[1]

- Abdominal aorta
- Superior and inferior mesenteric arteries
- Renal arteries
- Splenic artery
- Hepatic artery
- Iliac arteries
- Hepatic portal system
- Inferior vena cava

All abdominal organs and vascular structures are susceptible to injury. Quick recognition of injury, emergency care, and rapid transport for definitive care can tremendously alter morbidity and mortality.

Mechanisms of Abdominal Injury

Abdominal injury may result from blunt or penetrating trauma. As a rule, penetrating trauma results

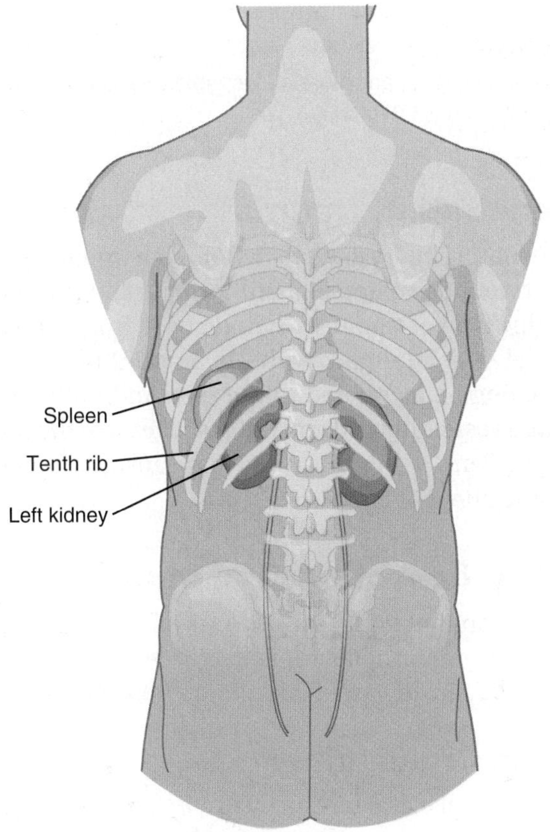

FIGURE 42-2 Surface projection of the spleen. Posterior view of a man.

BOX 42-1 Signs of Abdominal Trauma

Findings that raise the suspicion for abdominal trauma include the following:

- Mechanism of injury consistent with rapid deceleration or significant compression forces
- Bent steering wheel
- Soft-tissue injuries to the abdomen, flank, or back
- Shock without an obvious cause
- Level of shock greater than explained by other injuries
- "Seat belt signs"
- Peritoneal signs

Modified from: National Association of Emergency Medical Technicians. *PHTLS: Prehospital Trauma Life Support*. 8th ed. Burlington, MA: Jones & Bartlett Learning; 2014.

in a higher mortality rate than does blunt trauma; however, both are leading causes of morbidity and mortality among all age groups. Blunt trauma is also often accompanied by injury to multiple organ systems. BOX 42-1 lists some signs of abdominal trauma.

When evaluating a patient with abdominal trauma, the paramedic should be keenly aware of the kinematics and the mechanism of injury and the estimated or actual speed of travel. For example, in the case of a motor vehicle crash, the paramedic should note the extent of damage to the car, the patient's location within the car, whether the patient struck the steering wheel or dash, and whether personal restraints were used properly. In the case of penetrating injury, the type, size, and direction of the penetrating object, the posture or position of the victim during the injury, and the amount of blood loss at the scene can provide valuable information to the receiving hospital.

Regardless of the organ injured, management usually is limited to securing the airway with spinal precautions, providing ventilatory support, providing wound management, managing shock with judicious fluid use, and rapidly transporting the patient for definitive care (BOX 42-2).

Blunt Trauma

Blunt trauma to abdominal organs usually is caused by compression or shearing forces. Compression forces may cause the abdominal organs to be crushed between solid objects (eg, between the steering column and the spinal vertebrae). Shearing forces may cause a tear or rupture of the solid organs or blood vessels when the tissues are stretched at their points of attachment (stabilizing ligaments or blood vessels, respectively). The severity of injury usually depends on the degree and duration of force applied as well as the type of abdominal structure injured (fluid filled, gas filled, solid, or hollow).

BOX 42-2 Prehospital Care for Abdominal Injury

1. Use measures for spinal motion restriction if indicated.
2. Secure the airway.
3. Administer oxygen to maintain oxygen saturation, as measured by a pulse oximeter, at 95% or greater.
4. Provide ventilatory support if needed.
5. Control external hemorrhage with direct pressure.
6. Provide wound management.
7. Manage shock with judicious fluid replacement, based on the patient's mental status and overall appearance.
8. Rapidly transport the patient for definitive care.

Blunt abdominal trauma may be caused by motor vehicle and motorcycle crashes (including injuries that result from the use of personal restraints), pedestrian injuries, falls, assaults, and blast injuries. The motor vehicle is the major cause of blunt abdominal trauma (**FIGURE 42-3**). Motor vehicle collisions (eg, a crash involving two cars) and pedestrian–motor vehicle collisions have been cited as causes in 50% to 75% of abdominal trauma cases, blows to the abdomen in approximately 15% of cases, and falls in 6% to 9% of cases.[2]

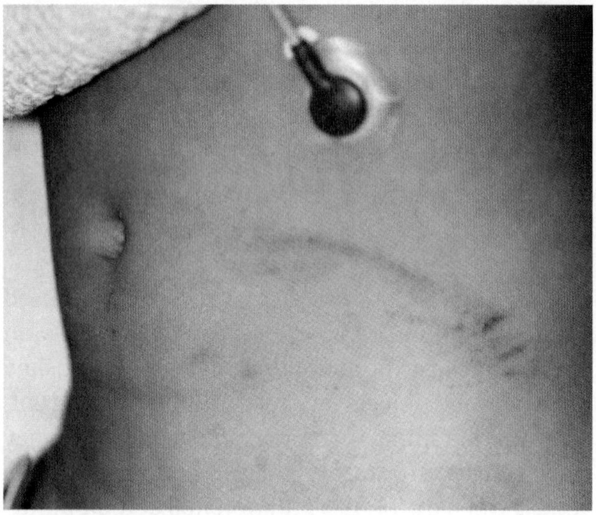

FIGURE 42-3 Marks of impact on the front-seat passenger in a car crash.

Courtesy of Peter T. Pons, MD, FACEP.

CRITICAL THINKING

Young children are more susceptible to abdominal injuries than are adults. Why?

Penetrating Trauma

Penetrating injury may result from stab wounds, gunshot wounds, or impalement. A major complication of this type of trauma is hemorrhage from a major vessel or solid organ, with the amount of internal bleeding being related to the type and number of blood vessels injured and the vascularity of the solid organ. Penetrating injury also may cause perforation of a segment of bowel.

Specific Abdominal Injuries

An abdominal injury may be classified as an injury to a solid organ, hollow organ, retroperitoneal organ, pelvic organ, or vascular structure (**FIGURE 42-4**).

Solid Organ Injury

Injury to solid organs usually results in rapid and significant blood loss. The two solid organs most often injured are the liver and the spleen, both of which can

CRITICAL THINKING

When does shock associated with injury to the liver or spleen develop?

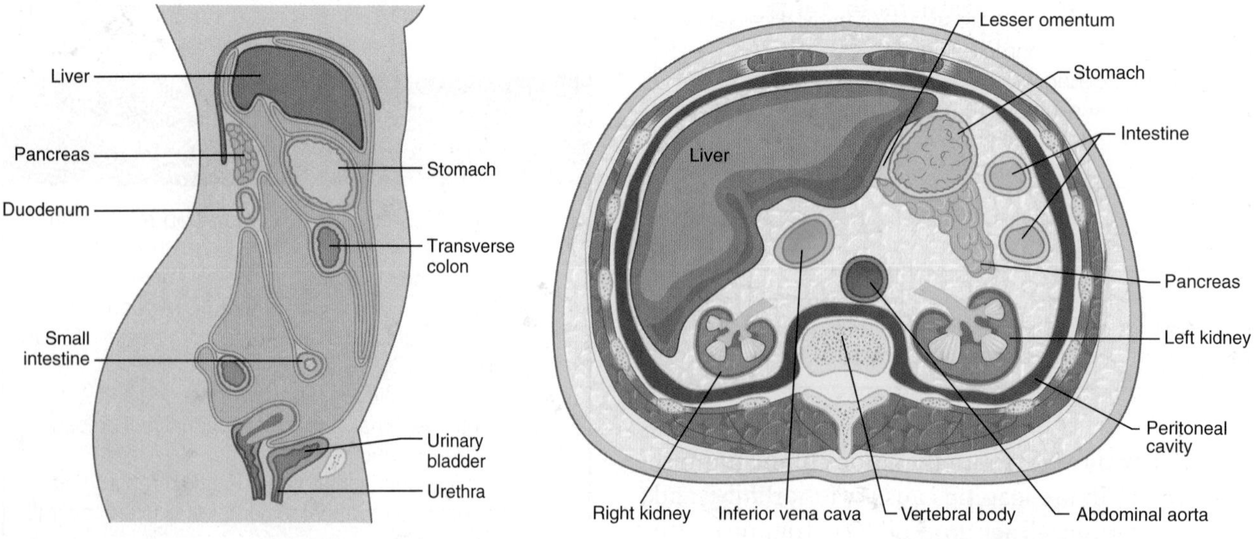

FIGURE 42-4 Hollow, solid, retroperitoneal, and pelvic organs.

be sources of life-threatening hemorrhage. Not all injuries to solid organs require surgical intervention, and many of these injuries are observed carefully in the hospital because bleeding often stops on its own.[3]

Liver

The liver is the largest organ in the abdominal cavity. Because of its location, it often is injured by trauma to the 8th through 12th ribs on the right side of the body as well as by trauma to the upper central part of the abdomen. Injury to the liver should be suspected in any patient with a steering wheel injury, lap belt injury, or history of epigastric trauma. After an injury to the liver, blood and bile escape into the peritoneal cavity, resulting in the signs and symptoms of shock and peritoneal irritation (abdominal pain, referred pain to the right shoulder, tenderness, rigidity).

The liver is the second-most commonly injured intra-abdominal organ, after the spleen. The liver is damaged in approximately 35% to 45% of blunt abdominal trauma cases,[3] and in approximately 30% of cases involving penetrating abdominal trauma.[3] The main cause of liver injury–related death is uncontrolled bleeding, which is associated with a mortality rate of 54%.[4]

Spleen

The spleen lies in the upper left quadrant of the abdomen. It is slightly protected by the organs that surround it medially and anteriorly, and by the lower portion of the rib cage. Injury to the spleen often is associated with other intra-abdominal injuries. Notably, such injury should be suspected in motor vehicle crashes and in falls or sports injuries involving an impact to the lower left chest or flank or to the upper left abdomen. The spleen is damaged in approximately 40% to 55% of cases of blunt abdominal trauma[3] and in approximately 7% of cases of penetrating trauma.[5]

Approximately 40% of patients with splenic injuries have no symptoms. Some may complain of pain in the left shoulder (**Kehr sign**). Pain in the left shoulder or left upper abdomen or generalized abdominal pain is thought to be referred pain that results from irritation of the adjacent diaphragm by a splenic hematoma or **hemoperitoneum**.

Hollow Organ Injury

Injuries to the hollow organs of the abdomen may result in sepsis, wound infection, and abscess formation, particularly if trauma to the intestine remains undiagnosed for an extended period. With injuries to solid organs, hemorrhage is the major cause of symptoms. In contrast, injury to the hollow organs results in spillage of their contents, which may then lead to **peritonitis** (BOX 42-3). Peritonitis usually is acute and quite painful, though its development may be delayed for hours or days after injury to a hollow viscus organ.

Stomach

Because of its protected location in the abdomen, the stomach is not often injured by blunt trauma. Penetrating trauma, however, may cause gastric transection or laceration. Patients with either of these injuries may show signs of peritonitis rather quickly as a result of leakage of acidic gastric contents. The diagnosis of injury to the stomach usually is confirmed during surgery or when nasogastric drainage returns blood. Injuries to the stomach following blunt trauma are associated with the highest mortality of all hollow viscus injuries.[6]

Colon and Small Intestine

The colon and small intestine, like the stomach and duodenum, are more likely to be injured as a result of

BOX 42-3 Peritoneal Irritation

When enzymes, acids, and bacteria spill into the abdominal cavity, they cause chemical irritation of the peritoneum—the membrane that lines the wall of the abdomen and covers the abdominal organs. The pain of peritonitis (inflammation of the peritoneum) usually is localized (via somatic nerve fibers) but may also be diffuse. Signs and symptoms of peritonitis include the following:

- Pain
- Tenderness on percussion, palpation, or cough
- Involuntary guarding or rigidity
- Diminished or absent bowel sounds
- Fever (if untreated)

Note: The adult abdomen can accommodate 3 pints (1.5 L) of fluid without the belly looking bloated (abdominal distention).

Modified from: Daley BJ. Peritonitis and abdominal sepsis. Medscape website. https://emedicine.medscape.com/article/180234-overview. Updated January 11, 2017. Accessed March 15, 2018; and Hertzler AE. Coagulated blood acts as a chemical irritant. In: *The Peritoneum*. Vol 2. St. Louis, MO: C. V. Mosby; 1919:441.

penetrating trauma than through blunt trauma.[3] For example, such an injury may be caused by a gunshot wound to the abdomen or buttocks. In addition, the large bowel and small bowel may be injured by compression forces in high-speed motor vehicle crashes and may sustain deceleration injuries associated with the wearing of personal restraints. Considerable force is required to cause an injury to the colon or small intestine, so other injuries usually are present. Peritoneal contamination with bacteria is a common problem when these organs are ruptured. With blunt abdominal trauma, the colon is damaged in 2% to 5% of cases and the small intestine in 5% to 15% of cases. Intra-abdominal injuries from gunshot wounds tend to involve the small bowel (50%), colon (40%), liver (30%), and abdominal vascular structures (25%).[7]

Retroperitoneal Organ Injury

Injury to the retroperitoneal organs—the kidneys, adrenal glands, ureters, pancreas, duodenum, and esophagus—may occur as a result of blunt or penetrating trauma to the anterior abdomen, posterior abdomen (particularly the flank area), or thoracic spine. Hemorrhage within the retroperitoneal area may be massive and usually results from pelvic or lumbar fractures. Retroperitoneal structures are damaged in approximately 9% of blunt abdominal injury cases and in approximately 11% of cases involving penetrating trauma.[8]

NOTE

Bruising of the flanks (**Grey Turner sign**) or around the umbilicus (**Cullen sign**) may indicate a number of possible problems, including retroperitoneal hemorrhage (**FIGURE 42-5**). These signs usually do not appear immediately, but rather are delayed 12 hours to several days.

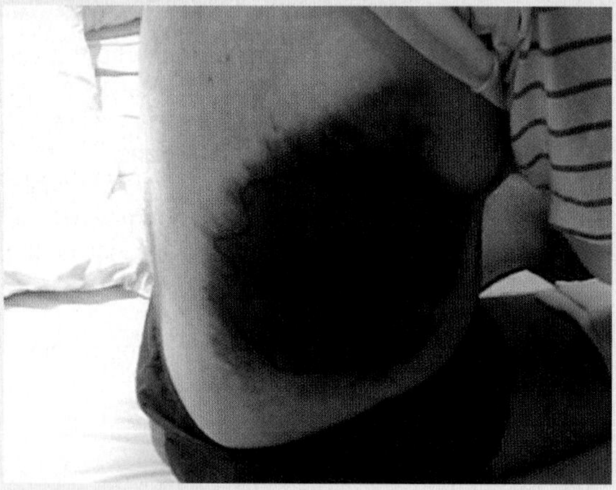

FIGURE 42-5 Bruising caused by rupture of the liver and right kidney.

Reproduced from: Teh, R.W., & Tsoi, D. T. (2012). Acute Disseminated Intravascular Coagulation in Neuroendocrine Carcinoma. Case Reports in Oncology, 5(3), 524–529. http://doi.org/10.1159/000338401

Kidneys

The kidneys are solid organs that lie in the retroperitoneal space; because of their location, they may be injured by abdominal trauma. Such trauma may cause minor lacerations and contusions (**FIGURE 42-6**) as well as major lacerations and fractures to the organ (**FIGURE 42-7**). These injuries can result in hemorrhage, extravasation of urine, or both. Contusions usually are

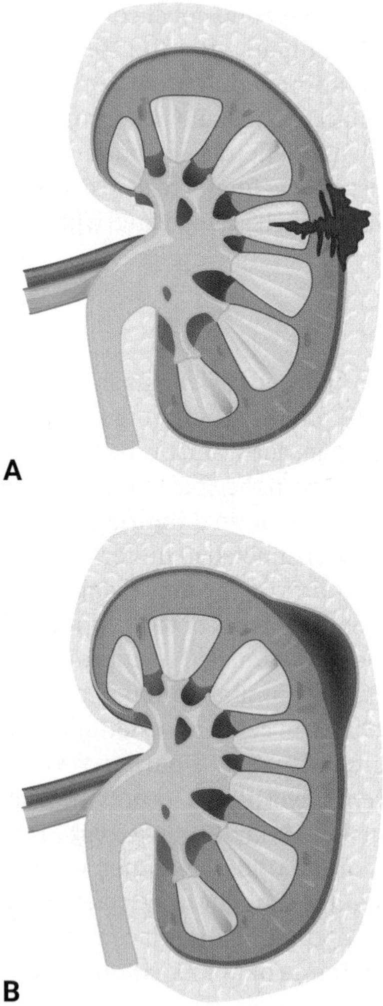

FIGURE 42-6 Minor renal injuries. **A.** Minor renal laceration. **B.** Renal contusion.

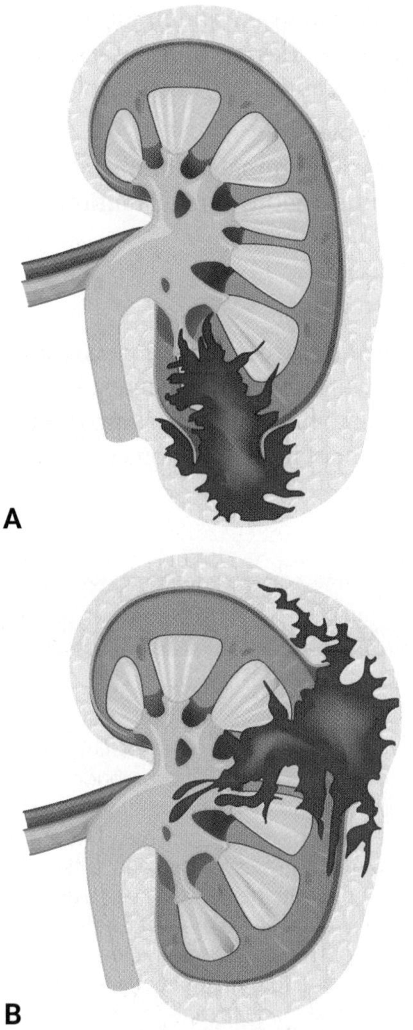

FIGURE 42-7 Major renal lacerations. **A.** Deep medullary laceration. **B.** Laceration into collecting system.

self-limiting and heal with bed rest and forced fluids. Organ fractures and lacerations are more severe and may require surgical repair, depending on which part of the kidney is damaged.

Ureters

The ureters are hollow organs that, because of their flexible structure, are rarely injured by blunt trauma. When injury occurs, it usually is the result of penetrating abdominal or flank wounds (eg, stab wounds, gunshot wounds).

Pancreas

The pancreas is a solid organ that lies within the retroperitoneal space. Injury to the pancreas is rare. When it occurs, it usually is caused by compression or penetrating forces on the upper left quadrant, as in steering wheel and bicycle handlebar impalement. The pancreas more often is injured by penetrating trauma (particularly gunshots) than by blunt trauma.

> CRITICAL THINKING
>
> Which functions of the pancreas may be disrupted after injury? What might be the effects of spillage of pancreatic juices into the abdominal cavity?

Duodenum

The duodenum, which lies across the lumbar spine, is seldom injured. It is largely protected due to its location in the retroperitoneal area, near the pancreas. When great force from blunt trauma or a penetrating injury occurs, however, the duodenum may be crushed or lacerated. Injury to this organ usually is associated with concurrent pancreatic trauma; it is confirmed through surgery.

Pelvic Organ Injury

Injury to pelvic organs (bladder, urethra) usually results from motor vehicle crashes that cause pelvic fractures. Other, less frequent causes of pelvic organ injury are penetrating trauma, straddle-type injuries from falls, pedestrian injuries, and some sexual acts. The pelvis supports and protects multiple organ systems, so the risk of associated injury—especially to the urinary bladder and urethra—is high when it is damaged. Fractures of the pelvis often are associated with severe retroperitoneal hemorrhage. The mortality rate for pelvic fractures ranges from 6.4% to 19%, depending on the severity of the fracture.[8] (Pelvic fractures are further described in Chapter 43, *Orthopaedic Trauma.*)

Urinary Bladder

The urinary bladder is a hollow organ that may be ruptured by blunt trauma, penetrating trauma, or pelvic fracture. Rupture is more likely if the bladder is distended at the time of injury. With rupture, the integrity of the peritoneum may be disrupted so that urine enters the peritoneal cavity. Bladder injury should be suspected in inebriated patients who suffer trauma to the lower abdomen. Gross

hematuria (blood in the urine) may be present, and the patient may complain of being unable to void. The urinary bladder and surrounding structures are damaged in approximately 6% of all cases of abdominal trauma.[8]

Urethra

A tear in the urethra occurs more often in men than in women, and usually results from blunt trauma associated with pelvic fracture. The patient may complain of abdominal pain and of being unable to urinate. Blood at the meatus is highly suggestive of urethral injury. Passage of an indwelling urinary catheter is contraindicated in these patients.

Vascular Structure Injuries

Injuries to arterial and venous vessels in the abdomen can be life threatening because of their potential for massive hemorrhage. These injuries usually are caused by penetrating trauma but also may result from compression or deceleration forces applied to the abdomen. Like solid organ injury, vascular injury usually is marked by hypovolemia. In some cases, vascular injuries are associated with a palpable abdominal mass.

The major vessels most often injured are the aorta, the inferior vena cava, and the renal, mesenteric, and iliac arteries and veins. Injury to these vessels has a high mortality rate, and immediate surgical repair or embolization is often required to save the patient's life.

> CRITICAL THINKING
> How can you attempt to manage shock when major vessels have been injured as a result of a severe pelvic fracture?

Assessment of Abdominal Trauma

The most significant sign of severe abdominal trauma is unexplained shock. The mechanism of injury and the classic presentation of hypovolemia are important indicators that abdominal trauma may have occurred. Other signs and symptoms that should alert the paramedic to the possibility of severe abdominal trauma include abdominal wall injuries (eg, bruising and discoloration of the abdomen, abrasions) and the following:

- Obvious bleeding
- Pain and abdominal tenderness or guarding
- Abdominal rigidity and distention
- **Evisceration** (BOX 42-4)
- Rib fractures
- Pelvic fractures

However, the absence of these signs and symptoms does not rule out an abdominal injury. The paramedic must maintain a high degree of suspicion based on the mechanism of injury.

BOX 42-4 Evisceration

Evisceration is the protrusion of an internal organ or the peritoneal contents through a wound or surgical incision, especially in the abdominal wall (**FIGURE 42-8**). The presence of an evisceration from abdominal trauma generally is associated with major abdominal injury.

In the prehospital setting, this type of wound is managed by covering the eviscerated contents with sterile gauze moistened with normal saline or a dressing with an occlusive outer cover to prevent further contamination and drying. The moist dressing should be covered with a dry dressing to maintain body temperature. No attempt should be made to replace eviscerated organs into the peritoneal cavity, as doing so would increase the risk of infection and complicate surgical evaluation of the injury.

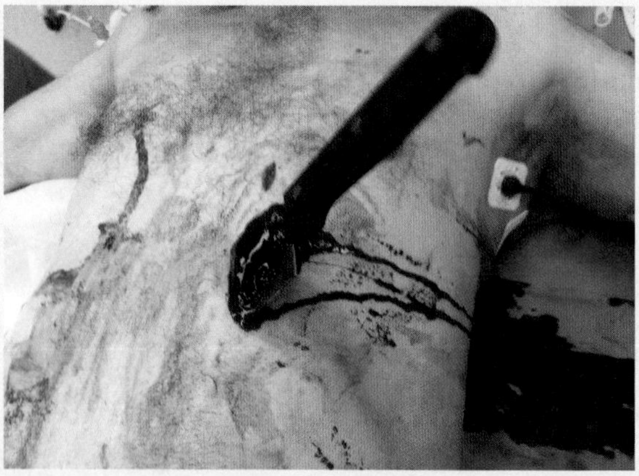

FIGURE 42-8 Abdominal contents that emerged through a stab wound to the abdomen.

Courtesy of Lance Stuke, MD, MPH.

NOTE

Assessment and management of abdominal trauma in children and older adults basically follow the same principles outlined in this chapter. Specific care considerations for pediatric and geriatric patients are presented in Chapter 47, *Pediatrics*, and Chapter 48, *Geriatrics*, respectively. Trauma care considerations for pregnant patients are discussed in Chapter 45, *Obstetrics*. Trauma that results from sexual assault is covered in Chapter 49, *Abuse and Neglect*.

Focused History

When possible, a focused history should be obtained from the patient or a reliable source. Historical facts that may be important include events before the injury (eg, use of seat belts, patient's location in the vehicle), alcohol or other drug use, and underlying medical problems such as diabetes, cardiovascular disease, respiratory disease, or seizure disorder. Medication use (eg, anticoagulants) and drug allergies can also be important in the course of the patient's care.

DID YOU KNOW?

Ultrasonography uses sound waves to make an image (known as a sonogram) of internal organs and structures. This technology is used in the emergency department to view the peritoneal cavity for the presence of fluid or blood. Advantages of ultrasonography are that it can be rapidly performed at the patient's bedside, it does not interfere with resuscitation, and it is noninvasive and less costly than computed tomography. Ultrasonography also does not use ionizing radiation.

The focused assessment with sonography for trauma (FAST) examination is used to rapidly detect intra-abdominal or intrathoracic bleeding. Although this test cannot differentiate the types of fluids that are present, any fluid in the trauma patient is presumed to be blood. The presence of fluid in one or more areas is considered a positive scan. These areas appear black on the monitor screen (**FIGURE 42-9**).

Studies are underway to evaluate the efficacy of sonogram technology in the prehospital setting. Flight nurses and paramedics were found to have moderate accuracy in interpreting the extended FAST (eFAST) examination. In 2014, 4.1% of EMS medical directors reported using ultrasonography within their systems.

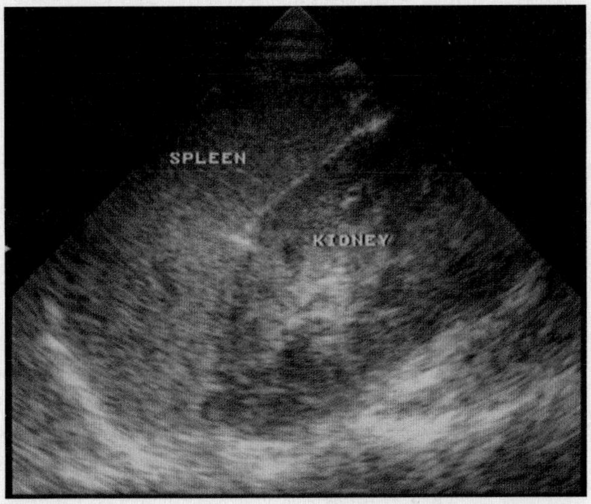

A

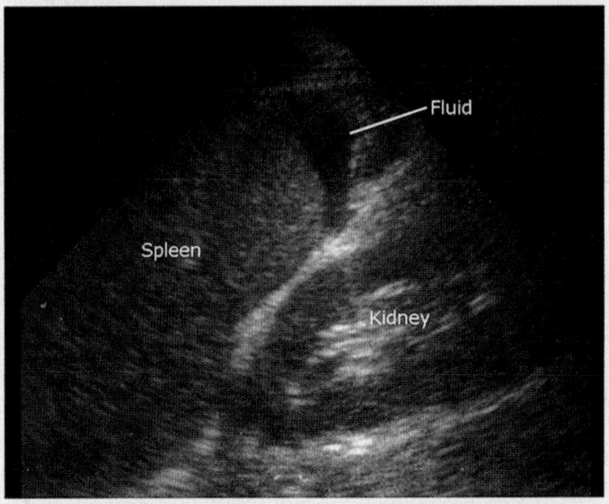

B

FIGURE 42-9 Abdominal ultrasonograms indicating trauma. **A.** Normal splenorenal view. **B.** The presence of fluid (black stripe next to spleen presumed to be blood).

Courtesy of John Kendall, MD.

Modified from: O'Dochartaigh D, Douma M. Prehospital ultrasound of the abdomen and thorax changes trauma patient management: a systematic review. *Injury.* 2015;46(11):2093-2102; Press GM, Miller SK, Hassan IA, et al. Prospective evaluation of prehospital trauma ultrasound during aeromedical transport. *J Emerg Med.* 2014;47(6):638-645; and Taylor J, McLaughlin K, McRae A, Lang E, Anton A. Use of prehospital ultrasound in North America: a survey of emergency medical services medical directors. *BMC Emerg Med.* 2014;14:6.

Management of Abdominal Trauma

Emergency care of patients with abdominal trauma usually is limited to two courses of action: (1) stabilizing the patient's condition and (2) rapidly transporting the patient to a hospital for physician evaluation and surgical repair of the injury.

Oxygen saturation should be maintained at 100% by nonrebreathing mask. The goal of fluid resuscitation for a patient with abdominal injury and hypotension is to maintain a systolic blood pressure between 80 and 90 mm Hg (mean arterial pressure of 60–65 mm Hg).[3] Because aggressive fluid replacement in these patients can reinitiate bleeding in the abdomen from sites that had stopped bleeding as a result of blood clots and hypotension, paramedics should strive to balance perfusion to vital organs without restoring blood pressure to normal limits.

En route to the hospital, a full physical examination and ongoing assessment can be performed. These procedures should include vital signs assessment (and reassessment) and inspection, percussion, and palpation of the abdomen. Auscultation of the abdomen for the presence of bowel sounds can establish a baseline measurement for hospital personnel. This assessment is difficult and time-consuming in the prehospital setting, however, and should never delay patient transport.

SHOW ME THE EVIDENCE

German researchers analyzed data from patients older than 16 years in their trauma registry to evaluate the effects of low-volume versus high-volume fluid resuscitation on patients with solid organ abdominal trauma. In the study, 68 patients were assigned to a low-volume fluid administration group (1–1,000 mL) and 68 patients to the high-volume fluid administration group (≥1,500 mL). The researchers used a matched-pairs method to group pairs based on pattern of injury for solid organs, date of injury, systolic blood pressure at the site of injury, age, intubation status, mode of transport, and transport time. Patients in the high-volume group had significantly lower hemoglobin and platelet counts and were more likely to receive more than 10 units of packed red blood cells than were patients in the lower-volume group. More patients from the high-volume group died in the hospital, although there was not a significant difference.

Modified from: Heuer M, Hussmann B, Lefering R, et al. Prehospital fluid management of abdominal organ trauma patients: a matched pair analysis. *Langenbeck Arch Surg.* 2015;400(3):371-379.

NOTE

Hemodilution is an increase in the fluid content of the blood that results in a lowered concentration of formed elements and lowered blood viscosity. Hemodilution can occur from aggressive intravenous fluid therapy and can affect or disrupt clot formation. After hospital arrival, fluid resuscitation will be guided by serial hematocrit measurements.

Summary

- Blunt trauma to abdominal organs usually results from compression or shearing forces.
- Penetrating injury may result from stab wounds, gunshot wounds, or impaled objects.
- The two solid organs most commonly injured are the liver and the spleen. Both of these organs are primary sources of death from hemorrhage.
- Injuries to the hollow abdominal organs may result in sepsis, wound infection, and abscess formation.
- Injury to the retroperitoneal organs (kidneys, ureters, pancreas, duodenum) may cause massive hemorrhage.
- Injury to the pelvic organs (bladder, urethra) usually results from motor vehicle crashes that produce pelvic fractures.
- Injuries to abdominal vascular structures may be life threatening due to their potential for massive hemorrhage.
- The most significant sign of severe abdominal trauma is the presence of unexplained shock.
- Emergency care of patients with abdominal trauma usually is limited to two courses of action: (1) stabilizing the patient and (2) rapidly transporting the patient to a hospital for surgery to repair the injury.

References

1. National Highway Traffic Safety Administration. *The National EMS Education Standards.* Washington, DC: US Department of Transportation, National Highway Traffic Safety Administration; 2009.
2. Walls R, Hockberger R, Gausche-Hill M. *Rosen's Emergency Medicine: Concepts and Clinical Practice*. 9th ed. Philadelphia, PA: Elsevier; 2017.

3. National Association of Emergency Medical Technicians. *PHTLS: Prehospital Trauma Life Support.* 8th ed. Burlington, MA: Jones & Bartlett Learning; 2014.
4. Slotta JE, Justinger C, Kollmar O, Kollmar C, Schäfer T, Schilling MK. Liver injury following blunt abdominal trauma: a new mechanism-driven classification. *Surg Today.* 2014;44(2): 241-246.
5. Waseem M, Bjerke S. Splenic injury. In: *StatPearls* [Internet]. National Center for Biotechnology Information website. https://www.ncbi.nlm.nih.gov/books/NBK441993/. Updated June 26, 2017. Accessed March 15, 2018.
6. Aboobakar MR, Singh JP, Maharaj K, Mewa Kinoo S, Singh B. Gastric perforation following blunt abdominal trauma. *Trauma Case Rep.* 2017;10:12-15.
7. Offner P. Penetrating abdominal trauma. Medscape website. https://emedicine.medscape.com/article/2036859-overview. Updated January 13, 2017. Accessed March 15, 2018.
8. Peitzman AB, Schwab CW, Yealy DM, Rhodes M, Fabian TC, eds. *The Trauma Manual: Trauma and Acute Care Surgery.* 4th ed. Philadelphia, PA: Lippincott; 2013.

Suggested Readings

Chenoweth JA, Diercks DB. ACEP clinical policy: blunt abdominal trauma. ACEP Now website. http://www.acepnow.com/article/acep-clinical-policy-blunt-abdominal-trauma. Published May 1, 2011. Accessed March 15, 2018.

Hodnick R. Penetrating trauma wounds challenge EMS providers. *JEMS* website. http://www.jems.com/articles/print/volume-37/issue-4/patient-care/penetrating-trauma-wounds-challenge-ems.html. Published March 30, 2012. Accessed March 15, 2018.

Moore E, Feliciano D, Mattox KL. *Trauma*. 8th ed. New York, NY: McGraw-Hill; 2017.

Ruesseler M, Kirschning T, Breitkreutz R, et al. Prehospital and emergency department ultrasound in blunt abdominal trauma. *Eur J Trauma Emerg Surg.* 2009;35:341-346.

Zygowicz WM. Anything but routine: responders answer unprecedented evisceration call. *JEMS* website. http://www.jems.com/articles/print/volume-33/issue-7/patient-care/anything-routine-responders-an.html. Published December 31, 2007. Accessed March 15, 2018.

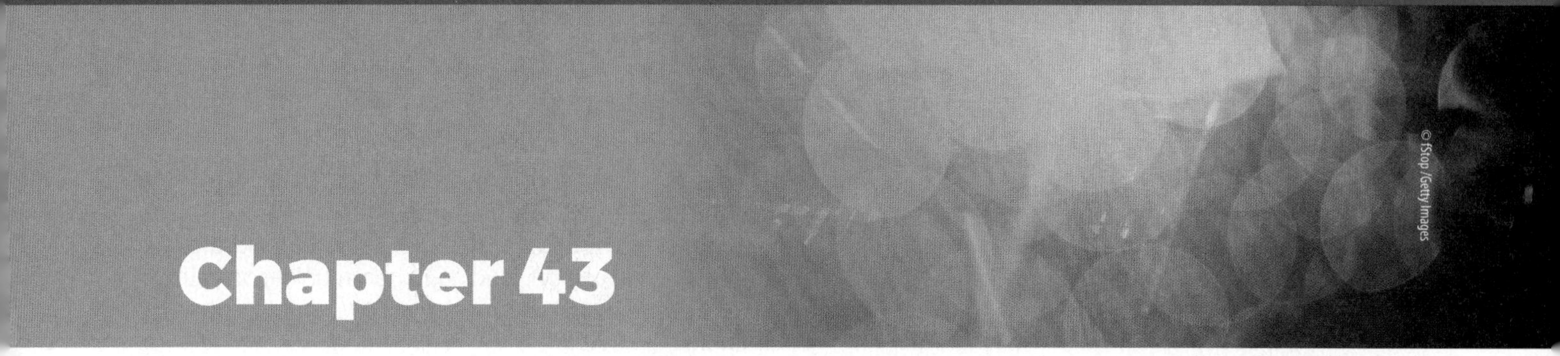

Chapter 43

Orthopaedic Trauma

NATIONAL EMS EDUCATION STANDARD COMPETENCIES

Trauma

Integrates assessment findings with principles of epidemiology and pathophysiology to formulate a field impression to implement a comprehensive treatment/disposition plan for an acutely injured patient.

Orthopaedic Trauma

Recognition and management of
- Open fractures (pp 1522–1523, 1538–1540)
- Closed fractures (pp 1522–1523, 1525–1538)
- Dislocations (pp 1524–1525, 1527–1530, 1532–1537, 1540)
- Amputations (see Chapter 37, *Bleeding and Soft-Tissue Trauma*)

Pathophysiology, assessment, and management of
- Upper and lower extremity orthopaedic trauma (pp 1528–1538)
- Open fractures (pp 1523, 1538–1540)
- Closed fractures (pp 1522–1523, 1525–1538)
- Dislocations (pp 1524–1525, 1527–1530, 1532–1537, 1540)
- Sprains/strains (pp 1522, 1524)
- Pelvic fractures (p 1534)
- Amputations/replantation (see Chapter 37, *Bleeding and Soft-Tissue Trauma*)
- Compartment syndrome (pp 1530, 1537)
- Pediatric fractures (see Chapter 47, *Pediatrics*)
- Tendon laceration/transection/rupture (Achilles and patellar) (p 1537)

Medicine

Integrates assessment findings with principles of epidemiology and pathophysiology to formulate a field impression and implement a comprehensive treatment/disposition plan for a patient with a medical complaint.

Nontraumatic Musculoskeletal Disorders

Anatomy, physiology, pathophysiology, assessment, and management of
- Nontraumatic fractures (see Chapter 32, *Nontraumatic Musculoskeletal Disorders*)

Anatomy, physiology, epidemiology, pathophysiology, psychosocial impact, presentations, prognosis, and management of common or major nontraumatic musculoskeletal disorders, including
- Disorders of the spine (see Chapter 40, *Spine and Nervous System Trauma*)
- Joint abnormalities (see Chapter 32, *Nontraumatic Musculoskeletal Disorders*)
- Muscle abnormalities (see Chapter 32, *Nontraumatic Musculoskeletal Disorders*)
- Overuse syndromes (see Chapter 32, *Nontraumatic Musculoskeletal Disorders*)

OBJECTIVES

Upon completion of this chapter, the paramedic student will be able to:
1. Describe the features of each class of musculoskeletal injury. (pp 1522–1524)
2. Describe the signs and symptoms of musculoskeletal injuries. (p 1525)
3. Outline the prehospital assessment and management of musculoskeletal injuries. (pp 1525–1528)
4. Outline general principles of splinting. (p 1526)
5. Describe the significance and prehospital management principles for selected upper extremity injuries. (pp 1528–1532)
6. Describe the significance and prehospital management principles for selected lower extremity injuries. (pp 1532–1538)
7. Identify prehospital management priorities for open fractures. (pp 1538–1540)
8. Describe the limited circumstances in which an attempt to realign an angular fracture or dislocation might be made. (p 1540)

KEY TERMS

Achilles tendon The largest tendon in the body; connects the calf muscle to the heel bone; also known as the tendon calcaneus.

Achilles tendon rupture A complete tear through the Achilles tendon.

appendicular skeleton The bones of the upper and lower extremities.

axial skeleton The bones of the head, neck, and torso.

boxer's fracture Fracture of the fifth metacarpal bone at the distal metaphysis from direct trauma to a closed fist.

buddy splinting Immobilization of an injured finger or toe to an adjoining finger or toe with padding and tape, such that the uninjured digit acts as a splint; also known as buddy wrapping.

Colles fracture A fracture of the radius at the epiphysis within 1 inch (3 cm) of the joint of the wrist, resulting in an upward (posterior) displacement of the radius and obvious deformity.

epiphyseal fracture A fracture involving the epiphyseal plate of a long bone.

epiphyseal plate The site of bone elongation; also known as the growth plate.

fall on an outstretched hand A common mechanism of injury that occurs when people attempt to break a fall by catching themselves with the palm of their hand, resulting in hand, wrist, elbow, or shoulder injury.

false movement An unnatural movement of an extremity, usually associated with fracture.

first-degree sprain An injury in which there is stretching of a ligament without joint disability. There is minimal, if any, associated swelling.

fracture A break in the continuity of bone.

joint dislocation An injury that occurs when the normal articulating ends of two or more bones are displaced.

luxation A complete dislocation.

nursemaid's elbow Subluxation of the radial head that generally occurs in children from the time they start to walk to early school age (2 to 5 years of age).

open fracture A break in a bone that has penetrated the soft tissue or skin, leading to communication with the outside environment; formerly known as compound fracture.

poikilothermia The inability to maintain a constant core temperature independent of ambient temperature.

rigid splint A splint in which the shape cannot be changed.

second-degree sprain An injury that results from some stretching and tearing of ligaments. Swelling and pain are more pronounced.

soft splint A splint that can be molded into a variety of shapes and configurations to accommodate the injured body part.

sprain An injury to a ligament due to mechanical force.

strain An injury to the muscle or its tendon from overexertion or overextension.

subluxation A partial dislocation.

third-degree sprain An injury that results from severe stretching and tearing of ligaments such that the ligament is completely ruptured with significant associated swelling and possible joint dislocation.

torus fracture The buckling of the cortex of bone due to a unicortical fracture in immature bone.

traction splint A splinting device, most commonly used for femoral fractures, that provides a counterpull to reduce pain, realign the fracture, and minimize bleeding complications.

Volkmann contracture A serious, persistent flexion contraction of the forearm and hand caused by posttraumatic ischemia specifically as a result of compartment syndrome.

Orthopaedic trauma and related complications are very common complaints. These injuries account for a large number of the more than 100 million patients in the United States who seek emergency department care each year.[1] Trauma to an extremity is seldom life threatening, but early recognition and management may prevent long-term disability.

Review of the Musculoskeletal System

As described in Chapter 10, *Review of Human Systems*, the musculoskeletal system and associated neurovascular structures are made up of bones, nerves, vessels, muscles, tendons, ligaments, and joints. To review, the skeletal system contains 206 individual bones, which are organized into two categories: the axial skeleton and the appendicular skeleton (**FIGURE 43-1**). The **axial skeleton** consists of the skull, hyoid bone, vertebral column, and thoracic cage.

The **appendicular skeleton** consists of the bones of the upper and lower extremities plus the girdles, by which the extremities are attached to the body.

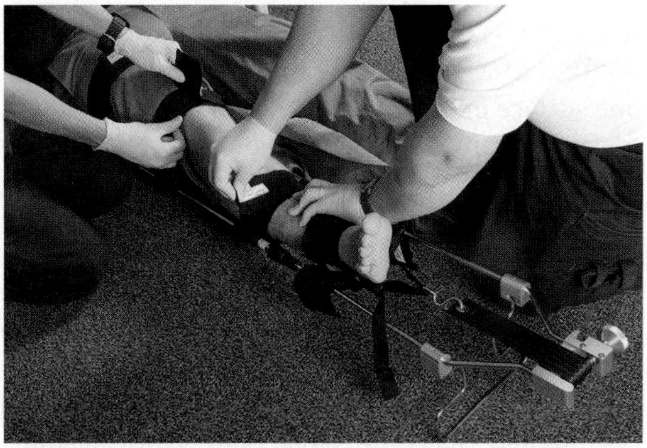

The muscular system provides for movement, postural maintenance (muscle tone), and heat production. The major types of muscles are skeletal, cardiac, and smooth. Skeletal muscle—the most common type of muscle in the body—is the focus of this chapter (**FIGURE 43-2**).

NOTE

Extremity trauma often results from motor vehicle crashes, falls, acts of violence, and contact sports. Prevention strategies include proper sports training (working with athletic trainers on the use of protective equipment), use of personal restraints, gun safety education, and fall prevention (eg, high-rise window guards) (see Chapter 3, *Injury Prevention, Health Promotion, and Public Health*).

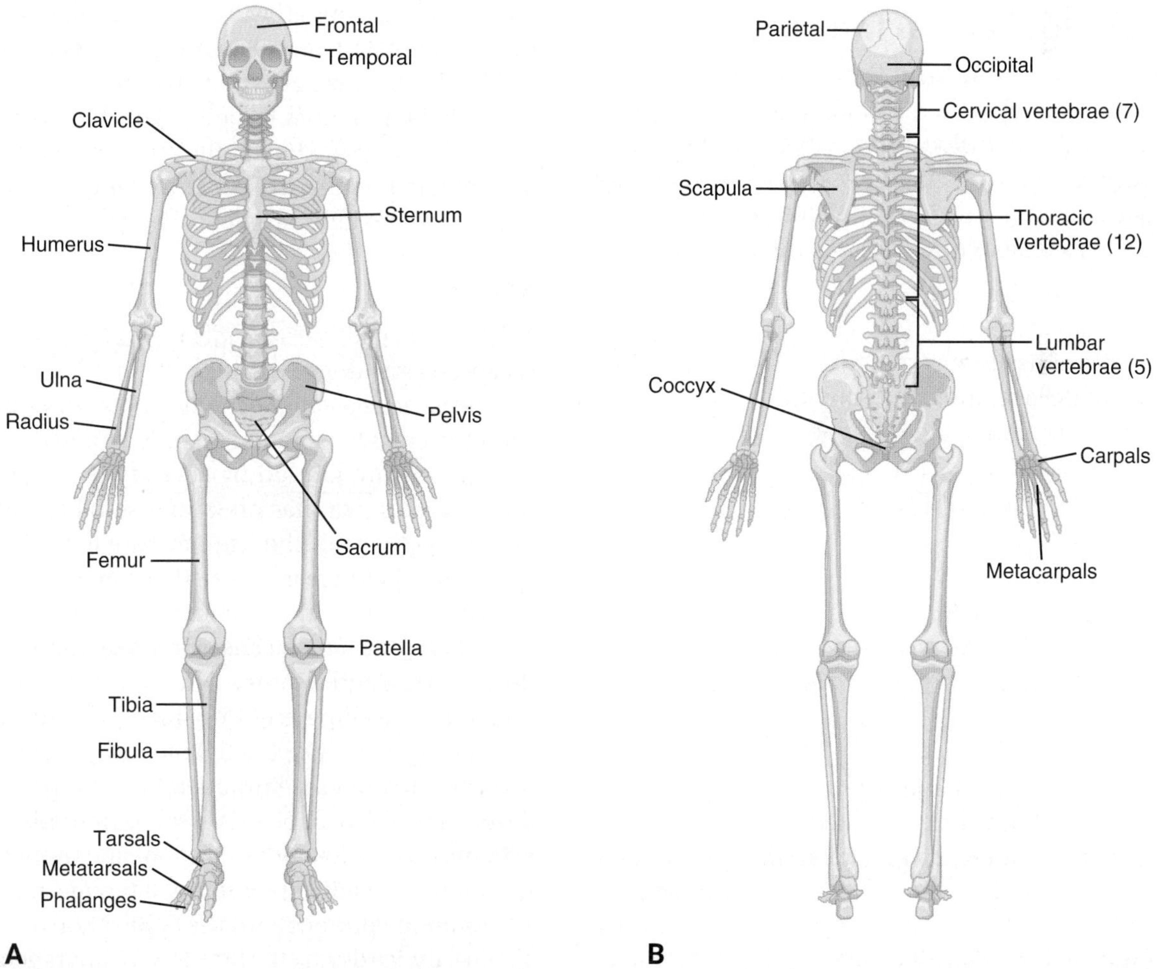

FIGURE 43-1 The axial (blue) and appendicular (bone color) skeleton. **A.** Anterior view. **B.** Posterior view.

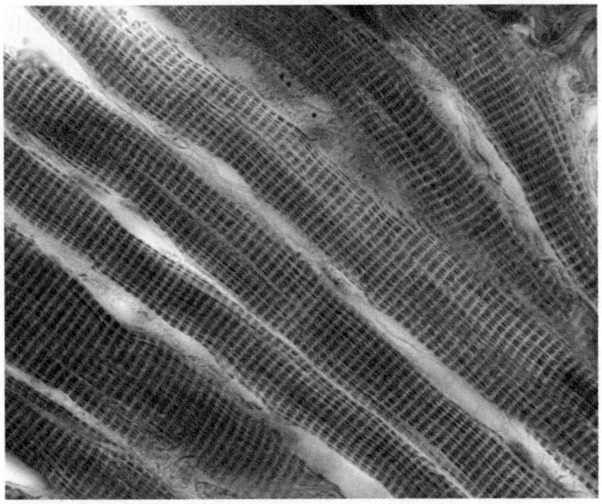

FIGURE 43-2 Skeletal muscle.

Classifications of Musculoskeletal Injuries

Injuries that result from traumatic forces to the musculoskeletal system include fractures, sprains, strains, and joint dislocations. Patients suspected of having trauma to an extremity should be managed as though a fracture exists. Problems associated with musculoskeletal injuries include the following:

- Hemorrhage
- Instability
- Loss of tissue
- Simple laceration and contamination
- Interruption of blood supply
- Nerve damage
- Long-term disability

> CRITICAL THINKING
> How could long-term disability result from a musculoskeletal injury?

Musculoskeletal injuries can result from direct trauma (eg, blunt force applied to an extremity), indirect trauma (eg, a vertical fall that produces a spinal fracture distant from the site of impact), or pathologic conditions such as some forms of arthritis and malignancy (described in Chapter 32, *Nontraumatic Musculoskeletal Disorders*). Paramedics should consider kinematics when caring for a patient with a musculoskeletal injury and carefully evaluate the scene and the mechanism of injury (see Chapter 36, *Trauma Overview and Mechanism of Injury*).

Fractures

A **fracture** is any break in the continuity of bone (**FIGURE 43-3**). It may be complete (traversing from one surface of bone to another) or incomplete (not traversing from one surface of bone to another). Fractures also are classified as open or closed, depending on the fracture and communication with the outside environment (BOX 43-1). Fractures of long bones may result in moderate to severe hemorrhage within the first 2 hours. As much as 550 mL of blood may be released in the lower leg from a tibial or fibular fracture, 1,000 mL of blood in the thigh from a femoral fracture, and 2,000 mL of blood from a pelvic fracture.[1]

As described in Chapter 10, *Review of Human Systems*, the head of long bones in children is separated from the shaft of the bone by the **epiphyseal plate** until the bone stops growing. A fracture that involves the epiphyseal plate, called an **epiphyseal fracture**, can be serious because it involves the growth plate and has the potential for joint growth deformity. A **torus fracture** (buckling of the cortex of bone) is an incomplete fracture in immature long bone and is generally of no long-term consequence.

Sprains

A **sprain** is an injury of a ligament (**FIGURE 43-4**), which is caused by sudden twisting or stretching of a joint beyond its normal range of motion (**FIGURE 43-5**). Two common areas for sprains are the knee and the ankle.

Sprains are graded by severity (BOX 43-2). A **first-degree sprain** has no joint instability, because only a few fibers of the ligament are torn. Swelling and hemorrhage are minimal. (Repeated first-degree sprains can result in stretching of the ligaments.) A **second-degree sprain** causes more disruption than does a first-degree injury. The joint usually is still intact, but swelling and bruising are increased. In a **third-degree sprain**, the ligaments are completely torn. If third-degree sprains are accompanied by dislocation, nerve or blood vessel compromise to the extremity is possible. Some second- and third-degree sprains have a similar presentation to some fractures.

Although protocols for the application of ice to a sprain vary, ice during the first 24 to 72 hours generally reduces the pain and swelling associated with this type of injury. After that time, heat (eg, warm soaks) often is prescribed to increase circulation and reduce stiffness.

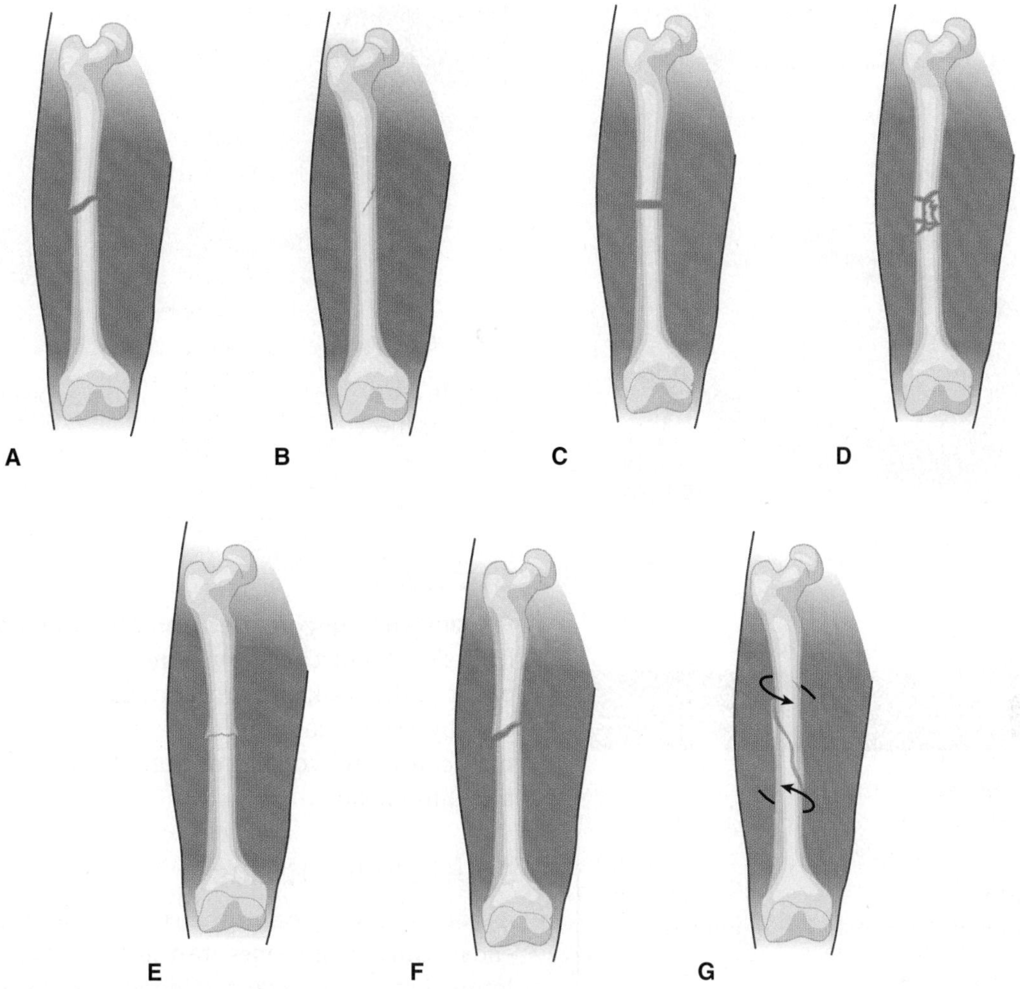

FIGURE 43-3 Types of bone fractures. **A.** Complete. **B.** Incomplete. **C.** Transverse. **D.** Comminuted. **E.** Impacted. **F.** Oblique. **G.** Spiral.

BOX 43-1 Classification of Fractures

- **Open.** A break in which a protruding bone or penetrating object causes a soft-tissue injury that communicates with the fracture.
- **Closed.** A break in the bone that has not yet penetrated the soft tissue or skin.
- **Comminuted.** A fracture that involves several breaks in the bone, resulting in multiple bone fragments. This is a rare occurrence in children.
- **Greenstick.** A break in which the bone is bent but only broken on the outside of the bend (common in children).
- **Spiral.** A break caused by a rotational force applied to the long axis of a bone where the broken bone resembles a corkscrew on radiography. This twisted or circular break affects the length rather than the width. It is seen frequently in child abuse.
- **Oblique.** A break that occurs at a diagonal or slanting angle between the horizontal and perpendicular planes of the bone.
- **Transverse.** A break or fracture line that occurs at right angles to the long axis of the bone.
- **Stress.** A break (especially in one or more of the foot bones) caused by repeated, long-term, or abnormal stress.
- **Pathologic.** A fracture through abnormal bone from a force that would not be expected break normal bone, such as a break through osteoporotic bone.
- **Epiphyseal.** A break that involves the epiphyseal growth plate of a child's long bone; it may result in permanent angulation or growth arrest or deformity and may cause premature arthritis.

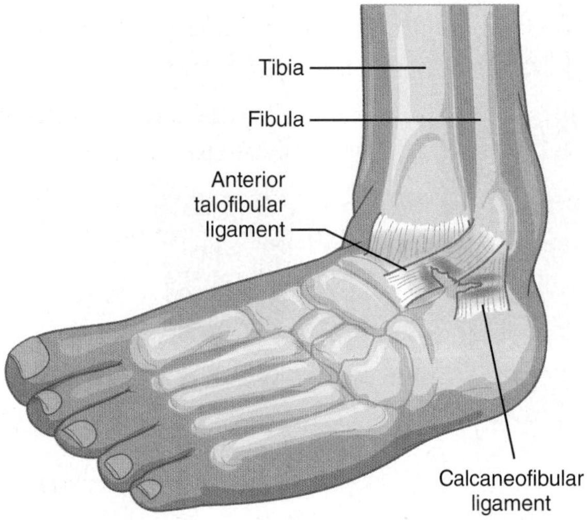

FIGURE 43-4 Ankle sprain.

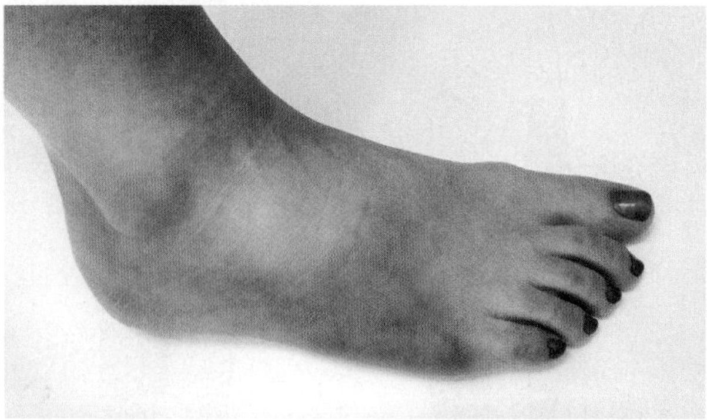

FIGURE 43-5 Swelling and bruising from a sprain of a lateral ligament.

BOX 43-2 Grading of Sprains by Severity

First-Degree Sprain
No joint instability
Minimal swelling/hemorrhage

Second-Degree Sprain
Joint usually intact
Increased swelling/ecchymosis

Third-Degree Sprain
Total disruption of ligaments
Possible nerve or vascular compromise

NOTE

Ice should be placed in a plastic bag and applied, through gauze or a cloth, for 20-minute periods to the injury site, removed for 20 minutes, and then reapplied. If ice is not available, refreezable packs of gelled solution can be used in the short term and may provide some comfort and reduce swelling. Ice should never be applied directly to the skin.

Strains

A **strain** is an injury to the muscle or its tendon from overexertion or overextension. Strains commonly occur in the back and arms and may be accompanied by a significant loss of function. Severe strains may cause an avulsion of bone from the tendon attachment site.

Joint Dislocations

A **joint dislocation** occurs when the normal articulating ends of two or more bones are displaced (**FIGURE 43-6**). Joints that are especially vulnerable to dislocations include those of the shoulders, elbows, fingers, hips, knees, and ankles. Dislocation should be suspected when a joint is deformed or does not move with normal range of motion. A complete dislocation is called a **luxation**; an incomplete dislocation is called a **subluxation**. All dislocations can result in great damage and instability.

CRITICAL THINKING

Why do dislocations have a high rate of vascular or nerve damage?

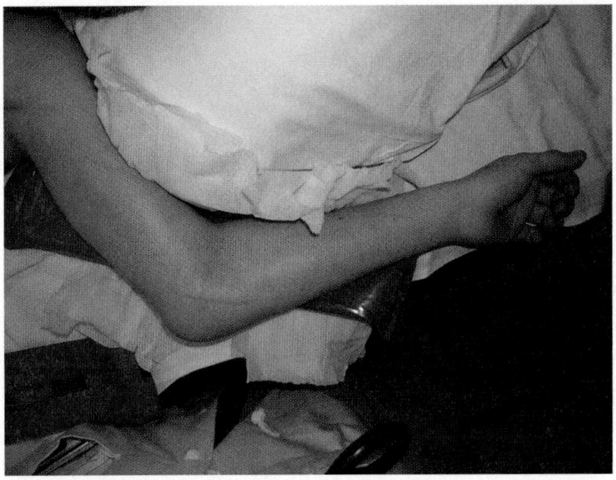

FIGURE 43-6 Clinical appearance of an elbow dislocation.

Signs and Symptoms of Extremity Trauma

The signs and symptoms of trauma to an extremity vary from subtle complaints of discomfort to obvious deformity or open fracture. Field evaluation should be rapid, with the paramedic assuming the patient has a significant injury. Common signs and symptoms of extremity trauma include the following:

- Pain on palpation or movement
- Swelling or deformity
- Crepitus
- Decreased range of motion
- **False movement** (unnatural movement of an extremity)
- Decreased or absent sensory perception or circulation distal to the injury (evidenced by alterations in skin color and temperature, distal pulses, and capillary refill)

CRITICAL THINKING

How can a paramedic differentiate a serious sprain from a fracture in the prehospital setting?

Assessment and Management of Musculoskeletal Injuries

For the purposes of musculoskeletal assessment, patients can be categorized into four classes:

- Those with life- or limb-threatening injuries or conditions, including life- or limb-threatening musculoskeletal trauma
- Those with other life- or limb-threatening vascular injuries and only simple musculoskeletal trauma
- Those with no other life- or limb-threatening injuries but with life- or limb-threatening musculoskeletal trauma
- Those with only isolated injuries that are not life or limb threatening

The paramedic should perform a primary survey to determine whether the patient has any conditions that pose a threat to life. Such conditions must be dealt with first. Paramedics must never overlook musculoskeletal trauma. In addition, a grotesque, but noncritical, musculoskeletal injury should never distract from the priorities of care.

NOTE

Orthopaedic trauma can be very painful. Ideally, the paramedic should address pain prior to moving the patient. Protocols established by medical direction for the use of analgesics to manage pain in patients of all ages are an important aspect of care for these patients.

Modified from: Kiviehan S, Friedman BT, Mercer MP. Orthopedic injuries. In: Brice J, Delbriddge TR, Meyers JB, eds. *Emergency Services Clinical Practice and Systems Oversight.* Vol 1. West Sussex, UK: John Wiley & Sons; 2015:272-279.

Evaluation of an injured extremity should always include checking the "six Ps": pain, pallor, paresthesia, pulselessness, paralysis, and **poikilothermia** (BOX 43-3). The paramedic also should evaluate an extremity's neurovascular status by assessing the distal pulse, motor

SHOW ME THE EVIDENCE

Baltimore researchers retrospectively examined the records of children from birth to age 18 years transferred to their tertiary pediatric center from community hospitals. They attempted to identify risk factors for secondary transfer of stable pediatric patients to their facility as compared to a control group. The three top diagnoses were seizure, orthopaedic injuries, and asthma and/or respiratory distress. Of the patients with orthopaedic injuries who were transferred, 69% had a deformity. The median transport distance to the community hospital was 4.7 miles (7.6 km), whereas the median transfer distance to the pediatric specialty hospital was 16.8 miles (27.0 km). If the patient had been transported directly to the pediatric specialty hospital, the median distance would have been 16.9 miles (27.2 km). The median time to deciding to transfer was 108 minutes, and the median wait time until EMS personnel arrived for the transfer was 90 minutes. Almost one-half of the children had duplicated diagnostic tests at the pediatric specialty center. Older age was associated with decreased interfacility transfer of orthopaedic injuries. The authors suggest that more-specific direct transport protocols be developed within their EMS systems.

Modified from: Fishe JN, Psoter KJ, Klein BL, Anders JF. Retrospective evaluation of risk factors for pediatric secondary transport. *Prehosp Emerg Care.* 2018;22(1):41-49.

BOX 43-3 Six Ps of Musculoskeletal Assessment

- **P**ain or tenderness
- **P**allor (pale skin or poor capillary refill)
- **P**aresthesia (pins-and-needles sensation)
- **P**ulselessness (diminished or absent)
- **P**aralysis (inability to move)
- **P**oikilothermia

function, and sensation (before and after movement or splinting). In addition, the injury should be inspected and palpated for surface trauma, tenderness, and swelling. If possible, the assessment should include comparison with the opposite, uninjured extremity. If trauma to an extremity is suspected, the extremity should be splinted (**FIGURE 43-7**).

NOTE

This text presents methods to immobilize fractures and dislocations for isolated extremity injuries. As noted earlier, seldom does trauma to an extremity pose a threat to life. Therefore patients with multiple-system traumatic injury should first be managed for conditions that compromise the airway, breathing, and circulation (including internal and external hemorrhage in the extremities) and spinal stability. Rapid transport may be indicated based on the patient's condition or mechanism of injury. In these extreme situations, injured extremities can be stabilized by fully immobilizing the patient on a long backboard.

General Principles of Splinting

The goal of splinting is to immobilize the injured body part. Immobilization by splinting helps alleviate pain; decreases tissue injury, bleeding, and contamination of an open wound; and simplifies and facilitates transport of the patient. The general principles of splinting are listed in **BOX 43-4**. Note that the principles of splinting and immobilization are the same for both children and adults. Special considerations for managing pediatric and geriatric patients are addressed in Chapter 47, *Pediatrics*, and Chapter 48, *Geriatrics*, respectively.

Types of Splints

A wide variety of splints and splinting materials are available. Splints can be broadly categorized as rigid splints, soft or formable splints, and traction splints.

The shape of a **rigid splint** cannot be changed; thus, the body part must be positioned to fit the splint's design. Examples of rigid splints include board splints, contoured metal and plastic splints, and some cardboard splints (**FIGURE 43-8**). Rigid splints should be padded before use to accommodate the shape of the injured body part and to decrease patient discomfort.

A **soft splint** or formable splint can be molded into a variety of shapes and configurations to accommodate the injured body part. Examples of soft or formable splints include pillows, blankets, slings and swathes, vacuum splints, some cardboard splints,

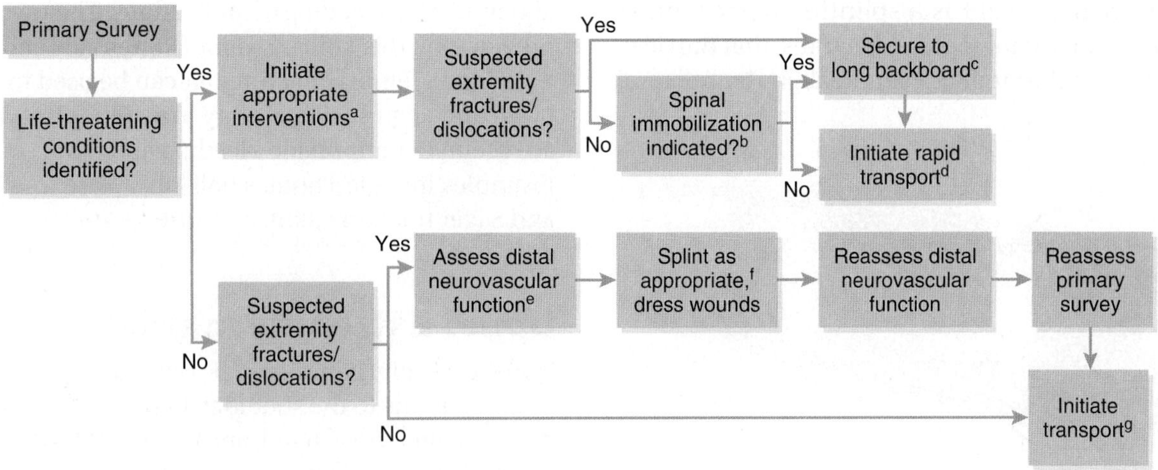

[a]Airway management, ventilatory support, shock therapy.
[b]See Indications for Spinal Immobilization algorithm.
[c]Injured extremities are immobilized in anatomic position by securing to long backboard.
[d]Transport to closest appropriate facility (trauma center, if available); assess distal neurovascular function and apply traction splint (if suspected femur fracture) as time permits.
[e]Assess perfusion (pulses and capillary refilling) and neurologic function (motor and sensory) distal to the suspected fracture or dislocation.
[f]Use appropriate splinting technique to immobilize suspected fracture or dislocation; if suspected midshaft femur fracture, apply traction splint.
[g]Transport to closest appropriate facility.

FIGURE 43-7 Evaluating extremity trauma.

BOX 43-4 General Principles of Splinting

1. Splint joints and bone ends above and below the injury.
2. Immobilize open and closed fractures in the same manner.
3. Cover open fractures to minimize contamination.
4. Check and document pulses, sensation, and motor function before and after splinting. Recheck frequently.
5. Stabilize the extremity with gentle in-line traction to a position of normal alignment.
6. Immobilize a long bone extremity in a straight position that can be splinted easily.
7. Immobilize dislocations in a position of comfort; ensure good vascular supply.
8. Immobilize joints as found; joint injuries are aligned only if no distal pulse is felt.
9. Apply cold to reduce swelling and pain. Give analgesics per protocol.
10. Apply compression to reduce swelling.
11. Elevate the extremity if possible.

Note: Immobilization requires a minimum of two rescuers. All splints should be well padded for patient comfort. *These principles should be employed in caring for all types of extremity trauma described in this chapter.*

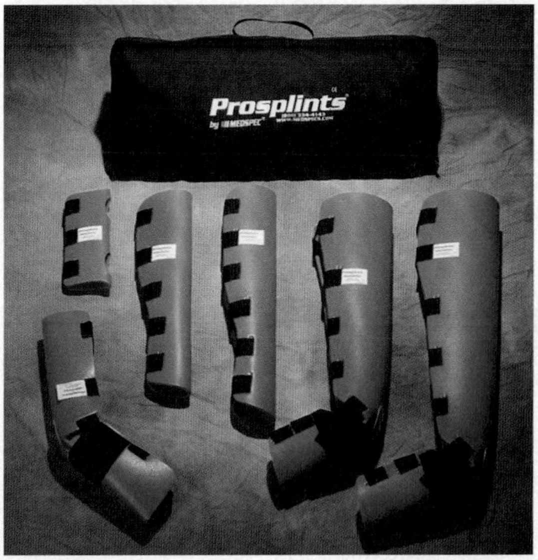

FIGURE 43-8 Rigid splints.

wire ladder splints, and padded, flexible aluminum splints (**FIGURE 43-9**). Inflatable air splints also are considered soft or formable splints, but they are not designed to be used for injuries to the knee or elbow.

A **traction splint** is a splinting device, most commonly used for femoral fractures, that provides a counterpull to reduce pain, realign the fracture, and minimize bleeding complications. The traction provided by this kind of splint is often not enough to reduce a femoral fracture but can be used to stabilize and align such an injury. Traction splints also are useful to tamponade bleeding and reduce pain. Examples include Thomas half-ring, Hare traction, and Sager traction splints (**FIGURE 43-10**).

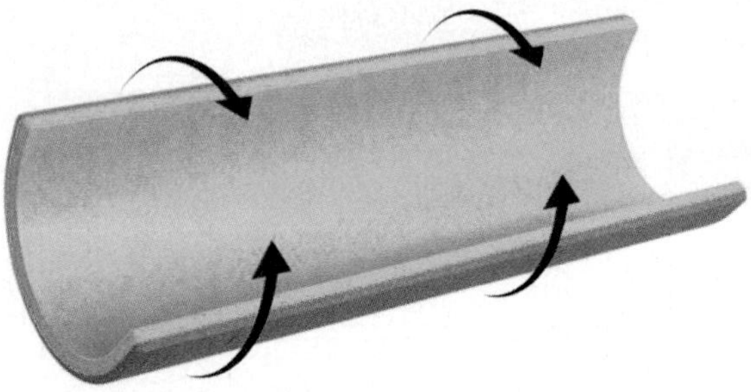

FIGURE 43-9 Formable splints.

Upper Extremity Injuries

Upper extremity injuries can be classified as fractures or dislocations to the shoulder, humerus, elbow, radius and ulna, wrist, hand, and finger (**FIGURE 43-11**). Clavicular injury is discussed in Chapter 41, *Chest Trauma.* Most upper extremity injuries can be adequately immobilized with a sling and swathe.

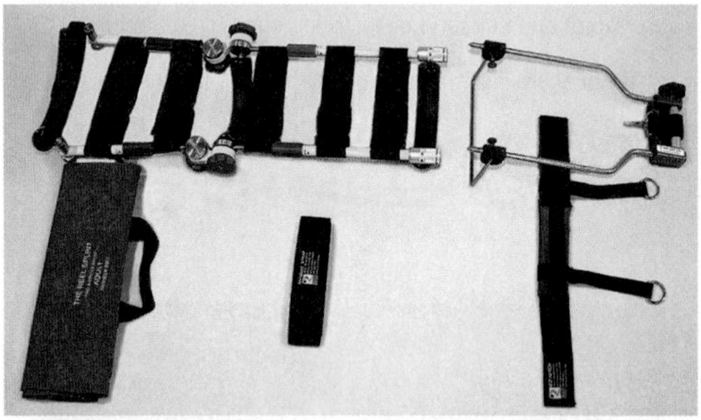

A

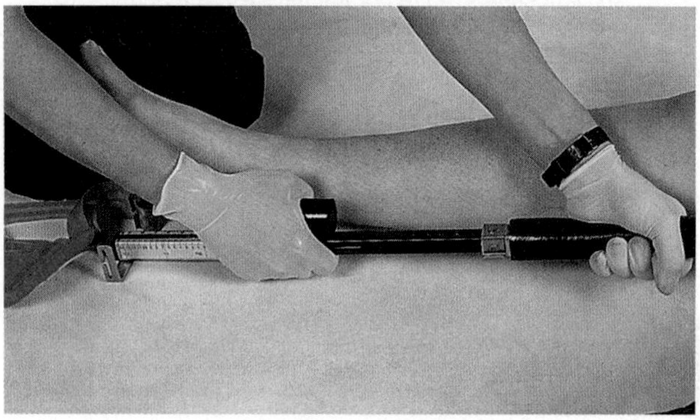

B

FIGURE 43-10 **A.** Traction splints. **B.** Unipolar traction splint.

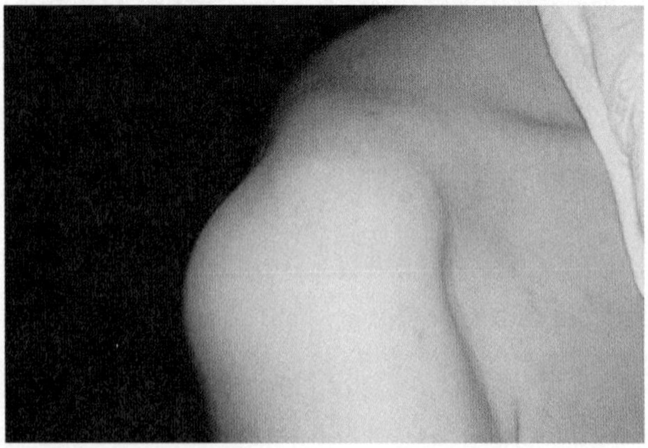

A

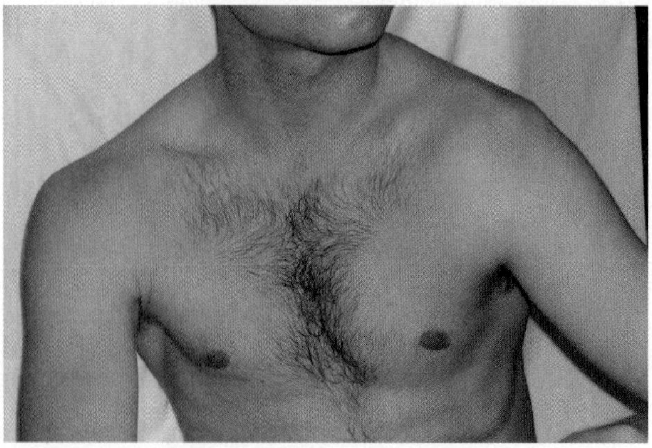

B

FIGURE 43-11 **A.** Complete separation of the right acromioclavicular joint. **B.** Anterior dislocation of the left shoulder.

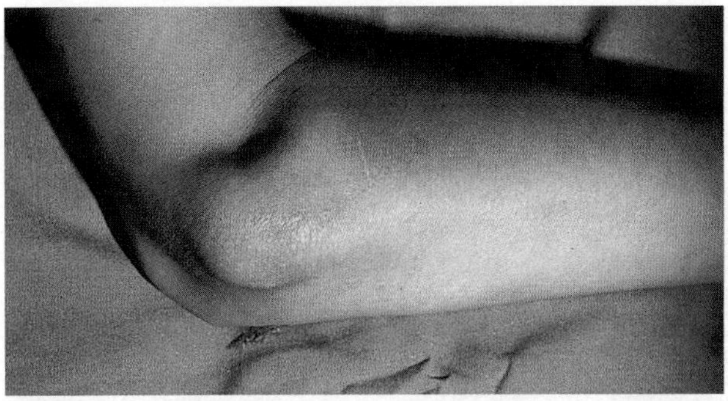

C

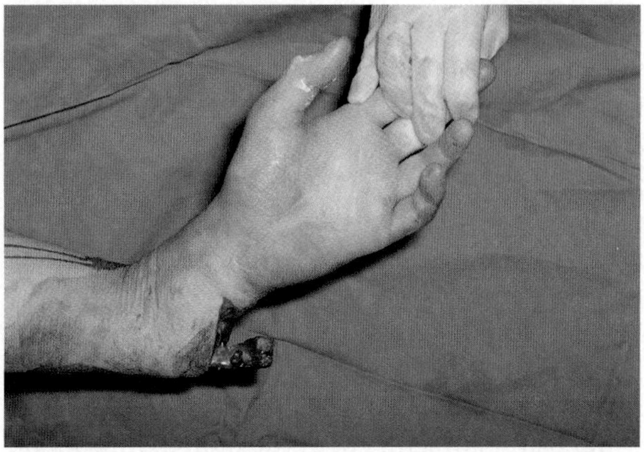

D

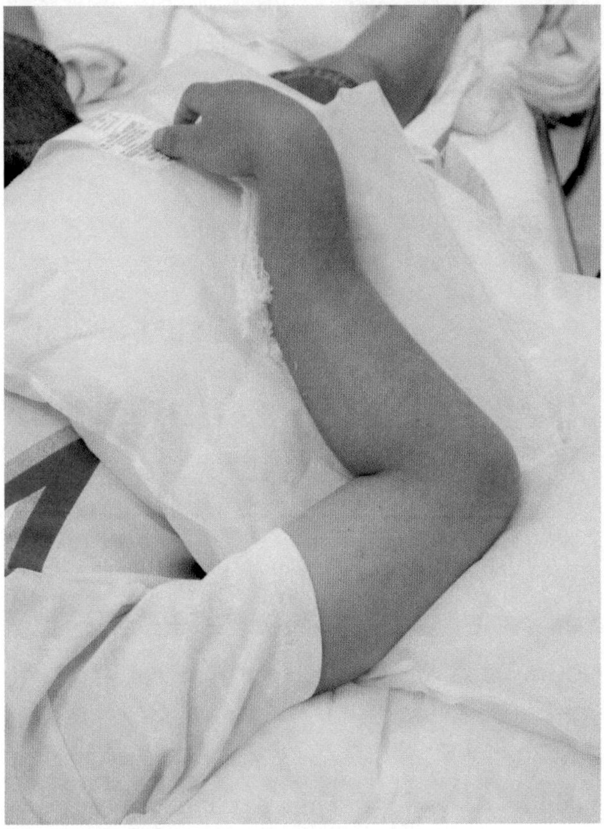

E

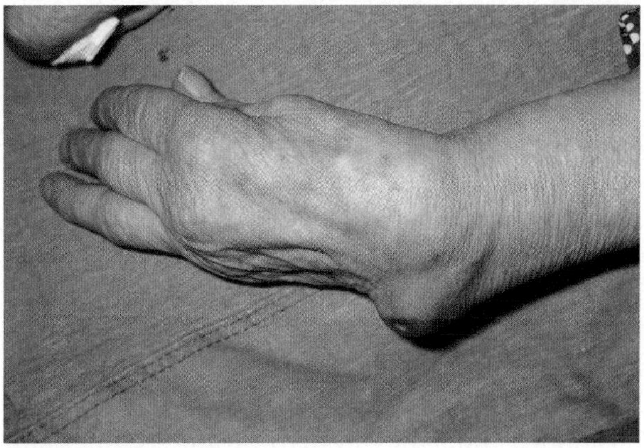

F

FIGURE 43-11 (Continued) **C.** Posterior dislocation of the elbow joint with marked deformity. **D.** Severe open fracture of the forearm. **E.** Greenstick fracture with marked deformity. **F.** Fracture of the distal radius

Shoulder Injury

Shoulder injuries are common in older adults due to their generally weaker bone structure. Shoulder injuries often result from a **fall on an outstretched hand**. In patients with an anterior fracture or dislocation (90% of shoulder dislocations are anterior[2]), the affected arm and shoulder may be held close to the chest (with the lateral aspect of the shoulder appearing flat instead of rounded). In addition, a deep depression between the head of the humerus and the acromion laterally ("hollow shoulder") may be visible. Patients with posterior fracture or dislocation may be found with the arm above the head.

Other injuries that may affect the shoulder include sternoclavicular strain (which results from a direct blow or twisting of an extended arm) and rotator cuff tendon injuries. Rotator cuff injuries can be acute or chronic and can lead to abnormal activation of the deltoid muscle. Injury to the rotator cuff can result from a violent pull on the arm, abnormal rotation of the shoulder, or a fall on an outstretched arm that tears and ruptures shoulder tendons.

Management of shoulder injuries includes application of a sling and swathe (**FIGURE 43-12**). Based on the position of the affected arm and shoulder, a makeshift splint may need to be devised to hold the injury in place. For example, with some fractures or dislocations, the paramedic may need to use a rolled blanket with a cravat at the center. The blanket roll is positioned under the elevated arm and secured like a sling. The arm is then swathed to prevent movement. If the patient's arm is positioned above the head, it should be splinted in position.

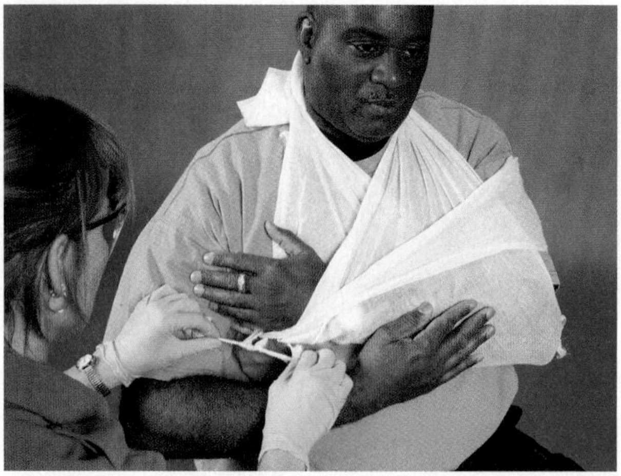

FIGURE 43-12 Immobilization of the shoulder.

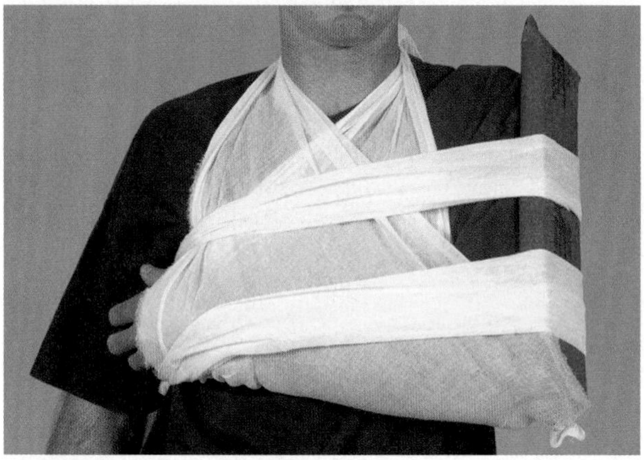

FIGURE 43-13 Immobilization of the humerus.

Humeral Injury

Midshaft humeral fractures are common in older adults and active young men. Radial nerve injury may be present if a fracture occurs in the middle or distal portion of the humeral shaft; such an injury can cause limited or decreased active wrist or finger extension and abnormal sensation in the first dorsal web space.[3] A fracture of the humeral neck may cause axillary nerve damage that affects deltoid function and sensation to the lateral aspect of the shoulder. Internal hemorrhage into the joint also may be a complication.

Management includes application of a rigid splint and sling and swathe (**FIGURE 43-13**). Note that midshaft humeral fractures are often difficult to stabilize. A lateral short board splint can be applied to the medial upper arm for added stability.

Elbow Injury

Elbow injuries are common in children (in whom they are especially dangerous[3]) and athletes. Indeed, the elbow is the third most frequently dislocated joint overall, after the shoulder and knee. The mechanism of injury usually involves a fall on an outstretched hand or flexed elbow. Such injuries may lead to vascular disruption and result either from vessel kinking for a prolonged time or from development of a compartment syndrome, which can lead to ischemic contracture (**Volkmann contracture**) with serious deformity of the forearm and a clawlike hand if not treated promptly.

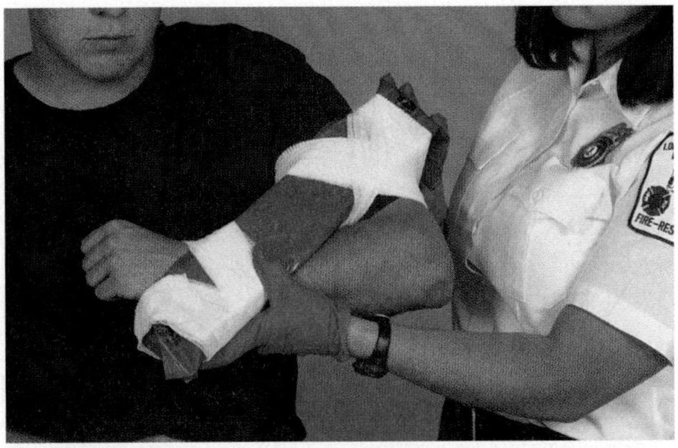

FIGURE 43-14 Immobilization of the elbow.
© Jones & Bartlett Learning. Courtesy of MIEMSS.

Frank laceration of the brachial artery and additional nerve damage can occur as well.

In general, reduction of these injuries is not attempted in the field. If there is a severely angulated fracture or significant neurovascular compromise distal to the injury, medical direction should be consulted regarding the need for gentle reduction. If reduction is attempted, a posterior moldable splint should be used to splint the elbow at 90° with the forearm supinated.[3] Management includes splinting in the position found with a pillow, blanket, rigid splint, or sling and swathe (**FIGURE 43-14**).

Radial, Ulnar, or Wrist Injury

As with most other upper extremity injuries, injuries to the radius, ulna, and wrist usually are the result of a fall on an outstretched hand. Wrist injuries may involve the distal radius, the ulna, or any of the eight carpal bones. The most common wrist injury is a fracture with a "silver fork" deformity of the distal radius with

> **NOTE**
>
> Subluxation of the radial head (**nursemaid's elbow**) accounts for approximately 20% of upper extremity injuries in children and is seen in children ages 6 months to 5 years, most often in children in the 1- to 3-year-old age group. History of a pull on the arm or a fall is often reported. The child usually refuses to use the arm but does not seem to be in pain or distress until movement of the elbow is attempted (either actively or passively).
>
> ---
>
> *Modified from*: Hammond B, Zimmerman P, eds. *Sheehy's Emergency Nursing: Principles and Practice*. 7th ed. Philadelphia, PA: Elsevier; 2013.

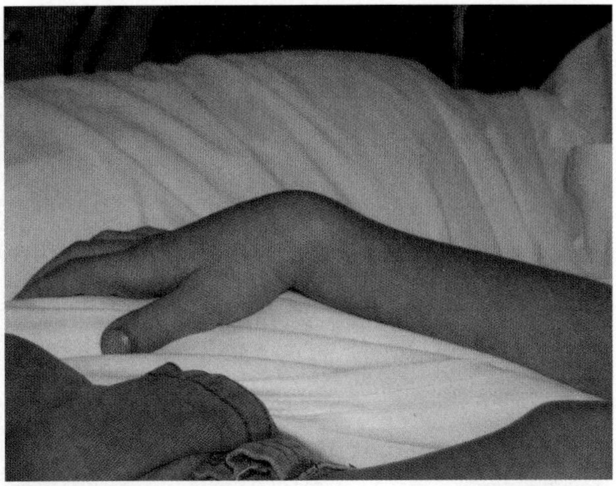

FIGURE 43-15 Colles fracture.
© E.M. Singletary, M.D. Used with permission.

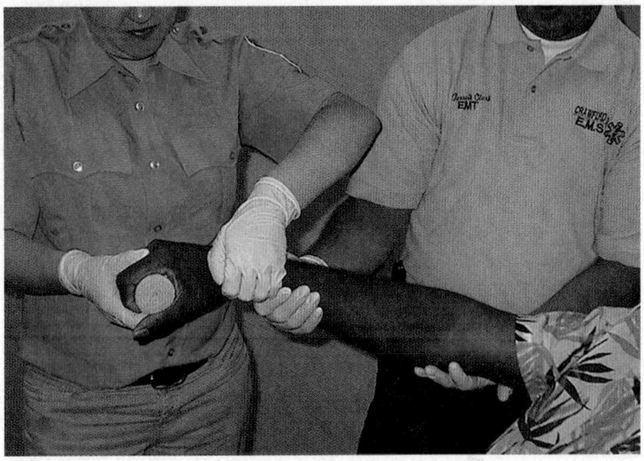

FIGURE 43-16 Immobilization of the forearm.
© Jones & Bartlett Learning. Courtesy of MIEMSS.

dorsal angulation (**Colles fracture**) (**FIGURE 43-15**). Forearm injury is common in both children and adults. These injuries are managed in the same way as elbow injuries (**FIGURE 43-16**).

> **CRITICAL THINKING**
>
> What effect does a cold pack have on musculoskeletal injuries?

Hand (Metacarpal) Injury

Injury to the hand often results from contact sports, violence (fighting), and work-related crushing injuries. A common metacarpal injury is **boxer's fracture**, which

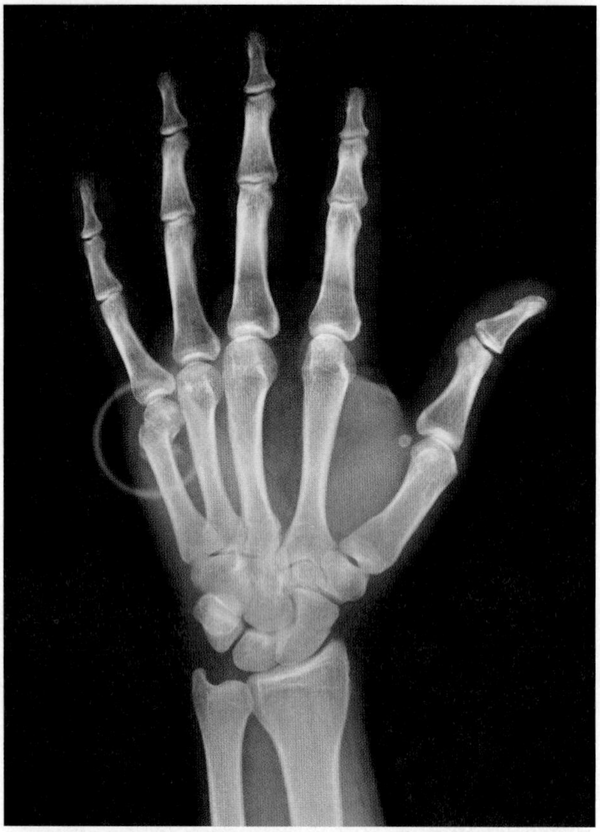

FIGURE 43-17 Boxer's fracture (circled).
© Scott Camazine/Medical Images.

results from direct trauma to a closed fist, leading to fracture of the fifth metacarpal bone at the distal metaphysis (**FIGURE 43-17**). These injuries also may be associated with hematomas and open wounds. Boxer's fracture is the most common metacarpal fracture, but any of the metacarpals can be fractured, depending on the mechanism of injury.

Management includes applying a rigid or formable splint (pillow, blanket) in the position of function. Hand injuries should be temporarily splinted in the position of function (as with a hand grasping a soda can). Rigid or formable splints (previously described for radial, ulnar, and wrist injury) may be used.

Finger (Phalangeal) Injury

Finger injuries are common—but they should not be considered trivial. Serious injuries include fractures of the thumb as well as any open or markedly comminuted fractures of the hand or fingers. These injuries should be managed by splinting as previously described.

Injured fingers may be immobilized with foam-filled aluminum splints or tongue depressors (**FIGURE 43-18**).

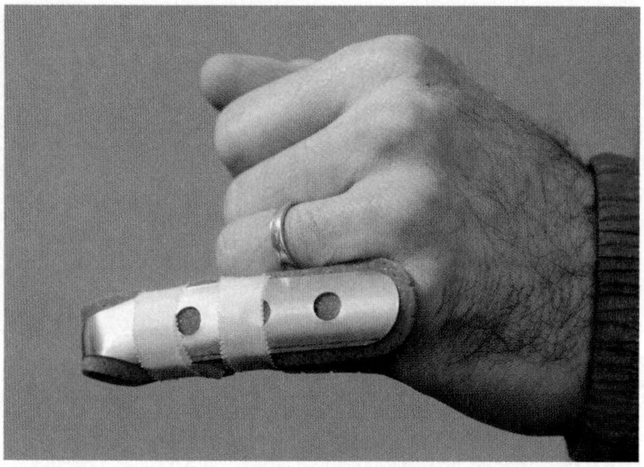

FIGURE 43-18 Immobilization of the finger.
© CTK/Alamy Stock Photo.

They also may be immobilized simply by taping the injured finger to an adjacent one ("buddy splinting").

NOTE
Buddy splinting (also known as buddy wrapping) refers to immobilizing an injured finger or toe to an adjoining finger or toe with padding and tape. In essence, the uninjured digit acts as a splint. This principle of stabilization can also be applied to lower leg injuries (buddy splinting the leg to the uninjured leg) if other splinting material is not readily available.

Lower Extremity Injuries

Lower extremity injuries include fractures of the pelvis and fractures or dislocations of the hip, femur, knee and patella, tibia and fibula, ankle and foot, and phalanx (**FIGURE 43-19**). Compared with upper extremity injuries, lower extremity injuries are associated with greater forces and more significant blood loss. They are more difficult to manage in patients with multiple injuries, and may be life threatening (eg, femoral and pelvic fractures). Serious injuries require the following management:

- Administration of high-concentration oxygen to maintain oxygen saturation (Spo_2), as measured by pulse oximeter, of 95% or greater
- Gentle movement, comfort measures, and appropriate analgesics
- Regular monitoring of vital signs
- Fluid replacement, if needed to manage hypovolemia
- Rapid transport

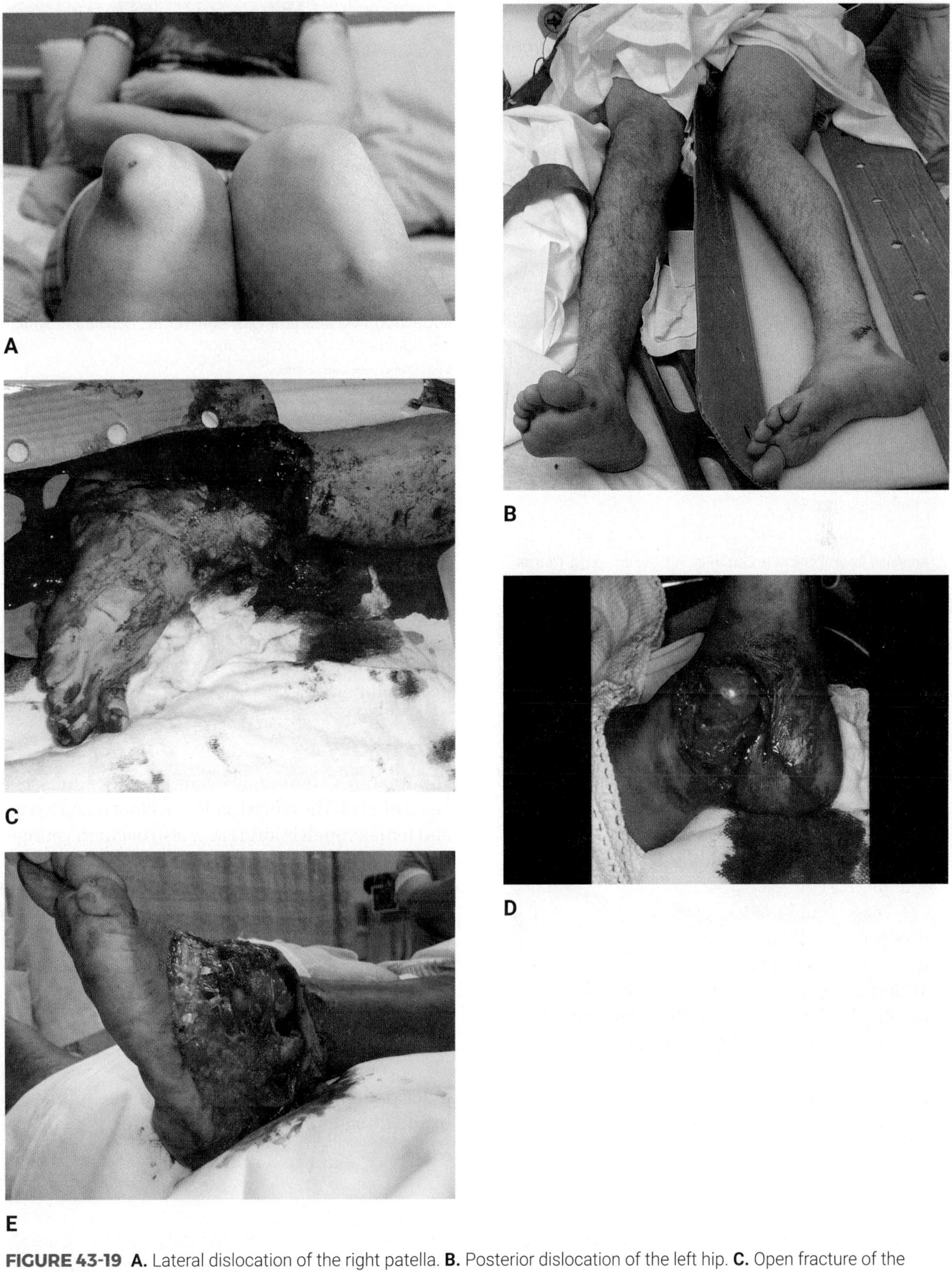

FIGURE 43-19 **A.** Lateral dislocation of the right patella. **B.** Posterior dislocation of the left hip. **C.** Open fracture of the lower leg. **D.** Subtalar dislocation. **E.** Open fracture of the ankle.

Pelvic Fracture

As described in Chapter 42, *Abdominal Trauma*, blunt or penetrating injury to the pelvis may result in fracture, severe hemorrhage, and associated injury to the urinary bladder and urethra. Injuries typically result from high-speed motor vehicle crashes, pedestrian–motor vehicle collisions, and falls. The pelvis is surrounded by heavy muscles and other soft tissues, so a deformity in this area may be difficult to see. Thus, injury to the pelvis should be suspected based on the mechanism of injury or tenderness on palpation of the iliac crests. Trauma to the abdomen and pelvic area may be complicated by pregnancy (further described in Chapter 45, *Obstetrics*). Management includes the use of a padded, long backboard or scoop stretcher to minimize movement from the point of injury to the ambulance stretcher, and the application of a pelvic binder.

> **NOTE**
>
> Commercial pelvic stabilization devices ("pelvic binders") immobilize unstable pelvic fractures. Research indicates their use may reduce mortality. Examples include the Trauma Pelvic Orthotic Device (T-POD) and the SAM Pelvic Sling (**FIGURE 43-20**). When possible, the pelvic binder should be applied prior to moving the patient when injury is suspected.
>
> *Modified from*: Gerecht R, Larrimore A, Steurerwald M. Critical management of deadly pelvic injuries. *J Emerg Med Serv.* 2014;39(12):28-35.

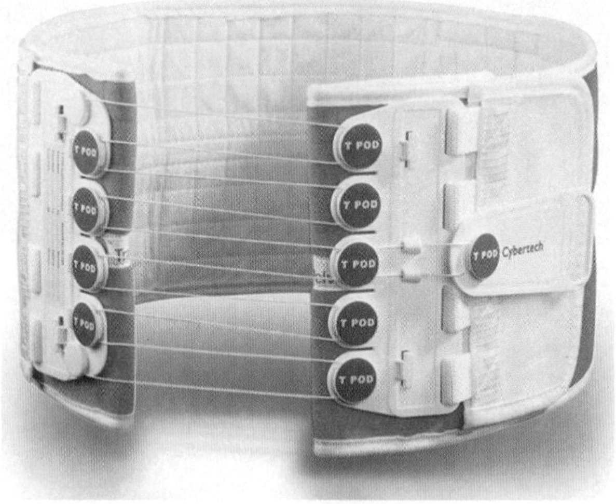

FIGURE 43-20 Pelvic stabilization device.

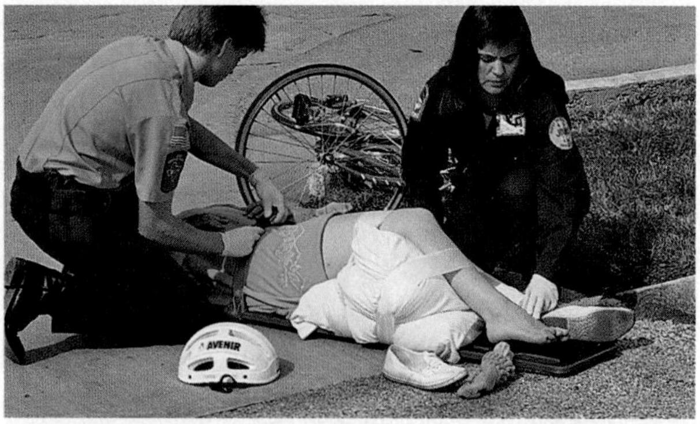

FIGURE 43-21 Young woman with internal rotation, adduction, and shortening of right femur, consistent with her right posterior hip dislocation.

Hip Injury

Hip fractures commonly occur in older adults as a result of a fall. The typical patient is older than 75 years and female. Such injuries may also occur in younger patients who experience major trauma. Usually the hip is fractured at the femoral head and neck, and the affected leg is shortened and externally rotated. By comparison, with hip dislocation, the affected leg is usually shortened and internally rotated (**FIGURE 43-21**). Fractures closer to the head of the femur may manifest similar to an anterior hip dislocation, with a shortened and internally rotated leg.

Hip fractures are serious injuries, especially in older patients. Complications from the injury can be life threatening, with approximately 20% to 30%

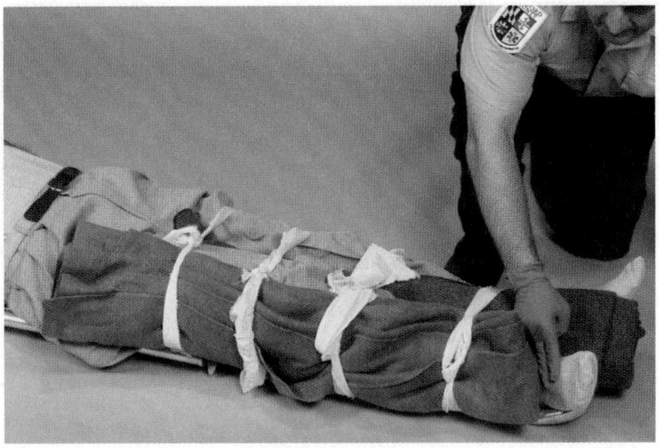

FIGURE 43-22 Immobilization of the hip.

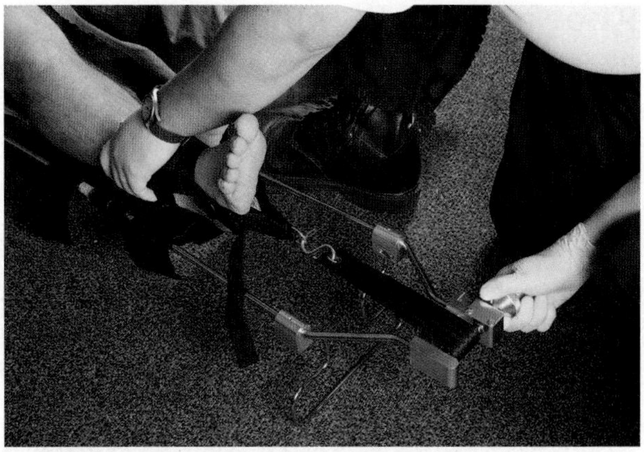

FIGURE 43-23 Application of a traction splint.

of older patients dying within the first year following hip fracture.[4] Many of these deaths result from venous thromboembolism, pneumonia, and infection. Many patients who sustain a hip fracture will require prolonged specialized care, such as in a long-term nursing or rehabilitation facility. Nearly 40% of patients who sustain a fractured hip will return to their preinjury level of activity.[5]

Hip dislocation is usually caused by large forces from motor vehicle crashes—forces that are usually associated with other major injuries.[3] Most hip dislocations are posterior dislocations of the femoral head.

Prehospital management of hip fracture includes use of a long backboard or scoop stretcher (**FIGURE 43-22**) to minimize hip motion when moving the patient from the point of injury to the stretcher and generously padding the patient for comfort during transport.[3] Slight flexion of the knee or padding beneath the knee may improve patient comfort.

Femoral Injury

Injury to the femur usually results from major trauma, such as may occur with motor vehicle crashes and pedestrian injuries. It also is a fairly common result of child abuse, accounting for 30% of femur fractures in children younger than 1 year.[6]

Fractures of the femur result in powerful thigh muscle contractions, which then cause the bone fragments to move back and forth over each other. The patient generally has a shortened leg that is externally rotated and midthigh swelling from hemorrhage, which can be life threatening. Femoral fractures should be immobilized in the field with a traction splint (**FIGURE 43-23**).

NOTE

Traction splints are used only to immobilize midshaft femoral fractures. They should not be used with fractures of the lower third of the leg, pelvic fractures, hip injury, knee injury, or avulsion or amputation of the ankle and foot. Transport should not be delayed to apply these splints if the patient has life-threatening injuries. Instead, the patient should be secured on a long backboard and rapidly transported for definitive care.

Modified from: National Association of Emergency Medical Technicians. *PHTLS: Prehospital Trauma Life Support*. 8th ed. Burlington, MA: Jones & Bartlett Learning; 2014.

Knee and Patellar Injury

Fractures of the knee (supracondylar fracture of the femur, intra-articular fracture of the femur or tibia) and fractures and dislocations of the patella commonly result from motor vehicle crashes, pedestrian injuries, contact sports, and falls on a flexed knee (**FIGURE 43-24**). (The popliteal artery is located close to the knee joint and, therefore, may experience an associated injury, especially with posterior dislocations.) Other common knee and patellar injuries involve nearby ligaments and tendons (**BOX 43-5**).

Management of knee and patellar injury includes splinting in the position found with a rigid or formable splint that effectively immobilizes the thigh and ankle. Traction splints should not be used to immobilize a

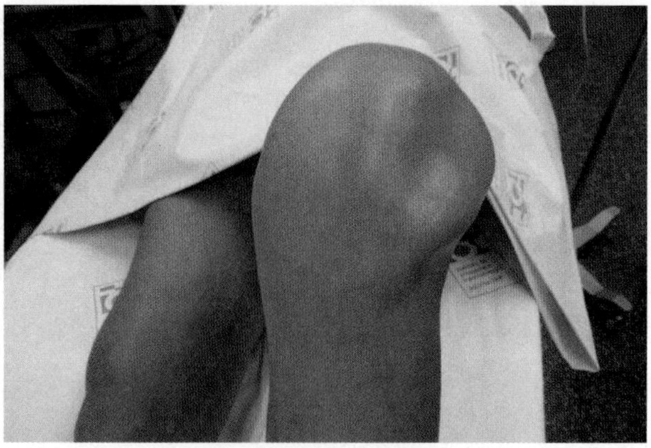

FIGURE 43-24 Left anterior knee dislocation.

Reproduced from: Junqueira JJ, Helito CP, Bonadio MB, Pécora JR, Demange MK. Total knee arthroplasty with subvastus approach in patient with chronic post-traumatic patellar dislocation. *Rev Bras Ortop*. 2016;51(5):614-618.

BOX 43-5 Ligament Injuries of the Knee

Injuries to the ligaments around the knee can result from direct blows, from hyperextension, and (more commonly) from twisting or torsion of the knee (eg, in sports activities). The ligaments outside the knee are the medial collateral ligament and the lateral collateral ligament. They provide the stability for the knee and limit the knee's movement from side to side. The medial collateral ligament is on the inner side of the knee and is taut when the leg is straight. Though a strong ligament, it can be sprained or completely ruptured (torn) if the straightened knee is twisted at the same time the knee is forced sideways (eg, during a football tackle). The lateral collateral ligament runs on the outer side of the knee. It connects the distal end of the femur to the top of the fibula. Injury to this ligament seldom occurs as an isolated event. If injured, it is usually associated with another damaged ligament.

The ligaments inside the knee are the anterior cruciate ligament and the posterior cruciate ligament. These ligaments cross over each other—a formation that provides additional stability to the knee, particularly in forward and backward movements of the knee joint (**FIGURE 43-25**).

Ligament injuries are managed with rest, ice, compression, and elevation (RICE); anti-inflammatories and analgesics; and physical therapy. In some cases, surgical repair is required.

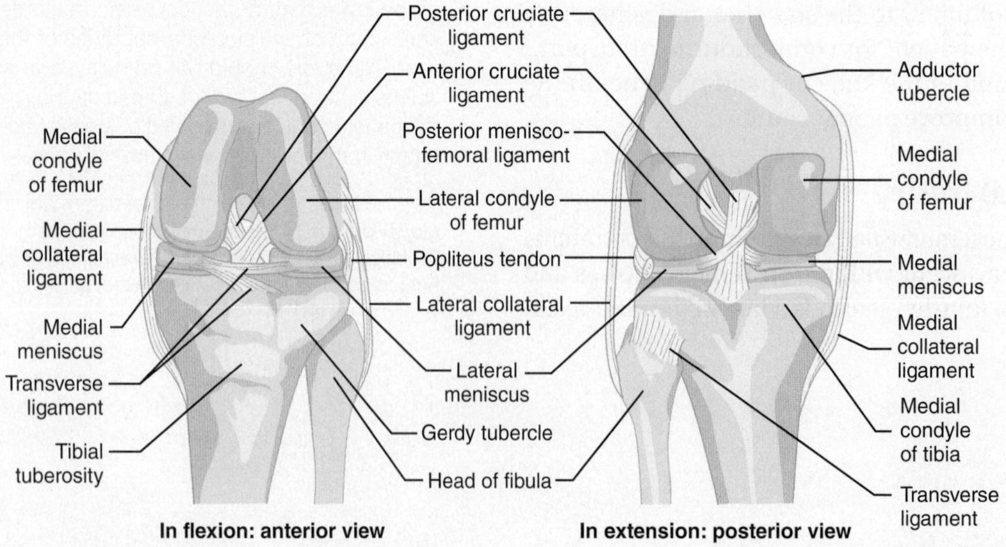

FIGURE 43-25 Anterior and posterior view of the right knee.

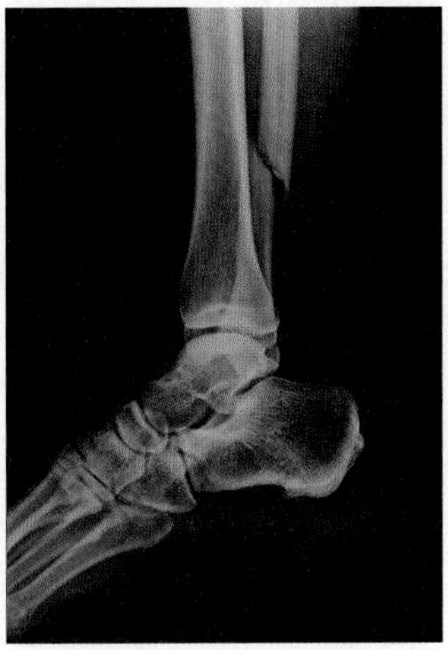

FIGURE 43-26 Isolated fibular fracture.

knee or patellar injury. Ice and elevation should be applied.

Tibial and Fibular Injury

The tibia is the most frequently fractured long bone. Fractures of the tibia often are associated with fibular fracture (**FIGURE 43-26**) because of the amount of force transmitted to the injured leg. Of these two bones, the tibia is the only weight-bearing bone. Injuries to the tibia and fibula may result from direct or indirect trauma or from twisting injury. If the injury is associated with the knee, popliteal vascular injury should be suspected. Management includes splinting with a rigid or formable splint (**FIGURE 43-27**) (including the knee and ankle on the same side).

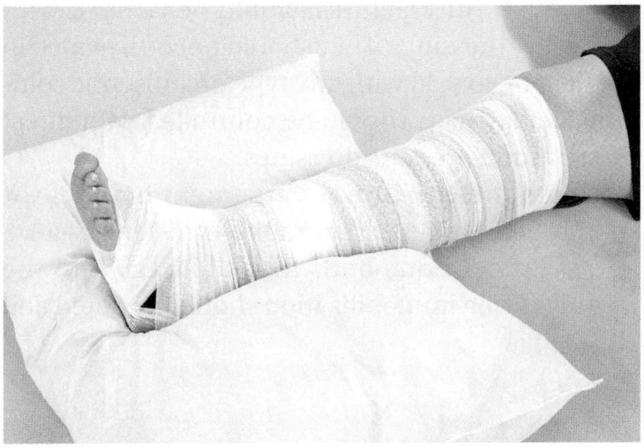

FIGURE 43-27 Immobilization of the lower leg.

NOTE

Compartment syndrome is a common complication of tibial and fibular injuries. As described in Chapter 37, *Bleeding and Soft-Tissue Trauma*, and Chapter 54, *Rescue Awareness and Operations*, compartment syndrome occurs when an extremity injury causes swelling to the point of obstructing the extremity's blood supply. Compartment syndrome is suggested by the presence of the "six Ps" (pain, pallor, paresthesia, pulselessness, paralysis, and poikilothermia [normalization of the body part's temperature with the surrounding environment]). These signs, except for pain, are all late signs of compartment syndrome and may herald irreversible damage. The hallmarks of compartment syndrome are pain out of proportion to the apparent injury and pain on passive stretching of the muscles in the involved compartment.

Surgical intervention in the form of a fasciotomy to relieve tension or pressure is urgently needed to prevent permanent disability or even loss of the limb. These patients require rapid transport.

Foot and Ankle Injury

Fractures and dislocations of the foot and ankle may result from a crush injury, a fall from a height, or a violent rotating or twisting force (**FIGURE 43-28**). Injuries to nearby tendons also can occur (BOX 43-6). The

BOX 43-6 Achilles Tendon Rupture

A fairly common injury to the ankle is a tear or rupture of the Achilles tendon. The **Achilles tendon**, or tendon calcaneus, is a fibrous, ropelike band of tissue that is the largest tendon in the human body. It serves to connect the calf muscle to the calcaneus (heel bone). The Achilles tendon pulls the heel when it contracts, for example in physical movement such as pointing the foot or running.

An **Achilles tendon rupture** occurs when the tendon rips completely. This injury typically occurs when playing sports. The location of injury is usually 2 inches (5 cm) above the heel. This injury usually results from excessive dorsiflexion of the foot. It is common in middle-age male athletes ("weekend warriors"), in older people, and in those with arthritis and diabetes. Use of corticosteroids and quinolone antibiotics also increases the risk for this injury. Treatment may include surgical and nonsurgical therapies as well as foot and ankle casts or braces to prevent movement while the tendon heals.

Modified from: Nannini CC. Achilles tendon rupture. emedicinehealth website. https://www.emedicinehealth.com/achilles_tendon_rupture/article_em.htm. Accessed June 1, 2018.

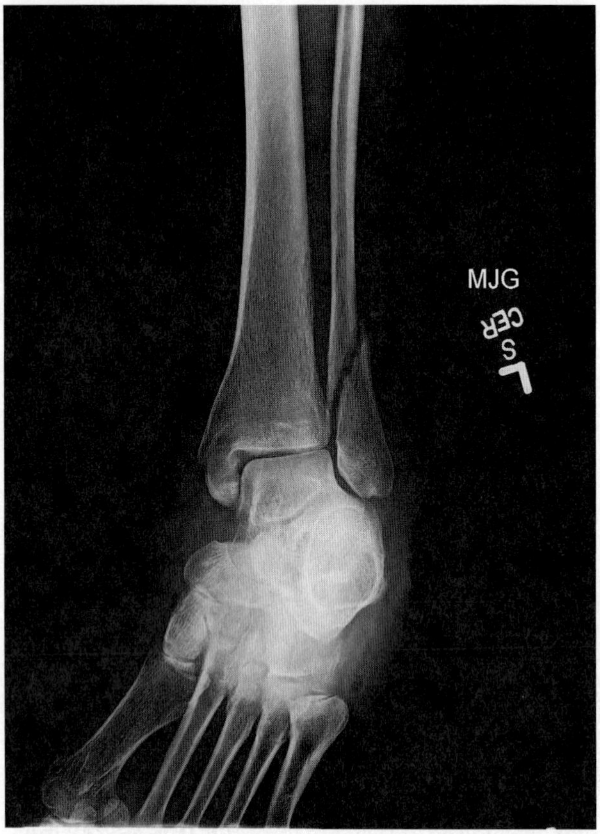

FIGURE 43-28 Bimalleolar ankle fracture which required surgical fixation of both fractures.

Courtesy of Andrew N. Pollak, MD, FAAOS. Used with permission.

patient with foot or ankle injury usually complains of reports point tenderness and may be hesitant to bear weight on the extremity. Management includes application of a formable splint, such as a pillow, blanket, or air splint (**FIGURE 43-29**).

Phalangeal Injury

Toe injuries often are caused by "stubbing" the toe on an immovable object. These injuries usually are managed by buddy taping the toe to an adjacent toe to support and immobilize the injury.

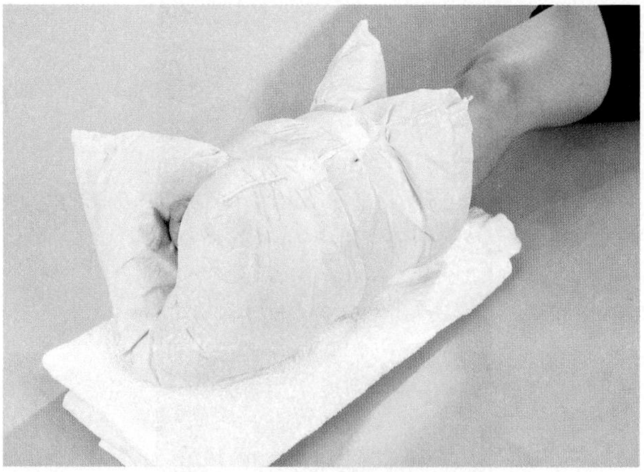

FIGURE 43-29 Immobilization of the foot and ankle.

© Jones & Bartlett Learning.

Open Fractures

Patients with an **open fracture** require special care and evaluation by the paramedic. Fractures may be opened in two ways: from within, as when a bone fragment pierces the skin, or from without, such as in an automobile crash. An open fracture also may have made contact with the skin some distance from the fracture site.

Although most open fractures are obvious because of associated hemorrhage, a small puncture wound may not be immediately apparent, and bleeding may be minimal. Therefore, the paramedic must consider any soft-tissue wound in the area of a suspected fracture to be evidence of an open fracture.

Open fractures are treated with surgical debridement relatively urgently because of the potential for infection. Most authorities agree that open wounds associated with fractures should be covered with sterile, dry dressings. They should not be irrigated in the field or soaked with any type of antiseptic solution. Hemorrhage should be controlled with direct pressure and pressure dressings.

If a bone end or bone fragment is visible, it should be covered with a saline-moistened gauze and splinted. Bone ends that slip back into the wound during immobilization should be noted and reported to the receiving hospital so that the bone can be cleaned in surgery.

Stages of Fracture Healing

The healing of most fractures proceeds in several different stages. In the earliest stage following the fracture, a hematoma forms at the fracture site. This is followed by the formation of fibrovascular tissue (fibrous tissue) that replaces the hematoma and stabilizes the fracture area. Genes and proteins in the bone marrow then stimulate the production of osteoblasts (immature bone cells) and chondrocytes (cartilage cells). Next, the membrane around the bone and the immature bone cells form a callus at the fracture site. Newly formed cartilage cells begin to replace the scar tissue. In the final stage of healing, the immature bone cells held in place by the membrane grow and mature. When this newly formed bone replaces the cartilage (remodeling), the healing is considered complete (**FIGURE 43-30**).

The time required for healing depends on how severe and how large the fracture is, where it occurs, how the broken bone is used, and how strong the bone was before the fracture. Some small fractures in the hands heal in a few weeks. Large fractures in the legs or pelvis may take many months to heal. Most

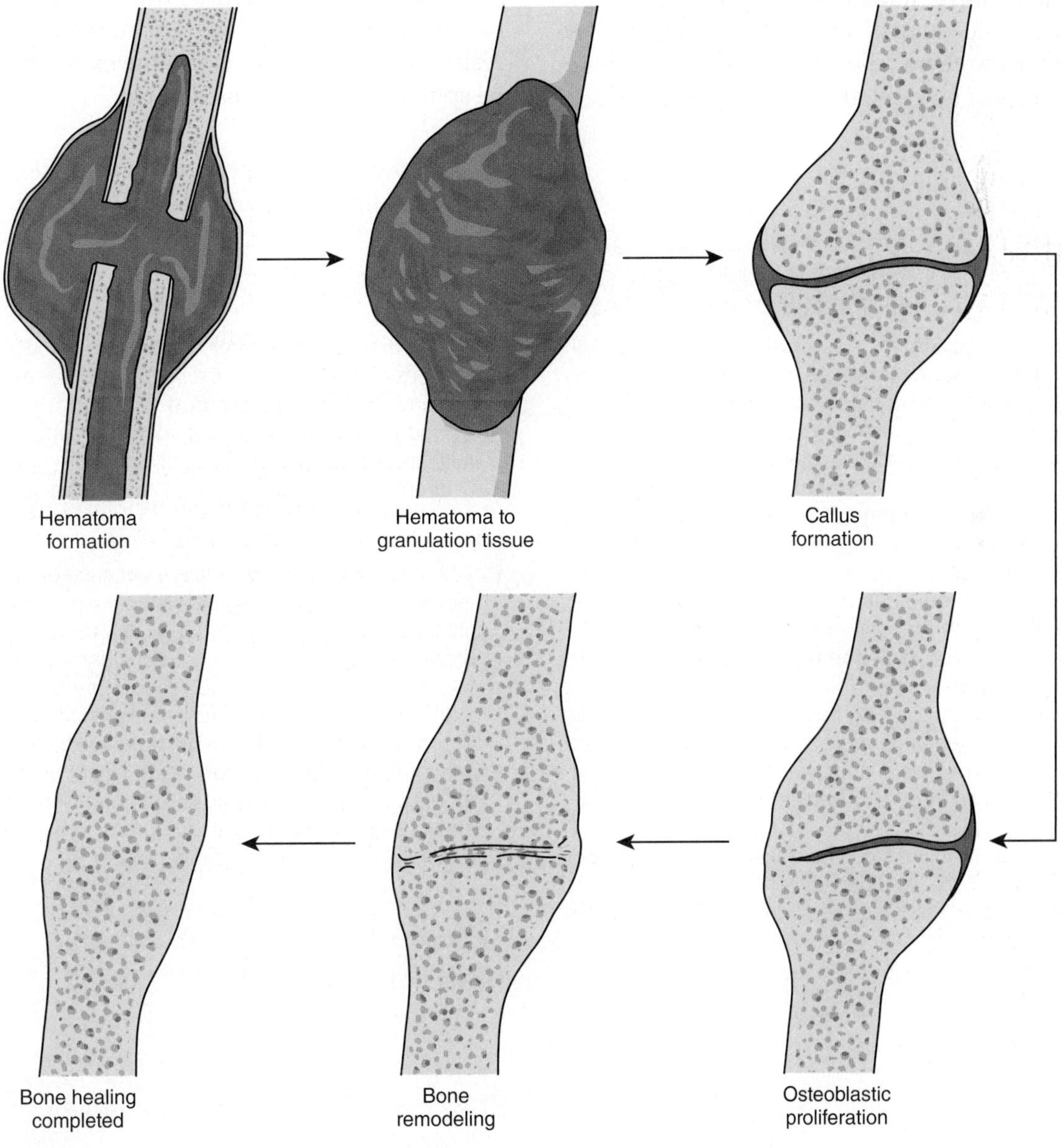

FIGURE 43-30 Stages of fracture healing.

fractured bones are immobilized with casts, braces, or surgical fixation devices while they heal. Even after healing, possible complications of fractures include nonunion and osteomyelitis.

Straightening Angular Fractures and Reducing Dislocations

Angular fractures and dislocations may pose significant problems in splinting and, in some situations, in patient extrication and transport. When manipulation of a fracture is required to aid in transport or to improve circulation to the injured extremity, the paramedic should consult with medical direction. Limb-threatening injuries include knee dislocation, fracture or dislocation of the ankle, and subcondylar fractures of the elbow. These serious injuries require rapid transport for evaluation by a physician.

As a rule, fractures and dislocated joints should be immobilized in the position of injury, and the patient should be transported as quickly as possible to the emergency department for radiography and realignment (reduction). In that setting, radiographs are often taken of the affected limb to rule out bone fragments or other fractures that may complicate reduction.

If transport is to be delayed and if circulation is compromised, medical direction may authorize a single attempt to reposition a grossly deformed fracture or dislocated joint that does not involved the elbow. (An elbow should never be manipulated in the prehospital setting.) Repositioning should be accomplished using gentle, firm traction applied in the direction of the long axis of the extremity. If resistance to alignment is felt, the extremity should be splinted without repositioning.

Summary

- Injuries that can result from traumatic force on the musculoskeletal system include fractures, sprains, strains, and joint dislocations. Problems associated with musculoskeletal injuries include hemorrhage, instability, loss of tissue, simple laceration and contamination, interruption of blood supply, and long-term disability.
- Common signs and symptoms of extremity trauma include pain on palpation or movement, swelling or deformity, crepitus, decreased range of motion, false movement, and decreased or absent sensory perception or circulation distal to the injury.
- Once the paramedic has assessed for life-threatening conditions, the extremity injury should be examined for the "six Ps": pain, pallor, paresthesia, pulselessness, paralysis, and poikilothermia.
- Immobilization by splinting helps alleviate pain; reduces tissue injury, bleeding, and contamination of an open wound; and simplifies and facilitates transport of the patient. Splints can be categorized as rigid, soft or formable, and traction splints.
- Upper extremity injuries can be classified as fractures or dislocations of the shoulder, humerus, elbow, radius and ulna, wrist, hand, and finger. Most upper extremity injuries can be adequately immobilized by application of a sling and swathe.
- Lower extremity injuries include fractures of the pelvis and fractures or dislocations of the hip, femur, knee and patella, tibia and fibula, ankle and foot, and toes.
- Compartment syndrome is a common complication of tibial and fibular injuries. The hallmarks of compartment syndrome are pain out of proportion to the apparent injury and pain on passive stretching of the muscles in the involved compartment.
- Most open fractures are obvious because of associated hemorrhage, although a small puncture wound may not be initially apparent and may produce only minimal bleeding. Therefore the paramedic must consider any soft-tissue wound in the area of a suspected fracture to be evidence of an open fracture. Open fractures are usually treated with surgical debridement due to the potential for infection.
- Only *one* attempt at realignment should be made and should be done *only* with medical control consultation when severe neurovascular compromise is present (eg, extremely weak or absent distal pulses).

References

1. Marx J, Hockberger R, Walls R. *Rosen's Emergency Medicine.* 8th ed. St. Louis, MO: Saunders; 2014.
2. Frontera WR, Herring SA, Micheli LJ, Silver JK. *Clinical Sports Medicine: Medical Management and Rehabilitation*. St. Louis, MO: Saunders; 2006.
3. Kiviehan S, Friedman BT, Mercer MP. Orthopedic injuries. In: Brice J, Delbriddge TR, Meyers JB, eds. *Emergency Services Clinical Practice and Systems Oversight*. Vol 1. West Sussex, UK: John Wiley & Sons; 2015:272-279.
4. Johnson K, Lie D. Hip fracture increases 1-year mortality rate in elderly women. Medscape website. https://www.medscape.org/viewarticle/750611. Accessed March 28, 2018.
5. Riemen AHK, Hutchison JD. The multidisciplinary management of hip fractures in older patients. *Orthopaed Trauma.* 2016;30(2):117-122.
6. Hubbard E, Rocco A. Pediatric orthopedic trauma: an evidence-based approach. *Orthoped Clin North Am.* 2018;49(2):195-210.

Suggested Readings

Gausche-Hill M, Brown KM, Oliver ZJ, et al. An evidence-based guideline for prehospital analgesia in trauma. *Prehosp Emerg Care.* 2014;18(suppl 1):25-34.

Gerecht R, Larrimore A, Steurerwald M. Critical management of deadly pelvic injuries. *J Emerg Med Serv.* 2014;39(12):28-35.

John R, Dhillon M, Raj G. Can biochemical indices supplement clinical examination in decision making regarding limb salvageability in lower limb musculoskeletal trauma with doubtful viability? A prospective outcome analysis study. *Bone Joint J.* 2017;99-B(suppl 17):11.

Montorfano MA, Montorfano LM, Quirante FP, Rodriguez F, Vera L, Neri L. The FAST D protocol: a simple method to rule out traumatic vascular injuries of the lower extremities. *Crit Ultrasound J.* https://doi.org/10.1186/s13089-017-0063-2. Published March 21, 2017. Accessed March 28, 2018.

Schmidt AH, Bosse MJ, Frey KP, et al. Predicting acute compartment syndrome (PACS): the role of continuous monitoring. *J Orthopaed Trauma.* 2017;31:S40-S47.

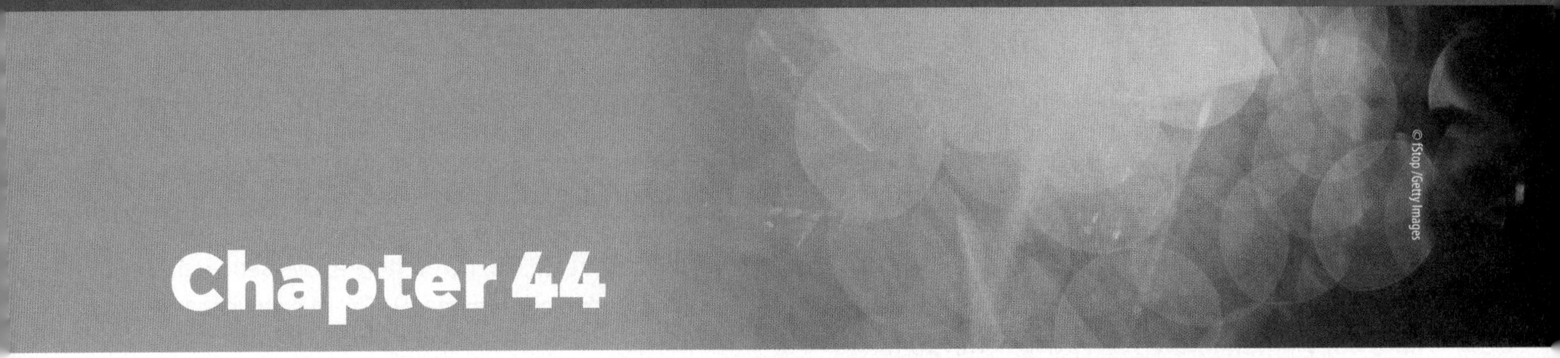

Chapter 44

Environmental Conditions

NATIONAL EMS EDUCATION STANDARD COMPETENCIES

Trauma

Integrates assessment findings with principles of epidemiology and pathophysiology to formulate a field impression to implement a comprehensive treatment/disposition plan for an acutely injured patient.

Environmental Emergencies

Recognition and management of
- Submersion incidents (pp 1556–1559)
- Temperature-related illness (pp 1548–1556)

Pathophysiology, assessment, and management of
- Near drowning (pp 1556–1559)
- Temperature-related illness (pp 1547–1556)
- Bites and envenomations (Chapter 37, *Bleeding and Soft-Tissue Trauma* and Chapter 33, *Toxicology*)
- Dysbarism
  - High-altitude (pp 1564–1567)
  - Diving injuries (pp 1559–1564)
- Electrical injury (Chapter 38, *Burns*)
- Radiation exposure (Chapter 38, *Burns*)
- High-altitude illness (pp 1564–1567)

OBJECTIVES

Upon completion of this chapter, the paramedic student will be able to:
1. Describe the physiology of thermoregulation. (pp 1545–1547)
2. Discuss the risk factors, pathophysiology, assessment findings, and management of specific hyperthermic conditions. (pp 1548–1550)
3. Discuss the risk factors, pathophysiology, assessment findings, and management of specific hypothermic conditions and frostbite. (pp 1551–1556)
4. Discuss the risk factors, pathophysiology, assessment findings, and management of submersion and drowning. (pp 1556–1559)
5. Identify the mechanical effects of atmospheric pressure changes on the body based on knowledge of the basic properties of gases. (pp 1559–1560)
6. Discuss the risk factors, pathophysiology, assessment findings, and management of diving emergencies and high-altitude illness. (pp 1561–1566)

KEY TERMS

acute mountain sickness (AMS) A common high-altitude illness that results when an unacclimatized person rapidly ascends to high altitudes.

afterdrop phenomenon A sudden return of cold blood and waste products to the core of the body as a result of rewarming methods used to treat hypothermia.

air embolism The presence of air bubbles in the bloodstream.

barotrauma A physical injury sustained as a result of exposure to increased atmospheric or environmental pressure; also known as dysbarism.

barotrauma of ascent A diving illness that occurs through the reverse process of descent; also known as "reverse squeeze."

barotrauma of descent A diving illness that results from the compression of gas in enclosed spaces as the ambient pressure increases with descent under water; also known as "squeeze."

Boyle's law A gas law that states pressure and volume are inversely related, assuming a constant temperature.

central thermoreceptors Nerve endings located in or near the anterior hypothalamus that are sensitive to subtle changes in core temperatures.

conduction The direct movement of heat from a warmer object to a cooler one (simple transfer).

convection The transfer of heat by mass motion of a fluid such as air or water.

core body temperature (CBT) The temperature of deep structures of the body as compared with the temperatures of peripheral tissues.

Dalton's law A law stating that the total pressure exerted by a mixture of gases is equal to the sum of the partial pressure of gases.

decompression sickness A multisystem disorder that results when nitrogen in compressed air (dissolved into tissues and blood from the increase in the partial pressure of the gas at depth) converts back from solution to gas. This process results in the formation of bubbles in the tissues and blood.

demarcation The visible boundary between living tissue and necrotic tissue.

drowning The process of experiencing respiratory impairment from submersion/immersion in liquid.

dysbarism Illness that results directly or indirectly from changes in ambient atmospheric pressure and the pressure of gases within the body.

frostbite A localized injury that results from freezing of body tissues.

frostnip A cold injury manifested by transient numbness and tingling that resolves after rewarming.

heat cramps Brief, intermittent, and often severe muscular cramps that frequently occur in muscles fatigued by heavy work or exercise.

heat exhaustion A form of heat illness characterized by dizziness, nausea, headache, and a mild to moderate increase in the core body temperature.

heatstroke The end stage of the heat illness spectrum that occurs when the thermoregulatory mechanisms normally in place to meet the demands of heat stress break down entirely. As a result, mental status becomes altered, and the core body temperature increases to extreme levels. Multisystem tissue damage and physiologic collapse also occur.

Henry's law A law stating that at a constant temperature, the amount of gas that dissolves in a liquid is directly proportional to the partial pressure of that gas in equilibrium with that liquid.

high-altitude cerebral edema (HACE) The most severe form of acute high-altitude illness. It is characterized by a progression of global cerebral signs in the presence of acute mountain sickness.

high-altitude illness Illness that principally occurs at altitudes 8,200 feet (2,500 m) or more above sea level.

high-altitude pulmonary edema (HAPE) A high-altitude illness thought to be caused at least partly by an increase in pulmonary artery pressure that develops in response to hypoxia.

hyperthermia Abnormal elevation of body temperature.

hypothermia An abnormal body temperature below 95°F (35°C).

mammalian diving reflex A reflex stimulated by cold water that shunts blood to the brain and heart from the skin, gastrointestinal tract, and extremities.

nitrogen narcosis An illness associated with scuba diving in which divers feel intoxicated when nitrogen becomes dissolved in solution as a result of greater than normal atmospheric pressure; also known as rapture of the deep.

Osborn wave A positive deflection at the J point on an electrocardiogram, characteristically seen in hypothermia; also known as a J wave.

peripheral thermoreceptors Nerve endings sensitive to temperature, located in the skin and some mucous membranes. They usually are categorized as cold or warm receptors.

pulmonary overpressurization syndrome (POPS) A condition that results from expansion of trapped air in the lungs. It may lead to alveolar rupture and extravasation of air into extra-alveolar locations.

radiation The direct release of body heat to cooler surroundings.

recompression The use of elevated pressure (including hyperbaric oxygen therapy) to treat conditions within the body caused by a rapid decrease in pressure.

submersion The act or state of being under water (or liquid) for any amount of time.

thermogenesis The production of heat, especially by the cells of the body.

thermolysis The dissipation of heat by means of radiation, evaporation, conduction, or convection.

thermoregulation The maintenance of body temperature, even under a variety of external conditions.

trench foot A foot injury that occurs from prolonged exposure to cold, but not freezing, water.

Exposure to elements in the environment can produce many types of emergencies. Paramedics must be prepared to recognize and manage these conditions. This requires being knowledgeable about the causative factors and the pathophysiology of specific disorders.

Thermoregulation

Thermoregulation is the maintenance of body temperature, even under a variety of external conditions. Body temperature is regulated in the brain by a thermoregulatory center. This center is located in the posterior hypothalamus. It receives information from **central thermoreceptors** in or near the anterior hypothalamus and from **peripheral thermoreceptors** in the skin and some mucous membranes. Peripheral thermoreceptors are nerve endings usually categorized as cold receptors and warm receptors. Cold receptors are stimulated by lower skin-surface temperatures. Warm receptors are stimulated by higher skin-surface temperatures. Information from these receptors is transmitted by the spinal cord to the posterior hypothalamus. The posterior hypothalamus responds with appropriate signals to help the body reduce heat loss and increase heat production (cold receptor stimulation) or increase heat loss and reduce heat production (warm receptor stimulation).

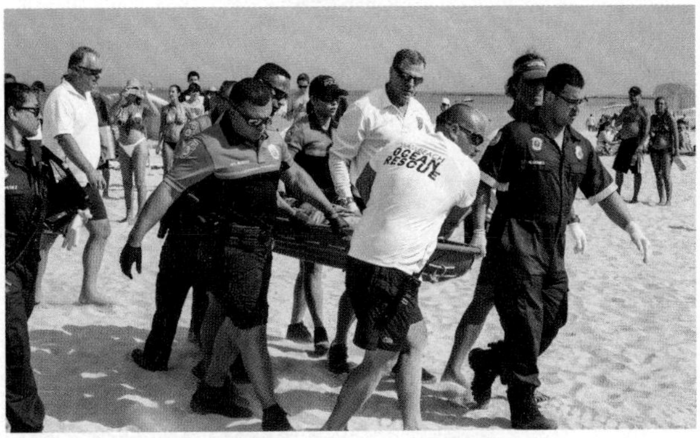

Central thermoreceptors are neurons that are sensitive to changes in temperature. These neurons react directly to changes in the temperature of the blood. They send messages to the skeletal muscle through the central nervous system (CNS). They affect vasomotor tone, sweating, and the metabolic rate through sympathetic nerve output to skin arterioles, sweat glands, and the adrenal medulla.

The thermoregulatory center has an inherent set point. This set point maintains a relatively constant **core body temperature (CBT)** of 98.6°F (37°C). To maintain an optimum environment for normal cell metabolism (homeostasis), the body must keep the CBT fairly constant, even when external and internal conditions tend to raise or lower it. Body temperature can be increased or decreased in two ways. One way is through the regulation of heat production (**thermogenesis**). The other way is through the regulation of heat loss (**thermolysis**).

Regulating Heat Production

The body can generate heat in response to cold. It does this through mechanical, chemical, metabolic, and endocrine activities. Several physiologic and biochemical factors affect the direction and magnitude of these compensatory responses. Such factors include the person's age, general health, and nutritional status.

Heat is controlled chemically by cellular metabolism (oxidation of energy sources). Every tissue contributes to this type of heat production. However, skeletal muscles produce the largest amount of heat, particularly when shivering occurs. Along with

CRITICAL THINKING

The body has many more cold receptors than it has heat receptors. Why do you think this is so?

CRITICAL THINKING

What fuels does the body need to increase heat production through the mechanism of shivering?

shivering, which is often associated with chattering of the teeth, vasoconstriction occurs to conserve as much heat as possible. Shivering is the body's best defense against cold. It can increase heat production by as much as 400%.[1]

Endocrine glands also regulate heat production. They do this through the release of hormones from the thyroid gland and adrenal medulla. Sympathetic discharge of epinephrine and norepinephrine (along with the activity of sympathetic nerves that lead to adipose tissue) increases metabolism, resulting in an increase in heat production. BOX 44-1 presents examples of ways the body regulates heat production.

Regulating Heat Loss

Heat is lost from the body to the external environment through the skin, lungs, and excretions. The skin is the most important of these in regulating heat loss. Radiation, conduction, convection, and evaporation are the major mechanisms of heat loss (**FIGURE 44-1**).

Radiation is the direct release of body heat to cooler surroundings. The surface of the human body constantly emits heat in the form of infrared rays. If the surface of the body is warmer than the environment, heat is lost through radiation.

BOX 44-1 Compensatory Mechanisms for Regulating Heat Production

Mechanisms That Decrease Heat Loss

Peripheral vasoconstriction
Reduction of surface area by body position (or clothing)
Piloerection (not effective in humans)

Mechanisms That Increase Heat Production

Shivering
Increased voluntary activity
Increased hormone secretion
Increased appetite

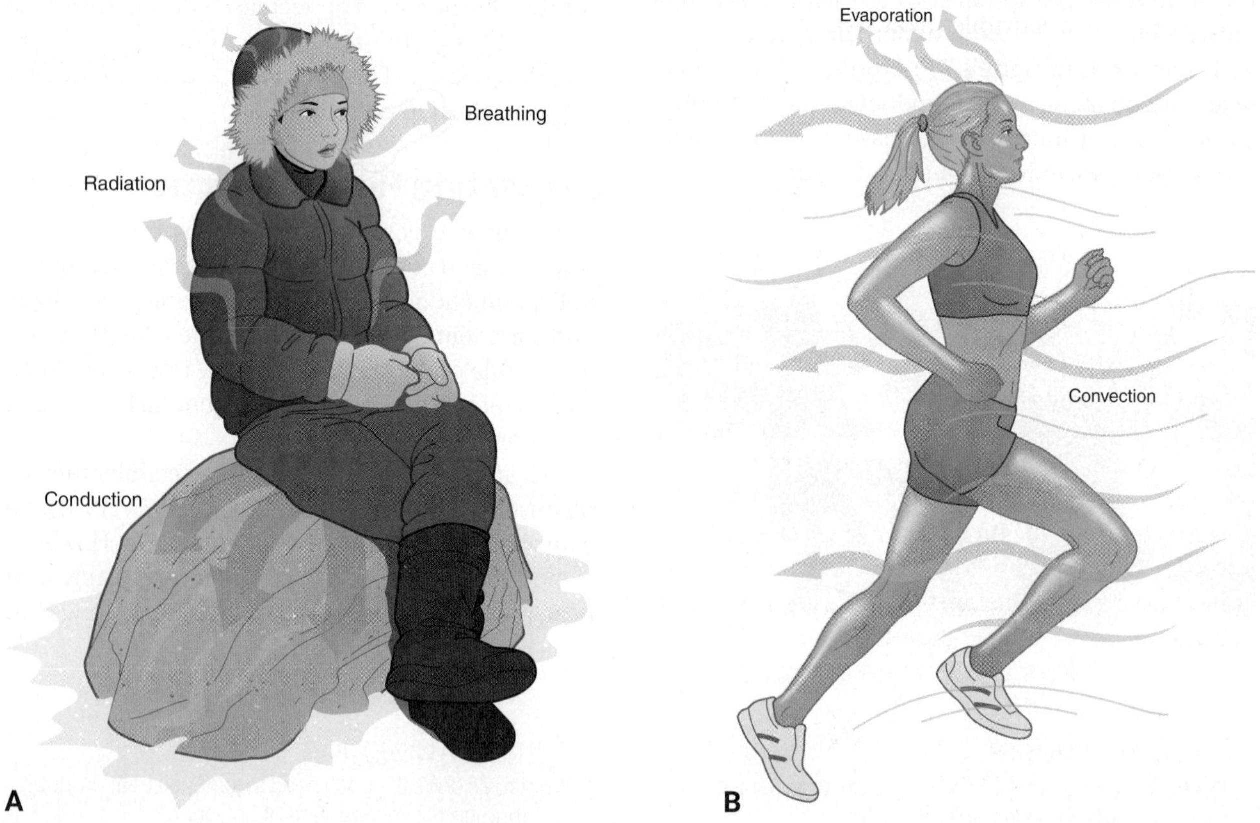

FIGURE 44-1 Mechanisms of heat loss. **A.** Conduction, radiation, and breathing are shown. **B.** Evaporation and convection are shown.

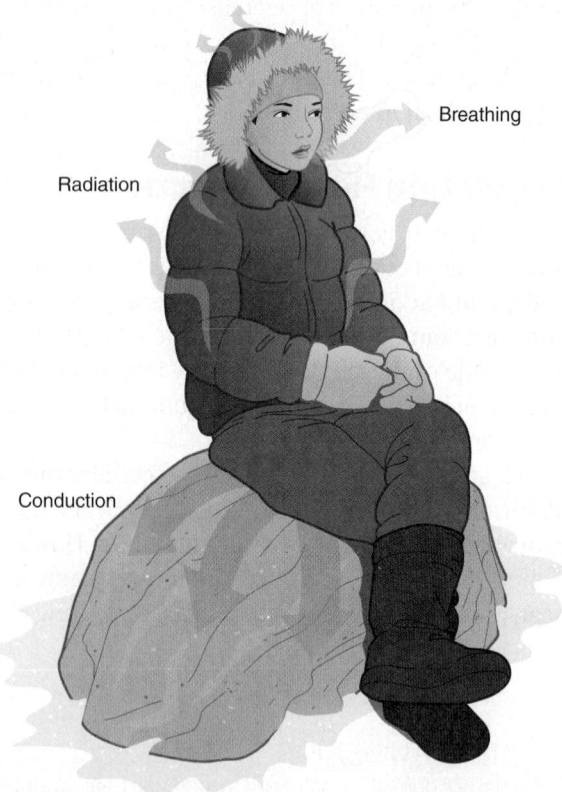

Conduction is the direct movement of heat from a warmer object to a cooler one (simple transfer). Heat moves from a higher temperature to a lower temperature. Thus the body surface loses or gains heat by direct contact with cooler or warmer surfaces, including air. If the ambient air temperature is lower than the skin temperature, body heat is lost to the surrounding air by conduction. The greater the temperature difference between two objects, the more quickly heat is transferred between them.

Convection is similar to conduction; however, in convection the two objects in contact are also moving relative to one another. It is heat transfer by mass motion of a fluid such as air or water. For example, if air or water next to the body is heated, moves away, and is replaced by cool air or water, heat loss occurs by convection. Convection can be greatly aided by external forces such as wind or fans. It promotes conductive heat exchange by continuously maintaining a supply of cool air. Factors that contribute to the cooling effects of convection are the speed of air currents and the temperature of the air. Doubling the wind speed quadruples heat loss.[2]

CRITICAL THINKING

How does wearing the fully enclosed hazardous materials suit affect your body's ability to regulate temperature?

Evaporation is a process by which fluid changes from a liquid to a gas and lowers the temperature on the surface where the evaporation occurred. When fluid evaporates, it absorbs heat from surrounding objects and air. This mechanism removes heat rapidly from the body regardless of the ambient temperature. Therefore, while it helps cool a person when the weather is hot, it hastens hypothermia during frigid conditions.[2] The temperature of the surrounding air and the relative humidity greatly affect the amount of heat lost as a result of evaporation of moisture from the skin or the respiratory tract (breathing). The relative humidity is 100% when the air is fully saturated with moisture. Sweating can markedly increase evaporative heat loss as long as the humidity is low enough to allow the sweat to evaporate. At humidity levels above 75%, evaporation decreases. At levels approaching 90%, evaporation essentially ceases.[3]

BOX 44-2 Compensatory Mechanisms for Regulating Heat Loss

Mechanisms That Increase Heat Loss

Vasodilation of skin vessels
Sweating

Mechanisms That Decrease Heat Production

Decreased muscle tone and voluntary activity
Decreased hormone secretion
Decreased appetite

SHOW ME THE EVIDENCE

Researchers performed a systematic review of cooling techniques and practices among firefighters and hazardous materials operators to identify strategies for fireground rehabilitation. They reviewed 27 published articles meeting their criteria, concluding that cooling devices do not appear to be needed if ambient temperature and humidity are close to room temperature and protective garments can be removed, which includes baring the arms. In hot and humid conditions, cooling devices are needed; hand/forearm immersion is considered the best method. Options such as cooling vests and liquid- or air-cooled suits that cool during exertion are under investigation. Such equipment adds weight to the firefighters, making it less desirable.

Modified from: McEntire SF, Suyama J, Hostler D. Mitigation and prevention of exertional heat stress in firefighters: a review of cooling strategies for structural firefighting and hazardous materials responders. *Prehosp Emerg Care*. 2013;17(2):241-260.

BOX 44-2 presents other examples of ways the body regulates heat loss.

External Environmental Factors

Some factors in the environment can contribute to a medical emergency. They also may affect rescue and transport. These elements include the climate, season, weather, atmospheric pressure, and terrain. When the potential for an environmental emergency exists, the paramedic must consider the following factors:

- Localized prevailing weather norms and any deviations
- Characteristics of seasonal variation in climate

- Weather extremes (wind, rain, snow, humidity)
- Barometric pressure (eg, at altitude or under water)
- Terrain that can complicate injury or rescue

The patient's health also is a factor related to environmental stressors and can worsen other medical or traumatic conditions. Examples include the patient's age, predisposing medical conditions, use of prescription and over-the-counter medications, use of alcohol or recreational drugs, and previous rate of exertion.

Hyperthermia

Hyperthermia, or heat illness, is actually a broad spectrum of problems that results from one of two basic causes: One cause is temperature-regulating mechanisms that are overwhelmed by high temperatures in the environment or, more commonly, by excessive exercise in moderate to extremely high temperatures. The second cause is temperature-regulating centers that fail, usually in older adults or in ill or incapacitated patients. Either cause can result in heat illness such as heat cramps, heat exhaustion, and heatstroke.

Heat Cramps

Heat cramps are brief, intermittent, and muscular cramps that occur in hot environments. They often affect leg or abdominal wall muscles fatigued by heavy work or exercise. The primary cause of heat cramps is sodium and water loss.

People who suffer from heat cramps sweat profusely and drink water without adequate salt. During times of high environmental temperatures, 1 to 3 L of water per hour can be lost through sweating.[3] Each liter contains 30 to 50 mEq of sodium chloride. The water and sodium deficiency together is believed to cause muscle cramping. This cramping normally occurs in the most heavily exercised muscles, including the calves and arms, although any muscle can be involved. The patient is usually alert and has hot, sweaty skin, tachycardia, and a normal blood pressure. The CBT is normal.

Heat cramps are easily managed by removing the patient from the hot environment. Also, sodium and water should be replaced. Stretching or massaging the affected areas may provide some relief. In more serious cases, medical direction may recommend intravenous (IV) infusion of normal saline. Oral salt additives (eg, salt tablets) are not recommended. They can cause gastrointestinal irritation, ulceration, and vomiting. Paramedics should follow local protocol with regard to providing a carbohydrate- and salt-containing beverage (eg, Gatorade, Powerade) to help rehydrate patients.

Heat Exhaustion

Heat exhaustion is a more severe form of heat illness. It is characterized by more severe cramps, dizziness, nausea, headache, and mild to moderate elevation of the CBT (up to 103°F [39.4°C]). In severe cases, dizziness caused by significant intravascular volume loss, as well as fainting, may occur. This orthostatic dizziness occurs when the patient changes from a lying position to a sitting or standing position.

Like heat cramps, heat exhaustion more often is associated with a hot environment and results in profuse sweating. The person usually recovers rapidly when removed from the hot environment, given replacement fluids, and cooled with a cool water spray. Patients with significant fluid loss or orthostatic hypotension may require IV administration of a balanced sodium chloride solution. Heat exhaustion can progress to heatstroke if left untreated.[3]

Heatstroke

Heatstroke occurs when the body's temperature-regulating mechanisms break down entirely and mental status becomes affected. As a result of this failure, the body temperature rises to 104°F (40°C) or higher, which destroys protein quickly, leading to cellular destruction, a severe inflammatory response, and disruption of the coagulation cascade.[4] Heatstroke is a serious medical emergency. The syndrome commonly is classified into two types: classic heatstroke and exertional heatstroke.

> **NOTE**
>
> Increased body temperature caused by failure of the temperature-regulating mechanisms should not be confused with fever associated with a response to inflammation or infection. With fever, the effect on the hypothalamus is caused by endogenous pyrogens released by phagocytic leukocytes. Antipyretic drugs can reverse these effects, returning the set point of the hypothalamus to normal.

Classic heatstroke occurs during periods of sustained high ambient temperatures and humidity. The illness commonly affects the very young, older adults, and those who live in poorly ventilated homes without air conditioning. An example is a young child left in an enclosed car on a hot afternoon. Another example is an older person confined to a hot room during a heat wave. Victims of classic heatstroke also often suffer from chronic diseases, including diabetes, heart disease, alcoholism, or psychiatric disorders. These diseases predispose the person to the syndrome. Many patients who are susceptible to classic heatstroke take prescribed medications for other conditions. These medications may include diuretics, antihypertensives, psychotropics (antipsychotics, phenothiazines), antihistamines, and anticholinergics. These drugs further impair a person's ability to tolerate heat stress. In these patients, the illness develops from poor dissipation of environmental heat.

> NOTE
>
> The autoimmune neuropathy associated with diabetes can interfere with vasodilation, perspiration, and thermoregulatory input. Some cardiac drugs (eg, anticholinergics, beta blockers, diuretics) can predispose a patient to dehydration, can interfere with vasodilation, and can reduce the body's ability to increase the heart rate in response to a volume loss.

In contrast to patients with classic heatstroke, patients with exertional heatstroke are usually young and healthy. Athletes, military recruits, hazardous materials technicians, and firefighters who work or exercise in the heat and humidity often are affected. In these situations, heat builds up more rapidly in the body than it can be dispersed into the environment. Preventive measures to reduce the risk of exertional heat illness for all age groups include the following:

- Avoiding or limiting exercise in hot environments, especially on consecutive days
- Maintaining an adequate fluid intake
- Achieving acclimatization, which results in more perspiration with a lower salt concentration, thereby increasing fluid volume in the body

Clinical Manifestations

As described previously, the temperature-regulating centers in the brain receive their information largely from the temperature of circulating blood in the deep and superficial veins and from the skin. In response to hypothalamic stimulation, a number of physiologic events occur: (1) The respiratory rate quickens to increase heat loss through exhaled air, (2) cardiac output increases to provide more blood flow through skin and muscle to enhance heat radiation, and (3) sweat gland activity increases to enhance evaporative heat loss.[5] These compensatory mechanisms require a normally functioning CNS to properly respond to the temperature extreme. They also require a working cardiovascular system to move excess heat from the core to the surface of the body. Problems in either or both of these systems lead to a rapidly increasing CBT.

CNS Manifestations. The CNS manifestations of heatstroke vary. Some patients may be in frank coma. Others may show confusion and irrational behavior before collapse. Convulsions are common and can occur early or late in the course of the illness. Because the brain stores little energy, it depends on a constant supply of oxygen and glucose. Decreased cerebral perfusion pressure results in cerebral ischemia and acidosis. Increased temperatures markedly increase the metabolic demands of the brain as well. The extent of brain damage depends on the severity and duration of the hyperthermic episode. Fever from illness (eg, infection) and an increased CBT from heatstroke produce similar symptoms, especially in the CNS. The paramedic should obtain a thorough history (if available) to distinguish between the two

> NOTE
>
> Heat syncope refers to a brief loss of consciousness and quick return to normal mental status that appears to be caused by heat exposure.
>
> *Modified from*: National Association of EMS Officials. *National Model EMS Clinical Guidelines*. Version 2.0. National Association of EMS Officials website. https://www.nasemso.org/documents/National-Model-EMS-Clinical-Guidelines-Version2-Sept2017.pdf. Published September 2017. Accessed February 13, 2018.

> CRITICAL THINKING
>
> What other conditions can demonstrate the types of mental status changes seen with heatstroke?

syndromes. If unsure of the cause, the paramedic should treat the patient for heatstroke.

Cardiovascular Manifestations. A rise in skin temperature reduces the thermal gradient between the core and the skin. This causes an increase in skin blood flow (peripheral vasodilation), which gives the skin a flushed appearance. About 50% of victims of exertional heatstroke have persistent sweating,[3] which results from increased release of catecholamines. In classic heatstroke, sweating usually is absent because of dehydration, drug use that impairs sweating, direct thermal injury to sweat glands, or sweat gland fatigue. Therefore the presence of sweating does not rule out the diagnosis. Also, the cessation of sweating is not the cause of heatstroke. Peripheral vasodilation results in decreased vascular resistance and shunting as the illness progresses. High-output cardiac failure is common, manifested by extreme tachycardia and hypotension. Cardiac output initially can be four to five times that of normal. However, as temperatures continue to rise, myocardial contractility begins to decrease and the central venous pressure rises. In any age group, the presence of hypotension and decreased cardiac output points to a poor prognosis. Other systemic manifestations associated with heatstroke include the following:

- Pulmonary edema (accompanied by systemic acidosis, tachypnea, hypoxemia, and hypercapnia)
- Myocardial dysfunction
- Cardiac dysrhythmias
- Gastrointestinal bleeding
- A reduction in renal function (secondary to hypovolemia and hypoperfusion)
- Hepatic injury
- Clotting disorders
- Electrolyte abnormalities

Management

Heatstroke almost invariably leads to death if left untreated. The factors most important to a successful outcome are initiation of basic life support (BLS) and advanced life support (ALS) measures, rapid recognition of the heat illness, and rapid cooling of the patient. The paramedic should manage the patient with heatstroke as follows:[6]

1. Move the patient to a cool and shaded environment and remove restrictive clothing. If available, use hyperthermic thermometers (eg, rectal probes) to monitor the CBT. Take and record the temperature at least every 5 minutes during the cooling process. This continued monitoring ensures adequate rates of cooling. It also helps to prevent inadvertent (rebound) hypothermia. Rebound hypothermia can best be avoided by stopping the cooling measures when the patient's CBT reaches about 102°F (38.9°C).
2. Begin cooling by fanning the patient while keeping the skin wet. Continue lowering the body temperature by this method en route to the hospital. If the patient has altered mental status with a temperature greater than 104°F (40°C), begin active cooling. If available, use complete immersion techniques by placing the victim in an ice bath up to the chin.[7] Alternatively, spraying tepid water (60°F [15.6°C]) over the body surface while fanning the patient is also effective. Shivering should be controlled with IV midazolam, lorazepam, or diazepam. Although less effective, ice packs may be applied to the trunk over pulse points. The ice packs should not be placed directly over the skin. Do not apply wet cloths or wet clothing, as they can trap heat and limit the evaporative cooling process.[7]
3. If hypovolemia is present, administer cool IV fluids in 20-mL/kg boluses. Reduce to a 10-mL/kg per hour infusion when vital signs stabilize. In most patients, the blood pressure rises to a normal range during the cooling process as large volumes of blood from the skin move back to the central circulation. Rapid cooling directly improves cardiac output. Be very cautious with fluid replacement. Also, closely monitor the patient for signs of fluid overload. The administration of too much fluid can cause pulmonary edema, especially in older adults.
4. If seizures occur, midazolam, lorazepam, or diazepam are indicated.
5. Blood glucose should be assessed early. If the patient is hypoglycemic, glucose should be administered.
6. Cardiac dysrhythmias are associated with heatstroke; continuous electrocardiographic (ECG) monitoring is indicated. When dysrhythmias are present, they are treated per American Heart Association (AHA) guidelines.

Hypothermia

Hypothermia (CBT less than 95°F [35°C]), sometimes referred to as accidental hypothermia, can result from a decrease in heat production, an increase in heat loss, or a combination of these two processes. At a temperature of less than 82°F (27.8°C), healthy naked humans no longer produce enough heat to maintain body temperature at rest.[2]

Hypothermia can have metabolic, neurologic, traumatic, toxic, and infectious causes. However, it most often is seen in cold climates and in exposure to extremely cold conditions in the environment. Failure to recognize and properly treat hypothermia can increase the rate of morbidity and mortality.

Pathophysiology

Exposure to cold produces a chain of events in the body aimed at conserving core heat. Initially, immediate vasoconstriction in the peripheral vessels occurs. At the same time, the rate of metabolism by the CNS increases. The blood pressure and the heart and respiratory rates also increase dramatically. As cold exposure continues, muscle tone increases. The body generates heat in the form of shivering. Shivering continues until the CBT reaches about 86°F (30°C), glucose or glycogen is depleted, or insulin is no longer available for glucose transfer. When shivering stops, cooling is rapid. A general decline then begins in the function of all body systems.

With continued cooling, respirations decline slowly, the pulse rate and blood pressure decrease, the blood pH drops, and significant electrolyte imbalances emerge. Hypovolemia can develop from a shift of fluid out of the vascular space, with increased loss of fluid through urination (cold diuresis). After early tachycardia, progressive bradycardia develops. This process often does not respond to atropine. Significant ECG changes occur, including prolonged PR, QRS, and QT intervals and obscure or absent P waves.[3] In addition, the J wave (**Osborn wave**) may be present at the junction of the QRS complex and ST segment (**FIGURE 44-2**). These events generally are followed by cardiac and respiratory arrest as the CBT approaches 68°F (20°C).

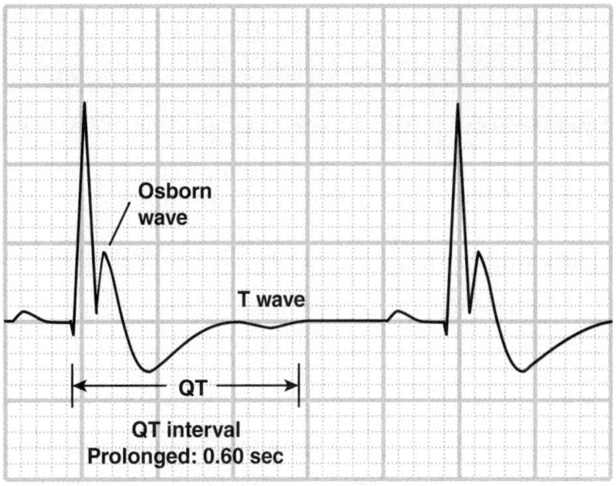

FIGURE 44-2 Osborn wave of hypothermia.

The progression of clinical signs and symptoms of hypothermia is divided into three classes based on the CBT: mild, moderate, and severe.[8] Mild hypothermia is classified as a CBT between 95°F (35°C) and 89.8°F (32.1°C); moderate hypothermia as a CBT between 89.7°F (32.1°C) and 82.5°F (28.1°C); and severe hypothermia as a CBT below 82.4°F (28°C).[8] The signs and symptoms of the three classes of hypothermia are listed in **TABLE 44-1**.

Those at increased risk for developing unintentional hypothermia are outdoor enthusiasts such as campers, hikers, hunters, and fishermen. Urban hypothermia is likely to occur in older adults, the very young, and people with concurrent medical or psychiatric illness. The homeless are particularly vulnerable. Thermoregulatory mechanisms also can be impaired by brain damage caused by trauma, hemorrhage, hypoxia, and CNS depression from drug overdose or intoxicants. Drugs known to impair thermoregulation include alcohol, antidepressants, antipyretics, phenothiazines, sedatives, and various pain medicines (including aspirin, acetaminophen, and nonsteroidal anti-inflammatory drugs [NSAIDs]). Acid–base imbalances, such as those that occur during ketoacidosis, can cause a decrease in heat production or an increase in heat loss, which can affect the body's ability to stabilize body temperature.

> CRITICAL THINKING
> What factors make homeless people especially vulnerable to hypothermia?

Management

The first step in managing hypothermia is to maintain a high degree of suspicion for its presence. When the

TABLE 44-1 Progression of Clinical Signs and Symptoms of Hypothermia[a]

Classification	Core Body Temperature	Signs and Symptoms
Mild	95°F–89.8°F (35°C–32.1°C)	Increased metabolic rate, maximum shivering, thermogenesis Impaired judgment, slurred speech
Moderate	89.7°F–82.5°F (32.1°C–28.1°C)	Respiratory depression, myocardial irritability, bradycardia, atrial fibrillation, Osborn waves
Severe	<82.4°F (<28°C)	Basal metabolic rate 50% of normal, loss of deep tendon reflexes, fixed and dilated pupils, spontaneous ventricular fibrillation

[a]Often no reliable correlation is seen between clinical signs and symptoms and a specific core body temperature.

Modified from: National Association of EMS Officials. *National Model EMS Clinical Guidelines*. Version 2.0. National Association of EMS Officials website. https://www.nasemso.org/documents/National-Model-EMS-Clinical-Guidelines-Version2-Sept2017.pdf. Published September 2017. Accessed February 14, 2018.

exposure is obvious (eg, a victim involved in an avalanche or cold water immersion), diagnosis is simple. However, in some situations, signs and symptoms may be subtle (eg, hunger, nausea, chills, dizziness). When hypothermia is suspected, the paramedic's immediate action is to extricate and evacuate the patient to a site of warm shelter, remove cold, wet clothing, prevent a further drop in the patient's CBT, survey for traumatic injuries, cover the patient with warm blankets and increase the temperature in the ambulance, and rapidly and gently transport the patient for definitive care.

Rewarming techniques for managing patients with hypothermia are classified as passive, active external, and active internal. Passive rewarming includes measures such as moving the patient to a warm environment, removing wet clothing, and applying warm blankets. If the patient cannot be moved immediately, a vapor barrier should be used over the warmed dry blankets. Large heat packs or heat blankets can be applied (never directly against patient's skin or burns may occur). The risk of burns increases when using heat packs that generate temperatures greater than 113°F (45°C). If available, forced air warming blankets are effective for rewarming. Application of a battery-operated charcoal vest that blows warm air from a tube wrapped around the patient's torso has been found to increase body temperature while avoiding afterdrop.[2]

Active rewarming techniques refer to heating methods or devices such as radiant heat, forced hot air, and warm water packs. Active internal rewarming is invasive. Some of these procedures can be performed in the field, such as administering warmed IV fluids and providing warm, humidified oxygen to a maximum temperature of 104°F to 108°F (40°C to 42.2°C). Other procedures are reserved for in-hospital care. Examples include peritoneal and/or pleural lavage with warm fluids, use of esophageal rewarming tubes, cardiopulmonary bypass (active core rewarming), and extracorporeal circulation (extracorporeal membrane oxygenation [ECMO]).

> NOTE
>
> Rewarming methods such as hot water immersion can cause hypotension from peripheral vasodilation (rewarming shock) and a sudden return of cold, acidotic blood and waste products to the body's core (**afterdrop phenomenon**). Therefore, active rewarming techniques in the prehospital setting generally are avoided unless patient transport will be markedly delayed.

Mild Hypothermia

In mild cases of hypothermia, removal of the victim from the cold environment and passive rewarming may be the only steps necessary to manage the cold exposure. The paramedic should remove the patient's wet clothing (wet clothes allow five times as much heat loss as dry clothes) and wrap the patient in a dry blanket to prevent further chilling and help retain body heat. If the victim is conscious, warm drinks and sugar sources can support a gradual rise in CBT and help correct any dehydration present. Patients should not be permitted to smoke, which causes vasoconstriction; to drink alcoholic beverages, which produce peripheral vasodilation and increase heat loss from the skin; or to drink caffeine-containing beverages, which cause vasoconstriction and diuresis. These patients may be lethargic and somewhat dulled mentally but generally are oriented with no marked mental derangements. Consider vascular access if indicated. If fluids are needed, normal saline boluses warmed to 107.6°F (42°C) are recommended.[7]

Moderate Hypothermia

At CBTs below 89.8°F (32.1°C), mental derangements are invariably present and include disorientation, confusion, and lethargy proceeding to stupor and coma. Patients with moderate hypothermia usually have lost their ability to shiver, and their uncoordinated physical activity renders them unable to perform meaningful tasks. Management of patients with moderate hypothermia begins with ensuring adequate airway, ventilatory, and circulatory support and maintaining body temperature. Hyperventilation should be avoided.[8] Hypocarbia may increase the risk of ventricular fibrillation. The paramedic should first employ passive rewarming techniques and should not permit these patients to move about independently or physically exert themselves. Even minor physical activity can trigger dysrhythmias, including ventricular fibrillation. Active external rewarming (eg, heated blankets, forced air, warmed IV infusion) and rapid and gentle transport for definitive care are indicated for these patients. Careful monitoring of the patient's mental status, ECG, and vital functions is crucial.

> NOTE
>
> Temperature measurement with an esophageal probe is preferred after the airway is secured. If this device is not available, an epitympanic thermometer with an isolating ear cap is recommended. If neither of these devices is available, or if the patient's condition prohibits their use, rectal temperature may be obtained once the patient is in the warmed ambulance.

Severe Hypothermia

If the patient's CBT is below 82.4°F (28°C), he or she usually is unconscious.[9] The patient should be gently moved to a warm environment if vital signs are present. To avoid increasing return of cold blood to the heart, maintain the patient horizontal and avoid moving the extremities. The paramedic should institute passive and active external rewarming, administer warm, humidified oxygen, and transport the patient to an appropriate medical facility.

Hypothermic Cardiac Arrest

If the patient with moderate-to-severe hypothermia is in cardiac arrest (ventricular fibrillation or pulseless ventricular tachycardia), the paramedic should begin cardiopulmonary resuscitation (CPR) and attempt defibrillation. If VT or VF persists after a single shock, the value of deferring subsequent defibrillations until a target temperature is achieved is uncertain.[10] It may be reasonable to perform further defibrillation attempts according to the standard BLS algorithm concurrent with rewarming strategies. Care should be focused on providing effective CPR, rewarming the patient, and ensuring rapid transport to the emergency department. In-hospital active internal rewarming will be required for these patients. If defibrillation is not successful and the patient remains in ventricular fibrillation with a temperature greater than 86°F (30°C), then routine advanced cardiac life support (ACLS) care should be continued.[8,9] It may be reasonable to consider administration of a vasopressor during cardiac arrest according to the standard ACLS algorithm concurrent with rewarming strategies.[10]

If a patient with severe hypothermia is pulseless and cyanotic, with fixed and dilated pupils, prolonged resuscitation can be beneficial and CPR may still be indicated unless the chest wall is frozen, making compressions impossible.[11] If the initial rhythm is organized (not ventricular fibrillation or ventricular tachycardia) without pulses, the patient should be monitored without initiating CPR.[7,8] Some physicians will not presume a hypothermic patient to be dead until a near-normal CBT has

BOX 44-3 Determining Death of a Hypothermic Patient

The aphorism that "no one is dead until they are warm and dead" is based on the difficulty of diagnosing death in a hypothermic patient in the field. However, some patients really are cold and dead. General contraindications to attempted resuscitation in the field include obvious fatal injuries, such as decapitation, open head injury with loss of brain matter, truncal transection, incineration, or a chest wall that is so stiff that compressions are not possible.

Modified from: Paal P, Milani M, Brown D, Boyd J, Ellerton J. Termination of cardiopulmonary resuscitation in mountain rescue. *High Alt Med Biol*. 2012;13:200-208.

been achieved and resuscitation efforts are still unsuccessful (BOX 44-3). If there is no advanced airway, the patient should be ventilated, per AHA guidelines. When an advanced airway is in place, ventilation should be delivered at one-half the AHA's recommended rate. When possible, these patients are transported to a hospital capable of performing cardiac bypass or ECMO.

Special Care Considerations for Patients With Hypothermia

Prehospital care for patients with hypothermia should focus on airway, breathing, and circulation, with the following modifications in approach:[8]

1. Pulse and respirations may be difficult to detect. These vital signs (including ECG readings) should be assessed for 60 seconds to confirm the need for CPR. If there is any doubt about the presence of a pulse, begin CPR immediately.
2. For unresponsive patients and those in arrest, advanced airway management is indicated. This will serve two purposes: (1) It will enable provision of effective ventilation with warm, humidified oxygen (if available), and (2) it will isolate the airway to reduce the likelihood of aspiration.
3. The hypothermic heart may be unresponsive to cardiovascular drugs. In addition, drug metabolism may be reduced, allowing for toxic accumulation of the drug in the peripheral tissues. For these reasons, antidysrhythmic drugs are often withheld when the CBT is less than 86°F (30°C). Once the patient is rewarmed to at least 86°F (30°C), it may be reasonable to consider administration of standard ACLS medications, concurrent with rewarming strategies, at an interval twice as long as in normothermic patients (Class IIc).[12]
4. Sinus bradycardia may be protective in severe hypothermia. This rhythm may maintain sufficient oxygen delivery when hypothermia is present. Cardiac pacing usually is not indicated or successful.

Frostbite

Frostbite is a localized injury that results from freezing of body tissues. It often occurs in the lower extremities, particularly the toes and feet. Less often it occurs in the upper extremities (the fingers and hands). Frostbite also occurs on the ears, nose, and other body areas not protected from environmental extremes.

Pathophysiology

Frostbite occurs as ice crystals form in tissue. This crystal formation produces macrovascular and microvascular damage and direct cellular injury. The freezing depth depends on the intensity and duration of cold exposure. Severe freezing can also occur in tissue exposed to volatile hydrocarbons (eg, from industrial injuries) at low temperatures.

Under most conditions of frostbite, ice crystals form in the extracellular tissue, drawing water out of the cells and into the extravascular spaces. As a result, the electrolyte concentration in the cell can reach toxic levels. The ice crystals can also expand and cause direct mechanical destruction of tissue, leading to damage to blood vessels (particularly the endothelial cells), partial shrinkage and collapse of the cell membrane, loss of vascular integrity, local edema, and disruption of nutritive blood flow. Ischemia often produces the most damaging effects of frostbite.

When frozen tissue thaws, blood flow through the capillaries is initially restored. However, blood flow declines within minutes after thawing. This decreased blood flow occurs as the arterioles and venules constrict and release emboli, which travel through the small vessels. Progressive tissue loss results from thrombosis and hypoxia. The endothelium is damaged and results in deterioration of the microvasculature and dermal necrosis. The process of thawing and refreezing is more harmful to tissue than is allowing the frostbitten part to remain frozen until it can be warmed with minimal risk of refreezing. In addition to extreme temperature, wind, and humidity, predisposing factors for frostbite include the following:[13]

- Lack of protective clothing
- Poor nutrition
- Preexisting injury or medical or psychiatric illness
- Fatigue
- Decrease in local tissue perfusion
- Tobacco use
- Atherosclerosis
- Tight, constrictive clothing (especially socks and boots)
- Increased vasodilation
- Alcohol or other drug consumption in hypothermic patients
- Use of medications
- History of previous cold injury

Classifications and Symptoms

Cold injury can be subdivided into a number of classifications. For example, cold injury commonly is divided into two categories: frostnip and frostbite. Initial evaluation of the severity of the frostbite is difficult because the injury does not always reflect the underlying vascular changes.[3] Regardless of the depth of injury, the area may appear to be frozen. Palpation may help the paramedic to distinguish between superficial and deep injury. With superficial injury, the underlying tissue springs back on compression. With deep injury, the underlying tissue is hard and cannot be compressed.

Frostnip

Frostnip is manifested by transient numbness and tingling that resolves after rewarming. This cold injury does not represent true frostbite, because no tissue destruction has occurred. The initial symptoms are coldness and numbness in the affected area.

Frostbite

Frostbite can be graded as first-, second-, third-, and fourth-degree injury, based on the severity of exposure.[14] Affected areas may include the dermal and shallow subcutaneous layers as well as the subdermal layers and deep tissues. Third- and fourth-degree injuries involve at least some tissue loss. The disrupted nutritional capillary flow is compromised to the damaged tissue. With severe injuries, the affected area remains cold, mottled, and blue or gray after rewarming. After rewarming, edema usually appears within 3 hours. This edema is followed by the formation of vesicles within 3 to 24 hours (**FIGURE 44-3**). The blisters begin to resolve within 1 week, after which the skin blackens into a hard eschar. Eventually, the blackened tissue peels away (**demarcation**) (**FIGURE 44-4**), revealing shiny, red skin beneath. This tissue is sensitive to heat and cold and often remains susceptible to repeated frostbite injury.[14]

Since the four degrees of injury are based on acute physical examination findings coupled with advanced imaging after rewarming, this classification scheme is less useful for the field provider. To simplify classification, either in the field or before rewarming and/or diagnostic imaging (ie, thermography,

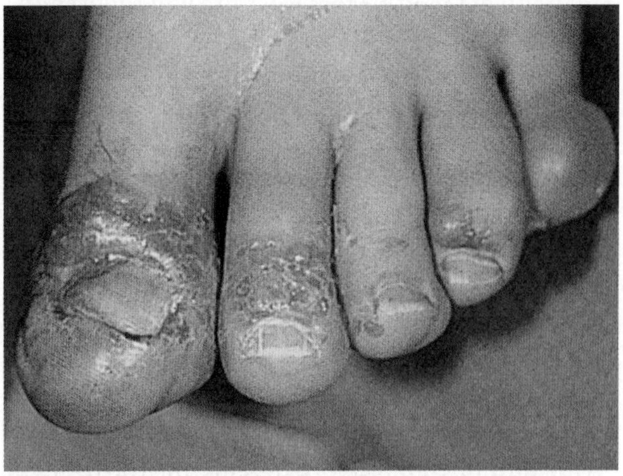

FIGURE 44-3 Edema and blister formation 24 hours after frostbite injury in an area covered by a tightly fitting boot.

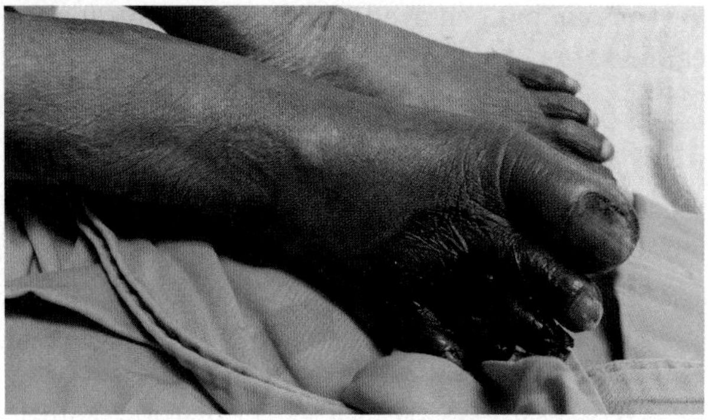

FIGURE 44-4 Gangrene developing after a frostbite injury.

angiography, plethysmography, radioisotope bone scanning; vascular and bone imaging) to determine tissue viability, the following two-tier classification scheme may be more practical:

- **Superficial.** No or minimal anticipated tissue loss; corresponding to first- and second-degree injury
- **Deep.** At least some anticipated tissue loss; corresponding to third- and fourth-degree injury

Management

Prehospital care for frostbite is limited to support of the patient's vital functions, elevation and protection of the affected extremity (jewelry should be removed), pain management, and rapid transport to a medical facility. Most frostbite will thaw spontaneously and should be allowed to do so if rapid rewarming cannot be readily achieved.[14] Vigorous rubbing or massage is ineffective and harmful. Partial, slow rewarming with blankets or other warm objects can worsen the injury. If the frostbite involves the patient's lower extremities, the person should not be allowed to walk. During transport, all restrictive and wet clothing should be removed from the patient and replaced with warm, dry clothing and blankets to guard against hypothermia. The patient should not be permitted to consume alcohol or smoke tobacco. Rapid rewarming of the frozen part by immersion in circulating warm water (98.6°F to 102°F [37°C to 38.9°C]) is the most effective therapeutic measure for preserving viable tissue if refreezing can be prevented.[7] In some settings (eg, backwoods rescue, natural disasters), this method of rewarming should not be used because of the risk of refreezing. After rewarming, the affected areas should be covered with loose sterile dressings. Blisters that are causing severe pain may be aspirated but should not be unroofed. Appropriate analgesia should be administered to manage the patient's pain.

> NOTE
>
> **Trench foot** (immersion foot) is a cold injury to the foot. However, the tissue does not freeze. It occurs from prolonged exposure to cold, but not freezing, water or air. Onset occurs within a day if the feet are wet and takes several days if they are dry. The signs and symptoms of this condition occur in phases and include painless blanched swollen skin that later becomes hot, red, swollen, and painful. The formation of blisters is serious and may signal the onset of gangrene. The paramedic should cover the affected area with sterile dressings and keep it dry and warm.
>
> *Modified from*: Busko J. Cold exposure illness and injury. In: Brice J, Delbridge TR, Meyers JB, eds. *Emergency Services: Clinical Practice and Systems Oversight*. Vol 1. 2nd ed. West Sussex, England: John Wiley & Sons; 2015:351-357.

Submersion

Drowning was the fifth-leading cause of unintentional death in the United States in 2015. It was the second-leading cause of unintentional injury or death among children and youths.[15] Drowning occurs more often in children younger than 5 years and between the ages of 15 and 24 years. Children younger than 1 year tend to drown in bathtubs, buckets, and toilets. Older children and young adults, however, are more likely to drown in outdoor water sources.[16]

Classifications

As recommended by the AHA, the World Health Organization, and the Utstein definition and style of data reporting, the term drowning is defined as "a process resulting in primary respiratory impairment from submersion/immersion in liquid."[8] (The term **submersion** usually refers to the head being below water, whereas *immersion* refers to the head being above water. The two terms often are used interchangeably.[17]) Nonfatal drowning refers to patients rescued from drowning. Fatal drowning indicates any death in the acute or subacute phase after injury that results from the drowning.[7] The definition further requires that a liquid–air interface be present at the entrance of the victim's airway, preventing the victim from breathing air. According to this definition, the victim may live or die after this process, but whatever the outcome, he or she has been involved in a drowning event. There are only three possible outcomes to drowning: fatality, survival with morbidity, and survival without morbidity.[18]

Pathophysiology

Drowning begins with intentional or unintentional submersion. After submersion, the victim realizes he or she is in distress. An example of this is a nonswimmer who panics or a swimmer who becomes fatigued. Drowning begins with the conscious victim taking in several deep breaths. This reaction is an attempt to store oxygen before breath-holding (**FIGURE 44-5**). The victim holds the breath until breathing reflexes override the breath-holding effort. As water is aspirated, laryngospasm occurs. Laryngospasm and aspiration produce severe hypoxia. This lack of oxygen to the tissue results in serious hypoxemia and acidosis, which lead to cardiac dysrhythmias and CNS anoxia. The physiologic events that follow are partly determined by the type and amount of water aspirated. Regardless of the type of water aspirated, the pathophysiology of drowning is characterized by

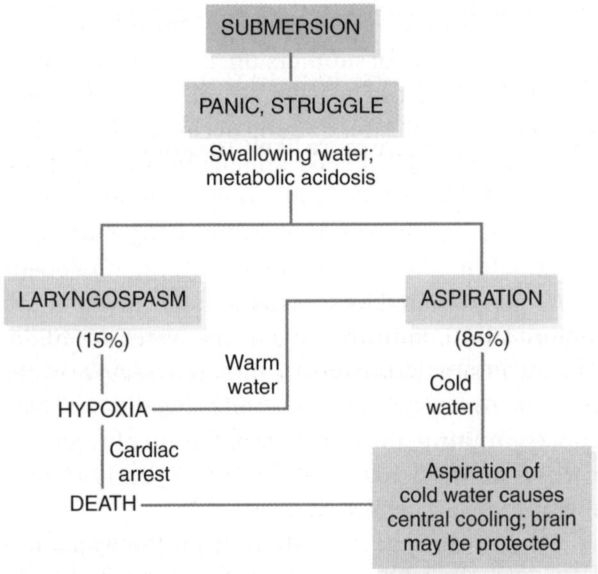

FIGURE 44-5 Progression of the drowning incident.

hypoxia, hypercapnia, and acidosis, which result in cardiac arrest.

> CRITICAL THINKING
> Do other swimmers or onlookers often "hear" a person who is drowning?

Drowning can occur in almost any type of water. Victims of drowning may aspirate saltwater or freshwater, tap water, or contaminated water (such as water containing sewage, chemicals, algae, bacteria, or sand). In theory, different fluids have different effects. However, these differences are not clinically significant in prehospital care. They should not be considered in the initial management of drowning patients. It is, however, important to relay such information in the transfer of care. The most important factors that determine outcome are the duration of submersion and the duration and severity of hypoxia.[19]

Pulmonary Pathophysiology Secondary to Drowning

Respiratory failure, hypoxia, and acidosis are the life-threatening complications of drowning. Hypoxia can result from the following factors:

- Fluid in the alveoli and interstitial spaces
- Loss of surfactant
- Contaminant particles in the alveoli and tracheobronchial tree
- Damage to the alveolar-capillary membrane and vascular endothelium

Poor perfusion and hypoxemia lead to metabolic acidosis in most patients. In those who survive the incident, acute respiratory failure may occur, including the development of acute respiratory distress syndrome (ARDS). ARDS (described in Chapter 23, *Respiratory*) reduces lung compliance and increases ventilation/perfusion mismatches and intrapulmonary shunting. The onset of symptoms can be delayed for as long as 24 hours after the submersion (secondary drowning).[20]

In addition to pulmonary effects, drowning can affect other body systems. For example, cardiovascular derangements can occur as a result of hypoxia and acidosis, leading to dysrhythmias and decreased cardiac output. CNS dysfunction and nerve damage result from cerebral edema and anoxia. The paramedic also must be suspicious of spinal injury in drowning victims. Renal dysfunction is not a common complication. However, when it does occur, it can progress to acute renal failure. Renal dysfunction is usually the result of hypoxic injury or hemoglobinuria, leading to acute tubular necrosis.

Factors That Affect the Clinical Outcome

The following four factors can affect the clinical outcome of a drowning incident:

1. **Duration of submersion.** The longer the patient is submersed, the less likely he or she is to survive. When rescue takes longer than 30 minutes, victims rescued from warm water in summer months or in warm southern waters usually do not survive. Submersion in cold water for up to 66 minutes in children has been associated with survival, including intact brain function. (Most children rescued from cold water should receive resuscitation even with prolonged submersion.) Resuscitation is indicated for all patients unless physical evidence of death is present (eg, putrefaction, dependent lividity, and rigor mortis). Drowning victims who have spontaneous circulation and breathing when they reach the hospital usually recover, with good outcomes.[8]
2. **Cleanliness of the water.** Contaminants in water have an irritant effect on the pulmonary system that may lead to bronchospasm and poor gas exchange. These effects can cause a secondary pulmonary infection with delayed severe respiratory compromise.
3. **Temperature of the water.** Submersion in cold water can have beneficial and negative effects. The rapid onset of hypothermia can act as a protective function, especially in the case of brain viability in patients who have undergone prolonged submersion. An incident in which a child was submerged for 66 minutes in a creek with a water temperature of 37°F (2.8°C) is the longest documented submersion with a good neurologic outcome.[21] This phenomenon is not fully understood. A contributing factor may be the **mammalian diving reflex** in infant and child submersions. This reflex is stimulated by cold water. It shunts blood to the brain and heart from the skin, gastrointestinal tract, and extremities. This reflex occurs in seals and lower mammals. It also occurs in humans to some extent. Hypothermia may slow brain cell death and organ demise that can lead to permanent neurologic damage. Likewise, hypothermia can contribute to neurologic recovery after prolonged submersion by reducing the metabolic needs of the brain. (Hypothermia also may develop secondary to submersion and later heat loss through evaporation during attempts at resuscitation. In these cases, the hypothermia is not protective.) In a submersion incident when the water temperature is less than 43°F (6°C) and the patient is in cardiac arrest, resuscitation should be attempted if submersion time is less than 90 minutes.[7] In cases where the water temperature is greater than 43°F (6°C) and the patient is in cardiac arrest, resuscitation should be attempted if submersion time is less than 30 minutes.[7] The relative contributions of the diving reflex and hypothermia are not clear. The adverse effects of submersion in cold water include severe ventricular dysrhythmias.
4. **Age of the victim.** The younger the victim, the better the chance for survival.

Management

At the site of a drowning incident, the safety of the EMS crew is paramount. Only personnel trained in water rescue should try to intervene (see Chapter 54, *Rescue Awareness and Operations*). Depending on the type and duration of submersion, the patient's symptoms may vary from an asymptomatic presentation to cardiac arrest. After gaining access to the victim, the paramedic should take spinal precautions while the victim is still in the water only if spinal injury is suspected (eg, diving injury, water skiing, surfing or watercraft incidents). Rescue breathing (if needed) should be initiated as soon as possible (even in the water). Chest compressions in the water are futile. The use of subdiaphragmatic thrusts to remove water from the airways is ineffective and dangerous and may cause vomiting and aspiration. Subdiaphragmatic thrusts are indicated only if foreign body airway obstruction is suspected.[3]

After removing the patient from the water, the paramedic should evaluate the patient to ensure an adequate airway. Administration of high-concentration oxygen is indicted if oxygen saturation (Spo_2) as measured by a pulse oximeter is less than 92% to achieve oxygen saturations of 94% to 98%. Positive pressure ventilation is considered for patients with severe dyspnea. The initial ventilations may be difficult due to increased resistance from water in the airway. Continuous positive airway pressure is considered for awake patients who have respiratory distress.[7] ECG monitoring and vascular access are indicated. Patients who are in cardiac arrest should be managed with standard BLS and ALS protocols.

Victims of submersion incidents often are at risk for hypothermia; heat loss in water can be up to 32 times greater than that in air.[22] Hypothermia can make resuscitation more difficult. It requires special consideration with regard to gentle handling, the administration of drugs, and defibrillation. The paramedic should remove the patient's wet clothing, as with all other victims of hypothermia, and should dry and wrap the patient in blankets to conserve body heat. External warming and the administration of heated, humidified oxygen at the scene and during transport should be considered. All patients suspected of having hypothermia should be managed as described earlier.

According to the AHA, "All victims of drowning who require any form of resuscitation (including rescue breathing alone) should be transported to the hospital."[8] Asymptomatic patients also require transport for physician evaluation because symptom onset may be delayed by 2 or 3 hours. There has never been a case published in the medical literature of a patient initially without symptoms who later deteriorates and dies. People who have drowned and have minimal symptoms will either get better or worse within 2 to 3 hours.[23] They should be given oxygen and carefully monitored to guard against aspiration pneumonia and undetected hypoxia that can result from submersion. Oxygen is the most important treatment needed by drowning victims.

CRITICAL THINKING

What are the risks to rescuers on a call involving submersion victims?

Diving Emergencies

The United States has more than 3 million recreational scuba divers,[24] and more than 200,000 new sport divers are certified each year.[25] Emergencies unique to pressure-related diving include those caused by the mechanical effects of pressure (barotrauma), air embolism, and the breathing of compressed air (decompression sickness and nitrogen narcosis).

NOTE

The term *scuba* is actually an acronym for self-contained underwater breathing apparatus. This equipment allows divers to breathe underwater. Scuba gear typically consists of one or two compressed air tanks. These tanks are strapped to the diver's back and connected by a hose to a regulator.

Basic Properties of Gases

The weight of the atmosphere exerts a pressure of 14.7 pounds per square inch (psi) of force at sea level (14.7 psi is equal to 760 mm Hg). This means that a 1-inch column of air as tall as the atmosphere would weigh 14.7 pounds. This weight is commonly referred to as 1 atmosphere of pressure (1 atm). One atm is referred to as ambient pressure or absolute pressure. Water weighs considerably more than air and can exert much more pressure. For example, a 1-inch column of seawater needs to be only 33 feet tall to weigh 14.7 pounds. Thus, at a depth of 33 feet, the total pressure is 29.4 psi, or 2 atm of pressure (1 atm from the air and 1 atm from the 33 feet of water [$2 \times 14.7 = 29.4$]). Every additional 33 feet of seawater adds another 14.7 pounds of pressure, or another 1 atm.

Laws Pertaining to Gases

Three laws of the properties of gases underpin all pressure diving-related emergencies (and some high-altitude illnesses): Boyle's law, Dalton's law, and Henry's law.[26] The following properties of gases can aid comprehension of these laws:

- Increased pressure dissolves gases into the blood.
- Oxygen metabolizes.
- Nitrogen dissolves.

NOTE

The term **dysbarism** describes illnesses that result directly or indirectly from changes in ambient atmospheric pressure and the pressure of gases within the body.

Boyle's Law. Boyle's law states that, if temperature remains constant, the volume of a given mass of gas is inversely proportional to the absolute pressure; that is, when the pressure is doubled, the volume of gas is halved (compressed into a smaller space), and vice versa. This law can be expressed by the equation $PV = k$, in which P is pressure, V is volume, and k is a constant. Boyle's law explains the "popping" or "squeezing" sensation in the ears that a person may feel when traveling by air. It is the basic mechanism for all types of barotrauma: trapped gases expand as pressure decreases. For example, when a diver uses a scuba tank of pressurized air, the lung volumes remain constant at various depths. If the diver ascends but does not exhale, water pressure decreases and the gas in the lungs expands, greatly increasing the pressure in the lungs (**FIGURE 44-6**).

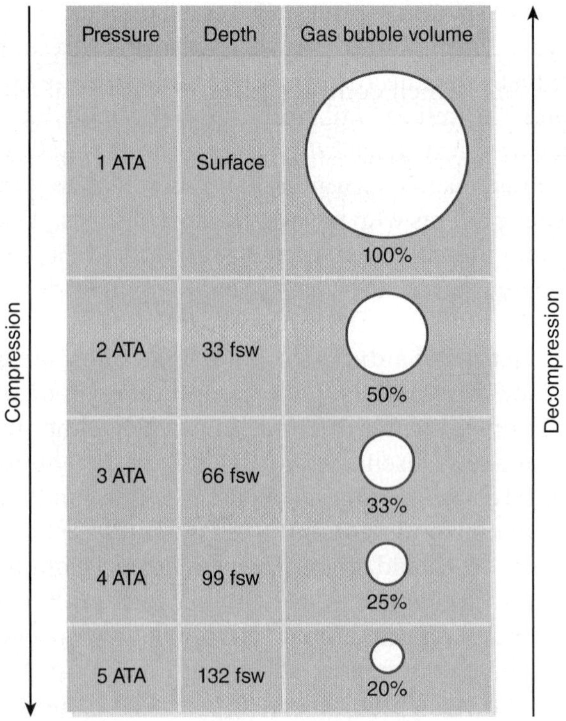

Pressure
Depth
Gas bubble volume
1 ATA
Surface
100%
2 ATA
33 fsw
50%
3 ATA
66 fsw
33%
4 ATA
99 fsw
25%
5 ATA
132 fsw
20%
Compression
Decompression

FIGURE 44-6 Boyle's law.

Reproduced from Frank AJ. Diving injury. In: Brice J, Delbridge TR, Meyers JB, eds. *Emergency Services: Clinical Practice and Systems Oversight*. Vol 1. 2nd ed. West Sussex, England: John Wiley & Sons Ltd; 2015:372-380.

NOTE

Gas expands as pressure decreases. This fact applies to increases in altitude that occur during air transport. For example, in a patient transported by air, gas can expand in the respiratory system, gastrointestinal system, or sinuses as altitude increases and pressure decreases. Medical equipment also can be affected by an increase in air volume. Examples include endotracheal tube cuffs and air splints.

Dalton's Law. Dalton's law states that the pressure exerted by each gas in a mixture of gases is the same pressure that the gas would exert if it alone occupied the same volume. However, the total pressure of a mixture of gases equals the sum of the partial pressures that make up the mixture. This law is expressed by the equation $P_t = Po_2 + PN_2 + Px$, where P_t is the total pressure, Po_2 is the partial pressure of oxygen, PN_2 is the partial pressure of nitrogen, and Px is the partial pressure of the remaining gases in the mixture.

To simplify, the air we breathe is about 80% nitrogen and 20% oxygen; that is, about 80% of the pressure of the air (ie, the gas mixture) is exerted by the nitrogen in the mixture. About 20% of the pressure is exerted by the oxygen in the mixture. This means that at sea level, the pressure exerted on us by the nitrogen in the air is 80% of 14.7, or 11.76 psi; the pressure from the oxygen is 20% of 14.7, or 2.94 psi. Together, these gases account for the 14.7 psi of pressure at the surface. Even though the gas mixtures remain with normal percentages of nitrogen and oxygen, the partial pressures of these gases change at different altitudes above sea level or at depths below sea level. The principles of this law explain problems that can arise from the breathing of compressed air: Gas expansion causes the partial pressure of oxygen to drop as gas molecules move farther apart, reducing the available oxygen.

Henry's Law. Henry's law states that, at a constant temperature, the solubility of a gas in a liquid solution is proportionate to the partial pressure of the gas. Thus, more gas can be dissolved into a liquid at a higher pressure, and less gas can be dissolved into the liquid when that pressure is released. For example, when a container of a carbonated beverage (pressurized with dissolved carbon dioxide gas) is opened, a "pop" is heard and bubbles form on the liquid. This reaction occurs because the pressure in the container is no longer great enough to hold the dissolved gas inside. Henry's law is expressed by the following equation: $\% X = Px / P_t \times 100$, where $\% X$ is the amount of gas dissolved in a liquid, Px is the partial pressure of the gas, and P_t is the total atmospheric pressure. This law explains why more nitrogen, which makes up almost 80% of air, dissolves in a diver's body as ambient pressure increases with descent. This dissolved nitrogen is released from the tissues on ascent as pressure decreases.

Barotrauma

Barotrauma is tissue injury caused by a change in pressure, which compresses or expands gas contained in various body structures. The type of barotrauma depends on whether the diver is in descent or ascent. Barotrauma is the most common injury of scuba divers. Many factors influence dive-related injuries. The paramedic should attempt to identify the following:[7]

- Water temperature
- Dive history
  - Number of dives in recent days
  - Bottom time in dives
  - Dive profiles
  - Maximum depth
  - Rate of ascent
  - Safety stops (if used)
  - Dive gas (air versus mixed gases such as nitrox, heliox, or trimix)
- Time of symptom onset
- History of air travel after dive
- Other injuries or exposures

General management for patients with dive-related illness is primarily supportive. Administer oxygen to achieve oxygen saturation as measured by arterial blood sampling (Sao_2) of 94% to 98%. If decompression illness is suspected, administer oxygen regardless of Sao_2. Assess the patient for hypothermia and treat if indicated. Establish vascular access and infuse fluids if needed.

Consult with medical direction regarding the need for hyperbaric oxygen therapy (HBOT). The detailed dive history will be needed in addition to physical examination findings to determine whether HBOT is indicated.

Barotrauma of Descent

Barotrauma of descent (also known as squeeze) results from the compression of gas in enclosed spaces as the ambient pressure increases with descent under water. Air trapped in noncollapsible chambers is compressed, leading to a vacuum-type effect that results in severe, sharp pain caused by the distortion, vascular engorgement, edema, and hemorrhage of the exposed tissue (BOX 44-4). As a rule, squeeze usually results from a blocked eustachian tube or from failure

BOX 44-4 Signs and Symptoms of Diving-Related Conditions

Squeeze
Pain
Sensation of fullness
Headache
Disorientation
Vertigo
Nausea
Bleeding from the nose or ears

Pulmonary Overpressurization Syndrome (POPS)
Gradually increasing chest pain
Hoarseness
Neck fullness
Dyspnea
Dysphagia
Subcutaneous emphysema

Air Embolism
Focal paralysis or sensory changes (strokelike symptoms)
Aphasia
Confusion
Blindness or other visual disturbances
Convulsions
Loss of consciousness
Dizziness
Vertigo
Abdominal pain
Cardiac arrest

Decompression Sickness
Shortness of breath
Itching
Rash
Joint pain
Crepitus
Fatigue
Vertigo
Paresthesias
Paralysis
Seizures
Unconsciousness

Nitrogen Narcosis
Impaired judgment
Sensation of alcohol intoxication
Slowed motor response
Loss of proprioception
Euphoria

of the diver to clear (open) the eustachian tube with exhalation during descent. The ears and paranasal sinuses are most likely to be affected. Squeeze occurs in the ears, sinuses, lungs and airways, gastrointestinal tract, thorax, teeth (pulp decay, recent extraction of sockets or fillings), or added air spaces (face mask or diving suit).

The management of barotrauma of descent involves slowly returning the diver to shallower depths. Prehospital care is mainly supportive. After the patient has been evaluated by a physician, definitive care may include bed rest with the head elevated, avoidance of strain and strenuous activity, use of decongestants and possibly antihistamines and antibiotics, and perhaps surgical repair.

CRITICAL THINKING

What preexisting illness can make a diver more susceptible to squeeze?

Barotrauma of Ascent

Barotrauma of ascent occurs through the reverse process of descent ("reverse squeeze"). Assuming that the air-filled cavities of the body have equalized pressure during the diver's descent, the volume of air trapped in this pressurized space expands as ambient pressure decreases with ascent (Boyle's law). If air is not allowed to escape because of obstruction (eg, breath-holding, bronchospasm, mucus plug), the expanding gases distend the tissues surrounding them. The most common cause of this type of barotrauma is breath-holding during ascent.

Problems from reverse squeeze are rare. However, one type of reverse squeeze, **pulmonary overpressurization syndrome (POPS)**, can occur as a result of the expansion of trapped air in the lungs and can lead to alveolar rupture. It also can lead to leakage of air into areas outside the alveoli. The clinical syndromes associated with barotrauma of ascent include pneumomediastinum, subcutaneous emphysema, pneumopericardium, pneumothorax, pneumoperitoneum, and systemic arterial air embolism. Except for tension pneumothorax (a rare complication that may require needle or tube decompression) and air embolism, which may require hyperbaric recompression therapy (BOX 44-5), POPS usually requires only administration of oxygen, observation, and transport for evaluation by a physician.

BOX 44-5 Hyperbaric Oxygen Therapy

Altering the surrounding air pressure for medical treatment is a practice that dates back to the 17th century. At that time, "fevers and inflammations" were treated in crude chambers that were pressurized using hand bellows. Today, HBOT is carried out in single-person chambers called monoplace chambers. The treatment also can be done in larger chambers, called multiplace chambers, which can house several patients and the attending hyperbaric health care workers. HBOT has proved to be effective in the treatment of a wide variety of medical disorders, including air embolism and decompression sickness; carbon monoxide poisoning and smoke inhalation; carbon monoxide poisoning complicated by cyanide poisoning; clostridial myonecrosis (gas gangrene); crush injury, and other acute traumatic ischemias; intracranial abscesses; and thermal burns. It also has been shown to enhance the healing of certain problem wounds.

Modified from: Latham E. Hyperbaric oxygen therapy. Medscape website. https://emedicine.medscape.com/article/1464149-overview. Updated December 11, 2017. Accessed February 14, 2018.

Air Embolism

Air embolism is the most serious complication of pulmonary barotrauma. It is a major cause of death and disability among sport divers.[6] Divers risk this condition when they ascend too rapidly or hold their breath during ascent. The classic description of a dive causing an air embolism is rapidly ascending to the surface because of panic.

Air embolism results as the expanding air disrupts tissues and air is forced into the circulatory system. The air bubbles pass through the left side of the heart and become lodged in small arterioles, thus occluding distal circulation. The syndrome usually manifests as the diver surfaces and exhales. Exhaling releases the high intrapulmonic pressure that resulted from lung overexpansion. With the decrease in intrathoracic pressure, bubbles advance into the left side of the heart and enter the systemic arterial supply. This process results in a dramatic presentation. The clinical manifestations depend on the site of systemic arterial occlusion. The most common presentation of air embolism is similar to that of stroke and includes vertigo, confusion, loss of consciousness, visual disturbances, and focal neurologic deficits.

Air embolism should be suspected if a diver suddenly loses consciousness immediately after surfacing. Paramedics should begin BLS and ALS measures, and the patient should be rapidly transported for recompression treatment. Also, the patient should be thoroughly evaluated for signs of POPS, such as a pneumothorax.

A patient suspected of having an air embolism should be transported in the left lateral recumbent position.[25] Formerly, the Trendelenburg position was recommended; however, it may increase cerebral edema.[3] If air transport is to be used, the patient should be transported by an aircraft that is pressurized to sea level to prevent existing intra-arterial air bubbles from expanding further. The flight altitude must be as low as possible if the internal cabin pressure cannot be maintained at sea level. Ideally, it should never be over 1,000 feet (300 m) above sea level. The patient also can be transported by a rotary wing aircraft that flies at low altitude.

Recompression. **Recompression** is the use of elevated pressure (including HBOT) to treat conditions within the body caused by a rapid decrease in pressure (eg, air embolism). Recompression takes place in a hyperbaric oxygen chamber (**FIGURE 44-7**). As described in Chapter 32, *Nontraumatic Musculoskeletal Disorders*, hyperbaric chambers allow for the delivery of oxygen at a higher than normal atmospheric pressure. The process is used to overcome the natural limit of oxygen solubility in blood. It thus reduces the intravascular bubble volume and restores tissue perfusion. Slow decompression helps to prevent bubbles from re-forming. Paramedics should know the location of the nearest hyperbaric treatment facility and should follow the protocol established by medical direction. Ground transport to a hyperbaric facility is preferred over air transport; air transport is avoided because the increase in altitude lowers the ambient pressure and allows microbubbles to expand. Recompression is not required for diving injuries such as ear or facial barotrauma, nitrogen narcosis, pneumothorax, pneumomediastinum, or subcutaneous emphysema.[3]

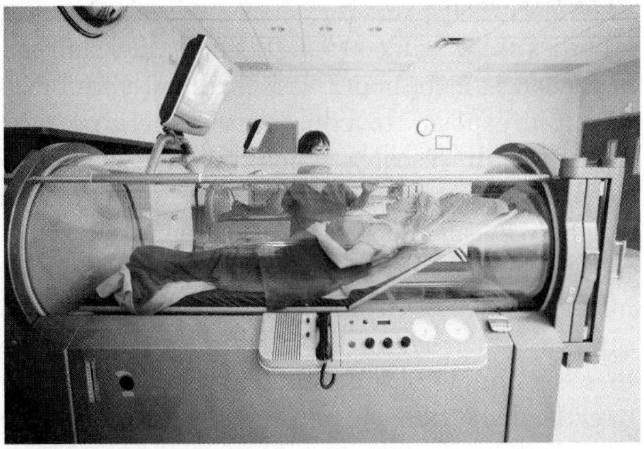

FIGURE 44-7 Hyperbaric oxygen chamber.

CRITICAL THINKING

Where is the nearest hyperbaric chamber in your area?

NOTE

The Divers Alert Network, a nonprofit organization operated by Duke University Medical Center, specializes in diving-related illnesses. It offers consultation and referral services. Their emergency telephone number is 1-919-684-9111.

Decompression Sickness

Decompression sickness is also known as the bends, dysbarism, caisson disease, and diver's paralysis. It is a multisystem disorder that results when nitrogen in compressed air (dissolved into tissues and blood from the increase in the partial pressure of the gas at depth) converts back from solution to gas. This conversion back to gas results in the formation of bubbles in the tissues and blood. The syndrome occurs when the ambient pressure decreases (Henry's law) as a result of ascending too rapidly. In such an ascent, the balance between the dissolved nitrogen in tissue and blood and the partial pressure of nitrogen in the inspired gas cannot be reached. Because the nitrogen bubbles can form in any tissue, lymphedema (the accumulation of lymph in soft tissues), cellular distention, and cellular rupture also can occur. The net effect of all these processes is poor tissue perfusion and ischemia. The joints and the spinal cord are most often affected. Signs and symptoms of decompression sickness may initially include rashes, itching, and a complaint of "bubbles under the skin." Pulmonary complaints may include chest pain, cough, and shortness of breath.

Failure to make recommended decompression "stops" during ascent usually causes decompression sickness. (Stops are based on diving tables and charts that consider depth, the duration of the dive, and previous dives completed.) Making stops during the ascent allows more time for safe off-gassing. Many hyperbaric professionals advise a 3- to 5-minute safety stop at 15 to 20 feet (5 to 6 m) for any dive.[27] For dives below 60 feet (18 m), another safety stop at 30 feet (9 m) may be of value. If possible, the paramedic should ask the diver about safety stops made during ascent.

> NOTE
>
> Compressed gas at 33 feet (10 m; 2 atmospheres) doubles in volume when the diver moves to the surface (1 atmosphere). This expansion occurs because the pressure is half of 33 feet (10 m). The last 6 feet (2 m) of ascent have the greatest potential for volume expansion. This is considered the most dangerous depth.

The paramedic should suspect decompression sickness in any patient who has symptoms within 48 hours after a scuba dive.[25] Patients who travel by air within 24 hours are particularly vulnerable.[7] The symptoms cannot be explained by other conditions. An example is a patient with unexplained joint pain who had been diving within the previous 24 hours. Prehospital care includes support of vital functions, administration of high-concentration oxygen, fluid resuscitation, and rapid transport for recompression. The patient transport and air evacuation guidelines described for air embolism should also be used with these patients.

Nitrogen Narcosis

Nitrogen narcosis ("rapture of the deep") is a condition in which nitrogen becomes dissolved in the blood. This condition is caused by a higher than normal partial pressure of nitrogen. Dissolved nitrogen crosses the blood–brain barrier. It produces depressant effects similar to those of alcohol, which can seriously impair the diver's thinking and lead to lethal errors in judgment. Symptoms of nitrogen narcosis usually become evident at depths of 75 to 100 feet (23 to 30 m).[28] At depths below 300 feet (91 m), with standard air (an oxygen–nitrogen mixture), the diver loses consciousness. Nitrogen narcosis affects all divers but is better tolerated by experienced divers. It is more likely to occur if the diver is cold, fatigued, or frightened. Helium–oxygen mixtures are used to improve the nitrogen complication (improving mental clarity) for deep dives. Examples of these mixtures are trimix and heliox. The narcotic effects of nitrogen are reversed with ascent.

> NOTE
>
> The depressant effect of pressurized nitrogen has been compared to drinking one dry martini on an empty stomach every 10 minutes (the "martini rule"). The theory is that being 50 feet (15 m) under water is equivalent to drinking one martini; at 100 feet (30 m), two martinis; at 150 feet (45 m), three martinis, and so on.
>
> *Modified from*: Szpilman D, Orlowski JP. Sports related to drowning. *Eur Respir Rev*. 2016;25:348-359.

Nitrogen narcosis is a common factor in diving accidents, and it may be responsible for memory loss. Prehospital care is mainly supportive. The paramedic should assess the patient for injuries that may have occurred during the dive, and the patient should be transported for evaluation by a physician.

> NOTE
>
> Less common diving-related illnesses may result from oxygen toxicity (usually seen with prolonged exposure to oxygen or exposure to excessive concentrations of oxygen), breathing of contaminated gases (eg, carbon monoxide in the compressed air), hypercapnia, and hyperventilation.

High-Altitude Illness

High-altitude illness principally occurs at altitudes 8,200 feet (2,500 m) or more above sea level.[3] However, altitudes as low as 5,000 feet (1,500 m) cause physiologic changes in the body.[29] This condition is attributed directly to exposure to reduced atmospheric pressure (described previously), which results in hypobaric hypoxia. So, despite the fact that the percentage of oxygen in the air remains fairly fixed at 21%, at an altitude of about 11,500 feet (3,500 m) a person breathes in only about 60% as much oxygen with each breath due to the low pressure.[29] Activities associated with these syndromes include mountain climbing, aircraft or glider flight, riding in hot air balloons, and the use of low-pressure or vacuum chambers.

The high-altitude syndromes discussed in this chapter are acute mountain sickness, high-altitude cerebral edema, and high-altitude pulmonary edema. Emergency care for all forms of high-altitude illness

NOTE

Worldwide, it is estimated that about 40 million people live above 8,000 feet (2,400 m), and 25 million live above 12,000 feet (3,700 m). Most cases of high-altitude illness are not associated with these groups, which are acclimated to high altitudes. Those most affected by illness from high altitudes are people who occasionally ascend into mountainous regions, such as mountain sport enthusiasts and tourists.

Modified from: Marx J, Hockberger R, Walls R. *Rosen's Emergency Medicine*. 8th ed. St. Louis, MO: Elsevier; 2013; Venugopalan P. High altitude pulmonary hypertension. Medscape website. https://emedicine.medscape.com/article/901668-overview. Updated August 1, 2016. Published February 13, 2018.

DID YOU KNOW?

Normal Pao_2 at High Altitude

Altitude also affects the normal, expected partial pressure of oxygen, arterial (Pao_2). High altitude decreases barometric pressure and therefore the Po_2 level. Up to an altitude of 10,000 feet (3,000 m) above sea level, barometric pressure decreases about 24 mm Hg per 1,000 feet (300 m) of elevation. For example, in Denver, Colorado, where the elevation is 5,280 feet (1,600 m), barometric pressure is about 633 mm Hg. At an elevation of 10,000 feet (3,000 m), barometric pressure is only 523 mm Hg. The general formula for changing observed sea-level Pao_2 values to Pao_2 values at a different barometric pressure is as follows:

Expected Pao_2 at high altitude = (High-altitude barometric pressure/760 mm Hg) × Sea-level Po_2

According to this calculation, if a normal person's sea-level Pao_2 is 95 mm Hg, the Pao_2 in Denver is about 79 mm Hg; at an elevation of 10,000 feet (3,000 m), it is only 65 mm Hg.

Modified from: Beachey W. *Respiratory Care Anatomy and Physiology: Foundations for Clinical Practice*. 4th ed. St. Louis, MO: Elsevier; 2018.

includes airway, ventilatory, and circulatory support and descent to a lower altitude. In addition, a physician should evaluate all patients with high-altitude illness. Strategies for preventing high-altitude illness include the following:[30]

1. Gradual ascent (days)
2. Limited exertion
3. Decreased sleeping at altitude
4. Adequate fluid intake to prevent dehydration
5. High-carbohydrate diet
6. Medications (all are controversial)
   - Acetazolamide (to speed acclimatization and reduce the incidence of acute mountain sickness)
   - Nifedipine (used solely by those with a history of high-altitude pulmonary edema to prevent recurrence upon ascent)
   - Steroids

Exposure to high altitude can worsen chronic medical conditions, even in the absence of apparent altitude sickness. Examples of such medical conditions include angina pectoris, congestive heart failure, chronic obstructive pulmonary disease, sickle cell disease, and hypertension. Chronic medical conditions can worsen as a result of a low partial pressure of oxygen. A low partial pressure of oxygen means that less oxygen is inhaled with each normal respiratory volume.

Acute Mountain Sickness

Acute mountain sickness (AMS) is a common high-altitude illness. It results when an unacclimatized person ascends rapidly to altitudes greater than 5,000 to 7,000 feet (1500–2100 m).[7] The illness usually develops within 4 to 6 hours of reaching a high altitude and reaches maximum severity within 24 to 48 hours (BOX 44-6). It abates on the third or fourth day after exposure with gradual acclimatization.

The physical findings with AMS vary. They include headache, anorexia, nausea, vomiting, weakness, dizziness, fatigue, difficulty sleeping, tachycardia, bradycardia, postural hypotension, and ataxia (impaired ability to coordinate movement). Ataxia is a key sign of the progression of the illness to high-altitude cerebral edema (HACE). As AMS becomes severe, the victim may experience alterations in consciousness, disorientation, and impaired judgment. Emergency care includes administration of oxygen to maintain Spo_2 of at least 90%. The person should stop his or her ascent and if possible descend to a lower altitude. Treatment may also include ibuprofen or acetaminophen for pain, ondansetron to manage nausea and vomiting, acetazolamide to speed acclimation, or, if symptoms are severe, dexamethasone. Hydrate the patient orally if tolerated, or establish IV access and infuse fluids.

High-Altitude Cerebral Edema

High-altitude cerebral edema (HACE) is the most severe form of acute high-altitude illness. It is characterized by a progression of global cerebral signs in the presence of AMS. These signs probably are related

BOX 44-6 Signs and Symptoms of High-Altitude Illness

Acute Mountain Sickness

Headache (most common symptom) attributed to subacute cerebral edema or to spasm or dilation of cerebral blood vessels secondary to hypocapnia or hypoxia
Malaise
Anorexia
Vomiting
Dizziness or lightheadedness
Irritability
Fatigue
Difficulty sleeping
Dyspnea on exertion

High-Altitude Pulmonary Edema

Shortness of breath
Dyspnea
Cough (with or without frothy sputum)
Crackles
Hypoxia
Generalized weakness
Lethargy
Disorientation

High-Altitude Cerebral Edema

Headache
Ataxia
Altered consciousness
Confusion
Hallucinations
Drowsiness
Stupor
Coma

to an increase in intracranial pressure caused by cerebral edema and swelling. Therefore the distinctions between AMS and HACE are inherently blurred, and HACE is often considered just the end stage of AMS.[31] The progression from mild AMS to ataxia and unconsciousness associated with HACE can occur quickly (ie, within 12 hours). However, it usually requires 1 to 3 days of exposure to high altitudes (greater than 8,000 feet [2,400 m]).[7]

HACE must be managed promptly, because without treatment the syndrome rapidly progresses to stupor, coma, and death. As with other forms of high-altitude illness, emergency care focuses on airway, ventilatory, and circulatory support and descent to a lower altitude. Establish vascular access and consider fluid bolus to achieve a systolic blood pressure of 90 mm Hg followed by an infusion of 125 mL/hr once the patient is rehydrated. Dexamethasone and acetazolamide can be administered in these patients as well.[7]

NOTE

The symptoms of mild AMS are similar to a "hangover" and usually include headache and slurred speech. Patients with HACE will have symptoms of mild AMS plus ataxia (an impaired ability to coordinate movements) and mental status changes.

Modified from: Bope ET, Kellerman RD. *Conn's Current Therapy*. St. Louis, MO: Elsevier; 2015.

High-Altitude Pulmonary Edema

High-altitude pulmonary edema (HAPE) is caused at least partly by increased pulmonary artery pressure that develops in response to hypoxia. The increased pressure results in the release of leukotrienes. Leukotrienes increase the permeability of pulmonary arterioles. The increased pressure also results in the leakage of fluid into extravascular space. The initial symptoms of HAPE usually begin 24 to 72 hours after the exposure to high altitudes. It is the most lethal of the altitude illnesses.[32] The symptoms often are preceded by vigorous exercise.

Physical findings in patients with HAPE include progressive cough, hypoxia, hyperpnea, and weakness at altitudes greater than 8,000 feet (2,400 m). As the illness progresses, the patient may develop crackles, rhonchi, tachycardia, and cyanosis. Emergency care includes administration of oxygen to increase arterial oxygenation and reduce pulmonary artery pressure. Descent to an altitude at least 500 to 1,000 feet (150 to 300 m) lower is essential. Adjunctive treatments that can be used with descent include nifedipine. If nifedipine is not available, either tadalafil (Cialis) or sildenafil (Viagra) may be used. Noninvasive positive pressure ventilation with continuous positive airway pressure or bag-mask may improve the patient's condition. Establish vascular access and consider fluid bolus to achieve a systolic blood pressure of 90 mm Hg followed by an infusion of 125 mL/hr once the patient is rehydrated.[7]

Portable hyperbaric chambers (eg, Gamow bag, Gamow tent) are commercially available. These may temporarily reverse the effects of HAPE and HACE. They are used by some EMS agencies in high-risk areas when immediate descent is not possible.

Summary

- Body temperature is regulated by a thermoregulatory center in the posterior hypothalamus. The body temperature can be increased or decreased in two ways:
  - Thermogenesis, the regulation of heat production
  - Thermolysis, the regulation of heat loss
- Heat illness results from one of two basic causes:
  - First, the normal temperature-regulating functions can be overwhelmed by conditions in the environment. These conditions can include heat stress. More often, though, they involve excessive exercise in moderate to extreme environmental conditions.
  - The other cause is failure of the body's thermoregulatory mechanism, which may occur in older adults or in people who are ill or debilitated.
- Heat illnesses can be classified as heat cramps, heat exhaustion, and heatstroke:
  - Heat cramps are brief, intermittent, and often severe. They are muscular cramps that occur in muscles fatigued by heavy work or exercise.
  - Heat exhaustion is characterized by dizziness, nausea, headache, and a mild to moderate rise in the core body temperature (CBT) (up to less than 103°F [39.4°C]).
  - Heatstroke occurs when mental status becomes altered because the temperature-regulating functions break down entirely. This failure results in body temperature increasing to 104°F (40°C) or higher. Temperatures this high damage all tissues and lead to collapse.
- Hypothermia (a CBT lower than 95°F [35°C]) can result from a decrease in heat production, an increase in heat loss, or a combination of these two factors. The progression of clinical signs and symptoms of hypothermia is divided into three classes based on the CBT: mild (CBT between 95°F [35°C] and 89.8°F [32.1°C]), moderate (CBT between 89.7°F [32.1°C] and 82.5°F [28.1°C]), and severe (CBT below 82.4°F [28°C]). Severely hypothermic patients have no vital signs, including respiratory effort, pulse, and blood pressure.
- Frostbite is a localized injury. It results from freezing of body tissues, which leads to damage to blood vessels. Ischemia often produces the most damaging effects of frostbite.
- Drowning is a process that results in primary respiratory impairment from submersion/immersion in a liquid medium. Outcomes of drowning are fatality, survival with morbidity, or survival without morbidity.
- The three laws pertaining to the basic properties of gases that are involved in all pressure-related diving emergencies are Boyle's law, Dalton's law, and Henry's law. Increased pressure dissolves gases into blood; oxygen metabolizes, and nitrogen dissolves.
- Barotrauma is tissue damage resulting from compression or expansion of gas spaces when the gas pressure in the body differs from the ambient pressure. The type of barotrauma depends on whether the diver is in descent or ascent. Air embolism is the most serious complication of pulmonary barotrauma. It is a major cause of death and disability among sport divers.
- High-altitude illness results from exposure to reduced atmospheric pressure, which results in hypoxia. Forms of high-altitude illness include acute mountain sickness, high-altitude pulmonary edema, and high-altitude cerebral edema.

References

1. Potter PA, Perry AG. *Potter and Perry's Fundamentals of Nursing*. 9th ed. St. Louis, MO: Mosby Elsevier; 2016.
2. Busko J. Cold exposure illness and injury. In: Brice J, Delbridge TR, Meyers JB, eds. *Emergency Services: Clinical Practice and Systems Oversight*. Vol 1. 2nd ed. West Sussex, England: John Wiley & Sons; 2015:351-357.
3. Marx J, Hockberger R, Walls R. *Rosen's Emergency Medicine*. 8th ed. St. Louis, MO: Elsevier; 2013.
4. Bertran G. Heat-related illnesses. In: Brice J, Delbridge TR, Meyers JB, eds. *Emergency Services: Clinical Practice and Systems Oversight*. Vol 1. 2nd ed. West Sussex, England: John Wiley & Sons; 2015:358-362.
5. US Department of Transportation, National Highway Traffic Safety Administration. *EMT-Paramedic: National Standard Curriculum*. EMS.gov website. https://www.ems.gov/pdf/education/Emergency-Medical-Technician-Paramedic/Paramedic_1998.pdf. Accessed February 14, 2018.
6. Auerbach PS, Cushing T, Harris NS. *Wilderness Medicine*. 7th ed. Philadelphia, PA: Elsevier; 2016.
7. National Association of EMS Officials. *National Model EMS Clinical Guidelines*. Version 2.0. National Association of EMS Officials website. https://www.nasemso.org/documents/National-Model-EMS-Clinical-Guidelines-Version2-Sept2017.pdf. Published September 2017. Accessed February 14, 2018.
8. Vanden Hoek TL, Morrison LJ, Shuster M, et al. Cardiac arrest in special situations: 2010 American Heart Association guidelines for cardiopulmonary resuscitation and emergency cardiovascular care science. *Circulation*. 2010;122(18):S829-S861.
9. Zafren K, Giesbrech GG, Danzl DF, et al. Wilderness Medical Society practice guidelines for the out-of-hospital evaluation and treatment of accidental hypothermia. *Wilderness Environ Med*. 2014;25:425-445.
10. Link MS, Berkow LC, Kudenchuk PJ, Halperin HR, Hess EP, Moitra VK, Neumar RW, O'Neil BJ, Paxton JH, Silvers SM, White RD, Yannopoulos D, Donnino MW. Part 7: adult advanced cardiovascular life support: 2015 American Heart Association Guidelines Update for Cardiopulmonary Resuscitation and Emergency Cardiovascular Care. *Circulation*. 2015;132(suppl 2):S444–S464.
11. Paal P, Milani M, Brown D, Boyd J, Ellerton J. Termination of cardiopulmonary resuscitation in mountain rescue. *High Alt Med Biol*. 2012;13:200-208.
12. Danzl D. Accidental hypothermia. In: Auerbach PS, ed. *Wilderness Medicine*. 6th ed. Philadelphia, PA: Elsevier; 2012:116-142.
13. Zonnoor B. Frostbite. Medscape website. https://emedicine.medscape.com/article/926249-overview. Updated June 2, 2017. Accessed February 14, 2018.

14. McIntosh SE, Hamonko M, Freer L, et al. Wilderness Medical Society Guidelines for the prevention and treatment of frostbite. *Wildern Environ Med*. 2011;22(2):156-166.
15. National Safety Council. *Injury Facts*. Itasca, IL: National Safety Council; 2017.
16. Centers for Disease Control and Prevention. Gateway to Health Communication and Social Marketing Practice. Centers for Disease Control and Prevention website. https://www.cdc.gov/healthcommunication/toolstemplates/entertainmented/tips/Drowning.html. Updated September 15, 2017. Accessed February 14, 2018.
17. Szpilman D, Bierens JJ, Handley AJ, Orlowski JP. Drowning. *N Engl J Med*. 2012;366(22):2102-2110.
18. Hawkins SC. *Wilderness EMS*. Philadelphia, PA: Wolters Kluwer; 2017.
19. Cantwell GP. Drowning. Medscape website. https://emedicine.medscape.com/article/772753-overview. Updated May 18, 2017. Accessed February 14, 2018.
20. Chandy D, Weinhouse GL. Drowning (submersion injuries). UpToDate website. https://www.uptodate.com/contents/drowning-submersion-injuries. Updated December 11, 2017. Accessed February 14, 2018.
21. Bolte RG, Black PO, Bowers RS, et al. The use of extracorporeal rewarming in a child submerged for 66 minutes. *JAMA*. 1988;260:377.
22. Cold water survival. US Search and Rescue Task Force website. http://www.ussartf.org/cold_water_survival.htm. Accessed February 14, 2018.
23. Hawkins SC, Sempsrott J, Schmidt A. Drowning in a sea of misinformation. *Emerg Med News*. 2017;39(8):1:39-40.
24. Fast facts: recreational scuba diving and snorkeling. Diving Equipment and Marketing Association website. http://www.dema.org/store/download.asp?id=7811B097-8882-4707-A160-F999B49614B6. Published 2017. Accessed February 14, 2018.
25. Frank AJ. Diving injury. In: Brice J, Delbridge TR, Meyers JB, eds. *Emergency Services: Clinical Practice and Systems Oversight*. Vol 1. 2nd ed. West Sussex, England: John Wiley & Sons; 2015:372-380.
26. Martin L. Scuba diving explained: questions and answers on physiology and medical aspects of scuba diving. Flagstaff, AZ: Best Publishing; 1997.
27. Richardson D, Shreeves K. *Open Water Diver Manual*. Rancho Santa Margarita, CA: Professional Association of Diving Instructors; 2010.
28. National Oceanic and Atmospheric Administration. *NOAA Diving Program: Diving Medical Technician Course*. Office of Marine and Aviation Operations website. https://www.omao.noaa.gov/sites/default/files/documents/DMT%202016%20Student%20Handouts.pdf. Published 2016. Accessed February 14, 2018.
29. Moy HP. High-altitude illnesses. In: Brice J, Delbridge TR, Meyers JB, eds. *Emergency Services: Clinical Practice and Systems Oversight*. Vol 1. 2nd ed. West Sussex, England: John Wiley & Sons; 2015:363-367.
30. Frazier MS, Drzymkowski J. *Essentials of Human Diseases and Conditions*. 6th ed. Philadelphia, PA: Saunders; 2016.
31. Jensen AD, Vincent AL. Altitude illness, cerebral syndromes, high altitude cerebral edema (HACE). National Center for Biotechnology Information website. https://www.ncbi.nlm.nih.gov/books/NBK430916/. Published 2017. Accessed February 14, 2018.
32. Gunga HC. *Human Physiology in Extreme Environments*. Philadelphia, PA: Elsevier; 2015.

Suggested Readings

Auerbach PS, Constance B, Freer L. *Field Guide to Wilderness Medicine: Expert Consult*. 4th ed. Philadelphia, PA: Elsevier; 2013.

Heil K, Thomas R, Robertson G, Porter A, Milner R, Wood A. Freezing and non-freezing cold weather injuries: a systematic review. *Br Med Bull*. 2016;117(1):79-93.

Hostler D. Recognizing and treating injuries caused by SCUBA diving. *JEMS* website. http://www.jems.com/articles/print/volume-40/issue-8/features/recognizing-and-treating-injuries-caused-by-scuba-diving.html. Published August 17, 2015. Accessed February 14, 2018.

Iserson KV. *Improvised Medicine: Providing Care in Extreme Environments*. 2nd ed. McGraw Hill; 2016.

Peters B. Cold injuries. Medscape website. https://emedicine.medscape.com/article/1278523-overview. Updated January 05, 2018. Accessed February 14, 2018.

Sport Diver Editors. Ten scuba diving safety rules for avoiding emergencies. Sport Diver website. https://www.sportdiver.com/how-to-avoid-scuba-diving-emergencies. Published August 9, 2017. Accessed February 14, 2018.

Stöppler MC. High altitude sickness symptoms. MedicineNet website. https://www.medicinenet.com/altitude_sickness_symptoms/views.htm. Accessed February 14, 2018.

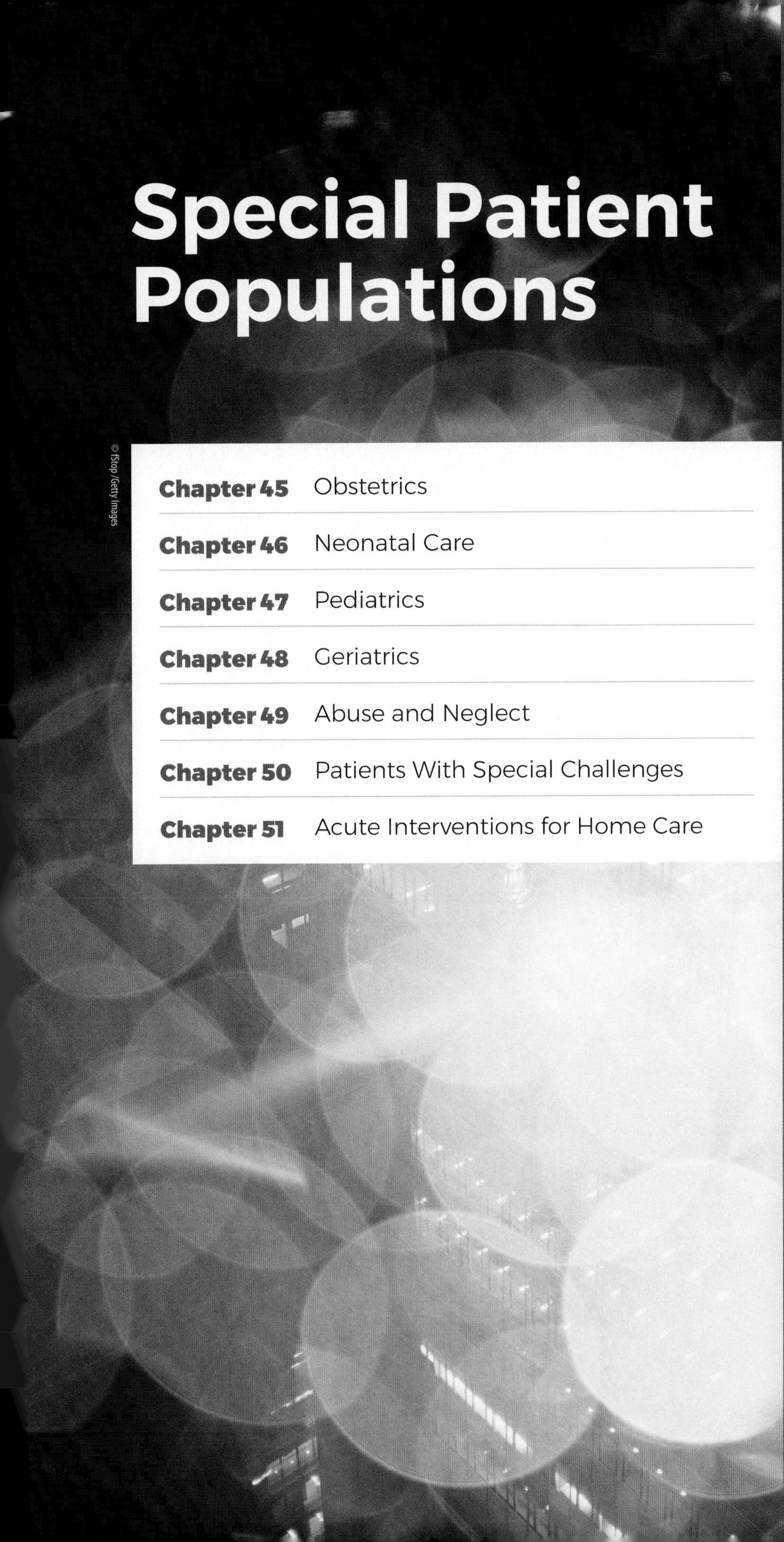

PART 10

Special Patient Populations

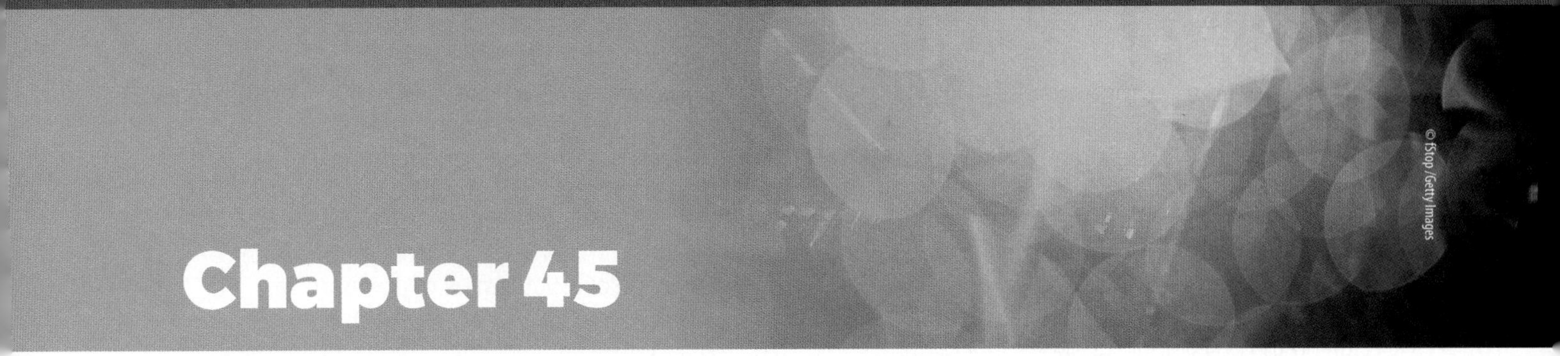

Chapter 45

Obstetrics

NATIONAL EMS EDUCATION STANDARD COMPETENCIES

Special Patient Populations

Integrates assessment findings with principles of pathophysiology and knowledge of psychosocial needs to formulate a field impression and implement a comprehensive treatment/disposition plan for patients with special needs.

Obstetrics

- Recognition and management of
  - Normal delivery (pp 1592–1599)
  - Vaginal bleeding in the pregnant patient (pp 1589–1592)
- Anatomy and physiology of normal pregnancy (pp 1574–1577)
- Pathophysiology of complications of pregnancy (pp 1583–1592)
- Assessment of the pregnant patient (pp 1580–1583)
- Psychosocial impact, presentations, prognosis, and management of
  - Normal delivery (pp 1592–1599)
  - Abnormal delivery (pp 1599–1605)
    - Nuchal cord (p 1596)
    - Prolapsed cord (p 1603)
    - Breech delivery (pp 1600–1602)
  - Third-trimester bleeding (pp 1590–1592)
    - Placenta previa (pp 1591–1592)
    - Abruptio placentae (pp 1590–1592)
  - Spontaneous abortion/miscarriage (p 1589)
  - Ectopic pregnancy (p 1590)
  - Preeclampsia/eclampsia (pp 1585–1587)
  - Antepartum hemorrhage (pp 1589–1592)
  - Pregnancy-induced hypertension (pp 1585–1587)

Trauma

Integrates assessment findings with principles of epidemiology and pathophysiology to formulate a field impression to implement a comprehensive treatment/disposition plan for an acutely injured patient.

Special Considerations in Trauma

Recognition and management in trauma in
- Pregnant patient (pp 1607–1608)
- Pediatric patient (see Chapter 47, *Pediatrics*)
- Geriatric patient (see Chapter 48, *Geriatrics*)

Pathophysiology, assessment, and management of trauma in the
- Pregnant patient (pp 1607–1608)
- Pediatric patient (see Chapter 47, *Pediatrics*)
- Geriatric patient (see Chapter 48, *Geriatrics*)
- Cognitively impaired patient (see Chapter 50, *Patients With Special Challenges*)

OBJECTIVES

Upon completion of this chapter, the paramedic student will be able to:

1. Describe the basic anatomy and physiology of the reproductive system during pregnancy. (pp 1574–1577)
2. Outline fetal development from ovulation through birth. (pp 1577–1579)
3. Explain normal maternal physiologic changes that occur during pregnancy and describe how they influence prehospital patient care and transport. (pp 1580–1581)
4. Describe appropriate information to be elicited during the obstetric patient's history. (pp 1581–1582)
5. Describe specific techniques for physical assessment of the pregnant patient. (pp 1582–1583)
6. Describe the general prehospital care of the pregnant patient. (p 1583)
7. Recognize and begin treatment for complications of pregnancy such as hyperemesis gravidarum, Rh sensitization,

diabetes mellitus, and infection. (pp 1583–1585, 1587–1588)
8. Describe the assessment and management of patients with preeclampsia and eclampsia. (pp 1585–1587)
9. Explain the pathophysiology, signs and symptoms, and management of vaginal bleeding in pregnancy. (pp 1589–1592)
10. Outline the physiologic changes that occur during the stages of labor. (pp 1592–1594)
11. Describe the role of the paramedic during normal labor and delivery. (pp 1592–1599)
12. Compute an Apgar score. (pp 1596–1598)
13. Discuss the identification, implications, and prehospital management of complicated deliveries. (pp 1599–1605)
14. Describe assessment and management of postpartum hemorrhage. (pp 1605–1606)
15. Describe characteristics of postpartum depression. (pp 1606–1607)
16. Discuss the special implications of trauma in pregnancy. (pp 1607–1608)
17. Outline principles of care for a pregnant patient in cardiac arrest. (pp 1608–1609)

KEY TERMS

abruptio placentae A partial or full detachment of a normally implanted placenta at more than 20 weeks' gestation; also known as placental abruption.

amniotic fluid Fluid in the amniotic sac.

amniotic fluid embolism An embolism that occurs when amniotic fluid gains access to maternal circulation during labor or delivery or immediately after delivery.

amniotic sac A thin-walled bag that contains the fetus and amniotic fluid during pregnancy.

Apgar score The evaluation of a newborn's physical condition, performed at 1 minute and 5 minutes after birth, including heart rate, respiratory effort, muscle tone, reflex irritability, and color.

Braxton-Hicks contractions Irregular tightening of the pregnant uterus that may begin as early as the second trimester and increases in frequency, duration, and intensity as the pregnancy progresses.

breech presentation The intrauterine position of the fetus in which the buttocks or feet present, rather than the head.

cephalopelvic disproportion An obstetric condition in which a newborn's head is too large or a mother's birth canal is too small to permit a normal vaginal delivery.

cesarean delivery A surgical procedure in which the abdomen and uterus are incised and the baby is delivered transabdominally.

chorioamnionitis An inflammatory reaction in the amniotic membranes caused by infection in the amniotic fluid.

crowning The phase at the end of labor in which the fetal head is seen at the opening of the vagina.

ductus arteriosus A blood vessel in the fetus that connects the pulmonary artery directly to the proximal descending aorta.

ductus venosus A vascular shunt unique to the fetal and neonatal circulations. In fetal life, the ductus venosus allows variable portions of the umbilical and portal venous blood flows to bypass the liver microcirculation.

eclampsia The onset of seizures in a woman with preeclampsia.

ectopic pregnancy A pregnancy that occurs when a fertilized ovum implants anywhere other than the uterus.

embryo The stage of prenatal development that begins with fertilization and continues until the end of the 8th week of gestation.

erythroblastosis fetalis Hemolytic anemia in the fetus caused by maternal antibodies directed against the fetus's erythrocytes, secondary to ABO or Rh incompatibility between the mother and the fetus.

estimated date of confinement Predicted delivery date for the fetus based on either last menstrual period or ideally ultrasonography performed in the first trimester.

fetus A stage in prenatal development. In humans this stage is between the embryonic stage (end of 10th week) and birth.

first stage of labor The stage of labor that begins with contractions and ends when the cervix is fully dilated at 10 cm. It is divided into early labor, active labor, and transition.

foramen ovale An opening in the septum between the right and left atria in the fetal heart that provides a bypass for blood that would otherwise flow to the fetal lungs.

fundal massage The application of external pressure to the uterus to decrease postpartum bleeding.

gestation The period from fertilization of the ovum until birth.

gestational diabetes mellitus (GDM) A disorder characterized by impaired ability to metabolize carbohydrates, usually caused by a deficiency of insulin. It occurs in pregnancy and disappears after delivery but in some cases returns years later.

gestational hypertension Hypertension (defined as a blood pressure of 140/90 mm Hg) that develops in a pregnant woman after 20 weeks' gestation without any other features of preeclampsia and resolves during the postpartum period.

gravida The number of all current and past pregnancies.

HELLP syndrome A severe form of preeclampsia that involves H, hemolysis; EL, elevated liver enzymes; and LP, low platelet count.

hydrops fetalis A fetal condition characterized by the accumulation of fluid throughout body tissues, including the lungs, heart, and abdominal organs.

hyperemesis gravidarum (HG) A condition of pregnancy characterized by severe nausea, vomiting, weight loss, and electrolyte disturbance.

lochia A normal postpartum vaginal discharge that contains blood, mucus, and placental tissue from the lining of the uterus.

mucus plug A collection of cervical mucus that fills and seals the cervical canal during pregnancy. It is discharged from the vagina prior to childbirth.

multiple gestation A pregnancy with more than one fetus.

ovum An egg in the ovary of a female.

para The number of past pregnancies that have remained viable to delivery.

parturition The process by which a fetus is born.

placenta A highly vascular fetal–maternal organ through which the fetus absorbs oxygen, nutrients, and other substances and excretes carbon dioxide and other wastes.

placenta previa Placental implantation in the lower uterine segment partially or completely covering the cervical opening.

postpartum depression Depression that occurs during or after pregnancy that is caused by a combination of sudden hormonal changes and psychological and environmental factors.

postpartum hemorrhage Blood loss of more than 500 mL after delivery of the newborn.

precipitous delivery A rapid, spontaneous delivery of less than 3 hours from onset of labor to birth. This childbirth occurs with such speed that usual preparations cannot be made. It results from overactive uterine contractions and little maternal soft-tissue or bony resistance.

preeclampsia An abnormal disease of pregnancy characterized by the onset of acute hypertension associated with either proteinuria after the 20th week of gestation or other abnormalities like thrombocytopenia, renal insufficiency, impaired liver function, pulmonary edema, or cerebral or visual symptoms.

premature newborn A newborn who is born before 37 weeks' gestation.

premature rupture of membranes (PROM) Rupture of the amniotic sac before the onset of labor, regardless of gestational age.

Rh disease An immune disorder that develops in a fetus, when IgG antibodies directed against Rh-positive red blood cells are produced by the mother and pass through the placenta.

Rh sensitization A condition that can occur during pregnancy if an Rh-negative woman is pregnant with a baby who has Rh-positive blood. If this occurs, the immune system reacts to the Rh factor by producing antibodies to destroy it.

second stage of labor The stage of labor that is measured from full dilation of the cervix to delivery of the newborn.

shoulder dystocia An obstacle to delivery that occurs when the fetal shoulders press against the maternal symphysis pubis, blocking shoulder delivery.

shoulder presentation A delivery presentation that results when the long axis of the fetus lies perpendicular to that of the mother; also known as transverse presentation.

spontaneous abortion Noninduced termination of pregnancy that usually occurs before 20 weeks' gestation; also known as miscarriage.

third stage of labor The stage of labor that begins with delivery of the newborn and ends when the placenta is expelled and the uterus has contracted.

third-trimester bleeding Vaginal bleeding that occurs in the third trimester of pregnancy. Common causes include abruptio placentae, placenta previa, or uterine rupture.

tocolytic A medication given to temporarily reduce the frequency and intensity of uterine contractions.

TORCH infections An acronym for a special group of infections that may be acquired by a woman during pregnancy: Toxoplasmosis, Other infections (namely, hepatitis B, syphilis, and herpes zoster), Rubella, Cytomegalovirus, Herpes simplex virus.

trimesters Periods of approximately 3 months into which pregnancy is divided. There are a total of three such periods in one pregnancy.

umbilical cord A flexible structure connecting the umbilicus of the fetus with the placenta. It contains the umbilical arteries and vein and is the key structure in delivery of oxygen and nutrients to the developing fetus.

umbilical cord prolapse A presentation that occurs when the cord passes through the cervix at the same time or in advance of the presenting part of the fetus.

uterine atony The lack of uterine tone.

uterine inversion A rare event in which the uterus turns inside out after birth.

uterine rupture A spontaneous or traumatic rupture of the uterine wall.

zygote The developing ovum from the time it is fertilized until it is implanted in the uterus as a blastocyst.

Childbirth is common in the prehospital setting. Most often, paramedics only assist in this natural process. However, obstetric emergencies can develop suddenly and have life-threatening consequences. The paramedic must be prepared to recognize and manage these events and sometimes assist in abnormal deliveries. This chapter presents the causes and treatment of obstetric emergencies. It also discusses the normal and abnormal events associated with childbirth.

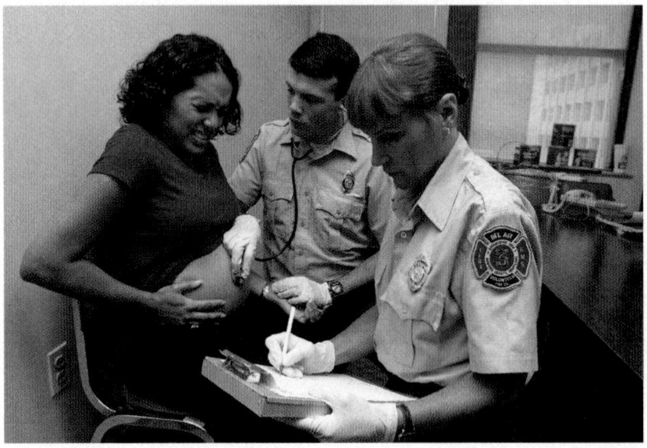

Review of Female Reproductive Anatomy

As described in Chapter 10, *Review of Human Systems*, and in Chapter 30, *Gynecology*, the female reproductive system is composed of external and internal anatomic structures that allow for pregnancy. To review, the external genitalia are the labium minora and majora, the vagina, and the clitoris. The internal organs that lie within the pelvis include the uterus, ovaries, uterine (or fallopian) tubes, and cervix (**FIGURE 45-1**).

The female reproductive cycle (described in Chapter 30, *Gynecology*) is under the control of the

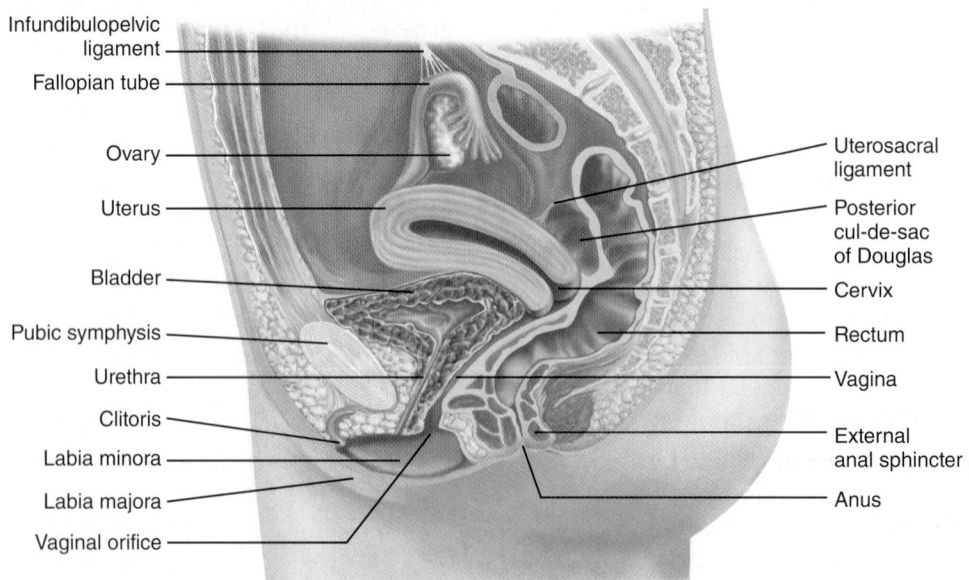

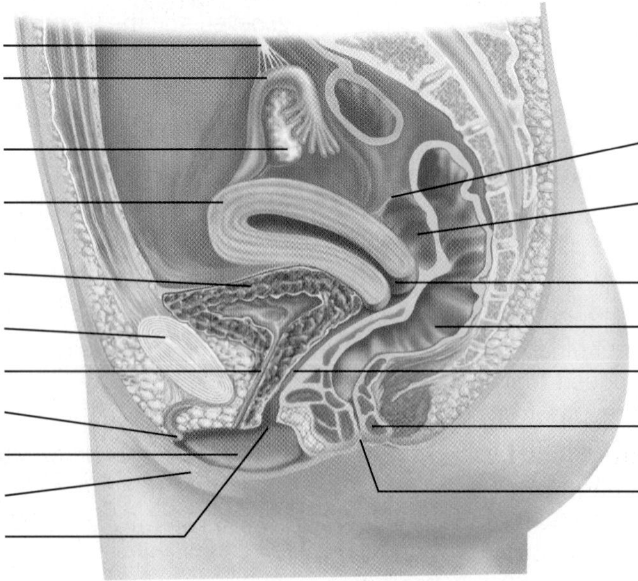

FIGURE 45-1 Organs of the female reproductive system.

endocrine system and its hormones. For women of childbearing age, the cycle usually is a monthly event that begins with menstruation (shedding of the endometrium or uterine lining). The cycle ends with pregnancy or, in the absence of fertilization, with another menstrual cycle.

NOTE

In 2015, there were 229,715 births to mothers aged 15 to 19 years in the United States (a birth rate of 22.3 live births per 1,000 women in this age group). Despite the fact that the birth rate for teenagers has fallen continuously since 1991, teen birth rates in the United States are considerably higher than in most other developed countries. The possibility of pregnancy should always be considered when caring for patients of childbearing age.

Modified from: Hamilton BE, Mathews TJ; Centers for Disease Control and Prevention, National Center for Health Statistics. Continued declines in teen births in the United States, 2015. Centers for Disease Control and Prevention website. https://www.cdc.gov/nchs/products/databriefs/db259.htm. Updated September 9, 2016. Accessed April 21, 2018.

DID YOU KNOW?

Cultural Values May Affect Childbirth

Pregnancy is a universal event that is embedded in a cultural context, both from expectant parents and from surrounding family members. Common to all cultures is the fear that there may be a negative outcome from the pregnancy or that the baby or woman may die during childbirth. A universal ideal of pregnancy is that the baby will be born healthy and eager to thrive. Given that cultural values may affect medical care, the beliefs of all pregnant women should be respected. Because cultural influences are one of the many influences on how a woman and her family experience pregnancy, it is important for the paramedic to be familiar with the cultures in his or her area.

Normal Events of Pregnancy

Fertilization normally occurs in the fallopian tube when the head of a sperm penetrates a mature **ovum**. After penetration, the nuclei of the sperm and ovum fuse and the newly fertilized ovum becomes a **zygote**. The zygote undergoes repeated cell divisions as it passes down the fallopian tube. After a few days of rapid cell division, a ball of cells called a morula is formed with cell differentiation between the inner layer of cells (blastocyst cells) and the outer layer of cells (trophoblast cells). Trophoblast cells attach to the endometrium lining of the uterus. Implantation begins within 7 days after fertilization. Implantation is completed when the trophoblast cells make contact with maternal circulation (which is about day 12). Trophoblast cells go on to make various life support systems for the embryo (placenta, amniotic sac, **umbilical cord**); blastocyst cells develop into the embryo itself (**FIGURE 45-2**).

Specialized Structures of Pregnancy

The placenta, the umbilical cord, and the amniotic sac and its fluid provide nutrients for the developing embryo. They also are part of fetal circulation.

Placenta

The trophoblast cells continue to develop and form the placenta for about 14 days after ovulation. The **placenta** is a disklike organ composed of interlocking fetal and maternal tissues. The placenta is the organ of exchange between the mother and the fetus and is responsible for the following five functions:

1. **Transfer of gases.** The diffusion of oxygen and carbon dioxide through the placental membrane is similar to the diffusion that occurs in the lungs. Dissolved oxygen in maternal blood passes through the placenta into fetal blood. This transfer results from the increase in the partial pressure of oxygen in the mother's blood compared with that of the fetus. Conversely, as the fetal partial pressure of carbon dioxide (P_{CO_2}) level increases, a low-pressure gradient of carbon dioxide develops across the placental membrane. The carbon dioxide then diffuses from the fetal blood to the maternal blood.
2. **Transport of nutrients.** Other metabolic substrates that the fetus needs diffuse into fetal blood in the same manner as oxygen. For example, glucose levels in fetal blood are about 20% to 30% lower than those in maternal blood. This results in a rapid diffusion of glucose to the fetus. Diffusion also transports other substrates, such as fatty acids, potassium, sodium, and chloride. The placenta also actively absorbs some nutrients from maternal blood.

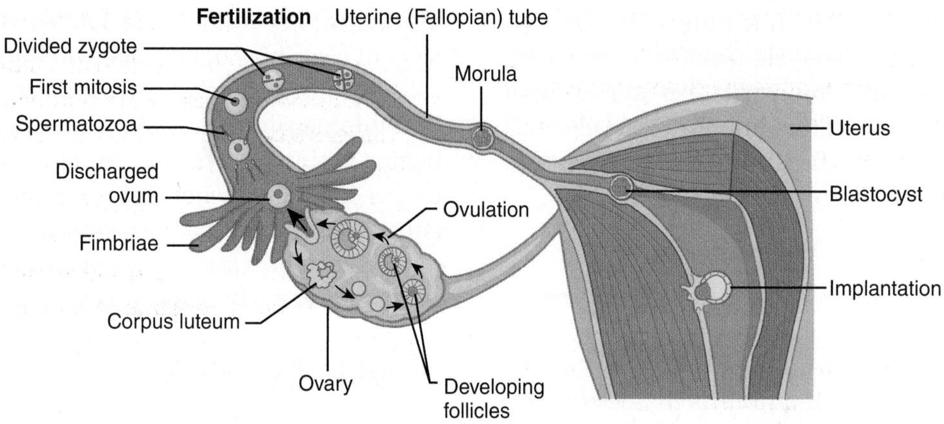

FIGURE 45-2 Fertilization and implantation. At ovulation, the ovary releases an ovum, which begins its journey through the uterine tube. While the ovum is in the tube, a sperm fertilizes the ovum to form the single-cell zygote. After a few days of rapid cell division, a ball of cells called a morula forms. After the morula develops into a hollow ball (blastocyte), implantation occurs.

3. **Excretion of wastes.** Waste products diffuse from fetal blood into maternal blood. Examples of such products are urea, uric acid, and creatinine. They are excreted with the waste products of the mother. Wastes transfer from fetal circulation to maternal circulation by moving osmotically from a higher concentration to a lower concentration, in the same manner as carbon dioxide.
4. **Hormone production.** The placenta becomes a temporary endocrine gland. It secretes estrogen and progesterone. By the third month of fetal development, the corpus luteum on the ovary no longer is needed to sustain the pregnancy. Estrogen, progesterone, and other hormones maintain the uterine lining, prevent the occurrence of menses, and stimulate changes in the pregnant woman's breasts, vagina, cervix, and pelvis that prepare her body for delivery and lactation.
5. **Formation of a barrier.** The placenta forms a barrier against some harmful substances in the mother's circulation (eg, bacteria, certain drugs). The placental barrier is only partially selective and does not fully protect the fetus. Certain medications cross the placenta. Among these are steroids, narcotics, anesthetics, and some antibiotics.

CRITICAL THINKING

What happens to diffusion of gases if the pregnant woman becomes hypoxic?

Fetal Circulation

Fetal circulation is physically separated but dependent on the maternal circulation. Well-oxygenated blood from the placenta returns to the fetus via the umbilical vein. The **ductus venosus**, a continuation of the umbilical cord, serves as a shunt to allow most blood returning from the placenta to bypass the immature liver of the embryo. As a result, blood empties directly into the inferior vena cava, which empties into the right atrium. Because the fetal lungs are fluid-filled and collapsed, oxygenated blood bypasses the fetal lungs in one of two ways. Blood moves from the right atrium directly to the left atrium through an opening called the **foramen ovale**. Oxygenated blood passes from the left atrium into the left ventricle and into the aorta, where it is pumped to the body. In addition, blood that passes from the right atrium into the right ventricle is pumped into the pulmonary arteries. The **ductus arteriosus** connects the pulmonary artery to the aorta, again directing blood away from the lungs. Mixed blood from the aorta returns to the placenta via the umbilical arteries, where waste products such as carbon dioxide are taken up by the maternal circulation. At birth, the various arteriovenous shunts close in most newborns in response to inflation of the lungs and dramatic lowering of the vascular resistance in the pulmonary circulation (**FIGURE 45-3**).

Amniotic Sac and Amniotic Fluid

The **amniotic sac** completely surrounds the embryo. It contains **amniotic fluid**, which is primarily produced by the placenta, and later by fetal urine. The fluid is continually produced. It amounts to about 175 to 225 mL by the 15th week of pregnancy and about 1 L at birth. The amniotic sac may rupture during labor, at which point there may be a large loss of fluid (gross rupture) or a small trickle (leaking of membranes). If the amniotic sac ruptures 1 hour or more prior to the onset of labor, this is premature and puts both the mother and the fetus at risk for complications.

Fetal Growth and Development

The developing ovum is called an **embryo** during the first 8 weeks of pregnancy. Thereafter and until birth, it is called a **fetus**. The period during which the fetus grows and develops within the uterus is known as **gestation**. Gestation averages 40 weeks from the time of fertilization to delivery of the newborn. Gestation is divided into **trimesters**. The calculated delivery date is referred to as the **estimated date of confinement**. Rapid fetal growth and development characterize the period of gestation (**FIGURE 45-4** and **BOX 45-1**).

Newborn Adaptations After Birth

At birth, the newborn loses the placental connection with the mother. The fetal circulation changes almost immediately to permit adequate blood flow through the lungs. A newborn usually begins to breathe spontaneously at birth. Breathing occurs when the chest exits the birth canal or with some external stimulation.

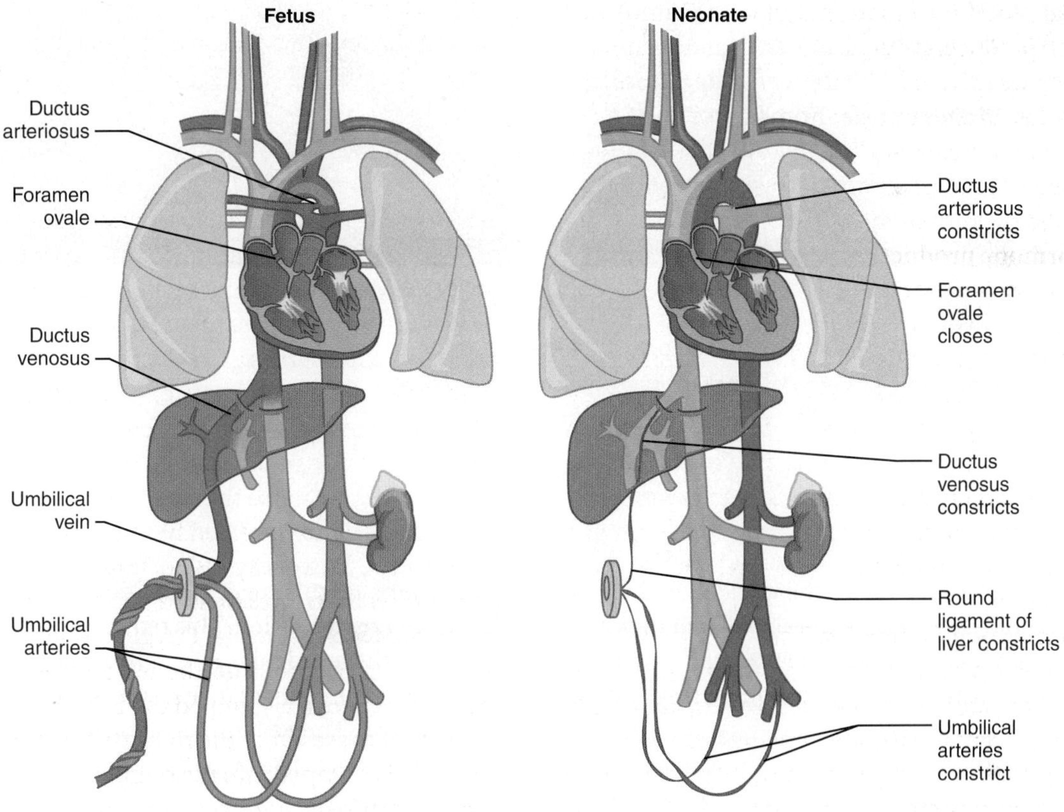

FIGURE 45-3 Fetal circulation and changes in circulation after birth.

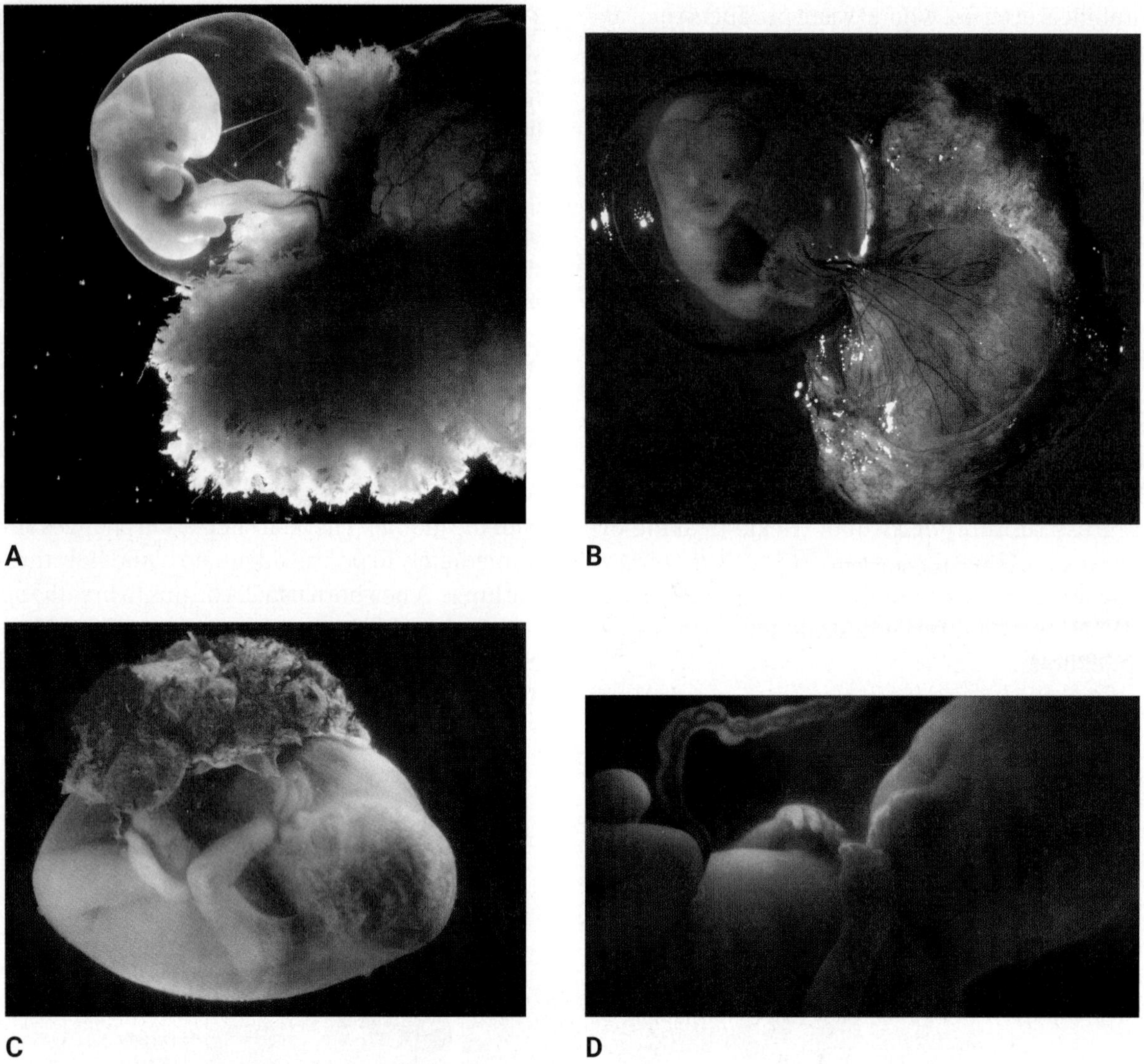

FIGURE 45-4 A-D. Development of the embryo and fetus.

A: © Joo Lee/Corbis Documentary/Getty Images; **B:** © VideoSurgery/Science Source; **C:** © Petit Format/Science Source; **D:** © Jellyfish Pictures/Science Source

At birth, the surface tension of the viscid fluid that fills the alveoli holds the walls of the alveoli together. The newborn's first breaths need to be powerful enough to open the alveoli and to allow subsequent respirations to occur with less effort.

The ductus venosus, ductus arteriosus, and foramen ovale allow blood flow to bypass the immature liver and lungs of the developing fetus. When blood flow through the placenta ceases at birth, systemic vascular resistance increases, as does pressure in the aorta, left ventricle, and left atrium. In addition, pulmonary vascular resistance decreases greatly because of lung expansion. This reduces the pulmonary arterial, right ventricular, and right atrial pressures. As a result of these changes in pressure, the arteriovenous shunts close. They eventually close completely and are covered with a growth of fibrous tissue.

CRITICAL THINKING

Do newborn heart tones sound normal if you auscultate them immediately after birth?

BOX 45-1 Embryo and Fetal Development in Utero for Each Lunar Month (28 Days)

First Lunar Month

- Foundations form for the nervous system, genitourinary system, skin, bones, and lungs.
- Buds of arms and legs begin to form.
- Rudiments of eyes, ears, and nose appear.

Second Lunar Month

- The head is disproportionately large because of brain development.
- Sex differentiation begins.
- The centers of bones begin to ossify.

Third Lunar Month

- Fingers and toes are distinct.
- The placenta is complete.
- Fetal circulation is complete.

Fourth Lunar Month

- Sex is differentiated.
- Rudimentary kidneys secrete urine.
- Heartbeat is present.
- Nasal septum and palate close.

Fifth Lunar Month

- Fetal movements are felt by the mother.
- Heart sounds are perceptible by auscultation.

Sixth Lunar Month

- The skin appears wrinkled.
- Eyebrows and fingernails develop.

Seventh Lunar Month

- The skin is red.
- The pupillary membrane disappears from the eyes.

Eighth Lunar Month

- The fetus is viable if born.
- The eyelids open.
- Fingerprints are set.
- Vigorous fetal movement occurs.

Ninth Lunar Month

- The face and body have a loose, wrinkled appearance because of subcutaneous fat deposits.
- Amniotic fluid decreases slightly.

Tenth Lunar Month

- Skin is smooth.
- Eyes are uniformly slate colored.
- The bones of the skull are ossified and nearly together at sutures.

BOX 45-2 Obstetric Terminology

- **Antepartum.** The maternal period before delivery.
- **Grand multipara.** A woman who has had five deliveries or more.
- **Multigravida.** A woman who has had two or more pregnancies.
- **Multipara.** A woman who has had two or more deliveries.
- **Nullipara.** A woman who has never delivered.
- **Perinatal.** Occurring at or near the time of birth.
- **Postpartum.** The maternal period after delivery.
- **Prenatal.** Existing or occurring before birth.
- **Primigravida.** A woman who is pregnant for the first time.
- **Primipara.** A woman who has given birth only once.
- **Term.** A pregnancy that has reached 40 weeks' gestation.

Pregnancy Terminology (GTPAL)

GTPAL is an acronym that stands for Gravida, Term, Preterm, Abortions, and Living. **Gravida** is the number of times a woman has been pregnant. Term is the number of term deliveries. Preterm is the number of preterm deliveries. Abortions is the number of spontaneous or induced abortions. Living is the number of living children.

Pregnant patients are described by their gravid and parous states. As just stated, gravida refers to the number of times the woman has been pregnant, including the present pregnancy. **Para** refers to the number of infants born after 20 weeks' gestation. For example, a woman who is pregnant for the first time is gravida 1, para 0 (BOX 45-2). A woman who has had two or more deliveries is multipara. A woman who has never delivered a child is nullipara.

Patient Assessment

The paramedic must be familiar with the normal physiologic changes that occur in the pregnant woman. This will help the paramedic to assess a pregnant patient.

Maternal Changes During Pregnancy

In addition to cessation of menstruation and obvious enlargement of the uterus, the pregnant woman undergoes many other physical changes. These changes affect the genital tract, breasts, gastrointestinal system, cardiovascular system, respiratory system, and metabolism.[1,2]

Genital Tract

Uterus

- Uterus grows from 70 g (nongravid) to 1,000 g by term.
- The uterus triples in size and weight by 8 weeks of pregnancy.
- The uterus occupies the entire pelvic cavity. It may be palpated suprapubically by 12 weeks of pregnancy.
- The uterus becomes an abdominal organ, and the top of the uterus (fundus) reaches the level of the umbilicus by 20 weeks' gestation.
- The uterine fundus descends a little when the fetus descends into the pelvis. This occurs close to term between 38 and 40 weeks' gestation.

Cervix

- Increased uterine blood volume and lymphatic fluid cause pelvic congestion and edema. This results in softening and blue discoloration of the cervix.

Vagina

- The vagina develops a violet color from increased vascularity.
- The vaginal mucosa increases in thickness, and vaginal secretions increase.
- The pH of vaginal secretions decreases to about 3.5 because of the increased production of lactic acid from glycogen in the vaginal epithelium. Acidic pH reduces the growth of some pathogens.

Bladder

- Early in the first trimester, frequency of urination occurs mainly from pressure of the expanding uterus on the bladder. Physiologic increases in blood volume and cardiac output of the mother may also play a role.
- Smooth muscle relaxation of the ureters increases the risk for urinary tract infection that can progress to pyelonephritis.

Breasts

- The breasts become tender in the early weeks of pregnancy.
- The breasts increase in size as a result of hypertrophy of the mammary alveoli by the second month of pregnancy.
- The nipples become larger, more deeply pigmented, and usually more erectile early in pregnancy.
- As breast glands proliferate, the nipples may secrete a clear fluid by the 10th week of pregnancy if stimulated.

Gastrointestinal System

- Nausea and vomiting early in pregnancy are often referred to as morning sickness because these symptoms tend to begin early in the day; however, they may occur at any time. They usually begin by the 6th week and abate by the 14th week of pregnancy. The cause of morning sickness is unknown but may be related to the high serum levels of chorionic gonadotropin in early pregnancy.
- The enlarging uterus displaces the mother's stomach and intestines upward and laterally. This may cause indigestion and gastroesophageal reflux disease and may increase the risk for aspiration in unconscious patients.
- The liver is displaced backward, upward, and to the right.
- The tone and motility of the gastrointestinal tract decrease, leading to prolonged gastric emptying and relaxation of the pyloric sphincter. Heartburn and constipation are common.

> CRITICAL THINKING
>
> Consider an unconscious pregnant woman who has sustained trauma. What are problems associated with the gastrointestinal changes of pregnancy?

Cardiovascular System

Heart

- Elevation of the diaphragm displaces the heart to the left and upward. Flat ST segments or negative T waves may be present in inferior and precordial leads on the electrocardiogram (ECG) as well as left axis deviation.

- Dysrhythmias occur, such as supraventricular tachycardia, atrial fibrillation or flutter, and rarely ventricular tachycardia.
- Cardiac output increases by 30% by the 34th week of pregnancy.
- The pulse rate may increase 15 to 20 beats/min above baseline late in the third trimester.
- Pulmonic systolic and apical systolic murmurs are common because lowered blood viscosity and increased flow lead to turbulence in the great vessels.

Circulation

- Total blood volume increases by 30%. Plasma volume increases by 50%. As a result, hemodilutional anemia is possible beginning at 28 weeks.
- Blood pressure decreases 10 to 15 mm Hg during the second trimester. This is because of the reduction in peripheral resistance. Blood pressure gradually increases to prepregnancy levels toward term.
- The enlarged uterus interferes with venous return from the legs, resulting in peripheral edema in the ankles. Hemorrhoids and varicose veins may be present.
- The supine position may cause the uterus to compress the inferior vena cava. This can produce decreased cardiac filling and decreased cardiac output (supine hypotension syndrome).

Blood

- The leukocyte count increases.
- Fibrinogen levels increase by 50% because of the influence of estrogen and progesterone.
- The risk for the development of venous thromboembolism increases four to five times.[3]

Respiratory System

- Tidal volume and minute ventilation increase by 30% to 40% in late pregnancy.
- Functional residual capacity decreases by about 25%.
- Oxygen consumption is increased by 30% to 60%.[4]
- The respiratory rate may be normal or may increase because of elevation of the diaphragm by the enlarged uterus.
- The Pco_2 level normally decreases because of an increased respiratory rate. Pco_2 changes from 40 to 30 mm Hg to provide a gradient for fetal carbon dioxide. This may cause dizziness and a sensation of shortness of breath for the pregnant woman.

Metabolism

- The pregnant woman normally will experience a weight gain of 15 to 30 pounds (7 to 14 kg).
- Increased water retention produces an increase in hydrostatic pressure within the capillaries. This favors filtration from the vascular bed and can result in edema.
- The metabolic rate and caloric demand (especially for protein) increase.
- Glucose escapes into the urine because of increased glomerular filtration.
- Maternal gestational diabetes mellitus (GDM) may result from an impaired ability to metabolize carbohydrates. GDM is further described later in this chapter.
- Fetal demands for calcium and iron may deplete maternal stores if the patient does not supplement them through diet.

History

When obtaining a history from an obstetric patient, the paramedic first should gather details about the chief complaint. This complaint may not be related to the pregnancy. If possible, the paramedic should solicit information about the onset of signs and symptoms and examine the patient in an area that provides privacy. After ruling out life-threatening illness or injury, the paramedic should interview the patient to obtain relevant information. The history for a pregnant patient must incorporate the following:

- Obstetric history
  - Length of gestation
  - Parity and gravidity
  - Previous cesarean delivery
  - Maternal lifestyle (alcohol or other drug use, smoking history)
  - Infectious disease status
  - History of previous gynecologic or obstetric complications (eg, eclampsia, GDM, premature labor, ectopic pregnancy)
- Presence of pain
  - Onset (gradual or sudden)
  - Character
  - Duration and evolution over time
  - Location and radiation
- Presence, quantity, and character of vaginal bleeding
- Presence of abnormal vaginal discharge
- Presence of "show" (expulsion of the mucus plug in early labor) or rupture of membranes

- Current general health and prenatal care (none, physician, nurse, midwife)
- Allergies and medications taken (especially the use of narcotics in the last 4 hours)
- Maternal urge to bear down or sensation of imminent bowel movement, indicating imminent delivery

NOTE

Pregnancy can worsen certain medical conditions and diseases, including hypertension, diabetes mellitus, infection, neuromuscular disorders, and cardiovascular disease. These conditions and diseases should be considered as part of the paramedic's differential diagnosis. Some medications (eg, antihypertensive agents, oral hypoglycemic drugs) used to manage these disorders cannot be taken by the mother during her pregnancy because of the potential harm to the fetus. Pregnancy can also cause diagnostic uncertainty and delay in some conditions, such as acute appendicitis and acute cholecystitis, even though their clinical presentation is relatively similar to the nonpregnant patient. Thus, a thorough patient history is vital and will help the paramedic anticipate care that may be required at the scene and during patient transport.

Physical Examination

The patient's chief complaint determines the extent of the examination. The goal in examining an obstetric patient is to identify acute life-threatening conditions rapidly. A part of this goal is to identify imminent delivery. If delivery is near, the paramedic must take the proper management steps.

The paramedic should assess the patient's general appearance and skin color. If she is very pale, hemorrhage should be suspected. Sunken cheeks, cracked lips, or hollow eyes with a history of vomiting indicate dehydration. Vital signs should be monitored often during the care. Orthostatic vital signs may indicate the early presence of significant bleeding or fluid loss. The paramedic should recall that normal physiologic changes in the pregnant patient can produce variations in vital signs. Examples are mild tachycardia, a slight fall in systolic and diastolic blood pressures, and an increase in the respiratory rate.

The patient's abdomen should be examined for scars and gross deformities. Gentle palpation may reveal the presence of masses, enlarged organs, intestinal distention, or a distended bladder. However, in late pregnancy, these signs may be difficult to recognize. During the examination, it may be possible to discern peritoneal irritation. Peritoneal irritation is diagnosed by the presence of tenderness, guarding, or rebound tenderness. If the patient is obviously pregnant, the paramedic may need to assess uterine size and monitor the fetus.

Evaluation of Uterine Size

The uterine contour usually is irregular between 8 and 10 weeks' gestation. Thus, early uterine enlargement may not be symmetrical and may be deviated to one side. The uterus is above the symphysis pubis at 12 to 16 weeks' gestation. The uterus is at the level of the umbilicus at 20 weeks and near the xiphoid process at term. **FIGURE 45-5** shows changes in fundal height at the various weeks of gestation.

Fetal Monitoring

Fetal heart sounds can be auscultated by using a Doppler probe (**FIGURE 45-6**) starting at 12 weeks'

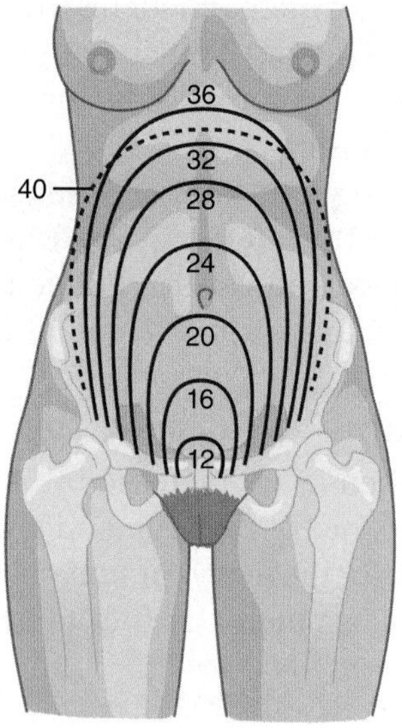

FIGURE 45-5 Changes in fundal height during pregnancy. Weeks 10 to 12: The uterus is within the pelvis, and the fetal heartbeat can be detected with a Doppler probe. Week 12: The uterus is palpable just above the symphysis pubis. Week 16: The uterus is palpable just between the symphysis pubis and the umbilicus. Week 20: The uterine fundus is at the lower border of the umbilicus. A fetal heartbeat can be auscultated with a Doppler probe. Weeks 24 to 26: The uterus becomes ovoid, and the fetus is palpable. Week 28: The uterus is about halfway between the umbilicus and the xiphoid process, and the fetus is easily palpable. Week 32: The uterine fundus is just below the xiphoid. Week 40: Fundal height drops as the fetus begins to engage in the pelvis.

gestation. The purpose of checking heart tones is to assess fetal well-being. If using a Doppler, it should be placed below the umbilicus on the side of the fetal back (**FIGURE 45-7**). The fetal heart rate is measured in beats per minute. Note: Patient transport should not be delayed, because fetal heart tones are often difficult to hear.

The normal fetal heart rate is 120 to 160 beats/min. A fetal heart rate that remains above 160 beats/min (fetal tachycardia) or below 110 beats/min (fetal bradycardia) for more than 60 seconds may be an early sign of fetal distress. It also may be a sign of fetal or maternal hypoxia. Intermittent, short-term increases or decreases in the fetal heart rate usually are normal. Short-term periodic changes in fetal heart rate are common during fetal sleep, fetal movement, and contractions associated with labor and delivery.

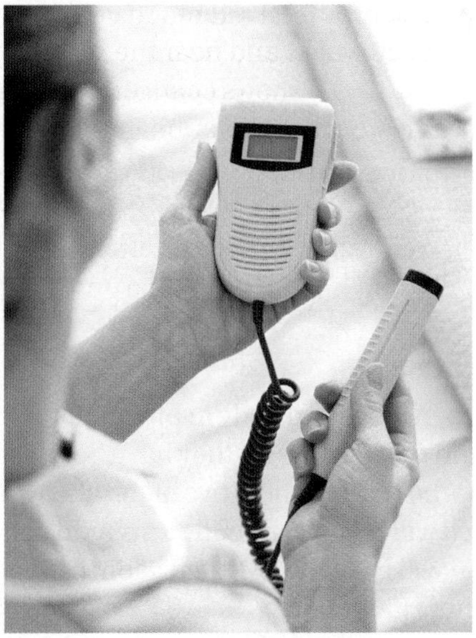

FIGURE 45-6 Doppler probe.

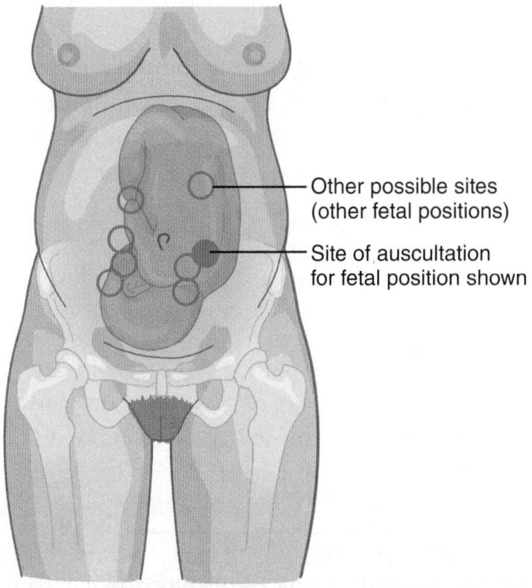

FIGURE 45-7 Sites for auscultation of fetal heart tones.

General Management of the Obstetric Patient

If birth is not imminent, care for the healthy patient should be limited to basic treatment modalities (airway, ventilatory, and circulatory support) and transport for physician evaluation. In the absence of distress or injury, the patient should be transported in a comfortable position (which is usually left lateral recumbent). Monitor the fetus based on patient assessment and vital sign determinations. Medical direction may advise intravenous (IV) access in some patients.

Complications of Pregnancy

Complications of pregnancy can be categorized as antepartum (disorders occurring before childbirth), intrapartum (complications associated with labor and delivery), and postpartum (disorders occurring after childbirth). **BOX 45-3** lists the complications and disorders of pregnancy discussed in this chapter.

BOX 45-3 Complications and Disorders of Pregnancy

- Antepartum disorders
  - Hyperemesis gravidarum
  - Rh sensitization
  - Pregnancy-induced hypertensive disorders
  - GDM
  - Infection
  - Pulmonary embolism
  - Premature rupture of membranes
  - Bleeding complications
  - Third-trimester bleeding
  - Abruptio placentae
  - Placenta previa
  - Uterine rupture
- Intrapartum complications
  - Labor and delivery
  - Delivery complications
- Postpartum disorders
  - Postpartum hemorrhage
  - Amniotic fluid embolism

Antepartum Disorders

Hyperemesis Gravidarum

Hyperemesis gravidarum (HG) is a condition of pregnancy characterized by severe nausea, vomiting, weight loss, ketosis, and electrolyte disturbance (especially hypokalemia).[3] It is sometimes referred to as "a severe case of morning sickness." In women who have HG, symptoms begin within 2 to 5 weeks after conception. The nausea and vomiting generally ease after the first trimester and typically stop before 20 weeks' gestation. About 10% to 20% of mothers will have nausea and vomiting until delivery, although they are usually less severe. HG in previous pregnancies often follows a similar pattern of duration and severity in future pregnancies.

The exact cause of HG is unknown. However, it is likely the result of several factors that may include the following:[4]

- Pregnancy hormone imbalances
- Vitamin B deficiency, hyperthyroidism
- Gastroesophageal reflux occurring in association with abnormalities in the electrical properties of muscles affecting the stomach (gastric dysrhythmias)
- *Helicobacter pylori* infections
- Psychological factors
- Disturbances in carbohydrate metabolism

Management

HG can lead to dehydration, weight loss, and malnutrition that can harm both the mother and the fetus. HG is usually managed with antiemetics to control the nausea and vomiting, rehydration, and electrolyte replacement. Severe cases may require hospitalization and IV fluid therapy to manage dehydration. Prehospital care is primarily supportive.

Rh Sensitization

As described in Chapter 11, *General Principles of Pathophysiology*, people with Rh-negative blood do not carry the Rh marker on their red blood cells; people with Rh-positive blood do carry the marker. Rh sensitization can occur during pregnancy if an Rh-negative woman is pregnant with a baby who has Rh-positive blood. If this occurs, the immune system reacts to the Rh factor by producing antibodies to destroy it (**Rh sensitization**). During the first pregnancy, Rh sensitization usually does not pose a problem for the mother or baby. This is because the first exposure of fetal blood to maternal blood normally does not occur until delivery, which then becomes the sensitizing event. Maternal antibodies take some time to develop. However, if the mother was sensitized before the pregnancy (eg, as a result of a previous abortion, ectopic pregnancy, or amniocentesis that caused bleeding into the uterus) or if there is a subsequent pregnancy with an Rh-positive fetus, maternal antibodies can destroy fetal red blood cells.

> **NOTE**
>
> If the pregnant woman is Rh-negative and the father is Rh-positive, the newborn has a 50% chance of being Rh-positive, and blood Rh sensitization can occur. If both parents have Rh-negative blood, the newborn will have Rh-negative blood. Sensitization will not occur.

Women are tested early in pregnancy for their Rh factor and to determine if they have been sensitized. Women who have Rh-negative blood and who are not sensitized will require antibody tests until delivery; the newborn will have blood tested at birth. Injections of Rh immune globulin (eg, RhoGAM) are usually given to prevent Rh sensitization. (One injection is given at 26 to 28 weeks, and a second injection is given within 72 hours of birth if the child is Rh positive. This process will need to be repeated with each pregnancy.) Women who are sensitized will need careful monitoring and serial blood testing to measure antibody levels during their pregnancy. Doppler studies and amniocentesis may be performed to monitor the fetus. If fetal anemia is severe, the baby may need blood transfusions before birth (intrauterine transfusion) and immediately after birth. Early cesarean delivery is common in these cases.

Rh Disease

Newborns with **Rh disease** may have no symptoms of the illness. Other newborns can have a serious and life-threatening blood disorder known as **erythroblastosis fetalis**. The most common form of erythroblastosis fetalis is ABO incompatibility. The less common form is Rh incompatibility. Symptoms of the disease include anemia, jaundice, edema, an enlarged liver or spleen, and **hydrops fetalis** (the accumulation of fluid throughout body tissues, including the lungs, heart, and abdominal organs). Rh disease is treated with blood transfusion.

Pregnancy-Induced Hypertensive Disorders

Pregnancy-induced hypertensive disorders occur in about 6% to 8% of pregnancies in the United States; they increase the risk to the mother and the fetus. Pregnancy-induced hypertensive disorders are generally divided into three categories: gestational hypertension, preeclampsia, and eclampsia.[5]

Gestational Hypertension

Gestational hypertension occurs during pregnancy and resolves during the postpartum period. It is recognized by a new blood pressure reading of 140/90 mm Hg or higher. This condition is thought to result from immunologic dysfunction as well as a host of other factors and can be an early sign of preeclampsia.

Preeclampsia and Eclampsia

Preeclampsia is gestational hypertension after 20 weeks' gestation and at least one of the following:[6]

- Proteinuria (most common)
- Thrombocytopenia (low platelets)
- Impaired liver function
- Renal insufficiency
- Pulmonary edema
- Visual or cerebral disturbances

The hypertension can be mild or severe. Severe forms are characterized by systolic blood pressures greater than 160 mm Hg or a diastolic blood pressure greater than 110 mm Hg. The progression of preeclampsia to eclampsia is unpredictable and can occur rapidly.[5] The pathophysiology of preeclampsia, which does not reverse until after delivery, is characterized by vasospasm, endothelial cell injury, increased capillary permeability, and activation of the clotting cascade. The signs and symptoms of preeclampsia result from hypoperfusion to the tissue or organs involved (BOX 45-4). Generalized edema is a possible sign of preeclampsia, although it may occur both in a normal pregnancy and in a pregnancy complicated by another disorder (**FIGURE 45-8**). In

BOX 45-4 Signs and Symptoms of Preeclampsia

Cerebrum
Headache
Confusion
Hyperreflexia

Retina
Blurred vision
Diplopia

Gastrointestinal System
Right upper quadrant or epigastric pain and tenderness

Renal System
Proteinuria
Azotemia
Oliguria
Anuria

Vasculature or Endothelium
Hypertension
Edema
Activation of the clotting cascade

Placenta
Abruptio placentae
Fetal distress

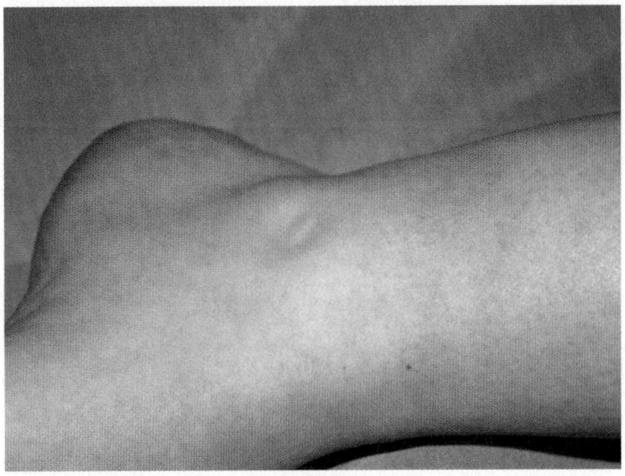

FIGURE 45-8 Pitting edema of the lower leg. Generalized edema is a possible sign identified with preeclampsia, although it may occur both in a normal pregnancy and in a pregnancy complicated by another disorder.

addition to a first-time pregnancy, factors associated with preeclampsia include advanced maternal age, chronic hypertension, chronic renal disease, vascular diseases such as diabetes mellitus and systemic lupus, and multiple gestation. When preeclampsia is suspected, most patients are hospitalized.

Eclampsia is the occurrence of seizures in a patient with other signs of preeclampsia. It is most common in patients with severe preeclampsia. It is a disease of unknown origin that primarily affects previously healthy, normotensive women in their first pregnancy. The disease occurs after 20 weeks' gestation, often near term, but may occasionally be seen postpartum. It can occur up to 4 weeks postpartum, although it is rare after 48 hours.[7] Preeclampsia is dangerous for the expectant mother and fetus for two reasons: (1) It can develop and progress rapidly, and (2) the early symptoms are often unnoticed by the woman or may be attributed to other causes.[8]

DID YOU KNOW?

HELLP Syndrome

The most severe form of preeclampsia is **HELLP syndrome** (H, hemolysis; EL, elevated liver enzymes; LP, low platelet count). HELLP syndrome is a true obstetric emergency that affects about 10% of pregnant women who have preeclampsia or eclampsia. Signs and symptoms of HELLP syndrome include headache, worsening nausea and vomiting, upper abdominal pain, and vision disturbances. When the disease is not treated early, serious complications develop in up to 25% of women. Without treatment, a small number of women die. The death rate among babies born to mothers with HELLP syndrome varies and depends on birth weight and the development of the baby's organs, especially the lungs. Definitive treatment is to deliver the newborn as soon as possible. The disease affects blood clotting abilities and liver function, with consequences that can be harmful to both the mother and the child.

HELLP syndrome often is asymptomatic, with vague complaints made by the patient of "feeling unwell" related to severe preeclampsia. It often presents without elevated blood pressure or proteinuria. The prominent symptom of HELLP syndrome is pain in the right upper quadrant, the lower chest, or epigastric area. There may be tenderness because of liver distention. It is important to avoid traumatizing the liver by abdominal palpation and to use care in transporting the patient. A sudden increase in intra-abdominal pressure, including that caused by a seizure, could lead to rupture of a subcapsular hematoma, resulting in internal bleeding and hypovolemic shock.

Modified from: How many women are affected by or at risk of preeclampsia? National Institutes of Health website. https://www.nichd.nih.gov/health/topics/preeclampsia/conditioninfo/risk. Accessed April 22, 2018; Queenan JT, Spong CY, Lockwood CJ. *Protocols for High-Risk Pregnancies: An Evidence-Based Approach*. 6th ed. West Sussex, England: Wiley Blackwell; 2015.

Management

Not all hypertensive patients have preeclampsia. Also, not all preeclamptic patients have hypertension. The illness has many serious complications. Thus, the paramedic should always suspect preeclampsia or eclampsia when hypertension or headache, visual changes, or epigastric pain present in late pregnancy or within 2 weeks postpartum. If preeclampsia or eclampsia is suspected, prehospital care is directed at preventing or controlling seizures and treating hypertension (under the guidance of medical direction).

Seizure activity in eclampsia most often is characterized by tonic–clonic activity (described in Chapter 24, *Neurology*). The seizure often begins around the mouth in the form of twitching. Eclampsia may be associated with apnea during the seizure. Labor can begin suddenly and progress rapidly. The regimen for managing severe preeclampsia is as follows:[7]

- Place the patient in a left lateral recumbent position to help maintain or improve uteroplacental blood flow. It also will help to lessen the risk of insult to the fetus.
- Administer high-concentration oxygen and monitor oxygen saturation. Assist respirations as needed.
- Initiate vascular access with a saline lock or IV with normal saline or lactated Ringer solution to keep the vein open. Maximum rate of fluid infusion is 80 mL/h.[7]
- Anticipate seizures at any moment. Be prepared to provide airway, ventilatory, and circulatory support.
- If seizures occur, administer magnesium sulfate, 4 grams (50% solution) over 10 to 20 minutes.[7] Follow this dose with 1 g/h IV infusion if possible. Contact medical control for further magnesium orders if seizures persist.
- If seizures do not stop after magnesium administration, administer midazolam, lorazepam, or diazepam. Monitor the patient closely for

respiratory depression and a precipitous fall in blood pressure. Fetal circulation may be jeopardized. Closely monitor vital signs and gently transport the patient to a proper medical facility.

If the patient has severe hypertension (systolic blood pressure >160 mm Hg or diastolic blood pressure >110 mm Hg) that lasts more than 15 minutes with other signs or symptoms of preeclampsia, the goal is to reduce the mean arterial pressure by 20% to 25%.[7] The following treatments may be implemented:

- Labetalol 20 mg IV over 2 minutes
  - May repeat every 10 minutes twice if severe symptomatic hypertension persists
  - Goal is to reduce mean arterial pressure by 20% to 25%
  - Heart rate must be greater than 60 beats/min prior to administration

or

- Hydralazine 5 mg IV
  - May repeat 10 mg after 20 minutes if severe symptomatic hypertension persists

or

- Nifedipine 10 mg orally
  - May repeat 10 to 20 mg orally every 20 minutes twice if severe symptomatic hypertension persists

and

- Magnesium sulfate 4 g IV (20% solution) over 20 minutes
  - Followed by 1 g/h IV infusion if possible

Observe the patient for signs of hypermagnesemia, such as hypotension, followed by these developments:

- Loss of deep tendon reflexes, then
- Drowsiness and slurred speech, then
- Respiratory paralysis, then
- Cardiac arrest

Treat hypermagnesemia by stopping magnesium administration. Administer calcium gluconate if severe respiratory depression with imminent arrest is noted. Note: The risk of eclampsia decreases if severe preeclampsia is treated early with magnesium and antihypertensives. Consult local protocols.

Gestational Diabetes Mellitus

Gestational diabetes mellitus (GDM) is diabetes caused by pregnancy. The condition occurs in about 2% to 10% of all pregnancies in the United States each year.[9] GDM is thought to be related to an inability of the pregnant woman to metabolize carbohydrates. This may be caused by a deficiency of the woman's insulin or by placental hormones that block the action of the insulin (insulin resistance). As a result, the woman's body is not able to produce or use all of the insulin it needs during the pregnancy. Excessive amounts of her glucose are transmitted to the fetus, where the glucose is stored as fat. Treatment for GDM includes regular glucose monitoring, dietary modification, and exercise. In some cases, pregnant women will need insulin injections to manage the condition. GDM usually subsides after pregnancy. However, it may return in later years or with future pregnancies.

Most women with GDM are aware of their condition through prenatal care and have healthy pregnancies and healthy babies. Without treatment, however, they often have very large babies. This results in a more difficult labor and delivery (with increased risk for fetal and maternal injury) and a longer recovery. In addition, children whose mothers had GDM are at higher risk for certain health problems. Examples of such are respiratory distress syndrome, obesity, and related health issues as children or adults. These children also have an increased risk for the development of type 2 diabetes during their lifetime.[10]

Management

Prehospital care for patients with insulin-dependent GDM may include airway, ventilatory, and circulatory support; glucose testing; management of hypoglycemia with IV fluids and dextrose; or management of hyperglycemia with the administration of IV fluids and insulin (per medical direction) (see Chapter 25, *Endocrinology*).

Infection

Numerous infections can pose problems for the pregnant mother, and some can be spread to the developing fetus and newborn. Examples include HIV infection (described in Chapter 27, *Infectious and Communicable Diseases*) and TORCH infections. Infectious diseases that may affect a woman's pregnancy, fetus, or newborn are listed in **BOX 45-5**.

BOX 45-5 Pregnancy and Infection

Urinary tract infection
Vaginal infection
Sexually transmitted disease
- Gonorrhea
- Human papillomavirus
- Syphilis
- Trichomoniasis
- Chlamydia

Bacterial vaginosis
Candidiasis

TORCH Infections

TORCH is an acronym for a special group of infections (**TORCH infections**) that may be acquired by a woman during pregnancy and result in fetal anomalies or death. "TORCH" stands for the following infections:[11]

Toxoplasmosis
Other infections: namely, hepatitis B, syphilis, and herpes zoster (the virus that causes chickenpox)
Rubella (formerly known as German measles)
Cytomegalovirus
Herpes simplex virus (the cause of genital herpes)

TORCH infections can be passed to the fetus in the womb, resulting in fetal death or serious complications for the newborn. These complications include the following:

- Miscarriage
- Congenital heart disease or heart defects (rare)
- Hearing impairment, including deafness
- Intellectual disability or other learning, behavioral, or emotional problems
- Anemia
- Liver or spleen enlargement
- Pneumonia
- Microcephaly (small head and brain size)
- Jaundice
- Low birth weight or poor growth inside the womb
- Blindness or other vision problems, such as cataracts (a clouding of the lens of the eye)
- Skin rash or scarring

Most TORCH infections can be prevented through immunization, good personal hygiene, and safe sex practices. In the case of toxoplasmosis, prevention includes avoidance of raw meat and exposure to cats and their wastes, which can sometimes carry the disease.

Pulmonary Embolism

The development of pulmonary embolism during pregnancy, labor, or the postpartum period is a significant cause of maternal death.[12] Venous stasis, hypercoagulability, and blood vessel injury are key factors that cause blood clot formation; the first two of these causes exist during normal pregnancy, and the third can occur at birth. The embolus often results from a blood clot in the lower extremity or pelvic circulation (venous thromboembolism).[12] It can also consist of amniotic fluid in the postpartum patient. There is a slight increased risk of pulmonary embolus with cesarean versus vaginal delivery.[12] The patient often has classic signs and symptoms that include sudden dyspnea, chest pain, tachycardia, tachypnea, crackles, hemoptysis, and sometimes hypotension. Large pulmonary emboli can lead to cardiac arrest. If the embolism occurs in the prehospital setting, emergency care should be focused on airway, ventilatory, and circulatory support; ECG monitoring; and rapid transport for physician evaluation.

NOTE

The incidence of pulmonary embolism during pregnancy and the postpartum period has been estimated to be 5.5 to 6 times higher than in the general female population. Pregnancy causes changes in the coagulation and fibrinolytic systems that persist into the postpartum period. During pregnancy, the levels of many coagulation factors are elevated. In addition, the fibrinolytic system is suppressed. Together, these factors hinder clot disintegration (lysis). The result is that factors that promote clot formation are increased to prevent maternal hemorrhage and factors that prevent clot formation are decreased, explaining the higher risk for thrombus formation during pregnancy and the postpartum period.

Modified from: Lee MY, Kim MY, Han JY, Park JB, Lee KS, Ryu HM. Pregnancy-associated pulmonary embolism during the peripartum period: an 8-year experience at a single center. *Obstet Gynecol Sci*. 2014;57(4):260-265; and McKinney ES, James SR, Murray SS, Ashwill JW. *Maternal-Child Nursing*. 3rd ed. Philadelphia, PA: Saunders; 2008.

Premature Rupture of Membranes

Premature rupture of membranes (PROM) is a rupture of the amniotic sac before the onset of labor. The condition is called preterm (PPROM) if the fetal age is less than 37 weeks. The risk to the fetus is highest when this occurs before 34 weeks. Premature rupture occurs in about 3% of pregnancies.[12] In 10% to 15% of all cases, the fetus is at or near term.[5] Signs and symptoms include a history of a trickle or sudden gush of fluid from the vagina. The paramedic should transport patients for physician evaluation. The medical facility will prepare for delivery if the patient begins labor. Delivery is required if an infection of fetal membranes is diagnosed (**chorioamnionitis**). Infection is more likely when more than 24 hours have elapsed since PROM. The infection generally is accompanied by maternal fever, chills, and uterine pain. Infection is treated with antibiotics. The definitive treatment for this infection is the delivery of the fetus.

Bleeding Complications Related to Pregnancy

Although most pregnancies are successful events, complications can and do occur. Vaginal bleeding during pregnancy can result from spontaneous abortion (miscarriage), ectopic pregnancy, abruptio placentae, placenta previa, uterine rupture, or postpartum hemorrhage. Patients with vaginal bleeding have varying degrees of blood loss. Some require aggressive resuscitation.

CRITICAL THINKING

When a mother loses blood from vaginal hemorrhage, how is the fetus affected?

Spontaneous Abortion

Spontaneous abortion, or miscarriage, is the noninduced termination of pregnancy from any cause before 20 weeks' gestation.[13] (Between 21 and 36 weeks' gestation, it is known as a preterm birth.) Abortion is the most frequent cause of vaginal bleeding in pregnant women. Spontaneous abortion occurs in 10% to 25% of all clinically recognized pregnancies.[14] BOX 45-6 lists common classifications of abortion.

BOX 45-6 Classifications of Abortion

- **Complete abortion.** An abortion in which the patient has passed all of the products of conception.
- **Elective abortion.** The elective termination of a pregnancy for nonmedical reasons.
- **Incomplete abortion.** An abortion in which the patient has passed some but not all of the products of conception.
- **Induced abortion.** An abortion in which the pregnancy is terminated intentionally.
- **Missed abortion.** The retention of the fetus in utero for 4 or more weeks after fetal death.
- **Septic abortion.** An abortion that results from infection of the placenta and fetus. Associated factors include fever, endometritis, parametritis, and pelvic disease.
- **Spontaneous abortion.** An abortion that usually occurs before the 12th week of gestation (also known as miscarriage). (Predisposing factors include acute or chronic illness in the mother, abnormalities in the fetus, and abnormal attachment of the placenta. Often the cause is unknown).
- **Therapeutic abortion.** A pregnancy terminated for reasons of maternal well-being.
- **Threatened abortion.** An abortion in which a patient has some uterine bleeding with an intrauterine pregnancy in which the internal cervical os is closed. A threatened abortion may stabilize and end in normal delivery or progress to an incomplete or complete abortion.

Most spontaneous abortions occur in the first trimester, usually before the 10th week. The patient often is anxious and apprehensive and complains of vaginal bleeding with pain. Bleeding may be slight (dime- or quarter-size spotting) or profuse. The pain may be referred to the lower back and is often described as cramplike and similar to the pain of labor or menstruation. In addition, the patient may have suprapubic pain. When obtaining a history, the paramedic should ascertain the time of onset of pain and bleeding, the amount of blood loss (a soaked sanitary pad suggests 20 to 30 mL of blood loss), and whether the patient passed any tissue with the blood. If the patient passed tissue during bleeding episodes, the tissue should be collected and transported with the patient for analysis.

Management. The assessment of all first-trimester bleeding should include close observation for signs of significant blood loss and hypovolemia. The paramedic should measure vital signs often during transport. Depending on the patient's hemodynamic status, IV fluid therapy may be indicated. All patients with suspected abortion should receive emotional support and transport for physician evaluation.

Ectopic Pregnancy

An **ectopic pregnancy** occurs when a fertilized ovum implants anywhere other than the uterus. Ectopic gestation occurs in about 2% of all pregnancies; it is the leading cause of first-trimester death and accounts for more than 6% of all maternal deaths in the United States.[5] Death from ectopic pregnancy usually results from hemorrhage.

Ectopic pregnancy has many causes. Most involve factors that delay or prevent the passage of the fertilized ovum to its normal site of implantation. Predisposing factors include pelvic inflammatory disease, adhesions from previous surgery, tubal ligation, previous ectopic pregnancy, and possibly the presence of intrauterine contraceptive devices. About 50% of women have no risks.[15] Thus, obtaining a full gynecologic history is important in risk assessment. Although the time from fertilization to rupture varies, most ruptures occur by 2 to 12 weeks' gestation.

The signs and symptoms of ectopic pregnancy often are difficult to distinguish from those of a ruptured ovarian cyst, pelvic inflammatory disease, appendicitis, or abortion (thus the name "the great imitator"). The classic triad of symptoms includes abdominal pain, vaginal bleeding, and amenorrhea (absence of menstruation); however, vaginal bleeding may be absent, spotty, or minimal, and amenorrhea may be replaced by oligomenorrhea (scanty flow). The variable presentation of this type of pregnancy is one reason for its high risk profile. Other symptoms of ectopic pregnancy include referred pain to the shoulder and signs of early pregnancy, which include nausea, vomiting, syncope, and the classic signs of shock.

Management. A ruptured ectopic pregnancy is a serious emergency. It calls for initial resuscitation measures and rapid transport for surgical intervention. The patient may become unstable quickly. If the paramedic suspects an ectopic pregnancy, the patient should be managed like any victim of hemorrhagic shock—with airway, ventilatory, and circulatory support and titrated IV fluid resuscitation. When the diagnosis is made prior to rupture, medical management versus surgery may be a possible solution.[16]

Third-Trimester Bleeding

Third-trimester bleeding occurs in 4% of all pregnancies and is never normal.[5] About one-half of bleeding episodes are a result of abruptio placentae, placenta previa, or uterine rupture. **TABLE 45-1** differentiates among abruptio placentae, placenta previa, and uterine rupture.

Abruptio Placentae. **Abruptio placentae** (also referred to as placental abruption) is partial or full detachment of a normally implanted placenta at more than 20 weeks' gestation. It occurs in about 1% of all pregnancies and is severe enough to result in fetal death in about 15% of cases of abruption.[17] Predisposing factors to abruptio placentae include maternal hypertension, preeclampsia, multiple pregnancies, cigarette smoking, trauma, and previous abruption.

> **NOTE**
>
> Maternal use of cocaine, which causes vasoconstriction in the endometrial arteries, is a leading cause of abruptio placentae and can lead to severe bleeding, preterm birth, and fetal death. Cocaine use during pregnancy is also associated with other poor outcomes such as spontaneous abortion and congenital anomalies.
>
> *Modified from*: Organization of Teratology Information Specialists. Cocaine and pregnancy. Cite Seer X website. http://citeseerx.ist.psu.edu/viewdoc/download;jsessionid=64D6E3820BAA4940979F5EF9394701D5?doi=10.1.1.370.5156&rep=rep1&type=pdf. Accessed April 23, 2018.

> **CRITICAL THINKING**
>
> Why is abruptio placentae associated with such a high fetal death rate?

The common presentation of abruptio placentae is sudden third-trimester vaginal bleeding and pain. The incidence peaks at 24 to 26 weeks and declines as delivery nears.[17] The vaginal bleeding may be minimal. The degree of shock may be out of proportion to the visible blood loss in cases when much of the hemorrhage is concealed behind the placenta. The severity of the patient's signs and symptoms is determined by the location of the abruption, the degree of the abruption, and whether the blood is escaping through the vagina or concealed behind the uterus. The more extensive the separation, the greater the

TABLE 45-1 Differentiation of Abruptio Placentae, Placenta Previa, and Uterine Rupture

History	Bleeding	Abnormal Pain	Abdominal Examination
Abruptio Placentae			
Association with severe hypertension, toxemia of pregnancy, and methamphetamine or cocaine use	Often absent or scant episode of dark vaginal bleeding	Present	Localized uterine tenderness Rigid uterus Fetal heart rate slows after contractions Absent fetal heart tones
Placenta Previa			
Previous cesarean section Grand multiparity	Bleeding after intercourse Classic bleeding pattern: • 1 bleed in early second trimester • 1 bleed in late second or early third trimester • 1 severe bleed after onset of labor	Absent unless in labor	Lack of uterine tenderness Labor Fetal heart tones
Uterine Rupture			
Previous cesarean section Tetanic contraction	Possible vaginal bleeding	Severe pain usually present and associated with sudden onset of nausea and vomiting	Diffuse abdominal tenderness Sudden cessation of labor Bradycardia

uterine irritability, resulting in a tender abdomen and rigid uterus. Contractions may be present. The absence of fetal heart tones or a bradycardic fetal heart rate suggests severe abruptio placentae, and fetal death is likely.

Placenta Previa. **Placenta previa** is placental implantation in the lower uterine segment partially or completely covering the cervical opening. It occurs in about 5 in 1,000 deliveries.[18] The incidence is higher in preterm births. The condition is characterized by painless (usually), bright red bleeding with or without uterine contraction. The bleeding may occur in episodes and may be slight to moderate. In addition, bleeding may become more profuse if active labor begins. Fetal heart rate slows because of hypoxia.

Placenta previa is strongly associated with the number of previous cesarean sections. Other risk factors are increasing maternal age, multiple pregnancies, cocaine use, and previous placenta previa episodes.[19] Recent sexual intercourse can lead to bleeding.

Uterine Rupture. **Uterine rupture** is a spontaneous or traumatic rupture of the uterine wall. It most frequently results from reopening of a previous uterine scar (eg, a previous cesarean section). It also may result from a prolonged or obstructed labor, or direct trauma. Uterine rupture is very rare. It carries a 0% to 1% maternal mortality rate and a 2% fetal mortality rate in developed countries.[20]

Uterine rupture is characterized by sudden abdominal pain described as steady and "tearing," active labor, early signs of shock (complaints of weakness, dizziness, anxiety), and bleeding, which may not be visible. On examination, the abdomen usually is rigid. The patient complains of diffuse abdominal pain. Fetal parts may be felt easily through the abdominal wall.

Management. The prehospital management of a patient with third-trimester bleeding is aimed at preventing shock. The paramedic should not try to examine the patient vaginally; doing so may increase hemorrhage and precipitate labor. Emergency care measures should include the following:

1. Provide adequate airway, ventilatory, and circulatory support as needed (with spinal precautions if indicated).
2. Place the patient in a left lateral recumbent position.
3. Begin transport immediately.
4. Initiate IV access in the event that volume-expanding fluid is indicated.
5. Apply a fresh perineal pad. Note the time of application to assess bleeding during transport.
6. Check fundal height. Document it for baseline measurement.
7. Closely monitor the patient's vital signs en route to the medical facility.
8. Closely monitor fetal heart rate if possible.

Intrapartum Complications

Labor and Delivery

Parturition is the process by which the fetus is born. Near the end of pregnancy, the uterus becomes increasingly irritable and exhibits occasional contractions. These contractions become stronger and more frequent until parturition begins. During and as a result of these contractions, the cervix begins to dilate. As uterine contractions increase, complete cervical dilation occurs to about 10 cm; the amniotic sac usually ruptures; and the fetus, and shortly thereafter the placenta, is expelled from the uterus through the vaginal canal (**FIGURE 45-9**). When the onset of labor to birth is less than 3 hours, this is considered a **precipitous delivery**.

Stages of Labor

Labor follows several distinct stages. The lengths of these stages vary depending on whether the mother is nullipara or multipara (BOX 45-7). Thus, the paramedic should use the stages of labor only as a guideline in assessing labor progression in the average pregnancy.

First Stage of Labor. The **first stage of labor** begins with contractions and ends when the cervix is fully dilated at 10 cm. This stage of labor is divided into early labor, active labor, and transition.

> NOTE
>
> About 2 to 3 weeks before the onset of active labor, the cervix undergoes the process of softening, effacement (thinning), and dilation. During this timeframe, the fetus may move into the mother's pelvis. This is commonly called lightening. Lightening is characterized by relief of pressure in the mother's upper abdomen and a simultaneous increase in pressure in her pelvis. **Braxton-Hicks contractions** refer to irregular tightening of the pregnant uterus. These begin in the first trimester (before 30 weeks' gestation). They are usually benign and painless. They often subside with walking or other exercise. Many patients are not aware of Braxton-Hicks contractions. They may perceive them as a slight uterine hardening. As the pregnancy continues, the Braxton-Hicks contractions increase in frequency and duration.

Early labor is defined by cervical dilation of 0 to 3 cm and contractions occurring every 5 to 20 minutes and lasting 30 to 45 seconds. In this stage of labor, the mother typically notices backache and mild discomfort. The contractions progress over time, becoming longer, stronger, and closer together. Between contractions, the woman feels relatively normal and pain free. For first-time mothers, this stage of labor may last 8 to 20 hours. With subsequent births, the stage lasts 6 to 8 hours or less.

Active labor is defined by cervical dilation of 4 to 8 cm, and contractions 4 to 5 minutes apart, lasting about 60 seconds. This stage marks the beginning of intense contractions. Between contractions, the woman may experience trembling, nausea, and vomiting. Coached relaxation and slowed breathing between contractions often is comforting. This stage of labor usually lasts 1 to 2 hours.

Transition is defined by cervical dilation of 8 to 10 cm. During transition, contractions are about 2 to 3 minutes apart and last for about 60 to 90 seconds. The contractions are intense and may occur with little rest for the woman. They may be accompanied by rectal pressure if the baby's head is positioned low. In many pregnancies, the amniotic sac ruptures (rupture of membranes) toward the end of the first stage of labor. The period of transition lasts only 15 to 30 minutes on average (BOX 45-8).

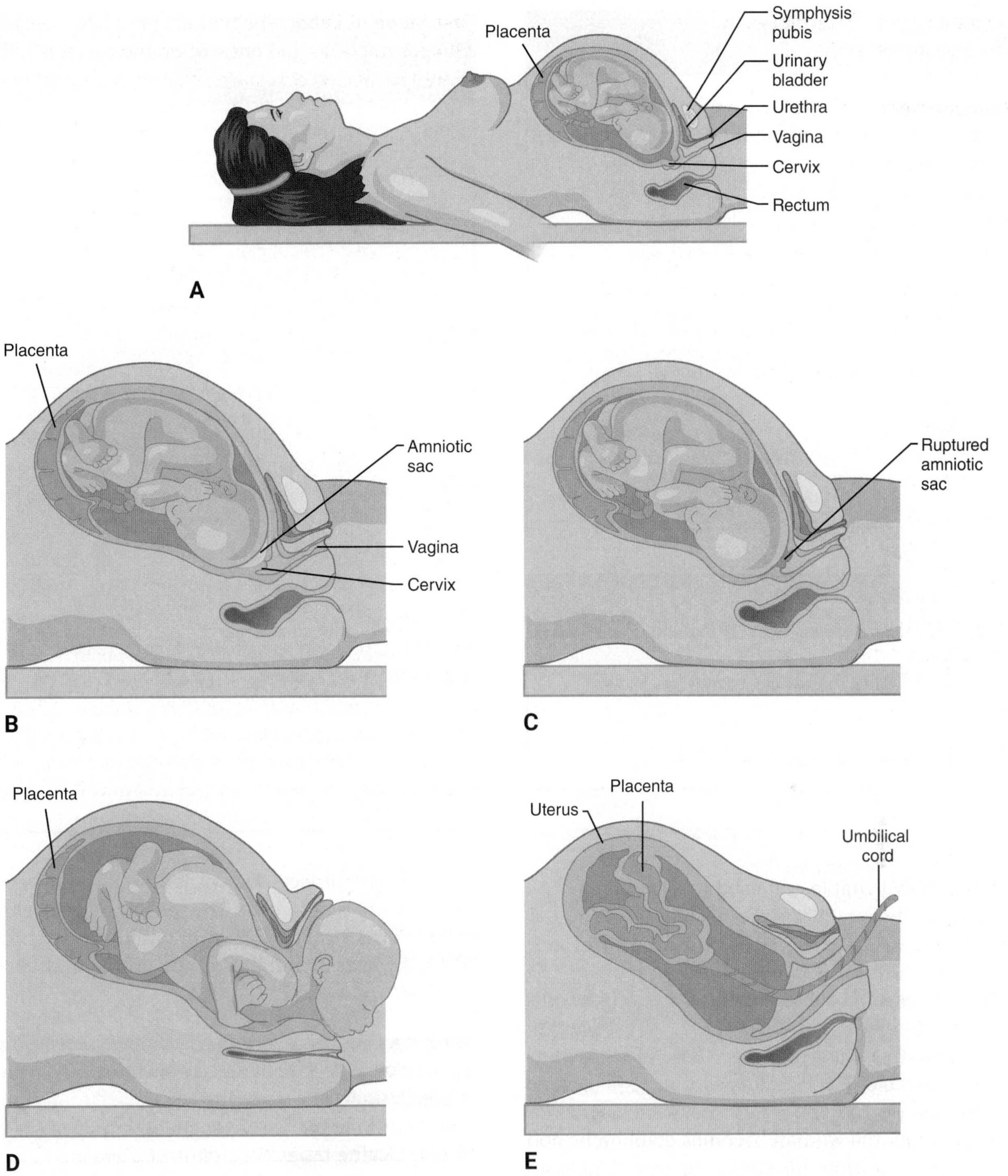

FIGURE 45-9 Parturition. **A.** The relation of the fetus to the mother. **B.** The fetus moves into the birth canal. **C.** Dilation of the cervix is complete. **D.** The fetus is expelled from the uterus. **E.** The placenta is expelled.

BOX 45-7 Stages of Labor

Stage 1

- Onset of regular contractions to complete cervical dilation
- Average time: Early labor 8 to 20 hours in primipara, 6 to 8 hours or less in multipara
- Active labor 1 to 2 hours
- Transition 15 to 30 minutes on average

Stage 2

- Full dilation of cervix to delivery of the newborn
- Average time: 1 to 2 hours in primipara, 30 minutes or less in multipara

Stage 3

- Immediately after delivery of the baby until expulsion of the placenta
- Average time: 5 to 60 minutes regardless of parity

BOX 45-8 Premonitory Signs of Labor

Lightening
Braxton-Hicks contractions
Cervical changes
Bloody show
Rupture of membranes

CRITICAL THINKING

What comfort measures can you use during transport for the patient who is in the first stage of labor?

Second Stage of Labor. The **second stage of labor** is measured from full dilation of the cervix to delivery of the newborn. During this stage, the fetal head enters the birth canal. The woman's contractions become more intense and frequent (usually 2 to 3 minutes apart); often the woman becomes diaphoretic and tachycardic during this stage. She experiences an urge to bear down with each contraction and may express the need to have a bowel movement. This sensation is normal, caused by pressure of the fetal head against the woman's rectum. During this stage a **mucus plug** (sometimes mixed with blood, thus the name *bloody show*) is expelled from the dilating cervix and discharged from the vagina. (The mother may not notice passage of the plug.) The presenting part of the fetus (usually the head) emerges from the vaginal opening. This process, known as **crowning**, indicates that delivery is imminent. The second stage of labor usually lasts 1 to 2 hours in the nullipara woman. It usually lasts 30 minutes or less in the multipara mother (BOX 45-9).

BOX 45-9 Cardinal Movements: Positional Changes During Birth

The fetus must make several positional changes (cardinal movements) during the birth process. These movements are deliberate and precise changes made by the fetus so that passage through the bony pelvis can occur. These positional changes are descent, flexion, internal rotation, extension, external rotation, and expulsion.

Descent is the movement of the baby's head into the pelvic cavity. Babies enter the birth canal with their head in the transverse position, with the occiput either to the right or to the left. Flexion occurs during descent as the head encounters resistance. This causes the baby's head to flex so that the chin meets the chest. As the head reaches the pelvic floor, it rotates to an anterior-posterior position (internal rotation) to accommodate for the smallest diameter of the birth canal between the ischial spines. Extension occurs as the fetus stops flexion of the head when the baby's head, face, and chin are born. Following extension, the baby must rotate (external rotation) from an anterior-posterior position to a transverse position (facing one of the mother's thighs). This movement (also known as restitution) allows for the shoulders to pass under the mother's pubic arch. After external rotation, the shoulders are born. This is followed by full delivery of the newborn (expulsion).

Modified from: Hagood Milton S. Normal labor and delivery. Medscape website. https://emedicine.medscape.com/article/260036-overview?. Updated November 16, 2017. Accessed April 23, 2018.

Third Stage of Labor. The **third stage of labor** begins with delivery of the baby and ends when the placenta is expelled and the uterus has contracted (described later in this chapter). The length of this stage varies from 5 to 60 minutes, regardless of parity.

Signs and Symptoms of Imminent Delivery

The following signs and symptoms indicate that delivery is imminent. When they occur, the paramedic should prepare for childbirth at the scene:

- Regular contractions lasting 45 to 60 seconds at 1- to 2-minute intervals. Intervals are measured from the beginning of one contraction to the

beginning of the next. If contractions are more than 5 minutes apart, there generally is time to transport the mother to a receiving hospital.
- The mother has an urge to bear down or has a sensation of a bowel movement.
- There is a large amount of bloody show.
- Crowning occurs.
- The mother believes that delivery is imminent.

If any of these signs and symptoms are present, the EMS crew should prepare for delivery. With the exception of cord presentation (described later in this chapter), the paramedic should not try to delay delivery. If complications are anticipated or an abnormal delivery occurs, medical direction may recommend expedited transport of the patient to a medical facility.

NOTE

A precipitous delivery is a rapid spontaneous delivery with less than 3 hours from onset of labor to birth. Precipitous delivery results from overactive uterine contractions and insignificant maternal soft-tissue or bony resistance. A precipitous delivery most often occurs in a mother who is grand multipara. It can be associated with soft-tissue injury and uterine rupture (rare). Precipitous delivery has an increased perinatal mortality rate because of trauma and hypoxia. The main danger to the fetus during this kind of delivery is from cerebral trauma or tearing of the umbilical cord.

If the paramedic expects a precipitous delivery, attempts should be made to prevent an explosive one. This can be done by providing gentle counterpressure to the fetal head; however, the paramedic should not attempt to detain fetal head descent. After delivery, the newborn should be kept dry and warm to prevent heat loss. The mother should be examined for perineal tears that often accompany a rapid birth.

Preparation for Delivery

When preparing for delivery, the paramedic should try to provide an area of privacy. The mother should be positioned on a bed, stretcher, or table. The surface should be long enough to project beyond the mother's vagina. The delivery area should be as clean as possible. It should be covered with absorbent material to guard against staining and contamination by blood and fecal material.

A pregnant woman should be placed on her back. Her knees should be flexed and widely separated (or in another position preferred by the woman). The vaginal area should be draped appropriately. If delivery occurs in a car, the woman should be instructed to lie on her back across the seat with one leg flexed on the seat and the other leg resting on the floorboard. A pillow or blanket, if available, should be placed beneath the mother's buttocks. This will aid in the delivery of the newborn's head. The paramedic should evaluate the woman's baseline vital signs. The fetal heart rate may be monitored for signs of fetal distress. Per protocol and medical direction, the paramedic should consider maternal oxygen administration and IV access for fluid administration or postdelivery administration of oxytocin if needed.

The woman should be coached to bear down and push during contractions and to rest between contractions to conserve strength. If the woman finds it difficult to refrain from pushing, she should be encouraged to breathe deeply or "pant" through her mouth between contractions. Deep breathing and panting help decrease the force of bearing down and promote rest.

NOTE

In 2011, the majority of newborns in the United States were delivered in hospitals (98.7%). Of the less than 2% of newborns not delivered in the hospital, 66.2% were born in a residence. Therefore, it is likely that paramedics will assist with newborn deliveries during their career. In the majority of births, the paramedic will only assist in delivery of the newborn.

Modified from: Martin JA, Hamilton BE, Ventura SJ, Osterman MJK, Mathews TJ; Division of Vital Statistics. Births: final data for 2011. *Natl Vital Stat Rep*. 2013 June 28;62(1). www.cdc.gov/nchs/data/nvsr/nvsr62/nvsr62_01.pdf. Accessed April 23, 2018.

Delivery Equipment. Prehospital delivery equipment ("OB kit") generally includes the following components (**FIGURE 45-10**):

- Surgical scissors
- Cord clamps or umbilical tape
- Towels
- Surgical masks
- 4 × 4–inch gauze sponges
- Sanitary napkins
- Bulb syringe and meconium suction kit
- Baby blanket and baby stocking cap
- Plastic bag for placental transport
- Neonatal resuscitation equipment
- IV fluid supplies

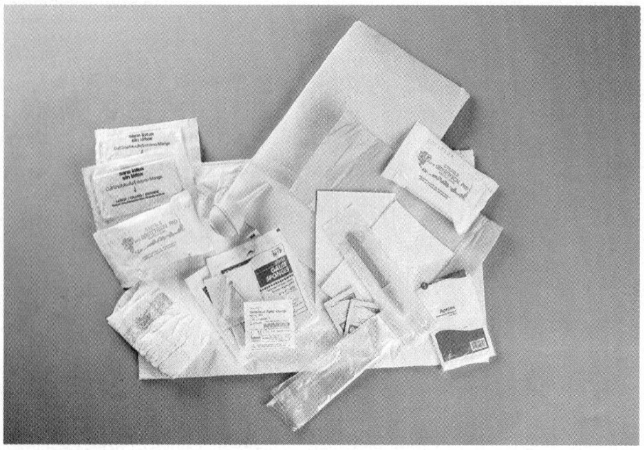

FIGURE 45-10 Prehospital delivery equipment.

Personal protective measures should be used when assisting in a delivery. Sterile technique should be used when handling equipment.

Assistance With Delivery

In most cases, the paramedic only assists in the natural events of childbirth. The chief duties of the EMS crew are to prevent an uncontrolled delivery and protect the newborn from cold and stress after the birth. The following are steps to be taken in assisting the mother with a normal delivery (**FIGURE 45-11**):

1. Observe standard precautions.
2. When crowning occurs, apply gentle palm counterpressure to the fetal head to prevent an explosive delivery and tearing of the mother's perineum. If membranes are still intact, tear the sac with finger pressure to allow escape of amniotic fluid.
3. After delivery of the head, examine the fetal neck for a looped (nuchal) umbilical cord. If the cord is looped around the neck, gently slip it over the head.
4. Grasp the head with hands over the ears to support the fetal head as it rotates for shoulder presentation. Most fetuses present facedown. The fetus usually rotates to the left or right so that the shoulders present in an anterior-posterior position.
5. If the shoulders do not spontaneously deliver with the next contraction, using gentle pressure, guide the fetal head downward to deliver the anterior shoulder and then upward to release the posterior shoulder. The rest of the baby is delivered quickly by smooth uterine contraction.
6. Be careful to grasp and support the baby as he or she emerges, using a dry towel or clean piece of clothing. Hold the newborn with his or her head dependent to aid drainage of secretions. Place the newborn on the mother's abdomen if she is able to hold her baby.
7. Clear the newborn's airway of any secretions with sterile gauze. Suction the newborn's mouth and then the nose if there is coarse gurgling.
8. Dry the newborn with sterile towels and cover the newborn (especially the head) to reduce heat loss.
9. Record the newborn's sex and time of birth.

CRITICAL THINKING

How do you think you will feel after attending a birth of a healthy baby?

Evaluation of the Newborn

After delivery, the newborn should be positioned on the side or with padding under the back if needed. The paramedic should clear the airway and provide tactile stimulation to initiate respirations. If there is no need for resuscitation, the paramedic should assign an **Apgar score** at 1 minute and 5 minutes to evaluate the newborn (**TABLE 45-2**). Criteria for computing the Apgar score include appearance (color), pulse (heart rate), grimace (reflex irritability to stimulation), activity (muscle tone), and respiratory effort. Each criterion is rated from 0 to 2. The numbers are added for a total Apgar score.

NOTE

Newborns who do not require resuscitation can generally be defined by a rapid assessment of the following four characteristics:

- Was the baby born after a full-term gestation?
- Is the amniotic fluid clear of meconium and evidence of infection?
- Is the baby breathing or crying?
- Does the baby have good muscle tone?

If the answer to all four of these questions is "yes," the baby does not need resuscitation and should not be separated from the mother. If the answer to any of these questions is "no," the baby should be resuscitated (see Chapter 46, *Neonatal Care*).

Modified from: Weiner GM, ed. *Textbook of Neonatal Resuscitation*. 7th ed. Elk Grove Village, IL: American Academy of Pediatrics; 2016.

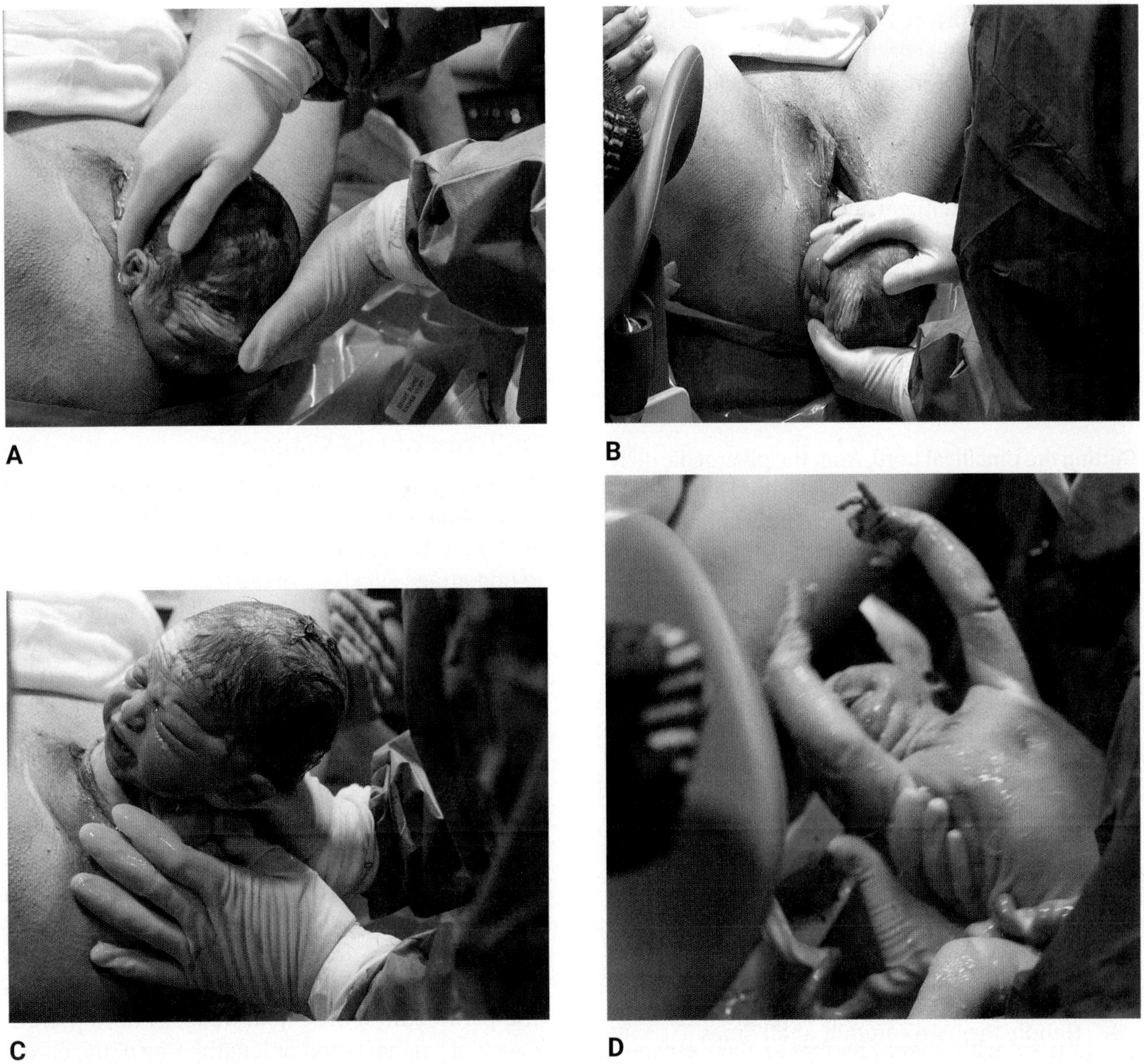

FIGURE 45-11 Normal delivery. **A.** As the newborn's head begins to emerge from the vagina, it will start to turn. Support the newborn's head as it turns. **B.** Guide the neonate's head downward to deliver the anterior shoulder. **C.** Guide the neonate's head upward to release the posterior shoulder. **D.** Once the shoulders are delivered, the newborn's trunk and legs will follow rapidly.

TABLE 45-2 The Apgar Scoring System

Sign	0	1	2
Appearance (skin color)	Blue, pale	Body pink, blue extremities	Completely pink
Pulse rate (heart rate)	Absent	<100 beats/min	>100 beats/min
Grimace (irritability)	No response	Grimace	Cough, sneeze, cry
Activity (muscle tone)	Limp	Some flexion	Active motion
Respirations (respiratory effort)	Absent	Slow, irregular	Good, crying

An Apgar score of 10 indicates that the baby is in the best possible condition, 7 to 9 indicates that the baby is generally normal, 4 to 6 indicates that the baby is moderately depressed, and 0 to 3 indicates that the baby is severely depressed. Most newborns have an Apgar score of 7 to 9 at 1 minute after birth. Newborns with an Apgar score of less than 6 generally require resuscitation; however, the paramedic should remember that the Apgar score is not used to determine the need for initial resuscitation, what resuscitation steps are necessary, or when to use them.[21] (Neonatal resuscitation is presented in Chapter 46, *Neonatal Care.*)

Cutting the Umbilical Cord. After the paramedic delivers and evaluates the baby and the cord has stopped pulsing, the umbilical cord should be clamped (or tied with umbilical tape) and cut (**FIGURE 45-12**). Clamping or cutting the cord should be delayed for at least 30 seconds to 1 minute in term and preterm newborns not requiring resuscitation.[22] The paramedic should take the following steps to manage the umbilical cord:

1. Clamp the cord about 4 to 6 inches (10 to 15 cm) away from the newborn in two places.
2. Cut between the two clamps with sterile scissors or a scalpel.
3. Examine the cut ends of the cord to ensure that there is no bleeding. If the cut end attached to the newborn is bleeding, clamp the cord proximal to the previous clamp and reassess for bleeding. Do not remove the first clamp.
4. Handle the cord carefully at all times.

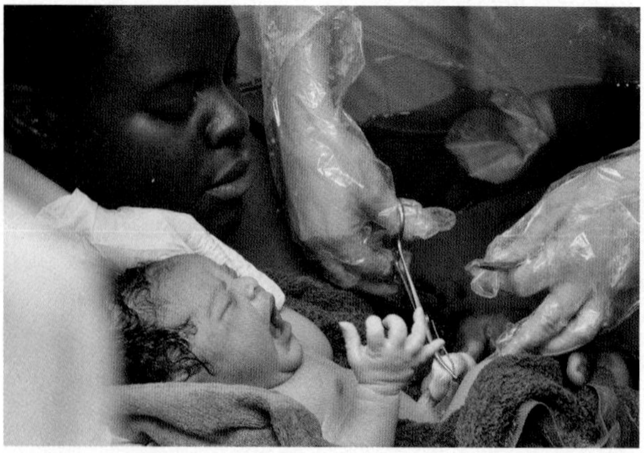

FIGURE 45-12 After delivery and evaluation of the newborn, the paramedic clamps and cuts the cord.

NOTE

In newborns who do not require resuscitation, delayed cord clamping is associated with less intraventricular hemorrhage, higher blood pressure and blood volume, less need for transfusion after birth, and less necrotizing enterocolitis (death of a portion of the bowel). However, if placental circulation is compromised (eg, abruptio placentae), the cord should be clamped immediately.

Modified from: Weiner GM, ed. *Textbook of Neonatal Resuscitation*. 7th ed. Elk Grove Village, IL: American Academy of Pediatrics; 2016.

Delivery of the Placenta

If the baby and mother are in good condition and if the mother is agreeable, place the baby skin-to-skin on the mother's abdomen and chest (kangaroo care) to encourage suckling. Breastfeeding will stimulate the release of oxytocin, which will lead to decreased blood loss. The placenta normally is delivered within 20 minutes of the newborn. Thus, transport should not be delayed for placental delivery. Placental delivery is characterized by episodes of contractions, a palpable rise of the uterus within the abdomen, lengthening of the umbilical cord protruding from the vagina, and a sudden gush of vaginal blood.

After birth of the newborn and clamping of the cord, the mother should be told to bear down with contractions. The paramedic should place one hand lightly on the mother's abdomen and should grasp the cord with the other hand, without pulling on it. The paramedic should hold the cord until there is a gush of vaginal blood or lengthening of the cord.

NOTE

The hand that is placed on the mother's abdomen may feel the rise of the uterus with cord lengthening or the gush of vaginal blood. This can indicate that the placenta is ready to deliver or only partly separated from the uterine wall. At this time, the paramedic should ask the mother to bear down with the next contraction. If there is no immediate progress (further lengthening of the cord), the paramedic should wait for spontaneous cord lengthening to occur. Again, placental delivery should not delay patient transport.

When the placenta is expelled, it should be placed in a plastic bag or other container and transported with the mother and newborn to the receiving hospital.

At the hospital, the placenta will be examined for abnormality and completeness. Pieces of placenta retained in the uterus can cause persistent hemorrhage and infection. After the delivery of the placenta, the paramedic should assess the mother's perineum for tears. If tears are present, the bleeding should be managed by applying sanitary napkins to the area and maintaining direct pressure. The paramedic should initiate fundal massage (described later in the chapter) to promote uterine contraction and monitor the mother during transport for signs of hemorrhage or shock. Medical direction also may prescribe oxytocin to manage postpartum bleeding, if needed.

SHOW ME THE EVIDENCE

Researchers in Melbourne, Australia, reported on the clinical and sociodemographic factors of pregnant women not yet in labor over a period of 12 months. In that year, their EMS system responded to 2,098 pregnant women ranging in age from 14 to 48 years. Most were multigravidas (86%). Just over half of calls (54%) related to obstetric problems. Vaginal bleeding was the most frequent pregnancy-related complaint (84%), with 60% occurring during the first trimester. Nonpregnancy-related calls were for abdominal pain unrelated to labor and without vaginal bleeding (30%); nausea, vomiting, and diarrhea (15%); fainting (6%); infection (5%); seizures (2%); and dizziness (5%). An additional 10.8% of women had traumatic injuries, with causes including motor vehicle crashes, falls, and strains from lifting. Fewer than one-half of the 62 women who were injured by interpersonal violence were victims of domestic violence. Almost 1 in 10 patients had preexisting mental health issues. Less than half of all patients needed an intervention.

It is important that paramedics understand normal findings in pregnant women so that abnormal findings associated with pregnancy or other conditions can be detected quickly and managed effectively.

Modified from: McLelland G, McKenna L, Morgans A, Smith K. Antenatal emergency care provided by paramedics: a one-year clinical profile. *Prehosp Emerg Care*. 2016;20(4):531-538.

Delivery Complications

As stated previously, most women have uncomplicated pregnancies. Prehospital deliveries seldom present any significant problems for the mother, newborn, or paramedic crew. The delivery complications discussed in this chapter include cephalopelvic disproportion, abnormal presentation, premature birth, multiple gestation, uterine inversion, pulmonary embolism, and fetal membrane disorders. BOX 45-10 lists factors that should alert the paramedic to anticipate an abnormal delivery.

BOX 45-10 Factors Associated With High-Risk Delivery

Maternal Factors

- Maternal age: very young or very old
- Absence of prenatal care
- Maternal lifestyle: alcohol, tobacco, or drug usage
- Preexisting maternal illness, including diabetes mellitus, chronic hypertension, or Rh sensitization
- Previous obstetric history of the following:
  - Premature delivery
  - Previous malformed neonate
  - Previous multiple births
  - Previous cesarean delivery
- Intrapartum disorders
  - Preeclampsia
  - Prolonged rupture of membranes
  - Prolonged labor
  - Abnormal presentation
  - Abruptio placentae
  - Placenta previa

Fetal Factors

- Lack of fetal well-being
  - History of decreased fetal movement
  - Hydramnios (excess amniotic fluid)
  - History of heart rate abnormalities
  - Evidence of fetal distress
- Fetal immaturity: prematurity as established by dates, ultrasound, uterine size, amniocentesis
- Fetal growth: history of poor intrauterine growth or postdate delivery; fetal macrosomia (birth weight more than 8 pounds [3.6 kg])
- Specific fetal malformation detected by ultrasonography: diaphragmatic hernia or omphalocele

Cephalopelvic Disproportion

Cephalopelvic disproportion is a condition in which the newborn's head is too large or the mother's birth canal is too small to allow normal labor or birth. The woman often is pregnant with her first child and having strong, frequent contractions for a prolonged period. Prehospital care is limited to maternal oxygen administration, IV access for fluid resuscitation if needed, and rapid transport to the receiving hospital.

Abnormal Presentation

Most babies are born headfirst (cephalic or vertex presentation). But sometimes a presentation is abnormal. These include shoulder dystocia, a breech presentation, shoulder presentation, and a cord presentation (umbilical cord prolapse).

Shoulder Dystocia. Shoulder dystocia occurs when the fetal shoulders are wedged against the maternal symphysis pubis, blocking shoulder delivery. In this presentation, the head delivers normally but then pulls back tightly against the maternal perineum (the *turtle sign*) and the shoulders fail to deliver after at least 60 seconds.[23] Shoulder dystocia is a common condition in pregnancy, occurring in 1 in 300 deliveries.[5] Complications include brachial plexus damage, fractured clavicle, and fetal anoxia from cord compression. Fifty percent of shoulder dystocia cases occur in women without risk factors.

Shoulder dystocia delivery requires dislodging one shoulder and then rotating the fetal shoulder girdle at an angle into the wider part of the pelvic opening. Because the shoulder is pressing against the pelvis, cord compression could occur. Thus, the paramedic should deliver the anterior shoulder immediately after the head. The paramedic should administer high-concentration oxygen to the woman.

Several maneuvers can help the paramedic successfully deliver a newborn when shoulder dystocia arises.[7] The following steps represent one approach to shoulder dystocia:

1. Position the woman supine with the hips hyperflexed in the McRoberts maneuver (**FIGURE 45-13**). This position increases the diameter of the pelvis.
2. Apply gentle pressure to the suprapubic area to attempt to dislodge the shoulder. Do *not* apply fundal pressure; doing so can make delivery more difficult. Try to guide the baby's head downward to allow the anterior shoulder to slip under the pubic symphysis. Avoid excessive force or manipulation.
3. External manipulation techniques, such as the McRoberts maneuver, in combination with suprapubic pressure usually resolve a shoulder issue. If this approach is unsuccessful, internal manipulation techniques may be attempted.[24] Internal manipulation techniques include the following:
   - Woods corkscrew and reverse corkscrew maneuver: Place a hand on the surface of the posterior shoulder and rotate the baby to free the anterior shoulder.
   - Manual delivery of the posterior shoulder: Place pressure in the baby's posterior axilla and flex the arm across the chest and pull out.

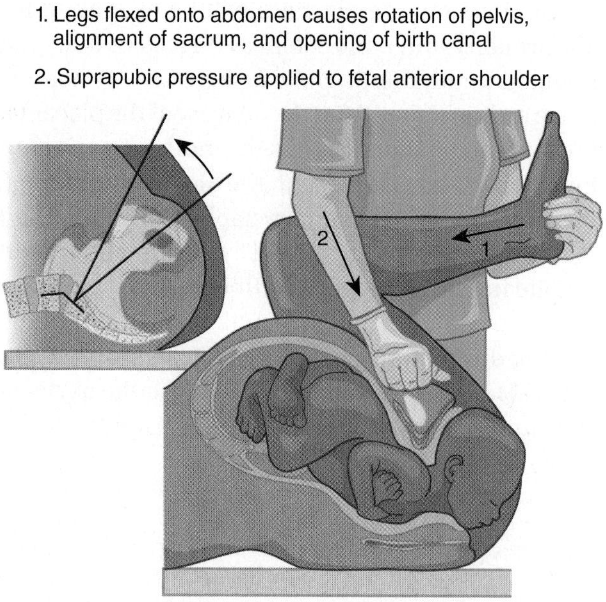

1. Legs flexed onto abdomen causes rotation of pelvis, alignment of sacrum, and opening of birth canal
2. Suprapubic pressure applied to fetal anterior shoulder
2
1

FIGURE 45-13 McRoberts maneuver.

If these methods are unsuccessful, the woman can be turned over and placed on her hands and knees ("all fours") to allow the posterior shoulder to descend. After delivery, the paramedic should continue with resuscitative measures as needed. If unable to deliver the shoulders, transport should begin as soon as possible. The paramedic should contact medical direction for advice.

Breech Presentation. In a breech presentation, the largest part of the fetus (the head) is delivered last. Breech presentation occurs in 3% to 4% of deliveries at term.[25] It is more common with multiple births and when labor occurs before 32 weeks' gestation. Categories of breech presentation include the following (**FIGURE 45-14**):[25]

- **Frank breech.** The fetal hips are flexed and the legs extend in front of the fetus. The buttocks are the presenting part. Frank breech accounts for about 60% to 65% of breech presentations.
- **Complete breech.** The fetus has both knees and hips flexed. The buttocks are the presenting part. Complete breech accounts for about 5% of breech presentations.

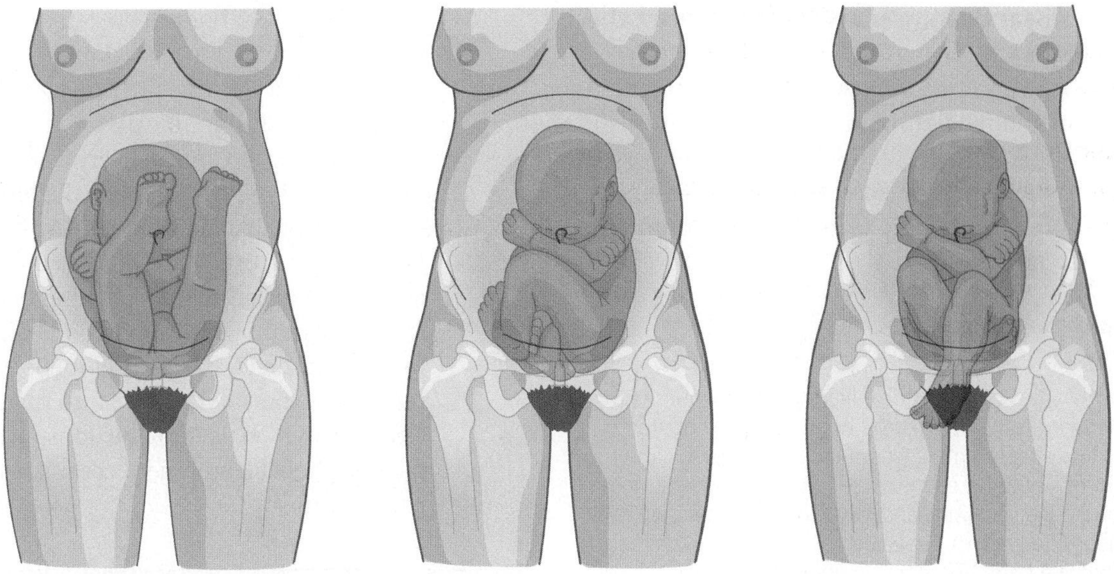

FIGURE 45-14 Types of breech presentation. **A.** Front or back. **B.** Complete. **C.** Incomplete.

- **Incomplete breech.** The fetus has one or both hips incompletely flexed. This results in presentation of one or both lower extremities (often a foot). Incomplete breech accounts for about 25% to 30% of breech presentations.

> CRITICAL THINKING
>
> What resources can you use to assist in a delivery with an abnormal presentation?

A newborn in a breech presentation is best delivered in a hospital where emergency cesarean section is immediately available. Sometimes, however, the paramedic must assist in a breech delivery.[26] If a breech delivery is reported and there is no fetus visible or leg/buttocks only are visible, the paramedic should proceed as follows:

- Tell the woman not to push.
- Begin rapid transport. This is the most important step with impending breech delivery.
- Call for assistance.
- Administer oxygen to the woman.
- Place a hand in the vagina and attempt to prevent the fetus from delivering. (Note: Placing a hand in the vagina to take pressure off the cord is not effective.) This should always be done in the context of online medical direction.
- Consider anticontraction drugs (tocolytic agents), if available.

If delivery is imminent and rapid transport to an emergency department is not an option, the paramedic should do the following:

- Instruct the woman to push forcefully.
- Do not assist with delivery until the fetal umbilicus is visible.

Although paramedics are not trained to perform the following procedures during a breech delivery, they should be familiar with certain procedures that might be performed by obstetricians or emergency physicians in breech deliveries:

- The Pinard maneuver (to rotate the fetal thigh and pelvis to assist delivery):
  - With the back of the fetus facing up, grasp the hips (not abdomen) by placing thumbs on the sacrum and the fingers on the anterior superior iliac crests.
  - Rotate the fetus 90° clockwise until the left shoulder is at the symphysis pubis.
  - Slide a finger under the fetal axilla and sweep toward the fetal antecubital fossa to deliver the left arm.
  - Once the first arm is delivered, grasp the hips and rotate the fetus 180° clockwise until the right arm is at the symphysis pubis.

- Repeat the preceding steps to release the right arm.
- Gently rotate the fetus so the back is oriented up (umbilicus toward the woman's buttocks).
- At this point the Mauriceau maneuver is used to deliver the head while another member of the health care team applies suprapubic pressure.

NOTE

Generally, the Pinard maneuver and the Mauriceau maneuver are performed by board-certified obstetricians and rarely by midwives, but not paramedics. EMS personnel must be educated to identify complications during labor and delivery and how to manage them, which includes knowledge of specialty centers in the area that can provide appropriate treatment.

- The Mauriceau maneuver (to keep the fetal head flexed to allow for delivery) (**FIGURE 45-15**):
  - Insert a gloved hand into the vagina, with the index and middle fingers on the fetal maxilla (not mandible) to flex the head of the fetus.
  - Rest the fetal body on the forearm, with the nondominant hand on the fetal shoulders.
  - Encourage the mother to push while downward traction is applied until the back of the head is visible.

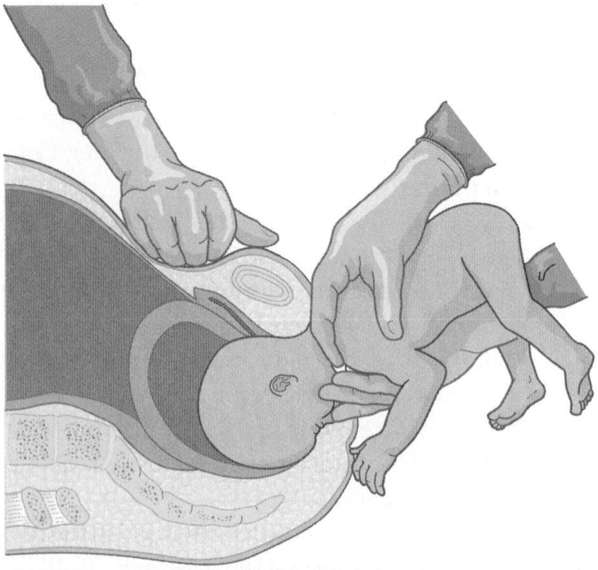

FIGURE 45-15 Mauriceau maneuver.

  - Elevate the lower body of the fetus, tipping it up toward the maternal abdomen while another member of the health care team continually applies suprapubic pressure and keeps the head in flexion until delivery is completed.
- The Zavanelli maneuver (to push the fetal head back into the birth canal) (**FIGURE 45-16**):
  - During transport, if the head is entrapped after the Mauriceau maneuver has been performed, as a final option, medical direction may recommend that an attempt be made to replace the born fetal parts into the uterus. The patient then needs to be transported to a facility where an emergent cesarean section can be done.

Shoulder Presentation. Shoulder presentation *(transverse presentation)* results when the long axis of the fetus lies perpendicular to that of the mother. This position usually results in the fetal shoulder lying over the pelvic opening. The fetal arm or hand may

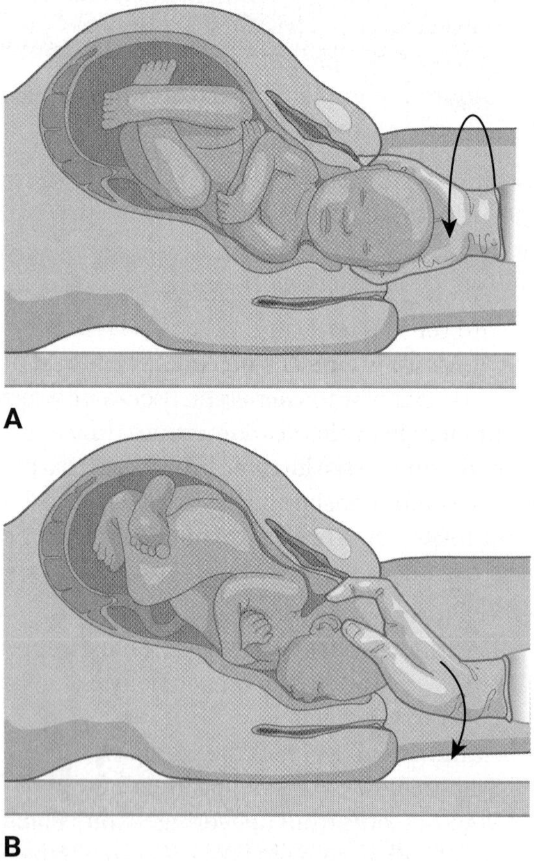

FIGURE 45-16 Zavanelli maneuver. **A.** Positioning the fetal head. **B.** Pushing the fetus back into the birth canal.

be the presenting part. This abnormal presentation occurs in only 0.3% of deliveries but occurs in 10% of second twins.[5]

Normal delivery of a shoulder presentation is not possible. The paramedic should provide the mother with adequate oxygen, ventilatory, and circulatory support and then provide rapid transport to the hospital. A cesarean delivery is required regardless of the condition of the fetus.

Umbilical Cord Prolapse. **Umbilical cord prolapse** occurs when the cord passes through the cervix at the same time or in advance of the presenting part of the fetus, after the amniotic membranes have ruptured. (If the membranes are intact, the condition is known as a cord presentation or funic presentation.) With umbilical cord prolapse, the umbilical cord is compressed against the presenting part of the fetus, which diminishes fetal oxygenation from the placenta. A prolapsed cord occurs in about 1 in 10 deliveries.[27] When fetal distress is present, the paramedic should suspect a prolapsed cord. Predisposing factors include breech presentation, lack of prenatal care, twinning, gestational diabetes with large baby, and preterm labor.[23]

Fetal asphyxia can ensue rapidly if circulation through the cord is not reestablished and maintained until delivery. If the paramedic can see or feel the umbilical cord in the vagina, the following steps should be taken:

1. With a gloved hand, gently push the fetus back into the vagina. Elevate the presenting part to relieve pressure on the cord. Assess for cord pulsation using care not to apply additional pressure on the cord. The cord may retract spontaneously. However, the paramedic should not try to reposition the cord.
2. Maintain this hand position during rapid transport to the hospital. The definitive treatment is a cesarean delivery.
3. Position the mother with hips elevated as much as possible. The Trendelenburg or knee–chest position may relieve pressure on the cord.
4. Administer oxygen to the woman.
5. If help is available, apply moist sterile dressings to the exposed cord. This will minimize temperature changes that may cause umbilical artery spasm.
6. Instruct the woman to pant with each contraction to prevent bearing down.

Other Abnormal Presentations. Other abnormal presentations include *face* or *brow (military) presentation* and *occiput posterior presentation.* In these presentations, the newborn's head is delivered face up instead of facedown. Face up presentations result in increased risks to the fetus because of difficult labor and delivery. Thus, early recognition of potential complications, maternal support and reassurance, and rapid transport for definitive care are the goals of prehospital management.

Premature Birth

A **premature newborn** is born before 37 weeks' gestation (**FIGURE 45-17**).[28] Low birth weight (less than 5.5 pounds [2.5 kg]) also determines prematurity,

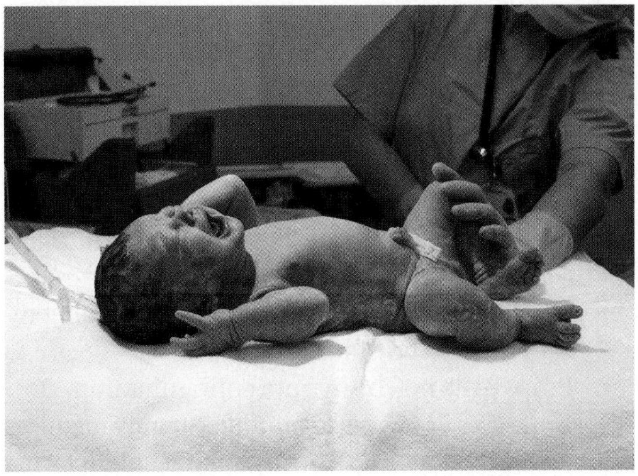

A

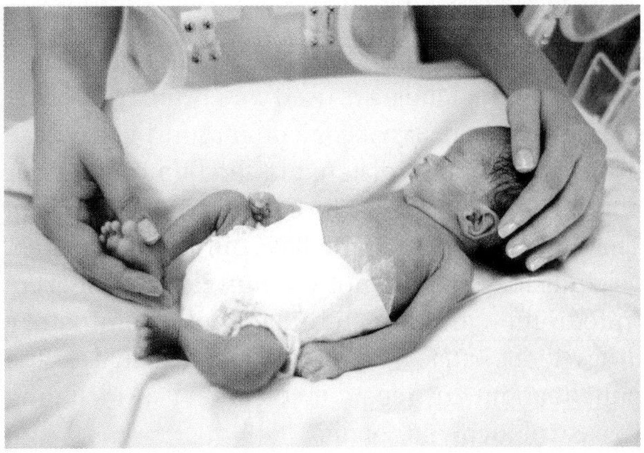

B

FIGURE 45-17 **A.** A healthy full-term newborn. **B.** A premature newborn.

although the conditions are not synonymous. Premature deliveries occur in about 1 in 10 pregnancies.[29] After a preterm labor, the newborn is at increased risk for hypothermia because of a high ratio of body surface to body mass and is at increased risk for cardiorespiratory distress because of the prematurely developed cardiovascular system. (Neonatal resuscitation is presented in Chapter 46, *Neonatal Care.*) Therefore, these newborns require special care and observation. After delivery, prehospital management for a premature baby includes the following:

- Keep the newborn warm. Dry the newborn, wrap the newborn in a warm blanket, place the newborn on the mother's abdomen, and cover the mother and newborn. If transport time is delayed, very small newborns (weighing less than 3.3 pounds [1.5 kg]) should be wrapped in food-grade heat-resistant plastic wrap and placed under radiant heat in addition to other warming methods.[22]
- Suction secretions if they occlude the newborn's mouth and nares.
- Carefully monitor the cut end of the umbilical cord for oozing. If bleeding is present, manage as described previously.
- Administer humidified free-flow oxygen through a makeshift oxygen tent. Aim oxygen flow toward the top of the tent; do not allow it to flow directly into the newborn's face.
- Protect the newborn from contamination. Don a mask and gown, and minimize family member (except the mother) and bystander contact with the newborn.
- Gently transport the mother and newborn to the receiving hospital.

One should note that **tocolytic** agents (drugs used to inhibit labor) are used widely today by some mothers who are at risk for a premature birth. These drugs may be administered in the home setting or administered before or during interfacility transfer. They include magnesium sulfate, nitroglycerin (patch, gel, infusion), salbutamol, calcium channel blockers (nifedipine), and nonsteroidal anti-inflammatory drugs (indomethacin).[30] The paramedic should ask the patient about any recent medication use, including the use of tocolytic agents.

Multiple Gestation

A **multiple gestation** is a pregnancy with more than one fetus. Historically, twin births usually occurred in only 1% of all deliveries. Because of the increasing use of fertility treatments, about 30% of every 1,000 live births are now multiple births (BOX 45-11).[31] Multiple gestation places more stress on the maternal system and also is accompanied by an increased complication rate. Associated complications include premature labor and delivery (30% to 50% of twin deliveries are premature), PROM, abruptio placentae, postpartum hemorrhage, and abnormal presentation. A mother who has not received prenatal care may be unaware of her multiple pregnancy.

BOX 45-11 Twin Terminology

Fraternal twins result from the fertilization of two ova by two spermatozoa. Each fraternal twin has a separate placenta. Each also is separated by individual amniotic membranes. Fraternal twins are not identical in appearance. They are often of different sex.

Identical twins result from the fertilization of a single ovum. They may share a common placenta and amniotic sac or have separate placental structures. Identical twins are less common than fraternal twins, occurring in one out of three twin conceptions. Unlike fraternal twins, identical twins look the same, are of the same sex, and are genetically identical.

CRITICAL THINKING

Do you have enough supplies on your ambulance to manage more than one delivery?

Delivery Procedure. First-twin delivery is identical to single delivery with the same presentation. However, up to 50% of second-twin deliveries are not in a normal presentation position. Fetuses are smaller in multiple births.

After the delivery of the first twin, the paramedic should cut and clamp (or tie) the umbilical cord as described earlier. Within 5 to 10 minutes after delivery of the first twin, labor begins again. The delivery of the second twin usually occurs within 30 to 45 minutes. Medical direction may recommend transport before the delivery of the second twin (depending on transport time). Usually both twins are born before the delivery of the placenta.

Newborns in multiple births often are smaller than newborns in single-term births. The paramedic should give special attention to keeping these babies warm, well oxygenated, and free from unnecessary contamination, as described for premature babies. Postpartum hemorrhage may be more severe after multiple births. Hemorrhage may require fluid resuscitation, uterine massage, and oxytocin infusion to control bleeding.

Uterine Inversion

Uterine inversion is an infrequent complication of childbirth in which the uterus turns "inside out." The condition is reported to occur in about 1 in 1,200 to 57,000 deliveries.[32] Uterine inversion is a serious condition. The resultant postpartum hemorrhage is associated with a maternal mortality rate of around 15%.[33]

Although the exact cause of uterine inversion after childbirth is not well understood, it has been associated with excessive pulling on the umbilical cord and **fundal massage** as well as other predisposing factors.[34] The risk is elevated when the placenta has implanted high in the uterus. Uterine inversion is incomplete if the uterine fundus does not extend beyond the cervix; it is complete if the fundus does protrude through the cervix; and it is prolapsed if the entire uterus protrudes through the vaginal ring. Signs and symptoms of uterine inversion include postpartum hemorrhage and sudden and severe lower abdominal pain. The hemorrhage may be profuse. Hypovolemic shock may develop quickly.

Management. Prehospital care for a patient with uterine inversion includes airway, ventilatory, and circulatory support and rapid transport for physician evaluation. Medical direction may recommend that the paramedic attempt manual replacement of the uterus only if the cervix has not yet constricted. The technique for manual replacement is as follows:

1. Place the patient in a supine position.
2. Do not attempt to remove the placenta if it has not already been delivered. Doing so is likely to increase hemorrhage.
3. Apply pressure with the fingertips and palm of a gloved hand and push the fundus upward and through the cervical canal. If this is ineffective, cover all protruding tissues with moist sterile dressings and rapidly transport the patient.

Manual replacement of the uterus may be painful to the patient. Medical direction may indicate the use of analgesics. The paramedic should explain the need for the procedure to the patient.

Postpartum Disorders

Postpartum Hemorrhage

Postpartum hemorrhage is characterized by more than 500 mL of blood loss after the delivery of the newborn. (The actual volume of blood loss is difficult to estimate with accuracy.) Hemorrhage often occurs within the first 24 hours after delivery (primary hemorrhage). Yet it can be delayed up to several weeks.[23] Postpartum hemorrhage occurs in about 5% of all deliveries and accounts for up to 25% of obstetric deaths.[5] Hemorrhage often results from ineffective or incomplete contraction of the interlacing uterine muscle fibers. Other causes of postpartum hemorrhage include retained pieces of placenta or membranes in the uterus. Hemorrhage can also be caused by vaginal or cervical tears during delivery. Risk factors associated with postpartum hemorrhage include **uterine atony** (lack of uterine tone) from prolonged or tumultuous labor, grand multiparity, twin pregnancy, placenta previa, and a full bladder.

NOTE

Lochia is postpartum vaginal discharge that contains blood, mucus, and placental tissue from the lining of the uterus. This discharge is normal and typically continues for about 2 to 4 weeks after childbirth. Lochia is similar to menstrual bleeding, but initially heavier, and then diminishes. The discharge usually begins as bright red and will later become pink or yellow-white in color.

Management

Postpartum hemorrhage can occur in the prehospital setting after a field delivery, home delivery, or delivery at an independent birthing center. The assessment and management are similar to those described for third-trimester bleeding. In addition, the paramedic should take the following measures to encourage uterine contraction:

1. **Massage the uterus.** Palpate the uterus for firmness or loss of tone. If the uterus does not feel firm, apply fundal pressure by supporting the lower uterine segment with the edge of one hand just above the symphysis and massaging the fundus in a circular motion with the other

hand. Continue massaging until the uterus feels firm. Reevaluate the patient every 10 minutes; note the location of the fundus in relation to the level of the umbilicus, the degree of firmness, and vaginal flow.

2. **Encourage the newborn to breastfeed.** If the conditions of the mother and newborn are stable and the mother agrees, place the newborn skin-to-skin against the mother and with the newborn's mouth to her breast to encourage breastfeeding. Stimulation of the breasts may promote uterine contraction.
3. **Administer oxytocin.** Per medical direction and after ensuring that a second fetus is not present in the uterus, add 10 units of oxytocin to 1,000 mL of lactated Ringer solution. Infuse at 20 to 30 drops/min via microdrip tubing (titrated to the severity of hemorrhage and uterine response or as ordered by medical direction). Continue with fluid resuscitation as indicated by the patient's vital signs.

NOTE

The paramedic should manage external bleeding from a perineal tear with direct pressure. There should be no attempts at vaginal examination or vaginal packing to control hemorrhage. These patients should be rapidly transported for physician evaluation.

Amniotic Fluid Embolism

When amniotic fluid enters the maternal circulation during labor or delivery or immediately after delivery, an **amniotic fluid embolism** can occur. Probable routes of entry include lacerations of the endocervical veins during cervical dilation, the lower uterine segment or placental site, and uterine veins at sites of uterine trauma. Particulate matter in the amniotic fluid (eg, meconium, lanugo hairs, fetal squamous cells) forms an embolus and obstructs the pulmonary vasculature. Amniotic fluid embolism is rare, occurring in 6 to 14.8 per 100,000 primigravid and multiparous deliveries, respectively.[35] The condition most often is seen in multiparous women late in the first stage of labor. Other conditions that can increase the incidence of this severe complication are placenta previa, abruptio placentae, and intrauterine fetal death. The maternal mortality rate is high. The signs and symptoms of amniotic fluid embolism are the same as those described for pulmonary embolism.

Postpartum Depression

Postpartum depression affects 10% to 15% of mothers.[36] The depression most likely is caused by a combination of sudden hormonal changes and psychological and environmental factors. It is a period of depression lasting at least 2 weeks beginning during pregnancy or within 4 weeks of childbirth. Several features characterize postpartum depression: a change in appetite or weight, sleep, or psychomotor activity; decreased energy; feeling worthless or guilty; difficulty thinking, concentrating, or making decisions; and recurrent thoughts of death or suicide with or without suicide plans or attempts.[37] Postpartum depression is more likely to occur after the first pregnancy. Other risk factors for postpartum depression include the following:

- Adverse socioeconomic conditions
- Depression during pregnancy or previous postpartum depression
- Complicated pregnancy or delivery
- Fetal complications
- Family history of depression, mental illness, or alcoholism
- Poor marital adjustment
- Anger or ambivalence about the pregnancy
- Single parent or young maternal age
- Lack of social or financial support
- Recent life stressors

NOTE

Postpartum blues ("baby blues"), characterized by mild depression after childbirth, affects more than 75% of new mothers. During this period, women experience anxiety, insomnia, fatigue, tearfulness, and altered mood. Postpartum blues begins in the first week and ends within 2 weeks. This condition is not the same as postpartum depression or postpartum psychosis—both of which require intensive therapy for optimum recovery.

Modified from: Tepper NK, Boulet S, Whiteman M, et al. Postpartum venous thromboembolism. *Obstet Gynecol*. 2014;123:987-996.

Recognizing and treating postpartum depression is important for both child and maternal health. The depression can interfere with the bonding between the mother and baby. It also can seriously affect the mother's ability to care for her newborn. Many women with postpartum depression fear they will harm their babies. They often feel ashamed and guilty for these feelings. Sensitivity to the possibility of depression is necessary for successful diagnosis and treatment (see Chapter 34, *Behavioral and Psychiatric Disorders*).

Trauma During Pregnancy

About 1 in every 12 pregnancies is complicated by physical trauma.[38] When a pregnant woman is severely injured, the fetus is at high risk for death. The anatomic and physiologic changes of pregnancy can alter the pregnant woman's response to injury. This may necessitate modified assessment, treatment, and transport strategies.

Maternal Injury

The causes of maternal injury, in decreasing order of frequency, are vehicular crashes, interpersonal violence, and falls.[39] The severity of any injury depends on many factors and may involve multiple organ systems.

During pregnancy, the fetus is well protected within the uterus; amniotic fluid surrounds the fetus. This fluid serves as an excellent shock absorber. Because of this protection, the fetus rarely experiences physical trauma except as a result of direct penetrating wounds or extensive blunt trauma to the maternal abdomen. Although direct life-threatening fetal injury is uncommon in blunt trauma, in penetrating trauma direct injury to the fetus can cause fetal death, even if the woman's injuries are not life threatening. Severe abdominal injury can result in abruptio placentae, premature labor or abortion, or uterine rupture. The greatest risk of fetal death is from interruption of blood flow to the placenta from trauma, severe maternal hypotension, or death of the mother. This can cause fetal distress and intrauterine demise. Thus, when caring for a pregnant trauma patient, the paramedic promptly should assess and intervene on behalf of the woman.

Assessment and Management

The priorities in assessing and managing a pregnant trauma patient are the same as those for a nonpregnant patient: address exsanguinating hemorrhage, followed by adequate airway, oxygenation, ventilatory, and circulatory support with spinal precautions; and rapid assessment, stabilization, and rapid transport to a medical facility. Resuscitating a pregnant woman is key to her survival and survival of the fetus. Thus, during the first stages of assessment and management, the woman's status should be the focus.

The examination should be thorough. The paramedic must detect, identify, and manage injuries that contribute to hypovolemia or hypoxia. With the normal increase in maternal blood volume, a pregnant woman can tolerate more blood loss before showing signs and symptoms of shock. A 30% to 35% reduction in blood volume can produce minimal changes in blood pressure but reduce uterine blood flow by 10% to 20%.[39] Thus, a pregnant woman may maintain adequate blood pressure at the expense of the fetus. The true amount of blood loss may be difficult to detect. Fetal monitoring is the best available indicator of fetal well-being after trauma. However, patient transport should never be delayed to assess the fetal heart rate.

> NOTE
> Any traumatic injury to the uterus causing blood loss can result in massive hemorrhage much more quickly than in nonpregnant patients. Any vaginal bleeding after injury should be addressed immediately.

Accelerations of the fetal heart rate above baseline are associated with fetal movement and contractions. However, this also may be an early sign of fetal distress. Decreased fetal movement and increased fetal heart rate can indicate maternal shock.

Decelerations in fetal heart rates (below the baseline) result from a decrease in cardiac output and hypoxia. A hypoxic fetus in metabolic acidosis cannot accelerate his or her heart rate. Thus, the fetus becomes bradycardic (a heart rate of less than 100 beats/min). Sustained fetal bradycardia (lasting 10 minutes or more) may be a response to increased parasympathetic tone. The fetus can tolerate this only for a short time before becoming acidotic. Fetal bradycardia may be a late sign of maternal hypotension, hypoxia, or decreased maternal circulating volume. It also is a sign of fetal distress attributable to umbilical cord compression or prolonged decelerations in the heart rate.

> CRITICAL THINKING
> What might be some common feelings of pregnant patients who have experienced trauma?

Special Management Considerations

Special considerations in managing the pregnant trauma patient include oxygenation, volume replacement, and hemorrhage control. Labor is a complication of trauma in pregnancy. The paramedic crew should be ready to manage delivery or spontaneous abortion (described previously in this chapter).

Oxygenation

- Adequate maternal airway maintenance and oxygenation are essential to prevention of fetal hypoxemia. Pulse oximetry should be used to monitor oxygen saturation. Supplemental oxygen should be administered to maintain a maternal oxygen saturation of greater than 95%.[40]
- Maternal oxygen supplementation in labor should be reserved for maternal hypoxia and should not be considered an indicated intervention for evidence of fetal distress.[41]

Volume replacement

- Signs and symptoms of hypovolemia may not be present until the blood loss is large.
- Blood is shunted preferentially from the uterus to preserve maternal blood pressure.
- Bleeding also may occur inside the uterus. The pregnant uterus can sequester up to 2,000 mL of blood after separation of the placenta with little or no evidence of vaginal bleeding.[5]
- Crystalloid fluid replacement is indicated initially for maternal hypotension.
- Vasopressors generally are not recommended. They decrease uterine blood flow and fetal oxygen delivery. Vasodilators sometimes are given to patients with severe preeclampsia who are hypertensive.

Hemorrhage control

- External hemorrhage should be controlled by using the same techniques as for a nonpregnant patient.
- Vaginal bleeding may point to placental separation, placenta previa, or uterine rupture.
- Avoid a vaginal examination. It may increase bleeding and trigger delivery. This may be the case especially if unsuspected placenta previa is present (described previously in this chapter).
- Document the amount and color of vaginal bleeding.
- Collect and transport any expelled tissue with the patient to the facility.

Transport Strategies

Pregnant patients who are beyond 3 to 4 months' gestation should not be transported in a supine position because of the potential for supine hypotension. In the absence of suspected spinal injury, the patient should be transported in a left lateral recumbent position. If spinal injury is suspected, the patient should be prepared for transport in the following manner:[42]

1. Fully immobilize the patient on a long backboard or device recommended by medical direction.
2. After immobilization, carefully tilt the board on its left side by logrolling the secured patient 10° to 15°.
3. Place a blanket, pillow, or towel under the right side of the board to move the uterus to the left side.

Transport destination is an important consideration in the pregnant trauma patient. Because both maternal and fetal outcomes depend on adequate resuscitation of the mother, studies have demonstrated that outcomes improve with transport to a trauma center.[43] Indeed, pregnancies that are greater than 20 weeks' gestation fall under the "Special Considerations" portion of the Centers for Disease Control and Prevention's Guidelines for Field Triage of Injured Patients, suggesting that these patients should be transported to a trauma center.[44] Ideally, the trauma center would also have obstetric capability. Pregnant patients with major injury should be transported to a trauma unit or emergency department in lieu of a labor and delivery unit regardless of gestational age.[40]

> CRITICAL THINKING
> Which facilities in your community have both trauma center and obstetric capabilities?

Cardiac Arrest in the Pregnant Patient

Cardiac arrest can occur in pregnant women from a number of causes (BOX 45-12). However, many cardiovascular problems associated with pregnancy are related to changes in anatomy that produce a decrease in the return of venous blood.[45] The key to

BOX 45-12 Causes of Cardiac Arrest Associated With Pregnancy

Events That Occur at the Time of Delivery

Amniotic fluid embolism
Aspiration pneumonitis
Drug toxicity (eg, because of magnesium sulfate or epidural anesthetic)
Eclampsia

Events That Occur From Complex Physiologic Changes Associated With Pregnancy

Possible contributing factors (BEAU-CHOPS)
- **B**leeding or disseminated intravascular coagulation
- **E**mbolism (pulmonary, amniotic fluid)
- **A**nesthetic complications
- **U**terine atony
- **C**ardiac disease (myocardial infarction, ischemia, aortic dissection, or myocarditis)
- **H**ypertension, preeclampsia, or eclampsia
- **O**ther: differential diagnosis of standard advanced cardiac life support guidelines
- **P**lacenta previa or abruptio placentae
- **S**epsis

resuscitation of the fetus is often resuscitation of the pregnant woman. A woman cannot be resuscitated until blood flow to her right ventricle is restored.

The best chance for survival of mother and fetus is rapid maternal resuscitation. Therefore, good chest compressions with minimal interruption should be initiated immediately. Although consideration may be given to manual uterine displacement to enhance venous return, this intervention should be performed only if it can be done without compromising the quality of chest compressions. Shockable rhythms should be defibrillated as soon as possible. Standard drug and defibrillation doses apply.

If gestational age is greater than or equal to 23 weeks or fundal height is two or more fingerbreadths above the umbilicus, the patient should be transported as soon as possible to allow for perimortem **cesarean delivery**. The goal of perimortem cesarean delivery is not just to save the life of the fetus, but to save the life of the mother as well by improving blood flow back to the maternal coronary circulation. The goal is for a perimortem caesarean to be performed within 4 minutes of loss of maternal pulses.[40] Survival is poor if the time is longer than 30 minutes.[46] Alerting the emergency department staff of the possible need for an emergency cesarean section is crucial to newborn survival. If there is an on-scene EMS physician, it is possible that this person would perform an on-scene perimortem caesarean section because it may be within his or her scope of practice.[47]

NOTE

A cesarean delivery, or C-section, is the delivery of a newborn through a surgical incision in the abdominal wall and uterus. A cesarean delivery is performed for a variety of fetal and maternal indications that can complicate childbirth. Cesarean delivery occurs in about 32% of deliveries in the United States.

Modified from: Centers for Disease Control and Prevention, National Center for Health Statistics. Births—method of delivery. Centers for Disease Control and Prevention website. https://www.cdc.gov/nchs/fastats/delivery.htm. Updated March 31, 2017. Accessed April 23, 2018.

NOTE

Magnesium sulfate toxicity in pregnant patients may result in prolonged PR, QRS, and QT intervals, nodal block, bradycardia, hypotension, and cardiac arrest. Should toxicity occur, the magnesium sulfate drip should be discontinued, and calcium chloride should be administered.

Modified from: EMS physician-performed clinical interventions in the field position statement. National Association of EMS Physicians website. http://www.naemsp.org/Documents/Position%20Papers/EMS%20Physician-Performed%20Clinical%20Interventions%20in%20the%20Field.pdf#search=position%20statement. Published October 10, 2017. Accessed April 23, 2018.

Summary

- Fertilization of an ovum by a sperm forms a zygote that divides as it passes through the fallopian tube to become a morula. The trophoblast cells of the morula implant within 7 days after fertilization and transform into the life support systems of the embryo. The blastocyst cells develop into the embryo.
- The placenta is a disklike organ. It is composed of interlocking fetal and maternal tissues. It is the organ of exchange between the pregnant woman and the fetus. Blood flows from the fetus to the placenta through two umbilical arteries. These arteries carry deoxygenated blood. Oxygenated blood returns to the fetus through the umbilical vein. The amniotic sac is a fluid-filled bag. It completely surrounds and protects the embryo.
- The developing ovum is known as an embryo during the first 8 weeks of pregnancy. After that time and until birth, it is called a fetus. Gestation (fetal development) usually averages 40 weeks from the time of fertilization to the delivery of the newborn.
- The arteriovenous shunts present in the fetus close at birth.
- Gravida is the total number of current and past pregnancies. Para refers to past pregnancies that resulted in a live birth.
- The pregnant woman undergoes many physiologic changes that affect the genital tract, breasts, gastrointestinal system, cardiovascular system, respiratory system, and metabolism.
- The patient history should include obstetric history; presence of pain; presence, quantity, and character of vaginal bleeding; presence of abnormal vaginal discharge; presence of "bloody show"; current general health and prenatal care; allergies and medications taken; and maternal urge to bear down.
- The goal in examining an obstetric patient is to rapidly identify acute life-threatening conditions. A part of this involves recognizing imminent delivery. Then the paramedic must take the proper management steps. In addition to the routine physical examination, the paramedic should assess the abdomen, uterine size, and fetal heart sounds.
- If birth is not imminent, the paramedic should limit prehospital care for the healthy patient to basic treatment modalities and transport for physician evaluation.
- Hyperemesis gravidarum presents with severe nausea, vomiting, weight loss, and electrolyte disturbance. Fluid therapy is indicated if there are signs of dehydration.
- Rh sensitization occurs if the pregnant woman has Rh-negative blood and the baby has Rh-positive blood. It can cause anemia, jaundice, edema, enlarged liver or spleen, and hydrops fetalis.
- Gestational hypertension is the onset of blood pressure greater than 140/90 mm Hg during pregnancy. It can indicate preeclampsia.
- Preeclampsia occurs after 20 weeks' gestation. The criteria for diagnosis include hypertension plus one other abnormality, such as protein in the urine, thrombocytopenia, renal insufficiency, impaired liver function, pulmonary edema, or cerebral or visual symptoms. Eclampsia is characterized by new-onset seizures in a woman with preeclampsia.
- Gestational diabetes mellitus is diabetes caused by pregnancy.
- Infection during pregnancy can place the woman and fetus at risk. TORCH is an acronym for infections the woman can pass to the fetus that cause fetal death or complications. It stands for Toxoplasmosis, Other infections, Rubella, Cytomegalovirus, and Herpes simplex virus.
- The development of pulmonary embolism during pregnancy, labor, or the postpartum period is a significant cause of maternal death.
- Premature rupture of membranes is a rupture of the amniotic sac before the onset of labor, regardless of gestational age.
- Vaginal bleeding during pregnancy can result from spontaneous abortion (miscarriage), ectopic pregnancy, abruptio placentae, placenta previa, uterine rupture, or postpartum hemorrhage. Abortion is the termination of pregnancy from any cause before 20 weeks' gestation. Ectopic pregnancy occurs when a fertilized ovum implants anywhere other than the uterus. Abruptio placentae is partial or complete detachment of the placenta at more than 20 weeks' gestation. Placenta previa is placental implantation in the lower uterine segment partially or completely covering the cervical opening. Uterine rupture is a spontaneous or traumatic rupture of the uterine wall.
- The first stage of labor begins with the onset of regular contractions. It ends with complete dilation of the cervix. The second stage of labor is measured from full dilation of the cervix to delivery of the fetus. The third stage of labor begins with delivery of the fetus and ends when the placenta is expelled and the uterus has contracted.
- One of the primary responsibilities of the EMS crew is to prevent an uncontrolled delivery. The other is to protect the newborn from cold and stress.
- Criteria for computing the Apgar score include appearance (color), pulse (heart rate), grimace (reflex irritability), activity (muscle tone), and respiratory effort.
- Paramedics should be alert to factors that point to a possible abnormal delivery.
- Cephalopelvic disproportion produces a difficult labor because of the presence of a small pelvis, an oversized uterus, or fetal abnormalities. Most babies are born headfirst (cephalic or vertex presentation). However, sometimes a presentation is abnormal. In breech presentation, the largest part of the fetus (the head) is delivered last. Shoulder dystocia occurs when the fetal shoulders impact against the maternal symphysis pubis, blocking shoulder delivery. Shoulder presentation (transverse presentation) results when the long axis of the fetus lies perpendicular to that of the mother. The fetal arm or hand may be the presenting part. Cord presentation occurs when the cord slips down into the vagina or presents externally.
- A premature newborn is born before 37 weeks' gestation.
- A multiple gestation is a pregnancy with more than one fetus. It is accompanied by an increased complication rate.

- Uterine inversion is a rare complication of childbirth. It is a serious complication. With this condition, the uterus turns "inside out."
- More than 500 mL of blood loss after the delivery of the newborn is called a postpartum hemorrhage. It often results from ineffective or incomplete contraction of the uterus.
- An amniotic fluid embolism may occur when amniotic fluid enters the maternal circulation during labor or delivery or immediately after delivery.
- Causes of fetal death from maternal trauma include death of the mother, separation of the placenta, maternal shock, uterine rupture, and fetal head injury.
- The paramedic should treat a critically ill pregnant patient as follows: Administer high-concentration oxygen. Place the patient in a left lateral position. Administer intravenous fluid if there are signs of shock. Aggressively resuscitate the mother in an attempt to save the baby.
- Cardiac arrest can occur from a number of causes. Rapid transport is indicated.

References

1. Soma-Pillay P, Nelson-Piercy C, Tolppanen H, Mebazaa A. Physiological changes in pregnancy. *Cardiovasc J Afr*. 2016;27(2):89-94.
2. Datta S, Kodali BS, Segal S. *Obstetric Anesthesia Handbook*. 5th ed. New York, NY: Springer; 2010.
3. Hirsch DJ. Physiology of pregnancy: EMS implications. In: Cone D, Brice JH, Delbridge TR, Myers JB, eds. *Emergency Medical Services: Clinical Practice and Systems Oversight*. 2nd ed. West Sussex, England: John Wiley & Sons; 2015:307-311.
4. Hyperemesis gravidarum. National Organization of Rare Disorders website. https://rarediseases.org/rare-diseases/hyperemesis-gravidarum/. Accessed April 23, 2018.
5. Rosen P, Barkin R. *Emergency Medicine: Concepts and Clinical Practice*. 7th ed. St. Louis, MO: Mosby; 2010.
6. *Hypertension in Pregnancy*. Washington, DC: American College of Obstetricians and Gynecologists; 2013. https://www.acog.org/~/media/Task%20Force%20and%20Work%20Group%20Reports/public/HypertensioninPregnancy.pdf. Accessed April 23, 2018.
7. National Association of EMS Officials. *National Model EMS Clinical Guidelines*. Version 2.0. National Association of EMS Officials website. https://www.nasemso.org/documents/National-Model-EMS-Clinical-Guidelines-Version2-Sept2017.pdf. Published September 2017. Accessed April 23, 2018.
8. McKinney ES, James SR, Murray SS, Ashwill JW. *Maternal-Child Nursing*. 3rd ed. Philadelphia, PA: Saunders; 2008.
9. Centers for Disease Control and Prevention. Gestational diabetes. Centers for Disease Control and Prevention website. https://www.cdc.gov/diabetes/basics/gestational.html. Updated July 15, 2017. Accessed April 23, 2018.
10. Ware J, Yerkes A; Women's Health Consultants with the National Association of Chronic Disease Directors. *Gestational Diabetes Collaborative Better Data Better Care*. Department of Health and Human Resources website. https://dhhr.wv.gov/hpcd/FocusAreas/wvdiabetes/Documents/Gest%20Diab%20Mgt_Collaborative_Final_S.pdf. Published 2016. Accessed April 23, 2018.
11. Stegmann BJ, Carey JC. TORCH infections. Toxoplasmosis, Other (syphilis, varicella-zoster, parvovirus B19), Rubella, Cytomegalovirus (CMV), and Herpes infections. *Curr Womens Health Rep*. 2002;2(4):253-258.
12. Murray SS, McKinney ES. *Foundations of Maternal-Newborn and Women's Health Nursing*. 6th ed. Philadelphia, PA: Saunders; 2018.
13. Gaufberg SV. Early pregnancy loss in emergency medicine. Medscape website. https://emedicine.medscape.com/article/795085-overview. Updated January 3, 2017. Accessed April 23, 2018.
14. Miscarriage. American Pregnancy Association website. Americanpregnancy.org/pregnancy-complications/miscarriage/. Accessed April 25, 2018.
15. Gilmore FS. Emergencies of pregnancy. In: Cone D, Brice JH, Delbridge TR, Myers JB, eds. *Emergency Medical Services: Clinical Practice and Systems Oversight*. 2nd ed. West Sussex, England: John Wiley & Sons; 2015:312-317.
16. Argyropoulos Bachman E, Barnhard K. Medical management of ectopic pregnancy: a comparison of regimens. *Clin Obstet Gynecol*. 2012:55(2):440-447.
17. Callahan T, Caughey A. *Blueprints Obstetrics and Gynecology*. 6th ed. New York, NY: Lippincott Williams & Wilkins; 2013.
18. Räisänen S, Kancherla V, Kramer MR, Gissler M, Heinonen S. Placenta previa and the risk of delivering a small-for-gestational-age newborn. *Obstet Gynecol*. 2014;124(2 Pt 1):285-291.
19. Macones GA, Sehdev HM, Parry S, Morgan MA, Berlin JA. The association between maternal cocaine use and placenta previa. *Am J Obstet Gynecol*. 1997;177(5):1097-1100.
20. Nahum GG. Uterine rupture in pregnancy. Medscape website. https://reference.medscape.com/article/275854-overview?pa=lCFhtK5CmNbtlB7pp083SQ3anR19l6pHtpTgHonaHV4HkTWC4AvAwEUf36jX7etDX8MwC0EECwzp432Skuf9qw%3D%3D#a6. Updated March 25, 2016. Accessed April 23, 2018.
21. De Caen AR, Berg MD, Chameides L, et al. Part 12: pediatric advanced life support. 2015 American Heart Association guidelines update for cardiopulmonary resuscitation and emergency cardiovascular care. *Circulation*. 2015;132:S526-S542.
22. Weiner GM, Zaichkin J, eds. *Textbook of Neonatal Resuscitation (NRP)*. 7th ed. Elk Grove Village, IL: American Academy of Pediatrics; 2016.
23. Jameson AM, Campbell M. Childbirth emergencies. In: Cone D, Brice JH, Delbridge TR, Myers JB, eds. *Emergency Medical Services: Clinical Practice and Systems Oversight*. 2nd ed. West Sussex, England: John Wiley & Sons; 2015:322-324.
24. Silver DW, Sabatino F. Precipitous and difficult deliveries. *Emerg Med Clin*. 2012;30(4):961-975.
25. Fischer R. Breech presentation. Medscape website. https://emedicine.medscape.com/article/262159-overview. Updated June 15, 2016. Accessed April 23, 2018.
26. Robertson JF, Braude DA, Stonehocker J, Moreno J. Prehospital breech delivery with fetal head entrapment: a case report and review. *Prehosp Emerg Care*. 2015;19(3):451-456.
27. Umbilical cord prolapse. American Pregnancy Association website. http://americanpregnancy.org/pregnancy-complications/umbilical-cord-prolapse/. Updated August 2015. Accessed April 23, 2018.
28. Part 13: neonatal resuscitation. Web-based integrated 2010 and 2015 American Heart Association guidelines for cardiopulmonary

resuscitation and emergency cardiovascular care. American Heart Association website. https://eccguidelines.heart.org/index.php/circulation/cpr-ecc-guidelines-2/part-13-neonatal-resuscitation/. Accessed April 23, 2018.
29. National Center for Chronic Disease Prevention and Health Promotion. CDC features: premature birth. Centers for Disease Control and Prevention website. https://www.cdc.gov/features/prematurebirth/index.html. Updated November 6, 2017. Accessed April 23, 2018.
30. McCubbin K, Moore S, MacDonald R, Vaillancourt C. Medical transfer of patients in preterm labor: treatments and tocolytics. *Prehosp Emerg Care.* 2015;19(1):103-109.
31. Centers for Disease Control and Prevention, National Center for Health Statistics. Multiple births. Centers for Disease Control and Prevention website. https://www.cdc.gov/nchs/fastats/multiple.htm. Updated March 31, 2017. Accessed April 23, 2018.
32. Repke JT. Puerperal uterine inversion. UpToDate website. https://www.uptodate.com/contents/puerperal-uterine-inversion#H3. Updated September 25, 2017. Accessed April 23, 2018.
33. Coad SL, Dahlgren LS, Hutcheon JA. Risks and consequences of puerperal uterine inversion in the United States, 2004 through 2013. *Am J Obstet Gynecol.* 2017;217(3):377.e1-377.e6.
34. Dorr P, Khouw F, Chervenak A, et al. (eds). Pathology of labor and labor and delivery. In: *Obstetric Interventions.* Cambridge, England: Cambridge University Press; 2017:79-224.
35. Liao CY, Luo FJ. Amniotic fluid embolism with isolated coagulopathy: a report of two cases. *J Clin Diagn Res.* 2016;10(10):QD03-QD05.
36. Murray SS, McKinney ES. *Foundations of Maternal-Newborn and Women's Health Nursing.* 6th ed. Philadelphia, PA: Saunders; 2018.
37. Postpartum depression: what is postpartum depression and anxiety? American Psychological Association website. http://www.apa.org/pi/women/resources/reports/postpartum-depression.aspx. Accessed April 23, 2018.
38. AAP Committee on Fetus and Newborn and ACOG Committee on Obstetric Practice. *Guidelines for Perinatal Care.* 8th ed. Washington, DC: American Academy of Pediatrics; 2017.
39. Walls R, Hockberger R, Gausche-Hill M. *Rosen's Emergency Medicine: Concepts and Clinical Practice.* 9th ed. Philadelphia, PA: Elsevier; 2017.
40. Jain V, Chari R, Maslovitz S, et al. Guidelines for the management of a pregnant trauma patient. *J Obstet Gynaecol Canada.* 2015;37(6):553-571.
41. Hamel MS, Anderson BL, Rouse DJ. Oxygen for intrauterine resuscitation: of unproved benefit and potentially harmful. *Am J Obstet Gynecol.* 2014;211(2):124-127.
42. Chang AK. Pregnancy trauma treatment and management. Medscape website. https://emedicine.medscape.com/article/796979-treatment. Updated May 12, 2015. Accessed April 23, 2018.
43. Distelhorst JT, Krishnamoorthy V, Schiff MA. Association between hospital trauma designation and maternal and neonatal outcomes after injury among pregnant women in Washington state. *J Am Coll Surg.* 2016;222(3):296-302.
44. Centers for Disease Control and Prevention. Guidelines for field triage of injured patients: recommendations of the National Expert Panel of Field Triage. *Morb Mortal Wkly Rep.* 2009; 58(RR-1). https://www.cdc.gov/mmwr/pdf/rr/rr5801.pdf. Accessed April 23, 2018.
45. Jeejeebhoy FM, Zelop CM, Lipman S, et al. Cardiac arrest in pregnancy. *Circulation.* 2015;132:1747-1773.
46. American Heart Association. 2010 American Heart Association guidelines for cardiopulmonary resuscitation and emergency cardiovascular care. *Circulation.* 2010;122(18 suppl):S639-S946.
47. EMS physician-performed clinical interventions in the field position statement. National Association of EMS Physicians website. http://www.naemsp.org/Documents/Position%20Papers/EMS%20Physician-Performed%20Clinical%20Interventions%20in%20the%20Field.pdf#search=position%20statement. Published October 10, 2017. Accessed April 23, 2018.

Suggested Readings

Cone D, Brice JH, Delbridge TR, Myers JB, eds. *Emergency Medical Services: Clinical Practice and Systems Oversight.* 2nd ed. West Sussex, England: John Wiley & Sons; 2015.

Cooney DR. *Cooney's EMS Medicine.* New York, NY: McGraw-Hill Education; 2016.

Girerd PH. Breech delivery treatment and management. Medscape website. https://reference.medscape.com/article/797690-treatment?pa=r6DZtK2YJEkggzL7bpPq59Zb47ahrqFuaOG4TKMAydTVwLATgtXNleSoYEbU%2FIFPs7CF3wx2Tu1U792SxywYLg%3D%3D. Updated December 28, 2015. Accessed April 23, 2018.

Hodgson R. Legal and professional boundaries: a case study. *J Paramed Pract.* 2016;8(2). HTTPS://DOI.ORG/10.12968/JPAR.2016.8.2.90.

Lee M, Todd HM, Bowe A. The effects of magnesium sulfate infusion on blood pressure and vascular responsiveness during pregnancy. *Am J Obstet Gynecol.* 1984;149(7):705-708.

McLelland G, McKenna L, Morgans A, Smith K. Antenatal emergency care provided by paramedics: a one-year clinical profile. *Prehosp Emerg Care.* 2016;20(4):531-538.

Mowry M. Case study: obstetrical trauma with maternal death and fetal survival. *Crit Care Nurs Q.* 2017;40(1):36-40.

National Institute for Health and Clinical Excellence. Ectopic pregnancy and miscarriage: diagnosis and initial management in early pregnancy of ectopic pregnancy and miscarriage. National Institute for Health and Care Excellence website. https://www.nice.org.uk/guidance/cg154/resources/ectopic-pregnancy-and-miscarriage-diagnosis-and-initial-management-pdf-35109631301317. Published December 12, 2012. Accessed April 23, 2018.

New Guidelines in Preeclampsia Diagnosis and Care Include Revised Definition of Preeclampsia. Preeclampsia Foundation website. https://www.preeclampsia.org/es/noticias/144-research-news/299-new-guidelines-in-preeclampsia-diagnosis-and-care-include-revised-definition-of-preeclampsia. Accessed April 25, 2018.

Robertson JF, Braude DA, Stonehocker J, Mareno J. Prehospital breech delivery with fetal head entrapment—a case report and review. Published February 9, 2015. Accessed June 28, 2018.

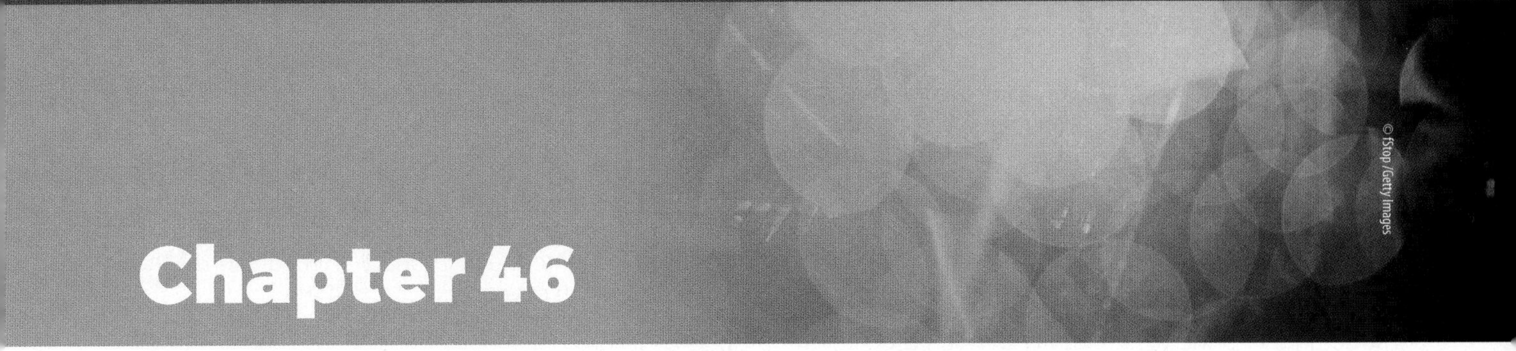

Chapter 46

Neonatal Care

NATIONAL EMS EDUCATION STANDARD COMPETENCIES

Special Patient Populations

Integrates assessment findings with principles of pathophysiology and knowledge of psychosocial needs to formulate a field impression and implement a comprehensive treatment/disposition plan for patients with special needs.

Neonatal Care

Anatomy and physiology of neonatal circulation (see Chapter 45, *Obstetrics*)
Assessment of the newborn (pp 1618–1622)
Presentation and management (pp 1618–1628)

- Newborn (pp 1618–1622)
- Neonatal resuscitation (pp 1622–1628)

OBJECTIVES

Upon completion of this chapter, the paramedic student will be able to:

1. Identify risk factors associated with the need for neonatal resuscitation. (pp 1615–1617)
2. Describe physiologic adaptations at birth. (pp 1617–1618)
3. Outline the prehospital assessment and management of the newborn. (pp 1618–1622)
4. Describe resuscitation of the distressed newborn. (pp 1622–1627)
5. Identify postresuscitative management and transport. (pp 1627–1628)
6. Describe appropriate interventions to manage the emotional needs of the newborn's family. (p 1629)
7. Describe signs and symptoms and prehospital management of specific newborn resuscitation situations. (pp 1629–1634)
8. Describe the signs and symptoms of sepsis in the newborn. (p 1633)
9. Identify injuries associated with birth. (pp 1633–1634)
10. Describe the pathophysiology and implications of selected genetic anomalies present in some newborns. (pp 1634–1644)

KEY TERMS

antepartum The period before labor and delivery.

apnea An absence of spontaneous respirations.

atrial septal defect (ASD) A congenital anomaly in which an opening exists between the heart's two upper chambers.

central cyanosis Cyanosis of the tongue and mucous membranes; usually reflects decreased saturation of the hemoglobin in arterial blood.

choanal atresia A bony or membranous occlusion that blocks the passageway between the nose and pharynx. It can result in serious ventilation problems in the newborn.

cleft lip An incomplete closure of the newborn's lip that occurs when one or more fissures fail to fuse in the embryo.

cleft palate An incomplete closure in the soft/hard palate of the roof of the mouth that runs along its midline; occurs when one or more fissures fail to fuse in the embryo.

coarctation of the aorta (CoA) A congenital defect in which there is narrowing or constriction of the aorta.

cold stress A condition that occurs when the body is unable to warm itself.

congenital anomalies Defects that occur during fetal development.

diaphragmatic hernia A herniation of abdominal structures into the pleural cavity through a defect in the diaphragm. Often caused by the improper fusion of pleuroperitoneal membranes that separate the chest from the abdomen during fetal development.

esophageal atresia The incomplete formation or abnormal development of the esophagus.

gastroschisis An abdominal wall defect in which the anterior abdomen does not close properly, allowing the intestines to protrude outside the fetus.

hypoplastic left heart syndrome A condition in which the heart's left side, including the aorta, aortic valve, left ventricle, and mitral valve, is underdeveloped.

intestinal malrotation A congenital defect caused by abnormal rotation of the intestine around the superior mesenteric artery during embryonic development.

intrapartum The period during labor and delivery.

meconium aspiration The inhalation of meconium by the fetus or newborn. The inhaled meconium can block air passages and result in failure of the lungs to expand or cause other pulmonary dysfunction

meconium staining A green coloration of amniotic fluid as a result of fetal in utero passage of meconium.

newborn A person in the first 28 days of life; also known as a neonate.

newborn jaundice A yellow discoloration of the eye, skin, and mucous membranes in a newborn as a result of high bilirubin levels.

omphalocele A type of hernia in which the newborn's intestines or other abdominal organs protrude through the umbilicus; results during fetal development when the muscles in the abdominal wall do not close properly.

patent ductus arteriosus (PDA) A persistent communication between the descending thoracic aorta and the pulmonary artery that results from failure of normal physiologic closure of the fetal ductus; common congenital heart defect.

peripheral cyanosis Cyanosis that is confined to the extremities (common in the first few minutes of life); also known as acrocyanosis.

Pierre Robin sequence A complex of congenital anomalies including a small mandible, a tongue that is placed farther back than normal and causes airway obstruction, and a cleft palate.

premature newborn A newborn who is born before 37 weeks' gestation.

pulmonary atresia A life-threatening congenital anomaly in which the pulmonary valve is replaced with a membrane, preventing blood from flowing from the right ventricle into the pulmonary artery and on to the lungs to pick up oxygen.

pulmonary hypoplasia A congenital malformation characterized by incomplete development of lung tissue.

pyloric stenosis A congenital defect in which there is narrowing of the pylorus (the opening from the stomach into the small intestine) caused by thickening of the muscles in the pyloric wall. It is the most common cause of intestinal obstruction in infancy.

single-ventricle defects Complex defects that occur in the embryonic stage and result when one of the ventricles is underdeveloped.

spina bifida A neural tube defect (congenital) with incomplete closing of the spine, spinal cord, and membranes around the spine.

tetralogy of Fallot (ToF) A congenital cardiac anomaly that consists of four defects: pulmonic stenosis, ventricular septal defect, malposition of the aorta so that it rises from the septal defect or the right ventricle, and right ventricular hypertrophy.

total anomalous pulmonary venous return (TAPVR) A congenital heart defect in which the four pulmonary veins that transport oxygen-rich blood back to the heart from the lungs are not properly attached to the left atrium and instead may connect to the right atrium.

tracheoesophageal fistula An abnormal connection between the esophagus and the trachea that results from a failed fusion of the tracheoesophageal ridges during fetal development.

transposition of the great arteries (TGA) A congenital defect in which the positions of the great arteries are reversed; the aorta arises from the right ventricle and the pulmonary artery from the left ventricle; may be a ductal-dependent lesion.

tricuspid atresia A congenital defect in which there is absence or abnormal development of a tricuspid valve.

truncus arteriosus A rare type of congenital heart disease characterized by a large ventricular septal defect over which a large, single great vessel (truncus) arises.

ventricular septal defect (VSD) A congenital anomaly in which an opening exists between the heart's two lower chambers.

About 10% of newborns require some assistance to begin breathing at birth, and about 1% require extensive resuscitation.[1] This chapter addresses risk factors that may lead to the need for resuscitation in the **newborn**. *It also describes initial care that may be required for the newborn.*

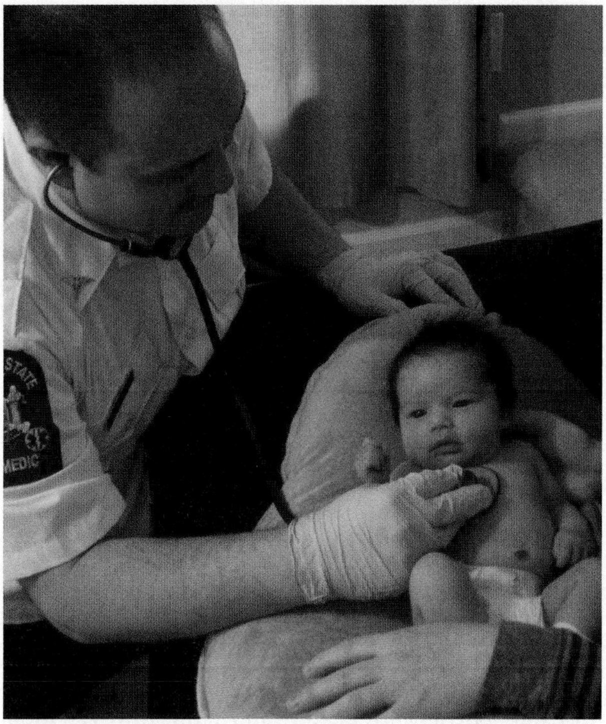

Courtesy of Howard E. Huth, III, BA, EMT-P.

> DID YOU KNOW?
>
> The average newborn birth weight in the United States had increased for decades but has been decreasing each year since 1997. Reasons for this trend are unknown but might be explained by an accumulation of risk factors, such as hypertension and obesity in pregnancy. An older age among women giving birth may also be a factor. Known causes of lower newborn birth weight include absent or inadequate prenatal care, poor nutrition, stress, smoking, anemia, diabetes mellitus, short intervals between pregnancies, and poor weight gain required for child and maternal health. Recent studies suggest that health and nutritional background, coupled with the care provided during pregnancy, are the factors that most influence a baby's birth size. The average term newborn weighs about 7.5 pounds (3.6 kg). The incidence of complications increases as birth weight decreases.
>
> *Modified from*: Catov JM, Lee M, Roberts JM, Xu J, Simhan HN. Race disparities and decreasing birth weight: are all babies getting smaller? *Am J Epidemiol*. 2016;183(1):15-23; and Mathur R, Grundy E, Smeeth L. National Centre for Research Methods Working Paper. January 2013. Availability and use of UK based ethnicity data for health research. National Centre for Research Methods website. http://eprints.ncrm.ac.uk/3040/1/Mathur-_Availability_and_use_of_UK_based_ethnicity_data_for_health_res_1.pdf. Published March 2013. Accessed May 10, 2018.

Risk Factors Associated With the Need for Resuscitation

Most term newborns require no resuscitation beyond maintenance of temperature and mild stimulation.[1] Yet, about 4% to 10% of newborns need positive pressure ventilation to begin breathing at birth.[1] Few newborns (1 to 3 in 1,000) require chest compressions or resuscitation medications.[1] Resuscitation is much more likely in newborns with low birth weight and those born to mothers with antepartum or intrapartum risk factors.[1] Resuscitation is also more likely in babies who are born prematurely.

The various **antepartum** (before labor and delivery) and **intrapartum** (during labor and delivery) risk factors that may affect the need for resuscitation include those listed in BOX 46-1.[1] When antepartum or intrapartum risk factors are present and delivery is imminent, the paramedic should prepare equipment and drugs that may be needed for neonatal resuscitation. Medical direction should be advised of the situation so the appropriate destination hospital can be determined. In addition, the pregnant woman should be asked the following questions to assess the need for resuscitation:

1. When is the baby due? (assess for prematurity)
2. If the membranes have ruptured, was the amniotic fluid clear?
3. How many babies are expected?
4. Are there other possible risk factors?

Prematurity

Preterm birth is childbirth that occurs between 20 and 37 weeks of pregnancy. It is a concern because babies who are born too early may not be fully developed and

BOX 46-1 Antepartum and Intrapartum Risk Factors

Antepartum

- Gestational age <36 or >41 weeks
- Multiple gestation
- Inadequate prenatal care
- Maternal preeclampsia, eclampsia, hypertension, diabetes mellitus
- Deficiency of amniotic fluid (oligohydramnios) or excess amniotic fluid (polyhydramnios)
- Fetus >8.8 pounds (4 kg)
- Intrauterine growth restriction
- Fetal anemia
- Fetal hydrops (abnormal fluid in fetal body compartments)
- Significant fetal malformations

Intrapartum

- Emergency cesarean delivery
- Forceps or vacuum used at delivery
- Meconium-stained amniotic fluid
- Use of narcotics within 4 hours of delivery
- Abnormal presentation (eg, breech)
- Shoulder dystocia
- Abnormal fetal heart rate pattern
- Maternal anesthesia or magnesium sulfate
- Chorioamnionitis (inflammation of fetal membranes from infection)
- Prolonged labor or precipitous delivery
- Prolapsed cord
- Hemorrhage (eg, abruptio placentae, uterine atony, genital tract lacerations)

may have serious and lifelong health problems. Factors that increase the risk for a preterm birth include:[2,3]

- Urinary tract infections
- Sexually transmitted diseases
- Certain vaginal infections, such as bacterial vaginosis and trichomoniasis
- Hypertension
- Vaginal bleeding
- Developmental abnormalities in the fetus
- Pregnancy resulting from in vitro fertilization
- Placenta previa
- Diabetes mellitus and gestational diabetes
- Blood clotting problems
- Maternal age (younger than 18 years; older than 35 years)
- Previous preterm birth
- A short cervix
- A short interval between pregnancies
- Lifestyle factors such as low pregnancy weight or obesity, smoking during pregnancy, and substance abuse during pregnancy

A **premature newborn** is commonly referred to as a preemie. The weight of these newborns often is 1.5 to 5 pounds (0.5 to 2.2 kg). Healthy premature newborns who weigh more than 3.7 pounds (1.7 kg) have a survivability and outcome about equal to those of full-term newborns. The mortality rate decreases weekly with gestation beyond the onset of fetal viability (currently around 23 to 24 weeks' gestation).[4] Premature newborns have an increased risk for respiratory depression, hypothermia, and brain injury from hypoxemia. They are also especially vulnerable to changes in blood pressure, intraventricular hemorrhage, and fluctuations in serum chemistry, such as changes in blood glucose and electrolyte levels. The degree of immaturity determines how the newborn appears physically (based on estimated due date and size for gestational age). However, most premature newborns have short extremities, less subcutaneous fat than full-term newborns, and thin, nonkeratinized skin that appears translucent. Their chest muscles are weak, and they have pliable ribs.[5] The lack of surfactant in their lungs makes them more difficult to ventilate and increases their risk of complications from positive pressure ventilation. Premature newborns have some telltale physical findings, including lanugo (**FIGURE 46-1**) and characteristic changes in the ears (**FIGURE 46-2**) and in muscle tone (**FIGURE 46-3**).[1]

The prehospital care for premature newborns is the same as for any other newborn. It may include airway and circulatory support. Special care must be taken to maintain the newborn's body temperature and to prevent hypothermia. Examples include wrapping the baby in plastic wrap with a cap, administering warm, humidified oxygen, and applying radiant heat. Temperature greater than 100.4°F (38°C) should be avoided.[6] Transport to a facility with special services for newborns with low birth weight may be indicated.

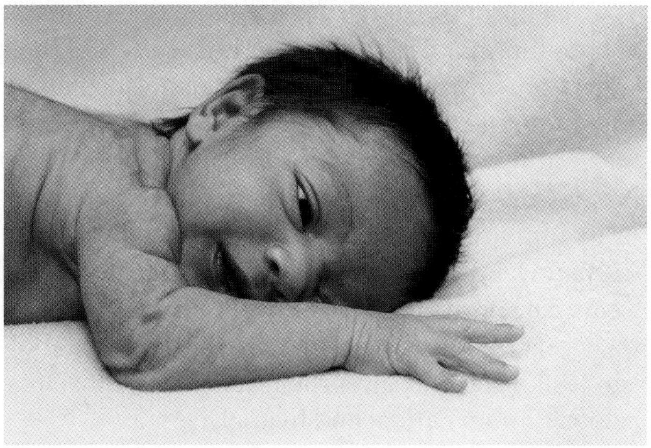

FIGURE 46-1 Newborns at gestational age 20 to 28 weeks are covered with fine hair all over the body called lanugo.

© Suzanne Tucker/Shutterstock

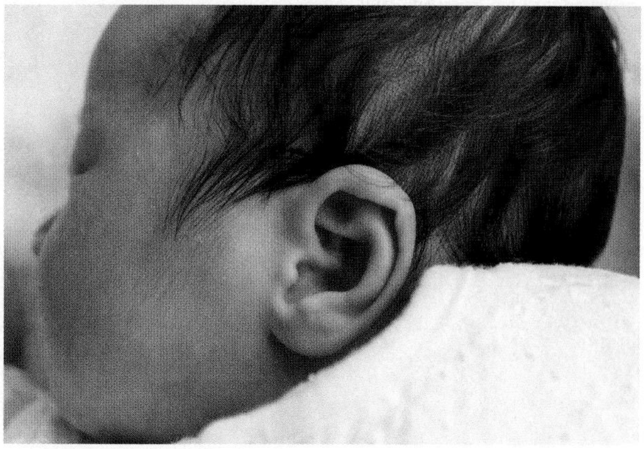

A

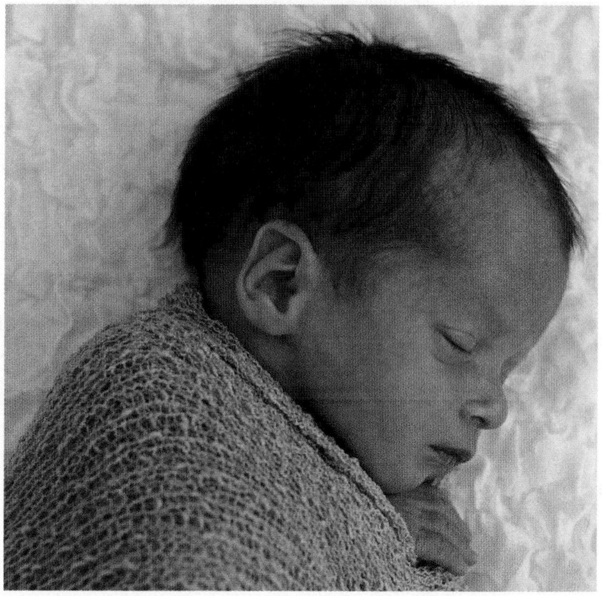

B

FIGURE 46-2 Ear maturation. **A.** Full-term newborn. **B.** Preterm newborn.

A: © Nanako Yamanaka/Shutterstock; **B:** © Sarahbean/Shutterstock

Physiologic Adaptations at Birth

As described in Chapter 45, *Obstetrics*, newborns make three major physiologic adaptations at birth that are necessary for survival: (1) emptying fluids from their lungs and beginning ventilation, (2) changing their circulatory pattern, and (3) maintaining body temperature.[7] When the umbilical cord is clamped, the baby transitions from maternal oxygenation to its own spontaneous breathing.

During labor, adrenalin activates the sodium channels and produces an increase in catecholamine levels that trigger the clearance of lung fluid.[8] The secretory chloride channels turn off and the sodium resorption begins. Water is resorbed with sodium and causes approximately one-third of fetal lung fluid to be cleared prior to delivery. Further clearance occurs during vaginal delivery when the newborn's chest is compressed, which forces fluid from the lungs into the mouth and nose. The newborn takes the first breath in response to chemical changes (exposure to air) and changes in temperature. As air enters the alveoli, the pulmonary capillaries dilate in response to oxygen, allowing the pulmonary pressure to fall and the blood to flow into the lungs. Circulation transitions to a normal pathway and the foramen ovale begins to close. A normal newly born baby may not reach an oxygen saturation level, as measured by a pulse oximeter (Spo_2), of 90% for 10 minutes.[1] It may take several hours to completely absorb alveolar fluid and several days for the ductus arteriosus and foramen ovale to close.

NOTE

Oxyhemoglobin saturation may normally remain in the 70% to 80% range for several minutes following birth, thus resulting in the appearance of cyanosis during that time. Other studies have shown that clinical assessment of skin color is a very poor indicator of oxyhemoglobin saturation during the immediate neonatal period.

Modified from: Weiner GM, Zaichkin J, eds. *Textbook of Neonatal Resuscitation.* 7th ed. Elk Grove, IL: American Academy of Pediatrics and American Heart Association; 2016.

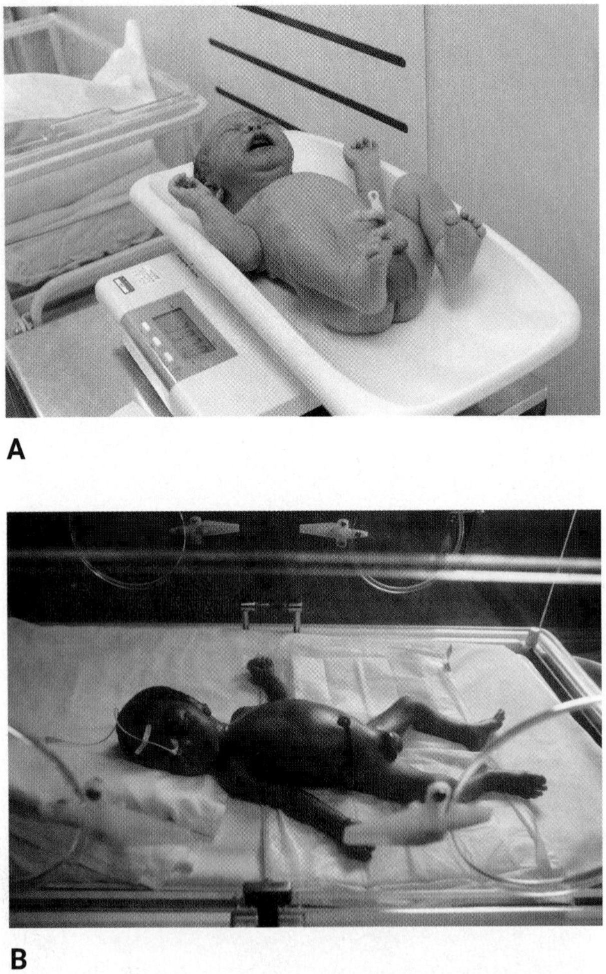

FIGURE 46-3 A. The full-term newborn shows flexion of the arms and legs. Note the acrocyanosis of the hands and feet. **B.** The preterm newborn holds extremities in extension, exposing more of the body surface area to the environment. This factor contributes to the development of cold stress and difficulty with thermoregulation.

Newborns are sensitive to hypoxia. Significant and irreversible brain injury can occur from prolonged hypoxemia. Causes of hypoxia include compression of the cord, difficult labor and delivery, maternal hemorrhage, maternal drug use, airway obstruction, hypothermia, newborn blood loss, and immature lungs in the premature newborn. Cardiovascular anomalies (described later) also may result in hypoxia.

Newborns are at risk for the rapid development of hypothermia. This risk factor is the result of their larger body surface area, decreased tissue insulation, and immature temperature regulatory mechanisms. Maximum heat loss in newborns is via evaporative losses, and they should be delivered in a warm, draft-free area when possible and dried off with warm towels or blankets with the head covered with a cap. Newborns try to conserve body heat through vasoconstriction and an increase in their metabolism. This response places them at risk for hypoxemia, acidosis, bradycardia, and hypoglycemia.

Assessment and Management of the Newborn: The Golden Minute

To prepare for delivery, the paramedic should have a standard obstetrics kit prepared, along with neonatal resuscitation equipment. Following delivery (see Chapter 45, *Obstetrics*), the initial steps of assessment and management of any newborn, especially those who require resuscitation, should follow the recommendations of the American Heart Association and the American Academy of Pediatrics. The initial goal of care is that the newborn should be breathing well or receiving ventilation within 60 seconds.[1,9] Note: 60 seconds (the "Golden Minute") are allotted for completing the initials steps, reevaluating, and beginning ventilation, if required (BOX 46-2).

Immediately following delivery, evaluation of the newborn should begin by answering these

BOX 46-2 The Golden Minute

- Emphasis is placed on the initial 60 seconds.
  - Complete the initial steps.
  - Evaluate the newborn.
- Begin ventilation (if required). Avoid unnecessary delay in initiating ventilation; this is *the most important* step for successful resuscitation of the newborn that has not responded to the initial steps.
- The decision to progress beyond the initial steps is based on a simultaneous assessment of two vital characteristics:
  - Respirations (apnea, gasping, or labored or unlabored breathing)
  - Heart rate (less than 100 beats/min)

questions: Is the newborn term? Does the newborn have good tone? Is the newborn breathing or crying? If the answer to all three questions is "yes," then the newly born baby may stay with the mother for routine care. Routine care means the newborn is dried, placed skin to skin with the mother, and covered with dry linen to maintain normal temperature. Observation of breathing, activity, and color must be ongoing.[1]

If the answer to any of the assessment questions is "no," then the newborn should receive one or more of the following four actions, in sequence:[1]

1. Perform initial steps in stabilization.
   - Warm and maintain normal temperature, position, clear secretions only if copious and obstructing the airway, dry, and stimulate.
2. Ventilate and oxygenate.
3. Initiate chest compressions.
4. Administer epinephrine and/or volume.

The decision to progress beyond the initial steps is based on a simultaneous assessment of two vital characteristics:

- Respirations (apnea, gasping, or labored or unlabored breathing)
- Heart rate (less than 100 beats/min)

Following these steps enables the paramedic to immediately recognize a newborn in need of resuscitation. It also leads to efficient and effective emergency care delivery (**FIGURE 46-4**).[1,10]

> **NOTE**
> Standard precautions are recommended during delivery of a newborn. Gloves and other appropriate protective barriers (including gowns and goggles) should be worn when handling the newborn or contaminated equipment.

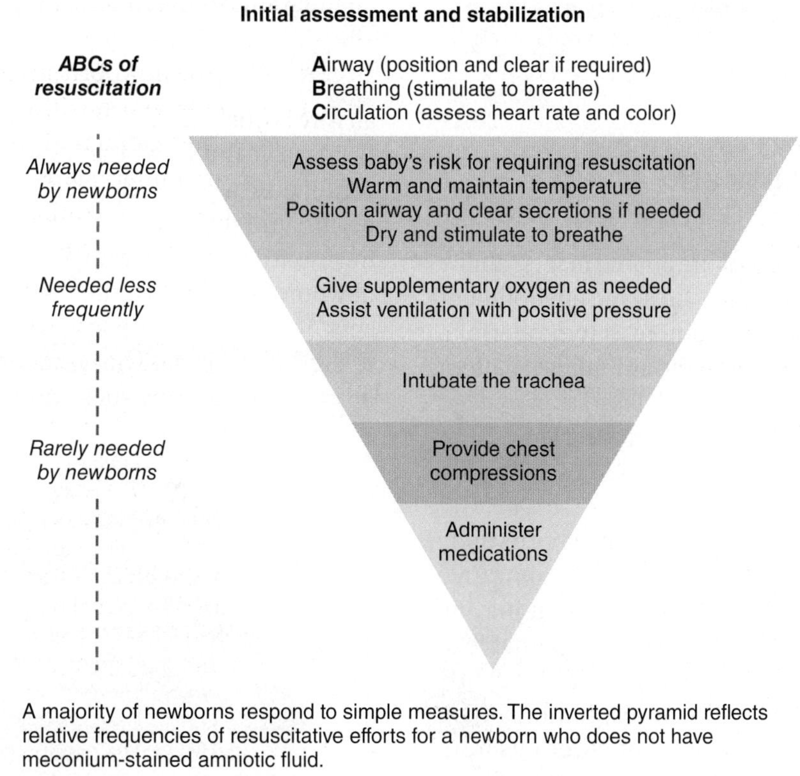

FIGURE 46-4 Initial assessment and stabilization.

SHOW ME THE EVIDENCE

Researchers in Oregon conducted a 4-year retrospective chart review of "lights and sirens" transports of newborns 30 days of age or older in a metropolitan area. Their aim was to quantify and characterize patient safety events during high-risk neonatal transports. A total of 26 neonatal transports were analyzed. Just over one-half (53.8%) were less than 24 hours old. Most calls were for cardiac arrest (30.8%) or respiratory distress (30.8%). The authors found safety events in almost 75% of the calls (19), and there were safety events that could potentially cause permanent injury, harm, or death (severe) in 38% of the cases. Safety events related to the following factors: medication administration, 90% (70% severe); resuscitation, 64.7% (47.1% severe); procedures, 64.7% (35.3% severe); fluid administration, 50% (25% severe); clinical assessment or decision making, 50% (30.8% severe); airway management, 47.6% (28.6% severe); equipment use, 25.5% (10% severe); and systems processes, 19.2% (7.7% severe). Safety events included failure to administer medication that was indicated, and there were several 10-fold epinephrine overdoses. The researchers concluded that although these calls occur infrequently in their EMS system, they are associated with a high risk of safety events.

Modified from: Duby R, Hansen M, Meckler G, Skarica B, Lambert W, Guise JM. Safety events in high risk prehospital neonatal calls. *Prehosp Emerg Care*. 2018;22(1):34-40.

Prevent Heat Loss and Avoid Hypothermia

Even healthy term newborns are limited in their ability to conserve heat when exposed to a cold environment and are at risk for the development of hypothermia. Therefore, the temperature in the ambulance patient compartment should be increased. The recommended ambient temperature for newly born, nonasphyxiated babies is 97.7°F to 99.5°F (36.5°C to 37.5°C) and for preterm newborns is 72°F to 77.9°F (22.2°C to 25.5°C).[1] Then, immediately after delivery, the newborn's body and head should be dried to prevent evaporative heat loss and metabolic derangements that may be instigated by **cold stress** (when the body is unable to warm itself). The act of drying also provides gentle stimulation, which may initiate respirations. Care should be taken to remove any wet coverings from the newborn and cover the newborn with dry wrappings and a cap. Most heat loss can be prevented by covering the newborn's head (which accounts for 20% of the newborn's body surface area). Other methods described earlier to prevent hypothermia should be observed.

CRITICAL THINKING

What other measures can you take to warm the newborn?

Clear the Airway

After the newborn has been dried and covered, the next step is to establish an open airway. This is achieved by placing the newborn supine, with the head in a sniffing position. Care should be taken to prevent hyperextension or flexion, which may compromise the airway. The heads of newborns are relatively large compared with their bodies. Placing a blanket or towel under the newborn's shoulders (thereby elevating the torso 0.75 to 1 inch [2 to 2.5 cm]) can help maintain the correct position (**FIGURE 46-5**).

CRITICAL THINKING

Do newborns breathe through their noses or mouths?

Once the newborn has been properly positioned, most newborns will breathe without difficulty. If the airway is obstructed by secretions or clear amniotic fluid, or if the newborn needs positive pressure ventilation, a bulb syringe can be used to suction the mouth and then the nose. It is preferable to suction the mouth first to prevent aspiration in the event the newborn gasps when the nose is cleared.[1] The process of suction should last no more than 5 seconds to prevent hypoxia. The newborn's heart rate should be monitored during suctioning, and time should be

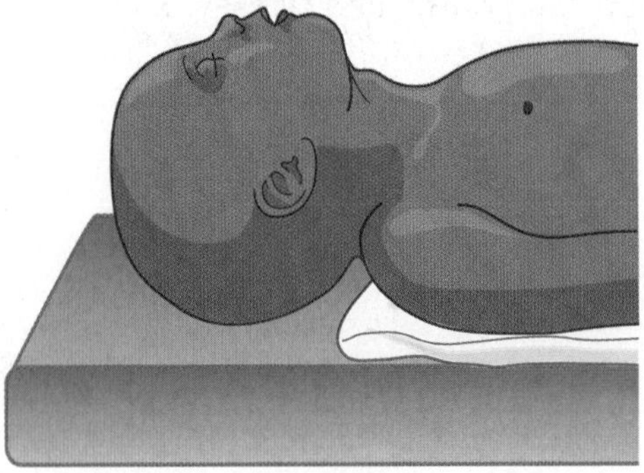

FIGURE 46-5 Positioning the newborn to open the airway.

provided during suction attempts for spontaneous ventilation.

NOTE

Suctioning the airway at birth can stimulate the posterior pharynx and can produce a vagal response that results in bradycardia, apnea, or both. Therefore, suctioning should be reserved for newborns with obvious obstruction that prevents spontaneous breathing and who require positive pressure ventilation. Supplemental oxygen delivery should be guided by electrocardiogram (ECG) and pulse oximetry results.

Modified from: Weiner GM, Zaichkin J, eds. *Textbook of Neonatal Resuscitation.* 7th ed. Elk Grove, IL: American Academy of Pediatrics and American Heart Association; 2016.

Meconium Staining

Meconium staining is the presence of fetal stool in the amniotic fluid. It occurs in utero or intrapartum and in about 12% of all deliveries.[11] Meconium staining becomes more common in postterm and small-for-gestational-age newborns. It is also common in those newborns in whom fetal distress develops during labor and delivery. Meconium staining is associated with increased perinatal mortality, hypoxemia, aspiration pneumonia, pneumothorax, and pulmonary hypertension. The appearance of meconium depends on the amount of meconium particles and amniotic fluid. Meconium staining may appear as only a slight yellow or light green staining that is thin and watery, or it may have a thick, pea-soup appearance that is dark green or black (**FIGURE 46-6**).

A newborn with meconium-stained amniotic fluid usually presents with poor muscle tone and inadequate breathing efforts. Positive pressure ventilation is the priority and should be initiated if the newborn is not breathing or has a heart rate of less than 100 beats/min after the initial steps are completed. Routine intubation for tracheal suctioning is no longer recommended. The emphasis should be to initiate ventilation within the first minute of life in nonbreathing or ineffectively breathing newborns. However, intubation equipment and the most experienced paramedic should be readily available if intubation is needed.[1]

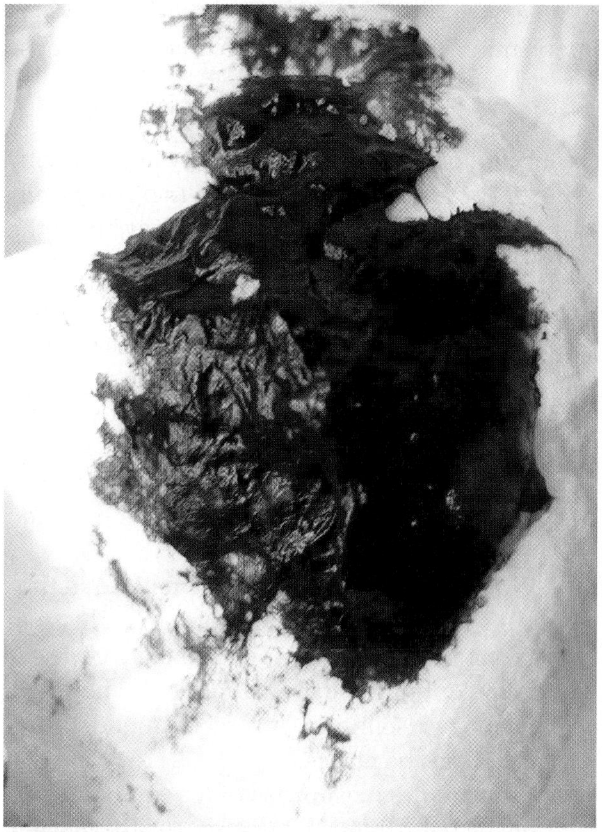

FIGURE 46-6 Meconium.

Courtesy of Jeremy Kemp.

DID YOU KNOW?

Meconium can be used to test for maternal drug use during pregnancy. Compared to urine, it has greater sensitivity and positive findings persist longer.

Modified from: Farst KJ, Valentine JL, Hall RW. Drug testing for newborn exposure to illicit substances in pregnancy: pitfalls and pearls. *Int J Pediatr*. 2011;2011:951616.

NOTE

Meconium aspiration is the inhalation of meconium by the fetus or newborn. When aspiration occurs, it can block air passages and result in failure of the lungs to expand or cause other pulmonary dysfunction, such as pneumonitis/inflammation of lung tissue. Death can result from hypoxia, hypercapnia, and acidosis.

Provide Tactile Stimulation to Initiate Breathing

If drying does not induce respirations in the newborn, additional tactile stimulation should be provided. The appropriate method of tactile stimulation is to gently rub the newborn's back, trunk, or extremities.[1] This intervention should not last more than 30 seconds.

Further Evaluate the Newborn

Drying and positioning are necessary in every baby at birth. These maneuvers are used to open the airway and initiate breathing. To further evaluate the newborn, the paramedic should follow these steps:

1. Observe and evaluate the newborn's respirations. If they are normal (eg, crying), continue the evaluation. A neonatal pulse oximetry probe should be placed on the right upper extremity (usually the newborn's wrist or medial surface of the palm) to monitor oxygen saturation. Target Spo_2 readings after birth are provided in **BOX 46-3**.
2. Evaluate the newborn's heart rate by stethoscope or palpation of the pulse in the base of the umbilical cord. If it is greater than100 beats/min, continue the evaluation. If the newborn needs resuscitation, it is recommended that ECG leads be placed.
3. Evaluate the newborn's color. Peripheral cyanosis (acrocyanosis) is common in the first few minutes of life and does not indicate hypoxemia. If the newborn's color is normal ("pinking up") and the Spo_2 readings are increasing, continue the evaluation by obtaining the Apgar score.

BOX 46-3 Target Spo_2 Readings After Birth

Resuscitation should be initiated with air (21%) or blended oxygen if available (21% to 30% for preterm newborns <35 weeks' gestation). For both term and preterm newborns, the goal is to titrate oxygen concentrations to achieve an Spo_2 level in the target range, described in the following table. Initiating resuscitation of preterm newborns with high oxygen (>65%) is not recommended.

1 minute	60–65%
2 minutes	65–70%
3 minutes	70–75%
4 minutes	75–80%
5 minutes	80–85%
10 minutes	85–95%

Modified from: Weiner GM, Zaichkin J, eds. *Textbook of Neonatal Resuscitation.* 7th ed. Elk Grove, IL: American Academy of Pediatrics and American Heart Association; 2016.

NOTE

Cyanosis can be divided into two types: central and peripheral. **Central cyanosis** is usually caused by a reduction in arterial oxygen saturation from heart or lung disease. Less commonly, it results from an increased amount of abnormal hemoglobin. Central cyanosis is usually apparent in the tongue and mucous membranes. **Peripheral cyanosis** is confined to the extremities. This type of cyanosis reflects an increase in the extraction of oxygen from hemoglobin by the peripheral tissues. Peripheral cyanosis is visible in the hands and feet and is expected and considered normal in newborns.

Modified from: Eichenwald EC. Overview of cyanosis in the newborn. UpToDate website. https://www.uptodate.com/contents/overview-of-cyanosis-in-the-newborn. Updated February 28, 2018. Accessed May 10, 2018.

Apgar Score

The Apgar score (see Chapter 45, *Obstetrics*) enables rapid evaluation of a newborn's condition at specific intervals after birth. It routinely is assessed at 1 and 5 minutes of age. Although the Apgar score is a useful tool to evaluate the newborn, it should not be used alone in determining the need for resuscitation. To review, an Apgar evaluates Appearance, Pulse rate, Grimace, Activity, and Respirations. A score of 7 to 10 is considered normal, a score of 4 to 6 identifies a moderately distressed newborn who requires oxygen and stimulation, and a score of less than 4 identifies a severely distressed newborn who requires resuscitation.

Resuscitation of the Distressed Newborn

Newborns who are full term, have an airway that is clear of meconium or have no evidence of infection, are breathing and crying, and have good muscle tone usually do not require resuscitation. As described earlier, this assessment should be completed within 60 seconds. If resuscitation is required because of inadequate respirations or heart rate, the newborn will need one or more of the following interventions, in sequence (**FIGURE 46-7**).[1]

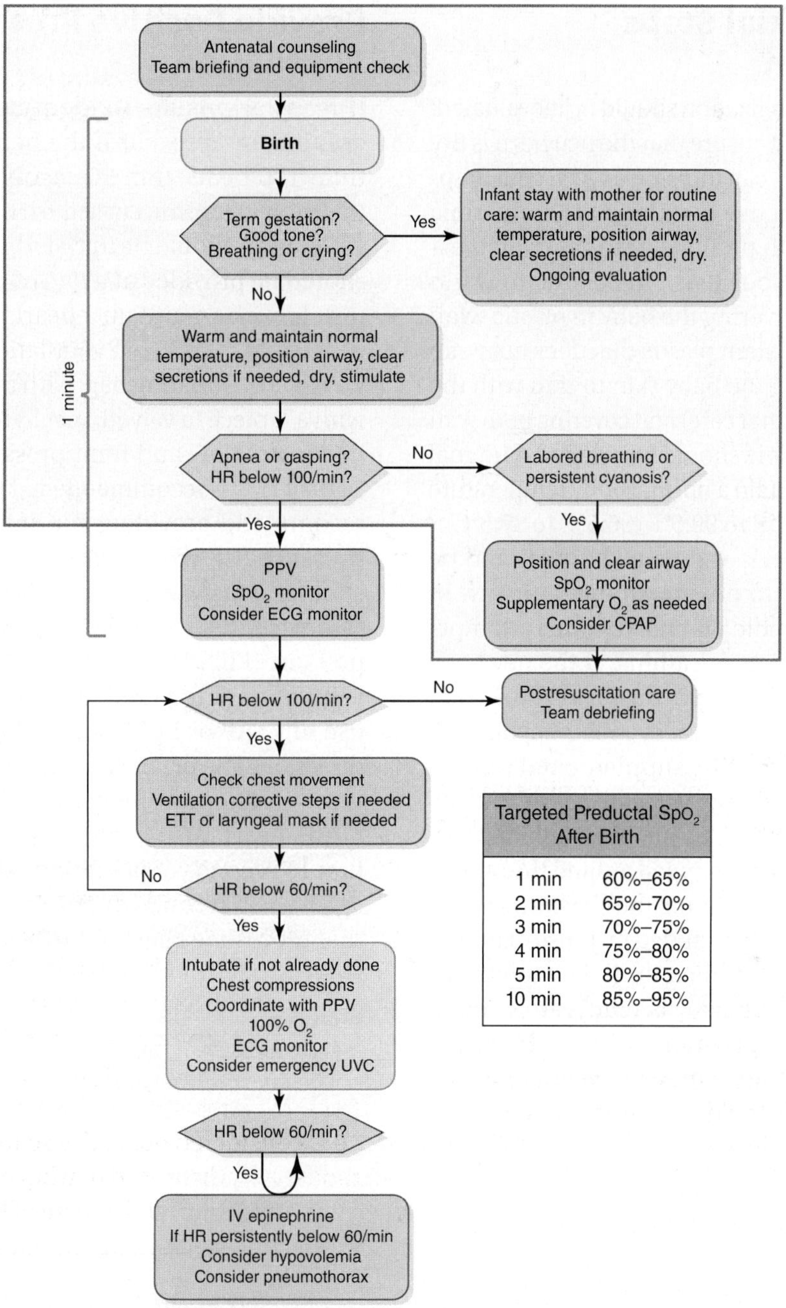

Targeted Preductal SpO_2 After Birth	
1 min	60%–65%
2 min	65%–70%
3 min	70%–75%
4 min	75%–80%
5 min	80%–85%
10 min	85%–95%

FIGURE 46-7 Neonatal Resuscitation Program/American Heart Association Neonatal Resuscitation Algorithm 2015.

NOTE

The vital role of establishing adequate ventilations must be emphasized. The newborn should have a normal respiratory rate and good effort/crying that are sufficient to improve color, achieve target Spo_2 ranges, and maintain a heart rate of greater than 100 beats/min. In addition, use of three-lead ECG is recommended for the rapid and accurate measurement of a newborn's heart rate. The use of the ECG does not replace the need for pulse oximetry to evaluate the newborn's oxygenation.

Modified from: Weiner GM, Zaichkin J, eds. *Textbook of Neonatal Resuscitation.* 7th ed. Elk Grove, IL: American Academy of Pediatrics and American Heart Association; 2016.

Reevaluate Initial Steps in Stabilization

The initial steps in stabilization should be reevaluated. The paramedic should ensure that the newborn is dry and warm. (Cold stress can increase oxygen consumption and impede effective breathing.) Hypothermia can be associated with perinatal respiratory depression. Additional methods that can be used to warm a newborn include covering the baby in plastic wrap (food-grade, heat-resistant plastic that does not wrap the head) and placing the baby skin to skin with the mother (kangaroo mother care) and covering both with a blanket. Hyperthermia should be avoided. The goal is to achieve and maintain a normal body temperature for the newborn: 97.7°F to 99.5°F (36.5°C to 37.5°C).

The head and neck of the newborn should be properly positioned to ensure an open airway. In addition, the paramedic can make other attempts at stimulation to initiate breathing. If the newborn is breathing, but color and SpO_2 do not improve soon after birth or if there is central cyanosis beyond the first 5 to 10 minutes of life, supplemental oxygen should be given. Free-flow oxygen mixed with air can be applied through a face mask and flow-inflating bag, an oxygen mask, or a hand cupped around the oxygen tubing (held 2 inches [5 cm] from the newborn's nose). Oxygen therapy should be guided by pulse oximetry measurements and continued until the target SpO_2 range is achieved. If the baby is bradycardic (heart rate of less than 60 beats/min) after 90 seconds of resuscitation with positive pressure ventilation, oxygen concentration should be increased until there is recovery of a normal heart rate.[1]

> NOTE
>
> Positive pressure ventilation of both premature and term newborns begins with room air. Healthy babies born at term have an initial oxygen saturation of less than 60% and can require more than 10 minutes to reach saturations above 90%. Preterm newborns and term newborns in need of resuscitation may take longer to achieve adequate oxygen saturation. It is important to provide adequate ventilation and to titrate the fraction of inspired oxygen based on the oxygen saturation targets in Box 46-3. Hyperoxia can be toxic to newborns, especially preterm newborns.
>
> *Modified from*: Weiner GM, Zaichkin J, eds. *Textbook of Neonatal Resuscitation.* 7th ed. Elk Grove, IL: American Academy of Pediatrics and American Heart Association; 2016.

Provide Positive Pressure Ventilation

If respirations are inadequate with bradypnea, gasping, or apnea or if the heart rate remains less than 100 beats/min 30 seconds after completing the initial steps discussed earlier, positive pressure ventilation should be initiated. Assisted ventilations should be provided at a rate of 40 to 60 breaths/min to achieve or maintain a heart rate greater than 100 beats/min.[2,3] Assisted ventilations can be delivered with a flow-inflating bag, with a self-inflating bag, or with a T-piece (a valved, mechanical device designed to control flow and limit pressure). Approximately 5 cm of H_2O is recommended.[1] Medical direction may recommend providing continuous positive airway pressure (CPAP) to newborns who are breathing spontaneously, but with difficulty, following birth. (A device that can provide positive end-expiratory pressure [PEEP] is preferable when positive pressure ventilation is required for a preterm newborn.) The use of CPAP or PEEP should be guided by medical direction. The primary measure of initial ventilation is prompt improvement in the heart rate.[1] The newborn's heart rate should initially be assessed in the first 15 seconds of positive pressure ventilation and again at 30 seconds of positive pressure ventilation that moves the chest (**FIGURE 46-8**).[12]

> NOTE
>
> Hypoxia is nearly always present in a newly born baby who requires resuscitation.

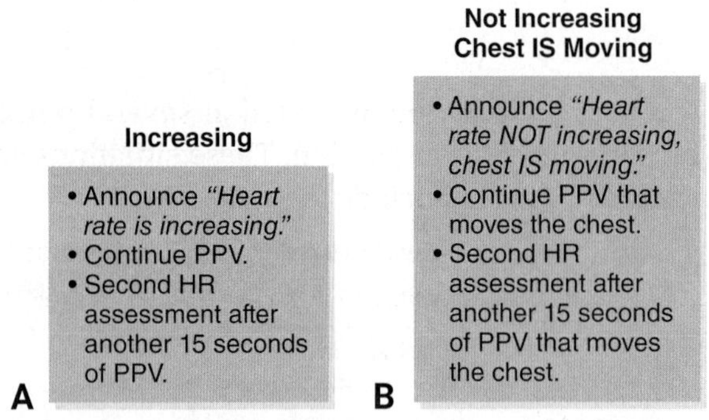

Chest IS Moving

• Continue PPV.

• Announce "Heart rate NOT increasing, chest IS moving."

Abbreviations: HR, heart rate; PPV, positive pressure ventilation

FIGURE 46-8 A. First assessment. Heart rate after 15 seconds of positive pressure ventilation. **B.** Second assessment. Heart rate after 30 seconds of positive pressure ventilation that moves the chest.

From Gary M. Weiner, MD,FAAP and Jeanette Zaichkin, RN,MN,NNP-BC. Textbook of Neonatal Resuscitation (NRP), 7th Ed. Elk Grove Village, IL: American Academy of Pediatrics; 2016:1-328. Copyright © 2016. American Academy of Pediatrics. Reproduced with permission.

NOTE

The lungs of a preterm newborn can be easily injured by large-volume inflations immediately after birth. Therefore, high pressures during assisted ventilation should be avoided with newborns who are premature. High inflation pressures may be evident by excessive chest wall movement. Inflation pressure should be monitored; an initial inflation pressure of 20 cm H_2O may be effective, but 30 to 40 cm H_2O may be required in some term newborns without spontaneous ventilation.

Modified from: Weiner GM, Zaichkin J, eds. *Textbook of Neonatal Resuscitation.* 7th ed. Elk Grove, IL: American Academy of Pediatrics and American Heart Association; 2016.

Laryngeal Mask Airway

The laryngeal mask airway (LMA) can achieve effective ventilation in term and preterm newborns at 34 weeks or more of gestation weighing more than 3.3 pounds (1.5 kg). The LMA may be considered as an alternative to tracheal intubation if face mask ventilation is unsuccessful and appropriate LMA sizes are available.[13] The LMA is also recommended during resuscitation of term and preterm newborns at 34 weeks or more of gestation when tracheal intubation is unsuccessful or not feasible. (See Chapter 15, *Airway Management, Respiration, and Artificial Ventilation.*)

Troubleshooting Ventilation Problems

Several corrective steps should be taken when ventilation is ineffective. These steps can be remembered with the mnemonic MR. SOPA, described in BOX 46-4.

ET Intubation

ET intubation may be indicated at several points during neonatal resuscitation. These situations are extremely rare and include the following:[1]

- When tracheal suctioning of meconium is required
- If bag-mask ventilation is ineffective or prolonged
- When chest compressions are performed
- For special resuscitation circumstances, such as congenital diaphragmatic hernia or extremely low birth weight (less than 2.2 pounds [1 kg])

Before the paramedic considers intubation or pharmacologic therapy, the corrective steps and actions of ventilation problems (MR. SOPA) should be reviewed.

The paramedic should verify tube placement visually during intubation and by using primary and secondary confirmation methods (see Chapter 15, *Airway Management, Respiration, and Artificial Ventilation*). Exhaled carbon dioxide detection is effective and is the most reliable method to confirm ET tube placement in newborns with adequate cardiac ouput.[1] (False-negative readings can occur if the newborn has poor or absent pulmonary flow.) A prompt increase in heart rate after ET intubation and administration of intermittent positive pressure ventilation is a good indicator of correct tube placement.

BOX 46-4 Troubleshooting Ventilation Problems Using MR. SOPA

Mask adjustment. Reapply the mask. Consider the two-hand technique.
Reposition the airway. Place the head in a neutral or slightly extended position.

Try positive pressure ventilation and reassess chest movement.

Suction mouth and nose. Use a bulb syringe or suction catheter.
Open the mouth. Open the mouth and lift the jaw forward.

Try positive pressure ventilation and reassess chest movement.

Pressure increase. Increase pressure in 5- to 10-cm H_2O increments (maximum, 40 cm H_2O).
Alternative airway. Place an endotracheal (ET) tube or laryngeal mask.

Try positive pressure ventilation and assess chest movement and breath sounds.

Modified from: Reed C. *Neonatal Resuscitation Program, 2015.* 7th ed. Elk Grove, IL: American Academy of Pediatrics; 2015:25.

Provide Chest Compressions

Chest compressions are indicated if the newborn's heart rate is less than 60 beats/min despite adequate ventilation. (The paramedic should ensure that assisted ventilations are effective before initiating chest compressions.) Chest compressions should be coordinated with ventilations to avoid simultaneous delivery. The chest should be allowed to re-expand fully during relaxation, but the rescuer's thumbs should not leave the chest. Compressions and ventilations should be delivered at a ratio of 3:1 at a rate of 120 per minute. This will achieve about 90 compressions and 30 breaths per minute (1-2-3-breathe). Compressions should be continued for 60 seconds before reassessing heart rate (>60 beats/min). Frequent interruptions of compressions should be avoided because they will compromise artificial maintenance of systemic perfusion and maintenance of coronary blood flow.[1]

NOTE

Intubation is strongly recommended prior to beginning chest compressions. Oxygen concentration should be increased to 100% whenever chest compressions are provided.

Modified from: Weiner GM, Zaichkin J, eds. *Textbook of Neonatal Resuscitation.* 7th ed. Elk Grove, IL: American Academy of Pediatrics and American Heart Association; 2016.

The two-thumb–encircling-hands chest compression is the preferred technique for chest compressions for newly born babies and older infants who are full term. This technique generates higher blood pressures and coronary perfusion pressure with less rescuer fatigue. Compressions should be performed just below the nipple line with the thumbs on the lower third of the sternum. Depth of compression should be approximately one-third of the anterior–posterior diameter of the chest and should be sufficiently deep to generate a palpable pulse.[1]

CRITICAL THINKING

Why would compressions be initiated when the newborn still has a pulse?

Administer Epinephrine and/or Volume Expanders

Drugs are rarely indicated in the resuscitation of the newly born baby. As a rule, drugs should be administered only if the heart rate remains below 60 beats/min, despite adequate ventilation with 100% oxygen and effective chest compressions.[1] Drug therapy that may be indicated includes the administration of epinephrine and volume expanders. Other drugs are rarely useful (**TABLE 46-1**).

Important points for the paramedic to remember when administering drugs or volume expanders include the following:[1,14]

1. All medications and fluids should be infused through intravenous (IV) access if possible. The recommended dose for IV administration is 0.01 to 0.03 mg/kg per dose (preferred route). The recommended dose for ET administration is 0.05 to 0.1mg/kg per dose. The concentration of epinephrine for either route should be 1:10,000 (0.1 mg/mL).
2. Volume expanders (0.9% saline) should be considered when blood loss is known or suspected. They should also be considered if the

TABLE 46-1 Medications for Neonatal Resuscitation

Medication	Dose/Route	Concentration	Weight (kg)	Total (mL)	Precautions
Epinephrine[a,b]	0.01–0.03 mg/kg IV/IO	0.1 mg/mL	1 2 3 4	0.1–0.3 0.2–0.6 0.3–0.9 0.4–1.2	Give rapidly. Repeat every 3–5 min.
Volume expanders, normal saline, or blood	10 mL/kg IV over 5–10 min		1 2 3 4	10 20 30 40	Reassess after each bolus.

[a]Epinephrine also may be given endotracheally 0.05–0.1 mg/kg (not preferred).

[b]The ET tube dose may not result in effective plasma concentration of the drug, so vascular access should be established as soon as possible. Drugs administered by ET tube should be diluted to a volume of 3 to 5 mL before instillation. Drugs given ET require higher dosing than when given IV/IO.

Abbreviations: ET, endotracheal; IO, intraosseous; IV, intravenous newborn appears to be in shock (pale skin, poor perfusion, rapid, weak pulse) and when the newborn's heart rate has not responded to other resuscitative measures. (End-organ perfusion should be evaluated by comparing the strength of central versus peripheral pulses and through capillary refill tests.) Volume expanders should be given slowly and with caution when resuscitating premature newborns. The recommended dose is 10 mL/kg, which may need to be repeated. Rapid infusions of large volumes of volume expanders have been associated with intracerebral ventricular hemorrhage.

> NOTE
>
> Bradycardia in the newborn is usually the result of inadequate lung inflation or hypoxemia. Therefore, establishing adequate ventilation is the most important step to correct it.

Routes of Drug Administration

Venous access in the prehospital setting is rarely needed in newborns. Resuscitation is largely focused on airway management and breathing.[15] If needed, the IV route is the preferred route for drug therapy in the newborn. Other methods that may be considered include the ET route and the intraosseous (IO) route (see Chapter 14, *Medication Administration*). During cardiopulmonary resuscitation (CPR) or treatment of severe shock, IO access should be established when venous access cannot be rapidly achieved.[1]

> NOTE
>
> Venous access through the umbilical cord is usually not recommended in the prehospital setting. The procedure carries serious risks similar to other central vein access procedures and requires special training and authorization from medical direction. Accessing the umbilical vein is described in the Appendix B, *Advanced Practice Procedures for Critical Care Paramedics*.
>
> *Modified from*: Tintinalli JE, Stapczynsk JS, Ma JO, Yealy DM, Meckler GD, Cline DM. *Tintinalli's Emergency Medicine: A Comprehensive Study Guide*. 8th ed. New York, NY: McGraw-Hill; 2016.

Postresuscitation Care

The three most common complications of the postresuscitation period are ET tube migration (including dislodgment), tube occlusion by mucus or meconium, and pneumothorax (BOX 46-5).[2,3] These complications should be suspected in the presence of the following:

> **BOX 46-5** DOPE Mnemonic
>
> **D**islodgement (ET tube is misplaced; right mainstem bronchus, esophagus)
> **O**bstruction (secretions obstructing the tube)
> **P**neumothorax (decreased or absent breath sounds on the affected side)
> **E**quipment failure (such as ventilator malfunction or disconnect)

- Decreased chest wall movement
- Diminished breath sounds
- Return of bradycardia
- Unilateral decrease in chest expansion
- Altered intensity to pitch of breath sounds
- Increased resistance to hand ventilation

Corrective management in the prehospital setting for these postresuscitative complications may include adjustment of the ET tube (exhaled carbon dioxide devices are recommended for monitoring tracheal tube placement), reintubation, and suction. Needle decompression to manage a suspected pneumothorax (see Chapter 41, *Chest Trauma*) must be guided carefully by medical direction.

> CRITICAL THINKING
>
> How much movement would it take to dislodge an ET tube from a newborn?

Induced Therapeutic Hypothermia

It is recommended that newborns born at more than 36 weeks' gestation with evolving moderate to severe hypoxic-ischemic encephalopathy should be offered therapeutic hypothermia under clearly defined protocols.[1] Induced therapeutic hypothermia is instituted in the hospital setting under physician supervision.

Neonatal Transport

Once effective ventilation and/or the circulation has been established, the newborn and mother should be transported to an appropriate facility where close monitoring and anticipatory care can be provided.

During transport, it is important to maintain the newborn's body temperature and prevent hypothermia. In addition, it is crucial to maintain oxygen levels and to support the newborn's ventilations. In the initial prehospital phase of care, transport strategies usually are limited to providing a warm ambulance, administering oxygen if appropriate (warmed if available), covering the baby's head, and applying warm blankets to prevent hypothermic complications. Specialized transport equipment, such as isolettes and radiant heating units, often is used for interhospital transfers. These devices require special training. Highly trained newborn transport teams consisting of paramedics, nurses, respiratory therapists, and physicians are part of well-organized regional referral systems throughout the United States (**FIGURE 46-9**).

Neonatal Resuscitation, Postresuscitation, and Stabilization

A newborn's heart generally is healthy and strong. However, disorders in the conduction system of the heart may occur. Most often the disorders occur as a result of hypoxemia and respiratory arrest. The outcome for these newborns is poor if interventions are not initiated quickly. In addition, the likelihood for brain and end-organ injury is increased in newborns who require resuscitation. The paramedic should continually assess and monitor newborns with respiratory distress for treatable causes.

Asystole and pulseless cardiac arrest are uncommon in the newborn. Like bradycardia, they usually are the result of hypoxia. Cardiac arrest also can be caused by primary and secondary apnea, unresolved bradycardia, and persistent fetal circulation (persistent pulmonary hypertension). Assessment findings may include peripheral cyanosis, inadequate respiratory effort, and an ineffective or absent heart rate. Risk factors associated with cardiac arrest in the newborn include the following:

- Congenital malformations
- Congenital neuromuscular disease
- Drugs administered to or taken by the mother
- Intrapartum hypoxemia
- Intrauterine asphyxia

Emergency care for newborns with asystole or pulseless arrest is described in Chapter 47, *Pediatrics*. Resuscitation includes airway, ventilatory, and circulatory support; pharmacologic therapy (epinephrine); and rapid transport to an appropriate medical facility.

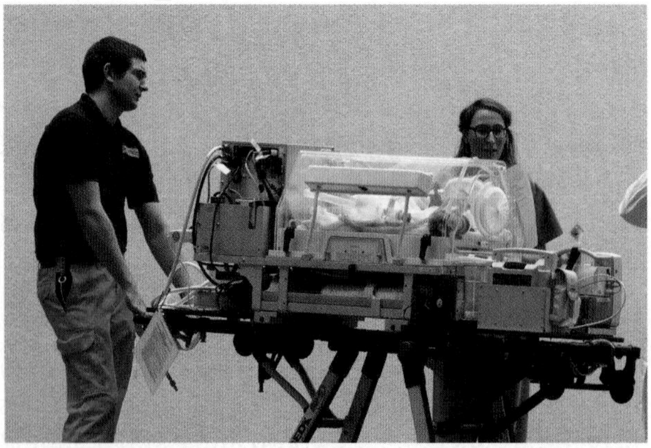

FIGURE 46-9 Neonatal transport.

NOTE

The decision to withhold resuscitation or to discontinue resuscitation efforts in the prehospital setting must be guided by the parents' wishes and medical direction. Resuscitation may not be indicated in newborns of less than 25 weeks' gestation and in those with some congenital malformation and chromosomal anomalies. It is also considered ethical to provide compassionate palliative care and not initiate resuscitation if intensive medical care will not improve chances of survival or poses an unacceptable burden on the child. An Apgar score of 0 at 10 minutes is a strong predictor of mortality and morbidity in late preterm and term newborns. In newborns with an Apgar score of 0 after 10 minutes of resuscitation and no detectable pulse, it may be reasonable to stop assisted ventilation.

Modified from: Weiner GM, Zaichkin J, eds. *Textbook of Neonatal Resuscitation*. 7th ed. Elk Grove, IL: American Academy of Pediatrics and American Heart Association; 2016; Preterm (premature) labor and birth. FAQ087. American College of Obstetricians and Gynecologists website. https://www.acog.org/Patients/FAQs/Preterm-Premature-Labor-and-Birth. Published November 2016. Accessed May 10, 2018; and What are the risk factors for preterm labor and birth? National Institutes of Health website. https://www.nichd.nih.gov/health/topics/preterm/conditioninfo/who_risk. Reviewed January 31, 2017. Accessed May 10, 2018.

CRITICAL THINKING

How will you feel if you deliver a critically ill or dead baby?

Psychological and Emotional Support

The paramedic must be aware of the normal feelings and reactions of parents, siblings, other family members, and caregivers while providing emergency care to an ill or injured child. (These events also are often highly charged and emotional for the emergency crew.) The paramedic should keep those at the scene abreast of all procedures being performed and should inform family members of the necessity of the procedures.

> NOTE
> After delivery, the mother continues to be a patient. She still has physical and emotional needs.

As a rule, emergency responders should never discuss the newborn's chances of survival with a parent or family member. They also should not give false hope about the newborn's condition. The paramedic should assure the family that everything that can be done for the newborn is being done. The paramedic also should assure the family that the newborn will receive the best possible care during transport and at the hospital. The hospital will have support personnel who can assist family members and loved ones.

Specific Situations

Specific situations may call for advanced life support for the newborn. These situations include apnea, bradycardia, respiratory distress and cyanosis, hypovolemia, seizures, fever, hypothermia, hypoglycemia, vomiting and diarrhea, newborn jaundice, sepsis, and common birth injuries. While providing advanced life support in these and other situations, the paramedic must consider the emotional needs of the mother and family. The paramedic should explain what is being done for the newborn and why a procedure is necessary.

Apnea

Apnea is an absence of spontaneous respirations. Primary apnea is a self-limited condition controlled by partial pressure of carbon dioxide levels. It is a common event immediately after birth. Secondary apnea is described as apnea that exceeds 20 seconds without spontaneous breathing occurring. This condition can lead to hypoxemia and bradycardia. Secondary apnea is common in the preterm newborn. It often results from hypoxia or hypothermia. Secondary apnea also may be caused by conditions that include maternal use of narcotics or central nervous system (CNS) depressants, prolonged or difficult labor and delivery, airway and respiratory muscle weakness, septicemia, metabolic disorders, and CNS disorders.[15] Presence of secondary apnea necessitates initiation of positive pressure ventilation and resuscitation. It cannot be reversed with stimulation.

Emergency care for a newborn with prolonged apnea begins with stimulating the newborn to breathe. This is done by flicking the soles of the feet or rubbing the back. If needed, a bag device (with a disabled pop-off valve) should be used while applying the least amount of pressure that produces adequate chest rise. The paramedic should suction secretions from the newborns airway as needed and maintain the newborn's body temperature to prevent hypothermia. Respiratory support with an LMA or ET intubation and circulatory support may be required if central cyanosis persists despite adequate ventilations.[16] Apnea that is treated early and aggressively is key to a good outcome.[17]

Bradycardia

Bradycardia is described as a heart rate of less than 100 beats/min. As described earlier, bradycardia in the newborn is most commonly caused by inadequate ventilation. Other risk factors include prolonged suctioning and the use of airway or any invasive procedures during resuscitation that may cause vagal stimulation. Bradycardia is a minimal risk to life in newborns if it is corrected quickly. The management of bradycardia in the newborn was described earlier

> NOTE
> Metabolic acidosis should be considered if bradycardia persists after resuscitation measures. Medical direction may recommend the administration of a fluid bolus (10 mL/kg normal saline) to improve perfusion. The goal of treatment is to address the underlying cause. The administration of sodium bicarbonate for neonatal metabolic acidosis is not currently recommended.
>
> *Modified from*: Weiner GM, Zaichkin J, eds. *Textbook of Neonatal Resuscitation*. 7th ed. Elk Grove, IL: American Academy of Pediatrics and American Heart Association; 2016.

in the chapter and may include chest compressions and drug therapy.

Respiratory Distress and Cyanosis

Prematurity is the most common cause of respiratory distress and cyanosis in the newborn.[18] These conditions occur most often in newborns weighing less than 2.5 pounds (1.2 kg) and aged less than 30 weeks' gestation.[18] These problems may be related to the newborn's immature lungs and central respiratory control center. The premature newborn's center is affected more easily by environmental and metabolic changes than is that of the full-term newborn. Other risk factors for respiratory distress and cyanosis in the newborn include multiple gestations, prenatal maternal complications, and newborns born with the following conditions:

- Birth defects
- CNS disorders
- Diaphragmatic hernia
- Esophageal atresia
- Lung or heart disease
- Meconium or amniotic fluid aspiration
- Metabolic acidosis
- Mucus obstruction of nasal passages
- Pneumonia
- Primary pulmonary hypertension
- Shock and sepsis
- Tracheoesophageal fistula

Respiratory distress and cyanosis can lead to cardiac arrest in the newborn. The situation necessitates immediate actions to improve breathing and support respirations. Assessment findings may include tachypnea, paradoxical breathing, intercostal retractions, nasal flaring, expiratory grunting, and central cyanosis. As described earlier, respiratory insufficiency in the newborn generally is managed with stimulation, positioning of the airway, prevention of heat loss and hypothermia, oxygenation and positive pressure ventilation, and if needed, suction and intubation with ventilatory support.

Hypovolemia

Hypovolemia in newborns may result from dehydration, hemorrhage, trauma, or sepsis. Signs and symptoms of hypovolemia include mottled or pale color, cool skin, tachycardia, diminished peripheral pulses, and delayed capillary refill despite normal ambient temperature. Shock may be present despite a normal blood pressure. Prompt and effective treatment of early signs of compensated shock may prevent the development of hypotension (decompensated shock) and associated high morbidity and mortality.[2] Prehospital care is always directed at ensuring adequate airway, ventilatory, and circulatory support; ensuring volume repletion (including control of external hemorrhage); and providing rapid transport to an appropriate facility.

When signs of hypovolemia are present, the paramedic should give a fluid bolus (10 mL/kg over 5 to 10 minutes of isotonic crystalloid) immediately after obtaining IV access and then reassess the newborn.[1] If signs of shock persist, the paramedic should give a second 10-mL/kg bolus. Further boluses should be given as needed and under the guidance of medical direction.

Seizures

Seizures occur in a small percentage of newborns. When present, they usually are a sign of an underlying abnormality (BOX 46-6). Prolonged seizures or frequent seizures may result in metabolic changes and cardiopulmonary difficulties. As described in Chapter 24, *Neurology*, seizures are classified as focal onset seizures, generalized onset seizures, and unknown onset seizures.

Emergency care for managing neonatal seizures includes providing airway, ventilatory, and circulatory support and maintaining the newborn's body temperature. Phenobarbital is the first-line drug for seizures in newborns. If seizures persist, phenytoin should be added. Persistent seizures may require the use of an IV benzodiazepine, such as lorazepam or midazolam.[19] Dextrose may also be prescribed by medical direction to treat hypoglycemia. Seizure activity

BOX 46-6 Causes of Neonatal Seizures

- Developmental abnormalities
- Drug withdrawal
- Hypoglycemia
- Hypoxic ischemic encephalopathy
- Intracranial hemorrhage
- Meningitis or encephalopathy
- Metabolic disturbances

is always considered pathologic; rapid transport for physician evaluation is needed.

Fever

Fever in newborns is described as a rectal temperature greater than 100.4°F (38°C). Fever in newborns usually is a cause for concern and often is a response to an acute viral or bacterial infection, including neonatal sepsis.[20] Fever also may result from a change in the newborn's limited ability to control body temperature or be an effect of dehydration. The rise in core temperature increases oxygen demands and increases glucose metabolism. These increases may lead to metabolic acidosis. Assessment findings in the newborn may include rashes and petechiae, and warm or hot skin. In these cases, it is important to obtain maternal prenatal history with attention to risk for infection.

The prehospital care for febrile newborns mainly is supportive. As a rule, cooling procedures and the use of antipyretics will be delayed until the newborn has arrived at the hospital. Febrile seizures may be present when caring for the newborn. All febrile newborns require immediate transport for physician evaluation.

Hypothermia

As described in Chapter 44, *Environmental Conditions*, hypothermia is a core body temperature below 95°F (35°C). Hypothermia may result from a decrease in heat production, an increase in heat loss (through evaporation, conduction, convection, or radiation), or a combination of both. Newborns are sensitive to the effects of hypothermia because of their increased surface-to-volume ratio. This risk is especially high when they are wet (eg, after delivery). The associated increase in metabolic demand to maintain body temperature can cause metabolic acidosis, pulmonary hypertension, and hypoxemia.[21] Hypothermia also may be a sign of sepsis in the newborn.[22] Assessment findings may include the following:

- Pale color
- Cool skin (especially in the extremities)
- Respiratory distress
- Apnea
- Bradycardia
- Central cyanosis
- Acrocyanosis (cyanosis of the extremities)
- Irritability (initially)
- Lethargy (in the late stage)
- Absence of shivering (variable)

The prehospital care for these patients may include provision of basic and advanced cardiac life support, depending on the severity of hypothermia. The care also consists of rapid transport to an appropriate facility. Other therapeutic measures include ensuring that the newborn is dry and warm, warming the hands before touching the newborn, and perhaps administering dextrose to treat hypoglycemia and IV therapy with warm fluids. The patient should be transported in a heated ambulance.

Hypoglycemia

A blood glucose measurement of less than 40 mg/dL for term newborns (<30 mg/dL for preterm newborns) indicates hypoglycemia (see Chapter 25, *Endocrinology*).[1] The condition should be determined by blood glucose screening on all sick newborns. Hypoglycemia may be the result of inadequate glucose intake or increased use of glucose. Risk factors associated with hypoglycemia include asphyxia, toxemia, being the smaller twin, CNS hemorrhage, being born to a mother with diabetes mellitus, and sepsis. Assessment findings may include the following:

- Twitching or seizure
- Hypotonia
- Lethargy
- Irritability
- Eye rolling
- High-pitched crying
- Apnea
- Irregular respirations
- Cyanosis (possibly)

> NOTE
>
> Small newborns/infants and chronically ill children have limited glycogen stores. These stores may be depleted rapidly during stress events. In newborns, prolonged hypoglycemia can depress myocardial function and is associated with an increased risk for brain injury, while increased glucose levels may be protective. IV glucose infusion should be considered as soon as practical after resuscitation, with the goal of avoiding hypoglycemia.
>
> *Modified from*: Reed C. *Neonatal Resuscitation Program, 2015.* 7th ed. Elk Grove, IL: American Academy of Pediatrics; 2015.

The prehospital care is directed at ensuring adequate airway, ventilatory, and circulatory support; maintaining body temperature; providing rapid transport; and possibly administering IV dextrose 10% (per medical direction). A dextrose dose of 0.2 g/kg, followed by 5 mL/kg per hour via IV/IO infusion, may be repeated in 30 minutes if needed.[2,3] All hypoglycemic newborns should be transported immediately to a medical facility. As described in Chapter 25, *Endocrinology*, dextrose is available in a number of concentrations. A 10% solution is the only concentration to be given to newborns.

Vomiting and Diarrhea

Occasional vomiting or diarrhea is not unusual in the newborn. For example, vomiting mucus that may be streaked with blood is common in the first few hours of life. Five to six stools per day is considered normal in newborns, especially if the newborn is breastfeeding. Persistent vomiting (bilious vomiting that is dark green) may indicate small bowel obstruction and is a surgical emergency. Persistent diarrhea should be considered a warning sign of serious illness.

Vomiting

Persistent or projectile vomiting in the first 24 hours of life suggests an obstruction in the upper digestive tract or perhaps increased intracranial pressure.[23] Vomit that contains non–bile-stained fluid or bilious vomiting that is dark green may indicate anatomic or functional obstruction and is a surgical emergency. Vomit that contains dark blood usually is a sign of life-threatening illness. Assessment findings may include a distended stomach and signs of infection, dehydration, and increased intracranial pressure. The paramedic also should consider that the vomiting may be a result of drug withdrawal (if the mother has an opiate substance abuse disorder).

The prehospital care usually requires maintaining an airway that is clear of vomit and ensuring adequate oxygenation. In severe cases, medical direction may advise that IV fluid therapy be initiated before transport. Fluid therapy treats dehydration and any bradycardia that may develop from vagal stimulation. If possible, newborns should be transported on their sides to help prevent aspiration.

DID YOU KNOW?

Neonatal abstinence syndrome (NAS) is a withdrawal syndrome that occurs when a newborn has been exposed to drugs such as opioids, alcohol, benzodiazepines, barbiturates, and some antidepressants (SSRIs) while in the mother's womb. NAS can also result from the discontinuation of medications, such as fentanyl or morphine, used for pain therapy in the newborn. The severity of symptoms will depend on the type and amount of drug used by the mother, how long the drug was used the drug, and how the mother metabolized the drug. Symptoms in the newborn may include high-pitched cry, seizures, fever, vomiting, and diarrhea. Care for newborns with severe NAS may include drug therapy (including opioids, phenobarbital, methadone). These drugs will allow the infant to feed, sleep, and gain weight during the period of withdrawal. The drug therapy is gradually decreased as the withdrawal is controlled. The length of hospitalization varies.

Naloxone is not recommended for narcotic-related respiratory depression because it may precipitate seizures in the neonate. Care should be directed at providing ventilatory and circulatory support and rapid transport. Medical direction may considered IV or intramuscular (IM) naloxone after heart rate and color are restored

Modified from: Hamdan AH. Neonatal abstinence syndrome. Medscape website. https://emedicine.medscape.com/article/978763-overview. Updated December 20, 2017. Accessed May 10, 2018; McQueen K, Murphy-Oikonen J. Neonatal abstinence syndrome. *N Engl J Med*. 2016;375:2468-2479; Preterm (premature) labor and birth. FAQ087. American College of Obstetricians and Gynecologists website. https://www.acog.org/Patients/FAQs/Preterm-Premature-Labor-and-Birth. Published November 2016. Accessed May 10, 2018; and What are the risk factors for preterm labor and birth? National Institutes of Health website. https://www.nichd.nih.gov/health/topics/preterm/conditioninfo/who_risk. Reviewed January 31, 2017. Accessed May 10, 2018.

Diarrhea

Persistent diarrhea can lead to serious dehydration and electrolyte imbalance in the newborn. The diarrhea often is associated with a bacterial or viral infection. Other possible causes include the following:

- Bacterial enteritis (*Clostridium difficile, Salmonella, Shigella*)
- Cystic fibrosis
- Lactose intolerance
- NAS (drug withdrawal)
- Thyrotoxicosis
- Viral gastroenteritis (rotavirus)

Assessment findings often include the presence of loose stools, decreased urinary output, and signs of dehydration. Treatment consists of supporting the newborn's vital functions, IV fluid therapy (per medical direction), and rapid transport to the receiving hospital.

Newborn Jaundice

Newborn jaundice occurs when an infant has a high level of bilirubin in the blood. As described in Chapter 31, *Hematology*, bilirubin is made during the normal breakdown of red blood cells. It is usually processed by the liver, recycled, and eliminated in the stool. Hyperbilirubinemia produces a yellowing of the infant's skin, mucous membranes, and eyes. Newborn jaundice is common, affecting about 3 in 5 newborns (physiologic jaundice).[24] The jaundice usually resolves as the liver matures within 2 weeks. Other, more serious causes of newborn jaundice include Rh disease, sepsis or other infection, liver dysfunction (e.g., hepatitis, cystic fibrosis), and G6PD (enzyme) deficiency.

Risk factors associated with newborn jaundice include prematurity, difficult delivery, bruising, sibling history of jaundice, and infants of East Asian or Mediterranean descent.[25] Newborn jaundice requires physician evaluation and testing. Jaundice that does not resolve may require phototherapy treatment, an exchange transfusion, and IV immunoglobulin to prevent possible neurologic complications. Prehospital care is primarily supportive.

Sepsis

Healthy newborns are vulnerable to several conditions that can require hospital treatment. Examples include jaundice, which results from physiologic immaturity of bilirubin metabolism, dehydration, which can lead to serious electrolyte abnormalities, and sepsis. In addition, newborns are highly susceptible to infection because of diminished nonspecific (inflammatory) and specific (humoral) immunity.

Sepsis in the newborn usually is caused by viral infections (eg, cytomegalovirus, hepatitis, herpes) and bacterial infections (eg, Group B streptococcus, *Escherichia coli*, gonorrhea, chlamydia).[26] Late-onset sepsis occurs between 8 and 28 days after birth. Signs and symptoms of sepsis may be minimal and nonspecific. (There is a common expression in neonatal care: "In the newborn, anything can be a sign of anything.") Examples of signs and symptoms of sepsis in the newborn include the following:

- Temperature instability (only 50% have temperature above 100°F (37.8°C)
- Respiratory distress
- Feeding changes
- Apnea
- Cyanosis
- Parent feels child is not well
- Gastrointestinal changes (eg, vomiting, distention, diarrhea, anorexia)
- CNS features (eg, irritability, lethargy, weak suck)

Risk factors for late sepsis include prematurity and low birth weight. The diagnosis generally is confirmed after physician evaluation by a positive blood, urine, or cerebrospinal fluid culture.

Common Birth Injuries

Birth injury occurs in about 2% of neonatal deaths and stillbirths in the United States.[27] The injuries range from minor problems, such as bruises, to severe injuries that can cause death. Higher rates are reported when there is maternal obesity, abnormal fetal presentation, and newborn weight of more than 8.8 pounds (4 kg).[28]

Cranial injuries may include molding of the head and overriding of the parietal bones, soft-tissue injuries from forceps delivery, subconjunctival and retinal hemorrhage, subperiosteal hemorrhage, and skull fracture. Intracranial hemorrhage can occur from trauma or asphyxia. Spine and spinal cord injury can result from strong traction or a lateral pull during delivery. Other birth injuries include peripheral nerve injury, liver or spleen injury, adrenal hemorrhage, clavicle or extremity fracture, and brain or soft-tissue injury from hypoxia-ischemia. The assessment findings vary by the nature of the injury. They may include the following:

- Diffuse, sometimes ecchymotic, edematous swelling of the soft tissues of the scalp
- Nasal septum dislocation
- Mild eye injuries
- Paralysis below the level of spinal cord injury (very rare)

- Paralysis of the upper arm with or without paralysis of the forearm
- Fractured clavicle, humerus, femur
- Paralysis of the diaphragm
- Movement on only one side of the face when the newborn cries
- Shock

The goal of prehospital care for a newborn with a birth injury is to support the vital functions. This can be done by ensuring adequate oxygenation, ventilation, and circulatory support and administering fluid or drug therapy (if indicated). These babies are high-risk newborns. They require rapid transport to a proper medical facility.

Congenital Anomalies

Congenital anomalies are birth defects that occur during fetal development. (Most develop within the first trimester.) They are present in about 3% of all births and are responsible for 20% of all newborn deaths.[29] Thus, the presence of congenital anomalies may be a factor in the need for neonatal resuscitation. Congenital anomalies may be heritable; caused by maternal infection, alcohol, or other drug use during pregnancy (teratogens); and other factors.[30] Congenital defects presented in this chapter include anomalies of the airway, heart, and abdomen and lower back.

> NOTE
> Prehospital care for babies born with congenital anomalies requires early assessment to control and protect the airway, positioning to improve respirations, suction to clear the airway if it is obstructed, oxygen administration, and careful monitoring with pulse oximetry to ensure adequate ventilation. Advanced airway equipment should be readily available.

Anomalies of the Airway

Choanal Atresia

Choanal atresia is a bony or tissue occlusion that blocks the passageway between the nose and the pharynx (**FIGURE 46-10**). (Atresia is a condition in which an orifice or passage in the body is closed or absent.) The defect is thought to occur during fetal development when the thin tissue that separates the nose and mouth remains after birth. Choanal atresia is the most common nose abnormality in newborns, affecting about 1 in 5,000 to 7,000 live births.[31] It is often associated with other congenital anomalies.

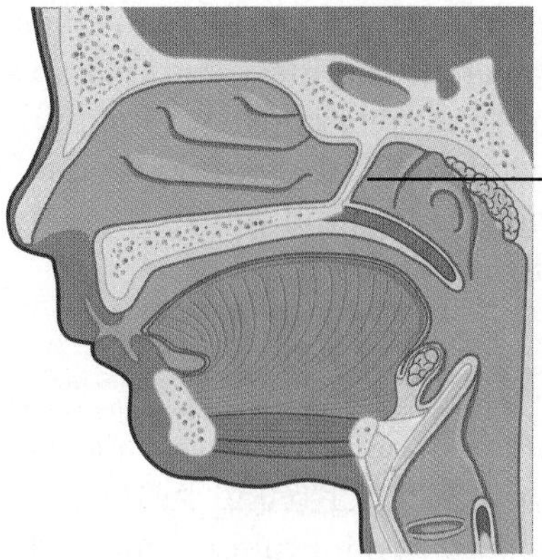

FIGURE 46-10 Choanal atresia.

> NOTE
> Newborns generally breathe through their nose unless they are crying. Therefore, babies born with choanal atresia have difficulty breathing unless they are crying. Resuscitation, including tracheal intubation, may be required.

Choanal atresia may affect one or both sides of the nasal cavity and may require surgical repair. Bilateral obstruction can result in serious ventilation problems. Depending on the degree of obstruction, symptoms may include the following:

- Chest wall retraction (unless the newborn is breathing through the mouth or crying)
- Dyspnea, which may result in cyanosis (unless the newborn is crying)
- Inability to nurse and breathe at the same time
- Persistent one-sided nasal blockage or discharge

Insertion of an oropharyngeal airway may improve the newborn's respiratory status until arrival at a health care facility.[1]

Tracheoesophageal Fistula

Tracheoesophageal fistula is a congenital disorder that occurs in about 1 in every 4,300 live births.[32] It is an abnormal connection between the esophagus and trachea that results from a failed fusion of the tracheoesophageal ridges during fetal development. It

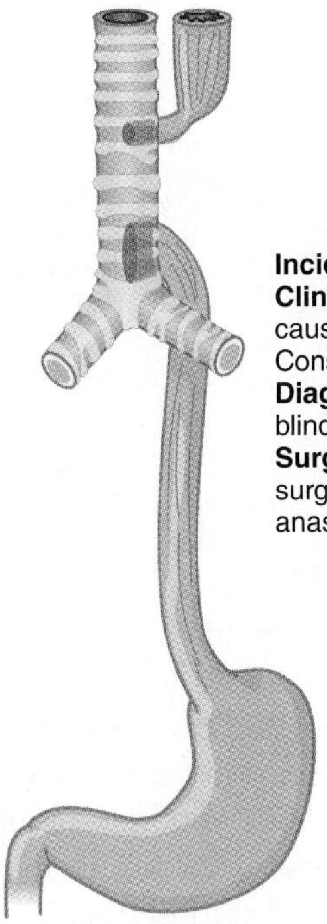

Incidence: 85%–88%
Clinical manifestations: Feeding causes regurgitation and coughing. Constant flow of saliva. Gastric distention.
Diagnostic findings: Contrast reveals blind pouch. Air on abdominal radiograph.
Surgical treatment: One-stage surgical repair to ligate fistula and anastomose esophagus.

FIGURE 46-11 Esophageal atresia with distal tracheoesophageal fistula.

commonly occurs along with **esophageal atresia** (the incomplete formation of the esophagus) (**FIGURE 46-11**). If not surgically corrected, both conditions can allow for food and fluid in the esophagus to enter the trachea and lungs. The defect can also allow for air in the trachea to enter the esophagus. Signs and symptoms of both disorders in the newborn include the following:

- Copious salivation
- Choking
- Coughing
- Regurgitation during feeding
- Cyanosis

Many babies born with tracheoesophageal fistula or esophageal atresia have other congenital anomalies, including heart, kidney, and limb deformities (often occurring together). These newborns are unable to feed properly. Once diagnosed, early surgery is required.

Cleft Lip and Cleft Palate

A **cleft lip** is incomplete closure of the newborn's lip. It occurs when one or more fissures fail to fuse in the embryo. It is visible at birth as a vertical, usually off-center split in the upper lip that may extend to the

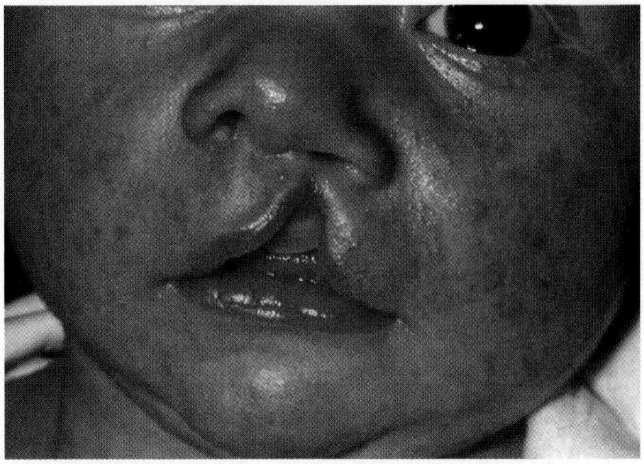

FIGURE 46-12 Cleft lip.

nose (**FIGURE 46-12**). A **cleft palate** is a fissure in the hard palate of the roof of the mouth that runs along its midline. Both conditions can occur with other congenital anomalies. A cleft palate may involve one or both sides of the roof of the mouth and can extend through the hard and soft palates into the nasal cavity. A cleft lip or cleft palate can cause nasal deformity and difficulty in feeding and speech and is associated with frequent ear infections. Annually, about 4,440 babies are born in the United States with cleft lip, with or without a cleft palate.[33] A cleft lip or cleft palate can lead to failure to thrive, misaligned teeth, and difficulties with speech. The defect is corrected with one or more surgeries, usually beginning in the first year of life.

Pierre Robin Sequence

Pierre Robin sequence (formerly Pierre Robin syndrome) is a rare complex of congenital anomalies including a small mandible, a tongue that is placed farther back in the oral cavity and may obstruct the airway, and often a cleft palate. Additional craniofacial abnormalities and defects of the eyes and ears may be present with this syndrome (**FIGURE 46-13**). Symptoms of the disorder include a high-arched palate, a receding chin, a tongue that appears large for the jaw, and teeth that are present at birth (natal teeth). Pierre Robin sequence occurs in 1 in every 8,500 to 14,000 people.[34]

Complications associated with Pierre Robin sequence include breathing difficulties, poor feeding early in life, cerebral hypoperfusion, pulmonary hypertension, and heart failure. Death can result from

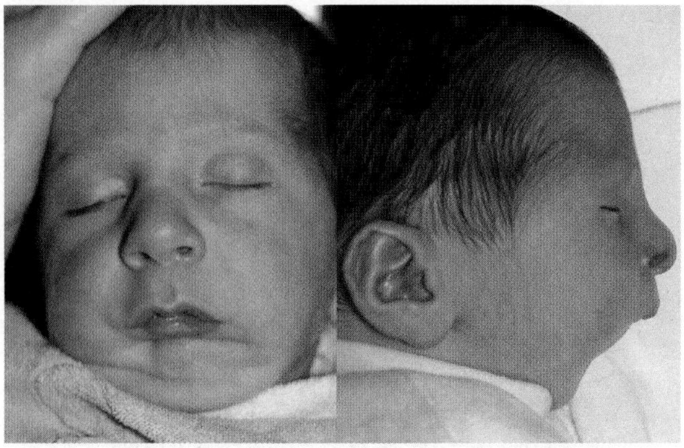

FIGURE 46-13 Pierre Robin sequence.

Reproduced from: Sesenna, E., Magri, A. S., Magnani, C., Brevi, B. C., & Anghinoni, M. L. (2012). Mandibular distraction in neonates: indications, technique, results. Italian journal of pediatrics, 38(1)7.

respiratory failure, secondary to airway obstruction. The condition is managed with surgical repair of the cleft palate and other methods to prevent breathing difficulties and episodes of choking. Most children have some relief from the effects of the Pierre Robin sequence as the jaw grows and allows more space for the tongue. Newborns who are dyspneic in the field should be positioned prone.[35] This positioning allows the tongue to move forward in some cases, improving the newborn's condition. If this intervention fails, a small (2.5-mm) ET tube may be inserted through the nose and advanced in the posterior pharynx behind the tongue but not past the vocal cords. In this case, the tube is not in the trachea. If resuscitation is needed, bag-mask ventilation and intubation are often very difficult. If an appropriately sized laryngeal airway is available, it can be inserted as a rescue device.[1]

NOTE

As a rule, oral airways are rarely indicated for airway control in newborns. However, in newborns with birth defects that affect the airway, an oral airway should be inserted. Examples include newborns with bilateral choanal atresia, Pierre Robin sequence, and unusual enlargement of the tongue (macroglossia). Newborns with these and other craniofacial defects are prone to airway obstruction and choking. They should not be placed supine.

Anomalies of the Heart

Congenital heart abnormalities refer to defects in the heart's structure (**FIGURE 46-14**). These defects occur during embryonic development and are present at birth (**BOX 46-7**). Congenital heart defects are the most common type of birth defect. They affect about 40,000 newborns, with 25% of these defects producing hemodynamic effects from altered cardiac function. About 1 million American children and 1.4 million adults live with a congenital heart abnormality.[36]

Causes of congenital heart defects are often unknown. Genetics may play a role in some heart defects. For example, a parent who has a congenital heart defect may be more likely than the average population to have a child with the condition. In rare cases, more than one child in a family is born with a heart defect. Children who have genetic disorders often have congenital heart defects. One-half of all babies who have Down syndrome have congenital heart defects. Smoking during pregnancy also has

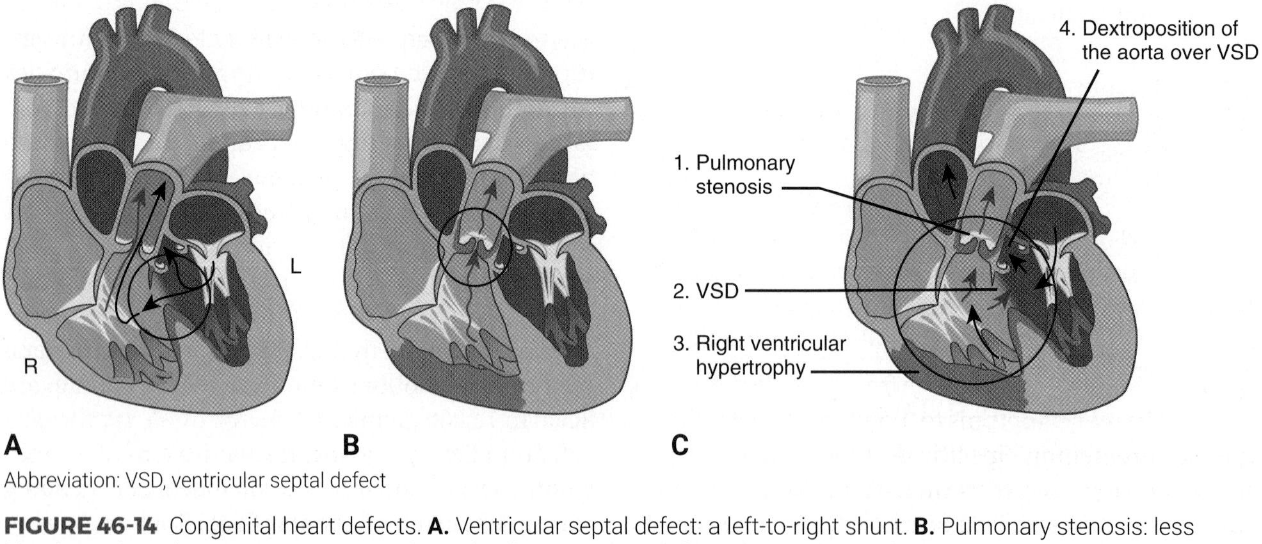

Abbreviation: VSD, ventricular septal defect

FIGURE 46-14 Congenital heart defects. **A.** Ventricular septal defect: a left-to-right shunt. **B.** Pulmonary stenosis: less blood into the pulmonary artery. **C.** Tetralogy of Fallot: a cyanotic defect with a right-to-left shunt.

BOX 46-7 Congenital Heart Defects

Congenital heart defects can be classified as critical and noncritical.

Critical Congenital Heart Defects

- Coarctation of the aorta
- Double outlet right ventricle
- Ebstein anomaly
- Hypoplastic left heart syndrome
- Interrupted aortic arch
- Pulmonary atresia
- Single ventricle
- Tetralogy of Fallot
- Total anomalous pulmonary venous return
- Transposition of the great arteries
- Tricuspid artresia
- Truncus ateriosus
- Other critical congenital heart defects requiring treatment in the first year of life

Noncritical Congenital Heart Defects

- Hemoglobinopathy
- Hypothermia
- Infection, including sepsis
- Lung disease (congenital or acquired)
- Noncritical congenital heart defect
- Persistent pulmonary hypertension
- Other hypoxic conditions not otherwise specified

Modified from: Division of Birth Defects and Developmental Disabilities, Centers for Disease Control and Prevention. Congenital heart defects (CHDs): information for healthcare providers. Centers for Disease Control and Prevention website. https://www.cdc.gov/ncbddd/heartdefects/hcp.html. Updated January 8, 2018. Accessed May 11, 2018.

been linked to several congenital heart defects,[37] including septal defects.[36] Other possible causes of congenital heart defects include maternal rubella and maternal ingestion of alcohol or other drugs and certain medications.[38]

Congenital heart defects can involve the interior walls of the heart, the heart valves, or the arteries and veins that carry blood to the heart and other body tissues. These defects can range from "simple defects" with no signs or symptoms to "complex defects" that are life threatening. Specific diseases discussed in this section include left-to-right shunt abnormalities, valvular defects, single-ventricle defects, transposition, and congenital dysrhythmias. Prehospital care for these patients may be limited to providing only comfort measures and transport to an appropriate medical facility. In some cases, complete support of vital functions will be needed. Babies who are born with congenital heart defects often require surgery within the first week of life. Additional surgeries may also be needed through adulthood. Medication therapy and long-term physician care are required.[39]

NOTE

Signs and symptoms of congenital heart defects depend on the number, type, and severity of the defects. In newborns, signs and symptoms may include tachypnea, cyanosis, poor circulation, and fatigue (eg, tiring easily when feeding). Older children who have congenital heart defects may tire easily or be short of breath during physical activity. In severe cases (and in adults), signs and symptoms of heart failure may develop. Congenital heart defects do not cause chest pain. A heart murmur may or may not be present and is not diagnostic. (Many healthy children have heart murmurs.)

Modified from: Johnson WH Jr, Moller JH. *Pediatric Cardiology: The Essential Pocket Guide*. Hoboken, NJ: John Wiley and Sons; 2014.

Left-to-Right Shunt

The most common physiology seen in patients with congenital heart disease involves a left-to-right shunt.[40] The physiologic effect of a left-to-right shunt is that oxygenated blood is shunted from the left (systemic) side to the right (pulmonary) side to be oxygenated again, creating a redundant circulation. This process leads to an increased venous return from the lungs, via the pulmonary veins, to the left atrium and the left ventricle. The associated volume overload on the left ventricle and the pulmonary circulation decreases cardiac output. Left-to-right shunts are classified according to their hemodynamic effects.

Coarctation of the Aorta. Coarctation of the aorta (CoA) is a narrowing or constriction of the aorta (**FIGURE 46-15**). The defect usually occurs at the point of curvature of the aorta just beyond where the arteries branch to the head and arms, close to where the ductus arteriosus attaches. (The ductus arteriosus is a blood vessel that is normally present in a fetus and that normally closes or contracts in the first hours of life.) Coarctation may be caused by the presence of extra ductal tissue that extends into the adjacent aorta, resulting in aortic

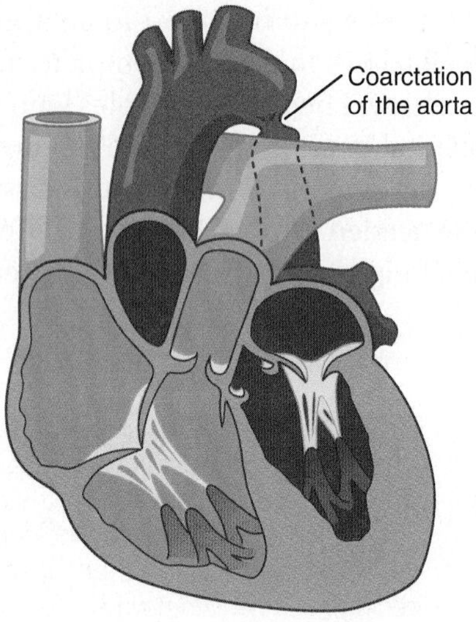

FIGURE 46-15 Coarctation of the aorta.

narrowing. Coarctation may also occur along with other cardiac defects, typically involving the left side of the heart (eg, left septal defect).[41] In the presence of a coarctation, the left ventricle has to work harder to force blood through the narrow segment of the aorta to the lower part of the body.

CoA is common in children with some chromosomal abnormalities, such as Turner syndrome.[42] Coarctation usually presents in the first month of life. It is suspected when the caregiver is unable to feel (or feels weak) pulses in the groin or the legs of a newborn or when the lower body is cyanotic. (A murmur may also be present.) Patients with CoA are at increased risk for hypertension, ruptured aorta, aortic aneurysm, and stroke.[43] Initially, the management may be focused on keeping the ductus open. Overall management is aimed at improving ventricular function and improving circulation to the lower extremities with various drugs. Surgical repair is frequently needed.

Septal Defects. Septal defects (a "hole in the heart") may involve the atrium or ventricle. With an **atrial septal defect (ASD)**, the opening between the heart's two upper chambers persists after birth. This condition lets some blood from the left atrium return via the hole to the right atrium instead of flowing through the left ventricle, out the aorta, and to the body. Many children with ASD have few, if any, symptoms.[44] Closing the atrial defect by open heart surgery in childhood can prevent serious problems later in life.

With a **ventricular septal defect (VSD)**, an opening exists between the heart's two lower chambers. Some blood that has returned from the lungs and been pumped into the left ventricle flows to the right ventricle through the hole instead of being pumped into the aorta. Because the heart has to pump extra blood and is overworked, the heart may become enlarged. Pulmonary hypertension also can develop. If a septal defect is large, surgery may be needed to close the hole. The hallmark of a septal defect is a loud heart murmur.[45]

Patent Ductus Arteriosus. Patent ductus arteriosus (PDA) allows blood to mix between the pulmonary artery and the aorta. As described previously, before birth an open passageway (the ductus arteriosus) exists between these two blood vessels. Normally this closes within a few hours of birth. When closure does not occur, some blood that should flow through the aorta and on to nourish the body returns to the lungs. (This condition is quite common in premature newborns but rather rare in full-term babies.[46]) If the ductus arteriosus is large, a child may become fatigued quickly, grow slowly, and be prone to pulmonary infection, especially pneumonia. If the ductus arteriosus is small, the child often seems healthy. Surgery is sometimes needed to close the ductus arteriosus and restore normal circulation. Some ductus arteriosus can be stimulated to close with nonsteroidal anti-inflammatory drugs or, more recently, acetaminophen.[47]

Truncus Arteriosus. Truncus arteriosus is a rare type of congenital heart disease. It is characterized by a large VSD over which a large, single great vessel (truncus) arises. It occurs when a single blood vessel (the truncus) arises from the right and left ventricles, instead of the normal two vessels (the pulmonary artery and the aorta).[48] This single great vessel carries blood both to the body and to the lungs. The truncus sits over a large opening or hole in the wall between the two pumping chambers (VSD). A decrease in peripheral vascular resistance at birth causes a left-to-right shunt with evidence of heart failure early in life. These children have a very high incidence of pulmonary hypertension and vascular disease.[49] Children with this defect may experience shortness of breath, decreased exercise endurance, and sometimes headaches and dizziness. Surgical repair is needed to close the VSD and separate blood flow to the body from blood flow to the lungs.

Valvular Defects

Some children are born with defective heart valves that occurred during embryonic development. These defects may present at birth or during childhood, or not become apparent until adulthood. Valvular heart disease is characterized by damage to or a defect in one of the four heart valves: the mitral, aortic, tricuspid, or pulmonary.

As described in Chapter 10, *Review of Human Systems*, the mitral and tricuspid valves control the flow of blood between the atria and the ventricles. The pulmonary valve controls the flow of blood from the heart to the lungs. The aortic valve governs blood flow between the heart and the aorta. The mitral and aortic valves are most frequently affected by valvular heart disease. Valves that function normally ensure that blood flows with proper force in the proper direction at the proper time. In valvular heart disease, the valves may become stenotic, preventing them from opening fully or completely closing (incompetent).[50]

A stenotic valve forces blood to back up in the adjacent heart chamber, whereas an incompetent valve allows blood to regurgitate (leak) back into the chamber it previously exited (**FIGURE 46-16**). To compensate for poor pumping action, the heart muscle enlarges and thickens, thereby losing elasticity and efficiency. In addition, in some cases, blood pooling in the chambers of the heart has a greater tendency to clot, increasing the risk of stroke or pulmonary embolism.[51]

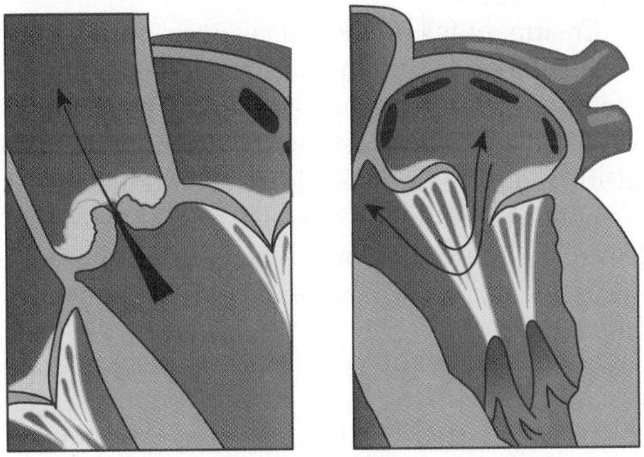

A B

FIGURE 46-16 Types of valve disease. **A.** Stenosis: valve does not open all the way, not enough blood passes through. **B.** Regurgitation: valve does not close all the way, blood leaks backwards.

The severity of valvular heart disease varies. In mild cases there may be no symptoms, whereas in advanced cases, valvular heart disease may lead to heart failure and other complications. Symptoms may be acute or develop slowly, and include palpitations, mild chest pain, fatigue, dizziness or fainting, fever (with bacterial endocarditis), and rapid weight gain. Treatment depends on the extent of the disease. Prehospital care is primarily supportive. Transport for physician evaluation is indicated.

Single-Ventricle Defects

Single-ventricle defects are complex and rare. They occur in the embryonic stage and result when one of the ventricles is underdeveloped. The most common types of single-ventricle defects are tricuspid atresia, pulmonary atresia, and hypoplastic left heart syndrome.[52] In the prehospital setting, standard resuscitation procedures should be followed in newborns, infants, and children with single-ventricle anatomy. It should be noted, however, that end-tidal carbon dioxide measurements in these children may not be a reliable indicator of CPR quality because in children with single-ventricle anatomy, pulmonary blood flow changes rapidly and will not always reflect cardiac output during CPR.[2,3] Modifications in the care of these patients will be provided in the in-hospital setting.

Tricuspid Atresia. **Tricuspid atresia** is the absence or abnormal development of a tricuspid valve. This condition prevents the normal flow of blood from the right atrium to the right ventricle and results in a right ventricle that is small and not fully developed. Ultimately, the blood cannot enter the lungs for oxygenation. The survival of these patients depends on the presence of an ASD and usually a VSD. Because there is no atrioventricular pathway, an ASD must be present to maintain blood flow. Likewise, because there is an underdeveloped right ventricle, there must be a way to pump blood into the pulmonary arteries through a VSD.[53] (A PDA is also usually formed to increase pulmonary flow.) Cyanosis and shortness of breath are usually present in these newborns until surgical repair is made. Surgery is required to repair the connection between the arteries to the body and the arteries to the lungs.

Pulmonary Atresia. In **pulmonary atresia**, no pulmonary valve exists. Blood cannot flow from the right ventricle into the pulmonary artery and on to the lungs. (The right ventricle and tricuspid valve also are often poorly developed.) In these patients, an opening in the atrial septum lets blood exit the right atrium, so low-oxygen blood mixes with the oxygen-rich blood in the left atrium. The left ventricle pumps this mixture of oxygen-poor blood into the aorta and out to the body. As a result, the newborn appears cyanotic. Often, the only source of blood flow to the lung is the PDA.[54] Surgical repair is required.

Hypoplastic Left Heart Syndrome. **Hypoplastic left heart syndrome** is a condition in which the heart's left side, including the aorta, aortic valve, left ventricle, and mitral valve, is underdeveloped. Blood returning from the lungs must flow through an opening in the wall between the atria (ASD). The right ventricle pumps the blood into the pulmonary artery, and blood reaches the aorta through a PDA. As with other single-ventricular defects, surgical repair is required.

Tetralogy of Fallot

Tetralogy of Fallot (ToF) is a rare congenital heart defect that affects about 1 out of every 2,518 babies born in the United States annually.[36] ToF involves four heart defects:

1. A large VSD
2. Pulmonary stenosis
3. Right ventricular hypertrophy
4. An overriding aorta

The VSD allows oxygen-rich blood from the left ventricle to mix with oxygen-poor blood from the right ventricle. Pulmonary stenosis causes the heart to work harder than normal to pump blood through the narrowed pulmonary valve, causing right ventricular hypertrophy. In ToF, the aorta is between the left and right ventricles (an overriding aorta), directly over the VSD. (In healthy hearts, the aorta is directly attached to the left ventricle.) As a result, oxygen-poor blood from the right ventricle flows directly into the aorta instead of into the pulmonary artery to the lungs. Together, these four defects prevent much of the blood from reaching the lungs for oxygenation. As a result, oxygen-poor blood flows out to the body, resulting in cyanosis. (Other signs and symptoms of ToF include a heart murmur, delayed growth and development, and clubbing of the fingers.) Although the cause of the defect is often unknown, contributing factors that may occur during pregnancy include the following:[55]

- German measles (rubella) and some other viral illnesses
- Poor nutrition
- Alcohol use
- Age (mother older than 40 years)
- Diabetes mellitus

Heredity may also play a role in causing ToF. An adult who has ToF is at an increased risk of having a baby with the condition. Children who have certain genetic disorders, such as Down syndrome and DiGeorge syndrome, often have congenital heart defects, including ToF. Surgical repair of the four defects is required early in life. Babies who have unrepaired ToF sometimes have hypoxic "tet spells" (a sudden drop in blood oxygen).[56] When blood oxygen levels rapidly drop, severe cyanosis (variable) can develop, often in response to an activity such as crying, feeding, or having a bowel movement. In acute hypoxic episodes, the baby may have shortness of breath; may be limp, unresponsive to voice or touch, or irritable; or may lose consciousness. Tet spells are potentially lethal and unpredictable.[57]

Treatment for prolonged cyanosis during a tet spell includes having the parent hold the child to attempt to calm him or her. The child's knees should be tucked up under him or her to decrease vascular return and increase systemic vascular resistance. If the child is supine, the knees should be flexed up toward the chest. Oxygen is unlikely to help because the problem is caused by a reduction of pulmonary blood flow.[58]

Transposition of the Great Arteries

In a healthy heart, the aorta and pulmonary artery are properly positioned and aligned with the appropriate ventricle. If this positioning is reversed (transposed), the aorta arises from the right ventricle and the pulmonary artery from the left ventricle. This congenital heart defect is known as **transposition of the great arteries (TGA)**. TGA results in the systemic and pulmonary circulations being in parallel rather than in series.[59] As a result, oxygen-poor blood returning from the body to the right atrium and right ventricle is pumped out to the aorta and to the body. Oxygen-rich blood returning from the lungs to the left atrium and ventricle is sent back to the lungs via the pulmonary artery. Like other heart defects, survival of these patients before surgical repair depends on the presence of an ASD, a VSD, and/or a PDA. TGA was once considered a fatal disease with 90% mortality in the first year. Today with treatment, the survival rate is greater than 90%.[60]

Total Anomalous Pulmonary Venous Return

Total anomalous pulmonary venous return (TAPVR) is a congenital heart defect in which the four pulmonary veins that carry oxygen-rich blood back to the heart from the lungs are not properly attached to the left atrium. Instead, they are improperly attached to another area (usually the superior vena cava). With this defect, oxygen-rich blood that should return to the left atrium—and then the left ventricle, the aorta, and the body—instead mixes with the oxygen-poor blood flowing into the right side of the heart. In other words, blood simply circles to and from the lungs, and never to the body.

To survive before corrective surgery, a large ASD or patent foramen ovale (a passage between the left and right atria) must exist to allow oxygenated blood to flow to the left side of the heart and the rest of the body. Newborns with TAPVR may appear critically ill with the following symptoms:[61]

- Lethargy
- Poor feeding
- Rapid breathing
- Poor growth
- Frequent respiratory tract infections
- Cyanosis

Congenital Dysrhythmias

Many children born with congenital heart disease now live well into adulthood. Although dysrhythmias can develop within any of these groups, the incidence is highest for patients in the moderate and severe categories.

Malfunctions in embryonic development that are responsible for congenital heart defects can directly impact the development of the heart's conduction system (especially displacement of the atrioventricular node and bundle of His).[62] This makes these patients more vulnerable to many dysrhythmias, including atrial fibrillation, atrial flutter, reentry tachycardia, and heart blocks. Standards of care for patients with dysrhythmias that result from congenital heart disease follow the same treatments guidelines as for other children (see Chapter 47, *Pediatrics*).

Anomalies of the Abdomen and Lower Back

Several abdominal and lower back anomalies can occur during embryonic development, including (among others) intestinal malrotation, pyloric stenosis, diaphragmatic hernia, abdominal wall defects, and spina bifida.

Intestinal Malrotation

Intestinal malrotation is caused by abnormal rotation of the intestine around the superior mesenteric artery during embryonic development. It is a congenital defect that can cause a serious bowel obstruction. The condition occurs in about 1 in every 500 live births.[63] Malrotation is commonly seen with other birth defects, such as omphalocele, diaphragmatic hernia, and Hirschsprung disease (a disorder of the distal colon that causes functional obstruction). The condition usually becomes evident within the first week of life; 90% of cases are diagnosed within the first 12 months.[64] The illness may be acute or chronic. The primary presenting sign in acute malrotation is emesis that contains bile (bilious emesis). This condition is a surgical emergency.

Features of chronic malrotation include recurrent bouts of abdominal pain and diarrhea (alternating with constipation), intolerance of solid food, jaundice, lower gastrointestinal tract bleeding, and gastroesophageal reflux. If symptoms persist, shock may develop, including poor perfusion, decreased urine output, and hypotension. Malrotation requires surgical repair.

Pyloric Stenosis

Pyloric stenosis is narrowing of the pylorus (the opening from the stomach into the small intestine). It is the most common cause of intestinal obstruction in the newborn or infant.[65] The narrowing occurs from muscles around the pylorus that have grown too

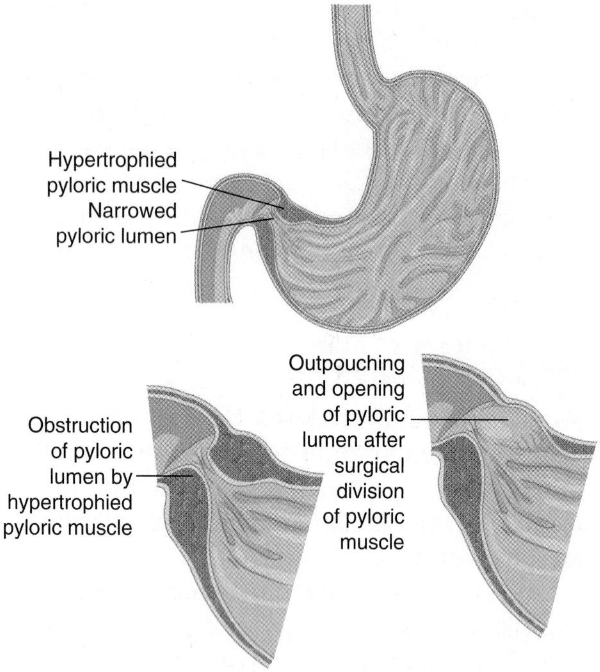

FIGURE 46-17 In pyloric stenosis, the pyloric muscle hypertrophies and obstructs the passage of stomach contents into the intestines.

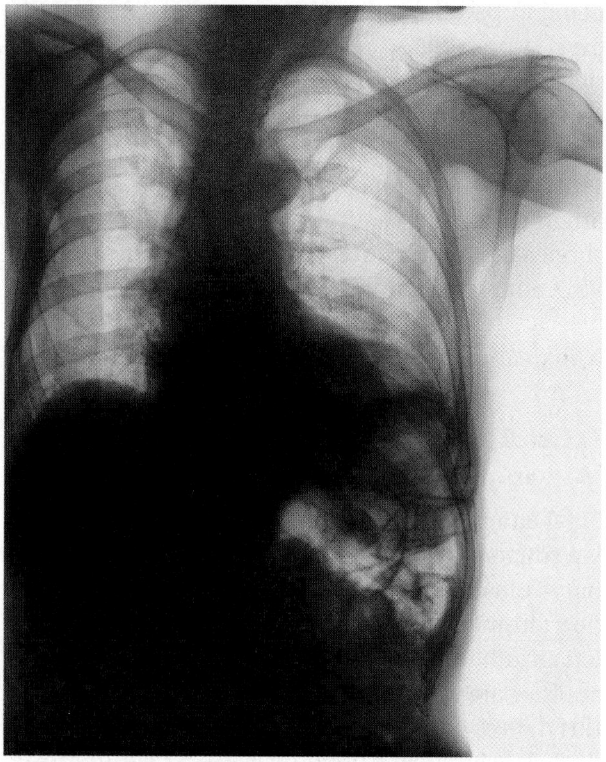

FIGURE 46-18 Left-side congenital diaphragmatic hernia. Note the loops of bowel present in the thoracic cavity.

large (**FIGURE 46-17**). The diagnosis is usually made when the baby presents with a history of progressive, forceful vomiting. This usually begins within the second or third week of life. Parents may complain that the baby is "spitting up" more. They often have tried a different formula in formula-fed babies without any change being noted. Signs and symptoms are related to dehydration and may include dry mucous membranes, slow capillary refill, sunken fontanels, and decreased urine output (dry diapers for several hours). After diagnosis, surgery will be required to dilate the muscles around the pyloric valve of the stomach.

Diaphragmatic Hernia

Diaphragmatic hernia is caused by the malformation of the diaphragm during fetal development. Diaphragmatic hernia may occur on the right, left, or both sides, but the left side is most common. It results from a defect (hole) in the diaphragm muscle. The opening allows abdominal organs, such as the stomach, bowel, liver, and spleen, to enter the chest cavity (**FIGURE 46-18**). As a result, the lung on the affected side does not develop normally (**pulmonary hypoplasia**), reducing lung capacity. Other organs can be damaged as well, including the heart. A significant prenatal shift in the mediastinum may indicate some degree of pulmonary hypoplasia on the contralateral side.[66] The newborn's head and thorax should be elevated to assist with downward displacement of the abdominal organs. Immediate intubation is indicated to prevent the air-filled stomach from compressing the lung further.

In the case of diaphragmatic hernia, respiratory distress usually develops shortly after birth. Other symptoms include cyanosis that is unresponsive to ventilations, tachypnea, and tachycardia. On examination, the newborn may have irregular chest wall movement, displaced heart sounds, decreased breath sounds on the affected side (mimicking pneumothorax), and bowel sounds in the chest cavity.[67] In addition, the abdomen may be scaphoid (flat). Medical direction may recommend placement of an orogastric tube (see Chapter 47, *Pediatrics*), with low periodic suction to decompress the stomach and to improve ventilation.[68] In most cases, tracheal intubation is needed. The use of a bag-mask device with positive pressure ventilation is not recommended because it may cause gastric distention and worsen the condition.[69] Intubation should be performed as soon as possible. Surgery is required to repair the hernia and to place the abdominal organs in their normal location. If the condition is diagnosed during pregnancy, fetal surgery may be indicated.

Abdominal Wall Defects

Congenital abdominal wall defects are among the more common neonatal surgical conditions and comprise both gastroschisis and omphalocele. Although the two conditions are considered similar and have some overlap and management, they are distinct conditions.[70]

Gastroschisis is a relatively uncommon condition that occurs in approximately 1 in 5,000 live births.[71] The defect occurs early in gestation and is characterized by an opening in the abdominal wall of the fetus. The opening allows the intestine and other abdominal organs to herniate through the abdominal wall and to spill out into the amniotic fluid around the fetus (**FIGURE 46-19**). This opening is usually found to the right of the naval where the unprotected intestine becomes irritated, causing it to swell and shorten. Gastroschisis occurs more often in babies born to younger mothers. For unknown reasons, the incidence of gastroschisis is increasing worldwide.[72]

An **omphalocele** is caused by different errors in fetal development. It occurs when the intestines do not recede back into the abdomen, but remain in the umbilical cord (**FIGURE 46-20**). The defect affects about 2 in every 10,300 live births. Up to 25% to 40% of newborns with an omphalocele will have another (often more serious) congenital anomaly.[29]

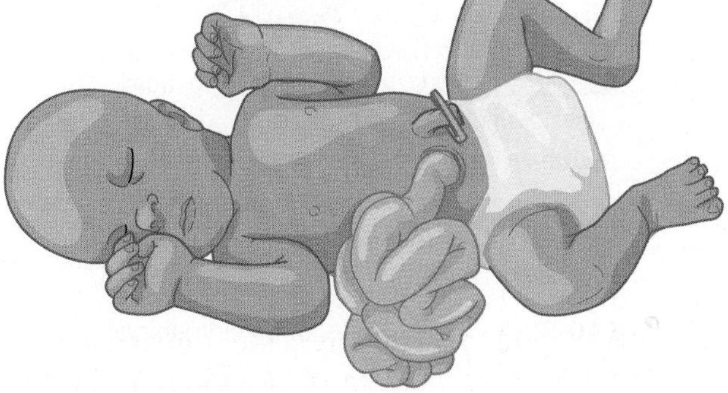

FIGURE 46-19 Gastroschisis.

Reproduced from Centers for Disease Control and Prevention. National Center on Birth Defects and Developmental Disabilities.

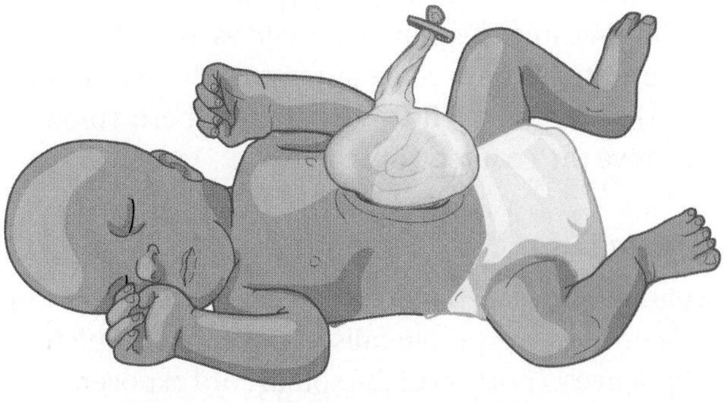

FIGURE 46-20 Omphalocele in membranous sac.

Reproduced from Centers for Disease Control and Prevention. National Center on Birth Defects and Developmental Disabilities.

The omphalocele usually is first seen on ultrasonography during prenatal care.

Both gastroschisis and omphaloceles will often be visible at birth. With gastroschisis, there is no sac or amnion that covers the viscera and protects it from the amniotic fluid as seen with an omphalocele. Omphalocele size has much more variability and the location on the abdomen may differ (epigastric, umbilical, or hypogastric). A ruptured omphalocele can be difficult to differentiate from a gastroschisis. Sterile drapes and gloves should be used during resuscitation. The newborn should be placed on his or her side to prevent kinking of the bowel loops.[73] Exposed tissue should be protected and covered with moist (soaked in warm normal saline or sterile water), sterile gauze pads immediately after birth to prevent injury and infection.

NOTE

An umbilical cord that appears unusually large in diameter should be examined for the presence of a small omphalocele before it is clamped and cut as part of the delivery process. If suspected, the cord should not be clamped or cut. The paramedic should consult with medical direction.

Modified from: Mirza B, Ali W. Distinct presentations of hernia of umbilical cord. *J Neonatal Surg*. 2016;5(4):53.

Simple abdominal wall defects are usually successfully repaired with surgery. Complicated defects have a much higher morbidity and mortality.[70] As part of the surgery, the exposed tissues will be covered and held in place with a special plastic pouch (silo) that over time squeezes the exposed tissue back into the newborn's abdomen. Surgical repair of the newborn's abdominal muscles may be needed as well. The tissue will eventually be covered by the growth of surrounding skin, after which surgery can be performed to improve the cosmetic outcome.

Spina Bifida

Spina bifida is a congenital defect in which part of one or more vertebrae fails to develop completely. This leaves a portion of the spinal cord exposed. The condition can occur anywhere on the spine. However, it is most common in the lower back. Each year, about 1,500 babies are born with spina bifida.[74] It is more likely to occur with extremes of maternal age. A woman who has given birth to one child with spina bifida is 10 times more likely than the average woman to give birth to another affected child (indicating the need for genetic counseling). The incidence of both anencephaly and spina bifida have decreased by 20% to 30% since the 1990s, when the US Public Health Service began to recommend that women of childbearing age and pregnant women take folic acid supplements, and the Food and Drug Administration required all grain products labeled as enriched have folic acid added to them.[74]

The severity of spina bifida depends on how much nerve tissue is exposed after the neural tube has closed. The four types of spina bifida are spina bifida occulta, meningocele, myelomeningocele, and encephalocele. Currently, the condition has no cure. Treatment includes surgery, medications, and physical therapy. Most patients with spina bifida live into adulthood.

Spina bifida occulta is the most common and least serious form. There is little external evidence of the defect. Meningocele (**FIGURE 46-21**) is a type of spina bifida in which the nerve tissue of the spinal cord usually is intact and covered with a membranous sac of skin. Meningocele usually does not cause functional problems. However, it requires surgical repair early in life. Myelomeningocele (Figure 46-21) is the severest form of spina bifida. The child often is severely handicapped. This type of spina bifida is marked by a raw swelling over the spine and a malformed spinal cord that may or may not be contained in a membranous sac. The legs of these children often are deformed. Also, the condition causes partial or complete paralysis and loss of sensation in all areas below the level of the defect. Associated abnormalities of myelomeningocele include hydrocephalus (excess cerebrospinal fluid in the skull) with brain damage, cerebral palsy, epilepsy, and developmental delay. In the fourth and very rare type of spina bifida, encephalocele, the protrusion occurs through the skull. Severe brain damage is common with this condition.

At delivery, the defect should be covered with sterile gauze soaked in sterile normal saline. The newborn should be resuscitated and handled using nonlatex sterile gloves.

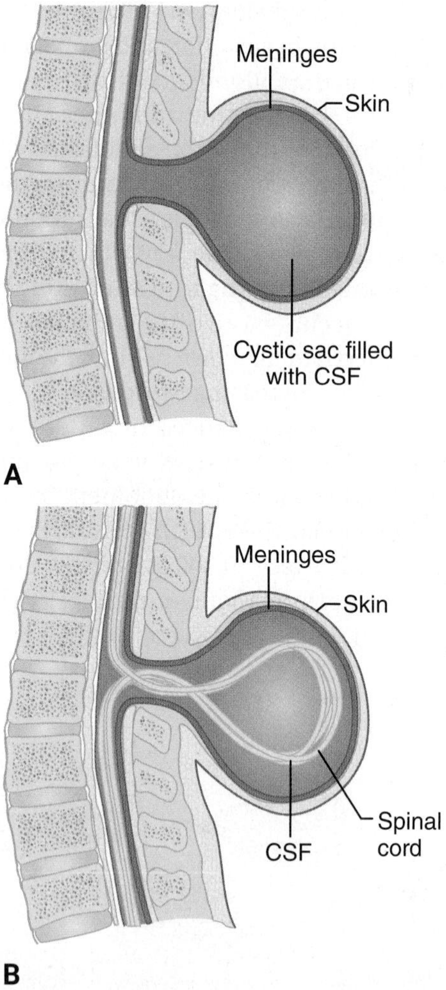

Abbreviation: CSF, cerebrospinal fluid

FIGURE 46-21 **A.** Meningocele. **B.** Myelomeningocele.

Summary

- Low birth weight, prematurity, and a variety of antepartum and intrapartum risk factors affect the need for resuscitation.
- Some of the more common congenital anomalies include choanal atresia, tracheobronchial fistula and atresia, Pierre Robin sequence, cleft lip and cleft palate, congenital heart anomalies, pyloric stenosis, diaphragmatic hernia, omphalocele, and spina bifida.
- At birth, newborns make three major physiologic adaptations necessary for survival: (1) emptying fluids from their lungs and beginning ventilation, (2) changing their circulatory pattern, and (3) maintaining body temperature.
- The initial steps of neonatal resuscitation (except for those born through meconium) are to prevent heat loss, clear the airway by positioning and suctioning, if needed provide tactile stimulation and initiate breathing if necessary, and further evaluate the newborn to ensure adequate ventilation.
- If neonatal resuscitation is needed, the paramedic should reevaluate the initial steps of stabilization (warm, position, clear airway, dry, stimulate, reposition). If there is no change, resuscitation proceeds in 30-second increments with ventilation, chest compressions, and, if needed, epinephrine administration.
- The three most common complications during the postresuscitation period are endotracheal tube position change (including dislodgment), tube occlusion by mucus or meconium, and pneumothorax. During transport of the newborn, it is important to maintain body temperature, oxygen administration, and ventilatory support.
- Specific situations that may require advanced life support for the newborn include meconium staining, apnea, diaphragmatic hernia, bradycardia, premature newborns, respiratory distress and cyanosis, hypovolemia, seizures, fever, hypothermia, hypoglycemia, vomiting and diarrhea, and birth injuries.
- Primary apnea is common immediately after birth and is self-limiting, resolved by tactile stimulation. Secondary apnea is a pause in breathing that exceeds 20 seconds; this condition requires ventilatory support.
- Bradycardia is a heart rate of less than 100 beats/min. It is most often caused by hypoxia. Positive pressure ventilation must be initiated for bradycardia.
- Premature newborns have an increased risk of respiratory suppression, hypothermia, and head and brain injury. In addition to low birth weight, various antepartum and intrapartum risk factors may affect the need for resuscitation.
- Prematurity is the most common cause of respiratory distress in the newborn.
- Hypovolemia in newborns may result from dehydration, hemorrhage, trauma, or sepsis.
- Seizures in the newborn signal an underlying abnormality.
- A temperature greater than 100.4°F (38°C) in a newborn is a fever and often signals viral or bacterial infection.
- Hypothermia is a core body temperature below 95°F (35°C). It increases metabolic demand and can cause metabolic acidosis, pulmonary hypertension, and hypoxemia.
- A blood glucose level of less than 40 mg/dL indicates hypoglycemia in the newborn.
- Injuries at birth may include cranial trauma, intracranial hemorrhage or brain injury, spine and spinal cord injury, peripheral nerve injury, spleen or liver injuries, fractures, or soft-tissue injury.
- The paramedic should be aware of the normal feelings and reactions of parents, siblings, other family members, and caregivers while providing emergency care to an ill or injured child.
- Specific situations may call for advanced life support for the newborn. These situations include apnea, bradycardia, respiratory distress and cyanosis, hypovolemia, seizures, fever, hypothermia, hypoglycemia, vomiting and diarrhea, newborn jaundice, sepsis, and common birth injuries.
- Congenital anomalies may be heritable; caused by maternal infection, alcohol, or other drug use during pregnancy (teratogens); and other factors. Anomalies that the paramedic may encounter include disorders of the airway, heart, and abdomen and lower back.

References

1. Weiner GM, Zaichkin J, eds. *Textbook of Neonatal Resuscitation.* 7th ed. Elk Grove, IL: American Academy of Pediatrics and American Heart Association; 2016.
2. Preterm (Premature) Labor and Birth. FAQ087. American College of Obstetricians and Gynecologists website. https://www.acog.org/Patients/FAQs/Preterm-Premature-Labor-and-Birth. Published November 2016. Accessed May 10, 2018.
3. What are the risk factors for preterm labor and birth? National Institutes of Health website. https://www.nichd.nih.gov/health/topics/preterm/conditioninfo/who_risk. Reviewed January 31, 2017. Accessed May 10, 2018.
4. Glass HC, Costarino AT, Stayer SA, Brett C, Cladis F, Davis PJ. Outcomes for extremely premature infants. *Anesth Analg.* 2015;120(6):1337-1351.
5. Chiocca EM. *Advanced Pediatric Assessment.* Baltimore, Maryland: LWW Publishing; 2011.
6. Wyckoff MH, Aziz K, Escobedo MB, et al. Part 13: Neonatal Resuscitation. 2015 American Heart Association Guidelines Update for Cardiopulmonary Resuscitation and Emergency Cardiovascular Care. *Circulation.* 2015;132:S543-S560.

7. Walls R, Hockberger R, Gausche-Hill M. *Rosen's Emergency Medicine: Concepts and Clinical Practice*. 9th ed. St. Louis, MO: Elsevier; 2017.
8. Hooper SB, Polglase GR, Roehr CC. Cardiopulmonary changes with aeration of the newborn lung. *Paediatr Respir Rev*. 2015;16(3):147-150.
9. Helping Babies Breathe. American Academy of Pediatrics website. https://www.aap.org/en-us/advocacy-and-policy/aap-health-initiatives/helping-babies-survive/Pages/Helping-Babies-Breathe.aspx. Accessed May 11, 2018.
10. American Heart Association. *2015 Handbook of Emergency Cardiovascular Care for Healthcare Providers*. Dallas, TX: American Heart Association; 2015.
11. Rodríguez-Fernandez V, Nicolas López C, Cajal R, Marin-Ortiz E, Couceiro-Naveira E. Intrapartum and perinatal results associated with different degrees of staining of meconium stained amniotic fluid. *Euro J Obstet Gynecol Reprod Biol*. 2018. https://doi.org/10.1016/j.ejogrb.2018.03.035.
12. Reed C. *Neonatal Resuscitation Program, 2015*. 7th ed. Elk Grove, IL: American Academy of Pediatrics; 2015.
13. Bansal SC, Dempsey E, Trevisanuto D, Roehr CC. The laryngeal mask airway and its use in neonatal resuscitation: a critical review of where we are in 2017/2018. *Neonatology*. 2018;113(2):152-161.
14. American Heart Association. *Pediatric Advanced Life Support*. Dallas, TX: American Heart Association; 2007.
15. American Academy of Pediatrics. *Pediatric Education for Prehospital Professionals (PEPP)*. 3rd ed. Burlington, MA: Jones and Bartlett Learning; 2014.
16. Rocker JA. Pediatric apnea. Medscape website. https://emedicine.medscape.com/article/800032-overview?pa=7E%2FcuUB0nk%2BHE9%2Fa9CZSRJIUlZ1xl0TinLezUNCBYg3Xm6RdvO2OCkBb%2B%2BXhVb7XLCEJNCrbkqLWYvqLrhntWA%3D%3D. Updated February 13, 2018. Accessed May 11, 2018.
17. Elzouki AY, Harfi HA. *Textbook of Clinical Pediatrics*. 2nd ed. Berlin, Germany: Springer; 2012.
18. Reuter S, Moser C, Baack M. Respiratory distress in the newborn. *Pediatr Rev*. 2014;35(10):417-428.
19. Sheth RD. Neonatal seizures medication. Medscape website. https://emedicine.medscape.com/article/1177069-medication#1. Updated September 6, 2017. Accessed May 11, 2018.
20. Simonsen KA, Anderson-Berry AL, Delair SF, Davies HD. Early-onset neonatal sepsis. *Clin Microbiol Rev*. 2014;27(1):21-47.
21. Gleason CA, Devaskar S. *Avery's Diseases of the Newborn*. 9th ed. St. Louis, MO: Elsevier; 2012.
22. Santhanam S. Pediatric sepsis. Medscape website. https://emedicine.medscape.com/article/972559-overview. Updated August 21, 2017. Accessed May 11, 2018.
23. Parashette KR, Croffie J. Vomiting. *Pediatr Rev*. 2013;34(7):307-319.
24. Ullah S, Rahman K, Hedayati M. Hyperbilirubinemia in neonates: types, causes, clinical examinations, preventive measures and treatments: a narrative review article. *Iran J Public Health*. 2016;45(5):558-568.
25. Centers for Disease Control and Prevention. Facts about jaundice and kernicterus. Centers for Disease Control and Prevention website. https://www.cdc.gov/ncbddd/jaundice/facts.html. Updated February 23, 2015. Accessed May 11, 2018.
26. Murray SS, McKinney ES. *Foundations of Maternal-Newborn and Women's Health Nursing*. 6th ed. Philadelphia, PA: Saunders; 2018.
27. McKee-Garrett TM. Neonatal birth injuries. UpToDate website. https://www.uptodate.com/contents/neonatal-birth-injuries. Updated October 31, 2017. Accessed May 11, 2018.
28. Vinturache AE, McDonald S, Slater D, Tough S. Perinatal outcomes of maternal overweight and obesity in term infants: a population-based cohort study in Canada. *Sci Rep*. 2015;5:9334.
29. Division of Birth Defects and Developmental Disabilities, NCBDDD, Centers for Disease Control and Prevention. Birth defects: data and statistics. Centers for Disease Control and Prevention website. https://www.cdc.gov/ncbddd/birthdefects/data.html. Updated April 30, 2018. Accessed May 11, 2018.
30. Overview of birth defects. Stanford Children's Health website. http://www.stanfordchildrens.org/en/topic/default?id=overview-of-birth-defects-90-P02113. Accessed May 11, 2018.
31. Hall BD. Factsheet about choanal atresia or stenosis. Charge Syndrome Foundation website. https://www.chargesyndrome.org/factsheet-about-choanal-atresia-or-stenosis/. Accessed May 11, 2018.
32. Division of Birth Defects and Developmental Disabilities, NCBDDD, Centers for Disease Control and Prevention. Birth defects: facts about esophageal atresia. Centers for Disease Control and Prevention website. https://www.cdc.gov/ncbddd/birthdefects/esophagealatresia.html. Updated December 4, 2017. Accessed May 11, 2018.
33. Cleft lip and palate. National Institute of Dental and Craniofacial Research website. https://www.nidcr.nih.gov/health-info/cleft-lip-palate/more-info. Reviewed February 2018. Accessed May 11, 2018.
34. Isolated Pierre Robin sequence. Genetics Home Reference website. https://ghr.nlm.nih.gov/condition/isolated-pierre-robin-sequence#statistics. Reviewed December 2016. Accessed May 11, 2018.
35. Kaiser G. *Symptoms and Signs in Pediatric Surgery*. Berlin, Germany: Springer; 2012.
36. Division of Birth Defects and Developmental Disabilities, Centers for Disease Control and Prevention. Congenital heart defects (CHDs): information for healthcare providers. Centers for Disease Control and Prevention website. https://www.cdc.gov/ncbddd/heartdefects/hcp.html. Updated January 8, 2018. Accessed May 11, 2018.
37. Bergstrom S, Carr H, Petersson G, et al. Trends in congenital heart defects in infants with Down syndrome. *Pediatrics*. 2016;138(1):e20160123.
38. Congenital heart defects (CHDs). American Pregnancy Association website. http://americanpregnancy.org/birth-defects/congenital-heart-defects/. Accessed May 11, 2018.
39. Understanding congenital heart defects into adulthood. American College of Cardiology website. https://www.cardiosmart.org/Heart-Conditions/Congenital-Heart-Defects/Content/Adult-CHD. Accessed May 15, 2018.
40. Yun SW. Congenital heart disease in the newborn requiring early intervention. *Korean J Pediatr*. 2011;54(5):183-191.
41. Coarctation of the aorta. Cincinnati Children's website. https://www.cincinnatichildrens.org/health/c/coarctation. Accessed May 15, 2018.

42. Shankar RK, Backeljauw PF. Current best practice in the management of Turner syndrome. *Ther Adv Endocrinol Metab*. 2018;9(1):33-40.
43. Hockenberry M, Wilson D. *Wong's Nursing Care of Infants and Children*. 10th ed. New York, NY: Elsevier; 2015:1251-1285.
44. Atrial septal defect (ASD). American Heart Association website. http://www.heart.org/HEARTORG/Conditions/Congenital-HeartDefects/AboutCongenitalHeartDefects/Atrial-Septal-Defect-ASD_UCM_307021_Article.jsp. Accessed May 11, 2018.
45. Ventricular septal defect (VSD). American Heart Association website. http://www.heart.org/HEARTORG/Conditions/CongenitalHeartDefects/AboutCongenitalHeartDefects/Ventricular-Septal-Defect-VSD_UCM_307041_Article.jsp. Accessed May 11, 2018.
46. Artman M, Mahony L, Teitel DF. *Neonatal Cardiology*. 3rd ed. New York, NY: McGraw-Hill Education; 2017.
47. Mehta SK, Younoszai A, Pietz J, Achanti BP. Pharmacological closure of the patent ductus arteriosus. *Paediatr Cardiol*. 2003;5(1):1-15.
48. Facts about truncus arteriosus. Centers for Disease Control and Prevention website. https://www.cdc.gov/ncbddd/heartdefects/truncusarteriosus.html. Accessed May 15, 2018.
49. Dimopoulos K, Wort SJ, Gatzoulis MA. Pulmonary hypertension related to congenital heart disease: a call for action. *Eur Heart J*. 2014;35(11):691-700.
50. Heart and Vascular Institute. Valvular heart disease. Johns Hopkins Medicine website. https://www.hopkinsmedicine.org/heart_vascular_institute/conditions_treatments/conditions/valvular_heart_disease.html. Accessed May 11, 2018.
51. Papadakis MA, McPhee SJ, Rabow MW. *Current Medical Diagnosis and Treatment*. New York, NY: McGraw-Hill; 2017.
52. Critical congenital heart disease. Genetics Home Reference website. https://ghr.nlm.nih.gov/condition/critical-congenital-heart-disease. Accessed May 11, 2018.
53. Butany J, Buja ML (eds). *Cardiovascular Pathology*. 4th ed. New York, NY: Elsevier; 2016.
54. Pulmonary atresia/intact ventricular septum. American Heart Association website. http://www.heart.org/idc/groups/heart-public/@wcm/@hcm/documents/downloadable/ucm_307665.pdf. Accessed May 15, 2018.
55. Tetralogy of Fallot. National Heart, Lung, and Blood Institute website. https://www.nhlbi.nih.gov/health-topics/tetralogy-fallot. Accessed May 11, 2018.
56. Tetralogy of Fallot. University of California San Francisco website. https://pediatricct.surgery.ucsf.edu/conditions--procedures/tetralogy-of-fallot.aspx. Accessed May 15, 2018.
57. Bhimji S. Tetralogy of Fallot clinical presentation. Medscape website. https://emedicine.medscape.com/article/2035949-clinical. Updated December 21, 2017. Accessed May 11, 2018.
58. Bhimji S. Tetralogy of Fallot treatment and management. Medscape website. https://emedicine.medscape.com/article/2035949-treatment#d11. Updated December 21, 2017. Accessed May 11, 2018.
59. Frescura C, Thiene G. The spectrum of congenital heart disease with transposition of the great arteries from the Cardiac Registry of the University of Padua. *Front Pediatr*. 2016;4:84.
60. Charpie JR. Transposition of the great arteries. Medscape website. https://emedicine.medscape.com/article/900574-overview. Updated April 11, 2017. Accessed May 11, 2018.
61. Division of Birth Defects and Developmental Disabilities, Centers for Disease Control and Prevention. Facts about total anomalous pulmonary venous return or TAPVR. Centers for Disease Control and Prevention website. https://www.cdc.gov/ncbddd/heartdefects/tapvr.html. Updated September 26, 2016. Accessed May 11, 2018.
62. Fuster V, Walsh RA, Harrington RA. *Hurst's The Heart*. 13th ed. New York, NY: McGraw-Hill; 2011.
63. Nath J, Corder A. Delayed presentation of familial intestinal malrotation with volvulus in two adult siblings. *Ann R Coll Surg Engl*. 2012;94(6):e191-e192.
64. Husberg B, Salehi K, Peters T, et al. Congenital intestinal malrotation in adolescent and adult patients: a 12-year clinical and radiological survey. *SpringerPlus*. 2016;5:245.
65. Subramaniam S. Pediatric pyloric stenosis. Medscape website. https://emedicine.medscape.com/article/803489-overview. Updated October 24, 2017. Accessed May 11, 2018.
66. Hedrick HL, Adzick S. Congenital diaphragmatic hernia in the neonate. UpToDate website. https://www.uptodate.com/contents/congenital-diaphragmatic-hernia-in-the-neonate?search=diaphragmatic%20hernia&source=search_result&selectedTitle=1~88&usage_type=default&display_rank=1. Updated April 4, 2014. Accessed May 11, 2018.
67. Vyas PK, Godbole C, Bindroo SK, Mathur RS, Akula B, Doctor N. Case-based discussion: an unusual manifestation of diaphragmatic hernia mimicking pneumothorax in an adult male. *Int J Emerg Med*. 2016;9(1):11.
68. Steinhorn RH. Pediatric congenital diaphragmatic hernia treatment and management. Medscape website. https://emedicine.medscape.com/article/978118-treatment. Updated April 25, 2014. Accessed May 11, 2018.
69. Kumar VHS. Current concepts in the management of congenital diaphragmatic hernia in infants. *Indian J Surg*. 2015;77(4):313-321.
70. Islam S, Gollin G, Koehler S, Wagner AJ. Gastroschisis. Pediatric Surgery Library website. https://www.pedsurglibrary.com/apsa/view/Pediatric-Surgery-NaT/829060/all/Gastroschisis. Updated March 19, 2018. Accessed May 11, 2018.
71. Gastroschisis. Children's Hospital of Philadelphia website. http://www.chop.edu/conditions-diseases/gastroschisis. Accessed May 11, 2018.
72. Centers for Disease Control and Prevention. Increasing prevalence of gastroschisis—14 states, 1995–2012. *Morb Mortal Wkly Rep*. 2016;65(2):23-26.
73. Gardner S, Carter BS, Hines ME, Hernandez JA. *Merenstein and Gardner's Handbook of Neonatal Intensive Care*. 8th ed. St. Louis, MO: Elsevier; 2016.
74. National Center on Birth Defects and Developmental Disabilities, Centers for Disease Control and Prevention. Spina bifida: data and statistics. Centers for Disease Control and Prevention website. https://www.cdc.gov/ncbddd/spinabifida/data.html. Updated December 21, 2017. Accessed May 11, 2018.

Suggested Readings

Bansal SC, Caoci S, Dempsey E, Trevisanuto D, Roehr CC. The laryngeal mask airway and its use in neonatal resuscitation: a critical review of where we are in 2017/2018. *Neonatology*. 2018;113(2):152-161.

Children's Hospital and Medical Center. Neonatal emergencies and transport. Semantic Scholar website. https://pdfs.semanticscholar.org/presentation/785e/c791aeeb7bea40a17948cdf6b5e2f52bdf0b.pdf. Accessed May 11, 2018.

Cloherty JP, Eichenwald EC, Hansen AR, Stark AR. *Manual of Neonatal Care*. 7th ed. New York, NY: Lippincott; 2016.

Collopy KT. Prehospital stabilization of unstable neonates. EMS World website. https://www.emsworld.com/article/12088865/prehospital-stabilization-of-unstable-neonates. Published July 1, 2015. Accessed May 11, 2018.

Duby R, Hansen M, Meckler G, Skarica B, Lambert W, Guise J-M. Safety events in high risk prehospital neonatal calls. *Prehosp Emerg Care*. 2018;22(1). https://doi.org/10.1080/10903127.2017.1347222.

Liberman RF, Getz KD, Lin AE, et al. Delayed diagnosis of critical congenital heart defects: trends and associated factors. *Pediatrics*. 2014;134(2). http://pediatrics.aappublications.org/content/134/2/e373. Accessed May 11, 2018.

Payne E. A brief history of advances in neonatal care. Neonatal Intensive Care Unit Awareness website. https://www.nicuawareness.org/blog/a-brief-history-of-advances-in-neonatal-care. Published January 5, 2016. Accessed May 11, 2018.

Pierro M, Ciralli F, Colnaghi M, et al. Oxygen administration at birth in preterm infants: a retrospective analysis. *J Matern Fetal Neonatal Med*. 2016;29(16):2675-2680.

Tappero EP, Honeyfield ME. *Physical Assessment of the Newborn: A Comprehensive Approach to the Art of Physical Examination*. 5th ed. Berlin, Germany: Springer; 2014.

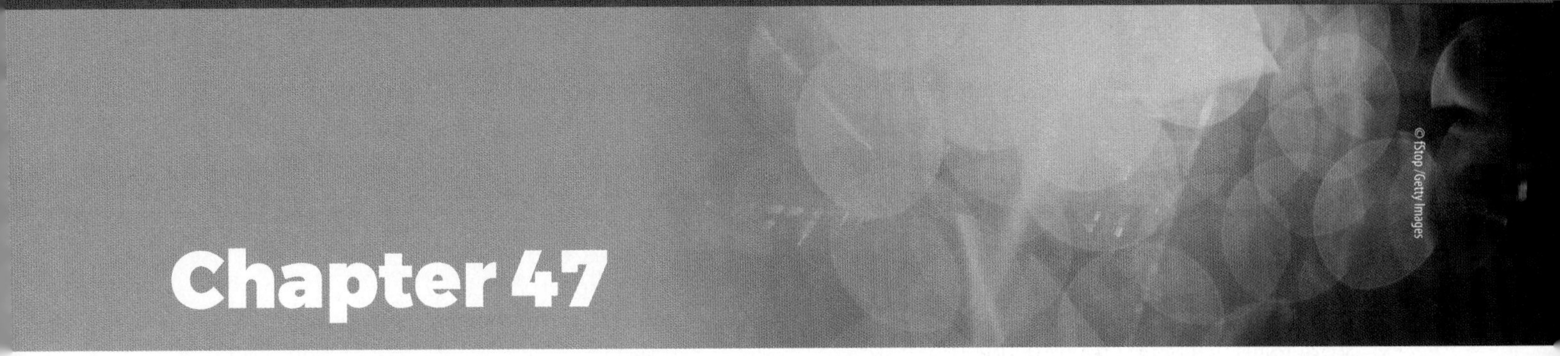

Chapter 47

Pediatrics

NATIONAL EMS EDUCATION STANDARD COMPETENCIES

Special Patient Populations

Integrates assessment findings with principles of pathophysiology and knowledge of psychosocial needs to formulate a field impression and implement a comprehensive treatment/disposition plan for patients with special needs.

Pediatrics

Age-related assessment findings, age-related anatomic and physiologic variations, age-related and developmental stage related assessment and treatment modifications of the pediatric-specific major or common diseases and/or emergencies:

- Foreign body (upper and lower) airway obstruction (p 1666)
- Bacterial tracheitis (p 1669)
- Asthma (p 1669)
- Bronchiolitis (p 1670)
  - Respiratory syncytial virus (RSV) (p 1670)
- Pneumonia (p 1670)
- Croup (pp 1666–1668)
- Epiglottitis (pp 1667–1669)
- Respiratory distress/failure/arrest (pp 1664–1666)
- Shock (pp 1671–1675)
- Seizures (pp 1685–1687)
- Sudden infant death syndrome (SIDS) (pp 1695–1697)
- Hyperglycemia (pp 1687–1688)
- Hypoglycemia (p 1687)
- Pertussis (pp 1670–1671)
- Cystic fibrosis (see Chapter 50, *Patients With Special Challenges*)
- Bronchopulmonary dysplasia (see Chapter 51, *Acute Interventions for Home Care*)
- Congenital heart diseases (see Chapter 46, *Neonatal Care*)
- Hydrocephalus and ventricular shunts (pp 1684–1685)

Patients With Special Challenges

Recognizing and reporting abuse and neglect (see Chapter 49, *Abuse and Neglect*)

Healthcare implications of

- Abuse (pp 1697–1700, and see Chapter 49, *Abuse and Neglect*)
- Neglect (pp 1697–1700, and see Chapter 49, *Abuse and Neglect*)
- Homelessness (see Chapter 50, *Patients With Special Challenges*)
- Poverty (see Chapter 50, *Patients With Special Challenges*)
- Bariatrics (see Chapter 50, *Patients With Special Challenges*)
- Technology dependent (see Chapter 51, *Acute Interventions for Home Care*)
- Hospice/terminally ill (see Chapter 51, *Acute Interventions for Home Care*)
- Tracheostomy care/dysfunction (pp 1701–1702, and see Chapter 51, *Acute Interventions for Home Care*)
- Home care (see Chapter 51, *Acute Interventions for Home Care*)
- Sensory deficit/loss (see Chapter 50, *Patients With Special Challenges*)
- Developmental disability (see Chapter 50, *Patients With Special Challenges*)

Trauma

Integrates assessment findings with principles of epidemiology and pathophysiology to formulate a field impression to implement a comprehensive treatment/disposition plan for an acutely injured patient.

Special Considerations in Trauma

Pathophysiology, assessment, and management of trauma in the

- Pregnant patient (see Chapter 45, *Obstetrics*)
- Pediatric patient (pp 1691–1695)
- Geriatric patient (see Chapter 48, *Geriatrics*)

- Cognitively impaired patient (see Chapter 50, *Patients With Special Challenges*)

OBJECTIVES

Upon completion of this chapter, the paramedic student will be able to:

1. Identify the role of the Emergency Medical Services for Children program. (pp 1651–1652)
2. Identify age-related illnesses and injuries in pediatric patients. (pp 1652–1658)
3. Identify modifications in patient assessment techniques that assist in the examination of patients at different developmental levels. (pp 1653, 1656–1658)
4. Outline the general principles of assessment and management of the pediatric patient. (pp 1658–1664)
5. Describe the pathophysiology, signs and symptoms, and management of selected pediatric respiratory emergencies. (pp 1664–1671)
6. Describe the pathophysiology, signs and symptoms, and management of shock in the pediatric patient. (pp 1671–1675)
7. Describe the pathophysiology, signs and symptoms, and management of selected pediatric dysrhythmias. (pp 1675, 1677–1682)
8. Describe the pathophysiology, signs and symptoms, and management of meningitis and blood and gastrointestinal disorders. (pp 1682–1684, 1688–1689)
9. Describe the pathophysiology, signs and symptoms, and management of pediatric seizures. (pp 1685–1687)
10. Describe the pathophysiology, signs and symptoms, and management of hypoglycemia and hyperglycemia in the pediatric patient. (pp 1687–1688)
11. Describe the pathophysiology, signs and symptoms, and management of infectious pediatric emergencies. (p 1690)
12. Identify common causes of poisoning and toxic exposure in the pediatric patient. (p 1690)
13. Describe special considerations for assessment and management of specific injuries in children. (pp 1691–1694)
14. Outline the pathophysiology and management of sudden infant death syndrome. (pp 1695–1697)
15. Describe the risk factors, key signs and symptoms, and management of injuries or illness resulting from child abuse and neglect. (pp 1697–1700)
16. Identify prehospital considerations for the care of infants and children with special needs. (pp 1699, 1701–1703)

KEY TERMS

asthma A respiratory disorder characterized by recurring episodes of paroxysmal dyspnea, coughing, and wheezing caused by constriction of the bronchi and viscous mucoid bronchial secretions.

bacterial tracheitis A bacterial infection of the upper airway and subglottic trachea; characterized by fever, barking cough, stridor, and respiratory distress.

brief resolved unexplained event (BRUE) Event lasting less than 1 minute in an infant younger than 1 year characterized by one or more of the following: cyanosis or pallor; absent, decreased, or irregular breathing; marked change in muscle tone (hypertonia or hypotonia); altered level of consciousness. Child is well-appearing at time of presentation.

bronchiolitis An inflammatory bronchial reaction in young children and infants that causes congestion in the small airways (bronchioles) of the lung.

child abuse The physical, sexual, or emotional maltreatment of a child.

croup A childhood infection of the upper airways (larynx, trachea, bronchial tubes) that causes a distinctive "seallike" barking cough. It is usually caused by a virus (most commonly parainfluenza) but rarely can be bacterial. Also known as laryngotracheobronchitis.

emetic center An area located in the reticular formation of the brainstem; thought to be the control center for vomiting.

epiglottitis Inflammation of the epiglottis; a severe form of the condition that affects primarily children is characterized by fever, sore throat, stridor, croupy cough, drooling, respiratory distress, and an erythematous epiglottis.

febrile seizure A seizure that results from fever. It most commonly occurs in children between ages 6 months and 5 years.

hydrocephalus A pathologic condition characterized by an abnormal accumulation of cerebrospinal fluid, usually under increased pressure, within the cranial vault, resulting in dilation of the cerebral ventricles.

pediatric trauma score An injury severity index that grades six components commonly seen in pediatric trauma patients: size (weight), airway, central nervous system, systolic blood pressure, open wound, and skeletal injury.

pertussis An acute, highly contagious respiratory disease characterized by paroxysmal coughing that ends in a loud, whooping inspiration; also known as whooping cough.

pneumonia An acute inflammation of the lungs, usually caused by infection with a bacterium, virus, or fungus.

shunt A tube or device surgically implanted in the body to redirect body fluid from one cavity or vessel to another. A common example is the ventriculoperitoneal shunt, which is a tube that drains fluid from the cerebral ventricle into the abdominal peritoneum in patients with hydrocephalus.

sudden infant death syndrome (SIDS) The unexpected and sudden death of an apparently normal and healthy infant that occurs during sleep and has no cause found even after a full investigation (including autopsy, investigation of the death scene, and review of clinical history). SIDS is one type of sudden unexpected infant death.

sudden unexpected infant death (SUID) Sudden and unexpected death of a baby younger than 1 year in which the cause was not obvious before investigation.

Emergencies involving pediatric patients account for fewer than 10% of EMS responses.[1] However, caring for these patients has unique challenges related to physical size and intellectual maturation, and diseases specific to newborns, infants, and children. This chapter addresses the anatomic and physiologic changes associated with normal growth and development, medical emergencies common to children, and initial assessment and management strategies that may be key in providing care to these patients.

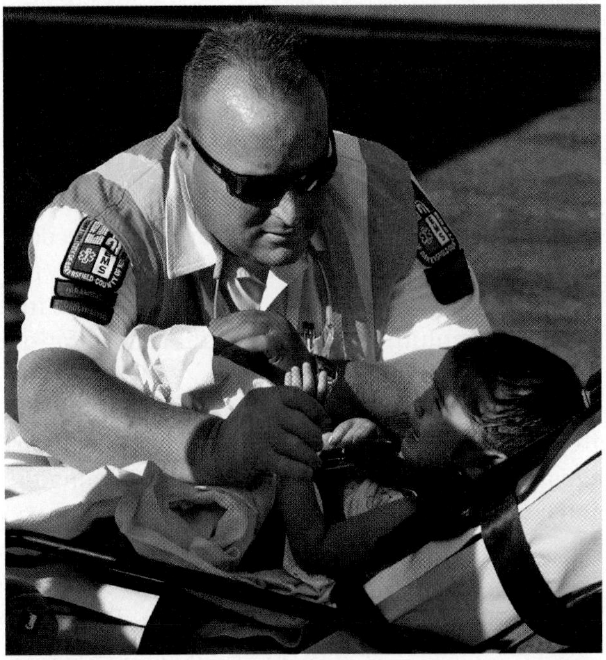

The Paramedic's Role in Caring for Pediatric Patients

Paramedics play an important role in the care of infants and children. They provide prehospital care and interfacility transfer and can help to reduce mortality and morbidity for pediatric patients. Paramedics can also play a key role in health care and injury prevention by becoming active participants in school, community, and parent education programs. In addition, paramedics provide documentation for prehospital trauma registries, epidemiologic research, and surveillance (see Chapter 3, *Injury Prevention, Health Promotion, and Public Health*). Numerous educational programs are available for those involved in pediatric care. A sampling of these programs includes the following:

- Neonatal Advanced Life Support
- Neonatal Resuscitation Program
- Emergency Pediatric Care
- Pediatric Advanced Life Support
- Pediatric Education for Prehospital Professionals
- Pediatric International Trauma Life Support
- Teaching Resource for Instructors of Prehospital Pediatrics

Other ways to enhance continuing education and clinical skills include reading textbooks and journals, participating in Internet study programs, attending regional conferences and seminars, and working or volunteering at pediatric emergency departments (EDs), pediatric hospitals, or a pediatrician's office.

EMS for Children

In 1985 the Emergency Medical Services for Children (EMSC) Demonstration Program was established through grants provided by the Maternal and Child Health Bureau of the US Department of Health and Human Services and by the National Highway Traffic Safety Administration, a division of the US Department of Transportation. This program, which was designed to enhance and expand EMS for acutely ill and injured children, defined 12 basic components of an effective EMSC system:[2]

1. System approach
2. Education
3. Data collection
4. Quality improvement
5. Injury prevention
6. Access
7. Prehospital care
8. Emergency care
9. Definitive care
10. Rehabilitation
11. Finance
12. Continual health care from birth to young adulthood

CRITICAL THINKING

Are you familiar with any EMSC injury prevention programs in your area?

EMSC grants and the organizational efforts aimed at improving emergency care for children have resulted in specific efforts targeted to prehospital care providers. These efforts include continuing education programs, educational resources for instructors, equipment guidelines, protocols for prehospital management, quality improvement procedures for evaluating prehospital care for children, research networks or node centers such as PECARN (Prehospital Emergency Care Applied Research Network), interagency agreements with federal partners, an EMSC data center, an EMSC innovation and improvement center, and designation of facilities with special capabilities for pediatric care.

As stated in *Emergency Medical Services for Children: A Report to the Nation*, published in 1991 by the National Center for Education in Maternal and Child Health:[3]

> The lives of many infants, children, and young adults . . . can be saved through implementation of emergency medical services for children. Outcomes for critically ill and injured children can be influenced by the provision of timely care by health care professionals who are well trained and equipped for pediatric emergency and critical care.

Pediatric Growth and Development

As described in Chapter 12, *Life Span Development*, children have unique anatomic, physiologic, and psychological characteristics that change during their development. The following is a review of growth and development by age group. Special considerations and approach strategies that must be considered when caring for pediatric patients are provided in BOX 47-1 (see Chapter 19, *Secondary Assessment and Reassessment*).

CRITICAL THINKING

How comfortable are you talking to a "normal" well child?

Newborns (Younger Than 1 Month)

Most newborns require no intervention at birth and begin extrauterine life without incident. Assessment and care for the newborn are described in Chapter 46, *Neonatal Care*. Resuscitation of the newborn (if needed) should follow the recommendations established by the American Heart Association, including those found in the curriculum for the Neonatal Resuscitation Program (**TABLE 47-1**).

Illnesses that may be encountered in these age groups include respiratory problems, cardiac problems, jaundice, vomiting, fever, sepsis, meningitis, and complications from prematurity.

Infants (1 to 12 Months)

By 12 months of age, infants are typically able to hold their head up, crawl, and babble. During this period, a significant amount of development occurs. Infants, however, cannot communicate their needs or feelings verbally. It is important to respect a caregiver's perception that something is wrong with the infant.

Common illnesses typically affect the respiratory, gastrointestinal (GI), and central nervous systems. They manifest as respiratory distress; nausea, vomiting, and diarrhea with dehydration; and seizures, respectively. Other illnesses that may be encountered in this age group include sepsis, meningitis, and sudden infant death syndrome (SIDS). SIDS (described later) is a type of sudden unexpected infant death, or SUID. In addition, the older infant (6 to 12 months of age) may

BOX 47-1 Developmental Stages and Approach Strategies for Pediatric Patients

Infants

Major Fears

Separation and strangers

Approach Strategies

Provide consistent caregivers

Reduce parents' anxiety, because it is transmitted to the infant

Minimize separation from parents

Toddlers

Major Fears

Separation and loss of control

Characteristics of Thinking

Primitive

Unable to recognize views of others

Little concept of body integrity

Approach Strategies

Keep explanations simple

Choose words carefully

Let toddler play with equipment (stethoscope)

Minimize separation from parents

Preschoolers

Major Fears

Bodily injury and mutilation

Loss of control

The unknown and the dark

Being left alone

Characteristics of Thinking

Highly literal interpretation of words

Unable to engage in abstract thinking

Primitive ideas about the body (eg, fear that all blood will "leak out" if a bandage is removed)

Approach Strategies

Keep explanations simple and concise

Choose words carefully

Emphasize that a procedure will help the child be healthier

Be honest

School-Age Children

Major Fears

Loss of control

Bodily injury and mutilation

Failure to live up to expectations of others

Death

Characteristics of Thinking

Vague or false ideas about physical illness and body structure and function

Able to listen attentively without always comprehending

Reluctant to ask questions about something they think they are expected to know

Increased awareness of significant illness, possible hazards of treatments, lifelong consequences of injury, and the meaning of death

Approach Strategies

Ask children to explain what they understand

Provide as many choices as possible to increase the child's sense of control

Reassure the child that he or she has done nothing wrong and that necessary procedures are not punishment

Anticipate and answer questions about long-term consequences (eg, what the scar will look like and how long activities may be curtailed)

Adolescents

Major Fears

Loss of control

Altered body image

Separation from peer group

Characteristics of Thinking

Able to think abstractly

Tendency toward hyperresponsiveness to pain (reactions not always in proportion to event)

Little understanding of the structure and workings of the body

Approach Strategies

When appropriate, allow adolescents to be a part of decision making about their care

Give information sensitively

Express how important their compliance and cooperation are to their treatment

Be honest about consequences

Use or teach coping mechanisms such as relaxation, deep breathing, and self-comforting talk

DID YOU KNOW?

Failure to thrive (weight faltering) is an abnormally slow rate of growth and development of an infant. It results from conditions that interfere with normal metabolism, appetite, and activity. Causative factors include chromosomal abnormalities; organ system illness that leads to deficiency or malfunction; systemic disease or acute illness; physical or nutritional deprivation related to inadequate calorie intake, insufficient breast milk, poverty, or poor knowledge of nutrition; and various psychosocial factors. Failure to thrive can result in permanent and irreversible delay in physical, mental, or social development. Any suspicions of failure to thrive should be documented carefully and reported to medical direction.

TABLE 47-1 Normal Vital Signs at Various Ages

Age	Pulse Rate (beats/min)	Respirations (breaths/min)	Blood Pressure (mm Hg)	Temperature
Newborn (0 to 1 month)	Awake: 100–205 Asleep: 90–160	30–60	Systolic: 67–84 Diastolic: 35–53 Mean arterial pressure: 45–60	98°F–100°F (37°C–38°C)
Infant (1 month to 1 year)	Awake: 100–180 Asleep: 90–160	30–53	Systolic: 72–104 Diastolic: 37–56 Mean arterial pressure: 50–62	96.8°F–99.6°F (36°C–37.5°C)
Toddler (1 to 2 years)	Awake: 98–140 Asleep: 80–120	22–37	Systolic: 86–106 Diastolic: 42–63 Mean arterial pressure: 49–62	96.8°F–99.6°F (36°C–37.5°C)
Preschool age (3 to 5 years)	Awake: 80–120 Asleep: 65–100	20–28	Systolic: 89–112 Diastolic: 46–72 Mean arterial pressure: 58–69	98.6°F (37°C)
School age (6 to 12 years)	Awake: 75–118 Asleep: 58–90	18–25	Systolic: 97–120 Diastolic: 57–80 Mean arterial pressure: 66–79	98.6°F (37°C)
Adolescent (12 to 18 years)	Awake: 60–100 Asleep: 50–90	12–20	Systolic: 110–131 Diastolic: 64–83 Mean arterial pressure: 73–84	98.6°F (37°C)
Early adult (19 to 40 years)	60–100	12–20	Systolic: 90–140	98.6°F (37°C)
Middle adult (41 to 60 years)	60–100	12–20	Systolic: 90–140	98.6°F (37°C)
Older adult (≥61 years)	60–100	12–20	Systolic: 90–140	98.6°F (37°C)

Modified from: American Heart Association (AHA). Vital signs in children. In: *Pediatric Advanced Life Support*. Dallas, TX: American Heart Association; 2015.

experience bronchiolitis, croup, foreign body airway obstruction, and physical injury from sexual abuse, neglect, falls, and motor vehicle crashes.

Toddlers (1 to 2 Years)

Children in this age group may struggle between dependence on their caregivers and their developing independence. They are also not capable of reasoning. Paramedics may need the assistance of a caregiver during examination to avoid separation anxiety.

Illnesses in this age group may cause respiratory distress (eg, from asthma, bronchiolitis, foreign body aspiration, or croup), vomiting and diarrhea with dehydration, febrile seizures, sepsis, and meningitis. Toddlers who are learning to walk are prone to falls. They also may find themselves in dangerous environments without proper supervision or barriers (eg, baby gates). Physical injuries also occur from poisonings from accidental ingestions, physical/sexual abuse, drowning, and motor vehicle crashes (**TABLE 47-2**).

TABLE 47-2 Ten Leading Causes of Death by Age Group, United States—2016

Rank	<1 Year	1-4 Years	5-9 Years	10-14 Years	15-24 Years
1	Congenital anomalies 4,816	Unintentional injury 1,261	Unintentional injury 787	Unintentional injury 847	Unintentional injury 13,895
2	Short gestation 3,927	Congenital anomalies 433	Malignant neoplasms 449	Suicide 436	Suicide 5,723
3	SIDS 1,500	Malignant neoplasms 377	Congenital anomalies 203	Malignant neoplasms 431	Homicide 5,172
4	Maternal pregnancy complications 1,402	Homicide 339	Homicide 139	Homicide 147	Malignant neoplasms 1,431
5	Unintentional injury 1,219	Heart disease 118	Heart disease 77	Congenital anomalies 146	Heart disease 949
6	Placenta cord membranes 841	Influenza and pneumonia 103	Chronic low respiratory disease 68	Heart disease 111	Congenital anomalies 388
7	Bacterial sepsis 583	Septicemia 70	Influenza and pneumonia 48	Chronic low respiratory disease 75	Diabetes mellitus 211
8	Respiratory distress 488	Perinatal period 60	Septicemia 40	Cerebrovascular 50	Chronic low respiratory disease 206
9	Circulatory system disease 460	Cerebrovascular 55	Cerebrovascular 38	Influenza and pneumonia 39	Influenza and pneumonia 189
10	Neonatal hemorrhage 398	Chronic low respiratory disease 51	Benign neoplasms 31	Septicemia 31	Complicated pregnancy 184

Abbreviation: SIDS, sudden infant death syndrome

Modified from: Centers for Disease Control and Prevention. 10 Leading Causes of Death by Age Group, United States, 2016. https://www.cdc.gov/injury/wisqars/pdf/leading_causes_of_death_by_age_group_2016-508.pdf. Accessed May 9, 2018.

Preschoolers (3 to 5 Years)

During the preschool years, children experience advances in gross and fine motor and verbal skills. Children in this age group can understand plain-language explanations of what is happening and descriptions of the treatment that is being provided.

Illnesses and injuries that may be encountered in this age group include those mentioned for toddlers. Preschoolers are more likely to experience injuries from thermal burns and pedestrian accidents and to experience submersion incidents or drowning. These children are curious and often have an urge to explore. Many have a minimal concept of danger.

School Age (6 to 12 Years)

During the school-age years, children display an increased ability to concentrate and learn quickly and experience the onset of puberty. School, popularity, and peer pressure are important components of school-age children.

Most illnesses in school-age children are caused by viral infection. Injuries become more common in this age group because of increased physical activity. These injuries include injuries from bicycle crashes, fractures from falls, and sport-related injuries.

> NOTE
>
> Unintentional injuries cause about one-third of the deaths in children aged 1 to 19 years. Suicide was ranked second (after unintentional harm) in children aged 13 to 18, and third for children aged 11 and 12 years. Assault ranked second (after unintentional injuries) as a cause of death in children aged 2 and 3 years and third for those aged 1, 6, 15, and 18 years.
>
> *Modified from*: National Safety Council. *Injury Facts*. Itasca, IL: National Safety Council; 2017.

Adolescents (13 to 18 Years)

During adolescence, final changes in growth and development occur, including struggles with issues of independence, body image, sexuality, and peer pressure. Adolescents interact more with friends and less with family. Experimentation and risk-taking behaviors occur.

Paramedics may encounter behavioral emergencies associated with alcohol or other drug use, eating disorders, depression, suicide and suicide gestures, sexually transmitted diseases, pregnancy, and sexual assault.

Anatomy and Physiology

As stressed throughout this text, physical differences in infants and children set them apart from the adult patient. The following is a review of anatomy and physiology by body region. Also included are special emergency care implications for the pediatric patient.

Head

Up until the age of 8 years, a child's head is proportionally large. It accounts for about 25% of the total body weight in newborns. Children also have a larger occipital region and a smaller face relative to adults. Because of these anatomic features, a high percentage of blunt trauma in children involves the head and face. The prominent occiput of the child predisposes the neck to slight flexion when the child is placed on a flat surface. To prevent this, a backboard with an occipital well or blankets placed under the child's torso can maintain a neutral position of the neck.[4]

To accommodate for brain growth in the infant, the anterior fontanel remains open for 9 to 18 months after birth. The anterior fontanel is usually level or slightly below the surface of the skull. A tight or bulging fontanel suggests increased intracranial pressure (ICP; as seen with meningitis or brain injury); a sunken fontanel indicates possible dehydration. The paramedic should assess the anterior fontanel in infants and young children who are ill or injured. This area is best assessed when the child is upright and not crying.

Airway

The airway structures of children are narrower and less stable at all levels than are those of adults. As a result, the airways of pediatric patients are more easily blocked by secretions, obstructions, and injury or inflammation. In addition, the larynx is higher (at the level of cervical vertebrae C3-C4) and more anterior, extending into the pharynx. The trachea is bifurcated at a higher level. The tracheal cartilage also is softer and smaller in length and diameter. The cricoid ring is the narrowest part of the airway in young children, whereas in adults the narrowest part of the airway is the vocal cords. The jaw is proportionally small, and the tongue is proportionally large, which increases the likelihood of airway obstruction by the tongue in the unconscious child. The epiglottis in infants is omega-shaped and extends into the airway at a 45° angle. The epiglottic folds also have softer cartilage and can become "floppy," causing airway obstruction. As described in Chapter 15, *Airway Management, Respiration, and Artificial Ventilation*, and later in this chapter, management considerations for these patients include the following:

- Placing padding under the shoulders of small children to maintain a neutral position of the airway

- Avoiding hyperflexion or hyperextension of the neck, which can obstruct the airway
- Using suction to clear the airway if secretions and particulate matter are present
- Modifying tracheal intubation techniques by ensuring a gentle touch to the soft tissue of the airway, which is easily injured and inflamed; using a straight blade that lifts the epiglottis; choosing an appropriately sized endotracheal (ET) tube; and constantly monitoring the airway for proper ET tube placement with continuous capnography[5]

The paramedic also should remember that infants breathe mainly through the nose during the first month of life. Obstruction of the small nares by secretions can result easily in respiratory insufficiency. Thus assessment and suction of the nares as needed are important, particularly in infants younger than 6 months.

Respiratory System

The tidal volume of infants and young children is proportionally smaller than that of adolescents and adults. The metabolic oxygen requirements for normal breathing are about double those of adolescents and adults. Pediatric patients also have smaller functional residual capacity and thus proportionally smaller oxygen reserves. Because of these factors, hypoxia can develop rapidly in infants and young children. Muscles are the main support for the chest wall and can tire easily during respiratory distress, which in turn can lead to respiratory failure and ultimately arrest. The paramedic should anticipate respiratory failure if any of the following signs are present:[4]

- An increased respiratory rate, particularly with signs of distress (eg, increased respiratory effort including nasal flaring, retractions, seesaw breathing, or grunting)
- An inadequate respiratory rate, effort, or chest excursion (eg, diminished breath sounds or gasping), especially if mental status is depressed
- No distal air movement
- Cyanosis or low oxygen saturation despite supplementary oxygen
- Decreasing consciousness
- Extreme tachycardia or rapidly decreasing heart rate

Cardiovascular System

Cardiac output is rate-dependent in infants and small children: The faster the heart rate, the greater the cardiac output. Children are less able than adults are to increase the contractility and stroke volume of the heart and their circulating blood volume is proportionally larger. Yet the child's absolute blood volume is smaller. The ability of children to use vasoconstriction to decrease size of the vessels allows them to maintain blood pressure longer than adults. However, early intervention is required to prevent irreversible or decompensated shock. Special considerations in managing these patients include the following:

- Cardiovascular reserve is vigorous, but limited.
- Loss of small absolute volumes of fluid and blood can cause shock.
- A child may be in shock despite a normal blood pressure.
- Bradycardia is often a response to hypoxia.

As described in Chapter 35, *Shock*, and later in this chapter, hypotension is a late sign of shock in a child. Thus the assessment of shock must be based on clinical signs of tissue perfusion, including level of consciousness, skin color, oxygen saturation, and capillary refill. The paramedic should suspect shock in any ill or injured children who have tachycardia and evidence of decreased perfusion.

Nervous System

The nervous system develops throughout childhood and developing neural tissue is fragile. However, compared to adults, there is a greater cerebrospinal fluid (CSF) space around the neural tissues in children, which buffers blunt forces. Their spinal column also is more pliable. As a result, spinal cord injury in children is rare, occurring in only 1% to 2% of blunt injuries.[6]

Because the anterior and posterior fontanels remain open for a period after birth, direct trauma to the head can lead to brain injuries that are devastating in young children.

Abdomen

Like the chest wall, the immature muscles of the abdomen in a child offer less protection to internal organs. In addition, the abdominal organs are closer together. The liver and spleen are also proportionally larger and more vascular. These features allow for multiple organ injuries to be more common following abdominal trauma. The liver and spleen also are injured more often than in adults.

Chest and Lungs

As stated earlier, the chest muscles children are immature and can fatigue easily. The use of these muscles for breathing also requires higher metabolic and oxygen consumption rates than in older children and adults. This increases a pediatric patient's susceptibility to the accumulation of lactic acid in the blood. The ribs of a child are more pliable and are positioned horizontally, and the mediastinum is more mobile. Therefore the chest wall offers less protection to internal organs. It allows for significant internal injury to occur without external signs of trauma. Rib fractures are less common in children, but do occur with abuse and other forms of trauma.

The limited protection provided by the chest wall makes pulmonary contusions from trauma and pneumothorax from barotrauma common in this age group.[7] When evaluating a pediatric patient who has sustained major trauma, it should be recalled that infants and children are diaphragmatic breathers and are prone to gastric distention, and that the mobile mediastinum may have a greater shift with a tension pneumothorax. In addition, the thin chest wall easily transmits breath sounds, which may complicate the assessment of a pneumothorax or ET tube placement. As a result, auscultation of breath sounds from the axillary regions in addition to the anterior and posterior thorax often is helpful.

Extremities

As described in Chapter 10, *Review of Human Systems,* bones in children are softer and more porous until adolescence. As long bones mature, hormones act on the cartilage in growing bones, replacing the soft cartilage with hard bones. Epiphyseal plates (growth plates) are located at the distal and proximal ends of the long bones and allow for lengthening during growth. These plates are a point of relative weakness and can easily be injured and disrupt growth if not properly managed.

Because of the soft composition of bones in pediatric patients, all strains and sprains should be considered to be possible fractures and immobilized. In addition, paramedics should be wary of injuries to the growth plate that may disrupt bone growth. Careful technique during intraosseous (IO) infusion procedures is crucial; improper insertion into the growth plate can potentially disrupt future bone growth (see Chapter 14, *Medication Administration*).

Skin and Body Surface Area

The skin in children is thinner and more elastic than is the skin of adults. In addition, most children younger than 2 years have less subcutaneous fat. Children also have larger body surface area–to–body mass ratios than adults. These factors can affect injury and illness in children in several ways. For example, the thinner skin of a child allows for deeper injury to occur from heat or cold exposure. The lack of subcutaneous fat and the larger surface area also reduces the child's ability to regulate body temperature. This increases the likelihood of hypothermia, hyperthermia, and dehydration from fluid loss.

Metabolic Differences

The way in which children and adults expend energy differs in many ways. For example, infants and children have limited glycogen and glucose stores. Their blood glucose levels can drop very quickly in response to illness or injury. Pediatric patients can experience rapid and significant volume loss from vomiting and diarrhea. They are also prone to hypothermia because of their increased body surface area. Newborns also have limited capacity to shiver or sweat to maintain body temperature. For these reasons, it is important to assess a severely ill or injured child for hypoglycemia or hypoperfusion, to minimize heat loss, and to keep all children warm during treatment and transport.

CRITICAL THINKING

Why is it important to know which injuries and illnesses are commonly seen in specific age groups?

General Principles of Pediatric Assessment

The general principles of assessment for pediatric patients are very similar to those for adult patients. Approach strategies and medical equipment will differ in some ways because of the patient's age, maturity, and physical development. The following is a brief overview of the general principles of pediatric assessment, including evaluation of the scene (scene size-up), primary survey, vital functions, transition phase, focused history, secondary assessment, and reassessment. Specific differences in providing care to a child are presented later in this chapter by subject matter.

Evaluation of the Scene (Scene Size-up)

As with all other patient care events, the paramedic should begin the physical assessment of a child with a quick scene survey, noting any potential hazards. Any visible mechanism of injury or nature of the illness should be noted. For example, the presence of pills, medication bottles, or household chemicals may indicate the possibility of toxic ingestion. Injury and a history that do not coincide with the stated mechanism of injury may indicate child abuse. In addition, the paramedic should observe the relationship between the parent, guardian, or caregiver and the child to determine the appropriateness of their interaction. For example, does the interaction demonstrate concern, anger, or indifference? Other important assessments to be made during the scene size-up include the orderliness, cleanliness, and safety of the home and the general appearance of other children in the family.

> NOTE
>
> Initial patient evaluation for children should include observing the patient and involving the parent or guardian in the assessment. The parent or guardian often can help make the child more comfortable during the assessment and can usually offer key details about the child's medical history. The parent also may know whether aspects of the child's behavior or response to the illness or injury are normal or abnormal.

> CRITICAL THINKING
>
> Would you want to comment to the parents about an unsafe situation on the scene before transport? Why or why not?

Primary Survey

The primary survey begins with the paramedic forming a general impression of the patient. This assessment

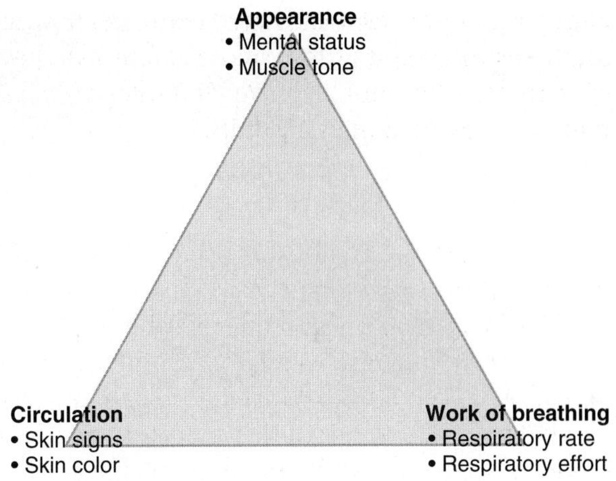

FIGURE 47-1 Pediatric assessment triangle.

Used with permission of the American Academy of Pediatrics, *Pediatric Education for Prehospital Professionals* © American Academy of Pediatrics; 2000.

should focus on the details most valuable for determining whether life-threatening conditions exist. The pediatric assessment triangle (**FIGURE 47-1**) is a tool that allows the paramedic to quickly assess a child and form an impression of clinical status.[8] The assessment triangle has three components: appearance (mental status and muscle tone), work of breathing (respiratory rate and effort), and circulation (skin signs and skin color). If the child's condition is urgent, care should proceed with rapid assessment of airway, breathing, and circulation; management; and rapid transport. If the child's condition is nonurgent, care can proceed with a focused history and detailed physical examination. Assessing the child's appearance can also be performed using the TICLS mnemonic:[8]

Tone. Is movement vigorous or limp?
Interactiveness. Is the child alert?
Consolability. Can the child be comforted?
Look/gaze. Does the child look at the caregiver or paramedic?
Speech/cry. Is there a strong cry or voice?

> CRITICAL THINKING
>
> Think about one abnormal finding in each area of the assessment triangle. Would any single finding influence your triage decision?

Vital Functions

The AVPU scale (Awake and alert, responsive to Verbal stimuli, responsive to Pain, Unresponsive) or the

TABLE 47-3 Pediatric Glasgow Coma Scale

Activity	Score	Infant	Score	Child
Eye opening	4	Open spontaneously	4	Open spontaneously
	3	Open to speech or sound	3	Open to speech
	2	Open to painful stimuli	2	Open to painful stimuli
	1	No response	1	No response
Verbal	5	Coos, babbles	5	Oriented conversation
	4	Irritable cry	4	Confused conversation
	3	Cries to pain	3	Cries; inappropriate words
	2	Moans to pain	2	Moans; incomprehensive words/sounds
	1	No response	1	No response
Motor	6	Normal spontaneous movement	6	Obeys verbal commands
	5	Localizes pain	5	Localizes pain
	4	Withdraws from pain	4	Withdraws from pain
	3	Abnormal flexion (decorticate)	3	Abnormal flexion (decorticate)
	2	Abnormal extension (decerebrate)	2	Abnormal extension (decerebrate)
	1	No response (flaccid)	1	No response (flaccid)

Modified from: Davis RJ, et al. Head and spinal cord injury. In: Rogers MC, ed. *Textbook of Pediatric Intensive Care*. Baltimore, MD: Williams & Wilkins; 1987; James H, Anas N, Perkin RM. *Brain Insults in Infants and Children*. New York, NY: Grune & Stratton; 1985; and Morray JP, et al. Coma scale for use in brain-injured children. *Crit Care Med.* 1984;12:1018.

modified Glasgow Coma Scale (GCS; **TABLE 47-3**) can be used to determine the child's level of consciousness and to assess for signs of inadequate oxygenation.

Airway and Breathing

The child's airway should be patent, and breathing should be associated with adequate chest rise and fall. Signs of respiratory compromise include the following:

- Abnormal breath sounds
- Absent breath sounds
- Apnea or bradypnea
- Grunting
- Head bobbing
- Irregular breathing pattern
- Nasal flaring
- Tachypnea
- Use of accessory muscles

Circulation

Circulation is assessed by comparing the strength and quality of central and peripheral pulses. Blood pressure should be measured in children older than 3 years, and in *all* children who are seriously ill or injured, with an appropriately sized cuff. The skin should be evaluated for color, temperature, moisture, turgor, and capillary refill (**FIGURE 47-2**). Any signs of visible hemorrhage should be managed appropriately. See Table 47-1 for normal vital signs for each age group.

Transition Phase

The transition phase is integrated throughout assessment. This phase allows the child to become more familiar with the paramedic crew and medical equipment (eg, "get to know you" conversations and playing with stethoscope) (see Chapter 19, *Secondary Assessment and Reassessment*). Use of this phase depends on the seriousness of the patient's condition and is appropriate only for a conscious child who is not acutely ill.

Focused History

When obtaining the focused history for an infant, a toddler, or a preschooler, the paramedic often must elicit information from the parent, guardian, or caregiver. School-age and adolescent patients can provide most information. If possible, children and adolescents should be questioned in private (away from parents or family members) about sexual activity, pregnancy, alcohol or other drug use, or suspicion of child abuse (if appropriate for the complaint). The focused history can be obtained using the methods described in Chapter 17, *History Taking*.

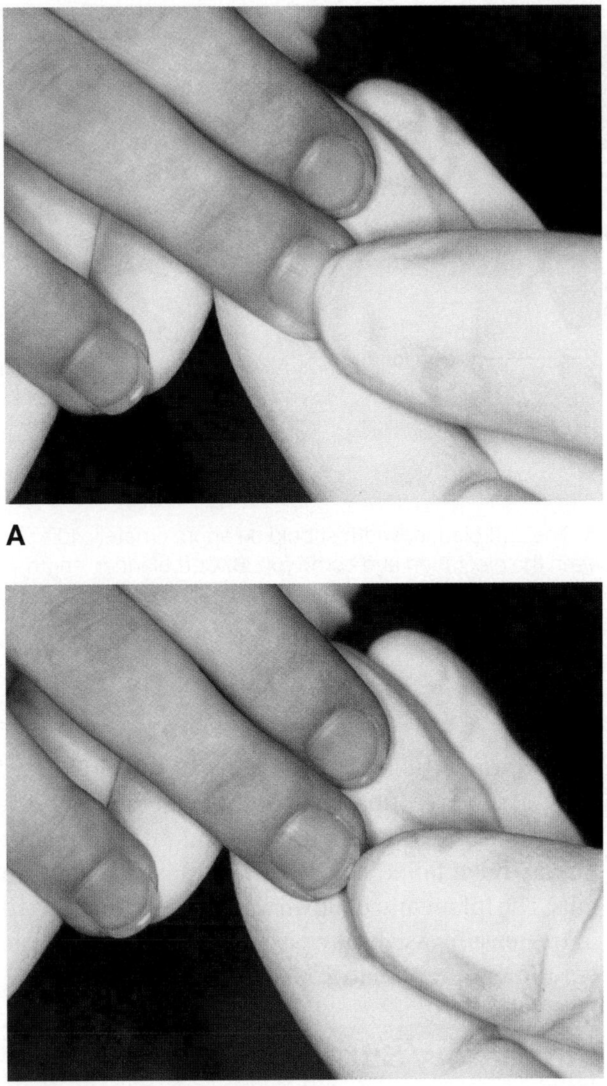
A

B

FIGURE 47-2 A. To test for capillary refill, compress the fingertip for 5 seconds using moderate pressure. **B.** Release the fingertip, and count the number of seconds it takes for the normal color to return to the nail bed. If the patient has dark skin, capillary refill time may need to be assessed in the pulp of the fingertip or on the palm of the hand.

Secondary Assessment

The detailed secondary assessment was described in Chapter 19, *Secondary Assessment and Reassessment.* The examination should proceed from head to toe in older children. In younger children, the paramedic should assess key areas first and then proceed from toe to head.[9] The patient's condition and the severity of injury or illness will determine the appropriateness and depth of the assessment performed at the scene.

NOTE

When assessing a pediatric patient who is ill, it is important to note the presence or absence of fever, nausea, vomiting, diarrhea, and frequency of urination.

If time allows and the patient's condition warrants, noninvasive monitoring of vital signs can provide useful information. Examples include the use of pulse oximetry to measure perfusion and oxygen saturation, blood pressure assessment, and measurement of body temperature. In addition, all seriously ill or injured children should receive continuous electrocardiographic (ECG) monitoring. Measurement tools (eg, blood pressure cuffs, electrodes) should be appropriate for the size of the child (**FIGURE 47-3**).

Reassessment

Reassessment should be ongoing and is appropriate for all patients. The purpose of reassessment is to monitor the patient for changes in respiratory effort, skin color and temperature, mental status, and vital signs (including pulse oximetry measurements). An ill or injured child's condition can change rapidly. Thus, vital signs should be assessed every 15 minutes in a child who is not in critical condition. They should be assessed every 5 minutes in a child who is seriously ill or injured.

CRITICAL THINKING

Why is ongoing assessment so important when caring for the young child?

General Principles of Patient Management

The general principles of patient management for children are similar to those of adult patients. The following discussion will serve as a brief review.

Basic Airway and Ventilation Management

Basic and advanced airway management procedures for pediatric patients are presented in detail in Chapter 15, *Airway Management, Respiration, and Artificial Ventilation.* These procedures may include manually positioning the airway; removing a foreign body airway obstruction with back blows,

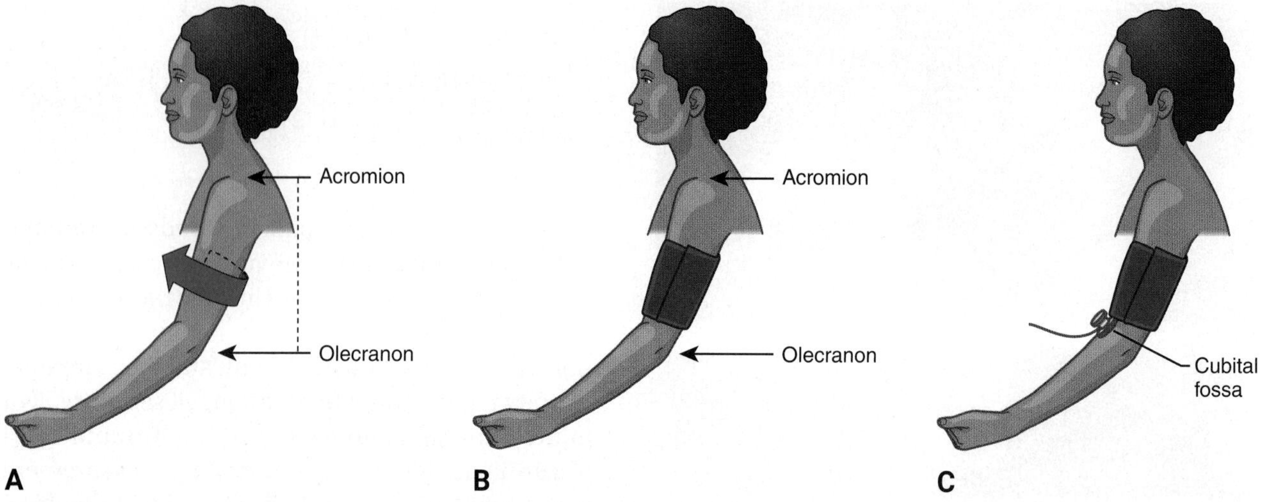

FIGURE 47-3 Determination of proper blood pressure cuff size. **A.** The cuff bladder width should be approximately 40% of the circumference of the arm measured at a point midway between the olecranon and acromion. **B.** Cuff bladder length should cover 80% to 100% of the circumference of the arm. **C.** Blood pressure should be measured with the cubital fossa at heart level. The arm should be supported. The stethoscope bell is placed over the brachial artery pulse, proximal and medial to the cubital fossa, and below the bottom edge of the cuff.

chest compressions, or abdominal thrusts; suctioning secretions from the airway; providing supplemental oxygen; using oral or nasal airway adjuncts; and assisting ventilation with a bag-valve device.

Advanced Airway Management

Advanced airway management procedures may be needed when caring for a child who is acutely ill or seriously injured. These techniques include removing a foreign body airway obstruction under direct visualization with Magill forceps, placement of a supraglottic airway, ET intubation (including drug-assisted intubation), and needle cricothyroidotomy when other methods to maintain a patent airway have failed or when bag-mask ventilation fails. The infant and child airway should be managed in the least invasive way possible.[10] **TABLE 47-4** lists equipment for pediatric ET intubation.

NOTE

Both cuffed and uncuffed ET tubes are acceptable for intubating infants and children. Cuffed ET tubes may decrease the risk of aspiration. If cuffed ET tubes are used, cuff inflating pressure should be monitored and limited according to the manufacturer's instructions (usually less than 20 to 25 cm H_2O).

Modified from: de Caen AR, Maconochie IK, Aickin R, et al.; Pediatric Basic Life Support and Pediatric Advanced Life Support Chapter Collaborators. Part 6: pediatric basic life support and pediatric advanced life support: 2015 International Consensus on Cardiopulmonary Resuscitation and Emergency Cardiovascular Care Science With Treatment Recommendations. *Circulation.* 2015;132(suppl 1):S177-S203.

Circulatory Support

Circulatory support may be required in an ill or injured child. In addition to providing basic life support with cardiopulmonary resuscitation (CPR), vascular access may be required for drug therapy and fluid resuscitation. Methods to obtain vascular access in pediatric patients are described in Chapter 14, *Medication Administration,* and later in this chapter. These methods may include peripheral venous cannulation and IO infusion.

Pharmacologic Therapy

Drug therapy may be required when caring for pediatric patients. Examples include therapy for pain management; drug-assisted intubation; and care for patients with respiratory, cardiac, endocrine, or neurologic conditions. Drug doses specific to pediatric emergencies are found in Appendix A, *Emergency Drug Index.* The incidence of medication error in

TABLE 47-4 Pediatric Resuscitation Supplies Based on Color-Coded Resuscitation Tape

Equipment	Gray (3–5 kg)[a]	Pink, Small Infant (6–7 kg)	Red, Infant (8–9 kg)	Purple, Toddler (10–11 kg)	Yellow, Small Child (12–14 kg)	White, Child (15–18 kg)	Blue, Child (19–23 kg)	Orange, Large Child (24–29 kg)	Green, Adult (30–36 kg)
Resuscitation bag		Infant/child	Infant/child	Child	Child	Child	Child	Child	Adult
Oxygen mask (NRB)		Pediatric	Pediatric	Pediatric	Pediatric	Pediatric	Pediatric	Pediatric	Pediatric/adult
Oral airway (mm)		50	50	60	60	60	70	80	80
LMA (size)	1	1.5	1.5	1.5–2.0	2.0	2.0	2.0–2.5	2.5	3
Laryngoscope blade (size)		1 Straight	1 Straight	1 Straight	2 Straight	2 Straight	2 Straight or curved	2 Straight or curved	3 Straight or curved
ET tube (mm)[b]		3.5 Uncuffed 3.0 Cuffed	3.5 Uncuffed 3.0 Cuffed	4.0 Uncuffed 3.5 Cuffed	4.5 Uncuffed 4.0 Cuffed	5.0 Uncuffed 4.5 Cuffed	5.5 Uncuffed 5.0 Cuffed	6.0 Cuffed	6.5 Cuffed
ET tube insertion length (cm)	3 kg, 9–9.5 4 kg, 9.5–10 5 kg, 10–10.5	10.5–11	10.5–11	11–12	13.5	14–15	16.5	17–18	18.5–19.5
Suction catheter (F)		8	8	10	10	10	10	10	10–12
BP cuff	Neonatal #5/infant	Infant/child	Infant/child	Child	Child	Child	Child	Child	Small adult
IV catheter (ga)		22–24	22–24	20–24	18–22	18–22	18–20	18–20	16–20
IO (ga)		18/15	18/15	15	15	15	15	15	15
NG tube (F)		5–8	5–8	8–10	10	10	12–14	14–18	16–18
Urinary catheter (F)	5	8	8	8–10	10	10–12	10–12	12	12
Chest tube (F)		10–12	10–12	16–20	20–24	20–24	24–32	28–32	32–38
Stylet (F)	6	6	6	6	6	6	6	14	14

[a]For gray column, use pink or red equipment sizes if no size is listed.

[b]Per *2005 AHA Guidelines*, in the hospital, cuffed or uncuffed tubes may be used.

Abbreviations: BP, blood pressure; ET, endotracheal; F, French; ga, gauge; IO, intraosseous; IV, intravenous; LMA, laryngeal mask airway; NG, nasogastric; NRB, nonrebreathing

Modified from: American Heart Association. *2015 Handbook of Emergency Cardiovascular Care for Healthcare Providers.* Dallas, TX: American Heart Association; 2015.

SHOW ME THE EVIDENCE

A literature review was conducted to assess the methods of pediatric weight estimation. This review assessed the outcomes of accuracy (proportion within 10% of actual weight), mean percentage error, and mean bias. Eighty studies were included. The review found parent estimation to be the most accurate to predict actual body weight. Length-based methods that adjusted for habitus (using published growth data or midarm circumference) were next best. Regular length-based systems underestimated weight for children who were obese and overestimated for malnourished children. Broselow length-based tape had 54% accuracy (to within 10% of actual weight). Age-based formulas tended to underestimate actual weight and were less accurate with older, heavier children. Health care worker estimation was not accurate.

Modified from: Young KD, Korotzer NC. Weight estimation methods in children: a systematic review. *Ann Emerg Med.* 2016;68(4): 441-451.e10.

pediatric patients is very high.[11-14] When possible, electronic or printed decision aids should be used to verify dose. It is advisable to use a cross-check procedure to have another caregiver verify the dose and medication prior to administration.

Additional Therapy

Additional therapies may be indicated depending on the type of illness or injury. These include spinal motion restriction for trauma patients, hemorrhage control and bandaging and splinting, and electrical therapy (described later in this chapter). Maintaining body temperature with blankets and warm clothing may be needed because infants and young children are at increased risk of hypothermia.

Transport Considerations

Some pediatric patients will need transport to a specialty care medical facility. Examples of specialty care facilities are pediatric trauma centers, high-risk newborn care facilities, and pediatric burn centers. In addition decisions to provide rapid transport versus providing on-scene care, and the use of ground or air ambulance or specialty care transport teams may need to be considered.

Psychological Support

Providing psychological support to pediatric patients and to a patient's family or caregivers is important. Pediatric emergencies often are emotionally charged events. Helpful strategies for approaching and communicating with pediatric patients and their caregivers are described in Chapter 16, *Therapeutic Communications.*

Specific Pathophysiology, Assessment, and Management

The conditions discussed in this section are specific to major body systems and associated illness or injury. In addition, shock, toxicology, abuse and neglect, and SIDS are discussed. Other considerations for specialized care (eg, children with cystic fibrosis, muscular dystrophy, cerebral palsy, Down syndrome) are presented in Chapter 50, *Patients With Special Challenges.*

Respiratory Compromise

Respiratory distress can be caused by many conditions that affect the upper and lower airways. These include upper and lower foreign body airway obstruction, upper airway disease (croup, epiglottitis, and bacterial tracheitis), and lower airway disease (asthma, bronchiolitis). Other causes of respiratory compromise include pneumonia, pertussis, and cystic fibrosis. Most cases of cardiac arrest in children occur because of respiratory insufficiency (asphyxial arrest).[4] For this reason, respiratory emergencies require rapid assessment and management. The severity of respiratory compromise may be classified as respiratory distress, respiratory failure, and respiratory arrest.

Respiratory distress is the mildest form of respiratory compromise. Respiratory distress is evident by an increase in the rate and depth of breathing and by the use of accessory muscles to assist ventilation (**FIGURE 47-4**). These changes cause a slight decrease in arterial carbon dioxide levels in the blood as respiratory rate increases. As respiratory distress increases,

NOTE

The paramedic should attempt to calm and reassure a child with respiratory compromise. It is important not to agitate the conscious patient or lay the child down (into a supine position). Doing so may aggravate the airway condition and lead to life-threatening airway obstruction. When possible, allow the parent or other caregiver to stay with the child. The receiving hospital should be advised of the patient's status as soon as possible so that arrangements can be made for appropriate medical personnel.

the patient becomes exhausted. The partial pressure of carbon dioxide level gradually increases as the patient's condition worsens and the child becomes fatigued. Signs and symptoms of respiratory distress include the following:

- A change in mental status from normal to irritable or anxious
- Tachypnea
- Retractions (accessory muscle use)
- Nasal flaring
- Poor muscle tone
- Tachycardia
- Head bobbing
- Grunting
- Cyanosis that improves with supplemental oxygen

If left untreated, respiratory distress may rapidly progress to respiratory failure.

As described in Chapter 23, *Respiratory*, respiratory failure results from poor ventilation or lack of oxygenation. It occurs when the heart and lungs do not exchange enough oxygen and carbon dioxide, causing a decrease in the partial pressure of oxygen level and an increase in the partial pressure of carbon dioxide level (leading to respiratory acidosis). Signs and symptoms of respiratory failure include the following:

- Irritability deteriorating to lethargy
- Marked tachypnea deteriorating to bradypnea
- Marked retractions deteriorating to agonal respirations
- Marked tachycardia deteriorating to bradycardia
- Central cyanosis

Respiratory failure in any patient is an ominous sign. Without immediate intervention, respiratory arrest can occur.

Respiratory arrest is the cessation of breathing. Good outcomes can be expected with early treatment that protects the airway and provides adequate

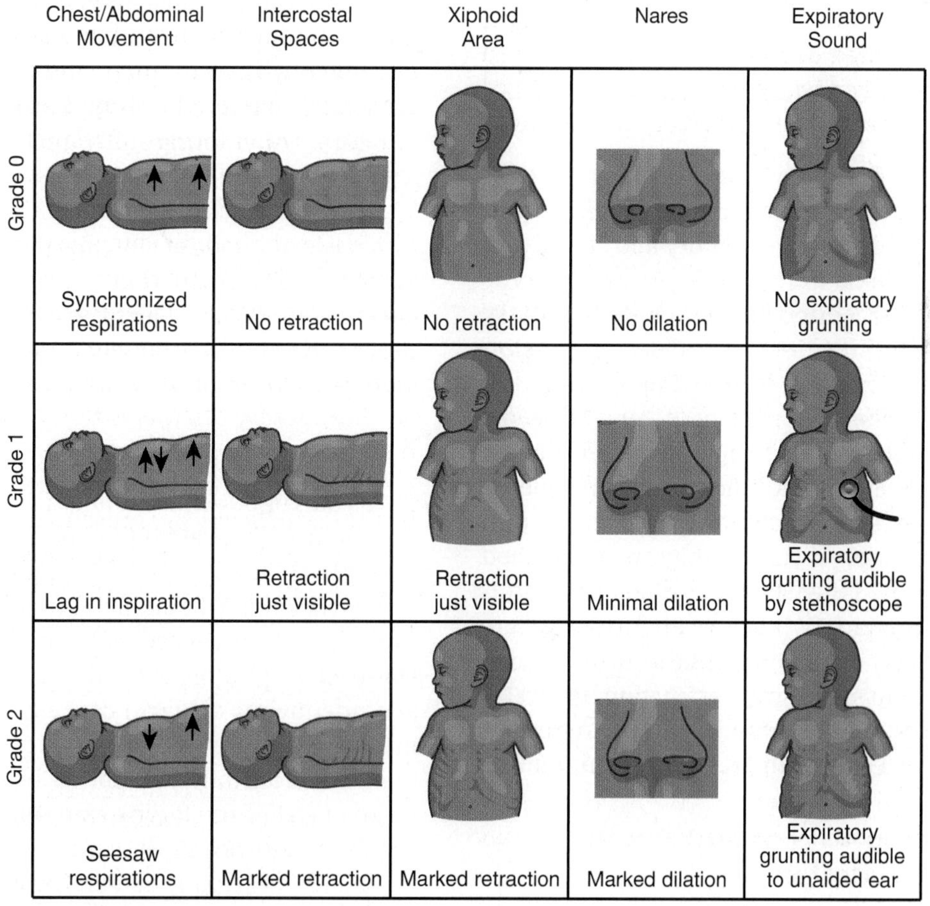

FIGURE 47-4 Assessment of respiratory distress. The Silverman-Anderson index is used to score the infant's degree of respiratory difficulty. The score for individual criteria matches the grade, with a total possible score of 10 indicating severe distress.

BOX 47-2 Assessment Information for Respiratory Compromise

History

Age
Preceding symptoms
Progression of symptoms (acute onset versus gradual progression)
Choking episode
Underlying disease
Recent exposure to illness
Exposure to toxins
Prematurity
Trauma

Physical Findings

Mental status
Respiratory rate
Work of breathing
Presence of stridor or wheezes
Skin color
Heart rate
Tidal volume
Pulse oximetry
Capnography

ventilation and oxygenation. However, failure to treat respiratory arrest can lead to cardiopulmonary arrest.

Providing aggressive ventilatory and circulatory support for patients in respiratory distress is crucial. Airway interventions may include bag-mask ventilation, ET intubation, gastric decompression (if abdominal distention is impeding ventilation), needle decompression for pneumothorax, and needle cricothyrotomy for complete upper airway obstruction that cannot be relieved by other means. In general, vascular access is not recommended for children who have respiratory distress if they are not in need of intravenous (IV) medication or fluid administration for dehydration. IV therapy can further agitate the child and may increase the child's distress, which can lead to complete airway obstruction. BOX 47-2 provides assessment information that is important when caring for a child with respiratory compromise.

Upper and Lower Foreign Body Airway Obstruction

Obstruction of the upper or lower airway by a foreign body may cause a partial or complete foreign body airway obstruction. About 80% of pediatric foreign body airway obstruction episodes occur in children younger than 3 years.[15] Children have narrow airways and develop molars around age 3 years, but they do not chew well. As a result, obstruction can be caused by foods such as peanuts, seeds, popcorn, hot dogs, or grapes. Other causes of upper airway obstruction include small toys or objects such as coins and balloons. The paramedic should suspect foreign body aspiration in an otherwise healthy child with sudden onset of respiratory compromise.

NOTE

Using inflated balloons or an inflated examination glove to entertain or distract a young child while providing care should be avoided. This practice can create a choke hazard for young children. In addition, parents and other caregivers should be advised to keep deflated balloons and broken balloon pieces away from children.

If a child with a partial obstruction is conscious and has adequate movement of air, the paramedic should not agitate the child; doing so can convert a partial obstruction into a complete obstruction. Rather, the paramedic should provide continuous respiratory monitoring and immediate transport for physician evaluation.

If a complete airway obstruction cannot be relieved with basic methods of clearing, direct laryngoscopy to identify the obstruction and removal with Magill forceps are indicated. Basic and advanced methods of clearing the airway are presented in Chapter 15, *Airway Management, Respiration, and Artificial Ventilation.*

Croup

Croup (laryngotracheobronchitis) is a common infection (usually viral) of the upper airway. It usually occurs in children between the ages of 6 months and 4 years and during the late fall and early winter months. Croup usually is caused by the parainfluenza virus. However, respiratory syncytial virus (RSV), rubeola, and adenovirus also can cause croup. Croup may involve the entire respiratory tract, with symptoms that result from inflammation in the subglottic region (at the level of the larynx extending to the cricoid cartilage) (**FIGURE 47-5**).

A child with croup usually has a history of recent upper respiratory tract infection and a low-grade fever. The patient may have hoarseness, inspiratory stridor (from subglottic edema), and a barking cough. Stridor mainly occurs on inspiration, but symptoms

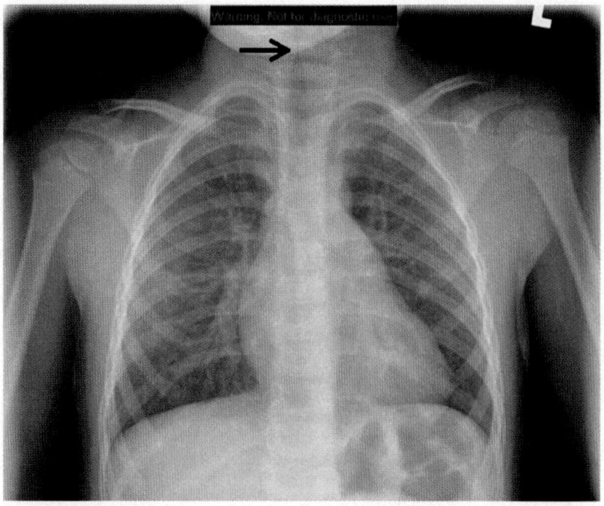

FIGURE 47-5 Frontal radiograph of neck of a child with croup. Notice the narrowing of the upper airway showing the "steeple" sign.

Case courtesy of Dr Andrew Ho, Radiopaedia.org, rID: 22936.

BOX 47-3 Stages of Croup

Stage 1. Fever, hoarse, croupy cough, inspiratory stridor
Stage 2. Continuous stridor, intercostal retractions, labored breathing
Stage 3. Signs of hypoxia and hypercapnia with pallor, sweating, tachypnea
Stage 4. Cyanosis, apnea

may be present on expiration if the lower airways are involved. Most often, the emergency episode occurs at night after the child has gone to bed. On EMS arrival, a patient with severe croup may have all the classic signs of respiratory distress. The child may be sitting upright and leaning forward to aid breathing (variable). Nasal flaring, intercostal retractions, and cyanosis (a late sign of respiratory insufficiency) may also be present. Children with severe croup are at risk of serious airway obstruction from the narrowed diameter of the trachea (BOX 47-3).

Prehospital management of croup includes maintaining the airway and transporting the patient in a position of comfort. Cool mist or humidified or nebulized oxygen may help minimize symptoms.[16] Nebulized racemic epinephrine is indicated to reduce upper airway edema (if not available, nebulized epinephrine) (BOX 47-4). (See Appendix A, *Emergency Drug Index*.) Vascular access is not indicated except in the case of dehydration or when IV medication is needed. The paramedic should make all efforts to keep the child comfortable and at ease.

BOX 47-4 Treatment for Children With Stridor at Rest

- Nebulized racemic epinephrine—peak effect 20 minutes. Signs and symptoms can reappear after 2 hours, when duration of effect is complete. If racemic epinephrine is not available, nebulized epinephrine (epinephrine 5 mL of 0.1 mg/mL [0.5 mg]) is administered, and may be repeated at this dose with unlimited frequency for ongoing distress.
- Cool mist therapy may be helpful, unless it provokes anxiety.
- Intubation is rarely needed.
- If available, dexamethasone 0.6 mg/kg oral, IV, or intramuscular (IM) is administered, to maximum dose of 16 mg.

Modified from: National Association of State EMS Officials. *National Model EMS Clinical Guidelines*, Version 2.0. September 2017; and American Heart Association. *Pediatric Advanced Life Support*. Dallas, TX: American Heart Association; 2016.

CRITICAL THINKING

Why would albuterol not be helpful in treating croup?

Epiglottitis

Epiglottitis is inflammation of the epiglottis caused by a bacterial infection of the upper airway. Although uncommon, epiglottitis can progress rapidly and become life threatening. It can occur at any age. The disease may be associated with *Haemophilus influenzae* type b, but other *H influenzae*, *Streptococcus*, and *Staphylococcus* organisms also have been implicated.[17] The bacterial infection causes edema and occlusion from swelling of the epiglottis and supraglottic structures (pharynx, aryepiglottic folds, and arytenoid cartilage). Epiglottitis is a true emergency that requires prompt, expert airway management. The *H influenzae* type b (Hib) vaccine has dramatically reduced the number of cases of epiglottitis in children.[18]

Epiglottitis usually begins suddenly. Typically, the child goes to bed without any symptoms and wakes up complaining of a sore throat and pain on swallowing. The child may have fever, a muffled voice, sometimes referred to as "hot potato voice" (from edema of the mucosal covering of the vocal cords), and drooling from the pooled saliva that occurs because of difficult and painful swallowing (an ominous sign

TABLE 47-5 Comparison of the Symptoms of Croup and Epiglottitis

Characteristics	Croup	Epiglottitis
Occurrence	6 months to 4 years	Median pediatric age 6 to 12 years
Onset	Slow; frequently at night	Rapid
Comfortable position	Patient may lie down or sit upright	Patient prefers to sit upright
Cough	Barking cough; may have inspiratory stridor	No barking cough; may have inspiratory stridor
Drooling	No drooling	Drooling, pain on swallowing
Temperature	<104°F (40°C)	>104°F (40°C)
Cause	Viral	Bacterial

Modified from: Woods CR. Epiglottitis (supraglottitis): clinical features and diagnosis. UpToDate website. https://www.uptodate.com/contents/epiglottitis-supraglottitis-clinical-features-and-diagnosis?source=see_link. Updated May 3, 2017. Accessed March 30, 2018.

of impending airway obstruction). Differentiating epiglottitis from croup in the prehospital setting may be difficult. **TABLE 47-5** lists the different characteristics of these illnesses.

On arrival, the paramedic usually finds a child with epiglottitis sitting upright (**FIGURE 47-6**). Often the child is leaning forward with the head hyperextended (tripod position) to aid in breathing. The tongue may be protruding, or the child may have inspiratory stridor. These children usually do not cry or struggle because all of their attention and energy is being used to maximize air exchange. Inspiratory stridor with a characteristic rattle often is present. The child also may be gasping or gulping for air. Classic signs of respiratory distress usually are present. The preferred

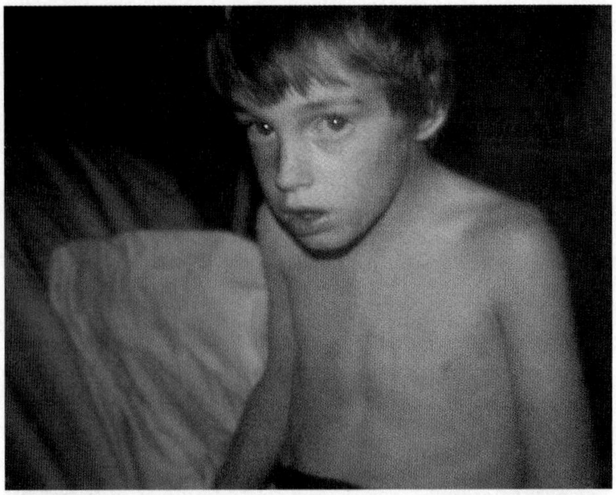

FIGURE 47-6 Acute epiglottitis at presentation.

Courtesy of Health Resources and Services Administration (HRSA), Maternal and Child Health Bureau (MCHB), Emergency Medical Services for Children (EMSC) Program.

and definitive care for epiglottitis is in-hospital intubation and parenteral antibiotic therapy.

Children with acute epiglottitis are in danger of full airway obstruction and respiratory arrest. Occlusion of the airway can occur suddenly. Occlusion may be caused by anxiety, stress, or minor irritation of the throat. For these reasons, gentle handling of a child suspected of having epiglottitis is essential. The following guidelines in prehospital management should be observed:

- Do not attempt to lay the child down or to change the position of comfort.
- Do not attempt to visualize the airway if the child is still ventilating adequately.
- Advise medical direction of the suspicion of epiglottitis so that appropriate personnel and resources can be made available.
- Administer supplemental oxygen by mask unless it provokes agitation.
- *Do not* attempt vascular access.
- Have the correct-size emergency airway equipment selected and ready.
- If advanced airway management may become necessary, have needle cricothyrotomy equipment readily available.
- Transport the child to the hospital in the position of comfort.

If intubation is required, it may be difficult because the vocal cords are likely to be hidden by swollen tissues. (An uncuffed ET tube one to two sizes smaller than normal may be recommended by some medical

CRITICAL THINKING

What other childhood respiratory problems (traumatic and nontraumatic) can manifest with stridor?

direction physicians.) The paramedic should locate the opening to the larynx by looking for mucous bubbles in the cleft between the edematous aryepiglottic folds and the swollen epiglottis. (Chest compressions during glottic visualization may produce a bubble at the tracheal opening.) In the rare instance that intubation cannot be achieved and the child cannot be ventilated adequately by a bag-mask device, medical direction may advise needle cricothyrotomy. Often a child's lungs can be ventilated through the occlusive crisis of epiglottitis by bag-mask ventilation using a tight facial seal. This may require two people—one to maintain the seal and the other to ventilate.

Bacterial Tracheitis

Bacterial tracheitis is a rare infection (often caused by *Staphylococcus*) of the upper airway and subglottic trachea that may occur after a viral respiratory illness such as croup. It generally occurs in children younger than 6 years but also can occur in older children. Bacterial tracheitis can lead to severe airway obstruction and respiratory arrest.[19] The signs and symptoms of bacterial tracheitis are those of respiratory distress or failure (depending on the severity) and may include the following:

- Respiratory distress
- Cough that produces pus or mucus
- Fever
- Hoarseness
- Inspiratory or expiratory stridor

Emergency care is directed at providing airway, ventilatory, and circulatory support and rapid transport for evaluation by a physician. If airway obstruction, respiratory failure, or respiratory arrest develops, bag-mask ventilation is indicated. ET intubation may be required with tracheal suction to remove mucus or pus. In-hospital care includes IV antibiotics that are specific for the causative organism. These will be given after the child's airway has been stabilized.

Asthma

As described in Chapter 23, *Respiratory*, **asthma** is a chronic inflammatory disorder of the airways that may cause recurrent episodes of wheezing, breathlessness, chest tightness, and cough. Asthma is characterized by inflammation, bronchoconstriction, and mucus production that obstructs the lower airways. It results from autonomic dysfunction or exposure to sensitizing agents. Asthma is common among children older than 2 years but can be difficult to diagnose. (Other respiratory conditions in children can cause similar signs and symptoms.) It affects about 8% of those younger than 18 years. In 2015, there were an estimated 6.2 million children with asthma in the United States.[20]

The hallmarks of an acute exacerbation are anxiety, dyspnea, tachypnea, and audible expiratory (and when severe, inspiratory) wheezes with a prolonged expiratory phase. (A silent chest indicates impending respiratory failure.) An acute exacerbation may be triggered by infection, changes in temperature, physical exercise, emotional response, and exposure to allergens. Exercise-induced asthma produces bronchospasm only when the child exercises. Risk factors for childhood asthma include allergies, family history, frequent respiratory infections, low birth weight, exposure to secondhand smoke before/after birth, and living in a low-income urban setting.[21]

CRITICAL THINKING

What other signs or symptoms would lead you to believe that a child with asthma is decompensating?

The goals of prehospital management include ventilatory assistance (as needed), administration of humidified oxygen, pharmacologic reversal of the bronchospasm, and rapid transport for evaluation and treatment. Severe asthma may be life threatening and can progress rapidly to respiratory failure. The paramedic should be ready to initiate airway management along with ventilatory and circulatory support. Depending on local protocol and prior medication use, drug therapy may include aerosolized bronchodilators (albuterol, ipratropium, or levalbuterol), subcutaneously administered epinephrine with severe respiratory distress or failure, and corticosteroids (eg, methylprednisolone, dexamethasone).[22] Continuous positive airway pressure or bilevel positive airway pressure can be used for patients with severe distress. If signs of respiratory failure develop, magnesium sulfate or IM epinephrine (0.01 mg/kg of 1 mg/mL solution to a maximum of 0.3 mg) can be given and bag-mask ventilation considered.[10] If the patient requires tracheal intubation, medical direction may advise low tidal volumes (5 to 8 mL/kg) and prolonged expiratory times to reduce the potential for barotrauma.

Bronchiolitis

Bronchiolitis (like asthma) manifests with tachypnea and wheezing. The illness is caused by a viral infection (eg, from RSV) that can cause inflammation of the lower airway. Bronchiolitis usually affects children younger than 2 years, often occurring in the winter months, and generally is associated with upper respiratory tract infection. Bronchiolitis sometimes is unresponsive to therapy aimed at relieving bronchospasm. **TABLE 47-6** lists key features that may aid in the differential diagnosis.

Bronchiolitis generally is not serious, and recovery is uneventful. However, sometimes it may become life threatening. Infants are at greater risk of developing respiratory failure from this condition because of the small diameter of the bronchioles. The prehospital care includes administration of supplemental oxygen, escalating from a nasal cannula to a nonrebreathing mask as needed to maintain normal oxygenation. The nose or mouth should be suctioned using a bulb syringe or a hard- or soft-tip suction catheter if the patient has excessive secretions. When coarse breath sounds are present and the patient does not improve despite oxygen and suctioning, nebulized epinephrine (3 mg in 3 mL of normal saline) is indicated. Continuous positive airway pressure or high-flow nasal cannula can be administered for severe respiratory distress. If respiratory failure develops, the patient should be ventilated with a bag-mask device.[9] IV therapy should only be initiated in children with respiratory distress for clinical concerns of dehydration, or when administering IV medications.[10]

NOTE

RSV is highly contagious. Most people infected with RSV have mild symptoms of upper respiratory infection. However, severe infection with bronchiolitis and/or pneumonia can also occur. Severe infection is most common in children younger than 2 years and usually occurs epidemically in the winter months.

Modified from: Respiratory syncytial virus infection (RSV). Centers for Disease Control and Prevention website. www.cdc.gov/rsv/index.html. Updated March 7, 2017.

TABLE 47-6 Differentiation of Bronchiolitis and Asthma

Clinical Features	Bronchiolitis	Asthma
Age of occurrence	Usually <2 years	Any age
Season	Winter, spring	Any time
Family history of asthma	Usually absent	Usually present
Cause	Virus	Allergy, infection, exercise, virus
Response to drugs	Some reversal of bronchospasm with beta agonists	Reversal of bronchospasm

Pneumonia

As described in Chapter 23, *Respiratory*, **pneumonia** is an acute infection of the lower airway and lungs that involves the alveolar walls or the alveoli. Pneumonia commonly is caused by a bacterial or viral infection. Children with pneumonia may have a history of recent airway infection, such as influenza or pertussis. They also may have respiratory distress or failure (depending on the severity) and any of the following:

- Decreased breath sounds in the affected area
- Fever
- Pain in the chest
- Crackles localized to the affected area
- Rhonchi (localized or diffuse)
- Tachypnea

Most children with pneumonia have only mild signs and symptoms and require no immediate treatment or airway support. However, when respiratory distress is present, stabilization of the airway and provision of oxygenation are the highest priority. In severe cases, bronchodilators may be indicated. Assisted ventilations via a bag-mask device or intubation of the trachea also may be required.

Pertussis

Pertussis primarily affects infants and young children. It is an infectious disease caused by the bacterium *Bordetella pertussis*. It is spread by direct contact with discharges from mucous membranes contained in airborne droplets. Pertussis causes inflammation of the entire respiratory tract. The major complications of pertussis in infants are pneumonia (younger than 6 months) and apnea (younger than 2 months). Other possible complications include weight loss, sleep disturbance, and seizures. The incidence of complications is highest in children younger than 1 year.

Pertussis is commonly associated with episodes of violent and productive coughing with an inspiratory "whoop" or gasp. High coughing pressure may cause pneumothorax, epistaxis, subconjunctival hemorrhage, and rib fracture.[23] Symptoms of pertussis can last 1 to 2 months. Most children are vaccinated for this disease through a series of pertussis vaccines given in combination with diphtheria and tetanus (DTaP). Children do not receive the vaccine until 2 months of age. Due to droplet transmission risk, respiratory protection for both the patient and the EMS crew is required.

Shock

As described in Chapter 35, *Shock*, shock is an abnormal condition characterized by inadequate delivery of oxygen to meet the metabolic demands of tissues. The condition may occur with increased, normal, or decreased blood pressure. Shock is categorized as compensated (shock without hypotension) or decompensated (shock with hypotension), and can be further categorized as cardiogenic and noncardiogenic. Cardiogenic shock is characterized by adequate intravascular volume, but myocardial dysfunction limits stroke volume and cardiac output. Noncardiac shock is caused by conditions that reduce preload. It can be hypovolemic shock from loss of volume. It may also be distributive shock (septic, neurogenic, or anaphylactic) or obstructive shock (eg, tension pneumothorax, pulmonary embolism).

Important considerations when caring for a child in shock include circulating blood volume, body surface area and hypothermia, cardiac reserve, respiratory fatigue, vital signs, and assessment.

Circulating Blood Volume

In adults, blood volume accounts for 5% to 6% of total body weight, or 50 to 60 mL/kg of body weight; in children, blood volume accounts for 7% to 8% of total body weight, or 70 to 80 mL/kg of body weight.[24] Although the percentage of circulating blood volume in a child is greater than that in an adult, a child's actual blood volume is considerably lower than an adult's. Therefore, a relatively small absolute loss of blood may be devastating. For example, a blood loss of 100 mL in an adult is a 2% loss; a 100-mL loss in an infant is a 15% to 20% loss.

A child with a blood or fluid deficit will maintain a normal blood pressure until all compensatory mechanisms fail (**TABLE 47-7**). At that point, shock progresses rapidly, with serious deterioration. These efficient compensatory mechanisms can mask a potentially life-threatening condition. Thus the paramedic must maintain a high degree of suspicion, based on the patient's complaint or clinical presentation. Early recognition, stabilization (airway control, fluid replacement), and rapid transport to a proper facility are crucial when caring for children in shock. Treatment must be focused on ventilation, fluid administration, and improvement of the pumping action of the heart.

CRITICAL THINKING

How comfortable are you with starting an IV infusion for an infant or young child?

Body Surface Area and Hypothermia

Young children have a large body surface area in proportion to body weight. Their compensatory mechanisms (eg, shivering and sweating) also are not well developed. Children in shock quickly can develop hypothermia from exposure and concurrent metabolic acidosis, increased vascular resistance, respiratory depression, and myocardial dysfunction. Hypothermia makes resuscitation and drug therapy

TABLE 47-7 Systolic Blood Pressure Characterizing Hypotension in the Pediatric Patient

Age	Systolic Blood Pressure
Term newborns (birth to 28 days of age)	<60 mm Hg
Infants (1–12 months)	<70 mm Hg
Children (1–10 years)	<70 mm Hg plus (2 × age in years)
Older than 10 years	<90 mm Hg

Modified from: Part 13: pediatric basic life support: 2010 American Heart Association Guidelines for Cardiopulmonary Resuscitation and Emergency Cardiovascular Care. *Circulation*. 2010 Nov 2;122(18)(suppl 3):S862-S875.

less effective. Thus, the paramedic should maintain the patient's body temperature by increasing the temperature in the ambulance patient compartment, using blankets, covering the child's head, and warming IV fluids when possible.

Cardiac Reserve

Infants and children already have high metabolic needs. As a result, they have less cardiac reserve than adults for stressful situations such as shock. An important step is to reduce the energy and oxygen requirements of a child in shock as much as possible. This can be accomplished by providing ventilatory support, reducing anxiety, and maintaining moderate ambient temperatures.

Vital Signs and Assessment

The paramedic must consider many factors when evaluating a child's vital signs. For example, blood pressure and pulse rate vary greatly with age, body temperature, and degree of agitation. The paramedic should measure vital signs as baseline assessments, even though they may be of limited value in assessing the circulation of a child in shock. The most effective assessment is constant monitoring of the child's mental and physical status and the response to therapy. The following should be evaluated when assessing a child in shock:

Level of Consciousness
- Ability to make eye contact
- Ability to recognize family members
- Agitation
- Anxiety

Skin
- Color
- Moisture
- Temperature
- Turgor

Mucous Membranes
- Color
- Moisture

Nail Beds
- Capillary refill (in children younger than 6 years)
- Color

Peripheral Circulation
- Collapse
- Distention

Cardiac
- ECG findings
- Location of pulses
- Quality of pulses
- Rate
- Rhythm

Respiration
- Depth
- Rate

Blood Pressure (in children older than 3 years, using appropriately sized cuff)

Body Temperature

> NOTE
>
> Sustained tachycardia in the absence of obvious causes such as fever, pain, and agitation may be an early sign of cardiovascular compromise. Bradycardia, however, may be a preterminal cardiac rhythm indicating advanced shock and often is associated with hypotension.
>
> *Modified from*: American Heart Association. *Pediatric Advanced Life Support*. Dallas, TX: American Heart Association; 2016.

Hypovolemia

One common cause of hypovolemia in children is dehydration resulting from vomiting and diarrhea. Another is blood loss resulting from trauma or internal bleeding. Children are also at risk of intravascular volume depletion as a result of burns (see Chapter 38, *Burns*).

Dehydration. Profound fluid and electrolyte imbalances can occur in children as a result of vomiting, diarrhea, poor fluid intake, fever, or burns. Cardiac output and systemic perfusion are compromised if the child loses the fluid equivalent of 5% or more of total body weight. For the adolescent, losses of 5% to 7% of total body weight can compromise perfusion (**FIGURE 47-7**).[25] If allowed to progress, dehydration can result in renal failure, shock, and death. The severity of the dehydration and fluid loss can be estimated from a history of the child's weight loss and the physical examination. **TABLE 47-8** provides signs and symptoms related to degrees of dehydration.

Airway and ventilatory support (if needed) are the initial steps in treatment for a dehydrated child. Next, treatment is directed at replacing and maintaining blood volume and perfusion. IV therapy should be initiated with isotonic crystalloids such as lactated Ringer solution or normal saline to maintain adequate perfusion.[26,27]

CRITICAL THINKING

What are some ways to determine the child's weight for fluid and drug dosing?

Blood Loss. As stated before, even a small amount of blood loss can be serious for the pediatric patient (**TABLE 47-9**). After the paramedic achieves control of external hemorrhage (if present), secures the patient's airway, and provides high-concentration oxygen, the child's circulatory status may require support with IV therapy.

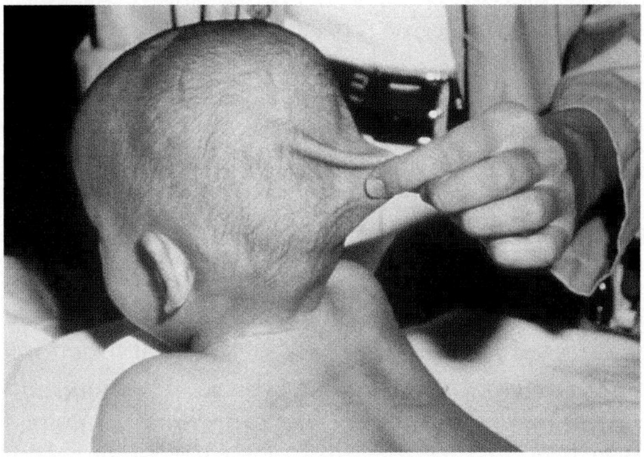

FIGURE 47-7 Severe dehydration.

Courtesy of Ronald Dieckmann, M.D.

Prehospital fluid resuscitation must take mental status into consideration. Blood transfusion may be indicated at the hospital, but the prehospital goal of care for pediatric hemorrhage is to control the bleeding (if possible), administer enough crystalloid to maintain mental status or perfusion, and transport as quickly as possible to a trauma center.[27,28]

NOTE

Establishing an IV line in a child through a peripheral vein (see Chapter 14, *Medication Administration*) can be difficult even in the most controlled settings. As a result, the paramedic may need to establish an IO infusion for the child in shock.

Distributive Shock

As described previously, *distributive shock* refers to septic shock, neurogenic shock, and anaphylactic shock. This type of shock results in peripheral pooling because of decreased vasomotor tone. The vasodilation that occurs causes the blood pressure to fall. Vasodilation also allows plasma to leak from the vascular space.

Septic shock usually is caused by a systemic infection. Toxins released by the pathogen affect arterioles, capillaries, and venules, altering microcirculatory pressure and capillary permeability. Children

TABLE 47-8 Assessment of Degree of Dehydration

Clinical Parameters	Mild	Moderate	Severe
Body weight loss	5% (50 mL/kg)	10% (100 mL/kg)	15% (150 mL/kg)
Skin turgor	Slightly decreased	Moderately decreased	Greatly decreased
Fontanel (infant)	Possibly flat or depressed	Depressed	Significantly depressed
Mucous membranes	Dry	Very dry	Parched
Skin perfusion	Warm with normal color	Cool (extremities), pale	Cold (extremities), mottled or gray
Heart rate	Mildly tachycardic	Moderately tachycardic	Extremely tachycardic
Peripheral pulses	Normal	Diminished	Absent
Blood pressure	Normal	Normal	Reduced
Sensorium	Normal or irritable	Irritable or lethargic	Unresponsive

TABLE 47-9 Classification of Hemorrhagic Shock in Pediatric Trauma Patients Based on Systemic Signs

System	Mild Blood Volume Loss (<30%)	Moderate Blood Volume Loss (30–45%)	Severe Blood Volume Loss (>45%)
Cardiovascular	Increased heart rate; weak, thready peripheral pulses; normal systolic blood pressure (80–90 + 2 × age in years); normal pulse pressure	Markedly increased heart rate; weak, thready central pulses; absent peripheral pulses; low normal systolic blood pressure (70–80 + 2 × age in years); narrowed pulse pressure	Tachycardia followed by bradycardia; very weak or absent peripheral pulses; hypotension (<70 + 2 × age in years); undetectable diastolic blood pressure (or widened pulse pressure)
Central nervous system	Anxious; irritable; confused	Lethargic; dulled response to pain[a]	Comatose
Skin	Cool, mottled; prolonged capillary refill	Cyanotic; markedly prolonged capillary refill	Pale and cold
Urine output[b]	Low to very low	Minimal	None

Abbreviation: IV, intravenous

[a]The child's dulled response to pain with this degree of blood loss (30%–45%) may be indicated by a decreased response to IV catheter insertion.

[b]After initial decompression by urinary catheter. Low normal is 2 mL/kg per hour (infant), 1.5 mL/kg per hour (younger child), 1 mL/kg per hour (older child), and 0.5 mL/kg per hour (adolescent). IV contrast can falsely elevate urinary output.

Modified from: American Heart Association. *2015 Handbook of Emergency Cardiovascular Care for Healthcare Providers*. Dallas, TX: American Heart Association; 2015:91.

experiencing septic shock usually appear very ill. They may have signs and symptoms that include those of decompensated shock. Characteristic findings in septic shock include skin that is warm in the early stages, and skin that is cool in the late stages of the illness.

Neurogenic shock results from sudden peripheral vasodilation caused by a traumatic injury to the spinal cord. The loss of sympathetic impulses and resultant vasodilation increase the size of the vascular compartment. The normal intravascular volume is not enough to fill the vascular compartment and to perfuse tissues. Characteristic findings in neurogenic shock include warm skin, bradycardia, and impaired neurologic function.

Anaphylactic shock occurs when a person is exposed to a substance that produces a severe allergic reaction (see Chapter 26, *Immune System Disorders*). Common causes of allergic reactions include antibiotic agents, foods, and insect stings. The bodily response to the antigen causes a release of histamine. This release results in peripheral vasodilation and the leakage of intravascular fluid into the interstitial space, resulting in a decrease in intravascular volume. Characteristic findings in anaphylactic shock include a rapid onset of skin signs (hives, allergic rash, and erythema), upper airway obstruction or dyspnea, signs of shock, and GI distress.

Emergency care for children with distributive shock is directed at ensuring the patient's vital functions through airway, ventilatory, and circulatory support and providing rapid transport to an appropriate medical facility. Fluid therapy for all types of distributive shock includes isotonic crystalloid bolus of 20 mL/kg over 5 to 20 minutes. Drugs are indicated to manage specific forms of distributive shock. For example, antibiotics are administered as soon as possible for septic shock; epinephrine is given before other treatments for anaphylactic shock; and epinephrine or norepinephrine drips are infused if fluid boluses do not improve septic or neurogenic shock.[4] Estimates of child weights are often inaccurate, so it is advisable to use a dosing aid to improve accuracy. These aids include the Pedi-Wheel, Broselow tape, and the Handtevy system (see Chapter 14, *Medication Administration*).

Heart Failure. Heart failure in children may result from cardiomyopathy, myocarditis, and congenital heart diseases. (Congenital heart defects are presented in Chapter 46, *Neonatal Care*.) Myocarditis is inflammation of the heart. Cardiomyopathy refers to degeneration of the heart muscle that causes a reduction in the force of heart contractions. Both conditions decrease the force of contractions and the amount of blood circulated to the lungs and to the rest of the body. In children, heart failure usually results from viral infection or congenital abnormalities that affect both ventricles of the heart (described in the following sections). Symptoms include fatigue, chest pain, and dysrhythmias. In severe cases, they include signs of heart failure and cardiogenic shock, such as the following:

- Crackles
- Hypotension
- Jugular venous distention (difficult to determine in young children)
- Peripheral edema
- Tachycardia
- Tachypnea

Patients in stable condition are managed with supportive care, oxygen administration, and transport for evaluation by a physician. IV fluid therapy should be given to children in cardiogenic shock in small boluses of 5 to 10 mL/kg slowly over 10 to 20 minutes.[4] Monitor breath sounds carefully.

Cardiac Emergencies and Resuscitation

Most children are born with healthy hearts. When rhythm disturbances occur, they usually are the result of hypoxia, acidosis, hypotension, or structural heart disease.[4] The most common dysrhythmias in pediatric patients are sinus tachycardia, supraventricular tachycardia, bradycardia, and asystole. Pulseless ventricular tachycardia or ventricular fibrillation is the initial rhythm in 5% to 15% of pediatric cardiac arrests.[4] The recommended management for these dysrhythmias is outlined in the following sections. Pediatric advanced life support drugs are listed in **TABLE 47-10**. Specific guidelines for use of airway equipment during pediatric life support were addressed earlier in this chapter.

Dysrhythmias and basic and advanced life support procedures (including CPR) are addressed in Chapter 21, *Cardiology*. The reader should refer to that chapter for review. The following discussions outline the unique aspects of abnormal rhythms in children.[4]

NOTE

Even though short-term initial resuscitation rates for infants and children in cardiac arrest have improved, survival to hospital discharge remains very low, at about 8%.

Modified from: American Heart Association. *Pediatric Advanced Life Support*. Dallas, TX: American Heart Association; 2016.

DID YOU KNOW?

Many intensive care units use scoring systems such as the Pediatric Emergency Warning Score (PEWS) for early identification of high-risk children who are likely to deteriorate and require resuscitation. The PEWS evaluates three categories of an ill child: behavior, cardiovascular, and respiratory symptoms. Scores in each category can range from 0 to 3 points. Additionally, 2 points are added for respiratory nebulizer treatments that are continuous or provided every 15 minutes, and 2 points for persistent vomiting following surgery. The total score can range from 0 to 13, with the higher number reflecting a child at increased risk of requiring advanced-level care. The AHA has concluded that the use of scoring systems might help to identify such patients sufficiently early to enable effective intervention. However, it has not been established that the use of PEWS outside of the pediatric intensive care unit setting reduces hospital mortality.

Modified from: Parshuram CS, Hutchinson J, Middaugh K. Development and initial validation of the Bedside Paediatric Early Warning System score. *Crit Care*. 2009;13:R135; DeVita MA, Hillman K, Bellomo R. *Textbook of Rapid Response Systems: Concept and Implementation*. 2nd ed. New York, NY: Springer; 2017; and Web-based integrated guidelines for cardiopulmonary resuscitation and emergency cardiovascular care. Part 12: pediatric advanced life support. American Heart Association website. https://eccguidelines.heart.org/index.php/circulation/cpr-ecc-guidelines-2/part-12-pediatric-advanced-life-support/. Accessed April 2, 2018.

Rhythm Disturbances

Bradydysrhythmias. Clinically significant bradycardia is defined as a heart rate less than 60 beats/min (or a rapidly dropping heart rate) associated with poor systemic perfusion. This bradycardia occurs despite adequate oxygenation and ventilation. Primary bradycardia is related to congenital heart defects, surgical injury, cardiomyopathy, or myocarditis. Secondary bradydysrhythmias may be caused by hypoxemia, acidosis, hypotension, hypoglycemia, central nervous system (CNS) injury, hypothermia, toxicity, or excessive vagal stimulation (eg, from ET intubation or pharyngeal suctioning). In infants and children, sinus bradycardia, and atrioventricular block are the most common bradydysrhythmias. All symptomatic bradycardias require treatment. Important ECG findings include the following:

- Heart rate is less than 60 beats/min.
- P waves may or may not be visible.
- QRS complex duration may be normal or prolonged.
- The P wave and QRS complex often are unrelated.

TABLE 47-10 Medications for Pediatric Resuscitation

Medication	Dose	Remarks
Adenosine	0.1 mg/kg (maximum 6 mg) Second dose: 0.2 mg/kg (maximum 12 mg)	Monitor ECG. Administer rapid IV/IO bolus with flush.
Amiodarone	5 mg/kg IV/IO; may repeat twice up to 15 mg/kg Maximum second dose: 300 mg	Monitor ECG and blood pressure; adjust administration rate to urgency (IV push during cardiac arrest, more slowly: over 20–60 min with perfusing rhythm). Expert consultation is strongly recommended prior to use when patient has a perfusing rhythm. Use caution when administering with other drugs that prolong QT (obtain expert consultation).
Atropine	0.02 mg/kg IV/IO 0.04–0.06 mg/kg ET[a] Repeat once if needed Maximum single dose: 0.5 mg	Higher doses may be used with organophosphate poisoning.
Calcium chloride (10%)	20 mg/kg IV/IO (0.2 mL/kg) Maximum single dose: 2 g	Administer slowly.
Epinephrine	0.01 mg/kg (0.1 mL/kg 1:10,000) IV/IO 0.1 mg/kg (0.1 mL/kg 1:1,000) ET[a] Maximum dose: 1 mg IV/IO; 2.5 mg ET	May repeat every 3–5 min.
Glucose	0.5–1 g/kg IV/IO	Newborn: 5–10 mL/kg $D_{10}W$ Infants and young children: 2–4 mL/kg $D_{25}W$ Adolescents: 1–2 mL/kg $D_{50}W$
Lidocaine	Bolus: 1 mg/kg IV/IO Infusion: 20–50 mcg/kg per min	
Magnesium sulfate	25–50 mg/kg IV/IO over 10–20 min; faster in torsades de pointes Maximum dose: 2 g	
Naloxone	Full Reversal: <5 years or ≤ 44 pounds (20 kg): 0.1 mg/kg IV/IO/ET[a] ≥ 5 years or >44 pounds (20 kg): 2 mg IV/IO/ET[a]	Use lower doses to reverse respiratory depression associated with therapeutic opioid use (1–5 mcg/kg titrated to effect).
Procainamide	15 mg/kg IV/IO	Monitor ECG and blood pressure. Give slowly—over 30–60 min. Use caution when administering with other drugs that prolong QT (obtain expert consultation).
Sodium bicarbonate	1 mEq/kg per dose IV/IO slowly	Provide after adequate ventilation.

[a]Flush with 5 mL of normal saline and follow with 5 ventilations.

Abbreviations: $D_{XX}W$, dextrose in specified percentage of water; ECG, electrocardiogram; ET, endotracheal; IO, intraosseous; IV, intravenous

Modified from: Medications for pediatric resuscitation. American Heart Association website. https://eccguidelines.heart.org/index.php/tables/2010-medications-for-pediatric-resuscitation. Accessed May 14, 2018.

The initial management of bradycardia should ensure that breathing is adequate and the patient is receiving supplemental oxygen (**FIGURE 47-8**). (Mechanical problems with oxygen delivery should be assessed before drug administration.) If pulses, perfusion, and respirations are adequate, no emergency treatment is necessary.[4] Monitor and proceed with evaluation. If drug therapy is required, epinephrine

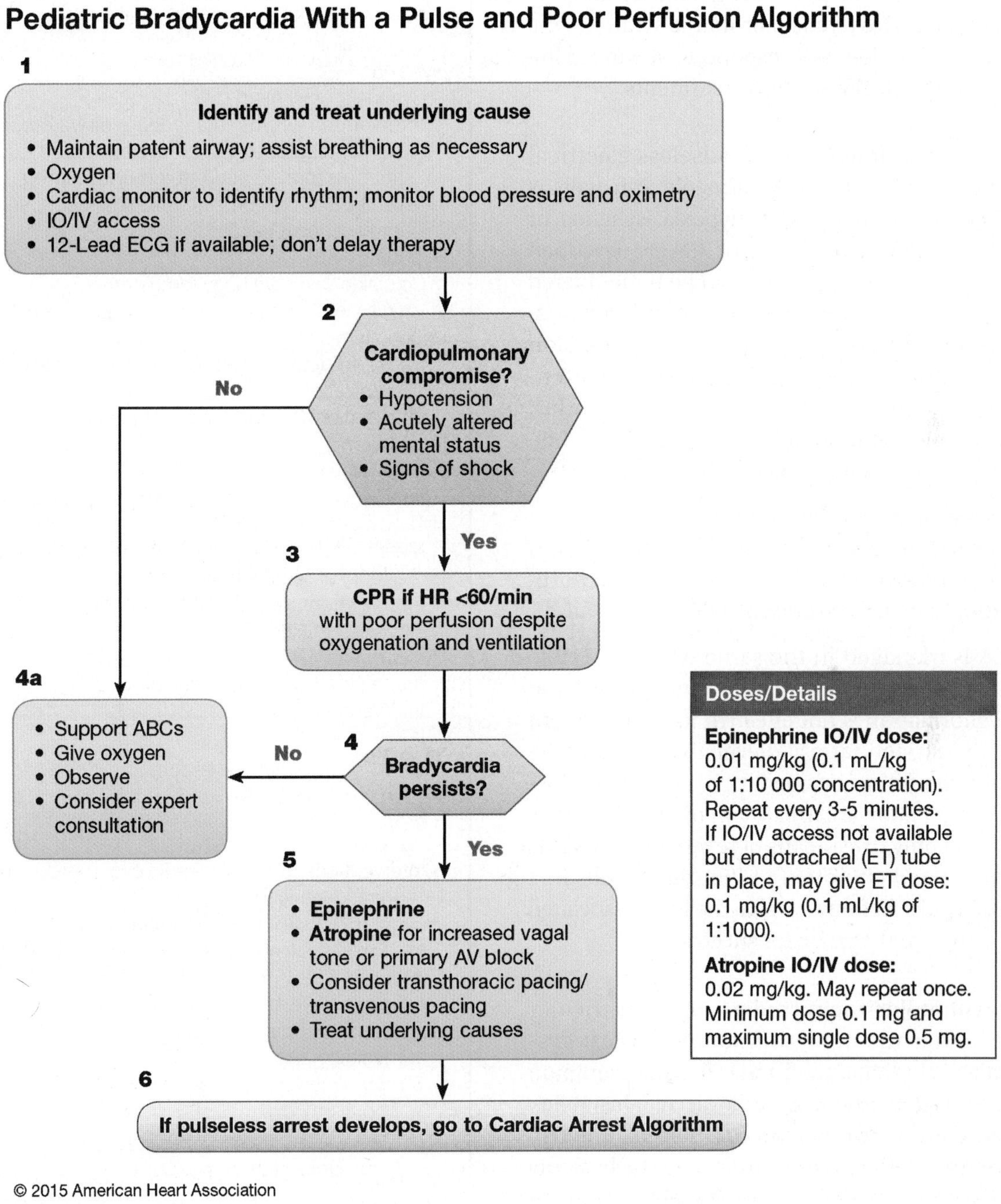

Abbreviations: ABCs, airway, breathing, and circulation; AV, atrioventricular; CPR, cardiopulmonary resuscitation; ECG, electrocardiogram; ET, endotracheal; HR, heart rate; IO, intraosseous; IV, intravenous

FIGURE 47-8 Pediatric advanced life support tachycardia algorithm for infants and children with a pulse and poor perfusion.

Modified from: Web-based Integrated 2015 American Heart Association Guidelines for CPR and ECC—Part 12: Pediatric Advanced Life Support © 2015 American Heart Association, Inc.

is the drug of choice. Bradycardia caused by primary atrioventricular heart block or increased vagal tone (both of which are rare in pediatric patients) should be managed with atropine. In cases where bradycardia is caused by dysfunction in the sinus node, or complete heart block, external cardiac pacing may be lifesaving.[4] External cardiac pacing is uncomfortable. Its use in children is reserved for profound symptomatic bradycardia that does not respond to advanced life support and basic life support treatments.

Pulseless Electrical Activity. Pulseless electrical activity (PEA) often precedes asystole. It usually is caused by prolonged periods of hypoxia, ischemia, or hypercapnia. Reversible causes of PEA are described in Chapter 21, *Cardiology*, and can be remembered as the "Hs and Ts." The Hs are hypovolemia, hypoxia, hypothermia, hyper-/hypokalemia, hydrogen ion excess (acidosis), and hypoglycemia. The Ts are tension pneumothorax, pericardial tamponade, toxins, and thrombosis (pulmonary, coronary) (**BOX 47-5**). Important ECG findings include the following:

- A slow, wide-complex rhythm
- The presence of some electrical activity (other than ventricular tachycardia/ventricular fibrillation) and the absence of a detectable pulse

PEA is managed in the same way as asystole (**FIGURE 47-9**), with drug therapy (epinephrine) and CPR. Defibrillation is not effective in the treatment of PEA and asystolic arrest.[4] Reversible causes of the condition should be considered and corrected if possible. Identification and treatment of the underlying cause is the only true means of reversing PEA. Early recognition and treatment of PEA that results in a return of a pulse before arrival in the ED is associated with an improved chance for survival.

Supraventricular Tachycardia. Supraventricular tachycardia is the most common nonarrest dysrhythmia during childhood and is the most common dysrhythmia that produces cardiovascular instability during infancy.[4] Two factors can help distinguish supraventricular tachycardia from sinus tachycardia caused by shock: patient history (eg, dehydration or hemorrhage associated with shock) and heart rate. With sinus tachycardia, heart rate is usually less than 220 beats/min in infants and less than 180 beats/min in children. Heart rate is usually greater than these

BOX 47-5 The Hs and Ts: Potentially Reversible Causes of PEA

The Hs

Hypovolemia
- Poor skin color, rapid heart rate, flat neck veins
- Intervention: Rapid 20-mL/kg bolus of isotonic crystalloid

Hypoxia
- Cyanosis, slow heart rate
- Intervention: Oxygenate; secure airway (consider DOPE: displaced ET tube, obstructed ET tube, pneumothorax, and equipment failure such as ventricular malfunction or disconnect); ventilate and suction if needed

Hypothermia
- Cold skin, low core body temperature
- Intervention: Rapid rewarming techniques; warm IV fluids

Hyperkalemia
- Peaked T waves, history of renal disease, crush syndrome
- Intervention: Calcium, sodium bicarbonate, albuterol

Hypokalemia
- Flat T waves
- Intervention: In-hospital infusion of potassium

Hydrogen ion excess
- Metabolic acidosis: Small-amplitude QRS, may have history of renal disease
- Intervention: In-hospital correction of underlying cause of acidosis

Hypoglycemia
- Altered level of consciousness
- Intervention: Dextrose

The Ts

Tension pneumothorax
- Deviated trachea, jugular venous distention, absent breath sounds
- Interventions: Thoracic needle decompression

Tamponade (pericardial)
- Jugular venous distention, rapid heart rate
- Intervention: Volume bolus; in-hospital pericardiocentesis

Toxins
- Drug overdose, bradycardia, tachycardia
- Intervention: Specific to toxin

Thrombosis
- ST-segment elevation (rare in children) or pulmonary embolism

Modified from: Clinical and Practice Guidelines: Guidelines for Care of Children in the Emergency Department. American College of Emergency Physicians website. https://www.acep.org/Clinical---Practice-Management/Guidelines-for-Care-of-Children-in-the-Emergency-Department/#sm.0000vyjqgsa95e2uwy91hykef6zea. Accessed March 28, 2018.

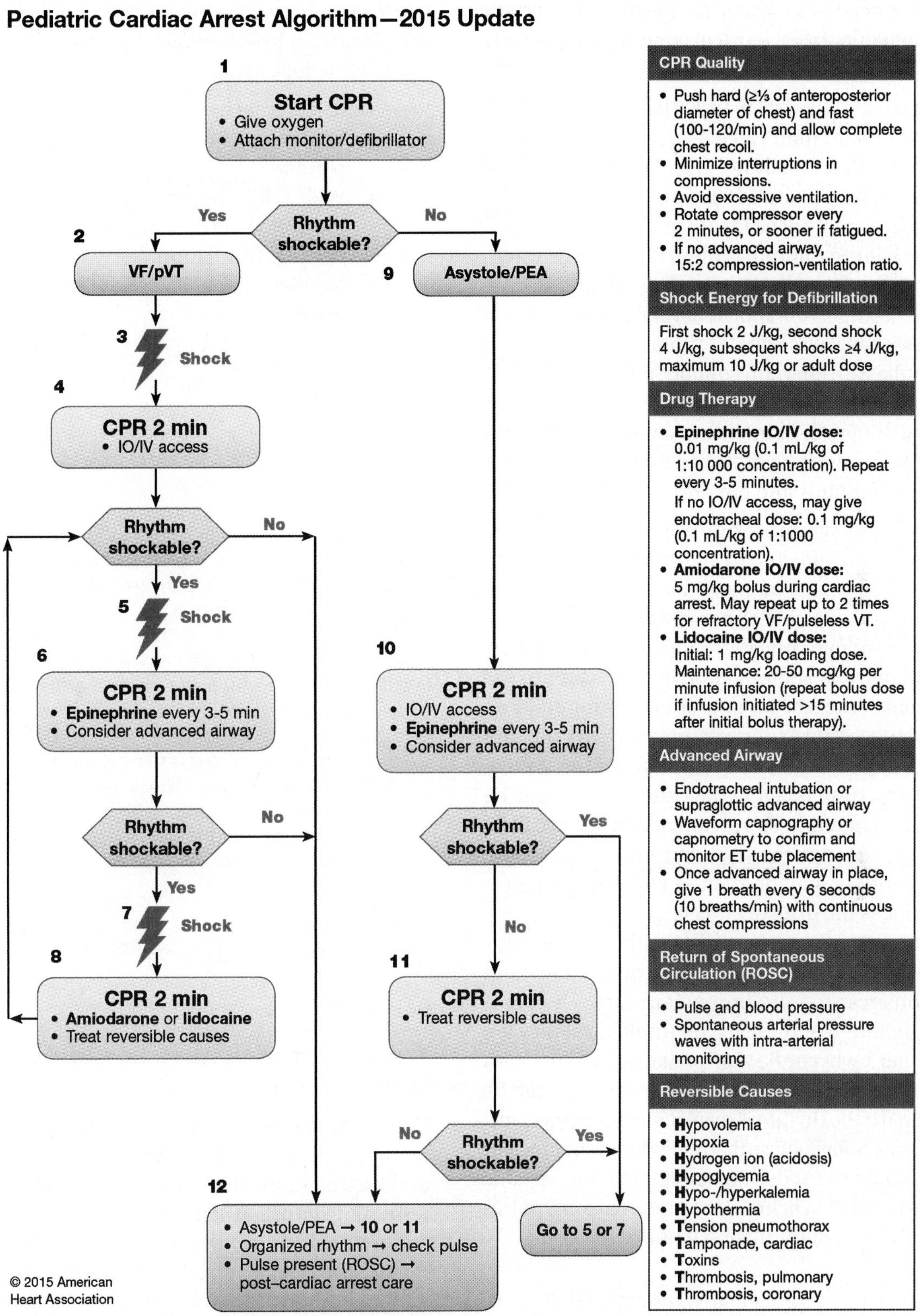
Pediatric Cardiac Arrest Algorithm—2015 Update
1
Start CPR
• Give oxygen
• Attach monitor/defibrillator
Rhythm shockable?
Yes
No
2
VF/pVT
3
Shock
4
CPR 2 min
• IO/IV access
Rhythm shockable?
No
Yes
5
Shock
6
CPR 2 min
• Epinephrine every 3-5 min
• Consider advanced airway
Rhythm shockable?
No
Yes
7
Shock
8
CPR 2 min
• Amiodarone or lidocaine
• Treat reversible causes
9
Asystole/PEA
10
CPR 2 min
• IO/IV access
• Epinephrine every 3-5 min
• Consider advanced airway
Rhythm shockable?
Yes
No
11
CPR 2 min
• Treat reversible causes
No
Rhythm shockable?
Yes
12
• Asystole/PEA → 10 or 11
• Organized rhythm → check pulse
• Pulse present (ROSC) → post–cardiac arrest care
Go to 5 or 7
© 2015 American Heart Association
CPR Quality
• Push hard (≥⅓ of anteroposterior diameter of chest) and fast (100-120/min) and allow complete chest recoil.
• Minimize interruptions in compressions.
• Avoid excessive ventilation.
• Rotate compressor every 2 minutes, or sooner if fatigued.
• If no advanced airway, 15:2 compression-ventilation ratio.
Shock Energy for Defibrillation
First shock 2 J/kg, second shock 4 J/kg, subsequent shocks ≥4 J/kg, maximum 10 J/kg or adult dose
Drug Therapy
• Epinephrine IO/IV dose: 0.01 mg/kg (0.1 mL/kg of 1:10 000 concentration). Repeat every 3-5 minutes.
If no IO/IV access, may give endotracheal dose: 0.1 mg/kg (0.1 mL/kg of 1:1000 concentration).
• Amiodarone IO/IV dose: 5 mg/kg bolus during cardiac arrest. May repeat up to 2 times for refractory VF/pulseless VT.
• Lidocaine IO/IV dose: Initial: 1 mg/kg loading dose. Maintenance: 20-50 mcg/kg per minute infusion (repeat bolus dose if infusion initiated >15 minutes after initial bolus therapy).
Advanced Airway
• Endotracheal intubation or supraglottic advanced airway
• Waveform capnography or capnometry to confirm and monitor ET tube placement
• Once advanced airway in place, give 1 breath every 6 seconds (10 breaths/min) with continuous chest compressions
Return of Spontaneous Circulation (ROSC)
• Pulse and blood pressure
• Spontaneous arterial pressure waves with intra-arterial monitoring
Reversible Causes
• Hypovolemia
• Hypoxia
• Hydrogen ion (acidosis)
• Hypoglycemia
• Hypo-/hyperkalemia
• Hypothermia
• Tension pneumothorax
• Tamponade, cardiac
• Toxins
• Thrombosis, pulmonary
• Thrombosis, coronary

Abbreviations: CPR, cardiopulmonary resuscitation; ET, endotracheal; IO, intraosseous; IV, intravenous; PEA, pulseless electrical activity; pVT, pulseless ventricular tachycardia; ROSC, return of spontaneous circulation; VF, ventricular fibrillation; VT, ventricular tachycardia

FIGURE 47-9 Pediatric advanced life support pulseless arrest algorithm.

Modified from: Web-based Integrated 2015 American Heart Association Guidelines for CPR and ECC—Part 12: Pediatric Advanced Life Support © 2015 American Heart Association, Inc.

rates with supraventricular tachycardia. Important ECG findings in supraventricular tachycardia include the following:

- Heart rate is greater than 220 beats/min in infants and greater than 180 beats/min in children.
- The rhythm usually is regular because associated atrioventricular block is rare.
- P waves may not be identifiable, especially when the ventricular rate is high. If present, P waves usually are negative in leads II, III, and aV_F.
- QRS complex duration is normal in most children (less than 0.09 second).[4] Supraventricular tachycardia with aberrant conduction (wide-complex supraventricular tachycardia) may be difficult to distinguish from ventricular tachycardia (but wide-complex supraventricular tachycardia is rare in infants and children).

Signs and symptoms during supraventricular tachycardia are affected by the child's age, duration of supraventricular tachycardia, prior ventricular function, and ventricular rate (**FIGURE 47-10**). If the child is hemodynamically stable and cooperative, vagal maneuvers such as applying ice/water to the upper half of the face for infants and young children may be successful in terminating the rhythm, and in older children, blowing through a straw, vagal maneuvers, or massaging the carotid sinus may be effective.[4] Unstable supraventricular tachycardia is best managed with synchronized cardioversion. Stable patients may be treated with drug therapy. Adenosine is the drug of choice.

Wide-complex tachycardias with signs of compromised tissue perfusion and impaired level of consciousness require immediate care. The paramedic should treat these dysrhythmias as if they are ventricular tachycardia. For pediatric patients with stable, wide-complex tachycardia, adenosine can be considered if the rhythm is regular and monomorphic. If adenosine is ineffective, then amiodarone or procainamide should be used. Urgent treatment for unstable patients includes synchronized cardioversion if pulses are present and defibrillation if pulses are absent.

Ventricular Tachycardia and Ventricular Fibrillation. As stated before, ventricular tachycardia and ventricular fibrillation are uncommon in children. If present, the paramedic should consider causes of these dysrhythmias that include congenital heart disease, cardiomyopathies, myocarditis, metabolic causes (eg, hypoglycemia), or reversible causes (ie, drug toxicity or hypothermia). Important ECG findings include the following:

- Ventricular tachycardia
  - Ventricular rate at least 120 beats/min and regular
  - Wide QRS complex
  - P waves that often are unidentifiable
- Ventricular fibrillation
  - No identifiable P wave, QRS complex, or T wave
  - Ventricular fibrillation activity that may be coarse or fine

NOTE

Automated external defibrillators (AEDs) with pediatric cable/pad systems with a dose attenuator have been approved by the Food and Drug Administration. They may be used in infants and children up to 8 years of age. In infants younger than 1 year, a manual defibrillator is preferred. If a manual defibrillator is not available, an AED with a dose attenuator may be used. An AED without a dose attenuator may be used if neither a manual defibrillator nor a defibrillator with a dose attenuator is available. Pads should be positioned so they do not touch each other. The lone rescuer responding to a child with no signs of circulation should perform 2 minutes of CPR before activating EMS or retrieving an AED. When the arrest is witnessed, the lone rescuer should call 9-1-1 or retrieve the AED and then commence CPR.

Modified from: American Heart Association. *Pediatric Advanced Life Support*. Dallas, TX: American Heart Association; 2016.

Treatment of Ventricular Tachycardia With a Pulse

Hemodynamically stable ventricular tachycardia should be managed under the advice of medical direction and with caution. The initial efforts are aimed at determining the origin of the tachycardia and obtaining a thorough history. Adenosine may be considered if the rhythm is regular and monomorphic. In-hospital administration of amiodarone or procainamide may be considered. (These drugs should not routinely be administered together.) Ventricular tachycardia that produces a palpable pulse and signs of shock (low cardiac output, poor perfusion) requires immediate synchronized cardioversion.

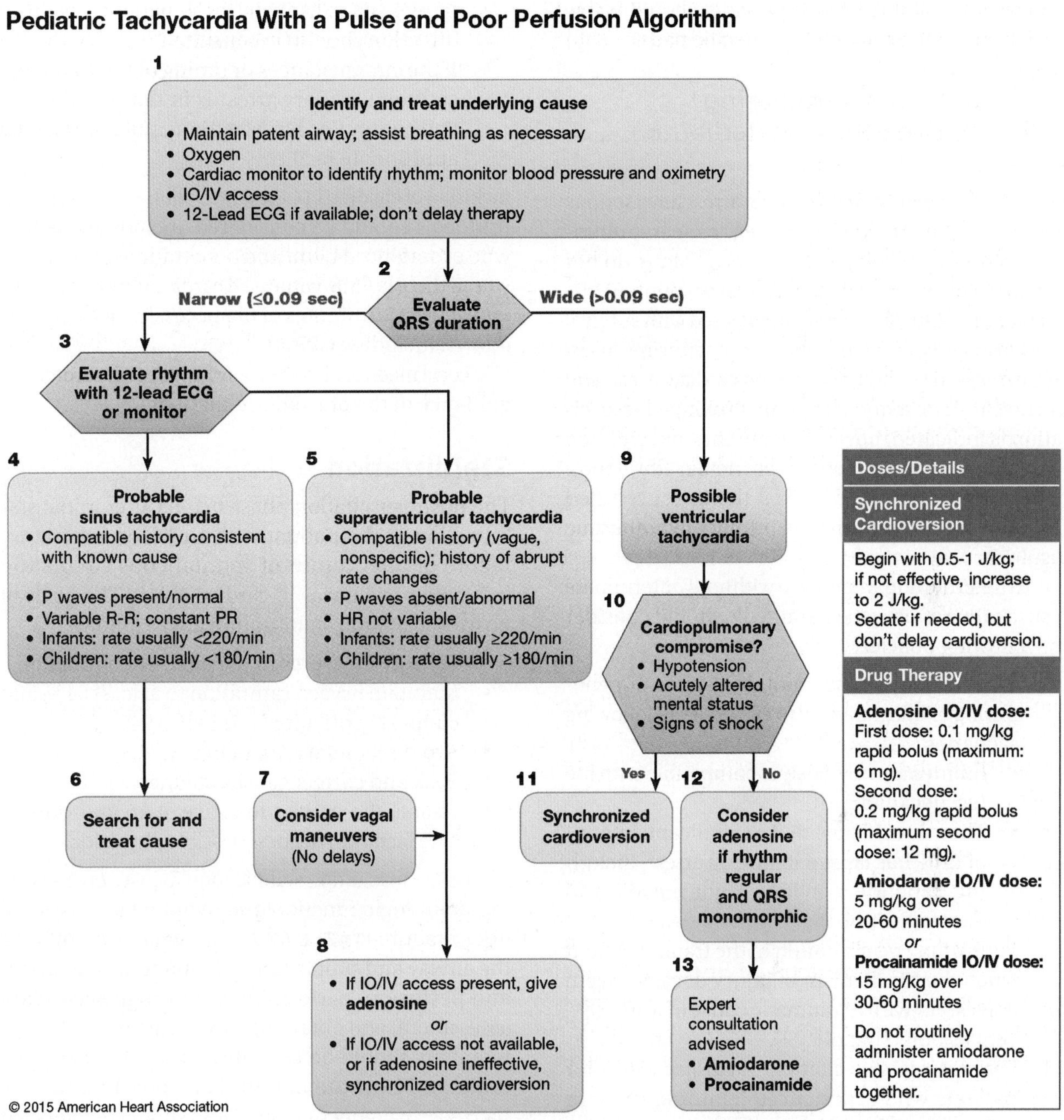

Abbreviations: ABCs, airway, breathing, circulation; ECG, electrocardiogram; HR, heart rate; IO, intraosseous; IV, intravenous

FIGURE 47-10 Pediatric advanced life support tachycardia algorithm for infants and children with a pulse and poor perfusion.

Treatment of Pulseless Ventricular Tachycardia and Ventricular Fibrillation

Pulseless ventricular tachycardia and ventricular fibrillation are managed with immediate defibrillation, CPR, advanced airway with ventilatory support, and drug therapy (eg, epinephrine and amiodarone or lidocaine).[29] Infant patches generally should be used during defibrillation for infants up to about 1 year of age or weighing less than 22 pounds (10 kg). Adult patches are used for all other children. Size recommendations vary by manufacturer, so the provider should follow the instructions on the device-specific pads.[4]

Withholding or Terminating Resuscitative Efforts in Pediatric Patients

Most children who suffer a cardiac arrest have serious preexisting health conditions (eg, cancer, pulmonary, cardiac, neurologic disorders).[30] Many do not survive, even with a transient return of spontaneous circulation. Clinical variables associated with survival include length of CPR, number of epinephrine doses, age, witnessed versus unwitnessed cardiac arrest, and the first and subsequent rhythm. Prolonged resuscitation is indicated, however, in infants and children with recurring or refractory ventricular fibrillation or ventricular tachycardia or if the arrest resulted from toxic drug exposure or a primary hypothermic insult.[4,31]

In determining whether to withhold or terminate resuscitative efforts, the paramedic should consider the following policies:[31]

1. Withholding resuscitation in victims of penetrating or blunt trauma in either of the following scenarios:
   - Injuries are obviously incompatible with life (eg, decapitation).
   - There is evidence that a significant amount of time has lapsed following arrest, including dependent lividity, rigor mortis, and decomposition.
2. Performing resuscitation in the trauma patient when the mechanism of injury does not seem consistent with a traumatic cause of arrest (except as noted in policy 1).
3. Performing resuscitation in cardiac arrest for patients who experienced lightning strike or drowning with hypothermia (except as noted in policy 1).
4. Providing immediate transport to an ED for patients in whom signs of life were observed prior to arrest and when CPR has been ongoing or started within 5 minutes in the field. Airway management and vascular access should be performed during transport.
5. Terminating resuscitation after 30 minutes for patients with blunt and penetrating trauma in cases where there was an unwitnessed traumatic cardiopulmonary arrest. A longer period of hypoxia is likely in these patients. Medical direction should be consulted.
   - If the circumstances or timing of the traumatic cardiopulmonary arrest is in doubt, initiating and continuing resuscitation until arrival at the appropriate facility.

Inclusion of children in state termination-of-resuscitation protocols should be considered, including children who experienced blunt and penetrating trauma or in whom there is EMS-witnessed cardiopulmonary arrest and at least 30 minutes of unsuccessful resuscitative efforts, including CPR.

Local medical direction may have specific protocols/guidance in the preceding situations.

Stabilization

The postresuscitation phase begins after initial stabilization of the patient with shock or respiratory failure or after return of spontaneous circulation in a patient who was in cardiac arrest. The goals of postresuscitation stabilization are as follows:[4]

- Identify measures to preserve brain function.
- Maintain oxygen saturation to at least 94%, and support ventilation and perfusion.
- Avoid secondary organ injury.
- Seek and correct causes of illness.
- Enable the patient to arrive at an appropriate care facility in the best possible physiologic state.

Postresuscitation stabilization focuses on preserving neurologic function and avoiding multisystem organ failure (**TABLE 47-11**). It includes stabilizing the airway and supporting oxygenation, ventilation, and perfusion; performing a thorough secondary assessment; and obtaining a medical history. Family members should be kept abreast of what has been done and how the patient is responding to care (**BOX 47-6**). Frequent reports also should be provided to the receiving hospital.

Meningitis

As described in Chapter 27, *Infectious and Communicable Diseases*, meningitis is inflammation of the fluid-containing membranes (meninges) that surround the brain and spinal cord. Meningitis normally occurs as a complication of bacterial or viral infection. Meningitis can be life threatening (there were 500 deaths reported between 2003 and 2007).[32] This infection can rapidly progress to permanent brain damage,

TABLE 47-11 Summary of Postresuscitation Care

Vital Function	Intervention
Airway	Perform tracheal intubation with confirmation of tube position and repeat confirmation on movement/transport (continuous $ETCO_2$ monitoring mandatory).
	Perform gastric decompression if no spontaneous respiration occurs.
Breathing	Titrate inspired oxygen for SpO_2 to 94% to 99%.
	Provide mechanical ventilation, targeting normal ventilation goals (PCO_2 35–45 mm Hg).
Circulation	Ensure adequate intravascular volume: Infuse 20-mL/kg boluses of isotonic crystalloid IV/IO to treat shock (10 mL/kg if cardiogenic shock is suspected).
	Optimize myocardial function and systemic perfusion if shock persists despite fluid boluses (eg, epinephrine, dopamine, norepinephrine infusions).
	Monitor capillary refill, blood pressure, continuous electrocardiogram, and urine output; measure arterial blood gas and lactate to assess degree of acidosis, if available.
	Ideally, maintain two routes of functional vascular access.
Disability	Perform secondary assessment, including brief neurologic assessment.
	Avoid hyperglycemia; treat hypoglycemia (monitor glucose).
	If seizures are observed, medicate with anticonvulsant agents.
	Control pain with analgesics (eg, fentanyl, morphine) and anxiety with sedatives (eg, midazolam, lorazepam).
Exposure	Avoid and correct hyperthermia (monitor temperature).
	Consider therapeutic hypothermia.

Abbreviations: $ETCO_2$, end-tidal carbon dioxide; PCO_2, partial pressure of carbon dioxide; SpO_2, oxygen saturation

Modified from: American Heart Association. Pediatric Advanced Life Support. Dallas, TX: American Heart Association; 2016; Frydland M, Kjaergaard J, Erlinge D, et al. Target temperature management of 33°C and 36°C in patients with out-of-hospital cardiac arrest with initial non-shockable rhythm—a TTM sub-study. *Resuscitation*. 2015;89:142-148; Mahmoud A, Elgendy IY, Bavry AA. Use of targeted temperature management after out-of-hospital cardiac arrest: a meta-analysis of randomized controlled trials. *Am J Med*. 2016;129(5):522-527.e2; and Part 12: Pediatric Advanced Life Support: Web-Based Integrated Guidelines for Cardiopulmonary Resuscitation and Emergency Cardiovascular Care. American Heart Association website. https://eccguidelines.heart.org/index.php/circulation/cpr-ecc-guidelines-2/part-12-pediatric-advanced-life-support/. Accessed May 14, 2018.

BOX 47-6 Interacting With the Family During Resuscitative Efforts

In cases where there is an impending or recent child death, effective measures to interact with family members include the following:

1. Provide rapid coordinated care.
2. Allow family to witness resuscitation.
3. Provide continuous communication about what is happening and why.
4. Give concrete forms of help, such as calling family or clergy, allowing the family to spend time with the child after the death, giving emotional support, and performing appropriate follow-up gestures.

If the resuscitation is not successful, it is important that the EMS crew be offered options for counseling. The death of a child is never a routine occurrence.

Modified from: Fallat ME, Barbee AP, Forest R, et al. Family centered practice during pediatric death in an out of hospital setting. *Prehosp Emerg Care*. 2016;20(6):798-807.

impaired vision or hearing, neurologic dysfunction, and death. The highest incidence of meningitis is 6 months to 2 years of age, with the greatest time for risk when an infant is younger than 1 year, followed by a second peak in adolescence.[33] Most commonly, meningitis develops over 1 to 4 days. However, in severe cases, a child who looks healthy can rapidly become seriously ill within a day.

The signs and symptoms of meningitis depend on the child's age and are not always obvious. Classic symptoms in infants younger than 3 months include decreased liquid intake, vomiting, irritability, lethargy, fever, bulging fontanel, and seizures. Signs and symptoms for older children and adults include nausea and vomiting, headache, photophobia, fever, altered mental status, lethargy, seizures, and neck stiffness (nuchal rigidity) or pain. Other classic presentations that may aid in diagnosis include the following:

- **Brudzinski sign.** The child's knees automatically move up toward the body when the neck is bent forward, or pain is experienced in the legs when bent.
- **Kernig sign.** Child is unable to extend the knees because of pain when the thigh is flexed on the abdomen.
- **Rash.** Petechial or purpuric rash may appear if meningococcus is the causative agent.

Prehospital care is primarily supportive. Droplet precautions should be employed. A surgical mask should be applied to the patient and EMS provider while providing care and during transport. In some cases, seizure control or IV fluid replacement will be necessary. Infuse fluids if sepsis is present, and follow local guidelines for hospital sepsis alert activation. In-hospital care will be based on the causative agent.

Hydrocephalus

Hydrocephalus is a condition in which there is excessive accumulation of CSF around the brain. CSF is normally absorbed into the bloodstream through small protrusions of the arachnoid (arachnoid villi) near the top and midline of the brain. From there, CSF is absorbed and filtered by the kidneys and liver. If this normal process fails, the excess CSF cannot drain, causing abnormal widening of the ventricles and increased pressure on brain tissues.

Hydrocephalus may be congenital or acquired. Congenital hydrocephalus is present at birth and can be caused by events during fetal development or by genetic abnormalities. An estimated 1 to 2 newborns in every 1,000 births has congenital hydrocephalus.[34] Acquired hydrocephalus can occur any time after birth. This form of hydrocephalus can affect people of all ages and may be caused by injury or disease (eg, head injury, CNS tumor, meningitis).

Congenital or acquired hydrocephalus is diagnosed through neurologic evaluation and by using ultrasonography, computed tomography, magnetic resonance imaging, or pressure-monitoring techniques. Hydrocephalus is most often treated by surgically inserting a shunt system into a ventricle to drain excess fluid. Shunts use catheters and flow-valve devices to divert the flow of CSF from the CNS to another area of the body (often the abdominal cavity), where it can be absorbed into the bloodstream. Complications include mechanical failure, obstructions, and infection. The shunts are likely to require replacement after several years and require frequent monitoring and follow-up.

In infancy, the most obvious indication of hydrocephalus is often a rapid increase in head circumference or an unusually large head size (**FIGURE 47-11**). Other symptoms may include vomiting, sleepiness, irritability, downward deviation of the eyes ("sun setting"), and seizures. Older children and adults with hydrocephalus may also experience headache, blurred or double vision, memory loss, poor coordination, sudden falls, gait disturbance, and urinary incontinence. Changes in personality or cognition may also occur.

Prehospital care for patients with hydrocephalus is primarily supportive. The signs and symptoms of shunt obstruction or displacement are those of increased ICP (headaches, nausea and vomiting, visual disturbances, seizures). Cushing triad (elevated systolic pressure, irregular respirations, and bradycardia) can indicate increased pressure on the

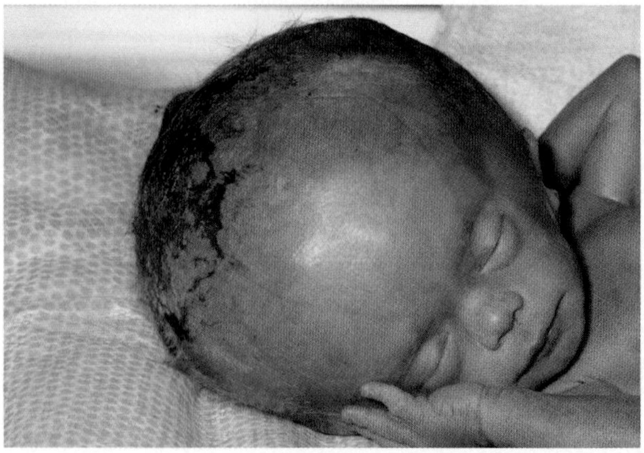

FIGURE 47-11 Infant with hydrocephalus.

brainstem. The paramedic first should ensure adequate airway, ventilatory, and circulatory support for these patients. Medical direction may recommend ET intubation and controlled hyperventilation to lower ICP.[35] These patients are prone to respiratory arrest. They need immediate transport to a proper facility for evaluation by a physician. If possible, the patient's head should be elevated during transport.

Shunt Systems

A **shunt** is a tube or device that is implanted surgically in the body and redirects body fluid from one cavity or vessel to another. Shunts are sometimes used to reroute excess fluid to the abdomen (ventriculoperitoneal or lumboperitoneal shunt), the lung (ventriculopleural shunt), and the heart (ventriculoatrial shunt).

The ventriculoperitoneal shunt for hydrocephalus consists of two catheters, a reservoir, and a valve to prevent backflow (**FIGURE 47-12**). The first catheter is inserted through the skull. It drains fluid from the ventricles of the brain. The second catheter is passed into another body cavity (usually the abdomen, chest, or right atrium of the heart through the jugular vein), where the excess fluid is absorbed. The two catheters are connected by a reservoir and valve, which is placed under the scalp. The reservoir usually can be palpated over the mastoid area, just behind the ear.

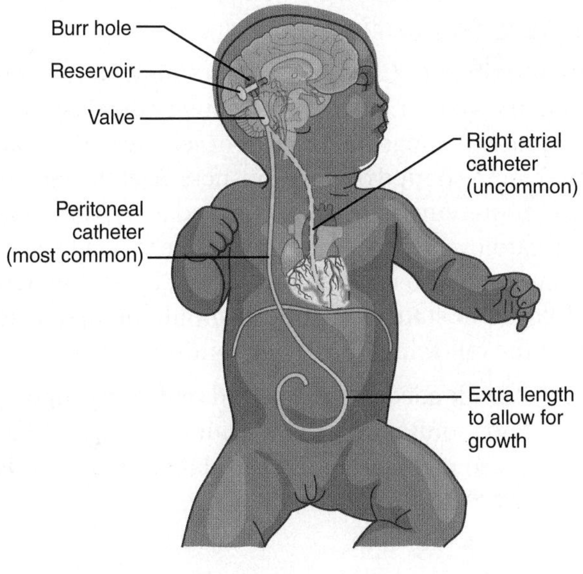

FIGURE 47-12 Ventriculoperitoneal shunt for drainage of symptomatic hydrocephalus.

Shunt systems can be either programmable or nonprogrammable.[36] The valves in programmable systems can be changed noninvasively or adjusted automatically (flow-regulated devices). Complications of shunt systems include obstruction from clotted blood or fluid and catheter displacement.

Seizures

A seizure (described in Chapter 24, *Neurology*) is an episode of sudden abnormal electrical activity in the brain. It results in abnormalities in motor, sensory, or autonomic function, usually associated with abnormal behavior, changes in level of consciousness, or both (**BOX 47-7**). Common causes of seizure in adults and children include noncompliance with a drug regimen for the treatment of epilepsy, head trauma, intracranial infection, brain tumor, metabolic disturbance, or poisoning. The most common cause of new onset of seizure in children is fever.

Febrile Seizures

A **febrile seizure** is a seizure associated with fever but without evidence of intracranial infection or other

BOX 47-7 Causes of Afebrile Seizures in Children

Idiopathic (50% of Cases)

Childhood and juvenile absence epilepsy
Benign epilepsy (childhood seizures that involve twitching, numbness, or tingling of the face or tongue)
Juvenile myoclonic epilepsy

Symptomatic or Probably Symptomatic (50% of Cases)

Malformations of brain development
Neurocutaneous syndromes (neurologic disorders that cause cutaneous manifestations)
Vascular malformation
Congenital or acquired CNS infection
Hypoxic ischemic brain injury
Stroke
Traumatic brain injury
Tumor
Inborn error of metabolism (inability to properly turn food into energy)

Reproduced from the BC Medical Journal (Reprinted from *BC Med J.* 2011;53[6]:275).

definable cause; such seizures usually occur between the ages of 6 months and 5 years.[19] About 2% to 5% of healthy children experience a febrile seizure. Of those, only 2% to 7% develop epilepsy. About 30% of those who have a febrile seizure experience recurrence.[19] Major risk factors for febrile seizure include age younger than 1 year, and a fever of short duration (<24 hours). Febrile seizures are most likely to occur with greater than 102°F (38.9°C), but may also occur with milder fevers. The seizures usually are associated with an underlying viral infection (most often of the upper respiratory tract), gastroenteritis, roseola, otitis media, or another febrile illness.

Febrile seizures often manifest with generalized tonic–clonic activity, but they can have a more subtle presentation. As a rule, classic febrile seizures are of short duration and usually last less than 5 minutes and no longer than 15 minutes. They also have an uncomplicated and short postictal period. Seizures that last longer than 15 minutes are considered febrile status epilepticus and require extensive investigation. These seizures should never be considered benign. Regardless of the suspected cause, children who have experienced a seizure should be transported for evaluation by a physician per protocol.

Assessment and Management of Seizures. In most cases the seizure has stopped before EMS arrives. In many instances, the child is in a postictal state. As in any emergency, the first priorities are airway management and ventilatory support. This includes airway positioning, suctioning of the airway, and administration of oxygen. Repeated assessment of the adequacy of ventilation is necessary. Special emphasis should be placed on respiratory rate and depth. If the airway cannot be maintained with manual maneuvers, airway adjuncts should be used.

After initial stabilization of the patient's condition, the paramedic should assess vital signs and obtain a history. Important elements of the history which may need to be obtained for the parent or caregiver include the following:

- Previous seizures
- Number of seizures in this episode
- Duration and description of seizure activity
- Presence of vomiting during the seizure (aspiration risk)
- Color change during seizure
- Eye movements during the seizure
- Condition of the child when first found
- Recent illness
- Potential for toxic ingestion
- Potential head injury (as primary cause or secondary complication)
- Significant medical conditions
- Recent headache or nuchal rigidity (suggestive of meningitis)
- Medication use and compliance with anticonvulsant medication

During transport to the ED, the paramedic should continuously monitor the child and be alert for recurrent seizures. The paramedic should prepare to treat seizure as for status epilepticus (discussed next). The characteristics of the postictal period (level of consciousness, movement, speech, sensory or motor impairment) should be noted. Medical direction may advise that a febrile patient be given an antipyretic if the patient is alert. The antipyretic may reduce the fever en route to the receiving hospital. The paramedic should not apply ice or submerge the patient in a cool bath in an effort to reduce fever.

Status Epilepticus

As described in Chapter 24, *Neurology*, status epilepticus is continuous seizure activity that lasts 4 to 5 minutes or longer or a recurrent seizure without an intervening period of consciousness. A status seizure is a serious emergency that can lead to hypotension and cardiovascular, respiratory, and renal failure. The seizure can also result in permanent brain damage. Children in status epilepticus should be managed with the following initial interventions:

1. Provide adequate airway and ventilatory support and monitor oxygen saturation as measured by pulse oximeter and end-tidal carbon dioxide ($ETCO_2$) levels.

2. Measure the blood glucose level to screen for hypoglycemia. If the value is less than 60 mg/dL, establish vascular access and administer dextrose 10%, or dextrose 25% (per medical direction).[37] Hypoglycemia also can be treated with an IM injection of glucagon if IV or IO access cannot be established.
3. If seizures do not stop, administer midazolam, lorazepam (intranasal, IM, or IV/IO) or diazepam (IV/IO).
4. Attach a cardiac monitor. Observe for rhythm or conduction abnormalities that may suggest hypoxia.

Hypoglycemia

As described in Chapter 25, *Endocrinology*, hypoglycemia is an abnormally low concentration of glucose in the blood. In children, hypoglycemia is usually the result of excessive response to glucose absorption, illness, physical exertion, or decreased dietary intake. Because children's insulin requirements vary as they grow, careful monitoring is needed. Diabetic children often have hypoglycemia related to an excessive insulin dose, a delayed or missed meal, or vigorous physical activity. In the prehospital setting, hypoglycemia is most frequently seen in infants and children with type 1 diabetes. About 132,000 children in the United States younger than 18 years have been diagnosed with type 1 diabetes.[38]

The signs and symptoms of hypoglycemia can be classified as mild, moderate, and severe. Mild symptoms include hunger, weakness, tachypnea, and tachycardia. Moderate symptoms include sweating, tremors, irritability, vomiting, mood disorders, blurred vision, stomachache, headache, and dizziness. Severe symptoms include decreased level of consciousness and seizure activity, requiring prompt treatment with dextrose to prevent brain damage.

Prehospital care is directed first at ensuring adequate airway and ventilatory support. A blood glucose measurement should be obtained in any child with an altered level of consciousness that has no explainable cause. Conscious children who are mildly hypoglycemic should receive an oral glucose solution or paste. Unconscious children or those with moderate or severe hypoglycemia require IV/IO dextrose or IM glucagon administration. This should be followed by a repeat blood glucose measurement in 10 to 15 minutes. All children with signs and symptoms of hypoglycemia should be transported for physician evaluation.

Hyperglycemia

Hyperglycemia is an abnormally high concentration of glucose in the blood. It results from an absence of or resistance to insulin. The low insulin level prevents glucose from entering the cells, causing glucose to build up in the blood. If not treated, hyperglycemia can lead to dehydration, diabetic ketoacidosis (DKA), coma, and death. DKA is the leading cause of morbidity and mortality in children with type 1 diabetes.[39] Although less common, it also occurs in pediatric patients with type 2 diabetes. In children diagnosed with type 1 diabetes, the condition often is the result of an insulin dose that is insufficient in relation to food intake, failure to take insulin, illness, or a malfunctioning insulin-delivery system (eg, insulin pump). Some children present with signs of hyperglycemia and no history of diabetes because it has not yet been diagnosed. In some of these cases, the patients are critically ill.

The signs and symptoms of hyperglycemia are classified as early or late. Early signs and symptoms include (polydipsia, polyphagia, and polyuria). Weight loss also is considered an early sign of the illness. Late signs and symptoms associated with dehydration and early ketoacidosis include weakness, abdominal pain, generalized aches, loss of appetite, nausea, vomiting, signs of dehydration (with the exception of urinary output), altered mental status, fruity breath odor, tachypnea, hyperventilation, and tachycardia. If untreated, Kussmaul respirations and coma may occur.

Children suspected of having hyperglycemia should receive adequate airway, ventilatory, and circulatory support. Blood glucose will be greater than 200 mg/dL. These patients require IV fluid therapy if signs of dehydration are present. Fluid resuscitation begins with 10 mL/kg normal saline or lactated Ringer solution (maximum 1,000 mL) over 1 hour.[40] If there are severe signs of circulatory compromise, the fluid boluses may begin at 20 mL/kg.[39] The administration of insulin usually is reserved as an in-hospital procedure.

CRITICAL THINKING

Why do you think type 1 diabetes may stay undetected until a child is seriously ill?

Blood Disorders

As described in Chapter 31, *Hematology*, there are a number of conditions and diseases that can cause blood disorders in children and adults. These disorders may affect the oxygen-carrying capacity of hemoglobin, blood-clotting mechanisms, immune function, and infection risk. Common blood disorders in children include sickle cell disease (presenting as acute chest syndrome, splenic sequestration, vaso-occlusive crisis, and priapism in males), bleeding disorders (eg, thrombocytopenia, hemophilia, von Willebrand disease), leukemia, leukopenia, lymphoma, and others.

DID YOU KNOW?

Childhood Leukemia

Leukemia in children often is described as being acute or chronic. Almost all childhood leukemia is acute. The two main types of acute leukemia in children are *acute lymphocytic leukemia* (ALL) and *acute myelogenous leukemia* (AML), both of which can be further divided into subtypes. Of the estimated 3,500 children (ages birth to 14 years) who will develop leukemia in the United States each year, about 3 out of 4 will be diagnosed with ALL. Most of the remaining cases will be diagnosed as AML.

ALL starts from the lymphoid cells in the bone marrow. ALL is most common in early childhood, peaking between 2 and 4 years of age. AML is most common during the first 2 years of life, and again during teenage years. The 5-year survival rate for children with ALL is now greater than 85%. The 5-year survival rate for children with AML is now 60% to 70%.

Modified from: What are the key statistics for childhood leukemia? American Cancer Society website. https://www.cancer.org/cancer/leukemia-in-children/about/key-statistics.html. Updated February 3, 2016. Accessed May 14, 2018.

Important findings (often provided by the parent or caregiver) include the following:[41]

- Nosebleeds that occur often or last more than 10 minutes
- Bruising (at least five bruises greater than 1 cm on exposed skin)
- Bleeding from minor wounds lasting more than 10 minutes
- Bleeding gums
- Hematuria
- Signs of shock
- GI bleeding
- Swollen, painful joints
- Swollen glands
- Fever

Depending on the condition of the patient and nature of the illness, prehospital care may include oxygen administration, fluid resuscitation, bleeding control, pain control, and transport for physician evaluation.

GI Disorders

Abnormalities in the GI tract can lead to illnesses in the pediatric patient that can cause vomiting and bleeding. These abnormalities may result from malformation of the GI tract during fetal development. They may also result from illness and infection. Important

DID YOU KNOW?

Malfunction of the GI Tract During Development

The primitive gut forms during the fourth week of gestation into the *midgut, foregut,* and *hindgut*. The midgut gives rise to the distal duodenum, jejunum, ileum, appendix, ascending colon, and proximal transverse colon. Errors in midgut development include omphaloceles (protrusion of the intestines through the umbilicus), umbilical hernias, and gastroschisis (extrusion of the viscera without involving the umbilicus).

The foregut develops into the pharynx, lower respiratory system, esophagus, stomach, proximal duodenum, liver and biliary tree, and pancreas. Errors in foregut development include esophageal atresia and tracheoesophageal fistula.

The hindgut matures into the distal transverse colon, descending colon, sigmoid colon, rectum, and proximal anal canal. Although rare, the most common error in hindgut development is neonatal bowel obstruction (*Hirschsprung disease*) attributable to improper muscle movement in the bowel.

components of the patient's history for children with GI disorders include the following:

- Onset and duration of GI signs and symptoms
- Blood or bile in emesis
- Epistaxis
- Presence and nature of pain
- Diarrhea
- Constipation
- Fever
- Medications
- Prematurity
- ABO incompatibility
- Liver disease

Depending on the cause of the child's illness, physical findings may include an elevation or decrease in heart rate and blood pressure, signs of dehydration (dry mucous membranes, absence of tears, decreased urinary output, delayed capillary refill), jaundice, abdominal distention or abdominal mass, pain, hepatomegaly (enlarged liver), and pallor.

GI Disorders That Cause Vomiting

Vomiting is a protective mechanism that removes toxic materials from the GI tract before they are absorbed. Vomiting is controlled by the **emetic center**, located in the reticular formation of the brainstem. The emetic center can be stimulated by chemoreceptors, cranial nerves, vagal and enteric input, and the CNS. Causes of vomiting vary according to the age of the child. Gastroenteritis, gastroesophageal reflux disease, and infection cause vomiting in children of all ages. In infants, vomiting often stems from overfeeding, obstruction, infection, pertussis, or otitis. The child may vomit because of gastritis, toxic ingestion, pertussis, medication, sinusitis, otitis, obstruction, or esophagitis. Causes of vomiting in the adolescent often relate to toxic ingestion, gastritis, gastroenteritis, sinusitis, inflammatory bowel disease, appendicitis, migraine, pregnancy, medications, bulimia, or concussion.[19]

As described in Chapter 28, *Abdominal and Gastrointestinal Disorders*, gastroenteritis is inflammation of the stomach and intestines that can accompany many conditions of the GI tract. In infants and children, gastroenteritis is most often due to viral infections that can cause diarrhea, with or without vomiting. Gastroenteritis can cause life-threatening dehydration that may require volume replacement therapy, especially in infants and young children. Age-appropriate antiemetic therapy (eg, ondansetron, metoclopramide) can be administered to relieve nausea and vomiting.

GI Disorders That Cause Bleeding

Bleeding can occur from the upper and lower GI tract in children of all ages and can have many etiologies (BOX 47-8). The child's condition, signs, and symptoms will be related to the site and cause of the bleeding. Prehospital care may range from supportive care and transport for physician evaluation to providing advanced life support for the management of shock and hypovolemia.

BOX 47-8 Common Causes of GI Bleeding

Newborns

Swallowed maternal or nasopharyngeal blood
Anal fissure
Necrotizing enterocolitis
Malrotation
Hirschsprung disease
Coagulopathy

Infants and Toddlers

Allergic colitis
Infectious enteritis
Intussusception
Swallowed maternal blood
Lymphonodular hyperplasia

School-Age Children

Infectious enteritis
Anal fissure
Intussusception
Peptic ulcer/gastritis
Juvenile polyps
Prolapse gastropathy (inflamed gastric mucosa in esophageal lumen after vomiting)
Mallory-Weiss syndrome

Adolescents

Infectious diarrhea
Juvenile polyps
Peptic ulcer/gastritis
Prolapse gastropathy
Anal fissure
Inflammatory bowel disease

Modified from: Kliegman R, Stanton B, St. Geme JW, et al. *Nelson Textbook of Pediatrics*. 20th ed. Philadelphia, PA: Elsevier; 2016.

Infection

Children with infection may have a variety of signs and symptoms. The symptoms depend on the source and extent of infection and the length of time since the patient was exposed (BOX 47-9). Often, the parent or caregiver provides a history of recent illness. This history may include, for example, fever, upper respiratory tract infection, or otitis media. When caring for any patient who may have an infectious disease, the paramedic must strictly adhere to standard precautions because of the unknown cause of the infection.

Most children with infection need only supportive care while being transported for evaluation by a physician. However, in very sick children, support of the airway, ventilation, and circulation may be needed. If signs of decompensated shock are present, IV therapy may be indicated. Active seizure activity may require the use of anticonvulsant agents. When possible, a child in stable condition should be transported in the child's position of comfort. The child also should be transported in the company of the parent or caregiver.

Poisoning and Toxic Exposure

As discussed in Chapter 33, *Toxicology*, most poisonings in the United States involve children. Poisoning is a major cause of preventable death in children younger than 5 years, with the highest incidence in 1- and 2-year-olds.[42] Common sources of poisoning, typically through unintentional or intentional ingestion, include the following:

- Cosmetic and personal care products
- Cleaning substances
- Analgesics
- Foreign bodies, including toys and other objects
- Topical preparations
- Vitamins
- Antihistamines
- Pesticides
- Dietary supplements

From 2012 to 2016, the top 10 products implicated in deaths of children younger than 6 years were as follows:[42]

1. Fumes/gases/vapors
2. Analgesics
3. Unknown drug
4. Batteries
5. Cardiovascular drugs
6. Antihistamines
7. Stimulants and street drugs
8. Antidepressants
9. Cleaning substances (household)
10. Sedatives/hypnotics/antipsychotics

The signs and symptoms of poisoning vary, depending on the toxic substance and the length of time since the child was exposed. These signs and symptoms may include cardiac and respiratory depression, CNS stimulation or depression, seizures, GI irritation, and behavioral changes. Emergency care should be directed first at ensuring adequate airway, ventilatory, and circulatory support. The paramedic should contact medical direction and the poison control center for specific treatments. All pills, substances, and containers associated with the poisoning should be transported with the child to the receiving hospital. As described in Chapter 33, *Toxicology*, no efforts should be made in the prehospital setting to induce vomiting.

BOX 47-9 Signs and Symptoms of Infection in Pediatric Patients

Bulging fontanel, if meningitis (infants)
Chills
Cool or clammy skin
Cough
Dehydration
Fever
Hypoperfusion
Hypothermia (newborns)
Irritability
Lethargy
Malaise
Nasal congestion
Poor feeding
Respiratory distress
Seizure
Severe headache
Sore throat
Stiff neck
Tachycardia
Tachypnea
Vomiting or diarrhea (or both)

CRITICAL THINKING

For what key signs or symptoms of poisoning should you be alert?

Pediatric Trauma

Blunt trauma and penetrating trauma are major causes of injury and death in children.[43] These and other significant injuries in children often result from falls, motor vehicle crashes, pedestrian–motor vehicle collisions, drowning/submersion incidents, penetrating injuries, burns, and abuse. The following common injuries highlight the value of injury prevention programs (see Chapter 3, *Injury Prevention, Health Promotion, and Public Health*):

Falls. Falls are the single most common cause of nonfatal injuries in children from birth to age 9 years, and they rank second for children 10 years and older.[43] Fortunately, serious injury or death from truly unintentional falls is uncommon—unless from a significant height.

Motor vehicle crashes. Motor vehicle crashes are the leading cause of death in children aged 1 to 4 years and older than 15 years. Among infants younger than 1 year, death from motor vehicle crashes is second only to mechanical suffocation.[43]

Pedestrian–motor vehicle collisions. Pedestrian–motor vehicle collisions that result in serious injury or death in children usually is caused by impact with the vehicle. (The vehicle most often impacts the child's extremity or trunk.) The child usually is thrown from the force of the first impact, producing an additional injury (eg, head and spine) upon a second impact with other objects. These objects may include the ground, another vehicle, or nearby objects (see Chapter 36, *Trauma Overview and Mechanism of Injury*).

Drowning/submersion. Drowning/submersion incidents are the second-leading cause of death in children from 1 to 14 years of age. About one in five people who die from drowning are aged 14 years or younger. For each pediatric drowning death, another five are treated in the hospital for nonfatal submersion injuries.[44]

Penetrating injuries. Although blunt trauma is more common, penetrating injuries are a major cause of trauma in children. They are most likely to occur during adolescence. Penetrating injuries that are intentional (eg, from violent crime) are more common in inner cities; however, unintentional penetrating injuries in rural areas also occur. Stab wounds and firearm injuries make up about 10% to 15% of all pediatric trauma admissions.[45] As with penetrating injuries to adults, the appearance of the external wounds cannot be used to determine the extent of internal injury in children.

Burns. More than 300 US children aged 0 to 19 years sustain burns requiring medical care each day.[46] These burns primarily relate to contact with hot substances such as scalds from food or drinks; scalds from tap water; and contact with hot objects such as irons, curling irons, or cooking ranges. Other burn sources in children include fireworks, gasoline, and cigarettes or other tobacco products.[47] Survival from burn trauma is determined by the size and depth of the burn, the presence of inhalation injury, and the nature of other injuries that may have occurred during the event (see Chapter 38, *Burns*).

> CRITICAL THINKING
> What types of situations in the home cause burn injuries in children?

Child abuse. Injuries to children may result from physical abuse, sexual abuse, emotional abuse, and child neglect. Physical abuse often is associated with domestic disturbances, younger-aged parents, substance abuse, and community violence. (Child abuse is described later in this chapter.)

Special Considerations for Specific Injuries

Special considerations for managing pediatric injury are addressed in the chapters of Section 9, *Trauma*. The following list is a review of some of the important elements in assessment and management for children with head and neck injury, traumatic brain injury, chest injury, abdominal injury, extremity injury, and burns.

Head and Neck Injury

- The larger relative mass of the head and lack of neck muscle strength provide increased momentum in acceleration–deceleration injuries.
- The fulcrum of cervical mobility in the younger child is at the C2-C3 level (the majority of fractures in children younger than 6 years occur in C1 or C2).[48]
- Head injury is the most common cause of death in pediatric trauma patients.[48]

- Diffuse head injuries are common in children; focal injuries are rare.
- Soft tissues, the skull, and the brain are more pliable in children than in adults.
- Because of open fontanels and sutures, children up to 12 to 18 months of age may be more tolerant to increased ICP and can have delayed signs.
- Subdural bleeding in an infant can produce hypotension (rare).
- Significant blood loss can occur through scalp lacerations, and such bleeding should be controlled immediately.
- The modified GCS should be used for assessing infants and young children.

Traumatic Brain Injury

- Early recognition and aggressive management can reduce mortality and morbidity.
- The modified GCS should be used for assessing infants and young children.
- Signs of increased ICP include elevated blood pressure, bradycardia, irregular respirations progressing (Cushing triad) to Cheyne-Stokes respirations, and bulging fontanel in infants.
- Signs of herniation include asymmetrical pupils and abnormal posturing.
- Management includes the following:
  - Administer high-concentration oxygen for mild to moderate head injury (GCS score of 9 to 15). Monitor pulse oximetry.
  - Intubate and ventilate at normal breathing rate with 100% oxygen for severe head injury (GCS score less than 8).[4]
  - Hyperventilate only with signs of increased ICP. Hyperventilation should be mild with a goal $ETCO_2$ of 30 to 35 mm Hg.
  - The use of lidocaine to blunt a rise in ICP should be guided by medical direction.

CRITICAL THINKING

What are some early signs of increasing ICP in a child?

Chest Injury

- Chest injuries in children younger than 14 years usually are the result of blunt trauma.[49]
- Because of flexibility of the chest wall, severe intrathoracic injury (such as severe pulmonary contusion) can be present without signs of external injury such as rib fractures.
- Tension pneumothorax is an immediate threat to life.
- Flail segment is an uncommon injury in children; when noted without a significant mechanism of injury, child abuse should be suspected.
- Many children with cardiac tamponade have no physical signs other than hypotension.

Abdominal Injury

- Musculature is minimal and poorly protects the viscera.
- Organs most commonly injured are the liver, kidneys, and spleen.
- Onset of symptoms may be rapid or gradual.
- Because of the small size of the abdomen, palpation should be performed in one quadrant at a time.
- Any child who is hemodynamically unstable without an obvious source of blood loss should be considered to have an abdominal injury until it is proved otherwise.
- The majority of children with abdominal injury have abdominal bruising or ecchymosis.

Extremity Injury

- Extremity injury is relatively more common in children than in adults.
- Growth plate injuries are common.
- Compartment syndrome is an emergency.
- Management includes the following:
  - Control any sites of active bleeding.
  - Perform splinting to prevent further injury and blood loss.
  - Use of a pelvic immobilizer may be helpful for an unstable pelvic fracture with hypotension (per protocol).
- Most femur fractures result from falls or other unintentional injuries; however, child abuse should be considered.

Burns

- Burns may be thermal, chemical, or electrical.
- Management priorities include the following:
  - Prompt management of the airway is required because swelling can develop rapidly.
  - If intubation is indicated, a smaller-size ET tube may be required due to significant airway edema.[50]
  - Suspect musculoskeletal injuries in electrical burn patients, and perform spine immobilization. (Spinal cord injury can be present in children without vertebral abnormality.)

Trauma Management Considerations for Pediatric Patients

In addition to the general patient care guidelines appropriate for all injured people, injured children require special consideration for airway control, immobilization techniques, fluid management, and pain relief. The following discussion reviews the highlights of management guidelines presented in the chapters of Section 9, *Trauma.*

Airway Control. The airway of an injured child should be maintained in an in-line or neutral position. The sniffing position is appropriate for older children and adults. Padding may need to be placed under the shoulders in some children. This will help to maintain a neutral airway position. High-concentration oxygen should be given if indicated. Jaw-thrust positioning and suctioning may be needed for airway patency. If necessary, a supraglottic airway should be placed. ET intubation (followed by insertion of a gastric tube) should be performed when airway and ventilation remain inadequate despite other airway measures. When tracheal intubation is required, ET tube placement should be confirmed by monitoring exhaled carbon dioxide. Cricothyroidotomy rarely is indicated for traumatic upper airway obstruction.

Spinal Motion Restriction. An extensive discussion of spinal immobilization appears in Chapter 40, *Spine and Nervous System Trauma.* Spinal motion restriction devices must be sized appropriately for infants and children. Equipment that may be used includes the following:[51]

- Child safety seat
- Long backboard
- Padding
- Pediatric immobilization device
- Rigid cervical collar
- Straps, cravats, tape
- Towel/blanket roll
- Vest-type/short backboard

NOTE

Backboards are extrication devices meant to assist emergency personnel in moving patients. As a stand-alone device, a backboard does not provide adequate immobilization of the spine and is not considered a treatment of spine injury.

A cervical collar is applied when substantial mechanism of nonpenetrating injury is present or in the following situations:

- The child complains of midline neck or spine pain.
- There is any midline neck or spinal tenderness with palpation.
- The patient is "unreliable":
  - GCS score of less than 15
  - Alcohol or drug intoxication
  - Other painful or distracting injury present
  - Communication barrier
- There are focal or neurologic deficits.
- Torticollis is present.

When an infant or toddler is restrained in a car seat with harness, the child should be extricated in the seat. If a backboard is used to move the child, the child should remain on the board and the board should be secured to the stretcher.[10]

The patient should be placed supine (unless positioned in an infant carrier) and immobilized in a neutral, in-line position. Because children have proportionally larger heads than adults have, more padding may be required under the torso to allow the head to lie in a neutral position on the board. The padding should be firm and should extend the full length and width of the torso from the buttocks to the top of the shoulders to prevent movement and misalignment of the spine. In addition to providing enhanced stabilization, padding improves patient comfort during transport. Alternatively, the appropriate position may be achieved by using a backboard with a recess for the head or an appropriately sized vacuum splint.

Fluid Management. Management of exsanguinating hemorrhage as well as the child's airway and breathing takes priority over management of circulation. (Circulatory compromise is less common in children than in adults.) The paramedic should remember that blood pressure may be normal in a child with compensated shock but may decline rapidly when the child decompensates. Like the other signs, hypotension must be interpreted within the context of the entire clinical picture, including nature of injury, vital signs, and level of consciousness. When vascular access is indicated, the paramedic should consider the following:[4]

- IV catheters should be inserted into large peripheral veins.

- Transport should not be delayed to obtain vascular access.
- IO access in children should be considered if IV access fails.
- An initial fluid bolus of up to 20 mL/kg of lactated Ringer solution or normal saline should be given in small increments with frequent ongoing assessment to help manage volume depletion.[52]
- Vital signs should be reassessed. Fluid therapy to maintain adequate perfusion should be guided by medical direction.

NOTE

Large fluid boluses are no longer recommended for treating hemorrhagic shock, as they can contribute to worsened outcomes. Potential complications include coagulopathy from dilution of clotting factors, hypothermia, an increase in blood pressure that can accelerate bleeding, and acidosis. The current recommendation for managing hemorrhagic shock in pediatric patients is a "permissive hypotension" with small fluid bolus increments that are just enough to maintain adequate perfusion.

Modified from: Tosounidis TH, Giannoudis PV. Paediatric trauma resuscitation: an update. *Eur J Trauma Emerg Surg*. 2016;42:297-301; and Hawnwan PM. Evidence-based EMS: permissive hypotension in trauma. EMS World website. www.emsworld.com/article/12163910/evidence-based-ems-permissive-hypotension-in-trauma. Published January 29, 2016. Accessed April 4, 2018.

Pain Relief. The relief of pain caused by an injury should be a priority when providing care to an injured child (see BOX 47-10). Drugs that may be used to manage some forms of pain and to alter the emotional response in pediatric patients include fentanyl, ketamine, ketorolac, morphine, or, in the absence of hemorrhage, nitrous oxide.[53] Other indications for pain relief or sedation in pediatric patients include some airway management procedures (eg, drug-assisted intubation), entrapment requiring extended extrication time, or other uncomfortable procedures.

BOX 47-10 Pain Management

Children do not always express their pain as clearly as adults do. As a result, they are less likely to receive appropriate pain therapy in an emergency situation. Thus the paramedic should perform a systematic pain assessment. A memory aid for one type of pain assessment is QUESTT:

Question the child about his or her pain, using age-appropriate language (eg, "owie" or "boo-boo" for young children).

Use pain rating scales (eg, the Faces Pain Rating Scale for young children, a numeric pain scale from 0 to 10 for older children).

Evaluate the child's behavior (eg, facial grimace, rigidity, crying, anxious behavior).

Secure the parent or caregiver's involvement in assessing the child's pain. (The parent will have seen the child in pain or discomfort before and will be aware of subtle changes.)

Take the cause of the pain into account (eg, type of injury and expected intensity of pain).

Take action to provide comfort and to relieve pain (eg, narcotic and nonnarcotic drugs, comfort measures such as application of cold, elevation, and distraction techniques).

Modified from: Wong D, Hess C. *Clinical Manual of Pediatric Nursing*. 5th ed. St. Louis, MO: Mosby; 2000.

Pediatric Trauma Score

The **pediatric trauma score** grades six characteristics commonly seen in pediatric trauma patients: size (weight), airway, CNS (consciousness), systolic blood pressure, skeletal injury(fracture), and open wound (cutaneous injury) (**TABLE 47-12**). The pediatric trauma score has a significant inverse linear relationship with patient mortality. A child with a pediatric trauma score of less than 8 should be cared for in an appropriate pediatric trauma center.[54]

A description of the pediatric assessment score follows:

- **Size.** Patient size (weight) is one of the first parameters to assess. The smaller the child, the greater the risk for severe injury because of an increased ratio of body surface to volume. The risk also is greater because of the potential for limited physiologic reserve.
- **Airway.** The child's airway is scored by potential difficulty in management. Scoring also is by the type of care required to ensure adequate ventilation and oxygenation. Respiratory failure is the main cause of death in most pediatric patients. Careful attention should be given to ensure that pediatric trauma patients are adequately ventilated and oxygenated early during their care using the least invasive means necessary to accomplish such management.
- **Consciousness.** As with adult patients, assessing and recording changes in the level of

TABLE 47-12 Pediatric Trauma Score

Component	+2	+1	−1
Size	Child/adolescent >44 pounds (20 kg)	Toddler 24–44 pounds (11–20 kg)	Infant <22 pounds (10 kg)
Airway	Normal	Assisted: oxygen mask, cannula	Intubated: endotracheal tube, cricothyroidotomy
Consciousness	Awake	Obtunded, lost consciousness	Coma, unresponsive
Systolic blood pressure	>90 mm Hg Good peripheral pulses, perfusion	50–90 mm Hg Carotid, femoral pulse palpable	<50 mm Hg Weak or no pulse
Fracture	None seen or suspected	Single closed fracture anywhere	Open or multiple fractures
Cutaneous injury	No visible injury	Confusion, abrasion, laceration <3 inches (8 cm) through fascia	Tissue loss, any gunshot wound or stab through fascia

Modified from: National Association of Emergency Medical Technicians. *PHTLS: Prehospital Trauma Life Support*. 8th ed. Burlington, MA: Jones & Bartlett Learning; 2014.

consciousness is very important. Any change in the level of consciousness will reduce this score—no matter how brief the duration.

- **Systolic blood pressure.** The assessment of systolic blood pressure in the pediatric patient is crucial because the circulating volume is notably less than that of the adult. Because of a normal child's healthy heart and excellent reserve capacity, children often do not show classic signs of shock until they have lost about 25% of their circulating volume. Any child who has a systolic blood pressure of less than 50 mm Hg is in obvious jeopardy.[55]
- **Fracture.** A child's skeleton is more pliable than an adult's is. It allows traumatic forces to be sent through the body and to the organs. A fracture in a child therefore is a sign that serious injury may have occurred.
- **Cutaneous injury.** Cutaneous injury in a pediatric patient can be a potential contributor to mortality and disability as well depending on the degree. These injuries include open and visible wounds and penetrating trauma.

The following is an example calculation of the pediatric trauma score: A head-injured child is 8 years old and weighs 75 pounds (34 kg) (+2). The child has spontaneous respirations (+2), is unresponsive (−1), has a systolic blood pressure of 86 mm Hg with palpable femoral pulses (+1), has no visible fractures (+2), and has an abrasion on the head with minimal bleeding (+1). The pediatric trauma score for this patient is 7.

Sudden Unexpected Infant Death

Sudden unexpected infant death (SUID) describes the sudden and unexpected death of a child younger than 1 year in which the cause was not obvious before investigation. SUID includes **sudden infant death syndrome (SIDS)**, unknown (ill-defined) cause, and accidental suffocation and strangulation in bed. It is the leading cause of death in US infants younger than 1 year.[56] The syndrome is defined as the sudden death of a seemingly healthy infant that remains unexplained by history and an autopsy. There were about 3,700 SUIDs in 2015. About 1,600 were caused by SIDS, 1,200 were from unknown causes, and 900 were related to accidental suffocation and strangulation in bed.[56] The syndrome cannot be predicted or prevented. However, positioning during sleep may be a factor (BOX 47-11).

SIDS occurs during periods of sleep. The typical age for SIDS is the first year of life, but most SIDS deaths occur between 2 and 4 months.[19] The infant often has a history of minor illness, such as a cold, within 2 weeks before death. Signs that may be present include lividity; frothy, blood-tinged drainage from

BOX 47-11 Sleep Positions and Other Factors That May Reduce the Risk of SIDS

In 1994 the Association of SIDS and Infant Mortality Programs joined with the US Public Health Service, the American Academy of Pediatrics, the SIDS Alliance, and others to launch a national public health campaign titled *Back to Sleep* to reduce the risk of SIDS. This initiative was based on research reports from Australia, New Zealand, England, Norway, and the United States. The data indicated that placing healthy newborns to sleep on the back or side was a means of reducing the risk of SIDS. In 1996 this recommendation was revised to endorse "back sleeping" as the best position for infants. This campaign significantly reduced the SIDS rate in the 1990s, but that decline has leveled off. Based on current evidence, the 2016 guidelines from the American Academy of Pediatrics recommend the following:

- Obtain medically recommended prenatal care.
- Position infants so they sleep lying flat on their backs for all sleep until 1 year of age.
- Use a firm sleep surface.
- Avoid drugs, alcohol, and smoking during and after pregnancy.
- Avoid smokers and places where people smoke.
- Breastfeed when possible.
- Room-share with the infant on a separate sleep surface (do not co-sleep).
- Keep soft objects and loose bedding away from the infant's sleep area.
- Consider offering a pacifier at sleep times.
- Avoid overheating the baby.
- Maintain regular well-baby health visits.
- Obtain immunizations on schedule. (The Recommended Immunization Schedule for Children and Adolescents Aged 18 Years or Younger, United States, 2018, can be located at https://www.cdc.gov/vaccines/schedules/hcp/imz/child-adolescent.html.)
- Do not use home cardiorespiratory monitors as a strategy to reduce SIDS.
- Have supervised, awake time with the infant placed on his or her stomach to promote normal development.
- Place the baby to sleep on a firm mattress, avoiding the use of beanbag cushions; water beds; soft, fluffy blankets; comforters; sheepskins; pillows; stuffed toys; or other soft materials.

Paramedics can play an important role in prevention by conveying this information to parents, other caregivers, and family members.

Modified from: AAP Task Force on Sudden Infant Death Syndrome. SIDS and other sleep-related infant deaths: updated 2016 recommendations for a safe infant sleeping environment. *Pediatrics*. 2016;138(5):e20162938

NOTE

Infants may experience an episode termed a **brief resolved unexplained event (BRUE)** (formerly described as an apparent life-threatening event [ALTE]). BRUEs occur when infants (usually younger than 12 months) experience absent, decreased, or irregular breathing, color change (cyanosis or pallor), muscle tone changes (rigid or floppy), or altered level of responsiveness. BRUE is a diagnosis of exclusion. The paramedic should conduct a thorough history and physical examination to rule out other potential life-threatening causes of the patient's reported signs and symptoms.

About 11% of infants with BRUE have been found to be victims of abuse. It is recommended that all infants with suspected BRUE be transported to a hospital with pediatric care capabilities. Transport to a facility with pediatric critical care capabilities should also be considered for patients with high-risk criteria such as the following:

- Younger than 2 months
- History of prematurity (32 weeks' gestation or less, or corrected gestational age of 45 weeks or less)
- More than one BRUE, now or in the past

Modified from: National Association of State EMS Officials. *National Model EMS Clinical Guidelines*. Version 2.0. www.nasemso.org/documents/National-Model-EMS-Clinical-Guidelines-Version2-Sept2017.pdf. Published September 18, 2017. Accessed April 5, 2018.

the nose and mouth; and rigor mortis. With most SIDS cases, no external signs of injury are found. Often evidence indicates that the baby was active just before the death (eg, rumpled bed clothes, unusual position or location in the bed).

Pathophysiology

The cause of SIDS is unknown. Studies have failed to confirm a number of physiologic, environmental, genetic, and social factors as causes. The studies have confirmed, however, that SIDS is not caused by external suffocation, regurgitation or aspiration of vomitus, hereditary factors, or allergies. (A small percentage of SIDS deaths are thought to be abuse related.[57]) Various physiologic aspects that have been suggested to explain SIDS include immaturity of the CNS following a prenatal event, idiopathic apnea, brainstem abnormalities, upper airway obstruction, hyperactive upper airway reflexes, cardiac conduction disorders, abnormal responses to hypoxia and hypercapnia, abnormal responses to hyperthermia, and alterations in fat metabolism. Although no specific cause has been identified, a number of risk factors have been associated with the syndrome. These factors include the following:[19]

- Maternal smoking
- Young maternal age (younger than 20 years) and limited education
- Intrauterine hypoxia or fetal growth restriction
- Infants of mothers who received poor or no prenatal care
- Infants born with low levels of serotonin
- Low socioeconomic status
- Premature births and low-birth-weight infants
- Male infant
- Inadequate immunization
- Soft sleep surface
- Bed sharing with adult or other children
- Overheating
- Infants of mothers who used cocaine, methadone, or heroin during pregnancy

SIDS is confirmed by excluding other causes of death. Autopsy findings that occur in some SIDS deaths include lung, brain, and hormonal changes.

Management

EMS providers can do little to help the suspected SIDS infant. The main role of the paramedic is to offer emotional support for parents or other caregivers and loved ones. If the infant possibly could be viable, resuscitation should proceed as for any other infant in cardiac arrest even though resuscitation most likely will be unsuccessful.[58] It is important for the parents or other caregivers to see that everything possible is being done for their child. The paramedic should follow pediatric resuscitation protocols and should consult with medical direction on decisions to initiate or continue efforts.

A variety of grief reactions should be expected from those who witness the event (parents, family members, neighbors, babysitters). These reactions may vary from shock and disbelief to anger, rage, and self-blame. Arrangements should be made for a relative or neighbor to stay with the family or accompany them to the hospital so that they are not left alone. Many areas have SIDS resource services. These services provide immediate counseling and support for the family of an infant who dies of SIDS.

SIDS victims may appear to have been abused or neglected. The mysterious nature of SIDS deaths and classic signs such as postmortem lividity and frothy fluid in the infant's nose and mouth give such an appearance. Regardless of the circumstances, the paramedic should avoid comments or questions that may imply a suspicion of improper child care. Determining the cause of death is not the duty of the EMS crew. However, careful scene observation is crucial. The paramedic should document all findings objectively, accurately, and completely. Medical direction and other authorities (per protocol) should be advised if inappropriate child care is suspected.

Rescuers commonly have a range of emotional reactions after a SIDS death. Some EMS systems, working with medical direction and SIDS resource agencies, provide counseling and formal debriefing programs. If these services are not available, the EMS crew should discuss the event openly with others involved in the response (eg, coworkers, law enforcement officers). This may help relieve normal feelings of anxiety and stress.

> CRITICAL THINKING
> What factors do you think influence the reactions of each crew member to a child who dies from SIDS?

Child Abuse and Neglect

More than 3 million cases of suspected **child abuse** and neglect are reported each year in the United States. These cases can include multiple children. In 2016, an estimated 676,000 US children were victims of maltreatment.[59] Of those maltreated, about three-fourths were neglected, 18.2% were physically abused, and 8.5% were sexually assaulted.[59] In the United States, child abuse and neglect result in about 1,750 deaths per year; almost one-half of deaths are children younger than 3 years.[59] Agencies that may be involved in cases of child abuse or neglect include state, regional, and local child protection services. Also included are hospital-based social service departments and child protection programs. Factors of child abuse are described in detail in Chapter 49, *Abuse and Neglect.*

Child abuse or neglect is a crime that, by law, must be reported in all 50 states. In almost all states, health care workers have a legal duty to report child abuse or neglect (mandated reporter).[60] Notifying receiving hospital personnel of suspected abuse does not satisfy mandatory reporting requirements to state officials in many states. Paramedics should follow local protocol in reporting suspected abuse. Failure to report these cases may result in criminal prosecution and may be punishable by fine or imprisonment or both. As a rule, reporting in good faith provides immunity from legal liability as a consequence of reporting.

Elements of Child Abuse

Child abuse and neglect is the maltreatment of children by their parents, guardians, or other caregivers. Forms of maltreatment include infliction of physical injury (battered child syndrome, shaken baby syndrome), sexual exploitation, and infliction of emotional pain and neglect (medical neglect, safety neglect, nutritional and social deprivation). A number of factors come into play in the potential for child abuse, including a caregiver with the potential to abuse, a child with particular characteristics that place him or her at risk for abuse, and an element of crisis.

Characteristics of Abusers. Child abuse usually reflects a pattern of unstable behavior. It is typically not a single act of violence. In many cases the abuser is the child's parent; however, other caregivers may be responsible. For example, abusers may include family members, a boyfriend or girlfriend of the child's mother or father, an unrelated babysitter, or a sibling of the abused child.

Characteristics of an Abused Child. Abused children often have certain characteristics that increase their risk for abuse.[61] Common traits include demanding and difficult behavior, decreased level of functioning (eg, a child with a disability or preterm infant requiring extra parenting), hyperactivity, and precociousness with intellectual ability equal to or superior to the parent's. Often the parent sees the abused child as "special" or "different" from other siblings. Other factors that tend to increase the potential for child abuse are age (the child is usually younger than 4 years), sex (boys are involved more often than girls), and not being the biologic offspring of the abuser.

Crises That May Precipitate Abuse. Physical abuse or neglect can occur constantly during a child's life. More often, though, abuse and neglect are intermittent and unpredictable. The abuse often is triggered by stressors in the adult caregiver's life, especially when the caregiver expects the child to fill emotional needs created by the stress. Failure of the child to respond in an ideal way to the caregiver's needs may lead to abuse.

History of Injuries Suspicious for Abuse

Physical abuse or neglect often is hard to determine. The ultimate diagnosis usually begins with suspicions based on unexplained injuries, discrepant history, delays in seeking medical care, and repeated episodes of suspicious injuries. If at any time an injured child indicates that an adult caused him or her physical harm, the paramedic should take this report seriously and advise medical direction and contact proper authorities. In many cases these accusations are true. Possible indicators of abuse include the following:[62]

- Any obvious or suspected fractures in a child younger than 2 years
- Injuries in various stages of healing, especially burns and bruises
- Injuries inconsistent with age (eg, femur fracture in a child not yet walking)
- More injuries than are usually seen in other children of the same age
- Injuries scattered on many areas of the body
- Bruises or burns in patterns that suggest intentional infliction
- Suspected increased ICP in an infant
- Suspected intra-abdominal trauma in a young child
- Any injury that does not fit the description of the cause
- An accusation that the child injured himself or herself intentionally
- Long-standing skin infections
- Extreme malnutrition
- Extreme lack of cleanliness
- Inappropriate clothing for the situation
- Child who withdraws from parent
- Child who responds inappropriately to the situation (eg, quiet, distant, withdrawn)

Physical Findings Suggestive of Abuse

Some physical findings, such as welts, burns, and multiple, widely dispersed bruises, are suggestive of abuse. Such physical findings, along with a vague history or delays in seeking medical care for the child, should alert the paramedic to the possibility of abuse or neglect (**FIGURE 47-13**). It is imperative that the paramedic fully expose the child for examination; key indicators of abuse can be hidden by clothing, including hats and headbands.

Injuries Related to Physical Abuse

Subdural Hematoma. Abusive head trauma is the leading cause of traumatic death in children under 2 years of age.[63] The various pathologic lesions include cerebral contusions, intraparenchymal hemorrhage, and subdural or even epidural hematomas. Subdural hematomas are among the most common injuries associated with intentionally inflicted head injury in children. They should be suspected in any young child who is in a coma or having convulsions, particularly if the child has no history of seizure disorder. In many cases, bleeding into the brain tissue occurs as a result of skull fractures or scalp bruises. These injuries commonly result from a direct blow from a hand or by being thrown against a wall or door.

Subdural hematomas also can result from vigorous shaking of the child (shaken baby syndrome). The acceleration and deceleration forces on the brain associated with shaking cause tearing of the bridging cerebral veins, which leads to bleeding into the subdural space. Signs and symptoms of the shaken baby syndrome include retinal hemorrhages, irritability, altered level of consciousness, vomiting, and a full or bulging fontanel.

CRITICAL THINKING

Why is it crucial that your documentation be clear, objective, and complete in cases of suspected abuse?

Abdominal Visceral Injury. Intra-abdominal injuries are the second most common cause of death in battered children.[64] These injuries usually are produced by a blunt force such as a punch or blow to the abdomen. Children with an abdominal injury often have recurrent vomiting, abdominal distention, absent bowel sounds, and localized tenderness with or without abdominal bruising. Caregivers routinely deny a history of trauma to the child's abdomen in these cases.

Bone Injury. More than 20% of physically abused children have a positive result on radiologic bone survey from previous abusive episodes.[49] Injuries that may be obvious only through radiography include fractures of the ribs, lateral portion of the clavicle, scapula, sternum, and extremities. Multiple fractures in various stages of healing are highly suspicious for physical abuse.

Injuries From Sexual Abuse

Sexual abuse of a child usually is associated with physical or emotional neglect or abuse. Sexual abuse may include vaginal intercourse, sodomy, oral–genital contact, or molestation (eg, fondling, masturbation, exposure). Abuse occurs to children of both sexes. More than one-half of sexually abused children are younger than 12 years at the time of the first offense.[65] Physical findings suggestive of sexual abuse include the following:

- Pregnancy or venereal disease in a child 12 years of age or younger
- Painful urination or defecation
- Tenderness or lacerations of the perineal area
- Bleeding from the rectum or vagina
- Presence of dried blood, semen, or pubic hair in the genital area of a child

Emergency care for children who have been sexually abused should be limited to managing injuries that pose a threat to life and giving emotional support during transport. These children undergo extensive interviews and examination by the ED physician and others. The paramedic should carefully document any statements made by the patient, family member, or caregiver. These children require compassionate support. A sexually abused child should never be made to feel that he or she is responsible for any of the abuse. The child also should not be given the impression that discussion of the event is inappropriate. If possible, a paramedic of the same sex should interview and care for the child.

Infants and Children With Special Needs

Some infants and children are born with or develop conditions that require special medical equipment to sustain life. Examples of these conditions include

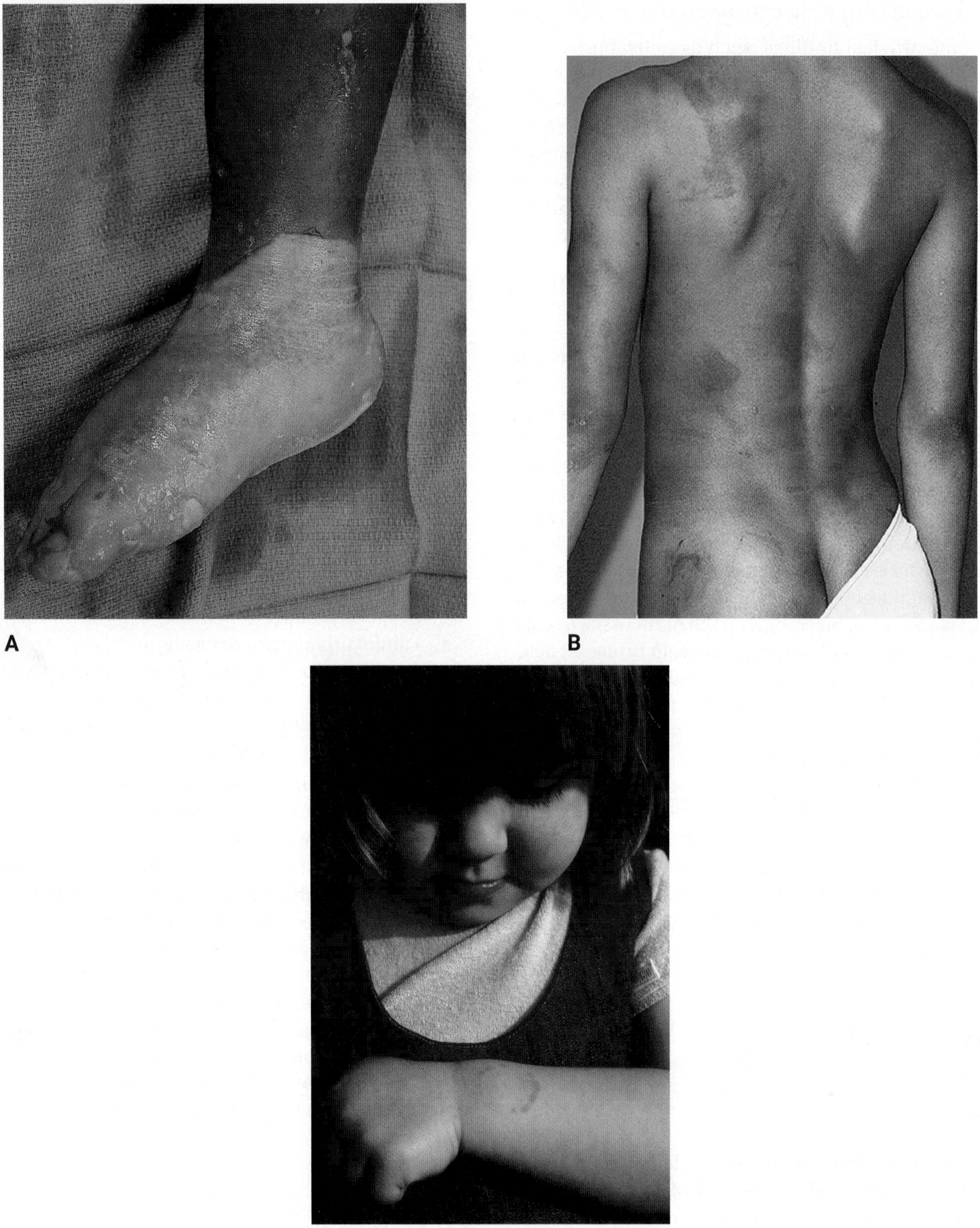

A

B

C

FIGURE 47-13 Cutaneous manifestations of child abuse. **A.** Dunking/submersion burns of the feet. **B.** Welts and abrasions as a result of an electrical cord. **C.** Human bites.

A: Courtesy of Dr. Jeffrey Guy; **B:** Courtesy of Ronald Dieckmann, M.D.; **C:** © ian west/Alamy Stock Photo premature birth, altered functions from birth, and chronic or acute disease of the lung, heart, or CNS. The number of children who are cared for at home by family has grown from 12.8% in 2001 to 15% in 2013.[66] Many are dependent on special medical equipment such as tracheostomy tubes, home ventilators, central venous lines, gastrostomy tubes, and shunts (see Chapter 51, *Acute Interventions for Home Care*). The parents and other family members of a child with special medical needs often are "experts" in caring for the child and maintaining the required medical equipment. Their knowledge, skills, and experience are valuable. The paramedic should use the skills and expertise of these parents when managing these emergencies.

The American College of Emergency Physicians recommends that there be a standardized emergency information form for children with special health needs.[67] It provides an easy means for the paramedic to find key information when a parent or caregiver is unable to provide it. On arrival at the scene, the paramedic should ask for the form. These children also typically have a "go bag." The go bag contains equipment needed during an emergency (eg, replacement tracheostomy, emergency medications).

NOTE

Cardinal Glennon Children's Hospital (CGCH) in St. Louis, Missouri, has established a system to communicate the needs of children with critical health needs to their local EMS agencies called the Special Needs Tracking and Awareness Response (STARS) program. Each ambulance district has a STARS coordinator. When a new "star" is identified, the patient is assigned a star number. The ambulance coordinator visits the family and gathers health information that is entered into a standardized form and shared with dispatch. When an emergency occurs, the family notifies dispatch of the child's STAR number. That way individualized information is shared with the crew en route so they can anticipate the care for the child. In smaller communities, EMS crews arrange visits with their STARS to observe the children and their needs before a crisis occurs. This system coupled with training provided to EMS agencies by pediatric specialists helps promote optimal care for children with special needs.

Modified from: STARS: Special Needs Tracking and Awareness Response. SSM Health website. https://www.ssmhealth.com/for-health-professionals/stars-for-special-needs-kids. Accessed April 6, 2018.

CRITICAL THINKING

How can an EMS agency prepare crews to care for children with special needs before a call is even received?

Tracheostomy Tubes

In a patient with a complete tracheostomy, the airway surgically bypasses the larynx at the level of the trachea. Modern tracheostomy tubes are flexible and relatively comfortable for the patient and have few associated risks (**FIGURE 47-14**). Complications that can occur with the tracheostomy tube and lead to inadequate ventilation include obstruction, air leak, bleeding, dislodgment, and infection. (Bleeding around a tracheostomy usually occurs within 24 hours of the surgery and is not commonly seen in the prehospital setting.[49]) Aseptic technique and respiratory support are always high priorities in caring for these patients.

Management

The tracheostomy tube may become blocked or dislodged. In these cases, the paramedic should first attempt ventilation with a bag-mask device. If the airway does not clear, suctioning the tube with sterile water or saline is performed. If both attempts fail, the tracheostomy must be removed and reinserted as described in Chapter 15, *Airway Management, Respiration, and Artificial Ventilation*, and Chapter 51, *Acute Interventions for Home Care.* (If no replacement tracheostomy tube is available, medical direction may advise that a tracheostomy tube be replaced with an ET tube.) Most patients have a replacement tracheostomy tube with them at all times.

NOTE

There are many videos on the Internet that demonstrate the procedure to replace a tracheostomy tube. The paramedic must be familiar with this procedure and be prepared to do it immediately if it is needed. Because it is an infrequently performed skill, it is wise to review the procedure periodically.

Home Ventilators

Home ventilators can simulate the normal movement of the diaphragm and thoracic cage. The type of home ventilator used depends on the patient's

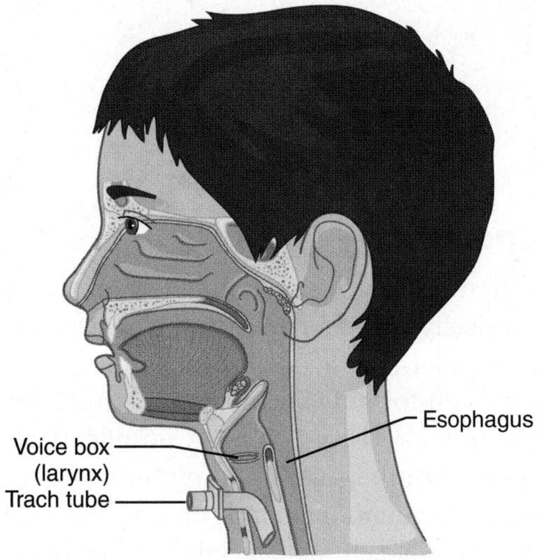

FIGURE 47-14 Pediatric tracheostomy tube.

© Jones & Bartlett Learning.

specific needs. Ventilators are classified by function, depending on the amount of air and pressure they are set to deliver during certain phases of the respiratory cycle. Complications can occur from malfunction of the machine or its alarm notifications, airway obstruction, and respiratory distress (**TABLE 47-13**).

Management

The different varieties of home ventilators and their individual settings can make it difficult for the paramedic to troubleshoot a malfunction problem. The paramedic should remove the child from the ventilator and manually ventilate the patient until the problem is resolved. If an appropriate pediatric transport ventilator is available, it should be used during transport. Steps in managing a patient with a home artificial ventilator problem are presented in Chapter 51, *Acute Interventions for Home Care*.

Central Venous Lines

Some patients with chronic illnesses need prolonged and frequent access to venous circulation for drug or

TABLE 47-13 Complications Seen With Home Ventilators

Complication	Possible Cause
Airway obstruction	Bronchospasm, mucus or secretions, tracheostomy or endotracheal tube malfunction, patient cough, fear, anxiety
Barotrauma	High PEEP/excessive volumes
Pneumothorax	High-pressure volumes
Atelectasis	Mucus plugging, poor suctioning, right mainstem intubation
Cardiovascular impairment	Reduction in venous return to heart caused by positive intrathoracic pressure, which compresses pulmonary circulation
Gastrointestinal complications	Swallowing air, gastrointestinal bleeding, gastric distention
Tracheal trauma	Cuff pressure on trachea
Respiratory tract infection (pneumonia, tracheitis)	Bypass of natural defenses of upper airway, poor aseptic technique

Modified from: Mahmood NA, Chaudry FA, Azam H, et al. Frequency of hypoxic events in patients on a mechanical ventilator. *Int J Crit Illn Inj Sci.* 2013;3(2):124-129.

fluid therapy. This access is made possible through vascular access devices. These devices are seen often in the prehospital setting in child and adult patients who are cared for in the home. Vascular access devices include surgically implanted medication delivery devices (eg, Port-A-Cath), peripheral vascular access devices (eg, peripherally inserted central catheters, Intracath), and central venous access devices (eg, Broviac, Groshong, Hickman) (see Chapter 14, *Medication Administration*, and Chapter 51, *Acute Interventions for Home Care*). Complications that may occur with

Pharynx

Nasogastric
tube

Esophagus

Stomach

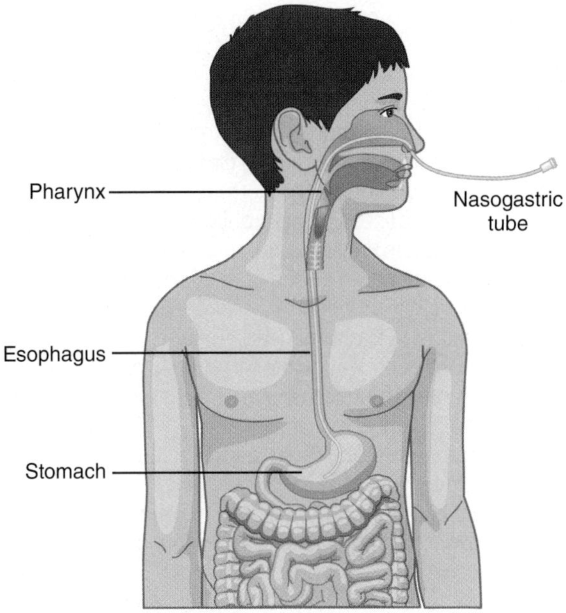

FIGURE 47-15 Nasogastric tube.

© Jones & Bartlett Learning.

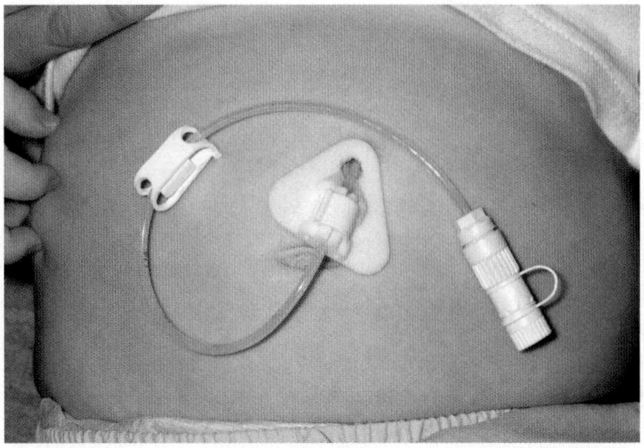

FIGURE 47-16 Gastrostomy tube.

© Dr P. Marazzi/Science Source

vascular access devices include a cracked line, air embolism, bleeding, obstruction, and local infection. Patients with vascular access devices often have a serious illness such as cancer or acquired immuno-deficiency syndrome. The effects of these illnesses may complicate the assessment and management of emergencies associated with central venous lines.

Gastric Tubes and Gastrostomy Tubes

A gastric tube (**FIGURE 47-15**) is used as a temporary measure to provide liquid feeding to a patient who cannot swallow or absorb nutrients (often used for feeding premature newborns). The tubes are inserted through the nose or mouth into the stomach and can cause irritation to the nasal and mucous membranes. They are designed for short-term use.

A gastrostomy tube (**FIGURE 47-16**) provides a permanent route for gastric feeding in patients who usually cannot be fed by mouth. The tube is surgically placed into the stomach and is often visible in the upper left quadrant of the abdomen. The opening (stoma) has a flexible, silicone "button" (which is covered with a protective cap). The stoma allows for regular feedings. Management is described in Chapter 51, *Acute Interventions for Home Care*.

> **NOTE**
>
> **Conditions That May Require a Gastrostomy Tube**
> - Congenital defects of the mouth, esophagus, stomach, or intestines
> - Sucking and swallowing disorders, often related to prematurity, brain injury, developmental delay, or some neuromuscular conditions (eg, severe cerebral palsy)
> - Failure to thrive
> - Extreme difficulty taking medications
> - Facial injuries or burns

Summary

- Paramedics must continually maintain their knowledge of pediatric emergency care.
- The Emergency Medical Services for Children (EMSC) program was designed to enhance and expand EMS for acutely ill and injured children. The program has defined 12 basic components of an effective EMSC system.
- Children have unique anatomic, physiologic, and psychological characteristics, which change during their development.
- Airway structures of children are narrower and less stable than are those of adults. This increases the risk of upper and lower airway obstruction related to injury or illness.
- Principles of child assessment are similar to those used for adults, but pediatric-sized equipment and specific adaptations to the examination should be made.
- Some childhood diseases and disabilities can be predicted by age group.
- Many elements of the initial evaluation can be done by observing the child. The child's parent or guardian also should be involved in the initial evaluation. The three components of the pediatric assessment triangle are appearance, work of breathing, and circulation.
- Paramedics must recognize and distinguish between respiratory distress, respiratory failure, and respiratory arrest.
- Obstruction of the upper or lower airway by a foreign body usually occurs in children younger than 3 years. Obstruction may be partial or complete.
- Croup is a common inflammatory respiratory illness. It usually is seen in children between the ages of 6 months and 4 years. Symptoms are caused by inflammation in the subglottic region.
- Epiglottitis is a rapidly progressive, life-threatening bacterial infection. It causes edema and swelling of the epiglottis and supraglottic structures. It often affects children between 6 and 12 years of age.
- Bacterial tracheitis is an infection of the upper airway and subglottic trachea usually seen in children younger than 6 years. It often occurs with or after croup.
- Asthma is common in children. Asthma is characterized by bronchoconstriction that results from autonomic dysfunction or exposure to sensitizing agents.
- Bronchiolitis is a viral disease frequently caused by respiratory syncytial virus infection of the lower airway. It usually affects children younger than 2 years.
- Pneumonia is an acute infection of the lower airways and lungs involving the alveolar walls and the alveoli.
- Pertussis is a bacterial respiratory tract infection associated with a long course of illness, a violent cough with a characteristic "whoop," and a risk of pneumonia.
- Several special differences must be remembered when caring for a child in shock, including circulating blood volume, body surface area and hypothermia, cardiac reserve, and vital signs and assessment. A child in shock may appear normal and stable until all compensatory mechanisms fail. At that point, pediatric shock progresses rapidly.
- When dysrhythmias occur in children, they usually result from hypoxia or structural heart disease.
- Goals of postresuscitation stabilization in children include preserving brain function; maintaining oxygen saturation, ventilation, and perfusion; avoiding secondary injury; identifying causes of illness; and transporting to an appropriate facility.
- Meningitis is inflammation of the meninges. It can lead to neurologic damage, hearing or vision impairment, and death.
- Common causes of seizure in adult and pediatric patients are noncompliance with a drug regimen for the treatment of epilepsy, head trauma, intracranial infection, metabolic disturbance, and poisoning. The most common cause of new onset of seizure in children is fever.
- Hypoglycemia and hyperglycemia should be suspected whenever a child has an altered level of consciousness with no explainable cause. Consider diabetes as a possible cause in children even in the absence of a history of diabetes.
- Blood disorders that may affect children include sickle cell disease, leukemia, clotting disorders, and others.
- Gastrointestinal disorders in children can lead to serious illness, including life-threatening dehydration and death.
- Children with infection may have a variety of signs and symptoms. These depend on the source and extent of infection and the length of time since the patient was exposed.
- Most poisoning events in the United States involve children. Signs and symptoms of accidental poisoning vary, depending on the toxic substance and the length of time since the child was exposed.
- Blunt and penetrating trauma is a chief cause of injury and death in children. Head injury is the most common cause of death in pediatric trauma patients. Early recognition and appropriate management can reduce morbidity and mortality caused by traumatic brain injury in children.
- Because of the pliability of the chest wall, severe intrathoracic injury can be present without signs of external injury. The liver, kidneys, and spleen are the most frequently injured abdominal organs. Extremity injuries are more common in children than in adults.
- Sudden infant death syndrome is the leading cause of death in US infants younger than 1 year. The syndrome is

defined as the sudden death of a seemingly healthy infant. The death cannot be explained by history and an autopsy.
- Child abuse or neglect is the maltreatment of children. Forms of maltreatment include infliction of physical injury, sexual exploitation, and infliction of emotional pain and neglect.
- Some infants and children are born with or develop conditions that pose special needs. These children may require special medical equipment to sustain life. Often these children are cared for at home. Many are dependent on specialized medical equipment such as tracheostomy tubes, home artificial ventilators, central venous lines, gastrostomy tubes, and shunts. They may have emergencies associated with airway obstruction, impaired ventilation, infection, or increased intracranial pressure.

References

1. Page D. EMS interventions and pediatric outcomes: studies examine outcomes of EMS response and treatment. JEMS website. http://www.jems.com/articles/print/volume-36/issue-10/patient-care/ems-interventions-pediatric-outcomes.html. Published September 30, 2011. Accessed May 22, 2018.
2. Durch J, Lohr K, eds. *The Institute of Medicine Report, EMSC Report Summary*. Washington, DC: National Academy Press; 1993:5.
3. National Center for Education in Maternal and Child Health. *Emergency Medical Services for Children: A Report to the Nation*. Washington, DC: National Center for Education in Maternal and Child Health; 1991.
4. American Heart Association. *Pediatric Advanced Life Support*. Dallas, TX: American Heart Association; 2016.
5. de Caen AR, Maconochie IK, Aickin R, et al.; Pediatric Basic Life Support and Pediatric Advanced Life Support Chapter Collaborators. Part 6: pediatric basic life support and pediatric advanced life support: 2015 International Consensus on Cardiopulmonary Resuscitation and Emergency Cardiovascular Care Science With Treatment Recommendations. *Circulation*. 2015;132(suppl 1):S177-S203.
6. Hannon M, Mannix R, Dorney K, et al. Pediatric cervical spine injury evaluation after blunt trauma: a clinical decision analysis. *Ann Emerg Med*. 2014;65(3):239-247.
7. Schafermeyer R, Tenenbein M, Macias CG, Sharieff GQ, Yamamoto LG. *Strange and Schafermeyer's Pediatric Emergency Medicine*. 4th ed. New York, NY: McGraw-Hill; 2015.
8. Fuchs S, Klein BL, eds. *Pediatric Education for Prehospital Professionals*. Revised 3rd ed. Burlington, MA: Jones & Bartlett Learning; 2016:6.
9. Fuchs S. The special needs of children. In: Brice J, Delbridge TR, Myers JB, eds. *Emergency Services: Clinical Practice and Systems Oversight*. 2nd ed. West Sussex, England: John Wiley & Sons; 2015:381-385.
10. National Association of State EMS Officials. National Model EMS Clinical Guidelines, Version 2.0. https://www.nasemso.org/documents/National-Model-EMS-Clinical-Guidelines-Version2-Sept2017.pdf. Published September 2017. Accessed May 15, 2018.
11. Bernius M, Thibodeau B, Jones A, et al. Prevention of pediatric drug calculation errors by prehospital care providers. *Prehosp Emerg Care*. 2008;12(4):486-494.
12. Hoyle JD Jr, Crowe RP, Bentley MA, et al. Pediatric prehospital medication dosing errors: a national survey of paramedics. *Prehosp Emerg Care*. 2017;21(2):185-191.
13. Hoyle JD Jr, Davis AT, Putman KK, et al. Medication dosing errors in pediatric patients treated by emergency medical services. *Prehosp Emerg Care*. 2012;16:59-66.
14. Vilke GM, Tornabene SV, Stepanski B, et al. Paramedic self-reported medication errors. *Prehosp Emerg Care*. 2007;11(1):80-84.
15. Ruiz FE. Airway foreign bodies in children. UpToDate website. https://www.uptodate.com/contents/airway-foreign-bodies-in-children#H2. Updated May 31, 2017. Accessed May 15, 2018.
16. Defendi GL. Croup treatment and management. Medscape website. https://emedicine.medscape.com/article/962972-treatment. Updated November 14, 2017. Accessed May 23, 2018.
17. Owusu-Ansah S. Emergent management of pediatric epiglottitis. Medscape website. https://emedicine.medscape.com/article/801369-overview. Updated August 17, 2017. Accessed May 15, 2018.
18. National Center for Immunization and Respiratory Diseases. Epidemiology and prevention of vaccine-preventable diseases: *Haemophilus influenzae* type b. Centers for Disease Control and Prevention website. https://www.cdc.gov/vaccines/pubs/pinkbook/hib.html. Updated September 29, 2015. Accessed May 15, 2018.
19. Kliegman R, Stanton B, St. Geme JW, et al. *Nelson Textbook of Pediatrics*. 20th ed. Philadelphia, PA: Elsevier; 2016.
20. National Center for Environmental Health. *Most recent asthma data*. Centers for Disease Control and Prevention website. https://www.cdc.gov/asthma/most_recent_data.htm. Updated February 13, 2018. Accessed May 15, 2018.
21. *Childhood asthma*. American Academy of Allergy, Asthma, and Immunology website. https://www.aaaai.org/conditions-and-treatments/conditions-a-to-z-search/Childhood-(pediatric)-Asthma. Accessed May 15, 2018.
22. Knapp B, Wood C. The prehospital administration of intravenous methylprednisolone lowers hospital admission rates for moderate to severe asthma. *Prehosp Emerg Care*. 2003;7(4):423-426.
23. National Center for Immunization and Respiratory Diseases, Division of Bacterial Diseases. Pertussis (whooping cough): clinical complications. Centers for Disease Control and Prevention website. https://www.cdc.gov/pertussis/clinical

/complications.html. Updated August 7, 2017. Accessed May 23, 2018.
24. Thibodeau GA, Patton KT. *Anatomy and Physiology*. 8th ed. St. Louis, MO: Mosby Elsevier; 2013.
25. Hazinski MF. *Nursing Care of the Critically Ill Child*. 3rd ed. St. Louis, MO: Elsevier; 2013.
26. Revell M, Greaves I, Porter K. Endpoints for fluid resuscitation in hemorrhagic shock. *J Trauma Acute Care Surg*. 2003;54(5): S63-S67.
27. Hawnwan PM. Evidence-based EMS: permissive hypotension in trauma. EMS World website. https://www.emsworld.com/article/12163910/evidence-based-ems-permissive-hypotension-in-trauma. Published January 29, 2016. Accessed May 15, 2017.
28. Tosounidis TH, Giannoudis PV. Paediatric trauma resuscitation: an update. *Eur J Trauma Emerg Surg*. 2016;42:297-301.
29. McBride ME, Marino BS, Webster G, et al. Amiodarone versus lidocaine for pediatric cardiac arrest due to ventricular arrhythmias: a systematic review. *Pediatr Crit Care Med*. 2017;18(2):183-189.
30. Tress EE, Kochanek PM, Saladino RA, Manole MD. Cardiac arrest in children. *J Emerg Trauma Shock*. 2010;3(3):267-272.
31. American College of Surgeons Committee on Trauma, American College of Emergency Physicians Pediatric Emergency Medicine Committee, National Association of EMS Physicians, et al. Withholding or termination of resuscitation in pediatric out-of-hospital traumatic cardiopulmonary arrest. *Pediatrics*. 2014;133(4):504-515.
32. National Center for Immunization and Respiratory Diseases. Bacterial meningitis. Centers for Disease Control and Prevention website. https://www.cdc.gov/meningitis/bacterial.html. Updated January 25, 2017. Accessed May 15, 2018.
33. National Center for Immunization and Respiratory Diseases. Meningococcal disease: technical and clinical information. Centers for Disease Control and Prevention website. https://www.cdc.gov/meningococcal/clinical-info.html. Updated July 6, 2017. Accessed May 15, 2018.
34. Facts and stats. Hydrocephalus Association website. https://www.hydroassoc.org/about-us/newsroom/facts-and-stats-2/. Accessed May 15, 2018.
35. Freeman WD. Management of intracranial pressure. *Continuum (Minneap Minn)*. 2015 Oct;21(5 Neurocritical Care):1299-1323.
36. Dulebohn SC, Mesfin FB. Ventriculoperitoneal shunt. In: *StatPearls* [Internet]. https://www.ncbi.nlm.nih.gov/books/NBK459351/. Updated March 4, 2018. Accessed May 15, 2018.
37. Kappy MS, Allen DB, Geffner ME. *Pediatric Practice: Endocrinology*. 2nd ed. New York, NY: McGraw-Hill; 2014.
38. US Diabetes Surveillance System. National diabetes statistics report, 2017. CDC Publication CS279910-A. Centers for Disease Control and Prevention website. https://www.cdc.gov/diabetes/pdfs/data/statistics/national-diabetes-statistics-report.pdf. Accessed May 15, 2018.
39. Haymond MW. Treatment and complications of diabetic ketoacidosis in children and adolescents. UpToDate website. https://www.uptodate.com/contents/treatment-and-complications-of-diabetic-ketoacidosis-in-children-and-adolescents. Updated January 24, 2017. Accessed May 15, 2018.
40. Long B, Koyfman A. Emergency medicine myths: cerebral edema in pediatric diabetic ketoacidosis and intravenous fluids. *J Emerg Med*. 2017;53(2):212-221.
41. Neutze D, Roque J. Clinical evaluation of bleeding and bruising in primary care. *Am Fam Physician*. 2016;15(93):279-286.
42. Poison statistics: national data 2016. National Capital Poison Center website. https://www.poison.org/poison-statistics-national. Accessed May 15, 2018.
43. National Safety Council. *Injury Facts*. Itasca, IL: National Safety Council; 2017.
44. Centers for Disease Control and Prevention, National Center for Injury Prevention and Control, Division of Unintentional Injury Prevention. Unintentional drowning: get the facts. Centers for Disease Control and Prevention website. https://www.cdc.gov/homeandrecreationalsafety/water-safety/waterinjuries-factsheet.html. Updated April 28, 2016. Accessed May 15, 2018.
45. Sheehan B, Nigrovic LE, Dayan PS, Kuppermann N, et al. Informing the design of clinical decision support services for evaluation of children with minor blunt head trauma in the emergency department: a sociotechnical analysis. *J Biomed Informatics*. 2013;46(5):905-913.
46. Centers for Disease Control and Prevention, National Center for Injury Prevention and Control, Division of Unintentional Injury Prevention. Protect the ones you love: child injuries are preventable; burn prevention. Centers for Disease Control and Prevention website. Updated April 28, 2016. Accessed May 23, 2018.
47. Pediatric burn fact sheet. Burn Foundation website. http://www.burnfoundation.org/programs/resource.cfm?c=1&a=12. Accessed May 15, 2018.
48. Miller MD, Thompson SR. *Miller's Review of Orthopaedics*. 7th ed. St. Louis, MO: Elsevier; 2015:655-705.
49. Marx J, Hockberger R, Walls R. *Rosen's Emergency Medicine: Concepts and Clinical Practice*. 8th ed. St. Louis, MO: Elsevier; 2014.
50. Lonie S, Prassas G. Anaesthetic management for burns in children. *JSM Burns Trauma*. 2017;2(3):1022.
51. Leonard J. Cervical spine injury. *Pediatr Clin N Am*. 2013;60: 1123-1137.
52. *Part 12: Pediatric Advanced Life Support: Web-Based Integrated 2010 and 2015 American Heart Association Guidelines for Cardiopulmonary Resuscitation and Emergency Cardiovascular Care*. American Heart Association website. https://eccguidelines.heart.org/wp-content/themes/eccstaging/dompdf-master/pdffiles/part-12-pediatric-advanced-life-support.pdf. Accessed May 15, 2018.
53. Park JW, Piknova B, Nghiem K, et al. Inhibitory effect of nitrite on coagulation processes demonstrated by thrombelastography. *Nitric Oxide*. 2014;40:45-51.
54. Brain Trauma Foundation. *Guidelines for the Management of Severe Traumatic Brain Injury*. 4th ed. Brain Trauma Foundation: New York, NY; 2016.
55. National Association of Emergency Medical Technicians. *PHTLS: Prehospital Trauma Life Support*. 8th ed. Burlington, MA: Jones & Bartlett Learning; 2014.

56. Division of Reproductive Health, National Center for Chronic Disease Prevention and Health Promotion. Sudden unexpected infant death and sudden infant death syndrome. Centers for Disease Control and Prevention website. https://www.cdc.gov/sids/index.htm. Updated January 10, 2018. Accessed May 15, 2018.
57. Giardino AP, Lyn MA. *A Practical Guide to the Evaluation of Child Physical Abuse and Neglect*. 2nd ed. New York, NY: Springer; 2010.
58. Smith MP, Kaji A, Young KD, et al. Presentation and survival of prehospital apparent sudden infant death syndrome. *Prehosp Emerg Care*. 2005;9(2):181-185.
59. Department of Health and Human Services. *Child Maltreatment 2016*. Washington, DC: Department of Health and Human Services; 2016.
60. Child Welfare Information Gateway. *Mandatory Reporters of Child Abuse and Neglect.* Washington, DC: US Department of Health and Human Services, Children's Bureau; 2016.
61. National Center for Injury Prevention and Control, Division of Unintentional Injury Prevention. Violence prevention: child abuse and neglect: risk and protective factors. Centers for Disease Control and Prevention website. https://www.cdc.gov/violenceprevention/childmaltreatment/riskprotectivefactors.html. Updated April 18, 2017. Accessed May 15, 2018.
62. *Indications of child abuse and maltreatment.* Childabuse.com website. www.childabuse.com/help.htm. Accessed May 15, 2010.
63. Colbourne M. Abusive head trauma: evolution of a diagnosis. *BC Med J.* 2015;57(8):331-335.
64. Kondolot M, Yağmur F, Yıkılmaz A, Turan C, Öztop DB, Oral R. A life-threatening presentation of child physical abuse: jejunal perforation. *Pediatr Emerg Care*. 2011 Nov;27(11):1075-1077.
65. Scope of the problem: statistics. RAINN website. https://www.rainn.org/statistics/scope-problem. Accessed May 15, 2018.
66. Cone D, Brice JH, Delbridge TR, Myers B. *Emergency Medical Services: Clinical Practice and Systems Oversight*. 2nd ed. Hoboken, NJ: Wiley; 2015:397-400.
67. American College of Emergency Physicians. Policy statement: emergency form for children with special health care needs. *Ann Emerg Med*. 2010;56:4.

Suggested Readings

Berdan EA. Sato TT. Pediatric airway and esophageal foreign bodies. *Surg Clin North Am*. 2017;97(1):85-91.

Committee on Pediatric Emergency Medicine, Council on Injury, Violence, and Poison Prevention, Section on Critical Care, et al. Management of pediatric trauma. *Pediatrics*. 2016;138(2):e20161569.

Giardino AP. Physical child abuse. Medscape website. https://emedicine.medscape.com/article/915664-overview. Updated April 24, 2017. Accessed May 15, 2018.

Lynne EG, Gifford EJ, Evans KE, et al. Barriers to reporting child maltreatment: do emergency medical services professionals fully understand their role as mandatory reporters? *N C Med J*. 2015; 76(1):13-18.

Marshall M. *Barriers to Asthma Education and Management Among Pediatric Respiratory Care Practitioners* [dissertation]. Capella University, ProQuest Dissertations Publishing; 2017:10254567.

Sandhu N, Eppich W, Mikrogianakis A, et al. Postresuscitation debriefing in the pediatric emergency department: a national needs assessment. *Can J Emerg Med*. 2014;16(5):383-392.

Silverman EC, Sporer KA, Lemieux JM, et al. Prehospital care for the adult and pediatric seizure patient: current evidence-based recommendations. *West J Emerg Med*. 2017;18(3):419-436.

Tiyyagura GK, Gawel M, Alphonso A, et al. Barriers and facilitators to recognition and reporting of child abuse by prehospital providers. *Prehosp Emerg Care*. 2017;21(1):46-53.

Walsh EE. Respiratory syncytial virus infection. *Clin Chest Med*. 2017;38(1):29-36.

Zanello E, Calugi S, Sanders LM, et al. Care coordination for children with special health care needs: a cohort study. *Ital J Pediatr*. 2017;43:18.

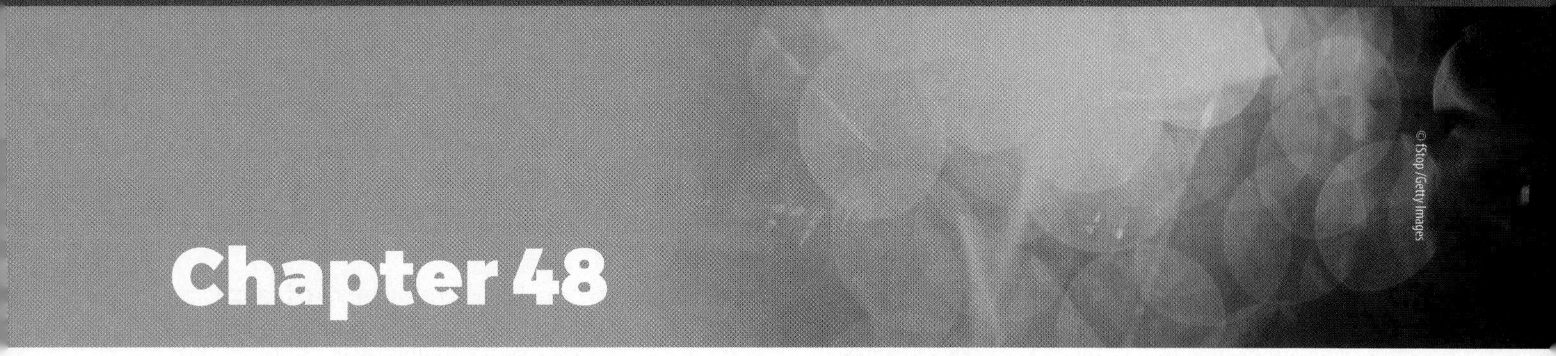
© fStop/Getty Images

Chapter 48

Geriatrics

NATIONAL EMS EDUCATION STANDARD COMPETENCIES

Special Patient Populations

Integrates assessment findings with principles of pathophysiology and knowledge of psychosocial needs to formulate a field impression and implement a comprehensive treatment/disposition plan for patients with special needs.

Geriatrics

Impact of age-related changes on assessment and care (pp 1718–1719)

Changes associated with aging, psychosocial aspects of aging, and age-related assessment and treatment modifications for the major or common geriatric diseases and/or emergencies

- Cardiovascular diseases (p 1715)
- Respiratory diseases (p 1715)
- Neurologic diseases (p 1716)
- Endocrine diseases (pp 1726–1727)
- Alzheimer disease (pp 1724–1725)
- Dementia (pp 1724–1726)
- Fluid resuscitation in older adults (p 1725)

Normal and abnormal changes associated with aging, pharmacokinetic changes, psychosocial and economic aspects of aging, polypharmacy, and age-related assessment and treatment modifications for the major or common geriatric diseases and/or emergencies

- Cardiovascular diseases (pp 1720–1722)
- Respiratory diseases (pp 1719–1720)
- Neurologic diseases (p 1722)
- Endocrine diseases (pp 1726–1727)
- Alzheimer disease (pp 1724–1725)
- Dementia (pp 1724–1726)
  - Acute confusional state (pp 1723–1724)
- Fluid resuscitation in older adults (p 1725)
- Herpes zoster (see Chapter 27, *Infectious and Communicable Diseases*)
- Inflammatory arthritis (p 1731)

OBJECTIVES

Upon completion of this chapter, the paramedic student will be able to:

1. Explain the physiology of the aging process as it relates to major body systems and homeostasis. (pp 1712–1718)
2. Describe general principles of assessment specific to older adults. (pp 1718–1719)
3. Describe the pathophysiology, assessment, and management of specific illnesses that affect selected body systems in the geriatric patient. (pp 1719–1740)
4. Identify specific problems with sensations experienced by some geriatric patients. (pp 1731–1732)
5. Discuss effects of drug toxicity and alcoholism in the older adult. (pp 1733–1734)
6. Identify factors that contribute to environmental emergencies in the geriatric patient. (pp 1734–1735)
7. Discuss prehospital assessment and management of depression and suicide in the older adult. (pp 1735–1736)
8. Describe epidemiology, assessment, and management of trauma in the geriatric patient. (pp 1736–1740)
9. Identify characteristics of elder abuse. (p 1740)

KEY TERMS

adverse drug event (ADE) An injury resulting from the use of a drug.

Alzheimer disease A disease characterized by confusion, memory failure, disorientation, speech disturbances, and inability to carry out purposeful movements.

biliary disease Disorders of the liver and gallbladder caused by abnormalities in bile composition, biliary anatomy, or function.

cataract A loss of transparency of the lens of the eye that results from changes in the delicate protein fibers within the lens.

cerebral atrophy Reduction in the size of brain tissue.

confabulation The invention of stories to make up for gaps in memory.

continence The ability to control bladder or bowel function.

delirium A medical emergency characterized by an abrupt disorientation for time and place, usually with delusions and hallucinations; may be reversible if causative etiology is identified.

dementia A slow, progressive loss of awareness of time and place. It usually involves an inability to learn new things or recall recent events.

elder abuse The infliction of physical pain, injury, debilitating mental anguish, unreasonable confinement, or willful deprivation by a caregiver of services that are necessary to maintain the mental and physical health of a geriatric person.

fecal impaction An accumulation of hardened feces in the rectum or sigmoid colon that the person is unable to move.

frailty A geriatric syndrome characterized by exhaustion, slowed performance, weakness, weight loss, and low physical activity.

gerontology The study of the special needs and restrictions associated with aging.

glaucoma A condition in which intraocular pressure increases and causes damage to the optic nerve.

hyperthyroidism A condition characterized by increased activity of the thyroid gland.

hypothyroidism A condition characterized by decreased activity of the thyroid gland.

incontinence The inability to control bladder or bowel function.

kyphosis An abnormal condition of the vertebral column characterized by increased convexity in the curvature of the thoracic spine as viewed from the side.

Lewy body disease Dementia associated with abnormal deposits of a protein called alpha-synuclein in the brain with neurons; also called Lewy body dementia.

organic brain dysfunction Abnormal cognition that results from primarily physical functional disorders (as opposed to psychological disorders).

osteoarthritis A form of arthritis in which one or many joints undergo degenerative changes.

osteoporosis A disorder characterized by a reduction in bone density. It occurs most often in postmenopausal women.

Parkinson disease A degenerative neurologic disease affecting dopaminergic neurons in the brain causing motor function deterioration. Manifestations include resting tremor, rigidity, slowed movements, and gait abnormality.

Parkinson disease dementia Parkinson disease that later progresses into dementia.

polypharmacy The simultaneous use of multiple drugs by a single patient for one or more conditions.

pressure ulcers Sores or ulcers in the skin usually over a bony prominence that occur most frequently on the sacrum, elbows, heels, outer ankles, inner knees, hips, and shoulder blades of high-risk patients, especially in older adults or people who are obese or suffering from chronic diseases, infections, injuries, or a poor nutritional state.

retinopathy A group of noninflammatory eye disorders often caused by diabetes mellitus, hypertension, and atherosclerotic vascular disease.

tinnitus A ringing sound in the ears.

vascular dementia A reduction in cognitive function caused by conditions that block or reduce circulation in the brain.

The "graying" of American society includes the prospect that the health care needs of older adults will continue to increase in all areas. This includes prehospital care. About 25% of Americans will be 65 years of age or older by the year 2030, and this age group will represent 49% of all ambulance transports.[1] This chapter addresses anatomic and physiologic changes that accompany the aging process, special considerations in assessing and managing geriatric patients, and common emergencies that may result from normal aging and chronic illness.

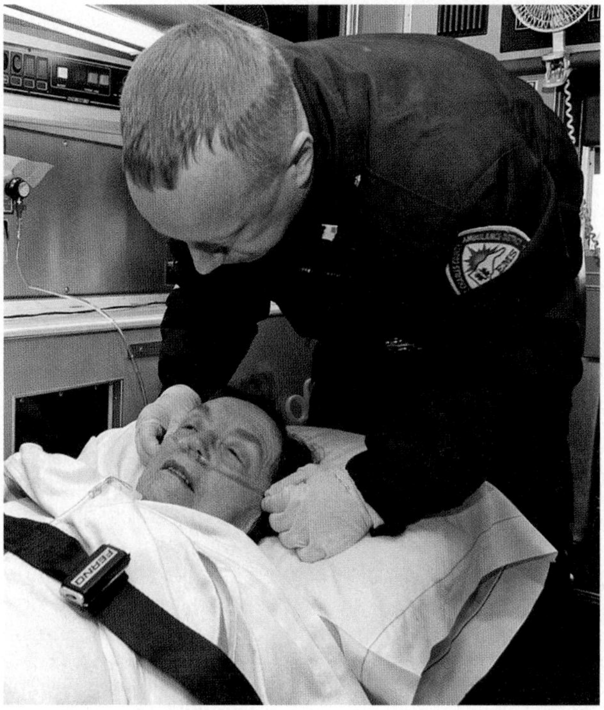

Courtesy of Ray Kemp, St. Charles, MO.

Demographics, Epidemiology, and Societal Issues

In 2015, more than 47 million Americans (14.5% of the US population) were aged 65 years or older.[2] This number is growing rapidly and is expected to reach 98 million by 2060.[2] By 2050, 92.8 million Americans are projected to be enrolled in Medicare.[3] This rapid growth creates many challenges. Society will need to provide quality, cost-effective health care and support the increasing health and living expenses for the older adult population. To meet the needs of this aging population properly, society must achieve the following:[4]

- The public must become better educated about the needs of older adults because caregiving often becomes the responsibility of families and friends.
- Current and new health care professionals must be educated on the special needs of the aging population.
- The aging of the US population demands continued and expanded research efforts into chronic diseases that affect older adults and their families.
- Health care professionals need to reform heath care financing, delivery, and administrative structures to accommodate the predominance of chronic illness among the aging population.
- Health care professionals must develop solutions for the long-term care needs of the growing aging population. These solutions must address the emotional and financial needs of older adults and their families. They also must address the financial influence of long-term care in the United States.

Other key issues to consider in caring for the aging population include legal ones, such as advance directives, durable power of attorney, do not resuscitate orders, and physician orders for life-sustaining treatment (POLST). Ethical principles of autonomy and self-determination often also come into play when caring for older adults. These issues are discussed in Chapter 5, *EMS Communications*, and Chapter 6, *Medical and Legal Issues*. Practicing person-centered care is key when caring for older adults. The American Geriatrics Society defines person-centered care as "providing care that is respectful of and responsive to individual patient preferences, needs, and values, and ensuring that patient values guide all clinical decisions."[5]

Research on national EMS data suggests that over 40% of adult EMS responses were for older adults.[6] In this population, complaints of syncope, cardiac arrest or rhythm disturbance, stroke, and shock were more likely compared with EMS calls for younger adults. This population demands a significant amount of EMS skill and resources to meet their needs. Repeated EMS transport of adults aged 65 years or older within 30 days of a previous response has been reported to be as high as 17%.[7] Dispatch reports indicate that complaints associated with an increased likelihood of repeat transport were psychiatric problems, back pain, breathing problems, problems related to diabetes, and falls.

Living Environments and Referral Sources

Many older Americans enjoy independent living. They enjoy this lifestyle with the help of spousal or family support and home health care programs. Others live dependently in nursing care facilities, assisted-living environments, and nursing homes. Older adults often receive assistance in independent and dependent living environments. They receive this help through local, state, and national programs and other resource agencies (BOX 48-1). The paramedic should be familiar with the programs in the community that offer assistance to older adults.

Physiologic Changes of Aging

Gerontology is the study of the problems of all aspects of aging. The aging process proceeds at different rates in different people. In addition, organ systems age at differing rates within the person. However, in certain areas, predictable functional declines occur in all people with increasing age. As a general guideline, these changes begin to occur at a rate of 5% to 10% for each decade of life after age 30 years.[8] The aging process affects all body systems. However, the effects on specific organ systems particularly relevant to the older adult occur in the respiratory, cardiovascular, renal, nervous, and musculoskeletal systems (**TABLE 48-1**). These are highly variable by person.

BOX 48-1 Sampling of Support and Assistance Programs for the Geriatric Patient

- Community-based services
- Home health care services
- Hospice programs
- In-home services
- Institutional services
- Mobile integrated health care services
- Multipurpose senior centers
- Nutrition services
- Religious and pastoral services
- State advisory councils
- State and national aging organizations
- Volunteer organizations

CRITICAL THINKING

Consider your family members and friends who are in their 60s, 70s, or 80s. What age-related changes have you noticed as they have gotten older?

NOTE

Frailty is defined as a state of heightened vulnerability to functional dependence or death in response to a stressor. It is a biologic syndrome of decreased reserve and resistance to stressors, resulting from cumulative declines across multiple physiologic systems and causing vulnerability to adverse outcomes. This concept distinguishes frailty from physical disability that is associated with advancing age.

Characteristics of frailty are low physical activity, muscle weakness, slowed performance, fatigue or poor endurance, impaired mobility, and unintentional weight loss. Most frail older adults are women (partly because women outlive men), are older than 80 years, and often receive care from an adult child. Frailty is associated with poor health outcomes, increased risk of hospitalization, and limited life span. Because of the rapid rate of growth in the population aged 65 years and older, the number of frail older people is increasing every year.

Modified from: Morley JE, Vellas B, van Kan GA, et al. Frailty consensus: a call to action. *J Am Med Dir Assoc*. 2013;14(6):392-397; Freid LP, Tangen CM, Walston J, et al. Frailty in older adults: evidence of a phenotype. *J Gerontol A Biol Sci Med Sci.* 2001;56(3):M146-M156; Mauk K. *Gerontological Nursing.* 4th ed. Burlington, MA: Jones & Bartlett Learning; 2018; and Knickman JR, Snell EK. The 2030 problem: caring for aging baby boomers. *Health Serv Res*. 2002;37(4):849-884.

TABLE 48-1 Physiologic Changes of Aging

Structural Changes	Changes in Function
Skin	
Loss of elasticity	Wrinkling, thinning of skin
Loss of collagen	Increased susceptibility to injury
Decreased turnover of epidermal keratinocytes slows rate of exfoliation replacement of dead cells; decreased melanocytes	Risk of skin cancer and infection increases; slower wound repair
Decreased sweat glands and skin vascularity	Dryness, increased risk of injury, less able to adapt to temperature change, less sweat production

TABLE 48-1 Physiologic Changes of Aging *(continued)*

Structural Changes	Changes in Function
Cardiovascular System	
Decreased myocardial cells (including pacemaker cells); increased myocardial cell size; stiffening of arteries; decreased vascular tone; increased left ventricle thickness; increased elastin and collagen levels; increased left atrial size	Hypertension (systolic); decreased diastolic filling; decreased reaction to beta-adrenergic stimulus; longer muscle contraction and relaxation phases Increased risk of stroke or heart attack Dysrhythmias
No changes in ejection fraction, stroke volume, overall systolic function	
Pulmonary System	
Decreased elasticity Decreased respiratory muscle strength; weakened diaphragm; overall loss of muscle mass	Diminished breathing capacity (decreased tidal volume, inspiratory reserve volume, expiratory reserve volume, forced expiratory volume, vital capacity) Increased residual volume and functional residual capacity
Decreased compliance and surface area: decreased alveolar surface area	Decreased maximal oxygen uptake
Decreased ciliary activity	Increased risk of infection/toxicity
No change in total lung capacity	
Gastrointestinal Tract	
Decreased gastric acid secretion (about one-third of older adults)	Decreased absorption of vitamin D, zinc, and calcium
Delay in intestinal motility in colon	Longer colonic transit time
Fewer taste buds and decreased sense of smell	Decreased appetite, increased risk of food poisoning
Stiffening of the esophageal wall	Difficulty swallowing
Tooth loss; atrophy of muscles and bones of jaw and mouth; absent gag reflex (about 40% of older adults)	Increased choking risk
Decreased liver size and perfusion	Risk of toxicity from drugs because of increased drug clearance time in some older adults
Decline in gallbladder emptying rates	Increased risk of gallstones
Decrease in GI immunologic function	Increased risk of GI infection
Central Nervous System	
Decreased cortical cell count; brain size and weight decrease	Prone to subdural hematoma
Decreased cerebral blood flow	Decreased cognitive function
Decreased nerve conduction velocity because of myelin degradation	Slower psychomotor skills Increased reflex time leading to risk of falling
Development of neurofibrillary tangles, beta-amyloid plaques, free radicals	Risk of Alzheimer disease, dementia
Decline in some neurotransmitters (acetylcholine, dopamine, serotonin)	Possible cognitive or motor changes, depression
Spinal cord cells decrease	Decline in motor and/or sensory function

(continued)

TABLE 48-1 Physiologic Changes of Aging *(continued)*

Structural Changes	Changes in Function
Endocrine System	
Decreased growth hormone	Loss of muscle mass; decreased bone formation, reduced protein synthesis, reduced tissue repair, decline in immune function
Decreased melatonin	Sleep disturbances
Decreased aldosterone	Impaired sodium regulation
Impaired adrenal medulla function	Decreased ability to secrete epinephrine in response to stress
Increased insulin	Predisposition for hypoglycemia
Alterations in estrogen and progesterone	Menopause (usually by age 51years)
Vision	
Thickening of collagen fibers, muscle loss, loss of aqueous and vitreous humor in eyes	Decreased focusing ability, color and depth perception, and peripheral vision; hyperopia (farsightedness), reduced night vision
Cataract deposition in eyes	Opacification of vision
Balance and Proprioception	
Decrease in number and altered structure of touch receptors	Loss of sensation and proprioception, increasing risk of falls
Hearing	
Ossicle degeneration, atrophy (shrinkage) of cochlear hair cells and auditory neurons, atrophy (shrinkage) of auditory meatus	Loss of high-frequency range of hearing, decreased keenness and pitch discrimination, decreased sense of balance
Renal Function	
Shrinking of kidneys; decline in glomerular function	Functional ability is usually retained until stressed; more difficulty regulating body water, sodium, and potassium
Decreased renal blood flow	Increased risk of toxicity from all drugs and toxins processed in kidneys
Genitourinary System	
Bladder filling capacity and ability to withhold voiding declines	Urinary dysfunction, including nocturia
Prostate enlargement (about 50% of men)	Urinary retention; increased risk of infection
Musculoskeletal System	
Decreased muscle mass	Loss of strength
Increased joint/tendon breakdown	Arthritis, stiffness, loss of flexibility; increased risk of falls
Bone loss	Increased risk of fracture
Immune System	
Loss of T cell function	Increased infection

Abbreviation: GI, gastrointestinal

Modified from: Mauk K. *Gerontological Nursing.* 4th ed. Burlington, MA: Jones & Bartlett Learning; 2018.

Respiratory System Changes

Respiratory function in the older adult generally declines as the lung tissue ages. Reduced pulmonary function results from changes in lung and chest wall compliance, decreased elastic recoil of the lung, and diminishing respiratory muscle strength.[9] With aging, the chest wall becomes stiffer as the bony thorax becomes more rigid. Lung elastic recoil also decreases. Despite the loss of elasticity, which would tend to increase total lung capacity, total lung capacity remains the same because of the opposing loss of chest wall compliance and weakened respiratory muscles. The alveoli become flatter and shallower and their surface area decreases.[9] The distal airways tend to collapse on expiration. These changes lead to an increase in residual volume and a decrease in vital capacity. Consequently, by age 75 years, vital capacity may decrease by as much as 50%.[10]

The arterial partial pressure of oxygen (Pao_2) also slowly decreases with age, but arterial carbon dioxide pressure stays the same. (This is most likely related to the much greater reserve in carbon dioxide elimination than in oxygen absorption.) At age 30 years, the Pao_2 level of a healthy person breathing ambient air at sea level is about 90 mm Hg. Predicted Pao_2 values for aging vary widely. In an 85-year-old man, the Pao_2 value could range from 63 to 84 mm Hg.[10] These findings, along with the normal decline in chemoreceptor function, produce a diminished ventilatory response to hypoxia and hypercapnia.

Other factors that affect the respiratory system are the loss of cilia in the airways and a diminished cough reflex and impaired gag reflex. These changes can impair the bodily defense against inhaled bacteria and particulate matter. The decline in these defense mechanisms makes infectious pulmonary diseases of the older adult more common. It also makes these infections harder to resolve.

Cardiovascular System Changes

Cardiac function declines with age as a result of nonischemic physiologic changes and the high incidence of atherosclerotic coronary artery disease. Differentiation of the changes that are solely the result of aging from those that are associated with ischemia is difficult because coronary artery disease is so prevalent in the older adult. However, even with aging alone, structural and physiologic changes occur that limit cardiac function in the cardiovascular system. These changes include a diminished ability to raise the heart rate even in response to exercise or stress, a decrease in compliance of the ventricle, a prolonged duration of contraction, and a decreased responsiveness to catecholamine stimulation. Myocardial hypertrophy, coronary artery disease, and hemodynamic changes predispose the geriatric patient to dysrhythmias, heart failure, and sudden cardiac arrest when the cardiovascular system is placed under unexpected stress.

Changes also occur in the electrical conduction pathways of the heart. These changes occur as cells in the sinoatrial and atrioventricular nodes and the rest of the conduction system lose the ability to function. These physiologic changes often lead to dysrhythmias, including chronic atrial fibrillation, sick sinus syndrome, and various types of bradycardias and heart blocks. All of these conditions can contribute to the decline in cardiac output.

CRITICAL THINKING

What lifestyle choices can slow down these physiologic changes of aging?

Renal System Changes

Structural and functional changes in the kidneys occur during the aging process. For example, renal blood flow decreases an average of 10% per decade beginning at age 20 years.[9] This reduction in renal blood flow is associated with a proportional decrease in the glomerular filtration rate that is measurable by the time people reach their 30s.[9] Renal mass decreases from 150 to 200 grams at age 30 years to 110 to 150 grams at age 90 years. The steady decline in kidney function places the geriatric patient at greater risk for renal failure from trauma, obstruction, infection, and vascular occlusion.

As the patient ages, significant impairment develops in renal concentrating ability, sodium conservation, free water clearance (diuresis), glomerular filtration, and renal plasma flow. Hepatic blood flow decreases as well, limiting the effectiveness of liver metabolism. Decreases in kidney and liver function and loss of muscle and body water make the geriatric patient more susceptible to electrolyte disturbances. They also make the geriatric patient more likely to experience problems with medications or drugs.

DID YOU KNOW?

Beers List

In 1993 a gerontologist named Mark H. Beers developed a national guideline and reference guide for pharmacists and physicians to improve medication use in the older adult population. (The list is updated frequently based on current evidence.) This guide is known as the Beers list. The Beers criteria includes several tables that identify individual medications or classes of medications to avoid or use within specified dose and duration ranges in older patients. The list helps clinicians avoid prescribing medicines that can cause complications such as falls or delirium in older adults. The application of the Beers criteria for identifying potentially inappropriate medication use helps physicians and pharmacists to plan interventions for decreasing both drug-related costs and overall costs and thus minimize drug-related problems.

Modified from: American Geriatrics Society 2015 updated Beers criteria for potentially inappropriate medication use in older adults. *J Am Geriatr Soc.* 2015;63(11);2227-2246.

Adverse Drug Events in Older Adults

An **adverse drug event (ADE)**, including a reaction or an interaction, is a common cause of hospital admission in older people and is an important cause of morbidity and death. Even after excluding errors in drug administration, noncompliance, overdose, drug abuse, therapeutic failures, and possible ADEs, the overall incidence of serious ADEs in the general hospitalized population in the United States is believed to be as high as 10%.[11] Studies suggest that many ADEs causing admission or occurring in the hospital are dose-related. Therefore, many ADEs are predictable and some are potentially avoidable. Cardiovascular medications, followed by diuretics, nonopioid or opioid analgesics, hypoglycemics, and anticoagulants are some of the most common medication categories associated with preventable ADEs. The most frequent ADEs causing hospital admission in older patients are typically gastrointestinal (GI) disorders, cardiovascular events, and metabolic/endocrine complications. Electrolyte/renal, GI tract, hemorrhagic, metabolic/endocrine, and neuropsychiatric events were the most common types of preventable ADEs.[12]

It is important for paramedics to recognize the need to reduce the dose of specific drugs (eg, midazolam), sometimes by as much as 50%, when giving them to older adults. Other drugs (eg, hydromorphone) should be used with caution in older adults because they are more likely to cause adverse effects.[13]

Nervous System Changes

Although it was long thought that mental dysfunction in the geriatric patient was caused solely by senility, it is now well known that intellectual functioning deteriorates selectively and may result from many organic causes.[14] For example, beginning at about age 55 years, the total number of neurons in certain cortical areas decreases gradually, so by age 70 years, an 11% reduction in brain weight has occurred.[9] These factors, decreased cerebral blood flow, and changes in the location and amounts of specific neurotransmitters probably contribute to changes in the central nervous system (CNS). The velocity of nerve conduction in the peripheral nervous system decreases with aging as well. This may lead to changes in motor or position sense and delays in reaction time and motor responses. Other gradual changes in the patient's nervous system can result in decreased visual acuity and auditory keenness. They also can result in changes in sleep patterns.

Toxic or metabolic factors that can affect mental functioning include the use of medications (eg, anticholinergics, antihypertensives, antidysrhythmics, analgesics); electrolyte imbalances; hypoglycemia; acidosis; alkalosis; hypoxia; liver, kidney, and lung failure; pneumonia; heart failure; cardiac dysrhythmias; infection; and the development of benign or malignant tumors.

Musculoskeletal System Changes

As the body ages, muscles shrink, muscles and ligaments calcify, and intervertebral disks become thin. Osteoporosis is common in geriatric patients (especially in women). Many geriatric patients show some degree of **kyphosis** (also called humpback posture) (**FIGURE 48-1**). These musculoskeletal changes result in a decrease in total muscle mass, a decrease in height of 2 to 3 inches (5 to 8 cm), widening and weakening of certain bones, and a posture that impairs mobility and alters the balance of the body. As a result, falls are common.

CRITICAL THINKING

Consider a patient who has significant kyphosis. What aspects of care will you need to alter to immobilize the spine of this patient?

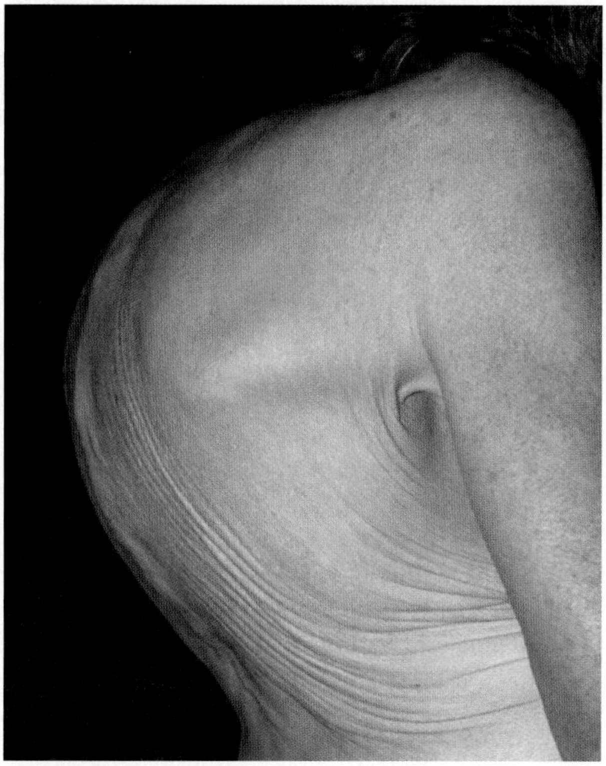

FIGURE 48-1 Kyphosis.

Other Physiologic Changes

Other physiologic changes that occur with aging include a decrease in lean body mass, an increase in body fat, a decrease in total body water, a decreased ability to maintain internal homeostasis, a decrease in the function of immunologic mechanisms, nutritional disorders, and decreases in hearing and visual acuity.

As a person approaches age 65 years, lean body mass may decrease as much as 25%, and fat tissue may increase as much as 35%.[15] These changes in body composition can affect the dosage and frequency of administration of fat-soluble drugs. This is because there is more drug per weight of metabolically active tissue and a larger reservoir for accumulation of the drug. Likewise, the decrease in total body water is likely to increase the concentration of water-soluble drugs.

The ability of the body to maintain normal temperature through thermoregulatory mechanisms declines over time. The decline begins at about age 30 years. As a result, the geriatric patient is at greater risk for cold- and heat-related conditions, including hypothermia, heat exhaustion, and hyperthermia. Several factors contribute to the increased risk of thermoregulatory disorders, including impaired sympathetic nervous system function, causing decreased capacity for peripheral vasoconstriction, lowered metabolic rate, poor peripheral circulation, and chronic illness. Because of the decline in many body functions, including blood pressure, cardiac output, and temperature regulation, a specific illness or injury often puts the geriatric patient "over the edge" without adequate compensatory mechanisms to manage the event.

Aging causes a decrease in primary antibody response and cellular immunity and elevations in the amount of abnormal immunoglobulins and immune complexes.[16] These physiologic changes increase the risk of infection, autoimmune disorders, and perhaps cancer. In addition, infections may not produce the usual signs and symptoms.

NOTE

Changes in the immunologic systems of older adults make them more prone to infections and exacerbations of chronic disease processes. As the thymus ages, T cell production is reduced and leukocytes are not activated. As a result, infections may not produce fever that would normally be seen in younger patients with viral, bacterial, or occult infection.

Age is the greatest risk factor for the development of cancer; 60% of people who have cancer are aged 65 or older.[17] In younger patients, cancer often is the main or only disease from which they suffer. However, geriatric patients often have more than one disease and disability. Thus, signs and symptoms such as a change in bowel habits, rectal bleeding, malaise, fatigue, weight loss, and anorexia may result from other maladies. Treatment with chemotherapy often results in immunosuppression. This increases the risk of infection and often masks the typical signs and symptoms associated with infection.

Many geriatric patients consume less than the minimum daily requirement of most vitamins, which may be a result of loneliness and depression, decreased sensitivity to taste, decreased appetite, financial difficulties, physical infirmity, decreased vision, or a combination of these elements. All of these elements may act to reduce the motivation to shop for and prepare fresh food. Other factors associated with poor nutrition are poor dentition and reduced mastication, decreased esophageal motility, frequent hypochlorhydria (low stomach acid secretion), and decreased intestinal secretions that reduce absorption. Geriatric patients easily can become victims of malnutrition. Malnutrition in turn can cause dehydration, hypoglycemia, and numerous other complications.

CRITICAL THINKING
What effects can poor nutrition have on body function?

General Principles in Assessment of the Geriatric Patient

Normal physiologic changes and underlying acute or chronic illness may make evaluation of an ill or injured geriatric patient a challenge. In addition to the components of a normal physical assessment (described in Chapter 20, *Assessment-Based Management and Clinical Decision Making*), the paramedic should consider special characteristics of geriatric patients that can complicate the clinical evaluation:

- Geriatric patients are likely to suffer from more than one illness at a time.
- Chronic problems can make assessment for acute problems difficult.
- Signs or symptoms of chronic illness can be confused with signs or symptoms of an acute problem.
- Aging can affect a person's response to illness or injury.
- Pain may be diminished or absent.
- The patient or paramedic can underestimate the severity of a condition.
- Social and emotional factors may have a greater influence on health in geriatric patients than in any other age group.
- The patient fears losing autonomy.
- The patient fears the hospital environment.
- The patient has financial concerns about health care.

Patient History

Gathering a history from a geriatric patient may take more time than with younger patients (see Chapter 18, *Scene Size-up and Primary Assessment*). In addition to a longer medical history because of the patient's age, chronic illness, and medication use, the geriatric patient may have physical impediments such as hearing loss and visual impairment. Questioning a patient who is fatigued or easily distracted also may lengthen the interview process. The paramedic should use the following techniques when communicating with geriatric patients:

- Always identify yourself.
- Speak at eye level to ensure that the patient can see you as you communicate.
- Locate a hearing aid, eyeglasses, and dentures (if needed).
- Turn on lights.
- Speak slowly, distinctly, and respectfully.
- Use the patient's surname, unless the patient requests otherwise.
- Listen closely.
- Be patient.
- Preserve dignity.
- Use gentleness.

CRITICAL THINKING
Why should you ask geriatric patients to bring all of their medications to the hospital?

Physical Examination

When conducting the physical examination of a geriatric patient, the paramedic should consider the following:

1. The patient may tire easily.
2. Geriatric patients often wear many layers of clothing for warmth. This may hamper the examination.
3. Respect the patient's modesty and need for privacy unless it interferes with the care.
4. Explain actions clearly before examining all geriatric patients. Keeping the patient informed of what is happening is important with patients with diminished sight.
5. Be aware that the patient may minimize or deny his or her symptoms. Denial may be caused by a fear of being bedridden or institutionalized or losing self-sufficiency.
6. Try to distinguish symptoms of chronic disease from acute problems.

If time allows, the paramedic should assess the geriatric patient's immediate surroundings for evidence of alcohol or medication use (eg, insulin syringes, "vial of life," or MedicAlert information), presence of food, general condition of housing, and signs of adequate personal hygiene. These and other observations help provide information to the physician about the patient's general health and ability for self-care after release from the hospital.

The paramedic should question friends or family members who are present about the patient's appearance and responsiveness now versus the patient's normal appearance, responsiveness, and other characteristics. The paramedic also should discreetly ask about advance directives and initiation of care for the patient (described in Chapter 6, *Medical and Legal Issues*). If these documents are available, the paramedic should obtain them and convey the information to medical direction. Finally, the paramedic should ensure gentle handling and padding for patient comfort if transport is needed.

System Pathophysiology, Assessment, and Management

This section describes the pathophysiology, assessment, and management of specific illnesses in relation to cognitive function, the pulmonary system, the cardiovascular system, the CNS, the endocrine system, the GI system, the integumentary system, the musculoskeletal system, and sensory function. Toxicology, environmental considerations, behavioral and psychiatric disorders, trauma, and elder abuse also are discussed in this section.

Cognitive Function

Impaired cognition is found in as many as 10% of older adults.[18] It is important to establish the patient's cognition early in the examination. The six-item screener is a reliable tool to identify cognitive impairment and is relatively easy to perform in the prehospital setting (BOX 48-2).

BOX 48-2 Six-Item Screener for Cognitive Impairment

Say to the patient: "I would like to ask you some questions that ask you to use your memory. I am going to name three objects. Please wait until I say all three words, then repeat them. Remember what they are because I am going to ask you to name them again in a few minutes. Please repeat these words for me: apple, table, penny." (The paramedic can repeat the words up to three times). If the patient cannot repeat the words correctly, the test cannot continue.

Questions	One Point for Each Correct Answer
1. What year is this?	______
2. What month is this?	______
3. What is the day of the week?	______
What were the three objects I asked you to remember?	
• Apple	
• Table	
• Penny	
Total score:	______

The patient receives one point for each correct answer. Three or more errors indicates possible dementia.

Modified from: Callahan CM, Unverzagt FW, Hui SL, Perkins AJ, Hendrie HC. Six-item screener to identify cognitive impairment among potential subjects for clinical research. *Med Care.* 2002;40(9):771-781.

Pulmonary System

Specific illnesses of the pulmonary system that are common in older patients include bacterial pneumonia and chronic obstructive pulmonary disease (COPD). These conditions are described in Chapter 23, *Respiratory.* They are presented here as a review.

Bacterial Pneumonia

About 85% of all pneumonia and influenza deaths occur in patients aged 65 years and older.[19] This age group has a risk of death from pneumonia that is 5 to 10 times greater than that in younger adults.[9] They also are more susceptible to several respiratory pathogens (eg, gram-negative bacilli). This susceptibility, associated with the presence of chronic disease, impairs respiratory tract clearance. It also allows germs to grow in the throat that then may travel to or be aspirated into the lungs. Because of the decreased lung function, pneumonia often may be associated with respiratory failure needing ventilator support, sepsis, and longer duration of treatment. Risk factors for bacterial pneumonia include institutional environments, feeding tubes, chronic diseases, and compromise of the immune system.

Unlike in younger patients with bacterial pneumonia, the usual clinical picture of fever, productive cough, dyspnea, pleurisy, chest pain, sweating, and signs of pulmonary congestion may be absent or diminished in the geriatric patient. Confusion or delirium may be the only early indicator of pneumonia.[9] This atypical presentation is responsible for the common delay in diagnosis.

Geriatric patients with pneumonia may be too weak to cough or produce sputum. They also may not be able to breathe deeply. Therefore, breath sounds may be misleading because of preexisting emphysema or chronic heart failure. Tachycardia and tachypnea often are the most reliable indicators of bacterial pneumonia in the prehospital setting.

Emergency care for geriatric patients with bacterial pneumonia focuses on managing life threats, maintaining oxygenation, and providing transport for physician evaluation. Pneumonia generally is managed with antibiotics.

CRITICAL THINKING

Why is flu season linked to an increase in pneumonia in older adults?

Chronic Obstructive Pulmonary Disease

COPD in the geriatric patient is a major health problem in the United States. COPD is a common finding in the geriatric patient with a history of smoking. It usually is associated with various diseases that result in reduced expiratory airflow. (Examples of such diseases are asthma, emphysema, and chronic bronchitis.) An exacerbation of COPD often follows an acute respiratory tract infection that causes airway edema, bronchial smooth muscle irritability, and increased mucus secretion. These airway abnormalities may lead to factors associated with acute decompensation, including the following:

- Limited airflow
- Increased work of breathing
- Dyspnea
- Ventilation/perfusion mismatching
- Hypoxemia
- Respiratory acidosis
- Hemodynamic compromise

Older adults with COPD often struggle with activities of daily living. They may become socially isolated. Smoking cessation, energy conservation techniques, prescribed exercise, and pneumonia vaccines can decrease their risk of illness and improve their quality of life. Treatment of the COPD patient with an acute emergency is described in Chapter 23, *Respiratory.*

Cardiovascular System

Cardiovascular disorders were described in Chapter 21, *Cardiology.* Specific disorders reviewed in this section include myocardial infarction (MI), heart failure, dysrhythmias, abdominal and thoracic aneurysm, and hypertension.

Myocardial Infarction

Chest pain as a symptom of MI becomes less frequent by age 70 years. Only 45% of patients older than 85 years with MI have this complaint. Lack of typical chest pain can cause MI to be unrecognized in the geriatric patient.[20] The following are major risk factors that the paramedic should evaluate when assessing a patient for MI:

1. Previous MI
2. Angina
3. Diabetes mellitus
4. Hypertension
5. High cholesterol level
6. Smoking

Some geriatric patients have chest pain or discomfort. However, many complain only of vague symptoms. Examples of such symptoms include dyspnea (the most common sign in patients aged 85 years and older), abdominal pain or indigestion, epigastric distress, unexplained jaw pain, and fatigue. Women may not have classic chest pain; instead they may report nonspecific symptoms such as sharp pain, fatigue, or weakness.[9]

In patients aged 85 years and older, atypical presentation for MI should be anticipated.[21] For many

CRITICAL THINKING

What other conditions have similar cardiovascular signs and symptoms?

geriatric patients, the event is totally "silent." This lack of perceived symptoms may be a result of decreased visceral sensory function or a higher incidence of mental deterioration in this age group. Silent MIs are almost always marked by an atypical complaint,which may include fatigue, breathlessness, nausea, or abdominal pain. Thus, the paramedic must maintain a high index of suspicion for MI in older patients with unusual warning signs or symptoms. A 12-lead electrocardiogram (ECG) is indicated if the patient has these issues. The patient should be transported for physician evaluation.

CRITICAL THINKING

What hormonal change in older women increases their risk for heart disease?

Heart Failure

Heart failure is the leading cause of hospitalizations for people aged 65 years and older.[22] The condition is common in the older adult population and contributes to about 5% of all emergency hospital admissions.[23] Heart failure occurs when one or both ventricles cannot pump effectively. The risk of heart failure doubles in older adults whose blood pressure is greater than 160/90 mm Hg.[24] Other major risk factors are diabetes mellitus and MI. Optimal care of heart failure involves taking multiple medications daily. The older adult may fail to follow this treatment regimen because of memory impairment, poor vision, or inability to pay for the medicines. Increasing shortness of breath often indicates the heart failure is not being controlled adequately. Follow the standard treatment described in Chapter 23, *Respiratory*, to manage older adult patients with heart failure.

NOTE

Dyspnea is a hallmark symptom of heart failure; however, many patients living with heart failure do not experience this symptom. Older patients with heart failure and those with lower levels of anxiety are less likely to report dyspnea. Paramedics must learn to evaluate symptoms other than dyspnea as signs of heart failure severity and potentially exacerbations.

Modified from: Jurgens CY, Masterson Creber RM, Lee CS. Abstract 17942: identifying heart failure patients less likely to report dyspnea. *Circulation*. 2016;134:A17942.

CRITICAL THINKING

How do continuous positive airway pressure, nitroglycerin, and morphine work to relieve the signs and symptoms of heart failure?

Dysrhythmias

A common cause of dysrhythmias in the geriatric patient is hypertensive heart disease.[25] However, any condition that decreases blood flow to the heart can cause rhythm irregularities. When assessing dysrhythmias in the geriatric patient, the paramedic should consider the following:

- Premature ventricular contractions are common in most adults older than 80 years.
- Atrial fibrillation is the most common dysrhythmia.
- Dysrhythmias may result from electrolyte imbalances.

In addition to the serious implications of some dysrhythmias, associated complications may include traumatic injury from falls that result from cerebral hypoperfusion, transient ischemic attack, and heart failure. Serious dysrhythmias should be managed as described in Chapter 21, *Cardiology*.

Abdominal and Thoracic Aneurysms

Atherosclerotic disease is a common cause of abdominal and thoracic aneurysm. Abdominal aortic aneurysm affects about 4% to 8% of older men.[26] Acute dissecting aortic aneurysm is more common than is abdominal aneurysm and is associated with a high mortality rate. Signs and symptoms vary according to the site of rupture or the extent of blood vessels affected by dissection (BOX 48-3).

The goals of prehospital care are gentle handling, blood pressure control, relief of pain, and immediate transport to a hospital. Airway, ventilatory, and circulatory support may be required (see Chapter 21, *Cardiology*).

Hypertension

Geriatric patients who have atherosclerosis also frequently have hypertension (**FIGURE 48-2**). Associated risk factors for hypertension include advanced age, diabetes mellitus, and obesity. Hypertension often is defined as a resting blood pressure consistently greater than 130/80 mm Hg.[27] Hypertensive crisis occurs when the blood pressure exceeds 180/120 mm Hg.

BOX 48-3 Signs and Symptoms of Abdominal and Thoracic Aneurysm

Absent or reduced pulses
Acute MI
Chest pain
Diminished distal pulses
Heart failure
Hypotension
Low back pain or flank pain
Pericardial tamponade
Pulsatile, tender mass
Stroke
Sudden onset of abdominal or back pain
Syncope
Unexplained hypotension

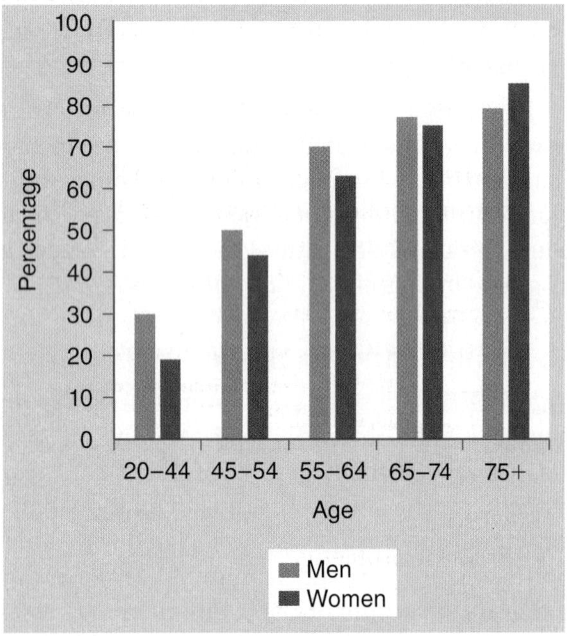

FIGURE 48-2 Percentage of different age groups of the US population with a diagnosis of high blood pressure.

Chronic hypertension is associated with many medical conditions, including the following:

- Aneurysm formation
- Blindness
- Cardiac hypertrophy and left ventricular failure
- Kidney failure
- Myocardial ischemia and infarction
- Peripheral vascular disease
- Stroke

NOTE

New blood pressure guidelines defining hypertension as a blood pressure of greater than 120/80 mm Hg were released in fall of 2017. The new guidelines suggest that almost half of the adult population (46%) are hypertensive. Concerns were expressed that drug treatment for the new targets could increase the risk of falls in older adults. This concern was balanced with studies that indicated that mobile patients not in a nursing home achieved great benefits from the lower blood pressure. The incidence in heart attack, heart failure, stroke, or death from cardiovascular disease decreases by nearly one-third in those who observe the new blood pressure guidelines.

Modified from: Whelton PK, Carey RM, Aronow WS, et al. 2017 ACC/AHA/AAPA/ABC/ACPM/AGS/APhA/ASH/ASPC/NMA/PCNA guideline for the prevention, detection, evaluation, and management of high blood pressure in adults. Executive summary: a report of the American College of Cardiology/American Heart Association Task Force on Clinical Practice Guidelines. *Hypertension*. 2017 Nov 13.

Paramedics who discover nonemergent hypertension in an older adult should explain the risks and advise the person to seek care. After physician evaluation, the patient with chronic hypertension often is managed with oral medications, dietary sodium reduction, weight loss, and exercise.

Nervous System

Neurologic disorders are described in Chapter 24, *Neurology*. Many of these illnesses cause cognitive impairment in the older adult, which often significantly affects their quality of life and ability to remain independent. It is estimated that about 13% of older adults transported by EMS have some degree of cognitive impairment.[28] Specific disorders described in this section for review include cerebral vascular disease, delirium, dementia, Alzheimer disease, and Parkinson disease. Possible assessment findings in patients with neurologic disorders are provided in BOX 48-4.

Cerebral Vascular Disease

Stroke is a leading cause of death in the United States.[29] As described in Chapter 24, *Neurology*, the neurologic impairment is caused by an ischemic or hemorrhagic interruption in the blood supply to the

BOX 48-4 Possible Assessment Findings in Patients With Neurologic Disorders

Changes in peripheral, core, and neurovascular perfusion
Changes in response of pupils
Changes in response to motor tests
Dysrhythmias
Adventitious breath sounds

BOX 48-5 Possible Complications of Stroke

Hemiplegia
Hemiparesis
Visual and perceptual deficits
Language or speech deficits
Emotional changes
Swallowing dysfunction
Bowel and bladder dysfunction
Dysphagia

Modified from: Mauk K. *Gerontological Nursing.* 4th ed. Burlington, MA: Jones & Bartlett Learning; 2018.

brain. Associated risk factors for cerebral vascular disease in the older adult include hypertension, diabetes mellitus, atherosclerosis, hyperlipidemia, polycythemia, and heart disease. Over three-fourths of people with a stroke had a blood pressure of greater than 140/90 mm Hg, and heavy smoking doubles the risk.[9] Almost 4 out of 10 people who have had a stroke have another one within 10 years.[30] Signs and symptoms and treatment of stroke are discussed in Chapter 24, *Neurology.* Aftereffects of stroke vary widely. Deficits that remain after a stroke can greatly impact a patient's life and may be permanent, leading to social isolation and depression. BOX 48-5 describes possible complications of stroke.

CRITICAL THINKING
Why might a person who has already had one stroke delay calling 9-1-1 if he or she is having another one?

Delirium

As described in Chapter 34, *Behavioral and Psychiatric Disorders,* **delirium** is an abrupt onset of confusion, inattention, disordered thinking, and altered mentation occurring because of a medical condition that has the potential to be reversed.[9] It usually includes illusions and hallucinations. In the hyperactive form of delirium, the patient's mind may "wander," speech may be incoherent, hallucinations and agitation may be present, and the patient may be in a state of mental confusion. Other patients are hypoactive and tend to present with an altered level of consciousness or coma. Older adults are at increased risk, as are people with preexisting dementia, sensory or functional impairment, medical problems, or alcohol abuse. Signs and symptoms vary according to personality, environment, and severity of the illness. Causes of delirium are associated with **organic brain dysfunction**: abnormal cognition that results from primarily physical functional disorders (as opposed to psychological disorders). As a reminder of the severity of conditions that can cause delirium, the I WATCH DEATH acronym can be used to consider differential diagnoses:[31]

Infection (encephalitis, meningitis, urinary tract infection, pneumonia)
Withdrawal (alcohol, barbiturate, sedative-hypnotic)
Acute metabolic condition (acidosis, alkalosis, electrolyte imbalance, liver or renal failure)
Trauma (head injury, heatstroke, severe burns)
CNS problem (abscess, hemorrhage, hydrocephalus, subdural hematoma, infection, seizures, stroke, tumors, cancer metastases, encephalitis, meningitis, syphilis)
Hypoxia (anemia, carbon monoxide poisoning, pulmonary or cardiac failure)
Deficiencies (vitamin B_{12}, folate, niacin, thiamine)
Endocrine problems (hyper- or hypoadrenocorticism, hyper- or hypoglycemia, myxedema, hyperparathyroidism)
Acute vascular (hypertensive encephalopathy, stroke, arrhythmia, shock)
Toxins/drugs (prescription or illicit drugs, pesticides, solvents)
Heavy metals (lead, manganese, mercury)

Delirium can be life threatening and requires emergency care. The condition may be reversible if it is diagnosed early. However, delirium can progress to chronic mental dysfunction. Prehospital care includes the following measures:

1. Ensure an adequate airway, breathing, and circulatory support, including assessment of blood glucose.

2. Identify and manage the underlying cause, when possible.
3. Reduce agitation and anxiety.
   - Manage pain if present.
   - Minimize visual and auditory stimuli.
4. Avoid patient injury and ensure personal safety.
   - Restrain the patient if needed, per protocol.
   - Sedate the patient in consultation with medical direction.
   - Recall that dose reduction is often needed for older adults.
5. Transport the patient for physician evaluation.

Dementia

Dementia is defined as the loss of intellectual functions (such as thinking, remembering, and reasoning) of sufficient severity to interfere with a person's daily functioning.[32] The condition is usually slow and progressive and causes impaired memory, concentration, language, reasoning, and ability to identify visual and spatial relationships among objects. It usually involves an inability to learn new things or recall recent events. Dementia may accompany certain diseases, as discussed in the following sections, and more than one type of dementia can occur simultaneously (mixed dementia). Dementia generally is considered irreversible. It is not a normal consequence of aging. It eventually results in full dependence on others as a result of the progressive loss of cognitive functioning. During the course of the disease, patients often try to "cover up" their memory loss by **confabulation** (fabricating stories to fill gaps in memory). Sudden outbursts or embarrassing conduct may be the first clear signs of dementia. Some patients eventually regress to a "second childhood." At that point, they need full-time care for feedings, toileting, and physical activity. Dementia is present in about 9% of people aged 65 years and older, and in about 38% of people older than 85 years.[33,34]

Dementia can be difficult to differentiate from delirium in the prehospital setting. The key difference between the two is that delirium is new with rapid onset, and dementia is progressive (**TABLE 48-2**). Thus, a history of the event from a reliable witness (eg, friend or family member) is the best source of information. A history provided by the patient may be unreliable. If a good witness is not available, the paramedic should manage the patient for delirium that may be a life-threatening emergency.

TABLE 48-2 Differential Diagnosis for Delirium and Dementia

	Delirium	Dementia
Onset	Abrupt	Gradual
Characteristics	Reduced attention span	Attention usually preserved
	Mentation and cognition fluctuate	Fairly constant mentation
	Potentially reversible	Irreversible

Modified from: Mauk K. *Gerontological Nursing.* 4th ed. Burlington, MA: Jones & Bartlett Learning; 2018.

> NOTE
>
> Dementia is not a disease in itself, but rather a group of symptoms that may accompany certain diseases or physical conditions. Some of the more well-known diseases that produce dementia include Alzheimer disease, Parkinson disease, diffuse Lewy body disease, frontotemporal disease, vascular (multi-infarct) dementia, and depression. Others include normal pressure hydrocephalus, Huntington disease, and Creutzfeldt-Jakob disease. Medical conditions that may cause or mimic dementia include depression, brain tumors, nutritional deficiencies, head injuries, hydrocephalus, infections (human immunodeficiency virus, meningitis, syphilis), drug reactions, and thyroid problems.
>
> *Modified from*: Dementia. Alzheimer's Community Care website. https://www.alzcare.org/dementia. Accessed April 11, 2018; Mauk K. *Gerontological Nursing.* 4th ed. Burlington, MA: Jones & Bartlett Learning; 2018.

Alzheimer Disease

Alzheimer disease is a condition in which nerve cells in the cerebral cortex die and the brain substance shrinks (see Chapter 24, *Neurology*). The disease is the single most common cause of dementia and is responsible for one-third of cases in people older than 85 years.[34] Alzheimer disease does not cause death directly: Patients ultimately stop eating and become malnourished and immobilized; they are then susceptible to intercurrent infections (infections that occur during another infection).

The exact cause of Alzheimer disease is not known. Risk factors include age, family history, history of head trauma, vascular disease, and some brain infections. Microscopic buildup of beta-amyloid plaques and neurofibrillary tangles are observed in the brain of patients with Alzheimer disease.[9] The primary disorder is in the nerve cells, not the blood vessels.

Early symptoms of Alzheimer disease mainly are related to memory loss, especially the ability to make and recall new memories (BOX 48-6). As the disease progresses, agitation, violence, and impairment of abstract thinking occur. Judgment and cognitive abilities begin to interfere with work and social relations. In the advanced stages of Alzheimer disease, patients often become bedridden and totally unaware of their surroundings. Once the patient is bedridden, pressure ulcers (bed sores), feeding problems, and pneumonia shorten the patient's life.

No specific treatment exists for Alzheimer disease. Some medications such as cholinesterase inhibitors (eg, donepezil [Aricept], galantamine [Razadyne], rivastigmine [Exelon]), or N-methyl-D-aspartate receptor antagonists (memantine [Namenda], memantine/donepezil [Namzaric]) may help delay progression of the disease and lessen associated symptoms. Treatment primarily consists of nursing and social care for the patient and relatives.

BOX 48-6 Ten Early Warning Signs of Alzheimer Disease

1. Memory loss that interferes with daily activities (eg, forgets recently learned information)
2. Difficulty with planning or solving problems (eg, has trouble following directions or paying bills)
3. Difficulty completing daily tasks at home, at work, or at leisure (eg, trouble finding a familiar place)
4. Confusion with time or place (eg, forgets where he or she is or how he or she got there)
5. Trouble understanding visual images and spatial relationships (eg, difficulty reading or determining color)
6. Difficulty speaking or writing (eg, has difficulty participating in a conversation, calls things by the wrong name)
7. Losing things and inability to retrace steps (eg, placing objects in unusual places, accuses others of stealing)
8. Decreased or poor judgment (eg, less attention to hygiene; easily tricked with money)
9. Withdrawal from work or social activities (eg, removes self from hobbies, sports)
10. Changes in mood or personality (eg, may be confused, paranoid, fearful, anxious)

Modified from: Ten early signs and symptoms of Alzheimer's. Alzheimer's Association website. https://www.alz.org/10-signs-symptoms-alzheimers-dementia.asp. Accessed April 11, 2018.

Vascular Dementia

Vascular dementia is a reduction in cognitive function caused by conditions that block or reduce circulation in the brain. It can be caused suddenly after a stroke in a major blood vessel. Alternately, vascular dementia may be a progressive decline in cognition related to multiple minor strokes. The changes vary from minor to severe depending on the amount of brain tissue impaired from low flow. Memory loss may or may not be a significant symptom. Common early signs of widespread small vessel disease include impaired planning and judgment, uncontrolled laughing and crying, declining ability to pay attention, impaired function in social situations, and difficulty finding the right words. Vascular dementia is widely considered the second-most common cause of dementia after Alzheimer disease, accounting for 10% of cases.[35]

Parkinson Disease Dementia

The average time of onset of Parkinson disease to developing dementia (**Parkinson disease dementia**) is about 10 years.[36] As described in Chapter 24, *Neurology*, **Parkinson disease** is a brain disorder caused by degeneration of or damage to nerve cells in the basal ganglia. The disease causes muscle tremor, stiffness, and weakness. Characteristic signs of Parkinson disease are resting tremors and shaking (usually beginning in one hand, arm, or leg), a rigid posture and muscle stiffness, slow movements, and a shuffling, unbalanced walk. These effects increase the patient's risk for falls. Other signs and symptoms include:

- Difficulty swallowing and chewing
- Impaired speech
- Impaired cognitive function
- Urinary problems
- Excessive sweating
- Depression
- Sleep difficulties
- Masklike facial expression

> **NOTE**
> Some patients with Parkinson disease "freeze" when trying to walk or stand up from a sitting position or walking through a doorway, especially if it is narrow. When assisting a patient to ambulate, the paramedic can have the patient rock from side to side to begin motion or count to begin motor movement.

Approximately 60,000 Americans are diagnosed with Parkinson disease each year.[37] Parkinson disease affects more than 1% of the population older than 60 years and 5% of the population older than 85 years.[38] If left untreated, the disease progresses over 10 to 15 years to severe weakness and incapacity. Patients with Parkinson disease dementia struggle with memory, attention, judgment, and planning steps to complete tasks.

Lewy Body Disease Dementia

Dementia associated with **Lewy body disease** (or Lewy body dementia) occurs in patients who have abnormal deposits of a protein called alpha-synuclein in their brains. Often these patients are initially misdiagnosed with Parkinson disease; however, they do not respond to dopaminergic medicines used to treat Parkinson disease.

Signs and symptoms of Lewy body dementia that distinguish it from Alzheimer disease are motor symptoms and hallucinations early in the disease and a fluctuating mental status.

Frontotemporal Lobe Dementia

Dementia can result from disease of the frontotemporal lobe, referred to as frontotemporal lobe dementia (FTLD). FTLD (formerly called Pick disease) refers to a group of disorders caused by progressive nerve cell loss in the brain's frontal lobes. The patient who has FTLD often has a fairly intact memory but struggles to plan or make decisions. The disease often begins around age 50 or 60 years but may not occur until the patient is in his or her 80s. There are three primary types of FTLD. In the first type, the person's personality changes and his or her conduct, judgment, empathy, and foresight deteriorate. Language skills, speaking, writing, and comprehension decline in the second type of FTLD. Motor decline characterizes the third type of FTLD. These patients may experience weakness, trouble walking, falls, and incoordination.[9,39]

Endocrine System

Two common endocrine disorders are often seen in geriatric patients. These disorders are type 2 diabetes mellitus and thyroid disease (described in Chapter 25, *Endocrinology*). The following is a review of these conditions.

Diabetes Mellitus

About 25% of adults older than 60 years have diabetes mellitus.[40] Roughly 90% of older patients with diabetes have type 2 diabetes, especially when the person is overweight.[9] This statistic is true even though people diagnosed with type 1 diabetes mellitus now have longer life spans.

Diagnosis of diabetes in older adults often occurs when hyperglycemia is found during blood work for routine care or evaluation for other illnesses. Geriatric patients do not always have classic signs of hyperglycemia, such as increased thirst, increased urination, or weight loss. The initial presentation may be related to evaluation for a fall, confusion, fatigue, or urinary incontinence.[9]

A combination of dietary measures, weight reduction, oral hypoglycemic agents, and, in some cases, insulin can often keep type 2 diabetes under control. However, if not controlled, diabetes can lead to complications. These complications may include **retinopathy** (disorder of the retina caused by vascular disease), peripheral neuropathy (ulcers on the feet are common), autonomic neuropathy causing GI symptoms, genitourinary symptoms, cardiovascular symptoms, sexual dysfunction, and kidney damage. Early warning signs of hypoglycemia, such as tremors, sweating, and tachycardia, may not be as reliable in older adults because of the age-related changes in the sympathetic nervous system. Emergency care for diabetic patients is outlined in Chapter 25, *Endocrinology*.

> **NOTE**
> Hyperglycemia is defined as a blood glucose level greater than 200 mg/dL or a fasting level greater than 126 mg/dL.
>
> *Modified from*: Diagnosing diabetes and learning about prediabetes. American Diabetes Association website. http://www.diabetes.org/diabetes-basics/diagnosis/. Updated November 21, 2016. Accessed April 11, 2018.

Hyperglycemic hyperosmolar nonketotic syndrome (HHNS), or hyperglycemic hyperosmolar state (HHS), described in Chapter 25, *Endocrinology*, is a serious complication that primarily occurs in older adults with type 2 diabetes. It presents with many of the same signs and symptoms as diabetic ketoacidosis. The patient with HHNS typically has a higher blood glucose level and does not have an acetone odor on the breath. If HHNS is suspected, the paramedic should ensure adequate airway, ventilatory, and circulatory support; search vigorously for an underlying cause; initiate intravenous (IV) therapy to manage dehydration; and rapidly transport the patient for physician evaluation.

NOTE

HHNS coma is a complication of type 2 diabetes in older adults. Unlike in diabetic ketoacidosis, the elevated blood glucose level in HHNS coma does not result in ketosis. Instead, it leads to osmotic diuresis and a fluid shift to the intravascular space that result in dehydration.

CRITICAL THINKING

What finding is present in the patient with diabetic ketoacidosis but is absent in the patient with HHNS coma?

Hypothyroidism

Hypothyroidism is common in geriatric patients and may be related to the aging process.[41] The classic signs and symptoms of thyroid disorders (eg, fullness in the neck, goiter, muscle or joint pain) often are not present in the geriatric patient. Thus, the paramedic should suspect thyroid dysfunction in any geriatric patient who complains of fatigue and weakness.

NOTE

Hyperthyroidism is less common in older adults, affecting only 0.5% to 4% of this population. Graves disease is the most common cause. Hyperthyroidism is discussed in Chapter 25, *Endocrinology*.

Modified from: Papaleontiou M, Haymart MR. Approach to and treatment of thyroid disorders in the elderly. *Med Clin North Am*. 2012;96(2):297-310.

As described in Chapter 25, *Endocrinology*, hypothyroidism results from the destruction of thyroid tissue over time. The disease leads to an insufficient amount of thyroid hormone in the blood. The older patient often attributes the signs and symptoms of hypothyroidism to "growing old." Common complaints include nonspecific musculoskeletal complaints and confusion. More serious conditions associated with this disorder include heart failure, anemia, hyponatremia, depression, dementia, seizures, and coma. Other signs and symptoms associated with hypothyroidism include the following:

- Cold intolerance
- Fatigue
- Weight gain
- Poor cognitive function
- Scaly dry skin and hair loss
- Peripheral and facial edema
- Depression
- Trouble breathing or swallowing

Emergency care mainly is supportive to ensure vital functions. The physician evaluates the patient with thyroid disease and treats the patient with various thyroid drugs, radioactive iodine treatments, and sometimes surgery. Myxedema coma is a severe complication from hypothyroidism (described in Chapter 25, *Endocrinology*).

GI System

GI emergencies (described in Chapter 28, *Abdominal and Gastrointestinal Disorders*) are common in older adults. The paramedic should always consider abdominal pain a serious complaint in a geriatric patient. Common GI complaints in older adults relate to gastroesophageal reflux disease, peptic ulcer disease, diverticulitis, and cancers. Life-threatening causes of abdominal pain in this age group include abdominal aortic aneurysm, appendicitis, GI hemorrhage, ruptured viscus, dead or ischemic bowel, and acute bowel obstruction. Specific disorders discussed in this section are GI hemorrhage, bowel obstruction, problems with continence, and problems with elimination. Possible assessment findings in patients with GI disorders are provided in **BOX 48-7**.

DID YOU KNOW?

The symptoms of appendicitis in older adults are often atypical, causing a delay in diagnosis and treatment. Classic symptoms of fever, anorexia, an elevated white blood cell count, and right lower quadrant pain or tenderness may not be present. Therefore, appendicitis may be more difficult to diagnose in older patients, resulting in high morbidity and mortality.

Modified from: Tazkarji MB. Abdominal pain among older adults. *Geriatr Aging*. 2008;11(7):410-415.

BOX 48-7 Possible Assessment Findings in Patients With GI Disorders

Heartburn or indigestion
Pain when swallowing
Fullness or belching
Nausea or vomiting
Vomiting of blood
Bloody stool
Diffuse abdominal tenderness, distention, guarding, or masses
Orthostatic blood pressure changes
Hypovolemia
Jaundice
Fever
Tachycardia
Dyspnea

GI Hemorrhage

GI bleeding most commonly affects patients older than 60 years.[42] Possible causes of GI bleeding include peptic ulcer disease, esophageal varices, stomach and esophageal cancer, diverticulitis, bowel obstruction, and cirrhosis of the liver. The older the patient, the higher the risk of death. GI bleeding in patients older than 85 years is associated with a mortality rate of about 20%. This high risk is because of the following:[43]

- Geriatric patients are less able to compensate for acute blood loss.
- They are less likely to feel symptoms and therefore seek treatment at later stages of disease.
- They are more likely to be taking aspirin or nonsteroidal anti-inflammatory drugs (NSAIDs), which places them at higher risk for ulcer disease and bleeding.
- They are at higher risk for colon cancer, intestinal vascular abnormalities, and diverticulitis.
- They are more likely to be taking anticoagulants such as warfarin (Coumadin).

Signs and symptoms of GI bleeding include vomiting of blood or coffee-ground emesis; blood-tinged or black, tarry stools; agitation; weakness; syncope; pain; jaundice; and constipation or diarrhea. If the paramedic suspects or confirms bleeding in a patient with signs and symptoms of shock, ensure the patient has an adequate airway, ventilatory, and circulatory support. The paramedic also should transport the patient rapidly for definitive care.

Bowel Obstruction

Bowel obstruction generally occurs in patients with prior abdominal surgeries or hernias. Obstruction occurs in those with colon cancer as well. Most patients complain of constipation, abdominal cramping, and an inability to pass gas. Other signs and symptoms include protracted vomiting of food or bile and vomiting of fecal material. The patient's heart rate and blood pressure measurements often are in normal ranges. The abdomen also may be mildly distended and tender in all four quadrants. (Abdominal pain is variable.)

Prehospital care mainly is supportive to ensure vital functions. After physician evaluation, patient care may include bowel rest, nasogastric suction, and volume replacement. Some patients may need surgery to lyse the offending adhesions. Surgery may result in a cycle of new scarring and obstruction. Patients also may need surgery for hernia repair (most often in men).

NOTE

Biliary disease refers to disorders of the liver and gallbladder. It describes a wide spectrum of disorders caused by abnormalities in bile composition, biliary anatomy, or function. The disease can result from primary liver disease, heart failure, gallstones, cholecystitis, and medications that adversely affect the liver. Like other GI disorders, biliary disease may be accompanied by jaundice, fever, and vomiting. There often is right upper quadrant abdominal pain that radiates to the upper back and shoulder.

Problems With Continence

Continence is the ability to control bladder or bowel function. It requires anatomically correct GI and genitourinary tracts, competent sphincter mechanisms, cognitive and physical function, and motivation. Some factors associated with continence are affected by age. These factors include a decrease in bladder capacity, involuntary bladder contractions, decreased ability to postpone voiding, and medications that can affect bladder and bowel control. **Incontinence** of urine or bowel is abnormal. Both cause complications and negatively impact the patient's quality of life.

Urinary incontinence can vary in severity. It can be mild incontinence (the escape of small amounts of urine). Or it can be total incontinence, with complete loss of bladder control. Causes of urinary incontinence include injury or disease of the urinary tract, prolapse of the uterus, a decline in sphincter muscle control

BOX 48-8 Possible Causes of Urinary Tract Infection

Cystocele (fallen bladder in women)
Diabetes mellitus
Indwelling urinary catheters
Kidney obstruction
Medications (immunosuppressive drugs and chemotherapy)
Prostatitis (inflammation of the prostate gland)
Urethrocele (urethra prolapse in women)

surrounding the urethra (common in older adults), CNS injury or disease, pelvic fracture, prostate cancer, and dementia.

Bowel incontinence in the geriatric patient is often the result of **fecal impaction**. With fecal impaction, feces lodged in the rectum irritate and inflame the lining. This allows fecal fluid and small feces to pass involuntarily. Other causes of bowel incontinence include severe diarrhea, injury to anal muscles (from childbirth or surgery), CNS injury or disease, and dementia.

Incontinence is embarrassing for the patient. If incontinence is chronic, it can lead to skin irritation, tissue breakdown, and urinary tract infection (**BOX 48-8**). Some cases are managed with surgery to restore sphincter function. Patients with mild cases often wear absorptive undergarments to relieve discomfort and embarrassment.

CRITICAL THINKING

Consider the incontinent patient. How can you minimize the patient's embarrassment and discomfort?

Problems With Elimination

Causes of difficulty in urination usually result from enlargement of the prostate (in men), urinary tract infection, urethral strictures, and acute or chronic renal failure. Difficulty in bowel elimination often is associated with medications, diverticular disease, constipation, and colorectal cancer. Problems with elimination can cause acute pain and anxiety for geriatric patients. The paramedic should take their complaints seriously. These conditions call for physician evaluation to identify the cause and to select the appropriate therapy.

NOTE

Chronic kidney disease (the inability of the kidneys to excrete waste, concentrate urine, or control electrolyte balance in the body) is described in Chapter 29, *Genitourinary and Renal Disorders*. Chronic kidney disease may be the result of diabetes mellitus, congenital disorders, pyelonephritis, hypertension, autoimmune disorders, glomerulonephritis, or medications that have an adverse effect on the kidneys (eg, antibiotics, NSAIDs, anticancer drugs).

Integumentary System

As people age, the skin gradually becomes dry, transparent, and wrinkled. These integumentary changes are associated with a loss of elasticity, uneven pigmentation, and various benign and malignant lesions. In addition, aging results in a gradual decrease in epidermal cellular turnover and a reduced rate of nail and hair growth. The associated loss of deep, dermal vessels and capillary circulation leads to common complaints such as dry, itchy skin, changes in thermal regulation, and skin-related complications. Some of these complications include the following:

- Slow healing
- Increased risk of secondary infection
- Increased risk of fungal or viral infections
- Increased susceptibility to abrasions and tears

The paramedic should always be gentle with the skin of a geriatric patient. Examples include use of aseptic technique during wound management, gentle placement and removal of ECG electrodes, and selection of the appropriate device for securing IV catheters or tubing.

CRITICAL THINKING

Consider a geriatric patient who has a burn injury. How do these changes influence the patient's recovery?

Pressure Ulcers

Pressure ulcers are common in geriatric patients (**FIGURE 48-3**). They often develop on the skin of patients who are bedridden or immobile. Most pressure ulcers occur in the lower legs, back, and buttocks, and over bony areas such as the greater trochanter or the sacrum. They often affect victims of brain or spinal cord injury, stroke, or other illnesses that result in a loss or change in the sensation of pain. Skin exposure to moisture (eg, from incontinence), poor nutrition, and friction or shear also may be factors for the development of pressure ulcers. Other causes of pressure ulcers in geriatric patients include vascular and metabolic disorders (eg, venous stasis and diabetes), trauma, and cancer.

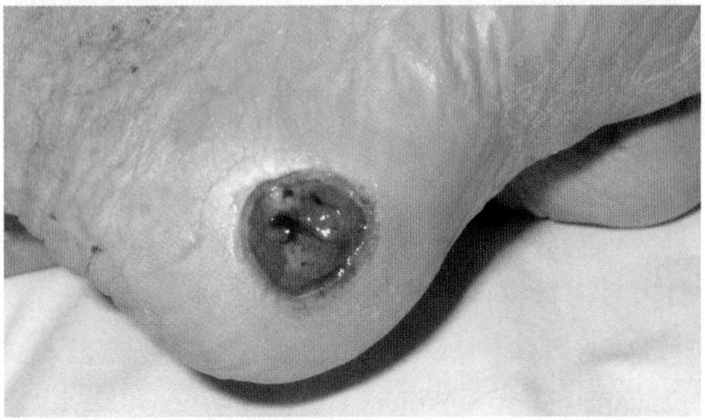

FIGURE 48-3 Pressure ulcers.

Pressure ulcers result from tissue hypoxia related to pressure. They can develop from 1 to 24 hours after the original injury. The severity of injury depends on how much pressure was applied, the duration of the pressure, and the ability of the skin to resist injury.[9] The ulcers generally start as red, nonblanching painful areas leading to blisters or ulcers followed by exposure of adipose tissue and finally full-thickness skin injury. In some cases, bones, muscle, or tendons are visible.[44] Once the integrity of the skin has been breached, the sores often become infected and then are slow to heal (**FIGURE 48-4**). Pressure ulcers should be covered with a sterile dressing using aseptic technique. The paramedic should transport the patient for physician

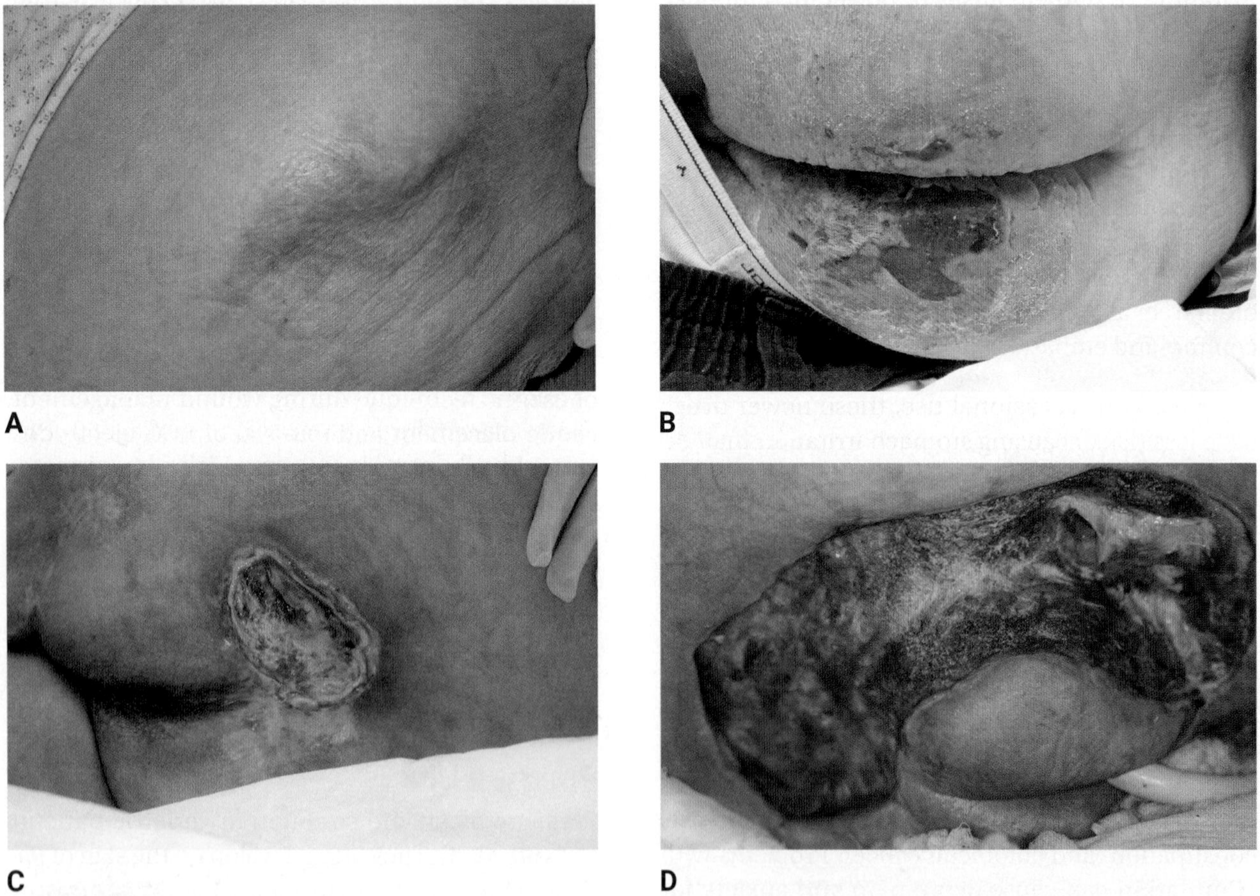

FIGURE 48-4 A pressure ulcer develops when pressure compromises the blood supply, and thus oxygenation, to an area of tissue. **A.** Stage 1. At this stage, the sore is not an open wound; the skin appears reddened or discolored. **B.** Stage 2. In this stage, the skin breaks open and looks like a scrape. At this stage, skin may be permanently damaged. **C.** Stage 3. At this stage, the sore has deepened to the beneath the skin. **D.** Stage 4. At this stage, the sore has extended into muscle, tendon, or bone.

evaluation and wound care to facilitate healing. The patient is also assessed for pain; analgesics are administered if indicated.

Musculoskeletal System

As described in Chapter 11, *General Principles of Pathophysiology*, and earlier in this chapter, musculoskeletal changes occur as part of the aging process. Two musculoskeletal conditions that are common in older adults are osteoarthritis and osteoporosis. (These and other forms of arthritis are described in Chapter 32, *Nontraumatic Musculoskeletal Disorders*.)

Osteoarthritis

Osteoarthritis is a common form of arthritis in geriatric patients. It is a degenerative condition that results from cartilage loss and wear and tear on the joints (**FIGURE 48-5**). This condition leads to pain, stiffness, and sometimes loss of function of the affected joint. Often, the affected joint becomes large and distorted from outgrowths of new bone (osteophytes) that tend to develop at the margins of the joint surface. Osteoarthritis evolves in the middle years. It occurs to some extent in almost all people older than 65 years. However, some people have no symptoms. After physician evaluation, treatment may include medications (analgesics, NSAIDs, corticosteroids), physical therapy, and sometimes joint replacement surgery. Newer drugs (cyclooxygenase-2 inhibitors) relieve the inflammation and pain associated with arthritis. With occasional use, these newer drugs have less risk of causing stomach irritation than do traditional medications such as aspirin, NSAIDs (eg, ibuprofen), or celecoxib (Celebrex). However, regular or long-term use of any of these medications in older patients may result in serious GI complications.[45]

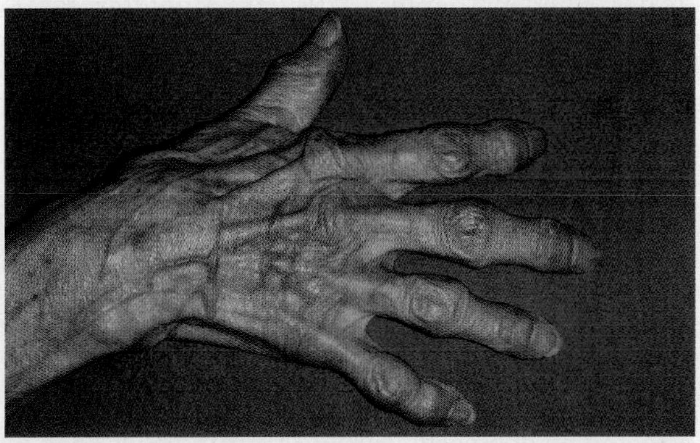

FIGURE 48-5 Osteoarthritis.

Osteoporosis

Osteoporosis is a disease that decreases bone density. It is especially common in older women after menopause. This is because of a decrease in the hormone estrogen, which helps maintain bone mass. Osteoporosis is present in most people by age 70 years, by which time the density of the skeleton has diminished by one-third. Most people with osteoporosis have some degree of kyphosis. Risk factors that may affect the progression of the disease include genetics, smoking, exercise habits, thin frame, anorexia nervosa, medications (steroids, some anticonvulsants), and calcium or vitamin D deficiency.

The loss of bone density causes bones to become brittle. Brittle bones can fracture easily, which often is the first sign of osteoporosis. Typical sites for fractures are just above the wrist, at the head of the femur, and at one of several vertebrae (often a spontaneous fracture). Osteoporosis is treated with preventive measures, including a diet high in calcium, calcium supplements, weight-bearing exercise, bisphosphonates, and hormone replacement therapy after menopause (controversial because of potential links to breast cancer, heart disease, and stroke).[46]

Sensory Impairments

As people age, they may experience problems with vision, hearing, and speech.

Problems With Vision

Vision changes begin to occur at around age 40 years and gradually increase over time. Vision impairments can severely limit daily activities. They can lead to a loss of independence in geriatric patients. The following are some effects of aging on vision:

- Reading or driving difficulties
- Poor depth perception
- Poor adjustment of the eyes to variations in distance
- Altered color perception
- Sensitivity to light
- Decreased visual acuity

Two common eye conditions that develop with age are cataracts and glaucoma. A **cataract** is a loss of transparency of the lens of the eye. It results from changes in the delicate protein fibers within the lens (**FIGURE 48-6**). A cataract never causes full blindness; however, clarity and detail of an image progressively are lost. Cataracts usually occur in both eyes. In most

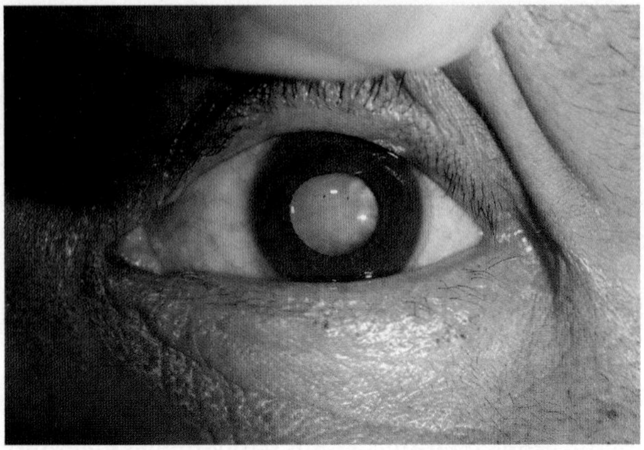

FIGURE 48-6 Appearance of an eye with a cataract.

cases, though, one eye is affected more severely than the other is. About one-half of adults older than 65 years have some degree of cataract.[9] They are most prevalent in people older than 75 years. Surgery to remove the cataract is a common procedure in the United States.

Glaucoma is a condition in which intraocular pressure increases. This pressure causes damage to the optic nerve. The result is nerve fiber destruction and partial or full loss of peripheral and central vision. Glaucoma may result from aging (rarely seen before age 40 years), a congenital abnormality, or trauma to the eye. Glaucoma is the most common major eye disorder in people older than 60 years and is the leading cause of visual impairment and the second-leading cause of blindness in the United States.[9] Symptoms of acute glaucoma include dull, severe, aching pain in and above one eye; reddened eye; fogginess of vision; nausea and vomiting; and the perception of "rainbow rings" (halos) around lights at night. Testing for glaucoma is part of most eye examinations in adults. If detected early, the condition can be treated with oral medications and eyedrops to relieve pressure.

CRITICAL THINKING

Consider the patient who has glaucoma. What prehospital cardiac medication should not be given to this patient?

Problems With Hearing

Not all geriatric patients have hearing loss. However, overall hearing tends to decrease with age. This results from degeneration of the hearing mechanism (sensorineural deafness). Ménière disease (increased fluid pressure in the labyrinth), certain drugs (eg, NSAIDs, antibiotics, diuretics), tumors, and some viral infections also can cause hearing problems. Hearing loss can interfere with the ability to perceive speech. Thus, it can limit the ability to communicate. Hearing aid devices and surgical implants sometimes can restore or improve hearing.

Tinnitus is the perception of noise in the ear (eg, ringing, buzzing, whistling). It can occur as a symptom of many ear disorders. The noise in the ear sometimes may change in nature and intensity. However, in most cases it is present at all times with intermittent awareness by the person. Tinnitus is almost always associated with hearing loss, especially hearing loss that develops from aging.

CRITICAL THINKING

What common analgesic, when taken in excess, can cause tinnitus?

Problems With Speech

Speech is the most often used method of communication. Common problems with speech in geriatric patients often are associated with difficulty in word retrieval, decreased fluency of speech, slowed rate of speech, and changes in voice quality. These disorders may occur from damage to the language centers of the brain (usually as a result of stroke, Parkinson disease, head injury, or brain tumor), degenerative changes in the nervous system, hearing loss, disorders of the larynx, and poor-fitting dentures.

Toxicology

As described in Chapter 13, *Principles of Pharmacology and Emergency Medications*, geriatric patients are at increased risk for adverse drug reactions. This vulnerability is the result of age-related changes in body composition as well as drug absorption, distribution, metabolism, and excretion.

Age-related changes that affect absorption include increased gastric pH and decreased GI motility. Both of these changes may increase or decrease the absorption of various drugs (depending on the chemical properties of the drug). Drug distribution may be affected by decreased cardiac output (eg, as seen in heart failure), decreased total body water, changes in the ratio of lean mass to fat, and increased body fat. Metabolic changes may result from decreased liver blood flow; diseases such as thyroid disease, heart failure, and cancer; smoking; and drug interactions. (Drug-induced metabolic changes are especially significant in older adults, because they often take several different drugs for multiple diseases and conditions. This further increases their risk for adverse drug reactions.) Renal function decreases with age in most adults, which can lead to an accumulation of drugs that normally are cleared through the renal system. In addition, the action of drugs affecting the CNS (eg, benzodiazepines, anesthetics, narcotics) and the cardiovascular system (eg, beta blockers, calcium channel blockers, diuretics) often is altered in older adults. Because of these changes, drugs may not produce the desired effect or may cause major drug toxicity in older adults. Drugs that commonly cause toxicity in the geriatric patient include the following:

- Analgesics
- Angiotensin-converting enzyme inhibitors
- Antidepressants
- Antihypertensives
- Beta blockers
- Digitalis
- Diuretics
- Psychotropics

The adverse reactions associated with these and other drugs often result from "accidents" or "mishaps" in the prescribed drug regimen. Other common reasons for drug-induced illness in the geriatric patient include dispensing errors, noncompliance, confusion, forgetfulness, vision impairment, and the self-selection of drugs. Changes in habits regarding alcohol intake, diet, and exercise also can affect drug metabolism and increase the risk for adverse drug reactions.

Older adults commonly have prescriptions from more than one physician, improperly resume using an old medication in addition to a newly prescribed one, or take prescribed medications along with over-the-counter drugs that may have synergistic or cumulative effects. This simultaneous use of multiple drugs is referred to as **polypharmacy**. Polypharmacy can lead to significant medication-related problems, particularly in the older adult who is living alone or has cognitive impairment and multiple chronic illnesses. The risk is compounded as the number of medicines and the number of caregivers and pharmacies supplying the medications increases. Lack of coordinated care can result in unnecessary prescriptions and increased adverse events in older adults.

The emergency care for geriatric patients with adverse drug reactions varies. Care may range from transport only to full advanced cardiac life support measures. When transporting the older adult, all of the patient's medicines should be delivered to the emergency department (ED) with the patient or brought by a family member.[47] BOX 48-9 lists symptoms of drug toxicity and adverse reactions that can occur in the geriatric patient.

Substance Abuse

As described in Chapter 33, *Toxicology*, substance abuse involving alcohol and other drugs is common in the older adult population. Over 1 million US citizens aged 65 years and older were estimated to be addicted to substances in 2014. This total included over 900,000 with alcohol use disorder and over 150,000 with an illicit drug use disorder.[48]

Substance abuse in the geriatric patient often is attributed to severe stress as the primary risk factor. This stress may result from life changes such as age-related changes in health or appearance, loss of

BOX 48-9 Symptoms of Drug Toxicity and Adverse Drug Reactions in the Geriatric Patient

Acute delirium
Akathisia (movement disorder characterized by a feeling of inner restlessness and inability to stay still)
Altered vision
Bradycardia
Cardiac dysrhythmias
Chorea
Coma
Confusion
Constipation
Fatigue
Glaucoma
Hypokalemia
Orthostatic hypotension
Paresthesias
Psychological disturbances
Pulmonary edema
Severe bleeding
Tardive dyskinesia
Urinary hesitancy

BOX 48-10 Signs of Substance Abuse

Alcohol Abuse
Anorexia
Confusion
Denial
Frequent falling
Hostility
Insomnia
Mood swings

Note: Ingestion of even small amounts of alcohol by the geriatric patient can cause intoxication.

Other Drug Abuse
Altered level of consciousness
Falling
Hallucinations
Memory changes
Orthostatic hypotension
Poor coordination
Restlessness
Weight loss

Note: People often have a history of alcohol and other drug abuse.

employment, loss of a spouse or life partner, illness, malnutrition, loneliness, loss of independent living arrangements, and others. BOX 48-10 lists signs of substance abuse.

If the paramedic suspects substance abuse, friends and family members at the scene should be discreetly interviewed about the patient's alcohol or other drug use. The cornerstones of therapy for these patients are identifying the problem and arranging referral to a physician for treatment. Treatment for the acutely intoxicated patient is described in Chapter 33, *Toxicology*, and may include resuscitative measures to manage the patient's airway, ventilation, and circulation. In addition, the paramedic should carefully assess the geriatric patient for occult trauma and any underlying medical conditions when signs and symptoms of alcohol or other drug intoxication are present. These conditions may include hypoglycemia, cardiomyopathy, and dysrhythmias (such as atrial fibrillation), GI bleeding, polydrug use (especially barbiturates and tranquilizers), and ethylene glycol or methanol ingestion.

Environmental Considerations

Older adults are at risk for the development of illness from extremes in the environment as a result of the aging process and other factors (see Chapter 44, *Environmental Conditions*). Two emergencies that relate to the environment and are most common in geriatric patients are hypothermia and hyperthermia.

Hypothermia

Patients who are younger are often at risk for the development of hypothermia from extremes in the environment. In contrast, hypothermia may develop in an older patient while indoors. This condition may occur as a result of cold surroundings and/or an illness that alters heat production or conservation. This increase risk of developing hypothermia is due in part to the following characteristics of older adults:

- They are less able to compensate for environmental heat loss.
- They have a decreased ability to sense changes in temperature.
- They have less total body water to store heat.
- They are less likely to develop tachycardia to increase cardiac output in response to cold stress.
- They have a decreased ability to shiver to increase body heat.

In addition to these physical changes, geriatric patients are more prone to the development of hypothermia as a result of socioeconomic factors. For example, a fixed income may inhibit an older person from paying for the cost of properly heating and insulating his or her home. Poor nutrition that results in a decrease in fat stores may contribute to hypothermia in geriatric patients who live alone. The following are other medical causes of hypothermia in geriatric patients:

- Arthritis
- Drug overdose
- Hepatic failure
- Hypoglycemia
- Infection
- Parkinson disease
- Stroke
- Thyroid disease
- Uremia

The signs and symptoms of hypothermia may be subtle. They may include an altered mental status, slurred speech, ataxia, and dysrhythmias. In severe cases, coma without signs of life may be present. Hypothermia in the geriatric patient carries a high mortality rate. The paramedic should manage these patients as described in Chapter 44, *Environmental Conditions.*

Hyperthermia

Hyperthermia in the geriatric patient is less common than is hypothermia; however, hyperthermia carries a significant mortality rate. The condition most likely results from exposure to high temperatures. These temperatures most likely continue for several days (eg, during a heat wave). As in hypothermia, geriatric patients are unable to control body temperature even in moderate heat. Hyperthermia also may result from medical conditions such as hypothalamic dysfunction and spinal cord injury. Alcohol and certain medications (eg, amphetamines, anticholinergics, antihistamines, beta blockers, diuretics) can increase the risk of hyperthermia. They do this by various mechanisms, including altering heat awareness and judgment, inhibiting heat dissipation, increasing motor activity, and impairing cardiovascular function.

As described in Chapter 44, *Environmental Conditions,* hyperthermic illness may present as heat cramps, heat exhaustion, or heatstroke. Emergency care includes removing the patient from the warm environment, cooling the patient, and ensuring the patient's vital functions through airway, ventilatory, and circulatory support. Rapid transport for physician evaluation is indicated to manage the problems resulting from serious heat-related illness.

Behavioral and Psychiatric Disorders

It is estimated that about one-fifth of people older than 55 years have some type of mental health concern.[49] In addition to the neurologic disorders, such as dementia and Alzheimer disease, anxiety, depression, and suicide are common in geriatric patients.

Depression

Depression is a serious illness that requires physician evaluation. In the geriatric patient, depression can result from physiologic and psychological causes. Research suggests that about 15% of older adult patients cared for by EMS are moderately or severely depressed.[50] Examples include cognitive disorders with physical causes (eg, dementia) and various personality disorders such as schizophrenia (see Chapter 34, *Behavioral and Psychiatric Disorders*).

BOX 48-11 Common Causes of Depression in the Geriatric Patient

Physiologic
Dehydration
Electrolyte imbalance
Fever
Hyponatremia
Hypoxia
Medications
Metabolic disturbances
Organic brain disease
Reduced cardiac output
Thyroid disease

Psychological
Fear of dying
Financial insecurity
Loss of a spouse
Loss of independence
Significant illness

BOX 48-11 lists other physiologic and psychological causes of depression in the geriatric patient. The signs and symptoms of depression vary by person. They may include the following:

- Decreased libido
- Deep feelings of worthlessness and guilt
- Extreme isolation
- Feelings of hopelessness
- Irritability
- Loss of appetite
- Loss of energy (fatigue)
- Recurrent thoughts of death
- Significant weight loss
- Sleeplessness
- Suicide attempts

CRITICAL THINKING
What endocrine disorder can produce signs or symptoms that are similar to those of depression?

A major goal of care is to identify the patient who may be depressed. These patients need to be evaluated by a physician. The physician will rule out medical illness—especially thyroid disease, stroke, malignancy, and dementia—or medication use (eg, beta blockers) that may be responsible for the patient's depression. After determining that there are no physical threats to life, the paramedic should try to establish a rapport with the patient who is depressed. The patient should be encouraged to talk openly about his or her feelings, especially any thoughts of suicide. If possible, the paramedic should interview the family about the patient's mental state and question family members about any history of depression in the patient.

Suicide

Patients older than 65 years account for about 18% of all suicides in the United States.[51] The rate of completed suicides for geriatric patients is higher than that of the general population, and most of these people visited their primary care physician in the month before the suicide.[52] Most were suffering from their first episode of major depression, which was only moderately severe, yet the depressive symptoms were unrecognized and untreated. Thus, the paramedic should be aware of the increased risk for suicide when evaluating geriatric patients who are depressed. Clues and indicators for suicide in the geriatric patient that may be obtained through a patient history or observed by friends and family include the following:[53]

- Talking about or seeming to be preoccupied with death and "getting affairs in order"
- Giving away prized possessions (eg, family heirlooms, photographs, keepsakes)
- Taking unnecessary risks (eg, walking alone in unsafe areas or driving without personal restraints)
- Using an increased amount of alcohol or other drugs
- Not adhering to the medical regimen (eg, failure to take prescribed medications)
- Acquiring a weapon, especially firearms

As described in Chapter 34, *Behavioral and Psychiatric Disorders*, there is no evidence that asking a person questions about suicidal thoughts and feelings increases the risk of suicide. Many depressed people are willing to discuss their suicidal thoughts; therefore, the paramedic should question the patient about suicidal thoughts if he or she suspects that the patient is at high risk. The following questions are appropriate for the paramedic to ask the patient:

1. Do you have thoughts about killing yourself?
2. Have you ever tried to kill yourself?
3. Have you thought about how you might kill yourself?

Most suicides committed by older adults involve firearms.[54] Therefore, the safety of those at the scene and the EMS crew is a priority when caring for a patient with suicidal tendencies. When indicated, law enforcement personnel should be available at the scene. After assessing the risk for suicidal tendencies, the patient should be transported for physician evaluation.

Trauma

Trauma is the sixth-leading cause of death for people older than 65 years. Despite this significant concern, older adults tend to be undertriaged to trauma centers.[55] Just over 25% of traumatic deaths in people aged 65 to 74 years are caused by vehicular trauma, and 33% result from falls. In people older than 67 years, falls are the leading cause of unintentional injury or death.[55] Burns also are a major cause of disability and death in geriatric patients. Contributing factors that increase the severity of traumatic injury in geriatric patients include the following:

- Osteoporosis and muscle weakness that increase the likelihood of falls and fractures
- Reduced cardiac reserve that decreases the ability to compensate for blood loss
- Decreased respiratory function that increases the likelihood of adult respiratory distress syndrome
- Impaired renal function that decreases the ability to adapt to fluid shifts

SHOW ME THE EVIDENCE

Researchers in London, Ontario, investigated 804 calls from 2013 where a person needed help with mobilization, referred to as lift assist (LA) calls, and was not transported to the hospital. They evaluated the 14-day morbidity and mortality of these patients and found that 116 patients (28%) had more than one LA call. Mean patient age was 74.8 years (14.1). They identified 169 ED visits (21%), 93 hospital admissions (11.6%), and 9 deaths (1.1%) within 14 days of the LA call. Hospital admissions were related to infection (33%), fall (12%), cancer complication or new diagnosis (9.7%), fracture (8.6%), and other (36.6%). Patient age ($P = 0.006$) predicted hospital admission. They concluded that LA calls are associated with short-term morbidity and mortality.

Modified from: Leggatt L, Van Aarsen K, Columbus M, et al. Morbidity and mortality associated with prehospital "lift-assist" calls. *Prehosp Emerg Care.* 2017;21(5):556-562.

Falls

One in four Americans older than 65 years falls each year.[56] Aside from the deaths they cause, falls result in 2.8 million injuries requiring care in EDs annually.[56] Most are preventable. Falls represent more than just physical injury. After a fall, geriatric patients may experience fear and deterioration in function, and in some cases, these effects can lead to institutionalization.[18] A reduction in function resulting in declining activities and social interactions can cause depression, social isolation, and feelings of helplessness.

Fractures are the most common fall-related injuries in older adults—the hip being the fracture that most often results in hospitalization. Mortality risk persists at 20% to 30% after 1 year with hip fractures.[57] In those patients who survive hip fracture, most will have significant problems with walking and moving about. They may become more dependent on others for help and unable to continue living on their own. Falls that do not result in physical injury may lead to self-imposed immobility from the fear of falling again. When immobility is strict and prolonged, joint contractures, pressure sores, urinary tract infection, muscle atrophy, depression, and functional dependency may result.

The National Council on Aging and Centers for Disease Control and Prevention have developed an evidence-based program to reduce the incidence of falls in older adults. Evidence suggests that this type of program increases scene time slightly but is safe and increases referrals. Some EMS systems have integrated their STEADI (Stopping Elderly Accidents, Deaths, and Injuries) program into community education programs.[58] The program describes how to identify risk factors for falls in older adults, how to perform a fall risk assessment, and strategies to reduce falls.

The fall assessment begins with three questions:

1. Have you fallen in the past year?
2. Do you feel unsteady when standing or walking?
3. Do you worry about falling?

An answer of yes to any of these questions indicates an increased fall risk.

Some risk factors for falls are easy to assess. These include lower body weakness, gait and balance problems, postural dizziness, a history of falls, and home safety or environmental hazards. Other fall risk factors may be more difficult to detect. They include poor vision, problems with feet or shoes, recent major life changes, mental health problems, chronic conditions (arthritis, stroke, incontinence, diabetes mellitus, Parkinson disease, dementia), urinary incontinence, or high-risk medications (**TABLE 48-3**).

Interventions include distribution of educational materials related to measures to reduce falls, a safety checklist, a brochure about postural hypotension, and instructions for exercise.

Prevention strategies (described in Chapter 3, *Injury Prevention, Health Promotion, and Public Health*) that can decrease injuries associated with falls include the following:

- Using assistive devices (eg, walker or cane)
- Removing scatter rugs and securing loose carpeting
- Removing items that may cause tripping
- Providing and using handrails
- Ensuring adequate lighting, including night lights
- Removing clutter from the environment
- Arranging furniture for walking ease
- Using nonslip stickers in the bathtub or shower

TABLE 48-3 Medications Associated With Falls

Psychoactive Medications
Anticonvulsants
Antidepressants
Antipsychotics
Benzodiazepines
Opioids
Sedative-hypnotics
Medications Associated With Dizziness, Sedation, Confusion, Blurred Vision, or Orthostatic Hypotension
Anticholinergics
Antihistamines
Blood pressure medications
Muscle relaxants

Modified from: Medications linked to falls. Centers for Disease Control and Prevention website. https://stacks.cdc.gov/view/cdc/50341/cdc_50341_DS1.pdf. Accessed April 15, 2018.

- Providing handrails on bathtubs, showers, and commodes
- Suggesting patients consult with their physician regarding medicines if they are taking medication that increases the risk of falls

Vehicular Trauma

More than 40 million licensed drivers are older than 65 years. In 2015, more than 6,800 deaths in this age group were attributed to motor vehicle crashes.[59] Fatal crashes increase among drivers aged 70 to 74 years and are highest among people aged 85 years and older. Most of the deaths are related to increased risk of injury and medical complications of aging, rather than an increased risk of crash involvement. The driving ability of some older adults is negatively affected by impaired cognitive function, changes in vision, and physical changes.[59] A large number of older adults are injured as drivers or passengers in moving vehicles. In 2015, more than 1,021 pedestrian fatalities among older adults occurred in the United States. This total accounts for 19% of all pedestrian deaths from trauma.[60]

Older trauma patients have increased morbidity and mortality and sustain more severe injury than do younger adults as a result of comorbid disease and the independent effects of aging.[61] Older patients also are less capable of an appropriate, protective physiologic response. Prompt identification of injuries and sources of hemorrhage is critical in any trauma patient but is especially important in the geriatric patient. The geriatric patient has much less cardiac reserve and will succumb more quickly to shock.

Burns

More than 1,200 older adults die from fires and burns in the United States each year.[62] The increased risk of morbidity and mortality from burn trauma in older adults is caused by preexisting disease, skin changes that result in increased burn depth, impaired nutrition, and decreased ability to fight infection. The initial care and resuscitation of geriatric patients with thermal injury is described in Chapter 38, *Burns*. Geriatric burn patients need special approaches to fluid therapy to prevent damage to the kidneys. The patient's fluid status will need to be assessed in the initial hours after a burn injury by monitoring pulse and blood pressure, and striving to maintain a urine output of at least 50 to 60 mL/h.

Head Trauma

A head injury with loss of consciousness in geriatric patients often has a poor outcome. The brain becomes smaller in size with age (**cerebral atrophy**). This atrophy produces an increase in distance between the surface of the brain and the skull. As veins are stretched across this space, they are more easily torn, resulting in subdural hematomas. The extra space within the skull often allows a large amount of bleeding to occur before signs and symptoms of increased intracranial pressure are seen.

Geriatric patients also are at high risk for injuries of the cervical spine because of the arthritic and degenerative changes associated with aging. These structural changes lead to increased stiffening and decreased flexibility of the spine with narrowing of the spinal canal. As a result, the spinal cord is at a much greater risk for damage from fairly minor trauma.

> CRITICAL THINKING
> Consider geriatric patients with head trauma. What home medications also can lead to an increased risk of intracerebral bleeding in these patients?

Chest Injuries

Any mechanism of injury that produces thoracic trauma in a geriatric patient can be potentially lethal. The aged thorax is less elastic. Thus, the thorax is more susceptible to injury. The pulmonary system also has marginal reserve because of a reduced alveolar surface area, decreased patency of small airways, and diminished chemoreceptor response.

Injuries to the heart, aorta, and major vessels are a greater risk to geriatric patients than they are to younger patients. Again, this is because of decreased functional reserve in older patients. It also is caused by anatomic changes that make injury in these areas of greater significance. Myocardial contusion may be a complication of blunt injury to the chest. If severe, myocardial contusion may result in pump failure or life-threatening dysrhythmias. Rarely, cardiac tamponade occurs after blunt thoracic trauma. Cardiac rupture, valvular injury (eg, flail valves), and aortic dissection also may occur with significant blunt chest injury. The first two entities are rare but rapidly fatal. When the mechanism of injury produces rapid deceleration, the paramedic should always consider the possibility of dissecting aortic aneurysm. Aortic dissections often are not immediately fatal. Proper evaluation and treatment can be lifesaving (see Chapter 21, *Cardiology*).

CRITICAL THINKING

Consider the patient who has a dissecting aortic aneurysm. What specific signs and symptoms may the paramedic see in this patient?

In geriatric patients, the heart cannot respond as effectively to increased demand for oxygen as in a younger person. This shortage of oxygen coupled with a slowed conduction system may cause ischemia and dysrhythmias when the geriatric patient has a significant trauma. These problems may occur even if the heart has not been damaged directly by the trauma. The patient's oxygenation and circulatory status must be closely monitored.

Abdominal Injuries

Abdominal injuries in geriatric patients have serious consequences. Abdominal injuries often are less obvious; therefore, they require a high degree of suspicion. The geriatric patient is less likely to tolerate abdominal surgery well. This patient is more likely to be at risk for the development of pulmonary complications and infection following abdominal surgery.

Musculoskeletal Injuries

The osteoporotic bones of geriatric patients are more at risk for fractures, even with mild trauma. Pelvic fractures are highly lethal in this age group, even in the absence of the severe hemorrhage and soft-tissue injury often associated with mortality in younger patients. When assessing for skeletal trauma, the paramedic should recall that the geriatric patient may have decreased pain perception. Often these patients have amazingly little tenderness with major fractures. Even with proper care, the mortality rate for geriatric patients with musculoskeletal injury is increased by delayed complications, such as adult respiratory distress syndrome, sepsis, acute kidney injury, and pulmonary embolism.

Trauma Management Considerations

The priorities of trauma care for geriatric patients are similar to those for all trauma patients. However, the paramedic should give special consideration to transport strategies and the geriatric patient's cardiovascular, respiratory, and renal systems.

Cardiovascular System

Special considerations for cardiovascular problems include the following:

- Recent or past MI contributes to the risk of dysrhythmias and heart failure.
- Adjustment of heart rate and stroke volume may be decreased in response to hypovolemia.
- Geriatric patients may need higher arterial pressures than do younger patients for perfusion of vital organs. This is because of atherosclerotic peripheral vascular disease.
- Rapid IV fluid administration to geriatric patients may cause volume overload. The paramedic must take care not to overhydrate these patients. Older adults as a group are more susceptible to heart failure. However, hypovolemia and hypotension are also poorly tolerated. Paramedics should consider hypovolemia in any geriatric patient whose systolic blood pressure is less than 120 mm Hg. Tachycardia may be blunted or simply may not occur if the patient takes beta blockers. The paramedic should monitor lung sounds and vital signs carefully and frequently during fluid administration.

Respiratory System

Special considerations for respiratory problems include the following:

- Physical changes decrease chest wall compliance and movement. Thus, they diminish vital capacity as well.
- Pa_{O_2} level decreases with age.
- Lower partial pressure of oxygen (P_{O_2}) level at the same fractional inspired oxygen concentration occurs with each passing decade.
- All organ systems have less tolerance to hypoxia.
- COPD (common in geriatric patients) requires that the paramedic carefully adjust airway management and ventilation support for appropriate

oxygenation and carbon dioxide removal. High-concentration oxygen may suppress the hypoxic drive in some patients. However, oxygen should never be withheld from a patient with clinical signs of hypoxemia such as cyanosis. The paramedic may need to remove the patient's dentures for adequate airway and ventilation management.

Renal System

Special considerations for renal problems include the following:

- The kidneys have decreased ability to maintain normal acid–base balance and a decreased ability to compensate for fluid changes.
- Kidney disease may further decrease the ability of the kidneys to compensate.
- Decreased kidney function (along with decreased cardiac reserve) places the injured geriatric patient at risk for fluid overload and pulmonary edema following IV fluid therapy.

Transport Strategies

Special considerations for transporting geriatric patients include the following:

- Positioning, immobilization, and transport of a geriatric trauma patient may require modifications to accommodate physical deformities (eg, arthritis, spinal abnormalities).
- Packaging should include bulk and extra padding to support and give comfort to the patient.
- The paramedic can prevent hypothermia by keeping the patient warm.

Elder Abuse

Elder abuse refers to the infliction of physical pain, injury, debilitating mental anguish, unreasonable confinement, or willful deprivation by a caregiver of services that are necessary to maintain mental and physical health of a geriatric person. Elder abuse has become more and more recognized as a growing problem in the United States. It is estimated to affect 1 in 10 older adults each year.[63]

Elder abuse takes many forms, including physical abuse, sexual abuse, emotional or psychological abuse, neglect, abandonment, financial or material exploitation, and self-neglect. It may occur in the home or in a residential care facility. BOX 48-12 lists the types of elder abuse, as defined by the National Center on Elder Abuse.

All 50 states have elder abuse statutes, and the reporting of suspected elder abuse is mandatory. If the paramedic suspects abuse or neglect of an older adult, procedures that are established by local protocol should be followed. Abuse and neglect are discussed further in Chapter 49, *Abuse and Neglect.*

BOX 48-12 Types of Elder Abuse and Neglect

Physical Abuse
Infliction of physical pain or injury

Financial Exploitation
Misuse or withholding of an older adult's resources by another person

Sexual Abuse
Touching, fondling, intercourse, or any sex act with an older adult who is unable to understand, does not consent, or is threatened or physically forced

Emotional Abuse
Verbal assaults, threats of harm, harassment, or intimidation

Passive Neglect
Failure to provide an older adult with essential requirements such as food, clothing, shelter, or medical care

Willful Deprivation
Denying an older adult medication, shelter, food, medical care, or other assistance that exposes the person to physical, mental, or emotional harm (unless the older adult expressed a wish to forgo such care)

Confinement
Restraining or isolating an older adult (except for medical reasons)

Modified from: Elder abuse facts: what is elder abuse. National Council on Aging website. https://www.ncoa.org/public-policy-action/elder-justice/elder-abuse-facts/. Accessed April 12, 2018.

Summary

- The aging process proceeds at different rates in different people.
- Normal changes with aging and existing illnesses may make evaluation of an ill or injured geriatric patient a challenge.
- Pneumonia is a leading cause of death in the geriatric age group. It often is fatal in frail adults.
- Chronic obstructive pulmonary disease (COPD) is a common finding in the geriatric patient who has a history of smoking. The disease usually is associated with various other diseases that result in reduced expiratory airflow.
- A lack of typical chest pain can cause a myocardial infarction to be unrecognized in the geriatric patient. Heart failure is more frequent in geriatric patients and has a larger incidence of noncardiac causes. The most common cause of dysrhythmias in the geriatric patient is hypertensive heart disease.
- Abdominal aortic aneurysm affects 2% to 4% of the US population older than 50 years. This type of aneurysm is most prevalent in people aged 60 to 70 years. The incidence of hypertension in the geriatric patient increases when atherosclerosis is present.
- Risk factors for cerebral vascular disease in the older adult include smoking, hypertension, diabetes mellitus, atherosclerosis, hyperlipidemia, polycythemia, and heart disease.
- Delirium is an abrupt disorientation to time and place. Delirium is commonly a result of physical illness.
- Dementia is a slow, progressive loss of awareness of time and place. It usually involves an inability to learn new things or remember recent events. This condition often is a result of brain disease. Alzheimer disease is the most common cause of dementia. Alzheimer disease is a condition in which nerve cells in the cerebral cortex die and the brain substance shrinks.
- Parkinson disease is a brain disorder. It causes muscle tremor, stiffness, weakness, and dementia.
- About 20% of older adults have diabetes mellitus. Almost 40% have some impaired glucose tolerance. Hyperglycemic hyperosmolar nonketotic coma is a serious complication in older adults with type 2 diabetes. It has a mortality rate of 20% to 50%. Thyroid disease is more common in geriatric patients. It may not present in the classic manner.
- Gastrointestinal bleeding most often affects patients between the ages of 60 and 90 years. Bowel obstruction often occurs in patients with prior abdominal surgeries or hernias. It also occurs in those with colon cancer. Some geriatric patients may have problems with continence or with elimination as well.
- Aging results in a gradual decrease in epidermal cellular turnover. It also results in loss of deep and dermal vessels. Alterations in capillary circulation lead to changes in thermal regulation and skin-related complications.
- Osteoarthritis is a common form of arthritis in geriatric patients. It results from cartilage loss and wear and tear on the joints. The loss in bone density from osteoporosis causes bones to become brittle. These bones may fracture easily.
- As people age, they may experience problems with vision, hearing, and speech.
- Geriatric patients are at an increased risk for adverse drug reactions because of age-related changes in body composition and drug distribution. It also is the result of metabolism and excretion. Moreover, the risk for adverse drug reactions often stems from multiple prescribed drugs. Alcohol abuse is a common problem in geriatric patients.
- Hypothermia may develop in the geriatric patient while indoors. This condition may be the result of cold surroundings and/or an illness that alters heat production or conservation. Hyperthermia most likely results from exposure to high temperatures that continue for several days.
- Depression is common in geriatric patients. It can result from physiologic and psychological causes. The rate of completed suicides for geriatric patients is higher than that of the general population.
- One-third of traumatic deaths in people aged 65 to 74 years result from vehicular trauma. Twenty-five percent result from falls. In those older than 80 years, falls account for 50% of injury-related deaths. The risk of fatality from multiple trauma is estimated to be three times greater at age 70 years than at age 20 years.
- Elder abuse is classified as physical abuse, psychological abuse, financial or material abuse, and neglect.

References

1. Platts-Mills TF, Leacock B, Cabanas JG, Shofer FS, McLean SA. Emergency medical services use by the elderly: analysis of a statewide database. *Prehosp Emerg Care*. 2010;14(3):329-333.
2. Facts for features: older Americans month: May 2017. Release Number: CB17-FF.08. US Census Bureau website. https://www.census.gov/newsroom/facts-for-features/2017/cb17-ff08.html. Published April 10, 2017. Accessed April 12, 2018.
3. Tips for selecting Medicare and Social Security. Aging in Place, National Council for Aging Care, website. http://www.aginginplace.org/how-to-select-medicare-social-security/. Published March 22, 2017. Accessed April 12, 2018.
4. American Geriatrics Society Foundation for Health in Aging. Health and aging facts. American Geriatrics Society website. http://www.healthinagingfoundation.org/. Accessed April 12, 2018.
5. The American Geriatrics Society Expert Panel on Person-Centered Care. Person-centered care: a definition and essential elements. *J Am Geriatr Soc*. 2016;64(1):15-18.
6. Duong HV, Herrera LN, Moore JX, et al. National characteristics of emergency medical services responses for older adults in the United States. *Prehosp Emerg Care*. 2018;22(1):7-14.

7. Evans CS, Platts-Mills TF, Fernandez AR, et al. Repeated emergency medical services use by older adults: analysis of a comprehensive statewide database. *Ann Emerg Med.* 2017;70(4):506-515.e3.
8. Perceptions of aging during each decade of life after 30. Westhealth Institute, NORC at the University of Chicago, website. http://www.norc.org/PDFs/WHI-NORC-Aging-Survey/Brief_WestHealth_A_2017-03_DTPv2.pdf. Published March 2017. Accessed April 12, 2018.
9. Mauk K. *Gerontological Nursing.* 4th ed. Burlington, MA: Jones & Bartlett Learning; 2018.
10. Beachey W. *Respiratory Care Anatomy and Physiology.* 4th ed. St. Louis, MO: Elsevier; 2018.
11. Lavan AH, Gallagher P. Predicting risk of adverse drug reactions in older adults. *Ther Adv Drug Saf.* 2016;7(1):11-22.
12. Parameswaran Nair N, Chalmers L, Peterson GM, Bereznicki B, Castelino RL, Bereznicki L. Hospitalization in older patients due to adverse drug reactions—the need for a prediction tool. *Clin Interv Aging.* 2016;11:497-505.
13. National Association of EMS Officials. *National Model EMS Clinical Guidelines*. Version 2.0. National Association of EMS Officials website. https://www.nasemso.org/documents/National-Model-EMS-Clinical-Guidelines-Version2-Sept2017.pdf. Published September 2017. Accessed April 12, 2018.
14. Rosen P, Barkin R. *Emergency Medicine: Concepts and Clinical Practice.* 8th ed. St. Louis, MO: Elsevier; 2014.
15. Pathy M, Sinclair A, Morley J. *Principles and Practice of Geriatric Medicine.* 5th ed. Hoboken, NJ: Wiley Blackwell; 2012.
16. Bosker G, Schwartz GR, Jones JS, et al. *Geriatric Emergency Medicine.* St. Louis, MO: Mosby; 1990.
17. Aging and cancer. Cancer.net website. https://www.cancer.net/navigating-cancer-care/older-adults/aging-and-cancer. Published September 2016. Accessed April 12, 2018.
18. Caprio TV, Shah MA. Approach to the geriatric patient. In: Brice J, Delbridge TR, Meyers JB, eds. *Emergency Services: Clinical Practice and Systems Oversight.* 2nd ed. West Sussex, England: John Wiley & Sons; 2015.
19. American Lung Association, Epidemiology and Statistics Unit Research and Health Education Division. *Trends in Pneumonia and Influenza Morbidity and Mortality*. American Lung Association website. Published November 2015. Accessed April 12, 2018.
20. Ochiai ME, Lopes NH, Buzo CG, Pierri H. Atypical manifestation of myocardial ischemia in the elderly. *Arquivos brasileiros de cardiologia*. 2014;102(3):31-33.
21. Engberding N, Wenger NK. Acute coronary syndromes in the elderly. *F1000Res*. 2017;6:1791.
22. Azad N, Lemay G. Management of chronic heart failure in the older population. *J Geriatr Cardiol.* 2014;11(4):329-337.
23. Cowie MR, Anker SD, Cleland JGF, et al. Improving care for patients with acute heart failure: before, during and after hospitalization. *ESC Heart Fail.* 2014;1(2):110-145.
24. Marín-García J. *Heart Failure: Bench to Bedside.* Berlin, Germany: Springer Science+Business Media; 2010.
25. Ham RJ, Sloane PD, Warshaw GA, Potter JF, Flaherty E. *Ham's Primary Care Geriatrics: A Case-Based Approach.* 6th ed. Philadelphia, PA: Elsevier; 2013.
26. Dalman RL, Mell M. Overview of abdominal aortic aneurysm. UpToDate website. https://www.uptodate.com/contents/overview-of-abdominal-aortic-aneurysm. Updated July 24, 2017. Accessed April 12, 2018.
27. Whelton PK, Carey RM, Aronow WS, et al. 2017 ACC/AHA/AAPA/ABC/ACPM/AGS/APhA/ASH/ASPC/NMA/PCNA guideline for the prevention, detection, evaluation, and management of high blood pressure in adults. Executive summary: a report of the American College of Cardiology/American Heart Association Task Force on Clinical Practice Guidelines. *Hypertension*. 2017 Nov 13.
28. Shah MN, Jones CMC, Richardson TM, Conwell Y, Katz P, Schneider SM. Prevalence of depression and cognitive impairment in older adult emergency medical services patients. *Prehosp Emerg Care.* 2011;15(1):4-11.
29. American Heart Association. *Advanced Cardiac Life Support*. Dallas, TX: American Heart Association; 2016.
30. Preventing a second stroke. Stroke Foundation website. https://strokefoundation.org.au/About-Stroke/Preventing-stroke/Preventing-a-second-stroke. Accessed April 12, 2018.
31. Terminology and mnemonics. ICU Delirium website. http://www.icudelirium.org/terminology.html. Accessed April 12, 2018.
32. Dementia. Alzheimer's Community Care website. https://www.alzcare.org/dementia. Accessed April 12, 2018.
33. Langa KM, Larson EB, Crimmins EM, et al. A comparison of the prevalence of dementia in the United States in 2000 and 2012. *JAMA Intern Med*. 2017;177(1):51-58.
34. 2017 Alzheimer's statistics. Alzheimers.net website. https://www.alzheimers.net/resources/alzheimers-statistics/. Accessed April 12, 2018.
35. Alzheimer's and dementia: vascular dementia. Alzheimer's Association website. https://www.alz.org/dementia/vascular-dementia-symptoms.asp. Accessed April 12, 2018.
36. Alzheimer's and dementia: Parkinson's disease dementia. Alzheimer's Association website. https://www.alz.org/dementia/parkinsons-disease-symptoms.asp. Accessed April 12, 2018.
37. Statistics. Parkinson' Foundation website. http://parkinson.org/Understanding-Parkinsons/Causes-and-Statistics/Statistics. Accessed April 12, 2018.
38. Reeve A, Simxoc E, Turnbull D. Ageing and Parkinson's disease: why is advancing age the biggest risk factor? *Aging Res Rev*. 2014;14:19-30.
39. Alzheimer's and dementia: frontotemporal dementia (FTD). Alzheimer's Association website. https://www.alz.org/dementia/fronto-temporal-dementia-ftd-symptoms.asp. Accessed April 12, 2018.
40. Older adults. American Diabetes Association. http://www.diabetes.org/in-my-community/awareness-programs/older-adults/. Updated November 21, 2017. Accessed April 12, 2018.
41. Kim MI. Hypothyroidism in the elderly. In: De Groot LJ, Chrousos G, Dungan K, et al., eds. *Endotext* [Internet]. South Dartmouth, MA: MDText.com; 2000. https://www.ncbi.nlm.nih.gov/books/NBK279005/. Accessed April 12, 2018.
42. Yeo CJ, McFadden DW, Pemberton JH, Peters JH, Matthews JB. *Shackelford's Surgery of the Alimentary Tract.* 7th ed. Philadelphia, PA: Elsevier; 2013.
43. Kozieł D, Matykiewicz J, Głuszek S. Gastrointestinal bleeding in patients aged 85 years and older. *Pol Przegl Chir.* 2011;83(11):606-613.
44. Snyder DR, Shah MA, eds. *Geriatric Education for Emergency Services*. 2nd ed. Burlington, MA: Jones & Bartlett Learning; 2016.
45. Celebrex® celecoxib capsules. Pfizer. https://www.accessdata.fda.gov/drugsatfda_docs/label/2008/020998s026lbl.pdf. LAB-0036-11. Revised January 2008. Accessed May 30, 2018.

46. Sood R, Faubion SS, Kuhle CL, Thielen JM, Shuster LT. Prescribing menopausal hormone therapy: an evidence-based approach. *Int J Womens Health*. 2014;6:47-57.
47. Chan EW, Taylor SE, Marriott J, Barger B. An intervention to encourage ambulance paramedics to bring patients' own medications to the ED: impact on medications brought in and prescribing errors. *Emerg Med Australas*. 2010;22(2):151-158.
48. Center for Behavioral Health Statistics and Quality. *Results From the 2014 National Survey on Drug Use and Health: Detailed Tables*. Rockville, MD: Substance Abuse and Mental Health Services Administration; 2015.
49. Centers for Disease Control and Prevention, National Association of Chronic Disease Directors. *The State of Mental Health and Aging in America: Issue Brief 1: What Do the Data Tell Us?* Atlanta, GA: Centers for Disease Control and Prevention; 2008. https://www.cdc.gov/aging/agingdata/data-portal/mental-health.html. Accessed April 12, 2018.
50. Shah MN, Jones CMC, Richardson TM, Conwell Y, Katz P, Schneider SM. Prevalence of depression and cognitive impairment in older adult emergency medical services patients. *Prehosp Emerg Care*. 2011;15(1):4-11.
51. Caruso K. Elderly suicide. Suicide.org website. http://www.suicide.org/elderly-suicide.html. Accessed April 12, 2018.
52. US Department of Health and Human Services, Substance Abuse and Mental Health Services Administration. Depression and older adults: key issues. Substance Abuse and Mental Health Services Administration website. https://store.samhsa.gov/shin/content/SMA11-4631CD-DVD/SMA11-4631CD-DVD-KeyIssues.pdf. Published 2011. Accessed April 12, 2018.
53. Evans GD, Radunovich HL. *Suicide and the Elderly: Warning Signs and How to Help*. Gainesville, FL: Department of Family, Youth and Community Sciences, UF/IFAS Extension; September 2017. Doc FCS2184.
54. Cohen D, Eisdorfer C. *Integrated Textbook of Geriatric Mental Health*. Baltimore, MD: John Hopkins University Press; 2011.
55. Garwe T, Stewart K, Stoner J, et al. Out-of-hospital and inter-hospital under-triage to designated tertiary trauma centers among injured older adults: a 10-year statewide geospatial-adjusted analysis. *Prehosp Emerg Care*. 2017;21(6):734-743.
56. Falls prevention facts. National Council on Aging website. https://www.ncoa.org/news/resources-for-reporters/get-the-facts/falls-prevention-facts/. Accessed April 12, 2018.
57. Panula J, Pihlajamäki H, Mattila VM, et al. Mortality and cause of death in hip fracture patients aged 65 or older: a population-based study. *BMC Musculoskelet Disord*. 2011(May 20);12:105.
58. Snooks HA, Carter BL, Dale J, et al. Support and assessment for fall emergency referrals (SAFER 1): cluster randomised trial of computerised clinical decision support for paramedics. *PLoS One*. 2014;9(9):e106436.
59. Centers for Disease Control and Prevention, National Center for Injury Prevention and Control, Division of Unintentional Injury Prevention. Older adult drivers. Centers for Disease Control and Prevention website. https://www.cdc.gov/motorvehiclesafety/older_adult_drivers/. Updated November 30, 2017. Accessed April 12, 2018.
60. Centers for Disease Control and Prevention, National Center for Injury Prevention and Control, Division of Unintentional Injury Prevention. Pedestrian safety. Centers for Disease Control and Prevention website. https://www.cdc.gov/motorvehiclesafety/pedestrian_safety/index.html. Updated August 9, 2017. Accessed April 12, 2018.
61. Marx J, Hockberger R, Walls R. *Rosen's Emergency Medicine: Concepts and Clinical Practice*. 8th ed. Philadelphia, PA: Elsevier; 2014.
62. Collins J. Preventing burn trauma. *Today Geriatr Med*. 2015;8(5):28.
63. Elder abuse facts. National Council on Aging website. https://www.ncoa.org/public-policy-action/elder-justice/elder-abuse-facts/. Accessed April 12, 2018.

Suggested Readings

Aoyama M, Suzuki Y, Kuzuya M. Muscle strength of lower extremities related to incident falls in community-dwelling older adults. *J Gerontol Geriatr Res*. 2015;4:2.

Basu R, Zeber JE, Copeland LA, Stevens AB. Role of co-existence of multiple chronic conditions on the longitudinal decline in cognitive performance among older adults in the US. *J Gerontol Geriatr Res*. 2015.

Murdoch I, Turpin S, Johnson B, MacLullich A, Losman E. *Geriatric Emergencies*. Hoboken, NJ: Wiley Blackwell; 2015.

Paolo D. Neurological illnesses and older people: what are the effects? *J Gerontol Geriatr Res*. 2015:247.

Récoché I, Lebaudy C, Cool C, et al. Potentially inappropriate prescribing in a population of frail elderly people. *Int J Clin Pharm*. 2017;39(1):113-119.

Sylvester J. Delirium screening in emergency department admission: a comparison with nice guidelines. *J Gerontol Geriatr Res*. 2016.

Weber JM, Jabolonski RA, Penrod J. Missed opportunities: under-detection of trauma in elderly adults involved in motor vehicle crashes. *J Emerg Nurs*. 2010;36(1):6-9.

Wei F, Hester AL. Gender difference in fall among adults treated in emergency departments and outpatient clinics. *J Gerontol Geriatr Res*. 2014:152.

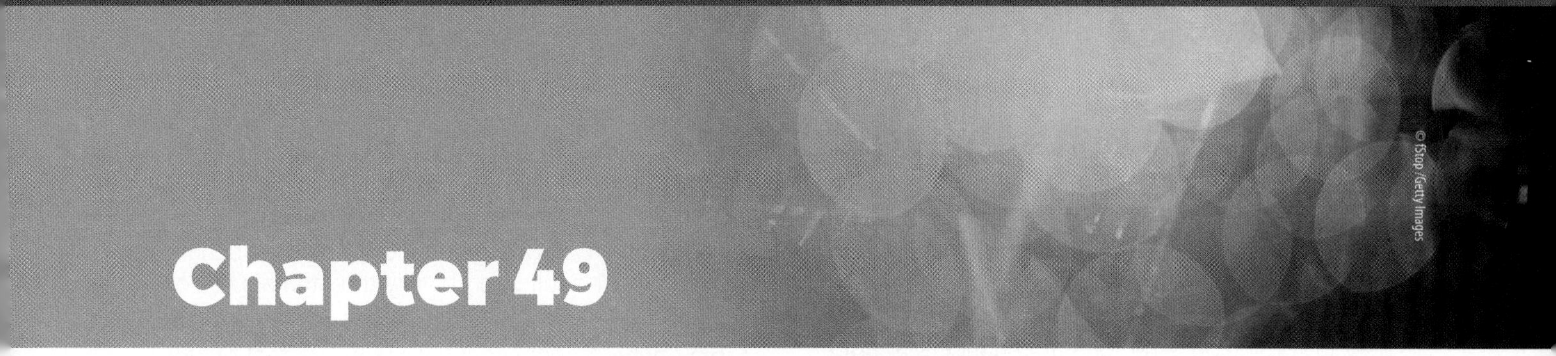

Chapter 49

Abuse and Neglect

NATIONAL EMS EDUCATION STANDARD COMPETENCIES

Special Patient Populations

Integrates assessment findings with principles of pathophysiology and knowledge of psychosocial needs to formulate a field impression and implement a comprehensive treatment/disposition plan for patients with special needs.

Patients With Special Challenges

Recognizing and reporting abuse and neglect (pp 1750–1751, 1753, 1756–1757, 1760)
Health care implications of
- Abuse (pp 1749–1750)
- Neglect (pp 1751–1757)
- Homelessness (see Chapter 50, *Patients With Special Challenges*)
- Poverty (see Chapter 50, *Patients With Special Challenges*)
- Bariatrics (see Chapter 50, *Patients With Special Challenges*)
- Technology dependent (see Chapter 51, *Acute Interventions for Home Care*)
- Hospice/terminally ill (see Chapter 50, *Patients With Special Challenges*)
- Tracheostomy care/dysfunction (see Chapter 51, *Acute Interventions for Home Care*)
- Home care (see Chapter 51, *Acute Interventions for Home Care*)
- Sensory deficit/loss (see Chapter 50, *Patients With Special Challenges*)
- Developmental disability (see Chapter 50, *Patients With Special Challenges*)

Trauma

Integrates assessment findings with principles of epidemiology and pathophysiology to formulate a field impression to implement a comprehensive treatment/disposition plan for an acutely injured patient.

Special Considerations in Trauma

Pathophysiology, assessment, and management of trauma in the
- Pregnant patient (see Chapter 45, *Obstetrics*)
- Pediatric patient (see Chapter 47, *Pediatrics*)
- Geriatric patient (see Chapter 48, *Geriatrics*)
- Cognitively impaired patient (see Chapter 50, *Patients With Special Challenges*)

OBJECTIVES

Upon completion of this chapter, the paramedic student will be able to:

1. Define intimate partner violence (IPV). (p 1747)
2. Describe the characteristics of abusive relationships. (p 1749)
3. Outline findings that indicate IPV. (p 1749)
4. Describe prehospital considerations when responding to and caring for patients who have experienced IPV. (pp 1749–1750)
5. Identify types of elder abuse. (pp 1751–1753)
6. Discuss legal considerations related to all forms of abuse. (pp 1750–1751, 1753, 1756–1757, 1760)
7. Describe characteristics of abused children and their abusers. (pp 1753–1755)
8. Outline the physical examination of the abused child. (pp 1755–1756)
9. Describe the characteristics of sexual assault. (pp 1758–1759)
10. Outline prehospital patient care considerations for the patient who has been sexually assaulted. (pp 1759–1760)

KEY TERMS

battering Repeated violence from physical and mental abuse (and other forms of abuse); may include establishing control and fear in a relationship.

economic abuse Making or attempting to make a person financially dependent by maintaining total control over financial resources, withholding a person's access to money, or forbidding a person's attendance at school or employment.

elder abuse The infliction of physical pain, injury, debilitating mental anguish, unreasonable confinement, or willful deprivation by a caregiver of services that are necessary to maintain mental and physical health of a geriatric person.

emotional abuse The infliction of anguish, pain, or distress through verbal or nonverbal acts.

human trafficking The illegal exploitation of a person.

intimate partner violence (IPV) A type of violence that occurs between two people in an intimate relationship, whether opposite- and same-sex partners.

neglect The refusal or failure of the caregiver to fulfill obligations or duties to a person.

patterned injuries Injuries that result from an identifiable object.

physical abuse The use of physical force that may result in bodily injury, physical pain, or impairment.

physical assault An intentional act by one person that creates apprehension in another person of an imminent harmful or offensive contact.

self-neglect A type of elder abuse in which the behaviors of an older adult intentionally threaten his or her own personal health or safety.

sexual abuse Nonconsensual sexual contact of any kind.

sexual assault Any genital, anal, oral, or manual penetration of a person's body by way of force and without the person's consent.

shaken baby syndrome (SBS) A serious form of child abuse that describes injuries to infants that occur after being shaken violently.

spiritual abuse The act of preventing a person from practicing his or her religion or forcing a person to practice another religion.

stalking A pattern of repeated and unwanted attention, harassment, contact, or any other course of conduct directed at a specific person that would cause a reasonable person to feel fear.

verbal abuse The use of degrading remarks, characterized by underlying anger and hostility, that attack a person's self-esteem. An example is name-calling.

Partner, elder, and child abuse are growing problems in the United States. Paramedics will encounter abused or maltreated patients in their careers. Abuse and neglect can result in mental and physical illness or injury, and even death. Education programs for paramedics must include information about these violent crimes. This information includes identification of abused and maltreated patients, special aspects of care, scene safety, and documentation requirements. This chapter addresses the types of abuse and neglect, the personality traits of those who abuse, and legal considerations in providing emergency care.

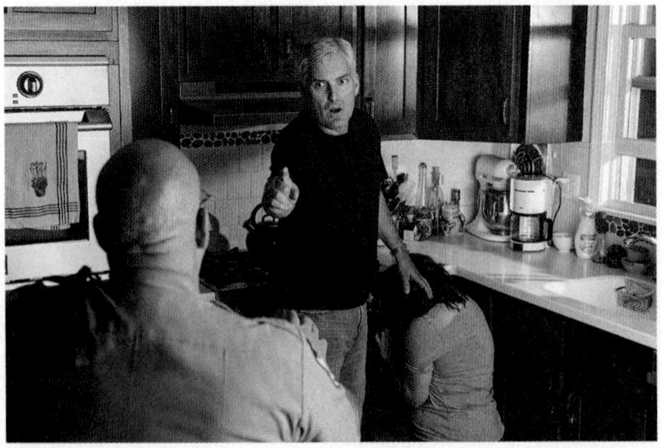

Abuse and Maltreatment

The term *abuse and maltreatment* broadly describes an "act or series of acts of commission or omission by a caregiver or person in a position of power over the patient that results in harm, potential for harm, or threat of harm to a patient."[1] This umbrella term includes intimate partner violence, elder abuse, child abuse, sexual assault, and human trafficking. While each of these types of abuse and maltreatment has distinct elements, there are some common features related to power and control that surround them all (**FIGURE 49-1**).

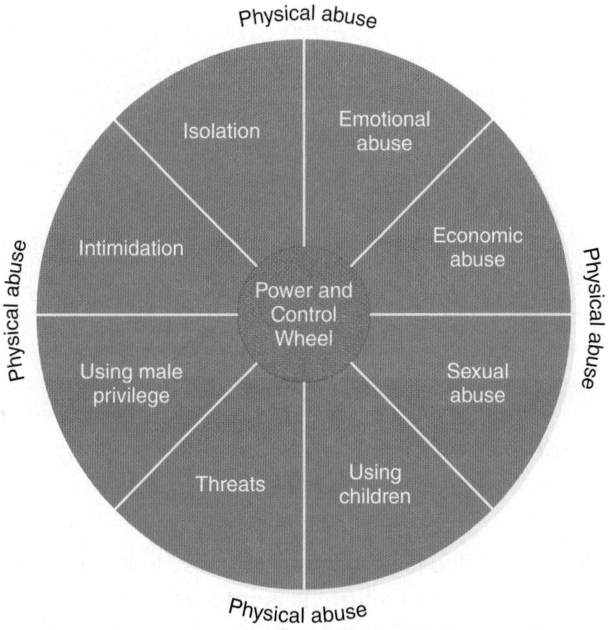

FIGURE 49-1 Relationship of violence to use of power and control.

Reproduced from Peace Over Violence. www.peaceoverviolence.org/iii-the-cycle-of-violence-and-power-and-control/

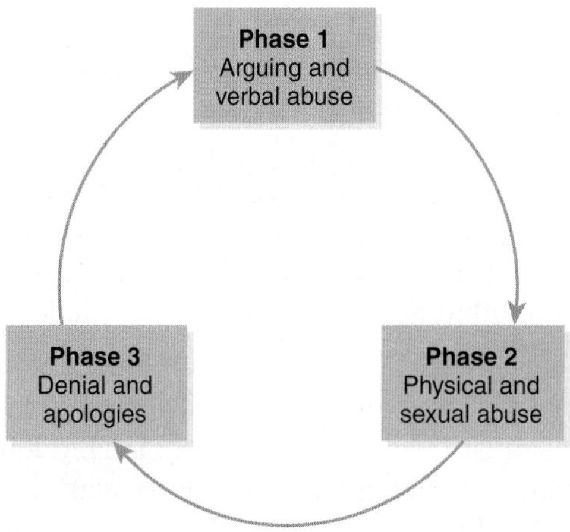

FIGURE 49-2 Cycle of violence.

Intimate Partner Violence

Intimate partner violence (IPV) is known by a variety of terms, including domestic violence. This type of violence occurs between two people in an intimate relationship, and includes opposite- and same-sex partners. It involves relationships where there is the intentional use of tactics to gain and maintain power and control over the thoughts, beliefs, and conduct of an intimate partner.[2] About 20% of homicides are committed by an intimate partner. Domestic violence follows a cycle of three phases (**FIGURE 49-2**).[2] Phase 1 involves arguing and verbal abuse; phase 2 progresses to physical and sexual abuse; and phase 3 consists of denial and apologies (the honeymoon phase). The paramedic best achieves intervention in phase 2 or 3. The cycle repeats itself without intervention and usually increases in frequency and severity. Understanding this cycle of violence will help the paramedic assess the situation and care for the patient.

The paramedic may encounter various types of abuse, including the following:

- **Physical abuse.** Hitting, slapping, shoving, grabbing, pinching, biting, and hair-pulling, for example. Physical abuse also includes denying a partner medical care or forcing alcohol and/or drug use.
- **Verbal abuse.** Attacking the person's self-esteem by degrading name-calling.
- **Sexual abuse.** Coercing or attempting to coerce any sexual contact or behavior without consent.
- **Emotional abuse.** Undermining a person's sense of self-worth and/or self-esteem. This abuse may include, but is not limited to, constant criticism, diminishing one's abilities, making threats, name-calling, or damaging one's relationship with his or her children.

NOTE

Although not usually considered a form of abuse, **stalking** can be defined as a pattern of repeated and unwanted attention, harassment, contact, or any other course of conduct directed at a specific person that would cause a reasonable person to feel fear. Like domestic violence, stalking is a crime of power and control. Each year, 6.6 million people are stalked in the United States. During their lifetimes, 1 in 6 women and 1 in 19 men in the United States will be stalked by an intimate partner. During the course of their careers and when assisting law enforcement personnel at emergency scenes, paramedics will likely encounter people who have been stalked.

Modified from: Stalking. Network of Victim Assistance website. http://www.novabucks.org/otherinformation/stalking/. Accessed April 13, 2018; Centers for Disease Control and Prevention, Division of Violence Prevention. *National Intimate Partner and Sexual Violence Survey: 2010 Summary Report.* Atlanta, GA: Centers for Disease Control and Prevention; 2011. https://www.cdc.gov/violenceprevention/pdf/nisvs_executive_summary-a.pdf. Accessed April 13, 2018.

- **Spiritual abuse.** Preventing a person from practicing his or her religion or forcing him or her to practice another religion.
- **Economic abuse.** Making or attempting to make a person financially dependent by maintaining total control over financial resources; withholding access to money, food, or medications; or forbidding attendance at school or employment.

The violence associated with IPV may not happen often, yet repeated violence from physical and mental abuse (also called **battering**) is a hidden and constant terrorizing factor in some relationships. Over time, the beatings usually become more severe and frequent and often occur without provocation. If children are present in a marriage or relationship, often the violence eventually turns toward them. People involved in abusive relationships often fail to see other options and feel powerless to change the situation.

Women

It is estimated that domestic violence accounts for 4% to 15% of emergency department visits by women. Of women in violent relationships, 77% who present to the ED do so for reasons other than trauma. The percentage of women with domestic violence-related symptoms who present to an ED with any complaint ranges from 22% to 35%, including patients requesting nontrauma, prenatal, or psychiatric care.[3] About one in four women have experienced physical violence by their intimate partner on one or more occasions: many go unreported for the following reasons:[2]

1. Fear for herself or for her children
2. Belief that the offender's behavior will change (abusers often appear charming and loving after the incident of repeated violence)
3. Lack of financial and/or emotional support
4. Belief that she is the cause of the violent behavior
5. Belief that repeated violence is a part of the marriage that must be endured to keep the family together

Women of all cultures, races, occupations, income levels, and ages suffer repeated violence from their past and present husbands, boyfriends, and intimate partners. Because a woman's departure from the abusive relationship can be dangerous, it is important to provide helpful resources for ways to effectively and safely leave the abuser. Approximately 75% of women who are killed by their batterers are murdered when they attempt to leave or after they have left an abusive relationship. Therefore, it is important to provide resources regarding ways to effectively and safely leave the abuser, as described later (**FIGURE 49-3**).[4]

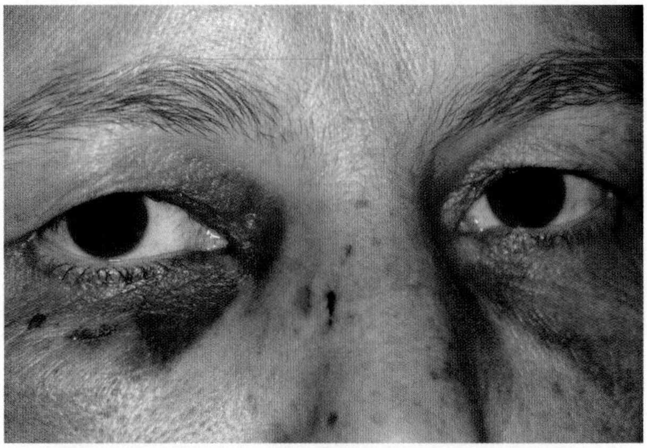

FIGURE 49-3 A woman who has been struck in the face.

NOTE

In 2010, IPV in the United States resulted in the murder of 241 males and 1,095 females. Other consequences of IPV include health conditions such as asthma, cardiovascular disease, gastrointestinal disorders, central nervous system disorders, and reproductive disorders. There is a strong association between IPV and psychological illness such as anxiety, depression, low self-esteem, and suicidal behaviors.

Modified from: National Center for Injury Prevention and Control, Division of Violence Prevention. Violence prevention: intimate partner violence: consequences. Centers for Disease Control and Prevention website. https://www.cdc.gov/violenceprevention/intimatepartnerviolence/consequences. Updated August 22, 2017. Accessed April 13, 2018.

Men

In the United States, one in nine men has experienced severe physical violence by an intimate partner,[5] and one in 71 has experienced rape during their lifetimes. Approximately 8% of men have experienced sexual violence other than rape (forced to penetrate someone, sexual coercion, unwanted sexual contact, and noncontact unwanted sexual experiences) by an intimate partner at some point in their lives (**FIGURE 49-4**).[6] Men report physical violence by a spouse or partner less often than women do, which may be the result of humiliation, guilt, and/or fear to admit loss of control.

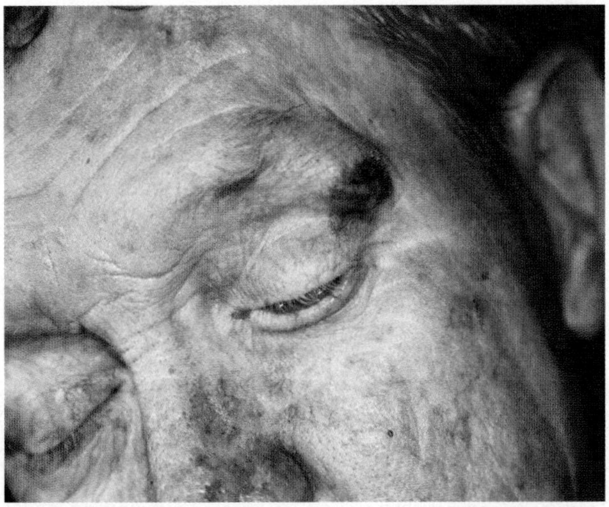

FIGURE 49-4 Soft-tissue injuries from blows to the face.
Courtesy of Rhonda Hunt.

In addition, society may seem to be less empathetic toward men who experience IPV than toward women who experience this type of violence. Communities generally have fewer resources for support.

Characteristics of People in Abusive Relationships

IPV exists among all societal groups and takes place in all settings.[7] However, certain personality traits may draw people into abusive relationships. The following are characteristics of one or both people in an abusive relationship:[8]

1. Alcohol or other drug dependence
2. Low income and unemployment
3. Background of exposure to physical, emotional, or sexual abuse
4. Belonging to a social group of aggressive peers
5. Early aggression, antisocial behavior, and hostility
6. Being a member of a minority group

It is important to note that men and women are equally likely to perpetrate IPV, but men are more likely to use more physical aggression and to cause injuries requiring treatment.[8]

Identifying IPV

The paramedic may have difficulty identifying IPV. Often the description of the injuries may be incorrect, inaccurate, and protective of the attacker. Injuries that are unintentional often involve the extremities and the periphery of the body; however, injuries from domestic violence often involve contusions and lacerations of the face, head, neck, upper arm, breast, and abdomen. Bruises and lacerations may appear to be of varying stages of healing. This presentation is because many people in abusive relationships suffer ongoing abuse but do not always seek medical help for their injuries. Other clues of domestic violence are the following:

- Excessive delays between injury and treatment
- Repeated requests for EMS assistance
- Injuries during pregnancy
- Substance abuse
- Frequent suicide gestures

Scene Safety

The paramedic must ensure scene and personal safety in domestic violence events. If dispatch reveals that the scene involves domestic violence, the paramedic should summon law enforcement personnel. The EMS crew also should not enter the scene until it has been secured. If domestic violence was not suspected until after arriving at the scene, the patient should be removed from the area as soon as possible. Because violence may be directed at EMS personnel, they should avoid confronting the abuser. Situational awareness should be maintained at all times.

Care of the Patient

All injuries should be managed according to established protocols. The abuser often is unwilling to allow the patient to give a history or allow the patient to be alone with EMS personnel; therefore the paramedic should attempt to avoid questioning the patient about possible violence in the presence of the abuser. No display of sympathy should be shown until the patient is in the ambulance or has been separated from the suspected abuser. Special attention should be directed to the emotional needs of the patient.

> CRITICAL THINKING
> If you suspect abuse, what can you say to encourage the patient to talk about it?

The history of the events that led to physical injury should be obtained by using direct questions. Often the patient will avoid eye contact and be hesitant or evasive about details of an injury. Some may offer clues by saying, "Things haven't been going

BOX 49-1 Encouraging Disclosure of IPV

First ask questions such as the following:

- "I am concerned that this injury may have been caused by someone hurting you. Did someone hurt you?"
- "I noticed your partner does not like to leave you alone. How do you feel about that?"
- "Violence against women has become a health care issue; therefore, I ask all my female patients if they have ever experienced abuse/violence as a child, adolescent, or adult."

If the patient answers yes, appropriate follow-up questions must include the following:

- "Are you safe now?"
- "Would you like to talk about it?"
- "Have you talked to anyone else about this?"
- "What do you need right now?"

Modified from: Norris P. Intimate partner violence. In: Brice J, Delbridge TR, Meyers JB, eds. *Emergency Services Clinical Practice and Systems Oversight.* West Sussex, England: John Wiley & Sons, Ltd.; 2015:423-429.

BOX 49-2 National Domestic Violence Hotline

In 1996, the US government established the National Domestic Violence Hotline, a 24-hour toll-free help hotline, through the Violence Against Women Act of 1994. The voice number for the hotline is 1-800-799-SAFE. The TTY (teletypewriter) number for the hard of hearing is 1-800-787-3224. Callers can also live chat in English or Spanish on the National Domestic Violence Hotline's website (www.thehotline.org). The hotline is available 365 days a year and operates throughout the United States, Puerto Rico, and the Virgin Islands. It is staffed by trained advocates who offer crisis intervention, support, and referrals to local services in the caller's community.

Other components of the act include allocating funds for training prosecutors and police, maintaining shelters, and providing educational programs in schools and communities. These programs work with the hotline to treat domestic violence as a serious crime. They also help to prevent domestic violence before it starts.

well lately," or "There have been problems at home" (BOX 49-1). The paramedic should convey to the patient his or her suspicions of repeated violence. The patient may be relieved to know that someone else is aware of the abuse.

During the patient interview, it is important to be nonjudgmental and to avoid comments such as "How awful" or "Why don't you leave?" The paramedic should listen carefully to the patient and offer emotional support. The patient should be strongly encouraged to be transported. These patients should not be left alone at the scene; law enforcement should be advised if transport is refused. Access to community resources should be provided to the patient. These resources include local resources, as well as the Administration for Children and Family's Family Violence Prevention and Services program, the National Women's Health Information Center, the US Department of Justice Office for Victims of Crime, and the US Department of Justice Office on Violence Against Women (BOX 49-2).[9]

CRITICAL THINKING

How would you feel if you were to respond to a call in which a woman has been injured by an abuser but chooses not to leave?

Some patients who have suffered abuse eventually leave the abusive relationship. This act often is made possible by first aid providers and support agency personnel who do the following:

- Treat the patient in a sensitive and sympathetic manner.
- Confirm that the patient is not at fault and does not deserve to be abused.
- Ensure the patient's safety (involve law enforcement).
- Become agents of change in helping provide the support needed for the patient to leave the abusive environment.

Legal Considerations

Physical assault is an intentional act by one person that creates apprehension in another of an imminent harmful or offensive contact. Physical assault is a crime that may be a misdemeanor or a felony, depending on state law, the amount of injury inflicted, and devices that the attacker uses during the assault. Often the attacker is arrested but is released from custody within hours on his or her own recognizance. If early release from custody is likely, the patient must be made aware of this and encouraged to take personal safety precautions.

Many states and local authorities have domestic abuse reporting requirements. Paramedics should be aware of the requirements in their state. EMS personnel are bound professionally to advise medical direction of their suspicions and observations about acts of violence.

Documentation is key. It should include a precise account of injuries, a description of the reported mechanisms of injuries, and a depiction of the behavior of the patient and alleged abuser. Using body diagrams in the patient care report may be helpful. The paramedic should record the patient's own words in quotation marks as part of the narrative when possible and record the names of police officers and witnesses at the scene. These details are important in cases of litigation (see Chapter 4, *Documentation*).

NOTE

The paramedic should document the event as objectively as possible and without bias. This can be done by quoting the patient and/or witnesses, rather than making generalized statements.

Elder and Vulnerable Adult Abuse

Elder abuse (abuse, neglect, exploitation of the older adult) was introduced in Chapter 48, *Geriatrics*. Elder abuse is a prevalent medical and social problem in the United States. Although it is difficult to estimate how many older Americans are abused, neglected, or exploited, studies suggest that as many as 1 in 10 adults aged 60 years and older have experienced some type of elder abuse, but most are never reported.[10] Older adults who are isolated, convalescent, or disabled are more likely to be abused. Almost one-half of those with dementia have experienced some kind of abuse.[11] Perpetrators include children, other family members, and spouses, as well as staff at nursing homes, assisted living facilities, and other facilities. Some risk factors for perpetration include the following:[12]

- Caregiving at an early age
- Inadequate coping skills
- Exposure to abuse as a child

CRITICAL THINKING

Do you think that the problem of elder abuse will increase or decrease during your career in EMS? Why?

Vulnerable Adults

Vulnerable adults are people older than 18 years who have impaired ability to protect themselves from violence, abuse, or neglect. A wide range of people fit within this definition, including people with physical, mental, emotional, or intellectual impairments and people with brain damage. Vulnerable adults include anyone living in a care facility or who is receiving in-home services through a health care agency, hospice, or individual caregiver. Because these people depend on others, and in some cases lack decision-making capacity, they are at risk for abuse or maltreatment similar to the older adult.

Types of Elder and Vulnerable Adult Maltreatment and Abuse

According to the National Center on Elder Abuse, elder abuse may be classified as physical abuse, sexual abuse, emotional/psychological abuse, neglect, abandonment, financial or material exploitation, and self-neglect (**FIGURE 49-5**).[13] (**Self-neglect** refers to behaviors of an older adult that threaten personal health or safety, such as poor nutrition and noncompliance with prescribed drugs.) The person may self-report the abuse, or the paramedic may observe warning signs (**BOX 49-3**). Elder abuse also is classified by where it occurs: in domestic settings or in institutions.

Although physical abuse may include bruising, many older adults frequently have accidental bruising; therefore, the paramedic should recognize some key features that can help distinguish accidental versus

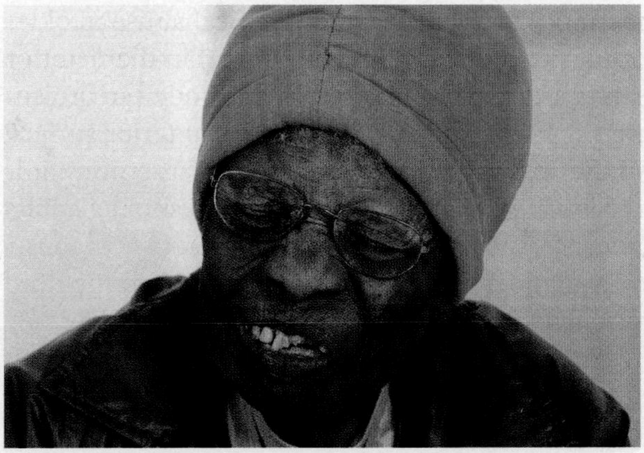

FIGURE 49-5 Signs of self-neglect include evidence of lack of hygiene, poor dental hygiene, and poor nutrition.

BOX 49-3 Signs and Symptoms of Elder Abuse

Signs of Physical Abuse

Bruises
Broken bones
Burns
Abrasions
Pressure marks
Odd explanations for injuries

Signs of Neglect

Dirty clothes
Soiled diapers
Bedsores
Unusual weight loss
A home that is unusually messy, especially if it was not before
Lack of needed medical aids, such as hearing aid, cane, glasses

Signs of Verbal or Emotional Abuse

Withdrawal and apathy
Unusual behavior, such as biting or rocking
Nervous or fearful behavior, especially around the caregiver
Strained or tense relationship between the caregiver and the older adult
Caregiver who is snapping or yelling at the older adult
Forced isolation by the family member or caregiver

Signs of Sexual Abuse

Bruises around the breasts
Bruises around the genital area
Evidence of venereal disease
Vaginal or rectal bleeding
Difficulty walking or standing
Depressed or withdrawn behavior
Flirtation or touchiness by the caregiver

Signs of Financial Exploitation

Bills not being paid
Money disappearing and unaccounted for
Caregiver taking money for a purchase that does not arrive
Unusual purchases
Increased use of credit cards
More frequent withdrawals of cash
Adding someone new to bank accounts or credit cards

Reproduced from: Speicher J. Five signs of elder abuse: five red flags that could signal neglect, mistreatment, or abuse. Caring.com website. https://www.caring.com/articles/signs-of-elder-abuse. Accessed April 13, 2018.

intentional bruising in the older adult. With regard to accidental bruising, color does not indicate the age of the injury, and about 90% of accidental bruises are on the extremities. Less than one-fourth of older adults can recall how they sustained an accidental bruise. More bruising is likely when an adult takes anticoagulant medication, such as dabigatran or warfarin. Bruises related to physical abuse in older adults are typically 2 inches (5 cm) in diameter or larger and can be anywhere on the body, but bruises on the lateral side of the face, the anterior surface of the arm, or the back require special scrutiny. It is essential, when possible, to privately ask older adults how they sustained their bruises. In the case of abuse, 90% of older adults, including those with memory problems and dementia, are able to report how they received the bruises.[14]

Domestic Settings

In a domestic setting, the average age of an abused older adult is about 78 years. The National Center on Elder Abuse provides data regarding types of elder abuse in domestic settings.[15] The abused older adult usually has multiple, chronic health conditions that make him or her dependent on others for care. Widows older than 75 years carry the greatest risk of elder abuse. Neglect is the most common form of elder abuse in domestic settings; unexplained trauma is the most common finding. Evidence suggests that elder abuse is associated more with the personality of the abuser than with the burden of caring for a sick, dependent person. Almost 60% of elder abuse is committed by a family member. Of these, two-thirds are adult children or spouses.[16] Because of this familial relationship, many older adults do not report the abuse, and many also do not seek medical care for their injuries.

Researchers have adapted a number of existing theories of interpersonal violence to supplement the study of elder abuse and have proposed a range of explanations, including the following:[17]

1. Abusers have learned from the behavior of others around them that violence is a way to solve problems or obtain a desired outcome.
2. Abusers feel they do not receive enough benefit or recognition from their relationship with the

older person, so they resort to violence in an effort to obtain their fair share.

3. A combination of background and current factors, such as recent conflicts and a family history of solving problems through violence, influences the relationship.
4. Abusers use a pattern of coercive tactics to gain and maintain power and control in a relationship.
5. Many factors in elder abuse arise through individual, relationship, community, and societal influences.
6. Elder abuse can be attributed to both the patient's and the abuser's social and biomedical characteristics, the nature of their relationship, and power dynamics within their shared environment of family and friends.

DID YOU KNOW?

About 1.5 million adults 65 years or older are lesbian, gay, bisexual, or transgender. This group is more likely to be abused or maltreated and, conversely, is less likely to ask for or accept help. In one survey of older adults who are lesbian, gay, or bisexual, 65% reported being harassed and 29% had been physically attacked. Some older adults have not disclosed their sexual identity, which subjects them to risk of blackmail and financial exploitation. Abuse related to caregiver homophobia was reported to be 8.3% in one study. The risk appears to be even higher in transgender patients.

Modified from: National Center on Elder Abuse. *Mistreatment of Lesbian, Gay, Bisexual, and Transgender (LGBT) Elders.* Alhambra, CA: National Center on Elder Abuse; 2013. https://ncea.acl.gov/resources/docs/Mistreatment-LGBT-NCEA-2013.pdf. Accessed April 13, 2018.

Institutional Settings

In 2014, there were an estimated 1.4 million residents in US nursing homes. Another 835,200 lived in residential care facilities. These numbers are expected to rise dramatically with the aging baby boomers. Residents in these settings are at risk for intentional harm, physical violence, verbal aggression, or neglect from other residents and paid caregivers, staff, and professionals. It has been reported that one of every three nursing homes in the United States has been cited for an abuse violation, and 2,500 of those caused harm to residents.[18] Clues that may indicate institutional abuse are listed in **TABLE 49-1**.

Legal Considerations

All 50 states have elder abuse statutes. Reporting of suspected elder abuse is mandatory under law in most states. If the paramedic suspects any form of elder abuse, all findings should be carefully documented and reported to the appropriate authorities. Medical direction should be advised, and procedures established by local protocol should be followed.

Child Abuse

In 2016, it was estimated that 1,750 children died because of abuse or neglect in the United States.[19] That same year, child protective service agencies investigated almost 3.5 million reports alleging maltreatment of children, with an estimated 676,000 substantiated. Of the substantiated reports, about three-fourths of the children were neglected, 18.2% were physically abused, and 8.5% were sexually assaulted. US federal law defines child abuse and neglect as "any recent act or failure to act on the part of a parent or caretaker which results in death, serious physical or emotional harm, sexual abuse or exploitation; or an act or failure to act, which presents an imminent risk of serious harm."[18]

NOTE

Young children are the most vulnerable to maltreatment. The Department of Health and Human Services reported that most maltreated children were younger than 3 years of age; the rate of maltreatment was highest for children younger than 1 year.

Modified from: Child maltreatment 2016. US Department of Health and Human Services, Administration for Children and Families, Administration on Children, Youth and Families, Children's Bureau website. https://www.acf.hhs.gov/cb/research-data-technology/statistics-research/child-maltreatment. Accessed April 16, 2018.

Neglect is the most common form of child abuse; however, many children suffer more than one type of abuse. Neglect is the failure to provide physical care (eg, medical care, nutrition, shelter, clothing) or the failure to provide emotional care (ie, indifference and disregard). Most substantiated reports of child abuse or neglect come from professional sources (educators, social services, law enforcement, lawyers, social services staff, and medical personnel).

Characteristics of Abusers

The characteristics of abusers are not related to social class or level of education. Over 90% of child abuse

TABLE 49-1 Characteristics of Abuse and Neglect in Long-Term Care Facilities

Category	Specific Characteristics
Physical condition and quality of care	• Documented but untreated injuries • Undocumented injuries • Multiple, untreated, or undocumented pressure sores • Medical orders not followed • Poor oral care, poor hygiene, and lack of cleanliness of residents • Malnourished residents that have no documentation for low weight • Bruising on nonambulatory residents or bruising that occurs in unusual locations • Family statements and facts concerning poor care • Deficient level of care for residents with nonattentive family members
Facility characteristics	• Unchanged linens • Strong odors (such as urine or feces) • Trash cans that have not been emptied • Food issues (such as smells that come from the cafeteria at all hours or food that has been left on trays) • Past problems • Excessive use of restraints (tied to a wheelchair) • Locking patient in room
Inconsistencies	• Between medical records, statements made by staff members, or observations made by the investigator • Between statements given by different groups • Between the reported time of death and condition of body
Staff behaviors	• Unnecessarily close oversight of the investigator by staff members • Lack of knowledge or concern about a resident • Evasiveness, unintended or purposeful, verbal or nonverbal • Unwillingness of the facility to release medical records

Modified from: Potential markers for elder mistreatment. National Institute of Justice website. https://nij.gov/topics/crime/elder-abuse/pages/potential-markers.aspx. Published January 8, 2008. Accessed April 13, 2018.

involves at least one of the child's parents, relatives, partner of the parent (male partner is most common), family friends, or caregivers.[19,20] Most abusers are between 18 and 44 years of age. Just over one-half are female (usually the child's mother). Neglect often is attributed to female perpetrators, whereas sexual abuse most often is attributed to males.[21] Almost one-half of perpetrators are Caucasian (49.8%), about 20% are African American, and 20% are Hispanic.[18] BOX 49-4 provides other characteristics of child abusers.

BOX 49-4 Characteristics of Child Abusers

- Poor parenting skills
- History of child maltreatment in their family
- Substance abuse or mental health issues
- Young age, low income, single parent, large number of dependent children
- Nonbiologic, transient caregivers in the home (eg, mother's male partner)
- Parental thoughts or emotions that support or justify maltreatment
- Social isolation

Modified from: National Center for Injury Prevention and Control, Division of Violence Prevention. Violence prevention: child abuse and neglect: risk and protective factors. Centers for Disease Control and Prevention website. https://www.cdc.gov/violenceprevention/childmaltreatment/riskprotectivefactors.html. Updated April 18, 2017. Accessed April 13, 2018.

CRITICAL THINKING

How does it make you feel when you hear a story about child abuse on the news? Think about how you will manage those feelings when you are at a scene with a child who has been abused.

Because many abusers were severely punished and beaten as children by their parents, they often prefer to use other forms of discipline for their children. But the stresses of child rearing eventually culminate in some parents regressing to the earliest patterns of discipline that they experienced as a child. The abusive adult sometimes is aware of this cyclical nature and may try to seek help to prevent abusive behavior toward his or her children. During this preabuse state, the following pattern often occurs:

1. The adult makes several calls for help within a 24-hour period to 9-1-1 or support agencies.
2. The adult frequently calls EMS for inconsequential symptoms.
3. The adult begins to exhibit behavior of being unable to handle an impending crisis.

The preabuse state is important in identifying the potential for abuse. The pattern is often repetitive and results in frequent calls for EMS to visit the patient's home. The paramedic should remember that this behavior indicates the adult's awareness that child abuse is likely to occur. It also means that the adult is actively seeking help to prevent the abuse.

SHOW ME THE EVIDENCE

Researchers in Connecticut had 28 EMS providers (16 emergency medical technicians and 12 paramedics) participate in a simulation exercise that involved a seizing infant with bruising over the ear and back. After the simulation, participants were interviewed. The researchers' goal was to explore barriers and facilitators to the recognition and reporting of child abuse and neglect. The EMS providers described three main tasks when caring for a child whom they suspect to have been maltreated: (1) providing medical management, (2) evaluating the scene and family interactions for indicators of child abuse or neglect, and (3) creating a safety plan (including notification of suspicions of abuse). The barriers to reporting included discomfort with caring for children, difficulty distinguishing between unintentional injury and child abuse, fear of being wrong, fear of caregiver reactions, and working in a fast-paced environment. The people who felt more comfortable reporting suspected child abuse and neglect were those who understood their mandated reporter role, who could talk about it with peers, and who had supervisor support.

Modified from: Tiyyagura GK, Gawel M, Alphonso A, Koziel J, Bilodeau K, Bechtel K. Barriers and facilitators to recognition and reporting of child abuse by prehospital providers. *Prehosp Emerg Care.* 2017;21(1):46-53.

Characteristics of Abused Children

Abused children often display behavior that provides important clues about abuse and neglect (BOX 49-5). Although this behavior may be age related, the paramedic should carefully observe the child younger than 6 years who is excessively passive, the child older than 6 years who is excessively aggressive, and the child of any age with the following characteristics:

- Does not mind if his or her parents leave the room
- Cries hopelessly during treatment or cries very little when crying would be expected
- Does not look at parents for reassurance
- Is wary of physical contact
- Is extremely apprehensive
- Appears constantly on the alert for danger
- Constantly seeks favors, food, or comfort items (eg, blankets, toys)

Physical Examination

Injuries during childhood are common. Most injuries are unintentional and not the result of abuse. Distinguishing between an intentional and an unintentional injury can be challenging for the paramedic. The most important clues can be obtained by observing the child and his or her relationship with the parent or caregiver and by matching the history of the event

BOX 49-5 Who Are the Abused Children?

- Most abused children are younger than 4 years.
- In regard to age, infants younger than 1 year experience the highest rate of abuse.
- In regard to race/ethnicity, American Indian or Alaska Native children experience the highest rate of victimization.
- Children with special needs such as disabilities, mental health problems, or chronic physical illness are at high risk of abuse.

Modified from: Department of Health and Human Services. *Child Maltreatment 2016*. Washington, DC: Department of Health and Human Services; 2018. https://www.acf.hhs.gov/sites/default/files/cb/cm2016.pdf. Accessed April 13, 2018; and National Center for Injury Prevention and Control, Division of Violence Prevention. Violence prevention: child abuse and neglect: risk and protective factors. Centers for Disease Control and Prevention website. https://www.cdc.gov/violenceprevention/childmaltreatment/riskprotectivefactors.html. Updated April 18, 2017. Accessed April 13, 2018.

to the injury. If the child volunteers the history of the event without hesitation and matches the history that the parent provides (and the history is suitable for the injury), child abuse is unlikely.

NOTE

"Imposters of abuse" include bruises that are common in active children, are associated with disease, or occur from a cultural healing practice such as coin-rubbing or scraping, cupping, and spooning; inflamed tissue from common diaper rash; and variants that may mimic child sexual abuse, such as impetigo and perianal streptococcal infection.

Modified from: Block RW. Child abuse—controversies and imposters. *Curr Probl Pediatr*. 1999 Oct;29(9):249-272.

Infant abuse is more likely to be detected if the baby's clothing is removed or lifted so all skin can be visualized. Additionally, it is essential to complete a thorough head-to-toe examination.

Legal Considerations

When possible, the paramedic should partner with another colleague when performing the examination of a child who is a suspected to have suffered abuse. This approach will help verify that the note taking is objective. The examination also will help ensure that assumptions and personal perceptions do not taint findings. The report must be succinct and legible. The paramedic should document all relevant findings and observations, which includes any statements relevant to the situation that are made by others on the scene—especially other children. Child abuse is a crime that is reportable under law in all 50 states. Paramedics should follow local protocol in reporting suspected child abuse. The requirement for reporting may not be satisfied by the hand-off report at the medical facility. The paramedic attending the child may be required to contact the state abuse hotline to make a report. The paramedic's actions and documentation may be subject to review and evidentiary discovery. As such, the record of the event must clear, objective, and made without bias.

Common Types of Injuries

Common types of injuries associated with child abuse include the following:

- **Soft-tissue injuries.** Soft-tissue injuries are the most common injury seen in cases of child abuse and are often found in early abuse. They may present in various forms, such as multiple bruises and ecchymosis, especially if bruises are extensive and are a mixture of bruises in various stages of healing. Defensive wounds may be found in multiple body planes. There often are **patterned injuries** that result from an identifiable object (eg, bites, loop marks from a cord or belt [**FIGURE 49-6**], cigarette burns, or bristle marks from a hairbrush). In addition, scalds are a common form of abuse in the young and old (**FIGURE 49-7**).
- **Fractures.** Fractures are the second most common injury in cases of child abuse. They often are caused by twisting and jerking forces and may be different ages (new and healed), indicating repeated injury. Rib fractures and multiple fractures are common findings.

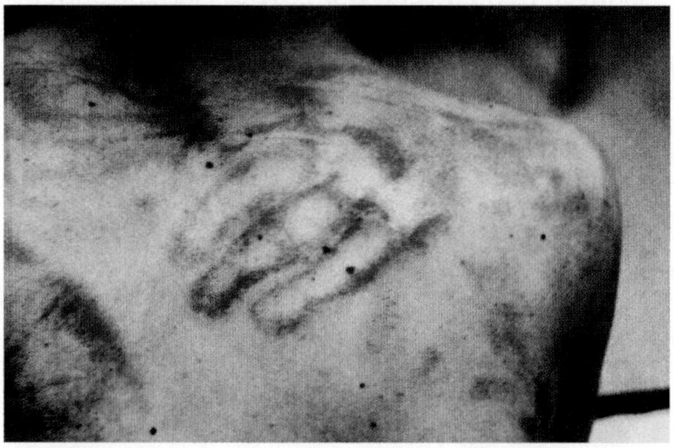

FIGURE 49-6 Patterned injury on a child's back.

Courtesy of Moose Jaw Police Service.

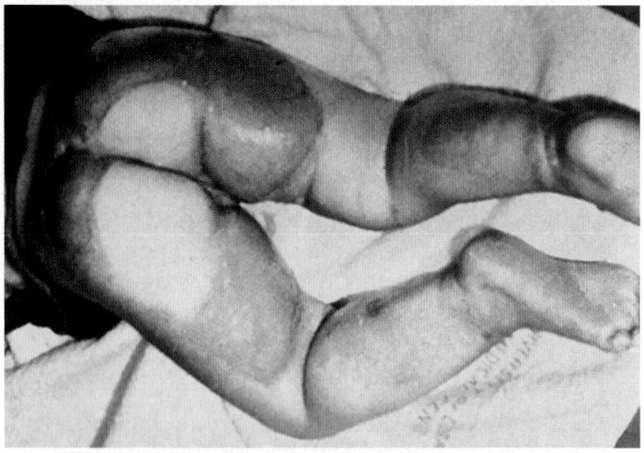

FIGURE 49-7 Bath dipping typically produces scalds on the buttocks and feet with distinct marks.

Courtesy of Health Resources and Services Administration (HRSA), Maternal and Child Health Bureau (MCHB), Emergency Medical Services for Children (EMSC) Program.

- **Head injuries.** Head injury is the most common cause of death in cases of child abuse, and children who survive head injury often have permanent disability. Often, there is a visible progression of injury that begins at the child's trunk and extremities and moves toward the head. Associated injuries include scalp wounds, skull fractures, subdural or subgaleal hematomas, and repeated concussions. Hidden injuries such as bruising behind the ears or in the mouth and a torn frenulum can be easily overlooked.
- **Abdominal injuries.** Abdominal injuries in cases of child abuse are less common than are those injuries just described; however, they often are serious. Blunt trauma to the abdomen may lead to rupture of the liver, spleen, and kidneys as well as injuries to the intestines and mesentery.

Children Who Die From Abuse and Neglect

As stated earlier in this chapter, more than 1,750 children die from child abuse and neglect in the United States each year.[19] Fatal injuries from maltreatment result from many different acts, including the following:

- Severe head trauma (especially in infants)
- Shaken baby syndrome
- Trauma to the abdomen from kicks and punches
- Scalding
- Drowning
- Suffocation
- Poisoning
- Starvation and dehydration

> NOTE
>
> **Shaken baby syndrome (SBS)** is a serious form of child abuse that describes injuries to infants that occur after being violently shaken for as little as 5 seconds. These rapid shakes can cause cerebral hemorrhage, brain damage, blindness, paralysis, and death. SBS most often occurs before 6 months of age but may be seen up to age 5 years. The shaking episode usually results from inconsolable crying. About 1,300 cases of SBS occur in the United States each year. About 25% of those children die, and 80% suffer lifelong disabilities.
>
> *Modified from*: Carbaugh SF. Understanding shaken baby syndrome. *Adv Neonatal Care*. 2004;4(2):105-114; National Center on Shaken Baby Syndrome website. https://www.dontshake.org/learn-more. Accessed April 13, 2018.

Types of neglect that can result in death include the following:

1. **Supervision neglect.** This type of neglect may involve a crucial moment in which the parent or caregiver is absent and the child is killed by a suddenly arising danger (eg, leaving a child unattended in a bathtub).
2. **Chronic neglect.** This type of neglect may result from slowly building problems (eg, malnutrition).
3. **Child physical abuse.** This type of neglect involves fatal parental or caregiver assaults on infants and children. These assaults are triggered by events such as inconsolable crying, feeding difficulties, failed toilet training, exaggerated perceptions of acts of disobedience, and unrealistic expectations for the child's behavior for the child's age group.

Another factor that increases a child's risk of death is living in a home where spouse or partner abuse occurs. Acts of domestic violence toward an adult often are transferred to children living in the household. Studies have shown that frequently an abusive parent who kills a child shares similar characteristics to all abusers.

> CRITICAL THINKING
>
> How can you calm yourself after caring for a child killed by abuse before writing a patient care report that likely will be used as evidence in court?

Sexual Assault

Sexual assault (sexual violence) is a serious crime. It refers to sexual activity when consent is not obtained or not given freely.[22] The number of reported sexual assaults has fallen by more than 50% in recent years. Even so, 324,500 patients aged 12 years or older reported a sexual assault in 2015, and it is estimated that every 98 seconds someone in the United States is sexually assaulted.[23] Approximately 60% of all assaults are not reported to law enforcement personnel.[24] Sexual assault can result in mental or physical injury and death.

Legal Aspects of Sexual Assault

Each state has different interpretations of sexual assault. The term generally refers to any genital, anal, oral, or manual penetration of the person's body by

DID YOU KNOW?

Who Are the Victims of Sexual Assault?

- In the United States, one woman out of every six has experienced an attempted or completed rape in her lifetime.
- In the United States, 17.7 million women have experienced an attempted or completed rape.
- About 3% of men have been sexually assaulted.
- Over one-half of the patients are 18 to 34 years of age.
- Male college students are about five times more likely than are nonstudents of the same age to be raped or sexually assaulted.
- Rates of sexual assault in sexual minority college students are higher than are rates in either male or female heterosexual college students.
- American Indians have double the risk of rape or sexual assault compared to all other races.
- In 2014, 18,900 military personnel experienced unwanted sexual contact.

Effects of Rape

Long-term effects of sexual violence on people include the following:

- People who experience sexual violence are three times more likely to suffer from depression.
- Of women who are raped, 94% experience symptoms of acute stress disorder during the 2 weeks following the rape; in 30%, it persists at 9 months after the rape.
- Of women who are raped, 13% attempt suicide.
- People who have been sexually assaulted are more likely to abuse drugs.
- Of people who have sustained sexual violence, 38% experience work or school problems.

Modified from: About sexual assault. RAINN (Rape, Abuse & Incest National Network) website. https://www.rainn.org/about-sexual-assault. Accessed April 13, 2018.

way of force and without the person's consent. Lack of consent includes the inability to give consent, which may be a result of impaired mental function caused by alcohol and other drugs (flunitrazepam [Rohypnol], gamma-hydroxybutyrate, ketamine), sleep, or unconsciousness. Those cases are referred to as drug-facilitated sexual assault. If a person reports a sexual assault, the paramedic should accept the person's story as accurate. The patient should be encouraged to seek medical care. Ideally, the patient should be transported to a medical facility with specialized personnel (sexual assault nurse examiner) so that evidence of the assault can be collected. In addition, the patient should be accompanied by a local support advocacy group representative, if available.

In many cases, sexual assault is a felony crime that must be proved by evidence. Both the location of the assault and the patient's body are part of the crime scene. Legal considerations for providing care to a patient who has been sexually assaulted include the following:

1. Take steps to preserve evidence.
2. Discourage the patient from urinating or defecating, douching, brushing the teeth, or bathing.
3. Do not give the patient anything to eat or drink.
4. Do not remove evidence from any part of the body that was subjected to sexual contact unless necessary to provide urgent medical care.
5. If clothing or other evidence is removed, place each individual item in a separate paper bag and remain in possession until custody of the evidence is formally turned over to law enforcement.
6. Notify law enforcement personnel as soon as possible, if the patient consents.
7. Be aware that there will be a chain of evidence with specific requirements of proof.
8. Follow local and state requirements in reporting these cases. Consult with medical direction and follow established protocols.

NOTE

In most states, it is the prerogative of the patient whether to report a sexual assault (unless a firearm is involved). If the patient does not want police to be involved and the paramedic summons law enforcement, the paramedic may be violating the patient's rights under the Health Insurance Portability and Accountability Act (see Chapter 6, *Medical and Legal Issues*).

Characteristics of Sexual Assault

Anyone can be sexually assaulted at any age. The person often knows the assailant, and sometimes the person feels shame and personal responsibility for the attack. The methods that the assailant uses to gain control over a person include entrapment, intimidation, and physical force. The assailant may use threats of harm and a weapon to gain submission, particularly when males are assaulted. Males are more likely to suffer significant physical trauma from sexual assault by other males than are females.

The following are common injuries that result from sexual assault:

- Abrasions and bruises on the upper limbs, head, and neck
- Forcible signs of restraint (eg, rope burns and mouth injuries)
- Petechiae of the face and conjunctiva caused by choking
- Human bites
- Broken teeth, swollen jaw or cheekbone, and eye injuries from being punched or slapped in the face
- Anogenital trauma (bruises, abrasions, lacerations)
- Muscle soreness or stiffness in the shoulder, neck, knee, hip, or back from restraint in postures that allow sexual penetration

CRITICAL THINKING

How do you feel when you hear others say, "That woman who was raped brought it on herself"?

Psychosocial Aspects of Care

The trauma of sexual assault creates physical and psychological distress. Some people who have been sexually assaulted may be surprisingly calm and seem in control of their emotions. In contrast, others may be agitated, apprehensive, distraught, or tearful. The paramedic, after managing all threats to life, should proceed with care by providing emotional support to the person. As described in Chapter 30, *Gynecology*, the paramedic should not question patients of sexual assault in detail about the incident in the prehospital setting. Rather, the patient history should be limited to only what is required to provide care. The paramedic's initial contact with the patient should include the following:

- Nonjudgmental and supportive attitude
- Empathetic and sensitive comments
- Quiet speech
- Slow movements
- Considerate gestures (ensure privacy and respect modesty)

The paramedic should move the patient to a safe and quiet environment, which will help to avoid further exposure and embarrassment. When possible, a paramedic of the same sex should provide care. If this is not possible, a chaperone should be present. The patient should not be left unattended. The paramedic should ask for permission to call a friend, family member, or sexual assault crisis advocate. Concerns of the patient about pregnancy and contracting human immunodeficiency virus and other sexually transmitted diseases should be relayed to medical direction. After the patient recovers from physical injury, the goal of treatment is for the patient to regain control of his or her life. Often, doing so requires long-term counseling and support.

Children Who Are Sexually Assaulted

Children are particularly vulnerable to sexual assault and usually have frequent contact with the assailant. Often the assault occurs in a trusted person's home. Most sexual assaults involve a male assailant and a female victim. About 30% of acquaintance sexual assaults occur when the child is between 11 and 17 years of age.[25] Many young children do not think of their experience as a sexual assault because they often are fondled or physically explored without intercourse. As a result, they rarely report the attack and often assume they are to blame. (Many times, children will conceal sexual assault out of fear of punishment.) Children involved in a same-sex assault also are unlikely to report the incident because of confusion or embarrassment. For these reasons, most children who have been sexually assaulted do not receive proper treatment, including prophylaxis and counseling.

Assessment and Patient Care Considerations

Assessment of children who have been sexually assaulted should proceed as described earlier for other patient populations who have been sexually assaulted. The assessment should include age-related considerations that are appropriate for all children. The paramedic should be aware of the following symptoms when caring for any child. These symptoms may indicate behavior or physical manifestations as a result of sexual assault:

- Abrupt behavior changes
- Sleep difficulties, sleep disorders, and nightmares
- Withdrawal from and avoidance of friends and family

- Low self-esteem or a desire to be invisible
- Phobias related to the offender
- Hostility
- Self-destructive behaviors
- Mood swings, depression, and anxiety
- Regression (eg, bed-wetting)
- Truancy
- Eating disorders
- Alcohol or other drug use

The attitude and behavior of adults, including first aid providers, greatly influence a child's impression of the assault. The paramedic should try to lessen the emotional influence of the assault by reassuring the child that he or she is not responsible for the attack. The child should also be assured that he or she did nothing wrong. The child should be encouraged to talk openly about the assault and any concerns that he or she may have.

Legal Considerations

If sexual assault is suspected or confirmed, the paramedic must follow laws that apply to the crime. Local and state laws affect the confidentiality of children. Paramedics should be aware of the regulations in their community and consult with medical direction. It is worth noting that paramedics have a high likelihood of being called to serve as a witness to the event. Because the paramedic is usually one of the first medical providers who assessed the patient, his or her testimony can be very influential. For this reason, solid, defendable documentation is essential.

Human Trafficking

Human trafficking is the illegal exploitation of a person. It is considered modern-day slavery. Human trafficking occurs when a person is exploited through force, fraud, or coercion. People are forced into sex trafficking, forced labor, and domestic servitude. Trafficking can happen in urban, suburban, and rural areas and involve people of either sex and any age or nationality. Paramedics are in a position to detect and report cases of suspected human trafficking, as they may encounter people being exploited at truck stops, rest areas, or workplaces, or in private homes. When it is suspected, the paramedic should not confront the suspected trafficker and should notify law enforcement.

Signs of human trafficking are subtle and may include the following:[26]

- A person who has recently been disconnected from his or her family or social network
- A child who stops attending school
- A child younger than 18 years who is involved in commercial sex acts
- Signs of mental or physical abuse
- A child who seems fearful, timid, or submissive
- Signs of physical or medical neglect

Questions a paramedic might consider when evaluating a person whom he or she suspects is involved in human trafficking include the following:

- Does the person appear to be controlled by another person?
- Does the person seem to be coached about what to say?
- Are the living conditions inappropriate?
- Does the person appear to lack personal possessions?
- Does the person not appear to be free to move about or leave (ie, existence of surveillance equipment or unusual locks or security measures)?

The Department of Homeland Security has developed awareness and educational materials through its Blue Campaign. It also provides support hotlines, which are available by calling 1-888-373-7888 or by texting HELP or INFO to BeFree (233733).

Summary

- Abuse and maltreatment broadly describes an "act or series of acts of commission or omission by a caregiver or person in a position of power over the patient that results in harm, potential for harm, or threat of harm to a patient." This phrase includes intimate partner violence (IPV), elder abuse, child abuse, sexual assault, and human trafficking.
- IPV (also known as domestic violence) follows a cycle of three phases. Phase 1 involves arguing and verbal abuse. Phase 2 progresses to physical and sexual abuse. Phase 3 consists of denial and apologies. Certain personality traits may predispose a person to abusive relationships.
- The paramedic may have a hard time identifying a patient who has experienced IPV. Injuries from domestic violence often involve contusions and lacerations of the face, neck, head, breast, and abdomen.
- The paramedic must ensure scene and personal safety in domestic violence events. If a scene involves domestic violence, the paramedic should summon law enforcement personnel and not enter the scene until it has been secured.
- In domestic violence events, the paramedic should not question the patient in the presence of the abuser. No display of sympathy should be shown until the patient has been separated from the suspected abuser. The paramedic should direct special attention toward the emotional needs of the patient.
- Elder abuse is classified into seven categories: physical abuse, sexual abuse, emotional/psychological abuse, neglect, abandonment, financial or material exploitation, and self-neglect.
- All 50 states have elder abuse statutes. Reporting of suspected elder abuse also is mandatory under law in most states.
- Ninety percent of child abuse involves at least one of the child's parents, relatives, partner of the parent, family friends, or caregivers. Abused children often exhibit behavior that provides key clues about abuse and neglect. The paramedic should carefully observe the child younger than 6 years who is passive or the child older than 6 years who is aggressive.
- If the child volunteers the history of the event without hesitation and matches the history that the parent provides (and the history is suitable for the injury), child abuse is unlikely.
- Injuries may include soft-tissue injuries, fractures, head injuries, and abdominal injuries.
- Sexual assault generally refers to any genital, anal, oral, or manual penetration of the person's body by way of force and without the person's consent.
- After managing all threats to life, the paramedic should provide emotional support to the patient. The paramedic should deliver care in a way that preserves evidence.
- Human trafficking occurs when a person is exploited through force, fraud, or coercion. It involves people of either sex and any age or nationality. When human trafficking is suspected, the paramedic should notify law enforcement.
- Documentation is essential for the paramedic, because he or she may serve in legal proceedings.

References

1. National Association of EMS Officials. *National Model EMS Clinical Guidelines*. Version 2.0. National Association of EMS Officials website. https://www.nasemso.org/documents/National-Model-EMS-Clinical-Guidelines-Version2-Sept2017.pdf. Published September 2017. Accessed April 13, 2018.
2. Norris P. Intimate partner violence. In: Brice J, Delbridge TR, Meyers JB, eds. *Emergency Services Clinical Practice and Systems Oversight.* West Sussex, England: John Wiley & Sons; 2015;423-429.
3. Barkley Burnett L. Domestic violence. Medscape website. http://www.emedicine.medscape.com/article/805546-overview. Updated June 28, 2017. Accessed April 16, 2018.
4. Domestic violence 101. Building Futures website. http://www.bfwc.org/pdf/DV%20101.pdf. Accessed April 13, 2018.
5. National Center for Injury Prevention and Control, Division of Violence Prevention. Violence prevention: facts everyone should know about intimate partner violence, sexual violence, and stalking. Centers for Disease Control and Prevention website. https://www.cdc.gov/violenceprevention/nisvs/infographic.html. Updated April 28, 2017.
6. Male victims of intimate partner violence. National Coalition Against Domestic Violence website. https://www.speakcdn.com/assets/2497/male_victims_of_intimate_partner_violence.pdf. Accessed April 16, 2018.
7. Understanding and addressing violence against women: Intimate Partner Violence. World Health Organization. http://apps.who.int/iris/bitstream/handle/10665/77432/WHO_RHR_12.36_eng.pdf;jsessionid=A0767951D98A74EDEE2741C78C9D50BD?sequence=1. 2012. WHO/RHR/12.36. Accessed May 30, 2018.
8. Capaldi DM, Knoble NB, Shortt JW, Kim HK. A systematic review of risk factors for intimate partner violence. *Partner Abuse*. 2012;3(2):231-280.
9. National Center for Injury Prevention and Control, Division of Violence Prevention. Violence prevention: intimate partner violence: additional resources. Centers for Disease Control and Prevention website. https://www.cdc.gov/violenceprevention/intimatepartnerviolence/resources.html. Updated January 9, 2018. Accessed April 13, 2018.
10. Elder abuse facts: what is elder abuse? National Council on Aging website. https://www.ncoa.org/public-policy-action/elder-justice/elder-abuse-facts/. Accessed April 13, 2018.
11. Research: statistics/data. National Center on Elder Abuse website. https://ncea.acl.gov/whatwedo/research/statistics.html. Accessed April 13, 2018.
12. National Center for Injury Prevention and Control, Division of Violence Prevention. Violence prevention: elder abuse: risk and protective factors. Centers for Disease Control and

Prevention website. https://www.cdc.gov/violenceprevention/elderabuse/riskprotectivefactors.html. Updated June 8, 2017. Accessed April 13, 2018.

13. Frequently asked questions: types of elder abuse. National Center on Elder Abuse website. https://ncea.acl.gov/faq/abusetypes.html. Accessed April 13, 2018.
14. National Center on Elder Abuse. *Research to Practice Translation: Bruising on Older Adults: Accidental Bruising and Bruising From Physical Abuse.* Alhambra, CA: National Center on Elder Abuse; 2014. https://ncea.acl.gov/resources/docs/Research-Translation-bruising-NCEA-2014.pdf. Accessed April 13, 2018.
15. National Center on Elder Abuse. *Types of Elder Abuse in Domestic Settings.* Alhambra, CA: National Center on Elder Abuse; 1999. https://ncea.acl.gov/whatwedo/research/statistics.html#impact. Accessed April 13, 2018.
16. Elder abuse facts: what is elder abuse? National Council on Aging website. https://www.ncoa.org/public-policy-action/elder-justice/elder-abuse-facts/. Accessed April 13, 2018.
17. Causes and characteristics of elder abuse. National Institute of Justice website. https://www.nij.gov/topics/crime/elder-abuse/Pages/understanding-causes.aspx. Published January 7, 2013. Accessed April 13, 2018.
18. Carroll R, American Society for Healthcare Risk Management. *Risk Management Handbook for Health Care Organizations.* Hoboken, NJ: John Wiley & Sons; 2011.
19. Department of Health and Human Services. *Child Maltreatment 2016.* Washington, DC: Department of Health and Human Services; 2016. https://www.acf.hhs.gov/sites/default/files/cb/cm2016.pdf. Accessed April 13, 2018.
20. Centers for Disease Control and Prevention. *Child Maltreatment: Facts at a Glance.* Atlanta, GA: Centers for Disease Control and Prevention; 2014. https://www.cdc.gov/violenceprevention/pdf/childmaltreatment-facts-at-a-glance.pdf. Accessed April 13, 2018.
21. Alexander LL, LaRosa JH, Bader H, Garfield S. *New Dimensions in Women's Health.* 5th ed. Burlington, MA: Jones & Bartlett Learning; 2010.
22. National Center for Injury Prevention and Control, Division of Violence Prevention. Violence prevention: sexual violence. Centers for Disease Control and Prevention website. https://www.cdc.gov/violenceprevention/sexualviolence/index.html. Updated April 10, 2018. Accessed April 13, 2018.
23. Scope of the problem: statistics. Rape, Abuse & Incest National Network (RAINN) website. https://www.rainn.org/statistics/scope-problem. Accessed April 13, 2018.
24. Rape and sexual assault. Bureau of Justice Statistics website. https://www.bjs.gov/index.cfm?ty=tp&tid=317. Accessed April 13, 2018.
25. National Sexual Violence Resource Center. *Statistics About Sexual Violence.* Harrisburg, PA: National Sexual Violence Resource Center; 2015. https://www.nsvrc.org/sites/default/files/publications_nsvrc_factsheet_media-packet_statistics-about-sexual-violence_0.pdf. Accessed April 13, 2018.
26. About the Blue Campaign. US Department of Homeland Security website. https://www.dhs.gov/blue-campaign/about-blue-campaign. Accessed April 13, 2018.

Suggested Readings

Breckman R, Burnes D, Ross S, et al. When helping hurts: nonabusing family, friends, and neighbors in the lives of elder mistreatment victims. *Gerontologist.* 2017.

Burnes D, Lachs MS, Burnette D, Pillemer K. Varying appraisals of elder mistreatment among victims: findings from a population-based study. *J Gerontol Ser B.* 2017.

Campbell JC, Messing JT. *Assessing Dangerousness: Domestic Violence Offenders and Child Abusers.* 3rd ed. New York, NY: Springer Publishing; 2017.

Clark JR. Reporting abuse. *Air Med J.* 2017;36(6):287-289.

Harning AT. (2015) Provide emotional first aid when responding to sexually assaulted patients. *JEMS* website. http://www.jems.com/articles/print/volume-40/issue-10/features/provide-emotional-first-aid-when-responding-to-sexually-assaulted-patients.html. Published September 28, 2015. Accessed April 13, 2018.

McGregor MJ, Wiebe E, Marion SA, Livingstone C. Why don't more women report sexual assault to the police? *CMAJ.* 2000;162(5):659-660.

Patten SB, Gatz YK, Jones B, Thomas DL. Posttraumatic stress disorder and the treatment of sexual abuse, social work. *McGill J Med.* 1989;34(3):111-118.

Rosen T, Lien C, Stern ME, et al. Emergency medical services perspectives on identifying and reporting victims of elder abuse, neglect, and self-neglect. *J Emerg Med.* 2017 Oct;53(4):573-582.

Stevens AL, Herrenhohl TI, Mason WA, Smith GL, Klevens J, Merrick MT. Developmental effects of childhood household adversity, transitions, and relationship quality on adult outcomes of socioeconomic status: effects of substantiated child maltreatment. *Child Abuse Negl.* 2018;79:42-50.

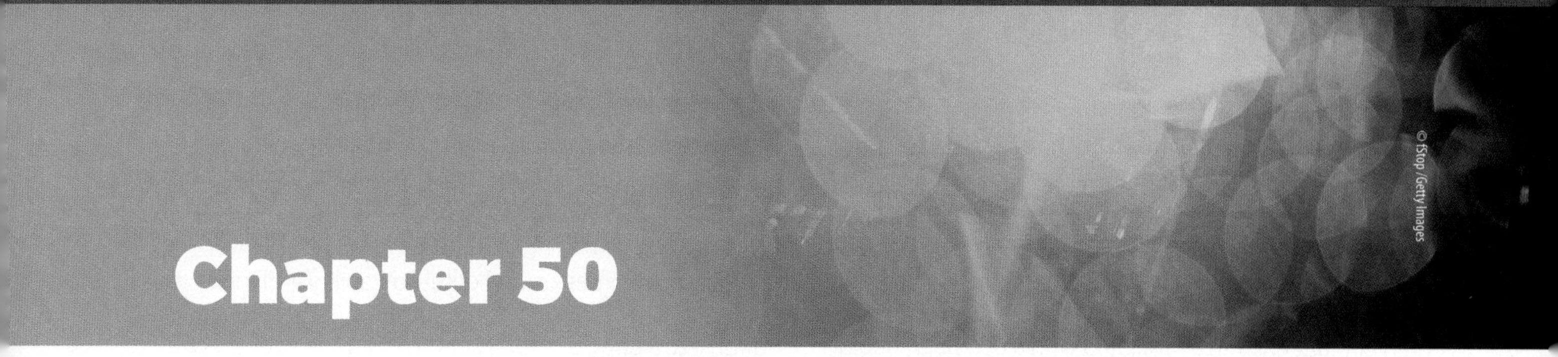

Chapter 50

Patients With Special Challenges

NATIONAL EMS EDUCATION STANDARD COMPETENCIES

Special Patient Populations

Integrates assessment findings with principles of pathophysiology and knowledge of psychosocial needs to formulate a field impression and implement a comprehensive treatment/disposition plan for patients with special needs.

Patients With Special Challenges

Recognizing and reporting abuse and neglect (see Chapter 49, *Abuse and Neglect*)
Health care implications of
- Abuse (see Chapter 49, *Abuse and Neglect*)
- Neglect (see Chapter 49, *Abuse and Neglect*)
- Homelessness (p 1781)
- Poverty (pp 1780–1781)
- Bariatrics (pp 1768–1772)
- Technology dependent (see Chapter 51, *Acute Interventions for Home Care*)
- Hospice/terminally ill (see Chapter 51, *Acute Interventions for Home Care*)
- Tracheostomy care/dysfunction (see Chapter 51, *Acute Interventions for Home Care*)
- Homecare (see Chapter 51, *Acute Interventions for Home Care*)
- Sensory deficit/loss (pp 1765–1768, 1772, 1777)
- Developmental disability (pp 1772–1776)

Trauma

Integrates assessment findings with principles of epidemiology and pathophysiology to formulate a field impression to implement a comprehensive treatment/disposition plan for an acutely injured patient.

Special Considerations in Trauma

Pathophysiology, assessment, and management of trauma in the
- Pregnant patient (see Chapter 45, *Obstetrics*)
- Pediatric patient (see Chapter 47, *Pediatrics*)
- Geriatric patient (see Chapter 48, *Geriatrics*)
- Cognitively impaired patient (pp 1777–1779)

OBJECTIVES

Upon completion of this chapter, the paramedic student will be able to:
1. Identify considerations in prehospital management related to physical challenges such as hearing, visual, and speech impairments; obesity; and paraplegia or quadriplegia. (pp 1765–1772)
2. Identify considerations in prehospital management of patients who have emotional impairment, mental illness, developmentally disability, or intellectual disability. (pp 1772–1776)
3. Describe special considerations for prehospital management of patients with selected pathologic challenges. (pp 1776–1779)
4. Outline considerations in management of culturally diverse patients. (pp 1779–1780)
5. Describe special considerations in the prehospital management of patients with financial challenges. (pp 1780–1781)
6. Outline characteristics and intervention strategies for high EMS system utilizers. (pp 1781–1782)

KEY TERMS

amblyopia A condition in which the brain favors use of one eye over the eye, potentially causing vision problems and disuse of the unfavored eye; the most common cause of eye vision problems in children; also known as lazy eye.

aphasia A neurologic syndrome that affects a person's ability to express and/or understand written and spoken language; often associated with a cerebrovascular accident or head trauma.

astigmatism A vision condition that causes blurred vision attributable either to the irregular shape of the cornea (the clear front cover of the eye) or sometimes to the curvature of the lens inside the eye. Astigmatism is not distance dependent.

ataxia Failure of muscle coordination.

athetosis A neuromuscular condition characterized by slow, continuous, and involuntary movement of the extremities; a possible consequence of cerebral palsy or other central nervous system abnormality.

bariatrics The field of medicine that focuses on the treatment and control of obesity and diseases associated with obesity.

cataract A loss of transparency of the lens of the eye that results from changes in the delicate protein fibers within the lens.

central hearing loss A hearing impairment caused by damage to the central nervous system rather than to the ear or its structures.

cerebral palsy A developmental disorder that occurs in utero or in the first year of life, in which disturbances in the brain result in issues with movement and posture and limit a person's activity. This disorder may also affect sensation, perception, cognition, communication, and behavior.

chorea A movement disorder that causes involuntary, unpredictable body movements ranging from minor fidgeting to severe, uncontrolled contractions that interfere markedly with gross motor function.

conductive hearing loss The faulty transportation of sound from the outer to the inner ear. This type of deafness often is curable.

cortical vision impairment A temporary or permanent visual impairment caused by the disturbance of the posterior visual pathways and/or the occipital lobes of the brain; the most common cause of permanent visual impairment in children.

cystic fibrosis An inherited metabolic disease of the lungs and digestive system that manifests in childhood; also known as mucoviscidosis.

deafness Profound hearing loss that results in the inability to understand speech even when amplified.

diversity Differences of any kind, including race, class, religion, sex, sexual preference, personal habitat, and physical ability.

Down syndrome A congenital condition characterized by varying degrees of intellectual disability and multiple defects. The cause of this condition is the presence of an extra copy of the 21st chromosome in every cell (trisomy 21).

glaucoma A condition in which intraocular pressure increases and causes damage to the optic nerve.

hearing impairment Any degree of hearing loss that is caused by disruption of the auditory system.

high system utilizer A patient who frequents the emergency department or repeatedly has inpatient stays.

hyperopia A vision condition in which distant objects are seen clearly but close ones do not come into proper focus; also known as farsightedness.

intellectual disability A disorder characterized by below-average intellectual function with deficits or impairments in the ability to learn and adapt socially.

mental illness Any form of psychiatric disorder.

mixed hearing loss A hearing impairment in which damage to both the outer/middle ear systems and the inner ear or auditory nerve results in a combination of sensorineural and conductive hearing loss.

myopia A vision condition in which near objects are seen clearly but distant objects do not come into proper focus; also known as nearsightedness.

obesity A condition in which a person's body weight is 30% over the ideal body weight.

optic nerve atrophy A permanent visual impairment caused by damage to the optic nerve.

optic nerve hypoplasia A congenital condition in which the optic nerve has not developed properly and is too small.

paraplegia Weakness or paralysis of both legs and sometimes part of the trunk.

poverty The scarcity or the lack of a certain amount of material possessions or money.

quadriplegia Weakness or paralysis of all four extremities and the trunk.

retinopathy A group of noninflammatory eye disorders often caused by diabetes mellitus, hypertension, and atherosclerotic vascular disease.

sensorineural hearing loss A type of deafness in which sounds that reach the inner ear fail to be transmitted to the brain because of damage to the structures within the ear or to the acoustic nerve; often incurable.

strabismus A condition of misalignment of the eyes. Both eyes do not properly align with each other when looking at an object.

trisomy 21 A genetic failure where there is a triplet of chromosome 21 rather than the usual pair; the cause of Down syndrome.

Paramedics often provide care to patients with special challenges. The patient groups to be discussed in this chapter include people who have physical, emotional, or pathologic challenges; people who are culturally diverse; and people with financial challenges that may hinder access to health care.

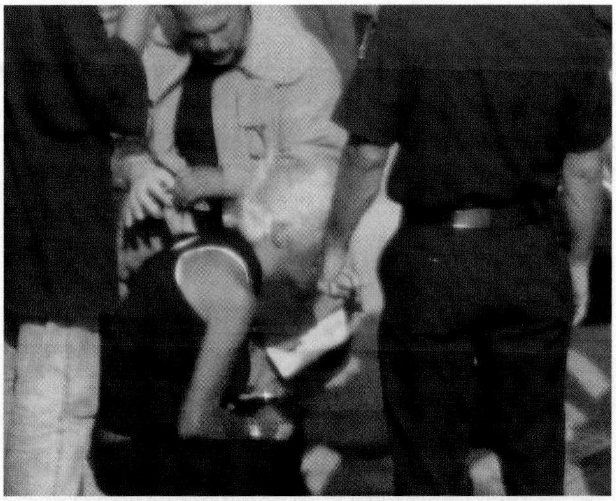

DID YOU KNOW?

- About 20% of Americans (48 million) report some degree of hearing loss.
- At age 65 years, one out of three people has a hearing loss.
- 60% of the people with hearing loss are either in the work force or in educational settings.
- While people in the workplace with the mildest hearing losses show little or no drop in income compared to their peers with normal hearing, as the hearing loss increases, so does the reduction in compensation.
- About 2 to 3 of every 1,000 children in the United States are born with hearing loss that is detectable in one or both ears.
- Almost 15% of children ages 6 to 19 years have some degree of hearing loss.

Reproduced with permission from Hearing Loss Association of America. Accessed at http://www.hearingloss.org/content/basic-facts-about-hearing-loss.

Physical Challenges

Patients who are physically challenged may require special considerations in patient assessment and management. The physical challenges presented in this chapter include hearing, visual, and speech impairments; obesity; and paraplegia or quadriplegia.

Hearing Impairments

Hearing impairment refers to any degree of hearing loss that is caused by disruption of the auditory system.[1] The degree of hearing impairment varies by person and can affect volume and clarity of sound. **Deafness** is a profound hearing loss that results in the inability to understand speech—even when it is amplified. Total deafness is rare and usually congenital. Partial hearing loss may range from mild to severe. It most commonly results from an ear disease, injury, or degeneration of the hearing mechanism that occurs with age. There are four types of hearing loss: conductive, sensorineural, combined conductive and sensorineural (mixed), and central.[2]

Conductive hearing loss refers to the faulty transportation of sound from the outer to the inner ear. This type of hearing loss often is curable. In adults, conductive hearing loss commonly results from the buildup of earwax that blocks the outer ear canal. It can also result from a foreign body, tumor, infection (eg, otitis media), and injury to the eardrum or middle ear (eg, from barotrauma). These causes alter the loudness, but not the clarity, of sound. If correcting the underlying problem does not improve hearing, a hearing aid may be prescribed.

Sensorineural hearing loss often is incurable. In this type of hearing loss, sounds that reach the inner ear fail to be transmitted to the brain. It occurs from damage to the structures within the inner ear or to the acoustic nerve. Sensorineural hearing loss that is present in early life may be congenital. It also can result from a birth injury or from damage to the developing fetus (eg, from premature birth or a mother who has syphilis during pregnancy). Sensorineural hearing loss that occurs in later life may be caused by prolonged exposure to loud noise, disease (eg, Ménière disease), tumors, medications, viral infections, or natural degeneration of the cochlea or labyrinth in old age (presbycusis).

Mixed hearing loss occurs when there is damage to both the outer/middle ear systems and the inner ear or auditory nerve, resulting in a combination of sensorineural and conductive hearing loss. The sensorineural component is permanent, while the conductive component can be either permanent or temporary. For example, a mixed hearing loss can occur when a person with presbycusis also has an ear infection.

Central hearing loss is caused by damage to the central nervous system rather than to the ear or its structures. Conditions such as brain trauma and stroke can lead to central hearing loss.

NOTE

Auditory neuropathy (AN) affects a small group of patients with hearing loss and speech difficulties that are out of proportion with their hearing loss. The ear detects sound but cannot send the sound to the brain. The exact cause of the disease is unknown. Theories include axonal damage to the auditory nerve, damage to inner sensory hair cells in the inner ear, or genetic abnormalities. AN is most common in children but is also diagnosed in adults. In children, AN may lead to developmental speech and language delays (auditory processing deficit) that can affect all levels of learning.

Modified from: Auditory neuropathy. National Institute on Deafness and Other Communication Disorders website. https://www.nidcd.nih.gov/health/auditory-neuropathy. Updated January 26, 2018. Accessed May 3, 2018.

Special Considerations

The paramedic can use several helpful techniques for recognizing a patient who has a hearing impairment. These include noting the presence of hearing-assistive devices and observing the patient for poor diction or the inability to respond to questions in the absence of direct eye contact. Accommodations that may be needed to aid in communication include retrieving the patient's hearing aid or other amplified listening device, and providing paper and pen.

Hearing Assistive Devices. Hearing aids can amplify sound, process signals for speech, and reduce noise, among other features. Several styles are available, including those that fit in or around one or both ears. Surgical interventions to improve hearing (eg, cochlear implants) can be helpful in some patients. All hearing aids have four components: a microphone to detect sound, an amplifier to make sounds louder, a receiver to transmit sounds to the ear, and a battery. Whenever possible, the patient's hearing aids should be transported with the patient. Other assistive devices include telephone or radio amplifiers, telecommunication display devices (TDDs), and hardwired listening devices (to listen to radio or television).

Speech Reading. Speech reading (lipreading) is used by some people with hearing impairment to improve communication. The person interprets speech by observing the speaker's lip movements and nonverbal cues such as facial expression. (Only about one-third of the words in the English language can be recognized through movement of the lips [speech reading].[3]) To promote maximum understanding when caring for a patient who is a speech reader, the paramedic should do the following:

- Assure good lighting.
- Face the patient.
- Be close enough so the patient can see the paramedic's lips clearly.
- Use a natural speaking voice and expression (avoid exaggeration).
- Speak at a normal pace and volume.
- When possible, have a caregiver without a beard or mustache communicate with the patient.
- Avoid distracting movements.
- Avoid chewing anything, including gum, while speaking.
- Assure the patient is looking at the paramedic before the paramedic begins to speak.

Sign Language. Sign language uses hand configurations to convey language. A person with hearing impairment may use several types of sign language to convey speech. American Sign Language has no written form and communicates concepts rather than specific words. Signed English uses hand signals that follow the same structure as the English language. While a person makes the hand signals, he or she mouths the corresponding words. Cued speech uses hand shapes to convey speech sounds. No single type of sign language is universal; different sign languages are used in different countries or regions.[4]

The paramedic must notify the hospital as soon as possible if the patient has profound hearing loss.

Personnel with special training (eg, a certified sign language interpreter) may need to be summoned to assist with patient care. To protect patient privacy, assistance from a trained professional, when available, is preferred to assistance from family or friends.

Visual Impairments

It is estimated that nearly 1.3 million Americans aged 40 years or older are legally blind and that nearly 4.2 million are visually impaired, even with the best correction.[5] Normal vision depends on the uninterrupted passage of light from the front of the eye to the light-sensitive retina at the back. Any condition that obstructs the passage of light from the retina can cause vision loss. Vision impairment may be present at birth from a congenital disorder or result from a number of other causes, including the following:

- Cataracts
- Degeneration of the eyeball, optic nerve, or nerve pathways
- Diseases such as diabetes and hypertension
- Eye or brain injury (eg, trauma, chemical burns, stroke)
- Infections such as those that are caused by cytomegalovirus, herpes simplex virus, and bacterial ulcers
- Vitamin A deficiency in children living in developing countries

Patients with visual impairments may be totally blind or have a partial loss of vision that affects color vision, night vision, binocular vision, central vision, and/or peripheral vision (BOX 50-1). A patient who has central loss of vision is usually aware of the condition. In contrast, loss of peripheral vision often remains unnoticed by the person until it is well advanced. As a result, the paramedic may not recognize this patient's condition as easily.

BOX 50-1 Types of Visual Impairments

amblyopia. A condition in which the brain favors use of one eye over the eye, potentially causing vision problems and disuse of the unfavored eye; the most common cause of eye vision problems in children; also known as lazy eye.

astigmatism. A vision condition that causes blurred vision attributable either to the irregular shape of the cornea (the clear front cover of the eye) or sometimes to the curvature of the lens inside the eye.

cataract. A cloudy or opaque area in the normally clear lens of the eye; most common in people older than 55 years.

cortical vision impairment. A temporary or permanent visual impairment caused by the disturbance of the posterior visual pathways and/or the occipital lobes of the brain; the most common cause of permanent visual impairment in children.

glaucoma. An eye disease in which the internal pressure in the eyes increases enough to damage the nerve fibers in the optic nerve, causing vision loss.

hyperopia. A vision condition in which distant objects are seen clearly but close ones do not come into proper focus; also called farsightedness.

myopia. A vision condition in which near objects are seen clearly but distant objects do not come into proper focus; also called nearsightedness.

optic nerve atrophy. A permanent visual impairment caused by damage to the optic nerve.

optic nerve hypoplasia. A congenital condition in which the optic nerve has not developed properly and is too small.

retinopathy. A general term that refers to some form of noninflammatory damage to the retina of the eye; one of many retinal diseases.

strabismus. A condition of misalignment of the eyes. Both eyes do not properly align with each other when looking at an object.

Modified from: Eye and vision problems. American Optometric Association website. https://www.aoa.org/patients-and-public/eye-and-vision-problems. Accessed May 3, 2018.

Special Considerations

Techniques in assessing and managing patients with vision loss are described in Chapter 16, *Therapeutic Communications.* To review, accommodations that may be necessary for these patients include retrieving visual aids, describing all procedures before performing them, and providing sensory information (eg, location of obstacles) as needed. The paramedic should guide ambulatory patients by "leading," not by "pushing." If possible and appropriate, a patient's guide dog should be permitted to accompany the patient to the hospital. The paramedic should advise medical direction of the patient's special needs so that appropriate personnel can be made available.

Speech Impairments

Speech impairments include disorders of language, articulation, voice production, or fluency (blockage of speech). All of these can lead to an inability to communicate well (BOX 50-2).

BOX 50-2 Types of Speech Impairments

Language Disorders
Brain tumor
Delayed development
Emotional disturbance
Head injury
Hearing loss
Lack of stimulation
Stroke

Articulation Disorders
Damage to nerve pathways passing from the brain to muscles in the larynx, mouth, or lips
Delayed development from hearing problems
Slow maturation of nervous system

Voice Production Disorders
Disorders affecting closure of vocal cords
Hormonal or psychiatric disturbance
Severe hearing loss

Fluency Disorders
Stuttering (for example)
Patient is not fully understood

Language disorders result from damage to the language centers of the brain. They usually result from stroke, head injury, or brain tumor. These patients often exhibit **aphasia** (loss of power of speech) with a slowness to understand speech and problems with vocabulary and sentence structure. Aphasia can affect children and adults. It may affect their ability to speak and to comprehend written or spoken words. Delayed development of language in a child may result from hearing loss, lack of stimulation, or emotional disturbance. It also may result from pragmatic language impairment, a developmental disorder related to autism and Asperger syndrome (described in Chapter 34, *Behavioral and Psychiatric Disorders*).

An articulation disorder is an inability to produce speech sounds. The disorder sometimes is referred to as dysarthria or motor speech disorder. These disorders result from damage to nerve pathways passing from the brain to the muscles of the larynx, mouth, or lips. Often the patient's speech will be slurred, indistinct, slow, or nasal. Disorders of articulation may result from brain injury or from diseases such as multiple sclerosis and Parkinson disease. In children, articulation disorders commonly result from delayed development from hearing problems. Phonologic process disorder is a type of articulation disorder in which there are difficulties with "rules of language," such as combinations of words and syllables. Examples include "top" for "stop," "daw" for "dog," and "tee" for "three."

CRITICAL THINKING

What may cause a paramedic to become impatient when caring for a patient with an articulation disorder?

Voice production disorders are characterized by hoarseness, harshness, inappropriate pitch, and abnormal nasal resonance. They often result from disorders that affect closure of the vocal cords. Some disorders are caused by hormonal or psychiatric disturbances and by severe hearing loss.

Fluency disorders are not well understood. They are marked by repetitions of single sounds or whole words and by the blocking of speech. An example of a fluency disorder is stuttering.

Special Considerations

Once speech impairment has been identified, history taking and assessment need to be modified. Methods include allowing extra time for the patient to respond to questions, clarifying what the patient says or asking the patient to repeat an answer if it was not clearly understood, and offering appropriate aids (eg, pen and paper) to assist in communications. If the patient speech reads, the paramedic should employ the techniques discussed earlier for patients with a hearing impairment. The hospital also should be advised if a patient has a severe speech impairment, so that appropriate personnel (eg, audiologist, speech specialist) can be made available.

Obesity

Obesity is defined as being 30% above ideal body weight. The disease affects more than one-third of the adult American population, and obesity-related diseases such as heart disease, stroke, diabetes, and cancer are among the top causes of mortality in the United States each year.[6] In addition, obesity in US children and teenagers ranges from about 9% in toddlers and preschoolers to between 17% and

20% in adolescents and teenagers.[7] As discussed in Chapter 2, *Well-Being of the Paramedic*, the body mass index (BMI) is used to define ideal body weight, overweight, and obesity ranges. An adult who has a BMI between 25 and 29.9 is considered overweight; a BMI of 30 or higher is considered obese.[8]

Obesity is an abnormally high proportion of fat and cells, mainly in the viscera and the subcutaneous tissues of the body. Although reasons for obesity in some people are unclear, known causes for the condition include the following:

- Caloric intake that exceeds calories expended
- Low basal metabolic rate
- Genetic disposition for obesity

The complications of obesity are many (BOX 50-3). Obesity increases a person's chance of becoming seriously ill. For example, obesity is associated with an increased risk for low quality of life and hypertension, stroke, heart disease, diabetes, and some cancers. Osteoarthritis also is aggravated by increased body weight. The condition is treated with weight-loss programs, exercise, counseling, medications, and sometimes surgery. The goal of treatment is lasting weight loss. The field of medicine that focuses on the treatment and control of obesity and diseases associated with it is known as **bariatrics**.

BOX 50-3 Medical Complications of Obesity

- High low-density lipoprotein cholesterol, low high-density lipoprotein cholesterol, or high triglyceride levels
- Cancer, including endometrial, breast, colon, kidney, gallbladder, and liver
- Depression and anxiety
- Gallbladder disease
- Body pain and difficulty with physical functions
- Heart disease
- High blood pressure
- Osteoarthritis
- Skin problems, such as intertrigo and impaired wound healing
- Sleep apnea and breathing problems
- Stroke
- Type 2 diabetes

Modified from: Division of Nutrition, Physical Activity, and Obesity, National Center for Chronic Disease Prevention and Health Promotion. The health effects of overweight and obesity. Centers for Disease Control and Prevention website. https://www.cdc.gov/healthyweight/effects/index.html. Updated June 5, 2015. Accessed May 3, 2018.

CRITICAL THINKING

How would you respond if a crew member were to make an insensitive remark about a patient's obesity within hearing range of the patient or the patient's family?

Bariatric Surgery

A variety of surgical procedures and intragastric balloon devices can assist the bariatric patient to lose weight (**FIGURE 50-1**). This weight loss can reduce or eliminate a significant number of the health problems associated with morbid obesity. Each procedure has advantages and disadvantages (**TABLE 50-1**). Complications that may initiate an EMS response to the patient's home soon following surgery are most likely related to pain, vomiting or dehydration, electrolyte imbalances, gastric obstruction, reflux or distention, wound infection, sepsis, bleeding, pulmonary embolism, respiratory failure, or pneumonia.[9-11] The incidence of cholecystitis is higher, as is the risk of fractures in many of these patients.

Special Considerations

Obtaining a thorough history is important when caring for a patient with obesity. The history often will be extensive because of associated health problems. The paramedic should be aware that symptoms the patient may credit to obesity (eg, fatigue, shortness of breath at rest or on exertion) may be a sign of an acute illness (eg, heart failure or myocardial infarction).

The examination of a patient with obesity may require some modifications. These may include using large blood pressure cuffs, positioning the patient to better allow for hearing breath sounds, and placing electrocardiogram leads on areas of the body with less fat (eg, the arms and thighs versus the chest wall). When establishing vascular or intraosseous access, a longer catheter or needle may be needed. Advanced airway management procedures may be difficult in patients with morbid obesity. For example, patients with obesity require much greater elevation of their head, neck, and

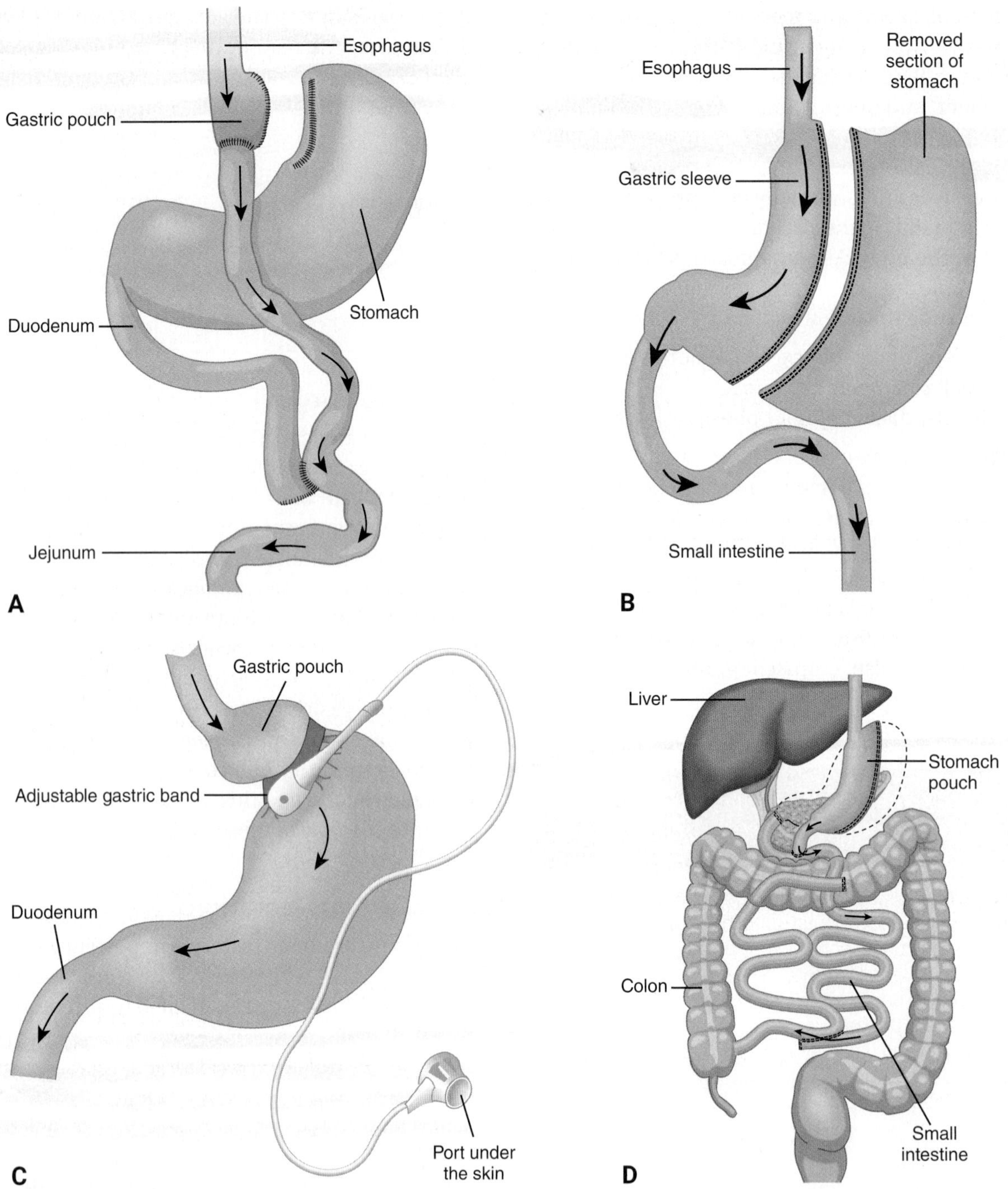

FIGURE 50-1 Types of bariatric weight-reduction procedures. **A.** Gastric bypass (Roux-en-Y gastric bypass). **B.** Sleeve gastrectomy. **C.** Adjustable gastric band (the *band* or the *lap-band*). **D.** Biliopancreatic diversion with duodenal switch.

shoulders to produce the same alignment of axes for intubation.[12] In addition, more personnel and special equipment may be needed to assist with moving the patient for transport (**FIGURE 50-2**). Stretchers that can accommodate excessive weight and wide girth, ambulances equipped with a winch system, and ramps to load and offload the patient safely may be required. Using appropriate lifting devices protects both the patient and the EMS crew. Patients with obesity often are self-conscious about their weight.

TABLE 50-1 Advantages and Disadvantages of Bariatric Weight-Reduction Procedures

Surgery Type	Procedure	Advantages	Disadvantages
Gastric bypass (Roux-en-Y gastric bypass)	A small stomach pouch is created and a piece of the small intestine is attached to the new pouch superiorly and to the rest of the small intestine inferiorly.	60%–80% excess weight loss Limits food consumption Reduces appetite and enhances sense of fullness Often maintains >50% excess weight loss	Complicated surgery with more complications Vitamin/mineral deficiencies (B_{12}, iron, calcium, folate)
Sleeve gastrectomy	About 80% of stomach is removed, and a new banana-sized pouch is created.	Reduces amount of food stomach can hold Decreases hunger, increases sense of fullness Weight loss of >50% with maintenance of >50% Short hospital stay	Nonreversible Potential for long-term vitamin deficiencies Higher earlier complication rate than adjustable gastric band
Adjustable gastric band (band or lap-band)	Inflatable band placed around upper portion of the stomach creates a small pouch above the band.	Reduces amount of food stomach can hold Weight loss 40%–50% No cutting of stomach or intestines Short hospital stay Reversible and adjustable Lowest rate of early postoperative complications and mortality Lowest risk of vitamin/mineral deficiencies	Slower weight loss than other procedures Small risk that band will slip or erode into stomach Esophagus may dilate if patient overeats Need to strictly adhere to dietary restrictions High rate of reoperation
Biliopancreatic diversion with duodenal switch	Size of the stomach is reduced and about three-fourths of the small intestine is bypassed.	60%–70% weight loss Eventually can eat "near normal" meals Reduces fat absorption by 70% Reduces appetite and improves satiety Most effective against diabetes	Highest complication rate Longer hospital stay Greater deficiencies in protein and iron, calcium, zinc, fat-soluble vitamins (eg, vitamin D) Follow-up essential to minimize complications

Modified from: Edwards ED, Jacob BP, Gagner, M, et al. Presentation and management of common post-weight loss surgery problems in the emergency department. *Ann Emerg Med*. 2006;47(2):160-166.

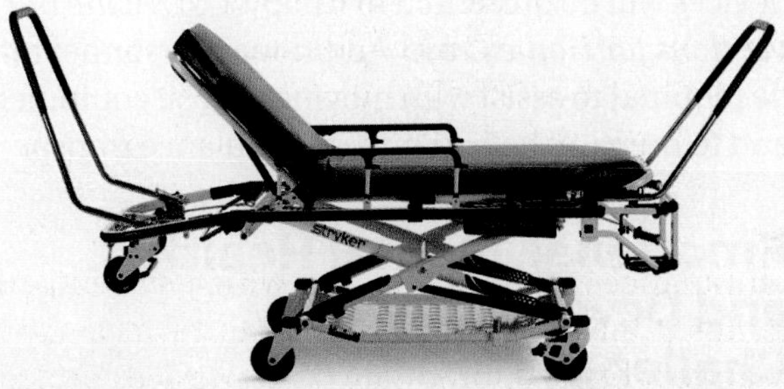

FIGURE 50-2 Bariatric stretcher.

NOTE

Weight limits vary widely for helicopters. When requesting an emergency rotary aircraft flight, the paramedic should inform the dispatcher if the patient has obesity and, to the extent possible, the patient's height and weight. The dispatch center can then consult with the aeromedical service to determine whether the patient can be transported safely by air.

They may worry about the hardships they place on the EMS crew and other rescuers. Paramedics should be sensitive to these concerns.

Patients With Paraplegia/ Quadriplegia

Paraplegia is weakness or paralysis of both legs and sometimes part of the trunk; **quadriplegia** (or tetraplegia) is weakness or paralysis of all four extremities and the trunk. The conditions result from nerve damage in the brain and/or spinal cord usually caused by a vehicle crash, sports injury, fall, or gunshot or stabbing wound. Medical illnesses such as lupus, multiple sclerosis, and stroke also can result in temporary or permanent weakness and paralysis. Paraplegia and quadriplegia often are accompanied by a loss of sensation and loss of bowel and urinary control. Breathing difficulties may be encountered with higher-level injuries. Priapism may be present in some male patients. Complications requiring EMS transport for these patients may include the following:

- Urinary tract infections leading to sepsis
- Pressure injuries from being immobile for prolonged periods
- Deep venous thrombosis and pulmonary emboli
- Respiratory emergencies (pneumonia or other respiratory infections)
- Autonomic dysreflexia (bradycardia, diaphoresis, headache, and extreme hypertension associated with a noxious stimulus [pain, full bladder] that is resolved when the stimulus is relieved)
- Muscle spasticity
- Unrecognized injuries (because of loss of sensation)

NOTE

When performing the physical assessment, the application of pressure that would be appreciated by patients with normal sensation may not be recognized in patients who have weakness or paralysis.

Special Considerations

Patients with extremity and trunk paralysis may require accommodations in patient care. For example, the patient may have a halo traction device to stabilize the spine (**FIGURE 50-3**). Or the patient may rely on a home ventilator to assist with breathing. Both of these situations can complicate airway management and can make patient transport more difficult. Some patients who are paralyzed will have special equipment (eg, walkers, wheelchairs); ostomies for the trachea, bladder, or colon; and medical devices that rely on electricity or a battery supply. (Technology-assisted devices will be presented in Chapter 51, *Acute Interventions for Home Care.*) Additional personnel may be required to assist with moving special equipment and to prepare the patient for ambulance transport.

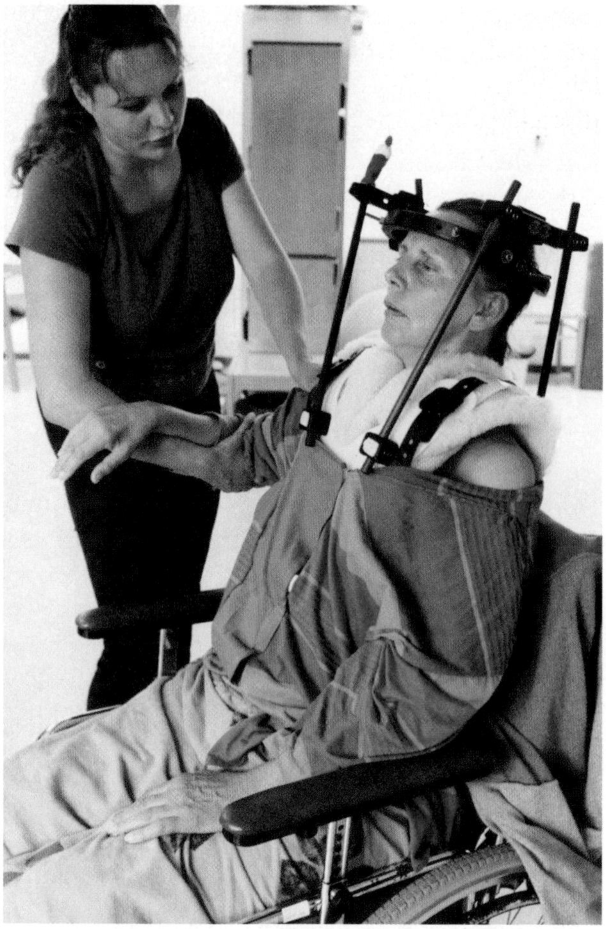

FIGURE 50-3 Halo ring with attached vest.

Emotional, Mental Health, and Developmental Challenges

People who have emotional, behavioral, psychological, psychiatric, or developmental conditions often have increased health needs. The specific patient groups presented in this section include those with emotional impairments, mental health conditions, developmental disabilities, and intellectual disabilities.

Emotional Impairment

People with emotional impairments often have anxiety disorders. These disorders are described in Chapter 34, *Behavioral and Psychiatric Disorders*. They can result in a wide range of physical or mental symptoms attributed to mental stress.

Special Considerations

Distinguishing between symptoms produced by stress and those that indicate serious medical illness may be difficult. Thus management should always focus on the presenting complaint. The paramedic also should assume the most serious cause. As described in Chapter 34, *Behavioral and Psychiatric Disorders*, signs and symptoms that may result from emotional impairment include somatic complaints such as chest discomfort, tachycardia, dyspnea, choking, and syncope. Hence, the paramedic must gather a full history from the patient. A thorough examination also is essential to rule out serious illness. The prehospital care for these patients (in the absence of serious illness) mainly is supportive. It includes calming measures and transport for physician evaluation.

Mental Illness

Mental illness refers to any form of psychiatric disorder. As described in Chapter 34, *Behavioral and Psychiatric Disorders*, most forms of mental illness result from biologic, psychosocial, or sociocultural causes. A person's mental illness may result from more than one of these factors. To review, biologic causes of mental illness result from biochemical imbalance or from organic causes such as trauma, illness, and dementia; examples of these conditions are schizophrenia and depression. Psychosocial causes of mental illness can result from childhood trauma, child abuse or neglect, a dysfunctional family structure, or other issues that cause an inability to resolve situational conflicts in a person's life. Sociocultural causes of mental illness may be related to personal relationships, family stability, economic status, and other factors that result in situational stress.

Special Considerations

Recognizing a patient with mental illness may be difficult. Other patients with more serious disorders may have signs and symptoms that are consistent with mental illness. (An example is paranoid behavior in patients with schizophrenia.) When obtaining the patient history, the paramedic should not hesitate to ask about the following:

- History of mental illness
- Prescribed medications
- Compliance with prescribed medications
- Use of over-the-counter herbal products (eg, St. John's wort)
- Concomitant use of alcohol or other drugs

If the patient is anxious, the paramedic should ask the patient's permission before performing any assessment or procedure. Ask, "What happened to you?" instead of "What's wrong with you?" This will help to establish rapport and trust during the care. Unless the call is related specifically to the mental illness, care should proceed in the same manner as for any other patient. Patients with mental illness experience medical illness at a higher rate than do other patient groups.[13] If the patient acts aggressively or combatively, the paramedic should retreat from the scene and request law enforcement personnel to secure the scene.

Developmental Disability

A person who is developmentally disabled has impaired or insufficient development of the brain. This condition may cause an inability to learn at the usual rate (developmental delay), to develop language skills, and to develop age-appropriate physical milestones or behaviors. Developmental delay has many causes, including the following:

- Use of alcohol or other drugs by the mother during pregnancy[14]
- Lack of stimulation (as seen with child abuse or neglect)
- Infection in utero or after birth
- Genetic and chromosomal defects
- Untreated jaundice after birth
- Brain damage before, during, or after birth

People who are developmentally disabled may function well with daily activities, hold jobs, and live independently (or with their family or in residential group homes). However, some developmental delays may be severe and may affect any or all of the major areas of human achievement: walking upright; fine eye–hand coordination; listening, language, and speech; and social interaction. About 1 in 6 children aged 3 to 17 years in the United Sates has one or more developmental disabilities, including the following:[14]

- Attention-deficit/hyperactivity disorder
- Autism spectrum disorder
- Cerebral palsy
- Hearing loss
- Intellectual disability
- Learning disability
- Vision impairment
- Other delays

The accommodations that may be needed when caring for these patients will vary depending on the severity of disability. The paramedic should allow extra time for obtaining a history and performing an examination. Additional time should also be allotted for preparing the patient for transport. When possible, a member of the patient's family or a caregiver should remain with the patient during the care.

CRITICAL THINKING

Do you think a patient with developmental disability should have any input into his or her own care? Why?

Down Syndrome

Down syndrome results from an abnormal complement of chromosomes. This abnormality causes mild to severe intellectual impairment and a characteristic physical appearance (**FIGURE 50-4**). The child with Down syndrome has features that typically include the following:

- Eyes that slope upward at the outer corners
- Folds of skin on either side of the nose that cover the inner corners of the eyes
- A small face and small facial features
- A large and protruding tongue
- Flattening on the back of the head
- Hands that are short and broad and may have only one palmar crease

In most cases, Down syndrome occurs from the failure of the two chromosomes numbered 21 in a parent cell to go into separate daughter cells during the first stage of sperm or egg cell formation. This results in a triplet of chromosome 21 (**trisomy 21**) rather than the usual pair. The extra number 21 chromosome is passed on to the child and leads to Down syndrome. The incidence of affected fetuses increases with increased maternal age (mothers older than 35 years). It also increases with a family history of Down syndrome.[15]

FIGURE 50-4 Child with Down syndrome.

NOTE

In the general population, trisomy 21 occurs in about 1 of about 700 live births. It is the most common chromosomal disorder. Because older maternal age increases the risk of having a child with Down syndrome, pregnant women older than 35 years are tested to assess for the abnormality.

Modified from: Division of Birth Defects and Developmental Disabilities, National Center on Birth Defects and Developmental Disabilities, Centers for Disease Control and Prevention. Birth defects: data and statistics. Centers for Disease Control and Prevention website. https://www.cdc.gov/ncbddd/birthdefects/downsyndrome/data.html. Updated June 27, 2017. Accessed May 3, 2018.

People with Down syndrome now have life expectancies of 60 or more years. Adults with Down syndrome are at age-related increased risk for dementia, skin and hair changes, early onset menopause, visual and hearing impairments, adult-onset seizure disorder, thyroid dysfunction, diabetes, obesity, sleep apnea, and musculoskeletal problems.[16] Many are cared for at home, and others live in assisted care facilities. About 50% of children born with Down syndrome

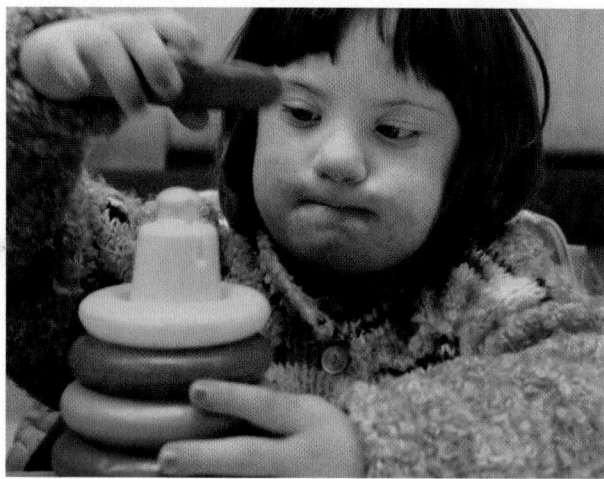

have a heart defect at birth. Many have congenital intestinal disorders, hearing defects, and other illnesses. The degree of mental disability varies, with an intelligence quotient (IQ) that ranges from 35 to 70.[17] People with Down syndrome are often friendly and engaging. Extra time might be needed for obtaining a history and for performing assessment and patient care procedures. About 15% of people who have Down syndrome have atlantoaxial instability of the spine, which increases the risk of cervical spinal injury after trauma.[18]

The airway in a person with Down syndrome is narrow, and although the face is smaller, the tongue is larger. These characteristics make intubation more difficult. If preparing to intubate the patient with Down syndrome, the paramedic should do the following:[19]

1. Preoxygenate. This patient will be more prone to hypoxia because of smaller functional residual capacity.
2. Consider a slight reverse Trendelenburg position (feet lower than head) if possible, especially if the patient has obesity.
3. Maintain in-line cervical stabilization (if possible with atlantoaxial instability).
4. Use an endotracheal tube two sizes smaller than recommended for people without Down syndrome. The airway and trachea are smaller in a patient with Down syndrome.
5. Observe for bradycardia.

Intellectual Disability

Intellectual disability is a disability in which intellectual functioning and ability to learn and adapt socially are significantly limited. It originates before age 18 years.[20] It is classified further with IQ assessment as mild (IQ 55 to 70), moderate (IQ 40 to 54), severe (IQ 25 to 39), and profound (IQ less than 25).[21] More severe grades of intellectual disability usually have a specific physical cause (eg, brain damage, Down syndrome). In contrast, mild intellectual disability often has no specific cause. However, poverty, malnutrition, and heredity may play a role (BOX 50-4). Approximately 1% of the population has an intellectual disability.

DID YOU KNOW?

In October 2010, US Congress passed Rosa's Law, which changed references to "mental retardation" in specified federal laws to "intellectual disability," and references to "a mentally retarded individual" to "an individual with an intellectual disability." Under the law, the terms "mental retardation" and "mentally retarded" were stripped from federal health, education, and labor policy.

Modified from: Colvin CW. Change in terminology: "mental retardation" to "intellectual disability." Federal Register website. https://www.federalregister.gov/documents/2013/08/01/2013-18552/change-in-terminology-mental-retardation-to-intellectual-disability. Published July 26, 2013. Accessed May 3, 2018.

BOX 50-4 Causes of Intellectual Disabilities

Genetic Conditions

Phenylketonuria (a single-gene disorder causing an enzyme deficiency)
Chromosomal disorder (eg, Down syndrome)
Fragile X syndrome (a single-gene disorder on the Y chromosome; the leading inherited cause of intellectual disability)

Problems During Pregnancy

Use of alcohol or other drugs by the mother
Use of tobacco
Malnutrition
Certain environmental toxins
Illness and infection (toxoplasmosis, cytomegalovirus, rubella, syphilis, human immunodeficiency virus [HIV])

Problems at Birth

Delivery problems
Oxygen deprivation
Brain injury
Prematurity
Low birth weight

Problems After Birth

Childhood diseases (whooping cough, chickenpox, measles, *Haemophilus influenzae* type b [Hib] disease)
Injury (eg, head injury or near drowning)
Exposure to lead, mercury, and other environmental toxins

Poverty and Cultural Deprivation

Malnutrition
Childhood diseases
Inadequate health care
Environmental health hazards
Understimulation

Modified from: Causes and prevention of intellectual disability. The Arc website. https://www.thearc.org/what-we-do/resources/fact-sheets/causes-and-prevention. Revised March 1, 2011. Accessed May 3, 2018.

Approximately 85% of this group have mild intellectual disability.[22]

Special Considerations

Changes to normal patient care vary based on the patient's level of intellectual disability. Many with mild disability show no symptoms other than slowness in carrying out mental tasks. Others with moderate to severe disability may have limited to absent speech. Neurologic problems are common. These patients may require extra time and care in patient assessment, management, and transport.

Pathologic Challenges

Certain pathologic conditions may require special assessment and management skills. Specific pathologic conditions presented in this section include cancer, cerebral palsy, cystic fibrosis, and previous head injury. The following discussion will provide a brief review.

Cancer

Cancer is a group of diseases that allow for an unrestrained growth of cells in one or more of the body organs or tissues. The malignant tumors most often develop in major organs, including the lungs, breasts, intestine, skin, stomach, and pancreas. However, they also may occur in cell-forming tissues of the bone marrow and in the lymphatic system, muscle, or bone (see Chapter 31, *Hematology*). The course of individual cancer progression and the treatments vary widely. Aside from the physical effects of their disease and treatment, patients often experience stress, anxiety related to waiting on test results and biopsy reports, lack of information, and uncertainty.

Special Considerations

Patients with cancer often are very ill. The signs and symptoms of their disease depend on the site of origin of the cancer (BOX 50-5). Often no signs of the disease are visible. However, medical treatment (eg, chemotherapy, radiation) for many of the cancers can produce obvious signs and symptoms and various illnesses that may initiate an EMS response. (Patients with metastatic cancer are also at increased risk for pulmonary embolism.[23]) Signs and symptoms associated with chemotherapy and radiation include the following:

- Anorexia
- Depression
- Dyspnea
- Fatigue
- Gastrointestinal upset
- General malaise
- Loss of appetite
- Loss of hair (alopecia)
- Fever (associated with neutropenia)
- Pain

Requests for EMS for patients with advanced cancer often are related to the patient's pain medication. An example is a patient whose pain is no longer relieved by the medicine. Another example is a patient who has taken an accidental overdose of pain medicine. This may result in an altered level of consciousness or respiratory depression. If the patient's pain is not being well managed, the paramedic should consult with medical direction. Larger-than-normal doses may need to be given to provide pain relief. If an overdose is suspected, the paramedic should initiate the standard care for narcotic overdose.

A full patient history should be obtained, including a list of all medications. Many cancer patients take anticancer drugs and pain medications through transdermal skin patches that contain analgesic agents and through surgically implanted devices (eg, MediPorts). If intravenous therapy is necessary, additional time should be allotted to access the patient's peripheral veins or medication port. Strict aseptic technique and additional training are important when treating these patients. They often are immunocompromised as a result of the treatment for their disease. As described

BOX 50-5 Common Examples of Site of Origin Classifications for Cancer

Adenocarcinoma: Originates in glandular tissue
Blastoma: Originates in embryonic tissue of organs, or precursor or undifferentiated cells
Carcinoma: Originates in epithelial tissue (ie, tissue that lines organs and tubes)
Leukemia: Originates in tissues that form blood cells
Lymphoma: Originates in lymphatic tissue
Myeloma: Originates in bone marrow
Sarcoma: Originates in connective or supportive tissue (eg, bone, cartilage, muscle)

in Chapter 14, *Medication Administration*, paramedics should consult with medical direction and follow protocols before using a surgically implanted port for fluid or drug therapy.

The course of the disease and the medical regimen of care for cancer patients can be devastating for the patient, family, and loved ones. The paramedic must provide emotional support for all involved. It is also essential to ensure the patient's comfort. Finally, when possible, patients should be transported to the hospital where they are being treated for their cancer.

Cerebral Palsy

Cerebral palsy is a general term for nonprogressive disorders of movement and posture that cause activity limitation. It is attributed to nonprogressive disturbances that occurred in the developing fetal or infant brain. The motor disorders are often accompanied by sensory, perceptual, cognitive, communication, and behavioral problems, and by epilepsy and secondary motor disorders (BOX 50-6). The most common cause of cerebral palsy is cerebral dysgenesis (abnormal cerebral development) or cerebral malformations.[24] Less common causes include fetal hypoxia, birth trauma, maternal infection, kernicterus (excessive fetal bilirubin, associated with hemolytic disease), and postpartum encephalitis, meningitis, or head injury. Cerebral palsy often is diagnosed during the child's first year of life when parents notice unusual muscle tone during holding or feeding difficulties. Although, no cure exists for the disease, people with moderate disability may live with relative independence and have a near-normal life expectancy.[25]

Types of Cerebral Palsy

Cerebral palsy is classified in several ways, including by severity, motor function, and topographic distribution. The severity level describes the patient's functional level. It ranges from mild, in which the patient moves without assistance and does not have limitations in activities of daily living, to severe, in which the patient is in a wheelchair and has significant challenges with activities of living. Patients with severe cerebral palsy are also more likely to have cognitive impairments and quadriplegia. Motor function is classified as spastic or nonspastic. Several types of movement irregularities are associated with cerebral palsy: spasticity, ataxia, and others (athetosis and chorea) (BOX 50-7).

BOX 50-6 Causes of Cerebral Palsy

Disorders During Pregnancy That May Cause Cerebral Palsy

1. Exposure to toxic chemicals
2. Infectious diseases
3. Rh or ABO blood type incompatibility between mother and fetus
4. Lack of oxygen to the fetal brain before birth (umbilical cord strangulation, abruptio placentae, prolonged labor)
5. Low birth weight
6. Prematurity

Disorders During Birth or Shortly After Birth

1. Birth trauma injuring the infant's skull
2. Fetal anoxia

Disorders After Birth That May Cause Cerebral Palsy

1. Infections such as meningitis and encephalitis
2. Exposure to toxic chemicals
3. Head injury following falls, vehicle crashes, or abuse
4. Anoxia related to drowning or carbon monoxide

Modified from: Falvo D, Holland BE. *Medical and Psychosocial Aspects of Chronic Illness and Disability*. Burlington, MA: Jones & Bartlett Learning; 2018.

CRITICAL THINKING

How can you determine the patient's normal level of functioning?

Special Considerations

Weakness, paralysis, and developmental delay vary by the type and severity of disease. For example, most children with mild cerebral palsy attend regular schools. Others with more severe forms of the disease never learn to walk or communicate well. They may require lifelong skilled nursing care. Accommodations that may be needed while providing care include allowing extra scene time for the physical examination and extra resources and personnel to aid transport.

Cystic Fibrosis

Cystic fibrosis (mucoviscidosis) is an inherited metabolic disease of the lungs, sweat glands (sudoriferous, or

BOX 50-7 Types of Cerebral Palsy

Spasticity is common and produces abnormal stiffness and contraction of groups of muscles. It can be very painful. With this type of cerebral palsy, the child may be categorized as diplegic, hemiplegic, or quadriplegic. With diplegia, all four limbs are affected. The legs are affected more severely than the arms are. With hemiplegia, the limbs on only one side of the body are affected. The arm is usually more severe than the leg is. With quadriplegia, all four limbs are severely affected, not necessarily symmetrically.

Athetosis produces involuntary writhing movements and a loss of coordination and balance. Hearing defects, epilepsy, and other central nervous system disorders are often present with the disease. Although some with athetosis and diplegia are highly intelligent, 30% to 50% of all people with cerebral palsy have intellectual disability. Most people with quadriplegia are severely intellectually disabled.

Ataxia in patients with cerebral palsy causes a disturbed sense of balance and depth perception. These patients usually have poor muscle tone (hypotonic), a staggering walk, and unsteady hands. Ataxia results from damage to the cerebellum, the brain's major center for balance and coordination. Chorea are involuntary, unpredictable body movements. Dystonias are involuntary, often repetitive movements in the presence of an abnormal sustained posture.

Modified from: Odding E, Roebroeck ME, Stam HJ. The epidemiology of cerebral palsy: incidence, impairments and risk factors. *Disabil Rehabil*. 2006;28(4):183-191.

sudoriparous, glands), and digestive and reproductive systems that manifests in childhood. The disease is caused by a defective, recessive gene that is inherited from each parent. The defective gene causes the glands in the lining of the bronchi to retain excessive sodium and chloride. As a result, the bronchi draw in water and produce excessive amounts of thick mucus. This condition predisposes the person to chronic lung infections. In addition, the pancreas of a patient with cystic fibrosis fails to produce the enzymes required for the breakdown of fats and their absorption from the intestine. These alterations in metabolism cause classic symptoms of cystic fibrosis that include pale, greasy-looking, foul-smelling stools (often noticeable soon after birth); persistent productive cough and breathlessness; and lung infections that often develop into pneumonia, bronchiectasis, and bronchitis.[26] Other features of the disease include stunted growth and sweat glands that produce abnormally salty sweat. In some cases, the child with cystic fibrosis may fail to thrive. Many patients survive into adulthood, although poor health is common.

NOTE

In the United States, among various ethnic groups, cystic fibrosis is more common within the Caucasian population, with a prevalence of 1 in 2,500 to 3,500 newborns in this group. Among African Americans, the prevalence is approximately 1 in 17,000; among Asian Americans, it is 1 in 31,000. If only one defective gene is inherited, that person will be a carrier of the disease. However, the person will have no symptoms. Often, people are unaware that they carry the defective gene. Genetic counseling and testing are appropriate for people who have a family history of cystic fibrosis.

Modified from: Cystic fibrosis. Genetics Home Reference website. https://ghr.nlm.nih.gov/condition/cystic-fibrosis#statistics. Published May 1, 2018. Accessed May 3, 2018.

Special Considerations

Older patients (and parents of children) with cystic fibrosis generally are aware of their disease. Some may be oxygen dependent. They may need respiratory support with noninvasive positive pressure ventilation, nebulized normal saline, and suctioning to clear the airway of mucus and secretions. Many use inhalants. The paramedic should expect a lengthy history and physical examination because of the nature of the disease and associated medical problems. Some patients will have received heart and lung transplants. They may require transfer to specialized medical facilities for treatment. If parents are unaware of the possibility of cystic fibrosis in the presence of signs and symptoms described previously, the paramedic should advise the physician at the hospital of his or her suspicions.

Previous Head Injury

Traumatic brain injury can result from many types of trauma (see Chapter 40, *Spine and Nervous System Trauma*). These injuries can affect many cognitive, physical, and psychological skills. Physical deficit can include ambulation, balance and coordination, fine motor skills, strength, and endurance. Cognitive deficits of language and communication, information processing, memory, and perceptual skills are common. Psychological status often is altered (**TABLE 50-2**).

TABLE 50-2 Traumatic Brain Injury Deficits

Injury	Injury Deficits in the Cerebral Cortex
Cerebral Cortex	
Frontal lobes	Paralysis of various body parts Inability to plan a sequence of complex movements Inability to focus on tasks Mood changes Personality changes Inability to express language
Parietal lobes	Inability to name an object Problems with reading and writing Difficulty in distinguishing right from left Difficulty with math skills Difficulty with hand–eye coordination
Occipital lobes	Defects in vision Production of hallucinations Visual illusions Inability to recognize words Difficulties in reading and writing
Temporal lobes	Difficulty in recognizing faces Difficulty in understanding spoken words Short-term memory loss Interference with long-term memory Persistent talking Aggressive behavior
Brainstem	Decreased vital capacity Difficulty in swallowing food and water Difficulty with organization Problems with balance and movement Dizziness and nausea Sleeping difficulties
Cerebellum	Loss of ability to coordinate fine movements Loss of ability to walk Tremors Dizziness Slurred speech

Modified from: Lehr RP. Brain function. Centre for Neuro Skills website. https://www.neuroskills.com/brain-injury/brain-function.php. Accessed May 3, 2018.

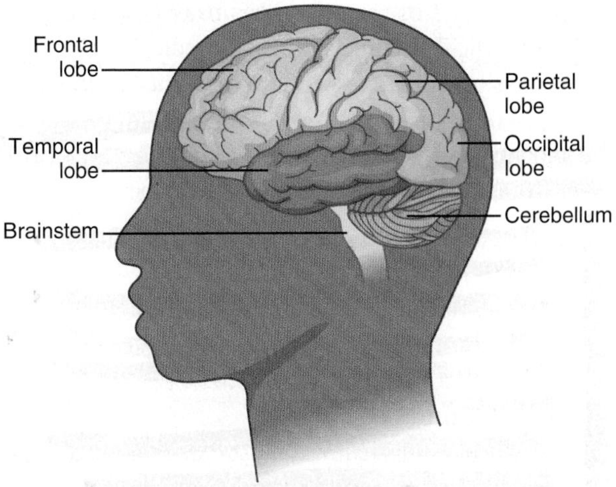

FIGURE 50-5 Areas of injury.

Special Considerations

Depending on the patient's area of brain injury, obtaining a history and performing assessment and care may be difficult (**FIGURE 50-5**). Some patients may need to be restrained. Family and other caregivers should be involved in managing the patient (when appropriate). The paramedic also should interview them to determine whether the patient's actions and responses are "normal" or "baseline" for the patient. Additional time should be allotted at the scene to provide care to these patients.

> CRITICAL THINKING
> Why is this group of patients at high risk for injury?

Culturally Diverse Patients

As described in Chapter 16, *Therapeutic Communications*, people vary in many ways, and huge diversity exists in populations of all cultures. Diversity refers to differences of any kind. These differences include age, race, class, religion, sex, sexual preference, personal habitat, and physical ability. Good health care depends on sensitivity toward these differences.

> CRITICAL THINKING
> What kinds of diversity are there in your classroom? How do you feel about that diversity?

Experiences of health and illness vary widely as a result of different beliefs, behaviors, and past experiences. These experiences may conflict with learned medical practice of the paramedic. By revealing awareness of cultural issues, the paramedic conveys interest, concern, and respect. When interacting with patients from different cultures, the paramedic should remember the following eight key points:[27]

1. The patient is the "foreground" and the culture is the "background."
2. Different generations and people within the same family may have different sets of beliefs.
3. Not all people identify with their ethnic cultural background.
4. All people share common problems or situations.
5. Respect the integrity of cultural beliefs.
6. Realize that people may not share your explanations of the causes of their ill health but may accept conventional treatments. (You do not have to "convert" a patient to your way of thinking to get the desired result.)
7. You do not have to agree with every aspect of another person's culture, nor does the person have to accept everything about yours for effective and culturally sensitive health care to occur.
8. Recognize your personal cultural assumptions, prejudices, and belief systems. Do not let them interfere with patient care.

Special Considerations

Regardless of the patient's cultural background, education, occupation, or ability to speak English, most patients will be anxious during an emergency event. If the paramedic does not speak the patient's language, communication should begin using English first. The patient may understand or speak some English words or phrases. (Bystanders, coworkers, or family members may be available to assist.) In some areas, special translator devices (eg, a telephone language line, a computer-generated Internet or cell phone application) for non–English-speaking patients are available. If the patient does not speak or understand English, the paramedic should try to communicate with signs or gestures. Some pocket guides and computer applications have tools for limited translation until other resources are available. The hospital should be notified as soon as possible so that arrangements for an interpreter can be made.

If time allows, the paramedic should perform all assessment procedures slowly and with the patient's permission. The paramedic should be aware that "private space" is culturally defined (see Chapter 16, *Therapeutic Communications*). Therefore the best approach is to point to the area of the body to be examined before touching the patient. The patient's need for modesty and privacy at the scene and during transport should be respected. Women and men of some cultures have very strict religious beliefs regarding personal modesty and the appropriateness of being touched, especially by strangers. When possible, every effort should be made to honor their wishes, protect their privacy, and ensure their comfort.

Financial Challenges

At the end of 2016, more than 28 million Americans were estimated to have no health insurance.[28] This represented a decline from 44 million uninsured in 2013. Millions of poor adults are in a coverage gap and unable to secure insurance. Financial challenges for health care can quickly result from loss of a job and depletion of savings. Financial challenges that are combined with medical conditions that require uninterrupted treatment (eg, cancer, tuberculosis, HIV/AIDS, diabetes, hypertension, mental disorders) or that occur in the presence of unexpected illness or injury can deprive the patient of basic health care. Most medical personnel and health care facilities recognize their ethical duty to provide services immediately, without regard to payment, in emergencies.

Poverty

Poverty is the scarcity or the lack of a certain amount of material possessions or money. Poverty is a multifaceted concept that may include social, economic,

SHOW ME THE EVIDENCE

California researchers merged over 88,000 EMS calls with community data related to poverty to determine whether there was an association between frequency of 9-1-1 ambulance calls when the patient severity was taken into account. They found that poverty was significantly and positively associated with 9-1-1 ambulance calls. A 10% point increase in tract-level poverty (concentrated areas of poverty) was associated with a 45% increase in ambulance contacts. There were significant positive correlations in low-, medium-, and high-severity calls.

Modified from: Seim J, English J, Sporer K. Neighborhood poverty and 9-1-1 ambulance contacts. *Prehosp Emerg Care.* 2017;21(6):722-728.

and political elements. In 2016, more than 40 million people were living below the poverty line in the United States. Of those, 13.3 million were children.[29] Poverty has a negative effect on education, child development, crime, social mobility, and social spending.[30] Efforts to reduce poverty are focused on modifying social and economic conditions through public policy interventions.[31]

Homelessness

Homelessness is closely associated with poor health and multiple health problems. The homeless are high utilizers of EMS.[32] Chronic illness, frostbite, leg ulcers, and respiratory tract infections are common and often are the direct result of homelessness. Homeless people are also at greater risk for trauma from muggings, beatings, and rape. Homelessness precludes good nutrition, good personal hygiene, and basic first aid. In some cases these people seek emergency care largely because of hunger, fear for safety, or lack of shelter.[32,33] Some homeless people with mental disorders may use alcohol or other drugs. Those with addictive disorders often are at risk of HIV and other communicable diseases. Paramedics should be familiar with services in their community for the homeless. They should know where to refer the homeless for food and shelter.

NOTE

It is estimated that approximately 500,000 people in the United States were homeless in 2017. New York City and Los Angeles recorded the highest homeless populations in the United States.

Modified from: McCarthy N. The US cities with the most homeless people. Statista website. https://www.statista.com/chart/6949/the-us-cities-with-the-most-homeless-people/. January 26, 2018. Accessed May 3, 2018.

CRITICAL THINKING

Consider patients with chronic illness and no insurance. How do you think financial pressures influence medication compliance in these patients?

Special Considerations

People with financial challenges often are anxious about seeking medical care. According to *Emergency Medical Services: Agenda for the Future*, "The focus of public access is the ability to secure prompt and appropriate EMS care regardless of socioeconomic status, age, or special need. For all those who contact EMS with a perceived requirement for care, the subsequent response and level of care provided must be commensurate with the situation."[34] When caring for a patient with financial challenges who is concerned about the cost of receiving needed health care, the paramedic should explain the following:

1. The patient's ability to pay should never be a factor in obtaining emergency care.
2. Federal law requires that care be provided, regardless of the patient's ability to pay.
3. Payment programs for health care services are available in most hospitals.
4. Government services are available to help patients in paying for health care.
5. There are some free (or near-free) health care services available through local, state, and federally funded organizations.

When patients refuse transport because they do not have insurance coverage and fear the high cost of a hospital visit, the paramedic should advise the patient of appropriate alternative facilities for health care. As an example, the paramedic should provide an approved list of alternative health care sites (eg, a minor-emergency center or health clinic) that can provide medical care at costs that are much less than those charged by emergency departments. However, patients who have serious illness or injury should be encouraged to have EMS transport for evaluation in the emergency department. Patients who refuse transport should be encouraged to call again for EMS assistance if needed.

High System Utilizers

In almost every EMS system, a small group of patients constitutes a disproportionate number of the annual call volume. This excess use of the EMS system is often associated with a lack of access to other health care resources. There are still barriers to adequate health care access, particularly related to mental health.[35,36] When these patients use 9-1-1 services frequently, it places a burden on the system without meeting the patient's underlying health needs.

An acute high system utilizer often has short-term health or social service needs. These patients may include older adults who are struggling to remain independent in their homes, recently discharged patients, or patients at the end of life who are not yet connected to appropriate short-term home health or social service resources. The needs of these patients are typically acute for a limited time. EMS personnel can help direct these patients to appropriate resources and decrease their need for 9-1-1 support.

The definition of chronic high system utilizers (super-users, super-utilizers, frequent-users) varies by system and can be from 10 or more calls per year up to 4 to 5 calls per month. Factors associated with high system use include male sex, age between 40 and 60 years, homelessness, behavioral illness, and alcohol abuse.[37,38] Complaints vary, often involving alcohol or substance abuse, abdominal pain, chest pain, seizure, head or neck trauma, respiratory distress and altered mental status related to diabetes, and other causes. Reducing 9-1-1 calls in this population is more complex and requires a multidisciplinary approach.

A variety of interventions have been attempted and have produced significant reductions in calls; however, in each case, there were patients who were resistant to interventions.[39] These interventions include specialized response teams to direct patients to alternative destinations, development of patient-specific case management, and programs to provide stable housing (BOX 50-8).[32,38,40] These teams may be part of a department's mobile integrated health care program. Alternately, the high utilizer program may involve a community partnership involving local EMS, fire, mental health, public health, public housing, and health care partners.

BOX 50-8 Ongoing Programs That Have Reduced the Number of High EMS System Utilizers

- 2013—Michigan counties of Ingham, Muskegon, and Saginaw partnered with local medical providers to refer patients to Michigan Pathways to Better Health, a community health program that connects patients to appropriate resources.
- 2009—The Area Metropolitan Ambulance Authority (MedStar) in Fort Worth, Texas, implemented mobile health care paramedics to visit high utilizers, reducing their 9-1-1 calls.
- 2008—The City of San Diego EMS system implemented the Resource Access Program to identify frequent callers at the call intake point. The paramedic coordinator works with community stakeholders to address the caller's health needs.

The need to reduce the use of EMS for nonurgent conditions has been identified as a high priority by the US Agency for Healthcare Research and Quality (AHRQ). The AHRQ has identified three aims to achieve this goal:[41]

1. Identify nonurgent high utilizers of emergency services.
2. Improve coordination between emergency services, emergency departments, primary care, and behavioral health and social services.
3. Appropriately reduce nonurgent high utilization of emergency services by exploring appropriate service delivery models to meet the target population's needs.

Summary

- Certain accommodations may be needed for patients with a hearing impairment. These include helping with a patient's hearing aid and providing paper and pen to aid in communication. Personnel with special training may be needed; notify the hospital as soon as possible.
- When caring for the visually impaired patient, the paramedic should help the patient use his or her glasses or other visual aids. The paramedic also should describe all procedures before performing them.
- The paramedic should allow extra time for the history of a patient with speech impairment. If appropriate, aids such as a pen and paper can assist in communication.
- When caring for a patient with obesity, the paramedic should use the proper-sized diagnostic devices. The patient's head, neck, and shoulders will require greater elevation to achieve alignment during intubation. Also, extra personnel may be needed to move the patient for transport.
- When transporting patients with paraplegia or quadriplegia, extra personnel may be needed to move special equipment.
- Once rapport and trust have been established with a patient who has mental illness, the paramedic should proceed with care in the standard manner.
- The challenge in assessing patients with emotional impairment is distinguishing between symptoms produced

by stress and those caused by serious medical illness. The paramedic should focus on the chief complaint.

- In people with Down syndrome, the airway is narrower and the tongue is larger, making intubation more difficult. Also, there is atlantoaxial instability, which increases the risk of cervical spine injury after trauma.
- Intellectual disability refers to significant limitation of intellectual functioning and ability to learn and adapt socially.
- When caring for a patient with developmental or intellectual disability, the paramedic should allow enough time to obtain a history, perform an assessment, deliver care, and prepare for transport.
- Pathologic conditions include cancer, cerebral palsy, cystic fibrosis, and previous head injury, among others. Patients with these conditions may require special assessment and management skills. The paramedic should ask about current medications and the patient's normal level of functioning. Some of these patients may require extra resources and personnel to aid transport.
- Diversity refers to differences of any kind. These include race, class, religion, sex, sexual preference, personal habitat, and physical ability. Good health care depends on sensitivity toward these differences.
- Financial challenges can deprive a patient of basic health care services. These patients may be reluctant to seek care for illness or injury. The patient's ability to pay should never be a factor in providing emergency care. If the patient refuses transport, the paramedic should advise the patient of appropriate alternative facilities for health care.
- High system utilizers are patients who use 9-1-1 services frequently. This use may be associated with a lack of access to other health care resources. Addressing this population's health care needs requires a multidisciplinary approach that may involve specialized response teams, community partnership, and housing efforts.

References

1. Basic facts about hearing loss. Hearing Loss Association of America website. http://www.hearingloss.org/content/basic-facts-about-hearing-loss. Accessed May 4, 2018.
2. Centers for Disease Control and Prevention, National Center on Birth Defects and Developmental Disabilities. Types of hearing loss. Centers for Disease Control and Prevention website. https://www.cdc.gov/ncbddd/hearingloss/types.html. Updated February 18, 2015. Accessed May 4, 2018.
3. Auditory neuropathy. National Institute on Deafness and Other Communication Disorders website. https://www.nidcd.nih.gov/health/auditory-neuropathy. Updated January 26, 2018. Accessed May 4, 2018.
4. American Sign Language. National Institute on Deafness and Other Communication Disorders website. https://www.nidcd.nih.gov/health/american-sign-language. Updated April 25, 2017. Accessed May 4, 2018.
5. Eye health statistics. American Academy of Ophthalmology website. https://www.aao.org/newsroom/eye-health-statistics. Accessed May 4, 2018.
6. Adult Obesity Facts. Centers for Disease Control and Prevention website. https://www.cdc.gov/obesity/data/adult.html. Updated March 5, 2018. Accessed May 4, 2018.
7. Division of Nutrition, Physical Activity, and Obesity, National Center for Chronic Disease Prevention and Health Promotion. Childhood obesity facts. Centers for Disease Control and Prevention website. https://www.cdc.gov/obesity/data/childhood.html. Updated April 10, 2017. Accessed May 4, 2018.
8. Division of Nutrition, Physical Activity, and Obesity, National Center for Chronic Disease Prevention and Health Promotion. Defining adult overweight and obesity. Centers for Disease Control and Prevention website. https://www.cdc.gov/obesity/adult/defining.html. Updated June 16, 2016. Accessed May 4, 2018.
9. Kiebel W, Hawkins D, Meyers L, et al. 98: Management of the bariatric surgery patient in the emergency department. *Ann Emerg Med*. 2009;54(3):S32.
10. Bariatric surgery and devices (obesity, severe obesity). Obesity Action Coalition website. http://www.obesityaction.org/obesity-treatments/bariatric-surgery. Accessed May 4, 2018.
11. Edwards ED, Jacob BP, Gagner M, et al. Presentation and management of common post-weight loss surgery problems in the emergency department. *Ann Emerg Med*. 2006;47(2):160-166.
12. Myatt J, Haire K. Airway management in obese patients. *Curr Anaesth Crit Care*. 2010;21:9-15.
13. De Hert M, Correll CU, Bobes J, et al. Physical illness in patients with severe mental disorders. I. Prevalence, impact of medications and disparities in health care. *World Psychiatry*. 2011;10(1):52-77.
14. National Center on Birth Defects and Developmental Disabilities, Centers for Disease Control and Prevention. Facts about developmental disabilities. Centers for Disease Control and Prevention website. https://www.cdc.gov/ncbddd/developmentaldisabilities/facts.html. Updated April 17, 2018. Accessed May 4, 2018.
15. Down syndrome. National Down Syndrome Society website. https://www.ndss.org/about-down-syndrome/down-syndrome/. Accessed May 4, 2018.
16. Esbensen AJ. Health conditions associated with aging and end of life of adults with Down syndrome. *Int Rev Res Ment Retard*. 2010;39(C):107-126.
17. Weijerman ME, de Winter JP. Clinical practice: the care of children with Down syndrome. *Eur J Pediatr*. 2010;169(12):1445-1452.
18. Altlantoaxial instability and Down syndrome. National Down Syndrome Society website. https://www.ndss.org/resources/atlantoaxial-instability-syndrome/. Accessed May 4, 2018.
19. Fox S. Down syndrome airway. Pediatric EM Morsels website. http://pedemmorsels.com/down-syndrome-airway/. Updated February 7, 2017. Accessed May 4, 2018.
20. Definition of intellectual disability. American Association on Intellectual and Developmental Disabilities website. http://aaidd.org/intellectual-disability/definition. Accessed May 4, 2018.
21. American Psychiatric Association. *Diagnostic and Statistical Manual of Mental Disorders*. 5th ed. Washington, DC: American Psychiatric Association; 2013.
22. Parekh R. What is intellectual disability? American Psychiatric Association website. https://www.psychiatry.org/patients-families/intellectual-disability/what-is-intellectual-disability. Reviewed July 2017. Accessed May 4, 2018.

23. Abdel-Razeq HN, Mansour AH, Ismael YM. Incidental pulmonary embolism in cancer patients: clinical characteristics and outcome—a comprehensive cancer center experience. *Vasc Health Risk Manag*. 2011;7:153-158.
24. Cerebral palsy: hope through research. NIH Publication 13-159. National Institute of Neurological Disorders and Stroke website. https://www.ninds.nih.gov/Disorders/Patient-Caregiver-Education/Hope-Through-Research/Cerebral-Palsy-Hope-Through-Research. Updated February 12, 2018. Accessed May 4, 2018.
25. Cremer N, Hurvitz EA, Peterson MD. Multimorbidity in middle-aged adults with cerebral palsy. *Am J Med*. 2017;130(6):744.e9-744.e15.
26. Cystic fibrosis. National Heart, Lung, and Blood Institute website. https://www.nhlbi.nih.gov/health-topics/cystic-fibrosis. Accessed May 20, 2018.
27. US Department of Transportation, National Highway Traffic Safety Administration. *National Emergency Medical Services Education Standards*. DOT HS 811 077E. 2009:24-25. EMS.gov website. www.ems.gov/pdf/811077a.pdf. Accessed May 4, 2018.
28. Key facts about the uninsured population. Henry J Kaiser Family Foundation website. https://www.kff.org/uninsured/fact-sheet/key-facts-about-the-uninsured-population/. Updated November 29, 2017. Accessed May 4, 2018.
29. Proctor BD, Semega JL, Kollar MA. Income and poverty in the United States: 2015. United States Census Bureau website. Report Number P60-256. 2016:50-55, Table B-2. https://www.census.gov/library/publications/2016/demo/p60-256.html. Published September 13, 2016. Accessed May 4, 2018.
30. Seim J, English J, Sporer K. Neighborhood poverty and 9-1-1 ambulance contacts. *Prehosp Emerg Care*. 2017;21(6):722-728.
31. Cosgrove S, Curtis B. *Understanding Global Poverty: Causes, Capabilities and Human Development*. New York, NY: Taylor & Francis; 2018.
32. Mackelprang JL, Collins SE, Clifasefi SL. Housing first is associated with reduced use of emergency medical services. *Prehosp Emerg Care*. 2014;18(4):476-482.
33. Rodriguez RM, Fortman J, Chee C, et al. Food, shelter and safety needs motivating homeless persons' visits to an urban emergency department. *Ann Emerg Med*. 2008;53(5):598-602.
34. US Department of Transportation, National Highway Traffic Safety Administration, US Department of Health and Human Services. *Emergency Medical Services: Agenda for the Future*. Washington, DC: US Department of Transportation; 1996.
35. National Center for Health Statistics. Chapter III: overview of midcourse progress and health disparities. In: *Healthy People 2020 Midcourse Review*. Hyattsville, MD: National Center for Health Statistics; 2016.
36. Tangherlini N, Villar J, Brown J, et al. The HOME team: Evaluating the effect of an EMS-based outreach team to decrease the frequency of 911 use among high utilizers of EMS. *Prehosp Disaster Med*. 2016;31(6):603-607.
37. Sanko SG, Eckstein M. Characteristics of the most frequent "super-users" of emergency medical services. *Ann Emerg Med*. 2013;62(4):S145.
38. Villar J, Tangherlini N, Friedman B, et al. Targeted intervention reduces use in frequent users of emergency medical services. *Ann Emerg Med*. 2013;62(4):S48.
39. Tadros AS, Castillo EM, Chan TC, et al. Effects of an emergency medical services–based resource access program on frequent users of health services. *Prehosp Emerg Care*. 2012;16(4):541-547.
40. Bronsky ES, McGraw C, Johnson R, et al. CARES: a community-wide collaboration identifies super-utilizers and reduces their 9-1-1 call, emergency department, and hospital visit rates. *Prehosp Emerg Care*. 2017;21(6):693-699.
41. Reducing non-urgent emergency services: an innovations exchange learning community. Agency for Healthcare Research and Quality website. https://innovations.ahrq.gov/learning-communities/reducing-non-urgent-emergency-services. Accessed May 4, 2018.

Suggested Readings

Beebe R. Treating and transporting bariatric patients. *JEMS* website. www.jems.com/article/patient-care/treating-and-transporting-bari. Published January 1, 2010. Accessed May 4, 2018.

Communicating comfortably. American Foundation for the Blind website. http://www.afb.org/info/friends-and-family/etiquette/communicating-comfortably/235. Accessed May 4, 2018.

Corrigan PW, Kraus DL, Pickett SA, et al. Using peer navigators to address the integrated health care needs of homeless African Americans with serious mental illness. American Psychiatric Association Publishing website. https://ps.psychiatryonline.org/doi/abs/10.1176/appi.ps.201600134. Published January 17, 2017. Accessed May 4, 2018.

Harvey A. Being deaf in EMS. EMSWorld website. https://www.emsworld.com/article/218355/being-deaf-ems. August 2, 2017. Accessed May 4, 2018.

Johnson TL, Rinehart DJ, Durfee J, et al. For many patients who use large amounts of health care services, the need is intense yet temporary. *Health Affairs*. 2015;34(8): Variety Issue. https://www.healthaffairs.org/doi/abs/10.1377/hlthaff.2014.1186. Accessed May 4, 2018.

Lim A, Mazurek A, Updike A, et al. Hearing-impaired patients require special consideration during a disaster. *JEMS* website. http://www.jems.com/articles/print/volume-39/issue-9/features/hearing-impaired-patients-require-specia.html. Published September 15, 2014. Accessed May 4, 2018.

Long W, McGary B, Jauch EC. EMS challenges with bariatric patients. *Carolina Fire Rescue EMS Journal* website. http://www.carolinafirejournal.com/Articles/Article-Detail/articleid/1586/ems-challenges-with-bariatric-patients. Published July 5, 2011. Accessed May 4, 2018.

Ohio Coalition for the Education of Children With Disabilities. *A Guide for Parents and Educators of Deaf or Hearing Impaired Children*. Ohio Coalition for the Education of Children with Disabilities website. https://www.ocecd.org/Downloads/A%20Guide%20for%20Parents%20Educ%20Deaf%20or%20HI%20Book%20Rev%2012%202015.pdf. Revised December 2015. Accessed May 4, 2018.

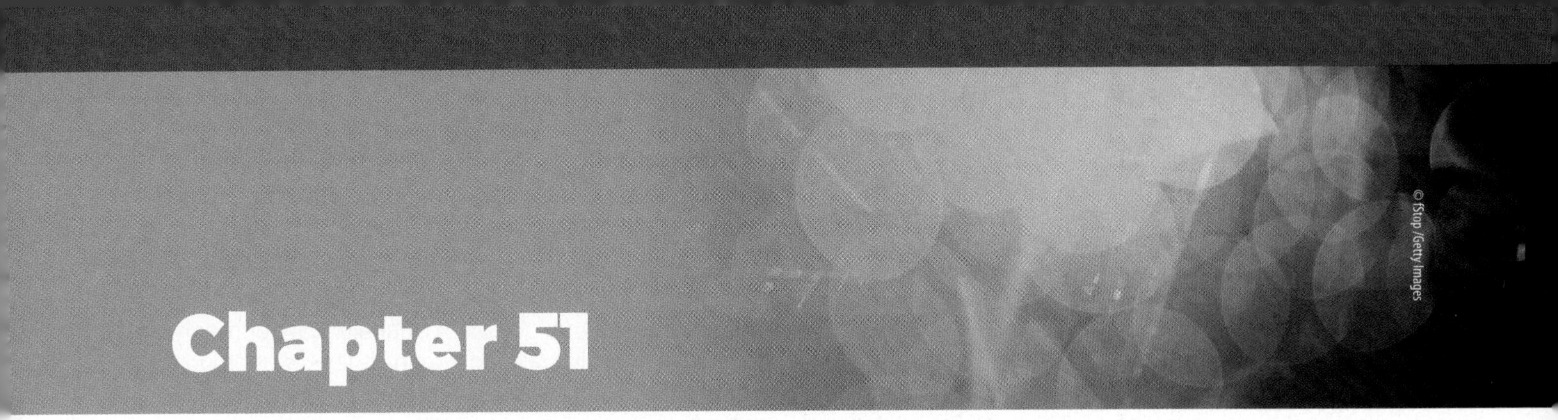

Chapter 51

Acute Interventions for Home Care

NATIONAL EMS EDUCATION STANDARD COMPETENCIES

Special Patient Populations

Integrates assessment findings with principles of pathophysiology and knowledge of psychosocial needs to formulate a field impression and implement a comprehensive treatment/disposition plan for patients with special needs.

Patients With Special Challenges

Recognizing and reporting abuse and neglect (see Chapter 49, *Abuse and Neglect*)

Health care implications of

- Abuse (see Chapter 49, *Abuse and Neglect*)
- Neglect (see Chapter 49, *Abuse and Neglect*)
- Homelessness (see Chapter 50, *Patients With Special Challenges*)
- Poverty (see Chapter 50, *Patients With Special Challenges*)
- Bariatrics (see Chapter 50, *Patients With Special Challenges*)
- Technology dependent (pp 1787–1788, 1790–1797)
- Hospice/terminally ill (pp 1806–1808)
- Tracheostomy care/dysfunction (pp 1790–1794)
- Home care (pp 1786–1789)
- Sensory deficit/loss (see Chapter 50, *Patients With Special Challenges*)
- Developmental disability (see Chapter 50, *Patients With Special Challenges*)

OBJECTIVES

Upon completion of this chapter, the paramedic student will be able to:

1. Discuss general issues related to the home health care patient. (pp 1786–1789)
2. Outline general principles of assessment and management of the home health care patient. (pp 1789–1790)
3. Describe medical equipment, assessment, and management of the home health care patient with inadequate respiratory support. (pp 1790–1794)
4. Identify assessment findings and acute interventions for problems related to vascular access devices in the home health care setting. (pp 1794–1800)
5. Describe medical equipment, assessment, and management of the patient with a gastrointestinal or genitourinary crisis in the home health care setting. (pp 1800–1805)
6. Identify key assessments and principles of wound care management in the home health care patient. (pp 1805–1806)
7. Describe medical therapy associated with hospice and comfort care in the home health care setting. (pp 1806–1808)

KEY TERMS

bladder catheterization Passage of a catheter (typically through the urethra) into the bladder for the purpose of drainage.

colostomy A surgical opening into the large intestine.

gastric tube A device that is inserted into the stomach to remove fluids and gas by suction or gravity, to instill irrigation solutions or medications, and to administer gastric feedings.

hospice care A type of care and philosophy of care that includes supportive social, emotional, and spiritual services for terminally ill patients and their families; occurs when the patient is at the end of life and the decision has been made to stop active treatment and only provide measures that decrease the severity of symptoms.

ileostomy A surgical opening into the small intestine.

ostomy An artificial opening into the urinary tract, gastrointestinal tract, or trachea; any surgical procedure in which an opening is created between two hollow organs or between a hollow viscus and the abdominal wall.

palliative care A unique form of health care primarily directed at providing relief to terminally ill people through symptom management and pain management; can occur at the same time as active treatment.

sleep apnea A disorder characterized by abnormal pauses in breathing or episodes of abnormally slow breathing during sleep.

urosepsis Sepsis due to infection from a genitourinary source.

vascular access device A device used to provide nutritional support and to administer medications in patients who need long-term vascular access.

The cost-driven allocation of health care resources and advances in technology have led to shortened hospital stays. These trends have also allowed many patients to be treated in the home setting. An estimated 12 million people in the United States require home health care services because of acute illness, long-term health conditions, personal preference, permanent disability, or terminal illness.[1] Paramedics likely will play a key role in providing acute interventions to these patients.

Overview of Home Health Care

Home health care began in the United States in the late 1800s as a direct result of growth in urban populations and an increase in the number of immigrants moving into large cities.[2] During this era, the emphasis of home health care was on personal hygiene and preventive care. The health services were provided by visiting nurses, who often worked in tenements to assist the poor; such nurses also cared for wealthy and middle-class families after births or discharges from hospitals. Few physicians were associated with most of these growing home health care groups.

Until the mid-1960s, home health care in the United States continued to focus on the poor, with the remainder of the population receiving care in hospitals and physicians' offices. With the passage of the Social Security Act Amendments (which established the Medicaid and Medicare programs) in 1965, home health care became a benefit to older adult patients covered by Medicare—a trend that greatly accelerated the growth of this industry. In 1973, coverage of home health care services was extended to certain disabled younger Americans; hospice benefits were added in 1983. In 2015, an estimated 55 million people were covered by Medicare,[3] and in January 2018, an estimated 68 million people were covered by Medicaid.[4] In 2016, 3.5 million Medicare recipients received more than 110 million home health care visits.[5] These health care programs are funded by Medicare, Medicaid, the Older Americans Act, Title XX Social Services block grants, the Veterans Administration, TRICARE for military personnel (formerly called the Civilian Health and Medical Program of the Uniformed Services

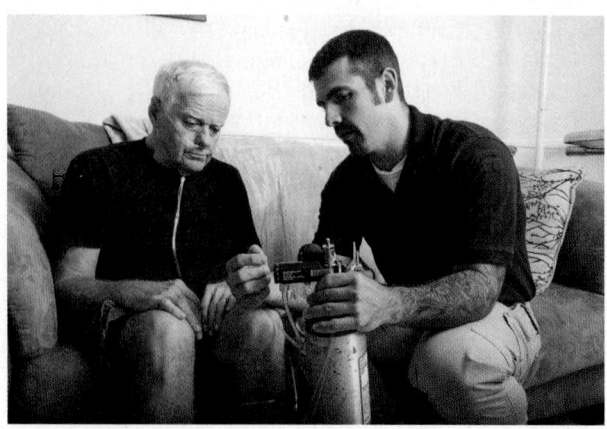

[CHAMPUS]), private insurance, and managed care organizations.

The paramedic may be the first provider to recognize the need for home care for a patient. The EMS agency should have a resource list to appropriately refer patients. Referral to home care services has been shown to decrease 9-1-1 calls and ambulance transports to the emergency department.[6]

Currently, home health care incorporates a wide variety of health and social services that are provided at home to people who are recovering, disabled, or chronically or terminally ill and who need medical, nursing, social, or therapeutic treatment and help with the essential activities of daily living. The following is a sampling of services provided to home health care patients:

- Skilled nursing services
- Physical and occupational therapy
- Medical social services
- Assistance with activities of daily living
  - Homemaker services
  - Dietary counseling

> NOTE
>
> The number of children with special needs, including those who are dependent on technology, is growing (see Chapter 47, *Pediatrics*). These children have frequent hospitalizations, and when they are sent home from the hospital, almost half of them rely on some type of technology. Medical devices often used by children in the home include gastrostomy or jejunostomy tubes, central venous catheters, medication nebulizers, ventriculoperitoneal cerebrospinal fluid shunts, and tracheostomy tubes. Although most home interventions for these children involve primarily basic life support (BLS) skills, the paramedic must be prepared to provide key advanced life support (ALS) interventions and to troubleshoot equipment problems when they arise.
>
> Using resources on the scene, such as consulting the caregiver and reviewing any printed emergency information sheets, is essential. Although most caregivers are very familiar with the child's history and medical needs, one case series found that almost 30% were not knowledgeable about the child's medications. Regardless of the child's condition, when these children are transported, their information sheets and any accessory medical equipment or "go bag" should be transported with them.
>
> *Modified from*: Kaziny BD, Shah MA. Technology-dependent children. In: Brice J, Delbridge TR, Myers JB, eds. *Emergency Medical Services: Clinical Practice and Systems Oversight*. Vol 1. 2nd ed. West Sussex, UK: John Wiley & Sons; 2015:397-400.

- Intravenous (IV) or nutritional therapy
  - Wound care
  - Patient or caregiver education
  - Injections
  - Monitoring of chronic health conditions

The Medical Home

A newer concept referred to as the medical home model is emerging as a means to manage care for patients with complex health needs that involves collaboration and coordination of primary and specialty care services. The tenets of the medical home model are as follows:[7]

- Comprehensive care, both physical and mental, using a team of caregivers
- Patient-centered care oriented toward the patient's individual needs based on culture, values, and preferences
- Coordinated care at home and during transitions from inpatient care to the home
- Accessible services eliminating barriers and delays to access of urgent health needs
- Quality and safety by using evidence-based practices and clinical decision-making tools to manage patient care

The American College of Emergency Physicians (ACEP) supports this concept of the medical home, provided the patient has a primary physician to coordinate care and is able to choose specialists and access emergency care when needed. Specifically, ACEP wants to ensure that patients in a medical home can seek emergency care when they think they have an urgent condition and that the emergency department is included in the network of the medical home so it can access the patient's electronic medical record during emergency situations.[8] Patients in properly managed medical homes may seek emergency care less frequently.[9] When the patient's condition permits, the paramedic may attempt to contact the patient's coordinator within the medical home to determine the appropriate plan of care.

ALS Response to Home Health Care Patients

Approximately 21% of home health care patients have conditions related to diseases of the circulatory system as their primary diagnosis.[10] (People with heart disease, including heart failure, constitute about half of this group.) Other common diagnoses of home health

BOX 51-1 Sampling of Home Health Care Conditions

Situations Requiring Aftercare by a Home Health Care Practitioner or Physician

Cardiopulmonary care
Catheter management and IV therapy infusion
Chemotherapy
Dermatologic and wound care
Gastroenterologic and ostomy care
Hospice care
Infectious disease
Organ transplantation
Orthopaedic care
Pain management
Rehabilitative care
Specimen collection
Urologic and renal care

Home Health Care Situations Requiring Acute Intervention

Acute cardiac events
Acute infections
Acute respiratory events
Equipment failure
Gastrointestinal/genitourinary crisis
Hospice/comfort care
Inadequate respiratory support
Maternal/child conditions
Vascular access complications

care patients include cancer, diabetes, chronic lung disease, renal failure/dialysis, and hypertension. Thus, emergency responses for home health care patients are likely to be provided by EMS agencies. Typical emergencies may include respiratory failure, cardiac decompensation, septic complications, equipment malfunction, and other conditions that worsen in the home health care setting (BOX 51-1).

Injury Control and Prevention in the Home Health Care Setting

The scientific approach to illness and injury prevention as a means to minimize morbidity and mortality is discussed in Chapter 3, *Injury Prevention, Health Promotion, and Public Health.* Readers should refer to that chapter to review primary prevention, acute care, and rehabilitation (tertiary prevention); their concepts; and their strategies.

As with all other patient encounters, the paramedic should practice infection control in the home health care setting. Infection control includes using standard precautions and body substance isolation (or transmission-based precautions) when indicated (Chapter 2, *Well-Being of the Paramedic*). Equipment that may be found in the home health care setting includes containers of medical waste, ostomy collection bags, tracheostomy tubes, sharps, soiled dressings, and other equipment (eg, emesis basins, walkers, wheelchairs) that may be contaminated with the patient's body fluids. In addition to personal precautions, the EMS crew should ensure that any infectious waste found in the home is contained properly and disposed of according to protocol.

The Occupational Safety and Health Administration (OSHA), Centers for Disease Control and Prevention (CDC), and Environmental Protection Agency (EPA) recommend the same infection control standards for the treatment of home health care patients as for acute care patients. Equipment proposed by these agencies for infection control in the home setting includes the following:

- Mask
- Gown
- Goggles, glasses, or face shield
- Resuscitation mask
- Specimen bags
- EPA-approved disinfectant effective against hepatitis B virus, human immunodeficiency virus (HIV), and tuberculosis
- Soap and water or hand sanitizers
- Disposable paper towels
- Impervious trash bags and labels

This text assumes that the proper personal protection will be utilized by paramedics. The nature of the emergency and the patient's condition will dictate which protection the paramedic should use.

CRITICAL THINKING

Which factors decrease the risk of spreading infection within a home health care setting compared with a hospital setting?

Types of Home Care Patients

The need to reduce the costs of health care and the technologic advances in medicine have allowed many types of patients to receive home care. Many EMS agencies ask their communities to notify them when someone is part of a complex home health care program. Many of these agencies will visit the home before the onset of an emergency, so that personnel can become familiar with the patient's condition and special equipment.

There are many classifications of home health care patients. Examples include those with the following conditions:

- Pathologic conditions of the airway causing inadequate pulmonary toileting or inadequate alveolar ventilation and/or oxygenation
- Circulatory pathologic conditions causing alterations in central circulation (eg, heart failure) or peripheral circulation (eg, pressure ulcers, delayed healing, infection)
- Neurologic conditions such as stroke, traumatic brain injury, spinal cord injury
- Orthopaedic trauma or surgery that requires rehabilitation (eg, fractured hip, hip or knee replacement)
- Gastrointestinal/genitourinary conditions requiring special devices such as ostomies, feeding catheters, and special equipment needed for home dialysis
- Infection from cellulitis or systemic illness (eg, sepsis)
- Wounds that require care (eg, surgical wound closure, decubitus wounds, surgical drains)

Other types of patients whom the paramedic may encounter in the home health care setting include patients receiving palliative or hospice care (described later in this chapter), expectant or new mothers, patients with dementia or other conditions that require psychological support for the patient or family, patients receiving chemotherapy or home care for chronic pain, and patients with organ transplants or those who are waiting for organ transplantation (transplant candidates).

General Principles and Management

Scene Size-up

When paramedics arrive at the scene of a home health care patient, the scene size-up should include the usual elements of scene safety, along with an assessment of the patient's environment (environmental setting).

Scene Safety

Whenever an EMS response is made to a person's home, the paramedic should evaluate the scene for the presence of dangerous pets, firearms and other home protection devices, and any home-related hazards (eg, inadequate lighting, icy sidewalks, steep stairwells). For the safety of the EMS crew, the patient, and others at the scene, all potential hazards found in a home must be contained or remedied. For example, it may be necessary to request law enforcement personnel to help with unruly or hostile bystanders. In addition, extra personnel and equipment may be needed to help move a patient down a flight of steps for transport or to manage technology-assisted patient care devices. If the paramedic is visiting a patient at home as part of a mobile health care program or department follow-up, it is advisable to establish a procedure to notify dispatch on arrival and departure from the scene.

Environmental Setting

The paramedic should assess the setting in terms of the patient's ability to maintain a healthy environment. Examples of factors considered include cleanliness of the home, evidence of basic nutritional support, and the needs of heat, water, shelter, and electricity. The EMS crew also should note any signs of abuse or neglect. Other factors to note are the cleanliness and condition of any medical devices—for example, clean oxygen and ventilation equipment and wheelchairs and hospital beds that are in good repair.

Patient Assessment

The primary survey should focus on life-threatening illness or injury, and appropriate measures should be taken as indicated (see Chapter 18, *Scene Size-up and Primary Assessment*). After the primary survey, a focused history should be obtained and the secondary assessment performed. The paramedic should make use of any medical documents found in the home, such as patient records kept by home health care providers and do not resuscitate (DNR) orders. In addition, information should be gathered from family and health care professionals (eg, a home care nurse, physical or respiratory therapist) who may be present at the scene.

Critical findings should alert the paramedic to forgo a detailed assessment and proceed with resuscitation measures and rapid transport for physician evaluation. If there are no critical findings, the paramedic should perform a physical examination that considers the possibility of medication interactions, compliance with the treatment regimen, and the possibility of dementia or a metabolic disturbance in a patient with an altered mental status.

Management and Treatment Plan

Depending on the patient's condition, the home health care treatment may need to be replaced with ALS measures. These measures may include airway, ventilatory, and circulatory support and pharmacologic and nonpharmacologic therapy (eg, electric therapy).

Some patients with acute illness or injury need to be transported to the hospital for evaluation. When transport is required, the paramedic must give special consideration for patient packaging and for moving the patient's equipment. Examples include properly securing IV catheters, urinary catheters, and feeding tubes, and ensuring sufficient personnel are available to assist with moving patient care devices such as ventilation equipment. Family members at the scene often are well versed in the use of the patient's medical devices, and they are usually eager to help when asked by the EMS crew. If there are no family members at the scene, the paramedic should attempt to contact a family member or caregiver and advise this person of the patient's condition and hospital destination. Backup supplies such as batteries and equipment in the patient's "go bag" should be transported with the patient.

Other patients do not need transport, but only home care follow-up by home health care practitioners, or perhaps a referral to other public service agencies. The paramedic should follow the local protocol and consult with medical direction about referrals and the need for notifying private physicians or home health care agencies. Regardless of the need for EMS transport, all findings and any care provided should be thoroughly documented on the patient care report.

Note that some home care patients who rely on medical devices have an emergency number to call in case of problems. If there is no life threat, the paramedic should call the emergency number to see if the patient's issue can be resolved, eliminating the need for transport.

CRITICAL THINKING

Which feelings may a patient's family member (or caregiver) in the home setting experience if there is a problem and the patient's condition worsens?

Specific Acute Home Health Care Interventions

Acute home health care emergencies may occur from equipment failure or malfunction, drug reactions, complications related to home treatment, and worsening medical conditions. This section discusses acute interventions for respiratory support, cardiovascular support, vascular access devices, gastrointestinal/genitourinary crisis, acute infections, and hospice/palliative care.

Respiratory Support

Each year, many patients with diseases of the respiratory system are discharged to home health care. These patients are at increased risk for airway infections. The progression of some respiratory diseases also may lead to increased respiratory demand, such that the patient's current support becomes inadequate. Examples of chronic pathologic conditions that require home respiratory support include the following:

- Asthma
- Awaiting lung transplantation
- Bronchopulmonary dysplasia
- Chronic lung disease

DID YOU KNOW?

Sleep Apnea

Sleep apnea is a disorder characterized by abnormal pauses in breathing or episodes of abnormally slow breathing during sleep. The pauses often occur 5 to 30 times, or even more often, each hour. This common condition affects approximately 18 million Americans. Untreated, sleep apnea can increase the risk of hypertension, stroke, myocardial infarction, worsening heart failure, and dysrhythmias; it also is related to obesity and diabetes.

Once diagnosed, the most common treatment for sleep apnea in adults is application of continuous positive airway pressure (CPAP) during sleep. Other treatment therapies include lifestyle changes (eg, weight loss, positional therapy, smoking cessation, limited alcohol use), alterations in sleep positioning, and the use of mouthpieces designed to maintain an open airway during sleep. Surgical alteration of the soft tissues of the airway may be indicated for some patients.

Modified from: Sleep apnea. National Sleep Foundation website. https://sleepfoundation.org/sleep-disorders-problems/sleep-apnea. Accessed May 9, 2018.

- Cystic fibrosis
- Infection causing exacerbation of the condition
- Sleep apnea

Acute interventions may be required for these patients. Any patient with respiratory distress should receive appropriate amounts of oxygen, pulse oximetry and end-tidal carbon dioxide monitoring, and ventilatory support as priorities in care. Problems that may lead to a request for EMS assistance include increased respiratory demand, increased bronchospasm, increased secretions, obstructed or malfunctioning respiratory devices, or improper application of medical devices to support respirations.

NOTE

Premature babies who have been released to home from a neonatal intensive care unit ("preemie grads") often have complicated medical issues. These conditions may include heart and respiratory problems (bronchopulmonary dysplasia is common), intraventricular hemorrhage, inadequate body temperature control, anemia and newborn jaundice, and problems associated with metabolism and infection. Premature babies are often released to home care with special health needs and a dependence on technology. These children and their families often require the involvement of professionals from multiple medical, rehabilitative, psychological, and social services subspecialties.

Respiratory Care in the Home Setting

Oxygen therapy in the home is typically provided by compressed gas, liquid oxygen, or oxygen concentrator.[11] As described in Chapter 15, *Airway Management, Respiration, and Artificial Ventilation,* compressed gas is oxygen stored under pressure in oxygen cylinders equipped with a regulator that controls flow rate. Liquid oxygen is cold and is stored in a container similar to a thermos. When released, the liquid is converted to gas, which may then be used like compressed gas. An oxygen concentrator is an electrically powered device that separates oxygen from air, concentrates it, and stores it (**FIGURE 51-1**). This system does not have to be resupplied and is not as costly as liquid oxygen. A cylinder of oxygen must be available as a backup, however, in case of power failure. With any of these systems, oxygen is ultimately delivered to the patient via a nasal cannula or oxygen mask, a tracheostomy collar (a device that delivers high humidity and oxygen to patients with surgical airways), or a home ventilator.

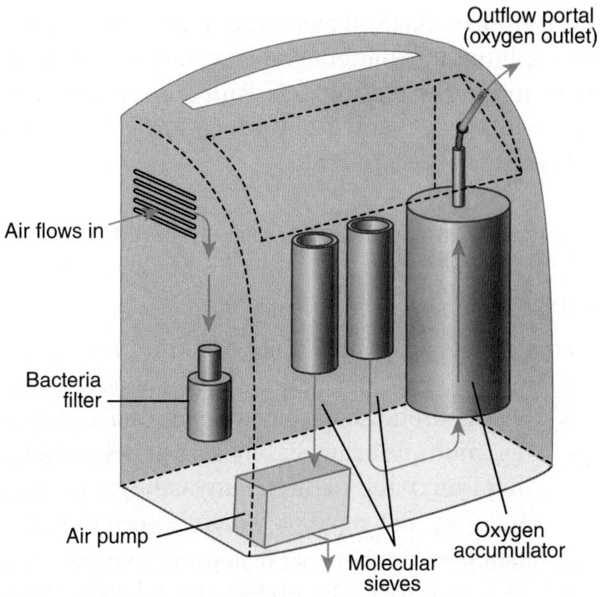

FIGURE 51-1 Oxygen concentrator.

CRITICAL THINKING

Which safety precautions for administering oxygen should be in place in the home setting?

Some patients may require CPAP delivered by ventilatory support systems through mask CPAP, nasal CPAP, or bilevel positive airway pressure (BPAP). Collectively, these types of ventilatory support are known as noninvasive positive pressure ventilation (NIPPV). As described in Chapter 23, *Respiratory,* the BPAP ventilatory support system (designed for mask-applied ventilation in the home) delivers two different levels of positive airway pressure, cycling spontaneously between preset levels of inspiratory positive airway pressure and expiratory positive airway pressure. The BPAP ventilatory support system is intended only to augment the patient's breathing; it does not meet the patient's total ventilatory requirements. A BPAP system is used by some patients with sleep apnea or chronic obstructive pulmonary disease (COPD).

Unlike continuous-flow oxygen systems, demand-flow (pulsed-dose) oxygen delivery devices use a flow sensor to trigger oxygen delivery as the patient inspires. This oxygen delivery method produces oxygen saturation levels equal to those achieved with traditional continuous-flow devices such as a nasal cannula. Demand-flow devices use 60% less oxygen than do continuous-flow devices and, therefore, are desirable for home use. On the downside, demand-flow devices are large, require batteries, and are more costly than the continuous-flow models. Patients must balance these advantages and disadvantages when selecting home oxygen equipment.[11]

Home Ventilatory Support. Patients needing home ventilatory support typically fall into one of three categories:[11]

1. Patients who are unable to maintain adequate ventilation for long periods. These patients usually have neuromuscular and thoracic wall disorders (eg, multiple sclerosis, chest wall deformities, diaphragmatic paralysis, myasthenia gravis), and they may need only nighttime ventilation support.
2. Patients who need continuous ventilator support to survive. Examples include patients with high spinal cord injuries, apneic encephalopathies, severe COPD, or severe muscular dystrophy.
3. Terminally ill patients, such as those with lung cancer, end-stage COPD, or cystic fibrosis.

Home ventilatory support may be noninvasive or invasive. Invasive ventilation in the home setting is always provided by tracheostomy.

TABLE 51-1 describes requirements for home ventilation. Most home ventilators have a number of controls and ventilator settings. They are electrically controlled but should have battery backup that will last several hours. When transporting the patient on a home ventilator using the patient's own ventilator, connect the device to the ambulance's power supply, but bring the patient's spare batteries. Do not change the patient's standard settings unless adjustment is needed to improve oxygenation or ventilation.

TABLE 51-1 Home Ventilator Requirements

Requirement	Details
Fraction of inspired oxygen	Should be <0.40
Positive end-expiratory pressure	Should be ≤10 cm H_2O
Tracheostomy	Should be mature
Care plan	Should specify: • Ventilator settings • Equipment function and configuration
Monitoring	Should be performed: • If ventilator settings or ventilation type is changed • After moving patient • At intervals specified in care plan
Backup ventilator	Should be available if: • Patient cannot spontaneously ventilate for 4 hours or more • Replacement ventilator is not available within 2 hours (eg, because of patient's location) • Patient needs ventilator when mobile

Types of Ventilators. Home ventilators can be classified as pressure ventilators or volume ventilators. Pressure-preset ventilators are pressure-cycled devices that terminate inspiration when a preset pressure is achieved. When the preset pressure is reached, the gas flow stops and the patient passively exhales. These ventilators most often are used for patients whose ventilatory resistance is not likely to change.

Volume-preset ventilators (volume-assured ventilators) deliver a predetermined volume of gas with each cycle, after which inspiration is terminated. These types of ventilators provide a constant tidal volume regardless of changes in airway resistance or compliance of the lungs and thorax. The volume remains the same unless very high peak airway pressures are reached, at which point safety release valves stop the flow.

Negative pressure ventilators create negative pressure within the chest so that air flows into the lungs. These types of ventilators are rarely used, though they may be encountered with patients who cannot use NIPPV. Such a ventilator is more difficult to apply and is not tolerated as well as NIPPV. In addition, the negative pressure ventilator limits patient mobility and may worsen upper airway obstruction in some patients.[11] Examples of this type of ventilator are the chest cuirass (rigid shell) and wrap-type systems.

Ventilator Alarms. Ventilators are equipped with alarms that alert the patient/caregiver if there is a problem with the ventilator (**TABLE 51-2**). For example, there are alarms for loss of power, frequency alarms (indicating changes in respiratory rate), volume alarms (indicating low exhaled volume or low/high minute ventilation), and low- and high-pressure alarms. A useful mnemonic for identifying possible causes of ventilator malfunction is DOPE: Displacement of the tube, Obstruction of the tube, Pneumothorax, and Equipment failure.

If a ventilator alarm is activated, the paramedic should consult with medical direction. Acute interventions specified by medical direction may include providing temporary ventilation assistance with a bag-mask device, repositioning the endotracheal tube, correcting poor ventilator tube connections, emptying water from the tube or water traps, suctioning the airway, decompressing the thorax, and possibly sedating the patient.

NOTE

The paramedic should always ensure that powered airway equipment is working properly, that oxygen is flowing, and that the equipment is connected to the power source (battery or electrical current). Equipment that is connected properly and still not working may result from a power outage in the home (eg, failed fuse or circuit breaker).

Assessment Findings

When caring for a patient who requires oxygen therapy, the paramedic should evaluate the patient's work of breathing, tidal volume, peak flow, oxygen saturation, and quality of breath sounds. This assessment can be performed with visual inspection (chest rise and fall), peak-flow meters, pulse oximetry, and auscultation

TABLE 51-2 Ventilator Alarms

Alarm Type	Cause	Intervention
High pressure	Increased secretions	Suction secretions from patient.
High pressure	Kinked tubing	Unkink tubing.
High pressure	Water in tubing	Disconnect tubing and allow it to drain.
High pressure	Anxiety	Decrease anxiety by providing a calm environment and eliminating reversible medical causes of anxiety such as clogged tubing or hypoxia.
Low pressure	Disconnected tubing	Reconnect tubing.
Low pressure	Cuff leak	Add 1 mL of air at a time to the pilot balloon of the tracheostomy tube.
Low pressure	Tracheostomy tube displaced	Reinsert new tracheostomy tube.
Oxygen delivery	Insufficient oxygen supply	Manually ventilate the patient's lungs and prepare for transport.
Ventilator not operating	Power failure	Manually ventilate the patient's lungs and prepare for transport.

(described in Chapter 15, *Airway Management, Respiration, and Artificial Ventilation,* and Chapter 23, *Respiratory*). The paramedic should be alert for signs and symptoms of hypoxia. Oxygen saturation and end-tidal carbon dioxide levels (if the patient has ventilator support) should be monitored.

Management

Management goals for a patient receiving oxygen therapy who requires acute intervention are to improve airway patency, ventilation, and oxygenation.

Improving Airway Patency. To improve airway patency, the paramedic first should reposition any airway device (eg, a NIPPV mask) to ensure it is applied properly and is well fitted. Any secretions that obstruct airflow from the airway should be cleared with suction, and sterile water should be used to clean airway devices. If needed, the home airway device should be replaced with a new device. A tracheostomy tube that has become blocked and cannot be cleared will need to be replaced with another tracheostomy tube to ensure adequate ventilation (**FIGURE 51-2**), or the tube can be replaced temporarily with an appropriately sized endotracheal tube (see Chapter 14, *Medication Administration*).

Improving Ventilation and Oxygenation. If ventilation does not improve after providing a patent airway, the paramedic should remove the home ventilator care device. The patient's ventilations should then be assisted with positive pressure ventilation via a bag-valve device and supplemental oxygen. Oxygen saturation should be monitored with pulse oximetry. The paramedic also should administer supplemental oxygen as needed to maintain oxygen saturation at 90% or higher or at the patient's normal oxygen saturation levels if that information is available. Medical direction may advise adjusting the settings of a home care device or changing the flow rate of an oxygen delivery device to improve ventilation and oxygenation. Extra personnel may be needed to assist in moving the patient who has a ventilator device to the ambulance for transport.

Psychological Support and Communication Strategies

Difficulty breathing can be a terrifying experience for the patient, especially for a patient who depends on a ventilator. The paramedic crew should try to calm the patient and family. They should be assured that respirations will be supported adequately by other means while at the scene and during transport.

Some patients with tracheostomies have special valves attached to the tracheostomy tube ("talking trachs"), such as the Passy Muir valve, Shikani valve, or Bivona tracheostomy tube. These valves or tubes redirect exhaled air around the tracheostomy tube, through the vocal cords, and out of the mouth and nose to allow for speech. (Such valves or tubes must be removed for suctioning and positive pressure ventilation.) Loss of verbal communication is a major source of anxiety in patients who have tracheostomies. The ability to communicate with these patients will be based on the patient's cognition, level of consciousness, language, and fine and gross motor skills. Methods of communication may include signing and writing on notepads. The paramedic should enlist the help of family and other caregivers in communicating with the patient.

Cardiovascular Support

Nearly 5 million Americans have heart failure,[12] a diagnosis that accounts for billions of dollars of health care expenditures annually.[13] The population with this condition is expected to grow over the next 20 years.

Patients discharged to home care with a diagnosis of heart failure may have an implanted device to monitor cardiovascular function. In addition, these patients may have a variety of technologic devices to aid in care or to prevent life threats. Implanted therapeutic electrical devices such as pacemakers or implantable cardioverter defibrillators (ICDs) also typically have the ability to monitor and transmit patient data (**TABLE 51-3**).

> NOTE
>
> As described in Chapter 21, *Cardiology*, it is likely that paramedics will encounter patients who have a left ventricular assist device (LVAD). The patient groups who most commonly use LVADs are heart transplant candidates, heart surgery patients during recovery, and patients with severe heart failure.

When a patient has a problem with a cardiovascular support device, the paramedic should contact the emergency number provided with it. Any external go bag or other accessories should be transported to the hospital with the patient. In addition to checking for device failure, the paramedic should observe for

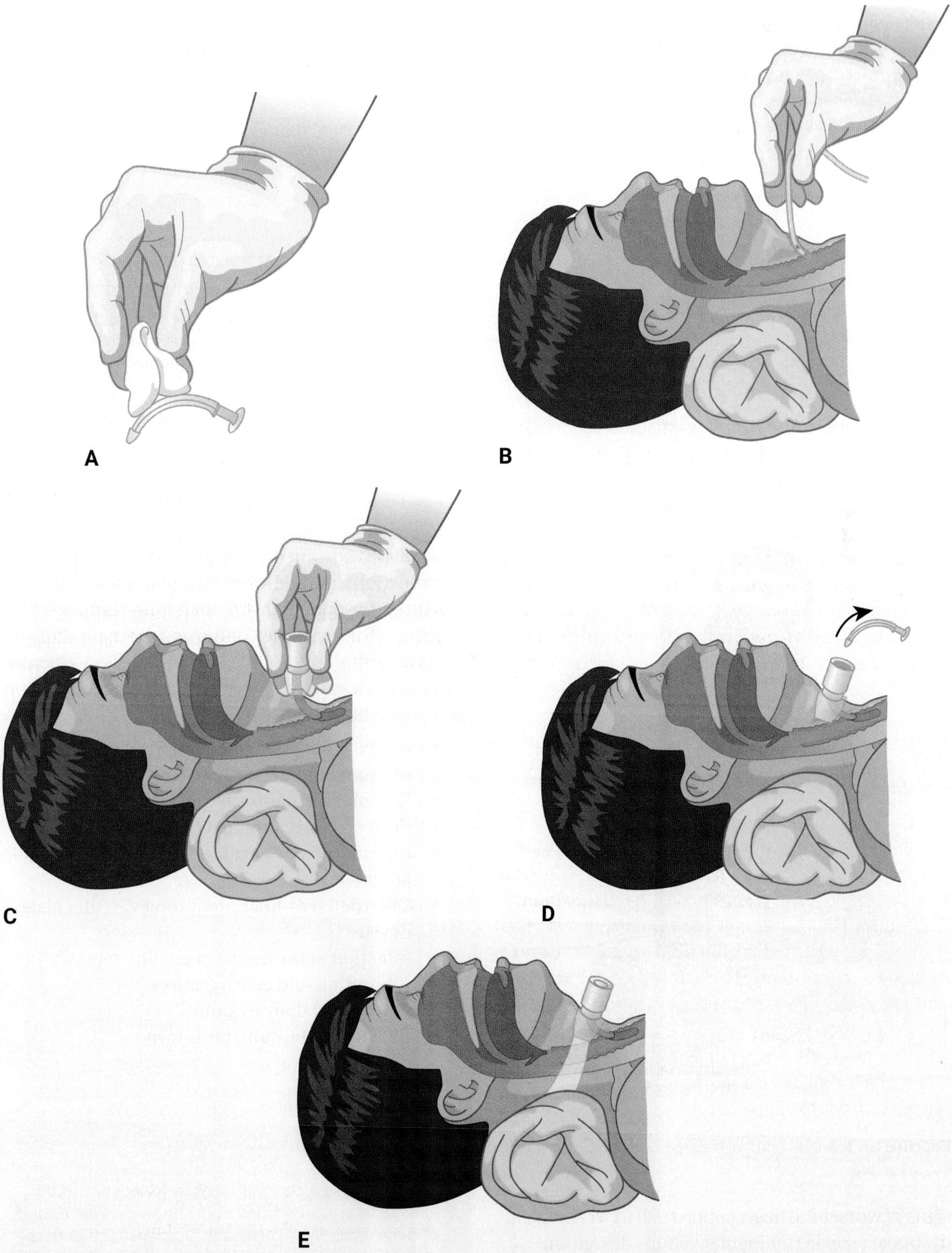

FIGURE 51-2 Replacement of a tracheostomy tube in an adult. **A.** Select a tube that is the same size or one size smaller than the one removed, and moisten it with sterile, water-soluble lubricant. **B.** Suction the stoma and trachea before inserting the new tube. **C.** Insert the tube gently into the trachea with the curve pointing downward. **D.** If the tube has an obturator, remove it; if it is a cuffed tube, inflate the cuff. **E.** Assess for correct tube placement and secure the tube.

TABLE 51-3 Types of Cardiovascular Support Devices[a]

Device	Purpose
Permanent pacemaker	Maintain adequate heart rate.
ICD	Detect and cardiovert life-threatening tachycardias.
CRT device	A biventricular pacemaker used to ensure the ventricles beat in unison when a bundle branch block causes asynchronous contraction.
Defibrillation vest	An external device worn as a vest that detects lethal ECG rhythms and cardioverts. It is used as a temporary measure while the patient awaits ICD placement in patients with low ejection fraction.
VAD, LVAD	A mechanical support device usually implanted in the left ventricle to improve ejection fraction (**FIGURE 51-3**). It receives blood from the ventricle and helps deliver it to the rest of the body. It is used as a bridge device to transplant or a destination (permanent) device in those who do not want or are not eligible for transplant.

[a]Pacemakers, ICDs, LVADs, and defibrillator vests are described in detail in Chapter 21, *Cardiology*. Some of these devices are combined (eg, pacemaker and ICD).

Abbreviations: CRT, cardiac resynchronization therapy; ECG, electrocardiogram; ICD, implantable cardioverter defibrillator; LVAD, left ventricular assist device; VAD, ventricular assist device

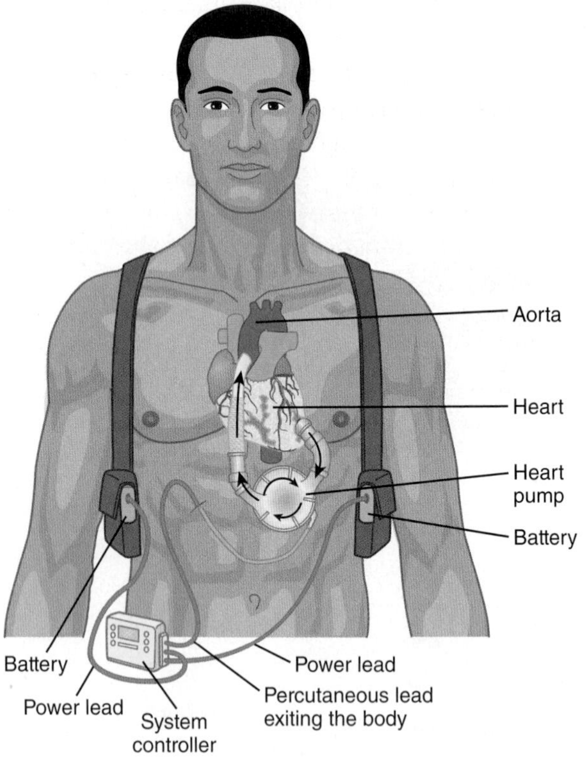

FIGURE 51-3 A left ventricular assist device.

signs of worsening heart failure such as weight gain, dyspnea, crackles, or jugular venous distention.

Many patients in the home care setting have an indwelling **vascular access device**. Such a device is used to provide nutritional support or to administer medications. In addition, vascular access devices are used for patients who need long-term vascular access—for example, patients receiving dialysis or chemotherapy. People with indwelling vascular access devices may experience problems, including the following:

- Anticoagulation associated with percutaneous or implanted devices
- Embolus formation associated with indwelling devices, stasis, and inactivity
- Air embolus associated with central vascular access devices
- Obstructed or malfunctioning vascular access devices
- Infection at the access site ("line sepsis")
- Infiltration and extravasation
- Obstructed dialysis shunts
- Bleeding if the catheter is torn

NOTE

Heart failure is a common reason for hospitalization. Paramedics may encounter patients with heart failure who are receiving medications (eg, dopamine, dobutamine, milrinone) intravenously through a vascular access device in the home setting.

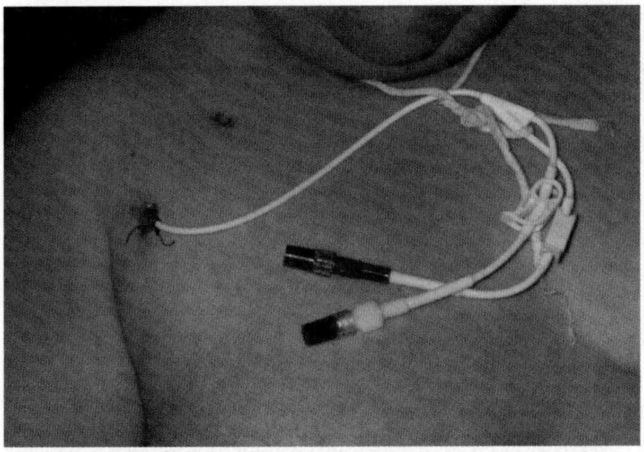

FIGURE 51-4 External venous catheter.

Types of Vascular Access Devices

As described in Chapter 14, *Medication Administration*, there are a variety of vascular access devices. They include medication delivery devices (eg, Port-a-Caths, MediPorts), peripherally inserted central catheters (PICCs), midline catheters, central venous tunneled catheters (eg, Hickman, Groshong, Broviac), and dialysis shunts (**FIGURE 51-4**).

Assessment Findings and Acute Interventions

Certain assessment findings may require acute interventions in patients with vascular access devices. These findings include infection, hemorrhage, hemodynamic compromise from circulatory overload or embolus, obstruction of the device, catheter breakage, and leakage of medication (eg, chemotherapeutic agents) (**TABLE 51-4**).

Infection. Home health care patients who have vascular access devices generally are instructed to regularly examine the area for infection. They also are instructed to change the dressings based on the type of dressing—every 24 hours for dry dressings and every 7 days for occlusive dressings (unless soiled).[14] As a rule, this changing is done by family members and home health care practitioners. All types of dressings must be changed immediately if they become wet, soiled, contaminated, or nonocclusive.

A common problem with these devices is infection near the entry site, tunnel, or port. Signs and symptoms of localized site infection include pain, redness, warmth, and purulence. Signs and symptoms of systemic infection (which may result from a site infection) include fever, tachycardia, general weakness, malaise, mental status changes, body aches, and possibly septicemia. If the patient has any evidence of systemic signs of infection, he or she should be transported to the hospital.

General principles in managing the site of infection are as follows:

1. Wash your hands.
2. Put on nonsterile gloves and remove the old dressing.
3. Discard the dressing and gloves.
4. Open the dressing change kit and don sterile gloves.
5. Inspect the site for signs of swelling, redness, or other complications.
6. Clean the site vigorously, using a side-to-side cleaning motion. Chlorhexidine gluconate in 70% alcohol is the antiseptic of choice; consider use of an aqueous solution of chlorhexidine gluconate if alcohol use is not permitted for the specific catheter.[14]
7. Do not apply ointment unless you are removing the catheter.
8. Cover with a transparent dressing.

> CRITICAL THINKING
> Will it always be possible to identify the catheter as the source of sepsis while on the scene?

Hemorrhage. Bleeding at the site of a vascular access device should be controlled by applying gentle, direct pressure with aseptic technique. Blood loss from a broken or dislodged device can be significant, enough

TABLE 51-4 Correcting Common Problems With Vascular Access Devices

Complication	Signs and Symptoms	Prehospital Interventions
Mechanical Problems		
Occluded IV catheter	Slow or interrupted flow rate, resistance to flushing and blood withdrawal	Reposition the patient. Have the patient cough. Raise the patient's arm overhead.[a] Attempt to aspirate the clot. If unsuccessful, transport for fibrinolytic therapy or removal and replacement.
Cracked or broken tubing	Fluid leaking from tubing	Apply padded hemostat near the insertion site to prevent air from entering the line, and change the tubing (with orders from medical direction). Cover the hole with sterile gauze.
Dislodged catheter	Catheter displaced from vein	Apply pressure to the site with a sterile gauze pad.
Too-rapid infusion	Flushing, erythema, pruritus, shortness of breath; sometimes hypotension, as can be seen in vancomycin infusion	Adjust the infusion rate, and if applicable, check the infusion pump. Contact medical direction about the need to transport.
Other Problems		
Air embolism	Apprehension, chest pain, tachycardia, hypotension, cyanosis, seizures, loss of consciousness, and cardiac arrest	Aspirate air and fluid. Clamp the catheter if the leak persists. Place the patient in a steep, left-lateral Trendelenburg position. Give oxygen as ordered.
Extravasation	Swelling, burning, or pain around the insertion site	Stop the infusion. Assess the patient for cardiopulmonary abnormalities. Apply warm or cold compresses based on the infusion. Notify medical direction for further advice.
Phlebitis	Pain, tenderness, redness, and warmth	Apply gentle heat to the area; elevate the insertion site if possible.
Pneumothorax and hydrothorax	Dyspnea, chest pain, cyanosis, and decreased breath sounds	If signs and symptoms of tension pneumothorax are present, consider needle decompression after consulting with medical direction.
Septicemia	Red and swollen catheter site, chills, fever	Follow sepsis protocol. Transport for physician evaluation.
Thrombosis	Erythema and edema at the insertion site; ipsilateral swelling of the arm, neck, face, and upper chest; pain at the insertion site and along the vein; malaise; fever; tachycardia	Apply warm compresses to the insertion site; elevate the affected extremity. Transport the patient.
Hemorrhage	Bleeding at the site of a vascular access device or from broken device	Apply pressure to the site. Clamp the vascular access device and treat for shock.

[a]Perry AG, Potter P, Ostendorf WR, Laplante N. *Clinical Nursing Skills and Techniques.* 9th ed. St. Louis, MO: Elsevier; 2018.

Abbreviation: IV, intravenous

that medical direction may recommend that the damaged catheter be clamped. If blood loss is severe, the patient should be treated for hemorrhagic shock. All patients with hemorrhage need to be transported for physician evaluation.

Hemodynamic Compromise. Hemodynamic compromise may result from circulatory overload or embolus. Circulatory overload can develop from too much IV fluid being delivered too fast. Signs and symptoms of circulatory overload include a rise in blood pressure, distended neck veins, pulmonary congestion (crackles and wheezes), and dyspnea. If circulatory overload is suspected, the paramedic should do the following:

1. Slow the infusion to a keep-open rate.
2. Provide high-concentration oxygen and monitor oxygen saturation.
3. Elevate the patient's head.
4. Maintain body warmth. This will both promote peripheral circulation and ease the stress on the central veins.
5. Monitor vital signs.
6. Consult with medical direction for patient management and disposition.

CRITICAL THINKING

Which drug(s) may the physician order in case of hemodynamic compromise in a patient with a vascular access device?

Displacement of a surgically implanted catheter or port is rare but may be associated with an embolus that occurs from air, thrombus, or plastic or catheter tip entering the circulation (BOX 51-2). Signs and symptoms of an embolus include dyspnea; hypoxia; hypotension; cyanosis; weak, rapid pulse; and loss of consciousness. A patient suspected of having an embolism should be managed as described in Table 51-4 and Chapter 14, *Medication Administration.*

NOTE

Accessing a vascular access device requires special needles and adapters. Only paramedics with special training and authorization from medical direction should attempt to access these devices.

BOX 51-2 Causes of Embolus Formation

Air Embolism

IV fluid containers that run dry
Air in IV tubing
Loose connections in catheter tubing
Catheter tears and breakage

Thrombus

Clot formation from inactivity or stasis

Plastic or Catheter Tip Migration

Plastic or catheter fragment from tugging or shearing forces
Wire from central line placement

Flushing and Irrigation. Vascular access devices and medication ports require regular irrigation with normal saline (Groshong) or heparin for nonvalved catheters. The solution used depends on the type of device, and the frequency of irrigation depends on the specific device and on the frequency of medication administration. To flush a device, the paramedic should consult with medical direction and follow these steps:[15]

1. Explain the procedure to the patient.
2. Establish a sterile field and use strict aseptic technique.
3. Prepare prescribed irrigation solutions (normal saline or heparin).
4. Clean the injection cap(s) with an antiseptic (per protocol) and allow it to air dry.
5. Release the clamp from the catheter (if present).
6. Irrigate the lumen with an appropriate volume of solution using only a 10-mL syringe (no faster than 0.5 mL/sec). If resistance is persistent, stop the irrigation; otherwise the catheter may rupture. Note: The paramedic must never try to force or dislodge a clot or other obstruction, as the application of force could dislodge the obstruction and cause it to enter the circulatory system or damage the catheter. Fibrinolytic agents may be required instead.
7. Aspirate blood back into the syringe; doing so removes clots or fibrin sheaths.
8. Flush with normal saline (10 to 20 mL) to clear the system.
9. Use a heparin (10 units/mL) flush if necessary (eg, Broviac, Hickman, or PICC). Volume is determined by the manufacturer and device and ranges from 1.5 mL for central venous catheters to 2.5 mL for specialty catheters.[16]
10. Clamp the catheter if needed.
11. Loop the catheter with the cap pointing upward on the dressing. Secure with tape.
12. Properly dispose of all equipment.

Anticoagulant Therapy. At times, a medication port or other vascular access device may require declotting with fibrinolytic agents (eg, tissue plasminogen activator). Flushing with fibrinolytic agents should be performed by specialized personnel. A radiograph may be needed before administration of these agents.

Other Complications. If you are unable to aspirate blood from the central line, or if the patient or family reports that the length of the catheter that was visible has changed, do not administer fluid or drugs through it. The patient will need transport for further evaluation.

For subclavian and internal jugular catheters, a decrease in the length of the catheter coupled with a sudden onset of tachycardia can mean that the catheter has moved into the right atrium. If the patient hears bubbling in the ear when the catheter is flushed, or has a sudden earache on the side of the body where the catheter is inserted, the catheter may have advanced into the jugular vein. In all of these situations, a radiograph will be needed to determine the location of the catheter.

Catheter Damage. A damaged (eg, cracked or torn) catheter can allow fluids or medications to infiltrate into the surrounding tissues and lead to an air embolism. Signs and symptoms of a damaged catheter include leaking fluid, complaint of a burning sensation, or swollen and tender skin near the insertion site. If catheter damage is suspected, the infusion should be stopped immediately. The catheter should be clamped between the crack or tear in the catheter and the patient. These patients are managed with high-concentration oxygen and pulse oximetry, IV access through a peripheral vein, and transport for physician evaluation. A patient in whom an altered level of consciousness develops (indicating a possible air embolism) should be positioned on the left side. The head should be slightly lowered. This positioning will help to prevent the embolism from traveling to the brain.[17]

Gastrointestinal/Genitourinary Crisis

Many patients with diseases of the digestive or genitourinary system are discharged to home health care each year. Some of these patients have medical devices such as urinary catheters or urostomies, indwelling nutritional support devices (eg, percutaneous endoscopic gastrostomy tube, jejunostomy tube), colostomy bags, and nasogastric tubes (BOX 51-3). Acute interventions that may be required for these patients can result from urinary tract infection (UTI), **urosepsis**, urinary retention, and problems with gastric emptying or feeding.

BOX 51-3 Medical Therapy Found in the Home Setting for Patients With Gastrointestinal/Genitourinary Disease

Devices for Gastric/Intestinal Emptying or Feeding

Colostomy bag
Gastrostomy or jejunostomy tube
Nasogastric tube

Devices for the Urinary Tract

External urinary catheter (eg, condom catheter, Texas catheter)
Indwelling urinary catheter (eg, Foley catheter, coudé catheter)
Surgical urinary catheter (eg, suprapubic catheter)
Urostomy

UTI, Urosepsis, and Urinary Retention

UTIs are common, occurring in all age groups and both sexes (see Chapter 29, *Genitourinary and Renal Disorders*). The organisms most often associated with UTI are the gram-negative organisms normally found in the gastrointestinal tract—for example, *Escherichia coli, Klebsiella, Proteus, Enterobacter*, and *Pseudomonas*. These bacteria frequently are introduced from the hands of health care personnel at the time of bladder catheterization.[17] Approximately 75% of UTIs are the result of urinary catheter,[18] so sterile technique during these procedures is crucial. Other factors that increase the risk of UTI include the following:

- Obstructions (eg, enlarged prostate, urethral strictures, calculi, tumors, blood clots)
- Trauma (eg, abdominal injury, ruptured bladder, local trauma related to sexual activity)
- Congenital anomalies (eg, polycystic kidneys, horseshoe kidney, spina bifida)
- Abdominal or gynecologic surgery
- Acute or chronic renal failure
- Immunocompromised state (eg, patients with HIV infections, older adults)
- Postpartum state
- Aging changes, particularly in women
- Reduced mobility

If UTI is allowed to progress, it may lead to urosepsis. This disease is managed with antibiotics.

Urinary retention may result from urethral stricture, inflammation, enlarged prostate, central nervous system dysfunction, foreign body obstruction, and use of certain drugs, such as parasympatholytic or anticholinergic agents. These patients need to be evaluated by a physician to determine the cause of the retention. If the cause is not easily correctable, the patient may need to be hospitalized.

Indwelling Urinary Catheter Insertion

Some patients with urinary retention may require **bladder catheterization** with an indwelling Foley catheter device. In addition, bladder catheterization using a urinary (Foley) catheter may be indicated to replace an indwelling urinary catheter that is not functioning or to measure urine output in critical patients. This invasive procedure carries some associated risks: the introduction of bacteria, which may lead to UTI; hematuria; and the creation of a false urethral passage, which may result in significant blood loss and the need for surgical repair.

To insert a Foley catheter, the paramedic should prepare the required equipment (eg, urinary catheter insertion set). The paramedic must closely follow the manufacturer's recommendations (BOX 51-4). Most patients will be anxious and frightened of the procedure. The paramedic should fully explain the procedure, reassure the patient, and make every effort to ensure privacy.

BOX 51-4 Equipment for Bladder Catheterization

- Personal protective equipment
- Urinary catheterization set containing the following:
  - Sterile gloves
  - Antiseptic solution
  - Sterile cleansing sponges
  - Sterile drapes or towels
  - Syringe containing 5 mL sterile water
  - Connecting tubing and collection bag
  - Water-soluble sterile lubricant
- Urinary catheter with 5-mL balloon
  - Catheter usually is a 16 French for males and a 14 French for females.
- Standard length is 18 inches (46 cm).

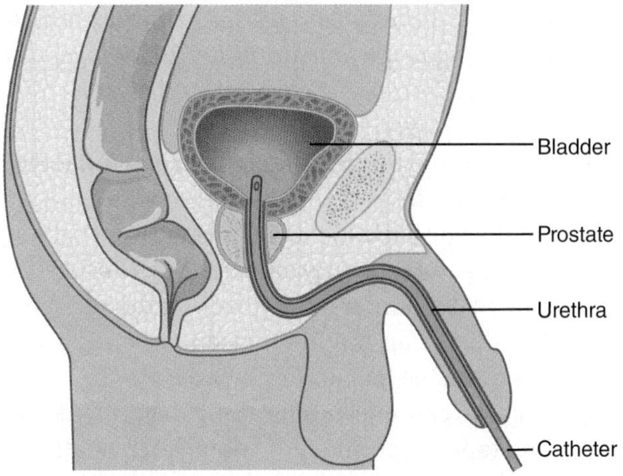

FIGURE 51-5 Male bladder catheterization.

Male Catheterization (FIGURE 51-5).

1. Explain the procedure to the patient.
2. Place the patient in the supine position and remove the patient's pants and undergarments.
3. Wash hands.
4. Open the catheterization set using sterile technique.
5. Don sterile gloves.
6. Place one sterile drape under the patient's penis and another above the penis to cover the abdomen.
7. Open a package of antiseptic solution and saturate sterile sponges (or cotton balls).
8. Attach the syringe to the catheter and test the balloon to make sure it inflates.
9. Open a package of water-soluble lubricant and lubricate the first several inches of the catheter.
10. Grasp the patient's penis with one hand and retract the foreskin (if present).
11. With the other hand, cleanse the glans with a sterile sponge (maintaining hand sterility) and then discard the sponge. Repeat the procedure.
12. Raise the shaft of the penis upright to straighten the penile urethra and pass the tip of the catheter through the meatus.
13. Continue passing the catheter with gentle, steady pressure, advancing the catheter 7 to 9 inches (18 to 23 cm) or until urine flows out the distal end of the catheter. Once urine appears, advance the catheter another 2 inches (5 cm). If mild resistance is felt at the external sphincter, slightly increase traction on the penis and continue with steady, gentle pressure on the

catheter. *If significant resistance is met prior to achieving urine flow from the bladder into the tube, withdraw the catheter and consult with medical direction.*

14. Attach the syringe to the catheter and inflate the balloon with 3 to 5 mL of sterile saline.
15. Gently pull back on the catheter until the balloon rests against the prostatic urethra. (Resistance will be encountered.) Reposition the retracted foreskin of an uncircumcised patient. Attach the drainage bag to the catheter.
16. Run the catheter tubing along the patient's leg and tape the connecting tubing to the patient's thigh. Do not place any tension on the catheter.
17. Attach the collection bag to the bed or stretcher at a level below that of the patient to facilitate drainage by gravity.

Female Catheterization (FIGURE 51-6).

1. Prepare the patient and equipment as described in steps 1 through 5 and 7 through 9 of the male catheterization procedure. Female patients should be positioned with knees bent, hips flexed, and feet resting approximately 24 inches (61 cm) apart. The patient should be draped appropriately by placing one sterile drape just under the patient's buttocks; position the fenestrated drape over the perineum, exposing the labia.
2. With one hand, separate the patient's labia to expose the urethral meatus.
3. Cleanse the surrounding area with a sterile sponge or cotton ball (maintaining hand sterility) in downward strokes from anterior to posterior. Discard the sponge. Repeat the procedure.

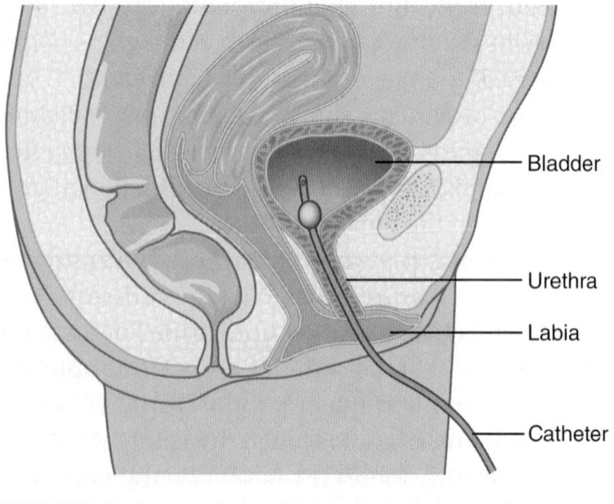

FIGURE 51-6 Female bladder catheterization.

4. Introduce the tip of the well-lubricated catheter into the urethra using aseptic technique. Continue to advance the catheter 2 to 3 inches (5 to 8 cm) with gentle, steady pressure until urine flows out of the distal end of the catheter. Once urine appears, advance the catheter another 2 inches (5 cm).
5. Attach a syringe to the catheter. Inflate the balloon with 3 to 5 mL of sterile saline.
6. Gently pull on the catheter until resistance is encountered.
7. Attach the collection tubing and bag to the catheter and secure the collection tubing to the patient's thigh as described in step 17 of the male catheterization procedure. Position the collection bag to facilitate drainage.

CRITICAL THINKING

What measure should you take to protect yourself legally when inserting a urinary catheter into a patient in a home?

Problems With Gastric Emptying or Feeding

A **gastric tube** used in the home health care setting is a device that is inserted into the stomach or intestines (**FIGURE 51-7**). It is used to remove fluids and gas by suction or gravity, to instill irrigation solutions or medications, and to administer enteral feedings (through feeding tubes) (**TABLE 51-5**). Two common problems with gastric tubes are aspiration of gastric contents and malfunction of gastric devices.

NOTE

Flexible feeding tubes (such as the Dobhoff feeding tube) are commonly used in patients who cannot take nourishment by mouth. The feeding tubes may be inserted orally or nasally so that the tip of the tube is placed in either the stomach or the duodenum. These tubes generally have a weighted tungsten tip and have a guidewire to prevent them from curling up in the back of the patient's throat.

Aspiration of Gastric Contents. Aspiration of gastric contents may occur in the home health care patient as a result of a nonpatent gastric tube, improper nutritional support via a feeding tube, or patient positioning with these medical devices. The patients

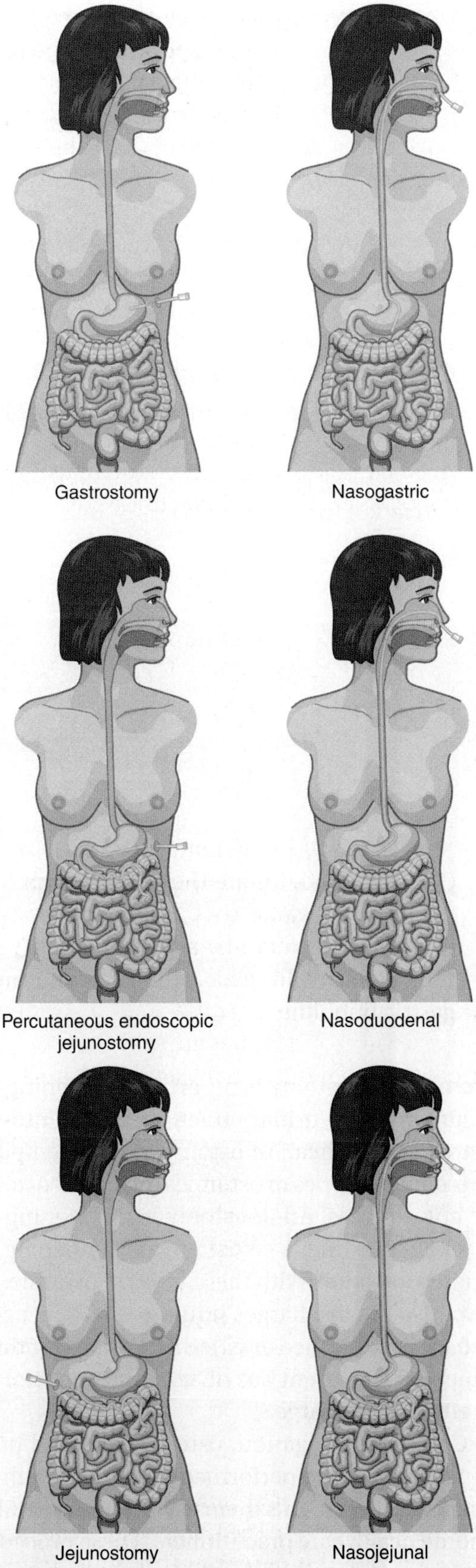

FIGURE 51-7 Tube-feeding sites.

TABLE 51-5 Feeding Tubes: Types and Placement

Type of Tube	Placement
Nasogastric	Passed via nose into stomach
Nasointestinal	Passed via nose into intestine
Esophagostomy	Passed into esophagus through a surgically created opening in the anterior neck
Gastrostomy	Passed directly into stomach through an opening created in the abdominal wall
Jejunostomy, percutaneous endoscopic gastrostomy tube	Passed into jejunum through an opening created in the abdominal wall

at greatest risk for aspiration of tube feedings are those with the following characteristics:

- Are unconscious
- Are confused
- Are seriously debilitated
- Are older adults
- Have tracheostomies or large-bore feeding tubes
- Have impaired gag reflexes
- Cannot sit upright

The paramedic should monitor patients with feeding tubes closely for signs of increased respiratory effort. Lung sounds should be clear on auscultation. Respiratory difficulty or tachypnea may indicate developing aspiration pneumonitis. Other problems that can occur in patients with feeding tubes include diarrhea, choking, irritable bowel syndrome, and bowel obstruction. Position patients with feeding tubes upright at a minimum of 30°, preferably 45°,[15] unless otherwise contraindicated.

Obstruction or Malfunction of Gastric Devices. A gastric device may become obstructed or malfunction for different reasons. For example, there may be a kinked or clogged tube, or a surgically implanted feeding tube may become displaced. Acute interventions that the nurse, paramedic, patient, or caregiver may use to solve home tube-feeding problems include unkinking a tube, irrigating a clogged tube, and reinserting a displaced tube, per medical direction (**TABLE 51-6**).

TABLE 51-6 Managing Tube-Feeding Problems

Complication	Interventions
Aspiration of gastric secretions	Discontinue feeding immediately and elevate the head of the bed. Perform tracheal suction of aspirated contents if possible. Notify the physician. To prevent this complication, check the tube placement before feeding
Tube obstruction	Attempt to verify tube placement. Place the patient in semi-Fowler position. Flush the tube with warm water. If necessary, replace the tube. Flush the tube with 30 mL of water after each feeding to remove excess sticky formula, which could occlude the tube.
Nasal or pharyngeal irritation or necrosis	Provide frequent oral hygiene using 0.12% oral chlorhexidine rinse or swabs with 1.5% hydrogen peroxide to remove plaque. Use petroleum jelly on cracked lips/nasal passages. Change the position of the tube. If necessary, replace the tube.
Vomiting, bloating, diarrhea, or cramps	Reduce the flow rate. Warm the formula. Assess for signs of infection. Notify the physician. The physician may reduce the amount of formula being given during each feeding.

Time is of the essence in correcting a malfunctioning gastric device, and immediate transport for definitive care is indicated. When transporting a patient with a gastric device, the paramedic must ensure patient comfort. The device should be positioned to allow for proper drainage and to prevent reflux.

If a gastrostomy tube comes out, the paramedic may be able to replace it if the local protocol permits such action and the paramedic is qualified to do so.[19] When possible, the paramedic should use the patient's replacement tube. If one is not available, the paramedic should cleanse the used tube in a gentle solution, rinse it, and reuse it (a Foley catheter may also be used). To replace the gastrostomy tube, the paramedic should do the following:

1. Inspect the site, ensuring the stoma is open and noting any tears.
2. Cleanse secretions or debris from the site.
3. Check that the gastrostomy tube balloon is intact and inflates.
4. Lubricate the tube with water-soluble gel.
5. Insert the gastrostomy tube into the stoma using light pressure. Stop insertion if resistance is met.
6. Once inserted, inflate the balloon with 3 to 5 mL saline or water.
7. Confirm placement by aspirating gastric contents and instilling air while auscultating for gastric bubbling.

Ostomies. An **ostomy** is an artificial opening into the lumen of the urinary tract, the gastrointestinal tract, or the trachea. An ostomy may be temporary or permanent. Types of ostomies include ileostomies and colostomies. An **ileostomy** is an opening into the small intestine; a **colostomy** is an opening into the large intestine. With these types of ostomies, the bowel usually discharges liquid or solid feces into the bag (pouch) once or twice a day; the bag then is changed. The patient has no voluntary control over the effluent discharge.

Colostomy irrigation, ostomy care, and pouch changes usually are performed for home health care patients by the patients themselves, family members, or home health care practitioners. These procedures require special training but usually are not considered an acute intervention for paramedic practice.

Bowel perforation and significant fluid/electrolyte imbalances may accidentally occur from colostomy irrigation performed by the patient or caregiver. Other potential complications associated with ostomies include infection, hemorrhage, obstruction, and stoma problems (eg, necrosis, retraction, stenosis, prolapse).

Assessment and Management of Patients With Gastrointestinal/Genitourinary Crisis

The paramedic should evaluate a patient with gastrointestinal/genitourinary complaints by obtaining a focused history and performing a physical examination to determine the need for immediate transport for physician evaluation. Depending on the patient's chief complaint, the physical examination may include assessment for the following:

- Abdominal distention
- Abdominal pain
- Aspiration
- Fever
- Intestinal obstruction
- Peritonitis
- UTI
- Urinary retention

Acute Infections

Patients with chronic diseases, poor nutrition, or an inability to perform self-care are at increased risk for infection and impaired healing. Home health care patients with acute infections have an increased death rate from sepsis and severe peripheral infections. They also may have a decreased ability to perceive pain or perform self-care.

During the time patients are in home health care, approximately 3.5% experience infections serious enough to seek emergency care or to require hospitalization.[20] Conditions that may result in the need for acute interventions in the home health care population include the following:[21]

- Airway infections in the immunocompromised patient
- Delayed healing and increased peripheral infection from poor peripheral perfusion
- Skin breakdown and peripheral infections from immobility or sedentary lifestyle
- Infection and sepsis from implanted medical devices
- Wounds and incisions
- Abscesses
- Cellulitis

Open Wounds

Patients with open wounds who are discharged to home health care may have a variety of dressings, wound packings, and drains that permit drainage of fluid or air. They also may have a variety of wound closure devices (BOX 51-5). The various dressings, packings, and wound closure devices can become contaminated; drains can become occluded or displaced.

Wound healing greatly depends on wound management. The patient must be made aware of the importance of taking all prescribed medications, but especially antibiotics. The patient also should be informed of the importance of completing all wound care procedures. Wound repair generally is believed to be enhanced by the following:

- Moist environment
- Wound bed free of necrotic tissue, eschar, and environmental contamination or infection

BOX 51-5 Wound Care Devices Found in Home Health Care Patients

Dressings and Wound Packing Material

Combination dressings
Cotton dressings (gauze)
Exudate absorptive dressings
Negative pressure wound therapy sponges
Hydrocolloid dressings
Hydrogel dressings
Impregnated cotton dressings
Alginate (highly absorptive)
Transparent film (adhesive or nonadhesive)

Drains

Jackson-Pratt drains
Penrose drains

Wound Closure Techniques

Skin adhesive
Staples
Sutures
Tape
Wires

- Adequate blood supply to meet metabolic demands for tissue generation
- Sufficient oxygen and nutrition for cellular metabolism and tissue generation

General Principles in Wound Care Management

Wound care requires assessment of the wound and the surrounding tissues as well as evaluation for infection or sepsis. General principles in wound care management include an assessment for the following:[22]

1. **Location, type, and size of wound.**
2. **Color of the wound bed.** A red or pink granular wound bed indicates healing. A green, yellow, or black wound bed suggests infection or necrosis (tissue death).
3. **Drainage.** Clear or blood-tinged drainage is common in a healing wound. Green or yellow drainage suggests infection.
4. **Wound odor.** A sweet smell may indicate decay. A foul smell may indicate infection.
5. **Surrounding skin.** The paramedic should assess the skin for redness, inflammation, or signs of tissue breakdown. If the dressing is wet or contaminated, the paramedic should change it after wound evaluation. Medical direction may advise cleaning the wound with normal saline and/or antiseptic solution before re-dressing it. The debridement of necrotic tissue may be required. Mechanical debridement is achieved by gently rubbing the tissue with a gauze pad moistened with sterile, normal saline. Some patients may require transport for physician evaluation if severe infection or sepsis is suspected.
6. **Pain.** Use a pain scale to assess the patient's wound-related pain.

Care for Life-Limiting and Terminal Illness

A number of programs have been developed to assist patients and their families in dealing with life-limiting illness and end-of-life care. Two of these programs are hospice care and palliative care. Both programs rely on the combined knowledge and skill of a team of professionals that includes physicians, nurses, medical social workers, therapists, counselors, chaplains, and volunteers. This team works together to provide a personal plan of care for each patient and family.

> SHOW ME THE EVIDENCE
>
> EMS providers in Atlanta, Georgia, were surveyed to assess their knowledge, attitudes, and experience with patients enrolled in hospice care. There were 182 responses. Of those, 84.1% had cared for a hospice patient. Only 29% reported having formal education on the care of hospice patients. More than one-third believed that a DNR order was required for hospice patients. Communicating with family was a theme that emerged, as well as conflicts related to the DNR.
>
> *Modified from*: Barnette Donnelly C, Armstrong KA, Perkins MM, Moulia D, Quest TE, Yancey AH. Emergency medical services provider experiences of hospice care. *Prehosp Emerg Care.* 2018;22(2):237-243.

Hospice Care

Hospice care serves more than 1.6 million patients throughout the United States each year.[23] Hospice services include supportive social, emotional, and spiritual services for the terminally ill patient. Patients are enrolled in hospice care when they have a diagnosis that predicts death within 6 months. Enrollment means the patient and family have agreed to stop therapy to cure or sustain life.

Hospice care may be delivered in the patient's home, a long-term care facility, or an inpatient hospice facility. A patient receiving hospice care may be receiving medication delivery for the relief of pain (eg, narcotic infusion devices) (BOX 51-6).[23] The patient may have medical and legal documents such as DNR orders and advance directives such as physician orders for life-sustaining treatment (POLST) (see Chapter 6, *Medical and Legal Issues*), though not all patients who receive hospice care will have a DNR order.[23] The paramedic should discuss any concerns about effective pain management, overmedication, or interpreting medical or legal documents with medical direction.

Despite their understanding of the terminal nature of the illness, and despite the fact that hospice personnel are on call 24 hours a day, these patients or their families frequently call EMS.[24] Family members are often alarmed by the patient's signs and symptoms and fear for their comfort. Calls may be related to complaints such as dyspnea, pain, oral secretions, hematemesis, or hemoptysis.

Paramedics and EMTs report difficulty in communicating with the family during such calls for

BOX 51-6 The Dying Person's Bill of Rights

1. I have the right to be treated as a living human being until I die.
2. I have the right to maintain a sense of hopefulness, however changing its focus may be.
3. I have the right to be cared for by those who can maintain a sense of hopefulness, however changing this might be.
4. I have the right to express my feelings and emotions about my approaching death in my own way.
5. I have the right to participate in decisions concerning my care.
6. I have the right to expect continuing medical and nursing attention, even though "cure" goals must be changed to "comfort" goals.
7. I have the right not to die alone.
8. I have the right to be free from pain.
9. I have the right to have my questions answered honestly.
10. I have the right not to be deceived.
11. I have the right to have help from and for my family in accepting my death.
12. I have the right to die in peace and dignity.
13. I have the right to retain my individuality and not be judged for my decisions, which may be contrary to beliefs of others.
14. I have the right to discuss and enlarge my religious and/or spiritual experiences, whatever these may mean to others.
15. I have the right to expect that the sanctity of the human body will be respected after death.
16. I have the right to be cared for by caring, sensitive, knowledgeable people who will attempt to understand my needs and will be able to gain some satisfaction in helping me face my death.

Modified from: Created at a workshop, "The Terminally Ill Patient and the Helping Person," in Lansing, Michigan, sponsored by the Southwestern Michigan Inservice Education Council and conducted by Amelia Barbus (1975), Associate Professor of Nursing, Wayne State University, Detroit. In: Whitman HH, Lukes S. Behavior modification for terminally ill patients. *Am J Nurs.* 1975;75(1):99.

hospice patients, largely due to the families' lack of understanding about hospice. The DNR or lack thereof often represents a source of conflict—for example, when the family disagrees with the patient's wishes for no resuscitation,[23] or when the family states there is a DNR but it cannot be found or is not properly executed. EMS personnel also report emotional distress and a sense of helplessness as they comfort the dying patient and family. Having proper training and a protocol that addresses these issues can help EMS personnel manage these difficult situations.

Palliative Care

Palliative care is a unique form of health care primarily directed at providing relief to terminally ill people through symptom management and pain management and can be a component of hospice care (**FIGURE 51-8**). Palliative care can also be a separate area of medical practice while the patient is receiving treatment and is not subject to any time restrictions; a terminal illness diagnosis is not required. Palliative care can be delivered over a period of weeks, months, or even years, and can work alongside a long-term treatment plan. Such care is directed at improving quality of life for patients with serious illness (comfort care) through symptom management and pain management. Like hospice care, this specialty focuses on the spiritual, physical, psychological, and social needs of the patient and family stemming from the diagnosis of a life-threatening illness such as cancer until death or cure.[23] A chief goal of palliative care is to improve the quality of a person's life as the person experiences his or her illness.

Palliative care may be delivered in hospice (BOX 51-7), home care settings, and hospitals. Medical needs vary depending on the disease. Thus, specialized palliative care programs exist for common conditions, such as cancer, heart failure, and severe respiratory symptoms.[25]

EMS and medical direction should work closely with the families and physicians of terminally ill patients receiving palliative care services so that they will make the best use of the EMS system—for instance, to ensure they know when to call 9-1-1. Very few agencies have palliative care protocols.[26] Even though resuscitation may not be indicated, paramedics may be needed to manage pain, treat acute medical illness or traumatic injury, and provide transport to a hospital. If the patient is not to receive medical intervention to prolong life, the paramedic should provide measures of comfort to the patient and emotional support to family members and loved ones (see Chapter 2, *Well-Being of the Paramedic*).

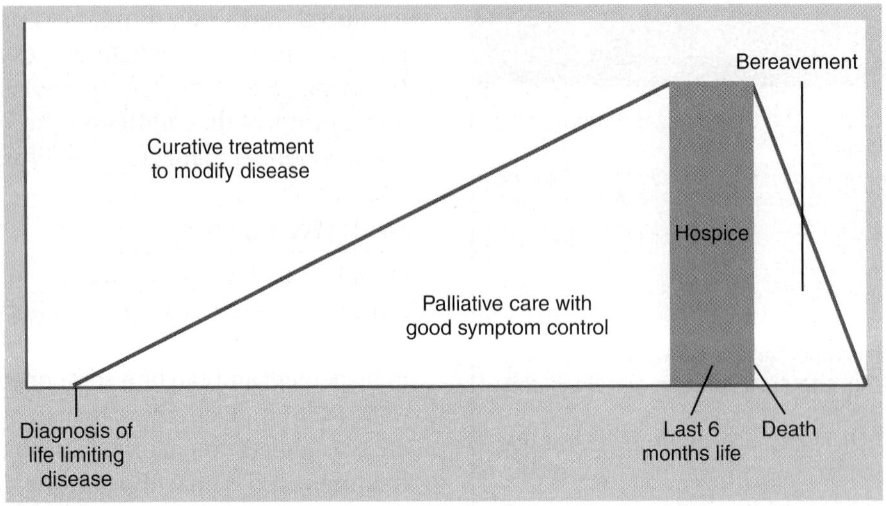

FIGURE 51-8 Optimal continuum of care on diagnosis of a life-limiting illness.

Reproduced from: Lamba S, Schmidt TA, Chan GK, et al. Integrating palliative care in the out-of-hospital setting: four things to jump-start an EMS-palliative care initiative. *Prehosp Emerg Care*. 2013;17(4):511-520.

BOX 51-7 Essential Elements of Hospice Palliative Care Programs

Hospice palliative care is an accepted specialty of medicine and nursing that concentrates on the total care of patients suffering from any form of terminal illness. Its development, as part of the health care services, is acknowledgment that dying is a normal consequence of living. Principles for all aspects of hospice palliative care are as follows:

1. Each person has intrinsic value as an autonomous and unique individual.
2. Life is valuable, death is a natural process, and both life and death provide opportunities for growth and self-actualization.
3. Patients' and families' suffering, expectations, needs, hopes, and fears must be addressed.
4. Care is provided only when the patient and/or family is prepared to accept it.
5. Care is guided by quality of life as defined by the patient.
6. Caregivers enter into a therapeutic relationship with patients and families based on dignity and integrity.
7. A unified response to suffering strengthens communities.

Modified from: Canadian Hospice Palliative Care Association. *Applying* A Model to Guide Hospice Palliative Care*: An Essential Companion Toolkit for Planners, Policy Makers, Caregivers, Educators, Managers, Administrators and Researchers*. Ontario, Canada: Canadian Hospice Palliative Care Association; 2005. http://www.chpca.net/media/7458/Applying_a-Model-to-Guide-Hospice-Palliative-Care-Toolkit.pdf. Accessed May 9, 2018.

Summary

- The medical home model is emerging as a means to coordinate care for patients with complex health needs to support their medical needs while they remain in their home. It involves collaboration and coordination of primary and specialty care services, including EMS.
- Approximately 21% of home health care patients have diseases of the circulatory system as their primary diagnosis. Other common diagnoses of home health care patients include cancer, diabetes, chronic lung disease, renal failure/dialysis, and hypertension. Typical EMS calls to a home health care setting may include respiratory failure, cardiac decompensation, septic complications, equipment malfunction, and other medical problems.
- After arrival at the scene of a home health care patient, the scene size-up should include standard precautions, elements of scene safety, and environmental setting. The

initial assessment should focus on illness or injury that poses a threat to life. The paramedic should take appropriate measures as indicated.

- Patients with diseases of the respiratory system being cared for at home are at increased risk for airway infections. In addition, the progression of their illnesses may lead to increased respiratory demand, such that the patient's current respiratory support becomes inadequate. Any patient with respiratory distress should receive appropriate amounts of oxygen, pulse oximetry and end-tidal carbon dioxide monitoring, and ventilatory support as priorities in care.
- Assessment findings that may require acute interventions in patients with vascular access devices include infection, hemorrhage, hemodynamic compromise from circulatory overload or embolus, obstruction of the vascular access device, and catheter damage with leakage of medication.
- Patients with diseases of the digestive or genitourinary system may have medical devices such as urinary catheters or urostomy tubes, indwelling nutritional support devices (eg, percutaneous endoscopic gastrostomy tube or gastrostomy tube), colostomy bags, and nasogastric tubes. Acute interventions required for these patients can result from urinary tract infection, urosepsis, urinary retention, and problems with gastric emptying or feeding.
- Home health care patients with acute infections have an increased death rate from sepsis and severe peripheral infections. Many also have a decreased ability to perceive pain or perform self-care.
- Hospice services include supportive social, emotional, and spiritual services for terminally ill patients, as well as support for the patient's family. Palliative care is directed mainly at providing relief to a person with a terminal or life-limiting illness; it focuses on symptom and pain management.

References

1. National Association for Home Care and Hospice. Basic statistics about home care. Washington, DC: National Association for Home Care and Hospice; 2010. http://www.nahc.org/wp-content/uploads/2017/10/10hc_stats.pdf. Accessed May 9, 2018.
2. Humphrey CJ, Milone-Nuzzo P. *Orientation to Home Care Nursing*. New York, NY: Aspen; 1996.
3. Boards of Trustees, Federal Hospital Insurance, Federal Supplementary Medical Insurance Trust Funds. *2016 Annual Report of the Boards of Trustees of the Federal Hospital Insurance and Federal Supplementary Medical Insurance Trust Funds*. Centers for Medicare and Medicaid Services website. https://www.cms.gov/Research-Statistics-Data-and-Systems/Statistics-Trends-and-Reports/ReportsTrustFunds/Downloads/TR2016.pdf. Published June 22, 2016. Accessed May 10, 2018.
4. Medicaid. Medicaid.gov website. https://www.medicaid.gov/medicaid/index.html. Published January 2018. Accessed May 10, 2018.
5. Home health quality initiative. Centers for Medicare and Medicaid Services website. https://www.cms.gov/Medicare/Quality-Initiatives-Patient-Assessment-Instruments/HomeHealthQualityInits/index.html. Updated January 10, 2018. Accessed May 10, 2018.
6. Verma AA, Klich J, Thurston A, et al. Paramedic-initiated home care referrals and use of home care and emergency medical services. *Prehosp Emerg Care.* 2018;22(3):379-384.
7. Defining the PCMH. Agency for Healthcare Research and Quality website. https://pcmh.ahrq.gov/page/defining-pcmh. Accessed May 10, 2018.
8. American College of Emergency Physicians. The patient-centered medical home model. *Ann Emerg Med.* 2009;53(2):289-291.
9. Pines JM, Keyes V, van Hasselt M, McCall N. Emergency department and inpatient hospital use by Medicare beneficiaries in patient-centered medical homes. *Ann Emerg Med.* 2015;65(6):652-660.
10. Roger VL, Go AS, Lloyd-Jones DM, et al.; American Heart Association Statistics Committee and Stroke Statistics Subcommittee. Heart disease and stroke statistics—2012 update. *Circulation.* 2012;125:e2-e220.
11. Kacmarek RM, Stoller JK, Heuer AJ. *Egan's Fundamentals of Respiratory Care.* 11th ed. St. Louis, MO: Elsevier; 2017.
12. National Center for Chronic Disease Prevention and Health Promotion, Division for Heart Disease and Stroke Prevention. Heart failure fact sheet. Centers for Disease Control and Prevention website. https://www.cdc.gov/dhdsp/data_statistics/fact_sheets/fs_heart_failure.htm. Updated June 16, 2016. Accessed May 10, 2018.
13. Good heart failure care follows patients home. Institute for Healthcare Improvement website. http://www.ihi.org/resources/Pages/ImprovementStories/GoodHeartFailureCareFollowsPatientsHome.aspx. Accessed May 10, 2018.
14. National Clinical Guideline Centre. *Infection: Prevention and Control of Healthcare-Associated Infections in Primary and Community Care: Partial Update of NICE Clinical Guideline 2. NICE Clinical Guidelines, No. 139.* London, UK: Royal College of Physicians; March 2012. https://www.ncbi.nlm.nih.gov/books/NBK115270/. Accessed May 10, 2018.
15. Perry AG, Potter P, Ostendorf WR, Laplante N. *Clinical Nursing Skills and Techniques.* 9th ed. St. Louis, MO: Elsevier; 2018.
16. Goossens GA. Flushing and locking of venous catheters: available evidence and evidence deficit. *Nurs Res Pract.* 2015;985686. http://doi.org/10.1155/2015/985686.
17. Marx J, Hockberger R, Walls R. *Rosen's Emergency Medicine.* 8th ed. St. Louis, MO: Saunders; 2014.
18. Centers for Disease Control and Prevention, National Center for Emerging and Zoonotic Infectious Diseases, Division of Healthcare Quality Promotion. Catheter-associated urinary tract infections (CAUTI). Centers for Disease Control and Prevention website. https://www.cdc.gov/HAI/ca_uti/uti.html. Updated July 19, 2017. Accessed May 10, 2018.

19. Kaziny BD, Shah MA. Technology-dependent children. In: Brice J, Delbridge TR, Myers JB, eds. *Emergency Medical Services: Clinical Practice and Systems Oversight.* Vol 1. 2nd ed. West Sussex, UK: John Wiley & Sons; 2015:397-400.
20. Shang J, Larson E, Liu J, Stone P. Infection in home health care: results from national Outcome and Assessment Information Set data. *Am J Infect Control.* 2015;43(5):454-459.
21. US Department of Transportation, National Highway Traffic Safety Administration. *The National EMS Education Standards.* Washington, DC: US Department of Transportation, National Highway Traffic Safety Administration; 2009.
22. Swezey L. Wound assessment: wound drainage and odor. WoundEducators.com website. https://woundeducators.com/wound-drainage-and-odor/. Published October 14, 2014. Accessed May 10, 2018.
23. Barnette Donnelly C, Armstrong KA, Perkins MM, Moulia D, Quest TE, Yancey AH. Emergency medical services provider experiences of hospice care. *Prehosp Emerg Care.* 2018;22(2): 237-243.
24. Case A, Zive D, Cook J, Schmidt TA. End-of-life issues. In: Brice J, Delbridge TR, Myers JB, eds. *Emergency Medical Services: Clinical Practice and Systems Oversight.* Vol 1. 2nd ed. West Sussex, UK: John Wiley & Sons; 2015:439-443.
25. Smith AK, Thai JN, Bakitas MA, et al. The diverse landscape of palliative care clinics. *J Palliat Med.* 2013;16(6):661-668.
26. Ausband SC, March JA, Brown LH. National prevalence of palliative care protocols in emergency medical services. *Prehosp Emerg Care.* 2002;6(1):36-41.

Suggested Readings

Beck E, Craig A, Beeson J, et al. Mobile integrated healthcare practice: a healthcare delivery strategy to improve access, outcomes, and value. American College of Emergency Physicians website. https://www.acep.org/uploadedFiles/ACEP/Practice_Resources/disater_and_EMS/MIHP_whitepaper%20FINAL1.pdf. Accessed May 10, 2018.

Carron P-N, Dami F, Diawara F, Hurst S, Hugli O. Palliative care and prehospital emergency medicine: analysis of a case series. Eroglu A, ed. *Medicine.* 2014;93(25):e128.

Harris-Kojetin L, Sengupta M, Park-Lee E, et al. Long-term care providers and services users in the United States: data from the National Study of Long-Term Care Providers, 2013–2014. National Center for Health Statistics. *Vital Health Stat.* 2016;3(38):x-xii, 1-105.

Improving palliative care in emergency services (IPAL-EM). Center to Advance Palliative Care website. https://www.capc.org/ipal/ipal-emergency-medicine/. Accessed May 10, 2018.

Marrelli TM. Update on home health care: how it's changing. *Am Nurs Today.* 2014;9(6). https://www.americannursetoday.com/update-on-home-health-care-how-its-changing/. Accessed May 10, 2018.

Punchik B, Komarov R, Gavrikov D, et al. Can home care for homebound patients with chronic heart failure reduce hospitalizations and costs? *PLoS One.* July 28, 2017. https://doi.org/10.1371/journal.pone.0182148.

Taigman M. Rescuing hospice patients. California Health Care Foundation website. https://www.chcf.org/blog/rescuing-hospice-patients/. Updated December 20, 2016. Accessed May 10, 2018.

Werdin F, Tennenhaus M, Schaller H-E, Rennekampff H-O. Evidence-based management strategies for treatment of chronic wounds. *Eplasty.* 2009;9:e19. https://www.ncbi.nlm.nih.gov/pmc/articles/PMC2691645/. Accessed May 10, 2018.

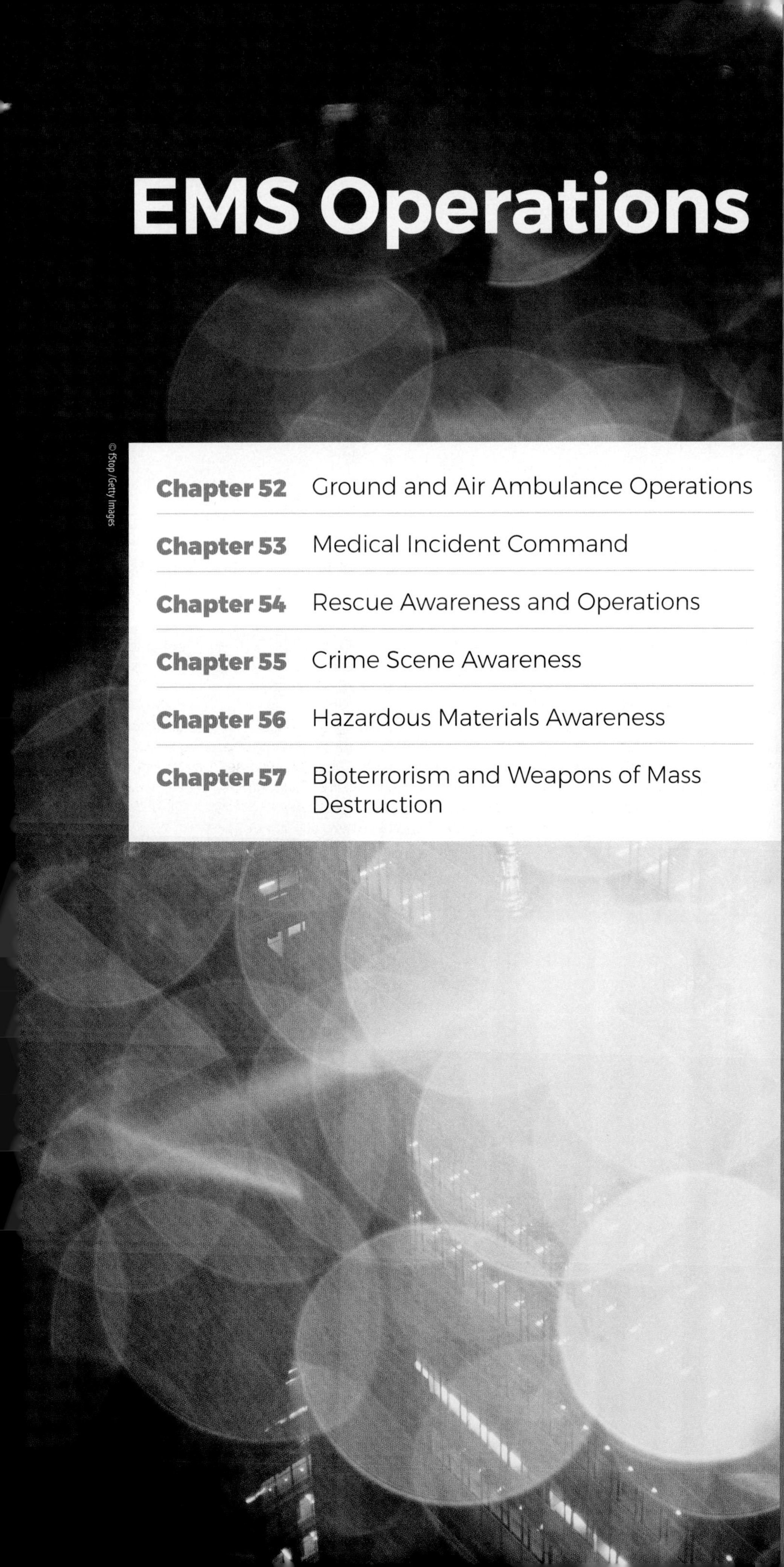

© fStop/Getty Images

PART 11

EMS Operations

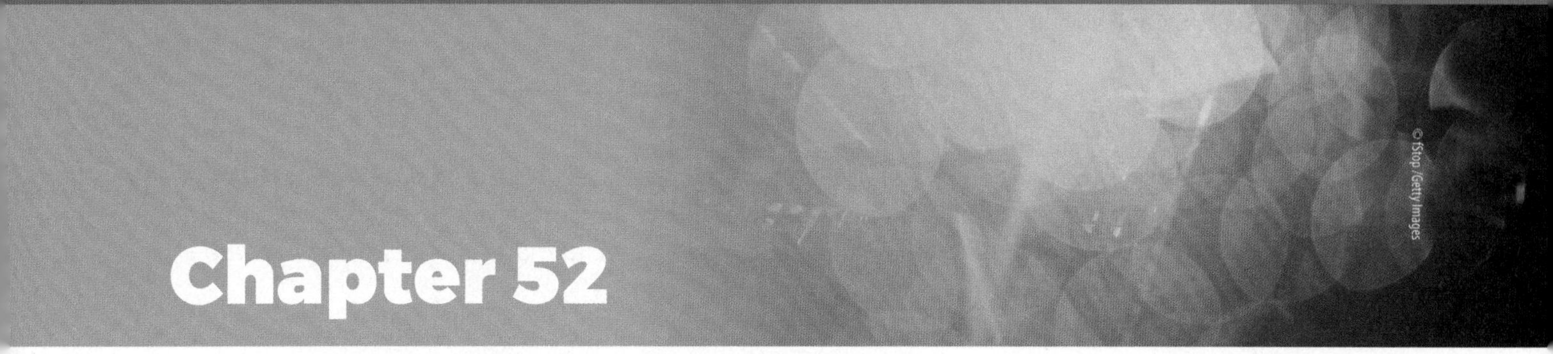

© fStop/Getty Images

Chapter 52

Ground and Air Ambulance Operations

NATIONAL EMS EDUCATION STANDARD COMPETENCIES

EMS Operations

Knowledge of operational roles and responsibilities to ensure patient, public, and personnel safety.

Principles of Safely Operating a Ground Emergency Vehicle

- Risks and responsibilities of emergency response (pp 1814–1822)
- Risks and responsibilities of transport (pp 1816–1822)

Air Medical

- Safe air medical operations (pp 1822–1823)
- Criteria for utilizing air medical response (pp 1823–1826)
- Medical risks/needs/advantages (pp 1823–1826)

OBJECTIVES

Upon completion of this chapter, the paramedic student will be able to:

1. Identify standards that govern ambulance performance and specifications. (pp 1814–1815)
2. Discuss the tracking of equipment, supplies, and maintenance on an ambulance. (p 1815)
3. Outline the considerations for appropriate stationing of ambulances. (pp 1815–1816)
4. Describe measures that can influence safe operation of an ambulance. (pp 1816–1822)
5. Identify aeromedical crew members and training. (pp 1822–1823)
6. Describe the appropriate use of aeromedical services in the prehospital setting. (pp 1823–1826)

KEY TERMS

ambulance A generic term that describes the various land-based emergency vehicles used by EMS personnel, including basic and advanced life support units, paramedic units, mobile intensive care units, and others.

fend-off position Positioning of the ambulance diagonally about 50 feet (15 m) in front of the scene for safety, so as to divert and avert oncoming traffic.

Ground Vehicle Standard for Ambulances (GVS v.1.0) The standard that identifies the minimum requirements for new ground ambulances built on a manufacturer's chassis. It applies to new vehicles only.

landing zone (LZ) An area prepared for the landing of an aircraft; generally 100 by 100 feet (30 by 30 m).

NFPA 1917, *Standard for Automotive Ambulances* The standard that defines the minimum requirements for the design, performance, and testing of new automotive ambulances intended for use under emergency conditions to transport sick or injured people to appropriate medical facilities; developed with consideration of the federal standards.

type I ambulance An ambulance design based on the chassis-cabs of light-duty pickup trucks.

type II ambulance An ambulance design based on modern passenger/cargo vans.

type III ambulance An ambulance design based on chassis-cabs of light-duty vans.

The modern ***ambulance*** *is more than just a vehicle for transporting a patient to the hospital. Today's ambulance is a well-equipped and efficiently organized vehicle or aircraft. It has advanced communications and technology that bring needed medical supplies, personnel, and advanced life support care to the emergency scene.*

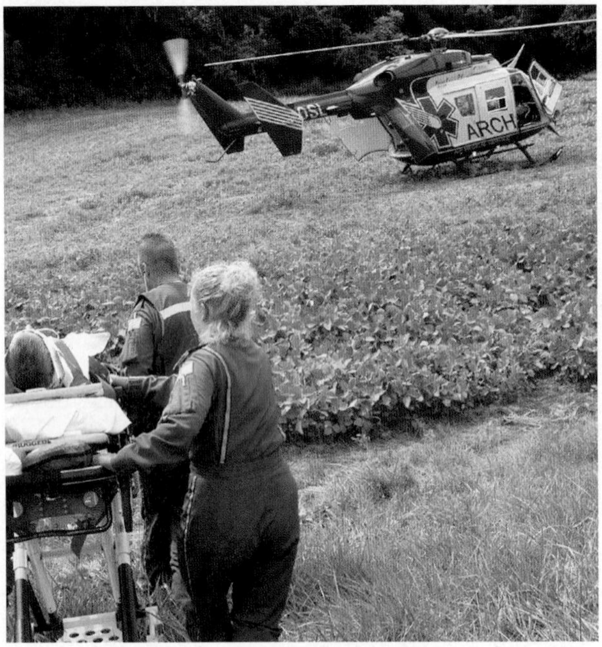

Courtesy Ray Kemp. St. Charles, MO

Ambulance Standards

In 1968, the National Academy of Sciences–National Research Council (NAS-NRC) recommended ambulance design standards that covered the size, shape, color, electrical systems, and emergency equipment to be carried on these vehicles. These standards eventually led to the development of the federal specifications that many states now use as ambulance standards. Collectively, the national standards developed by NAS-NRC and the National Highway Traffic Safety Administration (NHTSA) are known as the federal standards. These standards and their revisions provide the basis for uniformity in the design of ambulance vehicles. They cover the three basic ambulance designs: type I, type II, and type III (**FIGURE 52-1**). Also, because of the extra weight of equipment used in rescue and emergency care and the space needed for this equipment, the standards include additional-duty (AD) vehicles—namely, type I-AD and type III-AD (an ambulance mounted on a large chassis) (**BOX 52-1**). Fire service vehicles

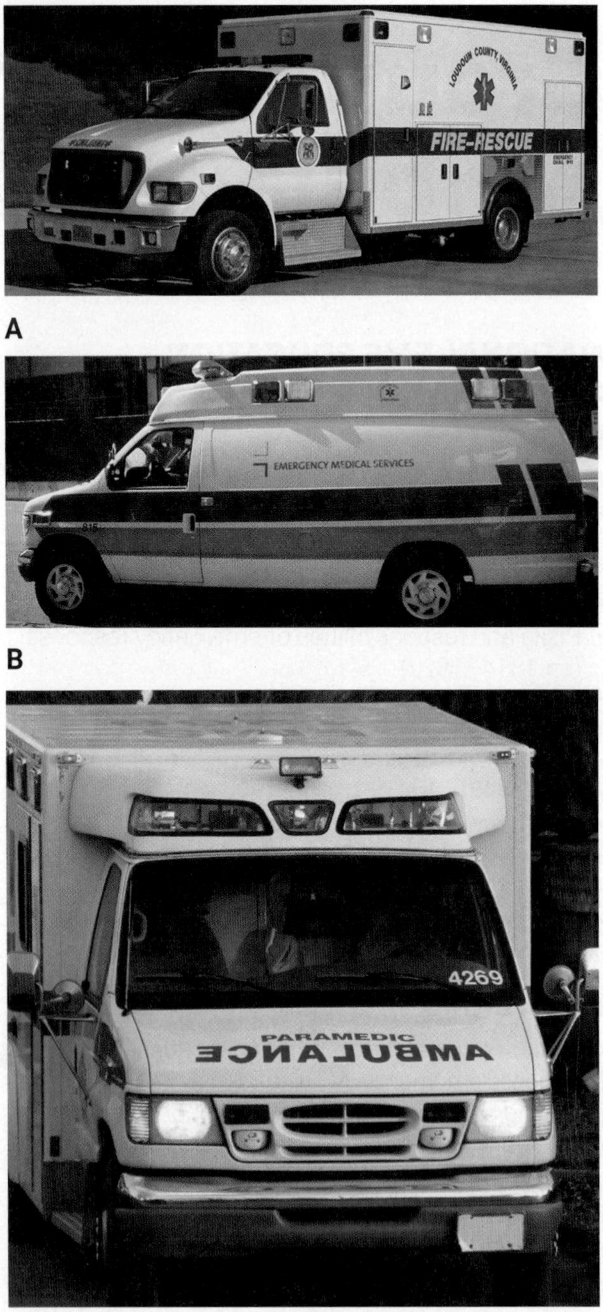

A

B

C

FIGURE 52-1 Basic ambulance designs. **A.** Type I. **B.** Type II. **C.** Type III.

A: © Jones & Bartlett Learning. Courtesy of MIEMSS; B: Courtesy of Captain David Jackson, Saginaw Township Fire Department; C: © Kevin Norris/Shutterstock.

BOX 52-1 Ambulance Types

- The **type I ambulance** design is based on the chassis-cabs of light-duty pickup trucks.
- The **type II ambulance** design is based on modern passenger/cargo vans.
- The **type III ambulance** design is based on the chassis-cabs of light-duty vans.

There are also AD versions of both type I and type III designs. They include large-chassis vehicles that allow for increased storage and payload capacity.

(eg, pumpers, rescue units, fire trucks) also carry EMS equipment.

Beginning in October 2016, the federal standards were replaced[1-3] by other national standards of design and performance for ambulance vehicles, such as **NFPA 1917, *Standard for Automotive Ambulances***,[4] of the National Fire Protection Association (NFPA) and **Ground Vehicle Standard for Ambulances (GVS v.1.0)** of the Commission on Accreditation of Ambulance Services.[5] States may require that ground ambulance services follow one or more of these standards. These standards are augmented by other state and local requirements that influence ambulance design, equipment, and staffing. These additional requirements include the following:

- Air ambulance standards
- Operational staffing standards
- Operational driver standards
- Operational driving standards
- Operational equipment standards

CRITICAL THINKING

Consider your state or regional standards. What do they require for ambulance design, performance, and equipment?

Checking Ambulances

Completing an equipment and supply checklist at the beginning of every work shift is essential for safety, patient care, and risk management. It also helps to ensure proper handling and safekeeping of scheduled medications. Either paper checklists or special computer software can be used for this purpose. Some equipment (eg, glucometers, defibrillators) requires routine maintenance, testing, and cleaning to ensure its safe and effective operation (**BOX 52-2**). Some disposable items—such as medications, electrocardiogram patches, defibrillation pads, and glucose check strips—lose their effectiveness over time and should be checked monthly to ensure they are still within their appropriate shelf life.

The procedures for vehicle maintenance vary by EMS agency but are always intended to improve the vehicles' reliability and extend their useful life. The paramedic should follow all agency guidelines and procedures for checking vehicles, equipment, and supplies.

BOX 52-2 Examples of Equipment Checks on an EMS Vehicle

General Operations

Airway equipment (basic and advanced)
Burn supplies
Drug inventory
Extrication/rescue supplies
Infection control supplies
Immobilization equipment
Obstetric/childbirth supplies
Patient assessment equipment
Stretchers and related equipment
Vehicle safety and operations
Wound care supplies

Specific Medical Equipment

Transport ventilator
Cardiac monitor/defibrillator
Glucometer/lactate monitor
Pulse oximetry and end-tidal carbon dioxide monitors
Telemedicine equipment

Ambulance Stationing

In the 1970s, the methods for estimating the need for ambulance service and where these vehicles should be stationed in a community were based on the availability of ambulances as well as on the average response time to the emergency scene. Since then, methods for estimating needs have shifted toward determining the percentage of compliance (standard of reliability) in providing EMS within time frames that meet national guidelines. All of the following factors may affect an EMS system's standard of reliability:

- Geographic area
- Population and patient demand
- Traffic conditions
- Time of day
- Appropriate placement of emergency vehicles

Strategies for ambulance stationing often are based on which areas have the highest volume of calls (peak load). These strategies take into consideration the day of the week and the time of day. Computers, global positioning systems, and other technology may be used to formalize strategic unit deployment and reduce response times.

Deployment strategies vary by EMS agency. They range from simple deployment of one vehicle stationed in the middle of a response area to comprehensive automated deployment plans for each hour of the day and each day of the week. The comprehensive plans include "mini-deployment" plans within each hour, depending on the number of ambulances left in the system (system status management). The optimal deployment system usually is a compromise between these two extremes.[6]

Safe Ambulance Operation

An estimated 4,500 vehicle crashes involving an ambulance occur each year. In 2015, there were 28 fatalities in crashes involving occupied ambulances.[7] Eleven (39%) of these deaths were ambulance occupants, and 17 (61%) were occupants of the other vehicle, cyclists, or pedestrians. These numbers are consistent with NHTSA's finding that there are, on average, 29 fatal ambulance crashes resulting in 33 deaths each year.[7-9] Work-related fatality rates among US paramedics and emergency medical technicians (EMTs) are higher than the national average for all occupations. Between 2003 and 2007, there were 59 fatalities of EMS personnel. Of those fatalities, 51 (86%) were transportation related.[10]

Safe operation of ambulances is essential for the safety of patients, the EMS crew, and others in the vicinity of a response. Most EMS agencies require their personnel to take an emergency driving course, and many also require those same personnel to undergo periodic evaluations of their emergency driving skills and knowledge (BOX 52-3). In addition to the size and weight of the emergency vehicle and the driver's experience, a number of factors influence the safe operation of an ambulance:

BOX 52-3 Guidelines for Safe Ambulance Driving

1. *Primum non nocere*—first do no harm.
2. Be tolerant and observant of other motorists and pedestrians.
3. Always use occupant safety restraints (both driver and passenger).
4. Be familiar with the characteristics of the emergency vehicle.
5. Be alert to changes in weather and road conditions.
6. Exercise caution in the use of audible and visual warning devices.
7. Drive within the speed limit except in circumstances allowed by law.
8. Select the fastest and most appropriate route to and from the incident scene.
9. Maintain a safe following distance.
10. Drive with due regard for the safety of all others.
11. Always drive in a manner consistent with managing acceptable levels of risk.

- Appropriate use of personal restraints
- Appropriate use of escorts
- Environmental conditions
- Appropriate use of warning devices
- Proceeding safely through intersections
- Parking at the emergency scene
- Operating with due regard for the safety of others
- Safely moving a patient into and out of the ambulance

CRITICAL THINKING
How would you feel if you struck another vehicle while driving an ambulance?

Maintaining ambulance safety for the EMS provider and the patient is complex and multifactorial. During a consensus conference on EMS safety in 2010, EMS and safety experts used a Haddon matrix (described in Chapter 3, *Injury Prevention, Health Promotion, and Public Health*) in an attempt to capture the host, agent, physical environment, and social environment factors contributing to injury during the pre-event, event, and post event phases of EMS response (**TABLE 52-1**).

TABLE 52-1 Haddon Matrix for EMS Provider and Patient Safety During Response and Transport

Phase	Host	Agent	Physical Environment	Social Environment
Pre-event	Physical fitness Shift length Substance abuse Education Knowledge Skill proficiency Capability Risk threshold	Vehicle design Equipment design Vehicle testing Equipment testing Ergonomic considerations Vehicle maintenance Equipment maintenance	Hands-free devices Ergonomic design of vehicle interior	Public expectation for response times Call prioritization Driver training Culture of seat belt use Emphasis on speed Emphasis on lights and siren use Availability of (lack of) consensus on vehicle design standards Availability of (lack of) driver training standards
Event	Distracted EMS driver Fatigue Seat belt use Risk-taking behavior	Speed Lights and siren use Stability of vehicle in transit	Weather Agitated or violent patients Character of interior surfaces Road conditions Traffic Curious onlookers	Seat belt use Driving habits Willingness to recognize error
Post-event	Preexisting conditions Physical fitness	Prevention of fire risk Escapability of the cabin Crash information collection Stability of the vehicle after crash	Post hoc analysis of event Root-cause analysis Availability of emergency responders (for ambulance crash)	Error recognition Error reporting Behavior change Human factor analysis

Reproduced from: Brice JH, Studnek JR, Bigham BL, et al. EMS provider and patient safety during response and transport: proceedings of an Ambulance Safety Conference. *Prehosp Emerg Care*. 2012;*16*(1):3-19.

DID YOU KNOW?

A major safety factor in ambulance operations is the overuse of lights and siren. With technological advances through emergency medical dispatching, oftentimes the 9-1-1 communications specialist can obtain sufficient medical information to determine whether the medical call warrants an emergent response. Studies have shown that the effectiveness and necessity for the use of lights and siren are very limited. It is estimated that patients would benefit from lights and siren response in 5% or fewer ambulance responses—namely, time-sensitive conditions such as cardiac or respiratory arrest, airway problems, unconsciousness, severe trauma with shock, and obstetric emergencies. The use of lights and siren increases the risk for not only the ambulance crew, but also the patient and any pedestrians or cyclists.

Despite this research, in 2015, National EMS Information System data indicated that in 74% of 9-1-1 responses to the scene, responders used lights and siren—a percentage virtually identical to that found in the 2010 data. However, lights and siren use from the scene of the 9-1-1 response to the patient destination declined from 27% in 2010 to 21.6% in 2015. Interestingly, 14% of EMS agencies respond to calls with lights and siren 100% of the time. Paramedics should consider the risk versus benefit when deciding whether to use lights and siren.

Modified from: Kupas DF. *Lights and Siren Use by Emergency Medical Services (EMS): Above All Do No Harm*. Washington, DC: National Highway Traffic Safety Administration; 2017. Contract DTNB2-14-F-00579.

Appropriate Use of Personal Restraints

According to NHTSA, during ambulance crashes, 84% of EMS providers in the patient compartment were not restrained.[8,9] Injury severity and mortality were substantially higher in the unrestrained EMS providers. Many of these injuries might have been prevented with the appropriate use of personal restraints. Many EMS agencies incorporate into their standard procedures the following guidelines in an effort to protect patients, passengers, and EMS personnel during transports:

- All operators and front-seat passengers of ambulance service vehicles must use seat belts when the vehicle is in motion.
- Any patient on a stretcher must be secured at all times when the vehicle is in motion or the stretcher is being moved. All lap and shoulder straps recommended by the manufacturer should be used.
- All equipment in the ambulance must be secured to prevent it from becoming a "missile" during a crash.
- All EMS personnel in the patient compartment must use seat belts when not attending to a patient and when the vehicle is in motion.
- All non-EMS personnel in the patient compartment must use seat belts when not attending to a patient and when the vehicle is in motion.
- Whenever possible, children who are not injured or ill (ie, children who are not patients, but rather passengers) should be transported in vehicles other than an emergency ground ambulance using a size-appropriate child restraint system.[11]
- If the child is the patient but does not require continuous or intensive medical monitoring or interventions, he or she should be appropriately secured onto the stretcher with a size-appropriate child restraint that complies with the injury criteria established by NHTSA.[11,12]
- In the case when a child is critical or requires intensive monitoring or interventions and the otherwise recommended restraint cannot be achieved, secure the child to the cot head first with three horizontal restraints across the torso and one vertical restraint across each shoulder.

More detailed recommendations related to child restraint can be found in a report prepared by the US Department of Transportation (DOT) and NHTSA, titled *Working Group Best-Practice Recommendations for the Safe Transportation of Children in Emergency Ground Ambulances.*[11]

The emergency vehicle should not be put in motion until the driver, EMS personnel, and all passengers are seated safely and wearing seat belts. (Every occupant of an emergency vehicle must be seat belted.) In addition, the emergency vehicle should be completely stopped before anyone unbuckles the seat belt and exits the ambulance.

Appropriate Use of Escorts

Police escorts during an emergency response can sometimes be dangerous. Collisions can occur as a result of confusion when motorists in the area wrongly assume that only one emergency vehicle is on the road. As a rule, paramedics should use escorts only when the EMS crew is responding to a scene in an unfamiliar area. Even then, the EMS driver should keep a safe distance between the ambulance and the escort. The use of lights and siren during escorts should be guided by local protocol. If the paramedic uses these warning devices, the ambulance and the police escort should use different siren tones (per protocol), thereby alerting other motorists to the fact that a second emergency vehicle is in the area.

Some communities use a tiered response system, in which several units and sometimes several agencies respond to emergency calls. A tiered response system allows for a safer emergency response and helps to ensure that the proper resources and personnel are available during an emergency. As an example, suppose a fire service unit staffed with basic-level EMTs responds to a car crash with full use of lights and siren. The EMTs determine that the patient's injury is minor and request a basic life support (BLS) ambulance (either public or private) to respond to the scene in a nonemergency mode (at normal speed and without lights and siren). On its arrival, the BLS ambulance crew assumes care of the patient and provides transport to the hospital.

Environmental Conditions

Environmental factors that can affect safe ambulance operation include poor road and weather conditions, such as fog and heavy rain that reduce visibility, and slippery pavement caused by ice, snow, mud, oil, or water that can cause the ambulance to hydroplane. When such conditions are present, the driver of the emergency vehicle should proceed at a safe speed—that is, a speed appropriate for the road and weather conditions. The driver should use low-beam headlights during all responses, as their use increases visibility for the EMS crew and makes it easier for other motorists to recognize the ambulance.

Dry roads and clear weather do not guarantee a safe response, however. Approximately 69% of all emergency vehicle crashes occur on dry roads, and 77% occur during clear weather.[13]

NOTE

It is important for EMS providers to arrive at an emergency scene safely so that they can aid the patient who called for assistance. A traffic incident that occurs en route to the scene not only delays patient care, but also creates another incident to be managed by other EMS personnel.

Appropriate Use of Warning Devices

As noted earlier, during an emergency response and patient transport, lights and siren should be used according to the agency's protocol and the state's motor vehicle laws. The driver is responsible for determining the mode of response to the scene based on local policy, the dispatch category, and information obtained from the dispatcher. When transporting a patient, the EMS provider with the highest level of training determines whether lights and siren will be used during transport. This decision should be made based on the patient's condition and the benefit that may be derived from potential time saved by using lights and siren.[14] In these cases, both lights and siren should be used simultaneously. (If one is indicated, so is the other.) The use of these warning devices during patient transport usually is reserved for patients with limb- or life-threatening illness or injury that would benefit from a shorter transport time. During either response to the scene or transport, the lights and siren response should be downgraded if it is no longer indicated.

When using lights and siren, paramedics should keep in mind that motorists who drive with the car windows rolled up or who are using an audio device, air conditioning, or the heating system may not be able to hear the sirens or air horns. For this reason, the EMS crew should always proceed with caution. They should never assume that the vehicle's lights, sirens, and air horns provide an absolute right-of-way or privileged immunity to proceed; rather, use of those devices simply indicate a request for permission to proceed.

EMS agencies using a lights and siren response should avoid using continuous siren tones when traveling unimpeded and not asking for emergency vehicle privileges. This approach will allow for improved communication for the response and patient care.[14]

Regardless of the decision to use emergency lights and siren, operation of other lighting can improve safety. Daytime running lights, which increase the vehicle's visibility, should be manually activated (if not automatic on the ambulance) anytime the ambulance is moving. The EMS crew should avoid using flashing white lights after dark, as they may blind oncoming traffic.

It is important to recognize situations when, regardless of the patient's condition or the use of lights and siren, the ambulance does not have privileges for the right-of-way in most states. For example, the ambulance is not allowed to pass a school bus with loading lights and arm activated. Likewise, an ambulance typically is not permitted to exceed the posted speed limit in school zones. In both cases, the potential benefit for the patient being transported is overridden by the risk of harm to children.

Rail crossings are another situation in which the ambulance emergency response does not grant right-of-way. In this case, the reason is largely practical because a train requires a very long stopping distance due to its weight. The ambulance should come to a complete stop, and the driver should look in both directions at noncontrolled railway crossings.[15]

CRITICAL THINKING

In which types of situations do you think the crew member driving an ambulance may be tempted to drive too fast?

Proceeding Safely Through Intersections

Reports estimate that between 43% and 53% of ambulance crashes in the United States occur in intersections where an ambulance proceeds against a red light.[16] Given this obvious danger, it is important that the driver of an emergency vehicle stop at all controlled intersections. The driver should try to make eye contact with all motorists before proceeding through the intersection. Another safety measure when going through an intersection is alternating the siren's "yelp" and "wail" modes to alert nearby traffic of the ambulance's presence.[14] Some emergency vehicles now have traffic signal preempting devices that can change the traffic light at an intersection to green (in the ambulance's direction of travel). Although these devices provide an additional safeguard during ambulance response, they are not a replacement for other intersection safety measures.

Similar strategies should be employed when proceeding against the flow of traffic. In this case it is recommended that ambulance speed be limited to less than 20 miles per hour (32 km/h).

SHOW ME THE EVIDENCE

During a 2-day ambulance safety conference held in 2010, experts in EMS and safety met to outline the nature of ambulance safety problems. Goals of the conference were to introduce a framework to describe the problem, get expert opinion, and develop an action plan to address the safety issues they identified. A partial list of their recommendations follows:

- Regulate uniform reporting for all ambulance crashes.
- Involve key stakeholders (employee and governmental leaders) to develop regulations governing safe ambulance design.
- Implement real-time driver monitoring and feedback systems.
- Implement hands-free technology (radios, telephones).
- Fund research for safe ambulance engineering.
- Develop rigorous hiring standards.
- Require driver training programs.
- Reinforce the concept of "due regard" for the safety of others.
- Identify measures to minimize the risk of impaired drivers (fatigue, medications).
- Reduce lights and siren responses.
- Foster a culture of safety.

Modified from: Brice JH, Studnek JR, Bigham BL, et al. EMS provider and patient safety during response and transport: proceedings of an Ambulance Safety Conference. *Prehosp Emerg Care.* 2012;16(1):3-19.

Parking at the Emergency Scene

When parking the ambulance at a scene, the paramedic should make sure the vehicle's location allows for traffic flow around the area. If law enforcement and fire service personnel have secured the scene, the paramedic should position the ambulance about 100 feet (30 m) past the scene, on the same side of the road. The ambulance should be positioned uphill (about 200 feet [60 m]) and should be positioned upwind if the presence of hazardous materials is suspected. If law enforcement and fire service personnel have not secured the scene, the paramedic should position the ambulance diagonally about 50 feet (15 m) in front of the scene in the **fend-off position** (**FIGURE 52-2**). In this position, the emergency vehicle can deflect and avert from the scene other vehicles that may strike the ambulance or providers.

Other safety precautions a paramedic can take when parking an ambulance at an emergency scene include the following:[14]

- Use emergency lighting when the vehicle blocks traffic. Set the lighting pattern to draw attention, yet not blind other drivers. Do not use headlights or flashing white lights. If the ambulance is not being used to block the scene, consider turning off distracting flashing emergency lights.
- Consider using amber directional signals to direct traffic away from the scene or hazards.
- Use scene floodlights to illuminate the scene and the work area around the ambulance.
- Set the parking brake. (Setting the parking brake before putting the transmission in "Park" allows the entire weight of the vehicle to be

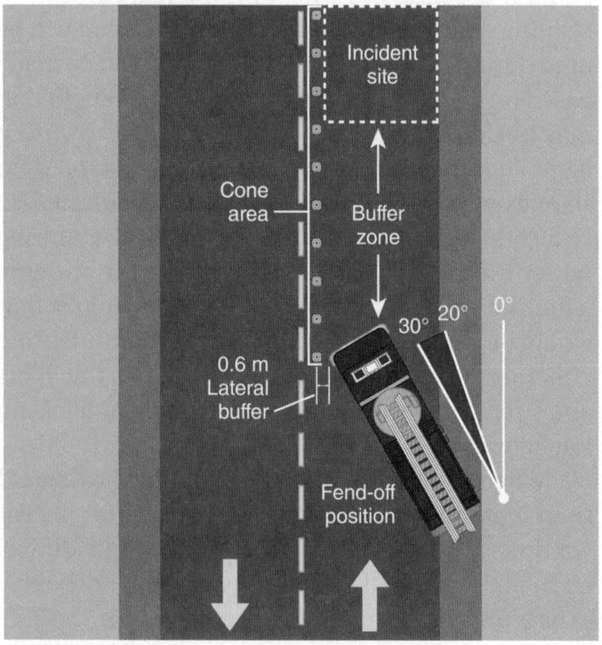

FIGURE 52-2 The "fend-off" position.

shared between the emergency brake and the transmission.)
- Ask another person to help guide the vehicle when it is backing up. This person should be visible in the vehicle mirrors at all times while the ambulance is slowly backing up.
- Wear reflective gear when working near the roadway.

When choosing a parking area for the ambulance, the paramedic also should consider the possibility of collapsing structures, fires, explosive hazards, and downed electrical wires.

Operating With Due Regard for the Safety of All Others

As previously discussed, most states allow privileges for drivers of emergency vehicles, but use of these privileges must take into consideration the safety of all people using the roads. This includes maintaining a safe following distance to avoid rear-end collisions (BOX 52-4). This "due regard for the safety of all others" carries legal responsibility. The paramedic and the EMS agency can incur liability if damage, injury, or death results from failure to observe this principle (see Chapter 6, *Medical and Legal Issues*). The paramedic should be aware of local and state

NOTE

Crashes involving emergency vehicles represent more than half of the claims paid by insurers of EMS systems.

Modified from: Cone D, Brice JH, Delbridge TR, Myers JB, eds. *Emergency Medical Services: Clinical Practice and Systems Oversight*. 2nd ed. Hoboken, NJ: John Wiley & Sons; 2015.

BOX 52-4 The 2-Second Rule and Braking Distance Chart

Most rear-end collisions are caused by drivers who follow too closely behind the vehicle in front of them. For this reason, it is important that the paramedic keep enough space (following distance) between the emergency vehicle and the vehicle in front to avoid a crash if the car in front brakes suddenly.

A quick method for gauging the recommended distance is the 2-second rule. It works like this:

1. You (the driver of the emergency vehicle) note an object by the side of the road (eg, a tree or sign) that the vehicle in front of you will soon pass.
2. Count "one thousand and one, one thousand and two." If you reach the object before the phrase is complete, you are too close to the vehicle in front of you.
3. This rule applies with good road and weather conditions. One to three additional seconds should be added to the stopping distance if a condition exists, such as nighttime, poor visibility, or wet pavement.

Braking distance is based on average reaction time, average vehicle weight, average road conditions, and average brakes. Wet roadways, poor brakes, poor tires, heavy vehicle weight, and poor reaction times may all lengthen the braking distance. The following chart shows braking distance at various speeds.

The stopping distances in this figure relate to police cars. Be aware that ambulances, especially larger emergency vehicles (eg, those mounted on a freightliner-type chassis) have different handling characteristics and longer braking and stopping distances than do conventional type I, II, or III emergency vehicles.

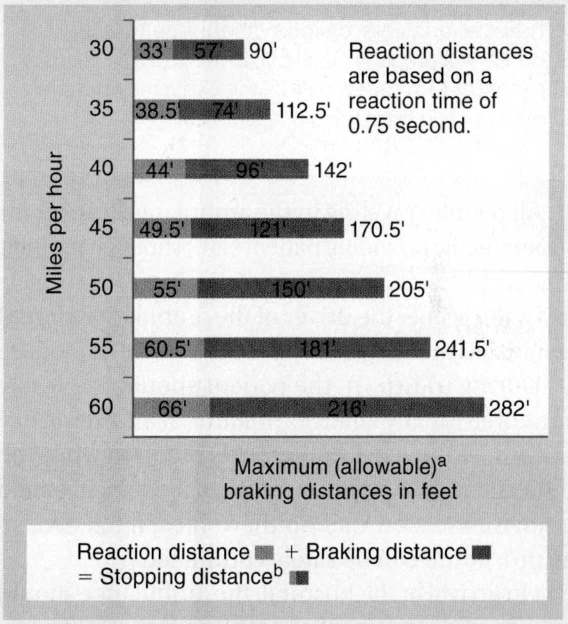

[a]Federal Motor Vehicle Safety Standard (FMVSS) #105-76 requires all new passenger cars to brake to a stop no more than the distances above from these speeds.

[b]Total Stopping Distance is made up of Perception Distance + Reaction Distance + Braking Distance. Average perception distance for an alert, sober driver is 0.25 to 0.5 second.

Reproduced from Los Angeles Unified School District Police Department: Braking Distance Chart. Los Angeles, CA: Los Angeles Police Department; 1999.

Modified from: New Yukon driver's basic handbook. Yukon Government website. http://www.hpw.gov.yk.ca/mv/newhandbook.html. Accessed April 19, 2018.

laws and regulations that cover the operation of an emergency vehicle.

Safely Moving a Patient Into and Out of an Ambulance

After initial stabilization at the scene, the patient must be packaged and safely placed in the emergency vehicle for transport. The paramedic crew should use safe lifting practices to help to prevent personal injury (see Chapter 2, *Well-Being of the Paramedic*). These techniques also ensure that the patient is positioned securely on the ambulance stretcher. The patient compartment of the ambulance is equipped with locking devices that prevent the stretcher from moving while the ambulance is in motion.

Unnecessary equipment should be stowed before transport. Also, objects such as monitors should be secured in a locking device to minimize the risk of injuries in a crash.

> NOTE
>
> Whenever possible, children should be transported secured in a properly sized child safety seat. Except in the most critical cases, care can be delivered effectively when the child is restrained in this way.

All people traveling in the ambulance (except for the paramedic providing patient care) should have their personal restraints securely fastened. Before the vehicle leaves the scene, the driver of the ambulance should be signaled that it is safe to put the vehicle in motion.

During transport, the patient should be closely monitored for any changes in status. If an emergency care procedure (eg, intubation) is required while the ambulance is in motion, the driver of the vehicle should be advised to slow or stop the vehicle if needed, so the procedure can be safely completed.

On arrival at the hospital, the ambulance should come to a full stop. At that point, personal restraints can be removed and the vehicle can be exited. All patient care equipment (eg, immobilization devices, intravenous lines, and airway adjuncts) must be secured before the stretcher is released from the locking device. Using safe lifting techniques, the patient's stretcher should be removed from the ambulance. The patient should be appropriately transferred to health care personnel at the facility.

Aeromedical Transport

Like many other aspects of prehospital emergency care, air evacuation is rooted in military history. During the Prussian siege of Paris in 1870, soldiers and civilians were evacuated by a hot-air balloon. In 1928, a Marine pilot used an engine-powered aircraft to evacuate the wounded in Nicaragua.[17] However, the first full-scale use of aircraft for medical evacuation did not occur until 1950, during the Korean conflict. The experience gained in Korea formed the basis for helicopter rescue in Vietnam. In Vietnam, nearly 1 million casualties were transported by air.[18] In the more recent military confrontations involving the United States in Panama, Grenada, and the Middle East, massive advanced aeromedical support capabilities and plans were on site before the conflicts began. Air evacuation of wounded soldiers was used in the Persian Gulf. Air medical evacuation has also been used during the course of military engagements in Afghanistan and Iraq.[19]

Currently, more than 300 air medical service programs using fixed-wing aircraft (**FIGURE 52-3**) and/or rotary-wing (helicopter) aircraft (**FIGURE 52-4**) have been established throughout the United States.[20] Fixed-wing aircraft services are not usually as high profile as helicopters. Often they are used for interhospital transfers of patients and to deliver organs for transplantation when the distance is greater than 100 miles (160 km).

Aeromedical Crew Members and Training

The staffing of air ambulances includes a pilot and various health care professionals—for example,

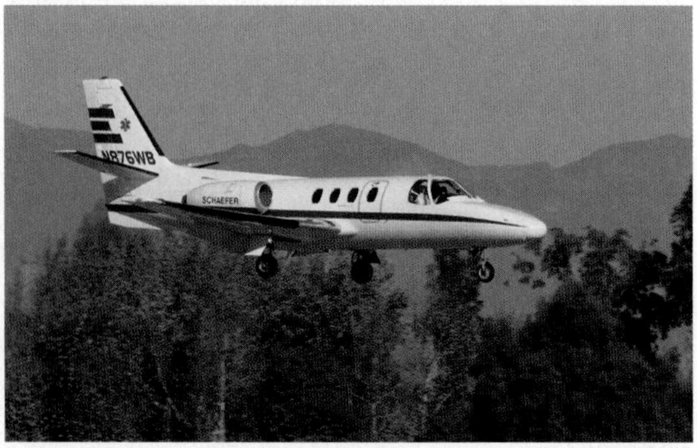

FIGURE 52-3 Fixed-wing aircraft.

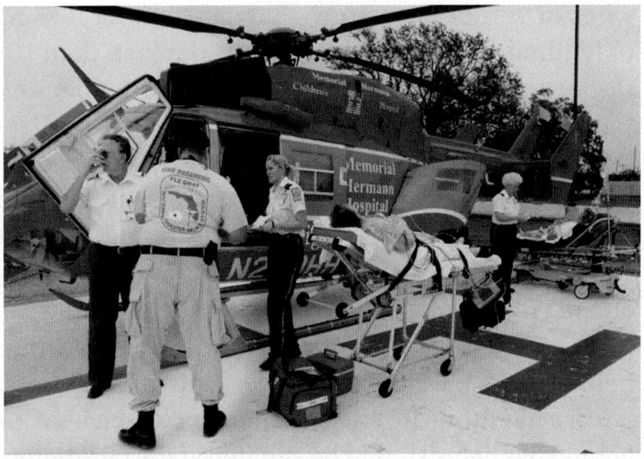

FIGURE 52-4 Rotary-wing aircraft.

Courtesy of Ed Edahl/FEMA.

EMTs, paramedics, respiratory therapists, nurses, physicians, and others. Air ambulance crews undergo specialized training in flight physiology and advanced medical equipment and procedures. The American College of Surgeons Committee on Trauma and the Association of Air Medical Services have established guidelines for personnel qualifications. The DOT and NHTSA funded the development of the Air Medical Crew National Standard Curriculum (AMC) in 1988. Many flight programs have used this curriculum as well as the Air Medical Crew Core Curriculum (AMCCC) to teach flight physiology, aircraft components and construction, safety regulations, aviation and navigation terminology, and operational safety (BOX 52-5).

BOX 52-5 Selected Organizations Associated With the Air Medical Industry

Aerospace Medical Association (AsMA)
Air Medical Operators Association (AMOA)
Air Medical Physicians Association (AMPA)
Air and Surface Transport Nurses Association (ASTNA)
Association of Air Medical Services (AAMS)
Commission on the Accreditation of Medical Transport Services (CAMTS)
International Association of Flight and Critical Care Paramedics (IAFCCP)
International Association of Medical Transport Communications Specialists (IAMTCS)
National EMS Pilots Association (NEMSPA)

NOTE

According to the National Transportation Safety Board, there were seven EMS-related aviation fatal accidents in the United States during 2015. It was reported that "many of these could have been prevented with simple corrective actions, including oversight, flight risk evaluations, improved dispatch procedures, and the incorporation of available technologies." Between 2006 and 2015, there were 92 aeromedical crashes that resulted in 90 fatalities.

Modified from: US HEMS accident rates 2006–2015. Aerossurance website. http://aerossurance.com/helicopters/us-hems-accident-2006-2015/. Accessed April 19, 2018.

Use of Aeromedical Services

The local EMS system develops the criteria for requesting aeromedical services' response to the scene of an emergency. When determining whether to use aeromedical resources, the decision should be supported by appropriate triage and evaluation of the scene. As described in Chapter 36, *Trauma Overview and Mechanism of Injury*, the paramedic generally should consider air transport when the situation involves one or more of the following factors:

- The time needed to transport a patient by ground to an appropriate facility would pose a threat to the patient's survival and recovery.
- Weather, road, or traffic conditions would seriously delay the patient's access to advanced life support.
- Critical care personnel and specialized equipment are needed to care for the patient adequately during transport (BOX 52-6).

Notification of Aeromedical Services

Most aeromedical transportation providers accept requests for medical services from physicians, EMS and fire service personnel, or other on-scene public service agency personnel. Local and state guidelines cover aeromedical activation. The paramedic should consult with medical direction and follow all state laws, administrative rules, and city, county, and district ordinances and standards when using aeromedical services.

When notified that an aeromedical response may be needed, the flight crews of some services begin to prepare for the flight and move to the aircraft so

BOX 52-6 Advantages and Disadvantages of Air Medical Services

Advantages

- Transports are rapid and usually smooth.
- Access to accident sites is quick.
- Traffic, trains, mountains, ship canals, and other barriers can be avoided.
- Travel is still possible when road conditions are poor.
- Sophisticated communication equipment is available.
- Quality of care is improved in rural areas where only BLS is available.

Disadvantages

- In urban settings, ground ambulances are usually faster within a 30-mile (48-km) range.
- If the helicopter is on another flight, no other aircraft may be available.
- Inclement weather may prevent the aircraft from traveling.
- Space and weight restrictions may limit access to the patient and restrict the crew, patients, and equipment that can be carried.
- Helicopter transports are significantly more expensive than are transports by ground ambulance. Helicopter crashes have fewer survivors.

Modified from: Thomas SH, Arthur AO. Helicopter EMS: research endpoints and potential benefits. *Emerg Med Int*. 2012;698562.

that they are ready for the flight. (They are placed on stand-by.) If paramedics determine that the situation does not require an aeromedical response, the appropriate agency should be notified as soon as possible, so as to make the crew available for other flights.

If paramedics request air service for medical, trauma, or search and rescue events, they should advise the flight crew of the type of emergency response, the number of patients, the location of a **landing zone (LZ)**, and any prominent landmarks and hazards (eg, vertical structures or power lines). Direct ground-to-air communication must be available between a designated LZ officer and the aeromedical staff on the responding aircraft. If possible, the fire department should be dispatched to the LZ to provide fire-suppression support. Law enforcement personnel also should be available for securing the scene.

Landing Site Preparation

The ideal space requirement for a helicopter LZ generally is 100 by 100 feet (30 by 30 m) with no overhead wires or vertical structures that can hamper takeoff or landing.[21] It should be relatively flat (less than 10° slope) and free of high grass, crops, or other factors that can conceal uneven terrain or hinder access. The LZ also should be free of debris that can injure people or damage structures or the helicopter. If patients are close to the LZ, the paramedic should provide protection by covering their wounds and eyes. Rescue personnel close to the landing site should wear protective equipment such as reflective clothing, helmets with lowered face shields, and safety glasses.

If a nighttime LZ is used, emergency vehicles with lighted bar lights should be situated at the perimeters of the LZ. If white lights are used, they should be directed down toward the center of the LZ as spotlights, because white lights (spotlights or headlights) directed toward the aircraft can temporarily blind the pilot. Rescue personnel should never be used to identify the LZ; cones or strobes should be used for such purposes. Flares should not be used because the helicopter rotor wash can blow the flares from the site and create a fire hazard. A fire crew should wet down dusty LZs, especially if vehicle traffic is moving in the area. This action prevents the pilot and vehicle drivers from being temporarily blinded by the dust.

Helpful radio communications with the pilot include notification of wind direction and any possible obstructions or hazards. Wind direction can be determined by throwing grass or dirt, by wetting a finger, or by observing smoke patterns from smoke canisters. If hazardous materials are present, the paramedic should advise the flight crew of the substance, the location of the hazardous materials site, and the possibility of patient contamination. Unless otherwise requested, patient status and clinical information should not be relayed to the aeromedical crew until they have landed and made contact with the ground crew.

The pilot generally does not land the aircraft until all danger of fire or explosion has been eliminated. (The pilot has the final decision to use or change an LZ to another location.) When the aircraft is coming in to land, one emergency responder should stand facing the LZ so that the pilot will see the landing area. LZ hand signals that may be useful to the pilot are shown in **FIGURE 52-5**.

Safety Precautions

Everyone should be clear of the landing area during takeoffs and landings. A distance of 100 to 200 feet

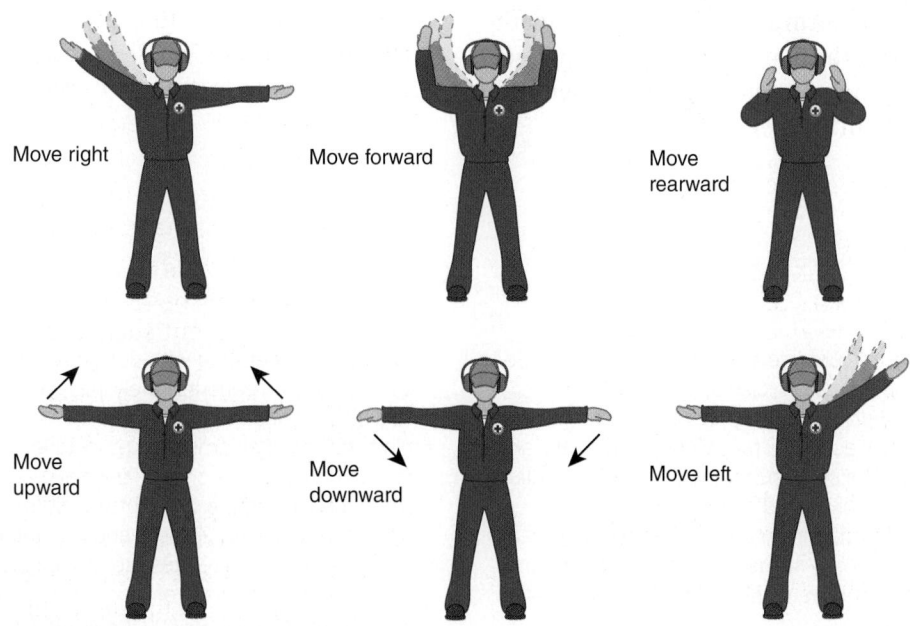

FIGURE 52-5 Landing zone hand signals.

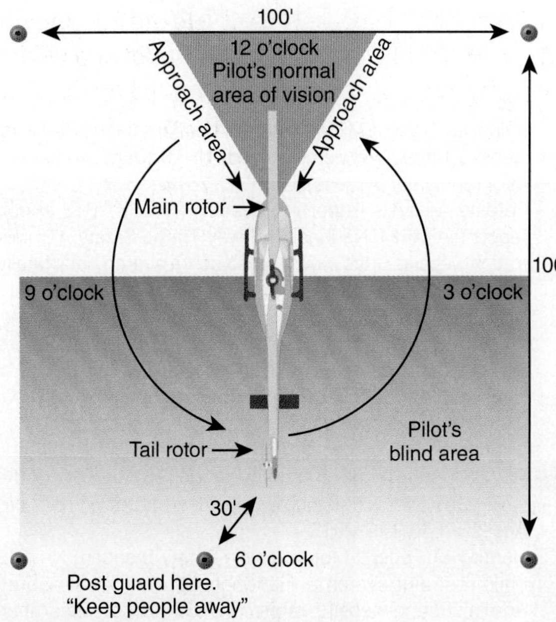

FIGURE 52-6 Safe-approach zones.

(30 to 60 m) is best (**FIGURE 52-6**). In addition, paramedics should take the following precautions:[22]

- Never allow ground personnel to approach the helicopter unless the pilot or flight crew asks them to do so.
- Allow only necessary personnel to help load or unload patients.
- Secure any loose objects or clothing that could be blown by rotor downwash (eg, stretcher, sheets, blankets).
- Do not allow smoking.
- After the aircraft is parked, make eye contact with the pilot, move to the front beyond the perimeter of the rotor blades, and *wait for a signal from the pilot* to approach.
- Approach the helicopter in a crouched position, staying in view of the pilot or other crew members.
- *Never approach the rear of the aircraft from any direction.* The tail rotors on most aircraft are near the ground and spin at 3,400 revolutions per minute, which makes them virtually invisible. Tail rotor injuries are often fatal.
- Carry long objects horizontally and no higher than waist high.
- Depart the helicopter from the front and within view of the pilot.

Patient Preparation

Preparing a patient for air transport requires special measures. Some medical procedures must be done *before* the patient is loaded into the aircraft. For example, the patient's airway should be established and secured before loading, as should application of a traction splint. Special equipment must be positioned according to the aircraft's configuration. Most aeromedical crews perform a brief patient assessment before liftoff to verify the patient's condition. Patients who are combative may require physical or chemical restraint during flight.

CRITICAL THINKING

How do you think an alert patient would feel while waiting for helicopter transport?

Summary

- The federal standards provide a consistent foundation for the design of ambulance vehicles.
- Completing an equipment and supply checklist at the start of every work shift is essential for safety, patient care, and risk management. It also helps to ensure proper handling and safekeeping of scheduled medications.
- The methods for estimating ambulance service needs and placement in a community are usually based on compliance in providing EMS services within time frames that meet national standards.
- Factors that influence safe ambulance operation include proper use of escorts, awareness of environmental conditions, proper use of warning devices, proceeding safely through intersections, correct parking at the emergency scene, and operating with due regard for the safety of all others. Moving patients safely in and out of the ambulance is also essential.
- The staffing of air ambulances includes a pilot and various health care professionals. These crew members undergo specialized training in flight physiology and the use of special medical equipment and procedures.
- When paramedics request aeromedical service, the flight crew should be advised of the type of emergency response, the number of patients, and the location of the landing zone as well as the presence of any prominent landmarks and hazards. Paramedics should always follow strict safety measures during helicopter landings to prevent injury to the air medical crew, ground crew, patient, and bystanders.

References

1. Ludwig G. EMS: understanding ambulance safety specs. Firehouse website. https://www.firehouse.com/safety-health/article/12186423/ems-understanding-ambulance-safety-specs. Published May 1, 2016. Accessed April 19, 2018.
2. Hampson J. Federal specification for the star-of-life ambulance KKK-A-1822F. Change notice 10GSA. Kentucky Board of Emergency Medical Services website. https://kbems.kctcs.edu/media/news-and-events/2018-event-folder/KKK-A-1822F%20change%20notice%2010%201July2017%20DRAFT%205-10.pdf. Published August 1, 2007. Accessed April 19, 2018.
3. SAE International (Society of Automotive Engineers). SafeAmbulances.org website. http://www.safeambulances.org/organizations/sae/. Accessed April 19, 2018.
4. National Fire Protection Association. *NFPA 1917: Standard for Automotive Ambulances*. Quincy, MA: National Fire Protection Association; 2016. https://www.nfpa.org/codes-and-standards/all-codes-and-standards/list-of-codes-and-standards/detail?code=1917. Accessed April 19, 2018.
5. CAAS releases ground vehicle standard for ambulances. Commission on Accreditation of Ambulance Services website. http://www.caas.org/2016/03/28/caas-releases-ground-vehicle-standard-for-ambulances/. Published March 28, 2016. Accessed April 19, 2018.
6. Penner J, Studnek JR. Debunking the myths of system status management. EMS World website. https://www.emsworld.com/article/219000/debunking-myths-system-status-management. Published October 30, 2017. Accessed April 19, 2018.
7. National Highway Traffic Safety Administration, National Center for Statistics and Analysis. *Traffic Safety Facts 2015*. Washington, DC: US Department of Transportation; 2015. DOT HS 812 384. https://crashstats.nhtsa.dot.gov/Api/Public/Publication/812384. Published 2015. Accessed April 19, 2018.
8. National Highway Traffic Safety Administration. When ambulances crash: EMS provider and patient safety. EMS.gov website. https://www.ems.gov/pdf/NHTSAOEMSAmbulanceInfographic.pdf. Accessed April 19, 2018.
9. Fatality Analysis Reporting System (FARS). 2013 annual report file (ARF). National Highway Traffic Safety Administration website. https://www.nhtsa.gov/research-data/fatality-analysis-reporting-system-fars. Accessed April 19, 2018.
10. Maguire BJ, Smith S. Injuries and fatalities among emergency medical technicians and paramedics in the United States. *Prehosp Disaster Med.* 2013;28(4):376-382.
11. National Highway Traffic Safety Administration. *Working Group Best-Practice Recommendations for the Safe Transportation of Children in Emergency Ground Ambulances*. Washington, DC: US Department of Transportation; 2012. DOH HS 811 677. https://www.nhtsa.gov/staticfiles/nti/pdf/811677.pdf. Accessed April 19, 2018.
12. Huntley M. Federal Motor Vehicle Safety Standard No. 213: child restraint systems. National Highway Traffic Safety Administration website. https://www.nhtsa.gov/sites/nhtsa.dot.gov/files/mhuntley_sae2k2.pdf. Published May 15, 2002. Accessed April 19, 2018.
13. National Safety Council. *Injury Facts*. Itasca, IL: National Safety Council; 2010.
14. Kupas DF. *Lights and Siren Use by Emergency Medical Services (EMS): Above All Do No Harm*. Washington, DC: National Highway Traffic Safety Administration; 2017. Contract DTNB2-14-F-00579. https://www.ems.gov/pdf/Lights_and_Sirens_Use_by_EMS_May_2017.pdf. Accessed April 19, 2018.
15. Boone CM, Malone TB. *A Research Study of Ambulance Operations and Best Practice Considerations for Emergency Medical Services Personnel*. Washington, DC: US Department

of Homeland Security; March 2015. https://www.naemt.org/docs/default-source/ems-health-and-safety-documents/health-safety-grid/ambulance-driver-(operator)-best-practices-report.pdf?sfvrsn=2. Accessed April 19, 2018.

16. Ballam E. Ambulance crash roundup: a review of emergency vehicle crashes during 2010. *EMS World.* 2011;40(3):74-75.
17. Hurd WW, Thompson NJ, Jernigan JG, et al. *Aeromedical Evacuation: Management of Acute and Stabilized Patients.* New York, NY: Springer Verlag; 2003.
18. Frame C. Modern EMS practices have their roots in Vietnam medical rescues. American Homefront Project website. http://americanhomefront.wunc.org/post/modern-ems-practices-have-their-roots-vietnam-medical-rescues. Published September 25, 2017. Accessed April 19, 2018.
19. Robert J, Tourtier JP, Vitalis V, Coste S, Gaspard W, Bourrilhon C. Air medical-evacuated battle injuries: french army 2001 to 2014 in Afghanistan. *Air Med J.* 2017;36(6):327-331.
20. CUBRC, Public Safety and Transportation Group. *Atlas and Database of Air Medical Services*. 15th ed. ADAMS website. http://www.adamsairmed.org/pubs/atlas_2017.pdf. Published September 2017. Accessed April 19, 2018.
21. Landing zone guidelines. https://www.uwmedicine.org/airlift-nw/Documents/v220170925LandingZone_final.pdf. Airlift Northwest website. Accessed April 19, 2018.
22. Federal Aviation Administration. *Rotorcraft Flying Handbook.* Washington, DC: US Department of Transportation; 2010. FAA-H-8083-21. https://www.faa.gov/regulations_policies/handbooks_manuals/aircraft/media/faa-h-8083-21.pdf. Accessed April 19, 2018.

Suggested Readings

Boone CM, Malone TB. *A Research Study of Ambulance Operations and Best Practice Considerations for Emergency Medical Services Personnel*. Washington, DC: US Department of Homeland Security; March 2015. https://www.naemt.org/docs/default-source/ems-health-and-safety-documents/health-safety-grid/ambulance-driver-(operator)-best-practices-report.pdf?sfvrsn=2. Accessed April 19, 2018.

Division of Occupational Health, Safety, and Medicine; International Association of Fire Fighters, AFL-CIO, CLC. *Best Practices for Emergency Vehicle and Roadway Operations Safety in the Emergency Services.* Washington, DC: US Department of Homeland Security; 2010. http://www.iaff.org/hs/evsp/best%20practices.pdf. Accessed April 19, 2018.

Emergency vehicle and roadway operations safety. US Fire Administration website. https://www.usfa.fema.gov/operations/ops_vehicle.html. Published May 25, 2017. Accessed April 19, 2018.

Federal Aviation Administration. *Advisory Circular: Helicopter Air Ambulance Operations*. Washington, DC: US Department of Transportation; March 26, 2015. AC No. 135-14B. https://www.faa.gov/documentLibrary/media/Advisory_Circular/AC_135-14B.pdf. Accessed April 19, 2018.

Federal Aviation Administration. *Helicopter Flying Handbook.* Washington, DC: US Department of Transportation; 2014. FAA-H-8083-21A. https://www.faa.gov/regulations_policies/handbooks_manuals/aviation/helicopter_flying_handbook/media/helicopter_flying_handbook.pdf. Accessed April 19, 2018.

Federal Emergency Management Agency. *US Fire Administration Emergency Vehicle Safety Initiative.* Washington, DC: US Department of Homeland Security; February 2014. FA-336. https://www.usfa.fema.gov/downloads/pdf/publications/fa_336.pdf. Accessed April 19, 2018.

LeCroix B. A profound impact. EMS World website. https://www.emsworld.com/article/12095290/a-profound-impact. Published July 3, 2015. Accessed April 19, 2018.

Reichard AA, Marsh SM, Tonozzi TR, et al. Occupational injuries and exposures among emergency medical services workers. *Prehosp Emerg Care.* 2017;21(4):420-431.

Smith N. A national perspective on ambulance crashes and safety: guidance from the National Highway Traffic Safety Administration on ambulance safety for patients and providers. EMS World website. https://www.emsworld.com/article/12110600/a-national-perspective-on-ambulance-crashes-and-safety. Published September 3, 2015. Accessed April 19, 2018.

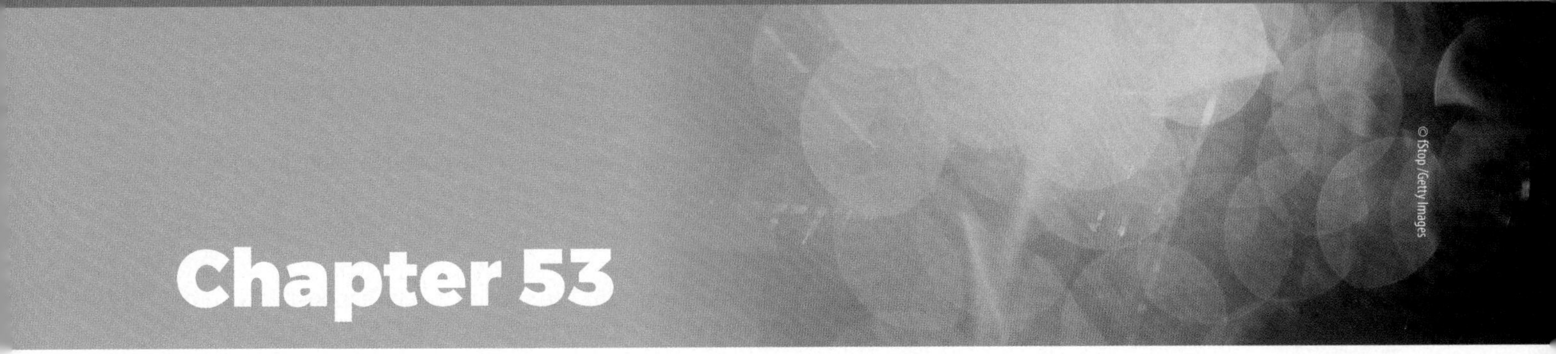

Chapter 53

Medical Incident Command

NATIONAL EMS EDUCATION STANDARD COMPETENCIES

EMS Operations

Knowledge of operational roles and responsibilities to ensure patient, public, and personnel safety.

Incident Management

Establish and work within the incident management system. (pp 1832–1833)

Multiple Casualty Incidents

- Triage principles (pp 1843–1848)
- Resource management (p 1848)
- Triage (pp 1843–1848)
  - Performing (pp 1844–1847)
  - Retriage (p 1847)
  - Destination decisions (p 1848)
  - Posttraumatic and cumulative stress (p 1848)

OBJECTIVES

Upon completion of this chapter, the paramedic student will be able to:

1. Identify situations that may be classified as major incidents. (p 1837)
2. Identify the components of an effective incident command system. (pp 1832–1833)
3. Identify the five major components of the incident command system. (p 1833)
4. List command responsibilities during a major incident response. (pp 1833–1834)
5. Describe the steps necessary to establish and operate the incident command system. (p 1833)
6. Describe the section responsibilities in the incident command system. (pp 1834–1837)
7. Outline the components that define a major incident. (p 1837)
8. Outline the activities of the preplanning, scene management, and postdisaster follow-up phases of an incident. (pp 1837–1838)
9. Given a major incident, describe the groups and/or divisions that would need to be established and the responsibilities of each. (pp 1839–1841)
10. List common problems related to the incident command system and to mass-casualty incidents. (pp 1842–1843)
11. Outline the principles and technology of triage. (pp 1843–1848)
12. Identify resources for the management of critical incident stress. (p 1848)

KEY TERMS

casualty collection areas Areas where ill or injured people are gathered for triage, treatment, or transport.

command The act of directing, ordering, or controlling by virtue of explicit, statutory, regulatory, or delegated authority.

command post The physical location of on-scene incident command and management organization.

communications center A facility used to dispatch emergency equipment and coordinate communications between field units and personnel.

disaster A term that usually is associated with a human-made or natural event that involves damage across a large area or to a community's infrastructure.

disaster management The mobilization of resources and the methods used to meet the needs of a disaster response.

divisions Geographic areas sometimes used to break command into more manageable chunks.

emergency operations center (EOC) The main communications center where representatives of emergency response organizations, government agencies, and sometimes private organizations gather to coordinate their response to an emergency event.

extrication/rescue group The group responsible for managing patients who are trapped. Responsibilities of this group may include search, rescue, initial triage, tagging, and in situ treatment before transfer of the patients to the treatment group.

finance/administration section The section responsible for tracking costs and reimbursement.

groups Resources, including people, apparatus, and equipment, assembled to perform a specific function, regardless of geographic area; sometimes used to break a command into more manageable chunks.

incident action plan (IAP) A mental, oral, or written plan of the general objectives and overall strategy for managing an incident. The IAP often identifies operational resources, assignments, time frames, and other information important for the management of the incident over one or more operational periods.

incident command system (ICS) A universal framework designed to improve coordination and efficient control of emergency response operations and resources.

incident commander (IC) The person responsible for all incident activities, including the development of strategies and tactics and the ordering and release of resources. The IC has overall authority and responsibility for conducting incident operations and is responsible for the management of all incident operations at the incident site.

infrastructure The basic physical and organizational framework needed for the operation of a society or enterprise, such as communication systems, power supplies, water systems, sewer systems, and roads and transportation systems.

intelligence/investigations function Determines the source or cause of the incidence to control its impact; may fall within a section or be a separate general staff section.

interoperability The ability of multiple organizations to communicate and coordinate effectively.

lifesaving interventions Priority care using rapid assessments and interventions to stop the dying process, such as controlling major hemorrhage, opening the airway, and providing rescue breathing, chest decompression, and auto-injector antidotes.

local/regional threshold The point at which the number of casualties or the nature of the event overwhelms the available resources of local emergency response agencies.

logistics section The section that is responsible for providing supplies and equipment, facilities, services, food, and communications support. The main function of this section is to provide gear and support to the responders.

major incident An event for which immediately available resources are insufficient to manage the nature of the emergency.

mass-casualty incident (MCI) An event for which immediately available resources are insufficient to manage the number of casualties.

mutual aid An agreement with neighboring emergency agencies to exchange equipment and personnel when necessary.

operations section The section that directs and coordinates all emergency scene operations. It also ensures the safety of all personnel. EMS functions generally fall under this section.

planning section The section responsible for providing past, present, and future information about the incident and the status of resources.

postdisaster follow-up An after-action review of an incident that includes the lessons learned from the incident and methods of improvement.

preplan The process of preparing for response to a major incident; also refers to the document that results from this process.

primary triage Triage performed at the incident site to rapidly categorize patient conditions for treatment and roughly identify the number and severity of patients.

rehabilitation area A part of the major incident response plans of many fire and EMS agencies. This area usually is set up outside the operational area. It allows rescue personnel to get physical and psychological rest.

SALT triage A method of triage that uses a four-step process—Sort, Assess, Lifesaving interventions, Treatment and/or Transport—to categorize patients.

scene management Control of all or part of the incident area.

secondary triage The more detailed and specific prioritization of patients based on the severity of their illness or injuries and their potential to survive.

section chiefs Those in charge of the major functional areas of the incident command system. Examples of major functional areas that may be established based on need include operations, logistics, planning, and finance/administration.

sections A broad organizational level of the incident command system at which the following functions are typically defined: planning, operations, logistics, and/or finance/administration.

single command An incident coordination system in which one person is responsible for the entire operation.

size-up The systematic process of gathering information about an incident and evaluating it in comparison to incident management goals and available resources. (Differs from scene size-up, which is an assessment of the scene to ensure scene safety for the paramedic crew, patient[s], bystanders; a quick assessment to determine the resources needed to manage the scene adequately.)

SMART tag system A method of triage that uses four color triage coding cards that have military bar codes for tracking patients.

span of control The number of people one supervisor is responsible for and can coordinate most effectively. This number is typically five to seven but should be as few as three if operations are especially challenging.

staging areas Designated areas where incident-assigned vehicles are directed and held until needed.

standard operating procedures (SOPs) Guidelines establishing the preferred method for operations to be carried out, as well as the framework (eg, line of authority, communications, coordination) to achieve these goals.

support branch The section that is in charge of gathering and distributing equipment and supplies at a major incident.

tracking log A system of record keeping that includes patient identification, transporting unit, patient priority, and medical facility destination.

transportation group The group that communicates with the receiving medical facilities, ambulances, and air medical services for patient transport during a major incident.

treatment group The group that provides advanced care and stabilization until the patients are transported to a medical facility. Most paramedics and medical facility personnel are assigned to this group.

triage A method used to sort patients and prioritize care based on the severity of their illness or injuries and their potential to survive.

triage tagging system A system of tags, tapes, ribbons, or labels used to indicate a patient's priority and triage category.

unified command An application of the incident command system used when there is more than one agency with incident jurisdiction. Agencies designate representatives to work together through unified command to establish a common set of objectives and strategies and a single incident action plan.

A **major incident** *is an event for which the available resources are insufficient to manage the number of casualties or the type of emergency. Major incidents can include highway crashes, air crashes, major fires, train derailments, building collapses, acts of violence or terrorism, search-and-rescue operations, hazardous materials releases, and natural disasters. These incidents stress and may overwhelm local, regional, state, and even national and international resources.*

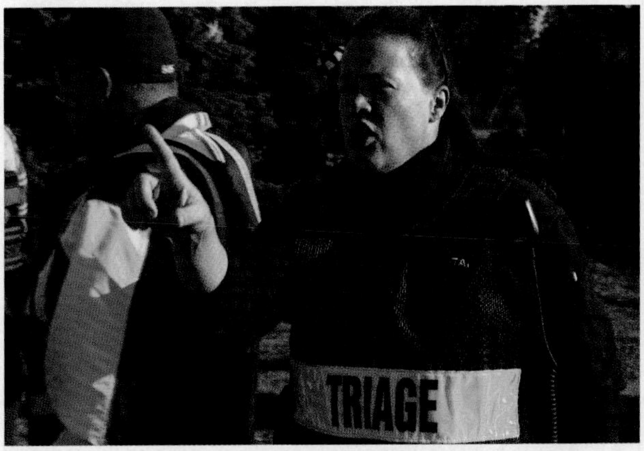

© Nancy G Fire Photography, Nancy Greifenhagen/Alamy Stock Photo

NOTE

The term **disaster** usually is associated with a human-made or natural event that involves damage across a large area or to a community's **infrastructure** (eg, roads, power, communications, housing). A subcategory of a disaster is a **mass-casualty incident (MCI)**, which involves many injuries and/or fatalities. The mobilization of resources and the methods used to meet the needs of a disaster response constitute **disaster management**.

CRITICAL THINKING

What effect do you think lack of effective coordination of emergency responders could have on rescue operations, scene safety, patient care, and transportation in a major incident?

Incident Command System

Historically, emergency management of a major incident often resulted in the response of many different agencies (EMS, fire service, rescue organizations, law enforcement, and others). Often, each of these agencies operated independently with little or no interagency organization, which made it difficult to determine who was in charge of the scene. It also made it difficult to determine what emergency services were needed or were being provided. In some cases, different agencies were wasting resources by duplicating efforts. In others, responders were even working against each other's goals.

The **incident command system (ICS)** was developed in the 1970s following a series of catastrophic fires in California that resulted in millions of dollars in property damage and a large loss of life. Evaluation of the emergency response to these fires showed that problems resulted from poor coordination and management more often than from any other reason.

The ICS organizes and coordinates emergency response functions and responsibilities. In 2004, the ICS was included as part of the National Incident Management System (NIMS) of the Department of Homeland Security (BOX 53-1). All emergency response agencies at every level of government are required to use the ICS at *all* incidents regardless of the type, size, or complexity.[1]

The ICS provides for a number of arrangements: (1) single jurisdiction and single agency involvement, (2) single jurisdiction and multiagency involvement, and (3) multijurisdiction and multiagency involvement. This structure allows the ICS to be adapted to the needs of any agency or to the size, nature, or geographic location of a particular incident requiring emergency management. The ICS also must be expandable from dealing with a nonmajor incident to a major one in a logical way. Use of the ICS as standard operating procedure for small incidents allows a smooth transition when a major incident occurs. Other components of the ICS include common elements of organization, terminology (BOX 53-2), and procedures. The use of ICS components on small incidents helps develop necessary emergency response muscle memory for improved response to larger incidents and disasters.

The ICS system can easily be used at a minor incident in which the units dispatched to the scene are sufficient to handle the event. It can be expanded if more units are needed for a minor incident that becomes a major one. Use of the ICS is crucial whenever it becomes apparent that the demands of the incident will overwhelm available resources. (An example is an event that involves many patients, a wide geographic or multijurisdictional area, or one that may last several hours to days.)

Federal law now requires use of the ICS in response to all types of incidents. The ICS is a flexible system. It is used in both public and private sectors in all incidents. Much of the success of the ICS is as

BOX 53-1 National Incident Management System (NIMS) Concepts

NIMS provides an organized set of scalable and standardized operational structures. This design is crucial for allowing various organizations and agencies to work together in a predictable, coordinated manner. NIMS can be described as follows:

- NIMS defines a comprehensive, nationwide systematic approach to incident management.
- NIMS represents a core set of concepts, principles, terminology, and organizational processes for all threats, hazards, and events. It is not a response plan.
- NIMS is scalable, flexible, and adaptable so it may be used for all incidents (from day-to-day operations to large-scale events).
- NIMS defines essential principles for communications and information management.
- NIMS defines standardized resource management procedures for coordination among different jurisdictions and organizations.

Modified from: Federal Emergency Management Agency. *National Incident Management System.* 3rd ed. Washington, DC: US Department of Homeland Security; 2017.

BOX 53-2 Important Terminology for Medical Incident Command Systems

- Apparatus
- Command
- Command post
- Communications center
- Divisions
- Groups
- Medical direction
- Mutual aid
- Staging area

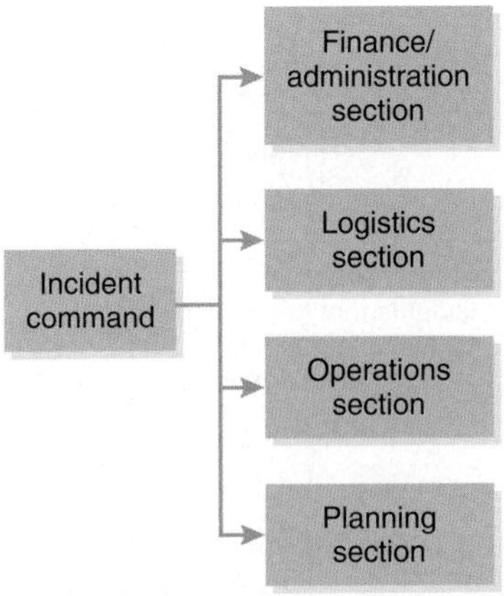

FIGURE 53-1 Incident command system organization.

a result of its standardized application of a common organizational structure and key principles. While they are not all needed at every incident, the following five major components (sometimes abbreviated C-FLOP) compose the ICS (**FIGURE 53-1**)[1]:

1. Command
2. Finance/administration
3. Logistics
4. Operations
5. Planning

Command Function

Command must be established immediately. At most incidents, the responsibility of command should belong to one person who assumes the function of **incident commander (IC)**. The commander must be clearly identified. Also, all others at the scene must know who is in command.

The initial command should be determined by a preplanned system of arriving emergency units and personnel (eg, the first or second arriving EMS, fire, or law enforcement unit). The IC must be familiar with ICS structure and also be familiar with the operating procedures of other responding agencies. The IC need not be the person with the highest rank or the most training (although this is commonly the case); rather, the IC should be the person best able to manage the emergency scene effectively.

In some cases, as a more qualified person arrives, command may be transferred to this person according to **standard operating procedures (SOPs)**. This transfer of command is usually done face to face and transmitted via radio to all units.

Once established, command should take the following steps:

- Perform a **size-up** of the situation.
- Assume an effective command mode and position.
- Transmit a brief initial report by radio including key points of the size-up and identifying the location of the **command post**.
- Develop an **incident action plan (IAP)**.
- Provide assignments and request additional resources as needed.

Whenever possible, command should also take the following steps:

- Implement a personal accountability and safety system.
- Control and assign **divisions** and/or **groups** as required (these should be consistent with the needs of the incident, SOPs, or disaster plans); also, provide these units with operating objectives.
- Provide ongoing effective command and progress reports until relieved by a higher-ranking person.
- Develop the command organization by delegating authority to subordinates. (This step helps to accomplish incident needs and objectives.)
- Review and evaluate the effectiveness of site operations and revise these operations as needed.
- Return units to service and end command when appropriate.

Types of Command

Command may take a single or unified form (**BOX 53-3**). With **single command**, one person is responsible for

> **BOX 53-3** Single and Unified Command Structures
>
> - **Single command structure.** A single IC is solely responsible (within the confines of authority) for establishing objectives and for devising the overall management strategy for the incident. The IC is directly responsible for follow-through and must ensure that all functional area actions are directed toward accomplishment of the strategy. Implementation of the overall strategy is the responsibility of a single person (section chief) who reports directly to the IC.
> - **Unified command structure.** The personnel designated by their jurisdictions (or by departments within a jurisdiction) must jointly determine objectives, strategies, and priorities. As in the single command structure, the section chief is responsible for carrying out the plan.

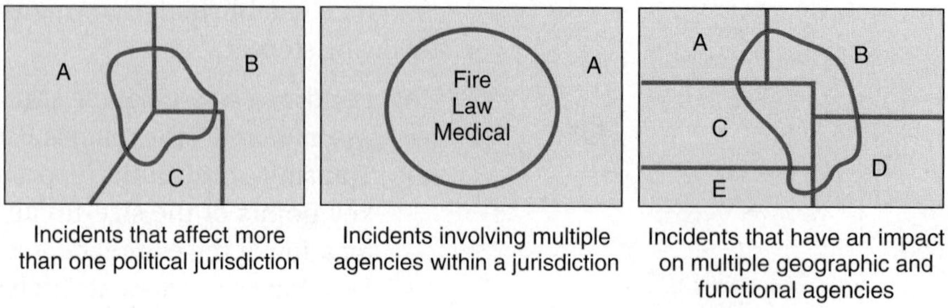

FIGURE 53-2 Application of unified command.

the entire operation. This type of command often works well for incidents with limited jurisdictions or responsibilities. It also works best in small events of short duration.

Unified command may be needed in large events or as a small incident evolves. In unified command, specialized organizations are identified (eg, EMS, fire, police, health department, American Red Cross), and personnel unify to complement command. This type of command stimulates cooperation (the right agency leads command at the right time) and provides for balanced decision making. It also facilitates **interoperability** (the ability of multiple organizations to communicate effectively) when many different communication frequencies and communications equipment are used by responding agencies. The concept of unified command allows agencies with different legal, geographic, and functional authorities and responsibilities to work together effectively. This interoperability occurs without affecting individual agency authority, responsibility, or accountability (**FIGURE 53-2**).[2] Unified command may be indicated in incidents such as those with the following characteristics:

- More than one political jurisdiction
- Multiple agencies within a jurisdiction
- Multiple geographic and functional agencies

CRITICAL THINKING

Where do you think command should be located in a major incident that is confined to one area?

In either single or unified command, the IC may delegate authority for certain activities by activating additional **sections** (operations, planning, logistics, or finance/administration). These sections help to meet the needs of the situation. The IC bases the decision to expand (or contract) the ICS organization on three major incident priorities:[3]

1. **Life safety.** The IC's first priority is *always* the safety of the responders and the public.
2. **Incident stability.** The IC is responsible for deciding on strategies to minimize the effect of the incident on the area. These strategies also should maximize the response effort while using resources effectively.
3. **Property conservation.** The IC is responsible for minimizing damage to property and the environment while achieving the incident objectives.

When expansion of command is required, the IC establishes the other general staff positions (**FIGURE 53-3**).

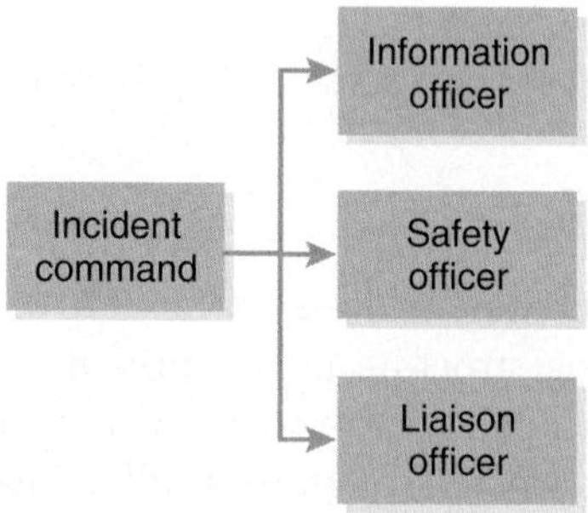

FIGURE 53-3 Command staff positions. The information officer handles all media inquiries and coordinates the release of information to the media with the public affairs officer at the emergency operations center. The safety officer monitors safety conditions and develops measures for ensuring the safety of all assigned personnel. The liaison officer is the on-scene contact for other agencies assigned to the incident.

Section Responsibilities

In the ICS, a manageable **span of control** (the number of people one section chief can manage effectively)

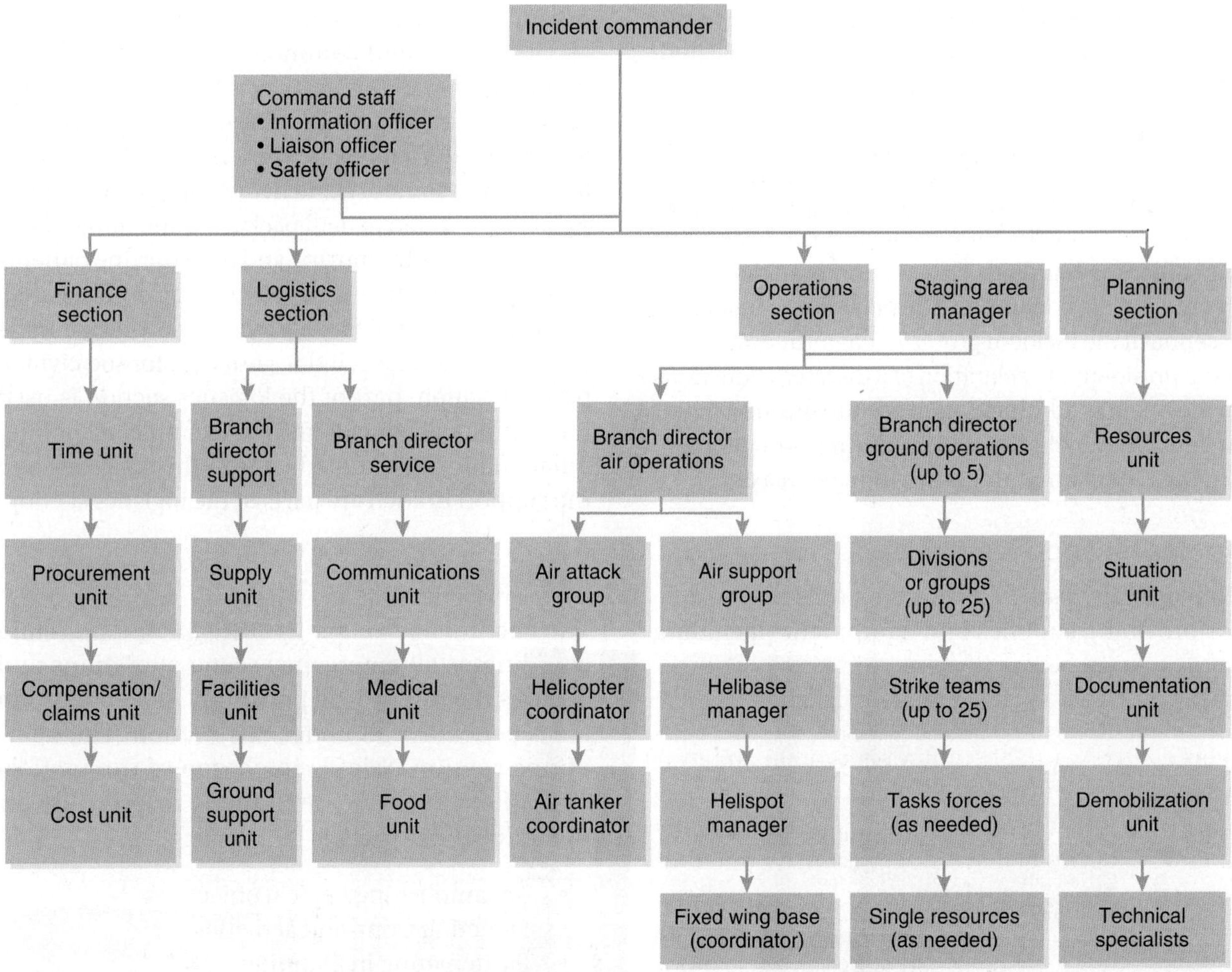

FIGURE 53-4 Command section organizational plan.

falls within the range of three to seven. Maintaining adequate span of control throughout the ICS organization is key to effective and efficient incident management.

In some cases, the span of control indicates that the incident organization must be expanded to allow effective management of the situation. In such cases, the IC assigns one or more of the general staff sections (planning, operations, logistics, and/or finance/administration) to **section chiefs**. Section chiefs must be strong supervisors and managers. Their principal role in the ICS is to make things happen. They enact the plans and strategies of the IC and also ensure that all rescuers in their sections are working toward a common goal. The section that may be needed varies, depending on the scope of the incident. The IC makes this determination (**FIGURE 53-4**).

Section chiefs should not become involved in physical tasks (eg, carrying litters, operating rescue equipment). Committing to such tasks impairs their ability to maintain control and supervise the section. General responsibilities of section chiefs include the following:

- Accomplishing the objectives set by command
- Monitoring work progress
- Redirecting activities as necessary
- Coordinating related activities with other sections
- Requesting additional resources as needed for the section
- Monitoring the welfare of personnel from each section
- Providing command with frequent reports
- Reallocating resources within the section

The section chief should report to command when a job is assigned, when a job is accomplished, or if a job cannot be accomplished.

Finance/Administration Section

The **finance/administration section** (**FIGURE 53-5**) is important for tracking costs and the way reimbursement is handled. This section is seldom used in small-scale incidents; however, it is considered essential if the incident grows in magnitude and costs (eg, a presidential declaration of a disaster). Functions of the finance/administration section during a major incident may include time accounting, procurement, payment of claims, and estimation of costs.

Logistics Section

The **logistics section** (**FIGURE 53-6**) is responsible for providing supplies and equipment (including personnel to operate the equipment), facilities, services, food, and communications support. The main function of this section is to provide gear and support to the responders. The essential equipment for supporting a medical incident includes supplies for airway, respiratory, and hemorrhage control, burn management, and patient packaging and immobilization. Resources for moving and transporting patients (people, ambulances, buses) also may be needed. The medical unit of the logistics section cares for the incident responders; it does not care for the civilian patients. Often, part of the logistics section is used for routine daily incidents. For example, responder rehabilitation (described later in this chapter) and the support branch are parts of the logistics section.

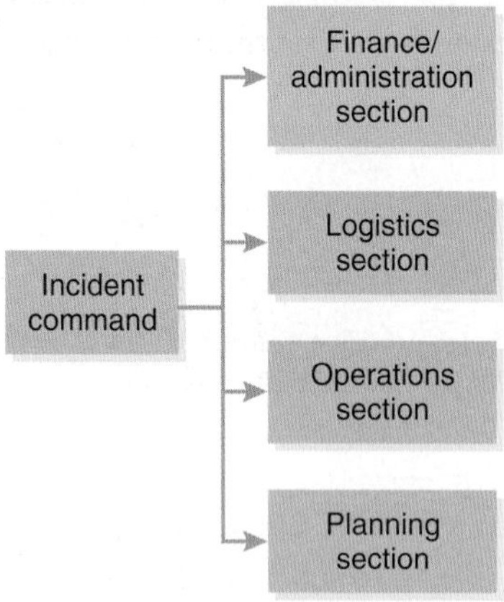

FIGURE 53-5 Finance/administration section.

Operations Section

The **operations section** (**FIGURE 53-7**) directs and coordinates all emergency scene operations and ensures the safety of all personnel. EMS operation areas generally fall under this section. The operations section chief is in charge of the tactical operations at an incident and is responsible for the following activities:

- Accomplishing tactical objectives
- Directing front-end activities
- Participating in planning
- Modifying action plans as needed
- Maintaining discipline
- Accounting for personnel
- Updating command on the progress or lack of progress of an operation

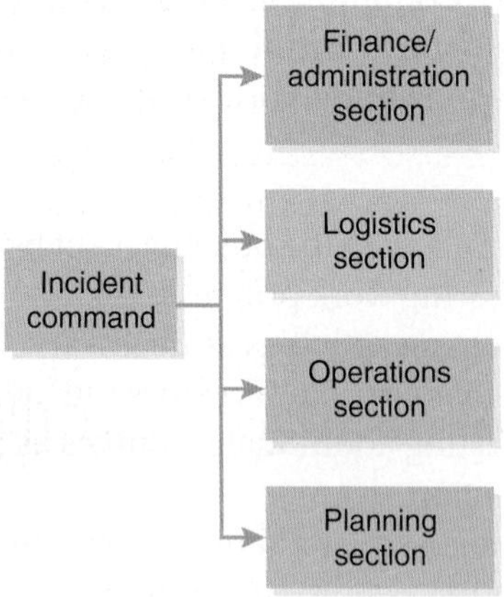

FIGURE 53-6 Logistics section.

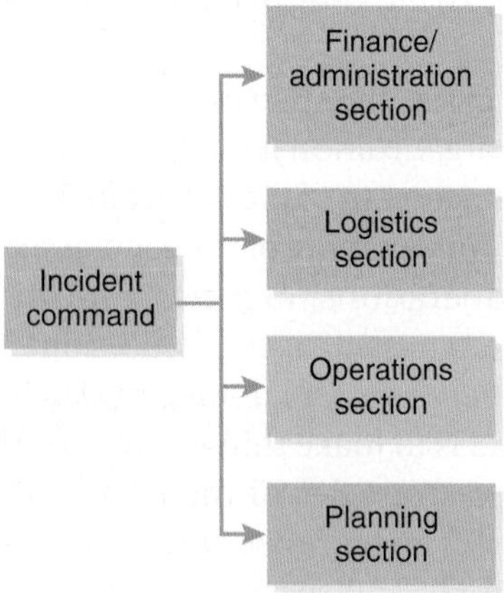

FIGURE 53-7 Operations section.

Planning Section

The staff function of the **planning section** (**FIGURE 53-8**) is to provide past, present, and future information about the incident and the status of resources. This section's duties also may include the creation of a written or verbal IAP. (The IC determines the need for an IAP.) The IAP defines the response activities and use of resources for a specified period. These operational periods can vary in length; however, they should be no longer than 24 hours (12-hour operational periods are common for large-scale incidents). IAPs may be indicated when (1) resources from several agencies are used, (2) several jurisdictions are involved, (3) the incident is complex, or (4) the incident extends past one operational period.

NOTE

In some incidents, such as disease outbreaks, fire, complex coordinated attacks, or cyber incidents, a special **intelligence/investigations function** may be needed. This function is tasked to find the source of the incident, to control its effect or to prevent its reoccurrence. The intelligence/investigations function is typically performed in the planning section, but it may fall under the operations section or command staff or may be a separate general staff section depending on the nature and size of the incident.

Declaring a Major Incident

Declaring a major incident is a crucial phase of the response. If an EMS unit is dispatched to a scene that has this potential, the crew should be advised or should declare (per established protocol) that they are responding to a possible major incident or MCI and will confirm on arrival. This information allows other agencies to be contacted, and those agencies can be placed on standby. It also allows time for determination of the availability of other resources. Medical direction and area medical facilities should also be alerted. The receiving medical facilities need information on the number of patients and the severity of injuries as soon as possible. That way, they can begin to prepare for the patients' arrival. A possible major incident should be declared in the following situations:

- More than two ambulance units are required for adequate treatment, particularly in rural areas where communities may have only one ambulance.
- Hazardous or radioactive materials or chemicals in significant quantity are involved.
- An MCI results in a large number of patients and requires special EMS resources, such as helicopters, rescue teams, or several rescue or extrication units.

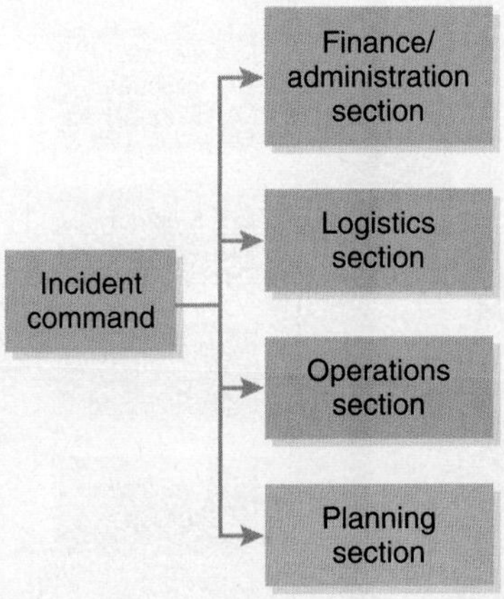

FIGURE 53-8 Planning section.

Preparing for a Major Incident

Preparation for a major incident involves three phases: preplanning, scene management, and postdisaster follow-up (or after-action review).[3]

Phase 1: Preplanning. Phase 1 of the preparation for a major incident is preplanning. Efforts by agencies to work together and to plan ahead are crucial to the management of a major incident. All agencies that will be called upon in an incident must agree to the **preplan**. The preplan also must address common goals and the specific duties of each group. Multiagency efforts succeed as a result of frequent meetings and practice sessions or exercises (drills or tabletop exercises). The preplan should include a system of sorting or prioritizing care, treatment, and transportation.

NOTE

The details of a disaster preparedness plan can be found through the community's local emergency disaster planning committee.

Another component of the disaster is the identification of hazards in a community (a risk assessment). Such hazards may include the manufacture, storage, and transport of hazardous materials; fire threats; the population base at various times of the day; and violence and other potential social problems. An inventory of resources that may be needed during a major incident includes the following:

- Shelter and mass feeding
- Air evacuation
- Medical equipment and supplies
- Heavy equipment, power generators, and lighting
- Communications equipment
- Law enforcement personnel
- Specialized rescue services

Phase 2: Scene Management. Phase 2 of preparation involves the development of a strategy to manage the incident scene (**scene management**). Some major incidents can be managed with local resources and personnel (closed or contained incidents); however, other incidents may affect large geographic areas and many jurisdictions (open or uncontained incidents). In these incidents, many federal, state, and local agencies become involved. Regardless of the size of the incident or the number of agencies involved, scene management calls for a coordinated effort. This effort must ensure an effective response and the efficient and safe use of resources.

NOTE

The procedure for managing a major multiagency, multijurisdictional incident is outlined in the federal NIMS. This procedure should be adopted for local use.

Phase 3: Postdisaster Follow-Up. Phase 3 involves a **postdisaster follow-up** (or after-action review). This review includes the lessons learned from the incident and methods of improvement, such as improvement of emergency response, planning, and community protection. This phase also should assess stress-related anxiety and illness among emergency workers that may have resulted from the incident.

Mass-Casualty Incidents

The ICS at an MCI is expanded when the number of casualties or the nature of the event overwhelms the available resources (the **local/regional threshold**). In communities where the local threshold is low, frequent use of the ICS for practice is encouraged. For example, it can be used when an incident involves more than one patient. When an MCI is identified, command must quickly determine how best to expand the ICS to meet the needs of the event. In other words, sections, groups, and divisions must be put into place according to the size and scope of the incident.

Typically, initial expansion of the ICS for an MCI requires the establishment of a medical group (including triage and treatment subcomponents, called units), a transportation group, and an extrication/rescue group for disentanglement and/or removal of patients from hazardous areas. If more than five groups (or divisions, if assigned geographically) are activated, an operations section typically is established (**FIGURE 53-9**).

CRITICAL THINKING

How do you think you will feel when you arrive first on the scene of an MCI?

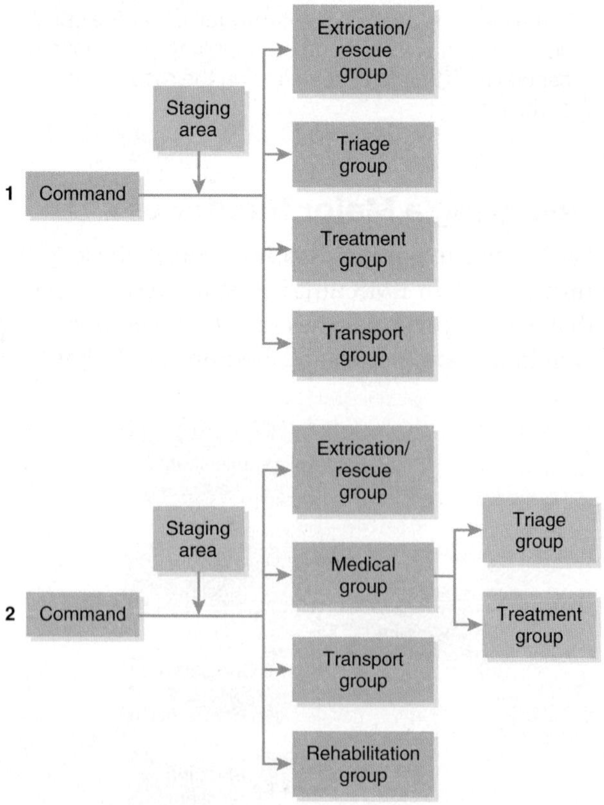

FIGURE 53-9 Two examples of incident command systems for mass-casualty incidents.

Scene Assessment

The first EMS unit to arrive at the scene should make a quick and rapid assessment (size-up) of the situation. If the arriving unit is a two-paramedic crew, one paramedic assumes the function of command; the second paramedic begins triage. A more precise and full assessment should be performed as soon as safety and time allow. This fuller assessment should include the following:

- The type of incident and the potential duration
- Whether entrapment or special rescue resources may be needed
- The number of patients in each triage category (described later in this chapter)
- Initial assignments for incoming units
- The need for any additional resources to manage the incident

> NOTE
> The scene assessment must be updated continually. This updating helps in the identification of specific or changing needs.

Communications

Command must immediately establish radio contact with the main **communications center** or the **emergency operations center (EOC)**. Most jurisdictions maintain an EOC as part of their community's preparedness program. This is the main communications center where representatives of emergency response organizations, government agencies, and sometimes private organizations gather to coordinate their response to an emergency event. Command and the EOC share similar goals; however, they function at different levels of responsibility. The IC is responsible for on-scene activities, while the EOC is responsible for the entire community-wide response to the event. Radio traffic can be very distracting; therefore, incident personnel must observe strict radio and/or phone procedures, they should use clear, plain English, and all transmissions should be short and to the point.

> NOTE
> Runners (messengers), cell phones, and satellite phones (SAT phones) are used when radio communications fail (eg, in a large-scale disaster). Communications is often considered the biggest problem in major incidents.

Obtaining Resources

More units should be requested as soon as the need has been identified or anticipated. (The communications center should have a written SOP for requesting **mutual aid**.) Support may include obtaining food, shelter, and clothing for patients. The IC is responsible for providing instructions for the deployment of the resources. (Personnel should stay with their vehicle until instructions are received.) Staging techniques that may be used to deploy resources effectively include the following:

- Lining vehicles up at the scene to facilitate egress
- Staging away from a limited-access highway
- Identifying a formal staging area with an assigned staging officer

The toolbox theory of strategic deployment of resources can be used. It involves identifying the resources (tools) specific to the incident, using only the needed resources, and issuing instructions for the deployment of resources.

Group or Division Functions

As stated previously, the number of groups or divisions needed at a major medical incident varies. Common groups and their responsibilities include extrication/rescue, treatment, and transportation. The staging area, rehabilitation area, and support branch are also important parts of an incident organization.

Extrication/Rescue Group

The **extrication/rescue group** is responsible for managing patients who are trapped or need extrication from a hazardous situation at the incident. Responsibilities of this group may include search, rescue, initial triage, tagging, and limited in situ treatment before transfer of the patients to the treatment group. Patient care for this group includes only identification and treatment of life-threatening injuries, such as the need to open the airway, control severe bleeding, and cover open chest wounds. In addition, the extrication/rescue group is responsible for site safety and personnel safety (eg, supplying self-contained breathing apparatus and protective clothing, atmospheric monitoring if indicated for explosive or oxygen-deficient atmospheres) and for evaluating and directing the resources needed for extrication and rescue. Extrication/rescue group responsibilities include the following:

- Determining whether triage and the primary treatment will be conducted on site or in the treatment group area
- Attaching tagging assignments to injured patients
- Evaluating the resources needed for extrication of trapped patients and for their delivery to the treatment group
- Ensuring site safety
- Evaluating resources needed for triage and the primary treatment of patients
- Communicating resource requirements to command
- Allocating assigned resources
- Supervising assigned personnel and resources
- Collecting, assembling, and assessing the walking wounded
- Reporting progress to command
- Reporting all clear to command when all patients have been extricated and delivered to the treatment group
- Coordinating with other groups

CRITICAL THINKING

What difficult decisions might you face in doing triage at an MCI?

Treatment Group

The **treatment group** works closely with the extrication/rescue group in patient care. As patients are delivered, they are recategorized according to their needs. The treatment group provides advanced care and stabilization until the patients are transported to a medical facility. Most paramedics and medical facility personnel are assigned to this group.

With a large number of patients, the area usually is further divided into immediate and delayed treatment zones. This categorization helps in the determination of priorities for patient transport. Immediate treatment patients include those with life-threatening injuries; delayed treatment patients include the walking wounded and those whose care and transport can be delayed if necessary. It should be noted that triage monitoring is a function of all groups involving ill or injured patients. It is a continuing component of the ICS. Treatment group responsibilities include the following:

- Locating a suitable treatment area that satisfies hazardous materials concerns, if applicable (eg, uphill/upwind/upstream), and reporting that location to the extrication/rescue group and command
- Evaluating resources required for patient treatment and reporting these needs to command
- Providing secondary triage of patients arriving in the treatment area; tagging patients if not already done
- Providing suitable immediate and delayed treatment areas
- Allocating resources
- Assigning, supervising, and coordinating personnel in the group
- Reporting progress to command
- Coordinating with other divisions and groups

On-Scene Physicians. Physicians who are on scene can provide valuable help during an MCI. The roles of the physicians may include performing triage, performing emergency surgery to facilitate extrication, performing specialized invasive procedures at the scene, and obtaining a more detailed patient assessment. In addition, they may provide direction for specific treatments that may be beyond the scope of normal paramedic practice.

Disposition of the Deceased. Depending on the scale of the incident, personnel may be assigned to disposition of the deceased. Their duties may include the following:

- Working with the medical examiner, coroner, law enforcement personnel, and other appropriate agencies to coordinate disposition
- Assisting in the establishment of an appropriate and secure area for a morgue, if needed

When possible, the deceased should be left in the location in which they were found until a plan has been made for removal and storage of the bodies.

Transportation Group

The **transportation group** communicates with the receiving medical facilities, ambulances, and air medical services for patient transport. This group must work closely with the treatment group. They help to determine appropriate destinations for injured patients. Also, the arrival and departure of transfer vehicles must be coordinated with the staging area. Transportation group responsibilities include the following:

- Determining patient transport needs and obtaining appropriate transportation
- Evaluating resources required to manage patient transport
- Establishing an ambulance staging area (if command has not already done so) and patient loading areas
- Establishing and operating a helicopter landing zone
- Communicating with medical facilities to determine medical facility surge capacity and capability to handle specialty patients
- Coordinating patient transport allocations with the treatment group and medical facilities
- Tracking patients leaving the site with a written log (including patient identification, the transporting unit, and the destination facility)
- Reporting resource requirements to command
- Coordinating with other divisions and groups
- Advising command when the last patient has been transported

Staging Area

Staging areas are needed for large incidents. They help to prevent vehicle congestion and delays in response. All emergency vehicles (fire, law enforcement, and EMS) should report to this area for direction. Other agencies, such as disaster relief services and news media, also may be supervised by the staging area manager. The responsibilities of the staging area manager include the following:

- Coordinating with law enforcement personnel to block streets, intersections, and other areas to allow the establishment of a staging area
- Ensuring that all equipment and vehicles are parked in an appropriate manner
- Maintaining a log of all equipment in the staging area and an inventory of all specialized equipment and medical equipment that may be needed
- Reviewing with command the resources that must be maintained in staging, as well as coordinating this request with the dispatching center
- Assuming a visible position for incoming equipment and vehicles (eg, leaving emergency lights operating on one vehicle and wearing an identification vest)
- Coordinating with other divisions and groups

Rehabilitation Area

A **rehabilitation area** (rehab area) is part of the major incident response plans of many fire and EMS agencies. This area usually is set up outside the operational area. It allows rescue personnel to get physical and psychological rest and to monitor their physical condition. With smaller incidents, the rehab unit leader usually reports directly to command. In large-scale incidents or whenever a logistics section is established, the rehab unit leader reports to the logistics chief. In large-scale incidents, more than one rehab area may be needed.

One duty of the rehab unit leader is to ensure that personnel receive medical care and treatment as needed. Another duty is to keep accurate logs of those who enter and leave the area. Records of medical care and treatments are kept for each person who enters the rehab area. (Medical care of rescue personnel is further addressed in Chapter 56, *Hazardous Materials Awareness.*)

> CRITICAL THINKING
> Why do you think establishing responder rehabilitation is important?

Support Branch

The **support branch** is in charge of gathering and distributing equipment and supplies. This branch may be responsible for obtaining medical supplies from area medical facilities, rescue supplies, and other equipment needed at the incident. Support branch responsibilities include the following:

- Determining the medical supply needs of other divisions and groups
- Establishing a suitable location for supply operations
- Coordinating procurement of medical supplies from medical facilities with the transportation group

- Coordinating procurement of medical supplies that are not available from medical facilities
- Reporting additional resource requirements to command
- Allocating supplies and equipment as needed
- Reporting progress to command
- Coordinating with other divisions and groups

NOTE

Often only specific parts of the logistics section are needed at an incident. One of these parts is the rehabilitation unit; the other is the support branch. Depending on the span of control, these two units can be implemented without the establishment of a logistics section chief; they report directly to command.

Identification and Communication

When an ICS is in place, all responders must know its organizational structure and the lines of radio communication. Although clothing and identification vary by system, the following guidelines usually apply:

- Color-coded vests identify personnel. For example, the commander may wear a white vest; EMS group managers, blue vests; fire group managers, red; law enforcement group managers, green; and so on.
- With the exceptions of command and division/group communications, most communications are face to face. Radio use is intended for command operations.
- Radio communications use operation titles instead of personal or unit names. For example, a responder may say, "Treatment group to command," or, "Extrication/rescue group to treatment group." This system ensures that all participants can reach the appropriate position (rather than person) by one radio designation. In longer incidents, the person may change, but the position remains stable.

Radio Communications

Communications is a key function during a major incident. Preplanning includes identifying the radio frequencies to be used in major incident responses. It also includes planning for the ways these frequencies are to be used. For example, all responding units should have multichannel radios that use a common frequency. Within this common frequency, separate frequencies should be used for EMS, fire, and other support operations. Division and group officers should have portable radios set on a channel that permits direct communication with command. These channels may be assigned in advance or by the dispatching agency at the time of the incident. In addition, state, regional, and local communications systems should undergo a periodic review. This review should include the controls for activating communications, system frequencies, and portable and mobile radio equipment. Other communications considerations include the following:

- Radio traffic must be clear, concise, and in plain English.
- Messages should be thoughtfully prepared before transmission.
- The speaker should clearly identify the unit number or division or group.
- All radio traffic should be minimized.
- Face-to-face communication is preferable and encouraged.

NOTE

One approach to keep radio communications concise is to use the UCAN format: Identify your Unit or ICS assignment; briefly state the Conditions you find; identify the Actions that you are taking to resolve the situation; and request any additional Needs that you have.

Common Problems at MCIs

In addition to common failures of the ICS (BOX 53-4), there are common problems specific to MCIs, including the following:[3]

- Failure to adequately provide widespread notification of the event
- Failure to provide rapid initial stabilization of all patients
- Failure to move, collect, and organize patients quickly in a treatment area
- Failure to provide proper triage
- Provision of overly time-consuming care
- Premature transport of patients
- Improper use of personnel in the field

BOX 53-4 Common Failures in the ICS

Incident Command Failures

- To establish a single, unified command
- To establish staging
- To request additional resources early
- To delegate authority

Dispatch Failure

- To coordinate the response of on-duty and off-duty emergency personnel to the scene

Communications Failures

- To designate a single radio channel for disaster operations
- To adopt SOPs that limit radio traffic during incident operations

Staging Operation Failures

- To establish a central staging area (command)
- To select a large or easily accessible staging area (staging manager)
- To frequently inventory specialized equipment and personnel (staging manager)

General Division/Group Failures

- To provide adequate progress reports to command
- To become involved in physical tasks, such as carrying litters or operating rescue equipment (division/group supervisor)
- To control the perimeter (law enforcement)
- To advise command of available personnel

Extrication/Rescue Group Failures

- To triage and tag patients
- To treat patients where they are found (as opposed to stabilizing them and moving them to a treatment area) (rescuers)
- To provide adequate safety precautions

Treatment Group Failures

- To collect patients into an organized treatment area
- To establish a sufficiently large treatment area
- To organize the treatment area and monitor patients
- To effectively coordinate transportation arrangements with the transportation group

Transportation Group Failures

- To establish adequate access and egress routes for vehicles
- To have adequate personnel to assist in transportation
- To alert or update medical facilities
- To advise medical facilities when the last patient has been transported

Support Branch Failures

- To plan for the medical supply needs of MCIs
- To provide rapid transport of supplies to the scene

- Failure to properly distribute patients to medical facilities
- Failure to communicate with local medical facilities regarding patient flow and medical facility capacity
- Lack of proper preplanning and lack of adequate training for all personnel

Principles and Technology of Triage

Triage is a method of categorizing patients based on an assessment of the severity of injury versus the resources required to care for the patient (BOX 53-5). This process often includes an appraisal of mental status including the ability to follow commands, the patient's ability to walk, and abnormal physiologic signs. It should be stressed that triage is an ongoing process during a major incident. Constant monitoring of the patient's condition may reveal a need to change the initial grouping and priority of treatment. The criteria for triage classifications are determined by the size of the incident, the number of injured patients, and the available personnel.

BOX 53-5 Primary Versus Secondary Triage

The process of triage will often have multiple phases. **Primary triage**, known in the SALT (Sort, Assess, Lifesaving interventions, Treatment and/or Transport) triage system as group sorting, is used to rapidly categorize patients according to the severity of their injuries and the resources that will be needed to treat them. Primary triage is also used to rapidly assess and report the number of patients and the severity of their injuries.

Secondary triage, known in SALT as individual assessment, is used at the treatment area, where patients are triaged again. They are labeled (usually with paper tags) to assign priorities of care. Secondary triage often is not needed at small-scale incidents.

National guidelines have been established for field triage,[4] and many other triage models exist, but no model has been definitively shown to be superior to any other. The paramedic must be familiar with local methods of triage categorization.

SALT Triage

SALT triage (Sort, Assess, Lifesaving interventions, Treatment and/or Transport) was developed as a national all-hazards mass-casualty initial triage standard for all patients (eg, adults, children, special populations). SALT is endorsed by leading EMS associations, including the American College of Emergency Physicians, the National Association of EMS Physicians, and the American College of Surgeons Committee on Trauma.[5] SALT was designed to allow providers to rapidly prioritize patient care, apply lifesaving interventions early, and group patients accurately and quickly.[6]

Step 1: Sort

SALT begins with a global sorting of patients, prioritizing them for individual assessment. All patients are first asked to walk to a designated area; for example, rescuers say something like, "Follow the sound of my voice if you need help." Patients who voluntarily ambulate will be the last priority for individual assessment. Those who remain, should be asked to wave (ie, follow a command) or be observed for purposeful movement. Those who do not move (ie, are still) and those with obvious life threats should be assessed first because they are the most likely to need lifesaving interventions. This sorting process results in the following patient prioritization:

- Priority 3: Can walk
- Priority 2: Can wave or makes purposeful movement
- Priority 1: Does not move or has obvious life threat

The S in SALT, global sorting, recognizes that some patients may be relatively uninjured but may elect to stay with another patient who cannot move (eg, a mother with an injured child). Likewise, some patients will be unable to walk on their own even though their injuries are not life threatening (eg, a patient with a nail through the foot). The purpose of global sorting is to identify and group the patients who should be first to receive the assessment and lifesaving intervention steps in SALT. The sorting step does not involve placing any kind of tag or marker on patients.

Step 2: Assess

The individual assessment should begin with limited rapid lifesaving interventions:

- Controlling major hemorrhage through the use of direct pressure provided by other patients, tourniquets, or other devices
- Opening the airway through positioning or basic airway adjuncts (no advanced airway devices should be used)
- If the patient is a child, giving two rescue breaths, if indicated
- Providing chest decompression
- Administering auto-injector antidotes

Step 3: Lifesaving Interventions

All **lifesaving interventions** should be performed rapidly and only within the responder's scope of practice. The paramedic should not stop to fetch additional equipment or supplies.

Step 4: Treatment and/or Transport

Patients are initially categorized into five categories: dead, immediate, expectant, delayed, or minimal. The appropriate color tag is applied.

Dead (Black Triage Tape or Tag). First, the paramedic should assess the following:

- If an adult, is the patient breathing after opening the airway?
- If a child, is the patient breathing after opening the airway and giving two breaths?

If the answer to this question is no, then the patient should be tagged *dead*. In the presence of an MCI, taking one responder away to continuously ventilate an apneic patient will rapidly break down the care system for all patients.

Immediate (Red Triage Tape or Tag). Next, the paramedic should rapidly assess the following:

- Does the patient follow commands or make purposeful movements?
- Does the patient have a peripheral pulse?

- Is the patient not in respiratory distress?
- Is hemorrhage controlled?

If the answer to *any* of these questions is no and the paramedic believes the patient is likely to survive given the available resources, then the patient should be tagged *immediate*. Immediate patients receive priority care and move forward first.

Expectant (Gray, White, or Blue Triage Tape or Tag, Depending on the Tag System). If the answer to *any* of the previous questions about pulse, breathing, hemorrhage, and mental status is no and the paramedic believes the patient is unlikely to survive given the available resources, then the patient is tagged *expectant*. These patients should not receive resources that are more likely to save immediate patients, but may receive treatment after all immediate patients have been moved forward.

Delayed (Yellow Triage Tape or Tag). Patients with serious injuries that will require eventual definitive treatment but not immediate forward movement and care are tagged *delayed*. In determining this classification, the paramedic should consider the following:

- Does the patient have a peripheral pulse?
- Is the patient not in respiratory distress?
- Is hemorrhage controlled?
- Does the patient follow commands or make purposeful movements?

If the answer is yes to *all* of these questions but the injuries are significant, then the patient is tagged as *delayed*.

Minimal (Green Triage Tape or Tag). If the answer to *all* of the preceding questions about pulse, breathing, hemorrhage, and mental status is yes and the injuries appear minor, then the patient should be tagged *minimal*. Minimal patients will typically be the last to be assessed because they will be in the group of ambulatory patients who were able to walk to a collection area during global sorting. Minimal patients may be able to help care for or move other patients.

Using the Tags. After immediate patients have received care, patients designated expectant, delayed, or minimal should be reassessed as soon as possible with the expectation that some patients will have improved and others will have decompensated. In general, treatment and/or transport should be provided for immediate patients first, then delayed, and then minimal. Expectant patients should be provided with treatment and/or transport when resources permit. Efficient use of transportation assets may include mixing categories of patients and using alternate forms of transportation. Some patients may require only treatment at the scene and not transport (**FIGURE 53-10**).

> NOTE
>
> In some MCIs, **casualty collection areas** are established. These areas provide a safe place away from hazards where ill or injured patients can be gathered for triage, treatment, or transport, or can be temporarily located until a specific branch, such as treatment, can be established.

START Triage

The simple triage and rapid treatment (START) system was developed by Hoag Memorial Presbyterian Hospital in Newport Beach, California. It is a 60-second assessment that focuses on the patient's ability to walk, respiratory effort, pulses/perfusion, and mental status (**FIGURE 53-11**). This assessment is used to classify a patient's status as minor, delayed, immediate, or dead. The START system allows rescuers to quickly identify patients at greatest risk of early death.

The paramedic should first assess the patient's ability to walk. Patients who can walk and understand basic commands are categorized as minor (walking wounded). They will be further triaged and tagged as more rescuers arrive. Patients who are minor should be directed to remain in their location for further assistance or to walk to a treatment or transportation site. The initial START triage is directed toward patients who cannot walk.

Patients who meet the 30-2-can-do (BOX 53-6) criteria but who cannot walk are categorized as delayed. Patients who are unconscious, have rapid breathing, have delayed or absent capillary refill, or have an absent radial pulse are categorized as immediate. Patients who are not breathing and resume spontaneous respiration after having their airway opened are considered immediate (tagged as red). If breathing does not resume after opening the airway, the patient is categorized as dead.

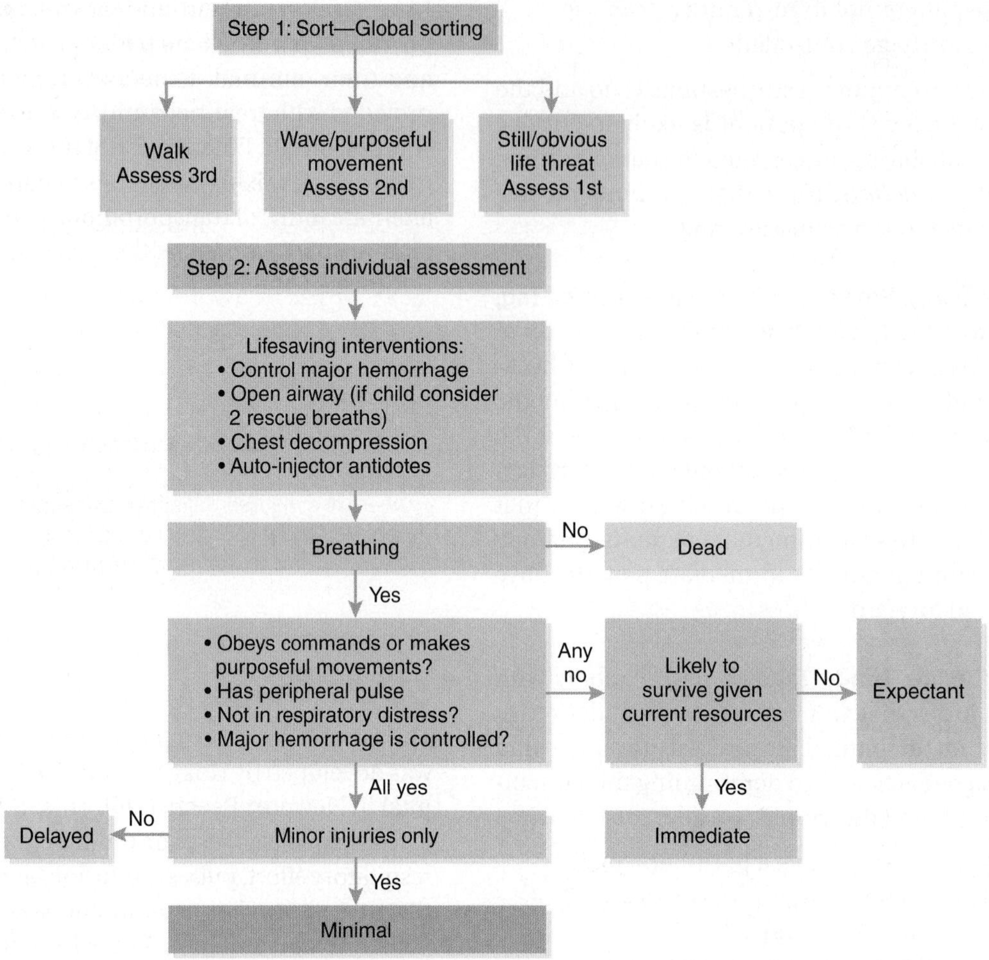

FIGURE 53-10 The Sort, Assess, Lifesaving interventions, and Treatment and/or Transport (SALT) Triage Scheme.

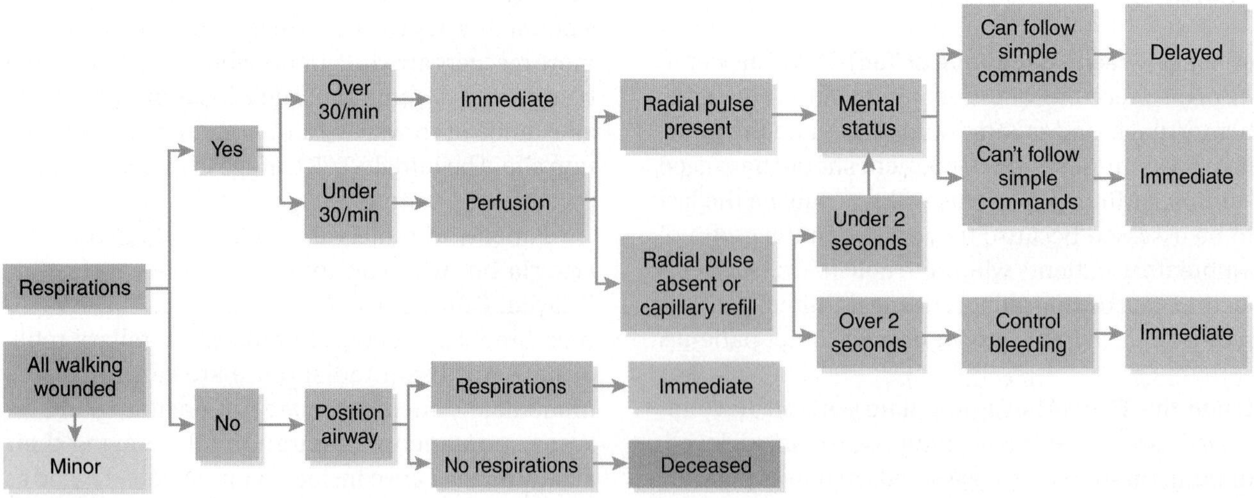

FIGURE 53-11 The Simple Triage And Rapid Treatment (START) system sorts patients into critical or delayed categories. Patients are quickly removed from the scene according to their triage group.

BOX 53-6 30-2-Can-Do

The mnemonic 30-2-can-do is used as the START triage prompt. The *30* refers to the patient's respiratory rate, *2* refers to capillary refill time, and *can-do* refers to the patient's ability to follow commands. A respiratory rate of fewer than 30 breaths/min, a capillary refill time of less than 2 seconds, and the ability to walk and follow commands are the criteria for a minor patient.

CRITICAL THINKING

What emergent conditions might a patient have if the respiratory rate is fewer than 10 or more than 30 breaths/min?

SHOW ME THE EVIDENCE

Researchers sought to assess the accuracy of the SALT and the START triage systems by comparing them to a published reference standard. In a field simulation MCI using patients categorized with a published reference standard, it was found that SALT provided overall more accurate triage when compared to the reference standard (r = 0.860, P <0.001). Both SALT and START agreed 100% on black and green patient categories. SALT had significantly less undertriage, at 9% (95% confidence interval [CI], 2–15) than did START, at 20% (95% CI, 11–28). There was no significant difference in overtriage rates. The researchers concluded that SALT triage was a more accurate triage method.

Modified from: Silvestri S, Field A, Mangalat N, et al. Comparison of START and SALT triage methodologies to reference standard definitions and to a field mass casualty simulation. *Am J Disaster Med.* 2017;12(1):27-33.

Triage Tagging/Labeling

Many types of tags, tapes, ribbons, and labels are used to indicate a patient's triage category (**triage tagging system**). Two commonly used labeling methods are the METTAG system and the **SMART tag system**.

The METTAG (which stands for Medical Emergency Triage Tags) system uses the international agreement on color coding and priorities to alert emergency care personnel and staff members of the receiving medical facility to the patient's category (**TABLE 53-1**). Red identifies the patients who are most critically injured; yellow, those less critically injured; green, those with injuries that are not life or limb threatening; and black, patients who have died or whose injuries preclude survival. Triage tags and labels should be used routinely for practice so that EMS crews become familiar with their use.

The SMART tag system uses four color triage coding cards that have military bar codes for tracking patients (**FIGURE 53-12**):

1. Priority 1 (red) indicates immediate treatment.
2. Priority 2 (yellow) indicates urgent treatment.
3. Priority 3 (green) indicates delayed treatment.
4. Black cards indicate death.

Regardless of the labeling system used, categorization must identify the priority of the patient's condition, prevent retriage of the same patient, and serve

TABLE 53-1 International Color Coding and Priorities[a]

Patient Status	Color Code	Priority
Immediate	Red	Priority 1 (P-1)
Delayed	Yellow	Priority 2 (P-2)
Hold	Green	Priority 3 (P-3)
Deceased	Black	Priority 0 (P-0)

[a]This field triage decision scheme, originally developed by the American College of Surgeons Committee on Trauma, was revised by an expert panel representing EMS, emergency medicine, trauma surgery, and public health. The panel was convened by the Centers for Disease Control and Prevention, with support from the National Highway Traffic Safety Administration.

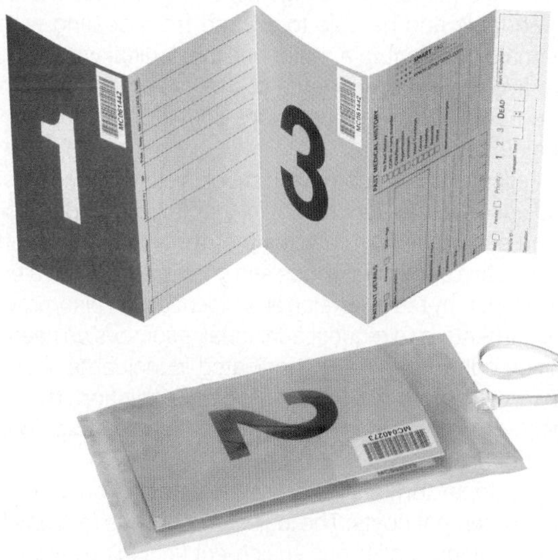

FIGURE 53-12 SMART triage tag with bar code.

as a tracking system during treatment and transport. For these reasons, all tags and labels should have the following characteristics:

- Be easy to use.
- Rapidly identify the patient's priority.
- Allow for easy tracking.
- Allow room for some documentation.
- Prevent patients from retriaging themselves.

Tracking Systems for Patients

As described previously, the transportation group officer must keep a tracking or destination log that integrates the triage tagging system. In addition, the log should have the patient's name or triage label identification number. A **tracking log** is similar to a shipping manifest and must have the following information:

- Patient identification
- Transporting unit
- Patient priority
- Medical facility destination

Patient Transport

The way patients are transported depends on their triage priority and situation. Ambulances typically are used; however, buses may be used to transport a large number of stable patients. Air ambulances are usually reserved for the transport of patients in critical condition.

Critical Incident Stress Management

As described in Chapter 2, *Well-Being of the Paramedic*, critical incident stress is a potential hazard for rescue personnel. For this reason, support services should be available to help manage the stress of a traumatic event. Depending on the nature and scale of the incident, these services may include structured stress debriefings, employee assistance programs, counseling, spouse support programs, family life programs, pastoral services, and periodic stress evaluations.[7]

Summary

- Major incidents are events for which available resources are insufficient to manage the number of casualties or the type of emergency.
- The incident command system (ICS) organizational structure should be adaptable to any agency or to any incident requiring emergency management. The ICS also must be expandable and be able to expand from dealing with a nonmajor incident to a major one in a logical way.
- The five major components of the ICS organization are command, planning, operations, logistics, and finance/administration.
- The responsibility of command should belong to one person who assumes the function of incident commander. Command should perform a size-up of the situation, assume an effective command mode and position, transmit a brief initial report by radio, develop an incident action plan, provide assignments, and request additional resources as needed.
- Unified command may be indicated in incidents such as those with more than one political jurisdiction, multiple agencies within a jurisdiction, or multiple geographic and functional agencies.
- The finance/administration section tracks incident and reimbursement costs. The logistics section is responsible for providing supplies and equipment (including personnel to operate the equipment), facilities, services, food, and communications support. The operations section directs and coordinates all emergency scene operations. It also ensures the safety of all personnel. The planning section should provide past, present, and future information about the incident and the status of resources.
- All participating response agencies must agree to the preplan (phase 1 of the ICS). The preplan must address common goals and the specific duties of each group. Phase 2 involves the development of a strategy to manage the emergency scene (scene management). Phase 3 includes a postdisaster review of lessons learned from the incident and the determination of ways to improve the response effort.
- The need to expand the ICS at a medical incident is based on the number of casualties and the nature of the event.
- The first EMS unit to arrive at the scene should make a quick and rapid assessment of the situation. Command must immediately establish radio contact with the communications center or emergency operations center. Additional units should be requested as soon as the need has been identified.
- Common divisions or groups that may need to be established include extrication/rescue, treatment, and transportation. The extrication/rescue group is responsible for managing patients who are trapped or need extrication from a hazardous situation at the incident. The treatment group provides advanced care and stabilization until the patients

are transported to a medical facility. The transportation group communicates with the receiving medical facility, ambulances, and air medical services for patient transport.
- The staging area, rehabilitation area, and support branch are also important parts of an incident organization. The staging area is used in large incidents to prevent vehicle congestion and delays in response. The rehabilitation area allows rescue personnel to receive physical and psychological rest and to monitor their physical condition. The support branch coordinates the gathering and distribution of equipment and supplies for all divisions and groups.
- Problems of mass-casualty incidents and ICS stem from numerous issues related to communication, resource allocation, and delegation.
- Triage is a method used to categorize patients for priorities of treatment. SALT (Sort, Assess, Lifesaving interventions, Treatment and/or Transport) triage uses rapid sorting and assessment questions to manage the scene and prioritize deployment of patient care resources. START (simple triage and rapid treatment) triage focuses on the patient's ability to walk, respiratory effort, pulses/perfusion, and mental status to quickly identify patients at greatest risk of early death.
- There are many types of tags, tapes, ribbons, and labels used to indicate a patient's triage category. The METTAG system uses the international agreement on color coding and priorities to alert emergency care personnel and staff members of the receiving medical facility to the patient's category. The SMART tag system uses four color triage coding cards that have military bar codes for tracking patients.
- Support services should be available to help manage the stress of a traumatic event. Depending on the nature and scale of the incident, these services may include structured stress debriefings, employee assistance programs, counseling, spouse support programs, family life programs, pastoral services, and periodic stress evaluations.

References

1. Federal Emergency Management Agency. *National Incident Management System*. 3rd ed. Washington, DC: US Department of Homeland Security; 2017.
2. Pennsylvania Emergency Management Agency. *ICS-400-Advanced ICS Student Manual*. Harrisburg, PA: Pennsylvania Emergency Management Agency; 2013.
3. US Department of Homeland Security. *National Incident Management System*. Washington, DC: US Department of Homeland Security; 2008.
4. McCoy CE, Chakravarthy B, Lotfipour S. Guidelines for field triage of injured patients: in conjunction with the *Morbidity and Mortality Weekly Report* published by the Centers for Disease Control and Prevention. *West J Emerg Med*. 2013;14(1):69-76.
5. SALT mass casualty triage: concept endorsed by the American College of Emergency Physicians, American College of Surgeons Committee on Trauma, American Trauma Society, National Association of EMS Physicians, National Disaster Life Support Education Consortium, and State and Territorial Injury Prevention Directors Association. *Disaster Med Public Health Prep*. 2008;2(4):245-246.
6. Lerner EB, Schwartz RB, Coule PL, et al. Mass casualty triage: an evaluation of the data and development of a proposed national guideline. *Disaster Med Public Health Prep*. 2008;2(S1):S25-S34.
7. Mitchell JT, Bray GP. *Emergency Services Stress*. Englewood Cliffs, NJ: Brady Publishing; 1990.

Suggested Readings

Biddinger PD, Baggish A, Harrington L, et al. Be prepared—the Boston Marathon and mass-casualty events. *N Engl J Med*. 2013;368:1958-1960.

Culley JM, Svendsen E. A review of the literature on the validity of mass casualty triage systems with a focus on chemical exposures. *Am J Disaster Med*. 2014;9(2):137-150.

Donofrio JJ, Kaji AH, Claudius IA, et al. Development of a pediatric mass casualty triage algorithm validation tool. *Prehosp Emerg Care*. 2016 May-Jun;20(3):343-353.

Edgerly D. The basics of mass casualty triage. *JEMS* website. http://www.jems.com/articles/print/volume-41/issue-5/departments-columns/back-to-basics/the-basics-of-mass-casualty-triage.html. Published May 1, 2016. Accessed March 29, 2018.

Gore TA. Posttraumatic stress disorder treatment and management. Medscape website. https://emedicine.medscape.com/article/288154-treatment. Updated March 7, 2018. Accessed March 29, 2018.

Russo C. Healing first responders through critical incident stress management interventions: critical incident stress management is a short-term, psychological first-aid intervention strategy that can help mitigate long-term mental health issues. EMS1.com website. https://www.ems1.com/ems-products/fitness-health/articles/225253048-Healing-first-responders-through-critical-incident-stress-management-interventions/. Published March 27, 2017. Accessed March 29, 2018.

Silvestri S, Field A, Mangalat N, et al. Comparison of START and SALT triage methodologies to reference standard definitions and to a field mass casualty simulation. *Am J Disaster Med*. 2017 Winter;12(1):27-33.

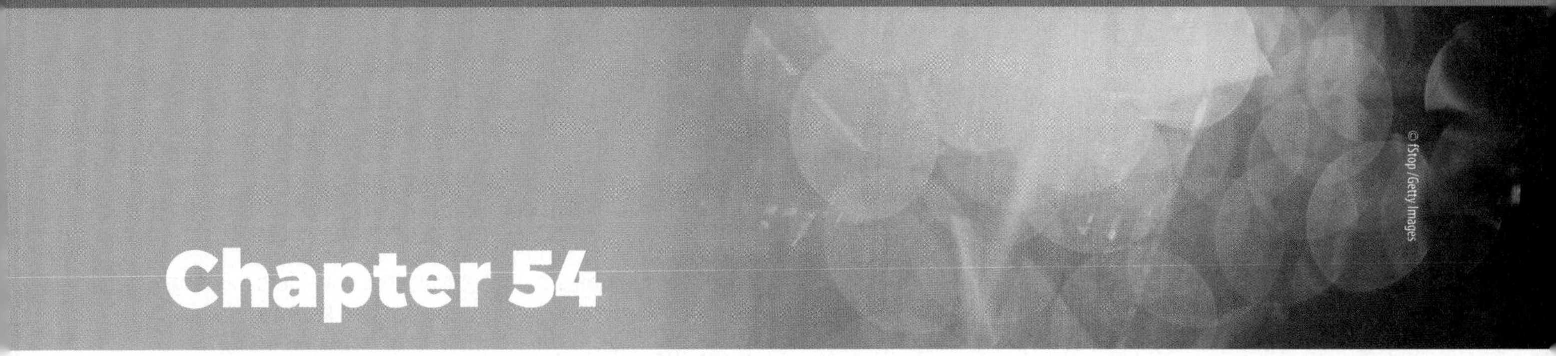

Chapter 54

Rescue Awareness and Operations

NATIONAL EMS EDUCATION STANDARD COMPETENCIES

EMS Operations

Knowledge of operational roles and responsibilities to ensure patient, public, and personnel safety.

Vehicle Extrication

- Safe vehicle extrication (pp 1854–1857, 1866–1869)
- Use of simple hand tools (pp 1855, 1866–1867)

OBJECTIVES

Upon completion of this chapter, the paramedic student will be able to:

1. Describe factors that must be considered to ensure appropriate timing of medical and mechanical skills during a rescue. (p 1853)
2. Contrast and compare each phase of a rescue operation. (pp 1854–1857)
3. Identify the appropriate personal protective equipment to work in proximity to rescue operations. (p 1857)
4. Describe important considerations for EMS crews in a surface water rescue. (pp 1858–1860)
5. Discuss important considerations for EMS crews in rescues associated with hazardous atmospheres, including confined spaces and trench or cave-in situations. (pp 1860–1864)
6. Describe hazards that may be present during an EMS rescue operation on a highway. (pp 1864–1869)
7. Describe important considerations for EMS crews in a rescue involving hazardous terrain. (pp 1869–1871)
8. Assess special considerations for prehospital assessment and management during a rescue operation. (pp 1871–1873)

KEY TERMS

basket stretcher A litter designed of a rigid frame made of wire, mesh, or plastic.

confined spaces Spaces that have limited access or egress and are not designed for ongoing human occupancy or habitation.

cross-trained personnel Emergency personnel who are trained in more than one type of emergency service (eg, fire, rescue, EMS, law enforcement).

disentanglement The process of making a pathway through the wreckage of an accident and removing wreckage from patients.

dynamic rope "High-stretch" rope that is designed to stretch as much as 20% to 50% under load (eg, when stopping a falling rescuer), which reduces the chance of rope breakage as well as the shock to the rescuer.

egress An exit pathway.

engulfment Mechanical entrapment that places a person in a confined space.

flat-terrain rescue A type of rescue involving the movement of a victim up or down a grade of approximately 0° to 20° of elevation or decline that may involve various obstructions. An example of this terrain is level land with large rocks, loose soil, and beds of water or creeks.

hazard control The phase of rescue that involves managing, reducing, and minimizing risks from uncontrollable hazards; ensuring scene safety; and providing personal protective equipment appropriate for the incident.

hazardous atmospheres Oxygen-deficient, toxic, or explosive environments that may occur in confined spaces.

high-angle rescue A type of rescue involving the movement of a victim up or down a grade of greater than 60°, typically requiring a high degree of specialized equipment, techniques, and training.

kernmantle rope A type of rope used in life-safety rescue operations that provides for minimal stretch (a low elongation factor). It is constructed with an interior synthetic fiber core protected by a woven exterior sheath, and designed to optimize strength, abrasion resistance, and flexibility.

lock-out process The disabling and securing of any kind of energized equipment to prevent any unauthorized person from entering the area or gaining access to the controls that have been shut off.

low-angle rescue A type of rescue involving the movement of a victim up or down a grade of approximately 35°, often requiring the use of specialized equipment, techniques, and training.

oxygen-deficient atmospheres Confined spaces in which there is an inadequate concentration of oxygen.

patient packaging Completion of the emergency care procedures needed to transfer a patient from the scene to the emergency vehicle.

personal flotation device (PFD) A safety device worn in water to reduce the risk of drowning.

power take-off (PTO) A splined driveshaft, usually on a tractor or other farm machinery, used to provide power to an attachment or separate machine.

rappelling A controlled descent by rope.

rescue The act of delivery from danger or imprisonment.

rescue versus body recovery The chance to save a human life (rescue) versus body recovery without the goal of saving a human life.

risk–benefit analysis An analysis that considers personal safety before rescue is attempted. It asks the question, "Does the risk outweigh the benefit, or vice versa?"

safety officer In a rescue operation, the official who remains alert to the stress of the operation on the rescuers.

static rope "Low-stretch" rope, which is designed to stretch typically less than 10% under load when used in rescue operations.

steep-angle rescue A type of rescue involving the movement of a victim up or down a grade of approximately 35° to 65°. The weight of the rescuer is distributed between the rope and the ground.

supplemental restraint system A safety device in a vehicle, such as an impact sensor, airbags, and seat belt pre-tensioners, that deploys to prevent driver/occupant injury.

supplied-air (air-line) breathing apparatus (SABA) A device that provides a nearly unlimited supply of air from a source located outside the confined space.

surface water rescue The rescue of a patient who is afloat on the surface of a body of water.

traffic incident management The process of coordinating the resources of a number of different partner agencies and private-sector companies to detect, respond to, and clear traffic incidents as quickly as possible so as to reduce the impacts of incidents on safety and congestion, while protecting the safety of on-scene rescuers.

Rescue *is defined as "the act of delivery from danger or imprisonment." Many of the day-to-day activities of EMS personnel and other public service agencies are encompassed within this definition when they respond to an emergency where people have been traumatized or trapped. Rescue requires specialized medical and mechanical skills, with the right amount of each being applied at the appropriate time.*

NOTE

Rescue skills have become highly specialized. National Fire Protection Association (NFPA) 1006, *Standard for Technical Rescuer Personnel Professional Qualifications*, lists 19 different rescue specializations, including vehicle, confined space, trench, tower, mine and tunnel, helicopter, ice, floodwater, and wilderness search and rescue, just to name a few. Each of these rescue specialties has three defined levels of competency: (1) awareness—a basic understanding of safety and the need to call for specialized rescue crews; (2) operations—basic rescue services and support for rescue technicians; and (3) technician—the highest level of rescue knowledge and skills. This chapter focuses on concepts that are basic to all rescue operations.

Modified from: National Fire Protection Association. *NFPA 1006: Standard for Technical Rescue Personnel Professional Qualifications.* Quincy, MA: National Fire Protection Association; 2017. https://www.nfpa.org/codes-and-standards/all-codes-and-standards/list-of-codes-and-standards/detail?code=1006. Accessed April 15, 2018.

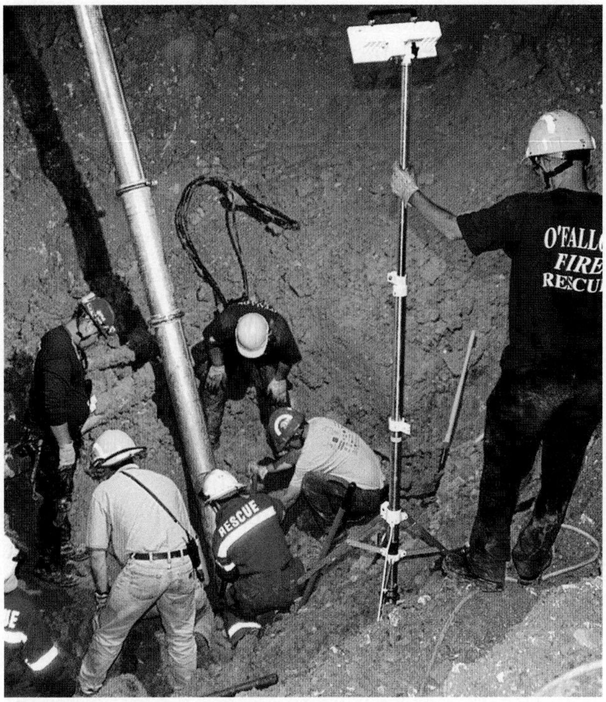

Courtesy of Ray Kemp, St. Charles, MO.

Appropriate Training for Rescue Operations

Rescue work requires training and expertise so that medical and mechanical skills are carefully balanced. This preparation helps to ensure that patients receive both effective treatment and timely extrication. The rescue effort must be driven by the patient's needs, both medical and physical. The success of any rescue depends on a coordinated effort between medical care and specialized rescue efforts, which allows for the following outcomes:

- Patient access and assessment for treatment needs
- Initiation of treatment at the site
- Release of the patient from entrapment or imprisonment
- Continuous medical care throughout the incident

Role of the Paramedic in Rescue Operations

Most rescues in the United States are accomplished with extrication performed by fire service personnel, specialized units, or both. Patient care is the duty of EMS personnel. In another type of rescue system, rescue services are provided by fire, EMS, or law enforcement agencies that have **cross-trained personnel**. In this system, the roles and responsibilities for rescue and patient care are shared.

The primary role of the paramedic in rescue operations is to have proper training and appropriate personal protective equipment (PPE) that allow for safe access to the patient and treatment at the site and throughout the incident. Paramedics often are the first responders to many scenes that require rescue. Therefore they should have the following abilities:

- Understand the hazards associated with various environments.
- Know when it is safe to gain access or attempt rescue.
- Have the skills to perform a rescue when it is safe and necessary.
- Understand the rescue process and know when certain techniques are indicated or contraindicated.
- Be skilled in patient packaging techniques to allow safe and efficient extrication and medical care.

CRITICAL THINKING

Are there times when provider safety can be compromised for the sake of performing a rescue?

NOTE

Medical monitoring and rehabilitation (rehab) of other rescuers at the scene are important functions of the paramedic. Medical monitoring and rehab are further addressed in Chapter 56, *Hazardous Materials Awareness*.

Safety

Safety during any rescue operation is paramount because of the potential for associated risks. For example, rescues may involve hazardous materials, inclement weather, temperature extremes, fire, electrical hazards, toxic gases, unstable structures, heavy equipment, road hazards, and sharp edges and fragments. Initial scene assessment for hazards, use of personal protective measures, and constant monitoring throughout the operation are essential for every rescue response.

The priorities for safety in any rescue are (1) personal safety, (2) the safety of the crew, (3) the safety of bystanders, and (4) rescue of the trapped and injured. The reasons for this order of priority are as follows:

- When well-trained and properly equipped rescuers act safely, remaining vigilant for hazards, they minimize the risk of personal injury and of complicating the scene by becoming another patient who requires care and possibly extrication.
- The crew is the support team for the rescuer, so crew safety is essential to ensure an effective rescue and to provide mutual support for each team member. Operating with disregard for the safety of fellow team members both increases the risk of injuries and complicates the operation.
- Uninvolved people must be evacuated and kept clear of hazards. Bystanders or untrained "helpers" increase the risk of additional injuries and may complicate the rescue operation.
- Rescue of the trapped or injured is the last priority. Simply put, these people are already trapped or injured. Carrying out the first three priorities safely maximizes the chance for a successful rescue.

Phases of a Rescue Operation

A rescue operation has seven phases: (1) arrival and scene size-up, (2) hazard control, (3) gaining access to the patient, (4) medical treatment, (5) disentanglement, (6) patient packaging, and (7) transport. As is stressed throughout this text, paramedics should not enter a scene until it has been secured and made safe by trained personnel. Personal safety is always the top priority.

Arrival and Scene Size-up

The first phase of a rescue is the arrival and scene size-up. This phase requires the paramedic to determine what is needed at a specific emergency event. It involves quickly gathering facts about the situation, analyzing the problems, and determining the appropriate response. During this phase, the EMS crew must focus on the following concerns:

- Understand the environment and risks.
- Establish command and conduct a scene assessment.
- Determine the number of patients, and triage them as necessary.
- Determine whether the situation is a search, a rescue, or a body recovery.
- Perform a risk–benefit analysis that considers personal safety before rescue is attempted.
- Request additional information, if needed.
- Make a realistic time estimate by accessing and evaluating patients or other people at the scene.

Scene size-up is an ongoing evaluation of the emergency scene. It begins when the call is received and when information is obtained from the dispatch center. Throughout the response, however, the paramedic must constantly be alert to situations that may change the needs of that particular incident. If power lines are downed during an extrication, for example, electrical utility services may be needed that were not initially required. Three elements of the assessment phase are response, other factors, and resources.

Response. During the initial response to a scene, the information available often is limited. En route, the EMS crew and the dispatcher should gather as much detail about the situation as possible. Essential information includes the exact location of the incident, the type of occupancy or location (manufacturing, residence), the number of victims, the type of situation, and the hazards involved. Weather conditions (eg, extreme heat or cold, rising water, rain, high winds) also can affect rescue attempts, the patient's status, and the need to expedite the operation.

As described in Chapter 18, *Scene Size-up and Primary Assessment*, standardized dispatch protocols guide the initial emergency response. This predetermined system is based on the level of the reported emergency. For example, if the event is a single-vehicle crash, a first-responder fire company and EMS unit may be dispatched. If the event involves a bus wreck with many patients, several fire companies and EMS units may respond. As the dispatch center receives information about the actual severity of the event, the dispatch protocol upgrades or downgrades the response as needed. The center advises the responding units of the updated reports.

> CRITICAL THINKING
>
> Are there disadvantages to sending "too much" emergency equipment to a scene?

Other Factors. Other factors to be considered in determining the type of response needed are the description of the scene and the time of day. An emergency in a highly populated area may call for special vehicles and equipment for extrication and fire suppression.

Examples of such scenes would include incidents in a high-rise apartment, a school, or a shopping mall. An emergency in a rural or wilderness setting may require helicopter rescue or other resources. If hazardous materials are present, special response and decontamination equipment may be needed for bystanders, patients, and rescue personnel.

The time of day may affect on-scene needs. For example, rush-hour traffic and crowd control may be a concern; extra lighting may be needed for early morning, evening, or night rescue. These and other factors determine the personnel requirements and the scene management operations.

Resources. The ability to assess an emergency quickly and correctly requires preplanning as well as the development of a systems approach to the response. Indeed, the available resources are a crucial part of any response, because the responding crew may not always have the personnel, training, or expertise to handle the event. Resources that may be required include the following:

- Additional emergency transport vehicles for a large number of patients
- Assessment of area hospital capacity to receive patients
- Assessment of specialty hospital capabilities
- Aeromedical services
- Law enforcement personnel
- Fire service responders for vehicle extrication, fire suppression, or lighting
- Water rescue teams, teams with self-contained underwater breathing apparatus (scuba), and other specialized rescue units
- Hazardous materials teams
- Urban search and rescue teams

Hazard Control

Hazard control is the phase of rescue in which on-scene dangers are quickly identified and managed by the first-arriving crew. This aspect of the response involves minimizing risks from uncontrollable hazards, making sure the scene is as safe as possible, and ensuring that all personnel are equipped with PPE appropriate for the incident. Examples of possible hazards at a scene include fire, unstable structures, confined spaces, swift water, poisonous substances, dangerous animals, and unruly crowds. Hazard control for specific types of incidents is discussed throughout this chapter.

Gaining Access to the Patient

The ability to rapidly access an ill or injured patient who requires extrication or rescue can be crucial to the patient's eventual outcome. For patients who have multisystem trauma, assessment, stabilization, and extrication should be rapid—but must be accomplished while maintaining the safety of both the patient and the rescue team as a top priority. To safely gain access, the paramedic must determine the best method of reaching the patient, deploy appropriate personnel to the patient, and stabilize the patient's physical location.

Specialty rescue tools and equipment (**FIGURE 54-1**) can cause injuries. To reduce the risk from their use, paramedics should apply the least amount of force needed and should clear the area of unnecessary people. An assigned **safety officer** should remain alert to the stress of the operation on the rescuers as well as potential safety hazards for bystanders and victims.

Although paramedics may not directly take part in freeing the patient, they have the chief responsibility for patient care. In addition, they serve a key role as observers for potentially hazardous procedures. The "team concept" is the most important element in any rescue system or operation. Teamwork using crew resource management maximizes safety, efficiency, and effectiveness. A basic element of prehospital care, this approach also has powerful implications for the safety of responders.

Medical Treatment

After the team has gained access to the patient, medical treatment can begin. The paramedic should perform a rapid primary survey to identify and manage any life-threatening situations. Although the ability to

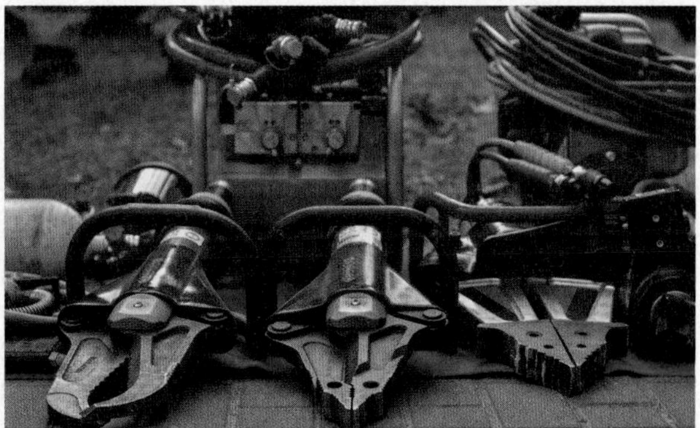

FIGURE 54-1 Hydraulic rescue tools.

provide specific care measures may be limited by the circumstances and the physical working area, the paramedic may be able to initiate some stabilization procedures, such as spinal immobilization, airway management, oxygen administration, and intravenous (IV) fluid therapy. If the paramedic recognizes that the conditions could be rapidly fatal or potentially fatal to the patient, a "load and go" approach must be taken. In these cases, rapid extrication and transport are indicated.

A physical examination should be performed after the primary survey has been completed and life-threatening conditions have been managed. Another crew member may perform the examination at the same time of the primary survey if it does not interrupt the initial assessment and emergency care.

Disentanglement

Disentanglement involves making a pathway through the wreckage of an incident and removing wreckage from the patient. The main responsibilities of the paramedic during disentanglement are to release the patient from entrapment and to perform a **risk–benefit analysis** by asking the question, "Does the risk outweigh the benefit?" This analysis should take personal safety into account. This phase of the rescue is driven by the needs of the patient. Because specialized rescue personnel and equipment may be required for disentanglement, paramedics should be aware of the available resources in their area and know how to mobilize them. Disentanglement often is time-consuming, so the EMS crew should be prepared to spend extended time at the scene.

CRITICAL THINKING

Which rescue teams are available to your community?

Patient Packaging

Stabilizing a patient physically and preparing the person for transport is known as **patient packaging**. This phase of the rescue may require special capabilities. For instance, the patient may need to be moved over hazardous terrain or lifted by hoist to a helicopter. As with all other aspects of rescue, the coordination of activities and the sharing of patient care responsibilities among the various agencies offer the greatest chance of a successful outcome.

It is the paramedic's responsibility to ensure the patient is ready to be removed from the scene. It also is the paramedic's duty to protect the patient from additional injury during disentanglement and **egress** (movement along the exit pathway). The patient should be covered with blankets or tarpaulins and provided with ear and eye protection. In addition, a face mask with supplemental oxygen or air should be applied; this measure protects the patient from toxic fumes, if present.

For minimum packaging for transport, the patient's airway and cervical spine must be stabilized, IV lines and oxygen tubing must be secured, and spinal motion restriction should be employed when indicated. When time allows, extremity fractures should be immobilized and open wounds covered with sterile dressings and secured with bandages. A scene delay for a patient who requires rapid stabilization and transport may reduce the patient's chances of survival.

Use of other patient care equipment should be considered as the patient is removed from the area of entrapment. Communication and coordination with other rescuers must continue during this process. The exit pathway must be clear and secure. No additional danger for the patient or the rescuers should exist during the removal phase.

During disentanglement and patient packaging, the paramedic should consider the patient's emotional needs. Patients often are anxious and frightened by the rescue operations. When possible, paramedics should maintain a good rapport with the patient by (1) providing reassurance that the patient is receiving good care, (2) preparing the patient for unexpected movements or procedures that may cause discomfort, and (3) explaining all rescue maneuvers.

Transport

If the patient is to be transported immediately to the ambulance, a wheeled stretcher, basket stretcher, scoop stretcher, soft stretcher, or long backboard should be available. While the patient is transported to the emergency vehicle, the terrain, equipment, and personnel requirements for moving the patient should be considered (eg, the need for air evacuation, specialized resources, and extra personnel). The ambulance should be appropriately warmed or cooled, based on the patient's needs and the rescue setting.

The rescue is considered complete once the patient is en route to the hospital. As in any other patient transport, the EMS crew continues emergency care during this transport, and medical direction is advised of the patient's status.

Rescuer PPE

PPE for EMS personnel historically has been adapted from other fields (eg, the fire service). The standards for protective clothing and PPE established by the NFPA[1] and the federal Occupational Safety and Health Administration (OSHA)[2] have been adopted by many fire and EMS agencies, including a number of municipal and industrial fire services throughout the United States. It generally is agreed that, at a minimum, EMS providers involved in rescue should have access to the following basic PPE:

- Impact-resistant protective helmet with ear protection and chinstrap
- Safety goggles with elastic strap and vents to prevent fogging
- Lightweight, puncture-resistant outer coat and pants or jumpsuit
- Slip-resistant, waterproof gloves
- Boots with steel insoles and steel toe protection

Of course, the same PPE is not appropriate in all situations. Adequate protection depends on the level of rescuer involvement and the nature of the incident. Other types of PPE may be appropriate in some rescue events (BOX 54-1).

Personal Protection from Bloodborne Pathogens

OSHA has established criteria for workplace protection from bloodborne and airborne diseases.[3,4] These measures for personal protection (described in Chapter 2, *Well-Being of the Paramedic*) should be observed whenever the potential exists for exposure to a patient's body fluids or to communicable diseases.

BOX 54-1 Supplemental PPE

Head Protection That Meets Safety Standards for the Appropriate Use

- Compact firefighters' helmet that meets NFPA standards for most vehicle/structural applications
- American National Standards Institute (ANSI)–rated helmets for confined-space and technical rescue uses
- Padded rafting/kayaking helmet for water rescue

Eye Protection

- Adequate face shield (face shields on most fire helmets are inadequate)
- ANSI-approved safety glasses or goggles with solid shields (preferred)

Hearing Protection

- Required for high-noise areas
- Ear plugs or ear muffs should be available

Hand Protection

- Gloves that allow adequate dexterity and protect against cuts and punctures

Foot Protection

- Gear that provides ankle support to limit the range of motion
- Tread that provides traction and prevents slips
- Insulation from environmental extremes
- Steel toe/shank that meets safety requirements

Flame/Flash Protection (When Fire Is Possible)

- Nomex, polybenzimidazole, or flame-retardant cotton to provide limited flash protection, turnout clothing, jumpsuits/flyers/coveralls (Note: This clothing does not provide complete protection from punctures or cuts. The thermal protection offered by turnout clothing may increase heat stress.)

Personal Flotation Device (When Operating on or Around Water)

- Meets Coast Guard standards for flotation
- Type II or type III (preferred for most water rescue work)
- Attached whistle and strobe light
- Attached knife for cutting

Visibility

- Reflective trim on all outerwear
- Orange clothing or safety vests for use during highway operations

Extended, Remote, or Wilderness Protection

- Additional or different PPE, if needed, for adverse weather conditions not normally encountered (eg, cold, rain, snow, wind)
- Personal drinking water and snacks
- Possible shelter needs

Surface Water Rescue

Surface water rescue is the rescue of a patient who is afloat on the surface of a body of water. People are drawn to moving water for recreation, but many—including rescuers—underestimate the power and hazards of water. The hydraulics of moving water are affected by several variables, such as the depth and velocity of water and any obstructions to flow. Water rescue is very dangerous and requires special training and skills; it should never be attempted by a single rescuer or by an untrained one.

Obstructions to Flow

Water that moves over a uniform obstruction can create recirculating currents ("drowning machines") that can trap victims and make escape difficult (**FIGURE 54-2**). Recirculating currents commonly are found in rivers and on low-head dams, and often appear harmless at first glance. (The height of the dam is no indication of the degree of hazard.) The force of the moving water is very deceptive and makes for a hazardous rescue. Trapped victims often succumb to fatigue, hypothermia, and drowning.

Strainers are obstructions (eg, trees, grating wire, mesh) that allow current to flow through but can trap objects such as boats or people. The force of the water against the victim makes escape difficult. Rescue teams must approach strainers cautiously to avoid becoming entrapped themselves.

Foot or Extremity Entrapment

It generally is considered unsafe to walk in fast-moving water that is more than knee-high in depth. Doing so may lead to entrapment of an extremity in a strainer, and the victim can be dragged under the water's surface. If a foot or extremity entrapment, it is crucial to remember that *the body part must be extricated in the same way it became trapped.*

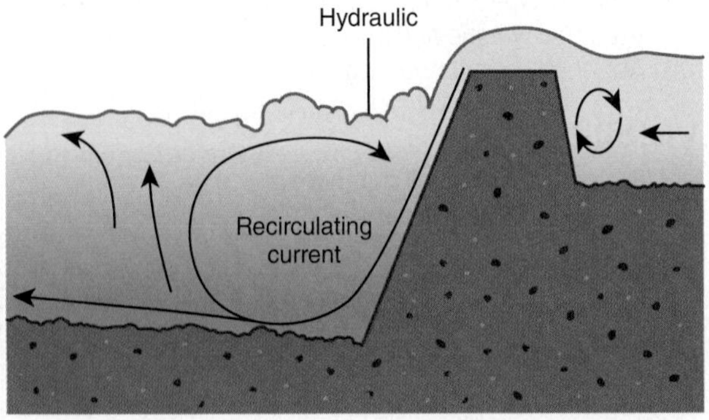

FIGURE 54-2 Low-head dams range in height from 6 inches (15 cm) to 10 feet (3 m). They can create dangerous hydraulics.

Flat Water

Approximately 3,500 deaths occur each year in the United States in flat (static) water (eg, lakes, ponds, marshes) as a result of drowning.[5] Factors that contribute to these deaths include alcohol or other drug use as well as a cool water temperature, which can lead to hypothermia. These factors can quickly incapacitate a victim and result in drowning.

Most people who drown never planned on being in the water. Routinely wearing a properly fastened **personal flotation device (PFD)** when on or around the water can save lives by reducing the likelihood of drowning. For all responders, PFDs are required during water rescue operations. Type I or type II PFDs are preferred for water rescue work, while specialty types III, IV (not worn by responders, but used in the rescue), and V are suitable for some rescue situations.

NOTE

Uses of Different Types of Flotation Devices

- **Type I.** Off-shore life jacket
- **Type II.** Near-shore buoyant vests
- **Type III.** Flotation aids
- **Type IV.** Throwable devices
- **Type V.** Special use devices

Water Temperature

As described in Chapter 44, *Environmental Conditions*, immersion in water with a temperature less than 98°F (36.7°C) can cause hypothermia. A person cannot maintain body heat when the water temperature is less than 92°F (33.3°C). Water causes heat loss 25 times faster than does exposure to air at the same temperature. Moreover, the colder the water, the faster the rate of heat loss. Hypothermia will become a significant contributor to death in a person immersed in cold water for 30 to 60 minutes.[6]

Sudden immersion in cold water may trigger laryngospasm, which can lead to aspiration, severe hypoxia, and unconsciousness. In water cold enough to produce the reflexive gasping termed cold shock

(50°F to 60°F [10°C to 16°C]), loss of hand coordination may occur within 60 seconds and loss of the ability to use arms within 5 minutes. If hypothermia develops, the victim often is unable to follow directions (eg, grab a safety device) or help himself or herself to safety. PFDs lessen both heat loss and the energy required for flotation. In cases of sudden immersion, a single victim should assume a fetal position (the heat escape–lessening posture [HELP]). Multiple victims should huddle together to reduce heat loss (**FIGURE 54-3**).

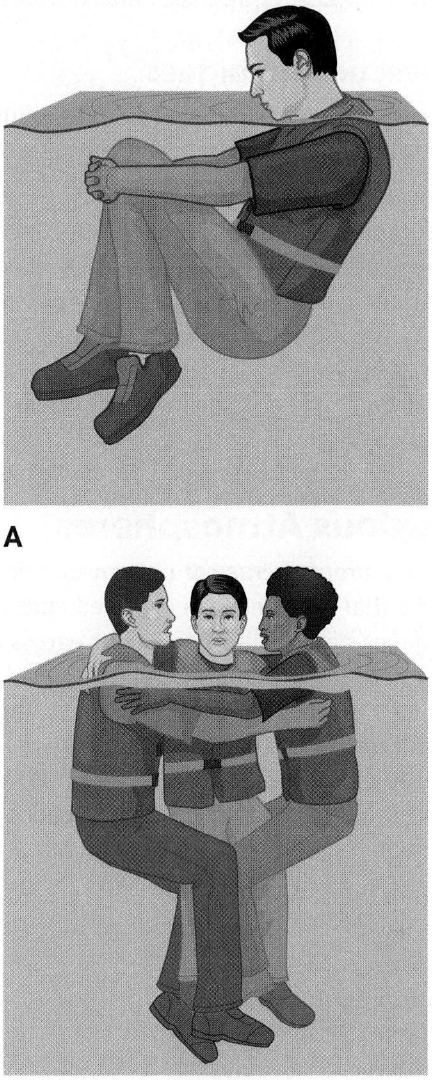

A

B

FIGURE 54-3 Heat escape–lessening posture (HELP) and huddle. When a person is floating in cold water, body heat can be conserved by using a body position that reduces the escape of heat. **A.** If the person is alone, the HELP position should be used. **B.** If several people are present, they should huddle together.

Cold-Protective Response

The cold-protective response, also known as the mammalian diving reflex (see Chapter 44, *Environmental Conditions*), increases a person's chance of survival in cold water. This protective response includes parasympathetic stimulation from immersion of the face in cold water. It leads to bradycardia, peripheral vasoconstriction that shunts blood to the core, and hypotension. The effectiveness of this protective response depends on the person's age, posture in the water, and lung volume, as well as the water temperature.

The rapid development of hypothermia sometimes can improve brain viability in patients who suffer prolonged submersion. Therefore hypothermic patients should be presumed salvageable. ("A victim is never cold and dead—only warm and dead.") The patient must be rewarmed in a hospital before an accurate assessment can be made.

Rescue Versus Body Recovery

Rescue versus body recovery refers to the chance to save a human life (rescue) versus recovering a body without the goal of saving a human life. In addition to temperature, other factors affect the outcome of a patient who has been submerged in water: the length of time the victim has been submerged, known or possible trauma, environmental conditions, the victim's age and physical condition, and the time until rescue or removal is achieved.[7] In temperatures 41°F (5°C) or below, resuscitation should be tried up to 90 minutes. In temperatures greater than 43°F (6°C) with submersion times longer than 30 minutes, resuscitation may not be started or terminated on scene.

In-Water Spinal Immobilization

Routine stabilization of the cervical spine is indicated only in patients with a known or suspected mechanism of injury (eg, diving incident, alcohol-related injury).[8] Only rescuers trained in water rescue should enter the water. General guidelines include providing manual support of the patient's head in a neutral position and limiting angular movement, providing rescue breathing if indicated and if it does not delay removal of the patient from the water, placing a buoyant backboard under the patient, securing the patient with straps, and rapidly extricating the patient from the water.[9] Following extrication, the patient should be covered to prevent hypothermia. (See Chapter 40, *Spine and Nervous System Trauma*.) If needed, ventilatory and circulatory support should be initiated. No attempt should be made to clear the airway of water.[10] Spinal immobilization should not take priority over initial resuscitation of a patient with severe respiratory distress who requires aggressive airway management.[11]

SHOW ME THE EVIDENCE

In a cross-over manikin study, researchers had 21 lifeguards and 21 laypeople perform two rescue procedures in an indoor swimming pool to determine the effectiveness and safety of in-water resuscitation (IWR). One rescue was performed with in-water ventilation and the other without. In both groups, IWR was associated with longer duration of rescue. Aspiration of water by the victim and physical effort were greater in both groups when IWR was performed. The lifeguards were faster and had fewer negative effects than did the laypeople. The researchers concluded that IWR delays rescue and results in considerable aspiration, even when performed under optimal conditions. They suggested that laypeople be advised not to attempt IWR.

Modified from: Winkler BE, Eff AM, Ehrmann U, et al. Effectiveness and safety of in-water resuscitation performed by lifeguards and laypersons: a crossover manikin study. *Prehosp Emerg Care*. 2013;17(3):409-415.

Overview of Rescue Techniques

As previously stated, rescuers should never underestimate the power of moving water. Also, they should never attempt water rescue without highly specialized training. The recommended water rescue model is reach, throw, row, go.

- **Reach.** If the victim is close to shore, the paramedic should try to reach out to the person. An oar, a large branch, a pole, or some other rescue device should be used for this purpose. Before a rescue attempt, paramedics should don a PFD. They also should make sure their footing is secure so that they are not pulled into the water by the victim.
- **Throw.** While the paramedic remains on the shore, a flotation device (eg, a water throw bag attached to polypropylene rope) should be thrown to the victim. That way, the victim can be pulled to shore.
- **Row.** If reach and throw methods are unsuccessful or if the victim is unconscious, trained rescuers should row out to the victim in a boat if one is available.
- **Go.** If a boat is unavailable and reach and throw methods are not viable options, trained rescuers should go to the patient by wading or swimming.

A shore-based rescue attempt by a first responder, either by coaching the victim in self-rescue or by reaching or throwing, is the method of choice. Boat-based or "go" techniques require specialized training.

Self-Rescue Techniques

If paramedics inadvertently enter dangerous water, they should use self-rescue techniques as follows:

1. Cover your mouth and nose during entry.
2. Protect your head and keep your face out of the water.
3. If in flat water, assume the HELP position.
4. If in moving water, do not attempt to stand up.
5. Float on your back with your feet downstream and your head pointed toward the nearest shore at a 45° angle.

Hazardous Atmospheres

Hazardous atmospheres are oxygen-deficient environments that may occur in **confined spaces**. Confined spaces have limited access or egress and are not designed for human occupancy or habitation. According to the National Institute for Occupational Safety and Health, nearly 60% of the deaths associated with confined spaces are people attempting rescue of a victim.[12] Examples of confined spaces include the following:

- Grain bins and silos
- Wells and cisterns
- Storage tanks
- Pumping stations
- Drainage culverts
- Underground vaults
- Trenches and cave-ins

Hazards Associated With Confined Spaces

According to OSHA, there are six major hazards associated with confined spaces: oxygen-deficient atmospheres, chemical/toxic exposure or explosion, engulfment, machinery entrapment, electricity, and structural concerns.

Oxygen-Deficient Atmospheres

Oxygen-deficient atmospheres are not a visible hazard, so rescuers must not presume that an atmosphere is safe based on the appearance of the air. Oxygen may be displaced by other neutral or toxic gases that are also colorless and often odorless—and, therefore, undetectable by human senses (BOX 54-2). The available oxygen in confined spaces must be tested by trained personnel using atmospheric monitoring at the top, middle, and bottom of a confined space before entry. Any confined space that has an oxygen concentration less than 19.5% must be considered an oxygen-deficient, atmospheric hazard.[13] An oxygen level that is extremely high (greater than 22%) in a confined space may support rapid combustion, so it is also a serious safety hazard.

NOTE

A common misconception is that a person in an atmosphere with inadequate oxygen will know it because he or she will sense a desperate urge to breathe. Unfortunately, rescuers may become victims themselves as they become debilitated by the lack of oxygen before they can sense the danger and react.

Chemical/Toxic Exposure or Explosion

Oxygen can be removed from the atmosphere by certain chemical reactions. Examples include reactions that occur during the formation of rust on steel structures and while pouring concrete, and natural decaying processes that displace oxygen by producing dangerous gases (eg, methane). In addition, the presence of some chemicals and gases can lead to toxic exposure (see Chapter 56, *Hazardous Materials Awareness*) (BOX 54-3). They also may pose a high risk of explosion. Some dusts and particulate materials found in grain bins, silos, and storage tanks can be highly explosive when mixed with air. Many gases are heavier than air, so they are found in higher concentrations at the bottom of storage vessels. As with oxygen content, trained personnel should monitor for toxic or explosive gases in confined spaces using an appropriate testing device.

BOX 54-2 Gases That Can Displace Oxygen

Acetylene
Argon
Carbon dioxide
Ethane
Ethylene
Helium
Hydrogen
Methane
Neon
Nitrogen
Propane
Propylene

BOX 54-3 Toxic Gases That May Be Found in Confined Spaces

Ammonia
Carbon dioxide
Carbon monoxide
Chlorine
Hydrogen sulfide
Low or high oxygen concentrations
Methane
Nitrogen dioxide

CRITICAL THINKING

Why can workers and laypeople easily become disabled in situations that may involve exposure to toxic gases?

NOTE

Some silos are designed to produce oxygen-limiting conditions, which aids the fermentation process. These silos usually can be identified by their blue exteriors.

Engulfment

Mechanical entrapment can occur when earth, grain, coal, or any other dry material that can flow engulfs a person in a confined space. **Engulfment** can lead to an oxygen-deficient atmosphere and subsequent suffocation. In addition, those trapped by engulfment may be victims of physical (crushing) injury. They also are at an increased risk from explosive hazards.

Machinery Entrapment

Some structures, such as grain bins and silos, have augers, screws, conveyors, and other machinery to move the material stored in them. These and other mechanical devices can entrap a person, requiring extrication. Before rescue is attempted, trained and experienced personnel should identify and secure all such devices.

> DID YOU KNOW?
>
> **The Power Take-Off**
>
> A **power take-off (PTO)** is a splined driveshaft, usually found on a tractor or other farm machinery, that is used to provide power to an attachment or separate machine. The power transfer shaft that connects to the PTO can be a safety hazard to both farm workers and emergency responders at the scene. Rescue personnel should never approach a PTO shaft until the machinery has been shut off, disengaging the PTO. In addition, it is important never to step over a rotating PTO shaft; responders should walk around the machinery instead.
>
> The PTO shaft is responsible for many farm injuries. Clothing, such as shirt sleeves and long pant legs, and long hair can easily get caught on the shaft. Typical injuries resulting from getting caught in an open PTO shaft are amputations, severe lacerations, multiple fractures, spine and neck injuries, or complete body destruction. Broken arms, broken legs, and severe facial lacerations are common. Spine and neck injuries can occur when a person is rotated around the shaft.
>
> *Modified from*: Power take off safety. National Ag Safety Database website. http://nasdonline.org/49/d001617/power-take-off-safety.html. Accessed April 16, 2018.

Electricity

Electrical hazards from the power supply of motors and materials-management equipment may be present in some situations. Like machinery, all electrical devices—including electrical boxes and switches—must be identified and secured by experienced personnel to ensure the safety of the rescuers. This **lock-out process** must prevent any unauthorized person from entering the area or gaining access to the controls that have been disconnected. Motors and other electrical devices can store power that can lead to entrapment or injury. Chemical, steam, and water lines also must be secured or blocked by trained personnel during all rescues.

Structural Concerns

The supporting structures of a confined space must be identified before rescuers' entry to ensure safe rescue and extrication. For example, most cylindrical structures are supported by central I-beams, which allow relatively easy maneuvering. In contrast, noncylindrical structures may have L-, T-, and X-shaped spaces. These designs can affect entry and rescue procedures and can complicate the extrication pathway.

Crush Compartment Syndromes Secondary to Entrapment

As described in Chapter 37, *Bleeding and Soft-Tissue Trauma*, compartment syndrome can be caused by crushing mechanisms, which lead to ischemic muscle damage, tissue necrosis, and crush syndrome. These injuries are associated with rupture of internal organs, major fractures, and hemorrhagic shock. The severity of the injury produced by the crushing force depends on four elements: (1) the amount of pressure applied to the body, (2) the surface area over which that pressure or force is applied, (3) the length of time the pressure is exerted on the body, and (4) the specific body region where the injury occurs. A massive crush injury to vital organs may cause immediate death.

Patients with crush syndrome of significant duration are victims of compressive forces that crush tissue, causing prolonged hypoxia. The patient may appear stable for hours or days, as long as the compressive forces remain in place. When the patient is released from the entrapment, however, the reperfusion of the trapped body part may lead to detrimental processes—for example, volume loss into the tissue and the release of myoglobin, lactic acid, and other toxins into the circulation. As described in Chapter 37, *Bleeding and Soft-Tissue Trauma*, these events occur simultaneously and may ultimately lead to death. If the patient's condition or the mechanism of injury is suspicious for compartment syndrome or crush injury, the paramedic should consult with medical direction. Prehospital care must be supervised by a medical direction physician familiar with this pathologic process.

Emergencies in Confined Spaces

OSHA requires a permit to be issued before workers may enter a confined space.[13] This standard has forced industrial, municipal, and government response teams to be better prepared to manage confined-space incidents. Requirements for obtaining a permit are that the area must be made safe or workers must wear PPE, fall-arresting and retrieval devices must be in place, and environmental monitoring must be available at the site before entry. Sites without permits at which no atmospheric monitoring is performed are likely locations for emergencies. At these sites, rescuers often may encounter oxygen-deficient atmospheres. Other types of emergencies that can occur in confined spaces (in both permitted and nonpermitted locations) include the following:

- Falls
- Medical emergencies
- Explosion
- Entrapment
- Exposure to toxic gases and chemicals

Safe Entry for Rescuers

As previously stated, safe entry for rescuers in a confined-space operation requires specialized training. No rescuer should enter the space until a rescue team has made the area safe. Safe entry cannot be made without the following measures being put in place:[14]

- Proper and thorough training in confined-space rescue
- Atmospheric monitoring to determine the oxygen concentration, hydrogen sulfide level, carbon monoxide level, explosive limits, flammable atmosphere, and toxic air contaminants
- Proper ventilation
- Secured electrical systems (lock-out/tag-out of all power)
- Dissipation of stored energy
- Disconnection of all pipes (blinding/blanking) to prevent flow into the site
- Appropriate respiratory protection

Supplied-Air Breathing Apparatus. Close quarters make access and extrication difficult in confined-space rescue. In these conditions, use of the typical "bottle on back" self-contained breathing apparatus (SCBA) is not practical. Such a device provides a limited air supply, can cause entrapment, and may have to be removed to reach the victim. Instead, the **supplied-air (air-line) breathing apparatus (SABA)** is preferred in confined-space operations (**FIGURE 54-4**).

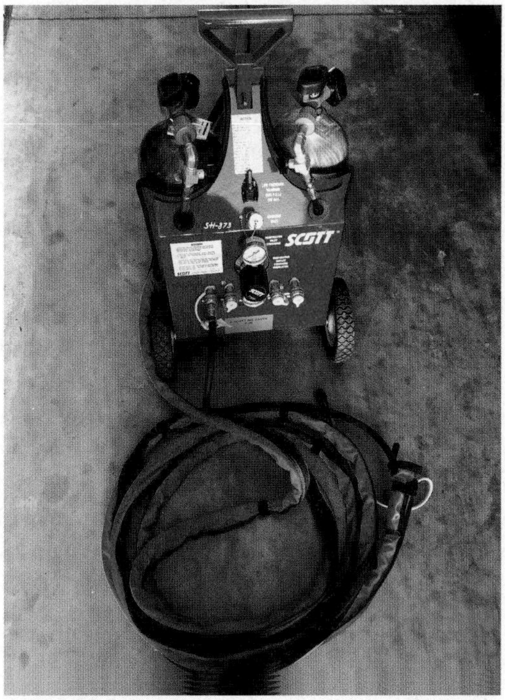

FIGURE 54-4 Supplied-air (air-line) breathing apparatus.

Courtesy of Kim McKenna.

These lightweight devices provide a nearly unlimited supply of air from a device located outside the confined space, along with an "escape bottle" similar to a regular SCBA unit, only much smaller.

Potential complications of the SABA include equipment malfunction, damaged or entangled air lines, and limitations imposed by the length of the air hose.

Arriving at the Scene

An EMS crew that arrives at the scene of a confined-space emergency should proceed as follows:

1. Perform a scene size-up and determine the nature of the emergency by obtaining a copy of the OSHA permit for the site from the permit/entry supervisor, if available. Determine the number of workers (victims) in the confined space.
2. Request specialized rescue teams.
3. Establish a safe perimeter away from the incident. Allow only rescue team members to enter the space.
4. Assist workers at the site with any remote retrieval devices they may be using without entry into the confined space.

Scene safety is of prime importance for all involved in the rescue. Only specialized rescue personnel should directly perform rescue activities. EMS personnel who are not trained in specialized rescue should assist the rescue team only if they can do so safely without entering the space.

Rescue From Trenches and Cave-Ins

Most trench collapses occur in trenches less than 12 feet (4 m) deep and 6 feet (2 m) wide. Federal law requires either shoring or a trench box for evacuations that are 5 feet (3 m) or deeper.[15] Often these types of collapses occur when contractors forsake safety measures because of the increased cost of providing them. Factors that contribute to collapse include the following:

- Cave-in of lips on one or both sides of the trench
- Walls that shear away and cave in
- Piling of excavated dirt too close to the edge, causing collapse
- The presence of intersecting trenches
- Ground vibrations
- Water seepage

NOTE

One cubic foot (0.03 m^3) of soil weighs 100 pounds (45 kg); 2 feet (0.6 m) of soil on a person's chest or back is equal to 700 to 1,000 pounds (318 to 454 kg) of pressure, which can cause burial and can rapidly lead to suffocation.

Modified from: OSHA sites [sic] company following trench death. ROCO Rescue website. http://www.rocorescue.com/roco-rescue-blog/osha-sites-company-following-trench-death. Published August 13, 2010. Accessed April 16, 2018.

Arrival at the Scene

On arrival at the scene of a collapse that has resulted in burial, paramedics should keep in mind that a second collapse is likely and should not approach the lip. EMS personnel should not attempt a rescue unless the trench is less than waist deep. Instead, they should secure the scene, establish command, and secure a safe perimeter; shut down nonessential equipment that can cause vibrations; request specialized rescue teams; and prevent entry into the trench or cave-in area.

Access to the patient should be attempted by trained personnel only after proper shoring is in place. The process of shoring and excavating can be labor and time intensive, but scene safety is always necessary for a successful rescue or recovery.

CRITICAL THINKING

If you are unable to enter a confined space to perform a rescue for safety reasons, what other options may be available?

Highway Operations

Traffic flow is a major hazard in EMS highway operations. Factors associated with highway hazards include emergency responses to limited- and unlimited-access highways, emergency vehicle crashes, and the backup of traffic that impedes flow to and from the scene. Because of the potential problems in traffic flow, EMS personnel must work closely with law enforcement personnel to help ensure a safe response. It is crucial to coordinate **traffic incident management** between police, fire, and EMS responders to provide safe traffic flow for civilians and a safe area of operation for emergency responders. Paramedics can take the following steps to reduce traffic hazards:

- Position an apparatus (pumper, rescue, or other emergency vehicle) across the traffic direction in the fend-off position (a vehicle angled toward the opposing traffic to protect the scene and deflect drivers away from the incident). This positioning protects the scene from traffic hazards.
- Stage unnecessary apparatus off the highway (this is essential on limited-access highways); establish a staging area away from the scene.
- Position an apparatus to reduce traffic flow and provide for a safe ambulance loading area.
- Use only essential warning lights so that drivers are not distracted or confused. Consider the use of amber scene lighting, and turn off headlights that might blind nearby motorists.
- Use traffic cones and flares to redirect traffic away from workers and to create a safe zone. Use flares safely in proximity to the scene; do not extinguish them once they have been ignited.
- Make sure all rescuers wear high-visibility clothing (eg, orange highway vests, reflective trim).

Other scene hazards associated with highway operations include fuel and fire hazards, electrical power, unstable vehicles, airbags and supplemental restraint systems, and hazardous cargoes.

Fuel and Fire Hazards

Gasoline spills from crashes are a common fire hazard encountered by EMS providers. The chances that flammable liquids will ignite can be reduced by turning off the vehicle ignition switch, forbidding smoking, and avoiding use of flares near the spill. EMS personnel should approach the scene with fire extinguishers and should keep those extinguishers readily available throughout extrication (BOX 54-4). Ideally, a fire apparatus with a charged hose line should be at the scene.

BOX 54-4 Fire Extinguishers

Portable fire extinguishers are classified by their anticipated effectiveness in suppressing five classes of fires:

- **Class A.** Ordinary combustibles
- **Class B.** Flammable liquids
- **Class C.** Energized electrical equipment
- **Class D.** Combustible metals
- **Class K.** Kitchen fires (combustible cooking fluids)

EMS crews should carry ABC multi-purpose extinguishers, which are suitable for more than one class of fire. These dry chemical extinguishers can be used to suppress fires of ordinary combustible materials, flammable liquids, and electrical equipment. Class D extinguishers are designed for combustible metals. Class K extinguishers are dry and wet extinguishers designed for kitchen fires.

Class A and Class B fire extinguishers are given a numeric rating in addition to the letter classification. This rating designates the size of fire the extinguisher can be expected to suppress. A 20-B extinguisher generally extinguishes 20 times as much fuel as a 1-B extinguisher.

Fire suppression agents work by reducing heat and eliminating the oxygen needed to maintain combustion. Eliminating oxygen may present a danger to the rescuer and patient; therefore, paramedics must work carefully in confined spaces. In addition, crew members and patients should avoid undue exposure to the fumes of any fire suppression agent. All rescuers should use an appropriate breathing apparatus.

Modified from: US Department of Labor, Occupational Safety and Health Administration. Evacuation plans and procedures eTool: portable fire extinguishers: extinguisher basics. Occupational Safety and Health Administration website. https://www.osha.gov/SLTC/etools/evacuation/portable_about.html. Accessed April 16, 2018.

The vehicle involved in the incident should be put in park, and the engine stopped immediately after gaining access to it. The battery of a crashed car generally should be left connected so that power electric door locks, windows, seat mechanisms, and trunks can be operated. However, if the battery is to be disabled, the ground cable should be disconnected first to reduce the chance of sparking. Sparking may ignite spilled fuel or leaking battery gases. Most newer American cars have positive ground cables that can be identified by battery markings or by locating the ground wires attached to the frame, engine, or body of the vehicle. The battery cable can be cut with wire cutters or disconnected with battery pliers. The disconnected cable should be folded back onto itself, then securely taped to insulate it from any bare metal contact that might reestablish the electrical ground to the system. Both cables should be disconnected and secured.

Vehicle fires associated with crashes usually are caused by ruptured fuel tanks and fuel lines ignited during the crash. (Catalytic converters are capable of igniting spilled fuel.) Paramedics should not try to fight fully involved vehicle fires unless they have been trained and are properly equipped to do so. If fire suppression units have not yet arrived and victims are in a burning vehicle, the EMS crew should quickly determine whether the victims can be safely removed. If the victims are trapped and the vehicle is not fully engulfed by flames, an attempt should be made to stop the fire from spreading, by using fire extinguishers.

Burning vehicles present very serious potential hazards. They may explode with deadly force at any time. All actions must be directed toward rescuer safety and protection. When paramedics must approach a burning vehicle, they should crouch low and approach from the side, staying clear of bumpers that may fly off during explosions. PPE also should be worn to guard against dangerous and caustic smoke.

Alternative Fuel Systems

Some vehicles operate with alternative fuel systems. Examples include cars that are powered by natural gas, high-voltage electrical storage cells, ethanol and flex fuel, biodiesel, and dimethyl ester. Hybrid vehicles use a combination of fuel sources. All of these alternative fuel sources are capable of producing fire hazards and injury from explosion of high-pressure cylinders and storage cells. Electric vehicles also carry enough voltage to cause serious burns, electrical shock, and death. Hybrid vehicles often can be identified by a hybrid label and the presence of orange sleeves that cover components under the hood, in the rear, and under the car.

Each vehicle manufacturer has specific guidelines for emergency personnel to follow when working at a crash scene involving a vehicle using an alternative fuel. The following are general guidelines for rescue:[16,17]

- Remain a safe distance from the vehicle if it is on fire.
- Always power down windows, open locks and latches, and move electric seats before disabling any vehicle. Put the vehicle in park. Chock the wheels as soon as possible in case a car in the "sleep mode" has its gas pedal depressed inadvertently by a driver.
- Verify that the vehicle is absolutely not under any power. *Always assume the vehicle is powered up, even in the absence of engine noises.* Shutting the vehicle off shuts down the hybrid system, shuts down the fuel pump, stops the electrical flow to airbags, and isolates the high-voltage current from the battery pack. (Many conventional and hybrid vehicles use a keyless entry/start ignition/start system.) High-voltage capacitors can store a voltage current for up to 10 minutes, even after the vehicle is shut down. During this "drain time," the vehicle should be considered unsafe.
- Never touch, cut, or open any orange cable or components protected by orange sleeves. Always consider a high-voltage cable to be live or hot.

NOTE

The term *alternative fuel* describes any of the various power sources that are used in place of conventional fuels. Each type of alternative fuel can pose unique hazards to rescue personnel. Special training programs have been designed by vehicle manufacturers and fire service organizations to develop response procedures and safety strategies when responding to these emergencies.

Electrical Power

Downed electrical wires are dangerous in any setting, including highway operations. Modern transformers are programmed to retest broken circuits at certain time intervals, so the supposedly "dead" lines can suddenly surge with lethal current. Rescuers must be familiar with the power system in their area. They should check with the local power company for information and the availability of training sessions for the response team. Only utility workers and trained rescuers using proper equipment should secure downed electrical wires.

Rescuers should never approach the patient until the scene is safe. Rescuers who experience tingling sensations in the soles of the feet, legs, or thorax as they enter an area should not proceed, but rather should retreat from the area. Victims inside a vehicle that is in contact with downed wires should be advised to remain inside unless they are at additional risk of injury (eg, explosion, fire). Leaving the vehicle is dangerous and poses a significant risk of electrical injury.

When it is absolutely necessary to touch a patient who is in contact with a source of electricity, trained personnel may use nonconductive equipment such as leather gauntlets, wooden poles, polypropylene rope, and other specially designed equipment. However, none of these measures provides absolute safety from electrical injury.

Unstable Vehicles

Unstable vehicles are a common hazard in rescue events. All unstable vehicles must be stabilized before access is gained. The mechanism of the crash, the position and number of vehicles, and the environment of the scene must all be considered when assessing the stability of vehicles.

Some vehicles are obviously unstable—for example, a vehicle positioned on its side or on its roof. However, even a car on its wheels that appears to be stable may be unstable from possible movement of the tires and swaying of the vehicle's suspension system. Thus, all wrecked vehicles should be approached cautiously.

Standard methods of stabilizing vehicles include supporting the vehicle with wooden cribbing, wheel chocks, and air bags, and securing the vehicle with ropes, cables, and chains to poles, trees, and other vehicles and structures (**FIGURE 54-5**). **FIGURE 54-6** shows some of the equipment used to stabilize vehicles. Specialized training is required for paramedics involved in this aspect of rescue management.

Airbags and Supplemental Restraint Systems

Airbags that serve as a **supplemental restraint system** are required safety features in all cars manufactured

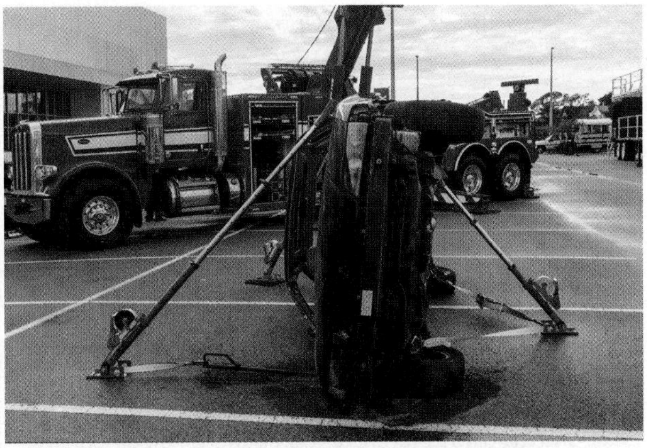

FIGURE 54-5 Vehicle stabilization with a strut.

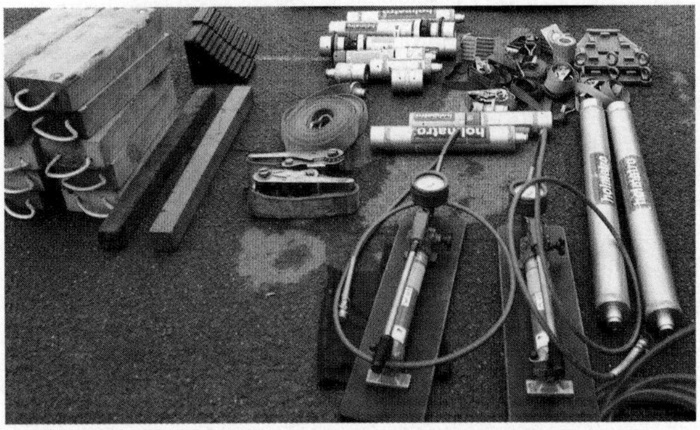

FIGURE 54-6 Equipment used to stabilize vehicles.

in the United States. The three main types of airbags are frontal-impact, side-impact, and head protection bags. These devices can be located in numerous places inside the vehicle. Airbags generally are considered an effective safety device in crashes, but children and small adults in the passenger seat have been fatally injured after their deployment.[18]

NOTE

Most airbags are designed to automatically deploy in the event of a vehicle fire when temperatures reach 300°F to 400°F (149°C to 204°C). This safety feature helps to ensure that such temperatures do not cause an explosion of the inflator unit within the airbag module.

Modified from: What you need to know about airbags? Canadian Express Card website. http://www.licensingoffice.com/Road Safety/Airbags.html. Accessed April 16, 2018.

Once deployed, airbags are not dangerous, although they do produce a residue that can cause minor, temporary skin or eye irritation. This irritation can be avoided by wearing gloves and eye protection, by keeping the residue away from the patient's eyes and wounds, and by thoroughly washing after exposure.

Emergency personnel should be trained in detection of supplemental restraint systems and management of these scenes. Rescue guidelines for airbag-equipped cars have been provided by the National Highway Traffic Safety Administration and by vehicle and airbag manufacturers, in coordination with the US Fire Administration (BOX 54-5).

Hazardous Cargoes

Most hazardous substances transported in the United States travel by road, so paramedics should be suspicious of crashes that involve commercial vehicles. Methods that can be used to identify carriers of hazardous cargoes (eg, United Nations class identification number and North American number [UN/NA number] and placards) and the management of hazardous materials incidents are discussed in Chapter 56, *Hazardous Materials Awareness.*

Vehicle Anatomy

Vehicle rescue operations require a basic understanding of the anatomy of vehicles (**FIGURE 54-7**). The following are several important features:

- **Construction, roof, and support posts.** Most vehicles are of unibody rather than frame construction. The support posts (A, B, C, and D posts), floor firewall, and trunk are integral to the integrity of unibody construction. Cutting the support posts can threaten the stability of these vehicles.
- **Firewall and engine compartment.** A firewall separates the engine and occupant compartments. This structure often collapses onto the occupant's legs during high-speed, head-on collisions. The vehicle's battery is usually located in the engine compartment.
- **Glass.** Safety glass is composed of both glass-plastic and laminated glass and is usually found in the windshield. It is designed to stay intact when the glass is broken or shattered (it fractures into long strands). Tempered glass has high tensile strength and may not remain intact when it is shattered or broken (it fractures into small pieces).

BOX 54-5 Rescue Guidelines for Airbag-Equipped Cars

Fontal and side-impact air bags are designed to deploy in moderate to severe crashes. Once deployed, the airbags are not dangerous and cannot deploy again. However, these safety devices operate independently and may not deploy simultaneously in every crash. The 5-10-20 rule should be observed by rescuers to reduce possible injury from the force of unexpected deployment of an airbag. The 5-10-20 rule for safe distancing to reduce the risk of injury is as follows:

- 5: Maintain a minimum distance of 5 inches (13 cm) from side-impact curtain and airbags.
- 10: Maintain a minimum distance of 10 inches (25 cm) from driver-side frontal airbags.
- 20: Maintain a minimum distance of 20 inches (51 cm) from passenger-side frontal airbags.

In addition, rescuers should not place any hard board or device between an airbag and a patient or rescuer.

Incident With an Undeployed Airbag

Airbags that deploy during a rescue can be dangerous to both the patient and the rescuer. Therefore, battery power should be deactivated as soon as possible, especially if the patient is in close proximity to an undeployed airbag. Once it has been determined that battery power will not be needed for patient access (power seats, electric doors, and windows), the battery should be deactivated as follows:

1. Turn off all power devices and the ignition switch. Disconnect the negative cable and then the positive cable.
2. If the cables need to be but cut, they should be cut in two places to prevent creating an electrical arc. Prevent the terminals from making contact with other metal parts of the car. Do not attempt turn on the vehicle ignition; rather, test the headlights to confirm the battery is disconnected.
3. Observe the 5-10-20 rule near undeployed airbags for additional safety measures.

If fire is present, follow normal procedures for containment. Be aware that heat can cause an airbag to deploy, but will not trigger the activation unit.

Modified from: Shaw R. New auto safety technology, part 2. Fire Engineering website. http://www.fireengineering.com/articles/print/volume-157/issue-7/departments/extraction-tactics/new-auto-safety-technology-part-2.html. Published July 1, 2004. Accessed April 16, 2018.

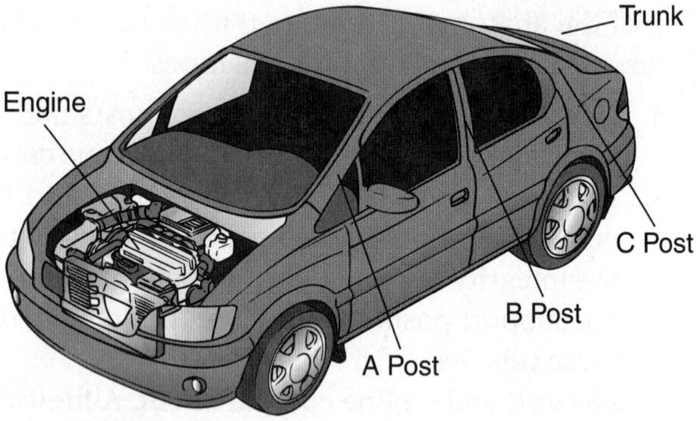

FIGURE 54-7 Anatomy of a car.

- **Doors.** Most car doors contain a reinforcing bar; thus, they are designed to provide structural integrity to the vehicle and protection to the occupants during front-impact and side-impact collisions. Doors also have a case-hardened steel "Nader" pin or latch that is designed to prevent the car door from opening during impact. If the pin is engaged, it may be difficult to pry open the door; it must be disengaged first.

Rescue Strategies

Rescue strategies for vehicle crashes should begin during the initial scene size-up. They sometimes can be based on the details provided by the dispatching center before arrival. On arriving at the scene, the EMS crew should begin hazard control, establish command, and call for appropriate backup. Important elements of the scene size-up include the following:

- Scene safety (including protecting the scene from traffic hazards)
- Location of the crash
- Vehicle stability
- Electrical hazards
- Fire hazards
- Hazardous materials
- Special rescue needs
- Number and location of patients

After performing the initial scene size-up and ensuring scene safety, the responding crew should assess the degree of entrapment and determine the fastest means of extrication. The paramedic should try to gain access to trapped victims by first trying

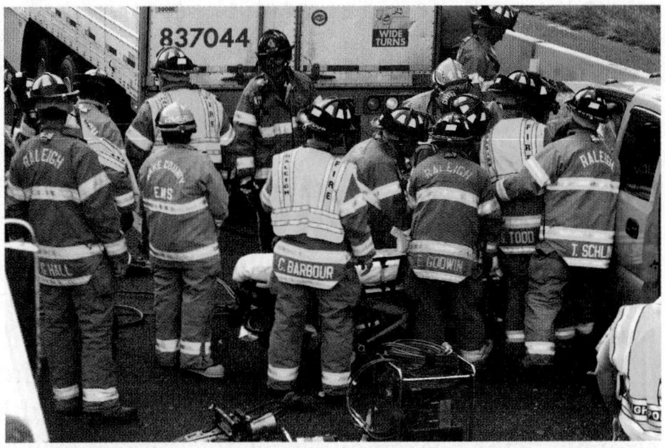

FIGURE 54-8 Patient care should occur simultaneously with extrication.
© Mike Legeros. Used with permission.

to open all car doors. When a door cannot be readily opened by the patient or rescuer, another option is the side windows. (Glass windows can be shattered by striking the glass in a lower corner or by using a spring-loaded center punch; people trapped in a vehicle should be protected during this and other phases of the extrication.) Initial care can then be provided until the patient has been extricated. Trained rescue personnel with extrication tools can gain access to the patient by door removal, roof removal, front or rear windshield openings, or a dash roll-up maneuver.

Paramedics involved in the rescue or who are near the site should wear PPE that provides adequate hand, eye, and body protection. Clothing with reflective striping improves safety during day and night operations (**FIGURE 54-8**).

Hazardous Terrain

Hazardous terrain can pose major difficulties during rescue operations. An example is a car crash that occurs on an embankment. Other examples are rescues of sports enthusiasts, such as rock climbers, snow skiers, and mountain bikers, which may require operating in inhospitable terrain.

Three common classifications of hazardous terrain are low angle, high angle, and flat terrain with obstructions (BOX 54-6). Highly specialized training and equipment are required for rescues in both low-angle (weight supported by ground) and high-angle (weight supported by rope) environments.

The term *low angle* (steep slope) refers to terrain that can be walked on without the use of the hands. However, secure footing may be difficult on steep slopes, which makes it hazardous to carry a

> **BOX 54-6** Terms and Definitions Related to Rescue Over Hazardous Terrain
>
> - **Anchoring.** Attaching a high-angle rope to a secure point.
> - **Belay.** A method of attaching a safety rope and controlling the rope so that if the person or load starts to fall, the belay rope prevents the fall.
> - **High angle.** A type of rescue involving the movement of a victim up or down a grade of greater than 60°, typically requiring a high degree of specialized equipment, techniques, and training.
> - **Low angle.** A type of rescue involving the movement of a victim up or down a grade of approximately 35°, often requiring the use of specialized equipment, techniques, and training.
> - **Rappelling.** A method of descent that involves lowering oneself with a rope.
> - **Scrambling.** Movement over rough terrain that is not steep enough to require the use of a rope.

FIGURE 54-9 Low-angle rescue.
© Ashley Cooper/Alamy Stock Photo

litter, even with several rescuers. In these situations, low-angle rescue is used to prevent falls and tumbles through the use of ropes to counteract gravity during litter carrying (**FIGURE 54-9**).

The term *high angle* (vertical) typically describes terrain that is so steep the hands must be used to maintain balance (eg, cliffs, sides of buildings); this terrain has a slope of more than 60°. In these situations, rescuers are completely dependent on rope or aerial apparatus for litter movement. High-angle rescue may require rappelling (controlled descent by a rope) by trained personnel to retrieve victims. In such an environment, falls are likely to result in serious injury or death (**FIGURE 54-10**). BOX 54-7 and **FIGURE 54-11** discuss ropes and basic knots used in rescue.

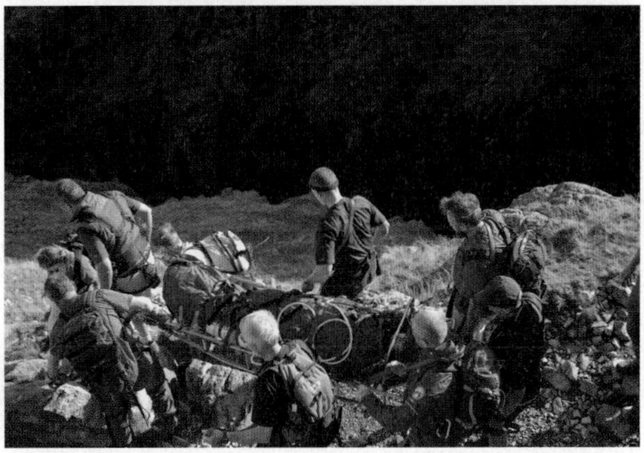

CRITICAL THINKING

Which factors in the environment can increase the danger of **steep-angle rescue**?

Flat-terrain rescue may include various obstructions that can make rescue difficult. Examples include level land with large rocks, loose soil (loose small rocks), and beds of water or creeks. In these situations, extra personnel and resources may be needed to extricate a victim safely and to ensure safe litter movement.

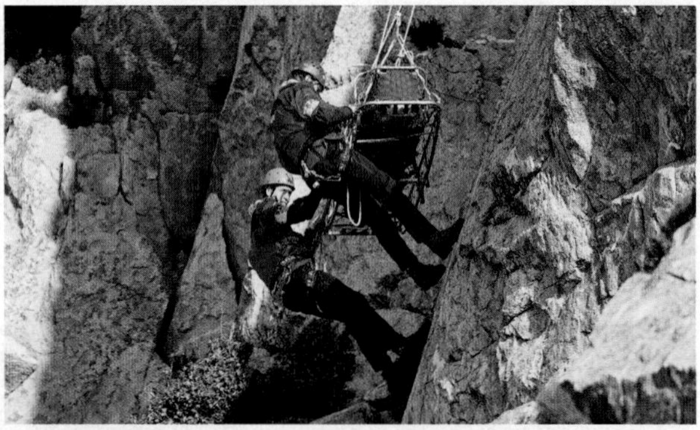

FIGURE 54-10 High-angle rescue.

Patient Packaging With Litters

The **basket stretcher** is the standard for rough-terrain evacuation. The rigid frame of this device offers protection for the victim. It also is relatively easy to carry with adequate personnel. Patients generally are secured on a long backboard and strapped in the basket. Alternative spinal immobilization devices (eg, vest-type devices) also can be used in conjunction with the basket stretcher.

Basket stretchers have two basic designs: wire mesh (Stokes) and plastic. Wire mesh generally is the stronger of the baskets and is relatively inexpensive. This design allows for air and water to flow through the device. As such, the Stokes basket is ideal in water rescue when used with supplemental flotation. Plastic basket stretchers generally are weaker than steel mesh, but they provide better protection for the patient. (Plastic bottoms with steel frames are considered superior designs.) Most basket stretchers are equipped with adequate restraints. Nevertheless, all require additional strapping or lacing (eg, harness, leg stirrups) to prevent movement of the patient within the basket, as well as padding for rough-terrain evacuation or extraction. A plastic helmet or litter shield should be available to protect the patient.

BOX 54-7 Ropes and Knots

There are generally two types of rope used for life-safety rope: **static rope** and **dynamic rope**. The preferred rope used for life-safety rescue operations is static **kernmantle rope** (*kern* means core, and *mantle* means sheath), which provides for minimal stretch (a low elongation factor). Dynamic rope is usually used when climbing toward or above an anchor point; it is designed to stretch (a higher elongation factor). All ropes used for rescue operations should meet the NFPA 1983 minimum standards for life-safety rope. These ropes will have a minimum safety factor of 15:1 for a two-person load.

Knots are used in rescue operations to fasten and secure a rope by tying or interweaving the rope. Although many different knots are used in rescue operations, the most common knots belong to the figure-eight family (see Figure 54-11):

- Figure eight
- Figure eight on a bight
- Figure eight follow-through
- Double-loop figure eight
- Figure eight bend
- Inline figure eight

A common phrase used by rescue personnel when teaching the tying of knots is "If you can't tie a knot, tie a lot!" Wrapping and rewrapping ropes around a stable structure often can provide stability.

Modified from: Fran J, ed. *Rope Rescue Manual*. 5th ed. Goleta, CA: CMC Rescue; 2017; National Fire Protection Association. *NFPA 1983: Standard on Life Safety Rope and Equipment for Emergency Services*. Quincy, MA: National Fire Protection Association; 2017. https://www.nfpa.org/codes-and-standards/all-codes-and-standards/list-of-codes-and-standards/detail?code=1983. Accessed April 16, 2013.

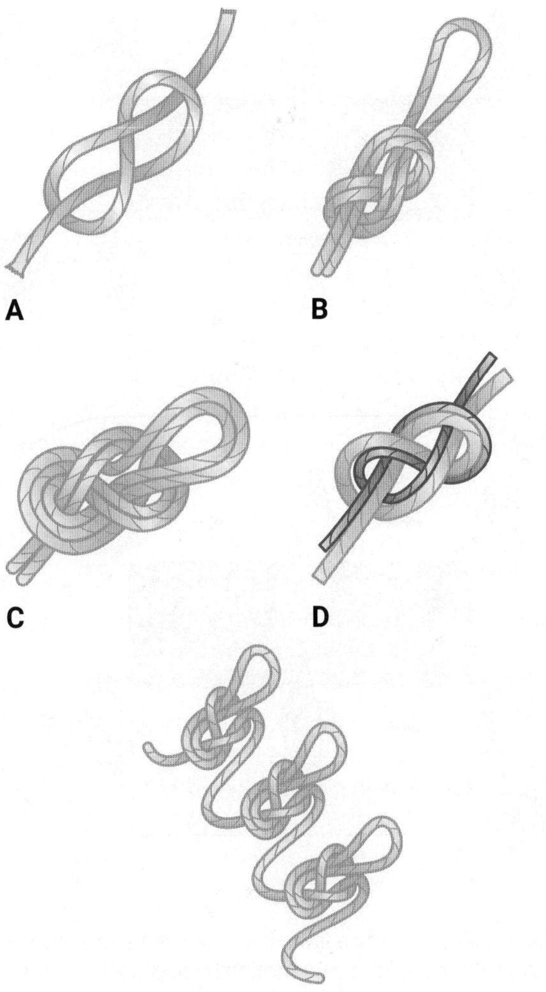

FIGURE 54-11 Knots. **A.** Figure eight. **B.** Figure eight on a bight/figure eight follow-through. These two knot types have the same end result, but the way they are created differs. **C.** Double-loop figure eight. **D.** Figure eight bend. **E.** Inline figure eight.

Patient Movement

Methods of moving a patient over rough terrain may include evacuation and litter-carrying over flat terrain. However, special rescue equipment may be required for low-angle and high-angle evacuation. Such equipment may include load-lifting straps, anchors, and rope-lowering and rope-hauling systems. In addition, the use of aerial apparatus (eg, tower-ladder or bucket trucks, aerial ladders) may be required in some high-angle rescue operations. Moving a patient during low-angle and high-angle evacuations requires specialized knowledge and skills.

Litter-Carrying Procedures

Carrying a litter across rough, flat terrain requires a minimum of six rescuers: four to carry the litter and two to observe or "scout" for potential hazards (eg, loose rocks, holes, tree branches). Team members should be matched in height, thereby ensuring that equal weight is shared and that the litter remains level. Load-lifting straps sometimes are used to spread the weight of the load over other parts of the rescuer's body (eg, around the rescuer's shoulders and back). As described in Chapter 2, *Well-Being of the Paramedic*, proper lifting techniques should be used to protect and support the rescuer's back. **FIGURE 54-12** shows a basic litter-carrying sequence.

Helicopter Use in Hazardous-Terrain Rescue

As described in Chapter 52, *Ground and Air Ambulance Operations*, helicopters can be used for transport and for rescues. When they are used for rescue, the helicopter team (civilian and military) is geared toward performing the rescue rather than providing medical care and transport. The rescue helicopter team has the specialized knowledge and skills needed to hover or land in tight places and to transport people and equipment. Special rescue techniques that these helicopters use may include cable hoisting to extract people from the ground and short-haul (sling load) operations that allow personnel and equipment to be carried beneath the helicopter as an external load. Rescue helicopters have the same safety concerns and limitations as those used for medical transport described in Chapter 52, *Ground and Air Ambulance Operations*. All personnel at the scene should be familiar with the elements of scene safety, hazards, and restrictions for helicopter use.

Assessment Procedures During Rescue

Patient assessment during rescue operations often is complicated by factors such as weather and temperature extremes, patient access challenges, equipment limitations, patient entrapment, and cumbersome PPE that affects rescuer mobility. Other factors that can affect the paramedic's ability to perform a thorough

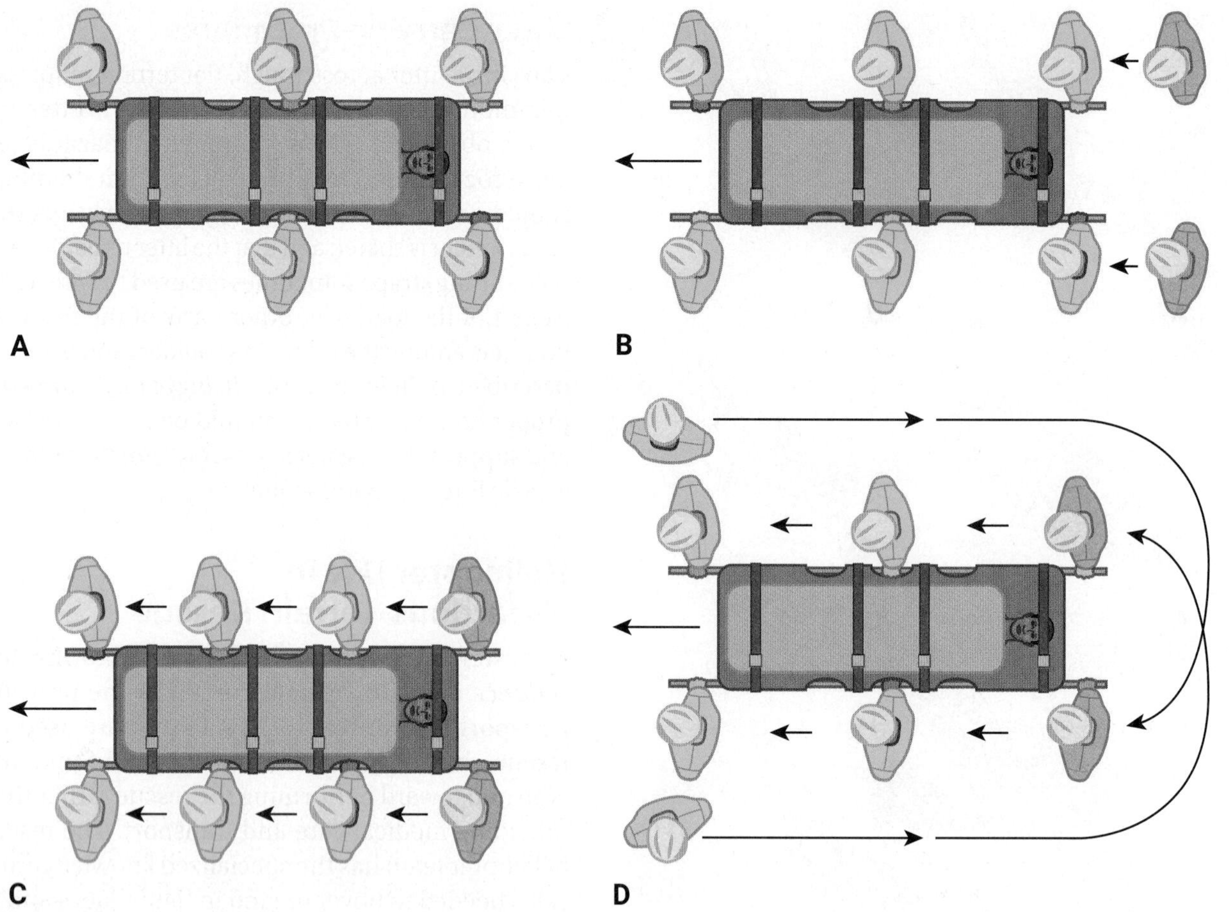

FIGURE 54-12 Litter-carrying sequence. **A.** Six rescuers are usually required to carry a litter; they may need relief over long distances (more than 1 mile). **B.** Relief rescuers can rotate into position while the litter is in motion by approaching from the rear. As relief rescuers move forward, others progressively move forward **(C)** until the forward-most rescuers can release the litter (peel out) and move to the rear **(D)**. Rescuers in the rear can rotate sides so that they can alternate carrying arms. Carrying straps (webbing) can also be used to distribute the load over the rescuers' shoulders. In most cases, the litter is carried feetfirst, with a medical attendant at the head monitoring the patient's airway, breathing, level of consciousness, and so on.

assessment and that can result in a compromised physical examination include the following:

- Difficulty completely exposing a patient
- Restrictive clothing and PPE required for personal safety
- Working in a cramped space
- Limited lighting
- Difficulty transporting medical equipment to the patient

Specific Assessment and Management Considerations

During rescues, paramedics may need to downsize the medical equipment they carry, as they may not be able to carry the normal bags and "street packaging." Ideally, paramedics should be able to carry the equipment while keeping their hands free. In addition to ensuring adequate lighting to perform assessment and treatment, paramedics should have access to the equipment listed in BOX 54-8.

Exposure of Patients

Patients who need to be rescued may be at high risk for developing hypothermia. They should be covered to ensure thermal protection. Also, the patient should be protected with shields (eg, backboards or blankets) to prevent injury from equipment and debris during the extrication.

BOX 54-8 Paramedic Equipment

Airway
Oral and nasal airways
Manual suction device
Intubation equipment

Breathing
Thoracic decompression device
Small oxygen tank and regulator
Masks and cannulae
Pocket mask and bag-mask device

Circulation
Bandages and dressings
Triangular bandages
Occlusive dressings
IV fluid administration set
Blood pressure cuff and stethoscope

Disability
Extrication collars

Exposure of Body Surface
Scissors

Miscellaneous
Headlamp and flashlight
Space blanket
Pneumatic splints

Personal Protective Equipment
Leather gloves
Latex gloves
Eye shields
Other equipment as indicated

Advanced Life Support Measures

Advanced life support (ALS) measures should be provided only if necessary. In contrast, good basic life support (BLS) techniques are mandatory. As a rule, ALS equipment such as IV lines, endotracheal tubes, and electrocardiographic leads will complicate the extrication process. Advanced airway support and volume replacement, however, may be essential in some cases. Airway control with administration of supplemental oxygen must always be a priority during the rescue.

Patient Monitoring

Monitoring of the patient's vital signs and level of consciousness is necessary throughout the rescue. In high-noise and tight spaces, blood pressure may need to be measured by palpation. It also may be necessary to use compact devices such as a pulse oximeter.

Paramedics should create and maintain a rapport with the patient when possible. Throughout the rescue process, they should explain which procedures are being performed and why they are necessary. Providing emotional support during the rescue is crucial.

Improvisation

Because of space and equipment limitations, some patient care may have to be improvised during a rescue. For example, an upper-extremity fracture can be temporarily stabilized by tying it to the patient's torso; a lower-extremity fracture can be tied to the patient's uninjured leg (buddy splinting). Formable splints (eg, SAM [structural aluminum malleable] splints) also can be very useful for securing extremity fractures or dislocations.

Pain Control

Pain control for patients who require rescue may include drug therapy (sedatives, anxiolytics, analgesics, antiemetics) and other methods. Examples of nondrug therapy to manage pain include splinting and positioning, distraction (talking to the patient and asking questions), and methods such as creating sensory stimuli (eg, mildly scratching the patient) when a painful procedure or maneuver is performed. Pain medication can alter a patient's level of consciousness, so the paramedic should follow the established protocol regarding the use of drug therapy in these situations.

Summary

- Rescue is a patient-driven event that requires specialized medical and mechanical skills, with the right amount of each being applied at the right time. The paramedic must have the proper training and the appropriate personal protective equipment (PPE) to safely access the patient and provide treatment at the site and throughout the incident.
- The seven phases of a rescue operation are arrival and scene size-up, hazard control, gaining access to the patient, medical treatment, disentanglement, patient packaging, and transport.
- The standards for protective clothing and personal protection equipment established by the National Fire Protection Association and the Occupational Safety and Health Administration have been adopted by many fire and EMS agencies. The appropriate PPE depends on the level of rescuer involvement and the nature of the incident.
- Water rescue should never be attempted by a single rescuer or by one who is untrained.
- Water hazards include obstructions to flow and foot or extremity pins that can trap victims and drag them under water. Factors that contribute to flat-water drownings include alcohol or other drug use and cool water temperatures.
- Hazardous atmospheres include environments with low oxygen, which can occur in confined spaces. The six major hazards associated with confined spaces are oxygen-deficient atmospheres, chemical/toxic exposure and explosion, engulfment, machinery entrapment, electricity, and structural concerns.
- Traffic flow is the biggest hazard in EMS highway operations. Other scene hazards associated with highway operations include fuel or fire hazards, electrical power, unstable vehicles, airbags and supplemental restraint systems, and hazardous cargoes.
- Hazardous terrain can create major difficulties during rescue events. Three common classifications of hazardous terrain are low angle, high angle, and flat terrain with obstructions.
- Paramedics must continue patient assessment during rescue operations, often while facing complications such as weather and temperature extremes, patient access challenges, equipment limitations, patient entrapment, and cumbersome PPE that affects rescuer mobility.

References

1. National Fire Protection Association. *NFPA 1999: Standard on Protective Clothing and Ensembles for Medical Operations*. Quincy, MA: National Fire Protection Association; 2018. https://www.nfpa.org/codes-and-standards/all-codes-and-standards/list-of-codes-and-standards/detail?code=1999. Accessed April 17, 2018.
2. US Department of Labor, Occupational Safety and Health Administration. Hazardous waste operations and emergency response (HAZWOPER), Standard 1910.120. Occupational Safety and Health Administration website. https://www.osha.gov/pls/oshaweb/owadisp.show_document?p_table=standards&p_id=976. Published 2003. Revised 2013. Accessed April 17, 2018.
3. US Department of Labor, Occupational Safety and Health Administration. Occupational exposure to bloodborne pathogens. 29 CFR 1910.1030. Occupational Safety and Health Administration website. https://www.osha.gov/pls/oshaweb/owadisp.show_document?p_table=standards&p_id=10051. Published 2001. Revised 2012. Accessed April 17, 2018.
4. US Department of Labor, Occupational Safety and Health Administration. Enforcement policy and procedures for occupational exposure to tuberculosis. Occupational Safety and Health Administration website. https://www.osha.gov/pls/oshaweb/owadisp.show_document?p_table=DIRECTIVES&p_id=1586. Published 1995. Revised 2004. Accessed April 17, 2018.
5. Centers for Disease Control and Prevention, National Center for Injury Prevention and Control, Division of Unintentional Injury Prevention. Home recreational safety: unintentional drowning: get the facts. Centers for Disease Control and Prevention website. https://www.cdc.gov/homeandrecreationalsafety/water-safety/waterinjuries-factsheet.html. Updated April 28, 2016. Accessed April 17, 2018.
6. Auerbach P. *Auerbach's Wilderness Medicine*. 7th ed. St. Louis, MO: Elsevier-Mosby; 2016.
7. American Heart Association. *Advanced Cardiac Life Support*. Dallas, TX: American Heart Association; 2015.
8. National Association of Emergency Medical Technicians. *PHTLS: Prehospital Trauma Life Support*. 8th ed. Burlington, MA: Jones & Bartlett Learning; 2016.
9. Changes to an important lifesaving technique. Royal Life Saving website. https://royallifesavingwa.com.au/news/lifesaving/changes-to-an-important-lifesaving-technique. Published May 11, 2016. Accessed April 17, 2018.
10. American Heart Association, American Red Cross. Part 15: first aid. Web-based integrated 2010 and 2015 American Heart Association and American Red Cross guidelines for first aid. American Heart Association website. https://eccguidelines.heart.org/wp-content/themes/eccstaging/dompdf-master/pdffiles/part-15-first-aid.pdf. Accessed April 17, 2018.
11. Schmidt AC, Sempsrot JR, Hawkins SC, Auerbach PS. Wilderness Medical Society practice guidelines for the prevention and treatment of drowning. *Wilderness Environ Med.* 2016; 27(2):236-251.
12. National Institute for Occupational Safety and Health, Education and Information Division. Preventing occupational fatalities in confined spaces. Centers for Disease Control and Prevention website. https://www.cdc.gov/niosh/docs/86-110/default.html. Updated June 6, 2014. Accessed April 17, 2018.
13. US Department of Labor, Occupational Safety and Health Administration. Permit-required confined spaces for general industry. 29 CFR 1910.146. Occupational Safety and Health Administration website. https://www.osha.gov/pls/oshaweb/owadisp.show_document?p_table=standards&p_id=979. Published 1998. Revised 2011. Accessed April 17, 2018.

14. US Department of Labor, Occupational Safety and Health Administration. Protecting construction workers in confined spaces: small entity compliance guide. OSHA 3825-09. Occupational Safety and Health Administration website. https://www.osha.gov/Publications/OSHA3825.pdf. Published 2015. Accessed April 17, 2018.
15. US Department of Labor, Occupational Safety and Health Administration. OSHA fact sheet: trenching and excavation safety. Occupational Safety and Health Administration website. https://www.osha.gov/Publications/trench_excavation_fs.html. Accessed April 17, 2018.
16. First responder guides, rescue sheets, and quick reference sheets. Service Technical College website. https://www.gmstc.com/FirstResponder.aspx. Updated December 1, 2016. Accessed April 17, 2018.
17. Electric vehicle safety training for emergency responders. National Fire Protection Association website. https://energy.gov/sites/prod/files/2014/03/f11/arravt036_ti_klock_2011_p.pdf. Published May 11, 2011. Accessed April 17, 2018.
18. US Department of Transportation, National Highway Traffic Safety Administration. Air bags and on-off switches: information for an informed decision. DOT HS 811 264. SaferCar.gov website. www.safercar.gov/staticfiles/safercar/pdf/811264.pdf. Accessed April 17, 2018.

Suggested Readings

Hunter J. *Swiftwater and Flood Rescue Field Guide.* Burlington, MA: Jones and Bartlett Learning; 2012.

International Fire Service Training Association. *Principles of Vehicle Extrication.* 4th ed. Stillwater, OK: International Fire Service Training Association, Fire Protection Publications; 2017.

LaBelle T. Firefighter survival: 10 ways to stay safe: Houston's "Rules of Survival" offer take-home messages for every firefighter. Fire Rescue 1 website. https://www.firerescue1.com/columnists/Tom-LaBelle/articles/763410-Firefighter-survival-10-ways-to-stay-safe/. Published February 22, 2010. Accessed April 17, 2018.

Merrell G. A swift water primer for EMS providers. *JEMS* website. http://www.jems.com/articles/print/volume-42/issue-6/features/a-swift-water-rescue-primer-for-ems-providers.html. Published May 31, 2017. Accessed April 17, 2018.

National Institute for Occupational Safety and Health, Office of the Director. Emergency response resources: guidance for supervisors at disaster rescue sites. Centers for Disease Control and Prevention website. https://www.cdc.gov/niosh/topics/emres/emhaz.html. Updated October 12, 2016. Accessed April 17, 2018.

Osvaldova LM, Petho M. Occupational safety and health during rescue activities. *Procedia Manufacturing.* 2015;3:4287-4293.

Richardson S. *Technical Rescue: Trench Levels I and II.* Boston, MA: Cengage Learning; 2009.

Sullivan J. Ten tips for firefighter safety at highway incidents. Firehouse website. http://www.firehouse.com/article/12249789/tips-for-firefighter-safety-at-highway-and-roadway-incidents-firefighter-training. Published August 29, 2016. Accessed April 17, 2018.

Treinish S. *Water Rescue: Principles and Practice to NFPA 1006 and 1670: Surface, Swiftwater, Dive, Ice, Surf, and Flood.* 2nd ed. Quincy, MA: National Fire Protection Association; 2017.

Zimmerman D. *Firefighter Safety and Survival.* Boston, MA: Delmar Cengage Learning; 2012.

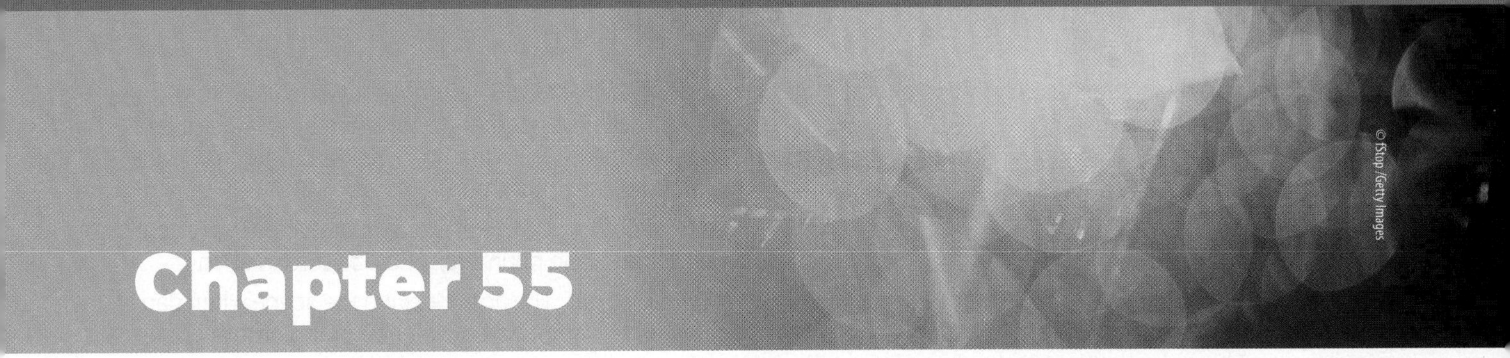
© fStop /Getty Images

Chapter 55

Crime Scene Awareness

NATIONAL EMS EDUCATION STANDARD COMPETENCIES

EMS Operations

Knowledge of operational roles and responsibilities to ensure patient, public, and personnel safety.

OBJECTIVES

Upon completion of this chapter, the paramedic student will be able to:

1. Explain general techniques for determining whether a scene is violent and choosing the appropriate response to a violent scene. (pp 1878–1879)
2. Outline techniques for recognizing and responding to potentially dangerous residential calls. (pp 1879–1880)
3. Outline techniques for recognizing and responding to potentially dangerous calls on the highway. (p 1880)
4. Identify signs of danger and appropriate EMS response to violent street incidents. (pp 1880–1881)
5. Identify characteristics of and appropriate EMS response to situations involving gangs, clandestine drug labs, and domestic violence. (pp 1881–1884)
6. Examine general safety tactics that EMS personnel can use if they find themselves in a dangerous situation. (pp 1884–1886)
7. Examine special EMS considerations when providing tactical patient care. (pp 1886–1888)
8. Discuss EMS documentation and preservation of evidence at a crime scene. (pp 1888–1889)

KEY TERMS

audible and visual warning (AVW) devices Safety devices used in emergency responses to make vehicle presence known. Examples include lights, sirens, and horns.

avoidance The act of keeping away from someone, something, or a situation, or of preventing the occurrence of something. It requires the paramedic to continually be aware of the scene by remaining observant and being knowledgeable about warning signs that may indicate a dangerous situation.

backlighting A type of lighting in which a person or object is positioned such that a light source from behind silhouettes the person or object; this is a safety hazard in the context of a hostile threat, by making a provider easier to see.

clandestine drug lab A place of illegal drug manufacturing.

concealment A means of keeping out of sight; does not necessarily provide ballistic protection.

contact provider The person who initiates and provides direct patient care.

cover A device or structure that offers ballistic protection; may or may not also provide concealment.

cover provider The person whose role is to ensure scene safety for the contact providers while they provide patient care.

crime scene A location where any part of a criminal act has occurred, or a location where evidence relating to a crime may be found.

distraction A self-defense measure in which a diversion is created to attract a person's attention.

evasive tactics A self-defense measure in which an aggressor's moves and actions are anticipated and unconventional pathways are used during retreat for personal safety.

gang Any group of people who engage in socially disruptive or criminal behavior.

graffiti Gang markings that usually indicate territorial boundaries; also known as tagging.

hot zone In tactical response, the area inside the scene perimeter where a direct threat exists and is immediately apparent.

soft body armor Clothing that provides protection from some blunt and penetrating trauma; also known as bullet-proof vests. The vest must be designed and rated to provide protection from edged weapons.

special weapons and tactics (SWAT) operations Violent and dangerous incidents; may include emergency medical personnel.

staging A tactical response to avoid danger by waiting at a safe distance from the scene until the area has been secured by the appropriate authorities.

tactical EMS (TEMS) Emergency medical support provided by EMS personnel who are specially trained and equipped to provide prehospital emergency care in tactical environments.

tactical patient care Patient care activities that occur inside the scene perimeter of a dangerous scene.

tactical retreat The act of leaving the scene when danger is observed or when violence or indicators of violence are displayed; requires immediate and decisive action.

turf Territorial boundaries established by gangs.

warm zone In tactical response, the area inside the scene perimeter where threats are indirect or possible but not immediately apparent.

Many violent crimes require an EMS response, and often EMS crews arrive at the scene before law enforcement personnel. Consequently, awareness and avoidance of dangerous situations are issues of concern for emergency responders. Violence against EMS personnel is a significant occupational risk that causes physical injury, higher stress levels, decreased job satisfaction, anxiety, avoidance behavior, adverse effects on personal relationships, and death.[1,2] *Personal safety and crime scene awareness must be top priorities on every call of this nature.*

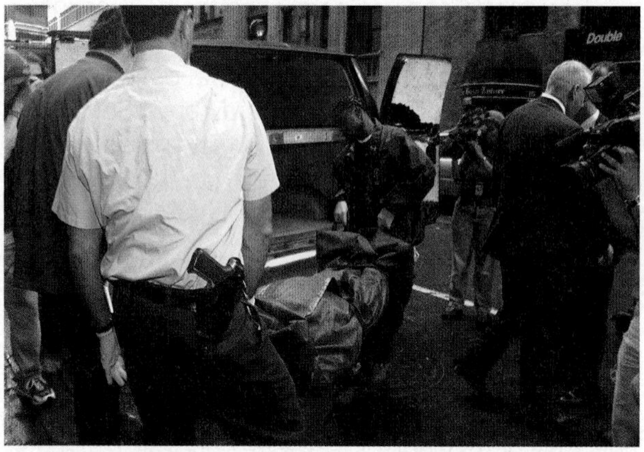

CRITICAL THINKING

Why is it not always possible to identify incident dangers before arriving at the scene?

Approaching the Scene

For paramedics and other responders, determining personal safety is a basic part of analyzing a scene. It begins before paramedics arrive at the scene with information provided by a dispatching center. A key point in ensuring personal safety is to identify and respond to potential dangers before they threaten. Information may be available from a dispatching center that should alert the EMS crew to possible dangers. Such information includes known locations of unsafe scenes (eg, through computer-aided dispatch systems) and/or the presence of the following:

- Large crowds
- People under the influence of alcohol or other drugs
- On-scene violence
- Weapons

Other information can sometimes be gathered en route to the scene from crew members, dispatchers, and other emergency responders monitoring the call who have had previous experience with a particular area or address. The paramedic also should be aware of additional inherent hazards that may exist at the scene. Examples include downed power lines, busy roadways, toxic substances, the potential for fire, dangerous pets, and vehicle hazards and dangers. If the scene is not safe, the EMS crew should retreat. The crew should stage at a safe location to await the arrival of law enforcement and/or other rescuers.

When responding to a scene with a potential for danger, the EMS crew should begin observation several blocks from the scene. They also should use **audible and visual warning (AVW) devices** that are appropriate for the call. For example, responding with AVW devices to an urban scene may draw a crowd of bystanders; lights generally are required for safety at highway scenes. As described in Chapter 52, *Ground and Air Ambulance Operations*, joint responses involving fire services, EMS, and law enforcement should be defined through preplanning. For example, for a given scenario, fire services and EMS may initiate an emergency response with full use of AVW devices while law enforcement responds without AVW devices and at normal speed.

Scene safety considerations for all types of danger must continue throughout the EMS response. A scene that has been made safe can become unsafe, even when the police are present. This can happen if violence erupts or resumes, crowds gather or turn violent, or other people enter the scene. Violence against EMS providers also may occur if they are mistaken for police officers (because of uniform colors or badges) or when they exit an emergency vehicle that has AVW devices. The paramedic crew must be familiar with local protocols when intervening in violent situations. They also must have a strategic escape plan ready.

Scenes Known to Be Violent

If the scene is known to be violent, the EMS crew should remain at a safe, out-of-sight distance from the area until it has been secured ("out of sight, out of scene"). Remaining at a safe staging area away from a violent scene is important for several reasons:

- If paramedics can be seen, people will come to them.
- Entering an unsafe scene adds one or more potential victims.
- Paramedics may be injured or killed.
- Paramedics may be taken hostage.
- Paramedics may become additional patients in a scene that is already a multiple-casualty incident.

It must be stressed that if the scene is unsafe, the EMS crew should not enter. Rather, they should retreat to a staging area and wait for resource personnel who can provide scene safety.

SHOW ME THE EVIDENCE

A cross-sectional mixed-methods study was conducted in two Canadian provinces to describe violence experienced by ground paramedics within the prior 12 months. Verbal violence was most common (67%), followed by intimidation (41%), physical assault (26%), sexual harassment (14%), and sexual assault (3%). Patients were the most frequent perpetrators of the violence. Female paramedics were physically and sexually assaulted more often than males were. Paramedics felt the assault affected their emotions and decreased their empathy.

Modified from: Bigham BL, Jensen JL, Tavares W, et al. Paramedic self-reported exposure to violence in the emergency medical services (EMS) workplace: a mixed-methods cross-sectional survey. *Prehosp Emerg Care.* 2014;18(4):489-494.

Weapons at the Scene

Paramedics will likely respond to emergency calls where weapons are present. If there is a question of scene safety, paramedics should retreat when there are weapons on the scene. All weapons should be secured by or under the supervision of law enforcement personnel if officers are present at the scene. If law enforcement is not present and no imminent danger exists, the paramedic should request that a weapon at the scene be safely secured, preferably in the patient's home or vehicle. If this is not possible, the paramedic should manage the weapon according to department policy and procedure. This request should be explained as an additional safety measure for the EMS crew, patient, and any bystanders (see Chapter 18, *Scene Size-up and Primary Assessment.*)

Dangerous Residence

A response to a residence is an everyday occurrence for most EMS personnel. However, even calls that appear "routine" require a scene size-up that begins before the EMS crew leaves the emergency vehicle. Warning signs of danger in residential calls include the following:

- A history of problems or violence
- A known drug or gang area
- Loud noises (eg, screams, items breaking, possible gunshots)
- Seeing or hearing acts of violence
- The presence of alcohol or other drug use

- The smell of chemicals or the presence of empty chemical containers
- Evidence of dangerous pets (eg, exotic snakes and reptiles, breeds of dogs that are often trained to be vicious)
- Unusual silence or darkened residence

If any of these or other warning signs are present, the EMS crew should retreat from the scene and call for law enforcement assistance.

When approaching a suspicious residence, the EMS crew should choose tactics that match the threat or situation. For example, avoiding the use of AVW devices, taking unconventional pathways (rather than using the sidewalk, for example), and avoiding a position between the ambulance lights and residence (**backlighting**) are safety measures that should be considered. In addition, paramedics should listen for sounds indicating danger before announcing their presence or entering the home. They should stand on the side of the entry door opposite the hinges (doorknob side). If danger becomes evident, paramedics should immediately retreat from the scene.

Dangerous Highway Encounters

As with calls to residences, a response to a traffic incident should never be considered routine. Such calls involve inherent dangers associated with traffic flow, emergency vehicle positioning, and extrication. Also, the danger of violence may exist. For example, a vehicle's occupants may be armed and wanted by law enforcement or may have an altered mental state because of alcohol or drug intoxication (**BOX 55-1**).

When approaching a vehicle, a one-person approach is recommended. This method allows the partner who remains in the ambulance to notify dispatch of the situation, location, license plate number, and state registration of suspicious vehicles. (Because the ambulance is elevated, it provides greater visibility of the vehicle.) At night, ambulance lights should be used to illuminate the interior of the vehicle and the surrounding area.

The paramedic who approaches the vehicle should do so from the passenger side of the vehicle. Doing so provides protection from vehicle traffic. Furthermore, it usually is the opposite approach a driver would expect from law enforcement personnel. As another safety precaution, the paramedic should not walk between the ambulance and the other vehicle to avoid being trapped and injured if the vehicle backs up. The paramedic should walk around the rear of the ambulance and then to the passenger side of the vehicle.

Car posts A, B, and C (see Chapter 54, *Rescue Awareness and Operations*) may provide the better ballistic protection as opposed to windows and doors. The paramedic should observe for unusual activity in the rear seat and not move forward of the post nearest the threat unless no threats exist in these areas. The paramedic should observe the front seat from behind post B and move forward only after ensuring it safe to do so (**FIGURE 55-1**). If signs of danger are present (eg, weapons, suspicious behavior or movements in the vehicle, arguing or fighting among passengers), paramedics should immediately retreat to a safe staging area. From that area, they should request the help of law enforcement, if not already present at the scene.

BOX 55-1 Street-Smart Safety Tips

- When working in vehicle traffic, always wear reflective clothing and make sure you can leave the scene quickly and safely if required.
- At night, use the ambulance lights to illuminate a vehicle's interior.
- Before approaching a vehicle, consider using the public address system to get a response from passengers in the vehicle.
- If your ambulance is approaching a vehicle in which a passenger is adjusting the side- or rearview mirror as you approach, retreat to safety. (This is a sign of danger.)
- Open or unlatched trunks may indicate that people are hiding or have been restrained in the compartment. If the trunk is slightly open, slam it shut without opening it further.
- Retreat to the ambulance (or another place of safety) at the first sign of danger.

Violent Street Incidents

Murder, assault, and robbery are common occurrences in the United States. Many of these crimes involve dangerous weapons. Violence may be directed toward EMS personnel from perpetrators at the scene (or who return to the scene). The violence may even come from injured and distraught patients. In

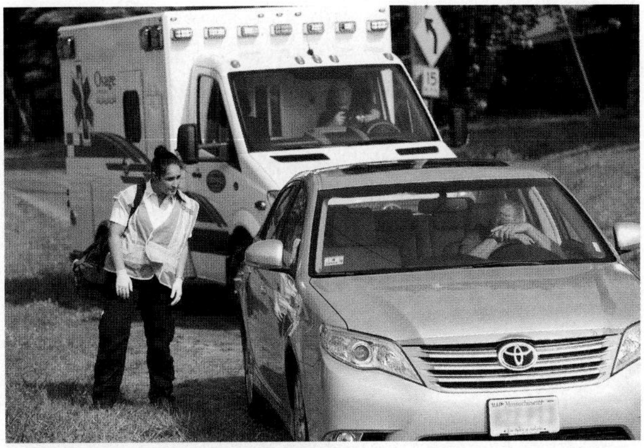

FIGURE 55-1 Paramedic approaching while partner calls dispatch and closely observes.

addition, dangerous crowds and bystanders quickly can become large in number and volatile. They may direct violence toward everyone and everything in the surrounding area. Warning signs of potential danger in violent street incidents include the following:

- Voices that become louder, escalating in tone
- Pushing and shoving
- Hostility toward people at the scene (eg, perpetrator, police, victim)
- Destruction of property
- A rapid increase in the size of the crowd
- The use of alcohol or other drugs by people at the scene
- Inability of law enforcement personnel to control the crowd

Paramedic crews should constantly monitor crowds and retreat from the scene if necessary. The location and careful parking of the emergency vehicle are important for personal safety. The EMS crew should position the ambulance so that it cannot be blocked by other vehicles (allowing for easy retreat from the scene). When possible and when it is safe to do so, the patient should be removed from the scene as the crew retreats. Doing so may eliminate the need to return to the scene.

CRITICAL THINKING

In your community, what type of EMS calls routinely merit a law enforcement response?

Violent Groups and Situations

According to the Federal Bureau of Investigation, more than 1.4 million gang members currently belong to more than 33,000 violent gangs throughout the United States and Puerto Rico (BOX 55-2).[3] Most gangs and other threat groups operate through intimidation and extortion (BOX 55-3).

Gang Characteristics

A **gang** can be defined as any group of people who engage in socially disruptive or criminal behavior. They usually are territorial and are often but not always of the same sex. Gangs also operate by creating an atmosphere of fear in a community. The gang may

CRITICAL THINKING

In addition to consulting police sources and familiarizing yourself with gang markings, dress, and colors, how can you obtain information about gang activity in your community?

BOX 55-2 Short History of Gangs

Modern-era gangs first emerged in the United States in the late 1960s. Two of the best known gangs, the Crips and the Bloods, started in Compton, California, when two rival high schools began to sport their school colors. The Bloods wore red to denote their gang affiliation; the Crips wore blue. Other gangs' ancestries originated in the prison system. The Black Gangster Disciples (now known as the Gangster Disciples) was the most noteworthy of these. This gang started in the Chicago prison system and competed for the drug market in that city. In recent years, gangs have evolved to include all ethnic origins and backgrounds (eg, Asian, Hispanic, Latin, white threat groups). Most operate in secrecy with codes of honor and pledges that frequently involve acts of violence. Gang membership often is a lifetime commitment. Gangs operate in the streets, in prisons, and even in the military. Social media has gained increased use for gang communication.

Modified from: Howell JC, Moore JP. *History of Street Gangs in the United States*. Washington, DC: Institute for Intergovernmental Research on behalf of the National Gang Center; 2010; National Gang Intelligence Center. *2015 National Gang Report*. Federal Bureau of Investigation website. https://www.fbi.gov/file-repository/national-gang-report-2015.pdf/view. Accessed April 18, 2018.

BOX 55-3 Sampling of Street Gangs and Other Threat Groups in the United States

18th Street Gang
Artistas Asesinos
Banditos
Barrio Azteca
Black Mob
Bloods (many subchapters)
Chosen Few
Cossacks
Crips (many subchapters)
Gangster Disciples
Hell's Angels
Hell's Lovers
Latin Kings (Almighty Latin King and Queen Nation)
Lincoln Park
Mara Salvatrucha 13 (MS-13)
Mexican Mafia
Mongols
Norteños
Outcasts
Outlaws
Pagans
Paisa
Queen Nation
Scanless
Sin City Deciples
Skin Heads
Sons of Silence
Sureños
Taliban
Tango Blast
Texas Syndicate
Thunderguards
Vagos
Wheels of Soul
Young 'n' Thuggin'

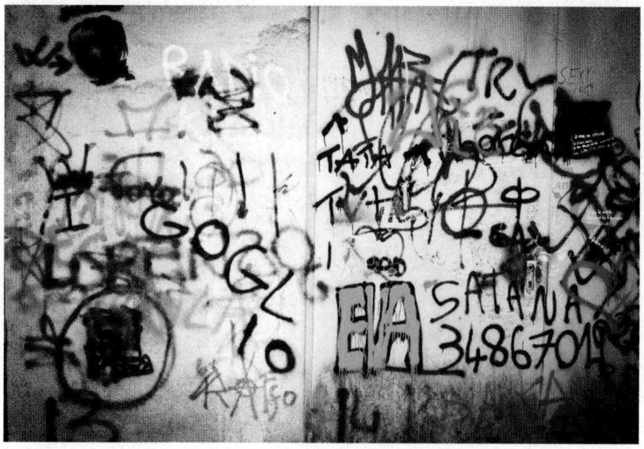

FIGURE 55-2 Graffiti on a wall in Los Angeles.

choose a name, logo, specific color, or method of dress to identify its own members and counterparts.

Graffiti and Clothing

Graffiti (often referred to as tagging) is probably the most visible sign of gang criminal activity. It can be seen in neighborhood parks and on the back and side walls of stores, fences, retaining walls, and any other prominent structure that is paintable (**FIGURE 55-2**). Gang graffiti usually marks territorial boundaries, known as **turf**. Gang-related clothing often is unique and specific to a group. It is worn to identify affiliation and rank. Gang-related clothing and styles vary widely across the country and even within regions.[4] Some examples are listed in **BOX 55-4**.

Safety Issues in Gang Areas

Common gang activities include fighting, vandalism, armed robbery, weapon offenses, automobile theft, battery, human trafficking, alien smuggling, prostitution, and drug dealing or transport. (Not all gang members are engaged in illegal activities.) A significant number of gangs are affiliated with domestic extremist

BOX 55-4 Gang Clothing and Styles

- **Beads.** Beads may be found on necklaces, key chains, rosaries, and any other jewelry. The colors found on the item can be linked to the gang, and the order of the beads may indicate the person's status in the group and/or the activities he or she has engaged in.
- **Tattoos/markings.** Markings on a person may be as simple as the gang's name or may be symbols associated with the gang (eg, crowns, numbers, pitchforks, dots). Markings may be applied with pens or markers to be easily removed and prevent detection by law enforcement.
- **Clothing.** Colors are used to show association with the gang. Apparel may have numbers or acronyms related to the group (very common with sports apparel). Members may wear a colored fabric belt that may have a buckle with the gang name. Clothing may be altered to identify the gang (such as gang-themed T-shirts). Bandanas are the most common piece of clothing members use to represent the gang.
- **Personal appearance/grooming.** Hairstyles and eyebrows may have covert numbers or symbols (eg, lines or symbols shaved in eyebrows or hair). Pants worn up on one leg, hat tilted to a certain side, and unusual hand gestures may also be used.

Modified from: Armstrong K, Phillips T. Street gangs in our schools: what to look for and what you can do to address them. Region One ESC website. www.esc1.net/cms/lib/TX21000366/Centricity/Domain/89/Gangspowrpt.pdf. Published June 2008. Accessed April 18, 2018.

groups.[5] The criminal activity usually is committed for status or monetary benefit, either for the gang in general or for a single member. The likelihood for those violent acts and the fact that EMS personnel often "look like" law enforcement officials require that paramedics be very cautious about personal safety when working in gang areas.

Clandestine Drug Labs

As described in Chapter 33, *Toxicology,* the illegal manufacture of drugs can pose significant hazards for emergency personnel. Activities that take place in a **clandestine drug lab** include creating drugs (synthesis) from chemical precursors (eg, lysergic acid diethylamide [LSD], methamphetamine [meth]). Also, a drug's form can be changed (conversion). For example, cocaine hydrochloride may be changed to a base form. The processes of drug synthesis and conversion can produce oxygen-depleted atmospheres. They also can create highly explosive and toxic gases (eg, phosgene).

DID YOU KNOW?

Shake-and-Bake Meth

A popular way to manufacture small quantities of meth is called the shake-and-bake or "one-pot" method. The method uses one sealed container, such as a soft drink bottle. The container is usually flipped upside down to cause the chemical reaction needed to turn the ingredients into meth. The chemical reaction causes an extremely high pressure inside the container after being shaken. This is one of the most dangerous ways to produce the drug because the pressure can cause a large explosion. The shake-and-bake method is fast and portable. The method is often "cooked" while driving an automobile. Driving while making meth releases the fumes from the chemical process into the air. Once the drug is produced, the container is then thrown from the car. EMS personnel must be aware of the explosive danger of this method of meth production when approaching an automobile or the trunk of a car. Explosions also pose a hazard to children, who naturally want to explore things they find on the ground. EMS personnel should not investigate these containers and should alert law enforcement if found.

Modified from: National Drug Intelligence Center. Methamphetamine laboratory identification and hazards: fast facts. US Department of Justice website. https://www.justice.gov/archive/ndic/pubs7/7341/7341p.pdf. Accessed April 19, 2018.

These gases can readily be absorbed through the skin in amounts that can be fatal. Toxic solvents involved in drug-making processes also can lead to lab explosions and exposure to dangerous chemicals.

Other safety hazards that are associated with clandestine drug labs include booby traps that can maim or kill an intruder. In addition, people who operate these labs are sometimes armed or otherwise violent. Clandestine labs usually are located in an area that ensures privacy. They generally are well ventilated. They also usually have access to water, electric, and gas utilities, which are required for the drug-making process. Suspicious people, activities, and deliveries often can be observed at the site.

When responding to a scene that may be a site of illegal drug manufacture, storage, or transport, EMS crews should be alert for suspicious signs. These signs may include chemical odors and the presence of chemical equipment (eg, glassware, chemical containers, heating mantles, burners). If a drug lab is identified, the EMS crew should do the following:

1. Leave the area at once.
2. Notify law enforcement and request appropriate agencies and personnel (eg, hazardous materials teams, fire service personnel, chemistry specialists).
3. Initiate an incident command system and hazardous materials procedures per protocol.
4. Assist law enforcement personnel to evacuate the surrounding area in an orderly fashion to ensure public safety.

NOTE

EMS crews should never touch anything found in or around a clandestine drug lab. Only specially trained personnel should try to alter drug-making equipment or stop chemical reactions in a drug lab.

Domestic Violence

As described in Chapter 49, *Abuse and Neglect,* domestic violence is violence that occurs between people in a relationship. The perpetrator may be male or female. Those involved may be in an opposite-sex or same-sex relationship. Domestic violence results in physical, emotional, sexual, verbal, or economic abuse. It may occur in several combinations. To review, many signs indicate domestic violence and abuse, including the following:

- Apparent fear of a household member
- Different or conflicting accounts by parties at the scene
- One party preventing another from speaking
- A patient who is reluctant to speak
- Injuries that do not match the reported mechanism of injury
- Unusual or unsanitary living conditions or personal hygiene

EMS personnel who respond to a scene of domestic violence should be aware that acts of violence may be directed toward them by the perpetrator. They should take all safety precautions. If the scene is considered safe for the EMS crew, paramedics should treat the patient's injuries. They also should notify medical direction and other authorities consistent per standard procedures and protocol. (Mandatory reporting may be required.) To help ensure scene safety for the crew and the abused person, paramedics should not be judgmental about the relationship. They should not direct accusations toward the abuser or the patient. When appropriate, paramedics should supply the patient with phone numbers for domestic violence hotlines, community support programs, and available shelters.

Safety Tactics

Tactics that help ensure personal safety include avoidance, tactical retreat, cover and concealment, and distraction and evasive maneuvers. Many programs in the United States teach tactics for safety and patient care. Some EMS providers are specially trained and equipped to work in tactical law enforcement settings (BOX 55-5).

Avoidance

Avoidance is the act of keeping away from a dangerous situation or preventing the development of a dangerous situation. Avoidance is always preferable to confrontation. To practice avoidance, paramedics must continually be aware of the scene. They can stay aware by being observant and by being knowledgeable about warning signs that may indicate a dangerous

BOX 55-5 Tactical Emergency Medical Support

Tactical emergency medical support (TEMS) refers to EMS personnel who are specially trained and equipped to provide prehospital medical care in support of tactical law enforcement operations. Such settings may include hostage-barricaded situations, high-risk search warrants, and other adverse situations involving law enforcement and/or rescue operations in which standard EMS units may be inappropriate.

The concept of training emergency medical technicians (EMTs) and paramedics in TEMS started in the late 1980s. It has since expanded nationwide. Forward-thinking law enforcement departments have adopted TEMS programs as a way to increase the safety of their special weapons and tactics (SWAT) officers and the innocent hostage or bystander. They also are a means of addressing liability exposure. Tactical training for EMS personnel also is recognized as a valuable tool for personal safety when EMS personnel find themselves in an unsafe situation.

Many tactical medical teams use the Counter Narcotics and Terrorism Operational Medical Support (CONTOMS) program for initial training of their personnel. CONTOMS is a joint federal program supported by the US Department of Health and Human Services, US Department of Homeland Security, and US Park Police, with assistance from the Department of Justice as well as many state and local law enforcement agencies. The CONTOMS program leads to certification as an EMT-Tactical (EMT-T) or SWAT medic. The focus of the training is to integrate specific skills to complement an agency's standard operating procedures. These skills include the ability to do the following:

- Assess and plan for preventive medicine needs in sustained operations.
- Provide preventive medical care in sustained operations.
- Recognize and treat unique wound patterns resulting from deliberate interpersonal aggression.
- Use medical care skills appropriate to hostile and austere environments.
- Explain medical and physiologic parameters that lead to performance decrement and implement plans that minimize those effects.
- Develop and apply injury-control strategies.
- Access and analyze medical information and make a medical threat assessment.
- Apply special law enforcement principles to the delivery of medical care.

Modified from: Rinnert KJ, Hall WL. Tactical emergency medical support. *Emerg Med Clin N Am*. 2002;20:929-952; United States Park Police: CONTOMS. National Park Service website. https://www.nps.gov/subjects/uspp/contoms.htm. Accessed April 17, 2018; and Counter Narcotics and Terrorism Operational Medical Support website. https://contoms.chepinc.org. Accessed April 17, 2018.

situation. In addition, they must be knowledgeable about tactical responses for avoiding danger or for dealing with danger that cannot be avoided. An example of avoidance is **staging**. With staging, the dispatching center learns of danger and advises the EMS crew not to approach the scene until it has been secured by the appropriate authorities.

Tactical Retreat

Tactical retreat describes leaving the scene when danger is observed or when violence or indicators of violence are displayed. Tactical retreat requires immediate and decisive action. Retreat on foot or by vehicle (in a calm, safe manner) involves choosing the mode and route of retreat that provides the least exposure to danger. During tactical retreat, the EMS crew should be aware that the risks they faced are now located behind them. They must stay alert for associated dangers. Of course, the required distance from danger for a safe tactical retreat must be guided by the nature of the incident. In general, a safe distance is judged by the following conditions:

- Protects the crew from any potential danger
- Keeps the crew out of the immediate line of sight
- Protects the crew from gunfire (ie, provides cover)
- Keeps the crew far enough away to give them time to react if danger reappears

CRITICAL THINKING

Could the EMS crew be charged with abandonment if they make a tactical retreat and leave the patient?

Once tactical retreat has been achieved, the EMS crew must notify other responding units and agencies of the danger. They notify other units using interagency EMS and law enforcement standard operating procedures and agreements. (Interagency procedures that deal with violent situations should be established in the preplanning stages so that each agency is aware of its specific duties.)

Documentation also is essential to reducing liability if injuries or deaths occur. Thorough documentation should include observations of danger at the scene, names of people notified of the danger, actions at the scene, and accurate times that retreat or return to the scene occurred. Most legal authorities do not consider tactical retreat for appropriate circumstances to be patient abandonment.

Cover and Concealment

Cover and **concealment** provide protection from injury. Cover provides ballistic protection and is often in the form of large, heavy structures. Examples of such structures include large trees, telephone poles, and a vehicle's engine block. Concealment hides the body. However, it offers little or no ballistic protection. Examples of concealment include bushes, wallboards, and the doors of vehicles.

Cover and concealment should be integrated into tactical retreat or used when the EMS crew is "pinned down" (eg, by gunfire) or in other dangerous settings. When the need for cover or concealment arises, paramedics should do the following:

- Maintain constant awareness of their surroundings.
- Be aware that "stepping off" cover may actually provide more protection than "hugging" cover (**FIGURE 55-3**).

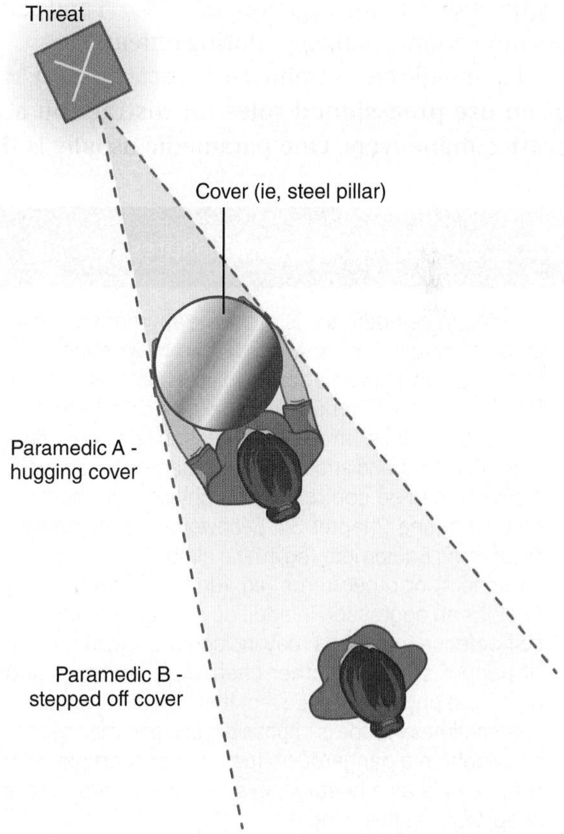

FIGURE 55-3 At times, stepping off cover provides more protection than hugging cover. Paramedic B is less exposed and must expose far less of himself/herself to visualize the threat if needed compared with paramedic A.

- Constantly look for ways to improve protection and location.
- Be aware of reflective clothing (eg, trim, badges) that may draw attention or serve as a target.

CRITICAL THINKING

What parts of your ambulance provide cover?

Distraction and Evasive Tactics

Distraction and **evasive tactics** can be used as self-defense measures during retreat. They also can be used when retreat and cover and concealment are not available options (BOX 55-6). For example, equipment may be used to provide distraction (eg, a stretcher may be wedged in a doorway to block an aggressor), or equipment may be thrown to trip or slow a pursuer. These actions may allow the EMS crew to make a safe retreat or gain adequate cover and concealment. Evasive tactics involve anticipating the moves of the aggressor (BOX 55-7) and using unconventional pathways during retreat.

Paramedic crews trained in **tactical EMS (TEMS)** often use preassigned roles for distraction and evasive maneuvers. One paramedic usually is the **contact provider**. This person initiates and provides direct patient care, including patient assessment and most elements of interpersonal scene contact. Another crew member serves as the **cover provider**. In a tactical context, the cover provider's role is to ensure scene safety for the contact providers while they provide patient care. This role includes monitoring the scene for danger. The cover provider generally does not perform patient care duties that would prevent observation of the scene. The cover provider also may be responsible for ensuring the safekeeping of equipment, drugs, and supplies while at the scene.

Methods of communication between the contact and cover providers should be developed in advance. That way, they can alert team members of potential dangers without alerting the aggressor. This communication often can be done with subtle verbal and nonverbal signals, such as using coded terms, scratching the neck, or rubbing the nose. It is crucial in these situations to maintain radio contact with the dispatching center. The crew also should involve the dispatcher in the danger signal process. For example, if the dispatcher hears a coded term that means danger, a priority response of the proper personnel can be initiated.

BOX 55-6 Self-Defense Measures

Training in self-defense is probably appropriate for all emergency responders. Avoidance is always superior to confrontation. However, some violent situations may call for self-defense. Examples include physical attacks that cannot be avoided, armed confrontation or robbery, hostage situations, and encounters with dangerous animals. A person can be controlled with physical or chemical restraints (see Chapter 34, *Behavioral and Psychiatric Disorders*). Equipment (eg, metal clipboards, jump kits, stretchers) or other items (eg, furniture) can be used to block an aggressor. In addition to these techniques, self-defense measures may include training in the use of pepper sprays or other chemical deterrents and defensive physical maneuvers that can allow escape.

Sometimes escape is impossible, and paramedics may be caught in a dangerous situation. For example, they may be held as a hostage. In such cases, paramedics should do the following:

- Remain as calm as possible.
- Avoid any confrontation.
- Play an active role with the captor in resolving the incident.
- Focus on a peaceful resolution and escape.

BOX 55-7 Warning Signs of Possible Violent Aggression

A person escalating toward violence may exhibit subtle warning signs, such as the following:

- Conspicuously ignores emergency responders
- Is verbally abusive
- Invades the responder's personal space
- Has a violent history or background
- Shifts body weight from side to side or foot to foot (boxer stance)
- Clenches the fists
- Tightens the muscles (eg, has stiff arms and/or shoulders)
- Engages in physical or verbal intimidation; parrots (repeats) a provider's questions rather than answering them
- Maintains eye contact by staring

Tactical Patient Care

The term **tactical patient care** describes patient care activities that occur inside the scene perimeter where there is a direct or indirect threat. An area where a direct threat exists is known as the **hot zone**. Very little, if any, medical care takes place in the hot zone because the main objective is for law enforcement to address the immediate danger, thus allowing medical personnel to extract the patient to an area of relative safety where threats are indirect and medical interventions may resume or be initiated. This area where no immediate threat exists but risk of danger remains is known as the **warm zone**. The provision of tactical patient care inside the perimeter requires special training and authorization, body armor and a tactical uniform, compact and functional equipment, and, in some operations, personal defensive weapons. Tactical EMS often requires risks not taken in standard EMS situations. Tactical medics provide immediate medical care to the injured during a **special weapons and tactics (SWAT) operation**. These medics treat the injured on site or stabilize them and extract them from the scene. Tactical medics generally work alongside law enforcement officers. They have specialized training with unique attributes and skills (**TABLE 55-1**).

Some agencies use personnel who are cross-trained in law enforcement and tactical EMS (**FIGURE 55-4**).

TABLE 55-1 Knowledge and Roles of Tactical Paramedics

TEMS Provider Knowledge	TEMS Provider Roles
• Tactical operations • Risks and effects of tactical team of weapons and deterrent devices • Hazards common to crime scenes • Recognizing, collecting, and preserving evidence • Identifying situations that might cause illness or injury to team members during prolonged operations • Tactical equipment use and removal • Principles of patient care in hostile situations	• Advises tactical commander about health hazards • Evaluates local medical resources • Assesses inaccessible victims from a distance • Assesses/treats team members with tactical equipment • Provides care in combat (hot) zone, tactical field care (warm zone), and combat casualty evacuation care (cold zone) • Performs gross decontamination

Modified from: Tan DK, Bozeman W, FitzGerald D. Tactical EMS. In: Brice J, Delbridge TR, Meyers JB, eds. *Emergency Services: Clinical Practice and Systems Oversight.* 2nd ed. West Sussex, England: John Wiley & Sons; 2015:355-362.

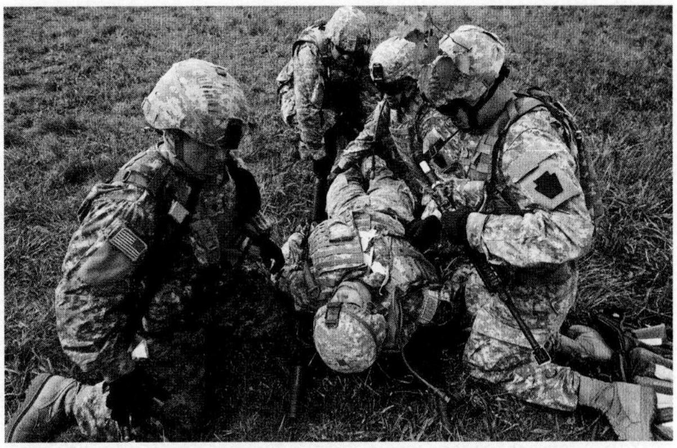

FIGURE 55-4 Tactical patient care.

In 2011, a consensus document was developed by the National Tactical Officers Association in collaboration with the American College of Surgeons Tactical Emergency Medicine section for TEMS. These competencies further define the role of the TEMS operator, medic, team commander, and medical director.[6]

Body Armor

As described in Chapter 36, *Trauma Overview and Mechanism of Injury*, **soft body armor** (also known as ballistic vests) offers protection from some blunt and penetrating trauma. It absorbs and distributes the impact of a ballistic missile. This equipment is effective against most handgun bullets. However, the equipment does not protect against knives or pointed, sharp objects.[7] In addition, the equipment does not provide protection from high-velocity rifle bullets or thin or edged weapons (eg, ice picks). Different levels of body armor provide various levels of protection. Like all other protective clothing, body armor is effective only when it is properly worn. It also must be in good condition and stored according to the manufacturer's instructions. Some body armor (eg, Kevlar) degrades with age. This armor may carry a ballistic expiration date that should be observed. Wet or worn vests do not provide optimum protection. A type III or higher level of protection generally is recommended for tactical EMS providers.

When wearing body armor, paramedics should take care not to develop a false sense of security. A general rule is, "Never try a maneuver that would not normally be done without body armor." Also, paramedics should keep in mind that body armor does not cover the entire body. Severe injury can still result from the forces of blunt trauma (in the absence of penetration) even when the vest is properly worn. This "back-face signature" (transmitted impact energy) is variable according to the type of vest and projectile.

NOTE

Calling for Help

Some EMS and fire portable radios (walkie-talkies) have a panic button. In most cases, this button must be pushed and held for several seconds to signal the dispatcher that there is a unit in distress. The panic signal should trigger a fixed response from local law enforcement and other appropriate resources. This process should be established in policy to ensure that the proper resources are automatically dispatched in these situations.

EMS Care in the Tactical Environment

As previously stated, the provision of EMS care in tactical situations calls for special training and authorization. Most tactical medics (EMT-Ts and SWAT medics) are trained in the following:[8]

- Team health and management
- Care under fire
- Officer rescue
- Medical operations preplanning and medical intelligence
- Responding to the active shooter
- Special medical gear for tactical operations
- Personal protective gear
- Special needs for extended operations
- Preventive medicine
- Management of weapons of mass destruction and toxic hazards

Most programs involve training exercises, which sometimes include the following:

- Physical assessment under sensory deprivation/overload conditions
- Medical threat assessment
- Advanced medical–tactical techniques
- Field-expedient decontamination
- New technologies for safe searches
- Management of dental injuries
- "Officer down" rescue and extraction
- Aeromedical evacuation
- Medical management of clandestine drug lab raids
- Safe search techniques
- Remote physical assessment

Patient care in dangerous settings involves a number of special concerns, including the frequent need to remove a patient from the area safely, the frequent care of trauma patients, the need to modify patient care, and the need to coordinate medical and transport actions with the incident commander. Often tactical EMS providers work under protocols and standing orders that differ from those of "standard" EMS practice. These medical direction issues regarding patient care are dictated by the nature of the event. They also are determined by the uncontrolled and hazardous scene in which emergency medical services are provided. Awareness programs are available for those who supervise or manage personnel assigned to a tactical team. Programs are also available for physicians (and others) who provide medical direction for rescuers who work with tactical law enforcement teams. Quality assurance programs and direct physician involvement at the local level are recommended.

NOTE

Of 110 EMS systems in North Carolina, 33% have TEMS programs. They serve about two-thirds of the state's population base. Only a small number of the TEMS personnel (12%) are sworn law enforcement officers.

Modified from: Bozeman WP, Morel BM, Black TD, Winslow JE. Tactical emergency medical support programs: a comprehensive statewide survey. *Prehosp Emerg Care*. 2012;16(3):361-365.

EMS at Crime Scenes

A **crime scene** is a location where any part of a criminal act has occurred. It also can be a location where evidence relating to a crime may be found. Important physical evidence that may be found at a crime scene includes fingerprints, footprints, and blood and other body fluids. Fingerprints and footprints are unique to a person. No two people have identical prints. These ridge characteristics often are left behind on a surface, along with oil and moisture from the skin. Blood and other body fluids can be tested for deoxyribonucleic acid (DNA) and ABO blood typing; they also have characteristics that may be unique to the person. In addition, particulate evidence (eg, hair, carpet, clothing fibers) can provide useful information and is considered valuable at a crime scene.

The paramedic's observations at a crime scene are important. They should be documented carefully on the patient care report or other appropriate form. For example, victims' positions and injuries and conditions at the scene may be helpful to law enforcement personnel in solving the crime. Documentation also should include any statements made by the patient or other people at the scene and any dying declarations. Paramedics should be careful to (1) record their observations objectively, (2) record patients' or bystanders' words in quotes, and (3) avoid personal opinions that are not relevant to patient care. Paramedics must keep in mind that patient care reports are legal documents; they may be used in court. Paramedics should avoid labeling ballistic injuries as "entrance" or "exit" wounds. Rather, the wound and characteristics of the wound should be described and documented in the patient care report.

NOTE

A dying declaration is a statement or statements made by a person who believes he or she is about to die. The statement concerns the cause or circumstances surrounding his or her impending death. An example is an assault victim who makes a dying declaration implicating a certain person as being his or her attacker.

Preserving Evidence

Patient care is the paramedic's ultimate priority, even at crime scenes. However, evidence can be protected while caring for the patient. This can be accomplished by being careful not to disturb the scene unnecessarily or destroy evidence. For example, paramedics should be observant of the scene and surroundings; they should touch only what is required for patient care; and they should wear medical gloves for infection control and to avoid leaving additional fingerprints at the scene. Other measures that aid crime scene preservation are listed in BOX 55-8.

BOX 55-8 Considerations for Crime Scene Preservation

Paramedics should observe the following rules when called to a known or a possible crime scene:

1. Approach no crime scene until it has been made relatively safe by law enforcement personnel.
2. Park your vehicle as far away as conveniently possible to preserve skid marks, tire prints, or other evidence.
3. Survey and assess the scene before proceeding to the victim.
4. Try to approach the victim from a route different from the assailant's probable route.
5. Follow the same path to and from the victim.
6. Avoid stepping on blood stains or spatter if possible.
7. Disturb the victim and the victim's clothing as little as possible while performing your assessment and during treatment.
8. When cutting clothing from a victim, try to do it in a way that preserves the points of wounding.
9. Report your actions and any disturbances you make to the crime scene investigator.
10. Keep all unnecessary people away from the victim.
11. Do not smoke or eat at the crime scene.
12. Do not touch any evidence if at all possible.
13. Make no comments to bystanders about the situation.
14. Save the victim's clothes and personal items in a paper bag. The bag should be labeled, sealed, and turned over to law enforcement personnel.
15. Be alert to any dying declarations the patient makes.
16. Keep accurate, detailed records.
17. Keep in mind that law enforcement personnel are in charge of the crime scene; you are in charge of the patient.

Modified from: Vollrath R. Crime scene preservation: it's everybody's concern. *J Emerg Med Serv.* 1995;20(1):53.

CRITICAL THINKING

If the main goal is caring for the patient, why should a paramedic be concerned about preserving evidence?

Summary

- A key point in ensuring scene safety is to identify and respond to dangers before they threaten. If the scene is known to be violent, the EMS crew should remain at a safe and out-of-sight distance from the area. They should remain at this distance until the scene has been made safe by law enforcement personnel.
- The paramedic should look for warning signs of violence during response to a residence. He or she should retreat from the scene if danger becomes evident.
- A response to a highway incident may present the dangers associated with traffic and extrication. However, it may present danger from violence as well. For example,

a vehicle's occupants may be armed and wanted by law enforcement or may have an altered mental state because of alcohol or drug intoxication.

- The paramedic should monitor for warning signs of danger in violent street incidents. He or she should retreat from the scene if necessary.
- A gang is any group of people who take part in socially disruptive or criminal behavior. Some gangs are involved in violent criminal activities. EMS personnel often look like law enforcement officers. Thus, they should be cautious about personal safety when working in gang areas.
- Clandestine drug lab activities can produce explosive and toxic gases. Other risks include booby traps that can maim or kill an intruder, and armed or violent occupants.
- EMS personnel who respond to a scene of domestic violence should be aware that acts of violence may be directed toward them by the perpetrator; they should take all safety precautions.
- Tactics for safety include avoidance, tactical retreat, cover and concealment, and distraction and evasive maneuvers.
- Tactical patient care refers to care activities that occur inside the scene perimeter in which direct and indirect threats exist. Zones of care within this perimeter are dynamic, and providers must always remain alert for changing circumstances in such a scene. Providing care in this area calls for special training and authorization, body armor and a tactical uniform, compact and functional equipment, and, in some operations, personal defensive weapons.
- The paramedic's observations at a crime scene are important. They should be carefully documented. Evidence should be protected while caring for the patient. This can be done by not unnecessarily disturbing the scene or destroying evidence.

References

1. Maguire BJ, O'Meara P, O'Neill B, Brightwell R. Violence against emergency medical services personnel: a systematic review of the literature. *Am J Ind Med.* 2017;61(2):167-180.
2. Reichard AA, Marsh SM, Tonozzi TR, Konda S, Gormley MA. Occupational injuries and exposures among emergency medical services workers. *Prehosp Emerg Care.* 2017;21(4):420-431.
3. What we investigate: gangs. Federal Bureau of Investigation website. https://www.fbi.gov/investigate/violent-crime/gangs. Accessed April 18, 2018.
4. Armstrong K, Phillips T. Street gangs in our schools: what to look for and what you can do to address them. Region One ESC website. www.esc1.net/cms/lib/TX21000366/Centricity/Domain/89/Gangspowrpt.pdf. Published June 2008. Accessed April 18, 2018.
5. National Gang Intelligence Center. *2015 National Gang Report.* Federal Bureau of Investigation website. https://www.fbi.gov/file-repository/national-gang-report-2015.pdf/view. Accessed April 18, 2018.
6. Schwartz RB, McManus JG, Croushorn J, et al. Tactical medicine—competency-based guidelines. *Prehosp Emerg Care.* 2011; 15(1):67-82.
7. Mukasey MB, Sedgwick JL, Hagy DW. *Ballistic Resistance of Body Armor.* Washington, DC: US Department of Justice, Office of Justice Programs; 2008. NIJ Standard-0101.06.
8. Counter Narcotics and Terrorism Operational Medical Support website [homepage]. https://contoms.chepinc.org. Accessed April 18, 2018.

Suggested Readings

Carhart E. Developing protocols for tactical EMS care. EMS World website. https://www.emsworld.com/article/10615988/developing-protocols-tactical-ems-care. Published January 19, 2012. Accessed April 18, 2018.

Grubbs TC. Preserving crime scene evidence when treating patients at an MCI. *JEMS* website. http://www.jems.com/articles/print/volume-39/issue-5/features/preserving-crime-scene-evidence-when-tre.html. Published May 5, 2014. Accessed April 18, 2018.

Karels SR. *Legal Considerations for Tactical Medical Officers*. High Mark website. https://highmarkblog.com/wp-content/uploads/2016/04/Legal-Considerations-for-Tactical-Medical-Officers-Article-Format.pdf. Published 2015. Accessed April 18, 2018.

Llewellyn CH. The symbiotic relationship between operational military medicine, tactical medicine, and wilderness medicine: a view through a personal lens. *Wilderness Environ Med.* 2017;28(2S):S6-S11.

Marino M, Delaney J, Atwater P, Smith R. To save lives and property: high threat response. Homeland Security Affairs website. https://www.hsaj.org/articles/4530. Published June 2015. Accessed April 18, 2018.

Protecting the protectors. Officer.com website. https://www.officer.com/tactical/swat/article/12231650/from-the-battlefield-to-special-operations-tactical-medics-save-lives. Published July 13, 2016. Accessed April 18, 2018.

Tan DK, Bozeman W, FitzGerald D. Tactical EMS. In: Brice J, Delbridge TR, Meyers JB, eds. *Emergency Services: Clinical Practice and Systems Oversight*. 2nd ed. West Sussex, England: John Wiley & Sons; 2015:355-362.

Waldman M, Shapira SC, Richman A, Haughton BP, Mechem CC. Tactical medicine: a joint forces field algorithm. *Milit Med.* 2014;179(10):1056-1061.

Wolfsburg D. Pro bono: violence against EMS providers. *JEMS* website. http://www.jems.com/articles/print/volume-42/issue-8/departments/pro-bono/pro-bono-violence-against-ems-providers.html. Published August 1, 2017. Accessed April 18, 2018.

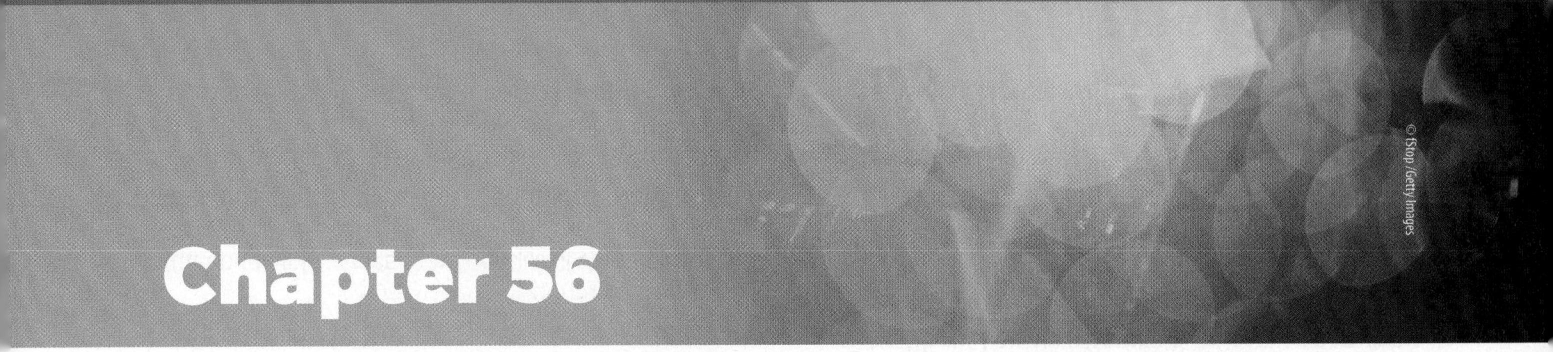

Chapter 56

Hazardous Materials Awareness

NATIONAL EMS EDUCATION STANDARD COMPETENCIES

EMS Operations

Knowledge of operational roles and responsibilities to ensure patient, public, and personnel safety.

Hazardous Materials Awareness

Risks and responsibilities of operating in a cold zone at a hazardous materials or other special incident. (pp 1910–1911)

OBJECTIVES

Upon completion of this chapter, the paramedic student will be able to:

1. Define hazardous materials (hazmat) terminology. (pp 1893, 1908)
2. Identify legislation about hazardous materials that influences emergency health care workers. (pp 1893–1896)
3. Describe resources to assist in identification and management of hazmat incidents. (pp 1896–1900)
4. Identify the protective clothing and equipment needed to respond to selected hazmat incidents. (pp 1900–1903)
5. Describe the pathophysiology and signs and symptoms of internal damage caused by exposure to selected hazardous materials. (pp 1904–1907)
6. Identify the pathophysiology, signs and symptoms, and prehospital management of selected hazardous materials that produce external damage. (p 1907)
7. Outline the prehospital response to a hazmat emergency. (pp 1907–1911)
8. Describe medical monitoring and rehabilitation of rescue workers who respond to a hazmat emergency. (pp 1911–1912)
9. Describe emergency decontamination and management of patients who have been contaminated by hazardous materials. (pp 1913–1915)
10. Outline the eight steps to decontaminate rescue personnel and equipment at a hazmat incident. (p 1915)

KEY TERMS

asphyxiants Gases that displace the oxygen in the air (simple asphyxiants) or disable the chemistry of cellular respiration despite adequate oxygen levels in the blood (chemical asphyxiants).

carcinogens Cancer-causing agents.

cardiotoxins Hazardous materials that can cause myocardial ischemia and dysrhythmias.

cold zone A safety zone in a hazmat response that typically surrounds the warm zone; usually considered safe, requiring only minimal protective clothing.

corrosives Hazardous materials that are either strong acids or strong bases (alkaline).

cryogens Refrigerant liquid gases that can freeze human tissue on contact.

decontamination The process of making patients, rescuers, equipment, and supplies safe by eliminating harmful substances.

dose response The physical change or effect caused by exposure to a chemical. The response depends on the concentration of the chemical to which the person was exposed.

formal product identification A method of identifying a hazardous material through written means.

hazard and risk assessment An analysis of the consequences and probability that exposure to a chemical may cause danger or peril.

hazardous material (hazmat) Any item or agent (biologic chemical, radiologic and/or physical) that has the potential to cause harm to humans, animals, or the environment, either by itself or through interaction with other factors.

hemotoxins Hazardous substances that may cause the destruction of red blood cells.

hepatotoxins Hazardous substances that damage the liver.

hot zone The area of a hazmat incident that presents an immediate danger to life or health and typically includes the hazardous material itself.

informal product identification A method of identifying a hazardous material through unwritten means.

irritants Chemicals that are not corrosives, but which can cause a reversible inflammatory effect on living tissue at the site of skin, mucous membrane, respiratory system, or eye contact.

liquefaction Conversion of solid tissues to a fluid or semifluid state.

medical monitoring The ongoing evaluation of rescuers who are at risk for illness or injury from operations at the incident.

nephrotoxins Hazardous materials that are especially destructive to the kidneys.

nerve poisons Poisonous substances that act on the nervous system; generally refers to nerve gas.

neurotoxins Substances that alter the structure or function of the nervous system.

placards Four-sided, diamond-shaped signs displayed on hazardous materials containers that usually are yellow, orange, white, or green. They have a four-digit United Nations identification number and a legend to indicate the contents of the container.

primary contamination Exposure to a hazardous substance that is harmful only to the person exposed and that poses little risk of exposure to others.

rehabilitation Activities that are provided at an incident to sustain the energy of rescuers, improve performance, and decrease the likelihood of on-scene injury or death; also known as rehab.

riot control/tear agents Chemicals that can produce sensory irritation or disabling physical effects that disappear within a short time after termination of exposure.

safe distance factor The minimum safe distance for personal safety from hazardous materials as outlined in the reference guides.

safety data sheet (SDS) Written product identification as required by the Occupational Safety and Health Administration for each chemical produced, stored, or used in the United States.

secondary contamination Exposure to a hazardous substance whereby liquid and particulate substances are transferred easily to others by touching.

self-contained breathing apparatus (SCBA) A respiratory protection device that provides an enclosed system of air.

shipping papers Descriptions of the hazardous materials that include the substance name, classification, shipper's certification, emergency response telephone number, emergency response information, and United Nations identification number.

supplied-air breathing apparatus (SABA) A device that provides a nearly unlimited supply of air from a source located outside the confined space.

synergistic effects The effects of one chemical enhancing the effects of a second chemical.

UN/NA number The United Nations class (or division) identification number and North American number for a hazardous material. The numbers are identical.

warm zone In a hazmat incident, a buffer area that surrounds the hot zone with "cold" and "hot" end corridors; usually considered a safer environment for workers than the hot zone.

Hazardous materials (hazmat) incidents create added responsibilities for EMS personnel. Large incidents may involve a number of political jurisdictions. In addition, cooperation in mass evacuations and mass decontamination may be required. Specialized roles and responsibilities include, among others, recognition and identification of hazardous materials, scene safety, responsibilities to stage at major scenes, containment and cleanup of the material, extrication and decontamination of exposed people, provision of emergency care, and continual medical monitoring of team members involved in the incident.

Scope of Hazardous Materials

A **hazardous material (hazmat)** is defined as any substance or material capable of posing a risk to health, safety, and property.[1] More than 50 billion tons of hazardous materials are made in the United States each year. About 2.5 billion tons are shipped within the United States.[1] The US Department of Transportation (DOT) reports there were almost 17,000 hazmat incidents reported in 2017.[2] They resulted in 138 injuries and 3 deaths. Most of the injuries, and all of the deaths, were related to highway incidents. Emergency responses to vehicular crashes are common; thus, the potential for exposure to hazardous materials is great. Other possible causes of hazmat incidents include mishaps in the storage of materials and manufacturing operations, illicit drug manufacturing (eg, "meth labs"), and acts of terrorism (see Chapter 57, *Bioterrorism and Weapons of Mass Destruction*).

CRITICAL THINKING

Consider the industries in your area. Do any of these have the potential for a hazardous materials exposure?

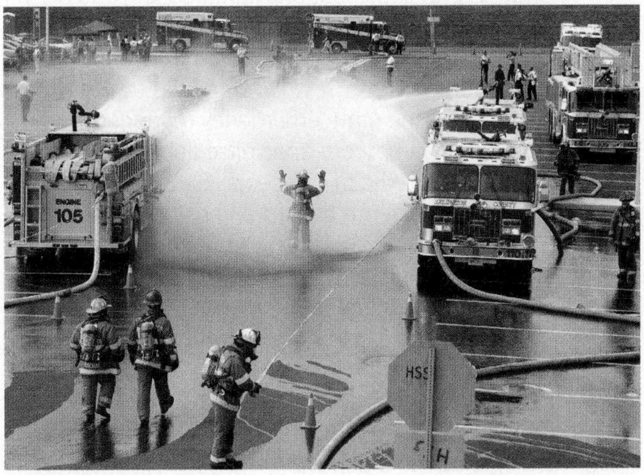

Courtesy of Master Sgt. Jim Varhegy/U.S. Air Force.

As described in Chapter 33, *Toxicology*, injury or illness can also result from exposure to household chemicals, pesticides, and industrial toxins. Most schools, stores, and homes have low quantities of chemicals that can be stable on their own; however, if these chemicals are mixed, the result can be a hazmat incident. For example, mixing bleach with other products, such as ammonia or toilet bowl cleaners, can produce toxic vapors. There were 39,807 chemical exposures reported to US poison control centers in 2016.[3]

Laws and Regulations

As more and more chemicals are created and used in the United States, much focus has been placed on the handling of these hazardous materials. Major incidents have attracted the attention of employee and citizen groups. These incidents also have drawn the attention of local, state, and federal officials. Some of these incidents include the Union Carbide disaster in Bhopal, India (1984); the Chernobyl nuclear accident in the Soviet Union (1986); the Three Mile Island incident in the United States (1979); and the Fukushima Daiichi nuclear disaster in Japan (2011).[4] This attention has resulted in more laws and regulations to ensure strict control of hazardous materials.

The Superfund Amendments and Reauthorization Act (the Superfund Act) of 1986 established requirements for federal, state, and local governments and industry regarding emergency planning and the reporting of hazardous materials–related incidents.[5] This act was intended to help communities better manage a chemical emergency. The Superfund Act helped increase public knowledge about hazardous materials in communities and helped to improve public access to this information. The act required owners and operators of facilities using or storing any of the extremely hazardous substances identified by the Environmental Protection Agency (EPA) to notify the local fire department, the local emergency managers, and the state emergency response commission.

In 1989, the Occupational Safety and Health Administration (OSHA) and the EPA published rules to govern training requirements, emergency plans, medical checkups, and other safety precautions for workers at uncontrolled hazardous waste sites and for those responding to hazardous chemical releases or spills.[6] The Superfund Act mandates that states adopt these rules. The training requirements from OSHA, commonly referred to as the Hazardous Waste Operations and Emergency Response (HAZWOPER) standards, apply to five groups of people who may respond to an emergency that involves hazardous materials (BOX 56-1). The minimum level of training for EMS workers and all first responders is the first

BOX 56-1 Overview of Training Requirements for EMS Personnel Responding to a Hazmat Incident, as Established by OSHA and the EPA

1. **First responder awareness.** This category pertains to people who are likely to witness or discover a hazardous substance release but who do not have emergency response duties pertaining to hazardous materials as part of their job functions. People in this category must have sufficient training to demonstrate the following:
   - An understanding of what hazardous substances are and the risks associated with them in an incident
   - An understanding of the potential outcomes associated with an emergency created when hazardous substances are present
   - The ability to recognize the presence of hazardous substances in an emergency
   - The ability to identify the hazardous substance, if possible
   - An understanding of the first responder awareness role in the employer's emergency response plan, including site security and control, and the DOT's *Emergency Response Guidebook (ERG)*
   - The ability to realize the need for additional resources and to make appropriate notifications to the communications center
2. **First responder operations.** People are included in this category if they respond to hazmat incidents to protect nearby people, property, or the environment without trying to stop the hazardous release. Firefighters and EMS personnel are in this category. In addition to the knowledge base of first responder awareness, these responders must have training to do the following:
   - Implement hazard and risk assessment techniques
   - Select and use proper personal protective equipment (PPE) provided at the first responder operational level
   - Understand basic hazmat terms
   - Perform basic control, containment, and/or confinement operations within the capabilities of the resources and PPE available with their unit
   - Implement basic decontamination procedures
   - Understand the relevant standard operating procedures and termination procedures
3. **Hazmat technicians.** People in this category respond to hazmat emergencies for the purpose of stopping the release. Hazmat technicians usually are considered members of a hazmat response team. These responders have additional training that allows them to do the following:
   - Know how to implement the employer's emergency response plan
   - Know the classification, identification, and verification of known and unknown materials by using field survey instruments and equipment
   - Function within an assigned role in the incident command system
   - Select and use proper specialized chemical PPE provided to the hazmat technician
   - Understand hazard and risk assessment techniques
   - Perform advance control, containment, and/or confinement operations within the capabilities of the resources and PPE available with the unit
   - Understand and implement decontamination procedures
   - Understand termination procedures
   - Understand basic chemical and toxicologic terminology and behavior
4. **Hazmat specialists.** The duties of these responders require specific knowledge of the various hazardous materials. Hazmat specialists respond with and provide support to hazmat technicians and act as site liaisons with federal, state, and local government authorities. In addition to the knowledge base of the hazmat technician, hazmat specialists have training to do the following:
   - Implement the local emergency response plan
   - Understand classification, identification, and verification of known and unknown materials by using advanced survey instruments and equipment
   - Understand the state emergency response plan
   - Select and use proper specialized chemical PPE provided to the hazmat specialist
   - Implement in-depth hazard and risk techniques
   - Perform specialized control, containment, and/or confinement operations within the capabilities of the resources and PPE available
   - Determine and implement decontamination procedures
   - Develop a site safety and control plan
   - Understand chemical, radiologic, and toxicologic terminology and behavior
5. **On-scene incident commander.** The on-scene incident commander is trained to assume control of a hazmat event. In addition to the first responder awareness level of training, the on-scene incident commander's responsibilities include the following:
   - Knowing and being able to implement the employer's incident command system
   - Knowing how to implement the employer's emergency response plan
   - Knowing and understanding the hazards and risks associated with employees working in chemical protective clothing

BOX 56-1 Overview of Training Requirements for EMS Personnel Responding to a Hazmat Incident, as Established by OSHA and the EPA *(continued)*

- Knowing how to implement the local emergency response plan
- Knowledge of the state emergency response plan and familiarity with the Federal Regional Response Team
- Knowing and understanding the importance of decontamination procedures

Note: The NFPA has also set competencies for EMS personnel responding to hazmat/weapon of mass destruction (WMD) incidents. These standards were designed to provide guidance for the roles and responsibilities of basic life support (BLS) and advanced life support (ALS) responders at hazmat and WMD incidents and to recognize that these incidents present unique challenges for EMS.

In brief, the goal of the competencies in NFPA 473 at the BLS responder level is to define the knowledge and skills necessary to safely deliver BLS medical care at hazmat/WMD incidents. The competencies defined for a BLS responder include the following:

- Analysis of a hazmat/WMD incident to determine potential health hazards
- Development of a plan to deliver BLS to any exposed patient within the scope of practice
- Implementation of the prehospital treatment plan within the scope of practice by determining the nature of the hazmat/WMD incident

The competencies defined for an ALS responder include all competencies required of a BLS responder plus the following:

- A more detailed analysis of a hazmat/WMD incident to determine the potential health hazards, including an assessment of health risks and identification of patients who may be candidates for advanced clinical care
- The development of a plan to deliver ALS to any exposed patient within the responder's scope of practice, including identification of supplemental regional and national resources
- Implementation of an enhanced prehospital treatment plan within the responder's scope of practice by determining the nature of the hazmat/WMD incident, including an assessment of available equipment and evaluation of the need for advanced clinical care

NFPA 473 provides additional information on these competencies.

Modified from: Regulations (Standards—29 CFR)—table of contents. Occupational Safety and Health Administration website. https://www.osha.gov/pls/oshaweb/owadisp.show_document?p_table=STANDARDS&p_id=9765. Accessed April 30, 2018; and National Fire Protection Association. *NFPA 473: Standard for Competencies for EMS Personnel Responding to Hazardous Materials/Weapons of Mass Destruction Incidents*. Quincy MA: National Fire Protection Association; 2018.

responder awareness level. At the awareness level, responders must be able to do the following:[7]

- Evaluate the incident and identify that a hazardous material or a WMD incident exists.
- Call for appropriate resources.
- Identify the name, United Nations/North American identification number, placard type, or other identifying markings on the hazardous materials.
- Gather information from the DOT's *ERG* related to the hazard.
- Begin measures to maintain a safe perimeter around the incident.

In addition to these training levels outlined by OSHA, the National Fire Protection Association (NFPA) has published standards that address competencies for EMS personnel at hazmat scenes.[8] According to NFPA 473, *Standard for Competencies for EMS Personnel Responding to Hazardous Materials/Weapons of Mass Destruction Incidents*, paramedics responding to a hazmat scene should be able to do the following:

1. Analyze the scene to determine potential health risks to everyone on the scene.
2. Deliver ALS to patients.
3. Implement a prehospital treatment plan for patients who have been exposed, and begin care after appropriate decontamination.

Paramedics involved in containment or other activities beyond simply calling for additional resources and securing an area should be additionally trained to the hazmat operations level. Personnel who expect to take offensive action to mitigate a hazmat incident or an incident involving chemical, biologic, radiologic, nuclear, or explosive (CBRNE) agents are typically certified to the hazmat technician level, consisting of intensive training up to 80 hours in length.

The ALS care provided by paramedics at the scene of a hazmat incident depends on the medical protocols of the medical director in the authority having jurisdiction, as well as generally accepted practices of hasty decontamination and mitigation recommendations set forth in the safety data sheet (SDS) or the *ERG* for a known hazardous material exposure.

Identification of Hazardous Materials

At the center of dealing with hazardous materials is identifying the substance. Two methods used to identify such materials are **informal product identification** and **formal product identification**.

Informal Product Identification

Arriving emergency personnel may be able to determine the presence and type of hazardous materials at the scene. Informal methods of identification include the following:[9]

- Visual inspection of the scene with binoculars before entering the site
- Verbal reports by bystanders or other responsible people
- Occupancy type (intended use of a particular structure, such as fuel storage or pesticide plant)
- Incident location (probable location for presence of hazardous materials)
- Location within a building (what is stored in that area)
- Visual indicators (vapor clouds, smoke, leakage)
- Vehicle types (named carriers or company)
- Container characteristics (size, shape, color, deformed containers)
- Senses (peculiar smell reported by bystanders)
- Signs and symptoms of people who have been exposed

These informal ways to identify a product should be used as a quick means to determine the presence of any hazardous materials. The paramedic should always identify a product formally before taking any action that may pose a threat to the safety of all responders.

NOTE

Personal safety is the number one priority when responding to a hazmat incident. If the scene is not safe, the EMS crew should retreat and not enter the scene until it has been made safe by trained personnel.

Formal Product Identification

Traditionally, hazardous materials have been labeled by one or more of the following six systems:[10]

1. The American National Standards Institute uses a label to identify a specific hazard (eg, explosives, flammable liquids, radioactive materials) rather than a specific chemical.
2. DOT uses labels and placards with pictographs and printed hazard categories. In addition, DOT requires specific information on shipping manifests.
3. The Globally Harmonized System of Classification and Labeling of Chemicals, which is managed by the United Nations, uses pictographs, symbols, or both, similar to those used by DOT, to identify a specific hazard rather than a specific chemical.
4. The International Air Transport Association uses the United Nations pictographs and indicates written emergency precaution measures in case of an incident.
5. The NFPA uses color and a numeric rating scale (NFPA 704 System) to identify the degree of hazard for health, fire, and reactivity. Many state and local fire codes require the diamond-shaped identification symbols on fixed facilities (**FIGURE 56-1**). The numbering system rates each category from 1 (least harmful) to 4 (most harmful).
6. OSHA's Hazard Communication Standard requires SDSs for hazardous chemicals that are stored, handled, or used in the workplace (**FIGURE 56-2**).

CRITICAL THINKING

The next time you are on the highway, see if you can easily spot the placards on large trucks.

Placards and Shipping Papers

A number of identification systems may be used. However, hazardous materials usually are identified by **placards** (**FIGURE 56-3**) and **shipping papers**.

The United Nations class (or division) identification number and the North American number (**UN/NA number**) may be displayed on the bottom of a placard, or the number may be displayed on the shipping paper after the listed shipping name or names. In certain cases, this class or division number may replace the written name of the hazard class in

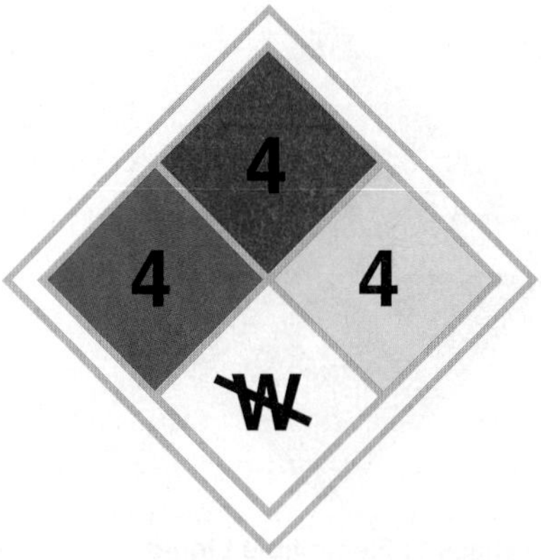

FIGURE 56-1 The National Fire Protection Association placard. It consists of four diamonds within a larger diamond. Reading the placard as a clock, the red (flammability) diamond is at 12 o'clock, the yellow (instability) diamond is at 3 o'clock, the white (special hazards) diamond is at 6 o'clock, and the blue (health hazard) diamond is at 9 o'clock. The degree of hazard severity is indicated by a numeric rating that ranges from 4, indicating the most severe hazard, to 0, indicating no hazard. Special hazards are indicated in the white section and refer to chemicals that react with water (W) and those that are oxidizers (OX).

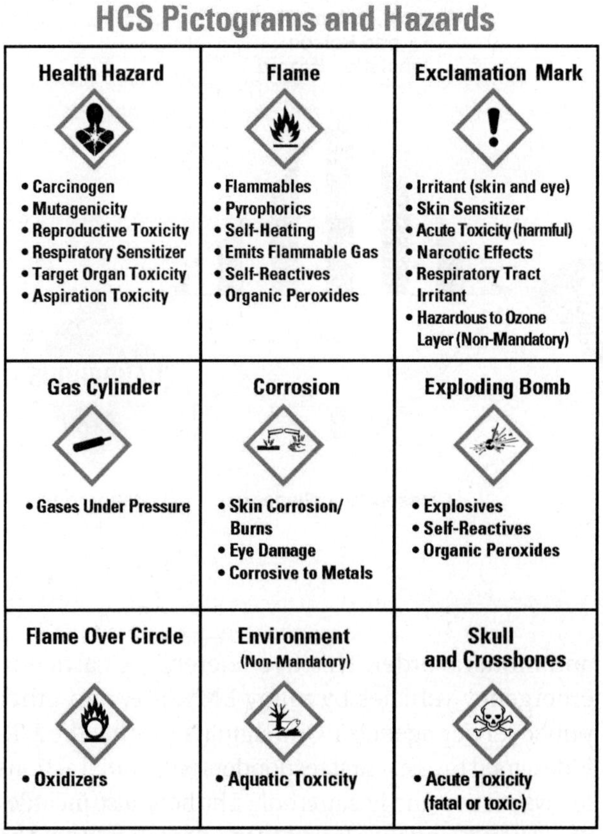
HCS Pictograms and Hazards
Health Hazard
• Carcinogen
• Mutagenicity
• Reproductive Toxicity
• Respiratory Sensitizer
• Target Organ Toxicity
• Aspiration Toxicity
Flame
• Flammables
• Pyrophorics
• Self-Heating
• Emits Flammable Gas
• Self-Reactives
• Organic Peroxides
Exclamation Mark
• Irritant (skin and eye)
• Skin Sensitizer
• Acute Toxicity (harmful)
• Narcotic Effects
• Respiratory Tract Irritant
• Hazardous to Ozone Layer (Non-Mandatory)
Gas Cylinder
• Gases Under Pressure
Corrosion
• Skin Corrosion/ Burns
• Eye Damage
• Corrosive to Metals
Exploding Bomb
• Explosives
• Self-Reactives
• Organic Peroxides
Flame Over Circle
• Oxidizers
Environment (Non-Mandatory)
• Aquatic Toxicity
Skull and Crossbones
• Acute Toxicity (fatal or toxic)

FIGURE 56-2 Pictograms and hazards.

From Occupational Safety and Health Administration. Hazard Communication Standard: Labels and Pictograms.

the shipping paper description. **TABLE 56-1** shows the meanings of the class and division numbers.

The location and type of paperwork that identifies hazardous materials vary according to the mode of transport. Most shipping papers are kept near the operator (eg, driver, pilot, captain) of the vehicle, aircraft, train, or ship. Several chemical agents may have the same UN/NA number. Thus, it is important to refer to specific guidelines for the hazardous material by chemical name in addition to this number.

NOTE

Shippers are responsible for tracking hazardous loads in transit. If shipping papers are difficult to obtain or too dangerous to recover, law enforcement personnel or the dispatch agency can contact the shipper by phone with a description of the vehicle (eg, truck or car number and license plate number). The shipping will then help identify the type of hazardous material.

Safety Data Sheets

A **safety data sheet (SDS)** is required by OSHA for each chemical produced, stored, or used in the United States. SDSs are supplied by the manufacturer. They contain information for the safe and proper handling and storage of the material. They also have information on emergency actions needed following exposure. SDSs also classify the potential of significant health hazards from exposure to a material.

The potential health hazard of a material may be defined in a number of different ways. This may depend on the degree of inherent toxicity and type of exposure. SDSs provide useful information. However, they should not be used as the sole source of chemical information, information on health risks, or treatment recommendations. Paramedics should consult with medical direction, a poison control center, or another appropriate authority.

Other Sources of Information on Hazardous Materials

A number of information references are available for hazardous materials. These references include books, telephone support through emergency hazmat agencies, computer databases, phone apps, and Internet sources. Product information should be referenced through more than one source. (Preferably three sources should be used, if time and availability permit.)

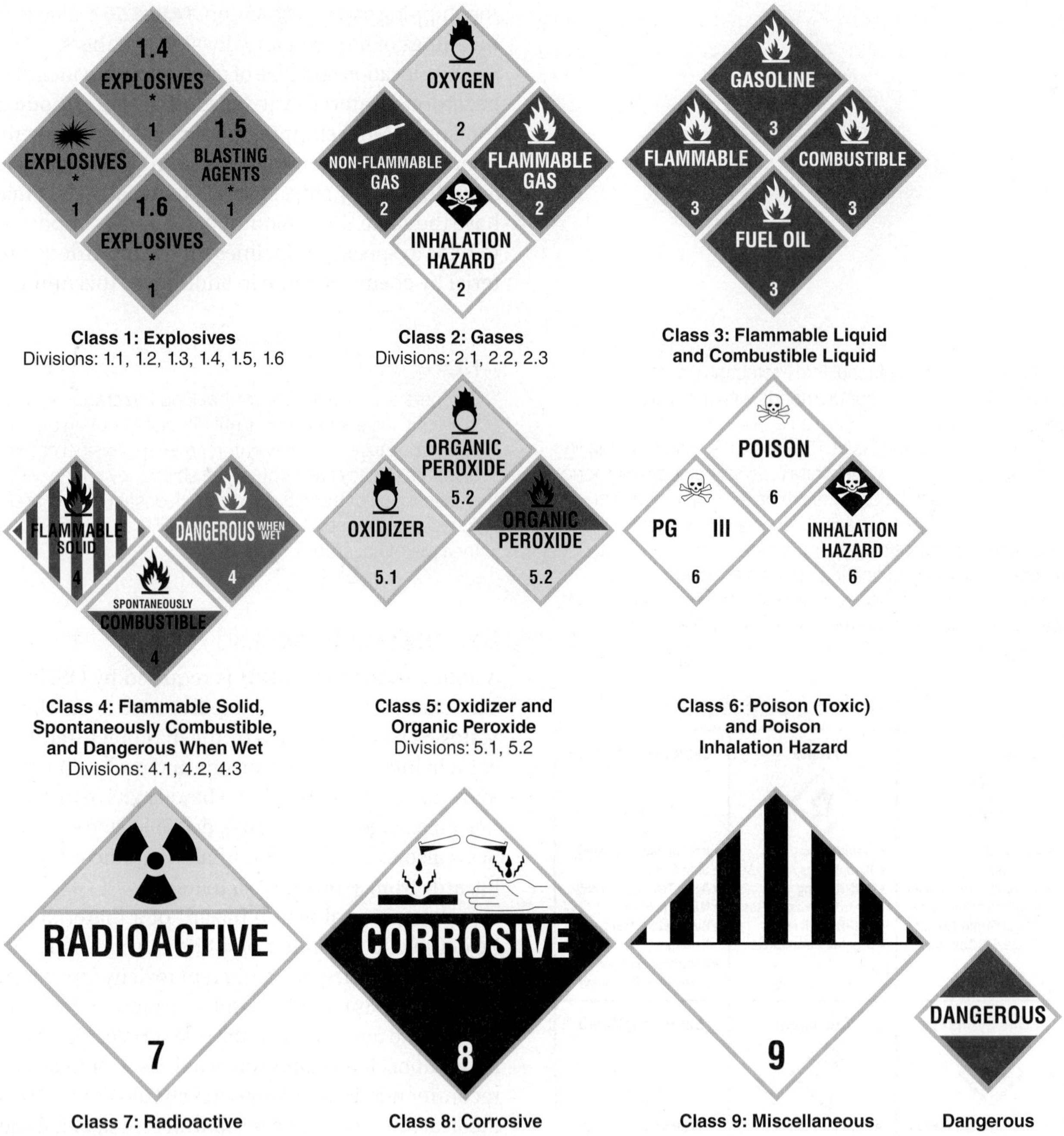

FIGURE 56-3 Hazmat warning placards and labels.

Courtesy of the US Department of Transportation.

One such reference is the *ERG* published by the DOT, Transport Canada, and the Secretariat of Communications and Transportation of Mexico. This guidebook lists more than 1,000 hazardous materials. It also lists the basic first aid procedures for managing an exposure. It includes names and identification numbers of substances. Materials discussed in the book and online resource are cross-referenced in alphabetical and numeric order. This free reference is carried in emergency vehicles by many EMS, fire, and other public service agencies. One should note that the *ERG* is designed to assist first responders with initial actions for evacuation and hazards only. The book also includes the distance and area from the incident that should be evacuated. The book is not the only guide that should be referenced when dealing with hazmat emergencies.

TABLE 56-1 International Classification System for Hazardous Materials

Class 1[a]	**Explosives**
Division 1.1	Explosives with a mass explosion hazard
Division 1.2	Explosives with a projection but not mass explosion hazard
Division 1.3	Explosives with predominantly a fire hazard and either a minor blast or a projection hazard
Division 1.4	Explosives with no significant blast hazard
Division 1.5	Very insensitive explosives with a mass explosion hazard
Division 1.6	Extremely insensitive explosive articles (do not have a mass explosion hazard)
Class 2	**Gases**
Division 2.1	Flammable gases
Division 2.2	Nonflammable, nontoxic gases
Division 2.3	Toxic (poisonous) gases
Class 3	**Flammable and Combustible Liquids**
Division 3.1	Flashpoint $<0°F$ ($-18°C$)
Division 3.2	Flashpoint $\geq 0°F$ ($-18°C$) but $<73°F$ ($23°C$)
Division 3.3	Flashpoint $\geq 73°F$ ($23°C$) but $<142°F$ ($61°C$)
Class 4	**Flammable Solids, Spontaneously Combustible Materials, Materials That Emit Flammable Gases on Contact With Water**
Division 4.1	Flammable solids, self-reactive substances, and solid desensitized explosives
Division 4.2	Materials that are liable to spontaneously combust
Division 4.3	Materials that emit flammable gases when in contact with water
Class 5	**Oxidizers and Organic Peroxides**
Division 5.1	Oxidizers
Division 5.2	Organic peroxides
Class 6	**Poisonous and Infectious Materials**
Division 6.1	Toxic (poisonous) substances
Division 6.2	Infectious materials
Class 7	**Radioactive Materials**
Class 8	**Corrosives**
Class 9	**Miscellaneous Hazardous Materials/Goods and Articles**

[a]Class or division numbers may be displayed in the bottom of placards, or they may be displayed in the hazardous materials description on shipping papers. In certain cases, a class or division number may replace the written name of the hazard class description on the shipping paper.

Modified from: US Department of Transportation. *Emergency Response Guidebook*. Washington, DC: Department of Transportation; 2016; and Environmental health and safety. Carnegie Mellon University website. https://www.cmu.edu/ehs/Laboratory-Safety/chemical-safety/shipping-dangerous-goods.html. Accessed April 30, 2018.

NOTE

When a hazardous substance cannot be precisely identified, trained personnel may use sophisticated devices to ensure scene safety and to aid in product identification. These devices include air and gas monitoring equipment and special equipment for pH testing, chemical testing, water detection, and colorimetric tube testing.

As described in Chapter 33, *Toxicology*, regional poison control centers have been established throughout most of the United States. They are a valuable asset in any EMS system. Many of these centers are available 24 hours a day. They are staffed with specialists who provide information, consultation, treatment recommendations, patient follow-up, and data collection. Poison control centers are linked to many agencies that deal with toxic substances. In addition, they are tied closely to all area hospitals. These centers maintain a listing of more than 350,000 drugs, toxic substances, and other products. The Universal Poison Control number is 1-800-222-1222.

The Chemical Transportation Emergency Center (CHEMTREC) is a public service of the American Chemistry Council. The center provides immediate advice to on-scene personnel about the management of known or unknown hazardous materials. The agency also contacts the shipper of the material for more information or assistance when needed. The Chemical Transportation Emergency Center operates 24 hours a day, 7 days a week. The center can be reached in the United States and the Virgin Islands through the emergency toll-free number 1-800-424-9300. The paramedic should contact CHEMTREC as soon as possible during a hazmat incident. EMS personnel should provide the center with the name of the substance, its identification number, and the nature of the problem. Involving CHEMTREC in the management of a hazmat incident is usually part of the standard operating procedure of any emergency response team.

ChemTel is an emergency response communications center. It serves the United States and Canada. Carriers transporting hazardous materials are required to have a 24-hour hotline for information when hazardous cargo is being shipped. The office can provide specific product information. It also can provide referral to the proper state and federal authorities for incidents that involve hazardous materials. ChemTel can be reached 24 hours a day, 7 days a week, through the toll-free number 1-888-255-3924.

Computer-aided management of emergency operations (CAMEO) systems are designed to assist emergency responders quickly in the management of hazmat incidents. These systems use computer modeling to predict the effects of chemical spills and toxins released in plumes of smoke and use geospatial information on a map to see if the hazards will impact specific locations in the community. The systems, which are available to municipalities, help communities prepare emergency response plans. CAMEO currently provides information on thousands of chemicals and contains more than 80,000 chemical synonyms and identification numbers that can be quickly searched to identify unknown substances during an incident. **BOX 56-2** lists other government and private sector agencies that may assist in a hazmat incident.

Many Internet sources are available for hazmat identification and management. These sources include federal, state, and local governmental agencies; colleges and universities; businesses and industry; trade associations; and nonprofit groups that have established easily accessible websites. In addition, several free applications can be downloaded to a portable electronic device for reference on emergency scenes. **TABLE 56-2** gives free applications for hazmat reference.

Personal Protective Clothing and Equipment

The potential for injury from exposure to hazardous materials is related to the toxicity, flammability, and reactivity of a particular substance. Use of the right protection is crucial for anyone dealing with hazardous materials. Key considerations include proper respiratory protection and protective clothing.

Protective Respiratory Devices

The potential for exposure of the respiratory system to hazardous materials is of paramount importance to the emergency responder. The respiratory system can be protected by air purification devices and by equipment that supplies clean air (atmosphere supplying device).

Air purification relies on respirators or filtration devices. These devices remove particulate matter, gases, or vapors from the atmosphere. They do not use a separate source of air. They also require constant monitoring for contaminants and oxygen levels. As a rule, they are not recommended for use in a hazmat release and must be fitted to the wearer. Filtration devices are material-specific (ie, "must match the gas"). They are not used in the presence of multiple

BOX 56-2 Agencies That Assist in Hazmat Incidents[a]

Federal Agencies

Centers for Disease Control and Prevention
DOT
EPA
Federal Aviation Administration
National Response Center
- Armed Forces (Army, Navy, Air Force, Marines)
- Coast Guard
- Department of Energy

Regional and State Agencies

National Guard
State emergency management agencies
State environmental protection agency
State health departments
State police

Local Agencies

Emergency management
Fire service (hazmat units)
Law enforcement agencies
Poison control center
Public utilities
Sewage and treatment facilities

Commercial Agencies

American Petroleum Institute
Association of American Railroads and Hazardous Materials Systems
Chemical Manufacturers Association
Chevron (provides assistance with Chevron products)
HELP (the Union Carbide Emergency Response System for company shipments)
Local industry
Local contractors
- Local: carriers and transporters
- Railway industry

[a]This box lists only a sampling of the agencies; the list is not all-inclusive.

types of chemicals. These devices cannot be used in an environment with a low oxygen concentration.

Atmosphere-supplying devices rely on a separate source of positive pressure to supply air. They provide the highest level of respiratory protection. Two basic types are available: the **self-contained breathing apparatus (SCBA)** and the **supplied-air breathing apparatus (SABA)**, or air lines. The use of either requires training, recertification, and testing for proper fit as governed by regulations from OSHA.

TABLE 56-2 Free Applications for Hazmat Reference

Application	Description
Emergency Response Guidebook: https://www.phmsa.dot.gov/hazmat/erg/erg2016-mobileapp	Helps identify hazardous materials Lists primary threat from hazardous materials Defines health threats associated with toxin Specifies initial evacuation distance from source
WISER (Wireless Information System for Emergency Responders) substance list: https://wiser.nlm.nih.gov/substances.html	Helps identify hazardous materials Describes physical characteristics of hazardous materials Gives human health information related to hazards Provides containment and suppression advice

The SCBA provides respiratory protection in oxygen-deficient and toxic atmospheres. Only SCBAs that maintain positive pressure in the facepiece during inhalation and exhalation should be used when working with hazardous materials. The SCBA usually is considered excellent protection in hazardous environments. However, the rescuer should be aware of potential facepiece penetration and contamination by certain toxic substances, such as methyl bromide and ethyleneimine.

The SABA supplies air to the rescuer via an air-line hose away from the scene. These devices often are used at hazmat sites when extended working times are required. The SABA must have an escape capability for operations in atmospheres classified as immediately dangerous to life and health. Respiratory protection devices that combine SCBAs and air-line hose units are available. However, because of their dependence on air supply via a line, they limit the distance entry personnel can enter into a contaminated area (hot zone).

Classifications of Protective Clothing

Protective clothing is categorized in two ways: disposable or reusable. The clothing is made from a variety of materials that are designed specifically for certain chemical exposures. (Training in the use of this clothing should take place in a safe environment before it is used at emergency scenes.) Examples of this material include Tyvek/Saranex, nitrile rubber, Teflon, and Viton. No single material is compatible with all chemicals. Thus, the manufacturer's guidelines and recommendations must be followed (BOX 56-3). Protective clothing is classified in several ways. The classifications defined by OSHA and the EPA follow:[11]

Level A. Level A provides the highest level of skin, respiratory, and eye protection (**FIGURE 56-4**). Level A equipment typically is used by hazmat teams for entry into the incident site. Level A equipment includes a positive-pressure (pressure demand), full-facepiece SCBA or positive-pressure supplied air respirator with escape SCBA, approved by the National Institute of Occupational Safety and Health (NIOSH). This level of protection also includes a totally encapsulating (gastight) chemical protective suit, coveralls, long underwear (optional), outer and inner gloves that are chemical resistant, cooling mechanism (optional), an undersuit hard hat (optional), and a disposable protective suit (including gloves and steel-toed boots) that may be worn over a totally encapsulating suit. (Unless specified by the manufacturer, these disposable suits are not to be worn in flammable atmospheres.) All level A suits are mandated to have 2-way radio communication, preferably voice activated and integrated within the suit.

Level B. Level B provides the highest level of respiratory protection. However, it provides a lower level of skin protection (**FIGURE 56-5**). Level B protection typically is worn by the decontamination team. It includes positive-pressure, full-facepiece SCBA or positive-pressure supplied air respirator with escape SCBA (NIOSH approved); hooded, chemical-resistant clothing (overalls, long-sleeved jacket, coveralls, one-or two-piece chemical splash suit, disposable chemical overalls); coveralls (optional); cooling mechanism (optional); inner and outer chemical-resistant gloves; chemical-resistant boots with steel toe and shank; outer chemical-resistant boot covers

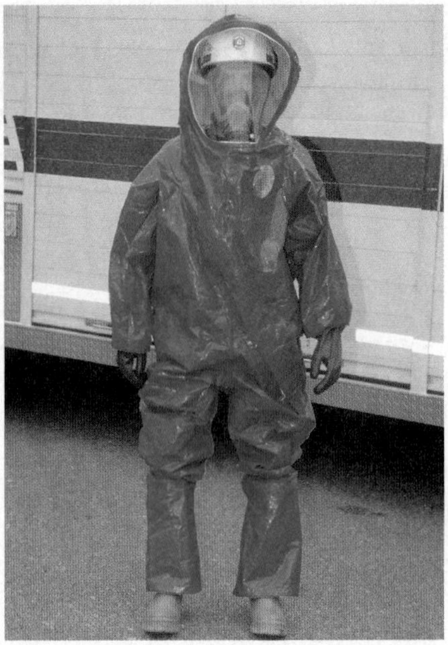

FIGURE 56-4 Level A protective clothing. It offers the highest levels of skin, eye, and respiratory protection.

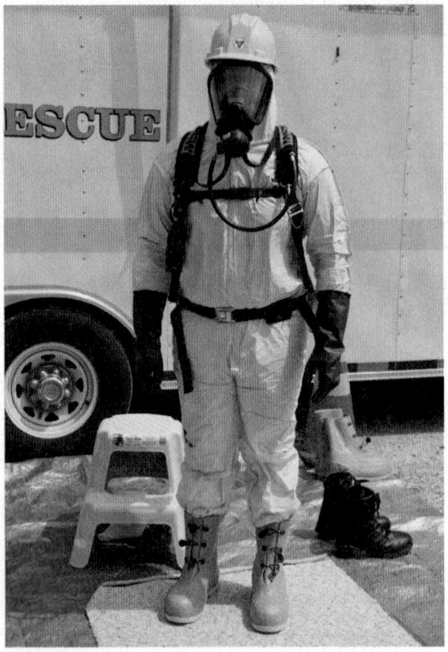

FIGURE 56-5 Level B protective clothing. It offers the highest level of respiratory protection and a higher level of skin protection than level C protective clothing.

BOX 56-3 Forms of Chemical Intrusion

- **Degradation.** The physical destruction or decomposition of a clothing material caused by exposure to chemicals, use, or ambient conditions.
- **Penetration.** The flow of a hazardous liquid chemical through zippers, stitched seams, pinholes, or other imperfections in a material.
- **Permeation.** The process by which a hazardous liquid chemical moves through a material on a molecular level.

(optional); and an optional hard hat and face shield. All level B suits are mandated to have 2-way radio communication.

Level C. Level C protection is used during the transport of contaminated patients. Level C protection is used when the concentration and type of airborne substance (or substances) is known and the criteria for using air-purifying respirators are met. Level C equipment includes full-face or half-mask air-purifying respirators (NIOSH approved); hooded, chemical-resistant clothing (overalls, two-piece chemical splash suit, disposable chemical-resistant overalls); coveralls (optional); outer and inner chemical-resistant gloves; outer chemical-resistant boots with steel toe and shank (optional); disposable outer chemical-resistant boot covers (optional); and optional escape mask and face shield.

Level D. Level D is a work uniform that affords minimal protection (used for nuisance contamination only; **FIGURE 56-6**). Level D protection commonly is known as firefighter "turnout" gear. (Turnout gear with SCBA may be considered level B protection for some chemicals that do not pose a danger for skin contact or absorption.) Level D equipment includes coveralls; optional gloves; chemical-resistant boots or shoes with steel toe and shank; disposable outer chemical-resistant boots (optional); safety glasses or chemical splash goggles; and optional hard hat, escape mask, and face shield.

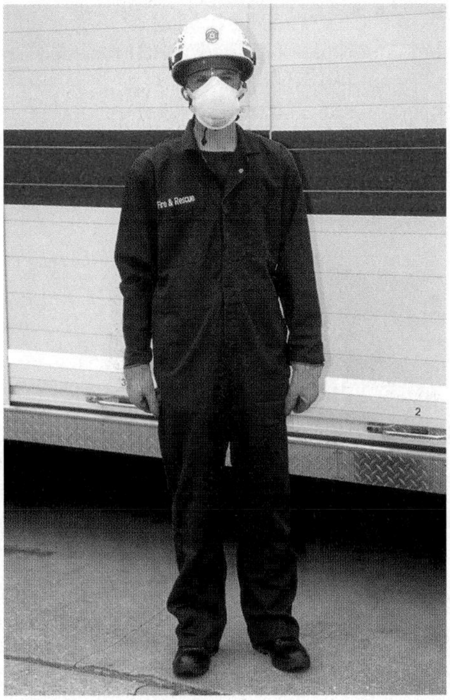

FIGURE 56-6 Level D protective clothing.

CRITICAL THINKING

What types of patient care do you think you will be able to provide when wearing each of the levels of hazmat protective gear?

Regardless of the type of PPE used during a hazmat incident, all avenues through which hazardous materials can enter the body must be protected. The following points should be of particular concern to any rescuer involved in hazmat response:

- Protective clothing should not be affected adversely by the hazardous materials involved.
- Protective clothing should seal all exposed skin.
- Contact with the hazardous materials should be of the absolute minimal duration required.
- Protective clothing and equipment should be decontaminated or discarded properly.
- The safety standards and methods for cleaning and disposing of clothing and equipment should be followed strictly.
- Contaminated patient clothing should be left at the scene for proper and safe disposal. It should not be transported with the patient. This approach will limit the contamination of the ambulance.

NOTE

Regardless of which level of hazmat PPE a responder wears, there will be some limitations and health concerns that the paramedic should consider. Often the responder in PPE experiences decreased peripheral vision, making him or her more prone to falls. The environment should be considered, especially in warmer temperatures, when the responder is easily overheated in the level A and level B suits. Paramedics assigned to rehabilitation should be prepared for fluid loss and heat-related emergencies in these situations.

Health Hazards

As described in Chapter 33, *Toxicology*, hazardous materials may enter the human body by inhalation, ingestion, injection, and absorption. Entry by means of any of these routes may result in internal and external damage to the rescuer. Exposure to dangerous substances may affect the body in several different ways. It may produce numerous injuries or illnesses.

Exposure to poisons can produce acute toxicity, delayed toxicity, and local and systemic effects. The body's response depends on the concentration of the chemical to which the body is exposed (also called the **dose response**). The paramedic also should be aware that drug treatment can result in **synergistic effects** (ie, the effects of one chemical enhancing the effects of a second chemical). Thus, all treatment methods must be guided by medical direction, a poison control center, or other appropriate authority.

Internal Damage

Internal damage to the human body from exposure to hazardous materials may involve the respiratory tract, the central nervous system, or other internal organs. Some substances injure all cells on contact. Others have a more direct effect on specific organs (target organs), such as the kidneys and liver.

Depending on the hazardous materials, the physical injury may vary. It may range from minor irritation to more serious complications, including cardiorespiratory compromise and death. Chronic illness (eg, chronic obstructive pulmonary disease) and various forms of cancer also may result. Some substances can cause abnormal fetal development and changes in gene structure. For example, penetrating radiation (described in Chapter 38, *Burns*) can lead to cell and chromosomal changes and can cause genetic changes, cell death, and sterility.

Irritants

Irritants that affect the respiratory system are a common complaint of rescuers and patients who have been exposed to hazardous materials. Chemical irritants emit vapors that affect the mucous membranes of the body, including the surfaces of the eyes, nose, mouth, and throat. As these irritants combine with moisture, acidic or alkaline reactions may occur. Exposure to these irritants may result in damage to the upper, lower, and deep respiratory tract. Examples of chemical irritants are hydrochloric acid, halogens, and ozone.

Self-defense chemical sprays used by some civilians and law enforcement officers are common and can present a hazard to responders. These sprays are

DID YOU KNOW?

Riot control/tear agents are solid chemicals with low vapor pressure that are dispersed in the air as fine particles. They produce sensory irritation or disabling physical effects that disappear within a short time after termination of exposure. Riot control agents (eg, Mace, pepper spray) often are referred to as "tear gas" and sometimes are used in military exercises, by law enforcement personnel for crowd control, and by the general public for personal protection. Paramedics and other emergency responders likely will encounter exposure to these agents during their careers. PPE is needed to guard against the effects of these agents.

The most common riot control agent compounds are chloroacetophenone and chlorobenzylidenemalononitrile. Riot control agents cause irritation to the area of contact (eg, eyes, skin, nose) within seconds of exposure. Signs and symptoms vary, depending on the location of exposure (open versus enclosed spaces) and the duration of contact with the agent, and may include some or all of the following:

- Eyes: excessive tearing, burning, blurred vision, redness
- Nose: runny nose, burning, swelling
- Mouth: burning, irritation, difficulty swallowing, drooling
- Lungs: chest tightness, coughing, choking sensation, wheezing, shortness of breath
- Skin: burns, rash
- Gastrointestinal system: nausea and vomiting

Although most effects from exposure to riot control agents are minor and last only 15 to 30 minutes, exposure to large doses or exposure in an enclosed area rarely may result in blindness, glaucoma, severe burns to airway structures, and life-threatening respiratory failure. Emergency care consists of moving people away from the source to fresh air and removing contaminated clothing when possible. The patient should remove contact lenses if the eyes are involved. Eye irrigation with water or saline may help resolve skin and ocular symptoms. If the patient is wheezing, follow guidelines to manage bronchospasm.

Modified from: National Center for Emerging and Zoonotic Infectious Diseases. Riot control agents/tear gas: facts about riot control agents. Centers for Disease Control and Prevention website. https://emergency.cdc.gov/agent/riotcontrol/factsheet.asp. Updated March 21, 2013. Accessed April 30, 2018; and National Association of EMS Officials. *National Model EMS Clinical Guideline*. Version 2.0. National Association of EMS Officials website. https://www.nasemso.org/documents/National-Model-EMS-Clinical-Guidelines-Version2-Sept2017.pdf. Published September 2017. Accessed April 30, 2018.

irritants and produce excessive tearing of the eyes. They include chloroacetophenone (known as CN gas or Mace), orthochlorobenzalmalononitrile (known as CS or tear gas), and oleoresin capsicum (pepper spray).

Asphyxiants

Asphyxiants are substances that displace oxygen in the air or prevent cellular uptake of oxygen despite adequate availability in the blood. Gases that displace the oxygen in the air are simple asphyxiants and include carbon dioxide, methane, and propane. Other gases not only displace oxygen in the air but also interfere with tissue oxygenation at the cellular level. These gases are referred to as blood poisons or chemical asphyxiants. They tend to interrupt the transport or use of oxygen by tissue cells. Through various mechanisms, these toxic gases deprive body tissue of needed oxygen. Examples include hydrogen cyanide, carbon monoxide, and hydrogen sulfide (BOX 56-4).

Nerve Poisons, Anesthetics, and Narcotics

Nerve poisons, anesthetics, and narcotics act on the nervous system. These agents affect either the cardiorespiratory mechanisms of the brain or the ability to transmit impulses required for adequate heart and lung function.

Nerve poisons were developed by the military. They often are referred to as war gases, nerve gases, or nerve agents (see Chapter 57, *Bioterrorism and Weapons of Mass Destruction*). Similar substances are used in solid pesticides. Exposure to these chemicals may result in fatal complications. Examples of these poisons include carbamates, organophosphates, parathion, and malathion. Anesthetics and narcotics are less hazardous than are nerve poisons. However, continuous exposure or exposure to large concentrations may result in unconsciousness or death. Examples include ethylene oxide, nitrous oxide, and ethyl alcohol.

Hepatotoxins

Hepatotoxins are substances that damage the liver. The poisons accumulate in the body and destroy the ability of the liver to function. Examples include chlorinated and halogenated hydrocarbons.

Cardiotoxins

Cardiotoxins are hazardous materials that can cause myocardial ischemia and dysrhythmias. Examples include some nitrates and ethylene glycol. Acute myocardial infarction and sudden death have been reported in healthy young people who were exposed to these substances. Short-term exposure to fluorocarbons and other halogenated hydrocarbons also has been known to cause cardiac abnormalities.

BOX 56-4 Hydrogen Sulfide

Hydrogen sulfide is considered a poison that affects several systems of the body, mostly the nervous system. It is a colorless, flammable, and extremely hazardous gas with a rotten egg smell. Hydrogen sulfide is similar to cyanide, and it is second only to carbon monoxide as a cause of inhalational deaths. Exposure to the gas can be lethal within a few minutes.

Hydrogen sulfide can be easily produced by combining common household chemicals. It is sometimes used as a method of suicide (detergent or chemical suicide). Most of these suicides in the United States have involved young adults who make the hydrogen sulfide in confined spaces such as closets, bathrooms, or cars. Another chemical used in these suicides is hydrogen cyanide. All rescuers working in a confined space or responding to a possible suicide in a confined space (eg, automobile, closet) should take appropriate precautions:

- Be aware of the possibility of poisonous gas.
- Remember that hydrogen sulfide has a pungent odor similar to rotten eggs.
- Retreat to a safe area and use PPE and SCBA if hydrogen sulfide is suspected.
- Be aware that confined spaces will temporarily continue to discharge noxious gas.
- Know that a person and his or her clothing will release the gas for a brief period.
- Expect the need for decontamination of the chemicals spilled.
- Request hazmat support with a cyanide antidote kit.

Modified from: Jiang J, Chan A, Ali S, et al. Hydrogen sulfide—mechanisms of toxicity and development of an antidote. *Sci Rep*. 2016;6:20831; and US Department of Health and Human Services. Chemical suicides: the risk to emergency responders. Chemical Hazards Emergency Medical Management website. https://chemm.nlm.nih.gov/chemicalsuicide.htm. Updated November 10, 2017. Accessed April 30, 2018.

Nephrotoxins

Nephrotoxins are hazardous materials that are especially destructive to the kidneys. Examples include carbon disulfide, lead, high concentrations of organic solvents, and inorganic mercury. Exposure to carbon tetrachloride, used as a solvent for dry cleaning or as a fire-extinguishing agent, can damage the kidneys.

Neurotoxins

Neurotoxins are poisons that affect the nervous system. Neurologic and behavioral toxicity may result from exposure to hazardous substances such as arsenic, lead, mercury, and organic solvents. In some cases, cerebral hypoxia may occur as a result of decreased oxygen in the blood.

Hemotoxins

Hemotoxins are hazardous substances that may cause the destruction of red blood cells. This destruction can result in hemolytic anemia (see Chapter 31, *Hematology*). Substances that can produce hemolytic anemia include aniline, naphthol, quinones, lead, mercury, arsenic, and copper. Pulmonary edema and cardiac and liver injury also may be caused by hemotoxin exposure.

Carcinogens

Carcinogens are cancer-causing agents. Many hazardous materials are carcinogenic or are suspected carcinogens. The exact amount of hazardous materials exposure required for cancer to develop is unknown. However, short-term exposure to specific agents is known to produce long-term effects. Disease and complications have been reported 30 years after exposure to some hazardous materials.[12]

Of particular interest to rescuers involved in firefighting is that all fossil and organic fuels produce dioxins when they are burned. Dioxin is a general term that describes a group of hundreds of chemicals that are highly persistent in the environment. These chemicals are an unintentional by-product of many industrial processes (eg, waste incineration, pesticide manufacturing). Many of the dioxins are carcinogens. (For example, burning wood produces carcinogenic formaldehyde.) Dioxins and other toxins, such as asbestos, are associated with the increased incidence of respiratory and some other cancers in firefighters.[13] Even with appropriate structural firefighting gear, toxic smoke absorbs into the skin. Intense heat increases this risk, with a reported 400% increase in skin absorption occurring with each five degrees of increased body temperature. A positive-pressure SCBA is the most important piece of protective equipment to protect against these carcinogenic vapors and respiratory poisons. Additional measures to reduce the risk of exposure to hazardous carcinogens include performing gross decontamination when leaving fire operations, wiping soot off the skin with moistened towelettes immediately after removing gear, showering as soon as possible after the incident, washing uniform clothing at the station immediately after the incident, cleaning gear as soon as possible, and not keeping contaminated gear near living areas or sleeping areas, or in the home.[14]

> NOTE
>
> An important sign of a critical exposure is several people having the same symptoms at the same time. Anytime two or more members of the team report that they "feel" similar symptoms, a toxic gas or agent should be suspected. Emergency personnel should immediately report the onset of symptoms to their crew members and other emergency responders at the scene.

General Symptoms of Exposure

Health effects from exposure to hazardous materials vary by each person. The effects also depend on the chemical involved, the concentration of the chemical, the duration of exposure, the number of exposures, and the route of entry (inhalation, ingestion, injection, absorption). In addition, a person's age, sex, general health, allergies, smoking habits, alcohol consumption, and medication use influence how that person is affected.

Various symptoms may result from exposure to hazardous materials. Some symptoms may be delayed or masked by common illnesses, such as influenza, or by smoke inhalation. If any of the following symptoms is present after exposure to hazardous materials, the rescuer or patient should seek immediate medical attention:

- Changes in skin color or flushing
- Chest tightness
- Confusion, light-headedness, anxiety, dizziness
- Coughing or painful respiration
- Diarrhea and involuntary urination or defecation (or both)

- Dim, blurred, or double vision; photophobia
- Loss of coordination
- Nausea, vomiting, abdominal cramping
- Salivation, drooling, rhinorrhea
- Seizure
- Shortness of breath, burning of the upper airway
- Tingling or numbness of extremities
- Unconsciousness

CRITICAL THINKING

Two rescuers complain of similar symptoms on the scene of a rescue that may involve hazardous materials. What actions should be taken immediately?

External Damage

Body surface tissue may be injured by hazardous materials. Many substances have corrosive properties or become corrosive when mixed with water. Exposure to these substances may produce chemical burns and severe tissue damage. Examples include hydrochloric acid, hydrofluoric acid, and caustic soda.

Soft-Tissue Damage

Corrosives are strong acids or strong bases (alkaline). Exposure to either may cause pain on contact. However, alkalis generally burn more extensively than do acids. Exposing human tissue to a base corrosive such as lye may result in **liquefaction** (a breakdown of fatty tissue) that produces a greasy or slick feeling to the skin. These signs should alert the rescuer to decontaminate immediately and seek medical attention. Unless the substance is identified or deemed corrosive when mixed with water, decontamination should begin by brushing off the dry powder and flushing the skin with copious amounts of water. (Different areas of the skin absorb chemicals at different rates.) Paramedics should never try to neutralize an acid or base; doing so could produce great heat and cause further burns. The area should be flushed copiously with water, and the patient should be transported for care. Rescuers should be aware of possible "off-gassing" or fumes resulting from the decontamination of a wound site and take appropriate protective measures.

Cryogens are refrigerant liquid gases that can freeze human tissue on contact. These liquids vaporize as soon as they are released from their containers. They may cause tissue damage. Extreme caution should be used when near any refrigerated liquids. They can produce freeze burns, frostbite, and other cold-related injuries. Examples include Freon, liquid oxygen, and liquid nitrogen.

Chemical Exposure to the Eyes

Chemical exposure to the eyes (described in Chapter 38, *Burns*) may cause damage ranging from superficial inflammation to severe burns. Patients with these conditions have local pain, visual disturbance, tearing, edema, and redness of surrounding tissues. Basic management guidelines include immediately flushing the eyes with water. This should be done using a mild flow from a hose, intravenous (IV) tubing, water from a container, or irrigation lens (per protocol). A rapid assessment of visual acuity is important. However, assessment should not delay flushing or irrigation of the eyes.

Response to Hazmat Emergencies

When an EMS crew is dispatched to a scene involving the potential for hazardous materials, decisions must be made about rescuer safety, the type and degree of the potential hazard, the involvement of other agencies, and protection for the general public. As discussed in Chapter 53, *Medical Incident Command*, preplanning and early coordination of activities in these major incidents are important. In addition, medical direction should be advised of the incident as soon as possible to prepare personnel and facilities. Not all hazmat incidents are large-scale events. Sometimes, a single event involving only one patient may require a full hazmat response.

The first rescue personnel to arrive at the scene of a hazmat incident may not be the most qualified or best equipped. However, most communities look to the first responders to provide immediate safety and direction. Thus, the EMS crew must be capable of the initial management of hazmat incidents.

Hazard and Risk Assessment

While en route to the scene, EMS personnel should begin to research hazmat references. They also should begin a **hazard and risk assessment**. In hazmat incidents, hazards are the chemical properties of a material that may cause danger or peril (BOX 56-5).

BOX 56-5 Hazmat Terminology and Definitions

Toxicologic Terms Used to Determine Toxicity of a Compound

- **IDLH (immediately dangerous to life and health).** Any atmosphere that poses an immediate hazard to life or that produces immediate, irreversible debilitating effects on health.
- **LD_{50} (lethal dose, 50% kill).** The amount of a dose that, when administered to laboratory animals, kills 50% of them.
- **PEL (permissible exposure limit).** The maximum time-weighted concentration at which 95% of exposed, healthy adults suffer no adverse effects over a 40-hour workweek.
- **ppm/ppb.** Parts per million/parts per billion.
- **TLV-C (threshold limit value, ceiling level).** The maximum concentration that should not be exceeded even instantaneously.
- **TLV-STEL (threshold limit value, short-term exposure limit).** A 15-minute, time-weighted average exposure that should not be exceeded at any time or repeated more than four times a day, with 60-minute rest periods required between each STEL exposure.

Specific Terminology for Medical Hazmat Operations

- **Alpha radiation.** Large radioactive particles that have minimal penetrating ability.
- **Beta radiation.** Small radioactive particles that can penetrate subcutaneous tissue and usually enter the body through damaged skin, ingestion, or inhalation.
- **Boiling point.** The temperature at which a liquid changes to a vapor or a gas; the temperature at which the pressure of the liquid equals atmospheric pressure.
- **Flammable range.** The range of gas or vapor concentration that will burn or explode if an ignition source is present.
- **Flashpoint.** The minimum temperature at which a liquid disperses enough vapors to ignite and flash over but not to continue to burn without additional heat.
- **Gamma radiation.** The most dangerous form of penetrating radiation, which can produce internal and external hazards.
- **Ignition temperature.** The minimum temperature required to ignite gas or vapor without a spark or flame being present.
- **Specific gravity.** The weight of a material as compared with the weight of an equal volume of water.
- **Vapor density.** The weight of a pure vapor or gas compared with the weight of an equal volume of dry air at the same temperature and pressure.
- **Vapor pressure.** The pressure exerted by the vapor within the container against the sides of a container.

Modified from: Schnepp R. *Hazardous Materials: Awareness and Operations*. 2nd ed. Burlington, MA: Jones & Bartlett Learning; 2016.

Risk refers to the possibility of suffering harm or loss. Risk levels vary and are influenced by several factors, including the following (**FIGURE 56-7**):[15]

- Hazardous nature of the material involved
- Worst-case scenario situations
- Quantity of the material involved
- Weather conditions that might affect the scene adversely
- Containment system and type of stress applied to the container
- Proximity of exposures (eg, schools, nursing homes, shopping centers)
- Level of available resources
- Lead time for mutual aid

A hazard and risk assessment also includes consideration of the potential hazards to the public and environment, the potential risk of **primary contamination** to patients, and the potential risk for **secondary contamination** to rescuers (**BOX 56-6**).

If the product can be identified through hazmat references, the EMS crew members should familiarize themselves with potential health hazards, recommended PPE, initial first aid, and the **safe distance factor** (the minimum safe distance for personal safety) as outlined in the *ERG* or other approved reference guides. Most emergency response guides offer only general management actions. After formal product identification, the appropriate hazmat agencies (eg, CHEMTREC and poison control) can give more exact information.

Approaching the Scene

The paramedic should approach the scene cautiously from uphill and upwind or upstream. The EMS crew should be alert to environmental clues, including wind direction, unusual odors, leakage, and vapor clouds. Other environmental clues that are good indicators for the presence of hazardous materials include affected or afflicted wildlife and plant life (eg, dead

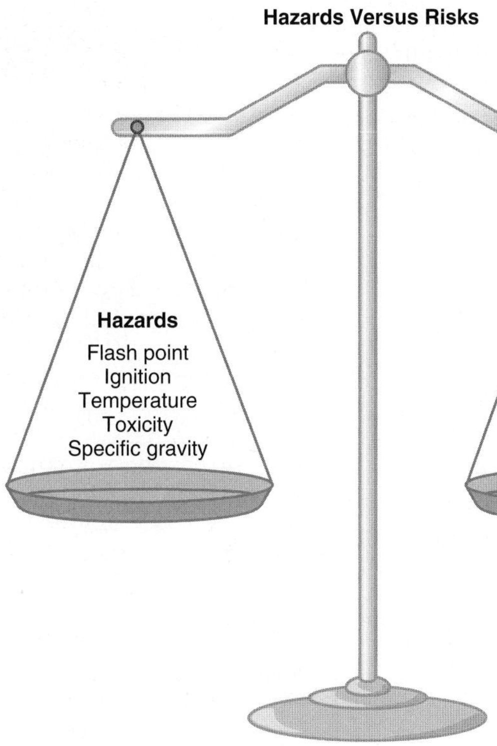

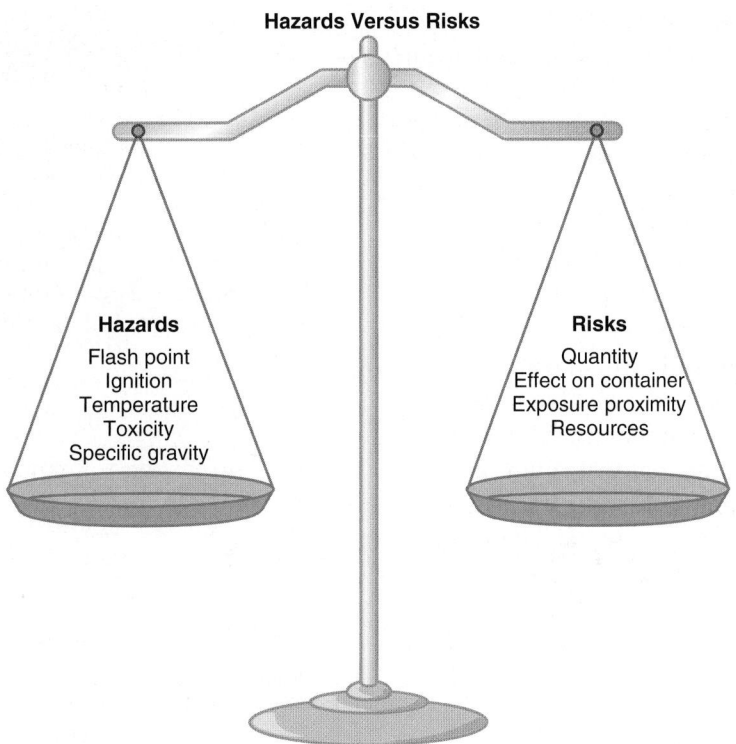

FIGURE 56-7 Hazards versus risks.

BOX 56-6 Types of Contamination

Primary Contamination

Exposure to substance
Substance harmful only to exposed person
Little chance of exposure to others

Secondary Contamination

Exposure to substance
Liquid and particulate substances easily transferred by touching

birds, wilted or discolored plants). Paramedics can use binoculars initially to observe the scene from a safe distance. Emergency vehicles should never be driven through leakage, vapor clouds, or smoke. In addition, personnel should not enter the incident area until it has been determined to be safe. In addition to these guidelines, rescuers should do the following as recommended in the *ERG*:[9]

- **Approach cautiously.** Resist the urge to rush into the incident area; you cannot help others until you know what you are facing. Park a safe distance from the scene. Stay clear of vapor, fumes, smoke, and spills.
- **Identify the hazards.** Placards, container labels, shipping papers, and knowledgeable people on the scene are valuable sources of information. Evaluate all of them and then consult the recommended guide page before you place yourself or others at risk. Do not be alarmed if new information from a CHEMTREC expert changes some of the emphasis or details of the guide page warnings. You must remember that the guide page provides only the most important information for your initial response with a family or class of hazardous materials. As more accurate, material-specific information becomes available, your response becomes more appropriate for the situation.
- **Secure the scene.** Without entering the immediate hazard zone, do what you can to isolate the area and ensure the safety of people and the environment. Move and keep nonaffected people away from the scene and the perimeter. Allow enough room to move and remove your own equipment.

- **Assess the situation.** Note whether the hazard involves a fire, spill, or leak. Consider the weather, especially the wind. Observe the terrain. Attempt to identify who or what is at risk in the situation. Consider additional resources that may be needed.
- **Obtain help.** Advise your dispatch center to notify responsible agencies and call for assistance from trained experts through CHEMTREC and the National Response Center.
- **Respond based on your level of training.** Any efforts you make to rescue people or protect property or the environment must be weighed against the possibility that you could become part of the problem. Enter the area with the appropriate protective gear (if trained to do so). Establish command if you are first on the scene. Above all, do not walk into or touch spilled material. Avoid inhaling fumes, smoke, and vapors, even if no hazardous materials are known to be involved. Do not assume that gases or vapors are harmless because of lack of smell.

CRITICAL THINKING

Which of these guidelines would it be easy for the first arriving crew to miss?

Control of the Scene

The first agency to arrive at the scene has several responsibilities. Its members must detect and identify the materials involved, assess the risk of exposure to rescue personnel and others, consider the potential risk of fire or explosion, gather information from on-site personnel or other sources, and confine and control the incident. In addition, a command post should be established per the preplanned incident command structure. Members also must define the safety distances and zones that can be obtained using the information provided in the *ERG*.

Safety Zones

After the presence of hazardous materials has been confirmed, the scene should be separated into hot, warm, and cold zones (**FIGURE 56-8**). These zones should have access and egress corridors between them. (Corridors provide control points. They also allow responders working in the zones to know where they should exit and enter for decontamination, accountability, and debriefing.) Safety zones should be established and enforced early in the incident (BOX 56-7). The dispatch center and responding units should be advised of the location of the hot zone and safe approach directions.

The **hot zone** is the area of the incident that includes the hazardous material. It also includes any surrounding area that may be exposed to gases, vapors, mist, dust, or runoff. All rescue personnel and vehicles should be stationed outside this zone. Anyone entering this zone must wear high-level PPE. Only specifically trained EMS personnel should attempt patient care activities in this area. Some EMS agencies and incident command system structures

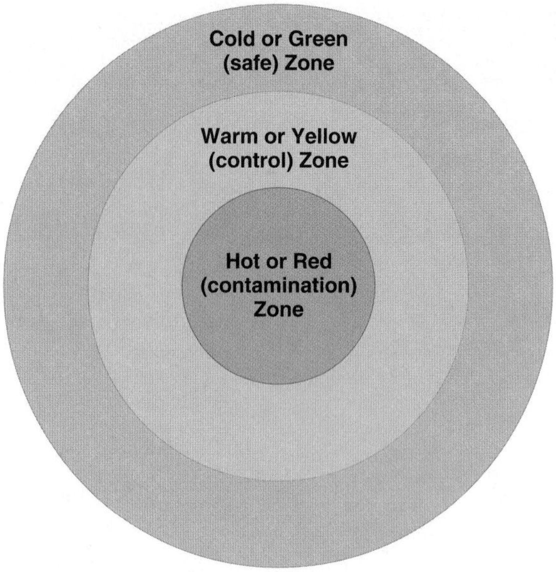

Hot or Red (contamination) Zone
- Contamination is actually present.
- Personnel must wear appropriate protective gear.
- Number of rescuers limited to those absolutely necessary.
- Bystanders never allowed.

Warm or Yellow (control) Zone
- Area surrounding the contamination zone.
- Vital to preventing spread of contamination.
- Personnel must wear appropriate protective gear.
- Lifesaving emergency care and decontamination are performed.

Cold or Green (safe) Zone
- Normal triage, stabilization, and treatment are performed.
- Rescuers must shed contaminated gear before entering the cold zone.

FIGURE 56-8 Zones at a hazmat incident.

BOX 56-7 Hazmat Zones

Hot Zone

Contamination present
Site of incident
Entry with high-level PPE
Entry limited

Warm Zone

Buffer zone outside hot zone
Contains decontamination corridor with "hot" and "cold" end

Cold Zone

Safe area
Staging area for personnel and equipment
Site of medical monitoring
One end of corridor

refer to the hot zone as the exclusion zone, a restricted area, or the red zone.

The **warm zone** is a larger buffer area that surrounds the hot zone with "cold" and "hot" end corridors. Although it is usually considered one level lower than the hot zone, protective clothing is required because if the hot zone becomes unstable, the warm zone may be exposed to the hazardous materials. This zone is where decontamination and limited patient care are performed. Some agencies refer to this zone as the limited-access zone, the containment reduction corridor, or the yellow zone.

The **cold zone** is the area that surrounds the warm zone. This zone is where most EMS care is provided; however, it also is restricted to emergency personnel. This area usually is considered safe, requiring minimal or no protective clothing. The cold zone contains the command post and other support agencies necessary to control the incident. This area is referred to by some agencies as a support zone or the green zone.

Rehabilitation and Medical Monitoring

The safety of rescue personnel is of prime importance in any emergency. Thus, a rehabilitation and medical monitoring program should be part of any incident where rescue personnel may be at risk for physical and emotional stress. In addition, the US Fire Administration and the NFPA recommend and require rehabilitation and medical monitoring at all emergency scenes where personnel exceed a safe level of physical or mental endurance.[16,17]

Rehabilitation

The purpose of **rehabilitation** (often referred to simply as rehab) is to sustain the energy of rescuers, improve performance, and decrease the likelihood of on-scene injury or death. As described in Chapter 53, *Medical Incident Command*, rehabilitation is part of the incident command structure and is a responsibility of command. The rehabilitation area (or areas) usually is established near the incident, but away from operations. The location must ensure safety and must provide for rest and recuperation. Depending on weather and the nature of the incident, these areas may be outdoors, in a building, or in a specially designed rehabilitation vehicle. Activities that may take place in a rehabilitation sector include the following:[17]

- Relief from environmental extremes (active or passive cooling or warming)
- Rest and recovery
- Rehydration
- Calorie and electrolyte replacement
- Medical monitoring
- EMS treatment
- Accountability and release
- Postincident rehabilitation

NOTE

In most management systems, emergency medical procedures are not performed in the rehabilitation area. If emergency care is needed for a rescuer, that care is provided by EMS personnel in the treatment sector, located away from or in a separate part of the rehabilitation area.

Medical Monitoring

Medical monitoring is the ongoing evaluation of rescuers who are at risk for illness or injury from operations at the incident. Medical monitoring should not be confused with treatment. The purpose of medical monitoring in the rehabilitation area is to identify personnel who may need treatment (provided in the treatment sector) or transport. In hazmat operations, medical monitoring may also include accountability, record keeping, and periodic evaluation of the surveillance program.

NOTE

OSHA requires medical examinations for members of hazmat response teams and employees who may have been exposed to hazardous substances during an emergency.

Medical monitoring should include assessment protocols that involve a "presuit" examination before entering a hazardous area. The purpose of the examination is to establish a health history and baseline vital signs for any rescuer who will be exposed to a hazardous substance. During the pre-suit examination, rescuers should be advised of the expected symptoms of illness or exposure before entering the hazardous area. In addition to injury from exposure, responders working in protective clothing and equipment can become dehydrated and heat illnesses can develop. Rescue protective suits protect, but they also prevent cooling through evaporation, conduction, convection, or radiation. Heat-stress factors are affected by the prehydration of the rescuer, degree of physical fitness, ambient air temperature, and degree and duration of physical activity. The parameters of the presuit evaluation should include the following:

- Temperature, pulse, respiration, and blood pressure measurements
- Cardiac rhythm
- Body weight
- Cognitive and motor skills
- Hydration
- Significant recent medical history (eg, medications, illnesses)

After entry into the hazardous area, medical monitoring should note the amount of time a rescuer has been in protective clothing. Rescuers should be observed for any signs of heat-related illness or exposure (described in Chapter 44, *Environmental Conditions*). Responders exposed to smoke should also be assessed for carboxyhemoglobin to detect carbon monoxide exposure. If illness or injury occurs to any team member, all entry team members should be removed from the hot zone for treatment. A backup team should be ready to assist the entry team members in the hot zone at all times.

After the incident, rescue personnel should be reevaluated in the "rehab sector," using the same parameters as in the pre-suit examination. This examination determines the rescuer's ability to be released to reenter the operation if needed. As a rule, rescuers are not allowed to reenter the site until vital signs and hydration level are normal. Body weight generally is used to estimate fluid loss and the need for oral or IV fluid replacement (per protocol) (**FIGURE 56-9**).

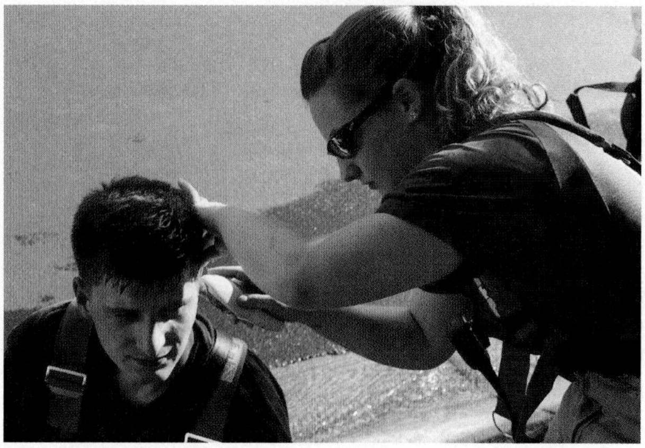

FIGURE 56-9 Rehabilitation branch.

CRITICAL THINKING

What might prevent personnel from seeking emergency medical services for medical monitoring unless there is a strict procedure to guarantee they are monitored?

SHOW ME THE EVIDENCE

A team of researchers conducted a systematic review of cooling techniques and practices among firefighters and hazmat operators to describe the evidence and provide recommendations for fireground rehabilitation. They searched five electronic databases and found 72 articles meeting their criteria. Two of the researchers reviewed the articles to answer predetermined questions. They concluded that cooling devices are not routinely needed if the ambient temperature and humidity are close to room temperature and the protective gear can be removed. However, active cooling devices are needed in hot or humid conditions. Hand/forearm immersion in cold water appears to be the best method for active cooling in these situations. It is relatively inexpensive and is simple to implement. This method appears to be supported by evidence and is considered to be the most practical and effective means to cool firefighters and hazmat technicians in hot and humid environments.

Modified from: McEntire SJ, Suyama J, Hostler D. Mitigation and prevention of exertional heat stress in firefighters: a review of cooling strategies for structural firefighting and hazardous materials responders. *Prehosp Emerg Care*. 2013;17(2):241-260.

Documentation

Detailed records are a necessary part of hazmat medical monitoring and rehabilitation. At a minimum, records should include the following:

- The name of the hazardous substance
- The toxicity and danger of secondary contamination
- Use of appropriate PPE and any permeation ("breakthrough") that occurred
- The level of decontamination performed or required
- Use of antidotes and other medical treatment
- The method of transport and destination

Baseline statistics from preentry and postentry screenings also should be included in the records. (Many agencies use preprinted forms for this information.)

Emergency Management of Contaminated Patients

Patient care activities, triage, and evacuation should be part of a preplanned incident command system structure. Identifying a specific hazardous substance may take some time. Thus, rescue efforts, decontamination, possible evacuation, and timely treatment of toxic exposures are important. The primary goals of **decontamination** are to reduce the patient's dosage of material, decrease the threat of secondary contamination, and reduce the risk of rescuer injury. The specific substance and route of contamination affect triage and decontamination methods. The following guidelines for rapid decontamination are general. They should not supersede any organizational approach in scene management of hazmat incidents or treatment recommendations for chemical exposures:

1. The paramedic should not enter a contaminated area or initiate care without adequate PPE. The paramedic also must possess training that is specific to the incident. Victims who can walk should be encouraged to extricate themselves from the scene. They should be advised to stay together for treatment or until they are escorted individually to decontamination.
2. Patients who cannot walk should be removed from the hot zone by trained personnel. Removal usually is performed by fire service personnel, specialized hazmat teams, or both. Patient care activities in the hot zone should be limited to initial airway management and hemorrhage control. Decontamination and further patient care should be done in the warm zone by a properly equipped decontamination team.
3. All patients exposed to the hot zone should be considered contaminated. They should be treated as such until they have been properly assessed, triaged, and decontaminated.
4. Patient care provisions of airway, breathing, and circulatory support should begin as soon as the patient is contacted and conditions allow. The rescuer safety information received from hazmat agencies should be used when performing BLS procedures.
5. IV therapy should be administered only under a physician's direction. This and other invasive procedures may allow the hazardous materials to enter the patient if initiated prior to decontamination.
6. Decontamination procedures should avoid any unnecessary exposure to the rescuer. EMS personnel assisting in decontamination should be well protected with two or three layers of gloves, head coverings, positive-pressure SCBA, and proper protective clothing. Decontamination teams or anyone working in the warm zone should be wearing the same PPE (or no less than one protection level down) as those working in the hot zone.
7. When the hazardous material is a dry agent, the material should be lightly brushed from the patient, with care to not introduce the dry agent into the patient's airway. Cutting or removing clothing often removes most of the contaminating material. After the dry agent has been removed, the decontamination should continue as follows:
   - Wash the patient with copious amounts of water and mild detergent soap. Make sure all water and runoff is contained in the warm zone. Depending on the exposure, other patient decontamination procedures may be warranted. Pay special attention to irrigation of the eyes, hair, ears, underarms, and pubic areas and thorough cleaning of the body creases of the neck, groin, elbows, and knees. Be careful not to abrade the skin, which may promote absorption of the material involved.
   - Leave all patient clothing, rescuer clothing, and decontamination equipment in the decontamination area. Safely move the patient to the support zone for further triage, treatment, and transport.

NOTE

Water is considered the universal decontamination solution to dilute the concentration of a substance. Water generally does not alter the chemical structure of a compound. Degradation solutions may be recommended for some exposures. These include water and mild soap, isopropyl alcohol, and vegetable oil (among others). These solutions should be used only when advised by medical direction or other appropriate authority. They should not be applied directly to the skin and should not be used for exposures to chemicals that react with water. The best universal liquid decontamination agent for chemical exposures is 0.5% hypochlorite solution. It is prepared by diluting household bleach to 1⁄10 strength (ie, nine parts water or saline to one part bleach).

Modified from: Kumar V, Goel R, Chawla R, Silambarasan M, Sharma RK. Chemical, biological, radiological, and nuclear decontamination: recent trends and future perspective. *J Pharm Bioallied Sci*. 2010;2(3):220-238.

The field decontamination procedures described represent only a gross decontamination. The resources needed for full decontamination usually are not available at the scene. Thus, the patient should be isolated from the environment, which will help to contain any contamination that has been missed during these procedures. Isolation is accomplished by placing the patient in a body bag (or similar containment) to the neck and covering the patient's hair. In the absence of body bags, the patient may be packaged for transport by folding one side of a sheet or blanket over the patient and using the other side to overlap and package the patient. If necessary, the patient's arm may be exposed through an opening in the sheet for vital sign assessment and fluid and drug administration.

NOTE

Rapid decontamination is a two-step process. In the first step, remove the patient from danger. In the second step, provide gross decontamination.

Decontamination Decision Making

Hazmat incidents often are "fast breaking" and may require rapid decision making. For example, a group of walking, contaminated people at the scene may be trying to reach rescuers; others self-rescue by walking out of the hot zone; and some may become impatient and leave the hot zone while waiting for rescue teams to arrive. In these situations, the paramedic crew must be prepared for quick gross decontamination and treatment, rapid application of PPE, and quick transport and isolation procedures.

If the patient's condition is critical (and it is unknown if the exposure involved a life-threatening material), the paramedic should perform decontamination and treatment simultaneously. This is done by removing the patient's clothing, treating life-threatening problems, performing lavage of the patient with copious amounts of water, and providing for isolation and transport. Patients who are not in critical condition can be managed in the same manner, with a more contemplative approach, particularly if the hazardous substance is known.

A hazmat incident that is well controlled (not a fast-breaking event) can be managed over longer duration. In these cases, rescue should not be attempted for patients in the hot zone. Rather, the paramedic crew should wait for a hazmat team and for a decontamination corridor to be established (**FIGURE 56-10**). (This may take an hour or more.) Events of longer duration allow for more thorough decontamination, better use of PPE, less chance of secondary contamination, and better environmental protection.

CRITICAL THINKING

What type of hazmat response resources does your community have?

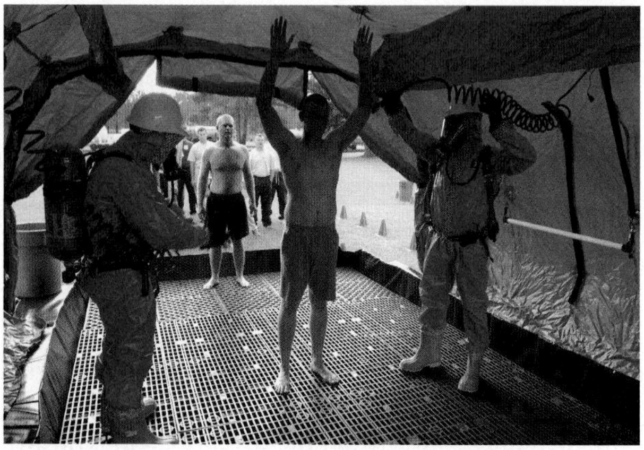

FIGURE 56-10 Decontamination corridor at a hazmat incident.

Preparing the Ambulance for Patient Transfer

Contamination of ambulances and equipment can be minimized by preparing the vehicle before transporting a partly decontaminated patient. These measures include using as much disposable equipment as necessary. They also include removing all items that will not be needed for patient use from cabinets. Ideally, the patient should be isolated completely in a stretcher decontamination pool. This should be covered in plastic and secured to the stretcher. Immediate notification of the hospital staff that they will be receiving contaminated patients is crucial. The emergency department will need time to prepare and manage the patients adequately and efficiently.

On arrival at the hospital, the EMS crew should follow the decontamination protocols of the hospital. The crew should not return to regular service until rescue personnel, the vehicle, and equipment have been monitored for contamination. Equipment decontamination should follow the recommendations of local, state, and federal authorities or standard operating procedures of medical direction. Specific solutions may be required for a particular hazardous material exposure. However, most equipment can be cleaned adequately and made ready for use with soap and water.

Decontamination of Rescue Personnel and Equipment

Decontamination procedures of rescue personnel vary by agency, protocol, and primary hazard. Decontamination typically involves a series of steps, which can vary in number, and begins in the decontamination corridor (**FIGURE 56-11**). An example of the decontamination process includes the following:[18]

1. An entry point is established at the "hot" end of the corridor where "dirty" personnel and equipment are set up to start the decontamination process. When more than one first responder needs decontamination, the responder who has a lower SCBA air level, a medical need, or any tears in his or her suit should be put through the decontamination first.
2. A tool drop is designated. Outer gloves and boots are removed and placed in a receptacle.
3. Gross surface contamination is removed. Generally, this is done by washing with copious amounts of water. The goal of this procedure is to make the PPE safe to remove.
4. Protective clothing is removed and handled (stored, decontaminated) as required.
5. Once the protective clothing has been removed, the responder can then remove the SCBA and mask to allow for maximum airway protection until the final step.
6. Other clothing is removed. This step depends on the seriousness of the hazardous materials involved.
7. Personnel wash their bodies using overhead showers. Usually two washings are required. Personnel dry off and receive new or clean, uncontaminated clothing.
8. Personnel going through the decontamination system receive medical evaluation.

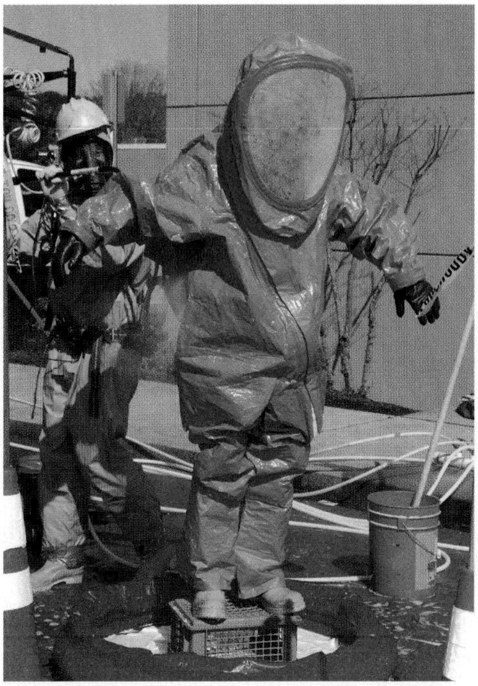

FIGURE 56-11 Rescuers in a decontamination corridor.

In addition, the following safety precautions should be followed by any rescuer exposed to hazardous materials:

- Do not touch the face, mouth, nose, or genital area before full-body decontamination.
- Shower first with a cold rinse (no scrubbing) to wash off potential contaminants without opening pores of the skin, and then thoroughly wash with warm water, surgical soap, sponge,

and brush. Pay particular attention to hair, body orifices (especially the ears), and any body parts that come in contact with each other (arms and chest, thighs, fingers, toes, and buttocks). Repeat shower and rinse.
- Shampoo hair several times and rinse thoroughly.

CRITICAL THINKING

Why do you think that extensive preplanning and drills are needed to make this system work well?

Care and Maintenance of Clothing and Equipment

After the hazmat incident, the rescuer should take the following precautions:

- Properly dispose of any protective clothing that has been torn or worn through.
- Properly and thoroughly clean all clothing and equipment. This will reduce the risk of chemical reactions at future incidents. It also will lessen the potential for chronic exposure to absorbed chemicals. Some hazardous materials can destroy or penetrate protective clothing and equipment. For this reason, product compatibility tables should be evaluated during the decontamination procedure. Decontamination provides no assurance that protective clothing is clean or that the process of chemical penetration has stopped.
- Do not wash or dispose of clothing or equipment at home. This helps to avoid exposing family members and contaminating home articles.
- Follow all local codes and laws regarding disposal or decontamination of equipment and clothing.
- Carefully maintain personal SCBA.

When the incident is over, all personnel operating at the scene (in any capacity) should be debriefed. The debriefing session should include identification and explanation of the substances. It also should include information regarding possible acute and chronic health issues that may arise and any associated signs and symptoms. Information describing follow-up procedures for long-term effects also should be provided. The documentation for possible work-related exposures should follow standard department/company policies.

Summary

- A hazardous material is any substance or material that is capable of posing an unreasonable risk to health, safety, and property.
- The Superfund Amendments and Reauthorization Act of 1986 established requirements for federal, state, and local governments and industry regarding emergency planning and the reporting of hazardous materials–related incidents. In 1989 the Occupational Safety and Health Administration and the Environmental Protection Agency published rules to govern training requirements, emergency plans, medical checkups, and other safety precautions for workers at uncontrolled hazardous waste sites and for those responding to hazardous chemical spills. In addition, the National Fire Protection Association has published standards that address competencies for EMS workers at hazmat scenes.
- Two methods are used to identify hazardous materials. One is informal product identification, which includes visual, olfactory, and verbal clues. The other is formal product identification, which includes, for example, placards and shipping papers. Information references for hazardous materials include the US Department of Transportation's *Emergency Response Guidebook*, regional poison control centers, CHEMTREC, ChemTel, and CAMEO.
- It is crucial that anyone dealing with hazardous materials use proper protection. This includes using the proper respiratory devices and wearing protective clothing. Protective clothing is made of a variety of materials and is designed for certain chemical exposures; thus, the manufacturer's guidelines must be followed.
- Hazardous materials may enter the body through inhalation, ingestion, injection, and absorption. Internal damage to the human body from hazardous materials exposure may involve the respiratory tract, central nervous system, or other internal organs. Chemicals producing internal damage include irritants, asphyxiants, nerve poisons, anesthetics, narcotics, hepatotoxins, cardiotoxins, nephrotoxins, neurotoxins, and carcinogens.
- Exposure to hazardous materials may result in burns. It also may result in severe tissue damage.
- The first agency to arrive at the scene of a hazmat incident must detect and identify the materials involved, assess the risk of exposure to rescue personnel and others, consider the potential risk of fire or explosion, gather information from on-site personnel or other sources, and confine and control the incident.
- A hazmat medical monitoring program may include medical examination for members of hazmat response teams, provision of medical care, record keeping, and periodic evaluation of the surveillance program.

- The primary goals of decontamination are to reduce the patient's dosage of material, decrease the threat of secondary contamination, and reduce the risk of rescuer injury.
- Rescuers should follow strict protocols for proper decontamination of themselves, their clothing, and any contaminated equipment.

References

1. Hazardous materials fatalities, injuries, accidents, and property damage data. Bureau of Transportation Statistics website. https://www.bts.dot.gov/content/hazardous-materials-fatalities-injuries-accidents-and-property-damage-data. Accessed May 1, 2018.
2. Hazmat intelligence portal: 10-year incident summary reports. US Department of Transportation website. https://hip.phmsa.dot.gov/analyticsSOAP/saw.dll?Dashboard. Accessed May 1, 2018.
3. Gummin DD, Mowry JB, Spyker DA, Brooks DE, Fraser MO, Banner W. 2016 Annual Report of the American Association of Poison Control Centers' National Poison Data System (NPDS): 34th Annual Report. *Clin Toxicol (Phila)*. 2017;55(10):1072-1254.
4. Kaszeta D. *CBRN and Hazmat Incidents at Major Public Events: Planning and Response*. Hoboken, NJ: John Wiley & Sons; 2013.
5. The Superfund Amendments and Reauthorization Act (SARA). Environmental Protection Agency website. https://www.epa.gov/superfund/superfund-amendments-and-reauthorization-act-sara. Accessed May 1, 2018.
6. Regulations (Standards—29 CFR)—table of contents. Occupational Safety and Health Administration website. https://www.osha.gov/pls/oshaweb/owadisp.show_document?p_table=STANDARDS&p_id=9765. Accessed May 1, 2018.
7. Schnepp R. *Hazardous Materials: Awareness and Operations*. 2nd ed. Burlington, MA: Jones & Bartlett Learning; 2016.
8. National Fire Protection Association. *NFPA 473: Standard for Competencies for EMS Personnel Responding to Hazardous Materials/Weapons of Mass Destruction Incidents*. Quincy, MA: National Fire Protection Association; 2018.
9. US Department of Transportation. *Emergency Response Guidebook (ERG)*. Washington, DC: Department of Transportation; 2016.
10. How to comply with federal hazardous materials regulations. Federal Motor Carrier Safety Administration website. https://www.fmcsa.dot.gov/regulations/hazardous-materials/how-comply-federal-hazardous-materials-regulations. Updated April 18, 2018. Accessed May 1, 2018.
11. US Department of Health and Human Services, Occupational Safety and Health Administration. *General Description and Discussion of the Levels of Protection and Protective Gear*. Washington, DC: Occupational Safety and Health Administration; 2004. 20 CFR, 1910.120, Appendix B.
12. Dikshith TS. *Hazardous Chemicals: Safety Management and Global Regulations*. Boca Raton, FL: CRC Press; 2013.
13. Daniels RD, Kubale TL, Yiin JH. Mortality and cancer incidence in a pooled cohort of US firefighters from San Francisco, Chicago and Philadelphia (1950–2009). *Occup Environ Med.* 2014;71(6):388-397.
14. Fire Service Occupational Cancer Alliance. *The Fire Service Cancer Toolkit*. National Fire Protection Administration website. https://www.nfpa.org/-/media/Files/News-and-Research/Resources/Fire-service/CancerToolkitv6.ashx?la=en. Published September 2017. Accessed May 1, 2018.
15. Noll G, Hildebrand M, Schnepp R. *Hazardous Materials: Managing the Incident*. 4th ed. Burlington, MA: Jones & Bartlett Learning; 2012.
16. US Fire Administration. *Emergency Incident Rehabilitation*. Washington, DC: US Department of Homeland Security; February 2008. www.usfa.dhs.gov/downloads/pdf/publications/fa_314.pdf. Accessed May 1, 2018.
17. National Fire Protection Association. *NFPA 1584: Standard on the Rehabilitation Process for Members During Emergency Operations and Training Exercises*. Quincy, MA: National Fire Protection Association; 2015.
18. Decontamination. Occupational Safety and Health Administration website. https://www.osha.gov/SLTC/hazardouswaste/training/decon.html. Accessed May 1, 2018.

Suggested Readings

Calams S. Fact or fiction: transdermal fentanyl exposure. For opioid toxicity to occur the drug must enter the blood and brain from the environment. EMS1.com website. https://www.ems1.com/opioids/articles/291433048-Fact-or-fiction-Transdermal-fentanyl-exposure/. Published July 16, 2017. Accessed May 1, 2018.

Califano F. EMS and hazmat: when your ambulance becomes the hot zone. Fire Engineering website. http://www.fireengineering.com/articles/print/volume-166/issue-8/departments/fireems/ems-and-hazmat-when-your-ambulance-becomes-the-hot-zone.html. Published August 6, 2013. Accessed May 1, 2018.

Haar RJ, Iacopino V, Ranadive N, Weiser SD, Dandu M. Health impacts of chemical irritants used for crowd control: a systematic review of the injuries and deaths caused by tear gas and pepper spray. BMC Public Health website. https://bmcpublichealth.biomedcentral.com/articles/10.1186/s12889-017-4814-6. Published October 19, 2017. Accessed May 1, 2018.

Hostler D, McEntire SJ, Rittenberger JC. Emergency incident rehabilitation: resource document to the position statement of the National Association of EMS Physicians. *Prehosp Emerg Care.* 2016;20(2):300-306.

Jagminas L. CBRNE—chemical decontamination. Medscape website. https://emedicine.medscape.com/article/831175-overview?pa=7uXkkbS0E30nGO8feeMBYDu58BJGcrq5pUKkxkWejs8R%2BYHjkNKwC%2FEUuMrkHsngcFrqow%2Bf2%2F37XuRaZT6JAA%3D%3D. Updated August 26, 2015. Accessed May 1, 2018.

Occupational Safety and Health Administration. *Best Practices for Protecting EMS Responders During Treatment and Transport of Victims of Hazardous Substance Releases*. Washington, DC: Occupational Safety and Health Administration; 2009. OSHA 3370-11.

Purvis MV, Rooks H, Young Lee J, Longerich S, Kahn SA. Prehospital hydroxocobalamin for inhalation injury and cyanide toxicity in the United States—analysis of a database and survey of EMS providers. *Ann Burns Fire Disaster*. 2017;30(2):126-128.

Radiation Emergency Assistance Center/Training Site (REAC/TS). Oak Ridge Institute for Science and Education website. https://orise.orau.gov/reacts/index.html. Accessed May 1, 2018.

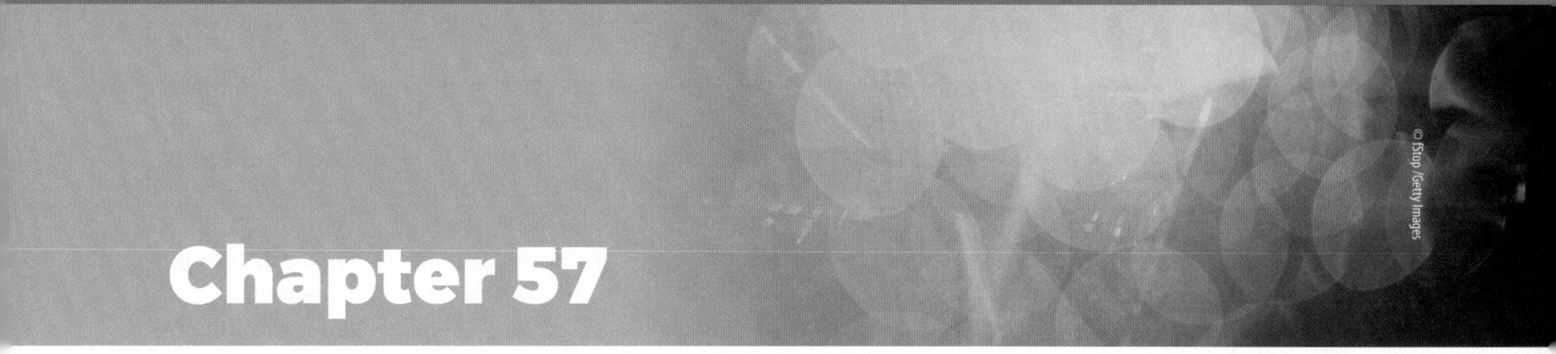

Chapter 57

Bioterrorism and Weapons of Mass Destruction

NATIONAL EMS EDUCATION STANDARD COMPETENCIES

EMS Operations

Knowledge of operational roles and responsibilities to ensure patient, public, and personnel safety.

Mass-Casualty Incidents Due to Terrorism and Disaster

Risks and responsibilities of operating on the scene of a natural or human-made disaster. (pp 1938–1939)

OBJECTIVES

Upon completion of this chapter, the paramedic student will be able to:

1. List five types of weapons of mass destruction (WMDs). (p 1922)
2. Identify actions, signs and symptoms, methods of distribution, and management of biologic WMDs. (pp 1922–1928)
3. Identify actions, signs and symptoms, methods of distribution, and management of nuclear WMDs. (pp 1928–1929)
4. Identify actions, signs and symptoms, methods of distribution, and management of chemical WMDs. (pp 1929–1934)
5. Describe security threat alerts as defined by the Department of Homeland Security. (p 1937)
6. Identify measures to be taken by paramedics who respond to incidents with suspected WMD involvement. (pp 1938–1939)

KEY TERMS

anthrax An acute infectious disease caused by the spore-forming bacterium *Bacillus anthracis*.

bioterrorism The use of biologic agents, such as pathogenic organisms or agricultural pests, for the express purpose of causing death or disease, to instill a sense of fear and panic in the victims, and to intimidate governments or societies for political, financial, or ideologic gain.

botulism A rare but life-threatening form of food poisoning caused by the bacillus *Clostridium botulinum*.

CBRNE An abbreviation for the categories of weapons of mass destruction: Chemical, Biologic, Radiologic, Nuclear, and Explosive agents.

chlorine A poisonous, yellow-green gas with an odor that has been described as a mixture of pineapple and pepper.

cutaneous anthrax Anthrax that affects the skin, caused by the spore-forming bacterium *Bacillus anthracis*.

Ebola An infectious viral hemorrhagic fever.

explosive A bomb, which can be made from a variety of dangerous materials.

foodborne botulism Illness that results from eating foods that contain the bacillus *Clostridium botulinum*.

improvised explosive device (IED) A "homemade" bomb constructed of explosives attached to a detonator; an example is a roadside bomb.

incendiary devices Devices used as weapons, that can ignite a fire via a chemical reaction of a flammable substance; also called firebombs.

infant botulism Illness caused by consumption of the spores of the botulinum bacteria, which then grow in the intestines and release toxin.

inhalational anthrax Anthrax caused by inhaling the spore-forming bacterium *Bacillus anthracis*.

intestinal anthrax Anthrax caused from consuming meat contaminated with the bacterium *Bacillus anthracis*.

Marburg An infectious viral hemorrhagic fever.

nerve agents Chemicals that disrupt the nerve transmissions in the central and peripheral nervous systems.

phosgene A poisonous gas that appears as a gray-white cloud and smells like newly mowed hay.

plague A disease caused by the bacterium *Yersinia pestis*, found in rodents (eg, chipmunks, prairie dogs, ground squirrels, mice) and their fleas in many areas around the world.

pneumonic plague An infectious pulmonary disease caused by exposure to the bacterium *Yersinia pestis*.

radiologic dispersion device (RDD) A nuclear explosive device; also known as a "dirty nuke" or "dirty bomb."

ricin A potent protein cytotoxin derived from the beans of the castor plant (*Ricinus communis*).

sarin A clear, colorless, and tasteless liquid that has no odor in its pure form; may be used as a nerve agent.

smallpox A highly contagious viral disease caused by the variola virus; characterized by fever, prostration, and a vesicular, pustular rash.

soman A clear, colorless, tasteless liquid with a slight camphor odor; may be used as a nerve agent.

tabun A clear, colorless, tasteless liquid with a faint fruity odor; may be used as a nerve agent.

tularemia A serious illness that is caused by the bacterium *Francisella tularensis* found in animals (especially rodents, rabbits, and hares).

vesicants Chemicals with severely irritating properties that produce blisters on the skin and damage to the eyes, lungs, and other mucous membranes.

viral hemorrhagic fevers (VHFs) A group of illnesses caused by several distinct families of viruses that include Ebola.

VX A human-made thick, amber-colored, odorless liquid that resembles motor oil; a chemical warfare agent classified as a nerve agent.

weapons of mass destruction (WMDs) Conventional biologic, nuclear, incendiary, chemical, or explosive weapons that have the ability to cause death and/or destruction on a widespread or massive scale.

wound botulism Botulism caused by toxins produced from a wound infected with *Clostridium botulinum*.

International conventions have long prohibited the use of chemicals and biologic agents during war and bar any country from making or acquiring biologic weapons.[1] *A number of countries and terrorist groups, however, maintain them. This chapter serves as an overview of* **bioterrorism** *and* **weapons of mass destruction (WMDs)**. *Bioterrorism is the intentional release of biologic products to cause illness or death. WMDs are weapons that can kill or bring harm to a large number of people. The chapter also provides general guidelines for emergency response.*

History of Biologic Weapons

The use of biologic agents as weapons has occurred throughout history, dating back at least as far as 184 BC when Hannibal ordered that pots filled with venomous snakes be thrown onto the decks of enemy ships (BOX 57-1).[2] However, many countries agreed to stop biologic weapons research and development in 1972. Some of these countries included the United States, the former Soviet Union, Canada, and the United Kingdom. Some countries, however, continue to have biologic warfare programs, and recently "non-state actors" have used WMD agents in acts of terrorism. A non-state actor is a political, social, or religious nongovernmental group that is trying to promote a cause.[3] The serious reality of

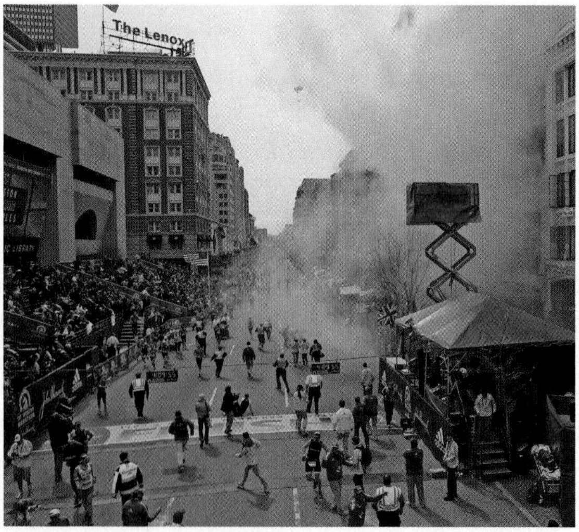

BOX 57-1 Timeline of Suspected or Reported Use of Biologic Weapons

Early Examples

- The Tartar army catapulted bodies of plague victims into the city of Caffa in 1346.
- In 1763, the British army provided the Delaware Indians with blankets that had been used by smallpox patients.

Pre–World War II

- The British used biologic warfare against Native Americans during the siege of Fort Pitt in the 1700s.
- The Germans used various human and animal pathogens as agents of germ warfare in Europe during World War I. They are reported to have shipped horses, sheep, and cattle inoculated with *Bacillus anthracis* and *Pseudomonas pseudomallei* to the United States and other countries.
- Germany was accused of spreading cholera in Italy and plague in Russia in 1915.

World War II

- The Japanese used germ warfare against the Chinese and the Soviets by scattering *Yersinia pestis*–contaminated rice and fleas–by airplane. This act was followed by an outbreak of bubonic plague in those areas.
- The Japanese experimented with biologic agents by exposing prisoners of war to anthrax, botulism, brucellosis, cholera, dysentery, gas gangrene, meningococcal infection, and plague. More than 1,000 prisoners died from the experiments.
- The British performed trials with *B anthracis* off the coast of Scotland.
- The United States prepared about 5,000 anthrax bombs at Camp Detrick, Maryland, in 1942 (although none were used during the war).

Post–World War II

- The United States dispersed aerosols over large areas around US cities from 1949 to 1968 to simulate a bacteriologic attack.
- The United States exposed willing volunteer members of the Seventh-day Adventist Church (who were conscientious objectors to warfare but still wanted to serve their country) to aerosols of *Francisella tularensis* and *Coxiella burnetii* in 1953. (No deaths occurred, and all recovered.)
- An unintentional release of anthrax spores from a biologic warfare facility in the Soviet Union resulted in at least 66 deaths from inhalational anthrax in 1979.

The Gulf War

- The Iraqi government admitted that it had conducted research into the offensive use of *B anthracis*, *Clostridium botulinum* toxin, and *Clostridium perfringens* and had filled warheads with biologic agents.

The Aum Shinrikyo

- The religious cult intentionally contaminated the Tokyo subway system with sarin in 1995, resulting in 5,500 health care visits and 12 deaths.
- Several successful attempts were made to release anthrax or botulinum toxin to other areas around Tokyo, but the strain of anthrax was not pathogenic in humans so no one became ill.

Recent Terrorist Group Activities

- In 1984, a religious commune deliberately contaminated several community salad bars in the United States with *Salmonella typhimurium*, resulting in more than 750 illnesses.
- Anthrax-laden envelopes were sent via US mail in 2001, resulting in 11 cases of inhalational anthrax (including 5 deaths) and 12 cases of cutaneous anthrax.

Recent Terrorist Wartime Activities

- More than 90% of all recent terrorist attacks occurred in countries engaged in violent conflicts. In 2014, there were 13,463 terrorist attacks worldwide. The majority of terrorism acts have been located in Middle Eastern countries such as Iraq, Afghanistan, and Pakistan.
- In 2015, four groups were responsible for 74% of all deaths from terrorism: Islamic State of Iraq and ash-Sham (ISIL), Boko Haram, the Taliban, and al-Qa'ida.
- In 2016, Iraq was the country with the most terrorist attacks and the most fatalities due to terrorism worldwide. A reported 9,764 people died due to terrorist attacks in Iraq that year. That same year, a total number of 1,340 terrorist attacks were registered in Afghanistan.

Modified from: Darling RG, Eitzen EM, Mothershead JL, Waeckerie JF, eds. *Bioterrorism: The May 2002 Issue of the Emergency Medicine Clinics of North America*. Philadelphia, PA: Saunders; 2002; *Global Terrorism Index 2016*. Institute for Economics and Peace website. http://economicsandpeace.org/wp-content/uploads/2016/11/Global-Terrorism-Index-2016.2.pdf. Published 2016. Accessed April 27, 2018; and Terrorism—statistics and facts. Statista website. https://www.statista.com/topics/2267/terrorism/. Accessed April 27, 2018.

> NOTE
>
> Acts of terrorism can pose significant risk to civilian populations. If airplanes were to spray chemical and biologic agents on a city on a clear, breezy night, thousands and perhaps millions of people would be killed. For example, 200 pounds (91 kg) of anthrax sprayed over a city the size of Omaha, Nebraska, would kill as many as 2.5 million people; 200 pounds of botulinum toxin would kill as many as 40,000 people in an area the size of Minnesota's Mall of America; and 200 pounds of VX sprayed over an area the size of Disneyland in California would kill about 12,500 people.
>
> *Modified from*: van der Steeg J. Bioterrorism and weapons of mass destruction. StudyLib website. https://studylib.net/doc/15411799/bio-terrorism-and-wmd. Accessed April 28, 2018.

bioterrorism became clear in the United States in 2001 when anthrax cases occurred following exposure to contaminated mail in New York, New Jersey, and Washington, DC.

Critical Biologic Agents and Responder Databases

The Centers for Disease Control and Prevention (CDC) has published a list of biologic agents.[4] The list is divided into categories A, B, and C (BOX 57-2).

Category A agents are the highest priority and pose a risk to national security. These agents can be easily disseminated or transmitted from person to person. Because these agents cause a high death rate and have the potential to cause a major public health problem, they might cause public panic and disruption. Category A agents require special action for public health preparedness. An example of a category A agent is *B anthracis* (anthrax).

Category B agents are the second-highest priority. They are fairly easy to disseminate. They cause moderate illnesses and have a lower death rate than do category A agents. These agents require specific enhancements of diagnostic capacity and disease surveillance. An example of a category B agent is *C burnetii* (Q fever).

Category C agents are the third-highest priority. They include new pathogens that could be engineered for mass dissemination in the future. These agents are widely available and are easy to produce and dispense. They have the potential to cause a high rate of death and sickness. An example of a category C agent is Nipah virus.

CBRNE Science Database

CBRNE is an abbreviation for the categories of WMDs: Chemical, Biologic, Radiologic, Nuclear, and Explosive agents. The US Department of Health and Human Services, Office of the Assistant Secretary for

BOX 57-2 Critical Biologic Agents

Category A

Anthrax (*B anthracis*)
Botulism (*C botulinum* toxin)
Plague (*Y pestis*)
Smallpox (variola major)
Tularemia (*F tularensis*)
Viral hemorrhagic fevers (VHFs) (filoviruses [eg, Ebola, Marburg] and arenaviruses [eg, Lassa, Machupo])

Category B

Brucellosis (*Brucella* species)
Epsilon toxin of *C perfringens*
Food safety threats (eg, *Salmonella* species, *Escherichia coli* O157:H7, *Shigella*)
Glanders (*Burkholderia mallei*)
Melioidosis (*Burkholderia pseudomallei*)
Psittacosis (*Chlamydia psittaci*)
Q fever (*C burnetii*)
Ricin toxin from *Ricinus communis* (castor beans)
Staphylococcal enterotoxin B
Typhus fever (*Rickettsia prowazekii*)
Viral encephalitis (alphaviruses [eg, Venezuelan equine encephalitis, eastern equine encephalitis, western equine encephalitis])
Water safety threats (eg, *Vibrio cholerae*, *Cryptosporidium parvum*)

Category C

Nipah virus
Hantaviruses

Modified from: NIAID emerging infectious diseases/pathogens. National Institute of Allergy and Infectious Diseases website. https://www.niaid.nih.gov/research/emerging-infectious-diseases-pathogens. Accessed April 28, 2018.

NOTE

Biosurveillance is a process of gathering, integrating, interpreting, and communicating essential information that might relate to disease activity and threats to human, animal, or plant health. Biosurveillance is conducted at local, state, and national levels of government. The goal of this surveillance is to improve the sharing of information between the health care system and government agencies to rapidly detect, respond to, and counter biologic, chemical, and agricultural threats. In the United States, the Department of Homeland Security (DHS), in conjunction with the CDC, is in charge of this process through the National Biosurveillance Integration Center (NBIC). The NBIC includes the following programs:

- Enhanced Passive Surveillance Program to identify endemic, transboundary, and emerging disease outbreaks in livestock
- BioThreat Awareness APEX Program to develop affordable, effective, and rapid detection systems and architectures to provide advance warning of a biologic attack at indoor, outdoor, and national security events
- Biosurveillance Information and Knowledge Integration Program to develop a Community of Practice platform prototype that integrates multiple data streams to support decision making during a biologic event and clinical practice guidelines for responders

Modified from: Biosurveillance. National Association of County and City Health Officials website. http://archived.naccho.org/topics/emergency/biosurveillance/index.cfm. Accessed April 28, 2018; and CBD focus areas—biosurveillance. US Department of Homeland Security website. https://www.dhs.gov/science-and-technology/biosurveillance. Accessed April 28, 2018.

Preparedness and Response (ASPR), has developed a program, called ASPR CBRNE Science, to bring experiential, evidence-based science and medicine to the process of preparing for and responding to CBRNE incidents. This program uses small teams, working groups, and task groups in an ongoing effort to meet the following objectives:[5]

- To provide coordinated strategic, technical, and operational leadership, advice, and guidance for all levels of the medical response, with focus on medical and public health impacts and interventions relating to CBRNE incidents
- To improve overall public health emergency preparedness by having systems prepared, responsive, and resilient to limit the adverse health impacts of CBRNE emergencies
- To apply evidence-based decision making to preparedness planning for, response to, and recovery from a CBRNE incident

The ASPR CBRNE Science website offers resources to enhance national preparedness and "just-in-time" response, with a focus on medical management, for the following groups of incidents:

- Radiation emergencies
- Chemical emergencies
- Nuclear detonation (state and local planning)

Methods of Dissemination

Most biologic agents used in bioterrorism are designed to enter the body through one of three ways. One way is the inhalation of small particles into the lungs. Another is through the ingestion of contaminated food or water. The third way is by contamination of the skin that allows for absorption of the toxins. A rarer type of exposure is by injection. Anthrax has been reported in northern European heroin users who inject drugs.[6] Because all category A agents, including weaponized botulism, can be disseminated through aerosolization, the inhalation route is of greatest concern.

Aerosols can be delivered in wet or dry form in closed or open spaces. Equipment that may be used to disseminate aerosols includes crop-dusting planes for open spaces, aerosol-generating devices for enclosed areas (eg, subways, enclosed malls), ventilation systems in buildings, and contamination of items in the environment with fine powders that are aerosolized easily when disrupted. The last example is the method of dispersal that occurred in the 2001 anthrax cases in the United States; dispersal was caused by opening contaminated mail.

CRITICAL THINKING

Why would aerosolized agents of mass destruction pose a great risk to first responders?

Specific Biologic Threats

Hundreds of biologic and chemical agents can be used in a bioterrorism attack. This section provides a brief overview of a few of these agents. The agents described in the following sections are considered most likely to be used as a threat to civilian populations. The most common biologic threats are thought to be anthrax, botulism, plague, ricin, tularemia, smallpox, and VHFs.[7]

NOTE

Like all other hazardous materials incidents, it is assumed that all responders will wear the proper PPE. It also is assumed that they will take standard precautions at the scene and during patient care. EMS personnel should not enter a scene with known or suspected biologic or chemical threats until the scene has been made safe by the proper personnel.

Anthrax

Anthrax is an acute infectious disease caused by the spore-forming bacterium *B anthracis*. Anthrax most often occurs in warm-blooded animals. However, it also can infect humans. Symptoms of disease vary. Usually, though, symptoms appear within 7 days after exposure. The most common form of anthrax is **cutaneous anthrax**. It results from direct contact with spores or bacilli. (Cutaneous anthrax also can occur from exposure to contaminated soil and is not necessarily associated with a WMD incident.) Cutaneous anthrax causes localized itching. This symptom is followed by a papular lesion that turns vesicular with subsequent development of black eschar within 7 to 10 days of the initial lesion (**FIGURE 57-1**). Symptoms of **inhalational anthrax** often resemble a common cold in the initial stages. This presentation is followed by severe respiratory distress and sepsis (**FIGURE 57-2**). Inhalational anthrax has very high death

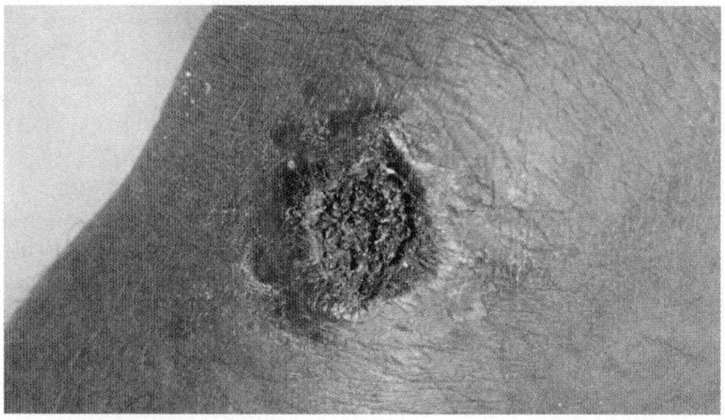

FIGURE 57-1 Cutaneous anthrax.

Courtesy of James H. Steele/CDC.

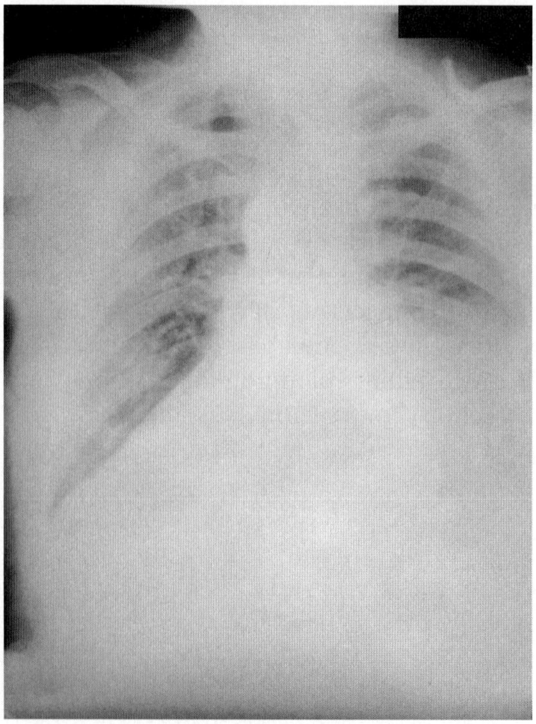

FIGURE 57-2 Respiratory distress and sepsis in anthrax.

Courtesy of Centers for Disease Control and Prevention.

rates.[8] Other, less common forms of anthrax include **intestinal anthrax** from consuming contaminated meat and oropharyngeal anthrax when the mouth and throat are infected (rare).

Treatment

Direct person-to-person spread of anthrax usually does not occur. Only rare cases of person-to-person transmission have been reported when there has been exposure to discharge from open lesions of cutaneous anthrax.[9] Thus, immunization or treatment of people who have come in contact with a patient (eg, household members, friends, coworkers) is unnecessary. These people do not need to be treated unless they also were exposed to the aerosol at the time of the attack. The disease is diagnosed by isolating *B anthracis* from the blood, skin lesions, or respiratory tract secretions or by measuring specific antibodies in the blood of suspected cases. Treatment with antibiotics should be early; if left untreated, the disease can be fatal. Human anthrax vaccines (controversial) are available and are reported to be 93% effective against cutaneous anthrax.[6] Vaccination to protect against anthrax is recommended only for those at high risk.[10] This group includes, for example, some military personnel, some people who handle animals or animal products, and workers in research laboratories who routinely handle anthrax bacteria.[11]

Botulism

As described in Chapter 33, *Toxicology*, **botulism** is a rare but serious paralytic illness. The bacterium *C botulinum* produces a nerve toxin that causes paralysis. Botulinum toxin is one of the most potent and lethal known substances. There are several types of botulism. One type is **foodborne botulism**, which is caused by eating foods that contain the botulism toxin. The second type is **wound botulism** (**FIGURE 57-3**), which is caused by toxin produced from a wound infected with *C botulinum*. The third type is **infant botulism**. This type is caused by consumption of the spores of the botulinum bacteria, which then grow in the intestines and release toxin. All forms of botulism can be fatal and are considered medical emergencies.

In a bioterrorism attack, inhaling the toxin as an aerosol weapon or ingesting the toxin via contaminated food or water are the most likely routes of exposure for serious illness. Foodborne botulism can be especially dangerous because small amounts of the bacterium in contaminated food can poison many people. Signs and symptoms of the illness include nausea, dry mouth, blurred vision, dysphagia, fatigue, and dyspnea that may begin several hours to several days after the exposure.

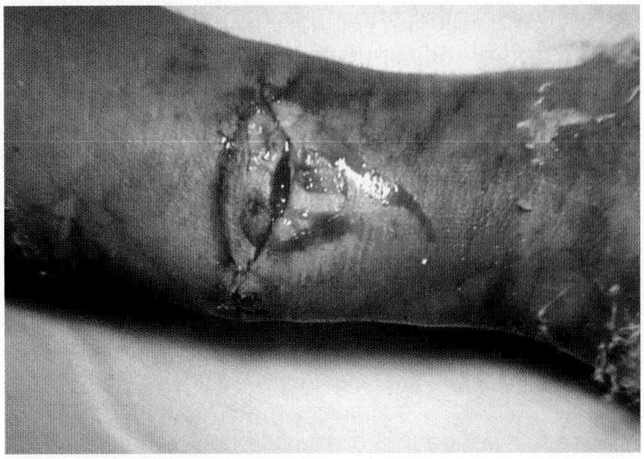

FIGURE 57-3 Wound botulism.

Courtesy of Centers for Disease Control and Prevention.

Treatment

Botulism is not spread from person to person. If diagnosed early, foodborne and wound botulism can be treated with an antitoxin. The antitoxin blocks the action of toxin circulating in the blood. Recovery may take several weeks. As a result of the paralysis and respiratory failure that occur with botulism, the patient may be placed on a ventilator.

> CRITICAL THINKING
> What kind of resources would your community need to support hundreds of patients who need care on a ventilator?

Plague

Plague is caused by the bacterium *Y pestis*. This bacterium is found in rodents (eg, chipmunks, prairie dogs, ground squirrels, rats, mice) and their fleas in many areas of the world. It also can be grown in large amounts and disseminated by aerosol in a bioterrorism attack. Such an attack would result in an epidemic of the pneumonic form of the disease (**pneumonic plague**) with the potential for secondary contamination. Signs and symptoms include fever, extreme weakness, shortness of breath, chest pain, cough, and bloody sputum. Gastrointestinal symptoms are often present, including nausea, vomiting, abdominal pain, and diarrhea. The illness can lead to septic shock within 2 to 4 days.[12] Without treatment, plague has a high mortality rate.

> NOTE
>
> There are three types of pneumonic plague arising from the lungs, all of which are caused by the bacterium *Y pestis.* Bubonic plague arises in the lymph nodes and leads to swelling that produces buboes. Septicemic plague occurs when the lymph infection spreads to the bloodstream.

A bioterrorism attack with the bacteria would be characterized by pneumonic plague occurring at the same time in people following a common exposure. A secondary outbreak of illness would occur in others who had close contact with an infected person's respiratory droplets.

Treatment

The disease is diagnosed through testing for the bacteria. Plague should be treated early (within 24 hours) with antibiotic or antimicrobial agents. People who have been in close contact with the patient should be identified. These people must be evaluated for post-exposure drug therapy. Pneumonic plague is spread through the respiratory droplets of an infected person. Thus, patients with the disease should be isolated. Standard precautions and personal respiratory protection for all caregivers are crucial.

> CRITICAL THINKING
>
> Your service notices a sudden increase in patients with severe respiratory distress. These patients also have pneumonia-like signs and symptoms. Would you initially consider bioterrorism as a cause of the outbreak?

Ricin

Ricin is a potent protein cytotoxin, a chemical that is derived from the beans of the castor plant (*R communis*) (**FIGURE 57-4**). Castor beans are widely available throughout the world. The toxin also is relatively easy to extract. Ricin can be made into a mist, powder, or pellet. When ricin is inhaled as an aerosol, it results in pulmonary toxicity with severe respiratory symptoms within 8 hours. This is followed by acute hypoxic respiratory failure in 36 to 72 hours.[13] (Nonspecific findings of weakness, fever, vomiting, cough, hypoxemia, hypothermia, and hypotension in large numbers of patients might suggest exposure to several respiratory pathogens.) If ricin is ingested, severe gastrointestinal symptoms occur, with rapid onset of nausea, vomiting, abdominal cramps, and severe diarrhea. This reaction is followed by vascular collapse and death.

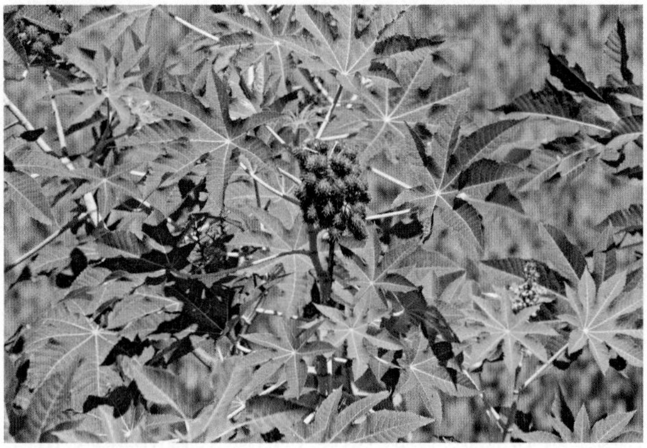

FIGURE 57-4 The seed pods of the castor bean plant are used to manufacture ricin.

Treatment

No antidote exists for ricin poisoning. Treatment is aimed at avoiding exposure and eliminating the toxin from the body as quickly as possible. Patients who have inhaled ricin should be moved to an area with fresh air, clothing contaminated with the toxin should be removed, and the patient should be decontaminated (see Chapter 56, *Hazardous Materials Awareness*). The prehospital care may include airway, ventilatory, and circulatory support. Seizures, hypotension, and respiratory failure should be anticipated.

Smallpox

Smallpox was declared extinct by the World Health Organization in 1980 because of near-universal vaccination. However, the virus could be used as a biologic weapon and has been in the past. The variola virus that causes smallpox is fairly stable, and the infectious dose is small. Moreover, an aerosol release of the virus would be widely spread. The incubation

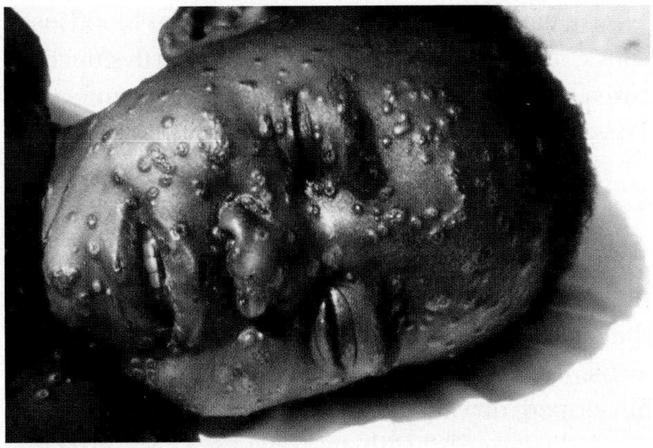

FIGURE 57-5 Smallpox lesions.

Courtesy of Centers for Disease Control and Prevention.

period for smallpox is about 12 days following exposure. The virus usually is spread by an infected person releasing infected saliva from the mouth into the air. People in close or prolonged contact with the infected person inhale the virus. Smallpox also can be spread through direct contact with infected body fluids or contaminated objects, such as bedding or clothing. Signs and symptoms of the disease include high fever, fatigue, headache, and backache. These are followed within 2 to 3 days with the smallpox rash and skin lesions. These lesions finally form crusts. On healing, the lesions leave depressed, depigmented scars (**FIGURE 57-5**). Permanent joint deformities and blindness may follow recovery. The death rate from smallpox is about 30% in unvaccinated people.[14]

Vaccine immunity may prevent or modify the illness. At this time, however, the federal government does not recommend prophylactic vaccination for health care workers or the general public because of the possibility of severe reactions.[15] If an attack is known or imminent, smallpox response teams whose members have received the vaccine will administer the vaccine to others. They also will care for victims who have been exposed. Currently, the United States has enough smallpox vaccine in storage to vaccinate everyone in the country who might need it in the event of an emergency.[16]

Treatment

There is no proven treatment for smallpox. However, several antiviral drugs are being studied. Patients with smallpox should receive supportive care provided by vaccinated personnel. The personnel must use standard precautions, including appropriate respiratory protection. Objects that come in contact with the patient require disinfection. Examples of such objects are bed linens, clothing, ambulances, and equipment. This disinfection must be by fire, steam, or sodium hypochlorite solution.

> CRITICAL THINKING
>
> Your employer asks you to get the smallpox vaccination after a terrorist attack causes an outbreak. Where can you look to find information about the side effects and risks of immunization with this vaccine?

Tularemia

Tularemia is a serious illness caused by the bacterium *F tularensis.* This bacterium is found in animals (especially rodents, rabbits, and hares). (The illness can be caused by skinning the fresh carcass of rabbits ["rabbit fever"], if the bacterium is introduced through broken skin. Rubber gloves should be worn when handling animals that might harbor the bacterium.) The disease is highly infectious. Some strains are resistant to antibiotics. The bacterium responsible for tularemia can be delivered in a bioterrorism attack by aerosol. Infection may result from inhalation of the aerosol. It also may result from the skin, mucous membranes, respiratory tract, or gastrointestinal tract (via contaminated soil, water, food, or animals) being exposed to the virus. Transmission of the disease from person to person does not occur. The development of signs and symptoms varies widely (from 1 day to 2 weeks). A person's reaction is based on the strength of the strain and the route of exposure. Following a bioterrorism attack with the agent, patients may complain of an abrupt onset of an acute febrile illness (headache, chills, general malaise). They also may complain of gastrointestinal illness that includes nausea, vomiting, and diarrhea. If left untreated, septic tularemia may lead to disseminated intravascular coagulation with bleeding, acute respiratory failure, and death.

Treatment

The disease is managed with antibiotics. The patient may require airway, ventilatory, and circulatory support. Until recently, a tularemia vaccine was available for laboratory workers. The safety of the vaccine is being reviewed and is not available at this time.[17]

Viral Hemorrhagic Fevers

Viral hemorrhagic fevers (VHFs) refer to a group of illnesses caused by several distinct families of viruses that include arenaviruses, filoviruses, bunyaviruses, paramyxoviruses, and flaviviruses. The VHFs have limited geographic ranges and are found mostly across eastern and southern Africa, South America, and the Pacific islands.[18] In the 2014–2015 outbreak of the Ebola virus in West Africa, almost 29,000 cases were reported, leaving about 11,000 dead. Four Ebola cases were reported in the United States in 2014, and one patient died.[19] Most hemorrhagic fevers are highly infectious if spread as an aerosol. These viruses naturally reside in animals (eg, cotton rat, deer mouse) or arthropods (eg, ticks, mosquitoes). The viruses are fully dependent on these living hosts for reproduction and survival. Viruses that cause hemorrhagic fever usually are transmitted to humans during contact with urine, fecal matter, saliva, or other body excretions from an infected rodent or by a bite from an infected mosquito or tick. Some VHFs (eg, **Ebola** and **Marburg**) also can spread from person to person following an initial infection. This type of infection most often results from close contact with infected people through their body tissues and fluids.

> **DID YOU KNOW?**
>
> Diseases named after regions are capitalized. For example, Ebola is named after the Ebola river in Zaire, where the virus surfaced in humans. The Marburg virus was named after a city in Germany where two large outbreaks of hemorrhagic fever (in Marburg and Frankfurt) occurred in laboratory workers.
>
> *Modified from*: Centers for Disease Control and Prevention, National Center for Emerging and Zoonotic Infectious Diseases, Division of High-Consequence Pathogens and Pathology, Viral Special Pathogens Branch. Marburg hemorrhagic fever (Marburg HF). Centers for Disease Control and Prevention website. https://www.cdc.gov/vhf/marburg/index.html. Updated December 1, 2014. Accessed April 28, 2018.

VHFs cause a multisystem syndrome. The syndrome is characterized by hemorrhage and life-threatening disease. Signs and symptoms vary by the type of VHF. However, they often include fever, fatigue, dizziness, muscle aches, loss of strength, and exhaustion. Patients with severe cases of VHF may bleed from mucous membranes, from internal organs, or from the mouth, eyes, or ears. (Death rarely results from this blood loss.) Shock, renal failure, central nervous system dysfunction, coma, and seizures may develop with severe infection. These conditions may lead to a fatal outcome.

Treatment

Therapy for patients with VHFs is supportive. With the exception of yellow fever and Argentine hemorrhagic fever, and more recently dengue and Rift Valley virus, for which experimental vaccines have been developed, no vaccines exist that can protect against these diseases.[20,21] Clinical trials for a safe, effective vaccine for Ebola continue. The goals of therapy are to maintain vital functions. This may allow recovery in some patients.

Nuclear and Radiologic Threats

Nuclear explosions can cause deadly effects from blinding light, intense heat (thermal radiation), initial nuclear radiation, blast, fires started by the heat pulse, and secondary fires caused by destruction. A **radiologic dispersion device (RDD)** is also called a "dirty nuke" or "dirty bomb." The use of such a device as a terrorist weapon is considered far more likely than use of a true nuclear device. (A true nuclear device uses weapons-grade uranium or plutonium.[22]) These dirty bombs appeal to terrorists. They require little technical knowledge to build and deploy compared with that of a true nuclear device. These radioactive materials also are used widely in medicine, agriculture, industry, and research. They are readily available and easy to obtain.

> **NOTE**
>
> Radiologic attacks are a credible threat. However, they would not result in the hundreds of thousands of deaths that could be caused by a crude nuclear weapon that requires a fission reaction. A radiologic attack, however, could cause serious illness in people in the immediate area, contaminate several city blocks, and require costly cleanup (if even possible). Thus, they are sometimes referred to as a "weapon of mass *disruption*."

The main type of RDD combines an explosive, such as dynamite, with a radioactive material. The extent of contamination would depend on a number of factors, such as the size of the explosive, the amount and type of radioactive material used, and weather conditions (eg, wind). The detonation of an RDD releases radioactive fallout, which could cause radiation sickness, severe burns, and long-term cancer fatalities. In most cases, the conventional explosive itself would result in more deaths than would exposure to the radioactive material.[23] A second type of RDD might involve a powerful radioactive source hidden in a public place. It may be hidden, for example, in a trash can in a busy train or subway station in which people passing close to the source might receive a significant dose of radiation.

> CRITICAL THINKING
> What EMS groups or divisions should you consider setting up if there is a report of a dirty bomb explosion?

Emergency Care

As described in Chapter 38, *Burns*, the principles of time, distance, and shielding should be used for personal protection and for the protection of others:

1. Limit the amount of time at a radiologic scene. Fallout radiation loses its intensity fairly rapidly. Use or wear radiation detection monitors. Remove clothing and shower if exposed to radioactive dust or sand (fallout).
2. Increase the distance between you and the scene.
3. Shield yourself with appropriate PPE, geographic features of the terrain (mountains, hills, depressions), or structural materials whenever possible. Your protection increases in proportion to the number of heavy, dense materials located between you and the fallout particles.

After dealing with the initial blast, the top priorities are the treatment of radiation sickness, the containment and monitoring of radioactive fallout, evacuation, and decontamination.

Incendiary Threats

Incendiary devices are weapons that produce heat and fire through the chemical reaction of a flammable substance.[24] They are often referred to as firebombs. Terrorists may choose to use an improvised incendiary device because most are inexpensive and can be easily made from materials purchased at the hardware or grocery store.[25] These devices range from a simple Molotov cocktail (a bottle containing a rag soaked in gasoline that is ignited) to much larger and sophisticated devices containing napalm, thermite, or chlorine trifluoride. Their main use in terrorism is to generate panic (a weapon of mass disruption). However, they are also capable of causing loss of life and property damage from fire. Depending on the severity of the attack, primary concerns may include the following:

- The possibility for large numbers of burn victims, inhalation injuries, and fatalities
- Significant damage to buildings and the infrastructure of a community
- Overwhelming of local resources (emergency response agencies, hospitals, mental health agencies)
- The involvement of law enforcement at local, state, and federal levels because of the criminal nature of the event
- The closing of workplaces and schools
- Possible restrictions on domestic and international travel
- The need for evacuation and extended cleanup
- Public fear that can continue for a prolonged period

White Phosphorus

Incendiary devices built with white phosphorus present special concerns. White phosphorus ignites when exposed to oxygen at temperatures above 84°F (30°C). As it burns, it produces a thick smoke. White phosphorus is highly soluble in human fat. Exposure causes deep thermal and chemical burns. If fragments of the chemical remain, they can reignite when bandages are removed because of the reexposure to oxygen.

Emergency Care

Emergency care depends on the nature of the attack. Care may include providing care for burns or inhalation injuries at a small-scale event. However, care also may include managing a scene with multiple patients at a large-scale event (see Chapter 53, *Medical Incident Command*). As with any emergency response, EMS crews should not approach the scene until it has been made safe by the proper personnel. Following the initial explosion, detonation of a second device is possible. The second device may be designed to injure or kill emergency response personnel or bystanders. In addition, biologic, chemical, or nuclear materials may have been used in the explosion.

Thus, it is crucial to personal safety not to enter the scene until the area is determined to be safe.

Specific Chemical Threats

Specific chemicals that may be used in war and acts of terrorism include nerve agents, poisonous gases, and blister agents. The deliberate release of these chemicals in gas, liquid, or solid form can poison people or the environment.

Nerve Agents

Nerve agents were used in military conflicts in the Persian Gulf in the 1980s. They also were used in terrorist attacks in Japan in 1995 and in Syria in 2017. They are the most toxic and rapidly acting of the known chemical warfare agents.[26] Nerve agents are similar to organophosphates in terms of their mechanism of action and the kinds of harmful effects they cause. (However, they are more potent [see Chapter 33, *Toxicology*].) Nerve agents inhibit the effects of acetylcholinesterase, which causes a cholinergic "overdrive" (cholinergic crisis) that disrupts the nerve transmissions in the central and peripheral nervous systems. The extent of poisoning caused by nerve agents depends on the amount, route, and length of exposure. Mildly or moderately exposed people usually recover fully. Severely exposed people are not likely to survive. The nerve agents discussed in this chapter are sarin, soman, tabun, and VX.

NOTE

Allied forces in World War II coined these nerve agents as "G" series. They were so named because they were first developed by German scientists during the war.

Modified from: Nerve agents. Organisation for the Prohibition of Chemical Weapons website. https://www.opcw.org/about-chemical-weapons/types-of-chemical-agent/nerve-agents/. Accessed April 28, 2018.

Sarin (also known as BG) is a clear, colorless, and tasteless liquid that has no odor in its pure form. However, sarin can evaporate into a vapor (gas) and spread into the environment. The agent also mixes easily with water, creating a contamination risk for those who touch or drink the water. Symptoms may begin within minutes to hours after exposure.

CRITICAL THINKING

Would you expect a fast or slow heart rate if the patient has been exposed to a nerve agent?

They may include headache, salivation, chest pain, abdominal cramps, wheezing, fasciculations (ie, muscle twitching), seizure, and respiratory failure that possibly can lead to death.

Soman (also known as GD) is a clear, colorless, tasteless liquid with a slight camphor odor. The odor is similar to the smell of a topical cough suppressant (eg, Vicks VapoRub) or rotting fruit. The agent can vaporize if heated. Compared with other nerve agents, soman is more volatile than VX but less volatile than sarin. (The higher the volatility of a chemical, the more likely it will evaporate and disperse into the environment.) People can be exposed to the vapor even if they do not come in contact with the liquid form. Symptoms may begin within seconds to hours after exposure. They include headache, salivation, chest pain, abdominal cramps, wheezing, fasciculations, seizure, and respiratory failure that possibly can lead to death.

Tabun (also known as GA) is a clear, colorless, tasteless liquid with a faint fruity odor. The chemical can vaporize if heated. Thus, people can be exposed to the nerve agent by skin or eye contact or by inhalation. The agent also mixes easily with water, allowing for possible cutaneous exposure and exposure to the gastrointestinal tract if contaminated food or water is ingested. Moreover, secondary contamination is possible, as would occur from coming into contact with clothing or personal articles that have been contaminated by tabun vapor. Symptoms generally appear within a few seconds after exposure to tabun vapor and within 18 hours after exposure to liquid tabun.[27] Signs and symptoms of mild to moderate exposure to tabun include watery eyes, blurred vision, headache, weakness, cough, drooling, polyuria, excessive sweating, fasciculations, hypotension or hypertension, and cardiac abnormalities. With severe exposure, patients may experience loss of consciousness, seizures, and cardiorespiratory arrest. Severely poisoned patients are not likely to survive.

VX is a thick, amber-colored, odorless liquid. It resembles motor oil and is the most potent of all nerve agents. VX is considered to be much more toxic when absorbed through the skin and somewhat more toxic by inhalation than are other nerve agents. VX is primarily a liquid exposure hazard. However, if heated to very high temperatures, it can turn into small amounts of vapor. Following release of VX into the air, people can be exposed through skin contact, eye contact, or inhalation. VX also can be released into the water, enabling exposure by ingestion or absorption. Symptoms will appear within a few seconds after exposure to the vapor form of VX. They will appear within a few minutes to up to 18 hours after exposure to the liquid form. Signs and symptoms of exposure are the same as those for other nerve agents.

Treatment

Treatment for exposure to nerve agents consists of quickly removing the agent from the body and supporting the patient's vital functions. If vapor exposure has occurred, the patient should be moved quickly to an area with fresh air. If the exposure occurred in an open-air environment, the patient should be moved uphill and upwind from the contamination site. Many nerve agents are heavier than air and will settle in low-lying areas. The patient's clothing should be removed, and the patient should be decontaminated by trained personnel. A person's clothing and other contaminated surfaces can release nerve agents for about 30 minutes after exposure.[28] Thus, secondary contamination is possible.

Atropine and pralidoxime chloride are antidotes for nerve agent toxicity (**TABLE 57-1**). They are available in autoinjector kits (eg, MARK I, Antidote Treatment Nerve Agent Auto-injector [ATNAA], DuoDote kits). They work by blocking the effects of acetylcholine (see Chapter 33, *Toxicology*, and Appendix A, *Emergency Drug Index*). Large doses of these drugs and repeated administration may be required. Midazolam, diazepam, or lorazepam may be indicated if seizures are present. The paramedic should consider administering one of these drugs if muscle twitching is present. Diazepam autoinjectors are available for these emergencies. Once seizures begin, they can be almost impossible to stop. Caring for patients who have ingested a nerve agent should be guided by medical direction, a poison control center, or other authority.

NOTE

The federal government has distributed caches of nerve agent antidotes throughout the country in CHEMPACK containers. EMS CHEMPACK containers contain a sufficient number of autoinjectors to treat about 450 patients. Each CHEMPACK contains Mark-1 or ATNAA autoinjector kits, atropine sulfate, pralidoxime, AtroPens, diazepam (solution and autoinjectors), and sterile water. When needed, designated EMS or law enforcement officials will transport the CHEMPACK to the incident site.

Modified from: National Association of EMS Officials. *National Model EMS Clinical Guidelines*. Version 2.0. National Association of EMS Officials website. https://www.nasemso.org/documents/National-Model-EMS-Clinical-Guidelines-Version2-Sept2017.pdf. Published September 2017. Accessed April 12, 2018.

SHOW ME THE EVIDENCE

Researchers hypothesized that intraosseous (IO) injections of drug antidotes into swine bone marrow would provide a more rapid means to treat exposure to nerve agents as compared to standard intramuscular (IM) injections. They compared IM and IO administration of pralidoxime chloride during normovolemia and hypovolemia, as well as their combined administration during normovolemia in swine. They randomly administered 2 mL, 660 mg pralidoxime chloride via the IM or IO route to 10 normovolemic and to 8 hypovolemic swine. IM injection achieved therapeutic levels (4 mcg/mL) in 2 minutes, whereas IO infusion achieved these levels in less than 15 seconds. In the hypovolemic swine, IM injection achieved therapeutic levels in 4 minutes compared with less than 15 seconds in the IO group. The researchers concluded that the IO route for delivery of pralidoxime chloride may provide greater initial therapy. Note: A limitation to their findings is that autoinjector medications may be administered only by the IM route.

Modified from: Uwaydah NI, Hoskins SL, Bruttig SP, et al. Intramuscular versus intraosseous delivery of nerve agent antidote pralidoxime chloride in swine. *Prehosp Emerg Care.* 2016;20(4):485-492.

Poisonous Gases

Poisonous gases were popular weapons during World War I. They are produced in large quantities worldwide for use in the industrial sector and are widely available.[29] Thus, use of these gases for acts of terrorism is a possibility. The choking agents, chlorine and phosgene, are the best known among this class.[30]

Chlorine is a yellow-green gas with an odor that has been described as a mixture of pineapple and pepper. Chlorine gas can be pressurized and condensed to change it into a liquid. In liquid form, chlorine can be shipped and stored. When liquid chlorine is released, it quickly vaporizes into a gas that stays close to the

TABLE 57-1 Recommendations for Prehospital Nerve Agent Therapy

Patient Category	Antidotes[a] Mild/Moderate Symptoms[b]	Antidotes[a] Severe Symptoms[c]	Notes
Infant (birth to 2 years)	Atropine: 0.05 mg/kg IM; 2-PAM-Cl: 15 mg/kg IM	Atropine: 0.1 mg/kg IM; 2-PAM-Cl: 45 mg/kg IM	For severe exposures, assisted ventilation should be started after administration of antidotes. Overdose of pralidoxime chloride can cause neuromuscular weakness and respiratory depression in children.
Child (3–7 years) (29–55 pounds [13–25 kg])	Atropine: 1 mg IM; 2-PAM-Cl: 15 mg/kg IM	Atropine: 0.1 mg/kg or 2 mg IM; 2-PAM-Cl: 45 mg/kg IM	Autoinjectors may be used.
Child (8–14 years) (56–110 pounds [26–50 kg])	Atropine: 2 mg IM; 2-PAM-Cl: 15 mg/kg IM	Atropine: 4 mg IM; 2-PAM-Cl: 45 mg/kg IM	Repeat atropine until secretions have diminished and breathing is comfortable or airway resistance has returned to near normal. Excessive doses of pralidoxime in adults (especially older adults) may cause severe hypertension, weakness, headache, tachycardia, and visual impairment.
Adolescent, adult, pregnant women	Atropine: 2–4 mg IM; 2-PAM-Cl: 600 mg IM *Or* One autoinjector kit (600 mg) IM	Atropine: 6 mg IM; 2-PAM-Cl: 1,800 mg IM *Or* Three autoinjector kits (1,800 mg) IM	
Older adult, frail condition	Atropine: 1 mg IM; 2-PAM-Cl: 10 mg/kg IM	Atropine: 2–4 mg IM; 2-PAM-Cl: 25 mg/kg IM	If the older adult has underlying medical conditions (renal function impairment or hypertension), a lower dose of pralidoxime should be considered.

[a]2-PAM-Cl solution must be prepared from an ampule containing 1 g of desiccated 2-PAM-Cl: The paramedic injects 3 mL of saline and 5% distilled or sterile water into the ampule and shakes well. The resulting solution is 3.3 mL of 300 mg/mL 2-PAM-Cl.
[b]Mild to moderate symptoms include localized sweating, muscle fasciculations, nausea, vomiting, weakness, and dyspnea.
[c]Severe symptoms include unconsciousness, convulsions, apnea, and flaccid paralysis.

Abbreviations: IM, intramuscular; 2-PAM-Cl, 2-pralidoxime chloride

Modified from: Agency for Toxic Substances and Disease Registry. Toxic substances portal: medical management guidelines (MMGs). Agency for Toxic Substances and Disease Registry website. https://www.atsdr.cdc.gov/mmg/index.asp. Updated March 3, 2011. Accessed April 27, 2018; and National Association of EMS Officials. *National Model EMS Clinical Guidelines*. Version 2.0. National Association of EMS Officials website. https://www.nasemso.org/documents/National-Model-EMS-Clinical-Guidelines-Version2-Sept2017.pdf. Published September 2017. Accessed April 27, 2018.

ground and spreads rapidly. If chlorine is released into the air, people may be exposed to chlorine gas through skin or eye contact or by inhalation. If chlorine liquid is released into water, exposure can occur by touching or drinking contaminated water or by ingesting food that was prepared with the contaminated water. Like other chemical agents, the extent of poisoning depends on the amount, route, and duration of exposure to the agent. Signs and symptoms may include cough; chest pain; burning sensation in the nose, eyes, or throat; watery eyes; blurred vision; gastrointestinal disturbances; dermal burns from skin contact; and shortness of breath and dyspnea. Pulmonary edema can develop within 2 to 4 hours following inhalation of the gas.[31]

Phosgene (also known as CG) is a poisonous gas that appears as a gray-white cloud and smells like newly mowed hay. With cooling and pressure, the gas can be condensed into a liquid so that it can be shipped and stored. When liquid phosgene is released, it quickly vaporizes into a gas that stays close to the ground and spreads rapidly. Inhaled phosgene damages the lungs, producing a burning sensation, cough, and labored breathing. Pulmonary edema with frothy sputum production may develop. Cutaneous exposure to the gas can result in skin or eye injury. Exposure also can occur by touching or drinking water contaminated with the gas or by ingesting food that was prepared with the contaminated water. In addition to the signs and symptoms noted previously for chlorine exposure, phosgene poisoning may cause hypotension and heart failure. In lethal doses, death can occur within 48 hours.[32]

NOTE

From December 1915 to August 1916, casualties from phosgene exposure during World War I occurred in 4.1% of gas-exposed troops, with 0.7% fatalities. During this war, phosgene was often combined with chlorine in liquid-filled shells. Total casualties from chemical gas exposure occurred in 1.2 million troops and caused 100,000 deaths. Phosgene accounted for an estimated 80% of these cases.

Modified from: Gresham C, LoVecchio F. Industrial toxins. Tintinalli JE, Stapczynski JS, Cline DM, Ma OJ, Cydulka RK, Meckler GD, eds. *Tintinalli's Emergency Medicine: A Comprehensive Guide*. 7th ed. New York, NY: McGraw-Hill; 2011.

Treatment

No antidotes exist for chlorine or phosgene poisoning. Treatment for exposure to these gases consists of removing them from the body as soon as possible and providing supportive medical care. All patients should be moved to an area of fresh air and to the highest ground possible (if exposure occurred in an open air space). The patient's clothing should be removed. The patient should then be decontaminated by trained personnel. Depending on severity of symptoms, additional therapy may include bronchodilators, high-dose steroids, nebulized sodium bicarbonate, and ventilatory and circulatory support.

Blister Agents

Blister agents or **vesicants** are chemicals with highly irritating properties that produce fluid-filled pockets on the skin and damage to the eyes, lungs, and other mucous membranes. In addition to cutaneous effects from exposure to these agents, blister agents also can cause loss of vision, convulsions, and respiratory failure. The gastrointestinal system, central nervous system, and bone marrow also can be affected through systemic absorption. Symptoms of exposure may be delayed until hours after exposure. The major chemicals in this category are sulfur mustard, nitrogen mustard, and lewisite. Phosgene oxime is more of an urticant, producing irritation without blisters. However, the gas still is classified as a vesicant.

Mustard (sulfur mustard and nitrogen mustard) is an oily liquid that comes in a variety of colors ranging from brown to yellow. It may smell like garlic, onion, horseradish, or mustard itself. Lewisite is an oily, odorless liquid. It is more volatile than mustard and smells like geraniums in its gaseous state. (Unlike mustard, in which symptoms may be delayed, lewisite causes immediate pain and irritation on contact.) Phosgene oxime is a colorless solid or yellow-brown liquid. It may have a peppery or pungent odor. Like lewisite, this agent causes immediate pain and irritation on contact with the skin or mucous membranes.

Treatment

After ensuring personal safety (including the use of appropriate PPE), the initial assessment and treatment of the patient should begin with airway, ventilatory, and circulatory support, as needed.

Immediate decontamination may reduce damage to tissue. All skin exposures should be treated with standard burn care. Advanced cardiac life support protocols should be followed for any patient with cardiac or respiratory problems. Advanced trauma life support protocols should be followed for any trauma patient. The signs and symptoms may not develop for several hours following exposure to some blister agents. Thus, a patient with a significant exposure should be evaluated by a physician. Patients who have only mild symptoms should be advised to seek physician evaluation if signs and symptoms worsen.

Explosive Threats

An **explosive** is a bomb. Bombs can be made from a variety of dangerous materials and can be made in a variety of sizes, weighing several ounces to several thousand pounds. The United States has historically experienced about 200 injuries or deaths annually related to bombings. Explosives are categorized as follows:[33,34]

- Low-order explosives
  - Explode with velocities of less than 3,300 feet/s (1,000 m/s)
  - Examples: gunpowder, fireworks, natural gas, flammable gas–air mixtures
- High-order explosives
  - Explode with velocities of 10,000 to 30,000 feet/s (3,000 to 9,000 m/s)
  - Examples: plastic explosives (C4 and Semtex), ANFO (ammonium nitrate/fuel oil), TNT (trinitrotoluene), military bombs
- Improvised explosive devices
  - Either low- or high-order explosives
  - Contain a fuel, an oxidizer (eg, ANFO), and projectiles
  - Examples: pipe bombs, letter bombs, backpack or satchel bombs, vest bombs, dirty bombs, vehicle bombs

NOTE

In January 2018, at least 103 people were killed and over 200 injured when an ambulance packed with explosives by a Taliban suicide bomber detonated in central Kabul, Afghanistan, near several government offices.

Modified from: Faiez R. Officials say 103 killed, 235 wounded in Afghan car bombing. NBC 6 South Florida website. https://www.nbcmiami.com/news/national-international/Afghanistan-Car-Bomb-Attack-Kabul-471405624.html. Published January 22, 2018. Accessed April 28, 2018.

The CDC has issued required resource guidelines and recommendations for EMS response to terrorist bombing attacks (BOX 57-3).

BOX 57-3 Recommendations for EMS Response to Terrorist Bombing Attacks

- Personnel must:
  1. Be trained, equipped, and knowledgeable about explosive devices and personal protection.
  2. Be prepared to institute ICS if needed and to initiate triage.
  3. Be trained in managing blast-related injuries for all age groups.
- Personnel must have:
  1. A system in place to effectively communicate with other emergency personnel (command, fire, law enforcement, other EMS agencies), and with receiving hospitals.
  2. Rapid access to sufficient medical equipment to and transport vehicles to manage large numbers of critically injured patients.
  3. A demobilization plan that includes access to mental health professionals.

Modified from: Hunt RC, Kapil V, Basavaraju SV, et al. Updated: in a moment's notice: surge capacity for terrorist bombings. Centers for Disease Control and Prevention. 2010:21-22. CDC-INFO Pub ID 220190. https://stacks.cdc.gov/view/cdc/5713. Accessed June 12, 2018.

NOTE

The term **improvised explosive device (IED)** originated during the Iraq war. These devices are "homemade" bombs constructed of explosives attached to a detonator. An example is a roadside bomb. IEDs are used in terrorist actions, by criminals or vandals, or in unconventional warfare. In 2007, these devices were responsible for nearly two-thirds of the American combat deaths in Iraq. The amount of damage and injury caused by an IED depends on its size and explosive capacity, the nature of the projectiles in the device, and where it is detonated (**TABLE 57-2**). Explosions in outdoor areas will produce different injury patterns and numbers of casualties than those in confined spaces, such as subway tunnels.

TABLE 57-2 Damage Radius for Different Types of Bombs

Threat	Explosive Capacity	Building Evacuation Distance	Outdoor Evacuation Distance
Small package or letter	1 lb (0.5 kg)	40 ft (12 m)	900 ft (274 m)
Pipe bomb	5 lb (2 kg)	70 ft (21 m)	1,200 ft (366 m)
FedEx package	10 lb (5 kg)	90 ft (27 m)	1,080 ft (329 m)
Vest or container bombs	20 lb (9 kg)	110 ft (30 m)	1,700 ft (518 m)
Parcel (box) package	50 lb (23 kg)	150 ft (46 m)	1,850 ft (564 m)
Compact car	500 lb (228 kg)	320 ft (98 m)	1,900 ft (579 m)
Full-size car or minivan	1,000 lb (454 kg)	400 ft (122 m)	2,400 ft (732 m)
Van, SUV, or pickup truck	4,000 lb (1,814 kg)	640 ft (195 m)	3,800 ft (1,158 m)
Delivery truck	10,000 lb (4,536 kg)	860 ft (262 m)	5,100 ft (1,554 m)

Modified from: National Academies, US Department of Homeland Security. IED attack: improvised explosive devices. News and Terrorism website. https://www.dhs.gov/sites/default/files/publications/prep_ied_fact_sheet.pdf. Accessed April 28, 2018.

Modified from: Virginia Department of Emergency Management. Terrorism information index chart. Terrorism information: the facts—how to prepare—how to respond. Scribd website. https://www.scribd.com/document/45194236/Terrorism-Information-Chart. Accessed April 28, 2018.

Active Shooter Incidents

Between 2000 and 2016, the United States experienced 1,486 casualties from 220 active shooter incidents. Of these, 661 people died and 825 were wounded.[35] Almost 70% of the incidents ended in 5 minutes or less. Although they occurred in a variety of locations, all involved a single shooter (**TABLE 57-3**).[36] As of this writing, only two mass-casualty attacks in the United States have been at the hands of multiple shooters: the Columbine High School massacre in Littleton, Colorado, in 1999, and the Inland Regional Center shootings in San Bernardino, California, in December 2015.[37] Other countries, however, have had coordinated attacks—in Paris, Mumbai, and Moscow—in which paramedics were killed.

TABLE 57-3 Location of 220 Active Shooter Incidents in the United States Between 2000 and 2016

Location	Number
Commerce	95 (42.3%)
Education	48 (21.8%)
Government properties	23 (10.5%)
Open space	29 (13.2%)
Residences	11 (10.5%)
Houses of worship	8 (3.6%)
Health care facilities	6 (2.7%)

NOTE

Some groups and organizations are advocating that the term mass-casualty attacker be used in place of active shooter. This change recognizes that a growing number of incidents involve weapons other than firearms (eg, knives, cars, buses).

Modified from: Mass casualty attacker (active shooter) prevention, preparedness, and response. Violence Prevention Agency website. https://www.violencepreventionagency.com/activeshooterpreparedness. Accessed April 28, 2018.

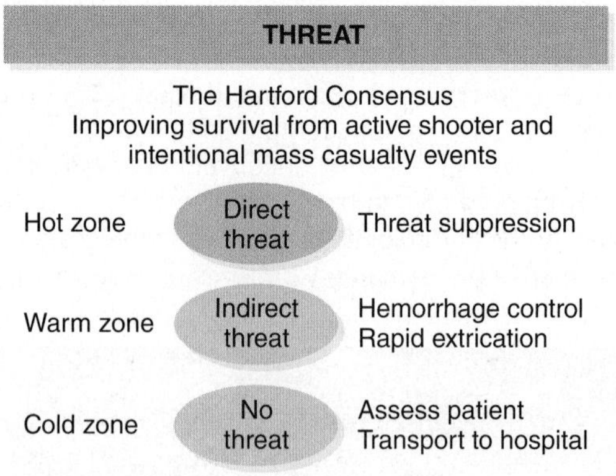

FIGURE 57-6 Zones of care for the THREAT acronym.

NOTE

Hartford Consensus

In April 2013, the American College of Surgeons and the Federal Bureau of Investigation formed the Joint Committee to Create a National Policy to Enhance Survivability From Intentional Mass Casualty and Active Shooter Events following the Sandy Hook Elementary School active shooter massacre. Their mission was to improve survival from active shooter and mass-casualty events, such as the Boston Marathon bombing. In the work they conducted at four meetings in Hartford, Connecticut, they concluded that most preventable deaths in these incidents resulted from uncontrolled bleeding. Together with stakeholders from health care, the military, and first responder agencies, they produced reports containing recommendations for citizen and first responder training for bleeding control and better coordination among emergency responders.

Modified from: The Joint Committee to Create a National Policy to Enhance Survivability From Intentional Mass Casualty and Active Shooter Events. Hartford Consensus. Strategies to enhance survival in active shooter and intentional mass casualty events: a compendium. *Bull Am Coll Surg.* 2015;100(15):1-88.

Emergency Care

The Hartford Consensus used the THREAT acronym to describe zones of care during mass shooter and other intentional mass-casualty events. The THREAT acronym stands for Threat suppression, Hemorrhage control, Rapid Extrication, Assess patient, and Transport to the hospital (**FIGURE 57-6**). The consensus recommendations advocate that the traditional zones of treatment in these situations consisting of red (hot—immediate/direct threat), yellow (warm—indirect threat), and green (cold—no known threat) be compressed from that in the past. This recommendation was derived from data in past incidents showing that if the immediate risk for danger was contained, rescuers could move to the yellow zone to provide lifesaving care before it was definitively and repeatedly cleared of all danger. Strategies to educate the public to become immediate responders (traditionally described as bystanders) were outlined. As soon as feasible, properly trained and equipped emergency responders could then move patients through access corridors secured by law enforcement to casualty collection points or directly to transporting ambulances for further assessment, care, and transport to hospitals for definitive care.[38]

When responding to IED or mass-casualty attacks, paramedics should be mindful of strategies for concealment and cover discussed in Chapter 55, *Crime Scene Awareness*. Tactical emergency medical support teams should be deployed with law enforcement if they are readily available. Because these resources are not accessible in many areas, additional measures should be employed by other EMS crews when providing care within areas not fully secured (yellow zone). Measures include wearing body armor and helmets if available to provide some protection from some weapons, IED fragments, and shock waves (although most nonmilitary tactical vests and helmets do not provide blast protection). Principles of the National Incident Management System (NIMS) should be employed for effective interagency cooperation and coordination.

Like the incendiary devices described earlier, the care for victims of an explosion may vary. Although treatment may require only minor wound care for several people, treatment could be extensive and involve a large-scale event. The incident may involve secondary explosions and chemical and biologic threats. Chapter 36, *Trauma Overview and Mechanism of Injury*, describes care of injuries that result from explosive forces, including primary, secondary, tertiary, and quaternary blast injuries.

In active shooter or explosive incidents, care begins with hemorrhage control. The DHS suggests the following interventions following an IED or active shooter incident:[39]

1. Tourniquets to control bleeding
2. Hemostatic gauze when bleeding control by tourniquet is not possible at the site
3. Nasopharyngeal airway if facial trauma is not present
4. Positioning in recovery position if possible when bleeding into the airway related to facial trauma is present
5. Spinal precaution if indicated and feasible for blunt trauma patients
6. IV access if indicated and provider is qualified and authorized to do so (IV access is not routinely needed in the initial phase of care.)
7. Surgical airway if "sit up and lean forward" posture is not possible in patients with face or neck trauma
8. IO access for medications or fluids if IV access is not possible
9. IV morphine, oral transmucosal fentanyl citrate lozenges, and ketamine for analgesia

Department of Homeland Security

Following the terrorist attacks on the World Trade Center in New York City on September 11, 2001, the DHS was established through the Homeland Security Act of 2002 (HR 5005).[40] The missions of the DHS are to (1) prevent terrorism and enhance security, (2) ensure resilience to disasters, (3) enforce and administer immigration laws, (4) safeguard and secure cyberspace, and (5) secure and manage the borders.[41] To help meet these goals, the Homeland Security Advisory System (HSAS) was developed to inform federal agencies, state and local officials, and the private sector of terrorist threats and appropriate protective actions. In 2011, the color-coded alerts of the HSAS were replaced with the National Terrorism Advisory System (NTAS), designed to more effectively communicate information about terrorist threats by providing timely, detailed information to the American public as follows[41]:

> "The NTAS establishes two types of advisories: bulletins and alerts. NTAS bulletins permit the Secretary of Homeland Security to communicate important terrorism information that, while not necessarily indicative of a specific threat against the United States, can reach Homeland Security partners or the public quickly, thereby allowing recipients to implement necessary protective measures. NTAS alerts are issued only when there is specific, credible information about a terrorist threat against the United States. Using available information, the alerts provide a concise summary of the potential threat, information about actions being taken to ensure public safety, and recommended steps that people, communities, businesses, and governments can take to help prevent, mitigate, or respond to the threat. The NTAS alerts are be based on the nature of the threat: in some cases, alerts are sent directly to law enforcement or affected areas of the private sector, while in others, alerts are issued more broadly to the American people through both official and media channels.[42] NTAS alerts contain a sunset provision indicating a specific date when the alert expires; there will not be a constant NTAS alert or blanket warning that there is an overarching threat. If threat information changes for an alert, the Secretary of Homeland Security may announce an updated NTAS alert. All changes, including the announcement that cancels an NTAS alert, are distributed the same way as the original alert (BOX 57-4)."

BOX 57-4 National Terrorism Advisory System

- **Imminent alert.** Warns of a credible, specific, and impending terrorist threat against the United States.
- **Elevated alert.** Warns of a credible terrorist threat against the United States.
- **Bulletin.** Describes current trends or developments related to terrorist threats.

Modified from: National terrorism advisory system: NTAS frequently asked questions. US Department of Homeland Security website. https://www.dhs.gov/ntas-frequently-asked-questions. Published January 25, 2018. Accessed April 28, 2018.

General Guidelines for Emergency Response

General guidelines for responding to a scene that may involve hazardous materials are described in

CRITICAL THINKING

Why will correct, prompt information to the media be crucial during a WMD event?

DID YOU KNOW?

Presidential Directives to Combat Terrorism in the 21st Century

The Federal Response Plan and Terrorism Incident Annex

In June 1995, the White House issued Presidential Decision Directive 39 (PDD-39), titled United States Policy on Counter-terrorism. PDD-39 directs that federal agencies will provide support to states and localities to reduce vulnerability to acts of terrorism. The directive also provides support in identifying the *crisis management* and *consequences management* activities of terrorist-related use of WMDs.

Crisis management activities include those used to anticipate, acquire, and plan for the necessary resources to prevent and/or resolve a threat or act of terrorism. Crisis management is mainly a law enforcement response. These activities may be supported at the same time by technical operations and by federal consequence management activities as shown in **FIGURE 57-7**.

Consequence management activities include those used to protect public health and safety; to alleviate suffering on lives and property; and to restore essential government services. These activities also provide emergency relief to governments and businesses affected by terrorist acts. State governments are primarily responsible for these consequence management activities, but may receive additional assistance from the federal government as required by the nature and scope of the event.

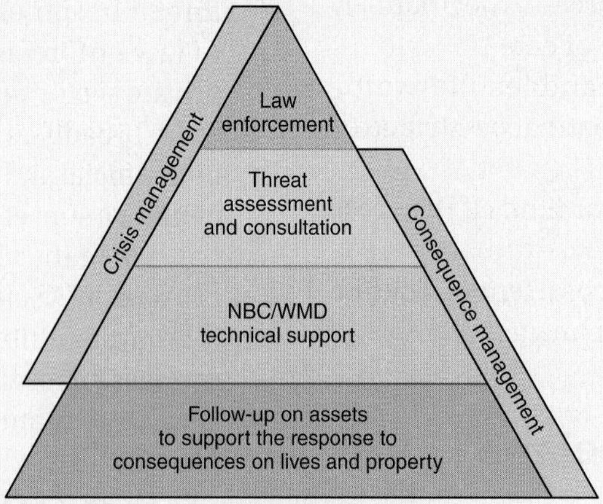

Abbreviations: NBC, nuclear, biologic, chemical; WMD, weapon of mass destruction

FIGURE 57-7 Relationship between crisis and consequence management.

Combating Terrorism: Presidential Decision Directive 62

Presidential Decision Directive 62 (PDD-62), titled Combating Terrorism, was signed on May 22, 1998, by President Bill Clinton. The Directive provided a more defined structure for counter terrorism and identified fighting terrorism as a security priority of the federal government. PDD-62 Section 3 of the directive states:

> We shall have the ability to respond rapidly and decisively to terrorism directed against us wherever it occurs, to protect Americans, arrest or defeat the perpetrators, respond with all appropriate instruments against the sponsoring organizations and governments, and provide recovery relief to victims, as permitted by law.

PDD-62 established the office of the National Coordinator for Security, Infrastructure Protection and Counter-Terrorism. The office was to facilitate interagency activities, policies, and programs to enhance the capability for counter-terrorism response.

Modified from: Federal Emergency Management Agency. Terrorism incident annex. Air University website. http://www.au.af.mil/au/awc/awcgate/frp/frpterr.htm. Updated June 3, 1999. Accessed April 28, 2018; and White House, Office of the Press Secretary. Combatting terrorism: Presidential Decision Directive 62. Wayback Machine website. https://web.archive.org/web/20161125235012/http://www.au.af.mil/au/awc/awcgate/ciao/62factsheet.htm. Published May 22, 1998. Accessed April 28, 2018.

Chapter 56, *Hazardous Materials Awareness*. Many aspects of a WMD incident are comparable to other medical, trauma, and hazardous materials incidents. However, there are some significant differences: (1) Terrorists have been known to time secondary events (eg, booby traps, additional bombs, armed resistance) to injure emergency responders. These events occur more commonly abroad (eg, with ISIL). (2) A terrorist act is a criminal event. As such, the site becomes a crime scene, and everything is considered evidence of the crime. Fear and panic can be expected from the public, patients, and emergency responders. This makes scene safety, security, and crowd control major issues with which to contend. (3) Contingency plans for emergency responders at the scene and at destination facilities will need to be in place. These plans will help emergency responders to deal with the large numbers of upset, agitated, frightened, and injured patients. Large-scale events will likely involve local, state, and federal agencies.

Emergency Responder Guidelines

Emergency responder guidelines have been established by the Office of Justice Program, Office for Domestic Preparedness, to prepare for and respond to incidents of domestic terrorism. These incidents may involve chemical and biologic agents and nuclear, radioactive, and explosive devices. Recommended guidelines for EMS providers are as follows:[43]

- Recognize hazardous materials incidents.
- Know the protocols used to detect the potential presence of WMD agents or materials.
- Know and follow self-protection measures for WMD events and hazardous materials events.
- Know procedures for protecting a potential crime scene.
- Know and follow agency/organization scene security and control procedures for WMD and hazardous material events.
- Possess and know how to use equipment properly to contact dispatchers or higher authorities to report information collected at the scene and to request additional assistance or emergency response personnel. Know how to characterize a WMD event and be able to identify available response assets within the affected jurisdiction(s).

The roles of first responders fall within several broad categories: information gathering, assessment, and dissemination; scene management; saving and protecting life; and securing additional specialist support. Effective management of these roles requires a system of care and preplanning to ensure that all elements of the response are prepared, coordinated, and accessible during a CBRN event.[44]

Finally, EMS agencies must be prepared to implement incident operations, provide personal and public safety measures, perform appropriate decontamination, and provide emergency medical care specific to the incident.

Summary

- There are five categories of weapons of mass destruction (WMDs), which can be remembered with the CBRNE mnemonic: Chemical, Biologic, Radiologic, Nuclear, and Explosive.
- Biologic agents include anthrax, botulism, plague, ricin, tularemia, and smallpox.
- Person-to-person spread is possible in patients who are infected with plague or smallpox.
- Nerve agents include sarin, soman, tabun, and VX. Exposure causes a cholinergic overdrive. The antidotes for nerve agent exposure are atropine and pralidoxime chloride.
- Poisonous gases, such as chlorine and phosgene, cause severe respiratory problems. They also can cause skin and eye injury. Paramedics must move exposed patients to safety, remove their clothing, and treat their symptoms.
- Dirty bombs could cause heat damage and radiation sickness, severe burns, and cancer.
- The Department of Homeland Security's National Terrorism Advisory System advisories communicate information about terrorist threats by providing timely, detailed information to the public, government agencies, first responders, public sector organizations, airports, and other transportation hubs.
- Emergency responders at a WMD incident should recognize hazardous materials incidents, know protocols to detect WMDs, use personal protective equipment, know crime scene procedures, know how to activate more resources, and implement incident operations.

References

1. Bureau of International Security and Nonproliferation. Convention on the Prohibition of the Development, Production and Stockpiling of Bacteriological (Biological) and Toxin Weapons and on Their Destruction (BWC). US Department of State website. https://www.state.gov/t/isn/4718.htm. Accessed April 29, 2018.
2. Osterholm MT, Schwartz J. *Living Terrors: What America Needs to Know to Survive the Coming Bioterrorist Catastrophe.* New York, NY: Delacorte Press; 2000.
3. Burstein JL. Weapons of mass destruction. In: Brice J, Delbridge TR, Myers JB, eds. *Emergency Services: Clinical Practice and Systems Oversight.* 2nd ed. West Sussex, UK: John Wiley & Sons; 2015:349-354.
4. NIAID Emerging Infectious Diseases/Pathogens. National Institute of Allergy and Infectious Diseases website. https://www.niaid.nih.gov/research/emerging-infectious-diseases-pathogens. Accessed April 29, 2018.
5. ASPR CBRNE Science. Public Health Emergency website. https://www.phe.gov/about/aspr/Pages/CBRNE-Science.aspx. Accessed April 29, 2018.
6. Centers for Disease Control and Prevention, National Center for Emerging and Zoonotic Infectious Diseases. Anthrax. Centers for Disease Control and Prevention website. https://www.cdc.gov/anthrax/index.html. Updated January 31, 2017. Accessed April 29, 2018.
7. Kortepeter MG, Parker GW; Centers for Disease Control and Prevention, National Center for Emerging and Zoonotic Infectious Diseases, Office of the Director. Potential biological weapons threats. https://wwwnc.cdc.gov/eid/article/5/4/99-0411_article. Centers for Disease Control and Prevention website. Updated December 13, 2010. Accessed April 29, 2018.
8. Frieden TR, Jaffe HW, Cono J, Richards CI, Iademarco MF. Clinical framework and medial countermeasure use during an anthrax mass-casualty incident. *MMWR Recomm Rep.* 2015;64(4):1-22. https://www.cdc.gov/mmwr/pdf/rr/rr6404.pdf. Accessed April 29, 2018.
9. Centers for Disease Control and Prevention, National Center for Emerging and Zoonotic Infectious Diseases. How people are infected. Centers for Disease Control and Prevention website. https://www.cdc.gov/anthrax/basics/how-people-are-infected.html. Updated September 1, 2015. Accessed April 29, 2018.
10. Centers for Disease Control and Prevention. Use of anthrax vaccine in response to terrorism: supplemental recommendations of the Advisory Committee on Immunization Practices. *MMWR.* 2002;51(45):1024-1026.
11. Centers for Disease Control and Prevention, National Center for Emerging and Zoonotic Infectious Diseases. Antibiotics. Centers for Disease Control and Prevention website. https://www.cdc.gov/anthrax/medical-care/prevention.html. Updated February 14, 2018. Accessed April 29, 2018.
12. Centers for Disease Control and Prevention, National Center for Emerging and Zoonotic Infectious Diseases, Division of Vector-Borne Diseases. Frequently asked questions: what is plague? Centers for Disease Control and Prevention website. https://www.cdc.gov/plague/faq/index.html. Accessed April 29, 2018.
13. National Center for Emerging and Zoonotic Infectious Diseases. Ricin toxin from *Ricinus communis* (castor beans). Centers for Disease Control and Prevention website. https://emergency.cdc.gov/agent/ricin/facts.asp. Updated November 18, 2015. Accessed April 29, 2018.
14. Centers for Disease Control and Prevention, National Center for Emerging and Zoonotic Infectious Diseases, Division of High-Consequence Pathogens and Pathology. Clinical disease: ordinary smallpox (variola major). Centers for Disease Control and Prevention website. https://www.cdc.gov/smallpox/clinicians/clinical-disease.html. Updated December 5, 2016. Accessed April 29, 2018.
15. Centers for Disease Control and Prevention, National Center for Emerging and Zoonotic Infectious Diseases, Division of High-Consequence Pathogens and Pathology. Smallpox: vaccine basics. Centers for Disease Control and Prevention website. https://www.cdc.gov/smallpox/vaccine-basics/index.html. Updated July 12, 2017. Accessed April 29, 2018.
16. Centers for Disease Control and Prevention, National Center for Emerging and Zoonotic Infectious Diseases, Division of High-Consequence Pathogens and Pathology. Prevention and treatment: smallpox vaccine. Centers for Disease Control and Prevention website. https://www.cdc.gov/smallpox/prevention-treatment/index.html. Updated June 7, 2016. Accessed April 29, 2018.
17. Centers for Disease Control and Prevention, National Center for Emerging and Zoonotic Infectious Diseases, Division of Vector-Borne Diseases. Tularemia: prevention. Centers for Disease Control and Prevention website. https://www.cdc.gov/tularemia/prevention/index.html. Updated October 26, 2015. Accessed April 29, 2018.
18. Schmidt-Chanasit J, Schmiedel S, Fleischer B, Burchard GD. Viruses acquired abroad: what does the primary care physician need to know? *Dtsch Ärztebl Int.* 2012;109(41):681-692.
19. Centers for Disease Control and Prevention, National Center for Emerging and Zoonotic Infectious Diseases, Division of High-Consequence Pathogens and Pathology, Viral Special Pathogens Branch. 2014 Ebola outbreak in West Africa: case counts. Disease Control and Prevention website. https://www.cdc.gov/vhf/ebola/outbreaks/2014-west-africa/case-counts.html. Updated April 14, 2016. Accessed April 29, 2018.
20. Centers for Disease Control and Prevention. Viral hemorrhagic fevers: fact sheet. Centers for Disease Control and Prevention website. https://www.cdc.gov/ncidod/dvrd/spb/mnpages/dispages/fact_sheets/viral_hemorrhagic_fevers_fact_sheet.pdf. Accessed April 29, 2018.
21. Falzarano D, Feldmann H. Vaccines for viral hemorrhagic fevers—progress and shortcomings. *Curr Opin Virol.* 2013;3(3):343-351.
22. National Center for Environmental Health (NCEH)/Agency for Toxic Substances and Disease Registry (ATSDR), National

Center for Injury Prevention and Control (NCIPC). Radiation emergencies. Centers for Disease Control and Prevention website. https://emergency.cdc.gov/radiation/. Updated February 5, 2018. Accessed April 29, 2018.
23. Fact sheet on dirty bombs. US Nuclear Regulatory Commission website. https://www.nrc.gov/reading-rm/doc-collections/fact-sheets/fs-dirty-bombs.html. Updated December 12, 2014. Accessed April 29, 2018.
24. An overdue review: addressing incendiary weapons in the contemporary context. Human Rights Watch website. https://www.hrw.org/news/2017/11/20/overdue-review-addressing-incendiary-weapons-contemporary-context. Published November 20, 2017. Accessed April 29, 2018.
25. Department of Homeland Security. Terrorist use of improvised incendiary devices and attack methods. Public Intelligence website. https://publicintelligence.net/ufouo-dhs-terrorist-use-of-improvised-incendiary-devices-and-attack-methods/. Published March 16, 2010. Accessed April 29, 2018.
26. National Center for Emerging and Zoonotic Infectious Diseases. Sarin (GB): facts about Sarin. Centers for Disease Control and Prevention website. https://emergency.cdc.gov/agent/sarin/basics/facts.asp. Updated November 18, 2015. Accessed April 29, 2018.
27. National Center for Emerging and Zoonotic Infectious Diseases. Nerve agents: tabun (GA). Centers for Disease Control and Prevention website. https://emergency.cdc.gov/agent/tabun/index.asp. Updated February 12, 2013. Accessed April 29, 2018.
28. National Center for Emerging and Zoonotic Infectious Diseases. VX: facts about VX. Centers for Disease Control and Prevention website. https://emergency.cdc.gov/agent/vx/basics/facts.asp. Updated November 18, 2015. Accessed April 29, 2018.
29. Urbanetti JS. Medical aspects of chemical and biological warfare. In: *Textbook of Military Medicine.* New Haven, CT: Yale University of Medicine; 1997:247-270.
30. Brief description of chemical weapons. Organisation for the Prohibition of Chemical Weapons website. https://www.opcw.org/about-chemical-weapons/what-is-a-chemical-weapon/. Accessed April 29, 2018.
31. Chlorine—emergency department/hospital management: acute management overview. Chemical Hazards Emergency Medical Management website. https://chemm.nlm.nih.gov/chlorine_hospital_mmg.htm. Updated September 29, 2017. Accessed April 29, 2018.
32. National Center for Emerging and Zoonotic Infectious Diseases. Phosgene (CG): facts about phosgene. Centers for Disease Control and Prevention website. https://emergency.cdc.gov/agent/phosgene/basics/facts.asp. Accessed April 29, 2018.
33. Westrol MS, Donovan CM, Kapitanyan R. Blast physics and pathophysiology of explosive injuries. *Ann Emerg Med.* 2017;69(1):S4-S9.
34. Virginia Department of Emergency Management. Terrorism information index chart. Terrorism information: the facts—how to prepare—how to respond. Scribd website. https://www.scribd.com/document/45194236/Terrorism-Information-Chart. Accessed April 28, 2018.
35. Quick look: 220 active shooter incidents in the United States between 2000–2016. Federal Bureau of Investigation website. https://www.fbi.gov/about/partnerships/office-of-partner-engagement/active-shooter-incidents-graphics. Accessed April 29, 2018.
36. Blair JP, Schweit K. *A Study of Active Shooter Incidents Between 2000 and 2013.* Washington, DC: Texas State University, Federal Bureau of Investigation, US Department of Justice; 2014. https://www.fbi.gov/file-repository/active-shooter-study-2000-2013-1.pdf. Accessed April 29, 2018.
37. Mass casualty shootings. *2017 National Crime Victims' Rights Week Resource Guide: Crime and Victimization Fact Sheets.* Office for Victims of Crime website. https://ovc.ncjrs.gov/ncvrw2017/images/en_artwork/Fact_Sheets/2017NCVRW_MassShootings_508.pdf. Accessed April 29, 2018.
38. The Joint Committee to Create a National Policy to Enhance Survivability from Intentional Mass Casualty and Active Shooter Events. Hartford Consensus. Strategies to enhance survival in active shooter and intentional mass casualty events: a compendium. *Am Coll Surg.* 2015;100(15):1-88.
39. Department of Homeland Security, Office of Health Affairs. *First Responder Guide for Improving Survivability in Improvised Explosive Device and/or Active Shooter Incidents*. Department of Homeland Security website. https://www.dhs.gov/sites/default/files/publications/First%20Responder%20Guidance%20June%202015%20FINAL%202.pdf. Published June 2015. Accessed April 29, 2018.
40. HR 5005, 107th Cong, 2nd Sess (2002).
41. Mission. US Department of Homeland Security website. https://www.dhs.gov/mission. Published August 29, 2016. Accessed April 29, 2018.
42. NTAS guide: National Terrorism Advisory System public guide. US Department of Homeland Security website. https://www.dhs.gov/xlibrary/assets/ntas/ntas-public-guide.pdf. Published April 2011. Accessed April 29, 2018.
43. US Department of Homeland Security, Office of Domestic Preparedness. *Emergency Responder Guidelines.* Washington, DC: Office of Domestic Preparedness; August 2002.
44. NATO Civil Emergency Planning, Civil Protection Group. Guidelines for first responders to a CBRN incident. North Atlantic Treaty Organization website. https://www.nato.int/nato_static_fl2014/assets/pdf/pdf_2016_08/20160802_140801-cep-first-responders-CBRN-eng.pdf. Updated August 1, 2014. Accessed April 29, 2018.

Suggested Readings

Britton S. EMS preparation and response to complex coordinated attacks. *JEMS* website. http://www.jems.com/articles/print/volume-42/issue-9/features/ems-preparation-and-response-to-complex-coordinated-attacks.html. Published September 1, 2017. Accessed April 29, 2018.

Champion HR, Holcomb JB, Young LA. Injuries from explosions: physics, biophysics, pathology, and required research focus. *J Trauma.* 2009;66(5):1468-1477.

National strategy for chemical, biological, radiological, nuclear, and explosives (CBRNE) standards. US Department of Homeland Security website. https://www.dhs.gov/national-strategy-chemical-biological-radiological-nuclear-and-explosives-cbrne-standards. Published June 22, 2017. Accessed April 29, 2018.

Thompson J, Rehn M, Lossius HM, Lockey D. Risks to emergency medical responders at terrorist incidents: a narrative review of the medical literature. *Crit Care.* 2014;18(5):521.

Westrol MS, Donovan C, Kapitanyan R. Blast physics and pathophysiology of explosive injuries. *Ann Emerg Med.* 2017;69(1):S4-S9.

Appendix A Emergency Drug Index

Pregnancy Category Ratings for Drugs

Drugs have been categorized by the Food and Drug Administration (FDA) according to the level of risk to the fetus. In 2015, the FDA began phasing out the categories identified in this section in favor of a more comprehensive description of the impact of medications on the pregnant mother and fetus, lactation, and any fertility risks for both males and females. Medications approved prior to June 30, 2015, continue to use the following pregnancy categories during a gradual transition period. Medications approved prior to 2001 are not affected by this change.[1,2] These categories are listed for each drug in this index under "Pregnancy safety" and are interpreted as follows:

- **Category A.** Controlled studies in women fail to demonstrate a risk to the fetus in the first trimester, and there is no evidence of risk in later trimesters; the possibility of fetal harm appears to be remote.
- **Category B.** Either (1) animal reproductive studies have not demonstrated a fetal risk but there are no controlled studies in pregnant women or (2) animal reproductive studies have shown an adverse effect (other than decreased fertility) that was not confirmed in controlled studies

on women in the first trimester and there is no evidence of risk in later trimesters.

- **Category C.** Either (1) studies in animals have revealed adverse effects on the fetus and there are no controlled studies in women or (2) studies in women and animals are not available. Drugs in this category should be given only if the potential benefit justifies the risk to the fetus.
- **Category D.** Positive evidence of human fetal risk exists, but the benefits for pregnant women may be acceptable despite the risk, as in life-threatening diseases for which safer drugs cannot be used or are ineffective. An appropriate statement must appear in the "Warnings" section of the labeling of drugs in this category.
- **Category X.** Studies in animals or humans have demonstrated fetal abnormalities, there is evidence of fetal risk based on human experience, or both; the risk of using the drug in pregnant women clearly outweighs any possible benefit. The drug is contraindicated in women who are or may become pregnant. An appropriate statement must appear in the "Contraindications" section of the labeling of drugs in this category.

Acetaminophen (Tylenol), Intravenous Acetaminophen (Ofirmev)

Class

Analgesic, antipyretic

Description

Acetaminophen is a widely used nonprescription analgesic and antipyretic medication for mild to moderate pain and fever. Unlike other common analgesics such as aspirin and ibuprofen, it has no anti-inflammatory properties or effects on platelet function, and it is not a member of the class of drugs known as nonsteroidal anti-inflammatory drugs (NSAIDs). Acetaminophen is thought to act primarily in the central nervous system (CNS), increasing the pain threshold by inhibiting the isoforms of cyclooxygenase (COX-1, COX-2, and COX-3), enzymes that are involved in prostaglandin synthesis. The antipyretic properties of acetaminophen are likely due to direct effects on the heat-regulating centers of the hypothalamus resulting in peripheral vasodilation, sweating, and, consequently, heat dissipation.

Onset and Duration

Onset: Orally (per os [PO]): 10–30 minutes; Intravenous (IV): 3–5 minutes
Duration: PO: 3–4 hours; IV: 4–6 hours

Indications

Temporary relief of fever, mild to moderate pain

Contradictions

Hypersensitivity to drug
Hepatic impairment
Renal impairment (long-term use)
Hypovolemia, severe
Chronic alcohol use

Adverse Reactions

Nausea/vomiting
Rash
Headache
Anemia
Thrombocytopenia

Drug Interactions

Avoid with concurrent use of ethanol, isoniazid, and over-the-counter drugs that contain acetaminophen.

How Supplied

325 mg, 500 mg (capsule); 325 mg, 500 mg, 650 mg (tablet); 20 mg/5 mL, 160 mg/5 mL (suspension); 160 mg/5 mL, 500 mg/15 mL (solution)

Dosage and Administration

Adults: Mild pain/fever: 325–1,000 mg PO every (q) 4–6 hours as needed (prn)
Infants and children: Mild pain/fever: 10–15 mg/kg PO q 4–6 hours prn; same as adult for children ≥12 years
IV dose (infuse over at least 15 minutes):
  Adults/adolescents (>13 years) >110 pounds (50 kg): 1,000 mg q 6 hours or 650 mg q 4 hours, with a maximum (max) single dose of 1,000 mg, a minimum dosing interval of 4 hours, and a max daily dose of

acetaminophen of 4,000 mg/d; <110 pounds (50 kg): 15 mg/kg q 6 hours or 12.5 mg/kg q 4 hours, with a max single dose of 15 mg/kg, a minimum dosing interval of 4 hours, and a max daily dose of acetaminophen of 75 mg/kg per day.

Children (2–12 years): 15 mg/kg q 6 hours or 12.5 mg/kg q 4 hours, with a max single dose of 15 mg/kg, a minimum dosing interval of 4 hours, and a max daily dose of acetaminophen of 75 mg/kg per day.

Special Considerations

Pregnancy safety: Category B

Harmless at low doses, acetaminophen has direct hepatotoxic potential when taken as an overdose and can cause acute liver injury and death from acute liver failure. Even in therapeutic doses, acetaminophen can cause transient serum aminotransferase elevations. Reduced dose and/or dosage interval may be warranted in older adults with decreased renal or hepatic function. Dosing errors can cause liver failure and death.

Acetazolamide (Diamox Sequels)

Class

Carbonic anhydrase inhibitor; anticonvulsant, diuretic

Description

Acetazolamide is used for acute mountain sickness. Additional uses include edema, chronic heart failure, glaucoma, and certain seizure disorders. It inhibits hydrogen ion excretion in the kidneys, causing increased excretion of bicarbonate, sodium, and potassium.

Onset and Duration

Onset: Tablets: 1–2 hours; IV: 2–10 minutes

Duration: Tablets: 24 hours; IV: 4–5 hours

Indications

Acute mountain sickness, altitude sickness prophylaxis

Contraindications

Hypersensitivity to acetazolamide or sulfa drugs

Hyponatremia

Hypokalemia

Known metabolic acidosis

Liver or renal disease

Noncongestive angle-closure glaucoma (chronic use only)

Adverse Reactions

Tinnitus

Nausea and vomiting

Diarrhea

Metabolic acidosis

Various electrolyte imbalances

Drug Interactions

May cause insoluble precipitate in urine when administered with methenamine

May increase toxicity from cisapride

How Supplied

125-mg and 500-mg tablets

Dosage and Administration

Adult and pediatric: 2.5 mg/kg per dose up to 250 mg PO q 12 hours

Special Considerations

Pregnancy safety: Category C

Acetazolamide has similar adverse reaction risks as sulfonamide derivative medications, including Stevens-Johnson syndrome and toxic epidermal necrosis. It is not recommended as acute mountain sickness prophylaxis in pediatric patients except in certain high-risk situations.

n-Acetylcysteine (Mucomyst, Acetadote)

Class

Antidote, mucolytic

Description

Acetylcysteine is the primary and most effective treatment for an acetaminophen (Tylenol) overdose.[3] It restores liver glutathione and may remove free radicals and prevent delayed hepatotoxicity. Depending on the setting and particular circumstances, it may be administered either PO or IV in repeated doses over 72 hours. Acetylcysteine is most effective when administered within 8 hours following acetaminophen overdose and becomes minimally effective >24 hours after overdose. Additionally, acetylcysteine is administered as a mucolytic agent to patients with thick pulmonary secretions from a variety of lung conditions.

Onset and Duration

Peak: PO: 1–2 hours
Duration: 5.6-hour half-life

Indications

Acetaminophen overdose

Contraindications

Hypersensitivity, acute asthma

Adverse Reactions

Nausea and vomiting
Edema
Flushing
Tachycardia
Hypotension

Drug Interactions

None

How Supplied

10% and 20% oral solutions; 20% IV solution (30 mL)

Dosage and Administration (Adults and Pediatrics)

Oral: 140-mg/kg loading dose, followed by 70 mg/kg q 4 hours for 17 additional doses (72 hours total).

IV: 300 mg/kg in three doses over 21 hours: a loading dose of 150 mg/kg in 200 mL of 5% dextrose over 1 hour, followed by a second dose of 50 mg/kg in 500 mL over 4 hours, and a third dose of 100 mg/kg in 1,000 mL infused over 16 hours. This regimen ("3-bag method") delivers 300 mg/kg acetylcysteine over 21 hours.[4]

Note: Consult a poison control center for dosing for children ≤20 kg.

Special Considerations

Pregnancy safety: Category B
Consult with online medical control or toxicologist prior to administration, as many acetaminophen overdose situations either do not require acetylcysteine or require additional treatment and monitoring. Activated charcoal may prevent toxic levels of acetaminophen reaching the bloodstream if administered within 1 hour of ingestion and make acetylcysteine administration unnecessary.[3] Nausea and vomiting frequently occur with oral administration; consider using antiemetic medications and other strategies to facilitate oral administration and absorption.

Activated Charcoal (Actidose-Aqua, Actidose, Liqui-Char)

Class

Adsorbent, antidote

Description

Activated charcoal is a fine black powder with a massive microscopic surface area that binds and adsorbs ingested toxins. Once the drug binds to the activated charcoal, the combined complex is excreted in the feces. Activated charcoal also possesses the novel ability to extract certain medications and chemicals from the bloodstream as they are circulated near the digestive tract. This ability allows activated charcoal to adsorb certain select medications even if they were administered parenterally.

Onset and Duration

Onset: Immediate
Duration: Continual while in gastrointestinal (GI) tract; reaches equilibrium once saturated

Indications

Many oral poisonings and medication overdoses

Contraindications

Corrosives, caustics, petroleum distillates (relatively ineffective and may induce vomiting)

Unprotected airway
Intestinal obstruction

Adverse Reactions

May indirectly induce nausea and vomiting
May cause constipation or mild, transient diarrhea

Drug Interactions

Syrup of ipecac (adsorbed by activated charcoal and will result in vomiting of the charcoal)

How Supplied

25 g (black powder); 25 g/125-mL bottle (200 mg/mL)
50 g (black powder); 50 g/240-mL bottle (200 mg/mL)
Other sizes include 15 g and 30 g, bottles and squeeze tubes. Most products come premixed (not powder) with water (aqueous preparations).

Dosage and Administration

From 1 g/kg body mass (larger amounts if food is also present), prepared in a slurry and administered PO or slowly via nasogastric or orogastric tube
- Adult: 30–100 g
- Pediatric (1–12 years): 15–30 g or 1–2 g/kg
- Infant (<1 year): 1 g/kg

Special Considerations

Pregnancy safety: Category C
Charcoal frequently is administered to pregnant patients, and the potential benefit versus risk is very high. Because charcoal remains within the GI tract, its risk to the fetus virtually is eliminated, unless the charcoal and other stomach contents are aspirated.
Activated charcoal also may be known as "AC."
Activated charcoal is relatively insoluble in water.
Activated charcoal may blacken feces.
Activated charcoal must be stored in a closed container. Different charcoal preparations may have varying adsorptive capacity.
Activated charcoal does not adsorb all drugs and toxic substances (eg, phenobarbital, aspirin, cyanide, lithium, iron, lead, and arsenic).

Adenosine (Adenocard)

Class

Endogenous nucleoside, miscellaneous antidysrhythmic

Description

Adenosine primarily is formed from the breakdown of adenosine triphosphate. Adenosine triphosphate and adenosine are found in every cell of the human body and have a wide range of metabolic roles. Adenosine slows supraventricular tachycardias (SVTs) by decreasing electrical conduction through the atrioventricular (AV) node without causing negative inotropic effects. It also acts directly on sinus pacemaker cells and vagal nerve terminals to decrease chronotropic (heart rate [HR]) activity. Adenosine is the first drug of choice for most forms of stable, narrow-complex SVT. It may be considered for unstable narrow-complex reentry tachycardia while preparing for cardioversion. Adenosine does not convert atrial fibrillation, atrial flutter, or ventricular tachycardia (VT).

Onset and Duration

Onset: Immediate
Duration: 10 seconds

Indications

First drug for most forms of narrow-complex paroxysmal SVT and dysrhythmias associated with bypass tracts such as Wolff-Parkinson-White (WPW) syndrome in adults and pediatric patients.
In undifferentiated regular stable wide-complex tachycardia, IV adenosine may be considered relatively safe. It may convert the rhythm to sinus and may help diagnose the underlying rhythm.

Contraindications

Drug-induced tachycardia
Second- or third-degree AV block
Hypersensitivity to adenosine
Atrial flutter, atrial fibrillation, VT, WPW with atrial fibrillation/flutter (Adenosine is not effective in converting these rhythms to sinus rhythm.)

Adverse Reactions

Facial flushing
Light-headedness
Paresthesias
Headache
Diaphoresis
Palpitations
Chest pain
Flushing

Hypotension
Shortness of breath
Transient periods of sinus bradycardia, sinus pause, or bradyasystole
Ventricular ectopy (fibrillation, flutter, tachycardia, torsades de pointes)
Nausea
Metallic taste

Drug Interactions

Methylxanthines (eg, caffeine, theophylline) antagonize the action of adenosine.
Dipyridamole potentiates the effect of adenosine; reduction of adenosine dose may be required.
Carbamazepine may potentiate the AV-nodal blocking effect of adenosine.

How Supplied

Parenteral for IV injection
3 mg/mL in 2-mL and 4-mL flip-top vials

Dosage and Administration

Adult: Initial dose: 6-mg rapid IV bolus over 1–3 seconds, followed by a 20-mL saline bolus; then elevate extremity. A second dose (12 mg) may be given in 1–2 minutes if needed.
Injection technique: Place patient in mild reverse Trendelenburg position before drug administration. Record electrocardiogram (ECG) during drug administration. Administer adenosine as rapidly as possible either diluted or followed by a flush.
Pediatric: Initial dose 0.1 mg/kg IV or intraosseous (IO) (max single dose: 6 mg); second dose 0.2 mg/kg IV/IO rapid push; followed with 5–10 mL normal saline (NS) flush.

Special Considerations

Pregnancy safety: Category C
A brief period of asystole (up to 15 seconds) following conversion, followed by normal sinus rhythm, is common after administration.
Reduce initial dose to 3 mg in patients receiving dipyridamole or carbamazepine, in heart transplant patients, or if given by central venous access.
Patients taking theophylline or caffeine may require larger doses of adenosine. Deterioration (including hypotension) may result if given for irregular, polymorphic wide-complex tachycardia/VT.
Adenosine may produce bronchoconstriction in patients with asthma and in patients with bronchopulmonary disease.

Albuterol (Proventil and Others)

Class

Sympathomimetic, bronchodilator, beta-2 agonist

Description

Albuterol is a sympathomimetic that is selective for beta-2 adrenergic receptors. It relaxes smooth muscles of the bronchial tree and peripheral vasculature by stimulating adrenergic receptors of the sympathetic nervous system.

Onset and Duration

Onset: 5–8 minutes after inhalation
Duration: 2–6 hours after inhalation

Indications

Relief of bronchospasm in patients with reversible obstructive airway disease
Prevention of exercise-induced bronchospasm
Anaphylaxis
Hyperkalemia

Contraindications

Prior hypersensitivity reaction to albuterol or levalbuterol
Cardiac dysrhythmias associated with tachycardia (precaution)

Adverse Reactions

Usually dose-related
Restlessness, apprehension
Dizziness
Palpitations, tachycardia
Dysrhythmias
Tremors

Drug Interactions

Other sympathomimetics may exacerbate adverse cardiovascular effects.
Monoamine oxidase (MAO) inhibitors and tricyclic antidepressants may potentiate effects on the vasculature (vasodilation).

Beta blockers may antagonize albuterol.
Albuterol may potentiate diuretic-induced hypokalemia.

How Supplied

Metered-dose inhaler (MDI): 90 mcg/metered spray (17-g canister with 200 inhalations)
Solution for aerosolization: 0.5% (5 mg/mL); 0.083% (2.5 mg) in 3-mL unit dose/nebulizer

Dosage and Administration

Bronchial Asthma/Allergy-Induced Bronchospasm/Hyperkalemia

Adult:

Solution: 2.5–5 mg (0.5–1 mL of 0.5% solution) diluted to 3 mL with 0.9% NS (0.083% solution); administer over 5–15 minutes; 3–4 times/d by nebulizer

MDI: 1–2 inhalations (90–180 mcg) q 4–6 hours (wait 5 minutes between inhalations); max 12 inhalations/d

Note: In settings of severe asthma exacerbation, 6 inhalations or 5 mg in 2.5–3 mL is indicated.

Pediatric:

Solution: 0.1–0.2 mg/kg per dose diluted in 2 mL of 0.9% NS; may be repeated q 20 minutes.

Nebulized albuterol: <44 pounds (20 kg): 2.5 mg/dose (inhalation); >44 pounds (20 kg): 5 mg/dose (inhalation)

MDI: 4–8 puffs (inhalation) prn, with spacer if not intubated.

Note: Use of MDIs without a spacer is essentially ineffective.

Special Considerations

Pregnancy safety: Category C
Albuterol may precipitate angina pectoris and dysrhythmias.
Albuterol should be used with caution in patients with diabetes mellitus, hyperthyroidism, prostatic hypertrophy, seizure disorder, or cardiovascular disorder.

Alteplase (t-PA)

Class

Fibrinolytic

Description

Tissue plasminogen activator is a naturally occurring enzyme that has been mass-produced using recombinant DNA technology. The enzyme binds to fibrin-bound plasminogen at the site of an arterial clot, converting plasminogen to plasmin. Plasmin digests the fibrin strands of the clot, causing clot lysis and restoration of perfusion to the occluded artery. In prehospital care, fibrinolytic agents are used in treating selected patients with acute evolving myocardial infarction (MI). (Other indications include ischemic stroke, deep venous thrombosis, peripheral artery embolism, and IV catheter occlusion.)

Onset and Duration

Onset: Clot lysis often occurs within 30 minutes.
Duration: 30–45 minutes (80% cleared in 10 minutes).

Indications

Acute evolving MI
Massive pulmonary emboli
Arterial thrombosis and embolism
To clear arteriovenous cannulae
Acute ischemic stroke

Contraindications

Active bleeding or known bleeding disorder
Recent surgery (within 2–3 weeks)
Recent stroke
History of intracranial hemorrhage
Prolonged cardiopulmonary resuscitation (CPR)
Recent intracranial or intraspinal surgery
Recent significant trauma (particularly head trauma)
Seizure at onset of stroke symptoms
Uncontrolled hypertension
Recent GI bleeding

Adverse Reactions

Bleeding (GI, genitourinary, intracranial, other sites)
Allergic reactions
Hypotension
Chest pain
Reperfusion dysrhythmias
Angioedema

Drug Interactions

Acetylsalicylic acid may increase risk of bleeding (and may be beneficial in improving overall effectiveness).
Heparin and other anticoagulants also may increase risk of bleeding and improve overall effectiveness.

How Supplied

50, 100 mg/vial with 50, 100 mL, and 2 mg (Cathflo) of diluent, respectively. May dilute further with equal amounts of 0.9% sodium chloride or 5% dextrose in water (D_5W).

Dosage and Administration (Based on Patient's Weight)

Adult ST segment elevation myocardial infarction (STEMI): Give 15-mg IV bolus, then 0.75 mg/kg over 30 minutes (not to exceed 50 mg), and then 0.5 mg/kg over 60 minutes (not to exceed 35 mg); max total dose 100 mg. (Other doses may be prescribed by medical direction; different dosing is indicated for stroke and massive acute pulmonary embolism.)
Pediatric: Safety not established.

Special Considerations

Pregnancy safety: Category C
Obtain blood sample for coagulation studies before administration.
Gently roll—do not shake—the vial to mix powder with liquid.
Closely monitor vital signs.
Observe for bleeding.
Do not administer intramuscular (IM) injections to patients receiving fibrinolytic drugs.
No arterial blood gas specimens should be drawn on potential fibrinolytic therapy candidates due to bleeding tendency.
Use caution when moving patient to avoid bleeding or bruising.
Use one IV line exclusively for fibrinolytic administration.

Amiodarone (Cordarone)

Class

Class III antidysrhythmic

Description

Amiodarone is a unique antidysrhythmic agent with multiple mechanisms of action. The drug prolongs the duration of the action potential and the effective refractory period, and when given short-term IV, probably includes noncompetitive beta adrenergic receptor and calcium channel blocker activity.

Onset and Duration

Onset: Within minutes
Duration: Variable

Indications (IV Use)

Initial treatment and prophylaxis of frequently recurring ventricular fibrillation (VF) and hemodynamically unstable VT in patients unresponsive to shock delivery, CPR, and vasopressors
Recurrent hemodynamically unstable VT
Treatment of some stable atrial and ventricular dysrhythmias

Contraindications

Pulmonary congestion
Cardiogenic shock
Severe sinus node dysfunction
Second- or third-degree AV block if no pacemaker present
Bradycardia
Hypersensitivity to amiodarone or iodine
Hyperkalemia

Adverse Reactions

Hypotension
Prolonged QT interval
Dizziness
Bradycardia
AV conduction abnormalities
Cardiac arrest
Torsades de pointes
Pain at IV site
Liver function abnormalities
Heart failure
Abnormal thyroid function

Drug Interactions

May potentiate bradycardia and hypotension with beta blockers and calcium channel blockers.
May increase risk of AV block and hypotension with calcium channel blockers.
May increase anticoagulant effects of warfarin.
May decrease metabolism and increase serum levels of phenytoin, procainamide, quinidine, and theophyllines. Routine use in combination with drugs that prolong the QT interval is not recommended.
Y-site incompatibilities with furosemide, heparin, and sodium bicarbonate.

How Supplied

50-mg/mL vials

Dosage and Administration

Adult:

Pulseless arrest unresponsive to CPR, shocks, and epinephrine: 300 mg IV/IO push. If needed, second dose of 150 mg IV/IO push.

Life-threatening dysrhythmias: Max cumulative dose: 2.2 g IV per 24 hour. May be given as rapid infusion 150 mg IV over first 10 minutes (15 mg/min) repeated q 10 minutes if VT recurs. Slow infusion: 360 mg IV over 6 hours (1 mg/min). Maintenance infusion: 540 mg IV over 18 hours (0.5 mg/min).

Pediatric:

Refractory VF, pulseless VT: 5 mg/kg rapid IV/IO bolus; can be repeated to total dose of 15 mg/kg (2.2 g in adolescents) IV per 24 hour; max single dose: 300 mg.

Perfusing supraventricular and ventricular dysrhythmias: Loading dose 5 mg/kg IV/IO over 20–60 minutes (max single dose: 300 mg); can repeat to a max of 15 mg/kg (2.2 g in adolescents) per day IV.

Special Considerations

Pregnancy safety: Category D

Rapid infusion may cause hypotension.

Continuous ECG monitoring is required. Slow infusion or discontinue if bradycardia or AV block occurs.

Do not give with other drugs that prolong QT interval (eg, procainamide).

Maintain at room temperature and protect from excessive heat.

Amyl Nitrite

Class

Antidote, vasodilator

Description

Amyl nitrite is a first-line (immediate) antidote to cyanide poisoning. It is supplied as 0.3-mL ampules designed to be crushed onto gauze and administered as an inhalational agent while waiting for or establishing IV access for more definitive treatment with sodium nitrite, sodium thiosulfate, or hydroxocobalamin (preferred). Amyl nitrite (and sodium nitrite) is contraindicated when there is concurrent or suspected carbon monoxide toxicity, as it may worsen tissue hypoxia with potentially lethal consequences. When administered by inhalation, amyl nitrite induces a condition in the blood known as methemoglobinemia; the resulting binding with cyanide molecules creates a less-toxic substance called cyanomethemoglobin.[5] The amyl nitrite has the additional beneficial effect of causing vasodilation, which improves hepatic (liver) circulation and promotes cyanide metabolism.

Onset and Duration

Onset: Rapid

Duration: 2–3 minutes per ampule

Indications

Cyanide poisoning

Contraindications

Concurrent carbon monoxide exposure

Known methemoglobinemia (>40%)

Hypotension (relative)

Not generally used for cyanide poisoning when hydroxocobalamin is readily available

Adverse Reactions

Hypotension

Methemoglobinemia

Flushing

Dizziness

Nausea and vomiting

Drug Interactions

Methylene blue may reverse desired methemoglobinemia

How Supplied

0.3-mL glass ampule; older cyanide antidote kits may contain 2 to 12 ampules.

Dosage and Administration

Crush ampule into gauze or similar material. Place material under the patient's nose or within the bag-mask device or endotracheal (ET) tube system. Alternate 30 seconds of inhalation with 30 seconds of respirations/ventilations without amyl nitrite. Continue only until IV access is established and other antidotes can be administered.

Special Considerations

Pregnancy safety: No FDA category established. Amyl nitrite may cause harmful effects on the fetus, but this risk may be outweighed by the potential benefits of a successful maternal resuscitation.

This is no longer the preferred treatment for toxic cyanide exposures.[5]

Aspirin (ASA, Bayer, Ecotrin, St. Joseph, Others)

Class

Analgesic, anti-inflammatory, antipyretic, antiplatelet

Description

Aspirin decreases inflammation (analgesic effect not limited to effects in CNS), dilates peripheral vessels, and decreases platelet aggregation. The use of aspirin is strongly recommended for all patients with acute coronary syndrome (ACS).

Onset and Duration

Onset: 15–30 minutes

Duration: 4–6 hours; antiplatelet effects may persist 4–10 days[6]

Indications

Mild to moderate pain or fever

Prevention of platelet aggregation in ischemia and thromboembolism

All patients with ACS

Any patient with symptoms of ischemic chest pain

Unstable angina

Prevention of MI or reinfarction

Contraindications

Hypersensitivity to salicylates

GI bleeding

Active ulcer disease or acute asthma (relative contraindication)

Hemorrhagic stroke

Bleeding disorders

Children with flulike symptoms

Adverse Reactions

Stomach irritation

Heartburn or indigestion

Nausea or vomiting

Allergic reaction

Drug Interactions

Decreased effects with antacids and steroids

Increased effects with anticoagulants, insulin, oral hypoglycemics, fibrinolytic agents

How Supplied

Tablets (65, 81, 325, 500, 650, 975 mg)

Capsules (325, 500 mg)

Controlled-release tablets (800 mg)

Suppositories (varies from 60 mg to 1.2 g)

Dosage and Administration

Adult: Mild pain and fever: 325–650 mg PO q 4 hours

ACS: 160–325 mg PO non–enteric-coated tablet (chewing is preferable to swallowing); may use rectal suppository for patients who cannot take orally

Pediatric: Not indicated in prehospital setting

Special Considerations

Pregnancy safety: Category D in third trimester, Category C in first and second trimesters

Is given as soon as possible to the patient with ACS. Aspirin is not routinely used as an *analgesic* in the prehospital setting.

Atropine Sulfate (Atropine and Others)

Class

Anticholinergic agent

Description

Atropine sulfate (a potent parasympatholytic) inhibits actions of acetylcholine at postganglionic parasympathetic (primarily muscarinic) receptor sites. Small doses inhibit salivary and bronchial secretions; moderate doses dilate pupils and increase HR. Large doses decrease GI motility, inhibit gastric acid secretion, and may block nicotinic receptor sites at the autonomic ganglia and at the neuromuscular junction. Blocked vagal effects result in increased

HR and enhanced AV conduction with limited or no inotropic effect. In emergency care, atropine primarily is used to increase the HR in life-threatening or symptomatic bradycardia and to antagonize excess muscarinic receptor stimulation caused by organophosphate insecticides or chemical nerve agents (eg, sarin, soman).

Onset and Duration

Onset: Rapid
Duration: 2–6 hours

Indications

Hemodynamically significant bradycardia
Organophosphate or nerve gas poisoning

Contraindications

Tachycardia
Hypersensitivity to atropine
Use with caution in patients with myocardial ischemia and hypoxia
Avoid in hypothermic bradycardia
Obstructive disease of GI tract
Obstructive uropathy
Unstable cardiovascular status in acute hemorrhage with myocardial ischemia
Narrow-angle glaucoma
Thyrotoxicosis

Adverse Reactions

Tachycardia
Paradoxical bradycardia when pushed too slowly or when adult dose is <0.5 mg
Palpitations
Dysrhythmias
Headache
Dizziness
Anticholinergic effects (dry mouth/nose/skin, photophobia, blurred vision, urinary retention, constipation)
Nausea and vomiting
Flushed, hot, dry skin
Allergic reactions

Drug Interactions

Use with other anticholinergic agents may increase vagal blockade.
Potential adverse effects may occur when administered with digitalis, cholinergics, or neostigmine.
The effects of atropine may be enhanced by antihistamines, procainamide, quinidine, antipsychotics and antidepressants, and thiazides.
Increased toxicity may occur with amantadine.

How Supplied

Parenteral: There are various injection preparations.
In emergency care, atropine usually is supplied in prefilled syringes containing 1 mg in 10 mL of solution.

Dosage and Administration

Bradydysrhythmia (With or Without ACS)

Adult: 0.5 mg q 3–5 minutes for desired response (max total dose: 3 mg); use shorter dosing intervals (3 minutes) and higher doses in severe clinical conditions.

Pediatric: 0.02 mg/kg IV/IO; minimum dose: 0.1 mg; max single dose of 0.5 mg; may be repeated once; max total dose for a child: 1 mg; for adolescent: 3 mg; ET dose is 0.04–0.06 mg/kg.

Anticholinesterase Poisoning

Adult: 1–2 mg IV push q 5–15 minutes until atropine effects are observed; then q 1–4 hours for at least 24 hours; extremely large doses (2–4 mg or more) may be needed. See Chapter 57, *Bioterrorism and Weapons of Mass Destruction*, for IM dosing.

Pediatric: <12 years: 0.05 mg/kg/dose IV/IO; may be repeated, doubling the dose q 20–30 minutes until muscarinic symptoms reverse; ≥12 years: 1 mg IV/IO; then doubling the dose IV/IO q 5 minutes until muscarinic symptoms reverse.

Special Considerations

Pregnancy safety: Category C
Atropine dilates pupils, rendering them nonreactive.
Atropine is not effective in heart transplantation patients.

Calcium Chloride

Class

Electrolyte

Description

Calcium is an essential component for the functional integrity of the nervous and muscular systems, for normal cardiac contractility, and for the coagulation of blood. Calcium chloride contains 27.2% elemental calcium. Calcium chloride is a hypertonic solution and should be administered only IV (slowly, not exceeding 1 mL/min).

Onset and Duration

Onset: 5–15 minutes
Duration: Dose-dependent (effects may persist for 4 hours after IV administration)

Indications

Hyperkalemia (except when associated with digitalis toxicity)
Hypocalcemia (eg, after multiple blood transfusions)
Calcium channel blocker toxicity
Hypermagnesemia
To prevent hypotensive effects of calcium channel–blocking agents (eg, IV verapamil and diltiazem)

Contraindications

VF during cardiac resuscitation
Patients with digitalis toxicity
Hypercalcemia

Adverse Reactions

Bradycardia (may cause asystole)
Hypotension
Metallic taste
Severe local necrosis and sloughing following IM use or IV infiltration

Drug Interactions

Calcium may worsen dysrhythmias caused by digitalis.
Calcium may antagonize the peripheral vasodilatory effects of calcium channel blockers.

How Supplied

10% solution in 10-mL (100 mg/mL) ampules, vials, and prefilled syringes

Dosage and Administration

Hyperkalemia and Calcium Channel Blocker Overdose

Adult: Typical dose is 500–1,000 mg (5–10 mL of a 10% solution); may be repeated prn.

Pediatric: 20 mg/kg (0.2 mL/kg) IV of 10% solution slow IV/IO; may repeat if documented or clinical indication persists (eg, toxicologic problem); dose should not exceed adult dose.

Special Considerations

Pregnancy safety: Category C
Calcium may produce vasospasm in coronary and cerebral arteries.
Do not use routinely in cardiac arrest. Hypertension and bradycardia may occur with rapid administration.
Monitor hemodynamic changes and IV site during administration.

> NOTE
> It is important to flush the IV line between administration of calcium chloride and sodium bicarbonate to avoid precipitation.

Calcium Gluconate (Cal-Glu)

Class

Electrolyte, antidote

Description

Calcium is an essential component for the functional integrity of the nervous and muscular systems, for normal cardiac contractility, and for the coagulation of blood. A 10% calcium gluconate solution contains one-third the amount of elemental calcium found in a 10% calcium chloride solution, making it generally preferred for IV administration. Calcium gluconate can be administered in a variety of other routes (eg, intradermal, intra-arterial) for treatment of severe, local hydrofluoric acid exposures.

Onset and Duration

Onset: 5–15 minutes
Duration: Dose-dependent (effects may persist for 4 hours after IV administration)

Indications

Hyperkalemia (except when associated with digitalis toxicity)
Hypocalcemia (eg, after multiple blood transfusions)
Calcium channel blocker toxicity
Hypermagnesemia

Contraindications

VF during cardiac resuscitation
Patients with digitalis toxicity

Hypercalcemia
Hypersensitivity
Sarcoidosis

Adverse Reactions

Bradycardia (may cause asystole)
Hypotension
Metallic taste
Severe local necrosis and sloughing following IV infiltration

Drug Interactions

Calcium may worsen dysrhythmias caused by digitalis.
Calcium may antagonize the peripheral vasodilatory effects of calcium channel blockers.

How Supplied

10% solution in 10-mL (100 mg/mL) ampules and vials

Dosage and Administration

Hyperkalemia and Calcium Channel Blocker Overdose

Adult: Typical dose is 1–2 g (10–20 mL of a 10% solution); may be repeated prn.

Pediatric: 60 mg/kg (0.6 mL/kg) IV of 10% solution slow IV/IO; may repeat if documented or clinical indication persists (eg, toxicologic problem); dose should not exceed adult dose.

Special Considerations

Pregnancy safety: Category C
Calcium may produce vasospasm in coronary and cerebral arteries.
Do not use routinely in cardiac arrest. Hypertension and bradycardia may occur with rapid administration.
Monitor hemodynamic response and IV site during administration.

Cimetidine (Tagamet)

Class

Histamine-2 (H_2) receptor antagonist

Description

Cimetidine blocks H_2 receptors and is used primarily to reduce gastric acid secretion in a variety of GI conditions. H_2 receptor antagonists are also used to augment diphenhydramine in the setting of severe allergic reactions and anaphylaxis.

Onset and Duration

Peak: 1–3 hours
Duration: 4–5 hours

Indications

Adjunctive treatment in allergic reactions
GI ulcers and gastric hypersecretory conditions

Contraindications

Hypersensitivity to cimetidine or other H_2 receptor antagonists

Adverse Reactions

Hypotension
Cardiac arrhythmias
Vasculitis
Confusion

Drug Interactions

Inhibits CYP1A2, CYP3A4, and other related enzymes, requiring dose reduction for a wide variety of medications.

How Supplied

300-, 400-, and 900-mg premixed solutions; 200-, 300-, 400-, and 800-mg oral doses.

Dosage and Administration

Adults: 200–400 mg IV or PO
Pediatric: 20–40 mg/kg per day (divided q 6 hours) for most conditions. Give daytime doses with food.
Infants: 10–20 mg/kg per day PO divided q 6–12 hours. Give daytime doses with food.
Neonates: 5–10 mg/kg per day PO divided q 8–12 hours. Give daytime doses with food.

Special Considerations

Pregnancy safety: Category B

Dexamethasone (Decadron, Hexadrol, and Others)

Class

Glucocorticoid

Description

Dexamethasone is a synthetic steroid that is related chemically to the natural hormones secreted by the adrenal cortex. The drug suppresses acute and chronic inflammation, potentiates the relaxation of vascular and bronchial smooth muscle by beta adrenergic agonists, and possibly alters airway hyperreactivity. In emergency care, dexamethasone generally is used in the treatment of allergic reactions and asthma and to reduce swelling in the CNS.

Onset and Duration

Onset: 4–8 hours after parenteral administration
Duration: 24–72 hours

Indications

Endocrine, rheumatic, and hematologic disorders
Allergic states
Septic shock
Chronic inflammation

Contraindications

Hypersensitivity to the product
Active untreated infections (relative)

Adverse Reactions

Decreased wound healing
Hypertension
GI bleeding
Hyperglycemia

Drug Interactions

Barbiturates and phenytoin can decrease dexamethasone effects.

How Supplied

Common preparations used in emergency care are for IV administration and are as follows:
- 4 mg/mL in 1-, 5-, 10-, 25-, 30-mL vials
- 10 mg/mL in 10-mL vials, 1-mL syringe, 1-mL ampule
- 20 mg/mL in 5-mL vials (IV or IM), 5-mL syringe (IV)
- 24 mg/mL (IV only) in 5- and 10-mL vials

Dosage and Administration

Adult: There is considerable variance in recommended dexamethasone doses. The usual range in emergency care is 0.6 mg/kg (max dose 16 mg) IV. Some physicians may prefer significantly higher doses (up to 100 mg) for unusual indications.

Pediatric: 1 dose of 0.6 mg/kg PO/IM/IV (max dose 16 mg).

Special Considerations

Pregnancy safety: Category C. Dexamethasone crosses the placenta and may cause fetal damage.
The medication should be protected from heat.
Because of its slow onset of action (4–8 hours), dexamethasone should not be considered a first-line medication for allergic reactions.

Dextrose 50%, 25%, 10%

Class

Carbohydrate, hypertonic solution

Description

The term *dextrose* is used to describe the six-carbon sugar D-glucose, the principal form of carbohydrate used by the body. The 50% dextrose solution is used in emergency care to treat hypoglycemia and in the management of coma of unknown origin.

Onset and Duration

Onset: 1 minute
Duration: Depends on the degree of hypoglycemia

Indications

Hypoglycemia (documented or strongly suspected)
Altered level of consciousness
Coma of unknown origin
Seizure of unknown origin

Contraindications

Intracranial or intraspinal hemorrhage
Increased intracranial pressure
Known or suspected stroke in the absence of hypoglycemia
Dehydrated patients with delirium

Adverse Reactions

Warmth, pain, or burning from medication infusion
Hyperglycemia
Thrombophlebitis

Drug Interactions

None significant

How Supplied

50%: 25 g/50 mL in prefilled syringe (500 mg/mL)
25%: 2.5 g/10 mL (250 mg/mL)
10%: 25 g/250 mL or 50 g/500 mL (100 mg/mL)

Dosage and Administration

Adult: 12.5–25 g slow IV (25–50 mL 50% dextrose; 50–100 mL 25% dextrose; or 125–250 mL 10% dextrose); may repeat to max dose
Pediatric:
- 0.5–1 g/kg IV/IO (max recommended concentration: 25%)
- 2–4 mL/kg 25% dextrose
- 5–10 mL/kg 10% dextrose
- Use 10% dextrose solution for infants >1 month and neonates

Special Considerations

Pregnancy safety: Category C
Draw blood sample before administration if possible. Perform blood glucose analysis before administration if possible.
Extravasation may cause tissue necrosis; use large vein and aspirate occasionally to ensure route patency.
Prolonged carbohydrate administration without thiamine supplementation in deficient patients has been reported to precipitate Wernicke encephalopathy, but there are *no* reported instances of a single glucose administration causing Wernicke encephalopathy.[7] Therefore, the paramedic should never delay glucose administration in a hypoglycemic patient to administer thiamine first.

Diazepam (Valium and Others)

Class

Benzodiazepine

Description

Diazepam is a frequently prescribed medication to treat anxiety and stress. In emergency care, it is used to treat alcohol withdrawal and generalized onset seizure activity. Diazepam acts on the limbic, thalamic, and hypothalamic regions of the CNS to potentiate the effects of inhibitory neurotransmitters, raising the seizure threshold in the motor cortex. It also may be used in conscious patients during cardioversion and transcutaneous pacing to induce amnesia and sedation. Its use as an anticonvulsant may be short-lived because of rapid redistribution from the CNS. Rapid IV administration may be followed by respiratory depression and excessive sedation, particularly in older adults.

Onset and Duration

Onset: IV: 1–5 minutes; IM: 15–30 minutes
Duration: IV: 15–60 minutes; IM: 15–60 minutes

Indications

Acute anxiety states
Acute alcohol withdrawal
Skeletal muscle relaxation
Seizure activity
Premedication before synchronized cardioversion or transcutaneous pacing

Contraindications

Hypersensitivity to the drug
Substance abuse (use with caution)
Coma (unless the patient has seizures or severe muscle rigidity or myoclonus)
Shock
CNS depression as a result of head injury
Respiratory depression

Adverse Reactions

Hypotension
Reflex tachycardia (rare)
Respiratory depression
Ataxia
Psychomotor impairment
Confusion
Nausea
Dizziness
Drowsiness
Blurred vision

Drug Interactions

Diazepam may precipitate CNS depression and psychomotor impairment when the patient is taking other CNS depressant medications.
Diazepam should not be administered with other drugs because of possible precipitation (incompatible

with most fluids; should be administered into an IV of NS solution).

How Supplied

Parenteral: 5-mg/mL vials, ampules, Tubex

Dosage and Administration

Seizure Activity

Adult: 0.1 mg/kg (or 5 mg) over 2 minutes IV q 10–15 minutes prn (max dose 30 mg) or 10 mg IM

Pediatric: Dose for infants 30 days to 5 years is 0.2–0.5 mg slow IV q 2–5 minutes to max 5 mg; dose for children ≥5 years is 1 mg q 2–5 minutes to max 10 mg slow IV

Premedication for Cardioversion or Transcutaneous Pacing

Adult: 5–15 mg IV, 5–10 minutes before procedure

Rapid-Sequence Induction in Children

0.2–0.3 mg/kg IV/IO; max single dose 10 mg

Special Considerations

Pregnancy safety: Category D
Diazepam may cause local venous irritation.
Diazepam has short duration of anticonvulsant effect. Reduce dose by 50% in older adults.
If no other route is available, rectal administration can be used at a higher dose.

Diltiazem (Cardizem) Injectable

Class

Calcium channel blocker or calcium channel antagonist

Description

Diltiazem is a calcium channel–blocking agent that slows conduction, increases refractoriness in the AV node, and causes coronary and peripheral vasodilation. The drug is used to control ventricular response rates in patients with atrial fibrillation, atrial flutter, and multifocal atrial tachycardias. Use after adenosine to treat refractory reentry SVT in patients with narrow QRS complex and adequate blood pressure (BP).

Onset and Duration

Onset: 2–5 minutes
Duration: 1–3 hours

Indications

To control ventricular rate in atrial fibrillation and atrial flutter
Multifocal atrial tachycardias
Paroxysmal SVT

Contraindications

Wide QRS tachycardias of unknown origin or poison- or drug-induced tachycardia
Sick sinus syndrome
Second- or third-degree AV block (except with a functioning pacemaker)
Hypotension (<90 mm Hg)
Cardiogenic shock
Hypersensitivity to diltiazem
Rapid atrial fibrillation or atrial flutter associated with WPW syndrome or a short PR interval syndrome
Lown-Ganong-Levine syndrome
VT
Acute MI

Adverse Reactions

Atrial flutter
First- and second-degree AV block
Bradycardia
Hypotension
Chest pain
Heart failure
Peripheral edema
Syncope
Ventricular dysrhythmias
Sweating
Nausea and vomiting
Dizziness
Dry mouth
Dyspnea
Headache
Rash

Drug Interactions

Caution is warranted in patients receiving medications that affect cardiac contractility and/or sinoatrial or AV node conduction.
Diltiazem is incompatible with simultaneous furosemide injection.

How Supplied

25 mg (5-mL vial); 50 mg (10-mL vial)

Dosage and Administration

Acute rate control: 0.25 mg/kg (15–20 mg for the average patient) IV over 2 minutes; may be repeated in 15 minutes (0.35 mg/kg; 20–25 mg for the average patient) IV over 2 minutes

Maintenance infusion: Dilute 125 mg (25 mL) in 100 mL of solution (NS or D_5W); infuse 5–15 mg/h, titrated to HR

Pediatric: Off-label use only

Special Considerations

Pregnancy safety: Category C

Use with caution in patients with impaired renal or hepatic function.

Hypotension occasionally may result (more common with verapamil); carefully monitor vital signs.

Concurrent IV administration with IV beta blockers can cause severe hypotension and AV block. Use caution in patients taking oral beta blockers.

Premature ventricular contractions may be present on conversion of paroxysmal SVT to sinus rhythm.

Shelf-life at room temperature is 1 month.

Diphenhydramine (Benadryl)

Class

Antihistamine

Description

Antihistamines prevent the physiologic actions of histamine by blocking histamine-1 (H_1; eg, diphenhydramine, cimetidine) and H_2 (eg, cimetidine, ranitidine, famotidine) receptor sites. Antihistamines are indicated for conditions in which histamine excess is present (eg, acute urticaria) and are used as adjunctive therapy (eg, with epinephrine) in the treatment of anaphylactic shock. Antihistamines also are effective in the treatment of certain extrapyramidal (dystonic) reactions and for relief of upper respiratory tract and sinus symptoms associated with allergic reactions.

Onset and Duration

Onset: Max effects 1–3 hours

Duration: 6–12 hours

Indications

Moderate to severe allergic reactions

Anaphylaxis (after epinephrine)

Acute extrapyramidal (dystonic) reactions

Contraindications

Patients taking nonselective MAO inhibitors (now increasingly rare)

Hypersensitivity

Narrow-angle glaucoma (relative)

Newborns and nursing mothers (per manufacturer)

Adverse Reactions

Dose-related drowsiness

Disturbed coordination

Hypotension

Palpitations

Tachycardia, bradycardia

Thickening of bronchial secretions

Dry mouth and throat

Paradoxical excitement in children

Drug Interactions

CNS depressants may increase depressant effects.

MAO inhibitors may prolong and intensify anticholinergic effects of antihistamines.

How Supplied

Parenteral: 10- and 50-mg/mL vials, prefilled syringe

Dosage and Administration

Adult: 1 mg/kg (max dose 50 mg), IM/PO or slow IV

Pediatric: 1 mg/kg IM/IV/PO (max dose 25 mg)

Special Considerations

Pregnancy safety: Category C

Use cautiously in patients with CNS depression or lower respiratory tract diseases such as asthma.

Dopamine (Intropin)

Class

Sympathomimetic

Description

Dopamine is related chemically to epinephrine and norepinephrine. It acts primarily on alpha-1 and beta-1 adrenergic receptors in a dose-dependent fashion. At moderate doses ("cardiac doses"), dopamine stimulates beta adrenergic receptors, causing enhanced myocardial contractility, increased cardiac output, and a rise in BP. At high doses ("vasopressor doses"), dopamine has an alpha adrenergic effect, producing peripheral arterial and venous constriction. Dopamine is a second-line drug for symptomatic bradycardia (after atropine). It commonly is used in the treatment of hypotension (systolic blood pressure [SBP] <70–100 mm Hg) with signs and symptoms of shock.

Onset and Duration

Onset: 2–4 minutes
Duration: 10–15 minutes

Indications

Hemodynamically significant hypotension in the absence of hypovolemia
Symptomatic bradycardia (second-line drug after atropine)

Contraindications

Hypersensitivity
Tachydysrhythmias
VF
Patients with pheochromocytoma

Adverse Reactions

Dose-related tachydysrhythmias
Hypertension
Increased myocardial oxygen demand (eg, ischemia)
Headache
Anxiety
Nausea and vomiting

Drug Interactions

Dopamine may be deactivated by alkaline solutions (sodium bicarbonate and furosemide).
MAO inhibitors may potentiate the effect of dopamine. Sympathomimetics and phosphodiesterase inhibitors exacerbate the dysrhythmia response.
Beta adrenergic antagonists may blunt the inotropic response. When dopamine is administered with phenytoin, hypotension, bradycardia, and seizures may develop.

How Supplied

200, 400, or 800 mg in 5-mL prefilled syringe and ampule for IV infusion (IV piggyback)

Dosage and Administration

Adult: Usual infusion rate 2–20 mcg/kg per minute; titrate to response; taper slowly. For hypotension after return of spontaneous circulation, 5–10 mcg/kg per minute.
Pediatric: 2–20 mcg/kg per minute IV/IO, titrated to patient response; if infusion dose >20 mcg/kg per minute is required, consider an alternative adrenergic agent (eg, epinephrine/norepinephrine).

Special Considerations

Pregnancy safety: Category C
Infuse through a large, stable vein to avoid the possibility of extravasation injury.
Use an infusion pump to ensure precise flow rates.

Droperidol (Inapsine)

Class

Antipsychotic, antiemetic

Description

Droperidol is a potent antipsychotic and antiemetic medication. In December 2001, the FDA required a "black box warning" suggesting that unexpected cardiovascular deaths could occur at normal therapeutic doses of droperidol. While subsequent studies have found these fears unsubstantiated,[8-10] droperidol is infrequently used in EMS. The drug is thought to block dopamine (type 2) receptors in the brain, altering mood and behavior. In emergency care, it may be administered IM or IV, depending on the circumstances and condition of the patient.

Onset and Duration

Onset: IV: 20 minutes; IM: 20 minutes
Duration: 2–4 hours, up to 10 hours

Indications

Acute psychotic episodes
Emergency sedation of severely agitated or delirious patients

Contraindications

CNS depression
Hypersensitivity to this drug or related drugs (eg, haloperidol)

Pregnancy
Severe liver or cardiac disease
Known or suspected prolonged QT interval; QTc interval >450 ms in females or >440 ms in males

Adverse Reactions

Dose-related extrapyramidal reactions: pseudoparkinsonism, akathisia, dystonias
Hypotension
Orthostatic hypotension
Nausea and vomiting
Allergic reactions
Blurred vision
Drowsiness

Drug Interactions

Other CNS depressants may potentiate effects.
Droperidol has a wide variety of interactions with other medications; careful consideration is essential prior to administration.

How Supplied

2.5 mg/mL (2-mL vial)

Dosage and Administration

Adult: 2.5 mg IV or 5 mg IM
Pediatric: Not routinely recommended

Special Considerations

Pregnancy safety: Category C
Use with caution in patients with bradycardia, cardiac disease, MAO inhibitors, Class I and Class III dysrhythmics, or drugs that prolong the QT interval.

Epinephrine (Adrenaline)

Class

Sympathomimetic

Description

Epinephrine is an endogenous catecholamine that directly stimulates alpha, beta-1, and beta-2 adrenergic receptors in a dose-related fashion. Epinephrine is the initial drug of choice for treating bronchoconstriction and hypotension resulting from anaphylaxis and all forms of cardiac arrest. It is useful in the management of reactive airway disease, but beta adrenergic agents usually are considered the drugs of choice in such cases because they are inhaled and have fewer side effects. Rapid injection produces a rapid increase in BP, ventricular contractility, and HR. In addition, epinephrine causes vasoconstriction in the arterioles of the skin, mucosa, and splanchnic areas, and antagonizes the effects of histamine.

Onset and Duration

Onset: Subcutaneously: 5–10 minutes; IV/ET tube: 1–2 minutes
Duration: IM: 5–10 minutes

Indications

Acute allergic reaction (anaphylaxis)
Cardiac arrest
Pulseless electrical activity
VF and pulseless VT unresponsive to initial defibrillation
Symptomatic bradycardia
Severe hypotension accompanied by bradycardia when pacing and atropine fail
Bronchial asthma

Contraindications

Hypersensitivity (not an issue especially in emergencies; the dose should be lowered or given slowly in non–cardiac arrest patients with heart disease)
Hypovolemic shock (as with other catecholamines, correct hypovolemia before use)
Dilated cardiomyopathy

Adverse Reactions

Tachycardia
Headache
Nausea and vomiting
Restlessness
Weakness
Dysrhythmias, including VT and VF
Hypertension
Precipitation of angina pectoris

Drug Interactions

MAO inhibitors may potentiate the effect of epinephrine. Beta adrenergic antagonists may blunt inotropic response.

Sympathomimetics and phosphodiesterase inhibitors may exacerbate dysrhythmia response.

May be deactivated by alkaline solutions (sodium bicarbonate, furosemide).

How Supplied

Parenteral: 1-mg/mL, 0.1-mg/mL ampule or vial and prefilled syringe

Autoinjector (EpiPen): 1 mg/mL

Dosage and Administration

Profound Bradycardia or Hypotension

Adult: 2–10 mcg/min infusion; titrate to patient response.

Pediatric: 0.01 mg/kg (0.1 mL/kg of 0.1 mg/mL solution); continuous infusion: 0.1–1 mcg/kg per minute; higher doses may be effective.

All ET doses: 0.1 mg/kg (0.1 mL/kg of 1 mg/mL solution).

Pulseless Arrest

Adult: IV/IO dose: 1 mg (10 mL of 0.1 mg/mL solution) IV/IO push or ET tube (2–2.5 mg diluted in 10 mL of NS), repeated q 3–5 minutes during resuscitation (follow each IV dose with a 20-mL saline flush); elevate arm for 20–30 seconds after dose; higher doses (up to 0.2 mg/kg) may be used for specific indications (eg, beta blocker or calcium channel blocker overdose; poison- or drug-induced shock).

Pediatric:

IV/IO dose: 0.01 mg/kg (0.1 mL/kg of 0.1 mg/mL solution) q 3–5 minutes during arrest; max dose 1 mg.

All ET doses: 0.1 mg/kg of 1 mg/mL solution (0.1 mL/kg) q 5 minutes of arrest until IV/IO access; then begin with first IV/IO dose.

Anaphylactic Reaction or Bronchoconstriction

Adult:

Mild: 0.3–0.5 mL (1 mg/mL solution) IM (preferred for anaphylaxis) or subcutaneously; repeat in 5–15 minutes if needed.

IV infusion at rates of 0.5 mcg/kg per minute may be indicated if shock persists despite repeated doses of IM epinephrine (with rapid isotonic fluid boluses).

Pediatric: Severe: 0.01 mg/kg (0.01 mL/kg of 1 mg/mL solution) IM (subcutaneously for asthma); max single dose 0.3 mg; repeat in 15 minutes prn; if hypotension persists despite fluids and IM injection, IV infusion 0.1–1 mcg/kg per minute.

Stridor or Bronchospasm

Anaphylaxis: 5 mL (0.1 mg/mL) nebulized[11]

Bronchiolitis: 3 mg in 3 mL NS

Croup: 0.5 mg (5 mL of 0.1 mg/mL) nebulized

Special Considerations

Pregnancy safety: Category C

Do not use prefilled syringes for epinephrine infusions. Syncope has occurred following epinephrine administration to asthmatic children.

Epinephrine may increase myocardial oxygen demand.

Epinephrine is safe for anaphylaxis when given at the correct dose by IM injection.[12]

NOTE

Complications of IV administration of epinephrine are significant and include the development of uncontrolled systolic hypertension, vomiting, seizures, dysrhythmias, and myocardial ischemia. This route should be used only in patients with a critical life-threatening condition. IV administration of epinephrine rarely is performed in conscious patients. IV administration is performed with extreme caution in rare circumstances and only with authorization from medical direction. The vast majority of reported cardiovascular adverse events with epinephrine occurred with IV dosing, highlighting the need to proceed with caution if considering epinephrine by this route for anaphylaxis. *Epinephrine 1:1000 (1 mg/mL) should never be given undiluted as an IV bolus.*

Epinephrine Racemic (Micronefrin)

Class

Sympathomimetic

Description

As with other forms of epinephrine, racemic epinephrine acts as a bronchodilator that stimulates beta-2 receptors in the lungs, resulting in relaxation of bronchial smooth muscle. This alleviates bronchospasm, increases vital capacity, and reduces airway resistance. Racemic epinephrine is also useful in treating laryngeal edema. It inhibits the release of histamine.

Onset and Duration

Onset: Within 5 minutes
Duration: 1–3 hours

Indications

Bronchial asthma
Treatment of bronchospasm
Croup (laryngotracheobronchitis)
Laryngeal edema

Contraindications

Hypertension
Underlying cardiovascular disease
Epiglottitis

Adverse Reactions

Tachycardia
Dysrhythmias

Drug Interactions

MAO inhibitors may potentiate the effect of epinephrine. Beta adrenergic antagonists may blunt the bronchodilating response.
Sympathomimetics and phosphodiesterase inhibitors may exacerbate the dysrhythmia response.

How Supplied

MDI: 0.16–0.25 mg/spray
Solution: 7.5, 15, 30 mL in 1%, 2.25% solution

Dosage and Administration

MDI

Adult: 2–3 inhalations, repeat once in 5 minutes prn

Solution

Adult: Dilute 0.5 mL (1% or 2.25%) in 5 mL of saline, administer over 15 minutes
Pediatric: 2.25% inhalation solution (0.25–0.5 mL nebulized) diluted in 3 mL NS; may be repeated in 2 hours if severe symptoms persist.[13]

Special Considerations

Pregnancy safety: Category C
Racemic epinephrine may produce tachycardia and other dysrhythmias.
Monitor vital signs closely.
Excessive use may cause bronchospasm.
Rebound exacerbation of severe croup may occur following drug administration.

Esmolol (Brevibloc)

Class

$Beta_1$ blocker

Description

Esmolol is an extremely short-acting cardioselective beta blocker. Unlike other beta-1 selective beta blockers (eg, metoprolol, atenolol), esmolol is administered via continuous IV infusion. It has a short duration of action, making it useful for acute control of hypertension or certain supraventricular dysrhythmias, such as sinus tachycardia, atrial flutter, and/or atrial fibrillation in the emergency setting. Nonapproved indications include short-term control of perioperative hypertension, management of tachydysrhythmias complicating acute MI, and minimization of acute myocardial ischemia secondary to acute MI or unstable angina.

Onset and Duration

Onset: Rapid
Duration: <10 minutes; some effects may persist up to 30 minutes after cessation of infusion.

Indications

To convert to normal sinus rhythm or to slow ventricular response (or both) in supraventricular tachydysrhythmias (reentry SVT, atrial fibrillation, or atrial flutter)
To reduce myocardial ischemia in acute MI patients with elevated HR, BP, or both
Refractory VF or pulseless VT (off-label) after conventional therapy fails

Contraindications

Hemodynamically unstable patients
STEMI if signs of heart failure, low cardiac output, or increased risk for cardiogenic shock are present

Relative contraindications include PR interval >0.24 second, second- or third-degree heart block, active asthma, reactive airway disease, severe bradycardia, SBP <100 mm Hg

Adverse Reactions

Myocardial depression
AV block
Bradycardia
Cardiac arrest
Diaphoresis
Dizziness
Headache
Hyperglycemia
Hypoglycemia
Hypotension
Nausea or vomiting

Drug Interactions

A potentially clinically significant interaction between esmolol and digoxin may exist because of their additive effects on the AV node.
Esmolol can potentiate the suppressive effects of diltiazem and verapamil on AV nodal conduction.
Depression of AV nodal conduction and myocardial function is possible when used in combination with adenosine, disopyramide, or other antidysrhythmics or drugs, especially in patients with preexisting left ventricular dysfunction.
Careful titration of esmolol is prudent when it is given with morphine.

How Supplied

Solution: 10 mg/mL; 20 mg/mL

Dosage and Administration

0.5 mg/kg (500 mcg/kg) over 1 minute, 0.05 mg/kg (50 mcg/kg) per minute infusion; max: 0.3 mg/kg (300 mcg/kg) per minute.
If inadequate response after 5 minutes, may repeat 0.5-mg/kg (500 mcg/kg) bolus and then titrate infusion up to 0.2 mg/kg (200 mcg/kg) per minute. Higher doses are unlikely to be beneficial.
Has a short half-life (2–9 minutes).

Special Considerations

Pregnancy safety: Category C
Administration of esmolol can exacerbate Raynaud disease or peripheral vascular disease.
Use with caution in patients with poorly controlled diabetes mellitus or renal disease.
Avoid extravasation of esmolol during IV administration. Sloughing of the skin and necrosis have been reported following infiltration and extravasation of IV esmolol infusions.

Etomidate (Amidate)

Class

Nonbarbiturate hypnotic, anesthetic

Description

Etomidate is a short-acting drug that acts at the level of the reticular activating system to produce anesthesia. It may be administered for conscious sedation to relieve apprehension or impair memory before tracheal intubation or cardioversion.

Onset and Duration

Onset: <1 minute
Duration: 5–10 minutes

Indications

Premedication for tracheal intubation or cardioversion

Contraindications

Hypersensitivity to etomidate
Labor/delivery

Adverse Reactions

Nausea and vomiting
Dysrhythmias
Breathing difficulties
Hypotension
Hypertension
Involuntary muscle movement
Pain at injection site
Cortisol suppression

Drug Interactions

Effects may be enhanced when given with other CNS depressants.

How Supplied

2-mg/mL vials

Dosage and Administration for Rapid-Sequence Induction

Adult: 0.2–0.6 mg/kg (often 0.3 mg/kg) IV over 30–60 seconds; limit to 1 dose.
Pediatric (>10 years): 0.2–0.4 mg/kg for sedation infused over 30–60 seconds; max dose: 20 mg.

Special Considerations

Pregnancy safety: Category C
Carefully monitor vital signs.
Etomidate can suppress adrenal gland production of steroid hormones, which can cause temporary gland failure.

Famotidine (Pepcid)

Class

H_2 receptor antagonist

Description

Famotidine blocks H_2 receptors and is used primarily to reduce gastric acid secretion in a variety of GI conditions. H_2 receptor antagonists are also used to augment diphenhydramine in the setting of severe allergic reactions and anaphylaxis.

Onset and Duration

Onset: 30 minutes
Peak: 1–3 hours
Duration: 10–12 hours

Indications

Adjunctive treatment in allergic reactions
GI ulcers and gastric hypersecretory conditions

Contraindications

Hypersensitivity

Adverse Reactions

Dizziness
Headache
Constipation
Diarrhea

Drug Interactions

Use with caution in patients taking medications known to prolong the QT interval.

How Supplied

20-mg/50 mL and 10-mg/mL IV solutions; 10-, 20-, 40-mg tablets

Dosage and Administration

Adults: 20 mg IV over 15–30 minutes or PO q 12 hours
Pediatric: 0.25–0.5 mg/kg (max dose 20 mg) infused over 20 minutes for most conditions

Special Considerations

Pregnancy safety: Category B

Fentanyl (Sublimaze)

Class

Opioid analgesic

Description

Fentanyl (like other opioids) combines with receptor sites in the brain to produce potent analgesic effects. This drug often is given in combination with benzodiazepines for conscious sedation.

Onset and Duration

Onset: IV: 1–2 minutes
Duration: 30–60 minutes

Indications

Pain control
Sedation for invasive airway procedures (eg, rapid-sequence induction)

Contraindications

Respiratory depression
Hypotension
Head injury
Cardiac dysrhythmias
Myasthenia gravis
Hypersensitivity to other opiates (relative)

Adverse Reactions

Respiratory depression
Bradycardia
Hypotension or hypertension
Nausea and vomiting
Chest wall muscle rigidity

Drug Interactions

Effects may be increased when this drug is given with other CNS depressants or skeletal muscle relaxants.

How Supplied

0.05- to 0.1-mg/mL ampules

Dosage and Administration

Adult: 1 mcg/kg IV, intranasal (IN), or IM (max initial dose 100 mcg); alternatively, use 0.05–0.1 mg (50–100 mcg) slow IV over 1–2 minutes q 1–2 hours prn to control pain

Child: 1–2 mcg/kg

Rapid-Sequence Induction

2–5 mcg/kg IV/IO

End-of-Life Care (Palliative or Hospice)

Adult: 25 mcg in 2 mL NS nebulized

Special Considerations

Pregnancy safety: Category C

Fentanyl is a Schedule II drug with the potential for abuse.

Fentanyl should be used with caution in older adults and in people who are pregnant, are using other CNS depressants, or have severe respiratory disorders, seizure disorders, cardiac disorders, head injury, suspected GI obstruction, or hypotension. Naloxone or nalmefene should be available to reverse respiratory depression.

Furosemide (Lasix)

Class

Loop diuretic

Description

Furosemide is a potent diuretic that inhibits the reabsorption of sodium and chloride in the proximal tubule and loop of Henle. IV doses also can reduce cardiac preload by increasing venous capacitance.

Onset and Duration

Onset: IV: Diuretic effects within 15–20 minutes; vascular effects within 5 minutes

Duration: 2 hours

Indications

Acute pulmonary edema in patients with a SBP >90–100 mm Hg (without signs and symptoms of shock)

Hypertensive emergencies

Hyperkalemia

Contraindications

Anuria (although loop diuretics can be used in patients with reduced creatinine clearance)

Hypersensitivity

Hypovolemia/dehydration

Known hypersensitivity to sulfonamides (caution)

Severe electrolyte depletion (hypokalemia)

Adverse Reactions

Hypotension

ECG changes associated with electrolyte disturbances

Dry mouth

Hypochloremia

Hypokalemia

Hyponatremia

Hypocalcemia

Hyperglycemia

Hearing loss can occur rarely after too-rapid infusion of large doses, especially in patients with renal impairment

Drug Interactions

Digitalis toxicity may be potentiated because of potassium depletion, which can result from furosemide administration.

Furosemide increases the ototoxic potential of aminoglycoside antibiotics.

Lithium toxicity may be potentiated because of sodium depletion.

Furosemide may potentiate the therapeutic effect of other antihypertensive drugs.

How Supplied

Parenteral: 10 mg/mL in 2-, 4-, 8-mL ampule, 10 mg/mL in 10-mL vial

Dosage and Administration

IV: 0.5–1 mg/kg over 1–2 minutes (or 20–40 mg) IV; if no response, double dose up to 2 mg/kg given slowly over 1–2 minutes; for new-onset pulmonary edema with hypovolemia, give <0.5 mg/kg.

Pediatric: 1 mg/kg per dose (max total dose: 6 mg/kg)
Hyperkalemia (adult): 40–80 mg IV

Special Considerations

Pregnancy safety: Category C. Furosemide has been known to cause fetal abnormalities.
Protect from light and store at room temperature; do not use if the solution is discolored or yellow.

Glucagon

Class

Pancreatic hormone, antihypoglycemic agent

Description

Glucagon is a protein secreted by the alpha cells of the pancreas. When it is released, glucagon results in blood glucose elevation by increasing the breakdown of glycogen to glucose (glycogenolysis) and stimulating glucose synthesis (gluconeogenesis). The drug is effective in treating hypoglycemia only if liver glycogen is available; therefore, it may be ineffective in patients in chronic states of hypoglycemia, starvation, and adrenal insufficiency. In addition, glucagon exerts a positive inotropic action on the heart and decreases renal vascular resistance. For this reason, glucagon also is used in managing patients with beta blocker and calcium channel blocker cardiotoxicity who do not respond to saline infusions or other conventional therapy.

Onset and Duration

Onset: Within 1 minute
Duration: 60–90 minutes

Indications

Hypoglycemia
Calcium channel blocker or beta blocker toxicity

Contraindications

Hypersensitivity (allergy to proteins); pheochromocytoma, insulinoma

Adverse Reactions

Tachycardia
Hypotension
Nausea and vomiting, especially with IV use
Urticaria

Drug Interactions

Effect of anticoagulants may be increased if given with glucagon.
Do not mix with saline.

How Supplied

Glucagon must be reconstituted (with provided diluent) before administration. Dilute 1 unit (1 mg) of white powder in 1 mL of diluting solution (1 mg/mL).

Dosage and Administration

Hypoglycemia

Adult: 1 mg IM/IN; may repeat in 7–10 minutes.
Pediatric: For ≥44 pounds (20 kg) or ≥5 years, give 1 mg IM/IN; for <44 pounds (20 kg) or <5 years, give 0.5 mg IM/IN.

Calcium Channel Blocker or Beta Blocker Toxicity

Adult: 3–10 mg slow IV over 3–5 minutes, followed by infusion at 3–5 mg/h.
Pediatric: 1 mg IV push (25–40 kg) q 5 minutes if needed; 0.5 mg IV push (<25 kg) q 5 minutes as necessary.

Special Considerations

Pregnancy safety: Category B
Glucagon is not a first-line choice for hypoglycemia.
May cause vomiting and hyperglycemia at higher doses.
Ineffective if the patient does not respond to a second dose.
Do not use the provided diluent to mix continuous infusions.

Haloperidol Lactate (Haldol)

Class

Antipsychotic/neuroleptic

Description

Haloperidol has pharmacologic properties similar to those of the phenothiazines. The drug is thought to block dopamine (type 2) receptors in the brain, altering mood and behavior. In emergency care, haloperidol usually is administered IM.

Onset and Duration

Onset: IM: 30–60 minutes
Duration: 12–24 hours

Indications

Acute psychotic episodes
Emergency sedation of severely agitated or delirious patients

Contraindications

CNS depression
Coma
Hypersensitivity
Pregnancy
Neuroleptic malignant syndrome
Poorly controlled seizure disorder
Parkinson disease
Severe liver or cardiac disease

Adverse Reactions

Dose-related extrapyramidal reactions: pseudoparkinsonism, akathisia, dystonias
Hypotension
Orthostatic hypotension
Nausea and vomiting
Allergic reactions
Blurred vision
Drowsiness

Drug Interactions

Other CNS depressants may potentiate haloperidol's effects.
Haloperidol may inhibit vasoconstrictor effects of epinephrine.

How Supplied

5 mg/mL

Dosage and Administration

Adult: 5 mg IV or 10 mg IM
Pediatric (6–12 years): 1–3 mg IM (max dose 0.15 mg/kg)

Special Considerations

Pregnancy safety: Category C
Continuous cardiac monitoring is needed if administering IV.

Heparin

Low-Molecular-Weight Heparin (Enoxaparin)

Class

Anticoagulant

Description

Heparin is available as low-molecular-weight heparin (LMWH [Enoxaparin]) and unfractionated heparin (UFH). Both inhibit the clotting cascade by activating specific plasma proteins. Natural heparin (heparin sodium) consists of molecular chains of varying lengths or molecular weights. LMWHs consist of only short chains of low molecular weight and produce a more predictable coagulation response than does UFH. The use of LMWH has been approved for both the prevention and the treatment of acute deep venous thrombosis and acute pulmonary embolism, and for the treatment of ACS.

Onset and Duration

Onset: IV: Immediate; Subcutaneous: 20–60 minutes
Peak: 3–5 hours
Duration: Approximately 12 hours

Indications

ACS
Acute deep venous thrombosis
Acute pulmonary embolism

Contraindications

Same as for fibrinolytic therapy
Renal insufficiency
Active bleeding or low platelet count
Hypersensitivity to heparin or pork products
Recent intracranial, intraspinal, or eye surgery
Severe hypertension
Heparin-induced thrombocytopenia

Adverse Reactions

Allergic reaction (chills, fever, back pain)
Thrombocytopenia
Hemorrhage
Bruising
Rash

Drug Interactions

None noted

Salicylates, ibuprofen, dipyridamole, and hydroxychloroquine may increase risk of bleeding.

How Supplied

Concentrations range from 30 mg to 150 mg in various mL of solution for subcutaneous or IV administration.

Dosage and Administration

STEMI Protocol

Age <75 years: Initial bolus 30 mg IV, with second dose 15 minutes later of 1 mg/kg subcutaneous (max 100 mg dose for first 2 doses).

Age ≥75 years: Eliminate initial IV bolus; give 0.75 mg/kg subcutaneously q 12 hours (max 75 mg dose for first 2 doses).

Should use UFH if early cardiac catheterization (within 12 hours) is planned.

Pulmonary Embolism Protocol

Adults: 1 mg/kg subcutaneously q 12 hours or 1.5 mg/kg subcutaneously q 24 hours.

Special Considerations

Pregnancy safety: Category B

The platelet count should be monitored in patients receiving enoxaparin.

Always follow the institutional protocol regarding heparin administration.

Multiple-dose vials of enoxaparin contain benzyl alcohol (1.5%) as a preservative and should be avoided in patients with benzyl alcohol hypersensitivity.

Do not administer IM.

Enoxaparin cannot be used interchangeably (unit for unit) with heparin sodium or other LMWHs.

Do not mix with other products or infusion fluids.

Heparin Sodium

Unfractionated Heparin

Class

Anticoagulant

Description

Heparin inhibits the clotting cascade by activating specific plasma proteins. The drug is used in the prevention and treatment of all types of thromboses and emboli, disseminated intravascular coagulation, arterial occlusion, and thrombophlebitis and is used prophylactically to prevent clotting before surgery. Heparin is considered part of the antithrombotic package (along with aspirin and fibrinolytic agents) administered to patients with STEMI, unstable angina or non–ST segment elevation myocardial infarction (NSTEMI), and ACS.

Onset and Duration

Onset: IV: immediate; Subcutaneous: 20–60 minutes

Duration: 4–8 hours

Indications

Acute MI

Unstable angina/NSTEMI

STEMI

Prophylaxis and treatment of thromboembolic disorders (eg, pulmonary emboli, deep venous thrombosis)

Contraindications

Same as for fibrinolytic therapy

Hypersensitivity

Active bleeding

Recent intracranial, intraspinal, or eye surgery

Severe hypertension

Bleeding tendencies

Severe thrombocytopenia

Adverse Reactions

Allergic reaction (chills, fever, back pain)

Thrombocytopenia

Hemorrhage

Bruising

Rash

Drug Interactions

Salicylates, ibuprofen, dipyridamole, and hydroxychloroquine may increase the risk of bleeding.

How Supplied

Concentrations range from 1,000 to 40,000 units/mL.

Dosage and Administration

IV infusion: STEMI and unstable angina/NSTEMI: Initial bolus of 60 units/kg (max bolus: 4,000 units); continue with infusion of 12 units/kg per hour, round to the nearest 50 units (max initial rate: 1,000 units/h).

Special Considerations

Pregnancy safety: Category C

Dosing should be guided by laboratory analysis of platelet count and partial thromboplastin time. Always follow the institutional protocol regarding heparin administration.

Hydralazine (Apresoline)

Class

Antihypertensive; vasodilator

Description

Decreases systemic vascular resistance and BP by direct vasodilator action on arterioles.

Onset and Duration

Onset: 10–80 minutes
Duration: Up to 12 hours

Indications

Hypertension (severe) in pregnancy

Contraindications

Hypersensitivity
Coronary artery disease
Hypotension
Mitral valve rheumatic heart disease

Adverse Reactions

Hypotension
Paradoxical hypertension
Tachycardia
Flushing
Dizziness
Headache

Drug Interactions

Use with caution with other medications prone to causing hypotension and with stroke.

Many medications are known to increase serum levels of hydralazine.

How Supplied

IV: 20 mg/mL (1-mL vial)
Oral: 10-, 25-, 50-, 100-mg tablets

Dosage and Administration

Adult: 5–10 mg IV, repeated prn q 20–30 minutes.
Pediatric: Not indicated.

Special Considerations

Pregnancy safety: Category C

Administer by slow IV push while monitoring HR and BP.

Hydrocortisone (Solu-Cortef, Cortef)

Class

Corticosteroid

Description

Hydrocortisone is a systemic corticosteroid used for a wide variety of endocrine and inflammatory conditions. Hydrocortisone has mineralocorticoid actions that cause sodium retention. This medication has many overlapping indications with methylprednisolone and dexamethasone.

Onset and Duration

Onset: 1–2 hours
Duration: >24 hours

Indications

Cerebral edema
Multiple sclerosis exacerbations
Bronchodilator-unresponsive asthma
Thyroid storm (off-label)
Septic shock (controversial/off-label)
Adrenal insufficiency

Contraindications

Use with caution in patients with GI bleeding, diabetes mellitus, or severe untreated infection.

Idiopathic thrombocytopenic purpura

Adverse Reactions

Depression
Hypertension

Sodium and water retention
Nausea and vomiting

Drug Interactions

Hypoglycemic responses to insulin and oral hypoglycemic agents may be blunted.
Potassium-depleting agents may potentiate hypokalemia induced by corticosteroids.

How Supplied

IV powder for reconstitution: 100-mg, 250-mg, 500-mg, 1,000-mg vials

Dosage and Administration

Adult: Variable; usually within the range of 50–500 mg IV depending on indication and severity.
Patients with history of adrenal insufficiency or long-term steroid dependence: 2 mg/kg (max 100 mg) IV/IM
Pediatric: 0.56–10 mg/kg per day, depending on indication and severity.

Special Considerations

Pregnancy safety: Category C
Numerous adverse effects related to long-term use.
Avoid confusion with methylprednisolone (Solu-Medrol versus Solu-Cortef).
Administer by slow IV push or intermittent infusion depending on dose ordered and indication.

Hydromorphone (Dilaudid)

Class

Analgesic; opiate agonist

Description

Hydromorphone is a semisynthetic analog of morphine used to relieve moderate to severe pain in cancer, surgery, trauma, burn, and cardiac patients. The drug works at opioid receptors to produce analgesia and euphoria. It may also produce respiratory depression, miosis, decreased GI motility, and physical dependence. Hydromorphone is a Schedule II controlled substance.

Onset and Duration

Onset: IV/IM: 5 minutes
Duration: 3–5 hours in nondependent patients

Indications

Moderate to severe pain
Analgesia
Preoperative medication

Contraindications

Asthma
GI obstruction
Hypersensitivity to narcotics
Ileus
Respiratory depression
Status asthmaticus

Adverse Reactions

Respiratory depression
Nausea and vomiting
Euphoria
Delirium
Agitation
Hallucination
Seizures
Headache
Hypotension
Visual disturbances
Coma
Facial flushing
Circulatory collapse
Dysrhythmias
Allergic reaction
Drowsiness
Rash

Drug Interactions

Respiratory depression, hypotension, or sedation may be potentiated by CNS depressants.
Therapeutic doses of hydromorphone have caused additive CNS or respiratory depression and hypotension in patients taking MAO inhibitors.

How Supplied

Solution for injection: 1 mg/mL, 2 mg/mL, 4 mg/mL

Dosage and Administration

Adult: 0.015 mg/kg (max initial dose 2 mg) subcutaneously/IM (IM use discouraged) or slow IV/IO (max cumulative dose 4 mg).

Pediatric (>110 pounds [50 kg]): 1 mg IV/subcutaneously q 4 hours; pediatric (<110 pounds [50 kg] or >6 months): 0.015–0.02 mg/kg IV/subcutaneously q 2–4 hours; titrate to pain relief.

Special Considerations

Pregnancy safety: Category C
High potential for abuse.
Use with extreme caution in patients with head trauma, increased intracranial pressure, or a preexisting seizure disorder.
Use with caution in patients with cardiac dysrhythmias, hypotension, circulatory shock, or hypovolemia. Older adults may be more susceptible to adverse reactions.
Can induce vasovagal syncope or orthostatic hypotension.
Naloxone should be readily available.

Hydroxocobalamin (Cyanokit)

Class

Vitamin; antidote

Description

Hydroxocobalamin is a parenteral preparation of vitamin B_{12}; specifically, it is the hydroxylated active form of vitamin B_{12}. Hydroxocobalamin is used to treat known or suspected cyanide toxicity.

Onset and Duration

Onset: Rapid
Duration: Greater than 24 hours

Indications

Known or suspected cyanide poisoning

Contraindications

Known hydroxocobalamin hypersensitivity

Adverse Reactions

Allergic reaction/anaphylaxis
Elevated BP
Headache
Hypertension
Injection site reaction
Nausea
Photophobia
Red-colored urine and skin

Drug Interactions

None

How Supplied

Powder for injection: 5 g
Solution: 1,000 mcg/mL

Dosage and Administration

Adult: Initially, 5 g (two 2.5-g vials) IV infused over 15 minutes. A second 5-g dose infused over 15 minutes to 2 hours (depending on patient status), for a total of 10 g, may be administered based on clinical response and severity of cyanide poisoning.
Pediatric: Doses of 70 mg/kg IV have been used; not FDA approved.

Special Considerations

Pregnancy safety: Category C
Treatment of cyanide poisoning includes symptomatic management in addition to the use of hydroxocobalamin.
Solution is bright red.

Ibuprofen (Motrin, Advil, and Others)

Class

NSAID

Description

Ibuprofen slows prostaglandin synthesis by inhibiting COX-1 and -2 enzymes. Inflammation is also decreased through other mechanisms. Ibuprofen is administered for its antipyretic (fever-reducing), analgesic, and anti-inflammatory properties. NSAIDs have a variety of warnings and precautions, primarily related to the GI system and kidneys. Ibuprofen's primary route of administration is oral, but an IV form is also available.

Onset and Duration

Onset: 30–60 minutes
Duration: 6–8 hours

Indications

Short-term management (<5 days) of moderate to severe pain
Fevers
Various rheumatoid and inflammatory disorders

Contraindications

Hypersensitivity to the drug, aspirin, or other NSAIDs
Bleeding disorders
Renal failure or disease
Active peptic ulcer disease
Preterm infants with infection
Congenital heart disease dependent on patent ductus arteriosus

Adverse Reactions

Anaphylaxis from hypersensitivity
Edema
Sedation
Bleeding disorders
Rash
Nausea
Headache

Drug Interactions

Avoid concomitant administration with other NSAIDs.
Ibuprofen may antagonize effects of angiotensin-converting enzyme (ACE) inhibitors, beta blockers, angiotensin-receptor antagonist medications, salicylates, and certain classes of diuretic medications.

How Supplied

100 mg/mL IV solution; numerous oral forms and concentrations frequently combined with other medications

Dosage and Administration

Adult: 400–800 mg q 6–8 hours
Pediatric: 10 mg/kg (up to 400 mg) q 4–6 hours

Special Considerations

Pregnancy safety: Category B during first two trimesters; Category D during third trimester.
Monitor renal function, bleeding, bruising, and GI effects with longer-term use or higher dosing regimens.

Ipratropium (Atrovent)

Class

Anticholinergic; bronchodilator

Description

Ipratropium inhibits interaction of acetylcholine at receptor sites on bronchial smooth muscle, resulting in decreased levels of cyclic guanosine monophosphate and bronchodilation.

Onset and Duration

Onset: <15 minutes
Duration: 2–4 hours

Indications

Persistent bronchospasm
Chronic obstructive pulmonary disease exacerbation

Contraindications

Hypersensitivity to ipratropium, atropine, alkaloid, soybean protein, or peanuts

Adverse Reactions

Nausea and vomiting
Cramps
Coughing
Worsening of symptoms
Headache
Tachycardia
Dry mouth
Blurred vision
Anxiety

Drug Interactions

None reported

How Supplied

MDI: 17 mcg/activation
Nebulizer solution: 0.02% (2.5 mL)

Dosage and Administration

Adult: 0.5 mg nebulized; repeated twice. Nebulized ipratropium can be simultaneously administered with the first three doses of albuterol[14] or started after the first dose of albuterol. Can be administered as 1–2 inhalations via MDI.

Pediatric: 250–500 mcg (by nebulizer or MDI) q 20 minutes times 3 doses.

Special Considerations

Pregnancy safety: Category B
Shake well before use.
Use with caution in patients with urinary retention.

Ketamine (Ketalar)

Class

Nonbarbiturate anesthetic

Description

Ketamine acts on the limbic system and cortex to block afferent transmission of impulses associated with pain perception. It produces short-acting amnesia without muscular relaxation. Ketamine is a derivative of a drug of abuse, phencyclidine.

Onset and Duration

Onset: Within 30 seconds
Duration: 5–10 minutes up to 1–2 hours

Indications

Analgesia, either as initial agent or when severe pain is refractory to other treatments[15]
Treatment of severe agitation[16]
Procedural sedation
As an adjunct to nitrous oxide

Contraindications

Stroke
Increased intracranial pressure (controversial)
Severe hypertension
History of schizophrenia, even if symptoms are well controlled
Cardiac decompensation
Hypersensitivity to ketamine

Adverse Reactions

Hypertension
Increased HR
Hallucinations, delusions, explicit dreams
Less common side effects: hypotension, bradycardia, and respiratory depression

Drug Interactions

Ketamine may increase effects from ethyl alcohol (ethanol), opioid medications, CNS depressant medications, and selective serotonin reuptake inhibitors.

How Supplied

10-, 50-, and 100-mg/mL vials

Dosage and Administration

Excited Delirium

Adult: 2 mg/kg IV over 1 minute or 4 mg/kg IM or IN
Child (>2 years): 1 mg/kg IV over 1 minute or 3 mg/kg IM

Pain Management

Moderate pain: 0.5 mg/kg IN (max initial dose 25 mg; max cumulative dose 100 mg)
Severe pain: 0.25 mg/kg IM, IV, IO (max initial dose 25 mg; max cumulative dose 100 mg)

Special Considerations

Pregnancy safety: Category C
Ketamine may increase BP, muscle tone, and HR.
As with any anesthetic, the dosage needs to be individualized. Dose selection for older adults should be cautious, usually starting at the low end of the dosing range.[17]
Keep the patient in a quiet environment (if possible). Overdose may lead to panic attacks, aggressive behavior, and rarely seizures. Administration of IV benzodiazepines such as midazolam will reduce or prevent "emergence" reactions, a feeling of terror as sedation from ketamine wanes.

Ketorolac Tromethamine (Toradol)

Class

NSAID

Description

Ketorolac tromethamine is an anti-inflammatory drug that also exhibits peripherally acting nonnarcotic analgesic activity by inhibiting prostaglandin synthesis.

Onset and Duration

Onset: Within 10 minutes
Duration: 6–8 hours

Indications

Short-term management (<5 days) of moderate to severe pain

Contraindications

Hypersensitivity to the drug
Patients with allergies to aspirin or other NSAIDs
Bleeding disorders
Renal failure
Active peptic ulcer disease

Adverse Reactions

Anaphylaxis from hypersensitivity
Edema
Sedation
Bleeding disorders
Rash
Nausea
Headache

Drug Interactions

Ketorolac may increase bleeding time when administered to patients taking anticoagulants.
Avoid concomitant administration with aspirin or other NSAIDs.

How Supplied

15 or 30 mg in 1 mL
60 mg in 2 mL

Dosage and Administration

Adult:
IM: 1 dose of 30 mg; 1 dose of 15 mg for patients who are >65 years, have renal impairment, and/or weigh <110 pounds (50 kg)
IV: 15 mg over 1 minute
Pediatric (2–16 years) (off-label): 0.5 mg/kg IM or IV (max dose 15 mg) q 6 hours.[18]

Special Considerations

Pregnancy safety: Category C
Solution is clear and slightly yellow.
Use with caution and reduce dose when administering to older adults. Use with caution or avoid use in patients with hepatic disease, renal disease, many GI conditions, or bleeding disorders.

Labetalol (Trandate, Normodyne)

Class

Alpha and beta adrenergic blocker

Description

Labetalol is a competitive alpha-1 receptor blocker and a nonselective beta receptor blocker that is used for lowering BP in hypertensive crises. Labetalol is a more potent beta blocker than alpha blocker. BP is reduced without reflex tachycardia, and total peripheral resistance is decreased, helping maintain cardiac output. In emergency care, labetalol is administered IV.

Onset and Duration

Onset: Within 5 minutes
Peak: 15 minutes
Duration: Up to 18 hours

Indications

Hypertensive emergencies
Hypertensive emergencies in pregnancy (off-label)
Useful as an adjunctive agent with fibrinolytic therapy (may reduce nonfatal reinfarction and recurrent ischemia)

Contraindications

Hemodynamically unstable patients
Bradycardia
Hypotension
Heart block greater than first degree
Asthma or obstructive airway disease
STEMI if signs of heart failure, low cardiac output, or increased risk for cardiogenic shock are present

Adverse Reactions

Hypotension
Bradycardia
Headache
Dizziness
Edema
Fatigue
Vertigo
Ventricular dysrhythmias
Dyspnea

Allergic reaction
Facial flushing
Diaphoresis
Dose-related orthostatic hypotension (most common)
Nausea and vomiting
Tinnitus

Drug Interactions

Bronchodilator effects of beta adrenergic agonists may be blunted by labetalol.
Nitroglycerin may augment hypotensive effects.

How Supplied

5 mg/mL in 4-, 8-, 20-, and 40-mL vials

Dosage and Administration

Adult: 10–20 mg IV over 2 minutes. May repeat or double labetalol q 10 minutes to a max dose of 200 mg.
Pediatric: Safety has not been established.

Special Considerations

Pregnancy safety: Category C
BP, pulse rate, and ECG should be monitored continuously.
Observe for signs of heart failure, bradycardia, and bronchospasm.
Labetalol should be administered only with the patient in a supine position.
May worsen CNS depression in patients with myasthenia gravis, psoriasis, or psychiatric illness.

Lidocaine (Xylocaine)

Class

Antidysrhythmic (Class IB), local anesthetic

Description

Lidocaine decreases phase 4 diastolic depolarization (which decreases automaticity) and has been shown to be effective in suppressing premature ventricular complexes. In addition, lidocaine is used as an alternative to amiodarone to treat cardiac arrest from VT or VF. Lidocaine also raises the VF threshold.

Onset and Duration

Onset: 45–90 seconds
Duration: 10–20 minutes

Indications

Cardiac arrest from VT or VF
Stable monomorphic VT with preserved ventricular function
Stable polymorphic VT with normal baseline QT interval and preserved left ventricular function after correction of ischemia and electrolyte balance
Stable polymorphic VT with baseline-prolonged QT interval if torsades de pointes is suspected
Wide-complex tachycardia of uncertain origin
Significant ventricular ectopy in the setting of myocardial ischemia/infarction

Contraindications

Prophylactic use in acute MI
Hypersensitivity to lidocaine or amide-type anesthetic
Stokes-Adams syndrome
Second- or third-degree heart block in the absence of an artificial pacemaker
WPW syndrome

Adverse Reactions

Light-headedness
Confusion
Blurred vision
Hypotension
Bradycardia
Cardiovascular collapse
Altered level of consciousness, irritability, muscle twitching
Headache
Seizures

Drug Interactions

Metabolic clearance of lidocaine may be decreased in patients taking beta adrenergic blockers or in patients with decreased cardiac output or liver dysfunction.
Cardiac depression may occur if lidocaine is given concomitantly with IV phenytoin.
Additive neurologic effects may occur with procainamide and tocainide.

How Supplied

Prefilled syringes: 100 mg in 5 mL of solution; 1- and 2-g additive syringes
Ampules: 100 mg in 5 mL of solution; 1- and 2-g vials in 30 mL of solution; 5 mL containing 100 mg/mL

Dosage and Administration

Cardiac Arrest From VT/VF

Adult: 1–1.5 mg/kg IV/IO bolus or ET tube (at 2–2.5 times the IV dose); for refractory VF, may give additional 0.5–0.75 mg/kg IV push; repeat in 5–10 minutes; max 3 doses or total of 3 mg/kg.

Pediatric: 1 mg/kg IV/IO loading dose; ET dose: 2–3 mg/kg.

Perfusing Dysrhythmia (Stable VT; Wide-Complex Tachycardia of Uncertain Type; Significant Ectopy)

Adult: 0.5–0.75 mg/kg (up to 1–1.5 mg/kg may be used). Repeat 0.5–0.75 mg/kg q 5–10 minutes; max total dose 3 mg/kg.

Pediatric: 1 mg/kg IV/IO. ET dose is 2–3 mg/kg.

Maintenance Infusion

Adult: 1–4 mg/min (30–50 mcg/kg per minute); reduce maintenance dose (not loading dose) if impaired liver function or left ventricular dysfunction.

Pediatric: Initial loading dose of 1 mg/kg IV/IO, followed by infusion of 20–50 mcg/kg per minute.

RSI (or Drug-Assisted Intubation) in Head-Injured Patient

1–2 mg/kg IV/IO (max 100 mg).

Local Pain Control After IO insertion for Infusion-Related Bone Pain

0.5 mg/kg (0.1 mg/mL) to max 40 mg IO.

Special Considerations

Pregnancy safety: Category B

A 75- to 100-mg bolus will maintain adequate blood levels for only 20 minutes (in the absence of shock).

If bradycardia occurs along with premature ventricular contractions, always treat the bradycardia first with atropine.

Discontinue the infusion immediately if signs of toxicity develop.

Decrease the dose in older adults.

Avoid lidocaine for reperfusion dysrhythmias following fibrinolytic therapy.

Use extreme caution in patients with hepatic disease, heart failure, marked hypoxia, severe respiratory depression, hypovolemia or shock, incomplete heart block, or bradycardia and atrial fibrillation.

Lorazepam (Ativan)

Class

Benzodiazepine

Description

Lorazepam is a benzodiazepine with antianxiety and anticonvulsant effects. When given by injection, it appears to suppress the propagation of seizure activity produced by foci in the cortex, thalamus, and limbic areas.

Onset and Duration

Onset: IV: 2–10 minutes

Duration: 6–8 hours

Indications

Seizures

Agitation requiring sedation

Initial control of status epilepticus or severe recurrent seizures

Severe alcohol withdrawal

Severe anxiety

Contraindications

Hypersensitivity to the drug

Narrow-angle glaucoma

Substance abuse (relative)

Coma (unless seizing)

Severe hypotension or respiratory depression

Sleep apnea

Shock

Preexisting CNS depression

Adverse Reactions

Respiratory depression

Tachycardia/bradycardia

Hypotension

Excessive sedation

Ataxia

Psychomotor impairment

Confusion

Blurred vision

Drug Interactions

Lorazepam may precipitate CNS depression and psychomotor impairment when the patient is taking CNS depressant medications.

How Supplied

2- and 4-mg/mL concentrations in 1-mL vials; 0.5-, 1-, 2-mg tablets

Dosage and Administration

Before IV administration, lorazepam must be diluted with an equal volume of sterile water or sterile saline. When given IM, lorazepam is not to be diluted.

Adult: 0.1 mg/kg or 1–4 mg IM/IV; may be repeated in 15–20 minutes to a max dose of 8 mg.

Pediatric (not FDA-approved): 0.05–0.1 mg/kg slow IV/IO/IM over 2 minutes; may be repeated once in 5–10 minutes to a max dose of 4 mg; 0.1–0.2 mg/kg (rectal dose); 0.1 mg/kg IN to max dose of 4 mg.

Special Considerations

Pregnancy safety: Category D

Monitor respiratory rate and BP during administration.

Have suction and intubation equipment available.

Lorazepam expires in 6 weeks when not refrigerated; do not use if discolored or if solution contains precipitate.

Magnesium Sulfate

Class

Electrolyte, anticonvulsant

Description

Magnesium sulfate reduces striated muscle contractions and blocks peripheral neuromuscular transmission by reducing acetylcholine release at the myoneural junction. In emergency care, this drug is used in the management of seizures associated with toxemia of pregnancy. Other uses of magnesium sulfate include uterine relaxation (to inhibit contractions of premature labor), as a bronchodilator after beta agonist and anticholinergic agents have been used, and as replacement therapy for magnesium deficiency. Magnesium sulfate is recommended for use in cardiac arrest only if torsades de pointes or suspected hypomagnesemia is present.

Onset and Duration

Onset: IV: Immediate; IM: 3–4 hours

Duration: IV: 30 minutes; IM: 3–4 hours

Indications

Seizures of eclampsia (toxemia of pregnancy)

Cardiac arrest only if torsades de pointes is suspected or hypomagnesemia is present

Life-threatening ventricular dysrhythmias attributable to digitalis toxicity

Suspected hypomagnesemia

Status asthmaticus not responsive to beta adrenergic drugs

Contraindications

Heart block or myocardial damage

Hypermagnesemia or hypercalcemia

Diabetic coma

Adverse Reactions

Diaphoresis

Facial flushing

Hypotension

Depressed reflexes

Hypothermia

Bradycardia

Circulatory collapse

Respiratory depression/arrest

Diarrhea

Nausea and vomiting

Drug Interactions

CNS depressant effects may be enhanced if the patient is taking other CNS depressants.

Serious changes in cardiac function may occur with cardiac glycosides (avoid excess magnesium administration).

How Supplied

10%, 12.5%, 50% solution in 40, 80, 100, and 125 mg/mL

Dosage and Administration

Seizure Activity Associated With Pregnancy

Adult: 4 g diluted in D_5W or NS for IV piggyback load over 15–20 minutes, followed by continuous infusion of 1 to 2 g/h; max dose of 30–40 g/d.

Pulseless Arrest (for Hypomagnesemia or Torsades de Pointes), Status Asthmaticus

Adult: 1–2 g (2–4 mL of a 50% solution) diluted in 10 mL of D_5W IV/IO push.

Pediatric: 25–50 mg/kg IV/IO (max 2 g) over 10–20 minutes; over 15–30 minutes for status asthmaticus.

Torsades de Pointes With Pulse or Acute MI With Hypomagnesemia

Adult: Loading dose of 1–2 g in 50–100 mL of D_5W over 5–60 minutes IV; follow with 0.5–1 g/h IV (titrate dose to control torsades de pointes).
Pediatric: Same as pulseless arrest.

Special Considerations

Pregnancy safety: Category A. Magnesium sulfate is administered for the treatment of toxemia of pregnancy. It is recommended that the drug not be administered in the 2 hours before delivery, if possible. IV calcium gluconate or calcium chloride should be available as an antagonist to magnesium if needed.

Convulsions may occur up to 48 hours after delivery, necessitating continued therapy.

The "cure" for toxemia is delivery of the baby.

Magnesium must be used with caution in patients with renal failure because it is cleared by the kidneys and can reach toxic levels easily in those patients.

Methylprednisolone (Solu-Medrol)

Class

Glucocorticoid

Description

Methylprednisolone is a synthetic steroid that suppresses acute and chronic inflammation. In addition, it potentiates vascular smooth muscle relaxation by beta adrenergic agonists and may alter airway hyperactivity. Methylprednisolone is frequently used as adjunctive treatment for various types of reactive airway diseases. It also shares a large number of potential uses with dexamethasone and hydrocortisone for a variety of inflammatory and endocrine conditions.[19]

Onset and Duration

Onset: 1–2 hours
Duration: 8–24 hours

Indications

Anaphylaxis
Bronchodilator-unresponsive asthma
Shock (controversial)
Adrenal insufficiency (hydrocortisone [Solu-Cortef] also may be used)

Contraindications

Use with caution in patients with GI bleeding, diabetes mellitus, or severe infection. IM route is contraindicated in patients with idiopathic thrombocytopenic purpura.

Adverse Reactions

Headache
Hypertension
Sodium and water retention
Hypokalemia
Alkalosis

Drug Interactions

Hypoglycemic responses to insulin and oral hypoglycemic agents may be blunted.

Potassium-depleting agents may potentiate hypokalemia induced by corticosteroids.

How Supplied

20, 40, 80 mg/mL; 125 mg/2 mL

Dosage and Administration

Adult: 2 mg/kg up to 125 mg IV, or 40–125 mg IV
Pediatric: Loading dose: 2 mg/kg IV (max 60 mg)

Special Considerations

Pregnancy safety: Category C

Metoclopramide (Metozolv ODT, Octamide, Reglan)

Class

Antiemetic, GI stimulant

Description

Metoclopramide enhances GI motility. The drug is chemically related to procainamide but has no anesthetic or antidysrhythmic properties. Metoclopramide was originally developed to treat nausea during pregnancy but is also useful in the treatment of chemotherapy-induced nausea and vomiting.

Onset and Duration

Onset: PO: 30–60 minutes; IV: 1–3 minutes; IM: 10–15 minutes
Duration: 1–2 hours

Indications

Nausea
Vomiting

Contraindications

Hypersensitivity to the drug or procainamide
GI obstruction, bleeding, or perforation
History of seizures
Pheochromocytoma
Use of other drugs causing extrapyramidal symptoms

Adverse Reactions

CNS effects may occur
Confusion
Depression
Drowsiness
Cardiac conduction disturbances
Fatigue
Headache
Hypotension
Hypertension
Nausea
Insomnia
Tardive dyskinesia
Extrapyramidal signs or symptoms

Drug Interactions

Metoclopramide can increase the rate or extent of absorption of other drugs (acetaminophen, aspirin) because of accelerated gastric emptying.
Digoxin absorption and bioavailability may be diminished in some patients.

How Supplied

Tablet: 5, 10 mg
Oral solution: 5 mg/mL
Solution for injection: 5 mg/mL

Dosage and Administration

Nausea and Vomiting

Adults: 10 mg IV/IM, severe situations may require 0.5–2 mg/kg IV; may be repeated twice at 2-hour intervals. Consider reduced doses in pregnant patients and older adults.

Children >2 years and >26 pounds (12 kg): 0.1 mg/kg, or 2.5–5 mg IV; max 10 mg IV.

Special Considerations

Pregnancy safety: Category B
Use with caution in patients with renal disease, such as renal failure or renal impairment, owing to possible accumulation and toxicity.
Not recommended for patients with Parkinson disease.
Concurrent use of ethanol can increase the CNS depressant effects of metoclopramide.
Combined use of metoclopramide and other CNS depressants, such as anxiolytics, sedatives, and hypnotics, can increase possible sedation.
Use caution if patients are taking medications prone to causing tardive dyskinesia or extrapyramidal symptoms.

Metoprolol (Lopressor)

Class

Beta blocking agent

Description

Beta adrenergic blocking agents compete with beta-adrenergic agonists for available beta receptor sites on the membrane of cardiac muscle, bronchial smooth muscle, and the smooth muscle of blood vessels. The beta-1 blocking action on the heart decreases HR, conduction velocity, myocardial contractility, and cardiac output. Metoprolol is used to control ventricular response in supraventricular tachydysrhythmias (paroxysmal SVT, atrial fibrillation, atrial flutter). Metoprolol is considered a second-line agent after adenosine or diltiazem.

Onset and Duration

Onset: 1–2 minutes
Peak: 20 minutes
Duration: 6–8 hours[20]

Indications

All patients with suspected MI and unstable angina in the absence of contraindications (can reduce the incidence of VF)

Useful as an adjunctive agent with fibrinolytic therapy (may reduce nonfatal reinfarction and recurrent ischemia)
To convert to normal sinus rhythm or to slow ventricular response (or both) in supraventricular tachydysrhythmias (reentry SVT, atrial fibrillation, or atrial flutter)
To reduce myocardial ischemia in acute MI patients with elevated HR, BP, or both

Contraindications

Hypersensitivity
Hemodynamically unstable patient
Bradycardia
Second- or third-degree heart block
STEMI if signs of heart failure, low cardiac output, or increased risk for cardiogenic shock are present
Relative contraindication: PR interval >0.24 second
Reactive airway disease

Adverse Reactions

Bradycardia
AV conduction delays
Hypotension
Palpitations
Nausea and vomiting

Drug Interactions

Metoprolol may potentiate bradycardia or antihypertensive effects when given to patients taking calcium channel blockers or MAO inhibitors.
Catecholamine-depleting drugs may potentiate hypotension.
Sympathomimetic effects may be antagonized; signs of hypoglycemia may be masked.

How Supplied

Ampule: 1 mg/mL, 5 mg/5 mL

Dosage and Administration

Adult: 5 mg slow IV at 5-minute intervals to a total of 15 mg
Pediatric: Oral dosing only

Special Considerations

Pregnancy safety: Category C
Metoprolol must be given slowly IV over 5 minutes. Concurrent IV administration with IV calcium channel blockers such as verapamil or diltiazem can cause severe hypotension.
Metoprolol should be used with caution in people with liver or renal dysfunction.

Midazolam Hydrochloride (Versed)

Class

Short-acting benzodiazepine

Description

Midazolam hydrochloride is a water-soluble benzodiazepine that may be administered for conscious sedation to relieve apprehension or impair memory before tracheal intubation or cardioversion. The drug may also be used in the management of seizures in children.

Onset and Duration

Onset: IV: 1–3 minutes; dose dependent
Duration: 2–6 hours; dose dependent

Indications

Premedication for tracheal intubation, cardioversion, or other painful procedures
Seizures in children when other benzodiazepines are not effective

Contraindications

Hypersensitivity to midazolam
Glaucoma (relative)
Shock
Alcohol intoxication (relative; may be used for alcohol withdrawal)
Depressed vital signs
Concomitant use of barbiturates, alcohol, narcotics, or other CNS depressants (relative, midazolam is often given with analgesic agents for procedural sedation or similar purpose)

Adverse Reactions

Respiratory depression
Hiccups
Cough

Oversedation
Pain at the injection site
Nausea and vomiting
Headache
Blurred vision
Fluctuations in vital signs
Hypotension
Respiratory arrest

Drug Interactions

Sedative effect of midazolam may be accentuated by concomitant use of barbiturates, alcohol, or narcotics; therefore, the drug should not be used in patients who have taken CNS depressants unless for procedural sedation or similar purpose in a controlled setting.

How Supplied

2-, 5-, 10-mL vials (1 mg/mL)
1-, 2-, 5-, 10-mL vials (5 mg/mL)

Dosage and Administration

Adult:
- 0.1 mg/kg IV up to 10 mg. Consider starting with 1–2.5 mg by slow IV push in adults, as smaller doses are often effective in many situations, including older adults and patients taking CNS depressant medications or substances.
- 0.2 mg/kg (max dose 10 mg) IN or IM.

Children:
- 0.05–0.1 mg/kg per dose.
- May also be administered by IM, IN (off-label), or rectal routes (off-label).

Excited Delirium
- Adult: 5 mg IV/IM/IN.
- Pediatric: 0.05–0.1 mg/kg IV (max dose 5 mg); 0.1–0.15 mg/kg IM (max dose 5 mg); 0.3 mg/kg IN (max dose 5 mg).

End-of-Life (Palliative or Hospice) Care
- Adult: Severe respiratory distress: 2–5 mg IV.

Special Considerations

Pregnancy safety: Category D
Midazolam has been associated with respiratory depression and respiratory arrest when used for sedation. Its use requires continuous monitoring of respiratory and cardiac function. Emergency airway equipment should be readily available.

Morphine Sulfate (Astramorph PF and Others)

Class

Opioid analgesic

Description

Morphine sulfate is a natural opium alkaloid that has a primary effect of analgesia. It also increases peripheral venous capacitance and decreases venous return. Morphine sulfate causes euphoria and respiratory and CNS depression. Secondary pharmacologic effects of morphine include depressed responsiveness of alpha adrenergic receptors (producing peripheral vasodilation) and baroreceptor inhibition. In addition, because morphine decreases preload and afterload, it may decrease myocardial oxygen demand. The properties of this medication make it extremely useful in emergency care. Morphine sulfate is a Schedule II drug.

Onset and Duration

Onset: 5–10 minutes
Peak: 20 minutes
Duration: 4–5 hours[21]

Indications

Chest pain associated with ACS unresponsive to nitrates
Acute cardiogenic pulmonary edema (with adequate BP), with or without associated pain
Moderate to severe acute or chronic pain

Contraindications

Hypersensitivity to narcotics
Hypovolemia
Hypotension
Head injury
Increased intracranial pressure
Severe respiratory depression
Patients who have taken MAO inhibitors within 14 days
Use with caution in right ventricular infarction

Adverse Reactions

Respiratory depression
Hypotension in volume-depleted patients
Tachycardia

Bradycardia
Palpitations
Syncope
Facial flushing, diaphoresis, pruritus
Euphoria
Bronchospasm
Dry mouth
Allergic reaction

Drug Interactions

CNS depressants may potentiate effects of morphine (respiratory depression, hypotension, sedation).
Phenothiazines may potentiate analgesia.
MAO inhibitors may cause paradoxical excitation.

How Supplied

Morphine is supplied in tablets, suppositories, and solution. In emergency care, morphine sulfate usually is administered IV.
Parenteral preparations are available in many strengths. A common preparation is 2 mg, 4 mg, or 10 mg in 1 mL of solution, ampules, and Tubex syringes.

Dosage and Administration

Adult:
- STEMI: 2–4 mg IV; may give additional doses of 2–8 mg IV at 5- to 15-minute intervals
- Unstable angina/NSTEMI: 1–5 mg IV only if symptoms not relieved by nitrates or if symptoms recur (use with caution)
- Pain: 0.1 mg/kg IM (moderate pain) (max dose 15 mg) or IV or IO (severe pain) (max dose 10 mg)

Pediatric: 0.1–0.2 mg/kg dose IV (max total dose: 15 mg)

Special Considerations

Pregnancy safety: Category B (if not used for prolonged periods or in high doses at term); narcotics rapidly cross the placenta.
Safety in neonates has not been established.
Use with caution in older adults, in those with asthma, and in those susceptible to CNS depression. Morphine should be used with caution in chronic pain syndromes.
Morphine may worsen bradycardia or heart block in inferior MI (vagotonic effect).
Naloxone (0.4–2 mg IV) should be readily available.

Naloxone (Narcan)

Class

Opioid antagonist

Description

Naloxone is a competitive narcotic antagonist used in the management of known or suspected overdose caused by narcotics. Naloxone antagonizes all actions of morphine. It is the preferred first-line agent in suspected opioid overdose unresponsive to oxygen and support of ventilation.

Onset and Duration

Onset: Within 2 minutes
Duration: 30–120 minutes

Indications

For the complete or partial reversal of CNS and respiratory depression induced by opioids including the following:

Narcotic Agonists
- Morphine sulfate
- Heroin
- Hydromorphone
- Methadone
- Fentanyl citrate
- Oxycodone
- Codeine

Narcotic Agonists/Antagonists
- Butorphanol tartrate
- Buprenorphine/naloxone (Suboxone)
- Pentazocine
- Nalbuphine

Decreased Level of Consciousness Coma of Unknown Origin

Contraindications

Hypersensitivity
Use with caution in narcotic-dependent patients who may experience withdrawal syndrome (including neonates of narcotic-dependent mothers).
Avoid use in meperidine-induced seizures.

Adverse Reactions

Withdrawal (opiate)
Tachycardia

Hypertension
Dysrhythmias
Nausea and vomiting
Diaphoresis
Blurred vision

Drug Interactions

Incompatible with bisulfite and alkaline solutions

How Supplied

0.4 mg/mL (1, 10 mL); 1-mg/mL (2-mL) vials

Dosage and Administration

Adult:

Typical IV dose: 0.4 mg; titrate until ventilation is adequate. Use higher doses (up to 2 mg) for complete narcotic reversal. Can administer up to 6–10 mg over short period (<10 minutes).

For respiratory depression from sedation: Smaller doses of 0.4 mg repeated q 2–3 minutes may be used.

For chronic opioid-addicted patients: Use smaller doses and titrate slowly.

When IV access has not been established, consider IM, IN, or subcutaneous routes.

Pediatric:

Infants and children from birth to 5 years or 44 pounds (20 kg) of body weight: 0.1 mg/kg.

Children >5 years or >44 pounds (20 kg): 2 mg.

Doses may be repeated as needed to maintain opiate reversal.

Special Considerations

Pregnancy safety: Category C

Some research has demonstrated the efficacy of IN naloxone administration; however, the optimal dose for the IN route has not been established.

Seizures have been reported (no causal relationship has been established).

Naloxone may not reverse hypotension.

Exercise caution and use smaller doses when administering naloxone to narcotic addicts (may precipitate withdrawal with hypertension, tachycardia, and violent behavior).

Naloxone may make intubation, airway adjunct placement, or prolonged assisted-ventilation unnecessary. Administer naloxone and assess for response prior to attempting ET intubation in apneic patients with a suspected opioid overdose.

Rare anaphylactic reactions have been reported.

Nifedipine (Procardia, Adalat, Nifedical)

Class

Calcium channel blocker or calcium channel antagonist

Description

Nifedipine is a calcium channel blocker medication that is used as adjunctive therapy for high-altitude pulmonary edema (HAPE) when descent and supplemental oxygen are impossible or unavailable. Nifedipine relaxes cardiac and vascular smooth muscle tone. In the setting of HAPE, nifedipine decreases systemic vascular resistance, lowers BP, lowers pulmonary vascular resistance, and lowers pulmonary artery pressure.

Onset and Duration

Onset: 20–60 minutes[22]

Duration: Extended-release formulations are administered q 12 hours

Indications

HAPE

Used in other settings for management of hypertension, angina, or vasospasm

Contraindications

Hypersensitivity to nifedipine or other calcium channel blockers

Severe hypotension or cardiogenic shock

Adverse Reactions

Heart failure
Hypotension
Peripheral edema
Dizziness
Fatigue
Headache

Drug Interactions

Caution is warranted in patients receiving medications that affect cardiac contractility and/or sinoatrial or AV node conduction.

Efficacy is reduced when given to patients who take CYP3A4 inhibitors (eg, rifampin, rifabutin, phenobarbital, phenytoin, carbamazepine, St. John's wort).
Avoid simultaneous use of multiple medications that dilate pulmonary blood vessels.

How Supplied

Extended- or immediate-release oral preparations: 10 mg, 20 mg, 30 mg, 60 mg, 90 mg

Dosage and Administration

Adult HAPE: 30 mg extended-release PO q 12 hours.

Special Considerations

Pregnancy safety: Category C
Prompt descent and supplemental oxygen are the treatment priorities for HAPE.
Avoid simultaneous use of sildenafil or tadalafil with nifedipine.

Nitroglycerin (Nitrostat and Others)

Class

Vasodilator

Description

Nitrates and nitrites dilate arterioles and veins in the periphery (and coronary arteries in high doses). The resultant reduction in preload, and to a lesser extent in afterload, decreases the workload of the heart and lowers myocardial oxygen demand. Nitroglycerin can be administered by sublingual, topical, and IV routes.

Onset and Duration

Onset: 1–3 minutes
Duration: IV: 3–5 minutes; Sublingual: Approximately 25 minutes

Indications

Ischemic chest pain
Heart failure
Acute MI (large anterior wall infarction, persistent or recurrent ischemia, hypertension)
Hypertensive emergencies with ACS
As local vasodilator as treatment for extravasation of vasopressor medications

Contraindications

Volume depletion
Hypersensitivity
Hypotension (SBP <90 mm Hg or ≥ 30 mm Hg below baseline)
Head injury
Extreme bradycardia (HR <50 beats/min)
Extreme tachycardia (HR >100 beats/min) in the absence of heart failure
Right ventricular infarction
Cerebral hemorrhage
Recent use of tadalafil (Cialis), vardenafil (Levitra), or sildenafil (Viagra)
Aortic stenosis

Adverse Reactions

Transient headache
Reflex tachycardia
Hypotension
Nausea and vomiting
Postural syncope
Diaphoresis
Flushing

Drug Interactions

Other vasodilators may have additive hypotensive effects. Do not mix with other drugs.

How Supplied

Tablets: 0.15 mg (1/400 gr), 0.3 mg (1/200 gr), 0.4 mg (1/150 gr), 0.6 (1/100 gr), and extended-release capsules and transdermal preparations
Metered spray: 0.4 mg per spray (do not shake)
Parenteral: 5 mg/mL; 10, 20, 40 mg/100 mL

Dosage and Administration

Adult:

Tablet: 0.4 mg sublingually; may repeat for a total of 3 doses at 3- to 5-minute intervals.
Metered spray: 1–2 sprays (0.4 mg/dose) for 0.5–1 second at 5-minute intervals; max 5 sprays within 15 minutes if SBP remains >100 mm Hg.

Pulmonary edema: In severe distress, consider 0.8 mg (2 tabs) if SBP >160 mm Hg or 1.2 mg (3 tabs) if SBP >200 mm Hg q 5 minutes.
Infusion: Begin at a rate of 10 mcg/min; increase by 10 mcg/min q 3–5 minutes until desired effect is achieved; ceiling dose of 200 mcg/min is commonly used.
Pediatric (continuous infusion): Initial dose 0.25–0.5 mcg/kg per minute; titrate by 1 mcg/kg at least q 15–20 minutes; typical dose range: 1–5 mcg/kg per minute. Max 20 mcg/kg per minute.[23]

Special Considerations

Pregnancy safety: Category C
Nitroglycerin is associated with increased susceptibility to hypotension in older adults.
Nitroglycerin decomposes when exposed to light or heat. Must be kept in airtight containers.
The active ingredient of nitroglycerin will "sting" when administered sublingually.
Use with caution in patients with inferior acute MI with possible right ventricular involvement.[24]
Administer IV nitroglycerin by infusion pump to ensure precise flow rate.
Polyvinyl chloride (PVC) tubing may absorb up to 80% of available drug; non-PVC tubing should be used.

Nitrous Oxide/Oxygen (50:50) (Nitronox)

Class

Gaseous analgesic/anesthetic

Description

Nitrous oxide/oxygen is a blended mixture of 50% nitrous oxide and 50% oxygen. When inhaled, nitrous oxide/oxygen depresses the CNS, causing analgesia without the need for full anesthesia. It is theorized that nitrous oxide activates endogenous opioid function, producing analgesia. In addition, the high concentration of oxygen delivered along with the nitrous oxide increases oxygen tension in the blood, thereby reducing hypoxia.[25] Nitrous oxide/oxygen is self-administered.

Onset and Duration

Onset: 2–5 minutes
Duration: 2–5 minutes

Indications

Moderate to severe pain
Anxiety
Apprehension

Contraindications

Impaired level of consciousness
Head injury
Chest trauma (pneumothorax)
Inability to comply with instructions
Decompression sickness (nitrogen narcosis, air embolus, air transport)
Undiagnosed abdominal pain or marked distention
Bowel obstruction
Hypotension
Shock
Chronic obstructive pulmonary disease (with history or suspicion of carbon dioxide retention)

Adverse Reactions

Dizziness
Apnea
Cyanosis
Nausea and vomiting
Malignant hyperthermia (rare but dangerous)

Drug Interactions

None significant

How Supplied

D and E cylinders (blue and white in Canada, blue and green in United States) of 50% nitrous oxide and 50% oxygen compressed gas

Dosage and Administration

Adult: Invert cylinder several times before use; instruct the patient to inhale deeply through a patient-held mask or mouthpiece.
Pediatric: Same as adult.

Special Considerations

Pregnancy safety: Nitrous oxide has been shown to increase the incidence of spontaneous abortion.
Nitrous oxide is 34 times more soluble than nitrogen is and will diffuse into pockets of trapped gas in the patient (intestinal obstruction, pneumothorax, blocked middle ear).

As the nitrogen leaves and is replaced by larger amounts of nitrous oxide, increased pressures or volumes may cause serious damage—for example, intestinal rupture.
Nitrous oxide is a nonexplosive gas.
Patient must hold mask and self-administer.

> NOTE
> When delivering nitrous oxide and oxygen from a single tank, the paramedic must ensure that enough oxygen remains in the tank to provide adequate oxygenation. Inverting the cylinder several times to mix the gases is important for this reason. Monitoring of oximetry during administration of nitrous oxide also is reasonable.

Norepinephrine (Levophed)

Class

Sympathomimetic

Description

Norepinephrine is an alpha and beta-1 adrenergic agonist. It is a potent vasoconstrictor that also increases myocardial contractility. Because this drug tends to constrict the renal and mesenteric blood vessels, it rarely is used in the prehospital setting. It is administered as a continuous infusion in many critical care environments for hypotension and shock states not caused by hypovolemia.

Onset and Duration

Onset: 1–3 minutes
Duration: 5–10 minutes

Indications

Severe cardiogenic shock
Neurogenic shock
Inotropic support
Hemodynamically significant hypotension (SBP <70 mm Hg) with low total peripheral resistance refractory to other sympathomimetic amines

Contraindications

Hypersensitivity
Hypotensive patients with hypovolemia

Adverse Reactions

Headache
Dysrhythmias
Tachycardia
Reflex bradycardia
Angina pectoris
Hypertension

Drug Interactions

Norepinephrine can be deactivated by alkaline solutions. Alkaline solutions may deactivate the drug when infused in the same IV line.
MAO inhibitors and bretylium may potentiate the effects of catecholamines.
Beta adrenergic antagonists may blunt inotropic response.
Sympathomimetics and phosphodiesterase inhibitors may exacerbate dysrhythmia response.
This drug is a vesicant that can cause severe tissue damage if extravasation occurs.

How Supplied

1 mg/mL, 4-mL ampule

Dosage and Administration

Adult: Dilute 4 mg in 250 mL of D_5W or D_5NS (16 mcg/mL); begin infusion at 0.05–0.5 mcg/kg per minute (up to 30 mcg/min) titrated to desired effect (average adult dose is 7–35 mcg/min). Many settings begin infusions at 2–4 mcg/min and titrate upward to a max of 30 mcg/min. Poison- or drug-induced hypotension may require higher doses to achieve adequate perfusion.
Pediatric: Begin at 0.05–0.1 mcg/kg per minute IV/IO; adjust infusion rate to achieve desired change in BP and systemic perfusion. Max dose is 2 mcg/kg per minute.

Special Considerations

Pregnancy safety: Category C. Norepinephrine may cause fetal anoxia when used in pregnancy.
Infuse norepinephrine through a large, stable vein to avoid extravasation and tissue necrosis.
Use an infusion pump to ensure precise flow rate.
Do not administer in the same IV line as alkaline solutions.
May induce dysrhythmias.

Olanzapine (Zyprexa)

Class

Antipsychotic

Description

Olanzapine is an atypical antipsychotic medication that antagonizes certain serotonin, alpha adrenergic, histamine, dopamine, and other receptors. This receptor antagonism improves symptoms in patients with schizophrenia and bipolar disorder. Olanzapine can be administered IM to EMS patients experiencing a behavioral emergency. Simultaneous administration of olanzapine and benzodiazepine medications is discouraged.

Onset and Duration

Onset: 15–45 minutes
Duration: 2–4 hours

Indications

Severe agitation
Schizophrenia or bipolar disorder

Contraindications

Hypersensitivity

Adverse Reactions

Hypertension
Hypotension
Prolonged QT interval
Sedation
Delirium
Extrapyramidal symptoms

Drug Interactions

Increased effects of CNS depressant medications including opioids and ethyl alcohol.
Increase risk for QT prolongation when combined with other medications that prolong the QT interval.

How Supplied

IM: 10 mg and other longer-acting formulations
Oral: 2.5 mg, 5 mg, 10 mg, 15 mg, 20 mg

Dosage and Administration

Adult: 10 mg IM
Pediatric:
- 6–11 years: 5 mg IM
- 12–18 years: 10 mg IM

Special Considerations

Pregnancy safety: Category C
Use extreme caution when attempting to administer an IM injection to an agitated or combative patient.
Severe sedation may occur when administered to a patient taking benzodiazepines.

Ondansetron (Zofran, Zuplenz)

Class

Antiemetic

Description

Ondansetron is an oral and parenteral antiemetic agent. It was the first selective serotonin-blocking agent to be marketed. The primary use of the drug is to manage nausea and vomiting in postoperative patients and in those undergoing chemotherapy. Ondansetron preferentially blocks the serotonin 5-HT_3 receptors; these receptors are found centrally in the chemoreceptor trigger zone and peripherally at vagal nerve terminals in the intestines. Ondansetron can be administered PO, IV, and IM and with an orally disintegrating tablet (ODT).

Onset and Duration

Onset: Within 30 minutes
Duration: 3–6 hours

Indications

Nausea
Vomiting

Contraindications

Hypersensitivity to the drug
Administration with apomorphine
Liver disease
GI obstruction
Prolonged QT syndrome

Adverse Reactions

Generally well tolerated
ECG irregularities (rare)
Hiccups

Pruritus
Flushing
Chills
Headache
Dizziness
Drowsiness
Extrapyramidal symptoms
Shivering
Hypoxia

Drug Interactions

None significant in emergency care

How Supplied

Tablet: 4, 8, 24 mg
Dissolving film and tablets: 4, 8 mg
Oral solution: 4 mg/5 mL
Solution for injection: 2 mg/mL

Dosage and Administration

Adult:

IV: Up to 4 mg may be given undiluted; inject over 30 seconds (2–5 minutes preferred); up to 16 mg max IV for emetogenic chemotherapy vomiting.

Infusion (available in a premix or dilute dose in 50 mL of D_5W): Infuse over 15 minutes.

IM: 4 mg, single injection in well-developed muscle.

Oral film and tablets: 4 mg (up to 16 mg) PO for postoperative nausea and vomiting.

Pediatric (>6 months to 14 years): 0.15 mg/kg per dose IV or PO, up to 4 mg max.

Special Considerations

Pregnancy safety: Category B
The use of ondansetron may mask the symptoms of adynamic ileus, GI obstruction, or gastric distention after abdominal surgery.
Tablets should be gently removed from the foil, not pushed through the package.
Allow ODT to dissolve on tongue with saliva.
Caution: May prolong QT interval.

Oxytocin (Pitocin)

Class

Pituitary hormone

Description

Oxytocin is a synthetic hormone named for the natural posterior pituitary hormone. It stimulates uterine smooth muscle contractions and helps expedite the normal contractions of a spontaneous labor. As with all significant uterine contractions, a transient reduction in uterine blood flow occurs. Oxytocin also stimulates the mammary glands to increase lactation, without increasing the production of milk. The drug is administered in the prehospital setting to control postpartum bleeding.

Onset and Duration

Onset: IV: Immediate; IM: Within 3–5 minutes
Duration: IV: 20 minutes after the infusion is stopped; IM: 30–60 minutes

Indications

Postpartum hemorrhage after infant and placental delivery

Contraindications

Hypertonic or hyperactive uterus
Presence of a second fetus
Fetal distress

Adverse Reactions

Hypotension
Tachycardia
Hypertension
Dysrhythmias
Angina pectoris
Anxiety
Seizure
Nausea and vomiting
Allergic reaction
Uterine rupture (from excessive administration)

Drug Interactions

Vasopressors may potentiate hypertension

How Supplied

10 USP units/1-mL ampule (10 units/mL) and prefilled syringe
5 USP units/1-mL ampule (5 units/mL) and prefilled syringe

Dosage and Administration

Control of Postpartum Hemorrhage

IM: 3–10 units IM following delivery of placenta

Bleeding Following Incomplete or Elective Abortion

IV: Mix 10–40 units (1–4 mL) in 1,000 mL of NS or lactated Ringer solution; infuse at 10–40 milliunits/min via microdrip tubing, titrated to severity of bleeding and uterine response

Special Considerations

Pregnancy safety: Category X

Vital signs and uterine tone should be monitored closely.

Oxytocin should be administered only in the prehospital setting after delivery of all fetuses.

Potassium Iodide (Thyrosafe, Thyroshield, SSKI)

Class

Antidote; antithyroid agent

Description

Potassium iodide performs the novel function of protecting the thyroid gland from uptake of radioactive iodine, protecting against the development of thyroid cancer. The thyroid gland is the only part of the body that absorbs and concentrates iodine. The concentration of iodine in the thyroid can be many times the circulating serum concentration. Potassium iodide is administered to block or limit thyroid update of radioactive isotopes of iodine, particularly in the setting of nuclear radiation exposure. It also functions as an expectorant (promotes ejection of mucus) and is used in other thyroid conditions and procedures.

Onset and Duration

Onset: Gradual over 24 hours

Duration: 24 hours in radiation exposures, longer during other treatment regimens[26]

Indications

Exposure to radioactive material

Contraindications

Hypersensitivity to iodine
Hyperkalemia
Hyperthyroidism
Respiratory failure

Adverse Reactions

Diarrhea
Nausea and vomiting
Hypothyroidism
Confusion

Drug Interactions

Monitor for increased potassium in patients taking potassium-sparing diuretics, ACE inhibitors, potassium supplements, and other medications known to increase potassium.

How Supplied

Solution: 1 g/mL, 65 mg/mL
Tablet: 130 mg, 65 mg

Dosage and Administration

Radiation Exposure

Adults: 130 mg PO

Pediatric:

Birth to 1 month: 16 mg PO
1 month to 3 years: 32 mg PO
3–18 years: 65 mg PO

Special Considerations

Pregnancy safety: Category D

Pralidoxime (2-PAM, Protopam)

Class

Cholinesterase reactivator and antidote

Description

Pralidoxime reactivates the enzyme acetylcholinesterase, which allows acetylcholine to be degraded, thus relieving the parasympathetic overstimulation caused by excess acetylcholine. This drug is sometimes combined with atropine in an autoinjector such as the Mark 1 or DuoDote autoinjector kit.

Onset and Duration

Onset: Within minutes
Duration: Variable

Indications

Organophosphate poisoning (after atropine)

Contraindications

Hypersensitivity to pralidoxime

Adverse Reactions

Tachycardia
Hypertension
Laryngospasm
Hyperventilation
Muscle weakness
Nausea

Drug Interactions

Pralidoxime should not be mixed in the same syringe or solution with any other drug.

How Supplied

Emergency single-dose kit containing a 20-mL vial of 1 g of the sterile drug, a 20-mL ampule of sterile diluent, and a 20-mL syringe with needle.

Dosage and Administration

Adult: 600 mg IM (usually by autoinjector) q 15 minutes for up to 3 doses, or 1–2 g IV over 15–30 minutes. See Chapter 57, *Bioterrorism and Weapons of Mass Destruction*, for detailed dosing information.
Pediatric: 20–50 mg/kg IV over 15–30 minutes

Special Considerations

Pregnancy safety: Category C
Each 1 g of sterile powder is diluted with 20 mL of sterile water for injection.
Pralidoxime should be diluted further in 100 mL of NS and given as an IV infusion. Use promptly after reconstitution.
Medical direction may recommend the almost simultaneous administration of atropine.
Pralidoxime is not recommended in carbamate poisoning.
Reduce the dosage in cases of known renal insufficiency.

Procainamide (Pronestyl, Procan SR)

Class

Antidysrhythmic (Class IA)

Description

Procainamide suppresses phase 4 depolarization in normal ventricular muscle and Purkinje fibers, reducing the automaticity of ectopic pacemakers. It also suppresses reentry dysrhythmias by slowing intraventricular conduction. Procainamide may be effective in treating premature ventricular contractions and recurrent VT that cannot be controlled with lidocaine.

Onset and Duration

Onset: 10–30 minutes
Peak: 25–60 minutes
Duration: 3–4 hours

Indications

Numerous dysrhythmias, including stable monomorphic VT with normal QT interval and preserved left ventricular function
Reentry SVT uncontrolled by adenosine and vagal maneuvers if normotensive
Stable wide-complex tachycardia of unknown origin
Atrial fibrillation with rapid ventricular response in WPW syndrome

Contraindications

Hypersensitivity
Second- and third-degree AV block (without functioning artificial pacemaker)
Digitalis toxicity
Torsades de pointes
Systemic lupus erythematosus
Tricyclic antidepressant toxicity
QT prolongation (relative)

Adverse Reactions

Hypotension in patients with impaired left ventricular function
Bradycardia
Reflex tachycardia
AV block
Widened QRS complex
Prolonged PR or QT interval
Premature ventricular contractions
VT, VF, asystole
CNS depression
Confusion
Seizure

Drug Interactions

Increases effects of skeletal muscle relaxants.
Increases plasma/*N*-acetylprocainamide (active metabolites) concentrations with cimetidine, ranitidine, beta blockers, amiodarone, trimethoprim, and quinidine.
Use with caution with other drugs that prolong the QT interval (eg, amiodarone).

How Supplied

1 g in 10-mL vial (100 mg/mL)
1 g in 2-mL vials (500 mg/mL) for infusion

Dosage and Administration

Adult:
20 mg/min IV infusion until one of the following occurs: dysrhythmia resolves, hypotension, QRS widens by >50% of original width, total dose of 17 mg/kg.
Maintenance: Infusion (after resuscitation from cardiac arrest): mix 1 g in 250 mL of solution in D_5W or NS (4 mg/mL), infuse at 1–4 mg/min.
Pediatric: Loading dose 15 mg/kg IV/IO; infuse over 30–60 minutes.

Special Considerations

Pregnancy safety: Category C
Procainamide has potent vasodilating and negative inotropic effects.
Rapid injection may cause procainamide-induced hypotension.
Monitor vital signs and ECG (a small amount of QRS complex widening is expected). Reduce dose in patients with cardiac or renal dysfunction to max total dose of 12 mg/kg and maintenance infusion to 1–2 mg/min.
Administer cautiously to patients with asthma, digitalis-induced dysrhythmias, acute MI, or cardiac, hepatic, or renal insufficiency.

NOTE
Discontinue if the dysrhythmia is suppressed, hypotension develops, the QRS complex is widened by 50% of its original width, or a total of 1 g has been administered.

Prochlorperazine (Compazine)

Class

Phenothiazine, antiemetic, antipsychotic

Description

Prochlorperazine blocks postsynaptic dopamine receptors in the chemoreceptor trigger zone of the brain and also blocks release of various hormones, including those that induce emesis. Prochlorperazine has antipsychotic properties but is primarily used as an antiemetic agent; it is particularly useful treating migraine and other types of headaches.[27,28]

Onset and Duration

Onset: IV: Rapid
Peak: 10–30 minutes
Duration: 3–4 hours

Indications

Nausea and vomiting
Motion sickness
Headaches
Anxiety

Contraindications

Hypersensitivity (to prochlorperazine or other phenothiazines)
Comatose states
CNS depression from alcohol, barbiturates, or narcotics
Signs associated with Reye syndrome

Adverse Reactions

Sedation
Dizziness
May impair mental and physical ability
Allergic reactions
Dysrhythmias
Nausea and vomiting
Hyperexcitability
Dystonias

Drug Interactions

Concomitant use of CNS depressants may have an additive sedative effect.
Numerous medication interactions that increase effects of prochlorperazine or where prochlorperazine

increases effect of other medications. Use with caution when considering administration to patients taking higher-risk medications.

How Supplied

5 mg/mL in 2-mL vials; 25-mg rectal suppositories; 5-mg and 10-mg tablets

Dosage and Administration

Adult: 5–10 mg IV/IM; standard dose is 10 mg IV
Pediatric (>2 years and >26 pounds [12 kg]): 0.1 mg/kg slow IV or deep IM

Special Considerations

Pregnancy safety: Category C
Administer by slow IV push (<5 mg/min) or by intermittent IV infusion. Rapid infusion may cause hypotension.
Monitor HR, BP, and patient's level of consciousness during and after administration.
May cause akathisia (restlessness) and extrapyramidal effects; have diphenhydramine available for treatment if needed.

Promethazine (Phenergan)

Class

Phenothiazine, antihistamine

Description

Promethazine is an H_1 receptor antagonist that blocks the actions of histamine by competitive antagonism at the H_1 receptor. In addition to antihistaminic effects, promethazine possesses sedative, antiemetic, and considerable anticholinergic activity. Promethazine often is administered with analgesics, particularly narcotics, to potentiate their effects, although the occurrence of potentiation is controversial.

Onset and Duration

Onset: IV: Rapid
Duration: 4–12 hours

Indications

Nausea and vomiting
Motion sickness
Preoperative and postoperative, obstetric (during labor) sedation
To potentiate the effects of analgesics
Allergic reactions

Contraindications

Hypersensitivity
Comatose states
CNS depression from alcohol, barbiturates, or narcotics

Adverse Reactions

Sedation
Dizziness
May impair mental and physical ability
Allergic reactions
Dysrhythmias
Nausea and vomiting
Hyperexcitability
Dystonias
Extravasation may cause massive local tissue injury
Use in children may cause hallucinations, convulsions, and sudden death

Drug Interactions

Concomitant use of CNS depressants may have an additive sedative effect.
Increased incidence of extrapyramidal or anticholinergic effects occurs when given with other phenothiazines, anticholinergic medications, and MAO inhibitors.

How Supplied

25, 50 mg/mL in 1-mL ampules and Tubex syringes
12.5-, 25-, and 50-mg suppositories
12.5- and 50-mg tablets

Dosage and Administration

Adult: 12.5–25 mg IV (dilute in 9 mL of NS and give 25 mg or less over 10–15 minutes) or deep IM (undiluted)
Pediatric (>2 years): Use with extreme caution; 0.25 to 1 mg/kg per dose (max dose 25 mg)

Special Considerations

Pregnancy safety: Category C. Generally considered safe for use during labor.

Use caution in patients with asthma, peptic ulcer, and bone marrow depression.
Take care to avoid accidental intra-arterial injection. Deep IM injections are the preferred route of administration.
Dilute into >10 mL NS and give slow IV administration over 1 minute or longer through a running IV line while monitoring carefully for signs of infiltration. Avoid veins in the hands or wrists.

Reteplase (Retavase)

Class

Fibrinolytic

Description

Reteplase is a recombinant plasminogen activator. Fibrinolytic action occurs by generating plasmin from plasminogen. Plasmin degrades the fibrin matrix of a thrombus. The drug is used in the management of acute MI in adults, for the improvement of ventricular function following acute MI, and for a reduction in the incidence of heart failure. Treatment with reteplase should be initiated as soon as possible after the onset of acute MI symptoms.

Onset and Duration

Onset: Causes reperfusion within 90 minutes for most patients
Duration: Variable

Indications

Management of acute MI in adults (must be confirmed with 12-lead ECG)

Contraindications

Active internal bleeding
History of stroke
Recent intracranial or intraspinal surgery or trauma
Intracranial neoplasm, AV malformation, or aneurysm
Bleeding disorders
Severe uncontrolled hypertension

Adverse Reactions

Bleeding (internal and at superficial sites)
Reperfusion dysrhythmias
Allergic reaction (rare)
Nausea and vomiting
Hypotension

Drug Interactions

Risk of bleeding will be increased if used concurrently with drugs that alter platelet function.
Risk of bleeding with concomitant use of heparin or vitamin K antagonist (eg, warfarin) is greatly increased.
Reteplase is incompatible with heparin; do not administer in the same IV line.

How Supplied

Supplied in kit with components for reconstitution: single-use reteplase vials (10.8 units each), single-use diluent vials of sterile water (10 mL each), sterile 10-mL syringes with 20-gauge needles, sterile dispensing pins, sterile 20-gauge needles for administration, and alcohol swabs. Reconstitute by withdrawing 10 mL of diluent; open the package containing the dispensing pin; remove the needle from the syringe and discard the needle; remove the connective cap from the dispensing pin and connect the syringe to the pin; remove the flip cap from one vial of reteplase; remove the protective cap from the spike end of the dispensing pin and insert the spike into the vial of reteplase; transfer the diluent through the dispensing pin into the vial of reteplase; with the dispensing pin and syringe still attached, swirl (do not shake) the vial gently to dissolve the reteplase; withdraw 10 mL of the reconstituted solution back into the syringe; detach the syringe from the dispensing pin; and attach a sterile 20-gauge needle. The 10-mL bolus dose is now ready to administer.

Dosage and Administration

Adult: Administer 10 units as IV bolus over 2 minutes; administer a second 10-unit IV bolus in 30 minutes. (Give NS flush before and after each bolus.) Heparin and aspirin should be administered concomitantly.
Pediatric: Safety not established.

Special Considerations

Pregnancy safety: Category C

Reteplase should be given in an IV line in which no other medication is being injected or infused simultaneously.
Protect the contents of the package from light.

Rocuronium (Zemuron)

Class

Nondepolarizing neuromuscular blocker

Description

Rocuronium competitively blocks acetylcholine at the neuromuscular junction, resulting in chemical paralysis. An increased initial dose of rocuronium causes a rapid onset of chemical paralysis, similar to that produced by succinylcholine. Rocuronium has a much longer duration of action than does succinylcholine but has fewer problematic side effects in many patient situations. Providers may use rocuronium in EMS systems that perform rapid-sequence induction or may use rocuronium for ongoing chemical paralysis of mechanically ventilated patients during interfacility transports. See "Special Considerations" for important information about overall patient care for patients receiving rocuronium

Onset and Duration

Onset: 1 minute
Peak: 4 minutes
Duration: 26–40 minutes[29]

Indications

Chemical paralysis for airway placement
Ongoing chemical paralysis for mechanically ventilated patients

Contraindications

Hypersensitivity
Consider risk versus benefit in patients with anticipated difficult/failed airways, chronic neuromuscular conditions such as myasthenia gravis, and in situations where neuromuscular blockade will prevent accurate clinical assessment or monitoring (eg, status epilepticus, head injury, severe stroke)

Adverse Reactions

Apnea
Tachycardia (assess for inadequate sedation or analgesia)
Hypertension (assess for inadequate sedation or analgesia)
Anaphylaxis
Dysrhythmias

Drug Interactions

Numerous medications have the potential to increase serum rocuronium levels, resulting in longer duration of action. Rocuronium may increase the effects of systemic corticosteroid and cardiac glycoside medications.

How Supplied

10 mg/mL solution 5-mL and 10-mL vials

Dosage and Administration

Adult: 0.6–1.2 mg/kg IV; often ordered as 1 mg/kg initially, then 0.5 mg/kg for subsequent doses.
Pediatric: Considered off-label for rapid-sequence induction despite numerous successful studies. 0.9–1.2 mg/kg; often ordered as 1 mg/kg (max 100 mg), then 0.5 mg/kg for subsequent doses.

Special Considerations

Pregnancy safety: Category C
Use only in settings where trained personnel and equipment for emergency airway management are immediately available.
Rocuronium has no sedative or analgesic properties, despite the patient appearing flaccid and unresponsive. Ongoing adjunctive analgesia and sedative medications are essential for patients receiving rocuronium. Rocuronium has a longer duration of action than do many sedative and opioid medications (particularly in hypermetabolic states and critically ill pediatric patients), potentially resulting in awake patients with intact awareness and sensation, without the ability to move or communicate.

Sildenafil (Viagra, Revatio)

Class

Phosphodiesterase-5 enzyme (PDE-5) inhibitor

Description

Sildenafil and other PDE-5 inhibitors increase local concentrations of cyclic guanosine monophosphate, which in turn causes vasodilation. This class of medications is prescribed for treatment of pulmonary artery hypertension and erectile dysfunction. In each of these conditions, symptoms are improved with smooth muscle relaxation, vasodilation, and improved blood flow. Sildenafil is available in oral and IV preparations. It is indicated for the prevention of HAPE[30] and may also be used for treatment of HAPE when neither oxygen nor descent is available as an option.

Onset and Duration

Onset: 60 minutes
Duration: Up to 8 hours

Indications

Pulmonary artery hypertension
Erectile dysfunction
HAPE prophylaxis

Contraindications

Hypersensitivity
Concurrent use of organic nitrate medications (nitroglycerin, isosorbide, "poppers")
Severe hepatic impairment
Recent history of stroke or MI

Adverse Reactions

Flushing
Dizziness
Headache
Visual disturbances

Drug Interactions

Avoid use with other PDE-5 inhibitors, alprostadil, amyl nitrite, and other vasodilators.
Numerous medications cause increased levels of effects from sildenafil.

How Supplied

10-mg/12.5 mL IV solution
10-mg/mL oral suspension
20-, 25-, 50-, and 100-mg oral tablets

Dosage and Administration

Adult (HAPE): 20 mg PO q 8 hours

Special Considerations

Pregnancy safety: Category B
Avoid use of sildenafil in patients taking nitrate medication or other vasodilator medications. Avoid vasodilator medications and nitroglycerin in patients taking sildenafil in the past 48 hours.

Sodium Bicarbonate

Class

Buffer, alkalinizing agent, electrolyte supplement

Description

Sodium bicarbonate reacts with hydrogen ions to form water and carbon dioxide, thereby buffering metabolic acidosis. As the plasma hydrogen ion concentration decreases, blood pH rises.

Onset and Duration

Onset: Rapid
Duration: 8–10 minutes

Indications

Tricyclic antidepressant overdose
Known preexisting hyperkalemia
Known preexisting bicarbonate-responsive acidosis
Alkalinization for treatment of specific intoxications/rhabdomyolysis
Management of metabolic acidosis
Diabetic ketoacidosis

Contraindications

Not effective in hypercarbic acidosis (eg, cardiac arrest and CPR without intubation)
Chloride loss from vomiting and GI suction
Alkalosis
Severe pulmonary edema
Abdominal pain of unknown origin
Hypocalcemia
Hypokalemia
Hypernatremia
When administration of sodium could be detrimental
Hypersensitivity

Adverse Reactions

Metabolic alkalosis
Hypoxia
Rise in intracellular partial pressure of carbon dioxide and increased tissue acidosis
Electrolyte imbalance (hypernatremia)
Heart failure exacerbations
Seizures
Tissue sloughing at injection site

Drug Interactions

Sodium bicarbonate may precipitate in calcium solutions.
Alkalinization of urine may shorten elimination half-lives of certain drugs.
Vasopressors may be deactivated.

How Supplied

50 mEq in 50 mL; 0.5, 0.6 mEq/mL

Dosage and Administration

Urgent Forms of Metabolic Acidosis/Severe Hyperkalemia
Adult: 1 mEq/kg IV
Pediatric:1 mEq/kg IV; infuse slowly and only if ventilations are adequate

Special Considerations

Pregnancy safety: Category C
Not recommended for routine use in patients with cardiac arrest.
When possible, blood gas analysis should guide bicarbonate administration.
Bicarbonate administration produces carbon dioxide, which crosses cell membranes more rapidly than does bicarbonate (potentially worsening intracellular acidosis).
Sodium bicarbonate may increase edematous or sodium-retaining states.
Sodium bicarbonate may worsen heart failure.
Maintain adequate ventilation (gas exchange).

Sodium Nitrite

Class

Antidote; vasodilator

Description

Sodium nitrate is the second step in an older approach to the management of cyanide poisoning. When administered, sodium nitrite typically follows inhalation of amyl nitrite, and is given as soon as IV access can be established. Sodium nitrite is contraindicated when there is concurrent or suspected carbon monoxide toxicity, as it may worsen tissue hypoxia with potentially lethal consequences. Sodium nitrite is significantly more effective than amyl nitrite is and also induces the condition in the blood known as methemoglobinemia, which in turn leads to binding with cyanide molecules, creating a less-toxic substance called cyanomethemoglobin.[5] Sodium nitrite has the additional beneficial effect of causing vasodilation, which improves hepatic (liver) circulation and promotes cyanide metabolism.

Onset and Duration

Onset: Rapid
Peak: 30–70 minutes[31]

Indications

Cyanide poisoning

Contraindications

Concurrent carbon monoxide exposure
Known methemoglobinemia (>40%)
Hypotension (relative)
Not generally used for cyanide poisoning when hydroxocobalamin is readily available

Adverse Reactions

Hypotension
Methemoglobinemia
Flushing
Dizziness
Nausea and vomiting

Drug Interactions

Methylene blue may reverse methemoglobinemia.

How Supplied

300 mg/10 mL IV solution

Dosage and Administration

Adults: 300 mg IV over 3–5 minutes
Pediatric: 0.15–0.33 mL/kg of 3% solution, diluted in 50–110 mL NS and given over 5 minutes

Special Considerations

Pregnancy safety: No FDA category established. Sodium nitrite may cause harmful effects on the fetus, but this may be outweighed by the potential benefits of a successful maternal resuscitation.

This is no longer the preferred treatment for toxic cyanide exposures.[5]

Sodium Thiosulfate

Class

Antidote

Description

Sodium thiosulfate is the third step in an older approach to the management of cyanide poisoning. When administered, sodium thiosulfate typically follows inhalation of amyl nitrite and IV administration of sodium nitrite. Sodium thiosulfate "donates" sulfur molecules and promotes conversion of cyanide to thiocyanate, a much less harmful substance.[32] Sodium thiosulfate can be administered to supplement the effects of hydroxocobalamin (preferred agent) or administered as part of the regimen with amyl nitrite and sodium nitrite (less desirable approach).

Onset and Duration

Onset: Rapid
Peak: 30–70 minutes[31]

Indications

Cyanide poisoning

Contraindications

Hypersensitivity

Adverse Reactions

Burning sensation during administration
Nausea and vomiting
Muscle cramping

Drug Interactions

None significant

How Supplied

10% 10-mL and 25% 50-mL IV solutions

Dosage and Administration

Adult: 12.5 g IV over 30 minutes
Pediatric: 0.5 g/kg of 25% solution (2 mL/kg) over 30 minutes

Special Considerations

Pregnancy safety: Category C

This is no longer the preferred treatment for toxic cyanide exposures.[5]

Succinylcholine (Anectine)

Class

Neuromuscular blocker (depolarizing)

Description

Succinylcholine has the quickest onset and briefest duration of action of all neuromuscular-blocking drugs. This rapid onset and short duration are desirable in many situations. Unfortunately, succinylcholine may exacerbate certain clinical conditions, making it inferior to nondepolarizing muscle relaxers in patients with these conditions (see "Contraindications"). Like nondepolarizing blockers, depolarizing drugs bind to the receptors for acetylcholine. However, because they cause depolarization of the muscle membrane, they often lead to fasciculations and some muscular contractions.

Onset and Duration

Onset: <1 minute
Duration: 5–10 minutes after single IV dose

Indications

To facilitate intubation
Terminating laryngospasm
Muscle relaxation

Contraindications

Burns or crush injuries >72 hours old
Hypersensitivity
Skeletal muscle myopathies (eg, muscular dystrophy)
Inability to control the airway and/or support ventilations with oxygen and positive pressure
Personal or family history of malignant hyperthermia
Acute rhabdomyolysis

Adverse Reactions

Hypotension
Respiratory depression
Bradycardias
Dysrhythmias
Initial muscle fasciculation
Excessive salivation
Malignant hyperthermia
Allergic reaction
Succinylcholine may exacerbate hyperkalemia in trauma patients (hours after trauma).

Drug Interactions

Oxytocin, beta blockers, chronic contraceptive use, and organophosphates may potentiate effects.
Diazepam may reduce duration of action.
Cardiac glycosides may induce dysrhythmias.

How Supplied

20, 100 mg/mL; 1-g multidose vial

Dosage and Administration

Adult: 0.3–1.1 mg/kg (25–75 mg) over 10–30 seconds IV; 0.04–0.07 mg/kg to maintain relaxation
Pediatric: 1–2 mg/kg dose rapid IV; max dose 150 mg
Rapid-Sequence Induction
Adult and pediatric: 1–1.5 mg/kg IV/IO
Infants: 2 mg/kg IV/IO

> NOTE
> If the patient is conscious, explain the effects of the medication before administration. Premedication with atropine should be considered. Sedation should be used in any conscious patient before undergoing neuromuscular blockade and during paralysis.

Special Considerations

Pregnancy safety: Category C
Carefully monitor the patient and be prepared to resuscitate. Administer with caution to patients with severe trauma, burns, and electrolyte imbalances (high potassium levels).
Brain or spinal cord injury may prolong effects.
Patients must have a patent or artificial airway and adequate sedation during paralysis.
Children are not as sensitive to succinylcholine on a weight basis as adults are and may require higher doses.
Succinylcholine has no effect on consciousness or pain.
Succinylcholine will not stop neuronal seizure activity.
Succinylcholine rarely may cause ventricular dysrhythmias/cardiac arrest in infants and children.

> NOTE
> Neuromuscular-blocking agents will produce respiratory paralysis. Therefore, intubation and ventilatory support must be readily available.

Tadalafil (Cialis, Adcirca)

Class

PDE-5 inhibitor

Description

Tadalafil and other PDE-5 inhibitors increase local concentrations of cyclic guanosine monophosphate, which in turn causes vasodilation. This class of medications is prescribed for treatment of pulmonary artery hypertension and erectile dysfunction. In each of these conditions, symptoms are improved with smooth muscle relaxation, vasodilation, and improved blood flow. Tadalafil is also indicated for benign prostatic hypertrophy, and works through a variety of potential mechanisms.[33]

Onset and Duration

Onset: 60 minutes
Peak: (Pulmonary hypertension) 75–90 minutes
Duration: Up to 36 hours

Indications

Pulmonary artery hypertension
Erectile dysfunction
HAPE prophylaxis
Benign prostatic hypertrophy

Contraindications

Hypersensitivity
Concurrent use of organic nitrate medications (eg, nitroglycerin, isosorbide, "poppers")
Severe hepatic impairment
Recent history of stroke or MI

Adverse Reactions

Flushing
Hypertension
Chest pain
CVA
Headache
Visual disturbances

Drug Interactions

Avoid use with other PDE-5 inhibitors, alprostadil, amyl nitrite, and other vasodilators.
Numerous medications cause increased levels of effects from sildenafil.

How Supplied

2.5-, 5-, 10-, and 20-mg oral tablets

Dosage and Administration

Adult (HAPE): 20–40 mg PO q 24 hours

Special Considerations

Pregnancy safety: Category B
Avoid use of tadalafil in patients taking nitrate medications or other vasodilator medications.
Avoid vasodilator medications and nitroglycerin in patients taking sildenafil in the past 48 hours.

Tetracaine (Pontocaine)

Class

Topical ophthalmic anesthetic

Description

Tetracaine is used for rapid, brief superficial anesthesia. The agent inhibits conduction of nerve impulses from sensory nerves.

Onset and Duration

Onset: Within 30 seconds
Duration: 10–15 minutes

Indications

Short-term relief from eye pain or irritation
Patient comfort before eye irrigation

Contraindications

Hypersensitivity to tetracaine
Open injury to the eye

Adverse Reactions

Burning or stinging sensation
Irritation

Drug Interactions

Incompatible with the mercury or silver salts often found in ophthalmic products

How Supplied

0.5% solution

Dosage and Administration

Adult: 1–2 drops
Pediatric: Same as adult

Special Considerations

Pregnancy safety: Category C
Tetracaine can cause epithelial damage and systemic toxicity.
Tetracaine is not recommended for prolonged use.

Thiamine (Betaxin)

Class

Vitamin (B_1)

Description

Thiamine combines with adenosine triphosphate to form thiamine pyrophosphate, a coenzyme necessary for carbohydrate metabolism. Most vitamins required by the body are obtained through diet; however, certain states such as alcoholism and malnourishment may affect the intake, absorption, and use of thiamine. The brain is extremely sensitive to thiamine deficiency.

Onset and Duration

Onset: Rapid
Duration: Depends on the degree of deficiency

Indications

Coma of unknown origin (with administration of dextrose 50% or naloxone)
Delirium tremens
Beriberi (rare)
Wernicke encephalopathy

Contraindications
None significant

Adverse Reactions
Hypotension (from rapid injection or large dose)
Anxiety
Diaphoresis
Nausea and vomiting
Allergic reaction (usually from IV injection; rare); angioedema

Drug Interactions
None significant

How Supplied
1-, 2-mL vials (100 mg/mL)

Dosage and Administration
Adult: 100 mg slow IV or IM
Pediatric: 10–25 mg IV or IM if needed, although not routinely administered in the prehospital setting

Special Considerations
Pregnancy safety: Category A; Category C if dose exceeds recommended daily allowance
Large IV doses may cause respiratory difficulties.
Anaphylactic reactions have been reported.

Tranexamic Acid (TXA, Cyklokapron, Lysteda)

Class
Antifibrinolytic agent; hemostatic agent

Description
Tranexamic acid is rapidly gaining popularity for the treatment of hemorrhage from trauma, surgery, and other conditions. It is a synthetic version of the enzyme lysine, which disrupts the cycle of clot formation and breakdown during bleeding episodes. Tranexamic acid binds with lysine sites on plasminogen, preventing plasminogen from converting to plasmin, and ultimately inhibiting the breakdown of fibrin.[34] Additionally, tranexamic acid may promote platelet function and decrease inflammation.

Onset and Duration
Onset: Unknown
Duration: 7–8 hours

Indications
Trauma
Hemorrhage following surgery or dental procedures
Excessive menstrual bleeding

Contraindications
Hypersensitivity
Thromboembolic disorders (prior or current)
Certain vision disorders

Adverse Reactions
Seizures
Headache
Visual changes
Hypotension
Thromboembolism
Thrombus (clot)

Drug Interactions
Use with caution in patients taking oral contraceptive hormones.
May increase blood clotting in patients taking clotting factor complexes.
May decrease the effectiveness of thrombolytic agents.

How Supplied
1,000 mg in 10-mL IV solution
650-mg oral tablets

Dosage and Administration
Adults: 10 mg/kg (up to 15 mg/kg in certain situations) IV
Pediatric: 10 mg/kg IV

Special Considerations
Pregnancy safety: Category B

Vecuronium

Class
Nondepolarizing neuromuscular blocker

Description

Vecuronium competitively blocks acetylcholine at the neuromuscular junction, resulting in chemical paralysis. Vecuronium has a slightly longer onset time than rocuronium has, making either rocuronium or succinylcholine the preferred agents for rapid-sequence induction procedures. Compared to succinylcholine, both vecuronium and rocuronium have fewer problematic side effects in many patient situations, but significantly longer durations of action. Providers may use vecuronium for ongoing chemical paralysis of mechanically ventilated patients during interfacility transports. See "Special Considerations" for important information about overall patient care for patients receiving vecuronium.

Onset and Duration

Onset: 2.5–3 minutes
Peak: 3–5 minutes
Duration: 30–40 minutes[35]

Indications

Chemical paralysis for airway placement, particularly in controlled situations and settings
Ongoing chemical paralysis for mechanically ventilated patients

Contraindications

Hypersensitivity
Consider risk versus benefit in patients with anticipated difficult/failed airways or chronic neuromuscular conditions such as myasthenia gravis, and in situations where neuromuscular blockade will prevent accurate clinical assessment or monitoring (eg, status epilepticus, head injury, severe CVA)

Adverse Reactions

Apnea
Tachycardia (assess for inadequate sedation or analgesia)
Hypertension (assess for inadequate sedation or analgesia)
Anaphylaxis
Dysrhythmias

Drug Interactions

Numerous medications have the potential to increase serum rocuronium levels, resulting in longer duration of action.
Rocuronium may increase the effects of systemic corticosteroid and cardiac glycoside medications.

How Supplied

1 mg/mL solution in 10-mL and 20-mL vials

Dosage and Administration

Adult: 0.08 to 0.1 mg/kg IV
Pediatric: Infants >7 weeks, children, and adolescents: IV: 0.08–0.1 mg/kg. *Note:* If intubation is performed using succinylcholine, the initial dose of vecuronium may be reduced to 0.04–0.06 mg/kg.

Special Considerations

Pregnancy safety: Category C
Use only in settings where trained personnel and equipment for emergency airway management are immediately available.
Vecuronium has no sedative or analgesic properties, despite the patient appearing flaccid and unresponsive. Ongoing adjunctive analgesia and sedative medications are essential for patients receiving vecuronium. Vecuronium has a longer duration of action than many sedative and opioid medications (particularly in hypermetabolic states and critically ill pediatric patients), potentially resulting in awake patients with intact awareness and sensation, without the ability to move or communicate.

Verapamil (Isoptin, Calan, Verelan)

Class

Calcium channel blocker (Class IV antidysrhythmic)

Description

Verapamil is used as an antidysrhythmic, antianginal, and antihypertensive agent. It works by inhibiting the movement of calcium ions across cell membranes. The slow calcium ion current blocked by verapamil is more important for the activity of the sinoatrial node and AV node than for many other tissues in the heart. By interfering with this current, calcium channel blockers achieve some selectivity of action. Verapamil decreases atrial automaticity, reduces AV conduction velocity, and prolongs the AV nodal refractory period. In addition, verapamil depresses myocardial contractility, reduces vascular smooth muscle tone, and dilates coronary arteries and arterioles in normal and ischemic tissues. Verapamil may be used as an alternative drug (after adenosine) to terminate reentry SVT with narrow QRS complex and adequate BP and preserved left ventricular function.

> NOTE
> Some physicians recommend slow IV administration of 500 mg of calcium chloride before the dose of verapamil to minimize the untoward results of hypotension and bradycardia.

Onset and Duration

Onset: 1–5 minutes
Duration: 30–120 minutes (may persist longer)

Indications

Give only to patients with narrow-complex reentry SVTs or known supraventricular dysrhythmias.
Atrial flutter with a rapid ventricular response
Atrial fibrillation with a rapid ventricular response
Multifocal atrial tachycardia
Vasospastic and unstable angina

Contraindications

Hypersensitivity
Sick sinus syndrome (unless the patient has a functioning pacemaker)
Second- or third-degree heart block
Sinus bradycardia
Hypotension
Cardiogenic shock
Severe heart failure
WPW syndrome with atrial fibrillation or flutter
Patients receiving IV beta blockers. Give with extreme caution to patients receiving oral beta blockers.
Wide-complex tachycardias of uncertain origin. VT can deteriorate into VF when calcium channel blockers are given.

Adverse Reactions

Dizziness
Headache
Nausea and vomiting
Hypotension
Bradycardia
Complete AV block
Peripheral edema

Drug Interactions

Verapamil increases the serum concentration of digoxin.
Beta adrenergic blockers may have additive negative inotropic and chronotropic effects.
Antihypertensives may potentiate hypotensive effects.

How Supplied

Parenteral: 5 mg/2 mL in 2-, 4-, 5-mL vials, or 2-, 4-mL ampules

Dosage and Administration

Adult:
- Initial dose: 2.5–5 mg slow IV bolus over 2 minutes (over 3 minutes in older patients).
- Repeat dose: 5- to 10-mg bolus in 15–30 minutes after initial dose if needed; or 5 mg bolus q 15 minutes until a desired response is achieved (max dose 30 mg).

Pediatric:
- 1–15 years: 0.1–0.3 mg/kg per dose IV.
- >15 years: Follow adult dosing.
- Not generally recommended for children <2 years.

Special Considerations

Pregnancy safety: Category C
Closely monitor patient's vital signs.
Be prepared to resuscitate.
AV block or asystole may occur because of slowed AV conduction.

Ziprasidone (Geodon)

Class

Antipsychotic agent

Description

Ziprasidone is used primarily for the management of schizophrenia and has additional uses for bipolar disorder, mania, and acute agitation episodes. It works by antagonizing alpha-2 adrenergic receptors and various dopamine and serotonin receptors. IM use is typically limited to acute agitation.

Onset and Duration

Onset: IV: Rapid
Duration: IV: >8 hours

Indications

Acute treatment of schizophrenia and bipolar I disorders
Acute management of agitation in schizophrenic patients
As an adjunct to lithium or valproate for maintenance treatment of bipolar I disorders

Contraindications

Hypersensitivity
Prolonged QT interval, or patient receiving medications causing QT prolongation
Recent MI
Heart failure

Adverse Reactions

Seizures
Headache
Drowsiness
Extrapyramidal symptoms
Orthostatic hypotension
Bradycardia
Nausea

Drug Interactions

Use with caution in patients taking antiarrhythmic medications.
Numerous medication interactions.

How Supplied

20-mg IV solution
20-, 40-, 60-, 80-mg oral tablets

Dosage and Administration

Behavioral Emergencies
Adults: 10 mg q 2 hours IM
Pediatric:
6–11 years: 5 mg IM
12–18 years: 10 mg IM
End-of-Life (Palliative) Care
Anxiety: 20 mg IM

Special Considerations

Pregnancy safety: Category C
Assess for patient medication history if possible.
QT interval prolongation and resulting ventricular arrhythmias are significant risks associated with ziprasidone administration.
Use extreme caution when attempting to administer an IM injection to an agitated or combative patient.

References

1. US Food and Drug Administration, US Department of Health and Human Services. *Content and Format of Labeling for Human Prescription Drug and Biological Products; Requirements for Pregnancy and Lactation Labeling.* 21 CFR Part 201. Amazon S3 website. https://s3.amazonaws.com/public-inspection.federalregister.gov/2014-28241.pdf. Accessed May 8, 2018.
2. FDA pregnancy categories. Drugs.com website. https://www.drugs.com/pregnancy-categories.html. Accessed May 8, 2018.
3. Heard K, Dart R. Acetaminophen (paracetamol) poisoning in adults: treatment. UpToDate website. https://www.uptodate.com/contents/acetaminophen-paracetamol-poisoning-in-adults-treatment?source=see_link. Updated March 16, 2018. Accessed May 8, 2018.
4. Chyka PA. Acetylcysteine and acetaminophen overdose: the many shades of gray. *J Pediatr Pharmacol Therap.* 2015;20(3):160-162.
5. Dasai S, Su M. Cyanide poisoning. UpToDate website. https://www.uptodate.com/contents/cyanide-poisoning#H22. Updated September 28, 2016. Accessed May 8, 2018.
6. Lee J, Kim JK, Kim JH, et al. Recovery time of platelet function after aspirin withdrawal. *Curr Therap Res Clin Exper.* 2014;76:26-31.
7. Hack JB, Hoffman RS. Thiamine before glucose to prevent Wernicke encephalopathy: examining the conventional wisdom. *JAMA.* 1998;279(8):583-584.
8. Mullins M, Van Zwieten K, Blunt JR. Unexpected cardiovascular deaths are rare with therapeutic doses of droperidol. Abstract presented as a platform presentation at the 2002 North American Congress of Clinical Toxicology, Palm Springs, CA, September 24, 2002. *Am J Emerg Med.* 2004;22(1):27-28.
9. Van Zweiten K, Mullins ME, Jang T. Droperidol and the black box warning. *Ann Emerg Med.* 2004;43(1):139-140.
10. Kao LW, Kirk MA, Evers SJ, Rosenfeld SH. Droperidol, QT prolongation, and sudden death: what is the evidence? *Ann Emerg Med.* 2003;41(4):546-558.
11. National Model EMS Clinical Guidelines Version 2.0. National Association of State EMS Officials website. www.nasemso.org. Revised September 18, 2017. Accessed April 5, 2018. Pg. 60.

12. Wood JP, Traub SJ, Lipinski C. Safety of epinephrine for anaphylaxis in the emergency setting. *World J Emerg Med.* 2013;4(4):245-251.
13. Bishop J, Enriquez B, Allard A, et al. Croup pathway. Seattle Children's Hospital website. http://www.seattlechildrens.org/pdf/croup-pathway.pdf. Updated August 2015. Accessed May 8, 2018.
14. Fanta CH. Management of acute exacerbations of asthma in adults. UpToDate website. https://www.uptodate.com/contents/management-of-acute-exacerbations-of-asthma-in-adults?search=Ipratropium%200.2mg,Salbutamol%201mg%2Fml&source=search_result&selectedTitle=6~150&usage_type=default&display_rank=6. Updated April 9, 2018. Accessed May 8, 2018.
15. Vadivelu N, Schermer E, Kodumudi V, et al. Role of ketamine for analgesia in adults and children. *J Anaesthesiol Clin Pharmacol.* 2016;32(3):298-306.
16. Riddell J, Tran A, Bengiamin R, et al. Ketamine as a first-line agent for severely agitated emergency department patients. *Am J Emerg Med.* 2017;35(7):1000-1004.
17. Lin M. Procedural sedation in the elderly. *Emerg Physicians Monthly* website. http://epmonthly.com/article/procedural-sedation-in-the-elderly/. Accessed May 8, 2018.
18. Ketorolac. Epocrates website. https://online.epocrates.com/u/102337/ketorolac/Pediatric+Dosing. Accessed May 8, 2018.
19. Evaniew N, Noonan VK, Fallah N, et al. Methylprednisolone for the treatment of patients with acute spinal cord injuries: a propensity score-matched cohort study from a Canadian multi-center spinal cord injury registry. *J Neurotrauma.* 2015;32(21):1674-1683.
20. Metoprolol. Davis's Drug Guide website. https://www.drugguide.com/ddo/view/Davis-Drug-Guide/51497/all/metoprolol. Accessed May 8, 2018.
21. Morphine. Davis's Drug Guide website. https://www.drugguide.com/ddo/view/Davis-Drug-Guide/51518/all/morphine. Accessed May 8, 2018.
22. Cohan JA, Checcio LM. Nifedipine in the management of hypertensive emergencies: report of two cases and review of the literature. *Am J Emerg Med.* 1985;3(6):524-530.
23. Nitroglycerin. Epocrates website. https://online.epocrates.com/u/102112/nitroglycerin/Pediatric+Dosing. Accessed May 8, 2018.
24. Robichaud L, Ross D, Proulx M-H, et al. Prehospital nitroglycerin safety in inferior ST elevation myocardial infarction. *Prehosp Emerg Care.* 2016;20(1):76-81.
25. Becker DE, Rosenberg M. Nitrous oxide and the inhalation anesthetics. *Anesthesia Prog.* 2008;55(4):124-131.
26. National Center for Environmental Health/Agency for Toxic Substances and Disease Registry, National Center for Injury Prevention and Control. Potassium iodide (KI). Centers for Disease Control and Prevention website. https://emergency.cdc.gov/radiation/ki.asp. Updated August 10, 2015. Accessed May 8, 2018.
27. Bajwa ZH, Smith JH. Acute treatment of migraine in adults. UpToDate website. https://www.uptodate.com/contents/acute-treatment-of-migraine-in-adults. Updated January 15, 2018. Accessed May 8, 2018.
28. Taylor F. Tension type headache in adults: acute treatment. UpToDate website. https://www.uptodate.com/contents/tension-type-headache-in-adults-acute-treatment. Updated January 24, 2017. Accessed May 8, 2018.
29. Rocuronium. Davis's Drug Guide website. https://www.drugguide.com/ddo/view/Davis-Drug-Guide/109873/all/rocuronium. Accessed May 8, 2018.
30. Gallagher SA, Hacket P. High altitude pulmonary edema. UpToDate website. https://www.uptodate.com/contents/high-altitude-pulmonary-edema#H19. Updated December 12, 2016. Accessed May 8, 2018.
31. DBL sodium nitrite injection. Medsafe website. http://www.medsafe.govt.nz/profs/Datasheet/d/dblSodiumNitriteinj.pdf. Published April 24, 2017. Accessed May 8, 2018.
32. Burkhardt C. Thiosulfate, sodium. In: *Poisoning and Drug Overdose.* 5th ed. New York, NY: McGraw-Hill; 2007:514-515.
33. Hatzimouratidis K. A review of the use of tadalafil in the treatment of benign prostatic hyperplasia in men with and without erectile dysfunction. *Therap Adv Urol.* 2014;6(4):135-147.
34. Reed R, Woolley T. Uses of tranexamic acid. *Cont Educ Anaesthesia Crit Pain.* 2015;15(1). https://doi.org/10.1093/bjaceaccp/mku009.
35. Vecuronium. Davis's Drug Guide website. https://www.drugguide.com/ddo/view/Davis-Drug-Guide/109869/all/vecuronium. Accessed May 8, 2018.

Appendix B Advanced Practice Procedures for Critical Care Paramedics

Some critically ill or injured patients require a level of care that is beyond the normal scope of the paramedic. For example, a patient may have special needs that require continuous medical supervision by one or more health professionals. These duties usually are provided by specialty personnel working in nursing, emergency medicine, respiratory care, and cardiovascular care. Supervision of the patient also can be provided by paramedics with advanced levels of training. This appendix addresses some of the advanced knowledge and patient care procedures that may be required of the paramedic who practices in critical care.

Critical Care and Critical Care Transport

Critical care is a specialty within professional health care that deals with patients who have life-threatening illness or injury. Historically, this level of care has been provided primarily by physicians, physician assistants, specially trained registered nurses, respiratory therapists, clinical nurse specialists, and nurse practitioners. In recent years, however, other health care professionals, including paramedics, have begun to provide such critical care. Paramedics who practice in critical care settings, including critical care transport (CCT), often have special training and advanced certifications. They also have additional experience working with critical care patients. Through this education, these paramedics are trained and credentialed in the critical decision making and advanced practice procedures that may be performed infrequently by most other prehospital personnel.

CCT is also known as specialty care transport (SCT). SCT is defined by the Centers for Medicare and Medicaid Services (CMS) as "the interfacility transportation of a critically injured or ill beneficiary by a ground ambulance vehicle, including the provision of medically necessary supplies and services, at a level of service beyond the scope of the EMT-Paramedic."[1] Most paramedics who are members of a CCT team have completed a training program and then passed an examination to achieve an advanced certification such as Certified Critical Care Paramedic (CCP-C) or

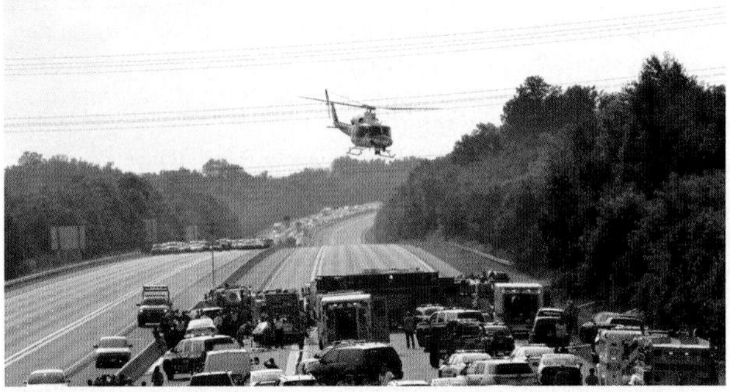

Certified Flight Paramedic (FP-C). These certifications are designed to attest that a paramedic possesses the competencies required to transport critically ill or specialty care patients from a community hospital to a tertiary care facility. This appendix serves as an introduction to knowledge and skills needed for these types of patients. Paramedics who routinely serve in this role should receive appropriate critical care training and credentialing.

Transport and Advanced Practice Procedures

Circumstances often arise when a paramedic without CCT or SCT training is called upon for an interfacility transport that may require some critical care knowledge. Unlike field responses, interfacility transfers are not always emergencies. They are sometimes scheduled or at least requested with some notice, include a list of equipment needed, and provide a patient diagnosis and reason for transport. With so much information, it would seem unlikely that problems could occur—yet CCT is a high-risk area of practice in EMS. Areas of exposure include accepting a patient for transport who requires care beyond the limitations of the EMS crew, failing to anticipate and prevent complications during transport, and not contacting medical control when issues arise (before or during transport). The American College of Emergency Physicians' policy statement on appropriate interfacility patient transfer[2] and the National Association of EMS Physicians' position paper on medical direction of interfacility transports[3] identify elements such as the following as key considerations in these kinds of transfers:

- Achieving the optimal health and well-being of the patient should be the principal goal of patient transfer.
- Hospital personnel should provide a medical screening examination (MSE) and stabilizing treatment within their capacity before transfer.
- The transferring facility should inform the patient or responsible party of the risks and benefits of transfer and obtain patient consent when possible.
- There should be dedicated personnel qualified to conduct the MSEs. These personnel will determine how the patient is to be transferred.
- The receiving hospital must agree to accept the patient.
- Patient records should accompany the patient or be transmitted electronically as soon as possible.
- Written transfer agreements should be in place with specialty centers.

Transport Choreography

Patients who are in an urgent care center, catheterization laboratory, doctor's office, clinic, or other medical facility are already at a health care setting. Thus, while their transfer may be time dependent, that factor should not cause a paramedic to accept an unstable patient or rush unnecessarily to move a patient. Adequate time should be allotted for packaging and initiating transport of a critically ill patient to definitive care.

On arrival to an interfacility transport, the paramedic should already have an understanding from dispatch information about the equipment needed, the diagnosis of the patient, and the reason for transfer. The transferring crew should note the route of ingress to the facility, keeping in mind that additional equipment added to and accompanying the patient has the potential to impede the egress.

If a two-paramedic team will provide the transport, one provider should get a report on the patient's condition from the bedside provider (preferably a nurse or physician), review pertinent lab tests and radiology reports, and prepare any needed equipment and the stretcher. The second provider should carefully review any pumps or machines in use or connected to the patient, assess the patient, and check and label all invasive lines. If either provider perceives that the condition of the patient is not stable for transport or if the anticipated care required exceeds the providers' scope of practice or local protocols, it is imperative to consult with online medical direction immediately. Questions or concerns can be solved between the transferring providers at the facility and the online medical director. In some instances, the risk of transfer outweighs any benefit and the transport should not be completed.[4]

Once these steps are complete, the patient is moved to the transport stretcher. When the patient is comfortably on the stretcher, equipment transfer begins. Most providers move the patient from the facility ventilator to the transport ventilator first and then switch intravenous (IV) infusions from facility pumps to the transport pumps. After these steps are completed, a quick reassessment should be performed, the patient reassured, and the family located to confirm that they know the transport destination.

In addition to assessing the patient's current condition, the transferring crew should anticipate some common issues that might occur to determine if they have the resources to manage them. For example, the crew needs appropriate equipment and skills to manage airway, breathing, or circulatory problems; loss of electrical or battery power; equipment failure or dislodgements; hypotension or hypertension; agitation, pain, nausea, or vomiting; and temperature changes. In addition, these providers should ensure they have adequate supplies of medication to last for the duration of the trip.

If the patient's airway is not secure or is anticipated to decline, it should be managed before departure.[4] Intubated patients should have their airway secured using a commercial device to prevent dislodgement of the airway equipment. Continuous waveform capnography is a standard of care in all patients with an advanced airway. Suction should be readily available.

If a temporary transvenous pacemaker is in use, the paramedic should determine when and why the pacemaker was inserted, what the underlying rhythm is, whether the patient is hemodynamically dependent on the pacemaker, and what the settings of the pacemaker are (eg, mA, rate, sensitivity, mode). All wires and connectors of the temporary pacemaker should be taped to prevent their disconnection, transcutaneous pads should be placed on the patient as a precaution, and a spare pacemaker battery should be obtained from the transferring facility.

SHOW ME THE EVIDENCE

To gather data needed to develop education and guide clinical practice, researchers randomly surveyed 1,991 paramedics practicing in the critical care environment. The 610 paramedic respondents (30.6% response rate) reported being the team lead for pediatric transports (75.2%); interpreting 12-lead electrocardiograms (ECGs) (66.3%); using IV infusion pumps (77%); managing mechanical ventilators (66.9%); and monitoring central lines (63.1%), chest tubes (71.8%), intra-aortic balloon pumps (79.2%), and intracranial pressure (ICP) monitors (64.9%). This care was, in some cases, rendered without additional training or education. The rate varied by procedure, but respondents reported no structured training on the following: chest tube management (11.8%), central venous line management (8.6%), arterial line management (9%), ICP monitoring (11%), neonatal isolette (14.3%), and blood or blood products (11.7%). The authors concluded that their findings should encourage development of standardized education and credentialing of paramedics to perform critical care.

Modified from: Raynovich W, Hums J, Stuhlmiller DF, et al. Critical care transportation by paramedics: a cross-sectional survey. *Air Med J.* 2013;32(5):280-288.

Advanced Practice Procedures

Most educational programs for critical care include advanced training and skill procedures that are based on body systems (eg, cardiac, respiratory, gastrointestinal, genitourinary, renal, and neurologic), surgical airway management, and drug therapy. *The descriptions of the advanced practice procedures presented in this appendix are intended as an overview. All procedures carry significant complications and risks. In addition, all procedures require advanced training and authorization from the program's medical director. Any advanced procedures performed should have a written advanced protocol.* Advanced practice procedures that are described here include the following:

- Central venous cannulation
- Accessing the umbilical vein
- Point-of-care testing (POCT)
- Invasive hemodynamic monitoring
- Monitoring of circulatory support devices
- ICP monitoring
- Blood administration
- Use of IV infusion pumps
- Tube thoracostomy
- Pericardiocentesis
- Use of ultrasound

Central Venous Cannulation

Central venous cannulation may be within the scope of paramedic practice in some critical care programs. Sites for central venous cannulation include the femoral vein, internal jugular vein, and subclavian vein (**FIGURES 1, 2,** and **3**). (Although the femoral vein is not truly a central vein, because the catheter is inserted in an area below the diaphragm, it is included in this section.)

The preparation for cannulation of the central vessels is similar to that for the peripheral veins (described in Chapter 14, *Medication Administration*); however, attention to providing and maintaining a sterile field during placement is especially important. Several factors affect the success of central venous cannulation, including the position of the patient's body, the paramedic's knowledge of anatomy, and the paramedic's familiarity with the procedure.

Cannulation of the central veins presents specific dangers in addition to the complications common to

NOTE

Central line placement is not routinely performed in the prehospital setting. Potential complications of this procedure include pneumothorax, arterial injury, air embolism, and abnormal placement. Critical care paramedics and paramedics who transport critical patients will be exposed to central lines and should be familiar with these devices.

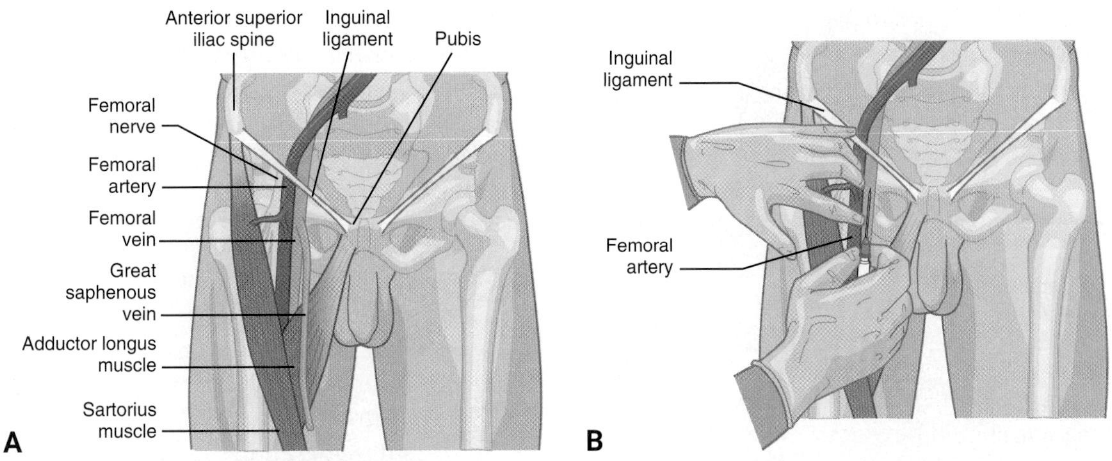

FIGURE 1 **A.** Anatomy of the femoral vein. **B.** Femoral venipuncture.

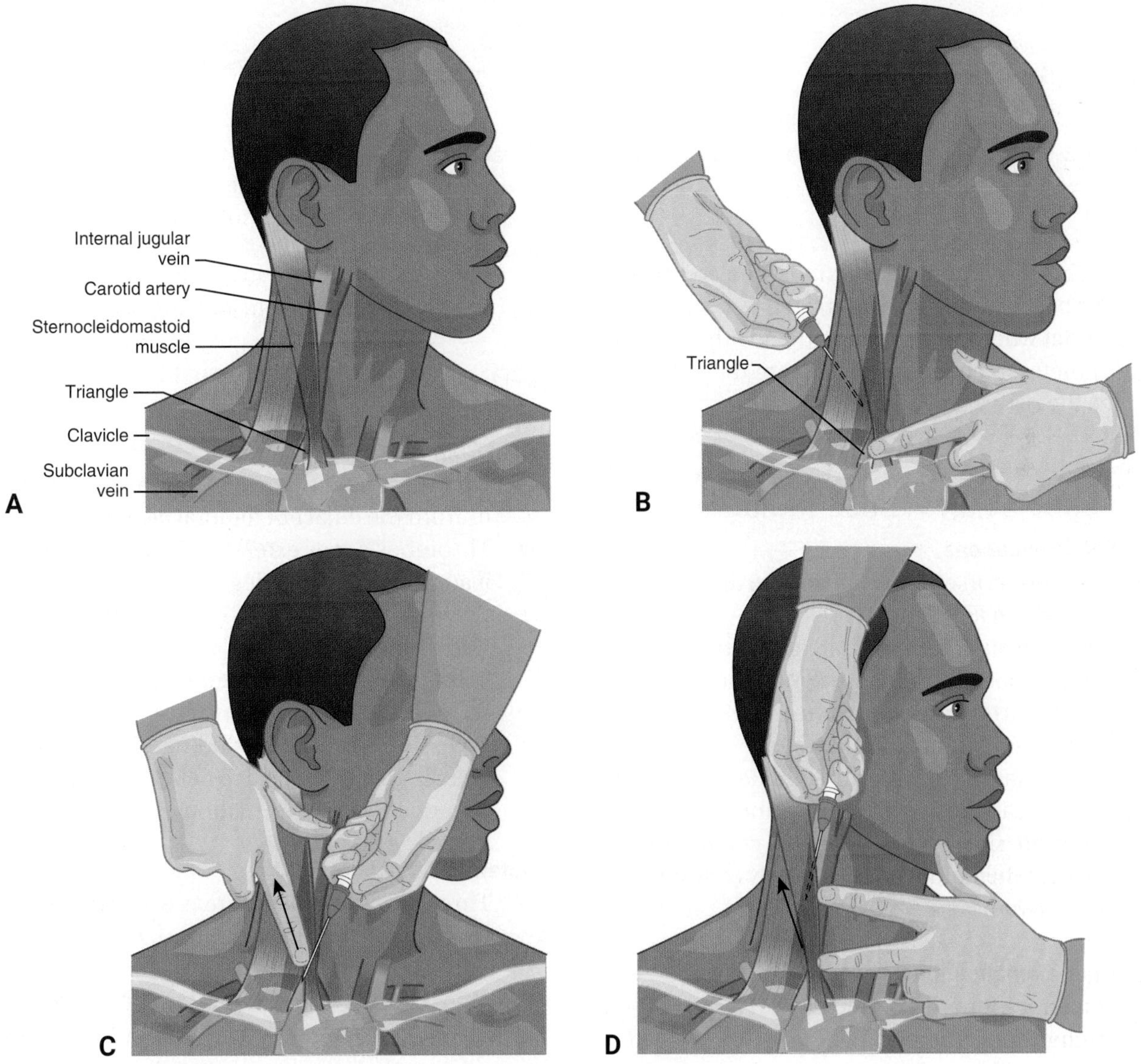

FIGURE 2 **A.** Anatomy of the internal jugular vein. **B.** Posterior approach for internal jugular venipuncture. **C.** Central approach for internal jugular venipuncture. **D.** Anterior approach for internal jugular venipuncture. (Arrows represent the direction of traction on the skin.)

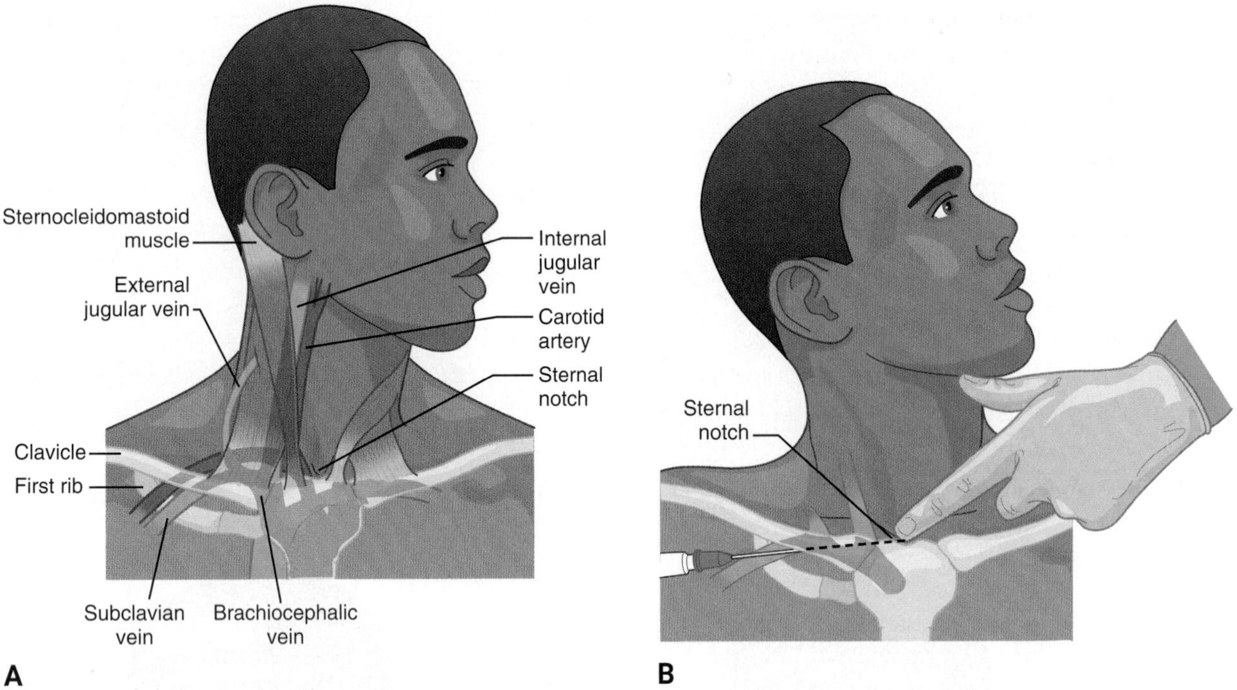

FIGURE 3 **A.** Anatomy of the subclavian vein. **B.** Infraclavicular subclavian venipuncture.

all IV techniques. The paramedic must be alert to these dangers because they can be fatal if unrecognized. It is essential when caring for a patient with a central vein catheter to eliminate all air from the tubing to reduce the risk of air embolism.

Complications of Internal Jugular and Subclavian Vein Cannulation

Local Complications.

- Hematoma may occur, either from the vein itself or from an adjacent artery.
- Damage may occur to an adjacent artery, nerve, or lymphatic duct. Inadvertent puncture of the carotid artery is not uncommon when jugular vein cannulation is attempted.
- If a hematoma occurs on one side of the neck, it is hazardous to attempt puncture on the opposite side, as this procedure could result in bilateral hematomas that severely compromise the airway.

Systemic Complications.

- Pneumothorax is common.
- Hemothorax can occur.
- Air embolism can occur.
- Fluid may infiltrate into the mediastinum or the pleural cavity from an extruded catheter.

Complications of Femoral Vein Cannulation

Local Complications.

- Hematoma may occur, either from the vein itself or from the adjacent femoral artery.
- Thrombosis may extend to the deep veins and lead to edema of the leg.
- Phlebitis may extend to the deep veins.
- Use of the femoral vein frequently precludes subsequent use of the saphenous vein.
- Inadvertent arterial puncture may lead to excessive bleeding (including retroperitoneal bleeding) and can lead to delayed aneurysm or pseudoaneurysm formation.

Systemic Complications.

- Thrombosis or phlebitis may occur and extend to the iliac veins or even the inferior vena cava.

Accessing the Umbilical Vein

As described in Chapter 45, *Obstetrics*, the umbilical cord contains three vessels: two arteries and one vein.

The vein in the umbilical cord has a thin wall and is larger than the arteries. The arteries are thick walled and usually paired.

To gain access to the umbilical vein, the paramedic who is credentialed by the medical director should take the following steps (**FIGURE 4**):

1. Set up IV fluid (per protocol) and tubing with a three-way stopcock.
2. Select a 3.5 French (for preterm neonates) or 5 French (for full-term neonates) umbilical catheter.
3. Connect the catheter to the stopcock and fill the catheter with IV fluid, which will remove any air. Leave the stopcock closed until the catheter is in the vein.
4. Cleanse the umbilical stump and surrounding skin with antibacterial solution (per protocol).
5. Loosely tie umbilical tape around the cord near the body so that pressure can be applied to control bleeding.
6. Hold the umbilical stump firmly and trim (with a scalpel) the cord several centimeters above the abdomen.
7. Locate the umbilical vein and insert the catheter until blood is freely obtained. Do not insert the catheter more than 1 to 2 cm (less than an inch) beyond the point at which good blood return is obtained. Insertion is approximately 2 inches (5 cm) in a full-term neonate. If the catheter is inserted farther, there is a risk of infusing solutions directly into the liver rather than the systemic circulation. Care should be taken to avoid introduction of air emboli into the umbilical vein. If resistance is met, loosening the umbilical tape or changing the angle of approach may help, but advancement must never be forced.
8. Draw blood for a sample, if needed.
9. Initiate the infusion and regulate the fluid flow per medical direction.
10. Secure the catheter in place with tape and cover with a sterile dressing.
11. Document the procedure.

The umbilical cord also may be cannulated by using a typical IV catheter. Insert the catheter-over-needle through the side of the proximal end of the cord into the vein, and advance it upward through the translucent wall. Start the infusion, adjust the fluid flow per medical direction, and secure the catheter in place with tape.

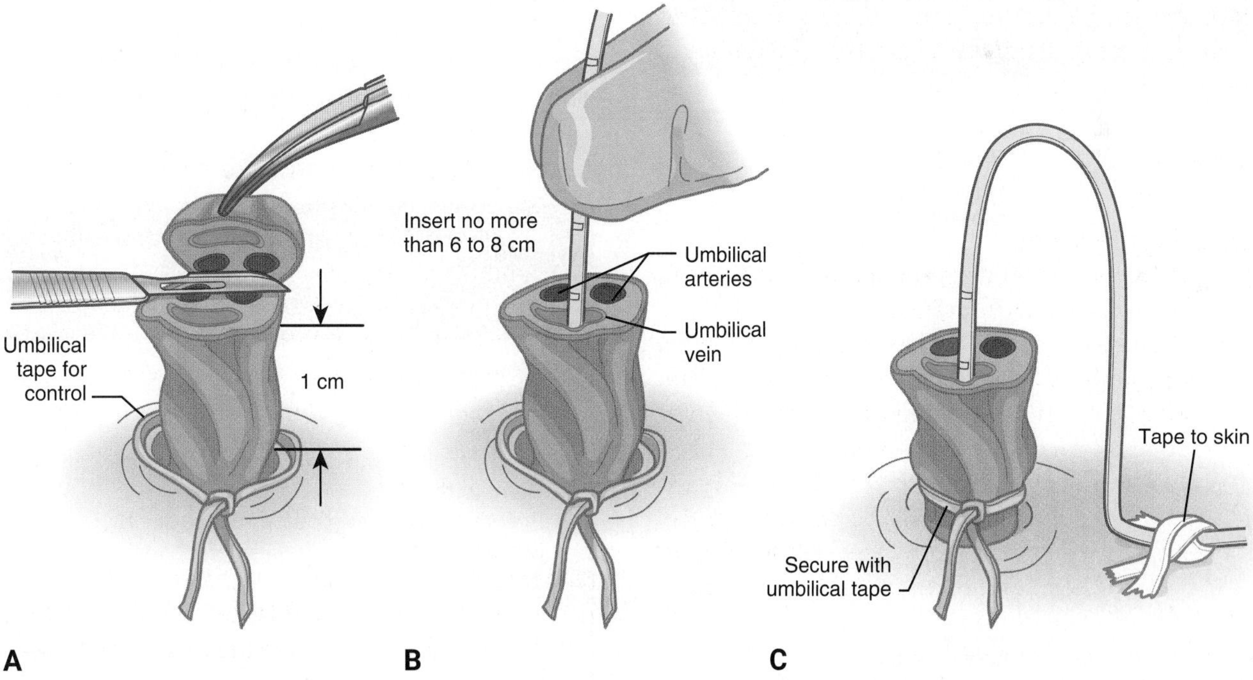

FIGURE 4 Umbilical vein cannulation procedure. **A.** Identify the umbilical vein after trimming the cord. **B.** Insert the umbilical catheter into the vein. **C.** Secure the base of the cord to hold the catheter in place and stabilize the catheter with tape.

Point-of-Care Testing

POCT refers to testing done outside of a traditional laboratory, often near where the patient is being cared for, with the results then being used to make decisions about patient care. Although many POCT devices exist, ranging from glucometers to complex blood gas, chemistry, and hematology instruments, use of POCT is highly regulated by CMS through the Clinical Laboratory Improvement Amendments (CLIA).[5] Further, each device to be used in patient care must be approved by the US Food and Drug Administration. These regulations protect patients from harm that could result if a test were done incorrectly, leading to inaccurate results.

Paramedics should use only POCT devices that they have been properly trained and credentialed to operate, keeping in mind that results from POCT units can affect patient care. Most EMS agencies are permitted to perform only point-of-care tests that have been granted CLIA-waived status (**TABLE 1**).

TABLE 1 Selected Tests Permitted by the Clinical Laboratory Improvement Amendments

Blood chemistries (specific devices only)	• Calcium • Carbon dioxide • Chloride • Creatinine • Glucose • Hemoglobin/Hematocrit • Potassium • Serum lactate • Sodium
Dipstick urinalysis	• Glucose • Hemoglobin • Ketone • Leukocytes • Nitrites • pH • Protein
Urine pregnancy test	

Modified from: Clinical Laboratory Improvement Amendments: categorization of tests. Centers for Medicare and Medicaid Services website. https://www.cms.gov/Regulations-and-Guidance/Legislation/CLIA/Categorization_of_Tests.html. Updated April 8, 2013. Accessed April 24, 2018.

Hemodynamic Monitoring

Hemodynamic monitoring is the measurement and interpretation of hemodynamic parameters in an effort to assess perfusion or the delivery of oxygen and nutrients to the tissues of the body. Conventional physical assessment of vital signs, skin color, mentation, and urine output provides clues about poor perfusion. Without more sophisticated monitoring, however, those assessments may lead providers to mistakenly believe that perfusion is adequate.

Traditionally, hemodynamic monitoring was invasive; that is, it required placement of a catheter (central venous line, arterial line) in a vein, artery, or heart chamber. Invasive hemodynamic monitoring is associated with significant risks (**BOX 1**). Thus, less invasive as well as noninvasive hemodynamic monitoring technologies are now beginning to replace the invasive devices of the past.

Hemodynamic monitoring has been considered useful for assessing and managing patients with severe hypertensive emergencies, profound shock, refractory pulmonary edema, vasopressor-resistant sepsis, and multiple-organ failure. Monitoring via pulmonary artery catheter (PAC) can help distinguish the various types of shock (cardiogenic, hypovolemic, and distributive). Invasive hemodynamic monitoring requires special equipment to produce visible waveforms on a pressure monitor (**FIGURE 5** and **BOX 2**). These waveforms reflect the phases of the cardiac

BOX 1 Possible Complications and Risks Associated With Invasive Hemodynamic Monitoring

- Air embolism
- Arterial spasm
- Bleeding
- Dysrhythmias (with heart chamber catheterization)
- Hematoma
- Pneumothorax (with chest insertion sites)
- Systemic infection
- Thrombosis
- Tissue and blood vessel injury

Modified from: Stathers CL, McEvoy M, Murphy M, et al., eds. *Critical Care Transport.* Burlington, MA: Jones & Bartlett Learning; 2011.

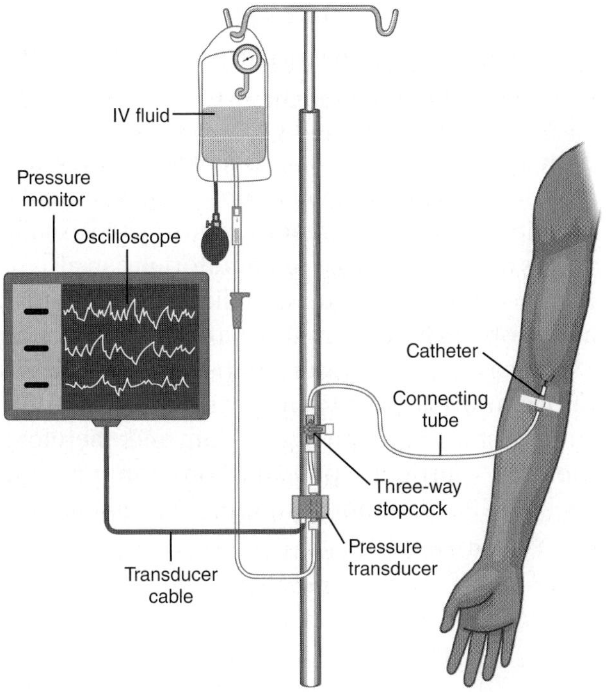

Abbreviation: IV, intravenous

FIGURE 5 Hemodynamic monitoring equipment.

BOX 2 Troubleshooting Monitors

All patient care monitors have a variety of user-configurable and mandatory alarms to alert clinicians of potential deterioration of the patient's condition. A systematic method of troubleshooting the alarms is to begin with the patient first, then look at the equipment:

1. Check the patient.
2. Check the insertion site.
3. Check the tubing or lead wire.
4. Check connections to the monitor.
5. Check the monitor.
6. Check the electrical connection or power source.

cycle and can be used to monitor arterial pressure, central venous pressure (CVP; also called right atrial pressure [RAP]), left atrial pressure (LAP), and pulmonary artery pressure (PAP) (**FIGURE 6**).

Pressure monitoring is accomplished by using a transducer connected to the area where pressure needs to be monitored. Pressure transducers are subject to two potential sources of interference, from the fluid in the pressure monitoring tubing and from the atmospheric pressure. In the case of a transducer connected to an arterial line or central venous catheter, fluid in the tubing between the transducer and the body could potentially cause a false increase or decrease in the measured pressures. This effect can be reliably eliminated by leveling the transducer to the phlebostatic axis, a landmark that equates to the level of the right atrium. The phlebostatic axis is located at the intersection of the fourth intercostal space and midaxillary line.[6,7] As the patient moves, so does the phlebostatic axis. Therefore, releveling is required whenever patient movement occurs. A predictable error is observed with inaccurate leveling: For every 1 inch (2.5 cm) the transducer is placed above the phlebostatic axis, observed readings will be 1.86 mm Hg lower than actual pressures; and for every 1 inch (2.5 cm) the transducer is leveled below the phlebostatic axis, the measured readings will be 1.86 mm Hg higher than the actual pressure.[8]

Atmospheric pressure at sea level is typically 760 mm Hg. Hemodynamic monitoring equipment must be "zeroed" prior to use by opening the transducer to atmospheric air and simultaneously pressing the "zero" button on the monitor to force the measured pressure to equal zero. Once this step is accomplished, the monitoring tubing can be redirected to measure the patient's pressure, allowing the previously measured atmospheric pressure not to interfere with the readings obtained. Zeroing needs to be done once at the time when the system is first assembled, whenever the cable from the transducer to the monitor is disconnected and reconnected, and whenever the values obtained are significantly questionable.

Arterial Pressure Monitoring

Arterial pressure monitoring is designed to measure systemic blood pressure. Such monitoring provides a continuous, accurate display of arterial pressure through the placement of an arterial line in an artery. It is indicated for any patient with shock who is unresponsive to initial therapy, including patients who are profoundly hypotensive, who are hypertensive, or who require multiple drug infusions with frequent titration to maintain their blood pressure.

Indwelling arterial catheters may be inserted into the radial, femoral, brachial, axillary, or (rarely) dorsalis pedis artery. The radial and brachial arteries are most commonly used for continuous blood pressure monitoring.

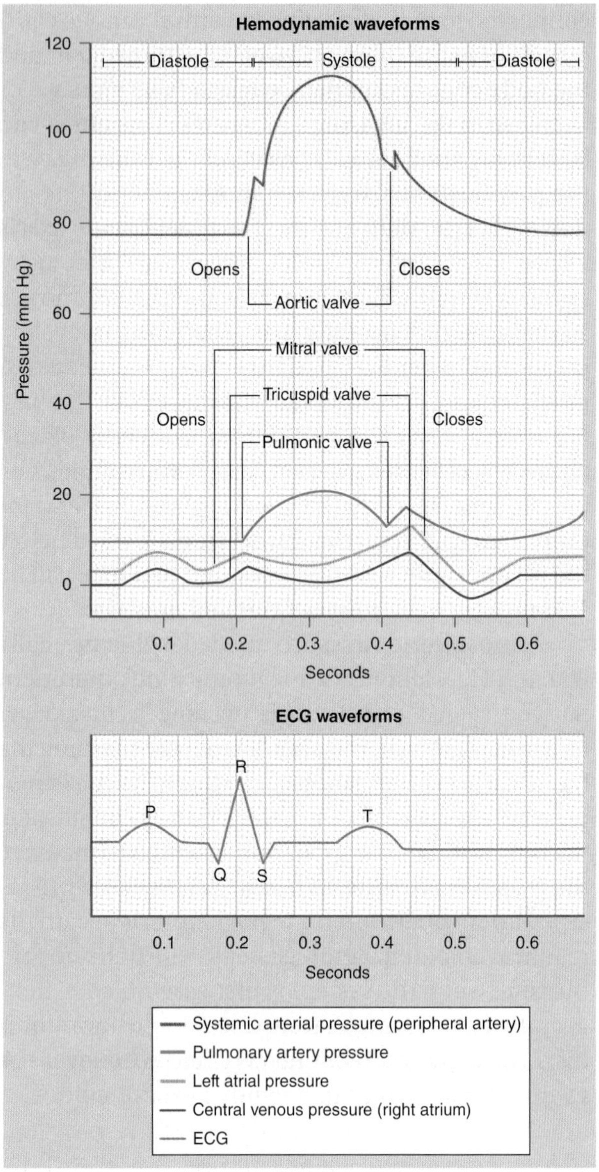

Abbreviation: ECG, electrocardiogram

FIGURE 6 How hemodynamic waveforms reflect the cardiac cycle.

Right Atrial Pressure Monitoring

CVP monitoring may be used to assess right ventricular preload in critically ill patients. CVP monitoring allows for direct measurement of pressure in the right atrium and reflects right ventricular pressure. It is used to monitor blood volume, right ventricular function, and central venous return. The vascular access device employed for monitoring can also be used to administer IV fluids, medications, and blood, and to obtain blood samples. Although monitoring CVP measures the pressure in the right atrium, this information is used to indirectly determine the volume of blood in the right atrium and, therefore, the right ventricular preload. Common insertion sites for CVP monitoring are the internal jugular and subclavian veins.

NOTE

CVP monitoring may reflect left ventricular preload but can be misleading, particularly in patients with right atrial or right ventricular dysfunction.

Left Atrial Pressure Monitoring

LAP monitoring measures the pressure of the blood as it returns to the left side of the heart. It is usually measured indirectly using the pulmonary capillary wedge pressure (PCWP), described later in this section. PCWP is a reliable indicator of left ventricular end-diastolic pressure and, therefore, left ventricular function. (This is true except in cases of severe mitral stenosis if LAP is obtained using PCWP.) In most settings, PCWP is monitored intermittently using a pulmonary artery catheter.

Pulmonary Artery Pressure Monitoring

PAP monitoring provides an indirect measurement of left ventricular function. The catheter used for PAP monitoring has four lumens (and sometimes a fifth proximal infusion port) that contain a balloon inflation port, proximal and distal injection ports, and a thermistor lumen for obtaining cardiac output measurements (**FIGURE 7**). Some PAP devices are also designed for transvenous pacing, assessment of oxygen saturation in the pulmonary artery, and/or electronic measurement of continuous cardiac output.

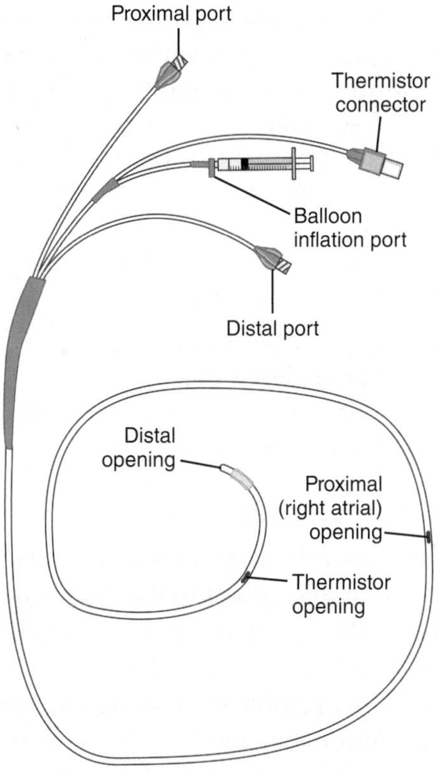

FIGURE 7 Number 7 French quadruple lumen, thermodilution pulmonary artery catheter.

Reproduced from: Darovic GO. *Hemodynamic Monitoring, Invasive and Noninvasive Clinical Application.* 3rd ed. Philadelphia, PA: Saunders; 2003.

The catheter is usually inserted in the subclavian or internal jugular vein and is passed through the right atrium and right ventricle into the pulmonary artery. PAP monitoring is used in patients who are hemodynamically unstable and is often employed for monitoring patients during and after cardiac surgery. The PAP indicates venous pressure in the lungs, the mean filling pressure for the left side of the heart, and left ventricular end-diastolic pressure (in the absence of mitral valve disease). In addition to measuring pulmonary artery pressure, PAP monitoring provides a measurement of CVP during insertion, PCWP, cardiac output, and mixed venous oxygen saturation.

Pulmonary Capillary Wedge Pressure. PCWP (also known as pulmonary artery wedge pressure) helps to determine left ventricular function. It is measured when the pulmonary balloon of the PAC is inflated and occludes a pulmonary artery branch, allowing the distal lumen in front of the balloon to register left heart pressure. Once the measurement is obtained, the balloon is deflated and the catheter floats back into the pulmonary artery. (The balloon is inflated only for PCWP readings; it remains deflated for continuous PAP monitoring and during patient transports.) PCWP usually is measured every 2 to 4 hours.

Cardiac Output. The thermistor lumen is a lumen on the pulmonary artery catheter that estimates cardiac output through a temperature thermistor. It does so by measuring the temperature change of fluid injected into the catheter. It also aids in assessing left ventricular function and the function of heart valves.

The cardiac output is estimated by injecting a solution called injectate at a known temperature (chilled or room temperature) into the proximal lumen port of the PAC that mixes with blood from the right atrium, thereby lowering the temperature of the heart's blood. The thermistor detects the change in temperature over time, and this change is analyzed by the computer to calculate cardiac output. Continuous cardiac output measurements are obtained by special catheters that send a coded temperature signal at specific intervals without injectate, calculating cardiac output in a continuous, serial fashion.

Mixed Venous Oxygen Saturation. Mixed venous oxygen saturation (Svo_2) is the direct measurement of the blended venous blood (from the inferior and superior vena cavae) usually sampled from the pulmonary artery. It reflects the balance between oxygen delivery and consumption in the tissues and can serve as an early indicator of low cardiac output. The Svo_2 level can be measured from a PAC when mixed venous blood from organs and tissues flows back to the lungs. This measurement is made by withdrawing blood from the pulmonary artery port of a PAC, or continuously by using fiberoptic catheters with an oximetry system displayed as an Svo_2 saturation on a bedside monitor. Normal values for Svo_2 are 60% to 80%.

Mixed central venous oxygen saturation ($Scvo_2$) is an alternative to Svo_2 for situations where a PAC is not in place but the patient has a central line (single- or multiple-lumen central venous catheter). The oxygen saturation of blood drawn from a central venous line also provides information about oxygen extraction requirements but, unlike the Svo_2, excludes blood returned from the lower part of the body. Normal values for $Scvo_2$ are 70% to 90%.

Less Invasive and Noninvasive Hemodynamic Monitoring. As part of the trend toward use of less invasive technologies, numerous hemodynamic platforms have been introduced into the critical care environment that use a variety of methods to assess fluid volume status, cardiac output, preload, afterload, and perfusion. Bedside ultrasound is also frequently employed by critical care practitioners to assess cardiac function and fluid volume status. The wide range of these monitoring platforms is beyond the scope of this text. Additionally, although practical and useful in the hospital setting, most of the newer less invasive and noninvasive hemodynamic monitoring devices are not portable, nor are they equipped with the battery power needed to accompany a patient during an interfacility transport.

Circulatory Support

Circulatory support devices are designed to augment cardiac output in patients with heart failure. These life-supporting therapies require the presence of experienced, specially trained, and credentialed operators throughout the course of their use. This operator will usually accompany the crew during transport of these patients.

Four circulatory support devices are commonly encountered in the CCT arena:

- Intra-aortic balloon pump (IABP)
- Continuous-flow pump
- Extracorporeal membrane oxygenation (ECMO)
- Ventricular assist device (VAD)

Intra-aortic Balloon Pump

An IABP is a mechanical cardiac assist device that benefits patients with actual or potentially life-threatening circulatory problems. Indications for its use include patients:

- Who are in cardiogenic shock, as a bridge to reperfusion therapy
- With ventricular septal defect and acute mitral regurgitation
- Who are candidates for cardiac transplant
- Who are high-risk surgical patients
- Who are high-risk patients and are undergoing angiography or angioplasty
- Who have refractory ventricular dysrhythmias complicating acute myocardial infarction
- Who have recurrent postinfarction angina

The catheter with the balloon usually is inserted in the patient's femoral artery and is advanced until the catheter lies in the aorta, just distal to the left subclavian artery. The balloon is found at the distal end of the catheter; when inflated by a computerized pump, it expands in the patient's descending thoracic aorta. The balloon inflates during diastole, causing blood in the aorta to be forced back proximally into the coronary arteries and forward distally into the renal arteries, thereby increasing coronary and renal artery flow. This allows for increased perfusion of the myocardium, helping to relieve myocardial ischemia. Just before systole, the balloon deflates, causing a decrease of the pressure in the aorta, making it easier for the left ventricle to expel blood during contraction. This results in decreased workload for the left ventricle, and increases cardiac output and perfusion of vital organs.

As a rule, the IABP is initially set to an inflation–deflation cycle for each cardiac cycle (1:1 ratio) and then is gradually reduced (2:1, 3:1 ratio), based on the patient's condition. Most IABP devices adapt the deflation automatically in the situation of ventricular ectopy or other dysrhythmias.

Modern IABP consoles are completely automatic and require few, if any, adjustments by the operator. Nevertheless, it is important to understand the timing of the IABP and the physiologic changes that occur (**TABLE 2** and **FIGURE 8**).

TABLE 2 Intra-aortic Balloon Pump Timing Errors

Timing Error	Effect
Early inflation	Premature closure of the aortic valve, causing aortic regurgitation
Late inflation	Suboptimal coronary perfusion
Early deflation	Retrograde coronary blood flow
Late deflation	Increase in the resistance that the balloon pumps against (afterload)

Modified from: Weigand DL, ed. *AACN Procedure Manual for High Acuity, Progressive, and Critical Care.* 7th ed. St. Louis, MO: Elsevier; 2017.

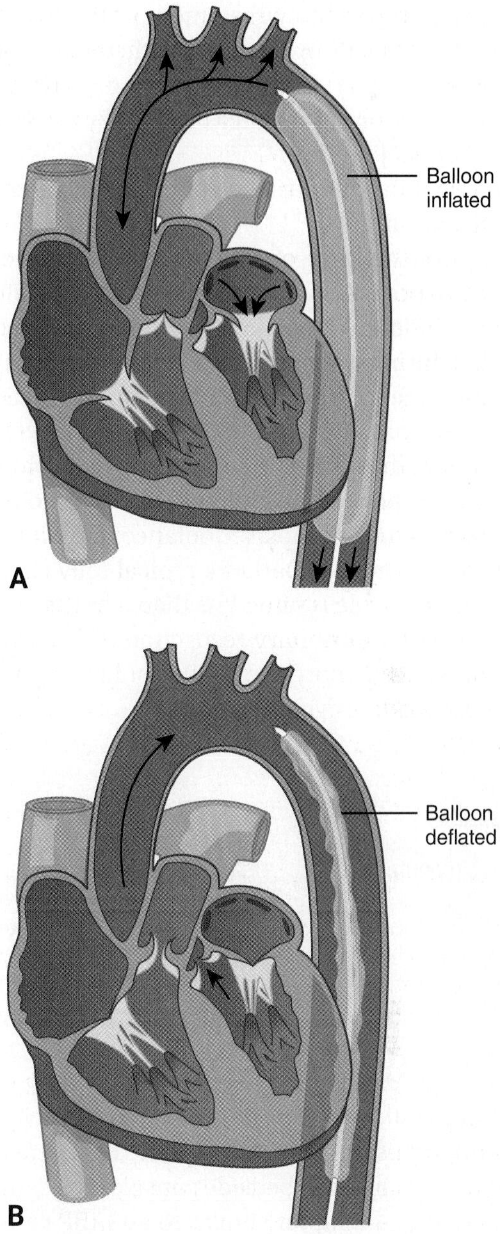

FIGURE 8 Mechanisms of action of the intra-aortic balloon pump. **A.** Diastolic balloon inflation augments coronary blood flow. **B.** Systolic balloon deflation decreases afterload.

Specific transport considerations for a patient with an IABP include the following:

- Carefully inspect the insertion site prior to transport to ensure the IABP catheter is secured in place. Note the length of the catheter at the insertion site so you can recognize any movement that might occur during transport.

- Perform periodic assessment of the insertion site for bleeding. The IABP catheter is inserted into an artery; thus, bleeding at the site can be serious. Control any such bleeding by application of direct pressure.
- Assess for the presence of pulses distal to the insertion site.
- Splint the knee on the insertion leg prior to transport. A knee splint serves as a helpful reminder to the patient not to flex the affected leg during transport. Leg flexion can result in movement of the IABP catheter and/or bleeding at the insertion site.
- Assure that the IABP console has been plugged into AC power and is fully charged prior to transport. Although most ambulances have inverter power, the life span of a typical fully charged IABP console is often less than 3 hours.
- If cardiopulmonary resuscitation is required during transport, the IABP should be switched to pressure triggering mode.

> NOTE
> Some manufacturers have adapters especially for transport in the event the transport team's pump is different from the model used at the referring facility. These adapters allow interfacing between the different pumps.

Continuous-Flow Pumps

Continuous-flow pumps provide temporary circulatory support using an axial flow pump connected to a catheter attached to a bedside console. The catheter is inserted in a manner similar to an IABP catheter (femorally) but, when used to support the left heart, is actually maneuvered up the aorta, across the aortic valve, and into the left ventricle. There, an inflow port pulls blood into the catheter, propelling it through an outflow port into the ascending aorta. The most commonly used continuous flow pump in the United States is the Impella heart pump. Currently there are Impella models available that are designed to provide flows from 2.5 L/min for the smallest catheter to 5 L/min for the largest model. A right heart Impella catheter is also available.

There are some transport considerations for paramedics accompanying a patient transported with an Impella continuous-flow device:[9]

- Securing the Impella console in the transport vehicle can be challenging. Although this console is designed with a bed mount on the back of its housing, this mount is not sufficient to secure the console for transport. The controller must be secured so that providers can see the screen, review alarms, and make adjustments as needed during transport.
- Proper patient positioning is crucial to operation of the Impella device. Patient movement—particularly upward and downward movement of the head of the stretcher—can result in malpositioning of the Impella catheter. Once the patient is comfortably positioned on the transport stretcher and the Impella device is functioning properly, the head of the stretcher should not be moved.
- Evaluation of Impella placement can be done during transport with echocardiography. Availability of a portable ultrasound machine with the appropriate probes and gel would be useful for Impella transport.
- The battery life of a fully charged Impella console is no more than 60 minutes. The console must be fully charged prior to transport and connected to a power source in the ambulance during transport.
- As with an IABP, the insertion site should be periodically assessed for bleeding, and any bleeding managed with direct pressure to the site.

Extracorporeal Membrane Oxygenation

ECMO is temporary support of a patient's heart and lung function by partial cardiopulmonary bypass (up to 75% of cardiac output). It is often used for patients who have reversible cardiopulmonary failure from pulmonary, cardiac, or other disease, and is often used in infants. There are several portable ECMO systems designed for transport use (**FIGURE 9**), though all rely on the same underlying principles.

An ECMO system is capable of providing blood flow as well as adding oxygen and removing carbon

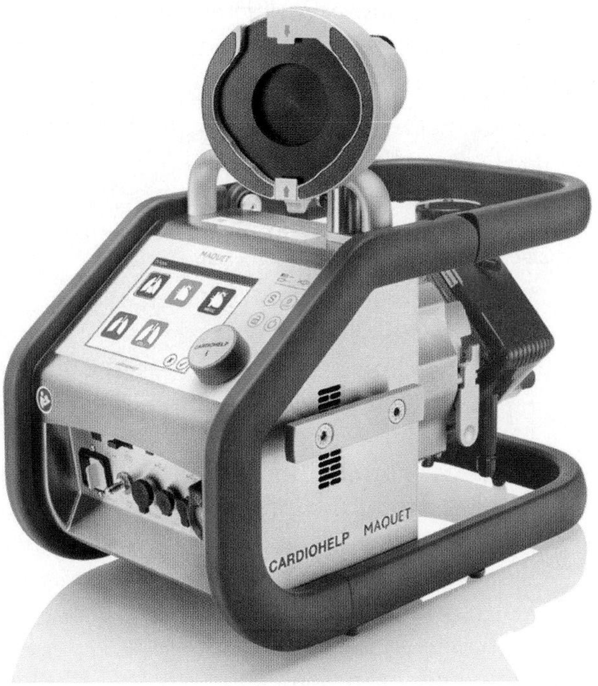

FIGURE 9 Portable extracorporeal membrane oxygenation systems can be used to provide temporary support of a patient's heart and lung function by partial cardiopulmonary bypass.

Reproduced from Maquet Cardiopulmonary GmbH, with permission.

dioxide from the blood. The circulatory function relies on a centrifugal pump, whereas the pulmonary function uses an artificial lung. The pump pushes the blood through a membrane gas exchanger (for oxygenation and carbon dioxide removal) and a warmer. The blood is then returned to the patient's circulation. ECMO requires anticoagulation of the patient usually with unfractionated heparin, guided by frequent measurements of activated clotting time.

There are three common configurations of ECMO circuits, depending on the reason for use:

- Venoarterial ECMO (VA-ECMO) bypasses the heart and lungs. VA-ECMO can be central, with blood being drained from the right atrium (via a right internal jugular venous catheter) and returned to the thoracic aorta (via a right carotid arterial catheter). It may also be peripheral, with the blood often being drained from a femoral artery and returned via a femoral vein approach into the inferior vena cava. VA-ECMO delivers circulatory and gas exchange support.
- Venovenous ECMO (VV-ECMO) returns blood prior to the lungs, providing gas exchange without circulatory support. It can also be central or peripheral. In central VV-ECMO, blood is drained from the right atrium (via side holes of a double-lumen catheter) and returned to the right atrium through the end hole of the catheter, which is directed toward the tricuspid valve. Peripheral VV-ECMO may involve the femoral artery to femoral vein approach; femoral vein to femoral vein approach; or femoral vein to internal jugular vein approach if circulation is intact. VV-ECMO requires good cardiac function and avoids cannulation of the carotid artery. With improved ECMO technology, the less invasive approaches are preferred when possible.
- Arteriovenous ECMO (AV-ECMO) employs the patient's own arterial pressure to circulate blood through an artificial lung.

The indications and reasons for ECMO support vary considerably among institutions. The Extracorporeal Life Support Organization is an excellent and authoritative source of information on uses and transport of ECMO. In general, ECMO is indicated for patients who fail to respond to conventional treatment for conditions that appear to be reversible:[10]

- Severe hypoxemic respiratory failure refractory to optimized ventilation
- Hypercapnic respiratory failure (pH <7.20) despite ventilator support
- Refractory cardiogenic shock
- Refractory septic shock (pediatric and neonate)
- Cardiac arrest
- Inability to wean from cardiopulmonary bypass
- Bridge to heart transplant or VAD placement

Bleeding (gastrointestinal, intracranial) is the most common complication of ECMO, given that ECMO cannulas are placed in large vessels and patients receiving such therapy are significantly anticoagulated. Other potential complications include thromboembolism, air embolism, limb ischemia, acute renal failure, and oxygenator failure. Transport of patients using ECMO systems should be done by specially trained transport teams using checklists designed to ensure that all the necessary equipment and supplies are carried in the transport unit.[7]

Ventricular Assist Devices

Ventricular assist devices (VADs) and left ventricular assist devices (LVADs) provide long-term support for patients with inadequate cardiac output. VADs are surgically implanted in patients with advanced heart failure who may or may not be candidates for transplant; they provide artificial circulatory support. LVADs are discussed in Chapter 21, *Cardiology*.

ICP Monitoring

As described in Chapter 39, *Head, Face, and Neck Trauma*, a rise in ICP can decrease cerebral perfusion. ICP monitoring is often used in patients with brain lesions, head trauma with bleeding or edema, hydrocephalus, encephalitis, and overproduction and/or insufficient absorption of cerebrospinal fluid. ICP can be monitored using an intraventricular cannula (the most common method), an epidural catheter, a subdural or subarachnoid monitoring device, or a fiberoptic transducer–tipped probe (**FIGURE 10**). All of these devices must be placed by a physician, and all monitoring systems require calibration (**BOX 3**).

The normal range for ICP in an adult is 5 to 15 mm Hg or less, but this can vary by person with position changes and activity level. For example, rotation of the head to either the right or the left and head-down positions can increase ICP significantly in both normal patients as well as those with head injury or stroke.[11] For patients with head trauma, the optimal positioning is not clear and varies by patient.[11]

Therapies that may be needed to control increasing ICP include the following:

- Maintain oxygenation to improve gas exchange.
- Avoid hypoxia and both hypocapnia and hypercapnia.
- Avoid maneuvers that might increase intrathoracic or intra-abdominal pressure (eg, coughing, Valsalva maneuver, patient movement, hip flexion).
- Prevent sudden variations in systemic blood pressure.
- Administer osmotic diuretics and/or steroids to reduce cerebral edema and inflammation.
- Restrict IV fluid therapy.
- Provide sedation to prevent agitation.
- Maintain normal body temperature.
- Avoid seizure activity.

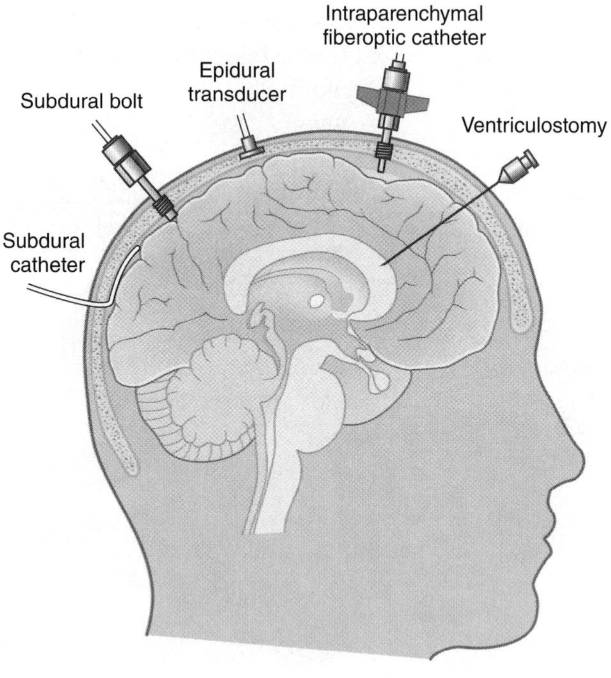

FIGURE 10 Intracranial pressure monitoring sites.

BOX 3 Important Considerations in ICP Monitoring

- Maintain sterile technique.
- Keep all stopcock ports capped unless one must be opened to expel air or to balance the transducer.
- Expel all air from the tubing or stopcock ports before connecting the line to the patient.
- Never flush any fluid into the patient's cranial cavity. Doing so will raise ICP and invite infection.

Blood Administration

As described in Chapter 11, *General Principles of Pathophysiology*, and Chapter 31, *Hematology*, blood replacement therapy may be indicated when caring for patients who have suffered acute blood loss and in some patients who have symptomatic anemia or other disorders. Blood products that commonly are administered to critically ill patients include packed red blood cells, fresh frozen plasma, and platelets. (Whole blood is not commonly available, but it is still used occasionally.) Because of the risk of transfusion reactions and the possible transmission of infectious disease, blood products should be given only when specifically indicated. The following steps help ensure safety when administering a blood transfusion:

1. The patient and blood product must be identified by two health care professionals.

2. Blood containing red blood cells must be compared to the patient's ABO group and Rh type. In extreme emergency situations, type-specific or O-negative (universal donor) blood may be transfused.[11]
3. The name and identification number on the patient's wristband must be compared to the slip on the blood bag.
4. The expiration date and time on the blood product must be identified. The blood bag should be turned upside down to gently mix it and inspect its contents for color and consistency.
5. The label must remain attached to the blood product until the transfusion is complete.

Blood and blood products can be safely administered through a peripheral IV line (18 gauge or larger is preferred), intraosseous, Portacath, and most central lines. Optimally, the tubing of the administration set should be connected directly to the access line and should not be piggybacked into an existing IV line (which can increase the risk of contamination). Peripheral IV access must be sufficient to maintain an adequate flow rate for the transfusion. Straight-type blood administration sets contain a standard filter in the tubing and are adequate for the administration of most blood products (**FIGURE 11**). Y-type blood/solution administration sets contain a standard filter in the tubing, with a Y-tubing segment above the filter to permit a dual connection for a blood component (eg, red blood cells) and saline.

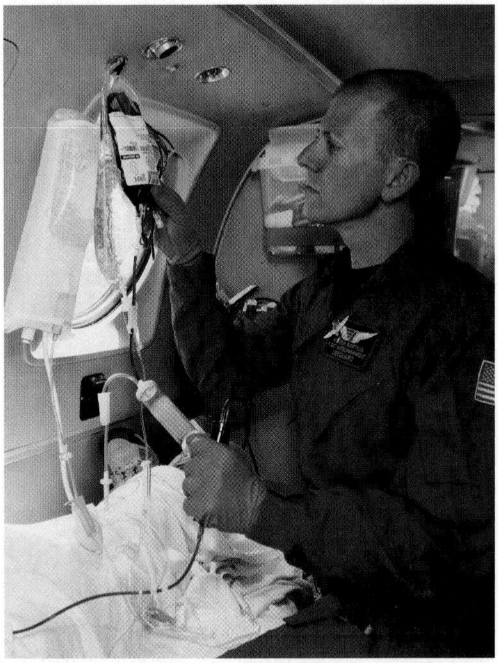

FIGURE 11 Blood administration set primed with normal saline.

> NOTE
> Paramedics who are considering blood administration should make sure administration of blood products falls within their state scope of practice. In some states, paramedics are permitted to monitor a blood transfusion that is already hanging but not initiate a new one.

IV Infusion Pumps

The standard of care for medication delivery during transport mandates use of an IV infusion pump for any continuously running medication. Infusion pumps maintain a more accurate flow rate when providing fluid and medication therapy compared to gravity systems. Many IV infusion pumps are available, and all require familiarity with the operating instructions for the specific device (**FIGURE 12**). Most models can be operated by battery as well as electric current. They incorporate warnings and alarms indicating low or high occlusion pressure, air in the tubing, infusion complete, and low battery power. All infusion pumps require frequent monitoring to ensure that they are accurately calibrated. During the infusion, a periodic assessment should include ensuring that the flow rate corresponds to the rate displayed on the IV infusion pump, and that the infusion site is patent. If any problems occur during IV therapy, the paramedic should check all alarms (per the manufacturer's instructions) and stop the IV infusion if necessary.

If the referring facility's IV pump tubing is not compatible with the transport unit's pump, it may be necessary to transfer the referring facility's medication into a syringe (for syringe pumps) or respike the referring facility's IV medication bag with the transport pump's tubing. The two greatest potential sources for error when using IV infusion pumps are as follows:

- Failing to check the medication concentration, dose, and rate to ensure the desired amount of medication is being properly administered to the patient
- Failing to confirm that sufficient medication is available to complete the transport

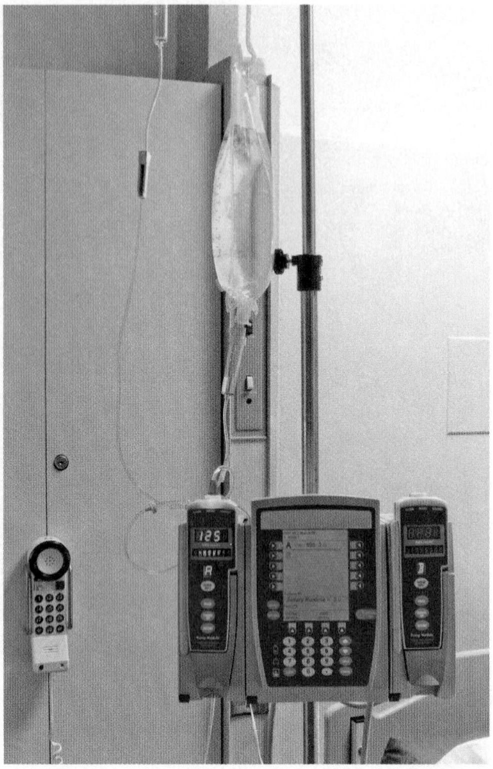

A

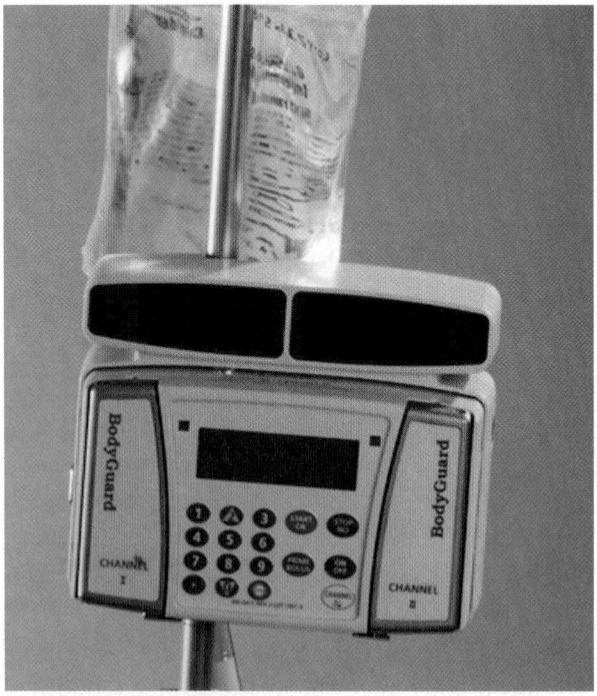

B

FIGURE 12 **A.** Electronic infusion device. **B.** Ambulatory infusion pump.

Prior to leaving the referring facility, it is important to address both of these needs.

Tube Thoracostomy

As described in Chapter 41, *Chest Trauma*, chest wall injury can result in pneumothorax, hemothorax, or hemopneumothorax. These potentially life-threatening conditions may need to be managed with pleural decompression, which can be achieved through needle thoracostomy (described in Chapter 41, *Chest Trauma*) or through tube thoracostomy.

Tube thoracostomy involves the insertion of a tube through the chest wall into the pleural space. The tube is usually secured to the chest wall with sutures and is further secured with an occlusive dressing and tape. It is then attached to suction to help with drainage.

Various chest wall drainage systems are available, but all work on the same principle as the original three-bottle system, described here for illustrative purposes (**FIGURE 13**). (Modern, rectangular plastic containers with three chambers have largely replaced the three-bottle system [**FIGURE 14**].) The first bottle or chamber collects the air, blood, or other fluid from the patient's pleural space through the chest tube. The second bottle or chamber is a water-seal bottle with a one-way valve that prevents air or fluid from moving backward into the first bottle. The third bottle contains water and is connected to suction. It controls the amount of suction either by a control valve or through a tube below the water surface. The higher the water level in the third bottle, the stronger the suction. (Some systems are waterless and contain a mechanical valve instead of water that allows drainage of blood or air.)

The chest tube remains in place until all or most of the air or fluid has been drained from the pleural space (usually a few days). Tube thoracostomy also is helpful in collecting infected fluid (eg, pus) that has accumulated in the pleural space from bacterial infection or tuberculosis. Components and management of chest drainage systems are outlined in **BOX 4**.

Care Considerations

After a chest tube is inserted, all tubing connections should be taped to minimize the risk of disconnection. Occlusive Vaseline gauze often is placed at the insertion site to minimize the risk of air leak. The chest drainage unit should be kept below the level of the

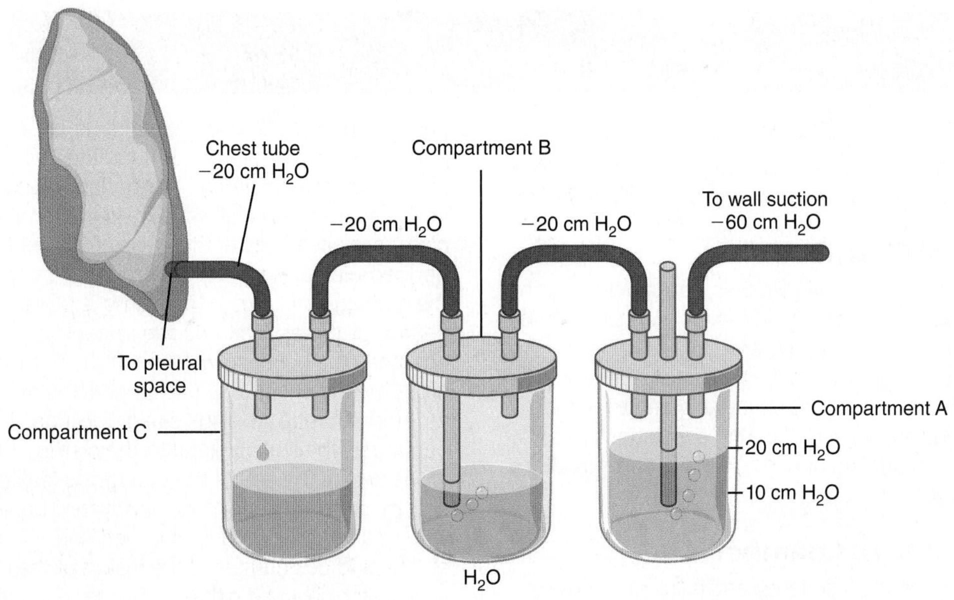

FIGURE 13 The standard three-bottle system is the basis for all commercial chest tube drainage systems. Pleural fluid and pleural air enter compartment C, which serves as a fluid collection trap so that the water-seal fluid volume will not rise (compartment B) and create resistance to air escaping the chest. Air cannot be inspired into the chest because of the water in compartment B. Open entrainment of room air through a submerged tube in compartment A buffers the amount of wall suction applied (−60 cm H_2O) to the height of the water column to standardize the pressure (−20 cm H_2O) transmitted to the chest.

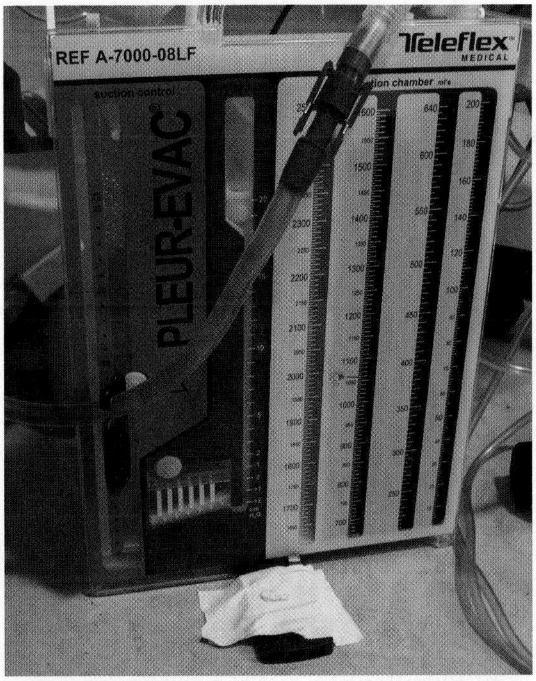

FIGURE 14 Chest tube drainage systems have three chambers: (1) a collection chamber, (2) a water-seal chamber, and (3) a suction control chamber. The suction control chamber requires a connection to a wall suction source that is dialed up higher than the prescribed suction for the suction to work.

chest when moving the patient, and the water-seal units should always be maintained in an upright position. Tubing must be monitored for accidental kinking. Initial chest tube drainage that is more than 50 ounces (1,500 mL) should be reported.

> **NOTE**
>
> If tube drainage stops suddenly, it is possible a clot has formed. If this occurs, the tube should be squeezed gently from its proximal end to its distal end. Avoid clamping the chest tube during transport: With some injuries, this action could lead to a tension pneumothorax. In some cases in which there is minimal drainage from the chest tube, a one-way valve may be attached to the tube during transport.
>
> *Modified from*: Weigand DL, ed. *AACN Procedure Manual for High Acuity, Progressive, and Critical Care*. 7th ed. St. Louis, MO: Elsevier; 2017.

During transport, all equipment should be assessed for air leaks and tube patency (BOX 5). Air leaks may be related to the chest drainage system, the injury to the lung, esophageal or bronchial injury, or a chest tube that is improperly placed. Persistent air leaks should be suspected if constant bubbling in the water-seal chamber is observed.

BOX 4 Chest Drainage Systems: Components and Management

Fluid Collection Chamber

Fluid drains from the patient through a long tube to a collection chamber, marked for assessment of drainage.

Water-Seal Chamber

Air is allowed to pass out, via bubbles, through the bottom of the chamber. It is often calibrated for measuring intrathoracic pressure and may have a float valve to protect the patient from high negativity. With the water-seal chamber, during spontaneous respirations, the water level should rise during inhalation and fall during exhalation. This oscillation is called tidaling and is one indicator of a patent pleural chest tube.

Suction Control Chamber

This chamber improves drainage and helps overcome the air leak. Suction control should be −10 to −20 cm H_2O. Dry suction control systems provide many advantages: Higher suction pressure levels can be achieved, setup is easy, no continuous bubbling provides for quiet operation, and there is no fluid to evaporate, which would decrease the amount of suction applied to the patient. Instead of regulating the level of suction with a column of water, dry suction units are controlled by a self-compensating regulator. Suction can be set at −10, −15, −20, −30, or −40 cm H_2O. The unit is preset at −20 cm H_2O when opened. Patient situations that may require higher suction pressures of −30 or −40 cm H_2O include a large air leak from the lung surface, empyema, a reduction in pulmonary compliance, or anticipated difficulty in expansion of the pulmonary tissue.

Paramedic Responsibilities

Secure and tape all connections prior to transport. Monitor catheters to prevent kinking. Monitor drainage output. Assess for air leaks. Maintain the unit in an upright position.

Assessing for Air Leaks

Look at the underwater seal. Leaks may originate with the patient or the drainage system. (Check the patient history. Would you expect a patient-source air leak?) For a patient receiving mechanical ventilation with positive end-expiratory pressure, leaking causes continuous bubbling. Note the pattern of the bubbling. If it fluctuates with respirations (ie, occurs on exhalation in a patient breathing spontaneously), the most likely source is the lung. Momentarily clamp the chest tube at the dressing site with a toothless/padded clamp. Move the clamp incrementally toward the drainage unit: When the clamp is placed between the source of the air leak and the water-seal/air-leak meter chamber, the bubbling will stop. If the bubbling stops the first time the chest tube is clamped, the air leak must be at the chest tube insertion site or the lung. If the bubbling continues, the leak is distal to the clamp. If the bubbling stops before the end of the tubing, the leak is in the tube, so it must be replaced. If the unit is still bubbling when the very end of the tubing is clamped, the unit has the leak and should be changed. If the leak is at the insertion site, remove the chest tube dressing and inspect the site. Make sure the catheter eyelets have not pulled out beyond the chest wall. Replace the dressing. Notify the physician of any new, increased, or unexpected air leaks that are not corrected by these actions.

Indications of Patency

The water level in the water seal should fluctuate with breathing, rising with inspiration and falling with expiration, and is an indicator of chest tube patency. If the patient is on mechanical ventilation, this pattern is reversed, because breaths are delivered under positive pressure. Fluctuations stop when the lung is fully reexpanded or when the tube is kinked or compressed.

Milking/Stripping the Tube

Vigorous milking or stripping can create dangerously high negative pressures, placing the patient at risk for mediastinal trauma.

To Clamp or Not to Clamp?

Never clamp a chest tube during patient transport unless the chest drainage system becomes disrupted during patient movement—and even then only if there is no air leak. Clamping the chest tube can create a tension pneumothorax.

Modified from: Weigand DL, ed. *AACN Procedure Manual for High Acuity, Progressive, and Critical Care*. 7th ed. St. Louis, MO: Elsevier; 2017.

Pericardiocentesis

Pericardiocentesis is an invasive procedure in which a needle is inserted in the pericardial sac to aspirate blood or fluid. The primary indication for pericardiocentesis is pericardial tamponade. Pericardiocentesis carries significant risk, including penetration through the surface of the heart. Other potential complications include laceration of a coronary artery, laceration of the lung or liver, cardiac dysrhythmias, and increased tamponade.

Ultrasound-guided pericardiocentesis is commonly used today, as it reduces the rate of complications. The

BOX 5 Checking for Air Leaks in a Chest Drainage System

1. Occlude the chest or drainage tube intermittently along the length of the system.
2. Reinforce the chest dressing and all connections.
3. If bubbling disappears when you occlude the tubing close to the drainage unit, this suggests an air leak is still present; consider replacing the unit if possible.

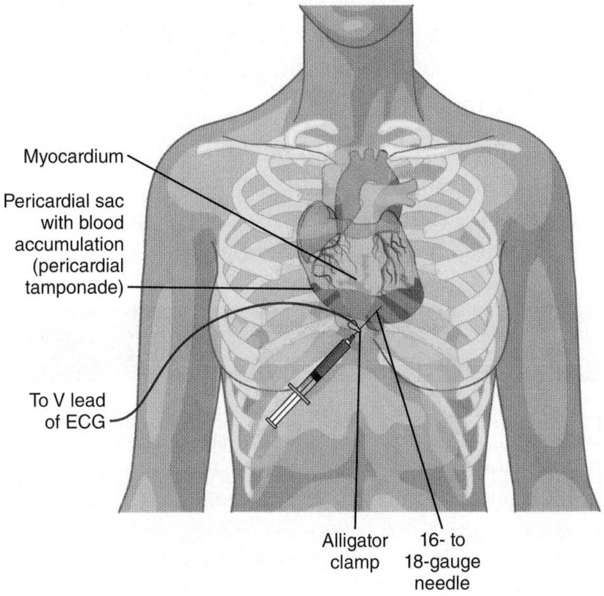

Abbreviation: ECG, electrocardiogram

FIGURE 15 Pericardiocentesis.

procedure for pericardiocentesis that is not guided by ultrasound is as follows (**FIGURE 15**):

1. Using aseptic technique, insert a 3-inch, 16- or 18-gauge needle (attached to a 50-cc syringe) at the angle of the xiphoid cartilage and the seventh rib.
2. Advance the needle at a 45° angle to the skin toward the left midclavicular line while aspirating the syringe with negative pressure. If the needle is advanced too far, a pulsation will be felt through the needle and syringe.
3. Aspirate as much fluid as possible. Fluid is usually encountered at a depth of 3 to 4 cm. (Removal of as little as 20 to 25 mL of blood from a distended pericardium may produce a dramatic blood pressure response.)
4. After withdrawing blood from the pericardial sac, attach a surgical clamp to the needle at the level of the skin to avoid accidental advancement of the needle.
5. If tamponade reoccurs, aspirate blood again if necessary.

Ultrasound

Ultrasound, or the use of high-frequency sound waves to image structures and fluids inside the body, has played an increasingly important role in medicine over the past decade. Portable, handheld ultrasound units can be used by transport crews for line placement, confirmation of tube and catheter placements, assessment of heart function and fluid volume status, and determination of the presence or absence of a pneumothorax (**FIGURE 16**). Use of ultrasound requires advanced training and frequent practice to maintain competency. It is likely that ultrasound will become a common prehospital tool of the future, given the many applications it has assumed in the critical care and emergency medicine environments.

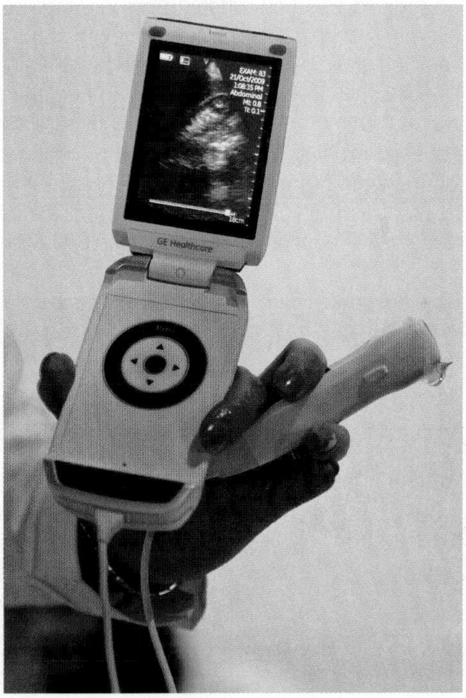

FIGURE 16 Portable, handheld ultrasound units can be used by transport crews for line placement, confirmation of tube and catheter placements, assessment of heart function and fluid volume status, and determination of the presence or absence of a pneumothorax.

Special Transport Considerations in Critical Care

Transporting patients with critical care needs can present special challenges for the paramedic, especially in regard to the unique equipment required for their care—equipment that is often unfamiliar to the EMS crew. Specific considerations that are discussed in this section are management of IV drug drips, use of push-dose pressors, and transport ventilators.

Managing IV Drug Drips

A number of IV drugs are administered via continuous infusion to critical care patients—for example, diltiazem, dobutamine, dopamine, fentanyl, furosemide, midazolam, norepinephrine, and vasopressin, among others (**BOX 6**) (see Appendix A, *Emergency Drug Index*). When preparing to transport a patient who is receiving an IV infusion of a drug that is unfamiliar to the paramedic, the paramedic should take the following steps:

1. Consult with the physician or nurse caring for the patient before transport.
2. Ensure that the prescribed drip rate is documented and clearly understood.

> **NOTE**
>
> Technical mishaps that are common in CCT include accidental extubation, ventilator disconnect, ECG monitor power failure, vasoactive drug interruption, and IV infiltration or disconnection.

> **DID YOU KNOW?**
>
> **Flight Paramedics**
>
> Flight paramedics (**FIGURE 17**) have played an important role in CCT since the 1970s. In 1986, these specialty care professionals united to form the National Flight Paramedic Association, which is now known as the International Association of Flight and Critical Care Paramedics. This organization focused attention on the need for quality improvements within the industry by helping found the Commission on Accreditation of Air Medical Services in 1990, now known as the Commission on Accreditation of Medical Transport Systems. Some flight paramedics have special training and certification in critical care procedures and flight physiology—namely, the FP-C certification. Air medical transport is further described in Chapter 52, *Ground and Air Ambulance Operations*.
>
>
>
> **FIGURE 17** Flight paramedics.
> © ZUMA Press, Inc./Alamy Stock Photo.
>
> ---
>
> *Modified from*: Holleran R, ed. *ASTNA Patient Transport: Principles and Practice*. 4th ed. St. Louis, MO: Mosby Elsevier; 2010.

BOX 6 IV Drugs Used in Critical Care[a]	
Abciximab	Infliximab
Alteplase	Insulin
Aminophylline	Ketamine
Amiodarone	Labetalol
Argatroban	Lepirudin
Atracurium	Lidocaine
Bivalirudin	Lorazepam
Bumetanide	Magnesium sulfate
Cisatracurium	Midazolam
Clevidipine	Milrinone
Dexmedetomidine	Nicardipine
Diltiazem	Nitroglycerin
Dobutamine	Nitroprusside
Dopamine	Norepinephrine
Epinephrine	Octreotide
Epoprostenol	Pantoprazole
Eptifibatide	Phenylephrine
Esmolol	Potassium chloride
Furosemide	Procainamide
Haloperidol	Propofol
Heparin	Reteplase
Hydromorphone	Tenecteplase
Ibutilide	Tirofiban HCl
Immune globulin	Vasopressin

[a]All infusions should be verified through medical direction or written protocol.

Modified from: Algozzine G, Lilly DJ, Algozzine R. *Critical Care Infusion Drug Handbook*. 3rd ed. St. Louis, MO: Mosby Elsevier; 2009.

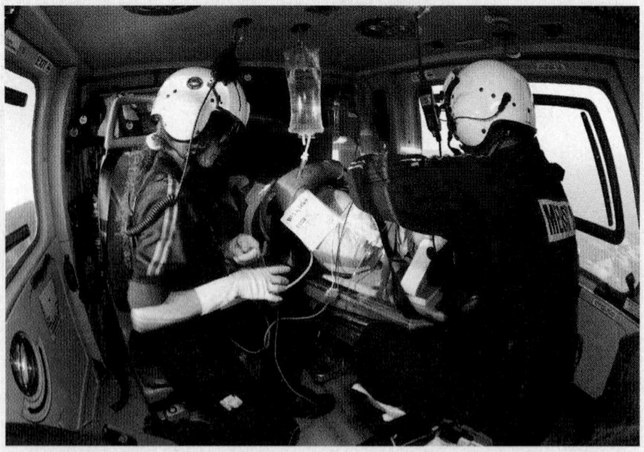

3. Ensure personal comfort with the operation of the infusion equipment and the meaning and management of any equipment alarms.
4. Ask about any suspected complications or possible adverse reactions associated with the drug.
5. Confirm there is sufficient volume of drug remaining to meet the needs of the patient during transport.

Paramedics who are transporting a patient who is receiving an unfamiliar drug(s) should have ready access to an infusion drip chart or electronic drug dose information source.

Intubated patients undergoing continuous sedation warrant particular attention from the paramedic. Although neuromuscular blocking agents (paralytics) are used to facilitate intubation, they are rarely used as continuous infusions except in the most critically ill patients. Any patient under the influence of a paralytic agent must also receive a sedative and/or analgesic. Currently, patients who are sedated for the purposes of facilitating continued mechanical ventilation often receive an infusion of a short-acting sedative such as propofol, dexmedetomidine, or midazolam, as well as a narcotic analgesic such as fentanyl or morphine. The synergistic effects of the two agents together mean that less drug is needed than when using either agent alone. Of particular importance to the paramedic is the extremely short duration of action of the sedative agents. The effects of propofol and dexmedetomidine diminish within minutes of stopping or decreasing the infusion. This could have untoward effects if a drip stops or runs out during transport, resulting in the patient rapidly awakening.

Sedation can also interfere with patients being able to communicate when they are in pain. The paramedic should be observant for signs such as increased respiratory rate, tachycardia, hypertension, and restlessness that may indicate painful conditions rather than a need for increased sedation. If possible, asking a patient who is awake enough to interact about his or her pain level will help with decision making about analgesia and sedative titration.

Push-Dose Pressors

Anesthesia providers have for many years drawn a syringe full of an available pressor infusion and used it to administer a bolus dose to treat hypotension.[12] The name push-dose pressors came from this practice, which is now widely used in critical care, emergency medicine, and some EMS systems. The two most commonly employed push-dose pressor medications are epinephrine and phenylephrine.

Indications for push-dose pressors include situations in which a patient with profound hypotension fails to respond to fluid boluses and vasopressors are either not yet mixed and infusing or fail to produce an increase in blood pressure. Patients who require push-dose pressors might include those with propofol-induced hypotension, postintubation hypotension, tachydysrhythmia-induced hypotension, or profound vasoplegia.

Push-dose pressors are very dilute. In the case of epinephrine, 0.1 mg (1 mL of 0.1 mg/mL solution) is mixed with 9 mL normal saline to make a total of 10 mL, yielding a concentration of 10 mcg/mL.[12] With an onset of action of approximately 1 minute, push doses of 0.5 to 2 mL (5 to 20 mcg) would be appropriate to administer every 1 to 5 minutes.

Phenylephrine, unlike epinephrine, has no beta effects. It is used for vasoconstriction and is usually mixed in a 100 mcg/mL solution. With an onset of action of approximately 1 minute, push doses of 0.5 to 2 mL (50 to 200 mcg) would be appropriate to administer every 1 to 5 minutes.

Vasopressor infusions warrant additional attention from the paramedic. Whenever possible, vasopressors should be infused into a central line to avoid the risks of extravasation that can occur with peripheral IV infusions. If the vasopressor is infusing through a peripheral line, the paramedic should assess the site initially and periodically during transport for signs of infiltration. It is imperative to note the rate of the infusion and plan for enough medication to continue the infusion throughout transport. The paramedic should consider also the potential need to increase the infusion rate and how much additional medication that might require.

Ideally, patients receiving pressor infusions should have their blood pressure monitored with an arterial line. When that is not available, electronic cuff pressures should be obtained at minimum every 5 minutes and, when titrating any vasoactive infusion, at 1-minute intervals.

Managing Transport Ventilators

During interfacility transport, it is recommended that a transport ventilator be used. Evidence shows that manual ventilation is not reliable because of the difficulty maintaining consistent depth and volume of ventilation.[13] Transitioning a patient from a hospital ventilator to a transport ventilator (and vice versa) is often a complicated procedure, which can be a source of anxiety for the patient and the paramedic crew. Although many different ventilator devices are used in both in-hospital and prehospital care, the same guidelines for transition between the devices should always be followed:[14]

1. Move the patient to the transport stretcher.
2. Prepare all necessary equipment and supplies.
3. Check that all equipment is functioning properly. Ensure sufficient oxygen is available for the duration of the transport by calculating the flow rate as well as the volume consumption versus the amount of available oxygen.
4. Ensure emergency airway equipment is readily available.
5. Assemble all equipment near the head of the stretcher.
6. Duplicate the settings of the transferring facility's ventilator on the transport unit's ventilator.
7. Disconnect the patient from the transferring facility's ventilator, attach the patient to the transport ventilator, and put the transferring facility's ventilator on standby.
8. During the transition, ensure that mechanical ventilation continues. The rate and depth of mechanical ventilation should closely simulate the rate and depth that were provided by the transferring facility's ventilator.
9. Closely observe the patient for tolerance of the change in mode of ventilation.

Ventilator Alarms

Ventilator alarms are set to warn of mechanical or physiologic problems. In turn, continuous monitoring of the patient and alarm parameters is important. During transport, ventilator alarms may be difficult to hear. They should be set to the maximum volume, and the ventilator should be positioned so that flashing warning lights are visible. BOX 7 provides guidelines for troubleshooting common ventilator alarms.

BOX 7 Troubleshooting Ventilator Alarms

1. Initial assessment:
   - **Airway.** Is the endotracheal (ET) tube in the correct position? Check ET tube insertion depth, end-tidal carbon dioxide, and breath sounds.
   - **Breathing.** Check breath sounds, look for chest excursion, check pulse oximetry and end-tidal carbon dioxide, check patient color.
   - **Circulation.** Check the pulse, ECG, and blood pressure.
2. Remove the patient from the ventilator and manually use a resuscitation bag if any compromise is found. Check for the following conditions:
   - Alarm
   - Cause
   - Management
   - Apnea
   - Insufficient spontaneous breathing by a nonintubated patient in continuous positive airway pressure or pressure-support mode
3. Switch the ventilator mode to one that provides a set rate of ventilations. Check for the following conditions:
   - High airway pressure
   - ET tube obstruction: sputum, kink, biting
   - Decreased compliance or increased resistance
   - Circumferential burns
   - Bronchospasm, lung collapse, pneumothorax, endobronchial intubation, worsening of lung process
   - Patient's anxiety, fear, pain, fighting of ventilator
   - Need to suction airway
4. Treat the cause of the resistance.
   - Adjust the mode or settings.
   - Rule out hypoxia and hypercapnia before treating agitation.
   - Change the ventilator mode to one that is better tolerated or provides sedation/analgesia.
   - Check for and remedy low airway pressure.
   - Check for and remedy ventilator disconnect.
   - Check for and remedy a leak in the ventilator system.
   - Check for and remedy a cuff leak.
   - Check for and remedy inadvertent extubation.
   - Ensure that all connections are intact and tight.
   - Troubleshoot the ET tube cuff.
   - Use a bag-mask device for ventilation if the ET tube was dislodged.
   - Check whether the oxygen pressure is too low.
   - Check whether the oxygen cylinder is empty.
   - Check for a closed cylinder valve.
   - Check for and remedy a unit that is not connected to the wall terminal.
   - Make sure the aircraft/ambulance oxygen flow is not in the off position.
   - Check the wall and cylinder connections.
   - Ventilate the patient with a bag-mask device until the problem is resolved.

Modified from: Holleran R, ed. *ASTNA Patient Transport: Principles and Practice.* 4th ed. St. Louis, MO: Mosby Elsevier; 2010.

References

1. Department of Health and Human Services, Centers for Medicare and Medicaid Services. *CMS Manual System*. Pub 100-02. Medicare Benefit Policy, Transmittal 130. Centers for Medicare and Medicaid Services website. https://www.cms.gov/Regulations-and-Guidance/Guidance/Transmittals/downloads/R130BP.pdf. Published July 29, 2010. Accessed April 25, 2018.
2. Clinical practice and management: appropriate interfacility transfer. American College of Emergency Physicians website. https://www.acep.org/Clinical---Practice-Management/Appropriate-Interfacility-Patient-Transfer/#sm.00017ocpq4y7l-crguyk1mzjca2nE. Published January 2016. Accessed April 25, 2018.
3. Shelton SL, Swor RA, Domeier RM, Lucas R. Position paper: medical direction of interfacility transports. *Prehosp Emerg Care.* October/December 2000;4(4):361-364. National Association of EMS Physicians website. http://www.naemsp.org/Documents/Position%20Papers/POSITION%20MedDirofInterfacilityTransports.pdf. Accessed April 25, 2018.
4. Keeperman JB. Interfacility transportation. In: Brice J, Delbridge TR, Meyers JB, eds. *Emergency Services: Clinical Practice and Systems Oversight.* Vol 2. 2nd ed. West Sussex, UK: John Wiley & Sons; 2015:29-35.
5. Collopy KT. What's the point of point-of-care testing? *EMS World* website. https://www.emsworld.com/article/11289724/whats-point-point-care-testing. Published January 6, 2014. Accessed April 17, 2018.
6. *Principles of Invasive Hemodynamics*. RN.com website. https://lms.rn.com/getpdf.php/1866.pdf. Updated December 18, 2016. Accessed April 25, 2018.
7. Weigand DL, ed. *AACN Procedure Manual for High Acuity, Progressive, and Critical Care.* 7th ed. St. Louis, MO: Elsevier; 2017.

8. American Academy of Orthopaedic Surgeons. *Critical Care Transport.* 2nd ed. Burlington, MA: Jones & Bartlett Learning; 2017.
9. *Patient Transport With the Automated Impella Controller.* Abiomed website. https://s3-us-west-2.amazonaws.com/abiomed-private/assets/files/Abiomed.com/IMP-1255-16+Patient+Transport+with+AIC+Brochure.pdf. Accessed April 17, 2018.
10. Lequier L, Lorusso R, MacLaren G, et al. *Extracorporeal Life Support: The ELSO Red Book.* Ann Arbor, MI: Extracorporeal Life Support Organization; 2017.
11. Sole ML, Klein DG, Moseley MJ. *Introduction to Critical Care Nursing.* 7th ed. St. Louis, MO: Elsevier; 2017.
12. Weingart S. Push-dose pressors for immediate blood pressure control. *Clin Exper Emerg Med.* 2015;2(2):131-132.
13. Blakeman TC, Branson RD. Inter- and intra-hospital transport of the critically ill. *Resp Care.* 2013;58(6):1008-1023.
14. Branson RD. Intrahospital transport of critically ill, mechanically ventilated patients. *Resp Care.* 1992;37:775-793.

Suggested Readings

Aguiar Carneiro T, da Paixão D, Tayse T, et al. Critical patient transport: a challenge for the 21st century. *J Nurs.* 2017;11(1):70-76.

Alabdali A, Trivedy C, Aljerian N, et al. Incidence and predictors of adverse events and outcomes for adult critically ill patients transferred by paramedics to a tertiary care medical facility. *J Health Specialties.* 2017;5(4):206-211.

Bergman LM, Pettersson ME, Chaboyer WP, et al. Safety hazards during intrahospital transport: a prospective observational study. *Crit Care Med.* 2017;45(10):e1043-e1049.

Biscotti M, Agerstrand C, Abrams D. One hundred transports on extracorporeal support to an extracorporeal membrane oxygenation center. *Ann Thorac Surg.* 2015;100(1):34-39; discussion 39-40.

Doyle GR, McCutcheon JA. Clinical procedures for safer patient care. British Columbia Institute of Technology website. 2015. https://open.bccampus.ca/find-open-textbooks/?uuid=fbbb4840-eda5-4265-9f1c-d6d8008402a9&contributor=&keyword=&subject=. Accessed April 17, 2018.

Francielli MPG, de Camargo WHB, Gomes ACB, et al. Analysis of adverse events during intrahospital transportation of critically ill patients. *Crit Care Res Pract.* 2017;2017:6847124.

Schartel SA, Yeh EL. Transport of critically ill patients. In: Criner G, Barnette R, D'Alonzo G, eds. *Critical Care Study Guide.* New York, NY: Springer; 2010.

Singh JM, MacDonald RD, Ahghari M. Critical events during land-based interfacility transport. *Ann Emerg Med.* 2014;64(1):9-15.

Wilcox SR, Saia MS, Waden H, et al. Mechanical ventilation in critical care transport. *Air Med J.* 2016;35(3):161-165.

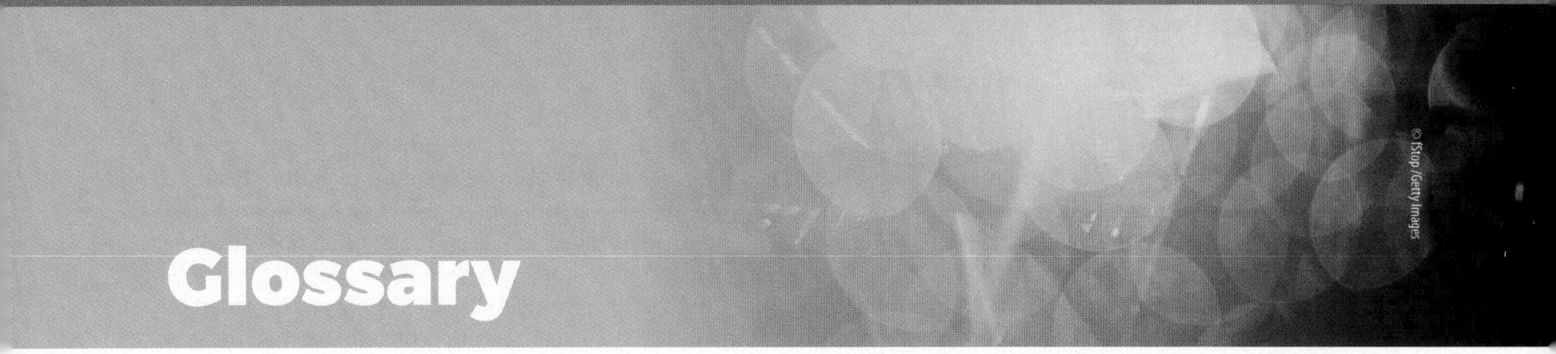

Glossary

abandonment The act of terminating medical care without legal excuse or of turning care over to personnel who do not have the training and expertise appropriate for the patient's medical needs.

abdominal aorta The portion of the descending aorta that passes from the aortic hiatus of the diaphragm into the abdomen, where it divides into the two common iliac arteries.

abdominal aortic aneurysm (AAA) A localized dilation and weakness of the wall of the abdominal aorta.

aberration The abnormal conduction of impulses through cardiac conduction pathways.

abrasion A partial-thickness injury caused by scraping or rubbing away of a layer or layers of skin.

abruptio placentae A partial or full detachment of a normally implanted placenta at more than 20 weeks' gestation; also known as placental abruption.

absence seizures Seizures characterized by brief lapses of consciousness without loss of posture; also known as petit mal seizures.

absolute refractory period The portion of the action potential during which the membrane is insensitive to subsequent electrical stimuli.

absorption The process by which drug molecules are moved from the site of entry into the body into the general circulation.

accelerated junctional rhythm A dysrhythmia that results from increased automaticity of the atrioventricular junction.

acceleration An increase in the velocity of a moving object.

accessory muscles Muscles that sometimes assist in breathing. They include the scalene muscles and the sternocleidomastoid, deep muscles of the neck and thorax, posterior neck and back muscles, pectoralis major, pectoralis minor, and abdominal muscles.

accountable care organization (ACO) Payment models in which a health insurance entity, most commonly Medicare but private insurance as well, shares financial responsibility for all the health care received by a defined patient population with providers or health care organizations.

acetabulum The large, cup-shaped articular cavity at the juncture of the ilium, the ischium, and the pubis that contains the ball-shaped head of the femur.

acetate A by-product of fatty acids in the liver.

acetylcholine A neurotransmitter, widely distributed in body tissues, with the primary function of mediating the synaptic activity of the nervous system.

Achilles tendon The largest tendon in the body; connects the calf muscle to the heel bone; also known as the tendon calcaneus.

Achilles tendon rupture A complete tear through the Achilles tendon.

acid–base balance The body's balance between acidity and alkalinity.

acidosis A condition marked by a high concentration of hydrogen ions (ie, a pH below 7.35).

acids Compounds that yield hydrogen ions when dissociated in solution.

acquired immunity Immunity that develops after exposure to specific antigens; also known as adaptive immunity.

action plan A plan of action based on the patient's condition and the environment.

action potential A change in membrane potential in an excitable tissue that acts as an electrical signal and is propagated in an all-or-none fashion.

active transport A carrier-mediated process that can move substances against a concentration gradient; assisted by enzymes and requires energy.

acute arterial occlusion A sudden blockage of arterial flow, most commonly caused by embolization or thrombosis.

acute chest syndrome A serious vaso-occlusive crisis in the pulmonary vasculature that often presents as an abnormal consolidation on a chest radiograph in a patient with sickle cell disease.

acute coronary syndrome (ACS) A spectrum of clinical disease that is the result of compromise of blood flow through the coronary arteries; includes acute myocardial infarction and unstable angina.

acute gastroenteritis Inflammation of the stomach and intestines with an associated sudden onset of vomiting and diarrhea.

acute kidney injury (AKI) A clinical syndrome that results from a sudden, significant decrease in filtration through the glomeruli, leading to the accumulation of salt, water, and nitrogenous wastes in the body; also known as acute renal failure.

acute lung injury (ALI) Acute onset of pulmonary inflammation with impaired gas exchange and radiologic appearance of pulmonary edema without evidence of heart failure; similar pathology to acute respiratory distress syndrome with less mortality.

acute mesenteric ischemia An abrupt interruption of intestinal blood flow. It may result from an embolism, thrombosis, or a low-flow state (decreased perfusion).

acute mountain sickness (AMS) A common high-altitude illness that results when an unacclimatized person rapidly ascends to high altitudes.

acute myocardial infarction (AMI) Blockage of blood flow within one or more of the coronary arteries causing tissue hypoxia and death of cardiac tissue.

acute prostatitis Inflammation of the prostate gland that develops suddenly.

acute psychosis A condition that refers to a patient who presents with one or more of the following criteria: a sudden onset of delusions that rapidly change; hallucinations; bizarre behavior and posture; or disorganized speech.

acute respiratory distress syndrome (ARDS) A fulminant form of respiratory failure characterized by acute lung inflammation and diffuse alveolar–capillary injury.

acute tubular necrosis The death of tubular cells, which form the tubule that transports urine to the ureters.

adaptation A cellular response to stress of any kind that seeks to escape and protect from injury; a central part of the response to changes in the physiologic condition.

addiction A compulsive, uncontrollable dependence on a substance, habit, or practice to such a degree that cessation causes severe emotional, mental, or physiologic reactions.

Addison disease A rare and potentially life-threatening disorder caused by a deficiency of the corticosteroid hormones normally produced by the adrenal cortex.

adenosine triphosphate (ATP) A nucleotide composed of adenosine, an organic base, with three phosphate groups attached to it. It stores energy in muscles.

adipose tissue A specialized connective tissue that stores lipids; also known as fat tissue.

administrative law Regulations developed by a government agency to provide details about the function and process of the law.

adolescent A person 13 to 18 years of age.

adrenaline An endogenous adrenal hormone that helps prepare the body for energetic action.

adrenergic Of or pertaining to the sympathetic nerve fibers of the autonomic nervous system, which use epinephrine or epinephrine-like substances as neurotransmitters.

adsorb To accumulate on a surface in a condensed layer.

advance directive A legal document in which a person specifies what should be done for his or her health if the person is unable to make medical decisions because of injury, illness, or lack of decision-making capacity.

advanced life support (ALS) A level of care provided by paramedics or allied health professionals that includes advanced airway management, defibrillation, intravenous therapy, and medication administration.

advanced old age A new age category that includes people older than 75 years.

adverse drug event (ADE) An injury resulting from the use of a drug.

aerobic Of or pertaining to the presence of air or oxygen.

aerobic oxidation A biochemical reaction that increases the positive charges on an atom or the loss of negative charges in the presence of oxygen.

affect An outward manifestation of a person's feelings or emotions.

afferent division The division of the peripheral nervous system that transmits impulses from the periphery to the central nervous system.

afferent neurons Neurons that carry action potentials from the periphery to the central nervous system.

afterdrop phenomenon A sudden return of cold blood and waste products to the core of the body as a result of rewarming methods used to treat hypothermia.

afterload The total resistance against which blood must be pumped; also known as peripheral vascular resistance.

agonist A drug that combines with receptors and initiates the expected response.

air embolism The presence of air bubbles in the bloodstream.

airborne precautions Steps taken to avoid infection spread by airborne droplet nuclei (typically 5 microns or smaller in size). Such steps include wearing an N95 respirator or powered air-purifying respirator.

albumin A water-soluble protein containing carbon, hydrogen, oxygen, nitrogen, and sulfur.

alcohol dependence A disorder characterized by chronic, excessive consumption of alcohol that results in injury to health or in inadequate social function and the development of withdrawal symptoms when the person suddenly stops drinking.

aldosterone A steroid hormone produced by the adrenal cortex to regulate the sodium and potassium balance in the blood.

algorithm A process or set of rules to be followed during a clinical scenario; commonly used format for clinical guidelines.

alkalosis A condition marked by a low concentration of hydrogen ions (ie, a pH above 7.45).

allergens Antigens that can produce hypersensitivity reactions in the body.

allergic reaction A hypersensitivity response to an allergen to which a person previously was exposed and to which the person has developed antibodies.

allergy A hypersensitivity reaction to intrinsically harmless antigens, most of which are environmental.

allografting The transplantation of cells, tissues, or organs between nonidentical (genetically unrelated) people.

alpha-adrenergic receptor Any one of the postulated adrenergic components of receptor tissues that responds to norepinephrine and to various blocking agents.

alternative time sampling Sampling to prevent bias by assigning a treatment group based on the day, week, or month in which patients are encountered in a study.

alveoli Minute air sacs in the lungs through which gas exchange takes place between alveolar air and pulmonary capillary blood.

Alzheimer disease A disease characterized by confusion, memory failure, disorientation, speech disturbances, and inability to carry out purposeful movements.

amblyopia A condition in which the brain favors use of one eye over the eye, potentially causing vision problems and disuse of the unfavored eye; the most common cause of eye vision problems in children; also known as lazy eye.

ambulance A generic term that describes the various land-based emergency vehicles used by EMS personnel, including basic and advanced life support units, paramedic units, mobile intensive care units, and others.

amino acids Organic chemical compounds composed of one or more basic amino groups and one or more acidic carboxyl groups.

ammonium ions The monovalent cations symbolized by NH_4^+.

amnesia Memory loss.

amniotic fluid Fluid in the amniotic sac.

amniotic fluid embolism An embolism that occurs when amniotic fluid gains access to maternal circulation during labor or delivery or immediately after delivery.

amniotic sac A thin-walled bag that contains the fetus and amniotic fluid during pregnancy.

amputation A complete or partial loss of a limb caused by mechanical force.

amyloidosis The accumulation of amyloid protein in tissues and organs of the body.

amyotrophic lateral sclerosis (ALS) One of a group of rare disorders in which the nerves that control muscular activity degenerate in the brain and spinal cord; also known as Lou Gehrig disease.

anaerobic Of or pertaining to the absence of oxygen.

anal abscess An infected, pus-filled cavity near the rectum.

anal fistula An abnormal passage between the end of the bowel and the cutaneous surface of the anus.

anaphylactic shock A form of distributive shock that occurs when the body is exposed to a substance that produces a severe, exaggerated, life-threatening hypersensitivity reaction to an antigen.

anaphylactoid reaction An allergic reaction that is not mediated by an antigen–antibody reaction. It presents exactly like anaphylaxis but does not require previous exposure.

anaphylaxis An exaggerated, life-threatening hypersensitivity reaction to an antigen.

anatomic dead space The volume of the conducting airways from the external environment down to the terminal bronchioles.

anatomic position The position of standing erect with the feet and palms facing the examiner.

anemia A decrease in the blood hemoglobin level.

aneurysm A weakening and localized dilation of a blood vessel wall.

angina pectoris Ischemic chest pain caused by insufficient blood flow to the myocardium usually as a result of atherosclerosis of the coronary arteries.

angioedema A localized edematous reaction of the deep dermal or subcutaneous or submucosal tissues that appears as giant wheals.

angioplasty A procedure to relieve blockage from a blood vessel.

angiotensin-converting enzyme (ACE) A circulating enzyme that participates in the body's renin-angiotensin system, which mediates extracellular volume and arterial vasoconstriction by converting angiotensin I to angiotensin II.

angiotensin I The inactive form of angiotensin, formulated by the stimulation of renin, which is converted to angiotensin II.

angiotensin II A potent vasoconstrictor that also acts to stimulate the secretion of antidiuretic hormone.

angle-closure glaucoma A form of glaucoma associated with a physically obstructed anterior chamber angle; may be chronic or acute; also known as acute glaucoma, chronic angle-closure glaucoma, or narrow-angle glaucoma.

anhedonia The inability to enjoy what is usually pleasurable.

anion An ion with a negative charge.

anisocoria A condition characterized by unequal pupil size; may be congenital or indicative of pathology.

ankylosing spondylitis (AS) A form of arthritis that primarily affects the spine, although other joints can become involved.

anorexia nervosa An emotional disturbance concerning body image manifested as an eating disorder characterized by a prolonged refusal to eat, resulting in emaciation, amenorrhea, and an abnormal fear of becoming obese.

antagonist An agent designed to inhibit or counteract the effects of other drugs or undesired effects caused by normal or hyperactive physiologic mechanisms.

antegrade amnesia The loss of memory for events that occurred immediately after recovery of consciousness.

antepartum The period before labor and delivery.

anterior The front, or ventral, surface.

anterior cord syndrome A spinal cord injury usually seen in flexion injuries; caused by damage to the anterior aspect of the spinal cord by a ruptured intervertebral disk or fragments of the vertebral body extruded posteriorly into the spinal canal or by damage to the anterior spinal artery.

anterior hemiblock Failure in conduction of the cardiac impulse in the anterior fascicle of the left bundle branch.

anthrax An acute infectious disease caused by the spore-forming bacterium *Bacillus anthracis.*

antibodies Proteins produced by the body that destroy or inactivate specific substances (antigens) that have entered the body.

anticholinergic Of or pertaining to the blocking of acetylcholine receptors, resulting in inhibition of transmission of parasympathetic nerve impulses.

antidiuretic hormone (ADH) A hormone produced in the posterior pituitary gland that regulates the balance of water in the body by accelerating the resorption of water.

antidote A drug or other substance that opposes the action of a poison.

antigen–antibody reaction The binding of an antibody with an antigen of the type that stimulated the formation of the antibody. This binding makes the antigen more susceptible to ingestion and destruction by phagocytes or neutralization of an exotoxin.

antigens Substances (usually proteins) that are capable of generating an immune response causing the formation of an antibody that reacts specifically with that antigen.

anuria The inability to urinate; the cessation of urine production; a diminished urinary output of less than 100 to 250 mL/d.

anus The distal end or outlet of the rectum.

anxiety A state or feeling of apprehension, uneasiness, agitation, uncertainty, or fear resulting from the anticipation of some threat or danger.

aorta The main and largest artery in the body.

aortic dissection Separation of layers within the wall of the aorta.

Apgar score The evaluation of a newborn's physical condition, performed at 1 minute and 5 minutes after birth, including heart rate, respiratory effort, muscle tone, reflex irritability, and color.

aphasia A neurologic syndrome that affects a person's ability to express and/or understand written and spoken language; often associated with a cerebrovascular accident or head trauma.

apical impulse A pulsation of the left ventricle of the heart that is palpable and sometimes visible at the fifth intercostal space to the left of the midline.

apnea An absence of spontaneous respirations.

apneustic center A group of neurons in the pons that has a stimulatory effect on the inspiratory center.

appendectomy Surgical removal of the appendix.

appendicitis Inflammation of the appendix.

appendicular region The region consisting of the limbs, or extremities.

appendicular skeleton The bones of the upper and lower extremities.

application of principles A component of critical thinking in which the examiner makes patient care decisions based on conceptual understanding of the situation and interpretation of data gathered from the patient.

aqueous humor The clear, watery fluid that circulates in the anterior and posterior chambers of the eye.

arachnoid layer The delicate, weblike, middle membrane that covers the brain.

areflexia A neurologic condition characterized by the absence of reflexes.

areola The circular, pigmented area surrounding the nipple.

areolar connective tissue A loose tissue that consists of delicate webs of fibers and a variety of cells embedded in a matrix of soft, sticky gel.

arterioles Small branches of arteries that lead into capillaries.

arteriovenous anastomoses Vessels that allow blood to flow from arteries to veins without passing through capillaries; also known as an arteriovenous shunts.

arteriovenous fistula An internal anastomosis between an artery and a vein.

arteriovenous graft A synthetic material grafted between the patient's artery and vein.

arteriovenous malformation An abnormal connection between veins and arteries. It is believed to arise during fetal development or soon after birth.

arthritis An inflammatory condition of the joints, characterized by pain and swelling.

artifact An abnormality in the electrocardiogram tracing produced by factors other than the electrical activity of the heart.

artificial pacemaker A rhythm that is generated by electrical stimulation of the heart through an electrode implanted in the heart.

ascites An abnormal intraperitoneal accumulation of fluid containing large amounts of protein and electrolytes.

asphyxiants Gases that displace the oxygen in the air (simple asphyxiants) or disable the chemistry of cellular respiration despite adequate oxygen levels in the blood (chemical asphyxiants).

aspiration pneumonia Inflammation of the lung tissue from foreign material entering the tracheobronchial tree.

asplenia Congenital absence or surgical removal of the spleen.

assault The act of creating apprehension or fear; also, unauthorized handling and treatment of a patient.

assessment-based management Comprehensive care that is based on patient assessment, the patient's history, and the physical examination.

asterixis Hand flapping during hand extension related to pathologic conditions such as hypercapnia, liver failure, or renal failure.

asthma A respiratory disorder characterized by recurring episodes of paroxysmal dyspnea, coughing, and wheezing caused by constriction of the bronchi and viscous mucoid bronchial secretions.

astigmatism A vision condition that causes blurred vision attributable either to the irregular shape of the cornea (the clear front cover of the eye) or sometimes to the curvature of the lens inside the eye. Astigmatism is not distance dependent.

asystole The absence of electrical and mechanical activity of the heart.

ataxia Failure of muscle coordination.

atelectasis An abnormal condition characterized by the collapse of lung tissue. It prevents respiratory exchange of oxygen and carbon dioxide.

atherosclerosis A common arterial disorder characterized by yellow plaques of cholesterol, lipids, and cellular debris in the inner layers of the walls of large and medium-size arteries.

athetosis A neuromuscular condition characterized by slow, continuous, and involuntary movement of the extremities; a possible consequence of cerebral palsy or other central nervous system abnormality.

atmospheric pressure The pressure of the gas around us, which varies with differences in altitude. At sea level, it is 760 mm Hg.

atonic seizures Seizures that cause an abrupt loss of muscle tone, loss of posture, or sudden collapse ("drop attacks").

atria The two upper chambers of the heart (singular, atrium).

atrial fibrillation (AF) An irregularly irregular heart rhythm that results from disorganized and rapid ectopic electrical impulses from the atria.

atrial flutter A dysrhythmia resulting from rapid atrial reentry of electrical impulses over a large, anatomically fixed circuit; characterized by rapid, regular activity at a rate of 180 to 350 beats/min.

atrial kick The priming force contributed by atrial contraction immediately before ventricular systole that acts to improve ventricular filling during diastole.

atrial natriuretic factor (ANF) A peptide released from the atria when atrial blood pressure is increased. It lowers blood pressure by increasing urine production, thereby reducing blood volume.

atrial natriuretic factor A peptide released from the atria when atrial blood pressure is increased. It lowers blood pressure by increasing urine production, thus reducing blood volume.

atrial septal defect (ASD) A congenital anomaly in which an opening exists between the heart's two upper chambers.

atrial tachycardia (AT) A rapid heart rhythm that originates in the atria.

atrioventricular (AV) dissociation Any situation in which the atria and the ventricles beat independently.

atrioventricular (AV) junction An area formed by the atrioventricular node and the bundle of His; serves as the normal electrical link between the atria and ventricles in a normal heart.

atrioventricular (AV) node An area of specialized cardiac muscle that receives the cardiac impulse from the sinoatrial node and conducts it to the bundle of His.

atrioventricular nodal reentrant tachycardia (AVNRT) A type of reentry supraventricular tachycardia in which the reentrant loop is formed by fast and slow pathways within the atrioventricular node. The most common cause of paroxysmal supraventricular tachycardia in adults.

atrioventricular node An area of specialized cardiac muscle that receives the cardiac impulse from the sinoatrial node and conducts it to the bundle of His.

atrioventricular reentrant tachycardia (AVRT) A type of reentry supraventricular tachycardia in which one limb of the reentrant loop is constituted by a bypass tract rather than separate fast and slow pathways within the atrioventricular node.

atrioventricular valve A valve in the heart through which blood flows from the atria to the ventricles.

atrophy Decrease in size (shrinkage) of a cell, which adversely affects cell function.

attachments Physical and emotional bonds that develop between infants and their family members or caregivers.

audible and visual warning (AVW) devices Safety devices used in emergency responses to make vehicle presence known. Examples include lights, sirens, and horns.

augmented limb leads Unipolar leads that record the difference in electrical potential in cardiac muscle.

aura A sensation that may precede a migraine or seizure activity.

auricle The part of the external ear that protrudes from the head; also known as the pinna.

auscultation A technique that requires the use of a stethoscope and is used to assess body sounds produced by the movement of various fluids or gases in organs or tissues.

autism spectrum disorder (ASD) A range of neurodevelopmental disorders characterized by three sets of behavioral features: (1) impairment in social interaction, (2) communication deficits (both verbal and nonverbal), and (3) restricted, repetitive behaviors, including decreased imaginative play, stereotyped behaviors, and inflexible adherence to routines.

autoimmune disease A condition that occurs when the immune system mistakenly attacks and destroys healthy body tissue.

autoimmunity An abnormal characteristic or condition in which the body reacts against constituents of its own tissues.

autolysis The spontaneous disintegration of tissues or cells by the action of their own autogenous enzymes.

automaticity A property of specialized excitable tissue that allows self-activation through spontaneous development of an action potential.

automatism Abnormal repetitive motor behavior (eg, lip smacking, chewing, swallowing) during which the patient is amnestic.

autonomic hyperreflexia syndrome Overactivity of the autonomic nervous system that causes an abrupt onset of extremely high blood pressure.

autonomic nervous system The part of the nervous system that regulates involuntary vital functions, including the activity of cardiac muscle, smooth muscle, and glands.

autonomic reflexes Any of a large number of normal reflexes governing and regulating the functions of the viscera.

autonomy The principle of self-determination; that is, a person's ability to make moral decisions, including those affecting personal medical care.

autophagia A condition in which the body obtains nutrition through consumption of its own tissues.

avoidance The act of keeping away from someone, something, or a situation, or of preventing the occurrence of something. It requires the paramedic to continually be aware of the scene by remaining observant and being knowledgeable about warning signs that may indicate a dangerous situation.

avulsion A full-thickness skin loss in which the wound edges cannot be approximated.

axial loading Vertical compression of the spine that results when direct forces are transmitted along the length of the spinal column.

axial region The region consisting of the head, neck, thorax, and abdomen.

axial skeleton The bones of the head, neck, and torso.

axis The major direction of the overall electrical activity of the heart.

axon The main process of a neuron that normally conducts action potentials away from the cell body of the neuron.

azotemia A condition marked by retention of excessive amounts of nitrogenous compounds in the blood.

B lymphocytes The lymphocytes responsible for antibodymediated immunity.

Babinski reflex A reflex movement in which the great toe bends upward when the outer edge of the sole is stroked.

backlighting A type of lighting in which a person or object is positioned such that a light source from behind silhouettes the person or object; this is a safety hazard in the context of a hostile threat, by making a provider easier to see.

bacteremia The presence of bacteria in the blood.

bacteria Single-celled microorganisms that cause an infection characteristic of that species.

bacterial endocarditis Inflammation and infection of the endocardium and one or more heart valves; also known as infective endocarditis.

bacterial meningitis A life-threatening illness that results from bacterial infection of the meninges.

bacterial pneumonia A type of pneumonia associated with a bacterial infection.

bacterial tracheitis A bacterial infection of the upper airway and subglottic trachea; characterized by fever, barking cough, stridor, and respiratory distress.

bariatrics The field of medicine that focuses on the treatment and control of obesity and diseases associated with obesity.

barotitis An inflammation of the ear caused by changes in atmospheric pressure.

barotrauma A physical injury sustained as a result of exposure to increased atmospheric or environmental pressure; also known as dysbarism.

barotrauma of ascent A diving illness that occurs through the reverse process of descent; also known as "reverse squeeze."

barotrauma of descent A diving illness that results from the compression of gas in enclosed spaces as the ambient pressure increases with descent under water; also known as "squeeze."

Bartholin abscess An accumulation of pus that forms a lump in one of the Bartholin glands. It results when blockage of the gland's duct allows infection to develop.

bases Chemical compounds that combine with acids to form salts; also known as alkalis.

basic life support (BLS) A level of care provided by people trained in first aid, cardiopulmonary resuscitation, and other noninvasive care.

basilar skull fracture A fracture, usually caused by substantial blunt force trauma, that involves at least one of the bones that compose the base of the skull; most commonly involves the temporal bones but may involve the occipital, sphenoid, ethmoid, and the orbital plate of the frontal bone.

basket stretcher A litter designed of a rigid frame made of wire, mesh, or plastic.

basophils White blood cells that promote inflammation.

battering Repeated violence from physical and mental abuse (and other forms of abuse); may include establishing control and fear in a relationship.

battery Physical contact with a person without consent and without legal justification.

Battle sign Bruising over the mastoid bone behind the ear, which may indicate a basilar skull fracture; also known as retroauricular ecchymosis or raccoon eyes.

Beck triad A combination of three signs that suggest the presence of cardiac tamponade: jugular venous distention, muffled heart sounds, and hypotension.

behavioral emergency A change in mood or behavior that cannot be tolerated by the involved person or others and that requires immediate attention.

Bell palsy A paralysis of the facial muscles caused by inflammation of the facial nerve (cranial nerve VII). The condition usually is one-sided and time-limited. It often develops suddenly.

beneficence A duty to confer benefits; the practice of good deeds; an obligation to benefit others or to seek their good.

benign Nonmalignant; generally considered less harmful.

benign paroxysmal positional vertigo (BPPV) A condition in which calcium carbonate crystals enter one (or several) of the semicircular canals of the ear and disturb the normal fluid movement, causing nystagmus and vertigo.

benign prostatic hypertrophy (BPH) Enlargement of the prostate gland.

beta-adrenergic receptor Any of the postulated adrenergic components of receptor tissues that respond to epinephrine and various blocking agents.

bias The tendency to make conclusions or decisions based on a preformed idea, assumption, or prejudice. In research, a systematic error introduced into sampling or testing that results in the deviation of the results of a study from the actual "truth."

bicarbonate An alkaline substance in the blood that participates in the transport of carbon dioxide and in the regulation of pH.

bicuspid valve One of the two atrioventricular valves located between the left atrium and the ventricle; also known as the mitral valve.

bifascicular block The blockage of two of three pathways (fascicles) for ventricular conduction.

bigeminy A cardiac rhythm disturbance characterized by a premature ventricular complex every other beat.

bile A bitter, yellow-green secretion of the liver that is stored in the gallbladder.

bilevel positive airway pressure (BPAP) Airway support that combines partial ventilatory support and continuous positive airway pressure; allows the pressure to vary during each breath cycle.

biliary disease Disorders of the liver and gallbladder caused by abnormalities in bile composition, biliary anatomy, or function.

bilirubin The orange-yellow pigment of bile, formed principally from the breakdown of hemoglobin in red blood cells after termination of their normal life span.

bioethics The systematic study of moral dimensions, including the moral vision, decisions, conduct, and policies of the life sciences and health care.

biologic disturbances Disorders that result from a physical rather than a purely psychological cause.

biologic half-life The time required to metabolize or eliminate half the total amount of a drug in the body.

bioterrorism The use of biologic agents, such as pathogenic organisms or agricultural pests, for the express purpose of causing death or disease, to instill a sense of fear and panic in the victims, and to intimidate governments or societies for political, financial, or ideologic gain.

biotransformation The process by which a drug is converted chemically to a metabolite.

biphasic reaction An anaphylactic reaction that resolves and then recurs hours later without further exposure to the trigger.

bipolar disorder A disorder marked by alternating periods of mania and depression; formerly known as manic-depressive disorder.

bipolar leads Leads composed of two electrodes of opposite polarity.

bivalent cation An ion with two positive charges.

bladder catheterization Passage of a catheter (typically through the urethra) into the bladder for the purpose of drainage.

blebs A small, thin-walled collection of air between the lung and visceral pleura that, when ruptured, results in a spontaneous pneumothorax.

blinding A research specification that dictates that parties are not made aware of the study, treatment, or outcome to be measured.

blood The fluid and its suspended, formed elements that circulate through the heart, arteries, capillaries, and veins.

blood clot The end result of the clotting process in blood. It normally consists of red blood cells, white blood cells, and platelets enmeshed in an insoluble fibrin network.

blood coagulation A process that results in the formation of a stable fibrin clot that entraps platelets, blood cells, and plasma.

blood–brain barrier An anatomic-physiologic feature of the brain thought to consist of walls of capillaries in the central nervous system and surrounding glial membranes. Its function is to prevent or slow the passage of chemical compounds from the blood into the central nervous system.

blowout fracture A fracture of the floor of the orbit caused by a blow that suddenly increases the intraocular pressure.

blunt trauma An injury produced by the wounding forces of compression and change of speed, both of which can disrupt tissue.

body lice Tiny parasites that concentrate around the waist, shoulders, axillae, and neck.

Bohr effect The property of hemoglobin by which an increasing concentration of protons and/or carbon dioxide reduces the oxygen affinity for hemoglobin.

bone A highly specialized form of hard, connective tissue. It consists of living cells and a mineralized matrix.

bone spurs Bony growths formed on normal bone.

bone tumor An abnormal growth of cells within a bone. It may be malignant or benign.

bony labyrinth Part of the inner ear. It contains the membranous labyrinth.

borrowed servant A legal doctrine that refers to a servant who serves two "masters" (eg, an emergency medical technician [EMT] who is employed by a municipality but who is supervised by a paramedic).

botulism A rare but life-threatening form of food poisoning caused by the bacillus *Clostridium botulinum.*

bowel obstruction An occlusion of the intestinal lumen that results in blockage of normal flow of intestinal contents.

Bowman capsule The expanded beginning of a renal tubule.

boxer's fracture Fracture of the fifth metacarpal bone at the distal metaphysis from direct trauma to a closed fist.

Boyle's law A gas law that states pressure and volume are inversely related, assuming a constant temperature.

bradycardia A heart rate of less than 60 beats/min.

brain abscess An accumulation of purulent material (pus) surrounded by a capsule within the brain.

brain lesion An abnormal area of the brain often reflective of traumatic injury.

brain tumors Masses, benign or malignant, in the cranial cavity.

Braxton-Hicks contractions Irregular tightening of the pregnant uterus that may begin as early as the second trimester and increases in frequency, duration, and intensity as the pregnancy progresses.

breach of duty A breach of a professional duty to act.

breech presentation The intrauterine position of the fetus in which the buttocks or feet present, rather than the head.

brief resolved unexplained event (BRUE) Event lasting less than 1 minute in an infant younger than 1 year characterized by one or more of the following: cyanosis or pallor; absent, decreased, or irregular breathing; marked change in muscle tone (hypertonia or hypotonia); altered level of consciousness. Child is well-appearing at time of presentation.

bronchial breath sounds Breath sounds heard only over the trachea. They are the highest in pitch.

bronchiectasis An abnormal dilation of the bronchi caused by congenital or acquired damage.

bronchioles Small branches of the bronchi.

bronchiolitis An inflammatory bronchial reaction in young children and infants that causes congestion in the small airways (bronchioles) of the lung.

bronchovesicular breath sounds Normal breath sounds heard over the major bronchi or in the posterior chest between the scapula.

Brown-Séquard syndrome A functional hemitransection of the spinal cord resulting in weakness of the upper and lower extremities on the same side and loss of pain and temperature sensation on the opposite side.

bruit An abnormal sound or murmur heard while auscultating an artery, organ, or gland caused by narrowing of the vessel.

buddy splinting Immobilization of an injured finger or toe to an adjoining finger or toe with padding and tape, such that the uninjured digit acts as a splint; also known as buddy wrapping.

bulbourethral glands Small glands located just below the prostate gland that lubricate the terminal portion of the urethra and contribute to seminal fluid; also known as the Cowper glands.

bulimia nervosa A disorder characterized by an insatiable craving for food, often resulting in episodes of binge eating followed by purging (through self-induced vomiting or use of laxatives), depression, and self-deprivation.

bullae Dilated air-filled spaces within the lung parenchyma; most commonly caused by chronic obstructive pulmonary disease.

bundle of His A band of fibers in the myocardium through which the cardiac impulse is rapidly transmitted from the atrioventricular node to the ventricles.

bundle of Kent Pathologic fibers that connect atrial muscle to ventricular muscle, bypassing the atrioventricular node; also known as Kent fibers.

burn shock A combination of hypovolemic and distributive shock that results from local and systemic responses to thermal trauma.

bursa A small sac containing synovial fluid that helps ease friction between a tendon and skin or between a tendon and bone.

bursitis An inflammation of the bursa, the connective tissue structure surrounding a joint.

***C diff* colitis** Inflammation of the colon caused by colonization and infection with the bacterium *Clostridium difficile.*

calcaneus The heel bone, the largest of the tarsal bones.

cancellous bone Lattice-like tissue normally present in the interior of many bones, where spaces usually are filled with marrow; also known as spongy bone.

cannon A waves Waves of pulse pressure that are visible in the jugular veins of a patient in ventricular tachycardia.

capillaries Tiny branching vessels that connect arterioles to venules; the site where most gas exchange occurs between the blood and tissues.

capillary network A complex, interconnected structure where a single blood cell traveling from an arteriole to a venule via a capillary bed passes through capillary segments.

capnography The combination of a capnometric reading (numeric value) and a capnogram (graph/drawing).

capsid A protein coat that encloses a virus.

carbonic acid An aqueous solution of carbon dioxide.

carbonic anhydrase The enzyme that converts carbon dioxide into carbonic acid.

carboxyhemoglobin A compound produced by the exposure of hemoglobin to carbon monoxide.

carcinogens Cancer-causing agents.

cardiac ejection fraction The percentage of blood volume ejected from the ventricle during a contraction.

cardiac muscle A special striated muscle of the myocardium that contains dark, intercalated disks at the junctions of the abutting fibers. It is characterized by special contractile abilities.

cardiac output The volume of blood pumped each minute by the ventricles.

cardiac sphincter A ring of muscle fibers at the juncture of the esophagus and the stomach.

cardiogenic shock A condition caused by loss of 40% or more of the functioning myocardium; the heart is no longer able to circulate sufficient blood to maintain adequate oxygen delivery.

cardiomyopathy Any disease that affects the myocardium.

cardiotoxins Hazardous materials that can cause myocardial ischemia and dysrhythmias.

carina A downward and backward projection of the lowest tracheal cartilage, forming a ridge between the openings of the right and the left primary bronchi.

carpal bones The bones of the carpus, or wrist.

carpal tunnel syndrome An entrapment neuropathy that occurs when the median nerve becomes pressed or squeezed at the wrist in the carpal tunnel.

carrier molecule A protein that combines with solutes on one side of a membrane, transporting the solute to the other side. It is used in mediated transport mechanisms.

carrier-mediated transport Movement that occurs across membranes to move substances against a concentration gradient, from areas of lower concentration to areas of higher concentration.

cartilage Firm, smooth, nonvascular connective tissue.

cartilaginous joints Joints that are slightly movable.

casualty collection areas Areas where ill or injured people are gathered for triage, treatment, or transport.

cataract A loss of transparency of the lens of the eye that results from changes in the delicate protein fibers within the lens.

cathartics Substances that accelerate defecation.

catheter fragment embolism The shearing or detachment of an intravenous catheter, allowing the embolus to travel in the bloodstream.

cation An ion with a positive charge.

cauda equina syndrome A rare disorder of the lumbar spine that affects the bundle of nerve roots at the lower end of the spinal cord. It is a surgical emergency.

cavitation A temporary or permanent opening produced by a force that pushes body tissues laterally away from the track of a projectile.

CBRNE An abbreviation for the categories of weapons of mass destruction: Chemical, Biologic, Radiologic, Nuclear, and Explosives agents.

cecum A cul-de-sac constituting the first part of the large intestine.

cell The functional basic unit of life.

cell body The part of the cell that contains the nucleus and surrounding cytoplasm, exclusive of any projections or processes. It is concerned more with metabolism of the cell than with a specific function.

cell-mediated immunity Immunity characterized by the formation of a population of lymphocytes that attack and destroy foreign material.

cellulitis An infectious condition of the skin resulting in inflammation that is characterized most commonly by local heat, redness, pain, and swelling, and occasionally by fever, malaise, chills, and headache.

centimeter A metric unit of length equal to 1⁄100 (ie, 0.01) of a meter, or 0.3937 inch.

central cord syndrome A spinal cord injury commonly seen with hyperextension cervical injuries; less commonly seen with flexion injuries; characterized by greater motor impairment of the upper extremities than of the lower extremities.

central cyanosis Cyanosis of the tongue and mucous membranes; usually reflects decreased saturation of the hemoglobin in arterial blood.

central hearing loss A hearing impairment caused by damage to the central nervous system rather than to the ear or its structures.

central nervous system (CNS) The system composed of the brain and spinal cord.

central nervous system ischemic response An increase in blood pressure caused by vasoconstriction that occurs when oxygen levels are too low, carbon dioxide levels are too high, or pH is too low in the medulla.

central retinal artery occlusion (CRAO) The blockage of blood supply to the arteries of the retina.

central retinal vein occlusion (CRVO) The blockage of blood supply to the main vein of the retina.

central thermoreceptors Nerve endings located in or near the anterior hypothalamus that are sensitive to subtle changes in core temperatures.

central vision The vision that results from images falling on the macula of the retina.

centrioles Usually paired organelles that lie in the centrosome.

centrosome A specialized zone of cytoplasm close to the nucleus that contains two centrioles.

cephalopelvic disproportion An obstetric condition in which a newborn's head is too large or a mother's birth canal is too small to permit a normal vaginal delivery.

cerebellum The second largest part of the brain. It plays an essential role in coordinating normal movements.

cerebral aneurysm A weak area in the wall of a blood vessel in the brain that dilates and is at risk of rupture, particularly with hypertension.

cerebral atrophy Reduction in the size of brain tissue.

cerebral blood flow (CBF) The volume of blood passing through a given amount of brain tissue per unit of time; a function of the cerebral perfusion pressure and the resistance of the cerebral vascular bed.

cerebral contusion Bruising of the brain in the area of the cortex or deeper within the frontal (most common), temporal, or occipital lobes.

cerebral cortex A thin layer of gray matter, made up of neuron dendrites and cell bodies, that comprises the surface of the cerebrum.

cerebral embolism An obstruction in a cerebral artery by an embolus, usually resulting in transient or permanent ischemic damage to brain tissue. As a result, it may cause impairment of cognitive, motor, or sensory function.

cerebral palsy A developmental disorder that occurs in utero or in the first year of life, in which disturbances in the brain result in issues with movement and posture and limit a person's activity. This disorder may also affect sensation, perception, cognition, communication, and behavior.

cerebral perfusion pressure (CPP) A measure of the amount of blood flow to the brain calculated by subtracting the intracranial pressure from the mean systemic arterial blood pressure.

cerebral thrombosis The formation of a blood clot (thrombus) in an artery or vein that supplies blood to the brain, resulting in ischemia to brain tissue.

cerebrospinal fluid (CSF) The fluid that fills the subarachnoid space in the brain and spinal cord and is found in the cerebral ventricles.

cerebrovascular accident A sudden interruption in blood flow to a portion of the brain resulting from occlusion of a cerebral artery by an embolus or thrombus, or a cerebral hemorrhage caused by vessel rupture; also known as a stroke.

cerebrum The largest and uppermost part of the brain. It controls consciousness, memory, sensations, emotions, and voluntary movements.

certification A process by which a status or level of achievement is recognized by the granting of a document attesting to that level of status or achievement.

cerumen A yellow or brown waxy secretion produced in the external ear canal; also known as earwax.

cervix The lower part of the uterus.

cesarean delivery A surgical procedure in which the abdomen and uterus are incised and the baby is delivered through the abdomen.

chalazion A small bump in the eyelid caused by the blockage of a tiny oil gland in the upper or lower eyelid.

chancre A painless ulcer, particularly one developing on the genitals as a result of a sexually transmitted disease.

chemical name The exact designation of a chemical structure as determined by the rules of chemical nomenclature.

chemical restraint The use of drugs to control behavior.

chemotactic factors Biochemical mediators that are important in activating the inflammatory response.

chickenpox An acute, highly contagious viral disease caused by a herpesvirus, varicella-zoster virus; also known as varicella. It occurs primarily during childhood and is characterized by crops of pruritic vesicular eruptions on the skin.

chief complaint A patient's primary complaint; usually the reason for the EMS response.

chief concern The paramedic's primary concern related to the patient condition.

Chikungunya virus A viral illness spread by mosquitoes that causes fever and joint pain, which is often severe and debilitating.

child abuse The physical, sexual, or emotional maltreatment of a child.

chlamydia A sexually transmitted disease caused by infection with the bacterium *Chlamydia trachomatis* that frequently causes of sterility.

chlorine A poisonous, yellow-green gas with an odor that has been described as a mixture of pineapple and pepper.

choanal atresia A bony or membranous occlusion that blocks the passageway between the nose and pharynx. It can result in serious ventilation problems in the newborn.

cholecystectomy Surgical removal of the gallbladder.

cholecystitis Inflammation of the gallbladder, most often associated with the presence of gallstones.

cholinergic Of or pertaining to the effects produced by the parasympathetic nervous system or drugs that stimulate or antagonize the parasympathetic nervous system.

chorea A movement disorder that causes involuntary, unpredictable body movements ranging from minor fidgeting to severe, uncontrolled contractions that interfere markedly with gross motor function.

chorioamnionitis An inflammatory reaction in the amniotic membranes caused by infection in the amniotic fluid.

chromatin granules The material within the cell nucleus from which chromosomes are formed.

chromosomes Organized structures of deoxyribonucleic acid (DNA) and protein that are found in cells.

chronic bronchitis Obstructive airway disease of the trachea and bronchi.

chronic fatigue syndrome (CFS) A debilitating and complex disorder, characterized by profound fatigue that is not improved by bed rest and that may be worsened by physical or mental activity.

chronic gastroenteritis Inflammation of the stomach and intestines that accompanies numerous gastrointestinal disorders.

chronic kidney disease (CKD) A progressive, irreversible systemic disease, caused by kidney dysfunction, that leads to abnormalities in blood counts and blood chemistry levels. Formerly known as chronic renal failure.

chyme The semifluid mass of partly digested food passed from the stomach into the duodenum.

cilia Small, hairlike processes on the outer surfaces of some cells.

circadian rhythm A pattern based on a 24-hour cycle, especially repetition of certain physiologic phenomena, such as sleeping and eating.

circle of Willis The circle of interconnected blood vessels at the base of the brain that allows for collateral blood flow to both hemispheres.

circumcision Surgical removal of the penile foreskin.

circumferential burns Burns that encircle a body part, producing a tourniquet-like effect that may quickly compromise circulation.

cirrhosis A chronic and progressive disease in which normal liver cells are replaced by fibrotic scar tissue.

civil law An area of law that deals with "private" complaints brought by one person (the plaintiff) against another person (the defendant); also known as tort law.

clandestine drug lab A place of illegal drug manufacturing.

cleft lip An incomplete closure of the newborn's lip that occurs when one or more fissures fail to fuse in the embryo.

cleft palate An incomplete closure in the soft/hard palate of the roof of the mouth that runs along its midline; occurs when one or more fissures fail to fuse in the embryo.

clinical decision making (clinical reasoning) A contextual, continuous, and evolving process, in which data are gathered, interpreted, and evaluated so as to select an evidence-based choice of action.

clinical judgment The outcome or conclusion a paramedic arrives at based on critical thinking and clinical decision making.

clinical reasoning Use of the results of questions to think about associated problems and body system changes related to the patient's complaint.

clitoris Erectile tissue in the vestibule of the vagina.

closed-ended questions Questions asked in a narrative form that can be answered with a "yes" or "no."

Clostridium difficile A bacterium that normally is present in small numbers in the intestines that may cause symptoms ranging from diarrhea to life-threatening inflammation of the colon when present in high numbers.

clotting cascade The blood clotting system or coagulation pathway.

clotting factors Substances in the blood that act in sequence to stop bleeding by forming a clot.

coarctation of the aorta (CoA) A congenital defect in which there is narrowing or constriction of the aorta.

coarse ventricular fibrillation (VF) Fibrillatory waves that are greater than 3 mm in amplitude; precedes fine ventricular fibrillation.

code of ethics A set of guidelines that are designed to set out acceptable behaviors for members of a particular group, association, or profession.

cognitive development The construction of thought processes, including remembering, problem solving, and decision making, from childhood through adolescence to adulthood.

cold stress A condition that occurs when the body is unable to warm itself.

cold zone A safety zone in a hazmat response that typically surrounds the warm zone; usually considered safe, requiring only minimal protective clothing.

collagen vascular disease An autoimmune disease characterized by inflammation in the connective tissues. It results in the accumulation of extra antibodies in the circulation.

Colles fracture A fracture of the radius at the epiphysis within 1 inch (3 cm) of the joint of the wrist, resulting in an upward (posterior) displacement of the radius and obvious deformity.

colloid solutions Solutions that contain molecules (usually proteins) that are too large to pass through the capillary membrane.

colostomy A surgical opening into the large intestine.

coma An abnormally deep state of unconsciousness from which the patient cannot be aroused by external stimuli.

combining vowel A vowel often used between root words and suffixes or between two or more root words.

command The act of directing, ordering, or controlling by virtue of explicit, statutory, regulatory, or delegated authority.

command post The physical location of on-scene incident command and management organization.

common law Law that comes from societal acceptance of customs or norms of behavior over time; also known as case law or judge-made law.

commotio cordis A dysrhythmia resulting from blunt-force chest trauma that often leads to cardiac arrest.

communicability period A stage of infection that begins when the latent period ends and continues as long as the agent is present and can spread to other hosts.

communicable disease An infectious disease that can be transmitted from one person to another.

communication The process by which one person or group transmits information to others.

communications center A facility used to dispatch emergency equipment and coordinate communications between field units and personnel.

communications systems The science and technology of communicating, especially by electronic means.

community health assessment An assessment of a target community to identify the needs and resources required to provide prevention and wellness promotion activities.

compact bone Hard, dense bone that usually is found at the surface of skeletal structures, as distinguished from cancellous bone.

compartment syndrome The result of an intolerably high pressure within a body space or cavity causing compromise of blood flow. It most commonly occurs in the extremities due to compressive forces or blunt trauma to muscle groups confined in tight fibrous sheaths, but may also be seen in overuse situations.

compensable damages Damages awarded in a lawsuit that may include medical expenses, lost earnings, conscious pain and suffering, and wrongful death.

compensated shock An early stage of shock in which the body is still able to maintain mean arterial blood pressure through compensatory changes in heart rate, stroke volume, or systemic vascular resistance.

compensatory pause A pause following a premature ventricular complex.

complement system A group of proteins that coat bacteria. The proteins then either help kill the bacteria directly or assist neutrophils (in the blood) and macrophages (in the tissues) to engulf and destroy the bacteria.

complex partial seizure A seizure that originates in the temporal lobe. It usually begins with an aura and is followed by repetitive motor behavior.

compliance The ease with which the lungs and thorax expand during pressure changes. The greater the compliance, the easier the expansion.

concealment A means of keeping out of sight; does not necessarily provide ballistic protection.

concentration gradient The concentration difference between two points in a solution divided by the distance between the points.

concept formation A component of critical thinking that refers to all elements that are gathered to form a general impression of the patient.

concussion A temporary loss or alteration of part or all of the brain's abilities to function without actual physical damage to the brain.

conduction The direct movement of heat from a warmer object to a cooler one (simple transfer).

conductive hearing loss The faulty transportation of sound from the outer to the inner ear. This type of deafness often is curable.
confabulation The invention of stories to make up for gaps in memory.
confidence interval An estimate of the range of likely values in the source population (the true value) based on the given study sample value, where a narrow range indicates more certainty about the value than does a wide range.
confined spaces Spaces that have limited access or egress and are not designed for ongoing human occupancy or habitation.
confounding variables Unmeasured variables that may affect the results of an experiment.
congenital Present at birth.
congenital anomalies Defects that occur during fetal development.
congenital rubella syndrome A serious disease that affects approximately 25% of infants born to women infected with rubella during the first trimester of pregnancy. It is associated with multiple congenital anomalies, mental retardation, and an increased risk of death.
conjunctiva A mucous membrane that covers the anterior surface of the eyeball and the lining of the eyelids.
conjunctivitis Inflammation of the conjunctiva caused by bacterial or viral infection, allergy, or environmental factors.
connective tissue Tissue that supports and binds other body tissues and parts.
consensual movement The movement of one eye acting in concert with the other.
contact precautions Steps taken to avoid infection spread by contact with a patient or contaminated items in a patient's room or surroundings. Such steps include wearing a gown and gloves while caring for a patient or while in the patient's room/surroundings.
contact provider The person who initiates and provides direct patient care.
contemplative approach An approach to patient care in which a history is obtained and a physical examination is performed before providing patient care.
contiguous leads Two or more electrocardiograph leads that are anatomically close together and that view the same general area of the heart.
continence The ability to control bladder or bowel function.
continuous positive airway pressure (CPAP) Airway support that transmits positive pressure into the airways of a spontaneously breathing patient throughout the respiratory cycle at a constant pressure.
continuous quality improvement (CQI) A management approach to organizational performance that includes constant monitoring, evaluation, decisions, and actions.
contracture deformity An abnormal, usually permanent condition of a joint characterized by flexion and fixation and caused by atrophy and shortening of muscle fibers or by loss of elasticity of the skin.
contraindications Medical or physiologic factors that make it harmful to administer a medication that would otherwise have a therapeutic effect.
contrecoup An injury that occurs at a site opposite the side of impact.
controlled substance Any drug defined in the categories of the Comprehensive Drug Abuse Prevention and Control Act (also known as the Controlled Substances Act) of 1970.
contusion A closed, soft-tissue injury characterized by swelling, discoloration, and pain.
convection The transfer of heat by mass motion of a fluid such as air or water.
convenience sampling The process of choosing the people who are easiest to reach, or sampling that is easily done. The sample does not represent the entire population.
conversion disorder A constellation of neurologic symptoms that are not consciously or deliberately produced and that cannot be explained by a physical examination. These disorders often cause clinically significant disruption in social or occupational functioning. Also referred to as functional neurologic disorder.
core body temperature (CBT) The temperature of deep structures of the body as compared with the temperatures of peripheral tissues.
cornea The convex, transparent, anterior part of the eye.
corneal abrasion A disruption or loss of cells in the top layer of the corneal epithelium.
coronary arteries The two arteries that arise from the base of the aorta and carry blood to the muscle of the heart.
corrosives Hazardous materials that are either strong acids or strong bases (alkaline).
cortical vision impairment A temporary or permanent visual impairment caused by the disturbance of the posterior visual pathways and/or the occipital lobes of the brain; the most common cause of permanent visual impairment in children.
cortisol A steroid hormone that occurs naturally in the body.
costal cartilages Cartilages that connect the sternum and the ends of the ribs. They allow the chest to move in respiration.
costochondral separation Separation of the costochondral cartilages from either the ribs or the sternum or both.

coup Local damage that occurs at the site of impact.

cover A device or structure that offers ballistic protection; may or may not also provide concealment.

cover provider The person whose role is to ensure scene safety for the contact providers while they provide patient care.

coxae The hip joints; the head of the femur and the acetabulum of the innominate bone.

crackle A fine, bubbling sound heard on auscultation of the lung. It is produced by air entering distal airways and alveoli that contain serous secretions.

cranial vault The eight skull bones that surround and protect the brain; the brain case.

creatinine A chemical waste molecule generated by muscle metabolism.

credentialing A local process that allows a paramedic to practice in a specific EMS agency (or setting) in accordance with his or her level of certification and licensure.

crepitus A grating sound or sensation that may be caused by bone fragments rubbing or other sources, such as a joint with inflammation.

cricoid cartilage The most inferior laryngeal cartilage.

cricothyroid membrane The membrane joining the thyroid and cricoid cartilages.

crime scene A location where any part of a criminal act has occurred, or a location where evidence relating to a crime may be found.

criminal law A type of law in which the federal, state, or local government prosecutes people for violating a law.

critical thinking The ability to quickly focus thinking to get the desired results depending on the situation.

Crohn disease A chronic, inflammatory bowel disease of unknown origin that usually affects the ileum, the proximal colon, or both, but may affect any part of the gastrointestinal tract.

cross-trained personnel Emergency personnel who are trained in more than one type of emergency service (eg, fire, rescue, EMS, law enforcement).

croup A childhood infection of the upper airways (larynx, trachea, bronchial tubes) that causes a distinctive "seallike" barking cough; also known as laryngotracheobronchitis. It is usually caused by a virus (most commonly parainfluenza) but rarely can be bacterial.

crowning The phase at the end of labor in which the fetal head is seen at the opening of the vagina.

crush injury Injury from exposure of tissue to a compressive force sufficient to interfere with the normal structure and metabolic function of the involved cells and tissues.

crush syndrome A life-threatening and sometimes preventable complication of prolonged immobilization or compressive forces; a pathologic process that causes destruction, alteration, or both of muscle tissue.

cryogens Refrigerant liquid gases that can freeze human tissue on contact.

crystalloid solutions Solutions created by dissolving crystals such as salts and sugars in water.

Cullen sign The appearance of irregularly formed hemorrhagic patches on the skin around the umbilicus.

cultural imposition The forcing of one's beliefs, values, and patterns of behavior on people from another culture.

cumulative action The effect that occurs when several doses of a drug are administered or when absorption occurs more quickly than removal by excretion or metabolism, or both.

current health status A focus on the patient's current state of health, environmental conditions, and personal habits.

Cushing reflex An attempt by the body to compensate for a decline in cerebral perfusion pressure by increasing the mean arterial pressure.

Cushing syndrome A condition caused by an abnormally high circulating level of corticosteroid hormones produced naturally by the adrenal glands.

Cushing triad Increased systolic blood pressure, bradycardia, and irregular respiratory rates that result from increased intracranial pressure.

cutaneous anthrax Anthrax that affects the skin, caused by the spore-forming bacterium *Bacillus anthracis.*

cystic fibrosis An inherited metabolic disease of the lungs and digestive system that manifests in childhood; also known as mucoviscidosis.

cystitis Inflammation of the urinary bladder and ureters.

cytochromes Proteins in the liver that play a role in drug detoxification.

cytoplasm All of the substance of a cell other than the nucleus.

cytoplasmic membrane The plasma membrane.

Dalton's law A law stating that the total pressure exerted by a mixture of gases is equal to the sum of the partial pressure of gases.

data interpretation A component of critical thinking in which the examiner gathers the necessary data to form a field impression and working diagnosis.

date rape Nonconsensual sex between people who are already acquainted (eg, friends, acquaintances, or people who are dating).

deafness Profound hearing loss that results in the inability to understand speech even when amplified.

deceleration A decrease in the velocity of a moving object.

decerebrate posturing A position that is also called abnormal extension posturing, in which a comatose patient's arms are extended and internally rotated and the legs are extended with the feet in forced plantar flexion; usually observed in patients who have compression of the brainstem.

deciliter A metric unit of volume equal to ¹⁄₁₀ (ie, 0.1) of a liter.

decision-making capacity Patients' ability to make their own health care decisions.

decoding The process by which the intended meaning of information is interpreted, either written or verbal.

decompression sickness A multisystem disorder that results when nitrogen in compressed air (dissolved into tissues and blood from the increase in the partial pressure of the gas at depth) converts back from solution to gas. This process results in the formation of bubbles in the tissues and blood.

decontamination The process of making patients, rescuers, equipment, and supplies safe by eliminating harmful substances.

decorticate posturing A position that is also called abnormal flexion posturing, in which the comatose patient's upper extremities are rigidly flexed at the elbows and at the wrists; usually observed in patients who have a lesion in the mesencephalic region of the brain.

deep fascia The dense layer of fibrous tissue beneath the dermis. It provides for insulation, cushioning, caloric reserve, and body substance and shape.

deep tendon reflexes Reflexes that examine the sensory and motor pathways of a nerve; often associated with muscle stretching.

deep vein thrombosis (DVT) Occlusion in any portion of the deep venous system by a thrombus; can be acute or chronic.

defamation Saying something untrue about a person's character or reputation without legal privilege or the person's consent.

defibrillation The delivery of electrical current through the myocardium to terminate ventricular fibrillation and pulseless ventricular tachycardia.

deficient ambient oxygen An oxygen concentration in the environment that is less than 21%.

degloving injury An injury usually involving the hand or finger, although it can occur anywhere in the body, in which the soft tissue is removed down to the bone.

degranulation A cellular process that releases antimicrobial substances from secretory vesicles (granules) found inside mast cells and basophils. It plays a role in allergic reactions.

dehydration An excessive loss of water from the body tissues. It may follow prolonged fever, diarrhea, vomiting, acidosis, and other conditions.

delirium A medical emergency characterized by an abrupt disorientation for time and place, usually with delusions and hallucinations; may be reversible if causative etiology is identified.

delirium tremens An acute and sometimes fatal psychotic reaction caused by cessation of excessive intake of alcohol over a long period of time; also known as DTs.

delta wave A slurring or notching of the onset of the QRS complex that is a diagnostic finding in Wolff-Parkinson-White syndrome.

delusions Persistent beliefs or perceptions held by a person despite evidence that refutes those beliefs (ie, false beliefs).

demarcation The visible boundary between living tissue and necrotic tissue.

dementia A slow, progressive, and irreversible loss of awareness of time and place. It usually involves an inability to learn new things or recall recent events.

dendrites The branching processes of a neuron that receive stimuli and conduct potentials toward the cell body.

dengue fever A mosquito-borne illness caused by dengue virus in tropical and subtropical areas; also known as breakbone fever. Symptoms include high fever, joint pain, and rash. Severe cases may result in hemorrhage and shock.

dental abscess A collection of pus in, around, or underneath a tooth.

dental malocclusion A misalignment of the teeth.

dentalgia The medical term for toothache.

deoxyribonucleic acid (DNA) A type of nucleic acid that makes up the genetic material of cells.

dependent practice A type of medical practice in which the provider offers a certain type of care that falls under the same scope of practice as a physician but that requires medical oversight.

depolarization A change in electrical charge difference across the cell membrane that causes the difference to be smaller or closer to 0 mV; a phase of the action potential in which the membrane potential moves toward zero or becomes positive.

deposition A testimony taken under oath in a location other than a courtroom.

depressed skull fracture Any fracture of the skull in which fragments are depressed below the normal surface of the skull.

depression A mood disturbance characterized by feelings of sadness, despair, and discouragement.

dermatomes Areas of skin surface supplied by a single spinal nerve.

dermatomyositis An inflammatory myopathy characterized by a skin rash that precedes or accompanies progressive muscle weakness.

dermis Dense, irregular connective tissue that forms the deep layer of the skin.

descriptive statistics A form of statistics that does not try to conclude (infer) anything about a subject that goes beyond the data; can be qualitative or quantitative.

designated infection control officer (DICO) A person who serves as a liaison between the public safety agency and community health agencies involved in monitoring and responding to communicable diseases.

diabetes insipidus (DI) A metabolic disorder characterized by extreme polyuria and polydipsia that is caused by deficient production or secretion of antidiuretic hormone or inability of the kidney tubules to respond to antidiuretic hormone.

diabetes mellitus A complex disorder of carbohydrate, fat, and protein metabolism that primarily results from partial or complete lack of insulin secretion by the beta cells of the pancreas or occurs because of defects in the insulin receptors.

diabetic ketoacidosis (DKA) An acute, life-threatening complication of uncontrolled diabetes characterized by hyperglycemia, hypovolemia, electrolyte imbalance, and a breakdown of free fatty acids, causing acidosis.

dialysate A solution used in dialysis.

dialysis A technique used to normalize blood chemistry in patients with acute or chronic renal failure and to remove blood toxins in some patients who have taken a drug overdose.

diaphragm The dome-shaped, musculofibrous partition that separates the thoracic and abdominal cavities.

diaphragmatic hernia A herniation of abdominal structures into the pleural cavity through a defect in the diaphragm. Often caused by the improper fusion of pleuroperitoneal membranes that separate the chest from the abdomen during fetal development.

diaphragmatic rupture Traumatic rupture of the diaphragm, which often results from sudden compression of the abdomen.

diaphysis The shaft of a long bone, consisting of a tube of compact bone that encloses the medullary cavity.

diastole The phase of the heartbeat in which the heart muscle relaxes and allows the chamber to fill with blood; separated into ventricular diastole and atrial diastole.

diastolic blood pressure The minimum level of blood pressure measured between contractions of the heart.

diastolic heart failure Failure of the ventricles to relax properly during diastole; also known as diastolic dysfunction.

diencephalon The parts of the brain between the cerebral hemispheres and the mesencephalon.

differential count A laboratory test that identifies the different types of leukocytes present in blood; also known as the diff.

differential diagnosis The process of weighing the probability of one disease versus that of other diseases possibly accounting for a patient's illness.

differentiation A process in which cells become specialized in one type of function or act in concert with other cells to perform a more complex task.

diffuse axonal injury (DAI) A disease process characterized by diffuse microscopic damage to the brain coupled with focal lesions that are the result of shear forces sustained in head trauma; a type of diffuse brain injury.

diffusion The process in which solid, particulate matter in a fluid moves from an area of higher concentration to an area of lower concentration, resulting in an even distribution of the particles in the fluid.

dilation and curettage (D&C) A gynecologic procedure in which the uterine cervix is widened and the endometrium of the uterus is scraped away.

direct medical oversight Physician-directed care provided in real time. The physician may be present on the scene or may provide direction through remote means; formerly known as online medical control.

disaster A term that usually is associated with a human-made or natural event that involves damage across a large area or to a community's infrastructure.

disaster management The mobilization of resources and the methods used to meet the needs of a disaster response.

discovery The judicial process in which documents are exchanged and depositions and interrogatives are taken.

disease period A stage of infection that follows the incubation period. The duration of this stage varies with the disease.

disentanglement The process of making a pathway through the wreckage of an accident and removing wreckage from patients.

disequilibrium syndrome A group of neurologic findings that sometimes occur during or immediately after dialysis. They are thought to result from a disproportionate decrease in the osmolality of the extracellular fluid compared with that of the intracellular compartment in the brain or cerebrospinal fluid.

disruptive, impulse-control, and conduct disorders A group of psychiatric conditions characterized by the inability to control emotions or to resist an impulse or a temptation to perform some act that is unlawful, socially unacceptable, or self-harmful.

disseminated intravascular coagulation (DIC) A grave coagulopathy that results from the overstimulation of the clotting and anticlotting processes in response to disease or injury.

dissociative disorders A group of psychological illnesses in which a particular mental function is separated (dissociated) from the mind as a whole.

distraction A spinal injury that occurs if spinal motion is stopped suddenly relative to body motion, causing the weight and momentum of the body to shift away from it; a pulling apart: also, a self-defense measure in which a diversion is created to attract a person's attention.

distress Negative, debilitating, or harmful stress.

distribution The transport of a drug through the bloodstream to various tissues of the body and ultimately to its site of action.

distributive shock Shock that occurs when peripheral vasodilation causes a decrease in systemic vascular resistance or as a result of impaired distribution of blood flow.

disulfiram-ethanol reaction A potentially life-threatening physiologic response caused by co-ingestion of disulfiram and ethanol that produces ill effects on the gastrointestinal, cardiovascular, and autonomic nervous systems; disulfiram is prescribed to some patients with alcohol use disorder to help them maintain abstinence.

diuretics Medicines that help increase excretion of water from the body.

diversity Differences of any kind, including race, class, religion, sex, sexual preference, personal habitat, and physical ability.

diverticulitis Inflammation of one or more diverticula.

diverticulosis The presence of pouchlike herniations through the muscular layer of the colon.

diverticulum A pouchlike herniation through the muscular wall of a tubular organ. It may be present in the stomach, small intestine, or, most commonly, the colon.

divisions Geographic areas sometimes used to break command into more manageable chunks.

dorsal root A sensory component that conveys afferent nerve processes to the spinal cord.

dose response The physical change or effect caused by exposure to a chemical. The response depends on the concentration of the chemical to which the person was exposed.

Down syndrome A congenital condition characterized by varying degrees of intellectual disability and multiple defects. The cause of this condition is the presence of an extra copy of the 21st chromosome in every cell (trisomy 21).

droplet precautions Steps taken to avoid infection spread in tiny droplets (typically greater than 5 microns in size and traveling no more than approximately 3 feet [1 m]). Such steps include wearing a surgical mask with face shield, gown, and gloves.

drowning The process of experiencing respiratory impairment from submersion/immersion in liquid.

drug Any substance taken by mouth; injected into a muscle, blood vessel, or cavity of the body; or applied topically to treat or prevent a disease or condition.

drug abuse Self-medication or self-administration of a drug in chronically excessive amounts, resulting in psychological or physical dependence (or both), functional impairment, and deviation from approved social norms.

drug interaction Modification of the effects of one drug by the previous or concurrent administration of another drug, thereby increasing or diminishing the pharmacologic or physiologic action of one or both drugs.

drug receptors Parts of a cell (usually an enzyme or large protein molecule) with which a drug molecule interacts to trigger its desired response or effect.

drug–protein complex A complex formed by the attachment of a drug to proteins, mainly albumin.

ductus arteriosus A blood vessel in the fetus that connects the pulmonary artery directly to the proximal descending aorta.

ductus deferens A thick, smooth muscular tube that allows sperm to exit from the epididymis through the ejaculatory duct; also known as the vas deferens.

ductus venosus A vascular shunt unique to the fetal and neonatal circulations. In fetal life, the ductus venosus allows variable portions of the umbilical and portal venous blood flows to bypass the liver microcirculation.

duodenum The first subdivision of the small intestine.

dura mater The outermost layer of the meninges.

duty to act The duty of a party to take necessary action to prevent harm to another party. This duty may be formal or contractual.

dynamic rope "High-stretch" rope that is designed to stretch as much as 20% to 50% under load (eg, when stopping a falling rescuer), which reduces the chance of rope breakage as well as the shock to the rescuer.

dysarthria Difficult and poorly articulated speech resulting from poor control over the muscles of speech.

dysbarism Illness that results directly or indirectly from changes in ambient atmospheric pressure and the pressure of gases within the body.

dysconjugate gaze Failure of the eyes to move with synchronized motion; may be diagnostic of a neurologic injury.

dysfunctional uterine bleeding (DUB) Abnormal bleeding that occurs because of changes in hormone levels.

dyskinesia A movement disorder characterized by involuntary muscle movements; often an adverse effect of prolonged use of antipsychotic medications.

dysmenorrhea Pain associated with menstruation.

dyspareunia Pain with intercourse.

dysphonia An abnormality in the speaking voice, such as hoarseness.

dysplasia Abnormal cellular growth.

dyspnea The sensation of shortness of breath.

dysrhythmias Variations from a normal rhythm.

dysthymia A form of depression that is chronic in nature, lasting as long as 2 years or more.

dystonia A condition characterized by local or diffuse changes in muscle tone, resulting in painful muscle spasms, unusually fixed postures, and strange movement patterns.

dysuria Difficult or painful urination.

early adulthood An age category that includes people 19 to 40 years of age.

Ebola An infectious viral hemorrhagic fever.

ecchymosis Skin discoloration (bruising) caused by the escape of blood into the tissues from ruptured blood vessels.

eclampsia The onset of seizures in a woman with preeclampsia.

economic abuse Making or attempting to make a person financially dependent by maintaining total control over financial resources, withholding a person's access to money, or forbidding a person's attendance at school or employment.

ectopic focus An excitable group of cells outside the normally functioning sinus node of the heart that initiates myocardial depolarization.

ectopic pregnancy A pregnancy that occurs when a fertilized ovum implants anywhere other than the uterus.

edema The accumulation of fluid in the interstitial spaces.

effective dose 50 (ED_{50}) The amount of drug that produces a therapeutic response in 50% of those who take it.

effector organs Muscles or glands that respond to nerve impulses from the central nervous system.

efferent division The division of the peripheral nervous system that transmits action potentials from the central nervous system to effector organs such as muscles and glands.

efferent neurons Neurons that carry impulses away from the central nervous system to the periphery.

egress An exit pathway.

ejection The forceful expulsion of blood from the ventricle of the heart.

elder abuse The infliction of physical pain, injury, debilitating mental anguish, unreasonable confinement, or willful deprivation by a caregiver of services that are necessary to maintain mental and physical health of a geriatric person.

electrical alternans Beat-to-beat variability in the amplitude of a patient's electrocardiographic waveforms. It is a rare finding in cardiac tamponade.

electrical capture Pacing capture in which a pacing stimulus precipitates a ventricular contraction.

electrocardiogram (ECG) A graphic representation of the electrical activity of the heart.

electrolytes Cations or anions in solution that conduct an electrical current.

electronic patient care report (ePCR) An electronic program used in the prehospital setting to record all patient care activities and circumstances related to an emergency response.

emancipation The state of being legally released from parental control and supervision.

embolus A blockage or free-moving thrombus in a blood vessel.

embryo The stage of prenatal development that begins with fertilization and continues until the end of the 8th week of gestation.

emergency medical services A national network of services coordinated to provide aid and medical assistance from primary response to definitive care. The network involves personnel trained in rescue, stabilization, transport, and advanced management of traumatic and medical emergencies.

emergency operations center (EOC) The main communications center where representatives of emergency response organizations, government agencies, and sometimes private organizations gather to coordinate their response to an emergency event.

emetic center An area located in the reticular formation of the brainstem; thought to be the control center for vomiting.

emotional abuse The infliction of anguish, pain, or distress through verbal or nonverbal acts.

empathy The ability to see a situation from the viewpoint of the person experiencing it.

emphysema An abnormal condition of the pulmonary system characterized by overinflation and destructive changes in the alveolar walls, resulting in a loss of lung elasticity, impaired gas exchange, and incomplete emptying of the alveoli during exhalation.

EMS communications The delivery of patient and scene information (either in person, in writing, or through communications technology) to other members of the emergency response team.

encephalitis Inflammation of the brain.

encoding The process by which information is organized in an understandable format (through a medium or channel), either written or verbal.

end-diastolic volume The volume of blood in either the left or the right ventricle at the end of ventricular filling (diastole).

endocarditis An inflammation of the endocardium (inner layer of the heart) typically caused by infection.

endocrine glands Glands that secrete hormones into the blood rather than through a duct.

endocrine system A collection of glands that produce and secrete hormones.

endometriosis An abnormal gynecologic condition characterized by ectopic growth and function of endometrial tissue. It is thought to result when fragments of endometrium from the lining of the uterus are regurgitated during menstruation backward through the fallopian tubes into the peritoneal cavity; there, they attach and grow as small cystic structures.

endometritis An inflammatory condition of the endometrium, usually caused by bacterial infection.

endometrium The mucous membrane lining of the uterus, which changes in thickness and structure with the menstrual cycle.

endoplasmic reticulum A network of connecting sacs or canals that wind through the cytoplasm of a cell, serving as a miniature circulatory system for the cell.

endorphins Peptides secreted in the brain that have pain-relieving effects similar to morphine.

endotoxins Toxins contained in the cell walls of some microorganisms, especially gram-negative bacteria.

end-stage renal disease Complete or near-complete failure of the kidneys to function.

engulfment Mechanical entrapment that places a person in a confined space.

enhanced automaticity An increase in the firing rate of myocardial cells beyond their inherent rate.

envenomation The injection of snake, arachnid, or insect venom into the body.

enzymes A protein produced by living cells that catalyzes chemical reactions in organic matter.

eosinophil chemotactic factor of anaphylaxis A group of active substances, including histamine and leukotrienes, that are released during an anaphylactic reaction.

eosinophils White blood cells that act as cellular mediators of inflammation; thought to play a key role in asthma and allergy as well as parasitic infections.

epicardium The portion of the serous pericardium that covers the heart's surface; also known as the visceral pericardium.

epidemic A widespread occurrence of an infectious disease in a community at a particular time (eg, influenza in the winter).

epidemiology The study of how disease is distributed within populations and the factors that influence that distribution.

epidermis The outer portion of the skin. It is formed of epithelial tissue that rests on or covers the dermis.

epididymis A tightly coiled tube, lying along the top of and behind the testes, where sperm matures.

epididymitis Inflammation of the epididymis, a tubular section of the male reproductive system that carries sperm from the testicle to the seminal vesicles.

epidural hematoma Accumulation of blood between the dura mater and the cranium.

epidural space The space above or on the dura.

epiglottis A lidlike cartilage that overhangs the entrance to the larynx.

epiglottitis Inflammation of the epiglottis; a severe form of the condition that affects primarily children is characterized by fever, sore throat, stridor, croupy cough, drooling, respiratory distress, and an erythematous epiglottis.

epilepsy A condition characterized by the tendency to have recurrent seizures (excluding those that arise from correctable or avoidable circumstances).

epiphyseal fracture A fracture involving the epiphyseal plate of a long bone.

epiphyseal plate The site of bone elongation; also known as the growth plate.

epistaxis Bleeding from the nose.

epithelial tissue The cellular covering of internal and external surfaces of the body, including the lining of vessels and other small cavities.

eponym A term that is derived from a person's name.

erection The condition of hardness, swelling, and elevation observed in the penis and to a lesser degree in the clitoris, usually caused by sexual arousal.

erythema Redness of the skin, caused by hyperemia of the capillaries in the lower layers of the skin.

erythroblastosis fetalis Hemolytic anemia in the fetus caused by maternal antibodies directed against the fetus's erythrocytes, secondary to ABO or Rh incompatibility between the mother and the fetus.

erythrocytes Red blood cells.

eschar A scab or dry crust of dead tissue resulting from a thermal or chemical burn.

escharotomy Surgical incision that splits an eschar to prevent or relieve compartment syndrome.

esophageal atresia The incomplete formation or abnormal development of the esophagus.

esophageal varices A complex of longitudinal, tortuous veins at the lower end of the esophagus that become enlarged and swollen as a result of portal hypertension.

esophagitis Inflammation of the esophagus.

esophagus The muscular canal extending from the pharynx to the stomach.

estimated date of confinement Predicted delivery date for the fetus based on either last menstrual period or ideally ultrasonography performed in the first trimester.

ethics The discipline relating to right and wrong, moral duty and obligation, moral principles and values, and moral character; a standard for honorable behavior designed by a group with expected conformity.

ethnocentrism The belief that one's own life is the most acceptable or best; acting in a superior manner toward another culture's way of life.

eukaryotes Cells with a true nucleus. They are found in all higher organisms and in some microorganisms.

eustachian tube The auditory canal, which extends from the middle ear to the nasopharynx; also known as the auditory tube.

eustress Positive, performance-enhancing stress.

evaluation A component of critical thinking in which the examiner assesses the patient's response to care.

evasive tactics A self-defense measure in which an aggressor's moves and actions are anticipated and unconventional pathways are used during retreat for personal safety.

event phase The phase of trauma that refers to the trauma event.

evidence-based medicine Medical practice that is based on current scientific evidence.

evisceration The protrusion of an internal organ or the peritoneal contents through a wound or surgical incision, especially in the abdominal wall.

excited delirium A sudden state of delirium, extreme psychomotor agitation, unusual strength, and hyperadrenergic autonomic dysfunction, typically in the setting of acute or chronic drug abuse or serious mental illness.

exclusion criteria Criteria that exclude a patient from eligibility for a particular research study; defined on a study-by-study basis.

excretion The elimination of toxic or inactive metabolites, primarily by the kidneys. The intestines, lungs, and mammary, sweat, and salivary glands also may be involved.

exocrine glands Glands that secrete chemicals and enzymes into a duct.

exotoxins Toxins secreted or excreted by a living organism.

expiration Breathing out (exhalation); normally a passive process.

expiratory reserve volume The amount of gas that can be forcefully exhaled after expiration of the normal tidal volume.

explosive A bomb, which can be made from a variety of dangerous materials.

exposure incident Any specific contact of the eyes, the mouth, other mucous membranes, or nonintact skin, or any parenteral contact, with blood, blood products, bloody body fluids, or other potentially infectious materials.

expressed consent Verbal or written consent to treatment.

extended (expanded) scope of practice The expansion of health care services provided by EMS personnel in the prehospital setting.

external barriers The surface of the body that is exposed to the environment, including the skin and the mucous membranes of the digestive, respiratory, and genitourinary tracts. The body's first line of defense against infection.

external ear The portion of the ear that includes the auricle and external auditory meatus. It terminates at the eardrum.

external respiration The transfer (diffusion) of oxygen and carbon dioxide between the inspired air and pulmonary capillaries.

extracellular Occurring outside a cell or cell tissues or in cavities or spaces between cell layers or groups of cells.

extracellular fluid The fluid found outside the cells, including that in the intravascular and interstitial compartments.

extracellular matrix Nonliving chemical substances located between connective tissue cells.

extravasation The passage or escape of blood, serum, or lymph into the tissues.

extrication/rescue group The group responsible for managing patients who are trapped. Responsibilities of this group may include search, rescue, initial triage, tagging, and in situ treatment before transfer of the patients to the treatment group.

extubation Removal of an endotracheal tube.

facilitated diffusion A carrier-mediated process that moves substances into or out of cells from a high to a low concentration.

factitious disorders A group of disorders in which symptoms are deliberately produced, feigned, or exaggerated to mimic a true illness. There is no motive for personal gain; the goal is merely to assume the role of a patient.

fall on an outstretched hand A common mechanism of injury that occurs when people attempt to break a fall by catching themselves with the palm of their hand, resulting in hand, wrist, elbow, or shoulder injury.

fallopian tubes A pair of ducts that open at one end into the uterus and at the other end into the peritoneal cavity, over the ovaries; also known as uterine tubes.

false imprisonment Intentional and unjustifiable detention of a person.

false movement An unnatural movement of an extremity, usually associated with fracture.

family history Illness or disease in a patient's family or family's background that may be relevant to the patient complaint.

fascia The loose areolar connective tissue found beneath the skin or dense connective tissue that encloses and separates muscle.

fasciitis Inflammation of the fascia.

Fc receptors Proteins found on the surface of certain cells that contribute to the protective functions of the immune system. These receptors bind to antibodies that are attached to infected cells or invading pathogens.

febrile seizure A seizure that results from fever. It most commonly occurs in children between ages 6 months and 5 years.

fecal impaction An accumulation of hardened feces in the rectum or sigmoid colon that the person is unable to move.

fecalith A hard, impacted mass of feces in the colon.

Federal Communications Commission (FCC) A federal agency that regulates interstate and international communications by radio, television, wire, satellite, and cable in all 50 states, the District of Columbia, and US territories.

female external genital organs The outer parts of the female genitalia; also known as the vulva. They consist of the labia majora, the labia minora, Bartholin glands, and the clitoris.

femur The thigh bone, which extends from the pelvis to the knee; the largest and strongest bone in the body.

fend-off position Positioning of the ambulance diagonally about 50 feet (15 m) in front of the scene for safety, so as to divert and avert oncoming traffic.

fetus A stage in prenatal development. In humans this stage is between the embryonic stage (end of 10th week) and birth.

fibrinogen A soluble blood protein that is converted into insoluble fibrin during clotting.

fibromyalgia A disorder that causes extreme fatigue; associated with "tender points" on the neck, shoulders, back, hips, arms, and legs.

fibrous connective tissue A connective tissue that consists mainly of bundles of strong, white collagenous fibers arranged in parallel rows.

fibrous joints Joints that are immovable.

fibula A bone of the lower leg, lateral to and smaller than the tibia.

Fick principle The assumption that the amount of oxygen delivered to an organ is equal to the amount of oxygen consumed by that organ plus the amount of oxygen carried away from that organ. This principle is used to determine cardiac output.

field impression An impression of the patient's condition that the paramedic makes based on pattern recognition that results from experience.

finance/administration section The section responsible for tracking costs and reimbursement.

fine ventricular fibrillation (VF) Fibrillatory waves less than 3 mm in amplitude.

first stage of labor The stage of labor that begins with contractions and ends when the cervix is fully dilated at 10 cm. It is divided into early labor, active labor, and transition.

first-degree atrioventricular (AV) block A benign dysrhythmia in which there is a delay in conduction, usually at the level of the atrioventricular node; seen as prolongation of the PR interval on an electrocardiogram to greater than 200 milliseconds.

first-degree sprain An injury in which there is stretching of a ligament without joint disability. There is minimal, if any, associated swelling.

first-pass metabolism The initial biotransformation of a drug during passage through the liver from the portal vein that occurs before the drug reaches the general circulation.

flail chest A chest wall injury in which two or more adjacent ribs are fractured in two or more places.

flat bones Bones that have a thin, flattened shape, such as certain skull bones, the ribs, the sternum, and the scapulae.

flat-terrain rescue A type of rescue involving the movement of a victim up or down a grade of approximately 0° to 20° of elevation or decline that may involve various obstructions. An example of this terrain is level land with large rocks, loose soil, and beds of water or creeks.

flexor tenosynovitis A pathologic state that causes a disruption of tendon function in the hand; usually the result of infection.

focal aware seizure A seizure during which the patient is aware of his or her surroundings.

focal impaired awareness seizure A seizure during which there is a change in the patient's level of awareness.

focal injury A specific, grossly observable brain lesion concentrated in one region of the brain.

focal onset seizure A seizure that begins within networks of one hemisphere of the brain (previously referred to as a partial seizure). These seizures usually arise from identifiable lesions in the motor or sensory cortex and may spread in an orderly way to surrounding areas (jacksonian march).

food poisoning Poisoning that results from food contaminated by toxic substances or by bacteria containing toxins.

foodborne botulism Illness that results from eating foods that contain the bacillus *Clostridium botulinum*.

foramen ovale An opening in the septum between the right and left atria in the fetal heart that provides a bypass for blood that would otherwise flow to the fetal lungs.

formal product identification A method of identifying a hazardous material through written means.

Fournier gangrene A life-threatening bacterial infection of the skin that affects the genitals and perineum in both men and women.

fracture A break in the continuity of bone.

frailty A geriatric syndrome characterized by exhaustion, slowed performance, weakness, weight loss, and low physical activity.

frostbite A localized injury that results from freezing of body tissues.

frostnip A cold injury manifested by transient numbness and tingling that resolves after rewarming.

full-thickness burn A burn injury in which the entire thickness of the epidermis and dermis is destroyed; also known as a third-degree burn.

fundal massage The application of external pressure to the uterus to decrease postpartum bleeding.

fusion beat A beat that occurs when supraventricular and ventricular electrical impulses act on the same region of the heart at the same time, producing a hybrid complex of intermediate width and morphology.

gag reflex A normal neural response triggered by touching the soft palate or posterior pharynx.

gait A manner of walking or moving on foot.

gallbladder A pear-shaped excretory sac on the visceral surface of the right lobe of the liver. It serves as a reservoir for bile.

gang Any group of people who engage in socially disruptive or criminal behavior.

ganglia A group of nerve cell bodies in the peripheral nervous system.

gangrene Dead or dying body tissues attributable to blood supply that is lost or inadequate.

gastric lavage Irrigation of the stomach with sterile water or normal saline.

gastric tube A device that is inserted into the stomach to remove fluids and gas by suction or gravity, to instill irrigation solutions or medications, and to administer gastric feedings.

gastroesophageal reflux disease (GERD) A condition in which the stomach contents leak backward from the stomach into the esophagus.

gastrointestinal decontamination The use of medical methods to empty the stomach of ingested toxins to prevent absorption.

gastroschisis An abdominal wall defect in which the anterior abdomen does not close properly, allowing the intestines to protrude outside the fetus.

gaze palsy Symmetric limitation of the movements of both eyes in the same direction (conjugate gaze).

general impression An immediate assessment of the environment and the patient's chief complaint used to determine whether the patient is ill or injured and the nature of illness or the mechanism of injury.

generalized onset seizure A seizure that begins within networks of both hemispheres of the brain.

generic name The official, established name assigned to a drug.

genitourinary system The system comprising the genital and reproductive organs.

gerontology The study of the special needs and restrictions associated with aging.

gestation The period from fertilization of the ovum until birth.

gestational diabetes mellitus A disorder characterized by impaired ability to metabolize carbohydrates, usually caused by a deficiency of insulin. It occurs in pregnancy and disappears after delivery but in some cases returns years later.

gestational hypertension Hypertension (defined as a blood pressure of 140/90 mm Hg) that develops in a pregnant woman after 20 weeks' gestation without any other features of preeclampsia and resolves during the postpartum period.

Glasgow Coma Scale (GCS) A standardized system for assessing the degree of impairment of consciousness in a critically ill patient and for predicting the duration and ultimate outcome of coma.

glaucoma A condition in which intraocular pressure increases and causes damage to the optic nerve.

globulins Simple proteins classified based on their solubility, mobility, and size.

glomerulus The mass of capillary loops at the beginning of each nephron.

glossopharyngeal neuralgia Irritation of the glossopharyngeal nerve (cranial nerve IX).

glottic opening The vocal cords and the space between them.

glucagon A hormone produced by the alpha cells in the islets of Langerhans that stimulates the conversion of glycogen to glucose in the liver.

gluconeogenesis The formation of glucose from fatty acids and proteins rather than carbohydrates.

glycogenolysis The breakdown of glycogen to glucose.

glycolysis An anaerobic process during which glucose is converted to pyruvic acid.

glycoproteins A large group of conjugated proteins in which the nonprotein substance is a carbohydrate.

Golgi apparatus Specialized endoplasmic reticulum that concentrates and packages materials for secretion from the cell.

gonorrhea A sexually transmitted disease that results from contact with the causative organism *Neisseria gonorrhoeae.*

Good Samaritan laws State laws that are passed to encourage people to help others in an emergency without fear of litigation (being sued), if not expressly abrogated by statute.

gout A disease associated with an inborn error of uric acid metabolism that increases production of or interferes with excretion of uric acid; also known as hyperuricemia.

graffiti Gang markings that usually indicate territorial boundaries; also known as tagging.

gram A metric unit of mass equal to $\frac{1}{1,000}$ (ie, 0.001) of a kilogram.

Graves disease A type of excessive thyroid activity characterized by generalized enlargement of the gland (goiter) that leads to a swollen neck and often to protruding eyes (exophthalmos).

gravida The number of all current and past pregnancies.

gray matter The gray tissue that makes up the inner core of the spinal column.

Grey Turner sign Bruising of the skin of the flanks or loin in retroperitoneal hemorrhage and acute hemorrhagic pancreatitis; also known as Turner sign.

Ground Vehicle Standard for Ambulances (GVS v.1.0) The standard that identifies the minimum requirements for new ground ambulances built on a manufacturer's chassis. It applies to new vehicles only.

groups Resources, including people, apparatus, and equipment, assembled to perform a specific function, regardless of geographic area; sometimes used to break a command into more manageable chunks.

growth hormone (GH) A polypeptide hormone produced and secreted by the anterior pituitary gland. It acts as an insulin antagonist.

Guillain-Barré syndrome (GBS) A rare disease associated with a viral infection or immunization that affects the peripheral nervous system, especially the spinal nerves, but also the cranial nerves.

half-duplex mode A communications mode in two frequencies that allows data to flow in one direction or the other, but not both at the same time.

hallucinations The apparent perception of sights, sounds, and other sensory phenomena that are not actually present.

hantavirus A virus that is carried by rodents and spread to humans through body fluids of rodents. Several strains can cause different forms of severe illness, such as hemorrhagic fever with renal syndrome and hantavirus pulmonary syndrome.

hazard and risk assessment An analysis of the consequences and probability that exposure to a chemical may cause danger or peril.

hazard control The phase of rescue that involves managing, reducing, and minimizing risks from uncontrollable hazards; ensuring scene safety; and providing personal protective equipment appropriate for the incident.

hazardous atmospheres Oxygen-deficient, toxic, or explosive environments that may occur in confined spaces.

hazardous material (hazmat) Any item or agent (biologic chemical, radiologic and/or physical) that has the potential to cause harm to humans, animals, or the environment, either by itself or through interaction with other factors.

head lice Tiny parasites that concentrate around the scalp (sometimes including the eyebrows and eyelashes).

hearing impairment Any degree of hearing loss that is caused by disruption of the auditory system.

heart failure An abnormal condition that reflects impaired ventricular filling (diastolic dysfunction) or blood volume ejection (systolic dysfunction); usually a result of myocardial infarction, ischemic heart disease, long-standing hypertension, or cardiomyopathy.

heart murmurs Abnormal heart sounds caused by altered blood flow into a chamber or through a valve.

heat cramps Brief, intermittent, and often severe muscular cramps that frequently occur in muscles fatigued by heavy work or exercise.

heat exhaustion A form of heat illness characterized by dizziness, nausea, headache, and a mild to moderate increase in the core body temperature.

heatstroke The end stage of the heat illness spectrum that occurs when the thermoregulatory mechanisms normally in place to meet the demands of heat stress break down entirely. As a result, mental status becomes altered, and the core body temperature increases to extreme levels. Multisystem tissue damage and physiologic collapse also occur.

HELLP syndrome A severe form of preeclampsia that involves H, hemolysis; EL, elevated liver enzymes; and LP, low platelet count.

hematemesis Vomiting of bright red blood, indicating upper gastrointestinal bleeding.

hematochezia The passage of red blood through the rectum.

hematology The scientific study of blood and blood-forming organs.

hematoma A closed injury characterized by blood vessel disruption and swelling beneath the epidermis.

hematoma formation The infiltration of blood into the tissues at the site of venipuncture.

hematopoietic tissue Tissue related to the process of formation and development of various types of blood cells.

hematuria The presence of blood in the urine.

hemifacial spasm A neuromuscular disorder characterized by frequent involuntary contractions of the muscles on one side of the face.

hemiparesis One-sided weakness; a possible complication of stroke.

hemodialysis A procedure in which impurities or wastes are removed from the blood. It is used in treating renal insufficiency and various toxic conditions.

hemodilution An increase in the fluid content of the blood that results in a lowered concentration of formed elements and lowered blood viscosity.

hemoglobin A complex protein–iron compound in the blood that carries oxygen to the cells from the lungs and carbon dioxide away from the cells to the lungs.

hemolysis The breakdown of red blood cells and the release of hemoglobin.

hemolytic anemia A condition in which delivery of oxygen to tissues is reduced because of an increase in hemolysis of erythrocytes.

hemoperitoneum The presence of extravasated blood in the peritoneal cavity.

hemophilia A group of hereditary bleeding disorders in which one of the factors necessary for blood coagulation is deficient.

hemophilia A A condition caused by a deficiency of coagulation factor VIII. It is considered the classic type of hemophilia.

hemophilia B A condition caused by a deficiency of coagulation factor IX.

hemopneumothorax A collection of air and blood in the pleural space; also known as a pneumohemothorax.

hemoptysis Coughing up of blood from the respiratory tract.

hemorrhage A disruption, or "leak," in the vascular system resulting in the flow of blood.

hemorrhagic stroke A stroke caused by a rupture of weakened blood vessels in the brain.

hemorrhoids Swollen, distended veins (internal, external, or both) in the rectoanal area.

hemostasis The cessation of bleeding by mechanical or chemical means or by substances that arrest the blood flow.

hemothorax The accumulation of blood and other fluids in the pleural space caused by bleeding from the lung parenchyma or damaged vessels.

hemotoxins Hazardous substances that may cause the destruction of red blood cells.

hemotympanum Blood behind the tympanic membrane often from fractures of the temporal bone.

Henry's law A law stating that at a constant temperature, the amount of gas that dissolves in a liquid is directly proportional to the partial pressure of that gas in equilibrium with that liquid.

hepatic artery The branch of the aorta that delivers blood to the liver.

hepatic encephalopathy A spectrum of neuropsychiatric dysfunction caused by liver disease and commonly associated with ammonia intoxication.

hepatitis Inflammation of the liver caused by viruses, trauma, toxins, autoimmune or metabolic disorders, genetic diseases, or fat deposits.

hepatotoxins Hazardous substances that damage the liver.

hereditary hemochromatosis An inherited condition in which the body absorbs and stores too much iron. The extra iron accumulates in several organs, especially the liver, heart, and pancreas.

Hering-Breuer reflex A reflex in which afferent impulses from stretch receptors in the lungs arrest inspiration. Expiration then occurs. Inflation and deflation reflexes are triggered to prevent overinflation of the lungs.

hernia Protrusion of any organ through an opening in the muscle or tissue holding it in place or where it normally resides.

herniated disk An injury in which all or part of a spinal disk is forced through a weakened part of the disk.

herpes simplex virus type 1 (HSV-1) An infection caused by the herpes simplex virus that tends to occur above the waist, particularly in the facial area, such as around the mouth and nose.

herpes simplex virus type 2 (HSV-2) An infection caused by the herpes simplex virus that usually is limited to the genital region.

hexaxial reference system The system of intersecting lines of the standard limb leads and three other intersecting lines of reference: aV_R, aV_L, and aV_F leads.

hiatal hernia Herniation of the stomach through the diaphragm and up into the chest.

high system utilizer A patient who frequents the emergency department or repeatedly has inpatient stays.

high-altitude cerebral edema (HACE) The most severe form of acute high-altitude illness. It is characterized by a progression of global cerebral signs in the presence of acute mountain sickness.

high-altitude illness Illness that principally occurs at altitudes 8,200 feet (2,500 m) or more above sea level.

high-altitude pulmonary edema (HAPE) A high-altitude illness thought to be caused at least partly by an increase in pulmonary artery pressure that develops in response to hypoxia.

high-angle rescue A type of rescue involving the movement of a victim up or down a grade of greater than 60°, typically requiring a high degree of specialized equipment, techniques, and training.

high-grade atrioventricular (AV) block Second-degree heart block with a P-to-QRS ratio of at least 3:1 or higher; distinguished from third-degree block because a conductive relationship between the atria and the ventricles still exists.

high-output heart failure A type of heart failure in which cardiac output remains high but is unable to meet the metabolic needs of the body because of increased demand.

histamine An amine released by mast cells and basophils that promotes inflammation.

history taking The process of gathering information during the patient interview.

Hodgkin lymphoma A malignant disorder of the lymphatic system characterized by the presence of Reed-Sternberg cells at biopsy. It is associated with pain and progressive enlargement of lymphoid tissue.

homeostasis A state of equilibrium in the body with respect to functions and composition of fluids and tissues.

homonym A word that has the same pronunciation as another word but a different meaning, and often a different spelling (in which case it can more specifically be referred to as a homophone).

hordeolum An acute infection of the oil gland; commonly known as a sty.

hormone receptors Receptors on target organs and body tissues that are able to respond to a particular hormone.

hormones Substances, usually peptides or a steroids, produced by one tissue and conveyed by the bloodstream to another to effect physiologic activity, such as growth or metabolism.

hospice care A type of care and philosophy of care that includes supportive social, emotional, and spiritual services for terminally ill patients and their families; occurs when the patient is at the end of life and the decision has been made to stop active treatment and only provide measures that decrease the severity of symptoms.

host The human or animal exposed to an infectious agent.

host susceptibility Factors of the host that contribute to prevention or continuation of infection.

hot zone The area of a hazmat incident that presents an immediate danger to life or health and typically includes the hazardous material itself.

household system A common system of measurement that includes the glass, cup, tablespoon, teaspoon, drop, quart, and pint.

human immunodeficiency virus (HIV) The viral agent responsible for acquired immunodeficiency syndrome.

human trafficking The illegal exploitation of a person.

humerus The largest bone of the upper arm, comprising a body, head, and condyle.

humoral immunity One of the two forms of immunity that respond to antigens such as bacteria and foreign tissue.

Huntington disease (HD) A rare, hereditary disease characterized by quick, involuntary movements, speech disturbances, and mental deterioration; also known as Huntington chorea. It is caused by degenerative changes in the cerebral cortex and basal ganglia.

hydrocele A fluid-filled sac along the spermatic cord in the scrotum.

hydrocephalus A pathologic condition characterized by an abnormal accumulation of cerebrospinal fluid, usually under increased pressure, within the cranial vault, resulting in dilation of the cerebral ventricles.

hydrogen ion The acidic element in a solution.

hydrops fetalis A fetal condition characterized by the accumulation of fluid throughout body tissues, including the lungs, heart, and abdominal organs.

hymen A mucous membrane that may partly or entirely occlude the vaginal outlet.

hyoid bone The U-shaped bone between the mandible and the larynx.

hypercalcemia A higher-than-normal concentration of calcium in the blood.

hyperemesis gravidarum (HG) A condition of pregnancy characterized by severe nausea, vomiting, weight loss, and electrolyte disturbance.

hyperemia An increase in organ blood flow.

hyperglycemia A greater-than-normal amount of glucose in the blood.

hyperkalemia A higher-than-normal concentration of potassium in the blood.

hypermagnesemia A higher-than-normal concentration of magnesium in the blood.

hypernatremic dehydration The loss of more water than sodium.

hyperopia A vision condition in which distant objects are seen clearly but close ones do not come into proper focus; also known as farsightedness.

hyperosmolar hyperglycemic nonketotic syndrome (HHNS) A diabetic state in which the level of ketone bodies is normal. It is caused by hyperosmolarity of extracellular fluid and results in dehydration of intracellular fluid.

hyperphosphatemia High levels of phosphate in the blood.

hyperplasia An excessive increase in the number of cells.

hypersensitivity An altered immunologic reactivity to an antigen.

hypersensitivity reactions A pathologic immune response to an antigen.

hypertension A disorder characterized by elevated blood pressure that persistently exceeds 130/80 mm Hg.

hypertensive encephalopathy A clinical syndrome of neurologic symptoms including headache, convulsions, and coma resulting from severe blood pressure elevation.

hyperthermia Abnormal elevation of body temperature.

hyperthyroidism A condition characterized by increased activity of the thyroid gland.

hypertonic A term used to describe a solution that has a greater concentration of solutes than does another solution, giving it a higher osmotic pressure than the pressure of body cells. Cells may shrink as water is pulled out of the cell into the area of higher solute concentration.

hypertonic solutions Solutions that have higher osmotic pressure than body cells have.

hypertrophic scar An excess accumulation of scar tissue within the original wound borders.

hypertrophy An increase in the size of a cell.

hyperventilation syndrome Abnormally deep or rapid breathing that leads to excessive loss of carbon dioxide, resulting in respiratory alkalosis.

hypocalcemia An abnormally low level of calcium in the blood.

hypocapnia A state of diminished carbon dioxide in the blood; also known as hypocarbia.

hypoglycemia A lower-than-normal amount of glucose in the blood.

hypokalemia A lower-than-normal concentration of potassium in the blood.

hypomagnesemia A lower-than-normal concentration of magnesium in the blood plasma.

hyponatremic dehydration The loss of more sodium than water.

hypoperfusion Severely inadequate circulation that results in insufficient delivery of oxygen and nutrients necessary for normal tissue and cellular function; may cause shock.

hypophosphatemia Low levels of phosphate in the blood.

hypoplastic left heart syndrome A condition in which the heart's left side, including the aorta, aortic valve, left ventricle, and mitral valve, is underdeveloped.

hypothalamus A portion of the diencephalon of the brain that activates, controls, and integrates the peripheral autonomic nervous system, endocrine processes, and many somatic functions, such as body temperature, sleep, and appetite.

hypothermia An abnormal body temperature below 95°F (35°C).

hypothesis A statement of the relationship between two or more variables.

hypothyroidism A condition characterized by decreased activity of the thyroid gland.

hypotonic A term used to describe a solution that has a lower concentration of solutes than does another solution.

hypovolemic shock A form of shock that is most frequently caused by inadequate circulating blood volume.

hypoxemia A lower than normal oxygen content of the blood as measured in an arterial blood sample.

hypoxia A state of decreased oxygen content at the tissue level.

hypoxic drive The low arterial oxygen pressure stimulus to respiration that is mediated through the carotid bodies.

hysterectomy The surgical removal of the uterus.

idiopathic Arising from an obscure or unknown cause.

idiosyncrasy An abnormal or peculiar response to a drug.

ileostomy A surgical opening into the small intestine.

ileum The distal portion of the small intestine.

ileus Cessation of peristalsis of the intestines, which may be paralytic or mechanical.

iliac crest The upper free margin of the ilium.

ilium One of the three bones that make up the innominate bone.

immune response A defense function of the body that produces antibodies to destroy invading antigens and malignancies.

immune system A complex network of cells, tissues, and organs that work together to protect the body against "attacks" by foreign substances.

immunoglobulin A (IgA) An antibody that plays a crucial role in mucosal immunity.

immunoglobulin D (IgD) An antibody present on the surface of most, but not all, B cells early in their development. It signals B cells to activate.

immunoglobulin E (IgE) An antibody that plays an important role in allergies. It is especially associated with type I anaphylactic reactions.

immunoglobulin G (IgG) The most abundant antibody. It is equally distributed in blood and tissue liquids.

immunoglobulin M (IgM) A basic antibody that produces B cells; the first antibody to appear in response to initial exposure to an antigen.

immunologic memory The body's ability to rapidly produce large numbers of specific immune cells after subsequent exposure to a previously encountered antigen.

immunology A broad branch of medical science that covers the study of the immune system.

immunosuppression Reduction in the activation or efficiency of the immune system. It often is caused by drugs or radiation administered to prevent the rejection of grafts or transplanted tissues or to control autoimmune disease.

implied consent The presumption that an unconscious or incompetent person would consent to lifesaving care.

improvised explosive device (IED) A "homemade" bomb constructed of explosives attached to a detonator; an example is a roadside bomb.

inadvertent hyperventilation Excessive ventilation that is thought to result in increased intrathoracic pressure and decreased coronary perfusion pressure; also known as rescuer hyperventilation.

incendiary devices Firebombs.

incident action plan (IAP) A mental, oral, or written plan of the general objectives and overall strategy for managing an incident. The IAP often identifies operational resources, assignments, time frames, and other information important for the management of the incident over one or more operational periods.

incident command system (ICS) A universal framework designed to improve coordination and efficient control of emergency response operations and resources.

incident commander (IC) The person responsible for all incident activities, including the development of strategies and tactics and the ordering and release of resources. The IC has overall authority and responsibility for conducting incident operations and is responsible for the management of all incident operations at the incident site.

inclusion criteria Criteria that a patient must meet to be eligible for a particular research study; defined on a study-by-study basis.

incontinence The inability to control bladder or bowel function.

incubation period The stage of infection during which an organism reproduces. It begins with invasion of the agent and ends when the disease process begins. The host is asymptomatic during this period.

indigenous flora Agents normally found on various sites of the body that could produce disease if allowed access to the interior of the body.

indirect medical oversight The oversight of all medical components of an EMS system, including provider credentialing and education, protocol development, standing orders, quality assurance, and continuous quality improvement; formerly known as off-line medical control.

infant A child 1 month to 1 year of age.

infant botulism Illness caused by consumption of the spores of the botulinum bacteria, which then grow in the intestines and release toxin.

infarction Tissue death from lack of oxygen.

infectious disease Any illness caused by a specific microorganism.

inferential statistics A form of statistics that enables the researcher to conclude (infer) whether the relationships seen in a sample are likely to occur in the larger population.

inferior Toward the feet; below a point of reference in the anatomic position.

inferior vena cava The vein that returns blood from the lower limbs and the greater part of the pelvic and abdominal organs to the right atrium.

infiltration The process by which a fluid passes into tissues.

inflammatory bowel disease (IBD) A general term that describes two diseases—ulcerative colitis and Crohn disease—that cause chronic inflammation of the digestive tract.

inflammatory myopathies A group of diseases that involve chronic muscle inflammation accompanied by muscle weakness.

inflammatory response A tissue reaction to injury or to an antigen. It may include pain, swelling, itching, redness, heat, and loss of function.

influenza A highly contagious infection of the respiratory tract transmitted by droplet spread. Researchers have identified three main types of the virus (types A, B, and C).

informal product identification A method of identifying a hazardous material through unwritten means.

informed consent Consent obtained from a patient after all facts necessary for the person to make a reasonable decision have been explained.

infrastructure The basic physical and organizational framework needed for the operation of a society or enterprise, such as communication systems, power supplies, water systems, sewer systems, and roads and transportation systems.

inguinal canal The passage through the lower abdominal wall that transmits the spermatic cord in the male and the round ligament in the female.

inhalation injury An upper and/or lower airway injury that results from thermal and/or chemical exposure.

inhalational anthrax Anthrax caused by inhaling the spore-forming bacterium *Bacillus anthracis.*

injury Intentional or unintentional damage inflicted on a person. Examples include falls, assault, burns, and frostbite.

injury risks Any situations that increase a person's risk for sustaining an injury.

injury surveillance The ongoing systematic collection, analysis, and interpretation of injury data essential to the planning, implementation, and evaluation of public health practice.

inner ear The part of the ear that contains the sensory organs for hearing and balance.

inspection A visual assessment of the patient and surroundings.

inspiration The act of drawing air into the lungs.

inspiratory reserve volume The maximum volume of air that can be inspired after inspiration of tidal volume.

institutional review board (IRB) A committee that performs critical oversight functions (scientific, ethical, and regulatory) for research conducted on human subjects.

insulin A hormone secreted by the pancreatic islets.

integumentary system The largest organ system in the body, consisting of the skin and accessory structures.

intellectual disability A disorder characterized by below-average intellectual function with deficits or impairments in the ability to learn and adapt socially.

intelligence/investigations function Determines the source or cause of the incidence to control its impact; may fall within a section or be a separate general staff section.

intercellular Occurring between or among cells.

intercostal muscles Internal and external muscles between the ribs that contract to raise the ribs, thereby increasing the front-to-back (anterior–posterior) and side-to-side dimensions of the chest cavity.

internal barriers Protection against germs provided by the inflammatory response and the immune response; the body's second line of defense against infection.

internal respiration The transfer (diffusion) of oxygen and carbon dioxide between the capillary red blood cells and the tissue cells.

interneurons Neurons that transmit impulses between other neurons, enabling communication between sensory or motor neurons and the central nervous system.

interoperability The ability of multiple organizations to communicate and coordinate effectively.

interrogative A set of questions about a lawsuit that is answered in consultation with the party's lawyer.

interstitial fluid Fluid that occupies the space outside the blood vessels and/or outside the cells of an organ or tissue.

interventricular septum The tissue that separates the right and left ventricles of the heart.

intestinal anthrax Anthrax caused from consuming meat contaminated with the bacterium *Bacillus anthracis.*

intestinal malrotation A congenital defect caused by abnormal rotation of the intestine around the superior mesenteric artery during embryonic development.

intimate partner violence (IPV) A type of violence that occurs between two people in an intimate relationship, whether opposite- and same-sex partners.

intracellular Occurring within cell membranes.

intracellular fluid The fluid found in all body cells.

intracerebral hematoma An accumulation of blood or fluid within the tissue of the brain.

intracerebral hemorrhage A type of intracranial bleed that occurs within the brain tissue or ventricles.

intracranial pressure (ICP) The pressure within the cranial vault.

intraocular pressure Pressure within the eye that keeps the eye inflated.

intrapartum The period during labor and delivery.

intrapulmonic pressure The pressure of the gas in the alveoli.

intrarenal disease Disease or damage within the kidney.

intrathoracic pressure The pressure in the pleural space; also known as the intrapleural pressure.

intussusception Telescoping of one portion of the intestine into another, which results in decreased blood supply of the involved segment.

invasion of privacy The release, without legal cause, of details about a patient's private life that might expose the person to ridicule, notoriety, or embarrassment.

involuntary consent Consent to treatment granted by authority of law.

involuntary guarding An unconscious rigid contraction of the abdominal muscles; a sign of peritoneal inflammation.

ions Atoms or groups of atoms that carry a charge of electricity by virtue of having gained or lost one or more electrons.

iris The colored contractile membrane of the eye that can be seen through the cornea.

iritis Inflammation of the iris of the eye.

iron-deficiency anemia Anemia caused by inadequate supplies of iron needed to synthesize hemoglobin.

irregular bones Bones that are not representative of the other three categories (long, short, or flat bones).

irreversible shock A stage of shock that results in cellular ischemia and necrosis and subsequent organ death, even once oxygenation and perfusion are restored.

irritants Chemicals that are not corrosives, but which can cause a reversible inflammatory effect on living tissue at the site of skin, mucous membrane, respiratory system, or eye contact.

ischemia A state of insufficient perfusion of oxygenated blood to a body organ or part.

ischemic stroke A stroke caused by blockage of a cerebral blood vessel; may be thrombotic or embolic in origin; also known as an occlusive stroke or dry stroke.

ischium One of the three parts of the hipbone. It joins the ilium and the pubis to form the acetabulum.

isografting The transplantation of cells, tissues, or organs between identical twins.

isoimmunity Production by an individual of antibodies from members of the same species, such as anti-Rh antibodies in an Rh-negative person; also known as alloimmunity.

isotonic A term used to describe a solution in which its solute concentration is the same as the solute concentration of another solution with which it is compared.

isotonic dehydration Excessive loss of sodium and water in equal amounts.

jacksonian march A transitory disturbance in motor, sensory, or autonomic function resulting from abnormal neuronal discharges in a localized part of the brain; also known as a focal seizure.

jejunum One of the three portions of the small intestine.

joint Any one of the connections between bones that are classified according to structure and mobility as fibrous, cartilaginous, or synovial. Fibrous joints are immovable, cartilaginous joints are slightly movable, and synovial joints are freely movable.

joint capsule A well-defined structure that encloses a joint.

joint dislocation An injury that occurs when the normal articulating ends of two or more bones are displaced.

joint disorder Any disease or injury that affects human joints.

joule A measurement of electrical energy. One joule is the product of 1 volt (potential) multiplied by 1 amp (current) multiplied by 1 second.

jugular notch The superior margin of the manubrium, which is palpated easily at the anterior base of the neck; also known as the suprasternal notch.

jugular venous distention (JVD) Engorgement of jugular veins caused by an increase in central venous pressure. It is estimated by positioning the head of a supine patient at a 45° angle and observing the neck veins.

junctional escape rhythm A rhythm that originates from the atrioventricular junction, usually at a rate of 40 to 60 beats/min. Complexes are narrow in morphology and are not related to any preceding atrial activity (P waves).

junctional hemorrhage Compressible bleeding in a location where a tourniquet cannot be placed (axilla, groin, base of neck).

junctional tachycardia A type of supraventricular tachycardia caused by a reentry mechanism in the junction of the atrioventricular node.

Kehr sign Pain in the left shoulder thought to be caused by referred pain secondary to irritation of the adjacent diaphragm.

keloid An excessive accumulation of scar tissue that extends beyond the original wound borders.

kernmantle rope A type of rope used in life-safety rescue operations that provides for minimal stretch (a low elongation factor). It is constructed with an interior synthetic fiber core protected by a woven exterior sheath, and designed to optimize strength, abrasion resistance, and flexibility.

ketogenesis The formation or production of ketone bodies.

ketone bodies The normal metabolic products of lipid and pyruvate within the liver. Excessive production leads to their excretion in the urine.

kidney One of the pair of organs that cleanse the body of the waste products continually produced by metabolism.

kilogram A metric unit of mass equal to 1,000 grams, or 2.2046 pounds.

kinematics The process of predicting injury patterns that can result from the forces and motions of energy.

Korsakoff psychosis A form of amnesia often seen in patients with alcohol use disorder, characterized by a loss of short-term memory and an inability to learn new skills.

Krebs cycle A sequence of enzymatic reactions, involving the metabolism of carbon chains of sugar, fatty acids, and amino acids, that yield carbon dioxide, water, and high-energy phosphate bonds.

kyphosis An abnormal condition of the vertebral column characterized by increased convexity in the curvature of the thoracic spine as viewed from the side.

labyrinthitis An ear disorder that involves irritation and swelling of the inner ear structure called the labyrinth.

laceration A torn or jagged wound.

lacrimal gland The tear gland located in the superolateral corner of the orbit.

lactate A salt of lactic acid.

lactic acidosis A disorder characterized by an accumulation of lactic acid in the blood, resulting in a lowered pH in muscle and serum.

lactose intolerance A sensitivity disorder that results in the inability to digest lactose because of a deficiency of or defect in the enzyme lactase.

laminectomy Surgery to remove a portion of a lamina of one or more vertebrae that is compressing the nerve in a herniated disk.

landing zone (LZ) An area prepared for the landing of an aircraft; generally 100 by 100 feet (30 by 30 m).

large intestine The portion of the digestive tract comprising the cecum; the appendix; the ascending, transverse, and descending colons; and the rectum.

large vessel occlusion (LVO) Acute ischemic stroke that involves a large blood vessel, such as vertebral, basilar, carotid, or middle and anterior cerebral arteries. LVO is often associated with worse prognosis.

laryngitis Inflammation of the larynx.

laryngopharynx The lowest part of the pharynx.

larynx The voice box, located just below the pharynx.

late adulthood An age category that includes people 61 to 75 years of age.

latent period A stage of infection that begins when a pathogenic agent invades the body and ends when the agent can be shed or communicated.

latent TB infection Tuberculosis that is not symptomatic or infectious. It must be treated to prevent active TB disease.

lateral recumbent A position in which the patient lies on the right or left side.

Le Fort fractures Classifications used to describe fracture patterns of the midface.

leading questions Questions that persuade the patient to respond in a particular way, usually in a way that confirms the paramedic's assumptions.

left atrium One of the four chambers of the human heart. It receives oxygenated blood from the lungs and pumps it into the left ventricle.

left axis deviation When the mean electrical axis of ventricular contraction is within the quadrant of $-30°$ and $-90°$.

left bundle branch A division in the bundle of His originating in the septum and extending into the left ventricle that provides pathways for impulse conduction.

left bundle branch block (LBBB) A conduction disturbance in the left bundle branch that alters normal septal activation and sends it in the opposite direction.

left main stem bronchus One of two main bronchi that branch from the trachea at the level of the carina.

left ventricular assist device (LVAD) A battery-operated mechanical device implanted into the left ventricle that augments blood flow in patients with severe systolic heart failure.

left-side heart failure A condition that occurs when the left ventricle fails to work as an effective forward pump, causing a back pressure of blood into the pulmonary circulation; also known as left ventricular failure.

legislation Laws made by legislative branches of government.

lens The crystalline portion of the eye.

leukemia A type of cancer in which an abnormal proliferation of white blood cells occurs, usually in the bone marrow.

leukocytes White blood cells.

leukocytosis An abnormal increase in the number of circulating white blood cells.

leukopenia A decrease in the number of white blood cells (most commonly neutrophils).

leukotrienes A class of biologically active compounds that occur naturally in leukocytes and that produce allergic and inflammatory reactions.

level of significance The likelihood that a finding in research data is due to chance; the probability of rejecting the null hypothesis if it is true.

Lewy body disease Dementia associated with abnormal deposits of a protein called alpha-synuclein in the brain with neurons; also known as Lewy body dementia.

libel False statements about a person with malicious intent or reckless disregard for the falsity of the statements; includes statements made in writing or through the mass media.

licensure A process by which a government entity regulates an occupation by granting authority (in the form of a license) to a person to take part in an activity.

lifesaving interventions Priority care using rapid assessments and interventions to stop the dying process, such as controlling major hemorrhage, opening the airway, and providing rescue breathing, chest decompression, and auto-injector antidotes.

ligaments Bands of white, fibrous tissue that connect bones.

limbic system The part of the brain involved with emotions and olfaction.

linear skull fracture A skull fracture that does not displace the bone tissue.

lipid bilayer The central layer of the cytoplasmic membrane. It is composed of a double layer of lipid molecules.

lipoproteins Conjugated proteins in which lipids form an integral part of the molecule. They are synthesized primarily in the liver.

liquefaction Conversion of solid tissues to a fluid or semifluid state.

liter A metric unit of capacity equal to 1 cubic decimeter, 61.025 cubic inches, or 1.0567 liquid quarts.

liver An organ in the upper abdomen that aids in digestion and removes waste products and cellular debris from the blood; the largest solid organ in the human body.

loading dose A large quantity of drug that temporarily exceeds the capacity of the body to excrete the drug.

lobules Small lobes or subdivisions of a lobe.

local/regional threshold The point at which the number of casualties or the nature of the event overwhelms the available resources of local emergency response agencies.

lochia A normal postpartum vaginal discharge that contains blood, mucus, and placental tissue from the lining of the uterus.

lock-out process The disabling and securing of any kind of energized equipment to prevent any unauthorized person from entering the area or gaining access to the controls that have been shut off.

logistics section The section that is responsible for providing supplies and equipment, facilities, services, food, and communications support. The main function of this section is to provide gear and support to the responders.

long bones Bones that are longer than they are wide, such as the humerus, ulna, radius, femur, tibia, fibula, and phalanges.

loop of Henle The U-shaped portion of the renal tubule.

lordosis An inward curvature in the lumbar spine that is normally present to some degree.

Los Angeles Motor Scale (LAMS) A brief stroke score derived from the Los Angeles Prehospital Stroke Screen that helps distinguish patients that have a large vessel occlusion.

Los Angeles Prehospital Stroke Screen (LAPSS) A prehospital stroke screening tool that enables the examiner to identify indications of a possible stroke and to rule out other causes of altered level of consciousness.

low-angle rescue A type of rescue involving the movement of a victim up or down a grade of approximately 35°, often requiring the use of specialized equipment, techniques, and training.

lower airway Airway structures below the glottis.

Ludwig angina A type of cellulitis that involves inflammation of the tissues of the floor of the mouth, under the tongue.

Lund and Browder chart A method to estimate burn injury that assigns specific numbers to each body part and that accounts for developmental changes in percentages of body surface area.

lung cancer A disease of uncontrolled cell growth in tissues of the lung.

luxation A complete dislocation.

Lyme disease An acute, recurrent inflammatory infection transmitted by a tick.

lymph nodes Encapsulated masses of lymphoid tissue found among lymph vessels.

lymph nodules Small, densely packed spherical nodes or aggregations of lymph cells embedded in the reticular meshwork of the lymphatic system. They are found mainly in the tonsils, spleen, and thymus.

lymphatic system The network of vessels, ducts, nodes, valves, and organs involved in protecting and maintaining the internal fluid environment of the body.

lymphocytes White blood cells formed in lymphoid tissue; the primary cells found in lymph fluid.

lymphoma A group of cancers of the immune system and white blood cells. The two main categories are Hodgkin lymphoma and non-Hodgkin lymphoma.

lysosomes Membranous-walled organelles that contain enzymes, which enable the lysosome to function as an intracellular digestive system.

macrophages Phagocytic cells in the immune system created from monocytes in the tissue.

maintenance dose The amount of a drug required to keep a desired steady state of drug concentration in tissues.

major depression A disabling condition that adversely affects a person's family, work, or school life, sleeping and eating habits, and general health; also known as major depressive disorder and clinical depression.

major incident An event for which immediately available resources are insufficient to manage the nature of the emergency.

malaise A vague feeling of weakness or discomfort.

malaria An infection spread by mosquitoes and caused by *Plasmodium* parasites. It results in fever, vomiting, headache.

malfeasance A wrongful or unlawful act.

malignant Having the ability to metastasize, as in a cancerous tumor; very dangerous or virulent; likely to cause death.

Mallory-Weiss syndrome A condition characterized by bleeding after a tear in the mucous membrane at the junction of the esophagus and the stomach; usually self-limited but may be severe.

mammalian diving reflex A reflex stimulated by cold water that shunts blood to the brain and heart from the skin, gastrointestinal tract, and extremities.

mammary glands External accessory sex organs in females; breasts.

managed care organization A network that provides patient care services to its members; includes health maintenance organizations and preferred provider organizations.

mandatory reporting The requirement by law that health care professionals report certain types of cases, such as abuse and neglect.

mania A mood disorder characterized by extreme excitement, hyperactivity, agitation, and sometimes violent and self-destructive behavior.

manubrium One of the three bones of the sternum. It has a broad, quadrangular shape that narrows caudally at its articulation with the superior end of the body of the sternum.

Marburg An infectious viral hemorrhagic fever.

mass-casualty incident (MCI) An event for which immediately available resources are insufficient to manage the number of casualties.

mast cells Specialized cells of the inflammatory response.

mean The arithmetic average of a group being studied.

mean arterial pressure (MAP) The arithmetic mean (the average) blood pressure in the arterial portion of the circulation; a measurement of perfusion; calculated as MAP = [(Diastolic blood pressure × 2) + Systolic blood pressure]/3.

mechanical capture Pacing capture that occurs when an associated pulse is generated with the electrical capture of an artificial pacemaker.

mechanism of injury The nature of the force exerted on the body that produced physical injury.

meconium aspiration The inhalation of meconium by the fetus or newborn. The inhaled meconium can block air passages and result in failure of the lungs to expand or cause other pulmonary dysfunction.

meconium staining A green coloration of amniotic fluid as a result of fetal in utero passage of meconium.

medial malleolus The rounded process on the medial side of the ankle joint.

median A descriptive statistic that is found by first arranging the measurements according to size from smallest to largest, then choosing the measurement in the middle; the midpoint of a distribution score.

mediastinal shift A shift in a patient's mediastinum that moves tissue and organs within the chest cavity to one side.

mediastinitis Inflammation of the mediastinum.

mediastinum The area of the body that includes the trachea, esophagus, thymus, heart, and great vessels.

mediated transport mechanisms Mechanisms that use carrier molecules to move large, water-soluble molecules or electrically charged molecules across cell membranes.

medical asepsis The removal or destruction of disease-causing organisms or infected material.

medical malpractice Professional negligence by act or omission by health care personnel in which the care provided deviates from accepted standards of practice in the medical community and causes injury to the patient.

medical malpractice insurance A type of professional liability insurance that protects health care professionals from medical acts and omissions that cause harm or injury.

medical monitoring The ongoing evaluation of rescuers who are at risk for illness or injury from operations at the incident.

medical oversight The ultimate responsibility and authority for the medical actions of an EMS system; usually provided by one or more physicians.

medical practice act A law that governs the practice of medicine.

medulla The lowest part of the brainstem, which controls vital functions; an enlarged extension of the spinal cord; also known as the medulla oblongata.

melena Abnormal black, tarry stools containing digested blood.

membrane permeability A quality of cell membranes that permits the passage of solvents and solutes into and out of cells.

memory cells Cells that remember a pathogen so that antibody production to the same pathogen can occur more rapidly with future exposures. They are produced by the division of B cells.

menarche The first menstruation and commencement of the cyclic menstrual function.

Ménière disease An abnormality of the inner ear that causes vertigo and tinnitus; associated with fluctuations in hearing loss and a sensation of pressure or pain in the affected ear.

meningitis Inflammation of the membranes (meninges) surrounding the brain and spinal cord.

meningococcal meningitis Meningitis caused by the bacterium *Neisseria meningitidis*; the deadliest form of meningitis, which is spread by respiratory droplets.

menopause The cessation of menses.

menstruation The periodic discharge through the vagina of a blood secretion containing tissue debris from the shedding of the endometrium from the nonpregnant uterus.

mental illness Any form of psychiatric disorder.

mental status examination (MSE) An evaluation tool that includes an assessment of appearance and behavior, speech and language, emotional stability, and cognitive abilities.

mesencephalon One of the three parts of the brainstem; also known as the midbrain.

mesentery A continuous abdominal organ composed of a double fold of peritoneum that holds other abdominal organs to the body wall.

metabolism The culmination of all chemical processes that take place in living organisms.

metacarpals The five bones that extend from the carpus to the phalanges.

metaplasia A change from one cell type to another that is better able to tolerate adverse conditions; a conversion into a form that is not normal for that cell.

metarterioles Small peripheral blood vessels that contain scattered groups of smooth muscle fibers in their walls. They are located between the arterioles and the true capillaries.

metastasis The movement or spreading of cancer cells from one organ or tissue to other locations in the body.

metatarsals The five bones that compose the metatarsus.

meter A metric unit of length equal to 1,000 millimeters.

methemoglobin Hemoglobin with ferrous iron in the oxidized (Fe^{3+}) state.

methemoglobinemia The presence of methemoglobin in the blood, causing cyanosis as a result of the inability of the red blood cells to release oxygen.

methicillin-resistant *Staphylococcus aureus* (MRSA) A *Staphylococcus* infection that is resistant to multiple antibiotics. It is spread by person-to-person contact.

metric system A system of measurement that includes the meter, liter, and gram.

microcirculation Circulation of blood in the smallest blood vessels, including arterioles, capillaries, shunts, and venules.

microdiskectomy The surgical removal of a disk using minimally invasive techniques.

microgram A metric unit of mass equal to $\frac{1}{1,000,000}$ (ie, 0.000001) of a gram.

microinfarcts Small infarcts caused by obstruction of circulation in capillaries, arterioles, or small arteries.

middle adulthood An age category that includes people 41 to 60 years of age.

middle ear An air-filled space in the temporal bone that contains the auditory ossicles.

migraine A severe headache that often is associated with nausea and photophobia, and may be preceded by visual auras.

mild DAI A Grade 1 axonal injury with microscopic changes of the cerebral hemispheres, the corpus callosum, the brainstem and, less commonly, the cerebellum; an example is a concussion.

military time A precise method of expressing time that is used by the armed forces and is based on a 24-hour clock.

milligram A metric unit of mass equal to $\frac{1}{1,000}$ (ie, 0.001) of a gram.

milliliter A metric unit of capacity equal to $\frac{1}{1,000}$ (ie, 0.001) of a liter.

millimeter A metric unit of length equal to $\frac{1}{1,000}$ (ie, 0.001) of a meter.

minute volume The amount of gas inhaled or exhaled in 1 minute. It is found by multiplying the tidal volume by the respiratory rate.

misfeasance A legal act that is performed in a manner that is harmful or injurious.

mitochondria Small, spherical, rod-shaped or thin filamentous structures in the cytoplasm of cells; a site of adenosine triphosphate production.

mitosis Cell division that results in two daughter cells with exactly the same number and type of chromosomes as the mother cell.

mittelschmerz Abdominal pain in the region of the ovary during ovulation. It usually occurs midway through the menstrual cycle.

mixed hearing loss A hearing impairment in which damage to both the outer/middle ear systems and the inner ear or auditory nerve results in a combination of sensorineural and conductive hearing loss.

mobile integrated health care (MIH) The provision of health care using patient-centered, mobile resources in the out-of-hospital environment that are integrated with the entire spectrum of health care and social service resources available in the local community.

mode The number that occurs more often than any other number in a set of data.

mode of transmission The way in which diseases are transmitted; may be direct or indirect contact.

moderate DAI A Grade 2 axonal injury that results in minute petechial bruising of brain tissue.

monocytes White blood cells found in lymph nodes, spleen, bone marrow, and loose connective tissue. These can differentiate into macrophages.

monomorphic ventricular tachycardia (VT) Ventricular tachycardia in which the QRS complex has the same morphology or fixed shape.

mononucleosis A viral infection that causes fever, sore throat, and swollen lymph glands, especially in the neck.

mons pubis The prominence caused by a pad of fatty tissue over the symphysis pubis in the female.

mood disorders Conditions in which the emotions that a person normally experiences in life (eg, happiness, depression, fear, anxiety) undergo undesirable and possibly distressing changes.

moral injury The psychological impact of witnessing events that conflict with one's personal morals, or acting in a way that contradicts one's morals.

morals The personal standards that a person uses to distinguish right from wrong.

Moro (startle) reflex A normal infant response elicited by a sudden loud noise. The infant flexes the legs, makes an embracing gesture with the arms, and usually gives a brief cry.

motor neurons Neurons that innervate muscle fibers.

motor onset seizure A seizure that produces a change in muscle activity, such as weakness, twitching, and stiffening of body parts.

mucus The viscous, slippery secretion of mucous membranes and glands.
mucus plug A collection of cervical mucus that fills and seals the cervical canal during pregnancy. It is discharged from the vagina prior to childbirth.
multifocal atrial tachycardia (MAT) An atrial tachycardia in which there are P waves of at least three different morphologies. Rates are often in the range of 120 to 150 beats/min.
multifocal premature ventricular complex (PVC) Premature ventricular complexes that originate from multiple sites in the ventricles.
multiple gestation A pregnancy with more than one fetus.
multiple myeloma A malignant neoplasm of plasma cells that tend to accumulate in the bone marrow, causing bone pain and pathologic fractures.
multiple organ dysfunction syndrome (MODS) The progressive failure of two or more organ systems after a severe illness or injury.
multiple sclerosis (MS) A progressive disease of the central nervous system in which scattered patches of myelin in the brain and spinal cord are destroyed.
multiplex mode A communications mode that allows multiple data streams to be aggregated onto a single carrier signal, which may then be transmitted via a single transmission medium, such as radio or telephone.
multitasking As it relates to interviewing, the ability to ask questions, take notes, and perform tasks while listening to the patient's answers.
mumps An acute viral disease characterized by swelling of the parotid glands.
Munchausen syndrome A self-imposed factitious disorder imposed in which the patient makes routine pleas for treatment and hospitalization for a symptomatic, but imaginary, illness to gain sympathy or attention.
Munchausen syndrome by proxy A factitious disorder imposed on another in which a person injures or induces illness in others (usually children) to gain sympathy or attention.
muscle strains Slight tears in a muscle or tendon.
muscle tone The constant tension produced by muscles of the body for long periods of time.
muscular dystrophy An inherited muscle disorder of unknown cause marked by a slow but progressive degeneration of muscle fibers.
muscular system The body system responsible for execution of movement and postural maintenance.
musculoskeletal system The body system that comprises bones, muscles, tendons and ligaments, and articulating surfaces (eg, joints, bursae, disks).
mutual aid An agreement with neighboring emergency agencies to exchange equipment and personnel when necessary.
myalgia Diffuse muscle pain, usually accompanied by malaise. It occurs in many infectious diseases.
mycoplasmal pneumonia A type of atypical pneumonia. It is caused by the bacterium *Mycoplasma pneumoniae.*
mycoplasmas A genus of microscopic organisms that lack rigid cell walls; considered the smallest free-living organisms.
myocardial contractility The intrinsic ability of the heart to contract.
myocardial contusion Trauma-induced damage to the heart that may range from a localized bruise to a full-thickness injury to the wall of the heart with hemorrhage and edema.
myocardial rupture Traumatic rupture of the myocardium that occurs when blood-filled chambers of the ventricles are compressed with enough force to rupture the chamber wall, septum, or valve.
myocarditis Inflammation of the heart muscle.
myoclonic seizures Seizures that cause brief muscle contractions, which usually occur at the same time and on both sides of the body.
myofilaments Extremely fine, molecular, threadlike structures that help form the myofibril of muscle. Thick myofibrils are formed of myosin, and thin myofilaments are formed of actin.
myopia A vision condition in which near objects are seen clearly but distant objects do not come into proper focus; also known as nearsightedness.
myositis Inflammation of the muscles; also known as inclusion body myositis.
myxedema A condition that results from a deficiency of thyroid hormone.
narrative The portion of the patient care report that allows a provider to describe events during a call often not captured in prepopulated check boxes or drop-down menus.
natural immunity Non–antigen-specific immunity that is present at birth; also known as innate immunity or nonspecific immunity.
nature of illness The principal characteristics and causes of an illness.
near-fatal asthma Acute asthma associated with respiratory arrest, a drop in blood pressure, and reduced cardiac output.
necrosis Death of a cell or group of cells as the result of disease or injury.
necrotizing fasciitis A rare but critical rapidly progressive inflammatory infection of the fascia with secondary necrosis of skin and subcutaneous tissues; requires urgent surgical intervention.
negative feedback mechanisms Mechanisms that tend to produce a response that balances a change in a system.
neglect The refusal or failure of the caregiver to fulfill obligations or duties to a person.
negligence Failure to use such care as reasonably prudent EMS personnel would use in similar circumstances.

nematocysts Capsules containing threadlike, venomous stinging cells found in some coelenterates.

neonate An infant from birth to 1 month of age.

neoplasia New and abnormal development of cells, which may be benign or malignant.

neoplasm An abnormal growth; may be malignant or benign.

nephron The functional unit of the kidney.

nephrotoxins Hazardous materials that are especially destructive to the kidneys.

nerve agents Chemicals that disrupt the nerve transmissions in the central and peripheral nervous systems.

nerve poisons Poisonous substances that act on the nervous system; generally refers to nerve gas.

neurocognitive disorder A disorder that results in a disturbance of cognitive functioning.

neurogenic shock A type of shock in which circulatory failure is caused by disruption of the nerves that control the size of the blood vessels, leading to widespread dilation; seen in patients with spinal cord injuries; also known as neurogenic hypotension.

neuroglia The supporting or nonneuronal tissue cells of the central and peripheral nervous system.

neurons The functional units of the nervous system, consisting of the nerve cell body, the dendrites, and the axon.

neurotoxins Substances that alter the structure or function of the nervous system.

neurotransmitters Chemicals that are released from neurons at the presynaptic nerve fiber.

neutrophils Small, phagocytic white blood cells, each of which has a lobed nucleus and small granules in the cytoplasm; the most abundant leukocytes in circulating blood.

newborn An infant within the first few hours of life.

newborn jaundice A yellow discoloration of the eye, skin, and mucous membranes in a newborn as a result of high bilirubin levels.

NFPA 1917, *Standard for Automotive Ambulances* The standard that defines the minimum requirements for the design, performance, and testing of new automotive ambulances intended for use under emergency conditions to transport sick or injured people to appropriate medical facilities; developed with consideration of the federal standards.

nitrogen narcosis An illness associated with scuba diving in which divers feel intoxicated when nitrogen becomes dissolved in solution as a result of greater than normal atmospheric pressure; also known as rapture of the deep.

nocturia Excessive urination at night.

nodes of Ranvier The short spaces in the myelin sheath of a nerve fiber between adjacent Schwann cells that allow rapid action potential conduction from one node to the next.

nonelectrolytes Substances with no electrical charge.

nonepileptic seizure A seizure that stems from psychological causes rather than from electrical disturbances in the brain. This type of seizure does not benefit from antiepileptic medication therapy.

nonfeasance Failure to perform a required act or duty.

non-Hodgkin lymphoma Cancer of the lymphocytes, which can accumulate in any tissue but particularly collect in the lymph nodes, spleen, and other organs of the immune system.

noninvasive positive pressure ventilation (NIPPV) Nonintubated application of positive airway pressure using either continuous positive airway pressure or bilevel positive airway pressure.

non–motor onset seizure A seizure that can affect any of the senses, causing changes in sensations of smell, taste, and hearing. The patient may also experience visual and/or auditory hallucinations.

nonselective beta-blocking agents Agents that block $beta_1$- and $beta_2$-receptor sites.

nonsteroid hormones Hormones synthesized chiefly from amino acids, such as insulin, parathyroid hormone, and others.

non–ST-segment elevation myocardial infarction (non-STEMI) A myocardial infarction in which there is no ST-segment elevation.

normal pressure hydrocephalus (NPH) Obstruction to flow or absorption of cerebrospinal fluid (CSF), resulting in increased CSF volume and potentially increased intracranial pressure.

nuchal rigidity Neck stiffness with flexion, which suggests meningeal irritation and possibly meningitis.

nucleoplasm The protoplasm of the nucleus, as contrasted with that of the cell.

nucleus The central controlling body within a living cell.

nuisance variables Variables that can make drawing accurate conclusions from a study difficult.

null hypothesis An exact statement that the results occur by chance (the opposite of the hypothesis).

number needed to harm (NNH) The number of patients, on average, who need to be exposed to a treatment or risk factor for one person to have an adverse effect.

number needed to treat (NNT) The number of patients, on average, who need to be treated to prevent one additional bad outcome.

nursemaid's elbow Subluxation of the radial head that generally occurs in children from the time they start to walk to early school age (2 to 5 years of age).

nystagmus Involuntary jerking movements of the eyes.

obesity A condition in which a person's body weight is 30% over the ideal body weight.

objective information Information based on observable facts, such as clinical signs.

obsessive-compulsive disorder (OCD) A psychiatric disorder in which a person feels stress or anxiety about thoughts or rituals over which the person has little control.

obstructive shock Shock that results from obstruction of forward blood flow.

obturator foramen A large opening on each side of the lower portion of the hipbone, formed posteriorly by the ischium, superiorly by the ilium, and anteriorly by the pubis.

oculomotor nerve The third cranial nerve, which contains sensory and motor fibers. It provides for movement of most of the muscles of the eye, for constriction of the pupil, and for accommodation of the eye to light.

official name The name of a drug that is followed by the initials USP (*United States Pharmacopeia*) or NF (*National Formulary*), denoting its listing in one of the official publications; usually the same as the generic name.

olfactory Of or pertaining to the sense of smell.

oliguria A condition marked by diminished capacity to form or pass urine.

omphalocele A type of hernia in which the newborn's intestines or other abdominal organs protrude through the umbilicus; results during fetal development when the muscles in the abdominal wall do not close properly.

oocytes Incompletely developed ova.

open-angle glaucoma (also known as wide-angle glaucoma) is the most common type of glaucoma. The structures of the eye appear normal, but fluid in the eye does not flow properly through the trabecular meshwork.

open fracture A break in a bone that has penetrated the soft tissue or skin, leading to communication with the outside environment; formerly known as compound fracture.

open pneumothorax A chest wall injury that exposes the pleural space to atmospheric pressure.

open vault fracture A fracture that results in direct communication between a scalp laceration and cerebral substance.

open-ended questions Questions asked in a narrative form that cannot be answered with a "yes" or "no."

opening questions Questions that determine why the patient is seeking medical care or advice.

operations section The section that directs and coordinates all emergency scene operations. It also ensures the safety of all personnel. EMS functions generally fall under this section.

opportunistic infections Infections that are pathogenic (disease-causing) only in immunocompromised hosts (eg, HIV-infected patients, patients receiving chemotherapy, patients following transplantation).

optic nerve The nerve that carries visual signals from the eye to the crossing of the optic tracts.

optic nerve atrophy A permanent visual impairment caused by damage to the optic nerve.

optic nerve hypoplasia A congenital condition in which the optic nerve has not developed properly and is too small.

oral candidiasis An infection of yeast fungi of the genus *Candida* on the mucous membranes of the mouth; also known as thrush.

orbital cellulitis An acute infection in the tissues posterior to the orbital septum often manifested as swelling of the eyelids, eyebrow, and cheek.

orchitis Painful inflammation of the testicle.

organ A structure made up of two or more kinds of tissues organized to perform a more complex function than any one tissue alone.

organ transplantation The replacement of a failing organ with a healthy one from a donor.

organelles Various particles of living substance that are bound within most cells, such as the mitochondria, the Golgi apparatus, the endoplasmic reticulum, the lysosomes, and the centrioles.

organic brain dysfunction Abnormal cognition that results from primarily physical functional disorders (as opposed to psychological disorders).

orphan drugs Medications that have been developed specifically to treat rare medical conditions.

Osborn wave A positive deflection at the J point on an electrocardiogram, characteristically seen in hypothermia; also known as a J wave.

osmolality The osmotic pressure of a solution.

osmosis The diffusion of solvent (water) through a membrane from a less concentrated solution to a more concentrated solution.

osmotic pressure The minimum pressure required to prevent the movement of a solution across a semipermeable membrane.

osteoarthritis A form of arthritis in which one or many joints undergo degenerative changes.

osteomyelitis Local or generalized infection of bone and bone marrow, usually caused by bacteria introduced by trauma or surgery.

osteoporosis A disorder characterized by a reduction in bone density. It occurs most often in postmenopausal women.

ostomy An artificial opening into the urinary tract, gastrointestinal tract, or trachea; any surgical procedure in which an opening is created between two hollow organs or between a hollow viscus and the abdominal wall.

otitis media Infection or inflammation of the middle ear.

ovarian follicles Spherical cell aggregations in the ovary that contain an oocyte.

ovarian torsion Twisting of an ovary around its vascular pedicle.

ovaries A pair of female gonads found on each side of the lower abdomen beside the uterus.

overflow incontinence A form of urinary incontinence in which urine is released from an overfull urinary bladder. The patient may or may not have the urge to urinate.

overhydration Water excess or water intoxication.

ovulation The release of an ovum or secondary oocyte from the vesicular follicle.

ovum An egg in the ovary of a female.

oxygen-deficient atmospheres Confined spaces in which there is an inadequate concentration of oxygen.

oxyhemoglobin Oxygenated hemoglobin.

P wave The first complex of the electrocardiogram, representing depolarization of the atria.

palliative care A unique form of health care primarily directed at providing relief to terminally ill people through symptom management and pain management; can occur at the same time as active treatment.

palmar grasp A normal infant response in which the infant curls the fingers in response to a touch on the palm of the hand.

palpation A technique in which an examiner uses the hands and fingers to gather information from a patient by touch.

palpitations The sensation of irregular or forceful beating of the heart.

pancreas A fish-shaped, nodular gland located across the posterior abdominal wall in the epigastric region of the body. It secretes various substances, including digestive enzymes, insulin, and glucagon.

pancreatitis Inflammation of the pancreas, which causes severe epigastric pain.

pandemic An infectious disease outbreak that affects large numbers of people worldwide.

panic disorder An anxiety disorder characterized by unexpected and repeated episodes of intense fear accompanied by physical symptoms that may include chest pain, heart palpitations, shortness of breath, dizziness, or abdominal distress.

papilledema Swelling of the head of the optic disc caused by a rise in intracranial pressure.

para The number of past pregnancies that have remained viable to delivery.

paradoxical motion Contrary movement of an injured segment of the chest wall with inspiration and expiration.

paralytic ileus A decrease in or the absence of intestinal peristalsis that can closely mimic bowel obstructions.

paramedic A person who has completed training consistent with the *National EMS Education Standards,* including advanced training in clinical decision making, patient assessment, cardiac rhythm interpretation, defibrillation, drug therapy, and airway management.

parameter An aspect of a population that is difficult or impossible to measure and so is estimated using a sample population.

paranoia A condition characterized by an elaborate, overly suspicious system of thinking.

paraphimosis A condition in uncircumcised men marked by the inability to pull the retracted foreskin back over the head of the penis.

paraplegia Weakness or paralysis of both legs and sometimes part of the trunk.

parasympathetic nervous system The subdivision of the autonomic nervous system, usually involved in activating vegetative functions such as digestion, defecation, and urination.

parenteral Of or pertaining to any medication route other than the alimentary canal.

paresthesia A sensation of numbness, tingling, or "pins and needles."

parietal peritoneum The serous membrane that covers the body cavity wall.

Parkinson disease A degenerative neurologic disease affecting dopaminergic neurons in the brain causing motor function deterioration. Manifestations include resting tremor, rigidity, slowed movements, and gait abnormality.

Parkinson disease dementia Parkinson disease that later progresses into dementia.

Parkland formula A formula used to calculate the fluid needs of a burn-injured patient over the first 24 hours after injury; also known as the consensus formula.

paronychia A common skin infection that occurs around the nails and that allows for an invasion of bacteria, yeast, or fungus.

paroxysmal atrial tachycardia (PAT) Atrial tachycardia that begins and ends abruptly.

paroxysmal nocturnal dyspnea Shortness of breath that awakens a person from sleep. It often is associated with left ventricular failure and pulmonary edema.

paroxysmal supraventricular tachycardia (PSVT) An ectopic rhythm usually faster than 170 beats/min that begins abruptly with a premature atrial or junctional beat and is supported by an atrioventricular nodal reentrant mechanism or by an atrioventricular reentry involving an accessory pathway.

partial pressure The pressure exerted by a single gas.

partial reabsorption Reabsorption from the renal tubule by passive diffusion.

partial-thickness burn A burn injury that extends through the epidermis to the dermis; also known as a second-degree burn. It is considered a superficial partial-thickness injury if it involves minimal papillary dermis; it is considered a deep partial-thickness injury if it extends to the reticular dermis.

parturition The process by which a fetus is born.

passive immunity Immunity acquired by transmission of antibodies from the mother, through placental transfer, to the fetus; a form of acquired immunity in which antibodies against disease are acquired naturally.

past medical history A patient's medical background, which may offer insight into the patient's current problem.

patella A flat, triangular bone at the front of the knee joint; the kneecap.

patent ductus arteriosus (PDA) A persistent communication between the descending thoracic aorta and the pulmonary artery that results from failure of normal physiologic closure of the fetal ductus; common congenital heart defect.

pathogen A disease-causing agent.

pathogenic microbe A microscopic pathogen, such as a bacterium, parasite, fungus, or virus, that can cause infection.

pathologic fracture A fracture through abnormally weak bone from a force that would not fracture a normal bone.

pathophysiology The abnormal functions and diseases of the human body.

patient care report (PCR) A document used in the prehospital setting to record all patient care activities and circumstances related to an emergency response.

patient handoff The effective communication and transfer of patient information from one health care provider to another as patient care is transferred.

patient management plan A plan of care that is based on principles and applications of findings in the patient assessment.

patient packaging Completion of the emergency care procedures needed to transfer a patient from the scene to the emergency vehicle.

pattern recognition The process of comparing gathered information with the paramedic's knowledge base of medical illness and disease.

patterned injuries Injuries that result from an identifiable object.

peak expiratory flow rate (PEFR) A measurement of how fast a person can exhale air.

pediatric trauma score An injury severity index that grades six components commonly seen in pediatric trauma patients: size (weight), airway, central nervous system, systolic blood pressure, open wound, and skeletal injury.

pelvic inflammatory disease (PID) Any inflammatory condition of the female pelvic organs, especially one caused by bacterial infection.

penetrating trauma An injury produced by crushing and stretching forces of a penetrating object that results in some form of tissue disruption.

penis The external reproductive organ of the male.

peptic ulcer disease An illness that results from a complex pathologic interaction among the acidic gastric secretions and proteolytic enzymes and the mucosal barrier.

percussion A surface tapping technique used to evaluate the presence of air or fluid in body tissues.

perforated tympanic membrane A hole or rupture in the eardrum; usually caused by trauma or infection.

perfusion The delivery of oxygen and nutrients to the cells, organs, and tissues of the body; also involves the removal of wastes.

pericardial friction rub A dry, grating sound heard with a stethoscope during auscultation; suggestive of pericarditis.

pericardial sac The sac that surrounds the heart.

pericardial tamponade Compression of the heart produced by the accumulation of fluid or blood in the pericardial sac.

pericarditis Inflammation of the pericardium.

perineum The pelvic floor and associated structures occupying the pelvic outlet, bounded anteriorly by the pubic symphysis, laterally by the ischial tuberosities, and posteriorly by the coccyx.

periodontal disease Disease that affects tissues that surround or support the teeth.

periosteum Tough connective tissue that covers the bone.

peripheral cyanosis Cyanosis that is confined to the extremities (common in the first few minutes of life); also known as acrocyanosis.

peripheral nervous system (PNS) The part of the nervous system that lies outside the brain and spinal cord; comprised of the somatic nervous system and the autonomic nervous system.

peripheral neuropathy Diseases and disorders that affect the peripheral nervous system, causing pain and unpleasant sensations in affected areas (often extremities).

peripheral thermoreceptors Nerve endings sensitive to temperature, located in the skin and some mucous membranes. They usually are categorized as cold or warm receptors.

peripheral vision The ability to see objects that reflect light waves on areas of the retina other than the macula.

peritoneal dialysis A dialysis procedure that uses the peritoneum as a diffusible membrane. It is performed to correct an imbalance of fluid or electrolytes in the blood or to remove toxins, drugs, or other wastes normally excreted by the kidney.

peritonitis Inflammation of the serous membrane that covers the abdominal wall (parietal peritoneum) or the abdominal organs (visceral peritoneum).

peritonsillar abscess A collection of pus in and around one or both tonsils; often caused by tonsillitis.

permissive hypotension A fluid resuscitation strategy in which fluid and blood products are restricted, in spite of lower than normal blood pressures, until bleeding has been controlled.

pernicious anemia Anemia that results from a vitamin B_{12} deficiency.

PERRL Acronym that indicates that the Pupils are Equal and Round, and Reactive to Light.

personal flotation device (PFD) A safety device worn in water to reduce the risk of drowning.

personal protective equipment (PPE) Clothing or specialized equipment that provides some protection to the wearer from environmental or infectious hazards.

personality disorders A large group of conditions distinguished by a failure to learn from experience or to adapt appropriately to changes; results in personal distress and impairment of social functioning.

pertinent negative findings Findings that warrant no medical care or intervention but that provide evidence of the thoroughness of the patient examination and the history of the event.

pertinent oral statements Statements made by the patient and other people at the scene.

pertinent positive findings Signs or symptoms that help substantiate the patient's condition.

pertussis An acute, highly contagious respiratory disease characterized by paroxysmal coughing that ends in a loud, whooping inspiration; also known as whooping cough.

pH An inverse logarithm of the hydrogen ion concentration.

phagocytosis The process by which cells ingest solid substances such as other cells, bacteria, bits of necrosed tissue, and foreign particles.

phalanges The bones of the fingers and toes.

pharmaceutics The science of dispensing drugs.

pharmacodynamics The study of how a drug acts on a living organism.

pharmacokinetics The study of how the body handles a drug over a period of time, including the processes of absorption, distribution, biotransformation, and excretion.

pharmacology The science of drugs used to prevent, diagnose, and treat disease.

pharyngitis Inflammation or infection of the pharynx.

phencyclidine psychosis A psychiatric emergency that may mimic schizophrenia.

phimosis Tightness of the prepuce (foreskin) of the penis that is unable to be retracted off the head of the penis.

phlebitis Inflammation of a vein, often accompanied by the formation of a clot; also known as thrombophlebitis.

phobia An anxiety disorder characterized by an obsessive, irrational, and intense fear of a specific object or activity.

phosgene A poisonous gas that appears as a gray-white cloud and smells of newly mowed hay.

phospholipids A class of compounds, widely distributed in living cells, that contain phosphoric acid, fatty acids, and a nitrogenous base.

photophobia Abnormal sensitivity to light.

phrenic nerve A nerve composed mostly of motor nerve fibers that produce contractions of the diaphragm; also provides sensory innervation for many components of the mediastinum and pleura.

physical abuse The use of physical force that may result in bodily injury, physical pain, or impairment.

physical assault An intentional act by one person that creates apprehension in another person of an imminent harmful or offensive contact.

physical examination An assessment of a patient that includes examination techniques, measurement of vital signs, an assessment of height and weight, and the skillful use of examination equipment.

physician orders for life-sustaining treatment (POLST) An approach to end-of-life planning that emphasizes patients' wishes regarding the medical treatment they receive.

physiologic dead space The sum of the anatomic dead space plus the volume of any nonfunctional alveoli.

pia mater The innermost layer of the meninges. It directly covers the brain.

Pierre Robin sequence A complex of congenital anomalies including a small mandible, a tongue that is placed farther back than normal and causes airway obstruction, and a cleft palate.

pitting edema Observable indentation of body tissues that persists after applying pressure to an area swollen from fluid accumulation.

pituitary gland A small gland attached to the hypothalamus. It supplies numerous hormones that govern many vital processes.

placards Four-sided, diamond-shaped signs displayed on hazardous materials containers that usually are yellow, orange, white, or green. They have a four-digit United Nations identification number and a legend to indicate the contents of the container.

placebo An inactive substance or a less-than-effective dose of a harmless substance. It is used in experimental drug studies to compare the effects of the inactive substance with those of the experimental drug.

placenta A highly vascular fetal–maternal organ through which the fetus absorbs oxygen, nutrients, and other substances and excretes carbon dioxide and other wastes.

placenta previa Placental implantation in the lower uterine segment partially or completely covering the cervical opening.

placental barrier A protective biologic membrane that separates the blood vessels of the mother and the fetus.

plague A disease caused by the bacterium *Yersinia pestis*, found in rodents (eg, chipmunks, prairie dogs, ground squirrels, mice) and their fleas in many areas around the world.

planning section The section responsible for providing past, present, and future information about the incident and the status of resources.

plasma The fluid portion of blood.

plasma membrane The outer covering of a cell that contains the cellular cytoplasm; also known as the cell membrane.

platelet plug A plug consisting of a mass of linked platelets that seals an injured vessel; part of the clotting process.

platelets Fragments of cells. These initiate the clotting process.

pleural cavity The area of the body that surrounds the lungs.

pleural friction rub A rubbing or grating sound that occurs as one layer of the pleural membrane slides over the other during breathing.

pleural space The potential space between the visceral layer and the parietal layer of the pleura.

pneumonia An acute inflammation of the lungs, usually caused by infection with a bacterium, virus, or fungus.

pneumonic plague An infectious pulmonary disease caused by exposure to the bacterium *Yersinia pestis*.

pneumoperitoneum The presence of air or gas within the peritoneal cavity of the abdomen.

pneumotaxic center A group of neurons in the pons that have an inhibitory effect on the inspiratory center.

poikilothermia The inability to maintain a constant core temperature independent of ambient temperature.

point of maximum impulse The location or area where the apical pulse is palpated the strongest, often in the fifth intercostal space of the thorax just medial to the left midclavicular line.

point-to-point movements Methods used to evaluate a patient's coordination.

poison Any substance that produces harmful physiologic or psychological effects.

polycythemia A condition characterized by an unusually large number of red blood cells in the blood as a result of their increased production by the bone marrow.

polymorphic ventricular tachycardia (VT) Ventricular tachycardia in which the QRS complex has varying morphology or shape.

polymyositis Slow but progressive muscle weakness that affects skeletal muscle on both sides of the body.

polypharmacy The simultaneous use of multiple drugs by a single patient for one or more conditions.

polysaccharides Carbohydrates that contain three or more molecules of simple carbohydrate.

polyuria Excessive excretion of urine.

pons The part of the brainstem between the medulla and the midbrain.

population A large group of people, places, or objects that are the main focus of a scientific query.

portal of entry The means by which the pathogenic agent enters a new host.

portal of exit The method by which a pathogenic agent leaves one host to invade another.

portal vein A vein in the liver that conveys the blood to the inferior vena cava through the hepatic veins.

positive end-expiratory pressure (PEEP) Airway support that maintains a degree of positive pressure at the end of exhalation.

postcapillary sphincter The smooth muscle sphincter at the venous end of a capillary that regulates blood flow out of the capillary.

postdisaster follow-up An after-action review of an incident that includes the lessons learned from the incident and methods of improvement.

posterior The back, or dorsal, surface.

posterior hemiblock Failure in conduction of the cardiac impulse in the posterior fascicle of the left bundle branch.

postevent phase The phase of trauma in which emergency care is delivered to injured patients.

postictal phase The period following a seizure in which the patient experiences drowsiness or unconsciousness. On regaining consciousness, the patient may be confused and fatigued.

postpartum depression Depression that occurs during or after pregnancy that is caused by a combination of sudden hormonal changes and psychological and environmental factors.

postpartum hemorrhage Blood loss of more than 500 mL after delivery of the newborn.

postrenal disease Disease that blocks the system that collects urine. It usually is caused by urinary tract obstruction.

posttraumatic stress disorder (PTSD) An anxiety disorder that can occur following a series of disturbing events or a single, emotionally traumatic incident.

postural maintenance The result of muscle tone responsible for keeping the back and legs straight, the head in an upright position, and the abdomen from bulging; also balances the distribution of body weight.

potassium ion channels Electrical channels in the cell membrane that allow for selective flow of potassium ions across the cell membrane.

potentiation Enhancement of the effect of a drug, caused by concurrent administration of two drugs in which one drug increases the effect of the other.

poverty The scarcity or the lack of a certain amount of material possessions or money.

power The ability of a study to detect difference if a difference really exists. It is based on the sample size (number of subjects) and effect size (difference in outcomes between the groups).

power take-off (PTO) A splined driveshaft, usually on a tractor or other farm machinery, used to provide power to an attachment or separate machine.

PR interval The time that elapses between the beginning of the P wave and the beginning of the QRS complex in the electrocardiogram.

precapillary sphincter The smooth muscle sphincter at the arterial end of a capillary that regulates blood flow into the capillary.

precipitous delivery A rapid, spontaneous delivery of less than 3 hours from onset of labor to birth. This childbirth occurs with such speed that usual preparations cannot be made. It results from overactive uterine contractions and little maternal soft-tissue or bony resistance.

precordial leads Unipolar chest leads used in 12-lead electrocardiographic monitoring that record the electrical activity of the heart in the horizontal plane.

precordial thump A technique to restore circulation in monitored, witnessed ventricular fibrillation or unstable ventricular tachycardia.

preeclampsia An abnormal disease of pregnancy characterized by the onset of acute hypertension associated with either proteinuria after the 20th week of gestation or other abnormalities like thrombocytopenia, renal insufficiency, impaired liver function, pulmonary edema, or cerebral or visual symptoms.

preevent phase The phase of trauma that refers to the prevention of intentional and unintentional trauma deaths.

preexcitation syndrome Anomalous or accelerated atrioventricular conduction associated with an abnormal conduction pathway between the atria and ventricles.

prefix A word part that appears at the beginning of a word. In the medical context, a prefix often describes location or intensity.

preload The amount of blood returning to the ventricle.

premature atrial complex (PAC) A cardiac dysrhythmia characterized by an atrial beat occurring before the expected excitation and indicated on the electrocardiogram as an early P wave of a different morphology.

premature junctional complex (PJC) An ectopic beat originating from the atrioventricular junction that occurs earlier than the next expected sinus beat.

premature newborn A newborn who is born before 37 weeks' gestation.

premature rupture of membranes (PROM) Rupture of the amniotic sac before the onset of labor, regardless of gestational age.

premature ventricular complex (PVC) A ventricular beat preceding the next expected electrical impulse. It has an early, wide QRS complex without a preceding related P wave.

preplan The process of preparing for response to a major incident; also refers to the document that results from this process.

prepuce In males, the free fold of skin that covers the glans penis; the foreskin. In females, the external fold of the labia minora that covers the clitoris.

prerenal disease Disease that compromises renal perfusion.

preschooler A child 3 to 5 years of age.

present illness The chief complaint. Identification of the present illness is supported by a full, clear, chronologic account of the symptoms.

pressure gradient The force produced by differences between atmospheric pressure, intrapulmonic pressure, and intrathoracic pressure.

pressure support A spontaneous mode of ventilation in which a ventilator delivers support with the preset pressure value for the patient's own respiratory rate.

pressure ulcers Sores or ulcers in the skin usually over a bony prominence that occur most frequently on the sacrum, elbows, heels, outer ankles, inner knees, hips, and shoulder blades of high-risk patients, especially in older adults or people who are obese or suffering from chronic diseases, infections, injuries, or a poor nutritional state.

priapism Painful, persistent erection of the penis.

primary assessment The combination of scene size-up and the initial patient evaluation used to establish scene safety and to recognize and manage life-threatening conditions.

primary brain injury The direct trauma to the brain and the associated vascular injuries that occurred from the initial injury.

primary contamination Exposure to a hazardous substance that is harmful only to the person exposed and that poses little risk of exposure to others.

primary injury prevention The practice of preventing an injury from occurring.

primary polycythemia A rare disorder of the bone marrow in which increased production of red blood cells causes the blood to thicken; also known as polycythemia vera.

primary survey A critical component of the primary assessment that focuses on the initial evaluation of a patient to recognize and manage life-threatening conditions.

primary triage Triage performed at the incident site to rapidly categorize patient conditions for treatment and roughly identify the number and severity of patients.

primary tumor A malignant tumor in the original site where it first arose.

priority patients Patients who need immediate care and transport.

private space The region surrounding a person that the person regards as his or hers; also known as personal space.

proarrhythmia A new or worsened rhythm disturbance seemingly generated by antidysrhythmic therapy.

prokaryotes Cells without a true nucleus; instead, nuclear material is scattered throughout the cytoplasm.

pronator drift test A test to evaluate balance and upper extremity weakness; performed by having the patient close the eyes and hold both arms out from the body.

prone A position in which the patient lies on the stomach (facedown).

prostate gland The gland that lies just below the male bladder. Its secretion is one of the components of semen.

protected health information (PHI) Any information about health status, provision of health care, or payment for health care that can be linked to a specific person.

prothrombin A chemical that is part of the clotting cascade; the precursor of thrombin.

prothrombin activator A substance that combines with an enzyme to increase its catalytic activity. It converts prothrombin to thrombin.

proximate cause Proof that a negligent act or lack of action caused an injury or worsened an existing injury.

pruritus A sensation that causes the desire or reflex to scratch.

pseudoaneurysm A condition resembling an aneurysm that is caused by enlargement and tortuosity of a vessel.

pseudogout Inflammation caused by calcium pyrophosphate crystals; often clinically indistinguishable from gout.

psychotic behavior Maladaptive behavior involving major distortions of reality.

puberty The period of life when the ability to reproduce begins.

pubic lice Tiny parasites that concentrate in the pubic area.

pubis One of a pair of pubic bones that, with the ischium and the ilium, form the hipbone and join the pubic bone from the opposite side at the pubic symphysis.

public health A field of medicine that deals with the physical and mental health of all people in a community.

pulmonary atresia A life-threatening congenital anomaly in which the pulmonary valve is replaced with a membrane, preventing blood from flowing from the right ventricle into the pulmonary artery and on to the lungs to pick up oxygen.

pulmonary contusion Bruising of the lung tissue that results in rupture of the alveoli and interstitial edema.

pulmonary edema The accumulation of extravascular fluid in lung tissues and alveoli.

pulmonary embolism The blockage of an artery in the lungs by a substance such as fat, air, tumor tissue, or a thrombus that has moved from elsewhere in the body, usually from a peripheral vein, through the bloodstream.

pulmonary hypoplasia A congenital malformation characterized by incomplete development of lung tissue.

pulmonary overpressurization syndrome (POPS) A condition that results from expansion of trapped air in the lungs. It may lead to alveolar rupture and extravasation of air into extra-alveolar locations.

pulmonary surfactant Certain lipoproteins that reduce the surface tension of pulmonary fluids, allowing the exchange of gases in the alveoli of the lungs and contributing to the elasticity of pulmonary tissue.

pulmonary trunk The large elastic artery that carries blood from the right ventricle of the heart to the right and left pulmonary arteries.

pulmonary veins The veins that carry oxygenated blood from the lung to the left atrium.

pulmonary ventilation The movement of air into and out of the lungs. This process brings oxygen into the lungs and removes carbon dioxide.

pulse deficit A condition that exists when the radial pulse is less than the ventricular rate; it indicates a lack of peripheral perfusion.

pulse pressure The difference between the systolic and diastolic blood pressures.

pulseless electrical activity (PEA) The absence of a detectable pulse in the presence of some type of organized electrical activity other than ventricular tachycardia; also known as electromechanical dissociation.

pulsus paradoxus An abnormal decrease in systolic blood pressure in which it drops more than 10 to 15 mm Hg during inspiration compared with expiration.

puncture wound A penetrating injury that is deeper than it is long.

punitive damages Damages awarded in a lawsuit that may be in excess of compensable damages; damages meant to punish the person at fault and to deter others from causing such harm in the future.

pupil The opening in the center of the iris that regulates the amount of light entering the eye.

Purkinje fibers Myocardial fibers that are a continuation of the bundle of His and that extend into the muscle walls of the ventricles.

pyelonephritis Inflammation of the kidney parenchyma caused by microbial infection.

pyloric stenosis A congenital defect in which there is narrowing of the pylorus (the opening from the stomach into the small intestine) caused by thickening of the muscles in the pyloric wall. It is the most common cause of intestinal obstruction in infancy.

QRS complex The principal deflection in the electrocardiogram, representing ventricular depolarization.

QT interval The time elapsing from the beginning of the QRS complex to the end of the T wave, representing the total duration of electrical activity of the ventricles.

quadriplegia Weakness or paralysis of all four extremities and the trunk.

qualitative analysis The non-numerical organization and interpretation of observations.

quantitative analysis Research data that are measured and analyzed numerically.

rabies An acute, usually fatal viral disease of the central nervous system of animals. It is transmitted from animals to human beings by infected blood, tissue, or, most commonly, saliva.

raccoon eyes Ecchymosis of one or both orbits with tarsal plate sparing caused by fracture of the base of the sphenoid sinus.

radiation The direct release of body heat to cooler surroundings.

radiologic dispersion device (RDD) A nuclear explosive device; also known as a "dirty nuke" or "dirty bomb."

radius One of the bones of the forearm. It lies parallel to the ulna.

random sample A subset from the larger population of a study chosen randomly and entirely by chance.

rape Nonconsensual sex or an attempt to force another person to have sex against his or her will. It includes intercourse in the vagina, anus, or mouth.

rapid sequence induction (RSI) The administration of a potent sedative or induction agent and a neuromuscular blocking agent at the same time to achieve optimal intubation conditions in less than 1 minute.

rappelling A controlled descent by rope.

Raynaud phenomenon A condition in which cold temperatures or strong emotions cause blood vessel spasms that block blood flow to the fingers, toes, ears, and nose.

reassessment The ongoing assessment that follows the paramedic's initial evaluation of the patient.

rebound tenderness Pain caused by the sudden release of fingertip pressure on the abdomen. It is a sign of peritoneal inflammation.

reciprocal socialization A term that refers to a child's temperament and the responses it elicits from adults and family members. This interaction forms the basis for early social interactions with others and with the child's environment.

reciprocity The practice of granting a person licensure or certification/registration based on licensure or certification/registration by another state, agency, or association.

recompression The use of elevated pressure (including hyperbaric oxygen therapy) to treat conditions within the body caused by a rapid decrease in pressure.

rectum The segment of the large intestine continuous with the descending sigmoid colon just proximal to the anal canal.

red bone marrow Specialized soft tissue found in many bones of infants and children, in the spongy bone of the proximal epiphyses of the humerus and femur; also known as red marrow. In adults, it is mostly found in the sternum, ribs, and vertebral bodies. It is essential in the manufacture of red blood cells.

red marrow Specialized soft tissue found in many bones of infants and children; in the spongy bone of the proximal epiphyses of the humerus and femur; also known as red bone marrow. In adults, it is mostly found in the sternum, ribs, and vertebral bodies. It is essential in the manufacture of red blood cells.

reentry The reactivation of tissue by a returning impulse; the sustaining mechanism in some cases of ventricular tachycardia and paroxysmal supraventricular tachycardia.

referred pain Pain felt at a site distant from its origin.

reflection on action A component of critical thinking (usually performed after the event) in which the examiner evaluates a patient care episode for possible improvement in similar future responses.

reflex An automatic response to a stimulus that occurs without conscious thought; produced by a reflex arc.

refractory period The period after effective stimulation during which excitable tissue will not respond to a stimulus of threshold intensity.

registration The act of enrolling one's name in a register or book of record.

regulations Standards promulgated by a government authority pursuant to a legislative grant that have the force and effect of law.

rehabilitation Activities that are provided at an incident to sustain the energy of rescuers, improve performance, and decrease the likelihood of on-scene injury or death; also known as rehab.

rehabilitation area A part of the major incident response plans of many fire and EMS agencies. This area usually is set up outside the operational area. It allows rescue personnel to get physical and psychological rest.

relative hypovolemia Inadequate preload as a result of vasodilation or shift of fluid out of the vascular space.

relative refractory period The portion of the action potential after the absolute refractory period during which another action potential can be produced with a greater-than-threshold stimulus strength.

renal pyramids Pyramidal masses seen on longitudinal section of the kidney. They contain part of the loop of Henle and the collecting tubules.

renin A proteolytic enzyme secreted by the kidneys that is involved in the release of angiotensin; plays an important role in the maintenance of blood pressure.

renin-angiotensin-aldosterone mechanism The mechanism for regulating levels of sodium and water.

repeater A device that is used to increase the effective communications range of handheld portable radios, mobile radios, and base station radios by retransmitting received radio signals.

repolarization The phase of the action potential in which the membrane potential moves from its maximum degree of depolarization toward the value of the resting membrane potential.

reproductive maturity The time at which a person has attained the ability to reproduce.

rescue The act of delivery from danger or imprisonment.

rescue versus body recovery The chance to save a human life (rescue) versus body recovery without the goal of saving a human life.

reservoir Any person, animal, plant, soil, or substance in which an infectious agent normally lives and multiplies. It typically harbors the infectious agent without injury to itself and serves as a source from which other people can be infected.

residual volume The volume of air remaining in the lungs after a maximum expiratory effort.

resistance The immune status of the host; the ability to ward off infection.

respiration The process of the molecular exchange of oxygen and carbon dioxide in the body's tissues.

respiratory acidosis An abnormal condition characterized by an increased arterial partial pressure of carbon dioxide, excess carbonic acid, and an increased plasma hydrogen ion concentration (pH).

respiratory alkalosis An abnormal condition characterized by decreased arterial partial pressure of carbon dioxide, decreased hydrogen ion concentration, and increased blood pH.

respiratory failure A syndrome in which the respiratory system fails in one or both of its gas exchange functions: oxygenation and carbon dioxide elimination.

respiratory membrane The membrane in the lungs, formed by the wall of an alveolus and the wall of a capillary, across which gas exchange with the blood occurs.

respiratory syncytial virus A viral infection of the lower respiratory tract that causes cold symptoms in most cases but can be severe with bronchiolitis. Premature babies and infants younger than 1 year are at risk of severe infection.

resting membrane potential The electrical charge difference inside a cell membrane measured relative to just outside the cell membrane.

resuscitative approach An approach to patient care that recognizes the need for immediate intervention for patients with life-threatening illness or injury.

resuscitative measures Lifesaving measures performed immediately, such as airway control, ventilatory assistance, control of severe bleeding, and cardiopulmonary resuscitation.

reticular activating system A functional system in the brain that is essential for wakefulness, attention, concentration, and introspection.

reticular formation A small, thick cluster of neurons nestled in the brainstem that controls breathing, the heartbeat, blood pressure, level of consciousness, and other vital functions.

reticuloendothelial system Part of the immune system composed of immune cells in the spleen, lymph nodes, liver, bone marrow, lungs, and intestines. It stores mature B and T cells until the immune system is activated.

retina The nervous tunic of the eye. It is continuous with the optic nerve.

retinal detachment A separation of the light-sensitive retina from its supporting layers.

retinal vascular occlusion Blockage of a vessel in the retina of the eye.

retinopathy A group of noninflammatory eye disorders often caused by diabetes mellitus, hypertension, and atherosclerotic vascular disease.

retrograde amnesia The loss of memory for events that occurred before the event that precipitated the amnesia.

retroperitoneal Behind the peritoneum.

return of spontaneous circulation (ROSC) Restoration of spontaneous circulation following a cardiac arrest that provides evidence of more than an occasional gasp, occasional fleeting palpable pulse, or arterial waveform.

Rh disease An immune disorder that develops in a fetus, when IgG antibodies directed against Rh-positive red blood cells are produced by the mother and pass through the placenta.

Rh factor An antigenic substance present in the erythrocytes of most people. A person lacking the Rh factor is Rh negative.

Rh sensitization A condition that can occur during pregnancy if an Rh-negative woman is pregnant with a baby who has Rh-positive blood. If this occurs, the immune system reacts to the Rh factor by producing antibodies to destroy it.

rhabdomyolysis An acute, sometimes fatal, disease characterized by destruction of skeletal muscle.

rheumatoid arthritis (RA) A chronic, sometimes deforming destructive collagen disease that has an autoimmune component.

rhinitis Inflammation of the mucous membranes of the nose.

rhonchi Abnormal, coarse, rattling respiratory sounds, usually caused by secretions in bronchial airways, muscular spasm, neoplasm, or external pressure.

ribonucleic acid (RNA) A nucleic acid found in the nucleus and the cytoplasm of cells that transmits genetic instructions from the nucleus to the cytoplasm. In the cytoplasm, RNA functions in the assembly of proteins.

ribosomes The "factories" in cells, in which protein is synthesized.

ricin A potent protein cytotoxin derived from the beans of the castor plant (*Ricinus communis*).

right atrium One of the four chambers of the human heart. It receives deoxygenated blood from the body through the venae cavae and pumps it into the right ventricle.

right axis deviation When the mean electrical axis of ventricular contraction falls between +90° and ±180°.

right bundle branch A division in the bundle of His responsible for depolarization of the right side of the heart.

right bundle branch block (RBBB) A conduction abnormality that occurs when transmission of the electrical impulse is delayed or not conducted along the right bundle branch.

right main stem bronchus One of two main bronchi that branch from the trachea at the level of the carina.

right-side heart failure Failure of the right ventricle to serve as an effective forward pump; also known as right ventricular failure.

rigid splint A splint in which the shape cannot be changed.

riot control/tear agents Chemicals that can produce sensory irritation or disabling physical effects that disappear within a short time after termination of exposure.

risk–benefit analysis An analysis that considers personal safety before rescue is attempted. It asks the question, "Does the risk outweigh the benefit, or vice versa?"

Rocky Mountain spotted fever A serious tick-borne infectious disease, characterized by chills, fever, severe headache, mental confusion, and rash.

Romberg test A test to evaluate stance and balance; performed by having the patient stand erect with eyes closed, feet together, and arms at the sides.

R-on-T phenomenon The occurrence of a ventricular depolarization during a vulnerable period of ventricular repolarization.

root word The foundation of a term. In the medical context, a root word may be combined with other word parts to describe a particular structure or condition.

rooting reflex A normal infant response elicited by touching or stroking the side of the cheek or mouth, causing the infant to turn the head toward that side and to begin to suck.

rubella A contagious viral disease characterized by fever, symptoms of mild upper respiratory tract infection, lymph node enlargement, and a diffuse, fine, red maculopapular rash; also known as German measles. It is spread by droplet infection. It results in congenital rubella syndrome in unborn babies of pregnant women infected with the disease.

rubeola An acute, highly contagious viral disease involving the respiratory tract. It is characterized by a spreading, maculopapular, cutaneous rash and occurs primarily in young children who have not been immunized. Complications include pneumonia, encephalitis, neurologic damage, and death. In pregnant women, this disease, also known as measles, can result in premature delivery and/or low birth weight of their unborn babies.

rule of nines A method to estimate burn injury that divides the total body surface area into segments that are multiples of 9%.

ruptured ovarian cyst A ruptured globular sac filled with fluid or semisolid material that develops in or on the ovary.

safe distance factor The minimum safe distance for personal safety from hazardous materials as outlined in the reference guides.

safe staging area An area away from the emergency scene that provides for safety.

safety data sheet (SDS) Written product identification as required by the Occupational Safety and Health Administration for each chemical produced, stored, or used in the United States.

safety officer In a rescue operation, the official who remains alert to the stress of the operation on the rescuers.

SALT triage A method of triage that uses a four-step process—Sort, Assess, Lifesaving interventions, Treatment and/or Transport—to categorize patients.

sampling error Error that results from observation of a sample rather than the whole population.

sarcomere The contractile unit of skeletal muscle. It contains thick and thin myofilaments.

sarin A clear, colorless, and tasteless liquid that has no odor in its pure form; may be used as a nerve agent.

scabies A contagious parasitic skin infection characterized by superficial burrows and intense pruritus; caused by the mite *Sarcoptes scabiei.*

scene management Control of all or part of the incident area.

scene size-up An assessment of the scene to promote scene safety for the paramedic crew, patient(s), and bystanders; includes determination of additional resources that may be needed to manage the scene adequately.

schizophrenia A group of disorders characterized by recurrent episodes of psychotic behavior.

school age An age category that includes children 6 to 12 years of age.

Schwann cells Cells that form a myelin sheath around each nerve fiber of the peripheral nervous system.

sciatica Pain that radiates along the path of the sciatic nerve.

sclera The opaque membrane covering the eyeball.

scleroderma A collagen vascular disease thought to arise when the immune system stimulates certain cells (fibroblasts) that cause increased production of collagen.

scoliosis A lateral curvature of the spine.

scope of practice Regarding EMS personnel, the range of duties and skills that paramedics are allowed and expected to perform when necessary.

scrotum The sac of skin that contains the testes.

sebaceous glands Glands of the skin, usually associated with a hair follicle, that produce sebum.

sebum The secretion of sebaceous glands. It prevents drying of the skin and protects against invasion by some bacteria.

secondary assessment An assessment that consists of physical examination techniques, measurement of vital signs, an assessment of body systems, and the skillful use of examination equipment.

secondary brain injury Brain injury that evolves over time from initial impact (primary injury) through intracellular and extracellular derangements contributing to further destruction of brain tissue.

secondary bronchi Branches from a primary bronchus that conduct air to each lobe of the lungs.

secondary contamination Exposure to a hazardous substance whereby liquid and particulate substances are transferred easily to others by touching.

secondary injury prevention Activities that minimize harm after an injury event occurs.

secondary polycythemia A condition of increased production of red blood cells caused by reduced air pressure and low oxygen concentration. It may be a natural response to chronic hypoxia.

secondary triage The more detailed and specific prioritization of patients based on the severity of their illness or injuries and their potential to survive.

secondary tumor A malignant tumor that originates in one area of the body and spreads to another area of the body.

second-degree atrioventricular (AV) block type I A conduction block that gradually prolongs the PR interval until a P wave is blocked from initiating a QRS complex; also known as Wenckebach.

second-degree atrioventricular (AV) block type II A conduction block with a constant PR interval where a P wave is blocked from initiating a QRS complex in a fixed or variable pattern.

second-degree sprain An injury that results from some stretching and tearing of ligaments. Swelling and pain are more pronounced.

second stage of labor The stage of labor that is measured from full dilation of the cervix to delivery of the newborn.

section chiefs Those in charge of the major functional areas of the incident command system. Examples of major functional areas that may be established based on need include operations, logistics, planning, and finance/administration.

sections A broad organizational level of the incident command system at which the following functions are typically defined: planning, operations, logistics, and/or finance/administration.

seizure A temporary change in behavior or consciousness caused by abnormal electrical activity in one or more groups of neurons in the brain.

selection bias A distortion of evidence or data that arises from the way the data are collected.

selective beta-blocking agents Agents that block $beta_1$ or $beta_2$ receptors.

self-concept The accumulation of knowledge about one's self, including beliefs regarding personality traits, physical characteristics, abilities, values, goals, and roles.

self-contained breathing apparatus (SCBA) A respiratory protection device that provides an enclosed system of air.

self-esteem A person's overall evaluation or appraisal of his or her own worth.

self-neglect A type of elder abuse in which the behaviors of an older adult intentionally threaten his or her own personal health or safety.

semen The male reproductive fluid.

seminal vesicle One of two glandular structures that empty into the ejaculatory ducts. Its secretion is one of the components of semen.

semipermeable membranes Membranes that allow some fluids and substances to pass through them but not others, usually dependent on size, shape, electrical charge, or other chemical properties of the substance or fluid.

sensitization An acquired reaction in which specific antibodies develop in response to an antigen.

sensorineural hearing loss A type of deafness in which sounds that reach the inner ear fail to be transmitted to the brain because of damage to the structures within the ear or to the acoustic nerve; often incurable.

sensory neurons Afferent neurons that transmit impulses to the spinal cord and brain from all parts of the body.

separation anxiety The anxiety that a child experiences when separated from the primary caregiver. It is a normal reaction during infancy.

sepsis Life-threatening organ dysfunction caused by a dysregulated host response to infection.

septic arthritis A condition that results from direct invasion of the joint space by various microorganisms; also known as infectious arthritis.

septic shock A subset of sepsis in which profound circulatory, cellular, and metabolic abnormalities cause severe compromise of end-organ perfusion. It carries a greater risk of mortality than does sepsis alone.

septum A thin wall dividing two cavities or masses of soft tissue.

serotonin syndrome A potentially life-threatening drug reaction; most often occurs when two or more drugs that affect serotonin levels are taken together.

serum Blood plasma without its clotting factors.

settlement An agreement to accept an amount of money in exchange for a promise not to pursue a legal claim.

severe acute respiratory syndrome (SARS) An infection caused by coronavirus, which resulted in a pandemic in 2003 with high mortality rates.

severe DAI A Grade 3 axonal injury that involves severe mechanical shearing of many axons in both cerebral hemispheres extending to the brainstem.

sexual abuse Nonconsensual sexual contact of any kind.

sexual assault The forcible perpetration of an act of sexual contact on the body of another person, male or female, without his or her consent.

sexually transmitted disease (STD) Any of a group of infections that are passed from one person to another through sexual contact.

sexually transmitted infection (STI) An infection (without symptoms) that has not yet developed into a disease.

sexually transmitted nonspecific urethritis A sexually transmitted disease characterized by inflammation or infection of the urethra in which the cause is not defined; also known as nongonococcal urethritis.

Sgarbossa criteria A set of electrocardiographic findings that can be used to identify myocardial infarction in the presence of a left bundle branch block or a ventricular paced rhythm.

shaken baby syndrome (SBS) A serious form of child abuse that describes injuries to infants that occur after being shaken violently.

shingles An acute infection caused by reactivation of the latent varicella-zoster virus; also known as herpes zoster. It is characterized by painful vesicular eruptions that follow a dermatome from a spinal root.

shipping papers Descriptions of the hazardous materials that include the substance name, classification, shipper's certification, emergency response telephone number, emergency response information, and United Nations identification number.

shock Hypoxia at the cellular level.

shock index A measurement calculated to detect shock by dividing heart rate by systolic blood pressure. Adult scales vary; typically a value of 0.9 or greater suggest shock in an adult; for pediatrics, there is an age-adjusted score.

short bones Bones that are approximately as broad as they are long, such as the carpal bones of the wrist and the tarsal bones of the ankle.

shoulder dystocia An obstacle to delivery that occurs when the fetal shoulders press against the maternal symphysis pubis, blocking shoulder delivery.

shoulder presentation A delivery presentation that results when the long axis of the fetus lies perpendicular to that of the mother; also known as transverse presentation.

shunt A tube or device surgically implanted in the body to redirect body fluid from one cavity or vessel to another. A common example is the ventriculoperitoneal shunt, which is a tube that drains fluid from the cerebral ventricle into the abdominal peritoneum in patients with hydrocephalus.

sickle cell anemia Low hemoglobin as a result of sickle cell disease.

sickle cell crisis An acute, episodic, vaso-occlusive condition causing severe pain. It occurs in people with sickle cell disease.

sickle cell disease A debilitating and unpredictable recessive genetic illness that produces an abnormal type of hemoglobin with an inferior oxygen-carrying capacity.

simple pneumothorax A collection of air or gas in the pleural space that causes the lung to collapse without exposing the pleural space to atmospheric pressure; also known as closed pneumothorax.

simplex mode A communications mode in which information can be transmitted or received in only one direction at a time on a single frequency. Simultaneous transmission cannot occur.

single command An incident coordination system in which one person is responsible for the entire operation.

single-ventricle defects Complex defects that occur in the embryonic stage and result when one of the ventricles is underdeveloped.

sinoatrial (SA) node An area of specialized heart tissue within the atria that serves as the endogenous cardiac pacemaker.

sinus arrest The failure of the sinus node, causing short periods of cardiac standstill.

sinus bradycardia Decreased heart rate that results from slowing of the pacemaker rate of the sinoatrial node to less than 60 beats/min in the typical adult.

sinus dysrhythmia A cardiac rhythm disturbance that often is related to the respiratory cycle and to changes in intrathoracic pressure.

sinus headache A headache characterized by pain in the forehead, nasal area, and eyes.

sinus tachycardia Increased heart rate of greater than 100 beats/min in the adult that results from an increase in the rate of the sinus node discharge.

sinuses The cavities in the bones of the skull that connect to the nasal cavities by small channels.

sinusitis Inflammation of one or more paranasal sinuses.

situational awareness A state of constant vigilance for changes in the scene or in the patient.

six cardinal fields of gaze A test to evaluate extraocular muscle function; performed by having the patient visually track an object in six visual fields in an H pattern.

size-up The systematic process of gathering information about an incident and evaluating it in comparison to incident management goals and available resources. (Differs from scene size-up, which is an assessment of the scene to ensure scene safety for the paramedic crew, patient[s], bystanders; a quick assessment to determine the resources needed to manage the scene adequately.)

skeletal muscle Muscle tissue that appears microscopically to consist of striped myofibrils; also known as striated muscle and voluntary muscle.

skeletal system The bony structures that provide support and protection for the body. It also provides a system of levers on which muscles act to produce body movement.

skin graft A portion of skin implanted to cover areas where skin has been lost through burns or injury or by the surgical removal of nonviable tissue.

slander False statements about a person.

sleep apnea A disorder characterized by abnormal pauses in breathing or episodes of abnormally slow breathing during sleep.

slipped capital femoral epiphysis A separation of the ball of the hip joint from the femur at the upper, growing end (growth plate) of the bone.

sloughing The separation of tissue.

small intestine The longest portion of the digestive tract. It is divided into the duodenum, jejunum, and ileum.

smallpox A highly contagious viral disease caused by the variola virus; characterized by fever, prostration, and a vesicular, pustular rash.

SMART tag system A method of triage that uses four color triage coding cards that have military bar codes for tracking patients.

smoke inhalation injury Inhalation injury caused by the accumulation of toxic by-products of combustion.

smooth muscle One of two kinds of muscle; also known as visceral muscle, involuntary muscle, and nonstriated muscle. It is composed of elongated, spindle-shaped cells in muscles not under voluntary control, such as smooth muscle of the intestines, stomach, and other visceral organs.

social determinants of health Factors that influence health, which include the conditions in which people are born, grow, work, live, and age and the conditions surrounding their daily life.

sodium ion channels Protein-lined channels in the cell membrane that allow sodium to enter the cell during rapid depolarization.

soft body armor Clothing that provides protection from some blunt and penetrating trauma; also known as bullet-proof vests. The vest must be designed and rated to provide protection from edged weapons.

soft splint A splint that can be molded into a variety of shapes and configurations to accommodate the injured body part.

solutes Substances dissolved in solution.

soman A clear, colorless, tasteless liquid with a slight camphor odor; may be used as a nerve agent.

somatic nervous system The part of the nervous system composed of nerve fibers that send impulses from the central nervous system to skeletal muscle.

somatic pain Pain that arises from skeletal muscles, ligaments, vessels, or joints.

somatic symptom disorders Any of a large group of neurotic disorders characterized by symptoms suggesting physical illness or disease, for which there are no organic or physiologic causes; also known as somatoform disorder.

somatomotor neurons Neurons that innervate skeletal muscles.

span of control The number of people one supervisor is responsible for and can coordinate most effectively. This number is typically five to seven but should be as few as three if operations are especially challenging.

special weapons and tactics (SWAT) operations Violent and dangerous incidents; may include emergency medical personnel.

spermatocele A benign cystic accumulation of sperm that arises from the head of the epididymis.

spermatogenesis The process of development of spermatozoa.

spermatozoa The male sex cells, which are composed of a head and a tail. Sperm contains genetic information transmitted by the male.

spina bifida A neural tube defect (congenital) with incomplete closing of the spine, spinal cord, and membranes around the spine.

spinal cord injury (SCI) Damage to the spinal cord; may result from direct injury to the cord itself or indirectly from damage to surrounding bones, tissues, or blood vessels.

spinal cord tumors Benign or malignant tumors that originate in the cells within or next to the spinal cord.

spinal nerves Thirty-one pairs of nerves formed by the joining of the dorsal and ventral routes that arise from the spinal cord.

spinal shock Temporary loss or depression of all or most spinal reflex activity below the level of the injury; may or may not include loss of sympathetic tone that causes hypotension.

spinal stenosis Narrowing of the spinal canal.

spiritual abuse The act of preventing a person from practicing his or her religion or forcing a person to practice another religion.

spleen A large, highly vascular lymphatic organ situated in the upper part of the abdominal cavity between the stomach and the diaphragm. It responds to foreign substances in the blood, destroys worn-out erythrocytes, and is a storage site for red blood cells.

spondylosis A condition of the spine characterized by fixation or stiffness of the vertebral joint.

spontaneous abortion Noninduced termination of pregnancy that usually occurs before 20 weeks' gestation; also known as miscarriage.

spontaneous pneumothorax A condition that results when a subpleural bleb ruptures, allowing air to enter the pleural space from within the lung.

sprain A partial tearing of a ligament caused by a sudden twisting or stretching of a joint beyond its normal range of motion.

ST segment The early part of repolarization in the electrocardiogram of the right and left ventricles measured from the end of the S wave to the beginning of the T wave.

staging A tactical response to avoid danger by waiting at a safe distance from the scene until the area has been secured by the appropriate authorities.

staging areas Designated areas where incident-assigned vehicles are directed and held until needed.

stalking A pattern of repeated and unwanted attention, harassment, contact, or any other course of conduct directed at a specific person that would cause a reasonable person to feel fear.

stance The position of the body while standing.

standard deviation An estimate of the average deviation from the mean, measured in the same units as the original data.

standard limb leads Bipolar electrocardiograph leads that record the difference in electrical potential between the left arm, the right arm, and the left leg electrodes.

standard of care The action and prudence that a reasonable person in the same or similar circumstances would exercise in providing care to a patient.

standard operating procedures (SOPs) Guidelines establishing the preferred method for operations to be carried out, as well as the framework (eg, line of authority, communications, coordination) to achieve these goals.

standard precautions Protective measures that have traditionally been developed by the Centers for Disease Control and Prevention for use in dealing with objects, blood, body fluids, or other potential exposure risks of communicable disease; considers all body fluids, except sweat, to present a possible risk.

standing orders Specific interventions or actions that must be taken in specific situations by prehospital emergency care personnel without the need for direct medical oversight.

Starling hypothesis The concept that describes the movement of fluid across the capillary wall (net filtration).

Starling law of the heart A rule that the stroke volume of the heart increases in response to an increase in end-diastolic volume.

static rope "Low-stretch" rope, which is designed to stretch typically less than 10% under load when used in rescue operations.

statistically significant A descriptive term used when the observed phenomenon represents a significant departure from what might be expected by chance alone.

statistics A summary of characteristics of numerical facts or data.

status asthmaticus A severe, prolonged asthma attack that has not been broken with repeated doses of bronchodilators.

status epilepticus Continuous seizure activity lasting 4 to 5 minutes or longer, or consecutive seizures without a return to consciousness between seizures.

statutes Formal written enactments of a legislative authority that governs a state, city, or county.

steep-angle rescue A type of rescue involving the movement of a victim up or down a grade of approximately 35° to 65°. The weight of the rescuer is distributed between the rope and the ground.

stellate wound A star-shaped wound.

sternal angle The point at which the manubrium joins the body of the sternum; also known as the angle of Louis.

sternal fracture Fracture of the sternum; usually results from a direct blow to the chest or from a massive crush injury.

sternoclavicular joint The double gliding joint between the sternum and the clavicle.

sternomanubrial joint The articulation between the upper two parts of the sternum, the manubrium and the sternal body.

sternum The elongated, flattened bone that forms the middle portion of the thorax.

steroid hormones Hormones synthesized by endocrine cells from cholesterol. They include cortisol, aldosterone, estrogen, progesterone, and testosterone.

strabismus A condition of misalignment of the eyes. Both eyes do not properly align with each other when looking at an object.

strain An injury to the muscle or its tendon from overexertion or overextension.

strep throat An infection of the throat caused by streptococcal bacteria.

stress A nonspecific mental or physical strain caused by any emotional, physical, social, economic, or other factor that initiates a physiologic response.

stridor An abnormal, high-pitched musical sound caused by obstruction in the trachea or larynx.

stroke volume The volume of blood ejected from one ventricle in a single heartbeat.

ST-segment elevation myocardial infarction (STEMI) A myocardial infarction in which there is ST-segment elevation.

subarachnoid hemorrhage A collection of blood or fluid in the subarachnoid space.

subarachnoid space The area below the arachnoid membrane but above the pia mater that contains cerebrospinal fluid.

subclavian vein The continuation of the axillary vein in the upper body. It extends from the lateral border of the first rib to the sternal end of the clavicle, where it joins the internal jugular to form the brachiocephalic vein.

subcutaneous emphysema The presence of air in the subcutaneous tissues.

subcutaneous tissue The adherent layer of adipose tissue just below the dermal layer; also known as the hypodermis.

subdural hematoma Accumulation of blood between the dura mater and the arachnoid mater.

subdural space The space between the dura mater and the arachnoid.

subgaleal hematoma Bleeding in the potential space between the skull periosteum and the scalp galea aponeurosis.

subjective information Information based on opinions expressed by patients or others or information based on subjective feelings of the patient, such as clinical symptoms.

subluxation A partial dislocation.

submersion The act or state of being under water (or liquid) for any amount of time.

sucking reflex A normal infant response in which touching the infant's lips with the nipple of a breast or bottle causes involuntary sucking movements.

sudden cardiac death A death that occurs within the first 2 hours after the onset of illness or injury.

sudden infant death syndrome (SIDS) The unexpected and sudden death of an apparently normal and healthy infant that occurs during sleep and has no cause found even after a full investigation (including autopsy, investigation of the death scene, and review of clinical history). SIDS is one type of sudden unexpected infant death.

sudden unexpected infant death (SUID) Sudden and unexpected death of a baby younger than 1 year in which the cause was not obvious before investigation.

suffix A word part that appears at the end of a word. In the medical context, a suffix often describes a patient's condition or diagnosis.

suicide The act of a human being intentionally causing his or her own death.

summation The combined effects of two drugs that equal the sum of the individual effects of each agent.

superficial burn A burn injury in which only a superficial layer of epidermal cells is destroyed; also known as a first-degree burn.

superficial reflexes Reflexes elicited by sensory afferents from skin.

superior Situated above or higher than a point of reference in the anatomic position.

superior vena cava The vein that returns blood from the head and neck, upper limbs, and thorax to the right atrium.

supine A position in which the patient lies on the back (faceup).

supplemental restraint system A safety device in a vehicle, such as an impact sensor, airbags, and seat belt pre-tensioners, that deploys to prevent driver/occupant injury.

supplied-air (air-line) breathing apparatus (SABA) A device that provides a nearly unlimited supply of air from a source located outside the confined space.

support branch The section that is in charge of gathering and distributing equipment and supplies at a major incident.

supraventricular tachycardia (SVT) A complex group of dysrhythmias that can be broadly defined as any tachycardia that originates above the level of the bundle of His.

surface tension The tendency of the surface of a liquid to minimize the area of its surface by contracting.

surface water rescue The rescue of a patient who is afloat on the surface of a body of water.

surfactant Lipoproteins that reduce the surface tension of pulmonary fluids.

sweat glands Glands that produce sweat or viscous organic secretions; also known as sudoriferous glands.

sympathetic nervous system A subdivision of the autonomic nervous system that usually is involved in preparing the body for physical activity.
sympathy The expression of one's feelings about another person's problem.
symphysis pubis The joint that connects the coxal bones of the pelvis.
synapse Any junction between nerve cells and other nerve cells, muscle cells, gland cells, or sensory receptors. It serves to transmit action potentials from one cell to another.
synchronized cardioversion An electrical countershock used to terminate dysrhythmias that is timed with the QRS complex. Synchronization is timed with the R wave of the cardiac cycle to avoid shock delivery during the relative refractory period of the cardiac cycle, which could cause ventricular fibrillation.
syncope A brief lapse in consciousness caused by transient cerebral hypoxia.
synergism The combined action of two drugs that is greater than the sum of each agent acting independently.
synergistic effects The effects of one chemical enhancing the effects of a second chemical.
synovial joints Joints that are freely movable.
syphilis A sexually transmitted disease characterized by distinct stages of effects over a period of years; may involve any organ system.
system Interconnected functions or organs in which a stimulus or an action in one area affects all other areas.
systematic sampling A statistical method that involves the selection of a population from an ordered sampling so as to ensure equal probability.
systemic lupus erythematosus (SLE) A chronic inflammatory autoimmune disease that affects many systems of the body. It is characterized by severe vasculitis, renal involvement, and lesions of the skin and nervous system.
systemic vascular resistance The total resistance against which blood must be pumped; also known as afterload.
systole Contraction of the atria and ventricles.
systolic blood pressure The blood pressure measured during the period of ventricular contraction.
systolic heart failure Failure of the ventricles to contract properly during systole; also known as systolic dysfunction.
T lymphocytes The lymphocytes responsible for cell-mediated immunity.
T wave A deflection in the electrocardiogram after the QRS complex, representing ventricular repolarization.
tabes dorsalis An abnormal condition characterized by the slow degeneration of all or part of the body and the progressive loss of peripheral reflexes; results from untreated syphilis infection that has spread to the spinal cord.
tabun A clear, colorless, tasteless liquid with a faint fruity odor; may be used as a nerve agent.
tachycardia A heart rate equal to or greater than 100 beats/min in an adult.
tactical EMS (TEMS) Emergency medical support provided by EMS personnel who are specially trained and equipped to provide prehospital emergency care in tactical environments.
tactical patient care Patient care activities that occur inside the scene perimeter of a dangerous scene.
tactical retreat The act of leaving the scene when danger is observed or when violence or indicators of violence are displayed; requires immediate and decisive action.
tardive dyskinesia A potentially irreversible neurologic disorder characterized by involuntary repetitious movements of the muscles of the face, limbs, and trunk.
tarsal bones The bones of the ankle.
taste buds The peripheral taste organs that are distributed over the tongue and the roof of the mouth.
TB disease Active tuberculosis.
teachable moment The time after an injury has occurred when the patient and observers remain acutely aware of what has happened and may be more receptive to being taught ways that the event or illness could have been prevented.
team dynamics The unseen forces that operate in a team between different groups of people; will enable a group of people to act as one.
telemedicine Technologic communications that allow the transmission of photographs, video, and other information directly from the scene to a hospital for physician evaluation and consultation.
temperament The characterization of a person's behavior, as defined by how the person interacts with the environment. It is the basis on which children develop relationships.
temporomandibular (TM) joint disorders A set of conditions that cause pain in the area of the TM joint. A TM joint is located on each side of the head in front of the ears where the mandible meets the temporal bones.
tendonitis An inflammatory condition of a tendon, usually caused by a sprain.
tendons Bands or cords of dense connective tissue that connect muscle to bone or other structures; characterized by strength and nonstretchability.
tension headache A headache caused by muscle contraction in the face, neck, and scalp.
tension pneumothorax An accumulation of air or gas in the pleural cavity that can lead to an increase in

intrathoracic pressure to the point of cardiorespiratory compromise or collapse.

terminal bronchioles The ends of the conducting airways.

terminal decline A theory that older adults experience an overall slowdown or gradual decline of cognitive abilities in the absence of dementia.

terminal drop A theory that a decline in intelligence in older adulthood may be caused by the person's conscious or unconscious perception of coming death.

tertiary injury prevention Activities that correct and prevent further deterioration of an illness or injury.

testes The male gonads, which produce the male sex cells, or sperm.

testicular mass An enlargement or growth on one or both testicles.

testicular torsion The twisting of a testicle on its spermatic cord, disrupting its blood supply.

tetanus An acute, potentially fatal infection of the central nervous system caused by the tetanus bacillus *Clostridium tetani.* It is characterized by muscle spasms and convulsions.

tetany The involuntary contraction of skeletal muscles.

tetralogy of Fallot (ToF) A congenital cardiac anomaly that consists of four defects: pulmonic stenosis, ventricular septal defect, malposition of the aorta so that it rises from the septal defect or the right ventricle, and right ventricular hypertrophy.

tetraplegia Weakness or paralysis of all four extremities and the trunk; also known as quadriplegia.

thalamus Tissue located just above the hypothalamus. It helps to produce sensations, associates sensations with emotions, and plays a part in arousal.

therapeutic action The desired, intended action of a drug.

therapeutic communications The use of communication techniques in a planned, professional manner to (1) foster a positive relationship with the patient and (2) facilitate a shared understanding of information between the patient and the paramedic. These two outcomes aid in the attainment of the desired patient care goals.

therapeutic index A measurement of the relative safety of a drug.

therapeutic range The range of plasma concentrations that is most likely to produce the desired drug effect with the least likelihood of toxicity; the range between minimal effective concentration and toxic level.

thermogenesis The production of heat, especially by the cells of the body.

thermolysis The dissipation of heat by means of radiation, evaporation, conduction, or convection.

thermoregulation The maintenance of body temperature, even under a variety of external conditions.

third stage of labor The stage of labor that begins with delivery of the newborn and ends when the placenta is expelled and the uterus has contracted.

third-degree atrioventricular (AV) block A condition that results from complete electrical block at or below the atrioventricular node; also known as complete heart block.

third-degree sprain An injury that results from severe stretching and tearing of ligaments such that the ligament is completely ruptured with significant associated swelling and possible joint dislocation.

third-trimester bleeding Vaginal bleeding that occurs in the third trimester of pregnancy. Common causes include abruptio placentae, placenta previa, or uterine rupture.

threshold potential The value of the membrane potential at which an action potential is produced as a result of depolarization in response to a stimulus.

thrills Fine vibrations felt by an examiner's hands over the site of an aneurysm or on the pericardium.

thrombin An enzyme formed in plasma as part of the clotting process. It causes fibrinogen to change to fibrin, which is essential in the formation of a clot.

thrombocytopenia An abnormal hematologic condition in which the number of platelets is reduced.

thromboembolism A condition in which a blood vessel is blocked by an embolus carried in the bloodstream from the site of formation of the clot.

thrombosis The formation of a blood clot (thrombus) in a blood vessel.

thromboxanes Antagonistic prostaglandin derivatives that are synthesized and released by degranulating platelets, causing vasoconstriction and promoting the degranulation of other platelets.

thymus A single, unpaired gland located in the mediastinum. The primary central gland of the lymphatic system.

thyroid membrane The fibrous membrane that joins the hyoid and the thyroid cartilages.

thyroid storm An acute life-threatening form of hyperthyroidism.

thyrotoxicosis Any toxic condition that results from thyroid hyperfunction.

tibia The second longest bone of the skeleton. It is located at the medial side of the leg.

tick paralysis A rare, progressive, reversible disorder caused by several species of ticks that release a neurotoxin that causes weakness, incoordination, and paralysis.

tidal volume The volume of air inspired or expired in a single, resting breath.

tinnitus A ringing sound in the ears.

tocolytic A medication given to temporarily reduce the frequency and intensity of uterine contractions.

Todd paralysis Temporary paralysis or weakness following a seizure that resolves within 48 hours; typically involves one side of the body.

toddler A child 1 to 2 years of age.

tolerance A physiologic response that requires that a drug dosage be increased to produce the same effect formerly produced by a smaller dose.

tonic–clonic seizures Generalized seizures involving the entire body; also known as grand mal seizures.

tonsillitis Inflammation of the tonsils.

tonsils Large collections of lymphatic tissue beneath the mucous membrane of the oral cavity and pharynx.

TORCH infections An acronym for a special group of infections that may be acquired by a woman during pregnancy: Toxoplasmosis, Other infections (namely, hepatitis B, syphilis, and herpes zoster), Rubella, Cytomegalovirus, Herpes simplex virus.

torr A non–Système International unit of pressure defined as 1 standard atmosphere divided by 760, or about 1 mm Hg.

torsades de pointes A type of polymorphic ventricular tachycardia occurring in the context of QT prolongation.

tort A personal harm or injury caused by civil versus criminal wrongs.

torticollis A twisting of the neck caused by injuries to the cervical spine that generate muscle spasms. This condition causes a painful fixed head tilt that is accompanied by shoulder elevation.

torus fracture The buckling of the cortex of bone due to a unicortical fracture in immature bone.

total anomalous pulmonary venous return (TAPVR) A congenital heart defect in which the four pulmonary veins that transport oxygen-rich blood back to the heart from the lungs are not properly attached to the left atrium and instead may connect to the right atrium.

total pressure The combination of pressures exerted by all the gases in any mixture of gas.

tourniquet A constricting or compressing device used to control venous and arterial bleeding in an extremity.

toxidromes Clinical syndromes grouped together for the successful recognition of poisoning patterns.

toxin A poison that is produced by a living organism.

toxoids Toxins that have been treated with chemicals or with heat to reduce their toxic effects but still retain their antigenic power.

trachea A cylindrical tube in the neck composed of cartilage and membrane. It conveys air to the lungs.

tracheal deviation Movement of the trachea from its midline position to the right or left.

tracheitis A bacterial infection of the upper airway and subglottic trachea.

tracheoesophageal fistula An abnormal connection between the esophagus and the trachea that results from a failed fusion of the tracheoesophageal ridges during fetal development.

tracking log A system of record keeping that includes patient identification, transporting unit, patient priority, and medical facility destination.

traction splint A splinting device, most commonly used for femoral fractures, that provides a counterpull to reduce pain, realign the fracture, and minimize bleeding complications.

trade name The trademark name of a drug, designated by the drug company that sells the medication.

traffic incident management The process of coordinating the resources of a number of different partner agencies and private-sector companies to detect, respond to, and clear traffic incidents as quickly as possible so as to reduce the impacts of incidents on safety and congestion, while protecting the safety of on-scene rescuers.

transcript A formal record of questions and answers that may be used during a trial.

transcutaneous cardiac pacing (TCP) The delivery of repetitive electrical currents to the heart through an external artificial pacemaker; also known as external cardiac pacing.

transdermal drug administration Administration of drugs that are absorbed through the skin.

transection A complete or incomplete lesion to the spinal cord.

transient ischemic attack (TIA) An acute episode of temporary neurologic dysfunction resulting from focal cerebral ischemia.

transportation group The group that communicates with the receiving medical facilities, ambulances, and air medical services for patient transport during a major incident.

transposition of the great arteries (TGA) A congenital defect in which the positions of the great arteries are reversed; the aorta arises from the right ventricle and the pulmonary artery from the left ventricle; may be a ductal-dependent lesion.

trauma centers Specialized medical facilities distinguished by the immediate availability of specialized personnel, equipment, and services to treat most severe and critical injuries.

traumatic aortic rupture Rupture of the aorta that is thought to be a result of shearing forces.

traumatic asphyxia A severe crushing injury to the chest and abdomen that causes an increase in the intrathoracic pressure. The increased pressure forces blood from the right side of the heart into the veins of the upper thorax, neck, and face.

traumatic brain injury (TBI) A traumatic insult to the brain capable of producing physical, intellectual, emotional, social, and vocational change.

traumatic hyphema A hemorrhage into the anterior chamber of the eye; usually is a result of blunt trauma.

traumatic perforation A tear or puncture of the tympanic membrane.

treatment group The group that provides advanced care and stabilization until the patients are transported to a medical facility. Most paramedics and medical facility personnel are assigned to this group.

treatment protocols Guidelines that define the scope of prehospital intervention practiced by emergency services personnel.

trench foot A foot injury that occurs from prolonged exposure to cold, but not freezing, water.

triage A method used to sort patients and prioritize care based on the severity of their illness or injuries and their potential to survive.

triage tagging system A system of tags, tapes, ribbons, or labels used to indicate a patient's priority and triage category.

tricuspid atresia A congenital defect in which there is absence or abnormal development of a tricuspid valve.

tricuspid valve The valve located between the right atrium and the right ventricle.

trigeminal neuralgia Infection or disease of the trigeminal nerve (cranial nerve V).

trigeminy An underlying rhythm that is interrupted by a ventricular complex after every two beats.

trimesters Periods of approximately 3 months into which pregnancy is divided. There are a total of three such periods in one pregnancy.

trismus Limited jaw range of motion commonly caused by muscle spasms of the jaw.

trisomy 21 A genetic failure where there is a triplet of chromosome 21 rather than the usual pair; the cause of Down syndrome.

truncus arteriosus A rare type of congenital heart disease characterized by a large ventricular septal defect over which a large, single great vessel (truncus) arises.

trunked radio system A sophisticated computer-controlled radio system that uses multiple frequencies and repeaters.

tuberculosis (TB) A chronic granulomatous infection caused by *Mycobacterium tuberculosis.* It usually affects the lungs and generally is transmitted by airborne spread.

tularemia A serious illness that is caused by the bacterium *Francisella tularensis* found in animals (especially rodents, rabbits, and hares).

tumor lysis syndrome A group of metabolic complications that can occur after treatment of cancer, usually non-Hodgkin lymphomas and acute leukemias. It results from the breakdown products of dying cancer cells being released into the bloodstream.

tunic One of the enveloping layers of a part; one of the coats of a blood vessel; one of the coats of the eye; one of the coats of the digestive tract.

tunnel vision A narrow outlook; the focusing of attention on a particular problem without proper regard for possible consequences or alternative approaches.

turf Territorial boundaries established by gangs.

tympanic membrane The cellular membrane that separates the external ear from the middle ear; also known as the eardrum.

tympany A hollow drumlike sound produced when a gas-containing cavity is percussed.

type 1 diabetes Diabetes characterized by inadequate production of insulin by the pancreas. It may occur any time after birth and requires lifelong treatment with insulin.

type 2 diabetes Diabetes usually characterized by a decrease in the production of insulin by the pancreatic beta cells and diminished tissue sensitivity to insulin (insulin resistance).

type I ambulance An ambulance design based on the chassis-cabs of light-duty pickup trucks.

type II ambulance An ambulance design based on modern passenger/cargo vans.

type III ambulance An ambulance design based on chassis-cabs of light-duty vans.

U wave A small deflection after the T wave in the electrocardiogram, seen in pathologic states such as hypokalemia.

ulcerative colitis An inflammatory condition of the large intestine characterized by severe diarrhea and ulceration of the mucosa of the colon and/or rectum.

ulna One of the bones of the forearm.

ulnar nerve entrapment An injury that occurs when the ulnar nerve in the arm becomes compressed.

ultrasonography A diagnostic test that uses sound waves to make images of internal organs and structures. It is often used in the emergency department to view the peritoneal cavity for the presence of fluid or blood. The resulting image is known as a sonogram.

umbilical cord A flexible structure connecting the umbilicus of the fetus with the placenta. It contains the umbilical arteries and vein and is the key structure in delivery of oxygen and nutrients to the developing fetus.

unblinding A research specification by which all parties are made aware of the study, treatment, and outcome to be measured.

uncompensated shock A stage of shock that occurs when the body is no longer able to maintain systemic blood pressure.

unethical Conduct that fails to conform to moral principles, values, or standards.

unified command An application of the incident command system used when there is more than one agency with incident jurisdiction. Agencies designate representatives to work together through unified command to establish a common set of objectives and strategies and a single incident action plan.

unifocal premature ventricular complex (PVC) A premature ventricular complex that originates from a single ectopic ventricular pacemaker site.

unipolar leads Augmented limb leads that record the difference in electrical potential, using one electrode for a positive pole, but having no distinct negative pole.

universal precautions Infection control practices in health care that are observed with every patient and procedure and that prevent exposure to bloodborne pathogens.

UN/NA number The United Nations class (or division) identification number and North American number for a hazardous material. The numbers are identical.

unstable angina An acute coronary syndrome associated with a pattern of ischemic chest pain that has changed in its ease of onset, frequency, intensity, duration, or quality.

unsynchronized cardioversion An electrical countershock used to terminate ventricular fibrillation and pulseless ventricular tachycardia, given without regard to where the shock occurs in the cardiac cycle; also known as defibrillation.

untoward effects Side effects that prove harmful to the patient.

upper airway Airway structures above the glottis.

upper respiratory tract infection Infection of the upper airway, affecting the nose, throat, sinuses, and larynx.

urea A nitrogen-containing waste product.

uremia A condition marked by an excess of urea and other nitrogenous wastes in the blood.

urethra A small tubular structure that drains urine from the bladder. In men, it also serves as a passageway for semen during ejaculation.

urethritis Inflammation of the urethra.

urinary bladder The muscular, membranous sac in the pelvis that stores urine for discharge through the urethra.

urinary calculi Solid particles in the urinary system, commonly known as kidney stones.

urinary retention Inability to empty the bladder.

urinary tract infection (UTI) Infection of one or more structures of the urinary tract.

urosepsis Sepsis due to infection from a genitourinary source.

urticaria A pruritic skin eruption characterized by transient wheals of various shapes and sizes that have well-defined margins and pale centers; also known as hives.

uterine atony The lack of uterine tone.

uterine inversion A rare event in which the uterus turns inside out after birth.

uterine prolapse The falling or sliding of the uterus from its normal position in the pelvic cavity into the vaginal canal.

uterine rupture A spontaneous or traumatic rupture of the uterine wall.

uterine tubes A pair of ducts that open at one end into the uterus and at the other end into the peritoneal cavity, over the ovary; also known as the fallopian tubes.

uterus The hollow, pear-shaped internal female organ of reproduction.

uvula The cone-shaped process hanging down from the soft palate that helps prevent food and liquid from entering the nasal cavities.

vagina The part of the female genitalia that forms a canal from the orifice through the vestibule to the uterine cervix.

vaginal bleeding The loss of blood through the vagina where the source of bleeding may be the uterus, the cervix, or the vaginal wall itself.

vaginitis Inflammation of the vaginal tissues.

vallecula A furrow between the glossoepiglottic folds on each side of the posterior oropharynx.

Valsalva maneuver A vagal maneuver used to slow the heart by stimulating postganglionic parasympathetic nerve fibers in the wall of the atria and specialized tissues of the sinoatrial and atrioventricular nodes via the vagus nerve.

valvular heart disease Any disease process that affects one or more valves of the heart: the mitral, aortic, tricuspid, or pulmonary valves.

vancomycin-resistant enterococcus (VRE) A type of bacteria that commonly live in the bowel and have become resistant to many antibiotics.

varicocele An abnormal enlargement of the veins that drain the testicle.

vascular access device A device used to provide nutritional support and to administer medications in patients who need long-term vascular access.

vascular dementia A reduction in cognitive function caused by conditions that block or reduce circulation in the brain.

vascular tunic The choroid, ciliary body, and iris.

vasovagal syncope A brief loss of consciousness that results from overstimulation of the vagus nerve.

venom A toxin that is injected from one living organism into another.

ventilation The mechanical movement of air into and out of the lungs that makes respiration possible.

ventilation/perfusion mismatch Any condition leading to interference of airflow at the alveolar level or blood flow at the pulmonary capillary level.

ventral root The nerve that conveys efferent nerve processes away from the spinal cord.

ventricles Small cavities; in the human systems context, this term usually refers to the right and left ventricles of the heart.

ventricular assist device An electromechanical pump to assist ventricular heart function and improve cardiac output.

ventricular escape complex A wide-complex beat originating in the ventricle that occurs when impulses from higher pacemakers fail to fire or to reach the ventricles. When firing at a rate of 30 to 40 beats/min, it is known as an idioventricular rhythm.

ventricular fibrillation (VF) A cardiac dysrhythmia marked by rapid, disorganized depolarization of the ventricular myocardium.

ventricular septal defect (VSD) A congenital anomaly in which an opening exists between the heart's two lower chambers.

ventricular tachycardia (VT) A tachycardia that usually originates in the Purkinje fibers.

verbal abuse The use of degrading remarks, characterized by underlying anger and hostility, that attack a person's self-esteem; an example is name-calling.

vertigo A sensation in which the patient feels as if he or she, or the objects around him or her, are moving in a circular or spinning motion, which causes difficulty in maintaining normal balance in a standing or seated position.

vesicants Chemicals with severely irritating properties that produce blisters on the skin and damage to the eyes, lungs, and other mucous membranes.

vesicular breath sounds Breath sounds heard over most of the lung fields; the major normal breath sound.

vicarious liability A form of liability in which an employer or supervisor is liable for the negligent actions of another person, even though the employer or supervisor was not directly responsible for the wrongdoing.

viral hemorrhagic fevers (VHFs) A group of illnesses caused by several distinct families of viruses that include Ebola.

viral meningitis Meningitis caused by viral infection (eg, enteroviral infection, herpesvirus infection, mumps, and, less commonly, influenza); also known as aseptic meningitis.

virulence The relative harmfulness or severity of a pathogen.

viruses Minute, parasitic microorganisms without independent metabolic activity that can replicate only within a cell of a living plant or animal host.

visceral pain Deep pain that arises from smooth vasculature or organ systems.

visceral peritoneum The serous membrane that covers the abdominal organs.

visceral reflexes Reflexes mediated by autonomic nerves and initiated in the viscera.

viscosity The physical property of a liquid. It is characterized by the degree of friction between its component molecules.

visual acuity A measurement of the clarity or sharpness of vision.

vitreous humor The transparent, jellylike material that fills the space between the lens and the retina of the eye.

vocal cords The two folds of elastic ligaments covered by mucous membrane that stretch from the thyroid cartilage to the arytenoid cartilage; also known as the true vocal cords. Vibration of these structures is responsible for voice production.

volatility The ability of a liquid to vaporize.

Volkmann contracture A serious, persistent flexion contraction of the forearm and hand caused by posttraumatic ischemia specifically as a result of compartment syndrome.

volvulus Twisting of the intestines.

vulva The external genitalia of the female.

VX A human-made thick, amber-colored, odorless liquid that resembles motor oil; a chemical warfare agent classified as a nerve agent.

wandering pacemaker An atrial arrhythmia that results from shifting of the pacemaker site between the sinoatrial node, atrioventricular node, and latent pacemaker sites within the atria.

warm zone In a hazmat incident, a buffer area that surrounds the hot zone with "cold" and "hot" end corridors; usually considered a safer environment for workers than the hot zone.

weapons of mass destruction (WMDs) Conventional biologic, nuclear, incendiary, chemical, or explosive weapons that have the ability to cause death and/or destruction on a widespread or massive scale.

Wernicke encephalopathy A stage of Wernicke-Korsakoff syndrome that usually develops suddenly, with the clinical manifestations of ataxia, nystagmus, disturbances of speech and gait, signs of neuropathy, stupor, or coma.

Wernicke-Korsakoff syndrome A disease that results from chronic thiamine deficiency combined with an inability to use thiamine because of a heritable disorder or because of a reduction in intestinal absorption and metabolism of thiamine by alcohol.

West Nile virus A virus spread by mosquitoes that can cause fever, headache, body aches, vomiting, diarrhea, and rash.

wheals Small areas of swelling of the skin that result from an allergic reaction.

wheeze A form of rhonchus characterized by a high-pitched, musical quality. It is caused by high-velocity airflow through narrowed airways.

Wolff-Parkinson-White (WPW) syndrome A syndrome of preexcitation of the ventricles of the heart; caused by an accessory pathway (bundle of Kent) that permits abnormal electrical communication from the atria to the ventricles.

wound botulism Botulism caused by toxins produced from a wound infected with *Clostridium botulinum.*

xiphoid process The smallest of three parts of the sternum. It articulates caudally with the body of the sternum and laterally with the seventh rib.

years of potential life lost The calculation obtained by subtracting the age of the victim's death from 65 (the average age of retirement); a measure of premature mortality.

yellow marrow Specialized soft tissue (mainly adipose) found in the compact bone of most adult epiphyses.

Zika A viral infection acquired from the bite of an infected mosquito or through blood or sexual contact with an infected person. Zika can spread from a pregnant woman to her fetus, which can result in microcephaly, severe brain malformations, and other birth defects.

zone of coagulation In a burn wound, the central area that has sustained the most intense contact with the thermal source. In this area, coagulation necrosis of the cells has occurred and the tissue is nonviable.

zone of hyperemia An area in which blood flow is increased as a result of the normal inflammatory response to injury. It lies at the periphery of the zone of stasis.

zone of stasis The area of burn tissue that surrounds the critically injured area. It consists of tissue that is potentially viable despite the serious thermal injury.

zygote The developing ovum from the time it is fertilized until it is implanted in the uterus as a blastocyst.

Index

Note: Page numbers followed by f indicate figures; t, tables; and b, boxes.

B

C

G

H

I

J

K

L

M

N

O

P

Q

R

T

U

W

X

Y

Z